POISONING
AND
TOXICOLOGY
HANDBOOK
FOURTH EDITION

POISONING AND TOXICOLOGY HANDBOOK

FOURTH EDITION

Jerrold B. Leikin, MD

Frank P. Paloucek, PharmD

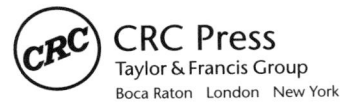

CRC Press
Taylor & Francis Group
Boca Raton   London   New York

CRC Press is an imprint of the
Taylor & Francis Group, an **informa** business

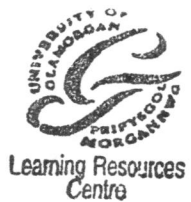
CRC Press
Taylor & Francis Group
6000 Broken Sound Parkway NW, Suite 300
Boca Raton, FL 33487-2742

Library of Congress Cataloging-in-Publication Data

Poisoning and toxicology handbook / editor (s) Jerrold B. Leikin and Frank P. Paloucek. -- 4th ed.
    p. cm.
  Includes bibliographical references and index.
  ISBN-13: 978-1-4200-4479-9 (alk. paper)
  ISBN-10: 1-4200-4479-6 (alk. paper)
  1. Toxicology--Handbooks, manuals, etc. I. Leikin, Jerrold B. II. Paloucek, Frank P. III. Title.

RA1215.P65 2007
615.9--dc22
                                                  2006100358

Visit the Taylor & Francis Web site at
http://www.taylorandfrancis.com

and the CRC Press Web site at
http://www.crcpress.com

TABLE OF CONTENTS

Section IV Herbal Agents

Section V Antidotes and Drugs Used in Toxicology

PREFACE

The term toxicology can today be defined as the assault, absorption, and adverse effects of foreign substances upon the human body. As such, toxicology is truly one of the most exciting and expanding fields in the medical sciences. The depth and scope of this discipline are increasing yearly with the discovery and the analysis of newer drugs, chemicals, or environmental toxins. Certainly, the areas of drug overdose, drug interactions, allergic reactions, street drug abuse, hazardous material accidents, radiation physics, industrial/occupational exposures, psychiatry, wilderness medicine, food safety, botany, virology, zoology, parasitology, mycology, teratology, analytical laboratory techniques, radiology, infectious agents, basic pharmacology, and just plain old detective investigational techniques are all encompassed within the field of toxicology.

Our sincere thanks goes out to the staff of the Illinois Poison Center, Evanston Northwestern Healthcare Omega, University of Illinois College of Pharmacy, Toxikon Consortium, and the many reviewers across the country who gave us immeasurable assistance in helping develop and enhance this book.

While preparing this reference book, we attempted to include as much information as possible. Quite often, all of the characteristics have not been delineated for every drug, chemical, or biological agent, and our clinical experience is truly in the embryonic stage for some of these toxins. Our goal is to provide the reader with our basic approach, incorporating these details to toxic management by using available pharmacological and clinical information along with our experience. Since the recent years have afforded us a literal explosion of information, the reader should realize that this reference still is representative of a beginning chapter in toxicology.

Jerrold B. Leikin, MD
Frank P. Paloucek, PharmD

ACKNOWLEDGMENTS

The *Poisoning & Toxicology Handbook* exists in its present form as the result of the concerted efforts of the following individuals: Robert D. Kerscher, publisher and president of Lexi-Comp Inc; Lynn D. Coppinger, managing editor; David C. Marcus, director of information systems; Matthew C. Kerscher, product manager; and Tracey J. Henterley, graphic designer.

Much of the material contained in this book is the result of contributions by pharmacists throughout the United States and Canada. Lexi-Comp has assisted many medical institutions to develop hospital-specific formulary manuals that contain clinical drug information as well as dosing. Working with these clinical pharmacists, hospital pharmacies and therapeutics committees, and hospital drug information centers, Lexi-Comp has developed an evolutionary drug database that reflects the practice of pharmacy in these major institutions. Information was derived from Lexi-Comp's Poisoning and Toxicology database (www.lexi.com) for this book.

The authors wish to thank their families, friends, and colleagues who supported them in their efforts to complete this book.

EDITORS

Jerrold Blair Leikin, MD, FACP, FACEP, FACMT, FAACT, FACOEM

Dr. Leikin is director of medical toxicology at Evanston Northwestern Healthcare-OMEGA, Glenbrook Hospital, located in Glenview, Illinois. He is associate director of the Toxikon Consortium based at Cook County Hospital in Chicago. He is also professor of medicine at Rush Medical College and professor of emergency medicine at Feinberg School of Medicine at Northwestern University in Chicago, Illinois.

Dr. Leikin received his medical doctorate degree from the Chicago Medical School in 1980 and completed a combined residency in internal medicine and emergency medicine at Evanston Hospital and Northwestern Memorial Hospital in 1984. He completed a fellowship in medical toxicology at Cook County Hospital in Chicago in 1987. He is also board-certified in the above specialties.

Dr. Leikin was the associate director of the emergency department from 1988 to 2001 at Rush-Presbyterian-St Luke's Medical Center in Chicago. He was medical director of the Rush Poison Control Center for 11 years and was the medical director of the United States Drug Testing Laboratory for 5 years. Dr. Leikin is also a consultant with the Illinois Poison Center and Wisconsin Poison Center. He is also medical director of PROSAR Drug Safety Call Center located in St. Paul, Minnesota.

Dr. Leikin has presented over 100 abstracts at national meetings and has published over 200 articles in peer-reviewed medical journals. He is coeditor of the *American Medical Association Handbook of First Aid and Emergency Care*. He has written chapters on the subjects of toxicology, emergency medicine, critical care medicine, internal medicine, and observational medicine in medical textbooks. Dr. Leikin is an active member of the American Academy of Clinical Toxicology, American College of Medical Toxicology, the American College of Emergency Physicians, and the American Medical Association.

Frank P. Paloucek, PharmD, DABAT, FASHP

Dr. Paloucek is a clinical associate professor of pharmacy practice and director of residency programs at the University of Illinois in Chicago. Dr. Paloucek received his BS degree in pharmacy from the University of Illinois in 1981 and his PharmD from the Philadelphia College of Pharmacy and Sciences in 1984. He completed a residency in pharmacy practice and a fellowship in clinical pharmacokinetics at the University of Illinois at Chicago.

He practices on the clinical toxicology service at the University of Illinois. He is an adjunct assistant professor in the emergency medicine program, has been a faculty member of the American Academy of Clinical Toxicology since 1989, and a Diplomate of the American Board of Applied Toxicology since 1991. He has been a director of a postdoctoral clinical toxicology fellowship program since 1991 and is now director of residency programs at the University of Illinois Hospital. In addition to numerous scientific posters and clinical toxicology publications, Dr. Paloucek is currently on the editorial board of *The Poison Review*. He is an acknowledged expert on the pharmacist's role in emergency medicine and the interpretation of drug-toxin concentrations in poisoning patients.

Dr. Paloucek is an active member of the American Society of Hospital Pharmacists and the American College of Clinical Pharmacy. His research interests are toxicokinetics of medications in overdose, drug misadventures in the emergency department, and theophylline toxicity.

CONTRIBUTORS

Steven E. Aks, DO, DABMT

Dr. Aks is the director at the Toxikon Consortium. He is an associate professor of emergency medicine at the Rush Medical College, Chicago, and an attending physician in the department of emergency medicine at John Stroger Hospital, Chicago, Illinois. He received his BA degree in biology and psychology at the University of Rochester and his DO degree from the New York College of Osteopathic Medicine. His internship was at the Brookdale Hospital Medical Center, his residency in emergency medicine at the Chicago College of Osteopathic Medicine Program in emergency medicine. He completed a fellowship in medical toxicology at the Toxikon Consortium at Cook County Hospital. Areas of interest include education, mushroom toxicity, cocaine toxicity, and clinical toxicology. He has recently completed work on drug and hallucinogenic mushroom use at rock concerts.

Anthony M. Burda, RPh, CSPI, DABAT

Anthony Burda is the chief specialist in poison information at the Illinois Poison Center in Chicago. He has become certified as a specialist in poison information through the American Association of Poison Control Centers (AAPCC) in 1983, 1988, 1993, and 2000. He became a diplomate of the American Board of Applied Toxicology in 1997. He is a 1978 graduate of the University of Illinois College of Pharmacy.

Mr. Burda is a clinical assistant professor of pharmacy practice at the University of Illinois College of Pharmacy, Chicago, and Chicago College of Pharmacy, Midwest University, Downers Grove, Illinois. He is an assistant professor in the department of pharmacology at Rush Medical College, Chicago. He serves as a rotation preceptor for a number of pharmacy colleges and emergency medicine and medical school clinical programs.

Mr. Burda's professional experiences include authoring continuing education programs for pharmacists, presenting lectures in pharmacology/medications courses for nurses, and serving as a technical advisor to the executive director of a pharmacy association.

Jack C. Clifton, MD

Following his PhD graduate study in the department of microbiology and immunology at the University of Illinois, Dr. Clifton attended medical school as a James Scholar at the University of Illinois College of Medicine. Subsequent to medical school, Dr. Clifton completed a combined internal medicine/pediatrics residency program at the University of Illinois, becoming chief resident during his final year. Having attended in the departments of pediatrics and internal medicine at the University of Chicago following his residency training, Dr. Clifton returned to graduate work in a combined PhD/pediatric critical care fellowship at the University of Chicago in the departments of pediatrics pathology and immunology. After accepting an attending position in the section of emergency medicine within the department of pediatrics at Rush Children's Hospital, Dr. Clifton then completed a fellowship in medical toxicology with the Toxikon Consortium at the University of Illinois, Cook County Hospital, and Rush-Presbyterian-St. Lukes Medical Center. In addition to being currently enrolled in a combined clinical pharmacology fellowship/master's of clinical research program at Rush, Dr. Clifton is presently an attending physician in the Toxikon Consortium at the University of Illinois, John Stroger Hospital, and Rush-Presbyterian-St. Luke's Medical Center.

Connie B. Fischbein, BA, CSPI

Connie Fischbein received her BS degree in chemistry from Northwestern University in Evanston, Illinois in 1977. She received her certification as a specialist in poison information from the AAPCC in 1985 and 1990. She has practiced as a certified specialist in poison information (CSPI) at the Intermountain Regional Poison Center in Salt Lake City, Utah, and at the Illinois Poison Center in Chicago (formerly at Rush-Presbyterian-St. Luke's Medical Center). She is an active member of the Illinois Mycological Association.

Christina E. Hantsch, MD

Dr. Hantsch is a medical director of the Illinois Poison Center and an assistant professor at Loyola University, Chicago. She practices both emergency medicine and medical toxicology at Loyola University Medical Center. She graduated from Northwestern University Medical School in Chicago in 1992. After finishing her internship at Northwestern University, she studied at the Medical College of Wisconsin for her emergency medicine residency. There, she was chief

Resident in 1995–1996. Dr. Hantsch completed a medical toxicology fellowship at the Center for Clinical Toxicology at Vanderbilt University. She is a member of several professional organizations including the American College of Medical Toxicology, the American Academy of Clinical Toxicology, and the European Association of Poisons Centres and Clinical Toxicologists.

Terry D. Jacobsen, PhD, FLS

Dr. Jacobsen received his BS degree from the College of Idaho and his MS and PhD degrees in systematic botany from Washington State University. In addition to his administrative and programmatic activities at the Institute, he teaches in the biological sciences department. He also is a research associate in the section of botany at the Carnegie Museum of Natural History and an adjunct scientist at the Pittsburgh Poison Center at Children's Hospital.

Dr. Jacobsen's main research interests include vascular taxonomy, especially *Allium* (onion, Liliaceae) in North America, and toxic plants and fungi.

Edward P. Krenzelok, PharmD, FAACT, ABAT

Dr. Krenzelok is director of the Pittsburgh Poison Center at Children's Hospital of Pittsburgh and a professor of pharmacy and pediatrics at the University of Pittsburgh. He received his BS degree in pharmacy from the University of Wisconsin in 1971 and his doctor of pharmacy degree from the University of Minnesota in 1974. Dr. Krenzelok is active in numerous professional toxicology and medically related societies and associations and is a past president of the American Academy of Clinical Toxicology. He is board certified in clinical toxicology by the American Board of Applied Toxicology and has been awarded the distinction of being a Fellow in the American Academy of Clinical Toxicology. Dr. Krenzelok is on the board of directors of the American Association of Poison Control Centers. He is a former chair of the United States Pharmacopeia Clinical Toxicology and Substance Abuse Committee, a former member of the Food and Drug Administration Nonprescription Drug Advisory Committee, on the editorial boards and review panels of numerous medical and toxicology journals, and the author of several hundred scientific publications and book chapters and the editor of three books.

Christine M. Moore, PhD

Dr. Moore is the vice president of Toxicology Research and Development for Immunalysis Corporation, a company specializing in the development of immunoassays for the testing of drugs in biological matrices. Additionally, she is the secretary of the Society of Hair Testing, and the treasurer of the Society of Forensic Toxicologists.

Following a PhD in forensic toxicology and postdoctoral work in Japan, Dr. Moore served as a research associate at the University of Illinois and as technical services manager of United Chemical Technologies, a manufacturer of solid-phases for use in clinical, drug testing, and pharmaceutical laboratories. She has also served as the associate scientific director of U.S. Drug Testing Laboratories, Chicago, a laboratory specializing in the detection of drugs in meconium, hair, and other less common sample matrices.

Lisa Sigg, BS, RPh

Lisa Sigg received her BS degree in pharmacy from Butler University in 1955 and became licensed to practice later that year. She is currently practicing community pharmacy in Chicago, Illinois.

Todd Sigg, PharmD, CSPI

Dr. Sigg received his doctor of pharmacy degree from the Purdue University College of Pharmacy in 1995. He then completed a pharmacy practice residency at Rush-Presbyterian-St. Luke's Medical Center in Chicago, Illinois. In 1998, the American Association of Poison Control Centers certified Dr. Sigg as a specialist in poison information. Presently he is employed by the Illinois Poison Center. He serves as affiliate faculty and preceptor for the University of Illinois College of Pharmacy and Midwestern University, Chicago College of Pharmacy.

Michael Wahl, MD, FACEP

Dr. Wahl received his medical degree from Case Western Reserve University in 1991. He completed residency at the University of Illinois, program in emergency medicine, in 1994. He completed a fellowship in toxicology in 1994 with the Toxikon Consortium in 1996. Dr. Wahl is board certified in both emergency medicine and toxicology. Current appointments include attending physician, Evanston and Glenbrook Hospitals, department of emergency medicine, and medical director, Illinois Poison Center since 1998.

Guy L. Weinberg, MD

Dr. Weinberg is a professor of anesthesiology at the University of Illinois at Chicago and is a diplomate of the American Boards of Internal Medicine, Medical Genetics, and Anesthesiology. He stumbled into the world of toxicology during experiments studying the effects of local anesthetics on fatty acid metabolism when he unexpectedly found that a lipid emulsion infusion prevented local anesthetic cardiac toxicity in rats. Since then, the clincal efficacy of lipid emulsion therapy for anesthetic-induced cardiac toxicity has been confirmed in many case reports. Current laboratory studies also point to its potential for treating other forms of poisoning. Dr. Weinberg's other research interests include cardiac metabolism, protection, and preservation. He has an abiding affection for intermediary metabolism and mitochondria in particular.

Larisa H. Cavallari, PharmD, BCPS
Assistant Professor, Section of Cardiology
University of Illinois
Chicago, Illinois

Harold L. Crossley, DDS, PhD
Associate Professor of Pharmacology
Baltimore College of Dental Surgery
Dental School
University of Maryland Baltimore
Baltimore, Maryland

Wayne R. DeMott, MD
Consultant in Pathology and Laboratory Medicine
Shawnee Mission, Kansas

Samir Desai, MD
Assistant Professor of Medicine
Department of Medicine
Baylor College of Medicine
Houston, Texas
Staff Physician
Veterans Affairs Medical Center
Houston, Texas

Andrew J. Donnelly, PharmD, MBA
Director of Pharmacy
and
Clinical Professor of Pharmacy Practice
University of Illinois Medical Center at Chicago
Chicago, Illinois

Thom C. Dumsha, DDS
Associate Professor and Chair
Dental School
University of Maryland Baltimore
Baltimore, Maryland

Michael S. Edwards, PharmD, MBA
Assistant Director, Weinberg Pharmacy
Johns Hopkins Hospital
Baltimore, Maryland

Vicki L. Ellingrod, PharmD, BCPP
Associate Professor
University of Iowa
Iowa City, Iowa

Kelley K. Engle, BSPharm
Pharmacotherapy Specialist
Lexi-Comp, Inc
Hudson, Ohio

Margaret A. Fitzgerald, MS, APRN, BC, NP-C, FAANP
President
Fitzgerald Health Education Associates, Inc.
North Andover, Massachusetts
Family Nurse Practitioner
Greater Lawrence Family Health Center
Lawrence, Massachusetts

Matthew A. Fuller, PharmD, BCPS, BCPP, FASHP
Clinical Pharmacy Specialist, Psychiatry
Cleveland Department of Veterans Affairs Medical Center
Brecksville, Ohio
Associate Clinical Professor of Psychiatry
Clinical Instructor of Psychology
Case Western Reserve University
Cleveland, Ohio
Adjunct Associate Professor of Clinical Pharmacy
University of Toledo
Toledo, Ohio

Morton P. Goldman, PharmD
Assistant Director, Pharmacotherapy Services
The Cleveland Clinic Foundation
Cleveland, Ohio

Julie A. Golembiewski, PharmD
Clinical Associate Professor
Colleges of Pharmacy and Medicine
Pharmacotherapist, Anesthesia/Pain
University of Illinois
Chicago, Illinois

Jeffrey P. Gonzales, PharmD
Critical Care Pharmacy Specialist
The Cleveland Clinic Foundation
Cleveland, Ohio

Barbara L. Gracious, MD
Assistant Professor of Psychiatry and Pediatrics
Case Western Reserve University
Director of Child Psychiatry and Training & Education
University Hospitals of Cleveland
Cleveland, Ohio

Larry D. Gray, PhD, ABMM
TriHealth Clinical Microbiology Laboratory
Bethesda and Good Samaritan Hospitals
Cincinnati, Ohio

James L. Gutmann, DDS
Professor and Director of Graduate Endodontics
The Texas A & M University System
Baylor College of Dentistry
Dallas, Texas

Tracey Hagemann, PharmD
Associate Professor
College of Pharmacy
The University of Oklahoma
Oklahoma City, Oklahoma

Charles E. Hawley, DDS, PhD
Professor Emeritus
Department of Periodontics
University of Maryland
Consultant on Periodontics
Commission on Dental Accreditation of the American Dental Association

Martin D. Higbee, PharmD
Associate Professor
Department of Pharmacy Practice and Science
The University of Arizona
Tucson, Arizona

Jane Hurlburt Hodding, PharmD
Director, Pharmacy
Miller Children's Hospital
Long Beach, California

Collin A. Hovinga, PharmD
Neuropharmacologist
Miami Children's Hospital
Miami, Florida

Darrell T. Hulisz, PharmD
Associate Professor
Department of Family Medicine
Case Western Reserve University
Cleveland, Ohio

David S. Jacobs, MD
President, Pathologists Chartered
Consultant in Pathology and Laboratory Medicine
Overland Park, Kansas

Polly E. Kintzel, PharmD, BCPS, BCOP
Clinical Pharmacy Specialist-Oncology
Spectrum Health
Grand Rapids, Michigan

Jill M. Kolesar, PharmD, FCCP, BCPS
Associate Professor of Pharmacy
University of Wisconsin
Madison, Wisconsin

Donna M. Kraus, PharmD, FAPhA
Associate Professor of Pharmacy Practice
Departments of Pharmacy Practice and Pediatrics
Pediatric Clinical Pharmacist
University of Illinois
Chicago, Illinois

Daniel L. Krinsky, RPh, MS
Director, Pharmacotherapy Sales and Marketing
Lexi-Comp, Inc
Hudson, Ohio

Kay Kyllonen, PharmD
Clinical Specialist
The Cleveland Clinic Children's Hospital
Cleveland, Ohio

Charles Lacy, RPh, PharmD, FCSHP
Vice President, Information Technologies
Professor, Pharmacy Practice
Professor, Business Leadership
University of Southern Nevada
Las Vegas, Nevada

Brenda R. Lance, RN, MSN
Program Development Director
Northcoast HealthCare Management Company
Northcoast Infusion Therapies
Oakwood Village, Ohio

Leonard L. Lance, RPh, BSPharm
Clinical Pharmacist
Lexi-Comp, Inc
Hudson, Ohio

Jerrold B. Leikin, MD, FACP, FACEP, FACMT, FAACT, FACOEM
Director, Medical Toxicology
Evanston Northwestern Healthcare-OMEGA
Glenbrook Hospital
Glenview, Illinois
Associate Director
Toxikon Consortium at Cook County Hospital
Chicago, Illinois
Professor of Emergency Medicine
Pharmacology and Health Systems Management
Rush Medical College
Chicago, Ilinois
Professor of Medicine
Feinberg School of Medicine
Northwestern University
Chicago, Ilinois

Jeffrey D. Lewis, PharmD
Pharmacotherapy Specialist
Lexi-Comp, Inc
Hudson, Ohio

Jennifer K. Long, PharmD, BCPS
Infectious Diseases Clinical Specialist
The Cleveland Clinic Foundation
Cleveland, Ohio

Laurie S. Mauro, BS, PharmD
Associate Professor of Clinical Pharmacy
Department of Pharmacy Practice
College of Pharmacy
The University of Toledo
Toledo, Ohio

Vincent F. Mauro, BS, PharmD, FCCP
Associate Professor of Clinical Pharmacy
College of Pharmacy
The University of Toledo
Adjunct Associate Professor of Medicine
College of Medicine
Medical University of Ohio at Toledo
Toledo, Ohio

Timothy F. Meiller, DDS, PhD
Professor
Diagnostic Sciences and Pathology
Baltimore College of Dental Surgery
Professor of Oncology
Greenebaum Cancer Center
University of Maryland Baltimore
Baltimore, Maryland

Franklin A. Michota, Jr, MD
Head, Section of Hospital and Preoperative Medicine
Department of General Internal Medicine
The Cleveland Clinic Foundation
Cleveland, Ohio

Michael A. Militello, PharmD, BCPS
Clinical Cardiology Specialist
Department of Pharmacy
The Cleveland Clinic Foundation
Cleveland, Ohio

J. Robert Newland, DDS, MS
Professor
Department of Diagnostic Sciences
University of Texas Health Science Center
Houston, Texas

Cecelia O'Keefe, PharmD
Pharmacotherapy Specialist
Lexi-Comp, Inc
Hudson, Ohio

Dwight K. Oxley, MD
Consultant in Pathology and Laboratory Medicine
Wichita, Kansas

Frank P. Paloucek, PharmD, DABAT
Clinical Associate Professor in Pharmacy Practice
Director, Residency Programs
University of Illinois
Chicago, Illinois

Christopher J. Papasian, PhD
Director of Diagnostic Microbiology and Immunology Laboratories
Truman Medical Center
Kansas City, Missouri

Alpa Patel, PharmD
Clinical Specialist, Infectious Diseases
Johns Hopkins Hospital
Baltimore, Maryland

Luis F. Ramirez, MD
Adjunct Associate Professor of Psychiatry
Case Western Reserve University
Cleveland, Ohio

A.J. (Fred) Remillard, PharmD
Assistant Dean, Research and Graduate Affairs
College of Pharmacy and Nutrition
University of Saskatchewan
Saskatoon, Saskatchewan

Martha Sajatovic, MD
Associate Professor of Psychiatry
Case Western Reserve University
Cleveland, Ohio

Todd P. Semla, PharmD, BCPS, FCCP
Clinical Pharmacy Specialist
Department of Veterans Affairs
Pharmacy Benefits Management
Associate Professor of Clinical Psychiatry
Feinberg School of Medicine
Northwestern University
Chicago, Illinois

Francis G. Serio, DMD, MS
Professor and Chairman
Department of Periodontics
University of Mississippi
Jackson, Mississippi

Dominic A. Solimando, Jr, MA, FAPhA, FASHP, BCOP
Oncology Pharmacist
President, Oncology Pharmacy Services, Inc
Arlington, Virginia

Joni Lombardi Stahura, BS, PharmD, RPh
Pharmacotherapy Specialist
Lexi-Comp, Inc
Hudson, Ohio

Carol K. Taketomo, PharmD
Pharmacy Manager
Children's Hospital Los Angeles
Los Angeles, California

Mary Temple, PharmD
Pediatric Clinical Research Specialist
Hillcrest Hospital
Mayfield Heights, Ohio

Elizabeth A. Tomsik, PharmD, BCPS
Pharmacotherapy Specialist
Lexi-Comp, Inc
Hudson, Ohio

Beatrice B. Turkoski, RN, PhD
Associate Professor, Graduate Faculty,
Advanced Pharmacology
College of Nursing
Kent State University
Kent, Ohio

David M. Weinstein, PhD, RPh
Pharmacotherapy Specialist
Lexi-Comp, Inc
Hudson, Ohio

Anne Marie Whelan, PharmD
Associate Professor
College of Pharmacy
Dalhouise University
Halifax, Nova Scotia

Richard L. Wynn, PhD
Professor of Pharmacology
Baltimore College of Dental Surgery
Dental School
University of Maryland Baltimore
Baltimore, Maryland

DESCRIPTION OF SECTIONS AND FIELDS USED IN THIS HANDBOOK

The *Poisoning & Toxicology Handbook* is divided into six sections, medicinal, nonmedicinal, biological, herbal, antidotal agents, and diagnostic tests and procedures. These sections (except for herbal agents) are introduced by essays from leaders in the field and are followed by monographs that list the numerical indices of the Chemical Abstract Services (CAS) registry numbers (internationally used) and the United Nations/United States Department of Transportation (DOT) numbers (used nationally). These monographs also contain the information described below. However, not all fields of information will appear for every monograph; only those fields that correspond to a particular type of agent will be given.

Abstract	A brief description of the test and its use
Additional Information	Information about sodium content and/or pertinent information about specific drug brands; or, additional information about a test/procedure and its uses
Administration	Specific instructions on proper procedure or information in relation to the administration of the drug
Admission Criteria/Prognosis	Clinical indicators of exposure used to determine if hospitalization is necessary (ie, symptoms, laboratory values, etc); may also include parameters that can impact on prognosis
Adverse Reactions	Side effects are listed by organ system affected. Symptoms reported in bold print have an incidence of 10% or greater.
Aftercare	Special instructions or warnings for medical personnel for the care of the patient after the procedure is performed
AHPA Botanical Safety Rating System	Relative safety rating of each herb as determined by the American Herbal Products Association (AHPA)
Antidote	Directs the reader to the drug and page where the antidote and its information can be located
Applies to	Refers to various sample sites or specimen types that follow the same procedure
Brand Names	Common trade names
CAS Number	Chemical Abstract Service Registry Number, the international nomenclature system
Causes for Rejection	Possible reasons why a specimen may be rejected by the laboratory
Collection	General and specific collection instructions that should be followed to obtain a proper and usable specimen
Container	Type of container required for acquiring and maintaining a usable specimen
Contraindications	Information pertaining to inappropriate use of a drug; or, reasons why a test should not be performed
Critical Values	Values that alert the medical staff that the patient has reached a range or value that may be hazardous
Diagnostic Tests/Procedures	Directs the reader to the page in the book for information on the tests and/or procedures which should be considered in the treatment of the patient
Dosage Forms	Information with regard to form, strength, and availability of the drug. This field is strung with the forms bolded and uses some abbreviations as follows: AERO: aerosol; AMP: ampul; CAP: capsule; CONC: concentration; CRM: cream; CRYST: crystal; ELIX: elixir; GRAN: granules; INF: infusion; INH: inhaler; INJ: injection; LIQ: liquid; LOZ: lozenge; OINT: ointment; SHAMP: shampoo; SOLN: solution; SUPP: suppository; SUSP: suspension; SYR: syrup; TOP: topical
Drug Interactions	Effects that may be potentially harmful or toxic when used with other medications
Equipment	Equipment needed to perform the named procedure
Impairment Potential	Possible effect on an individual's functional capacity; probability of increased risk of involvement in an accident
Limitations	Limits of the test/procedure
Mechanism of Action	How the drug works in the body to elicit a response
Mechanism of Toxic Action	How nontherapeutic agents elicit a toxic response
Methodology	Testing methodologies available
Minimum Volume	Minimum amount of specimen required to perform testing
Monitoring Parameters	Laboratory tests and patient physical parameters that should be monitored for safety and efficacy of drug therapy are listed when appropriate
Monograph Name	The generic (U.S. adopted) name is used for antidotes and medicinal agents. For the purpose of this publication antidotes are defined as [ANTIDOTE] after the monograph name.
Nursing Implications	Includes additional instructions for the administration of the drug and monitoring tips from the nursing perspective
Overdosage Treatment	Description of treatment modalities of adverse effects and overdosage presented in sections: Decontamination; Supportive therapy; Enhanced elimination
Pharmacodynamics/ Kinetics	The magnitude of a drug's effect depends on the drug concentration at the site of action. The pharmacodynamics are expressed in terms of onset of action and duration of action. Pharmacokinetics are expressed in terms of absorption, distribution (including appearance in breast milk and crossing of the placenta), protein binding, metabolism, bioavailability, half-life, time to peak serum concentration, and elimination.
Patient Preparation	Any special preparation that the patient must undergo prior to the procedure being performed
Possible Panic Range	Values that alert the medical staff that the patient has reached a range or value that may be hazardous
Pregnancy Implications	Includes the five categories established by the FDA to indicate the potential of a systemically absorbed drug for causing birth defects, as well as, information which may be critical in the treatment of a pregnant patient
Reference Range	Serves as a general guideline. Therapeutic and toxic serum concentrations are listed when appropriate. For diagnostic tests: See specific testing facility for their ranges.
Related Information	Cross-references to other tests or procedures, or the appendix, that are related to the named test and may be helpful to the user
Sampling Time	The time frame a specimen should be collected
Scientific Name	Taxonomic name
Signs & Symptoms of Acute Overdose	Primarily clinical effects of acute toxic exposure
Slang Name	"Street names" for drugs of abuse
Special Instructions	Specific instructions for the acquisition and handling of specimens
Specific References	Specific references used in the information of the monograph published since 2003. For references published before 2003, consult the Poisoning & Toxicology database or CD-ROM online version.
Specimen	Possible specimens that can be used for testing

Stability	Storage, refrigeration, and compatibility information
Storage Instructions	The appropriate storage of the specimen after collection but prior to testing
Technique	Explanation of how the procedure is performed
Test Commonly Includes	All laboratory tests or procedures that may occur when the named test is performed
Test Interactions	Listing of assay interferences when relevant; (B) = Blood; (S) = Serum; (U) = Urine
Toxicodynamics/Kinetics	The magnitude of a drug's effect depends on the drug concentration at the site of action. The toxicodynamics are expressed in terms of onset of action and duration of action. Toxicokinetics are expressed in terms of absorption, distribution (including appearance in breast milk and crossing of the placenta), protein binding, metabolism, bioavailability, half-life, time to peak serum concentration, and elimination.
UN Number	United Nations/United States Department of Transportation (D.O.T.) number. Identification nomenclature used for shipping in the United States; usually found on placard on side of vehicle.
U.S. Brand Names	Common United States trade names
Use	Information pertaining to appropriate indications of a drug; or common uses for a test/procedure
Usual Dosage	Information regarding the recommended final concentrations and rates for administration of the drug
Volume	Desirable amount of specimen needed for testing
Warnings	Hazardous conditions related to use of the drug and disease states or patient populations in which the drug should be cautiously used

FDA PREGNANCY CATEGORIES

In many of the drug monographs throughout this book there is a field labeled Pregnancy Implications and the letter A, B, C, D, or X immediately following which signifies a category. The FDA has established these five categories to indicate the potential of a systemically absorbed drug for causing birth defects. The key differentiation among the categories rests upon the reliability of documentation and the risk:benefit ratio. Pregnancy category X is particularly notable in that if any data exist that may implicate a drug as a teratogen and the risk:benefit ratio is clearly negative, the drug is contraindicated during pregnancy.

These categories are summarized as follows:

A	Controlled studies in pregnant women fail to demonstrate a risk to the fetus in the first trimester with no evidence of risk in later trimesters. The possibility of fetal harm appears remote.
B	Either animal-reproduction studies have not demonstrated a fetal risk but there are no controlled studies in pregnant women, or animal-reproduction studies have shown an adverse effect (other than a decrease in fertility) that was not confirmed in controlled studies in women in the first trimester and there is no evidence of a risk in later trimesters.
C	Either studies in animals have revealed adverse effects on the fetus (teratogenic or embryocidal effects or other) and there are no controlled studies in women, or studies in women and animals are not available. Drugs should be given only if the potential benefits justify the potential risk to the fetus.
D	There is positive evidence of human fetal risk, but the benefits from use in pregnant women may be acceptable despite the risk (eg, if the drug is needed in a life-threatening situation or for a serious disease for which safer drugs cannot be used or are ineffective).
X	Studies in animals or human beings have demonstrated fetal abnormalities, or there is evidence of fetal risk based on human experience, or both, and the risk of the use of the drug in pregnant women clearly outweighs any possible benefit. The drug is contraindicated in women who are or may become pregnant.

FDA NAME DIFFERENTIATION PROJECT: THE USE OF TALL-MAN LETTERS

Confusion between similar drug names is an important cause of medication errors. For years, the Institute for Safe Medication Practices (ISMP) has urged generic manufacturers use a combination of large and small letters as well as bolding (eg, chlorpro **MAZINE** and chlorpro **PAMIDE**) to help distinguish drugs with look-alike names, especially when they share similar strengths. Recently, the FDA's Division of Generic Drugs began to issue recommendation letters to manufacturers suggesting this novel way to label their products to help reduce this drug name confusion. Although this project has had marginal success, the method has successfully eliminated problems with products such as diphenhydr **AMINE** and dimenhy **DRINATE**. Hospitals should also follow suit by making similar changes on their own labels, preprinted order forms, computer screens and printouts, and drug storage location labels.

Lexi-Comp Medical Publishing, with this edition of the *Poisoning and Toxicology Handbook*, will begin using these "Tall-Man" letters for the drugs suggested by the FDA.

The following is a list of product names and recommended FDA revisions.

Drug Product	Recommended Revision
acetazolamide	aceta **ZOLAMIDE**
acetohexamide	aceto **HEXAMIDE**
bupropion	bu **PROP**ion
buspirone	bus **PIR**one
chlorpromazine	chlorpro **MAZINE**
chlorpropamide	chlorpro **PAMIDE**
clomiphene	clomi **PHENE**
clomipramine	clomi **PRAMINE**
cycloserine	cyclo **SERINE**
cyclosporine	cyclo **SPORINE**
daunorubicin	**DAUNO**rubicin
dimenhydrinate	dimenhy **DRINATE**
diphenhydramine	diphenhydr **AMINE**
dobutamine	**DOBUT**amine
dopamine	**DOP**amine
doxorubicin	**DOXO**rubicin
glipizide	glipi **ZIDE**
glyburide	gly **BURIDE**
hydralazine	hydr **ALAZINE**
hydroxyzine	hydr **OXY**zine
medroxyprogesterone	medroxy **PROGESTER**one
methylprednisolone	methyl **PREDNIS**olone
methyltestosterone	methyl **TESTOSTER**one
nicardipine	ni **CAR**dipine
nifedipine	**NIFE**dipine
prednisolone	predniso **LONE**
prednisone	predni **SONE**
sulfadiazine	sulfa **DIAZINE**
sulfisoxazole	sulfi **SOXAZOLE**

(Continued)

Drug Product	Recommended Revision
tolazamide	**TOLAZ**amide
tolbutamide	**TOLBUT**amide
vinblastine	vin **BLAS**tine
vincristine	vin **CRIS**tine

Institute for Safe Medication Practices. "New Tall-Man Lettering Will Reduce Mix-Ups Due to Generic Drug Name Confusion," *ISMP Medication Safety Alert*, September 19, 2001. Available at: http://www.ismp.org.

Institute for Safe Medication Practices. "Prescription Mapping Can Improve Efficiency While Minimizing Errors with Look-Alike Products," *ISMP Medication Safety Alert*, October 6, 1999. Available at: http://www.ismp.org.

U.S. Pharmacopeia, "USP Quality Review: Use Caution-Avoid Confusion," March 2001, No. 76. Available at: http://www.usp.org.

SAFE WRITING

Health professionals and their support personnel frequently produce handwritten copies of information they see in print; therefore, such information is subjected to even greater possibilities for error or misinterpretation on the part of others. Thus, particular care must be given to how drug names and strengths are expressed when creating written healthcare documents.

The following are a few examples of safe writing rules suggested by the Institute for Safe Medication Practices, Inc.*

1. There should be a space between a number and its units as it is easier to read. There should be no periods after the abbreviations mg or mL.

Correct	Incorrect
10 mg	10mg
100 mg	100mg

2. Never place a decimal and a zero after a whole number (2 mg is correct and 2.0 mg is **incorrect**). If the decimal point is not seen because it falls on a line or because individuals are working from copies where the decimal point is not seen, this causes a tenfold overdose.

3. Just the opposite is true for numbers less than one. Always place a zero before a naked decimal (0.5 mL is correct, .5 mL is **incorrect**).

4. Never abbreviate the word unit. The handwritten U or u looks like a 0 (zero), and may cause a tenfold overdose error to be made.

5. IU is not a safe abbreviation for international units. The handwritten IU looks like IV. Write out international units or use int. units.

6. Q.D. is not a safe abbreviation for once daily, as when the Q is followed by a sloppy dot, it looks like QID which means four times daily.

7. O.D. is not a safe abbreviation for once daily, as it is properly interpreted as meaning "right eye" and has caused liquid medications such as saturated solution of potassium iodide and Lugol's solution to be administered incorrectly. There is no safe abbreviation for once daily. It must be written out in full.

8. Do not use chemical names such as 6-mercaptopurine or 6-thioguanine, as sixfold overdoses have been given when these were not recognized as chemical names. The proper names of these drugs are mercaptopurine or thioguanine.

9. Do not abbreviate drug names (5FC, 6MP, 5-ASA, MTX, HCTZ, CPZ, PBZ, etc) as they are misinterpreted and cause error.

10. Do not use the apothecary system or symbols.

11. Do not abbreviate microgram as mic g instead use µg as there is less likelihood of misinterpretation.

12. When writing an outpatient prescription, write a complete prescription. A complete prescription can prevent the prescriber, the pharmacist, and/or the patient from making a mistake and can eliminate the need for further clarification.

    The legible prescriptions should contain:

    a. patient's full name
    b. for pediatric or geriatric patients: their age (or weight where applicable)
    c. drug name, dosage form, and strength; if a drug is new or rarely prescribed, print this information
    d. number or amount to be dispensed
    e. complete instructions for the patient, including the purpose of the medication
    f. when there are recognized contraindications for a prescribed drug, indicate to the pharmacist that you are aware of this fact (eg, when prescribing a potassium salt for a patient receiving an ACE inhibitor, write "K serum level being monitored")

*From "Safe Writing" by Davis NM, PharmD and Cohen MR, MS, Lecturers and Consultants for Safe Medication Practices, 1143 Wright Drive, Huntington Valley, PA 19006. Phone: (215) 947-7566.

GENERAL REFERENCES

The following is a list of references utilized in the production of the individual monographs contained in this book.

AMA: Basic Disaster Life Support Provider Manual, Version 2.5, *AMA*, 2004.

American College of Medical Toxicology, Medical Toxicology Board Review Course Syllabus 2006, Schaumberg, IL: ACMT, 2006.

Anderson PO, Knoben JE, and Troutman WG, *Handbook of Clinical Drug Data*, 9th ed, Stamford, CT: Appleton and Lange, 1999.

Auerbach PS, *Wilderness Medicine: Management of Wilderness and Environmental Emergencies*, 4th ed, St Louis, MO: Mosby, 2001.

Auerbach PS, *A Medical Guide to Hazardous Marine Life*, 2nd ed, St Louis, MO: Mosby, 1991.

Bartlett JC and Greenberg MI, *PDR Guide to Terrorism Response*, Montvale, NJ: Thomson PDR, 2005.

Baselt RC, *Drug Effects on Psychomotor Performance*, Foster City, CA: Biomedical Publications, 2001.

Baselt RC, *Disposition of Toxic Drugs and Chemicals in Man*, 7th ed, Foster City, CA: Biomedical Publications, 2004.

Benjamin DR, *Mushrooms: Poisons and Panaceas*, New York, NY: W.H. Freeman, 1995.

Billups NF, *American Drug Index*, 38th ed, St Louis, MO: Facts and Comparisons, 1994.

Bleecker ML and Hansen JA, *Occupational Neurology and Clinical Neurotoxicology*, Baltimore, MD: Williams and Wilkins, 1994.

Blumenthal M, Busse WR, Goldberg A, et al, eds, *The Complete German Commission E Monographs. Therapeutic Guide to Herbal Medicines*, Austin, TX: American Botanical Council; Boston, MA: Integrative Medicine Communications, 1998.

Bove AA, *Diving Medicine*, 3rd ed, Philadelphia, PA: W.B. Saunders, 1997.

Brent J, Wallace K, Burkhart KK, et al, *Critical Care Toxicology*, Philadelphia, PA: Elsevier Mosby, 2005.

Briggs GG, Freeman RK, and Yaffe SJ, *Drugs in Pregnancy and Lactation*, 6th ed, Baltimore, MD: Williams and Wilkins, 2002.

Bryson PD, *Comprehensive Review in Toxicology for Emergency Clinicians*, 3rd ed, Washington, DC: Taylor and Francis, 1996.

Ciottone GR, *Disaster Medicine*, Boston, MA: Elsevier Mosby, 2006.

Cooney DO, *Activated Charcoal in Medical Applications*, New York, NY: Marcel Dekker, Inc, 1995.

Dart RC, ed, *Medical Toxicology*, 4th ed, Philadelphia, PA: Lippincott, Williams, and Wilkins, 2004.

Derelank MJ and Hollinger MA, *CRC Handbook of Toxicology*, Boca Raton, FL: CRC Press, Inc, 1995.

Dorr RT and von Hoff DD, *Cancer Chemotherapy Handbook*, 2nd ed, Norwalk, CT: Appleton and Lange, 1994.

Drugdex System, Intranet Database, Thomson Micromedex, Version 5.1, Greenwood Village, CO: 2006.

Drummer OH and Odell M, *The Forensic Pharmacology of Drugs of Abuse*, London: Arnold, 2001.

Edmonds S and Stather R, *Reactions Weekly*, Langhorne, PA: Adis International Limited, 1995.

Ellis MD, *Dangerous Plants, Snakes, Arthropods, and Marine Life Toxicity and Treatment*, Hamilton, IL: Drug Intelligence Publications, Inc, 1978.

Emergency Response Guidebook, Washington DC: U.S. Department of Transportation (DOT), Labelmaster, 2000.

Fernandez H, *Heroin*, Center City, MN: Hazelden, 1998.

Ford MD, Delaney KA, Ling LJ, et al, *Clinical Toxicology*, Philadelphia, PA: W.B. Saunders, 2001.

Gardner DE, *Toxicology of the Lung*, 4th ed, Boca Raton, FL: CRC Press, Taylor & Francis Group, 2001.

Gilman AG, Rall TW, Nies AS, et al, eds, *Goodman and Gilman's The Pharmacological Basis of Therapeutics*, 8th ed, New York, NY: Pergamon Press, 1990.

Goldfrank LR, Flomenbaum NE, Hoffman RS, et al, *Goldfrank's Toxicologic Emergencies*, 8th ed, New York, NY: McGraw-Hill, 2006.

Goldstein SM and Wintroub BU, *Adverse Cutaneous Reactions to Medication*, CoMedica Inc., 1994.

Greenberg MI, Hamilton RJ, Phillips SD, and McCluskey GJ, *Occupational, Industrial, and Environmental Toxicology*, 2nd ed, St Louis, MO: CV Mosby Co, 2003.

Haddad LM, Shannon MW, and Winchester JF, *Clinical Management of Poisoning and Drug Overdose*, 3rd ed, Philadelphia, PA: WB Saunders Company, 1997.

Halstead BW and Halsted LG, *Poisonous and Venomous Marine Animals of the World*, revised edition, Princeton, NY: Darwin Press, Inc, 1978.

Hansten PD and Horn JR, *The Top 100 Drug Interactions: A Guide to Patient Management*, H & H Publications, 2000.

Hartman DE, *Neuropsychological Toxicology*, 2nd ed, New York, NY: Plenum Press, 1995.

Hayes WJ and Laws ER, *Handbook of Pesticide Toxicology*, San Diego, CA: Academic Press, Inc, 1991.

Henderson DA, Inglesby TV, and O'Toole T, eds, *Bioterrorism: Guidelines for Medical and Public Health Management*, Chicago, IL: American Medical Association Press, 2002.

Hodgson E and Levi PE, *A Textbook of Modern Toxicology*, New York, NY: Elsevier, 1987.

Huang KC, *The Pharmacology of Chinese Herbs*, Boca Raton, FL: CRC Press, 1993.

Janicak PG, Davis JM, Preskorn MD, et al, *Principles and Practice of Psychopharmacotherapy*, 4th ed, Baltimore, MD: Lippincott Williams & Wilkins, 2006.

Katzung BG, *Basic and Clinical Pharmacology*, 8th ed, New York, NY: Lange Medical Books, 2001.

Klaassen CD, *Casarett and Doull's Toxicology: The Basic Science of Poisons*, 6th ed, New York, NY: McGraw-Hill, 2001.

Koren G, *Maternal-Fetal Toxicology: A Clinician's Guide*, 3rd ed, New York, NY: Marcel Dekker, Inc, 2001.

Lampe KF and McCann MA, *AMA Handbook of Poisonous and Injurious Plants*, Chicago, IL: American Medical Association, 1985.

Lewis RJ, *Sax's Dangerous Properties of Industrial Materials*, 8th ed, New York, NY: Van Nostrand Reinhold, 1992.

Litt JZ, *Physician's Guide to Drug Eruptions*, New York, NY: The Parthenon Publishing Group, 1998.

Liu RH and Goldberger BA, *Handbook of Workplace Drug Testing*, Washington, DC: AACC Press, 1995.

Mandell GL, Bennett JE, and Dolin R, *Principles and Practice of Infectious Diseases*, 4th ed, New York, NY: Churchill Livingstone, 1995.

Marzulli F and Maibach HI, *Dermatotoxicology*, 5th ed, Washington, DC: Taylor and Francis, 1996.

McCunney RJ, ed, *A Practical Approach to Occupational and Environmental Medicine*, 3rd ed, Philadephia, PA: Lippincott Williams & Wilkins, 2003.

McEvoy GK, *AHFS 2001 Drug Information American Hospital Formulary Service*, Bethesda, MD: American Society of Health-System Pharmacists, 2001.

Newall CA, Anderson LA, and Phillipson JD, *Herbal Medicines, A Guide for Health Care Professionals*, London, England: Pharmaceutical Press, 1997.

Noji EK, Kelen GP, and Goessel TK, *Manual of Toxicologic Emergencies*, Chicago, IL: Yearbook Medical Publisher, Inc, 1989.

Olin BR, *Drug Facts and Comparisons*, St Louis, MO: Facts and Comparisons Inc, JB Lippincott Co, 2001.

Olin BR, *Lawrence Review of Natural Products*, St Louis, MO: Facts and Comparisons Inc, 1989–2001.

Penney DG, ed, *Carbon Monoxide Toxicity*, Boca Raton, FL; CRC Press, 2002.

Poisindex System: Intranet Database, Thomson Micromedex, Inc: Greenwood Village, CO; Poisindex Information System, Version 5.1, 2006.

Reigart JR and Roberts JR, *Recognition and Management of Pesticide Poisonings*, 5th ed, 1999. Available at: http://www.epa.gov/pesticides/safety/healthcare.

Reynolds JE, *Martindale The Extra Pharmacopoeia*, 32nd ed, London, England: Council of the Royal Pharmaceutical Society of Great Britain, 1999.

Russell RE, *Snake Venom Poisoning*, Philadelphia, PA: JB Lippincott Co, 1980.

Ryan RP and Terry CE, *Toxicology Desk Reference*, 4th ed, Taylor & Francis, 1997.

Schlesser JL, *1991 Drugs Available Abroad*, Detroit, MI: Medec Books/Gale Research Inc, 1991.

Segen JC, *Dictionary of Alternative Medicine*, Stamford, CT: Appleton and Lange, 1998.

Semla TP, Beizer JL, and Higbee MD, *Geriatric Dosage Handbook*, 8th ed, Hudson, OH: Lexi-Comp Inc, 2003.

Shulman ST, Phair JP, and Sommers HM, *The Biologic and Clinical Basis of Infectious Diseases*, 4th ed, Philadelphia, PA: WB Saunders Company, 1992.

Shults TF, *The Medical Review Officer Handbook*, 8th ed, Research Triangle Park, NC: Quadrangle Research, LLC, 2005.

Sidell FR, *Management of Chemical Warfare Agent Casualties: A Handbook for Emergency Medical Services*, Bel Air, MD: HB Publishing, 1995.

Sidell FR, Patrick III WC, Dashiell TR, et al, *Jane's Chem-Bio Handbook*, 2nd ed, Alexandria, VA: Jane's Information Group, 2002.

Smith RP, *A Primer of Environmental Toxicology*, Philadelphia, PA: Lea and Febiger, 1992.

Spandorfer M, Curtiss D, and Snyder J, *Making Art Safely*, New York, NY: Van Nostrand Reinhold, 1993.

Spencer PS, Schaumburg HH, and Ludloph AC, eds, *Experimental and Clinical Neurotoxicology*, New York, NY: 2000.

Spoerke DG and Rumack BH, *Handbook of Mushroom Poisoning, Diagnosis & Treatment*, Boca Raton, FL: CRC Press, 1994.

Spoerke DG and Smolinske SC, *Toxicity of Houseplants*, Boca Raton, FL: CRC Press, 1990.

Strange GR, Ahrens WR, Lelyveld S, et al, *Pediatric Emergency Medicine*, 2nd ed, American College of Emergency Physicians, McGraw-Hill, 2002.

Sullivan JB and Krieger GR, *Clinical Environmental Health and Toxic Exposures*, 2nd ed, Philadelphia, PA: Lippincott Williams and Wilkins, 2001.

Sweetman S, ed, *Martindale: The Complete Drug Reference*, Intranet Database, Verison 5.1, Lodon Pharmaceutical Press Electronic Version: Greenwood Village, CO: Thomson Micromedex, 2006.

Swotinsky R and Smith D, *The Medical Review Officer's Manual*, 3rd ed, Beverly Farms, MA: OEM Press, 2006.

Taketomo CK, Hodding JH, and Kraus DM, *Pediatric Dosage Handbook*, 9th ed, Hudson, OH: Lexi-Comp Inc, 2002–2003.

Tarcher AB, *Principles and Practice of Environmental Medicine*, New York, NY: Plenum Medical Book Company, 1992.

TOMES® System Intranet, Version 5.1, Greenwood Village, CO: Thomason Micromedex, 2006.

Trissel LA, *Handbook on Injectable Drugs*, 11th ed, Bethesda, MD: American Society of Hospital Pharmacists, 2001.

Turner NJ and Szczawinski AF, *Common Poisonous Plants and Mushrooms of North America*, Portland, OR: Timber Press, 1991.

Tyler VE, *Herbs of Choice: The Therapeutic Use of Phytomedicinals*, New York, NY: Pharmaceutical Products Press, 1994.

Tyler VE, *The Honest Herbal: A Sensible Guide to the Use of Herbs and Related Remedies*, 3rd ed, New York, NY: Pharmaceutical Products Press, 1993.

Upfal MJ, Krieger GR, Phillips SD, et al, *Clinics in Occupational and Environmental Medicine*, Vol 2, No 2, Philadelphia, PA: WB Saunders Co, 2003.

Walter FG, Klein R, Thomas RG, *Advance Hazmat Life Supoprt: for Chemical Burns and Toxic Products of Combustion*, Arizona Board of Regents, 2006.

POISON INFORMATION CENTERS

Updated from the American Association of Poison Control Centers (AAPCC). Available at: http://www.aapcc.org/certctrlst/certifie.html

(Certified centers are printed in italics.)

Centers in each state are listed alphabetically. Telephone numbers designated "TTY" are teletype lines for the hearing-impaired. "TDD" numbers reach a telecommunciation device for the deaf.

Note: As of June 2001, the National toll-free poison center number is (800) 222-1222 (automatically connects to caller's locale).

ALABAMA

Alabama Poison Center
2503 Phoenix Drive
Tuscaloosa, AL 35405
Emergency phone: (205) 345-0600

Regional Poison Control Center
Children's Hospital
1600 7th Avenue South
Birmingham, AL 35233
Emergency phone: (205) 933-4050
http://198.245.254.2/safetyzone/pcontrol.htm

ARIZONA

Arizona Poison and Drug Info Center
Arizona Health Sciences Center, Room 1156
1501 North Campbell Avenue
Tucson, AZ 85724
Emergency phone: (800) 362-0101; (AZ only): (520) 626-6016
http://www.pharmacy.arizona.edu

Banner Poison Center
901 East Willetta Street
Room 2701
Phoenix, AZ 85006

ARKANSAS

Arkansas Poison and Drug Information Center
University of Arkansas for Medical Sciences, College of Pharmacy
4301 W Markham, Mail Slot 522-2
Liffle Rock, AR 72205

CALIFORNIA

California Poison Control System

Fresno/Madera Division
Valley Children's Hospital
9300 Valley Children's Place
Madera, CA 93638-8762

Sacramento Division
UC Davis Medical Center
2315 Stockton Boulevard
Sacramento, CA 95817

San Diego Division
University of CA, San Diego, Medical Center
200 West Arbor Drive
San Diego, CA 92103-8925
http://health.ucsd.edu/poison/index.htm

San Francisco Division
UCSF
Box 1369
San Francisco, CA 94143-1369

COLORADO

Rocky Mountain Poison and Drug Center
777 Bannock Street
Mail Code 0180
Denver, CO 80204-4028
Emergency phone: (800) 332-3073 (CO only/outside metro area); (303) 739-1123 (Denver metro area)
http://www.rmpdc.org

CONNECTICUT

Connecticut Poison Control Center
University of Connecticut Health Center
263 Farmington Avenue
Farmington, CT 06030-5365

DELAWARE

The Poison Control Center
34th and Civic Center Blvd.
Philadelphia, PA 19104-4304
Emergency phone: (215) 386-2100; (215) 590-2100

DISTRICT OF COLUMBIA

National Capital Poison Center
3201 New Mexico Avenue, NW, Suite 310
Washington, DC 20016
Emergency phone: (202) 625-3333
TDD/TTY: (202) 362-8563 (TTY)
http://www.poison.org

FLORIDA

Florida Poison Information Center – Jacksonville
655 West Eighth Street
Jacksonville, FL 32209
Emergency phone: (904) 244-4480
http://ora.umc.ufl.edc/pcc/Pic_jax/htm/index.html

Florida Poison Information Center – Miami
University of Miami, Dept of Pediatrics
Jackson Memorial Medical Center
PO Box 016960 (R-131)
Miami, FL 33101
Emergency phone: (305) 585-5253
http://www.pediatrics.med.miami.edu/FPIC/index.html

Florida Poison Information Center – Tampa
Tampa General Hospital
PO Box 1289
Tampa, FL 33601
Emergency phone: (813) 253-4444

GEORGIA

Georgia Poison Center
Hughes Spalding Children's Hospital
Grady Health System
PO Box 26066
80 Jesse Hill Jr Drive, SE
Atlanta, GA 30335-3801
Emergency phone: (404) 616-9000
TDD/TTY: (404) 616-9287 (TDD)
http://www.georgiapoisoncenter.com/

ILLINOIS

Illinois Poison Center
222 S Riverside Plaza, Suite 1900
Chicago, IL 60606
Emergency phone: (312) 906-6186
TDD/TTY: (312) 906-6185
http://www.mchc.org/ipc/ipc.html

INDIANA

Indiana Poison Center
Methodist Hospital, Clarian Health Partners
I-65 at 21st Street
Indianapolis, IN 46206-1367
Emergency phone: (317) 929-23236
TDD/TTY: (317) 929-2336 (TTY)
http://www.clarian.com/CommunityServices/Poison/default.asp

IOWA

Iowa Statewide Poison Control Center
Iowa Health System
401 Douglas Street, Suite 402
Sioux City, IA 51101
Emergency phone: (712) 277-2222

KANSAS

Mid-America Poison Control Center
University of Kansas Medical Center
3901 Rainbow Boulevard, Room B-400
Kansas City, KS 66160-7231
Emergency phone: (913) 588-6633
TDD/TTY: (913) 588-6639 (TDD)

KENTUCKY

Kentucky Regional Poison Center
Medical Towers South, Suite 572
234 East Gray Street

Louisville, KY 40202
Emergency phone: (502) 589-8222
http://www.krpc.com

LOUISIANA

Louisiana Drug and Poison Information Center
1521 Wilkinson Street
Shreveport, LA 71103

MAINE

Maine Poison Control Center
Maine Medical Center
22 Bramhall Street
Portland, ME 04102
Emergency phone: (207) 871-2879

MARYLAND

Maryland Poison Center
University of MD at Baltimore, School of Pharmacy
20 North Pine Street, PH 772
Baltimore, MD 21201
Emergency phone: (410) 706-7701
TDD/TTY: (410) 706-1858 (TDD)
http://www.pharmacy.umaryland.edu/%7empc/

MASSACHUSETTS

Regional Center for Poison Control and Prevention Serving Massachusetts and Rhode Island
300 Longwood Avenue
Boston, MA 02115
Emergency phone: (617) 232-2120
TDD/TTY: (888) 244-5313
http://www.mapoison.org

MICHIGAN

Children's Hospital of Michigan
Regional Poison Control Center
4160 John R Harper Professional Office Building, Suite 616
Detroit, MI 48201
Emergency phone: (313) 745-5711

DeVos Children's Hospital
Regional Poison Center
1300 Michigan NE, Suite 203
Grand Rapids, MI 49503

MINNESOTA

Hennepin Regional Poison Center
Hennepin County Medical Center
701 Park Avenue
Minneapolis, MN 55415
TDD/TTY: (612) 904-4691 (TTY)
http://www.mnpoison.org/

MISSISSIPPI

Mississippi Regional Poison Control Center
University of Mississippi Medical Center
2500 N State Street
Jackson, MS 39216
Emergency phone: (601) 354-7660

MISSOURI

Cardinal Glennon Children's Hospital
Regional Poison Center
7980 Clayton Road, Suite 200
St Louis, MO 63117
(314) 772-5200

MONTANA

Rocky Mountain Poison & Drug Center
1010 Yosemite Circle, Building 752
Denver, CO 80230-6800

NEBRASKA

The Poison Center
Children's Hospital
8401 Dodge Street, Suite 115
Omaha, NE 68114
Emergency phone: (402) 955-5555
http://www.childrens-omaha.com/site/index.cgi

NEVADA

Oregon Poison Center
Oregon Health Sciences University
3181 SW Sam Jackson Park Road, CB550
Portland, OR 97201
Emergency phone: (503) 494-8968

Rocky Mountain Poison and Drug Center
1010 Yosemite Circle, Building 752
Denver, CO 80230-6800

NEW JERSEY

New Jersey Poison Information and Education System
140 Bergen Street
Newark, NJ 07101
TDD/TTY (973) 926-8008
http://njpies.org/index2.htm

NEW MEXICO

New Mexico Poison and Drug Information Center
MSC 09 5080
University of New Mexico
Albuquerque, NM 87131-0001
Emergency phone: (505) 272-2222

NEW YORK

Central New York Poison Center
750 East Adams Street
Syracuse, NY 13210
Emergency phone: (315) 476-4766

The Ruth A. Lawrence Poison and Drug Info Center
University of Rochester Medical Center
601 Elmwood Avenue
PO Box 321
Rochester, NY 14642
Emergency phone: (716) 275-3232
TDD/TTY: (716) 273-3854 (TTY)
http://www.urmc.rochester.edu/urmc/telemed/flrpc/

Long Island Regional Poison and Drug Information Center
Winthrop University Hospital
259 First Street
Mineola, NY 11501
Emergency phone: (516) 542-2323; (516) 663-2650
TTD/TTY: (516) 924-8811 (TDD Suffolk); (516) 747-3323 (TDD Nassau)

New York City Poison Control Center
NYC Department of Health
455 First Avenue, Room 123, Box 81
New York, NY 10016
Emergency phone: (212) 340-4494; (212) POI-SONS; (212) VEN-ENOS
TTD/TTY: (212) 689-9014 (TDD)

Western New York Regional Poison Control Center
Children's Hospital of Buffalo
219 Bryant Street
Buffalo, NY 14222
Emergency phone: (716) 878-7654

NORTH CAROLINA

Carolinas Poison Center
Carolinas Medical Center
PO Box 32861
Charlotte, NC 28232
Emergency phone: (704) 355-4000
http:/www.carolinas.org/services/poison

OHIO

Central Ohio Poison Center
Children's Hospital
700 Children's Drive, Room L032
Columbus, OH 43205
TDD/TTY: (614) 228-2272 (TTY)
http://www.childrenscolumbus.com/gen/numbers.cfm

Cincinnati Drug and Poison Information Center
Regional Poison Control System
3333 Burnet Avenue
Vernon Place - 3rd Floor
Cincinnati, OH 45229
Emergency phone: (513) 558-5111 (Local)

Greater Cleveland Poison Control Center
11100 Euclid Avenue
Cleveland, OH 44106-6007
Emergency phone: (216) 231-4455

OKLAHOMA

Oklahoma Poison Control Center
Children's Hospital of Oklahoma, Room 3512
940 NE 13th Street
Oklahoma City, OK 73104
Emergency phone: (405) 271-5454
TDD/TTY: (405) 271-1122

OREGON

Oregon Poison Center
Oregon Health Sciences University
3181 SW Sam Jackson Park Road, CB550
Portland, OR 97239
Emergency phone: (800) 452-7165 (OR only); (503) 494-8968

PENNSYLVANIA

Pittsburgh Poison Center
Children's Hospital of Pittsburgh
3705 Fifth Avenue
Pittsburgh, PA 15213
Emergency phone: (412) 681-6669

The Poison Control Center at the Children's Hospital of Philadelphia
34th and Civic Center Road
CHOP North Suite 985
Philadelphia, PA 19104-4304
Emergency phone: (215) 386-2100; (215) 590-2100

PUERTO RICO

Puerto Rico Poison Center
PO Box 367212
San Juan, PR

RHODE ISLAND

Regional Center for Poison Control and Prevention Serving Massachusetts and Rhode Island
300 Longwood Avenue
Boston, MA 02115
Emergency phone: (617) 232-2120

SOUTH CAROLINA

Palmetto Poison Center
University of South Carolina, College of Pharmacy
Columbia, SC 29208
Emergency phone: (803) 777-1117

SOUTH DAKOTA

Hennepin Regional Poison Center
Hennepin County Medical Center
701 Park Avenue
Minneapolis, MN 55415
TDD/TTY: (612) 904-4691 (TTY)

TENNESSEE

Tennessee Poison Center
501 Oxford House
1161 21st Avenue South
Nashville, TN 37232-4632
Emergency phone: (615) 936-2034 (greater Nashville)
TDD/TTY: (615) 936-2047 (TDD)
http://www.toxicology.mc.vanderbilt.edu/poison

TEXAS

Central Texas Poison Center
Scott and White Memorial Hospital
2401 South 31st Street
Temple, TX 76508
Emergency phone: (254) 724-7401
http://swinfo.tamu.edu/poison/ctpc.htm

North Texas Poison Center
Texas Poison Center Network
Parkland Health and Hospital System
5201 Harry Hines Boulevard
PO Box 35926
Dallas, TX 75235

South Texas Poison Center
The University of Texas Health Science Center - San Antonio
Department of Surgery, Mail Code 7849
7703 Floyd Curl Drive
San Antonio, TX 78229-3900

Southeast Texas Poison Center
The University of Texas Medical Branch
3.112 Trauma Building
Galveston, TX 77555-1175
Emergency phone: (409) 765-1420
http://www.utmb.edu/setpc/

Texas Panhandle Poison Center
1501 S Coulter
Amarillo, TX 79106

West Texas Regional Poison Center
Thomason Hospital
4815 Alameda Avenue
El Paso, TX 79905

UTAH

Utah Poison Control Center
585 Komas Drive, Suite 200
Salt Lake City, UT 84108-1208

Emergency phone: (801) 581-2151
http://lysine.pharm.utah.edu/upcc/html/index2.htm

VIRGINIA

Blue Ridge Poison Center
University of Virginia Health System
PO Box 800774
Charlottesville, VA 22908-0774
Emergency phone: (804) 924-5543

National Capital Poison Center
3201 New Mexico Avenue, NW, Suite 310
Washington, DC 20016
Emergency phone: (202) 625-3333
TDD/TTY: (202) 362-8563 (TTY)

Virginia Poison Center
Medical College of Virginia Hospitals
Virginia Commonwealth University
PO Box 980522
Richmond, VA 23298-0522
Emergency phone: (804) 828-9123

WASHINGTON

Washington Poison Center
155 NE 100th Street, Suite 400
Seattle, WA 98125-8011
Emergency phone: (206) 526-2121
TDD/TTY: (206) 517-2394 (TDD

WEST VIRGINIA

West Virginia Poison Center
3110 MacCorkle Avenue SE
Charleston, WV 25304
http://hsc.wvu.edu/charleston/wvpc

WISCONSIN

Children's Hospital of Wisconsin Poison Center
PO Box 1997, Mail Station 677A
Milwaukee, WI 53201-1997
Emergency phone: (414) 266-2222

WYOMING

The Poison Center
8301 Dodge Street
Omaha, NE 68114
Emergency phone: (402) 955-5555

ANIMAL POISON CENTER

ASPCA

National Animal Poison Control Center
1717 South Philo Road, Suite 36

Urbana, IL 61802
Emergency phone: (888) 426-4435; (900) 443-0000 ($55 one-time charge)
http://www.napcc.aspca.org
NSAL-PROSAR
(888) 232-8870 ($35 per incident)

CANADA

ALBERTA

Poison and Drug Information Service
Foothills Hospital
1403 29th Street NW
Calgary, Alberta T2N 2T9
(800) 332-1414 (Alberta only); (403) 670-1414
Fax: (403) 944-1472

BRITISH COLUMBIA

British Columbia Drug and Poison Information Centre
1081 Burrard Street
Vancouver, British Columbia V6Z 1Y6
(800) 567-8911; (604) 682-2344 (ext 2126)
Fax: (604) 806-8262
e-mail: daws@dpk.bcca

MANITOBA

Poison Control Center
Children's Hospital
685 Bannatyne Ave
Winnipeg, Manitoba R3E OWL
Emergency phone: (204) 787-2444

NOVA SCOTIA

Poison Information Centre
1 WK Children's Hospital
PO Box 3070
5850 University Avenue
Halifax, Nova Scotia B3J 3G9
(800) 565-8161 (Prince Edward Island); (902) 428-8161 (Nova Scotia); (902) 428-8132 (Administrative)

ONTARIO

Ontario Regional Poison Control Center
The Hospital for Sick Children
555 University Avenue
Toronto, Ontario M5G 1X8
(416) 813-5900
Fax: (416) 813-7489
http://www.sickkids.ca

Provincial Regional Poison Information Center
Children's Hospital
401 Smyth Road
Ottawa, Ontario KIH 8L1
(800) 267-1373 or (613) 737-1100

QUEBEC

Quebec Poison Control Centre
1050 Chemin Saite-Foy
Quebec G1S4L8, Canada
(418) 654-2731 (Administrative)

AUSTRALIA

The Children's Hospital at West Mead
Locked Bag 4001
West Mead SW 2145
Sydney, Australia
Emergency phone: 61-2-9845-3111
Fax: 61-2-9845-3597
http://www.chw.edu.au

NEW ZEALAND

National Poison Center
Dunedin School of Medicine
PO Box 913
Dunedin, New Zealand
64-3-479-7248
Emergency phone: 0800764-766
http://www.toxinz.com

GENERAL POISON INFORMATION SOURCES

Agency for Toxic Substances and Disease Registry (ATSDR)

1600 Clifton Road NE
Atlanta, GA 30333
(888) 42-ATSDR
(888) 422-8737
(404) 639-6300 (Division of Toxicology)
(404) 498-0093 (Fax)
http://www.atsdr.cdc.gov/

American Academy of Clinical Toxicology

777 East Park Drive
PO Box 8820
Harrisburg, PA 17105
(717) 558-7847
(717) 558-7841 (Fax)
http://www.clintox.org

American Association of Poison Control Centers

3201 New Mexico Avenue NW
Suite 330
Washington, DC 20016
(202) 362-7217
(202) 362-3240 (Fax)
e-mail: info@aapcc.org
http://www.aapcc.org

American Botanical Council

6200 Manor Road
Austin, TX 78723
(512) 926-4900
(512) 926-2345 (Fax)
http://www.herbalgram.org

American Chemical Society

1155 Sixteenth Street, NW
Washington, DC 20036
(800) 227-5558
e-mail: help@acs.org
http://www.chemistry.org

American College of Medical Toxicology

1901 North Roselle Road, Suite 920
Schaumburg, IL 60195
(847) 885-0674
(847) 885-8393 (Fax)
http://www.acmt.net
e-mail: info@acmt.net

American College of Occupational and Environmental Medicine

25 Northwest Point Blvd, Suite 700
Elk Grove Village, IL 60007-1030
(847) 818-1800
(847) 818-9266 (Fax)
http://www.acoem.org

American Parkinson's Disease Association

National Young-Onset Information and Referral Center
2100 Pfingston Road, Suite B100
Glenview, IL 60025
(847) 657-5787
(847) 657-5708 (Fax)
http://www.youngparkinsons.org

American Pharmacists Association

2215 Constitution Ave, NW
Washington, DC 20037-2985
(800) 237-2742
(202) 783-2351 (Fax)
http://www.aphanet.org

American Society of Addiction Medicine (ASAM)

4601 North Park Avenue
Upper Arcade, Suite 101
Chevy Chase, MD 20815
(301) 656-3920
(301) 656-3815 (Fax)
e-mail: email@asam.org
http://www.asam.org

American Society of Health-System Pharmacists

7272 Wisconsin Avenue
Bethesda, MD 20814
(301) 657-3000
http://www.ashp.org

Association of Occupational and Environmental Clinics

(888) 347-2632; (202)347-4976
1010 Vermont Avenue, NW #513
Washington, DC 20005
(800) 347-26326
http://www.aoec.org

Association of American Railroads

Bureau of Explosives
50 S Street, NW
Washington, DC
(719) 584-7159
(719) 585-1895
e-mail: BOE@aar.com

Biological Effects of Low Level Exposures (BELLE)

Northeast Regional Environmental Public Health Center
University of Massachusetts
Amherst, MA 01003
(413) 545-3164
(413) 545-4692 (Fax)
http://www.belleonline.com

Button Battery Hotline

Washington, DC
(202) 625-3333

Canadian Transportation Emergency Center (CANUTEC)

330 Sparks Street
Office 1415
Placedeville, Tower C
Ottawa, Canada, K14 0NS
(613) 996-6666
(613) 954-5101 (Fax)
e-mail: canutec@tc.gc.ca
http://www.tc.gc.ca

Cancer Information Service (National Cancer Institute) (ATSDR)

Office of Cancer Communication
NCI Building 31, Room 10A18
Bethesda, MD 20205
(800) 4-CANCER

Center for Disease Control

Atlanta, GA
(404) 639-3311
http://www.cdc.gov/cdc.html

Center for Substance Abuse Treatment (CSAT)

(800) 662-HELP

Chemical Abstract Service

2540 Olentangy River Road
P.O. Box 3012
Columbus, OH 43210
(614) 447-3600
(614) 447-3713 (Fax)
e-mail: help@cas.org

Chemical Transportation Emergency Center (CHEMTREC®)

1300 Wilson Blvd
Arlington, VA 22209
(800) 424-9300; Customer service: (800) 262-8200; (703) 741-6037 (Fax)
http://www.cmahq.com/chemtrec.nsf
e-mail: chemtrec@americanchemistry.com

Consumer Product Safety Commission

4330 East-West Highway
Bethesda, MD 20814
(800) 638-CPSC
(301) 504-0124 (Fax)
http://www.cpsc.gov

DES Action USA

(Diethylstilbestrol exposure)
158 South Stanwood Road
Columbus, OH 43209
(800) DES-9288
http://www.desaction.org/

Drug Abuse Warning Network (DAWN)

(Consumer Affairs)
Substance Abuse and Mental Health Services
Room 16-105
Rockville, MD 20857

(301) 443-7934 (Administration Office of Applied Studies)
http://www.dawninfo.samhsa.gov

EPA Indoor Air Quality Clearinghouse

PO Box 37133
Washington, DC 20013
(800) 438-4318
http://www.epa.gov/iaq/

EPA Office of Pesticide Programs

(800) 858-7378
(541) 737-0761 (Fax)
e-mail: npic@ace.orst.edu

EPA Safe Drinking Water Hotline

(800) 426-4791
(703) 412-3333 (Fax)
Monday-Friday, 9 AM – 5:30 PM (EST, except Federal holidays)

Food and Drug Administration

Drugs Information Line
(301) 827-4570
Emergency Operations for IND requests or an FDA emergency
(301) 443-1240

Food and Drug Administration

Office of Consumer Affairs (HFE-88)
5600 Fishers Lane
Rockville, MD 20857-0001
(888) INFO-FDA (463-6332)
Monday-Friday, 8 AM – 4:30 PM (EST)
http://www:fda;gov

Food and Safety Inspection Service

U.S. Department of Agriculture
Meat and Poultry Hotline
Washington, DC 20250
(800) 535-4555
Monday-Friday, 10 AM – 4 PM (EST)

Herb Research Foundation

4140 15th Street
Boulder, CO 80304
(303) 449-2265; (303) 449-7849 (Fax)
http://www.herbs.org

Institute for Drug Free Workplace

8614 Westwood Center Drive
Suite 950
Washington, DC 20005
(202) 842-7400; (202) 842-0022 (Fax)
http://www.drugfreeworkplace.org

Malignant Hyperthermia Association of the United States

PO Box 1069
11 E State Street
Sherburne, NY 13460
(607) 674-7901; (607) 674-7910 (Fax)

(800) 644-9737 (in U.S.); 0011 315-464-7079 (outside U.S.)
http://www.mhaus.org

MedWatch

U.S. Food and Drug Administration
5515 Security Lane
Suite 5100
Rockville, MD 20852
(800) 332-1088
http://www.fda.gov/medwatch

National Center for Complementary and Alternative Medicine (NCCAM) Clearinghouse

PO Box 7923
Gaithersburg, MD 20898
(888) 644-6226; (866) 464-3616 (Fax)
e-mail: info@nccam.nih.gov
http://www.nccam.nih.gov/

National Center for Environmental Health (NCEH)

Mailstop F29
4770 Buford Highway NE
Atlanta, GA 30341
(888) 422-8737
http://www.cdd.gov/nceh/

National Inhalant Prevention Coalition (NIPC)

322-A Thompson Street
Chattanooga, TN 37405
(800) 269-4237 or (423) 265-4662
e-mail: nipe@io.com
http://www.inhalants.org

National Institute of Occupational Safety and Health (NIOSH)

(Education and Information Division)
4676 Columbia Pkwy
Cincinnati, OH 45226
(800) 356-4674; (513) 533-8573 (Fax)
(513) 533-8328 (outside U.S.)
http://www.cdc.gov/niosh/homepage.html

National Lead Information Center Hotline

422 South Clinton Avenue
Rochester, NY 14620
(800) 424-5323; (585) 232-3111 (Fax)

National Organization on Fetal Alcohol Syndrome

900 17th Street NW, Suite 910
Washington, DC 20006
(800) 666-6327; (202) 466-6456 (Fax)
http://www.nofas.org

National Pesticide Information Center (NPIC)

Agricultural Chemistry Extension
Oregon State University
333 Weniger
Corvallis, OR 97331-6502
(800) 858-7378 (toll-free in U.S.); (541) 737-0761 (Fax)
Daily, 6:30 AM – 4:30 PM (PST)

http://www.npic.orst.edu/
e-mail: nptn@ace.ost.edu

National Response Center

U.S. Coast Guard Headquarters
2100 2nd Street SW, Rm 2611
Washington, DC 20593
(800) 424-8802; (202) 267-2165 (Fax)
24 hours
http://www.nrc.uscg.mil/terrorismtxt.htm

Neuroleptic Malignant Syndrome Hotline

PO Box 1069
11 East State Street
Sherburne, NY 13460-1069
(888) 667-8367
e-mail: info@nmsis.org
http://www.nmsis.org

Occupational Safety and Health Administration (OSHA)

US Dept of Labor
200 Constitution Avenue NW
Washington, DC 20210
800-321-6742
http://www.osha.gov/

Orphan Medical, Inc

13911 Ridgedale Drive, Suite 250
Minnetonka, MN 55305
(888) 867-7426; (952) 513-6900; (952) 541-9209 (Fax)

Paraquat/Diquat Information

Zeneca, Inc, Agriculture Products
Wilmington, DE
(800) 327-8633

ICI Chipman

Stony Creek, Ontario
(800) 561-3636

Poisindex-Thomson Micromedex, Inc

6200 S Syracuse Way, Suite 300
Greenwood Village, CO 80111-4740
(800) 525-9083
(303) 486-6400
(303) 486-6464 (Fax)
http://www.micromedex.com

Protherics, Inc (formerly Therapeutic Antibodies, Inc)

5214 Maryland Way, Suite 405
Brentwood, TN 37027
(615) 327-1027
615) 320-1212 (Fax)
http://www.protherics.com/wcomp_contact.html

Rabies Immune Globulin (RIG) Producers

Aventis Pharmaceuticals
(800) 822-2463

Bayer Pharmaceutical Division
(800) 288-8371

Radiation Emergency Assistance Center/Training Site (REAC/TS)

Oak Ridge Institute for Science and Education
PO Box 117
Oak Ridge, TN 37831
(865) 576-3131 (days)
(865) 576-1005 (24-hour hotline)
(865) 576-9522 (Fax)
http://www,oraau.gov/reacts/

Substance Abuse and Mental Health Services Administration (SAMHSA)

National Clearinghouse for Alcohol and Drug Information
PO Box 2345
Rockville, MD 20852
(800) 729-6686
http://www.samhsa.gov

Press Office
5600 Fishers Lane, Room 13-C-05
Rockville, MD 20857
(301) 443-8956; (800) 789-2647
http://www.samhsa.gov/

Toxikon

John Stroger, Jr. Hospital
1900 West Polk, Suite 500
Chicago, IL 60612
(312) 864-5520
http://toxikon.er.uic.edu/

United States Drug Testing Laboratories

(Meconium/Hair Drug Analysis)
1700 South Mount Prospect Road
Des Plaines, IL 60018
(847) 375-0770
(847) 375-0775 (Fax)

U.S. Department of Health and Human Services

200 Independence Ave SW
Washington, DC
(877) 696-6775
(202) 619-0257
http://www.os.dhhs.gov/

U.S. National Library of Medicine

8600 Rockville Pike
Bethesda, MD 20894
(888) 346-3656
(301) 402-1384 (Fax)
http://www.nlm.nih.gov/

Vaccine Adverse Event Reporting System (CDC and FDA)

P.O. Box 1100
Rockville, MD 20849-1100
(800) 822-7967, 8 AM - 5 PM (EST)
http://www.hhs.gov

Veterans Special Issue Hotline

(Gulf War veterans - agent orange exposure)
1-800-749-8387
Monday-Friday, 8 AM - 4 PM

White House Office of National Drug Control Policy (ONDCP): Drugs and Crime Clearing House

P.O. Box 6000
Rockville, MD 20849-6000
(800) 666-3332
(301) 519-5212 (Fax)
http://www.whitehousedrugpolicy.gov

TERATOLOGY INFORMATION SERVICES

Organization of Teratology Information Specialists
(866) 626-6847
http://www.otispregnancy.org

ARIZONA

Arizona Teratogen Information Program
(520) 626-3410 or (888) 285-3410
University of Arizona
1501 N. Campbell, Room 1156
Tucson, AZ 85724-5079
Geographic region served: AZ/national
Hours: 8 AM - 5 PM, M-F
Inquiries not handled: Breastfeeding
Accepts calls from: Public and healthcare professionals
Immediate information for most calls? Yes

ARKANSAS

Arkansas Teratogen Information Service
(501) 296-1700 or (800) 358-7229
University of Arkansas for Medical Sciences
Department of Obstetrics and Gynecology
Arkansas Genetics Program
4301 West Markam, Slot 506
Little Rock, AR 72205
Geographic region served: AR
Hours: 8 AM - 4:30 PM, M-F
Accepts calls from: Healthcare professionals only
Immediate information for most calls? No
Inquiries not handled: No public calls

CALIFORNIA

California Teratogen Information Service and Clinical Research Program
University of California, San Diego Medical Center
(619) 543-2131 or (800) 532-3749 (CA only)
UCSD Medical Center, Department of Pediatrics
200 W Arbor Dr. - Mail Stop 8446
San Diego, CA 92103-8446
Geographic region served: CA
Hours: 9 AM - 4 PM
Accepts calls from: Public and healthcare professionals
Immediate information for most calls? Yes
Inquiries not handled: Breastfeeding

CONNECTICUT

Connecticut Pregnancy Exposure Information Service
(800) 325-5391 (CT only) or (860) 679-8850
University of Connecticut Health Center
65 Kane Street
First floor genetics
West Hartford, CT 06119
Geographic region served: CT

Hours: 8 AM - 3:30 PM; W 12:30 - 3:30
Accepts calls from: Public and healthcare professionals
Immediate information for most calls? No
Inquiries not handled: Breastfeeding

ILLINOIS

Illinois Teratogen Information Service
(800) 252-4847 (IL only) or (312) 981-4354
680 N. Lakeshore Dr, Suite 1230
Chicago, IL 60611
Geographic region served: IL
Hours: 8:30 AM - 4:30 PM, M-F
Accepts calls from: Public and healthcare professionals
Immediate information for most calls? Yes

INDIANA / KENTUCKY / OHIO

Indiana Teratogen Information Service
(317) 274-1071
Indiana University Medical Center
Department of Medical and Molecular Genetics, IB130
975 W Walnut St
Indianapolis, IN 46202-5251
Geographic region served: Priority to IN callers; also serves IL, KY, OH
Hours: 8 AM - 4 PM, M-F
Accepts calls from: Public and healthcare professionals
Immediate information for most calls? Yes

MARYLAND

Sonia Tabacova
FDA Center for Drug Evaluation and Research
5600 Fishers Lane HFD 120, Room 4090
Rockville, MD 20857
Accepts inquiries from: Healthcare professionals

MASSACHUSETTS / MAINE / NEW HAMPSHIRE / RHODE ISLAND

Massachusetts Teratogen Information Service (MTIS)
(800) 322-5014 (MA only) or (781) 466-8474
Pregnancy Environmental Hotline
40 Second Ave, Suite 520
Waltham, MA 02451
Geographic region served: MA, ME, NH, RI
Hours: 9 AM - 4 PM, M-F
Accepts calls from: Public and healthcare professionals
Immediate information for most calls? Yes
Inquiries not handled: Breastfeeding

MICHIGAN

Michigan Teratogen Information Service
(313) 966-9368 or (877) 52-MITIS (64748)
Children's Hospital of Michigan
Division of Neonatology
3901 Beaubien Blvd.
Detroit, MI 48201
Accepts calls from: Healthcare professionals

MISSOURI

Missouri Teratogen Information Service
(573) 884-1345 or (800) 645-6164
University of Missouri Hospital and Clinics
One Hospital Dr, DC058.00
Columbia, MO 65212
Geographic region served: MO
Hours: 9 AM - 4 PM, M-F
Accepts calls from: Public and healthcare professionals
Immediate information for most calls? Yes

NEBRASKA

Nebraska Teratogen Project
(402) 559-5071
University of Nebraska Medical Center
985440 Nebraska Medical Center
Omaha, NE 68198-5440
Geographic region served: NE
Hours: 8:30 AM - 5:00 PM, M-F
Accepts calls from: Primarily healthcare professionals
Immediate information for most calls? Yes

NEW JERSEY / DELAWARE / PENNSYLVANIA

Pregnancy Healthline
(609) 665-6000 (NJ), (610) 222-9126 (Southeast PA)
(888) 722-2903 (NJ)
Southern New Jersey Perinatal Cooperative
2500 McClellan Ave, Suite 110
Pennsauken, NJ 08109-4613
Hours: 9:00 AM - 5:00 PM, M-F
Accepts calls from: Healthcare providers and patients in South NJ and South PA
Immediate information for most calls? Yes

NEW YORK

Pregnancy Risk Network
(800) 724-2454 (NY only)
124 Front Street
Binghamton, NY 13905
Caller's first contact: Teratology information specialist
Geographic region served: NY

PEDECS
(716) 275-3638
University of Rochester Medical Center
Department of Obstetrics and Gynecology
601 Elmwood Ave
Rochester, NY 14642-8668
Geographic region served: NY
Hours: 8 AM - 4 PM, M-F
Accepts calls from: Public and healthcare professionals
Immediate information for most calls? Yes

NORTH CAROLINA

North Carolina NCTIS Pregnancy Exposure Riskline
(800) 532-6302

Fullerton Genetics Center
14 Victoria Road, Suite 101
Asheville, NC 28801
Hours: 9:00 AM - 4:00 PM, M-F
Accepts calls from: Healthcare professionals
Immediate information for most calls? No

TEXAS

Texas Teratogen Information Service
(940) 565-3892 or (800) 733-4727
UNT Department of Biology
PO Box 305220
Denton, TX 76203-5220
Geographic region served: TX
Hours: 9 AM - 4:00 PM, M-F
Accepts calls from: Public and healthcare professionals
Immediate information for most calls? Yes

UTAH

Pregnancy Riskline
(801) 328-2229 or (800) 822-2229
Utah Department of Health
Box 144691
44 North Medical Drive
Salt Lake City, UT 84114-2106
Geographic region served: UT, MT
Healthcare professionals served only from ID, NM, WY
Hours: 8:30 AM - 4:30 PM, M-F
Accepts calls from: Public and healthcare professionals
Immediate information for most calls? Yes

VERMONT

Pregnancy Risk Information Service
(800) 932-4609 (press option 4) or (802) 847-4664
Vermont Regional Genetics Center
112 Colchester Avenue
Burlington, VT 05401
Hours: 8:30 AM - 4:30 PM, Tue and Thurs
Accept calls from: Healthcare professionals

WASHINGTON / ALASKA / IDAHO / OREGON

Care Northwest
(888) 616-8484
Box 357920
University of Washington
Seattle, WA 98195-7920
Geographic region served: AK, ID, OR, WA
Hours: 8:00 AM - 4:00 PM, M-F
Accepts calls from: Public and healthcare professionals

WEST VIRGINIA'

West Virginia School of Medicine
(800) 442-6692
OB/GYN Department
P.O. Box 9186
Robert C. Byrd Health Science Center
Morgantown, WV 26506
Hours: 8:30 AM - 5:00 PM
Accepts calls from: Public and healthcare professionals

FOREIGN

CANADA

IMAGE: Info-Medicaments en Allaitement et Grossesse
(514) 345-2333
Pharmacy Dept Ste Justine Hospital
Montreal, Quebec H3T IC5
Geographic Region: Province of Quebec
Hours: 9 AM - 12 noon, 1-4 PM
Accepts calls from: Healthcare professionals only
Immediate information available in most cases? Yes
Caller's first contact: Teratology information specialist (pharmacist)
Inquiries not handled: Disease – physical exposures

Motherisk Program
(416) 813-6780
Hospital for Sick Children
555 University Ave
Toronto, Ontario M5G 1X8
Geographic Region: Ontario (although we have accepted calls from across Canada)
Hours: 9 AM - 5 PM, M-F EST
Accepts calls from: Public and healthcare professionals
Immediate information available in most cases? Yes
Caller's first contact: Teratology information specialist

ISRAEL

Israel Teratogen Information Service
(927) 2 8243663/9
Lab of Teratology
Hebrew University - Hadassah Medical School
Jerusalem, Israel
Accepts calls from: Public and healthcare professionals

UNITED KINGDOM

The Breastfeeding Network
02392 598604
28 Green Lane, Clanfield
Waterboville, Hampshire, UK P08 0JU
Accepts calls from: Public and heathcare professionals

SECTION I

MEDICINAL AGENTS

APPROACH TO TOXICOLOGY

Jerrold B. Leikin, MD

Peter Mere Latham (1789-1875) is credited with the statement, "Poisons and medicines are oftentimes the same substance given with different intents." While this remark was penned in a bygone era, it is probably more true today than it was then. For confirmation of this fact, one can open any clinical pharmacology textbook (or even the *Physician's Desk Reference*) and note therapeutic agents that can lead to specific toxic syndromes or toxidromes.[1] There are few fields in medicine that demand such immediate, decisive, and definitive treatment strategy with as small an information base as in the area of toxicologic emergencies. Despite the potential for the wide range of clinical presentations due to a virtually unlimited amount of toxins, <0.05% of all poison exposures (about 2.5 million) annually called in to a Poison Control Center result in death.[2] In about 40% of these deaths, cardiac or respiratory arrest occurred in the prehospital setting.[1] Although this statistic may be somewhat misleading because of biased population sample, it is still evident that if one follows a consistent treatment algorithm of the poisoned patient, the outcome will be favorable in a vast majority of cases.[3-8]

Patterns of Mortality Risk from Drugs/Substance Overdose
A Theoretical Model

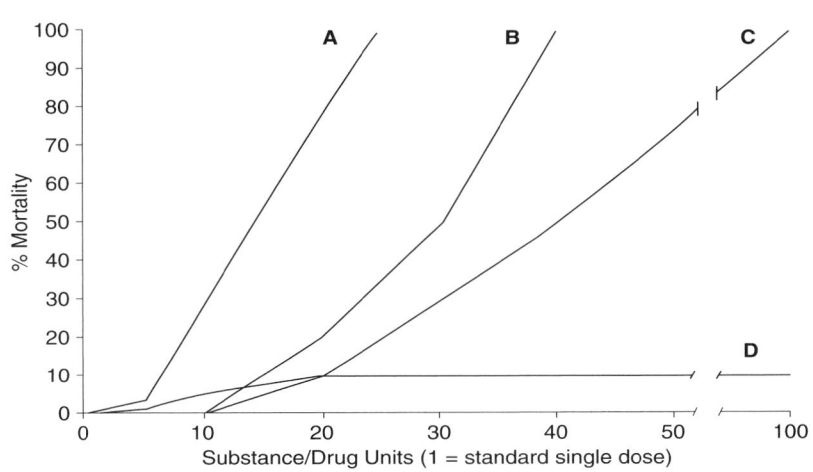

A — High toxicity: Digoxin, tricyclic antidepressant, theophylline, carbon monoxide, cyanide
B — Intermediate: Acetaminophen, salicylate, phenobarbital
C — Low: Propranolol (immediate-release)
D — Threshold for overdose effect: Atropine, phenylpropanolamine

Theoretical model of patterns of mortality risk from drug or substance overdose.
A = highly toxic substances that cause mortality with a dose-effect pattern (eg, digoxin, tricyclic antidepressants, theophylline, carbon monoxide, cyanide); B = other substances that react in a similar manner but require a larger dose or more time to reach 100% mortality (eg, acetaminophen, aspirin, iron); C = less toxic substances that act in a predictable dose-response relationship (eg, nonsteroidal anti-inflammatory drugs); D = substances that may cause mortality in a less predictable fashion where a clear dose-response relationship cannot be established (eg, atropine, phenylpropanolamine). (Courtesy of Yona Amitai, MD, Hadassah Medical Organization, Jerusalem, Israel)

Mortality from poisoning often follows two distinct patterns (see figure). Those toxins that cause mortality usually through cell necrosis by a dose-dependent mechanism are demonstrated in the figure by mortality curves A, B, and C. Highly toxic substances which can cause cellular damage and necrosis in a rapid dose-effect pattern are illustrated by mortality curve A. Moderately toxic agents, for which a higher dose is required to achieve 100% mortality, are illustrated by mortality curve B. Substances that are less toxic but whose dose-effect curve is more predictable (with a slope approaching 1) are illustrated by mortality curve C. Note that a definition of an antidote is any agent that moves a toxin mortality curve to the right. A second mechanism of toxin-induced mortality is demonstrated by curve D. This can be termed the "threshold effect", which is usually demonstrated by drugs that operate through a receptor mechanism (ie, atropine, beta-agonists, phenylpropanolamine). These drugs do not demonstrate a dose-dependent mortality curve but rather a plateau following a certain threshold dose whereupon maximal target organ response is achieved but no further mortality is expected to occur. These curves do not reflect the patterns of mortality risk for drugs that are metabolized to potentially lethal substances nor do they reflect death secondary to organ system failures in susceptible patients.

The recommended treatment plan for the poisoned patient is not unlike general treatment plans taught in advanced cardiac life support (ACLS) or advanced trauma life support (ATLS) courses. In this manner, the initial approach to the poisoned patient should be essentially similar in every case, irrespective of the toxin ingested, just as the initial approach to the trauma patient is the same irrespective of the mechanism of injury. This approach, which can be termed as routine poison management, essentially includes the following aspects:

- Stabilization: ABCs (airway, breathing, circulation); administration of glucose, thiamine, oxygen, and naloxone
- History, physical examination leading toward the identification of class of toxin (toxidrome recognition)
- Prevention of absorption (decontamination)
- Specific antidote, if available
- Removal of absorbed toxin (enhancing excretion)
- Support and monitoring for adverse effects
- If discharged, preventive education and environmental detoxification

Stabilization of the Patient

In the initial evaluation of a toxic patient, the treating physician must remember that the most common cause of airway obstruction in the unconscious patient is passive obstruction by the tongue. The neck lift with jaw thrust may be the first maneuver performed by the physician on the unconscious poisoned patient followed by endotracheal intubation. Indications for endotracheal intubation in the poisoned patient include protection of the airway in the obtunded or comatose patient with a depressed or absent gag reflex to prevent aspiration during gastric lavage; controlled ventilation in patients who demonstrate respiratory depression or failure; removal of secretions in patients who develop pulmonary edema secondary to a toxic substance; and institution of positive end-expiratory pressure (PEEP) therapy for those patients who are at risk for developing adult respiratory distress syndrome (ARDS). A chest film should be obtained to note the position of the endotracheal tube.

Following evaluation of airway and breathing, the circulatory status needs to be assessed. Hypotension in the toxic patient must be addressed as quickly as possible in order to avoid the sequelae of shock. While hypotension in this group of patients may arise from a variety of mechanisms (ranging from decreased cardiac output due to myocardial depression; to venous pooling; to decreased peripheral resistance; or to hemorrhage), the initial treatment is essentially the same: intravenous fluid administration. A fluid challenge of 100-200 mL of a crystalloid solution (10-20 mL/kg in pediatrics) is often given at this time while urine output is monitored (0.5-1 mL/kg/hour). At this time, if the patient's mental status is altered or if hypotension exists, four essentially innocuous drugs (oxygen, naloxone, glucose, and thiamine) are administered for a combination of diagnostic and therapeutic reasons. See the following table:

Drugs to Be Utilized in the Toxic Patient with Altered Mental Status		
Drug	**Effect**	**Comment**
25-50 g **dextrose** ($D_{50}W$) intravenously to reverse the effects of drug-induced hypoglycemia (adult) 1 mL/kg $D_{50}W$ diluted 1:1 (child).	This can be especially effective in patients with limited glycogen stores (ie, neonates and patients with cirrhosis).	Extravasation into the extremity of this hyperosmolar solution can cause Volkmann's contractures.
50-100 mg intravenous **thiamine**	Prevent Wernicke's encephalopathy	A water-soluble vitamin with low toxicity; rare anaphylactoid reactions have been reported.
Initial dosage of **naloxone** should be 2 mg in adult patients preferably by the intravenous route, although intramuscular, subcutaneous, intralingual, and endotracheal routes may also be utilized. Pediatric dose is 0.1 mg/kg from birth until 5 years of age. For potentially opioid-dependent patients with altered mental status, smaller doses (0.1-0.2 mg) could initially be used to increase arousal without producing withdrawal.	Specific opioid antagonist without any agonist properties.	It should be noted that some semisynthetic opiates (such as meperidine or propoxyphene) may require higher initial doses for reversal, so that a total dose of 6-10 mg is not unusual. If the patient responds to a bolus dose and then relapses to a lethargic or comatose state, a naloxone drip can be considered. This can be accomplished by administering two-thirds of the bolus dose that revives the patient per hour or injecting 4 mg naloxone in 1 L crystalloid solution and administering at a rate of 100 mL/hour (0.4 mg/hour); pediatric infusion rate: 0.16 mg/kg/hour.
Oxygen, utilized in 100% concentration	Useful for carbon monoxide, hydrogen, sulfide, and asphyxiants	While oxygen is antidotal for carbon monoxide intoxication, the only relative toxic contraindication is in paraquat intoxication (in that it can promote pulmonary fibrosis).

History and Physical Examination

While the history and physical examination is the cornerstone of clinical patient management, it takes on special meaning with regard to the toxic patient. While taking a history may be a more direct method of the determination of the toxin, often it is not reliable. Information obtained may prove minimal in some cases and could be considered partial or inaccurate in suicide gestures and addicts. A quick physical examination often leads to important clues about the nature of the toxin. These clues can be specific symptom complexes associated with certain toxins and can be referred to as "toxidromes." See the following table:

Examples of Toxidromes			
Toxidromes	**Pattern**	**Example of Drugs**	**Treatment Approach**
Anticholinergic	Fever, ileus, flushing, tachycardia, urinary retention, inability to sweat, visual blurring, and mydriasis. Central manifestations include myoclonus, choreoathetosis, toxic psychosis with lilliputian hallucinations, seizures, and coma	Antihistamines Atropine Baclofen Benztropine Jimson weed Methylpyroline Phenothiazines Propantheline Tricyclic antidepressants	Physostigmine for life-threatening symptoms*
Carbolic marasmus	Headache, dizziness, salivation, anorexia, and skin pigmentation changes	Phenol	Lavage/activated charcoal with cathartic Possible endoscopy
Cholinergic	Characterized by salivation, lacrimation, urination, defecation, gastrointestinal cramps, and emesis ("sludge"). Bradycardia and bronchoconstriction may also be seen	Carbamate Organophosphates Pilocarpine	Atropine* Pralidoxime for organophosphate insecticides*
Extrapyramidal	Choreoathetosis, hyperreflexia, trismus, opisthotonos, rigidity, and tremor	Haloperidol Phenothiazines	Diphenhydramine Benztropine
Hallucinogenic	Perceptual distortions, synesthesia, depersonalization, and derealization	Amphetamines Cannabinoids Cocaine Indole alkaloids Phencyclidine	Benzodiazepine
Metal fume fever	Pleuritic chest pain, cough, dyspnea, thirst, metallic taste, fever (temperature ranges from 102°-104°), tachycardia, chills, nausea, myalgia	Most common: Zinc and copper Also: Cadmium, mercury	Supportive (usually resolves within 2 days) Avoidance of further exposure
Monosodium glutamate symptom complex	Burning sensation of back of neck, forearm, and chest; numbness in back of neck radiating to arms and back; tingling, warmth, and weakness in facial area, temples, upper back, neck, and arms; facial pressure or tightness, chest pain, headache, nausea, tachycardia, bronchospasm, drowsiness, weakness	Monosodium glutamate	Usually self-limited; diphenhydramine may be useful
Narcotic	Altered mental status, unresponsiveness, shallow respirations, slow respiratory rate or periodic breathing, miosis, bradycardia, hypothermia	Opiates Dextromethorphan Pentazocine Propoxyphene	Naloxone*
Retinoic acid syndrome	Fever, dyspnea (60%), arrhythmias (23%), tachycardia, hypotension, cardiac failure (6%), respiratory distress, nausea, vomiting (57%), renal failure (seen in patients with acute promyelocytic leukemia treated with >45 mg/m^2/day of tretinoin)	Tretinoin	Dexamethasone (10 mg I.M. every 12 hours for 3 or more days)
Sedative/Hypnotic	Manifested by sedation with progressive deterioration of central nervous system function. Coma, stupor, confusion, apnea, delirium, or hallucinations may accompany this pattern	Anticonvulsants Antipsychotics Barbiturates Benzodiazepines Ethanol Ethchlorvynol Fentanyl Glutethimide Meprobamate Methadone Methocarbamol Opiates Quinazolines Propoxyphene	Naloxone* (opiates) Flumazenil* (benzodiazepines) Urinary alkalinization (barbiturates)

Examples of Toxidromes (*Continued*)

Toxidromes	Pattern	Example of Drugs	Treatment Approach
Epileptogenic†	May mimic stimulant pattern with hyperthermia, hyperreflexia, and tremors being prominent signs	Anticholinergics Camphor Chlorinated hydrocarbons Cocaine Isoniazid Lidocaine Lindane Nicotine Phencyclidine Strychnine Xanthines	Anticonvulsants (though generally not phenytoin) Pyridoxine for isoniazid* Extracorporeal removal of drug (ie, lindane, camphor, xanthines) Physostigmine for anticholinergic agents* Avoid phenytoin
Serotonin†	Confusion, myoclonus, hyperreflexia, diaphoresis tremor, facial flushing, diarrhea, fever, trismus	Clomipramine Fluoxetine Isoniazid L-tryptophan Paroxetine Phenelzine Sertraline Tranylcypromine Drug combinations include: MAO inhibitors with L-tryptophan Fluoxetine or meperidine Fluoxetine with carbamazepine or sertraline Clomipramine and meclobemide Trazadol and buspirone Paroxetine and dextromethorphan	Withdrawal of drug/benzodiazepine Beta-blocker (?) Cyproheptadine (?)
Solvent	Lethargy, confusion, dizziness, headache, restlessness, incoordination, derealization, depersonalization	Acetone Chlorinated hydrocarbons Hydrocarbons Naphthalene Trichloroethane Toluene	Avoid catecholamines
Stimulant	Restlessness, excessive speech and motor activity, tachycardia, tremor, and insomnia — may progress to seizure. Other effects noted include euphoria, mydriasis, anorexia, and paranoia	Amphetamines Caffeine (xanthines) Cocaine Ephedrine/pseudoephedrine Methylphenidate Nicotine Phencyclidine	Benzodiazepines
Uncoupling of oxidative phosphylation	Hyperthermia, tachypnea, diaphoresis, metabolic acidosis (usually)	Aluminum phosphide Aspirin/Salicylates Bromethalin 2,4-Dichlorophenol Di-n-Butyl Phthalate Dinitrophenols Dinitro cresols Glyphosate (?) Hexachlorobutadiene Phosphorus Pentachlorophenol Tin (?) Zinc phosphide	Sodium bicarbonate to treat metabolic acidosis Patient cooling techniques Avoidance of atropine or salicylate agents Hemodialysis may be required for acidosis treatment.

The term toxidromes was originated by Mofensen in 1974 to assist the clinician in identifying the classification of toxins by toxin-specific symptom complexes. With the clinician focusing on the patient's vital signs, sensorium, motor signs, ocular findings, and other clinical abnormalities (eg, odor on breath, discoloration of urine), clinical toxin-pattern recognition can be achieved and an initial treatment plan formalized.

Sensorium: Determine whether the patient is comatose, stuporous, lethargic, confused, or alert.

Behavior and hallucinations: Often the hallucinatory pattern of the patient can be specific for certain drugs. For example, with atropine the patient experiences lilliputian hallucinations; with cocaine, there is a simple visual hallucinatory pattern with objects appearing in the periphery of vision; with phencyclidine, complex hallucinations are often indistinguishable clinically from a paranoid psychosis; and with LSD, the patient experiences a combination of illusions (seeing objects in altered forms), hallucination (experiencing sensations without external stimuli), and pseudohallucinations (knowing when one is hallucinating).[9]

Motor signs: Tremors, hyporeflexia and hyperreflexia, and even the nature of seizures can be useful diagnostic tools. Like hallucinations, seizures caused by specific toxins can exhibit certain specific properties. For example, strychnine is unique in that it can cause generalized seizures while the patient is alert. This can be referred to as a "spinal seizure." Other drug-induced seizures will respond only to specific antidotal therapies and not to conventional antiseizure medication. Examples of this property include anticholinergic-induced seizures, which may respond to physostigmine, and isoniazid-induced seizures, which respond to pyridoxine. Additionally, theophylline-induced seizures rarely respond to phenytoin alone and often only to multidrug therapy.

Vital signs: Sympathomimetics and anticholinergics essentially cause an increase in all of the vital signs parameters. This is particularly true for cocaine intoxication, where it has been noted that hyperthermia may be a particularly ominous sign for mortality. Conversely, organophosphates, opiates, barbiturates, beta-blockers, benzodiazepines, alcohol, and clonidine toxicities result in hypothermia, respiratory depression, and bradycardia.

Ocular findings: This can be divided into categories: pupillary size and reactivity, and demonstration of nystagmus.

Pupillary signs: Both anticholinergic and sympathomimetic substances can result in mydriasis, but in cocaine intoxication, the pupils will respond to light, whereas with anticholinergics the pupils will not. Agents that contribute to miosis include organophosphate insecticides, narcotics, bromide, acetone, clonidine, and nicotine. Phencyclidine has been known to cause either mydriasis or miosis.

Nystagmus: Alcohols are probably the most common etiology of horizontal nystagmus, although lithium, carbamazepine, solvents, meprobamate, quinine, and primidone can also result in horizontal nystagmus. Phencyclidine can cause a combination of vertical, horizontal, and even rotary nystagmus, as can phenytoin and sedative-hypnotics.

Other findings: In addition to these physical signs, odors emanating from the patient may also provide important directions in management. For example, a garlic odor is often caused by arsenicals, phosphorus compounds, or organophosphates. A rotten egg odor can be associated with decomposition of organic materials (hydrogen sulfide) or disulfiram. Periodic gaze disturbances ("ping-pong" gaze) are associated with MAO inhibitor overdose.

Radiographs can be of some utility in toxic exposure analysis. Factors that influence radiodensity include molecular weight, atomic number, relative contrast to surrounding tissues, and compactness of the form of drug. Sustained-released medications can be more easily detected through digital enhancement of the radiograph.[10] Also, specific sustained-release dosage forms (bead-filled capsules) may appear as radiolucencies. It should be pointed out that this is not a reliable method for evaluating toxic exposure and should be utilized in only specific cases. These cases include evaluation of heavy metal exposure (including leaded paint chips), concretion formation of drugs (such as aspirin, meprobamate, glutethimide, barbiturates, iron, and sustained-release theophylline), and the body packing/stuffing phenomenon.

The clinical laboratory evaluation includes the evaluation of the "three gaps of toxicology": anion gap (usually a type A lactic acidosis due to tissue hypoxia), osmolar gap, and oxygen saturation gap. What these "gaps" have in common is that the toxic substance accounts for a difference between calculated and measured determination. The following drugs are known to cause these gaps.

Drugs/Toxins Causing Increased Anion Gap (>12 mEq/L)

Nonacidotic

Carbenicillin   Sodium salts

Metabolic Acidosis

Acetaminophen (ingestion >75-100 g)   Ammonium chloride
Acetazolamide   Ascorbic acid
Aluminum phosphate   Benzalkonium chloride
Amiloride   Bialaphos
4-Aminopyridine   2-Butanone

2-Butoxyethanol
Carbon monoxide
Centrimonium bromide
Chloramphenicol
Clozapine
Cobalt
Colchicine
Cotrimoxazole (I.V. high dose)
Cyanide
Dapsone
Dimethyl sulfate
Dinitrophenol
Endosulfan
Epinephrine (I.V. overdose)
Ethanol
Ethyl acetate
Ethylene dibromide
Ethylene glycol
Fenoprofen
Fluoroacetate
Formaldehyde
Fructose (I.V.)
Funnel web spiders
Glycol ethers
Glyphosate
Hydrogen sulfide
Ibuprofen (ingestion >300 mg/kg)
Inorganic acid
Iodine
Iron
Isoniazid
Ketamine
Ketoprofen
Lime sulfur
Margosa oil
Metaldehyde
Metformin

Methanol
Methenamine mandelate
Misoprostol
Monochloracetic acid
Nalidixic acid
Naproxen
Nefopam
Niacin
Papaverine
Paraldehyde
Pennyroyal oil
Pentaborane
Pentachlorophenol
Phenelzine
Phenformin (off the market)
Phenol
Phenylbutazone
Phosphoric acid
Polyethylene glycol (low molecular weight)
Propofol
Propylene glycol
Salicylates
Sodium Azide
Sorbitol (I.V.)
Strychnine
Sublimed sulfur
Sultiame
Surfactant herbicide
Tetracycline (outdated)
Tienilic acid
Toluene
Tranylcypromine
Vacor
Valproic acid
Verapamil
Zidovudine (chronic use >6 months)
Zinc phosphide

Drugs/Toxins Causing Decreased Anion Gap (<6 mEq/L)

Acidosis

Acetazolamide
Amiloride
Ammonium chloride
Amphotericin B
Bromide
Fialuridine (FIAU)
Iodide

Kombucha Tea
Lithium
Polymyxin B
Spironolactone
Sulindac
Toluene
Tromethamine

Toxins Causing Osmolar Gap (By Freezing-Point Depression, Gap is >10 mOsm from Baseline Value)

Ethanol
Ethylene glycol
Glycerol
Hypermagnesemia (>9.5 mEq/L)
Isopropanol (acetone)

Iodine (questionable)
Mannitol
Methanol
Sorbitol
Valproic acid (minor)

Toxins Associated With Oxygen Saturation Gap (>5% Difference Between Measured and Calculated Value)

Carbon monoxide
Cyanide (questionable)
Hydrogen sulfide (possible)

Methemoglobin
Nitrates

The Toxicology Laboratory is also very useful for determining levels of toxin in body fluids. Often these drug levels will guide therapy. For example, use of the Rumack-Matthew nomogram for acute acetaminophen poisoning can direct N-acetylcysteine therapy if the serum acetaminophen level falls above the treatment line.

Nomogram: Plasma or Serum Acetaminophen Concentration vs Time Post Acetaminophen Ingestion

Estimating potential for hepatotoxicity:
The following nomogram has been developed to estimate the probability that plasma levels in relation to intervals postingestion will result in hepatotoxicity.

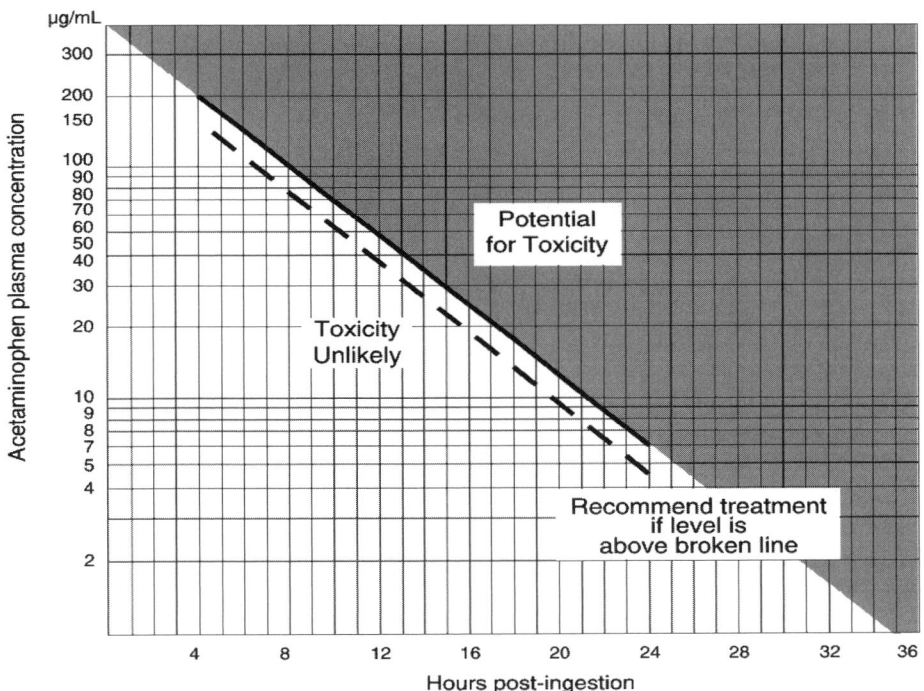

From Rumack BH and Matthew H, "Acetaminophen Poisoning and Toxicity," *Pediatrics,* June 1975, 55:871-6 with permission.

If the acetaminophen level determined at least 4 hours following an overdose falls above the broken line, administer the entire course of acetylcysteine treatment.

If the acetaminophen level, determined at least 4 hours following an overdose, falls below the broken line, acetylcysteine treatment is not necessary or if already initiated may be discontinued. Serum levels drawn before 4 hours may not represent peak levels.

Cautions for Use of this Chart:
1. The time coordinates refer to time postingestion.
2. The graph relates only to plasma levels following a single acute overdose ingestion.
3. The broken line, which represents a 25% allowance below the solid line, is included to allow for possible errors in acetaminophen plasma assays and estimated time from ingestion of an overdose.

Similarly, the Done nomogram is somewhat useful in predicting salicylate toxicity in pediatric patients; see the Serum Salicylate Toxicity Nomogram and the Ibuprofen Toxicity Nomogram. Neither nomogram should be utilized with chronic ingestions.

A nomogram has been devised for theophylline ingestion.

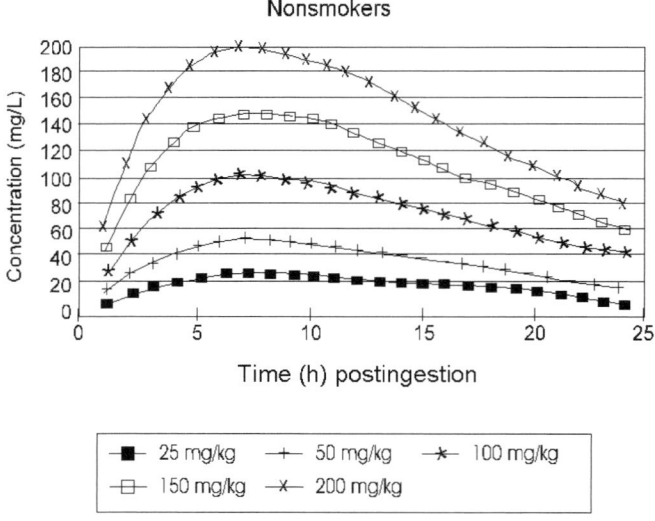

SERUM THEOPHYLLINE OVERDOSE
Nonsmokers

■ 25 mg/kg	+ 50 mg/kg	* 100 mg/kg
□ 150 mg/kg	× 200 mg/kg	

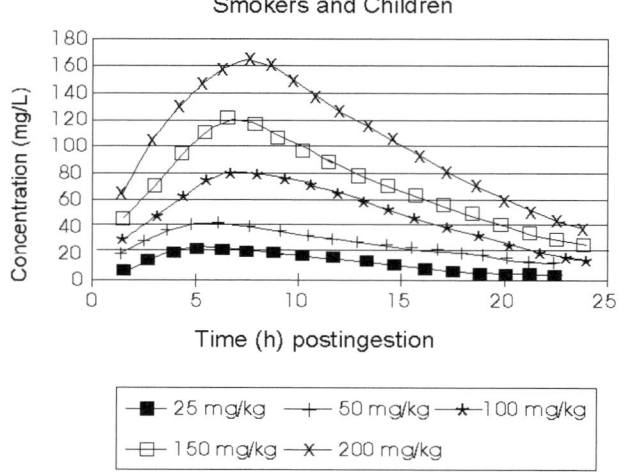

SERUM THEOPHYLLINE OVERDOSE
Smokers and Children

■ 25 mg/kg	+ 50 mg/kg	* 100 mg/kg
□ 150 mg/kg	× 200 mg/kg	

Nomogram for overdose of sustained-release theophylline in 1) nonsmoking adults, and 2) smokers and children. (Courtesy of Frank Paloucek, PharmD, College of Pharmacy, University of Illinois, Chicago.)

Additionally, certain serum levels demand immediate attention when they are obtained. For example, one should consider aggressive treatment in the setting of an acute exposure when one obtains a quantitative level of such toxins as a carboxyhemoglobin level >25% (hyperbaric oxygen), ethylene glycol >20 μg/dL (ethanol therapy with possible hemodialysis), methanol level >20 μg/dL (ethanol therapy with possible hemodialysis), lithium level >2.5 mEq/L (hemodialysis), iron level >350 μg/dL (deferoxamine), methemoglobin level >30% (methylene blue), salicylate level >100 mg/dL (hemodialysis), lead level >45 μg/dL (chelation), or mercury level >3 μg/dL (chelation).

Prevention of Absorption

Toxic substances can enter the body through the dermal, ocular, pulmonary, parenteral, and gastrointestinal routes. The basic principle of decontamination involves appropriate copious irrigation of the toxic substance relatable to the route of exposure. For example, with ocular exposure, this can be done with normal saline for 30-40 minutes through a Morgan therapeutic lens. With alkali exposures, the pH should be checked until the runoff of the solution is either neutral or slightly acidic. Skin decontamination involves removal of the toxin with nonabrasive soap. This should especially be considered for organophosphates, methylene chloride, dioxin, radiation, hydrocarbons, and herbicide exposure. Separate drainage areas should be obtained for the contaminated runoff.

Since >80% of incidents of accidental poisoning in children occur through the gastrointestinal tract, a thorough knowledge of gastric decontamination is essential. There are essentially four modes of gastric decontamination, of which three are physical removal (emesis, gastric lavage, and whole bowel irrigation). Activated charcoal is the fourth mode for preventing absorption.

Emesis: Emesis by means of syrup of ipecac (a derivative of the plant alkaloid emetine) has been a standard of gastric decontamination; utilized at a dose of 30 mL accompanied with 16 oz of fluid for adults (repeated in 20 minutes if no emesis). Dosage of 15 mL in children 1-12 years of age accompanied with 6-8 oz fluid, or 10 mL in infants 6-12 months of age with 4 oz fluid is virtually 100% effective in producing emesis. However, it is apparent that a 100% rate of emesis is not equitable to a 100% rate of removal of toxin. In ideal circumstances, only 30% to 40% removal can be achieved within 1-2 hours postingestion, although significantly higher removal rates can be achieved if emesis is obtained within 30 minutes postingestion. For this reason, home ipecac use is being discouraged. Its use as a method of gastric decontamination in the hospital setting is virtually zero[11,12]. The use of salt water, detergents, apomorphine, copper sulfate, and physical induction of emesis should be confined to the medical history books.

Gastric lavage: Gastric lavage through a 36- to 40-French single-use Ewald tube in adults (28- to 34-French in children) is another mode of physical removal of ingested toxin. With the patient in the left lateral decubitus position, feet elevated 20°, approximately 200-300 mL warm saline (38°C) is lavaged per run (10-15 mL/kg in children), with an additional 1-2 L used for irrigation after clearing. As with ipecac, 30% to 40% removal rate can be achieved. The contraindications are ingestion of caustic material, hydrocarbons, hemorrhagic diathesis, and seizures. Lavage should only be considered with an intubated airway with a cuffed endotracheal tube if the gag reflex is lost. Gastric lavage is not a routine procedure for all poisonings. Its use is reserved for life-threatening ingestions of selected agents within 1 hour of the ingestion. Complications of lavage include aspiration, laryngospasm, mechanical injury, and electrolyte imbalance.[13]

Activated charcoal: The use of activated charcoal has had a resurgence over the past 10 years, with several studies comparing it favorably to the other forms of physical gastric decontamination.[14,15] An inert, nontoxic adsorbent with a surface area as high as 3000 m^2/g, it is quite effective in binding high molecular weight compounds due to intermolecular attractions (van der Waals forces). The dose of activated charcoal commonly used is 0.5-1 g/kg in children and 25-100 g in adults (can be instilled through an Ewald tube), although data (with theophylline and salicylate) suggest that the optimum dose is 10 g of activated charcoal for every gram of toxin ingested. Doses in excess of 100 gms determined by a 10:1 ratio calculation must be split so that after the initial dose, no dose greater than 25 g be given every 2 hours. While children may not want to drink activated charcoal because it is black and gritty, mixing it with juice may bring a higher acceptance rate. Tablets of activated charcoal should not be used for gastric contamination.

Activated charcoal had been traditionally administered in conjunction with a cathartic to facilitate evacuation of the toxic substance. Cathartics most often administered are magnesium sulfate (15-20 g in a 10% solution), magnesium citrate (200-300 mL), sodium sulfate or sorbitol (100-150 mL in a 70% solution, or 0.5-3 mL/kg up to 50 g in pediatric patients). While cathartics may account for an additional 30% of more drug elimination, they should not be used in the presence of ileus.[16] Additionally, recent reports of hypermagnesemia, in the setting of magnesium-containing cathartic administration with renal insufficiency and emesis associated with increasing amounts of sorbitol, indicate that cathartics are not a benign medication and should not be used routinely.

Whole bowel irrigation: Whole bowel irrigation with the use of GoLYTELY® has been advocated for certain intoxications, most particularly iron, lead, lithium, sustained-release or enteric-coated medications, and the body packer phenomenon.[17] The patient should be seated or the head of the bed elevated 45°; the cathartic should be administered through a 12-French nasogastric tube. At an adult infusion rate of 1.5-2 L/hour (500-1000 mL/hour in children), it may take 4-6 hours (or 3 L) for complete bowel irrigation until the rectal effluent is clear. If emesis occurs, metoclopramide may be administered. Additionally, the infusion rate can be decreased by 50% for up to 1 hour and then returned to the original rate. It should be considered as a first-line decontamination procedure when one encounters a toxin that is not well adsorbed by activated charcoal within 2 hours of ingestion. Contraindications include adynamic ileus, hemorrhage, bowel obstruction, bowel perforation, unprotected airway, hemodynamic instability, or uncontrolled vomiting. Activated charcoal should not be administered with whole bowel irrigation.

Antidotes

One can use as a definition of an antidote any drug that increases the median lethal dose (LD_{50}) of a toxin. While certain drugs may modify symptoms produced by a toxin (eg, beta-blockers reducing heart rate in cocaine intoxication), only a relatively few toxins have specific antidotes. The reader should be referred to specific monographs for antidote utilization.

Enhancement of Elimination

Only recently has this aspect of poison management received more than cursory attention in practice and in the literature. The standard practice for enhancement of elimination consisted primarily of forced diuresis in order to excrete the toxin. However, the past 10 years experience has produced a radical change in the approach to this and therefore a more focused methodology to eliminating absorbed toxins. Essentially, there are three methods by which absorbed toxins may be eliminated: recurrent adsorption with multiple dosings of activated charcoal, use of forced diuresis in combination with possible alkalinization of the urine, and use of dialysis, charcoal hemoperfusion, or other extracorporeal methods to support renal function. Other methods such as exchange transfusions and plasmapheresis are used rarely.

Multiple dosing of activated charcoal ("pulse dosing") has been advocated as a method for removal of absorbed drug.[18] This procedure has been demonstrated to be efficacious in drugs that re-enter the gastrointestinal tract through enterohepatic circulation (eg, digitoxin, carbamazepine, glutethimide) and with drugs that diffuse from the systemic circulation into the gastrointestinal tract due to formation of a concentration gradient ("the infinite sink" hypothesis).

Toxins with Enhanced Elimination by Multiple Dosing of Activated Charcoal

Acetaminophen	Maprotiline
Amitriptyline	Methyprylon
Atrazine (?)	Nadolol
Baclofen (?)	Nortriptyline
Bupropion (?)	Phencyclidine (?)
Carbamazepine*	Phenobarbital*
Chlordecone	Phenylbutazone
Cyclosporine	Phenytoin (?)
Dapsone*	Piroxicam
Dextropropoxyphene	Propoxyphene
Diazepam (desmethyldiazepam)	Propranolol (?)
Digitoxin	Quinine*
Digoxin (with renal impairment)	Salicylates (?)
Disopyramide	Sotalol
Glutethimide	Theophylline*

* Recommended in American Academy of Clinical Toxicology Practice Guidelines.[18]

The following agents have been studied and have not been demonstrated to result in enhanced elimination.

Amiodarone	Meprobamate
Astemizole	Methotrexate
Chlorpropamide	Sodium Valproate
Doxepin	Tobramycin
Imipramine	Vancomycin

Essentially, this can be thought of as "intestinal dialysis." The toxins by which this method appears to be most efficacious are those with low volume of distribution (<1.0 L/kg), uncharged, lipophilic, low protein binding, long half-life, and that undergo enterohepatic circulation (although the latter property is not essential). Note that these are similar criteria required for a toxin to be removed by hemoperfusion.

Despite the above limitations, multiple dosing of activated charcoal is utilized quite often. The literature has demonstrated that the data on phenytoin and salicylates are somewhat equivocal due primarily to their high protein binding. The usual dosage of activated charcoal is 1 g/kg as the initial dose, followed by 0.5 g/kg every 2-4 hours. Usually at least three doses are required; cathartics should not be administered more than once daily. Multiple dosing of cholestyramine (4 g every 8 hours) resin may be useful in enhancing elimination of digitoxin, phenobarbital, warfarin, lorazepam, methotrexate, lindane, or chlordecone.

The practice of blindly overloading the toxic patient with intravenous fluids to promote diuresis has not been supported in the literature and is associated with an increased risk of pulmonary edema, hyponatremia, or increased intracranial pressure.[19,20] Patients who exhibit the syndrome of inappropriate secretion of antidiuretic hormone (SIADH) should not undergo a diuresis. Ion trapping techniques are useful to increase renal excretion of polar drugs with a dissociable group that will carry a charge at a pH that is distant from their pKa. Thus, most of the drug will be ionic (either acidic or alkali) in the distal tubular lumen and in its ionic form will not undergo tubular reabsorption and thus enhance urinary excretion. The use of this modality (with or without ion trapping) should be limited to the following drugs.

Toxins Eliminated by Saline Diuresis

Barium	Isoniazid (?)
Bromides	Meprobamate
Chromium	Methyl iodide
Cimetidine (?)	Mushrooms (Group I)
Cis-platinum	Nickel
Cyclophosphamide	Potassium chloroplatinite
Hydrazine	Thallium
Iodide	Valproic Acid (?)
Iodine	

Toxins Eliminated by Urine Alkalinization

2,4-D-chlorophenoxyacetic acid (Mecoprop)* (urine pH >8 and urine flow of 600 mL/h)	Methotrexate*
	2-Methyl-4-chlorophenoxyacetic acid (MCPA)
Barbital (?)	Orellanine (?)
Chlorpropamide*	Phenobarbital*
Diflunisal* (2-fold increase)	Primidone
Fluoride	Quinolones antibiotic
Iopanoic Acid (?)	Salicylates*
Isoniazid (?)	Sulfisoxazole
Mephobarbital	Uranium

* Confirmed in clinical studies

A urine flow of 3-5 mL/kg/hour should be achieved with a combination of isotonic fluids or diuretics. Alkalinization can be achieved by administration of 44-88 mEq of intravenous sodium bicarbonate per liter to titrate a urine pH of 7.5-8.5; 20-40 mEq/L of intravenous potassium chloride may also be required (potassium should not be administered in patients with renal insufficiency). Arterial pH should not exceed 7.50. In a child, the dose of I.V. sodium bicarbonate is 25-50 nmol (25 mL of an 8.4% solution) over one hour. It should be noted that urine alkalinization is most often for salicylates and phenobarbital; however, it should be noted that multiple dosing of activated charcoal is more efficient in phenobarbital elimination. Complications of urine alkalinization include hypokalemia, hypocalcemia, and systemic alkalinization. Although several drugs can exhibit enhanced elimination through an acidic urine (tranylcypromine, quinine, chlorpheniramine, fenfluramine, strychnine, cathinone or khat, amphetamines, phencyclidine, nicotine, bismuth, diethylcarbamazine citrate, ephedrine, flecainide, local anesthetics), the practice of acidifying the urine should be discouraged in that it can produce metabolic acidosis and promote renal failure in the presence of rhabdomyolysis.

Hemodialysis can be used to increase clearance with the following drugs:

Drugs and Toxins Removed by Hemodialysis

Acetaminophen
Acetazolamide
Acyclovir
Alkyl phosphate
Allopurinol
Aluminum
Amanita phalloides (?)
Amantadine (?)
Amikacin
Ammonia
Ammonium chloride
Amobarbital
Amoxicillin
Amphetamine
Ampicillin
Anilines
Antimony (Pentavalent) (?)
Arsenic (?)
Atenolol
Azathioprine
Azlocillin
Aztreonam
Bacitracin (?)
Baclofen
Barbital
Boric acid
Bretylium
Bromides
Bromisoval
Butalbital
Calcium
Captopril (?)
Carbamazepine
Carbenicillin
Carbromal
Carisoprodol
Cefaclor
Cefamandole
Cefazolin
Cefoperazone (?)
Cefotaxime
Cefoxitin
Ceftazidime
Cephalexin
Cephaloridine
Cephalothin

Cephapirin
Cephradine
Chloral hydrate
Chloramphenicol (?)
Chlordiazepoxide (?)
Chloride
Chlorpropamide
Chromic acid
Chromium
Cimetidine (?)
Ciprofloxacin (?)
Colistin
Cyclobarbital
Cyclophosphamide
Cycloserine
Dapsone
Demeton-S-methyl sulfoxide
Dextropropoxyphene
Diethyl pentenamide
Dimethoate
Dinitro-ortho-cresol
Diquat
Disopyramide
Enalapril (?)
Ergotamine
Erythromycin
Ethambutol
Ethanol
Ethchlorvynol (?)
Ethinamate
Ethosuximide (?)
Ethylene glycol
Eucalyptus oil
Famciclovir (Penciclovir)
Famotidine (?)
Flucytosine
Fluoride
Fluoridem chlorate
5-Fluorouracil (?)
Folic acid
Formaldehyde
Foscarnet sodium
Fosfomycin
Gabapentin
Gallamine triethiodide
Ganciclovir

Gentamicin
Glufosinate Ammonium
Glutethimide (?)
Glycol ethers
Hydrazine (?)
Hydrochlorothiazide
Imipenem/Cilastatin
Iodides
Isoniazid
Isopropanol
Kanamycin
Ketoprofen
Lead (with EDTA)
Lithium
Magnesium
Mannitol
Meprobamate
Meropenem
Metal-chelate compounds
Metformin (?)
Methanol
Methaqualone
Methotrexate
Methyldopa
Methylprednisolone (?)
Methylprylone
4-Methylpyrazole
Metronidazole
Mezlocillin
Monochloroacetic acid
Nadolol
Nafcillin
Neomycin
Netilmicin
Nitrates
Nitrite
Orellanine (?)
Ouabain (?)
Oxalic acid
Paraldehyde
Paraquat (?)
Pargyline
Penicillin G

Pentachlorophenol
Pentobarbital
Phenelzine (?)
Phenobarbital
Phosphate
Phosphoric acid
Piperacillin
Potassium Chloride
Potassium Dichromate
Practolol
Prednisone (?)
Primidone
Procainamide
Propoxyphene
Quinalbital
Quinidine
Ranitidine (?)
Rifabutin
Salicylates
Secobarbital (?)
Sodium chlorate
Sodium chloride
Sodium citrate
Sotalol
Streptomycin
Strychnine
Succimer (?)
Sulfamethoxazole
Sulfisoxazole
Tetracycline (?)
Thallium
Theophylline
Thiocyanates
Ticarcillin
Tobramycin
Tocainide
Topiramate
Tranylcypromine sulfate (?)
Trimethoprim
Valproic acid (?)
Vancomycin
Verapamil (?)
Vidarabine

Hemodialysis is especially effective in correcting metabolic acidosis induced by certain toxins such as salicylates. Criteria utilized for hemodialysis include water solubility of the toxin, low steady state volume of distribution (<1 L/kg), low protein binding ($<70\%$ to 80%), polarity, and low molecular weight (<500 daltons). Drugs in which hemodialysis is required at an early stage of intoxication include methanol, ethylene glycol, lithium, and boric acid.[21,22] Hemodialysis also should be definitely used after heavy metal chelation in patients with renal failure.

A lipid-based dialysis (used by adding soy bean oil to an aqueous bath) may be useful in enhancing the elimination of such lipid soluble toxins as ethchlorvynol, glutethimide, camphor, or N,N-diethyltoluamide (DEET), although clinical studies with this modality are minimal. Complications of hemodialysis include hypotension, bleeding (due to systemic anticoagulation), nosocomial infection, or air embolism. Peritoneal dialysis should not be considered for the enhancement of elimination of drugs with the possible exception of vancomycin or boric acid.

Charcoal hemoperfusion can increase clearances of toxins that are absorbed by an absorbent. Unlike hemodialysis, drug clearance through hemoperfusion is less dependent on water solubility, but on ability of the adsorbent to bind to the drug. Hemoperfusion is most efficacious for phenobarbital, glutethimide, theophylline, and paraquat. The complications of hemoperfusion are analogous to hemodialysis. Additionally, leukopenia, thrombocytopenia, or hypocalcemia may occur.[22]

Drugs and Toxins Removed by Hemoperfusion (Charcoal)

Amanita phalloides (?)	Meprobamate
Atenolol (?)	Methaqualone
Bromisoval	Methotrexate
Bromoethylbutyramide	Methsuximide
Caffeine	Methyprylon (?)
Carbamazepine	Metoprolol (?)
Carbon tetrachloride (?)	Nadolol (?)
Carbromal	Orellanine (?)
Chloral hydrate (trichloroethanol)	Oxalic acid (?)
Chloramphenicol	Paraquat
Chlorfenvinphos (?)	Parathion (?)
Chlorpropamide	Pentamidine
Cibenzoline succinate	Phenelzine (?)
Clonidine	Phenobarbital
Colchicine (?)	Phenol
Creosote (?)	Phenytoin
Dapsone	Podophyllin (?)
Demeton-S-methyl Sulfoxide	Procainamide (?)
Diltiazem (?)	Quinidine (?)
Dimethoate	Rifabutin (?)
Disopyramide	Sotalol (?)
Ethchlorvynol	Thallium
Ethylene oxide	Thyroglobulin/Thyroid hormone
Glutethimide	Theophylline
Levothyroxine (?)	Valproic acid
Lindane	Verapamil (?)
Liotrix	

Continuous arteriovenous hemofiltration has been used to treat lithium, paraquat, N-acetyl-procainamide, and vancomycin ingestions with varying results. It is capable of filtering molecules with a molecular weight up to 500 daltons, but some substances such as thallium and formaldehyde cannot be removed by this method despite their low molecular weight. High flux dialyzers can promote clearance of larger molecules (eg, vancomycin, valproic acid) and compounds bound to proteins (eg, carbamazepine). Hemodialysis can also correct systemic acidosis induced by salicylate, toxic alcohols, and metformin. Plasmaphoresis is a method for removal of plasma in exchange for albumin or fresh frozen plasma. With plasma exchange, the plasma concentration of drugs or toxins can theorectically be lowered if they are primarily in the intravascular compartment. Thus, toxins which are highly protein bound and have a high molecular weight can be removed. In reality, multiple plasma exchanges have only been demonstrated to be marginally useful in treating life-threatening exposure to *Amanita* mushroom (Group I) poisoning, botulism, pentachlorophenol, crotalid envenomation, and thyroxine and digoxin overdose.[23]

Exchange transfusion is a useful modality to enhance drug elimination in neonatal or infant drug toxicity. Usually double or triple volume exchanges are performed. It has been utilized to treat barbiturate, phenobarbital, acetaminophen, iron, caffeine, methyl salicylate, propafenone, ganciclovir, sodium nitrite, lead, phenazopyridine hydrochloride, Group I mushrooms, atropine, reserpine, pentachlorophenol, pine oil, theophylline overdose, and nitrate exposure in pediatric patients. Exchange transfusions (500-2000 mL) volume replacement have also been used to treat adults with 80-150 g ingestions of parathion.

EXCHANGE TRANSFUSIONS

Toxicants for Which Exchange Transfusions May Be Helpful

Parathion
Acetaminophen
Iron (serum levels >1000 mcg/dL)
Caffeine
Methyl salicylate
Propafenone
Ganciclovir/acyclovir
Methemoglobin producers[1]
Lead
Phenazopyridine hydrochloride
Pine oil
Theophylline (serum levels >90 mcg/mL)
Vancomycin
Plasmodium falciparum malaria
Halothane hepatitis
E. coli 0157:H7 associated Hemolytic-Uremic Syndrome

[1]Especially patients with G6PD or NADPH-dependent methemoglobin reductase deficiency and/or methylene blue therapy with methemoglobin levels >70%.

References

Cohen BL and Bovasso GJ Jr, "Acquired Methemoglobinemia and Hemolytic Anemia Following Excessive Pyridium (Phenazopyridine Hydrochloride) Ingestion," *Clin Pediatr (Phila),* 1971, 10(9):537-40.

de Monchy JG, Snoek WJ, Sluiter HJ, et al, "Treatment of Severe Parathion Intoxication," *Vet Hum Toxicol,* 1979, 21 Suppl:115-7.

Fural MA and Heineman SM, "Vancomycin Removal During a Plasma Exchange Transfusion," *Ann Pharmacother*, 2001, 35(11):1400-2.

McDonald LK, Tartaglione TA, Mendelman PM, et al, "Lack of Toxicity in Two Cases of Neonatal Acyclovir Overdose," *Pediatr Infect Dis J,* 1989, 8(8):529-32.

Perrin C, Debruyne D, Lacotte J, et al, "Treatment of Caffeine Intoxication by Exchange Transfusion in a Newborn," *Acta Paediatr Scand,* 1987, 76(4):679-81.

Sancak R, Kucukoduk S, Tasdemir HA, et al, "Exchange Transfusion Treatment in a Newborn With Phenobarbital Intoxication," *Pediatr Emerg Care,* 1999, 15(4):268-70.

Shannon M, Wernovsky G, and Morris C, "Exchange Transfusion in the Treatment of Severe Theophylline Poisoning," *Pediatrics,* 1992, 89(1):145-7.

Tauscher JW and Polich JJ, "Treatment of Pine Oil Poisoning by Exchange Transfusion," *Pediatr,* 1959, 55:511-5.

Wright RO, Lewander WJ, and Woolf AD, "Methemoglobinemia: Etiology, Pharmacology, and Clinical Management," *Ann Emerg Med,* 1999, 34(5):646-56.

Support and Monitoring for Adverse Effects

This aspect of poison management is the least studied. The usual disposition of the admitted poisoned patient is an intensive care unit bed or cardiac monitored bed to evaluate the late sequelae of the toxic agent. However, the practice of admitting the poisoned patient routinely to the intensive care unit is being questioned. A recent retrospective study identified eight clinical risk factors that predicted ICU interventions: (1) arterial carbon dioxide pressure ≥ 45 mm Hg, (2) need for emergency intubation, (3) seizures, (4) cardiac arrhythmia, (5) QRS duration ≥ 0.12 seconds, (6) systolic blood pressure < 80 mm Hg, (7) second- or third-degree atrioventricular block, and (8) unresponsiveness to verbal stimuli.[24] If a toxic patient did not exhibit any of these characteristics, no ICU interventions (such as intubation, antiseizure therapy, intravenous vasopressors, antiarrhythmics, and dialysis or hemoperfusion) were performed.

Additionally, other risk factors that should be considered for ICU admission include the need for emergent hemodialysis or hemoperfusion, increasing metabolic acidosis, and any tricyclic or phenothiazine overdose manifesting anticholinergic signs of cardiac abnormalities.[25,26] While many drugs (such as ibuprofen) will manifest their toxicity within 4 hours after ingestion, tricyclic overdoses are renowned for their incidence of delayed complications.[27] It has been noted that most of these patients exhibited cardiac or neurologic abnormality prior to the delayed arrhythmia. The following are suggested criteria for ICU admission.

Criteria for Admission of the Poisoned Patient to ICU

Respiratory depression (pCO$_2 > 45$ mm Hg)

Emergency intubation

Seizures

Cardiac arrhythmia

Hypotension (systolic blood pressure < 80 mm Hg)

Unresponsiveness to verbal stimuli

Second- or third-degree atrioventricular block

Emergent dialysis or hemoperfusion

Increasing metabolic acidosis

Tricyclic or phenothiazine overdose manifesting anticholinergic signs, neurologic abnormality, QRS duration > 0.12 second, or QT$_c$ duration > 0.5 seconds

Administration of pralidoxime in organophosphate toxicity

Pulmonary edema induced by drugs or toxic inhalation (ARDS)

Cerebral edema (from salicylate, lead, carbon monoxide, etc)

Drug-induced hypothermia or hyperthermia including neuroleptic malignant syndrome

Hyperkalemia secondary to digitalis overdose

Any use of digoxin-immune Fab fragments

Body packers and stuffers

Concretions secondary to drugs

Emergent surgical intervention

Monoamine oxidase inhibitor overdose

Antivenom administration in Crotalidae, coral snake, or arthropod envenomation

Significant aspiraiton pneumonitis in the elderly

Need for continuous infusion of naloxone

Need for extracorporeal membrane oxygenation (ECMO)

Continuous arteriovenous hemofiltration

Requirement for exchange transfusion

Sustained release beta-adrenergic blocker, calcium channel blocker overdose, bupropion, lithium, or oral hypoglycemic agent overdose

pCO_2 = carbon dioxide pressure

ARDS = adult respiratory distress syndrome

Adapted from Kulling P, Persson H, "Role of the Intensive Care Unit in the Management of the Poisoned Patient," *Med Toxicol*, 1986, 1:375-86, and Brett AS, Rothschild N, Gray R, et al, "Predicting the Clinical Course in Intentional Drug Overdose: Implication for Use of the Intensive Care Unit, *Arch Intern Med*, 1987, 147:133-7, and Callaham M, "Admission Criteria for Tricyclic Antidepressant Ingestion," *West J Med*, 1982, 137:425-9.

Extracorporeal membrane oxygenation (ECMO) has been used with varying success to treat hydrocarbon pneumonitis (primarily in pediatric exposures), tricyclic antidepressant, propranolol, paraquat, chlorine gas, or quinidine poisoning.[28-31] Prerequisites for its use include ability to survive until ECMO is applied (about 2 hours), high expected mortality (>75%) from cardiac or respiratory failure if ECMO is not used, and lack of long-term toxin sequelae. Peripheral cardiopulmonary bypass support has been shown to be useful in accidental lidocaine, aconitine, flecainide, bupivicaine, propranolol, and organophosphate overdoses.[32-34] Also, the use of partial liquid ventilation has been used successfully to treat severe pulmonary complications due to verapamil poisoning.[35]

Footnotes

1. Nice A, Leikin JB, Maturen A, et al, "Toxidrome Recognition to Improve Efficiency of Emergency Urine Drug Screens," *Ann Emerg Med*, 1988, 17(7):676-80.
2. Watson WA, Litovitz TL, Rodgers GC, et al, "2004 Annual Report of the American Association of Poison Control Centers Toxic Exposure Surveillance System," *Am J Emerg Med*, 2005, 23(5):589-666.
3. Noji EK and Kelen EK, eds, *Manual of Toxicologic Emergencies*, Chicago, IL: Year Book Medical Publishers, 1989.
4. Rumack BH, Hess AJ and Gelman CR, eds, *Poisondex* Information System, Englewood CO: Micromedex, Inc, Vol 93.
5. Goldfrank LR, ed, *Toxicologic Emergencies*, 8th ed, Philadelphia, PA: McGraw-Hill, 2006.
6. Ellenhorn MJ, *Medical Toxicology: Diagnosis and Treatment of Human Poisoning*, 2nd ed, Baltimore, MD: Williams & Wilkins, 1997.
7. Bryson PD, ed, *Comprehensive Review in Toxicology for Emergency Clinicians*, 3rd ed, Washington, DC: Taylor and Francis, 1996.
8. Kulig K, "Initial Management of Ingestions of Toxic Substances," *N Engl J Med*, 1992, 326(25):1677-81.
9. Leikin JB, Krantz A, Zell-Kanter M, et al, "Clinical Features and Management of Intoxication Due to Hallucinogenic Drugs," *Med Toxicol Adverse Drug Exp*, 1989, 4(5):324-53.
10. Tillman DJ, Ruggles DL, and Leikin JB, "Radiopacity Study of Extended-Release Formulations Using Digitalized Radiography," *Am J Emerg Med*, 1994, 12(3):310-4.
11. Merigian KS, Woodard M, Hedges JR, et al, "Prospective Evaluation of Gastric Emptying in the Self-Poisoned Patient," *Am J Emerg Med*, 1990, 8(6):479-83.
12. AACT/EAPCC: Position Paper, "Ipecac Syrup," *J Tox Clin Tox*, 2004, 42(2):133-43.
13. AACT/EAPCC: Position Paper, "Gastric Lavage" *J Tox Clin Tox*, 2004, 42(7):933-43.
14. AACT/EAPCC: Position Paper, "Single-Dose Activated Charcoal" *J Tox Clin Tox*, 2005, 43(2):61-87.
15. Bond GR, "The Role of Activated Charcoal and Gastric Emptying in Gastrointestinal Decontamination: A State of the Art Review," *Ann Emerg Med*, 2002, 39(3):273-86.
16. AACT/EAPCC: Position Paper, "Cathartics," *J Tox Clin Tox*, 2004, 42(3):243-53.
17. AACT/EAPCC: Position Paper, "Whole Bowel Irrigation," *J Tox Clin Tox*, 2004, 42(6):843-54.
18. AACT/EAPCC: "Position Statement and Practice Guidelines on the Use of Multi-Dose Activated Charcoal in the Treatment of Acute Poisoning," *Clin Toxicol*, 1999, 37(6):731-57.
19. Proudfoot AT, Krezelok EP, and Vale JA, "Position Paper on Urine Alkalinization," *J Tox Clin Tox*, 2004, 42(1):1-26.

20. Garrettson LK and Geller RJ, "Acid and Alkaline Diuresis: When Are They of Value in the Treatment of Poisoning?" *Drug Safety*, 1990, 5(3):220-32.

21. Zimmerman HE, Burkhart KK, and Donavan JW, "Ethylene Glycol and Methanol Poisoning: Diagnosis and Treatment," *J Emerg Nurs*, 1999, 25:116-20.

22. Cutler RE, Forland SC, St. John Hammond PG, Evans JR, "Extracorporeal Removal of Drugs and Poisons by Hemodialysis and Hemoperfusion," *Ann Rev Pharmacol Toxicol*, 1987, 27:169-91.

23. Larsen LS, Sterrett JR, Whitehead B, et al, "Adjunctive Therapy of Phenytoin Overdose - A Case Report Using Plasmaphoresis," *J Toxicol Clin Toxicol*, 1986, 24(1):37-49.

24. Brett AS, Rothschild N, Gray R, et al, "Predicting the Clinical Course in Intentional Drug Overdose: Implications for Use of the Intensive Care Unit," *Arch Intern Med*, 1987, 147(1):133-7.

25. Kulling P and Persson H, "Role of the Intensive Care Unit in the Management of the Poisoned Patient," *Med Toxicol*, 1986, 1(5):375-86.

26. Zimmerman JL, "Managing Acute Poisonings and Drug Overdoses in the ICU," *J Crit Illness*, 1997, 12(6):368-75.

27. Callaham M, "Admission Criteria for Tricyclic Antidepressant Ingestion," *West J Med*, 1982, 137(5): 425-9.

28. Klein MD and Whittlesey GC, "Extracorporeal Membrane Oxygenation," *Pediatr Clin N Am*, 1994, 4:365-84.

29. Goodwin DA, Lally KP, and Null DM Jr, "Extracorporeal Membrane Oxygenation Support for Cardiac Dysfunction From Tricyclic Antidepressant Overdose," *Crit Care Med*, 1993, 21:625-7.

30. Banner W Jr, Timmons OD, and Vernon DD, "Advances in the Critical Care of Poisoned Paediatric Patients," *Drug Safety*, 1994, 10:83-92.

31. Tecklenburg FW, Thomas NJ, and Webb SA, "Pediatric ECMO for Severe Quinidine Cardiotoxicity," *Ped Emerg Care*, 1997, 13:111-4.

32. Yasui RK, Culclasure TF, Kaufman D, et al, "Flecainide Overdose: Is Cardiopulmonary Support the Treatment?" *Ann Emerg Med*, 1997, 29:680-2.

33. Kamijo Y, Soma K, Uchimiya H, et al, "A Case of Serious Organophosphate Poisoning Treated by Percutaneous Cardiopulmonary Support" *Vet Human Toxicol*, 1999, 41(5):326-8.

34. Ohuchi S, Izumoto H, Kamata J, et al, "A Case of Aconitine Poisoning Saved With Cardiopulmonary Bypass," *Kyobu Geka*, 2000, 53(7):541-4.

35. Svekly LA, Thompson BT, and Woolf AD, "The Use of Partial Liquid Ventilation to Manage Verapamil-SR™ Poisoning," *J Toxicol Clin Toxicol*, 1997, 35:542-3.

CLINICAL TOXICOKINETICS

Frank P. Paloucek, PharmD

The common "no calculation" approach in the assessment of the poisoned patient is to obtain a history of the dose ingested (assuming the maximum value possible), converting to a weight-based value (mg/kg), and comparing it with published standards for either prognosis or treatment decisions. A limited number of agents including, but not limited to, acetaminophen, salicylate, theophylline, lithium, digoxin, phenytoin, and the toxic alcohols have reasonable, and timely, availability of serum concentration analysis. This leads to use of the magnitude of a serum concentration at the time of presentation, or subsequent peak value to predict outcome or serve as an indication for therapeutic decisions. Unfortunately, the common practice is to apply routine serum concentration analysis and monitoring practices to the overdose population.

Ideally, predictive pharmacokinetic calculations, based on the historical data, should include considerations for the continued absorption and distribution phases of an acute ingestion. Furthermore, the use of comparative analysis of predicted vs observed data should enhance the assessment and need-to-treat decisions. The use of these formulas should not provide sole or absolute criteria in patient management issues but should be combined with overall clinical assessments, preferably with the assistance of poison control centers or clinical toxicologists.

Initial assessment of any case prior to obtaining the results of the initial serum concentration determination should include calculation of the "worst case" scenario. The following formula can be used to predict the highest magnitude concentration ("worst case") for a specified dose and patient:

$$C_{peak} = dose/[V_d \text{ weight (kg)}] \tag{1}$$

where C_{peak} is the highest observed serum concentration, dose is the greatest possible ingested dose in mg, and V_d is the population value for the volume of distribution (in L/kg) of the ingested agent.

Observed values will vary from prediction on the basis of the accuracy of dose ingested, time between ingestion and serum sampling, and bioavailability (assumes F = 1.0), and ignores any reductions, or delay, in toxin dose due to the presence of a salt form (S = 1.0) or dosage form. Additionally, any intervening symptoms and/or treatments (vomiting or gastric decontamination) will also affect predictive performance. Thus, if the history is accurate, the calculation should nearly always be an overprediction.

Accounting for the passage of time between ingestion and serum sampling, the following formula is preferred to the formula above for a more precise prediction:

$$C_p = \{dose/[V_d \text{ weight (kg)}]\} \times e^{-(Ke \times t)} \tag{2}$$

or

$$C_p = (C_{peak}) (e^{-(Ke \times t)}) \tag{3}$$

where C_p is the serum concentration at any time (t, in hours) after an ingestion, dose and V_d are defined as above, and Ke is the population value for the elimination rate of the toxin (hr^1).

Formula 3 can be generalized to:

$$C_{p2} = (C_{p1}) (e^{-(Ke \times t)}) \tag{4}$$

where C_{p1} and C_{p2} are any two consecutive serum concentrations with time interval (t) between. This allows the ability to anticipate future sampling times and/or potential windows of threat/opportunity/resolution.

Once two consecutive declining serum samples have been determined, the elimination rate might be approximated by the following formula (which is a mere rearrangement of formula 4):

$$Ke = \{\ln (C_{p1}/C_{p2})\}/t \tag{5}$$

This can be compared with a known population value to assess the competency of the patient to eliminate the toxin and provide an etiology for the presentation. It should be noted that the value determined can be falsely diminished or in "normal" range (slower or equal to normal elimination) if sampling occurs during significant drug absorption. This would be common with sustained-releases preparations or in presence of a bezoar. Also, the calculated value determined can be falsely elevated (faster than normal elimination) if sampling occurs during significant tissue distribution, especially with drugs like digoxin or lithium. This technique is useful for determining the patient-specific impairment of underlying elimination, especially with chronic overdoses, as well as to access the impact of intervening treatment strategies and/or the need to add or continue elimination-enhancing modalities.

Elimination rates are best determined graphically with at least three values to determine a linear plot. The use of formula 5 and its frequent adaptation to calculate half-life (formula 6 below) assumes that the absorption and distribution processes are essentially complete, which is frequently not true of initial samplings in the evaluation of a poisoning. The elimination half-life is calculated using Ke by the following formula:

$$T_{1/2} = 0.693/Ke \tag{6}$$

The formulas above assume essentially complete and instantaneous absorption and hold limited value (consistently overpredicting) for predicting values in sustained-release dosage form overdoses. While consistent with the worst-case approach to evaluating patients, accounting for the absorption process can improve accuracy of predictions and may refine evaluation and need-to-treat decisions.

The following formula provides the potentially most accurate prediction of a serum concentration at any time for any toxin for which the parameters V_d, Ka, and Ke are available.

$$C_p = [dose/(V_d \times weight)] \times [Ka/(Ka \times Ke)] \times (e^{-(Ke \times t)} \, e^{-(Ka \times t)}) \tag{7}$$

Unfortunately, absorption rates (Ka) are rarely found in the common biomedical literature, limiting the application of this calculation and evaluation of its potential benefit in use.

In any event, when the initial prediction is compared to the actual concentration and a marked discrepancy is noted, reconsideration of the history must be undertaken. A reasonable approach would be to assume an inaccuracy of dose. Back calculation using the same formula and the observed concentration to determine the "actual" dose ingestion can be performed. Repeat calculations can be made for future serum concentration determinations based on the calculated "actual" dose ingested and assuming the time of ingestion history was accurate.

Explanations for Variations Between Predicted and Observed Values

Overpredictions for Initial Concentrations
- Inaccurate history of dose (historical dose used was too high)
- Inaccurate time interval (historical data too short)
- Early sampling with minimal time for product dissolution and absorption to occur
- Decreased absorption (positive outcomes from gastric emptying events)
- Delayed/incomplete absorption (bezoars, sustained-release, enteric-coated, highly compressed, or poorly water soluble products)

Overpredictions for Subsequent Concentrations
- Patient still in absorption-phase, or endogenous metabolism and/or elimination better than the specific average population parameter value chosen
- Calculation with V_d central compartment not postdistribution or steady-state V_d

Underpredictions for Initial Concentrations
- Inaccurate history of dose (historical data too low)
- Inaccurate time interval (historical data too long)
- Alterations in absorption (dose-dumping of sustained-release dosage forms)
- Early sampling during distribution phase, but C_p is calculated using postdistribution V_d

Overpredictions for Subsequent Concentrations
- Alterations in absorption (dose-dumping of sustained-release dosage forms)
- Bezoar dissolution endogenous metabolism and/or elimination is slower than known population values
- Calculated patient-specific Ke was peridistribution not during true elimination
- Ineffective decontamination or elimination-enhancement therapies, and/or unaccounted new administration

Potential Benefits in the Toxicokinetic Evaluation and/or Management of the Overdose Patient

- Differentiating the acute or acute-on-chronic overdose from a chronic intoxication
  Acute ingestions generally require higher serum concentrations for specific morbidity or mortality than acute-on-chronic or chronic. Conversely, aggressive treatment measures are indicated at lower serum concentrations in acute-on-chronics and chronics than for acute overdoses. Specific poisonings for which this is true include theophylline, lithium, salicylate, and digoxin. Acute-on-chronic overdoses could be characterized by increases in serum concentrations greater than expected from a maintenance dose, whereas a chronic intoxication would generally have a normal increase. Chronic intoxications frequently are associated with prolonged elimination half-lives. Differentiation assist in determining the need for psychiatric consult and for etiologies in the chronic.

- Clarifying the history
  Comparing predicted with observed values can lead to revised etiologies, which may reflect reversible process errors. Calculations can assist in suggesting prognosis and/or chronicity of exposure, as in the suspected acetaminophen ingestion without any history of time or dose. Calculations allow anticipation of future serum concentration changes. This could allow for prospective use of treatment measures vs traditional reactive implementation.

Suggested Reading

1. Ellenhorn MJ, "Elimination Enhancement," *Ellenhorn's Medical Toxicology*, 2nd ed, Baltimore, MD: Williams & Wilkins, 1997.
2. Ellenhorn MJ, "Toxicokinetics," *Ellenhorn's Medical Toxicology*, 2nd ed, Baltimore, MD: Williams & Wilkins, 1997.
3. Paloucek FP, "Clinical Toxicokinetics," *J Pharm Practice*, 1997, 10:271-7.
4. Paloucek FP, "Theophylline Toxicokinetics," *J Pharm Practice*, 1993, 6:57-62.
5. Pond SM, "Techniques to Enhance Elimination of Toxic Compounds," *Goldfrank's Toxicologic Emergencies*, 5th ed, Goldfrank LR, Flomembaum NE, Lewin NA, et al, eds, Norwalk, CT: Appleton & Lange, 1994.
6. Weisman RS, Howland MA, Reynolds JR, et al, "Pharmacokinetic and Toxicokinetic Principles," *Goldfrank's Toxicologic Emergencies*, 5th ed, Goldfrank LR, Flomembaum NE, Lewin NA, et al, eds, Norwalk, CT: Appleton & Lange, 1994.

HIGHLIGHTS OF RECENT REPORTS (2006) ON SUBSTANCE ABUSE AND MENTAL HEALTH

Reprinted from www.oas.samhsa.gov.

SAMHSA's National Survey on Drug Use and Health found that 2.4 million persons aged 12 and older initiated nonmedical use of prescription pain relievers (analgesics) such as OxyContin® within the past year in 2004. Among persons who initiated nonmedical use of pain relievers in the past year, 48.0% used Vicodin®, Lortab®, or Lorcet®, nonmedically; 34.3% had used Darvocet®, Darvon®, or Tylenol® with codeine nonmedically; and 20.0% had used Percocet®, Percodan®, or Tylox® nonmedically. Of the past year new users of nonmedical pain relievers, 73.8% had used another illicit drug prior to using pain relievers nonmedically. In 2004, about 615,000 persons began using OxyContin® nonmedically. Nearly all (99.1%) of the persons who first used OxyContin® nonmedically in the past year had used another illicit drug prior to using OxyContin® nonmedically (http://www.oas.samhsa.gov/2k6/pain/pain.cfm).

Based on SAMHSA's Treatment Episode Data Set (TEDS), young adults aged 18 to 25 accounted for 21% and youth aged 12 to 17 accounted for 8% of the 1.9 million admissions to substance abuse treatment reported to TEDS in 2004. Young adults aged 18-25 were less likely than youths aged 12-17 to be admitted with marijuana as their primary substance of abuse (27% vs. 64%). The criminal justice system was the principal source of referral to treatment for 47% of young adult admissions compared to 52% of youth admissions to substance abuse treatment. About 48% of all TEDS substance abuse treatment admissions in 2004 were in the 28 states that provided data on a psychiatric problem in addition to an alcohol or drug problem for their treatment admissions. Based on this TEDS supplemental data set, 17% of young adults had a psychiatric problem in addition to substance abuse compared with 20% of the youth admissions for substance abuse treatment (http://www.oas.samhsa.gov/2k6/youngTX/youngTX.cfm).

Based on SAMHSA's National Survey on Drug Use and Health combined data from 2002 to 2004, most of the young adults aged 18 to 25 who had used marijuana in the past year obtained their most recently used marijuana from a friend either free or by purchase. Among young adults who had used marijuana in the past year, 58.3% obtained their most recently used marijuana for free or shared someone else's and 40.0% bought their marijuana. Young adults who were daily marijuana users were more likely than nondaily marijuana users to have bought their most recently used marijuana (75.3% vs. 33.8%). Young adult users of marijuana in the past year who used marijuana daily were more likely than nondaily marijuana users to have gotten their most recently used marijuana inside a home, apartment, or dorm room and less likely to have gotten their marijuana from inside a public building or outside in a public area (http://www.oas.samhsa.gov/2k6/MJsource/MJsource.cfm).

SAMHSA's Drug Abuse Warning Network (DAWN) collects data on all deaths where drugs played a role, either directly (eg, overdose) or indirectly (eg, fatal car crash where drugs were involved). Drug misuse death is defined as a drug-related death caused by overmedication, all other accidental causes, homicide by drugs, and drug-related deaths where the cause could not be determined. Six states participate in the mortality component of the Drug Abuse Warning Network: Maine, Maryland, New Hampshire, New Mexico, Utah, and Vermont. The rates of opiate-related drug misuse deaths in 2003 ranged from 7.2 per 100,000 population in New Hampshire to 11.6 per 100,000 population in New Mexico. In each of these 6 states, most opiate-related drug misuse deaths involved multiple drugs. Three opiate pain medications as a group (oxycodone, hydrocodone, and methadone) were involved in 40% or more of the opiate misuse deaths in these states. The involvement of oxycodone ranged from 13% in New Mexico to 30% in Vermont; hydrocodone ranged from 3% in Maryland to 17% in Utah; and methadone ranged from 17% in New Mexico to 46% in Maine (http://www.oas.samhsa.gov/2k6/opiateDeaths.cfm).

Based on SAMHSA's National Survey on Drug Use & Health, 70.4% of students aged 12 to 17 reported that they had an A or B grade average in their last semester or grading period, while 29.6% had a C average or less. Younger students were more likely to report good grades than older students; for example, 75.6% of students aged 12 or 13 reported an A or B average compared with 68.3% of students aged 16 or 17. Students who did not use alcohol in the past month (72.5%) were more likely to have an A or B grade average than those drank alcohol but did not binge (67.1%) or those who binge drank alcohol in the past month (57.7%). Students who did not use marijuana in the past month (72.2%) were more likely to have an A or B grade average than those who used marijuana on 1 to 4 days in the past month (58.0%) or those using marijuana on 5 or more days in the past month (44.9%) (http://www.oas.samhsa.gov/2k6/academics/academics.cfm).

Based on SAMHSA's Drug Abuse Warning Network (DAWN), of the 1.3 million drug-related visits to emergency departments in 2004 that were associated with drug misuse or abuse, 30% involved illicit drugs only, 25% involved pharmaceuticals only, 15% involved illicit drugs and alcohol, 8% involved illicit drugs with pharmaceuticals, and 14% involved illicit drugs with pharmaceuticals and alcohol (http://dawninfo.samhsa.gov/pubs/edpubs/default.asp).

Among older adult admissions to substance abuse treatment reported to SAMHSA's Treatment Episode Data Set (TEDS), about half (48%) were admitted for abuse of alcohol only. Older adult alcohol-only admissions were less likely than other older adult admissions to be self/individual referrals (37% vs. 45%). Among older adult admissions alcohol-only admissions were more likely than other admissions to have entered treatment for the first time (45% vs. 33%) (http://www.oas.samhsa.gov/2k6/olderAdultsTX/olderAdultsTX.cfm).

Based on analysis of combined data from SAMHSA's 2002-2004 National Surveys on Drug Use & Health, 7.6% (18.2 million) persons aged 12 or older met the criteria for alcohol dependence or abuse in the past year. Alcohol abuse or dependence was more prevalent among adults aged 18 or older who were never married (16%) than adults who were divorced or separated (4.6%) or widowed (1.3%). Persons aged 12 or older who were dependent on or abused alcohol in the past year were more likely to have been treated in an emergency room at least once in the past year than those who did not meet alcohol dependence or abuse criteria (34.2% vs. 27.9%) (http://www.oas.samhsa.gov/2k6/alcDepend/alcDepend.cfm).

Provides latest data on treatment completion rates by type of substance abuse care (inpatient, outpatient, hospital, methadone maintenance, etc.). Among the 888,432 discharges from substance abuse treatment reported to SAMHSA's TEDS system, 42% were from outpatient treatment, 23% from detoxification, 12% were from intensive outpatient treatment, 8% from long-term residential treatment, 8% from short term residential treatment, 5% from methadone treatment, and 1% from hospital residential treatment. Overall, treatment was completed by 41% of the substance abuse treatment discharges. The treatment completion rate was highest from short-term treatment programs (69% of the discharges from hospital residential treatment completed treatment, 64% from short-term residential, and 55% from detoxification). The treatment completion rate was 41% for long-term residential treatment and 38% for outpatient treatment (http://wwwdasis.samhsa.gov/teds03/tedsdischweb2k3.pdf).

During 2004, an estimated 192,690 patients in drug-related emergency department visits were diagnosed with co-occurring substance use and mental disorders. When emergency department visits involved co-occurring disorders, 40.4% were treated and released home or referred to detoxification or other drug treatment and 42.2% were admitted to inpatient units including chemical dependency or detoxification units. Of the emergency department visits with co-occurring diagnosis, the drug most frequently reported were cocaine (31.8%), alcohol (29.3%), opiates/opioids (18.0%), and marijuana (16.3%) (http://dawninfo.samhsa.gov/pubs/shortreports/default.asp).

Opiates were the primary substance of abuse for 324,000 (18%) of the 1.8 million substance abuse treatment admissions reported to SAMHSA's Treatment Episode Data Set (TEDS) in 2003. Of these, 51,000 (3% of all admissions) were for a non-heroin opiate. Non-heroin opiates include methadone, codeine, Dilaudid, morphine, Demerol, opium, oxycodone, and any other drug with morphine-like effects. Non-heroin opiate admissions (40%) were more likely than heroin admissions (22%) to be entering treatment for the first time. Non-heroin opiate admissions were less likely than heroin admissions to report cocaine as their secondary substance of abuse (17% vs. 50%) and more likely than heroin admissions to report marijuana as their secondary substance of abuse (19% vs. 10%) (http://www.oas.samhsa.gov/2k6/opiatesTX/opiatesTX.cfm).

This report on underaged drinking (by persons aged 12 to 20) is based on state level data combined from 2 years of data, i.e. from SAMHSA's 2003 and 2004 National Surveys on Drug Use and Health. Data are annualized estimates, that is, an average per year estimate is calculated from the combined data years. In 2003-2004, past month alcohol use rates for persons aged 12 to 20 were among the lowest in Utah (18.6%) and Tennessee (22.3%) and among the highest in North Dakota (42.7%) and South Dakota (39.1%). Between 2002-2003 and 2003-2004, past month alcohol use increased in California (from 24.7 to 26.3%) and Wisconsin (from 34.7% to 38.3%), while binge alcohol drinking increased in Iowa (from 24.7% to 27.7%) and Oklahoma (from 19.1% to 21.5%). Past month alcohol drinking decreased between 2002-2003 and 2003-2004 in South Carolina (from 27.2% to 24.1%) and Michigan (from 31.8% to 30.2%), while binge alcohol drinking decreased in South Carolina and North Carolina (both from 18.0% to 15.9%) and in Tennessee (from 15.9% to 13.1%) (http://www.oas.samhsa.gov/2k6/StateUnderageDrinking/underageDrinking.cfm).

Between 1993 and 2003, the number of substance abuse treatment admissions increased from 1.62 million to 1.84 million treatment admissions. This increase in substance abuse treatment admissions was almost 14%. The proportion of admissions also increased between 1993 and 2003 for those reporting as their primary substance of abuse: marijuana (increased from 7% in 1993 to 16% in 2003), opiates (increased from 13% to 18%), or stimulants (increased from 2% to 7%). The proportion of admissions decreased during this decade for those reporting alcohol (57% to 41%) or cocaine (17% to 14%) as their primary substance of abuse. Substance abuse treatment admissions that were aged 25 to 34 decreased from 40% of admissions in 1993 to 25% of treatment admissions in 2003 (http://www.oas.samhsa.gov/2k6/TXtrends/TXtrends.cfm).

According to SAMHSA's Drug Abuse Warning Network (DAWN), in 2004 there were over 15,000 emergency department visits by adolescents aged 12 to 17 whose suicide attempts involved drugs. Pain medications were involved in about half of the suicide attempts. Almost three quarters of the drug, related suicide attempts were serious enough to merit the patient's admission to the same hospital or transfer to another health care facility. Antidepressants or other psychotherapeutic medications were involved in over 40% of the suicide attempts by adolescents who were admitted to the hospital (http://dawninfo.samhsa.gov/pubs/shortreports/).

In SAMHSA's 2002 to 2004 National Surveys on Drug Use & Health, an average of 598,000 youths aged 12 to 17 per year reported that they initiated inhalant use in the 12 months prior to being surveyed. The types of inhalants most frequently mentioned as having been used by recent initiates were: glue, shoe polish, or toluene (30.3%), gasoline or lighter fluid (24.9%), nitrous oxide or "whippets" (24.9%), and spray paints (23.4%). Among recent inhalants initiates, 19.4% used inhalants on 13 or more days in the past year. In 2002 to 2004, 59.7% of recent inhalant initiates aged 12 to 17 had used cigarettes prior to using inhalants, 67.6% had previously used alcohol, 42.4% had previously used marijuana, and 35.9% had used all three substances (cigarettes, alcohol, and marijuana) before they used inhalants (http://www.oas.samhsa.gov/2k6/inhalants/inhalants.cfm).

Based on SAMHSA's National Survey on Drug Use and Health (NSDUH), an estimated 43.9% of individuals who received alcohol or illicit drug use treatment in the past year paid at least a portion of the cost of their last or current treatment with their own savings or earnings. The majority (52.9%) of the individuals who received substance use treatment in the past year used two or more sources of payment for their last or current services. Among persons who received alcohol or illicit drug use treatment in the past year, females were more likely than males to have paid at least a portion of the costs for their last or current services with private insurance (30.9% vs. 23.5%), Medicaid (19.8% vs. 11.6%), and other public assistance (21.0% vs. 13.6%) (http://www.oas.samhsa.gov/2k6/pay/pay.cfm).

According to SAMHSA's Treatment Episode Data Set (TEDS), 47 of the 50 states distinguish between methamphetamines and amphetamines as primary substances of abuse in their reporting to TEDS. In these 47 states, methamphetamine was the primary drug in 86% of the combined methamphetamine/ amphetamine treatment admissions in 2003. Arkansas, Oregon, and Texas do not distinguish between amphetamine and methamphetamine in their reporting of primary substance of abuse in treatment admissions. Nationally, the rate of substance abuse treatment admissions for primary methamphetamine/amphetamine abuse increased between 1993 to 2003 from 13 per 100,000 to 56 admissions per 100,000 population aged 12 or older. In 2003, 18 states had rates in excess of the national rate (56 admissions per 100,000 population): 10 states were in the West, 6 were in the Midwest, and 2 were in the South; none were in the Northeast. The highest rates were in Oregon (251 admissions per 100,000), Hawaii (241 per 100,000), Iowa (213 per 100,000), California (212 per 100,000), Wyoming (209 per 100,000), Utah (186 per 100,000), Nevada (176 per 100,000), Washington State (143 per 100,000), Montana (133 per 100,000), Arkansas (130 admissions per 100,000 population), Nebraska (118 per 100,000), and Oklahoma (117 per 100,000). All the rates for the states in the Northeast were 5 or less per 100,000 population (http://www.oas.samhsa.gov/2k6/methTx/methTX.cfm).

Based on SAMHSA's National Survey on Drug Use and Health, an estimated 33.7% of youths aged 15 to 17 were employed either part- or full-time during the past week. Employed youths were more likely than youths who were not employed to have used alcohol (35.9% vs. 24.4%), to have engaged in binge alcohol use (24.6% vs. 15.2%), and to have used an illicit drug (19.4% vs. 15.6%) during the past month. Youths working 20 or more hours per week were more likely than those working 19 or fewer hours per week to have drunk alcohol (41.1% vs. 33.8%), to have binged on alcohol (29.0% vs. 23.1%), and to have used any illicit drug (22.3% vs. 18.5%) during the past month (http://www.oas.samhsa.gov/2k6/employedYouth/employedYouth.cfm).

Based on SAMHSA's Treatment Episode Data Set (TEDS) among the 29 states that reported retirement status in 2003, about twice as many substance abuse treatment admissions among retired persons (80%) than other admissions (44%) reported alcohol as the primary substance of abuse. Only 17% of substance abuse treatment admissions among retired persons reported a secondary substance of abuse compared to 52% of other admissions. Substance abuse treatment admissions who were retired persons were more likely to have some form of health insurance than other admissions (60% vs. 42%) (http://www.oas.samhsa.gov/2k6/retiredTX/retiredTX.cfm).

Based on SAMHSA's National Survey on Drug Use & Health, youths aged 12 to 17 who used an illicit drug in the past year were almost twice as likely to have engaged in a violent behavior as those who did not use an illicit drug (49.8% vs. 26.6%). Rates of past year violent behavior were higher among youths aged 13, 14, and 15 than those either younger or older. The likelihood of having engaged in violent behavior increased with the number of drugs used in the past year: 45.6% of youths who used one illicit drug engaged in violent behavior compared to 61.9% of youths who used three or more illicit drugs (http://www.oas.samhsa.gov/2k6/ youthViolence/youthViolence.cfm).

Based on SAMHSA's Treatment Episode Data Set (TEDS), the average age of first illicit drug use among admissions for substance abuse treatment changed between 1993 and 2003. The average age of first use of any illicit drug among substance abuse treatment admissions showed a slight decrease from age 18.8 in 1993 to age 18.6 in 2003. Among substance abuse treatment admissions whose earliest reported drug of abuse at admission was stimulants, opiates, or cocaine, the average age of first use rose between 1993 and 2003 (for stimulants from age 18.5 to age 19.7; for opiates from age 21.0 to age 22.1; and for cocaine from age 22.5 to age 22.7). For marijuana, however, it decreased. The average age of first use among substance abuse treatment admissions whose earliest reported drug of abuse was marijuana decreased from age 15.1 in 1993 to age 14.6 in 2003. While the average age of first use of any drug remained the same or decreased between 1993 and 2003 for all age groups, the percentage of substance abuse treatment admissions starting drug use before age 13 increased for all age groups except those age 18-24 at treatment admission. Criminal justice was the only admissions referral source that had a decrease in the average age of first use of any illicit drug. The average age of first use of any illicit drug for admissions referred by the criminal justice system decreased from age 17.6 in 1993 to age 16.8 in 2003 (http://www.oas.samhsa.gov/2k6/AgeDrugTX/AgeDrugTX.cfm).

SAMHSA's National Survey on Drug Use and Health in 2002 through 2004 assessed whether respondents met criteria for serious psychological distress during the month in the past year when respondents were at their worst emotionally. An estimated 10.3% of males aged 18 to 25 (1.6 million persons) experienced serious psychological distress during the past year. Divorced or separated males aged 18 to 25 (20.9%) were more likely to have experienced serious psychological distress during the past year than those who were married (7.3%) or never married (10.5%). Males aged 18 to 25 with serious psychological distress during the past year were more likely than those without past year serious psychological distress to have engaged in heavy alcohol use (27.2% vs. 20.7%), binge alcohol use (56.7% vs. 49.9%), and illicit drug use (35.6% vs. 22.1%) in the past month (http://www.oas.samhsa.gov/2k6/menMH/menMH.cfm).

Of the 13,454 facilities that responded to SAMHSA's National Survey of Substance Abuse Treatment Services (N-SSATS), 4756 facilities (35%) had special programs or groups for clients with co-occurring psychiatric and substance use disorders in 2004. Facilities operated by state governments were most likely to offer special programs or groups for clients with co-occurring substance abuse and psychiatric disorders (50%), followed by those operated by local governments (44%), the federal government (41%) and private nonprofit organizations (36%). Facilities operated by private-for-profit organizations (31%) and tribal governments (29%) were least likely to offer special programs or groups for clients with co-occurring substance abuse and psychiatric disorders. Facilities with special programs or groups for clients with co-occurring substance abuse and psychiatric disorders were more likely than those not offering such special programs or groups to offer a number of services, including family counseling (83% vs. 73%), Hepatitis B testing (30% vs. 19%), transitional social services (65% vs. 49%), domestic violence services (40% vs. 29%), and HIV testing (38% vs. 28%) (http://www.oas.samhsa.gov/2k6/DualTX/DualTX.cfm).

An estimated 142,701 alcohol-related emergency department (ED) visits reported to SAMHSA's Drug Abuse Warning Network (DAWN) system were made by patients aged 12 to 20. Nearly half (42%) of drug-related ED visits among patients aged 12 to 20 involved alcohol. Patients aged 18 to 20 were approximately 3 times as likely as patients aged 12 to 17 to have an alcohol-related ED visit. ED visits involving alcohol with other drugs were almost 2 times as likely as visits involving only alcohol to result in admission to the hospital for inpatient care (19% vs. 10%) (http://dawninfo.samhsa.gov/pubs/shortreports/default.asp).

LIPID EMULSION RESUSCITATION FOR LOCAL ANESTHETIC AND TOXIC CARDIAC ARREST

Guy L. Weinberg, MD

Background

Recent observations that lipid infusion is effective in treating cardiac arrest due to local anesthetic toxicity have suggested that this method could have wider application in clinical toxicology (1). Cardiovascular collapse induced by local anesthetic overdose is a rare but potentially devastating complication of regional anesthesia. The problem was first publicized thirty years ago by Albright in an editorial describing several cases of intractable cardiac arrest in patients receiving large doses of bupivacaine or etidocaine for neuraxial anesthesia (2). He proposed a link between the lipid solubility of these agents and fatal arrhythmias. Bupivacaine, the canonical cardio-toxic local anesthetic, is one of the most lipophilic of local anesthetics. It is also one of the most commonly used local anesthetics, in large part because of its potency and long duration of action (3).

Clinical Features of Local Anesthetic Toxicity

Inadvertent intravascular injection or excessive absorbtion, particularly of the lipophilic local anesthetics (e.g., bupivacaine, levo-bupivacaine, ropivacaine), causes CNS excitation or suppression of neural activity, resulting in agitation, seizures, obtundation, or loss of consciousness (4). Signs of cardiovascular toxicity may quickly follow and are typified by progressive hypotension, bradycardia, conduction blockade, malignant arrhythmias, and asystole. Typical of bupivacaine-related cardiac arrest is its resistance to standard resuscitative measures. Cases of successful resuscitation with cardiopulmonary bypass have been reported but, until recently, other modes have proven ineffective (5).

Animal Studies

An intravascular infusion (pre-treatment) of soy oil emulsion will render laboratory rats relatively resistant to bupivacaine cardiac toxicity (6). Furthermore, when given lipid during the resuscitation phase (post-treatment) rats will survive doses of bupivacaine that are uniformly fatal to control animals. Follow-up studies in dogs confirm that lipid infusion given during open-chest cardiac massage allows successful resuscitation from an overwhelming, otherwise fatal bupivacaine overdose, even after prolonged "down-times" (7).

Mechanisms

Several mechanisms are likely to play a role in lipid reversal of bupivacaine toxicity. Bupivacaine is highly lipophilic and exhibits a lipid:aqueous partition coefficient of ~11. Hence, the easiest mechanism to envision is that bupivacaine partitions into a lipemic phase, or "lipid sink", thereby lowering the concentration of free bupivacaine in the aqueous phase of blood. Weinberg et al observed in isolated rat hearts exposed to bupivacaine that adding lipid to the perfusion buffer resulted in more rapid decline of cardiac bupivacaine content than seen in controls (8). These data support the "lipid sink" mechanism. However, the rapidity of lipid reversal observed in experimental animals seems to belie a mechanism that requires bupivacaine to traverse several diffusion barriers in quickly re-establishing an equilibrium that favors the vascular space over cardiac tissue, all within minutes or less of the lipid injection. Another possible mechanism includes a positive metabolic effect of lipids (9). Cardiac lipid metabolism is strongly inhibited by bupivacaine and lipid infusion could overwhelm such inhibition (10). Lipids can also exhibit direct inotropy on isolated heart, suggesting that direct antagonism of bupivacaine contractile depression is possible. Dilution of plasma bupivacaine by volume expansion could also play a role. Elucidating the mechanism(s) of lipid rescue resuscitation remains an important goal for research on this topic.

Clinical Efficacy

The first reports of the clinical use of lipid infusion for treating local anesthetic-related cardiac arrest have recently been published. Rosenblatt et al reported a successful resuscitation from prolonged cardiac arrest after a brachial plexus block with bupivacaine and mepivacaine (11). The patient, a middle-aged man with a history of ischemic cardiac disease, remained in asystole and non-perfusing idioventricular rhythms for more than twenty minutes despite standard ACLS. The report describes a rapid return of normal rhythm and vital signs after injection of 100 mL of 20% lipid. Litz et al published a very similar case of cardiac arrest after injection of ropivaciane for brachial plexus block in an elderly lady with heart disease (12). Standard CPR was ineffective for fifteen minutes, but chest compressions were stopped shortly after infusion of lipid emulsion. Both patients recovered without evidence of cardiac damage and both were neurologically intact. Subsequently, there have been unpublished reports of several instances where CNS symptoms associated with regional anesthesia (obtundation, loss of consciousness) were rapidly reversed with lipid infusion (personal communications, Rainer Litz, Dresden; Andrew Spence, Bermuda; Harvey Woehlk, Wisconsin). Thus, lipid infusion appears to interrupt local anesthetic-induced toxicity for both cardiovascular and central nervous systems.

General Applicability of Lipid Rescue Resuscitation

The lipid sink mechanism suggests that lipid infusion could provide a general method for treating poisoning by any sufficiently lipophilic agent. Alternately, by assuming that the underlying mechanism is specific to local anesthetics, lipid infusion might work for overdose due to any of amphipathic sodium channel blocker. Together, these two classes encompass a wide array of potential toxins, including: tricyclic antidepressants, calcium channel blockers, cocaine, anti-convulsants, anti-depressants, organic solvents, and bio-weapons. In support of this prediction, lipid infusion has recently been shown by Harvey and colleagues to improve cardiac function in a rabbit model of chlomipramine overdose where all controls exhibited intractable pulseless electrical activity, while all rabbits in the treatment group maintained normal circulation (13).

Future Directions: Research and Practice

The future use of lipid emulsion therapy will be directed by the findings in basic laboratory research. The main goals of such efforts include identifying the underlying mechanisms of action of lipid rescue resuscitation, identifying optimized regimens of treatment, and determining the range of toxins it can be used to treat. The full scope and potential clinical application of this simple method has yet to be determined. Understanding the method will likely extend its use beyond the niche of treating a complication of regional anesthesia.

Recommendations

Lipid infusion is still in its infancy and since no data are available from human trials regarding its efficacy or safety, all guidelines are based on laboratory findings in animal models and upon a small number of reported clinical cases. While no official recommendations are published, the treatment has, nevertheless, proven life-saving in a number of cases of local anesthetic toxicity. Suggestions for its use are posted on an educational website: *www.lipidrescue.org*. This site is dedicated to disseminating information on the use of lipid infusion and providing a forum for physicians to exchange ideas and experiences related to this method. Typical suggestions include:

Stock. 500 mL of 20% lipid emulsion (e.g., Intralipid) at sites where large doses of local anesthetic are likely to be used.

Therapy. An initial intravenous dose of lipid (1.5 mL/kg) is given by bolus and followed by a continuous infusion of 0.25 mL/kg/min. CPR should continue throughout as the lipid will only work if it is circulated to the heart. The bolus can be repeated twice more at 3-5 minute intervals for persistent circulatory collapse. Once blood pressure is re-established, the infusion should be continued for 15 minutes and can be increased to 0.5 mL/kg for declining blood pressure.

This is a general guideline that will be amended as further clinical and laboratory studies indicate. Future changes in the regimen will lead to improved efficacy and safety.

References

1. Weinberg G, "Lipid Rescue Resuscitation from Local Anaesthetic Cardiac Toxicity," *Toxicol Rev*, 2006, 25:139-45.
2. Albright GA, "Cardiac Arrest Following Regional Anesthesia with Etidocaine or Bupivacaine," *Anesthesiology*, 1979, 51:285-7.
3. Corcoran W, Butterworth J, Weller RS, et al, "Local Anesthetic-induced Cardiac Toxicity: A Survey of Contemporary Practice Strategies Among Academic Anesthesiology Departments," *Anesth Analg*, 2006, 103:1322-6.

4. Weinberg GL, "Current Concepts in Resuscitation of Patients with Local Anesthetic Cardiac Toxicity," *Reg Anesth Pain Med*, 2002, 27:568-75.

5. Long WB, Rosenblum S, and Grady IP, "Successful Resuscitation of Bupivacaine-induced Cardiac Arrest Using Cardiopulmonary Bypass," *Anesth Analg*, 1989, 69:403-6.

6. Weinberg GL, VadeBoncouer T, Ramaraju GA, et al, "Pretreatment or Resuscitation with a Lipid Infusion Shifts the Dose-response to Bupivacaine-induced Asystole in Rats," *Anesthesiology*, 1998, 88:1071-5.

7. Weinberg G, Ripper R, Feinstein DL et al, "Lipid Emulsion Infusion Rescues Dogs from Bupivacaine-induced Cardiac Toxicity," *Reg Anesth Pain Med*, 2003, 28:198-202.

8. Weinberg GL, Ripper R, Murphy P et al, "Lipid Infusion Accelerates Removal of Bupivacaine and Recovery from Bupivacaine Toxicity in the Isolated Rat Heart," *Reg Anesth Pain Med*, 2006, 31:296-303.

9. Stehr SN, Ziegeler JC, Pexa A et al, "The Effects of Lipid Infusion on Myocardial Function and Bioenergetics in l-bupivacaine Toxicity in the Isolated Rat Heart," *Anesth Analg*, 2007, 104:186-92.

10. Weinberg GL, Palmer JW, VadeBoncouer TR et al, "Bupivacaine Inhibits Acylcarnitine Exchange in Cardiac Mitochondria," *Anesthesiology*, 2000, 92:523-8.

11. Rosenblatt MA, Abel M, Fischer GW et al, "Successful Use of a 20% Lipid Emulsion to Resuscitate a Patient after a Presumed Bupivacaine-related Cardiac Arrest," *Anesthesiology*, 2006, 105:217-8.

12. Litz RJ, Popp M, Stehr SN et al, "Successful Resuscitation of a Patient with Ropivacaine-induced Asystole after Axillary Plexus Block Using Lipid Infusion," *Anaesthesia*, 2006, 61:800-1.

13. Harvey M and Cave G, "Intralipid Outperforms Sodium Bicarbonate in a Rabbit Model of Clomipramine Toxicity," *Ann Emerg Med*, 2007, 49:178-85, 85 e1-4.

POSITION STATEMENT AND PRACTICE GUIDELINES ON THE USE OF MULTI-DOSE ACTIVATED CHARCOAL IN THE TREATMENT OF ACUTE POISONING

Reprinted from *American Academy of Clinical Toxicology; European Association of Poisons Centres and Clinical Toxicologists*, 1999, 37(6):731-51, by courtesy of Marcel Dekker, Inc.

SUMMARY STATEMENT

Introduction

- The challenge for clinicians managing poisoned patients is to identify at an early stage those who are most at risk of developing serious complications and who might potentially benefit, therefore, from elimination techniques.
- Multiple-dose activated charcoal therapy involves the repeated administration (more than two doses) of oral activated charcoal to enhance the elimination of drugs already absorbed into the body.
- No evidence has yet been published to demonstrate convincingly that multiple-dose activated charcoal reduces morbidity and mortality in poisoned patients.
- Further studies are required to establish its role and the optimal dosage regimen of charcoal to be administered.

Rationale

- Drugs with a prolonged elimination half-life following overdose and small volume of distribution (< 1 L/kg body weight) are particularly likely to have their elimination enhanced to a clinically significant degree by multiple-dose activated charcoal.
- Multiple-dose activated charcoal is thought to produce its beneficial effect by interrupting the enteroenteric and, in some cases, the enterohepatic and the enterogastric circulation of drugs. In addition, any unabsorbed drug still present in the gut will be absorbed to activated charcoal, thereby reducing drug absorption.

Animal Studies

- In animal studies multiple-dose activated charcoal has been shown to reduce the elimination half-life and increase the total body clearance of acetaminophen (paracetamol),[1] digoxin,[1] phenobarbital,[2] phenytoin,[3] and theophylline.[1] The elimination of salicylate[4] and valproic acid[1] was not enhanced by this means.

Volunteer Studies

- Studies in volunteers have demonstrated that multiple-dose activated charcoal increases the elimination of carbamazepine,[5] dapsone,[6] dextropropoxyphene,[7] digitoxin,[8,9] digoxin,[8-10] disopyramide,[11] nadolol,[12] phenobarbital,[5,13-15] phenylbutazone,[5] phenytoin,[16,17] piroxicam,[18] quinine,[19] sotalol,[20] and theophylline.[21-26]
- The elimination of salicylate was increased by multiple-dose activated charcoal in two studies,[27,28] but not in two other studies.[29,30] Although a statistically significant difference was shown, the treatment effect was small.
- Multiple-dose activated charcoal therapy did not increase the elimination of astemizole,[31] chlorpropamide,[32] sodium valproate,[33] tobramycin,[34,35] and vancomycin.[36]
- The elimination half-life of amitriptyline,[37] but not of doxepin[38] or imipramine,[39] was also reduced by multiple-dose activated charcoal in volunteer studies. Crome, et al,[40] showed a significant reduction in the area under the curve (AUC) of nortriptyline after multiple-dose activated charcoal. However, there are good pharmacokinetic reasons to suggest that in the case of tricyclic antidepressants, a clinically significant increase in body clearance is unlikely to result from the use of such treatment, even though the apparent half-life may be shortened.

Clinical Studies

- Clinical studies of multiple-dose activated charcoal consist only of case series and reports.
- Studies in poisoned patients have confirmed those studies in volunteers which demonstrate that the elimination of carbamazepine,[41,42] dapsone,[6,43] phenobarbital,[44-47] quinine,[48] and theophylline[23,26,49-55] is enhanced by multiple-dose activated charcoal.
- Clearance values achieved by multiple-dose activated charcoal in the case of carbamazepine,[89-91] dapsone,[43] and phenobarbital[96] are comparable to those produced by the more invasive techniques of hemodialysis and hemoperfusion.
- There is also some evidence to suggest that, contrary to the findings in one animal[4] and two volunteer studies,[29,30] multiple-dose activated charcoal may increase the elimination of salicylate[56,57]; these results need to be confirmed in further studies before this therapy can be recommended.
- Although the elimination of digoxin was enhanced by the use of multiple-dose activated charcoal in four experimental studies,[1,8,9,10] in three case reports,[58-60] and in one case series,[61] it is unlikely that the increase in body clearance of digoxin will be of clinical significance because of the large volume of distribution of digoxin. Moreover, severe digoxin poisoning may be treated effectively with digoxin-specific antibody fragments. There is also limited clinical evidence that multiple-dose activated charcoal may increase the clearance of digitoxin.[62]
- The elimination of dapsone was increased by multiple-dose activated charcoal in volunteer and clinical studies.[6,43]
- Although an experimental study[36] did not demonstrate enhanced clearance, two case reports[63,64] suggest that multiple-dose activated charcoal may increase vancomycin clearance.
- Multiple-dose activated charcoal does not appear to increase the clearance of meprobamate,[65,66] methotrexate,[67] phenytoin,[68-72] tricyclic antidepressants,[73,74] and valproic acid[75] in patients who have ingested or been administered these drugs.

Indications

- The use of multiple-dose activated charcoal should be considered if the patient has ingested a life-threatening amount of carbamazepine, dapsone, phenobarbital, quinine, or theophylline, and may obviate the need for invasive extracorporeal techniques in these cases.
- The ultimate decision to use multiple-dose activated charcoal therapy depends on:
  - the physician's clinical judgment regarding the expected outcome in a patient poisoned with carbamazepine, dapsone, phenobarbital, quinine, or theophylline;
  - the presence of a contraindication to the use of activated charcoal therapy;
  - the effectiveness of alternative methods of treatment.

Dosage Regimen

- The optimum dose of charcoal is unknown but it is recommended that after an initial dose of 50-100 g to an adult, activated charcoal should be administered at a rate of not less than 12.5 g/hour or equivalent. Lower doses (10-25 g) of activated charcoal may be employed in children less than 5 years of age as usually they have ingested smaller overdoses and their gut lumen capacity is smaller.
- Activated charcoal should be continued until the patient's condition and laboratory parameters, including plasma drug concentration, are improving.
- It may be difficult in clinical practice to administer substantial doses of activated charcoal because of drug-induced vomiting such as occurs with theophylline in overdose. Smaller doses (and therefore smaller volumes) of activated charcoal administered more frequently may reduce the likelihood of vomiting. However, it is often necessary to give an antiemetic intravenously to ensure satisfactory administration of charcoal, even by a nasogastric tube.

Coadministration of a Cathartic

- The need for concurrent administration of a cathartic, such as sorbitol, remains unproven and is not recommended. In particular, a cathartic should not be administered to young children because of the propensity to cause fluid and electrolyte imbalance.

Contraindications

Absolute

- An unprotected airway
- Presence of intestinal obstruction
- A gastrointestinal tract not anatomically intact

Relative

- Decreased peristalsis (decreased bowel sounds, abdominal distention, ileus) such as occurs following overdoses of drugs with opioid or anticholinergic properties.
- Multiple-dose charcoal should be administered cautiously in the presence of decreased peristalsis with careful monitoring for the development of obstruction and for the prevention of aspiration.

Complications of Use

- Treatment with multiple-dose activated charcoal is relatively free from serious side-effects, although transient constipation may occur if aqueous charcoal is administered in substantial dose, particularly in nonambulatory patients due to a depressed level of consciousness.
- Occasionally, bowel obstruction has been reported necessitating manual evacuation or surgical intervention.[107,108,110,111]
- Regurgitation, with subsequent aspiration into the lungs of gastric contents containing charcoal, or direct instillation of charcoal into the lungs as a result of a misplaced nasogastric tube, has led rarely to severe pulmonary complications and death.[112,117-119] Emesis of aqueous activated charcoal occurs infrequently. The incidence appears to be greater when activated charcoal is administered with sorbitol.

Supporting Documentation

Introduction

Charcoal is prepared from vegetable matter, usually peat, coal, wood, coconut shell, or petroleum. Charcoal is "activated" by heating it at high temperature in a stream of oxidizing gas (eg, steam, carbon dioxide, air) or with an activating agent such as phosphoric acid or zinc chloride, or by a combination of both. The process of activation creates a highly developed internal pore structure and thereby increases the surface area from 2-4 m^2/g to an area in excess of 1500 m^2/g. Medicinal activated charcoal must meet BP, USP, or similar standards and have a surface area of at least 900 m^2/g.

Multiple-dose activated charcoal therapy is the repeated administration (more than two doses) of oral activated charcoal with the intent of enhancing drug elimination.

Multiple-dose activated charcoal is perceived as a simple, inexpensive, and safe therapy which may avoid the need for more invasive procedures such as hemodialysis and hemoperfusion. While studies in volunteers demonstrate that its administration both reduces the elimination half-life and increases drug clearance of some drugs, most of the clinical data supporting the use of multiple-dose activated charcoal are anecdotal case reports. Controlled clinical studies are necessary to establish the role of this therapy.

Methodology

In preparing this Position Statement all relevant scientific literature was identified by searching Medline, Toxline, and EMBASE using the terms "activated charcoal," "multiple-dose activated charcoal," and "repeat dose activated charcoal." The original papers were obtained and reviewed critically by a group of clinical toxicologists chosen by the two sponsoring societies. A draft Position Statement was produced which went through multiple drafts before being approved by the boards of the two societies.

Rationale

Drugs with a prolonged elimination half-life following overdose are likely to have their elimination enhanced by multiple-dose activated charcoal.[1,76] Other relevant pharmacokinetic factors include volume of distribution (< 1 L/kg body weight), pKa, and protein binding. If multiple-dose activated charcoal therapy is initiated during a drug's distributive phase, particularly if it is long, it may have a considerable pharmacokinetic effect by interrupting drug distribution into tissues.[1] In addition, if a major route of elimination is no longer available due to the onset of organ failure, this treatment has the potential to make a contribution to total body clearance of the drug ingested which is clinically beneficial.

Mechanisms of Action

Multiple-dose activated charcoal is thought to produce its beneficial effects by:

1. Binding any drug which diffuses from the circulation into the gut lumen.[77] After absorption, a drug will reenter the gut by passive diffusion provided that the concentration there is lower than that in blood. The rate of passive diffusion depends on the concentration gradient and the intestinal surface area, permeability, and blood flow. Under these "sink" conditions, a concentration gradient is maintained and the drug passes continuously into the gut lumen where it is absorbed to charcoal. This process has been termed "gastrointestinal dialysis."[78] Animal studies have confirmed that activated charcoal significantly interrupts the enteroenteric circulation of phenobarbital.[79]

2. Interrupting the enterohepatic and the enterogastric circulation of drugs.

Animal Studies

Acetaminophen (Paracetamol). Acetaminophen 30 mg/kg was administered intravenously over 12 minutes with three other drugs (aminophylline, digoxin, valproic acid) to seven pigs with an indwelling gastrostomy tube.[1] Activated charcoal 25 g with sorbitol (48 g) was administered as the initial intervention at time zero and an aqueous slurry of activated charcoal (25 g) was administered at 2, 4, 6, 12, 18, 24, and 30 hours via the gastrostomy tube. The mean acetaminophen half-life was reduced significantly ($p < 0.01$) from $1.7 \pm$ (SD) 0.2 hours to 1.4 ± 0.3 hours and significantly increased ($p < 0.01$) the clearance from 4.57 ± 0.54 mL/minute/ kg to 5.41 ± 0.63 mL/minute/kg.

Aspirin. In a crossover study, six fasted pigs received aspirin 300 mg/kg intravenously followed by no treatment or activated charcoal 1 g/kg every hour for six doses [the first dose contained sorbitol (70%) 4 mL/kg] via a gastrostomy tube.[4] There were no statistical differences between the control and treatment arms. Mean peak serum salicylate concentrations were 474 ± 62 mg/L and 484 ± 3.9 mg/L, respectively ($p = 0.74$), and the AUC over 6 hours was $171,000 \pm 24,000$ mg times minutes/L in the control group and $188,000 \pm 18,000$ mg times minutes/L in the treatment group ($p = 0.22$).

Digoxin. Seven female pigs were administered digoxin 30 mcg/kg intravenously together with three other drugs (aminophylline, digoxin, valproic acid).[1] Activated charcoal (25 g) with sorbitol (48 g) was administered as the initial intervention at time zero and an aqueous slurry of activated charcoal (25 g) was administered at 2, 4, 6, 12, 18, 24, and 30 hours via an indwelling gastrostomy tube. The half-life was reduced significantly ($p < 0.001$) from a mean of $64.8 \pm$ (SD) 23.7 hours to 17.2 ± 5.6 hours. Clearance was increased from 2.33 ± 0.85 mL/minute/kg to 7.05 ± 1.42 mL/minute/kg ($p < 0.001$).

Phenobarbital (Phenobarbitone). Arimori and Nakano[2] administered phenobarbital 10 mg/kg body weight intravenously to five fasted Wistar strain male rats. Activated charcoal 300 mg was given orally at time zero and then in a dose of 150 mg at 1, 2, 3, 4, and 6 hours after dosing. The mean phenobarbital elimination half-life was reduced significantly ($p < 0.05$) from $8.52 \pm$ (SEM) 0.62 hours to 5.71 ± 0.35 hours and the mean total body clearance of phenobarbital was increased significantly ($p < 0.01$) from $50.2 \pm$ (SEM) 2.73 mL/kg/hour to 77.0 ± 1.21 mL/kg/hour. There was a significant ($p < 0.01$) reduction in the mean AUC of 64% from 184.2 ± 9.56 mcg times hour/mL to 118.7 ± 188 mcg times hour/mL.

Phenytoin. A reduction in the elimination half-life of phenytoin by multiple-dose activated charcoal was reported by Arimori and Nakano.[3] Five fasted Wistar strain rats were treated with activated charcoal 300 mg at time zero and 150 mg at 1, 2, 3, 4, and 6 hours after the administration of a single intravenous dose of phenytoin 10 mg/kg or 50 mg/kg body weight. There were no statistical differences between any parameters at 10 mg/kg. The mean elimination half-life at the 50 mg/kg dose fell significantly ($p < 0.05$) from $6.2 \pm$ (SEM) 0.73 hours to 4.77 ± 0.43 hours and the total body clearance increased significantly ($p < 0.01$) from $0.16 \pm$ (SEM) 0.01 L/kg/hour to 0.22 ± 0.01 L/kg/hour. The AUC was reduced significantly ($p < 0.01$) from 311.2 ± 19.3 mcg times hour/mL to 233.5 ± 12.4 mcg times hour/mL.

Theophylline. Arimori and Nakano[2] administered aminophylline 10 mg/kg body weight intravenously to five fasted Wistar strain rats. Activated charcoal 300 mg was given orally at time zero and then 150 mg was administered at 1, 2, 3, and 4 hours postdosing with aminophylline. The mean elimination half-life was reduced significantly (p < 0.05) from 4.63±(SEM) 0.49 hours to 2.84±0.20 hours and the mean total body clearance of theophylline was increased significantly (p < 0.05) from 66.7±(SEM) 9.03 mL/kg/hour to 101.2±9.77 mL/kg/hour. There was a significant (p < 0.02) reduction in the mean AUC from 138.1±17.5 mcg times hour/mL to 88.0±8.39 mcg times hour/mL.

Aminophylline was administered intravenously to five dogs in doses of 50-100 mg/kg followed by duodenal administration of activated charcoal 45-50 g every hour for 7 hours (eight doses).[80] Although mean AUC values were reduced in the charcoal-treated group, no statistical analysis was undertaken and the results are therefore uninterpretable.

Chyka, et al,[1] administered theophylline (as aminophylline) 8.9 mg/kg intravenously over 12 minutes to seven pigs that were also coadministered digoxin, acetaminophen, and valproic acid. Activated charcoal (25 g) with sorbitol (48 g) was administered as the initial intervention at time zero and an aqueous slurry of activated charcoal (25 g) was administered at 2, 4, 6, 12, 18, 24, and 30 hours via a gastrostomy tube after the initiation of the aminophylline infusion. The mean (±SD) theophylline half-life was reduced from 9.4±2.0 to 3.5±2.3 (p < 0.01) hours and the AUC from 168.9±34.3 mg/hour/L to 43.6±9.8 mg/hour/L (p < 0.001).

Valproic acid. Valproic acid was administered intravenously over 12 minutes with three other drugs (acetaminophen, aminophylline, digoxin) to seven pigs with an indwelling gastrostomy tube.[1] Activated charcoal (25 g) with sorbitol (48 g) was administered as the initial intervention at time zero and an aqueous slurry of activated charcoal (25 g) was administered at 2, 4, 6, 12, 18, 24, and 30 hours via the gastrostomy tube, but did not reduce significantly the half-life and AUC or increase the clearance of valproic acid.

Volunteer Studies

Aspirin. Barone et al[27] gave activated charcoal 50 g to ten fasted volunteers at 1, 5, and 9 hours after the administration of aspirin 1944 mg. There was a statistically significant reduction (p < 0.01) in the mean percent recovery of total salicylate from the urine (49.2%±12.48%) compared to controls [91.0±(SD) 6.12%]; serum salicylate concentrations were not measured.

Kirshenbaum et al[28] investigated the effect of multiple dose charcoal therapy in ten volunteers who were given aspirin 2880 mg (29-59 mg/kg body weight) orally, which produced a mean peak serum salicylate concentration of 192±(SD) 27.6 mg/L. During the treatment phase, between 4 and 10 hours postingestion, each received activated charcoal 25 g every 2 hours (total dose 100 g). A significant reduction (p < 0.05) in the AUC of 9% was observed in the treatment phase, with an 18% reduction (p < 0.01) in total urinary excretion of salicylate. While concluding that the "modest" effect of multiple dose charcoal on salicylate clearance suggested it was "of questionable value" in the treatment of acute salicylate poisoning, the authors acknowledged that the observed benefit would be potentially greater in severely intoxicated patients in whom the plasma concentrations would be significantly higher and the salicylate half-life substantially longer than in this study.

The administration of activated charcoal 25 g 4 hours after aspirin dosing (1300 mg orally) to six fasted adult volunteers, followed by three further doses of charcoal 10 g every 2 hours, did not result in a significant reduction in half-life or AUC.[29] Peak serum salicylate concentrations ranged from 55-136 mg/L.

Mayer et al[30] administered aspirin 2800 mg (33-44 mg/kg body weight) to nine volunteers and 4 hours later activated charcoal 25 g was given and repeated every 2 hours for four doses. Following charcoal treatment, no significant difference was observed in the mean peak serum salicylate concentrations: 160±(SD) 17 mg/L in the control group and 150±24 mg/L in the charcoal group. No significant differences in the AUCs were observed.

Astemizole. Laine et al[31] demonstrated that activated charcoal (12 g) administered twice daily (from 6 hours onwards) to seven volunteers for 8 days did not alter the rate of elimination or AUC (0-192 hours) of astemizole (30 mg).

Carbamazepine. In a randomized crossover study in five fasted volunteers given carbamazepine 400 mg orally, Neuvonen and Elonen[5] found the mean elimination half-life was reduced significantly (p < 0.05) from 32±(SEM) 3.4 hours to 17.6±2.4 hours following multiple-dose charcoal therapy (50 g at 10 hours postdosing: 17 g at 14, 24, 36, and 48 hours postdosing). The mean total body clearance was also increased significantly (p < 0.05) from 22.0±(SEM) 1.9 mL/minute to 40.0±2.7 mL/minute.

Chlorpropamide. Neuvonen and Kärkkäinen[32] demonstrated that the half-life of chlorpropamide was not reduced significantly by the use of multiple-dose activated charcoal (50 g at 6 hours followed by 12.5 g every 6 hours for 8 hours) following the administration of chlorpropamide 250 mg orally to six volunteers.

Dapsone. Neuvonen et al[6] administered dapsone 500 mg to five volunteers over 4 days (100 mg daily for 3 days and 100 mg twice daily on day 4) in a randomized crossover study. Ten hours after the last dose, subjects were given charcoal 50 g, then 17 g every 12 hours for an additional four doses. The dapsone elimination half-life was reduced significantly ($p < 0.01$) from $20.5 \pm$ (SEM) 2.0 hours during the control period to 10.8 ± 0.4 hours after charcoal. The half-life of the metabolic monoacetyldapsone was also reduced significantly ($p < 0.001$) during treatment.

Dextropropoxyphene. Kärkkäinen and Neuvonen[7] found that the elimination half-lives of dextropropoxyphene and its metabolite, norpropoxyphene, were reduced in six volunteers given activated charcoal 50 g 6 hours after the oral administration of dextropropoxyphene 130 mg; further doses of charcoal (12.5 g) were administered every 6 hours for eight doses. It should be noted that in the control phase, volunteers received activated charcoal 50 g 5 minutes after dextropropoxyphene dosing. The mean elimination half-life of dextropropoxyphene was reduced significantly ($p < 0.05$) from $31.1 \pm$ (SEM) 4.2 hours to 21.2 ± 3.1 hours and the mean elimination half-life of norpropoxyphene was reduced significantly ($p < 0.001$ from $34.4 \pm$ (SEM) 2.5 hours to 19.8 ± 3.4 hours.

Digitoxin and digoxin. Park et al[8] gave six adult volunteers intravenous infusions of digoxin (0.75 mg/70 kg body weight) or digitoxin (1 mg/70 kg body weight) followed either by water alone or activated charcoal (20 g immediately, then 20 g every 4 hours for 36 hours; a further 20 g dose was administered 48 hours postinfusion). The serum digoxin half-life was decreased significantly ($p < 0.05$) from $23.1 \pm$ (SEM) 1.7 hours to 17.0 ± 1.5 hours, but the increase in digoxin clearance was not statistically significant ($p > 0.1$). The half-life of digitoxin was decreased significantly ($p < 0.01$) from 110.6 ± 11.0 hours to 51.1 ± 4.5 hours and digitoxin clearance was increased significantly ($p < 0.001$) from 0.24 ± 0.01 to 0.47 ± 0.04 L/hour. The authors also reported a reduction in the digoxin elimination half-life from 93.3 to 29.3 hours in a volunteer with chronic renal failure; the total body clearance of digoxin increased from 3.6 L/hour to 10.1 L/hour.

Reissel and Manninen[9] found that during maintenance therapy with digoxin or digitoxin in six individuals aged 60-74 years, the administration of activated charcoal 6 g a day significantly decreased ($p < 0.001$) the mean plasma digoxin concentration by 31.2% and reduced significantly ($p < 0.05$) the mean serum digitoxin concentration by 18.3%.

Activated charcoal (225 g over 40 hours) was given to ten healthy volunteers after the intravenous administration of digoxin 10 mcg/kg. Charcoal increased significantly ($p < 0.005$) the total body clearance of digoxin from $12.2 \pm$ (SD) 2.0 L/hour to 18.0 ± 2.9 L/hour and the terminal half-life was reduced significantly ($p < 0.005$) from $36.5 \pm$ (SD) 11.8 hours to 21.5 ± 6.5 hours.[10]

Disopyramide. Arimori et al[11] administered activated charcoal (40 g at 4 hours and 20 g at 6, 8, and 12 hours) to six volunteers after they had been given disopyramide 200 mg orally. The mean elimination half-life was decreased significantly ($p < 0.05$) from $6.09 \pm$ (SEM) 0.48 hours to 4.11 ± 0.45 hours and the total body clearance increased significantly ($p < 0.01$) from $0.113 \pm$ (SEM) 0.017 L/hour/kg to 0.138 ± 0.019 L/hour/kg.

Naldolol. The elimination half-life of oral naldolol 80 mg in eight adult volunteers was reduced significantly ($p < 0.05$) from $17.3 \pm$ (SEM) 1.7 hours to 11.8 ± 1.6 hours by small doses (500 mg at 3 and 4 hours after dosing and then 250 mg hourly for a further 8 hours) of activated charcoal tablets.[12]

Phenobarbital (Phenobarbitone). Neuvonen and Elonen[5] gave five fasted volunteers activated charcoal 50 g at 10 hours and 17 g at 24, 36, and 48 hours after the oral administration of phenobarbital 200 mg and found that the mean phenobarbital elimination half-life was reduced significantly ($p < 0.05$) $110 \pm$ (SEM) 23 hours to 19.8 ± 1.0 hours. The total phenobarbital clearance was increased significantly ($p < 0.05$) from $4.6 \pm$ (SEM) 0.9 mL/min to 23.0 ± 3.0 mL/min.

Six volunteers were given activated charcoal 40 g at time zero and 20 g at 6, 12, 18, 24, 30, 42, and 66 hours following the intravenous administration of the phenobarbital 200 mg.[13] The mean phenobarbital half-life was reduced significantly ($p < 0.01$) from $110 \pm$ (SEM) 8 hours to 45 ± 6 hours, the mean total body clearance of phenobarbital was increased significantly ($p < 0.01$) from 4.4 ± 0.2 to 12.0 ± 1.6 mL/kg/hour, and the nonrenal clearance of phenobarbital was increased from 52% to 80% of the total body clearance.

In another study[14] the effects of charcoal alone and a charcoal-sorbitol mixture on phenobarbital elimination were investigated in six men. Following the intravenous administration of phenobarbital 200 mg/70 kg over 1 hour, either activated charcoal 105 g or activated charcoal 105 g with sorbitol was given over a 36-hour period (30 g at end of dosing; 15 g at 6, 12, 18, 24, and 36 hours after dosing). The mean phenobarbital elimination half-life ($T_{1/2}$ 3-60 hours) fell significantly ($p < 0.05$) from $72 \pm$ (SD) 7 hours (control) to 36 ± 4 hours (charcoal alone), and 30 ± 4 hours (charcoal-sorbitol). However, there was no significant difference in the terminal elimination half-life in each group: 102 ± 19 hours (control), 119 ± 22 hours (charcoal alone), and 116 ± 25 hours (charcoal-sorbitol). The apparent mean systemic clearance of phenobarbital increased significantly (but no p value was included) from 0.0895 ± 0.019 mL/minute (control) to 0.141 ± 0.029 mL/minute/kg (charcoal alone) and 0.146 ± 0.36 mL/minute/kg (charcoal-sorbitol).

Frenia et al[15] administered phenobarbital 5 mg/kg to ten volunteers. Each volunteer received six doses of activated charcoal: 50 g with sorbitol (50 g of 70%) 30 minutes after phenobarbital and five 25 g doses at 4.5, 8.5, 12.5, 16.5 and 20.5 hours; and a dose of sorbitol (25 g of 70%) was administered at 12.5 and 24.5 hours. The mean ($\pm$ SD) phenobarbital half-life was reduced significantly ($p = 0.005$) from 148.1 ± 332.1 hours to 18.87 ± 14.70 hours and the mean ($\pm$ SD) phenobarbital clearance was increased significantly ($p < 0.0005$) from 2.79 ± 9.69 mL/kg/hour (control group) to 19.95 ± 11.5 mL/kg/hour (charcoal group).

Phenylbutazone. Multiple-dose activated charcoal (50 g 10 hours postdosing; 17 g at 14, 24, 36, and 48 hours postdosing) reduced significantly ($p < 0.05$) the mean elimination half-life of phenylbutazone from $51.5 \pm$ (SEM) 7.6 hours to 36.7 ± 4.1 hours after the oral administration of phenylbutazone 200 mg.[5] The total phenylbutazone clearance was also increased significantly ($p < 0.05$) from $1.5 \pm$ (SEM) 0.16 mL/minute to 2.1 ± 0.23 mL/minute.

Phenytoin. The effect of multiple-dose activated charcoal on the elimination of intravenously administered phenytoin was studied in seven fasting volunteers by Mauro et al.[16] Each participant received phenytoin 15 mg/kg intravenously over 60 minutes which produced a mean C_{max} of approximately 22 mg/L. At the end of the phenytoin infusion, activated charcoal 60 g with sorbitol was given followed by 30 g (with random sorbitol administration) at 2, 4, 8, 12, 24, 30, 36, and 48 hours (total dose 300 g over 48 hours). Charcoal significantly reduced ($p < 0.001$) the mean phenytoin elimination half-life from $44.5 \pm$ (SD) 14.0 hours to 22.3 ± 6.9 hours.

In another study,[17] eight fasted volunteers received phenytoin 15 mg/kg intravenously over 1 hour followed by charcoal 140 g over 10 hours (40 g at end of the infusion; 20 g at 2, 4, 6, 8, and 10 hours after the infusion). Half of the subjects received sorbitol in their loading dose and with every other dose of activated charcoal. Administration of activated charcoal led to a significant increase ($p = 0.008$) in mean phenytoin clearance from 15.3 ± 3.8 mL/minute/1.73 m^2 to 20.9 ± 5.2 mL/minute/1.73 m^2. There was a nonsignificant decrease in half-life from 25.5 ± 9.8 hours to 23.6 ± 15.9 hours after charcoal. The addition of sorbitol to the treatment regimen did not change clearance values.

Piroxicam. In a study with a randomized crossover design and six volunteers, Laufen and Leitold[18] studied the use of multiple-dose activated charcoal following the administration of piroxicam 20 mg by either the oral or rectal route. In the oral drug administration phase, activated charcoal 50 g was administered at 10 hours postingestion followed by doses of 20-30 g for a total of 70 g every 24 hours up to 58 hours after piroxicam ingestion. The elimination half-life was reduced significantly ($p < 0.05$) from a mean ($\pm$ SD) of 40.2 ± 10.0 hours (control group) to 19.6 ± 5.9 hours (charcoal group). The mean apparent total clearance increased significantly ($p < 0.05$) from 3.46 ± 1.33 mL/minute to 5.66 ± 1.41 mL/minute. In the rectal administration phase, activated charcoal 30 g was administered at 2 hours after drug delivery and 20-30 g was given at varying intervals for a total of 70 g every 24 hours. The elimination half-life was reduced significantly from a mean ($\pm$ SD) of 40.7 ± 12.6 hours in the control group to 21.6 ± 6.4 hours in the charcoal group. There was also a significant ($p < 0.05$) increase in the mean ($\pm$ SD) apparent total clearance from 3.65 ± 1.19 mL/minute to 6.86 ± 2.23 mL/minute.

Quinine. The effect of multiple-dose activated charcoal on quinine elimination was studied following a therapeutic (600 mg) dose of quinine bisulphate to seven adult fasted volunteers.[19] Activated charcoal 50 g was administered 4 hours after quinine dosing and three further doses were given over the next 12 hours. Activated charcoal significantly lowered ($p < 0.001$) the quinine elimination half-life from $8.23 \pm$ (SD) 0.57 to 4.55 ± 0.15 hours and the clearance was significantly increased ($p < 0.001$) from $11.8 \pm$ (SD) 1.23 L/hour to 18.4 ± 2.8 L/hour.

Sotalol. The mean elimination half-life of sotalol was decreased significantly ($p < 0.01$) from $9.4 \pm$ (SEM) 0.4 hours to 7.6 ± 0.3 hours by the administration of activated charcoal (50 g at 6 hours, then 12.5 g every 6 hours for eight doses) to seven fasted adult volunteers who had received sotalol 160 mg orally.[20]

Theophylline. The effect of activated charcoal on theophylline kinetics when a sustained-release preparation was administered orally to 20 children in a dose of 10 mg/kg was studied by Lim et al.[81] Five children given activated charcoal 1 g/kg body weight (maximum 60 g) at 6, 9, and 12 hours postdosing had a 20.65% nonsignificant reduction in the AUC compared to controls.

Minton and Henry[82] administered three sustained-release theophylline 200 mg tablets to ten fasted volunteers. Activated charcoal 50 g was given at 6 hours, with two further 25 g doses at 10 hours and 14 hours. The AUC of theophylline in the control group was 152.8±(SD) 1.44 mg/L/hour and in the charcoal group was 65.3±1.33 mg/L/hour. No statistical calculations were undertaken.

Goldberg et al[83] demonstrated that the addition of sorbitol to charcoal significantly reduced (p < 0.01) the AUC (85.5±[SEM] 10.0 mg/hour/L) when compared to multiple-dose charcoal alone (113±5.7 mg/hour/L) and controls (304.6±18.8 mg/hour/L). In this study, charcoal, with or without sorbitol, was administered at 6, 7, 8, 10, and 12 hours after administration of slow release theophylline 1200 mg/70 kg to nine subjects.

The effect of multiple-dose charcoal on the kinetics of an intravenous dose of aminophylline (6 mg/kg body weight) administered to five volunteers was investigated by Berlinger et al.[21] Activated charcoal 40 g was given at time zero and 20 g at 2, 4, 6, 9, and 12 hours after completion of the theophylline infusion. Treatment with activated charcoal significantly decreased (p < 0.05) the mean elimination half-life from 6.4±(SEM) 1.2 hours to 3.3±0.4 hours. The AUC in the charcoal group was 42±4 mg times hour/L compared to 78±14 mg times hour/L in controls (p < 0.05).

Mahutte et al[23] administered an infusion of aminophylline 8 mg/kg to seven volunteers. Each then received activated charcoal 30 g at time zero and at 2, 4, and 6 hours. A significant reduction (p < 0.001) in the mean theophylline elimination half-life from 10.2±(SD) 2.1 hours to 4.6±1.3 hours was observed. The total body clearance of theophylline was also increased significantly (p < 0.001) by charcoal administration from 35.6±(SD) 7.3 mL/kg/hour to 72.6±17.0 mL/kg/hour.

The effect of different regimens of multiple-dose activated charcoal on the elimination of aminophylline 6 mg/kg given by infusion over 1 hour in six volunteers was investigated by Park et al.[24] A significant reduction (p < 0.01) in the mean theophylline elimination half-life from 9.1±(SEM) 0.7 hours was achieved either with charcoal 20 g every 2 hours for six doses (4.3±0.4 hours) or 10 g every hour for six doses (4.3±0.2 hours). Park et al[25] also gave eight volunteers aminophylline 5-6 mg/kg intravenously over 60 minutes. Immediately on discontinuing the aminophylline infusions, the volunteers received activated charcoal either 5 g or 20 g every 2 hours for six doses. The 20 g regimen produced a significant reduction (p < 0.01) in the half-life (4.9±[SEM] 0.2 hours) compared to the 5 g regimen (6.3±0.5 hours). The AUC was also reduced significantly (p < 0.01) from 88.9±8.4 (5 g regimen) mg/L/hour to 67.7±3.6 mg/L/hour (20 g regimen).

In another study,[26] six subjects with cirrhosis were given multiple-dose activated charcoal (40 g at time zero and 20 g at 2, 4, 6, 9, and 12 hours) following an infusion of aminophylline 6 mg/kg over 1 hour. The mean theophylline half-life during treatment was reduced significantly (p < 0.05) from 12.7±(SEM) 4.0 hours to 4.0±0.7 hours.

Five fasted volunteers received an infusion of aminophylline 8 mg/kg over 1 hour followed by various activated charcoal regimens: 12.5 g every hour for 8 hours; 25 g every 2 hours for 8 hours; 50 g every 4 hours for 8 hours.[22] Each dosage regimen was preceded by activated charcoal 50 g and each subject received a total of 150 g. The mean theophylline elimination half-life was reduced significantly (p < 0.05) for each charcoal regimen compared to controls, but there was no significant difference between the treatment groups. Similarly, the mean AUC for each charcoal regimen was significantly lower (p < 0.05) than controls, although there was no significant difference between the charcoal regimens.

Tobramycin. Davis et al[34] administered tobramycin 2.5 mg/kg intravenously over 30 minutes to six volunteers. Activated charcoal 50 g was given prior to tobramycin administration and subsequent doses of 15 g were administered at 2, 4, and 6 hours. There was no difference in the mean values for total body clearance of tobramycin compared to control.

Multiple-dose activated charcoal (10 g 2 hours prior to dosing, 10 g at zero time, and 10 g at 2, 6, and 8 hours after dosing) had no effect on the elimination of tobramycin 1.5 mg/kg administrated intravenously in five volunteers.[35]

Tricyclic antidepressants. Kärkkäinen and Neuvonen[37] studied the impact of activated charcoal on the elimination of amitriptyline 75 mg administered orally to six fasted volunteers. Activated charcoal 50 g was given 6 hours after amitriptyline dosing and further doses (12.5 g) of charcoal were administered at 12, 18, 24, 30, 36, 42, 48, and 54 hours. Charcoal shortened significantly (p < 0.05) the elimination half-life of amitriptyline from 27.4±(SEM) 4.8 hours (control) to 21.1±3.3 hours (charcoal group). The AUC (0-72 hours) was also reduced significantly (p < 0.05) in the charcoal group.

In a further study, eight volunteers were given doxepin 50 mg orally and then received activated charcoal 15 g 3 hours later, followed by charcoal 10 g at 6, 9, 12, and 24 hours after dosing.[38] The half-life in the activated charcoal group 16.2 ± SEM 2.3 hours was not significantly different from the control group (17.9 ± 4.3 hours) and the clearance of doxepin in the activated charcoal group 1.23 ± SEM 0.31 L/hour/kg was not significantly different from the control group (0.93 ± 0.03 L/hour/kg).

The effect of multiple-dose activated charcoal on the elimination of imipramine was studied in a randomized crossover trial.[39] Four fasted volunteers received imipramine 12.5 mg/70 kg intravenously over 1 hour followed by either water or 180 g activated charcoal over 24 hours (20 g at 0, 2, 4, 6, 9, 12, 16, 20, and 24 hours after dosing). There was no significant difference (p > 0.05) in imipramine half-life in controls [9.0 ± SEM 0.8 hours] compared to the charcoal treated group (10.9 ± 1.6 hours) or in the clearance values in the control group (992.2 ± 138.3 mL/minute/70 kg) and in the charcoal treated group (930.3 ± 101.9 mL/minute/70 kg).

Chrome et al[40] administered four separate doses of activated charcoal 5 g to six volunteers 30, 120, 240, and 360 minutes after they had been given nortriptyline 75 mg orally. There was a mean 72% (range 62% to 78%) reduction (p < 0.01) in peak nortriptyline concentrations and a significant reduction (mean 70%; range 58% to 76%; p < 0.01) in $AUC_{0-48\ hours}$ compared to control after multiple doses of charcoal. When only a single dose of activated charcoal 5 g was administered 30 minutes after nortriptyline, there was a mean 58% (range 30% to 81%) reduction in peak plasma nortriptyline concentrations and a mean 55% (range 32% to 67%) reduction in the $AUC_{0-48\ hours}$. The difference in peak nortriptyline concentrations and $AUC_{0-48\ hours}$ after single- and multiple-dose charcoal therapy was also significant (p < 0.05).

Valproic acid. Following the oral administration of sodium valproate 300 mg to seven volunteers, multiple-dose activated charcoal 20 g was administered at 4 hours; 10 g was given at 8, 12, 24, and 32 hours.[33] Activated charcoal did not significantly change the half-life of sodium valproate which was 20.0 ± (SD) 6.8 hours in the control group and 22 ± 9.2 hours in the charcoal group. The $AUC_{0-48\ hours}$ after activated charcoal was 408.0 ± (SD) 114.5 mg/L/hour which was not significantly different from control (398.1 ± 108.6 mg/L/hour).

Vancomycin. Davis et al[36] investigated the role of multiple-dose activated charcoal after the administration of vancomycin 1 g intravenously to six volunteers. Activated charcoal 50 g was administered before the infusion followed by 15 g doses at 2, 4, 6, and 8 hours after the start of the vancomycin infusion. Multiple-dose activated charcoal therapy did not enhance vancomycin clearance.

Clinical Studies

Clinical studies of multiple-dose activated charcoal consist only of case series and case reports.

Aspirin. Hillman and Prescott[56] described five patients with salicylate poisoning whose peak plasma salicylate concentrations were 425-655 mg/L. In two cases where the salicylate concentration exceeded 500 mg/L, alkaline diuresis was employed initially. All patients received multiple-dose activated charcoal (75 g, then 50 g every 4 hours) until their symptoms resolved. However, the charcoal preparation administered (Medicoal) contains substantial amounts of sodium bicarbonate and all patients developed an alkaline urine (personal communication) which may have further increased salicylate elimination. In a control group (selection criteria were not stated) of six patients with mild salicylate poisoning who were treated with oral fluids alone, the mean elimination half-life was 27 hours, whereas the mean half-life in the treatment group was less than 3.2 hours.

In seven patients, all of whom had salicylate concentrations greater than 500 mg/L and who received no other therapy, Vale[57] found the elimination half-life to be 9.7 ± (SD) 3.0 hours after each received at least 12.5 g/hour activated charcoal. However, no control data were included in this case series.

Conclusion. One animal study and two of four volunteer studies did not demonstrate increased salicylate clearance with multiple-dose charcoal therapy. Data in poisoned patients are insufficient to recommend the use of charcoal therapy.

Carbamazepine. After multiple-dose activated charcoal (mean total dose 203 ± 58 g), the mean elimination half-life in fifteen patients poisoned with carbamazepine was 8.6 ± (SD) 2.4 hours and the mean total body clearance was 113 ± (SD) 44 mL/minute,[41] whereas in two other series of patients treated only with supportive measures,[84,85] the mean elimination half-life was approximately 19 hours [19.0 ± (SD) 6.9 hours[84] and 18.9 ± (SD) 9.8 hours[85]].

Montoya-Cabrera et al[42] administered multiple-dose activated charcoal (1 g/kg every 4 hours) to eight patients (mean total dose 386 ± 72 g). The mean ($\pm$ SD) carbamazepine half-life was 9.5 ± 1.9 hours and the mean ($\pm$ SD) total body clearance was 105.13 ± 20.4 mL/minute/kg.

The role of multiple-dose charcoal in carbamazepine poisoning was questioned by Watson et al,[86] who reported on its use in two children with acute, and two (one with two episodes of poisoning) with acute-on-chronic, carbamazepine intoxication. The peak carbamazepine concentrations in this study were between 22.4 and 60.0 mg/L. The mean elimination half-life of carbamazepine was 23.3 hours (one case) without charcoal, 10.17 hours ($p < 0.05$) when activated charcoal 30-50 g was given (two episodes of poisoning), and 7.21 hours ($p < 0.05$) when more than 50 g of charcoal was used (three episodes of poisoning). The authors reported no benefit from multiple-dose charcoal in terms of time to complete recovery despite the effect on the plasma half-life of the drug. However, this conclusion has been criticized by Vale and Heath,[87] who stated that the study was too small to test reliably the hypothesis that there exists a relationship between the dose of activated charcoal and time to recovery.

Conclusion. There is good evidence from animal and volunteer studies and from poisoned patients that the total body clearance of carbamazepine is enhanced significantly by multiple-dose activated charcoal therapy. In terms of total body clearance, multiple-dose charcoal is comparable to charcoal hemoperfusion (Table 1). However, a reduction in morbidity has not yet been demonstrated by its use.

Table 1. Comparison of Elimination Techniques in Carbamazepine Poisoning		
Elimination	**Half-life (hours)**	**Clearance (mL/minute)**
Hemoperfusion	8.6-10.7[90]	80-129[89-91]
Multiple-dose charcoal	8.6 ± 2.4[41]	113 ± 44[41]
Multiple-dose charcoal	9.5 ± 1.9[41]	105.13 ± 20.4[41]

Dapsone. Neuvonen et al[6] described two patients with dapsone poisoning. One received activated charcoal 20 g every 6 hours on days 5 and 6 postingestion, with a reduction in the elimination half-life from 88 to 13.5 hours. The second patient received charcoal 20 g every 6 hours only on the third day postoverdose. A reduction in the dapsone elimination half-life from 33 to 11 hours approximately was observed. Workers from the same unit[43] reported a further three patients with dapsone poisoning. The initial dapsone concentrations measured between 16-17 hours after ingestion were 28.0, 23.6, and 17.5 mg/L, respectively. Oral activated charcoal 20 g every 6 hours was administered for 1-2 days beginning 2-4 days postingestion. The mean dapsone elimination half-life was reduced from $77 \pm$ (SEM) 23 hours to 12.7 ± 0.7 hours.

Conclusion. Volunteer studies demonstrate that multiple-dose activated charcoal increases dapsone elimination. Clinical data support this conclusion and the elimination half-life achieved by charcoal is comparable to that (10.4 ± 1.7 hours) during hemodialysis.[43] However, it has not been demonstrated that methemoglobinemia and hemolytic anemia are less likely to result after the use of charcoal therapy.

Digitoxin. Pond et al[62] advocated the use of multiple-dose charcoal in digitoxin poisoning, based on their experience of a patient with a peak plasma digitoxin concentration of 264 mcg/L who received activated charcoal 50 g initially, then 60 g (with magnesium citrate 250 mL) every 8 hours for 72 hours. Following charcoal, the digitoxin half-life was 18 hours compared to a half-life of 162 hours after discontinuation of charcoal.

Conclusion. Volunteer studies and one case report suggest that the clearance of digitoxin may be increased by multiple-dose activated charcoal, though clinical benefit has yet to be demonstrated. However, in severe cases of poisoning, digoxin-specific antibody fragments should be considered.

Digoxin. Boldy et al[58] described a 69-year-old man who had ingested a digoxin overdose and had a plasma digoxin concentration of 8.3 mcg/L, 14.5 hours postingestion. He received activated charcoal 100 g over 1 hour, then 50 g every 4 hours for a further seven doses. The plasma digoxin concentration fell to 1.0 mcg/L over the ensuing 48 hours with a terminal elimination half-life of 14 hours.

Lake et al[59] reported a 71-year-old woman with chronic renal failure and digoxin toxicity (peak plasma concentration 9 mcg/L) who was treated with activated charcoal 50 g followed by 25 g every 6 hours for 8 doses. The digoxin elimination half-lives calculated before, during, and after charcoal therapy were 7.3, 1.4, and 6.3 days, respectively.

Critchley and Critchley[60] described a 66-year-old male with an 8-year history of chronic renal failure who was suffering from digoxin toxicity (severe bradycardia and hypotension). The patient's serum digoxin concentration failed to decrease over 4 days despite the use of daily hemodialysis. On day 4, multiple-dose activated charcoal therapy was instituted (50 g every 6 hours for 48 hours). The serum digoxin concentration decreased from 2.1 mcg/L to 0.8 mcg/L within 48 hours. A second course of activated charcoal (50 g every 6 hours for 72 hours) was instituted from admission day 9 to 12, resulting in a decrease in the digoxin concentration from 0.8 mcg/L to 0.4 mcg/L. During each course of activated charcoal therapy, there was a precipitous reduction in the serum half-life of digoxin, but precise half-lives were not calculated.

Multiple-dose activated charcoal (dose not stated) increased the mean digoxin clearance in 23 patients to $98 \pm$ (SD) 34 mL/minute (mean clearance in sixteen nontreated patients 55 ± 17 mL/minute) and decreased the digoxin elimination half-life from $68 \pm$ (SD) 19 hours to 36 ± 14 hours (control group); all patients had plasma digoxin concentrations >2.5 mcg/L.[61]

Conclusion. The elimination half-life of digoxin was decreased by the use of multiple-dose activated charcoal in animal and volunteer studies, in two case reports and one case series. However, in severe cases of poisoning, digoxin-specific antibody fragments should be considered.

Meprobamate. Hassan[65] described a further two patients with meprobamate poisoning whose peak plasma concentrations were 320 mg/L and 240 mg/L. Each received oral activated charcoal 50 g every 4-6 hours for five doses after an initial loading dose (75 g in one patient). The elimination half-lives for meprobamate were 4.4 hours and 4.5 hours, respectively.

Three patients with meprobamate poisoning were treated with multiple-dose activated charcoal.[66] Peak meprobamate concentrations were 221 mg/L, 91 mg/L, and 80.5 mg/L, respectively, and all patients initially required mechanical ventilation. With charcoal therapy, the elimination half-lives for meprobamate were 4.0, 4.5, and 5.0 hours, respectively.

Conclusion. Reports of meprobamate poisoning managed without multiple-dose charcoal suggest an elimination half-life of about 13 hours[92] and thus charcoal therapy may be effective in increasing drug elimination though there are no volunteer studies to confirm this.

Methotrexate. Serum methotrexate concentrations were estimated after a 6-hour infusion of 1 g/m^2 methotrexate had been administered to seven patients.[67] Each received activated charcoal 25 g at 12, 18, 24, 36, and 48 hours after the infusion. The elimination half-life in the charcoal treated group was reduced, but not significantly, from $8.46 \pm$ (SEM) 0.47 hours (controls) to 7.6 ± 0.44 hours (charcoal group).

Conclusion. This single study does not support the clinical use of multiple-dose activated charcoal after high-dose methotrexate therapy.

Phenobarbital (phenobarbitone). Goldberg and Berlinger[44] gave multiple-dose activated charcoal to two patients poisoned with phenobarbital. The first patient (serum phenobarbital concentration 141 mg/L) received activated charcoal 40 g (with sodium sulfate 20 g) on admission and activated charcoal 40 g (with magnesium citrate 60 mL) every 4 hours for five additional doses. The second patient (serum concentration 107 mg/L) was given activated charcoal 30 g (and sodium sulfate 30 g) 6 hours after admission and this dose was continued every 6 hours for a total of six doses. The phenobarbital elimination half-lives in these two patients were approximately 24 hours.

A randomized study of ten comatose patients who required endotracheal intubation and mechanical ventilation was reported by Pond et al.[45] The control group (n = 5) who received only a single dose of activated charcoal (mean plasma phenobarbital concentration 121 ± 31 mg/L) and the treatment group (n = 5) who received multiple doses of activated charcoal (mean plasma phenobarbital concentration 132 ± 36 mg/L) both received activated charcoal 50 g with magnesium citrate 250 mL on presentation and, in addition, patients in the treatment group were given activated charcoal 17 g together with sorbitol 70 mL (70%) every 4 hours until they had recovered sufficiently to be extubated. Although the mean elimination half-life of phenobarbital was shortened ($36 \pm$ (SD) 13 hours) significantly ($p < 0.01$) in the multiple-dose charcoal group when compared to the single-dose charcoal group (93 ± 52 hours), the length of time that the patients in each group required mechanical ventilation did not differ significantly, nor did the time spent in the hospital. This trial has been criticized as being too small and having unevenly matched groups.[93,94]

In another series,[46] charcoal, in larger doses and given without cathartic, not only greatly enhanced the elimination of phenobarbital, but also decreased the time to recovery. Six patients with moderate to severe phenobarbital intoxication (mean peak plasma phenobarbital concentration 139.2 ± 76.8 mg/L) were treated with repeated oral doses of activated charcoal 50 g (in 3 cases the charcoal employed contained sodium bicarbonate) following an initial dose of 50-150 g (total dose 225-500 g). During and for up to 12 hours after treatment with activated charcoal, the mean phenobarbital half-life was 11.7 ± 3.5 hours. The mean total body clearance of the drug during and up to 12 hours after administration of charcoal was 84 ± 34 mL/minute. It is possible that in the three patients receiving sodium bicarbonate, renal clearance of phenobarbital may have been enhanced. It should be noted that only one-third of the patients in this series were receiving long-term anticonvulsant therapy, in contrast to 100% of patients in the study reported by Pond et al.[45]

The administration of six doses of activated charcoal (0.7 g/kg) to a severely brain-damaged neonate (weight 2.6 kg), treated with intravenous phenobarbital (50 mg/kg), decreased the serum phenobarbital half-life from a calculated 250 hours to 22 hours, enabling earlier initiation of brain-stem testing.[47]

Conclusion. There is good evidence from animal and volunteer studies and from poisoned patients that the total body clearance of phenobarbital is enhanced significantly by multiple-dose activated charcoal therapy. In terms of total body clearance, multiple-dose charcoal is comparable to other elimination techniques such as hemodialysis and hemoperfusion (Table 2).

Table 2. Comparison of Elimination Techniques in Phenobarbital Poisoning	
Elimination	**Clearance (mL/minute)**
Intrinsic clearance	4[95]
Alkaline diuresis	7[96]
Hemodialysis	49[97]
Hemoperfusion	77[96,98]
Multiple-dose charcoal	84[46*]
*Estimated	

Phenytoin. A 21-year-old woman presented 9 hours after allegedly ingesting phenytoin 20 g and was treated with three doses (amount not stated) of activated charcoal every 2 hours (time after overdose not stated). The phenytoin concentration fell from 41 mg/L on admission to 11 mg/L on day 5 postoverdose.[68]

Howard et al[69] reported the clinical course of a 36-year-old, hepatitis B-positive, chronic alcohol abuser receiving both phenobarbital and phenytoin long-term for epilepsy. Twenty-four hours before admission his plasma phenytoin concentration was 34 mg/L and on admission 47 mg/L, at which time features of phenytoin toxicity were present. He received activated charcoal 50 g with sorbitol 96 g every 6 hours for 4 doses. The phenytoin concentration decreased to 20 mg/L approximately 44 hours after admission. Since it is likely that this patient had taken an acute overdose of phenytoin and had induced hepatic enzymes, the benefit of multiple-dose activated charcoal is difficult to determine.

Ros and Black[70] described a 17-year-old epileptic whose serum phenytoin concentration at admission was 56 mg/L, rising to 69 mg/L after 24 hours. He was then treated with nine doses of activated charcoal 30 g every 4 hours. Thirty-eight hours after the first dose of charcoal, the serum phenytoin concentration had fallen to 22 mg/L. When charcoal was discontinued, the serum phenytoin concentration increased to 33 mg/L, then slowly declined.

Weichbrodt and Elliott[71] reported a 38-year-old woman on long-term phenytoin therapy who was treated with multiple-dose activated charcoal after an overdose of phenytoin 10-15 g. She received an initial dose of activated charcoal 30 g at 7 hours postoverdose, followed by 30 g every 6 hours for 4.5 days commencing some 30 hours after overdose (magnesium citrate 180 mL was coadministered with each dose). Her peak serum phenytoin concentration (52 mg/L) was reached within 42.5 hours and the phenytoin concentration fell to within the therapeutic range 6 days postoverdose.

A further case of chronic phenytoin intoxication in a patient with severe liver disease was reported by Weidle et al.[72] Seven days after commencing phenytoin 300 mg twice daily, the patient became agitated and incoherent and the serum phenytoin concentration was found to be 44.4 mg/L. Phenytoin was discontinued and 2 days later (phenytoin concentration 45.2 mg/L) she was commenced on a multiple-dose charcoal regimen of 30 g every 4 hours. After ten doses of charcoal, the serum phenytoin concentration was 11.4 mg/L. The authors estimated that the clearance had been increased by approximately 1.65 L/hour/1.78 m^2.

Conclusion. Although there is some evidence from animal and volunteer studies that multiple-dose activated charcoal may enhance phenytoin elimination, the five anecdotal case reports published to date do not confirm that this therapeutic approach is of clinical benefit.

Quinine. In five symptomatic patients with acute quinine poisoning, the mean elimination half-life was $8.1\pm$(SD) 1.1 hours after each had been administered activated charcoal 50 g every 4 hours.[48] This should be compared to a half-life of approximately 26 hours in poisoned patients treated supportively.[99]

Conclusion. A volunteer study has demonstrated that quinine elimination is enhanced significantly by multiple-dose activated charcoal and a single clinical study has confirmed this observation, even though the relatively large volume of distribution (>1-2.7 L/kg) and high protein binding (70% to 90%) do not favor the use of charcoal therapy. Further studies are required to demonstrate that the serious sequelae encountered in quinine poisoning are reduced or even abolished by charcoal therapy.

Theophylline poisoning. Mahutte et al[23] reported a 72-year-old man with theophylline poisoning (admission concentration 31 mg/L) in whom four doses of activated charcoal 30 g every 2 hours reduced the pre-treatment half-life from 34.4 to 5.7 hours. Workers from the same unit subsequently described four further patients [mean$\pm$(SD) pretreatment theophylline concentrations were 37.1 ± 11.25 mg/L] in whom multiple-dose charcoal reduced the mean serum theophylline half-life from $23.30\pm$(SD) 7.95 hours to 8.0 ± 3.95 hours.[35]

Five patients with moderate theophylline poisoning who were treated with multiple-dose charcoal were reported by Radomski et al.[26] The mean serum theophylline half-life (SEM) was 4.9 ± 0.8 hours with peak serum theophylline concentrations ranging from 32-59 mg/L.

Amitai et al[49] reported two patients (a 34-year-old woman and a 5-month-old infant) with theophylline poisoning (peak plasma concentrations 100 mg/L and 97 mg/L, respectively). With activated charcoal 15 g hourly for nine doses commencing 14 hours after overdose, the adult patient's theophylline elimination half-life fell to 3.7 hours. The infant received three doses of activated charcoal: 10 g at 4.5 hours, 5 g at 8 hours, and 2.5 g at 11 hours postoverdose. The initial elimination half-life of 19 hours decreased to 2.4 hours after charcoal.

Following a medical error,[50] a patient with a peak theophylline concentration of 42.5 mg/L was treated with multiple-dose activated charcoal 15 g every 2 hours for four doses and the elimination half-life was reduced from 7.5 to 2.2 hours.

A 23-year-old woman attempted suicide by ingesting theophylline and terbutaline tablets.[51] The peak (on admission) serum theophylline concentration was 111.4 mg/L. Treatment with multiple-dose activated charcoal 50 g every 6 hours led to a reduction in the theophylline half-life from 17.2 to 5.9 hours.

Two adolescents with serum theophylline concentrations >100 mg/L were treated with a continuous nasogastric infusion of activated charcoal at a maximum rate of 50 g/hour.[52] During the first 20 hours of charcoal therapy, the elimination half-life of theophylline was estimated as 7.7 and 13.5 hours, respectively, decreasing subsequently to 2.6 and 3.2 hours.

Sesler et al[53] reported fourteen cases of theophylline poisoning, ten of whom were treated with activated charcoal. Although several patients vomited charcoal, the mean theophylline half-life during charcoal therapy was $5.7\pm$(SD) 2.5 hours.

A further five cases, including one reported previously by Amitai et al,[49] of theophylline poisoning due to medical error in infants under 7 months old, were reported by Shannon et al.[54] Multiple-dose activated charcoal resulted in an elimination half-life of $8.3\pm$(SD) 4.7 hours (n = 4).

Conclusion. Patients poisoned severely with theophylline are invariably vomiting repeatedly, which makes administration of charcoal problematic, even via a nasogastric tube. In these circumstances, the use of an antiemetic intravenously should be considered. Studies in animals and volunteers confirm that the elimination of theophylline is enhanced by multiple-dose activated charcoal. Case reports also suggest that theophylline elimination is increased by this means although further studies are required to demonstrate that morbidity is reduced by multiple-dose charcoal therapy.

Tricyclic antidepressants. Swartz and Sherman[73] administered activated charcoal to three patients poisoned with amitriptyline. The first patient received two doses (50 g at 2 hours and 25 g at 10 hours postoverdose) of activated charcoal, the second patient received three doses (50 g at 2 hours, 25 g at 6 hours, and 25 g at 23 hours postoverdose), and the third patient received four doses (40 g at 1 hour, 20 g at 4 hours, 20 g at 9 hours, and 20 g at 21 hours postoverdose) of activated charcoal. Although the authors concluded that charcoal "greatly accelerated tricyclic elimination," this cannot be supported from the data.

Three patients poisoned with dothiepin received activated charcoal 100-200 g following overdose.[74] The mean elimination half-life was $12.1 \pm (SD)$ 1.3 hours, which is not substantially different from cases treated supportively in the same series.

Conclusion. A variable effect on the elimination half-life of amitriptyline, doxepin, and imipramine has been reported in volunteer studies. However, it would not be expected from the very large volume of distribution of tricyclic antidepressants that their elimination would be enhanced by activated charcoal.

Valproic acid. A 26-month-old infant ingested a minimum of 4.5 g enteric-coated valproic acid. On arrival at hospital, activated charcoal 20 g was administered (no detectable valproic acid in the serum) and following a marked clinical deterioration (serum valproic acid 315 mg/L), gastric infusion of 3 g/hour activated charcoal was given from 9 hours to 25 hours postoverdose.[75] The elimination half-life was 4.8 hours, which is shorter than the 23 hours reported by Dupuis et al.[100]

Conclusion. The elimination of sodium valproate was not enhanced in animal and volunteer studies by the use of multiple-dose charcoal therapy. It is possible that at higher plasma drug concentrations, when more free drug is likely to be present, such therapy could have greater benefit. Further studies are needed to confirm this.

Vancomycin. A 17-day-old neonate was administered vancomycin 500 mg intravenously. Multiple-dose activated charcoal 1 g/kg was administered 5 hours later and continued every 4 hours for 12 doses.[64] The half-life of vancomycin was calculated to be 9.4 hours.

A 47-day-old premature neonate received an overdose of vancomycin as a result of medical error. Exchange transfusion did not change the measured serum vancomycin concentration. Multiple doses of activated charcoal 1 g/kg were administered through a nasogastric tube every 4 hours (nine doses in all) beginning 5 hours after exchange transfusion. The calculated half-life prior to and after charcoal therapy was 35 hours and 12 hours, respectively. During therapy the serum vancomycin concentration fell from 230 mg/L to 42 mg/L.[63]

Conclusion. The elimination of vancomycin was not increased by multiple-dose activated charcoal in a volunteer study. The apparent greater benefit of this treatment in two case reports is suggestive of benefit but further studies are required to confirm efficacy.

Dosage Regimen

If multiple-dose activated charcoal is considered appropriate, it is essential that the staff undertaking the procedure are experienced in its use both to reassure the conscious patient and to reduce the risk of complications in the obtunded patient.

A patient should be told that large and repeated doses of activated charcoal need to be given and that its administration may lead to a faster recovery. If appropriate, the patient should be informed that the treatment is to be given via a nasogastric tube. Such an approach is mandatory if the patient is unconscious but may also be necessary if the individual is nauseated or vomiting.

If the patient has ingested a drug in overdose which induces nausea and vomiting, the administration of activated charcoal, particularly if it contains sorbitol, may produce emesis. In these circumstances it is appropriate to administer an antiemetic intravenously to ensure compliance. Alternatively, smaller more frequent doses of charcoal may be used but are not always retained.

The dose of administered charcoal is probably of greater importance than the surface area of the charcoal.[101] In a study involving six volunteers, activated charcoal 20 g, given every 2 hours, produced a significantly greater reduction in the half-life of theophylline than 5 g every 2 hours.[24] In addition, administering the same total dose of activated charcoal (120 g over 12 hours) in hourly doses rather than less frequently, resulted in a further reduction in half-life. Ilkhanipour et al[22] have also confirmed that activated charcoal 12.5 g every hour (total dose 150 g over 12 hours) produced the greatest reduction in theophylline elimination half-life. Moreover, the more frequent administration of smaller doses of activated charcoal tends to prevent regurgitation which commonly occurs when large doses are given. There is some evidence that a continuous gastric infusion of charcoal, at least after a large initial dose (50-100 g), may offer advantages.[52]

Clinical experience suggests that, after an initial dose of 50-100 g given to an adult, charcoal may be administered hourly, every 2 hours, or every 4 hours at a dose equivalent to 1.25 g/hour. In children, lower doses (10-25 g) of charcoal may be employed because smaller overdoses have usually been ingested and the capacity of the gut lumen is smaller.

Coadministration of a Cathartic

The role of cathartics such as sorbitol, mannitol and sodium, and magnesium sulfate remains controversial. They are often given at the same time as activated charcoal in order to increase palatability. Sorbitol sweetens the mixture but palatability is not relevant if administration is via a nasogastric tube. Some studies (but not others) suggest that the coadministration of a cathartic may not only reduce drug absorption to charcoal but, paradoxically, increase absorption by increasing the volume of intestinal fluid.[102] Furthermore, mannitol and sorbitol delay gastric emptying in man,[103] thereby reducing the amount of charcoal available to adsorb the drug in the small bowel. More recent evidence, however, indicates that in man the coadministration of a cathartic to charcoal may further hasten the elimination of phenobarbital[14] and of a slow-release theophylline preparation,[83] although the combined use of sorbitol and charcoal was not without adverse effects. Two of the nine volunteers in the latter study developed liquid stools, severe abdominal cramps, nausea, sweating, and hypotension. However, Al-Shareef et al[104] did not demonstrate an additional benefit from the use of a sorbitol-charcoal formulation in the management of theophylline poisoning. Cathartics theoretically decrease the risk of constipation and hence small bowel obstruction if very large doses of activated charcoal are administered.

The need for a cathartic as part of a multiple-dose activated charcoal regimen remains unproven and many clinical toxicologists have not found it necessary to employ cathartics in clinical practice. While the use of sorbitol produces a more rapid onset of catharsis without the development of hypermagnesemia associated with the use of magnesium-containing cathartics, it too has well-recognized complications. It is probable that the increased morbidity from its use will outweigh any potential benefit (see Position Statement on Cathartics[105]) and therefore the concurrent administration of a cathartic is not recommended. In particular, cathartics should not be administered to young children because of the propensity of laxatives to cause fluid and electrolyte imbalance.

Complications of Use

The administration of multiple-dose activated charcoal rarely produces clinically important side effects. Black stools and mild transient constipation are well recognized, but constipation is not usually severe enough to require treatment, even if a cathartic has not been coadministered.

Gastrointestinal Complications

An adult patient treated for carbamazepine poisoning with activated charcoal 240 g and magnesium citrate 600 mL developed an ileus which resolved with the administration of additional doses of magnesium citrate.[106] A further case of small bowel obstruction has been reported in a patient poisoned with amitriptyline who required a laparotomy 5 days after admission to remove a charcoal bezoar in the distal ileum; activated charcoal 30-60 g had been given every 4-6 hours for 5 days.[107]

Atkinson et al[108] have described a 24-year-old patient intoxicated with barbiturates and benzodiazepines, who required a limited right hemicolectomy after he developed small bowel obstruction due to a large bolus of inspissated charcoal in the cecum. A total of 125 g of activated charcoal was administered over 18 hours.

A rectal ulcer with massive hemorrhage followed the administration of activated charcoal 50 g, with magnesium sulfate 50 g in a 1000 mL slurry every 4-6 hours for 50 hours, to a patient with organophosphorous insecticide poisoning.[109] Bloody stools did not occur until 10 days after she had ingested fenitrothion and passed hard charcoal masses.

Goulbourne and Cisek[110] have reported the development of gastrointestinal obstruction 5 days after a patient poisoned with theophylline was given activated charcoal 350 g. The patient underwent laparotomy with lysis of low-grade adhesions at the ileocecal region, for which an ileotransverse colostomy was performed. On opening the bowel, several charcoal clumps were removed measuring $4.5 \times 5 \times 3$ cm.

An obstructing charcoal mass (120 g) was found at the site of an intestinal perforation in a 39-year-old female who was receiving maintenance methadone and who had ingested a modest overdose of amitriptyline.[111] Apart from lethargy, she was asymptomatic but was prescribed activated charcoal 50 g every 4 hours; she declined more than 100 g. Four days later after two enemas, perforation occurred.

Respiratory Complications

In some reports is is unclear whether the respiratory complications described were due to the well-recognized consequences of aspiration of gastric contents into the lung or the aspiration of activated charcoal specifically. In one instance the presence of povidone in the charcoal formulation was thought to be the major factor.[112]

Severe airway obstruction has been reported in one infant given charcoal after vomiting was induced by syrup of ipecac.[113] Accidental administration of activated charcoal into the lung produced an adult respiratory distress syndrome, but the patient recovered and was discharged home 14 days later.[114] Even if recovery results, cerebral anoxic damage may have occurred.[115] Bronchiolitis obliterans has followed aspiration of activated charcoal with fatal consequences.[116]

Six cases of fatal pulmonary aspiration of charcoal have been reported,[112,117-119] but in one case[112] this was probably due to the povidone in the formulation rather than to activated charcoal itself.

Fluid, Electrolyte, and Acid-Base Abnormalities

The coadministration of cathartics may produce hypernatremia,[120-122] hypokalemia, hypermagnesemia,[123-124] and metabolic acidosis, particularly in infants.

References

1. Chyka PA, Holley JE, Mandrell TD, et al, "Correlation of Drug Pharmacokinetics and Effectiveness of Multiple-Dose Activated Charcoal Therapy," *Ann Emerg Med*, 1995, 25:356-62.
2. Arimori K and Nakano M, "Accelerated Clearance of Intravenously Administered Theophylline and Phenobarbital by Oral Doses of Activated Charcoal in Rats," *J Pharmacobiodyn*, 1986, 9:437-41.
3. Arimori K and Nakano M, "The Intestinal Dialysis of Intravenously Administered Phenytoin by Oral Activated Charcoal in Rats," *J Pharmacobiodyn*, 1987, 10:157-65.
4. Johnson D, Eppler J, Giesbrecht E, et al, "Effect of Multiple-Dose Activated Charcoal on the Clearance of High-Dose Intravenous Aspirin in a Porcine Model," *Ann Emerg Med*, 1995, 26:569-74.
5. Neuvonen PJ and Elonen E, "Effect of Activated Charcoal on Absorption and Elimination of Phenobarbitone, Carbamazepine, and Phenyl butazone in Man," *Eur J Clin Pharmacol*, 1980, 17:51-7.
6. Neuvonen PJ, Elonen E, and Mattila MJ, "Oral Activated Charcoal and Dapsone Elimination," *Clin Pharmacol Ther*, 1980, 27:823-7.
7. Kärkkäinen S and Neuvonen PJ, "Effect of Oral Charcoal and Urine pH on Dextropropoxyphene Pharmacokinetics," *Int J Clin Pharmacol Ther*, 1985, 23:219-25.
8. Park GD, Goldberg MJ, Spector R, et al, "The Effects of Activated Charcoal on Digoxin and Digitoxin Clearance," *Drug Intell Clin Pharm*, 1985, 19:937-41.
9. Reissel P and Manninen V, "Effect of Administration of Activated Charcoal and Fibre on Absorption, Excretion and Steady State Blood Levels of Digoxin and Digitoxin: Evidence for Intestinal Secretion of the Glycosides," *Acta Med Scand*, 1982, 668(Suppl):88-90.
10. Lalonde RL, Deshpande R, Hamilton PP, et al, "Acceleration of Digoxin Clearance by Activated Charcoal," *Clin Pharmacol Ther*, 1985, 37:367-71.
11. Arimori K, Kawano H, and Nakano M, "Gastrointestinal Dialysis of Disopyramide in Healthy Subjects," *Int J Clin Pharmacol Ther Toxicol*, 1989, 27:280-4.
12. Du Souich P, Caillé G, and Larochelle P, "Enhancement of Nadolol Elimination by Activated Charcoal and Antibiotics," *Clin Pharmacother Ther*, 1983, 33:585-90.
13. Berg MJ, Berlinger WG, Goldberg MJ, et al, "Acceleration of the Body Clearance of Phenobarbital by Oral Activated Charcoal," *N Engl J Med*, 1982, 307:642-4.
14. Berg MJ, Rose JQ, Wurster DE, et al, "Effect of Charcoal and Sorbitol-Charcoal Suspension on the Elimination of Intravenous Phenobarbital," *Ther Drug Monit*, 1987, 9:41-7.
15. Frenia ML, Schauben JL, Wears RL, et al, "Multiple-Dose Activated Charcoal Compared to Urinary Alkalinization for the Enhancement of Phenobarbital Elimination," *J Toxicol Clin Toxicol*, 1996, 34:169-75.
16. Mauro LS, Mauro VF, Brown DL, et al, "Enhancement of Phenytoin Elimination by Multiple-Dose Activated Charcoal," *Ann Emerg Med*, 1987, 16:1132-5.
17. Rowden AM, Spoor JE, and Bertino JS, "The Effect of Activated Charcoal on Phenytoin Pharmacokinetics," *Ann Emerg Med*, 1990, 19:1144-7.
18. Laufen H and Leitold M, "The Effect of Activated Charcoal on the Bioavailability of Piroxicam in Man," *Int J Clin Pharmacol Ther*, 1986, 24:48-52.

19. Lockey D and Bateman DN, "Effect of Oral Activated Charcoal on Quinine Elimination," *Br J Clin Pharmacol*, 1989, 27:92-4.

20. Kärkkäinen S and Neuvonen PJ, "Effect of Oral Charcoal and Urine pH on Sotalol Pharmacokinetics," *Int J Clin Pharmacol Ther*, 1984, 22:441-6.

21. Berlinger WG, Spector R, Goldberg MJ, et al, "Enhancement of Theophylline Clearance by Oral Activated Charcoal," *Clin Pharmacol Ther*, 1983, 33:351-4.

22. Ilkhanipour K, Yealy DM, and Krenzelok EP, "The Comparative Efficacy of Various Multiple-Dose Activated Charcoal Regimens," *Am J Emerg Med*, 1992, 10:298-300.

23. Mahutte CK, True RJ, Michiels TM, et al, "Increased Serum Theophylline Clearance with Orally Administered Activated Charcoal," *Am Rev Respir Dis*, 1983, 128:820-2.

24. Park GD, Radomski L, Goldberg MJ, et al, "Effects of Size and Frequency of Oral Doses of Charcoal on Theophylline Clearance," *Clin Pharmacol Ther*, 1983, 34:663-6.

25. Park GD, Spector R, Goldberg MJ, et al, "Effect of the Surface Area of Activated Charcoal on Theophylline Clearance," *J Clin Pharmacol*, 1984, 24:289-92.

26. Radomski L, Park GD, Goldberg MJ, et al, "Model for Theophylline Overdose Treatment with Oral Activated Charcoal," *Clin Pharmacol Ther*, 1984, 35:402-8.

27. Barone JA, Raia JJ, and Huang YC, "Evaluation of the Effects of Multiple-Dose Activated Charcoal on the Absorption of Orally Administered Salicylate in a Simulated Toxic Ingestion Model," *Ann Emerg Med*, 1988, 17:34-7.

28. Kirshenbaum LA, Mathews SC, Sitar DS, et al, "Does Multiple-Dose Charcoal Therapy Enhance Salicylate Excretion?" *Arch Intern Med*, 1990, 150:1281-3.

29. Ho JL, Tierney MG, and Dickinson GE, "An Evaluation of the Effect of Repeated Doses of Oral Activated Charcoal on Salicylate Elimination," *J Clin Pharmacol*, 1989, 29:366-9.

30. Mayer AL, Sitar DS, Tenebein M, et al, "Multiple-Dose Charcoal and Whole-Bowel Irrigation Do Not Increase Clearance of Absorbed Salicylate," *Arch Intern Med*, 1992, 152:393-6.

31. Laine K, Kivistö KT, and Neuvonen PJ, "The Effect of Activated Charcoal on the Absorption and Elimination of Astemizole," *Hum Exp Toxicol*, 1994, 13:502-5.

32. Neuvonen PJ and Kärkkäinen S, "Effects of Charcoal, Sodium Bicarbonate, and Ammonium Chloride on Chlorpropamide Kinetics," *Clin Pharmacol Ther*, 1983, 33:386-93.

33. Al-Shareef A, Buss DC, Shetty HG, et al, "The Effect of Repeated-Dose Activated Charcoal on the Pharmacokinetics of Sodium Valproate in Healthy Volunteers," *Br J Clin Pharmacol*, 1997, 43:109-11.

34. Davis RL, Koup JR, Roon RA, et al, "Effect of Oral Activated Charcoal on Tobramycin Clearance," *Anitmicrob Agents Chemother*, 1998, 32:274-5.

35. Watson WA, Jenkins TC, Velasquez N, et al, "Repeated Oral Doses of Activated Charcoal and the Clearance of Tobramycin, a Non-Absorbable Drug," *J Toxicol Clin Toxicol*, 1987, 25:171-84.

36. Davis RL, Roon RA, and Koup JR, "Effect of Orally Administered Activated Charcoal on Vancomycin Clearance," *Antimicrob Agents Chemother*, 1987, 31:720-2.

37. Kärkkäinen S and Neuvonen PJ, "Pharmacokinetics of Amitriptyline Influenced by Oral Charcoal and Urine pH," *Int J Clin Pharmacol Ther*, 1986, 24:326-32.

38. Scheinin M, Virtanen R, and Iisalo E, "Effect of Single and Repeated Doses of Activated Charcoal on the Pharmacokinetics of Doxepin," *Int J Clin Pharmacol Ther*, 1985, 23:38-42.

39. Goldberg MJ, Park GD, Spector R, et al, "Lack of Effect of Oral Activated Charcoal on Imipramine Clearance," *Clin Pharmacol Ther*, 1985, 38:350-3.

40. Crome P, Dawling S., Braithwaite RA, et al, "Effect of Activated Charcoal on Absorption of Nortriptyline," *Lancet*, 1977, 2:1203-5.

41. Boldy DA, Heath A, Ruddock S, et al, "Activated Charcoal for Carbamazepine Poisoning," *Lancet*, 1987, 1:1027.

42. Montoya-Cabrera MA, Sauceda-Garcia JM, Escalante-Galindo P, et al, "Carbamazepine Poisoning in Adolescent Suicide Attempters: Effectiveness of Multiple-Dose Activated Charcoal in Enhancing Carbamazepine Elimination," *Arch Med Res*, 1996, 27:485-9.

43. Neuvonen PJ, Elonen E, and Haapanen EJ, "Acute Dapsone Intoxication: Clinical Findings and Effect of Oral Charcoal and Haemodialysis on Dapsone Elimination," *Acta Med Scand*, 1983, 214:215-20.

44. Goldberg MJ and Berlinger WG, "Treatment of Phenobarbital Overdose With Activated Charcoal," *JAMA*, 1982, 247:2400-1.

45. Pond SM, Olson KR, Osterloh JD, et al, "Randomized Study of the Treatment of Phenobarbital Overdose with Repeated Doses of Activated Charcoal," *JAMA*, 1984, 251:3104-8.

46. Boldy DA, Vale JA, and Prescott LF, "Treatment of Phenobarbitone Poisoning with Repeated Oral Administration of Activated Charcoal," *Q J Med*, 1986, 61:997-1002.

47. Veerman M, Espejo MG, Christopher MA, et al, "Use of Activated Charcoal to Reduce Elevated Serum Phenobarbital Concentration in a Neonate," *J Toxicol Clin Toxicol*, 1991, 29:53-8.

48. Prescott LF, Hamilton AR, and Heyworth R, "Treatment of Quinine Overdosage with Repeated Oral Charcoal," *Br J Clin Pharmacol*, 1989, 27:95-7.

49. Amitai Y, Yeung AC, Moye J, et al, "Repetitive Oral Activated Charcoal and Control of Emesis in Severe Theophylline Toxicity," *Ann Intern Med*, 1986, 105:386-7.

50. Davis R, Ellsworth A, Justus RE, et al, "Reversal of Theophylline Toxicity Using Oral Activated Charcoal," *J Fam Pract*, 1985, 20:73-4.

51. Gal P, Miller A, and McCue JD, "Oral Activated Charcoal to Enhance Theophylline Elimination in an Acute Overdose," *JAMA*, 1984, 251:3130-1.

52. Ohning BL, Reed MD, and Blumer JL, "Continuous Nasogastric Administration of Activated Charcoal for the Treatment of Theophylline Intoxication," *Pediatr Pharmacol*, 1986, 5:241-5.

53. Sessler CN, Glauser FL, and Cooper KR, "Treatment of Theophylline Toxicity with Oral Activated Charcoal," *Chest*, 1985, 87:325-9.

54. Shannon M, Amitai Y, and Lovejoy FH Jr, "Multiple Dose Activated Charcoal for Theophylline Poisoning in Young Infants," *Pediatrics*, 1987, 80:368-70.

55. True RJ, Berman JM, and Mahutte CK, "Treatment of Theophylline Toxicity with Oral Activated Charcoal," *Crit Care Med*, 1984, 12:113-4.

56. Hillman RJ and Prescott LF, "Treatment of Salicylate Poisoning with Repeated Oral Charcoal," *Br Med J*, 1985, 291:1472.

57. Vale JA, "Methods to Increase Poison Elimination," *New Clinical Applications: Nephrology, Drugs and the Kidney*, Catto GR, ed, Lancaster, PA: Kluwer Academic Publishers, 1990, 65-111.

58. Boldy DA, Smart V, and Vale JA, "Multiple Doses of Charcoal in Digoxin Poisoning," *Lancet*, 1985, 2:1076-7.

59. Lake KD, Brown DC, and Peterson CD, "Digoxin Toxicity: Enhanced Systemic Elimination During Oral Activated Charcoal Therapy," *Pharmacotherapy*, 1984 4:161-3.

60. Critchley JA and Critchly LA, "Digoxin Toxicity in Chronic Renal Failure: Treatment by Multiple Dose Activated Charcoal Intestinal Dialysis," *Hum Exp Toxicol*, 1997, 16:733-5.

61. Ibanez C, Carcas AJ, Frias J, et al, "Activated Charcoal Increases Digoxin Elimination in Patients," *Int J Cardiol*, 1995, 48:27-30.

62. Pond S, Jacobs M, Marks J, et al, "Treatment of Digitoxin Overdose with Oral Activated Charcoal," *Lancet*, 1981, 2:1177-8.

63. Burkhart KK, Metcalf S., Shurnas E, et al, "Exchange Transfusion and Multidose Activated Charcoal Following Vancomycin Overdose," *J Toxicol Clin Toxicol*, 1992, 30:285-94.

64. Kucukguclu S, Tuncok Y, Ozkan H, et al, "Multiple-Dose Activated Charcoal in an Accidental Vancomycin Overdose," *J Toxicol Clin Toxicol*, 1996, 34:83-6.

65. Hassan E, "Treatment of Meprobamate Overdose with Repeated Oral Doses of Activated Charcoal," *Ann Emerg Med*, 1986, 15:73-6.

66. Linden CH and Rumack BH, "Enhanced Elimination of Meprobamate by Multiple Doses of Activated Charcoal," *Vet Hum Toxicol*, 1984, 26(Suppl 2):47.

67. Gadgil SD, Damle SR, Advani SH, et al, "Effect of Activated Charcoal on the Pharmacokinetics of High-Dose Methotrexate," *Cancer Treat Rep*, 1982, 66:1169-71.

68. Griffiths ML, Kaplan H, and Monteagudo FS, "Phenytoin Overdose," *S Afr Med J*, 1987, 71:471.

69. Howard CE, Roberts RS, Ely DS, et al, "Use of Multiple-Dose Activated Charcoal in Phenytoin Toxicity," *Ann Pharmacother*, 1994, 28:201-3.

70. Ros SP and Black LE, "Multiple-Dose Activated Charcoal in Management of Phenytoin Overdose," *Pediatr Emerg Care*, 1989, 5:169-70.

71. Weichbrodt GD and Elliott DP, "Treatment of Phenytoin Toxicity with Repeated Doses of Activated Charcoal," *Ann Emerg Med*, 1987, 16:1387-9.

72. Weidle PJ, Skiest DJ, and Forrest A, "Multiple-Dose Activated Charcoal as Adjunct Therapy After Chronic Phenytoin Intoxication," *Clin Pharm*, 1991, 10:711-4.

73. Swartz CM and Sherman A, "The Treatment of Tricyclic Antidepressant Overdose with Repeated Charcoal," *J Clin Psychopharmacol*, 1984, 4:336-40.

74. Ilett KF, Hackett LP, Dusci JL, et al, "Disposition of Dothiepin After Overdose: Effects of Repeated-Dose Activated Charcoal," *Ther Drug Monit*, 1991, 13:485-9.

75. Farrar HC, Herold DA, and Reed MD, "Acute Valproic Acid Intoxication: Enhanced Drug Clearance with Oral-Activated Charcoal," *Crit Care Med*, 1993, 21:299-301.

76. Campbell JW and Chyka PA, "Physicochemical Characteristics of Drugs and Response to Repeat-Dose Activated Charcoal," *Am J Emerg Med*, 1992, 10:208-10.

77. McKinnon RS, Desmond PV, Harman PJ, et al, "Studies on the Mechanisms of Action of Activated Charcoal on Theophylline Pharmacokinetics," *J Pharm Pharmacol*, 1987, 39:522-5.

78. Levy G, "Gastrointestinal Clearance of Drugs With Activated Charcoal," *N Engl J Med*, 1982, 307:676-8.

79. Wakabayashi Y, Maruyama S, Hachimura K, et al, "Activated Charcoal Interrupts Enteroenteric Circulation of Phenobarbital," *J Toxicol Clin Toxicol*, 1994, 32:419-24.

80. Kulig KW, Bar-Or D, and Rumack BH, "Intravenous Theophylline Poisoning and Multiple-Dose Charcoal in an Animal Model," *Ann Emerg Med*, 1987, 16:842-6.

81. Lim DT, Singh P, Nourtsis S, et al, "Absorption Inhibition and Enhancement of Elimination of Sustained-Release Theophylline Tablets by Oral Activated Charcoal," *Ann Emerg Med*, 1986, 15:1303-7.

82. Minton NA and Henry JA, "Prevention of Drug Absorption in Simulated Theophylline Overdose," *J Toxicol Clin Toxicol*, 1995, 33:43-9.

83. Goldberg MJ, Spector R, Park GD, et al, "The Effect of Sorbitol and Activated Charcoal on Serum Theophylline Concentrations After Slow-Release Theophylline," *Clin Pharmacol Ther*, 1987, 41:108-11.

84. Hundt HK, Aucamp AK, and Müller FO, "Pharmacokinetic Aspects of Carbamazepine and Its Two Major Metabolites in Plasma During Overdosage," *Hum Toxicol*, 1983, 2:607-14.

85. Vree TB, Janssen TJ, Hekster YA, et al, "Clinical Pharmacokinetics of Carbamazepine and Its Epoxy and Hydroxy Metabolites in Humans After an Overdose," *Ther Drug Monit*, 1986, 8:297-304.

86. Wason S, Baker RC, Carolan P, et al, "Carbamazepine Overdose - The Effects of Multiple Dose Activated Charcoal," *J Toxicol Clin Toxicol*, 1992, 30:39-48.

87. Vale JA and Heath A, "Carbamazepine Overdose," *J Toxicol Clin Toxicol*, 1992, 30:481-2.

88. *Goodman and Gilman's The Pharmacological Basis of Therapeutics*, 9th ed, Hardman JG, Limbird LE, Molinoff PB, et al, eds, New York, NY: McGraw-Hill, 1996, 1721.

89. Nilsson C, Sterner G, and Idvall J, "Charcoal Hemoperfusion for Treatment of Serious Carbamazepine Poisoning," *Acta Med Scand*, 1984, 216:137-40.

90. De Groot G, van Heijst AN, and Maes RA, "Charcoal Hemoperfusion in the Treatment of Two Cases of Acute Carbamazepine Poisoning," *J Toxicol Clin Toxicol*, 1984, 22:349-62.

91. Leslie PJ, Heyworth R, and Prescott LF, "Cardiac Complications of Carbamazepine Intoxication: Treatment by Haemoperfusion," *Br Med J*, 1983, 286:1018.

92. Lobo PI, Spyker D, Surratt P, et al, "Use of Hemodialysis in Meprobamate Overdosage," *Clin Nephrol*, 1977, 7:73-5.

93. Goldberg MJ, Berlinger WG, and Park GD, "Activated Charcoal in Phenobarbital Overdose," *JAMA*, 1985, 253:1120-1.

94. Pond SM, Osterloh JD, Olson KR, et al, "Activated Charcoal in Phenobarbital Overdose," *JAMA*, 1985, 253:1121.

95. *Goodman and Gilman's The Pharmacological Basis of Therapeutics*, 9th ed, Hardman JG, Limbird LE, Molinoff PB, et al, eds, New York, NY: McGraw-Hill, 1996, 1770.

96. Jacobsen D, Wiik-Larsen E, Dahl T, et al, "Pharmacokinetic Evaluation of Haemoperfusion in Phenobarbital Poisoning," *Eur J Clin Pharmacol*, 1984, 26:109-12.

97. Verpooten GA, Heyndrickx, Zachee P, et al, "Comparison of Hemoperfusion and Hemodialysis Clearances During Combined and Prolonged Treatment of Severely Poisoned Patients," *Mechanisms of Toxicity and Hazard Evaluation*, Holmstedt B, Lauwerys R, Mercier M, et al, eds, Amsterdam, Netherlands: Elsevier/North-Holland Biomedical Press, 1980, 411-4.

98. Vale JA, "The Medical Management of Acute Poisoning: An Evaluation of Charcoal Haemoperfusion," MD Thesis, University of London, 1980.

99. Bateman DN, Blain PG, Woodhouse KW, et al, "Pharmacokinetics and Clinical Toxicity of Quinine Overdosage: Lack of Efficacy of Techniques Intended to Enhance Elimination," *Q J Med*, 1985, 54: 125-31.

100. Dupuis RE, Lichtman SN, and Pollack GM, "Acute Valproic Acid Overdose. Clinical Course and Pharmacokinetics Disposition of Valproic Acid and Metabolites," *Drug Saf*, 1990, 5:65-71.

101. Ilkhanipour K, Yealy DM, and Krenzelok EP, "Activated Charcoal Surface Area and Its Role in Multiple-Dose Charcoal Therapy," *Am J Emerg Med*, 1993, 11:583-5.

102. Van de Graaff WB, Leigh Thompson W, Sunshine I, et al, "Adsorbent and Cathartic Inhibition of Enteral Drug Absorption," *J Pharmacol Exp Ther*, 1982, 221:656-63.

103. Hunt JN and Stubbs DF, "The Volume and Energy Content of Meals as Determinants of Gastric Emptying," *J Physiol*, 1975, 245:209-25.

104. Al-Shareef AH, Buss DC, and Allen EM, "The Effects of Charcoal and Sorbitol (Alone and in Combination) on Plasma Theophylline Concentrations After a Sustained-Release Formulation," *Hum Exp Toxicol*, 1990, 9:179-82.

105. "AACT/EAPCCT Position Statement: Cathartics," *J Toxicol Clin Toxicol*, 1997, 35:743-52.

106. Watson WA, Cremer KF, and Chapman JA, "Gastrointestinal Obstruction Associated With Multiple-Dose Activated Charcoal," *J Emerg Med*, 1986, 4:401-7.

107. Ray MJ, Padin DR, Condie JD, et al, "Charcoal Bezoar. Small-Bowel Obstruction Secondary to Amitriptyline Overdose Therapy," *Dig Dis Sci*, 1988, 33:106-7.

108. Atkinson SW, Young Y, and Trotter GA, "Treatment with Activated Charcoal Complicated by Gastrointestinal Obstruction Requiring Surgery," *Br Med J*, 1992, 305:563.

109. Mizutani T, Naito H, and Oohashi N, "Rectal Ulcer With Massive Hemorrhage Due to Activated Charcoal Treatment in Oral Organophosphate Poisoning," *Hum Exp Toxicol*, 1991, 10:385-6.

110. Goulbourne KB and Cisek JE, "Small-Bowel Obstruction Secondary to Activated Charcoal and Adhesions," *Ann Emerg Med*, 1994, 24:108-10.

111. Gomez HF, Brent JA, Munoz DC, et al, "Charcoal Stercolith with Intestinal Perforation in a Patient Treated for Amitriptyline Ingestion," *J Emerg Med*, 1994, 12:57-60.

112. Menzies DG, Busuttil A, and Prescott LF, "Fatal Pulmonary Aspiration of Oral Activated Charcoal," *Br Med J*, 1988, 297:459-60.

113. Pollack MM, Dunbar BS, Holbrook PR, et al, "Aspiration of Activated Charcoal and Gastric Contents," *Ann Emerg Med*, 1981, 10:528-9.

114. Harris CR and Filandrinos D, "Accidental Administration of Activated Charcoal Into the Lung: Aspiration by Proxy," *Ann Emerg Med*, 1993, 22:1470-3.

115. Givens T, Holloway M, and Wason S, "Pulmonary Aspiration of Activated Charcoal After Tricyclic Antidepressant Overdose," *Vet Hum Toxicol*, 1990, 32:375.

116. Elliott CG, Colby TV, Kelly TM, et al, "Charcoal Lung. Bronchiolitis Obliterans After Aspiration of Activated Charcoal," *Chest*, 1989, 96:672-4.

117. Benson B, VanAntwerp M, and Hergott T, "A Fatality Resulting from Multiple Dose Activated Charcoal Therapy," *Vet Hum Toxicol*, 1989, 31:335.

118. Harsch HH, "Aspiration of Activated Charcoal," *N Engl J Med*, 1986, 314:318.

119. Rau NR, Nagaraj MV, Prakash PS, et al, "Fatal Pulmonary Aspiration of Oral Activated Charcoal," *Br Med J*, 1988, 297:918-9.

120. Allerton JP and Strom JA, "Hypernatremia Due to Repeated Doses of Charcoal-Sorbitol," *Am J Kidney Dis*, 1991, 17:581-4.

121. Farley TA, "Severe Hypernatremic Dehydration After Use of an Activated Charcoal-Sorbitol Suspension," *J Pediatr*, 1986, 109:719-22.

122. Gazda-Smith E and Synhavsky A, "Hypernatremia Following Treatment of Theophylline Toxicity with Activated Charcoal and Sorbitol," *Arch Intern Med*, 1990, 150:689-92.

123. Garrelts JS, Watson WA, Holloway KD, et al, "Magnesium Toxicity Secondary to Catharsis During Management of Theophylline Poisoning," *Am J Emerg Med*, 1989, 7:34-7.

124. Weber CA and Santiago RM, "Hypermagnesemia: A Potential Complication During Treatment of Theophylline Intoxication with Oral Activated Charcoal and Magnesium-Containing Cathartics," *Chest*, 1989, 95:56-9.

SUBSTANCE-RELATED DISORDERS

Adapted from Fuller MA and Sajatovic M, *Drug Information for Mental Health*, Hudson, OH: Lexi-Comp, Inc, 2001.

Substance-related disorders are conditions in which an individual uses/abuses a substance, leading to maladaptive behaviors and symptoms. In DSM-IV, substance-related disorders are further grouped into substance dependence and substance abuse. Substance abuse refers to a maladaptive pattern of substance use leading to clinically significant impairment or distress, manifested by at least one symptom that interferes with life functioning within a 12-month period. Diagnostic criteria for substance dependence requires at least three of the following within a 12-month period: development of tolerance to the substance, withdrawal symptoms, persistent desire/unsuccessful attempts to stop the substance, ingestion of larger amounts of substance than was intended, diminished life functioning, and persistent substance use in the phase of physical or psychological problems. Substance abuse and substance dependence are enormous societal problems. In the United States, the lifetime prevalence of substance abuse or dependence in adults is over 15%. Substance abuse prevalence is greatest among individuals 18-25 years of age. Substance abuse is also more common in men compared to women, and in urban residents compared to rural residents.

Over 50% of individuals with substance-related disorders have comorbid psychiatric disorders. Individuals with mental illness are about twice as likely to smoke as compared to the general population and to consume about 44% of cigarettes smoked nationally. The term "dual diagnosis" usually refers to individuals with concomitant substance abuse and psychiatric diagnosis. Comorbid psychiatric diagnoses, common in individuals who abuse substances, include major depression, personality disorder, particularly antisocial personality, anxiety disorders, and dysthymia. Genetic studies involving twins, adoptees, and siblings raised separately have suggested good evidence for familial patterns in alcohol abuse. Genetic patterns with other substances of abuse have not been well demonstrated.

General Treatment Recommendations

Individuals with substance abuse are often both physically and psychologically impaired. Management and treatment of substance abuse can be divided in the main areas of:

- treatment of acute intoxication/overdose
- treatment of withdrawal
- general treatments for psychological addiction/rehabilitation

Additionally, individuals who abuse substances frequently have comorbid psychiatric disorders which affect final outcome. Proper diagnosis and treatment of comorbid psychiatric disorders improve outcome in nearly all cases.

Psychosocial treatments include inpatient care (now increasingly rare in today's managed care settings), outpatient therapies which may be in individual or group settings, and self-help residential treatment programs (therapeutic communities).

Numerous studies have demonstrated that psychotherapy added to pharmacologic management promotes abstinence better than pharmacologic management alone.

Alcohol

Intoxication/Overdose (see Ethyl Alcohol)

Alcohol intoxication may be severe with extreme usage, potentially leading to respiratory depression, coma, and death. These individuals require close monitoring in an intensive care setting. An idiosyncratic reaction of severe behavioral symptoms occurring after relatively low level alcohol ingestion has been reported. Symptomatic support with environmental protection, and possibly the addition of low-dose antipsychotic medication, may be beneficial in these individuals (eg, haloperidol 1-2 mg orally or I.M.).

Withdrawal

Symptoms can begin within 6-48 hours postcessation and persist up to 5 days. About 5% of these patients will develop full-blown delirium tremens. The mortality rate for delirium tremens is 1% to 5%. Benzodiazepines are the most effective treatment for alcohol withdrawal. For tremor and mild agitation, an oral benzodiazepine such as lorazepam 1-2 mg every 4-6 hours is generally effective. Individuals with more severe agitation or hallucinations may require I.M. or I.V. medication. Chlordiazepoxide (25-100 mg orally) can be administered as an alternative to lorazepam. Phenobarbital (5 mg/kg I.V. or 15 mg of phenobarbital for each 30 mL "1 ounce" of 80-100 proof) may be used for resistant cases. Phenytoin is not useful in treating ethanol withdrawal seizures. Trazodone (50-150 mg orally at night) can be used as a sleep aid. Beta-adrenergic blockers should be utilized to treat hyperadrenergic symptoms, especially in the elderly. Individuals with delirium tremens (or DTs) should be in closely observed medical settings (hospitalized) and must receive maintenance benzodiazepine treatment (eg, diazepam 0.15 mg/kg at 2.5 mg/minute) until behavior and autonomic symptoms (tachycardia, hypertension) stabilize. Dosage should then be titrated as clinically indicated. In very resistant cases, a propofol infusion (40 mg I.V. followed by an infusion of 50 mcg/kg/minute) can be considered with ventilatory support. Sodium pentobarbital (with appropriate airway management) is also a reasonable alternative. The initial dose is 3-5 mg/kg I.V., followed by a 100 mg/hour infusion for sedation. Oral baclofen (30 mg/day in divided doses for 10 days) has also been utilized to treat withdrawal. Most cases of DTs may be avoided if treated with oral or I.M. benzodiazepines when the patient is in the early alcohol withdrawal phase. Vital signs should be closely monitored as an index of severity of withdrawal. Intravenous fluid hydration with D_5 0.9% NS at 300-1000 mL/hour should be instituted if dehydration is present. Other adjunctive agents to consider include clonidine, valproic acid (500 mg orally 3 times/day for 7 days), baclofen (10 mg every 8 hours), and carbamazepine. A supportive, nonthreatening and therapeutic environment is helpful as patients with alcohol withdrawal are often frightened and severely anxious. Treatment with benzodiazepines may be decreased in both dosage and frequency over the next several days as withdrawal symptoms resolve. The Clinical Institute Withdrawal Assessment for Alcohol Scale (CIWA) should be utilized to monitor withdrawal.

Acute alcoholic encephalopathy (Wernicke's syndrome) should be managed with thiamine 50 mg/day I.M. or 100 mg/day orally for 1-2 weeks. Serum glucose, phosphate, and magnesium should be monitored. The chronic amnestic syndrome associated with long-term alcohol abuse (Korsakoff's syndrome) may improve with thiamine 100 mg/day continued for 6-12 months, although most patients have limited cognitive recovery. Antipsychotics are generally best avoided in alcohol withdrawal as they may lower seizure threshold. However, in cases of failure of benzodiazepines to control paranoid behavioral symptoms or hallucinations, judicious use of antipsychotic medication may be helpful.

General Treatment

Most clinicians agree that complete abstinence from alcohol is the cornerstone of successful alcohol abuse treatment. Psychotherapy which focuses on drinking behavior and alternative behaviors is generally the most effective intervention. This includes individual, group, marital, and family therapies. Self-help groups such as Alcoholics Anonymous (AA) may be extremely helpful.

Specific biologic interventions that may be adjunctive in promoting alcohol abstinence are disulfiram, naltrexone, and some psychotropic drugs. Disulfiram competitively inhibits the enzyme aldehyde dehydro-genase, so that subsequent alcohol ingestion leads to serum acetaldehyde accumulation and resultant symptoms of flushing, feeling overheated, nausea, and general malaise. Dizziness, palpitations, and hypotension may occur. Symptoms generally persist for 30-60 minutes and may be useful in motivated, healthy patients in assisting with abstinence. Disulfiram must be taken daily, generally in the morning, and is usually prescribed at a dosage of 125-250 mg/day. Although some individuals benefit from the addition of disulfiram to an alcohol treatment regimen, its use must be weighed against the medical risks (severe hypotension, hypocalcemia, respiratory depression) if the individual continues to drink while on disulfiram.

Naltrexone, a narcotic antagonist, may also be a useful adjunct as part of an alcohol treatment regimen. Naltrexone at doses of 50 mg/day may reduce drinking in recovering alcoholics. Adverse effects may include hypertension, GI disturbance, and sedation. Rarely, liver functioning may become impaired, and hepatic screening and monitoring should be done concurrently.

Additional psychotropic medications that have been reported to be useful in alcohol treatment include antidepressants such as serotonin reuptake inhibitors and dopamine agonists. Additionally, treatment of existing comorbid psychiatric disorders such as major depression, bipolar disorder, or post-traumatic stress disorder (PTSD) will usually substantially improve outcome.

Cocaine

Intoxication/Overdose (see Cocaine)

The symptoms of cocaine intoxication are similar to alcohol. In cases of high-dose use or when intravenous route has been used, symptoms may be severe, including extreme anxiety, paranoia, and hallucinations. Severe hypertension, hyperthermia, and arrhythmias may occur. Management of autonomic hyperarousal may benefit from benzodiazepines. Phentolamine may be beneficial in hypertensive crisis. Other supportive measures include close monitoring of vital signs, maintenance of fluid status, and ambient cooling for hyperthermia.

Withdrawal

Cocaine withdrawal is characterized by three phases: 1) an initial "cocaine crash" phase (fatigue, insomnia, depression) lasting for 1-2 days; 2) withdrawal phase (dysphoria, anxiety); followed by 3) an extinction phase. An intense craving for cocaine can occur at any time. Cocaine withdrawal symptoms generally are managed supportively with no specific identified pharmacologic treatments. Intense cocaine cravings may lead individuals to self-medicate with cocaine or other illicit substances.

General Treatment

As with alcohol and other drugs of abuse, abstinence from cocaine is essential in maintaining successful treatment. Psychotherapy has been proven to be helpful while some pharmacotherapies (desipramine, amantadine) have suggested efficacy in some individuals with reduced cocaine craving, dysphoria, and drug use. Comorbid psychiatric illness should be treated as needed to optimize outcome.

Opioids

Intoxication/Overdose

Most individuals with self-induced opioid intoxication (as with other types of illicit substance intoxication) do not present for treatment unless distressing physical or behavioral symptoms occur. Overdosage situations, however, are relatively common among chronic opioid drug abusers. Anoxia, coma, and death may occur unless intervention treatment is initiated. Initial measures include airway protection, vital sign monitoring, and administration of naloxone, an opiate antagonist. Naloxone may be given at an adult dose of 0.4-2 mg I.V. and should reverse overdose symptoms within 2 minutes. Dosage may be repeated twice more at 5-minute intervals, if necessary. Alternatively, nalmefene at doses of 0.5-1 mg in up to ten boluses can reverse opioid toxicity rapidly. Treating clinicians should also be alert to the possibility of concomitant substance overdose (eg, barbiturates) or medical conditions that may contribute to respiratory depression (eg, traumatic head injury). Patients with good response to naloxone may require repeated dosing over the next several hours as duration of action of naloxone generally does not exceed 4 hours. Care should be taken when using naloxone to guard against precipitating a withdrawal reaction in opioid-dependent patients.

Withdrawal

Withdrawal symptoms occur within 6-12 hours after ingestion of last drug dose in opioid-dependent persons. Treatment of opioid dependence involves management of primarily acute physical symptoms in the acute phase. For acute phase withdrawal (detoxification), the synthetic opioid methadone has been used successfully by many clinicians who treat substance abuse disorders. In patients who begin to exhibit signs and symptoms of opioid withdrawal (hypertension, tachycardia, sweating, lacrimation, rhinorrhea), methadone 1 mg orally is given as needed over the next 24 hours for a maximum of 10-40 mg over the first day of detoxification treatment. Once maintenance dosage requirements are determined (total methadone dose required to contain symptoms over the first 24 hours of detoxification), this dose can be given for an additional 2 days, then a slow daily taper initiated until the individual is to be maintained off opioid drugs. Other minor tranquilizers such as chlordiazepoxide (25-50 mg orally twice daily) or clorazepate (3.75-7.5 mg orally twice daily) can be used to treat opiate withdrawal during the first 72 hours. Ultra-rapid opioid detoxification has been used since the 1980s with varying success. Using principles of general anesthesia in combination with an opiate antagonist, followed by naltrexone maintenance therapy, 1-month abstinence rates vary from 53% to 93%.

Some clinicians use the nonopioid antihypertensive clonidine to treat symptoms of acute opioid withdrawal. Clonidine may be used alone or concurrently with methadone. For acute detoxification, clonidine 0.4-2 mg/day may be used. Due to its antihypertensive properties, pulse and blood pressure must be closely monitored. Some patients experience excessive sedation with clonidine, which may be moderated by dosage adjustments. Gastrointestinal cramps can be treated with dicyclomine (20 mg orally every 4-6 hours as needed), while nausea can be safely treated with prochlorperazine (10 mg orally or I.M. every 6 hours as needed). Loose stools may respond to loperamide (2 mg orally as needed, to a maximum daily dose of 6 mg). Trazodone (50-150 mg orally at night) can be given as a sleep aid.

An alternative compound, buprenorphine, a partial opioid antagonist, may be useful in acute detoxification situations (dose is about 3 mg/day sublingual up to 8 mg/day with a gradual taper 10-36 days). Like methadone, dosage should be customized to the individual and tapered and eventually discontinued as tolerated.

General Treatment

Treatment of chronic opioid dependence involves both treatment of physical withdrawal symptoms and psychological dependence on the drug. Psychosocial and psychotherapeutic treatments are essential in promoting the lifestyle changes needed to prevent relapse.

Methadone maintenance has proven efficacy in some groups of opioid abusers. As with acute phase treatment, chronic methadone treatment dosage/format must be tailored to the individual. Usual daily oral dosage ranges from 40-120 mg/day. Generally, patients must come to the clinic daily (usually morning) to receive methadone. Other interventions involved in clinic treatment may include counseling, urine drug testing, vocational rehabilitation, etc. When used successfully, methadone maintenance reduces illegal drug use, and reduces the medical, legal, and societal ramifications associated with the illicit drug culture.

L-α-acetyl methadol (LAMM) is a long-acting opioid that has been successfully used to treat chronic opioid dependence. LAMM can be dosed at 30-80 mg 3 times/week and may eliminate the need for daily clinic visits, as is required for most methadone programs.

An alternative strategy in managing long-term opioid abuse treatment is the use of opioid antagonists. Naltrexone, a long-acting (72 hours) antagonist, blocks the euphoric effects of opioids, and may be taken 3 times/week at dosages of 100-150 mg. Theoretically, the use of naltrexone discourages persons from opioid use as it eliminates the subsequent CNS effects. Naltrexone works best with highly motivated individuals with good psychosocial support as there are no physical incentives (withdrawal symptoms) to continue taking opioid antagonist on a long-term basis.

Sedative/Hypnotic

Intoxication/Overdose

Severity of symptoms of sedative-hypnotic intoxication depends on drugs used, route administered, and tolerance of the individual to the drug. Sequelae of overdose are greatly worsened when alcohol or multiple sedative/hypnotics are combined. Respiratory depression is the major danger and successful management includes respiratory and cardiac support. Margin of safety in benzodiazepine overdose is much greater compared to barbiturate overdose where unintentional lethal dosing is not uncommon. In addition to standard supportive measures (vital sign monitoring, gastric lavage, hospitalization, etc), patients with overdose should be closely assessed for suicide risk and intent.

Withdrawal

As with toxicity, severity of withdrawal symptoms is dependent on a variety of clinical factors, including duration of drug use (usually maintenance of 1 month or longer for dependence to develop) and tolerance of the individual. Withdrawal of sedative-hypnotic is generally managed by either 1) gradual reduction of sedative substance or 2) substitution with a long-acting benzodiazepine or phenobarbital with subsequent taper and eventual discontinuation.

Gradual discontinuation from sedative-hypnotic is best accomplished with motivated patients in settings with good psychosocial supports. The rate of drug taper should be tailored to the individual, with slower titrations generally being most successful.

For benzodiazepine-dependent patients, substitution of an equivalent dose of long-acting benzodiazepine (eg, clonazepam) with gradual downward titration will promote reduction of withdrawal effects over time. As with other addiction treatments, concurrent psychosocial treatments will optimize clinical outcome.

For barbiturate-dependent individuals, the clinician should attempt to determine the patient's daily dose of barbiturates and stabilize withdrawal symptoms with the barbiturate. As many individuals who abuse sedative-hypnotics may be unreliable in providing accurate daily use information, the clinician may elect to assess barbiturate tolerance with a challenge dose of the short-acting barbiturate pentobarbital. This should be done in hospital settings. The patient undergoing sedative withdrawal is given 200 mg of pentobarbital and observed for resolution of withdrawal symptoms and mild intoxication. Patients in whom this occurs may then be maintained on pentobarbital 100-200 mg every 6 hours. Patients who are not intoxicated on the initial challenge dose of 200 mg are given an additional 100 mg pentobarbital every 2 hours (for a maximum of 500 mg) until mild toxicity develops. Maintenance pentobarbital dose is then determined based on total amount of barbiturate needed to cause mild intoxication. Once stabilization is achieved, the clinician can then taper the dose by 10% daily. Alternatively, phenobarbital, a long-acting barbiturate, may be substituted for pentobarbital. Phenobarbital has the advantages of less frequent dosing, fewer fluctuations in blood level, and anticonvulsant activity. The equivalent dosing of 30 mg phenobarbital as a barbiturate is 100 mg pentobarbital, 100 mg secobarbital, 100 mg amobarbital, or 60 mg butabarbital. Other sedative-hypnotic agents equivalent to 30 mg phenobarbital in the withdrawal state include: chloral hydrate 500 mg; ethchlorvynol 350 mg; glutethimide 250 mg; meprobamate 400 mg; methaqualone 300 mg; methyprylon 100 mg.

General Treatment

Psychotherapeutic interventions appear to be the most effective long-term treatments in sedation/hypnotic abuse.

Benzodiazepine

Intoxication

Central nervous system depression with hypotension due to vasodilation and concomitant respiratory depression are the predominant sequelae. The mainstay of therapy is supportive with particular attention to ventilatory and circulatory support. Flumazenil (Children: 0.005-0.2 mg/kg; Adults: 0.5-5 mg) infused over 3-5 minutes is effective in reversing CNS and respiratory depression.

Withdrawal

Tolerance can develop rapidly in benzodiazepine therapy and from 15% to 44% of chronic users experience withdrawal symptoms when their benzodiazepine dose is decreased. Patients who take benzodiazepines for greater than 3 months are at risk for withdrawal. The onset of symptoms may be as short as 1 day for the longer acting benzodiazepines (ie, diazepam). Symptoms may last for 6 weeks. Symptoms are due to neuronal excitation and may include anxiety, insomnia, fever, tremor, nausea, tinnitus, myalgias, seizures, vomiting, and diaphoresis. Treatment consists of reinstitution of a long acting benzodiazepine with a gradual taper (over a period of 6-8 weeks). In cases of severe symptomatology, an intravenous infusion of diazepam (at 20 mg/hour or more) in a monitored setting may be initially required. Barbiturates are reasonable alternatives to benzodiazepines in treating benzodiazepine withdrawal. Phenobarbital 30 mg equivalency for benzodiazepines includes: alprazolam 0.5 mg; clorazepate 7.5 mg; chlordiazepoxide 25 mg; diazepam 5 mg; flurazepam 30 mg; lorazepam 1 mg; oxazepam 15 mg; temazepam 60 mg; triazolam 0.5 mg; clonazepam 0.25 mg. One-fourth of this calculated dose is administered and the dose is increased as necessary. The phenobarbital dose can be tapered after the patient is stabilized for 48 hours at a rate of 10% of the dose daily. Propranolol (20 mg 3-4 times/day) can be instituted on day 5 and continued for 2 weeks as an adjunctive agent.

Gamma Hydroxybutyrate (GHB)/Gamma Butyrolactone (GBL)

Intoxication

Central nervous system predominates and the mainstay of management is respiratory support. Hypothermia, hypotension, and seizures may also occur. Atropine can be used to treat bradycardia. Sudden arousal is usually noted 5-8 hours postingestion.

Withdrawal

Withdrawal symptoms may occur with constant use for a period of over 2 months, especially if there is a recent dose escalation. Central nervous system hyperactivity such as insomnia, tremor, delirium, psychosis, and auditory/visual hallucinations occurs within 12 hours of cessation of doses. Duration of symptoms ranges from 5-15 days. Treatment is supportive with lorazepam and/or haloperidol (5 mg) effective for treatment of delirium or psychosis. Often large doses of benzodiazepines are required. Pentobarbital (initial dose 2.5-5 mg/kg I.V.) can also be given to treat resistant symptoms. Other agents utilized include propofol (initial dose: 1-2 mg/kg; maintenance: 2-10 mg/kg/hour) and droperidol (2.5 mg). Avoid flumazenil, physostigmine, and naloxone.

Stimulants

Intoxication/Overdose

Intoxication/overdose management involves reducing autonomic hyperactivity (tachycardia, hypertension) and managing CNS symptoms (agitation, psychosis/delirium, or seizures). Supportive measures such as appropriate hydration, vital sign monitoring, and cooling for hyperthermia are indicated. Anxiolytics or antipsychotics may be useful on a short-term basis, and a supportive, low-stimulation environment will reduce CNS irritability.

Withdrawal

Amphetamine withdrawal is generally treated supportively. The judicious use of antipsychotic medication may be of benefit to patients with post-amphetamine psychosis.

General Treatment

Psychotherapeutic interventions appear to be the most effective long-term treatment.

Caffeine

Intoxication

Treatment for caffeine intoxication is outlined in the caffeine monograph (see Caffeine).

Withdrawal

Physical dependency to caffeine does exist with withdrawal symptoms usually occurring within 12-24 hours following cessation and peaks at 20-51 hours and may last for one week. A daily dose over 235 mg (about 2.5 cups of coffee/day) can increase the risk for likelihood of withdrawal. While lethargy and weakness may occur, facial flushing and severe headaches predominate this syndrome and may last as long as 9 days. Symptoms correlate with the amount ingested prior to cessation. Treatment focuses on a gradual reduction of caffeine intake over several days. Caffeine tablets may be useful in headache treatment.

Hallucinogens

Intoxication

Individuals who experience toxic delirium, panic reactions, or psychosis associated with hallucinogens require a supportive environment (low stimulation with supervision) and may benefit from judicious dosing of anxiolytics (eg, diazepam 5-10 mg orally).

Withdrawal

Physical dependence and withdrawal symptoms have not been reported.

General Treatment

Psychotherapeutic interventions appear to be the most effective in long-term treatment.

Baclofen

Intoxication

Treatment of baclofen intoxication is outlined in the baclofen monograph (see Baclofen).

Withdrawal

Baclofen withdrawal syndrome usually occurs within 12-72 hours following dose cessation. The syndrome is similar to the sedative-hypnotic withdrawal syndrome with agitation, delusions, spasticity, rhabdomyolysis, paranoia, psychosis, pruritus, hallucinations, hypertonia, fever, and seizures. Benzodiazepines (diazepam 5-10 mg orally every 6-12 hours) are the mainstay of baclofen withdrawal therapy. For acute intrathecal baclofen withdrawal, baclofen (10-20 mg orally every 6 hours) and cyproheptadine (4-8 mg orally every 6-8 hours) can also be utilized with the latter agent particularly effective in treating pruritus.

Inhalants

Intoxication

CNS effects of intoxication usually resolve within minutes to hours of inhalant use. Toxic effects depend on the solvent used and may require emergency treatment for arrhythmias or CNS hyperactivity (seizures). Some agents (such as toluene) produce renal damage and renal functioning should be monitored. Intoxication treatment is generally supportive.

Withdrawal

Withdrawal reactions occur rarely as most inhalant use is relatively short-lived. Symptoms that may occur are generally treated supportively with concurrent psychosocial interventions.

General Treatment

Psychotherapeutic interventions are generally most effective. Due to the young age of most patients, family therapy is often also indicated.

Selective Serotonin Reuptake Inhibitors (SSRIs)

Intoxication/Overdose

See individual monographs.

Withdrawal

Withdrawal occurs most frequently upon abrupt cessation with paroxetine, sertraline, fluoxetine, and venlafaxine. Paroxetine appears to be the SSRI with the highest incidence of withdrawal reactions. Symptoms usually begin within 1-2 days and involve dizziness, ataxia, anorexia, diarrhea, flu-like symptoms, diaphoresis, parethesias, tremor, and sleep disturbances. Symptoms may last as long as 2-3 weeks. Temporary reinstitution of an SSRI with gradual tapering over several weeks is suggested. Ginger root, 1100 mg 3 times/day, for 1-2 weeks has been noted to be efficacious for sertraline withdrawal.

Synthesized Compounds

Intoxication/Overdose

PCP toxicity is best managed in a low-stimulation, secure environment. Benzodiazepines and careful use of antipsychotic medication may be helpful for the severe agitation/aggression sometimes seen in PCP intoxication. Some clinicians advocate promoting rapid drug excretion with ammonium chloride or ascorbic acid. Most PCP toxic reactions resolve within 1-3 days, but behavioral symptoms may persist for 2 weeks or more.

In acute intoxication situations, MDMA has been associated with cardiac arrhythmias suggesting a need for close intensive medical monitoring. Additionally, some designer drugs may contain contaminants which have been associated with chronic neurologic damage.

Withdrawal

Physical dependence on PCP generally does not occur, although psychological dependence may be associated with drug craving and relapse.

General Treatment

Psychotherapeutic interventions are generally most effective in the long term. Little is known about long-term treatment of designer drug abuse.

Marijuana

Intoxication

The incidence of acute adverse reactions to marijuana is quite low. In rare cases, individuals may experience acute panic, toxic delirium, or flashbacks. These generally remit spontaneously within 12-48 hours. Management may include anxiolytics of antipsychotics if behavioral symptoms are severe. Treatment is outlined in the marijuana monograph (see Marijuana (Cannabis)).

Withdrawal

Tolerance generally does not develop to marijuana, although heavy daily users may experience withdrawal symptoms of insomnia, diaphoresis, dysphoria, irritability, tremor, and nausea. Symptoms peak at 48 hours of abstinence and persist for 96 hours. There is no recognized withdrawal regimen.

General Treatment

As with other substance abuse disorders, individuals should receive psychosocial rehabilitation and there should be assessment and treatment of any coexisting psychiatric disorders.

Nicotine

Intoxication/Overdose

Nicotine intoxication from tobacco use is rare. Excess nicotine from nicotine replacement therapies used in smoking cessation (ie, nicotine gum) may occasionally cause adverse effects such as nausea, headaches, or cardiac abnormalities. Treatment is outlined in the nicotine monograph (see Nicotine).

Withdrawal

Withdrawal symptoms begin within 6-12 hours and generally peak 24-72 hours after smoking cessation. Most symptoms last for approximately 1 month, although craving can persist for 6 weeks or longer. Smoking cessation is associated with slowing on EEG, and decline in metabolic rate, including mean heart rate decline of 8 beats/minute. Blood levels of some antidepressants (eg, clomipramine, desipramine, doxepin, imipramine, and nortriptyline) may increase as may some antipsychotic medications (eg, clozapine, fluphenazine, haloperidol) and some anxiolytics (eg, oxazepam, desmethyldiazepam).

The most successful treatment of nicotine withdrawal frequently includes both psychosocial and pharmacological interventions. Patients must generally be committed to quitting, and most clinicians advocate abrupt cessation of tobacco rather than gradual reduction. Approximately 33% of adults who smoke make an attempt to stop smoking each year. Relapse is common, particularly among those who attempt to quit smoking on their own without formal treatment. Approximately 50% of smokers eventually quit, although individuals with histories of anxiety or mood disorders or of schizophrenia are less likely to stop smoking. Most smokers require 5-7 attempts at smoking cessation before they eventually quit for good. Psychosocial treatments include behavior therapies (relapse prevention, relaxation, stimulus control among other techniques), education (group or individual), and hypnosis. Pharmacotherapies include nicotine replacement therapy, nicotine antagonists, agents that mimic nicotine effects, aversive therapies, and symptomatic management. Nicotine replacement therapy and antidepressants for symptomatic management are among the most commonly utilized pharmacologic measures.

Nicotine replacement provides the nicotine-dependent patient with nicotine in a form that is not associated with the carcinogenic elements in tobacco. Nicotine gum, transdermal nicotine patches, nicotine nasal spray, and nicotine inhalers are available for smoking cessation. Nicotine gum, now available over-the-counter, consists of 2-4 mg of nicotine in a polacrilex resin designed to be slowly chewed for 20-30 minutes. Nicotine absorption peaks 30 minutes after initiation of gum use. Most common adverse effects are GI complaints (nausea, anorexia) and headache. Although nicotine replacement has been used for relief of withdrawal symptoms, some patients utilize these therapies long-term.

Nicotine patches consist of nicotine impregnated into an adhesive patch for transdermal application. Patches are applied daily each morning upon quitting smoking with starting dosages of 21-22 mg/24-hour patch and 15 mg/16-hour patch. Patients should not smoke cigarettes while on patches as nicotine toxicity may occur. Typical treatment duration is 6-8 weeks. The nicotine inhaler contains a replaceable component that delivers nicotine in inhaled air. Unlike cigarettes which deliver nicotine directly into the arterial blood in the lungs, the inhaler delivers nicotine into the buccal mucosa.

In addition to nicotine replacement, some antidepressants (bupropion, doxepin, and desipramine) have been shown to improve the chances of nicotine abstinence. Sustained-release bupropion hydrochloride has been approved by the FDA for smoking cessation (150 mg every morning for 3 days, then 150 mg twice daily beginning 1-2 weeks prequit) for a minimum of 7-12 weeks. In addition to reducing nicotine withdrawal symptoms, bupropion S-R may diminish weight gain. Some clinicians utilize both bupropion and nicotine replacement concurrently.

Other pharmacologic therapies that have been reported to be potentially useful in the management of tobacco cessation include nicotine antagonists (eg, mecamylamine) and aversive treatments such as silver acetate gum, although efficacy of these agents are not proven. Some clinicians utilize clonidine at dosages of 0.1-0.4 mg/day for nicotine withdrawal in individuals who fail or are unable to tolerate other symptomatic treatment or nicotine replacement.

General Treatment

A widely used intervention for practitioners in general medical settings for smoking cessation is the "4 As" strategy of the National Cancer Institute. This consists of the following:

1. **Ask** and record smoking status. In several surveys, only about 50% of physicians asked patients about their tobacco use.
2. **Advise** to stop. Direct recommendation from a physician produces quit rates of 7% to 10%.
3. **Assist** the patient in addressing cessation. Identifying a quit date may assist in obtaining commitment to quit. Patients who are unable or unwilling to commit to quitting may benefit from educational materials at this time.
4. **Arrange** follow-up. This should occur within 3 days as the first several days after quitting are a critical period in relapse risk.

Most pharmacotherapies are primarily utilized during the initial period of quitting tobacco use. Psychological treatments/lifestyle changes, while also utilized during nicotine withdrawal, must also become long-term interventions. Although biologic treatments do not require concurrent psychological therapies, best outcome is usually associated with combined treatment.

Psychiatric Emergencies - Violence

Violent and agitated behavior creates an emergency situation due to potential risk to patients, bystanders, and healthcare staff. Patients with both nonpsychiatric and psychiatric disorders presenting to emergency rooms may exhibit violent or agitated behavior. It has been reported that up to 80% of teaching hospital emergency rooms experience patient assault of staff members. The initial task in managing a potentially violent individual is to assess for signs of impending violence such as verbal or physical threats, presence of objects that may be used as weapons, signs of substance intoxication, and level of agitation or psychiatric symptoms such as psychosis. Serum glucose should be determined as hypoglycemia may lead to aggressive behavior. Serum cholesterol levels have also been associated with aggressive behavior. Patients who are a potential risk of harm to self or others should be placed in a protective environment with an attempt to de-escalate the situation. Police or security assistance is often essential, and a calm show of overwhelming force may commonly lead to abandonment of threatening behavior by the patient. The use of physical restraints may be necessary for continued agitated or violent behavior if other less restrictive measures are ineffective, and prompt pharmacotherapy of underlying psychiatric or medical disorders should be initiated. A reassuring, safe, and low-stimulation environment is optimum. In some acutely agitated individuals, rapid tranquilization and the use of antipsychotics and benzodiazepines to control severely disruptive behavior is indicated. Beta-blockers may also be useful to treat this entity. If violent, agitated patients are unable to take oral medications (such as risperidone 1-2 mg), many clinicians use a high potency I.M. antipsychotic such as haloperidol 5-10 mg P.O., I.V., or I.M., repeated every 10-30 minutes until desired effects are achieved (start elderly dosing at 2 mg P.O. or I.M.), and/or an injectable benzodiazepine such as lorazepam 0.5-2 mg I.M. or I.V. to quickly sedate the patient and stabilize disruptive behavior. Droperidol 2.5-10 mg I.M. (or 0.05 mg/kg), risperidone 2 mg/day (up to 6 mg/day) P.O., ziprasidone 5-20 mg I.M. every 4-6 hours, or olanzapine 5-10 mg I.M. (I.M. route not available in the U.S.) may also be useful in treating psychotic patients. (**Note**: On December 5, 2001 Akorn, Inc. announced the addition of a **Black Box Warning** and Updated Warnings/Precautions in the Inapsine® (droperidol) product labeling. Droperidol is contraindicated in patients with known or suspected QT prolongation. It should be used with caution in patients with risk factors (CHF, bradycardia, diuretic use, cardiac hypertrophy, hypokalemia, hypomagnesemia, concomitant use of medications known to prolong the QT interval, age older than 65 years, ethanol abuse, benzodiazepine use, volatile anesthetics, and I.V. opiates. In patients where droperidol treatment is appropriate, dosage should be started low and titrated upward. EKG monitoring should be done prior to treatment and continued for 2-3 hours after treatment to monitor for arrhythmias.) Patients at risk for acute extrapyramidal symptoms may receive a concomitant anticholinergic agent such as benztropine 2 mg I.M or diphenhydramine 25-50 mg I.M. The antipsychotic plus benzodiazepine combination may be repeated every 30-60 minutes, if needed, with antipsychotic haloperidol dosage generally not exceeding 20 mg/day, or the benzodiazepine may be given alternating with the antipsychotic. Avoid antipsychotic agents in anticholinergic-induced delirium. Rapid tranquilization should not be confused with rapid neuroleptization, a procedure that was used in the past where patients were treated with "mega" doses of neuroleptic, and were placed at risk of severe neurological side effects. If patients are able to take oral medications, antipsychotic options are increased to include atypical antipsychotics such as risperidone, olanzapine, or quetiapine. Benzodiazepines may also be given orally (eg, diazepam 5-10 mg). For nonpsychotic patients, some clinicians utilize benzodiazepine monotherapy (eg, lorazepam 1-2 mg orally every 1-4 hours).

For the long-term management of individuals with chronic or intermittent aggression, there are a variety of interventions including psychotherapy, treatment of underlying psychiatric illness if present, and pharmacotherapies that target aggressive behaviors. Drugs that may diminish aggressive behavior include mood-stabilizers such as lithium (target serum lithium level: 0.7-1 mM/L), valproate, cyproterone acetate [investigational] (doses up to 300 mg/day), pipamperone [investigational] (80-240 mg/day), and carbamazepine (300-800 mg/day). Antidepressants such as the SSRIs and trazodone may be useful as well as buspirone, and atypical antipsychotics such as clozapine.

Neuroleptic Malignant Syndrome

Neuroleptic malignant syndrome (NMS) is a condition characterized by progressive worsening (over 24-72 hours) of muscle rigidity, changes in consciousness, and autonomic instability. Symptoms of autonomic instability include sweating, fever, flushing, tachycardia, and labile blood pressure. Additionally, the white blood count (WBC) (in the range of 10,000-40,000 cells/mm^3) and creatine phosphokinase (CPK) (up to 60,000 IU/L) may be elevated. Severe CPK elevation may be associated with renal failure. True NMS is a medical emergency. Fortunately, NMS is relatively rare, occurring in <1% of patients on conventional antipsychotics. NMS appears to be extremely rare with atypical antipsychotics. Over 60% of cases of NMS occur during the first 2 weeks of antipsychotic therapy, with strongest risk factors being male gender and previous history of NMS. Mortality ranges from 4% to 22% and is usually due to renal failure due to rhabdomyolysis or respiratory pneumonia. Management consists of early diagnosis, immediate discontinuation of antipsychotic drugs, symptomatic treatment, including I.V. hydration, antipyretics, and cooling blankets. Close monitoring of clinical status/vital signs is essential. Bromocriptine at dosages of 5 mg 3-4 times/day (up to 40 mg/day) or dantrolene at dosages of 3-5 mg/kg I.V. 4 times/day may be beneficial in acute NMS. Alternative therapies include carbidopa/levodopa (25/100), amantadine, carbamazepine, and electroconvulsive therapy.

Catatonia

Catatonia is a syndrome associated with a variety of medical disorders such as encephalopathy and ketoacidosis, and a variety of psychiatric disorders such as schizophrenia and serious mood disorders. Catatonia produces cataplexy and waxy flexibility, mutism, intermittent agitation, and resistance to movement and/or instructions. There exists a lethal form of catatonia in which patients experience hyperthermia, rigidity, rhabdomyolysis, and autonomic instability. As its name implies, lethal catatonia has high mortality if untreated.

Patients with suspected catatonia should have a thorough medical evaluation to identify and make appropriate interventions for treatable medical disorders. Clinical entities such as aspiration pneumonia and neuroleptic malignant syndrome can exhibit catatonic behavior with a fever. In cases where no medical etiology can be identified, patients are generally treated in inpatient psychiatric settings. I.V. amobarbital sodium (50 mg/minute for a total dose up to 300 mg) may be used to assist in obtaining history from psychiatric patients with catatonia. However, amobarbital is not effective in treating catatonia as its effects are short-lived and there may be risk of respiratory depression. More recently, it has been demonstrated that parenteral or oral lorazepam is helpful in catatonia and may more safely facilitate the patient's ability to give a history. Lethal catatonia may improve with antipsychotics or dantrolene although most rapid treatment of catatonia generally occurs with ECT. Other therapies used successfully in treating catatonia include risperidone (4 mg twice daily), intravenous biperiden (5 mg every 30 minutes, not to exceed 3 doses), clonazepam (1-7 mg I.M. or I.V.), clozapine (350 mg orally), amantadine (200 mg every 6-7 hours for 3 doses), lithium carbonate (1.2-1.5 g/day orally), and diazepam (up to 40 mg/day orally). Lorazepam (2 mg I.M.) can be used to treat psychogenic catatonia.

Agents Known to Elicit Aggressive or Catatonic Behavior	
Aggression	**Catatonia**
Alprazolam	Allopurinol
Acetylcarnitine	Amantadine (withdrawal)
Amantadine	Baclofen
Amineptine	Bulbocapnine
Amitriptyline	Bupropion
Amphetamine	Chlorpromazine
Androstenedione	Cocaine
Clobazam	Cycloserine
Clomipramine	Cyclosporine
Cocaine	Diphenhydramine
Cyproheptadine	Disulfiram
Dapsone	Doxylamine
Dehydroepiandrosterone	Ecstasy (hallucinogenic amphetamine)
Donepezil	Fluphenazine
Ethyl alcohol	*Kyllinga brevifolia* Rottb. (extract)
Felbamate	Lead
Fluoxetine	Loxapine
Gabapentin	Lysergic acid diethylamide
Heroin	Marijuana (cannabis)
Imipramine	Morphine sulfate
Medazepam	Phencyclidine
Melarsoprol	Piperazine
Ketamine	Pipothiazine (injection)
Lamotrigine	Primidone
Lead	Prochlorperazine
Lorazepam	Risperidone
Midazolam	Sulthiamine
Morphine sulfate	Trifluoperazine
Nandrolone	
Omeprazole	
Oxandrolone	
Oxymetholone	
Peginterferon alfa 2b	
Phencyclidine	
Rivastigmine	
Sodium oxybate	
Stanozolol	
Temazepam	
Testosterone	
Valproic acid	
Vigabatrin	
Zopiclone	

Acute Extrapyramidal Syndromes (Eps)

Acute Dystonias

Acute dystonias are uncomfortable, involuntary muscle spasms of the face, neck, trunk, or extremities associated with antipsychotic treatment. Dystonias occur in 10% to 15% of patients on conventional antipsychotic medications, usually in the first several weeks of treatment. Acute dystonias are much rarer with atypical antipsychotic medications. Manifestations of acute dystonia include facial grimacing, tongue twisting, dysarthria and/or dysphagia, eye deviation, neck twisting (torticollis), and back spasm (opisthotonos). Acute laryngospasm may be life-threatening. Most prominent risk factors for acute dystonia include male gender, history of acute extrapyramidal symptoms, and adolescence. When dystonia occurs, intramuscular anticholinergic medication (eg, diphenhydramine 50 mg I.M. or benztropine 2 mg I.M.) usually brings rapid symptom reduction. Subsequently, the patient should receive maintenance anticholinergic/antiparkinsonian medication (eg, benztropine 1-2 mg twice daily). Laryngospasm requires immediate I.V. treatment (eg, diphenhydramine 25-50 mg I.V.) or benztropine 2 mg I.V.

When initiating conventional antipsychotic agents in those patients with strong risk factors for developing acute dystonias, it is reasonable to begin prophylactic anticholinergic treatment. For elderly patients, due to increased risk of anticholinergic toxicity and potential adverse effects on cognitive status, it is usually best to avoid prophylactic anticholinergic medication.

Geriatric patients generally require lower doses of anticholinergic drug. Adverse effects associated with anticholinergic medication include constipation, urinary retention, tachycardia, and blurred vision. Intraocular pressure may be increased, posing some danger for patients with narrow-angle glaucoma. In addition, some individuals, particularly elderly patients, may develop a delirium-like presentation associated with anticholinergics that is characterized by disorientation, hallucinations, behavioral lability, and cognitive impairment. Occasionally, patients may abuse anticholinergics.

Patients on anticholinergic medication should be reassessed on a regular basis to determine continued need for medication. A significant number of patients on antipsychotic medication exhibit spontaneous reduction or resolution of EPS during continued antipsychotic medication therapy, particularly during the first 3 months of treatment. Therefore, after this time period, one should consider tapering anticholinergic agent. Tolerance often develops to dystonic effects over the first month of treatment, and need for maintenance anticholinergic medication should be reassessed at that point.

Akathisia

Akathisia is a subjective feeling of restlessness seen in 20% to 40% of patients on typical antipsychotic medications. Patients may appear agitated, with frequent pacing and inability to keep their legs still. As with all acute extrapyramidal adverse effects, akathisia is significantly less common with atypical antipsychotic agents. Primary management is to lower antipsychotic dosage, or switch antipsychotic agents to either an atypical antipsychotic or to a typical agent with lower dopamine-blocking potency. Medication management of symptoms of akathisia include benzodiazepines such as clonazepam 1 mg twice daily, or alternatively benztropine 1-2 mg/day. Beta-blocking drugs (eg, propranolol, atenolol, pindolol) may be useful in EPS. Beta-blockers appear to be most effective in treating akathisia. Use of beta blockers (propranolol or nadolol at doses up to 80 mg/day) with a benzodiazepine may be quite efficacious. Patients on beta-blockers may experience hypotension or bradycardia, thus, blood pressure and pulse should be monitored during initial drug titration. Clonidine is another agent that may be effective in akathisia. Usual dosage for akathisia is 0.2-0.8 mg/day. As with beta-blockers, hypotension may occur, and blood pressure should be monitored during initial titration. Clonidine should generally be tried after failure of beta-blockers to control akathisia. Recognition and management of akathisia is important as the condition can be extremely stressful to patients, and there is a danger of misdiagnosis if the agitation of akathisia is mistakenly attributed to worsening of psychotic symptoms.

Drug-Induced Parkinsonism

Antipsychotic medication-associated parkinsonism is characterized by rigidity, bradykinesia, masked facies, drooling, and tremor. While not strictly an emergency, the disabling symptoms occur subacutely within the first month of therapy on 10% to 15% of patients on typical antipsychotics. Drug-induced parkinsonism is significantly less common with atypical antipsychotics. Strongest risk factors for parkinsonism are female gender and older age. Treatment is with antiparkinsonian agents such as trihexyphenidyl 2 mg twice daily or benztropine 1-2 mg twice daily. Some tolerance may develop to parkinsonian effects. Alternatively, reduction or resolution of parkinsonian symptoms may be achieved by decreasing antipsychotic medication dosage, switching to a lower potency typical agent, or switching to an atypical agent.

Dopaminergic agents, such as amantadine and levodopa, have also been reported to be useful in management of EPS. Amantadine has been reported to be beneficial in acute dystonia, akathisia, and drug-induced parkinsonism. As with anticholinergics, amantadine is believed to work by normalizing dopamine-acetylcholine balance in the striatum. Dosing of 100-400 mg/day in a once or twice daily pattern is usually used. Adverse effects with amantadine include orthostasis, peripheral edema, and a skin reaction called livedo reticularis (venous marbleization of the skin, usually lower extremities). Also, worsening of psychosis or delirium have been reported. Generally, amantadine should only be utilized after failure of anticholinergic agents. Levodopa is far less commonly used due to concern regarding worsening of psychotic illness.

References

1. Addolorato G, Leggio L, Abenavoli L, et al, "Baclofen in the Treatment of Alcohol Withdrawal Syndrome: A Comparative Study vs Diazepam," *Am J Med*, 2006, 119(3):276.
2. Breier A, Meehan K, Birkett M, et al, "A Double-Blind, Placebo-Controlled Dose-Response Comparison of Intramuscular Olanzapine and Haloperidol in the Treatment of Acute Agitation in Schizophrenia," *Arch Gen Psychiatry*, 2002, 59(5):441-8.
3. Calfee R and Fadale P, "Popular Ergogenic Drugs and Supplements in Young Athletes," *Psychopharmacology (Berl)*, 2004, 176(1):1-29.
4. Carbone JR, "The Neuroleptic Malignant and Serotonin Syndromes," *Emerg Med Clin North Am*, 2000, 18(2):317-25.
5. Craig K, Gomez HF, McManus JL, et al, "Severe Gamma-Hydroxybutyrate Withdrawal: A Case Report and Literature Review," *J Emerg Med*, 2000, 18(1):65-70.
6. *Diagnostic and Statistical Manual of Mental Disorders*, 4th ed revised, Washington, DC: American Psychiatric Press, 1994.
7. Dyer JE, Roth B, Hyma BA, "Gamma-Hydroxybutyrate Withdrawal Syndrome," *Ann Emerg Med*, 2001, 37(2):147-53.
8. Foy A, "The Pathophysiology, Diagnosis and Management of Alcohol Withdrawal," *J Toxicol Clin Toxicol*, 2000, 38(2):189-90.
9. Gelenberg AL and Bassuk EL, eds, *The Practitioners Guide to Psychoactive Drugs*, 4th ed, New York, NY: Plenum Medical Book Company, 1997, 291-363.
10. Hill S and Petit J, "The Violent Patient," *Emerg Med Clin North Am*, 2000, 18(2):301-15.
11. Hyman SE and Tesar GE, eds, *Manual of Psychiatric Emergencies,* 3rd ed, Boston, MA: Little, Brown, 1994.
12. Juliano LM and Griffiths RR, "A Critical Review of Caffeine Withdrawal: Empirical Validation of Symptoms and Signs, Incidence, Severity, and Associated Features," *Psychopharmacol*, 2004, 176(1):1-29.
13. Lasser K, Boyd JW, Woolhandler S, et al, "Smoking and Mental Illness: A Population-Based Prevalence Study," *JAMA*, 2000, 284(20):2606-10.
14. Leggio L, Abenavoli L, Caputo F, et al, "Baclofen Use in the Treatment of Alcohol Delirium Tremens," *Arch Intern Med*, 2005, 165(5):586.
15. Meythaler JM, Roper JF, and Brunner RC, "Cyproheptadine for Intrathecal Baclofen Withdrawal," *Arch Phys Med Rehabil*, 2003, 84(5):638-42.
16. Mullins ME and Fitzmaurice SC, "Lack of Efficacy of Benzodiazepines in Treating Gamma-Hydroxybutyrate Withdrawal," *J Emerg Med*, 2001, 20:418-9.
17. Munizza C, Furlan PM, d'Elia A, et al, "Emergency Psychiatry: A Review of the Literature," *Acta Psychiatr Scand Suppl*, 1993, 374:1-51.
18. O'Connor PG and Kosten TR, "Rapid and Ultrarapid Opioid Detoxification Techniques," *JAMA*, 1998, 279(3):229-34.
19. Olmedo R and Hoffman RS, "Withdrawal Syndromes," *Emerg Med North Am*, 2000, 18(2):273-88.
20. Olmedo RE, Nelson L, Howland M, et al, "Propofol Safely Controls Delirium Tremens," *J Toxicol Clin Toxicol*, 2000, 38(5):537.
21. Perry PJ, Alexander B, and Liskow BI, *Psychotropic Drug Handbook*, 7th ed, Washington, DC: American Psychiatric Press, 1997, 425-51.

22. Petty TL, "The Early Diagnosis of Lung Cancer," *Disease-a-Month*, 2001, 47(6):204-58.

23. Sadock BJ and Sadock VA, eds, *Kaplan & Sadock's Comprehensive Textbook of Psychiatry*, 7th ed, Philadelphia, PA: Lippincott Williams and Wilkins, 2000.

24. Sajatovic M and Schultz SC, "Schizophrenia," *Current Psychiatric Therapy II*, DL Dunner, ed, Philadelphia, PA: W.B. Saunders Company, 1997.

25. Schatzberg AF, Cole O, and DeBattista C, *Manual of Clinical Psychopharmacology*, 3rd ed, Washington, DC: American Psychiatric Press, 1997, 335-76.

26. Schechter JO, "Treatment of Disequilibrium and Nausea in the SRI Discontinuation Syndrome," *J Clin Psychiatry*, 1998, 59(8):431-2.

27. Shaw SC and Fletcher AP, "Aggression As an Adverse Drug Reaction," *Adverse Drug React Toxicol Rev*, 2000, 19(1):35-45.

28. Sivilotti ML, Burns MJ, and Aaron CK, "Pentobarbital for Control of Acute Delirium Due to Gamma-Butyrolactone Withdrawal," *Ann Emerg Med*, 2000, 35(5):S52-3.

29. Zajecka J, Tracy KA, and Mitchell S, "Discontinuation Symptoms After Treatment with Serotonin Reuptake Inhibitors: A Literature Review," *J Clin Psych*, 1997, 58(7):291-7.

Acarbose

Pronunciation (AY car bose)
CAS Number 56180-94-0
U.S. Brand Names Precose®
Use
  Monotherapy, as indicated as an adjunct to diet to lower blood glucose in patients with type 2 diabetes mellitus (noninsulin dependent, NIDDM) whose hyperglycemia cannot be managed on diet alone
  Combination with a sulfonylurea, metformin, or insulin in patients with type 2 diabetes mellitus (noninsulin dependent, NIDDM) when diet plus acarbose do not result in adequate glycemic control. The effect of acarbose to enhance glycemic control is additive to that of other hypoglycemic agents when used in combination.
Mechanism of Action Competitive inhibitor of pancreatic α-amylase and intestinal brush border α-glucosidases, resulting in delayed hydrolysis of ingested complex carbohydrates and disaccharides and absorption of glucose; dose-dependent reduction in postprandial serum insulin and glucose peaks; inhibits the metabolism of sucrose to glucose and fructose Competitive inhibitor of pancreatic α-amylase and intestinal brush border α-glucosidases, resulting in delayed hydrolysis of ingested complex carbohydrates and disaccharides and absorption of glucose; dose-dependent reduction in postprandial serum insulin and glucose peaks; inhibits the metabolism of sucrose to glucose and fructose
Adverse Reactions
  Central nervous system: Sleepiness, headache, vertigo
  Dermatologic: Erythema, urticaria
  Gastrointestinal: Abdominal pain and diarrhea tend to return to pretreatment levels over time, and the frequency and intensity of flatulence tend to abate with time; severe GI distress
  Hepatic: Elevated liver transaminases
  Neuromuscular & skeletal: Weakness
Signs and Symptoms of Overdose Overdose may result in transient increased flatulence, diarrhea, and abdominal discomfort which will subside shortly. Overdose will not result in hypoglycemia. However, acarbose may complicate the treatment of hypoglycemia from other causes, since it will inhibit the absorption of oral disaccharides (sucrose).
Pharmacodynamics/Kinetics
  Absorption: <2% as active drug
  Metabolism: Exclusively via GI tract, principally by intestinal bacteria and digestive enzymes; 13 metabolites identified
  Bioavailability: Low systemic bioavailability of parent compound; acts locally in GI tract
  Excretion: Urine (~34%)
Dosage
  Oral:
  Adults: Dosage must be individualized on the basis of effectiveness and tolerance while not exceeding the maximum recommended dose
    Initial dose: 25 mg 3 times/day with the first bite of each main meal
    Maintenance dose: Should be adjusted at 4- to 8-week intervals based on 1-hour postprandial glucose levels and tolerance. Dosage may be increased from 25 mg 3 times/day to 50 mg 3 times/day. Some patients may benefit from increasing the dose to 100 mg 3 times/day.
      Maintenance dose ranges: 50-100 mg 3 times/day.
    Maximum dose:
      ≤60 kg: 50 mg 3 times/day
      >60 kg: 100 mg 3 times/day
  Patients receiving sulfonylureas: Acarbose given in combination with a sulfonylurea will cause a further lowering of blood glucose and may increase the hypoglycemic potential of the sulfonylurea. If hypoglycemia occurs, appropriate adjustments in the dosage of these agents should be made.
  Dosing adjustment in renal impairment: Cl$_{cr}$ <25 mL/minute: Peak plasma concentrations were 5 times higher and AUCs were 6 times larger than in volunteers with normal renal function; however, long term clinical trials in diabetic patients with significant renal dysfunction have not been conducted and treatment of these patients with acarbose is not recommended
Stability Store at <25°C (77°F) and protect from moisture
Monitoring Parameters Postprandial glucose, glycosylated hemoglobin levels, serum transaminase levels should be checked every 3 months during the first year of treatment and periodically thereafter
Administration
  Should be administered with the first bite of each main meal
Contraindications Hypersensitivity to acarbose or any component of the formulation; patients with diabetic ketoacidosis or cirrhosis; patients with inflammatory bowel disease, colonic ulceration, partial intestinal obstruction, or in patients predisposed to intestinal obstruction; patients who have chronic intestinal diseases associated with marked disorders of digestion or absorption, and in patients who have conditions that may deteriorate as a result of increased gas formation in the intestine

Warnings
  Acarbose may increase the hypoglycemic potential of sulfonylureas. Oral glucose (dextrose) should be used in the treatment of mild-to-moderate hypoglycemia. Severe hypoglycemia may require the use of either intravenous glucose infusion or glucagon injection.
  Treatment-emergent elevations of serum transaminases (AST and/or ALT) occurred in 15% of acarbose-treated patients in long-term studies. These serum transaminase elevations appear to be dose related. At doses >100 mg 3 times/day, the incidence of serum transaminase elevations greater than 3 times the upper limit of normal was 2-3 times higher in the acarbose group than in the placebo group. These elevations were asymptomatic, reversible, more common in females, and, in general, were not associated with other evidence of liver dysfunction.
  When diabetic patients are exposed to stress such as fever, trauma, infection, or surgery, a temporary loss of control of blood glucose may occur. At such times, temporary insulin therapy may be necessary.
Dosage Forms Tablet: 25 mg, 50 mg, 100 mg
Overdosage/Treatment
  Decontamination: Activated charcoal/gastric lavage. Treatment is otherwise supportive.
  Oral glucose (dextrose) should be used in mild to moderate hypoglycemia; severe hypoglycemia should be treated with I.V. glucose.
Drug Interactions
  Calcium channel blocking agents: May decrease the efficacy of acarbose due to hyperglycemic effects.
  Corticosteroids: May decrease the efficacy of acarbose due to hyperglycemic effects.
  Digoxin: Acarbose decreases the bioavailability of digoxin, resulting in lower serum concentrations.
  Diuretics (including thiazides): May decrease the efficacy of acarbose due to hyperglycemic effects.
  Enzyme replacement (pancrelipase, amylase): May decrease the efficacy of acarbose due to effects on carbohydrate metabolism.
  Estrogens: May decrease the efficacy of acarbose due to hyperglycemic effects.
  Insulin: Acarbose may increase the hypoglycemic potential of insulin. Oral glucose (dextrose) should be used in the treatment of mild-to-moderate hypoglycemia; severe hypoglycemia may require the use of either intravenous glucose infusion or glucagon injection.
  Isoniazid: May decrease the efficacy of acarbose due to hyperglycemic effects.
  Nicotinic acid: May decrease the efficacy of acarbose due to hyperglycemic effects.
  Oral contraceptives: May decrease the efficacy of acarbose due to hyperglycemic effects.
  Phenothiazines: May decrease the efficacy of acarbose due to hyperglycemic effects.
  Sulfonylureas: Acarbose may increase the hypoglycemic potential of sulfonylureas. Oral glucose (dextrose) should be used in the treatment of mild-to-moderate hypoglycemia; severe hypoglycemia may require the use of either intravenous glucose infusion or glucagon injection.
  Thyroid hormones: May decrease the efficacy of acarbose due to hyperglycemic effects.
Pregnancy Risk Factor B
Pregnancy Implications Abnormal blood glucose levels are associated with a higher incidence of congenital abnormalities. Insulin is the drug of choice for the control of diabetes mellitus during pregnancy. It is not known whether acarbose is excreted in human milk
Lactation Excretion in breast milk unknown/use caution
Nursing Implications Administer acarbose 3 times/day at the start (with the first bite) of each main meal. It is important to continue to adhere to dietary instructions, a regular exercise program, and regular testing of urine and/or blood glucose. The risk of hypoglycemia, its symptoms and treatment, and conditions that predispose to its development should be well understood by patients and responsible family members. A source of glucose (dextrose) should be readily available to treat symptoms of low blood glucose when taking acarbose in combination with a sulfonylurea or insulin. If side effects occur, they usually develop during the first few weeks of therapy and are mild to moderate GI effects, such as flatulence, diarrhea, or abdominal discomfort and generally diminish in frequency and intensity with time.
Specific References
  Hsiao SH, Liao LH, Cheng PN, et al, "Hepatotoxicity Associated with Acarbose Therapy," *Ann Pharmacother*, 2006, 40(1):151-4.

Acebutolol

Pronunciation (a se BYOO toe lole)
Related Information
  ● Selected Properties of Beta-Adrenergic Blocking Drugs
CAS Number 34381-68-5; 37517-30-9
U.S. Brand Names Sectral®
Synonyms Acebutolol Hydrochloride
Impairment Potential Yes

Use Treatment of hypertension; ventricular arrhythmias; angina

Mechanism of Action Competitively blocks beta$_1$-adrenergic receptors with little or no effect on beta$_2$-receptors except at high doses. Exhibits membrane stabilizing and intrinsic sympathomimetic activity ("quinidine-like effect"); low lipid solubility, therefore, little crosses blood-brain barrier.

Adverse Reactions

Cardiovascular: Persistent bradycardia, hypotension, chest pain, edema, heart failure, exacerbation of Raynaud's phenomenon, sinus bradycardia, myocardial depression, palpitations, QT prolongation

Central nervous system: CNS depression, confusion, dizziness, **fatigue**, drowsiness, night terrors, insomnia, headache, electroencephalogram abnormalities

Dermatologic: Exanthema, erythema multiforme, alopecia, toxic epidermal necrolysis, xerosis, urticaria, onycholysis, pruritus, psoriasis, licheniform eruptions, cutaneous vasculitis

Gastrointestinal: Constipation, abdominal pain, diarrhea, nausea, vomiting

Genitourinary: Impotence

Hepatic: Elevated liver enzymes

Respiratory: Hypersensitivity pneumonitis, pleurisy, pulmonary granulomas, rhinitis

Miscellaneous: Hyperhidrosis, cold extremities, lupus syndrome

Signs and Symptoms of Overdose Asystole, ataxia, bradycardia, cardiovascular collapse, cough, depression, dyspepsia, dyspnea, electromechanical dissociation, first degree AV block, flatulence, heart failure, hyperglycemia, hypoglycemia, hypotension, impotence, insomnia, myalgia, myasthenia gravis (exacerbation or precipitation), nocturia, QRS prolongation, wheezing

Pharmacodynamics/Kinetics

Onset of action: 1-2 hours

Duration: 12-24 hours

Absorption: Oral: 40%

Protein binding: 5% to 15%

Metabolism: Extensive first-pass effect

Half-life elimination: 6-7 hours

Time to peak: 2-4 hours

Excretion: Feces (~55%); urine (35%)

Dosage

Oral:

Adults:

Hypertension: 400-800 mg/day (larger doses may be divided); maximum: 1200 mg/day; usual dose range (JNC 7): 200-800 mg/day in 2 divided doses

Ventricular arrhythmias: Initial: 400 mg/day; maintenance: 600-1200 mg/day in divided doses

Elderly: Initial: 200-400 mg/day; dose reduction due to age related decrease in Cl$_{cr}$ will be necessary; do not exceed 800 mg/day

Dosing adjustment in renal impairment:

Cl$_{cr}$ 25-49 mL/minute/1.73 m^2: Reduce dose by 50%.

Cl$_{cr}$ <25 mL/minute/1.73 m^2: Reduce dose by 75%.

Dosing adjustment in hepatic impairment: Use with caution.

Monitoring Parameters Blood pressure, orthostatic hypotension, heart rate, CNS effects, ECG

Administration

To discontinue therapy, taper dose gradually. May be administered without regard to meals.

Contraindications Hypersensitivity to beta-blocking agents; uncompensated congestive heart failure; cardiogenic shock; bradycardia or second- and third-degree heart block (except in patients with a functioning artificial pacemaker); sinus node dysfunction; pregnancy (2nd and 3rd trimesters)

Warnings Abrupt withdrawal of drug **should be avoided.** May result in an exaggerated cardiac responsiveness such as tachycardia, hypertension, ischemia, angina, myocardial infarction, and sudden death. It is recommended that patients be gradually tapered off beta-blockers (over a 2-week period) rather than via abrupt discontinuation. Although acebutolol primarily blocks beta$_1$-receptors, high doses can result in beta$_2$-receptor blockage. Use with caution in diabetic patients. Beta-blockers may impair glucose tolerance, potentiate hypoglycemia, and/or mask symptoms of hypoglycemia in a diabetic patient. Use with caution in bronchospastic lung disease and renal dysfunction (especially the elderly). Beta-blockers with intrinsic sympathomimetic activity do not appear to be of benefit in CHF and should be avoided. See Dosage - Renal/Hepatic Impairment.

Dosage Forms Capsule, as hydrochloride: 200 mg, 400 mg

Reference Range Acebutolol serum levels >13 mg/L associated with fatality

Overdosage/Treatment

Decontamination: Lavage (within 1 hour)/activated charcoal

Supportive therapy: Initiate support with fluids; epinephrine or dopamine may be useful; glucagon may be particularly effective for reversing cardiac manifestations; sympathomimetics (eg, epinephrine, dopamine, or amrinone), atropine, isoproterenol, glucagon, or a pacemaker may be used to treat the toxic bradycardia, asystole, and/or hypotension; acebutolol-induced ventricular tachycardia may respond to I.V. sodium bicarbonate (1-2 mEq/kg). The glucagon dose is 50-150 mcg/kg I.V. (~5-10 mg in adults) over 1 minute followed by continuous infusion of 1-5 mg/hour.

Enhancement of elimination: Multiple-dose activated charcoal may be effective; hemodialysis (4 hours) and extracorporeal oxygenation (12 hours) has been used successfully in one case

Test Interactions ↑ triglycerides, potassium, uric acid, cholesterol (S), glucose; ↓ HDL

Drug Interactions

Inhibits CYP2D6 (weak)

Alpha-blockers (prazosin, terazosin): Concurrent use of beta-blockers may increase risk of orthostasis.

Clonidine: Hypertensive crisis after or during withdrawal of either agent.

Drugs which slow AV conduction (digoxin): Effects may be additive with beta-blockers.

Glucagon: Acebutolol may blunt the hyperglycemic action of glucagon.

Insulin and oral hypoglycemics: Acebutolol masks the tachycardia from hypoglycemia.

NSAIDs (ibuprofen, indomethacin, naproxen, piroxicam) may reduce the antihypertensive effects of beta-blockers.

Salicylates may reduce the antihypertensive effects of beta-blockers.

Sulfonylureas: Beta-blockers may alter response to hypoglycemic agents.

Verapamil or diltiazem may have synergistic or additive pharmacological effects when taken concurrently with beta-blockers.

Pregnancy Risk Factor B (manufacturer); D (2nd and 3rd trimesters - expert analysis)

Pregnancy Implications Acebutolol crosses the placenta. Beta-blockers have been associated with persistent bradycardia, hypotension, and IUGR; IUGR is probably related to maternal hypertension. Available evidence suggests beta-blockers are generally safe during pregnancy (JNC-7). Cases of neonatal hypoglycemia have been reported following maternal use of beta-blockers at parturition or during breast-feeding.

Lactation Enters breast milk/use caution

Additional Information Since bioavailability has been shown to increase about twofold in the elderly, they may require lower maintenance doses; therefore, as serum and tissue concentrations increase, beta$_1$ selectivity diminishes.

Specific References

Chobanian AV, Bakris GL, Black HR, et al, "The Seventh Report of the Joint National Committee on Prevention, Detection, Evaluation, and Treatment of High Blood Pressure: The JNC 7 Report," *JAMA*, 2003, 289(19):2560-71.

Acetaminophen

Pronunciation (a seet a MIN oh fen)

Related Information

● Donor Victims of Poisoning in Whom Transplantation of Organs Occurred

CAS Number 103-90-2

U.S. Brand Names Acephen® [OTC]; Aspirin Free Anacin® Maximum Strength [OTC]; Cetafen Extra® [OTC]; Cetafen® [OTC]; Comtrex® Sore Throat Maximum Strength [OTC]; ElixSure™ Fever/Pain [OTC]; Feverall® [OTC]; Genapap® Children [OTC]; Genapap® Extra Strength [OTC]; Genapap® Infant [OTC]; Genapap® [OTC]; Genebs® Extra Strength [OTC]; Genebs® [OTC]; Mapap® Arthritis [OTC]; Mapap® Children's [OTC]; Mapap® Extra Strength [OTC]; Mapap® Infants [OTC]; Mapap® [OTC]; Redutemp® [OTC]; Silapap® Children's [OTC]; Silapap® Infants [OTC]; Tylenol® 8 Hour [OTC]; Tylenol® Arthritis Pain [OTC]; Tylenol® Children's [OTC]; Tylenol® Extra Strength [OTC]; Tylenol® Infants [OTC]; Tylenol® Junior Strength [OTC]; Tylenol® Sore Throat [OTC]; Tylenol® [OTC]; Valorin Extra [OTC]; Valorin [OTC]

Synonyms APAP; N-Acetyl-P-Aminophenol; Paracetamol

Use

Treatment of mild to moderate pain and fever (antipyretic/analgesic); does not have antirheumatic or anti-inflammatory effects

First used clinically in the United States in 1950

Mechanism of Action

Inhibits the synthesis of prostaglandin E$_2$ in the central nervous system and peripherally blocks pain impulse generation; produces antipyresis from inhibition of hypothalamic heat-regulating center

Exhibits Mild anti inflammatory effects via inhibition of peripheral COX-2

Adverse Reactions

Cardiovascular: Rare cardiomyopathy, bradycardia, cardiomegaly, pericardial effusion/pericarditis, Reye's-like syndrome, vasculitis, leukocytoclastic vasculitis

Central nervous system: Hypothermia

Dermatologic: Rash, toxic epidermal necrolysis, exanthema, pityriasis rosea-like reaction, erythema multiforme, acute generalized exanthematous pustulosis, alopecia, angioedema, urticaria, purpura, Stevens-Johnson syndrome, pruritus, erythema nodosum, exanthem, cutaneous vasculitis

Endocrine & metabolic: Elevated serum transaminases, hyponatremia, hypophosphatemia

Gastrointestinal: Vomiting, nausea, diarrhea, pancreatitis

Hematologic: Leukemoid reaction, thrombocytopenia

Hepatic: Hepatic encephalopathy, hepatitis (fulminant) with centrilobular necrosis (zone 3), jaundice, cirrhosis, liver transaminase rise may occur within 24 hours of ingestion, centrilobular hepatic necrosis, primary biliary cirrhosis, hepatic vasculitis

Ocular: Mydriasis, nystagmus, vision color changes (yellow tinge)

Renal: Renal injury with chronic use, acute tubular necrosis; renal failure (acute) is uncommon in overdose

Respiratory: Eosinophilic pneumonia, pulmonary vasculitis

Miscellaneous: Hypersensitivity reactions (rare), fixed drug eruption

Signs and Symptoms of Overdose The acute symptomatic presentation of acetaminophen toxicity can be divided into 4 phases:

Phase I (up to 1 day): Gastrointestinal irritability predominates with nausea, vomiting, and sweating. Large ingestions (>75 g in adults; >10 g in pediatric patients) can result in metabolic acidosis within 4 hours of ingestion. Cardiac effects (arrhythmias, bradycardia) may develop.

Phase II (1-3 days): Hepatic toxicity develops with elevation of hepatic enzymes, prothrombin time, and bilirubin. Amylase elevation may peak at 2 days. The patient may otherwise be asymptomatic. Oliguric renal failure may develop and may coincide with hepatic encephalopathy.

Phase III (3-5 days): Hepatic necrosis continues with disseminated intravascular coagulation, hepatic encephalopathy, portal hypertension, and icterus. The patient is at risk for hypoglycemia. Renal insufficiency may also be present.

Phase IV (5-14 days): Recovery with resolution of elevated hepatic enzymes usually occurs.

Admission Criteria/Prognosis Admit any patient with a 4 hour plasma acetaminophen level >150 mg/L or abnormal liver function tests, acidosis, or adult or adolescent ingestions >125 mg/kg

Pharmacodynamics/Kinetics

Onset of action: <1 hour

Duration: 4-6 hours

Absorption: Incomplete; varies by dosage form

Protein binding: 8% to 43% at toxic doses

Metabolism: At normal therapeutic dosages, hepatic to sulfate and glucuronide metabolites, while a small amount is metabolized by CYP to a highly reactive intermediate (acetylimidoquinone) which is conjugated with glutathione and inactivated; at toxic doses (as little as 4 g daily) glutathione conjugation becomes insufficient to meet the metabolic demand causing an increase in acetylimidoquinone concentration, which may cause hepatic cell necrosis

Half-life elimination: Prolonged following toxic doses

Neonates: 2-5 hours

Adults: 1-3 hours (may be increased in elderly; however, this should not affect dosing)

Time to peak, serum: Oral: 10-60 minutes; may be delayed in acute overdoses

Excretion: Urine (2% to 5% unchanged; 55% as glucuronide metabolites; 30% as sulphate metabolites)

Dosage

Oral, rectal:

Children <12 years: 10-15 mg/kg/dose every 4-6 hours as needed; do **not** exceed 5 doses (2.6 g) in 24 hours; alternatively, the following doses may be used. See table.

Acetaminophen Dosing

Age	Dosage (mg)	Age	Dosage (mg)
0-3 mo	40	4-5 y	240
4-11 mo	80	6-8 y	320
1-2 y	120	9-10 y	400
2-3 y	160	11 y	480

Note: Higher rectal doses have been studied for use in preoperative pain control in children. However, specific guidelines are not available and dosing may be product dependent. The safety and efficacy of alternating acetaminophen and ibuprofen dosing has not been established.

Adults: 325-650 mg every 4-6 hours or 1000 mg 3-4 times/day; do **not** exceed 4 g/day

Toxic dosage for hepatitis: 200 mg/kg

Dosing interval in renal impairment:

Cl_{cr} 10-50 mL/minute: Administer every 6 hours

Cl_{cr} <10 mL/minute: Administer every 8 hours (metabolites accumulate)

Dosing adjustment/comments in hepatic impairment: Appears to be well tolerated in cirrhosis; serum levels may need monitoring with long-term use

Nomogram: Plasma or Serum Acetaminophen Concentration vs Time Post Acetaminophen Ingestion

Estimating potential for hepatotoxicity:
The following nomogram has been developed to estimate the probability that plasma levels in relation to intervals postingestion will result in hepatotoxicity.

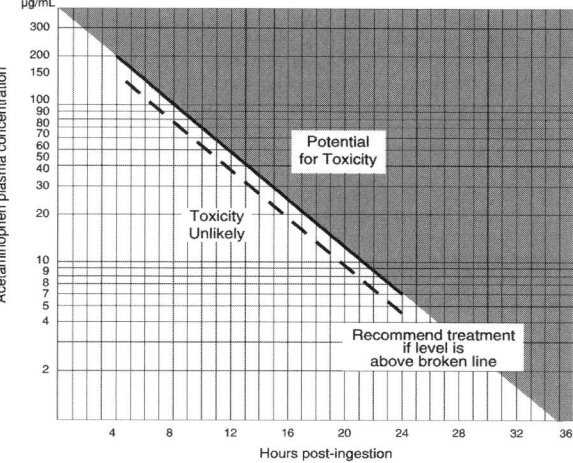

From Rumack BH and Matthew H, "Acetaminophen Poisoning and Toxicity," *Pediatrics*, June 1975, 55:871-6 with permission.

If the acetaminophen level determined at least 4 hours following an overdose falls above the broken line, administer the entire course of acetylcysteine treatment.

If the acetaminophen level, determined at least 4 hours following an overdose, falls below the broken line, acetylcysteine treatment is not necessary or if already initiated may be discontinued. Serum levels drawn before 4 hours may not represent peak levels.

Cautions for Use of this Chart:
1. The time coordinates refer to time postingestion.
2. The graph relates only to plasma levels following a single acute overdose ingestion.
3. The broken line, which represents a 25% allowance below the solid line, is included to allow for possible errors in acetaminophen plasma assays and estimated time from ingestion of an overdose.

Monitoring Parameters Relief of pain or fever

Administration Suppositories: Do not freeze.

Suspension, oral: Shake well before pouring a dose.

Contraindications Hypersensitivity to acetaminophen or any component of the formulation

Warnings

Limit dose to <4 g/day. May cause severe hepatic toxicity on acute overdose; in addition, chronic daily dosing in adults has resulted in liver damage in some patients. Use with caution in patients with alcoholic liver disease; consuming ≥3 alcoholic drinks/day may increase the risk of liver damage. Use caution in patients with known G6PD deficiency.

OTC labeling: When used for self-medication, patients should be instructed to contact healthcare provider if used for fever lasting >3 days or for pain lasting >10 days in adults or >5 days in children.

Dosage Forms

[DSC] = Discontinued product

Caplet: 500 mg

Cetafen Extra® Strength, Genapap™ Extra Strength, Genebs Extra Strength, Mapap Extra Strength, Tycolene Maximum Strength, Tylenol® Extra Strength: 500 mg

Caplet, extended release:

Tylenol® 8 Hour, Tylenol® Arthritis Pain: 650 mg

Capsule: 500 mg

Elixir: 160 mg/5 mL (120 mL, 480 mL, 3780 mL)

Apra Children's: 160 mg/5 mL (120 mL, 480 mL, 3780 mL) [alcohol free; contains benzoic acid; cherry and grape flavors]

Mapap Children's: 160 mg/5 mL (120 mL) [alcohol free; contains benzoic acid and sodium benzoate; cherry flavor]

Gelcap:

Mapap Extra Strength, Tylenol® Extra Strength: 500 mg

Geltab:

Tylenol® Extra Strength: 500 mg

Geltab, extended release:

Tylenol® 8 Hour: 650 mg

Liquid, oral: 500 mg/15 mL (240 mL)

Comtrex® Sore Throat Maximum Strength: 500 mg/15 mL (240 mL) [contains sodium benzoate; honey lemon flavor]

Genapap™ Children: 160 mg/5 mL (120 mL) [contains sodium benzoate; cherry and grape flavors]

Silapap®: 160 mg/5 mL (120 mL, 240 mL, 480 mL) [sugar free; contains sodium benzoate; cherry flavor]

Tylenol® Extra Strength: 500 mg/15 mL (240 mL) [contains sodium benzoate; cherry flavor]

Solution, oral: 160 mg/5 mL (120 mL, 480 mL)

Solution, oral drops: 80 mg/0.8 mL (15 mL) [droppers are marked at 0.4 mL (40 mg) and at 0.8 mL (80 mg)]

Genapap™ Infant: 80 mg/0.8 mL (15 mL) [fruit flavor]

Infantaire: 80 mg/0.8mL (15 mL, 30 mL)

Silapap® Infant's: 80 mg/0.8 mL (15 mL, 30 mL) [contains sodium benzoate; cherry flavor]

Suppository, rectal: 120 mg, 325 mg, 650 mg

Acephen™: 120 mg, 325 mg, 650 mg

FeverALL®: 80 mg, 120 mg, 325 mg, 650 mg

Mapap: 125 mg, 650 mg

Suspension, oral:

Mapap Children's: 160 mg/5 mL (120 mL) [contains sodium benzoate; cherry flavor]

Nortemp Children's: 160 mg/5 mL (120 mL) [alcohol free; contains sodium benzoate; cotton candy flavor]

Tylenol® Children's: 160 mg/5 mL (120 mL, 240 mL) [contains sodium benzoate; bubble gum yum, cherry blast, dye free cherry, grape splash, and very berry strawberry flavors]

Tylenol® Children's with Flavor Creator: 160 mg/5 mL (120 mL) [contains sodium 2 mg/5 mL and sodium benzoate; cherry blast flavor; packaged with apple (4), bubblegum (8), chocolate (4), & strawberry (4) sugar free flavor packets]

Suspension, oral drops:

Mapap Infants: 80 mg/0.8 mL (15 mL, 30 mL) [contains sodium benzoate; cherry flavor]

Tylenol® Infants: 80 mg/0.8 mL (15 mL, 30 mL) [contains sodium benzoate; cherry, dye free cherry, and grape flavors]

Syrup, oral:

ElixSure™ Fever/Pain: 160 mg/5 mL (120 mL) [bubble gum, cherry, and grape flavors] [DSC]

Tablet: 325 mg, 500 mg

Aspirin Free Anacin® Extra Strength, Genapap™ Extra Strength, Genebs Extra Strength, Mapap Extra Strength, Pain Eze, Tylenol® Extra Strength, Valorin Extra: 500 mg

Cetafen®, Genapap™, Genebs, Mapap, Tycolene, Tylenol®, Valorin: 325 mg

Tablet, chewable: 80 mg

Genapap™ Children: 80 mg [contains phenylalanine 6 mg/tablet; fruit and grape flavors]

Mapap Children's: 80 mg [contains phenylalanine 3 mg/tablet; bubble gum, fruit, and grape flavors]

Mapap Junior Strength: 160 mg [contains phenylalanine 12 mg/tablet; grape flavor]

Tylenol® Children's: 80 mg [fruit and grape flavors contain phenylalanine 3 mg/tablet; bubble gum flavor contains phenylalanine 6 mg/tablet] [DSC]

Tylenol® Junior: 160 mg [contains phenylalanine 6 mg/tablet; fruit and grape flavors] [DSC]

Tablet, orally disintegrating: 80 mg, 160 mg

Tylenol® Children's Meltaways: 80 mg [bubble gum, grape, and watermelon flavors]

Tylenol® Junior Meltaways: 160 mg [bubble gum and grape flavors]

Reference Range Patients with concentrations >150 mg/L before 4 hours can be empirically treated with acetylcysteine until repeat concentration after 4 hours has been obtained and interpreted; analgesic/antipyretic reference range: 10-30 mg/L (66-199 µmol/L); the antigenic biomarker (3-[cystein-s-yl]-APAP protein adducts [3-cys-A]) appearance in serum may be useful to confirm the diagnosis of acetaminophen-induced hepatic injury

Overdosage/Treatment

Decontamination: Lavage within 1 hour of overdose, activated charcoal if <2 hours following ingestion. While activated charcoal can decrease acetaminophen bioavailability by 30% when given within 1 hour postingestion, it does not appear useful if given at longer than 2 hours postingestion. Gastrointestinal decontamination may be more effective if more than 10 extended release tablets are ingested at 8 hours postingestion.

Supportive therapy: Acetylcysteine (antidote) indicated for:

Any patient with a serum concentration above probable risk line on Rumack-Matthew nomogram

Any patient presenting ≥24 hours following an ingestion with evidence of hepatic toxicity

Empirically for any ingestion of ≥200 mg/kg where availability of serum concentration results exceeds 8 hours following ingestion; N-acetylcysteine is given orally 140 mg/kg followed by 70 mg/kg every 4 hours for 17 doses; although shorter 20-48 intravenous courses can be used also

See Acetylcysteine [ANTIDOTE]. See flow chart.

Acetadote® Treatment Flowchart

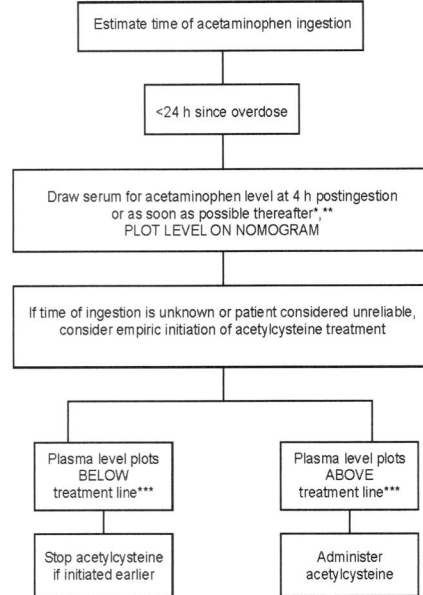

* Acetaminophen levels drawn <4 hours postingestion may be misleading.
** With the extended-release preparation, an acetaminophen level drawn <8 hours postingestion may be misleading. Draw a second level at 4-6 hours.
*** Acetylcysteine may be withheld until acetaminophen assay results are available as long as initiation of treatment is not delayed beyond 8 hours postingestion. If more than 8 hours postingestion, start acetylcysteine treatment immediately.

For persistent vomiting, metoclopramide (10 mg to 1 mg/kg I.V. or I.M. 30 minutes before N-acetylcysteine dose) can be used. Prochlorperazine (10 mg I.V.) can also be added to metoclopramide. Other agents which can be used include droperidol (1.25-2.5 mg I.V. in adult) or ondansetron (up to 0.15 mg/kg I.V.). If vomiting persists, a nasogastric tube or duodenal tube may need to be inserted and thus N-acetylcysteine can be infused over 30-60 minutes.

Combination antiemetic therapy, which is very effective, may include metoclopramide (10 mg I.V.) followed by ondansetron (0.15 mg/kg); granisetron (10 mcg/kg I.V.) given over 5 minutes may also be used; patients with INR >2 should receive prophylactic antibiotics and sucralfate; consider liver transplantation if serum pH is <7.3 (despite adequate fluid replacement), or PT is >50 seconds in U.S. (>100 seconds in Europe) and grade III/IV hepatic encephalopathy and creatinine >300 µmol/L (3.3 mg/dL). APACHE score >15 or serum phosphorous over 3.75 mg/dL are poor prognostic indicators.

Enhancement of elimination: Multiple dosing of activated charcoal may be effective, but is usually not required if N-acetylcysteine therapy is given; forced diuresis is of no benefit; hemodialysis removes significant amounts of acetaminophen especially in patients with severe hepatic and renal dysfunction; usually not required if acetylcysteine is given; moderately dialyzable (20% to 50%). Exchange transfusion has been used successfully.

Extracorporeal removal (by charcoal hemoperfusion and/or high-flux dialysis) can be considered if the patient has (1) not received N-acetylcysteine within first 15 hours postingestion and (2) is at high risk for severe liver damage according to the nomogram or has peak AST or ALT >5000 units/L

Antidote(s)
- Acetylcysteine [ANTIDOTE]

Diagnostic Procedures
- Acetaminophen, Serum

Test Interactions Can cause false elevation of urinary catecholamine and may interfere with blood glucose assays leading to false elevation of glucose; false-positive acetaminophen levels with hyperbilirubinemia >10 mg/L

Tylenol® Acetaminophen Extended Release

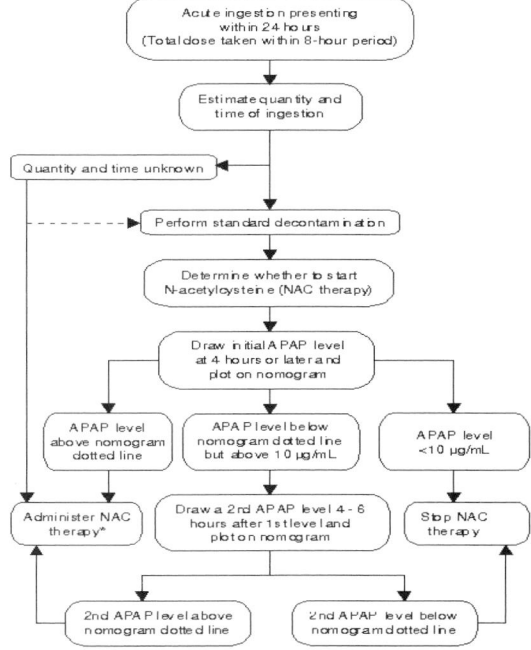

* See text for full discussion of NAC therapy, use of baseline LFTs, and other supportive care

Drug Interactions

Substrate (minor) of CYP1A2, 2A6, 2C9, 2D6, 2E1, 3A4; **Inhibits** CYP3A4 (weak)

Decreased effect: Barbiturates, carbamazepine, hydantoins, rifampin, sulfinpyrazone may decrease the analgesic effect of acetaminophen. Cholestyramine may decrease acetaminophen absorption (separate dosing by at least 1 hour).

Increased toxicity: Barbiturates, carbamazepine, hydantoins, isoniazid, rifampin, sulfinpyrazone may increase the hepatotoxic potential of acetaminophen. Chronic ethanol abuse increases risk for acetaminophen toxicity; effect of warfarin may be enhanced.

Pregnancy Risk Factor B

Pregnancy Implications Fetal liver toxicity can occur in overdose situations

Lactation Enters breast milk/compatible

Additional Information Toxic dosage for hepatitis: See Usual Dosage.

Cimetidine is not effective for hepatoprotection in acetaminophen overdose.

The 4-hour serum concentration can be approximated by 0.59 × the amount ingested as mg/kg in patients taking only acetaminophen; acetylcysteine is not useful for treatment of renal disease induced by acetaminophen. For extended relief product ingestions, draw an acetaminophen level at least 4 hours postingestion; a second and third acetaminophen level should be drawn every 4-6 hours after the initial level. These levels should be plotted on the Rumack-Matthew nomogram at the times each were drawn; if any of the plasma levels are above the hepatotoxic line on the Rumack-Matthew nomogram, the entire course of acetylcysteine treatment should be administered; or, if initiated, completed. There is increased risk of liver toxicity in individuals who ingest 3 or more ethanol-containing beverages daily. See Overdosage/Treatment flow chart (Tylenol® Acetaminophen Extended Release) . When sustained release acetaminophen and drugs that slow GI motility are coingested, prolonged monitoring of levels is justified. In an *in vitro* model, with ingestion of >10 tablets of extended release tablets there was an increase in the number of tablets that did not disintegrate at 8 hours.

A peak prothrombin time of 25 seconds at 2 days postingestion, or 40 seconds at 3 days, will usually be associated with hepatic encephalopathy (grade III) in acetaminophen overdose. Note that N-acetylcysteine can prolong clotting time. A normal initial prothrombin time correlates with a good outcome in acetaminophen overdose.

Predictors for fatal outcome include arterial pH <7.3, prothrombin time >50 seconds in the U.S. (>100 seconds in Europe), creatinine (least discriminating) >3.4 mg/dL (>300 µmol/L). The combination of prothrombin time >50 seconds (>100 seconds in Europe) and serum creatinine >3.4 mg/dL (>300 µmol/L), with grade III to IV hepatic encephalopathy, is the best predictor of death (predictive accuracy of

0.83). Other predictors of mortality include a plasma factor V concentration ≤10% of normal (especially in conjunction with a significant rise in factor VIII, leading to a factor VIII to factor V ratio >30, or severe hepatic coma within 72 hours of overdose). The above criteria may be useful in the selection for liver transplantation.

High-dose (>1 g) acetaminophen may cause bronchospasm in aspirin-sensitive asthmatic patients.

Watercress (*Nasturtium officinale*) can cause a decrease in oxidative metabolites of acetaminophen.

An increase of serum alpha-fetoprotein levels higher than 3.9 mcg/L on the day after the peak level of alanine aminotransferase may predict survival from severe acetaminophen-induced hepatotoxicity.

Specific References

Amato CS, Wang RY, Wright RO, et al, "Evaluation of Promotility Agents to Limit the Gut Bioavailability of Extended-Release Acetaminophen," *J Toxicol Clin Toxicol*, 2004, 42(1):73-7.

Amitai Y, Mitchell AA, McGuigan MA, et al, "Comment on Acetaminophen: The 150 mg/kg Myth," *Clin Toxicol (Phila)*, 2005, 43(3):217.

Anderson K, Dahl B, HbisA, et al, "Serious Liver Injury from an Acute Pediatric Acetaminophen Ingestion," *Clin Toxicol (Phila)*, 2005, 43:660.

Bailey B, Amre DK, and Gaudreault, "Fulminant Hepatic Failure Secondary to Acetaminophen Poisoning: A Systematic Review and Meta-Analysis of Prognostic Criteria Determining the Need for Liver Transplantation," *Crit Care Med*, 2003, 31(1):299-305.

Bailey JE, Bogdan GM, and Dart RC, "Liver Injury During Repeated Dosing of Acetaminophen (APAP): What Does the Medical Literature Really Say?" *Clin Toxicol*, 2005, 43:638.

Balit CR, Hartley V, Shieffelbien L, et al, "Acetaminophen Poisoning: An International Comparison," *J Toxicol Clin Toxicol*, 2003, 41(5):717-8.

Bartels SA, Crosby DL, Richard JI, et al, "Dos Maximal Therapeutic Dosing of Acetaminophen Perturb Hepatic Biomarkers in Recently Abstinent Alcoholics?" *Clin Toxicol (Phila)*, 2005, 43:680.

Bateman DN, Gorman DR, Bain M, et al, "Restricting Acetaminophen Pack Size - Does It Make a Difference?" *Clin Toxicol (Phila)*, 2005, 43:712.

Bentur Y, Basis F, and Keyes D, "The Reliability of History in Suicidal Patients: Is Routine APAP Screening Required?" *J Toxicol Clin Toxicol*, 2004, 42(5):743.

Beuhler MC and Curry SC, "False Positive Acetaminophen Levels Associated with Hyperbilirubinemia," *Clin Toxicol (Phila)*, 2005, 43(3):167-70.

Bogdan GM, Kuffner EK, Green JL, et al, "Evaluation of Hepatotoxicity in Alcoholic Patients from 3-Day Maximal Therapeutic Dosing of Acetaminophen (APAP)," *J Toxicol Clin Toxicol*, 2004, 42(5):798-9.

Bond GR, "A New Acetaminophen Nomogram with a Different Purpose," *Ann Emerg Med*, 2005, 46(3):272-4.

Bond GR, "Reduced Toxicity of Acetaminophen in Children: It's the Liver," *J Toxicol Clin Toxicol*, 2004, 42(2):149-52 (review).

Bond GR, Wiegand CB, and Hite LK, "The Difficulty of Risk Assessment for Hepatic Injury Associated with Supra-Therapeutic Acetaminophen Use," *Vet Hum Toxicol*, 2003, 45(3):150-3.

Bryant S, Bellamy L, Paloucek F, et al, "Acute Acetaminophen Poisoning in Children: Kids Aren't Just Little Adults," *J Emerg Med*, 2003, 24(4):472-3.

Burillo-Putze G, Mintegui S, and Munne P, "Changes in Pediatric Toxic Dose of Acetaminophen," *Am J Emerg Med*, 2004, 22(4):323.

Burkhart KK, Garcia M, and Donovan JW, "Coingestion of Iron May Enhance Acetaminophen Toxicity," *Int J Med Toxicol*, 2003, 6(2):9.

Daubert GP, Smolinske S, and White S, "Chronic Acetaminophen Exposure Resulting in Hepatorenal Failure in a Neonate Treated with Acetadote®," *Clin Toxicol*, 2005, 43:634.

Famularo G, De Maria S, Minisola G, et al, "Severe Acquired Hemophilia with Factor VIII Inhibition Associated with Acetaminophen and Chlorpheniramine," *Ann Pharmacother*, 2004, 38(9):1432-4.

Fosnocht DE and Caravati EM, "Does This Medication Contain Acetaminophen?" *Ann Emerg Med*, 2003, 42(4):S21.

Gelotte CK, Auiler JF, Temple Ar, et al, "Clinical Features of a Repeat-Dose Multiple-Day Pharmacokinetics Trial of Acetaminophen at 4, 6, and 8 g/Day," *J Toxicol Clin Toxicol*, 2003, 41(5):726.

Goklaney A, Mullins ME, Halcomb SE, et al, "Pharmacokinetic Effects of Co-Ingested Diphenhydramine or Oxycodone on Simulated Acetaminophen Overdose," *Acad Emerg Med*, 2003, 10:510a.

Goldman RD and Scolnik D, "Underdosing of Acetaminophen By Parents and Emergency Department Utilization," *Pediatr Emerg Care*, 2004, 20(2):89-93.

Graham GG and Scott KF, "Mechanism of Action of Paracetamol," *Am J Ther*, 2005, 12(1):46-55.

Green JL, Dart RC, and Bogdan GM, "Summary of Sustained-Release Acetaminophen (SR-APAP) Data from the American Association of Poison Control Centers (AAPCC)," *J Toxicol Clin Toxicol*, 2004, 42(5):738.

Green JL, Kuffner EK, Bogdan GM, et al, "Hepatic Function in Alcoholics Throughout 5 Days of Maximal Therapeutic Dosing of Acetaminophen (APAP)," *Clin Toxicol (Phila)*, 2005, 43:683.

Greene SL, Dargan PI, Leman P, et al, "Adherence to Legislation Limiting Acetaminophen Availability in the United Kingdom," *Clin Toxicol (Phila)*, 2005, 43:712.

Greene SL, Leman P, Kerins M, et al, "Paracetamol (Acetaminophen) Overdose in the United Kingdom; Where Do Patients Obtain the Tablets?" *J Toxicol Clin Toxicol*, 2003, 41(5):705.

Hodman MJ, Horn JF, Stork CM, et al, "Profound Metabolic Acidosis and Oxoprolinuria After Acetaminophen Use," *J Toxicol Clin Toxicol*, 2004, 42(5):719.

Hofbauer RD and Holger JS, et al, "The Use of Cholecystokinin as an Adjunctive Treatment for Toxin Ingestion," *J Toxicol Clin Toxicol*, 2004, 42(1):61-6.

Houle J, Ondiveeran HK, BeGora A, et al, "Hepatic Microvascular Response to Acetaminophen Toxicity," *Clin Toxicol (Phila)*, 2005, 43:681.

Hur C, Simon LS, and Gazelle GS, "Analysis of Aspirin-Associated Risks in Healthy Individuals," *Ann Pharmacother*, 2005, 39(1):51-7.

Kirages TJ, Sule HP, and Mycyk MB, "Severe Manifestations of Coricidin Intoxication," *Am J Emerg Med*, 2003, 21(6):473-5.

Koivusalo AM, Yildirim Y, Vakkuri A, et al, "Experience with Albumin Dialysis in Five Patients with Severe Overdoses of Paracetamol," *Acta Anaesthesiol Scand*, 2003, 47(9):1145-50.

Kurtovic J and Riordan SM, "Paracetamol-Induced Hepatotoxicity at Recommended Dosage," *J Intern Med*, 2003, 253(2):240-3.

Lai MW, Friedman D, Kalmowitz BD, et al, "Extracorporeal Removal of Acetaminophen," *J Toxicol Clin Toxicol*, 2004, 42(5):748.

Liu YP, Fang CC, Chen WJ, et al, "Fulminant Hepatic Failure Due to Chronic Acetaminophen Intoxication in an Infant," *Am J Emerg Med*, 2005, 23(1):94-5.

Losek JD, "Acetaminophen Dose Accuracy and Pediatric Emergency Care," *Pediatr Emerg Care*, 2004, 20(5):285-8.

Ly BT, Schneir AB, and Clark RF, "Effect of Whole Bowel Irrigation on the Pharmacokinetics of an Acetaminophen Formulation and Progression of Radiopaque Markers Through the Gastrointestinal Tract," *Ann Emerg Med*, 2004, 43(2):189-95.

Maloney GE, Rhee JW, Schuermann T, et al, "Fulminant Hepatic Failure After Using Reported Herbal Medication Containing High Levels of Acetaminophen," *Clin Toxicol (Phila)*, 2005, 43:760.

Marshall LL, "Angioedema Associated with Aspirin and Rofecoxib," *Ann Pharmacother*, 2005, 39(5):944-8.

Matsumoto T, Sano T, Matsuoka T, et al, "Simultaneous Determination of Carisoprodol and Acetaminophen in an Attempted Suicide by Liquid Chromatography-Mass Spectrometry with Positive Electrospray Ionization," *J Anal Toxicol*, 2003, 27(2):118-22.

Nikles CJ, Yelland M, Del Mar C, et al, "The Role of Paracetamol in Chronic Pain: An Evidence-Based Approach," *Am J Ther*, 2005, 12(1):80-91.

Osborne ZP and Bryant SM, "Patients Discharged with a Prescription for Acetaminophen-Containing Narcotic Analgesics Do Not Receive Appropriate Written Instructions," *Am J Emerg Med*, 2003, 21(1):48-50.

Palmer RB, Green JL, Kuffner EK, et al, "Plasma Reduced Glutathione (GSH) in Alcoholics Receiving Maximal Therapeutic Doses of Acetaminophen," *J Toxicol Clin Toxicol*, 2003, 41(5):726.

Prior MJ, Cooper K, Cummins P, et al, "Acetaminophen Availability Increases in Canada with No Increase in the Incidence of Reports of Inpatient Hospitalizations with Acetaminophen Overdose and Acute Liver Toxicity," *Am J Ther*, 2004, 11(6):443-52.

Rhee JW, Leikin JB, Akhter S, et al, "Survival Following Liver Transplants Performed Following Acetaminophen Toxicity," *Clin Toxicol (Phila)*, 2005, 43:682.

Rowden AK, Norvell J, Eldridge DL, et al, "Updates on Acetaminophen Toxicity," *Med Clin N Am*, 2005, 89(6):1145-59 (review).

Rumack BH and Spykert DA, "An Acetaminophen Dosing Error in a Child - Commentary," *Int J Med Toxicol*, 2003, 6(2):8.

Salhanick SD, Pavlides S, Orlow D, et al, "Early Acetaminophen Toxicity Is Independent of NOS$_3$-Derived Nitric Oxide," *SAEM Annual Meeting Abstracts*, 2004, 468.

Sato RL, Wong JJ, Sumida SM, et al, "Efficacy of Superactivated Charcoal Administered Late (3 Hours) After Acetaminophen Overdose," *Am J Emerg Med*, 2003, 21(3):189-91.

Schier JG, Nelson LS, and Hoffman RS, "An Acetaminophen Dosing Error in a Child," *Int J Med Toxicol)*, 2003, 6(2):7.

Sivilotti ML, Good AM, Yarema MC, et al, "A New Predictor of Toxicity Following Acetaminophen Overdose Based on Pretreatment Exposure," *Clin Toxicol (Phila)*, 2005, 43(4):229-34.

Sivilotti ML, Good AM, Juurlink DN, et al, "Construction of a Novel Predictor of Hepatotoxicity Following Acetaminophen Overdose: Beyond the Nomogram," *J Toxicol Clin Toxicol*, 2003, 41(5):642.

Sivilotti ML, Green TJ, Yarema MC, et al, "Multiplying the Aminotransferase by the Acetaminophen Concentration to Identify Overdose Patients at Risk for Hepatotoxicity," *Clin Toxicol (Phila)*, 2005, 43:683.

Sivilotti ML, Yarema MC, Juurlink DN, et al, "Predicting Hepatotoxicity Following Acetaminophen Overdose: A Nomogram for the Post-N-AC Era," *J Toxicol Clin Toxicol*, 2003, 41(5):724.

Spiller HA, "Evaluation of Impact of Activated Charcoal (AC) Use in Acute Acetaminophen Overdoses Treated with N-Acetylcysteine (NAC)," *Clin Toxicol (Phila)*, 2005, 43:672.

Spiller HA, Winter ML, Klein-Schwartz W, et al, "Late Activated Charcoal Use in Acetaminophen Overdose," *J Toxicol Clin Toxicol*, 2003, 41(5):725.

Spillum BJ, Tosterud M, Foss A, et al, "Fulminant Liver Failure from Moderate Paracetamol (Acetaminophen), Ferrous Sulphate, and Ethanol Overdose, Successfully Treated by Liver Transplantation: A Case Report," *Clin Toxicol (Phila)*, 2005, 43:742.

Temple AR, Lynch JM, Vena J, et al, "Amino Tranferase Activities in Healthy Subjects Receiving Three-Day Dosing of 4, 6 or 8 Grams per Day of Acetaminophen," *Clin Toxicol*, 2007, 45(1):36-44.

Tenenbein M, "Acetaminophen: The 150 mg/kg Myth," *J Toxicol Clin Toxicol*, 2004, 42(2):145-8 (review).

Toes MJ, Jones AL, and Prescott L, "Drug Interactions with Paracetamol," *Am J Ther*, 2005, 12(1):56-66.

Vale JA and Kulig K, "Position Paper: Gastric Lavage," *J Toxicol Clin Toxicol*, 2004, 42(7):933-43.

von Mach MA, Hermanns-Clausen M, Koch I, et al, "Experiences of a Poison Center Network with Renal Insufficiency in Acetaminophen Overdose: An Analysis of 17 Cases," *Clin Toxicol (Phila)*, 2005, 43(1):31-7.

Walgren JL, Mitchell MD, and Thompson DC, " Role of Metabolism in Drug-Induced Idiosyncratic Hepatotoxicity," *Critical Reviews in Toxicology*, 2005, 35:325-61.

Waseem M, Bomann S, Gernsheimer J, et al, "Unusual Presentation of Acetaminophen Toxicity," *Am J Emerg Med*, 2003, 21(1):88-9.

Watkins PB, Kaplowitz N, Slattery JT, et al, "Aminotransferase Elevations in Healthy Adults Receiving 4 Grams of Acetaminophen Daily - A Randomized Controlled Trial," *JAMA*, 2006, 296(1):87-93.

Whelton A, "Appropriate Analgesia: An Evidence-Based Evaluation of the Role of Acetaminophen in Pain Management," *Am J Ther*, 2005, 12(1):43-5.

AcetaZOLAMIDE

Pronunciation (a set a ZOLE a mide)

Related Information

- Dichlorphenamide

CAS Number 59-66-5

U.S. Brand Names Diamox® Sequels®

Use Treatment of glaucoma (chronic simple open-angle, secondary glaucoma, preoperatively in acute angle-closure); drug-induced edema or edema due to congestive heart failure (adjunctive therapy); centrencephalic epilepsies (immediate release dosage form); prevention or amelioration of symptoms associated with acute mountain sickness

Unlabeled/Investigational Use Urine alkalinization; respiratory stimulant in COPD; metabolic alkalosis

Mechanism of Action Reversible inhibition of the enzyme carbonic anhydrase resulting in reduction of hydrogen ion secretion at the renal tubule and an increased renal excretion of sodium, potassium, bicarbonate, and water to decrease production of aqueous humor; also inhibits carbonic anhydrase in the central nervous system to retard abnormal and excessive discharge from CNS neurons

Adverse Reactions

Frequency not defined.

Cardiovascular: Flushing

Central nervous system: Ataxia, confusion, convulsions, depression, dizziness, drowsiness, excitement, fatigue, headache, malaise

Dermatologic: Allergic skin reaction, photosensitivity, Stevens-Johnson syndrome, toxic epidermal necrolysis, urticaria

Endocrine & metabolic: Electrolyte imbalance, growth retardation (children), hyperglycemia, hypoglycemia, hypokalemia, hyponatremia, metabolic acidosis,

Gastrointestinal: Appetite decreased, diarrhea, melena, nausea, taste alternation, vomiting

Genitourinary: Crystalluria, glycosuria, hematuria, polyuria, renal failure

Hematologic: Agranulocytosis, aplastic anemia, leukopenia, thrombocytopenia, thrombocytopenic purpura

Hepatic: Cholestatic jaundice, fulminant hepatic necrosis, hepatic insufficiency, liver function tests abnormal

Neuromuscular & skeletal: Flaccid paralysis, paresthesia

Ocular: Myopia

Otic: Hearing disturbance, tinnitus

Miscellaneous: Anaphylaxis

Pharmacodynamics/Kinetics

Onset of action: Capsule, extended release: 2 hours; I.V.: 2 minutes

Peak effect: Capsule, extended release: 8-12 hours; I.V.: 15 minutes; Tablet: 2-4 hours

Duration: Inhibition of aqueous humor secretion: Capsule, extended release: 18-24 hours; I.V.: 4-5 hours; Tablet: 8-12 hours

Distribution: Erythrocytes, kidneys; blood-brain barrier and placenta; distributes into milk (~30% of plasma concentrations)

Excretion: Urine (70% to 100% as unchanged drug)

Dosage

Note: I.M. administration is not recommended because of pain secondary to the alkaline pH

Children:

Glaucoma:

Oral: 8-30 mg/kg/day or 300-900 mg/m^2/day divided every 8 hours

I.V.: 20-40 mg/kg/24 hours divided every 6 hours, not to exceed 1 g/day

Edema: Oral, I.V.: 5 mg/kg or 150 mg/m^2 once every day

Epilepsy: Oral: 8-30 mg/kg/day in 1-4 divided doses, not to exceed 1 g/day; sustained release capsule is not recommended for treatment of epilepsy

Adults:

Glaucoma:

Chronic simple (open-angle): Oral: 250 mg 1-4 times/day or 500 mg sustained release capsule twice daily

Secondary, acute (closed-angle): I.V.: 250-500 mg, may repeat in 2-4 hours to a maximum of 1 g/day

Edema: Oral, I.V.: 250-375 mg once daily

Epilepsy: Oral: 8-30 mg/kg/day in 1-4 divided doses; **sustained release capsule is not recommended for treatment of epilepsy**

Mountain sickness: Oral: 250 mg every 8-12 hours (or 500 mg extended release capsules every 12-24 hours)

Therapy should begin 24-48 hours before and continue during ascent and for at least 48 hours after arrival at the high altitude

Urine alkalinization (unlabeled use): Oral: 5 mg/kg/dose repeated 2-3 times over 24 hours

Respiratory stimulant in COPD (unlabeled use): Oral, I.V.: 250 mg twice daily

Elderly: Oral: Initial: 250 mg twice daily; use lowest effective dose

Dosing adjustment in renal impairment:

Cl$_{cr}$ 10-50 mL/minute: Administer every 12 hours

Cl$_{cr}$ <10 mL/minute: Avoid use (ineffective)

Hemodialysis: Moderately dialyzable (20% to 50%)

Peritoneal dialysis: Supplemental dose is not necessary

Monitoring Parameters Intraocular pressure, potassium, serum bicarbonate; serum electrolytes, periodic CBC with differential

Administration

Oral: May cause an alteration in taste, especially carbonated beverages; short-acting tablets may be crushed and suspended in cherry or chocolate syrup to disguise the bitter taste of the drug, do not use fruit juices, alternatively submerge tablet in 10 mL of hot water and add 10 mL honey or syrup

Contraindications Hypersensitivity to acetazolamide, sulfonamides, or any component of the formulation; hepatic disease or insufficiency; decreased sodium and/or potassium levels; adrenocortical insufficiency, cirrhosis; hyperchloremic acidosis, severe renal disease or dysfunction; severe pulmonary obstruction; long-term use in noncongestive angle-closure glaucoma

Warnings

Use in impaired hepatic function may result in coma. Use with caution in patients with respiratory acidosis and diabetes mellitus. Impairment of mental alertness and/or physical coordination may occur. Chemical similarities are present among sulfonamides, sulfonylureas, carbonic anhydrase inhibitors, thiazides, and loop diuretics (except ethacrynic acid). Use in patients with sulfonamide allergy is specifically contra-indicated in product labeling, however, a risk of cross-reaction exists in patients with allergy to any of these compounds; avoid use when previous reaction has been severe. Discontinue if signs of hypersensitivity are noted.

I.M. administration is painful because of the alkaline pH of the drug; use by this route is not recommended.

Drug may cause substantial increase in blood glucose in some diabetic patients; malaise and complaints of tiredness and myalgia are signs of excessive dosing and acidosis in the elderly.

Dosage Forms Capsule, extended release:

Diamox® Sequels®: 500 mg

Injection, powder for reconstitution: 500 mg

Tablet: 125 mg, 250 mg

Reference Range

Therapeutic range: 5-20 mg/L

Peak plasma level: 16 mcg/mL after 250 mg of acetazolamide

Overdosage/Treatment

Decontamination: Lavage (within 1 hour)/activated charcoal

Enhancement of elimination: Hemodialysis may remove as much as 30% of dose if performed prior to significant distribution

Test Interactions May cause false-positive results for urinary protein with Albustix®, Labstix®, Albutest®, Bumintest®; interferes with HPLC theophylline assay

Drug Interactions

Inhibits CYP3A4 (weak)

Amphetamines: Urinary excretion of amphetamine may be decreased; magnitude and duration of effects may be enhanced.

Carbamazepine: May increase serum concentrations of carbamazepine.

Cyclosporine trough concentrations may be increased resulting in possible nephrotoxicity and neurotoxicity.

Flecainide: May decrease excretion of flecainide.

Lithium: Serum concentrations may be decreased by acetazolamide; monitor.

Memantine: May decrease excretion of memantine.

Methenamine: Urinary antiseptic effect may be prevented by acetazolamide.

Phenytoin: Serum concentrations of phenytoin may be increased; incidence of osteomalacia may be enhanced or increased in patients on chronic phenytoin therapy.

Primidone serum concentrations may be decreased; carbonic anhydrase inhibitors may enhance the adverse/toxic effects of primidone.

Quinidine: Urinary excretion of quinidine may be decreased and effects may be enhanced.

Salicylate use (high dose) may result in carbonic anhydrase inhibitor accumulation and toxicity including CNS depression and metabolic acidosis. Salicylate toxicity might also be enhanced.

Pregnancy Risk Factor C

Pregnancy Implications Teratogenic in animal studies, however, there are no adequate and well-controlled studies in pregnant women.

Lactation Enters breast milk/not recommended (AAP rates "compatible")

Nursing Implications Tablet may be crushed and suspended in cherry or chocolate syrup to disguise the bitter taste of the drug

Additional Information Sodium content of 500 mg injection: 47.2 mg (2.05 mEq)

AcetoHEXAMIDE

CAS Number 968-81-0

Use Adjunct to diet for the management of mild to moderately severe, stable, noninsulin-dependent (type II) diabetes mellitus

Mechanism of Action Causes hypoglycemia by stimulating pancreatic islet cells to release insulin; stimulates insulin release from the pancreatic beta cells; reduces glucose output from the liver; insulin sensitivity is increased at peripheral target sites; produces a mild diuretic effect and increases the urinary excretion of uric acid

Adverse Reactions

Cardiovascular: Sinus tachycardia

Central nervous system: **Headache**, ataxia, **dizziness**

Dermatologic: Skin rash, hives, photosensitivity

Endocrine & metabolic: Severe hypoglycemia, hyponatremia, syndrome of inappropriate antidiuretic hormone, hyperinsulinemia

Gastrointestinal: Nausea, vomiting, **epigastric fullness**, abdominal pain, **heartburn**, **diarrhea**, **anorexia**, **constipation**

Hematologic: Aplastic anemia, hemolysis, bone marrow suppression, thrombocytopenia, leukopenia, neutropenia, agranulocytosis, granulocytopenia

Hepatic: Cholestatic jaundice, cirrhosis

Neuromuscular & skeletal: Fasciculations

Ocular: Diplopia, photophobia

Toxicodynamics/Kinetics

Onset of effect: 1 hour

Peak hypoglycemic effects: 8-10 hours

Duration: 12-24 hours, prolonged with renal impairment

Distribution: Into breast milk

Protein binding: 85% to 88%

Metabolism: In the liver to hydroxyhexamide (active metabolite)

Half-life: Parent compound: 0.8-2.4 hours; Metabolite: 5-6 hours

Elimination: Urinary excretion of <40% as unchanged drug; ~80% to 95% of dose excreted in urine within 24 hours; ~15% excreted in bile

Dosage

Adults: Oral (elderly patients may be more sensitive and should be started at a lower dosage initially): 250 mg to 1.5 g/day in 1-2 divided doses; doses >1.5 g/day are not recommended; if dose is ≤1 g, administer as a single daily dose

Dosing adjustment in renal impairment: Cl$_{cr}$ <50 mL/minute: Avoid use; prolonged hypoglycemia occurs in azotemic patients

Dosing adjustment in hepatic impairment: Initiate therapy at lower than recommended doses

Monitoring Parameters Blood (preferred) and urine glucose concentrations should be monitored when therapy is started; normally takes 7 days to determine therapeutic response

Reference Range Glucose fasting: Adults: 80-140 mg/dL; Elderly: 100-180 mg/dL

Overdosage/Treatment

Decontamination: Lavage (within 1 hour)/activated charcoal

Supportive therapy: Glucose (25 g I.V.) is mainstay of therapy. Glucagon (1-5 mg I.V., I.M., or SubQ) (0.03-0.1 mg/kg in pediatrics) will have limited benefit; diazoxide is a third-line agent (3-8 mg/kg/24 hours); octreotide (50 mcg every 12 hours SubQ) will suppress plasma insulin

Enhancement of elimination: Multiple dosing of activated charcoal may be effective. Peritoneal dialysis has been used with some success. Urine alkalinization is also useful.

Antidote(s)
- Dextrose [ANTIDOTE]
- Glucagon [ANTIDOTE]
- Octreotide [ANTIDOTE]

Test Interactions May cause a false elevation of serum creatinine due to interference with tubular secretion of creatinine

Pregnancy Risk Factor D

Pregnancy Implications Abnormal blood glucose levels are associated with a higher incidence of congenital abnormalities. Insulin is the drug of choice for the control of diabetes mellitus during pregnancy.

Nursing Implications Advise patient to avoid alcohol or products containing alcohol; blood and urine glucose concentrations should be monitored when therapy is started; normally takes 7 days to determine therapeutic response

Specific References
Johnson KK, Green DL, Rife JP, et al, "Sulfonamide Cross-Reactivity: Fact or Fiction?" *Ann Pharmacother*, 2005, 39(2):290-301.

Acrivastine and Pseudoephedrine

Pronunciation (AK ri vas teen & soo doe e FED rin)
CAS Number 87848-99-5
U.S. Brand Names Semprex®-D
Synonyms Pseudoephedrine Hydrochloride and Acrivastine
Impairment Potential Yes. Acrivastine may mildly affect driving performance at therapeutic doses
Use Allergic rhinitis, rash, atopic eczema, demographism
Mechanism of Action Analog of triprolidine, a potent antihistamine with sedative but no anticholinergic effects; histamine H_1-receptor antagonist
Adverse Reactions
Cardiovascular: Sinus tachycardia
Central nervous system: Lethargy, lightheadedness, **headache, drowsiness**, insomnia
Gastrointestinal: Xerostomia, nausea, diarrhea, dyspepsia
Pharmacodynamics/Kinetics
Pseudoephedrine: See Pseudoephedrine.
Acrivastine:
Metabolism: Minimally hepatic
Time to peak: ~1.1 hours
Excretion: Urine (84%); feces (13%)
Dosage Oral: 8 mg every 4-6 hours
Contraindications Hypersensitivity to pseudoephedrine, acrivastine (or other alkylamine antihistamines), or any component of the formulation; MAO inhibitor therapy within 14 days of initiating therapy; severe hypertension, severe coronary artery disease; renal impairment (Cl_{cr} ≤48 mL/minute)
Warnings Use with caution in patients >60 years of age. Use with caution in patients with high blood pressure, ischemic heart disease, diabetes, increased intraocular pressure, GI or GU obstruction, asthma, thyroid disease, or prostatic hyperplasia. Not recommended for use in children.
Dosage Forms Capsule: Acrivastine 8 mg and pseudoephedrine hydrochloride 60 mg
Reference Range After a 12 mg oral dose, peak serum level is ~179 ng/mL within 1 hour of ingestion
Overdosage/Treatment
Decontamination: Lavage (within 1 hour)/activated charcoal
Supportive therapy: There is no specific treatment for an antihistamine overdose, however, most of its clinical toxicity is due to anticholinergic effects. For anticholinergic overdose with severe life-threatening symptoms, physostigmine 1-2 mg (0.5 or 0.02 mg/kg for children) I.V., slowly may be given to reverse these effects in life-threatening situations.
Drug Interactions Decreased effect of guanethidine, reserpine, methyldopa, and beta-blockers
Increased toxicity with MAO inhibitors (hypertensive crisis), sympathomimetics, CNS depressants, ethanol (sedation)
Pregnancy Risk Factor B
Lactation Enters breast milk/contraindicated

Adalimumab

Pronunciation (a da LIM yoo mab)
U.S. Brand Names Humira™
Synonyms Antitumor Necrosis Factor Apha (Human); D2E7; Human Antitumor Necrosis Factor Alpha
Use Treatment of active rheumatoid arthritis (moderate to severe) in patients with inadequate response to one or more disease-modifying antirheumatic drugs (DMARDs)
Mechanism of Action Adalimumab is a recombinant monoclonal antibody that binds to human tumor necrosis factor alpha (TNF-alpha) receptor sites, thereby interfering with endogenous TNF-alpha activity. Elevated TNF levels in the synovial fluid are involved in the pathologic pain and joint destruction in rheumatoid arthritis. Adalimumab decreases signs and symptoms of rheumatoid arthritis and inhibits progression of structural damage.

Adverse Reactions
Cardiovascular: Hypertension, arrhythmias, atrial fibrillation, chest pain, congestive heart failure, coronary artery disorder, heart arrest, hypertensive encephalopathy, myocardial infarct, palpitations, pericardial effusion, pericarditis, peripheral edema, syncope, tachycardia, thrombosis (leg), vascular disorder
Central nervous system: **Headache**, confusion, fever, multiple sclerosis, pain in extremity, paresthesia, subdural hematoma, tremor
Dermatologic: **Rash**, cellulitis
Endocrine & metabolic: Hyperlipidemia, hypercholesterolemia, dehydration, menstrual disorder, parathyroid disorder
Gastrointestinal: Nausea, abdominal pain, esophagitis, gastroenteritis, gastrointestinal hemorrhage, vomiting
Genitourinary: Urinary tract infection, cystitis, pelvic pain
Hematologic: Agranulocytosis, granulocytopenia, leukopenia, pancytopenia, polycythemia
Hepatic: Cholecystitis, cholelithiasis, hepatic necrosis
Local: Injection site reaction
Neuromuscular & skeletal: Back pain, arthritis, bone fracture, bone necrosis, joint disorder, muscle cramps, myasthenia, pyogenic arthritis, synovitis, tendon disorder
Ocular: Cataract
Renal: Hematuria, kidney calculus, paraproteinemia, pyelonephritis
Respiratory: **Upper respiratory tract infection, sinusitis**, asthma, bronchospasm, dyspnea, lung function decreased, pleural effusion, pneumonia
Miscellaneous: **Accidental injury**, flu-like syndrome, adenoma, carcinoma (including breast, gastrointestinal, skin, urogenital), erysipelas, healing abnormality, herpes zoster, ketosis, lupus erythematosus syndrome, lymphoma, melanoma, sepsis, tuberculosis (reactivation of latent infection)

Pharmacodynamics/Kinetics
Distribution: V_d: 4.7-6 L; Synovial fluid concentrations: 31% to 96% of serum
Bioavailability: Absolute: 64%
Half-life elimination: Terminal: ~2 weeks (range 10-20 days)
Time to peak, serum: SubQ: 131±56 hours
Excretion: Clearance increased in the presence of antiadalimumab antibodies; decreased in patients 40 years and older
Dosage SubQ: Adults: Rheumatoid arthritis: 40 mg every other week; may be administered with other DMARDs; patients not taking methotrexate may increase dose to 40 mg/weekly
Monitoring Parameters Improvement of symptoms; signs of infection; place and read PPD before initiation
Administration
For SubQ injection; rotate injection sites. Do not use if solution is discolored. Do not administer to skin which is red, tender, bruised, or hard.
Contraindications Hypersensitivity to adalimumab or any component of the formulation
Warnings
[U.S. Boxed Warnings]: Patients should be evaluated for latent tuberculosis infection with a tuberculin skin test prior to therapy. Treatment of latent tuberculosis should be initiated before adalimumab is used. Tuberculosis (disseminated or extrapulmonary) has been reactivated while on adalimumab. Most cases have been reported within the first 8 months of treatment. **[U.S. Boxed Warning]: Patients with initial negative tuberculin skin tests should receive continued monitoring for tuberculosis throughout treatment; active tuberculosis has developed in this population during treatment.** Rare reactivation of hepatitis B has occurred in chronic virus carriers; evaluate prior to initiation and during treatment. Adalimumab may affect defenses against infections and malignancies.
[U.S. Boxed Warning]: Serious and potential fatal infections (including invasive fungal and other opportunistic infections) have been reported in patients receiving TNF-blocking agents, including adalimumab. Use caution with chronic infection, history of recurrent infection, or predisposition to infection. Do not give to patients with an active chronic or localized infection. Many of the serious infections have occurred in patients on concomitant immunosuppressive therapy. Other opportunistic infections included *Histoplasma*, *Aspergillus*, and *Nocardia*. Use caution in patients who have resided in regions where histoplasmosis is endemic. Patients who develop a new infection while undergoing treatment with adalimumab should be monitored closely. If a patient develops a serious infection or sepsis, adalimumab should be discontinued. Rare cases of lymphoma have also been reported in association with adalimumab. Impact on the development and course of malignancies is not fully defined.
May exacerbate pre-existing or recent-onset demyelinating CNS disorders. Worsening and new-onset CHF has been reported; use caution in patients with decreased left ventricular function. Use caution in patients with CHF. Patients should be brought up to date with all immunizations

before initiating therapy. No data are available concerning the effects of adalimumab on vaccination. Live vaccines should not be given concurrently. No data are available concerning secondary transmission of live vaccines in patients receiving adalimumab. Rare cases of pancytopenia (including aplastic anemia) have been reported with TNF-blocking agents; with significant hematologic abnormalities, consider discontinuing therapy. Positive antinuclear antibody titers have been detected in patients (with negative baselines) treated with adalimumab. Rare cases of autoimmune disorder, including lupus-like syndrome, have been reported; monitor and discontinue adalimumab if symptoms develop. May cause hypersensitivity reactions, including anaphylaxis; monitor. Safety and efficacy have not been established in pediatric patients.

Dosage Forms
Injection, solution [preservative free]:
Humira®: 40 mg/0.8 mL (1 mL) [prefilled glass syringe or Humira® pen; packaged with alcohol preps; needle cover contains latex]

Overdosage/Treatment Doses of up to 10 mg/kg have been tolerated in clinical trials. In case of overdose, treatment should be symptomatic and supportive.

Drug Interactions
Abatacept: Concurrent use may increase the risk of infection; avoid concurrent use.
Abciximab: Allergic reactions may be increased in patients who have received diagnostic or therapeutic monoclonal antibodies due to the presence of HACA; may also cause thrombocytopenia or decreased therapeutic effect.
Anakinra: Concomitant use may increase risk of infections; not recommended.
Vaccines (killed organism or component): Adalimumab may decrease the effect of vaccines; monitor.
Vaccines (live organism): Adalimumab may increase the risk of vaccinal infection; avoid concurrent use.

Pregnancy Risk Factor B

Pregnancy Implications Teratogenic effects were not observed in animal studies; however, there are no adequate and well-controlled studies in pregnant women. Use during pregnancy only if clearly needed.

Lactation Excretion in breast milk unknown/not recommended

Adenosine

Pronunciation (a DEN oh seen)
CAS Number 56-56-5; 58-61-7
U.S. Brand Names Adenocard®; Adenoscan®
Synonyms 9-Beta-D-Ribofuranosyladenine
Use Adenocard®: Treatment of paroxysmal supraventricular tachycardia (PSVT) including that associated with accessory bypass tracts (Wolff-Parkinson-White syndrome); when clinically advisable, appropriate vagal maneuvers should be attempted prior to adenosine administration; **not effective in atrial flutter, atrial fibrillation, or ventricular tachycardia**
Adenoscan®: Pharmacologic stress agent used in myocardial perfusion thallium-201 scintigraphy

Unlabeled/Investigational Use Adenoscan®: Acute vasodilator testing in pulmonary artery hypertension

Mechanism of Action Endogenous nucleoside; produces transient atrioventricular block and coronary vasodilatation; slows conduction time through the AV node, interrupting the re-entry pathways through the AV node, restoring normal sinus rhythm. No direct ventricular effect.

Adverse Reactions
Cardiovascular: **Facial flushing, palpitations, chest pain, hypotension**, fibrillation (atrial) may last for up to 5 hours, flutter (atrial), sinus bradycardia, angina, arrhythmias (ventricular), vasodilation, AV block
Central nervous system: Lightheadedness, dizziness, tingling in arms, numbness, fear, burning sensation, **headache**, heaviness in arms, neck and back, pain
Gastrointestinal: Nausea, metallic taste, tightness in throat, pressure in groin
Ocular: Blurred vision
Respiratory: **Dyspnea**, bronchospasm, chest pressure, hypoventilation
Miscellaneous: **Diaphoresis**

Signs and Symptoms of Overdose Arrhythmias, bradycardia, hypotension, lightheadedness, numbness, urine discoloration (milky), wheezing

Pharmacodynamics/Kinetics
Onset of action: Rapid
Duration: Very brief
Metabolism: Blood and tissue to inosine then to adenosine monophosphate (AMP) and hypoxanthine
Half-life elimination: <10 seconds

Dosage
Adenocard®: **Rapid I.V. push (over 1-2 seconds) via peripheral line:**
Infants and Children:
Manufacturer's recommendation:
<50 kg: 0.05 to 0.1 mg/kg. If conversion of PSVT does not occur within 1-2 minutes, may increase dose by 0.05 to 0.1 mg/kg. May repeat until sinus rhythm is established or to a maximum

single dose of 0.3 mg/kg or 12 mg. Follow each dose with normal saline flush.
≥50 kg: Refer to Adults dosing
Pediatric advanced life support (PALS): Treatment of SVT: I.V., I.O.: 0.1 mg/kg; if not effective, administer 0.2 mg/kg of PSVT; medium dose required: 0.15 mg/kg; maximum single dose: 12 mg. Follow each dose with normal saline flush.
Adults: 6 mg; if not effective within 1-2 minutes, 12 mg may be given; may repeat 12 mg bolus if needed
Maximum single dose: 12 mg
Follow each I.V. bolus of adenosine with normal saline flush
Note: Preliminary results in adults suggest adenosine may be administered via a central line at lower doses (ie, initial adult dose: 3 mg).
Adenoscan®: Continuous I.V. infusion via peripheral line: 140 mcg/kg/minute for 6 minutes using syringe or columetric infusion pump; total dose: 0.84 mg/kg. Thallium-201 is injected at midpoint (3 minutes) of infusion.
Hemodialysis: Significant drug removal is unlikely based on physiochemical characteristics.
Peritoneal dialysis: Significant drug removal is unlikely based on physiochemical characteristics.
Note: Higher doses may be needed for administration via peripheral versus central vein.

Monitoring Parameters ECG monitoring, heart rate, blood pressure

Administration
For rapid bolus I.V. use only; administer I.V. push over 1-2 seconds at a peripheral I.V. site as proximal as possible to trunk (not in lower arm, hand, lower leg, or foot); follow each bolus with normal saline flush. **Note:** Preliminary results in adults suggest adenosine may be administered via central line at lower doses (eg, adults initial dose: 3 mg)

Contraindications Hypersensitivity to adenosine or any component of the formulation; second- or third-degree AV block or sick sinus syndrome (except in patients with a functioning artificial pacemaker); atrial flutter, atrial fibrillation, and ventricular tachycardia (this drug is not effective in converting these arrhythmias to sinus rhythm). The manufacturer states that Adenoscan® should be avoided in patients with known or suspected bronchoconstrictive or bronchospastic lung disease.

Warnings
Adenosine decreases conduction through the AV node and may produce first-, second-, or third-degree heart block. Patients with pre-existing S-A nodal dysfunction may experience prolonged sinus pauses after adenosine; use caution in patients with first-degree AV block or bundle branch block; avoid use of adenosine for pharmacologic stress testing in patients with high-grade AV block or sinus node dysfunction (unless a functional pacemaker is in place). There have been reports of atrial fibrillation/flutter in patients with PSVT associated with accessory conduction pathways after adenosine. Rare, prolonged episodes of asystole have been reported, with fatal outcomes in some cases. Use caution in patients receiving other drugs which slow AV conduction (eg, digoxin, verapamil). Drugs which affect adenosine (theophylline, caffeine) should be withheld for five half-lives prior to adenosine use. Avoid dietary caffeine for 12-24 hours prior to pharmacologic stress testing.
Adenosine may also produce profound vasodilation with subsequent hypotension. When used as a bolus dose (PSVT), effects are generally self-limiting (due to the short half-life of adenosine). However, when used as a continuous infusion (pharmacologic stress testing), effects may be more pronounced and persistent, corresponding to continued exposure. Adenosine infusions should be used with caution in patients with autonomic dysfunction, stenotic valvular heart disease, pericarditis, pleural effusion, carotid stenosis (with cerebrovascular insufficiency), or uncorrected hypovolemia. Use caution in elderly patients; may be at increased risk of hemodynamic effects, bradycardia, and/or AV block.
A limited number of patients with asthma have received adenosine and have not experienced exacerbation of their asthma. Adenosine may cause bronchoconstriction in patients with asthma, and should be used cautiously in patients with obstructive lung disease not associated with bronchoconstriction (eg, emphysema, bronchitis).
Adenocard®: Transient AV block is expected. When used in PSVT, at the time of conversion to normal sinus rhythm, a variety of new rhythms may appear on the ECG. Administer as a rapid bolus, either directly into a vein or (if administered into an I.V. line), as close to the patient as possible (followed by saline flush).

Dosage Forms
Injection, solution [preservative free]: 3 mg/mL (2 mL, 4 mL)
Adenocard®: 3 mg/mL (2 mL, 4 mL)
Adenoscan®: 3 mg/mL (20 mL, 30 mL)

Reference Range 0.1-1.0 μmol/L

Overdosage/Treatment Supportive therapy: I.V. fluids for hypotensive effect; aminophylline may antagonize effects. External pacing may be required.

Drug Interactions
Carbamazepine may increase heart block.
Dipyridamole potentiates effects of adenosine; reduce dose of adenosine.

Theophylline and caffeine (methylxanthines) antagonize adenosine's effects; may require increased dose of adenosine.

Pregnancy Risk Factor C

Pregnancy Implications Reports of administration during pregnancy have indicated no adverse effects on fetus or newborn attributable to adenosine.

Lactation Excretion in breast milk unknown

Additional Information No negative inotropic effect; may be effective against theophylline-induced seizures

Specific References

Delacretaz E, "Clinical Practice: Supraventricular Tachycardia," *N Engl J Med*, 2006, 354(10):1039-51 (review).

Falk RH, "Adenosine-Induced Ventricular Flutter?" *Am J Emerg Med*, 2003, 21(3):249.

Albendazole

Pronunciation (al BEN da zole)

CAS Number 54965-21-8

U.S. Brand Names Albenza®

Use Treatment of parenchymal neurocysticercosis caused by *Taenia solium* and cystic hydatid disease of the liver, lung, and peritoneum caused by *Echinococcus granulosus*

Unlabeled/Investigational Use Albendazole has activity against *Ascaris lumbricoides* (roundworm), *Ancylostoma caninum*, *Ancylostoma duodenale* and *Necator americanus* (hookworms); cutaneous larva migrans; *Enterobius vermicularis* (pinworm); *Gnathostoma spinigerum*; *Gongylonema* sp; *Hymenolepis nana* sp (tapeworms); *Mansonella perstans* (filariasis); *Opisthorchis sinensis* and *Opisthorchis viverrini* (liver flukes); *Strongyloides stercoralis* and *Trichuris trichiura* (whipworm); visceral larva migrans (toxocariasis); activity has also been shown against the liver fluke *Clonorchis sinensis*, *Giardia lamblia*, *Cysticercus cellulosae*, and *Echinococcus multilocularis*. Albendazole has also been used for the treatment of intestinal microsporidiosis (*Encephalitozoon intestinalis*), disseminated microsporidiosis (*E. hellem*, *E. cuniculi*, *E. intestinalis*, *Pleistophora* sp, *Trachipleistophora* sp, *Brachiola vesicularum*), and ocular microsporidiosis (*E. hellem*, *E. cuniculi*, *Vittaforma corneae*).

Mechanism of Action Active metabolite, albendazole, causes selective degeneration of cytoplasmic microtubules in intestinal and tegmental cells of intestinal helminths and larvae; glycogen is depleted, glucose uptake and cholinesterase secretion are impaired, and desecratory substances accumulate intracellulary. ATP production decreases causing energy depletion, immobilization, and worm death; albendazole has activity against *Ascaris lumbricoides* (roundworm), *Ancylostoma duodenale* and *Necator americanus* (hookworms), *Enterobius vermicularis* (pinworm), *Hymenolepis nana* and *Taenia* sp (tapeworms), *Opisthorchis sinensis* and *Opisthorchis viverrini* (liver flukes), *Strongyloides stercoralis* and *Trichuris trichiura* (whipworm); activity has also been shown against the liver fluke *Clonorchis sinensis*, *Giardia lamblia*, *Cysticercus cellulosae*, *Echinococcus granulosus* and *multilocularis*, and *Toxocara* sp.

Adverse Reactions

N = Neurocysticercosis; H = Hydatid disease

>10%:

Central nervous system: Headache (11% - N; 1% - H)

Hepatic: LFTs Increased (~15% - H; <1% - N)

1% to 10%:

Central nervous system: Dizziness, vertigo, fever (≤1%); intracranial pressure increased (1% - N), meningeal signs (1% - N)

Dermatologic: Alopecia (2% - H; <1% - N)

Gastrointestinal: Abdominal pain (6% - H; 0% - N); nausea/vomiting (3% to 6%)

Hematologic: Leukopenia (reversible) (<1%)

Miscellaneous: Allergic reactions (<1%)

<1%: Acute renal failure, agranulocytopenia, allergic reactions, granulocytopenia, pancytopenia, rash, thrombocytopenia, urticaria

Pharmacodynamics/Kinetics

Absorption: <5%; may increase up to 4-5 times when administered with a fatty meal

Distribution: Well inside hydatid cysts and CSF

Protein binding: 70%

Metabolism: Hepatic; extensive first-pass effect; pathways include rapid sulfoxidation (major), hydrolysis, and oxidation

Half-life elimination: 8-12 hours

Time to peak, serum: 2-2.4 hours

Excretion: Urine (<1% as active metabolite); feces

Dosage

Oral:

Children:

Cysticercus cellulosae (unlabeled use): 15 mg/kg/day (maximum: 800 mg/day) in 2 divided doses for 8-30 days; may be repeated as necessary

Echinococcus granulosus (tapeworm) (unlabeled use): 15 mg/kg/day (maximum: 800 mg) divided twice daily for 1-6 months

Children and Adults:

Neurocysticercosis:

<60 kg: 15 mg/kg/day in 2 divided doses (maximum: 800 mg/day) for 8-30 days

≥60 kg: 400 mg twice daily for 8-30 days

Note: Give concurrent anticonvulsant and steroid therapy during first week.

Hydatid:

<60 kg: 15 mg/kg/day in 2 divided doses (maximum: 800 mg/day)

≥60 kg: 400 mg twice daily

Note: Administer dose for three 28-day cycles with a 14-day drug-free interval in between.

Ancylostoma caninum, *Ascaris lumbricoides* (roundworm), *Ancylostoma duodenale*, and *Necator americanus* (hookworms) (unlabeled use): 400 mg as a single dose

Clonorchis sinensis (Chinese liver fluke) (unlabeled use): 10 mg/kg for 7 days

Cutaneous larva migrans (unlabeled use): 400 mg once daily for 3 days

Enterobius vermicularis (pinworm) (unlabeled use): 400 mg as a single dose; may repeat in 2 weeks

Gnathostoma spinigerum (unlabeled use): 400 mg twice daily for 21 days

Gongylonemiasis (unlabeled use): 10 mg/kg/day for 3 days

Mansonella perstans (unlabeled use): 400 mg twice daily for 10 days

Visceral larva migrans (toxocariasis) (unlabeled use): 400 mg twice daily for 5 days

Adults:

Cysticercus cellulosae (unlabeled use): 400 mg twice daily for 8-30 days; may be repeated as necessary

Disseminated microsporidiosis (unlabeled use): 400 mg twice daily

Echinococcus granulosus (tapeworm) (unlabeled use): 400 mg twice daily for 1-6 months

Intestinal microsporidiosis (unlabeled use): 400 mg twice daily for 21 days

Ocular microsporidiosis (unlabeled use): 400 mg twice daily, in combination with fumagillin

Monitoring Parameters Monitor fecal specimens for ova and parasites for 3 weeks after treatment; if positive, retreat; monitor LFTs, and clinical signs of hepatotoxicity; CBC at start of each 28-day cycle and every 2 weeks during treatment

Administration

Administer with meals. Administer anticonvulsant and steroid therapy during first week of neurocysticercosis therapy.

Contraindications Hypersensitivity to albendazole or any component of the formulation

Warnings

Discontinue therapy if LFT elevations are significant; may restart treatment when decreased to pretreatment values. Becoming pregnant within 1 month following therapy is not advised.

Neurocysticercosis: Corticosteroids should be administered 1-2 days before albendazole therapy to minimize inflammatory reactions. Steroid and anticonvulsant therapy should be used concurrently during the first week of therapy to prevent cerebral hypertension. If retinal lesions exist, weigh risk of further retinal damage due to albendazole-induced changes to the retinal lesion vs benefit of disease treatment.

Dosage Forms Tablet: 200 mg

Reference Range Peak plasma albendazole sulphoxide level following an oral dose of 400 mg ranges from 0.04-0.14 mcg/mL

Overdosage/Treatment

Decontamination: Emesis within 30 minutes/lavage within 1 hour; activated charcoal

Enhanced elimination: Hemodialysis is not useful

Drug Interactions **Substrate** (minor) of CYP1A2, 3A4; **Inhibits** CYP1A2 (weak)

Pregnancy Risk Factor C

Pregnancy Implications Albendazole has been shown to be teratogenic in laboratory animals and should not be used during pregnancy, if at all possible. Women should be advised to avoid pregnancy for at least 1 month following therapy. Discontinue if pregnancy occurs during treatment.

Lactation Excretion in breast milk unknown/not recommended

Additional Information Should be taken with a high fat meal

Albuterol

Pronunciation (al BYOO ter ole)

Related Information

• Clenbuterol

CAS Number 18559-94-9

U.S. Brand Names AccuNeb™; Proventil® HFA; Proventil® Repetabs®; Proventil®; Ventolin® HFA; Ventolin® [DSC]; Volmax®; VoSpire ER™

Synonyms Albuterol Sulfate; Salbutamol

Use Bronchodilator in reversible airway obstruction due to asthma or COPD; prevention of exercise-induced bronchospasm

Mechanism of Action Relaxes bronchial smooth muscle by action on β_2-receptors with little effect on heart rate

Adverse Reactions

Cardiovascular: **Tachycardia** (slight), **palpitations**, hypertension, flushing, shortened P-R segment, lengthened QT segment, cardiac arrhythmias, fibrillation (atrial), flutter (atrial), chest pain, tachycardia (supraventricular), torsade de pointes, sinus tachycardia, **pounding heartbeat**

Central nervous system: Dizziness, psychosis, headache, **nervousness**, CNS stimulation, hyperactivity, insomnia, mania

Dermatologic: Maculopapular rash, pruritus

Endocrine & metabolic: Hypokalemia, hyperglycemia

Gastrointestinal: **GI upset**, **nausea**, xerostomia

Neuromuscular & skeletal: **Tremor**

Miscellaneous: Systemic lupus erythematosus

Signs and Symptoms of Overdose Agitation, angina, diplopia, hyperglycemia, hypertension, hypokalemia, hypomagnesemia, increased intraocular pressure, seizures, thrombocytopenia, tachycardia, tremor. Cardiac arrest and death may be associated with abuse of beta-agonist bronchodilators.

Pharmacodynamics/Kinetics

Onset of action: Peak effect:

Nebulization/oral inhalation: 0.5-2 hours

CFC-propelled albuterol: 10 minutes

Ventolin® HFA: 25 minutes

Oral: 2-3 hours

Duration: Nebulization/oral inhalation: 3-4 hours; Oral: 4-6 hours

Metabolism: Hepatic to an inactive sulfate

Half-life elimination: Inhalation: 3.8 hours; Oral: 3.7-5 hours

Excretion: Urine (30% as unchanged drug)

Dosage

Oral:

Children: Bronchospasm (treatment):

2-6 years: 0.1-0.2 mg/kg/dose 3 times/day; maximum dose not to exceed 12 mg/day (divided doses)

6-12 years: 2 mg/dose 3-4 times/day; maximum dose not to exceed 24 mg/day (divided doses)

Extended release: 4 mg every 12 hours; maximum dose not to exceed 24 mg/day (divided doses)

Children >12 years and Adults: Bronchospasm (treatment): 2-4 mg/dose 3-4 times/day; maximum dose not to exceed 32 mg/day (divided doses)

Extended release: 8 mg every 12 hours; maximum dose not to exceed 32 mg/day (divided doses). A 4 mg dose every 12 hours may be sufficient in some patients, such as adults of low body weight.

Elderly: Bronchospasm (treatment): 2 mg 3-4 times/day; maximum: 8 mg 4 times/day

Inhalation: MDI 90 mcg/puff:

Children ≤12 years:

Bronchospasm (acute): 4-8 puffs every 20 minutes for 3 doses, then every 1-4 hours; spacer/holding-chamber device should be used

Exercise-induced bronchospasm (prophylaxis): 1-2 puffs 5 minutes prior to exercise

Children >12 years and Adults:

Bronchospasm (acute): 4-8 puffs every 20 minutes for up to 4 hours, then every 1-4 hours as needed

Exercise-induced bronchospasm (prophylaxis): 2 puffs 5-30 minutes prior to exercise

Children ≥4 years and Adults: Bronchospasm (chronic treatment): 1-2 inhalations every 4-6 hours; maximum: 12 inhalations/day

NIH guidelines: 2 puffs 3-4 times a day as needed; may double dose for mild exacerbations

Nebulization:

Children ≤12 years:

Bronchospasm (treatment): 0.05 mg/kg every 4-6 hours; minimum dose: 1.25 mg, maximum dose: 2.5 mg

2-12 years: AccuNeb™: 0.63 mg or 1.25 mg 3-4 times/day, as needed, delivered over 5-15 minutes

Children >40 kg, patients with more severe asthma, or children 11-12 years: May respond better with a 1.25 mg dose

Bronchospasm (acute): Solution 0.5%: 0.15 mg/kg (minimum dose: 2.5 mg) every 20 minutes for 3 doses, then 0.15-0.3 mg/kg (up to 10 mg) every 1-4 hours as needed; may also use 0.5 mg/kg/hour by continuous infusion. Continuous nebulized albuterol at 0.3 mg/kg/hour has been used safely in the treatment of severe status asthmaticus in children; continuous nebulized doses of 3 mg/kg/hour $\pm$ 2.2 mg/kg/hour in children whose mean age was 20.7 months resulted in no cardiac toxicity; the optimal dosage for continuous nebulization remains to be determined.

Note: Use of the 0.5% solution should be used for bronchospasm (acute or treatment) in children <15 kg. AccuNeb™ has not been studied for the treatment of acute bronchospasm; use of the 0.5% concentrated solution may be more appropriate.

Children >12 years and Adults:

Bronchospasm (treatment): 2.5 mg, diluted to a total of 3 mL, 3-4 times/day over 5-15 minutes

NIH guidelines: 1.25-5 mg every 4-8 hours

Bronchospasm (acute) in intensive care patients: 2.5-5 mg every 20 minutes for 3 doses, then 2.5-10 mg every 1-4 hours as needed, **or** 10-15 mg/hour continuously

Hemodialysis: Not removed

Peritoneal dialysis: Significant drug removal is unlikely based on physiochemical characteristics

Monitoring Parameters FEV$_1$, peak flow, and/or other pulmonary function tests; blood pressure, heart rate; CNS stimulation; serum glucose, serum potassium; asthma symptoms; arterial or capillary blood gases (if patients condition warrants)

Administration

Inhalation: MDI: Shake well before use; prime prior to first use, and whenever inhaler has not been used for >2 weeks or when it has been dropped, by releasing 4 test sprays into the air (away from face)

Oral: Do not crush or chew extended release tablets.

Contraindications Hypersensitivity to albuterol, adrenergic amines, or any component of the formulation

Warnings

Optimize anti-inflammatory treatment before initiating maintenance treatment with albuterol. Do not use as a component of chronic therapy without an anti-inflammatory agent. Only the mildest forms of asthma (Step 1 and/or exercise-induced) would not require concurrent use based upon asthma guidelines. Patient must be instructed to seek medical attention in cases where acute symptoms are not relieved or a previous level of response is diminished. The need to increase frequency of use may indicate deterioration of asthma, and treatment must not be delayed.

Use caution in patients with cardiovascular disease (arrhythmia or hypertension or CHF), convulsive disorders, diabetes, glaucoma, hyperthyroidism, or hypokalemia. Beta agonists may cause elevation in blood pressure, heart rate, and result in CNS stimulation/excitation. β_2 agonists may increase risk of arrhythmia, increase serum glucose, or decrease serum potassium.

Do not exceed recommended dose; serious adverse events, including fatalities, have been associated with excessive use of inhaled sympathomimetics. Rarely, paradoxical bronchospasm may occur with use of inhaled bronchodilating agents; this should be distinguished from inadequate response. All patients should utilize a spacer device when using a metered-dose inhaler; in addition, face masks should be used in children <4 years of age.

Because of its minimal effect on β_1-receptors and its relatively long duration of action, albuterol is a rational choice in the elderly when an inhaled beta agonist is indicated. Oral use should be avoided in the elderly due to adverse effects. Patient response may vary between inhalers that contain chlorofluorocarbons and those which are chlorofluorocarbon-free.

Dosage Forms

Aerosol, for oral inhalation: 90 mcg/metered inhalation (17 g) [200 metered inhalations; contains chlorofluorocarbons]

Proventil®: 90 mcg/metered inhalation (17 g) [200 metered inhalations; contains chlorofluorocarbons]

Aerosol, for oral inhalation:

ProAir™ HFA: 90 mcg/metered inhalation (8.5 g) [200 metered inhalations; chlorofluorocarbon free]

Proventil® HFA: 90 mcg/metered inhalation (6.7 g) [200 metered inhalations; chlorofluorocarbon free]

Ventolin® HFA: 90 mcg/metered inhalation (18 g) [200 metered inhalations; chlorofluorocarbon free]

Solution for nebulization: 0.042% (3 mL); 0.083% (3 mL); 0.5% (0.5 mL, 20 mL)

AccuNeb® [preservative free]: 0.63 mg/3 mL (3 mL) [0.021%]; 1.25 mg/3 mL (3 mL) [0.042%]

Proventil®: 0.083% (3 mL) [preservative free]; 0.5% (20 mL) [contains benzalkonium chloride]

Syrup, as sulfate: 2 mg/5 mL (480 mL)

Tablet: 2 mg, 4 mg

Tablet, extended release:

VoSpire ER®: 4 mg, 8 mg

Reference Range Serum albuterol levels >25 ng/mL associated with increased cardiac toxicity; a level of 160 ng/mL was fatal

Overdosage/Treatment In cases of overdose, symptomatic and supportive therapies should be instituted, and prudent use of a cardioselective beta-adrenergic blocker (eg, atenolol or metoprolol) should be considered, keeping in mind the potential for induction of bronchoconstriction in an asthmatic individual. Adenosine may be effective in the management of tachycardia (ventricular); dialysis has not been shown to be of value in the treatment of an overdose with this agent.

Diagnostic Procedures

• Electrolytes, Blood

Drug Interactions

Substrate of CYP3A4 (major)

Beta-adrenergic blockers (eg, propranolol) antagonize albuterol's effects; avoid concurrent use.

CYP3A4 inducers may decrease the levels/effects of albuterol. Example inducers include aminoglutethimide, carbamazepine, nafcillin, nevirapine, phenobarbital, phenytoin, and rifamycins.

Halothane may increase risk of malignant arrhythmias; avoid concurrent use.

Inhaled ipratropium may increase duration of bronchodilation.

MAO inhibitors may increase side effects; monitor heart rate and blood pressure.

TCAs may increase side effects; monitor heart rate and blood pressure.

Sympathomimetics may increase side effects; monitor heart rate and blood pressure.

Pregnancy Risk Factor C

Pregnancy Implications
Albuterol crosses the placenta; tocolytic effects, fetal tachycardia, fetal hypoglycemia secondary to maternal hyperglycemia with oral or intravenous routes reported. Available evidence suggests safe use during pregnancy.

Lactation
Excretion in breast milk unknown/use caution

Nursing Implications
Before using, the inhaler must be shaken well; assess lung sounds, pulse, and blood pressure before administration and during peak of medication; observe patient for wheezing after administration, if this occurs, call physician

Specific References

Carroll CL and Goodman DM, "Endotracheal Albuterol Treatment of Acute Bronchospasm," *Am J Emerg Med*, 2004, 22(6):506-7.

Kelly HW, "What Is New with the β2-Agonists: Issues in the Management of Asthma," *Ann Pharmacother*, 2005, 39(5):931-8.

Kelly HW, Keim KA, and McWilliams BC, "Comparison of Two Methods of Delivering Continuously Nebulized Albuterol," *Ann Pharmacother*, 2003, 37(1):23-6.

Nowak R, Emerman C, Hanrahan JP, et al, "A Comparison of Levalbuterol with Racemic Albuterol in the Treatment of Acute Severe Asthma Exacerbations in Adults," *Am J Emerg Med*, 2006, 24:259-67.

Rivera ML, Kim TY, Stewart GM, et al, "Albuterol Nebulized in Heliox in the Initial ED Treatment of Pediatric Asthma: A Blinded, Randomized Controlled Trial," *Am J Emerg Med*, 2006, 24(1):38-42.

Schreck DM and Babin S, "Comparison of Racemic Albuterol and Levalbuterol in the Treatment of Acute Asthma in the ED," *Am J Emerg Med*, 2005, 23(7):842-7.

Spooner LM and Olin JL, "Paradoxical Bronchoconstriction with Albuterol Administered by Metered-Dose Inhaler and Nebulizer Solution," *Ann Pharmacother*, 2005, 39(11):1924-7.

Stein J and Levitt MA, "A Randomized, Controlled Double-Blind Trial of Usual-Dose Versus High-Dose Albuterol via Continuous Nebulization in Patients with Acute Bronchospasm," *Acad Emerg Med*, 2003, 10(1):31-6.

Aldesleukin

Pronunciation (al des LOO kin)

U.S. Brand Names Proleukin®

Synonyms
Epidermal Thymocyte Activating Factor; ETAF; IL-2; Interleukin-2; Lymphocyte Mitogenic Factor; NSC-373364; T-Cell Growth Factor; TCGF; Thymocyte Stimulating Factor

Use
Primarily investigated in tumors known to have a response to immunotherapy, such as melanoma and metastatic renal cell carcinoma; has been used in conjunction with LAK cells, TIL cells, IL-1, and interferon

Unlabeled/Investigational Use
Investigational: Multiple myeloma, HIV infection, and AIDS; may be used in conjunction with lymphokine-activated killer (LAK) cells, tumor-infiltrating lymphocyte (TIL) cells, interleukin-1, and interferons; colorectal cancer; non-Hodgkin's lymphoma; atopic eczema; chronic active Epstein-Barr infection

Mechanism of Action
Aldesleukin promotes proliferation, differentiation, and recruitment of T and B cells, natural killer (NK) cells, and thymocytes; aldesleukin also causes cytolytic activity in a subset of lymphocytes and subsequent interactions between the immune system and malignant cells; aldesleukin can stimulate lymphokine-activated killer (LAK) cells and tumor-infiltrating lymphocytes (TIL) cells. LAK cells (which are derived from lymphocytes from a patient and incubated in aldesleukin) have the ability to lyse cells which are resistant to NK cells; TIL cells (which are derived from cancerous tissue from a patient and incubated in aldesleukin) have been shown to be 50% more effective than LAK cells in experimental studies.

Adverse Reactions

Cardiovascular: **Hypotension (85%), dose-limiting, possibly fatal; sinus tachycardia (70%); arrhythmias (22%); edema (47%); angina**; capillary-leak syndrome, including peripheral edema, ascites, pulmonary infiltration, and pleural effusion, may be dose-limiting and potentially fatal; myocardial infarction, congestive heart failure

Central nervous system: **Mental status changes (transient memory loss, confusion, drowsiness) (73%); dizziness (17%); cognitive changes, fatigue, malaise, somnolence and disorientation (25%); headaches, insomnia, paranoid delusion**, seizures, coma

Dermatologic: **Macular erythematous rash (100% of patients on high-dose therapy); pruritus (48%); erythema (41%); rash (26%); exfoliative dermatitis (14%); dry skin (15%)**, alopecia

Endocrine & metabolic: **Fever and chills (89%); low electrolyte levels (magnesium, calcium, phosphate, potassium, sodium) (1% to 15%)**; hypo- and hyperglycemia, increased electrolyte levels (magnesium, calcium, phosphate, potassium, sodium), hypothyroidism

Gastrointestinal: **Nausea and vomiting (87%); diarrhea (76%); stomatitis (32%); GI bleeding (13%); weight gain (23%), anorexia (27%)**, pancreatitis

Hematologic: **Anemia (77%); thrombocytopenia (64%); leukopenia (34%)** - may be dose-limiting; **coagulation disorders (10%)**

Hepatic: **Transient elevations of bilirubin (64%) and enzymes (56%); jaundice**, ascites

Local: Injection site reactions (SubQ doses)

Neuromuscular & skeletal: **Weakness; rigors** - respond to acetaminophen, diphenhydramine, an NSAID, or meperidine; arthralgia, myalgia

Renal: **Oliguria/anuria (63%, severe in 5% to 6%), proteinuria; renal failure** (dose-limiting toxicity) manifested as oliguria noted within 24-48 hours of initiation of therapy; marked **fluid retention, azotemia, and increased serum creatinine** seen, which may return to baseline within 7 days of discontinuation of therapy; **hypophosphatemia**, hematuria, increased creatinine

Respiratory: **Congestion (54%), dyspnea (27% to 52%), edema**, pleural effusions

Miscellaneous: **Pain (54%), infection (including sepsis and endocarditis) due to neutrophil impairment (23%)**, allergic reactions

Pharmacodynamics/Kinetics

Distribution: V_d: 4-7 L; primarily in plasma and then in the lymphocytes

Bioavailability: I.M.: 37%

Half-life elimination: Initial: 6-13 minutes; Terminal: 80-120 minutes

Toxicodynamics/Kinetics

Absorption: Oral: Not absorbed; I.M., subcutaneous: 2% absorbed

Metabolism: Renal tubular catabolism

Dosage

Refer to individual protocols.

I.V.:

Renal cell carcinoma: 600,000 int. units/kg every 8 hours for a maximum of 14 doses; repeat after 9 days of rest for a total of 28 doses per course. Re-evaluate at 4 weeks. Retreat if needed 7 weeks after hospital discharge from previous course.

Melanoma:

Single-agent use: 600,000 int. units/kg every 8 hours for a maximum of 14 doses; repeat after 9 days of rest for a total of 28 doses per course. Re-evaluate at 4 weeks. Retreat if needed 7 weeks after hospital discharge from previous course.

In combination with cytotoxic agents: 24 million int. units/m^2 days 12-16 and 19-23

SubQ:

Single-agent doses: 3-18 million int. units/day for 5 days weekly and repeated weekly up to 6 weeks

In combination with interferon:

5 million int. units/m^2 3 times/week

1.8 million int. units/m^2 twice daily 5 days/week for 6 weeks

Investigational regimen: SubQ: 11 million int. units (flat dose) daily × 4 days per week for 4 consecutive weeks; repeat every 6 weeks

Stability

Store vials of lyophilized injection in a refrigerator at 2°C to 8°C (36°F to 46°F). Reconstitute vials with 1.2 mL SWFI. Gently swirl; do not shake. Further dilute with 50 mL of D$_5$W. Smaller volumes of D$_5$W should be used for doses <1.5 mg; avoid concentrations <30 mcg/mL and >70 mcg/mL (an increased variability in drug delivery has been seen). Reconstituted vials and solutions diluted for infusion are stable for 48 hours at room temperature or refrigerated, per the manufacturer. Solution diluted with D$_5$W to a concentration of 220 mg/mL and repackaged into tuberculin syringes was reported to be stable for 14 days refrigerated.

Note: Filtration will result in significant loss of bioactivity

Recommendations for aldesleukin dilution:

Final dilution concentration <30 mcg/mL (<0.49 10^6 int. units/mL): Albumin must be added to bag prior to addition of aldesleukin at a final concentration of 0.1% (1 mg/mL) albumin; stable at room temperature or at ≥32°C (89°F) for 6 days. Continuous infusion via ambulatory infusion device raises aldesleukin to this temperature. These solutions do not contain a preservative; use for more than 24 hours may not be advisable.

Final dilution concentration ≥30 mcg/mL and ≤70 mcg/mL (≥0.49 and ≤1.1 10^6 int. units/mL): Stable at room temperature for 6 days without albumin added or at ≥32°C (89°F) for 6 days only if albumin (0.1%) is added. (Continuous infusion via ambulatory infusion device raises aldesleukin to this temperature.) These solutions do not contain a preservative; use for more than 24 hours may not be advisable.

Final dilution concentration 70-100 mcg/mL (1.2-1.6 106int. units/mL): Unstable; avoid use.

Final dilution concentration >100-500 mcg/mL (1.7-8.2 10^6 int. units/mL): Stable at room temperature and at ≥32°C (≥89°F)for 6 days. Continuous infusion via ambulatory infusion pump or similar infusion device raises aldesleukin to this temperature. These solutions do not contain a preservative; use for more than 24 hours may not be advisable.

Monitoring Parameters: The following clinical evaluations are recommended for all patients prior to beginning treatment and then frequently during drug administration:

Standard hematologic tests including CBC, differential, and platelet counts; blood chemistries including electrolytes, renal and hepatic function tests

Chest x-rays

Monitoring during therapy should include vital signs (temperature, pulse, blood pressure, and respiration rate) and weight; in a patient with a decreased blood pressure, especially <90 mm Hg, cardiac monitoring for rhythm should be conducted. If an abnormal complex or rhythm is seen, an ECG should be performed; vital signs in these hypotension patients should be taken hourly and central venous pressure (CVP) checked.

During treatment, pulmonary function should be monitored on a regular basis.

Administration

Administer as I.V. infusion over 15 minutes; may be administered by SubQ injection

Management of symptoms related to vascular leak syndrome:

If actual body weight increases >10% above baseline, or rales or rhonchi are audible:

Administer furosemide at dosage determined by patient response

Administer dopamine hydrochloride 2-4 mcg/kg/minute to maintain renal blood flow and urine output

If patient has dyspnea at rest: Administer supplemental oxygen by face mask

If patient has severe respiratory distress: Intubate patient and provide mechanical ventilation; administer ranitidine (as the hydrochloride salt), 50 mg I.V. every 8-12 hours as prophylaxis against stress ulcers

Contraindications Hypersensitivity to aldesleukin or any component of the formulation; patients with abnormal thallium stress or pulmonary function tests; patients who have had an organ allograft; retreatment in patients who have experienced sustained ventricular tachycardia (≥5 beats), refractory cardiac rhythm disturbances, recurrent chest pain with ECG changes consistent with angina or myocardial infarction, intubation ≥72 hours, pericardial tamponade, renal dialysis for ≥72 hours, coma or toxic psychosis lasting ≥48 hours, repetitive or refractory seizures, bowel ischemia/perforation, GI bleeding requiring surgery

Warnings

Hazardous agent - use appropriate precautions for handling and disposal.

[U.S. Boxed Warning]: High-dose aldesleukin therapy has been associated with capillary leak syndrome (CLS) resulting in hypotension and reduced organ perfusion which may be severe and can result in death. Therapy should be restricted to patients with normal cardiac and pulmonary functions as defined by thallium stress and formal pulmonary function testing. Extreme caution should be used in patients with a history of prior cardiac or pulmonary disease. Patients must have a serum creatinine ≤1.5 mg/dL prior to treatment.

[U.S. Boxed Warning]: Should be administered under the supervision of an experienced cancer chemotherapy physician in a facility with cardiopulmonary or intensive specialists and intensive care facilities available. Adverse effects are frequent and sometimes fatal. May exacerbate pre-existing or initial presentation of autoimmune diseases and inflammatory disorders. Patients should be evaluated and treated for CNS metastases and have a negative scan prior to treatment. Mental status changes (irritability, confusion, depression) can occur and may indicate bacteremia, hypoperfusion, CNS malignancy, or CNS toxicity.

[U.S. Boxed Warning]: Impaired neutrophil function is associated with treatment; patients are at risk for sepsis, bacterial endocarditis, and central line-related gram-positive infections. Antibiotic prophylaxis which has been associated with a reduced incidence of staphylococcal infections in aldesleukin studies includes the use of oxacillin, nafcillin, ciprofloxacin, or vancomycin.

[U.S. Boxed Warning]: Withhold treatment for patients developing moderate-to-severe lethargy or somnolence; continued treatment may result in coma. Standard prophylactic supportive care during high-dose aldesleukin treatment includes acetaminophen to relieve constitutional symptoms and an H_2 antagonist to reduce the risk of GI ulceration and/or bleeding.

Dosage Forms Injection, powder for reconstitution: 22×10^6 int. units [18 million int. units/mL = 1.1 mg/mL when reconstituted]

Overdosage/Treatment Supportive therapy: Hypotension should be treated with I.V. crystalloid infusion; vasopressor therapy should be used for refractory hypotension; atropine can be used to treat symptomatic bradycardia; rigors can be treated with acetaminophen or ibuprofen and meperidine; droperidol can be used to control nausea and vomiting, while diphenoxylate/atropine can be used to treat diarrhea; pruritus can be treated with diphenhydramine and hydroxyzine; peptic ulcers can be treated with ranitidine

Drug Interactions

Beta-blockers and other antihypertensives may potentiate the hypotension seen with aldesleukin.

Corticosteroids: Have been shown to decrease toxicity of aldesleukin, but may decrease the efficacy of the lymphokine.

Increased toxicity: Concomitant administration of drugs possessing nephrotoxic (eg, aminoglycosides, indomethacin), myelotoxic (eg, cytotoxic chemotherapy), cardiotoxic (eg, doxorubicin), or hepatotoxic effects with aldesleukin may increase toxicity in these organ systems.

Iodinated contrast media: Acute reactions including fever, chills, nausea, vomiting, pruritus, rash, diarrhea, hypotension, edema, and oliguria have occurred within hours of contrast infusion; this reaction may occur within 4 weeks or up to several months after aldesleukin administration.

Psychotropic agents: Aldesleukin may affect central nervous function; therefore, interactions could occur following concomitant administration of psychotropic drugs (eg, narcotics, analgesics, antiemetics, sedatives, tranquilizers).

Pregnancy Risk Factor C

Pregnancy Implications There are no adequate and well-controlled studies in pregnant women; use during pregnancy only if benefits to the mother outweigh potential risk to the fetus. Contraception is recommended for fertile males or females using this medication.

Lactation Enters breast milk/contraindicated

Additional Information 1 Cetus unit = 6 int. units

1.1 mg = 18×10^6 int. units (or 3×10^6 Cetus units)

1 Roche unit (Teceleukin) = 3 int. units

Alendronate

Related Information

● Etidronate Disodium

CAS Number 121268-17-5; 66376-36-1

U.S. Brand Names Fosamax®

Synonyms Alendronate Sodium

Use Treatment and prevention of osteoporosis in postmenopausal females; treatment of osteoporosis in males; Paget's disease of the bone in patients who are symptomatic, at risk for future complications, or with alkaline phosphatase ≥2 times the upper limit of normal; treatment of glucocorticoid-induced osteoporosis in males and females with low bone mineral density who are receiving a daily dosage ≥7.5 mg of prednisone (or equivalent)

Mechanism of Action Aminobiphosphonate which inhibits osteoclastic bone resorption by binding to hydroxyapatite

Adverse Reactions

Note: Incidence of adverse effects increases significantly in patients treated for Paget's disease at 40 mg/day, mostly GI adverse effects.

Central nervous system: Headache

Dermatologic: Angioedema, photosensitivity (rare), pruritus, rash, urticaria, Stevens-Johnson syndrome, toxic epidermal necrolysis

Endocrine & metabolic: **Hypocalcemia** (transient, mild, 18%); **hypophosphatemia** (transient, mild, 10%), hypocalcemia (symptomatic)

Gastrointestinal: Abdominal pain, acid reflux, dyspepsia, nausea, flatulence, diarrhea, constipation, esophageal ulcer, gastroesophageal reflux disease, abdominal distension, gastritis, vomiting, dysphagia, gastric ulcer, melena, duodenal ulcer, esophageal erosions, esophageal perforation, esophageal stricture, esophagitis, taste perversion

Neuromuscular & skeletal: Musculoskeletal pain, muscle cramps

Ocular: Scleritis (rare), uveitis (rare)

Respiratory: Oropharyngeal ulceration

Miscellaneous: Hypersensitivity reactions

Pharmacodynamics/Kinetics

Distribution: 28 L (exclusive of bone)

Protein binding: ~78%

Metabolism: None

Bioavailability: Fasting: 0.6%; reduced 60% with food or drink

Half-life elimination: Exceeds 10 years

Excretion: Urine; feces (as unabsorbed drug)

Toxicodynamics/Kinetics

Absorption: Oral: ~1% (reduced in presence of calcium and food)

Elimination: Renal: 50%

Dosage Oral: Adults: **Note:** Patients treated with glucocorticoids and those with Paget's disease should receive adequate amounts of calcium and vitamin D.

Osteoporosis in postmenopausal females:

Prophylaxis: 5 mg once daily **or** 35 mg once weekly

Treatment: 10 mg once daily **or** 70 mg once weekly

Osteoporosis in males: 10 mg once daily **or** 70 mg once weekly

Osteoporosis secondary to glucocorticoids in males and females:
Treatment: 5 mg once daily; a dose of 10 mg once daily should be used in postmenopausal females who are not receiving estrogen.

Paget's disease of bone in males and females: 40 mg once daily for 6 months

Retreatment: Relapses during the 12 months following therapy occurred in 9% of patients who responded to treatment. Specific retreatment data are not available. Retreatment with alendronate may be considered, following a 6-month post-treatment evaluation period, in patients who have relapsed based on increases in serum alkaline phosphatase, which should be measured periodically. Retreatment may also be considered in those who failed to normalize their serum alkaline phosphatase.

Elderly: No dosage adjustment is necessary

Dosage adjustment in renal impairment:
Cl$_{cr}$ 35-60 mL/minute: None necessary
Cl$_{cr}$ <35 mL/minute: Alendronate is not recommended due to lack of experience

Dosage adjustment in hepatic impairment: None necessary

Monitoring Parameters Alkaline phosphatase should be periodically measured; serum calcium and phosphorus; monitor pain and fracture rate; hormonal status (male and female) prior to therapy; bone mineral density (should be done prior to initiation of therapy and after 6-12 months of combined glucocorticoid and alendronate treatment)

Administration
Alendronate must be taken with plain water (tablets 6-8 oz; oral solution 2 oz) first thing in the morning and ≥30 minutes before the first food, beverage, or other medication of the day. Patients should be instructed to stay upright (not to lie down) for at least 30 minutes **and** until after first food of the day (to reduce esophageal irritation). Patients should receive supplemental calcium and vitamin D if dietary intake is inadequate.

Contraindications Hypersensitivity to alendronate, other bisphosphonates, or any component of the formulation; hypocalcemia; abnormalities of the esophagus which delay esophageal emptying such as stricture or achalasia; inability to stand or sit upright for at least 30 minutes; oral solution should not be used in patients at risk of aspiration

Warnings
Use caution in patients with renal impairment (not recommended for use in patients with Cl$_{cr}$ <35 mL/minute); hypocalcemia must be corrected before therapy initiation; ensure adequate calcium and vitamin D intake. May cause irritation to upper gastrointestinal mucosa. Esophagitis, esophageal ulcers, esophageal erosions, and esophageal stricture (rare) have been reported; risk increases in patients unable to comply with dosing instructions. Use with caution in patients with dysphagia, esophageal disease, gastritis, duodenitis, or ulcers (may worsen underlying condition).

Bisphosphonate therapy has been associated with osteonecrosis, primarily of the jaw; this has been observed mostly in cancer patients, but also in patients with postmenopausal osteoporosis and other diagnoses. Risk factors include a diagnosis of cancer, with concomitant chemotherapy, radiotherapy, or corticosteroids; anemia, coagulopathy, infection, or pre-existing dental disease. Symptoms included nonhealing extraction socket or an exposed jawbone. There are no data addressing whether discontinuation of therapy reduces the risk of developing osteonecrosis; however, as a precautionary measure, dental exams and preventative dentistry should be performed prior to placing patients with risk factors on chronic bisphosphonate therapy. Invasive dental procedures should be avoided during treatment.

Infrequently, severe (and occasionally debilitating) bone, joint, and/or muscle pain have been reported during bisphosphonate treatment. The onset of pain ranged from a single day to several months. Symptoms usually resolve upon discontinuation. Some patients experienced recurrence when rechallenged with same drug or another bisphosphonate; avoid use in patients with a history of these symptoms in association with bisphosphonate therapy.

Safety and efficacy in children have not been established.

Dosage Forms
Note: Strength expressed as free acid
Solution, oral, as monosodium trihydrate:
Fosamax™: 70 mg/75 mL [contains parabens; raspberry flavor]
Tablet, as sodium:
Fosamax™: 5 mg, 10 mg, 35 mg, 40 mg, 70 mg

Reference Range After a 10 mg I.V. dose, peak serum level of alendronic acid is ~309 ng/mL

Overdosage/Treatment Supportive therapy: I.V. hydration; monitor urine flow and calcium and phosphorus level; for esophageal ulceration, discontinue the drug and give ranitidine 150 mg twice daily

Drug Interactions
Aminoglycosides: May lower serum calcium levels with prolonged administration. Concomitant use may have an additive hypocalcemic effect.
Antacids: May decrease the absorption of bisphosphonate derivatives; should be administered at a different time of the day. Antacids containing aluminum, calcium, or magnesium are of specific concern.

Calcium salts: May decrease the absorption of bisphosphonate derivatives. Separate oral dosing in order to minimize risk of interaction.
Iron salts: May decrease the absorption of bisphosphonate derivatives. Only oral iron salts and oral bisphosphonates are of concern.
Magnesium salts: May decrease the absorption of bisphosphonate derivatives. Only oral magnesium salts and oral bisphosphonates are of concern.
Nonsteroidal anti-inflammatory drugs (NSAIDs): May enhance the gastrointestinal adverse/toxic effects (increased incidence of GI ulcers) of bisphosphonate derivatives.
Phosphate supplements: Bisphosphonate derivatives may enhance the hypocalcemic effect of phosphate supplements.

Pregnancy Risk Factor C
Pregnancy Implications Safety and efficacy have not been established in pregnant women. Animal studies have shown delays in delivery and fetal/neonatal death (secondary to hypocalcemia). Bisphosphonates are incorporated into the bone matrix and gradually released over time. Theoretically, there may be a risk of fetal harm when pregnancy follows the completion of therapy. Based on limited case reports with pamidronate, serum calcium levels in the newborn may be altered if administered during pregnancy.

Lactation Excretion in breast milk unknown/use caution

Additional Information Better suited than etidronate for chronic therapy due to the fact that alendronic acid does not impair bone mineralization and thus does not increase the risk for osteomalacia. Rapid injection can lead to renal failure due to calcium biphosphonate formation in renal tubules. Alendronate is 200-1000 times more potent than etidronate. Should be taken with a full glass of water; should not lie down for 30 minutes after taking this drug

Specific References
French AE, Kaplan N, Lishner M, et al, "Taking Bisphosphonates During Pregnancy," *Can Fam Physician*, 2003, 49:1281-2.

Alfentanil

Pronunciation (al FEN ta nil)
CAS Number 64049-06-5; 70879-28-6; 71195-58-9
U.S. Brand Names Alfenta®
Synonyms Alfentanil Hydrochloride
Impairment Potential Yes
Use Analgesia; adjunct to anesthesia
Mechanism of Action Binds with stereospecific receptors at many sites within the CNS, increases pain threshold, alters pain perception, inhibits ascending pain pathways; is an ultra short-acting narcotic

Adverse Reactions
Cardiovascular: **Bradycardia**, **hypotension**, cardiac arrhythmias, hypotension (orthostatic), circulatory depression, sinus bradycardia, sinus tachycardia, **peripheral vasodilation**
Central nervous system: **Drowsiness**, confusion, CNS depression, seizures, agitation, paradoxical CNS excitation or delirium, dizziness, **sedation, increased intracranial pressure**, extrapyramidal symptoms
Dermatologic: Skin rash, hives, itching
Endocrine & metabolic: **Syndrome of inappropriate antidiuretic hormone release**
Gastrointestinal: **Nausea, vomiting**, biliary spasm, **constipation**
Genitourinary: Priapism
Neuromuscular & skeletal: Dysesthesia
Ocular: Blurred vision, **miosis**
Respiratory: Apnea, **respiratory depression** (at doses >1000 mcg), bronchospasm, sinus arrest, apnea, laryngospasm
Miscellaneous: Cold, clammy skin, physical and psychological dependence with prolonged use

Signs and Symptoms of Overdose Clammy skin, CNS depression, dysphagia, hiccups, miosis, respiratory depression, seizures, wheezing

Pharmacodynamics/Kinetics
Onset of action: Rapid
Duration (dose dependent): 30-60 minutes
Distribution: V$_d$: Newborns, premature: 1 L/kg; Children: 0.163-0.48 L/kg; Adults: 0.46 L/kg
Half-life elimination: Newborns, premature: 5.33-8.75 hours; Children: 40-60 minutes; Adults: 83-97 minutes

Toxicodynamics/Kinetics
Protein binding: 92%
Metabolism: Hepatic to noralfentanil

Dosage
Doses should be titrated to appropriate effects; wide range of doses is dependent upon desired degree of analgesia/anesthesia
Children <12 years: Dose not established
Adults: Dose should be based on ideal body weight. See table.

Alfentanil

Indication	Approx Duration of Anesthesia (min)	Induction Period (Initial Dose) (mcg/kg)	Maintenance Period (Increments/ Infusion)	Total Dose (mcg/kg)	Effects
Incremental injection	≤30	8-20	3-5 mcg/kg or 0.5-1 mcg/kg/min	8-40	Spontaneously breathing or assisted ventilation when required.
	30-60	20-50	5-15 mcg/kg	Up to 75	Assisted or controlled ventilation required. Attenuation of response to laryngoscopy and intubation.
Continuous infusion	>45	50-75	0.5-3 mcg/kg/min average infusion rate 1-1.5 mcg/kg/min	Dependent on duration of procedure	Assisted or controlled ventilation required. Some attenuation of response to intubation and incision, with intraoperative stability.
Anesthetic induction	>45	130-245	0.5-1.5 mcg/kg/min or general anesthetic	Dependent on duration of procedure	Assisted or controlled ventilation required. Administer slowly (over 3 minutes). Concentration of inhalation agents reduced by 30% to 50% for initial hour.

Stability Dilute in D_5W, normal saline, or LR

Monitoring Parameters Respiratory rate, blood pressure, heart rate

Administration
Administer I.V. slowly over 3-5 minutes or by I.V. continuous infusion

Contraindications Hypersensitivity to alfentanil hydrochloride, to narcotics, or any component of the formulation; increased intracranial pressure, severe respiratory depression

Warnings Use with caution in patients with drug dependence, head injury, acute asthma and respiratory conditions; hypotension has occurred in neonates with respiratory distress syndrome; use caution when administering to patients with bradyarrhythmias; rapid I.V. infusion may result in skeletal muscle and chest wall rigidity, impaired ventilation, or respiratory distress/arrest; inject slowly over 3-5 minutes; nondepolarizing skeletal muscle relaxant may be required. Alfentanil may produce more hypotension compared to fentanyl, therefore, be sure to administer slowly and ensure patient has adequate hydration.

Dosage Forms
Injection, solution [preservative free]: 500 mcg/mL (2 mL, 5 mL, 10 mL)
Alfenta®: 500 mcg/mL (2 mL, 5 mL, 10 mL, 20 mL)

Reference Range 100-340 ng/mL (depending upon procedure); 310-340 ng/mL adequate anesthesia for intra-abdominal surgery; 190 ng/mL adequate for skin closure; 100-200 ng/mL adequate for superficial surgery

Overdosage/Treatment
Decontamination: Lavage (within 1 hour)/activated charcoal for oral ingestion
Supportive therapy: Naloxone in large doses and/or a continuous infusion may be necessary

Antidote(s)
- Nalmefene [ANTIDOTE]
- Naloxone [ANTIDOTE]

Drug Interactions
Substrate of CYP3A4 (major)
Dextroamphetamine: May enhance the analgesic effect of morphine and other opiate agonists.
Increased toxicity with CNS depressants (eg, benzodiazepines, barbiturates, tricyclic antidepressants), erythromycin, reserpine, beta-blockers.
CYP3A4 inhibitors: May increase the levels/effects of alfentanil. Example inhibitors include azole antifungals, clarithromycin, diclofenac, doxycycline, erythromycin, imatinib, isoniazid, nefazodone, nicardipine, propofol, protease inhibitors, quinidine, telithromycin, and verapamil.

Pregnancy Risk Factor C

Pregnancy Implications Neonatal respiratory depression can occur

Additional Information Alfentanil may produce more hypotension compared to fentanyl; therefore, administer slowly and ensure adequate hydration. Half-life is increased in burn patients. Since the drug does not release histamine, it can be used safely in patients with pheochromocytoma.

Alglucerase

Pronunciation (al GLOO ser ase)

CAS Number 143003-46-7

U.S. Brand Names Ceredase®

Synonyms Glucocerebrosidase

Use Replacement therapy for Gaucher's disease (type 1)

Mechanism of Action Glucocerebrosidase is an enzyme prepared from human placental tissue. Gaucher's disease is an inherited metabolic disorder caused by the defective activity of beta-glucosidase and the resultant accumulation of glucosyl ceramide laden macrophages in the liver, bone, and spleen. The disease affects an estimated 10,000-15,000 people in the United States, primarily of Eastern European Jewish descent, with up to 5,000 being symptomatic and requiring treatment; Ceredase® acts by replacing the missing enzyme associated with Gaucher's disease.

Adverse Reactions
Frequency not defined.
Cardiovascular: Peripheral edema
Central nervous system: Chills, fatigue, fever, headache, lightheadedness
Endocrine & metabolic: Hot flashes, menstrual abnormalities
Gastrointestinal: Abdominal discomfort, diarrhea, nausea, oral ulcerations, vomiting
Local: Injection site: Abscess, burning, discomfort, pruritus, swelling
Neuromuscular & skeletal: Backache, weakness
Miscellaneous: Dysosmia; hypersensitivity reactions (abdominal cramping, angioedema, chest discomfort, flushing, hypotension, nausea, pruritus, respiratory symptoms, urticaria); IgG antibody formation (~13%)

Signs and Symptoms of Overdose No obvious toxicity detected following single doses of up to 234 units/kg

Pharmacodynamics/Kinetics Half-life elimination: ~3-11 minutes

Dosage I.V.: Children and Adults: Dosing is individualized based on disease severity; average dose: 60 units/kg every 2 weeks. Range: 2.5 units/kg 3 times/week to 60 units/kg 1-4 times/week. Once patient response is well established, dose may be reduced every 3-6 months to determine maintenance therapy.

Monitoring Parameters CBC, platelets, liver function tests, IgG antibody formation, acid phosphatase (AP)

Administration
I.V.: Infuse I.V. over 1-2 hours; use of an in-line filter is recommended; do not shake solution as it denatures the enzyme

Contraindications Hypersensitivity to any component of the formulation

Warnings
Prepared from pooled human placental tissue that may contain the causative agents of some viral diseases. Patients who develop IgG antibodies may be at a higher risk for developing hypersensitivity. Use caution with androgen-sensitive malignancies or prior allergies to hCG. May cause early virilization in males <10 years of age. Safety and efficacy have not been established in children <2 years of age.

Dosage Forms
[DSC] = Discontinued product
Injection, solution [preservative free]: 10 units/mL (5 mL) [DSC]; 80 units/mL (5 mL) [contains human albumin 1%]

Overdosage/Treatment Supportive therapy: Acetaminophen for fever therapy

Test Interactions False positive pregnancy tests

Pregnancy Risk Factor C

Pregnancy Implications Animal studies have not been conducted.

Lactation Excretion in breast milk unknown/use caution

Allopurinol

Pronunciation (al oh PURE i nole)
CAS Number 315-30-0
U.S. Brand Names Aloprim™; Zyloprim®
Synonyms Allopurinol Sodium
Use
 Oral: Prevention of attack of gouty arthritis and nephropathy; treatment of secondary hyperuricemia which may occur during treatment of tumors or leukemia; prevention of recurrent calcium oxalate calculi
 I.V.: Treatment of elevated serum and urinary uric acid levels when oral therapy is not tolerated in patients with leukemia, lymphoma, and solid tumor malignancies who are receiving cancer chemotherapy
Mechanism of Action Decreases the production of uric acid by inhibiting the action of xanthine oxidase, an enzyme that converts hypoxanthine to xanthine and xanthine to uric acid
Adverse Reactions
 Cardiovascular: Cerebral vasculitis, leukocytoclastic vasculitis, vasculitis
 Central nervous system: Drowsiness, neuritis, fever, hyperthermia, aseptic meningitis
 Dermatologic: **Pruritic maculopapular rash**, **exfoliative dermatitis**, erythema multiforme, toxic pustuloderma, pustulosis, generalized granuloma annulare, **Stevens-Johnson syndrome**, exanthema, angioedema, urticaria, onycholysis, licheniform eruptions, cutaneous vasculitis
 Gastrointestinal: GI irritation, stomatitis
 Hematologic: Leukocytosis, leukopenia, thrombocytopenia, eosinophilia, bone marrow suppression
 Hepatic: Hepatitis, centrilobular hepatic necrosis, granulomatous hepatitis, cholestasis
 Ocular: Cataracts, diplopia
 Renal: Renal impairment, proteinuria, acute tubular necrosis, renal vasculitis
 Miscellaneous: Systemic lupus erythematosus, fixed drug eruption, elevated antineutrophilic cytoplasmic antibodies (ANCA)
Signs and Symptoms of Overdose Most symptoms are from chronic use. Agranulocytosis, alopecia, cerebral edema, dysosmia, centrilobular hepatic necrosis, granulocytopenia, hematuria, hepatitis, hypersensitivity, hyperthermia, leukopenia, metallic taste, myoglobinuria, nausea, nephritis, neutropenia, paresthesia, pseudotumor cerebri, seizures, toxic epidermal necrolysis, vomiting, wheezing
Admission Criteria/Prognosis Admit ingestions >6 g.
Pharmacodynamics/Kinetics
 Onset of action: Peak effect: 1-2 weeks
 Absorption: Oral: ~80%; Rectal: Poor and erratic
 Distribution: V_d: ~1.6 L/kg; V_{ss}: 0.84-0.87 L/kg; enters breast milk
 Protein binding: <1%
 Metabolism: ~75% to active metabolites, chiefly oxypurinol
 Bioavailability: 49% to 53%
 Half-life elimination:
  Normal renal function: Parent drug: 1-3 hours; Oxypurinol: 18-30 hours
  End-stage renal disease: Prolonged
 Time to peak, plasma: Oral: 30-120 minutes
 Excretion: Urine (76% as oxypurinol, 12% as unchanged drug)
 Allopurinol and oxypurinol are dialyzable
Dosage
 Oral: Doses >300 mg should be given in divided doses.
  Children ≤10 years: Secondary hyperuricemia associated with chemotherapy: 10 mg/kg/day in 2-3 divided doses **or** 200-300 mg/m²/day in 2-4 divided doses, maximum: 800 mg/24 hours
   Alternative (manufacturer labeling): <6 years: 150 mg/day in 3 divided doses; 6-10 years: 300 mg/day in 2-3 divided doses
  Children >10 years and Adults:
   Secondary hyperuricemia associated with chemotherapy: 600-800 mg/day in 2-3 divided doses for prevention of acute uric acid nephropathy for 2-3 days starting 1-2 days before chemotherapy
   Gout: Mild: 200-300 mg/day; Severe: 400-600 mg/day; to reduce the possibility of acute gouty attacks, initiate dose at 100 mg/day and increase weekly to recommended dosage.
   Recurrent calcium oxalate stones: 200-300 mg/day in single or divided doses
  Elderly: Initial: 100 mg/day, increase until desired uric acid level is obtained
 I.V.: Hyperuricemia secondary to chemotherapy: Intravenous daily dose can be given as a single infusion or in equally divided doses at 6-, 8-, or 12-hour intervals. A fluid intake sufficient to yield a daily urinary output of at least 2 L in adults and the maintenance of a neutral or, preferably, slightly alkaline urine are desirable.
  Children ≤10 years: Starting dose: 200 mg/m²/day
  Children >10 years and Adults: 200-400 mg/m²/day (max: 600 mg/day)
Dosing adjustment in renal impairment: Must be adjusted due to accumulation of allopurinol and metabolites:
 Oral: Removed by hemodialysis; adult maintenance doses of allopurinol (mg) based on creatinine clearance (mL/minute): See table.

Adult Maintenance Doses of Allopurinol*

Creatinine Clearance (mL/min)	Maintenance Dose of Allopurinol (mg)
140	400 qd
120	350 qd
100	300 qd
80	250 qd
60	200 qd
40	150 qd
20	100 qd
10	100 q2d
0	100 q3d

*This table is based on a standard maintenance dose of 300 mg of allopurinol per day for a patient with a creatinine clearance of 100 mL/min.

 Hemodialysis: Administer dose posthemodialysis or administer 50% supplemental dose
  I.V.:
   Cl_{cr} 10-20 mL/minute: 200 mg/day
   Cl_{cr} 3-10 mL/minute: 100 mg/day
   Cl_{cr} <3 mL/minute: 100 mg/day at extended intervals
Monitoring Parameters CBC, serum uric acid levels, I & O, hepatic and renal function, especially at start of therapy
Administration
 Oral: Should administer oral forms after meals with plenty of fluid.
  I.V.: The rate of infusion depends on the volume of the infusion. Whenever possible, therapy should be initiated at 24-48 hours before the start of chemotherapy known to cause tumor lysis (including adrenocorticosteroids). I.V. daily dose can be administered as a single infusion or in equally divided doses at 6-, 8-, or 12-hour interval.
Contraindications Hypersensitivity to allopurinol or any component of the formulation
Warnings
 Do not use to treat asymptomatic hyperuricemia. Discontinue at first signs of rash. Caution in renal impairment, dosage adjustments needed. Use with caution in patients taking diuretics concurrently. Risk of skin rash may be increased in patients receiving amoxicillin or ampicillin. The risk of hypersensitivity may be increased in patients receiving thiazides, and possibly ACE inhibitors. Use caution with mercaptopurine or azathioprine.
Dosage Forms
 Injection, powder for reconstitution, as sodium (Aloprim™): 500 mg
 Tablet (Zyloprim®): 100 mg, 300 mg
Reference Range
 Allopurinol: Therapeutic: 3-9 mcg/mL
 Oxypurinol: Therapeutic: 4-8 mcg/mL
  Blood allopurinol level of 231 mcg/mL has been associated with fatal centrilobular hepatic necrosis in an overdose setting
 Serum uric acid: Adults: Male: 3.4-7.0 mg/dL (SI: 202-416 μmol/L) or slightly more; Female: 2.4-6.0 mg/dL (SI: 143-357 μmol/L) or slightly more
 An increase occurs during childhood. Values >7.0 mg/dL (SI: 416 μmol/L) are sometimes arbitrarily regarded as hyperuricemia, but there is no sharp line between normals on the one hand, and the serum uric acid of those with clinical gout. Normal ranges cannot be adjusted for purine ingestion, but high purine diet increases uric acid. Uric acid may be increased with body size, exercise, and stress. One fatal case was reported with levels of 230 mcg/mL; death is rare.
Overdosage/Treatment
 Decontamination: Emesis within 30 minutes in ingestions; lavage within 1 hour if indicated in ingestions >6 g; activated charcoal should be given
 Supportive therapy: If significant amounts of allopurinol are thought to have been absorbed, it is a theoretical possibility that oxypurinol stones could be formed but no record of such occurrence in overdose exists. Alkalinization of the urine and forced diuresis can help prevent potential xanthine stone formation. Steroids and antihistamines are useful for hypersensitivity.
 Enhancement of elimination: Removed by hemodialysis, but this modality is of unknown value in overdose
Test Interactions ↑ alkaline phosphatase, AST, ALT, bilirubin, eosinophils, BUN, creatinine; ↓ uric acid (S), cholesterol (S)
Drug Interactions
 Ampicillin, amoxicillin: Incidence of rash may be increased.
 Anticoagulants: Allopurinol may prolong the half-life of anticoagulants, effect seen with dicumarol; monitor.
 ACE inhibitors: Captopril may increase risk of hypersensitivity.
 Azathioprine: Metabolism inhibited by allopurinol; reduce azathioprine dose by $^1/_3$ or $^1/_4$.

Chlorpropamide: Half-life of chlorpropamide may be increased.
Cyclosporine: Allopurinol may increase cyclosporine serum levels.
Mercaptopurine: Metabolism inhibited by allopurinol; reduce mercapto-purine dose by $^1/_3$ or $^1/_4$.
Thiazide diuretics: Toxicity and risk of hypersensitivity may be increased.
Theophylline: Half-life of theophylline may be increased.
Vidarabine: Neurotoxicity may be enhanced.

Pregnancy Risk Factor C

Pregnancy Implications There are few reports describing the use of allopurinol during pregnancy; no adverse fetal outcomes attributable to allopurinol have been reported in humans; use only if potential benefit outweighs the potential risk to the fetus.

Lactation Enters breast milk/use caution (AAP rates "compatible")

Additional Information Skin rash occurs most often in patients taking diuretics concurrently; may predispose patient to ampicillin-induced rash; alcohol decreases effectiveness

Indications for desensitization in patients with allopurinol-induced maculopapular eruptions:
• Patients with gout and renal insufficiency rendering uricosurics ineffective
• Patients with gout and allergy or intolerance of uricosuric drugs
• Patients with gout, "overproduction" hyperuricemia, uricosuria, and uric acid nephrolithiasis
• Patients with malignancy-associated hyperuricemia caused by cytolytic therapy for myelo- or lymphoproliferative disorder

For standard allopurinol desensitization protocol: See table.

Specific References

Buie LW, Oertel MD, Cala, SO, "Allopurinol as Adjuvant Therapy in Poorly Responsive or Treatment Refractory Schizophrenia," *Ann Pharmacother*, 2006, 40(12):2200-2204.

Chao SC, Yang CC, and Lee JY, "Hypersensitivity Syndrome and Pure Red Cell Aplasia Following Allopurinol Therapy in a Patient with Chronic Kidney Disease," *Ann Pharmacother*, 2005, 39(9):1552-6.

Gomez-Cabrera MC, Pallardo FV, Sastre J, et al, "Allopurinol and Markers of Muscle Damage Among Participants in the Tour de France," *JAMA*, 2003, 289(19):2503-4.

Raebel MA, McClure DL, Simon SR, et al, "Frequency of Serum Creatinine Monitoring During Allopurinol Therapy in Ambulatory Patients," *Ann Pharmacother*, 2006, 40(3):386-91.

Alprazolam

Pronunciation (al PRAY zoe lam)

CAS Number 28981-97-7

U.S. Brand Names Alprazolam Intensol®; Xanax XR®; Xanax®

Impairment Potential Yes. Cognitive and psychomotor deficits occur in the elderly at doses of 0.25 mg and 0.5 mg. At the lower dose, the effect appears to last for 2.5 hours. (Pomara N, Tun H, DaSilva D, et al, "Benzodiazepine Use and Crash Risk in Older Patients," *JAMA*, 1998, 279(2):113-4.)

Use Treatment of anxiety disorder (GAD); panic disorder, with or without agoraphobia; anxiety associated with depression

Unlabeled/Investigational Use Anxiety in children

Mechanism of Action Binds at stereospecific receptors at several sites within the central nervous system, including the limbic system and reticular formation; effects may be mediated through GABA. Alprazolam is a triazolobenzodiazepine with some antidepressant activity.

Adverse Reactions

Cardiovascular: Hypotension

Central nervous system: **Drowsiness, fatigue, ataxia, lightheadedness, memory impairment, dysarthria, irritability, sedation, depression**, confusion, derealization, dizziness, disinhibition, akathisia, nightmares

Dermatologic: Dermatitis, rash

Endocrine & metabolic: **Libido decreased**, libido increased, **menstrual disorders**

Gastrointestinal: **Xerostomia, salivation decreased, appetite increased/decreased, weight gain/loss**, salivation increased, dyspepsia

Genitourinary: **Micturition difficulties**, sexual dysfunction, incontinence

Neuromuscular & skeletal: Rigidity, tremor, muscle cramps, ataxia, arthralgia

Otic: Tinnitus

Respiratory: Nasal congestion, dyspnea

Miscellaneous: Diaphoresis

Signs and Symptoms of Overdose Coma, combativeness, confusion, delirium, depression, dermatitis, diminished reflexes, hypotension, hypothermia, insomnia, lightheadedness, leukocytosis, mania, photosensitivity, respiratory depression, somnolence

Pharmacodynamics/Kinetics

Distribution: V_d: 0.9-1.2 L/kg; enters breast milk

Protein binding: 80%

Metabolism: Hepatic via CYP3A4; forms two active metabolites (4-hydroxyalprazolam and α-hydroxyalprazolam)

Bioavailability: 90%

Half-life elimination:
Adults: 11.2 hours (range: 6.3-26.9)

Elderly: 16.3 hours (range: 9-26.9 hours)
Alcoholic liver disease: 19.7 hours (range: 5.8-65.3 hours)
Obesity: 21.8 hours (range: 9.9-40.4 hours)

Time to peak, serum: 1-2 hours

Excretion: Urine (as unchanged drug and metabolites)

Dosage

Oral: **Note:** Treatment >4 months should be re-evaluated to determine the patient's continued need for the drug

Children: Anxiety (unlabeled use): Immediate release: Initial: 0.005 mg/kg/dose or 0.125 mg/dose 3 times/day; increase in increments of 0.125-0.25 mg, up to a maximum of 0.02 mg/kg/dose or 0.06 mg/kg/day (0.375-3 mg/day)

Adults:

Anxiety: Immediate release: Effective doses are 0.5-4 mg/day in divided doses; the manufacturer recommends starting at 0.25-0.5 mg 3 times/day; titrate dose upward; maximum: 4 mg/day

Anxiety associated with depression: Immediate release: Average dose required: 2.5-3 mg/day in divided doses

Ethanol withdrawal (unlabeled use): Immediate release: Usual dose: 2-2.5 mg/day in divided doses

Panic disorder:

Immediate release: Initial: 0.5 mg 3 times/day; dose may be increased every 3-4 days in increments ≤1 mg/day; many patients obtain relief at 2 mg/day, as much as 10 mg/day may be required

Extended release: 0.5-1 mg once daily; may increase dose every 3-4 days in increments ≤1 mg/day (range: 3-6 mg/day)

Switching from immediate release to extended release: Patients may be switched to extended release tablets by taking the total daily dose of the immediate release tablets and giving it once daily using the extended release preparation.

Dose reduction: Abrupt discontinuation should be avoided. Daily dose may be decreased by 0.5 mg every 3 days, however, some patients may require a slower reduction. If withdrawal symptoms occur, resume previous dose and discontinue on a less rapid schedule.

Elderly: Elderly patients may be more sensitive to the effects of alprazolam including ataxia and oversedation. The elderly may also have impaired renal function leading to decreased clearance. The smallest effective dose should be used. Titrate gradually, if needed.
Immediate release: Initial 0.25 mg 2-3 times/day
Extended release: Initial: 0.5 mg once daily

Dosing adjustment in hepatic impairment: Reduce dose by 50% to 60% or avoid in cirrhosis

Monitoring Parameters Respiratory and cardiovascular status

Administration Immediate release preparations: Can be administered sublingually with comparable onset and completeness of absorption.

Extended release tablet: Should be taken once daily in the morning; do not crush, break or chew.

Contraindications Hypersensitivity to alprazolam or any component of the formulation (cross-sensitivity with other benzodiazepines may exist); narrow-angle glaucoma; concurrent use with ketoconazole or itraconazole; pregnancy

Warnings

Rebound or withdrawal symptoms, including seizures, may occur 18 hours to 3 days following abrupt discontinuation or large decreases in dose (more common in patients receiving >4 mg/day or prolonged treatment). Dose reductions or tapering must be approached with extreme caution. Breakthrough anxiety may occur at the end of dosing interval. Use with caution in patients receiving concurrent CYP3A4 inhibitors, particularly when these agents are added to therapy. Has weak uricosuric properties, use with caution in renal impairment or predisposition to urate nephropathy. Use with caution in elderly or debilitated patients, patients with hepatic disease (including alcoholics), renal impairment, or obese patients.

Causes CNS depression (dose related) resulting in sedation, dizziness, confusion, or ataxia which may impair physical and mental capabilities. Patients must be cautioned about performing tasks which require mental alertness (eg, operating machinery or driving). Use with caution in patients receiving other CNS depressants or psychoactive agents. Effects with other sedative drugs or ethanol may be potentiated. Benzodiazepines have been associated with falls and traumatic injury and should be used with extreme caution in patients who are at risk of these events (especially the elderly). Use with caution in patients with respiratory disease or impaired gag reflex.

Use caution in patients with depression, particularly if suicidal risk may be present. Episodes of mania or hypomania have occurred in depressed patients treated with alprazolam. May cause physical or psychological dependence - use with caution in patients with a history of drug dependence. Acute withdrawal, including seizures, may be precipitated in patients after administration of flumazenil to patients receiving long-term benzodiazepine therapy.

Benzodiazepines have been associated with anterograde amnesia. Paradoxical reactions, including hyperactive or aggressive behavior, have been reported with benzodiazepines, particularly in adolescent/

pediatric or psychiatric patients. Does not have analgesic, antidepressant, or antipsychotic properties.

Benzodiazepines have the potential to cause harm to the fetus, particularly when administered during the first trimester. In addition, withdrawal symptoms may occur in the neonate following *in utero* exposure. Use of alprazolam during pregnancy should be avoided. In addition, symptoms of withdrawal, lethargy, and loss of body weight have been reported in infants exposed to alprazolam and/or benzodiazepines while nursing; use during breast-feeding is not recommended.

Dosage Forms
Solution, oral [concentrate]:
Alprazolam Intensol®: 1 mg/mL (30 mL)
Tablet: 0.25 mg, 0.5 mg, 1 mg, 2 mg
Xanax®: 0.25 mg, 0.5 mg, 1 mg, 2 mg
Tablet, extended release: 0.5 mg, 1 mg, 2 mg, 3 mg
Xanax XR®: 0.5 mg, 1 mg, 2 mg, 3 mg
Tablet, orally disintegrating [scored]:
Niravam™: 0.25 mg, 0.5 mg, 1 mg, 2 mg [orange flavor]

Reference Range
Therapeutic plasma level 20-30 ng/mL; postmortem levels average ~230 ng/mL in suicides; in the postmortem state, anatomical site concentration differences (ie, postmortem redistribution) may occur; postmortem levels in overdoses range from 122-390 mcg/L

Overdosage/Treatment
Decontamination: Lavage (within 1 hour)/activated charcoal
Supportive: Treatment for benzodiazepine overdose is supportive. Rarely is mechanical ventilation required. Flumazenil has been shown to selectively block the binding of benzodiazepines to CNS receptors, resulting in a reversal of benzodiazepine-induced CNS depression. Carbamazepine may be effective for withdrawal.
Enhancement of elimination: Multiple dosing of activated charcoal may be effective

Antidote(s)
● Flumazenil [ANTIDOTE]

Test Interactions ↑ alkaline phosphatase; Visine®, Drano®, bleach may cause false-negative urine tests; oxazepam may interfere giving falsely elevated glucose results

Drug Interactions
Substrate of CYP3A4 (major)
CNS depressants: Sedative effects and/or respiratory depression may be additive with CNS depressants. Includes ethanol, barbiturates, narcotic analgesics, and other sedative agents; monitor for increased effect.
CYP3A4 inducers: CYP3A4 inducers may decrease the levels/effects of alprazolam. Example inducers include aminoglutethimide, carbamazepine, nafcillin, nevirapine, phenobarbital, phenytoin, and rifamycins.
CYP3A4 inhibitors: May increase the levels/effects of alprazolam. Example inhibitors include azole antifungals, clarithromycin, diclofenac, doxycycline, erythromycin, imatinib, isoniazid, nefazodone, nicardipine, propofol, protease inhibitors, quinidine, telithromycin, and verapamil. Contraindicated with itraconazole and ketoconazole.
Fluoxetine: May increase plasma concentrations/effects of alprazolam.
Oral contraceptives: May increase serum levels/effects of alprazolam.
Theophylline: May partially antagonize some of the effects of benzodiazepines; monitor for decreased response; may require higher doses for sedation.
Tricyclic antidepressants: Plasma concentrations of imipramine and desipramine have been reported to be increased 31% and 20%, respectively, by concomitant administration; monitor.

Pregnancy Risk Factor D
Pregnancy Implications Benzodiazepines have the potential to cause harm to the fetus, particularly when administered during the first trimester. In addition, withdrawal symptoms may occur in the neonate following *in utero* exposure. Use during pregnancy should be avoided.
Lactation Enters breast milk/not recommended (AAP rates "of concern")
Nursing Implications Assist with ambulation during beginning therapy, raise bed rails and keep room partially illuminated at night; monitor for CNS respiratory depression
Additional Information Not intended for management of anxiety and minor distress associated with everyday life; treatment longer than 4 months should be re-evaluated to determine need for the drug; 1 mg of alprazolam is approximately equivalent in anxiolytic activity to 10 mg of diazepam

Specific References
Banerji S, Schiavoni A, Bronstein AC, et al, "Alprazolam Toxicity After Accidental Inhalation Exposure at a Pharmaceutical Plant," *J Toxicol Clin Toxicol*, 2004, 42(5):806.
Honey D, Mazarr-Proo S, Blackwell W, et al, "Increased Incidence of Alprazolam Usage Among New Mexico Drivers," *J Anal Toxicol*, 2006, 30:150.
Isbister GK, O'Regan L, Sibbritt D, et al, "Alprazolam Is Relatively More Toxic Than Other Benzodiazepines in Overdose," *J Toxicol Clin Toxicol*, 2003, 41(5):715.
Kraner JC, Lewis SA, and Jackson GF, "Unusually High Blood Concentration of Alprazolam Along with Fentanyl in a Case of Driving Impairment," *J Anal Toxicol*, 2003, 27(3):186.

Olnes MJ, Golding A, and Kaplan PW, "Nonconvulsive Status Epilepticus Resulting from Benzodiazepine Withdrawal," *Ann Intern Med*, 2003, 139(11):956-8

Alteplase

Pronunciation (AL te plase)
Related Information
● Reteplase
CAS Number 105857-23-6
U.S. Brand Names Activase®; Cathflo™ Activase®
Synonyms Alteplase, Recombinant; Alteplase, Tissue Plasminogen Activator, Recombinant; tPA
Use
Management of acute myocardial infarction for the lysis of thrombi in coronary arteries; management of acute massive pulmonary embolism (PE) in adults; acute ischemic stroke (within 3 hours after onset of symptoms and after exclusion of intracranial hemorrhage by a cranial computerized tomography scan or other diagnostic imaging modalities)
Acute myocardial infarction (AMI): Chest pain ≥20 minutes, ≤12-24 hours; S-T elevation ≥0.1 mV in at least two ECG leads
Acute pulmonary embolism (APE): Age ≤75 years: As soon as possible within 5 days of thrombotic event. Documented massive pulmonary embolism by pulmonary angiography or echocardiography or high probability lung scan with clinical shock.
Cathflo™ Activase®: Restoration of central venous catheter function
Unlabeled/Investigational Use Acute peripheral arterial occlusive disease
Mechanism of Action Initiates local fibrinolysis by binding to fibrin in a thrombus (clot) and converts entrapped plasminogen to plasmin; does not initiate systemic fibrinolysis in absence of a thrombus
Adverse Reactions
Cardiovascular: Hypotension, reperfusion arrhythmia (bradycardia, premature ventricular contraction), pericardial effusion/pericarditis, chest pain, sinus bradycardia, angina, arrhythmias (ventricular)
Central nervous system: Fever, seizures, intracranial hemorrhage
Dermatologic: Ecchymosis, angioneurotic edema (1 case)
Gastrointestinal: Gastrointestinal hemorrhage, nausea, vomiting, gingival hemorrhage
Genitourinary: GU hemorrhage
Local: Extravasation injury
Respiratory: Epistaxis, alveolar hemorrhage, pulmonary hemorrhage
Miscellaneous: Retroperitoneal hemorrhage, allergic reactions (rare), acute atraumatic compartment syndrome
Signs and Symptoms of Overdose Coagulopathy, GI bleeding, increased incidence of intracranial bleeding or peripheral bleeding, headache, hematuria, hemoptysis, ocular hemorrhage
Pharmacodynamics/Kinetics
Duration: >50% present in plasma cleared ~5 minutes after infusion terminated, ~80% cleared within 10 minutes
Excretion: Clearance: Rapidly from circulating plasma (550-650 mL/minute), primarily hepatic; >50% present in plasma is cleared within 5 minutes after the infusion is terminated, ~80% cleared within 10 minutes
Dosage
I.V.:
Coronary artery thrombi: Front loading dose (weight-based):
Patients >67 kg: Total dose: 100 mg over 1.5 hours; infuse 15 mg over 1-2 minutes. Infuse 50 mg over 30 minutes. See "Note."
Patients ≤67 kg: Total dose: 1.25 mg/kg; infuse 15 mg I.V. bolus over 1-2 minutes, then infuse 0.75 mg/kg (not to exceed 50 mg) over next 30 minutes, followed by 0.5 mg/kg over next 60 minutes (not to exceed 35 mg). See "Note."
Note: Concurrently, begin heparin 60 units/kg bolus (maximum: 4000 units) followed by continuous infusion of 12 units/kg/hour (maximum: 1000 units/hour) and adjust to aPTT target of 1.5-2 times the upper limit of control. Infuse remaining 35 mg of alteplase over the next hour.
Acute pulmonary embolism: 100 mg over 2 hours.
Acute ischemic stroke: Doses should be given within the first 3 hours of the onset of symptoms; recommended total dose: 0.9 mg/kg (maximum dose should not exceed 90 mg) infused over 60 minutes.
Load with 0.09 mg/kg (10% of the 0.9 mg/kg dose) as an I.V. bolus over 1 minute, followed by 0.81 mg/kg (90% of the 0.9 mg/kg dose) as a continuous infusion over 60 minutes. Heparin should not be started for 24 hours or more after starting alteplase for stroke.
Intracatheter: Central venous catheter clearance: Cathflo™ Activase®:
Patients ≥10 to <30 kg: 110% of the internal lumen volume of the catheter (≤2 mg [1 mg/mL]); retain in catheter for ≤2 hours; may instill a second dose if catheter remains occluded
Patients ≥30 kg: 2 mg (1 mg/mL); retain in catheter for ≤2 hours; may instill a second dose if catheter remains occluded
Intra-arterial: Acute peripheral arterial occlusive disease (unlabeled use): 0.02-0.1 mg/kg/hour for up to 36 hours

Advisory Panel to the Society for Cardiovascular and Interventional Radiology on Thrombolytic Therapy recommendation: ≤2 mg/hour and subtherapeutic heparin (aPTT <1.5 times baseline)

Stability
Activase®: The lyophilized product may be stored at room temperature (not to exceed 30°C/86°F), or under refrigeration; once reconstituted it must be used within 8 hours. Reconstitution:
50 mg vial: Use accompanying diluent (50 mL sterile water for injection); do not shake; final concentration: 1 mg/mL
100 mg vial: Use transfer set with accompanying diluent (100 mL vial of sterile water for injection); no vacuum is present in 100 mg vial; final concentration: 1 mg/mL Alteplase is **incompatible** with dobutamine, dopamine, heparin, and nitroglycerin infusions; physically **compatible** with lidocaine, metoprolol, and propranolol when administered via Y-site; **compatible** with either D_5W or NS. Standard dose: 100 mg/100 mL 0.9% NaCl (total volume: 200 mL)
Cathflo™ Activase®: Store lyophilized product under refrigeration; protect from excessive exposure to light when stored for extended periods of time. Reconstitution: Add 2.2 mL SWFI to vial; do not shake. Final concentration: 1 mg/mL. Once reconstituted, store at 2°C to 30°C (36°F to 86°F). Do not mix other medications into infusion solution.

Monitoring Parameters
When using for central venous catheter clearance: Assess catheter function by attempting to aspirate blood.
When using for management of acute myocardial infarction: Assess for evidence of cardiac reperfusion through resolution of chest pain, resolution of baseline ECG changes, preserved left ventricular function, cardiac enzyme washout phenomenon, and/or the appearance of reperfusion arrhythmias; assess for bleeding potential through clinical evidence of GI bleeding, hematuria, gingival bleeding, fibrinogen levels, fibrinogen degradation products, prothrombin times, and partial thromboplastin times.

Administration Activase®:
Bolus dose may be prepared by one of three methods:
1) removal of 15 mL reconstituted (1 mg/mL) solution from vial
2) removal of 15 mL from a port on the infusion line after priming
3) programming an infusion pump to deliver a 15 mL bolus at the initiation of infusion
Remaining dose may be administered as follows:
50 mg vial: Either PVC bag or glass vial and infusion set
100 mg vial: Insert spike of the infusion set through the same puncture site created by transfer device and infuse from vial
If further dilution is desired, may be diluted in equal volume of 0.9% sodium chloride or D_5W to yield a final concentration of 0.5 mg/mL AD
Cathflo™ Activase®: Intracatheter: Instill dose into occluded catheter. Do not force solution into catheter. After a 30-minute dwell time, assess catheter function by attempting to aspirate blood. If catheter is functional, aspirate 4-5 mL of blood to remove Cathflo™ Activase® and residual clots. Gently irrigate the catheter with NS. If catheter remains nonfunctional, let Cathflo™ Activase® dwell for another 90 minutes (total dwell time: 120 minutes) and reassess function. If catheter function is not restored, a second dose may be instilled.

Contraindications
Hypersensitivity to alteplase or any component of the formulation
Treatment of acute MI or PE: Active internal bleeding; history of CVA; recent intracranial or intraspinal surgery or trauma; intracranial neoplasm; arteriovenous malformation or aneurysm; known bleeding diathesis; severe uncontrolled hypertension
Treatment of acute ischemic stroke: Evidence of intracranial hemorrhage or suspicion of subarachnoid hemorrhage on pretreatment evaluation; recent (within 3 months) intracranial or intraspinal surgery; prolonged external cardiac massage; suspected aortic dissection; serious head trauma or previous stroke; history of intracranial hemorrhage; uncontrolled hypertension at time of treatment (eg, >185 mm Hg systolic or >110 mm Hg diastolic); seizure at the onset of stroke; active internal bleeding; intracranial neoplasm; arteriovenous malformation or aneurysm; known bleeding diathesis including but not limited to: current use of anticoagulants or an INR >1.7, administration of heparin within 48 hours preceding the onset of stroke and an elevated aPTT at presentation, platelet count <100,000/mm³.
Other exclusion criteria (NINDS recombinant tPA study): Stroke or serious head injury within 3 months, major surgery or serious trauma within 2 weeks, GI or urinary tract hemorrhage within 3 weeks, aggressive treatment required to lower blood pressure, glucose level <50 mg/dL or >400 mg/dL, arterial puncture at a noncompressible site or lumbar puncture within 1 week, clinical presentation suggesting post-MI pericarditis, pregnancy, breast-feeding.
Warnings Concurrent heparin anticoagulation may contribute to bleeding. Monitor all potential bleeding sites. Doses >150 mg are associated with increased risk of intracranial hemorrhage. Intramuscular injections and nonessential handling of the patient should be avoided. Venipunctures should be performed carefully and only when necessary. If arterial puncture is necessary, use an upper extremity vessel that can be

manually compressed. If serious bleeding occurs, the infusion of alteplase and heparin should be stopped.
For the following conditions, the risk of bleeding is higher with use of thrombolytics and should be weighed against the benefits of therapy: Recent major surgery (eg, CABG, obstetrical delivery, organ biopsy, previous puncture of noncompressible vessels), cerebrovascular disease, recent gastrointestinal or genitourinary bleeding, recent trauma, hypertension (systolic BP >175 mm Hg and/or diastolic BP >110 mm Hg), high likelihood of left heart thrombus (eg, mitral stenosis with atrial fibrillation), acute pericarditis, subacute bacterial endocarditis, hemostatic defects including ones caused by severe renal or hepatic dysfunction, significant hepatic dysfunction, pregnancy, diabetic hemorrhagic retinopathy or other hemorrhagic ophthalmic conditions, septic thrombophlebitis or occluded AV cannula at seriously infected site, advanced age (eg, >75 years), patients receiving oral anticoagulants, any other condition in which bleeding constitutes a significant hazard or would be particularly difficult to manage because of location.
Coronary thrombolysis may result in reperfusion arrhythmias. Treatment of patients with acute ischemic stroke more than 3 hours after symptom onset is not recommended Treatment of patients with minor neurological deficit or with rapidly improving symptoms is not recommended.
Cathflo® Activase®: When used to restore catheter function, use Cathflo® Activase® cautiously in those patients with known or suspected catheter infections. Evaluate catheter for other causes of dysfunction before use. Avoid excessive pressure when instilling into catheter.

Dosage Forms
Injection, powder for reconstitution, recombinant:
Activase®: 50 mg [29 million int. units; contains polysorbate 80; packaged with diluent]; 100 mg [58 million int. units; contains polysorbate 80; packaged with diluent and transfer device]
Cathflo® Activase®: 2 mg [contains polysorbate 80]

Reference Range Not routinely measured; literature supports therapeutic levels of 0.52-1.80 mcg/mL

Overdosage/Treatment Supportive therapy: Treat bleeding complications with transfusions of red blood cells, fresh frozen plasma, and cryoprecipitate; do not administer dextran; although human overdose data is lacking, administration of aminocaproic acid (Amicar®) at a dose of 3-5 g I.V. followed by an infusion rate of 1-1.25 g/hour may be useful

Test Interactions Decreases fibrinogen levels 16% to 36%

Drug Interactions
Aminocaproic acid (antifibrinolytic agent) may decrease effectiveness.
Drugs which affect platelet function (eg, NSAIDs, dipyridamole, ticlopidine, clopidogrel, IIb/IIIa antagonists) may potentiate the risk of hemorrhage; use with caution.
Heparin and aspirin: Use with aspirin and heparin may increase the risk of bleeding. However, aspirin and heparin were used concomitantly with alteplase in many patients in myocardial infarction or pulmonary embolism trials. This combination was prohibited in the NINDS tPA stroke trial.
Nitroglycerin may increase the hepatic clearance of alteplase, potentially reducing lytic activity (limited clinical information).
Warfarin or oral anticoagulants: Risk of bleeding may be increased during concurrent therapy.

Pregnancy Risk Factor C
Lactation Excretion in breast milk unknown/use caution
Nursing Implications Assess for hemorrhage during first hour of treatment
Additional Information
Allergic reactions are unlikely
Investigational for angina, deep vein thrombosis, catheter thrombosis, peripheral artery thrombosis, and thrombotic stroke; has been used to treat acute myocardial infarction in a heart transplant recipient
For acute ischemic stroke, patients treated with alteplase were at least 30% more likely to have minimal or no disability at 3 months when compared with placebo. Increased incidence of symptomatic intracerebral hemorrhage noted within 36 hours of onset of stroke in e-PA treated group (6.4% in t-AP treated group versus 0.6% in placebo)
Reimbursement Hotline: 1-800-879-4747
Professional Services (Genentech): 1-800-821-8590

Specific References
Khosla S, Jain P, Manda R, et al, "Acute and Long-Term Results After Intra-Arterial Thrombolysis of Occluded Lower Extremity Bypass Grafts Using Recombinant Tissue Plasminogen Activator for Acute Limb-Threatening Ischemia," *Am J Ther*, 2003, 10(1):3-6.
Le Conte P, Huchet L, Trewick D, et al, "Efficacy of Alteplase Thrombolysis for ED Treatment of Pulmonary Embolism with Shock," *Am J Emerg Med*, 2003, 21(5):438-40.
Morris DC, Silver B, Mitsias P, et al, "Treatment of Acute Stroke with Recombinant Tissue Plasminogen Activator and Abciximab," *Acad Emerg Med*, 2003, 10(12):1396-9.
National Institute of Neurological Disorders Stroke rt-PA Stroke Study Group, "Recombinant Tissue Plasminogen Activator for Minor Strokes: The National Institute of Neurological Disorders and Stroke rt-PA Stroke Study Experience," *Ann Emerg Med*, 2005, 46(3):243-52.

Schull MJ, Vermeulen M, Slaughter G, et al, "Emergency Department Crowding and Thrombolysis Delays in Acute Myocardial Infarction," *Ann Emerg Med*, 2004, 44(6):577-85.

Walker CA, Shirk MB, Tschampel MM, et al, "Intrapleural Alteplase in a Patient with Complicated Pleural Effusion," *Ann Pharmacother*, 2003, 37(3):376-9.

Zacharias JM, Weatherston CP, Spewak CR, et al, "Alteplase Versus Urokinase for Occluded Hemodialysis Catheters," *Ann Pharmacother*, 2003, 37(1):27-33.

Altretamine

CAS Number 645-05-6

U.S. Brand Names Hexalen®

Synonyms Hexamethylmelamine; HEXM; HMM; HXM; NSC-13875

Use Palliative treatment of persistent or recurrent ovarian cancer

Mechanism of Action Although altretamine clinical antitumor spectrum resembles that of alkylating agents, the drug has demonstrated activity in alkylator-resistant patients. The drug selectively inhibits the incorporation of radioactive thymidine and uridine into DNA and RNA, inhibiting DNA and RNA synthesis; reactive intermediates covalently bind to microsomal proteins and DNA; can spontaneously degrade to demethylated melamines and formaldehyde which are also cytotoxic.

Adverse Reactions

Central nervous system: **Peripheral sensory neuropathy, neurotoxicity** (21%; may be progressive and dose-limiting), seizures, depression, dizziness

Dermatologic: Alopecia, rash

Gastrointestinal: **Nausea/vomiting** (50% to 70%), **anorexia** (48%), **diarrhea** (48%), stomach cramps

Hematologic: **Anemia, thrombocytopenia** (31%), **leukopenia** (62%), **neutropenia**

Hepatic: Alkaline phosphatase increased, hepatotoxicity

Neuromuscular & skeletal: Tremor

Pharmacodynamics/Kinetics

Absorption: Well absorbed (75% to 89%)

Distribution: Highly concentrated hepatically and renally; low in other organs

Protein binding: 50% to 94%

Metabolism: Hepatic; rapid and extensive demethylation to active metabolites (pentamethylmelamine and tetramethylmelamine)

Half-life elimination: 13 hours

Time to peak, plasma: 0.5-3 hours

Excretion: Urine (90%, <1% as unchanged drug)

Dosage

Refer to individual protocols. Oral:

Adults: 4-12 mg/kg/day in 3-4 divided doses for 21-90 days

Alternatively: 240-320 mg/m²/day in 3-4 divided doses for 21 days, repeated every 6 weeks

Alternatively: 260 mg/m²/day for 14-21 days of a 28-day cycle in 4 divided doses

Alternatively: 150 mg/m²/day in 3-4 divided doses for 14 days of a 28-day cycle

Monitoring Parameters CBC with differential, liver function tests; neurologic examination

Administration

Administer total daily dose as 3-4 divided doses after meals and at bedtime.

Contraindications Hypersensitivity to altretamine or any component of the formulation; pre-existing severe bone marrow suppression or severe neurologic toxicity; pregnancy

Warnings Hazardous agent - use appropriate precautions for handling and disposal. **[U.S. Boxed Warning]: Peripheral blood counts and neurologic examinations should be done routinely before and after drug therapy.** Myelosuppression and neurotoxicity are common; use with caution in patients previously treated with other myelosuppressive drugs or with pre-existing neurotoxicity. Use with caution in patients with renal or hepatic dysfunction. **[U.S. Boxed Warning]: Should be administered under the supervision of an experienced cancer chemotherapy physician.** Safety and efficacy in children have not been established.

Dosage Forms

Gelcap:

Hexalen®: 50 mg

Reference Range Peak plasma levels after a 200-300 mg/m² dose range from 0.3-20.8 mg/L

Overdosage/Treatment

Decontamination: Lavage (within 1 hour)/activated charcoal

Supportive therapy: Pyridoxine can be used to treat neuropathy (peripheral), although this mode of therapy is unproven

Antidote(s)

• Pyridoxine [ANTIDOTE]

Drug Interactions

MAO inhibitors: Altretamine may enhance the orthostatic effect of MAO inhibitors.

Pyridoxine: May diminish the therapeutic effect of altretamine; concurrent use not recommended.

Tricyclic antidepressants: Altretamine may enhance the orthostatic effect of tricyclic antidepressants.

Pregnancy Risk Factor D

Pregnancy Implications Teratogenic effects were noted in animal studies. There are no adequate and well-controlled studies in pregnant women. Women of childbearing potential should avoid becoming pregnant while on therapy.

Lactation Excretion in breast milk unknown/not recommended

Additional Information Mucosal and dermal irritant

Aluminum Hydroxide

Pronunciation (a LOO mi num hye DROKS ide)

CAS Number 7429-90-5

UN Number 1309; 1396; 9260

U.S. Brand Names ALternaGel® [OTC]; Alu-Cap® [OTC]

Use Antacid; coloring agent in foods; antiperspirant; also found in sucralfate (207 mg aluminum per g dose)

Mechanism of Action Neutralizes hydrochloride in stomach to form Al(Cl)₃ salt + H₂O

Adverse Reactions

Frequency not defined.

Gastrointestinal: Constipation, stomach cramps, fecal impaction, nausea, vomiting, discoloration of feces (white speckles)

Endocrine & metabolic: Hypophosphatemia, hypomagnesemia

Signs and Symptoms of Overdose Toxicity is usually seen in the setting of water contamination used in hemodialysis, aluminum hydroxide toxicity in renal failure patients, and contamination of total parenteral nutrition. Aluminum antacids may cause constipation, phosphate depletion, bezoars or fecalith formation, and feces discoloration (black; white/speckling). In patients with renal failure, aluminum may accumulate to toxic levels; jaundice may also occur.

Toxicodynamics/Kinetics

Absorption: 12% gastric, <1% oral

Protein binding: 50%

Half-life: 276 minutes

Elimination: Renal clearance: 0.12 L/hour

Dosage

Oral:

Hyperphosphatemia:

Children: 50-150 mg/kg/24 hours in divided doses every 4-6 hours, titrate dosage to maintain serum phosphorus within normal range

Adults: Initial: 300-600 mg 3 times/day with meals

Antacid: Adults: 600-1200 mg between meals and at bedtime

Topical: Apply to affected area as needed; reapply at least every 12 hours

Monitoring Parameters Monitor phosphorous levels periodically when patient is on chronic therapy

Administration

Oral: Dose should be followed with water.

Contraindications Hypersensitivity to aluminum salts or any component of the formulation

Warnings

Oral: Hypophosphatemia may occur with prolonged administration or large doses; aluminum intoxication and osteomalacia may occur in patients with uremia. Use with caution in patients with CHF, renal failure, edema, cirrhosis, and low sodium diets, and patients who have recently suffered gastrointestinal hemorrhage; uremic patients not receiving dialysis may develop osteomalacia and osteoporosis due to phosphate depletion.

Elderly may be predisposed to constipation and fecal impaction. Careful evaluation of possible drug interactions must be done. When used as an antacid in ulcer treatment, consider buffer capacity (mEq/mL) to calculate dose.

Topical: Not for application over deep wounds, puncture wounds, infected areas, or lacerations. When used for self medication (OTC use), consult with healthcare provider if needed for >7 days or for use in children <6 months of age.

Dosage Forms

Ointment:

Dermagran®: 0.275% (120 g)

Suspension, oral: 320 mg/5 mL (473 mL)

ALternaGel®: 600 mg/5 mL (360 mL)

Reference Range Normal plasma aluminum levels are <10 mcg/L; levels >100 mcg/L are associated with toxicity; normal urinary aluminum level: 0.05-1 mg/L

Overdosage/Treatment

Supportive therapy: Diazepam can be used for seizure control. Consider deferoxamine for aluminum serum levels >60 mcg/L

Deferoxamine (15-20 mg/kg once weekly I.V.), traditionally used as an iron chelator, has been shown to increase urinary aluminum output

For dialysis patients: I.V.: 40-80 mg/kg once weekly prior to dialysis with reduction of dose to 20-60 mg/kg if a positive response occurs

Deferoxamine chelation of aluminum has resulted in improvements of clinical symptoms and bone histology. However, deferoxamine remains an experimental treatment for aluminum poisoning and has a significant potential for adverse effects.

Deferoxamine infused 1-2 hours at the end of dialysis; monitor iron levels carefully along with platelet counts

Enhancement of elimination: Hemodialysis or charcoal hemoperfusion will also remove aluminum; aluminum-desferrioxamine complex can be efficiently removed with high flux dialysate membranes

Drug Interactions

Decreased effect: Aluminum hydroxide may decrease the absorption of allopurinol, antibiotics (tetracyclines, quinolones, some cephalosporins), bisphosphonate derivatives, corticosteroids, cyclosporine, delavirdine, iron salts, imidazole antifungals, isoniazid, mycophenolate, penicillamine, phosphate supplements, phenytoin, phenothiazines, trientine.

Absorption of aluminum hydroxide may be decreased by citric acid derivatives.

Pregnancy Risk Factor C

Pregnancy Implications No data available on clinical effects on the fetus; available evidence suggests safe use during pregnancy and breast-feeding.

Lactation Excretion in breast milk unknown

Additional Information

Insoluble in water and alcohol; iron deficiency may increase aluminum absorption, possible association with dialysis, dementia, and renal osteodystrophy; aluminum comprises 8% of the earth's crust; bauxite is the main source of environmental aluminum

Aluminum only has one oxidation state (+3); background atmospheric aluminum levels range from 0.005-0.2 mg/m^3; baseline drinking water aluminum levels range from 0.003-1.6 mg/L; soil aluminum levels range from 700 mg/kg to over 100,000 mg/kg

Foods containing highest aluminum levels are ground coffee beans (52 mg/kg), salt (31-37 mg/kg), natural peanut butter (26-94 mg/kg), pumpernickel bread (13.2 mg/kg), chocolate cookie, Orea® (12.7 mg/kg), spinach (8.7 mg/kg), and lettuce (7.2 mg/kg). Calcium gluconate contains 38.8 mcg aluminum per 8 mL volume; potassium acid phosphate contains 2.8 mcg aluminum per 1.3 mL total volume.

Aluminum is not bioconcentrated in plants or terrestrial food chain; antacids/buffered aspirin can contain from 4-562 mg/kg of aluminum. Daily intake of aluminum is ~2-14 mg by food ingestion, 0.2 mg through drinking water, and 0.2 mg by inhalation; total body burden of aluminum is ~30-50 mg (50% in bone, 25% in lungs).

Specific References

Robinson RF, Casavant MJ, Nahata MC, et al, "Metabolic Bone Disease After Chronic Antacid Administration in an Infant," *Ann Pharmacother*, 2004, 38(2):265-8.

Amantadine

Pronunciation (a MAN ta deen)

Related Information

● Therapeutic Drugs Associated with Hallucinations

CAS Number 665-66-7

U.S. Brand Names Symmetrel®

Synonyms Adamantanamine Hydrochloride; Amantadine Hydrochloride

Use Prophylaxis and treatment of influenza A viral infection; treatment of parkinsonism; treatment of drug-induced extrapyramidal symptoms Creutzfeldt-Jakob disease

Mechanism of Action As an antiviral, blocks the uncoating of influenza A virus preventing penetration of virus into host; antiparkinsonian activity may be due to blocking the reuptake of dopamine into presynaptic neurons and causing direct stimulation of postsynaptic receptors

Adverse Reactions

Cardiovascular: Edema, hypotension (orthostatic), QT prolongation, sinus bradycardia, myocardial depression, sinus tachycardia, peripheral edema

Central nervous system: Dizziness, ataxia, confusion, insomnia, difficulty concentrating, anxiety, restlessness, irritability, visual hallucinations, auditory hallucinations, headache, akathisia, panic attacks, extrapyramidal symptoms, amnesia

Gastrointestinal: Nausea, anorexia, constipation, xerostomia

Genitourinary: Urinary retention

Neuromuscular & skeletal: Rhabdomyolysis, peripheral neuropathy

Signs and Symptoms of Overdose Anticholinergic symptoms, blurred vision, bradycardia, cardiac arrhythmias (including torsade de pointes), chorea (extrapyramidal), CNS depression followed by stimulation, coma, congestive heart failure, depression, drowsiness, dystonic reactions, fever, hyperthermia, insomnia, mania, memory loss, metabolic acidosis, myasthenia gravis (exacerbation or precipitation), nausea, neuroleptic malignant syndrome, neutropenia, night terrors, photosensitivity, psychosis, pulmonary edema, seizures, slurred speech, tachycardia, vomiting

Admission Criteria/Prognosis Admit any ingestion >1 g

Pharmacodynamics/Kinetics

Onset of action: Antidyskinetic: Within 48 hours

Absorption: Well absorbed

Distribution: V$_d$: Normal: 1.5-6.1 L/kg; Renal failure: 5.1±0.2 L/kg; in saliva, tear film, and nasal secretions; in animals, tissue (especially lung) concentrations higher than serum concentrations; crosses blood-brain barrier

Protein binding: Normal renal function: ~67%; Hemodialysis: ~59%

Metabolism: Not appreciable; small amounts of an acetyl metabolite identified

Bioavailability: 86% to 90%

Half-life elimination: Normal renal function: 16±6 hours (9-31 hours); End-stage renal disease: 7-10 days

Excretion: Urine (80% to 90% unchanged) by glomerular filtration and tubular secretion

Total clearance: 2.5-10.5 L/hour

Dosage

Oral:

Children:

Influenza A treatment:

1-9 years: 5 mg/kg/day in 2 divided doses (manufacturers range: 4.4-8.8 mg/kg/day); maximum dose: 150 mg/day

≥10 years and <40 kg: 5 mg/kg/day; maximum dose: 150 mg/day

10-12 years and ≥40 kg: 100 mg twice daily.

≥13 years: Refer to Adults dosing

Note: Initiate within 24-48 hours after onset of symptoms; discontinue as soon as possible based on clinical response (generally within 3-5 days or within 24-48 hours after symptoms disappear)

Influenza A prophylaxis: Refer to "Influenza A treatment" dosing

Note: Continue treatment throughout the peak influenza activity in the community or throughout the entire influenza season in patients who cannot be vaccinated. Development of immunity following vaccination takes ~2 weeks; amantadine therapy should be considered for high-risk patients from the time of vaccination until immunity has developed. For children <9 years receiving influenza vaccine for the first time, amantadine prophylaxis should continue for 6 weeks (4 weeks after the first dose and 2 weeks after the second dose)

Adults:

Drug-induced extrapyramidal symptoms: 100 mg twice daily; may increase to 300-400 mg/day, if needed

Parkinson's disease or Creutzfeldt-Jakob disease (unlabeled use): 100 mg twice daily as sole therapy; may increase to 400 mg/day if needed with close monitoring; initial dose: 100 mg/day if with other serious illness or with high doses of other anti-Parkinson drugs

Influenza A viral infection: 100 mg twice daily; initiate within 24-48 hours after onset of symptoms; discontinue as soon as possible based on clinical response (generally within 3-5 days or within 24-48 hours after symptoms disappear)

Influenza A prophylaxis: 100 mg twice daily

Note: Continue treatment throughout the peak influenza activity in the community or throughout the entire influenza season in patients who cannot be vaccinated. Development of immunity following vaccination takes ~2 weeks; amantadine therapy should be considered for high-risk patients from the time of vaccination until immunity has developed

Elderly:

Influenza A treatment: ≤100 mg/day; initiate within 24-48 hours after onset of symptoms; discontinue as soon as possible based on clinical response (generally within 3-5 days or within 24-48 hours after symptoms disappear)

Influenza A prophylaxis: ≤100 mg/day

Note: Continue treatment throughout the peak influenza activity in the community or throughout the entire influenza season in patients who cannot be vaccinated. Development of immunity following vaccination takes ~2 weeks; amantadine therapy should be considered for high-risk patients from the time of vaccination until immunity has developed.

Dosing interval in renal impairment:

Cl$_{cr}$ 30-50 mL/minute: Administer 200 mg on day 1, then 100 mg/day

Cl$_{cr}$ 15-29 mL/minute: Administer 200 mg on day 1, then 100 mg on alternate days

Cl$_{cr}$ <15 mL/minute: Administer 200 mg every 7 days

Hemodialysis: Administer 200 mg every 7 days

Peritoneal dialysis: No supplemental dose is needed

Continuous arterio-venous or venous-venous hemofiltration: No supplemental dose is needed

Monitoring Parameters Renal function, Parkinson's symptoms, mental status, influenza symptoms, blood pressure

Contraindications Hypersensitivity to amantadine, rimantadine, or any component of the formulation

Warnings Use with caution in patients with liver disease, history of recurrent and eczematoid dermatitis, uncontrolled psychosis or severe psychoneurosis, seizures, and in those receiving CNS stimulant drugs; reduce dose in renal disease. When treating Parkinson's disease, do not discontinue abruptly. In many patients, the therapeutic benefits of amantadine are limited to a few months. Elderly patients may be more susceptible to CNS effects (using 2 divided daily doses may minimize this effect). Has been associated with neuroleptic malignant syndrome (associated with dose reduction or abrupt discontinuation). Has not been shown to prevent bacterial infection or complications when used as prophylaxis or treatment of influenza A. Use with caution in patients with CHF, peripheral edema, or orthostatic hypotension. Avoid in angle closure glaucoma. Due to increased resistance, in June 2006, the CDC recommended that amantadine no longer be used for the treatment or prophylaxis of influenza A in the United States until susceptibility has been re-established.

Dosage Forms
Capsule, as hydrochloride: 100 mg
Syrup, as hydrochloride: 50 mg/5 mL (480 mL)
Tablet, as hydrochloride: 100 mg
  Symmetrel®: 100 mg

Reference Range
Therapeutic range: 0.7-1 mcg/mL; toxic and potentially fatal: 4-23 mcg/mL; highest survival reported level in overdose: 27 mcg/mL
In the postmortem state, anatomical site concentration differences (ie, postmortem redistribution) may occur

Overdosage/Treatment
Decontamination: Emesis not recommended due to potential for seizures; lavage (within 1 hour) recommended in early ingestions after seizure control; activated charcoal of value; multiple-dose activated charcoal not studied
Supportive therapy: If symptomatic, observe for 24-48 hours since cardiac symptoms are delayed. Treatment should be directed at reducing CNS stimulation and maintaining cardiovascular function. Seizures can be treated with diazepam or lorazepam 5-10 mg I.V. every 15 minutes as needed, up to a total of 30 mg in adults (0.25-0.4 mg/kg/dose I.V. every 15 minutes as needed up to a total of 10 mg for children). Lidocaine is the drug of choice for ventricular arrhythmias, followed by procainamide, propranolol (if arrhythmias are due to beta-adrenergic excess); MgSO$_4$ for torsade de pointes. Avoid class IA (other than procainamide), isoproterenol, and class II agents. Pulmonary edema may respond to corticosteroids. Norepinephrine may be effective for hypotension. Physostigmine has been used and is recommended only in severe, life-threatening anticholinergic symptoms. Ice baths, bromocriptine, and/or dantrolene may be effective for malignant hyperthermia, but clinical experience in this setting is limited. Since bicarbonate prevents renal elimination, this modality should be avoided if possible.
Enhancement of elimination: Hemodialysis is of minimal value, as is peritoneal dialysis; slightly dialyzable (5% to 20%)

Drug Interactions
Anticholinergics may potentiate CNS side effects of amantadine; monitor for altered response. Includes benztropine and trihexyphenidyl, as well as agents with anticholinergic activity such as quinidine, tricyclics, and antihistamines.
Thiazide diuretics: Hydrochlorothiazide has been reported to increase the potential for toxicity with amantadine (limited documentation); monitor response.
Triamterene: Has been reported to increase the potential for toxicity with amantadine (limited documentation); monitor response.
Trimethoprim: Has been reported to increase the potential for toxicity with amantadine (limited documentation); monitor for acute confusion.

Pregnancy Risk Factor C
Pregnancy Implications
Teratogenic effects were observed in animal studies; limited data in humans. Impaired fertility has also been reported during animal studies and during human in vitro fertilization.
Lactation
Enters breast milk/not recommended
Nursing Implications
If insomnia occurs, the last daily dose should be taken several hours before retiring; assess parkinsonian symptoms prior to and throughout course of therapy
Additional Information
Cardiac conduction disturbances may occur as long as 52 hours postingestion

Specific References
Arima H, Sobue K, So M, et al, "Transient and Reversible Parkinsonism After Acute Organophosphate Poisoning," J Toxicol Clin Toxicol, 2003, 41(1):67-70.
DeWitt C, Heard K, and Dart RC, "CNS and CV Effects in Acute Amantadine Overdoses in Children," J Toxicol Clin Toxicol, 2004, 42(5):750.
Michalski LS, Hantsch CE, and Hou SH, "Amantadine Toxicity in a Renal Transplant Patient," J Toxicol Clin Toxicol, 2003, 41(5):679.

Amiloride

Pronunciation (a MIL oh ride)
CAS Number 17440-83-4; 2016-88-8; 2609-46-3
U.S. Brand Names Midamor® [DSC]
Synonyms Amiloride Hydrochloride
Use Counteracts potassium loss induced by other diuretics in the treatment of hypertension or edematous conditions including CHF, hepatic cirrhosis, and hypoaldosteronism; usually used in conjunction with more potent diuretics such as thiazides or loop diuretics

Unlabeled/Investigational Use Investigational: Cystic fibrosis; reduction of lithium-induced polyuria
Mechanism of Action Interferes with potassium/sodium exchange in the distal renal tubule
Adverse Reactions
Cardiovascular: Hypotension (orthostatic), vasculitis
Central nervous system: Headache, dizziness
Dermatologic: Pruritus, photosensitivity, exanthema, alopecia, urticaria, purpura
Endocrine & metabolic: Hyperkalemia, hyponatremia
Gastrointestinal: Nausea, vomiting, abdominal pain, diarrhea, loss of taste perception, salt hypogeusia
Neuromuscular & skeletal: Leg ischemia, muscle cramps, paresthesia
Respiratory: Cough, dyspnea
Miscellaneous: Thirst

Signs and Symptoms of Overdose Constipation, cough, encephalopathy, hyperuricemia, hyponatremia, hypotension, impotence, numbness, photosensitivity

Pharmacodynamics/Kinetics
Onset of action: 2 hours
Duration: 24 hours
Absorption: ~15% to 25%
Distribution: V$_d$: 350-380 L
Protein binding: 23%
Metabolism: No active metabolites
Half-life elimination: Normal renal function: 6-9 hours; End-stage renal disease: 8-144 hours
Time to peak, serum: 6-10 hours
Excretion: Urine and feces (equal amounts as unchanged drug)

Dosage
Oral:
Children: Although safety and efficacy in children have not been established by the FDA, a dosage of 0.625 mg/kg/day has been used in children weighing 6-20 kg.
Adults: 5-10 mg/day (up to 20 mg)
  Hypertension (JNC 7): 5-10 mg/day in 1-2 divided doses
Elderly: Initial: 5 mg once daily or every other day
Dosing adjustment in renal impairment:
  Cl$_{cr}$ 10-50 mL/minute: Administer at 50% of normal dose.
  Cl$_{cr}$ <10 mL/minute: Avoid use.

Monitoring Parameters I & O, daily weights, blood pressure, serum electrolytes, renal function
Administration Administer with food or meals to avoid GI upset.
Contraindications Hypersensitivity to amiloride or any component of the formulation; presence of elevated serum potassium levels (>5.5 mEq/L); if patient is receiving other potassium-conserving agents (eg, spironolactone, triamterene) or potassium supplementation (medicine, potassium-containing salt substitutes, potassium-rich diet); anuria; acute or chronic renal insufficiency; evidence of diabetic nephropathy. Patients with evidence of renal impairment or diabetes mellitus should not receive this medicine without close, frequent monitoring of serum electrolytes and renal function.
Warnings May cause hyperkalemia (patients with renal impairment or diabetes and the elderly are at greatest risk). Should be stopped at least 3 days before glucose tolerance testing. Use caution in severely ill patients in whom respiratory or metabolic acidosis may occur.
Dosage Forms Tablet, as hydrochloride: 5 mg
Reference Range Peak serum amiloride level: 30-50 ng/mL after a 20 mg dose
Overdosage/Treatment
Decontamination: Ipecac within 30 minutes or lavage (within 1 hour)/activated charcoal
Supportive therapy: Hyperkalemia can be treated with glucose/insulin and sodium bicarbonate (1 mEq/kg); sodium polystyrene sulfonate can also be given; I.V. fluid administration of 0.45% sodium chloride with furosemide (1 mg/kg, up to 40 mg) can be used to promote urine flow
Test Interactions ↑ potassium (S)
Drug Interactions
Amoxicillin's absorption may be reduced; avoid concurrent use or observe for clinical response.
ACE inhibitors or angiotensin receptor antagonists can cause hyperkalemia, especially in patients with renal impairment, potassium-rich diets, or on other drugs causing hyperkalemia; avoid concurrent use or monitor closely.
Cyclosporine or tacrolimus: Risk of hyperkalemia may be increased by concurrent therapy.
NSAIDs: May decrease the effect of diuretics.
Potassium supplements may further increase potassium retention and cause hyperkalemia; avoid concurrent use.
Quinidine and amiloride together may increase risk of malignant arrhythmias; avoid concurrent use.

Pregnancy Risk Factor B

Lactation Excretion in breast milk unknown/contraindicated

Additional Information Amiloride is considered an alternative to triamterene or spironolactone. Unlike triamterene, renal stone formation does not occur; diminishes the potassium excretion effects of thiazide diuretics. Medication should be discontinued if potassium level exceeds 6.5 mEq/L.

Specific References

Chobanian AV, Bakris GL, Black HR, et al, "The Seventh Report of the Joint National Committee on Prevention, Detection, Evaluation, and Treatment of High Blood Pressure: The JNC 7 Report," *JAMA*, 2003, 289(19):2560-71.

Aminophylline

Pronunciation (am in OFF i lin)

Related Information

- Theophylline

CAS Number 317-34-0

Synonyms Theophylline Ethylenediamine

Use Bronchodilator in reversible airway obstruction due to asthma or COPD; increase diaphragmatic contractility

Mechanism of Action Causes bronchodilatation, diuresis, CNS and cardiac stimulation, and gastric acid secretion by blocking phosphodiesterase which increases tissue concentrations of cyclic adenine monophosphate (cAMP) which in turn promotes catecholamine stimulation of lipolysis, glycogenolysis, and gluconeogenesis and induces release of epinephrine from adrenal medulla cells

Adverse Reactions

Uncommon at serum theophylline concentrations ≤15 mcg/mL

Cardiovascular: Tachycardia

Central nervous system: Nervousness, restlessness, insomnia, irritability, seizures

Dermatologic: Skin rash

Gastrointestinal: Nausea, vomiting, gastric irritation

Neuromuscular & skeletal: Tremor

Miscellaneous: Allergic reactions

Signs and Symptoms of Overdose Delirium, diuresis, feces discoloration (black), hypercalcemia, hyperglycemia, hypokalemia, hypotension, insomnia, irritability, lactic acidosis, nausea, seizures, tachycardia, vomiting. Repetitive vomiting is an indication to hold theophylline therapy and rule out toxicity by serum concentrations.

Pharmacodynamics/Kinetics

Theophylline:

Absorption: Oral: Dosage form dependent

Distribution: 0.45 L/kg based on ideal body weight

Protein binding: 40%, primarily to albumin

Metabolism: Children >1 year and Adults: Hepatic; involves CYP1A2, 2E1, and 3A4; forms active metabolites (caffeine and 3-methylxanthine)

Half-life elimination: Highly variable and dependent upon age, liver function, cardiac function, lung disease, and smoking history

Time to peak, serum:

Oral: Immediate release: 1-2 hours

I.V.: Within 30 minutes

Excretion: Children >3 months and Adults: Urine (10% as unchanged drug)

Dosage

Treatment of acute bronchospasm: I.V.:

Loading dose (in patients not currently receiving aminophylline or theophylline): 6 mg/kg (based on aminophylline) administered I.V. over 20-30 minutes; administration rate should not exceed 25 mg/minute (aminophylline)

Approximate I.V. maintenance dosages are based upon **continuous infusions**; bolus dosing (often used in children <6 months of age) may be determined by multiplying the hourly infusion rate by 24 hours and dividing by the desired number of doses/day

6 weeks to 6 months: 0.5 mg/kg/hour

6 months to 1 year: 0.6-0.7 mg/kg/hour

1-9 years: 1 mg/kg/hour

9-16 years and smokers: 0.8 mg/kg/hour

Adults, nonsmoking: 0.5 mg/kg/hour

Older patients and patients with cor pulmonale: 0.3 mg/kg/hour

Patients with congestive heart failure: 0.1-0.2 mg/kg/hour

Dosage should be adjusted according to serum level measurements during the first 12- to 24-hour period. See table.

Guidelines for Drawing Theophylline Serum Levels

Dosage Form	Time to Draw Level
P.O. liquid, fast-release tab	Peak: 1 h post 4th dose; Trough: just before 4th dose
P.O. slow-release product	Peak: 4 h post 3rd dose; Trough: just before 3rd dose

Bronchodilator: Oral: Children ≥45 kg and Adults: Initial: 380 mg/day (equivalent to theophylline 300 mg/day) in divided doses every 6-8 hours; may increase dose after 3 days; maximum dose: 928 mg/day (equivalent to theophylline 800 mg/day)

Stability Store injection at room temperature, do not refrigerate; protect from heat and from freezing; use only clear solutions; stability of parenteral admixture at room temperature (25°C): 30 days

Administration

Dilute with I.V. fluid to a concentration of 1 mg/mL and infuse over 20-30 minutes; maximum concentration: 25 mg/mL; maximum rate of infusion: 0.36 mg/kg/minute, and no greater than 25 mg/minute. I.M. administration is not recommended. Oral and I.V. should be administered around-the-clock rather than 4 times/day, 3 times/day, etc (ie, 12-6-12-6, not 9-1-5-9) to promote less variation in peak and trough serum levels.

Contraindications Hypersensitivity to theophylline, ethylenediamine, or any component of the formulation

Warnings If a patient develops signs and symptoms of theophylline toxicity, a serum level should be measured and subsequent doses held. Due to potential saturation of theophylline clearance at serum levels within (or in some patients less than) the therapeutic range, dosage adjustment should be made in small increments (maximum: 25% reduction). Due to wide interpatient variability, theophylline serum level measurements must be used to optimize therapy and prevent serious toxicity. Use caution with peptic ulcer, hyperthyroidism, seizure disorder, hypertension, or tachyarrhythmias.

Dosage Forms

Injection, solution, as dihydrate: 25 mg/mL (10 mL, 20 mL)

Tablet, as dihydrate: 100 mg, 200 mg

Reference Range

Therapeutic (theophylline):

Neonatal apnea: 6-13 mcg/mL

Sample size: 0.5-1 mL serum (red top tube)

Toxic: >20 mcg/mL

Timing of serum samples: If toxicity is suspected, draw a level at any time; if lack of therapeutic effect, draw a trough immediately before the next oral dose

Overdosage/Treatment

Decontamination: **Do not** use ipecac; lavage should be performed if <1 hour after ingestion and if >50 mg/kg was ingested; activated charcoal should be given; whole bowel irrigation should be considered for significant sustained release preparation ingestion

Supportive therapy: Metoclopramide, ranitidine, or ondansetron can be used for vomiting; hypotension should be treated with I.V. normal saline hydration. Phenylephrine or levarterenol are preferred vasopressors that can be utilized for hypotension, although an I.V. beta-adrenergic blocker (propranolol or esmolol) can be utilized in patients with no history of bronchospastic disease. Seizures may require diazepam/ lorazepam along with phenobarbital; phenytoin is contraindicated. Lidocaine can be used for ventricular arrhythmias; must monitor for hypoglycemia.

Enhancement of elimination: Multiple doses of activated charcoal can halve the half-life of aminophylline/theophylline; do not use if an ileus is present. Charcoal hemoperfusion can increase the clearance of aminophylline/theophylline by approximately twofold to threefold over that of hemodialysis and is thus the extracorporeal modality of choice. Guidelines for charcoal hemoperfusion include a theophylline level >100 mcg/mL in an acute overdose setting (or 50 mcg/mL in a chronic setting), or the following signs if the level is >35 mcg/mL: ventricular arrhythmias, metabolic acidosis, hypotension, refractory to vasopressors or fluid therapy, seizures, ileus. If a sustained-release preparation is ingested or if the patient is >60 years of age, the threshold for using charcoal hemoperfusion should be lower. If the patient is experiencing fluid overload due to congestive heart failure, hemodialysis can be performed to remove both theophylline/aminophylline and fluid. Drug clearance rates for hemodialysis and hemoperfusion are 185 mL/kg/ hour and 295 mL/kg/hour, respectively.

Test Interactions In selected procedures, caffeine in high concentrations cross reacts as theophylline.

Drug Interactions

Substrate of CYP1A2 (major), 2E1 (minor), 3A4 (minor)

CYP1A2 inducers: May decrease the levels/effects of aminophylline. Example inducers include aminoglutethimide, carbamazepine, phenobarbital, and rifampin.

CYP1A2 inhibitors: May increase the levels/effects of aminophylline. Example inhibitors include ciprofloxacin, fluvoxamine, ketoconazole, norfloxacin, ofloxacin, and rofecoxib.

Pregnancy Risk Factor C

Pregnancy Implications Theophylline crosses the placenta; adverse effects may be seen in the newborn. Theophylline metabolism may change during pregnancy; monitor serum levels.

Lactation Enters breast milk/compatible (AAP rates "compatible")

Nursing Implications Encourage patient to drink adequate fluids (2 L/ day) to decrease mucous viscosity in airways; monitor vital signs, I & O, serum concentrations, and CNS effects (insomnia, irritability)

Additional Information Elderly, acutely ill, and patients with severe respiratory problems, pulmonary edema, or liver dysfunction are at greater risk of toxicity because of reduced drug clearance. Saliva levels are approximately equal to 60% of plasma levels. Charcoal-broiled foods may increase elimination, reducing half-life by 50%. Cigarette smoking may require a dosage increase of 50% to 100%. Aminophylline, 100 mg, is equivalent to theophylline, 79 mg. Aminophylline (2.5 mg/kg) has been used to treat methotrexate-induced neurotoxicity in children.

Specific References
Abu-Laban RB, McIntyre CM, Christenson JM, et al, "Aminophylline in Bradyasystolic Cardiac Arrest: A Randomized Placebo-Controlled Trial," *Acad Emerg Med*, 2004, 11(5):435.

Amiodarone

Pronunciation (a MEE oh da rone)
CAS Number 1951-25-3; 19774-82-4
U.S. Brand Names Cordarone®; Pacerone®
Synonyms Amiodarone Hydrochloride
Use

Oral: Management of life-threatening recurrent ventricular fibrillation (VF) or hemodynamically unstable ventricular tachycardia (VT)

I.V.: Initiation of treatment and prophylaxis of frequency recurring VF and unstable VT in patients refractory to other therapy. Also, used for patients when oral amiodarone is indicated, but who are unable to take oral medication

Unlabeled/Investigational Use Conversion of atrial fibrillation to normal sinus rhythm; maintenance of normal sinus rhythm

Prevention of postoperative atrial fibrillation during cardiothoracic surgery
Paroxysmal supraventricular tachycardia (SVT)
Control of rapid ventricular rate due to accessory pathway conduction in pre-excited atrial arrhythmias [ACLS guidelines]
Cardiac arrest with persistent ventricular tachycardia (VT) or ventricular fibrillation (VF) if defibrillation, CPR, and vasopressor administration have failed [ACLS/PALS guidelines]
Control of hemodynamically-stable VT, polymorphic VT with a normal QT interval, or wide-complex tachycardia of uncertain origin [ACLS/PALS guidelines]

Mechanism of Action Class III antiarrhythmic agent which inhibits adrenergic stimulation (alpha- and beta-blocking properties), affects sodium, potassium, and calcium channels, prolongs the action potential and refractory period in myocardial tissue; decreases AV conduction and sinus node function

Adverse Reactions

Cardiovascular: Atropine-resistant bradycardia, heart block, sinus arrest, myocardial depression, chest pain, congestive heart failure, paroxysmal tachycardia (ventricular), proarrhythmia, **hypotension** (I.V. 16%, refractory in rare cases), torsade de pointes with QT interval prolongation, angina, myocardial depression, pericardial effusion/pericarditis, sinus tachycardia, tachycardia (supraventricular), arrhythmias (ventricular), vasodilation, leukocytoclastic vasculitis, atrial fibrillation, acute intracranial hypertension (I.V.), vasculitis, nodal arrhythmia, sinus bradycardia, ventricular fibrillation

Central nervous system: (20% to 40% incidence): **Fatigue, malaise, psychosis, dizziness, encephalopathy, insomnia, night terrors, extrapyramidal reaction, fever, headache, restlessness, abulia, ataxia, parkinsonism, nightmares**, CNS depression, depression, proximal muscle asthenia, myelinopathy, pseudotumor cerebri, brainstem dysfunction, delirium

Dermatologic: Skin discoloration (slate blue), rash, alopecia, **photosensitivity**, cutaneous vasculitis, angioedema, toxic epidermal necrolysis, Stevens-Johnson syndrome, erythema multiforme

Endocrine & metabolic: Hypothyroidism (or less commonly hyperthyroidism), hyperglycemia, increased triglycerides, gynecomastia, Hashimoto's disease, Graves' disease, autoimmune thyroid disease, thyroiditis, SIADH

Gastrointestinal: **Nausea, vomiting, anorexia, constipation**, metallic taste, pancreatitis, lingua villosa nigra, diarrhea

Genitourinary: Scrotal pain, epididymal pain and edema, impotence, noninfectious epididymitis, loss of libido

Hematologic: Coagulation abnormalities, thrombocytopenia, aplastic anemia, bone marrow granuloma, hemolytic anemia, pancytopenia

Hepatic: Elevated liver enzymes, severe hepatic toxicity (potentially fatal), elevated bilirubin, increased serum ammonia, hepatic steatosis, cholestatic hepatitis, cirrhosis, increased ALT/AST, neutropenia

Local: Injection site reactions

Neuromuscular & skeletal: **Tremors, paresthesia, weakness**, abnormal gait, myopathy, dyskinesias, myoclonic jerks

Ocular: Visual disturbances, corneal microdeposits (occur in a majority of patients, but lead to visual disturbance in ~10%), diplopia; photophobia, optic neuropathy, cataract, optic neuritis

Renal: Abnormal renal function

Respiratory: Potentially fatal: **Interstitial pneumonitis**, hypersensitivity pneumonitis, **pulmonary fibrosis**; may present with cough, dyspnea, bronchiolitis obliterans, pleural effusion, organizing pneumonia, hemoptysis, pleuritis, pulmonary edema; **alveolitis**, bronchospasm, hypoxia, wheezing; ARDS has been reported in up to 2% of patients receiving I.V. amiodarone, and post-operatively in patients receiving oral amiodarone.

Miscellaneous: Diaphoresis, anaphylactic shock

Signs and Symptoms of Overdose Patients should be monitored for several days following ingestion. AV block, chest pain, cirrhosis, delirium, extension of pharmacologic effect, heart block, hemoptysis, hyperthyroidism, hypotension, hypothyroidism, insomnia, myopathy, night terrors, pseudotumor cerebri, photosensitivity, sinus bradycardia, sweating, syncope, thrombocytopenia, toxic epidermal necrolysis, QT prolongation

Admission Criteria/Prognosis Admit any patient with ECG abnormalities or any adult ingestion >3 g

Pharmacodynamics/Kinetics

Onset of action: Oral: 2 days to 3 weeks; I.V.: May be more rapid
Peak effect: 1 week to 5 months
Duration after discontinuing therapy: 7-50 days
Note: Mean onset of effect and duration after discontinuation may be shorter in children than adults

Distribution: V_d: 66 L/kg (range: 18-148 L/kg); crosses placenta; enters breast milk in concentrations higher than maternal plasma concentrations
Protein binding: 96%
Metabolism: Hepatic via CYP2C8 and 3A4 to active N-desethylamiodarone metabolite; possible enterohepatic recirculation
Bioavailability: Oral: ~50%
Half-life elimination: Terminal: 40-55 days (range: 26-107 days); shorter in children than adults
Excretion: Feces; urine (<1% as unchanged drug)

Dosage

Note: Lower loading and maintenance doses are preferable in women and all patients with low body weight.

Oral:

Children: Arrhythmias (unlabeled use):
Loading dose: 10-20 mg/kg/day in 1-2 doses for 4-14 days or until adequate control of arrhythmia or prominent adverse effects occur; alternative loading dose in children <1 year: 600-800 mg/1.73 m^2/day in 1-2 divided doses/day
Maintenance dose: Dose may be reduced to 5 mg/kg/day for several weeks (or 200-400 mg/1.73 m^2/day given once daily); if no recurrence of arrhythmia, dose may be further reduced to 2.5 mg/kg/day; maintenance doses may be given 5-7 days/week

Adults:
Ventricular arrhythmias: 800-1600 mg/day in 1-2 doses for 1-3 weeks, then when adequate arrhythmia control is achieved, decrease to 600-800 mg/day in 1-2 doses for 1 month; maintenance: 400 mg/day. Lower doses are recommended for supraventricular arrhythmias.

Prophylaxis of atrial fibrillation following open heart surgery (unlabeled use): 400 mg twice daily (starting in postop recovery) for up to 7 days. An alternative regimen of amiodarone 600 mg/day for 7 days prior to surgery, followed by 200 mg/day until hospital discharge, has also been shown to decrease the risk of postoperative atrial fibrillation. **Note:** A variety of regimens have been used in clinical trials.

Recurrent atrial fibrillation (unlabeled use): No standard regimen defined; examples of regimens include: Initial: 10 mg/kg/day for 14 days; followed by 300 mg/day for 4 weeks, followed by maintenance dosage of 100-200 mg/day (Roy D, 2000). Other regimens have been described and are used clinically (ie, 400 mg 3 times/day for 5-7 days, then 400 mg/day for 1 month, then 200 mg/day).

I.V.:

Children:
Arrhythmias (unlabeled use, dosing based on limited data): Loading dose: 5 mg/kg over 30 minutes; may repeat up to 3 times if no response. Maintenance dose: 2-20 mg/kg/day (5-15 mcg/kg/minute) by continuous infusion
Note: I.V. administration at low flow rates (potentially associated with use in pediatrics) may result in leaching of plasticizers (DEHP) from intravenous tubing. DEHP may adversely affect male reproductive tract development. Alternative means of dosing and administration (1 mg/kg aliquots) may need to be considered.
Pulseless VF or VT (PALS dosing): 5 mg/kg rapid I.V. bolus or I.O.; repeat up to a maximum dose of 15 mg/kg (300 mg)
Perfusing tachycardias (PALS dosing): Loading dose: 5 mg/kg I.V. over 20-60 minutes or I.O.; may repeat up to maximum dose of 15 mg/kg/day

Adults:
Breakthrough VF or VT: 150 mg supplemental doses in 100 mL D$_5$W over 10 minutes
Pulseless VF or VT: I.V. push: Initial: 300 mg in 20-30 mL NS or D$_5$W; if VF or VT recurs, supplemental dose of 150 mg followed by

infusion of 1 mg/minute for 6 hours, then 0.5 mg/minute (maximum daily dose: 2.1 g)

Prophylaxis of atrial fibrillation following open heart surgery (unlabeled use): 1000 mg infused over 24 hours (starting at postop recovery) for 2 days has been shown to reduce the risk of postoperative atrial fibrillation. **Note:** A variety of regimens have been used in clinical trials.

Stable VT or SVT (unlabeled use): First 24 hours: 1050 mg according to following regimen

Step 1: 150 mg (100 mL) over first 10 minutes (mix 3 mL in 100 mL D_5W)

Step 2: 360 mg (200 mL) over next 6 hours (mix 18 mL in 500 mL D_5W): 1 mg/minute

Step 3: 540 mg (300 mL) over next 18 hours: 0.5 mg/minute

Note: After the first 24 hours: 0.5 mg/minute utilizing concentration of 1-6 mg/mL

Note: When switching from I.V. to oral therapy, use the following as a guide:

<1-week I.V. infusion: 800-1600 mg/day
1- to 3-week I.V. infusion: 600-800 mg/day
>3-week I.V. infusion: 400 mg/day

Recommendations for conversion to intravenous amiodarone after oral administration: During long-term amiodarone therapy (ie, ≥4 months), the mean plasma-elimination half-life of the active metabolite of amiodarone is 61 days. Replacement therapy may not be necessary in such patients if oral therapy is discontinued for a period <2 weeks, since any changes in serum amiodarone concentrations during this period may **not** be clinically significant.

Elderly: No specific guidelines available. Dose selection should be cautious, at low end of dosage range, and titration should be slower to evaluate response.

Hemodialysis: Not dialyzable (0% to 5%); supplemental dose is not necessary.

Peritoneal dialysis effects: Not dialyzable (0% to 5%); supplemental dose is not necessary.

Dosing adjustment in hepatic impairment: Probably necessary in substantial hepatic impairment. No specific guidelines available.

Stability May precipitate in 0.9% saline solution, or when combined with flucloxacillin sodium, furosemide, quinidine, heparin sodium, aminophylline, cefamandole nafate, cefazolin sodium or mezlocillin sodium

Monitoring Parameters Blood pressure, heart rate (ECG) and rhythm throughout therapy; assess patient for signs of lethargy, edema of the hands or feet, weight loss, and pulmonary toxicity (baseline pulmonary function tests); liver function tests; monitor serum electrolytes, especially potassium and magnesium. Assess for thyroid dysfunction (thyroid function tests): Amiodarone partially inhibits the peripheral conversion of thyroxine (T_4) to triiodothyronine (T_3); serum T_4 and reverse triiodothyronine (rT_3) concentrations may be increased and serum T_3 may be decreased; most patients remain clinically euthyroid, however, clinical hypothyroidism or hyperthyroidism may occur.

Administration Oral: Administer consistently with regard to meals. Take in divided doses with meals if high daily dose or if GI upset occurs. If GI intolerance occurs with single-dose therapy, use twice daily dosing.

I.V.: Give I.V. therapy using an infusion pump through a central line or a peripheral line at a concentration of <2 mg/mL. Slow the infusion rate if hypotension develops. **Note:** I.V. administration at low flow rates (potentially associated with use in pediatrics) may result in leaching of plasticizers (DEHP) from intravenous tubing. DEHP may adversely affect male reproductive tract development. Alternative means of dosing and administration (1 mg/kg aliquots) may need to be considered.

Contraindications Hypersensitivity to amiodarone, iodine, or any component of the formulation; severe sinus-node dysfunction; second- and third-degree heart block (except in patients with a functioning artificial pacemaker); bradycardia causing syncope (except in patients with a functioning artificial pacemaker); pregnancy

Warnings

[U.S. Boxed Warning]: Only indicated for patients with life-threatening arrhythmias because of risk of toxicity. Monitor for pulmonary toxicity (hypersensitivity or interstitial/alveolar pneumonitis). Lung damage (abnormal diffusion capacity) may occur without symptoms. Pre-existing pulmonary disease does not increase risk of developing pulmonary toxicity, but if pulmonary toxicity develops then the prognosis is worse. Liver toxicity is common, but usually mild with evidence of increased liver enzymes. Severe liver toxicity can occur and has been fatal in a few cases.

Amiodarone can exacerbate the arrhythmia (including torsade de pointes), making it more difficult to tolerate or reverse. Other types of arrhythmias have occurred (eg, significant heart block, sinus bradycardia). Proarrhythmic effects may be prolonged. Use very cautiously and with close monitoring in patients with thyroid or liver disease. May cause hyper- or hypothyroidism. Hyperthyroidism may aggravate or cause breakthrough arrhythmias. May cause optic neuropathy and/or optic neuritis, usually resulting in visual impairment. Corneal microdeposits occur in a majority of patients, and may cause visual disturbances in some patients (blurred vision, halos); these are not generally considered a reason to discontinue treatment.

[U.S. Boxed Warning]: Alternative therapies should be tried first before using amiodarone. Patients should be hospitalized when amiodarone is initiated. Due to complex pharmacokinetics, it is difficult to predict when an arrhythmia or interaction with a subsequent treatment will occur following discontinuation of amiodarone.

Amiodarone is a potent inhibitor of CYP enzymes and transport proteins (including p-glycoprotein), which may lead to increased serum concentrations/toxicity of a number of medications. Particular caution must be used when a drug with QT_c-prolonging potential relies on metabolism via these enzymes, since the effect of elevated concentrations may be additive with the effect of amiodarone. Carefully assess risk:benefit of coadministration of other drugs which may prolong QT_c interval. Correct electrolyte disturbances, especially hypokalemia or hypomagnesemia, prior to use and throughout therapy.

May cause hypotension and bradycardia (infusion-rate related). Caution in surgical patients; may enhance hemodynamic effect of anesthetics; associated with increased risk of adult respiratory distress syndrome (ARDS) postoperatively. Injection contains benzyl alcohol, which has been associated with "gasping syndrome" in neonates. Safety and efficacy of amiodarone in children has not been fully established.

Dosage Forms

[DSC] = Discontinued product

Injection, solution, as hydrochloride: 50 mg/mL (3 mL, 9 mL, 18 mL) [contains benzyl alcohol and polysorbate (Tween®) 80]

Cordarone®: 50 mg/mL (3 mL) [contains benzyl alcohol and polysorbate (Tween®) 80]

Tablet, as hydrochloride [scored]: 200 mg, 400 mg

Cordarone®: 200 mg

Pacerone®: 100 mg [not scored], 200 mg, 300 mg [DSC], 400 mg

Reference Range

Therapeutic: 1.5-2.5 mg/L (SI: 1-4 μmol/L) (parent); desethyl metabolite is active and is present in equal concentration to parent drug

Toxic effects can be observed at levels >2.5 mg/L for parent compound or 1.5 mcg/mL for desethylamiodarone

Overdosage/Treatment

Decontamination: Lavage (within 1 hour)/activated charcoal; cholestyramine can also decrease absorption

Supportive therapy: Intoxication with amiodarone necessitates ECG monitoring. When bradycardia occurs atropine may be given, however, atropine resistant bradycardia has been reported. In cases of difficult to treat amiodarone-induced bradycardia, injectable isoproterenol or a temporary pacemaker may be required. Corticosteroids may be useful to treat amiodarone pulmonary toxicity; corticosteroid therapy can be used to treat amiodarone- induced pleural disease. Propylthiouracil (with lithium) has been used to treat amiodarone-induced thyrotoxicosis with normalization of T_4 levels within 5 weeks. Angiotensin amide may be useful in treating hypotension (refractory to other modalities) due to amiodarone toxicity. Amiodarone-induced ataxia can be successfully treated with acetazolamide (125-250 mg twice daily).

Enhancement of elimination: Multiple dose of activated charcoal may be useful. Cholestyramine (4 g/hour for 4 hours) may be useful to decrease half-life. Dialysis is not useful.

Test Interactions Thyroid function tests: Amiodarone partially inhibits the peripheral conversion of thyroxine (T_4) to triiodothyronine (T_3); serum T_4 and reverse triiodothyronine (rT_3) concentrations may be increased and serum T_3 may be decreased; most patients remain clinically euthyroid, however, clinical hypothyroidism or hyperthyroidism may occur; hyperglycemia. Causes a falsely increased free thyroxine level.

Drug Interactions

Substrate of CYP1A2 (minor), 2C8 (major at low concentrations), 2C19 (minor), 2D6 (minor), 3A4 (major); **Inhibits** CYP1A2 (weak), 2A6 (moderate), 2B6 (weak), 2C9 (moderate), 2C19 (weak), 2D6 (moderate), 3A4 (moderate)

Anesthetics (halogenated, inhaled): Amiodarone enhances the myocardial depressant and conduction effects of inhalation anesthetics; monitor.

Azole antifungals: May prolong QT_c, potentially leading to malignant arrhythmias; use caution.

Beta-blockers may cause excessive AV block; monitor response.

Calcium channel blockers (diltiazem, verapamil): May cause excessive AV block; monitor.

Cimetidine: May increase amiodarone blood levels.

Cholestyramine: May decrease amiodarone blood levels.

Cisapride: May prolong QT_c interval potentially leading to malignant arrhythmias.

Clonazepam effects may be increased by amiodarone.

Cyclosporine: Serum levels may be increased by amiodarone; monitor.

CYP2A6 substrates: Amiodarone may increase the levels/effects of CYP2A6 substrates. Example substrates include dexmedetomidine and ifosfamide.

CYP2C8 inducers: May decrease the levels/effects of amiodarone. Example inducers include carbamazepine, phenobarbital, phenytoin, rifampin, rifapentine, and secobarbital.

CYP2C8 inhibitors: May increase the levels/effects of amiodarone. Example inhibitors include atazanavir, gemfibrozil, and ritonavir.

CYP2C9 substrates: Amiodarone may increase the levels/effects of CYP2C9 substrates. Example substrates include bosentan, dapsone, fluoxetine, glimepiride, glipizide, losartan, montelukast, nateglinide, paclitaxel, phenytoin, warfarin, and zafirlukast.

CYP2D6 substrates: Amiodarone may increase the levels/effects of CYP2D6 substrates. Example substrates include amphetamines, selected beta-blockers, dextromethorphan, fluoxetine, lidocaine, mirtazapine, nefazodone, paroxetine, risperidone, ritonavir, thioridazine, tricyclic antidepressants, and venlafaxine.

CYP2D6 prodrug substrates: Amiodarone may decrease the levels/effects of CYP2D6 prodrug substrates. Example prodrug substrates include codeine, hydrocodone, oxycodone, and tramadol.

CYP3A4 inducers: CYP3A4 inducers may decrease the levels/effects of amiodarone. Example inducers include aminoglutethimide, carbamazepine, nafcillin, nevirapine, phenobarbital, phenytoin, and rifamycins.

CYP3A4 inhibitors: May increase the levels/effects of amiodarone. Example inhibitors include azole antifungals, clarithromycin, diclofenac, doxycycline, erythromycin, imatinib, isoniazid, nefazodone, nicardipine, propofol, protease inhibitors, quinidine, telithromycin, and verapamil.

CYP3A4 substrates: Amiodarone may increase the levels/effects of CYP3A4 substrates. Example substrates include benzodiazepines, calcium channel blockers, ergot derivatives, mirtazapine, nateglinide, nefazodone, tacrolimus, and venlafaxine.

Digoxin levels may be increased by amiodarone; consider reducing digoxin dose by 50% and monitor digoxin blood levels closely.

Fentanyl: Concurrent use may lead to bradycardia, sinus arrest, and hypotension.

Flecainide blood levels may be increased; consider reducing flecainide dose by 25% to 33% with concurrent use.

Fluoroquinolones (sparfloxacin, gatifloxacin, moxifloxacin): May result in additional prolongation of the QT interval; concurrent use of sparfloxacin is contraindicated.

HMG-CoA reductase inhibitors (lovastatin, simvastatin, and others dependent on CYP3A4 metabolism): Amiodarone inhibits metabolism of lovastatin and/or simvastatin and may increase the risk of myopathy and rhabdomyolysis. Concurrent use of lovastatin or simvastatin is not recommended, but if unavoidable, dose of lovastatin should not exceed 40 mg/day. The dose of simvastatin should not exceed 20 mg/day; consider alternative HMG-CoA reductase inhibitor.

Lidocaine: Amiodarone may increase serum levels/toxicity of lidocaine. Sinus bradycardia may occur with concurrent use.

Macrolide antibiotics: May prolong QT_c, potentially leading to malignant arrhythmias. Use caution and evaluate risk:benefit.

Metoprolol blood levels may be increased; monitor response.

Phenytoin blood levels may be increased by amiodarone; amiodarone blood levels may be decreased by phenytoin.

Procainamide and NAPA plasma levels may be increased; consider reducing procainamide dosage by 25% with concurrent use.

Propranolol blood levels may be increased.

Protease inhibitors (amprenavir, indinavir, ritonavir): May increase amiodarone blood levels and toxicity; concurrent use is contraindicated.

QT_c interval prolonging agents (including but may not be limited to amitriptyline, bepridil, disopyramide, erythromycin, haloperidol, imipramine, quinidine, pimozide, procainamide, sotalol, and thioridazine): Effect/toxicity increased; use with caution.

Quinidine blood levels may be increased; monitor quinidine trough concentration.

Rifampin may decrease amiodarone blood levels.

Theophylline blood levels may be increased.

Thyroid supplements: Amiodarone may alter thyroid function; monitor closely.

Warfarin: Hypoprothrombinemic response increased. Monitor INR closely when amiodarone is initiated or discontinued. Reduce warfarin's dose by $^1/_3$ to $^1/_2$ when amiodarone is started.

Pregnancy Risk Factor D

Pregnancy Implications May cause fetal harm when administered to a pregnant woman, leading to congenital goiter and hypo- or hyperthyroidism.

Lactation Enters breast milk/not recommended (AAP rates "of concern")

Nursing Implications Assess patient for signs of thyroid dysfunction, drowsiness, edema of the hands and feet, weight loss, and pulmonary toxicity

Additional Information

CNS symptoms normally develop within 7 days; muscle asthenia may present a significant hazard for ambulation; elevated erythrocyte sedimentation rate is found in >60% of patients with amiodarone-induced pulmonary disease. Grapefruit juice increases bioavailability of oral amiodarone by 50%; use should be avoided during therapy. Amiodarone contains iodine 37.3% by weight.

Rate of amiodarone-induced pulmonary disease is 5% to 10% with daily dosage >400 mg. Risk factors include pre-existing disease, radiographic abnormalities, history of lung resection, or history of pulmonary angiography.

Specific References

Barrueto F Jr, Chuang A, Hoffman RS, et al, "The Effect of Amiodarone on Amitriptyline Poisoned Mice," J Toxicol Clin Toxicol, 2003, 41(5):695.

Camus P, Martin WJ 2nd, and Rosenow EC 3rd, "Amiodarone Pulmonary Toxicity," Clin Chest Med, 2004, 25(1):65-75 (review).

Gillespie EL, Coleman CI, Sander S, et al, "Effect of Prophylactic Amiodarone on Clinical and Economic Outcomes After Cardiothoracic Surgery: A Meta-Analysis," Ann Pharmacother, 2005, 39(9):1409-15.

Graham MR, Wright MA, and Manley HJ, "Effectiveness of an Amiodarone Protocol and Management Clinic in Improving Adherence to Amiodarone Monitoring Guidelines," J Pharm Technol, 2004, 20(1):5-10.

Handschin AE, Lardinois D, Schneiter D, et al, "Acute Amiodarone-Induced Pulmonary Toxicity Following Lung Resection," Respiration, 2003, 70(3):310-2.

Juenke JM, Brown PI, McMillin GA, et al, "A Rapid Pocedure for the Monitoring of Amiodarone and N-Desethylamiodarone by HPLC-UV Detection," J Anal Toxicol, 2004, 28(1):63-6.

Lien WC, Huang CH, and Chen WJ, "Bidirectional Ventricular Tachycardia Resulting from Digoxin and Amiodarone Treatment of Rapid Atrial Fibrillation," Am J Emerg Med, 2004, 22(3):235-6.

Matsumoto K, Ueno K, Nakabayashi T, et al, "Amiodarone Interaction Time Differences with Warfarin and Digoxin," J Pharm Technol, 2003, 19:83-90.

Ott MC, Khoor A, Leventhal JP, et al, "Pulmonary Toxicity in Patients Receiving Low-Dose Amiodarone," Chest, 2003, 123(2):646-51.

Ren ZW, "The Pulmonary Toxicity of Amiodarone: Six-Case Report," Zhonghua Xin Xue Guan Bing Za Zhi, 2005, 33(1):66-8.

Roten L, Schoenenberger RA, Krahenbuhl S, et al, "Rhabdomyolysis in Association with Simvastatin and Amiodarone," Ann Pharmacother, 2004, 38(6):978-81.

Singh S, "Amiodarone-Induced Pulmonary Hemorrhage," South Med J, 2006, 99(4):329-30.

Skroubis G, Galiatsou E, Metafratzi Z, et al, "Amiodarone-Induced Acute Lung Toxicity in an ICU Setting," Acta Anaesthesiol Scand, 2005, 49(4):569-71.

Somberg JC, Cao W, Cvetanovic I, et al, "Pharmacology and Toxicology of a New Aqueous Formulation of Intravenous Amiodarone (Amio-Aqueous) Compared with Cordarone IV," Am J Ther, 2005, 12(1):9-16.

Amisulpride

CAS Number 71675-85-9

Use Schizophrenia; acute psychosis, tic disorders, infantile autism

Mechanism of Action A substituted benzamide with selective blockade of central dopamine (D_2) receptors; has antiemetic neuroleptic properties (not FDA approved in U.S.)

Adverse Reactions

Cardiovascular: Hypotension

Central nervous system: Lethargy, extrapyramidal reaction

Endocrine & metabolic: Amenorrhea, galactorrhea, gynecomastia, hyperprolactinemia

Genitourinary: Impotence

Signs and Symptoms of Overdose Coma, confusion, hyperthermia, mydriasis, seizures, tachycardia, QT prolongation on ECG

Toxicodynamics/Kinetics

Distribution: V_d: 13-16 L/kg

Protein binding: 17%

Metabolism: Hepatic to inactive metabolites

Half-life: 14.5-17.3 hours

Elimination: Renal (70% of drug is unchanged)

Dosage Oral: 50 mg to 1.2 g daily

Reference Range Peak plasma level after single oral dose of 200 mg: ~350 ng/mL; blood amisulpride level after 3 g ingestion (50 mg/kg) associated with seizures and light coma was 9.63 mcg/mL; a postmortem level of 41.7 mcg/mL was associated with suicide due to amisulpride overdose

Overdosage/Treatment

Decontamination: Lavage within 3 hours; activated charcoal

Supportive therapy: Benzodiazepines may be useful for seizure control

Amitriptyline

Pronunciation (a mee TRIP ti leen)

Related Information

- Anticholinergic Effects of Common Psychotropics
- Antidepressant Agents
- Butriptyline
- Dibenzepin
- Therapeutic Drugs Associated with Hallucinations

CAS Number 549-18-8

U.S. Brand Names Elavil® [DSC]

Synonyms Amitriptyline Hydrochloride; Elavil

Impairment Potential Yes. Doses of 50 mg can cause impairment; a greater than 5-times increased risk of injurious auto crash involvement following ingestion ≥125 mg amitriptyline in elderly drivers

Use Relief of symptoms of depression

Unlabeled/Investigational Use Analgesic for certain chronic and neuropathic pain; prophylaxis against migraine headaches; treatment of depressive disorders in children

Mechanism of Action Increases synaptic concentration of serotonin and/or norepinephrine in the central nervous system by inhibition of their reuptake by the presynaptic neuronal membrane

Adverse Reactions

Anticholinergic effects may be pronounced; moderate to marked sedation can occur (tolerance to these effects usually occurs).

Frequency not defined.

Cardiovascular: Orthostatic hypotension, tachycardia, nonspecific ECG changes, changes in AV conduction, cardiomyopathy (rare), MI, stroke, heart block, arrhythmias, syncope, hypertension, palpitations

Central nervous system: Restlessness, dizziness, insomnia, sedation, fatigue, anxiety, impaired cognitive function, seizures, extrapyramidal symptoms, coma, hallucinations, confusion, disorientation, impaired coordination, ataxia, headache, nightmares, hyperpyrexia

Dermatologic: Allergic rash, urticaria, photosensitivity, alopecia

Endocrine & metabolic: Syndrome of inappropriate ADH secretion

Gastrointestinal: Weight gain, xerostomia, constipation, paralytic ileus, nausea, vomiting, anorexia, stomatitis, peculiar taste, diarrhea, black tongue

Genitourinary: Urinary retention

Hematologic: Bone marrow depression, purpura, eosinophilia

Ocular: Blurred vision, mydriasis, ocular pressure increased

Otic: Tinnitus

Neuromuscular & skeletal: Numbness, paresthesia, peripheral neuropathy, tremor, weakness

Miscellaneous: Diaphoresis; withdrawal reactions (nausea, headache, malaise)

Postmarketing and/or case reports: Neuroleptic malignant syndrome (rare), serotonin syndrome (rare)

Signs and Symptoms of Overdose Agitation, bowel ischemia, confusion, decreased GI motility, delirium, dementia, dental erosion, ejaculatory disturbances, extrapyramidal reaction, fever, hallucinations, hyperacusis, hyperthermia, hyponatremia, hypotension, hypothermia, increased intraocular pressure, insomnia, lactation, memory loss, mania, myoglobinuria, neuroleptic malignant syndrome, nystagmus, paresthesia, periarteritis nodosa, photosensitivity, purpura, QRS prolongation, respiratory depression, seizures, tachycardia, urinary retention, urine discoloration (blue-green)

Admission Criteria/Prognosis Admit any patient who has any symptoms (including sinus tachycardia) 6 hours postingestion; admit any pediatric ingestion >5 mg/kg

Pharmacodynamics/Kinetics

Onset of action: Migraine prophylaxis: 6 weeks, higher dosage may be required in heavy smokers because of increased metabolism; Depression: 4-6 weeks, reduce dosage to lowest effective level

Distribution: Crosses placenta; enters breast milk

Metabolism: Hepatic to nortriptyline (active), hydroxy and conjugated derivatives; may be impaired in the elderly

Half-life elimination: Adults: 9-27 hours (average: 15 hours)

Time to peak, serum: ~4 hours

Excretion: Urine (18% as unchanged drug); feces (small amounts)

Dosage

Children:

Chronic pain management (unlabeled use): Oral: Initial: 0.1 mg/kg at bedtime, may advance as tolerated over 2-3 weeks to 0.5-2 mg/kg at bedtime

Depressive disorders (unlabeled use): Oral: Initial doses of 1 mg/kg/day given in 3 divided doses with increases to 1.5 mg/kg/day have been reported in a small number of children (n=9) 9-12 years of age; clinically, doses up to 3 mg/kg/day (5 mg/kg/day if monitored closely) have been proposed

Migraine prophylaxis (unlabeled use): Oral: Initial: 0.25 mg/kg/day, given at bedtime; increase dose by 0.25 mg/kg/day to maximum 1 mg/kg/day. Reported dosing ranges: 0.1-2 mg/kg/day; maximum suggested dose: 10 mg

Adolescents: Depressive disorders: Oral: Initial: 25-50 mg/day; may administer in divided doses; increase gradually to 100 mg/day in divided doses

Adults:

Depression:

Oral: 50-150 mg/day single dose at bedtime or in divided doses; dose may be gradually increased up to 300 mg/day

I.M.: 20-30 mg 4 times/day

Migraine prophylaxis (unlabeled use): Oral: Initial: 10-25 mg at bedtime; usual dose: 150 mg; reported dosing ranges: 10-400 mg/day

Pain management (unlabeled use): Oral: Initial: 25 mg at bedtime; may increase as tolerated to 100 mg/day

Elderly: Depression: Oral: Initial: 10-25 mg at bedtime; dose should be increased in 10-25 mg increments every week if tolerated; dose range: 25-150 mg/day

Dosing interval in hepatic impairment: Use with caution and monitor plasma levels and patient response

Hemodialysis: Nondialyzable

Stability Keep oral solution in refrigerator; remains stable for 7 days after preparation; protect injection and Elavil® 10 mg tablets from light

Monitoring Parameters Monitor blood pressure and pulse rate prior to and during initial therapy; evaluate mental status; monitor weight; ECG in older adults and patients with cardiac disease

Contraindications Hypersensitivity to amitriptyline or any component of the formulation (cross-sensitivity with other tricyclics may occur); use of MAO inhibitors within past 14 days; acute recovery phase following myocardial infarction; concurrent use of cisapride

Warnings

[U.S. Boxed Warning]: Antidepressants increase the risk of suicidal thinking and behavior in children and adolescents with major depressive disorder (MDD) and other depressive disorders; consider risk prior to prescribing. Closely monitor for clinical worsening, suicidality, or unusual changes in behavior; the child's family or caregiver should be instructed to closely observe the patient and communicate condition with healthcare provider. Such observation would generally include at least weekly face-to-face contact with patients or their family members or caregivers during the first 4 weeks of treatment, then every other week visits for the next 4 weeks, then at 12 weeks, and as clinically indicated beyond 12 weeks. Additional contact by telephone may be appropriate between face-to-face visits. Adults treated with antidepressants should be observed similarly for clinical worsening and suicidality, especially during the initial few months of a course of drug therapy, or at times of dose changes, either increases or decreases. A medication guide should be dispensed with each prescription. **Amitriptyline is not FDA-approved for use in children <12 years of age.**

The possibility of a suicide attempt is inherent in major depression and may persist until remission occurs. Monitor for worsening of depression or suicidality, especially during initiation of therapy or with dose increases or decreases. Worsening depression and severe abrupt suicidality that are not part of the presenting symptoms may require discontinuation or modification of drug therapy. Use caution in high-risk patients during initiation of therapy. Prescriptions should be written for the smallest quantity consistent with good patient care. The patient's family or caregiver should be alerted to monitor patients for the emergence of suicidality and associated behaviors such as anxiety, agitation, panic attacks, insomnia, irritability, hostility, impulsivity, akathisia, hypomania, and mania; patients should be instructed to notify their healthcare provider if any of these symptoms or worsening depression occur.

May worsen psychosis in some patients or precipitate a shift to mania or hypomania in patients with bipolar disorder. Monotherapy in patients with bipolar disorder should be avoided. Patients presenting with depressive symptoms should be screened for bipolar disorder. **Amitriptyline is not FDA approved for the treatment of bipolar depression.**

Often causes drowsiness/sedation, resulting in impaired performance of tasks requiring alertness (eg, operating machinery or driving). Sedative effects may be additive with other CNS depressants and/or ethanol. The degree of sedation is very high relative to other antidepressants. May cause hyponatremia/SIADH. May increase the risks associated with electroconvulsive therapy. Consider discontinuing, when possible, prior to elective surgery. Therapy should not be abruptly discontinued in patients receiving high doses for prolonged periods.

May cause orthostatic hypotension; the risk of this problem is very high relative to other antidepressants. Use with caution in patients at risk of hypotension or in patients where transient hypotensive episodes would be poorly tolerated (cardiovascular disease or cerebrovascular disease). The degree of anticholinergic blockade produced by this agent is very high relative to other cyclic antidepressants; use with caution in patients with urinary retention, benign prostatic hyperplasia, narrow-angle glaucoma, xerostomia, visual problems, constipation, or a history of bowel obstruction. May alter glucose control - use with caution in patients with diabetes.

Use with caution in patients with a history of cardiovascular disease (including previous MI, stroke, tachycardia, or conduction abnormalities). The risk of conduction abnormalities with this agent is high relative to other antidepressants. May lower seizure threshold - use caution in patients with a previous seizure disorder or condition predisposing to seizures such as brain damage, alcoholism, or concurrent therapy with other drugs which lower the seizure threshold. Use with caution in hyperthyroid patients or those receiving thyroid supplementation. Use with caution in patients with hepatic or renal dysfunction and in elderly patients.

Dosage Forms Tablet, as hydrochloride: 10 mg, 25 mg, 50 mg, 75 mg, 100 mg, 150 mg

Reference Range

Therapeutic:

Amitriptyline and nortriptyline: 100-250 ng/mL (SI: 360-900 nmol/L)

Nortriptyline: 50-150 ng/mL (SI: 190-570 nmol/L)

Toxic: >500 ng/mL; seizures can occur at levels >1000 ng/mL (SI: >3605 nmol/L)

In the postmortem state, anatomical site concentration differences (ie, postmortem redistribution) may occur

Overdosage/Treatment

Decontamination: Lavage within 2-3 hours/activated charcoal; **do not** induce emesis; multiple dosing of activated charcoal is more effective

Supportive therapy: Following initiation of essential overdose management, toxic symptoms should be treated. Ventricular arrhythmias and ventricular conduction defects often respond to concurrent systemic alkalinization (sodium bicarbonate 0.5-2 mEq/kg I.V.). Titrate to a serum pH of 7.45-7.55. Arrhythmias unresponsive to this therapy may respond to lidocaine 1 mg/kg I.V. followed by a titrated infusion. Phenytoin is also useful in treating ventricular dysrhythmias (15 mg/kg up to 1 g I.V.). Physostigmine (1-2 mg I.V. slowly for adults or 0.5 mg I.V. slowly for children) may be indicated for seizures or movement disorders but only as **a last resort**. Propranolol may also be utilized for supraventricular arrhythmias (rate: >160) at 1 mg/minute to a maximum of 5 mg in adults; pediatric dosage of 0.1 mg/kg/dose to 1 mg I.V.. Seizures usually respond to lorazepam or diazepam I.V. boluses (5-10 mg for adults up to 30 mg or 0.25-0.4 mg/kg/dose for children up to 10 mg/dose). If seizures are unresponsive or recur, phenytoin or phenobarbital may be required. Patients must be monitored for at least 24 hours if any signs or symptoms are exhibited. Dobutamine is preferred over dopamine for hypotension, although there is conflicting animal data. Norepinephrine appears effective in treating hypotension; glucagon (10 mg I.V.) can be given to treat hypotension. Vasopressin (initial dose: 0.04 units/minute) may be an effective vasopressor in treating hypotension. Flumazenil is contraindicated; magnesium has potentiated adverse cardiac effects (ie, asystole, decreased left ventricular pressure) in an animal model, although it was used successfully in treating refractory ventricular fibrillation at a dose of 20 nmol I.V. (a total of 2 doses). For treatment of lingua villosa nigra, discontinue causative agent. Clean the tongue with a toothbrush and rinse mouth with a half-strength solution of hydrogen peroxide or 10% carbamide peroxide. Oral symptoms should subside in a few days.

TCA ovine antibody fragments (TCA Fab, Protherics Inc) have been developed and used investigationally at a dose of 1-2 g over 30 minutes I.V.; if QRS was >100 msec or terminal deflection of QRS in lead aVR was >3 mm, a second dose (2 g over 30 min or 4 g over 1 hour) was given. If no response, a third infusion (4 g over 60 minutes or 8 g over 2 hours) was given.

Enhanced elimination: Multiple dosing of activated charcoal may be effective

Antidote(s)

• Sodium Bicarbonate [ANTIDOTE]

Test Interactions ↑ glucose, CPK, LDH, plasma catecholamine levels; cross reacts with phenothiazine levels

Drug Interactions

Substrate of CYP1A2 (minor), 2B6 (minor), 2C9 (minor), 2C19 (minor), 2D6 (major), 3A4 (minor); **Inhibits** CYP1A2 (weak), 2C9 (weak), 2C19 (weak), 2D6 (weak), 2E1 (weak)

Altretamine: Concurrent use may cause orthostatic hypertension.

Amphetamines: TCAs may enhance the effect of amphetamines; monitor for adverse CV effects.

Anticholinergics: Combined use with TCAs may produce additive anticholinergic effects.

Antihypertensives: Amitriptyline inhibits the antihypertensive response to bethanidine, clonidine, debrisoquin, guanadrel, guanethidine, guanabenz, guanfacine; monitor BP; consider alternate antihypertensive agent.

Beta-agonists: When combined with TCAs may predispose patients to cardiac arrhythmias.

Bupropion: May increase the levels of tricyclic antidepressants; based on limited information, monitor response.

Carbamazepine: Tricyclic antidepressants may increase carbamazepine levels; monitor.

Cholestyramine and colestipol: May bind TCAs and reduce their absorption; monitor for altered response.

Cisapride: May increase the risk of QT$_c$ prolongation and/or arrhythmia; concurrent use is contraindicated.

Clonidine: Abrupt discontinuation of clonidine may cause hypertensive crisis; amitriptyline may enhance the response (also see note on antihypertensives).

CNS depressants: Sedative effects may be additive with TCAs; monitor for increased effect; includes benzodiazepines, barbiturates, antipsychotics, ethanol, and other sedative medications.

CYP2D6 inhibitors: May increase the levels/effects of amitriptyline; example inhibitors include chlorpromazine, delavirdine, fluoxetine, miconazole, paroxetine, pergolide, quinidine, quinine, ritonavir, and ropinirole.

Epinephrine (and other direct alpha-agonists): Pressor response to I.V. epinephrine, norepinephrine, and phenylephrine may be enhanced in patients receiving TCAs. (**Note:** Effect is unlikely with epinephrine or levonordefrin dosages typically administered as infiltration in combination with local anesthetics.)

Fenfluramine: May increase tricyclic antidepressant levels/effects.

Hypoglycemic agents (including insulin): TCAs may enhance the hypoglycemic effects of tolazamide, chlorpropamide, or insulin; monitor for changes in blood glucose levels; reported with chlorpropamide, tolazamide, and insulin.

Levodopa: Tricyclic antidepressants may decrease the absorption (bioavailability) of levodopa; rare hypertensive episodes have also been attributed to this combination.

Linezolid: Hyperpyrexia, hypertension, tachycardia, confusion, seizures, and **deaths have been reported** with agents which inhibit MAO (serotonin syndrome); this combination should be avoided.

Lithium: Concurrent use with a TCA may increase the risk for neurotoxicity.

MAO inhibitors: Hyperpyrexia, hypertension, tachycardia, confusion, seizures, and **deaths have been reported** (serotonin syndrome); this combination should be avoided.

Methylphenidate: Metabolism of amitriptyline may be decreased.

Phenothiazines: Serum concentrations of some TCAs may be increased; in addition, TCAs may increase concentration of phenothiazines; monitor for altered clinical response.

QT$_c$ prolonging agents: Concurrent use of tricyclic agents with other drugs which may prolong QT$_c$ interval may increase the risk of potentially fatal arrhythmias; includes type Ia and type III antiarrhythmics agents, selected quinolones (sparfloxacin, gatifloxacin, moxifloxacin, grepafloxacin), cisapride, and other agents.

Ritonavir: Combined use of high-dose tricyclic antidepressants with ritonavir may cause serotonin syndrome in HIV-positive patients; monitor.

Sucralfate: Absorption of tricyclic antidepressants may be reduced with coadministration.

Sympathomimetics, indirect-acting: Tricyclic antidepressants may result in a decreased sensitivity to indirect-acting sympathomimetics; includes dopamine and ephedrine; also see interaction with epinephrine (and direct-acting sympathomimetics).

Tramadol: Tramadol's risk of seizures may be increased with TCAs.

Valproic acid: May increase serum concentrations/adverse effects of some tricyclic antidepressants.

Warfarin (and other oral anticoagulants): Amitriptyline may increase the anticoagulant effect in patients stabilized on warfarin; monitor INR.

Pregnancy Risk Factor D

Pregnancy Implications Teratogenic effects have been observed in animal studies. Amitriptyline crosses the human placenta; CNS effects, limb deformities and developmental delay have been noted in case reports.

Lactation Enters breast milk/not recommended (AAP rates "of concern")

Additional Information Plasma levels do not always correlate with clinical effectiveness. The desired therapeutic effect (for depression) may take as long as 3-4 weeks, at that point the dosage should be reduced to the lowest effective level. When used for migraine headache prophylaxis, the therapeutic effect may take as long as 6 weeks. Because of increased metabolism, a higher dosage may be required in heavy smokers.

Specific References

Aygoren O, Kalkan S, Akgun A, et al, "The Effects of Adenosine Receptor Antagonists on Amitriptyline-Induced Cardiovascular Toxicity in Rats," *J Toxicol Clin Toxicol*, 2003, 41(5):751.

Bailey B, Buckley NA, and Amre DK, "A Meta-Analysis of Prognostic Indicators to Predict Seizures, Arrhythmias or Death After Tricyclic Antidepressant Overdose," *J Toxicol Clin Toxicol*, 2004, 42(6):877-88.

Bania TC and Chu J, "Hemodynamic Effect of Intralipid in Amitriptyline Toxicity," *Acad Emerg Med*, 2006, 13(5):S177.

Barrueto F Jr, Chuang A, Cotter BW, et al, "Amiodarone Fails to Improve Survival in Amitriptyline-Poisoned Mice," *Clin Toxicol (Phila)*, 2005, 43(3):147-9.

Barrueto F Jr, Chuang A, Hoffman RS, et al, "The Effect of Amiodarone on Amitriptyline Poisoned Mice," *J Toxicol Clin Toxicol*, 2003, 41(5):695.

Bebarta VS, Phillips S, Eberhardt A, et al, "Incidence and Outcomes of Patients with the Brugada Pattern in a Large Case Series of Tricyclic Overdoses," *J Toxicol Clin Toxicol*, 2004, 42(5):714.

Bynum ND, Poklis JL, Gaffney-Kraft M, et al, "Postmortem Distribution of Tramadol, Amitriptyline, and Their Metabolites in a Suicidal Overdose," *J Anal Toxicol*, 2005, 29(5):401-6.

Crockett J, Ndon JA, Sahin E, et al, "Pharmacogenomics as an Adjunct in Death Certification of Amitriptyline, Nortriptyline, Clomipramine, and Fluoxetine," *J Anal Toxicol*, 2004, 28:278.

Eizadi-Mood N, Moein N, and Saghaei M, "Evaluation of Relationship Between Arterial and Venous Blood Gas Values in the Patients with Tricyclic Antidepressant Poisoning," *Clin Toxicol* , 2005, 43(5):357-60.

Franssen EJ, Kunst PW, Bet PM, et al, "Toxicokinetics of Nortriptyline and Amitriptyline: Two Case Reports," *Ther Drug Monit*, 2003, 25(2): 248-51.

Fukumoto M, Udagawa R, Yoshimura K, et al, "Evaluation of Plasma Levels for Predicting Clinical Outcomes in Tricyclic Antidepressant Overdose," *Clin Toxicol (Phila)*, 2005, 43:697.

Garg U, Frazee III CC, Beckenbach B, et al, "Interpreting Postmortem Tricyclic Antidepressant Levels in Vitreous Humor," *J Anal Toxicol*, 2004, 28:293-4.

Gorczynski LY and Rajotte JW, "Amitriptyline-Related Fatalities in Ontario," *J Anal Toxicol*, 2006, 30:152.

Greene SL, Dargan PI, Antoniades H, et al, "Delayed Clinical Effects in Modified-Release Amitriptyline Poisoning: A Case Report with Toxicokinetic Data," *J Toxicol Clin Toxicol*, 2002, 40(3):353-4.

Heard K, Dart RC, Bogdan G, et al, "A Preliminary Study of Tricyclic Antidepressant (TCA) Ovine FAB for TCA Toxicity," *J Toxicol Clin Toxicol*, 2006, 44:275-81.

Hollowell H, Mattu A, Perron AD, et al, "Wide-Complex Tachycardia: Beyond the Traditional Differential Diagnosis of Ventricular Tachycardia vs Supraventricular Tachycardia with Aberrant Conduction," *Am J Emerg Med*, 2005, 23(7):876-89.

Kalkan S, Aygoren O, Akgun A, et al, "Do Adenosine Receptors Play a Role in Amitriptyline-Induced Cardiovascular Toxicity in Rats?" *J Toxicol Clin Toxicol*, 2004, 42(7):945-54.

Kalkan S, Hocaogla N, Akgun A, et al, "Effects of the Adenosine Receptor Antagonists on Amitriptyline-Induced Vasodilation in Rat Isolated Aorta," *Clin Toxicol (Phila)*, 2005, 43:730.

Malik DJ, Rielly CD, Inman S, et al, "The Characterization and Development of Microstructured Carbons for the Treatment of Drug Overdose," *J Toxicol Clin Toxicol*, 2003, 41(5):694.

Martinez MA, De La Torre CS, and Almarza E, "A Comparative Solid-Phase Extraction Study for the Simultaneous Determination of Fluoxetine, Amitriptyline, Nortriptyline, Trimipramine, Maprotiline, Clomipramine, and Trazodone in Whole Blood By Capillary Gas-Liquid Chromatography with Nitrogen-Phosphorus Detection," *J Anal Toxicol*, 2003, 27(6):353-8.

O'Connor N, Greene S, Dargan P, et al, "Prolonged Clinical Effects in Modified-Release Amitriptyline Poisoning," *Clin Toxicol (Phila)*, 2006, 44(1):77-80.

Robert R, Frat JP, Veinstein A, et al, "Protective Effect of Medication Bezoar After a Massive Beta-Blocker, Digoxin, and Amitriptyline Poisoning," *Clin Toxicol*, 2005, 43(5):381-2.

Schaeffer TH, Phillips SD, Heard KJ, et al, "Terminal 40 ms R Wave Height vs Serum Levels in Tricyclic Antidepressant (TCA) Overdose: Is There a Correlation?" *Clin Toxicol (Phila)*, 2005, 43:732.

Seger DL, Hantsch C, Zavoral T, et al, "Variability of Recommendations for Serum Alkalinization in Tricyclic Antidepressant Overdose: A Survey of U.S. Poison Center Medical Directors," *J Toxicol Clin Toxicol*, 2003, 41(4):331-8.

Spiller HA, Baker SD, Krenzelok EP, et al, "Use of Dosage as a Triage Guideline for Unintentional Cyclic Antidepressant (UCA) Ingestions in Children," *Am J Emerg Med*, 2003, 21(5):422-4.

Amlodipine

Pronunciation (am LOE di peen)
Related Information
● Calcium Channel Blockers
CAS Number 111470-99-6; 88150-42-9; 88150-47-4
U.S. Brand Names Norvasc®
Synonyms Amlodipine Besylate
Use Treatment of hypertension and angina
Mechanism of Action A 1,4 dihydropyridine calcium channel blocking agent; a potent vasodilator
Adverse Reactions
Cardiovascular: Dose dependent **peripheral edema** (2% to 15%), flushing, palpitations, exacerbation of intracranial hypertension
Central nervous system: Headache, fatigue, dizziness, somnolence, intracranial hemorrhage
Dermatologic: Erythematous rash, pruritus, exanthema, erythema multiforme, alopecia, urticaria, purpura
Gastrointestinal: Nausea, gingival hyperplasia, xerostomia, weight gain/loss
Hematologic: Thrombocytopenia
Hepatic: Jaundice
Neuromuscular & skeletal: Arthralgias, myalgias
Signs and Symptoms of Overdose Bradycardia, conductive defects, hypotension, reflex tachycardia

Admission Criteria/Prognosis Admit any symptomatic (cardiovascular) patient or ingestions >1 mg/kg
Pharmacodynamics/Kinetics
Onset of action: Antihypertensive: 30-50 minutes
Duration of antihypertensive effect: 24 hours
Absorption: Oral: Well absorbed
Distribution: V_d: 21 L/kg
Protein binding: 93% to 98%
Metabolism: Hepatic (>90%) to inactive metabolite
Bioavailability: 64% to 90%
Half-life elimination: 30-50 hours; increased with hepatic dysfunction
Time to peak, plasma: 6-12 hours
Excretion: Urine (10% as parent, 60% as metabolite)
Dosage
Oral:
Children 6-17 years: Hypertension: 2.5-5 mg once daily
Adults:
Hypertension: Initial dose: 5 mg once daily; maximum dose: 10 mg once daily. In general, titrate in 2.5 mg increments over 7-14 days. Usual dosage range (JNC-7): 2.5-10 mg once daily.
Angina: Usual dose: 5-10 mg
Elderly: Dosing should start at the lower end of dosing range due to possible increased incidence of hepatic, renal, or cardiac impairment. Elderly patients also show decreased clearance of amlodipine.
Hypertension: 2.5 mg once daily
Angina: 5 mg once daily
Dialysis: Hemodialysis and peritoneal dialysis does not enhance elimination. Supplemental dose is not necessary.
Dosage adjustment in hepatic impairment:
Angina: Administer 5 mg once daily.
Hypertension: Administer 2.5 mg once daily.
Administration
May be administered without regard to meals.
Contraindications Hypersensitivity to amlodipine or any component of the formulation
Warnings Increased angina and/or MI has occurred with initiation or dosage titration of calcium channel blockers. Use caution in severe aortic stenosis. Use caution in patients with severe hepatic impairment. Dosage titration should occur after 7-14 days on a given dose.
Dosage Forms
Tablet:
Norvasc®: 2.5 mg, 5 mg, 10 mg
Reference Range Peak plasma amlodipine level after a 10 mg oral dose: ~5.9 mcg/L; postmortem peripheral blood amlodipine level after a 140 mg overdose was 2.7 mg/L; therapeutic range: 3-11 ng/mL. Serum level of amlodipine of 140 ng/mL associated with an 800 mg ingestion and hypotension. Postmortem heart blood amlodipine level >1 mg/L associated with fatal overdoses.
Overdosage/Treatment
Decontamination: Ipecac-induced emesis can hypothetically worsen calcium antagonist toxicity, since it can produce vagal stimulation. The potential for seizures precipitously following acute ingestion of large doses of a calcium antagonist may also contraindicate the use of ipecac. Lavage (within 1 hour)/activated charcoal is useful. Whole bowel irrigation for sustained release preparations.
Supportive therapy: I.V. fluids and Trendelenburg positioning should be initiated as intoxication may cause hypotension. Calcium (calcium chloride I.V. 1-3 g in adults or 10-30 mg/kg in children over 5-10 minutes with repeats as needed) has been used as treatment for acute intoxications and is considered as second line therapy for shock after traditional use of vasopressors. Hyperinsulinemic therapy with 0.5-1.0 unit I.V. insulin bolus with an infusion of 0.2-1 unit/kg/hour plus a glucose bolus of 25 g I.V. and dextrose infusion to maintain a serum glucose >100 mg/dL may reverse cardiogenic shock due to calcium blockers. Heart block may respond to isoproterenol, glucagon, atropine and/or calcium, although a temporary pacemaker may be required. Inamrinone or dopamine may be required for hypotension. Glucagon may increase myocardial contractility. High dose vasopressin (up to 4.8 units/hour) may be effective in treating hypotension.
Vasopressin (20 IU bolus I.V titrated by blood pressure to 4 to 5 IU/hour infusion) can increase systemic vascular resistence and cardiac output.
Enhancement of elimination: Multiple dosing of activated charcoal is useful
Drug Interactions
Substrate of CYP3A4 (major); **Inhibits** CYP1A2 (moderate), 2A6 (weak), 2B6 (weak), 2C8 (weak), 2C9 (weak), 2D6 (weak), 3A4 (weak)
Azole antifungals may inhibit calcium channel blocker metabolism; avoid this combination. Try an antifungal like terbinafine (if appropriate) or monitor closely for altered effect of the calcium channel blocker.
Calcium may reduce the calcium channel blocker's effects, particularly hypotension.
CYP1A2 substrates: Amlodipine may increase the levels/effects of CYP1A2 substrates. Example substrates include aminophylline, fluvoxamine, mexiletine, mirtazapine, ropinirole, theophylline, and trifluoperazine.

CYP3A4 inducers: CYP3A4 inducers may decrease the levels/effects of amlodipine. Example inducers include aminoglutethimide, carbamazepine, nafcillin, nevirapine, phenobarbital, phenytoin, and rifamycins.

CYP3A4 inhibitors: May increase the levels/effects of amlodipine. Example inhibitors include azole antifungals, clarithromycin, diclofenac, doxycycline, erythromycin, imatinib, isoniazid, nefazodone, nicardipine, propofol, protease inhibitors, quinidine, telithromycin, and verapamil.

Grapefruit juice: May modestly increase amlodipine levels.

Rifampin increases the metabolism of calcium channel blockers; adjust the dose of calcium channel blocker to maintain efficacy.

Sildenafil, tadalafil, vardenafil: Blood pressure-lowering effects are additive; use caution.

Pregnancy Risk Factor C

Pregnancy Implications Embryotoxic effects have been demonstrated in small animals. No well-controlled studies have been conducted in pregnant women. Use in pregnancy only when clearly needed and when the benefits outweigh the potential hazard to the fetus.

Lactation Excretion in breast milk unknown/not recommended

Specific References

Andersen J, Groshong T, and Tobias JD, "Preliminary Experience with Amlodipine in the Pediatric Population," *Am J Ther*, 2006, 13:198-204.

Benson BE, Spyker DA, Troutman WG, et al, "TESS-Based Amlodipine Dose-Response in Pediatric Exposures," *J Toxicol Clin Toxicol*, 2004, 42(5):753-4.

Israili ZH, "The Use of Calcium Antagonists in the Therapy of Hypertension in the Elderly," *Am J Ther*, 2003, 10(6):383-95.

Lund-Johansen P, Stranden E, Helberg S, et al, "Quantification of Leg Oedema in Postmenopausal Hypertensive Patients Treated with Lercanidipine or Amlodipine," *J Hypertens*, 2003, 21(5):1003-10.

Kamijo Y, Yoshida T, Ide A, et al, "Mixed Venous Oxygen Saturation Monitoring in Calcium Channel Blocker Poisoning Tissue Hypoxia Avoidance Despite Hypotension," *Am J Emerg Med*, 2006, 24:357-60.

Marquardt KA, Alsop JA, and Albertson TE, "Amlodipine Ingestions in Children Less Than Six Years Old," *Clin Toxicol (Phila)*, 2005, 43:644.

Marraffa JM, Stork CM, Medicis JJ, et al, "Massive Amlodipine Overdose Successfully Treated Using High-Dose Vasopressin," *J Toxicol Clin Toxicol*, 2004, 42(5):732.

Ohmori M, Arakawa M, Harada K, et al, "Stereoselective Pharmacokinetics of Amlodipine in Elderly Hypertensive Patients," *Am J Ther*, 2003, 10(1):29-31.

Rasmussen L, Husted SE, and Johnsen SP, "Severe Intoxication After an Intentional Overdose of Amlodipine," *Acta Anaesthesiol Scand*, 2003, 47(8):1038-40.

Sener D, Halil M, Yavuz BB, et al, "Anasarca Edema with Amlodipine Treatment," *Ann Pharmacother*, 2005, 39(4):761-3.

Sklerov JH, Levine B, Ingwersen KM, et al, "Two Cases of Fatal Amlodipine Overdose," *J Anal Toxicol*, 2006, 30:346-8.

Wood DM, Dargam PI, Greene SL, et al, "Metaraminol (Aramine®) in the Management of Significant Amlodipine Poisoning: A Case Report," *Clin Toxicol (Phila)*, 2005, 43:739.

Amoxapine

Pronunciation (a MOKS a peen)

Related Information

- Anticholinergic Effects of Common Psychotropics
- Antidepressant Agents
- Therapeutic Drugs Associated with Hallucinations

CAS Number 14028-44-5

Synonyms Asendin [DSC]

Use Treatment of neurotic and endogenous depression and mixed symptoms of anxiety and depression

Mechanism of Action Reduces the reuptake of serotonin and norepinephrine and blocks the response of dopamine receptors to dopamine; low effect on serotonin reuptake. Amoxapine is a metabolite of the antipsychotic agent loxapine.

Adverse Reactions

Anticholinergic: Extrapyramidal effects, tardive dyskinesia, blurred vision

Cardiovascular: Hypotension, sinus tachycardia, relatively low cardiac toxicity as compared to other tricyclic antidepressants, AV block, sinus tachycardia, tachycardia (supraventricular), arrhythmias (ventricular), vasculitis

Central nervous system: **Drowsiness**, restlessness, **dizziness**, nervousness, insomnia, seizures, Parkinson's-like symptoms, chorea (extrapyramidal), tardive dyskinesia, fever, visual hallucinations, neuroleptic malignant syndrome, electroencephalogram abnormalities, hyperthermia

Dermatologic: Rash, toxic epidermal necrolysis, exanthema, acne, acute generalized exanthematous pustulosis, alopecia, xerosis, purpura, pruritus, lingua villosa nigra

Endocrine & metabolic: Amenorrhea, galactorrhea, syndrome of inappropriate antidiuretic hormone

Gastrointestinal: **Constipation, xerostomia, nausea, unpleasant taste, weight gain**, pancreatitis, stomatitis

Hematologic: Leukopenia/neutropenia (agranulocytosis, granulocytopenia)

Neuromuscular & skeletal: Rhabdomyolysis, paresthesia

Ocular: Oculogyric crisis (extrapyramidal)

Signs and Symptoms of Overdose Acidosis, cognitive dysfunction, coma, dementia, depression, ejaculatory disturbances, extrapyramidal reaction, grand mal seizures, hematuria, hyperprolactinemia, impotence, incomplete right bundle-branch block, insomnia, mania, myoglobinuria, photosensitivity, neuroleptic malignant syndrome, nystagmus, supraventricular arrhythmias, renal failure (acute). Neurotoxic effects may be permanent.

Admission Criteria/Prognosis Admit any patient who is symptomatic (including sinus tachycardia) 6 hours postingestion; admit any pediatric ingestion >5 mg/kg

Pharmacodynamics/Kinetics

Onset of antidepressant effect: Usually occurs after 1-2 weeks, but may require 4-6 weeks

Absorption: Rapid and well absorbed

Distribution: V_d: 0.9-1.2 L/kg; enters breast milk

Protein binding: 80%

Metabolism: Primarily hepatic

Half-life elimination: Parent drug: 11-16 hours; Active metabolite (8-hydroxy): Adults: 30 hours

Time to peak, serum: 1-2 hours

Excretion: Urine (as unchanged drug and metabolites)

Dosage

Once symptoms are controlled, decrease gradually to lowest effective dose. Maintenance dose is usually given at bedtime to reduce daytime sedation. Oral:

Children <16 years: Not established

Adolescents: Initial: 25-50 mg/day; increase gradually to 100 mg/day; may give as divided doses or as a single dose at bedtime

Adults: Initial: 25 mg 2-3 times/day, if tolerated, dosage may be increased to 100 mg 2-3 times/day; may be given in a single bedtime dose when dosage <300 mg/day

Maximum daily dose:

Inpatient: 600 mg

Outpatient: 400 mg

Monitoring Parameters Monitor blood pressure and pulse rate prior to and during initial therapy evaluate mental status; monitor weight; ECG in older adults

Administration

May be administered with food to decrease GI distress.

Contraindications Hypersensitivity to amoxapine or any component of the formulation; use of MAO inhibitors within past 14 days; acute recovery phase following myocardial infarction

Warnings

[U.S. Boxed Warning]: Antidepressants increase the risk of suicidal thinking and behavior in children and adolescents with major depressive disorder (MDD) and other depressive disorders; consider risk prior to prescribing. Closely monitor for clinical worsening, suicidality, or unusual changes in behavior; the child's family or caregiver should be instructed to closely observe the patient and communicate condition with healthcare provider. Such observation would generally include at least weekly face-to-face contact with patients or their family members or caregivers during the first 4 weeks of treatment, then every other week visits for the next 4 weeks, then at 12 weeks, and as clinically indicated beyond 12 weeks. Additional contact by telephone may be appropriate between face-to-face visits. Adults treated with antidepressants should be observed similarly for clinical worsening and suicidality, especially during the initial few months of a course of drug therapy, or at times of dose changes, either increases or decreases. A medication guide should be dispensed with each prescription. **Amoxapine is not FDA approved for use in patients <16 years of age.**

The possibility of a suicide attempt is inherent in major depression and may persist until remission occurs. Monitor for worsening of depression or suicidality, especially during initiation of therapy or with dose increases or decreases. Worsening depression and severe abrupt suicidality that are not part of the presenting symptoms may require discontinuation or modification of drug therapy. Use caution in high-risk patients during initiation of therapy. Prescriptions should be written for the smallest quantity consistent with good patient care. The patient's family or caregiver should be alerted to monitor patients for the emergence of suicidality and associated behaviors such as anxiety, agitation, panic attacks, insomnia, irritability, hostility, impulsivity, akathisia, hypomania, and mania; patients should be instructed to notify their healthcare provider if any of these symptoms or worsening depression occur.

May worsen psychosis in some patients or precipitate a shift to mania or hypomania in patients with bipolar disorder. Monotherapy in patients with bipolar disorder should be avoided. Patients presenting with depressive symptoms should be screened for bipolar disorder. **Amoxapine is not FDA approved for the treatment of bipolar depression.**

May cause sedation, resulting in impaired performance of tasks requiring alertness (eg, operating machinery or driving). Sedative effects may be additive with other CNS depressants and/or ethanol. The degree of sedation is moderate relative to other antidepressants. May increase the risks associated with electroconvulsive therapy. Consider discontinuing, when possible, prior to elective surgery. Therapy should not be abruptly discontinued in patients receiving high doses for prolonged periods.

May cause extrapyramidal symptoms, including pseudoparkinsonism, acute dystonic reactions, akathisia, and tardive dyskinesia (risk of these reactions is low). May be associated with neuroleptic malignant syndrome.

May cause orthostatic hypotension (risk is moderate relative to other antidepressants) - use with caution in patients at risk of hypotension or in patients where transient hypotensive episodes would be poorly tolerated (cardiovascular disease or cerebrovascular disease). The degree of anticholinergic blockade produced by this agent is moderate relative to other cyclic antidepressants - use caution in patients with urinary retention, benign prostatic hyperplasia, narrow-angle glaucoma, xerostomia, visual problems, constipation, or history of bowel obstruction.

Use with caution in patients with a history of cardiovascular disease (including previous MI, stroke, tachycardia, or conduction abnormalities). The risk conduction abnormalities with this agent is moderate relative to other antidepressants. May lower seizure threshold - use caution in patients with a previous seizure disorder or condition predisposing to seizures such as brain damage, alcoholism, or concurrent therapy with other drugs which lower the seizure threshold. Use with caution in hyperthyroid patients or those receiving thyroid supplementation. Use with caution in patients with hepatic or renal dysfunction and in elderly patients.

Dosage Forms Tablet: 25 mg, 50 mg, 100 mg, 150 mg

Reference Range

Therapeutic:

Amoxapine 20-100 ng/mL (SI: 64-319 nmol/L)

8-OH-amoxapine: 150-400 ng/mL (SI: 478-1275 nmol/L)

Both: 200-500 ng/mL (SI: 637-1594 nmol/L)

Fatal: 261 ng/mL

In the postmortem state, anatomical site concentration differences (ie, postmortem redistribution) may occur

Overdosage/Treatment

Decontamination: Lavage (up to 8 hours postingestion)/activated charcoal; multiple dosing of activated charcoal may be effective; **do not** induce emesis

Supportive therapy: Following initiation of essential overdose management, toxic symptoms should be treated. Propofol (2.5 mg/kg bolus I.V. followed by infusion of 0.2 mg/kg/minute) has been effective in terminating amoxapine-induced seizures in a case report; ventricular arrhythmias often respond to phenytoin 15-20 mg/kg (adults) with concurrent systemic alkalinization (sodium bicarbonate 0.5-2 mEq/kg I.V.). Arrhythmias unresponsive to this therapy may respond to lidocaine 1 mg/kg I.V. followed by a titrated infusion. Seizures usually respond to diazepam I.V. boluses (5-10 mg for adults up to 30 mg or 0.25-0.4 mg/kg/dose for children up to 10 mg/dose). If seizures are unresponsive or recur, phenytoin or phenobarbital may be required. Use physostigmine only as **a last resort**. For treatment of lingua villosa nigra, discontinue causative agent. Clean the tongue with a toothbrush and rinse mouth with a half-strength solution of hydrogen peroxide or 10% carbamide peroxide. Symptoms should subside in a few days.

Antidote(s)

● Sodium Bicarbonate [ANTIDOTE]

Test Interactions ↑ glucose; may ↑ prolactin level

Drug Interactions

Substrate of CYP2D6 (major)

Anticholinergics: Combined use with TCAs may produce additive anticholinergic effects.

Altretamine: Concurrent use may cause orthostatic hypertension.

Amphetamines: TCAs may enhance the effect of amphetamines; monitor for adverse CV effects.

Antihypertensives: Amitriptyline inhibits the antihypertensive response to bethanidine, clonidine, debrisoquin, guanadrel, guanethidine, guanabenz, guanfacine; monitor BP; consider alternate antihypertensive agent.

Beta-agonists: When combined with TCAs, may predispose patients to cardiac arrhythmias.

Bupropion: May increase the levels of tricyclic antidepressants; based on limited information; monitor response.

Carbamazepine: Tricyclic antidepressants may increase carbamazepine levels; monitor.

Cholestyramine and colestipol: May bind TCAs and reduce their absorption; monitor for altered response.

Clonidine: Abrupt discontinuation of clonidine may cause hypertensive crisis; amitriptyline may enhance the response.

CNS depressants: Sedative effects may be additive with TCAs; monitor for increased effect; includes benzodiazepines, barbiturates, antipsychotics, ethanol, and other sedative medications.

CYP2D6 inhibitors: May increase the levels/effects of amoxapine. Example inhibitors include chlorpromazine, delavirdine, fluoxetine, miconazole, paroxetine, pergolide, quinidine, quinine, ritonavir, and ropinirole.

Epinephrine (and other direct alpha-agonists): Pressor response to I.V. epinephrine, norepinephrine, and phenylephrine may be enhanced in patients receiving TCAs. (**Note:** Effect is unlikely with epinephrine or levonordefrin dosages typically administered as infiltration in combination with local anesthetics).

Fenfluramine: May increase tricyclic antidepressant levels/effects.

Hypoglycemic agents (including insulin): TCAs may enhance the hypoglycemic effects of tolazamide, chlorpropamide, or insulin; monitor for changes in blood glucose levels; reported with chlorpropamide, tolazamide, and insulin.

Levodopa: Tricyclic antidepressants may decrease the absorption (bioavailability) of levodopa; rare hypertensive episodes have also been attributed to this combination.

Linezolid: Hyperpyrexia, hypertension, tachycardia, confusion, seizures, and **deaths have been reported** with agents which inhibit MAO (serotonin syndrome); this combination should be avoided.

Lithium: Concurrent use with a TCA may increase the risk for neurotoxicity.

MAO inhibitors: Hyperpyrexia, hypertension, tachycardia, confusion, seizures, and **deaths have been reported** (serotonin syndrome); this combination should be avoided.

Methylphenidate: Metabolism of amitriptyline may be decreased.

Phenothiazines: Serum concentrations of some TCAs may be increased; in addition, TCAs may increase concentration of phenothiazines; monitor for altered clinical response.

QT_c-prolonging agents: Concurrent use of tricyclic agents with other drugs which may prolong QT_c interval may increase the risk of potentially fatal arrhythmias; includes type Ia and type III antiarrhythmics agents, selected quinolones (sparfloxacin, gatifloxacin, moxifloxacin, grepafloxacin), cisapride, and other agents.

Ritonavir: Combined use of high-dose tricyclic antidepressants with ritonavir may cause serotonin syndrome in HIV-positive patients; monitor.

Sucralfate: Absorption of tricyclic antidepressants may be reduced with coadministration.

Sympathomimetics, indirect-acting: Tricyclic antidepressants may result in a decreased sensitivity to indirect-acting sympathomimetics; includes dopamine and ephedrine; also see interaction with epinephrine (and direct-acting sympathomimetics).

Tramadol: Tramadol's risk of seizures may be increased with TCAs.

Valproic acid: May increase serum concentrations/adverse effects of some tricyclic antidepressants.

Warfarin (and other oral anticoagulants): Amitriptyline may increase the anticoagulant effect in patients stabilized on warfarin; monitor INR.

Pregnancy Risk Factor C

Lactation Enters breast milk/contraindicated (AAP rates "of concern")

Nursing Implications May increase appetite and possibly a craving for sweets; recognize signs of neuroleptic malignant syndrome and tardive dyskinesia

Additional Information May take up to 2 weeks for full therapeutic effects to be apparent; maintenance dose is usually given at bedtime to reduce daytime sedation; tolerance develops in 1-3 months in some patients, close medical follow-up is essential

Amoxicillin

Pronunciation (a moks i SIL in)

CAS Number 26787-78-0; 34642-77-8; 61336-70-7

U.S. Brand Names Amoxil®; DisperMox™; Moxilin®; Trimox®

Synonyms p-Hydroxyampicillin; Amoxicillin Trihydrate; Amoxycillin

Use Treatment of otitis media, sinusitis, and infections caused by susceptible organisms involving the respiratory tract, skin, and urinary tract; prophylaxis of bacterial endocarditis in patients undergoing surgical or dental procedures; as part of a multidrug regimen for H. pylori eradication

Unlabeled/Investigational Use Postexposure prophylaxis for anthrax exposure with documented susceptible organisms

Mechanism of Action Interferes with bacterial cell wall synthesis during active multiplication, causing cell wall death and resultant bactericidal activity against susceptible bacteria

Adverse Reactions

Frequency not defined.

Central nervous system: Hyperactivity, agitation, anxiety, insomnia, confusion, convulsions, behavioral changes, dizziness

Dermatologic: Acute exanthematous pustulosis, erythematous maculopapular rash, erythema multiforme, Stevens-Johnson syndrome, exfoliative dermatitis, toxic epidermal necrolysis, hypersensitivity vasculitis, urticaria

Gastrointestinal: Nausea, vomiting, diarrhea, hemorrhagic colitis, pseudomembranous colitis, tooth discoloration (brown, yellow, or gray; rare)

Hematologic: Anemia, hemolytic anemia, thrombocytopenia, thrombocytopenia purpura, eosinophilia, leukopenia, agranulocytosis

Hepatic: Elevated AST (SGOT) and ALT (SGPT), cholestatic jaundice, hepatic cholestasis, acute cytolytic hepatitis

Signs and Symptoms of Overdose Many beta-lactam antibiotics have the potential to cause neuromuscular hyperirritability or convulsive seizures. Acute renal failure, hematuria, neuromuscular sensitivity, pemphigus

Pharmacodynamics/Kinetics

Absorption: Oral: Rapid and nearly complete; food does not interfere

Distribution: Widely to most body fluids and bone; poor penetration into cells, eyes, and across normal meninges

Pleural fluids, lungs, and peritoneal fluid; high urine concentrations are attained; also into synovial fluid, liver, prostate, muscle, and gallbladder; penetrates into middle ear effusions, maxillary sinus secretions, tonsils, sputum, and bronchial secretions; crosses placenta; low concentrations enter breast milk

CSF:blood level ratio: Normal meninges: <1%; Inflamed meninges: 8% to 90%

Protein binding: 17% to 20%

Metabolism: Partially hepatic

Half-life elimination:

Neonates, full-term: 3.7 hours

Infants and Children: 1-2 hours

Adults: Normal renal function: 0.7-1.4 hours

Cl_{cr} <10 mL/minute: 7-21 hours

Time to peak: Capsule: 2 hours; Suspension: 1 hour

Excretion: Urine (80% as unchanged drug); lower in neonates

Dosage

Oral:

Children ≤3 months: 20-30 mg/kg/day divided every 12 hours

Children: >3 months and <40 kg: Dosing range: 20-50 mg/kg/day in divided doses every 8-12 hours

Ear, nose, throat, genitourinary tract, or skin/skin structure infections:

Mild to moderate: 25 mg/kg/day in divided doses every 12 hours **or** 20 mg/kg/day in divided doses every 8 hours

Severe: 45 mg/kg/day in divided doses every 12 hours **or** 40 mg/kg/day in divided doses every 8 hours

Acute otitis media due to highly-resistant strains of *S. pneumoniae*: Doses as high as 80-90 mg/kg/day divided every 12 hours have been used

Lower respiratory tract infections: 45 mg/kg/day in divided doses every 12 hours **or** 40 mg/kg/day in divided doses every 8 hours

Subacute bacterial endocarditis prophylaxis: 50 mg/kg 1 hour before procedure

Anthrax exposure (unlabeled use): **Note:** Postexposure prophylaxis only with documented susceptible organisms:

<40 kg: 15 mg/kg every 8 hours

≥40 kg: 500 mg every 8 hours

Adults: Dosing range: 250-500 mg every 8 hours or 500-875 mg twice daily; maximum dose: 2-3 g/day

Ear, nose, throat, genitourinary tract or skin/skin structure infections:

Mild to moderate: 500 mg every 12 hours **or** 250 mg every 8 hours

Severe: 875 mg every 12 hours **or** 500 mg every 8 hours

Lower respiratory tract infections: 875 mg every 12 hours **or** 500 mg every 8 hours

Endocarditis prophylaxis: 2 g 1 hour before procedure

Helicobacter pylori eradication: 1000 mg twice daily; requires combination therapy with at least one other antibiotic and an acid-suppressing agent (proton pump inhibitor or H_2 blocker)

Anthrax exposure (unlabeled use): **Note:** Postexposure prophylaxis only with documented susceptible organisms: 500 mg every 8 hours

Dosing interval in renal impairment: The 875 mg tablet should not be used in patients with Cl_{cr} <30 mL/minute.

Cl_{cr} 10-30 mL/minute: 250-500 mg every 12 hours

Cl_{cr} <10 mL/minute: 250-500 mg every 24 hours

Dialysis: Moderately dialyzable (20% to 50%) by hemo- or peritoneal dialysis; approximately 50 mg of amoxicillin per liter of filtrate is removed by continuous arteriovenous or venovenous hemofiltration; dose as per Cl_{cr} <10 mL/minute guidelines

Monitoring Parameters With prolonged therapy, monitor renal, hepatic, and hematologic function periodically; assess patient at beginning and throughout therapy for infection; monitor for signs of anaphylaxis during first dose

Administration Administer around-the-clock to promote less variation in peak and trough serum levels. The appropriate amount of suspension may be mixed with formula, milk, fruit juice, water, ginger ale or cold drinks; administer dose immediately after mixing.

DisperMox™: Dissolve 1 tablet in ~10 mL of water immediately before administration. Rinse container with additional water and drink entire contents to ensure that complete dose is taken. Do not chew or swallow tablet whole.

Contraindications Hypersensitivity to amoxicillin, penicillin, or any component of the formulation

Warnings In patients with renal impairment, doses and/or frequency of administration should be modified in response to the degree of renal impairment. A high percentage of patients with infectious mononucleosis have developed rash during therapy with amoxicillin. A low incidence of cross-allergy with other beta-lactams and cephalosporins exists.

Dosage Forms

[DSC] = Discontinued product

Capsule, as trihydrate: 250 mg, 500 mg

Amoxil®: 500 mg

Trimox®: 250 mg, 500 mg [DSC]

Powder for oral suspension, as trihydrate: 125 mg/5 mL (80 mL, 100 mL, 150 mL); 200 mg/5 mL (50 mL, 75 mL, 100 mL); 250 mg/5 mL (80 mL, 100 mL, 150 mL); 400 mg/5 mL (50 mL, 75 mL, 100 mL)

Amoxil®: 200 mg/5 mL (5 mL, 50 mL, 75 mL, 100 mL) [contains sodium benzoate; bubble gum flavor]; 250 mg/5 mL (100 mL, 150 mL) [contains sodium benzoate; bubble gum flavor]; 400 mg/5 mL (5 mL, 50 mL, 75 mL, 100 mL) [contains sodium benzoate; bubble gum flavor]

Trimox®: 125 mg/5 mL (80 mL, 100 mL, 150 mL); 250 mg/5 mL (80 mL, 100 mL, 150 mL) [contains sodium benzoate; raspberry-strawberry flavor] [DSC]

Powder for oral suspension, as trihydrate [drops]:

Amoxil®: 50 mg/mL (30 mL) [contains sodium benzoate; bubble gum flavor]

Tablet, as trihydrate: 500 mg, 875 mg

Amoxil®: 500 mg, 875 mg

Tablet, chewable, as trihydrate: 125 mg, 200 mg, 250 mg, 400 mg

Amoxil®: 200 mg [contains phenylalanine 1.82 mg/tablet; cherry banana peppermint flavor]; 400 mg [contains phenylalanine 3.64 mg/tablet; cherry banana peppermint flavor]

Tablet, for oral suspension, as trihydrate:

DisperMox™: 200 mg [contains phenylalanine 5.6 mg; strawberry flavor]; 400 mg [contains phenylalanine 5.6 mg; strawberry flavor]; 600 mg [contains phenylalanine 11.23 mg; strawberry flavor] [DSC]

Reference Range After a 250 mg oral dose, peak plasma level of 5 mcg/mL and urine level >300 mcg/mL have been noted

Overdosage/Treatment

Decontamination: Emesis within 30 minutes or lavage within 1 hour (rarely necessary)/activated charcoal can be used

Supportive therapy: Allergic reactions can be treated with epinephrine, diphenhydramine, and corticosteroids. For treatment of lingua villosa nigra, discontinue causative agent. Clean the tongue with a toothbrush and rinse mouth with a half-strength solution of hydrogen peroxide or 10% carbamide peroxide. Symptoms should subside in a few days.

Enhancement of elimination: Hemodialysis or charcoal hemoperfusion can be useful in removing penicillin

Test Interactions Increases AST, ALT, protein

Drug Interactions

Allopurinol: Theoretically has an additive potential for amoxicillin rash.

Aminoglycosides: May be synergistic against selected organisms.

Methotrexate: Penicillins may increase the exposure to methotrexate during concurrent therapy; monitor.

Oral contraceptives: Anecdotal reports suggesting decreased contraceptive efficacy with penicillins have been refuted by more rigorous scientific and clinical data.

Probenecid, disulfiram: May increase levels of penicillins (amoxicillin).

Warfarin: Effects of warfarin may be increased.

Pregnancy Risk Factor B

Lactation Enters breast milk/compatible

Nursing Implications Assess patient at beginning and throughout therapy for infection; give around-the-clock rather than 3 times/day to promote less variation in peak and trough serum levels.

Additional Information

Food does not interfere with absorption; rash appearing after a few days of therapy may indicate hypersensitivity

Amoxil® chewable contains phenylalanine 1.82 mg per 200 mg tablet, phenylalanine 3.64 mg per 400 mg tablet. DisperMox™ contains phenylalanine 5.6 mg in each 200 mg and 400 mg tablet.

Amphotericin B

Pronunciation (am foe TER i sin bee con VEN sha nal)

CAS Number 1397-89-3

U.S. Brand Names Amphocin®; Fungizone®

Synonyms Amphotericin B Desoxycholate

Use Treatment of severe systemic infections and meningitis caused by susceptible fungi; fungal peritonitis; irrigant for bladder fungal infections; topically for cutaneous and mucocutaneous candidal infections

Unlabeled/Investigational Use Visceral leishmaniasis

Mechanism of Action Binds to ergosterol altering cell membrane permeability in susceptible fungi and causing leakage of cell components with subsequent cell death

Adverse Reactions

Cardiovascular: Hypotension, hypertension, cardiac arrest, tachycardia, dilated cardiomyopathy, flushing, myocarditis (hypersensitivity), fibrillation (atrial), flutter (atrial), sinus bradycardia, cardiomegaly, myocardial depression, myocarditis, sinus tachycardia

Central nervous system: **Fever, generalized pain, chills, headache, malaise**, delirium, seizures, psychosis, dysphoria, dizziness, parkinsonian symptoms, hyperthermia, hemiparesis, arachnoiditis, gustatory hallucinations, hypothermia, leukoencephalopathy

Dermatologic: Maculopapular rash, exanthema, exfoliative dermatitis, urticaria, purpura, pruritus

Endocrine & metabolic: **Hypokalemia, hypomagnesemia**, nephrogenic diabetes insipidus

Gastrointestinal: **Anorexia**, nausea, vomiting

Genitourinary: Urinary retention

Hematologic: **Anemia**, leukocytosis, coagulation defects, thrombocytopenia, agranulocytosis, leukopenia, bone marrow suppression

Hepatic: Acute liver failure

Local: Thrombophlebitis

Neuromuscular & skeletal: Myalgia, paresthesia, clonus, myoclonus, pain along lumbar nerves, rhabdomyolysis

Ocular: Vision changes, diplopia

Otic: Hearing loss

Renal: Acidosis (renal tubular), renal failure, **nephrotoxicity** (cortical ischemia), anuria, renal tubular acidosis type I

Respiratory: Dyspnea

Miscellaneous: Anaphylaxis

Signs and Symptoms of Overdose Anemia, anorexia, coagulopathy, congestive heart failure, encephalopathy, deafness, delirium, dysphoria, feces discoloration (black), fever, granulocytopenia, hematuria, hyperthyroidism, hypokalemia, hypomagnesemia, meningitis, myalgia, myoclonus, nausea, renal dysfunction, thrombocytopenia, tubular necrosis, vomiting

Pharmacodynamics/Kinetics

Distribution: Minimal amounts enter the aqueous humor, bile, CSF (inflamed or noninflamed meninges), amniotic fluid, pericardial fluid, pleural fluid, and synovial fluid

Protein binding, plasma: 90%

Half-life elimination: Biphasic: Initial: 15-48 hours; Terminal: 15 days

Time to peak: Within 1 hour following a 4- to 6-hour dose

Excretion: Urine (2% to 5% as biologically active form); ~40% eliminated over a 7-day period and may be detected in urine for at least 7 weeks after discontinued use

Dosage

The minimum dilution for amphotericin B infusions is 0.1 mg/mL for peripheral lines and 1 mg/mL for central lines

Infants and Children:

Test dose: I.V.: 0.1 mg/kg/dose to a maximum of 1 mg; infuse over 30-60 minutes. If the test dose is tolerated, the initial therapeutic dose is 0.25 mg/kg. The daily dose can then be gradually increased, usually in 0.25 mg/kg increments on each subsequent day until the desired daily dose is reached.

Maintenance dose: 0.25-1 mg/kg/day given once daily; infuse over 2-6 hours. Once therapy has been established, amphotericin B can be administered on an every other day basis at 1-1.5 mg/kg/dose.

I.T.: 25-100 mcg every 48-72 hours; increase to 500 mcg as tolerated

Adults: I.V.:

Test dose: 1 mg infused over 20-30 minutes. Institute therapy with 0.25 mg/kg administered over 2-6 hours; the daily dose can be gradually increased on subsequent days to the desired level

Maintenance dose: 0.25-1 mg/kg/day or 1.5 mg/kg every other day; do not exceed 1.5 mg/kg/day. If the test dose is tolerated, the initial therapeutic dose is 0.25 mg/kg. The daily dose can then be gradually increased, usually in 0.25 mg/kg increments on each subsequent day until the desired daily dose is reached.

Duration of therapy varies with nature of infection: Histoplasmosis, *Cryptococcus*, or blastomycosis may be treated with total dose of 2-4 g

I.T.: 25-300 mcg every 48-72 hours; increase to 500 mcg to 1 mg as tolerated

Children and Adults (doses up to 8 mg/kg in infants did not experience any permanent sequelae)

Bladder irrigation: 50 mg/day in 1 L of sterile water irrigation solution instilled over 24 hours for 2-7 days or until cultures are clear

Dialysate: 1-2 mg/L of peritoneal dialysis fluid either with or without low-dose I.V. amphotericin B (a total dose of 2-10 mg/kg given over 7-14 days)

Topical: Apply to affected areas 2-4 times/day for 1-4 weeks of therapy depending on nature and severity of infection

Visceral leishmaniasis unresponsive to antimony (investigational): 5-15 mg/kg/day for 5 days (in lipid complex)

Dosing adjustment in renal impairment: If renal dysfunction is due to the drug, the daily total can be decreased by 50% or the dose can be given every other day; I.V. therapy may take several months

Monitoring Parameters

Renal function (monitor frequently during therapy), electrolytes (especially potassium and magnesium), liver function tests, temperature, PT/PTT, CBC; monitor input and output; monitor for signs of hypokalemia (muscle weakness, cramping, drowsiness, ECG changes, etc)

Administration

Amphotericin is administered by I.V. infusion over 2-6 hours at a final concentration not to exceed 0.1 mg/mL. In patients unable to tolerate a large fluid volume, amphotericin B 0.25 mg/mL in D_5W given through a central venous catheter is the highest concentration reported to have been administered.

Contraindications Hypersensitivity to amphotericin or any component of the formulation

Warnings Anaphylaxis has been reported with other amphotericin B-containing drugs. During the initial dosing, the drug should be administered under close clinical observation. Avoid use with other nephrotoxic drugs; drug-induced renal toxicity usually improves with interrupting therapy, decreasing dosage, or increasing dosing interval. Infusion reactions are most common 1-3 hours after starting the infusion and diminish with continued therapy. Use amphotericin B with caution in patients with decreased renal function. Pulmonary reactions may occur in neutropenic patients receiving leukocyte transfusions; separation of the infusions as much as possible is advised.

Dosage Forms Injection, powder for reconstitution, as desoxycholate: 50 mg

Reference Range Therapeutic: 1.0-2.0 mcg/mL (SI: 1.0-2.2 μmol/L)

Overdosage/Treatment

Supportive therapy: Premedication with hydrocortisone, diphenhydramine, or nonsteroidal anti-inflammatory agents can decrease chills; phosphate buffer or heparin can be added to amphotericin B infusions to decrease thrombophlebitis; simultaneous use of mannitol (1 g/kg) or sodium supplements may decrease renal failure incidence; meperidine (50-75 mg) may be used to prevent or treat chills; coadministration of amiloride (5 mg twice daily) can decrease incidence of hypokalemia

Enhancement of elimination: Exchange transfusion has been used with limited success in infants; no significant effect on amphotericin B plasma levels on double exchange transfusion and thus this modality is not recommended; poorly dialyzed

Test Interactions ↑ BUN (S); ↓ magnesium, potassium (S), erythropoietin levels

Drug Interactions Increased nephrotoxicity: Aminoglycosides, cyclosporine, other nephrotoxic drugs.

Potentiation of hypokalemia: Corticosteroids, corticotropin.

Increased digitalis and neuromuscular-blocking agent toxicity due to hypokalemia.

Decreased effect: Pharmacologic antagonism may occur with azole antifungal agents (eg, miconazole, ketoconazole).

Pulmonary toxicity has occurred with concomitant administration of amphotericin B and leukocyte transfusions.

Pregnancy Risk Factor B

Lactation Excretion in breast milk unknown/contraindicated

Nursing Implications May premedicate patients with acetaminophen and diphenhydramine 30 minutes prior to the amphotericin infusion; meperidine (Demerol®) may help to reduce rigors

Additional Information Premedication with diphenhydramine and acetaminophen may reduce the severity of acute infusion-related reactions. Meperidine reduces the duration of amphotericin B-induced rigors and chilling. Hydrocortisone may be used in patients with severe or refractory infusion-related reactions. Bolus infusion of normal saline immediately preceding, or immediately preceding and following amphotericin B may reduce drug-induced nephrotoxicity. Risk of nephrotoxicity increases with amphotericin B doses >1 mg/kg/day. Infusion of admixtures more concentrated than 0.25 mg/mL should be limited to patients absolutely requiring volume restriction. Amphotericin B does not have a bacteriostatic constituent, subsequently admixture expiration is determined by sterility more than chemical stability.

Specific References

Burke D, Lal R, Finkel KW, et al, "Acute Amphotericin B Overdose," *Ann Pharmacotherapy*, 2006, 40(12):2254-2259.

Ampicillin

Pronunciation (am pi SIL in)

CAS Number 69-53-4

U.S. Brand Names Principen®

Synonyms Aminobenzylpenicillin; Ampicillin Sodium; Ampicillin Trihydrate

Use Treatment of susceptible bacterial infections (nonbeta-lactamase-producing organisms); susceptible bacterial infections caused by streptococci, pneumococci, nonpenicillinase-producing staphylococci, *Listeria*, meningococci; some strains of *H. influenzae*, *Salmonella*, *Shigella*, *E. coli*, *Enterobacter*, and *Klebsiella*

Mechanism of Action Interferes with bacterial cell wall synthesis during active multiplication, causing cell wall death and resultant bactericidal activity against susceptible bacteria

Adverse Reactions

Frequency not defined.

Central nervous system: Fever, penicillin encephalopathy, seizures

Dermatologic: Erythema multiforme, exfoliative dermatitis, rash, urticaria

Note: Appearance of a rash should be carefully evaluated to differentiate (if possible) nonallergic ampicillin rash from hypersensitivity reaction. Incidence is higher in patients with viral infections, *Salmonella* infections, lymphocytic leukemia, or patients that have hyperuricemia.

Gastrointestinal: Black hairy tongue, diarrhea, enterocolitis, glossitis, nausea, pseudomembranous colitis, sore mouth or tongue, stomatitis, vomiting

Hematologic: Agranulocytosis, anemia, hemolytic anemia, eosinophilia, leukopenia, thrombocytopenia purpura

Hepatic: AST increased

Renal: Interstitial nephritis (rare)

Respiratory: Laryngeal stridor

Miscellaneous: Anaphylaxis, serum sickness-like reaction

Signs and Symptoms of Overdose
Cholestatic jaundice, colitis, deafness, erythema multiforme, hypokalemia hypoprothrombinemia, myalgia, myocarditis, toxic epidermal necrolysis

Pharmacodynamics/Kinetics

Absorption: Oral: 50%

Distribution: Bile, blister, and tissue fluids; penetration into CSF occurs with inflamed meninges only, good only with inflammation (exceeds usual MICs)

Normal meninges: Nil; Inflamed meninges: 5% to 10%

Protein binding: 15% to 25%

Half-life elimination:

Children and Adults: 1-1.8 hours

Anuria/end-stage renal disease: 7-20 hours

Time to peak: Oral: Within 1-2 hours

Excretion: Urine (~90% as unchanged drug) within 24 hours

Dosage

Infants and Children:

Mild-to-moderate infections:

I.M., I.V.: 100-150 mg/kg/day in divided doses every 6 hours (maximum: 2-4 g/day)

Oral: 50-100 mg/kg/day in doses divided every 6 hours (maximum: 2-4 g/day)

Severe infections/meningitis: I.M., I.V.: 200-400 mg/kg/day in divided doses every 6 hours (maximum: 6-12 g/day)

Endocarditis prophylaxis: I.M., I.V.:

Dental, oral, respiratory tract, or esophageal procedures: 50 mg/kg within 30 minutes prior to procedure in patients unable to take oral amoxicillin

Genitourinary and gastrointestinal tract (except esophageal) procedures:

High-risk patients: 50 mg/kg (maximum: 2 g) within 30 minutes prior to procedure, followed by ampicillin 25 mg/kg (or amoxicillin 25 mg/kg orally) 6 hours later; must be used in combination with gentamicin.

Moderate-risk patients: 50 mg/kg within 30 minutes prior to procedure

Adults:

Susceptible infections:

Oral: 250-500 mg every 6 hours

I.M., I.V.: 250-500 mg every 6 hours

Sepsis/meningitis: I.M., I.V.: 150-250 mg/kg/24 hours divided every 3-4 hours (range: 6-12 g/day)

Endocarditis prophylaxis: I.M., I.V.:

Dental, oral, respiratory tract, or esophageal procedures: 2 g within 30 minutes prior to procedure in patients unable to take oral amoxicillin

Genitourinary and gastrointestinal tract (except esophageal) procedures:

High-risk patients: 2 g within 30 minutes prior to procedure, followed by ampicillin 1 g (or amoxicillin 1 g orally) 6 hours later; must be used in combination with gentamicin

Moderate-risk patients: 2 g within 30 minutes prior to procedure

Dosing interval in renal impairment:

Cl_{cr} >50 mL/minute: Administer every 6 hours

Cl_{cr} 10-50 mL/minute: Administer every 6-12 hours

Cl_{cr} <10 mL/minute: Administer every 12-24 hours

Hemodialysis: Moderately dialyzable (20% to 50%); administer dose after dialysis

Peritoneal dialysis: Moderately dialyzable (20% to 50%)

Administer 250 mg every 12 hours

Continuous arteriovenous or venovenous hemofiltration effects: Dose as for Cl_{cr} 10-50 mL/minute; ~50 mg of ampicillin per liter of filtrate is removed

Monitoring Parameters
With prolonged therapy monitor renal, hepatic, and hematologic function periodically; observe signs and symptoms of anaphylaxis during first dose

Administration
Ampicillin can be administered IVP over 3-5 minutes at a rate not to exceed 100 mg/minute or I.V. intermittent infusion over 15-30 minutes; final concentration for I.V. administration should not exceed 100 mg/mL (IVP) or 30 mg/mL (I.V. intermittent infusion)

Contraindications
Hypersensitivity to ampicillin, any component of the formulation, or other penicillins

Warnings
Dosage adjustment may be necessary in patients with renal impairment. A low incidence of cross-allergy with other beta-lactams exists. High percentage of patients with infectious mononucleosis have developed rash during therapy with ampicillin. Appearance of a rash should be carefully evaluated to differentiate a nonallergic ampicillin rash from a hypersensitivity reaction. Ampicillin rash occurs in 5% to 10% of children receiving ampicillin and is a generalized dull red, maculopapular rash, generally appearing 3-14 days after the start of therapy. It normally begins on the trunk and spreads over most of the body. It may be most intense at pressure areas, elbows, and knees.

Dosage Forms
Capsule: 250 mg, 500 mg

Injection, powder for reconstitution, as sodium: 125 mg, 250 mg, 500 mg, 1 g, 2 g, 10 g

Powder for oral suspension: 125 mg/5 mL (100 mL, 200 mL); 250 mg/5 mL (100 mL, 200 mL)

Overdosage/Treatment

Decontamination: Emesis within 30 minutes or lavage within 1 hour (rarely necessary)/activated charcoal can be used; whole bowel irrigation is effective in decreasing bioavailability by 67%

Supportive therapy: Allergic reactions can be treated with epinephrine, diphenhydramine, and corticosteroids

Enhancement of elimination: Hemodialysis or charcoal hemoperfusion can be useful in removing penicillin; moderately dialyzable (20% to 50%)

Test Interactions
Increases protein, urinary glucose (Benedict's solution, Clinitest®); positive Coombs' [direct]

Drug Interactions
Allopurinol: Theoretically has an additive potential for ampicillin/amoxicillin rash.

Aminoglycosides: May be synergistic against selected organisms.

Methotrexate: Penicillins may increase the exposure to methotrexate during concurrent therapy; monitor.

Oral contraceptives: Anecdotal reports suggesting decreased contraceptive efficacy with penicillins have been refuted by more rigorous scientific and clinical data.

Probenecid, disulfiram: May increase levels of penicillins (ampicillin).

Warfarin: Effects of warfarin may be increased.

Pregnancy Risk Factor
B

Pregnancy Implications
Teratogenic effects were not observed in animal studies. Ampicillin crosses the human placenta.

Lactation
Enters breast milk/use caution

Nursing Implications
Ampicillin and gentamicin should not be mixed in the same I.V. tubing or administered concurrently; give orally on an empty stomach (ie, 1 hour prior to, or 2 hours after meals) to increase total absorption. Give around-the-clock rather than 4 times/day to promote less variation in peak and trough serum levels.

Additional Information
Sodium content of 5 mL suspension (250 mg/5 mL): 10 mg (0.4 mEq); sodium content of 1 g: 66.7 mg (3 mEq)

Specific References

Köklü S, Köksal A, Asil M, et al, "Probable Sulbactam/Ampicillin-Associated Prolonged Cholestasis," *Ann Pharmacother*, 2004, 38(12): 2055-8.

Köklü S, Yüksel O, Filik L, et al, "Recurrent Cholestasis Due to Ampicillin," *Ann Pharmacother*, 2003, 37(3):395-7.

Amsacrine

Pronunciation (AM sah kreen)

Synonyms 4-(9-Acridinylamino)Methanesulfon-m-Anisidide; Acridinyl Anisidide; AMSA; m-AMSA; NSC-249992

Unlabeled/Investigational Use Investigational: Refractory acute lymphocytic and nonlymphocytic leukemias, Hodgkin's disease, and non-Hodgkin's lymphomas; head and neck tumors

Mechanism of Action Amsacrine has been shown to inhibit DNA synthesis by binding to, and intercalating with, DNA and inhibition of topoisomerase II activity.

Adverse Reactions

Cardiovascular: **ECG changes** (T-wave flattening, S-T wave alterations) consistent with anterolateral ischemia, ventricular fibrillation, ventricular extrasystoles, atrial tachycardia and fibrillation, congestive heart failure, cardiac arrest. Patients with hypokalemia, who have received >400 mg/m^2 of doxorubicin or daunorubicin (or the equivalent), >200 mg/m^2 of amsacrine within 48 hours, or a total dose of anthracycline + amsacrine >900 mg/m^2 have an increased risk of cardiac toxicity.

Central nervous system: Headache, dizziness, confusion, convulsions

Dermatologic: **Alopecia**

Endocrine & metabolic: Sperm production decreased

Gastrointestinal: **Nausea and vomiting (30%), diarrhea (30%), dose-limiting stomatitis (32%), oral ulceration**
Genitourinary: **Orange-red discoloration of the urine**
Hematologic: **Leukopenia** (nadir at 10 days); **thrombocytopenia** (nadir at 12-14 days), with recovery at 21-25 days, anemia
Hepatic: **Hyperbilirubinemia (30%), increased liver enzymes**
Local: **Phlebitis**
Neuromuscular & skeletal: Paresthesias
Ocular: Blurred vision
Miscellaneous: Allergic reactions

Pharmacodynamics/Kinetics
Distribution: V_d: 1.67 L/kg; minimal CNS penetration
Protein binding: 96% to 98%
Metabolism: Hepatic, to inactive metabolites (major metabolite is 5′ glutathione conjugate)
Half-life elimination: 1.4-5 hours; Terminal: 5.6-7.8 hours
Excretion: Bile; urine (2% to 10% as unchanged drug)

Dosage
Refer to individual protocols. I.V.:
Children: 125-150 mg/m²/day for 5 days
Adults: 60-160 mg/m²/day every 3-4 weeks; 5- to 7-day I.V. infusions of 40-120 mg/m²/day every 3-4 weeks have also been reported.
Dosage adjustment in renal impairment: BUN >20 or S_{cr} >1.5: Administer 25% of normal dose.
Dosage adjustment in hepatic impairment: Bilirubin >2 mg/dL: Administer 75% of normal dose.

Stability
Intact vials are stored at controlled room temperature 15°C to 30°C (59°F to 86°F). Reconstitute 1.5 mL of solution by adding 13.5 mL of lactic acid diluent (provided with the drug) to form a 5 mg/mL solution. Solutions diluted for administration are stable for up to 48 hours at room temperature. The addition of 1 mEq/L of sodium bicarbonate increases the stability to 96 hours. Reconstituted vials may be stored at room temperature for up to 48 hours.
Note: Use of glass syringes and avoidance of plastic filters to draw up undiluted amsacrine solutions is recommended since the N,N-dimethylacetamide solvent has been reported to dissolve plastic syringes and filters.

Administration
I.V.: Administer as a 30- to 90-minute infusion or a 24-hour continuous infusion. Use of glass syringes and avoidance of plastic filters to draw up undiluted amsacrine solutions is recommended since the N,N-dimethylacetamide solvent has been reported to dissolve plastic syringes and filters. The solution can be placed in plastic bags when diluted for I.V. infusion.

Contraindications Hypersensitivity to amsacrine or any component of the formulation; hypokalemia

Warnings Procedures for proper handling and disposal of antineoplastic agents should be considered. The drug should be used cautiously in patients who have underlying cardiac disease, severe renal or hepatic dysfunction, or who have received high cumulative doses of anthracyclines. **Do not administer amsacrine if serum potassium <4 mEq/L.**

Dosage Forms Injection, solution [preservative free]: 50 mg/1.5 mL (supplied with L-lactic acid 0.0353 M 13.5 mL)

Androstenedione

Related Information
• Testosterone

Synonyms Andro

Use Often used for performance enhancement in sports; also has been used for libido enhancement (neither use FDA approved)

Mechanism of Action Androstenedione is a weak androgenic steroid hormone. It is a product of natural gonadal and adrenal synthesis. As a precursor to testosterone; converted in the body to testosterone. Testosterone regulates the development and function of the reproductive organs, enhances development of muscle and bone mass, and increases muscular strength. Androstenedione is believed to facilitate faster recovery from exercise and to promote muscle development in response to training.

Mechanism of Toxic Action A precursor to testosterone (and estrone); elevates serum testosterone from 15% to 300%

Adverse Reactions
Central nervous system: Euphoria, cerebrovascular accident, psychosis, aggressive behavior
Dermatologic: **Edema, acne**, pruritus, exacerbation of psoriasis, hirsutism (increase in pubic hair growth)
Endocrine & metabolic: Gynecomastia, **amenorrhea**, hypercalcemia, increased libido, **virilism, breast soreness**, hypoprolactinemia
Gastrointestinal: GI irritation, nausea, vomiting
Genitourinary: Impotence, testicular atrophy, clitoral enlargement, **priapism**, azoospermia, prostatic hypertrophy, prostatic carcinoma, **epididymitis, bladder irritability**
Hematologic: Polycythemia, leukopenia

Hepatic: Hepatic dysfunction, hepatic necrosis (especially with water-based oral preparations), cholestatic hepatitis, hepatocellular carcinoma, aminotransferase level elevation (asymptomatic)
Neuromuscular & skeletal: Piloerection
Miscellaneous: Hypersensitivity reactions

Signs and Symptoms of Overdose Cholestatic jaundice, depression, gynecomastia, hirsutism, hypercalcemia, hypertension, hypertrichosis, impotence, jaundice, leukopenia or neutropenia (agranulocytosis, granulocytopenia), oligospermia

Toxicodynamics/Kinetics Duration of action: 1-2 hours

Dosage Forms Androstenedione (androstene, adriol), 4-androstenediol (4-AD, androdiol), 5-androstenediol (5-AD, 5-androdiol), norandrostenediol (norandrostene), 19-norandrostenedione (19-nordione), 19-nor-androstenediol (19-nordiol)

Reference Range
Male: 65-270 ng/dL; female, postmenopausal: <180 ng/dL; children, prepubertal: <60 ng/dL
While doses of 100 mg daily did not change serum testosterone or estradiol concentrations, doses of 300 mg daily did cause a significant increase in the above hormones

Overdosage/Treatment Decontamination: Oral: Ipecac within 30 minutes or lavage (within 1 hour)/activated charcoal

Additional Information First synthesized in 1935. Has both androgenic and anabolic properties. Available as tablet: 50 mg, 100 mg.

Specific References
Reilly CA and Crouch DJ, "Analysis of the Nutritional Supplement 1AD, Its Metabolites, and Related Endogenous Hormones in Biological Matrices Using Liquid Chromatography-Tandem Mass Spectrometry," *J Anal Toxicol*, 2004, 28(1):1-10.
Tseng YL, Kuo F-H, and Sun K-H, "Quantification and Profiling of 19-Norandrosterone and 19-Noretiocholanolone in Human Urine After Consumption of a Nutritional Supplement and Norsteroids," *J Anal Toxicol*, 2005, 29:124-34.

Aprotinin

Pronunciation (a proe TYE nin)
CAS Number 9087-70-1
U.S. Brand Names Trasylol®
Use Treatment of life-threatening hemorrhage caused by increased plasmin concentration; prophylactic use to reduce perioperative blood loss in patients undergoing cardiopulmonary bypass in repeat coronary artery bypass graft surgery; may be effective against streptokinase-induced bleeding

Mechanism of Action Serine protease inhibitor; inhibits plasmin, kallikrein, and platelet activation; a weak inhibitor of plasma pseudocholinesterase

Adverse Reactions Increase in postoperative renal dysfunction compared to placebo; anaphylactic reactions have been reported in of cases; such reactions are more likely to occur with repeated administration; bronchospasm and acute respiratory distress syndrome can result

Signs and Symptoms of Overdose Possible liver/tubular necrosis (acute) at a dose of 15 million KIU

Pharmacodynamics/Kinetics
Distribution: Extracellular space; renal phagolysomes
Metabolism: Aprotinin is slowly degraded by lysosomal enzymes.
Half-life elimination: 2.5 hours (plasma); terminal: 10 hours
Excretion: Urine (25% to 40%; <10% as unchanged drug)

Dosage
Test dose: **All** patients should receive a 1 mL I.V. test dose at least 10 minutes prior to the loading dose to assess the potential for allergic reactions
Regimen A:
2 million units (280 mg) loading dose I.V. over 20-30 minutes
2 million units (280 mg) into pump prime volume
500,000 units/hour (70 mg/hour) I.V. during operation
Regimen B:
1 million units (140 mg) loading dose I.V. over 20-30 minutes
1 million units (140 mg) into pump prime volume
250,000 units/hour (35 mg/hour) I.V. during operation

Stability Incompatible with corticosteroids, heparin, tetracyclines

Monitoring Parameters Bleeding times, prothrombin time, activated clotting time, platelet count, red blood cell counts, hematocrit, hemoglobin and fibrinogen degradation products; for toxicity also include renal function tests and blood pressure

Administration
Administer through a central line. Infuse loading dose over 20-30 minutes, then continuous infusion at 50 mL/hour (regimen A) or 25 mL/hour (regimen B). Rapid infusion (<20 minutes) can cause transient blood pressure decrease; to avoid incompatibility with heparin, add while recirculating the prime fluid of the cardiac bypass circuit.

Contraindications Hypersensitivity to aprotinin or any component of the formulation

Warnings [U.S. Boxed Warning]: Anaphylactic reactions are possible. Hypersensitivity reactions are more common with repeated use, especially when re-exposure is within 6 months. All patients should receive a test dose at least 10 minutes before loading dose. Patients with a history of allergic reactions to drugs or other agents may be more likely to develop a reaction. Epinephrine, steroids, and facilities for cardiopulmonary resuscitation should be available in case such a reaction occurs. Patients with a previous exposure to aprotinin (particularly when re-exposure is within 6 months) are at an increased risk for hypersensitivity reactions including anaphylactic or anaphylactoid reactions; pretreatment with an antihistamine and H_2 blocker before administration of the loading dose is recommended in these patients; delay the addition of aprotinin into the pump prime solution until the loading dose has been safely administered. Safety and efficacy in children have not been established.

Dosage Forms Injection, solution: 1.4 mg/mL [10,000 KIU/mL] (100 mL, 200 mL) [bovine derived]

Reference Range Plasma concentration of 250 KIU/mL in patients after receiving 2 million KIU I.V. loading dose

Overdosage/Treatment Supportive therapy: Bronchospasm can be treated with beta agonist therapy; anaphylaxis can be treated with epinephrine, antihistamines, and corticosteroids

Drug Interactions Captopril (and other ACE inhibitors): Antihypertensive effects may be blocked; monitor.
Fibrinolytic drugs may have poorer activity. Aprotinin blocks this fibrinolytic activity; monitor.

Pregnancy Risk Factor B

Pregnancy Implications Teratogenic effects were not observed in animal studies. There are no adequate and well-controlled studies in pregnant women.

Lactation Excretion in breast milk unknown

Arginine

Pronunciation (AR ji neen)
CAS Number 1119-34-2; 74-79-3
U.S. Brand Names R-Gene®
Synonyms Arginine Hydrochloride

Use Pituitary function test (growth hormone). Also used in treating ammonia intoxication in patients with cirrhosis.

Unlabeled/Investigational Use Management of severe, uncompensated, metabolic alkalosis (pH $\geq$7.55) **after** optimizing therapy with sodium and potassium supplements

Mechanism of Action Causes release of growth hormone, insulin, glucagon, and prolactin. Also has acidifying properties.

Adverse Reactions
Cardiovascular: Rapid I.V. infusion may produce flushing
Central nervous system: Headache
Endocrine & metabolic: Hyperkalemia
Gastrointestinal: Nausea, vomiting
Local: Venous irritation
Neuromuscular & skeletal: Numbness
Miscellaneous: Allergic reactions

Signs and Symptoms of Overdose Hyponatremia, hypotension due to vasodilation, hyperkalemia, increased intracranial pressure, metabolic acidosis, nausea, vomiting

Admission Criteria/Prognosis Admit ingestions over 30 g

Pharmacodynamics/Kinetics
Absorption: Oral: Well absorbed
Time to peak, serum: Oral: ~2 hours; I.V.: 20-30 minutes

Toxicodynamics/Kinetics
Duration of action: ~1 hour
Metabolism: Hepatic hydrolytic cleavage to urea and ornithine
Elimination: Renal

Dosage
I.V.: Pituitary function test:
Children: 500 mg kg/dose administered over 30 minutes
Adults: 30 g (300 mL of a 10% solution) administered over 30 minutes
Ammonia intoxication in cirrhotics: 37.5-100 g (4 doses in 10 days) followed by 50 g/day for 5 days
Metabolic alkalosis: Dose in grams = desired decrease in serum bicarbonate level (mEq/L) times patient weight (kg), divided by 9.6.
Acidifying agent: 10 g infused over 30 minutes
Oral: Oligospermia: 2-4 g/day

Monitoring Parameters Monitor acid-base status (arterial or capillary blood gases), serum electrolytes (sodium, potassium, chloride, HCO_3^-), BUN, glucose

Administration
May be infused without further dilution; maximum rate of I.V. infusion: 1 g/kg/hour (maximum: 60 g/hour).

Contraindications Hypersensitivity to arginine or any component of the formulation

Warnings Use caution with hepatic or renal impairment; use may lead to life-threatening hyperkalemia. Use caution with electrolyte imbalances or pediatric patients.

Dosage Forms Injection, solution, as hydrochloride: 10% [100 mg/mL = 950 mOsm/L] (300 mL) [contains chloride 0.475 mEq/mL]

Reference Range Normal serum arginine level: 40-150 nmol/mL; fatal arginine (plasma) level: 1314 nmol/mL following a 3.9 g/kg infusion

Overdosage/Treatment Supportive therapy: Epinephrine and antihistamines can be used for allergic reactions. Monitor and treat electrolyte disturbances.

Test Interactions May ↑ increase BUN and serum creatinine

Drug Interactions Increased toxicity: Estrogen-progesterone combinations (increase growth hormone response and decrease glucagon and insulin effects); spironolactone (potentially fatal hyperkalemia has been reported)

Pregnancy Risk Factor C

Pregnancy Implications Teratogenic effects were not observed in animal studies; however, the manufacturer does not recommend use of arginine during pregnancy.

Lactation Enters breast milk/use caution

Additional Information Chloride content of arginine is 47.5 mEq/100 mL (950 mOsmol/L); fatal I.V. dose: 3.9 g/kg

Aripiprazole

Pronunciation (ay ri PIP ray zole)
U.S. Brand Names Abilify®
Synonyms BMS 337039; OPC-14597

Use Treatment of schizophrenia; stabilization and maintenance therapy of bipolar disorder (with acute manic or mixed episodes)

Unlabeled/Investigational Use Depression with psychotic features

Mechanism of Action Aripiprazole is a quinolinone antipsychotic which exhibits high affinity for D_2, D_3, 5-HT$_{1A}$, and 5-HT$_{2A}$ receptors; moderate affinity for D_4, 5-HT$_{2C}$, 5-HT$_7$, alpha, and H_1 receptors. It also possesses moderate affinity for the serotonin reuptake transporter; has no affinity for muscarinic receptors. Aripiprazole functions as a partial agonist at the D_2 and 5-HT$_{1A}$ receptors, and as an antagonist at the 5-HT$_{2A}$ receptor.

Adverse Reactions
>10%:
Central nervous system: Headache (31%), agitation (25%), anxiety (20%), insomnia (20%), somnolence (12%), akathisia (15%). lightheadedness (11%)
Endocrine & metabolic: Weight gain (8% to 30%; highest frequency in patients with BMI <23), pancreatitis
Gastrointestinal: Nausea (16%), dyspepsia (15%), constipation (13%), vomiting (11%)
1% to 10%:
Cardiovascular: Edema (peripheral 2%), hypertension (2%), tachycardia, hypotension, bradycardia, chest pain
Central nervous system: Extrapyramidal symptoms (6%), fever, depression, nervousness, mania, confusion, hallucination, hostility, paranoid reaction, suicidal thought, delusion, abnormal dream
Dermatologic: Rash (6%), dry skin, skin ulcer
Endocrine & metabolic: Dehydration, hypothyroidism
Gastrointestinal: Salivation increased (3%), anorexia
Genitourinary: Urinary incontinence, pelvic pain
Hematologic: Anemia, bruising
Neuromuscular & skeletal: Weakness (8%), myalgia (4%), tremor (4%), neck pain, neck rigidity, muscle cramp, CPK increased, abnormal gait
Ocular: Blurred vision (3%), conjunctivitis
Respiratory: Rhinitis (4%), pharyngitis (4%), asthma, cough (3%), dyspnea, pneumonia, sinusitis
Miscellaneous: Accidental injury (6%), flu-like syndrome
<1% (Limited to important or life-threatening): Albuminuria, alkaline phosphatase increased, ALT increased, angina, apnea, arthralgia, arthrosis, aspiration pneumonia, AST increased, ataxia, atrial fibrillation, atrial flutter, AV block, bilirubinemia, bone pain, bradykinesia, BUN increased, bundle branch block, cardiomegaly, cardiopulmonary failure, cataract, cerebral ischemia, cerebrovascular accident, CHF, chest tightness, cholecystitis, cholelithiasis, colitis, cyanosis, cystitis, deafness, deep vein thrombosis, delirium, diabetes mellitus, duodenal ulcer, eosinophilia, extrasystoles, fecal impaction, hematemesis, hematuria, hemoptysis, hemorrhage, hepatitis, hepatomegaly, hypercholesterolemia, hyper-/hypoglycemia, hyper-/hypokalemia, hyper-/hyponatremia, hyperthyroidism, hyperuricemia, hypoesthesia, hypokinesia, hypotonia, hypoxia, intestinal obstruction, intestinal perforation, LDH increased, leukocytosis, leukopenia, maculopapular rash, Mendelson's syndrome, MI, migraine, moniliasis, myoclonus, myopathy, neuroleptic malignant syndrome, melena, neuropathy, oculogyric crisis, palpitation, pancreatitis, panic attack, peptic ulcer, phlebitis, pulmonary edema, pulmonary embolism, QT prolongation, renal calculus, renal failure, respiratory failure, rhabdomyolysis, seborrhea, serum creatinine increased, stroke, suicide attempt, tardive dyskinesia, throat tightness, thrombocythemia, thrombocytopenia, tongue edema, vesiculobullous rash
Postmarketing and/or case reports: Anaphylactic reaction, angioedema, laryngospasm

Signs and Symptoms of Overdose Lethargy, vomiting, salivation, hypotonia, coma (at ingestion of 17.1 mg/kg), ataxia, tremor

Admission Criteria/Prognosis Six-hour observation time is appropriate; asymptomatic patients can then be discharged

Pharmacodynamics/Kinetics
Onset: Initial: 1-3 weeks
Absorption: Well absorbed
Distribution: V_d: 4.9 L/kg
Protein binding: 99%, primarily to albumin
Metabolism: Hepatic, via CYP2D6, CYP3A4 (dehydro-aripiprazole metabolite has affinity for D2 receptors similar to the parent drug and represents 40% of the parent drug exposure in plasma)
Bioavailability: 87%
Half-life: Aripiprazole: 75 hours; CYP2D6 poor metabolizers: 146 hours; dehydro-aripiprazole: 94 hours
Time to peak, plasma: 3-5 hours
Delayed with high-fat meal: Aripiprazole: 3 hours; dehydro-aripiprazole: 12 hours
Excretion: Feces (55%), urine (25%); primarily as metabolites

Dosage
Oral: **Note:** Oral solution may be substituted for the oral tablet on a mg-per-mg basis, up to 25 mg. Patients receiving 30 mg tablets should be given 25 mg oral solution.
Adults:
Schizophrenia: 10-15 mg once daily; may be increased to a maximum of 30 mg once daily (efficacy at dosages above 10-15 mg has not been shown to be increased). Dosage titration should not be more frequent than every 2 weeks.
Bipolar disorder (acute manic or mixed episodes):
Stabilization: 30 mg once daily; may require a decrease to 15 mg based on tolerability (15% of patients had dose decreased); safety of doses >30 mg/day has not been evaluated
Maintenance: Continue stabilization dose for up to 6 weeks; efficacy of continued treatment >6 weeks has not been established
Dosage adjustment with concurrent CYP3A4 inducer therapy: with the addition of CYP3A4 inducers (eg, carbamazepine), aripiprazole dose should be doubled. If CYP3A4 inducers are withdrawn from therapy with aripiprazole, aripiprazole dose should be decreased by one-half.
Elderly: Refer to Adults dosing
Dosage adjustment in renal/hepatic impairment: No dosage adjustment required

Stability
Capsule: Store under refrigeration of 2°C to 8°C (36°F to 46°F); use within 6 months after opening
Tablet: Store at 25°C (77°F); excursions permitted to 15°C to 30°C (59°F to 86°F)

Monitoring Parameters Vital signs; fasting lipid profile and fasting blood glucose/Hgb A_{1c} (prior to treatment, at 3 months, then annually); BMI, personal/family history of diabetes, waist circumference; blood pressure; mental status, abnormal involuntary movement scale (AIMS), extrapyramidal symptoms (EPS). Weight should be assessed prior to treatment, at 4 weeks, 8 weeks, 12 weeks, and then at quarterly intervals. Consider titrating to a different antipsychotic agent for a weight gain ≥5% of the initial weight.

Administration
May be administered with or without food. Tablet and oral solution may be interchanged on a mg-per-mg basis, up to 25 mg. Doses using 30 mg tablets should be exchanged for 25 mg oral solution.

Contraindications Hypersensitivity to aripiprazole or any component of the formulation

Warnings
[U.S. Boxed Warning]: Patients with dementia-related behavioral disorders treated with atypical antipsychotics are at an increased risk of death compared to placebo. Aripiprazole is not approved for this indication.
May cause extrapyramidal symptoms, including pseudoparkinsonism, acute dystonic reactions, akathisia, and tardive dyskinesia (risk of these reactions is very low relative to typical/conventional antipsychotics, frequencies reported are similar to placebo). May be associated with neuroleptic malignant syndrome (NMS).
May be sedating, use with caution in disorders where CNS depression is a feature. May cause orthostatic hypotension (although reported rates are similar to placebo); use caution in patients at risk of this effect or those who would not tolerate transient hypotensive episodes (cerebrovascular disease, cardiovascular disease, or other medications which may predispose). Clinical data have demonstrated an increased incidence of serious, including fatal, cerebrovascular events in elderly patients.
Use caution in patients with Parkinson's disease; hemodynamic instability; bone marrow suppression; predisposition to seizures; subcortical brain damage; and severe cardiac, hepatic, renal, or respiratory disease. Esophageal dysmotility and aspiration have been associated with antipsychotic use; use caution in patients at risk of pneumonia (ie, Alzheimer's disease). May alter temperature regulation or mask toxicity

of other drugs due to antiemetic effects. Use caution in patients with a history of drug abuse.
Atypical antipsychotics have been associated with development of hyperglycemia; in some cases, may be extreme and associated with ketoacidosis, hyperosmolar coma, or death. Reports of hyperglycemia with aripiprazole therapy have been few and specific risk associated with this agent is not known. Use caution in patients with diabetes or other disorders of glucose regulation; monitor for worsening of glucose control.
The possibility of a suicide attempt is inherent in psychotic illness or bipolar disorder; use caution in high-risk patients during initiation of therapy. Prescriptions should be written for the smallest quantity consistent with good patient care. Safety and efficacy in pediatric patients have not been established.

Dosage Forms
Solution, oral: 1 mg/mL (150 mL) [contains sucrose 400 mg/mL and fructose 200 mg/mL; orange cream flavor]
Tablet: 2 mg, 5 mg, 10 mg, 15 mg, 20 mg, 30 mg

Reference Range
Following ingestion of 17.1 mg/kg, serum levels of aripiprazole and dehydroaripiprazole was 1420 ng/mL and 453 ng/mL, respectively
Mean peak plasma concentrations range from 74-452 ng/mL for 5-30 mg doses, respectively

Overdosage/Treatment
Decontamination: Activated charcoal and/or lavage
Supportive therapy: Mainstay of treatment

Drug Interactions
Substrate (major) of CYP2D6, 3A4
Acetylcholinesterase inhibitors (central): May increase the risk of antipsychotic-related extrapyramidal symptoms; monitor.
Carbamazepine: Carbamazepine may decrease aripiprazole levels. Manufacturer recommends a doubling of the aripiprazole dose when carbamazepine is added.
CYP2D6 inhibitors: May increase the levels/effects of aripiprazole. Example inhibitors include chlorpromazine, delavirdine, fluoxetine, miconazole, paroxetine, pergolide, quinidine, quinine, ritonavir, and ropinirole.
CYP3A4 inducers: CYP3A4 inducers may decrease the levels/effects of aripiprazole. Example inducers include aminoglutethimide, carbamazepine, nafcillin, nevirapine, phenobarbital, phenytoin, and rifamycins.
CYP3A4 inhibitors: May increase the levels/effects of aripiprazole. Example inhibitors include azole antifungals, clarithromycin, diclofenac, doxycycline, erythromycin, imatinib, isoniazid, nefazodone, nicardipine, propofol, protease inhibitors, quinidine, telithromycin, and verapamil.
Ketoconazole: Ketoconazole may increase aripiprazole levels. Manufacturer recommends a 50% reduction in dose during concurrent ketoconazole therapy.

Pregnancy Risk Factor C
Pregnancy Implications Aripiprazole demonstrated developmental toxicity in animal models. There are no adequate and well-controlled trials in pregnant women. Should be used in pregnancy only when potential benefit to mother outweighs possible risk to the fetus.
Lactation Excretion in breast milk unknown/not recommended
Specific References
Babu KM, Ganetsky M, Liang IE, et al, "Pancreatitis and Diabetic Ketoacidosis Associated with Aripiprazole Therapy," *Clin Toxicol*, 2005, 43:642.
Lackey GD, Alsop JA, and Albertson TE, "Aripiprazole: A 24-Motnh Review of Acute Overdoses in Adults," *Clin Toxicol*, 2005, 43:641.
Lackey GD, Alsop JA, and Albertson TE, "A Two-Year Review of Pediatric Aripiprazole Ingestions," *Clin Toxicol*, 2005, 43:642.
Levine M, Traub S, and Burns MJ, "The Pharmacology and Toxicology of Aripiprazole," *Int J Med Toxicol*, 2004, 7(1):5.
Lofton AL and Klein-Schwartz W, "Atypical Experience: A Case Series of Pediatric Aripiprazole Exposures," *Clin Toxicol (Phila)*, 2005, 43(3):151-3.
Lovecchio F, Watts D, and Winchell J, "One-Year Experience with Aripiprazole Exposures," *Am J Emerg Med*, 2005, 23(4):585-6.
Seifert SA, Schwartz MD, and Thomas JD, "Aripiprazole (Abilify) Overdose in a Child," *Clin Toxicol (Phila)*, 2005, 43(3):193-5.

Ascorbic Acid

CAS Number 50-81-7
U.S. Brand Names C-500-GR™ [OTC]; C-Gram [OTC]; Cecon® [OTC]; Cevi-Bid® [OTC]; Dull-C® [OTC]; Vita-C® [OTC]
Synonyms Vitamin C
Use Prevention and treatment of scurvy; urinary acidification; dietary supplementation; chromium nephrotoxicity/dermal burns due to chromium
Unlabeled/Investigational Use Investigational: In large doses, to decrease the severity of "colds"; dietary supplementation; a 20-year study was recently completed involving 730 individuals which indicates a

possible decreased risk of death by stroke when ascorbic acid at doses ≥45 mg/day was administered

Mechanism of Action Necessary for collagen formation and tissue repair in the body; involved in some oxidation-reduction reactions, as well as many other metabolisms

Adverse Reactions

Cardiovascular: Flushing, chest pain, angina

Central nervous system: Faintness, dizziness, headache, fatigue

Dermatologic: Systemic contact dermatitis

Gastrointestinal: Nausea, vomiting, heartburn, diarrhea, esophageal ulceration, esophagitis

Renal: Hyperoxaluria

Signs and Symptoms of Overdose Dental erosion, esophageal ulceration, hematuria, intestinal bezoar or concretion, renal insufficiency, nephropathy, nephrotoxicity

Pharmacodynamics/Kinetics

Absorption: Oral: Readily absorbed; an active process thought to be dose dependent

Distribution: Large

Metabolism: Hepatic via oxidation and sulfation

Excretion: Urine (with high blood levels)

Dosage

Oral, I.M., I.V., SubQ:

Children:

Scurvy: 100-300 mg/day in divided doses for at least 2 weeks

Urinary acidification: 500 mg every 6-8 hours

Dietary supplement: 35-45 mg

Adults:

Scurvy: 100-250 mg 1-2 times/day

Urinary acidification: 4-12 g/day in 3-4 divided doses

Dietary supplement: 50-60 mg/day

Prevention and treatment of cold: 1-3 g/day

Recommended daily allowance: 60 mg

Antioxidant: I.V.: 0.5-1 g

Severe chromium poisoning: I.V.: 1 g every 10-20 minutes, up to 3 g

Chromium dermal burns: 10% topical ascorbic acid along with 10 g of oral ascorbic acid

Stability Injectable form should be stored under refrigeration (2°C to 8°C); protect oral dosage forms from light; is rapidly oxidized when in solution in air and alkaline media

Monitoring Parameters Monitor pH of urine when using as an acidifying agent

Administration

Avoid rapid I.V. injection.

Warnings Patients with diabetes and patients prone to recurrent renal calculi (eg, dialysis patients) should not take excessive doses for extended periods of time.

Dosage Forms

Capsule: 500 mg, 1000 mg

C-500-GR™: 500 mg

Capsule, timed release: 500 mg

Crystal (Vita-C®): 4 g/teaspoonful (100 g)

Injection, solution: 250 mg/mL (2 mL, 30 mL); 500 mg/mL (50 mL)

Cenolate®: 500 mg/mL (1 mL, 2 mL) [contains sodium hydrosulfite]

Powder, solution (Dull-C®): 4 g/teaspoonful (100 g, 500 g)

Solution, oral (Cecon®): 90 mg/mL (50 mL)

Tablet: 100 mg, 250 mg, 500 mg, 1000 mg

C-Gram: 1000 mg

Tablet, chewable: 100 mg, 250 mg, 500 mg [some products may contain aspartame]

Tablet, timed release: 500 mg, 1000 mg, 1500 mg

Cevi-Bid®: 500 mg

Reference Range Normal serum level: 10 mcg/mL

Overdosage/Treatment Decontamination: Lavage (within 1 hour)/activated charcoal; dilution with milk or water may minimize chances of esophageal injury

Test Interactions False-positive urinary glucose with cupric sulfate reagent, false-negative urinary glucose with glucose oxidase method; false-negative stool occult blood 48-72 hours after ascorbic acid ingestion; Hemoccult® and Gastroccult® tests can be unreliable in detecting GI bleeding in iron overdoses treated with whole bowel irrigation (ferrous sulfate/ferrous gluconate: false-positive; ascorbic acid: false-negative); may cause a false elevation of serum creatinine through interference with laboratory determination

Drug Interactions

Decreased effect:

Aspirin (decreases ascorbate levels, increases aspirin)

Fluphenazine (decreases fluphenazine levels)

Warfarin (decreased effect)

Increased effect:

Iron (absorption enhanced)

Oral contraceptives (increased contraceptive effect)

Pregnancy Risk Factor A/C (dose exceeding RDA recommendation)

Lactation Enters breast milk/compatible

Nursing Implications Avoid rapid I.V. injection

Additional Information Sodium content of 1 g: ~5 mEq; >715 mg/day may result in slower progression of HIV illness (RR=0.55). Single doses of 40 g I.V. or chronic ingestions >2 g daily can result in renal toxicity.

Specific References

Cohen HA, Varsano I, Kahan E, et al, "Effectiveness of an Herbal Preparation Containing Echinacea, Propolis, and Vitamin C in Preventing Respiratory Tract Infections in Children: A Randomized, Double-Blind, Placebo-Controlled, Multicenter Study," *Arch Pediatr Adolesc Med*, 2004, 158(3):217-21.

Hajjar IM, George V, Sasse EA, et al, "A Randomized, Double-Blind, Controlled Trial of Vitamin C in the Management of Hypertension and Lipids," *Am J Ther*, 2002, 9(4):289-93.

Pimentel L, "Scurvy: Historical Review and Current Diagnostic Approach," *Am J Emerg Med*, 2003, 21(4):328-32.

Atenolol

Pronunciation (a TEN oh lole)

Related Information

• Selected Properties of Beta-Adrenergic Blocking Drugs

CAS Number 29122-68-7; 60966-51-0

U.S. Brand Names Tenormin®

Use Treatment of hypertension, alone or in combination with other agents; management of angina pectoris, postmyocardial infarction patients

Unlabeled/Investigational Use Acute ethanol withdrawal, supraventricular and ventricular arrhythmias, and migraine headache prophylaxis

Mechanism of Action Competitively blocks response to beta-adrenergic stimulation; more hydrophilic than propranolol; not lipid soluble

Adverse Reactions

Cardiovascular: Persistent bradycardia, hypotension, chest pain, edema, heart failure, AV block, exacerbation of Raynaud's phenomenon, sinus bradycardia, myocardial depression, QRS prolongation, vasculitis

Central nervous system: Dizziness, fatigue, insomnia, drowsiness, confusion, psychosis, CNS depression, headache, night terrors, memory impairment, paranoia

Dermatologic: Exacerbation of vitiligo, erythema multiforme, alopecia, toxic epidermal necrolysis, xerosis, urticaria, purpura, onycholysis, photosensitivity, pruritus; exanthema, licheniform eruptions, cutaneous vasculitis

Endocrine & metabolic: Sexual dysfunction, hyperprolactinemia

Gastrointestinal: Constipation, abdominal pain, diarrhea, nausea,

Genitourinary: Impotence, retroperitoneal fibrosis

Hepatic: Cholestasis

Respiratory: Dyspnea has occurred when daily dosage exceeds 100 mg/day, wheezing

Miscellaneous: Cold extremities, systemic lupus erythematosus

Signs and Symptoms of Overdose Ataxia, AV block, bradycardia, congestive heart failure, depression, dermatitis, dry eyes, dry mouth, hypoglycemia, hypotension, hypothermia, impotence, insomnia, night terrors, wheezing

Pharmacodynamics/Kinetics

Onset of action: Peak effect: Oral: 2-4 hours

Duration: Normal renal function: 12-24 hours

Absorption: Incomplete

Distribution: Low lipophilicity; does not cross blood-brain barrier

Protein binding: 3% to 15%

Metabolism: Limited hepatic

Half-life elimination: Beta:

Neonates: ≤35 hours; Mean: 16 hours

Children: 4.6 hours; children >10 years may have longer half-life (>5 hours) compared to children 5-10 years (<5 hours)

Adults: Normal renal function: 6-9 hours, prolonged with renal impairment; End-stage renal disease: 15-35 hours

Excretion: Feces (50%); urine (40% as unchanged drug)

Dosage

Oral:

Children: 1-2 mg/kg/dose given daily

Adults:

Hypertension: 25-50 mg once daily, may increase to 100 mg/day; doses >100 mg are unlikely to produce any further benefit

Angina pectoris: 50 mg once daily, may increase to 100 mg/day; some patients may require 200 mg/day

Postmyocardial infarction: Follow I.V. dose with 100 mg/day or 50 mg twice daily for 6-9 days postmyocardial infarction

I.V.: Postmyocardial infarction: Early treatment: 5 mg slow I.V. over 5 minutes; may repeat in 10 minutes; if both doses are tolerated, may start oral atenolol 50 mg every 12 hours or 100 mg/day for 6-9 days postmyocardial infarction

Dosing interval for oral atenolol in renal impairment:

Cl_cr 15-35 mL/minute: Administer 50 mg/day maximum

Cl_cr <15 mL/minute: Administer 50 mg every other day maximum

Hemodialysis: Moderately dialyzable (20% to 50%) via hemodialysis; administer dose postdialysis or administer 25-50 mg supplemental dose

Peritoneal dialysis: Elimination is not enhanced; supplemental dose is not necessary

Monitoring Parameters Acute cardiac treatment: Monitor ECG and blood pressure with I.V. administration; heart rate and blood pressure with oral administration

Administration

When administered acutely for cardiac treatment, monitor ECG and blood pressure. The injection can be administered undiluted or diluted with a compatible I.V. solution. May administer by rapid infusion (I.V. push) at a rate of 1 mg/minute or by slow infusion over ~30 minutes. Necessary monitoring for surgical patients who are unable to take oral beta-blockers (prolonged ileus) has not been defined. Some institutions require monitoring of baseline and postinfusion heart rate and blood pressure when a patient's response to beta-blockade has not been characterized (ie, the patient's initial dose or following a change in dose). Consult individual institutional policies and procedures.

Contraindications Hypersensitivity to atenolol or any component of the formulation; sinus bradycardia; sinus node dysfunction; heart block greater than first-degree (except in patients with a functioning artificial pacemaker); cardiogenic shock; uncompensated cardiac failure; pulmonary edema; pregnancy

Warnings Safety and efficacy in children have not been established. Administer cautiously in compensated heart failure and monitor for a worsening of the condition (efficacy of atenolol in heart failure has not been established). **[U.S. Boxed Warning]: Beta-blocker therapy should not be withdrawn abruptly (particularly in patients with CAD), but gradually tapered to avoid acute tachycardia, hypertension, and/or ischemia.** Use caution with concurrent use of beta-blockers and either verapamil or diltiazem; bradycardia or heart block can occur. Avoid concurrent I.V. use of both agents. Beta-blockers should be avoided in patients with bronchospastic disease (asthma). Atenolol, with B1 selectivity, has been used cautiously in bronchospastic disease with close monitoring. Use cautiously in peripheral arterial disease, especially if severe disease is present. Use cautiously in patients with diabetes - may mask hypoglycemic symptoms. May mask signs of thyrotoxicosis. May cause fetal harm when administered in pregnancy. Use cautiously in the renally impaired (dosage adjustment required). Use care with anesthetic agents which decrease myocardial function. Caution in myasthenia gravis.

Dosage Forms Injection, solution: 0.5 mg/mL (10 mL)
Tablet: 25 mg, 50 mg, 100 mg

Reference Range Peak plasma level of 1-2 mcg/mL 2-4 hours after 200 mg dose. Highest survivable atenolol (serum) level: 35 mcg/mL

Overdosage/Treatment

Decontamination: **Do not** use ipecac; lavage (within 1 hour)/activated charcoal is useful

Supportive therapy: Sympathomimetics (eg, epinephrine or dopamine), glucagon, atropine, or a pacemaker can be used to treat the toxic bradycardia, asystole, and/or hypotension. Initially, fluids may be the best treatment for toxic hypotension, with norepinephrine being used for refractory hypotension. Calcium chloride can be used to treat electromechanical dissociation caused by atenolol overdose.

Enhancement of elimination: Multiple dosing of activated charcoal may be useful; hemodialysis may be of some benefit (moderately dialyzable 20% to 50%); hemodialysis clearance: ~29-39 mL/minute (45% of drug can be fractionally removed during 4 hours of hemodialysis)

Test Interactions ↑ triglycerides, potassium, uric acid, cholesterol (S), glucose; ↓ HDL

Drug Interactions

Alpha-blockers (prazosin, terazosin): Concurrent use of beta-blockers may increase risk of orthostasis.

Ampicillin, in single doses of 1 gram, decreases atenolol's pharmacologic actions.

Antacids (magnesium-aluminum, calcium antacids or salts) may reduce the bioavailability of atenolol.

Clonidine: Hypertensive crisis after or during withdrawal of either agent.

Drugs which slow AV conduction (digoxin): Effects may be additive with beta-blockers.

Glucagon: Atenolol may blunt the hyperglycemic action of glucagon.

Insulin and oral hypoglycemics: Atenolol masks the tachycardia that usually accompanies hypoglycemia.

NSAIDs (ibuprofen, indomethacin, naproxen, piroxicam) may reduce the antihypertensive effects of beta-blockers.

Salicylates may reduce the antihypertensive effects of beta-blockers.

Sulfonylureas: Beta-blockers may alter response to hypoglycemic agents.

Verapamil or diltiazem may have synergistic or additive pharmacological effects when taken concurrently with beta-blockers.

Pregnancy Risk Factor D

Pregnancy Implications Atenolol crosses the placenta; beta-blockers have been associated with persistent bradycardia, hypotension, and IUGR; IUGR is probably related to maternal hypertension. Available evidence suggests beta-blockers are generally safe during pregnancy (JNC-7). Cases of neonatal hypoglycemia have been reported following maternal use of beta-blockers at parturition or during breast-feeding.

Lactation Enters breast milk/use caution

Nursing Implications Patient's therapeutic response may be evaluated by looking at blood pressure, apical and radial pulses, fluid I & O, daily weight, respirations, and circulation in extremities before and during therapy; modify dosage in patients with renal insufficiency

Additional Information Most effective for treating hypertension in older, white patients

Specific References

Chobanian AV, Bakris GL, Black HR, et al, "The Seventh Report of the Joint National Committee on Prevention, Detection, Evaluation, and Treatment of High Blood Pressure: The JNC 7 Report," *JAMA*, 2003, (19)289:2560-71.

Dupuis C, Gaulier JM, Pelissier-Alicot AL, et al, "Determination of Three Beta-blockers in Biofluids and Solid Tissues by Liquid Chromatography-Electrospray-Mass Spectrometry," *J Anal Toxicol*, 2004, 28(8):674-9.

Johnson RD and Lewis RJ, "Simultaneous Quantitation of Atenolol, Metoprolol, and Propranolol in Biological Matrices via LC-MS," *J Anal Toxicol*, 2006, 30:129.

Kelleher JA, "Atenolol-Induced Breast Pain in a Woman with Hypertension," *Ann Pharmacother*, 2006, 40(5):990-2.

Wax PM, Erdman AR, Chyka PA, et al, "Beta-Blocker Ingestion: An Evidence-Based Consensus Guideline for Out-of-Hospital Management," *Clin Toxicol (Phila)*, 2005, 43(3):131-46.

Atomoxetine

Pronunciation (AT oh mox e teen)

CAS Number 82248-59-7; 83015-26-3

U.S. Brand Names Strattera™

Synonyms Atomoxetine Hydrochloride; LY139603; Methylphenoxy-Benzene Propanamine; Tomoxetine

Use Treatment of attention deficit/hyperactivity disorder (ADHD)

Unlabeled/Investigational Use Treatment of depression

Mechanism of Action Selectively inhibits the reuptake of norepinephrine (Ki 4.5nM) with little to no activity at the other neuronal reuptake pumps or receptor sites. No anticholinergic effects.

Adverse Reactions

Percentages as reported in children and adults; some adverse reactions may be increased in "poor metabolizers" (CYP2D6).

Cardiovascular: Palpitations, tachycardia, systolic blood pressure increased, orthostatic hypotension

Central nervous system: **Headache**, fatigue/lethargy, irritability, somnolence, dizziness, mood swings, abnormal dreams, paresthesia, sleep disturbance, pyrexia, rigors, crying

Dermatologic: Dermatitis, rash, urticaria, angioedema

Endocrine & metabolic: Dysmenorrhea, libido decreased, menstruation disturbance, orgasm abnormal, weight loss

Gastrointestinal: **Xerostomia (4% to 21%), abdominal pain, insomnia, vomiting, anorexia, nausea**, dyspepsia, diarrhea, flatulence, constipation

Genitourinary: Erectile disturbance, ejaculatory disturbance, prostatitis, impotence

Neuromuscular & skeletal: Paresthesia, myalgia

Renal: Urinary retention/hesitation

Respiratory: **Cough**, rhinorrhea, sinus headache

Miscellaneous: Diaphoresis increased, sinusitis, ear infection, influenza, allergy

Hepatic: Hepatitis

Signs and Symptoms of Overdose Anorexia, dyspepsia, abdominal pain, rhabdomyolysis, tachycardia, agitation, hypertension, lethargy

Pharmacodynamics/Kinetics

Absorption: Rapid

Distribution: V$_d$: I.V.: 0.85 L/kg

Protein binding: 98%, primarily albumin

Metabolism: Hepatic, via CYP2D6 and CYP2C19; forms metabolites (4-hydroxyatomoxetine, active, equipotent to atomoxetine; N-desmethylatomoxetine in poor metabolizers, limited activity)

Bioavailability: 63% in extensive metabolizers; 94% in poor metabolizers

Half-life elimination: Atomoxetine: 5 hours (up to 24 hours in poor metabolizers); Active metabolites: 4-hydroxyatomoxetine: 6-8 hours; N-desmethylatomoxetine: 6-8 hours (34-40 hours in poor metabolizers)

Time to peak, plasma: 1-2 hours

Excretion: Urine (80%, as conjugated 4-hydroxy metabolite); feces (17%)

Dosage

Oral:

Children and Adolescents ≤70 kg: ADHD: Initial: 0.5 mg/kg/day, increase after minimum of 3 days to ~1.2 mg/kg/day; may administer as either a single daily dose or two evenly divided doses in morning and late afternoon/early evening. Maximum daily dose: 1.4 mg/kg or 100 mg, whichever is less. In patients receiving effective CYP2D6 inhibitors (eg, paroxetine, fluoxetine, quinidine), do not exceed 1.2 mg/kg.

Children and Adolescents >70 kg: Refer to Adults dosing

Adults:

ADHD: Initial: 40 mg/day, increased after minimum of 3 days to ~80 mg/day; may administer as either a single daily dose or two evenly divided doses in morning and late afternoon/early evening. May increase to 100 mg in 2-4 additional weeks to achieve optimal response. In patients receiving effective CYP2D6 inhibitors (eg, paroxetine, fluoxetine, quinidine), do not exceed 80 mg/day.

Depression (unlabeled use): 40-65 mg/day

Elderly: Use has not been evaluated in the elderly

Dosage adjustment in renal impairment: No adjustment needed

Dosage adjustment in hepatic impairment:

Moderate hepatic insufficiency (Child-Pugh class B): All doses should be reduced to 50% of normal

Severe hepatic insufficiency (Child-Pugh class C): All doses should be reduced to 25% of normal

Monitoring Parameters

Patient growth (weight/height gain in children); attention, hyperactivity, anxiety, worsening of aggressive behavior or hostility; blood pressure, pulse

Family members and caregivers need to monitor patient daily for emergence of irritability, agitation, unusual changes in behavior, and suicidal ideation. Pediatric patients should be monitored closely for suicidality, clinical worsening, or unusual changes in behavior, especially during the initial for months of therapy or at times of dose changes. Appearance of symptoms needs to be immediately reported to healthcare provider. Weekly office visits from patient or caregiver are necessary for the first 4 weeks, then every other week for the next 4 weeks, then at 12 weeks, and as clinically indicated beyond 12 weeks. Additional contact may be required between office visits.

Administration

May be administered with or without food.

Contraindications Hypersensitivity to atomoxetine or any component of the formulation; use with or within 14 days of MAO inhibitors; narrow-angle glaucoma

Warnings

[U.S. Boxed Warning]: Use caution in pediatric patients; may be an increased risk of suicidal ideation. Closely monitor for clinical worsening, suicidality, or unusual changes in behavior; the child's family or caregiver should be instructed to closely observe the patient and communicate condition with healthcare provider. Patients should be observed for, especially during the initial few months of a course of drug therapy, or at times of dose changes, either increases or decreases. Atomoxetine is not approved for major depressive disorder. Patients presenting with depressive symptoms should be screened for bipolar disorder. A medication guide should be dispensed with each prescription.

Use caution with hepatic (dosage adjustments necessary in hepatic impairment). Use may be associated with rare but severe hepatotoxicity; discontinue and do not restart if signs or symptoms of hepatotoxic reaction (eg, jaundice, pruritus, flu-like symptoms) are noted. Use caution in patients who are poor metabolizers of CYP2D6 metabolized drugs ("poor metabolizers"), bioavailability increases.

May cause increased heart rate or blood pressure; use caution with hypertension or other cardiovascular disease. Use caution with renal impairment. May cause urinary retention/hesitancy; use caution in patients with history of urinary retention or bladder outlet obstruction. Allergic reactions (including angioneurotic edema, urticaria, and rash) may occur.

Growth should be monitored during treatment. Height and weight gain may be reduced during the first 9-12 months of treatment, but should recover by 3 years of therapy. Safety and efficacy have not been evaluated in pediatric patients <6 years of age.

Dosage Forms

Capsule:

Strattera®: 10 mg, 18 mg, 25 mg, 40 mg, 60 mg, 80 mg, 100 mg

Reference Range Peak plasma atomoxetine level ranging from 315-1231 ng/mL noted following single 90 mg oral dose

Overdosage/Treatment

Effects of overdose unknown

Decontamination: Lavage and/or activated charcoal with ingestions exceeding 2 mg/kg

Drug Interactions

Substrate of CYP2C19 (minor), 2D6 (major)

β_2 agonists (albuterol): Atomoxetine may potentiate cardiovascular effects of albuterol.

CNS depressants: May enhance the adverse/toxic effect of atomoxetine.

CYP2D6 inhibitors: May increase the levels/effects of atomoxetine. Example inhibitors include chlorpromazine, delavirdine, fluoxetine, miconazole, paroxetine, pergolide, quinidine, quinine, ritonavir, and ropinirole. Dose adjustment may be needed when coadministered with CYP2D6 inhibitors in patients who are extensive metabolizers of CYP2D6.

Fluoxetine: CYP2D6 inhibitors (strong) may decrease the metabolism of CYP2D6 substrates such as atomoxetine. Manufacturer recommends dosage adjustment.

MAO inhibitors: Therapy with or within 2 weeks of atomoxetine may cause serious toxicity (eg, hyperthermia, rigidity, myoclonus, mental status changes, autonomic instability, NMS). Combined use is contra-indicated.

Paroxetine: May decrease the metabolism, via CYP isoenzymes, of atomoxetine. Manufacturer recommends dosage adjustment.

Quinidine: CYP2D6 inhibitors (strong) may decrease the metabolism of CYP2D6 substrates such as atomoxetine. Manufacturer recommends dosage adjustment.

Sympathomimetics (including epinephrine): Atomoxetine may increase heart rate or blood pressure. Use caution with pressor agents.

Pregnancy Risk Factor C

Pregnancy Implications No adequate and well-controlled studies in pregnant women; use only if potential benefit to the mother outweighs possible risk to fetus.

Lactation Excretion in breast milk unknown/use caution

Specific References

Audi J, Traub S, and Burns MJ, "The Pharmacology and Toxicology of Atomoxetine," *Int J Med Toxicol*, 2004, 7(1):6.

Barker MJ, Benitez JG, Ternullo S, et al, "Acute Oxcarbazepine and Atomoxetine Overdose with Quetiapine," *Vet Hum Toxicol*, 2004, 46(3):130-2.

Blair HW, Coco NP, Borys DJ, et al, "Review of the Clinical Effects Following Atomoxetine Exposure," *J Toxicol Clin Toxicol*, 2004, 42(5):734.

Bond GR, Garro AC, and Gilbert D, "Dyskinesia Associated with Atomoxetine in Combination with Other Psychoactive Drugs," *J Toxicol Clin Toxicol*, 2004, 42(5):731.

Cantrell FL and Nestor M, "Benign Clinical Course Following Atomoxetine Overdose," *Clin Toxicol (Phila)*, 2005, 43(1):57.

Forrester MB, "Adult Atomoxetine Ingestions Reported to Texas Poison Control Centers, 2003-2005," *Annals of Pharmacotherapy*, 2006, 40(12):2136-2141.

Kashani JS and Ruha AM, "Isolated Atomoxetine Overdose Resulting in Seizures," *Clin Toxicol (Phila)*, 2005, 43:733.

Kelleher JA, "Atenolol-Induced Breast Pain in a Woman with Hypertension," *Ann Pharmacother*, 2006, 40(5):990-2.

Lackey GD, Alsop JA, and Albertson TE, "24-Month Retrospective Review of Atomoxetine Ingestions in Children Less Than 6 Years Old," *Clin Toxicol (Phila)*. 2005, 43:653.

Lackey GD, Alsop JA, and Albertson TE, "24-Month Retrospective Study of Adult Atomoxetine Ingestions," *Clin Toxicol (Phila)*. 2005, 43:649.

LoVecchio F and Kashani J, "Isolated Atomoxetine (Strattera™) Ingestion Commonly Result in Toxicity," *J Toxicol Clin Toxicol*, 2004, 42(5):815.

Spiller HA, Lintner CP, and Winter ML, "Atomoxetine Ingestions in Children: A Report from Poison Centers," *Ann Pharmacother*, 2005, 39(6):1045-8.

Spiller HA, Lintner CP, and Winter ML, "Atomoxetine (Strattera®) Exposure in Children," *J Toxicol Clin Toxicol*, 2004, 42(5):720.

Stojanovski SD, Cassavant MS, Moosa HM, et al, "Atomoxetine Induced Hepatitis in a Child," *Clin Toxicol*, 2007, 45:51-5.

Stojanovski SD, Robinson RF, Baker SD, et al, "Children and Adolescent Exposures to Atomoxetine Hydrochloride Reported to a Poison Control Center," *Clin Toxicol*, 2006, 44:243-7.

Atorvastatin

Pronunciation (a TORE va sta tin)

CAS Number 134523-00-5; 134523-03-8

U.S. Brand Names Lipitor®

Use

Treatment of dyslipidemias or primary prevention of cardiovascular disease (atherosclerotic) as detailed below:

Primary prevention of cardiovascular disease (high-risk for CVD): To reduce the risk of MI or stroke in patients without evidence of heart disease who have multiple CVD risk factors or type 2 diabetes. Treatment reduces the risk for angina or revascularization procedures in patients with multiple risk factors.

Treatment of dyslipidemias: To reduce elevations in total cholesterol, LDL-C, apolipoprotein B, and triglycerides in patients with elevations of one or more components, and/or to increase HDL-C as present in Fredrickson type IIa, IIb, III, and IV hyperlipidemias; treatment of primary dysbetalipoproteinemia, homozygous familial hypercholesterolemia

Treatment of heterozygous familial hypercholesterolemia (HeFH) in adolescent patients (10-17 years of age, females >1 year postmenarche) having LDL-C ≥190 mg/dL or LDL ≥160 mg/dL with positive family history of premature cardiovascular disease (CVD) or with two or more CVD risk factors.

Mechanism of Action Inhibitor of 3-hydroxy-3-methylglutaryl coenzyme A (HMG-CoA) reductase, the rate limiting enzyme in cholesterol synthesis (reduces the production of mevalonic acid from HMG-CoA); this then results in a compensatory increase in the expression of LDL receptors on hepatocyte membranes and a stimulation of LDL catabolism

Adverse Reactions

Cardiovascular: Chest pain, peripheral edema, facial edema, edema, palpitations, vasodilation, postural hypotension, arrhythmia, angina, hypertension, syncope

Central nervous system: Headache, insomnia, dizziness, fever, malaise, somnolence, abnormal dreams, emotional lability, incoordination, depression, migraine

Dermatologic: Rash, photosensitivity, cheilitis, pruritus, alopecia, dry skin, urticaria, acne, eczema, seborrhea, skin ulcer, ecchymosis, Stevens-Johnson syndrome, erythema multiforme, petechiae, angioneurotic edema, bullous rashes, toxic epidermal necrolysis

Endocrine & metabolic: Hyperglycemia, gout, hypoglycemia

Gastrointestinal: Abdominal pain, constipation, diarrhea, dyspepsia, flatulence, nausea, gastroenteritis, colitis, vomiting, gastritis, xerostomia, rectal hemorrhage, esophagitis, eructation, glossitis, stomatitis, anorexia, increased appetite, duodenal ulcer, dysphagia, enteritis, melena, gingival hemorrhage, tenesmus, pancreatitis, taste loss, taste perversion, weight gain

Genitourinary: Urinary tract infection, decreased libido, cystitis, impotence, epididymitis, vaginal hemorrhage, dysuria, nocturia, abnormal urination

Hematologic: Anemia, immune thrombocytopenia

Hepatic: Elevated transaminases, hepatitis, cholestatic jaundice, biliary pain

Neuromuscular & skeletal: Arthralgia, myalgia, back pain, arthritis, paresthesia, peripheral neuropathy, torticollis, facial paralysis, hyperkinesia, hypesthesia, hypertonia, leg cramps, bursitis, myasthenia, myositis, tendinous contracture, rhabdomyolysis, myopathy, weakness

Ocular: Amblyopia, glaucoma

Otic: Tinnitus, deafness

Renal: Hematuria, nephritis

Respiratory: Sinusitis, bronchitis, dyspnea, epistaxis, pharyngitis, rhinitis

Miscellaneous: Infection, flu-like syndrome, allergic reaction, phlebitis, anaphylaxis, fibrocystic breast disease, lymphadenopathy

Additional class-related events or case reports (not necessarily reported with atorvastatin therapy): Myopathy, increased CPK ($>10 \times$ normal), rhabdomyolysis, renal failure (secondary to rhabdomyolysis), alteration in taste, impaired extraocular muscle movement, facial paresis, tremor, memory loss, vertigo, paresthesia, peripheral neuropathy, peripheral nerve palsy, anxiety, depression, psychic disturbance, hypersensitivity reaction, angioedema, anaphylaxis, systemic lupus erythematosus-like syndrome, polymyalgia rheumatica, dermatomyositis, vasculitis, purpura, thrombocytopenia, leukopenia, hemolytic anemia, positive ANA, increased ESR, eosinophilia, arthritis, urticaria, photosensitivity, fever, chills, flushing, malaise, dyspnea, rash, toxic epidermal necrolysis, erythema multiforme, Stevens-Johnson syndrome, pancreatitis, hepatitis, cholestatic jaundice, fatty liver, cirrhosis, fulminant hepatic necrosis, hepatoma, anorexia, vomiting, alopecia, nodules, skin discoloration, dryness of skin/mucous membranes, nail changes, gynecomastia, decreased libido, erectile dysfunction, impotence, cataracts, ophthalmoplegia, elevated transaminases, increased alkaline phosphatase, increased GGT, hyperbilirubinemia, thyroid dysfunction

Pharmacodynamics/Kinetics

Onset of action: Initial changes: 3-5 days; Maximal reduction in plasma cholesterol and triglycerides: 2 weeks

Absorption: Rapid

Distribution: V_d: 318 L

Protein binding: $\geq 98\%$

Metabolism: Hepatic; forms active ortho- and parahydroxylated derivates and an inactive beta-oxidation product

Half-life elimination: Parent drug: 14 hours

Time to peak, serum: 1-2 hours

Excretion: Bile; urine (2% as unchanged drug)

Dosage

Oral: **Note:** Doses should be individualized according to the baseline LDL-cholesterol levels, the recommended goal of therapy, and patient response; adjustments should be made at intervals of 2-4 weeks

Children 10-17 years (females >1 year postmenarche): HeFH: 10 mg once daily (maximum: 20 mg/day)

Adults: Hyperlipidemias: Initial: 10-20 mg once daily; patients requiring $>45\%$ reduction in LDL-C may be started at 40 mg once daily; range: 10-80 mg once daily

Primary prevention of CVD: 10 mg once daily

Dosing adjustment in renal impairment: No dosage adjustment is necessary.

Dosing adjustment in hepatic impairment: Do not use in active liver disease.

Monitoring Parameters

Lipid levels after 2-4 weeks; LFTs, CPK

It is recommended that liver function tests (LFTs) be performed prior to and at 12 weeks following both the initiation of therapy and any elevation in dose, and periodically (eg, semiannually) thereafter

Administration

May be administered with food if desired; may take without regard to time of day.

Contraindications

Hypersensitivity to atorvastatin or any component of the formulation; active liver disease; unexplained persistent elevations of serum transaminases; pregnancy

Warnings

Secondary causes of hyperlipidemia should be ruled out prior to therapy. May cause hepatic dysfunction. Use with caution in patients who consume large amounts of ethanol or have a history of liver disease. Monitoring is recommended. Rhabdomyolysis with acute renal failure has occurred. Risk is dose related and is increased with concurrent use of lipid-lowering agents which may cause rhabdomyolysis (gemfibrozil, fibric acid derivatives, or niacin at doses ≥ 1 g/day) or during concurrent use with potent CYP3A4 inhibitors (including amiodarone, clarithromycin, cyclosporine, erythromycin, itraconazole, ketoconazole, nefazodone, grapefruit juice in large quantities, verapamil, or protease inhibitors such as indinavir, nelfinavir, or ritonavir). Weigh the risk versus benefit when combining any of these drugs with atorvastatin. Discontinue in any patient experiencing an acute or serious condition predisposing to renal failure secondary to rhabdomyolysis. Safety and efficacy have not been established in patients <10 years of age or in premenarcheal girls.

Dosage Forms Tablet: 10 mg, 20 mg, 40 mg, 80 mg

Overdosage/Treatment

Decontamination: Consider gastric decontamination for acute ingestions >200 mg; activated charcoal or cholestyramine may be useful

Supportive therapy: Monitor for rhabdomyolysis; adequate hydration with 0.9% NS is appropriate

Drug Interactions

Substrate of CYP3A4 (major); **Inhibits** CYP3A4 (weak)

Antacids: Plasma concentrations may be decreased when given with magnesium-aluminum hydroxide containing antacids (reported with atorvastatin and pravastatin). Clinical efficacy is not altered, no dosage adjustment is necessary.

Bile acid sequestrants (cholestyramine and colestipol): Reduce absorption of several HMG-CoA reductase inhibitors; separate administration times by at least 4 hours. Cholesterol-lowering effects are additive.

Cyclosporine: May increase serum concentrations of atorvastatin, increasing the risk of myopathy; monitor.

CYP3A4 inhibitors: May increase the levels/effects of atorvastatin. Example inhibitors include azole antifungals, clarithromycin, diclofenac, doxycycline, erythromycin, imatinib, isoniazid, nefazodone, nicardipine, propofol, protease inhibitors, quinidine, telithromycin, and verapamil.

Digoxin: Plasma concentrations of digoxin may be increased by ~20%; monitor.

Fibric acid derivatives (clofibrate and fenofibrate): May increase the risk of myopathy and rhabdomyolysis.

Grapefruit juice: May inhibit metabolism of atorvastatin via CYP3A4; more likely to occur with lovastatin or simvastatin; avoid high dietary intake of grapefruit juice.

Niacin: May increase the risk of myopathy and rhabdomyolysis.

Pregnancy Risk Factor X

Pregnancy Implications A case of bone deformity, tracheoesophageal fistula, and anal atresia has been noted in a fetus after first trimester use of lovastatin and dextroamphetamine.

Lactation Enters breast milk/contraindicated

Additional Information Atorvastatin serum concentrations may be increased by grapefruit juice; avoid concurrent intake of large quantities (>1 quart/day). St John's wort may decrease atorvastatin levels.

Specific References

Sipe BE, Jones RJ, and Bokhart GH, "Rhabdomyolysis Causing AV Blockade Due to Possible Atorvastatin, Esomeprazole, and Clarithromycin Interaction," *Ann Pharmacother*, 2003, 37(6):808-11.

Azathioprine

Pronunciation (ay za THYE oh preen)

Related Information

- Mercaptopurine

CAS Number 446-86-6

U.S. Brand Names Azasan®; Imuran®

Synonyms Azathioprine Sodium

Use Adjunct with other agents in prevention of rejection of kidney transplants; also used in severe active rheumatoid arthritis unresponsive to other agents; other autoimmune diseases (ITP, SLE, MS, Crohn's disease)

Unlabeled/Investigational Use Adjunct in prevention of rejection of solid organ (nonrenal) transplants; steroid-sparing agent for corticosteroid-dependent Crohn's disease (CD) and ulcerative colitis (UC); maintenance of remission in CD; fistulizing Crohn's disease

Mechanism of Action Antagonizes purine metabolism and may inhibit synthesis of DNA, RNA, and proteins; may also interfere with cellular metabolism and inhibit mitosis

Adverse Reactions

Central nervous system: Fever, chills

Dermatologic: Alopecia, erythematous or maculopapular rash

Gastrointestinal: Nausea, vomiting, anorexia, diarrhea, aphthous stomatitis, pancreatitis

Hematologic: Leukopenia, thrombocytopenia, anemia, pancytopenia (bone marrow suppression may be determined, in part, by genetic factors, ie, patients with TPMT deficiency are at higher risk)

Hepatic: Hepatotoxicity, jaundice, hepatic veno-occlusive disease

Neuromuscular & skeletal: Arthralgias

Ocular: Retinopathy

Miscellaneous: Rare hypersensitivity reactions (including myalgias, rigors, dyspnea, hypotension, serum sickness, rash); secondary infections may occur secondary to immunosuppression

Signs and Symptoms of Overdose Diarrhea, leukopenia (in 2-3 days), vomiting

Pharmacodynamics/Kinetics

Distribution: Crosses placenta

Protein binding: ~30%

Metabolism: Hepatic, to 6-mercaptopurine (6-MP), possibly by glutathione S-transferase (GST). Further metabolism of 6-MP (in the liver and GI tract), via three major pathways: Hypoxanthine guanine phosphoribosyltransferase (to 6-thioguanine-nucleotides, or 6-TGN), xanthine oxidase (to 6-thiouric acid), and thiopurine methyltransferase (TPMT), which forms 6-methylmercaptopurine (6-MMP).

Half-life elimination: Parent drug: 12 minutes; mercaptopurine: 0.7-3 hours; End-stage renal disease: Slightly prolonged

Time to peak, plasma: 1-2 hours (including metabolites)

Excretion: Urine (primarily as metabolites)

Dosage I.V. dose is equivalent to oral dose

Children and Adults: Renal transplantation: Oral, I.V.: 2-5 mg/kg/day to start, then 1-3 mg/kg/day maintenance

Adults: Rheumatoid arthritis: Oral: 1 mg/kg/day for 6-8 weeks; increase by 0.5 mg/kg every 4 weeks until response or up to 2.5 mg/kg/day

Dosing adjustment in renal impairment:

Cl_{cr} 10-50 mL/minute: Administer 75% of normal dose

Cl_{cr} <10 mL/minute: Administer 50% of normal dose

Administer dose posthemodialysis

CAPD effects: Unknown

CAVH effects: Unknown

Stability Stability of parenteral admixture at room temperature (25°C): 24 hours

Stability of parenteral admixture at refrigeration temperature (4°C): 16 days

Stable in neutral or acid solutions, but is hydrolyzed to mercaptopurine in alkaline solutions

Monitoring Parameters CBC, platelet counts, total bilirubin, alkaline phosphatase

Administration

Can be administered IVP over 5 minutes at a concentration not to exceed 10 mg/mL or azathioprine can be further diluted with normal saline or D_5W and administered by intermittent infusion over 15-60 minutes

Contraindications Hypersensitivity to azathioprine or any component of the formulation; pregnancy

Warnings [U.S. Boxed Warning]: Chronic immunosuppression increases the risk of neoplasia and serious infections. Azathioprine has mutagenic potential to both men and women and with possible hematologic toxicities; hematologic toxicities are dose related and may be more severe with renal transplants undergoing rejection. Gastrointestinal toxicity may occur within the first several weeks of therapy and is reversible. Symptoms may include severe nausea, vomiting, diarrhea, rash, fever, malaise, myalgia, hypotension, and liver enzyme abnormalities. Use with caution in patients with liver disease, renal impairment; monitor hematologic function closely. Patients with genetic deficiency of thiopurine methyltransferase (TPMT) or concurrent therapy with drugs which may inhibit TPMT may be sensitive to myelosuppressive effects. Azathioprine is metabolized to mercaptopurine; concomitant use may result in profound myelosuppression and should be avoided.

Dosage Forms

Injection, powder for reconstitution: 100 mg

Tablet [scored]: 50 mg

Azasan®: 75 mg, 100 mg

Imuran®: 50 mg

Overdosage/Treatment

Decontamination: Ipecac within 30 minutes or lavage within 1 hour; give activated charcoal

Enhanced elimination: Hemodialysis (43% removed during 8 hours) can enhance azathioprine and its metabolites removal

Drug Interactions

ACE inhibitors: Concomitant therapy may induce anemia and severe leukopenia.

Allopurinol: May increase serum levels of azathioprine's active metabolite (mercaptopurine). Decrease azathioprine dose to $^1/_3$ to $^1/_4$ of normal dose.

Aminosalicylates (olsalazine, mesalamine, sulfasalazine): May inhibit TPMT, increasing toxicity/myelosuppression of azathioprine. Use caution.

Mercaptopurine: Azathioprine is metabolized to mercaptopurine; concomitant use may result in profound myelosuppression and should be avoided.

Warfarin: Effect may be decreased by azathioprine.

Pregnancy Risk Factor D

Pregnancy Implications Azathioprine was found to be teratogenic in animal studies; temporary depression in spermatogenesis and reduction in sperm viability and sperm count were also reported in mice. Azathioprine crosses the placenta in humans; congenital anomalies, immunosuppression, and intrauterine growth retardation have been reported. There are no adequate and well-controlled studies in pregnant women. Azathioprine should not be used to treat arthritis during pregnancy. The potential benefit to the mother versus possible risk to the fetus should be considered when treating other disease states.

Lactation Enters breast milk/not recommended

Additional Information Will not cause dermal toxicity if extravasation occurs

Specific References

Li AC, Warnakulasuriya S, and Thompson RP, "Neoplasia of the Tongue in a Patient with Crohn's Disease Treated with Azathioprine: Case Report," *Eur J Gastroenterol Hepatol*, 2003, 15(2):185-7.

Navarro JT, Ribera JM, Mate JL, et al, "Hepatosplenic T-Gammadelta Lymphoma in a Patient with Crohn's Disease Treated with Azathioprine," *Leuk Lymphoma*, 2003, 44(3):531-3.

Moretti ME, Verjee Z, Ito S and Koren G, "Breast-Feeding During Maternal Use of Azathioprine," *Ann of Pharmacotherapy*, 2006, 40(12):2269-72.

Azithromycin

Pronunciation (az ith roe MYE sin)

CAS Number 83905-01-5

U.S. Brand Names Zithromax®

Synonyms Azithromycin Dihydrate; Zithromax® TRI-PAK™; Zithromax® Z-PAK®

Use Treatment of acute otitis media due to *H. influenzae*, *M. catarrhalis*, or *S. pneumoniae*; pharyngitis/tonsillitis due to *S. pyogenes*; treatment of mild to moderate upper and lower respiratory tract infections, infections of the skin and skin structure, community-acquired pneumonia, pelvic inflammatory disease (PID), sexually-transmitted diseases (urethritis/cervicitis), pharyngitis/tonsillitis (alternative to first-line therapy), and genital ulcer disease (chancroid) due to susceptible strains of *C. trachomatis*, *M. catarrhalis*, *H. influenzae*, *S. aureus*, *S. pneumoniae*, *Mycoplasma pneumoniae*, and *C. psittaci*; acute bacterial exacerbations of chronic obstructive pulmonary disease (COPD) due to *H. influenzae*, *M. catarrhalis*, or *S. pneumoniae*; acute bacterial sinusitis

Unlabeled/Investigational Use Prevention of (or to delay onset of) or treatment of MAC in patients with advanced HIV infection; prophylaxis of bacterial endocarditis in patients who are allergic to penicillin and undergoing surgical or dental procedures; pertussis

Mechanism of Action Inhibits RNA-dependent protein synthesis at the chain elongation step; binds to the 50S ribosomal subunit resulting in blockage of transpeptidation

Adverse Reactions

Cardiovascular: Arrhythmias (ventricular)

Central nervous system: Headache, dizziness, fever, hypothermia

Dermatologic: Rash, angioedema, urticaria, photosensitivity, exanthema, cutaneous vasculitis

Endocrine & Metabolic: Inappropriate antidiuretic hormone secretion

Gastrointestinal: Diarrhea, nausea, abdominal pain, vomiting, cramping, hypertrophic pyloric stenosis, feces discoloration (greenish gray, white/speckling)

Hematologic: Eosinophilia

Hepatic: Elevation in hepatic enzymes, cholestatic jaundice

Local: Thrombophlebitis

Neuromuscular & skeletal: Myasthenia gravis, myalgia

Otic: Ototoxicity, tinnitus

Renal: Nephritis

Miscellaneous: Allergic reactions

Pharmacodynamics/Kinetics

Absorption: Rapid

Distribution: Extensive tissue; distributes well into skin, lungs, sputum, tonsils, and cervix; penetration into CSF is poor; I.V.: 33.3 L/kg; Oral: 31.1 L/kg

Protein binding (concentration dependent): 7% to 51%

Metabolism: Hepatic

Bioavailability: 38%, decreased by 17% with extended release suspension; variable effect with food (increased with immediate or delayed release oral suspension, unchanged with tablet)

Half-life elimination: Terminal: Immediate release: 68-72 hours; Extended release: 59 hours

Time to peak, serum: Immediate release: 2-3 hours; Extended release: 5 hours

Excretion: Biliary (major route); urine (6%)

Dosage

Note: Extended release suspension (Zmax™) is not interchangeable with immediate release formulations. Use should be limited to approved indications. All doses are expressed as immediate release azithromycin unless otherwise specified.

Oral:
Children <6 months: Pertussis (CDC guidelines): 10 mg/kg/day for 5 days
Children ≥6 months:
Community-acquired pneumonia, pertussis (CDC guidelines): 10 mg/kg on day 1 (maximum: 500 mg/day) followed by 5 mg/kg/day once daily on days 2-5 (maximum: 250 mg/day)
Bacterial sinusitis: 10 mg/kg once daily for 3 days (maximum: 500 mg/day)
Otitis media:
1-day regimen: 30 mg/kg as a single dose (maximum dose: 1500 mg)
3-day regimen: 10 mg/kg once daily for 3 days (maximum: 500 mg/day)
5-day regimen: 10 mg/kg on day 1 (maximum: 500 mg/day) followed by 5 mg/kg/day once daily on days 2-5 (maximum: 250 mg/day)
Children ≥2 years: Pharyngitis, tonsillitis: 12 mg/kg/day once daily for 5 days (maximum: 500 mg/day)
Children:
M. avium-infected patients with acquired immunodeficiency syndrome (unlabeled use): 5 mg/kg/day once daily (maximum dose: 250 mg/day) or 20 mg/kg (maximum dose: 1200 mg) once weekly given alone or in combination with rifabutin
Treatment and secondary prevention of disseminated MAC (unlabeled use): 5 mg/kg/day once daily (maximum dose: 250 mg/day) in combination with ethambutol, with or without rifabutin
Prophylaxis for bacterial endocarditis (unlabeled use): 15 mg/kg 1 hour before procedure
Uncomplicated chlamydial urethritis or cervicitis (unlabeled use): Children ≥45 kg: 1 g as a single dose
Adolescents ≥16 years and Adults:
Community-acquired pneumonia: Extended release suspension (Zmax™): 2 g as a single dose
Respiratory tract, skin and soft tissue infections, pertussis (CDC guidelines): 500 mg on day 1 followed by 250 mg/day on days 2-5 (maximum: 500 mg/day)
Alternative regimen: Bacterial exacerbation of COPD: 500 mg/day for a total of 3 days
Bacterial sinusitis: 500 mg/day for a total of 3 days
Extended release suspension (Zmax™): 2 g as a single dose
Urethritis/cervicitis:
Due to *C. trachomatis*: 1 g as a single dose
Due to *N. gonorrhoeae*: 2 g as a single dose
Chancroid due to *H. ducreyi*: 1 g as a single dose
Prophylaxis of disseminated *M. avium* complex disease in patient with advanced HIV infection (unlabeled use): 1200 mg once weekly (may be combined with rifabutin)
Treatment of disseminated *M. avium* complex disease in patient with advanced HIV infection (unlabeled use): 600 mg daily (in combination with ethambutol 15 mg/kg)
Prophylaxis for bacterial endocarditis (unlabeled use): 500 mg 1 hour prior to the procedure
I.V.: Adults:
Community-acquired pneumonia: 500 mg as a single dose for at least 2 days, follow I.V. therapy by the oral route with a single daily dose of 500 mg to complete a 7-10 day course of therapy
Pelvic inflammatory disease (PID): 500 mg as a single dose for 1-2 days, follow I.V. therapy by the oral route with a single daily dose of 250 mg to complete a 7-day course of therapy

Dosage adjustment in renal impairment: Use caution in patients with Cl_{cr} <10 mL/minute

Dosage adjustment in hepatic impairment: Use with caution due to potential for hepatotoxicity (rare). Specific guidelines for dosing in hepatic impairment have not been established.

Stability
Injection: Store intact vials of injection at room temperature. Reconstitute the 500 mg vial with 4.8 mL of sterile water for injection and shake until all of the drug is dissolved. Each mL contains 100 mg azithromycin. Reconstituted solution is stable for 24 hours when stored below 30°C/86°F.
The initial solution should be further diluted to a concentration of 1 mg/mL (500 mL) to 2 mg/mL (250 mL) in 0.9% sodium chloride, 5% dextrose in water, or lactated Ringer's. The diluted solution is stable for 24 hours at or below room temperature (30°C or 86°F) and for 7 days if stored under refrigeration (5°C or 41°F).
Other medications should not be infused simultaneously through the same I.V. line.
Suspension: Store dry powder below 30°C (86°F); following reconstitution, store suspension at 5°C to 30°C (41°F to 86°F).
Tablets: Store between 15°C to 30°C (59°F to 86°F).

Monitoring Parameters Liver function tests, CBC with differential

Administration I.V.: Infusate concentration and rate of infusion for azithromycin for injection should be either 1 mg/mL over 3 hours or 2 mg/mL over 1 hour. Other medications should not be infused simultaneously through the same I.V. line.

Oral: Immediate release suspension and tablet may be taken without regard to food; extended release suspension should be taken on an empty stomach (at least 1 hour before or 2 hours following a meal), within 12 hours of reconstitution.

Contraindications Hypersensitivity to azithromycin, other macrolide antibiotics, or any component of the formulation

Warnings Use with caution in patients with hepatic dysfunction; hepatic impairment with or without jaundice has occurred chiefly in older children and adults. It may be accompanied by malaise, nausea, vomiting, abdominal colic, and fever; discontinue use if these occur. May mask or delay symptoms of incubating gonorrhea or syphilis, so appropriate culture and susceptibility tests should be performed prior to initiating azithromycin. Pseudomembranous colitis has been reported with use of macrolide antibiotics; use caution with renal dysfunction. Prolongation of the QT_c interval has been reported with macrolide antibiotics; use caution in patients at risk of prolonged cardiac repolarization. Safety and efficacy have not been established in children <6 months of age with acute otitis media, acute bacterial sinusitis, or community-acquired pneumonia, or in children <2 years of age with pharyngitis/tonsillitis. Suspensions (immediate release and extended release) are not interchangeable.

Dosage Forms
Note: Strength expressed as base
Injection, powder for reconstitution, as dihydrate: 500 mg
Zithromax®: 500 mg [contains sodium 114 mg (4.96 mEq) per vial]
Microspheres for oral suspension, extended release, as dihydrate:
Zmax™: 2 g [single-dose bottle; contains sodium 148 mg per bottle; cherry and banana flavor]
Powder for oral suspension, immediate release, as dihydrate:
Zithromax®: 100 mg/5 mL (15 mL) [contains sodium 3.7 mg/ 5 mL; cherry creme de vanilla and banana flavor]; 200 mg/5 mL (15 mL, 22.5 mL, 30 mL) [contains sodium 7.4 mg/5 mL; cherry creme de vanilla and banana flavor]; 1 g [single-dose packet; contains sodium 37 mg per packet; cherry creme de vanilla and banana flavor]
Tablet, as dihydrate:
Zithromax®: 250 mg [contains sodium 0.9 mg per tablet]; 500 mg [contains sodium 1.8 mg per tablet]; 600 mg [contains sodium 2.1 mg per tablet]
Zithromax® TRI-PAK™ [unit-dose pack]: 500 mg (3s)
Zithromax® Z-PAK® [unit-dose pack]: 250 mg (6s)
Tablet, as monohydrate: 250 mg, 500 mg, 600 mg

Reference Range Peak serum levels: 0.4-0.6 mg/L following a 500 mg dose

Overdosage/Treatment
Decontamination: Lavage (within 1 hour)/activated charcoal
Enhancement of elimination: Multiple dosing of activated charcoal may be effective

Drug Interactions
Substrate of CYP3A4 (minor); **Inhibits** CYP3A4 (weak)
Cardiac glycosides: Macrolides may increase the serum concentrations of cardiac glycosides; monitor.
Colchicine: Macrolides may increase the adverse/toxic effects of colchicine.
Nelfinavir: May increase azithromycin serum levels; monitor for adverse effects.
Warfarin: Azithromycin and other macrolides may decrease metabolism, via CYP isoenzymes, of warfarin. Monitor for increased effects.

Pregnancy Risk Factor B
Pregnancy Implications Azithromycin has been shown to cross the placenta. It has been used as an alternative treatment of *Chlamydia* in late-term pregnancy. There are no adequate and well-controlled studies in pregnant women. Use during pregnancy only if clearly needed.

Lactation Enters breast milk/use caution

Additional Information Suggestion of improvement of cyclosporine-associated gingival hyperplasia with treatment of azithromycin

Specific References
Baciewicz AM, Al-Nimr A, and Whelan P, "Azithromycin-Induced Hepatoxicity," *Am J Med*, 2006, 118(12):1438-9.
Centers for Disease Control and Prevention (CDC), "Azithromycin Treatment Failures in Syphilis Infections - San Francisco, California, 2002-2003," *MMWR Morb Mortal Wkly Rep*, 2004, 53(9):197-8.
Cercek B, Shah PK, Noc M, et al, "Effect of Short-Term Treatment with Azithromycin on Recurrent Ischaemic Events in Patients with Acute Coronary Syndrome in the Azithromycin in Acute Coronary Syndrome (AZACS) Trial: A Randomised Controlled Trial," *Lancet*, 2003, 361(9360):809-13.
Law C and Amsden GW, "Single-Dose Azithromycin for Respiratory Tract Infections," *Ann Pharmacother*, 2004, 38(3):433-9.
Navarro JA, Villas F, Garcia JC, et al, "Macrolide-Induced Serum Sickness," *Allerg Clin Immunol Int*, 2000, (Suppl 2):158.
Page RL 2nd, Ruscin JM, Fish D, et al, "Possible Interaction Between Intravenous Azithromycin and Oral Cyclosporine," *Pharmacotherapy*, 2001, 21(11):1436-43.
Saha D, Karim MM, Khan WA, et al, "Single-Dose Azithromycin for the Treatment of Cholera in Adults," *N Engl J Med*, 2006, 354(23):2452-62.

Schissel DJ, Singer D, and David-Bajar K, "Azithromycin Eruption in Infectious Mononucleosis: A Proposed Mechanism of Interaction," *Cutis*, 2000, 65(3):163-6.

Stork CM, Marraffa JM, Ragosta K, et al, "Prophylactic Long-Term Antibiotic Induced Vitamin K Deficiency with Resultant Coagulopathy," *Clin Toxicol*, 2005, 43:637.

Bacitracin

CAS Number 1405-87-4; 1405-89-6

U.S. Brand Names AK-Tracin® [DSC]; Baciguent® [OTC]; BaciiM®

Use Treatment of susceptible bacterial infections (staphylococcal pneumonia and empyema); due to toxicity risks, systemic and irrigant uses of bacitracin should be limited to situations where less toxic alternatives would not be effective

Unlabeled/Investigational Use Oral administration: Successful in antibiotic-associated colitis; has been used for enteric eradication of vancomycin-resistant enterococci (VRE)

Mechanism of Action Inhibits bacterial cell wall synthesis by preventing transfer of mucopeptides into the growing cell wall

Adverse Reactions

Cardiovascular: Hypotension, tightness of chest, edema of lips and face

Central nervous system: Pain

Dermatologic: Rash, itching, contact dermatitis, urticaria, systemic contact dermatitis, immunologic contact urticaria

Gastrointestinal: Anorexia, nausea, vomiting, diarrhea, rectal itching and burning

Hematologic: Blood dyscrasias

Ocular: Diplopia

Otic: Ototoxicity

Renal: Nephrotoxic when given parenterally (tubular or glomerular necrosis); hematuria, albuminuria (reversible)

Miscellaneous: Anaphylactic shock, anaphylaxis following topical administration, diaphoresis

Signs and Symptoms of Overdose Hypokalemia, myasthenia gravis (exacerbation or precipitation), tubular necrosis (acute)

Pharmacodynamics/Kinetics

Duration: 6-8 hours

Absorption: Poor from mucous membranes and intact or denuded skin; rapidly following I.M. administration; not absorbed by bladder irrigation, but absorption can occur from peritoneal or mediastinal lavage

Distribution: CSF: Nil even with inflammation

Protein binding, plasma: Minimal

Time to peak, serum: I.M.: 1-2 hours

Excretion: Urine (10% to 40%) within 24 hours

Dosage

Do not administer I.V.:

Infants: I.M.:

≤2.5 kg: 900 units/kg/day in 2-3 divided doses

>2.5 kg: 1000 units/kg/day in 2-3 divided doses

Children: I.M.: 800-1200 units/kg/day divided every 8 hours

Adults: Oral:

Antibiotic-associated colitis: 25,000 units 4 times/day for 7-10 days

VRE eradication (unlabeled use): 25,000 units 4 times/day for 7-10 days

Children and Adults:

Topical: Apply 1-5 times/day

Ophthalmic, ointment: Instill $^1/_4$" to $^1/_2$" ribbon every 3-4 hours into conjunctival sac for acute infections, or 2-3 times/day for mild to moderate infections for 7-10 days

Irrigation, solution: 50-100 units/mL in normal saline, lactated Ringer's, or sterile water for irrigation; soak sponges in solution for topical compresses 1-5 times/day or as needed during surgical procedures

Stability Sterile powder should be stored in the refrigerator; once reconstituted, bacitracin is stable for 1 week under refrigeration (2°C to 8°C); bacitracin sterile powder should be dissolved in 0.9% sodium chloride injection containing 2% procaine hydrochloride for I.M. use; do not use diluents containing parabens; bacitracin zinc is more stable than bacitracin

Monitoring Parameters I.M.: Urinalysis, renal function tests

Administration

For I.M. administration only, **do not administer I.V.** Confirm any orders for parenteral use. pH of urine should be kept >6 by using sodium bicarbonate. Bacitracin sterile powder should be dissolved in 0.9% sodium chloride injection containing 2% procaine hydrochloride. Do not use diluents containing parabens.

Contraindications Hypersensitivity to bacitracin or any component of the formulation; I.M. use is contraindicated in patients with renal impairment

Warnings [U.S. Boxed Warning]: I.M. use may cause renal failure due to tubular and glomerular necrosis; monitor renal function daily. Prolonged use may result in overgrowth of nonsusceptible organisms. Do not administer intravenously because severe thrombophlebitis occurs.

Dosage Forms

[DSC] = Discontinued product

Injection, powder for reconstitution (BaciiM®): 50,000 units

Ointment, ophthalmic (AK-Tracin® [DSC]): 500 units/g (3.5 g)

Ointment, topical: 500 units/g (0.9 g, 15 g, 30 g, 120 g, 454 g)

Baciguent®: 500 units/g (15 g, 30 g)

Reference Range Doses of 200-300 units/kg every 6 hours (I.M.) produce plasma levels of 2 units/mL

Overdosage/Treatment Decontamination: Lavage (within 1 hour)/activated charcoal with oral ingestion; irrigate dermal exposure with soap and water

Drug Interactions Increased toxicity: Nephrotoxic drugs, neuromuscular blocking agents, and anesthetics (increases neuromuscular blockade).

Pregnancy Risk Factor C

Lactation Excretion in breast milk unknown/use caution

Nursing Implications For I.M. injection only, do **not** administer I.V.; confirm any orders for parenteral use; pH of urine should be kept >6 by using sodium bicarbonate

Additional Information 1 unit is equivalent to 0.026 mg

Baclofen

Related Information

- Substance-Related Disorders
- Therapeutic Drugs Associated with Hallucinations

CAS Number 1134-47-0

U.S. Brand Names Lioresal®

Impairment Potential Yes

Use Treatment of reversible spasticity associated with multiple sclerosis or spinal cord lesions; intractable hiccups

Treatment of intractable spasticity caused by spinal cord injury, multiple sclerosis, and other spinal disease (spinal ischemia or tumor, transverse myelitis, cervical spondylosis, degenerative myelopathy); alcohol withdrawal

Mechanism of Action Inhibits transmission of both monosynaptic and polysynaptic reflexes at the spinal cord level, possibly by hyperpolarization of primary afferent fiber terminals, with resultant relief of muscle spasticity; a gamma aminobutyric acid (GABA$_B$) agonist

Adverse Reactions

Withdrawal reactions have occurred with abrupt discontinuation (particularly severe with intrathecal use).

Cardiovascular: Hypotension, palpitations, chest pain, syncope

Central nervous system: **Drowsiness, vertigo, psychiatric disturbances, insomnia, slurred speech, ataxia, hypotonia,** confusion, euphoria, excitement, depression, fatigue, headache, hallucinations, psychosis

Dermatologic: Rash

Endocrine & metabolic: Impotence, inability to ejaculate

Gastrointestinal: Xerostomia, anorexia, abnormal taste, abdominal pain, nausea, vomiting, diarrhea

Genitourinary: Enuresis, dysuria, nocturia, hematuria, polyuria

Neuromuscular & skeletal: **Weakness,** paresthesia

Respiratory: Dyspnea

Signs and Symptoms of Overdose Angina, bradycardia or tachycardia (ventricular) [flutter (atrial)], coma, dementia, depression, diarrhea, drowsiness, dyspnea, encephalopathy, euphoria, hypertension or hypotension, hypothermia, insomnia, impotence, mania, muscle hypotonia, nystagmus, respiratory depression, salivation, seizures, vomiting, wheezing

Pharmacodynamics/Kinetics

Onset of action: 3-4 days

Peak effect: 5-10 days

Absorption (dose dependent): Oral: Rapid

Protein binding: 30%

Metabolism: Hepatic (15% of dose)

Half-life elimination: 3.5 hours

Time to peak, serum: Oral: Within 2-3 hours

Excretion: Urine and feces (85% as unchanged drug)

Dosage

Oral (avoid abrupt withdrawal of drug):

Children:

2-7 years: Initial: 10-15 mg/24 hours divided every 8 hours; titrate dose every 3 days in increments of 5-15 mg/day to a maximum of 40 mg/day

≥8 years: Maximum: 60 mg/day in 3 divided doses

Adults: 5 mg 3 times/day, may increase 5 mg/dose every 3 days to a maximum of 80 mg/day

Hiccups: Adults: Usual effective dose: 10-20 mg 2-3 times/day

Intrathecal:

Test dose: 50-100 mcg, doses >50 mcg should be given in 25 mcg increments, separated by 24 hours. A screening dose of 25 mcg may be considered in very small patients. Patients not responding to screening dose of 100 mcg should not be considered for chronic infusion/implanted pump.

Maintenance: After positive response to test dose, a maintenance intrathecal infusion can be administered via an implanted intrathecal pump. Initial dose via pump: Infusion at a 24-hour rate dosed at twice the test dose. Avoid abrupt discontinuation.

Alcohol withdrawal (investigational): Oral: 30 mg/day for 10 consecutive days

Elderly: Oral (the lowest effective dose is recommended): Initial: 5 mg 2-3 times/day, increasing gradually as needed; if benefits are not seen withdraw the drug slowly.

Dosing adjustment in renal impairment: It is necessary to reduce dosage in renal impairment but there are no specific guidelines available

Hemodialysis: Poor water solubility allows for accumulation during chronic hemodialysis. Low-dose therapy is recommended. There have been several case reports of accumulation of baclofen resulting in toxicity symptoms (organic brain syndrome, myoclonia, deceleration and steep potentials in EEG) in patients with renal failure who have received normal doses of baclofen.

Administration

Intrathecal: For screening dosages, dilute with preservative-free sodium chloride to a final concentration of 50 mcg/mL for bolus injection into the subarachnoid space. For maintenance infusions, concentrations of 500-2000 mcg/mL may be used.

Contraindications Hypersensitivity to baclofen or any component of the formulation

Warnings Use with caution in patients with seizure disorder or impaired renal function. **[U.S. Boxed Warning]: Avoid abrupt withdrawal of the drug; abrupt withdrawal of intrathecal baclofen has resulted in severe sequelae (hyperpyrexia, obtundation, rebound/exaggerated spasticity, muscle rigidity, and rhabdomyolysis), leading to organ failure and some fatalities.** Risk may be higher in patients with injuries at T-6 or above, history of baclofen withdrawal, or limited ability to communicate. Elderly are more sensitive to the effects of baclofen and are more likely to experience adverse CNS effects at higher doses.

Dosage Forms Injection, solution, intrathecal [preservative free] (Lioresal®): 50 mcg/mL (1 mL); 500 mcg/mL (20 mL); 2000 mcg/mL (5 mL)

Tablet: 10 mg, 20 mg

Reference Range Toxicity can occur at baclofen blood levels >1 mg/L; fatality associated with blood and urine baclofen levels of 17 mg/L and 760 mg/L, respectively

Overdosage/Treatment

Decontamination: Lavage within 1 hour for ingestions over 5 mg/kg; activated charcoal should also be used

Supportive therapy: Following initiation of essential overdose management, symptomatic and supportive treatment should be instituted; physostigmine can alleviate drowsiness when intrathecal baclofen toxicity is present; atropine can be utilized for bradycardia; diazepam or lorazepam can be used for seizure management; dantrolene (10 mg/kg) has been used to treat hyperthermia due to baclofen withdrawal; for intrathecal overdose, remove 30-50 mL of CSF fluid and treat supportively; flumazenil may be useful in reversing oral (but not intrathecal) baclofen-induced coma; flumazenil has been used to treat coma and respiratory depression with uneven results; caution should be used with flumazenil administration due to baclofen's inherent seizurgenic properties. In a single case report, 10 mg I.V. of ondansetron reversed coma in a baclofen overdose.

Cyproheptadine (4-8 mg every 6-8 hours) can assist with benzodiazepine and baclofen in treating intrathecal baclofen withdrawal.

Antidote(s)

- Atropine [ANTIDOTE]
- Physostigmine [ANTIDOTE]

Test Interactions ↑ alkaline phosphatase, AST, glucose, ammonia (B); ↓ bilirubin (S)

Drug Interactions

Increased effect: Opiate analgesics, benzodiazepines, hypertensive agents

Increased toxicity: CNS depressants and ethanol (sedation), tricyclic antidepressants (short-term memory loss), clindamycin (neuromuscular blockade), guanabenz (sedation), MAO inhibitors (decrease blood pressure, CNS, and respiratory effects)

Pregnancy Risk Factor C

Pregnancy Implications Crosses placenta

Lactation Enters breast milk (small amounts)/compatible

Nursing Implications Epileptic patients should be closely monitored; supervise ambulation; avoid abrupt withdrawal of the drug

Additional Information

Baclofen withdrawal syndrome usually occurs within 12-72 hours following dose cessation. The syndrome is similar to the sedative-hypnotic withdrawal syndrome with agitation, delusions, spasticity, rhabdomyolysis, paranoia, psychosis, pruritus, hallucinations, hypertonia, fever, and seizures. Benzodiazepines (diazepam 5-10 mg orally every 6-12 hours) are the mainstay of baclofen withdrawal therapy. For acute intrathecal baclofen withdrawal, baclofen (10-20 mg orally every 6 hours) and cyproheptadine (4-8 mg orally every 6-8 hours) can also be utilized with the latter agent particularly effective in treating pruritus.

Elderly are sensitive to this drug

Specific References

Addalorato G, Leggio L, Abenavoli L, et al, "Baclofen in the Treatment of Alcohol Withdrawal Syndrome: A Comparative Study vs Diazepam," *Am J Med*, 2006, 119(3):276.

Chawla JM, Sagar R, "Baclofen Induced Psychosis," *Ann Pharmacol*, 2006, 40(11):2071-2073.

Chen YC, Chang CT, Fang JT, et al, "Baclofen Neurotoxicity in Uremic Patients: Is Continuous Ambulatory Peritoneal Dialysis Less Effective Than Intermittent Hemodialysis?" *Ren Fail*, 2003, 25(2):297-305.

Drake RG, Davis LL, Cates ME, et al, "Baclofen Treatment for Chronic Posttraumatic Stress Disorder," *Ann Pharmacother*, 2003, 37(9):1177-81.

Greenberg MI and Hendrickson RG, "Baclofen Withdrawal Following Removal of an Intrathecal Baclofen Pump Despite Oral Baclofen Replacement," *J Toxicol Clin Toxicol*, 2003, 41(1):83-5.

Kao LW, Amin Y, Kirk MA, et al, "Intrathecal Baclofen Withdrawal Mimicking Sepsis," *J Emerg Med*, 2003, 24(4): 423-7.

Leung NY, Whyte IM, and Isbister GK, "Baclofen Overdose: Defining the Spectrum of Toxicity," *Emerg Med Australas*, 2006, 18(1):77-82.

Meythaler JM, Roper JF, and Brunner RC, "Cyproheptadine for Intrathecal Baclofen Withdrawal," *Arch Phys Med Rehabil*, 2003, 84(5):638-42.

Miksa IR and Poppenga RH, "Direct and Rapid Determination of Baclofen (Lioresal®) and Carisoprodol (Soma®) in Bovine Serum by Liquid Chromatography-Mass Spectrometry," *J Anal Toxicol*, 2003, 27(5): 275-83.

Pizon AF, Curry SC, and LoVecchio F, "Reversible Cardiomyopathy," *Clin Toxicol (Phila)*. 2005, 43:647.

Shirley KW, Kothare S, Piatt JH Jr, et al, "Intrathecal Baclofen Overdose and Withdrawal," *Pediatr Emerg Care*, 2006, 22(4):258-61.

Wiersma HE, Van Boxtel CJ, Butter JJ, et al, "Pharmacokinetics of a Single Oral Dose of Baclofen in Pediatric Patients with Gastroesophageal Reflux Disease," *Ther Drug Monit*, 2003, 25(1):93-8.

Wogoman H, Bultman S, Smith R, et al, "Increased Incidence of Gabapentin and Baclofen in Postmortem Casework, Both Alone and In Combination with Other Drugs," *J Anal Toxicol*, 2004, 28:301.

Yeh RN, Nypaver MM, Deegan TJ, et al, "Baclofen Toxicity in an 8-Year-Old with an Intrathecal Baclofen Pump," *J Emerg Med*, 2004, 26(2):163-7.

Belladonna

Pronunciation (bel a DON a)

Use Decrease gastrointestinal activity in functional bowel disorders and to delay gastric emptying as well as decrease gastric secretion

Mechanism of Action Belladonna is a mixture of the anticholinergic alkaloids atropine, hyoscyamine, and scopolamine (hyoscine). The belladonna alkaloids act primarily by competitive inhibition of the muscarinic actions of acetylcholine on structures innervated by postganglionic cholinergic neurons and on smooth muscle. The resulting effects include antisecretory activity on exocrine glands and intestinal mucosa and smooth muscle relaxation. The anticholinergic properties of scopolamine and atropine differ in that scopolamine has a more potent activity on the iris, ciliary body, and certain secretory glands; has more potent activity on the heart, intestine, and bronchial muscle, and a more prolonged duration of action; in contrast, hyoscyamine has actions similar to those of atropine, but is more potent in both its central and peripheral effects

Adverse Reactions

Cardiovascular: Hypotension (orthostatic), fibrillation (ventricular), tachycardia, palpitations, sinus tachycardia, tachycardia (supraventricular), arrhythmias (ventricular)

Central nervous system: Confusion, anxiety, lightheadedness, headache, loss of memory, hallucinations, drowsiness, tiredness, ataxia, paranoia, fever

Dermatologic: Skin rash, **dry skin**

Endocrine & metabolic: Breast milk (decreased flow)

Gastrointestinal: **Constipation, xerostomia and dry throat**, nausea, vomiting, bloated feeling, dysphagia

Genitourinary: Dysuria

Neuromuscular & skeletal: Weakness

Ocular: Blurred vision, photophobia, vision color changes (red tinge), intraocular pain (increased), increased intraocular pressure, sensitivity to light (increased)

Respiratory: **Dry nose**

Miscellaneous: Enuresis, **diaphoresis (decreased)**

Signs and Symptoms of Overdose Anticholinergic toxicity may be caused by strong binding of a belladonna alkaloid to cholinergic receptors. Anticholinesterase inhibitors reduce acetylcholinesterase, the enzyme that breaks down acetylcholine and thereby allows acetylcholine to accumulate and compete for receptor binding with the offending anticholinergic.

Dosage

Tincture: Oral:

Children: 0.03 mL/kg 3 times/day

Adults: 0.6-1 mL 3-4 times/day

Stability Store in tight, light-resistant container at 15°C to 30°C

Monitoring Parameters CNS depression

Contraindications Hypersensitivity to belladonna or any component of the formulation; glaucoma, elevated intraocular pressure; significant hepatic or renal disease; pulmonary insufficiency

Dosage Forms Tincture: Belladonna alkaloids (principally hyoscyamine and atropine) 0.3 mg/mL with alcohol 65% to 70% (120 mL, 480 mL, 3780 mL)

Overdosage/Treatment Decontamination: With life-threatening symptoms, physostigmine 1-2 mg (0.5 or 0.02 mg/kg for children) SubQ or I.V. slowly may be given to reverse these effects

Drug Interactions Phenothiazines, amantadine, antiparkinsonian drugs, glutethimide, meperidine, tricyclic antidepressants, antiarrhythmic agents, some antihistamines

Pregnancy Risk Factor C

Nursing Implications Assist patient with ambulation

Benazepril

Related Information
- Angiotensin Agents

CAS Number 86541-75-5

U.S. Brand Names Lotensin®

Synonyms Benazepril Hydrochloride

Use Treatment of hypertension, either alone or in combination with other antihypertensive agents

Mechanism of Action Competitive inhibition of angiotensin I being converted to angiotensin II, a potent vasoconstrictor, through the angiotensin I-converting enzyme (ACE) activity, with resultant lower levels of angiotensin II which causes an increase in plasma renin activity and a reduction in aldosterone secretion

Adverse Reactions

Cardiovascular: Hypotension, tachycardia, palpitations, sinus tachycardia, vasodilation

Central nervous system: Fatigue, headache, dizziness

Dermatologic: Rash, photosensitivity, angioedema, urticaria, pruritus, exanthema

Endocrine & metabolic: Hyperkalemia, hypoglycemia

Gastrointestinal: Nausea, pancreatitis

Hematologic: Leukopenia, eosinophilia

Neuromuscular & skeletal: Hypertonia, paresthesia

Renal: Proteinuria

Respiratory: Transient cough during early therapy, rhinitis

Miscellaneous: Hypersensitivity reaction

Signs and Symptoms of Overdose Agranulocytosis, dermatitis, drowsiness, granulocytopenia, hypertonia, impotence, leukopenia, myalgia, neutropenia, renal insufficiency, severe hypotension

Pharmacodynamics/Kinetics

Reduction in plasma angiotensin-converting enzyme (ACE) activity:
Onset of action: Peak effect: 1-2 hours after 2-20 mg dose
Duration: >90% inhibition for 24 hours after 5-20 mg dose

Reduction in blood pressure:
Peak effect: Single dose: 2-4 hours; Continuous therapy: 2 weeks

Absorption: Rapid (37%); food does not alter significantly; metabolite (benazeprilat) itself unsuitable for oral administration due to poor absorption

Distribution: V_d: ~8.7 L

Metabolism: Rapidly and extensively hepatic to its active metabolite, benazeprilat, via enzymatic hydrolysis; extensive first-pass effect

Half-life elimination: Benazeprilat: Effective: 10-11 hours; Terminal: Children: 5 hours, Adults: 22 hours

Time to peak: Parent drug: 0.5-1 hour

Excretion: Clearance: Nonrenal clearance (ie, biliary, metabolic) appears to contribute to the elimination of benazeprilat (11% to 12%), particularly patients with severe renal impairment; hepatic clearance is the main elimination route of unchanged benazepril

Dialysis: ~6% of metabolite removed within 4 hours of dialysis following 10 mg of benazepril administered 2 hours prior to procedure; parent compound not found in dialysate

Dosage

Oral: Hypertension:

Children ≥6 years: Initial: 0.2 mg/kg/day as monotherapy; dosing range: 0.1-0.6 mg/kg/day (maximum dose: 40 mg/day)

Adults: Initial: 10 mg/day in patients not receiving a diuretic; 20-40 mg/day as a single dose or 2 divided doses; the need for twice-daily dosing should be assessed by monitoring peak (2-6 hours after dosing) and trough responses.

Note: Patients taking diuretics should have them discontinued 2-3 days prior to starting benazepril. If they cannot be discontinued, then initial dose should be 5 mg; restart after blood pressure is stabilized if needed.

Elderly: Oral: Initial: 5-10 mg/day in single or divided doses; usual range: 20-40 mg/day; adjust for renal function; also see "Note" in Adults dosing.

Dosing interval in renal impairment: $Cl_{cr} <30$ mL/minute:

Children: Use is not recommended.

Adults: Administer 5 mg/day initially; maximum daily dose: 40 mg.

Hemodialysis: Moderately dialyzable (20% to 50%); administer dose postdialysis or administer 25% to 35% supplemental dose.

Peritoneal dialysis: Supplemental dose is not necessary.

Monitoring Parameters CBC, renal function tests, electrolytes

Contraindications Hypersensitivity to benazepril or any component of the formulation; angioedema or serious hypersensitivity related to previous treatment with an ACE inhibitor; bilateral renal artery stenosis; patients with idiopathic or hereditary angioedema; pregnancy (2nd and 3rd trimesters)

Warnings Anaphylactic reactions can occur. Angioedema can occur at any time during treatment (especially following first dose). Angioedema can occur at any time during treatment (especially following first dose). It may involve head and neck (potentially affecting the airway) or the intestine (presenting with abdominal pain). Prolonged monitoring may be required especially if tongue, glottis, or larynx are involved as they are associated with airway obstruction. Those with a history of airway surgery in this situation have a higher risk. Careful blood pressure monitoring with first dose (hypotension can occur especially in volume-depleted patients).

[U.S. Boxed Warning]: Based on human data, ACEIs can cause injury and death to the developing fetus when used in the second and third trimesters. ACEIs should be discontinued as soon as possible once pregnancy is detected. Dosage adjustment needed in renal impairment. Use with caution in hypovolemia; collagen vascular diseases; valvular stenosis (particularly aortic stenosis); hyperkalemia; or before, during, or immediately after anesthesia. Avoid rapid dosage escalation which may lead to renal insufficiency. Rare toxicities associated with ACE inhibitors include cholestatic jaundice (which may progress to hepatic necrosis) and neutropenia/agranulocytosis with myeloid hyperplasia. Hypersensitivity reactions may be seen during hemodialysis with high-flux dialysis membranes (eg, AN69). Deterioration in renal function can occur with initiation. Use with caution in unilateral renal artery stenosis and pre-existing renal insufficiency.

Dosage Forms Tablet, as hydrochloride: 5 mg, 10 mg, 20 mg, 40 mg

Lotensin®: 5 mg, 10 mg, 20 mg, 40 mg

Overdosage/Treatment

Decontamination: Emesis within 30 minutes or lavage (within 1 hour)/activated charcoal

Supportive therapy: Following initiation of essential overdose management, toxic symptom treatment and supportive treatment should be initiated. Hypotension usually responds to I.V. fluids or Trendelenburg positioning. If unresponsive to these measures, the use of a parenteral inotrope may be required (eg, norepinephrine 0.1-0.2 mcg/kg/minute titrated to response). Seizures commonly respond to lorazepam or diazepam (I.V. 5-10 mg bolus in adults every 15 minutes if needed up to a total of 30 mg; I.V. 0.25-0.4 mg/kg/dose up to a total of 10 mg in children) or to phenytoin or phenobarbital. For refractory hypotension, angiotensin amide infusion may be attempted.

Enhancement of elimination: Multiple dosing of activated charcoal may be effective; moderately dialyzable (20% to 50%); ~6% of metabolite was removed by 4 hours of dialysis following 10 mg of benazepril administered 2 hours prior to procedure; the parent compound was not found in the dialysate

Drug Interactions

α_1 blockers: Hypotensive effect increased.

Aspirin: The effects of ACE inhibitors may be blunted by aspirin administration, particularly at higher dosages, and/or increase adverse renal effects.

Diuretics: Hypovolemia due to diuretics may precipitate acute hypotensive events or acute renal failure.

Insulin: Risk of hypoglycemia may be increased.

Lithium: Risk of lithium toxicity may be increased; monitor lithium levels.

NSAIDs: May attenuate hypertensive efficacy; effect has been seen with captopril and may occur with other ACE inhibitors; monitor blood pressure. May increase adverse renal effects.

Potassium-sparing diuretics or potassium supplements (amiloride, potassium, spironolactone, triamterene): Increased risk of hyperkalemia.

Trimethoprim (high dose) may increase the risk of hyperkalemia.

Pregnancy Risk Factor C (1st trimester)/D (2nd and 3rd trimesters)

Pregnancy Implications Decreased placental blood flow, low birth weight, fetal hypotension, preterm delivery, and fetal death have been noted with the use of some ACE inhibitors (ACEIs) in animal studies. Neonatal hypotension, skull hypoplasia, anuria, renal failure, oligohydramnios (associated with fetal limb contractures, craniofacial deformities, hypoplastic lung development), prematurity, intrauterine growth retardation, and patent ductus arteriosus have been reported with the use of ACEIs, primarily in the 2nd and 3rd trimesters. The risk of neonatal toxicity has been considered less when ACEIs have been used in the 1st trimester; however, major congenital malformations have been reported. The cardiovascular and/or central nervous systems are most commonly affected. Unless alternative agents are not appropriate, ACEIs should be discontinued as soon as possible once pregnancy is detected.

Lactation Enters breast milk/compatible

Nursing Implications Watch for hypotensive effect within 1-3 hours of first dose or new higher dose; many patients complain of transient cough during early therapy

Specific References

Cooper W, Hernandez-Diaz S, Arbogast P, et al, "Major Congenital Malformations After First Trimester Exposure to ACE Inhibitors," *N Engl J Med*, 2006, 354:2443-51.

Mastrobattista J, "Angiontensin-Converting Enzyme Inhibitors in Pregnancy," *Semin Perinatol*, 1997, 21(2):124-34.

Quan A, "Fetopathy Associated with Exposure to Angiotensin-Converting Enzyme Inhibitors and Angiotensin Receptor Antagonists," *Early Hum Dev*, 2006, 82(1):23-8.

Benzalkonium Chloride

Pronunciation (benz al KOE nee um KLOR ide)

CAS Number 8001-54-5

U.S. Brand Names 3M™ Cavilon™ Skin Cleanser [OTC]; Benza® [OTC]; HandClens® [OTC]; Ony-Clear [OTC] [DSC]; Zephiran® [OTC]

Synonyms BAC

Use Surface antiseptic and germicidal preservative

Mechanism of Action Quaternary ammonium disinfectant (cationic)

Adverse Reactions

Cardiovascular: Hypotension

Central nervous system: Lethargy, seizures, pain

Dermatologic: Bullous or pustular reactions, contact dermatitis

Endocrine & metabolic: Inhibits sperm motility

Gastrointestinal (ingestion): Vomiting (hemetemesis), burning mouth/throat, salivation, esophageal burns

Ocular: Corneal damage

Otic: May be ototoxic

Miscellaneous: Hypersensitivity, **corrosive burn at concentrations**

Signs and Symptoms of Overdose Confusion, elevated liver function test results, hypotension, metabolic acidosis, muscle paralysis, myoclonus, profuse diarrhea, seizures

Dosage Thoroughly rinse anionic detergents and soaps from the skin or other areas prior to use of solutions because they reduce the antibacterial activity of BAC. To protect metal instruments stored in BAC solution, add crushed antirust tablets, 4 tablets/quart, to antiseptic solution, change solution at least once weekly. Not to be used for storage of aluminum or zinc instruments, instruments with lenses fastened by cement, lacquered catheters, or some synthetic rubber goods.

Stability Foams when shaken; **incompatible** with iodine, soaps, anionic detergent, iodides, citrates, salicylates, silver nitrate, fluorescein, nitrates, peroxide, lanolin, potassium permanganate, aluminum, caramel, kaolin, pine oil, zinc sulfate, zinc oxide, and yellow mercuric oxide

Contraindications Hypersensitivity to benzalkonium or any component of the formulation

Dosage Forms [DSC] = Discontinued product

Solution, topical:

Benza®: 1:750 (60 mL, 240 mL, 480 mL, 3840 mL)

HandClens®: 0.13% (120 mL, 480 mL, 800 mL)

Ony-Clear [DSC]: 1% (30 mL)

Zephiran®: 1:750 (240 mL, 3840 mL) [aqueous]

Solution, topical spray (3M™ Cavilon™ Skin Cleanser): 0.11% (240 mL)

Overdosage/Treatment

Decontamination: Oral: Activated charcoal may be useful, dilute with milk or water; **do not** induce emesis

Supportive therapy: Treat hypotension with isotonic saline; endoscopy may be required to evaluated gastrointestinal burns

Enhancement of elimination: Hemodialysis or forced diuresis is not useful

Pregnancy Risk Factor C

Benzbromarone

CAS Number 3562-84-3

Use Uricosuric agent which lowers uric acid concentrations; used for hyperuricemia, gout, and Lesch-Nyhan syndrome

Mechanism of Action Blocks proximal tubular reabsorption of uric acid; also increases gastrointestinal elimination of uric acid

Adverse Reactions

Dermatologic: Petechiae

Endocrine & metabolic: Gouty attacks

Gastrointestinal: Diarrhea, nausea

Genitourinary: Impotence

Hematologic: Porphyrinogenic

Hepatic: Elevated liver enzymes

Ocular: Allergic conjunctivitis

Renal: Elevated serum creatinine

Toxicodynamics/Kinetics

Onset of action: 3 hours

Peak effect: 8-12 hours

Duration: 15-21 hours

Absorption: Oral: 50%

Distribution: V_d: <0.3 L/kg

Protein binding: 99%

Metabolism: To benzarone and bromobenzarone

Half-life: 2.7 hours

Elimination: Feces (50%), renal

Dosage 50-200 mg/day

Reference Range Peak serum level of 1.84 mcg/mL after oral dose of 100 mg of benzbromarone

Overdosage/Treatment

Decontamination: Ipecac within 30 minutes or lavage (within 1 hour)/activated charcoal

Enhancement of elimination: Multiple dosage activated charcoal may be effective

Additional Information Investigational (phase II trials) in the U.S.

Benzocaine

CAS Number 94-09-7

U.S. Brand Names Americaine® Anesthetic Lubricant; Americaine® [OTC]; Anbesol® Baby [OTC]; Anbesol® Maximum Strength [OTC]; Anbesol® [OTC]; Babee® Teething® [OTC]; Benzodent® [OTC]; Chiggerex® [OTC]; Chiggertox® [OTC]; Cylex® [OTC]; Detane® [OTC]; Foille® Medicated First Aid [OTC]; Foille® Plus [OTC]; Foille® [OTC]; HDA® Toothache [OTC]; Hurricaine®; Lanacane® [OTC]; Mycinettes® [OTC]; Orabase®-B [OTC]; Orajel® Baby Nighttime [OTC]; Orajel® Baby [OTC]; Orajel® Maximum Strength [OTC]; Orajel® [OTC]; Orasol® [OTC]; Solarcaine® [OTC]; Trocaine® [OTC]; Zilactin® Baby [OTC]; Zilactin®-B [OTC]

Synonyms Ethyl Aminobenzoate

Use Local anesthetic

Mechanism of Action Blocks both the initiation and conduction of nerve impulses by decreasing the neuronal membrane's permeability to sodium ions, which results in inhibition of depolarization with resultant blockade of conduction; a group I (ester) anesthetic; low water solubility

Adverse Reactions

Cardiovascular: Sinus tachycardia

Dermatologic: Eczema, urticaria, nonimmunologic contact urticaria, systemic contact urticaria, immunologic contact urticaria, photoallergic reaction

Gastrointestinal: GI irritation, gagging, increased sour sensitivity taste

Hematologic: Methemoglobinemia in infants

Local: Burning, stinging, tenderness, rash, contact dermatitis, edema

Signs and Symptoms of Overdose Cyanosis, drowsiness, eczema, methemoglobinemia (within 1 hour), photosensitivity, tachycardia, tachypnea

Admission Criteria/Prognosis Admit ingestions >100 mg/kg, symptomatic methemoglobinemia or methemoglobin levels >30%; any patient with change in mental status or cardiopulmonary complaints should be admitted; asymptomatic patients with methemoglobin levels <30% may be considered for discharge after 6 hours of observation and if methemoglobin levels fall to <15%

Pharmacodynamics/Kinetics

Absorption: Topical: Poor to intact skin; well absorbed from mucous membranes and traumatized skin

Metabolism: Hepatic (to a lesser extent) and plasma via hydrolysis by cholinesterase

Excretion: Urine (as metabolites)

Dosage Mucous membranes: Dosage varies depending on area to be anesthetized and vascularity of tissues

Topical: Apply to affected area as needed

Administration

Avoid application to large areas of broken skin, especially in children. When possible, apply to clean, dry area.

Contraindications Hypersensitivity to benzocaine, other ester-type local anesthetics, or any component of the formulation; secondary bacterial infection of area; ophthalmic use; otic preparations are also contraindicated in the presence of perforated tympanic membrane

Warnings

Methemoglobinemia has been reported following topical use (rare). When applied as a spray to the mouth or throat, multiple sprays (or sprays of longer than indicated duration) are not recommended. Use caution with breathing problems (asthma, bronchitis, emphysema, in smokers), heart disease, children <6 months of age, and hemoglobin or enzyme abnormalities (glucose-6-phosphodiesterase deficiency, hemoglobin-M disease, NADH-methemoglobin reductase deficiency, pyruvate-kinase deficiency)

When used for self-medication (OTC), notify healthcare provider if condition worsens or does not improve within 7 days, or if swelling, rash, or fever develops. Do not use on open wounds. Avoid contact with the eyes.

Dosage Forms

Aerosol, oral spray (Hurricaine®): 20% (60 mL) [dye free; cherry flavor]

Aerosol, topical spray:

Americaine®: 20% (60 mL)

Dermoplast® Antibacterial: 20% (83 mL) [contains aloe vera, benzethonium chloride, menthol]

Dermoplast® Pain Relieving: 20% (60 mL, 83 mL) [contains menthol]

Foille®: 5% (92 g) [contains chloroxylenol 0.63% and corn oil]

Ivy-Rid®: 2% (83 mL)

Lanacane® Maximum Strength: 20% (120 mL) [contains alcohol]

Solarcaine®: 20% (120 mL) [contains triclosan 0.13%, alcohol 35%]

Combination package (Orajel® Baby Daytime and Nighttime):

Gel, oral [Daytime Regular Formula]: 7.5% (5.3 g)

Gel, oral [Nighttime Formula]: 10% (5.3 g)

Cream, oral:

Benzodent®: 20% (7.5 g, 30 g)

Orajel PM®: 20% (5.3 g, 7 g)

Cream, topical:

Lanacane®: 6% (30 g, 60 g)

Lanacane® Maximum Strength: 20% (30 g)

Gel, oral:

Anbesol®: 10% (7.5 g) [contains benzyl alcohol; cool mint flavor]

Anbesol® Baby: 7.5% (7.5 g) [contains benzoic acid; grape flavor]

Anbesol® Jr.: 10% (7 g) [contains benzyl alcohol; bubble gum flavor]

Anbesol® Maximum Strength: 20% (7.5 g, 10 g) [contains benzyl alcohol]

Dentapaine: 20% (11 g) [contains clove oil]

HDA® Toothache: 6.5% (15 mL) [contains benzyl alcohol]

Hurricaine®: 20% (5 g) [dye free; wild cherry flavor]; (30 g) [dye free; mint, pina colada, watermelon, and wild cherry flavors]

Kanka® Soft Brush™: 20% (2 mL) [packaged in applicator with brush tip]

Orabase® with Benzocaine®: 20% (7 g) [contains ethyl alcohol 48%; mild mint flavor]

Orajel®: 10% (5.3 g, 7 g, 9.4 g)

Orajel® Baby Teething: 7.5% (9.4 g, 11.9 g) [cherry flavor]

Orajel® Baby Teething Nighttime: 10% (5.3 g)

Orajel® Denture Plus: 15% (9 g) [contains menthol 2%, ethyl alcohol 66.7%]

Orajel® Maximum Strength: 20% (5.3 g, 7 g, 9.4 g, 11.9 g)

Orajel® Mouth Sore: 20% (5.3 g, 9.4 g, 11.9 g) [contains benzalkonium chloride 0.02%, zinc chloride 0.1%]

Orajel® Multi-Action Cold Sore: 20% (9.4 g) [contains allantoin 0.5%, camphor 3%, dimethicone 2%]

Orajel® Ultra Mouth Sore: 15% (9.4 g) [contains ethyl alcohol 66.7%, menthol 2%]

Zilactin®-B: 10% (7.5 g)

Gel, topical (Detane®): 7.5% (15 g)

Liquid, oral:

Anbesol®: 10% (9 mL) [cool mint flavor]

Anbesol® Maximum Strength: 20% (9 mL) [contains benzyl alcohol]

Hurricaine®: 20% (30 mL) [pina colada and wild cherry flavors]

Orajel® Baby Teething: 7.5% (13 mL) [very berry flavor]

Orajel® Maximum Strength: 20% (13 mL) [contains ethyl alcohol 44%, tartrazine]

Liquid, oral drop:

Dent's Maxi-Strength Toothache: 20% (3.7 mL) [contains alcohol 74%]

Rid-A-Pain Dental Drops: 6.3% (30 mL) [contains alcohol 70%]

Liquid, topical:

Chiggertox®: 2% (30 mL)

Outgro®: 20% (9 mL)

Skeeter Stik: 5% (14 mL) [contains menthol]

Tanac®: 10% (13 mL) [contains benzalkonium chloride]

Lozenge: 6 mg (18s) [contains menthol]; 15 mg (10s)

Cepacol® Sore Throat: 10 mg (18s) [contains cetylpyridinium, menthol; cherry, citrus, honey lemon, and menthol flavors]

Cepacol® Sore Throat: 10 mg (16s) [sugar free; contains cetylpyridinium, menthol; cherry and menthol flavors]

Cylex®: 15 mg [sugar free; contains cetylpyridinium chloride 5 mg; cherry flavor]

Mycinettes®: 15 mg (12s) [sugar free; contains sodium 9 mg; cherry or regular flavor]

Thorets: 18 mg (500s) [sugar free]

Trocaine®: 10 mg (40s, 400s)

Ointment, oral:

Anbesol® Cold Sore Therapy: 20% (7.1 g) [contains benzyl alcohol, allantoin, aloe, camphor, menthol, vitamin E]

Red Cross™ Canker Sore: 20% (7.5 g) [contains coconut oil]

Ointment, rectal (Americaine® Hemorrhoidal): 20% (30 g)

Ointment, topical:

Chiggerex®: 2% (50 g) [contains aloe vera]

Foille®: 5% (3.5 g, 14 g, 28 g) [contains chloroxylenol 0.1%, benzyl alcohol; corn oil base]

Pads, topical (Sting-Kill): 20% (8s) [contains menthol and tartrazine]

Paste, oral (Orabase® with Benzocaine): 20% (6 g)

Solution, otic drops (Oticaine, Otocaine™): 20% (15 mL)

Swabs, oral:

Hurricaine®: 20% (6s, 100s) [dye free; wild cherry flavor]

Orajel® Baby Teething: 7.5% (12s) [berry flavor]

Orajel® Medicated Mouth Sore, Orajel® Medicated Toothache: 20% (8s, 12s) [contains tartrazine]

Zilactin® Toothache and Gum Pain: 20% (8s) [grape flavor]

Swabs, topical (Sting-Kill): 20% (5s) [contains menthol and tartrazine]

Wax, oral (Dent's Extra Strength Toothache Gum): 20% (1 g)

Overdosage/Treatment

Decontamination: Lavage (within 1 hour)/activated charcoal; gastric decontamination should be considered for ingestions >100 mg/kg

Supportive therapy: Methemoglobinemia has been reported with benzocaine in oral overdose. Treatment is primarily symptomatic and supportive; termination of anesthesia by pneumatic tourniquet inflation should be attempted when the agent is administered by infiltration or regional injection. Methemoglobinemia may be treated with methylene blue, 1-2 mg/kg I.V. infused over several minutes. Seizures commonly respond to diazepam, while hypotension responds to I.V. fluids and Trendelenburg positioning. Bradyarrhythmias (when the heart rate is <60) can be treated with I.V., I.M., or SubQ atropine 15 mcg/kg. With the development of metabolic acidosis, I.V. sodium bicarbonate 0.5-2 mEq/kg and ventilatory assistance should be instituted.

Enhancement of elimination: Hyperbaric oxygen or exchange transfusion should be considered if the patient does not respond to methylene blue; exchange transfusion should be considered if methemoglobin levels >70%

Diagnostic Procedures

● Methemoglobin, Blood

Drug Interactions May antagonize actions of sulfonamides

Pregnancy Risk Factor C

Pregnancy Implications Reproduction studies have not been conducted.

Lactation Excretion in breast milk unknown/use caution

Specific References

Allen TL and Jolley SJ, "Iatrogenic Methemoglobinemia from Benzocaine Spray in Trauma," *Am J Emerg Med*, 2004, 22(3):226.

Leclaire AC, Mullett TW, Jahania MS, et al, "Methemoglobinemia Secondary to Topical Benzocaine Use in a Lung Transplant Patient," *Ann Pharmacother*. 2005, 39(2):373-6.

Saha SA, Kordouni MR, Siddiqui M and Arora RR, "Methemoglobinemia-induced Cardio-Respiratory Failure Secondary to Topical Anesthesia," *Am J Therapeutics*, 2006, 13:545-9.

Vidyarthi V, Manda R, Ahmed A, et al, "Severe Methemoglobinemia After Transesophageal Echocardiography," *Am J Ther*, 2003, 10(3):225-7.

Benzonatate

CAS Number 104-31-4

U.S. Brand Names Tessalon®

Use Symptomatic relief of nonproductive cough

Mechanism of Action Tetracaine congener with antitussive properties; suppresses cough by topical anesthetic action on the respiratory stretch receptors

Adverse Reactions

Cardiovascular: Chest numbness

Central nervous system: Sedation, headache, dizziness

Dermatologic: Rash

Gastrointestinal: GI upset

Neuromuscular & skeletal: Numbness in chest

Ocular: Burning sensation in eyes

Respiratory: Nasal congestion

Signs and Symptoms of Overdose Coma, CNS stimulation, disorientation, seizure, restlessness, tremor, ventricular tachycardia

Admission Criteria/Prognosis Admit any symptomatic patient or any pediatric ingestion.

Pharmacodynamics/Kinetics

Onset of action: Therapeutic: 15-20 minutes

Duration: 3-8 hours

Dosage Children >10 years and Adults: Oral: 100 mg 3 times/day or every 4 hours up to 600 mg/day

Monitoring Parameters Monitor patient's chest sounds and respiratory pattern

Administration

Swallow capsule whole (do not break or chew).

Contraindications Hypersensitivity to benzonatate, related compounds (such as tetracaine), or any component of the formulation

Dosage Forms

Capsule: 100 mg

Tessalon®: 100 mg, 200 mg

Reference Range Plasma benzonatate level of 2.5 mcg/mL associated with a 3.6 g ingestion and seizure development. Fatalities are associated with plasma levels >4 mcg/mL.

Overdosage/Treatment

Decontamination: Lavage within 1 hour/activated charcoal

Supportive therapy: Ventricular tachycardia may respond to direct current cardioversion (100 joules)

Drug Interactions No data reported

Pregnancy Risk Factor C

Lactation Excretion in breast milk unknown/use caution

Nursing Implications Change patient position every 2 hours to prevent pooling of secretions in lung; capsules are not to be crushed

Specific References

Boehm K, Caraccio TR, McGuigan MA, et al, "Benzonatate Overdose in an Infant and Review of Literature," *Clin Toxicol (Phila)*, 2005, 43:657.

Doyon S and Welsh C, "Life-Threatening Toxicity from Intravenous Injection of Benzonatate," *Clin Toxicol (Phila)*, 2005, 43:666.

Weber J, Scalzo A, Tabba M, et al, "Survival After Recreational I.V. Administration of Benzonatate," *J Toxicol Clin Toxicol*, 2003, 41(5):745.

Benztropine

Related Information
- Anticholinergic Effects of Common Psychotropics
- Therapeutic Drugs Associated with Hallucinations

CAS Number 86-13-5

U.S. Brand Names Cogentin®

Synonyms Benztropine Mesylate

Use Adjunctive treatment of all forms of parkinsonism; also used in treatment of drug-induced extrapyramidal effects (except tardive dyskinesia) and acute dystonic reactions

Mechanism of Action Thought to partially block striatal cholinergic receptors to help balance cholinergic and dopaminergic activity

Adverse Reactions

Cardiovascular: Tachycardia, sinus bradycardia, sinus tachycardia, tachycardia (supraventricular)

Central nervous system: Drowsiness, nervousness, visual hallucinations, restlessness, anxiety, extrapyramidal reaction, hyperthermia, coma, memory disturbance, mania, paranoia

Dermatologic: **Dry skin**, urticaria, pruritus, exanthema

Gastrointestinal: **Xerostomia, dry throat, constipation**, nausea, vomiting, ileus, esophageal atony

Genitourinary: Urinary retention

Neuromuscular & skeletal: Rhabdomyolysis, paresthesia

Ocular: Blurred vision, mydriasis

Respiratory: **Dry nose**

Miscellaneous: **Diaphoresis (decreased)**

Signs and Symptoms of Overdose Blurred vision, CNS depression, chorea (extrapyramidal), confusion, dementia, dizziness, fever, hallucinations, hyperthermia, impotence, nausea, nervousness, memory loss, seizures, vomiting

Pharmacodynamics/Kinetics

Onset of action: Oral: Within 1 hour; Parenteral: Within 15 minutes

Duration: 6-48 hours

Metabolism: Hepatic (N-oxidation, N-dealkylation, and ring hydroxylation)

Bioavailability: 29%

Dosage Use in children <3 years of age should be reserved for life-threatening emergencies

Drug-induced extrapyramidal reaction: Oral, I.M., I.V.:

Children >3 years: 0.02-0.05 mg/kg/dose 1-2 times/day

Adults: 1-4 mg/dose 1-2 times/day

Acute dystonia: Adults: I.M., I.V.: 1-2 mg

Parkinsonism: Oral:

Adults: 0.5-6 mg/day in 1-2 divided doses; if one dose is greater, administer at bedtime; titrate dose in 0.5 mg increments at 5- to 6-day intervals

Elderly: Initial: 0.5 mg once or twice daily; increase by 0.5 mg as needed at 5-6 days; maximum: 6 mg/day

Monitoring Parameters Symptoms of EPS or Parkinson's, pulse, anticholinergic effects

Contraindications Hypersensitivity to benztropine or any component of the formulation; pyloric or duodenal obstruction, stenosing peptic ulcers; bladder neck obstructions; achalasia; myasthenia gravis; children <3 years of age

Warnings Use with caution in older children (dose has not been established). Use with caution in hot weather or during exercise. May cause anhidrosis and hyperthermia, which may be severe. The risk is increased in hot environments, particularly in the elderly, alcoholics, patients with CNS disease, and those with prolonged outdoor exposure.

Elderly patients frequently develop increased sensitivity and require strict dosage regulation - side effects may be more severe in elderly patients with atherosclerotic changes. Use with caution in patients with tachycardia, cardiac arrhythmias, hypertension, hypotension, prostatic hyperplasia (especially in the elderly), any tendency toward urinary retention, liver or kidney disorders, and obstructive disease of the GI or GU tract. When given in large doses or to susceptible patients, may cause weakness and inability to move particular muscle groups.

May be associated with confusion or hallucinations (generally at higher dosages). Intensification of symptoms or toxic psychosis may occur in patients with mental disorders. Benztropine does not relieve symptoms of tardive dyskinesia.

Dosage Forms Injection, solution, as mesylate (Cogentin®): 1 mg/mL (2 mL)

Tablet, as mesylate: 0.5 mg, 1 mg, 2 mg

Reference Range Toxic serum levels: >25 ng/mL

Overdosage/Treatment Supportive therapy: Anticholinergic toxicity is caused by strong binding of the drug to cholinergic receptors. Anticholinesterase inhibitors reduce acetylcholinesterase, the enzyme that breaks down acetylcholine and thereby allows acetylcholine to accumulate and compete for receptor binding with the offending anticholinergic. For anticholinergic overdose with severe life-threatening symptoms, physostigmine 1-2 mg (0.5 or 0.02 mg/kg for children) SubQ or I.V., slowly may be given to reverse these effects.

Drug Interactions

Substrate of CYP2D6 (minor)

Amantadine, rimantadine: Central and/or peripheral anticholinergic syndrome can occur when administered with amantadine or rimantadine.

Anticholinergic agents: Central and/or peripheral anticholinergic syndrome can occur when administered with narcotic analgesics, phenothiazines and other antipsychotics (especially with high anticholinergic activity), tricyclic antidepressants, quinidine and some other antiarrhythmics, and antihistamines.

Atenolol: Anticholinergics may increase the bioavailability of atenolol (and possibly other beta-blockers); monitor for increased effect.

Cholinergic agents: Anticholinergics may antagonize the therapeutic effect of cholinergic agents; includes tacrine and donepezil.

Digoxin: Anticholinergics may decrease gastric degradation and increase the amount of digoxin absorbed by delaying gastric emptying.

Levodopa: Anticholinergics may increase gastric degradation and decrease the amount of levodopa absorbed by delaying gastric emptying.

Neuroleptics: Anticholinergics may antagonize the therapeutic effects of neuroleptics.

Pregnancy Risk Factor C

Pregnancy Implications May cross the placenta

Lactation Excretion in breast milk unknown/use caution

Nursing Implications No significant difference in onset of I.M. or I.V. injection, therefore, there is usually no need to use the I.V. route. Improvement is sometimes noticeable a few minutes after injection. Titrate dose in 0.5 mg increments at 5- or 6-day intervals.

Bepridil

CAS Number 49571-04-2; 64616-81-5; 64706-54-3; 74764-40-2

U.S. Brand Names Vascor® [DSC]

Use Treatment of chronic stable angina; only approved indication is hypertension, but may be used for congestive heart failure; doses should not be adjusted for at least 10 days after beginning therapy

Mechanism of Action Bepridil, a type 4 calcium antagonist, that possesses characteristics of the traditional calcium antagonist (nifedipine) but also possesses additional pharmacological properties. Similar to other calcium antagonists, bepridil relaxes vascular muscle, decreases pacemaker activity, and reduces cardiac muscle contractile force; however, a direct bradycardia effect of bepridil has been postulated, differing from calcium channel blockers. It is suggested that bradycardia effects arise out of direct action of bepridil on the S-A node; highly lipid soluble.

Adverse Reactions

Cardiovascular: Ventricular premature contractions, prolonged QT intervals, torsade de pointes, flattening or notched T waves, AV block, sinus bradycardia, QRS prolongation, sinus tachycardia, arrhythmias (ventricular), vasodilation

Central nervous system: **Headache, dizziness**

Dermatologic: Dermatitis, rash

Gastrointestinal: **Dyspepsia, nausea, abdominal pain, GI distress**, anorexia, GI upset, diarrhea, constipation, taste change

Genitourinary: Sexual difficulties

Hematologic: Agranulocytosis

Neuromuscular & skeletal: **Weakness**, tremors

Respiratory: Cough, nasal congestion, pharyngitis

Miscellaneous: Diaphoresis, flu-like syndrome

Signs and Symptoms of Overdose Bradycardia, asthenia, confusion, decreased cardiac output, drowsiness, gingival hyperplasia, hypotension, ileus, nausea, prolongation of QT interval, second or third degree AV block, torsade de pointes, tachycardia (ventricular)

Toxicodynamics/Kinetics

Distribution: V_d: 8.0 L/kg

Protein binding: 99%

Metabolism: Significant first-pass effect, metabolized to 4-hydroxyphenyl bepridil

Bioavailability: 59%

Half-life: Multiple doses: 42 hours; Single dose: 33 hours

Elimination: Renal: 66%; fecal: 22%

Dosage Adults: Oral: Initial: 200 mg/day, then adjust dose at 10-day intervals until optimal response is achieved; maximum daily dose: 400 mg

Monitoring Parameters ECG and serum electrolytes, blood pressure, signs and symptoms of congestive heart failure; elderly may need very close monitoring due to underlying cardiac and organ system defects

Reference Range Peak serum bepridil levels after a 400 mg dose: ~1631 ng/mL

Overdosage/Treatment

Decontamination: Lavage (within 1 hour)/activated charcoal

Supportive therapy: Fluids and vasopressors (dopamine, norepinephrine, or amrinone) are successful in treating hypotension and negative inotropic effects, calcium is often required to reverse chronotropic effects, ventricular arrhythmias should be treated with lidocaine or magnesium for torsade de pointes. Hyperinsulinemic therapy with 0.5-1.0 unit I.V. insulin bolus with an infusion of 0.2-1 unit/kg/hour plus a glucose bolus of 25 g I.V. and dextrose infusion to maintain a serum glucose >100 mg/dL may reverse cardiogenic shock due to calcium blockers.

Enhancement of elimination: Multiple dosing of activated charcoal may be effective

Antidote(s)

- Calcium Gluconate [ANTIDOTE]

Test Interactions ↑ aminotransferases, CPK, LDH

Pregnancy Risk Factor C

Betamethasone

Pronunciation (bay ta METH a sone)

Related Information

- Corticosteroids

U.S. Brand Names Beta-Val®; Celestone® Soluspan®; Celestone®; Diprolene® AF; Diprolene®; Luxiq®; Maxivate®

Synonyms Betamethasone Dipropionate, Augmented; Betamethasone Dipropionate; Betamethasone Sodium Phosphate; Betamethasone Valerate; Flubenisolone

Use Inflammatory dermatoses such as seborrheic or atopic dermatitis, neurodermatitis, anogenital pruritus, psoriasis, inflammatory phase of xerosis

Mechanism of Action Controls the rate of protein synthesis; depresses the migration of polymorphonuclear leukocytes, fibroblasts; reverses capillary permeability and lysosomal stabilization at the cellular level to prevent or control inflammation

Adverse Reactions

Systemic:

Cardiovascular: Congestive heart failure, edema, hyper-/hypotension

Central nervous system: Dizziness, headache, insomnia, intracranial pressure increased, lightheadedness, nervousness, pseudotumor cerebri, seizure, vertigo

Dermatologic: Ecchymoses, facial erythema, fragile skin, hirsutism, hyper-/hypopigmentation, perioral dermatitis (oral), petechiae, striae, wound healing impaired

Endocrine & metabolic: Amenorrhea, Cushing's syndrome, diabetes mellitus, growth suppression, hyperglycemia, hypokalemia, menstrual irregularities, pituitary-adrenal axis suppression, protein catabolism, sodium retention, water retention

Gastrointestinal: Abdominal distention, appetite increased, hiccups, indigestion, peptic ulcer, pancreatitis, ulcerative esophagitis

Local: Injection site reactions (intra-articular use), sterile abscess

Neuromuscular & skeletal: Arthralgia, muscle atrophy, fractures, muscle weakness, myopathy, osteoporosis, necrosis (femoral and humeral heads)

Ocular: Cataracts, glaucoma, intraocular pressure increased

Miscellaneous: Anaphylactoid reaction, diaphoresis, hypersensitivity, secondary infection

Topical:

Dermatologic: Acneiform eruptions, allergic dermatitis, burning, dry skin, erythema, folliculitis, hypertrichosis, irritation, miliaria, pruritus, skin atrophy, striae, vesiculation

Endocrine and metabolic effects have occasionally been reported with topical use.

Pharmacodynamics/Kinetics

Protein binding: 64%

Metabolism: Hepatic

Half-life elimination: 6.5 hours

Time to peak, serum: I.V.: 10-36 minutes

Excretion: Urine (<5% as unchanged drug)

Dosage

Base dosage on severity of disease and patient response

Children: Use lowest dose listed as initial dose for adrenocortical insufficiency (physiologic replacement)

I.M.: 0.0175-0.125 mg base/kg/day divided every 6-12 hours **or** 0.5-7.5 mg base/m²/day divided every 6-12 hours

Oral: 0.0175-0.25 mg/kg/day divided every 6-8 hours **or** 0.5-7.5 mg/m²/day divided every 6-8 hours

Topical:

≤12 years: Use is not recommended.

≥13 years: Use minimal amount for shortest period of time to avoid HPA axis suppression

Gel, augmented formulation: Apply once or twice daily; rub in gently. **Note:** Do not exceed 2 weeks of treatment or 50 g/week.

Lotion: Apply a few drops twice daily

Augmented formulation: Apply a few drops once or twice daily; rub in gently.

Note: Do not exceed 2 weeks of treatment or 50 mL/week.

Cream/ointment: Apply once or twice daily.

Augmented formulation: Apply once or twice daily.

Note: Do not exceed 2 weeks of treatment or 45 g/week.

Adolescents and Adults:

Oral: 2.4-4.8 mg/day in 2-4 doses; range: 0.6-7.2 mg/day

I.M.: Betamethasone sodium phosphate and betamethasone acetate: 0.6-9 mg/day (generally, ¹/₃ to ¹/₂ of oral dose) divided every 12-24 hours

Adults:

Intrabursal, intra-articular, intradermal: 0.25-2 mL

Intralesional: Rheumatoid arthritis/osteoarthritis:

Very large joints: 1-2 mL

Large joints: 1 mL

Medium joints: 0.5-1 mL

Small joints: 0.25-0.5 mL

Topical:

Foam: Apply to the scalp twice daily, once in the morning and once at night

Gel, augmented formulation: Apply once or twice daily; rub in gently.

Note: Do not exceed 2 weeks of treatment or 50 g/week.

Lotion: Apply a few drops twice daily

Augmented formulation: Apply a few drops once or twice daily; rub in gently.

Note: Do not exceed 2 weeks of treatment or 50 mL/week.

Cream/ointment: Apply once or twice daily

Augmented formulation: Apply once or twice daily.

Note: Do not exceed 2 weeks of treatment or 45 g/week.

Dosing adjustment in hepatic impairment: Adjustments may be necessary in patients with liver failure because betamethasone is extensively metabolized in the liver

Administration Oral: Not for alternate day therapy; once daily doses should be given in the morning.

I.M.: Do **not** give injectable sodium phosphate/acetate suspension I.V.

Topical: Apply topical sparingly to areas. Not for use on broken skin or in areas of infection. Do not apply to wet skin unless directed; do not cover with occlusive dressing. Do not apply very high potency agents to face, groin, axillae, or diaper area.

Foam: Invert can and dispense a small amount onto a saucer or other cool surface. Do not dispense directly into hands. Pick up small amounts of foam and gently massage into affected areas until foam disappears. Repeat until entire affected scalp area is treated.

Contraindications Hypersensitivity to betamethasone, other corticosteroids, or any component of the formulation; systemic fungal infections

Warnings

Topical use in patients ≤12 years of age is not recommended. May cause suppression of hypothalamic-pituitary-adrenal (HPA) axis, particularly in younger children or in patients receiving high doses for prolonged periods.

Very high potency topical products are not for treatment of rosacea, perioral dermatitis; not for use on face, groin, or axillae; not for use in a diapered area. Avoid concurrent use of other corticosteroids.

May suppress the immune system; patients may be more susceptible to infection. Use with caution in patients with systemic infections or ocular herpes simplex. Avoid exposure to chickenpox and measles.

Use with caution in patients with hypothyroidism, cirrhosis, ulcerative colitis; do not use occlusive dressings on weeping or exudative lesions and general caution with occlusive dressings should be observed; adverse effects may be increased. Discontinue if skin irritation or contact dermatitis should occur; do not use in patients with decreased skin circulation.

Dosage Forms

Note: Potency expressed as betamethasone base.

Cream, topical, as dipropionate: 0.05% (15 g, 45 g)

Maxivate®: 0.05% (45 g)

Cream, topical, as dipropionate augmented (Diprolene® AF): 0.05% (15 g, 50 g)

Cream, topical, as valerate (Beta-Val®): 0.1% (15 g, 45 g)

Foam, topical, as valerate (Luxiq®): 0.12% (50 g, 100 g, 150 g) [contains alcohol 60.4%]

Gel, topical, as dipropionate augmented: 0.05% (15 g, 50 g)

Injection, suspension (Celestone® Soluspan®): Betamethasone sodium phosphate 3 mg/mL and betamethasone acetate 3 mg/mL [6 mg/mL] (5 mL)

Lotion, topical, as dipropionate (Maxivate®): 0.05% (60 mL)

Lotion, topical, as dipropionate augmented (Diprolene®): 0.05% (30 mL, 60 mL)

Lotion, topical, as valerate (Beta-Val®): 0.1% (60 mL)

Ointment, topical, as dipropionate: 0.05% (15 g, 45 g)
 Maxivate®: 0.05% (45 g)

Ointment, topical, as dipropionate augmented (Diprolene®): 0.05% (15 g, 50 g)

Ointment, topical, as valerate: 0.1% (15 g, 45 g)

Syrup, as base (Celestone®): 0.6 mg/5 mL (118 mL)

Drug Interactions
Inhibits CYP3A4 (weak)

Phenytoin, phenobarbital, rifampin increase clearance of betamethasone. Potassium-depleting diuretics increase potassium loss.

Skin test antigens, immunizations: Betamethasone may decrease response and increase potential infections.

Insulin or oral hypoglycemics: Betamethasone may increase blood glucose.

Pregnancy Risk Factor C
There are no reports linking the use of betamethasone with congenital defects in the literature. Betamethasone is often used in patients with premature labor [26-34 weeks gestation] to stimulate fetal lung maturation.

Pregnancy Implications
Teratogenic effects were noted in animal studies. There are no reports linking the use of betamethasone with congenital defects in the literature. Betamethasone is often used in patients with premature labor [26-34 weeks gestation] to stimulate fetal lung maturation.

Lactation
Excretion in breast milk unknown/use caution

Additional Information
Very high potency: Augmented betamethasone dipropionate ointment, lotion

High potency: Augmented betamethasone dipropionate cream, betamethasone dipropionate cream and ointment

Intermediate potency: Betamethasone dipropionate lotion, betamethasone valerate cream

Betaxolol

Related Information
● Selected Properties of Beta-Adrenergic Blocking Drugs

CAS Number 63659-18-7; 63659-19-8

U.S. Brand Names Betoptic® S; Kerlone®

Synonyms Betaxolol Hydrochloride

Use Treatment of chronic open-angle glaucoma, ocular hypertension; management of hypertension

Mechanism of Action Competitively blocks beta$_1$-receptors, with little or no effect on beta$_2$-receptors; lipophilic; no membrane stabilizing effect

Adverse Reactions
Cardiovascular: Bradycardia, palpitations, edema, congestive heart failure, sinus bradycardia, myocardial depression, QRS prolongation, Raynaud's phenomenon, pericarditis

Central nervous system: Dizziness, psychosis, fatigue, drowsiness, headache, depression

Dermatologic: Exfoliative dermatitis, acne, alopecia, angioedema, toxic epidermal necrolysis, xerosis, urticaria, purpura, photosensitivity, psoriasis, exanthema

Gastrointestinal: Xerostomia

Local: Mild ocular stinging and discomfort, tearing, erythema, itching

Neuromuscular & skeletal: Paresthesia

Ocular: Photophobia, decreased corneal sensitivity, keratitis

Respiratory: Rhinitis

Miscellaneous: Cold extremities, systemic lupus erythematosus, lupus

Signs and Symptoms of Overdose Abdominal pain, ataxia, bradycardia, depression, hypotension, night terrors, photophobia

Pharmacodynamics/Kinetics
Onset of action: Ophthalmic: 30 minutes; Oral: 1-1.5 hours

Duration: Ophthalmic: ≥12 hours

Absorption: Ophthalmic: Some systemic; Oral: ~100%

Metabolism: Hepatic to multiple metabolites

Protein binding: Oral: 50%

Bioavailability: Oral: 89%

Half-life elimination: Oral: 12-22 hours

Time to peak: Ophthalmic: ~2 hours; Oral: 1.5-6 hours

Excretion: Urine

Dosage
Adults:

Ophthalmic: Instill 1 drop twice daily.

Oral: 5-10 mg/day; may increase dose to 20 mg/day after 7-14 days if desired response is not achieved. Initial dose in elderly: 5 mg/day.

Dosage adjustment in renal impairment: Administer 5 mg/day. Can increase every 2 weeks up to a maximum of 20 mg/day.

Cl$_{cr}$ <10 mL/minute: Administer 50% of usual dose.

Stability Avoid freezing ophthalmic forms

Monitoring Parameters Ophthalmic: Intraocular pressure. Systemic: Blood pressure, pulse

Administration
Ophthalmic: Shake suspension well before using. Tilt head back and instill in eye. Keep eye open and do not blink for 30 seconds. Apply gentle pressure to lacrimal sac for 1 minute. Wipe away excess from skin. Do not touch applicator to eye and do not contaminate tip of applicator.

Contraindications Hypersensitivity to betaxolol or any component of the formulation; sinus bradycardia; heart block greater than first-degree (except in patients with a functioning artificial pacemaker); cardiogenic shock; uncompensated cardiac failure; pulmonary edema; pregnancy (2nd and 3rd trimester)

Warnings Administer cautiously in compensated heart failure and monitor for a worsening of the condition. Beta-blocker therapy should not be withdrawn abruptly (particularly in patients with CAD), but gradually tapered to avoid acute tachycardia, hypertension, and/or ischemia. Use caution with concurrent use of beta-blockers and either verapamil or diltiazem; bradycardia or heart block can occur. Use caution in patients with PVD (can aggravate arterial insufficiency). In general, beta-blockers should be avoided in patients with bronchospastic disease. Betaxolol, with beta$_1$ selectivity, should be used cautiously in bronchospastic disease with close monitoring. Use cautiously in diabetics because it can mask prominent hypoglycemic symptoms. Can mask signs of thyrotoxicosis. Dosage adjustment required in severe renal impairment and in patients on dialysis. Use care with anesthetic agents which decrease myocardial function. Safety and efficacy in pediatric patients have not been established.

Dosage Forms
Solution, ophthalmic, as hydrochloride: 0.5% (5 mL, 10 mL, 15 mL) [contains benzalkonium chloride]

Suspension, ophthalmic, as hydrochloride (Betoptic® S): 0.25% (2.5 mL, 5 mL, 10 mL, 15 mL) [contains benzalkonium chloride]

Tablet, as hydrochloride (Kerlone®): 10 mg, 20 mg

Reference Range Oral dose of 20 mg produces a level of 42.6 ng/mL 4-6 hours after ingestion; postmortem blood level of 36,000 mcg/mL reported in a betaxolol-poisoned fatality

Overdosage/Treatment
Decontamination: Lavage (within 1 hour)/activated charcoal for oral ingestion

Supportive therapy: Sympathomimetics (eg, epinephrine or dopamine), atropine, glucagon, or a pacemaker can be used to treat the toxic bradycardia, asystole, and/or hypotension; initially, fluids may be the best treatment for toxic hypotension

Enhancement of elimination: Multiple dosing of activated charcoal may be effective

Drug Interactions
Substrate (major) of CYP1A2, 2D6; **Inhibits** CYP2D6 (weak)

Acetylcholinesterase inhibitors: May enhance the bradycardic effect of beta-blockers.

Alpha-/beta-agonists (direct-acting): Beta-blockers may enhance the vasopressor effect of alpha-/beta-agonists (direct-acting).

α_1-blockers: Beta-blockers may enhance the orthostatic effect of alpha$_1$-blockers. The risk associated with ophthalmic products is probably less than systemic products.

α_2-agonists: Beta-blockers may enhance the rebound hypertensive effect of α_2-agonists. This effect can occur when the alpha$_2$-agonist is abruptly withdrawn.

Aminoquinolines (antimalarial): May decrease the metabolism, via CYP isoenzymes, of beta-blockers.

Amiodarone: May enhance the bradycardic effect of beta-blockers.

Antipsychotic agents (phenothiazines): May enhance the hypotensive effect of beta-blockers. Either group may decrease the metabolism of the other.

Barbiturates: May increase the metabolism, via CYP isoenzymes, of beta-blockers.

β_2-agonists: May diminish the bradycardic effect of beta-blockers (β_1 selective).

Calcium channel blockers (nondihydropyridine): May enhance the hypotensive effect of beta-blockers; may also decrease the metabolism of beta-blockers.

Cardiac glycosides: Beta-blockers may enhance the bradycardic effect of cardiac glycosides.

CYP1A2 inducers: May decrease the levels/effects of betaxolol. Example inducers include aminoglutethimide, carbamazepine, phenobarbital, and rifampin.

CYP1A2 inhibitors: May increase the levels/effects of betaxolol. Example inhibitors include ciprofloxacin, fluvoxamine, ketoconazole, norfloxacin, ofloxacin, and rofecoxib.

CYP2D6 inhibitors: May increase the levels/effects of betaxolol. Example inhibitors include chlorpromazine, delavirdine, fluoxetine, miconazole, paroxetine, pergolide, quinidine, quinine, ritonavir, and ropinirole.

Dipyridamole: May enhance the bradycardic effect of beta-blockers.

Disopyramide: May enhance the bradycardic effect of beta-blockers.

Insulin: Beta-blockers may mask the hypoglycemic effect of insulin.

Lidocaine: Beta-blockers may decrease the metabolism of lidocaine.

Nonsteroidal anti-inflammatory agents (NSAIDs): May diminish the antihypertensive effect of beta-blockers.

Propafenone: May decrease the metabolism, via CYP isoenzymes, of beta-blockers. Propafenone possesses some independent beta-blocking activity.

Propoxyphene: May decrease the metabolism, via CYP isoenzymes, of beta-blockers.

Quinidine: May decrease the metabolism, via CYP isoenzymes, of beta-blockers.

Rifamycin derivatives: May increase the metabolism, via CYP isoenzymes, of beta-blockers.

Selective serotonin reuptake inhibitors (SSRIs): May enhance the bradycardic effect of beta-blockers.

Sulfonylureas: Beta-blockers may enhance the hypoglycemic effect of sulfonylureas; beta-blockers appear to mask tachycardia as an initial symptom of hypoglycemia. Ophthalmic beta-blockers are probably associated with lower risk than systemic agents.

Theophylline derivatives: Beta-blockers (beta$_1$ selective) may diminish the bronchodilatory effect of theophylline derivatives. this is true at higher beta-blockers doses where cardioselectivity is lost.

Pregnancy Risk Factor C (manufacturer); D (2nd and 3rd trimesters - expert analysis)

Pregnancy Implications Teratogenic effects were not observed in animal studies; however, there was drug-related postimplantation loss in rats and rabbits.

Lactation Oral: Enters breast milk/use caution

Additional Information Because of betaxolol's low lipid solubility, it is less likely to enter the CNS, decreasing the likelihood of CNS side effects.

Specific References

Chobanian AV, Bakris GL, Black HR, et al, "The Seventh Report of the Joint National Committee on Prevention, Detection, Evaluation, and Treatment of High Blood Pressure: The JNC 7 Report," *JAMA*, 2003, (19)289:2560-71.

Bethanechol

CAS Number 590-63-6; 674-38-4

U.S. Brand Names Urecholine®

Synonyms Bethanechol Chloride

Use Nonobstructive urinary retention and retention due to neurogenic bladder

Unlabeled/Investigational Use Treatment and prevention of bladder dysfunction caused by phenothiazines; diagnosis of flaccid or atonic neurogenic bladder; gastroesophageal reflux

Mechanism of Action Stimulates cholinergic receptors in the smooth muscle of the urinary bladder and GI tract resulting in increased peristalsis, increased gastrointestinal and pancreatic secretions, bladder muscle contraction, and increased ureteral peristaltic waves

Adverse Reactions

Cardiovascular: Flushed skin, hypotension, tachycardia

Central nervous system: Headache, malaise

Gastrointestinal: Abdominal cramps, diarrhea, eructation, nausea, salivation, vomiting

Genitourinary: Urinary urgency

Ocular: Lacrimation, miosis

Respiratory: Asthmatic attacks, bronchial constriction

Miscellaneous: Diaphoresis

Signs and Symptoms of Overdose Abdominal pain, AV block, defecation, diarrhea, drowsiness, flushing, headache, heart block, hypothermia, lacrimation, miosis, salivation, vomiting

Pharmacodynamics/Kinetics

Onset of action: 30-90 minutes

Duration: Up to 6 hours

Absorption: Variable

Dosage

Oral:

Children:

Urinary retention (unlabeled use): 0.6 mg/kg/day divided 3-4 times/day

Gastroesophageal reflux (unlabeled use): 0.1-0.2 mg/kg/dose given 30 minutes to 1 hour before each meal to a maximum of 4 times/day

Adults:

Urinary retention, neurogenic bladder, and/or bladder atony:

Oral: Initial: 10-50 mg 2-4 times/day (some patients may require dosages of 50-100 mg 4 times/day). To determine effective dose, may initiate at a dose of 5-10 mg, with additional doses of 5-10 mg hourly until an effective cumulative dose is reached. Cholinergic effects at higher oral dosages may be cumulative.

SubQ: Initial: 2.575 mg, may repeat in 15-30 minutes (maximum cumulative initial dose: 10.3 mg); subsequent doses may be given 3-4 times daily as needed (some patients may require more frequent dosing at 2.5- to 3-hour intervals). Chronic neurogenic atony may require doses of 7.5-10 every 4 hours.

Gastroesophageal reflux (unlabeled): Oral: 25 mg 4 times/day

Elderly: Use the lowest effective dose

Stability Store at room temperature of 15°C to 30°C (59°F to 86°F).

Monitoring Parameters Observe closely for side effects

Contraindications Hypersensitivity to bethanechol or any component of the formulation; mechanical obstruction of the GI or GU tract or when the strength or integrity of the GI or bladder wall is in question; hyperthyroidism, peptic ulcer disease, epilepsy, obstructive pulmonary disease, bradycardia, vasomotor instability, atrioventricular conduction defects, hypotension, or parkinsonism

Warnings Potential for reflux infection if the sphincter fails to relax as bethanechol contracts the bladder. Safety and efficacy in children have not been established.

Dosage Forms Tablet, as chloride: 5 mg, 10 mg, 25 mg, 50 mg

Overdosage/Treatment

Decontamination: Lavage (within 1 hour)/activated charcoal

Supportive therapy: Atropine (2-4 mg in adults or 0.04-0.08 mg/kg in children) should be given to control muscarinic symptoms; diazepam or lorazepam can be given for seizure control

Antidote(s)

• Atropine [ANTIDOTE]

Test Interactions ↑ lipase, amylase (S), bilirubin, aminotransferases (ALT, AST) (S)

Drug Interactions

Decreased effect: Procainamide, quinidine.

Increased toxicity: Bethanechol and ganglionic blockers may cause a critical fall in blood pressure. Cholinergic drugs or anticholinesterase agents may have additive effects.

Pregnancy Risk Factor C

Lactation Excretion in breast milk unknown/contraindicated

Nursing Implications Contraindicated for I.M. or I.V. use due to a likely severe cholinergic reaction; for SubQ injection only - should never be give I.M. or I.V.; observe closely for side effects; have bedpan readily available if administered for urinary retention

Additional Information Cardiac effects are less likely with bethanechol than acetylcholine chloride (Covochol®, Miochol®).

Biperiden

Related Information

• Dicyclomine

CAS Number 1235-82-1; 514-65-8

U.S. Brand Names Akineton®

Synonyms Biperiden Hydrochloride; Biperiden Lactate

Use Treatment of all forms of parkinsonism including drug-induced type (extrapyramidal symptoms)

Mechanism of Action Biperiden is a weak anticholinergic agent. The beneficial effects in Parkinson's disease and neuroleptic-induced extrapyramidal reactions are believed to be due to the inhibition of striatal cholinergic receptors.

Adverse Reactions

Cardiovascular: Hypotension (orthostatic), fibrillation (ventricular), tachycardia, palpitations

Central nervous system: Confusion, drowsiness, headache, loss of memory, ataxia, tiredness, euphoria, agitation, paranoia, delusions, visual hallucinations, cognitive dysfunction, hypothermia, extrapyramidal reaction

Dermatologic: **Dry skin**, skin rash, urticaria

Endocrine & metabolic: Decreased flow of breast milk

Gastrointestinal: **Constipation, xerostomia or dry throat**, dysphagia, bloated feeling, nausea, vomiting

Genitourinary: Dysuria

Neuromuscular & skeletal: Weakness, paresthesia

Ocular: Intraocular pain (increased), blurred vision, sensitivity to light (increased)

Respiratory: **Dry nose**

Miscellaneous: **Diaphoresis (decreased)**

Signs and Symptoms of Overdose Dry mouth, hyperthermia, hypertension, ileus, mydriasis, tachycardia, urinary retention

Admission Criteria/Prognosis Admit any patient with symptoms of anticholinergic toxicity

Pharmacodynamics/Kinetics

Bioavailability: 29%

Half-life elimination, serum: 18.4-24.3 hours

Time to peak, serum: 1-1.5 hours

Dosage

Children:

Extrapyramidal reaction:

I.M.: 0.04 mg/kg/dose

I.V.: 1-2 mg

Adults:

Parkinsonism: Oral: 2 mg 3-4 times/day

Extrapyramidal:

Oral: 2 mg 1-3 times/day

I.M., I.V.: 2 mg every 30 minutes up to 4 doses or 8 mg/day

Monitoring Parameters Symptoms of EPS or Parkinson's, pulse, anticholinergic effects (ie, CNS, bowel, and bladder function)

Administration
I.V. must be given slowly

Contraindications Hypersensitivity to biperiden or any component of the formulation; narrow-angle glaucoma; bowel obstruction, megacolon; myasthenia gravis

Warnings Use with caution in patients with narrow-angle glaucoma, peptic ulcer, urinary tract obstruction, and hyperthyroidism.

Dosage Forms Tablet, as hydrochloride: 2 mg

Reference Range After a 4 mg oral dose, peak plasma levels range from 3.9-6.3 ng/mL

Overdosage/Treatment
Decontamination: Lavage (within 1 hour)/activated charcoal
Supportive therapy: Physostigmine should be reserved for life-threatening anticholinergic effects; tachyarrhythmias can respond to physostigmine or I.V. beta-adrenergic blockers; agitation can be treated with benzodiazepines

Antidote(s)
- Physostigmine [ANTIDOTE]

Drug Interactions
Inhibits CYP2D6 (weak)
Amantadine, rimantadine: Central and/or peripheral anticholinergic syndrome can occur when administered with amantadine or rimantadine.
Anticholinergic agents: Central and/or peripheral anticholinergic syndrome can occur when administered with narcotic analgesics, phenothiazines and other antipsychotics (especially with high anticholinergic activity), tricyclic antidepressants, quinidine and some other antiarrhythmics, and antihistamines.
Atenolol: Anticholinergics may increase the bioavailability of atenolol (and possibly other beta-blockers); monitor for increased effect.
Cholinergic agents: Anticholinergics may antagonize the therapeutic effect of cholinergic agents; includes tacrine and donepezil.
Digoxin: Anticholinergics may decrease gastric degradation and increase the amount of digoxin absorbed by delaying gastric emptying.
Levodopa: Anticholinergics may increase gastric degradation and decrease the amount of levodopa absorbed by delaying gastric emptying.
Neuroleptics: Anticholinergics may antagonize the therapeutic effects of neuroleptics.

Pregnancy Risk Factor C

Nursing Implications No significant difference in onset of I.M. or I.V. injection, therefore, there is usually no need to use the I.V. route. Improvement is sometimes noticeable a few minutes after injection. Do not discontinue drug abruptly.

Bisacodyl

CAS Number 1336-29-4; 603-50-9

U.S. Brand Names Alophen® [OTC]; Bisac-Evac™ [OTC]; Bisacodyl Uniserts® [OTC]; Correctol® Tablets [OTC]; Doxidan® (reformulation) [OTC]; Dulcolax® [OTC]; Femilax™ [OTC]; Fleet® Bisacodyl Enema [OTC]; Fleet® Stimulant Laxative [OTC]; Gentlax® [OTC]; Modane Tablets® [OTC]; Veracolate [OTC]

Use Treatment of constipation; colonic evacuation prior to procedures or examination

Mechanism of Action Stimulates peristalsis by directly irritating the smooth muscle of the intestine, possibly the colonic intramural plexus; alters water and electrolyte secretion producing net intestinal fluid accumulation and laxation

Adverse Reactions
Endocrine & metabolic: Electrolyte and fluid imbalance (metabolic acidosis or alkalosis, hypocalcemia)
Gastrointestinal: Abdominal cramps, abdominal pain, nausea, vomiting, rectal burning

Signs and Symptoms of Overdose Abdominal pain, diarrhea, colonic atony, hypocalcemia, proctitis

Pharmacodynamics/Kinetics
Onset of action: Oral: 6-10 hours; Rectal: 0.25-1 hour
Absorption: Oral, rectal: Systemic, <5%

Dosage
Children:
Oral: >6 years: 5-10 mg (0.3 mg/kg) at bedtime or before breakfast
Rectal suppository:
<2 years: 5 mg as a single dose
>2 years: 10 mg
Adults:
Oral: 5-15 mg as single dose (up to 30 mg when complete evacuation of bowel is required)
Rectal suppository: 10 mg as single dose
Tannex:
Enema: 2.5 g in 1000 mL warm water
Barium enema: 2.5-5 g in 1000 mL barium suspension
Do not administer >10 g within 72-hour period

Administration Administer with a glass of water on an empty stomach for rapid effect. Do not administer within 1 hour of milk, any dairy products, or taking an antacid, to protect the coating.

Contraindications Hypersensitivity to bisacodyl or any component of the formulation; abdominal pain or obstruction, nausea, or vomiting

Dosage Forms
[DSC] = Discontinued product
Enema (Fleet® Bisacodyl Enema): 10 mg/30 mL (37 mL)
Suppository, rectal (Bisac-Evac™, Bisacodyl Uniserts®, Dulcolax®): 10 mg
Tablet, enteric coated (Alophen®, Bisac-Evac™, Correctol®, Dulcolax®, Femilax™, Fleet® Stimulant Laxative, Gentlax® [DSC], Modane®, Veracolate): 5 mg
Tablet, delayed release (Doxidan®): 5 mg

Reference Range Urinary bisacodyl diphenol level after a 10 mg oral dose ranges from 1-5 mcg/mL.

Overdosage/Treatment
Decontamination: Lavage (within 1 hour)/activated charcoal (no cathartic)
Supportive therapy: I.V. crystalloid hydration with potassium replacement

Drug Interactions Decreased effect: Milk, antacids; decreased effect of warfarin

Pregnancy Risk Factor C

Nursing Implications Administer tablets 2 hours prior to, or 4 hours after antacids; increased pH may dissolve the enteric coating leading to GI distress; do not crush enteric coated drug product

Bismuth Subgallate

CAS Number 7440-69-9

Use Symptomatic treatment of mild, nonspecific diarrhea; skin protectant; antacid; in industry, used in boiler plugs, electrical fuses, solders, and dental techniques

Mechanism of Action Binds with thiol-containing enzyme in cerebrum; antimicrobial action against *Helicobacter pylori*

Adverse Reactions
Central nervous system: Headache, drowsiness, malaise, memory disturbance, seizures, ataxia, encephalopathy
Dermatologic: Oral lesions, bluish gum line, erythema, alopecia
Gastrointestinal: **Feces discoloration (black), discoloration of the tongue (darkening)**, stomatitis, nausea, vomiting, fecal impaction, anorexia, bezoars, metallic taste
Hematologic: Methemoglobinemia
Neuromuscular & skeletal: Osteoporosis, tremors
Renal: Acute tubular necrosis

Signs and Symptoms of Overdose Confusion, dementia, fever, hyperactivity, hyperthermia, jaundice, memory loss, methemoglobinemia, proteinuria, seizures, stomatitis, sweating, tongue discoloration, tubular necrosis

Pharmacodynamics/Kinetics
Absorption: Bismuth is minimally absorbed across the GI tract while the salt (eg, salicylate) may be readily absorbed
Metabolism: Undergoes chemical dissociation to various bismuth salts after oral administration

Dosage Oral: 1-2 tablets 3 times/day with meals
Dosing adjustment in renal impairment: Should probably be avoided in patients with renal failure

Dosage Forms Tablet, chewable: 200 mg

Reference Range Plasma levels <5 mcg/dL are not toxic

Overdosage/Treatment
Decontamination: Emesis within 30 minutes or lavage (within 1 hour)/activated charcoal
Supportive therapy: D-penicillamine (15-40 mg/kg/day up to 250-500 mg 4 times/day in adults; 20-30 mg/kg/day orally in children before meals) has been tested in animal models; no human use experience. Alternatively, unithiol 250 mg I.V. every 4 hours within 6 hours of dialysis using a membrane with large pores. Continue dialysis until renal function is normal. Continue unithiol therapy with 500 mg/day in two divided doses for 2 weeks.

Antidote(s)
- Penicillamine [ANTIDOTE]
- Unithiol [ANTIDOTE]

Drug Interactions Decreased effect of tetracyclines
Increased toxicity of aspirin

Pregnancy Risk Factor C (D in 3rd trimester)

Nursing Implications Seek causes for diarrhea

Additional Information Bismuth subsalicylate (Pepto-Bismol®) contains 58% bismuth and 42% salicylate; do not exceed 4.2 g/day dosage; bismuth is radiopaque

Specific References
Dargan PI, Bailey CA, Greene SL, et al, "A Case of Severe Iatrogenic Bismuth Poisoning," *J Toxicol Clin Toxicol*, 2003, 41(5):738.

Bisoprolol

Related Information
- Atropine [ANTIDOTE]
- Glucagon [ANTIDOTE]
- Selected Properties of Beta-Adrenergic Blocking Drugs

CAS Number 104344-23-2; 66722-44-9; 66722-45-0

U.S. Brand Names Zebeta®

Synonyms Bisoprolol Fumarate

Use Treatment of hypertension, alone or in combination with other agents

Unlabeled/Investigational Use Angina pectoris, supraventricular arrhythmias, PVCs, CHF

Mechanism of Action Selective inhibitor of beta$_1$-adrenergic receptors; competitively blocks beta$_1$-receptors, with little or no effect on beta$_2$-receptors at doses <10 mg

Adverse Reactions

Cardiovascular: Bradycardia, palpitations, edema, CHF, reduced peripheral circulation, arrhythmias, chest pain, orthostatic hypotension, syncope, vasculitis

Central nervous system: **Drowsiness, insomnia**, mental depression, confusion (especially in the elderly), hallucinations, headache, nervousness

Dermatologic: Angioedema, exfoliative dermatitis, itching, psoriasiform eruption

Endocrine & metabolic: **Decreased sexual ability**

Gastrointestinal: Diarrhea or constipation, nausea, vomiting, stomach discomfort

Genitourinary: Peyronie's disease

Hematologic: Leukopenia, thrombocytopenia

Ocular: Mild ocular stinging and discomfort, tearing, photophobia, decreased corneal sensitivity, keratitis

Respiratory: Bronchospasm, dyspnea

Miscellaneous: Cold extremities

Signs and Symptoms of Overdose Ataxia, bradycardia, cold extremities, cough, hypoglycemia, hypotension, impotence, insomnia, night terrors, wheezing

Pharmacodynamics/Kinetics

Onset of action: 1-2 hours

Absorption: Rapid and almost complete

Distribution: Widely; highest concentrations in heart, liver, lungs, and saliva; crosses blood-brain barrier; enters breast milk

Protein binding: 26% to 33%

Metabolism: Extensively hepatic; significant first-pass effect

Half-life elimination: 9-12 hours

Time to peak: 1.7-3 hours

Excretion: Urine (3% to 10% as unchanged drug); feces (<2%)

Dosage

Oral:

Adults: 2.5-5 mg once daily, may be increased to 10 mg, and then up to 20 mg once daily, if necessary

Hypertension (JNC 7): 2.5-10 mg once daily

Elderly: Initial dose: 2.5 mg/day; may be increased by 2.5-5 mg/day; maximum recommended dose: 20 mg/day

Dosing adjustment in renal/hepatic impairment: Cl$_{cr}$ <40 mL/minute: Initial: 2.5 mg/day; increase cautiously.

Hemodialysis: Not dialyzable

Monitoring Parameters Blood pressure, ECG, neurologic status

Contraindications Hypersensitivity to bisoprolol or any component of the formulation; sinus bradycardia; heart block greater than first-degree (except in patients with a functioning artificial pacemaker); cardiogenic shock; uncompensated cardiac failure; pulmonary edema; pregnancy (2nd and 3rd trimesters)

Warnings Administer cautiously in compensated heart failure and monitor for a worsening of the condition. Beta-blocker therapy should not be withdrawn abruptly (particularly in patients with CAD), but gradually tapered to avoid acute tachycardia, hypertension, and/or ischemia. Use caution in patients with PVD (can aggravate arterial insufficiency). Use caution with concurrent use of beta-blockers and either verapamil or diltiazem; bradycardia or heart block can occur. In general, beta-blockers should be avoided in patients with bronchospastic disease. Bisoprolol, with B1 selectivity, should be used cautiously in bronchospastic disease with close monitoring. Use cautiously in diabetics because it can mask prominent hypoglycemic symptoms. Can mask signs of thyrotoxicosis. Can cause fetal harm when administered in pregnancy. Dosage adjustment is required in patients with significant hepatic or renal dysfunction. Use care with anesthetic agents which decrease myocardial function.

Dosage Forms Tablet, as fumarate: 5 mg, 10 mg

Reference Range Peak plasma level of 56 ng/mL after 10 mg dose and 445 ng/mL after 100 mg dose

Overdosage/Treatment

Decontamination: Lavage (within 1 hour)/activated charcoal; do **not** use ipecac

Supportive therapy: Glucagon (50-150 mcg/kg followed by continuous drip of 1-5 mg/hour) for positive chronotropic effect; atropine/isoproterenol can be utilized to increase heart rate; calcium chloride may also be effective; do **not** use epinephrine

Enhancement of elimination: Multiple dosing of activated charcoal is not likely to be of benefit; dialysis is not useful

Antidote(s)
- Atropine [ANTIDOTE]
- Glucagon [ANTIDOTE]

Test Interactions ↑ thyroxine (S), glucose; no effect on lipid profile

Drug Interactions

Substrate of CYP2D6 (minor), 3A4 (major)

Alpha-blockers (prazosin, terazosin): Concurrent use of beta-blockers may increase risk of orthostasis.

AV conduction-slowing agents (digoxin): Effects may be additive with beta-blockers.

Clonidine: Hypertensive crisis after or during withdrawal of either agent.

CYP3A4 inducers: CYP3A4 inducers may decrease the levels/effects of bisoprolol. Example inducers include aminoglutethimide, carbamazepine, nafcillin, nevirapine, phenobarbital, phenytoin, and rifamycins.

CYP3A4 inhibitors: May increase the levels/effects of bisoprolol. Example inhibitors include azole antifungals, clarithromycin, diclofenac, doxycycline, erythromycin, imatinib, isoniazid, nefazodone, nicardipine, propofol, protease inhibitors, quinidine, telithromycin, and verapamil.

Glucagon: Bisoprolol may blunt the hyperglycemic action of glucagon.

Insulin: Bisoprolol may mask tachycardia from hypoglycemia.

NSAIDs (ibuprofen, indomethacin, naproxen, piroxicam) may reduce the antihypertensive effects of beta-blockers.

Salicylates may reduce the antihypertensive effects of beta-blockers.

Sulfonylureas: Beta-blockers may alter response to hypoglycemic agents.

Pregnancy Risk Factor C (manufacturer); D (2nd and 3rd trimesters - expert analysis)

Pregnancy Implications No data available on whether bisoprolol crosses the placenta. Beta-blockers have been associated with persistent bradycardia, hypotension, and IUGR; IUGR is probably related to maternal hypertension. Available evidence suggests beta-blockers are generally safe during pregnancy (JNC-7). Cases of neonatal hypoglycemia have been reported following maternal use of beta-blockers at parturition or during breast-feeding.

Lactation Enters breast milk/use caution

Specific References

Chobanian AV, Bakris GL, Black HR, et al, "The Seventh Report of the Joint National Committee on Prevention, Detection, Evaluation, and Treatment of High Blood Pressure: The JNC 7 Report," *JAMA*, 2003, (19)289:2560-71.

Blasticidin S

CAS Number 2079-00-7

Synonyms BLA-s; Blaes-M

Use A contact fungicide used for control of rice blast (*Picicularia oryzae*) in Taiwan, Japan, Korea, Central and South America

Mechanism of Toxic Action A benzylamino benzene-sulfonate derived from fermentation of *Streptomyces griseochromogenes*, blasticidin S inhibits protein synthesis (spore protein polymerization). Can cause severe mucous membrane irritation.

Adverse Reactions

Cardiovascular: Hypotension, cyanosis, acrocyanosis

Central nervous system: Fever, headache

Dermatologic: Erythema

Endocrine & metabolic: Hyponatremia

Gastrointestinal: Vomiting (immediate and protracted), profuse watery diarrhea, abdominal pain, nausea

Ocular: Conjunctivitis, corneal ulcers, keratitis, blepharitis

Respiratory: Pharyngitis, dyspnea, cough, pulmonary edema, aspiration pneumonitis, bronchospasm, stridor

Admission Criteria/Prognosis Admit any symptomatic patient (other than with local irritation) or any ingestion >0.1 g

Monitoring Parameters ECG, electrolytes

Overdosage/Treatment

Decontamination: **Oral**: Dilute with water (4-8 ounces). **Do not** induce emesis. Lavage (within 1 hour)/activated charcoal or sodium polystyrene sulfonate (15 g of resin in adults or 1 g/kg in children every 6 hours). **Dermal**: Wash the exposed area with soap and water. **Inhalation**: Administer humidified oxygen. **Ocular**: Copiously irrigate with saline or water. The addition of calcium salts within 30 minutes of exposure may decrease eye irritation.

Supportive therapy: Treat hypotension with I.V. crystalloid replacement. Vasopressors can be used for refractory cases. Corticosteroids may be helpful in treating respiratory adverse effects.

Additional Information Lethal oral dose (LD$_{50}$): ~20 mg/kg. Conjunctivitis can be caused by as little as 1 mcg of ocular exposure while 20 mcg can cause keratitis. Conjunctivitis usually develops within 5 hours and may take 10 days to resolve.

Bleomycin

CAS Number 11056-06-7; 9041-93-4
U.S. Brand Names Blenoxane®
Synonyms Bleo; Bleomycin Sulfate; BLM; NSC-125066
Use Treatment of squamous cell carcinomas, melanomas, sarcomas, testicular carcinoma, Hodgkin's lymphoma, and non-Hodgkin's lymphoma
  Orphan drug: Sclerosing agent for malignant pleural effusion
Mechanism of Action Inhibits synthesis of DNA; binds to DNA leading to single- and double-strand breaks

Adverse Reactions
Cardiovascular: **Raynaud's phenomenon**
Central nervous system: **Chills**, hypersomnia, personality changes, memory impairment, thermal dysfunction, **mild febrile reaction, fever**
Dermatologic: Alopecia, hyperpigmentation, nailbed changes, vesiculation, radiation recall dermatitis, scleroderma, **pruritic erythema**
Gastrointestinal: **Stomatitis, anorexia, nausea, vomiting**, weight loss, loss of taste perception, **mucocutaneous toxicity**
Local: **Pain at tumor site, phlebitis**, extravasation injury
Respiratory: Dose related when total dose is >400 units or with single doses >30 units; pathogenesis is poorly understood, but may be related to damage of pulmonary, vascular, or connective tissue. Manifested as an acute or chronic interstitial pneumonitis with interstitial fibrosis, hypoxia, and death. Symptoms include cough, dyspnea, and bilateral pulmonary infiltrates noted on chest x-ray. It is controversial whether steroids improve symptoms of bleomycin pulmonary toxicity. Risk factors for development of pulmonary toxicity include cumulative dose >450 mg/m², age >70 years, pre-existing pulmonary disease, high oxygen therapy, concomitant chemotherapy, or thoracic irradiation. Bilateral lung opacities.
Miscellaneous: Patients may become febrile after intracavitary administration

Signs and Symptoms of Overdose Acrodynia, chills, cystitis (hemorrhagic), deafness, erythema, fever, hyperpigmentation, hyperthermia, hypocalcemia, pulmonary fibrosis, seizures, thrombocytopenia

Pharmacodynamics/Kinetics
Absorption: I.M. and intrapleural administration: 30% to 50% of I.V. serum concentrations; intraperitoneal and SubQ routes produce serum concentrations equal to those of I.V.
Distribution: V_d: 22 L/m²; highest concentrations in skin, kidney, lung, heart tissues; lowest in testes and GI tract; does not cross blood-brain barrier
Protein binding: 1%
Metabolism: Via several tissues including hepatic, GI tract, skin, pulmonary, renal, and serum
Half-life elimination: Biphasic (renal function dependent):
  Normal renal function: Initial: 1.3 hours; Terminal: 9 hours
  End-stage renal disease: Initial: 2 hours; Terminal: 30 hours
Time to peak, serum: I.M.: Within 30 minutes
Excretion: Urine (50% to 70% as active drug)

Dosage
Refer to individual protocols; 1 unit = 1 mg
May be administered I.M., I.V., SubQ, or intracavitary
Children and Adults:
  Test dose for lymphoma patients: I.M., I.V., SubQ: Because of the possibility of an anaphylactoid reaction, ≤2 units of bleomycin for the first 2 doses; monitor vital signs every 15 minutes; wait a minimum of 1 hour before administering remainder of dose; if no acute reaction occurs, then the regular dosage schedule may be followed
  Single-agent therapy:
    I.M./I.V./SubQ: Squamous cell carcinoma, lymphoma, testicular carcinoma: 0.25-0.5 units/kg (10-20 units/m²) 1-2 times/week
    CIV: 15 units/m² over 24 hours daily for 4 days
  Combination-agent therapy:
    I.M./I.V.: 3-4 units/m²
    I.V.: ABVD: 10 units/m² on days 1 and 15
    Maximum cumulative lifetime dose: 400 units
  Pleural sclerosing: 60-240 units as a single infusion. Dose may be repeated at intervals of several days if fluid continues to accumulate (mix in 50-100 mL of D₅W, NS, or SWFI); may add lidocaine 100-200 mg to reduce local discomfort.
  Dosing adjustment in renal impairment:
    Cl_{cr} 10-50 mL/minute: Administer 75% of normal dose
    Cl_{cr} <10 mL/minute: Administer 50% of normal dose

Monitoring Parameters Pulmonary function tests (total lung volume, forced vital capacity, carbon monoxide diffusion), renal function, chest x-ray, temperature initially

Administration Administer I.V. slowly over at least 10 minutes (no greater than 1 unit/minute) at a concentration not to exceed 3 units/mL; bleomycin for I.V. continuous infusion can be further diluted in normal saline (preferred) or D₅W

Contraindications Hypersensitivity to bleomycin or any component of the formulation; severe pulmonary disease; pregnancy

Warnings Hazardous agent - use appropriate precautions for handling and disposal. **[U.S. Boxed Warnings]: Occurrence of pulmonary fibrosis (commonly presenting as pneumonitis) is higher in elderly patients, patients receiving >400 units total lifetime dose or single doses >30 units, smokers, and patients with prior radiation therapy or receiving concurrent oxygen. A severe idiosyncratic reaction consisting of hypotension, mental confusion, fever, chills, and wheezing (similar to anaphylaxis) has been reported in 1% of lymphoma patients treated with bleomycin.** Since these reactions usually occur after the first or second dose, careful monitoring is essential after these doses. Follow manufacturer recommendations for administering O_2 during surgery to patients who have received bleomycin. Use caution with renal impairment, may require dose adjustment. May cause renal or hepatic toxicity. **[U.S. Boxed Warning]: Should be administered under the supervision of an experienced cancer chemotherapy physician.** Safety and efficacy in children have not been established.

Dosage Forms Injection, powder for reconstitution, as sulfate: 15 units, 30 units

Reference Range Steady-state levels for a dose of 20 units/day is from 50-200 milliunits/L

Overdosage/Treatment Supportive therapy: Use minimal amounts of oxygen; steroids are of uncertain benefit in preventing pulmonary fibrosis; use of 21-aminosteroids (U-74389 G; 10 mg/kg I.V.) to reduce pulmonary fibrosis is experimental

Test Interactions ↑ potassium (S)

Drug Interactions
Cisplatin: May decrease bleomycin elimination.
Digitalis glycosides: Bleomycin may decrease plasma levels of digoxin.
Phenytoin: Results in decreased phenytoin levels.

Pregnancy Risk Factor D
Pregnancy Implications Animal studies have demonstrated teratogenic and abortifacient effects. There are no adequate and well-controlled studies in pregnant women. Women of childbearing potential should avoid becoming pregnant during treatment.

Lactation Excretion in breast milk unknown/not recommended

Additional Information Myelosuppressive effects: **WBC**: Rare. **Platelets**: Rare. Onset (days): 7; Nadir (days): 14; Recovery (days): 21

Specific References
Burdick MD, Murray LA, Keane MP, et al. "CXCL11 Attenuates Bleomycin-Induced Pulmonary Fibrosis via Inhibition of Vascular Remodeling," *Am J Respir Crit Care Med*, 2005, 171(3):261-8.

Botulinum Toxin Type A

Related Information
  • Clostridium botulinum Food Poisoning
U.S. Brand Names Botox® Cosmetic; Botox®
Synonyms BTX-A
Use Treatment of strabismus and blepharospasm associated with dystonia (including benign essential blepharospasm or VII nerve disorders in patients ≥12 years of age); cervical dystonia (spasmodic torticollis) in patients ≥16 years of age; temporary improvement in the appearance of lines/wrinkles of the face (moderate to severe glabellar lines associated with corrugator and/or procerus muscle activity) in adult patients ≤65 years of age
  Orphan drug: Treatment of dynamic muscle contracture in pediatric cerebral palsy patients

Unlabeled/Investigational Use Treatment of oromandibular dystonia, spasmodic dysphonia (laryngeal dystonia) and other dystonias (ie, writer's cramp, focal task-specific dystonias); migraine treatment and prophylaxis

Mechanism of Action Botulinum A toxin is a neurotoxin produced by *Clostridium botulinum*, spore-forming anaerobic bacillus. Six distinct antigenic types of neurotoxins are generated by *Clostridium botulinum*, named from A to F, however, only the A toxin has been used clinically. Botulinum A toxin is a double-chain protein with a molecular weight of ~900,000; active portion of the molecule is the light chain and the heavy chain is inactive. The toxin appears to affect only one structure in humans, the presynaptic membrane of the neuromuscular junction, where it prevents calcium-dependent release of acetylcholine and produces a state of denervation. Following injection of the toxin into a muscle, the degree of resultant skeletal muscle asthenia or paralysis is dependent upon the dose administered. Muscle inactivation persists until new fibrils grow from the nerve and form junction plates on new areas of the muscle-cell walls. The antagonist muscle shortens simultaneously ("contracture"), taking up the slack created by agonist paralysis; following several weeks of paralysis, alignment of the eye is measurably changed, despite return of innervation to the injected muscle. In patients with sixth nerve palsy, the objective is to prevent contracture of the ipsilateral medial rectus muscle while the patient awaits recovery of the palsied lateral rectus muscle.

Adverse Reactions
Adverse effects usually occur in 1 week and may last up to several months.

Cardiovascular: Arrhythmia, myocardial infarction, syncope (blepharospasm)

Central nervous system: **Headache** (cervical dystonia, reduction of glabellar lines; can occur with other uses), dizziness (cervical dystonia, reduction of glabellar lines); speech disorder (cervical dystonia), fever (cervical dystonia), drowsiness (cervical dystonia), vertigo with nystagmus (reduction of glabellar lines)

Dermatologic: Ecchymoses (blepharospasm), erythema multiforme, pruritus, psoriasiform eruption, skin rash, urticaria

Gastrointestinal: **Dysphagia** (cervical dystonia), xerostomia (cervical dystonia), nausea (cervical dystonia, reduction of glabellar lines)

Local: Injection site reaction

Neuromuscular & skeletal: **Neck pain** (cervical dystonia), back pain (cervical dystonia); hypertonia (cervical dystonia); weakness (cervical dystonia, reduction of glabellar lines); facial pain (reduction of glabellar lines), stiffness (cervical dystonia, blepharospasm), numbness (cervical dystonia), facial weakness (blepharospasm), brachial plexopathy (cervical dystonia), focal facial paralysis (blepharospasm), exacerbation of myasthenia gravis (blepharospasm, reduction of glabellar lines)

Ocular: **Ptosis** (blepharospasm, strabismus, reduction of glabellar lines); vertical deviation (strabismus), dry eyes (blepharospasm), superficial punctate keratitis (blepharospasm), ectropion (blepharospasm), lagophthalmos (blepharospasm), eyelid edema (blepharospasm), tearing (blepharospasm), photophobia (blepharospasm); reduced blinking leading to corneal ulceration (blepharospasm), corneal perforation (blepharospasm); acute angle-closure glaucoma (blepharospasm), vitreous hemorrhage (blepharospasm), retrobulbar hemorrhage (strabismus), ciliary ganglion damage (strabismus), anterior segment eye ischemia (strabismus), retinal vein occlusion (reduction of glabellar lines), glaucoma (reduction of glabellar lines)

Otic: Abnormal hearing/hearing loss (reduction of glabellar lines)

Respiratory: **Upper respiratory infection** (cervical dystonia), cough (cervical dystonia), rhinitis (cervical dystonia), infection (reduction of glabellar lines), dyspnea (cervical dystonia), aspiration (cervical dystonia)

Miscellaneous: Flu syndrome (cervical dystonia, reduction of glabellar lines), allergic reactions

Signs and Symptoms of Overdose Blurred vision, conjunctivitis, corneal irritation, cranial nerve palsies, dermatitis, dry eyes, dry mouth, dysphagia, lacrimation, mydriasis, neuromuscular paralysis, photophobia

Pharmacodynamics/Kinetics

Onset of action (improvement):
Blepharospasm: ~3 days
Cervical dystonia: ~2 weeks
Strabismus: ~1-2 days
Reduction of glabellar lines (Botox® Cosmetic): 1-2 days, increasing in intensity during first week

Duration:
Blepharospasm: ~3 months
Cervical dystonia: <3 months
Strabismus: ~2-6 weeks
Primary axillary hyperhidrosis: 201 days (mean)
Reduction of glabellar lines (Botox® Cosmetic): Up to 3 months

Absorption: Not expected to be present in peripheral blood at recommended doses

Time to peak:
Blepharospasm: 1-2 weeks
Cervical dystonia: ~6 weeks
Strabismus: Within first week

Dosage

I.M.:

Children ≥16 years and Adults:
Achalasia: 80 units (20 units in each quadrant) injected directly into inferior esophageal sphincter through upper endoscopy

Cervical dystonia: For dosing guidance, the mean dose is 236 units (25th to 75th percentile range 198-300 units) divided among the affected muscles in patients previously treated with botulinum toxin. Initial dose in previously untreated patients should be lower. Sequential dosing should be based on the patient's head and neck position, localization of pain, muscle hypertrophy, patient response, and previous adverse reactions. The total dose injected into the sternocleidomastoid muscles should be ≤100 units to decrease the occurrence of dysphagia.

Axillary hyperhidrosis: 200 units injected into the axilla

Chronic anal fissure: 20 units through a 27 gauge needle near the fissure; after 2 months, can give second dose of 25 units of botulinum A

Children ≥12 years and Adults:
Blepharospasm: Initial dose: 1.25-2.5 units injected into the medial and lateral pretarsal orbicularis oculi of the upper and lower lid; dose may be increased up to twice the previous dose if the response from the initial dose lasted ≤2 months; maximum dose per site: 5 units; cumulative dose in a 30-day period: ≤200 units. Tolerance may occur if treatments are given more often than every 3 months, but the effect is not usually permanent.

Strabismus:

Initial dose:
Vertical muscles and for horizontal strabismus <20 prism diopters: 1.25-2.5 units in any one muscle
Horizontal strabismus of 20-50 prism diopters: 2.5-5 units in any one muscle
Persistent VI nerve palsy >1 month: 1.5-2.5 units in the medial rectus muscle

Re-examine patients 7-14 days after each injection to assess the effect of that dose. Subsequent doses for patients experiencing incomplete paralysis of the target may be increased up to twice the previous administered dose. The maximum recommended dose as a single injection for any one muscle is 25 units. Do not administer subsequent injections until the effects of the previous dose are gone.

Adults ≤65 years: Reduction of glabellar lines: An effective dose is determined by gross observation of the patient's ability to activate the superficial muscles injected. The location, size and use of muscles may vary markedly among individuals. Inject 0.1 mL dose into each of five sites, two in each corrugator muscle and one in the procerus muscle (total dose 0.5 mL).

Elderly: No specific adjustment recommended

Dosage adjustment in renal impairment: No specific adjustment recommended

Dosage adjustment in hepatic impairment: No specific adjustment recommended

Administration

Cervical dystonia: Use 25-, 27-, or 30-gauge needle for superficial muscles and a longer 22-gauge needle for deeper musculature; electromyography may help localize the involved muscles

Blepharospasm: Use a 27- or 30-gauge needle without electromyography guidance. Avoid injecting near the levator palpebrae superioris (may decrease ptosis); avoid medial lower lid injections (may decrease diplopia). Apply pressure at the injection site to prevent ecchymosis in the soft eyelid tissues.

Strabismus injections: Must use surgical exposure or electromyographic guidance; use the electrical activity recorded from the tip of the injections needle as a guide to placement within the target muscle. Local anesthetic and ocular decongestant should be given before injection. The volume of injection should be 0.05-0.15 mL per muscle. Many patients will require additional doses because of inadequate response to initial dose.

Reduction of glabellar lines (Botox® Cosmetic): Use a 30-gauge needle. Ensure injected volume/dose is accurate and where feasible keep to a minimum. Avoid injection near the levator palpebrae superioris. Medial corrugator injections should be at least 1 cm above the bony supraorbital ridge. Do not inject toxin closer than 1 cm above the central eyebrow.

Contraindications Hypersensitivity to albumin, botulinum toxin, or any component of the formulation; infection at the proposed injection site(s); pregnancy. Relative contraindications include diseases of neuromuscular transmission; coagulopathy including therapeutic anticoagulation; uncooperative patient.

Warnings

Higher doses or more frequent administration may result in neutralizing antibody formation and loss of efficacy. Product contains albumin and may carry a remote risk of virus transmission. Use caution if there is inflammation, excessive weakness, or atrophy at the proposed injection site(s). Have appropriate support in case of anaphylactic reaction. Use with caution in patients with neuromuscular diseases (such as myasthenia gravis), neuropathic disorders (such as amyotrophic lateral sclerosis), or patients taking aminoglycosides or other drugs that interfere with neuromuscular transmission. Ensure adequate contraception in women of childbearing years. Long-term effects of chronic therapy unknown.

Cervical dystonia: Dysphagia is common. It may be severe requiring alternative feeding methods. Risk factors include smaller neck muscle mass, bilateral injections into the sternocleidomastoid muscle, or injections into the levator scapulae. Dysphasia may be associated with increased risk of upper respiratory infection.

Blepharospasm: Reduced blinking from injection of the orbicularis muscle can lead to corneal exposure and ulceration.

Strabismus: Retrobulbar hemorrhages may occur from needle penetration into orbit. Spatial disorientation, double vision, or past pointing may occur if one or more extraocular muscles are paralyzed. Covering the affected eye may help. Careful testing of corneal sensation, avoidance of lower lid injections, and treatment of epithelial defects are necessary.

Primary axillary hyperhidrosis: Evaluate for secondary causes prior to treatment (eg, hyperthyroidism). Safety and efficacy for treatment of hyperhidrosis in other areas of the body have not been established.

Temporary reduction in glabellar lines: Do not use more frequently than every 3 months. Patients with marked facial asymmetry, ptosis, excessive dermatochalasis, deep dermal scarring, thick sebaceous skin, or the inability to substantially lessen glabellar lines by physically spreading them apart were excluded from clinical trials. Reduced blinking from injection of the orbicularis muscle can lead to corneal exposure and ulceration. Spatial disorientation, double vision, or past pointing may occur if one or more extraocular muscles are paralyzed.

Dosage Forms Injection, powder for reconstitution [preservative free]: *Clostridium botulinum* toxin type A 100 units [contains human albumin]

Overdosage/Treatment Supportive therapy: Treatment is entirely supportive; artificial ventilation may be required; antitoxins to botulism are of no benefit; neostigmine (intranasal: 3 puffs in each nostril prior to meals) has been used to treat dysphagia

Drug Interactions

Aminoglycosides: May increase neuromuscular blockade.

Neuromuscular-blocking agents: May increase neuromuscular blockade.

Other agents which may have neuromuscular-blocking activity: Calcium channel blockers, catecholamines, chloroquine, clindamycin, colistin, corticosteroids, digitalis glycosides, diuretics, inhalation anesthetics, lidocaine, lincomycin, magnesium salts, opioids, phenytoin, phenelzine, polymixin B, procainamide, propranolol, quinidine, and tetracyclines.

Pregnancy Risk Factor C (manufacturer)

Pregnancy Implications Decreased fetal body weight, delayed ossification, maternal toxicity, abortions, and fetal malformations were observed in animal studies. Human reproduction studies have not been conducted. Avoid use in pregnancy.

Lactation Excretion in breast milk unknown/not recommended

Nursing Implications To alleviate spatial disorientation or double vision in strabismic patients, cover the affected eye; inject using a 27- to 30-gauge needle

Specific References

American Medical Association; American Nurses Association-American Nurses Foundation; Centers for Disease Control and Prevention; Center for Food Safety and Applied Nutrition, Food and Drug Administration; Food Safety and Inspection Service, US Department of Agriculture, "Diagnosis and Management of Foodborne Illnesses: A Primer for Physicians and Other Health Care Professionals," *MMWR Recomm Rep*, 2004, 53(RR-4):1-33.

Anand KS, Prasad A, Singh MM, et al, "Botulinum Toxin Type A in Prophylactic Treatment of Migraine," *Am J Ther*, 2006, 13(3):183-7.

Lim EH, Ong BC, and Seet RS, "Botulinum Toxin-A Injections for Spastic Toe Clawing," *Parkinsonism and Related Disorders*, 2006, 12:43-7.

Mancini F, Zangaglia R, Cristina S, et al, "Double-Blind, Placebo-Controlled Study to Evaluate the Efficacy and Safety of Botulinum Toxin Type A in the Treatment of Drooling in Parkinsonism," *Mov Disord*, 2003, 18(6):685-8.

Marcus SM, "Clinical Botulism Syndrome in a Patient Receiving Unlicensed Botulinum Type A Toxin," *Clin Toxicol (Phila)*, 2005, 43:724.

Mejia NI, Vuong KD, and Jankovic J, "Long-Term Botulinum Toxin Efficacy, Safety, and Immunogenicity," *Mov Disord*, 2005, 20(5):592-7.

Simpson LL, "Identification of the Major Steps in Botulinum Toxin Action," *Annu Rev Pharmacol Toxicol*, 2004, 44:167-93.

Truong D, Duane DD, Jankovic J, et al, "Efficacy and Safety of Botulinum Type A Toxin (Dysport) in Cervical Dystonia: Results of the First US Randomized, Double-blind, Placebo-Controlled Study," *Mov Disord*, 2005, 20(7):783-91.

Tsutaoka BT and Olson KR, "Inadvertent Injection of Botulinum Toxin A (Botox™) Into the Infraorbital and Mental Nerves Resulting in Dysphagia," *J Toxicol Clin Toxicol*, 2003, 41(5):675.

Wong SM, Hui AC, Tong PY, et al, "Treatment of Lateral Epicondylitis with Botulinum Toxin: A Randomized, Double-Blind, Placebo-Controlled Trial," *Ann Intern Med*, 2005, 143(11):793-7.

Bromazepam

Pronunciation (broe MA ze pam)

CAS Number 1812-30-2

Impairment Potential Yes (with acute or chronic usage) at dosages >3 mg

Use Short-term, symptomatic treatment of anxiety

Mechanism of Action Binds to stereospecific benzodiazepine receptors on the postsynaptic GABA neuron at several sites within the central nervous system, including the limbic system, reticular formation. Enhancement of the inhibitory effect of GABA on neuronal excitability results by increased neuronal membrane permeability to chloride ions. This shift in chloride ions results in hyperpolarization (a less excitable state) and stabilization.

Adverse Reactions

Frequency not defined.

Cardiovascular: Hypotension (rare), palpitations, tachycardia

Central nervous system: Drowsiness, ataxia, dizziness, confusion, depression, euphoria, lethargy, slurred speech, stupor, headache, seizures, anterograde amnesia, dystonia. In addition, paradoxical reactions (including excitation, agitation, hallucinations, and psychosis) are known to occur with benzodiazepines.

Dermatologic: Rash, pruritus

Endocrine & metabolic: Hyperglycemia, hypoglycemia

Gastrointestinal: Xerostomia, nausea, vomiting

Genitourinary: Incontinence, libido decreased

Hematologic: Hemoglobin decreased, hematocrit decreased, WBCs increased/decreased

Hepatic: Transaminases increased, alkaline phosphatase increased, bilirubin increased

Neuromuscular & skeletal: Weakness, muscle spasm

Ocular: Blurred vision, depth perception decreased

Signs and Symptoms of Overdose Alkaline phosphatase increased, anterograde amnesia, ataxia, bilirubin increased, confusion, blurred vision, depression, depth perception decreased, dizziness, drowsiness, dystonia, euphoria, headache, hematocrit decreased, hemoglobin decreased, hyperglycemia, hypoglycemia, hypotension (rare), incontinence, lethargy, libido decreased, muscle spasm, nausea, palpitations, pruritus, rash, seizures, slurred speech, stupor, tachycardia, transaminases increased, vomiting, WBCs increased/decreased, weakness, xerostomia

Pharmacodynamics/Kinetics

Protein binding: 70%

Metabolism: Hepatic

Bioavailability: 60%

Half-life elimination: 20 hours

Excretion: Urine (69%), as metabolites

Dosage

Oral:

Adults: Initial: 6-18 mg/day in equally divided doses; initial course of treatment should not last longer than 1 week; optimal dosage range: 6-30 mg/day

Elderly/debilitated: Initial dose: Should not exceed 3 mg/day in divided doses

Stability Store at 20°C to 25°C (68°F to 77°F).

Administration

May be administered with or without food.

Contraindications Hypersensitivity to bromazepam or any component of the formulation (cross-sensitivity with other benzodiazepines may exist); myasthenia gravis; narrow-angle glaucoma; severe hepatic or respiratory disease; sleep apnea; pregnancy

Warnings

Rebound or withdrawal symptoms may occur following abrupt discontinuation or large decreases in dose. Dose reductions or tapering must be approached with caution. Use with caution in elderly or debilitated patients, patients with hepatic disease (including alcoholics), renal impairment, or obesity.

Causes CNS depression (dose related) resulting in sedation, dizziness, confusion, or ataxia which may impair physical and mental capabilities. Patients must be cautioned about performing tasks which require mental alertness (eg, operating machinery or driving). Use with caution in patients receiving other CNS depressants or psychoactive agents. Effects with other sedative drugs or ethanol may be potentiated. Benzodiazepines have been associated with falls and traumatic injury and should be used with caution in patients who are at risk of these events (especially the elderly).

Use with caution in patients with respiratory disease or impaired gag reflex. Use caution in patients with depression, especially if suicidal risk may be present. May cause physical or psychological dependence - use with caution in patients with a history of drug dependence. Acute withdrawal, including seizures, may be precipitated in patients after administration of flumazenil to patients receiving long-term benzodiazepine therapy.

Benzodiazepines have been associated with anterograde amnesia. Paradoxical reactions, including hyperactive or aggressive behavior, have been reported with benzodiazepines, particularly in adolescent/pediatric or psychiatric patients. Does not have analgesic, antidepressant, or antipsychotic properties. Safety and efficacy have not been established in patients <18 years of age.

Dosage Forms

[CAN] = Canadian brand name

Tablet: 1.5 mg, 3 mg, 6 mg [not available in the U.S.]

Reference Range Therapeutic serum range for anxiety: ~0.08-0.2 mcg/mL; serum levels >0.3 mcg/mL and >1 mcg/mL are associated with toxicity and coma, respectively

Overdosage/Treatment

Decontamination: Lavage/activated charcoal for ingestion >1 mg/kg

Supportive therapy: Rarely is mechanical ventilation required; flumazenil has been shown to selectively block the binding of benzodiazepines to CNS receptors, resulting in a reversal of benzodiazepine-induced CNS depression and respiratory depression

Enhancement of elimination: Multiple dose activated charcoal may be effective

Drug Interactions

Substrate of CYP3A4 (major); **Inhibits** CYP2E1 (weak)

CNS depressants: Sedative effects and/or respiratory depression may be additive with CNS depressants (includes ethanol, barbiturates, narcotic analgesics, and other sedative agent); monitor for increased effect.

CYP3A4 inducers: CYP3A4 inducers may decrease the levels/effects of bromazepam. Example inducers include aminoglutethimide, carbamazepine, nafcillin, nevirapine, phenobarbital, phenytoin, and rifamycins.

CYP3A4 inhibitors: May increase the levels/effects of bromazepam. Example inhibitors include azole antifungals, clarithromycin, diclofenac, doxycycline, erythromycin, imatinib, isoniazid, nefazodone, nicardipine, propofol, protease inhibitors, quinidine, telithromycin, and verapamil.

Levodopa: Therapeutic effects may be diminished in some patients following the addition of a benzodiazepine; limited/inconsistent data.

Oral contraceptives: May decrease the clearance of some benzodiazepines (those which undergo oxidative metabolism); monitor for increased benzodiazepine effect.

Theophylline: May partially antagonize some of the effects of benzodiazepines; monitor for decreased response; may require higher doses for sedation.

Pregnancy Risk Factor D (based on other benzodiazepines)

Pregnancy Implications Crosses the placenta. Oral clefts reported, however, more recent data does not support an association between drug and oral clefts; inguinal hernia, cardiac defects, spina bifida, urinary system abnormalities, dysmorphic facial features, skeletal defects, multiple other malformations reported; hypotonia and withdrawal symptoms reported following use near time of delivery

Lactation Enters breast milk/contraindicated (AAP rates other benzodiazepines "of concern")

Additional Information Not available in U.S.

Specific References

Mokhlesi B, Leikin JB, Murray P, et al, "Adult Toxicology in Critical Care: Part II: Specific Poisonings," *Chest*, 2003, 123(3):897-922.

Buflomedil

CAS Number 35543-24-9; 55837-25-7

Synonyms Buflomedil Hydrochloride; Buflomedilum

Use Dementia; diabetic nephropathy or retinopathy; claudication; Raynaud's phenomenon

Mechanism of Action A peripheral vasodilator (arterioles greater than veins)

Adverse Reactions

Cardiovascular: Hypotension, syncope, AV block, sinus tachycardia, arrhythmias (ventricular), vasodilation

Central nervous system: Dizziness

Dermatologic: Skin rash, pruritus, exanthema

Gastrointestinal: Nausea, diarrhea

Miscellaneous: Anaphylaxis

Signs and Symptoms of Overdose Asystole, coma, flattened T wave on ECG, hypokalemia, hypotension, mydriasis, myoclonus, pulmonary edema, QT and QRS interval prolongation, respiratory depression, seizures, tachycardia, ventricular fibrillation

Admission Criteria/Prognosis Admit any symptomatic ingestion to a cardiac monitored bed or admit any ingestion >500 mg

Pharmacodynamics/Kinetics

Distribution: V_d: 1.3-1.4 L/kg

Protein binding: 60% to 80%

Metabolism: Hepatic to para-desmethyl buflomedil

Bioavailability: 50% to 80%

Half-life: 1.5-4.3 hours

Elimination: Renal (primarily); fecal (6%); total body clearance: 15-40 L/hour

Dosage Oral: 300-600 mg in divided doses

I.V.: Up to 400 mg

I.M.: 50 mg 3 times/day up to 2 weeks

Monitoring Parameters EKG, electrolytes

Contraindications Hypersensitivity to buflomedil; immediate postpartum use; severe arterial bleeding; pregnancy; lactation; pediatric patients; following vascular surgery

Dosage Forms

Tablet, as hydrochloride: 150 mg, 300 mg, 600 mg

Drops, as hydrochloride: 150 mg/mL

Injection, as hydrochloride: 50 mg (ampul)

Reference Range Serum and urine buflomedil levels 3 hours after a 3 g overdose: 24.8 mg/L and 324.4 mg/L, respectively; plasma buflomedil levels >5 mg/L are toxic; seizures occur with plasma levels >10 mg/L

Overdosage/Treatment

Decontamination: **Do not** induce emesis; lavage within 1 hour any ingestion >1 g in adults/activated charcoal

Supportive therapy: In order to treat hypotension, a fluid challenge of isotonic saline (10-20 mL/kg) and placement in Trendelenburg position should first be performed; dopamine or norepinephrine can be given for refractory hypotension; ventricular arrhythmias may respond to serum alkalinization (pH 7.45-7.55) with sodium bicarbonate (1-3 mEq/kg); avoid quinidine, disopyramide and procainamide; lidocaine, phenytoin, or bretylium can be used for refractory cases; lorazepam or diazepam can be used for seizure control

Antidote(s)

• Sodium Bicarbonate [ANTIDOTE]

Test Interactions Can cause a positive tricyclic antidepressant urinary immunoassay.

Drug Interactions Enhanced hypotensive effect can occur with ethanol or calcium channel blockers

Additional Information Minimum lethal dose: 2.2 g; Toxic oral dose: 600 mg; Seizurgenic dose: 900 mg

Bumetanide

CAS Number 28395-03-1

U.S. Brand Names Bumex®

Use Management of edema secondary to congestive heart failure or hepatic or renal disease including nephrotic syndrome; may also be used alone or in combination with antihypertensives in the treatment of hypertension; can be used in furosemide-allergic patients (1 mg is equivalent to 40 mg furosemide)

Mechanism of Action Inhibits reabsorption of sodium and chloride in the ascending loop of Henle and distal renal tubule, interfering with the chloride-binding cotransport system, thus causing increased excretion of water, sodium, chloride, magnesium, and calcium

Adverse Reactions

Cardiovascular: Hypotension, angina

Central nervous system: Dizziness, headache, encephalopathy

Dermatologic: Stevens-Johnson syndrome, bullous pemphigoid

Endocrine & metabolic: **Hypokalemia, hyperuricemia, hypochloremia**, hyperglycemia,

Gastrointestinal: Cramps, nausea, vomiting

Hepatic: Altered liver function test results

Neuromuscular & skeletal: Weakness

Otic: Ototoxicity

Renal: Elevated serum creatinine, **azotemia**, decreased uric acid excretion

Signs and Symptoms of Overdose Agranulocytosis, asterixis, chest pain, dermatitis, diarrhea, electrolyte depletion, granulocytopenia, hyperglycemia, hyperuricemia, hypokalemia, hypomagnesemia, hyponatremia, leukopenia, nausea, neutropenia, volume depletion, vomiting, xerostomia

Pharmacodynamics/Kinetics

Onset of action: Oral, I.M.: 0.5-1 hour; I.V.: 2-3 minutes

Duration: 4-6 hours

Distribution: V_d: 13-25 L/kg

Protein binding: 95%

Metabolism: Partially hepatic

Half-life elimination: Neonates: ~6 hours; Infants (1 month): ~2.4 hours; Adults: 1-1.5 hours

Excretion: Primarily urine (as unchanged drug and metabolites)

Dosage

Oral, I.M., I.V.:

Neonates (see Warnings/Precautions): 0.01-0.05 mg/kg/dose every 24-48 hours

Infants and Children: 0.015-0.1 mg/kg/dose every 6-24 hours (maximum dose: 10 mg/day)

Adults:

Edema:

Oral: 0.5-2 mg/dose (maximum dose: 10 mg/day) 1-2 times/day

I.M., I.V.: 0.5-1 mg/dose; may repeat in 2-3 hours for up to 2 doses if needed (maximum dose: 10 mg/day)

Continuous I.V. infusion: 0.9-1 mg/hour

Hypertension: Oral: 0.5 mg daily (maximum dose: 5 mg/day); usual dosage range (JNC 7): 0.5-2 mg/day in 2 divided doses

Monitoring Parameters Blood pressure, serum electrolytes, renal function

Administration

Give I.V. slowly, over 1-2 minutes

Contraindications Hypersensitivity to bumetanide, any component of the formulation, or sulfonylureas; anuria; patients with hepatic coma or in states of severe electrolyte depletion until the condition improves or is corrected; pregnancy (based on expert analysis)

Warnings

Adjust dose to avoid dehydration. In cirrhosis, avoid electrolyte and acid/base imbalances that might lead to hepatic encephalopathy. Ototoxicity is associated with I.V. rapid administration, renal impairment, excessive doses, and concurrent use of other ototoxins. Hypersensitivity reactions can rarely occur. Monitor fluid status and renal function in an attempt to prevent oliguria, azotemia, and reversible increases in BUN and creatinine. Close medical supervision of aggressive diuresis required. Watch for and correct electrolyte disturbances. Coadministration of antihypertensives may increase the risk of hypotension.

Chemical similarities are present among sulfonamides, sulfonylureas, carbonic anhydrase inhibitors, thiazides, and loop diuretics (except ethacrynic acid). Use in patients with sulfonylurea allergy is specifically contraindicated in product labeling, however, a risk of cross-reaction exists in patients with allergy to any of these compounds; avoid use when previous reaction has been severe.

[U.S. Boxed Warning]: Loop diuretics are potent diuretics; excess amounts can lead to profound diuresis with fluid and electrolyte loss; close medical supervision and dose evaluation are requir-

ed. *In vitro* studies using pooled sera from critically-ill neonates have shown bumetanide to be a potent displacer of bilirubin; avoid use in neonates at risk for kernicterus.

Dosage Forms
Injection, solution: 0.25 mg/mL (2 mL, 4 mL, 10 mL) [contains benzyl alcohol]

Tablet (Bumex®): 0.5 mg, 1 mg, 2 mg

Reference Range Effective plasma level: 40-80 ng/mL

Overdosage/Treatment
Decontamination: Activated charcoal

Supportive therapy: Hydration with 0.9% saline

Test Interactions ↑ BUN, creatinine, ammonia (B), amylase (S), glucose, uric acid (S); ↓ sodium, calcium, chloride, potassium

Drug Interactions
ACE inhibitors: Hypotensive effects and/or renal effects are potentiated by hypovolemia.

Antidiabetic agents: Glucose tolerance may be decreased.

Antihypertensive agents: Hypotensive effects may be enhanced.

Cholestyramine or colestipol may reduce bioavailability of bumetanide.

Digoxin: Bumetanide-induced hypokalemia may predispose to digoxin toxicity; monitor potassium.

Indomethacin (and other NSAIDs) may reduce natriuretic and hypotensive effects of diuretics.

Lithium: Renal clearance may be reduced. Isolated reports of lithium toxicity have occurred; monitor lithium levels.

NSAIDs: Risk of renal impairment may increase when used in conjunction with diuretics.

Ototoxic drugs (aminoglycosides, cis-platinum): Concomitant use of bumetanide may increase risk of ototoxicity, especially in patients with renal dysfunction.

Peripheral adrenergic-blocking drugs or ganglionic blockers: Effects may be increased.

Salicylates (high dose) with diuretics may predispose patients to salicylate toxicity due to reduced renal excretion or alter renal function.

Thiazides: Synergistic diuretic effects occur.

Pregnancy Risk Factor C (manufacturer); D (expert analysis)

Lactation Excretion in breast milk unknown/use caution

Nursing Implications Be alert to complaints about hearing difficulty

Additional Information Patients with impaired hepatic function must be monitored carefully, often requiring reduced doses; larger doses may be necessary in patients with impaired renal function to obtain the same therapeutic response; can cause elevation of parathyroid hormone; patients allergic to sulfonamides may show allergy to bumetanide

Specific References
Chobanian AV, Bakris GL, Black HR, et al, "The Seventh Report of the Joint National Committee on Prevention, Detection, Evaluation, and Treatment of High Blood Pressure: The JNC 7 Report," *JAMA*, 2003, 289(19):2560-71.

Bunazosin

CAS Number 80755-51-7

Use Antihypertensive agent

Unlabeled/Investigational Use Investigational in the United States

Mechanism of Action Selective alpha$_1$-receptor blocking agent

Adverse Reactions
Cardiovascular: Syncope (first dose), postural hypotension, tachycardia, palpitations, chest pain, vasodilation

Central nervous system: Headache, fatigue, dizziness, confusion, depression

Dermatologic: Urticaria

Gastrointestinal: Nausea, xerostomia, constipation

Ocular: Miosis, ptosis

Otic: Tinnitus

Signs and Symptoms of Overdose Hypotension, miosis, oliguria, tachycardia

Toxicodynamics/Kinetics
Protein binding: 97%

Metabolism: Hepatic

Bioavailability: Oral: 45%

Half-life: 12 hours

Elimination: Fecal: 60%; Renal: 40%

Dosage
Renal insufficiency: Initial: 3 mg

Sustained release: 6 mg once daily; maximum dose: 12 mg/day

Reference Range Maximum plasma bunazosin level after 6 mg dose: ~6 ng/mL

Overdosage/Treatment
Decontamination: Ipecac within 30 minutes or lavage (within 1 hour)/ activated charcoal

Supportive therapy: Hypotension usually responds to I.V. fluids or Trendelenburg positioning. If unresponsive to these measures, the use of a parenteral vasoconstrictor may be required (eg, norepinephrine

0.1-0.2 mcg/kg/minute titrated to response). Treatment is primarily supportive and symptomatic.

Enhancement of elimination: Multiple dosing of activated charcoal may be effective

Pregnancy Implications No teratogenic effects noted

Bupivacaine

CAS Number 14252-80-3; 18010-40-7; 2180-92-9

U.S. Brand Names Marcaine® Spinal; Marcaine®; Sensorcaine®-MPF; Sensorcaine®

Synonyms Bupivacaine Hydrochloride

Use Local anesthetic (injectable) for peripheral nerve block, infiltration, sympathetic block, caudal or epidural block, retrobulbar block

Mechanism of Action Blocks both the initiation and conduction of nerve impulses by decreasing the neuronal membrane's permeability to sodium ions, which results in inhibition of depolarization with resultant blockade of conduction; a group II (amide) anesthetic

Adverse Reactions
Cardiovascular: Cardiac arrest, hypotension, bradycardia, palpitations, sinus bradycardia, arrhythmias (ventricular)

Central nervous system: Convulsions, restlessness, anxiety, dizziness, seizures

Gastrointestinal: Nausea, vomiting, metallic taste

Neuromuscular & skeletal: Weakness

Ocular: Blurred vision, diplopia, conjunctivitis

Otic: Ototoxicity, tinnitus

Respiratory: Apnea, rhinitis

Signs and Symptoms of Overdose Cardiac arrest, cardiac depression, coma, cyanosis, depression, disorientation, hypoglycemia, lightheadedness, myopathy, nystagmus, ototoxicity, ptosis, seizures, tinnitus

Pharmacodynamics/Kinetics
Onset of action: Anesthesia (route and dose dependent): 1-17 minutes

Duration (route and dose dependent): 2-9 hours

Protein binding: ~95%

Metabolism: Hepatic; forms metabolite (PPX)

Half-life elimination (age dependent): Neonates: 8.1 hours; Adults: 1.5-5.5 hours

Excretion: Urine (~6% unchanged)

Dosage
Dose varies with procedure, depth of anesthesia, vascularity of tissues, duration of anesthesia and condition of patient. Metabisulfites (in epinephrine-containing injection); do not use solutions containing preservatives for caudal or epidural block.

Local anesthesia: Maximum dose: 2 mg/kg

Local anesthesia with epinephrine: Maximum dose: 3 mg/kg

Caudal block (with or without epinephrine):
Children: 1-3.7 mg/kg
Adults: 15-30 mL of 0.25% or 0.5%

Epidural block (other than caudal block):
Children: 1.25 mg/kg/dose
Adults: 10-20 mL of 0.25% or 0.5%

Peripheral nerve block: 5 mL dose of 0.25% or 0.5% (12.5-25 mg); maximum: 2.5 mg/kg (plain); 3 mg/kg (with epinephrine); up to a maximum of 400 mg/day

Sympathetic nerve block: 20-50 mL of 0.25% (no epinephrine) solution

Stability Solutions with epinephrine should be protected from light

Monitoring Parameters Monitor fetal heart rate during paracervical anesthesia

Administration
Solutions containing preservatives should not be used for epidural or caudal blocks.

Contraindications Hypersensitivity to bupivacaine hydrochloride, amide-type local anesthetics, or any component of the formulation; obstetrical paracervical block anesthesia

Warnings Use with caution in patients with hepatic impairment. Not recommended for use in children <12 years of age. The solution for spinal anesthesia should not be used in children <18 years of age. **Do not use solutions containing preservatives for caudal or epidural block**. Local anesthetics have been associated with rare occurrences of sudden respiratory arrest; convulsions due to systemic toxicity leading to cardiac arrest have also been reported, presumably following unintentional intravascular injection. **[U.S. Boxed Warning]: The 0.75% is not recommended for obstetrical anesthesia.** A test dose is recommended prior to epidural administration (prior to initial dose) and all reinforcing doses with continuous catheter technique. Use caution with cardiovascular dysfunction. Use caution in debilitated, elderly, or acutely ill patients; dose reduction may be required.

Dosage Forms
Injection, solution, as hydrochloride [preservative free]: 0.25% [2.5 mg/mL] (10 mL, 20 mL, 30 mL, 50 mL); 0.5% [5 mg/mL] (10 mL, 20 mL, 30 mL); 0.75% [7.5 mg/mL] (10 mL, 20 mL, 30 mL)

Marcaine®: 0.25% [2.5 mg/mL] (10 mL, 30 mL); 0.5% [5 mg/mL] (10 mL, 30 mL); 0.75% [7.5 mg/mL] (10 mL, 30 mL)

Marcaine® Spinal: 0.75% [7.5 mg/mL] (2 mL) [in dextrose 8.25%]

Sensorcaine®-MPF: 0.25% [2.5 mg/mL] (10 mL, 30 mL); 0.5% [5 mg/mL] (10 mL, 30 mL); 0.75% [7.5 mg/mL] (10 mL, 30 mL)

Injection, solution, as hydrochloride (Marcaine®, Sensorcaine®): 0.25% [2.5 mg/mL] (50 mL); 0.5% [5 mg/mL] (50 mL) [contains methylparaben]

Reference Range Therapeutic plasma levels: <3 mcg/mL

Overdosage/Treatment

Supportive therapy: Treatment is primarily symptomatic and supportive. Termination of anesthesia by pneumatic tourniquet inflation should be attempted when the agent is administered by infiltration or regional injection. Seizures commonly respond to diazepam or lorazepam, while hypotension responds to I.V. fluids and Trendelenburg positioning. Bradyarrhythmias (when the heart rate is less than 60) can be treated with I.V., or SubQ atropine 15 mcg/kg. With the development of metabolic acidosis, I.V. sodium bicarbonate 0.5-2 mEq/kg and ventilatory assistance should be instituted.

Intravenous lipid infusions (100 ml of a 20% lipid infusion bolus) with one mg of atropine and one mg of epinephrine IV followed by a 0.5 ml/kg/min infusion over 2 hours has been used to resuscitate a patient successfully from a cardiac arrest. Propofol (100 mg I.V.) can be used as a secondary agent to treat seizures.

Drug Interactions Substrate (minor) of CYP1A2, 2C19, 2D6, 3A4

Pregnancy Risk Factor C

Pregnancy Implications Can result in fetal bradycardia and fetal death

Lactation Enters breast milk/not recommended

Additional Information Metabisulfites (in epinephrine-containing injection); do not use solutions containing preservatives for caudal or epidural block

Specific References

Weinberg G, Ripper R, Feinstein DL, et al, "Lipid Emulsion Infusion Rescues Dogs from Bupivacaine-Induced Cardiac Toxicity," *Reg Anesth Pain Med*, 2003, 28(3):198-202.

Rosenblatt MA, Abel M, Fischer GW, et al, "Successful Use of a 20% Lipid Emulsion to Resuscitate a Patient After a Presumed Bupivacaine-related Cardiac Arrest," *Anesthesiology*, 2006, 105(1):217-8.

Weinberg G, "Lipid Infusion Resuscitation for Local Anesthetic Toxicity: Proof of Clinical Efficacy," *Anesthesiology*, 2006, 105(1):7-8.

Buprenorphine

CAS Number 52485-79-7; 53152-21-9

U.S. Brand Names Buprenex®; Subutex®

Synonyms Buprenorphine Hydrochloride

Impairment Potential Yes

Use

Injection: Management of moderate to severe pain

Tablet: Treatment of opioid dependence

Unlabeled/Investigational Use Injection: Heroin and opioid withdrawal

Mechanism of Action Opiate agonist/antagonist that produces analgesia by binding to kappa and mu opiate receptors in the CNS

Adverse Reactions

Injection:

Cardiovascular: Bradycardia, cyanosis, flushing, hypertension, hypotension, pallor, tachycardia, Wenckebach block

Central nervous system: **Sedation**, agitation, coma, confusion, convulsion, depersonalization, depression, dizziness, dysphoria, euphoria, fatigue, hallucinations, headache, malaise, nervousness, psychosis, respiratory depression, slurred speech, vertigo

Dermatologic: Pruritus, rash, urticaria

Gastrointestinal: Appetite increased, constipation, flatulence, nausea, vomiting, xerostomia

Genitourinary: Urinary retention

Local: Injection site reaction

Neuromuscular & skeletal: Paresthesia, tremor, weakness

Ocular: Blurred vision, diplopia, miosis

Otic: Tinnitus

Respiratory: Apnea

Miscellaneous: Diaphoresis, allergic reaction

Tablet:

Central nervous system: **Anxiety**, chills, **depression** dizziness, fever, **headache**, **insomnia**, nervousness, **pain**, somnolence

Gastrointestinal: **Abdominal pain**, **constipation**, diarrhea, dyspepsia, **nausea**, vomiting

Neuromuscular & skeletal: **Back pain**, **weakness**, rhabdomydysis

Ocular: Lacrimation

Respiratory: Cough, pharyngitis, **rhinitis**

Miscellaneous: **Diaphoresis**, flu-like syndrome, **infection**, **withdrawal syndrome**

Signs and Symptoms of Overdose Bradycardia, CNS depression, depression, dysphoria, hypotension, pinpoint pupils

Pharmacodynamics/Kinetics

Onset of action: Analgesic: 10-30 minutes

Duration: 6-8 hours

Absorption: I.M., SubQ: 30% to 40%

Distribution: V_d: 97-187 L/kg

Protein binding: High

Metabolism: Primarily hepatic; extensive first-pass effect

Half-life elimination: 2.2-3 hours

Excretion: Feces (70%); urine (20% as unchanged drug)

Dosage Long-term use is not recommended

Note: These are guidelines and do not represent the maximum doses that may be required in all patients. Doses should be titrated to pain relief/prevention. In high-risk patients (eg, elderly, debilitated, presence of respiratory disease) and/or concurrent CNS depressant use, reduce dose by one-half. Buprenorphine has an analgesic ceiling.

Acute pain (moderate to severe):

Children 2-12 years: I.M., slow I.V.: 2-6 mcg/kg every 4-6 hours

Children ≥13 years and Adults:

I.M.: Initial: Opiate-naive: 0.3 mg every 6-8 hours as needed; initial dose (up to 0.3 mg) may be repeated once in 30-60 minutes after the initial dose if needed; usual dosage range: 0.15-0.6 mg every 4-8 hours as needed

Slow I.V.: Initial: Opiate-naive: 0.3 mg every 6-8 hours as needed; initial dose (up to 0.3 mg) may be repeated once in 30-60 minutes after the initial dose if needed

Elderly: 0.15 mg every 6 hours; elderly patients are more likely to suffer from confusion and drowsiness compared to younger patients

Heroin or opiate withdrawal (unlabeled use): Children ≥13 years and Adults: I.M., slow I.V.: Variable; 0.1-0.4 mg every 6 hours

Sublingual: Children ≥16 years and Adults: Opioid dependence:

Induction: Range: 12-16 mg/day (doses during an induction study used 8 mg on day 1, followed by 16 mg on day 2; induction continued over 3-4 days). Treatment should begin at least 4 hours after last use of heroin or short-acting opioid, preferably when first signs of withdrawal appear. Titrating dose to clinical effectiveness should be done as rapidly as possible to prevent undue withdrawal symptoms and patient drop-out during the induction period.

Maintenance: Target dose: 16 mg/day; range: 4-24 mg/day; patients should be switched to the buprenorphine/naloxone combination product for maintenance and unsupervised therapy

Stability Tablet: Store at room temperature of 25°C (77°F).

Injection: Protect from excessive heat of >40°C (>104°F) and light.

Monitoring Parameters Pain relief, respiratory and mental status, CNS depression, blood pressure

Administration

I.V.: Administer slowly, over at least 2 minutes.

Sublingual: Tablet should be placed under the tongue until dissolved; should not be swallowed. If 2 or more tablets are needed per dose, all may be placed under the tongue at once, or 2 at a time; to ensure consistent bioavailability, subsequent doses should always be taken the same way.

Contraindications Hypersensitivity to buprenorphine or any component of the formulation

Warnings

An opioid-containing analgesic regimen should be tailored to each patient's needs and based upon the type of pain being treated (acute versus chronic), the route of administration, degree of tolerance for opioids (naive versus chronic user), age, weight, and medical condition. The optimal analgesic dose varies widely among patients. Doses should be titrated to pain relief/prevention.

May cause respiratory depression - use caution in patients with respiratory disease or pre-existing respiratory depression. Potential for drug dependency exists; abrupt cessation may precipitate withdrawal. Use caution in elderly, debilitated, or pediatric patients. Use with caution in patients with depression or suicidal tendencies, or in patients with a history of drug abuse. Tolerance, psychological and physical dependence may occur with prolonged use. Use with caution in patients with hepatic, pulmonary, or renal function impairment. May cause CNS depression, which may impair physical or mental abilities. Patients must be cautioned about performing tasks which require mental alertness (eg, operating machinery or driving). Effects with other sedative drugs or ethanol may be potentiated. Elderly may be more sensitive to CNS depressant and constipating effects. Use with caution in patients with head injury or increased ICP, biliary tract dysfunction, pancreatitis, patients with history of ileus or bowel obstruction, glaucoma, hyperthyroidism, adrenal insufficiency, prostatic hyperplasia, urinary stricture, CNS depression, toxic psychosis, alcoholism, delirium tremens, or kyphoscoliosis. Partial antagonist activity may precipitate acute narcotic withdrawal in opioid-dependent individuals. Tablets, which are used for induction treatment of opioid dependence, should not be started until effects of withdrawal are evident.

Dosage Forms

Injection, solution (Buprenex®): 0.3 mg/mL (1 mL)

Tablet, sublingual (Subutex®): 2 mg, 8 mg

Additional dosage strength available in Canada: 0.4 mg

Reference Range

I.V. dose of 0.3 mg results in a plasma buprenorphine level of 0.5 mcg/L

Postmortem blood buprenorphine and norbuprenorphine levels in buprenorphine-related fatalities among opiate addicts ranged from 1.1-29 ng/mL (mean 8.4 ng/mL) and 0.2-12.6 ng/mL (mean 2.6 ng/mL), respectively.

Overdosage/Treatment

Decontamination: Lavage (within 1 hour)/activated charcoal for oral ingestion

Supportive therapy: Naloxone in large doses (5-10 mg) and/or a continuous infusion may be necessary to reverse respiratory depression. As much as 10 mg of naloxone may be required to reverse sedation.

Antidote(s)

- Nalmefene [ANTIDOTE]
- Naloxone [ANTIDOTE]

Test Interactions ↑ amylase, lipase

Drug Interactions

Substrate of CYP3A4 (major); **Inhibits** CYP1A2 (weak), 2A6 (weak), 2C19 (weak), 2D6 (weak)

Cimetidine: May increase sedation from narcotic analgesics; however, histamine blockers may attenuate the cardiovascular response from histamine release associated with narcotic analgesics.

CNS depressants: May produce additive respiratory and CNS depression; includes benzodiazepines, barbiturates, ethanol, and other sedatives. Respiratory and CV collapse was reported in a patient who received diazepam and buprenorphine.

CYP3A4 inducers: CYP3A4 inducers may decrease the levels/effects of buprenorphine. Example inducers include aminoglutethimide, carbamazepine, nafcillin, nevirapine, phenobarbital, phenytoin, and rifamycins.

CYP3A4 inhibitors: May increase the levels/effects of buprenorphine. Example inhibitors include azole antifungals, clarithromycin, diclofenac, doxycycline, erythromycin, imatinib, isoniazid, nefazodone, nicardipine, propofol, protease inhibitors, quinidine, and verapamil.

Naltrexone: May antagonize the effect of narcotic analgesics; concurrent use or use within 7-10 days of injection for pain relief is contraindicated.

Pregnancy Risk Factor C

Pregnancy Implications Withdrawal has been reported in infants of women receiving buprenorphine during pregnancy. Onset of symptoms ranged from day 1 to day 8 of life, most occurring on day 1.

Lactation Enters breast milk/not recommended

Nursing Implications Gradual withdrawal of drug is necessary to avoid withdrawal symptoms

Additional Information

Buprenorphine injection: 0.4 mg = 10 mg morphine or 75 mg meperidine, has longer duration of action than either agent

Subutex® (buprenorphine) should be limited to supervised use whenever possible; patients should be switched to Suboxone® (buprenorphine/naloxone) for maintenance and unsupervised therapy

Specific References

Baker JR, Best AM, Pade PA, et al, "Effect of Buprenorphine and Antiretroviral Agents on the QT Interval in Opioid-Dependent Patients," *Ann Pharmacother*, 2006, 40(3):392-6.

Cho CS, Calello DP, and Osterhoudt KC, "Exploratory Buprenorphine Ingestion in an Infant," *Ann Emerg Med*, 2006, 48(1):109.

Cirimele V, Kintz P, Lohner S, et al, "Enzyme Immunoassay Validation for the Detection of Buprenorphine in Urine," *J Anal Toxicol*, 2003, 27(2):103-5.

Doyon S, Klein-Schwartz W, and Welsh C, "Toxicity Following Buprenorphine Ingestion," *Clin Toxicol*, 2005, 43:640.

ElSohly MA, Gul W, Feng S, et al, "Hydrolysis of Conjugated Metabolites of Buprenorphine II: The Quantitative Enzymatic Hydrolysis of Norbuprenorphine-3-Beta-D-Glucuronide in Human Urine," *J Anal Toxicol*, 2005, 29:570-81.

Fox EJ, Tetlow VA, and Allen KR, "Quantitative Analysis of Buprenorphine and Norbuprenorphine in Urine Using Liquid Chromatography Tandem Mass Spectrometry," *J Anal Toxicol*, 2006, 30:238-44.

Gaulier JM, Charvier F, Monceaux F, et al, "Ingestion of High-dose Buprenorphine by a 4-Year-Old Child," *J Toxicol Clin Toxicol*, 2004, 42(7):993-5.

Huang W and Moody DE, "Simultaneous Determination of Buprenorphine, Norbuprenorphine, Buprenorphine-3-Glucuronide and Norbuprenorphine-3-Glucuronide in Human Plasma by Liquid Chromatography-Electrospray Ionization-Tandem Mass Spectrometry," *J Anal Toxicol*, 2004, 28:290.

Kintz P, Villain M, Tracqui A, et al, "Buprenorphine in Drug-Facilitated Sexual Abuse: A Fatal Case Involving a 14-Year-Old Boy," *J Anal Toxicol*, 2003, 27:527.

Kronstrand R, Selden TG, and Josefsson M, "Analysis of Buprenorphine, Norbuprenorphine, and Their Glucuronides in Urine by Liquid Chromatography-Mass Spectrometry," *J Anal Toxicol*, 2003, 27:464-70.

Malinoff HL, Barkin RL, and Wilson G, "Sublingual Buprenorphine is Effective in the Treatment of Chronic Pain Syndrome," *Am J Ther*, 2005, 12(5):379-84.

Miller EI, Torrance HJ, and Oliver JS, "Validation of the Immunalysis® Microplate ELISA for the Detection of Buprenorphine and Its Metabolite Norbuprenorphine in Urine," *J Anal Toxicol*, 2006, 30:153.

Moody DE and Chang Y, "Effect of Benzodiazepines on the *In Vitro* Metabolism of Buprenorphine in Human Liver Microsomes," *J Anal Toxicol*, 2004, 28:304.

Moody D and Slawson M, "Metabolism of Buprenorphine at Therapeutic Concentrations in Human Liver Microsomes and cDNA-Expressed Human Liver Cytochrome P450s," *J Anal Toxicol*, 2003, 27:198.

Scislowski M, Piekoszewski W, Kamenczak A, et al, "Simultaneous Determination of Buprenorphine and Norbuprenorphine in Serum by High-Performance Liquid Chromatography-Electrospray Ionization - Mass Spectrometry," *J Anal Toxicol*, 2005, 29(4):249-53.

Seet RS and Lin EH, "Intravenous Use of Buprenorphine Tablets Associated with Rhabdomyolysis and Compressive Sciatic Neuropathy," *Ann Emerg Med*, 2006, 47(4):396-7.

Sporer KA, "Buprenorphine: A Primer for Emergency Physicians," *Ann Emerg Med*, 2004, 43(5):580-4.

Stramesi C, Zucchella A, Vignali C, et al, "Determination of Buprenorphine and Norbuprenorphine in Hair by GC-MS," *Annale de Toxicologie Analytique*, 2005, 17(4):247-52.

Sung S and Conry JM, "Role of Buprenorphine in the Management of Heroin Addiction," *Ann Pharmacother*, 2006, 40(3):501-5.

BuPROPion

Related Information

- Antidepressant Agents
- Drugs Used in Addiction Treatment
- Therapeutic Drugs Associated with Hallucinations

CAS Number 31677-93-7; 34911-55-2

U.S. Brand Names Wellbutrin SR®; Wellbutrin XL™; Wellbutrin®; Zyban®

Use Treatment of depression; adjunct in smoking cessation

Unlabeled/Investigational Use Attention-deficit/hyperactivity disorder (ADHD); depression associated with bipolar disorder

Mechanism of Action Bupropion is an antidepressant structurally different from all other previously marketed antidepressants; like other antidepressants the mechanism of bupropion's activity is not fully understood; the drug is a weak blocker of serotonin and norepinephrine re-uptake, inhibits neuronal dopamine re-uptake and is not a monoamine oxidase A or B inhibitor

Adverse Reactions

Cardiovascular: Arrhythmias, atrioventricular block, chest pain, extrasystoles, facial edema, flushing, hypertension (may be severe), hypotension, myocardial infarction, pallor, palpitations, peripheral edema, postural hypotension, syncope, tachycardia, vasodilation

Central nervous system: **Dizziness, headache, insomnia**, akinesia, agitation, alopecia, amnesia, anxiety, aphasia, ataxia, coma, confusion, coordination abnormal, delirium, depersonalization, depression, derealization, dysphoria, dystonia, EEG abnormality, emotional lability, euphoria, extrapyramidal syndrome, fever with rash (and other symptoms suggestive of delayed hypersensitivity resembling serum sickness), hallucinations, hostility, hypesthesia, hypokinesia, hypomania, irritability, malaise, manic reaction, memory decreased, migraine, nervousness, paranoid reaction, seizure, sleep disturbance, somnolence, stroke, suicidal ideation, tardive dyskinesia, vertigo

Dermatologic: Angioedema, dry skin, ecchymosis, exfoliative dermatitis, hirsutism, maculopapular rash, photosensitivity, pruritus, rash, urticaria

Endocrine & metabolic: Gynecomastia, hot flashes, hyperglycemia, hypoglycemia, impotence, libido decreased, libido increased, menstrual complaints, SIADH

Gastrointestinal: **Nausea, xerostomia**, abdominal pain, anorexia, appetite increased, colitis, constipation, diarrhea, dyspepsia, dysphagia, esophagitis, gastric reflux, gastrointestinal hemorrhage, gingivitis, glossitis, gum hemorrhage, intestinal perforation, mouth ulcers, pancreatitis, salivation increased, stomach ulcer, stomatitis, taste perversion, tongue edema, vomiting

Genitourinary: Cystitis, dyspareunia, dysuria, ejaculation abnormality, enuresis, nocturia, painful erection, testicular swelling, urinary frequency, urinary incontinence, urinary retention, vaginal irritation, vaginitis

Hematologic: Anemia, leukocytosis, leukopenia, pancytopenia, thrombocytopenia

Hepatic: Hepatic damage, hepatitis, jaundice

Local: Phlebitis

Neuromuscular & skeletal: Arthralgia, arthritis, ballismus, dysarthria, dyskinesia, hyperkinesia, hypertonia, leg cramps, muscle rigidity, muscle weakness, myalgia, musculoskeletal chest pain, myoclonus, neck pain, neuralgia, neuropathy, paresthesia, rhabdomyolysis, tremor, twitching

Ocular: Accommodation abnormality, amblyopia, blurred vision, diplopia, dry eye, mydriasis

Otic: Auditory disturbance, deafness, tinnitus

Renal: Glycosuria, polyuria

Respiratory: **Pharyngitis**, bronchospasm, chills, cough increased, dyspnea, epistaxis, pulmonary embolism, sinusitis

Miscellaneous: Allergic reaction (including anaphylaxis, pruritus, urticaria), bruxism, frigidity, increased diaphoresis, infection, lymphadenopathy, salpingitis, sciatica, thirst

Note: Data for the immediate-release formulation of bupropion revealed a seizure incidence of 0.4% in patients treated at doses in the 300-450 mg/day range. The estimated seizure incidence increases almost tenfold between 450 mg and 600 mg per day. Data for the sustained release dosage form revealed a seizure incidence of 0.1% in patients treated at a dosage range of 100-300 mg/day, and increases to ~0.4% at the maximum recommended dose of 400 mg/day.

Signs and Symptoms of Overdose Arched back, ataxia, confusion, delirium, fever, hypokalemia, hypophosphatemia, impotence, insomnia, labored breathing, leukopenia, mania, muscle rigidity, Parkinson's-like symptoms, salivation, seizures (21%), sinus tachycardia, slurred speech, vomiting

Admission Criteria/Prognosis Asymptomatic pediatric ingestions <200 mg may be discharged.

Pharmacodynamics/Kinetics

Absorption: Rapid

Distribution: V_d: 19-21 L/kg

Protein binding: 82% to 88%

Metabolism: Extensively hepatic via CYP2B6 to hydroxybupropion; non-CYP-mediated metabolism to erythrohydrobupropion and threohydrobupropion. Metabolite activity ranges from 20% to 50% potency of bupropion.

Bioavailability: 5% to 20% in animals

Half-life:

Distribution: 3-4 hours

Elimination: 21 ± 9 hours; Metabolites: Hydroxybupropion: 20 ± 5 hours; Erythrohydrobupropion: 33 ± 10 hours; Threohydrobupropion: 37 ± 13 hours

Time to peak, serum: Bupropion: ~3 hours; bupropion extended release: ~5 hours

Metabolites: Hydroxybupropion, erythrohydrobupropion, threohydrobupropion: 6 hours

Excretion: Urine (87%); feces (10%)

Dosage

Oral:

Children and Adolescents: ADHD (unlabeled use): 1.4-6 mg/kg/day

Adults:

Depression:

Immediate release: 100 mg 3 times/day; begin at 100 mg twice daily; may increase to a maximum dose of 450 mg/day

Sustained release: Initial: 150 mg/day in the morning; may increase to 150 mg twice daily by day 4 if tolerated; target dose: 300 mg/day given as 150 mg twice daily; maximum dose: 400 mg/day given as 200 mg twice daily

Extended release: Initial: 150 mg/day in the morning; may increase as early as day 4 of dosing to 300 mg/day; maximum dose: 450 mg/day

Smoking cessation (Zyban®): Initiate with 150 mg once daily for 3 days; increase to 150 mg twice daily; treatment should continue for 7-12 weeks

Elderly: Depression: 50-100 mg/day, increase by 50-100 mg every 3-4 days as tolerated; there is evidence that the elderly respond at 150 mg/day in divided doses, but some may require a higher dose

Dosing adjustment/comments in renal impairment: Effect of renal disease on bupropion's pharmacokinetics has not been studied; elimination of the major metabolites of bupropion may be affected by reduced renal function. Patients with renal failure should receive a reduced dosage initially and be closely monitored.

Dosing adjustment in hepatic impairment:

Note: The mean AUC increased by ~1.5-fold for hydroxybupropion and ~2.5-fold for erythro/threohydrobupropion; median T_{max} was observed 19 hours later for hydroxybupropion, 31 hours later for erythro/threohydrobupropion; mean half-life for hydroxybupropion increased fivefold, and increased twofold for erythro/threohydrobupropion in patients with severe hepatic cirrhosis compared to healthy volunteers.

Mild to moderate hepatic impairment: Use with caution and/or reduced dose/frequency

Severe hepatic cirrhosis: Use with extreme caution; maximum dose:

Wellbutrin®: 75 mg/day

Wellbutrin SR®: 100 mg/day or 150 mg every other day

Wellbutrin XL™: 150 mg every other day

Zyban®: 150 mg every other day

Stability Store at controlled temperature of 20°C to 25°C (68°F to 77°F).

Monitoring Parameters Body weight; mental status for depression, suicidal ideation (especially at the beginning of therapy or when doses are increased or decreased), anxiety, social functioning, mania, panic attacks

Administration

May be taken without regard to meals. Sustained and extended release tablets should be swallowed whole; do not crush, chew, or divide. The insoluble shell of the extended-release tablet may remain intact during GI transit and is eliminated in the feces.

Contraindications Hypersensitivity to bupropion or any component of the formulation; seizure disorder; anorexia/bulimia; use of MAO inhibitors within 14 days; patients undergoing abrupt discontinuation of ethanol or sedatives (including benzodiazepines); patients receiving other dosage forms of bupropion

Warnings

[U.S. Boxed Warning]: Antidepressants increase the risk of suicidal thinking and behavior in children and adolescents with major depressive disorder (MDD) and other depressive disorders; consider risk prior to prescribing. Closely monitor for clinical worsening, suicidality, or unusual changes in behavior; the child's family or caregiver should be instructed to closely observe the patient and communicate condition with healthcare provider. Such observation would generally include at least weekly face-to-face contact with patients or their family members or caregivers during the first 4 weeks of treatment, then every other week visits for the next 4 weeks, then at 12 weeks, and as clinically indicated beyond 12 weeks. Additional contact by telephone may be appropriate between face-to-face visits. Adults treated with antidepressants should be observed similarly for clinical worsening and suicidality, especially during the initial few months of a course of drug therapy, or at times of dose changes, either increases or decreases. A medication guide should be dispensed with each prescription. **Bupropion is not FDA approved for use in children.**

The possibility of a suicide attempt is inherent in major depression and may persist until remission occurs. Monitor for worsening of depression or suicidality, especially during initiation of therapy or with dose increases or decreases. Worsening depression and severe abrupt suicidality that are not part of the presenting symptoms may require discontinuation or modification of drug therapy. Use caution in high-risk patients during initiation of therapy. Prescriptions should be written for the smallest quantity consistent with good patient care. The patient's family or caregiver should be alerted to monitor patients for the emergence of suicidality and associated behaviors such as anxiety, agitation, panic attacks, insomnia, irritability, hostility, impulsivity, akathisia, hypomania, and mania; patients should be instructed to notify their healthcare provider if any of these symptoms or worsening depression occur.

May worsen psychosis in some patients or precipitate a shift to mania or hypomania in patients with bipolar disorder. Monotherapy in patients with bipolar disorder should be avoided. Patients presenting with depressive symptoms should be screened for bipolar disorder. **Bupropion is not FDA approved for bipolar depression.**

The risk of seizures is dose-dependent and increased in patients with a history of seizures, anorexia/bulimia, head trauma, CNS tumor, severe hepatic cirrhosis, abrupt discontinuation of sedative-hypnotics or ethanol, medications which lower seizure threshold (antipsychotics, antidepressants, theophyllines, systemic steroids), stimulants, or hypoglycemic agents. Discontinue and do not restart in patients experiencing a seizure. May cause CNS stimulation (restlessness, anxiety, insomnia) or anorexia. May increase the risks associated with electroconvulsive therapy. Consider discontinuing, when possible, prior to elective surgery. May cause weight loss; use caution in patients where weight loss is not desirable. The incidence of sexual dysfunction with bupropion is generally lower than with SSRIs.

Use caution in patients with cardiovascular disease, history of hypertension, or coronary artery disease; treatment-emergent hypertension (including some severe cases) has been reported, both with bupropion alone and in combination with nicotine transdermal systems. Use with caution in patients with hepatic or renal dysfunction and in elderly patients; reduced dose recommended. Elderly patients may be at greater risk of accumulation during chronic dosing. May cause motor or cognitive impairment in some patients; use with caution if tasks requiring alertness such as operating machinery or driving are undertaken. Arthralgia, myalgia, and fever with rash and other symptoms suggestive of delayed hypersensitivity resembling serum sickness reported.

Extended release tablet: Insoluble tablet shell may remain intact and be visible in the stool.

Dosage Forms

Tablet, as hydrochloride (Wellbutrin®): 75 mg, 100 mg

Tablet, extended release, as hydrochloride:

Budeprion™ SR: 100 mg [contains tartrazine; equivalent to Wellbutrin® SR], 150 mg [equivalent to Wellbutrin® SR]

Buproban™: 150 mg [equivalent to Zyban®]

Wellbutrin XL™: 150 mg, 300 mg

Tablet, sustained release, as hydrochloride: 100 mg, 150 mg [equivalent to Wellbutrin® SR], 150 mg [equivalent to Zyban®]

Wellbutrin® SR: 100 mg, 150 mg, 200 mg

Zyban®: 150 mg

Reference Range Blood levels >170 ng/mL associated with seizures and therapeutic level is 50-100 ng/mL; level of 446 ng/mL associated with a fatality

Overdosage/Treatment
Decontamination: Lavage (within 12 hours)/activated charcoal
Supportive therapy: I.V. diazepam or lorazepam is useful in treating seizures
Enhancement of elimination: Multiple dose of activated charcoal may be useful

Test Interactions May lower serum potassium; fluoxetine can interfere with bupropion quantitation by HPLC analysis in plasma or serum

Drug Interactions
Substrate of CYP1A2 (minor), 2A6 (minor), 2B6 (major), 2C9 (minor), 2D6 (minor), 2E1 (minor), 3A4 (minor); **Inhibits** CYP2D6 (weak)
Note: Seizure threshold-lowering agents: Use with caution in individuals receiving other agents that may lower seizure threshold (antipsychotics, antidepressants, fluoroquinolones, theophylline, abrupt discontinuation of benzodiazepines, systemic steroids)
Amantadine: Concurrent use appears to result in a higher incidence of adverse effects; use caution.
CNS depressants: Concomitant use may increase adverse effects/toxicity.
CYP2B6 inducers: May decrease the levels/effects of bupropion. Example inducers include carbamazepine, nevirapine, phenobarbital, phenytoin, and rifampin.
CYP2B6 inhibitors: May increase the levels/effects of bupropion. Example inhibitors include desipramine, paroxetine, and sertraline.
Levodopa: Toxicity of bupropion is enhanced by levodopa.
MAO inhibitors: Toxicity of bupropion is enhanced by MAO inhibitors (phenelzine); concurrent use is contraindicated.
Nicotine: Treatment-emergent hypertension may occur; monitor BP in patients treated with bupropion and nicotine patch.
Selegiline: When used in low doses (<10 mg/day), risk of interaction is theoretically lower than with nonselective MAO inhibitors.
Tricyclic antidepressants: Serum levels may be increased by bupropion; in addition, these agents lower seizure threshold (see Note).

Pregnancy Risk Factor B
Pregnancy Implications A slight increase in malformations was observed in some animal studies. The manufacturer provides results from a retrospective database study conducted in women taking bupropion during pregnancy. The study showed no greater risk of congenital malformations following bupropion exposure in comparison to other antidepressant agents. There are no adequate and well-controlled studies in pregnant women. Bupropion should be used during pregnancy only if the potential benefit outweighs the possible risks. A registry has been established for women exposed to bupropion during pregnancy (800-336-2176).
Lactation Enters breast milk/not recommended (AAP rates "of concern")
Nursing Implications Be aware that drug may cause seizures

Specific References
Ai-Leng K, Lai-San T, Kang-Hoe L, et al, "Acute Liver Failure with Concurrent Bupropion and Carbimazole Therapy," *Ann Pharmacother*, 2003, 37(2):220-3.
Biswas AK, Zabrocki LA, Mayes KL, et al, "Cardiotoxicity Associated with Intentional Ziprasidone and Bupropion Overdose," *J Toxicol Clin Toxicol*, 2003, 41(1):79-82.
Colbridge MG, Dargan PI, and Jones AL, "Bupropion - The Experience of the National Poisons Information Service (London)," *J Toxicol Clin Toxicol*, 2002, 40(3):398-9.
Cumpston KL, Bryant SM, and Aks SE, "Gastric Decontamination, Enhanced Elimination, and Toxicokinetics in a Sustained-Release Bupropion Overdose," *Am J Emerg Med*, 2004, 22(3):231-2.
Curry S, Holubek W, and Kashani J, "Confirmed Isolated Bupropion OD Producing QRS Widening," *J Toxicol Clin Toxicol*, 2003, 41(5):680.
de Graaf L, Admiraal P, and van Puijenbroek EP, "Ballism Associated with Bupropion Use," *Ann Pharmacother*, 2003, 37(2):302-3.
Elko C, Bunce J, and Martin T, "The Dilemma of Delayed Symptom Onset After Bupropion Overdose," *J Toxicol Clin Toxicol*, 2004, 42(5):735.
Ginzburg R, Wong Y, and Fader JS, "Effect on Bupropion on Sexual Dysfunction," *Ann Pharmacother*, 2005, 39(12):2096-9.
Goldstein RA, Perez A, McKay CA, et al, "Delayed Onset of Seizures Following Wellbutrin SR® Overdose," *J Toxicol Clin Toxicol*, 2003, 41(5):676.
Isbister GK and Balit CR, "Bupropion Overdose: QTc Prolongation and Its Clinical Significance," *Ann Pharmacother*, 2003, 37(7-8):999-1002.
Jepsen F, Matthews J, and Andrews FJ, "Sustained Release Bupropion Overdose: An Important Cause of Prolonged Symptoms After an Overdose," *Emerg Med J*, 2003, 20(6):560-1.
LoVecchio F, Hilder R, and Ruha AM, "A Prospective Poison Center Experience of Sustained-Release Bupropion Over 40-Months in Children," *J Toxicol Clin Toxicol*, 2003, 41(5):655.
Malek-Ahmadi P, "Bupropion for Treatment of Interferon-Induced Depression," *Ann Pharmacother*, 2004, 38(7):1202-5.
Stang P, Young S, and Hogue S, "Better Patient Persistence with Once-Daily Bupropion Compared with Twice-Daily Bupropion," *Am J Ther*, 2007, 14:20-4.
Stremski E and Uherick L, "Seizures Following Bupropion Ingestion," *Clin Toxicol (Phila)*, 2005, 43:733.
Thundiyil JG, Kearney TK, and Olson KR, "Evolving Epidemiology of Drug-Induced Seizures Reported to a Poison Control Center System," *J Toxicol Clin Toxicol*, 2004, 42(5):730.
Tong EK, Carmody TP, and Simon JA, "Bupropion for Smoking Cessation," *Comp Ther*, 2006, 32(1)26-33.
Velez LI, Delaney KA, Rivera W, et al, "Delayed Status Epilepticus After a Sustained Release Bupropion Overdose," *J Toxicol Clin Toxicol*, 2002, 40(3):323-4.
Vogel R and Goetz R, "Time of Onset of Seizures After Bupropion Overdose," *J Toxicol Clin Toxicol*, 2004, 42(5):747-8.
White RS, "Sustained Release Bupropion: Overdose and Treatment," *Am J Emerg Med*, 2002, 20(4):388-9.
Wills B, Zell-Kanter M, and Aks S, "QRS Prolongation Associated with Bupropion Ingestion," *J Toxicol Clin Toxicol*, 2004, 42(5):724.

BusPIRone

CAS Number 33386-08-2; 36505-84-7
U.S. Brand Names BuSpar®
Synonyms Buspirone Hydrochloride
Use Management of generalized anxiety disorder (GAD); treat bruxism induced by serotonin reuptake inhibitors
Unlabeled/Investigational Use Management of aggression in mental retardation and secondary mental disorders; major depression; potential augmenting agent for antidepressants; premenstrual syndrome
Mechanism of Action Selectively antagonizes CNS serotonin 5-HT$_1$A receptors without affecting benzodiazepine-GABA receptors; an azaspirodecanedione derivative with lower potential for addition or sedation than other anxiolytics
Adverse Reactions
Cardiovascular: Bradycardia, sinus bradycardia, palpitations, sinus tachycardia
Central nervous system: Sedation, disorientation, excitation, **dizziness**, dysphoria (at doses >40 mg), extrapyramidal signs, **lightheadedness**, panic attacks, mania, fever, **headache**, ataxia, psychosis
Dermatologic: Rash, acne, alopecia, bullous skin disease, xerosis, urticaria, seborrheic dermatitis, pruritus, exanthema
Gastrointestinal: **Nausea**, vomiting, diarrhea, flatulence
Genitourinary: Urinary frequency
Hematologic: Leukopenia, eosinophilia
Hepatic: Elevated liver function test results
Neuromuscular & skeletal: Paresthesia, clonus, myoclonus
Ocular: Miosis
Respiratory: Nasal congestion
Signs and Symptoms of Overdose Agranulocytosis, bradycardia, depression, dizziness, drowsiness, dysphoria, dry mouth, extrapyramidal reaction, granulocytopenia, hyperprolactinemia, leukopenia, lightheadedness, memory loss, nausea, neutropenia, pinpoint pupils, seizures, vomiting
Pharmacodynamics/Kinetics
Absorption: Oral: ~100%
Distribution: V$_d$: 5.3 L/kg
Protein binding: 95%
Metabolism: Hepatic via oxidation; extensive first-pass effect
Bioavailability: ~4%
Half-life elimination: Mean: 2.4 hours (range: 2-11 hours)
Time to peak, serum: Within 0.7-1.5 hours
Excretion: Urine: 65%; feces: 35%; ~1% dose excreted unchanged
Dosage
Oral:
Generalized anxiety disorder:
Children and Adolescents: Initial: 5 mg daily; increase in increments of 5 mg/day at weekly intervals as needed, to a maximum dose of 60 mg/day divided into 2-3 doses
Adults: 15 mg/day (7.5 mg twice daily); may increase in increments of 5 mg/day every 2-4 days to a maximum of 60 mg/day; target dose for most people is 30 mg/day (15 mg twice daily)
Bruxism: 5 mg every night at bedtime
Dosing adjustment in renal or hepatic impairment: Buspirone is metabolized by the liver and excreted by the kidneys. Patients with impaired hepatic or renal function demonstrated increased plasma levels and a prolonged half-life of buspirone. Therefore, use in patients with severe hepatic or renal impairment cannot be recommended.
Monitoring Parameters Mental status, symptoms of anxiety
Contraindications Hypersensitivity to buspirone or any component of the formulation
Warnings Use in hepatic or renal impairment is not recommended; does not prevent or treat withdrawal from benzodiazepines. Low potential for

cognitive or motor impairment. Use with MAO inhibitors may result in hypertensive reactions.

Dosage Forms
Tablet, as hydrochloride: 5 mg, 7.5 mg, 10 mg, 15 mg, 30 mg
BuSpar®: 5 mg, 10 mg, 15 mg, 30 mg
Reference Range Peak plasma levels ≤6 ng/mL noted up to 90 minutes after a 20 mg dose

Overdosage/Treatment
Decontamination: Lavage (within 1 hour)/activated charcoal
Supportive therapy: There is no known antidote for buspirone and most therapies are supportive and symptomatic in nature; diazepam or lorazepam may be used for seizures
Enhancement of elimination: Multiple dosing of activated charcoal would not be expected to be useful

Test Interactions ↑ AST, ALT

Drug Interactions
Substrate of CYP2D6 (minor), 3A4 (major)
Calcium channel blockers: Diltiazem and verapamil may increase serum concentrations of buspirone; consider a dihydropyridine calcium channel blocker.
CYP3A4 inducers: CYP3A4 inducers may decrease the levels/effects of buspirone. Example inducers include aminoglutethimide, carbamazepine, nafcillin, nevirapine, phenobarbital, phenytoin, and rifamycins.
CYP3A4 inhibitors: May increase the levels/effects of buspirone. Example inhibitors include azole antifungals, clarithromycin, diclofenac, doxycycline, erythromycin, imatinib, isoniazid, nefazodone, nicardipine, propofol, protease inhibitors, quinidine, telithromycin, and verapamil.
MAO inhibitors: Buspirone should not be used concurrently with an MAO inhibitor due to reports of increased blood pressure; includes classic MAO inhibitors and linezolid (due to ability to inhibit MAO).
Nefazodone: Concurrent use may increase risk of CNS adverse events. Limit buspirone initial dose (eg, 2.5 mg/day).
Selegiline: Theoretically, risk of interaction with selective MAO type B inhibitor would be less than with nonselective inhibitors; however, this combination is generally best avoided.
SSRIs: Concurrent use of buspirone with SSRIs may cause serotonin syndrome. Some SSRIs may increase buspirone serum concentrations (see CYP3A4 inhibitors). Buspirone may increase the efficacy of fluoxetine in some patients; however, the anxiolytic activity of buspirone may be lost when combined with SSRIs (fluoxetine).
Trazodone: Concurrent use of buspirone with trazodone may cause serotonin syndrome.

Pregnancy Risk Factor B
Lactation Excretion in breast milk unknown/not recommended
Nursing Implications Monitor patient's mental status and for benzodiazepine withdrawal; food may increase the bioavailability of the drug
Additional Information Has shown little potential for abuse; related to ipsapirone; unpleasant taste; buspirone (15-60 mg/day) may be useful in treatment of sexual dysfunction during treatment with a selective serotonin reuptake inhibitor

Specific References
Clay PG and Adams MM, "Pseudo-Parkinson Disease Secondary to Ritonavir-Buspirone Interaction," *Ann Pharmacother*, 2003, 37(2): 202-5.

Busulfan

CAS Number 55-98-1
U.S. Brand Names Busulfex®; Myleran®
Use
Oral: Chronic myelogenous leukemia and bone marrow disorders, such as polycythemia vera and myeloid metaplasia, conditioning regimens for bone marrow transplantation
I.V.: Combination therapy with cyclophosphamide as a conditioning regimen prior to allogeneic hematopoietic progenitor cell transplantation for chronic myelogenous leukemia

Unlabeled/Investigational Use Oral: Bone marrow disorders, such as polycythemia vera and myeloid metaplasia; thrombocytosis

Mechanism of Action Reacts with N-7 position of guanosine and interferes with DNA replication and transcription of RNA (an alkylating agent). Busulfan has a more marked effect on myeloid cells (and is, therefore, useful in the treatment of CML) than on lymphoid cells. The drug is also very toxic to hematopoietic stem cells (thus its usefulness in high doses in BMT preparative regimens). Busulfan exhibits little immunosuppressive activity. Interferes with the normal function of DNA by alkylation and cross-linking the strands of DNA.

Adverse Reactions
Cardiovascular: Pericardial fibrosis, pericardial effusion/pericarditis, endocardial fibrosis
Central nervous system: Dizziness, seizures, **generalized or myoclonic seizures and loss of consciousness have been associated with high-dose busulfan (4 mg/kg/day)**
Dermatologic: **Hyperpigmentation**, **alopecia**, dermal irritant, rash, **urticaria, erythema**

Endocrine & metabolic: Addison-like syndrome, hyperuricemia, **amenorrhea, ovarian suppression, malignant tumors have been reported in patients on busulfan therapy**, **sterility**, ovarian failure
Gastrointestinal: **Nausea, vomiting, diarrhea**, mucositis
Genitourinary: Hemorrhagic cystitis, **azoospermia, testicular atrophy**
Hematologic: Porphyria; **myelosuppression with nadirs of 14-21 days for leukopenia** and **thrombocytopenia; anemia, severe pancytopenia, bone marrow suppression**; since this is a delayed effect (busulfan affects the stem cells), the drug should be discontinued temporarily at the first sign of a large or rapid fall in any blood element. Some patients may develop bone marrow fibrosis or chronic aplasia which is probably due to the busulfan toxicity. In large doses, busulfan is myeloablative and is used for this reason in BMT.
Hepatic: Hepatic dysfunction, hepatic veno-occlusive disease, elevated liver function test results
Ocular: Blurred vision, **cataract formation**
Respiratory: After long-term or high-dose therapy, a syndrome known as busulfan lung may occur; this syndrome is manifested by a diffuse interstitial pulmonary fibrosis and persistent cough, fever, rales, and dyspnea; may be relieved by corticosteroids
Miscellaneous: Kaposi's sarcoma

Signs and Symptoms of Overdose Agranulocytosis, cataract, cholestatic jaundice, CNS depression, erythema multiforme, granulocytopenia, hematuria, hyperuricemia, leukopenia, myoclonus, neutropenia, periarteritis nodosa, seizures, sexual dysfunction

Pharmacodynamics/Kinetics
Duration: 28 days
Absorption: Rapid and complete
Distribution: V_d: ~1 L/kg; into CSF and saliva with levels similar to plasma
Protein binding: ~14%
Metabolism: Extensively hepatic (may increase with multiple doses)
Half-life elimination: After first dose: 3.4 hours; After last dose: 2.3 hours
Time to peak, serum: Oral: Within 4 hours; I.V.: Within 5 minutes
Excretion: Urine (10% to 50% as metabolites) within 24 hours (<2% as unchanged drug)

Dosage
Busulfan should be based on adjusted ideal body weight because actual body weight, ideal body weight, or other factors can produce significant differences in busulfan clearance among lean, normal, and obese patients; refer to individual protocols
Children:
For remission induction of CML: Oral: 0.06-0.12 mg/kg/day OR 1.8-4.6 mg/m²/day; titrate dosage to maintain leukocyte count above 40,000/mm³; reduce dosage by 50% if the leukocyte count reaches 30,000-40,000/mm³; discontinue drug if counts fall to ≤20,000/mm³
BMT marrow-ablative conditioning regimen:
Oral: 1 mg/kg/dose (ideal body weight) every 6 hours for 16 doses
I.V.:
≤12 kg: 1.1 mg/kg/dose (ideal body weight) every 6 hours for 16 doses
>12 kg: 0.8 mg/kg/dose (ideal body weight) every 6 hours for 16 doses
Adjust dose to desired AUC [1125 μmol(min)] using the following formula:
Adjusted dose (mg) = Actual dose (mg) × [target AUC μmol(min) / actual AUC μmol(min)]
Adults:
For remission induction of CML: Oral: 4-8 mg/day (may be as high as 12 mg/day); Maintenance doses: Controversial, range from 1-4 mg/day to 2 mg/week; treatment is continued until WBC reaches 10,000-20,000 cells/mm³ at which time drug is discontinued; when WBC reaches 50,000/mm³, maintenance dose is resumed
BMT marrow-ablative conditioning regimen:
Oral: 1 mg/kg/dose (ideal body weight) every 6 hours for 16 doses
I.V.: 0.8 mg/kg (ideal body weight or actual body weight, whichever is lower) every 6 hours for 4 days (a total of 16 doses)
I.V. dosing in morbidly obese patients: Dosing should be based on adjusted ideal body weight (AIBW) which should be calculated as ideal body weight (IBW) + 0.25 times (actual weight minus ideal body weight)
AIBW = IBW + 0.25 × (AW - IBW)
Cyclophosphamide, in combination with busulfan, is given on each of two days as a 1-hour infusion at a dose of 160 mg/m² beginning on BMT day -3, 6 hours following the 16th dose of busulfan
Unapproved use:
Polycythemia vera: 2-6 mg/day
Thrombocytosis: 4-6 mg/day

Monitoring Parameters CBC with differential and platelet count, hemoglobin, liver function tests

Administration
Intravenous busulfan should be administered as a 2-hour infusion, every 6 hours for 4 consecutive days for a total of 16 doses.
BMT only: To facilitate ingestion of high oral doses, insert multiple tablets into gelatin capsules.
Contraindications Hypersensitivity to busulfan or any component of the formulation; failure to respond to previous courses; pregnancy

Warnings Hazardous agent - use appropriate precautions for handling and disposal. **[U.S. Boxed Warning]: May induce severe bone marrow hypoplasia.** Use caution in patients predisposed to seizures. Discontinue if lung toxicity develops. Busulfan has been causally related to the development of secondary malignancies (tumors and acute leukemias). Busulfan has been associated with ovarian failure (including failure to achieve puberty) in females. High busulfan area under the concentration versus time curve (AUC) values (>1500 µM/minute) are associated with increased risk of hepatic veno-occlusive disease during conditioning for allogenic BMT.

Dosage Forms
Injection, solution (Busulfex®): 6 mg/mL (10 mL)
Tablet (Myleran®): 2 mg

Reference Range Mean peak serum level of a busulfan dose of 1 mg/kg is ~1080 ng/mL

Overdosage/Treatment
Decontamination: Lavage (within 1 hour)/activated charcoal
Enhancement of elimination: Multiple dosing of charcoal may be effective

Antidote(s)
- Thrombopoietin [ANTIDOTE]

Drug Interactions Substrate of CYP3A4 (major)
CYP3A4 inducers: CYP3A4 inducers may decrease the levels/effects of busulfan. Example inducers include aminoglutethimide, carbamazepine, nafcillin, nevirapine, phenobarbital, phenytoin, and rifamycins.
CYP3A4 inhibitors: May increase the levels/effects of busulfan. Example inhibitors include azole antifungals, clarithromycin, diclofenac, doxycycline, erythromycin, imatinib, isoniazid, nefazodone, nicardipine, propofol, protease inhibitors, quinidine, telithromycin, and verapamil.
Itraconazole: May decrease busulfan clearance and increase risk of pulmonary toxicity; monitor.
Metronidazole: May increase busulfan plasma levels.
Other cytotoxic agents: Pulmonary toxicity may be additive.

Pregnancy Risk Factor D
Lactation Contraindicated
Nursing Implications Avoid I.M. injection if platelet count falls <100,000/mm³
Additional Information Moderately radiopaque; alopecia is dose related
Specific References
Connor TH, McDiarmid, MA, "Preventing Occupational Exposures to Antineoplastic Drugs in Health Care Settings," *CA Cancer J Clin*, 2006, 56:354-65
Hoffer E, Akria L, Tabak A, et al, "A Simple Approximation for Busulfan Dose Adjustment in Adult Patients Undergoing Bone Marrow Transplantation," *Ther Drug Monit*, 2004, 26(3):331-5.

Butorphanol

CAS Number 42408-82-2; 58786-99-5
U.S. Brand Names Stadol® NS; Stadol®
Synonyms Butorphanol Tartrate
Impairment Potential Yes
Use
Parenteral: Management of moderate to severe pain; preoperative medication; supplement to balanced anesthesia; management of pain during labor
Nasal spray: Management of moderate to severe pain, including migraine headache pain

Mechanism of Action Mixed narcotic agonist-antagonist with central analgesic actions; binds to opiate receptors in the CNS (limbic system), causing inhibition of ascending pain pathways, altering the perception of and response to pain; produces generalized CNS depression

Adverse Reactions
Cardiovascular: Hypotension, flushing of the face, hypertension, bradycardia or tachycardia, sinus tachycardia
Central nervous system: CNS depression, anxiety, **drowsiness**, dizziness, lightheadedness, headache, agitation, malaise, restlessness, night terrors, confusion, hallucinations, false sense of well being, paradoxical CNS stimulation, acute psychosis
Dermatologic: Skin rash, pruritus
Gastrointestinal: Anorexia, nausea, vomiting, stomach cramps, constipation, xerostomia
Genitourinary: Decreased urination, painful urination
Neuromuscular & skeletal: Weakness
Ocular: Blurred vision
Otic: Ototoxicity, tinnitus
Respiratory: Apnea, respiratory depression, dyspnea
Miscellaneous: Dependence with prolonged use, diaphoresis (increased)

Signs and Symptoms of Overdose Biliary tract spasm, confusion, coma, diplopia, euphoria, disorientation, lightheadedness, night terrors, pulmonary hypertension

Pharmacodynamics/Kinetics
Onset of action: I.M.: 5-10 minutes; I.V.: <10 minutes; Nasal: Within 15 minutes
Peak effect: I.M.: 0.5-1 hour; I.V.: 4-5 minutes
Duration: I.M., I.V.: 3-4 hours; Nasal: 4-5 hours
Absorption: Rapid and well absorbed
Protein binding: 80%
Metabolism: Hepatic
Bioavailability: Nasal: 60% to 70%
Half-life elimination: 2.5-4 hours
Excretion: Primarily urine

Dosage
Note: These are guidelines and do not represent the maximum doses that may be required in all patients. Doses should be titrated to pain relief/prevention. Butorphanol has an analgesic ceiling.
Adults:
Parenteral:
Acute pain (moderate to severe):
I.M.: Initial: 2 mg, may repeat every 3-4 hours as needed; usual range: 1-4 mg every 3-4 hours as needed
I.V.: Initial: 1 mg, may repeat every 3-4 hours as needed; usual range: 0.5-2 mg every 3-4 hours as needed
Preoperative medication: I.M.: 2 mg 60-90 minutes before surgery
Supplement to balanced anesthesia: I.V.: 2 mg shortly before induction and/or an incremental dose of 0.5-1 mg (up to 0.06 mg/kg), depending on previously administered sedative, analgesic, and hypnotic medications
Pain during labor (fetus >37 weeks gestation and no signs of fetal distress):
I.M., I.V.: 1-2 mg; may repeat in 4 hours
Note: Alternative analgesia should be used for pain associated with delivery or if delivery is anticipated within 4 hours
Nasal spray:
Moderate to severe pain (including migraine headache pain): Initial: 1 spray (~1 mg per spray) in 1 nostril; if adequate pain relief is not achieved within 60-90 minutes, an additional 1 spray in 1 nostril may be given; may repeat initial dose sequence in 3-4 hours after the last dose as needed
Alternatively, an initial dose of 2 mg (1 spray in each nostril) may be used in patients who will be able to remain recumbent (in the event drowsiness or dizziness occurs); additional 2 mg doses should not be given for 3-4 hours
Note: In some clinical trials, an initial dose of 2 mg (as 2 doses 1 hour apart or 2 mg initially - 1 spray in each nostril) has been used, followed by 1 mg in 1 hour; side effects were greater at these dosages
Dosage adjustment in renal impairment:
I.M., I.V.: Initial dosage should generally be ¹/₂ of the recommended dose; repeated dosing must be based on initial response rather than fixed intervals, but generally should be at least 6 hours apart
Nasal spray: Initial dose should not exceed 1 mg; a second dose may be given after 90-120 minutes
Dosage adjustment in hepatic impairment:
I.M., I.V.: Initial dosage should generally be ¹/₂ of the recommended dose; repeated dosing must be based on initial response rather than fixed intervals, but generally should be at least 6 hours apart
Nasal spray: Initial dose should not exceed 1 mg; a second dose may be given after 90-120 minutes
Elderly:
I.M., I.V.: Initial dosage should generally be ¹/₂ of the recommended dose; repeated dosing must be based on initial response rather than fixed intervals, but generally should be at least 6 hours apart
Nasal Spray: Initial dose should not exceed 1 mg; a second dose may be given after 90-120 minutes

Stability Store at room temperature, protect from freezing; **incompatible** when mixed in the same syringe with diazepam, dimenhydrinate, methohexital, pentobarbital, secobarbital, thiopental
Monitoring Parameters Pain relief, respiratory and mental status, blood pressure
Administration
Intranasal: Consider avoiding simultaneous intranasal migraine sprays; may want to separate by at least 30 minutes
Contraindications Hypersensitivity to butorphanol or any component of the formulation; avoid use in opiate-dependent patients who have not been detoxified, may precipitate opiate withdrawal; pregnancy (prolonged use or high doses at term)
Warnings An opioid-containing analgesic regimen should be tailored to each patient's needs and based upon the type of pain being treated (acute versus chronic), the route of administration, degree of tolerance for opioids (naive versus chronic user), age, weight, and medical condition. The optimal analgesic dose varies widely among patients. Doses should be titrated to pain relief/prevention. May cause CNS depression, which may impair physical or mental abilities. Effects with other sedative drugs or ethanol may be potentiated. Use with caution in patients with hepatic/renal dysfunction. Tolerance or drug dependence may result from extended use. Concurrent use of sumatriptan nasal spray and butorphanol nasal spray may increase risk of transient high blood pressure.

Dosage Forms

Injection, solution, as tartrate [preservative free] (Stadol®): 1 mg/mL (1 mL); 2 mg/mL (1 mL, 2 mL)

Injection, solution, as tartrate [with preservative] (Stadol®): 2 mg/mL (10 mL)

Solution, intranasal, as tartrate [spray]: 10 mg/mL (2.5 mL) [14-15 doses]

Reference Range 0.7-1.5 ng/mL

Overdosage/Treatment Supportive therapy: Naloxone hydrochloride (0.4-2 mg I.V., SubQ, or through an endotracheal tube); a continuous infusion (at $^2/_3$ the response dose/hour) may be required; naloxone (2 mg I.M.) has reversed intranasal butorphanol-induced apraxia

Antidote(s)

- Nalmefene [ANTIDOTE]
- Naloxone [ANTIDOTE]

Drug Interactions Increased toxicity: CNS depressants, phenothiazines, barbiturates, skeletal muscle relaxants, alfentanil, guanabenz, and MAO inhibitors.

Pregnancy Risk Factor C/D (prolonged use or high doses at term)

Pregnancy Implications Crosses the placenta; sinusoidal fetal heart rate pattern described in two cases

Lactation Enters breast milk/use caution (AAP rates "compatible")

Nursing Implications Raise bed rails; aid with ambulation

Butriptyline

CAS Number 35941-65-2; 5585-73-9

Synonyms Butriptyline Hydrochloride

Use Depression

Mechanism of Action Increases synaptic concentration of serotonin and/or norepinephrine in the central nervous system by inhibition of their reuptake by the presynaptic neuronal membrane

Adverse Reactions

Cardiovascular: Postural hypotension, cardiomyopathy, cardiac arrhythmias, tachycardia, sudden death, QT prolongation

Central nervous system: Sedation, fatigue, anxiety, confusion, insomnia, psychosis, impaired cognitive function, seizures, extrapyramidal reactions are possible, restlessness, moderate to marked sedation can occur (tolerance to these effects usually occur), neuroleptic malignant syndrome, acute polyradiculopathy, visual hallucinations, encephalopathy

Dermatologic: Photosensitivity, cutaneous pseudolymphomas

Endocrine & metabolic: Syndrome of inappropriate antidiuretic hormone (rarely)

Gastrointestinal: **Xerostomia, increased appetite, constipation**, adynamic ileus, lower esophageal sphincter tone may cause GE reflux, **weight gain**

Genitourinary: Urinary retention

Hematologic: Leukopenia (rarely), neutropenia, agranulocytosis, granulocytopenia, eosinophilia

Hepatic: Elevated liver enzymes, cholestatic jaundice

Neuromuscular & skeletal: Tremors, clonus, myoclonus, weakness

Ocular: Blurred vision, photophobia, diplopia, increased intraocular pressure, mydriasis

Respiratory: Hyperventilation, adult respiratory distress syndrome

Miscellaneous: Allergic reactions

Signs and Symptoms of Overdose Agitation, bowel ischemia, confusion, decreased gastrointestinal motility, delirium, dementia, dental erosion, ejaculatory disturbances, extrapyramidal reaction, fever, hallucinations, hyperacusis, hyperthermia, hyponatremia, hypotension, hypothermia, insomnia, increased intraocular pressure, lactation, mania, memory loss, myoglobinuria, neuroleptic malignant syndrome, nystagmus, paresthesia, periarteritis nodosa, photosensitivity, purpura, QRS prolongation, respiratory depression, seizures, tachycardia, urinary retention, urine discoloration (blue-green)

Pharmacodynamics/Kinetics

Absorption: 3 hours

Metabolism: Hepatic to n-desmethylbutriptyline

Dosage Oral: Initial: 25 mg 3 times/day (lower dose in elderly); maximum daily dose: 150 mg

Dosage Forms Tablet, as hydrochloride: 10 mg, 25 mg, 50 mg

Reference Range Peak plasma level after a single 75 mg oral dose: 0.024-0.11 mcg/mL; postmortem blood and urine butriptyline levels after an overdose estimated to be 3,425 g was 14.9 mg/L and 2.96 mg/L, respectively

Overdosage/Treatment

Decontamination: Lavage (within 2-3 hours)/activated charcoal; **do not** induce emesis; multiple dosing of activated charcoal is more effective

Supportive therapy: Following initiation of essential overdose management, toxic symptoms should be treated. Ventricular arrhythmias often respond to phenytoin 15-20 mg/kg (adults) with concurrent systemic alkalinization (sodium bicarbonate 0.5-2 mEq/kg I.V.). Arrhythmias unresponsive to this therapy may respond to lidocaine 1mg/kg I.V. followed by a titrated infusion. Physostigmine (1-2 mg I.V. slowly for adults or 0.5 mg I.V. slowly for children) may be indicated in seizures or movement disorders but should only be used as a last resort. Seizures usually respond to lorazepam or diazepam I.V. boluses (5-10 mg for adults up to 30 mg or 0.25-0.4 mg/kg/dose for children up to 10 mg/dose). If seizures are unresponsive or recur, phenytoin or phenobarbital may be required. Phenytoin is effective to decrease QRS complex interval. Do not use bretylium in hypotensive patients. Norepinephrine is effective for hypotension. Avoid procainamide or other type IA antiarrhythmics.

Additional Information Less sedation than amitriptyline

Caffeine

Related Information

- Substance-Related Disorders

CAS Number 5743-12-4; 58-08-2; 69-22-7

U.S. Brand Names Cafcit®; Caffedrine® [OTC]; Enerjets [OTC]; Lucidex [OTC]; No Doz® Maximum Strength [OTC]; Vivarin® [OTC]

Synonyms Caffeine and Sodium Benzoate; Caffeine Citrate; Sodium Benzoate and Caffeine

Use Central nervous system stimulant; treatment of idiopathic apnea of prematurity; has several advantages over theophylline in the treatment of neonatal apnea, half-life is ~3 times as long, allowing once daily dosing, drug levels do not need to be drawn at peak and trough; has a wider therapeutic window, allowing more room between an effective concentration and toxicity

Unlabeled/Investigational Use Caffeine and sodium benzoate: Treatment of spinal puncture headache; CNS stimulant; diuretic

Mechanism of Action Increases levels of 3-5-AMP by inhibiting phosphodiesterase; methyl xanthine, CNS stimulant which increases medullary respiratory center sensitivity to carbon dioxide, stimulates central inspiratory drive, and improves skeletal muscle contraction (diaphragmatic contractility)

Adverse Reactions

Cardiovascular: Flushing, chest pain, angina, palpitations, sinus tachycardia, tachycardia (supraventricular), arrhythmias (ventricular), vasodilation

Central nervous system: Headache, agitation, dizziness, delirium, hallucinations, insomnia, psychosis

Dermatologic: Urticaria

Gastrointestinal: Gastritis, decreased esophageal sphincter tone

Neuromuscular & skeletal: Fasciculations

Ocular: Miosis, increased intraocular pressure (>180 mg caffeine)

Renal: Diuresis (<250 mg/day)

Signs and Symptoms of Overdose Delirium, diarrhea, hallucinations, hypercholesterolemia, hyperglycemia, hyperthermia, hypokalemia, hyponatremia, insomnia, leukocytosis, muscle twitching, myoglobinuria, nausea, premature ventricular contractions, rhabdomyolysis, seizures, tachycardia, tachycardia (ventricular), tinnitus, tremors, vomiting

Admission Criteria/Prognosis Any patient with change in mental status, cardiopulmonary complaints, or ingestions >2 g should be admitted

Pharmacodynamics/Kinetics

Distribution: V_d:

Neonates: 0.8-0.9 L/kg

Children >9 months to Adults: 0.6 L/kg

Protein binding: 17% (children) to 36% (adults)

Metabolism: Hepatic, via demethylation by CYP1A2. **Note:** In neonates, interconversion between caffeine and theophylline has been reported (caffeine levels are ~25% of measured theophylline after theophylline administration and ~3% to 8% of caffeine would be expected to be converted to theophylline)

Half-life elimination:

Neonates: 72-96 hours (range: 40-230 hours)

Children >9 months and Adults: 5 hours

Time to peak, serum: Oral: Within 30 minutes to 2 hours

Excretion:

Neonates ≤1 month: 86% excreted unchanged in urine

Infants >1 month and Adults: In urine, as metabolites

Dosage

Apnea of prematurity: Oral:

Loading dose: 10-20 mg/kg as caffeine citrate (5-10 mg/kg as caffeine base). If theophylline has been administered to the patient within the previous 5 days, a full or modified loading dose (50% to 75% of a loading dose) may be given at the discretion of the physician.

Maintenance dose: 5-10 mg/kg/day as caffeine citrate (2.5-5 mg/kg/day as caffeine base) once daily starting 24 hours after the loading dose. Maintenance dose is adjusted based on patient's response, (efficacy and adverse effects), and serum caffeine concentrations.

Administration Oral: May be administered without regard to feedings or meals. May administer injectable formulation (caffeine citrate) orally.

Parenteral:

Caffeine citrate: Infuse loading dose over at least 30 minutes; maintenance dose may be infused over at least 10 minutes. May administer without dilution or diluted with D_5W to 10 mg caffeine citrate/mL.

Caffeine and sodium benzoate: I.V. as slow direct injection. For spinal headaches, dilute in 1000 mL NS and infuse over 1 hour. Follow with 1000 mL NS; infuse over 1 hour. May administer I.M. undiluted.

Contraindications Hypersensitivity to caffeine or any component of the formulation; sodium benzoate is not for use in neonates

Warnings

Use with caution in patients with a history of peptic ulcer, gastroesophageal reflux, impaired renal or hepatic function, seizure disorders, or cardiovascular disease. Avoid use in patients with symptomatic cardiac arrhythmias, agitation, anxiety, or tremor. Over-the-counter [OTC] products contain an amount of caffeine similar to one cup of coffee; limit the use of other caffeine-containing beverages or foods.

Caffeine citrate should not be interchanged with caffeine and sodium benzoate. Avoid use of products containing sodium benzoate in neonates; has been associated with a potentially fatal toxicity ("gasping syndrome") in neonates, including metabolic acidosis, respiratory distress, gasping respirations, seizures, intracranial hemorrhage, hypotension, and cardiovascular collapse. *In vitro* and animal studies have shown that benzoate also displaces bilirubin from protein-binding sites. Neonates receiving caffeine citrate should be closely monitored for the development of necrotizing enterocolitis. Caffeine serum levels should be closely monitored to optimize therapy and prevent serious toxicity.

Dosage Forms

Caplet (Caffedrine®, Vivarin®): 200 mg [OTC]

Injection, solution, as citrate [preservative free] (Cafcit®): 20 mg/mL (3 mL) [equivalent to 10 mg/mL caffeine base]

Injection, solution [with sodium benzoate]: Caffeine 125 mg/mL and sodium benzoate 125 mg/mL (2 mL); caffeine 121 mg/mL and sodium benzoate 129 mg/mL (2 mL)

Lozenge (Enerjets): 75 mg [OTC; Hazelnut coffee or mochamint flavor]

Solution, oral, as citrate (Cafcit®): 20 mg/mL (3 mL) [equivalent to 10 mg/mL caffeine base]

Tablet:

Lucidex: 100 mg [OTC]

NoDoz® Maximum Strength, Vivarin®: 200 mg [OTC]

Reference Range

Therapeutic: 8-14 mcg/mL for neonatal apnea

Toxic: >30 mcg/mL

Fatal: >80 mcg/mL

In the postmortem state, anatomical site concentration differences (ie, postmortem redistribution) may occur

Overdosage/Treatment

Decontamination: Lavage (within 1 hour)/activated charcoal; **do not** induce emesis

Supportive therapy: Vasopressin infusion can assist in raising blood pressure. Ventricular dysrhythmias and tachycardia (ventricular) with aberrancy have been successfully treated with procainamide in an adult (400 mg I.V. bolus followed by a 2 mg/minute infusion); esmolol or adenosine can be used to treat tachycardia

Seizures: If anticipated serum caffeine level is >20 mcg/mL or >2 g are ingested, pretreatment with phenobarbital (6-10 mg/kg I.V.) can be considered; midazolam or other benzodiazepine can be used to treat seizures

Enhancement of elimination: Multiple dosing of activated charcoal may be useful; exchange transfusion (in the neonate) hemodialysis or charcoal hemoperfusion for 4-5 hours can be useful

Test Interactions ↑ uric acid (S); slight increase in urine VMA, catecholamines; can cause false elevation of serum theophylline

Drug Interactions

Substrate of CYP1A2 (major), 2C9 (minor), 2D6 (minor), 2E1 (minor), 3A4 (minor); **Inhibits** CYP1A2 (weak), 3A4 (moderate)

Benzodiazepines: Caffeine may diminish the sedative or anxiolytic effects of benzodiazepines.

CYP1A2 inducers: May decrease the levels/effects of caffeine. Example inducers include aminoglutethimide, carbamazepine, phenobarbital, and rifampin.

CYP1A2 inhibitors: May increase the levels/effects of caffeine. Example inhibitors include fluvoxamine, ketoconazole, and rofecoxib.

Quinolone antibiotics (specifically ciprofloxacin, norfloxacin, ofloxacin): May increase the levels/effects of caffeine.

Pregnancy Risk Factor C

Pregnancy Implications Teratogenic effects in animal studies at caffeine doses >40 mg/day; association with increased rate of spontaneous abortion, low birthweight, and premature delivery; data is conflicting and no definitive association shown

Lactation Enters breast milk/use caution (AAP rates "compatible")

Additional Information

Lethal dose: Oral: 150-200 mg/kg; symptoms usually occur at a total caffeine dose of 500 mg

Coffee beans contain 1% to 2% caffeine; 40% of the bronchodilatory activity of theophylline; lithium blood levels increase during caffeine

withdrawal; analgesia from transcutaneous electrical nerve stimulation may be lessened with concomitant caffeine use; one 12 ounce glass of cola in a 40 pound child is equivalent to 4 glasses of coffee in a 160 pound adult; the average American adult ingests ~200 mg of caffeine/day

Caffeine content: Stimulants: 75-200 mg; Cold preparations: 30-75 mg

Coffee (5 oz): 100-150 mg/cup (brewed); 70 mg/cup (instant); Decaffeinated coffee: 4 mg/cup; Tea: 30-50 mg/cup

Cola drinks (12 oz): 35-55 mg (Maximal allowable content of caffeine in 12 oz of soft drink is 72 mg [0.02%].); Dr. Pepper®: 40 mg; MelloYellow®: 52 mg; Mountain Dew® (12 oz): 54 mg; Coca-Cola® (12 oz): 46 mg; Jolt® (12 oz): 71 mg; Pepsi-Cola®: 38 mg; Tab®: 46 mg; Water Joe® (16 oz): 70 mg

Dark chocolate bar (29 g): 20-25 mg/bar; Milk chocolate bar (29 g): 6 mg/bar; Guarana (800 mg): 24-40 mg; Cocoa (5 oz): 2-20 mg; Hot cocoa (6 oz): 2-20 mg; Chocolate milk (8 oz): 2-7 mg

Specific References

Andrenyak DM, Chen M, Slawson MH, et al, "Analysis of Caffeine and Metabolites by Liquid Chromatography-Mass Spectrometry," *J Anal Toxicol*, 2004, 28:289.

Gordon SM, Nanagas K, and Mowry JB, "Caffeine Elimination Half-Life During Peritoneal Dialysis in a Pediatric Overdose," *J Toxicol Clin Toxicol*, 2004, 42(5):742.

Haller C, Duan M, Benowitz NL, et al, "Concentrations of Ephedra Alkaloids and Caffeine in Commercial Dietary Supplements," *J Anal Toxicol*, 2004, 28:145-51.

Holstege CP, Hunter Y, Baer AB, et al, "Massive Caffeine Overdose Requiring Vasopressin Infusion and Hemodialysis," *J Toxicol Clin Toxicol*, 2003, 41(7):1003-7.

Jacob P, Haller CA, Duan M, et al, "Determination of Ephedra Alkaloid and Caffeine Concentrations in Dietary Supplements and Biological Fluids," *J Anal Toxicol*, 2004, 28:152-9.

Lindsey T, Mazarr-Proo S, Hwang RJ, et al, "Elevated Caffeine Levels in Two Postmortem Cases and a DUI Case in New Mexico," *J Anal Toxicol*, 2006, 30:157.

McCusker RR, Goldberger BA, and Cone EJ, "Caffeine Content of Energy Drinks, Carbonated Sodas, and Other Beverages," *J Anal Toxicol*, 2006, 30:112-4.

McCusker RR, Goldberger BA, and Cone EJ, "Caffeine Content of Specialty Coffees," *J Anal Toxicol*, 2003, 27:520-2.

McCusker RR, Merves ML, Goldberger BA, et al, "Café Noir, Café Au Lait, or Just Caffeine?" *J Anal Toxicol*, 2004, 28:277.

McCusker RR, Merves ML, Goldberger BA, et al, "Café Noir, Café Au Lait, or Just Caffeine? - Part 2," *J Anal Toxicol*, 2006, 30:157-8.

Pollak CP and Bright D, "Caffeine Consumption and Weekly Sleep Patterns in U.S. Seventh-, Eighth-, and Ninth-Graders," *Pediatrics*, 2003, 111(1):42-6.

Schmidt B, Roberts RS, Davis P, et al, "Caffeine Therapy for Apnea of Prematurity," *N Engl J Med*, 2006, 354:2112-21.

Winkelmayer WC, Stampfer MJ, Willett WC, et al. "Habitual Caffeine Intake and the Risk of Hypertension in Women," *JAMA*, 2005, 294(18):2330-5.

Calcitonin

CAS Number 12321-44-7; 47931-85-1; 60731-46-6; 9007-12-9

U.S. Brand Names Miacalcin®

Synonyms Calcitonin (Salmon)

Use Calcitonin (salmon): Treatment of Paget's disease of bone and as adjunctive therapy for hypercalcemia; also used in postmenopausal osteoporosis, cholecalciferol (vitamin D₃) induced hypercalcemia

Calcitonin (human): Treatment of Paget's disease of bone

Nasal spray (salmon calcitonin) has been used to treat postmenopausal osteoporosis in women >5 years postmenopause with a low bone mass.

Mechanism of Action Structurally similar to human calcitonin; regulates serum calcium concentration along with vitamin D and parathyroid hormone; acts on bone as well as kidneys and GI tract; directly inhibits osteoclastic bone resorption; promotes the renal excretion of calcium, phosphate, sodium, magnesium, and potassium by decreasing tubular reabsorption; increases the jejunal secretion of water, sodium, potassium, and chloride

Adverse Reactions

Cardiovascular: **Flushing of the face**, edema

Central nervous system: Dizziness, headache, chills

Dermatologic: Rash

Endocrine & metabolic: Hypocalcemia, hypophosphatemia, hyperprolactinemia

Gastrointestinal: **Nausea, anorexia, diarrhea**, metallic taste, salty taste, vomiting

Local: **Edema at injection site**

Neuromuscular & skeletal: Weakness, tingling of palms and soles

Renal: Diuresis, hypercalciuria

Respiratory: Dyspnea, nasal congestion

Miscellaneous: Shivering

Pharmacodynamics/Kinetics

Hypercalcemia: I.M. or SubQ:
Onset of action: ~2 hours
Duration: 6-8 hours
Absorption: Nasal: ~3% of I.M. level (range: 0.3% to 31%)
Distribution: Does not cross placenta
Half-life elimination: SubQ: 1.2 hours; Nasal: 43 minutes
Time to peak: Nasal: ~30-40 minutes
Excretion: Urine (as inactive metabolites)

Dosage

Dosage for calcitonin salmon is expressed in international units (int. units); dosage of calcitonin human is expressed in mg; dosage for children not established

Hepatic osteodystrophy:
Infants: 5-7 mcg/kg/day
Children and Adults: 20-100 mcg/kg/day or every other day, titrate to obtain normal serum calcium/phosphate levels

Calcitonin salmon:
Skin test: 1 unit/0.1 mL intracutaneously on the inner aspect of the forearm
The skin test is 0.1 mL of 10 int. units dilution of calcitonin (must be prepared) injected intradermally; observe injection site for 15 minutes for wheal or significant erythema
Paget's disease: SubQ: 100 units/day
Postmenopause osteoporosis:
I.M., SubQ: 100 units/day (concomitant therapy with supplemental calcium and vitamin D is recommended)
Nasal spray: 200 int. units/day (one actuation in one nostril); alternate nostrils daily
Hypercalcemia: I.M., SubQ: 4 units/kg every 12 hours, may increase to maximum of 8 units/kg every 6 hours

Calcitonin human: I.M., SubQ: Paget's disease: 0.5 mg/day initially; some patients require as little as 0.25 mg or 0.5 mg 2-3 times/week; some patients require up to 0.5 mg twice daily

Stability Refrigeration is recommended for calcitonin salmon, is stable for up to 2 weeks at room temperature; NS has been recommended for the dilution to prepare a skin test; protect from light; calcitonin human may be stored at room temperature

Monitoring Parameters Serum electrolytes and calcium; alkaline phosphatase and 24-hour urine collection for hydroxyproline excretion (Paget's disease); serum calcium

Administration Injection solution: Administer I.M. or SubQ; intramuscular route is recommended over the subcutaneous route when the volume of calcitonin to be injected exceeds 2 mL.
Nasal spray: Before first use, allow bottle to reach room temperature, then prime pump by releasing at least 5 sprays until full spray is produced. To administer, place nozzle into nostril with head in upright position. Alternate nostrils daily. Do not prime pump before each daily use. Discard after 30 doses.

Contraindications Hypersensitivity to calcitonin salmon or any component of the formulation

Warnings A skin test should be performed prior to initiating therapy of calcitonin salmon in patients with suspected sensitivity; have epinephrine immediately available for a possible hypersensitivity reaction. A detailed skin testing protocol is available from the manufacturers. Temporarily withdraw use of nasal spray if ulceration of nasal mucosa occurs. Safety and efficacy have not been established in pediatric patients.

Dosage Forms

Injection, solution, calcitonin-salmon: (Miacalcin®): 200 int. units/mL (2 mL)
Solution, nasal spray, calcitonin-salmon:
Fortical®: 200 int. units/0.09 mL (3.7 mL) [rDNA origin; contains benzyl alcohol; delivers 30 doses, 200 units/actuation]
Miacalcin®: 200 int. units/0.09 mL (3.7 mL) [contains benzalkonium chloride; delivers 30 doses, 200 units/actuation]

Reference Range Therapeutic: <19 pg/mL (SI: 19 ng/L) basal, depending on the assay

Overdosage/Treatment Supportive therapy: I.V. hydration; monitor urine flow and calcium and phosphorus level; oral pizotyline (0.5 mg 3 times/day) may prevent adverse GI effects (nausea, vomiting, anorexia) of calcitonin therapy

Test Interactions ↓ calcium (S)

Pregnancy Risk Factor C

Pregnancy Implications Decreased birth weight was observed in animal studies. Calcitonin does not cross the placental barrier. There are no adequate and well-controlled studies in pregnant women.

Lactation Excretion in breast milk unknown/not recommended

Nursing Implications I.M. route is preferred; skin test should be performed prior to administration of salmon calcitonin; refrigerate when volume exceeds 2 mL

Calfactant

U.S. Brand Names Infasurf®

Use
Prevention of respiratory distress syndrome (RDS) in premature infants at high risk for RDS and for the treatment ("rescue") of premature infants who develop RDS
Prophylaxis: Therapy at birth with calfactant is indicated for premature infants <29 weeks of gestational age at significant risk for RDS. Should be administered as soon as possible, preferably within 30 minutes after birth.
Treatment: For infants ≤72 hours of age with RDS (confirmed by clinical and radiologic findings) and requiring endotracheal intubation.

Mechanism of Action Endogenous lung surfactant is essential for effective ventilation because it modifies alveolar surface tension, thereby stabilizing the alveoli. Lung surfactant deficiency is the cause of respiratory distress syndrome (RDS) in premature infants and lung surfactant restores surface activity to the lungs of these infants.

Adverse Reactions
Cardiovascular: Bradycardia, cyanosis
Respiratory: Airway obstruction, reflux, requirement for manual ventilation, reintubation

Signs and Symptoms of Overdose There have been no known reports of overdosage. While there are no known adverse effects of excess lung surfactant, overdoses would result in overloading the lungs with an isotonic solution. Ventilation should be supported until clearance of the liquid is accomplished.

Pharmacodynamics/Kinetics No human studies of absorption, biotransformation, or excretion have been performed

Dosage Intratracheal administration **only**: Each dose is 3 mL/kg body weight at birth; should be administered every 12 hours for a total of up to 3 doses

Stability Gentle swirling or agitation of the vial of suspension is often necessary for redispersion. **Do not shake**. Visible flecks of the suspension and foaming at the surface are normal. Calfactant should be stored at refrigeration (2°C to 8°C/36°F to 46°F). Warming before administration is not necessary. Unopened and unused vials of calfactant that have been warmed to room temperature can be returned to refrigeration storage within 24 hours for future use. Repeated warming to room temperature should be avoided. Each single-use vial should be entered only once; the vial with any unused material should be discarded after the initial entry.

Monitoring Parameters Following administration, patients should be carefully monitored so that oxygen therapy and ventilatory support can be modified in response to changes in respiratory status

Administration
Should be administered intratracheally through an endotracheal tube. Dose is drawn into a syringe from the single-use vial using a 20-gauge or larger needle with care taken to avoid excessive foaming. Should be administered in 2 aliquots of 1.5 mL/kg each. After each aliquot is instilled, the infant should be positioned with either the right or the left side dependent. Administration is made while ventilation is continued over 20-30 breaths for each aliquot, with small bursts timed only during the inspiratory cycles. A pause, followed by evaluation of respiratory status and repositioning, should separate the two aliquots.

Warnings For intratracheal administration only; the administration of exogenous surfactants often rapidly improves oxygenation and lung compliance. Transient episodes of cyanosis, bradycardia, reflux of surfactant into the endotracheal tube, and airway obstruction were observed more frequently among infants treated with calfactant in clinical trials.

Dosage Forms Suspension, intratracheal [preservative free]: 35 mg/mL (6 mL)

Overdosage/Treatment Supportive therapy: Mechanical ventilation and reintubation may be required. Monitor for upper airway obstruction.

Candesartan

U.S. Brand Names Atacand®

Synonyms Candesartan Cilexetil

Use Alone or in combination with other antihypertensive agents in treating essential hypertension; treatment of heart failure (NYHA class II-IV)

Mechanism of Action Candesartan is an angiotensin receptor antagonist. Angiotensin II acts as a vasoconstrictor. In addition to causing direct vasoconstriction, angiotensin II also stimulates the release of aldosterone. Once aldosterone is released, sodium as well as water are reabsorbed. The end result is an elevation in blood pressure. Candesartan binds to the AT1 angiotensin II receptor. This binding prevents angiotensin II from binding to the receptor thereby blocking the vasoconstriction and the aldosterone secreting effects of angiotensin II.

Adverse Reactions
Cardiovascular: Flushing, chest pain, peripheral edema, tachycardia, palpitations, angina, myocardial infarction
Central nervous system: Dizziness, lightheadedness, drowsiness, fatigue, headache, vertigo, anxiety, depression, somnolence, fever

Dermatologic: Rash, angioedema
Endocrine & metabolic: Hyperglycemia, hypertriglyceridemia, hyperuricemia
Gastrointestinal: Nausea, diarrhea, vomiting, dyspepsia, gastroenteritis
Neuromuscular & skeletal: Back pain, arthralgia, paresthesias, increased CPK, myalgia, weakness
Renal: Hematuria
Respiratory: Upper respiratory tract infection, pharyngitis, rhinitis, bronchitis, cough, sinusitis, epistaxis, dyspnea
Miscellaneous: Diaphoresis (increased)
Signs and Symptoms of Overdose Hypotension and tachycardia
Pharmacodynamics/Kinetics
Onset of action: 2-3 hours
  Peak effect: 6-8 hours
Duration: >24 hours
Distribution: V_d: 0.13 L/kg
Protein binding: 99%
Metabolism: To candesartan by the intestinal wall cells
Bioavailability: 15%
Half-life elimination (dose dependent): 5-9 hours
Time to peak: 3-4 hours
Excretion: Urine (26%)
  Clearance: Total body: 0.37 mL/kg/minute; Renal: 0.19 mL/kg/minute
Dosage
Adults: Oral:
  Hypertension: Usual dose is 4-32 mg once daily; dosage must be individualized. Blood pressure response is dose-related over the range of 2-32 mg. The usual recommended starting dose of 16 mg once daily when it is used as monotherapy in patients who are not volume depleted. It can be administered once or twice daily with total daily doses ranging from 8-32 mg. Larger doses do not appear to have a greater effect and there is relatively little experience with such doses.
  Congestive heat failure: Initial: 4 mg once daily; double the dose at 2-week intervals, as tolerated; target dose: 32 mg
Elderly: No initial dosage adjustment is necessary for elderly patients (although higher concentrations (C_{max}) and AUC were observed in these populations), for patients with mildly impaired renal function, or for patients with mildly impaired hepatic function.
Dosage adjustment in hepatic impairment: No initial dosage adjustment required in mild hepatic impairment. Consider initiation at lower dosages in moderate hepatic impairment (AUC increased by 145%). No data available concerning dosing in severe hepatic impairment.
Monitoring Parameters Supine blood pressure, electrolytes, serum creatinine, BUN, urinalysis, symptomatic hypotension, and tachycardia
Contraindications Hypersensitivity to candesartan or any component of the formulation; hypersensitivity to other A-II receptor antagonists; bilateral renal artery stenosis; pregnancy (2nd and 3rd trimesters)
Warnings [U.S. Boxed Warning]: Based on human data, drugs that act on the angiotensin system can cause injury and death to the developing fetus when used in the second and third trimesters. Angiotensin receptor blockers should be discontinued as soon as possible once pregnancy is detected. Avoid use or use a smaller dose in patients who are volume depleted; correct depletion first. May be associated with deterioration of renal function and/or increases in serum creatinine, particularly in patients dependent on renin-angiotensin-aldosterone system; deterioration may result in oliguria, acute renal failure, and progressive azotemia. Small increases in serum creatinine may occur following initiation; consider discontinuation in patients with progressive and/or significant deterioration in renal function. Use with caution in unilateral renal artery stenosis, hepatic dysfunction, pre-existing renal insufficiency, or significant aortic/mitral stenosis. Use caution when initiating in heart failure; may need to adjust dose, and/or concurrent diuretic therapy, because of candesartan-induced hypotension. Although some properties may be shared between these agents, concurrent therapy with ACE inhibitor may be rational in selected patients.
Dosage Forms
Tablet, as cilexetil:
  Atacand®: 4 mg, 8 mg, 16 mg, 32 mg
Reference Range Therapeutic blood concentration: 34-183 ng/mL
Overdosage/Treatment
Decontamination: Lavage/activated charcoal
Supportive therapy: I.V. crystalloid fluids should be utilized for hypotension; norepinephrine or dopamine are vasopressors that can be used
Drug Interactions
Substrate of CYP2C9 (minor); **Inhibits** CYP2C8 (weak), 2C9 (weak)
Lithium: Risk of toxicity may be increased by candesartan; monitor lithium levels.
NSAIDs: May decrease angiotensin II antagonist efficacy; effect has been seen with losartan, but may occur with other medications in this class; monitor blood pressure.
Potassium-sparing diuretics (amiloride, spironolactone, triamterene): May increase risk of hyperkalemia.

Potassium supplements: May increase the risk of hyperkalemia.
Trimethoprim (high dose): May increase the risk of hyperkalemia.
Pregnancy Risk Factor C/D (2nd and 3rd trimesters)
Pregnancy Implications Candesartan should be discontinued as soon as possible when pregnancy is detected. Drugs which act directly on renin-angiotensin can cause fetal and neonatal morbidity and death. Fetal and neonatal toxicity have been reported in infants born to women treated with candesartan during pregnancy.
Lactation Enters breast milk/contraindicated
Specific References
Morton A, Muir J, and Lim D, "Rash and Acute Nephritic Syndrome Due to Candesartan," *BMJ*, 2004, 328(7430):25.

Cantharidin

Pronunciation (kan THAR e din)
CAS Number 56-25-7
U.S. Brand Names Verr-Canth™
Use Derived from the blister beetle (*Cantharis vesicatoria*), it has been used topically as a wart remover (at concentrations of 0.7% to 1%)
Unlabeled/Investigational Use Primary use is found today as an aphrodisiac
Mechanism of Action Cantharidin (an anhydride of cantharidic acid) is a dermal and mucosal vesicant; lipid soluble and thus systemic absorption can occur from dermal contact; a potent inhibitor of protein phosphatases types 1 and 2A
Adverse Reactions
Cardiovascular: Syncope
Central nervous system: Delirium, ataxia
Dermatologic: Dermal irritation, dermal burns, acantholysis
Gastrointestinal: GI hemorrhage, rectal bleeding, dysphagia
Genitourinary: Priapism
Hepatic: Fatty degeneration
Neuromuscular & skeletal: Hyperreflexia
Ocular: Conjunctivitis, iritis, keratitis
Renal: Proteinuria, hematuria
Respiratory: Burning of oropharynx
Signs and Symptoms of Overdose Abdominal pain, asystole, ataxia, coagulopathy, diarrhea, ECG abnormalities (S-T elevation), hyperreflexia, hypotension, renal failure (acute tubular necrosis), seizures (may last 36 hours), tachycardia, tachypnea, tenesmus, ventricular ectopy, ventricular tachycardia
Admission Criteria/Prognosis Admit any symptomatic patient to a cardiac monitored bed for at least 24 hours; any asymptomatic ingestion >10 mg (or 4 dried blister beetles) should be admitted
Toxicodynamics/Kinetics Absorption: Absorbed by oral and dermal routes
Contraindications Hypersensitivity to cantharidin or any component of the formulation
Overdosage/Treatment
Decontamination:
  Oral: **Do not** induce emesis; dilution with milk or water may be helpful; if no oral pathology is noted, cautious gastric lavage (if performed within 1 hour) with a soft nasogastric tube can be performed; although no studies as to its efficacy exist, activated charcoal can be administered
  Dermal: Irrigate with soap and water
  Ocular: Irrigate with copious amounts of saline
Supportive therapy: To treat hypotension, an isotonic crystalloid fluid challenge (10-20 mL/kg) can be performed with placement of patient in Trendelenburg position; refractory hypotension can be treated with dopamine or norepinephrine seizures can be treated with a benzodiazepine; refractory seizures can be treated with phenobarbital or phenytoin; a urine flow rate of >4 L/day should be maintained with fluids and mannitol
Pregnancy Risk Factor C
Additional Information Minimal fatal dose: Oral: ~30 mg

Capreomycin

CAS Number 11003-38-6; 1405-37-4
U.S. Brand Names Capastat® Sulfate
Synonyms Capreomycin Sulfate
Use Treatment of tuberculosis in conjunction with at least one other antituberculosis agent
Mechanism of Action Polypeptide antibiotic; bacteriostatic
Adverse Reactions
Central nervous system: Vertigo
Endocrine & metabolic: Hypokalemia
Hematologic: Eosinophilia (dose-related, mild), leukocytosis, thrombocytopenia (rare)
Local: Pain, induration, and bleeding at injection site

Otic: **Ototoxicity** [subclinical hearing loss (11%), clinical loss (3%)], **tinnitus**

Renal: **Nephrotoxicity** (36%, increased BUN), acute tubular necrosis, Bartter's syndrome

Miscellaneous: Hypersensitivity (urticaria, rash, fever)

Pharmacodynamics/Kinetics

Half-life elimination: Normal renal function: 4-6 hours

Time to peak, serum: I.M.: ~1 hour

Excretion: Urine (as unchanged drug)

Dosage

I.M., I.V.:

Infants and Children: 15-30 mg/kg/day, up to 1 g/day maximum

Adults: 1 g/day (not to exceed 20 mg/kg/day) for 60-120 days, followed by 1 g 2-3 times/week

Elderly: Refer to Adults dosing; use with caution due to the increased potential for pre-existing renal dysfunction or impaired hearing

Dosing interval in renal impairment: Adults:

Cl_{cr} >100 mL/minute: Administer 13-15 mg/kg every 24 hours

Cl_{cr} 80-100 mL/minute: Administer 10-13 mg/kg every 24 hours

Cl_{cr} 60-80 mL/minute: Administer 7-10 mg/kg every 24 hours

Cl_{cr} 40-60 mL/minute: Administer 11-14 mg/kg every 48 hours

Cl_{cr} 20-40 mL/minute: Administer 10-14 mg/kg every 72 hours

Cl_{cr} <20 mL/minute: Administer 4-7 mg/kg every 72 hours

Monitoring Parameters Audiometric measurements and vestibular function at baseline and during therapy; renal function at baseline and weekly during therapy; serum potassium; liver function tests

Administration

I.M.: Administer by deep I.M. injection into a large muscle mass.

I.V.: Administer over 60 minutes.

Contraindications Hypersensitivity to capreomycin sulfate or any component of the formulation

Warnings [U.S. Boxed Warning]: Use in patients with renal insufficiency or pre-existing auditory impairment must be undertaken with great caution, and the risk of additional eighth nerve impairment or renal injury should be weighed against the benefits to be derived from therapy. Since other parenteral antituberculous agents (eg, streptomycin) also have similar and sometimes irreversible toxic effects, particularly on eighth cranial nerve and renal function, simultaneous administration of these agents with capreomycin is not recommended. Use with nonantituberculous drugs (ie, aminoglycoside antibiotics) having ototoxic or nephrotoxic potential should be undertaken only with great caution. Use caution with renal dysfunction and in the elderly. **[U.S. Boxed Warning]: Safety in pregnant women or pediatric patients not established.**

Dosage Forms Injection, powder for reconstitution, as sulfate: 1 g

Reference Range 1 g administered I.M. gives a peak serum concentration of 30 mcg/mL; desired serum steady-state level is 10 mcg/mL

Overdosage/Treatment

Decontamination: Lavage for ingestions >1 g/activated charcoal

Enhancement of elimination: Hemodialysis if renal failure develops

Test Interactions ↑ BUN, WBCs; ↓ platelets, potassium

Drug Interactions Increased effect/duration of nondepolarizing neuromuscular blocking agents

Additive toxicity (nephrotoxicity and ototoxicity, respiratory paralysis): Aminoglycosides (eg, streptomycin)

Pregnancy Risk Factor C

Pregnancy Implications Capreomycin has been shown to be teratogenic in animal studies. There are no adequate and well-controlled studies in pregnant women; use during pregnancy only if the potential benefit to the mother outweighs the possible risk to the fetus.

Lactation Excretion in breast milk unknown/use caution

Nursing Implications Solution for injection may acquire a pale straw color and darken with time; this is not associated with a loss of potency or development of toxicity

Captopril

Related Information
- Angiotensin Agents

CAS Number 62571-86-2

U.S. Brand Names Capoten®

Synonyms ACE

Use Management of hypertension and treatment of congestive heart failure; increase circulation in Raynaud's phenomenon; idiopathic edema

Unlabeled/Investigational Use Treatment of hypertensive crisis, rheumatoid arthritis; diagnosis of anatomic renal artery stenosis, hypertension secondary to scleroderma renal crisis; diagnosis of aldosteronism, idiopathic edema, Bartter's syndrome, postmyocardial infarction for prevention of ventricular failure; increase circulation in Raynaud's phenomenon, hypertension secondary to Takayasu's disease; acute pulmonary edema

Mechanism of Action Competitive inhibitor of angiotensin-converting enzyme (ACE); prevents conversion of angiotensin I to angiotensin II, a potent vasoconstrictor; results in lower levels of angiotensin II which

causes an increase in plasma renin activity and a reduction in aldosterone secretion

Adverse Reactions

Cardiovascular: Hypotension, chest pain, tachycardia, pericardial effusion/pericarditis, angina, sinus tachycardia, vasodilation

Central nervous system: Psychosis, gustatory hallucinations

Dermatologic: Rash, pruritus, exfoliative dermatitis, hyperpigmentation in children, pemphigus, lichenoid eruptions, angioedema, hyperhidrosis, Stevens-Johnson syndrome, toxic epidermal necrolysis, xerosis, urticaria, purpura, exanthema, cutaneous vasculitis

Endocrine & metabolic: Hyperkalemia, hyponatremia, hypoglycemia

Gastrointestinal: Tongue irritation, altered taste, loss of taste perception, salty taste, esophagitis, aphthous stomatitis, xerostomia, scalded mouth syndrome, gastrointestinal vasculitis

Hematologic: Leukopenia/neutropenia (agranulocytosis, granulocytopenia), thrombocytopenia

Hepatic: Hepatitis, cholestatic hepatitis

Neuromuscular & skeletal: Paresthesia

Ocular: Phototoxic

Renal: Proteinuria, elevated BUN/serum creatinine, reversible renal failure, renal vasculitis

Respiratory: **Transient cough**, wheezing

Miscellaneous: Systemic lupus erythematosus, zinc depletion

Signs and Symptoms of Overdose Alopecia, atrial ectopy, bone marrow depression, bullous skin disease/pemphigoid, coagulopathy, cholestatic jaundice, diarrhea, drowsiness, dysosmia, eosinophilia, fever, hematuria, hyperkalemia, hyperthermia, hypoglycemia, hyponatremia, lichenoid eruptions, nephrotic syndrome, night terrors, oliguria, ototoxicity, Parkinson's-like symptoms, pemphigus, pericarditis, photosensitivity, renal insufficiency, seizures, severe hypotension, sweating, tinnitus, tubular necrosis, wheezing

Pharmacodynamics/Kinetics

Onset of action: Peak effect: Blood pressure reduction: 1-1.5 hours after dose

Duration: Dose related, may require several weeks of therapy before full hypotensive effect

Absorption: 60% to 75%; reduced 30% to 40% by food

Protein binding: 25% to 30%

Metabolism: 50%

Half-life elimination (renal and cardiac function dependent):

Adults, healthy volunteers: 1.9 hours; Congestive heart failure: 2.06 hours; Anuria: 20-40 hours

Excretion: Urine (95%) within 24 hours

Dosage

Note: Dosage must be titrated according to patient's response; use lowest effective dose. Oral:

Infants: Initial: 0.15-0.3 mg/kg/dose; titrate dose upward to maximum of 6 mg/kg/day in 1-4 divided doses; usual required dose: 2.5-6 mg/kg/day

Children: Initial: 0.5 mg/kg/dose; titrate upward to maximum of 6 mg/kg/day in 2-4 divided doses

Older Children: Initial: 6.25-12.5 mg/dose every 12-24 hours; titrate upward to maximum of 6 mg/kg/day

Adolescents: Initial: 12.5-25 mg/dose given every 8-12 hours; increase by 25 mg/dose to maximum of 450 mg/day

Adults:

Acute hypertension (urgency/emergency): 12.5-25 mg, may repeat as needed (may be given sublingually, but no therapeutic advantage demonstrated)

Hypertension:

Initial dose: 12.5-25 mg 2-3 times/day; may increase by 12.5-25 mg/dose at 1- to 2-week intervals up to 50 mg 3 times/day; maximum dose: 150 mg 3 times/day; add diuretic before further dosage increases

Usual dose range (JNC 7): 25-100 mg/day in 2 divided doses

Congestive heart failure:

Initial dose: 6.25-12.5 mg 3 times/day in conjunction with cardiac glycoside and diuretic therapy; initial dose depends upon patient's fluid/electrolyte status

Target dose: 50 mg 3 times/day

Maximum dose: 150 mg 3 times/day

LVD after MI: Initial dose: 6.25 mg followed by 12.5 mg 3 times/day; then increase to 25 mg 3 times/day during next several days and then over next several weeks to target dose of 50 mg 3 times/day

Diabetic nephropathy: 25 mg 3 times/day; other antihypertensives often given concurrently

Dosing adjustment in renal impairment:

Cl_{cr} 10-50 mL/minute: Administer at 75% of normal dose.

Cl_{cr} <10 mL/minute: Administer at 50% of normal dose.

Note: Smaller dosages given every 8-12 hours are indicated in patients with renal dysfunction; renal function and leukocyte count should be carefully monitored during therapy.

Hemodialysis: Moderately dialyzable (20% to 50%); administer dose postdialysis or administer 25% to 35% supplemental dose.

Peritoneal dialysis: Supplemental dose is not necessary.

Stability Unstable in aqueous solutions; to prepare solution for oral administration, mix prior to administration and use within 10 minutes

Monitoring Parameters BUN, serum creatinine, urine dipstick for protein, complete leukocyte count, and blood pressure

Administration

Unstable in aqueous solutions; to prepare solution for oral administration, mix prior to administration and use within 10 minutes.

Contraindications Hypersensitivity to captopril or any component of the formulation; angioedema related to previous treatment with an ACE inhibitor; idiopathic or hereditary angioedema; bilateral renal artery stenosis; pregnancy (2nd or 3rd trimester)

Warnings Anaphylactic reactions can occur. Angioedema can occur at any time during treatment (especially following first dose). It may involve head and neck (potentially affecting the airway) or the intestine (presenting with abdominal pain). Prolonged monitoring may be required especially if tongue, glottis, or larynx are involved as they are associated with airway obstruction. Those with a history of airway surgery in this situation have a higher risk. Careful blood pressure monitoring with first dose (hypotension can occur especially in volume-depleted patients). **[U.S. Boxed Warning]: Based on human data, ACEIs can cause injury and death to the developing fetus when used in the second and third trimesters. ACEIs should be discontinued as soon as possible once pregnancy is detected.** Dosage adjustment needed in renal impairment. Use with caution in hypovolemia; collagen vascular diseases; valvular stenosis (particularly aortic stenosis); hyperkalemia; or before, during, or immediately after anesthesia. Avoid rapid dosage escalation which may lead to renal insufficiency. Rare toxicities associated with ACE inhibitors include cholestatic jaundice (which may progress to hepatic necrosis) and neutropenia/agranulocytosis with myeloid hyperplasia. If patient has renal impairment, then a baseline WBC with differential and serum creatinine should be evaluated and monitored closely during the first 3 months of therapy. Hypersensitivity reactions may be seen during hemodialysis with high-flux dialysis membranes (eg, AN69). Deterioration in renal function can occur with initiation. Use with caution in unilateral renal artery stenosis and pre-existing renal insufficiency.

Dosage Forms Tablet: 12.5 mg, 25 mg, 50 mg, 100 mg

Reference Range Plasma level of 6 mcg/mL associated with hypotension while a level of 60 mcg/mL associated with fatality

Overdosage/Treatment

Decontamination: Ipecac within 30 minutes or lavage (within 1 hour)/ activated charcoal

Supportive therapy: Following initiation of essential overdose management, toxic symptom treatment and supportive treatment should be initiated. Hypotension usually responds to I.V. fluids or Trendelenburg positioning. If unresponsive to these measures, the use of a parenteral inotrope may be required (eg, norepinephrine 0.1-0.2 mcg/kg/minute titrated to response). Seizures commonly respond to lorazepam or diazepam (I.V. 5-10 mg bolus in adults every 15 minutes if needed up to a total of 30 mg; I.V. 0.25-0.4 mg/kg/dose up to a total of 10 mg in children) or to phenytoin or phenobarbital. Naloxone (2 mg) may reverse hypotension. Sulindac may be useful for captopril-induced cough. Inhaled sodium cromoglycate (total dose: 40 mg/day) can decrease ACE-inhibitor cough by 50%. For refractory hypotension, angiotensin amide infusion may be attempted.

Enhancement of elimination: Multiple dosing of activated charcoal or hemodialysis may be quite useful; moderately dialyzable (20% to 50%)

Antidote(s)

- Naloxone [ANTIDOTE]

Diagnostic Procedures

- Creatinine, Serum
- Urea Nitrogen, Blood

Test Interactions ↑ BUN, creatinine, potassium; positive Coombs' [direct]; ↓ cholesterol (S); may cause false-positive urine acetone determinations using sodium nitroprusside reagent

Drug Interactions

Substrate of CYP2D6 (major)

Allopurinol: Case reports (rare) indicate a possible increased risk of Stevens-Johnson syndrome when combined with captopril.

Alpha$_1$ blockers: Hypotensive effect increased.

Aspirin: The effects of ACE inhibitors may be blunted by aspirin administration, particularly at higher dosages and/or increase adverse renal effects.

CYP2D6 inhibitors: May increase the levels/effects of captopril. Example inhibitors include chlorpromazine, delavirdine, fluoxetine, miconazole, paroxetine, pergolide, quinidine, quinine, ritonavir, and ropinirole.

Diuretics: Hypovolemia due to diuretics may precipitate acute hypotensive events or acute renal failure.

Insulin: Risk of hypoglycemia may be increased.

Lithium: Risk of lithium toxicity may be increased; monitor lithium levels, especially the first 4 weeks of therapy.

Mercaptopurine: Risk of neutropenia may be increased.

NSAIDs: May attenuate hypertensive efficacy; effect has been seen with captopril and may occur with other ACE inhibitors; monitor blood pressure. May increase adverse renal effects.

Potassium-sparing diuretics (amiloride, potassium, spironolactone, triamterene): Increased risk of hyperkalemia.

Potassium supplements may increase the risk of hyperkalemia.

Trimethoprim (high dose) may increase the risk of hyperkalemia.

Pregnancy Risk Factor C (1st trimester)/D (2nd and 3rd trimesters)

Pregnancy Implications Decreased placental blood flow, low birth weight, fetal hypotension, preterm delivery, and fetal death have been noted with the use of some ACE inhibitors (ACEIs) in animal studies. Neonatal hypotension, skull hypoplasia, anuria, renal failure, oligohydramnios (associated with fetal limb contractures, craniofacial deformities, hypoplastic lung development), prematurity, intrauterine growth retardation, and patent ductus arteriosus have been reported with the use of ACEIs, primarily in the 2nd and 3rd trimesters. The risk of neonatal toxicity has been considered less when ACEIs have been used in the 1st trimester; however, major congenital malformations have been reported. The cardiovascular and/or central nervous systems are most commonly affected. Unless alternative agents are not appropriate, ACEIs should be discontinued as soon as possible once pregnancy is detected.

Lactation Enters breast milk/not recommended (AAP rates "compatible")

Nursing Implications Watch for hypotensive effect within 1-3 hours of first dose or new higher dose; many patients complain of transient cough during early therapy

Additional Information Most effective for treating hypertension in young, white patients; conversion factor from captopril to lisinopril is 5:1.

Specific References

Alkurtass DA and Al-Jazairi AS, "Possible Captopril-Induced Toxic Epidermal Necrolysis," *Ann Pharmacother*, 2003, 37(3):380-3.

Cheng RM, Mamdani M, Jackevicius CA, et al, "Association Between ACE Inhibitors and Acute Pancreatitis in the Elderly," *Ann Pharmacother*, 2003, 37(7-8):994-8.

Chobanian AV, Bakris GL, Black HR, et al, "The Seventh Report of the Joint National Committee on Prevention, Detection, Evaluation, and Treatment of High Blood Pressure: The JNC 7 Report," *JAMA*, 2003, 289(19):2560-71.

Cooper WO, Hernandez-Diaz S, Arbogast PG, et al, "Major Congenital Malformations After First-Trimester Exposure to ACE Inhibitors," *N Engl J Med*, 2006, 354(23):2443-51.

Mastrobattista J, "Angiontensin-Converting Enzyme Inhibitors in Pregnancy," *Semin Perinatol*, 1997, 21(2):124-34.

Quan A, "Fetopathy Associated with Exposure to Angiotensin-Converting Enzyme Inhibitors and Angiontensin Receptor Antagonists," *Early Hum Dev*, 2006, 82(1):23-8.

Yanturali S, Ergun N, Eminoglu O, et al, "Life Threatening Tongue Angioedema Associated with an Angiotensin-Converting Enzyme Inhibitor," *Vet Hum Toxicol*, 2004, 46(2):85-6.

Carbamazepine

Related Information

- Carbamazepine-10,11-Epoxide
- Therapeutic Drugs Associated with Hallucinations

CAS Number 298-46-4

U.S. Brand Names Carbatrol®; Epitol®; Tegretol®-XR; Tegretol®

Synonyms CBZ; SPD417

Use Partial seizures with complex symptomatology (psychomotor, temporal lobe); generalized tonic-clonic seizures (grand mal), mixed seizure patterns; pain relief of trigeminal or glossopharyngeal neuralgia

Unlabeled/Investigational Use Treatment of bipolar disorders and other affective disorders, resistant schizophrenia, ethanol withdrawal, restless leg syndrome, psychotic behavior associated with dementia, post-traumatic stress disorders

Mechanism of Action May depress activity in the nucleus ventralis of the thalamus or decrease synaptic transmission or to decrease summation of temporal stimulation leading to neural discharge by limiting influx of sodium ions across cell membrane or other unknown mechanisms; stimulates the release of ADH and potentiates its action in promoting reabsorption of water; chemically related to tricyclic antidepressants; in addition to anticonvulsant effects, carbamazepine has anticholinergic, antineuralgic, antidiuretic, muscle relaxant, and antiarrhythmic properties. May also decrease the turnover of γ-aminobutyric acid (GABA).

Adverse Reactions

Cardiovascular: Edema, congestive heart failure, syncope, bradycardia, hypertension or hypotension, AV block, arrhythmias, thrombophlebitis, thromboembolism

Central nervous system: Sedation, dizziness, fatigue, ataxia, confusion, headache, slurred speech, aseptic meningitis (case report)

Dermatologic: Rash, urticaria, toxic epidermal necrolysis, Stevens-Johnson syndrome, photosensitivity reaction, alterations in skin pigmentation, exfoliative dermatitis, erythema multiforme, purpura, alopecia, cutaneous vasculitis

Endocrine & metabolic: Hyponatremia, SIADH, fever, chills, hyperglycemia

Gastrointestinal: Nausea, vomiting, gastric distress, abdominal pain, diarrhea, constipation, anorexia, pancreatitis

Genitourinary: Urinary retention, urinary frequency, azotemia, renal failure, impotence

Hematologic: Aplastic anemia, agranulocytosis, eosinophilia, leukopenia, pancytopenia, thrombocytopenia, bone marrow suppression, acute intermittent porphyria, leukocytosis

Hepatic: Hepatitis, abnormal liver function tests, jaundice, hepatic failure, hepatic vasculitis

Neuromuscular & skeletal: Peripheral neuritis

Ocular: Blurred vision, nystagmus, lens opacities, conjunctivitis

Otic: Tinnitus, hyperacusis

Renal: Renal vasculitis

Respiratory: Eosinophilic pneumonia

Miscellaneous: Cutaneous T-cell lymphoma, hypersensitivity (including multiorgan reactions, may include vasculitis, disorders mimicking lymphoma, eosinophilia, hepatosplenomegaly), diaphoresis, lymphadenopathy

Signs and Symptoms of Overdose Agranulocytosis, agitation, alopecia, apnea, arrhythmias, ataxia, AV block, bone marrow depression, bradycardia, cholestatic jaundice, chorea (extrapyramidal), cognitive dysfunction, coma, cough, decreased GI motility, delirium, dizziness, drowsiness, dysosmia, encephalopathy, erythema multiforme, exfoliative dermatitis, extrapyramidal reaction, fever, flushing, gingival hyperplasia, granulocytopenia, hyperreflexia, hyperthermia, hypotension, hypothermia, hypothyroidism, hyponatremia, ileus, jaundice, leukocytosis, leukemoid reaction, leukopenia, lichenoid eruptions, lymphoma, mania, myoclonus, mydriasis, nausea, neuroleptic malignant syndrome, neutropenia, nystagmus, oliguria, photosensitivity, P-R prolongation, QRS prolongation, QT prolongation, seizures, toxic epidermal necrolysis, tremors, urinary retention, vomiting

Pharmacodynamics/Kinetics

Absorption: Slow

Distribution: V_d: Neonates: 1.5 L/kg; Children: 1.9 L/kg; Adults: 0.59-2 L/kg

Protein binding: Carbamazepine: 75% to 90%, may be decreased in newborns; Epoxide metabolite: 50%

Metabolism: Hepatic via CYP3A4 to active epoxide metabolite; induces hepatic enzymes to increase metabolism

Bioavailability: 85%

Half-life elimination:

Carbamazepine: Initial: 18-55 hours; Multiple doses: Children: 8-14 hours; Adults: 12-17 hours

Epoxide metabolite: Initial: 25-43 hours

Time to peak, serum: Unpredictable:

Immediate release: Suspension: 1.5 hour; tablet: 4-5 hours

Extended release: Carbatrol®, Equetro™: 12-26 hours (single dose), 4-8 hours (multiple doses); Tegretol®-XR: 3-12 hours

Excretion: Urine 72% (1% to 3% as unchanged drug); feces (28%)

Dosage

Oral (dosage must be adjusted according to patient's response and serum concentrations):

Children:

<6 years: Initial: 5 mg/kg/day; dosage may be increased every 5-7 days to 10 mg/kg/day; then up to 20 mg/kg/day if necessary; administer in 2-4 divided doses

6-12 years: Initial: 100 mg twice daily or 10 mg/kg/day in 2 divided doses; increase by 100 mg/day at weekly intervals depending upon response; usual maintenance: 20-30 mg/kg/day in 2-4 divided doses (maximum dose: 1000 mg/day)

Children >12 years and Adults: 200 mg twice daily to start, increase by 200 mg/day at weekly intervals until therapeutic levels achieved; usual dose: 400-1200 mg/day in 2-4 divided doses; maximum dose: 12-15 years: 1000 mg/day, >15 years: 1200 mg/day; some patients have required up to 1.6-2.4 g/day

Trigeminal or glossopharyngeal neuralgia: Initial: 100 mg twice daily with food, gradually increasing in increments of 100 mg twice daily as needed; usual maintenance: 400-800 mg daily in 2 divided doses; maximum dose: 1200 mg/day

Elderly: 100 mg 1-2 times daily, increase in increments of 100 mg/day at weekly intervals until therapeutic level is achieved; usual dose: 400-1000 mg/day

Dosing adjustment in renal impairment: $Cl_{cr} < 10$ mL/minute: Administer 75% of dose

Monitoring Parameters CBC with platelet count, reticulocytes, serum iron, liver function tests, urinalysis, BUN, serum carbamazepine levels, thyroid function tests, serum sodium; observe patient for excessive sedation, especially when instituting or increasing therapy

Administration

Suspension dosage form must be given on a 3-4 times/day schedule versus tablets which can be given 2-4 times/day. When carbamazepine suspension has been combined with chlorpromazine or thioridazine solutions a precipitate forms which may result in loss of effect. Therefore, it is recommended that the carbamazepine suspension dosage form not be administered at the same time with other liquid medicinal agents or

diluents. Damaged extended release tablets (without release portal) should not be administered.

Contraindications Hypersensitivity to carbamazepine, tricyclic antidepressants, or any component of the formulation; bone marrow depression; with or within 14 days of MAO inhibitor use; pregnancy

Warnings

Administer carbamazepine with caution to patients with history of cardiac damage, hepatic or renal disease. **[U.S. Boxed Warning]: Potentially fatal blood cell abnormalities have been reported following treatment.** Patients with a previous history of adverse hematologic reaction to any drug may be at increased risk. Early detection of hematologic change is important; advise patients of early signs and symptoms including fever, sore throat, mouth ulcers, infections, easy bruising, petechial or purpuric hemorrhage. Prescriptions should be written for the smallest quantity consistent with good patient care. The smallest effective dose is suggested for use in bipolar disorder to reduce the risk for overdose; high-risk patients should be monitored. Actuation of latent psychosis is possible.

Carbamazepine is not effective in absence, myoclonic, or akinetic seizures; exacerbation of certain seizure types have been seen after initiation of carbamazepine therapy in children with mixed seizure disorders. Abrupt discontinuation is not recommended in patients being treated for seizures. Dizziness or drowsiness may occur; caution should be used when performing tasks which require alertness (operating machinery or driving) until the effects are known. Coadministration of carbamazepine and delavirdine may lead to loss of virologic response and possible resistance. Elderly may have increased risk of SIADH-like syndrome. Carbamazepine has mild anticholinergic activity; use with caution in patients with increased intraocular pressure (monitor closely), or sensitivity to anticholinergic effects (urinary retention, constipation). Severe dermatologic reactions, including Lyell and Stevens-Johnson syndromes, although rarely reported, have resulted in fatalities. Drug should be discontinued if there are any signs of hypersensitivity.

Dosage Forms

Capsule, extended release (Carbatrol®, Equetro™): 100 mg, 200 mg, 300 mg

Suspension, oral: 100 mg/5 mL (10 mL, 450 mL)

Tegretol®: 100 mg/5 mL (450 mL) [citrus vanilla flavor]

Tablet (Epitol®, Tegretol®): 200 mg

Tablet, chewable (Tegretol®): 100 mg

Tablet, extended release (Tegretol®-XR): 100 mg, 200 mg, 400 mg

Reference Range

Therapeutic: 4-12 mcg/mL (SI: 17-51 μmol/L). Patients who require higher levels (8-12 mcg/mL) (SI: 34-51 μmol/L) should be watched closely. Side effects including CNS effects occur commonly at higher dosage levels. If other anticonvulsants are given, therapeutic range is 4-8 mcg/mL (SI: 17-34 μmol/L)

Ataxia and nystagmus is noted at levels >10 mcg/mL (SI: >42 μmol/L); levels >30 mcg/mL (SI: >127 μmol/L) associated with coma and respiratory depression

Fatal: Levels of 54 mcg/mL

Overdosage/Treatment

Decontamination: Lavage (within 1 hour)/activated charcoal is effective at binding certain chemicals and drugs, and this is especially true for carbamazepine

Supportive therapy: Other treatment is supportive/symptomatic; flumazenil has been reported to reverse coma although its use is contraindicated in patients with seizure disorder; flumazenil has been utilized to reverse carbamazepine induced coma (serum level 27.8 mg/L), but it should not be utilized in patients with an underlying seizure disorder. Furthermore, since carbamazepine may in itself be seizurgenic, it should probably not be used routinely in overdoses due to this agent. Lithium, diltiazem, miconazole, and metoclopramide use with carbamazepine has been associated with neurotoxicity. Do not use physostigmine.

Enhancement of elimination: Multiple dose of activated charcoal is effective; forced diuresis is not effective; clearance by hemoperfusion ranges from 80-129 mL/minute with 36% of the drug being removed during 4 hours; ~17% of the drug is normally excreted in 4 hours in a healthy person; charcoal hemoperfusion may be effective (hemoperfusion clearance is ~10 mL/hour/kg or ~5 times higher than intrinsic clearance)

Diagnostic Procedures

• Carbamazepine, Blood

Test Interactions ↑ BUN, AST, ALT, ammonia, bilirubin, alkaline phosphatase (S); ↓ calcium, T_3, T_4, sodium (S); may cause false-positive urine immunoassay for tricyclic antidepressants; produces sustained reduction of both free thyroxine and free triiodothyronine, at therapeutic levels

Drug Interactions

Substrate of CYP2C8 (minor), 3A4 (major); **Induces** CYP1A2 (strong), 2B6 (strong), 2C8 (strong), 2C9 (strong), 2C19 (strong), 3A4 (strong)

Acetaminophen: Carbamazepine may enhance hepatotoxic potential of acetaminophen; risk is greater in acetaminophen overdose.

Antimalarial drugs (chloroquine, mefloquine): Concomitant use with carbamazepine may reduce seizure control by lowering plasma levels; monitor.

Antipsychotics: Carbamazepine may enhance the metabolism (decrease the efficacy) of antipsychotics; monitor for altered response; dose adjustment may be needed.

Barbiturates: May reduce serum concentrations of carbamazepine; monitor.

Benzodiazepines: Serum concentrations and effect of benzodiazepines may be reduced by carbamazepine; monitor for decreased effect.

Calcium channel blockers: Diltiazem and verapamil may increase carbamazepine levels, due to enzyme inhibition (see below); other calcium channel blockers (felodipine) may be decreased by carbamazepine due to enzyme induction.

Chlorpromazine: **Note:** Carbamazepine suspension is incompatible with chlorpromazine solution. Schedule carbamazepine suspension at least 1-2 hours apart from other liquid medicinals.

Corticosteroids: Metabolism may be increased by carbamazepine.

Cyclosporine (and other immunosuppressants): Carbamazepine may enhance the metabolism of immunosuppressants, decreasing its clinical effect; includes both cyclosporine and tacrolimus.

CYP1A2 substrates: Carbamazepine may decrease the levels/effects of CYP1A2 substrates. Example substrates include aminophylline, estrogens, fluvoxamine, mirtazapine, ropinirole, and theophylline.

CYP2B6 substrates: Carbamazepine may decrease the levels/effects of CYP2B6 substrates. Example substrates include bupropion, efavirenz, promethazine, selegiline, and sertraline.

CYP2C8 Substrates: Carbamazepine may decrease the levels/effects of CYP2C8 substrates. Example substrates include amiodarone, paclitaxel, pioglitazone, repaglinide, and rosiglitazone.

CYP2C9 Substrates: Carbamazepine may decrease the levels/effects of CYP2C9 substrates. Example substrates include bosentan, celecoxib, dapsone, fluoxetine, glimepiride, glipizide, losartan, montelukast, nateglinide, paclitaxel, phenytoin, sulfonamides, trimethoprim, warfarin, and zafirlukast.

CYP2C19 substrates: Carbamazepine may decrease the levels/effects of CYP2C19 substrates. Example substrates include citalopram, diazepam, methsuximide, phenytoin, propranolol, proton pump inhibitors, sertraline, and voriconazole.

CYP3A4 inducers: CYP3A4 inducers may decrease the levels/effects of carbamazepine. Example inducers include aminoglutethimide, nafcillin, nevirapine, phenobarbital, phenytoin, and rifamycins. Carbamazepine may induce its own metabolism.

CYP3A4 inhibitors: May increase the levels/effects of carbamazepine. Example inhibitors include azole antifungals, clarithromycin, diclofenac, doxycycline, erythromycin, imatinib, isoniazid, nefazodone, nicardipine, propofol, protease inhibitors, quinidine, telithromycin, and verapamil.

CYP3A4 substrates: Carbamazepine may decrease the levels/effects of CYP3A4 substrates. Example substrates include benzodiazepines, calcium channel blockers, clarithromycin, cyclosporine, erythromycin, estrogens, mirtazapine, nateglinide, nefazodone, nevirapine, protease inhibitors, tacrolimus, and venlafaxine.

Danazol: May increase serum concentrations of carbamazepine; monitor.

Delavirdine: May lead to loss of virologic response and possible resistance.

Doxycycline: Carbamazepine may enhance the metabolism of doxycycline, decreasing its clinical effect.

Ethosuximide: Serum levels may be reduced by carbamazepine.

Felbamate: May increase carbamazepine levels and toxicity (increased epoxide metabolite concentrations); carbamazepine may decrease felbamate levels due to enzyme induction.

Immunosuppressants: Carbamazepine may enhance the metabolism of immunosuppressants, decreasing its clinical effect; includes both cyclosporine and tacrolimus.

Isoniazid: May increase the serum concentrations and toxicity of carbamazepine; in addition, carbamazepine may increase the hepatic toxicity of isoniazid (INH).

Isotretinoin: May decrease the effect of carbamazepine.

Lamotrigine: Increases the epoxide metabolite of carbamazepine resulting in toxicity; carbamazepine increases the metabolism of lamotrigine.

Lithium: Neurotoxicity may result in patients receiving concurrent carbamazepine.

Loxapine: May increase concentrations of epoxide metabolite and toxicity of carbamazepine.

Methadone: Carbamazepine may enhance the metabolism of methadone resulting in methadone withdrawal.

Methylphenidate: concurrent use of carbamazepine may reduce the therapeutic effect of methylphenidate; limited documentation; monitor for decreased effect.

Neuromuscular blocking agents, nondepolarizing: Effects may be of shorter duration when administered to patients receiving carbamazepine.

Oral contraceptives: Metabolism may be increased by carbamazepine, resulting in a loss of efficacy.

Phenytoin: Carbamazepine levels may be decreased by phenytoin. Metabolism of phenytoin may be altered by carbamazepine; phenytoin levels may be increased or decreased.

SSRIs: Metabolism may be increased by carbamazepine (due to enzyme induction).

Theophylline: Serum levels may be reduced by carbamazepine.

Thioridazine: **Note:** Carbamazepine suspension is incompatible with thioridazine liquid. Schedule carbamazepine suspension at least 1-2 hours apart from other liquid medicinals.

Thyroid: Serum levels may be reduced by carbamazepine.

Tramadol: Tramadol's risk of seizures may be increased with TCAs (carbamazepine may be associated with similar risk due to chemical similarity to TCAs).

Tricyclic antidepressants: May increase serum concentrations of carbamazepine; carbamazepine may decrease concentrations of tricyclics due to enzyme induction.

Valproic acid: Serum levels may be reduced by carbamazepine; carbamazepine levels may also be altered by valproic acid.

Warfarin: Carbamazepine may inhibit the hypoprothrombinemic effects of oral anticoagulants via increased metabolism; this combination should generally be avoided.

Pregnancy Risk Factor D

Pregnancy Implications Crosses the placenta. Dysmorphic facial features, cranial defects, cardiac defects, spina bifida, IUGR, and multiple other malformations reported. Epilepsy itself, number of medications, genetic factors, or a combination of these probably influence the teratogenicity of anticonvulsant therapy. Benefit:risk ratio usually favors continued use during pregnancy and breast-feeding.

Lactation Enters breast milk/not recommended (AAP rates "compatible")

Nursing Implications Observe patient for excessive sedation

Additional Information Suspension dosage form must be given on a 3-4 times/day schedule versus tablets which can be given 2-4 times/day; ECG changes do **not** correlate with serum carbamazepine levels; it is hypothesized that hematological toxicity and immune system toxicity is due to 9-acridine carboxyaldehyde metabolite. Carbamazepine (400-800 mg/day) has been used to treat cocaine dependence.

Specific References

Adams BK, Mann MD, Aboo A, et al, "Prolonged Gastric Emptying Half-time and Gastric Hypomotility After Drug Overdose," *Am J Emerg Med*, 2004, 22(7):548-554.

Askenazi DJ, Goldstein SL, Chang IF, et al, "Management of a Severe Carbamazepine Overdose Using Albumin-Enhanced Continuous Venovenous Hemodialysis," *Pediatrics*, 2004, 113(2):406-9.

Bates DE and Herman RJ, "Carbamazepine Toxicity Induced by Lopinavir/Ritonavir and Nelfinavir," *Ann Pharmacother*, 2006, 40(6):1190-5.

Cumpston KL, Skrupky R, Pallasch E, et al, "Hyperglycemia in a Pediatric Carbamazepine Overdose," *J Toxicol Clin Toxicol*, 2003, 41(5):677.

Doose DR, Wang SS, Padmanabhan M, et al, "Effect of Topiramate or Carbamazepine on the Pharmacokinetics of an Oral Contraceptive Containing Norethindrone and Ethinyl Estradiol in Healthy Obese and Nonobese Female Subjects," *Epilepsia*, 2003, 44(4):540-9.

Gül U, Kilic A, and Dursun A, "Carbamazepine-Induced Pseudo Mycosis Fungoides," *Ann Pharmacother*, 2003, 37(10):1441-3.

Hassan Y, Tan YT, Peh KK, et al, "Bioequivalence of Carpine Tablets Containing Carbamazepine," *J Pharm Technol*, 2003, 19:278-82.

Klys M, Bystrowska B, and Bujak-Gizycka B, "Postmortem Toxicology of Carbamazepine," *J Anal Toxicol*, 2003, 27(4):243-8.

Kuz GM and Manssourian A, "Carbamazepine-Induced Hyponatremia: Assessment of Risk Factors," *Ann Pharmacother*, 2005, 39(11):1943-6.

Carboplatin

CAS Number 41575-94-4

U.S. Brand Names Paraplatin®

Synonyms CBDCA; NSC-241240

Use Treatment of ovarian cancer

Unlabeled/Investigational Use Lung cancer, head and neck cancer, endometrial cancer, esophageal cancer, bladder cancer, breast cancer, cervical cancer, CNS tumors, germ cell tumors, osteogenic sarcoma, and high-dose therapy with stem cell/bone marrow support

Mechanism of Action Carboplatin is an alkylating agent which covalently binds to DNA; possible cross-linking and interference with the function of DNA

Adverse Reactions

Cardiovascular: Hypertension

Central nervous system: Neurotoxicity, malaise

Dermatologic: **Alopecia** (includes other agents in combination with carboplatin), urticaria, rash

Endocrine & metabolic: **Hypomagnesemia, hypokalemia, hyponatremia, hypocalcemia**; less severe than those seen after cisplatin (usually asymptomatic)

Gastrointestinal: **Nausea, vomiting, stomatitis**, diarrhea, anorexia

Hematologic: Myelosuppression is dose-related and is the dose-limiting toxicity; **thrombocytopenia** is the predominant manifestation, with a reported incidence of 37% in patients receiving 400 mg/m^2 as a single agent and 80% in patients receiving 520 mg/m^2; **leukopenia** has been reported in 27% to 38% of patients receiving carboplatin as a single agent; hemorrhagic complications

Nadir: ~21 days following a single dose

Hepatic: **Alkaline phosphatase increased, AST increased** (usually mild and reversible)

Local: Pain at injection site

Neuromuscular & skeletal: Peripheral neuropathy (4% to 6%; up to 10% in older and/or previously-treated patients)

Otic: Ototoxicity; **hearing loss at high tones** (above speech ranges, up to 19%); clinically-important ototoxicity is not usually seen

Renal: Nephrotoxicity, **increases in creatinine and BUN** have been reported; most of them are mild and they are commonly reversible; considerably less nephrotoxic than cisplatin

Miscellaneous: Secondary malignancies, anaphylaxis

Pharmacodynamics/Kinetics

Distribution: V_d: 16 L/kg; into liver, kidney, skin, and tumor tissue

Protein binding: 0%; platinum is 30% irreversibly bound

Metabolism: Minimally hepatic to aquated and hydroxylated compounds

Half-life elimination: Terminal: 22-40 hours; $Cl_{cr} > 60$ mL/minute: 2.5-5.9 hours

Excretion: Urine (~60% to 90%) within 24 hours

Dosage

Refer to individual protocols: **Note**: Doses are usually determined by the AUC using the Calvert formula

IVPB, I.V. infusion, intraperitoneal:

Children:

Solid tumor: 300-600 mg/m^2 once every 4 weeks

Brain tumor: 175 mg/m^2 weekly for 4 weeks every 6 weeks, with a 2-week recovery period between courses

Adults:

Ovarian cancer: 300-360 mg/m^2 I.V. every 3-4 weeks

Autologous BMT: I.V.: 1600 mg/m2 (total dose) divided over 4 days

Dosing adjustment in renal impairment: No guidelines are available.

Dosing adjustment in hepatic impairment: No guidelines are available.

Intraperitoneal: 200-650 mg/m^2 in 2 L of dialysis fluid have been administered into the peritoneum of ovarian cancer patients

Stability Store intact vials at room temperature of 15°C to 30°C (59°F to 86°F); protect from light. Reconstitute powder to yield a final concentration of 10 mg/mL which is stable for 5 days at room temperature (25°C). Aluminum needles should not be used for administration due to binding with the platinum ion. Further dilution to a concentration as low as 0.5 mg/mL is stable at room temperature (25°C) or under refrigeration for 8 days in D$_5$W.

Monitoring Parameters CBC (with differential and platelet count), serum electrolytes, creatinine clearance, liver function tests

Administration

Do not use needles or I.V. administration sets containing aluminum parts that may come in contact with carboplatin (aluminum can react causing precipitate formation and loss of potency)

Administer as IVPB over 15 minutes up to a continuous intravenous infusion over 24 hours; may also be administered intraperitoneally

Contraindications History of severe allergic reaction to cisplatin, carboplatin, other platinum-containing formulations, or any component of the formulation; pregnancy; breast-feeding

Warnings

Hazardous agent - use appropriate precautions for handling and disposal. High doses have resulted in severe abnormalities of liver function tests.

[U.S. Boxed Warning]: Bone marrow suppression, which may be severe, and vomiting are dose related; reduce dosage in patients with bone marrow suppression and impaired renal function. Clinically significant hearing loss has been reported to occur in pediatric patients when carboplatin was administered at higher than recommended doses in combination with other ototoxic agents.

[U.S. Boxed Warning]: Increased risk of allergic reactions in patients previously exposed to platinum therapy. When administered as sequential infusions, taxane derivatives (docetaxel, paclitaxel) should be administered before the platinum derivatives (carboplatin, cisplatin) to limit myelosuppression and to enhance efficacy. **[U.S. Boxed Warning]: Should be administered under the supervision of an experienced cancer chemotherapy physician.** Safety and efficacy in children have not been established.

Dosage Forms

Injection, powder for reconstitution: 50 mg, 150 mg, 450 mg

Injection, solution: 10 mg/mL (5 mL, 15 mL, 45 mL, 60 mL)

Reference Range Therapeutic plasma carboplatin levels: 10-25 mcg/mL

Overdosage/Treatment

Supportive therapy: Nausea and vomiting can be treated with standard antiemetic therapies; patients should be vigorously hydrated 3 hours before and after carboplatin treatment to prevent nephrotoxicity (I.V. normal saline at ~250 mL/hour)

Enhanced elimination: Hemodialysis can remove carboplatin at ~25% of the rate of intact kidney

Drug Interactions

Aminoglycosides may enhance the nephrotoxic and/or ototoxic effects of carboplatin, especially with higher doses of carboplatin.

Docetaxel, paclitaxel (taxane derivatives): When administered as sequential infusions, taxane derivatives should be administered before platinum derivatives to limit myelosuppression and to enhance efficacy.

Pregnancy Risk Factor D

Lactation Excretion in breast milk unknown/contraindicated

Carfentanil Citrate

Related Information

- Fentanyl

CAS Number 59708-52-0; 61380-27-6

Use Highly potent opioid analgesic usually used in veterinary medicine to immobilize large animals; used to study opiate receptors in brain imaging

Mechanism of Action Binds with stereospecific receptors at many sites within the CNS, increases pain threshold, alters pain reception, inhibits ascending pain pathways; a very specific mu-opioid agonist

Signs and Symptoms of Overdose Apnea, chest pain, coma, confusion, depression, dyspnea, exfoliative dermatitis, flatulence, hiccups, hypertension, hypertonia, hypotension, laryngospasm, pseudotumor cerebri, respiratory depression (especially with doses >200 mcg), seizures

Toxicodynamics/Kinetics Duration of action: 2-24 hours

Dosage Incapacitation of large animals: Oral, I.M.: 6.8-18.8 mcg/kg.

Stability 59°F to 86°F; protect from prolonged excessive heat

Administration

Inject deep into large muscle mass of shoulder, back, or hindquarter of animal (deer, elk, moose)

Additional Information 8000-10,000 times more potent than morphine and 100 times as potent as fentanyl; may be a chemical submissive agent when inhaled

Specific References

Wax PM, Becker CE, and Curry SC, "Unexpected 'Gas' Casualties in Moscow: A Medical Toxicology Perspective," *Ann Emerg Med*, 2003, 41(5):700-5.

Zilker TH, Pfab R, Eyer F, et al, "The Mystery About the Gas Used for the Release of the Hostages in the Moscow Musical Theater," *J Toxicol Clin Toxicol*, 2003, 41(5):661.

Carisoprodol

Related Information

- Meprobamate

CAS Number 78-44-4

U.S. Brand Names Soma®

Synonyms Carisoprodate; Isobamate

Impairment Potential Yes. Driving impairment can occur if combined serum levels of carisoprodol and meprobamate exceed 10 mg/L

Use Skeletal muscle relaxant

Mechanism of Action Precise mechanism is not yet clear, but many effects have been ascribed to its central depressant actions

Adverse Reactions

Cardiovascular: Hypotension, tachycardia, tightness in chest, flushing of face, sinus tachycardia

Central nervous system: Sedation, **drowsiness**, dizziness, fatigue, fainting, CNS depression, lightheadedness, headache, clumsiness, insomnia, ataxia

Dermatologic: Skin rash, hives, erythema multiforme

Gastrointestinal: Nausea, vomiting, stomach cramps

Hematologic: Aplastic anemia, eosinophilia, porphyrinogenic

Neuromuscular & skeletal: Trembling

Ocular: Diplopia, blurred vision, burning eyes, nystagmus

Respiratory: Dyspnea

Miscellaneous: Hiccups

Signs and Symptoms of Overdose Coma, CNS depression, depression, dizziness, erythema multiforme, insomnia, lightheadedness, nystagmus, respiratory depression, shock, stupor, hypotonia, agitation

Pharmacodynamics/Kinetics

Onset of action: ~30 minutes

Duration: 4-6 hours

Distribution: Crosses placenta; high concentrations enter breast milk

Metabolism: Hepatic, via CYP2C19 to active metabolite (meprobamate)

Half-life elimination: 2.4 hours; Meprobamate: 10 hours

Excretion: Urine, as metabolite

Dosage Adults: Oral: 350 mg 3-4 times/day; take last dose at bedtime; compound: 1-2 tablets 4 times/day

Monitoring Parameters Look for relief of pain and/or muscle spasm and avoid excessive drowsiness

Administration
Give with food to decrease GI upset.

Contraindications Hypersensitivity to carisoprodol, meprobamate, or any component of the formulation; acute intermittent porphyria

Warnings May cause CNS depression, which may impair physical or mental abilities. Effects with other sedative drugs or ethanol may be potentiated. Use with caution in patients with hepatic/renal dysfunction. Tolerance or drug dependence may result from extended use. Limit to 2-3 weeks; use caution in patients who may be prone to addiction. Idiosyncratic reactions and/or severe allergic reactions may occur. Idiosyncratic reactions occur following the initial dose and may include severe weakness, transient quadriplegia, euphoria, or vision loss (temporary). Has been associated (rarely) with seizures in patients with and without seizure history. Safety and efficacy in children <12 years of age have not been established.

Dosage Forms
Tablet: 350 mg
Soma®: 350 mg

Reference Range 600 mg oral dose can produce peak carisoprodol plasma level between 9-20 mg/L; plasma levels >30 mg/L associated with stupor, coma, or death

Overdosage/Treatment
Decontamination: Lavage (within 2 hours of ingestion)/activated charcoal
Supportive therapy: Benzodiazepines for seizure control; flumazenil at doses of 0.2 mg I.V. can reverse CNS depression due to carisoprodol. Hypotension should be treated with I.V. fluids and/or Trendelenburg positioning.
Enhancement of elimination: Forced diuresis is not helpful; multiple dosing of activated charcoal may be helpful.

Drug Interactions
Substrate of CYP2C19 (major)
CNS depressants (includes CNS depressants, benzodiazepines, and phenothiazines): Sedation may be increased; avoid concurrent use.
CYP2C19 inhibitors: May increase the levels/effects of carisoprodol. Example inhibitors include delavirdine, fluconazole, fluvoxamine, gemfibrozil, isoniazid, omeprazole, and ticlopidine.

Pregnancy Risk Factor C

Pregnancy Implications Reproduction studies have not been conducted.

Lactation Enters breast milk (high concentrations)/not recommended

Nursing Implications Raise bed rails; institute safety measures; assist with ambulation

Additional Information Minimal lethal dose: Children: 3.5 g

Specific References
Beebe FA, Barkin RL, and Barkin S, "A Clinical and Pharmacologic Review of Skeletal Muscle Relaxants for Musculoskeletal Conditions," *Am J Ther*, 2005, 12(2):151-71.

Bramness JG, Morland J, Sorlid HK, et al, "Carisoprodol Intoxications and Serotonergic Features," *Clin Toxicol (Phila)*, 2005, 43(1):39-45.

Forrester MB, "Carisoprodol Abuse in Texas, 1998-2003," *J Med Toxicol*, 2006, 2(1):8-13.

Matsumoto T, Sano T, Matsuoka T, et al, "Simultaneous Determination of Carisoprodol and Acetaminophen in an Attempted Suicide by Liquid Chromatography-Mass Spectrometry with Positive Electrospray Ionization," *J Anal Toxicol*, 2003, 27(2):118-22.

Miksa IR and Poppenga RH, "Direct and Rapid Determination of Baclofen (Lioresal®) and Carisoprodol (Soma®) in Bovine Serum by Liquid Chromatography-Mass Spectrometry," *J Anal Toxicol*, 2003, 27(5):275-83.

Siddiqi M and Jennings CA, "A Near-Fatal Overdose of Carisoprodol (SOMA): Case Report," *J Toxicol Clin Toxicol*, 2004, 42(2):239-40.

Carmustine

CAS Number 154-93-8
U.S. Brand Names BiCNu®; Gliadel®
Synonyms BCNU; bis-chloronitrosourea; Carmustinum; NSC-409962; WR-139021

Use
Injection: Treatment of brain tumors (glioblastoma, brainstem glioma, medulloblastoma, astrocytoma, ependymoma, and metastatic brain tumors), multiple myeloma, Hodgkin's disease, non-Hodgkin's lymphomas, melanoma, lung cancer, colon cancer
Wafer (implant): Adjunct to surgery in patients with recurrent glioblastoma multiforme; adjunct to surgery and radiation in patients with high-grade malignant glioma

Mechanism of Action Interferes with the normal function of DNA by alkylation and cross-linking the strands of DNA, and by possible protein modification

Adverse Reactions
Cardiovascular: **Hypotension is associated with HIGH-DOSE administration secondary to the high alcohol content of the diluent**, facial flushing is probably due to the ethanol used in reconstitution

Central nervous system: **Dizziness, ataxia**, headache, circumoral paresthesia, leukoencephalopathy
Dermatologic: **Hyperpigmentation of skin**, alopecia, dermatitis
Endocrine & metabolic: Gynecomastia, hyperprolactinemia
Gastrointestinal: **Nausea and vomiting occur within 2-4 hours after drug injection, dose-related**; stomatitis, diarrhea, anorexia, metallic taste
Genitourinary: Hemorrhagic cystitis
  Emetic potential:
    <200 mg: Moderately high (60% to 90%)
    ≥200 mg: High (>90%)
Hematologic: Anemia
  Myelosuppressive: Delayed, occurs 4-6 weeks after administration and is dose-related; usually persists for 1-2 weeks; thrombocytopenia is usually more severe than leukopenia. Myelofibrosis and preleukemic syndromes have been reported.
    WBC: Moderate; Platelets: Severe; Onset (days): 14; Nadir (days): 21-35; Recovery (days): 42-50
Hepatic: Reversible toxicity, **elevated liver function tests** in 20%, **hepatotoxicity (26%), hepatic necrosis (centrilobular)**
Local: **Burning at injection site; Irritant chemotherapy:** pain at injection site, extravasation injury
Ocular: **Ocular toxicity, retinal hemorrhages**, neuroretinopathy blindness
Renal: Azotemia, decrease in kidney size
Respiratory: Fibrosis occurs mostly in patients treated with prolonged total doses >1400 mg/m^2 or with bone marrow transplantation doses. Risk factors include a history of lung disease, concomitant bleomycin, or radiation therapy. PFTs should be conducted prior to therapy and monitored. Patients with predicted FVC or DLCO <70% are at a higher risk. Idiopathic pneumonia can occur when dose exceeds 475 mg/m^2.

Pharmacodynamics/Kinetics
Distribution: Readily crosses blood-brain barrier producing CSF levels equal to 15% to 70% of blood plasma levels; enters breast milk; highly lipid soluble
Metabolism: Rapidly hepatic
Half-life elimination: Biphasic: Initial: 1.4 minutes; Secondary: 20 minutes (active metabolites: plasma half-life of 67 hours)
Excretion: Urine (~60% to 70%) within 96 hours; lungs (6% to 10% as CO_2)

Dosage
I.V. (refer to individual protocols):
Children: 200-250 mg/m^2 every 4-6 weeks as a single dose
Adults: Usual dosage (per manufacturer labeling): 150-200 mg/m^2 every 6-8 weeks as a single dose or divided into daily injections on 2 successive days
Alternative regimens:
75-120 mg/m^2 days 1 and 2 every 6-8 weeks **or**
50-80 mg/m^2 days 1,2,3 every 6-8 weeks
  Primary brain cancer:
    150-200 mg/m^2 every 6-8 weeks as a single dose **or**
    75-120 mg/m^2 days 1 and 2 every 6-8 weeks **or**
    20-65 mg/m^2 every 4-6 weeks **or**
    0.5-1 mg/kg every 4-6 weeks **or**
    40-80 mg/m^2/day for 3 days every 6-8 weeks
  Autologous BMT: ALL OF THE FOLLOWING DOSES ARE FATAL WITHOUT BMT
    Combination therapy: Up to 300-900 mg/m^2
    Single-agent therapy: Up to 1200 mg/m^2 (fatal necrosis is associated with doses >2 g/m^2)
Implantation (wafer): Adults: Recurrent glioblastoma multiforme, malignant glioma: Up to 8 wafers may be placed in the resection cavity (total dose 62.6 mg); should the size and shape not accommodate 8 wafers, the maximum number of wafers allowed should be placed
Hemodialysis: Supplemental dosing is not required
Dosing adjustment in hepatic impairment: Dosage adjustment may be necessary; however, no specific guidelines are available

Stability Injection: Store intact vials under refrigeration; vials are stable for 36 days at room temperature. Initially, dilute with 3 mL of absolute alcohol. Further dilute with SWFI to a concentration of 3.3 mg/mL. Solutions are stable for 8 hours at room temperature (25°C) and 24 hours under refrigeration (2°C to 8°C) and protected from light. Further dilution in D$_5$W or NS is stable for 8 hours at room temperature (25°C) and 48 hours under refrigeration (4°C) in glass or Excel® protected from light.
Wafer: Store at or below -20°C (-4°F); may be kept at room temperature for up to 6 hours

Monitoring Parameters
CBC with differential and platelet count, pulmonary function, liver function, and renal function tests; monitor blood pressure during administration
Wafer: Complications of craniotomy (seizures, intracranial infection, brain edema)

Administration Injection: Significant absorption to PVC containers - should be administered in either glass or Excel® container. I.V. infusion over 1-2 hours is recommended; infusion through a free-flowing saline or dextrose infusion, or administration through a central catheter can alleviate venous pain/irritation

High-dose carmustine: Maximum rate of infusion of ≤ 3 mg/m^2/minute to avoid excessive flushing, agitation, and hypotension; infusions should run over at least 2 hours; some investigational protocols dictate shorter infusions.

Fatal doses if not followed by bone marrow or peripheral stem cell infusions.

Extravasation management: Elevate extremity. Inject long-acting dexamethasone (Decadron® LA) or by hyaluronidase (Wydase®) throughout tissue with a 25- to 37-gauge needle. Apply warm, moist compresses.

Contraindications Hypersensitivity to carmustine or any component of the formulation; myelosuppression; pregnancy

Warnings

Hazardous agent - use appropriate precautions for handling and disposal.

[U.S. Boxed Warning]: Bone marrow suppression (thrombocytopenia, leukopenia) is the major toxicity and may be delayed; monitor blood counts weekly for at least 6 weeks after administration. Myelosuppression is cumulative; consider nadir blood counts from prior dose for dosage adjustment. May cause bleeding (due to thrombocytopenia) or infections (due to neutropenia); monitor closely. Administer with caution to patients with depressed platelet, leukocyte, or erythrocyte counts; renal or hepatic impairment. Diluent contains significant amounts of ethanol; use caution with aldehyde dehydrogenase-2 deficiency or history of "alcohol flushing syndrome."

[U.S. Boxed Warning]: Dose-related pulmonary toxicity may occur; patients receiving cumulative doses >1400 mg/m^2 are at higher risk. Baseline pulmonary function tests are recommended. **[U.S. Boxed Warning]: Delayed onset of pulmonary fibrosis has occurred up to 17 years after treatment** in children (1-16 years) who received carmustine in cumulative doses ranging from 770-1800 mg/m^2 combined with cranial radiotherapy for intracranial tumors. May be associated with the development of secondary malignancies. **[U.S. Boxed Warning]: Should be administered under the supervision of an experienced cancer chemotherapy physician.** Safety and efficacy in children have not been established.

Dosage Forms

Injection, powder for reconstitution (BiCNu®): 100 mg [packaged with 3 mL of absolute alcohol as diluent]

Wafer (Gliadel®): 7.7 mg (8s)

Overdosage/Treatment Supportive therapy: Corticosteroids can be used to treat pulmonary toxicity; although its use is controversial, infiltration of 5 mL of 8.4% sodium bicarbonate (1 mM/mL solution) has been advocated for extravasation injuries

Antidote(s)

- Thrombopoietin [ANTIDOTE]

Drug Interactions

Cimetidine: Reported to cause bone marrow suppression.

Ethanol: Diluent for infusion contains alcohol; avoid concurrent use of medications that inhibit aldehyde dehydrogenase-2 or cause disulfiram-like reactions.

Etoposide: Reported to cause severe hepatic dysfunction with hyperbilirubinemia, ascites, and thrombocytopenia.

Pregnancy Risk Factor D

Pregnancy Implications Carmustine can cause fetal harm if administered to a pregnant woman.

Lactation Excretion in breast milk unknown/contraindicated

Additional Information Delayed onset pulmonary fibrosis occurring up to 17 years after treatment has been reported in patients who received cumulative >1400 mg/m^2. Avoid ethanol.

Carteolol

Related Information

- Selected Properties of Beta-Adrenergic Blocking Drugs

CAS Number 51781-06-7; 51781-21-6

U.S. Brand Names Cartrol®; Ocupress® [DSC]

Synonyms Carteolol Hydrochloride

Use Management of hypertension; treatment of chronic open-angle glaucoma and intraocular hypertension

Mechanism of Action Blocks both beta$_1$- and beta$_2$-receptors and has mild intrinsic sympathomimetic activity; has negative inotropic and chronotropic effects and can significantly slow AV nodal conduction

Adverse Reactions

Cardiovascular: Mesenteric arterial thrombosis, AV block, persistent bradycardia, hypotension, chest pain, edema, heart failure, exacerbation of Raynaud's phenomenon, myocardial depression, QRS prolongation

Central nervous system: Fatigue, dizziness, headache, insomnia, drowsiness, night terrors, CNS depression, confusion

Dermatologic: Purpura, exfoliative dermatitis, acne, alopecia, angioedema, xerosis, photosensitivity, pruritus, psoriasis

Gastrointestinal: Ischemic colitis, abdominal pain, constipation, nausea, diarrhea, xerostomia, exanthem

Genitourinary: Impotence

Hematologic: Thrombocytopenia

Neuromuscular & skeletal: Paresthesia

Ocular: Corneal irritation, blurred vision with eye drop use

Respiratory: Wheezing, rhinitis

Miscellaneous: Cold extremities, diaphoresis (excessive), systemic lupus erythematosus

Signs and Symptoms of Overdose Arrhythmias, ataxia, cardiovascular collapse, colitis, congestive heart failure, cough, heart/respiratory failure and wheezing, insomnia, impotence, mesenteric ischemia, night terrors, pulmonary edema, purpura, severe hypotension, sinus bradycardia

Pharmacodynamics/Kinetics

Onset of action: Oral: 1-1.5 hours

Peak effect: 2 hours

Duration: 12 hours

Absorption: Oral: 80%

Protein binding: 23% to 30%

Metabolism: 30% to 50%

Half-life elimination: 6 hours

Excretion: Urine (as metabolites)

Dosage

Adults:

Oral: 2.5 mg as a single daily dose, with a maintenance dose normally 2.5-5 mg once daily

Ophthalmic: Instill 1 drop in eye(s) twice daily

Monitoring Parameters Ophthalmic: Intraocular pressure; Systemic: Blood pressure, pulse, CNS status

Administration

Oral: Administer with meals.

Ophthalmic: Intended for twice daily dosing. Keep eye open and do not blink for 30 seconds after instillation. Wear sunglasses to avoid photophobic discomfort. Apply gentle pressure to lacrimal sac during and immediately following instillation (1 minute).

Contraindications Hypersensitivity to carteolol or any component of the formulation; sinus bradycardia; heart block greater than first-degree (except in patients with a functioning artificial pacemaker); cardiogenic shock; bronchial asthma, bronchospasm, or COPD; uncompensated cardiac failure; pulmonary edema; pregnancy (2nd and 3rd trimesters)

Warnings Avoid abrupt discontinuation in patients with a history of CAD; slowly wean while monitoring for signs and symptoms of ischemia. Use caution in patients with PVD (can aggravate arterial insufficiency). Use caution with concurrent use of beta-blockers and either verapamil or diltiazem; bradycardia or heart block can occur. Patients with bronchospastic disease should not receive beta-blockers. Use cautiously in diabetics because it can mask prominent hypoglycemic symptoms. Can mask signs of thyrotoxicosis. Can cause fetal harm when administered in pregnancy. Dosage adjustment is required in patients with renal dysfunction. Use care with anesthetic agents that decrease myocardial function. Beta-blockers with intrinsic sympathomimetic activity have not been demonstrated to be of value in CHF.

Dosage Forms

[DSC] = Discontinued product

Solution, ophthalmic, as hydrochloride: 1% (5 mL, 10 mL, 15 mL) [contains benzalkonium chloride]

Ocupress® [DSC]: 1% (5 mL, 10 mL, 15 mL) [contains benzalkonium chloride]

Tablet, as hydrochloride (Cartrol®): 2.5 mg, 5 mg

Overdosage/Treatment

Decontamination: Lavage (within 1 hour)/activated charcoal; **do not** use ipecac

Supportive therapy: Glucagon (50-150 mcg/kg followed by continuous drip of 1-5 mg/hour) for positive chronotropic effect; atropine/isoproterenol can be utilized to increase heart rate; calcium chloride may also be effective; do **not** use epinephrine

Enhancement of elimination: Multiple dosing of activated charcoal is not likely to be of benefit; dialysis is not useful

Drug Interactions

Substrate of CYP2D6 (minor)

Albuterol (and other beta$_2$ agonists): Effects may be blunted by nonspecific beta-blockers.

Alpha-blockers (prazosin, terazosin): Concurrent use of beta-blockers may increase risk of orthostasis.

Carteolol causes hypertension when used with local anesthetics (tetracaine, lidocaine, or bupivacaine) containing epinephrine.

Clonidine: Hypertensive crisis after or during withdrawal of either agent.

Drugs which slow AV conduction (digoxin): Effects may be additive with beta-blockers.

Glucagon: Carteolol may blunt the hyperglycemic action of glucagon.

Insulin: Carteolol may mask tachycardia from hypoglycemia.

NSAIDs (ibuprofen, indomethacin, naproxen, piroxicam) may reduce the antihypertensive effects of beta-blockers.

Salicylates may reduce the antihypertensive effects of beta-blockers.

Sulfonylureas: Beta-blockers may alter response to hypoglycemic agents.

Verapamil or diltiazem may have synergistic or additive pharmacological effects when taken concurrently with beta-blockers.

Pregnancy Risk Factor C (manufacturer); D (2nd and 3rd trimesters - expert analysis)

Lactation Excretion in breast milk unknown/use caution

Carvedilol

CAS Number 72956-09-3

U.S. Brand Names Coreg®

Use Mild to severe heart failure of ischemic or cardiomyopathic origin (usually in addition to standardized therapy); left ventricular dysfunction following myocardial infarction (MI); management of hypertension

Unlabeled/Investigational Use Angina pectoris

Mechanism of Action Noncardioselective beta-blocking agent with calcium channel blocking activity at higher dose ($\sim$30 times the normal dose); similar to labetalol in that there is some alpha$_1$-adrenergic antagonist effect, thus acting as a vasodilator; less alpha$_1$ effect than labetalol or prazosin

Adverse Reactions

Note: Frequency ranges include data from hypertension and heart failure trials. Higher rates of adverse reactions have generally been noted in patients with CHF. However, the frequency of adverse effects associated with placebo is also increased in this population. Events occurring at a frequency > placebo in clinical trials.

Cardiovascular: **Hypotension** (9% to 14%), **bradycardia** (2% to 10%), hypertension, AV block, angina, postural hypotension, syncope, dependent edema, palpitations, peripheral edema, generalized edema, cerebrovascular disorder, bundle branch block, myocardial ischemia, peripheral ischemia, tachycardia

Central nervous system: **Dizziness** (6% to 32%), **fatigue** (4% to 24%), headache, fever, paresthesia, somnolence, insomnia, malaise, hypesthesia, vertigo, abnormal thinking, aggravated depression, amnesia, convulsions, emotional lability, impaired concentration, migraine, nervousness, paranoia, paresis, sleep disorders

Dermatologic: Alopecia, erythematous rash, exfoliative dermatitis, maculopapular rash, photosensitivity, pruritus, psoriaform rash

Endocrine & metabolic: **Hyperglycemia** (5% to 12%), **weight gain** (10% to 12%), gout, hypercholesterolemia, dehydration, hyperkalemia, hypervolemia, hypertriglyceridemia, hyperuricemia, hypoglycemia, hyponatremia, diabetes mellitus, HDL-cholesterol decreased, hypokalemia, libido decreased (male)

Gastrointestinal: **Diarrhea** (2% to 12%), nausea, vomiting, melena, periodontitis, GI hemorrhage, xerostomia

Genitourinary: Hematuria, impotence, micturition (increased)

Hematologic: Thrombocytopenia, decreased prothrombin, purpura, anemia, atypical lymphocytes, leukopenia, pancytopenia

Hepatic: Increased transaminases, increased alkaline phosphatase, bilirubinemia

Neuromuscular & skeletal: **Weakness**, back pain, arthralgia, myalgia, muscle cramps, hypokinesis, neuralgia

Ocular: Blurred vision

Otic: Hearing decreased, tinnitus

Renal: Increased BUN, abnormal renal function, albuminuria, glycosuria, increased creatinine, kidney failure

Respiratory: Rhinitis, increased cough, asthma, bronchospasm, pulmonary edema, respiratory alkalosis

Miscellaneous: Injury, increased diaphoresis, allergy, sudden death, anaphylactoid reactions

Postmarketing and/or case reports: Aplastic anemia (rare): All events occurred in patients receiving other medications capable of causing this effect; Stevens-Johnson syndrome; cholestatic jaundice

Pharmacodynamics/Kinetics

Onset of action: 1-2 hours

Peak antihypertensive effect: $\sim$1-2 hours

Absorption: Rapid; food decreases rate but not extent of absorption; administration with food minimizes risks of orthostatic hypotension

Distribution: V$_d$: 115 L

Protein binding: >98%, primarily to albumin

Metabolism: Extensively hepatic, via **CYP2C9, 2D6,** 3A4, and 2C19 (2% excreted unchanged); three active metabolites (4-hydroxyphenyl metabolite is 13 times more potent than parent drug for beta-blockade); first-pass effect; plasma concentrations in the elderly and those with cirrhotic liver disease are 50% and 4-7 times higher, respectively

Bioavailability: 25% to 35%

Half-life elimination: 7-10 hours

Excretion: Primarily feces

Dosage

Oral: Adults: Reduce dosage if heart rate drops to <55 beats/minute.

Hypertension: 6.25 mg twice daily; if tolerated, dose should be maintained for 1-2 weeks, then increased to 12.5 mg twice daily. Dosage may be increased to a maximum of 25 mg twice daily after 1-2 weeks. Maximum dose: 50 mg/day

Congestive heart failure: 3.125 mg twice daily for 2 weeks; if this dose is tolerated, may increase to 6.25 mg twice daily. Double the dose every 2 weeks to the highest dose tolerated by patient. (Prior to initiating therapy, other heart failure medications should be stabilized and fluid retention minimized.)

Maximum recommended dose:

Mild to moderate heart failure:

<85 kg: 25 mg twice daily

>85 kg: 50 mg twice daily

Severe heart failure: 25 mg twice daily

Left ventricular dysfunction following MI: Initial 3.125-6.25 mg twice daily; increase dosage incrementally (ie, from 6.25 to 12.5 mg twice daily) at intervals of 3-10 days, based on tolerance, to a target dose of 25 mg twice daily. **Note:** Should be initiated only after patient is hemodynamically stable and fluid retention has been minimized.

Angina pectoris (unlabeled use): 25-50 mg twice daily

Dosing adjustment in renal impairment: None necessary

Dosing adjustment in hepatic impairment: Use is contraindicated in severe liver dysfunction.

Monitoring Parameters Heart rate, blood pressure (base need for dosage increase on trough blood pressure measurements and for tolerance on standing systolic pressure 1 hour after dosing); renal studies, BUN, liver function

Administration

Administer with food.

Contraindications Hypersensitivity to carvedilol or any component of the formulation; patients with decompensated cardiac failure requiring intravenous inotropic therapy; bronchial asthma or related bronchospastic conditions; second- or third-degree AV block, sick sinus syndrome, and severe bradycardia (except in patients with a functioning artificial pacemaker); cardiogenic shock; severe hepatic impairment; pregnancy (2nd and 3rd trimesters)

Warnings

Initiate cautiously and monitor for possible deterioration in patient status (including symptoms of CHF). Adjustment of other medications (ACE inhibitors and/or diuretics) may be required. In severe chronic heart failure, trial patients were excluded if they had cardiac-related rales, ascites, or a serum creatinine >2.8 mg/dL. Congestive heart failure patients may experience a worsening of renal function; risks include ischemic disease, diffuse vascular disease, underlying renal dysfunction; systolic BP <100 mm Hg. Patients should be advised to avoid driving or other hazardous tasks during initiation of therapy due to the risk of syncope. Avoid abrupt discontinuation (may exacerbate underlying condition), particularly in patients with coronary artery disease; dose should be tapered over 1-2 weeks with close monitoring.

Manufacturer recommends discontinuation of therapy if liver injury occurs (confirmed by laboratory testing). Use caution in patients with PVD (can aggravate arterial insufficiency). Use caution with concurrent use of verapamil or diltiazem; bradycardia or heart block can occur. Use caution in patients with bronchospastic disease. Use cautiously in diabetics because it can mask prominent hypoglycemic symptoms. May mask signs of thyrotoxicosis. Use care with anesthetic agents that decrease myocardial function. Safety and efficacy in children <18 years of age have not been established.

Dosage Forms Tablet: 3.125 mg, 6.25 mg, 12.5 mg, 25 mg

Reference Range Peak serum levels of $\sim$122 mcg/L achieved after oral 50 mg dose

Overdosage/Treatment

Decontamination: Gastric lavage (within 1 hour)/activated charcoal; **do not** use ipecac

Supportive therapy: Sympathomimetics (eg, epinephrine or dopamine), atropine, glucagon or a pacemaker can be used to treat the toxic bradycardia, asystole, and/or hypotension; inamrinone may also be effective for labetalol-induced hypotension; initially fluids may be the best treatment for toxic hypotension with norepinephrine being used for second-line therapy

Enhancement of elimination: Multiple dosing of activated charcoal may be useful; not dialyzable

Drug Interactions

Substrate of CYP1A2 (minor), 2C9 (major), 2D6 (major), 2E1 (minor), 3A4 (minor)

Alpha-blockers (prazosin, terazosin): Concurrent use of beta-blockers may increase risk of orthostasis.

Beta-agonists: Beta-blockers may counteract desired effects of beta-agonists.

Calcium channel blockers (nondihydropyridine): May enhance hypotensive effects of beta-blockers.

Cimetidine: May increase carvedilol serum levels.

CYP2C9 inducers: May decrease the levels/effects of carvedilol. Example inducers include carbamazepine, phenobarbital, phenytoin, rifampin, rifapentine, and secobarbital.

CYP2C9 Inhibitors may increase the levels/effects of carvedilol. Example inhibitors include delavirdine, fluconazole, gemfibrozil, ketoconazole, nicardipine, NSAIDs, sulfonamides and tolbutamide.

CYP2D6 inhibitors: May increase the levels/effects of carvedilol. Example inhibitors include chlorpromazine, delavirdine, fluoxetine, miconazole, paroxetine, pergolide, quinidine, quinine, ritonavir, and ropinirole.

Digoxin: Carvedilol may increase the serum levels of digoxin.

Disopyramide: May exacerbate heart failure or enhance bradycardic effect of beta-blockers.

Drugs which slow AV conduction (digoxin): Effects may be additive with beta-blockers.

Insulin and oral hypoglycemics: Carvedilol may mask symptoms of hypoglycemia.

NSAIDs (ibuprofen, indomethacin, naproxen, piroxicam) may reduce the antihypertensive effects of beta-blockers.

Rifampin: May increase the metabolism of carvedilol.

Salicylates: May reduce the antihypertensive effects of beta-blockers.

SSRIs: May decrease the metabolism of carvedilol.

Sulfonylureas: Beta-blockers may alter response to hypoglycemic agents.

Verapamil, diltiazem: May have synergistic or additive pharmacological effects when taken concurrently with beta-blockers.

Pregnancy Risk Factor C (manufacturer); D (2nd and 3rd trimesters - expert analysis)

Pregnancy Implications No data available on whether carvedilol crosses the placenta; beta-blockers have been associated with persistent bradycardia, hypotension, and IUGR; IUGR probably related to maternal hypertension. Cases of neonatal hypoglycemia have been reported following maternal use of beta-blockers at parturition or during breast-feeding. Use during pregnancy only if the potential benefit justifies the risk.

Lactation Excretion in breast milk unknown/contraindicated

Additional Information High concentrations of carvedilol (>1 μmol/L) can cause calcium channel blocking effect; not useful for pheochromocytoma; should be taken with food

Specific References

Horani MH, Haas MJ, and Mooradian AD, "Suppression of Hyperglycemia-Induced Superoxide Formation and Endothelin-1 Gene Expression by Carvedilol," *Am J Ther*, 2006, 13(1):2-7.

Castor Oil

CAS Number 8001-79-4

U.S. Brand Names Emulsoil® [OTC] [DSC]; Purge® [OTC]

Synonyms Oleum Ricini

Use Preparation for rectal or bowel examination or surgery; rarely used to relieve constipation; also applied to skin as emollient and protectant

Mechanism of Action Acts primarily in the small intestine; hydrolyzed to ricinoleic acid which reduces net absorption of fluid and electrolytes and stimulates peristalsis; oil is expressed from the seeds of *Ricinus communis*

Adverse Reactions

Frequency not defined.

Cardiovascular: Hypotension

Central nervous system: Dizziness

Endocrine & metabolic: Electrolyte disturbance

Gastrointestinal: Abdominal cramps, nausea, diarrhea

Genitourinary: Pelvic congestion

Pharmacodynamics/Kinetics Onset of action: 2-6 hours

Dosage

Oral:

Oil:

Children 2-11 years: 5-15 mL as a single dose

Children $\geq$12 years and Adults: 15-60 mL as a single dose

Emulsified (36.4%):

Children <2 years: 5-15 mL/dose

Children 2-11 years: 7.5-30 mL/dose

Children $\geq$12 years and Adults: 30-60 mL/dose

Stability Protect from heat (castor oil emulsion should be protected from freezing)

Administration

Do not administer at bedtime because of rapid onset of action.

Dosage Forms

[DSC] = Discontinued product

Emulsion, oral (Emulsoil® [DSC]): 95% (60 mL)

Oil, oral: 100% (60 mL, 120 mL, 480 mL, 3840 mL)

Purge®: 95% (30 mL, 60 mL) [lemon flavor]

Overdosage/Treatment

Decontamination: Lavage (within 1 hour)/activated charcoal without a cathartic

Supportive therapy: I.V. fluid and electrolyte replacement; restrict solid food

Drug Interactions No data reported

Pregnancy Risk Factor X

Pregnancy Implications Can cause uterine contractures

Nursing Implications Do not administer at bedtime because of rapid onset of action

Additional Information Yellow liquid

Ceftriaxone

CAS Number 104376-79-6; 73384-59-5; 74578-69-1

U.S. Brand Names Rocephin®

Synonyms Ceftriaxone Sodium

Use Treatment of lower respiratory tract infections, acute bacterial otitis media, skin and skin structure infections, bone and joint infections, intra-abdominal and urinary tract infections, sepsis and meningitis due to susceptible organisms; documented or suspected infection due to susceptible organisms in home care patients and patients without I.V. line access; treatment of documented or suspected gonococcal infection or chancroid; emergency room management of patients at high risk for bacteremia, periorbital or buccal cellulitis, salmonellosis or shigellosis, and pneumonia of unestablished etiology (<5 years of age); treatment of Lyme disease, depends on the stage of the disease (used in Stage II and Stage III, but not stage I; doxycycline is the drug of choice for Stage I)

Unlabeled/Investigational Use Treatment of chancroid, epididymitis, complicated gonococcal infections; sexually-transmitted diseases (STD); periorbital or buccal cellulitis; salmonellosis or shigellosis; atypical community-acquired pneumonia; Lyme disease; used in chemoprophylaxis for high-risk contacts and persons with invasive meningococcal disease; sexual assault

Mechanism of Action Inhibits bacterial cell wall synthesis by binding to one or more of the penicillin-binding proteins (PBPs) which in turn inhibits the final transpeptidation step of peptidoglycan synthesis in bacterial cell walls, thus inhibiting cell wall biosynthesis. Bacteria eventually lyse due to ongoing activity of cell wall autolytic enzymes (autolysins and murein hydrolases) while cell wall assembly is arrested.

Adverse Reactions

Cardiovascular: Flushing

Central nervous system: Chills, dizziness, seizures

Dermatologic: Rash, pruritus

Gastrointestinal: Diarrhea, dysgeusia, gallstones, nausea, vomiting, colitis, pseudomembranous colitis

Genitourinary: Vaginitis

Hematologic: Eosinophilia, thrombocytosis, leukopenia, agranulocytosis, anemia, basophilia, hemolytic anemia, leukocytosis, lymphocytosis, lymphopenia, monocytosis, neutropenia, thrombocytopenia

Hepatic: Elevated transaminases, jaundice, prolonged or decreased PT; increased alkaline phosphatase, increased bilirubin

Local: Pain, induration at injection site (I.V.); warmth, tightness, induration following I.M. injection, phlebitis

Renal: Increased BUN, glycosuria, hematuria, renal stones, urinary casts, nephrolithiasis, renal precipitations

Renal: Elevated creatinine

Respiratory: Bronchospasm, allergic pneumonitis

Miscellaneous: Anaphylaxis, candidiasis, serum sickness

Other reactions with cephalosporins include angioedema, aplastic anemia, asterixis, cholestasis, encephalopathy, erythema multiforme, hemorrhage, interstitial nephritis, neuromuscular excitability, pancytopenia, paresthesia, renal dysfunction, Stevens-Johnson syndrome, superinfection, toxic epidermal necrolysis, toxic nephropathy

Signs and Symptoms of Overdose Hypersensitivity and convulsions; many beta-lactam containing antibiotics have the potential to cause neuromuscular hyperirritability or convulsive seizures

Pharmacodynamics/Kinetics

Absorption: I.M.: Well absorbed

Distribution: Widely throughout the body including gallbladder, lungs, bone, bile, CSF (higher concentrations achieved when meninges are inflamed); crosses placenta; enters amniotic fluid and breast milk

Protein binding: 85% to 95%

Half-life elimination: Normal renal and hepatic function: 5-9 hours

Time to peak, serum: I.M.: 1-2 hours

Excretion: Urine (33% to 65% as unchanged drug); feces

Dosage

I.M., I.V.:

Neonates:

Postnatal age $\leq$7 days: 50 mg/kg/day given every 24 hours

Postnatal age >7 days:

$\leq$2000 g: 50 mg/kg/day given every 24 hours

>2000 g: 50-75 mg/kg/day given every 24 hours

Gonococcal prophylaxis: 25-50 mg/kg as a single dose (dose not to exceed 125 mg)

Gonococcal infection: 25-50 mg/kg/day (maximum dose: 125 mg) given every 24 hours for 10-14 days

Infants and Children: 50-75 mg/kg/day in 1-2 divided doses every 12-24 hours; maximum: 2 g/24 hours

Meningitis: 100 mg/kg/day divided every 12-24 hours, up to a maximum of 4 g/24 hours; loading dose of 75 mg/kg/dose may be given at start of therapy

Acute otitis media: I.M., I.V.: 50 mg/kg in a single dose (maximum dose: 1 g)

Persistent or relapsing acute otitis media: I.M., I.V.: 50 mg/kg once daily for 3 days (maximum dose: 1 g/day)

Uncomplicated gonococcal infections, sexual assault, and STD prophylaxis: I.M.: 125 mg as a single dose plus doxycycline

Complicated gonococcal infections:

Infants: I.M., I.V.: 25-50 mg/kg/day in a single dose (maximum: 125 mg/dose); treat for 7 days for disseminated infection and 7-14 days for documented meningitis

<45 kg: 50 mg/kg/day once daily; maximum: 1 g/day; for ophthalmia, peritonitis, arthritis, or bacteremia: 50-100 mg/kg/day divided every 12-24 hours; maximum: 2 g/day for meningitis or endocarditis

>45 kg: 1 g/day once daily for disseminated gonococcal infections; 1-2 g dose every 12 hours for meningitis or endocarditis

Acute epididymitis: I.M.: 250 mg in a single dose

Adults: 1-2 g every 12-24 hours (depending on the type and severity of infection); maximum dose: 2 g every 12 hours for treatment of meningitis

Uncomplicated gonorrhea: I.M.: 250 mg as a single dose

Surgical prophylaxis: 1 g 30 minutes to 2 hours before surgery

Dosing adjustment in renal or hepatic impairment: No change necessary

Hemodialysis: Not dialyzable (0% to 5%); administer dose postdialysis

Peritoneal dialysis: Administer 750 mg every 12 hours

Continuous arteriovenous or venovenous hemofiltration: Removes 10 mg of ceftriaxone per liter of filtrate per day

Stability Reconstituted solution (100 mg/mL) is stable for 3 days at room temperature and 3 days when refrigerated; for I.V. infusion in NS or D_5W solution is stable for 3 days at room temperature, 10 days when refrigerated, or 26 weeks when frozen; after freezing, thawed solution is stable for 3 days at room temperature or 10 days when refrigerated. Incompatible with vancomycin or pentamidine

Monitoring Parameters Observe for signs and symptoms of anaphylaxis

Administration

Do not admix with aminoglycosides in same bottle/bag.

I.M.: Inject deep I.M. into large muscle mass; a concentration of 250 mg/mL or 350 mg/mL is recommended for all vial sizes except the 250 mg size (250 mg/mL is suggested); can be diluted with 1:1 water and 1% lidocaine for I.M. administration.

I.V.: Infuse intermittent infusion over 30 minutes.

Contraindications Hypersensitivity to ceftriaxone sodium, any component of the formulation, or other cephalosporins; **do not use in hyperbilirubinemic neonates**, particularly those who are premature since ceftriaxone is reported to displace bilirubin from albumin binding sites

Warnings Modify dosage in patients with severe renal impairment. Prolonged use may result in superinfection. Use with caution in patients with a history of penicillin allergy, especially IgE-mediated reactions (eg, anaphylaxis, urticaria). May cause antibiotic-associated colitis or colitis secondary to *C. difficile*. Discontinue in patients with signs and symptoms of gallbladder disease.

Dosage Forms

Note: Contains sodium 83 mg (3.6 mEq) per ceftriaxone 1 g

Infusion [premixed in dextrose]: 1 g (50 mL); 2 g (50 mL)

Injection, powder for reconstitution: 250 mg, 500 mg, 1 g, 2 g, 10 g

Reference Range Peak plasma ceftriaxone levels of 40 mcg/mL and 80 mcg/mL have been reported after I.M. administration of 0.5 g and 1 g, respectively.

Overdosage/Treatment Supportive therapy: Hemodialysis may be helpful to aid in removal of the drug from blood; otherwise, treatment is supportive or symptom directed. Anaphylaxis can be treated with standard therapy.

Test Interactions Positive direct Coombs', false-positive urinary glucose test using cupric sulfate (Benedict's solution, Clinitest®, Fehling's solution), false-positive serum or urine creatinine with Jaffé reaction

Drug Interactions

Coumarin derivative (eg, dicumarol, warfarin): Cephalosporins may increase the anticoagulant effect of coumarin derivatives.

Uricosuric agents (eg, probenecid, sulfinpyrazone): Uricosuric agents may decrease the excretion of cephalosporin; monitor for toxic effects.

Pregnancy Risk Factor B

Lactation Enters breast milk/use caution (AAP rates "compatible")

Nursing Implications For I.M. injection, the maximum concentration is 250 mg/mL; ceftriaxone can be diluted with 1:1 water and 1% lidocaine for I.M. administration. Do not admix with aminoglycosides in same bottle/bag.

Additional Information Sodium content of 1 g: 60 mg (2.6 mEq)

Specific References

American Academy of Family Physicians and American Academy of Pediatrics, Clinical Care and Research, "Diagnosis and Management of Acute Otitis Media: Clinical Recommendations," available at: http://www.aafp.org/x26481.xml. Last accessed March 19, 2004.

Greenberg ML, Hendrickson RG, and Muller AA, "Occupational Exposure to Cephalosporins Leading to *Clostridium difficile* Infection," *J Toxicol Clin Toxicol*, 2003, 41(2):205-6.

Cefuroxime

CAS Number 64544-07-6

U.S. Brand Names Ceftin®; Zinacef®

Synonyms Cefuroxime Axetil; Cefuroxime Sodium

Use Treatment of infections caused by staphylococci, group B streptococci, *H. influenzae* (type A and B), *E. coli*, *Enterobacter*, *Salmonella*, and *Klebsiella*; treatment of susceptible infections of the lower respiratory tract, otitis media, urinary tract, skin and soft tissue, bone and joint, sepsis and gonorrhea

Mechanism of Action Inhibits bacterial cell wall synthesis by binding to one or more of the penicillin-binding proteins (PBPs) which in turn inhibits the final transpeptidation step of peptidoglycan synthesis in bacterial cell walls, thus inhibiting cell wall biosynthesis. Bacteria eventually lyse due to ongoing activity of cell wall autolytic enzymes (autolysins and murein hydrolases) while cell wall assembly is arrested.

Adverse Reactions

Central nervous system: Dizziness, fever, headache, seizures

Dermatologic: Cutaneous vasculitis, angioedema, erythema multiforme, rash, toxic epidermal necrolysis

Gastrointestinal: Colitis, diarrhea, GI bleeding, nausea, stomach cramps, vomiting, pseudomembranous colitis

Genitourinary: Vaginitis

Hematologic: Eosinophilia, **decreased hemoglobin and hematocrit**, leukopenia, neutropenia, hemolytic anemia, pancytopenia, prolonged PT/INR, thrombocytopenia

Hepatic: Increased transaminases, increased alkaline phosphatase, cholestasis

Local: Thrombophlebitis, pain at injection site

Renal: Increased BUN, increased creatinine, interstitial nephritis

Miscellaneous: Anaphylaxis

Reactions reported with other cephalosporins include agranulocytosis, aplastic anemia, asterixis, encephalopathy, hemorrhage, neuromuscular excitability, serum-sickness reactions, superinfection, toxic nephropathy

Signs and Symptoms of Overdose Symptoms of overdose include neuromuscular hypersensitivity and convulsions. Many beta-lactam containing antibiotics have the potential to cause neuromuscular hyperirritability or convulsive seizures.

Pharmacodynamics/Kinetics

Absorption: Oral (cefuroxime axetil): Increases with food

Distribution: Widely to body tissues and fluids; crosses blood-brain barrier; therapeutic concentrations achieved in CSF even when meninges are not inflamed; crosses placenta; enters breast milk

Protein binding: 33% to 50%

Bioavailability: Tablet: Fasting: 37%; Following food: 52%

Half-life elimination: Adults: 1-2 hours; prolonged with renal impairment

Time to peak, serum: I.M.: ~15-60 minutes; I.V.: 2-3 minutes

Excretion: Urine (66% to 100% as unchanged drug)

Dosage

Note: Cefuroxime axetil film-coated tablets and oral suspension are not bioequivalent and are not substitutable on a mg/mg basis

Children ≥3 months to 12 years:

Pharyngitis, tonsillitis: Oral:

Suspension: 20 mg/kg/day (maximum: 500 mg/day) in 2 divided doses for 10 days

Tablet: 125 mg every 12 hours for 10 days

Acute otitis media, impetigo: Oral:

Suspension: 30 mg/kg/day (maximum: 1 g/day) in 2 divided doses for 10 days

Tablet: 250 mg twice daily for 10 days

I.M., I.V.: 75-150 mg/kg/day divided every 8 hours; maximum dose: 6 g/day

Meningitis: Not recommended (doses of 200-240 mg/kg/day divided every 6-8 hours have been used); maximum dose: 9 g/day

Acute bacterial maxillary sinusitis:

Suspension: 30 mg/kg/day in 2 divided doses for 10 days; maximum dose: 1 g/day

Tablet: 250 mg twice daily for 10 days

Children ≥13 years and Adults:

Oral: 250-500 mg twice daily for 10 days (5 days in selected patients with acute bronchitis)

Uncomplicated urinary tract infection: 125-250 mg every 12 hours for 7-10 days

Uncomplicated gonorrhea: 1 g as a single dose

Early Lyme disease: 500 mg twice daily for 20 days

I.M., I.V.: 750 mg to 1.5 g/dose every 8 hours or 100-150 mg/kg/day in divided doses every 6-8 hours; maximum: 6 g/24 hours

Dosing adjustment in renal impairment:
Cl_{cr} 10-20 mL/minute: Administer every 12 hours
Cl_{cr} <10 mL/minute: Administer every 24 hours
Hemodialysis: Dialyzable (25%)
Continuous arteriovenous or venovenous hemodiafiltration effects: Dose as for Cl_{cr} 10-20 mL/minute

Stability Reconstituted solution is stable for 24 hours at room temperature and 48 hours when refrigerated; I.V. infusion in NS or D_5W solution is stable for 24 hours at room temperature, 7 days when refrigerated, or 26 weeks when frozen; after freezing, thawed solution is stable for 24 hours at room temperature or 21 days when refrigerated

Monitoring Parameters Observe for signs and symptoms of anaphylaxis during first dose; with prolonged therapy, monitor renal, hepatic, and hematologic function periodically; monitor prothrombin time in patients at risk of prolongation during cephalosporin therapy (nutritionally-deficient, prolonged treatment, renal or hepatic disease)

Administration Oral: Administer around-the-clock to promote less variation in peak and trough serum levels.
Oral suspension: Administer with food. Shake well before use.
I.M.: Inject deep I.M. into large muscle mass.
I.V.: Inject direct I.V. over 3-5 minutes. Infuse intermittent infusion over 15-30 minutes.

Contraindications Hypersensitivity to cefuroxime, any component of the formulation, or other cephalosporins

Warnings Modify dosage in patients with severe renal impairment. Prolonged use may result in superinfection. Use with caution in patients with a history of penicillin allergy, especially IgE-mediated reactions (eg, anaphylaxis, urticaria). May cause antibiotic-associated colitis or colitis secondary to *C. difficile*. May be associated with increased INR, especially in nutritionally-deficient patients, prolonged treatment, hepatic or renal disease. Tablets and oral suspension are not bioequivalent (do not substitute on a mg-per-mg basis).

Dosage Forms
Infusion, as sodium [premixed] (Zinacef®): 750 mg (50 mL); 1.5 g (50 mL) [contains sodium 4.8 mEq (111 mg) per 750 mg]
Injection, powder for reconstitution, as sodium (Zinacef®): 750 mg, 1.5 g, 7.5 g [contains sodium 4.8 mEq (111 mg) per 750 mg]
Powder for oral suspension, as axetil (Ceftin®): 125 mg/5 mL (100 mL) [contains phenylalanine 11.8 mg/5 mL; tutti-frutti flavor]; 250 mg/5 mL (50 mL, 100 mL) [contains phenylalanine 25.2 mg/5 mL; tutti-frutti flavor]
Tablet, as axetil (Ceftin®): 250 mg, 500 mg

Reference Range Peak plasma level: 27 mcg/mL achieved 45 minutes after 750 mg I.M. dose

Overdosage/Treatment Supportive therapy: Hemodialysis may be helpful to aid in removal of the drug from blood. Most treatment is supportive or symptom directed following GI decontamination.

Test Interactions Positive direct Coombs', false-positive urinary glucose test using cupric sulfate (Benedict's solution, Clinitest®, Fehling's solution), false-positive serum or urine creatinine with Jaffé reaction

Drug Interactions
Increased effect: High-dose probenecid decreases clearance.
Increased toxicity: Aminoglycosides increase nephrotoxic potential.

Pregnancy Risk Factor B

Lactation Enters breast milk/use caution

Nursing Implications Do not admix with aminoglycosides in same bottle/bag; obtain specimens for culture and sensitivity prior to the first dose

Additional Information Sodium content of 1 g: 54.2 mg (2.4 mEq)

Celecoxib

Related Information
- Nonsteroidal Anti-inflammatory Drugs

CAS Number 169590-42-5

U.S. Brand Names Celebrex®

Use Relief of the signs and symptoms of osteoarthritis; relief of the signs and symptoms of rheumatoid arthritis in adults; decreasing intestinal polyps in familial adenomatous polyposis (FAP); management of acute pain; treatment of primary dysmenorrhea

Mechanism of Action Inhibits prostaglandin synthesis by decreasing the activity of the enzyme, cyclooxygenase-2 (COX-2), which results in decreased formation of prostaglandin precursors.

Adverse Reactions
Cardiovascular: Peripheral edema, hypertension (aggravated), chest pain, myocardial infarction, palpitations, tachycardia, facial edema, vasculitis, torsade de pointes
Central nervous system: **Headache**, insomnia, dizziness, hallucinations (auditory)
Dermatologic: Skin rash, toxic epidermal necrolysis
Gastrointestinal: Dyspepsia, diarrhea, abdominal pain, nausea, flatulence
Neuromuscular & skeletal: Back pain
Renal: Increased BUN, increased creatinine, albuminuria, hematuria, renal calculi

Respiratory: Upper respiratory tract infection, sinusitis, pharyngitis, rhinitis
Miscellaneous: Accidental injury

Signs and Symptoms of Overdose Epigastric pain, drowsiness, lethargy, nausea, and vomiting; GI bleeding may occur. Rare manifestations include coma, hypertension, respiratory depression, and acute renal failure.

Pharmacodynamics/Kinetics
Distribution: V_d (apparent): 400 L
Protein binding: 97% to albumin
Metabolism: Hepatic via CYP2C9; forms inactive metabolites
Bioavailability: Absolute: Unknown
Half-life elimination: 11 hours (fasted)
Time to peak: 3 hours
Excretion: Urine (27% as metabolites, <3% as unchanged drug); feces (57%)

Dosage
Adults: Oral:
Acute pain or primary dysmenorrhea: Initial dose: 400 mg, followed by an additional 200 mg if needed on day 1; maintenance dose: 200 mg twice daily as needed
Familial adenomatous polyposis (FAP): 400 mg twice daily
Osteoarthritis: 200 mg/day as a single dose or in divided dose twice daily
Rheumatoid arthritis: 100-200 mg twice daily
Elderly: No specific adjustment is recommended. However, the AUC in elderly patients may be increased by 50% as compared to younger subjects. Use the lowest recommended dose in patients weighing <50 kg.

Dosing adjustment in renal impairment: No specific dosage adjustment is recommended; not recommended in patients with advanced renal disease

Dosing adjustment in hepatic impairment: Reduced dosage is recommended (AUC may be increased by 40% to 180%); decrease dose by 50% in patients with moderate hepatic impairment (Child-Pugh Class II)

Monitoring Parameters Periodic LFTs; in patients treated for FAP, continue routine endoscopic exams

Contraindications Hypersensitivity to celecoxib, sulfonamides, aspirin, other NSAIDs, or any component of the formulation; perioperative pain in the setting of coronary artery bypass surgery (CABG); pregnancy (3rd trimester)

Warnings
[U.S. Boxed Warning]: NSAIDs are associated with an increased risk of adverse cardiovascular events, including MI, and new onset or worsening of pre-existing hypertension. Risk may be increased with duration of use or pre-existing cardiovascular risk factors or disease. Carefully evaluate individual cardiovascular risk profiles prior to prescribing. Use caution with fluid retention, CHF, cerebrovascular disease, ischemic heart disease, or hypertension.

[U.S. Boxed Warning]: NSAIDs may increase risk of gastrointestinal irritation, ulceration, bleeding, and perforation. These events may occur at any time during therapy and without warning. Use caution with a history of GI disease (bleeding or ulcers), concurrent therapy with aspirin, anticoagulants and/or corticosteroids, smoking, use of alcohol, the elderly or debilitated patients. Use the lowest effective dose for the shortest duration of time, consistent with individual patient goals, to reduce risk of cardiovascular or GI adverse events. Alternate therapies should be considered for patients at high risk.

NSAIDs may cause serious skin adverse events including exfoliative dermatitis, Stevens-Johnson syndrome (SJS), and toxic epidermal necrolysis (TEN). Anaphylactoid reactions may occur, even without prior exposure; patients with "aspirin triad" (bronchial asthma, aspirin intolerance, rhinitis) may be at increased risk. Do not use in patients who experience bronchospasm, asthma, rhinitis, or urticaria with NSAID or aspirin therapy.

Use with caution in patients with dehydration, decreased renal or hepatic function. Use of NSAIDs can compromise existing renal function, especially when Cl_{cr} <30 mL/minute. Not recommended for use in severe renal or hepatic impairment.

Anaphylactoid reactions may occur, even with no prior exposure to celecoxib. Use caution in patients with known or suspected deficiency of cytochrome P450 isoenzyme 2C9. Safety and efficacy have not been established in patients <18 years of age. **[U.S. Boxed Warning]: Celecoxib is contraindicated for treatment of perioperative pain in the setting of coronary artery bypass surgery (CABG).**

Dosage Forms Capsule: 100 mg, 200 mg, 400 mg

Overdosage/Treatment
Decontamination: Activated charcoal
Supportive therapy: Symptomatic and supportive treatment. Forced diuresis, hemodialysis and/or urinary alkalinization may not be useful.

Drug Interactions
Substrate of CYP2C9 (major), 3A4 (minor); **Inhibits** CYP2C8 (moderate), 2D6 (weak)
ACE inhibitors: Antihypertensive effect may be diminished by celecoxib.

Aminoglycosides: Celecoxib may decrease excretion; monitor levels.

Aspirin: Low-dose aspirin may be used with celecoxib, however, monitor for GI complications.

Beta-blockers: Antihypertensive effect may be diminished by celecoxib.

Bile acid sequestrants: May decrease absorption of NSAIDs.

CYP2C8 Substrates: Celecoxib may increase the levels/effects of CYP2C8 substrates. Example substrates include amiodarone, paclitaxel, pioglitazone, repaglinide, and rosiglitazone.

Cyclosporine: NSAIDs may increase levels/nephrotoxicity of cyclosporine.

Fluconazole: Fluconazole increases celecoxib concentrations twofold. Lowest dose of celecoxib should be used.

Hydralazine: Antihypertensive effect may be diminished by celecoxib.

Lithium: Plasma levels of lithium are increased by ~17% when used with celecoxib. Monitor lithium levels closely when treatment with celecoxib is started or withdrawn.

Loop diuretics (bumetanide, furosemide, torsemide): Natriuretic effect of furosemide and other loop diuretics may be decreased by celecoxib.

Methotrexate: Severe bone marrow suppression, aplastic anemia, and GI toxicity have been reported with concomitant NSAID therapy. Selective COX-2 inhibitors appear to have a lower risk of this toxicity, however, caution is warranted.

Thiazide diuretics: Natriuretic effects of thiazide diuretics may be decreased by celecoxib.

Vancomycin: Celecoxib may decrease excretion; monitor levels.

Warfarin: Bleeding events (including rare intracranial hemorrhage in association with increased prothrombin time) have been reported with concomitant use. Monitor closely, especially in the elderly.

Pregnancy Risk Factor C/D (3rd trimester)

Pregnancy Implications In late pregnancy, this drug may cause premature closure of the ductus arteriosus.

Lactation Enters breast milk/not recommended (contraindicated in Canadian labeling)

Additional Information Cross-reactivity, including bronchospasm, between aspirin and other NSAIDs has been reported in aspirin-sensitive patients. The manufacturer suggests that celecoxib should not be administered to patients with this type of aspirin sensitivity and should be used with caution in patients with pre-existing asthma.

Specific References

Akhund L, Quinet RJ, and Ishaq S, "Celecoxib-Related Renal Papillary Necrosis," *Arch Intern Med*, 2003, 163(1):114-5.

Alper AB Jr, Tomlin H, Sadhwani U, et al, "Effects of the Selective Cyclooxygenase-2 Inhibitor Analgesic Celecoxib on Renal Carbonic Anhydrase Enzyme Activity: A Randomized, Controlled Trial," *Am J Ther*, 2006, 13(3):229-35.

Cohen JS, "How Celecoxib Could Be Safer, How Valdecoxib Might Have Been," *Ann Pharmacother*, 2005, 39(9):1542-5.

Jones SC, "Relative Thromboembolic Risks Associated with COX-2 Inhibitors," *Ann Pharmacother*, 2005, 39(7):1249-59.

Kaushik P, Zuckerman SJ, Campo NJ, et al, "Celecoxib-Induced Methemoglobinemia," *Ann Pharmacother*, 2004, 38(10):1635-8.

Moskowitz RW, Sunshine A, Brugger A, et al, "American Pain Society Pain Questionnaire and Other Pain Measures in the Assessment of Osteoarthritis Pain: A Pooled Analysis of Three Celecoxib Pivotal Studies," *Am J Ther*, 2003, 10(1):12-20.

Salo DF, Lavery R, Varma V, et al, "A Randomized, Clinical Trial Comparing Oral Celecoxib 200 mg, Celecoxib 400 mg, and Ibuprofen 600 mg for Acute Pain," *Acad Emerg Med*, 2003, 10(1):22-30.

Sanchez-Borges M, Capriles-Hulett A, and Caballero-Fonseca F, "Adverse Reactions to Selective Cyclooxygenase-2 Inhibitors (Coxibs)," *Am J Ther*, 2004, 11(6):494-500.

Spiegel BM, Targownik L, Dulai GS, et al, "The Cost-Effectiveness of Cyclooxygenase-2 Selective Inhibitors in the Management of Chronic Arthritis," *Ann Intern Med*, 2003, 138(10):795-806.

Verrico MM, Weber RJ, McKaveney TP, et al, "Adverse Drug Events Involving COX-2 Inhibitors," *Ann Pharmacother*, 2003, 37(9):1203-13.

Celiprolol

CAS Number 56980-93-9; 57470-78-7

Synonyms Celiprolol Hydrochloride

Unlabeled/Investigational Use Hypertension, angina

Mechanism of Action Selective beta$_1$-adrenergic blocking agent with weak alpha$_2$ receptor blocking activity; no negative inotropic effect; may also stimulate beta$_2$ receptors resulting in vasodilatation

Adverse Reactions

Cardiovascular: Bradycardia, AV block, Raynaud's syndrome, congestive heart failure, sinus bradycardia, myocardial depression

Central nervous system: Insomnia, dizziness, headache, depression

Gastrointestinal: Nausea, diarrhea, xerostomia

Neuromuscular & skeletal: Tremors

Signs and Symptoms of Overdose AV block, hypoglycemia, insomnia, wheezing

Pharmacodynamics/Kinetics

Absorption: 30% to 74%; reduced by food

Protein binding: 25%

Half-life elimination: 4-10 hours

Time to peak, plasma: 2-4 hours

Excretion: Urine (50%)

Dosage Oral: 200-600 mg once daily; no dosage alteration needed in elderly

Monitoring Parameters Monitor blood pressure, apical and radial pulses, I & O, daily weight, respirations, and circulation in extremities before and during therapy

Contraindications Hypersensitivity to celiprolol, any component of the formulation, or other beta-blocking agents; sinus bradycardia; heart block greater than first-degree (except in patients with a functioning artificial pacemaker); cardiogenic shock; uncompensated cardiac failure

Warnings Administer cautiously in compensated heart failure and monitor for a worsening of the condition. Avoid abrupt discontinuation in patients with a history of CAD; slowly wean while monitoring for signs and symptoms of ischemia. Use caution with concurrent use of beta-blockers and either verapamil or diltiazem; bradycardia or heart block can occur. In general, beta-blockers should be avoided in patients with bronchospastic disease. Use cautiously in PVD (can exacerbate arterial insufficiency). Can mask signs of thyrotoxicosis. Dosage adjustment is required in patients with renal dysfunction. Use care with anesthetic agents that decrease myocardial function.

Overdosage/Treatment

Decontamination: Lavage (within 1 hour)/activated charcoal; **do not** use ipecac

Supportive therapy: Glucagon (50-150 mcg/kg followed by continuous drip of 1-5 mg/hour) for positive chronotropic effect, inamrinone may need to be added; atropine/isoproterenol can be utilized to increase heart rate; calcium chloride may also be effective but this approach has not thoroughly been investigated; do **not** use epinephrine in that unopposed alpha effects may occur; pacemaker or intra-aortic balloon counter pulsation may be required

Enhancement of elimination: Multiple dosing of activated charcoal is not likely to be of benefit; dialysis is not useful; not dialyzable (0% to 5%)

Antidote(s)

- Glucagon [ANTIDOTE]

Drug Interactions

Expected interactions:

Alpha-blockers (prazosin, terazosin): Concurrent use of beta-blockers may increase risk of orthostasis.

Ampicillin, in single doses of 1 gram, decrease celiprolol's pharmacologic actions.

Antacids (magnesium-aluminum, calcium antacids or salts) may reduce the bioavailability of celiprolol.

Clonidine: Hypertensive crisis after or during withdrawal of either agent.

Drugs which slow AV conduction (digoxin): Effects may be additive with beta-blockers.

Glucagon: Celiprolol may blunt the hyperglycemic action of glucagon.

Insulin and oral hypoglycemics: Celiprolol masks the tachycardia that usually accompanies hypoglycemia.

NSAIDs (ibuprofen, indomethacin, naproxen, piroxicam) may reduce the antihypertensive effects of beta-blockers.

Salicylates may reduce the antihypertensive effects of beta-blockers.

Sulfonylureas: Beta-blockers may alter response to hypoglycemic agents.

Verapamil or diltiazem may have synergistic or additive pharmacological effects when taken concurrently with beta-blockers.

Additional Information Can cause decrease in serum cholesterol; HDL increases noted; can cause increase in thyroid function tests; reduction in fibrinogen levels have been described

Cephalexin

CAS Number 15686-71-2; 23325-78-2

U.S. Brand Names Biocef®; Keflex®

Synonyms Cephalexin Monohydrate

Use Treatment of susceptible bacterial infections, including those caused by group A beta-hemolytic *Streptococcus*, *Staphylococcus*, *Klebsiella pneumoniae*, *E. coli*, *Proteus mirabilis*, and *Shigella*; predominantly used for lower respiratory tract, urinary tract, skin and soft tissue, and bone and joint

Mechanism of Action Inhibits bacterial cell wall synthesis by binding to one or more of the penicillin-binding proteins (PBPs) which in turn inhibits the final transpeptidation step of peptidoglycan synthesis in bacterial cell walls, thus inhibiting cell wall biosynthesis. Bacteria eventually lyse due to ongoing activity of cell wall autolytic enzymes (autolysins and murein hydrolases) while cell wall assembly is arrested.

Adverse Reactions

Central nervous system: Dizziness, fatigue, headache

Dermatologic: Rash, toxic epidermal necrolysis, urticaria, pemphigus vulgaris, erythema multiforme, angioedema, purpura, Stevens-Johnson syndrome, pruritus, exanthem

Gastrointestinal: Nausea, diarrhea, vomiting, pseudomembranous colitis

Hematologic: Transient neutropenia, anemia, eosinophilia, hemolytic anemia

Hepatic: Transient elevation in liver enzymes

Ocular: Diplopia

Otic: Tinnitus

Miscellaneous: Fixed drug eruption

Signs and Symptoms of Overdose Crystalluria, seizures, toxic psychosis

Pharmacodynamics/Kinetics

Absorption: Delayed in young children

Distribution: Widely into most body tissues and fluids, including gallbladder, liver, kidneys, bone, sputum, bile, and pleural and synovial fluids; CSF penetration is poor; crosses placenta; enters breast milk

Protein binding: 6% to 15%

Half-life elimination: Adults: 0.5-1.2 hours; prolonged with renal impairment

Time to peak, serum: ~1 hour

Excretion: Urine (80% to 100% as unchanged drug) within 8 hours

Dosage

Oral:

Children: 25-50 mg/kg/day every 6 hours; severe infections: 50-100 mg/kg/day in divided doses every 6 hours; maximum: 3 g/24 hours

Adults: 250-1000 mg every 6 hours; maximum: 4 g/day

Dosing interval in renal impairment: Cl_{cr} <10 mL/minute: Administer every 8-12 hours

Stability Refrigerate suspension after reconstitution; discard after 14 days

Monitoring Parameters With prolonged therapy monitor renal, hepatic, and hematologic function periodically; monitor for signs of anaphylaxis during first dose

Administration

Take without regard to food. If GI distress, take with food. Give around-the-clock to promote less variation in peak and trough serum levels.

Contraindications Hypersensitivity to cephalexin, any component of the formulation, or other cephalosporins

Warnings Modify dosage in patients with severe renal impairment; prolonged use may result in superinfection. Use with caution in patients with a history of penicillin allergy, especially IgE-mediated reactions (eg, anaphylaxis, urticaria). May cause antibiotic-associated colitis or colitis secondary to *C. difficile*.

Dosage Forms

[DSC] = Discontinued product

Capsule: 250 mg, 500 mg

Biocef®: 500 mg

Keflex®: 250 mg, 333 mg, 500 mg, 750 mg

Powder for oral suspension: 125 mg/5 mL (100 mL, 200 mL); 250 mg/5 mL (100 mL, 200 mL)

Biocef®: 125 mg/5 mL (100 mL); 250 mg/5 mL (100 mL)

Keflex®: 125 mg/5 mL (100 mL, 200 mL); 250 mg/5 mL (100 mL, 200 mL)

Tablet, for oral suspension (Panixine DisperDose™): 125 mg [contains phenylalanine 2.8 mg; peppermint flavor], 250 mg [contains phenylalanine 5.6 mg; peppermint flavor] [DSC]

Reference Range Peak serum cephalexin levels after a 1 g oral dose: ~32 mg/mL; therapeutic range: 12-30 mg/mL; level >120 mg/mL associated with seizures

Overdosage/Treatment

Decontamination: Emesis within 30 minutes or lavage within 1 hour for ingestions >500 mg/kg; activated charcoal or cholestyramine can be used to decrease absorption

Supportive therapy: Seizures can be treated with benzodiazepines; phenobarbital or phenytoin can be used for refractory seizures

Enhanced elimination: Moderately dialyzable (20% to 50%); 58% of dose can be removed in a 6-hour dialysis

Test Interactions False-positive Coombs' test, may falsely elevate creatinine values when Jaffé reaction is used, may cause false-positive results in urine glucose tests using cupric sulfate (Benedict's solution, Clinitest®), false-positive urinary proteins and steroids; can result in false elevation of theophylline by HPLC method. The presence of this drug can result in a decrease of reactivity of urinary leukocyte esterase.

Drug Interactions Aminoglycosides: Increase nephrotoxic potential.

Probenecid: High-dose probenecid decreases clearance of cephalexin.

Typhoid vaccine: Antibiotics may diminish the efficacy of the live, attenuated Ty21a strain vaccine.

Pregnancy Risk Factor B

Pregnancy Implications Animal studies have not demonstrated fetal effects. There are no adequate and well-controlled studies in pregnant women. Use in pregnancy only if needed.

Lactation Enters breast milk (small amounts)/use caution

Nursing Implications Obtain specimens for culture and sensitivity prior to the first dose

Cephradine

CAS Number 31828-50-9; 38821-53-3; 58456-86-3

U.S. Brand Names Velosef®

Use Treatment of infections when caused by susceptible strains in respiratory, genitourinary, gastrointestinal, skin and soft tissue, bone and joint infections; treatment of susceptible gram-positive bacilli and cocci (never enterococcus); some gram-negative bacilli including *E. coli*, *Proteus*, and *Klebsiella* may be susceptible

Mechanism of Action Bactericidal antibiotic with a mechanism similar to that of penicillins; after penetrating the bacterial cell wall, it stops cell synthesis and thereby kills the organism

Adverse Reactions

Frequency not defined.

Central nervous system: Dizziness

Dermatologic: Rash, pruritus

Gastrointestinal: Diarrhea, nausea, vomiting, pseudomembranous colitis

Hematologic: Leukopenia, neutropenia, eosinophilia

Neuromuscular & skeletal: Joint pain

Renal: BUN increased, creatinine increased

Pharmacodynamics/Kinetics

Absorption: Well absorbed

Distribution: Widely into most body tissues and fluids including gallbladder, liver, kidneys, bone, sputum, bile, and pleural and synovial fluids; CSF penetration is poor; crosses placenta; enters breast milk

Protein binding: 18% to 20%

Half-life elimination: 1-2 hours; prolonged with renal impairment

Time to peak, serum: 1-2 hours

Excretion: Urine (~80% to 90% as unchanged drug) within 6 hours

Dosage

Oral:

Children ≥9 months: Usual dose: 25-50 mg/kg/day in divided doses every 6 hours

Otitis media: 75-100 mg/kg/day in divided doses every 6 or 12 hours (maximum: 4 g/day)

Adults: 250-500 mg every 6-12 hours

Dosing adjustment in renal impairment: Adults:

Cl_{cr} 10-50 mL/minute: 250 mg every 6 hours

Cl_{cr} <10 mL/minute: 125 mg every 6 hours

Monitoring Parameters Observe for signs and symptoms of anaphylaxis during first dose

Administration

Administer around-the-clock to promote less variation in peak and trough serum levels. Shake oral suspension well.

Contraindications Hypersensitivity to cephradine, any component of the formulation, or cephalosporins

Warnings Use caution with renal impairment; dose adjustment required. Prolonged use may result in superinfection; use with caution in patients with a history of penicillin allergy, especially IgE-mediated reactions (eg, anaphylaxis, urticaria). May cause antibiotic-associated colitis or colitis secondary to *C. difficile*.

Dosage Forms

[DSC] = Discontinued product

Capsule: 250 mg, 500 mg [DSC]

Powder for oral suspension: 250 mg/5 mL (100 mL) [fruit flavor]

Reference Range Oral doses of 1 g result in a peak plasma level of 24 mcg/mL; intramuscular dose of 1 g results in a peak plasma level of 14 mcg/mL

Overdosage/Treatment

Decontamination: Emesis within 30 minutes or lavage (within 1 hour)/activated charcoal

Supportive therapy: Anaphylaxis can be treated with epinephrine, antihistamines, and corticosteroids

Enhancement of elimination: Multiple dosing of activated charcoal may be effective; hemodialysis or hemoperfusion can help enhance elimination

Test Interactions False-positive Coombs' test, may falsely elevate creatinine values when Jaffé reaction is used, may cause false-positive results in urine glucose tests using cupric sulfate (Benedict's solution, Clinitest®), false-positive urinary proteins and steroids

Drug Interactions

Increased effect: High-dose probenecid decreases clearance.

Increased toxicity: Aminoglycosides may increase nephrotoxic potential.

Pregnancy Risk Factor B

Pregnancy Implications Crosses the placenta

Lactation Enters breast milk/use caution

Additional Information Sodium concentration: 6 mEq/g

Cetirizine

CAS Number 83881-51-0; 83881-52-1

U.S. Brand Names Zyrtec®

Synonyms Cetirizine Hydrochloride; P-071; UCB-P071

Impairment Potential Yes. Minimal mental performance changes may occur at doses of 20 mg (none at lower doses); may mildly affect driving performance at therapeutic doses

Use Perennial and seasonal allergic rhinitis and other allergic symptoms including urticaria; chronic idiopathic urticaria

Mechanism of Action Potent antihistamine (H_1 receptor antagonist) with little antimuscarinic effects. It is a carboxylated metabolite of hydroxyzine. Also inhibits inflammatory cell migration, and exhibits a mild bronchodilatory effect

Adverse Reactions

Cardiovascular: Cardiac failure, chest pain, edema, face edema, hypertension, hypotension, palpitations, syncope, tachycardia

Central nervous system: Abnormal thinking, aggressiveness, amnesia, anxiety, ataxia, dizziness (adults 2%), fatigue (adults 6%), **headache** (children 11% to 14%, placebo 12%), insomnia, malaise (4%), **somnolence** (adults 14%, children 2% to 4%), confusion, convulsions, coordination abnormal, depersonalization, depression, dysphonia, emotional lability, euphoria, fever, flushing, fussiness, hallucinations, hyperesthesia, hypertonia, hypoesthesia, impaired concentration, irritability, migraine, nervousness, pain, paroniria, rigors, sleep disorder, suicidal ideation, suicide, tremor, vertigo

Dermatologic: Acne, alopecia, angioedema, bullous eruption, dermatitis, dry skin, eczema, erythematosus rash, furunculosis, hyperkeratosis, hypertrichosis, maculopapular rash, pallor, photosensitivity, pruritus, purpura, rash, seborrhea, skin nodule, urticaria

Endocrine & metabolic: Breast pain (female), dehydration, diabetes mellitus, dysmenorrhea, hot flashes, intermenstrual bleeding, libido decreased, menorrhagia

Gastrointestinal: Abdomen enlarged, abdominal pain (children 4% to 6%), anorexia, appetite increased, diarrhea (children 2% to 3%), dry mouth (adults 5%), nausea (children 2% to 3%, placebo 2%), vomiting (children 2% to 3%) constipation, dyspepsia, eructation, flatulence, gastritis, hemorrhoids, melena, rectal hemorrhage, salivation increased, sputum increased, stomatitis, taste loss, taste perversion, tongue discoloration, tongue edema, ulcerative stomatitis, weight gain

Genitourinary: Cystitis, dysuria, leukorrhea, micturition frequency, urinary incontinence, urinary retention, urinary tract infection, vaginitis

Hepatic: Cholestasis, hepatitis, increased bilirubin, liver enzymes elevated (transient), abnormal liver function

Hematologic: Hemolytic anemia, thrombocytopenia

Neuromuscular & skeletal: Arthralgia, arthritis, arthrosis, back pain, hyperkinesia, leg cramps, leg edema, muscle weakness, myalgia, myelitis, orofacial dyskinesia, paralysis, paresthesia, twitching, weakness

Ocular: Accommodation loss, blindness, conjunctivitis, eye pain, glaucoma, ocular hemorrhage, periorbital edema, ptosis, visual field defect, xerophthalmia

Otic: Deafness, earache, ototoxicity, tinnitus

Renal: Glomerulonephritis, hematuria, polyuria

Respiratory: Bronchitis, bronchospasm (children 2% to 3%, placebo 2%) epistaxis (children 2% to 4%, placebo 3%), pharyngitis (children 3% to 6%, placebo 3%), dyspnea, hyperventilation, nasal polyp, pneumonia, rhinitis, sinusitis, upper respiratory tract infection

Miscellaneous: Anaphylaxis, lymphadenopathy, sweating, thirst, parosmia

Pharmacodynamics/Kinetics

Onset of action: 15-30 minutes

Absorption: Rapid

Protein binding, plasma: Mean: 93%

Metabolism: Limited hepatic

Half-life elimination: 8 hours

Time to peak, serum: 1 hour

Excretion: Urine (70%); feces (10%)

Dosage

Oral:

Children:

6-12 months: Chronic urticaria, perennial allergic rhinitis: 2.5 mg once daily

12 months to <2 years: Chronic urticaria, perennial allergic rhinitis: 2.5 mg once daily; may increase to 2.5 mg every 12 hours if needed

2-5 years: Chronic urticaria, perennial or seasonal allergic rhinitis: Initial: 2.5 mg once daily; may be increased to 2.5 mg every 12 hours **or** 5 mg once daily

Children ≥6 years and Adults: Chronic urticaria, perennial or seasonal allergic rhinitis: 5-10 mg once daily, depending upon symptom severity

Elderly (≥77 years): Initial: 5 mg once daily; adjust for renal impairment

Dosage adjustment in renal/hepatic impairment:

Children <6 years: Cetirizine use not recommended

Children 6-11 years: <2.5 mg once daily

Children ≥12 and Adults:

Cl_{cr} 11-31 mL/minute, hemodialysis, or hepatic impairment: Administer 5 mg once daily

Cl_{cr} <11 mL/minute, not on dialysis: Cetirizine use not recommended

Monitoring Parameters Relief of symptoms, sedation and anticholinergic effects

Administration

May be administered with or without food.

Contraindications Hypersensitivity to cetirizine, hydroxyzine, or any component of the formulation

Warnings Cetirizine should be used cautiously in patients with hepatic or renal dysfunction and the elderly. Use in breast-feeding women is not recommended. May cause drowsiness; use caution performing tasks which require alertness (eg, operating machinery or driving). Safety and efficacy in pediatric patients <6 months of age have not been established.

Dosage Forms

Syrup, as hydrochloride: 5 mg/5 mL (120 mL, 480 mL) [banana-grape flavor]

Tablet, as hydrochloride: 5 mg, 10 mg

Tablet, chewable, as hydrochloride: 5 mg, 10 mg [grape flavor]

Reference Range Peak levels after a 10 mg oral dose: ~341 ng/mL and 978 ng/mL in adults and pediatric patients, respectively

Overdosage/Treatment

Decontamination: Lavage (within 1 hour)/activated charcoal

Supportive therapy: Monitor respiratory status; physostigmine is probably **not** useful

Enhanced elimination: Hemodialysis removes <10% of the drug and is therefore **not** useful

Drug Interactions

Substrate of CYP3A4 (minor)

Increased toxicity: CNS depressants, anticholinergics

Pregnancy Risk Factor B

Pregnancy Implications Cetirizine was not shown to be teratogenic in animal studies, however, adequate studies have not been conducted in pregnant women. Use during pregnancy only if clearly needed.

Lactation Enters breast milk/not recommended

Specific References

Morgan MM, Khan DA, and Nathan RA, "Treatment for Allergic Rhinitis and Chronic Idiopathic Urticaria: Focus on Oral Antihistamines," *Ann Pharmacother*, 2005, 39(12):2056-63.

Pompili M, Basso M, Grieco A, et al, "Recurrent Acute Hepatitis Associated with Use of Cetirizine," *Ann Pharmacother*, 2004, 38(11):1844-7.

Chloral Hydrate

CAS Number 302-17-0; 480-30-8

U.S. Brand Names Aquachloral® Supprettes®; Somnote™

Synonyms Chloral; Hydrated Chloral; Trichloroacetaldehyde Monohydrate

Impairment Potential Yes

Use Short-term sedative and hypnotic (<2 weeks), sedative/hypnotic for dental and diagnostic procedures; sedative prior to EEG evaluations

Mechanism of Action Central nervous system depressant effects are due to its active metabolite trichloroethanol, mechanism unknown; highly lipid soluble

Adverse Reactions

Cardiovascular: Bigeminy, tachycardia (ventricular), hypotension, QT prolongation, sinus bradycardia, congestive heart failure, sinus tachycardia, arrhythmias (ventricular)

Central nervous system: Disorientation, sedation, excitation (paradoxical), dizziness, fever, headache, ataxia, tachycardia (ventricular, bidirectional)

Gastrointestinal: **GI irritation**, **nausea**, **vomiting**, **diarrhea**, flatulence, gastric perforation

Hematologic: Leukopenia, eosinophilia

Hepatic: Hepatotoxicity

Local: Corrosive to skin

Ocular: Miosis

Respiratory: Laryngeal edema, aspiration

Miscellaneous: Physical and psychological dependence may occur with prolonged use of large doses; pear-like odor; aneuploidy induction

Signs and Symptoms of Overdose Acetone breath, acne, agranulocytosis, alopecia, cardiac arrhythmias, coma, cough, eczema, granulocytopenia, hyporeflexia, hypotension, hypothermia, ileus, jaundice, laryngospasm, leukopenia, myocardial depression, myoglobinuria, neutropenia, nystagmus, ptosis, rhabdomyolysis, respiratory depression, tachycardia (ventricular), tachycardia (ventricular, bidirectional), thirst, torsade de pointes, ventricular ectopy

Admission Criteria/Prognosis Admit any patient with respiratory depression, cardiac abnormalities, or ingestion >3 g.

Pharmacodynamics/Kinetics

Onset of action: Peak effect: 0.5-1 hour

Duration: 4-8 hours

Absorption: Oral, rectal: Well absorbed

Distribution: Crosses placenta; negligible amounts enter breast milk

Metabolism: Rapidly hepatic to trichloroethanol (active metabolite); variable amounts hepatically and renally to trichloroacetic acid (inactive)

Half-life elimination: Active metabolite: 8-11 hours

Excretion: Urine (as metabolites); feces (small amounts)

Dosage

Neonates: Oral, rectal: 25 mg/kg/dose for sedation prior to a procedure or 50 mg/kg as hypnotic

Children:

Sedation or anxiety: Oral, rectal: 5-15 mg/kg/dose every 8 hours (maximum: 500 mg/dose)

Prior to EEG: Oral, rectal: 20-25 mg/kg/dose, 30-60 minutes prior to EEG; may repeat in 30 minutes to maximum of 100 mg/kg or 2 g total

Hypnotic: Oral, rectal: 20-40 mg/kg/dose up to a maximum of 50 mg/kg/24 hours or 1 g/dose or 2 g/24 hours

Conscious sedation: Oral, rectal: 50-75 mg/kg/dose 30-60 minutes prior to procedure; may repeat 30 minutes after initial dose if needed, to a total maximum dose of 120 mg/kg or 1 g total

Adults: Oral, rectal:

Sedation, anxiety: 250 mg 3 times/day

Hypnotic: 500-1000 mg at bedtime or 30 minutes prior to procedure, not to exceed 2 g/24 hours

Dosing adjustment/comments in renal impairment: Cl_{cr} <50 mL/minute: Avoid use

Hemodialysis: Dialyzable (50% to 100%); supplemental dose is not necessary

Dosing adjustment/comments in hepatic impairment: Avoid use in patients with severe hepatic impairment

Stability Sensitive to light; exposure to air causes volatilization; store in light-resistant, airtight container; **incompatible** with alkali, soluble barbiturates

Monitoring Parameters Vital signs, O_2 saturation and blood pressure with doses used for conscious sedation

Administration

Chilling the syrup may help to mask unpleasant taste. Do not crush capsule (contains drug in liquid form). Gastric irritation may be minimized by diluting dose in water or other oral liquid.

Contraindications Hypersensitivity to chloral hydrate or any component of the formulation; hepatic or renal impairment; gastritis or ulcers; severe cardiac disease

Warnings Use with caution in patients with porphyria. Use with caution in neonates. Drug may accumulate with repeated use; prolonged use in neonates associated with hyperbilirubinemia. Tolerance to hypnotic effect develops, therefore, not recommended for use >2 weeks. Taper dosage to avoid withdrawal with prolonged use. Trichloroethanol (TCE), a metabolite of chloral hydrate, is a carcinogen in mice; there is no data in humans. Chloral hydrate is considered a second line hypnotic agent in the elderly. Recent interpretive guidelines from the Centers for Medicare and Medicaid Services (CMS) discourage the use of chloral hydrate in residents of long-term care facilities.

Dosage Forms

Capsule (Somnote™): 500 mg

Suppository, rectal (Aquachloral® Supprettes®): 325 mg [contains tartrazine], 650 mg

Syrup: 500 mg/5 mL (480 mL) [contains sodium benzoate]

Reference Range Therapeutic: 2-12 mcg/mL of trichloroethanol; toxic serum trichloroethanol level: >100 mcg/mL, although 25 mcg/mL trichloroethanol has been correlated with fatalities

Overdosage/Treatment

Decontamination: Carefully lavage adult ingestions >2.4 g within 1 hour of ingestion, due to risk of perforation; activated charcoal should be utilized

Supportive therapy: Treatment is supportive and symptomatic; isoproterenol or atropine may be required for torsade de pointes; flumazenil has been used successfully in treating chloral hydrate overdose; ventricular arrhythmias may also respond to propranolol (2 mg I.V.) or metoprolol (5 mg I.V.) to titrate to a heart rate of 80-100 bpm.

Enhancement of elimination: Multiple dosing of activated charcoal may be effective; hemodialysis and/or charcoal hemoperfusion is effective; exchange transfusion also may be useful for neonatal intoxication; dialyzable (50% to 100%); clearance of trichloroethanol by hemodialysis is ~162 mL/minute with removal of 34% body stores over a 4-hour period; clearance by hemoperfusion is ~157-238 mL/minute with removal of 37% body stores during a 4-hour period

Test Interactions False-positive urine glucose using Clinitest® method; may interfere with fluorometric urine catecholamine and urinary 17-hydroxycorticosteroid tests; increases urine protein; well visualized on plain film x-ray; may interfere with BUN test

Drug Interactions

CNS depressants: Sedative effects and/or respiratory depression with chloral hydrate may be additive with other CNS depressants; monitor for increased effect; includes ethanol, sedatives, antidepressants, narcotic analgesics, and benzodiazepines.

Furosemide: Diaphoresis, flushing, and hypertension have occurred in patients who received I.V. furosemide within 24 hours after administration of chloral hydrate; consider using a benzodiazepine.

Phenytoin: Half-life may be decreased by chloral hydrate; limited documentation (small, single-dose study); monitor.

Warfarin: Effect of oral anticoagulants may be increased by chloral hydrate; monitor INR; warfarin dosage may require adjustment. Chloral hydrate's metabolite may displace warfarin from its protein binding sites resulting in an increase in the hypoprothrombinemic response to warfarin.

Pregnancy Risk Factor C

Pregnancy Implications Crosses the placenta

Lactation Enters breast milk/compatible

Nursing Implications Gastric irritation may be minimized by diluting dose in water or other oral liquid

Additional Information Tolerance to hypnotic effect develops, therefore, not recommended for use >2 weeks; taper dosage to avoid withdrawal with prolonged use; radiopaque; genotoxic; question of carcinogenesis is unanswered

Specific References

Caksen H, Odabas D, Uner A, et al, "Respiratory Arrest Due to Chloral Hydrate in an Infant," *J Emerg Med*, 2003, 24(3):342-3.

Tenenbein MS, Sitar DS, and Tenenbein M, "Post-Mortem Chloral Hydrate Disposition and Interpretation of Forensic Data," *J Toxicol Clin Toxicol*, 2004, 42(5):770.

Chlorambucil

CAS Number 305-03-3

U.S. Brand Names Leukeran®

Synonyms CB-1348; Chlorambucilum; Chloraminophene; Chlorbutinum; NSC-3088; WR-139013

Use Management of chronic lymphocytic leukemia, Hodgkin's and non-Hodgkin's lymphoma; breast and ovarian carcinoma; Waldenström's macroglobulinemia, testicular carcinoma, thrombocythemia, choriocarcinoma

Mechanism of Action Interferes with DNA replication and RNA transcription by alkylation and cross-linking the strands of DNA; derived from mustine (a nitrogen mustard)

Adverse Reactions

Central nervous system: **Confusion, agitation, rarely generalized or focal seizures,** drowsiness, psychosis, **hallucinations, ataxia,** drug fever

Dermatologic: Skin rashes, dermal irritant, toxic epidermal necrolysis, **Skin hypersensitivity**

Endocrine & metabolic: Hyperuricemia, ovotoxic, can produce amenorrhea in females

Gastrointestinal: **Diarrhea, oral ulcerations are infrequent**

Genitourinary: Has caused chromosomal damage in man, oligospermia, both reversible and permanent sterility have occurred in both sexes; cystitis, azoospermia

Hematologic: Possible porphyria; **use with caution when receiving radiation; bone marrow suppression frequently occurs and occasionally bone marrow failure has occurred; blood counts should be monitored closely while undergoing treatment; leukopenia** (at doses in excess of 6.5 mg/kg), lymphocytopenia, **thrombocytopenia, anemia**

Hepatic: **Hepatotoxicity,** hepatic necrosis, liver failure

Neuromuscular & skeletal: **Tremors,** muscular myoclonus, paresthesia, weakness

Ocular: Transient blindness (at 1.5 mg/kg/day), **keratitis**

Respiratory: **Pulmonary fibrosis** at doses of 40 mg/kg

Miscellaneous: Cardiotoxic

Signs and Symptoms of Overdose Azoospermia, agranulocytosis, ataxia, coma (at 5 mg/kg), convulsions, granulocytopenia, hyperuricemia, leukopenia, neutropenia, oligospermia, toxic epidermal necrolysis

Pharmacodynamics/Kinetics

Absorption: Rapid and complete

Distribution: V_d: 0.14-0.24 L/kg

Protein binding: ~99%

Metabolism: Hepatic; active metabolite, phenylacetic acid mustard

Bioavailability: Reduced 10% to 20% with food

Half-life elimination: ~1.5 hours; Phenylacetic acid mustard: 2.5 hours

Time to peak, plasma: Within 1 hour; Phenylacetic acid mustard: 1.2-2.6 hours

Excretion: Urine (15% to 60% primarily as metabolites, <1% as unchanged drug or phenylacetic acid mustard: 2.5 hours)

Dosage

Oral (refer to individual protocols):

Children:

General short courses: 0.1-0.2 mg/kg/day OR 4.5 mg/m²/day for 3-6 weeks for remission induction (usual: 4-10 mg/day); maintenance therapy: 0.03-0.1 mg/kg/day (usual: 2-4 mg/day)

Nephrotic syndrome: 0.1-0.2 mg/kg/day every day for 5-15 weeks with low-dose prednisone

Chronic lymphocytic leukemia (CLL):

Biweekly regimen: Initial: 0.4 mg/kg/dose every 2 weeks; increase dose by 0.1 mg/kg every 2 weeks until a response occurs and/or myelosuppression occurs

Monthly regimen: Initial: 0.4 mg/kg, increase dose by 0.2 mg/kg every 4 weeks until a response occurs and/or myelosuppression occurs

Malignant lymphomas:
Non-Hodgkin's lymphoma: 0.1 mg/kg/day
Hodgkin's lymphoma: 0.2 mg/kg/day

Adults: 0.1-0.2 mg/kg/day **or**
3-6 mg/m^2/day for 3-6 weeks, then adjust dose on basis of blood counts **or**
0.4 mg/kg and increased by 0.1 mg/kg biweekly or monthly **or**
14 mg/m^2/day for 5 days, repeated every 21-28 days

Hemodialysis: Supplemental dosing is not necessary
Peritoneal dialysis: Supplemental dosing is not necessary

Stability Protect from light

Monitoring Parameters Liver function tests, CBC, platelets, serum uric acid

Administration
Usually administered as a single dose; preferably on an empty stomach.

Contraindications Hypersensitivity to chlorambucil or any component of the formulation; hypersensitivity to other alkylating agents (may have cross-hypersensitivity); pregnancy

Warnings
Hazardous agent - use appropriate precautions for handling and disposal. Convulsions have been observed; use with caution in patients with seizure disorder; history of nephrotic syndrome and high pulse doses are at higher risk of seizures. **[U.S. Boxed Warning]: May cause bone marrow suppression;** reduce initial dosage if patient has received myelosuppressive or radiation therapy, or has a depressed baseline leukocyte or platelet count within the previous 4 weeks. Lymphopenia may occur. Avoid administration of live vaccines to immunocompromised patients. Rare instances of severe skin reactions (eg, erythema multiforme, Stevens-Johnson syndrome) have been reported; discontinue if a reaction occurs.

[U.S. Boxed Warning]: Affects human fertility; carcinogenic in humans and probably mutagenic and teratogenic as well; chromosomal damage has been documented. Secondary malignancies and acute myelocytic leukemia may be associated with chronic therapy. Safety and efficacy in pediatric patients have not been established.

Dosage Forms Tablet: 2 mg

Reference Range Peak plasma level after a dose of 0.6-1.2 mg/kg: 1 mcg/mL

Overdosage/Treatment
Decontamination: Lavage (within 1 hour)/activated charcoal
Supportive therapy: Replace blood products/diazepam or lorazepam for seizures
Enhancement of elimination: Multiple dosing of activated charcoal may be effective; probably not dialyzable

Drug Interactions Patients may experience impaired immune response to vaccines; possible infection after administration of live vaccines in patients receiving immunosuppressants

Pregnancy Risk Factor D

Pregnancy Implications Urogenital malformation seen in rodent studies

Lactation Excretion in breast milk unknown

Additional Information Myelosuppressive effects: **WBC**: Moderate. **Platelets**: Moderate. Onset (days): 7. Nadir (days): 14-21

Chloramphenicol

CAS Number 530-43-8; 56-75-7; 982-57-0

U.S. Brand Names Chloromycetin® Sodium Succinate

Use Treatment of serious infections due to organisms resistant to other less toxic antibiotics or when its penetrability into the site of infection is clinically superior to other antibiotics to which the organism is sensitive; useful in infections caused by *Bacteroides*, *H. influenzae*, *Neisseria meningitidis*, *Salmonella*, and *Rickettsia*; active against many vancomycin-resistant enterococci

Mechanism of Action Reversibly binds to 50S ribosomal subunits of susceptible organisms preventing amino acids from being transferred to growing peptide chains thus inhibiting protein synthesis

Adverse Reactions
Three (3) major toxicities associated with chloramphenicol include:
Aplastic anemia, an idiosyncratic reaction which can occur with any route of administration; usually occurs 3 weeks to 12 months after initial exposure to chloramphenicol
Bone marrow suppression is thought to be dose-related with serum concentrations >25 mcg/mL and reversible once chloramphenicol is discontinued; anemia and neutropenia may occur during the first week of therapy
Gray syndrome is characterized by circulatory collapse, cyanosis, acidosis, abdominal distention, myocardial depression, coma, and death; reaction appears to be associated with serum levels ≥50 mcg/mL; may

result from drug accumulation in patients with impaired hepatic or renal function

Additional adverse reactions, frequency not defined:
Central nervous system: Confusion, delirium, depression, fever, headache
Dermatologic: Angioedema, rash, urticaria
Gastrointestinal: Diarrhea, enterocolitis, glossitis, nausea, stomatitis, vomiting
Hematologic: Granulocytopenia, hypoplastic anemia, pancytopenia, thrombocytopenia
Ocular: Optic neuritis
Miscellaneous: Anaphylaxis, hypersensitivity reactions

Pharmacodynamics/Kinetics
Distribution: To most tissues and body fluids; readily crosses placenta; enters breast milk
CSF:blood level ratio: Normal meninges: 66%; Inflamed meninges: >66%
Protein binding: 60%
Metabolism: Extensively hepatic (90%) to inactive metabolites, principally by glucuronidation; chloramphenicol sodium succinate is hydrolyzed by esterases to active base
Half-life elimination:
Normal renal function: 1.6-3.3 hours
End-stage renal disease: 3-7 hours
Cirrhosis: 10-12 hours
Excretion: Urine (5% to 15%)

Dosage
Meningitis: I.V.: Infants >30 days and Children: 50-100 mg/kg/day divided every 6 hours
Other infections: I.V.:
Infants >30 days and Children: 50-75 mg/kg/day divided every 6 hours; maximum daily dose: 4 g/day
Adults: 50-100 mg/kg/day in divided doses every 6 hours; maximum daily dose: 4 g/day
Ophthalmic: Children and Adults: Instill 1-2 drops 4-6 times/day; increase interval between applications after 72 hours to 2-3 times/day; treatment should continue for ~7 days

Dosing adjustment/comments in hepatic impairment: Avoid use in severe liver impairment as increased toxicity may occur

Hemodialysis: Slightly dialyzable (5% to 20%) via hemo- and peritoneal dialysis; no supplemental doses needed in dialysis or continuous arteriovenous or veno-venous hemofiltration

Stability Injection: Store at room temperature prior to reconstitution; reconstituted solutions remain stable for 30 days; use only clear solutions; frozen solutions remain stable for 6 months
Ophthalmic: Refrigerate

Monitoring Parameters CBC with reticulocyte and platelet counts, periodic liver and renal function tests, serum drug concentration

Administration
Can be administered IVP over 5 minutes at a maximum concentration of 100 mg/mL, or I.V. intermittent infusion over 15-30 minutes at a final concentration for administration of ≤20 mg/mL

Contraindications Hypersensitivity to chloramphenicol or any component of the formulation

Warnings [U.S. Boxed Warning]: Serious and fatal blood dyscrasias have occurred after both short-term and prolonged therapy. Should not be used when less potentially toxic agents are effective. Prolonged use may result in superinfection. Use with caution in patients with impaired renal or hepatic function and in neonates. Reduce dose with impaired liver function. Use with care in patients with glucose 6-phosphate dehydrogenase deficiency.

Dosage Forms Injection, powder for reconstitution: 1 g [contains sodium ~52 mg/g (2.25 mEq/g)]

Reference Range
Timing of serum samples: Draw levels 1.5 hours and 3 hours after completion of I.V. or oral dose; trough levels may be preferred; should be drawn ≤1 hour prior to dose
Therapeutic: 10-25 mcg/mL; Toxic: >25 mcg/mL

Overdosage/Treatment
Decontamination: Emesis within 30 minutes or lavage within 1 hour (for doses >50 mg/kg)/activated charcoal
Supportive therapy: For optic neuropathy or paresthesia, give pyridoxine (vitamin B$_6$ 500 mg twice daily) and vitamin B$_{12}$ (0.5 mg/day) orally
Enhancement of elimination: Multiple dosing of activated charcoal may be effective; hemodialysis may be effective and can reduce half-life to under 1 hour; hemoperfusion may also be effective; exchange transfusion may be helpful in neonates; slightly dialyzable (5% to 20%)

Antidote(s)
• Pyridoxine [ANTIDOTE]

Diagnostic Procedures
• Iron and Total Iron Binding Capacity/Transferrin

Test Interactions ↑ iron (B), prothrombin time; ↓ urea nitrogen (B), total iron binding capacity (S)

Drug Interactions Inhibits CYP2C9 (weak), 3A4 (weak)

Decreased effect: Phenobarbital and rifampin may decrease concentration of chloramphenicol.

Increased toxicity: Chloramphenicol inhibits the metabolism of chlorpropamide, phenytoin, oral anticoagulants.

Pregnancy Risk Factor C

Pregnancy Implications Crosses placenta

Lactation Enters breast milk/not recommended (AAP rates "of concern")

Nursing Implications Give around-the-clock rather than 4 times/day to promote less variation in peak and trough serum levels

Additional Information Sodium content of 1 g (injection): 51.8 mg (2.25 mEq). Gray baby syndrome occurs when neonates are given large doses of chloramphenicol and cardiovascular collapse occurs; it is associated with plasma levels of 50-100 mcg/mL. Blood dyscrasias can occur with ocular use; no evidence of aplastic anemia with chloramphenicol eye drops

Chlordiazepoxide

Related Information
● Therapeutic Drugs Associated with Hallucinations

CAS Number 438-41-5; 58-25-3

U.S. Brand Names Librium®

Synonyms Methaminodiazepoxide Hydrochloride

Impairment Potential Yes. Brief or extended period (up to 1 year) of use is consistent with driving impairment in the elderly; impairment is greatest in the first 7 days of use

Use Management of anxiety disorder or for the short-term relief of symptoms of anxiety; withdrawal symptoms of acute alcoholism; preoperative apprehension and anxiety

Mechanism of Action Benzodiazepine anxiolytic sedative that produces CNS depression at the subcortical level, except at high doses, whereby it works at the cortical level

Adverse Reactions
Cardiovascular: Tachycardia, vasculitis

Central nervous system: **Drowsiness, ataxia, lightheadedness, dizziness, slurred speech,** euphoria, headache, mental depression, hallucinations, insomnia, convulsions, paranoid symptoms, confusion, dystonic reactions

Dermatologic: Erythema multiforme, alopecia, angioedema, urticaria, purpura, pruritus, erythema nodosum, exanthem

Endocrine & metabolic: Changes in libido, gynecomastia

Gastrointestinal: Nausea, xerostomia, vomiting, diarrhea, constipation, abdominal cramps

Hematologic: Thrombocytopenia, anemia, leukopenia, neutropenia, agranulocytosis

Hepatic: Liver dysfunction

Local: Phlebitis

Neuromuscular & skeletal: Paresthesia, muscle spasm, trembling

Ocular: Blurred vision, photophobia

Miscellaneous: Allergic reaction, drug dependence, diaphoresis (excessive), systemic lupus erythematosus, fixed drug eruption

Signs and Symptoms of Overdose Agranulocytosis, cardiac arrhythmias, coma, ejaculatory disturbances, galactorrhea, granulocytopenia, hiccups, hyperglycemia, hypotension, hypothermia, jaundice, lactation, leukopenia, myoglobinuria, neutropenia, photosensitivity, respiratory depression, rhabdomyolysis

Pharmacodynamics/Kinetics
Distribution: V_d: 3.3 L/kg; crosses placenta; enters breast milk

Protein binding: 90% to 98%

Metabolism: Extensively hepatic to desmethyldiazepam (active and long-acting)

Half-life elimination: 6.6-25 hours; End-stage renal disease: 5-30 hours; Cirrhosis: 30-63 hours

Time to peak, serum: Oral: Within 2 hours; I.M.: Results in lower peak plasma levels than oral

Excretion: Urine (minimal as unchanged drug)

Dosage
Children:
<6 years: Not recommended
>6 years: Anxiety: Oral, I.M.: 0.5 mg/kg/24 hours divided every 6-8 hours

Adults:
Anxiety:
Oral: 15-100 mg divided 3-4 times/day
I.M., I.V.: Initial: 50-100 mg followed by 25-50 mg 3-4 times/day as needed

Preoperative anxiety: I.M.: 50-100 mg prior to surgery

Ethanol withdrawal symptoms: Oral, I.V.: 50-100 mg to start, dose may be repeated in 2-4 hours as necessary to a maximum of 300 mg/24 hours

Note: Up to 300 mg may be given I.M. or I.V. during a 6-hour period, but not more than this in any 24-hour period.

Dosing adjustment in renal impairment: Cl_{cr} <10 mL/minute: Administer 50% of dose

Hemodialysis: Not dialyzable (0% to 5%)

Dosing adjustment/comments in hepatic impairment: Avoid use

Monitoring Parameters Respiratory and cardiovascular status, mental status, check for orthostasis

Administration I.M.: Administer by deep I.M. injection slowly into the upper outer quadrant of the gluteus muscle; use only the diluent provided for I.M. use; solutions made with SWFI or NS cause pain with I.M. administration

I.V.: Administer slowly over at least 1 minute; do not use the diluent provided for I.M. use; air bubbles form during reconstitution

Contraindications Hypersensitivity to chlordiazepoxide or any component of the formulation (cross-sensitivity with other benzodiazepines may also exist); narrow-angle glaucoma; pregnancy

Warnings
Active metabolites with extended half-lives may lead to delayed accumulation and adverse effects. Use with caution in elderly or debilitated patients, pediatric patients, patients with hepatic disease (including alcoholics) or renal impairment. Use with caution in patients with respiratory disease or impaired gag reflex. Use with caution in patients with porphyria.

Parenteral administration should be avoided in comatose patients or shock. Adequate resuscitative equipment/personnel should be available, and appropriate monitoring should be conducted at the time of injection and for several hours following administration. The parenteral formulation should be diluted for I.M. administration with the supplied diluent only. This diluent should not be used when preparing the drug for intravenous administration.

Causes CNS depression (dose related) resulting in sedation, dizziness, confusion, or ataxia which may impair physical and mental capabilities. Patients must be cautioned about performing tasks which require mental alertness (eg, operating machinery or driving). Use with caution in patients receiving other CNS depressants or psychoactive agents (lithium, phenothiazines). Effects with other sedative drugs or ethanol may be potentiated. Benzodiazepines have been associated with falls and traumatic injury and should be used with extreme caution in patients who are at risk of these events (especially the elderly).

Use caution in patients with depression, particularly if suicidal risk may be present. Use with caution in patients with a history of drug dependence. Benzodiazepines have been associated with dependence and acute withdrawal symptoms on discontinuation or reduction in dose. Acute withdrawal, including seizures, may be precipitated in patients after administration of flumazenil to patients receiving long-term benzodiazepine therapy.

Benzodiazepines have been associated with anterograde amnesia. Paradoxical reactions, including hyperactive or aggressive behavior have been reported with benzodiazepines, particularly in adolescent/pediatric or psychiatric patients. Does not have analgesic, antidepressant, or antipsychotic properties.

Dosage Forms
Capsule, as hydrochloride: 5 mg, 10 mg, 25 mg

Injection, powder for reconstitution, as hydrochloride: 100 mg [diluent contains benzyl alcohol, polysorbate 80, and propylene glycol]

Reference Range
Therapeutic: 0.1-3 mcg/mL (SI: 0-10 µmol/L)

Toxic: >20 mcg/mL (SI: >77 µmol/L); toxicity may be related to demoxepam levels >10 mcg/mL

Urine drug screens can remain positive for 30 days

In the postmortem state, anatomical site concentration differences (ie, postmortem redistribution) may occur

Overdosage/Treatment
Decontamination: Lavage (within 1 hour)/activated charcoal

Supportive therapy: Treatment for benzodiazepine overdose is supportive. Rarely is mechanical ventilation required. Flumazenil has been shown to selectively block the binding of benzodiazepines to CNS receptors, resulting in a reversal of benzodiazepine-induced CNS depression; do not use stimulants.

Enhancement of elimination: Multiple dosing of activated charcoal may be effective; not dialyzable (0% to 5%)

Antidote(s)
● Flumazenil [ANTIDOTE]

Test Interactions Visine®, Drano®, hand soap, or bleach can result in false-negative tests for benzodiazepines

Drug Interactions
Substrate of CYP3A4 (major)

CNS depressants: Sedative effects and/or respiratory depression may be additive with CNS depressants; includes ethanol, barbiturates, narcotic analgesics, and other sedative agents; monitor for increased effect.

CYP3A4 inducers: CYP3A4 inducers may decrease the levels/effects of chlordiazepoxide. Example inducers include aminoglutethimide, carbamazepine, nafcillin, nevirapine, phenobarbital, phenytoin, and rifamycins.

CYP3A4 inhibitors: May increase the levels/effects of chlordiazepoxide. Example inhibitors include azole antifungals, clarithromycin, diclofenac, doxycycline, erythromycin, imatinib, isoniazid, nefazodone, nicardipine, propofol, protease inhibitors, quinidine, telithromycin, and verapamil.

Levodopa: Therapeutic effects may be diminished in some patients following the addition of a benzodiazepine; limited/inconsistent data.

Oral contraceptives: May decrease the clearance of some benzodiazepines (those which undergo oxidative metabolism); monitor for increased benzodiazepine effect.

Theophylline: May partially antagonize some of the effects of benzodiazepines; monitor for decreased response; may require higher doses for sedation.

Pregnancy Risk Factor D

Pregnancy Implications Crosses the placenta

Lactation Enters breast milk/not recommended

Nursing Implications Up to 300 mg may be given I.M. or I.V. during a 6-hour period, but not more than this in any 24-hour period; do not use diluent provided with parenteral form for I.V. administration; dissolve with normal saline instead

Additional Information Often formulated with amitriptyline hydrochloride

Chlorhexidine Gluconate

Pronunciation (klor HEKS i deen GLOO koe nate)

CAS Number 18472-51-0; 55-56-1

U.S. Brand Names Avagard™ [OTC]; BactoShield® CHG [OTC]; Betasept® [OTC]; ChloraPrep® [OTC]; Chlorostat® [OTC]; Dyna-Hex® [OTC]; Hibiclens® [OTC]; Hibistat® [OTC]; Operand® Chlorhexidine Gluconate [OTC]; Peridex®; PerioChip®; PerioGard®

Synonyms 3M™ Avagard™ [OTC]; CHG

Use Skin cleanser for surgical scrub, cleanser for skin wounds, preoperative skin preparation, germicidal hand rinse, and as antibacterial dental rinse. Chlorhexidine is active against gram-positive and gram-negative organisms, facultative anaerobes, aerobes, and yeast.

Orphan drug: Peridex®: Oral mucositis with cytoreductive therapy when used for patients undergoing bone marrow transplant

Mechanism of Action Chlorhexidine, a cationic polybiguanide, is an antiseptic and antimicrobial drug with bactericidal activity. At physiologic pH, chlorhexidine salts dissociate releasing a positively charged component. The bactericidal effect of chlorhexidine is a result of the binding of this cationic molecule to negatively charged bacterial cell walls and extramicrobial complexes. At low concentrations, this causes an alteration of bacterial cell osmotic equilibrium and leakage of potassium and phosphorous resulting in a bacteriostatic effect; at high concentrations of chlorhexidine, the cytoplasmic contents of the bacterial cell precipitate and result in cell death.

Adverse Reactions

Cardiovascular: Sinus bradycardia, facial edema

Dermatologic: Dermal hypersensitivity, urticaria, contact dermatitis (8%), immunologic contact urticaria, desquamation

Endocrine & metabolic: Parotid gland edema with mouthwash

Gastrointestinal: **Staining of oral surfaces (mucosa, teeth, dorsum of tongue), increased tartar on teeth, altered taste,** tongue irritation, oral irritation, salt hypogeusia

Hematologic: Methemoglobinemia caused by conversion to parachloroaniline

Ocular: Corneal irritation

Respiratory: Dyspnea, nasal congestion

Signs and Symptoms of Overdose Bradycardia, deafness, esophageal ulceration, fatty degeneration of liver, gastritis, hemolysis with systemic absorption, methemoglobinemia on inhalation, pulmonary edema, tongue discoloration

Admission Criteria/Prognosis Any patient with change in mental status, GI symptoms, cardiopulmonary complaints, or methemoglobin levels >30% should be admitted; asymptomatic patients with methemoglobin levels <30% may be considered for discharge after 6 hours of observation and if methemoglobin levels fall to <15%

Pharmacodynamics/Kinetics

Topical hand sanitizer (Avagard™): Duration of antimicrobial protection: 6 hours

Oral rinse (Peridex®, PerioGard®):

Absorption: ~30% retained in the oral cavity following rinsing and slowly released into oral fluids; poorly absorbed

Time to peak, plasma: Oral rinse: Detectable levels not present after 12 hours

Excretion: Feces (~90%); urine (<1%)

Dosage

Adults:

Oral rinse (Peridex®, PerioGard®):

Precede use of solution by flossing and brushing teeth; completely rinse toothpaste from mouth. Swish 15 mL undiluted oral rinse around

in mouth for 30 seconds, then expectorate. Caution patient not to swallow the medicine. Avoid eating for 2-3 hours after treatment. (The cap on bottle of oral rinse is a measure for 15 mL.)

When used as a treatment of gingivitis, the regimen begins with oral prophylaxis. Patient treats mouth with 15 mL chlorhexidine, swishes for 30 seconds, then expectorates. This is repeated twice daily (morning and evening). Patient should have a re-evaluation followed by a dental prophylaxis every 6 months.

Cleanser:

Surgical scrub: Scrub 3 minutes and rinse thoroughly, wash for an additional 3 minutes

Hand sanitizer (Avagard™): Dispense 1 pumpful in palm of one hand; dip fingertips of opposite hand into solution and work it under nails. Spread remainder evenly over hand and just above elbow, covering all surfaces. Repeat on other hand. Dispense another pumpful in each hand and reapply to each hand up to the wrist. Allow to dry before gloving.

Hand wash: Wash for 15 seconds and rinse

Hand rinse: Rub 15 seconds and rinse

Periodontal chip: One chip is inserted into a periodontal pocket with a probing pocket depth ≥5 mm. Up to 8 chips may be inserted in a single visit. Treatment is recommended every 3 months in pockets with a remaining depth ≥5 mm. If dislodgment occurs 7 days or more after placement, the subject is considered to have had the full course of treatment. If dislodgment occurs within 48 hours, a new chip should be inserted.

Stability

Store at room temperature

Avagard™: Avoid excessive heat. Ethanol-containing products are flammable; keep away from flames or fire. Hand lotions and gel hand sanitizers are incompatible. The thickeners used in these products (eg, carbomer) react to form an insoluble salt and cause loss of antibacterial action.

Administration Hand sanitizer (Avagard™): To facilitate drying, continue rubbing hand prep into hands until dry.

Periodontal chip insertion: Pocket should be isolated and surrounding area dried prior to chip insertion. The chip should be grasped using forceps with the rounded edges away from the forceps. The chip should be inserted into the periodontal pocket to its maximum depth. It may be maneuvered into position using the tips of the forceps or a flat instrument. The chip biodegrades completely and does not need to be removed. Patients should avoid dental floss at the site of PerioChip® insertion for 10 days after placement because flossing might dislodge the chip.

Topical: Keep out of eyes, ears, and mouth. Do not routinely apply to wounds which involve more than superficial layers of skin.

Contraindications Hypersensitivity to chlorhexidine gluconate or any component of the formulation

Warnings

Oral: Staining of oral surfaces (mucosa, teeth, tooth restorations, dorsum of tongue) may occur; may be visible as soon as 1 week after therapy begins and is more pronounced when there is a heavy accumulation of unremoved plaque and when teeth fillings have rough surfaces. Stain does not have a clinically adverse effect, but because removal may not be possible, patient with frontal restoration should be advised of the potential permanency of the stain.

Topical: For topical use only. Keep out of eyes and ears. May stain fabric. There have been case reports of anaphylaxis following chlorhexidine disinfection. Not for preoperative preparation of face or head; avoid contact with meninges.

Dosage Forms

Chip, for periodontal pocket insertion (PerioChip®): 2.5 mg

Liquid, topical [surgical scrub]:

Avagard™: 1% (500 mL) [contains ethyl alcohol and moisturizers]

BactoShield® CHG: 2% (120 mL, 480 mL, 750 mL, 1000 mL, 3800 mL); 4% (120 mL, 480 mL, 750 mL, 1000 mL, 3800 mL) [contains isopropyl alcohol]

Betasept®: 4% (120 mL, 240 mL, 480 mL, 960 mL, 3840 mL) [contains isopropyl alcohol]

ChloraPrep®: 2% (0.67 mL, 1.5 mL, 3 mL, 10.5 mL) [contains isopropyl alcohol 70%; prefilled applicator]

Dyna-Hex®: 2% (120 mL, 960 mL, 3840 mL); 4% (120 mL, 960 mL, 3840 mL)

Hibiclens®: 4% (15 mL, 120 mL, 240 mL, 480 mL, 960 mL, 3840 mL) [contains isopropyl alcohol]

Operand® Chlorhexidine Gluconate: 2% (120 mL); 4% (120 mL, 240 mL, 480 mL, 960 mL, 3840 mL) [contains isopropyl alcohol]

Liquid, oral rinse: 0.12% (480 mL)

Peridex®: 0.12% (480 mL) [contains alcohol 11.6%]

PerioGard®: 0.12% (480 mL) [contains alcohol 11.6%; mint flavor]

Pad [prep pad] (Hibistat®): 0.5% (50s) [contains isopropyl alcohol]

Sponge/Brush (BactoShield® CHG): 4% per sponge/brush [contains isopropyl alcohol]

Reference Range Topical use (vaginal or dermal) as an antiseptic agent results in serum chlorhexidine levels ranging from 0.01-0.128 mcg/mL. Following inadvertent administration of 10 mL of a 20% chlorhexidine gluconate solution I.V., a patient developed cardiac arrest within 20 minutes; postmortem blood chlorhexidine level was 39.5 mcg/mL. Serum chlorhexidine level of 24.6 mcg/mL has been associated with an oral overdose, ARDS, and fatality.

Overdosage/Treatment

Decontamination: Lavage (within 1 hour)/dilution with milk or water (4-8 oz or 15 mL/kg); activated charcoal is not useful; irrigate skin/eyes

Supportive therapy: Methylene blue for methemoglobin toxicity

Test Interactions ↑ LFTs

Drug Interactions No data reported

Pregnancy Risk Factor B

Pregnancy Implications No teratogenic effects reported

Nursing Implications Inform patient that reduced taste perception during treatment is reversible with discontinuation of chlorhexidine

Chlormezanone

CAS Number 80-77-3

Use Anxiety; insomnia; muscle spasm

Mechanism of Action Precise mechanism is not yet clear, but many effects have been ascribed to its central depressant actions; an indirect GABA-A agonist

Adverse Reactions

Cardiovascular: Flushing, toxic epidermal necrosis

Central nervous system: Drowsiness, confusion, headache

Gastrointestinal: Nausea, xerostomia

Hematologic: Porphyrinogenic

Hepatic: Reversible jaundice, hepatitis

Neuromuscular & skeletal: Tremor, muscle weakness

Respiratory: Hyposmia

Signs and Symptoms of Overdose Ataxia, coma, hot dry skin, hypotension, hyporeflexia, mydriasis, tachycardia

Admission Criteria/Prognosis Admit any symptomatic patient or any adult ingestion >5 g

Toxicodynamics/Kinetics

Peak plasma level: 2 hours

Duration of action: >6 hours

Protein binding: ~50%

Metabolism: Hydrolysis in the stomach and then metabolized in the liver (4-chlorohippuric acid is the major metabolite)

Half-life: 19-53 hours

Elimination: Renal

Dosage

Oral:

Children >5 years: 50-100 mg 3-4 times/day

Adults:

Anxiety: 100-200 mg 3-4 times/day

Insomnia: 400 mg at bedtime (200 mg in elderly patients)

Muscle spasm: 200-400 mg 3-4 times/day

Reference Range Therapeutic range (in a steady state of 600 mg/day for 5 days): ~ 10-14 mcg/mL. Levels >18 mcg/mL are associated with mild toxicity (weakness, ataxia, tachycardia) while a postmortem blood and urine chlormezanone level in a fatality was 53 mcg/mL and 31 mcg/mL, respectively.

Overdosage/Treatment

Decontamination: Lavage (within 2 hours of ingestion)/activated charcoal

Supportive therapy: Benzodiazepines for seizure control

Enhancement of elimination: Forced diuresis is not helpful; multiple dosing of activated charcoal may be helpful. Following attempts to enhance drug elimination, hypotension should be treated with I.V. fluids and/or Trendelenburg positioning.

Chloroprocaine

CAS Number 133-16-4; 3858-89-7

U.S. Brand Names Nesacaine®-MPF; Nesacaine®

Synonyms Chloroprocaine Hydrochloride

Use Infiltration anesthesia and peripheral and epidural anesthesia

Mechanism of Action Ester local anesthetic similar to procaine produces conduction block at nerve cell membrane

Adverse Reactions

Cardiovascular: Myocardial depression, hypotension, bradycardia, cardiovascular collapse, edema, sinus bradycardia, congestive heart failure, sinus tachycardia

Central nervous system: Anxiety, restlessness, disorientation, confusion, psychosis, seizures, drowsiness, unconsciousness, chills

Dermatologic: Urticaria

Gastrointestinal: Nausea, vomiting

Local: Transient stinging or burning at injection site

Neuromuscular & skeletal: Tremors

Ocular: Blurred vision, diplopia, nystagmus

Otic: Ototoxicity, tinnitus

Respiratory: Respiratory arrest

Miscellaneous: Anaphylactoid reactions, shivering

Signs and Symptoms of Overdose Cardiac arrhythmias, coma, hypertension, mydriasis, seizures, tachycardia, tachypnea progressing to apnea

Pharmacodynamics/Kinetics

Onset of action: 6-12 minutes

Duration: 30-60 minutes

Distribution: V_d: Depends upon route of administration; high concentrations found in highly perfused organs such as liver, lungs, heart, and brain

Metabolism: Plasma cholinesterases

Excretion: Urine

Dosage

Dosage varies with anesthetic procedure, the area to be anesthetized, the vascularity of the tissues, depth of anesthesia required, degree of muscle relaxation required, and duration of anesthesia

Infiltration and peripheral nerve block: 1% to 2%

Infiltration, peripheral and central nerve block, including caudal and epidural block: 2% to 3%, without preservatives

Stability May contain sodium bisulfite

Monitoring Parameters Cardiovascular and respiratory status; mental status

Administration

Before injecting, withdraw syringe plunger to ensure injection is not into vein or artery.

Contraindications Hypersensitivity to chloroprocaine, other ester type anesthetics, or any component of the formulation; myasthenia gravis; do not use for subarachnoid administration

Warnings Use with caution in patients with hepatic impairment. **Do not use solutions containing preservatives for caudal or epidural block.** Local anesthetics have been associated with rare occurrences of sudden respiratory arrest; seizures due to systemic toxicity leading to cardiac arrest have also been reported, presumably following unintentional intravascular injection. A test dose is recommended prior to epidural administration (prior to initial dose) and all reinforcing doses with continuous catheter technique.

Dosage Forms

Injection, solution, as hydrochloride (Nesacaine®): 1% (30 mL); 2% (30 mL) [contains disodium EDTA and methylparaben]

Injection, solution, as hydrochloride [preservative free] (Nesacaine®-MPF): 2% (20 mL); 3% (20 mL)

Overdosage/Treatment

Decontamination: Lavage (within 1 hour)/activated charcoal for oral ingestions

Supportive therapy: Treatment is primarily symptomatic and supportive. Termination of anesthesia by pneumatic tourniquet inflation should be attempted when the agent is administered by infiltration or regional injection. Seizures commonly respond to diazepam or lorazepam, while hypotension responds to I.V. fluids and Trendelenburg positioning. Bradyarrhythmias (when the heart rate is less than 60) can be treated with I.V., I.M. or SubQ atropine 15 mcg/kg. With the development of metabolic acidosis, I.V. sodium bicarbonate 0.5-2 mEq/kg and ventilatory assistance should be instituted. Chlorpromazine may be used to treat acute psychosis.

Enhancement of elimination: Multiple dosing of activated charcoal may be effective for oral ingestions

Drug Interactions PABA (from ester-type anesthetics) may inhibit sulfonamides.

Pregnancy Risk Factor C

Pregnancy Implications Animal reproduction studies have not been conducted. Local anesthetics rapidly cross the placenta and may cause varying degrees of maternal, fetal, and neonatal toxicity. Close maternal and fetal monitoring (heart rate and electronic fetal monitoring advised) are required during obstetrical use. Maternal hypotension has resulted from regional anesthesia. Positioning the patient on her left side and elevating the legs may help. Epidural, paracervical, or pudendal anesthesia may alter the forces of parturition through changes in uterine contractility or maternal expulsive efforts. The use of some local anesthetic drugs during labor and delivery may diminish muscle strength and tone for the first day or two of life. Administration as a paracervical block is not recommended with toxemia of pregnancy, fetal distress, or prematurity. Administration of a paracervical block early in pregnancy has resulted in maternal seizures and cardiovascular collapse. Fetal bradycardia and acidosis also have been reported. Fetal depression has occurred following unintended fetal intracranial injection while administering a paracervical and/or pudendal block.

Lactation Excretion in breast milk unknown/use caution

Nursing Implications Before injecting, withdraw syringe plunger to ensure injection is not into vein or artery

Chloroquine

CAS Number 50-63-5

U.S. Brand Names Aralen®

Synonyms Chloroquine Phosphate

Use Suppression or chemoprophylaxis of malaria; treatment of uncomplicated or mild to moderate malaria; extraintestinal amebiasis Rheumatoid arthritis; discoid lupus erythematosus

Mechanism of Action Binds to and inhibits DNA and RNA polymerase; interferes with metabolism and hemoglobin utilization by parasites; inhibits prostaglandin effects; additionally has quinidine-like cardiac effects

Adverse Reactions

Frequency not defined.

Cardiovascular: Hypotension (rare), ECG changes (rare; including T-wave inversion), cardiomyopathy

Central nervous system: Fatigue, personality changes, headache, psychosis, seizures, delirium, depression

Dermatologic: Pruritus, hair bleaching, pleomorphic skin eruptions, alopecia, lichen planus eruptions, alopecia, mucosal pigmentary changes (blue-black), photosensitivity

Gastrointestinal: Nausea, diarrhea, vomiting, anorexia, stomatitis, abdominal cramps

Hematologic: Aplastic anemia, agranulocytosis (reversible), neutropenia, thrombocytopenia

Neuromuscular & skeletal: Rare cases of myopathy, neuromyopathy, proximal muscle atrophy, and depression of deep tendon reflexes have been reported

Ocular: Retinopathy (including irreversible changes in some patients long-term or high-dose therapy), blurred vision

Otic: Nerve deafness, tinnitus, reduced hearing (risk increased in patients with pre-existing auditory damage)

Signs and Symptoms of Overdose Doses of 20 mg/kg are considered toxic. Arrhythmias, AV block, cardiovascular collapse, disseminated intravascular coagulation, headache, hypotension in very rapid progression, hypoglycemia, hypokalemia, hypopigmented hair, methemoglobinemia, myasthenia gravis (exacerbation or precipitation), myopathy, nystagmus, ptosis, seizures, urine discoloration (brown; yellow-brown; milky; rust); visual changes including blindness, corneal microdeposits, and vision color changes (blue tinge; green tinge; yellow tinge)

Admission Criteria/Prognosis Any patient with change in mental status, cardiopulmonary complaints, or >3 g ingestion should be admitted; asymptomatic patients should be observed on an ECG monitor for 8 hours; predictors for fatality include QRS duration >0.12 seconds, ingested dose >6 g or chloroquine blood level >0.6 mg/L

Pharmacodynamics/Kinetics

Duration: Small amounts may be present in urine months following discontinuation of therapy

Absorption: Oral: Rapid (~89%)

Distribution: Widely in body tissues (eg, eyes, heart, kidneys, liver, lungs) where retention prolonged; crosses placenta; enters breast milk

Metabolism: Partially hepatic

Half-life elimination: 3-5 days

Time to peak, serum: 1-2 hours

Excretion: Urine (~70% as unchanged drug); acidification of urine increases elimination

Dosage

Suppression or prophylaxis of malaria: Oral:

Children: Administer 5 mg base/kg/week on the same day each week (not to exceed 300 mg base/dose); begin 1-2 weeks prior to exposure; continue for 4-6 weeks after leaving endemic area; if suppressive therapy is not begun prior to exposure, double the initial loading dose to 10 mg base/kg and administer in 2 divided doses 6 hours apart, followed by the usual dosage regimen

Adults: 500 mg/week (300 mg base) on the same day each week; begin 1-2 weeks prior to exposure; continue for 4-6 weeks after leaving endemic area; if suppressive therapy is not begun prior to exposure, double the initial loading dose to 1 g (600 mg base) and administer in 2 divided doses 6 hours apart, followed by the usual dosage regimen

Acute attack: Oral:

Children: 10 mg/kg (base) on day 1, followed by 5 mg/kg (base) 6 hours later and 5 mg/kg (base) on days 2 and 3

Adults: 1 g (600 mg base) on day 1, followed by 500 mg (300 mg base) 6 hours later, followed by 500 mg (300 mg base) on days 2 and 3

Extraintestinal amebiasis:

Children: Oral: 10 mg/kg (base) once daily for 2-3 weeks (up to 300 mg base/day)

Adults: Oral: 1 g/day (600 mg base) for 2 days followed by 500 mg/day (300 mg base) for at least 2-3 weeks

Rheumatoid arthritis, lupus erythematosus (unlabeled uses): Adults: 250 mg (150 mg base) once daily; reduce dosage following maximal response (taper to discontinue after response in lupus); generally requires 3-6 weeks

Note: Not considered first-line agent.

Dosing adjustment in renal impairment:

Cl_{cr} <10 mL/minute: Administer 50% of dose

Hemodialysis: Minimally removed by hemodialysis

Monitoring Parameters Periodic CBC, examination for muscular weakness, and ophthalmologic examination in patients receiving prolonged therapy

Administration

Chloroquine phosphate tablets have also been mixed with chocolate syrup or enclosed in gelatin capsules to mask the bitter taste.

Contraindications Hypersensitivity to chloroquine or any component of the formulation; retinal or visual field changes

Warnings

Use with caution in patients with liver disease, G6PD deficiency, alcoholism or in conjunction with hepatotoxic drugs. May exacerbate psoriasis or porphyria. Retinopathy (irreversible) has occurred with long or high-dose therapy; discontinue drug if any abnormality in the visual field or if muscular weakness develops during treatment. Use caution in patients with pre-existing auditory damage; discontinue immediately if hearing defects are noted. Use caution in patients with seizure disorders.

Dosage Forms

Tablet, as phosphate: 250 mg [equivalent to 150 mg base]; 500 mg [equivalent to 300 mg base]

Aralen®: 500 mg [equivalent to 300 mg base]

Reference Range

Average plasma concentration: up to 0.4 mg/L

Toxic plasma concentration: >0.6 mg/L

In the postmortem state, anatomical site concentration differences (ie, postmortem redistribution) may occur by a tenfold increase as compared to the antemortem state.

Overdosage/Treatment

Decontamination: Activated charcoal within 30 minutes, if available, for prehospital use clearly indicated; lavage within 1 hour if the patient is obtunded

Supportive therapy: Early administration of diazepam or lorazepam and epinephrine appears beneficial; avoid class I antiarrhythmics; 2 mg (I.V.) of clonazepam has terminated chloroquine-induced nonconvulsive status epilepticus; aqueous epinephrine and diazepam (bolus of 1 mg/kg in children followed by an infusion of 0.4 mg/kg/hour) should be given following return of circulation following cardiopulmonary arrest due to chloroquine; inamrinone can be used to treat refractory hypotension

Enhancement of elimination: Minimally removed by hemodialysis; hemoperfusion useful early in course of ingestion, but toxicities often prevent use; multiple doses of activated charcoal may be effective

Antidote(s)

• Epinephrine [ANTIDOTE]

Diagnostic Procedures

• Electrolytes, Blood

• Urinalysis

Test Interactions A high concentration of chloroquine in urine gives a positive result with amphetamine CEDIA reagent.

Drug Interactions

Substrate (major) of CYP2D6, 3A4; **Inhibits** CYP2D6 (moderate)

Ampicillin: Chloroquine may reduce the absorption of ampicillin; separate administration by 2 hours.

Antacids and kaolin: Chloroquine and other 4-aminoquinolones may be decreased due to GI binding with kaolin or magnesium trisilicate.

Cimetidine: Cimetidine increases levels of chloroquine and probably other 4-aminoquinolones.

Cyclosporine: Chloroquine may increase cyclosporine concentrations; monitor.

CYP2D6 inhibitors: May increase the levels/effects of chloroquine. Example inhibitors include chlorpromazine, delavirdine, fluoxetine, miconazole, paroxetine, pergolide, quinidine, quinine, ritonavir, and ropinirole.

CYP2D6 substrates: Chloroquine may increase the levels/effects of CYP2D6 substrates. Example substrates include amphetamines, selected beta-blockers, dextromethorphan, fluoxetine, lidocaine, mirtazapine, nefazodone, paroxetine, risperidone, ritonavir, thioridazine, tricyclic antidepressants, and venlafaxine.

CYP2D6 prodrug substrates: Chloroquine may decrease the levels/effects of CYP2D6 prodrug substrates. Example prodrug substrates include codeine, hydrocodone, oxycodone, and tramadol.

CYP3A4 inducers: CYP3A4 inducers may decrease the levels/effects of chloroquine. Example inducers include aminoglutethimide, carbamazepine, nafcillin, nevirapine, phenobarbital, phenytoin, and rifamycins.

CYP3A4 inhibitors: May increase the levels/effects of chloroquine. Example inhibitors include azole antifungals, clarithromycin, diclofenac, doxycycline, erythromycin, imatinib, isoniazid, nefazodone, nicardipine, propofol, protease inhibitors, quinidine, telithromycin, and verapamil.

Praziquantel: Chloroquine may decrease praziquantel concentrations.

Pregnancy Risk Factor C

Pregnancy Implications There are no adequate and well-controlled studies using chloroquine during pregnancy. However, based on clinical experience and because malaria infection in pregnant women may be more severe than in nonpregnant women, chloroquine prophylaxis may be considered in areas of chloroquine-sensitive *P. falciparum* malaria. Pregnant women should be advised not to travel to areas of *P. falciparum* resistance to chloroquine.

Lactation Enters breast milk/not recommended (AAP considers "compatible")

Additional Information Toxic dose: 5 mg/kg

Specific References
Davis TM, Syed DA, Ilett KF, et al, "Toxicity Related to Chloroquine Treatment of Resistant Vivax Malaria," *Ann Pharmacother*, 2003, 37(4):526-9.
Tagwireyi D, Gadaga L, Ball DE, et al, "A Simple Qualitative Procedure for the Detection of Chloroquine in Urine with Potential for Use in Clinical Analytical Toxicology in Developing Countries: A Preliminary Report," *Clin Toxicol (Phila)*, 2005, 43:687.
Telgt DS, van der Ven AJ, Schimmer B, et al, "Serious Psychiatric Symptoms After Chloroquine Treatment Following Experimental Malaria Infection," *Ann Pharmacother*. 2005, 39(3):551-4.

Chlorpheniramine

Related Information
- Therapeutic Drugs Associated with Hallucinations

CAS Number 113-92-8

U.S. Brand Names Aller-Chlor® [OTC]; Chlor-Trimeton® [OTC]; Chlorphen [OTC]; Diabetic Tussin® Allergy Relief [OTC]

Synonyms Chlorpheniramine Maleate; CTM

Impairment Potential Yes

Use Perennial and seasonal allergic rhinitis and other allergic symptoms including rash

Mechanism of Action Competes with histamine for H_1-receptor sites on effector cells in the GI tract, blood vessels, and respiratory tract

Adverse Reactions
Central nervous system: **Slight to moderate drowsiness**, headache, excitability, fatigue, nervousness, dizziness
Gastrointestinal: Nausea, xerostomia, diarrhea, abdominal pain, appetite increase, weight gain
Genitourinary: Urinary retention
Neuromuscular & skeletal: Arthralgia, weakness
Ocular: Diplopia, blepharospasm
Renal: Polyuria
Respiratory: **Thickening of bronchial secretions**, pharyngitis

Signs and Symptoms of Overdose Agranulocytosis, CNS depression, dry mouth, extrapyramidal reaction, flushing, granulocytopenia, leukopenia, mydriasis, neutropenia

Pharmacodynamics/Kinetics
Onset of action: 20-60 minutes
Duration: 8-12 hours
Absorption: Well from the GI tract; food in stomach delays absorption but does not affect bioavailability
Distribution: V_d: Children: 7 L/kg; Adults: 3.2 L/kg
Protein binding: 69% to 72%
Metabolism: In the liver
Half-life: Children: 13 hours; Adults: 20-24 hours; Renal failure: 280-330 hours
Time to peak serum concentration: 2-6 hours
Elimination: Metabolites and parent drug (3% to 4%) excreted in urine; 35% of total within 48 hours

Dosage
Children: Oral: 0.35 mg/kg/day in divided doses every 4-6 hours
2-6 years: 1 mg every 4-6 hours, not to exceed 6 mg in 24 hours
6-12 years: 2 mg every 4-6 hours, not to exceed 12 mg/day or sustained release 8 mg at bedtime
Children >12 years and Adults: Oral: 4 mg every 4-6 hours, not to exceed 24 mg/day or sustained release 8-12 mg every 8-12 hours, not to exceed 24 mg/day
Elderly: Oral: 4 mg once or twice daily. **Note:** Duration of action may be 36 hours or more when serum concentrations are low.
Hemodialysis: Supplemental dose is not necessary

Administration
Timed release oral forms are to be swallowed whole, not crushed or chewed.

Contraindications Hypersensitivity to chlorpheniramine maleate or any component of the formulation; narrow-angle glaucoma; bladder neck obstruction; symptomatic prostate hypertrophy; during acute asthmatic attacks; stenosing peptic ulcer; pyloroduodenal obstruction. Avoid use in premature and term newborns due to possible association with SIDS.

Warnings Causes sedation, caution must be used in performing tasks which require alertness (eg, operating machinery or driving). Sedative effects of CNS depressants or ethanol are potentiated. Use with caution in patients with angle-closure glaucoma, pyloroduodenal obstruction

(including stenotic peptic ulcer), urinary tract obstruction (including bladder neck obstruction and symptomatic prostatic hyperplasia), hyperthyroidism, increased intraocular pressure, and cardiovascular disease (including hypertension and tachycardia). High sedative and anticholinergic properties, therefore may not be considered the antihistamine of choice for prolonged use in the elderly. May cause paradoxical excitation in pediatric patients, and can result in hallucinations, coma, and death in overdose.

Dosage Forms
Capsule, variable release:
QDALL® AR: Chlorpheniramine maleate 12 mg [immediate release and sustained release]
Syrup, as maleate:
Aller-Chlor®: 2 mg/5 mL (120 mL) [contains alcohol 5%]
Diabetic Tussin® Allergy Relief: 2 mg/5 mL (120 mL) [alcohol free, dye free, sugar free]
Tablet, as maleate: 4 mg
Aller-Chlor®, Chlor-Trimeton®, Chlorphen, Teldrin® HBP: 4 mg
Tablet, extended release, as maleate:
Chlor-Trimeton®: 12 mg

Reference Range In the postmortem state, anatomical site concentration differences (ie, postmortem redistribution) may occur.

Overdosage/Treatment There is no specific treatment for an antihistamine overdose, however, most of its clinical toxicity is due to anticholinergic effects. Anticholinesterase inhibitors may be useful by reducing acetylcholinesterase. Anticholinesterase inhibitors include physostigmine, neostigmine, pyridostigmine, and edrophonium. For anticholinergic overdose with severe life-threatening symptoms, physostigmine 1-2 mg (0.5 or 0.02 mg/kg for children) I.V., slowly may be given to reverse these effects.

Drug Interactions
Substrate of CYP2D6 (minor), 3A4 (major); **Inhibits** CYP2D6 (weak)
Increased toxicity (CNS depression): CNS depressants, MAO inhibitors, tricyclic antidepressants, phenothiazines
CYP3A4 inhibitors: May increase the levels/effects of chlorpheniramine. Example inhibitors include azole antifungals, clarithromycin, diclofenac, doxycycline, erythromycin, imatinib, isoniazid, nefazodone, nicardipine, propofol, protease inhibitors, quinidine, telithromycin, and verapamil.

Pregnancy Risk Factor B

Additional Information Not effective for nasal stuffiness

ChlorproMAZINE

Related Information
- Anticholinergic Effects of Common Psychotropics
- Antipsychotic Agents
- Therapeutic Drugs Associated with Hallucinations
- Zuclopenthixol

CAS Number 50-53-3; 69-09-0

U.S. Brand Names Thorazine® [DSC]

Synonyms Chlorpromazine Hydrochloride; CPZ

Impairment Potential Yes

Use Control of mania; treatment of schizophrenia; control of nausea and vomiting; relief of restlessness and apprehension before surgery; acute intermittent porphyria; adjunct in the treatment of tetanus; intractable hiccups; combativeness and/or explosive hyperexcitable behavior in children 1-12 years of age and in short-term treatment of hyperactive children; Tourette's syndrome; tension and vascular headaches; LSD flashback control

Unlabeled/Investigational Use Management of psychotic disorders

Mechanism of Action Avoid rectal administration in immunocompromised patients. Blocks postsynaptic mesolimbic dopaminergic receptors in the brain; exhibits a strong alpha-adrenergic blocking effect and depresses the release of hypothalamic and hypophyseal hormones; strongly anticholinergic

Adverse Reactions
Cardiovascular: **Hypotension** (especially with I.V. use), **hypotension (orthostatic)**, **tachycardia**, **cardiac arrhythmias**, sinus tachycardia, vasodilation, torsade de pointes (5 cases)
Central nervous system: Sedation, drowsiness, restlessness, anxiety, extrapyramidal reactions, **pseudoparkinsonian** signs and symptoms, **akathisia, dystonias, dizziness, tardive dyskinesia**, neuroleptic malignant syndrome, seizures, altered central temperature regulation, fever, auditory and visual hallucinations, somnambulism
Dermatologic: Hyperpigmentation, pruritus, rash, photosensitivity, toxic epidermal necrolysis, pustulosis, immunologic contact urticaria, cutaneous vasculitis
Endocrine & metabolic: Amenorrhea, galactorrhea, gynecomastia, syndrome of inappropriate antidiuretic hormone
Gastrointestinal: GI upset, xerostomia, **constipation**, Ogilvie's syndrome, weight gain
Genitourinary: Urinary retention, impotence, priapism

Hematologic: Leukopenia/neutropenia (agranulocytosis, granulocytopenia) usually in patients with large doses for prolonged periods; thrombocytopenia, hemolysis, eosinophilia

Hepatic: Cholestatic jaundice (rare), cholestatic hepatitis, primary biliary cirrhosis

Neuromuscular & skeletal: Rhabdomyolysis, Meige syndrome

Ocular: **Retinal pigmentation** (>600 g total dosage), blurred vision, mydriasis, photophobia, nystagmus, diplopia, pigmentary deposits in the lens and cornea, epithelial keratopathy

Respiratory: **Nasal congestion**, eosinophilic pneumonia

Miscellaneous: Anaphylactoid reactions, systemic lupus erythematosus, **diaphoresis (decreased)**, antiphospholipid syndrome

Signs and Symptoms of Overdose Abnormal involuntary muscle movements, appetite (increased), coma, corneal microdeposits, deep sleep, delirium, ejaculatory disturbances, extrapyramidal reaction, hirsutism, hyperprolactinemia, hyperthermia, hypoglycemia, hypotension or hypertension, hypothermia, impotence, jaundice, myasthenia gravis (exacerbation or precipitation), neuroleptic malignant syndrome, night terrors, Parkinson's-like symptoms, photosensitivity, toxic epidermal necrolysis, QT prolongation, urine discoloration (pink; red; red-brown), vision color changes (brown tinge; yellow tinge)

Pharmacodynamics/Kinetics

Onset of action: I.M.: 15 minutes; Oral: 30-60 minutes

Absorption: Rapid

Distribution: V_d: 20 L/kg; crosses the placenta; enters breast milk

Protein binding: 92% to 97%

Metabolism: Extensively hepatic to active and inactive metabolites

Bioavailability: 20%

Half-life, biphasic: Initial: 2 hours; Terminal: 30 hours

Excretion: Urine (<1% as unchanged drug) within 24 hours

Dosage

Children ≥6 months:

Schizophrenia/psychoses:

Oral: 0.5-1 mg/kg/dose every 4-6 hours; older children may require 200 mg/day or higher

I.M., I.V.: 0.5-1 mg/kg/dose every 6-8 hours

<5 years (22.7 kg): Maximum: 40 mg/day

5-12 years (22.7-45.5 kg): Maximum: 75 mg/day

Nausea and vomiting:

Oral: 0.5-1 mg/kg/dose every 4-6 hours as needed

I.M., I.V.: 0.5-1 mg/kg/dose every 6-8 hours

<5 years (22.7 kg): Maximum: 40 mg/day

5-12 years (22.7-45.5 kg): Maximum: 75 mg/day

Rectal: 1 mg/kg/dose every 6-8 hours as needed

Adults:

Schizophrenia/psychoses:

Oral: Range: 30-2000 mg/day in 1-4 divided doses, initiate at lower doses and titrate as needed; usual dose: 400-600 mg/day; some patients may require 1-2 g/day

I.M., I.V.: Initial: 25 mg, may repeat (25-50 mg) in 1-4 hours, gradually increase to a maximum of 400 mg/dose every 4-6 hours until patient is controlled; usual dose: 300-800 mg/day

Intractable hiccups: Oral, I.M.: 25-50 mg 3-4 times/day

LSD flashback control: Oral, I.M.: 50-100 mg every 3-4 hours until a response is seen

Nausea and vomiting:

Tetanus adjunct (usually with a barbiturate): I.M.: 25-50 mg 3-4 times/day or continuous I.V. infusion: 1 mg/minute

Oral: 10-25 mg every 4-6 hours

I.M., I.V.: 25-50 mg every 4-6 hours

Rectal: 50-100 mg every 6-8 hours

Elderly: Behavioral symptoms associated with dementia: Initial: 10-25 mg 1-2 times/day; increase at 4- to 7-day intervals by 10-25 mg/day. Increase dose intervals (bid, tid, etc) as necessary to control behavior response or side effects; maximum daily dose: 800 mg; gradual increases (titration) may prevent some side effects or decrease their severity.

Dosing adjustment/comments in hepatic impairment: Avoid use in severe hepatic dysfunction

Stability Protect oral dosage forms from light; a slightly yellowed solution does not indicate potency loss, but a markedly discolored solution should be discarded; diluted injection (1 mg/mL) with NS and stored in 5 mL vials remain stable for 30 days; not soluble with alkali, aminophylline, ampicillin, chlorothiazide, methohexitone, phenobarbital, amphotericin, sulfadimidine

Monitoring Parameters Vital signs; lipid profile, fasting blood glucose/Hgb A_{1c}; BMI; mental status; abnormal involuntary movement scale (AIMS); extrapyramidal symptoms (EPS)

Administration Note: Avoid skin contact with oral solution or injection solution; may cause contact dermatitis.

Oral: Dilute oral concentrate solution in juice before administration. Chlorpromazine concentrate is not compatible with carbamazepine suspension; schedule dosing at least 1-2 hours apart from each other.

I.V.: Direct of intermittent infusion: Infuse 1 mg or portion thereof over 1 minute.

Contraindications Hypersensitivity to chlorpromazine or any component of the formulation (cross-reactivity between phenothiazines may occur); severe CNS depression; coma

Warnings

Highly sedating, use with caution in disorders where CNS depression is a feature. Use with caution in Parkinson's disease. Caution in patients with hemodynamic instability; bone marrow suppression; predisposition to seizures; subcortical brain damage, severe cardiac, hepatic, renal, or respiratory disease. Esophageal dysmotility and aspiration have been associated with antipsychotic use - use with caution in patients at risk of aspiration pneumonia (ie, Alzheimer's disease). Caution in breast cancer or other prolactin-dependent tumors (may elevate prolactin levels). May alter temperature regulation or mask toxicity of other drugs due to antiemetic effects. May alter cardiac conduction - life-threatening arrhythmias have occurred with therapeutic doses of neuroleptics. May cause orthostatic hypotension - use with caution in patients at risk of this effect or those who would tolerate transient hypotensive episodes (cerebrovascular disease, cardiovascular disease, or other medications which may predispose). Significant hypotension may occur, particularly with parenteral administration. Injection contains sulfites.

Phenothiazines may cause anticholinergic effects (confusion, agitation, constipation, xerostomia, blurred vision, urinary retention). Therefore, they should be used with caution in patients with decreased gastrointestinal motility, urinary retention, BPH, xerostomia, or visual problems. Conditions which also may be exacerbated by cholinergic blockade include narrow-angle glaucoma (screening is recommended) and worsening of myasthenia gravis. Relative to other neuroleptics, chlorpromazine has a moderate potency of cholinergic blockade.

May cause extrapyramidal symptoms, including pseudoparkinsonism, acute dystonic reactions, akathisia, and tardive dyskinesia (risk of these reactions is low-moderate relative to other neuroleptics). May be associated with neuroleptic malignant syndrome (NMS) or pigmentary retinopathy.

Dosage Forms

Injection, solution, as hydrochloride: 25 mg/mL (1 mL, 2 mL)

Tablet, as hydrochloride: 10 mg, 25 mg, 50 mg, 100 mg, 200 mg

Reference Range

Therapeutic: 50-300 ng/mL (SI: 157-942 nmol/L)

Toxic: >750 ng/mL (SI: >2355 nmol/L)

Overdosage/Treatment

Decontamination: Lavage (within 1 hour)/activated charcoal

Supportive therapy: Following initiation of essential overdose management, toxic symptom treatment and supportive treatment should be initiated. Hypotension usually responds to I.V. fluids or Trendelenburg positioning. If unresponsive to these measures, the use of a parenteral inotrope may be required (eg, norepinephrine 0.1-0.2 mcg/kg/minute titrated to response). Seizures commonly respond to lorazepam or diazepam (I.V. 5-10 mg bolus in adults every 15 minutes if needed up to a total of 30 mg; I.V. 0.25-0.4 mg/kg/dose up to a total of 10 mg in children) or to phenytoin or phenobarbital. Also critical cardiac arrhythmias often respond to I.V. phenytoin (15 mg/kg up to 1 g), while other antiarrhythmics can be used. Neuroleptics often cause extrapyramidal reaction (eg, dystonic reactions) requiring management with diphenhydramine 1-2 mg/kg (adults) up to a maximum of 50 mg I.V. slow push followed by a maintenance dose for 48-72 hours. When these reactions are unresponsive to diphenhydramine, benztropine mesylate I.V. 1-2 mg (adults) may be effective. These agents are generally effective within 2-5 minutes.

Enhancement of elimination: Not dialyzable (0% to 5%); multiple dosing of activated charcoal would not be expected to be useful

Test Interactions False-positive for phenylketonuria, amylase, uroporphyrins, urobilinogen; possible false-negative pregnancy urinary test; may cause positive direct Coombs', may interfere with BUN and vitamin B_{12} test determinations

Drug Interactions

Substrate of CYP1A2 (minor), 2D6 (major), 3A4 (minor); **Inhibits** CYP2D6 (strong), 2E1 (weak)

Acetylcholinesterase inhibitors (central): May increase the risk of antipsychotic-related extrapyramidal symptoms; monitor.

Aluminum salts: May decrease the absorption of phenothiazines; monitor

Amphetamines: Efficacy may be diminished by antipsychotics; in addition, amphetamines may increase psychotic symptoms; avoid concurrent use

Anticholinergics: May inhibit the therapeutic response to phenothiazines and excess anticholinergic effects may occur; includes benztropine, trihexyphenidyl, biperiden, and drugs with significant anticholinergic activity (TCAs, antihistamines, disopyramide)

Antihypertensives: Concurrent use of phenothiazines with an antihypertensive may produce additive hypotensive effects (particularly orthostasis)

Bromocriptine: Phenothiazines inhibit the ability of bromocriptine to lower serum prolactin concentrations

CNS depressants: Sedative effects may be additive with phenothiazines; monitor for increased effect; includes barbiturates, benzodiazepines, narcotic analgesics, ethanol and other sedative agents

CYP2D6 inhibitors: May increase the levels/effects of chlorpromazine. Example inhibitors include delavirdine, fluoxetine, miconazole, paroxetine, pergolide, quinidine, quinine, ritonavir, and ropinirole.

CYP2D6 substrates: Chlorpromazine may increase the levels/effects of CYP2D6 substrates. Example substrates include amphetamines, selected beta-blockers, dextromethorphan, fluoxetine, lidocaine, mirtazapine, nefazodone, paroxetine, risperidone, ritonavir, thioridazine, tricyclic antidepressants, and venlafaxine.

CYP2D6 prodrug substrates: Chlorpromazine may decrease the levels/effects of CYP2D6 prodrug substrates. Example prodrug substrates include codeine, hydrocodone, oxycodone, and tramadol.

Epinephrine: Chlorpromazine (and possibly other low potency antipsychotics) may diminish the pressor effects of epinephrine

Guanethidine and guanadrel: Antihypertensive effects may be inhibited by chlorpromazine

Levodopa: Chlorpromazine may inhibit the antiparkinsonian effect of levodopa; avoid this combination

Lithium: Chlorpromazine may produce neurotoxicity with lithium; this is a rare effect

Metoclopramide: May increase extrapyramidal symptoms (EPS) or risk.

Phenytoin: May reduce serum levels of phenothiazines; phenothiazines may increase phenytoin serum levels

Propranolol: Serum concentrations of phenothiazines may be increased; propranolol also increases phenothiazine concentrations

Polypeptide antibiotics: Rare cases of respiratory paralysis have been reported with concurrent use of phenothiazines

QT_c-prolonging agents: Effects on QT_c interval may be additive with phenothiazines, increasing the risk of malignant arrhythmias; includes type Ia antiarrhythmics, TCAs, and some quinolone antibiotics (sparfloxacin, moxifloxacin and gatifloxacin)

Sulfadoxine-pyrimethamine: May increase phenothiazine concentrations

Tricyclic antidepressants: Concurrent use may produce increased toxicity or altered therapeutic response

Trazodone: Phenothiazines and trazodone may produce additive hypotensive effects

Valproic acid: Serum levels may be increased by phenothiazines

Pregnancy Risk Factor C

Pregnancy Implications Crosses the placenta; may cause damage to fetal retina

Lactation Enters breast milk/not recommended (AAP rates "of concern")

Nursing Implications Dilute oral concentrate solution in juice before administration; avoid contact of oral solution or injection with skin (contact dermatitis); watch for hypotension when administering I.M. or I.V.

Additional Information Use decreased doses in elderly or debilitated patients. Extrapyramidal reaction may be more common in patients with hypocalcemia and in pediatric patients, especially those with dehydration or acute illnesses (viral or CNS infections). Avoid rectal administration in immunocompromised patients. May be useful in treating headaches due to meningitis.

ChlorproPAMIDE

CAS Number 99-20-2

U.S. Brand Names Diabinese®

Use Management of blood sugar in type 2 diabetes mellitus (noninsulin dependent, NIDDM)

Unlabeled/Investigational Use Neurogenic diabetes insipidus

Mechanism of Action Stimulates insulin release from the pancreatic beta cells; reduces glucose output from the liver; insulin sensitivity is increased at peripheral target sites

Adverse Reactions

Cardiovascular: Edema

Central nervous system: **Headache, dizziness**

Dermatologic: Skin rash, urticaria, photosensitivity, erythema multiforme, exfoliative dermatitis

Endocrine & metabolic: Disulfiram reaction, hypoglycemia, hyponatremia, SIADH

Gastrointestinal: **Anorexia, constipation, heartburn, epigastric fullness, nausea, vomiting, diarrhea**, proctocolitis

Hematologic: Agranulocytosis, aplastic anemia, bone marrow suppression, eosinophilia, hemolytic anemia, leukopenia, porphyria cutanea tarda, thrombocytopenia

Hepatic: Cholestatic jaundice

Signs and Symptoms of Overdose Agranulocytosis, ataxia, colitis, erythema multiforme, feces discoloration (black), granulocytopenia, hypoglycemia (may be prolonged), hyponatremia, jaundice, leukopenia, lichenoid eruptions, neutropenia, photosensitivity

Admission Criteria/Prognosis Admit all intentional adult overdoses. Pediatric patients should be observed in a medical setting through an overnight sleep cycle (and for a minimum of 8 hours). No intravenous glucose or dextrose should be given prophylactically. Asymptomatic pediatric patients should have a blood glucose determination at 3-6 hours postingestion or immediately when symptoms (hunger, irritability, lethargy, tremulousness, tachycardia, diaphoresis, or seizures) develop. Any borderline blood glucose reading (about 70 mg/dL) are repeated in one hour. Consider regular 2- to 3-hour interval blood glucose measurements during sleep. If no hypoglycemic events occur and prebreakfast blood glucose levels are normal, pediatric patients can be monitored by parental observation at home.

Pharmacodynamics/Kinetics

Onset of action: Peak effect: ~6-8 hours

Distribution: V_d: 0.13-0.23 L/kg; enters breast milk

Protein binding: 60% to 90%

Metabolism: Extensively hepatic (~80%)

Half-life elimination: 30-42 hours; prolonged in elderly or with renal impairment

End-stage renal disease: 50-200 hours

Time to peak, serum: 3-4 hours

Excretion: Urine (10% to 30% as unchanged drug)

Dosage

Oral: The dosage of chlorpropamide is variable and should be individualized based upon the patient's response

Initial dose:

Adults: 250 mg/day in mild to moderate diabetes in middle-aged, stable diabetic

Elderly: 100-125 mg/day in older patients

Subsequent dosages may be increased or decreased by 50-125 mg/day at 3- to 5-day intervals

Maintenance dose: 100-250 mg/day; severe diabetics may require 500 mg/day; avoid doses >750 mg/day

Dosing adjustment/comments in renal impairment: Cl_{cr} <50 mL/minute: Avoid use

Hemodialysis: Removed with hemoperfusion

Peritoneal dialysis: Supplemental dose is not necessary

Dosing adjustment in hepatic impairment: Dosage reduction is recommended. Conservative initial and maintenance doses are recommended in patients with liver impairment because chlorpropamide undergoes extensive hepatic metabolism.

Monitoring Parameters Fasting blood glucose, normal Hgb A_{1c} or fructosamine levels; monitor for signs and symptoms of hypoglycemia (fatigue, sweating, numbness of extremities); monitor urine for glucose and ketones

Contraindications Hypersensitivity to sulfonylureas, sulfonamides, or any component of the formulation; do not use with type 1 diabetes mellitus (insulin dependent, IDDM) or with severe renal, hepatic, thyroid, or other endocrine disease

Warnings

Patients should be properly instructed in the early detection and treatment of hypoglycemia; long half-life may complicate recovery from excess effects. Because of chlorpropamide's long half-life, duration of action, and the increased risk for hypoglycemia, it is not considered a hypoglycemic agent of choice in the elderly.

Chemical similarities are present among sulfonamides, sulfonylureas, carbonic anhydrase inhibitors, thiazides, and loop diuretics (except ethacrynic acid). Use in patients with sulfonylurea or sulfonamide allergy is specifically contraindicated in product labeling, however, a risk of cross-reaction exists in patients with allergy to any of these compounds; avoid use when previous reaction has been severe.

Product labeling states oral hypoglycemic drugs may be associated with an increased cardiovascular mortality as compared to treatment with diet alone or diet plus insulin. Data to support this association are limited, and several studies, including a large prospective trial (UKPDS) have not supported an association.

Dosage Forms Tablet: 100 mg, 250 mg

Reference Range

Glucose: Adults: 60-115 mg/dL

Elderly fasting glucose: 100-180 mg/dL

Chlorpropamide lethal level: >400 mcg/mL in nondiabetic patients

Overdosage/Treatment

Decontamination: Lavage (within 1 hour)/activated charcoal

Supportive therapy: Glucose (25 g I.V.) is mainstay of therapy. Glucagon (1-5 mg I.V., I.M., or SubQ) will have limited benefit (0.03-0.1 mg/kg in pediatrics); diazoxide is a third-line agent; octreotide (50 mcg SubQ every 12 hours) may be helpful in sulfonylurea overdose.

For pediatric patients with profound sulfonylurea-induced hypoglycemia: Give 0.5 g of dextrose per kg of body weight (5 mL/kg of 10% dextrose concentration of intravenous fluid, 2 mL/kg of D_{25} or 1 mL/kg of D_{50}).

Enhancement of elimination: Multiple dosing of activated charcoal is not useful; alkalinization of urine is useful; charcoal hemoperfusion may remove as much as 80% of the body burden of chlorpropamide

Antidote(s)

● Dextrose [ANTIDOTE]

● Octreotide [ANTIDOTE]

Drug Interactions

Substrate of CYP2C8/9 (minor)

Thiazides may decrease effectiveness of chlorpropamide

Possible interaction between chlorpropamide and fluoroquinolone antibiotics has been reported resulting in a potentiation of hypoglycemic action of chlorpropamide

Since this agent is highly protein bound, the toxic potential is increased when given concomitantly with other highly protein bound drugs (ie, phenylbutazone, oral anticoagulants, hydantoins, salicylates, NSAIDs, beta-blockers, sulfonamides) - increase hypoglycemic effect.

Ethanol increases disulfiram reactions.

Phenylbutazone can increase hypoglycemic effects.

Certain drugs tend to produce hyperglycemia and may lead to loss of control (ie, thiazides and other diuretics, corticosteroids, phenothiazines, thyroid products, estrogens, oral contraceptives, phenytoin, nicotinic acid, sympathomimetics, calcium channel blocking drugs, and isoniazid).

Possible interactions between chlorpropamide and coumarin derivatives have been reported that may either potentiate or weaken the effects of coumarin derivatives.

Pregnancy Risk Factor C

Pregnancy Implications Crosses the placenta; hypoglycemia, ear defects reported; other malformations reported but may have been secondary to poor maternal glucose control/diabetes. Insulin is the drug of choice for the control of diabetes mellitus during pregnancy. Prolonged hypoglycemia has been reported in neonates born to mothers who were receiving sulfonylureas (particularly long-acting drugs).

Lactation Enters breast milk/contraindicated

Nursing Implications

Patients who are anorexic or NPO may need to hold the dose to avoid hypoglycemia

Monitor fasting blood glucose, normal Hgb A_{1c}, or fructosamine levels; monitor for signs and symptoms of hypoglycemia (fatigue, sweating, numbness of extremities); monitor urine for glucose and ketones

Specific References

Calello D, Kelly A, and Osterhoudt KC, "Case Files of the Medical Toxicology Fellowship Training Program at the Childrens Hospital of Philadelphia: A Pediatric Exploratory Sulfonylurea Ingestion," *J Med Toxicol*, 2006, 2(1):19-26.

Johnson KK, Green DL, Rife JP, et al, "Sulfonamide Cross-Reactivity: Fact or Fiction?" *Ann Pharmacother*, 2005, 39(2):290-301.

Proudfoot AT, Krenzelok EP, Vale JA, et al, "AACT/EAPCCT Position Paper on Urine Alkalinization," *J Toxicol Clin Toxicol*, 2004, 42(1):1-26.

Chlorprothixene

CAS Number 113-59-7

Use Management of psychotic disorders, emotional disturbances

Mechanism of Action Low anticholinergic activity with similar properties as chlorpromazine

Adverse Reactions

Cardiovascular: **Hypotension** (especially with I.V. use), **hypotension (orthostatic)**, tachycardia, cardiac arrhythmias, QT prolongation, sinus bradycardia, sinus tachycardia

Central nervous system: **Tardive dyskinesia, pseudoparkinsonian signs and symptoms, dizziness, akathisia, dystonias**, sedation, drowsiness, restlessness, anxiety, extrapyramidal reactions, neuroleptic malignant syndrome, seizures, altered central temperature regulation, fever, hyperthermia

Dermatologic: Hyperpigmentation, pruritus, rash, photosensitivity

Endocrine & metabolic: Amenorrhea, galactorrhea, gynecomastia, hyperprolactinemia

Gastrointestinal: GI upset, xerostomia, **constipation**, weight gain

Genitourinary: Urinary retention, impotence

Hematologic: Leukopenia/neutropenia (agranulocytosis, granulocytopenia) usually in patients with large doses for prolonged periods; thrombocytopenia, hemolysis, eosinophilia

Hepatic: Cholestatic jaundice

Ocular: **Retinal pigmentation**, diplopia, blurred vision, mydriasis

Miscellaneous: **Diaphoresis (decreased)**, anaphylactoid reactions, systemic lupus erythematosus

Signs and Symptoms of Overdose Abnormal involuntary muscle movements, coma, deep sleep, dry eyes, ejaculatory disturbances, extrapyramidal reaction, hyperactivity, hypotension, impotence, jaundice, neuroleptic malignant syndrome, neutropenia, oliguria with azotemia, Parkinson's-like symptoms, photosensitivity

Pharmacodynamics/Kinetics

Absorption: Oral absorption results in peak concentrations between 2-4 hours. Absorption may be affected by the inherent anticholinergic action on the gastrointestinal tissue causing variable absorption. Absorption from tablets is erratic with less variation seen with solutions.

Distribution: Widely distributed in tissues with CNS concentrations exceeding that of plasma due to their lipophilic characteristics.

Protein binding: Antipsychotic agents are bound 90% to 99% to plasma proteins; highly bound to brain and lung tissue and other tissues with a high blood perfusion.

Elimination: Elimination occurs through hepatic metabolism (oxidation) where numerous active metabolites are produced; active metabolites excreted in urine; elimination half-lives of antipsychotics ranges from 20-40 hours which may be extended in elderly due to decline in oxidative hepatic reactions (phase I) with age. The biologic effect of a single dose persists for 24 hours. When the patient has accommodated to initial side effects (sedation), once daily dosing is possible due to the long half-life of antipsychotics.

Steady-state plasma levels are achieved in 4-7 days; therefore, if possible, do not make dose adjustments more than once in a 7-day period. Due to the long half-lives of antipsychotics, as needed (PRN) use is ineffective since repeated doses are necessary to achieve therapeutic tissue concentrations in the CNS.

Dosage

Children >6 years: Oral: 10-25 mg 3-4 times/day

Adults:

Oral: 25-50 mg 3-4 times/day, to be increased as needed; doses exceeding 600 mg/day are rarely required

I.M.: 25-50 mg up to 3-4 times/day

Monitoring Parameters Monitor for reduction of psychotic symptoms; hyperthermia, acute EPS, autonomic changes (irregular pulse/blood pressure, diaphoresis)

Administration

I.M. dose is 4-10 times the activity of oral dose

Contraindications Circulatory collapse, hypersensitivity to chlorprothixene or any component, comatose states due to central depressant drugs

Warnings Safety in children <6 months of age has not been established; use with caution in patients with cardiovascular disease or seizures; bone marrow depression, severe liver or cardiac disease; significant hypotension may occur, especially when the drug is administered parenterally; extended release capsules and injection contain benzyl alcohol; injection also contains sulfites which may cause allergic reaction

Dosage Forms

Injection, as hydrochloride: 12.5 mg/mL (2 mL)

Solution, oral concentrate, as lactate and hydrochloride: 100 mg/5 mL (480 mL) [fruit flavor]

Tablet: 10 mg, 25 mg, 50 mg, 100 mg

Reference Range

Therapeutic: 0.04-0.30 mcg/mL

Fatal: 1.00-2.00 mcg/mL

Overdosage/Treatment

Decontamination: Lavage (within 1 hour)/activated charcoal

Supportive therapy: Following initiation of essential overdose management, toxic symptom treatment and supportive treatment should be initiated. Hypotension usually responds to I.V. fluids or Trendelenburg positioning. If unresponsive to these measures, the use of a parenteral inotrope may be required. Seizures commonly respond to lorazepam or diazepam (I.V. 5-10 mg bolus in adults every 15 minutes if needed up to a total of 30 mg; I.V. 0.25-0.4 mg/kg/dose up to a total of 10 mg in children) or to phenytoin or phenobarbital. Also critical cardiac arrhythmias often respond to I.V. phenytoin (15 mg/kg up to 1 g), while other antiarrhythmics can be used. Neuroleptics often cause extrapyramidal reaction (eg, dystonic reactions) requiring management with benztropine mesylate I.V. 1-2 mg (adults) may be effective. These agents are generally effective within 2-5 minutes.

Enhancement of elimination: Multiple dosing of activated charcoal may be useful; combined hemodialysis/hemoperfusion over 4 hours may be beneficial; not dialyzable (0% to 5%)

Test Interactions ↑ cholesterol (S), glucose; ↓ uric acid (S)

Drug Interactions Decreased effect of guanethidine

Increased effect/toxicity: Ethanol, CNS depressants

Metoclopramide: May increase extrapyramidal symptoms (EPS) or risk.

Pregnancy Risk Factor C

Nursing Implications Observe for tremor and abnormal movement or posturing (extrapyramidal symptoms)

Additional Information Slight amine-like odor

Chlorthalidone

CAS Number 77-36-1

U.S. Brand Names Thalitone®

Synonyms Hygroton

Use Management of mild to moderate hypertension, used alone or in combination with other agents; treatment of edema associated with congestive heart failure, nephrotic syndrome, or pregnancy

Mechanism of Action Sulfonamide-derived diuretic that inhibits sodium and chloride reabsorption in the cortical-diluting segment of the ascending loop of Henle

Adverse Reactions

Cardiovascular: Hypotension, myocarditis (hypersensitivity), myocarditis

Dermatologic: Psoriasiform eruption, photosensitivity

Endocrine & metabolic: Hypokalemia, hypercalcemia, hypercholesterolemia, fluid and electrolyte imbalances (hypocalcemia, hypomagnesemia, hyponatremia), hyperuricemia, hyperglycemia

Gastrointestinal: Pancreatitis

Genitourinary: Impotence

Hematologic: Rarely blood dyscrasias (ie, neutropenia, thrombocytopenia), agranulocytosis

Neuromuscular & skeletal: Rhabdomyolysis

Renal: Prerenal azotemia

Miscellaneous: Periarteritis nodosa

Signs and Symptoms of Overdose Confusion, diuresis, hypermotility, hyperglycemia, hyperuricemia, hypocalcemia, hypokalemia, hypomagnesemia, hyponatremia, impotence, LDL (increased), lethargy, muscle weakness, myasthenia gravis (exacerbation or precipitation), myopia, nocturia, periarteritis nodosa, photosensitivity, vision color changes (yellow tinge)

Pharmacodynamics/Kinetics

Onset of action: Peak effect: 2-6 hours

Duration: 24-72 hours

Absorption: 65%

Distribution: Crosses placenta; enters breast milk

Metabolism: Hepatic

Half-life elimination: 35-55 hours; may be prolonged with renal impairment; Anuria: 81 hours

Excretion: Urine (~50% to 65% as unchanged drug)

Dosage

Oral:

Children (nonapproved): 2 mg/kg/dose 3 times/week or 1-2 mg/kg/day

Adults: 25-100 mg/day or 100 mg 3 times/week; usual dosage range (JNC 7): 12.5-25 mg/day

Elderly: Initial: 12.5-25 mg/day or every other day; there is little advantage to using doses >25 mg/day

Dosage adjustment in renal impairment: Cl_{cr} <10 mL/minute: Administer every 48 hours

Monitoring Parameters Assess weight, I & O records daily to determine fluid loss; blood pressure, serum electrolytes, renal function

Contraindications Hypersensitivity to chlorthalidone or any component of the formulation; cross-sensitivity with other thiazides or sulfonamides; anuria; renal decompensation; pregnancy

Warnings Use with caution in patients with hypokalemia, renal disease, hepatic disease, gout, lupus erythematosus, or diabetes mellitus. Use with caution in severe renal diseases. Correct hypokalemia before initiating therapy. Chemical similarities are present among sulfonamides, sulfonylureas, carbonic anhydrase inhibitors, thiazides, and loop diuretics (except ethacrynic acid). Use in patients with thiazide or sulfonamide allergy is specifically contraindicated in product labeling, however, a risk of cross-reaction exists in patients with allergy to any of these compounds; avoid use when previous reaction has been severe.

Dosage Forms

Tablet: 25 mg, 50 mg, 100 mg

Thalitone®: 15 mg

Reference Range Peak serum chlorthalidone level of 6.3 mg/L after a single 200 mg dose

Overdosage/Treatment

Decontamination: Lavage (within 1 hour)/activated charcoal

Supportive therapy: I.V. fluid and electrolyte replacement

Test Interactions ↑ creatine phosphokinase (CPK) (S), ammonia (B), amylase (S), calcium (S), cholesterol (S), glucose, increases acidity (S); ↓ chloride (S), magnesium, potassium (S), sodium (S)

Drug Interactions

ACE inhibitors: Increased hypotension if aggressively diuresed with a thiazide diuretic.

Beta-blockers increase hyperglycemic effects of thiazides in type 2 diabetes mellitus (noninsulin dependent, NIDDM)

Cyclosporine and thiazides can increase the risk of gout or renal toxicity; avoid concurrent use.

Digoxin toxicity can be exacerbated if a thiazide induces hypokalemia or hypomagnesemia.

Lithium toxicity can occur by reducing renal excretion of lithium; monitor lithium concentration and adjust as needed.

Neuromuscular blocking agents can prolong blockade; monitor serum potassium and neuromuscular status.

NSAIDs can decrease the efficacy of thiazides reducing the diuretic and antihypertensive effects.

Pregnancy Risk Factor B (manufacturer); D (expert analysis)

Pregnancy Implications Decreased birth weight, neonatal hypoglycemia, or neonatal thrombocytopenia can occur

Lactation Enters breast milk/use caution (AAP rates "compatible")

Nursing Implications Assess weight, I & O reports daily to determine fluid loss; take blood pressure with patient lying down and standing

Additional Information Recent studies have found chlorthalidone effective in the treatment of isolated systolic hypertension in the elderly

Specific References

Chobanian AV, Bakris GL, Black HR, et al, "The Seventh Report of the Joint National Committee on Prevention, Detection, Evaluation, and Treatment of High Blood Pressure: The JNC 7 Report," *JAMA*, 2003, (19)289:2560-71.

Chlorzoxazone

CAS Number 95-25-0

U.S. Brand Names Parafon Forte® DSC

Impairment Potential Yes

Use Musculoskeletal pain, muscle spasm

Mechanism of Action Precise mechanism is not yet clear, but many effects have been ascribed to its central depressant actions

Adverse Reactions

Central nervous system: **Drowsiness**, opisthotonos, amnesia, dizziness

Dermatologic: Petechiae

Genitourinary: Orange colored urine

Hematologic: Porphyrinogenic

Hepatic: Hepatotoxicity (including fatal hepatic necrosis) is idiosyncratic and unpredictable, centrilobular necrosis

Neuromuscular & skeletal: Torticollis

Admission Criteria/Prognosis Admit any symptomatic patient or any adult ingestion >5 g

Pharmacodynamics/Kinetics

Onset of action: ~1 hour

Duration: 6-12 hours

Absorption: Readily absorbed

Metabolism: Extensively hepatic via glucuronidation

Excretion: Urine (as conjugates)

Dosage

Children: 125-500 mg 3-4 times/day

Adult: 250-750 mg 3-4 times/day; maximum tolerated dose: 5 g

Monitoring Parameters Periodic liver functions tests

Contraindications Hypersensitivity to chlorzoxazone or any component of the formulation; impaired liver function

Dosage Forms

Caplet (Parafon Forte® DSC): 500 mg

Tablet: 250 mg, 500 mg

Reference Range Peak plasma levels following an oral 750 mg dose: ~36 mg/L at 38 minutes

Overdosage/Treatment

Decontamination: Lavage (within 2 hours of ingestion)/activated charcoal

Supportive therapy: Benzodiazepines for seizure control; for torticollis, 1-2 mg of benztropine can be given; flumazenil can reverse coma due to chlorzoxazone (the dose of flumazenil used was 0.1 mg initially followed by 0.25 mg); hypotension should be treated with I.V. fluids and/or Trendelenburg positioning.

Enhancement of elimination: Forced diuresis is not helpful; multiple dosing of activated charcoal may be helpful.

Test Interactions False-positive serum test for aprobarbital may be noted with Toxi-Lab Screen™

Drug Interactions

Substrate of CYP1A2 (minor), 2A6 (minor), 2D6 (minor), 2E1 (major), 3A4 (minor); **Inhibits** CYP2E1 (weak), 3A4 (weak)

CNS depressants: Effects may be increased by chlorzoxazone.

CYP2E1 inhibitors: May increase the levels/effects of chlorzoxazone. Example inhibitors include disulfiram, isoniazid, and miconazole.

Disulfiram: May increase chlorzoxazone concentration; monitor.

Isoniazid: May increase chlorzoxazone concentration; monitor.

Pregnancy Risk Factor C

Lactation Excretion in breast milk unknown/not recommended

Cholecalciferol

U.S. Brand Names Delta-D®; Quintox®; Rampage®

Synonyms: Oleovitamin D_3; Vitamin D_3

Use Rodenticide in grain bait

Mechanism of Toxic Action A vitamin D_3 compound (equipotent to vitamin D_2) which increases absorption of calcium and phosphorus from the gastrointestinal tract; usually found in concentrations of 0.075% (750 ppm)

Adverse Reactions

Cardiovascular: Hypertension

Central nervous system: Drowsiness, headache, confusion, dysosmia

Endocrine & metabolic: Hypercalcemia, hypomagnesemia, hyperphosphatemia, ectopic calcification

Gastrointestinal: Anorexia, nausea, vomiting, pancreatitis

Hematologic: Anemia

Neuromuscular & skeletal: Weakness

Ocular: Conjunctivitis, nystagmus

Renal: Azotemia, albuminuria, renal failure

Pharmacodynamics/Kinetics
Distribution: Primarily hepatic

Protein binding: Extensively to vitamin D-binding protein

Metabolism: Primary liver and kidney hydroxylation; glucuronidation (minimal)

Half-life elimination: 14 hours

Time to peak, plasma: 11 hours

Excretion: As metabolites, urine (2.4%) and feces (4.9%)

Monitoring Parameters Calcium, renal function tests

Contraindications Hypercalcemia; hypersensitivity to cholecalciferol or any component of the formulation; malabsorption syndrome; evidence of vitamin D toxicity

Dosage Forms
Tablet: 1000 int. units

Delta-D®: 400 int. units

Overdosage/Treatment
Decontamination: **Oral:** Lavage (within 1 hour); cholestyramine may be particularly effective (8 g twice daily) **Ocular:** Irrigate with saline.

Supportive therapy: Hypercalcemia can be treated with saline, diuresis, furosemide (20-40 mg I.V.), and hydrocortisone (100 mg I.V. every 6 hours). Calcitonin (4-8 int. units/kg I.M. every 6-12 hours) can be used for persistent or severe hypercalcemia. Hemodialysis can also be used for severe hypercalcemia.

Enhanced elimination: Forced saline diuresis (urine flow of 3 mL/kg/hour) - furosemide may be added as needed to maintain urine flow. Hemodialysis (against a calcium free dialysate) can be considered.

Drug Interactions Inhibits CYP2C9 (weak), 2C19 (weak), 2D6 (weak)

Thiazide diuretics, cholestyramine, colestipol, corticosteroids, mineral oil, orlistat, phenytoin, barbiturates, digitalis glycosides, antacids (magnesium)

Pregnancy Risk Factor A

Nursing Implications Do not administer more than the recommended amount. While taking this medication, your physician may want you to follow a special diet or take a calcium supplement. Follow this diet closely. Avoid taking magnesium supplements or magnesium containing antacids. Early symptoms of hypercalcemia include weakness, fatigue, somnolence, headache, anorexia, dry mouth, metallic taste, nausea, vomiting, cramps, diarrhea, muscle pain, bone pain, and irritability.

Additional Information 1 mg of cholecalciferol is equivalent to 40,000 int. units of vitamin D

Choline Magnesium Trisalicylate

CAS Number 64425-90-7

U.S. Brand Names Trilisate® [DSC]

Synonyms Tricosal

Use Management of osteoarthritis, rheumatoid arthritis, and other arthritis; acute painful shoulder

Mechanism of Action Inhibits prostaglandin synthesis; acts on the hypothalamus heat-regulating center to reduce fever; blocks the generation of pain impulses

Adverse Reactions
Cardiovascular: Edema

Central nervous system: Headache, lightheadedness, dizziness, drowsiness, lethargy, confusion, hallucinations

Dermatologic: Rash, pruritus, bruising, erythema multiforme

Gastrointestinal: **Nausea, vomiting, diarrhea, heartburn, dyspepsia, epigastric pain, constipation,** gastric ulceration, anorexia, weight gain, dysgeusia, duodenal ulceration, esophagitis

Hematologic: Occult bleeding

Hepatic: Hepatic enzymes increased

Otic: **Tinnitus,** hearing impairment, hearing loss (irreversible)

Renal: Increased BUN and creatinine

Respiratory: Epistaxis, asthma

Signs and Symptoms of Overdose Bezoars, cognitive dysfunction, drowsiness, GI bleeding, GI upset, hypoglycemia, hyponatremia, nausea, nephrotic syndrome, nystagmus, ototoxicity, tinnitus, vomiting, wheezing Severe poisoning can manifest with coma, feces discoloration (black; pink; red; tarry), hyperglycemia, hyperthermia, hypotension, irritability, metabolic acidosis, renal failure and/or hepatic failure, respiratory depression, seizures, urine discoloration (pink)

Pharmacodynamics/Kinetics
Onset of action: Peak effect: ~2 hours

Absorption: Stomach and small intestines

Distribution: Readily into most body fluids and tissues; crosses placenta; enters breast milk

Half-life elimination (dose dependent): Low dose: 2-3 hours; High dose: 30 hours

Time to peak, serum: ~2 hours

Dosage
Oral (based on total salicylate content):

Children <37 kg: 50 mg/kg/day given in 2 divided doses; 2250 mg/day for heavier children

Adults: 500 mg to 1.5 g 2-3 times/day **or** 3 g at bedtime; usual maintenance dose: 1-4.5 g/day

Elderly: 750 mg 3 times/day

Dosing adjustment/comments in renal impairment: Avoid use in severe renal impairment

Monitoring Parameters Serum magnesium with high dose therapy or in patients with impaired renal function; serum salicylate levels, renal function, hearing changes or tinnitus, abnormal bruising, weight gain and response (ie, pain)

Administration
Liquid may be mixed with fruit juice just before drinking. Do not administer with antacids. Take with a full glass of water and remain in an upright position for 15-30 minutes after administration.

Contraindications Hypersensitivity to salicylates, other nonacetylated salicylates, other NSAIDs, or any component of the formulation; bleeding disorders; pregnancy (3rd trimester)

Warnings
Salicylate salts may not inhibit platelet aggregation and, therefore, should not be substituted for aspirin in the prophylaxis of thrombosis. Use with caution in patients with impaired renal function, dehydration, erosive gastritis, asthma, or peptic ulcer. Discontinue use 1 week prior to surgical procedures. Children and teenagers who have or are recovering from chickenpox or flu-like symptoms should not use this product. Changes in behavior (along with nausea and vomiting) may be an early sign of Reye's syndrome; patients should be instructed to contact their healthcare provider if these occur.

Elderly are a high-risk population for adverse effects from NSAIDs. As many as 60% of elderly can develop peptic ulceration and/or hemorrhage asymptomatically. Use lowest effective dose for shortest period possible. Tinnitus or impaired hearing may indicate toxicity. Tinnitus may be a difficult and unreliable indication of toxicity due to age-related hearing loss or eighth cranial nerve damage. CNS adverse effects may be observed in the elderly at lower doses than younger adults.

Dosage Forms
Liquid: 500 mg/5 mL (240 mL) [choline salicylate 293 mg and magnesium salicylate 362 mg per 5 mL; cherry cordial flavor]

Tablet: 500 mg [choline salicylate 293 mg and magnesium salicylate 362 mg]; 750 mg [choline salicylate 440 mg and magnesium salicylate 544 mg]; 1000 mg [choline salicylate 587 mg and magnesium salicylate 725 mg]

Reference Range
Salicylate blood levels for anti-inflammatory effect: 10-30 mg/dL

Analgesia and antipyretic effect: Up to 10 mg/dL

Overdosage/Treatment
Decontamination: Lavage (within 1 hour)/activated charcoal may be most efficacious

Supportive therapy: Hypotension/dehydration can be managed with I.V. fluid therapy; acidosis should be treated with bicarbonates, seizures with benzodiazepines; antacids, blood products are indicated, as appropriate, for hemorrhage

Enhancement of elimination: Dialysis is indicated for secondary complications, acidosis, or renal failure and not toxin removal alone; multiple dosing of activated charcoal may be effective

Test Interactions False-negative results for Clinistix® urine test; false-positive results with Clinitest®

Drug Interactions
ACE inhibitors: Effects of ACE inhibitors may be decreased by concurrent therapy with NSAIDs.

Antacids: Concomitant use may lead to decreased salicylate concentration.

Warfarin: Concomitant use may increase the hypoprothrombinemic effect of warfarin.

Pregnancy Risk Factor C/D (3rd trimester)

Pregnancy Implications Animal reproduction studies have not been conducted. Due to the known effects of other salicylates (closure of ductus arteriosus), use during late pregnancy should be avoided.

Lactation Enters breast milk/use caution

Nursing Implications Liquid may be mixed with fruit juice just before drinking

---

Cidofovir

U.S. Brand Names Vistide®

Use Treatment of cytomegalovirus (CMV) retinitis in patients with acquired immunodeficiency syndrome (AIDS); currently under Phase I and II trials for systemic treatment of AIDS. **Note:** Should be administered with probenecid and intravenous saline in order to reduce nephrotoxicity.

Mechanism of Action As a nucleotide analog, cidofovir suppresses CMV replication by selective prevention of viral DNA synthesis through inhibition of CMV DNA polymerase; the active form is the intracellular metabolite, cidofovir diphosphate; cross-resistance to ganciclovir but not foscarnet has been demonstrated *in vitro*

Adverse Reactions

Cardiovascular: Hypotension, pallor, syncope, tachycardia

Central nervous system: **Infection, chills, fever, headache, amnesia, anxiety, confusion, seizures, insomnia,** dizziness, hallucinations, depression, somnolence, malaise

Dermatologic: **Alopecia, rash, acne, skin discoloration,** pruritus, urticaria

Endocrine & metabolic: Hyperglycemia, hyperlipidemia, hypocalcemia, hypokalemia, dehydration, nephrogenic diabetes insipidus

Gastrointestinal: **Nausea, vomiting, diarrhea, anorexia, abdominal pain, constipation, dyspepsia, gastritis,** abnormal taste, stomatitis

Genitourinary: Glycosuria, urinary incontinence, urinary tract infections

Hematologic: **Thrombocytopenia, neutropenia (not dose related), anemia**

Neuromuscular & skeletal: **Weakness, paresthesia,** skeletal pain

Ocular: **Amblyopia, conjunctivitis, ocular hypotony,** retinal detachment, iritis, uveitis, abnormal vision

Renal: **Tubular damage, proteinuria, Cr elevations,** hematuria

Respiratory: **Asthma, bronchitis, coughing, dyspnea, pharyngitis,** pneumonia, rhinitis, sinusitis

Miscellaneous: Diaphoresis, allergic reactions

Pharmacodynamics/Kinetics

The following pharmacokinetic data is based on a combination of cidofovir administered with probenecid:

Distribution: V_d: 0.54 L/kg; does not cross significantly into CSF

Protein binding: <6%

Metabolism: Minimal; phosphorylation occurs intracellularly

Half-life elimination, plasma: ~2.6 hours

Excretion: Urine

Dosage

Induction: 5 mg/kg I.V. over 1 hour once weekly for 2 consecutive weeks

Maintenance: 5 mg/kg over 1 hour once every other week

Administer with probenecid - 2 g orally 3 hours prior to the cidofovir dose and 1 g at 2 and 8 hours after completion of the infusion (total: 4 g)

Hydrate with 1 L of 0.9% normal saline I.V. prior to cidofovir infusion; a second liter may be administered over a 1- to 3-hour period immediately following infusion, if tolerated

Dosing adjustment in renal impairment:

Cl_{cr} 41-55 mL/minute: 2 mg/kg

Cl_{cr} 30-40 mL/minute: 1.5 mg/kg

Cl_{cr} 20-29 mL/minute: 1 mg/kg

Cl_{cr} <19 mL/minute: 0.5 mg/kg

If the Cr increases by 0.3-0.4 mg/dL, reduce the cidofovir dose to 3 mg/kg; DC therapy for increases ≥0.5 mg/dL or development of ≥3+ proteinuria

Stability Store admixtures under refrigeration for ≤24 hours; prepare admixtures in a class two laminar flow hood, wearing protective gear; dispose of cidofovir as directed; wash and flush skin thoroughly with water if contact with skin

Monitoring Parameters Renal function (Cr, BUN, UAs), LFTs, WBCs, intraocular pressure and visual acuity

Administration

For I.V. infusion only. Infuse over 1 hour. Hydrate with 1 L of 0.9% NS I.V. prior to cidofovir infusion. A second liter may be administered over a 1- to 3-hour period immediately following infusion, if tolerated.

Contraindications Hypersensitivity to cidofovir; history of clinically-severe hypersensitivity to probenecid or other sulfa-containing medications; serum creatinine >1.5 mg/dL; Cl_{cr} <55 mL/minute; urine protein ≥100 mg/dL (≥2+ proteinuria); use with or within 7 days of nephrotoxic agents; direct intraocular injection

Warnings [U.S. Boxed Warning]: Dose-dependent nephrotoxicity requires dose adjustment or discontinuation if changes in renal function occur during therapy (eg, proteinuria, glycosuria, decreased serum phosphate, uric acid or bicarbonate, and elevated creatinine). Neutropenia has been reported; monitor counts during therapy. Cases of ocular hypotony have also occurred; monitor intraocular pressure. Monitor for signs of metabolic acidosis. Safety and efficacy have not been established in children or the elderly. Administration must be accompanied by oral probenecid and intravenous saline prehydration. Prepare admixtures in a class two laminar flow hood, wearing protective gear; dispose of cidofovir as directed. **[U.S. Boxed Warning]: Indicated only for CMV retinitis treatment in HIV patients; possibly carcinogenic based on animal data.**

Dosage Forms Injection, solution [preservative free]: 75 mg/mL (5 mL)

Reference Range Peak serum cidofovir levels after I.V. dose of 5 mg/kg: ~12 mcg/mL; coadministration of probenecid may double peak serum cidofovir level

Overdosage/Treatment Decontamination: Ipecac within 30 minutes; lavage within 1 hour/activated charcoal

Drug Interactions

Nephrotoxic agents: Drugs with nephrotoxic potential (eg, amphotericin B, aminoglycosides, foscarnet, and I.V. pentamidine) should not be used with or within 7 days of cidofovir therapy.

Zidovudine: Due to concomitant probenecid administration, temporarily discontinue or decrease zidovudine dose by 50% on the day of cidofovir administration only.

Pregnancy Risk Factor C

Pregnancy Implications Although studies are inconclusive, adenocarcinomas have occurred in animal studies with cidofovir; use during pregnancy only if the potential benefit justifies the potential risk to the fetus.

Lactation Excretion in breast milk unknown/contraindicated

Nursing Implications Zidovudine (AZT) doses should be decreased or discontinued during cidofovir therapy since probenecid decreases its elimination; administration of probenecid with a meal may decrease associated nausea; acetaminophen and antihistamines may ameliorate hypersensitivity reactions; dilute in 100 mL 0.9% saline; administer probenecid and I.V. saline before each infusion; allow the admixture to come to room temperature before administration

Cimetidine

Related Information

- Therapeutic Drugs Associated with Hallucinations

CAS Number 51481-61-9

U.S. Brand Names Tagamet® HB 200 [OTC]; Tagamet®

Use Short-term treatment of active duodenal ulcers and benign gastric ulcers; long-term prophylaxis of duodenal ulcer; gastric hypersecretory states; gastroesophageal reflux; prevention of upper GI bleeding in critically-ill patients; labeled for OTC use for prevention or relief of heartburn, acid indigestion, or sour stomach

Unlabeled/Investigational Use Part of a multidrug regimen for *H. pylori* eradication to reduce the risk of duodenal ulcer recurrence

Mechanism of Action Competitive inhibition of histamine at H_2-receptors of the gastric parietal cells resulting in reduced gastric acid secretion

Adverse Reactions

Cardiovascular: Bradycardia, hypotension, AV block, sinus bradycardia

Central nervous system: Dizziness, mental confusion, agitation, drowsiness, psychosis, delirium, fatigue, auditory and visual hallucination, fever, headache, gustatory hallucinations

Dermatologic: Rash, pruritus, alopecia, erythema annulare centrifugum, Stevens-Johnson syndrome, exfoliative dermatitis, rash, cutaneous vasculitis, angioedema, toxic epidermal necrolysis, xerosis, urticaria, purpura, exanthem

Endocrine & metabolic: Gynecomastia, reduces parathyroid hormone, nephrogenic diabetes insipidus, parotitis, decreased libido

Gastrointestinal: Mild diarrhea, pancreatitis, lymphocytic colitis

Genitourinary: Impotence

Hematologic: Neutropenia, thrombocytopenia, granulocytopenia, aplastic anemia

Hepatic: Elevation of AST and ALT

Neuromuscular & skeletal: Myalgia

Ocular: Mydriasis, photophobia

Renal: Interstitial nephritis, elevated creatinine

Respiratory: Asthma, bronchospasm

Miscellaneous: Cutaneous lupus erythematosus, systemic lupus erythematosus, fixed drug eruption

Signs and Symptoms of Overdose Agranulocytosis, ataxia, AV block, bradycardia, cholestatic jaundice, coma, delirium, dementia, depression, disorientation, dry mouth, eosinophilia, erythema multiforme, extrapyramidal reaction, galactorrhea, granulocytopenia, hyperthermia, hyperprolactinemia, ileus, impotence, leukocytosis, leukopenia, mania, myalgia, mydriasis, myopathy, neutropenia, parotid pain, respiratory failure, slurred speech, sweating

Admission Criteria/Prognosis Admit any patient central nervous system or cardiovascular toxicity or any adult ingestion >3 g

Pharmacodynamics/Kinetics

Onset of action: 1 hour

Duration: 4-8 hours

Absorption: Rapid

Distribution: Crosses placenta; enters breast milk

Protein binding: 20%

Metabolism: Partially hepatic

Bioavailability: 60% to 70%

Half-life elimination: Neonates: 3.6 hours; Children: 1.4 hours; Adults: Normal renal function: 2 hours

Time to peak, serum: Oral: 1-2 hours

Excretion: Primarily urine (48% as unchanged drug); feces (some)

Dosage

Children: Oral, I.M., I.V.: 20-40 mg/kg/day in divided doses every 6 hours

Children ≥12 years and Adults: Oral: Heartburn, acid indigestion, sour stomach (OTC labeling): 200 mg up to twice daily; may take 30 minutes prior to eating foods or beverages expected to cause heartburn or indigestion

Adults:

Short-term treatment of active ulcers:

Oral: 300 mg 4 times/day or 800 mg at bedtime or 400 mg twice daily for up to 8 weeks

I.M., I.V.: 300 mg every 6 hours or 37.5 mg/hour by continuous infusion; I.V. dosage should be adjusted to maintain an intragastric pH ≥ 5

Patients with an active bleed: Administer cimetidine as a continuous infusion (see above)

Duodenal ulcer prophylaxis: Oral: 400-800 mg at bedtime

Gastric hypersecretory conditions: Oral, I.M., I.V.: 300-600 mg every 6 hours; dosage not to exceed 2.4 g/day

Helicobacter pylori eradication (unlabeled use): 400 mg twice daily; requires combination therapy with antibiotics

Dosing adjustment/interval in renal impairment: Children and Adults:

Cl_{cr} 20-40 mL/minute: Administer every 8 hours or 75% of normal dose

Cl_{cr} 0-20 mL/minute: Administer every 12 hours or 50% of normal dose

Hemodialysis: Slightly dialyzable (5% to 20%)

Dosing adjustment/comments in hepatic impairment: Usual dose is safe in mild liver disease but use with caution and in reduced dosage in severe liver disease; increased risk of CNS toxicity in cirrhosis suggested by enhanced penetration of CNS

Monitoring Parameters CBC, gastric pH, occult blood with GI bleeding; monitor renal function to correct dose.

Administration Oral: Administer with meals so that the drug's peak effect occurs at the proper time (peak inhibition of gastric acid secretion occurs at 1 and 3 hours after dosing in fasting subjects and approximately 2 hours in nonfasting subjects; this correlates well with the time food is no longer in the stomach offering a buffering effect)

Injection: May be administered as a slow I.V. push or preferably as an I.V. intermittent or I.V. continuous infusion. Administer each 300 mg (or fraction thereof) over a minimum of 5 minutes when giving I.V. push. Give intermittent infusion over 15-30 minutes for each 300 mg dose. Intermittent infusions are administered over 15-30 minutes at a final concentration not to exceed 6 mg/mL; for patients with an active bleed, preferred method of administration is continuous infusion.

Contraindications Hypersensitivity to cimetidine, any component of the formulation, or other H_2 antagonists

Warnings

Reversible confusional states, usually clearing within 3-4 days after discontinuation, have been linked to use. Increased age (>50 years) and renal or hepatic impairment are thought to be associated. Dosage should be adjusted in renal/hepatic impairment or in patients receiving drugs metabolized through the P450 system.

Over the counter (OTC) cimetidine should not be taken by individuals experiencing painful swallowing, vomiting with blood, or bloody or black stools; medical attention should be sought. A physician should be consulted prior to use when pain in the stomach, shoulder, arms or neck is present; if heartburn has occurred for >3 months; or if unexplained weight loss, or nausea and vomiting occur. Frequent wheezing, shortness of breath, lightheadedness, or sweating, especially with chest pain or heartburn, should also be reported. Consultation of a healthcare provider should occur by patients if also taking theophylline, phenytoin, or warfarin; if heartburn or stomach pain continues or worsens; or if use is required for >14 days. Pregnant or breast-feeding women should speak to a healthcare provider before use. OTC cimetidine is not approved for use in patients <12 years of age.

Dosage Forms

[DSC] = Discontinued product

Infusion, as hydrochloride [premixed in NS]: 300 mg (50 mL)

Injection, solution, as hydrochloride: 150 mg/mL (2 mL, 8 mL) [8 mL size contains benzyl alcohol]

Liquid, oral, as hydrochloride: 300 mg/5 mL (240 mL, 480 mL) [contains alcohol 2.8%; mint-peach flavor]

Tablet: 200 mg [OTC], 300 mg, 400 mg, 800 mg

Tagamet®: 300 mg; 400 mg [DSC]

Tagamet® HB 200: 200 mg

Reference Range Therapeutic: 0.25-1 mcg/mL (SI: 1-4 μmol/L); confusion occurs in levels >2 mcg/mL (SI: >8 μmol/L)

Overdosage/Treatment

Decontamination: Emesis within 30 minutes or lavage within 1 hour; activated charcoal

Supportive therapy: Treatment is primarily symptomatic and supportive; routine use of physostigmine is not advised, although it can be used for life-threatening anticholinergic; benzodiazepines can be used to treat seizures

Enhancement of elimination: Multiple dosing of activated charcoal may be beneficial; hemodialysis may be useful in reducing half-life; should be considered in patients experiencing severe toxicity or renal failure; slightly dialyzable (5% to 20%)

Test Interactions ↑ AST, ALT, creatinine (S); may cause a false elevation of serum creatinine due to interference with tubular secretion of creatinine

Drug Interactions

Inhibits CYP1A2 (moderate), 2C9 (weak), 2C19 (moderate), 2D6 (moderate), 2E1 (weak), 3A4 (moderate)

Note: There are many potential interactions. Listed are the most significant ones.

Alfentanil: Increased serum concentration; monitor for toxicity.

Amiodarone: Serum concentration of amiodarone is increased; avoid concurrent use.

Atazanavir: Absorption may be decreased by cimetidine; separate doses by 12 hours.

Benzodiazepines (except lorazepam, oxazepam, temazepam): Serum concentration of the benzodiazepine is increased; consider alternative H_2 antagonist or monitor for benzodiazepine toxicity.

Beta-blockers (except atenolol, betaxolol, bisoprolol, nadolol, penbutolol): Effects of the beta-blocker may be increased; use a renally-eliminated beta-blocker or alternative H_2 antagonist.

Calcium channel blockers (except amlodipine and nicardipine): Serum concentration of the CCB is increased; monitor for toxicity.

Carbamazepine: Plasma concentration of carbamazepine may increase transiently (1 week). Monitor for carbamazepine toxicity or use an alternative H_2 antagonist.

Carmustine: Myelotoxicity of carmustine is increased; avoid concurrent use.

Cefpodoxime, cefuroxime: Oral absorption of these agents may be reduced by increased pH; consider alternative antibiotic or separate dosing by at least 2 hours.

Cisapride: Bioavailability of cisapride is increased; avoid concurrent use.

Citalopram: Serum concentration of citalopram is increased; use an alternative H_2 antagonist or adjust citalopram dose.

Clozapine: Cimetidine may increase levels/effects; consider alternative H_2 antagonist

Cyclosporine: Serum concentration of cyclosporine may increase; monitor cyclosporine levels.

CYP1A2 substrates: Cimetidine may increase the levels/effects of CYP1A2 substrates. Example substrates include aminophylline, fluvoxamine, mexiletine, mirtazapine, ropinirole, theophylline, and trifluoperazine.

CYP2C19 substrates: Cimetidine may increase the levels/effects of CYP2C19 substrates. Example substrates include citalopram, diazepam, methsuximide, phenytoin, propranolol, and sertraline.

CYP2D6 substrates: Cimetidine may increase the levels/effects of CYP2D6 substrates. Example substrates include amphetamines, selected beta-blockers, dextromethorphan, fluoxetine, lidocaine, mirtazapine, nefazodone, paroxetine, risperidone, ritonavir, thioridazine, tricyclic antidepressants, and venlafaxine.

CYP2D6 prodrug substrates: Cimetidine may decrease the levels/effects of CYP2D6 prodrug substrates. Example prodrug substrates include codeine, hydrocodone, oxycodone, and tramadol.

CYP3A4 substrates: Cimetidine may increase the levels/effects of CYP3A4 substrates. Example substrates include benzodiazepines, calcium channel blockers, cyclosporine, mirtazapine, nateglinide, nefazodone, sildenafil (and other PDE-5 inhibitors), tacrolimus, and venlafaxine. Selected benzodiazepines (midazolam and triazolam), cisapride, ergot alkaloids, selected HMG-CoA reductase inhibitors (lovastatin and simvastatin), and pimozide are generally contraindicated with strong CYP3A4 inhibitors.

Delavirdine: Absorption of delavirdine is decreased; avoid concurrent use with H_2 antagonists.

Dofetilide: Cimetidine may increase the levels/effects of dofetilide; avoid concurrent use

Flecainide: Serum concentration of flecainide is increased, especially in patients with renal failure.

Ketoconazole, fluconazole, itraconazole (especially capsule): Decreased serum concentration; avoid concurrent use with H_2 antagonists.

Lidocaine: Serum concentration of lidocaine is increased; use alternative H_2 antagonist.

Metformin: Serum levels/effects may be increased by cimetidine; monitor for hypoglycemia.

Moricizine: Serum concentration of moricizine is increased; monitor for toxicity.

Phenytoin: Serum levels/effects may be increased by cimetidine; avoid concurrent use.

Procainamide: Cimetidine may increase levels/effects; monitor.

Propafenone: Serum concentration of propafenone is increased; monitor for toxicity.

Quinolones: Renal elimination of quinolone antibiotics may be decreased.

Selective serotonin reuptake inhibitors (eg, paroxetine, citalopram): Serum concentrations may be increased by cimetidine; monitor.

Sulfonylureas: Cimetidine may increase levels/effects; monitor for hypoglycemia

Tacrine: Plasma concentration of tacrine is increased; consider alternative H_2 antagonist.

TCAs: Serum concentration is increased; consider alternative H_2 antagonist or monitor for TCAs toxicity.

Theophylline: Serum concentration of theophylline is increased; consider alternative H_2 antagonist.

Thioridazine: Serum levels/effects may be increased by cimetidine; concurrent use contraindicated by manufacturer.

Warfarin: INR is increased; cimetidine's effect is dose related. Use an alternative H_2 antagonist if possible or monitor INR closely and adjust warfarin dose as needed.

Pregnancy Risk Factor B

Pregnancy Implications Crosses the placenta

Lactation Enters breast milk/not recommended

Additional Information Cimetidine is not effective for hepatoprotection in acetaminophen overdose; may inhibit absorption of cobalamin; may increase HDL cholesterol concentrations; may cause phytobezoar formation. At doses >1 g/day of cimetidine, the risk of developing gynecomastia is 40 times that of nonusers.

Ciprofloxacin

Related Information
- Levofloxacin

CAS Number 85721-33-1 (base); 86483-48-9 (hydrochloride)

U.S. Brand Names Ciloxan®; Cipro® XR; Cipro®; Proquin® XR

Synonyms Ciprofloxacin Hydrochloride

Use Treatment of documented or suspected infections of the lower respiratory tract, sinuses, skin and skin structure, bone/joints, and urinary tract (including prostatitis) due to susceptible bacterial strains; especially indicated for pseudomonal infections and those due to multidrug-resistant gram-negative organisms, chronic bacterial prostatitis, infectious diarrhea, complicated gram-negative and anaerobic intra-abdominal infections (with metronidazole) due to *E. coli* (enteropathic strains), *B. fragilis*, *P. mirabilis*, *K. pneumoniae*, *P. aeruginosa*, *Campylobacter jejuni* or *Shigella*; approved for acute sinusitis caused by *H. influenzae* or *M. catarrhalis*; also used in treatment of typhoid fever due to *Salmonella typhi* (although eradication of the chronic typhoid carrier state has not been proven), osteomyelitis when parenteral therapy is not feasible, acute uncomplicated cystitis in females, to reduce incidence or progression of disease following exposure to aerolized *Bacillus anthracis*, febrile neutropenia (with piperacillin), and sexually transmitted diseases such as uncomplicated cervical and urethral gonorrhea due to *Neisseria gonorrhoeae*; used ophthalmologically for superficial ocular infections (corneal ulcers, conjunctivitis) due to susceptible strains

Acute pulmonary exacerbations in cystic fibrosis (children); cutaneous/gastrointestinal/oropharyngeal anthrax (treatment, children and adults); disseminated gonococcal infection (adults); chancroid (adults); prophylaxis to *Neisseria meningitidis* following close contact with an infected person

Mechanism of Action Inhibits DNA-gyrase in susceptible organisms; inhibits relaxation of supercoiled DNA and promotes breakage of double-stranded DNA

Adverse Reactions

Cardiovascular: Fibrillation (atrial), flutter (atrial), hypertension, palpitations, syncope, tachycardia (infants), vasculitis

Central nervous system: Agitation, aseptic meningitis, CNS depression, confusion, delusions, delirium, dizziness, fever, headache, insomnia, malaise, mania, night terrors, psychosis, paranoia, restlessness, seizures

Dermatologic: Acne, angioedema, bullous skin disease, cutaneous vasculitis, epidermal necrolysis, erythema nodosum, exanthem, Henoch-Schönlein purpura, photosensitivity, somnambulism, Stevens-Johnson syndrome, exfoliative dermatitis, phototoxicity, pruritus, rash, toxic pustulosis, urticaria

Gastrointestinal: Dysphagia, gastritis; gastrointestinal vasculitis, fecal discoloration (greenish gray, white/speckling), nausea, pancreatitis, stomatitis, tooth discoloration, vomiting, xerostomia, diarrhea, abdominal pain

Genitourinary: Urinary retention

Hematologic: Anemia, eosinophilia, hemolytic anemia, methemoglobinemia, thrombocytopenia, hemolytic uremic syndrome

Hepatic: Aminotransferase level elevation (asymptomatic), cholestasis, cholestatic jaundice, elevated liver enzymes, jaundice, hepatic necrosis

Neuromuscular & skeletal: Arthralgia, dyskinesia, exacerbation of myasthenia gravis, hemiplegia, myalgia, tendon rupture, tremors, paresthesia, peripheral neuropathy

Ocular: Diplopia, photophobia, keratitis, keratopathy, visual disturbance

Otic: Tinnitus

Renal: Hematuria, interstitial nephritis, proteinuria, renal failure, renal vasculitis, serum creatinine increased

Respiratory: Hyposmia, pulmonary vasculitis, rhinitis (children 3%)

Miscellaneous: Anaphylactoid reaction (rate of 1.2/100,000 prescriptions), elevated antineutrophilic cytoplasmic antibodies (ANCA) fixed drug eruption, serum sickness, toxic shock syndrome

Signs and Symptoms of Overdose Acute renal failure; seizures

Admission Criteria/Prognosis Admit any patient with CNS or renal abnormalities, or any adult ingestion >8 g

Pharmacodynamics/Kinetics

Absorption: Oral: Immediate release tablet: Rapid ($\sim$50% to 85%)

Distribution: V_d: 2.1-2.7 L/kg; tissue concentrations often exceed serum concentrations especially in kidneys, gallbladder, liver, lungs, gynecological tissue, and prostatic tissue; CSF concentrations: 10% of serum concentrations (noninflamed meninges), 14% to 37% (inflamed meninges); crosses placenta; enters breast milk

Protein binding: 20% to 40%

Metabolism: Partially hepatic; forms 4 metabolites (limited activity)

Half-life elimination: Children: 2.5 hours; Adults: Normal renal function: 3-5 hours

Time to peak: Oral:
  Immediate release tablet: 0.5-2 hours
  Extended release tablet: Cipro® XR: 1-2.5 hours, Proquin® XR: 3.5-8.7 hours

Excretion: Urine (30% to 50% as unchanged drug); feces (15% to 43%)

Dosage Note: Extended release tablets and immediate release formulations are not interchangeable:

Children (see Warnings):
  Oral: Immediate release formulation: 20-30 mg/kg/day in 2 divided doses; maximum: 1.5 g/day
    Cystic fibrosis (unlabeled use): Children 5-17 years: 40 mg/kg/day divided every 12 hours administered following 1 week of I.V. therapy has been reported in a clinical trial; total duration of therapy: 10-21 days
    Anthrax:
      Inhalational (postexposure prophylaxis): 15 mg/kg/dose every 12 hours for 60 days; maximum: 500 mg/dose
      Cutaneous (treatment, CDC guidelines): 10-15 mg/kg every 12 hours for 60 days (maximum: 1 g/day); amoxicillin 80 mg/kg/day divided every 8 hours is an option for completion of treatment after clinical improvement. **Note:** In the presence of systemic involvement, extensive edema, lesions on head/neck, refer to I.V. dosing for treatment of inhalational/gastrointestinal/oropharyngeal anthrax
  I.V.:
    Complicated urinary tract infection or pyelonephritis: Children 1-17 years: 6-10 mg/kg every 8 hours for 10-21 days (maximum: 400 mg/dose)
    Cystic fibrosis (unlabeled use): Children 5-17 years: 30 mg/kg/day divided every 8 hours for 10-21 days (maximum: 400 mg/dose)
    Anthrax:
      Inhalational (postexposure prophylaxis): 10 mg/kg/dose every 12 hours for 60 days; do **not** exceed 400 mg/dose (800 mg/day)
      Inhalational/gastrointestinal/oropharyngeal (treatment, CDC guidelines): Initial: 10-15 mg/kg every 12 hours for 60 days (maximum: 500 mg/dose); switch to oral therapy when clinically appropriate; refer to Adults dosing for notes on combined therapy and duration

Adults: Oral:
  Urinary tract infection:
    Acute uncomplicated: Immediate release formulation: 250 mg every 12 hours for 3 days
    Acute uncomplicated pyelonephritis: Extended release formulation (Cipro® XR): 1000 mg every 24 hours for 7-14 days
    Uncomplicated/acute cystitis: Extended release formulation (Cipro® XR, Proquin® XR): 500 mg every 24 hours for 3 days
    Mild/moderate: Immediate release formulation: 250 mg every 12 hours for 7-14 days
    Severe/complicated:
      Immediate release formulation: 500 mg every 12 hours for 7-14 days
      Extended release formulation (Cipro® XR): 1000 mg every 24 hours for 7-14 days
  Lower respiratory tract, skin/skin structure infections: 500-750 mg twice daily for 7-14 days depending on severity and susceptibility
  Bone/joint infections: 500-750 mg twice daily for 4-6 weeks, depending on severity and susceptibility
  Infectious diarrhea: 500 mg every 12 hours for 5-7 days
  Intra-abdominal (in combination with metronidazole): 500 mg every 12 hours for 7-14 days
  Typhoid fever: 500 mg every 12 hours for 10 days
  Urethral/cervical gonococcal infections: 250-500 mg as a single dose (CDC recommends concomitant doxycycline or azithromycin due to developing resistance; avoid use in Asian or Western Pacific travelers)
  Disseminated gonococcal infection: 500 mg twice daily to complete 7 days of therapy (initial treatment with ceftriaxone 1 g I.M./I.V. daily for 24-48 hours after improvement begins)
  Chancroid: 500 mg twice daily for 3 days
  Sinusitis (acute): 500 mg every 12 hours for 10 days
  Chronic bacterial prostatitis: 500 mg every 12 hours for 28 days
  Anthrax:
    Inhalational (postexposure prophylaxis): 500 mg every 12 hours for 60 days
    Cutaneous (treatment, CDC guidelines): Immediate release formulation: 500 mg every 12 hours for 60 days. **Note:** In the presence of systemic involvement, extensive edema, lesions on head/neck,

refer to I.V. dosing for treatment of inhalational/gastrointestinal/oropharyngeal anthrax

Adults: I.V.:
Bone/joint infections:
Mild to moderate: 400 mg every 12 hours for 4-6 weeks
Severe or complicated: 400 mg every 8 hours for 4-6 weeks
Lower respiratory tract, skin/skin structure infections:
Mild to moderate: 400 mg every 12 hours for 7-14 days
Severe or complicated: 400 mg every 8 hours for 7-14 days
Nosocomial pneumonia (mild to moderate to severe): 400 mg every 8 hours for 10-14 days
Prostatitis (chronic, bacterial): 400 mg every 12 hours for 28 days
Sinusitis (acute): 400 mg every 12 hours for 10 days
Urinary tract infection:
Mild to moderate: 200 mg every 12 hours for 7-14 days
Severe or complicated: 400 mg every 12 hours for 7-14 days
Febrile neutropenia (with piperacillin): 400 mg every 8 hours for 7-14 days
Intra-abdominal infection (with metronidazole): 400 mg every 12 hours for 7-14 days
Anthrax:
Inhalational (postexposure prophylaxis): 400 mg every 12 hours for 60 days
Inhalational/gastrointestinal/oropharyngeal (treatment): 400 mg every 12 hours. **Note:** Initial treatment should include two or more agents predicted to be effective (per CDC recommendations). Agents suggested for use in conjunction with ciprofloxacin or doxycycline include rifampin, vancomycin, imipenem, penicillin, ampicillin, chloramphenicol, clindamycin, and clarithromycin. May switch to oral antimicrobial therapy when clinically appropriate. Continue combined therapy for 60 days.
Elderly: No adjustment needed in patients with normal renal function
Ophthalmic:
Solution: Children >1 year and Adults: Instill 1-2 drops in eye(s) every 2 hours while awake for 2 days and 1-2 drops every 4 hours while awake for the next 5 days
Ointment: Children >2 years and Adults: Apply a $^1/_2$" ribbon into the conjunctival sac 3 times/day for the first 2 days, followed by a $^1/_2$" ribbon applied twice daily for the next 5 days
Dosing adjustment in renal impairment:
Cl_{cr} 30-50 mL/minute: Oral: 250-500 mg every 12 hours
Cl_{cr} <30 mL/minute: Acute uncomplicated pyelonephritis or complicated UTI: Oral: Extended release formulation: 500 mg every 24 hours
Cl_{cr} 5-29 mL/minute:
Oral: 250-500 mg every 18 hours
I.V.: 200-400 mg every 18-24 hours
Dialysis: Only small amounts of ciprofloxacin are removed by hemo- or peritoneal dialysis (<10%); usual dose: Oral: 250-500 mg every 24 hours following dialysis
Continuous arteriovenous or venovenous hemodiafiltration effects: Administer 200-400 mg I.V. every 12 hours

Stability
Refrigeration and room temperature:
Prepared bags: 14 days
Premixed bags: Manufacturer expiration dating
Out of overwrap stability: 14 days

Monitoring Parameters Patients receiving concurrent ciprofloxacin, theophylline, or cyclosporine should have serum levels monitored

Administration
Oral: May administer with food to minimize GI upset; avoid antacid use; maintain proper hydration and urine output. Administer immediate release ciprofloxacin and Cipro® XR at least 2 hours before or 6 hours after, and Proquin® XR at least 4 hours before or 6 hours after antacids or other products containing calcium, iron, or zinc (including dairy products or calcium-fortified juices). Separate oral administration from drugs which may impair absorption (see Drug Interactions).
Oral suspension: Should not be administered through feeding tubes (suspension is oil-based and adheres to the feeding tube). Patients should avoid chewing on the microcapsules.
Nasogastric/orogastric tube: Crush immediate-release tablet and mix with water. Flush feeding tube before and after administration. Hold tube feedings at least 1 hour before and 2 hours after administration.
Tablet, extended release: Do not crush, split, or chew. May be administered with meals containing dairy products (calcium content <800 mg), but not with dairy products alone. Proquin® XR should be administered with a main meal of the day; evening meal is preferred.
Parenteral: Administer by slow I.V. infusion over 60 minutes to reduce the risk of venous irritation (burning, pain, erythema, and swelling); final concentration for administration should not exceed 2 mg/mL.

Contraindications Hypersensitivity to ciprofloxacin, any component of the formulation, or other quinolones; concurrent administration of tizanidine

Warnings
CNS stimulation may occur (tremor, restlessness, confusion, and very rarely hallucinations or seizures). Use with caution in patients with known or suspected CNS disorder. Potential for seizures, although very rare, may be increased with concomitant NSAID therapy. Use with caution in individuals at risk of seizures. Prolonged use may result in superinfection. Tendon inflammation and/or rupture have been reported with ciprofloxacin and other quinolone antibiotics. Risk may be increased with concurrent corticosteroids, particularly in the elderly. Discontinue at first sign of tendon inflammation or pain. Adverse effects, including those related to joints and/or surrounding tissues, are increased in pediatric patients and therefore, ciprofloxacin should not be considered as drug of choice in children (exception is anthrax treatment). Rare cases of peripheral neuropathy may occur.
Severe hypersensitivity reactions, including anaphylaxis, have occurred with quinolone therapy. Quinolones may exacerbate myasthenia gravis, use with caution (rare, potentially life-threatening weakness of respiratory muscles may occur). Use caution in renal impairment. Avoid excessive sunlight; may cause moderate-to-severe phototoxicity reactions.
Ciprofloxacin is a potent inhibitor of CYP1A2. Coadministration of drugs which depend on this pathway may lead to substantial increases in serum concentrations and adverse effects.

Dosage Forms
[DSC] = Discontinued product
Infusion [premixed in D_5W] (Cipro®): 200 mg (100 mL); 400 mg (200 mL) [latex free]
Injection, solution (Cipro®): 10 mg/mL (20 mL, 40 mL, 120 mL [DSC])
Microcapsules for oral suspension (Cipro®): 250 mg/5 mL (100 mL); 500 mg/5 mL (100 mL) [strawberry flavor]
Ointment, ophthalmic, as hydrochloride (Ciloxan®): 3.33 mg/g [0.3% base] (3.5 g)
Solution, ophthalmic, as hydrochloride (Ciloxan®): 3.5 mg/mL [0.3% base] (2.5 mL, 5 mL, 10 mL) [contains benzalkonium chloride]
Tablet: 250 mg, 500 mg, 750 mg
Cipro®: 100 mg, 250 mg, 500 mg, 750 mg
Tablet, extended release:
Cipro® XR: 500 mg [equivalent to ciprofloxacin hydrochloride 287.5 mg and ciprofloxacin base 212.6 mg]; 1000 mg [equivalent to ciprofloxacin hydrochloride 574.9 mg and ciprofloxacin base 425.2 mg]
Proquin® XR: 500 mg
Tablet, extended release [dose pack]:
Proquin® XR: 500 mg (3s)

Reference Range
Peak plasma concentrations after a 750 mg oral dose: 3.0 mcg/mL (9 μmol/g)
Therapeutic: 2.6-3.0 mcg/mL
Toxic: >5.0 mcg/mL

Overdosage/Treatment
Decontamination: Lavage (within 1 hour)/activated charcoal
Supportive therapy: Treatment should include adequate hydration and renal function monitoring. Magnesium or calcium-containing antacids may be given to decrease absorption of oral ciprofloxacin. Do **not** use flumazenil. Diazepam, phenobarbital, or phenytoin can be used for seizures.
Enhancement of elimination: Multiple dosing of activated charcoal may be effective; only small amounts of ciprofloxacin are removed by dialysis (<10%)

Test Interactions High urine concentrations of ciprofloxacin can invalidate EMIT urine drug screening procedures

Drug Interactions
Inhibits CYP1A2 (strong), 3A4 (weak)
Caffeine: Ciprofloxacin may decrease the metabolism of caffeine.
Corticosteroids: Concurrent use may increase the risk of tendon rupture, particularly in elderly patients (overall incidence rare).
CYP1A2 substrates: Ciprofloxacin may increase the levels/effects of CYP1A2 substrates. Example substrates include aminophylline, fluvoxamine, mexiletine, mirtazapine, ropinirole, tizanidine, and trifluoperazine.
Foscarnet: Concomitant use with ciprofloxacin has been associated with an increased risk of seizures.
Glyburide: Quinolones may increase the effect of glyburide; monitor.
Metal cations (aluminum, calcium, iron, magnesium, and zinc) bind quinolones in the gastrointestinal tract and inhibit absorption. Concurrent administration of most antacids, oral electrolyte supplements, quinapril, sucralfate, some didanosine formulations (chewable/buffered tablets and pediatric powder for oral suspension), and other highly-buffered oral drugs, should be avoided. Ciprofloxacin should be administered 2 hours before or 6 hours after these agents.
Methotrexate: Ciprofloxacin may decrease renal secretion of methotrexate; monitor.
Pentoxifylline: Monitor for headache during concomitant therapy.
Phenytoin: Ciprofloxacin may decrease phenytoin levels; monitor.
Probenecid: May decrease renal secretion of quinolones.
Ropivacaine: Ciprofloxacin may decrease the metabolism of ropivacaine.
Sevelamer: May decrease absorption of oral ciprofloxacin.

Theophylline: Serum levels may be increased by ciprofloxacin; in addition, CNS stimulation/seizures may occur at lower theophylline serum levels due to additive CNS effects.

Tizanidine: Ciprofloxacin may increase serum levels of tizanidine. Concurrent administration is contraindicated.

Warfarin: The hypoprothrombinemic effect of warfarin may be enhanced by ciprofloxacin; monitor INR.

Pregnancy Risk Factor C

Pregnancy Implications Reports of arthropathy (observed in immature animals and reported rarely in humans) has limited the use of fluoroquinolones in pregnancy. According to the FDA, the Teratogen Information System concluded that therapeutic doses during pregnancy are unlikely to produce substantial teratogenic risk, but data are insufficient to say that there is no risk. In general, reports of exposure have been limited to short durations of therapy in the first trimester. When considering treatment for life-threatening infection and/or prolonged duration of therapy (such as in anthrax), the potential risk to the fetus must be balanced against the severity of the potential illness.

Lactation Enters breast milk/not recommended (AAP rates "compatible")

Nursing Implications Hold antacids for 3-4 hours after giving

Additional Information

Tablets can be crushed and mixed with apple or fruit juice for pediatric administration.

A 12 g ingestion resulted in mild symptoms in an adult, but a 14 g ingestion resulted in acute renal failure

Not effective in eliminating typhoid carrier state; has been used unsuccessfully to treat infectious diarrhea due to *Pseudomonas aeruginosa* (500 mg twice daily for 10 days)

Food decreases the rate, but not the extent, of absorption. Ciprofloxacin serum levels may be decreased if taken with dairy products or calcium-fortified juices. Ciprofloxacin may increase serum caffeine levels if taken with caffeine. Avoid dong quai, St John's wort (may also cause photosensitization). Peak plasma ciprofloxacin levels are decreased when given concurrently with *Garcinia kola* seed extract.

Specific References

Bhavnani SM, Callen WA, Forrest A, et al, "Effect of Fluoroquinolone Expenditures on Susceptibility of *Pseudomonas aeruginosa* to Ciprofloxacin in U.S. Hospitals," *Am J Health Syst Pharm*, 2003, 60(19):1962-70.

Daya SK, Gowda RM, and Khan IA, "Ciprofloxacin- and Hypocalcemia-Induced Torsade de Pointes Triggered by Hemodialysis," *Am J Ther*, 2004, 11(1):77-9.

Geib A and Burns EM, "Increasing Sirolimus Levels in a Multiorgan Transplant Patient Related to Interaction with Ciprofloxacin," *Clin Toxicol*, 2005, 43:631.

Ho DY, Song JC, and Wang CC, "Anaphylactoid Reaction to Ciprofloxacin," *Ann Pharmacother*, 2003, 37(7-8):1018-23.

Roberge R, Comment on "Refractory Hypoglycemia from Ciprofloxacin and Glyburide Interaction," *Clin Toxicol (Phila)*, 2005, 43(3):213-4.

Cisapride

CAS Number 81098-60-4

U.S. Brand Names Propulsid®

Use

Investigational Limited Access Program:

Three treatment protocols:

- Adults: Gastroesophageal reflux disease (GERD), gastroparesis, pseudo-obstruction, and severe chronic constipation
- Pediatrics: Refractory GERD (associated with failure to thrive, asthma, bradycardia, apnea, or other serous conditions) or pseudo-obstruction
- Neonates: Feeding intolerance

For enrolling patients in the limited access program, physicians should call Janssen Pharmaceuticals at (800) 795-4247.

Cisapride should be handled as an investigational drug, with completion of FDA form 1572 and informed consent.

Mechanism of Action Enhances the release of acetylcholine at the myenteric plexus. *In vitro* studies have shown cisapride to have serotonin-4 receptor agonistic properties (similar to metoclopramide) without dopamine-blocking activity.

Adverse Reactions

Cardiovascular: Prolonged QT interval, chest pain, shock, angina

Central nervous system: Headache, insomnia, anxiety, nervousness, fever, dystonic reaction, extrapyramidal effects, motor akathisia, pain

Dermatological: Rash, pruritus, urticaria, exanthem

Gastrointestinal: Diarrhea, abdominal pain, nausea, constipation, flatulence, dyspepsia, vomiting, xerostomia

Ocular: Lacrimation

Respiratory: Rhinitis, sinusitis, coughing, upper respiratory tract infection

Miscellaneous: Increased incidence of viral infection

Signs and Symptoms of Overdose Abdominal cramping, diarrhea, insomnia, seizures

Admission Criteria/Prognosis Admit any ingestion >1 mg/kg or any symptomatic patient

Pharmacodynamics/Kinetics

Onset of action: 0.5-1 hour

Protein binding: 97.5% to 98%

Metabolism: Extensively hepatic to norcisapride

Bioavailability: 35% to 40%

Half-life elimination: 6-12 hours

Excretion: Urine and feces (<10%)

Dosage

Oral:

Children: Not recommended

Adults: Initial: 10 mg 4 times/day at least 15 minutes before meals and at bedtime; in some patients the dosage will need to be increased to 20 mg to obtain a satisfactory result; reduce dosage in half in patients with liver failure

Chronic idiopathic constipation: 5 mg 3 times/day to 20 mg twice daily for 8-12 weeks

Liquid suspension: 10 mL 4 times/day at least 15 minutes before meals and at bedtime; can increase dose to 20 mL as needed

Contraindications

Hypersensitivity to cisapride or any component of the formulations; GI hemorrhage, mechanical obstruction, GI perforation, or other situations when GI motility stimulation is dangerous

Serious cardiac arrhythmias including ventricular tachycardia, ventricular fibrillation, torsade de pointes, and QT prolongation have been reported in patients taking cisapride with other drugs that inhibit CYP3A4. Some of these events have been fatal. Concomitant oral or intravenous administration of the following drugs with cisapride may lead to elevated cisapride blood levels and is contraindicated:

Antibiotics: Oral or I.V. erythromycin, clarithromycin, troleandomycin

Antidepressants: Nefazodone

Antifungals: Oral or I.V. fluconazole, itraconazole, miconazole, oral ketoconazole

Protease inhibitors: Indinavir, ritonavir, amprenavir, atazanavir

Cisapride is also contraindicated for patients with a prolonged electrocardiographic QT intervals (QT_c >450 msec), a history of QT_c prolongation, or known family history of congenital long QT syndrome; clinically significant bradycardia, renal failure, history of ventricular arrhythmias, ischemic heart disease, and congestive heart failure; uncorrected electrolyte disorders (hypokalemia, hypomagnesemia); respiratory failure; and concomitant medications known to prolong the QT interval and increase the risk of arrhythmia, such as certain antiarrhythmics, certain antipsychotics, certain antidepressants, bepridil, sparfloxacin, and terodiline. The preceding lists of drugs are not comprehensive. Cisapride should not be used in patients with uncorrected hypokalemia or hypomagnesemia or who might experience rapid reduction of plasma potassium such as those administered potassium-wasting diuretics and/or insulin in acute settings.

Warnings

On March 24, 2000, the FDA announced that the manufacturer of cisapride would voluntarily withdraw its product from the U.S. market on July 14, 2000. This decision was based on 341 reports of heart rhythm abnormalities including 80 reports of deaths. The company will continue to make the drug available to patients who meet specific clinical eligibility criteria for a limited-access protocol (contact 1-800-JANSSEN).

[U.S. Boxed Warning]: Serious cardiac arrhythmias including ventricular tachycardia, ventricular fibrillation, torsade de pointes, and QT prolongation have been reported in patients taking this drug. Many of these patients also took drugs expected to increase cisapride blood levels by inhibiting the cytochrome P450 3A4 enzymes that metabolize cisapride. These drugs include clarithromycin, erythromycin, troleandomycin, nefazodone, fluconazole, itraconazole, ketoconazole, indinavir and ritonavir. Some of these events have been fatal. Cisapride is contraindicated in patients taking any of these drugs. **QT prolongation, torsade de pointes (sometimes with syncope), cardiac arrest and sudden death have been reported in patients taking cisapride without the above-mentioned contraindicated drugs.** Most patients had disorders that may have predisposed them to arrhythmias with cisapride. Cisapride is contraindicated for those patients with: history of prolonged electrocardiographic QT intervals; renal failure; history of ventricular arrhythmias, ischemic heart disease, and CHF; uncorrected electrolyte disorders (hypokalemia, hypomagnesemia); respiratory failure; and concomitant medications known to prolong the QT interval and increase the risk of arrhythmia, such as certain antiarrhythmics, including those of Class 1A (such as quinidine and procainamide) and Class III (such as sotalol); tricyclic antidepressants (such as amitriptyline); certain tetracyclic antidepressants (such as maprotiline); certain antipsychotic medications (such as certain phenothiazines and sertindole), protease inhibitors, bepridil, sparfloxacin and terodiline. (The preceding lists of drugs are not comprehensive.) Recommended doses of cisapride should not be exceeded.

Patients should have a baseline ECG and an electrolyte panel (magnesium, calcium, potassium) prior to initiating cisapride (see Contraindications). Potential benefits should be weighed against risks prior administration of cisapride to patients who have or may develop prolongation of cardiac conduction intervals, particularly QT_c. These include patients with conditions that could predispose them to the development of serious arrhythmias, such as multiple organ failure, COPD, apnea and advanced cancer. Cisapride should not be used in patients with uncorrected hypokalemia or hypomagnesemia, such as those with severe dehydration, vomiting or malnutrition, or those taking potassium-wasting diuretics. Cisapride should not be used in patients who might experience rapid reduction of plasma potassium, such as those administered potassium-wasting diuretics and/or insulin in acute settings. Safety and effectiveness in children have not been established.

Reference Range Single oral dose of 10 mg results in plasma level of 41-65 mg/L; therapeutic range (serum): 32-75 mcg/mL; 900 mg ingestion associated with a serum cisapride level of 143 mcg/mL

Overdosage/Treatment

Decontamination: Lavage (within 1 hour)/activated charcoal

Supportive therapy: Sinus tachydysrhythmias should be treated with esmolol (titrate to desired effect). Torsade de pointes can be treated with magnesium sulfate (Children: 25-50 mg/kg; Adults: 2 g), isoproterenol, or atrial overdrive pacing (at 130-150 beats/minute). Avoid class Ia and class III antiarrhythmic agents.

Enhancement of elimination: Multiple dosing of activated charcoal may be effective; hemodialysis is not useful

Drug Interactions

Substrate of CYP1A2 (minor), 2A6 (minor), 2B6 (minor), 2C9 (minor), 2C19 (minor), 3A4 (major); **Inhibits** CYP2D6 (weak), 3A4 (weak)

Azole antifungals (fluconazole, itraconazole, ketoconazole, miconazole) increase cisapride's concentration. Pre-existing cardiovascular disease or electrolyte imbalances increase the risk of malignant arrhythmias; concurrent use is contraindicated.

Bepridil increases the risk of malignant arrhythmias; concurrent use is contraindicated

Cimetidine increases the bioavailability of cisapride; use an alternative H_2 antagonist

Class Ia (quinidine, procainamide) and Class III (amiodarone, sotalol) antiarrhythmics increase the risk of malignant arrhythmias; concurrent use is contraindicated

CYP3A4 inhibitors: May increase the levels/effects of cisapride. Example inhibitors include azole antifungals, clarithromycin, diclofenac, doxycycline, erythromycin, imatinib, isoniazid, nefazodone, nicardipine, propofol, protease inhibitors, quinidine, telithromycin, and verapamil. Concurrent use of azole antifungals, clarithromycin, erythromycin, nefazodone, and protease inhibitors is contraindicated.

Grapefruit juice may increase the bioavailability of cisapride; concomitant use should be avoided.

Macrolides (clarithromycin, erythromycin, troleandomycin) increase serum concentrations of cisapride. Risk of arrhythmias; concurrent use is contraindicated.

Nefazodone and maprotiline may increase the risk of malignant arrhythmias; concurrent use is contraindicated

Phenothiazines (prochlorperazine, promethazine) may increase the risk of malignant arrhythmias; concurrent use is contraindicated

Pimozide may prolong the QT interval; concurrent use is contraindicated.

Protease inhibitors (amprenavir, atazanavir, indinavir, nelfinavir, ritonavir) increase cisapride's concentration. Increased risk of malignant arrhythmias; concurrent use is contraindicated.

Quinolone antibiotics: Sparfloxacin, gatifloxacin, moxifloxacin increase the risk of malignant arrhythmias; concurrent use is contraindicated

Sertindole may increase the risk of malignant arrhythmias; concurrent use is contraindicated

TCAs increase the risk of malignant arrhythmias; concurrent use is contraindicated

Warfarin: Isolated cases of increased INR; monitor closely

Pregnancy Risk Factor C

Pregnancy Implications Not associated with a major increase in risk of malformations or spontaneous abortions

Lactation Enters breast milk/use caution (AAP rates "compatible")

Additional Information In U.S., available via limited-access protocol only. Rate of torsade de pointes associated with cisapride: 1:120,000 patients

---

Cisplatin

Related Information
- Carboplatin

CAS Number 15663-27-1

U.S. Brand Names Platinol®-AQ

Synonyms CDDP

Use Treatment of bladder, testicular, and ovarian cancer

Unlabeled/Investigational Use Treatment of head and neck, breast, gastric, lung, esophageal, cervical, prostate and small cell lung cancer; Hodgkin's and non-Hodgkin's lymphoma; neuroblastoma; sarcomas, myeloma, melanoma, mesothelioma, and osteosarcoma

Mechanism of Action Inhibits DNA synthesis by the formation of DNA cross-links; denatures the double helix; covalently binds to DNA bases and disrupts DNA function; may also bind to proteins; the *cis*-isomer is 14 times more cytotoxic than the *trans*-isomer; both forms cross-link DNA but cis-platinum is less easily recognized by cell enzymes and, therefore, not repaired. Cisplatin can also bind two adjacent guanines on the same strand of DNA producing intrastrand cross-linking and breakage.

Adverse Reactions

Cardiovascular: Bradycardia, arrhythmias, tachycardia, sinus bradycardia, myocardial depression, sinus tachycardia

Central nervous system: **Neurotoxicity**, convulsions, fever, headache, visual hallucinations, Frey's syndrome, leukoencephalopathy

Dermatologic: Alopecia (mild), urticaria, scleroderma, acral erythema

Endocrine & metabolic: Hypomagnesemia, hypocalcemia, hyponatremia, hypokalemia, hypophosphatemia, **hyperuricemia**

Gastrointestinal: **Nausea, vomiting**, diarrhea, loss of taste perception, mouth sores

Hematologic: **Myelosuppression**, leukopenia, thrombocytopenia, **anemia**, neutropenia, hemolytic/uremic syndrome

Hepatic: Elevated liver enzymes (dose related)

Local: Phlebitis, extravasation injury

Neuromuscular & skeletal: Paresthesia, **neuropathy (peripheral)**, paralysis

Ocular: Papilledema, optic neuropathy, blurred vision, altered color vision, cortical blindness, visual field defects or loss

Otic: **Ototoxicity**, tinnitus (especially pronounced in children and the elderly)

Renal: **Nephrotoxicity** (dose-related proximal tubular defect usually seen in first month of treatment); **acute renal failure, azotemia, chronic renal dysfunction**; Fanconi syndrome

Miscellaneous: **Anaphylactoid reactions**, thirst

Signs and Symptoms of Overdose Bone marrow depression, congestive heart failure, cortical blindness, deafness, dermatitis, encephalopathy, Fanconi syndrome, hyperpigmented hair, hypertension, hyperthermia, hyperuricemia, hypocalcemia, hypokalemia, hypomagnesemia, hyponatremia, hypophosphatemia, hypopigmented hair, leukopenia or neutropenia (agranulocytosis, granulocytopenia), migraine headache (exacerbation), thirst, tubular necrosis

Pharmacodynamics/Kinetics

Distribution: I.V.: Rapidly into tissue; high concentrations in kidneys, liver, ovaries, uterus, and lungs

Protein binding: >90%

Metabolism: Nonenzymatic; inactivated (in both cell and bloodstream) by sulfhydryl groups; covalently binds to glutathione and thiosulfate

Half-life elimination: Initial: 20-30 minutes; Beta: 60 minutes; Terminal: ~24 hours; Secondary half-life: 44-73 hours

Excretion: Urine (>90%); feces (10%)

Dosage

Refer to individual protocols. **VERIFY ANY CISPLATIN DOSE EXCEEDING 100 mg/m² PER COURSE.**

Children (unlabeled uses):

Intermittent dosing schedule: 37-75 mg/m² once every 2-3 weeks or 50-100 mg/m² over 4-6 hours, once every 21-28 days

Daily dosing schedule: 15-20 mg/m²/day for 5 days every 3-4 weeks

Osteogenic sarcoma or neuroblastoma: 60-100 mg/m² on day 1 every 3-4 weeks

Recurrent brain tumors: 60 mg/m² once daily for 2 consecutive days every 3-4 weeks

Bone marrow/blood cell transfusion: Continuous Infusion: High dose: 55 mg/m²/day for 72 hours; total dose = 165 mg/m²

Adults:

Advanced bladder cancer: 50-70 mg/m² every 3-4 weeks

Head and neck cancer (unlabeled use): 100-120 mg/m² every 3-4 weeks

Malignant pleural mesothelioma in combination with pemetrexed (unlabeled use): 75 mg/m² on day 1 of each 21-day cycle; see Pemetrexed monograph for additional details

Metastatic ovarian cancer: 75-100 mg/m² every 3-4 weeks

Intraperitoneal: Cisplatin has been administered intraperitoneal with systemic sodium thiosulfate for ovarian cancer; doses up to 90-270 mg/m² have been administered and retained for 4 hours before draining

Testicular cancer: 10-20 mg/m²/day for 5 days repeated every 3-4 weeks

Dosing adjustment in renal impairment: The manufacturer(s) recommend that repeat courses of cisplatin should not be given until serum creatinine is <1.5 mg/100 mL and/or BUN is <25 mg/100 mL. There is no FDA-approved renal dosing adjustment guideline; the following guidelines have been used by some clinicians:

Kintzel, 1995:

Cl_{cr} 46-60 mL/minute: Reduce dose by 25%

Cl_{cr} 31-45 mL/minute: Reduce dose by 50%

Cl_{cr} <30 mL/minute: Consider use of alternative drug

Aronoff, 1999:

Cl_{cr} 10-50 mL/minute: Administer 75% of dose

Cl$_{cr}$ <10 mL/minute: Administer 50% of dose

Hemodialysis: Partially cleared by hemodialysis; administer dose post-hemodialysis

CAPD effects: Unknown

CAVH effects: Unknown

Stability Incompatible with sodium bicarbonate; do not infuse in solutions containing <0.2% sodium chloride; do not refrigerate reconstituted solutions since precipitation may occur; protect from light; aluminum needles should not be used to administer the drug due to binding with the platinum

Monitoring Parameters Renal function (serum creatinine, BUN, Cl$_{cr}$); electrolytes (particularly magnesium, calcium, potassium) before and within 48 hours after cisplatin therapy; hearing test, neurologic exam (with high dose); liver function tests periodically, CBC with differential and platelet count; urine output, urinalysis

Administration Needles, syringes, catheters, or I.V. administration sets that contain aluminum parts should not be used for administration of drug. Pretreatment hydration with 1-2 L of fluid is recommended prior to cisplatin administration; adequate hydration and urinary output (>100 mL/hour) should be maintained for 24 hours after administration.

I.V.: Rate of administration has varied from a 15- to 120-minute infusion, 1 mg/minute infusion, 6- to 8-hour infusion, 24-hour infusion, or per protocol; maximum rate of infusion of 1 mg/minute in patients with CHF

Extravasation management: Large extravasations (>20 mL) of concentrated solutions (>0.5 mg/mL) produce tissue necrosis. **Treatment is not recommended unless a large amount of highly concentrated solution is extravasated.** Mix 4 mL of 10% sodium thiosulfate with 6 mL sterile water for injection: Inject 1-4 mL through existing I.V. line cannula. Administer 1 mL for each mL extravasated; inject SubQ if needle is removed.

Recommendations for minimizing nephrotoxicity include:

Prepare cisplatin in saline-containing vehicles

Infuse dose over 24 hours

Vigorous hydration (125-150 mL/hour) before, during, and after cisplatin administration

Simultaneous administration of either mannitol or furosemide

Pretreatment with amifostine

Avoid other nephrotoxic agents (aminoglycosides, amphotericin, etc)

Contraindications Hypersensitivity to cisplatin, other platinum-containing compounds, or any component of the formulation (anaphylactic-like reactions have been reported); pre-existing renal insufficiency; myelosuppression; hearing impairment; pregnancy

Warnings Hazardous agent - use appropriate precautions for handling and disposal. **[U.S. Boxed Warning]: Doses > 100 mg/m^2 once every 3-4 weeks are rarely used and should be verified with the prescriber.** All patients should receive adequate hydration, with or without diuretics, prior to and for 24 hours after cisplatin administration. Reduce dosage in renal impairment. **[U.S. Boxed Warning]: Cumulative renal toxicity may be severe.** Elderly patients may be more susceptible to nephrotoxicity; select dose cautiously and monitor closely. **[U.S. Boxed Warnings]: Dose-related toxicities include myelosuppression, nausea, and vomiting. Ototoxicity, especially pronounced in children, is manifested by tinnitus or loss of high frequency hearing and occasionally, deafness.** Serum magnesium, as well as other electrolytes, should be monitored both before and within 48 hours after cisplatin therapy. When administered as sequential infusions, taxane derivatives (docetaxel, paclitaxel) should be administered before platinum derivatives (carboplatin, cisplatin). **[U.S. Boxed Warnings]: Anaphylactic-like reactions have been reported; may be managed with epinephrine, corticosteroids, and/or antihistamines. Should be administered under the supervision of an experienced cancer chemotherapy physician.**

Dosage Forms [DSC] = Discontinued product

Injection, solution: 1 mg/mL (50 mL, 100 mL, 200 mL)

Platinol®-AQ: 1 mg/mL (50 mL, 100 mL) [contains sodium 9 mg/mL] [DSC]

Reference Range

Plasma levels for cytotoxicity: 50 mg/L at 1 hour or 5 mg/L at 8 hours

Heart and peripheral blood concentrations of platinum overdosage of 750 mg were 1515 and 1253 µg/L, respectively. Concentrations in urine and bile were 1038 and 501 µg/L, respectively.

Overdosage/Treatment

Supportive therapy: Erythropoietin can be given to prevent anemia; ondansetron, droperidol, metoclopramide, or corticosteroids can be given for emesis; sodium thiosulfate (7.5 g/m^2 I.V. followed by 2.13 g/m^2/hour over 12 hours) or mannitol (12.5 g) and/or furosemide can decrease nephrotoxicity. Tachycardia can be treated with I.V. verapamil; allopurinol (600-800 mg/day in divided doses) may be useful in managing hyperuricemia. Amifostine (910 mg/m^2) pretreatment may be protective of drug-induced neutropenia, renal toxicity, or ototoxicity.

Enhancement of elimination: Hemodialysis is not effective

Antidote(s)

- Amifostine [ANTIDOTE]
- Mannitol [ANTIDOTE]
- Sodium Thiosulfate [ANTIDOTE]

Diagnostic Procedures

- Electrolytes, Blood

Drug Interactions

Amifostine: Theoretically inactivates drug systemically; has been used clinically to reduce nephrotoxicity and neutropenia associated with administration of cisplatin.

Bleomycin: Delayed bleomycin elimination with decreased glomerular filtration rate.

Ethacrynic acid: Has resulted in severe ototoxicity in animals.

Sodium thiosulfate: Theoretically inactivates drug systemically; has been used clinically to reduce systemic toxicity with intraperitoneal administration of cisplatin.

Taxane derivatives (docetaxel, paclitaxel): When administered as sequential infusions, taxane derivatives should be administered before platinum derivatives to limit myelosuppression and to enhance efficacy.

Pregnancy Risk Factor D

Pregnancy Implications May be toxic to fetal urogenital tract

Lactation Enters breast milk/contraindicated

Nursing Implications Needles, syringes, catheters, or I.V. administration sets that contain aluminum parts should not be used for administration of drug; perform pretreatment hydration with 1-2 liters of fluid infused for 8-12 hours prior to dose; monitor for possible anaphylactoid reaction

Additional Information

Sodium content: 9 mg/mL (equivalent to 0.9% sodium chloride solution)

Osmolality of Platinol®-AQ = 285-286 mOsm

Specific References

Charlier C, Kintz P, Dubois N, et al, "Fatal Overdosage with Cisplatin," *J Anal Toxicol*, 2004, 28(2):138-40.

Dietrich J, Marienhagen J, Schalke B, et al, "Vascular Neurotoxicity Following Chemotherapy with Cisplatin, Ifosfamide, and Etoposide," *Ann Pharmacother*, 2004, 38(2):242-6.

Pourrat X, Antier D, Crenn I, et al, "A Prescription and Administration Error of Cisplatin: A Case Report," *Pharm World Sci*, 2004, 26(2):64-5.

Citalopram

Related Information

- Antidepressant Agents

CAS Number 59729-32-7; 59729-33-8

U.S. Brand Names Celexa™

Synonyms Citalopram Hydrobromide; Nitalapram

Use Treatment of depression

Unlabeled/Investigational Use Treatment of dementia, smoking cessation, ethanol abuse, obsessive-compulsive disorder (OCD) in children, diabetic neuropathy

Mechanism of Action A bicyclic phthalane derivative, citalopram selectively inhibits serotonin reuptake in the presynaptic neurons

Adverse Reactions

Cardiovascular: Chest pain, QT prolonged, thrombosis, ventricular arrhythmia, torsade de pointes

Central nervous system: **Somnolence, insomnia,** anxiety, anorexia, agitation, yawning, akathisia, delirium, neuroleptic malignant syndrome, grand mal seizures

Dermatologic: Rash, pruritus, angioedema, bruising, epidermal necrolysis, erythema multiforme

Endocrine & metabolic: Sexual dysfunction, serotonin syndrome, SIADH, prolactinemia, spontaneous abortion

Gastrointestinal: **Nausea, xerostomia,** diarrhea, dyspepsia, vomiting, abdominal pain, weight gain, hemorrhage, pancreatitis

Genitourinary: Priapism

Hematologic: Hemolytic anemia, thrombocytopenia, prothrombin decreased

Neuromuscular & skeletal: Tremor, arthralgia, myalgia, choreoathetosis, dyskinesia, myoclonus, rhabdomyolysis

Ocular: Nystagmus

Renal: Acute renal failure

Respiratory: Cough, rhinitis, sinusitis

Miscellaneous: **Diaphoresis,** withdrawal syndrome, allergic reaction, anaphylaxis

Signs and Symptoms of Overdose Widened QRS complex at ingestions >600 mg. Coma, CNS depression, prolonged QT interval, rhabdomyolysis, seizures (within a few hours of ingestion), tachycardia

Admission Criteria/Prognosis Admit any ingestion >600 mg to a cardiac-monitored bed

Pharmacodynamics/Kinetics

Distribution: V$_d$: 12 L/kg

Protein binding, plasma: ~80%

Metabolism: Extensively hepatic, including CYP, to N-demethylated, N-oxide, and deaminated metabolites

Bioavailability: 80%

Half-life elimination: 24-48 hours; average 35 hours (doubled with hepatic impairment)

Time to peak, serum: 1-6 hours, average within 4 hours

Excretion: Urine (10% as unchanged drug)

Note: Clearance was decreased, while AUC and half-life were significantly increased in elderly patients and in patients with hepatic impairment. Mild-to-moderate renal impairment may reduce clearance (17%) and prolong half-life of citalopram. No pharmacokinetic information is available concerning patients with severe renal impairment.

Dosage

Oral:

Children and Adolescents: OCD (unlabeled use): 10-40 mg/day

Adults: Depression: Initial: 20 mg/day, generally with an increase to 40 mg/day; doses of more than 40 mg are not usually necessary. Should a dose increase be necessary, it should occur in 20 mg increments at intervals of no less than 1 week. Maximum dose: 60 mg/day; reduce dosage in elderly or those with hepatic impairment.

Monitoring Parameters Monitor patient periodically for symptom resolution; mental status for depression, suicidal ideation (especially at the beginning of therapy or when doses are increased or decreased), anxiety, social functioning, mania, panic attacks; akathisia

Contraindications Hypersensitivity to citalopram or any component of the formulation; hypersensitivity or other adverse sequelae during therapy with other SSRIs; concomitant use with MAO inhibitors or within 2 weeks of discontinuing MAO inhibitors

Warnings *Major psychiatric warnings:*

- **[U.S. Boxed Warning]: Antidepressants increase the risk of suicidal thinking and behavior in children and adolescents with major depressive disorder (MDD) and other depressive disorders;** consider risk prior to prescribing. Closely monitor for clinical worsening, suicidality, or unusual changes in behavior; the child's family or caregiver should be instructed to closely observe the patient and communicate condition with healthcare provider. A medication guide concerning the use of antidepressants in children and teenagers should be dispensed with each prescription. **Citalopram is not FDA approved for use in children.**

- The possibility of a suicide attempt is inherent in major depression and may persist until remission occurs. Patients treated with antidepressants should be observed for clinical worsening and suicidality, especially during the initial few months of a course of drug therapy, or at times of dose changes, either increases or decreases. Worsening depression and severe abrupt suicidality that are not part of the presenting symptoms may require discontinuation or modification of drug therapy. Use caution in high-risk patients during initiation of therapy.

- Prescriptions should be written for the smallest quantity consistent with good patient care. The patient's family or caregiver should be alerted to monitor patients for the emergence of suicidality and associated behaviors such as anxiety, agitation, panic attacks, insomnia, irritability, hostility, impulsivity, akathisia, hypomania, and mania; patients should be instructed to notify their healthcare provider if any of these symptoms or worsening depression or psychosis occur.

- May worsen psychosis in some patients or precipitate a shift to mania or hypomania in patients with bipolar disorder. Monotherapy in patients with bipolar disorder should be avoided. Patients presenting with depressive symptoms should be screened for bipolar disorder. **Citalopram is not FDA approved for the treatment of bipolar depression.**

Key adverse effects:

- Anticholinergic effects: Relatively devoid of these side effects.
- CNS depression: Has a low potential to impair cognitive or motor performance; caution operating hazardous machinery or driving.
- SIADH and hyponatremia: Has been associated with the development of SIADH; hyponatremia has been reported rarely, predominately in the elderly.

Concurrent disease:

- Hepatic impairment: Use caution; clearance is decreased and plasma concentrations are increased; a lower dosage may be needed.
- Platelet aggregation: May impair platelet aggregation, resulting in bleeding.
- Renal impairment: Use caution; clearance is decreased and plasma concentrations are increased; a lower dosage may be needed.
- Sexual dysfunction: May cause or exacerbate sexual dysfunction.

Concurrent drug therapy:

- Anticoagulants/Antiplatelets: Use caution with concomitant use of NSAIDs, ASA, or other drugs that affect coagulation; the risk of bleeding is potentiated.
- CNS depressants: Use caution with concomitant therapy.
- MAO inhibitors: Potential for severe reaction when used with MAO inhibitors; autonomic instability, coma, death, delirium, diaphoresis, hyperthermia, mental status changes/agitation, muscular rigidity, myoclonus, neuroleptic malignant syndrome features, and seizures may occur.

Special populations:

- Elderly: Use caution in elderly patients.
- Pregnancy: Use caution in pregnant patients; high doses of citalopram have been associated with teratogenicity in animals.

Special notes:

- Electroconvulsive therapy: May increase the risks associated with electroconvulsive therapy; consider discontinuing, when possible, prior to ECT treatment.
- Withdrawal syndrome: May cause dysphoric mood, irritability, agitation, dizziness, sensory disturbances, anxiety, confusion, headache, lethargy, emotional lability, insomnia, hypomania, tinnitus, and seizures. Upon discontinuation of citalopram therapy, gradually taper dose. If intolerable symptoms occur following a decrease in dosage or upon discontinuation of therapy, then resuming the previous dose with a more gradual taper should be considered.

Dosage Forms Solution, oral: 10 mg/5 mL (240 mL) [alcohol free, sugar free; peppermint flavor]

Tablet: 10 mg, 20 mg, 40 mg

Reference Range Following a 50 mg oral dose, peak serum citalopram levels range from 120-160 nmol/L

Overdosage/Treatment

Decontamination: Lavage within 2 hours/activated charcoal

Supportive therapy: Administer I.V. hypertonic sodium chloride ($\sim$440 mM in 2 hours) or sodium bicarbonate (1-3 mEq/kg) to normalize QRS duration on ECG; benzodiazepines can be used to treat seizures

Enhanced elimination: Due to possibility of enterohepatic recirculation, multiple dosing of activated charcoal may be effective

Drug Interactions

Substrate of CYP2C19 (major), 2D6 (minor), 3A4 (major); **Inhibits** CYP1A2 (weak), 2B6 (weak), 2C19 (weak), 2D6 (weak)

Aspirin: Concomitant use of citalopram and NSAIDs, aspirin, or other drugs affecting coagulation has been associated with an increased risk of bleeding; monitor.

Beta-blockers: Citalopram may increase levels of some beta-blockers (see Carvedilol and Metoprolol); monitor carefully.

Buspirone: Concurrent use of citalopram with buspirone may cause serotonin syndrome; avoid concurrent use.

Carbamazepine: May enhance the metabolism of citalopram.

Carvedilol: Serum concentrations may be increased; monitor carefully for increased carvedilol effect (hypotension and bradycardia).

Cimetidine: May inhibit the metabolism of citalopram.

CYP2C19 inducers: May decrease the levels/effects of citalopram. Example inducers include aminoglutethimide, carbamazepine, phenytoin, and rifampin.

CYP2C19 inhibitors: May increase the levels/effects of citalopram. Example inhibitors include delavirdine, fluconazole, fluvoxamine, gemfibrozil, isoniazid, omeprazole, and ticlopidine.

CYP3A4 inducers: CYP3A4 inducers may decrease the levels/effects of citalopram. Example inducers include aminoglutethimide, carbamazepine, nafcillin, nevirapine, phenobarbital, phenytoin, and rifamycins.

CYP3A4 inhibitors: May increase the levels/effects of citalopram. Example inhibitors include azole antifungals, clarithromycin, diclofenac, doxycycline, erythromycin, imatinib, isoniazid, nefazodone, nicardipine, propofol, protease inhibitors, quinidine, telithromycin, and verapamil.

Linezolid: Hyperpyrexia, hypertension, tachycardia, confusion, seizures, and **deaths have been reported** with agents which inhibit MAO (serotonin syndrome); this combination should be avoided.

MAO inhibitors: Hyperpyrexia, hypertension, tachycardia, confusion, seizures, and **deaths have been reported** with MAO inhibitors (serotonin syndrome); this combination should be avoided.

Meperidine: Combined use theoretically may increase the risk of serotonin syndrome.

Metoprolol: Citalopram may increase plasma levels of metoprolol; monitor for increased effect.

Moclobemide: Concurrent use of citalopram with moclobemide may cause serotonin syndrome; avoid concurrent use.

Nefazodone: Concurrent use of citalopram with nefazodone may cause serotonin syndrome.

NSAIDs: Concomitant use of citalopram and NSAIDs, aspirin, or other drugs affecting coagulation has been associated with an increased risk of bleeding; monitor.

Ritonavir: Combined use of citalopram with ritonavir may cause serotonin syndrome in HIV-positive patients; monitor.

Selegiline: Concurrent use with citalopram has been reported to cause serotonin syndrome; as an MAO type B inhibitor, the risk of serotonin syndrome may be less than with nonselective MAO inhibitors, and reports indicate that this combination has been well tolerated in Parkinson's patients.

Serotonin reuptake inhibitors: Concurrent use with other reuptake inhibitors may increase the risk of serotonin syndrome.

Sibutramine: May increase the risk of serotonin syndrome with SSRIs.

Sumatriptan (and other serotonin agonists): Concurrent use may result in toxicity; weakness, hyper-reflexia, and incoordination have been observed with sumatriptan and SSRIs. In addition, concurrent use may theoretically increase the risk of serotonin syndrome; includes sumatriptan, naratriptan, rizatriptan, and zolmitriptan.

Tramadol: Concurrent use of citalopram with tramadol may cause serotonin syndrome; avoid concurrent use.

Trazodone: Concurrent use of citalopram with trazodone may cause serotonin syndrome.

Venlafaxine: Combined use with citalopram may increase the risk of serotonin syndrome.

Pregnancy Risk Factor C

Pregnancy Implications Should be used in pregnancy only if potential benefit justifies potential risk

Lactation Enters breast milk/contraindicated

Specific References

Bania TC and Chu J, "Sucrose as a Potential Therapy for Chlorine-Induced Pulmonary Edema," *Acad Emerg Med*, 2006, 13(5):S177-8.

Burrows DL, Hagardorn AN, Harlan GC, et al, "GC-MS Method for the Detection of Citalopram in Biological Matrices," *J Anal Toxicol*, 2003, 27(3):179.

Cuenca PJ, Holt KR, and Hoefle JD, "Seizure Secondary to Citalopram Overdose," *J Emerg Med*, 2004, 26(2):177-81.

Duffull SB, Isbister GK, Dawson AH, et al, "Estimating Population Pharmacokinetic Parameters When Dose and Dose-Time Are Not Known Accurately," *J Toxicol Clin Toxicol*, 2003, 41(5):652.

Engebretsen KM, Harris CR, and Wood JE, "Cardiotoxicity and Late Onset Seizures with Citalopram Overdose," *J Emerg Med*, 2003, 25(2):163-6.

Ertel G and Nesbit T, "Citalopram-Related SIADH," *J Pharm Technol*, 2003, 19:91-3.

Hemels ME, Kasper S, Walter E, et al, "Cost-Effectiveness of Escitalopram Versus Citalopram in the Treatment of Severe Depression," *Ann Pharmacother*, 2004, 38(6):954-960.

Ho R, Norman RF, van Veen MM, et al, "A 3-Year Review of Citalopram and Escitalopram Ingestions," *J Toxicol Clin Toxicol*, 2004, 42(5):746.

Holmgren P, Carlsson B, Zackrisson AL, et al, "Enantioselective Analysis of Citalopram and Its Metabolites in Postmortem Blood and Genotyping for CYD2D6 and CYP2C19," *J Anal Toxicol*, 2004, 28(2):94-104.

Kelly CA, Dhaun N, Laing WJ, et al, "Comparative Toxicity of Citalopram and the Newer Antidepressants After Overdose," *J Toxicol Clin Toxicol*, 2004, 42(1):67-71.

Kelly CA, Upex A, Spencer EP, et al, "Adult Respiratory Distress Syndrome and Renal Failure Associated with Citalopram Overdose," *Hum Exp Toxicol*, 2003, 22(2):103-5.

Kugelberg FC, Druid H, Carlsson B, et al, "Postmortem Redistribution of the Enantiomers of Citalopram and Its Metabolites: An Experimental Study in Rats," *J Anal Toxicol*, 2004, 28(8):631-7.

Kugelberg FC, Kingback M, Carlsson B, et al, "Early-Phase Postmortem Redistribution of the Enantiomers of Citalopram and Its Demethylated Metabolites in Rats," *J Anal Toxicol*, 2005, 29(4):223-8.

Le Bloc'h Y, Woggon B, Weissenrieder H, et al, "Routine Therapeutic Drug Monitoring in Patients Treated with 10-360 mg/day Citalopram," *Ther Drug Monit*, 2003, 25(5):600-8.

Martínez MA, Sánchez de la Torre C, and Almarza E, "A Comparative Solid-Phase Extraction Study for the Simultaneous Determination of Fluvoxamine, Mianserin, Doxepin, Citalopram, Paroxetine, and Etoperidone in Whole Blood by Capillary Gas-Liquid Chromatography with Nitrogen-Phosphorus Detection," *J Anal Toxicol*, 2004, 28(4):174-80.

Masullo LN, Miller MA, Baker SD, et al, "Clinical Course and Toxicokinetic Data Following Isolated Citalopram Overdose in an Infant," *Clin Toxicol*, 2006, 44:165-8.

Rajotte JW and Warren RJ, "Association of Citalopram with Deaths in Northern Ontario: Comparison of Cases with the Literature," *J Anal Toxicol*, 2004, 28:301.

Reis M, Lundmark J, and Bengtsson F, "Therapeutic Drug Monitoring of Racemic Citalopram: A 5-Year Experience in Sweden, 1992-1997," *Ther Drug Monit*, 2003, 25(2):183-91.

Sagduyu A and Sentürk V, "Hypertension Associated with Citalopram," *J Pharm Technol*, 2003, 20:14-6.

Tarabar AF, Hoffman RS, and Nelson LS, "Citalopram Overdose: Late Presentation of Torsade de Pointes (TDP) with Cardiac Arrest," *J Toxicol Clin Toxicol*, 2003, 41(5):676.

Cladribine

CAS Number 4291-63-8

U.S. Brand Names Leustatin®

Synonyms 2-CdA; 2-Chlorodeoxyadenosine; NSC-105014

Use Treatment of hairy cell leukemia, chronic lymphocytic leukemia (CLL), chronic myelogenous leukemia (CML)

Unlabeled/Investigational Use Treatment of chronic lymphocytic leukemia (CLL), chronic myelogenous leukemia (CML), non-Hodgkin's lymphomas, progressive multiple sclerosis

Mechanism of Action A purine nucleoside analogue; prodrug which is activated via phosphorylation by deoxycytidine kinase to a 5'-triphosphate derivative. This active form incorporates into DNA to result in the breakage of DNA strand and shutdown of DNA synthesis. This also results in a depletion of nicotinamide adenine dinucleotide and adenosine triphosphate (ATP). Cladribine is cell-cycle nonspecific.

Adverse Reactions

Allergic: **Fever (70%), chills (18%); skin reactions (erythema, itching) at the catheter site (18%)**

Cardiovascular: Edema, tachycardia

Central nervous system: **Fatigue (17%),** **headache,** dizziness, pains, chills, malaise; severe infections, possibly related to thrombocytopenia

Dermatologic: **Rash,** pruritus, erythema

Gastrointestinal: Nausea (mild to moderate) usually not seen at doses <0.3 mg/kg/day, constipation, abdominal pain

Hematologic: **Myelosuppression** (common, dose-limiting), **leukopenia (70%), anemia (37%), thrombocytopenia**

Nadir: 5-10 days

Recovery: 4-8 weeks

Neuromuscular & skeletal: Myalgia, arthralgia, weakness, paraparesis, quadriplegia (reported at high doses)

Renal: Renal failure at high doses (>0.3 mg/kg/day)

Miscellaneous: Diaphoresis, delayed herpes zoster infections, tumor lysis syndrome, increased risk of opportunistic infection

Signs and Symptoms of Overdose Agranulocytosis, bone marrow suppression, granulocytopenia, insomnia, leukopenia, myalgia, neutropenia, quadriparesis, serum creatinine (increased)

Pharmacodynamics/Kinetics

Absorption: Oral: 55%; SubQ: 100%; Rectal: 20%

Distribution: V_d: 4.52±2.82 L/kg

Protein binding: 20%

Metabolism: Hepatic; 5'-triphosphate moiety-active

Half-life elimination: Biphasic: Alpha: 25 minutes; Beta: 6.7 hours; Terminal, mean: Normal renal function: 5.4 hours

Excretion: Urine (18% to 44%)

Clearance: Estimated systemic: 640 mL/hour/kg

Dosage I.V.: Refer to individual protocols.

Pediatrics: Acute leukemias: 6.2-7.5 mg/m^2/day continuous infusion for days 1-5; maximum tolerated dose was 8.9 mg/m^2/day.

Adults:

Hairy cell leukemia: Continuous infusion:

0.09-0.1 mg/kg/day days 1-7; may be repeated every 28-35 days **or** 3.4 mg/m^2/day SubQ days 1-7

Chronic lymphocytic leukemia: Continuous infusion:

0.1 mg/kg/day days 1-7 **or**

0.028-0.14 mg/kg/day as a 2-hour infusion days 1-5

Chronic myelogenous leukemia: 15 mg/m^2/day as a 1-hour infusion days 1-5; if no response increase dose to 20 mg/m^2/day in the second course.

Stability Store intact vials under refrigeration 2°C to 8°C (36°F to 46°F). Dilutions in 500 mL NS are stable for 72 hours. Stable in PVC containers for 24 hours at room temperature of 15°C to 30°C (59°F to 86°F) and 7 days in Pharmacia Deltec® cassettes. Solutions for 7-day infusion should be prepared in bacteriostatic NS.

Monitoring Parameters Monitor periodic assessment of peripheral blood counts, particularly during the first 4-8 weeks post-treatment, is recommended to detect the development of anemia, neutropenia, and thrombocytopenia and for early detection of any potential sequelae (ie, infection or bleeding)

Administration

I.V.: Administer as a 1- to 2-hour infusion or by continuous infusion

Contraindications Hypersensitivity to cladribine or any component of the formulation

Warnings Hazardous agent - use appropriate precautions for handling and disposal. **[U.S. Boxed Warnings]: Dose-dependent, reversible myelosuppression will occur; use with caution in patients with pre-existing hematologic or immunologic abnormalities. Neurologic toxicity has been reported, usually with higher doses, but may occur at normal doses. Acute renal toxicity has been reported with high doses; use caution when administering with other nephrotoxic agents.** Use caution with renal or hepatic impairment. Fever may occur, with or without neutropenia. Use caution in patients with high tumor burden; tumor lysis syndrome may occur. **[U.S. Boxed Warning]: Should be administered under the supervision of an experienced cancer chemotherapy physician.** Safety and efficacy in children have not been established.

Dosage Forms Injection, solution [preservative free]: 1 mg/mL (10 mL)

Reference Range Infusion of 8.9 mg/m^2/day for 5 days results in a plasma concentration range of 20-54 nmol/L

Overdosage/Treatment

Decontamination: Lavage (within 1 hour)/activated charcoal

Supportive therapy: Cladribine extravasation can be treated with subcutaneous administration of chondroitin sulfate or hyaluronidase

Pregnancy Risk Factor D

Pregnancy Implications Teratogenic effects and fetal mortality were observed in animal studies. There are no adequate and well-controlled studies in pregnant women. Women of childbearing potential should avoid becoming pregnant.

Lactation Excretion in breast milk unknown/not recommended

Clarithromycin

CAS Number 81103-11-9
U.S. Brand Names Biaxin® XL; Biaxin®
Use Treatment against most respiratory pathogens (eg, *S. pyogenes*, *S. pneumoniae*, *S. agalactiae*, *S. viridans*, *M. catarrhalis*, *C. trachomatis*, *Legionella* spp., *Mycoplasma pneumoniae*, *S. aureus*). Clarithromycin is highly active (MICs ≤0.25 mcg/mL) against *H. influenzae*, the combination of clarithromycin and its metabolite demonstrate an additive effect. Additionally, clarithromycin has shown activity against *C. pneumoniae* (including strain TWAR) and *M. avium* infection. Approved for pediatric use to treat *Mycobacterium avium* complex or otitis media. Clarithromycin may have some activity against *Cryptosporidium* and *Toxoplasma* encephalitis. Also used for disseminated *Mycobacterium avium* complex in advanced AIDs patients.

Unlabeled/Investigational Use Pertussis

Mechanism of Action Exerts its antibacterial action by binding to 50S ribosomal subunit resulting in inhibition of protein synthesis. The 14-OH metabolite of clarithromycin is twice as active as the parent compound against certain organisms.

Adverse Reactions

Cardiovascular: Tachycardia (ventricular), torsade de pointes, sinus tachycardia, arrhythmias (ventricular), vasculitis, leukocytoclastic vasculitis

Central nervous system: Headache, delirium, visual hallucinations, fever, psychosis

Dermatologic: Urticaria, pruritus, psoriasis, exanthem, cutaneous vasculitis

Gastrointestinal: Diarrhea, nausea, abnormal taste, dyspepsia, abdominal pain, pseudomembranous colitis, tooth discoloration, gastrointestinal vasculitis

Hematologic: Decreased white blood count, elevated prothrombin time, eosinophilia, thrombocytopenia, thrombocytopenic purpura

Hepatic: Elevation of AST, alkaline phosphatase, and bilirubin

Renal: Proteinuria, hematuria, elevated BUN/serum creatinine, interstitial nephritis

Respiratory: Respiratory tract infection

Miscellaneous: Loss of smell

Signs and Symptoms of Overdose Diarrhea, deafness with or without tinnitus or vertigo, eosinophilia, hematuria, jaundice, nausea, prostration, purpura, reversible pancreatitis, tachycardia (ventricular), vomiting

Pharmacodynamics/Kinetics

Absorption: Highly stable in presence of gastric acid (unlike erythromycin); food delays but does not affect extent of absorption

Distribution: Widely into most body tissues except CNS

Metabolism: Partially hepatic via CYP3A4; converted to 14-OH clarithromycin (active metabolite)

Bioavailability: 50%

Half-life elimination: Clarithromycin: 3-7 hours; 14-OH-clarithromycin: 5-9 hours

Time to peak: 2-4 hours

Excretion: Primarily urine

Clearance: Approximates normal GFR

Dosage

Oral:

Children ≥1 months: Pertussis (CDC guidelines): 15 mg/kg/day divided every 12 hours for 7 days; maximum: 1 g/day

Children ≥6 months:

Community-acquired pneumonia, sinusitis, bronchitis, skin infections: 15 mg/kg/day divided every 12 hours for 10 days

Mycobacterial infection (prevention and treatment): 7.5 mg/kg twice daily, up to 500 mg twice daily. **Note:** Safety of clarithromycin for MAC not studied in children <20 months.

Prophylaxis of bacterial endocarditis: 15 mg/kg 1 hour before procedure (maximum dose: 500 mg)

Adults:

Usual dose: 250-500 mg every 12 hours **or** 1000 mg (two 500 mg extended release tablets) once daily for 7-14 days

Upper respiratory tract: 250-500 mg every 12 hours for 10-14 days

Pharyngitis/tonsillitis: 250 mg every 12 hours for 10 days

Acute maxillary sinusitis: 500 mg every 12 hours **or** 1000 mg (two 500 mg extended release tablets) once daily for 14 days

Lower respiratory tract: 250-500 mg every 12 hours for 7-14 days

Acute exacerbation of chronic bronchitis due to:

M. catarrhalis and *S. pneumoniae*: 250 mg every 12 hours for 7-14 days **or** 1000 mg (two 500 mg extended release tablets) once daily for 7 days

H. influenzae: 500 mg every 12 hours for 7-14 days or 1000 mg (two 500 mg extended release tablets) for 7 days

H. parainfluenzae: 500 mg every 12 hours for 7 days or 1000 mg (two 500 mg extended release tablets) for 7 days

Pneumonia due to:

C. pneumoniae, *M. pneumoniae*, and *S. pneumoniae*: 250 mg every 12 hours for 7-14 days **or** 1000 mg (two 500 mg extended release tablets) once daily for 7 days

H. influenzae: 250 mg every 12 hours for 7 days **or** 1000 mg (two 500 mg extended release tablets) once daily for 7 days

Mycobacterial infection (prevention and treatment): 500 mg twice daily (use with other antimycobacterial drugs, eg, ethambutol, clofazimine, or rifampin)

Pertussis (CDC guidelines): 500 mg twice daily for 7 days

Prophylaxis of bacterial endocarditis: 500 mg 1 hour prior to procedure

Uncomplicated skin and skin structure: 250 mg every 12 hours for 7-14 days

Helicobacter pylori: Dual or triple combination regimen with bismuth subsalicylate, tetracycline, clarithromycin, and an H₂-receptor; or combination of omeprazole and clarithromycin; 500 mg every 8-12 hours for 10-14 days

Elderly: Pharmacokinetics are similar to those in younger adults; may have age-related reductions in renal function; monitor and adjust dose if necessary

Dosing adjustment in renal impairment:

Cl$_{cr}$ <30 mL/minute: Half the normal dose or double the dosing interval

In combination with ritonavir:

Cl$_{cr}$ 30-60 mL/minute: Decrease clarithromycin dose by 50%

Cl$_{cr}$ <30 mL/minute: Decrease clarithromycin dose by 75%

Dosing adjustment in hepatic impairment: No dosing adjustment is needed as long as renal function is normal

Administration

Clarithromycin may be given with or without meals. Give every 12 hours rather than twice daily to avoid peak and trough variation.

Biaxin® XL: Should be given with food. Do not crush or chew extended release tablet.

Contraindications Hypersensitivity to clarithromycin, erythromycin, or any macrolide antibiotic; use with ergot derivatives, pimozide, cisapride; combination with ranitidine bismuth citrate should not be used in patients with history of acute porphyria or Cl$_{cr}$ <25 mL/minute

Warnings Dosage adjustment required with severe renal impairment, decreased dosage or prolonged dosing interval may be appropriate; antibiotic-associated colitis has been reported with use of clarithromycin. Macrolides (including clarithromycin) have been associated with rare QT prolongation and ventricular arrhythmias, including torsade de pointes. The extended release formulation consists of drug within a nondeformable matrix; following drug release/absorption, the matrix/shell is expelled in the stool. The use of nondeformable products in patients with known stricture/narrowing of the GI tract has been associated with symptoms of obstruction. Safety and efficacy in children <6 months of age have not been established.

Dosage Forms

Granules for oral suspension (Biaxin®): 125 mg/5 mL (50 mL, 100 mL); 250 mg/5 mL (50 mL, 100 mL) [fruit punch flavor]

Tablet (Biaxin®): 250 mg, 500 mg

Tablet, extended release (Biaxin® XL): 500 mg

Reference Range Steady-state levels of 250 mg/dose of clarithromycin: ~1 mcg/mL

Overdosage/Treatment

Decontamination: Lavage (within 1 hour)/activated charcoal

Supportive therapy: Acute gastrointestinal irritation can be treated with milk or bismuth subsalicylate, lidocaine can be used for ventricular arrhythmias

Drug Interactions

Substrate of CYP3A4 (major); **Inhibits** CYP1A2 (weak), 3A4 (strong)

Alfentanil (and possibly other narcotic analgesics): Serum levels may be increased by clarithromycin; monitor for increased effect.

Benzodiazepines (those metabolized by CYP3A4, including alprazolam, midazolam, triazolam): Serum levels may be increased by clarithromycin; somnolence and confusion have been reported.

Bromocriptine: Serum levels may be increased by clarithromycin; monitor for increased effect.

Buspirone: Serum levels may be increased by clarithromycin; monitor.

Calcium channel blockers (felodipine, verapamil, and potentially others metabolized by CYP3A4): Serum levels may be increased by clarithromycin; monitor.

Carbamazepine: Serum levels may be increased by clarithromycin; monitor.

Cilostazol: Serum levels may be increased by clarithromycin; monitor.

Cisapride: Serum levels may be increased by clarithromycin; serious arrhythmias have occurred; concurrent use contraindicated.

Clopidogrel: Therapeutic effect may be decreased by clarithromycin; monitor.

Clozapine: Serum levels may be increased by clarithromycin; monitor.

Colchicine: Serum levels/toxicity may be increased by clarithromycin; monitor. Avoid use, if possible.

Cyclosporine: Serum levels may be increased by clarithromycin; monitor serum levels.

CYP3A4 inducers: CYP3A4 inducers may decrease the levels/effects of clarithromycin. Example inducers include aminoglutethimide, carbamazepine, nafcillin, nevirapine, phenobarbital, phenytoin, and rifamycins.

CYP3A4 inhibitors: May increase the levels/effects of clarithromycin. Example inhibitors include azole antifungals, diclofenac, doxycycline, erythromycin, imatinib, isoniazid, nefazodone, nicardipine, propofol, protease inhibitors, quinidine, telithromycin, and verapamil.

CYP3A4 substrates: Clarithromycin may increase the levels/effects of CYP3A4 substrates. Example substrates include benzodiazepines, calcium channel blockers, mirtazapine, nateglinide, nefazodone, tacrolimus, and venlafaxine. Selected benzodiazepines (midazolam and triazolam), cisapride, ergot alkaloids, selected HMG-CoA reductase inhibitors (lovastatin and simvastatin), and pimozide are generally contraindicated with strong CYP3A4 inhibitors.

Delavirdine: Serum levels may be increased by clarithromycin; monitor.

Digoxin: Serum levels may be increased by clarithromycin; digoxin toxicity and potentially fatal arrhythmias have been reported; monitor digoxin levels.

Disopyramide: Serum levels may be increased by clarithromycin; in addition, QT_c prolongation and risk of malignant arrhythmia may be increased; avoid combination.

Ergot alkaloids: Concurrent use may lead to acute ergot toxicity (severe peripheral vasospasm and dysesthesia).

Fluconazole: Increases clarithromycin levels and AUC by ~25%

HMG-CoA reductase inhibitors (atorvastatin, lovastatin, and simvastatin); Clarithromycin may increase serum levels of "statins" metabolized by CYP3A4, increasing the risk of myopathy/rhabdomyolysis (does not include fluvastatin and pravastatin). Switch to pravastatin/fluvastatin or suspend treatment during course of clarithromycin therapy.

Methylprednisolone: Serum levels may be increased by clarithromycin; monitor.

Phenytoin: Serum levels may be increased by clarithromycin; other evidence suggested phenytoin levels may be decreased in some patients; monitor.

Pimozide: Serum levels may be increased, leading to malignant arrhythmias; concomitant use is contraindicated.

Protease inhibitors (amprenavir, nelfinavir, and ritonavir): May increase serum levels of clarithromycin.

QT_c-prolonging agents: Concomitant use may increase the risk of malignant arrhythmias.

Quinidine: Serum levels may be increased by clarithromycin; in addition, the risk of QT_c prolongation and malignant arrhythmias may be increased during concurrent use.

Quinolone antibiotics (sparfloxacin, gatifloxacin, or moxifloxacin): Concurrent use may increase the risk of malignant arrhythmias.

Rifabutin: Serum levels may be increased by clarithromycin; monitor.

Sildenafil, tadalafil, vardenafil: Serum levels may be increased by clarithromycin. Do not exceed single sildenafil doses of 25 mg in 48 hours, a single tadalafil dose of 10 mg in 72 hours, or a single vardenafil dose of 2.5 mg in 24 hours.

Tacrolimus: Serum levels may be increased by clarithromycin; monitor serum concentration.

Theophylline: Serum levels may be increased by clarithromycin; monitor.

Thioridazine: Risk of QT_c prolongation and malignant arrhythmias may be increased.

Valproic acid (and derivatives): Serum levels may be increased by clarithromycin; monitor.

Vinblastine (and vincristine): Serum levels may be increased by clarithromycin.

Warfarin: Effects may be potentiated; monitor INR closely and adjust warfarin dose as needed or choose another antibiotic

Zidovudine: Peak levels (but not AUC) of zidovudine may be increased; other studies suggest levels may be decreased.

Zopiclone: Serum levels may be increased by clarithromycin; monitor.

Pregnancy Risk Factor C

Pregnancy Implications There are no adequate and well-controlled studies in pregnant women. Due to adverse fetal effects reported in animal studies, the manufacturer recommends that clarithromycin not be used in a pregnant woman unless there are no alternatives to therapy.

Lactation Excretion in breast milk unknown/use caution

Nursing Implications Give every 12 hours rather than twice daily to avoid peak and trough variation

Additional Information In comparative trials, clarithromycin has been shown to be as effective treatment as penicillin for streptococcal pharyngitis, amoxicillin for acute maxillary sinusitis, ampicillin or erythromycin for acute bacterial exacerbations of chronic bronchitis, erythromycin for community acquired pneumonia, and erythromycin or cefadroxil for skin infections. In small studies, clarithromycin has also demonstrated efficacy in the treatment of *M. pneumoniae*, *C. pneumoniae*, and *Legionella pneumophila* respiratory tract infections. Additionally, the data from a short-term trial involving only small numbers of patients suggest that clarithromycin has clear activity against *M. avium* and may benefit patients with AIDS and disseminated *M. avium* infection.

Specific References

Basyigit I, Yildiz F, Ozkara SK, et al, "The Effect of Clarithromycin on Inflammatory Markers in Chronic Obstructive Pulmonary Disease: Preliminary Data," *Ann Pharmacother*, 2004, 38(9):1400-5.

Carro, et al, "Acute Pancreatitis and Modified-Release Clarithromycin," *Ann Pharmacother*, 2004, 38:508-9.

Geronimo-Pardo M, Cuartero-Del-Pozo AB, Jimenez-Vizuete JM, et al, "Clarithromycin-Nifedipine Interaction as Possible Cause of Vasodilatory Shock," *Ann Pharmacother*, 2005, 39(3):538-42.

Giannattasi A, D'Ambrosi M, Volpicelli M, et al, "Steroid Therapy for a Case of Severe Drug-Induced Cholestasis," *Ann Pharmacother*, 2006, 40(6):1196-99.

Tanaka H, Matsumoto K, Ueno K, et al, "Effect of Clarithromycin on Steady-State Digoxin Concentrations," *Ann Pharmacother*, 2003, 37(2):178-81.

Tietz A, Heim MH, Eriksson U, et al, "Fulminant Liver Failure Associated with Clarithromycin," *Ann Pharmacother*, 2003, 37(1):57-60.

Clemastine

CAS Number 14976-57-9; 15686-51-8

U.S. Brand Names Dayhist® Allergy [OTC]; Tavist® Allergy [OTC]

Synonyms Clemastine Fumarate

Use Perennial and seasonal allergic rhinitis and other allergic symptoms including rash

Mechanism of Action Competes with histamine for H_1-receptor sites on effector cells in the GI tract, blood vessels, and respiratory tract

Adverse Reactions

Frequency not defined.

Cardiovascular: Palpitations, hypotension, tachycardia

Central nervous system: Dyscoordination, sedation, slight to moderate somnolence, sleepiness, confusion, restlessness, nervousness, insomnia, irritability, fatigue, headache, increased dizziness

Dermatologic: Rash, photosensitivity

Gastrointestinal: Diarrhea, nausea, xerostomia, epigastric distress, vomiting, constipation

Genitourinary: Urinary frequency, difficult urination, urinary retention

Hematologic: Hemolytic anemia, thrombocytopenia, agranulocytosis

Ocular: Blurred vision

Otic: Tinnitus

Respiratory: Thickening of bronchial secretions

Miscellaneous: Anaphylaxis

Pharmacodynamics/Kinetics

Onset of action: Peak effect: Therapeutic: 5-7 hours

Duration: 8-16 hours

Absorption: Almost complete

Metabolism: Hepatic

Excretion: Urine

Dosage

Oral:

Infants and Children <6 years: 0.05 mg/kg/day as **clemastine base** or 0.335-0.67 mg/day clemastine fumarate (0.25-0.5 mg base/day) divided into 2 or 3 doses; maximum daily dosage: 1.34 mg (1 mg base)

Children 6-12 years: 0.67-1.34 mg clemastine fumarate (0.5-1 mg base) twice daily; do not exceed 4.02 mg/day (3 mg/day base)

Children ≥12 years and Adults:

1.34 mg clemastine fumarate (1 mg base) twice daily to 2.68 mg (2 mg base) 3 times/day; do not exceed 8.04 mg/day (6 mg base)

OTC labeling: 1.34 mg clemastine fumarate (1 mg base) twice daily; do not exceed 2 mg base/24 hours

Elderly: Lower doses should be considered in patients >60 years

Monitoring Parameters Look for a reduction of rhinitis, urticaria, eczema, pruritus, or other allergic symptoms

Contraindications Hypersensitivity to clemastine or any component of the formulation; narrow-angle glaucoma

Warnings Safety and efficacy have not been established in children <6 years of age. Use caution with bladder neck obstruction, symptomatic prostate hypertrophy, asthmatic attacks, stenosing peptic ulcer, increased intraocular pressure, hyperthyroidism, cardiovascular disease, hypertension, and in the elderly. May cause drowsiness; use caution in performing tasks which require alertness.

Dosage Forms

Syrup, as fumarate [prescription formulation]: 0.67 mg/5 mL (120 mL) [0.5 mg base/5 mL; contains alcohol 5.5%; citrus flavor]

Tablet, as fumarate: 1.34 mg [1 mg base; OTC], 2.68 mg [2 mg base; prescription formulation]

Dayhist® Allergy, Tavist® Allergy: 1.34 mg [1 mg base]

Overdosage/Treatment Supportive therapy: There is no specific treatment for an antihistamine overdose, however, most of its clinical toxicity is due to anticholinergic effects. For anticholinergic overdose with severe life-threatening symptoms, physostigmine 1-2 mg (0.5 or 0.02 mg/kg for children) I.V., slowly may be given to reverse these effects.

Test Interactions May suppress wheal and flare response to antigen skin testing

Drug Interactions

Inhibits CYP2D6 (weak), 3A4 (weak)

Increased toxicity (CNS depression): CNS depressants, MAO inhibitors, tricyclic antidepressants, phenothiazines

Pregnancy Risk Factor B

Lactation Enters breast milk/not recommended

Nursing Implications Raise bed rails, institute safety measures, assist with ambulation

Additional Information Clemastine fumarate 1.34 mg = clemastine base 1 mg; offers no significant benefit over other antihistamines except that it may be dosed twice daily (in adults) as compared to other antihistamines with more frequent dosing

Clenbuterol

Related Information

● Albuterol

CAS Number 21898-19-1; 3714-27-9

Use Asthma/exercise-induced asthma; also has been utilized as an ergogenic acid (unapproved use); used illicitly in animal feed to enhance animal weight gain

Mechanism of Action A long-acting sympathomimetic agent with direct β-2 adrenergic properties and enhanced lipolytic effect

Adverse Reactions

Cardiovascular: Tachycardia, palpitations (25%)

Central nervous system: Dizziness, headache, tremors (11%), dyskinesia

Dermal: Contact dermatitis

Gastrointestinal: Nausea, dry mouth

Miscellaneous: Diaphoresis

Signs and Symptoms of Overdose Hyperglycemia, hypokalemia, tachycardia (usually without elevated blood pressure), tremor; symptoms may last for 6 days

Admission Criteria/Prognosis Admit any ingestion >3 mcg/kg, or any patient with tachycardia or electrolyte deficiencies

Toxicodynamics/Kinetics

Onset of action: Initial: 15 minutes

Duration of action: 4-12 hours

Metabolism: Liver (slight)

Bioavailability (oral): 70% to 80%

Half-life: 25-39 hours

Elimination: Renal (clearance 38-60 mL/minute)

Dosage

Oral: Adults: 20-40 mcg twice daily; ergogenic dose: up to 600 mcg/day

Inhalation: 20 mcg 3 times/day

Reference Range Steady-state clenbuterol serum level is ~293 pg/mL in doses of 20 mcg twice daily

Overdosage/Treatment

Decontamination: Oral: Activated charcoal (without cathartic)

Supportive therapy: Monitor and replace potassium as needed. Monitor cardiac status. Tachycardia can be treated with esmolol or metoprolol.

Pregnancy Implications A uterine relaxant

Additional Information May increase protein deposition in striated muscle by 20%, resulting in muscle hypertrophy (type II fibers).

Clobazam

CAS Number 22316-47-8

Impairment Potential Yes

Use Adjunctive treatment of epilepsy

Unlabeled/Investigational Use Monotherapy for epilepsy or intermittent seizures, antianxiety, anticonvulsant, and sedative agent

Mechanism of Action Facilitates gamma-aminobutyric acid neurotransmission; a 1,5 benzodiazepine derivative; weak hypnotic agent

Adverse Reactions

May induce systemic lupus erythematosus

Cardiovascular: Hypotension (orthostatic), syncope

Central nervous system: Sedation, dizziness, lightheadedness, headache, ataxia, CNS depression, depression, aggressive behavior

Dermatologic: Toxic epidermal necrolysis

Gastrointestinal: Xerostomia, weight gain

Signs and Symptoms of Overdose Confusion, dizziness

Pharmacodynamics/Kinetics

Absorption: Rapid

Protein binding: 85% to 91%

Metabolism: Hepatic via N-dealkylation (likely via CYP) to active metabolite (N-desmethyl), and glucuronidation

Bioavailability: 87%

Half-life elimination: 18 hours; N-desmethyl (active): 42 hours

Time to peak: 15 minutes to 4 hours

Excretion: Urine (90%), as metabolites

Dosage

Adults: 20-30 mg/day in divided doses or at night; maximum daily dose: 60 mg

Elderly: 10-20 mg/day

Administration

May be administered with food.

Contraindications Hypersensitivity to clobazam or any component of the formulation (cross sensitivity with other benzodiazepines may exist); myasthenia gravis; narrow-angle glaucoma; severe hepatic or respiratory disease; sleep apnea; history of substance abuse; use in pregnancy (particularly 1st trimester); breast-feeding is contraindicated per manufacturer

Warnings

Rebound or withdrawal symptoms may occur following abrupt discontinuation or large decreases in dose (more common with prolonged treatment). Cautiously taper dose if drug discontinuation is required. Use with caution in elderly or debilitated patients, patients with hepatic disease (including alcoholics), renal impairment, or obese patients.

Causes CNS depression (dose related) resulting in sedation, dizziness, confusion, or ataxia which may impair physical and mental capabilities. Patients must be cautioned about performing tasks which require mental alertness (eg, operating machinery or driving). Use with caution in patients receiving other CNS depressants or psychoactive agents. Effects with other sedative drugs or ethanol may be potentiated. Benzodiazepines have been associated with falls and traumatic injury and should be used with caution in patients who are at risk of these events (especially the elderly). Use with caution in patients with respiratory disease or impaired gag reflex.

Tolerance and loss of seizure control have been reported with chronic administration. Not recommended in patients with psychosis or depression (particularly if suicidal risk may be present). May cause physical or psychological dependence - avoid in patients with a history of drug dependence. Acute withdrawal, including seizures, may be precipitated in patients after administration of flumazenil to patients receiving long-term benzodiazepine therapy.

Benzodiazepines have been associated with anterograde amnesia. Paradoxical reactions, including hyperactive or aggressive behavior, have been reported with benzodiazepines, particularly in adolescent/pediatric or psychiatric patients. Does not have analgesic, antidepressant, or antipsychotic properties.

Dosage Forms

[CAN] = Canadian brand name

Tablet: 10 mg

Alti-Clobazam [CAN], Apo-Clobazam® [CAN], Clobazam-10 [CAN], Dom-Clobazam [CAN], Frisium® [CAN], Novo-Clobazam [CAN], PMS-Clobazam [CAN], ration-Clobazam [CAN]: 10 mg [not available in the U.S.]

Reference Range After a 40 mg oral dose, peak plasma levels are ~730 mcg/L

Overdosage/Treatment

Decontamination: Lavage (within 1 hour)/activated charcoal

Supportive therapy: Rarely is mechanical ventilation required; flumazenil has been shown to selectively block the binding of benzodiazepines to CNS receptors, resulting in a reversal of benzodiazepine-induced CNS depression and respiratory depression

Enhancement of elimination: Multiple dose of activated charcoal is effective

Antidote(s)

● Flumazenil [ANTIDOTE]

Drug Interactions

Substrate (major) of CYP2C19 and 3A4

Anticonvulsants (carbamazepine, phenytoin, valproate, phenobarbital): Clinically-significant interactions are rare, but reports of clobazam increasing levels of carbamazepine, phenytoin, valproate, and phenobarbital exist. Enzyme-inducing agents may decrease clobazam concentrations.

CNS depressants: Sedative effects and/or respiratory depression may be additive with CNS depressants. Includes ethanol, barbiturates, narcotic analgesics, and other sedative agents; monitor for increased effect.

CYP2C19 inhibitors: May increase the levels/effects of clobazam. Example inhibitors include delavirdine, fluconazole, fluvoxamine, gemfibrozil, isoniazid, omeprazole, and ticlopidine.

CYP3A4 inducers: CYP3A4 inducers may decrease the levels/effects of clobazam. Example inducers include aminoglutethimide, carbamazepine, nafcillin, nevirapine, phenobarbital, phenytoin, and rifamycins.

CYP3A4 inhibitors: May increase the levels/effects of clobazam. Example inhibitors include azole antifungals, clarithromycin, diclofenac, doxycycline, erythromycin, imatinib, isoniazid, nefazodone, nicardipine, propofol, protease inhibitors, quinidine, telithromycin, and verapamil.

Levodopa: Therapeutic effects may be diminished in some patients following the addition of a benzodiazepine; limited/inconsistent data.

Theophylline: May partially antagonize some of the effects of benzodiazepines; monitor for decreased response; may require higher doses for sedation.

Pregnancy Risk Factor Not assigned; similar agents rated D. Contraindicated in 1st trimester (per manufacturer).

Pregnancy Implications Clobazam crosses the placenta. Oral clefts reported with benzodiazepines, however, more recent data does not support an association between drug and oral clefts. Inguinal hernia, cardiac defects, spina bifida, dysmorphic facial features, skeletal defects, multiple other malformations also reported. Hypotonia and withdrawal symptoms reported following use during 3rd trimester or near time of delivery.

Lactation Enters breast milk/contraindicated (AAP rates other benzodiazepines "of concern"); clinical effects on infant include sedation

Additional Information Used to relieve phantom limb pain; similar efficacy as with buspirone in treatment of anxiety/panic disorders; oral ingestion of 300 mg has produced mental status changes; reduce dosage in elderly and cirrhosis

Clofibrate

CAS Number 637-07-0; 882-09-7
U.S. Brand Names Atromid-S® [DSC]
Use Adjunct to dietary therapy in the management of type III hyperlipidemias associated with high triglyceride levels
Mechanism of Action Mechanism is unclear but thought to reduce cholesterol synthesis and triglyceride hepatic-vascular transference (a fibric acid derivative)
Adverse Reactions
Cardiovascular: Angina, cardiac arrhythmias, cardiomyopathy, chest pain
Central nervous system: Headache, dizziness, fatigue
Dermatologic: Skin rash, pruritus, dry brittle hair, alopecia, Stevens-Johnson syndrome, desquamation (scaling), toxic epidermal necrolysis, exfoliative dermatitis, xerosis, urticaria, purpura, photosensitivity, exanthem
Endocrine & metabolic: Syndrome of inappropriate antidiuretic hormone, gynecomastia
Gastrointestinal: **Nausea** which usually decreases with continued therapy or reduction in dosage; diarrhea, vomiting, dyspepsia, flatulence, abdominal distress, gallstones, stomatitis
Genitourinary: Impotence
Hematologic: Anemia, eosinophilia, eosinophilic pneumonitis, leukopenia, neutropenia, agranulocytosis, granulocytopenia
Hepatic: Increased liver function tests, increased incidence of cholecystitis
Neuromuscular & skeletal: Myalgia, aching, muscle cramping, myopathy (associated with hypoalbuminemia), rhabdomyolysis, weakness
Ocular: Photophobia
Renal: Rhabdomyolysis-induced renal failure, renal insufficiency, renal toxicity
Miscellaneous: Systemic lupus erythematosus
Signs and Symptoms of Overdose Cardiomegaly, cholelithiasis, desquamation, dysuria, erythema multiforme, fever, hematuria, hyperthermia, hyponatremia, impotence, lethargy, myalgia, myoglobinuria, photophobia
Toxicodynamics/Kinetics
Absorption: Occurs completely; intestinal transformation is required to activate the drug
Distribution: V_d: 5.5 L/kg
Protein binding: 95% (75% in patients with nephrotic syndrome)
Metabolism: In the liver to an inactive glucuronide ester and an active metabolite (clofibric acid)
Half-life: 6-24 hours, increases significantly with reduced renal function; with anuria: 110 hours
Time to peak serum concentration: Within 3-6 hours
Elimination: 40% to 70% excreted in urine; clearance: 1.5-2.0 mL/minute
Dosage
Adults: Oral: 500 mg 4 times/day; some patients may respond to lower doses
  Dosing interval in renal impairment:
  Cl_{cr} 10-50 mL/minute: Administer every 12-18 hours
  Cl_{cr} <10 mL/minute: Avoid use
Monitoring Parameters Serum lipids, cholesterol and triglycerides, LFTs, CBC
Reference Range Therapeutic plasma level of parachlorophenoxyisobutyric acid: 80-150 mcg/mL
Overdosage/Treatment
Decontamination: Emesis within 30 minutes or lavage (within 1 hour)/activated charcoal
Enhancement of elimination: Multiple dosing of activated charcoal may be effective
Test Interactions ↑ creatine phosphokinase (CPK), aldolase, serum AST (S); ↓ alkaline phosphatase (S), cholesterol (S), glucose, uric acid (S), fibrinogen, plasma thyroxine
Pregnancy Risk Factor C
Pregnancy Implications Crosses the placenta
Additional Information Atromid-S® discontinued in January 2001; not available in the U.S.

ClomiPHENE

CAS Number 15690-55-8; 15690-57-0; 50-41-9; 7599-79-3; 7619-53-6; 911-45-5
U.S. Brand Names Clomid®; Serophene®
Synonyms Clomiphene Citrate
Use Treatment of ovulatory failure in patients desiring pregnancy
Unlabeled/Investigational Use Male infertility
Mechanism of Action Induces ovulation by stimulating the release of pituitary gonadotropins; triphenylethylene which binds to estrogen receptors; acts as an antagonist at low doses but is an estrogen agonist at doses >100 mg
Adverse Reactions
Central nervous system: Dizziness, psychosis, dementia, headache, ataxia, coma
Dermatologic: Alopecia (reversible), rash, neutrophilic dermatosis (Sweet's syndrome)
Endocrine & metabolic: **Ovarian enlargement**, ectopic pregnancy, gynecomastia, **hot flashes**, breast tenderness, diabetes insipidus, hypertriglyceridemia
Gastrointestinal: Gastric distention, bloating, nausea, vomiting, stomatitis, abdominal/pelvic pain, weight gain, pancreatitis
Ocular: **Blurring of vision**, photophobia, diplopia, cataract formation, palinopsia, color vision abnormalities
Renal: Polyuria
Miscellaneous: Anterior pituitary hemorrhage
Pharmacodynamics/Kinetics
Metabolism: Undergoes enterohepatic recirculation
Half-life elimination: 5-7 days
Excretion: Primarily feces; urine (small amounts)
Dosage Adults: Female: Oral: 50 mg/day for 5 days (first course); start the regimen on or about the fifth day of cycle; if ovulation occurs, do not increase dosage; if ovulation does not occur, increase next course to 100 mg/day for 5 days. Three courses of therapy are an adequate therapeutic trial. Further treatment is not recommended in patients who do not exhibit ovulation.
Contraindications Hypersensitivity to clomiphene citrate or any of its components; liver disease; abnormal uterine bleeding; enlargement or development of ovarian cyst; uncontrolled thyroid or adrenal dysfunction in the presence of an organic intracranial lesion such as pituitary tumor; pregnancy
Warnings Use with caution in patients unusually sensitive to pituitary gonadotropins (eg, polycystic ovary disease). Multiple pregnancies, blurring or other visual symptoms, ovarian hyperstimulation syndrome, and abdominal pain can occur.
Dosage Forms Tablet, as citrate: 50 mg
Overdosage/Treatment
Decontamination: Lavage (within 1 hour)/activated charcoal
Enhancement of elimination: Due to its enterohepatic recirculation, multiple dosing of activated charcoal may be effective
Test Interactions FSH/LH levels increase by ∼150%
Drug Interactions Decreased response when used with danazol; decreased estradiol response when used with clomiphene
Pregnancy Risk Factor X
Pregnancy Implications Multiple births occur in ∼10% of pregnancies with induced ovulation; increased frequency of delayed follicular rupture and ectopic pregnancy also noted
Lactation Excretion in breast milk unknown/contraindicated
Additional Information Has been associated with testicular cancer, ectopic pregnancy, ovarian cancer

ClomiPRAMINE

CAS Number 17321-77-6; 303-49-1
U.S. Brand Names Anafranil®
Synonyms Clomipramine Hydrochloride
Use Treatment of obsessive-compulsive disorder (OCD)
Unlabeled/Investigational Use Depression, panic attacks, chronic pain
Mechanism of Action Clomipramine appears to affect serotonin uptake while its active metabolite, desmethylclomipramine, affects norepinephrine uptake; a tricyclic tertiary amine antidepressant
Adverse Reactions
Cardiovascular: Hypotension (orthostatic), tachycardia, flushing, QRS prolongation, sinus tachycardia, tachycardia (supraventricular), vasculitis, cardiomyopathy, exacerbation of Brugada syndrome
Central nervous system: **Drowsiness, dizziness, headache**, neuroleptic malignant syndrome, convulsions, psychosis, serotonin syndrome (confusion, restlessness, diarrhea), aggressive behavior
Dermatologic: Photosensitivity, hypertrichosis, acne, alopecia, xerosis, urticaria, purpura, pruritus, psoriasis, exanthem
Endocrine & metabolic: Hyponatremia, syndrome of inappropriate antidiuretic hormone, spontaneous orgasm (when yawning) may occur, gynecomastia

Gastrointestinal: **Xerostomia, constipation, increased appetite, nausea, unpleasant taste, weight gain**, stomatitis, lingua villosa nigra

Hepatic: Acute hepatitis

Neuromuscular & skeletal: Hyperreflexia, clonus, myoclonus, paresthesia

Ocular: Amaurosis fugax, visual hallucinations

Respiratory: Eosinophilic pneumonia

Miscellaneous: Diaphoresis

Signs and Symptoms of Overdose Agitation, agranulocytosis, apnea, confusion, hallucinations, hyperprolactinemia, hyperthermia, hypotension, lactation, leukopenia, mania, memory loss, myoclonus, neuroleptic malignant syndrome, nystagmus, photosensitivity, seizures, tachycardia, thrombocytopenia, urinary retention

Admission Criteria/Prognosis Admit any patient who displays symptoms (including sinus tachycardia) 6 hours postingestion

Pharmacodynamics/Kinetics

Absorption: Rapid

Metabolism: Hepatic to desmethylclomipramine (active); extensive first-pass effect

Half-life elimination: 20-30 hours

Dosage

Oral: Initial:

Children: 25 mg/day and gradually increase, as tolerated, to a maximum of 3 mg/kg/day or 200 mg/day, whichever is smaller

Adults: 25 mg/day and gradually increase, as tolerated, to 100 mg/day the first 2 weeks, may then be increased to a total of 250 mg/day maximum

Monitoring Parameters Pulse rate and blood pressure prior to and during therapy; ECG/cardiac status in older adults and patients with cardiac disease

Contraindications Hypersensitivity to clomipramine, other tricyclic agents, or any component of the formulation; use of MAO inhibitors within 14 days; use in a patient during the acute recovery phase of MI

Warnings

[U.S. Boxed Warning]: Antidepressants increase the risk of suicidal thinking and behavior in children and adolescents with major depressive disorder (MDD) and other depressive disorders; consider risk prior to prescribing. Closely monitor for clinical worsening, suicidality, or unusual changes in behavior; the child's family or caregiver should be instructed to closely observe the patient and communicate condition with healthcare provider. Such observation would generally include at least weekly face-to-face contact with patients or their family members or caregivers during the first 4 weeks of treatment, then every other week visits for the next 4 weeks, then at 12 weeks, and as clinically indicated beyond 12 weeks. Additional contact by telephone may be appropriate between face-to-face visits. Adults treated with antidepressants should be observed similarly for clinical worsening and suicidality, especially during the initial few months of a course of drug therapy, or at times of dose changes, either increases or decreases. A medication guide should be dispensed with each prescription. **Clomipramine is FDA approved for the treatment of OCD in children ≥10 years of age.**

The possibility of a suicide attempt is inherent in major depression and may persist until remission occurs. Monitor for worsening of depression or suicidality, especially during initiation of therapy or with dose increases or decreases. Worsening depression and severe abrupt suicidality that are not part of the presenting symptoms may require discontinuation or modification of drug therapy. Use caution in high-risk patients during initiation of therapy. Prescriptions should be written for the smallest quantity consistent with good patient care. The patient's family or caregiver should be alerted to monitor patients for the emergence of suicidality and associated behaviors such as anxiety, agitation, panic attacks, insomnia, irritability, hostility, impulsivity, akathisia, hypomania, and mania; patients should be instructed to notify their healthcare provider if any of these symptoms or worsening depression occur.

May worsen psychosis in some patients or precipitate a shift to mania or hypomania in patients with bipolar disorder. Monotherapy in patients with bipolar disorder should be avoided. Patients presenting with depressive symptoms should be screened for bipolar disorder. **Clomipramine is not FDA approved for the treatment of bipolar depression.**

May cause seizures (relationship to dose and/or duration of therapy) - do not exceed maximum doses. Use caution in patients with a previous seizure disorder or condition predisposing to seizures such as brain damage, alcoholism, or concurrent therapy with other drugs which lower the seizure threshold. Has been associated with a high incidence of sexual dysfunction. Weight gain may occur. May cause sedation, resulting in impaired performance of tasks requiring alertness (eg, operating machinery or driving). Sedative effects may be additive with other CNS depressants and/or ethanol. The degree of sedation is very high relative to other antidepressants. May increase the risks associated with electroconvulsive therapy. Consider discontinuing, when possible, prior to elective surgery. Therapy should not be abruptly discontinued in patients receiving high doses for prolonged periods.

May cause orthostatic hypotension (risk is moderate to high relative to other antidepressants) - use with caution in patients at risk of hypotension or in patients where transient hypotensive episodes would be poorly tolerated (cardiovascular disease or cerebrovascular disease). The degree of anticholinergic blockade produced by this agent is very high relative to other cyclic antidepressants - use caution in patients with urinary retention, benign prostatic hyperplasia, narrow-angle glaucoma, xerostomia, visual problems, constipation, or history of bowel obstruction.

Use with caution in patients with a history of cardiovascular disease (including previous MI, stroke, tachycardia, or conduction abnormalities). The risk conduction abnormalities with this agent is high relative to other antidepressants. Use with caution in hyperthyroid patients or those receiving thyroid supplementation. Use with caution in patients with hepatic or renal dysfunction and in elderly patient.

Dosage Forms Capsule, as hydrochloride: 25 mg, 50 mg, 75 mg

Reference Range Level of 6560 ng/mL associated with fatality; serum levels may not peak until the fourth day; plasma levels >1 mg/L associated with serious toxicity

Overdosage/Treatment

Decontamination: Lavage (within 3 hours)/activated charcoal; multiple dosing of activated charcoal may be effective

Supportive therapy: Following initiation of essential overdose management, toxic symptoms should be treated. Ventricular arrhythmias often respond to phenytoin 15-20 mg/kg (adults) with concurrent systemic alkalinization (sodium bicarbonate 0.5-2 mEq/kg I.V.). Arrhythmias unresponsive to this therapy may respond to lidocaine 1 mg/kg I.V. followed by a titrated infusion. Physostigmine (1-2 mg I.V. slowly for adults or 0.5 mg I.V. slowly for children) may be indicated in reversing seizures or movement disorders, but **only as a last resort.** Seizures usually respond to lorazepam or diazepam I.V. boluses (5-10 mg for adults up to 30 mg or 0.25-0.4 mg/kg/dose for children up to 10 mg/dose). If seizures are unresponsive or recur, phenytoin or phenobarbital may be required. For treatment of lingua villosa nigra, discontinue causative agent. Clean the tongue with a toothbrush and rinse mouth with a half-strength solution of hydrogen peroxide or 10% carbamide peroxide. Symptoms should subside in a few days.

Test Interactions ↑ glucose, plasma catecholamine

Drug Interactions

Substrate of CYP1A2 (major), 2C19 (major), 2D6 (major), 3A4 (minor); **Inhibits** CYP2D6 (moderate)

Altretamine: Concurrent use may cause orthostatic hypertension.

Amphetamines: TCAs may enhance the effect of amphetamines; monitor for adverse CV effects.

Anticholinergics: Combined use with TCAs may produce additive anticholinergic effects.

Antihypertensives: TCAs inhibit the antihypertensive response to bethanidine, clonidine, debrisoquin, guanadrel, guanethidine, guanabenz, guanfacine; monitor BP; consider alternate antihypertensive agent.

Beta-agonists: When combined with TCAs may predispose patients to cardiac arrhythmias.

Bupropion: May increase the levels of tricyclic antidepressants; based on limited information; monitor response.

Carbamazepine: Tricyclic antidepressants may increase carbamazepine levels; monitor.

Cholestyramine and colestipol: May bind TCAs and reduce their absorption; monitor for altered response.

Clonidine: Abrupt discontinuation of clonidine may cause hypertensive crisis, amitriptyline may enhance the response.

CNS depressants: Sedative effects may be additive with TCAs; monitor for increased effect; includes benzodiazepines, barbiturates, antipsychotics, ethanol, and other sedative medications.

CYP1A2 inducers: May decrease the levels/effects of clomipramine. Example inducers include aminoglutethimide, carbamazepine, phenobarbital, and rifampin.

CYP1A2 inhibitors: May increase the levels/effects of clomipramine. Example inhibitors include ciprofloxacin, fluvoxamine, ketoconazole, norfloxacin, ofloxacin, and rofecoxib.

CYP2C19 inducers: May decrease the levels/effects of clomipramine. Example inducers include aminoglutethimide, carbamazepine, phenytoin, and rifampin.

CYP2C19 inhibitors: May increase the levels/effects of clomipramine. Example inhibitors include delavirdine, fluconazole, fluvoxamine, gemfibrozil, isoniazid, omeprazole, and ticlopidine.

CYP2D6 inhibitors: May increase the levels/effects of clomipramine. Example inhibitors include chlorpromazine, delavirdine, fluoxetine, miconazole, paroxetine, pergolide, quinidine, quinine, ritonavir, and ropinirole.

CYP2D6 substrates: Clomipramine may increase the levels/effects of CYP2D6 substrates. Example substrates include amphetamines, selected beta-blockers, dextromethorphan, fluoxetine, lidocaine, mirtazapine, nefazodone, paroxetine, risperidone, ritonavir, thioridazine, tricyclic antidepressants, and venlafaxine.

CYP2D6 prodrug substrates: Clomipramine may decrease the levels/effects of CYP2D6 prodrug substrates. Example prodrug substrates include codeine, hydrocodone, oxycodone, and tramadol.

Epinephrine (and other direct alpha-agonists): Pressor response to I.V. epinephrine, norepinephrine, and phenylephrine may be enhanced in patients receiving TCAs. (**Note:** Effect is unlikely with epinephrine or levonordefrin dosages typically administered as infiltration in combination with local anesthetics.)

Fenfluramine: May increase tricyclic antidepressant levels/effects.

Hypoglycemic agents (including insulin): TCAs may enhance the hypoglycemic effects of tolazamide, chlorpropamide, or insulin; monitor for changes in blood glucose levels; reported with chlorpropamide, tolazamide, and insulin.

Levodopa: Tricyclic antidepressants may decrease the absorption (bioavailability) of levodopa; rare hypertensive episodes have also been attributed to this combination.

Linezolid: Hyperpyrexia, hypertension, tachycardia, confusion, seizures, and **deaths have been reported** with agents which inhibit MAO (serotonin syndrome); this combination should be avoided.

Lithium: Concurrent use with a TCA may increase the risk for neurotoxicity.

MAO inhibitors: Hyperpyrexia, hypertension, tachycardia, confusion, seizures, and **deaths have been reported** (serotonin syndrome); this combination should be avoided.

Methylphenidate: Metabolism of some TCAs may be decreased.

Olanzapine: When used in combination, clomipramine and olanzapine have been reported to be associated with the development of seizures; limited documentation (case report).

Phenothiazines: Serum concentrations of some TCAs may be increased; in addition, TCAs may increase concentration of phenothiazines; monitor for altered clinical response.

QT_c-prolonging agents: Concurrent use of tricyclic agents with other drugs which may prolong QT_c interval may increase the risk of potentially fatal arrhythmias; includes type Ia and type III antiarrhythmics agents, selected quinolones (sparfloxacin, gatifloxacin, moxifloxacin, grepafloxacin), cisapride, and other agents.

Ritonavir: Combined use of high-dose tricyclic antidepressants with ritonavir may cause serotonin syndrome in HIV-positive patients; monitor.

Sucralfate: Absorption of tricyclic antidepressants may be reduced with coadministration.

Sympathomimetics, indirect-acting: Tricyclic antidepressants may result in a decreased sensitivity to indirect-acting sympathomimetics; includes dopamine and ephedrine; also see interaction with epinephrine (and direct-acting sympathomimetics).

Tramadol: Tramadol's risk of seizures may be increased with TCAs.

Valproic acid: May increase serum concentrations/adverse effects of some tricyclic antidepressants.

Warfarin (and other oral anticoagulants): TCAs may increase the anticoagulant effect in patients stabilized on warfarin; monitor INR.

Pregnancy Risk Factor C

Pregnancy Implications There are no adequate studies in pregnant women. Withdrawal symptoms (including dizziness, nausea, vomiting, headache, malaise, sleep disturbance, hyperthermia, and/or irritability) have been observed in neonates whose mothers took clomipramine up to delivery. Use in pregnancy only if the benefits to the mother outweigh the potential risks to the fetus.

Lactation Enters breast milk/contraindicated (AAP rates "of concern")

Nursing Implications Monitor pulse rate and blood pressure prior to and during therapy, evaluate mental status

Additional Information May also relieve depression, panic attacks, and chronic pain; may be unsafe to use in patients with porphyria; not effective for sleep apnea; radiopaque

Specific References

Avella J, Lehrer M, Katz M, et al, "Two Cases Involving Clomipramine Intoxication," *J Anal Toxicol*, 2004, 28(6):504-8.

Harvey M, and Cave G, "Intralipid Outperforms Sodium Bicarbonate in a Rabbit Model on Clomipramine Toxicity," *Ann Emerg Med*, 2007, 49:178-185.

Clonazepam

Related Information

- Flunitrazepam
- Nitrazepam
- Therapeutic Drugs Associated with Hallucinations

CAS Number 1622-61-3

U.S. Brand Names Klonopin®

Impairment Potential Yes. Plasma clonazepam levels >0.1 mg/L are consistent with impairment. Brief or extended period (up to 1 year) of use is consistent with driving impairment in the elderly; impairment is greatest in the first 7 days of use. (Baselt RC and Cravey RH, *Disposition of Toxic Drugs and Chemicals in Man*, 4th ed, Foster City, CA: Chemical Toxicology Institute, 1995.)

Use Alone or as an adjunct in the treatment of petit mal variant (Lennox-Gastaut), akinetic, and myoclonic seizures; petit mal (absence) seizures unresponsive to succimides; panic disorder with or without agoraphobia

Unlabeled/Investigational Use Restless legs syndrome; neuralgia; multifocal tic disorder; parkinsonian dysarthria; bipolar disorder; adjunct therapy for schizophrenia

Mechanism of Action Suppresses the spike-and-wave discharge in absence seizures by depressing nerve transmission in the motor cortex

Adverse Reactions

Reactions reported in patients with seizure and/or panic disorder. Frequency not defined.

Cardiovascular: Edema (ankle or facial), palpitations

Central nervous system: Amnesia, ataxia (seizure disorder ~30%; panic disorder 5%), behavior problems (seizure disorder ~25%), coma, confusion, depression, dizziness, drowsiness (seizure disorder ~50%), emotional lability, fatigue, fever, hallucinations, headache, hypotonia, hysteria, insomnia, intellectual ability reduced, memory disturbance, nervousness; paradoxical reactions (including aggressive behavior, agitation, anxiety, excitability, hostility, irritability, nervousness, nightmares, sleep disturbance, vivid dreams); psychosis, slurred speech, somnolence (panic disorder 37%), suicidal attempts, vertigo

Dermatologic: Hair loss, hirsutism, skin rash

Endocrine & metabolic: Dysmenorrhea, libido increased/decreased

Gastrointestinal: Abdominal pain, anorexia, appetite increased/decreased, coated tongue, constipation, dehydration, diarrhea, gastritis, gum soreness, nausea, weight changes (loss/gain), xerostomia

Genitourinary: Dysuria, ejaculation delayed, enuresis, impotence, micturition frequency, nocturia, urinary retention, urinary tract infection, colpitis

Hematologic: Anemia, eosinophilia, leukopenia, thrombocytopenia

Hepatic: Alkaline phosphatase increased (transient), hepatomegaly, serum transaminases increased (transient)

Neuromuscular & skeletal: Choreiform movements, coordination abnormal, dysarthria, muscle pain, muscle weakness, myalgia, tremor

Ocular: Blurred vision, eye movements abnormal, diplopia, nystagmus

Respiratory: Chest congestion, cough, bronchitis, hypersecretions, pharyngitis, respiratory depression, respiratory tract infection, rhinitis, rhinorrhea, shortness of breath, sinusitis

Miscellaneous: Allergic reactions, aphonia, dysdiadochokinesis, encopresis, "glassy-eyed" appearance, hemiparesis, lymphadenopathy

Signs and Symptoms of Overdose May produce ataxia, coma, confusion, cyanosis, depression, diminished reflexes, diplopia, dysarthria, hirsutism, hyperactivity, hypotension, neuroleptic malignant syndrome, purpura, somnolence; agranulocytosis, granulocytopenia, leukopenia, neutropenia

Pharmacodynamics/Kinetics

Onset of action: 20-60 minutes

Duration: Infants and young children: 6-8 hours; Adults: ≤12 hours

Absorption: Well absorbed

Distribution: Adults: V_d: 1.5-4.4 L/kg

Protein binding: 85%

Metabolism: Extensively hepatic via glucuronide and sulfate conjugation

Half-life elimination: Children: 22-33 hours; Adults: 19-50 hours

Time to peak, serum: 1-3 hours; Steady-state: 5-7 days

Excretion: Urine (<2% as unchanged drug); metabolites excreted as glucuronide or sulfate conjugates

Dosage

Oral:

Children <10 years or 30 kg: Seizure disorders:

Initial daily dose: 0.01-0.03 mg/kg/day (maximum: 0.05 mg/kg/day) given in 2-3 divided doses; increase by no more than 0.5 mg every third day until seizures are controlled or adverse effects seen

Usual maintenance dose: 0.1-0.2 mg/kg/day divided 3 times/day, not to exceed 0.2 mg/kg/day

Adults:

Seizure disorders:

Initial daily dose not to exceed 1.5 mg given in 3 divided doses; may increase by 0.5-1 mg every third day until seizures are controlled or adverse effects seen (maximum: 20 mg/day)

Usual maintenance dose: 0.05-0.2 mg/kg; do not exceed 20 mg/day

Panic disorder: 0.25 mg twice daily; increase in increments of 0.125-0.25 mg twice daily every 3 days; target dose: 1 mg/day (maximum: 4 mg/day)

Discontinuation of treatment: To discontinue, treatment should be withdrawn gradually. Decrease dose by 0.125 mg twice daily every 3 days until medication is completely withdrawn.

Elderly: Initiate with low doses and observe closely

Hemodialysis: Supplemental dose is not necessary

Monitoring Parameters CBC, liver function tests

Administration

Orally-disintegrating tablet: Open pouch and peel back foil on the blister; do not push tablet through foil. Use dry hands to remove tablet and place in mouth. May be swallowed with or without water. Use immediately after removing from package.

Contraindications Hypersensitivity to clonazepam or any component of the formulation (cross-sensitivity with other benzodiazepines may exist); significant liver disease; narrow-angle glaucoma; pregnancy

Warnings
Use with caution in elderly or debilitated patients, patients with hepatic disease (including alcoholics), or renal impairment. Use with caution in patients with respiratory disease or impaired gag reflex or ability to protect the airway from secretions (salivation may be increased). Worsening of seizures may occur when added to patients with multiple seizure types. Concurrent use with valproic acid may result in absence status. Monitoring of CBC and liver function tests has been recommended during prolonged therapy.

Causes CNS depression (dose related) resulting in sedation, dizziness, confusion, or ataxia which may impair physical and mental capabilities. Patients must be cautioned about performing tasks which require mental alertness (eg, operating machinery or driving). Use with caution in patients receiving other CNS depressants or psychoactive agents. Effects with other sedative drugs or ethanol may be potentiated. Benzodiazepines have been associated with falls and traumatic injury and should be used with extreme caution in patients who are at risk of these events (especially the elderly).

Use caution in patients with depression, particularly if suicidal risk may be present. Use with caution in patients with a history of drug dependence. Benzodiazepines have been associated with dependence and acute withdrawal symptoms, including seizures, on discontinuation or reduction in dose. Acute withdrawal, including seizures, may be precipitated in patients after administration of flumazenil to patients receiving long-term benzodiazepine therapy.

Benzodiazepines have been associated with anterograde amnesia. Paradoxical reactions, including hyperactive or aggressive behavior, have been reported with benzodiazepines, particularly in adolescent/pediatric or psychiatric patients. Does not have analgesic, antidepressant, or antipsychotic properties.

Dosage Forms
Tablet: 0.5 mg, 1 mg, 2 mg
Tablet, orally disintegrating [wafer]: 0.125 mg, 0.25 mg, 0.5 mg, 1 mg, 2 mg

Reference Range
Sample size: 2 mL serum or plasma
Therapeutic: 10-50 ng/mL
Toxic: >100 ng/mL
Timing of serum samples: Peak serum levels occur 1-3 hours after oral ingestion

Overdosage/Treatment
Decontamination: Lavage (within 1 hour)/activated charcoal
Supportive therapy: Treatment for benzodiazepine overdose is supportive. Rarely is mechanical ventilation required. Flumazenil has been shown to selectively block the binding of benzodiazepines to CNS receptors, resulting in a reversal of benzodiazepine-induced CNS depression.
Enhancement of elimination: Multiple dose of activated charcoal may be effective

Antidote(s)
• Flumazenil [ANTIDOTE]

Drug Interactions
Substrate of CYP3A4 (major)
CNS depressants: Sedative effects and/or respiratory depression may be additive with CNS depressants; includes ethanol, barbiturates, narcotic analgesics, and other sedative agents; monitor for increased effect.
CYP3A4 inducers: CYP3A4 inducers may decrease the levels/effects of clonazepam. Example inducers include aminoglutethimide, carbamazepine, nafcillin, nevirapine, phenobarbital, phenytoin, and rifamycins.
CYP3A4 inhibitors: May increase the levels/effects of clonazepam. Example inhibitors include azole antifungals, clarithromycin, diclofenac, doxycycline, erythromycin, imatinib, isoniazid, nefazodone, nicardipine, propofol, protease inhibitors, quinidine, telithromycin, and verapamil.
Disulfiram: Disulfiram may inhibit the metabolism of clonazepam; monitor for increased benzodiazepine effect.
Levodopa: Therapeutic effects may be diminished in some patients following the addition of a benzodiazepine; limited/inconsistent data.
Oral contraceptives: May decrease the clearance of some benzodiazepines (those which undergo oxidative metabolism); monitor for increased benzodiazepine effect.
Theophylline: May partially antagonize some of the effects of benzodiazepines; monitor for decreased response; may require higher doses for sedation.
Valproic acid: The combined use of clonazepam and valproic acid has been associated with absence seizures.

Pregnancy Risk Factor D
Pregnancy Implications Clonazepam was shown to be teratogenic in some animal studies. Clonazepam crosses the placenta. Benzodiazepine use during pregnancy is associated with increased risk of congenital malformations. Nonteratogenic effects (including neonatal flaccidity, respiratory and feeding problems, and withdrawal symptoms) during the postnatal period have also been reported with benzodiazepine use.

Epilepsy itself, number of medications, genetic factors, or a combination of these probably influence the teratogenicity of anticonvulsant therapy.
Lactation Enters breast milk/not recommended
Nursing Implications Observe patient for excess sedation, respiratory depression
Additional Information Ethosuximide or valproic acid may be preferred for treatment of absence (petit mal) seizures; clonazepam-induced behavioral disturbances may be more frequent in mentally handicapped patients; may be effective therapy for tinnitus will not usually give a positive urinary drug screen for benzodiazepines

Specific References
Burrows DL, Hagardorn AN, Harlan GC, et al, "A Fatal Drug Interaction Between Oxycodone and Clonazepam," *J Forensic Sci*, 2003, 48(5):683-6.
Cates ME, Bishop MH, Davis LL, et al, "Clonazepam for Treatment of Sleep Disturbances Associated with Combat-Related Post-Traumatic Stress Disorder," *Ann Pharmacother*, 2004, 38(9):1395-9.
Cheze M, Deveaux M, Lenoan A, et al, "Clonazepam, Bromazepam, and Zolpidem in Hair of Victims of Drug-Facilitated Crimes: Quantitative Analysis by LC-MS/MS and Correlation with Self-Report," *Annale de Toxicologie Analytique*, 2005, 17(4):269-74.
Hackett J and Elian AA, "Solid-Phase Extraction and Analysis of Clonazepam/7-Aminoclonazepam in Blood and Urine Using a Dual Internal Standard Methodology," *J Anal Toxicol*, 2006, 30:128.
Negrusz A, Bowen AM, Moore CM, et al, "Elimination of 7-Aminoclonazepam in Urine After a Single Dose of Klonopin™," *J Anal Toxicol*, 2003, 27(3):196-7.

Clonidine

Related Information
• Drugs Used in Addiction Treatment
• Therapeutic Drugs Associated with Hallucinations
CAS Number 4205-90-7; 4205-91-8
U.S. Brand Names Catapres-TTS®; Catapres®; Duraclon™
Synonyms Clonidine Hydrochloride
Impairment Potential Yes. Doses >0.3 mg are associated with sedation in first-time users. (Baselt RC and Cravey RH, *Disposition of Toxic Drugs and Chemicals in Man*, 4th ed, Foster City, CA: Chemical Toxicology Institute, 1995, 178.)
Use Management of mild to moderate hypertension; either used alone or in combination with other antihypertensives
Orphan drug: Duraclon™: For continuous epidural administration as adjunctive therapy with intraspinal opiates for treatment of cancer pain in patients tolerant to or unresponsive to intraspinal opiates
Unlabeled/Investigational Use Heroin or nicotine withdrawal; severe pain; dysmenorrhea; vasomotor symptoms associated with menopause; ethanol dependence; prophylaxis of migraines; glaucoma; diabetes-associated diarrhea; impulse control disorder, attention-deficit/hyperactivity disorder (ADHD), clozapine-induced sialorrhea, neonatal opiate withdrawal
Mechanism of Action Stimulates α_2-adrenoreceptors in the brain stem, thus activating an inhibitory neuron, resulting in reduced sympathetic outflow, producing a decrease in vasomotor tone and heart rate
Adverse Reactions
Cardiovascular: Exacerbation of Raynaud's phenomenon, hypotension, **bradycardia**, palpitations, tachycardia, congestive heart failure, AV block, transient paradoxical hypertension (at doses >7 mg/day), hypertension (at doses >7 mg/day), **hypertension (rebound)**, **hypotension (orthostatic)**, sinus bradycardia, myocardial depression, sinus tachycardia
Central nervous system: **Drowsiness**, **dizziness**, fatigue, insomnia, **anxiety**, auditory and visual hallucinations, headache, depression, psychosis, **confusion**
Dermatologic: Rash, pruritus, skin pigmentation after transdermal application, alopecia, angioedema, urticaria, exanthem
Endocrine & metabolic: Sodium and water retention, parotitis, parotid pain, hypoprolactinemia
Gastrointestinal: **Constipation**, anorexia, **xerostomia**, **nausea**, vomiting, Ogilvie's syndrome
Genitourinary: Impotence, **urinary tract infection**
Hepatic: Hepatitis
Local: Skin reactions with patch
Ocular: Miosis, diplopia
Miscellaneous: Anogenital cicatricial pemphigoid, systemic lupus erythematosus, pseudolymphoma
Signs and Symptoms of Overdose Apnea, ataxia, AV block, bradycardia (17% incidence in children), coma, CNS depression, delirium, dementia, diarrhea, dry eyes, heart block, hyperglycemia, hypoglycemia, hyponatremia, hyporeflexia, hypotension (15% incidence in children), hypothermia (usually resolves in 8 hours), hypotonia, impotence, insomnia, irritability, lethargy (80% incidence in children), miosis, nocturia, paralytic ileus, personality changes, respiratory depression (5% incidence in children), seizures, syncope

Admission Criteria/Prognosis Admit any symptomatic patient after a four hour observation or any pediatric ingestion over 0.2 mg

Pharmacodynamics/Kinetics

Onset of action: Oral: 0.5-1 hour; Transdermal: Initial application: 2-3 days

Duration: 6-10 hours

Distribution: V_d: Adults: 2.1 L/kg; highly lipid soluble; distributes readily into extravascular sites

Protein binding: 20% to 40%

Metabolism: Extensively hepatic to inactive metabolites; undergoes enterohepatic recirculation

Bioavailability: 75% to 95%

Half-life elimination: Adults: Normal renal function: 6-20 hours; Renal impairment: 18-41 hours

Time to peak: 2-4 hours

Excretion: Urine (65%, 32% as unchanged drug); feces (22%)

Dosage

Children:

Oral:

Hypertension: Initial: 5-10 mcg/kg/day in divided doses every 8-12 hours; increase gradually at 5- to 7-day intervals to 25 mcg/kg/day in divided doses every 6 hours; maximum: 0.9 mg/day

Clonidine tolerance test (test of growth hormone release from pituitary): 0.15 mg/m^2 or 4 mcg/kg as single dose

ADHD (unlabeled use): Initial: 0.05 mg/day; increase every 3-7 days by 0.05 mg/day to 3-5 mcg/kg/day given in divided doses 3-4 times/day (maximum dose: 0.3-0.4 mg/day)

Epidural infusion: Pain management: Reserved for patients with severe intractable pain, unresponsive to other analgesics or epidural or spinal opiates: Initial: 0.5 mcg/kg/hour; adjust with caution, based on clinical effect

Adults:

Oral:

Acute hypertension (urgency): Initial 0.1-0.2 mg; may be followed by additional doses of 0.1 mg every hour, if necessary, to a maximum total dose of 0.6 mg

Hypertension: Initial dose: 0.1 mg twice daily (maximum recommended dose: 2.4 mg/day); usual dose range (JNC 7): 0.1-0.8 mg/day in 2 divided doses

Nicotine withdrawal symptoms: 0.1 mg twice daily to maximum of 0.4 mg/day for 3-4 weeks

Transdermal: Hypertension: Apply once every 7 days; for initial therapy start with 0.1 mg and increase by 0.1 mg at 1- to 2-week intervals (dosages >0.6 mg do not improve efficacy); usual dose range (JNC 7): 0.1-0.3 mg once weekly

Neonatal opiate withdrawal: 0.5-1 mcg/kg (oral)

Epidural infusion: Pain management: Starting dose: 30 mcg/hour; titrate as required for relief of pain or presence of side effects; minimal experience with doses >40 mcg/hour; should be considered an adjunct to intraspinal opiate therapy

Elderly: Initial: 0.1 mg once daily at bedtime, increase gradually as needed

Dosing adjustment in renal impairment: Cl$_{cr}$ <10 mL/minute: Administer 50% to 75% of normal dose initially

Dialysis: Not dialyzable (0% to 5%) via hemo- or peritoneal dialysis; supplemental dose not necessary

Monitoring Parameters Blood pressure, standing and sitting/supine, mental status, heart rate

Administration Oral: Do not discontinue clonidine abruptly. if needed, gradually reduce dose over 2-4 days to avoid rebound hypertension

Transdermal patch: Patches should be applied weekly at bedtime to a clean, hairless area of the upper outer arm or chest. Rotate patch sites weekly. Redness under patch may be reduced if a topical corticosteroid spray is applied to the area before placement of the patch.

Contraindications Hypersensitivity to clonidine hydrochloride or any component of the formulation

Warnings

Gradual withdrawal is needed (over 1 week for oral, 2-4 days with epidural) if drug needs to be stopped. Patients should be instructed about abrupt discontinuation (causes rapid increase in BP and symptoms of sympathetic overactivity). In patients on both a beta-blocker and clonidine where withdrawal of clonidine is necessary, withdraw the beta-blocker first and several days before clonidine. Then slowly decrease clonidine.

Use with caution in patients with severe coronary insufficiency; conduction disturbances; recent MI, CVA, or chronic renal insufficiency. Caution in sinus node dysfunction. Discontinue within 4 hours of surgery then restart as soon as possible after. Clonidine injection should be administered via a continuous epidural infusion device. **[U.S. Boxed Warning]: Epidural clonidine is not recommended for perioperative, obstetrical, or postpartum pain.** It is not recommended for use in patients with severe cardiovascular disease or hemodynamic instability. In all cases, the epidural may lead to cardiovascular instability (hypotension, bradycardia). Transdermal patch may contain conducting metal (eg, aluminum); remove patch prior to MRI. Due to the potential for altered electrical conductivity, remove transdermal patch before cardioversion or defibrillation. Clonidine cause significant CNS depression and xerostomia. Caution in patients with pre-existing CNS disease or depression. Elderly may be at greater risk for CNS depressive effects, favoring other agents in this population.

Dosage Forms

Injection, epidural solution, as hydrochloride [preservative free] (Duraclon™): 100 mcg/mL (10 mL); 500 mcg/mL (10 mL)

Patch, transdermal [once-weekly patch]:

Catapres-TTS®-1: 0.1 mg/24 hours (4s)

Catapres-TTS®-2: 0.2 mg/24 hours (4s)

Catapres-TTS®-3: 0.3 mg/24 hours (4s)

Tablet, as hydrochloride (Catapres®): 0.1 mg, 0.2 mg, 0.3 mg

Reference Range

Therapeutic: 1-2 ng/mL (SI: 4.4-8.7 nmol/L); ingestion of a clonidine patch in a 14-month old girl resulted in a clonidine serum level of 4 ng/mL with major toxicity noted; ingestion of 2.9 mg/kg of clonidine resulted in a serum clonidine level of 64 ng/mL and severe toxicity in a 5-year-old

Peak clonidine plasma and cerebrospinal fluid levels following a 700 mcg bolus of epidural clonidine are ~4.4 and 418 ng/mL, respectively

Overdosage/Treatment

Decontamination: Lavage (within 1 hour)/activated charcoal; whole bowel irrigation (200 mL/hour of GoLYTELY® increased up to a rate of 500 mL/hour) has been used successfully in decontamination of ingested clonidine patch in a girl who was 14 months of age who had been symptomatic

Supportive therapy: Treatment is primarily supportive and symptomatic. Hypotension usually responds to I.V. fluids or Trendelenburg positioning. If unresponsive to these measures, the use of a parenteral vasoconstrictor may be required (eg, norepinephrine 0.1-0.2 mcg/kg/minute titrated to response). Naloxone may be utilized in treating the hypotension, CNS depression and/or apnea and should be given I.V. 0.01 mg/kg to 0.1 mg/kg, with repeats as needed. There is ~31% positive response rate to naloxone for clonidine toxicity and rebound hypertension does **not** occur. Atropine 15 mcg/kg I.V. may be needed for symptomatic bradycardia. Tolazoline may be utilized to treat hypotension and bradycardia refractory to above therapy (initial dose of tolazoline is 10 mg I.V.). Yohimbine (oral: 0.1 mg/kg) has been used successfully to reverse neurologic and cardiac effects.

Enhancement of elimination: Multiple dosing of activated charcoal may be effective; not dialyzable (0% to 5%); hemoperfusion may be helpful in removing clonidine

Antidote(s)

● Naloxone [ANTIDOTE]

Test Interactions ↑ sodium (S); ↓ catecholamines (U)

Drug Interactions

Antipsychotics: Concurrent use with antipsychotics (especially low potency) or nitroprusside may produce additive hypotensive effects.

Beta-blockers: May potentiate bradycardia in patients receiving clonidine and may increase the rebound hypertension of withdrawal; discontinue beta-blocker several days before clonidine is tapered.

CNS depressants: Sedative effects may be additive; monitor for increased effect; includes barbiturates, benzodiazepines, narcotic analgesics, ethanol, and other sedative agents.

Cyclosporine: Clonidine may increase cyclosporine (and perhaps tacrolimus) serum concentrations; cyclosporine dosage adjustment may be needed.

Hypoglycemic agents: Clonidine may decrease the symptoms of hypoglycemia; monitor patients receiving antidiabetic agents.

Levodopa: Effects may be reduced by clonidine in some patients with Parkinson's disease (limited documentation); monitor.

Local anesthetics: Epidural clonidine may prolong the sensory and motor blockade of local anesthetics.

Mirtazapine: Antihypertensive effects of clonidine may be antagonized by mirtazapine (hypertensive urgency has been reported following addition of mirtazapine to clonidine). In addition, mirtazapine may potentially enhance the hypertensive response associated with abrupt clonidine withdrawal. Avoid this combination; consider an alternative agent.

Narcotic analgesics: May potentiate hypotensive effects of clonidine.

Tricyclic antidepressants: Antihypertensive effects of clonidine may be antagonized by tricyclic antidepressants. In addition, tricyclic antidepressants may enhance the hypertensive response associated with abrupt clonidine withdrawal; avoid this combination; consider an alternative agent.

Verapamil: Concurrent administration may be associated with hypotension and AV block in some patients (limited documentation); monitor.

Pregnancy Risk Factor C

Pregnancy Implications Clonidine crosses the placenta. Caution should be used with this drug due to the potential of rebound hypertension with abrupt discontinuation.

Lactation Enters breast milk/not recommended

Nursing Implications Patches should be applied weekly at bedtime to a clean, hairless area of the upper outer arm or chest; rotate patch sites weekly

Additional Information Unsafe in patients with porphyria; rebound hypertension upon abrupt withdrawal usually occurs with doses >1.2 mg/day; appears to be the preferred "Mickey Finn" drug used by criminals in Moscow/Russia; addition of clonidine (75-150 mcg) increased duration of analgesia produced by epidural morphine (2 mg) for cesarean delivery

Specific References

Benson BE, Spyker DA, Troutman WG, et al, "TESS-Based Clonidine Dose-Response in Pediatric Exposures," *J Toxicol Clin Toxicol*, 2004, 42(5):751-2.

Blume C, Menendez J, and Scalzo A, "Unintentional Acute Catapres® Patch Ingestion in an Adult," *J Toxicol Clin Toxicol*, 2003, 41(5):652.

Chobanian AV, Bakris GL, Black HR, et al, "The Seventh Report of the Joint National Committee on Prevention, Detection, Evaluation, and Treatment of High Blood Pressure: The JNC 7 Report," *JAMA*, 2003, 289(19):2560-71.

Eddy O and Howell JM, "Are One or Two Dangerous? Clonidine and Topical Imidazolines Exposure in Toddlers," *J Emerg Med*, 2003, 25(3):297-302.

Matteucci MJ, "One Pill Can Kill: Assessing the Potential for Fatal Poisonings in Children," *Pediatr Ann. 2005 Dec;34(12):964-8*

Quail MT and Shannon M, "Severe Hypothermia Caused by Clonidine," *Am J Emerg Med*, 2003, 21(1):86.

Rowden AK, Buck ML, Eldridge DL, et al, "The Radiopacity of Ingested Transdermal Medicinal Patches in a Simulated Human Model," *Clin Toxicol (Phila)*, 2005, 43:695.

Simic J, Kishineff S, Goldberg R, et al, "Acute Myocardial Infarction as a Complication of Clonidine Withdrawal," *J Emerg Med*, 2003, 25(4): 399-402.

Simone K, Tomassoni A, Walsh LM, et al, "Cardiac Arrest and Withdrawal After Clonidine Overdose in a Toddler with ADHD," *J Toxicol Clin Toxicol*, 2004, 42(5):749.

Spiller HA, Colvin JM, Villalobos D, et al, "Clonidine Ingestion in Children," *J Toxicol Clin Toxicol*, 2003, 41(5):663.

Clorazepate

CAS Number 20432-69-3; 57109-90-7; 5991-71-9

U.S. Brand Names T-Tab®; Tranxene® SD™-Half Strength; Tranxene® SD™; Tranxene®

Synonyms Clorazepate Dipotassium; Tranxene T-Tab®

Impairment Potential Yes. Brief or extended period (up to 1 year) of use is consistent with driving impairment in the elderly; impairment is greatest in the first 7 days of use.

Use Treatment of generalized anxiety and panic disorders; management of alcohol withdrawal; adjunct anticonvulsant in management of partial seizures

Mechanism of Action Facilitates gamma aminobutyric acid (GABA)-mediated transmission inhibitory neurotransmitter action, depresses subcortical levels of CNS

Adverse Reactions

Cardiovascular: Decreased systolic blood pressure, vasculitis

Central nervous system: **Drowsiness**, headache, dizziness, mental confusion, nervousness

Dermatologic: Urticaria, purpura, pruritus, exanthem

Gastrointestinal: Xerostomia

Hematologic: Decreased hematocrit

Hepatic: Abnormal liver function test results

Neuromuscular & skeletal: Paresthesia

Ocular: Blurred vision

Renal: Abnormal kidney function tests

Signs and Symptoms of Overdose Ataxia, coma, confusion, diminished reflexes, somnolence

Pharmacodynamics/Kinetics

Onset of action: 1-2 hours

Duration: Variable, 8-24 hours

Distribution: Crosses placenta; appears in urine

Metabolism: Rapidly decarboxylated to desmethyldiazepam (active) in acidic stomach prior to absorption; hepatically to oxazepam (active)

Half-life elimination: Adults: Desmethyldiazepam: 48-96 hours; Oxazepam: 6-8 hours

Time to peak, serum: ~1 hour

Excretion: Primarily urine

Dosage

Oral:

Children 9-12 years: Anticonvulsant: Initial: 3.75-7.5 mg/dose twice daily; increase dose by 3.75 mg at weekly intervals, not to exceed 60 mg/day in 2-3 divided doses

Children >12 years and Adults: Anticonvulsant: Initial: Up to 7.5 mg/dose 2-3 times/day; increase dose by 7.5 mg at weekly intervals; not to exceed 90 mg/day

Adults:

Anxiety: 7.5-15 mg 2-4 times/day, or given as single dose of 11.25 or 22.5 mg at bedtime

Alcohol withdrawal: Initial: 30 mg, then 15 mg 2-4 times/day on first day; maximum daily dose: 90 mg; gradually decrease dose over subsequent days

Stability Unstable in water

Monitoring Parameters Respiratory and cardiovascular status, excess CNS depression

Contraindications Hypersensitivity to clorazepate or any component of the formulation (cross-sensitivity with other benzodiazepines may exist); narrow-angle glaucoma; pregnancy

Warnings

Not recommended for use in patients <9 years of age or patients with depressive or psychotic disorders. Use with caution in elderly or debilitated patients, patients with hepatic disease (including alcoholics), or renal impairment. Active metabolites with extended half-lives may lead to delayed accumulation and adverse effects. Use with caution in patients with respiratory disease or impaired gag reflex. Avoid use in patients with sleep apnea.

Causes CNS depression (dose related) resulting in sedation, dizziness, confusion, or ataxia which may impair physical and mental capabilities. Patients must be cautioned about performing tasks which require mental alertness (eg, operating machinery or driving). Use with caution in patients receiving other CNS depressants or psychoactive agents. Effects with other sedative drugs or ethanol may be potentiated. Benzodiazepines have been associated with falls and traumatic injury and should be used with extreme caution in patients who are at risk of these events (especially the elderly).

Use caution in patients with depression, particularly if suicidal risk may be present. Use with caution in patients with a history of drug dependence. Benzodiazepines have been associated with dependence and acute withdrawal symptoms on discontinuation or reduction in dose. Acute withdrawal, including seizures, may be precipitated in patients after administration of flumazenil to patients receiving long-term benzodiazepine therapy.

Benzodiazepines have been associated with anterograde amnesia. Paradoxical reactions, including hyperactive or aggressive behavior, have been reported with benzodiazepines, particularly in adolescent/pediatric or psychiatric patients. Does not have analgesic, antidepressant, or antipsychotic properties.

Dosage Forms

Tablet, as dipotassium: 3.75 mg, 7.5 mg, 15 mg

Tranxene® SD™: 22.5 mg [once daily]

Tranxene® SD™-Half Strength: 11.25 mg [once daily]

Tranxene® T-Tab®: 3.75 mg, 7.5 mg, 15 mg

Reference Range Therapeutic: 0.12-2.00 mcg/mL (SI: 0.36-6.02 μmol/L)

Overdosage/Treatment

Decontamination: Lavage (within 1 hour)/activated charcoal

Supportive therapy: Treatment for benzodiazepine overdose is supportive; rarely is mechanical ventilation required. Flumazenil (Romazicon™) has been shown to selectively block the binding of benzodiazepines to CNS receptors, resulting in a reversal of benzodiazepine-induced CNS depression.

Antidote(s)

• Flumazenil [ANTIDOTE]

Drug Interactions

Substrate of CYP3A4 (major)

CNS depressants: Sedative effects and/or respiratory depression may be additive with CNS depressants; includes ethanol, barbiturates, narcotic analgesics, and other sedative agents; monitor for increased effect.

CYP3A4 inducers: CYP3A4 inducers may decrease the levels/effects of clorazepate. Example inducers include aminoglutethimide, carbamazepine, nafcillin, nevirapine, phenobarbital, phenytoin, and rifamycins.

CYP3A4 inhibitors: May increase the levels/effects of clorazepate. Example inhibitors include azole antifungals, clarithromycin, diclofenac, doxycycline, erythromycin, imatinib, isoniazid, nefazodone, nicardipine, propofol, protease inhibitors, quinidine, telithromycin, and verapamil.

Levodopa: Therapeutic effects may be diminished in some patients following the addition of a benzodiazepine; limited/inconsistent data.

Oral contraceptives: May decrease the clearance of some benzodiazepines (those which undergo oxidative metabolism); monitor for increased benzodiazepine effect.

Theophylline: May partially antagonize some of the effects of benzodiazepines; monitor for decreased response; may require higher doses for sedation.

Pregnancy Risk Factor D

Pregnancy Implications Fetal malformations described with first trimester use; crosses the placenta

Lactation Excretion in breast milk unknown/not recommended

Nursing Implications Observe patient for excess sedation, apnea; raise bed rails, initiate safety measures, assist with ambulation

Additional Information Clorazepate offers no advantage over the other benzodiazepines; can cause fetal malformations

Clotrimazole

CAS Number 23593-75-1

U.S. Brand Names Cruex® Cream [OTC]; Gyne-Lotrimin® 3 [OTC]; Lotrimin® AF Athlete's Foot Cream [OTC]; Lotrimin® AF Athlete's Foot Solution [OTC]; Lotrimin® AF Jock Itch Cream [OTC]; Mycelex® Twin Pack [OTC]; Mycelex®-7 [OTC]; Mycelex®

Use Treatment of susceptible fungal infections, including oropharyngeal candidiasis, dermatophytoses, superficial mycoses, and cutaneous candidiasis, as well as vulvovaginal candidiasis; limited data suggest that clotrimazole troches may be effective for prophylaxis against oropharyngeal candidiasis in neutropenic patients

Mechanism of Action An imidazole agent which binds to phospholipids in the fungal cell membrane altering cell wall permeability resulting in loss of essential intracellular elements

Adverse Reactions

Central nervous system: Drowsiness, confusion, CNS depression, depression

Dermatologic: Contact dermatitis

Gastrointestinal: Nausea, vomiting, anorexia

Hepatic: **Abnormal liver function tests**

Local: Mild burning, irritation, stinging to skin or vaginal area

Pharmacodynamics/Kinetics

Absorption: Topical: Negligible through intact skin

Time to peak, serum:

Oral topical (troche): Salivary levels occur within 3 hours following 30 minutes of dissolution time

Vaginal cream: High vaginal levels: 8-24 hours

Vaginal tablet: High vaginal levels: 1-2 days

Excretion: Feces (as metabolites)

Dosage

Children >3 years and Adults:

Oral:

Prophylaxis: 10 mg troche dissolved 3 times/day for the duration of chemotherapy or until steroids are reduced to maintenance levels

Treatment: 10 mg troche dissolved slowly 5 times/day for 14 consecutive days

Topical (cream, solution): Apply twice daily; if no improvement occurs after 4 weeks of therapy, re-evaluate diagnosis

Children >12 years and Adults:

Vaginal:

Cream:

1%: Insert 1 applicatorful vaginal cream daily (preferably at bedtime) for 7 consecutive days

2%: Insert 1 applicatorful vaginal cream daily (preferably at bedtime) for 3 consecutive days

Tablet: Insert 100 mg/day for 7 days or 500 mg single dose

Topical (cream, solution): Apply to affected area twice daily (morning and evening) for 7 consecutive days

Monitoring Parameters Periodic liver function tests during oral therapy with clotrimazole lozenges

Administration Oral: Allow to dissolve slowly over 15-30 minutes.

Topical: Avoid contact with eyes. For external use only. Apply sparingly. Protect hands with latex gloves. Do not use occlusive dressings.

Contraindications Hypersensitivity to clotrimazole or any component of the formulation

Warnings Clotrimazole should not be used for treatment of systemic fungal infection. Safety and effectiveness of clotrimazole lozenges (troches) in children <3 years of age have not been established. When using topical formulation, avoid contact with eyes.

Dosage Forms

Combination pack (Mycelex®-7): Vaginal tablet 100 mg (7s) and vaginal cream 1% (7 g)

Cream, topical: 1% (15 g, 30 g, 45 g)

Cruex®: 1% (15 g)

Lotrimin® AF Athlete's Foot: 1% (12 g, 24 g)

Lotrimin® AF Jock Itch: 1% (12 g)

Cream, vaginal: 2% (21 g)

Mycelex®-7: 1% (45 g)

Solution, topical: 1% (10 mL, 30 mL)

Lotrimin® AF Athlete's Foot: 1% (10 mL)

Tablet, vaginal (Gyne-Lotrimin® 3): 200 mg (3s)

Troche (Mycelex®): 10 mg

Reference Range Peak serum levels after dermal cream application: <0.001 mcg/mL; after vaginal tablet application, serum levels range from 0.02-0.05 mcg/mL; peak serum levels after a 1.5 g oral dose ranges from 1-5 mcg/mL

Overdosage/Treatment

Decontamination: Ipecac within 30 minutes or gastric lavage (within 1 hour)/activated charcoal

Enhancement of elimination: Multiple dosing of activated charcoal may be effective

Drug Interactions

Inhibits CYP1A2 (weak), 2A6 (weak), 2B6 (weak), 2C8 (weak), 2C9 (weak), 2C19 (weak), 2D6 (weak), 2E1 (weak), 3A4 (moderate)

CYP3A4 substrates: Clotrimazole may increase the levels/effects of CYP3A4 substrates. Example substrates include benzodiazepines, calcium channel blockers, cyclosporine, mirtazapine, nateglinide, nefazodone, sildenafil (and other PDE-5 inhibitors), tacrolimus, and venlafaxine. Selected benzodiazepines (midazolam and triazolam), cisapride, ergot alkaloids, selected HMG-CoA reductase inhibitors (lovastatin and simvastatin), and pimozide are generally contraindicated with strong CYP3A4 inhibitors.

Pregnancy Risk Factor B (topical); C (troches)

Lactation Excretion in breast milk unknown

Additional Information Periodic assessment of hepatic function is advisable in patients with pre-existing hepatic impairment; re-evaluate topical therapy after one month

Clozapine

Related Information

- Anticholinergic Effects of Common Psychotropics
- Antipsychotic Agents
- Olanzapine

CAS Number 5786-21-0

U.S. Brand Names Clozaril®; Fazaclo™

Use Treatment of refractory schizophrenia; reduce risk of recurrent suicidal behavior in schizophrenia or schizoaffective disorder

Unlabeled/Investigational Use Schizoaffective disorder, bipolar disorder, childhood psychosis, severe obsessive-compulsive disorder

Mechanism of Action Tricyclic dibenzodiazepine structure; blocks dopamine receptors

Adverse Reactions

Cardiovascular: **Tachycardia**, angina, ECG changes, hypertension, hypotension, syncope, arrhythmias, cardiomyopathy (usually dilated), CHF, MI, myocarditis, pericardial effusion, pericarditis, thromboembolism

Central nervous system: **Drowsiness**, **dizziness**, akathisia, seizures, headache, nightmares, akinesia, confusion, insomnia, fatigue, myoclonic jerks, restlessness, agitation, lethargy, ataxia, slurred speech, depression, anxiety, neuroleptic malignant syndrome, tardive dyskinesia, stroke, status epilepticus

Dermatologic: Rash, photosensitivity

Endocrine & metabolic: Diabetes mellitus, hyperglycemia

Gastrointestinal: **Constipation**, **weight gain**, **sialorrhea**, abdominal discomfort, anorexia, diarrhea, heartburn, xerostomia, nausea, vomiting, fecal impaction, intestinal obstruction, paralytic ileus, salivary gland swelling

Genitourinary: **Urinary incontinence**, difficult urination, impotence

Hematologic: Eosinophilia, leukopenia, leukocytosis, agranulocytosis, granulocytopenia, thrombocytopenia

Hepatic: Liver function tests abnormal, cholestasis, hepatitis, jaundice

Neuromuscular & skeletal: Tremor, rigidity, hyperkinesia, weakness

Ocular: Visual disturbances, blurred vision, narrow-angle glaucoma

Respiratory: Rhinorrhea, pulmonary embolism, aspiration

Miscellaneous: Diaphoresis (increased), fever, ESR increased, systemic lupus erythematosus

See table.

Clozapine-Induced Side Effects		
INCIDENCE AND MANAGEMENT		
Effect	**Incidence**	**Management**
Sedation & fatigue	35%	Initiate split dosing with long-term goal to administer twice daily with larger portion at bedtime (appears to be dose-dependent). For chronic sedation, consider an empiric trial of methylphenidate 5-20 mg/day.
Sialorrhea	25%	Clozapine may affect the swallowing mechanism; behavioral approach may be best. Consider lowering the dose. Pharmacological management consists of clonidine 0.1-0.9 mg/day (monitor blood pressure) or benztropine 0.5-2 mg/day (monitor for increased anticholinergic side effects).
Weight gain	35%	Diet and exercise best. No pharmacological agent shown to be consistently useful; one study showed the addition of quetiapine to clozapine minimized weight gain; consider lowering dose.

Table   (Continued)

INCIDENCE AND MANAGEMENT

Effect	Incidence	Management
Urinary incontinence	25%	If patient receiving co-pharmacy with typical antipsychotic, consider discontinuing; pharmacological management consists of ephedrine 25-150 mg/d, oxybutynin 5 mg tid, or desmopressin.
Tachycardia	25%	Dose dependent. Beta-blocker; atenolol 50 mg/d or propranolol 10 mg tid (adjust for rate)
Constipation	20%	Discontinue other medications with anticholinergic activity, if possible. May need chronic psyllium and/or docusate.
Seizures	4%	Dose dependent. Valproic acid/valproate; initiate at 250 mg tid or 500 mg bid and titrate to serum level of at least 50 mcg/mL
Agranulocytosis	1%	Stop drug. Do not rechallenge. Consider filgrastim (G-CSF) or sargramostim (GM-CSF) during acute recovery phase.

Signs and Symptoms of Overdose Agitation, ataxia, coma, cognitive dysfunction, delirium, disorientation, enuresis, eosinophilia, extrapyramidal reaction, fasciculations, hypertension, hypoglycemia, hypotension, hypotonicity, impotence, inability to urinate, myoclonus, nausea, neuroleptic malignant syndrome, nystagmus, Parkinson's-like symptoms, salivation, seizures, torticollis, vomiting

Admission Criteria/Prognosis Admit any patient exhibiting acidosis or neurologic sequelae

Pharmacodynamics/Kinetics
Protein binding: 97% to serum proteins
Metabolism: Extensively hepatic; forms metabolites with limited or no activity
Bioavailability: 12% to 81% (not affected by food)
Half-life elimination: Steady state: 12 hours (range: 4-66 hours)
Time to peak: 2.5 hours (range: 1-6 hours)
Excretion: Urine (~50%) and feces (30%) with trace amounts of unchanged drug

Dosage
Oral: If dosing is interrupted for >48 hours, therapy must be reinitiated at 12.5-25 mg/day; may be increased more rapidly than with initial titration.
Children and Adolescents: Childhood psychosis (unlabeled use): Initial: 25 mg/day; increase to a target dose of 25-400 mg/day
Adults: Schizophrenia or to reduce risk of suicidal behavior: Initial: 12.5 mg once or twice daily; increased, as tolerated, in increments of 25-50 mg/day to a target dose of 300-450 mg/day after 2-4 weeks, may require doses as high as 600-900 mg/day for the treatment of schizophrenia; median dose to reduce risk of suicidal behavior is ~300 mg/day (range 12.5-900 mg)
Elderly: Schizophrenia: Dose selection and titration should be cautious
Note: In the event of planned termination of clozapine, gradual reduction in dose over a 1- to 2-week period is recommended. If conditions warrant abrupt discontinuation (leukopenia), monitor patient for psychosis and cholinergic rebound (headache, nausea, vomiting, diarrhea).

Monitoring Parameters
Mental status, ECG, WBC (see below), vital signs, fasting lipid profile and fasting blood glucose/Hgb A_{1c} (prior to treatment, at 3 months, then annually; BMI, personal/family history of obesity; waist circumference (weight should be assessed prior to treatment, at 4 weeks, 8 weeks, 12 weeks, and then at quarterly intervals. Consider titrating to a different antipsychotic agent for a weight gain ≥5% of the initial weight); blood pressure; abnormal involuntary movement scale (AIMS).
WBC and ANC should be obtained at baseline and at least weekly for the first 6 months of continuous treatment. If counts remain acceptable (WBC ≥3500/mm³, ANC ≥2000/mm³) during this time period, then they may be monitored every other week for the next 6 months. If WBC/ANC continue to remain within these acceptable limits after the second 6 months of therapy, monitoring can be decreased to every 4 weeks. (Note: The decease in monitoring to every 4 weeks is applicable in the United States. Blood monitoring requirements related to the use of clozapine have not changed in Canada). If clozapine is discontinued, a weekly WBC should be conducted for an additional 4 weeks or until WBC is ≥3500/mm³ and ANC is ≥2000/mm³. If clozapine therapy is interrupted due to moderate leukopenia, weekly WBC/ANC monitoring is required for 12 months in patients restarted on clozapine treatment. If therapy is interrupted for reasons other than leukopenia/granulocytopenia, the 6-month time period for initiation of biweekly WBCs may need to be reset. This determination depends upon the treatment duration, the length of the break in therapy, and whether or not an abnormal blood event occurred.
Consult full prescribing information for determination of appropriate WBC/ANC monitoring interval (http://www.clozaril.com/index.jsp).

Administration
Orally-disintegrating tablet: Should be removed from foil blister by peeling apart (do not push tablet through the foil). Remove immediately prior to use. Place tablet in mouth and allow to dissolve; swallow with saliva. If dosing requires splitting tablet, throw unused portion away. May be taken without regard to food. Fazaclo™ contains phenylalanine 1.75 mg per 25 mg tablet and phenylalanine 6.96 mg per 100 mg tablet.

Contraindications Hypersensitivity to clozapine or any component of the formulation; history of agranulocytosis or granulocytopenia with clozapine; uncontrolled epilepsy, severe central nervous system depression or comatose state; paralytic ileus; myeloproliferative disorders or use with other agents which have a well-known risk of agranulocytosis or bone marrow suppression

Warnings
[U.S. Boxed Warning]: Patients with dementia-related behavioral disorders treated with atypical antipsychotics are at an increased risk of death compared to placebo. Clozapine is not approved for this indication.

[U.S. Boxed Warning]: Significant risk of agranulocytosis, potentially life-threatening. Therapy should not be initiated in patients with WBC <3500 cells/mm³ or ANC <2000 cells/mm³ or history of myeloproliferative disorder. WBC testing should occur periodically on an on-going basis (see prescribing information for monitoring details) to ensure that acceptable WBC/ANC counts are maintained. Initial episodes of moderate leukopenia or granulopoietic suppression confer up to a 12-fold increased risk for subsequent episodes of agranulocytosis. WBCs must be monitored weekly for at least 4 weeks after therapy discontinuation or until WBC is ≥3500/mm³ and ANC is ≥2000/mm³. Use with caution in patients receiving other marrow suppressive agents. Eosinophilia has been reported to occur with clozapine and may require temporary or permanent interruption of therapy. Due to the significant risk of agranulocytosis, it is strongly recommended that a patient must fail at least two trials of other primary medications for the treatment of schizophrenia (of adequate dose and duration) before initiating therapy with clozapine.

Cognitive and/or motor impairment (sedation) is common with clozapine, resulting in impaired performance of tasks requiring alertness (eg, operating machinery or driving); use caution in patients receiving general anesthesia. **[U.S. Boxed Warning]: Seizures have been associated with clozapine use in a dose-dependent manner;** use with caution in patients at risk of seizures, including those with a history of seizures, head trauma, brain damage, alcoholism, or concurrent therapy with medications which may lower seizure threshold. Has been associated with benign, self-limiting fever (<100.4°F, usually within first 3 weeks). However, clozapine may also be associated with severe febrile reactions, including neuroleptic malignant syndrome (NMS). Clozapine's potential for extrapyramidal symptoms (including tardive dyskinesia) appears to be extremely low.

Deep vein thrombosis, myocarditis, pericarditis, pericardial effusion, cardiomyopathy, and CHF have also been associated with clozapine. **[U.S. Boxed Warning]: Fatalities due to myocarditis have been reported; highest risk in the first month of therapy, however, later cases also reported.** Myocarditis or cardiomyopathy should be considered in patients who present with signs/symptoms of heart failure (dyspnea, fatigue, orthopnea, paroxysmal nocturnal dyspnea, peripheral edema), chest pain, palpitations, new electrocardiographic abnormalities (arrhythmias, ST-T wave abnormalities), or unexplained fever. Patients with tachycardia during the first month of therapy should be closely monitored for other signs of myocarditis. Discontinue clozapine if myocarditis is suspected; do not rechallenge in patients with clozapine-related myocarditis. The reported rate of myocarditis in clozapine-treated patients appears to be 17-322 times greater than in the general population. Clozapine should be discontinued in patients with confirmed cardiomyopathy unless benefit clearly outweighs risk. Rare cases of thromboembolism, including pulmonary embolism and stroke resulting in fatalities, have been associated with clozapine.

May cause anticholinergic effects; use with caution in patients with urinary retention, benign prostatic hyperplasia, narrow-angle glaucoma, xerostomia, visual problems, constipation, or history of bowel obstruction. May cause hyperglycemia; in some cases may be extreme and associated with ketoacidosis, hyperosmolar coma, or death. Use with caution in patients with diabetes or other disorders of glucose regulation; monitor for worsening of glucose control. Use with caution in patients with hepatic disease or impairment; hepatitis has been reported as a consequence of therapy.

Use caution with cardiovascular, renal, or pulmonary disease. **[U.S. Boxed Warning]: May cause orthostatic hypotension (with or without syncope)** and tachycardia; use with caution in patients at risk of hypotension or in patients where transient hypotensive episodes would be poorly tolerated (cardiovascular disease or cerebrovascular disease). Concurrent use with benzodiazepines may increase the risk of severe cardiopulmonary reactions.

The possibility of a suicide attempt is inherent in psychotic illness or bipolar disorder; use caution in high-risk patients during initiation of therapy. Prescriptions should be written for the smallest quantity consistent with good patient care.

Medication should not be stopped abruptly; taper off over 1-2 weeks. If conditions warrant abrupt discontinuation (leukopenia, myocarditis, cardiomyopathy), monitor patient for psychosis and cholinergic rebound (headache, nausea, vomiting, diarrhea). Consider titrating to a different antipsychotic agent for a weight gain ≥5% of the initial weight). Elderly patients are more susceptible to adverse effects (including agranulocytosis, cardiovascular, anticholinergic, and tardive dyskinesia).

Dosage Forms

Tablet: 12.5 mg, 25 mg, 100 mg
  Clozaril®: 25 mg, 100 mg
Tablet, orally disintegrating (FazaClo®): 25 mg [contains phenylalanine 1.75 mg; mint flavor], 100 mg [contains phenylalanine 6.96 mg; mint flavor]

Reference Range Therapeutic: 200-400 ng/mL; levels >500 ng/mL associated with change in mental status in children; levels >2000 ng/mL associated with CNS changes in adults; highest survivable clozapine serum level of 5200 ng/mL followed a 3 g clozapine ingestion and deep coma.

Overdosage/Treatment

Decontamination: Lavage (within 1 hour)/activated charcoal
Supportive therapy: I.V. fluids for hypotension; lorazepam, diazepam, phenobarbital, or phenytoin for seizures; granulocyte colony-stimulating factor may be useful for agranulocytosis; clozapine-induced hypotension (orthostatic) can be treated with fludrocortisone 0.1 mg/day, with increasing doses to 0.3 mg/day over 2 weeks; desmopressin (intranasal: 10 mcg at bedtime) can be used to treat clozapine-induced enuresis; lithium (600-900 mg/day) can be given to treat clozapine-induced neutropenia; pirenzepine (25-100 mg/day) can be used to treat clozapine-induced hypersalivation; benztropine at a dose of 2 mg/day can be used to treat sialorrhea; diphenhydramine can be used to treat extrapyramidal symptoms; clozapine-induced incontinence may respond to ephedrine (up to 150 mg/day); intranasal ipratropium bromide may be useful in the treatment of clozapine-induced sialorrhea
Enhancement of elimination: Multiple dose of activated charcoal may be useful

Antidote(s)

- Filgrastim [ANTIDOTE]

Test Interactions Nitrazepam can cause false elevation (~15%) of serum clozapine

Drug Interactions

Substrate of CYP1A2 (major), 2A6 (minor), 2C9 (minor), 2C19 (minor), 2D6 (minor), 3A4 (minor); **Inhibits** CYP1A2 (weak), 2C9 (weak), 2C19 (weak), 2D6 (moderate), 2E1 (weak), 3A4 (weak)

Acetylcholinesterase inhibitors (central): May increase the risk of antipsychotic-related extrapyramidal symptoms; monitor.

Anticholinergics: Clozapine has potent anticholinergic effects. May potentiate the effects of anticholinergic agents.

Antihypertensives: Clozapine may potentiate the hypotensive effects of antihypertensive agents.

Benzodiazepines: In combination with clozapine, may produce respiratory depression and hypotension, especially during the first few weeks of therapy; monitor for altered response.

Carbamazepine: A case of neuroleptic malignant syndrome has been reported in combination with clozapine; in addition, carbamazepine may alter clozapine levels (see enzyme inducers); monitor.

Citalopram: May increase the levels/effects of clozapine; monitor.

CNS depressants: Sedative effects may be additive with other CNS depressants; includes ethanol, barbiturates, benzodiazepines, narcotic analgesics, and other sedatives.

CYP1A2 inducers: May decrease the levels/effects of clozapine. Example inducers include aminoglutethimide, carbamazepine, phenobarbital, and rifampin.

CYP1A2 inhibitors: May increase the levels/effects of clozapine. Example inhibitors include ciprofloxacin, fluvoxamine, ketoconazole, norfloxacin, ofloxacin, and rofecoxib.

CYP2D6 substrates: Clozapine may increase the levels/effects of CYP2D6 substrates. Example substrates include amphetamines, selected beta-blockers, dextromethorphan, fluoxetine, lidocaine, mirtazapine, nefazodone, paroxetine, risperidone, ritonavir, thioridazine, tricyclic antidepressants, and venlafaxine.

CYP2D6 prodrug substrates: Clozapine may decrease the levels/effects of CYP2D6 prodrug substrates. Example prodrug substrates include codeine, hydrocodone, oxycodone, and tramadol.

Epinephrine: Clozapine may reverse the pressor effect of epinephrine; use should be avoided in the treatment of drug-induced hypotension.

Metoclopramide: May increase extrapyramidal symptoms (EPS) or risk.

Omeprazole: May alter the concentrations/effects of clozapine; monitor.

Risperidone: Effects and/or toxicity may be increased when combined with clozapine; monitor.

Valproic acid: May cause reductions in clozapine concentrations; monitor for altered response.

Pregnancy Risk Factor B

Pregnancy Implications Teratogenic effects were not seen in animal studies; however, there are no adequate and well-controlled studies in pregnant women. Use during pregnancy only if clearly needed.

Lactation Enters breast milk/not recommended (AAP rates "of concern")

Additional Information May be useful in the treatment of neuroleptic-induced vomiting (in doses up to 500 mg/day); ECG effects include T-wave inverse, S-T depression and S-T segment elevation

Specific References

Ball MP, Hooper ET, Skipwith F, et al, "Clozapine-Induced Hyperlipidemia Resolved After Switch to Aripiprazole Therapy," *Ann Pharmacother*, 2005, 39(9):1570-2.

Borzutzky A, Avello E, Rumie H, et al, "Accidental Clozapine Intoxication in a Ten-Year-Old Child," *Vet Hum Toxicol*, 2003, 45(6):309-10.

Derenne JL and Baldessarini RJ, "Clozapine Toxicity Associated with Smoking Cessation," *Am J Ther*, 2005, 12:469-71.

Goossen RB, Freeman DJ, Satchell AM, et al, "Monitoring Clozapine: Are Fingerprick Blood and Plasma Clozapine Levels Equivalent to Arm Venipuncture Blood and Plasma Levels?" *Ther Drug Monit*, 2003, 25(4):469-72.

Hadley C, Griffith J, and Casavant M, "Mellow Yellow - Intentional Abuse of Clozapine," *J Toxicol Clin Toxicol*, 2003, 41(5):743.

Langman LJ, Kaliciak HA, and Boone SA, "Death Attributed to Chronic Cumulative Clozapine Toxicity," *J Anal Toxicol*, 2004, 28:280.

McKenna K, Einarson A, Levinson A, et al, "Significant Changes in Antipsychotic Drug Use During Pregnancy," *Vet Hum Toxicol*, 2004, 46(1):44-6.

Rami AF, Barkan D, Mevorach D, et al, "Clozapine-Induced Systemic Lupus Erythematosus," *Ann Pharamacother*, 2006, 40(5):983-5.

Razminia M, Salem Y, Devaki S, et al, "Clozapine Induced Myopericarditis Early Recognition Improves Clinical Outcome," *Am J Ther*, 2006, 13(3):274-6.

Schulte PF, "What Is an Adequate Trial with Clozapine? Therapeutic Drug Monitoring and Time to Response in Treatment-Refractory Schizophrenia," *Clin Pharmacokinet*, 2003, 42(7):607-18.

Thomas L and Pollak PT, "Delayed Recovery Associated with Persistent Serum Concentrations After Clozapine Overdose," *J Emerg Med*, 2003, 25(1): 61-6.

Ulrich S, Wolf R, and Staedt J, "Serum Level of Clozapine and Relapse," *Ther Drug Monit*, 2003, 25(2):252-5.

Cocaine

Related Information

- Donor Victims of Poisoning in Whom Transplantation of Organs Occurred
- Substance-Related Disorders

CAS Number 50-36-2; 53-21-4

Synonyms Cocaine Hydrochloride

Impairment Potential Yes. Positive qualitative urinary test for cocaethylene or the parent compound of cocaine is consistent with recent usage

Use Topical anesthesia for mucous membranes

Mechanism of Action Blocks both the initiation and conduction of nerve impulses by decreasing the neuronal membrane's permeability to sodium ions, which results in inhibition of depolarization with resultant blockade of conduction; interferes with the uptake of norepinephrine by adrenergic nerve terminals producing vasoconstriction; a type I antiarrhythmic

Adverse Reactions

Cardiovascular: Decreased heart rate with low doses, tachycardia with moderate doses, hypertension, cardiomyopathy, cardiac arrhythmias, myocarditis, QRS prolongation, Raynaud's phenomenon, cerebral vasculitis, thrombosis, fibrillation (atrial), flutter (atrial), sinus bradycardia, congestive heart failure, pulmonary hypertension, sinus tachycardia, tachycardia (supraventricular), arrhythmias (ventricular), vasoconstriction

Central nervous system: **CNS stimulation**, fever, nervousness, restlessness, euphoria, excitation, headache, psychosis, hallucinations, agitation, seizures, slurred speech, hyperthermia, dystonic reactions, cerebrovascular accident, vasculitis, clonic-tonic reactions, paranoia, sympathetic storm, aggressive behavior, leukoencephalopathy

Dermatologic: Skin infarction, pruritus, madarosis, bullous skin disease

Gastrointestinal: **Loss of taste perception**, nausea, anorexia, colonic ischemia

Genitourinary: Priapism, uterine rupture

Hematologic: Thrombocytopenia

Neuromuscular & skeletal: Chorea (extrapyramidal), paresthesia, tremors, fasciculations

Ocular: Mydriasis (peak effect at 45 minutes; may last up to 12 hours), sloughing of the corneal epithelium, ulceration of the cornea, iritis, mydriasis, chemosis

Renal: Myoglobinuria, necrotizing vasculitis

Respiratory: **Rhinitis, nasal congestion**, tachypnea, nasal mucosa damage (when snorting), hyposmia, bronchiolitis obliterans organizing pneumonia, acute respiratory distress syndrome, alveolar hemorrhage, pneumothorax, pneumomediastinum, eosinophilic pneumonia

Miscellaneous: **Loss of smell**, spontaneous bowel perforation, "washed-out" syndrome, asthma, Pott puffy tumor (PPT), acute atraumatic compartment syndrome

Signs and Symptoms of Overdose Abdominal pain, angina, apnea, ataxia, blurred vision, cardiomegaly, chest pain, CNS hemorrhage, colitis, coma, corneal irritation, delirium, dental erosion, depression, disorientation, dry mouth, dyspnea, epistaxis, euphoria, extrapyramidal reaction, hallucinations, hyperreflexia, hypertension, hyperthermia, impotence, insomnia, intracranial hemorrhage, lacrimation, mania, migraine headache (exacerbation), muscular spasm, myalgia, mydriasis, myocardial depression, myoglobinuria, nasal congestion, nystagmus, paroxysmal tachycardia (ventricular), photophobia, ptosis, rhabdomyolysis, respiratory alkalosis, respiratory depression, restlessness, seizures, sensory aberrations, sweating, tachycardia (ventricular), vomiting

Admission Criteria/Prognosis Patients with moderate to severe acute symptomatology (including chest pain, severe hyperadrenergic signs, hyperthermia, rhabdomyolysis, coagulopathy, mental status changes) should be admitted to an intensive care unit; patients with mild hyperadrenergic signs can be monitored for 6 hours and if resolving, can then be discharged; all body packers/body stuffers should be admitted even if asymptomatic (most complications occur within 4 hours).

Pharmacodynamics/Kinetics
Onset of action: Topical: Within 5 minutes following administration to mucosa; Inhalation: 3-5 seconds; I.V.: 10-60 seconds
Peak action: Inhalation: 1-3 minutes; I.V.: 3-5 minutes; Intranasal: 15-20 minutes
Duration: Inhalation: 5-15 minutes; I.V.: 20-60 minutes; Intranasal: 60-90 minutes
Absorption: Well absorbed through mucous membranes, limited by drug-induced vasoconstriction, and enhanced by inflammation
Distribution: V_d: 1.96-2.7 L/kg
Protein binding: ~90%
Metabolism: In the liver to benzoylecgonine, ecgonine methylester and norcocaine (active)
Bioavailability: Cocaine Smoked in glass pipes: 70%; Cocaine Smoked in corncob pipes: 60%; Intranasal route: Dose dependent: 25% to 94%; Oral: 30%
Half-life: (Benzoylecgonine from all 3 routes: 3.55-5.79 hours); During first week of life: Cocaine: 11.6 hours; Benzoylecgonine: 11.2 hours; Intravenous: 37-41 minutes; Smoked: 58-89 minutes; Intranasal: 73-207 minutes
Elimination: Excreted primarily in urine as metabolites (benzoylecgonine and ecgonine methylester) unchanged drug (<10%)

Dosage Topical application (ear, nose, throat, bronchoscopy): Dosage depends on the area to be anesthetized, tissue vascularity, technique of anesthesia, and individual patient tolerance; the lowest dose necessary to produce adequate anesthesia should be used; concentrations of 1% to 10% are used (not to exceed 1 mg/kg). Use reduced dosages for children, elderly, or debilitated patients.

Stability Store in well closed, light-resistant containers

Monitoring Parameters Vital signs

Administration
Topical: Use only on mucous membranes of the oral, laryngeal, and nasal cavities. Do not use on extensive areas of broken skin.

Contraindications Hypersensitivity to cocaine or any component of the topical solution; ophthalmologic anesthesia (causing sloughing of the corneal epithelium); pregnancy (nonmedicinal use)

Warnings For topical use only. Limit to office and surgical procedures only. Resuscitative equipment and drugs should be immediately available when any local anesthetic is used. Debilitated, elderly patients, acutely ill patients, and children should be given reduced doses consistent with their age and physical status. Use caution in patients with severely traumatized mucosa and sepsis in the region of the proposed application. Use with caution in patients with cardiovascular disease or a history of cocaine abuse. In patients being treated for cardiovascular complication of cocaine abuse, avoid beta-blockers for treatment.

Dosage Forms
Powder, as hydrochloride: 1 g, 5 g, 25 g
Solution, topical, as hydrochloride: 4% [40 mg/mL] (4 mL, 10 mL); 10% [100 mg/mL] (4 mL, 10 mL)

Reference Range
Therapeutic: 100-500 ng/mL (SI: 330 nmol/L)
Toxic: >1000 ng/mL (SI: >3300 nmol/L)
Blood cocaine levels in "bodypackers" may exceed 50,000 ng/mL
Average blood levels after smoking a standard dose of crack cocaine: 600-700 ng/mL
Average postmortem blood cocaine levels from deceased cocaine abusers: 2500 ng/mL
Highest postmortem cocaine level from bodypacker: 104,000 ng/mL
In the postmortem state, anatomical site concentration differences (ie, postmortem redistribution) may occur.
Topical ophthalmic cocaine (10%) will cause a positive urine cocaine screen of ~48 hours when applied therapeutically in the eye.

Overdosage/Treatment
Decontamination: Activated charcoal is useful for oral ingestion; whole bowel irrigation should be considered for body packers or body stuffers of cocaine packets; oral bicarbonate decreased gastrointestinal cocaine absorption for body packers/stuffers in an *in vitro* model
Supportive therapy: Since no specific antidote for cocaine exists, serious toxic effects are treated symptomatically. Seizures are treated with lorazepam or diazepam. Benzodiazepines may also be useful for life-threatening arrhythmias, agitation, and/or hypertension. Sodium bicarbonate may decrease QRS prolongation. Phentolamine can be used for cocaine-induced vasoconstriction therapy. Hypertension can be treated with nitroprusside (0.5-10 mcg/kg/minute), nitroglycerin (10 mcg/minute), phentolamine (5-10 mg I.V.), or enalaprilat (0.625-1.25 mg). Although lidocaine may promote cocaine-induced seizures, it is probably safe to use if used over 3 hours after cocaine use. Lidocaine and sodium bicarbonate are first-line agents for hemodynamically stable ventricular tachycardia or refractory ventricular fibrillation. The combination of esmolol and lorazepam has been advocated to treat hyperadrenergic crisis, but this combination has not been well studied. Labetalol or beta adrenergic blockers are not recommended to treat cocaine-associated myocardial ischemia. Nicardipine (50 mg/hour I.V.) has been used to control hypertension due to crack cocaine overdose. Active cooling measures should take place if core temperature exceeds 40°C. Thrombolytic agents (preferably by intracoronary administration) can be use to treat acute coronary syndrome if uncontrolled hypertension does not exist.
Enhancement of elimination: Butyrylcholinesterase is strictly investigational; bisacodyl, psyllium, hydrophilic mucilloid, saline, or emollient laxative can be used to enhance fecal excretion of body packages.

Antidote(s)
- Phentolamine [ANTIDOTE]

Drug Interactions
Substrate of CYP3A4 (major); **Inhibits** CYP2D6 (strong), 3A4 (weak)
Beta-blockers potentiate cocaine-induced coronary vasoconstriction (potentiate alpha-adrenergic effect of cocaine); avoid concurrent use.
CYP2D6 substrates: Cocaine may increase the levels/effects of CYP2D6 substrates. Example substrates include amphetamines, selected beta-blockers, dextromethorphan, fluoxetine, lidocaine, mirtazapine, nefazodone, paroxetine, risperidone, ritonavir, thioridazine, tricyclic antidepressants, and venlafaxine.
CYP2D6 prodrug substrates: Cocaine may decrease the levels/effects of CYP2D6 prodrug substrates. Example prodrug substrates include codeine, hydrocodone, oxycodone, and tramadol.
CYP3A4 inhibitors: May increase the levels/effects of cocaine. Example inhibitors include azole antifungals, clarithromycin, diclofenac, doxycycline, erythromycin, imatinib, isoniazid, nefazodone, nicardipine, propofol, protease inhibitors, quinidine, telithromycin, and verapamil.
Sympathomimetic amines may cause malignant arrhythmias; avoid concurrent use.

Pregnancy Risk Factor C/X (nonmedicinal use)

Pregnancy Implications Sustained arrhythmias may occur in the neonatal period; genitourinary abnormalities may occur; prenatal cocaine exposure can impair fetal growth in a dose-dependent manner; uterine rupture can occur during late gestation

Lactation Enters breast milk/contraindicated

Additional Information
May cause corneas to become clouded or pitted, therefore, normal saline should be used to irrigate and protect corneas during surgery; not for injection; converted to cocaine sulfate as a drug of abuse; may precipitate porphyria. Increased incidence of anticardiolipin antibody has been reported in cocaine abusers (especially with I.V. use); positive rheumatoid factor also has been noted in cocaine abusers. Incidence of acute myocardial infarction in patients with cocaine-associated chest pain is ~6%; initial ECG is only sensitive for 36% of acute myocardial infarction; ethanol plus cocaine use produces cocaethylene which has a longer half-life (~2 hours) than cocaine. While cocaethylene can produce tachycardia, myocardial depression, and is a competitive muscarinic antagonist, no direct effect on blood pressure is usually seen. Age, cardiac risk factors, inferior infarction, and bradydysrhythmias can predict underlying coronary artery disease in cocaine-induced myocardial infarctions.

In a rodent model, cocaethylene may continue to form after death, but hepatic postmortem cocaethylene production ceases 1 hour after death.

Cocaine is present on 79% of U.S. Currency analyzed in amounts >0.1 mcg and in 54% in amounts >1 mcg (highest amount recorded was 1327 mcg). Anticonvulsants (phenytoin, carbamazepine) have been used to treat cocaine dependence.

According to the Drug Abuse Warning Network, in 2004:
- Cocaine was involved in an estimated 383,350 Emergency Department (ED) visits.
- Cocaine and alcohol accounted for an estimated 83,816 ED visits.
- 46% of Cocaine ED visits involved. Seeking detox.
- 13,940 cocaine ED visits involved a suicide attempt.

U.S. retail price per gram: 1981: $500; 2000: $150. Production in certain countries in 2000: Columbia: 266 tons; Peru: 54 tons; Bolivia: 13 tons.

U.S. spending on illicit cocaine: 1988: 76 billion dollars; 2000: 36 billion dollars. Recovery rate from addiction is about 90%; about 21% of all U.S. drug users are dependent on cocaine (1999 data).

Specific References

Ananias DC, Zhao Y, Hoch DK, et al, "The Detection of Cocaine Metabolite in Urine with an ONLINE® DAT II Immunoassay," *J Anal Toxicol*, 2004, 28:303-4.

Bacis G, Papa P, Rocchi L, et al, "Cocaine Adultered with Atropine: An Epidemic Poisoning in Northern Italy in 2004," *Clin Toxicol (Phila)*, 2005, 43:664.

Borges CR, Roberts JC, Wilkins DG, et al, "Cocaine, Benzoylecgonine, Amphetamine, and *N*-Acetylamphetamine Binding to Melanin Subtypes," *J Anal Toxicol*, 2003, 27(3):125-34.

Brown WC, Setter CR, Kuntz DJ, et al, "Production of Benzoylecgonine with a Wash and Extraction Technique for Removing External Contamination of Cocaine on Hair," *J Anal Toxicol*, 2004, 28:283.

Campora P, Bermejo AM, Tabernero MJ, et al, "Quantitation of Cocaine and Its Major Metabolites in Human Saliva Using Gas Chromatography-Positive Chemical Ionization-Mass Spectrometry (GC-PCI-MS)," *J Anal Toxicol*, 2003, 27(5):270-4.

Catenacci MH and Tuckler VE, "Bilateral Central Retinal Artery Occlusion Secondary to Inhalation of Crack Cocaine," *Clin Toxicol (Phila)*, 2005, 43:661.

Clauwaert K, Decaestecker T, Mortier K, et al, "The Determination of Cocaine, Benzoylecgonine, and Cocaethylene in Small-Volume Oral Fluid Samples by Liquid Chromatography-Quadrupole-Time-of-Flight Mass Spectrometry," *J Anal Toxicol*, 2004, 28(8):655-9.

Cleveland N, DeWitt C, Marietta M, et al, "Ziprasidone is Protective in an Animal Model of Acute Cocaine Poisoning," *SAEM Annual Meeting Abstracts*, 2004, 472.

Cone EJ, Sampson-Cone AH, Darwin WD, et al, "Method for Detection of Cocaine Metabolite in Urine Below Conventional Cutoff Concentrations," *J Anal Toxicol*, 2004, 28:283.

Cooper G, Wilson L, Reid C, et al, "Validation of the Cozart® Microplate EIA for Cocaine and Metabolites in Oral Fluid," *J Anal Toxicol*, 2004, 28(6):498-503.

Cox RD, Koelliker DE, and Bradley KG, "Association Between Droperidol Use and Sudden Death in Two Patients Intoxicated with Illicit Stimulant Drugs," *Vet Hum Toxicol*, 2004, 46(1):21-3.

Crouch DJ, Cook RF, Dove DC, et al, "The Detection of Drugs of Abuse in Liquid Perspiration," *J Anal Toxicol*, 2004, 28:276-7.

Cumpston KL, Laeben L, and Crandall C, "Life-Threatening Toxicity in a Cocaine "Stuffer" Greater Than Fourteen Hours from Ingestion," *Clin Toxicol (Phila)*, 2005, 43:670.

Darwin WD, Shimomura ET, Lalani SA, et al, "Cocaine and Metabolites in Urine After Controlled Smoked, Intravenous, Intranasal, and Oral Cocaine Administration," *J Anal Toxicol*, 2006, 30:145-6.

DeWitt C, Heard K, Cleveland NJ, et al, "The Effect of Amiodarone in Mice with Acute Cocaine Toxicity," *J Toxicol Clin Toxicol*, 2004, 42(5):740.

Dhawan SS, and Wang BWE, "Four Extremity Gargrene Associated with Crack Cocaine Abuse," *Ann Emerg Med*, 2007, 49:186-9.

Fareed FN, Chan GM, and Hoffman RS, "Fatal Cocaine Metoprolol Interaction," *Clin Toxicol*, 2005, 43:641.

Forrester MB and Merz RD, "Risk of Selected Birth Defects with Prenatal illicit Drug Use, 1986-2002," *Clin Toxicol (Phila)*, 2005, 43:667.

Gehlhausen JM, Klette KL, and Stout PR, "Occupational Cocaine Exposure of Crime Laboratory Personnel Preparing Training Aids for a Military Working Dog Program," *J Anal Toxicol*, 2003, 27:453-8.

Ginsburg BY, Weinberg HR, Hoffman RS, et al, "Symptomatic Bilateral Adrenal Infarction Associated with Cocaine Use," *Clin Toxicol (Phila)*, 2005, 43:663.

Giroud C, Michaud K, Sporkert F, et al, "A Fatal Overdose of Cocaine Associated with Coingestion of Marijuana, Buprenorphine, and Fluoxetine: Body Fluid and Tissue Distribution of Cocaine and Its Metabolites Determined by Hydrophilic Interaction Chromatography-Mass Spectrometry (HILIC-MS)," *J Anal Toxicol*, 2004, 28(6):464-74.

Hill V, Schaffer M, and Cairns T, "Absence of Hair Color Effects in Hair Analysis Results for Cocaine, Benzoylecgonine, Morphine, 6-Monoacetylmorphine, Codeine, and 11-Nor-9-Carboxy-△9-THC in Large Workplace Populations," *Annale de Toxicologie Analytique*, 2005, 17(4):285-98.

Hoffman RS, Burkhart K, Chan G, et al, "Multistate Outbreak of Clenbuterol Contaminated Heroin and Cocaine," *Clin Toxicol (Phila)*, 2005, 43:683.

Hon K, Cordery R, Haase W, et al, "A Multicenter Evaluation of Roche ONLINE® DAT II Methadone, Cocaine, and Cannabinoid Assays," *J Anal Toxicol*, 2004, 28:295-6.

Honderick T, Williams D, Seaberg D, et al, "A Prospective, Randomized, Controlled Trial of Benzodiazepines and Nitroglycerine or Nitroglycerine Alone in the Treatment of Cocaine-Associated Acute Coronary Syndromes," *Am J Emerg Med*, 2003, 21(1):39-42.

Honey D, Mazarr-Proo S, and Kerrigan S, "Distribution of Cocaine and Benzoylecgonine in Postmortem Casework," *J Anal Toxicol*, 2004, 28:294.

Jones JH and Weir WB, "Cocaine-Associated Chest Pain," *Med Clin North Am*, 2005, 89(6):1323-42 (review).

Kacinko SL, Barnes AJ, Schwilke EW, et al, "Detection Rates, Dose-Concentration Relationships, and Reproducibility of Cocaine, Benzoylecgonine, and Ecgonine Methyl Ester in Human Sweat Following Controlled Cocaine Administration," *J Anal Toxicol*, 2006, 30:140.

Kolbrich EA, Kelly TL, Barnes AJ, et al, "Salive/Plasma Ratios of Cocaine, Ecgonine Methyl Ester, and Benzoylecgonine Following Controlled Cocaine Administration," *J Anal Toxicol*, 2006, 30:137.

Kolbrich EA, Kim I, Barnes AJ, et al, "Cozart® RapiScan Oral Fluid Drug Testing System: An Evaluation of Sensitivity, Specificity, and Efficiency for Cocaine Detection Compared with ELISA and GC-MS Following Controlled Cocaine Administration," *J Anal Toxicol*, 2003, 27:407-11.

Kontos MC, Jesse RL, Tatum JL, et al, "Coronary Angiographic Findings in Patients with Cocaine-Associated Chest Pain," *J Emerg Med*, 2003, 24(1):9-13.

Kupiec T, Spiehler V, Isenschmid D, et al, "Performance of a Microtiter Plate ELISA for Screening of Postmortem Blood for Cocaine and Metabolites," *J Anal Toxicol*, 2004, 28:299-300.

Langston CS and Pollack M, "Pseudo-Wellens Syndrome in a Cocaine User,'" *Am J Emerg Med*, 2006, 24(1):122-3.

Lester L, Uemura N, Ademola J, et al, "Disposition of Cocaine in Skin, Interstitial Fluid, Sebum, and Stratum Corneum," *J Anal Toxicol*, 2002, 26(8):547-53.

Liberty HJ, Johnson BD, and Fortner N, "Detecting Cocaine Use Through Sweat Testing: Multilevel Modeling of Sweat Patch Length-of-Wear Data," *J Anal Toxicol*, 2004, 28(8):667-73.

Logan BK, "Ecgonine Is an Important Marker for Cocaine Use in Inadequately Preserved Specimens," *J Anal Toxicol*, 2001, 25(3):219-20.

Long H, Greller H, Mercurio-Zappala M, et al, "Medicinal Use of Cocaine: A Shifting Paradigm over 25 Years," *J Toxicol Clin Toxicol*, 2003, 41(5):717.

Messinger DS, Bauer CR, Abhik D, et al, "The Maternal Lifestyle Study: Cognitive, Motor, and Behavioral Outcomes of Cocaine-Exposed and Opiate-Exposed Infants Through Three Years of Age," *Pediatrics*, 2004, 113(6):1677-85.

Moody DE, Spanbauer AC, Taccogno JL, et al, "Comparative Analysis of Sweat Patches for Cocaine (and Metabolites) by Radioimmunoassay and Gas Chromatography-Positive Ion Chemical Ionization-Mass Spectrometry," *J Anal Toxicol*, 2004, 28(2):86-93.

Moore C, Feldman M, Harrison E, et al, "Analysis of Cocaine and Metabolites in Hair, Oral Fluid, and Urine," *Annale de Toxicologie Analytique*, 2005, 17(4):221-8.

Moore C, Feldman M, Harrison E, et al, "Cocaine and Metabolites in Hair, Oral Fluid, and Urine," *J Anal Toxicol*, 2006, 30:148.

Moore KA, Levine B, and Fowler DR, "Prediction of Impairment from Urine Benzoylecgonine Concentrations," *J Anal Toxicol*, 2003, 27(6):383-4.

O'Connor AD, Rusyniak DE, and Bruno A., "Cerebrovascular and Cardiovascular Complications of Alcohol and Sympathomimetic Drug Abuse," *Med Clin North Am*, 2005, 89(6):1343-58 (review).

Pedersen-Bjergaard U, Reubsaet JL, Nielsen SL, et al, "Psychoactive Drugs, Alcohol, and Severe Hypoglycemia in Insulin-Treated Diabetes: Analysis of 141 Cases," *Am J Med*, 2005, 118(3):307-10.

Perrone J, Solari S, Milone M, et al, "New Etiology of Cocaine True Positive Drug Screen: Does South American Coca Tea Really Contain Cocaine?" *J Toxicol Clin Toxicol*, 2004, 42(5):795.

Pichini S, Ventura M, Pujadas M, et al, "Letter to the Editor: HAIRVEQ 2005: An External Quality Control Exercise for Drugs of Abuse Analysis in Hair in Cooperation with Society of Hair Testing," *Annale de Toxicologie Analytique*, 2005, 17(4):307-9.

Raes E and Verstraete AG, "Usefulness of Roadside Urine Drug Screening in Drivers Suspected of Driving Under the Influence of Drugs (DUID)," *J Anal Toxicol*, 2005, 29:632-42.

Robarge T, Edwards J, Phillips E, et al, "Positive Ion Chemical Ionization Gas Chromatography-Quadrupole Mass Spectrometry for Confirmation and Quantification of Benzoylecgonine in Oral Fluid," *J Anal Toxicol*, 2006, 30:142.

Runkle JL, Lowe RH, Abraham TT, et al, "Optimization of Glucuronide Hydrolysis for Improved Recovery of 11-Hydroxy-△9-Tetrahydrocannabinol in Urine," *J Anal Toxicol*, 2006, 30:143.

Schaffer M, Hill V, and Cairns T, "Hair Analysis for Focaine: The Requirement for Effective Wash Procedures and Effects of Drug Concentration and Hair Porosity in Contamination and Decontamination," *J Anal Toxicol*, 2005, 29(5):319-26.

Sellers KJ, Wittrig R, and Kowalski J, "Cocaine Analysis on a Bonded Pentafluorophenylpropyl High-Performance Liquid Chromatography Stationary Phase Using Mass Spectrometry," *J Anal Toxicol*, 2006, 30:144.

Seymour A, Black M, McFarlane JH, et al, "Death by Obstruction: Sudden Death Resulting from Impromptu Ingestion of Drugs," *Am J Forensic Med Pathol*, 2003, 24(1):17-21.

Shakleya DM, Plumley AE, Kraner JC, et al, "Presence of Methamphetamine and Cocaine-Pyrolytic Products in Light Bulb Trace Evidence and *Trans*-Phenylpropene as a Marker of Smoked Methamphetamine in Urine," *J Anal Toxicol*, 2006, 30:144.

Skanning PG and Christophersen AB, "Retroperitoneal Hemorrhage and Kidney Damage Due to Trauma Caused by Play-Fighting During a Cocaine High," *J Toxicol Clin Toxicol*, 2003, 41(5):661.

Spiehler V, Isenschmid DS, Matthews P, et al, "Performance of a Microtiter Plate ELISA for Screening of Postmortem Blood for Cocaine and Metabolites," *J Anal Toxicol*, 2003, 27(8):587-91.

Stephens BG, Jentzen JM, Karch S, et al, "Criteria for the Interpretation of Cocaine Levels in Human Biological Samples and Their Relation to the Cause of Death," *Am J Forensic Med Pathol*, 2004, 25(1):1-10.

Stephens BG, Jentzen JM, Karch S, et al, "National Association of Medical Examiners Position Paper on the Certification of Cocaine-Related Deaths," *Am J Forensic Med Pathol*, 2004, 25(1):11-13.

Stover M, Chang B. Jackson O, et al, "Vascular Occlusion and Digital Necrosis After Intra-Arterial Cocaine Injection," *Clin Toxicol (Phila)*, 2005, 43:669.

Tan-Laxa MA, Sison-Switala C, Rintelman W, et al, "Abnormal Auditory Brainstem Response Among Infants with Prenatal Cocaine Exposure," *Pediatrics*, 2004, 113(2):357.

Traub SJ, Hoffman RS, and Nelson LS, et al, "Body Packing - The Internal Concealment of Illicit Drugs," *N Engl J Med*, 2003, 349(26):2519-26.

Uemura N, Nath RP, Harkey MR, et al, "Cocaine Levels in Sweat Collection Patches Vary by Location of Patch Placement and Decline Over Time," *J Anal Toxicol*, 2004, 28:253-9.

Uhl M and Scheufler F, "Effects of Hair Colon on the Drug Incorporation Into Human Hair," *Annale de Toxicologie Analytique*, 2005, 17(4):279-84.

Wade NA, Mertens-Maxham D, McCall-Tackett K, et al, "Fatal Oral Ingestion of a Large Amount of Cocaine by a 1-Year-Old Child," *J Anal Toxicol*, 2006, 30:162.

Widmer-Girod C, Cognard E, and Staub C, "Validation of an Analytical Procedure for the Simultaneous Determination of Cocaine and Three of Its Metabolites in Hair by GC-Cl/MS^2 Using an Ion-Trap Detection," *Annale de Toxicologie Analytique*, 2005, 17(4):299-306.

Wiegand T, Schneider E, and Goldsmith S, "Cocaine-Associated Chest Pain and the Incidence of a Positive Troponin I Assay: A Two-Year Retrospective Review," *J Toxicol Clin Toxicol*, 2004, 42(5):826.

Wiener SW, Ravikumar PR, Hoffman RS, et al, "Cinnamoylecgonine in the Urine of Cocaine Users," *J Toxicol Clin Toxicol*, 2004, 42(5):797.

Wilson LD and Shelat C, "Electrophysiologic and Hemodynamic Effects of Sodium Bicarbonate in a Canine Model of Severe Cocaine Intoxication," *J Toxicol Clin Toxicol*, 2003, 41(6):777-88.

Wogoman HM and Marinetti L, "Vitreous Fluid Quantiation of Opiates and Cocaine: Comparison of Calibration Curves in Both Blood and Vitreous Matrix," *J Anal Toxicol*, 2006, 30:136.

Yao IC, Mazor SS, O'Koren K, et al, "Delayed Onset of Seizure in a Body Stuffer," *J Toxicol Clin Toxicol*, 2003, 41(5):650.

Codeine

CAS Number 1420-53-7; 1422-07-7; 41444-62-6; 52-28-8; 5913-76-8; 6854-40-6; 76-57-3

Synonyms Codeine Phosphate; Codeine Sulfate; Methylmorphine

Impairment Potential Yes. Serum codeine level >2.6 mg/L is consistent with driving impairment

Use Treatment of mild to moderate pain; antitussive in lower doses; dextromethorphan has equivalent antitussive activity but has much lower toxicity in accidental overdose

Mechanism of Action Binds to opiate receptors in the CNS, causing inhibition of ascending pain pathways, altering the perception of and response to pain; causes cough supression by direct central action in the medulla; produces generalized CNS depression; also has a dose-related histamine-releasing effect

Adverse Reactions

Cardiovascular: Palpitations, hypotension, bradycardia, peripheral vasodilation, sinus bradycardia

Central nervous system: CNS depression, psychosis, increased intracranial pressure, agitation, dizziness, **drowsiness**, sedation

Dermatologic: Pruritus, systemic contact dermatitis, exfoliative dermatitis, pityriasis rosea-like reaction, acute generalized exanthematous pustulosis, angioedema, bullous skin disease, toxic epidermal necrolysis, erythema nodosum, exanthem

Endocrine & metabolic: Antidiuretic hormone release

Gastrointestinal: Nausea, vomiting, **constipation**, adynamic ileus, biliary tract spasm, xerostomia, pancreatitis

Genitourinary: Urinary tract spasm, urinary incontinence

Neuromuscular & skeletal: Paresthesia

Ocular: Miosis

Respiratory: Apnea, respiratory depression, aspiration

Miscellaneous: Physical and psychological dependence, histamine release, fixed drug eruption

Signs and Symptoms of Overdose Ataxia, constipation, erythema multiforme, hallucinations, hypocalcemia, miosis, myasthenia gravis (exacerbation or precipitation), myoglobinuria, respiratory failure, rhabdomyolysis, somnolence, syncope, syndrome of inappropriate antidiuretic hormone (SIADH), urine discoloration (milky), vomiting

Pharmacodynamics/Kinetics

Onset of action: Oral: 0.5-1 hour; I.M.: 10-30 minutes
Peak effect: Oral: 1-1.5 hours; I.M.: 0.5-1 hour
Duration: 4-6 hours
Absorption: Oral: Adequate
Distribution: Crosses placenta; enters breast milk
Protein binding: 7%
Metabolism: Hepatic to morphine (active)
Half-life elimination: 2.5-3.5 hours
Excretion: Urine (3% to 16% as unchanged drug, norcodeine, and free and conjugated morphine)

Dosage

Note: These are guidelines and do not represent the maximum doses that may be required in all patients. Doses should be titrated to pain relief/prevention. Doses >1.5 mg/kg body weight are not recommended.

Analgesic:

Children: Oral, I.M., SubQ: 0.5-1 mg/kg/dose every 4-6 hours as needed; maximum: 60 mg/dose

Adults:

Oral: 30 mg every 4-6 hours as needed; patients with prior opiate exposure may require higher initial doses. Usual range: 15-120 mg every 4-6 hours as needed

Oral, controlled release formulation (Codeine Contin®, not available in U.S.): 50-300 mg every 12 hours. **Note:** A patient's codeine requirement should be established using prompt release formulations; conversion to long acting products may be considered when chronic, continuous treatment is required. Higher dosages should be reserved for use only in opioid-tolerant patients.

I.M., SubQ: 30 mg every 4-6 hours as needed; patients with prior opiate exposure may require higher initial doses. Usual range: 15-120 mg every 4-6 hours as needed; more frequent dosing may be needed

Antitussive: Oral (for nonproductive cough):

Children: 1-1.5 mg/kg/day in divided doses every 4-6 hours as needed: Alternative dose according to age:

2-6 years: 2.5-5 mg every 4-6 hours as needed; maximum: 30 mg/day

6-12 years: 5-10 mg every 4-6 hours as needed; maximum: 60 mg/day

Adults: 10-20 mg/dose every 4-6 hours as needed; maximum: 120 mg/day

Dosing adjustment in renal impairment:

Cl_{cr} 10-50 mL/minute: Administer 75% of dose
Cl_{cr} <10 mL/minute: Administer 50% of dose

Dosing adjustment in hepatic impairment: Probably necessary in hepatic insufficiency

Stability Store injection between 15°C to 30°C, avoid freezing; do not use if injection is discolored or contains a precipitate; protect injection from light

Monitoring Parameters Pain relief, respiratory and mental status, blood pressure, heart rate

Administration

Not approved for I.V. administration (although this route has been used clinically). If given intravenously, must be given slowly and the patient should be lying down. Rapid intravenous administration of narcotics may increase the incidence of serious adverse effects, in part due to limited opportunity to assess response prior to administration of the full dose. Access to respiratory support should be immediately available.

Contraindications Hypersensitivity to codeine or any component of the formulation; pregnancy (prolonged use or high doses at term)

Warnings

An opioid-containing analgesic regimen should be tailored to each patient's needs and based upon the type of pain being treated (acute versus chronic), the route of administration, degree of tolerance for opioids (naive versus chronic user), age, weight, and medical condition. The optimal analgesic dose varies widely among patients. Doses should be titrated to pain relief/prevention.

Use with caution in patients with hypersensitivity reactions to other phenanthrene derivative opioid agonists (morphine, hydrocodone, hydromorphone, levorphanol, oxycodone, oxymorphone); respiratory diseases including asthma, emphysema, COPD, or severe liver or renal insufficiency; some preparations contain sulfites which may cause allergic reactions; tolerance or drug dependence may result from extended use

Not recommended for use for cough control in patients with a productive cough; not recommended as an antitussive for children <2 years of age; the elderly may be particularly susceptible to the CNS depressant and confusion as well as constipating effects of narcotics

Not approved for I.V. administration (although this route has been used clinically). If given intravenously, must be given slowly and the patient should be lying down. Rapid intravenous administration of narcotics may increase the incidence of serious adverse effects, in part due to limited opportunity to assess response prior to administration of the full dose. Access to respiratory support should be immediately available

Dosage Forms
[CAN] = Canadian brand name

Injection, as phosphate: 15 mg/mL (2 mL); 30 mg/mL (2 mL) [contains sodium metabisulfite]

Tablet, as phosphate: 30 mg, 60 mg

Tablet, as sulfate: 15 mg, 30 mg, 60 mg

Tablet, controlled release (Codeine Contin®) [CAN]: 50 mg, 100 mg, 150 mg, 200 mg [not available in U.S.]

Reference Range
Therapeutic: 13-33 ng/mL

Toxic: Serum: >1.0 mcg/mL. In the postmortem state, anatomical site concentration differences (ie, postmortem redistribution) may occur.

Lethal: >1000 ng/mL

Methodology: Radioimmunoassay (RIA), gas chromatography (GC), high performance liquid chromatography (HPLC)

Peak codeine:morphine serum ratio: ~33:1

Overdosage/Treatment
Supportive therapy: Naloxone hydrochloride (0.4-2 mg I.V., SubQ, or through an endotracheal tube); a continuous infusion (at $^2/_3$ the response dose/hour) may be required

Enhancement of elimination: Multiple dosing of activated charcoal may be useful

Antidote(s)
- Nalmefene [ANTIDOTE]
- Naloxone [ANTIDOTE]

Test Interactions ↑ aminotransferases (ALT, AST) (S)

Drug Interactions
Substrate of CYP2D6 (major), 3A4 (minor); **Inhibits** CYP2D6 (weak)

CYP2D6 inhibitors: May decrease the effects of codeine. Example inhibitors include chlorpromazine, delavirdine, fluoxetine, miconazole, paroxetine, pergolide, quinidine, quinine, ritonavir, and ropinirole.

Decreased effect with cigarette smoking

Increased toxicity: CNS depressants, phenothiazines, TCAs, other narcotic analgesics, guanabenz, MAO inhibitors, neuromuscular blockers

Pregnancy Risk Factor C/D (prolonged use or high doses at term)

Pregnancy Implications Crosses the placenta

Lactation Enters breast milk/use caution (AAP rates "compatible")

Nursing Implications Observe patient for excessive sedation, respiratory depression, implement safety measures, assist with ambulation

Specific References
Barnes AJ, Kim I, Schepers R, et al, "Comparison of Cozart Oral Fluid Opiate ELISA and GC/MS Results Following Controlled Administration of Codeine Sulphate," *J Anal Toxicol*, 2003, 27:187.

Barnes AJ, Kim I, Schepers R, et al, "Sensitivity, Specificity, and Efficiency in Detecting Opiates in Oral Fluid with the Cozart® Opiate Microplate EIA and GC-MS Following Controlled Codeine Administration," *J Anal Toxicol*, 2003, 27:402-6.

Gasche Y, Daali Y, Fathi M, et al, "Codeine Intoxication Associated with Ultrarapid CYP2D6 Metabolism," *N Engl J Med*, 2004, 351(27): 2827-31.

Hill V, Cairns T, Cheng CC, et al, "Multiple Aspects of Hair Analysis for Opiates: Methodology, Clinical and Workplace Populations, Codeine, and Poppy Seed Ingestion," *J Anal Toxicol*, 2005, 29:696-703.

Kuo SC, Lin YC, Kao SM, et al, "Probable Codeine Phosphate-Induced Seizures," *Ann Pharmacother*, 2004, 38(11):1848-51.

Langille RM, "A Case of Nearly Uniform Post-Mortem Redistribution," *J Anal Toxicol*, 2006, 30:147.

Langille RM, "Aggressive Resuscitation as a Cause of Post-Mortem Redistribution," *J Anal Toxicol*, 2006, 30:157.

Rollins DE, Wilkins DG, Krueger GG, et al, "The Effect of Hair Color on the Incorporation of Codeine Into Human Hair," *J Anal Toxicol*, 2003, 27(8):545-51.

Colchicine

Related Information
- Autumn Crocus

CAS Number 64-86-8

Use Treatment of acute gouty arthritis attacks and prevention of recurrences of such attacks

Primary biliary cirrhosis; management of familial Mediterranean fever; pericarditis

Mechanism of Action Alkaloids from meadow saffron; mechanism of action is not completely understood; decreases leukocyte motility, decreases phagocytosis in joints, and lactic acid production, thereby reducing the deposition of urate crystals that perpetuates the inflammatory response; not an analgesic; antimitotic, may be responsible for toxicity

Adverse Reactions
Cardiovascular: Hypotension, sinus bradycardia, vasculitis

Central nervous system: Confusion, delirium, seizures

Dermatologic: Rash, alopecia (in 2 to 3 weeks) bullous skin disease, toxic epidermal necrolysis, urticaria, pruritus, axonopathy, licheniform eruptions, exanthem

Endocrine & metabolic: Dehydration

Gastrointestinal: **Nausea, vomiting, diarrhea, abdominal pain**, steatorrhea, fecal discoloration (gray), pancreatitis

Genitourinary: Azoospermia

Hematologic: Leukopenia (in 4-6 days) neutropenia, agranulocytosis (0.8 mg/kg), thrombocytopenia, granulocytopenia, aplastic anemia, methemoglobinemia, megaloblastic anemia

Hepatic: Hepatotoxicity

Neuromuscular & skeletal: Myopathy, peripheral neuritis, paralysis, rhabdomyolysis

Ocular: Diplopia

Renal: Hematuria, acute tubular necrosis

Respiratory: Apnea, respiratory depression, respiratory collapse

Miscellaneous: Aneuploidy induction, fixed drug eruption

Signs and Symptoms of Overdose Apnea, bradycardia, diabetes insipidus, diarrhea, dysosmia, feces discoloration (gray), fever, hematuria, hypernatremia, hyperthermia, hypocalcemia, hypothermia, leukocytosis, myasthenia gravis (exacerbation or precipitation), myoglobinuria, nausea, nephritis, oligospermia (doses over 0.5mg/kg) polyuria, ptosis, purpura, rhabdomyolysis, sexual dysfunction, vomiting (doses over 0.5 mg/kg)

Admission Criteria/Prognosis Admit any symptomatic patient or ingestion over 0.5 mg/kg.

Pharmacodynamics/Kinetics
Onset of action: Oral: Pain relief: ~12 hours if adequately dosed

Distribution: Concentrates in leukocytes, kidney, spleen, and liver; does not distribute in heart, skeletal muscle, and brain

Protein binding: 10% to 31%

Metabolism: Partially hepatic via deacetylation

Half-life elimination: 12-30 minutes; End-stage renal disease: 45 minutes

Time to peak, serum: Oral: 0.5-2 hours, declining for the next 2 hours before increasing again due to enterohepatic recycling

Excretion: Primarily feces; urine (10% to 20%)

Dosage
Familial Mediterranean fever (unlabeled use): Prophylaxis: Oral:
Children:
≤5 years: 0.5 mg/day
>5 years: 1-1.5 mg/day in 2-3 divided doses
Adults: 1-2 mg daily in divided doses (occasionally reduced to 0.6 mg/day in patients with GI intolerance)

Gouty arthritis: Adults:
Prophylaxis of acute attacks: Oral: 0.6 mg twice daily; initial and/or subsequent dosage may be decreased (ie, 0.6 mg once daily) in patients at risk of toxicity or in those who are intolerant (including weakness, loose stools, or diarrhea); range: 0.6 mg every other day to 0.6 mg 3 times/day

Acute attacks:
Oral: Initial: 0.6-1.2 mg, followed by 0.6 every 1-2 hours; some clinicians recommend a maximum of 3 doses; more aggressive approaches have recommended a maximum dose of up to 6 mg. Wait at least 3 days before initiating another course of therapy

I.V.: Initial: 1-2 mg, then 0.5 mg every 6 hours until response, not to exceed total dose of 4 mg. If pain recurs, it may be necessary to administer additional daily doses. The amount of colchicine administered intravenously in an acute treatment period (generally ~1 week) should not exceed a total dose of 4 mg. Do not administer more colchicine by any route for at least 7 days after a full course of I.V. therapy.

Note: Many experts would avoid use because of potential for serious, life-threatening complications. Should not be administered to patients with renal insufficiency, hepatobiliary obstruction, patients >70 years of age, or recent oral colchicine use. Should be reserved for hospitalized patients who are under the care of a physician experienced in the use of intravenous colchicine.

Recurrent pericarditis (with aspirin): 1-2 mg the first day and then 0.5-1 mg/day for 6 months

Surgery: Gouty arthritis, prophylaxis of recurrent attacks: Adults: Oral: 0.6 mg/day or every other day; patients who are to undergo surgical procedures may receive 0.6 mg 3 times/day for 3 days before and 3 days after surgery

Primary biliary cirrhosis (unlabeled use): Adults: Oral: 0.6 mg twice daily

Elderly: Reduce maintenance/prophylactic dose by 50% in individuals >70 years

Dosing adjustment in renal impairment: Gouty arthritis, acute attacks:

Oral: Specific dosing recommendations not available from the manufacturer:

Prophylaxis:
Cl_{cr} 35-49 mL/minute: 0.6 mg once daily
Cl_{cr} 10-34 mL/minute: 0.6 mg every 2-3 days
Cl_{cr} < 10 mL/minute: Avoid chronic use of colchicine. Use in serious renal impairment is contraindicated by the manufacturer.

Treatment: Cl_{cr} <10 mL/minute: Use in serious renal impairment is contraindicated by the manufacturer. If a decision is made to use colchicine, decrease dose by 75%.

Peritoneal dialysis: Supplemental dose is not necessary

Dosage adjustment in hepatic impairment: Avoid in hepatobiliary dysfunction and in patients with hepatic disease.

Monitoring Parameters CBC and renal function test

Administration
I.V.: Injection should be made over 2-5 minutes into tubing of free-flowing I.V. With compatible fluid. Do not administer I.M. or SubQ; severe local irritation can occur following SubQ or I.M. administration. Extravasation can cause tissue irritation.

Tablet: Administer orally with water and maintain adequate fluid intake.

Contraindications Hypersensitivity to colchicine or any component of the formulation; severe renal, gastrointestinal, hepatic, or cardiac disorders; blood dyscrasias; pregnancy (parenteral)

Warnings
Use with caution in debilitated patients or elderly patients; use caution in patients with mild-to-moderate cardiac, GI, renal, or liver disease. Severe local irritation can occur following SubQ or I.M. administration. Dosage reduction is recommended in patients who develop weakness or gastrointestinal symptoms (anorexia, diarrhea, nausea, vomiting) related to drug therapy.

Intravenous: Use only with extreme caution; potential for serious, life-threatening complications. Should not be administered to patients with renal insufficiency, hepatobiliary obstruction, patients >70 years of age, or recent oral colchicine use. Should be reserved for hospitalized patients who are under the care of a physician experienced in the use of intravenous colchicine.

Dosage Forms
Injection, solution: 0.5 mg/mL (2 mL)
Tablet: 0.6 mg

Reference Range Plasma colchicine level of 12 ng/mL achieved after a 0.96 mg/kg overdose ingestion; patient was severely symptomatic; postmortem femoral blood colchicine level of 62 ng/mL associated with a suicidal overdose; peak plasma colchicine level of 2.2 ng/mL achieved after 1 mg oral dose

Overdosage/Treatment
Decontamination: Emesis not recommended due to potential for seizures; lavage (within 1 hour) indicated if early in ingestion (control seizures with benzodiazepines prior to lavage); activated charcoal with sorbitol (first dose only) 1-2 g/kg at $^1/_2$ first dose every 2-6 hours until toxic symptoms abate and patient is stable

Supportive therapy: Granulocyte colony-stimulating factor (300 mcg/day SubQ) has been used to treat neutropenia; observe 2-12 hours due to latency of symptoms of toxicity; treat manifestations of toxicity accordingly; no specific antidote; supportive care is mainstay of treatment. Serum troponin I (TnI) elevation with echocardiographic abnormalities may be useful in predicting impending cardiovascular collapse.

Enhancement of elimination: Multiple dosing of activated charcoal may be useful; dialysis is not effective; not dialyzable (0% to 5%); colchicine specific antibodies are investigational

Antidote(s)
● Filgrastim [ANTIDOTE]

Test Interactions May cause false-positive urine tests for erythrocytes or hemoglobin; interferes with urine tests for hydrocorticoids

Drug Interactions Substrate of CYP3A4 (major); **Induces** CYP2C8 (weak), 2C9 (weak), 2E1 (weak), 3A4 (weak)

Cyclosporine: Concurrent use with colchicine may increase toxicity of colchicine.

CYP3A4 inhibitors: May increase the levels/effects of colchicine. Example inhibitors include azole antifungals, diclofenac, doxycycline, imatinib, isoniazid, nefazodone, nicardipine, propofol, protease inhibitors, quinidine, telithromycin, and verapamil.

Macrolide antibiotics (clarithromycin, erythromycin, troleandomycin): May decrease the metabolism of colchicine resulting in severe colchicine toxicity. Avoid, if possible.

Telithromycin: May decrease the metabolism of colchicine resulting in colchicine toxicity. Avoid, if possible.

Verapamil: May increase colchicine toxicity (especially nephrotoxicity).

Pregnancy Risk Factor C (oral); D (parenteral)

Lactation Enters breast milk/use caution (AAP rates "compatible")

Additional Information Colchicine-specific Fab fragments are prepared from goat antiserum with an affinity constant of 2×10^{10} M^{-1}; total plasma colchicine level may rise six- to tenfold after infusion of antibody fragment; this treatment may not prevent bone marrow depression, but can improve

hemodynamic status; colchicine may be useful in the treatment of Palmer fibromatosis.

Colchicine
Additional info: Probability of death due to ingestion of colchicine equals

$$\frac{e^{(0.964 \times 10^{-3} \times dose\ (mcg/kg)\ +\ 0.282\ (PT)\ +\ 0.265 \times 10^{-6}\ (WBC)\ +\ 0.611)}}{1 + e^{(0.964 \times 10^{-3} \times dose\ (mcg/kg)\ +\ 0.282\ (PT)\ +\ 0.265 \times 10^{-6}\ (WBC)\ +\ 0.611)}}$$

dose = ingested amount in mcg/kg
PT = lowest prothrombin time in % control
WBC = highest white blood cell count in cells per L

Fatal dose: About 0.8 mg/kg

Specific References
Abe E, LeMaire-Hurtel AS, Durvenevol C, et al, "A Novel LC-ESI-MS-MS Method for Sensitive Quantification of Colchicine in Human Plasma: Application to Two Case Reports," *J Anal Tox*, 2006, 30:210-5.

Arroyo MP, Sanders S, Yee H, et al, "Toxic Epidermal Necrolysis-Like Reaction Secondary to Colchicine Overdose," *Br J Dermatol*, 2004, 150(3):581-8 (review).

Flesch F, Krencker E, Mootien Y, et al, "Diagnosis Wandering in a Case of Accidental Poisoning by *Colchicum autumnale*," *J Toxicol Clin Toxicol*, 2002, 40(3):375-6.

Imazio M, Bobbio M, Cecchi E, et al, "Colchicine as First-Choice Therapy for Recurrent Pericarditis: Results of the CORE (Colchicine for Recurrent Pericarditis) Trial," *Arch Intern Med*, 2005, 165(17):1987-91.

Morris I, Varughese G, and Mattingly P, "Colchicine in Acute Gout," *BMJ*, 2003, 327(7426): 1275-6.

Rauber-Lüthy CH, Baer W, Rentsch K, et al, "Misdiagnosed Fatal Meadow Saffron Poisoning in a Toddler," *J Toxicol Clin Toxicol*, 2003, 41(5):728.

Rollot F, Pajot O, Chauvelot-Moachon L, et al, "Acute Colchicine Intoxication During Clarithromycin Administration," *Ann Pharmacother*, 2004, 38(12):2074-7.

Cortisone

Related Information
● Corticosteroids

CAS Number 50-04-4; 53-06-5

Synonyms Compound E; Cortisone Acetate

Use Management of adrenocortical insufficiency

Mechanism of Action Decreases inflammation by suppression of migration of polymorphonuclear leukocytes and reversal of increased capillary permeability

Adverse Reactions
Cardiovascular: Edema, hypertension, QT prolongation, cardiomegaly, cardiomyopathy

Central nervous system: **Insomnia, nervousness,** mood swings, vertigo, seizures, headache, psychosis, pseudotumor cerebri, delirium, hallucinations, euphoria, depression, mania

Dermatologic: Hirsutism, acne, skin atrophy, hyperpigmentation, bruising, telangiectasia, striae

Endocrine & metabolic: Diabetes mellitus, Cushing's syndrome, pituitary-adrenal axis suppression, growth suppression, glucose intolerance, hypokalemia, alkalosis, amenorrhea, sodium and water retention, hyperglycemia

Gastrointestinal: **Increased appetite, indigestion,** peptic ulcer, nausea, vomiting, black stools, abdominal distention, esophagitis ulceration, pancreatitis

Neuromuscular & skeletal: Muscle weakness, osteoporosis, fractures, arthralgia, muscle wasting, rhabdomyolysis

Ocular: Cataracts, glaucoma

Respiratory: Epistaxis

Miscellaneous: Hypersensitivity reactions

Signs and Symptoms of Overdose When consumed in excessive quantities for prolonged periods, systemic hypercorticism and adrenal suppression may occur. In those cases, discontinuation and withdrawal of the corticosteroid should be done judiciously. Cushingoid changes from continued administration of large doses results in acne, central obesity, diabetes, ecchymoses, electrolyte and fluid imbalance, hirsutism, hyperlipidemia, hypertension, increased susceptibility to infection, moon face, myopathy, osteoporosis, peptic ulcer, sexual dysfunction, and striae.

Pharmacodynamics/Kinetics
Onset of action: Peak effect: Oral: ~2 hours; I.M.: 20-48 hours
Duration: 30-36 hours
Absorption: Slow
Distribution: Muscles, liver, skin, intestines, and kidneys; crosses placenta; enters breast milk
Metabolism: Hepatic to inactive metabolites
Half-life elimination: 0.5-2 hours; End-stage renal disease: 3.5 hours
Excretion: Urine and feces

Toxicodynamics/Kinetics

Peak effect: Oral: Within 2 hours; I.M.: Within 20-48 hours

Duration of action: 30-36 hours

Absorption: Slow rate of absorption

Distribution: Crosses the placenta; appears in breast milk; distributes to muscles, liver, skin, intestines, and kidneys

Plasma binding: 90%

Metabolism: In the liver to inactive metabolites

Half-life: 30 minutes to 2 hours; End stage renal disease: 3.5 hours

Elimination: In bile and urine

Note: Insoluble in water; supplemental doses may be warranted during times of stress in the course of withdrawing therapy

Dosage

If possible, administer glucocorticoids before 9 AM to minimize adrenocortical suppression; dosing depends upon the condition being treated and the response of the patient; supplemental doses may be warranted during times of stress in the course of withdrawing therapy

Children:

Anti-inflammatory or immunosuppressive:

Oral: 2.5-10 mg/kg/day **or** 20-300 mg/m^2/day in divided doses every 6-8 hours

I.M.: 1-5 mg/kg/day **or** 14-375 mg/m^2/day in divided doses every 12-24 hours

Physiologic replacement:

Oral: 0.5-0.75 mg/kg/day **or** 20-25 mg/m^2/day in divided doses every 8 hours

I.M.: 0.25-0.35 mg/kg/day once daily **or** 12.5 mg/m^2/day

Stress coverage for surgery: I.M.: 1 and 2 days before preanesthesia, and 1-3 days after surgery: 50-62.5 mg/m^2/day; 4 days after surgery: 31-50 mg/m^2/day; 5 days after surgery, resume presurgical corticosteroid dose.

Adults: Oral, I.M.: 25-300 mg/day in divided doses every 12-24 hours

Hemodialysis effects: Supplemental dose is not necessary

Administration

Administer I.M. daily dose before 9 AM to minimize adrenocortical suppression

Contraindications Hypersensitivity to cortisone acetate or any component of the formulation; serious infections, except septic shock or tuberculous meningitis; administration of live virus vaccines; pregnancy

Warnings Use with caution in patients with hypothyroidism, cirrhosis, hypertension, CHF, ulcerative colitis, thromboembolic disorders, osteoporosis, convulsive disorders, peptic ulcer, diabetes mellitus, myasthenia gravis; prolonged therapy (>5 days) of pharmacologic doses of corticosteroids may lead to hypothalamic-pituitary-adrenal suppression, the degree of adrenal suppression varies with the degree and duration of glucocorticoid therapy; this must be taken into consideration when taking patients off steroids

Dosage Forms Tablet, as acetate: 25 mg

Overdosage/Treatment

Decontamination: Emesis within 30 minutes or lavage (within 1 hour)/activated charcoal; acute overdose does not require tapering of dose

Enhanced elimination: Its metabolite (prednisolone) is slightly dialyzable (5% to 20%)

Test Interactions May cause false elevation of digoxin by Abbott TDx method

Drug Interactions

Decreased effect:

Barbiturates, phenytoin, rifampin may decrease cortisone effects

Live virus vaccines

Anticholinesterase agents may decrease effect

Cortisone may decrease warfarin effects

Cortisone may decrease effects of salicylates

Increased effect: Estrogens (increase cortisone effects)

Increased toxicity:

Cortisone + NSAIDs may increase ulcerogenic potential

Cortisone may increase potassium deletion due to diuretics

Pregnancy Risk Factor D

Lactation Enters breast milk/use caution

Nursing Implications I.M. use only; shake vial before measuring out dose; withdraw gradually following long-term therapy

Additional Information Insoluble in water

Cromolyn

CAS Number 15826-37-6; 16110-51-3

U.S. Brand Names Crolom®; Gastrocrom®; Intal®; Nasalcrom® [OTC]; Opticrom®

Synonyms Cromoglycic Acid; Cromolyn Sodium; Disodium Cromoglycate; DSCG

Use

Inhalation: May be used as an adjunct in the prophylaxis of allergic disorders, including rhinitis, asthma; prevention of exercise-induced bronchospasm

Oral: Systemic mastocytosis

Ophthalmic: Treatment of vernal keratoconjunctivitis, vernal conjunctivitis, and vernal keratitis

Unlabeled/Investigational Use Oral: Food allergy, treatment of inflammatory bowel disease

Mechanism of Action Prevents the mast cell release of histamine, leukotrienes and slow-reacting substance of anaphylaxis by inhibiting degranulation after contact with antigens

Adverse Reactions

Cardiovascular: Pericardial effusion, pericarditis with pericardial tamponade

Central nervous system: Dizziness, headache

Dermatologic: Rash, eczema, angioedema, cutaneous vasculitis

Endocrine & metabolic: Parotitis

Gastrointestinal: **Unpleasant taste (inhalation aerosol)**, xerostomia, nausea, vomiting, diarrhea, throat irritation

Genitourinary: Dysuria

Hepatic: Hepatic vasculitis

Neuromuscular & skeletal: Arthralgia, myositis

Ocular: Ocular stinging, lacrimation, chemosis

Respiratory: **Coughing**, **hoarseness**, sneezing, stuffy nose, wheezing, eosinophilic pneumonia

Miscellaneous: Eosinophilic pneumonia, anaphylactic reaction, nasal burning, pulmonary infiltrates

Signs and Symptoms of Overdose Bronchospasm, dyspnea, dysuria, lacrimation, laryngeal edema, pericarditis, wheezing

Pharmacodynamics/Kinetics

Onset: Response to treatment:

Nasal spray: May occur at 1-2 weeks

Ophthalmic: May be seen within a few days; treatment for up to 6 weeks is often required

Oral: May occur within 2-6 weeks

Absorption:

Inhalation: ~8% reaches lungs upon inhalation; well absorbed

Oral: <1% of dose absorbed

Half-life elimination: 80-90 minutes

Time to peak, serum: Inhalation: ~15 minutes

Excretion: Urine and feces (equal amounts as unchanged drug); exhaled gases (small amounts)

Dosage

Oral:

Systemic mastocytosis:

Neonates and preterm Infants: Not recommended

Infants and Children <2 years: 20 mg/kg/day in 4 divided doses; may increase in patients 6 months to 2 years of age if benefits not seen after 2-3 weeks; do not exceed 30 mg/kg/day

Children 2-12 years: 100 mg 4 times/day; not to exceed 40 mg/kg/day

Children >12 years and Adults: 200 mg 4 times/day

Food allergy and inflammatory bowel disease:

Children <2 years: Not recommended

Children 2-12 years: Initial dose: 100 mg 4 times/day; may double the dose if effect is not satisfactory within 2-3 weeks; not to exceed 40 mg/kg/day

Children >12 years and Adults: Initial dose: 200 mg 4 times/day; may double the dose if effect is not satisfactory within 2-3 weeks; up to 400 mg 4 times/day

Once desired effect is achieved, dose may be tapered to lowest effective dose

Inhalation:

For chronic control of asthma, taper frequency to the lowest effective dose (ie, 4 times/day to 3 times/day to twice daily):

Nebulization solution: Children >2 years and Adults: Initial: 20 mg 4 times/day; usual dose: 20 mg 3-4 times/day

Metered spray:

Children 5-12 years: Initial: 2 inhalations 4 times/day; usual dose: 1-2 inhalations 3-4 times/day

Children ≥12 years and Adults: Initial: 2 inhalations 4 times/day; usual dose: 2-4 inhalations 3-4 times/day

Prevention of allergen- or exercise-induced bronchospasm: Administer 10-15 minutes prior to exercise or allergen exposure but no longer than 1 hour before:

Nebulization solution: Children >2 years and Adults: Single dose of 20 mg

Metered spray: Children >5 years and Adults: Single dose of 2 inhalations

Ophthalmic: Children >4 years and Adults: 1-2 drops in each eye 4-6 times/day

Nasal: Allergic rhinitis (treatment and prophylaxis): Children ≥2 years and Adults: 1 spray into each nostril 3-4 times/day; may be increased to 6 times/day (symptomatic relief may require 2-4 weeks)

Dosage in renal/hepatic impairment: Specific guidelines not available; consider lower dose of oral product.

Stability

Store at room temperature of 15°C to 30°C (59°F to 86°F); protect from light.

Nebulizer solution is **compatible** with metaproterenol sulfate, isoproterenol hydrochloride, 0.25% isoetharine hydrochloride, epinephrine hydrochloride, terbutaline sulfate, and 20% acetylcysteine solution for at least 1 hour after their admixture

Oral concentrate: Do not use if solution becomes discolored or forms a precipitate.

Monitoring Parameters Periodic pulmonary function tests

Administration

For oral use, cromolyn powder is dissolved in hot water and taken at least 30 minutes before meals

Contraindications Hypersensitivity to cromolyn or any component of the formulation; acute asthma attacks

Warnings Severe anaphylactic reactions may occur rarely; cromolyn is a prophylactic drug with no benefit for acute situations; caution should be used when withdrawing the drug or tapering the dose as symptoms may reoccur; use with caution in patients with a history of cardiac arrhythmias. Transient burning or stinging may occur with ophthalmic use. Dosage of oral product should be decreased with hepatic or renal dysfunction.

Dosage Forms

Aerosol, for oral inhalation, as sodium (Intal®): 800 mcg/inhalation (8.1 g) [112 metered inhalations; 56 doses], (14.2 g) [200 metered inhalations; 100 doses]

Solution for nebulization, as sodium (Intal®): 20 mg/2 mL (60s, 120s)

Solution, intranasal, as sodium [spray] (NasalCrom®): 40 mg/mL (13 mL, 26 mL) [5.2 mg/inhalation; contains benzalkonium chloride]

Solution, ophthalmic, as sodium (Crolom®, Opticrom®): 4% (10 mL) [contains benzalkonium chloride]

Solution, oral, as sodium (Gastrocrom®): 100 mg/5 mL (96s)

Reference Range Plasma levels not relatable to effect; peak plasma level after inhalation: ~15 ng/mL

Overdosage/Treatment

Decontamination: Oral: Lavage (within 1 hour)/activated charcoal

Supportive therapy: Treat inhalation exposure with 100% humidified oxygen; treat anaphylaxis with epinephrine and corticosteroids; albuterol can be given for bronchospasm

Drug Interactions Corticosteroids: Ophthalmic preparation may be used with ophthalmic corticosteroids

Pregnancy Risk Factor B

Pregnancy Implications No known teratogenic effect

Lactation Excretion in breast milk unknown/use caution

Nursing Implications Advise patient to clear as much mucus as possible before inhalation treatments

Additional Information Reserve systemic use in children <2 years of age for severe disease; avoid systemic use in premature infants

---

Cyanocobalamin

CAS Number 68-19-9

U.S. Brand Names Nascobal®

Synonyms Vitamin B₁₂

Use Treatment of pernicious anemia; vitamin B_{12} deficiency; increased B_{12} requirements due to pregnancy, thyrotoxicosis, hemorrhage, malignancy, liver or kidney disease; water-soluble vitamin with a wide margin of safety

Mechanism of Action Coenzyme for various metabolic functions, including fat and carbohydrate metabolism and protein synthesis, used in cell replication and hematopoiesis

Adverse Reactions

Cardiovascular: Peripheral vascular thrombosis

Dermatologic: Itching, rash

Endocrine & metabolic: Hypokalemia, hyperuricemia

Gastrointestinal: Diarrhea, bezoar formation

Miscellaneous: Allergic reactions, exacerbation of multiple myeloma

Signs and Symptoms of Overdose Hypokalemia

Pharmacodynamics/Kinetics

Absorption: Oral: Variable from the terminal ileum; requires the presence of calcium and gastric "intrinsic factor" to transfer the compound across the intestinal mucosa

Distribution: Principally stored in the liver and bone marrow, also stored in the kidneys and adrenals

Protein binding: To transcobalamin II

Metabolism: Converted in tissues to active coenzymes, methylcobalamin and deoxyadenosylcobalamin

Bioavailability: Intranasal:

Gel: 8.9% (relative to I.M.)

Solution: 6.1% (relative to I.M.)

Dosage

Recommended daily allowance (RDA):

Children 1-4 years: 3 mcg/day

Adults: 6 mcg/day

Nutritional deficiency: 25-250 mcg/day

Children:

Congenital pernicious anemia (if evidence of neurologic involvement): I.M.: 1000 mcg/day for at least 2 weeks; maintenance: 50 mcg/month

Vitamin B₁₂ deficiency: I.M., SubQ: 1-5 mg given in single or SubQ doses of 100 mcg/day over 2 or more weeks

Adults:

Pernicious anemia: I.M., SubQ: 100 mcg/day for 6-7 days

Vitamin B₁₂ deficiency:

Oral: Usually not recommended, maximum absorbed from a single oral dose is 2-3 mcg

I.M., SubQ: 30 mcg/day for 5-10 days, followed by 100-200 mcg/month

Stability Clear pink to red solutions are stable at room temperature; protect from light; **incompatible** with chlorpromazine, phytonadione, prochlorperazine, warfarin, ascorbic acid, dextrose, heavy metals, oxidizing or reducing agents

Monitoring Parameters Serum potassium, erythrocyte and reticulocyte count, hemoglobin, hematocrit

Administration

I.M./SubQ: I.M. or deep SubQ are preferred routes of administration

Intranasal: Nasal spray: Prior to initial dose, activate (prime) spray nozzle by pumping unit quickly and firmly until first appearance of spray, then prime twice more. The unit must be reprimed once immediately before each use.

I.V.: Not recommended due to rapid elimination

Oral: Not recommended due to variable absorption; however, oral therapy of 1000-2000 mcg/day has been effective for anemia if I.M./SubQ routes refused or not tolerated

Contraindications Hypersensitivity to cyanocobalamin or any component of the formulation, cobalt; hereditary optic nerve atrophy (Leber's disease)

Warnings I.M. route used to treat pernicious anemia; vitamin B₁₂ deficiency for >3 months results in irreversible degenerative CNS lesions; treatment of vitamin B₁₂ megaloblastic anemia may result in severe hypokalemia, sometimes fatal, due to intracellular potassium shift upon anemia resolution. B₁₂ deficiency masks signs of polycythemia vera; vegetarian diets may result in B₁₂ deficiency; pernicious anemia occurs more often in gastric carcinoma than in general population. Patients with Leber's disease may suffer rapid optic atrophy when treated with vitamin B₁₂; an intradermal test dose of parenteral B₁₂ is recommended prior to administration of intranasal product in patients suspected of cyanocobalamin sensitivity; do not use folic acid as substitute for vitamin B₁₂ in preventing anemia, as progression of spinal cord degeneration may occur; some parenteral products contain aluminum: use caution in neonates and patients with renal impairment.

Dosage Forms

[DSC] = Discontinued product

Gel, intranasal (Nascobal®): 500 mcg/0.1 mL (2.3 mL) [contains benzalkonium chloride; delivers 8 doses] [DSC]

Injection, solution: 1000 mcg/mL (1 mL, 10 mL, 30 mL) [may contain benzyl alcohol and/or aluminum]

Lozenge [OTC]: 100 mcg, 250 mcg, 500 mcg

Solution, intranasal spray (Nascobal®): 500 mcg/0.1 mL actuation (2.3 mL) [contains benzalkonium chloride; delivers 8 doses]

Tablet [OTC]: 50 mcg, 100 mcg, 250 mcg, 500 mcg, 1000 mcg, 5000 mcg

Twelve Resin-K: 1000 mcg [may be used as oral, sublingual, or buccal]

Tablet, extended release [OTC]: 1500 mcg

Tablet, sublingual [OTC]: 2500 mcg

Reference Range The lower limit of normal (critical to the diagnosis of B₁₂ deficiency/pernicious anemia) has not been firmly established; it is likely in the range of 100-250 pg/mL (SI: 74-185 pmol/L)

Overdosage/Treatment Supportive therapy: Allergic reactions can be treated with epinephrine, diphenhydramine, and corticosteroids

Test Interactions Methotrexate, pyrimethamine, and most antibiotics invalidate folic acid and vitamin B₁₂ diagnostic microbiological blood assays

Drug Interactions Neomycin, colchicine, anticonvulsants, and metformin may decrease oral absorption of B₁₂, chloramphenicol may decrease B₁₂ effects

Pregnancy Risk Factor A/C (dose exceeding RDA recommendation); C (nasal gel)

Lactation Enters breast milk/compatible

Nursing Implications I.M. or deep SubQ are preferred routes of administration; oral therapy is markedly inferior to parenteral therapy; monitor potassium concentrations during early therapy

Additional Information Radiopaque

Cyclizine

Pronunciation (SYE kli zeen)

CAS Number 303-25-3 (hydrochloride); 5897-19-8 (lactate); 82-92-8 (base)

U.S. Brand Names Marezine® [OTC]

Synonyms Cyclizine Hydrochloride; Cyclizine Lactate

Impairment Potential Yes

Use Prevention and treatment of nausea, vomiting, and dizziness associated with motion sickness; control of postoperative nausea and vomiting

Mechanism of Action Cyclizine is a piperazine derivative with properties of histamines. The precise mechanism of action in inhibiting the symptoms of motion sickness is not known. It may have effects directly on the labyrinthine apparatus and central actions on the labyrinthine apparatus and on the chemoreceptor trigger zone. Cyclizine exerts a central anticholinergic action.

Adverse Reactions

Cardiovascular: Palpitations, sinus tachycardia

Central nervous system: **Drowsiness**, dizziness, headache, euphoria, ataxia, paranoia

Dermatologic: Dermatitis

Gastrointestinal: Nausea, **xerostomia**

Genitourinary: Urinary retention

Hematologic: Blood dyscrasias, agranulocytosis

Hepatic: Hepatitis, cholestasis

Neuromuscular & skeletal: Weakness

Ocular: Diplopia

Renal: Polyuria

Signs and Symptoms of Overdose Cholestatic jaundice, CNS depression, diarrhea, dry mouth, dry nose, euphoria, extrapyramidal reaction, flushing, insomnia, mydriasis

Toxicodynamics/Kinetics Duration of action: 4-6 hours

Dosage

Children 6-12 years:
Oral: 25 mg up to 3 times/day
I.M.: Not recommended

Adults:
Oral: 50 mg taken 30 minutes before departure, may repeat in 4-6 hours if needed, up to 200 mg/day
I.M.: 50 mg every 4-6 hours as needed

Contraindications Hypersensitivity to cyclizine or any component of the formulation

Dosage Forms Tablet, as hydrochloride: 50 mg

Reference Range Peak serum concentrations of 69 ng/mL after a 50 mg oral dose

Overdosage/Treatment Decontamination: Lavage (within 1 hour)/activated charcoal

Drug Interactions Increased effect/toxicity with CNS depressants, ethanol

Pregnancy Risk Factor B

Nursing Implications Raise bed rails, institute safety measures, assist with ambulation

Additional Information Commonly abused with opiates for euphoric effects

---

Cyclobenzaprine

CAS Number 303-53-7; 6202-23-9

U.S. Brand Names Flexeril®

Synonyms Cyclobenzaprine Hydrochloride

Impairment Potential Yes

Use Treatment of muscle spasm associated with acute painful musculoskeletal conditions

Mechanism of Action Reduces tonic somatic motor activity influencing both alpha and gamma motor neurons; structurally related to amitriptyline

Adverse Reactions

Cardiovascular: Arrhythmia, facial edema, hypotension, palpitation, tachycardia

Central nervous system: **Drowsiness** (29% to 39%), **dizziness**, fatigue, confusion, headache, irritability, mental acuity decreased, nervousness, agitation, hallucinations, insomnia, malaise, psychosis, seizures, abnormal thinking, vertigo

Dermatologic: Angioedema, pruritus, rash, urticaria

Gastrointestinal: Abdominal pain, constipation, ageusia, diarrhea, dyspepsia, nausea, **xerostomia** (21% to 32%), anorexia, gastritis, tongue edema, vomiting

Genitourinary: Urinary frequency, urinary retention

Hepatic: Cholestasis, hepatitis (rare), jaundice, liver function tests abnormal

Neuromuscular & skeletal: Muscle weakness, hypertonia, paresthesia, tremors

Ocular: Blurred vision, diplopia

Otic: Tinnitus

Respiratory: Pharyngitis

Miscellaneous: Anaphylaxis

Signs and Symptoms of Overdose Mean time to onset of symptoms: 1.4 hours (all patients should be symptomatic within 4 hours). Ataxia, combativeness (13%), delirium, diaphoresis, fever, hallucinations, lethargy (54%), mania, muscular rigidity, myalgia, mydriasis, rhabdomyolysis, tachycardia (33%)

Admission Criteria/Prognosis Admit any pediatric ingestion over 100 mg or any patient symptomatic 4 hours postingestion

Pharmacodynamics/Kinetics

Onset of action: ~1 hour

Duration: 12-24 hours

Absorption: Complete

Metabolism: Hepatic via CYP3A4, 1A2, and 2D6; may undergo enterohepatic recirculation

Bioavailability: 33% to 55%

Half-life elimination: 18 hours (range: 8-37 hours)

Time to peak, serum: 3-8 hours

Excretion: Urine (as inactive metabolites); feces (as unchanged drug)

Dosage

Oral: **Note:** Do not use longer than 2-3 weeks

Adults: Initial: 5 mg 3 times/day; may increase to 10 mg 3 times/day if needed

Elderly: 5 mg 3 times/day; plasma concentration and incidence of adverse effects are increased in the elderly; dose should be titrated slowly

Toxic symptoms occur with ingestions >100 mg

Dosage adjustment in hepatic impairment:

Mild: 5 mg 3 times/day; use with caution and titrate slowly

Moderate to severe: Use not recommended

Contraindications Hypersensitivity to cyclobenzaprine or any component of the formulation; do not use concomitantly or within 14 days of MAO inhibitors; hyperthyroidism; congestive heart failure; arrhythmias; acute recovery phase of MI

Warnings Cyclobenzaprine shares the toxic potentials of the tricyclic antidepressants and the usual precautions of tricyclic antidepressant therapy should be observed; use with caution in patients with urinary hesitancy, angle-closure glaucoma, hepatic impairment, or in the elderly. Do not use concomitantly or within 14 days after MAO inhibitors; combination may cause hypertensive crisis, severe convulsions. Safety and efficacy have not been established in patients <15 years of age.

Dosage Forms

Tablet, as hydrochloride: 5 mg, 10 mg

Flexeril®: 5 mg, 10 mg

Reference Range Therapeutic serum levels following a 40 mg dose: 10-40 ng/mL; a serum level of 260 ng/mL was associated with lethality; cyclobenzaprine blood concentration of ≥ 0.8 mg/L may be associated with a fatal outcome

Overdosage/Treatment

Decontamination: Lavage (within 1 hour)/activated charcoal

Supportive therapy: Physostigmine can be utilized for severe life-threatening anticholinergic effects; hyperthermic states may require dantrolene and/or bromocriptine similar to the treatment of neuroleptic malignant syndrome

Enhancement of elimination: Multiple dosing of activated charcoal may be effective; dialysis is not useful

Antidote(s)

• Physostigmine [ANTIDOTE]

Test Interactions Cyclobenzaprine can falsely elevate serum amitriptyline; 5-fluorouracil can falsely elevate serum creatinine

Drug Interactions

Substrate of CYP1A2 (major), 2D6 (minor), 3A4 (minor)

Anticholinergics: Because of cyclobenzaprine's anticholinergic action, use with caution in patients receiving these agents.

CNS depressants: Effects may be enhanced by cyclobenzaprine.

CYP1A2 inhibitors: May increase the levels/effects of cyclobenzaprine. Example inhibitors include ciprofloxacin, fluvoxamine, ketoconazole, norfloxacin, ofloxacin, and rofecoxib.

Guanethidine: Antihypertensive effect of guanethidine may be decreased; effect seen with tricyclic antidepressants.

MAO inhibitors: Do not use concomitantly or within 14 days after MAO inhibitors.

Tramadol: May increase risk of seizure; effect seen with tricyclic antidepressants and tramadol.

Pregnancy Risk Factor B

Lactation Excretion in breast milk unknown/not recommended

Nursing Implications Raise bed rails, institute safety measures, assist with ambulation

Additional Information Has tricyclic antidepressant effect (similar to amitriptyline) at doses of 75-250 mg/day; some antidepressant effects include anticholinergic effects, sedation, reserpine antagonism and norepinephrine potentiation

Specific References

Beebe FA, Barkin RL, and Barkin S, "A Clinical and Pharmacologic Review of Skeletal Muscle Relaxants for Musculoskeletal Conditions," *Am J Ther*, 2005, 12(2):151-71.

Gordon A and Logan B, "Significance of Cyclobenzaprine in Death Investigation and Impaired Driving Cases in Washington State," *J Anal Toxicol*, 2003, 27:198.

Jufer RA, Levine BS, and Fowler DR, "Cyclobenzaprine (Flexeril®) Concentrations in Postmortem Cases," *J Anal Toxicol*, 2006, 30:156.

Ruha AM, Curry SC, Riley B, et al, "Cyclobenzaprine and Prolonged Anticholinergic Toxicity, Hypotension, and Mild Intraventricular Conduction Delay," *J Toxicol Clin Toxicol*, 2004, 42(5):721.

Spiller HA and Cutino L, "Death: Two Case Reports," *J Forensic Sci*, 2003, 48(4):883-4.

Van Hoey NM, "Effect of Cyclobenzaprine on Tricyclic Antidepressant Assays," *Ann Pharmacother*, 2005, 39(7):1314-7.

Cyclophosphamide

CAS Number 50-18-0; 6055-19-2
U.S. Brand Names Cytoxan®
Synonyms CPM; CTX; CYT; NSC-26271
Use

Oncologic: Treatment of Hodgkin's and non-Hodgkin's lymphoma, Burkitt's lymphoma, chronic lymphocytic leukemia (CLL), chronic myelocytic leukemia (CML), acute myelocytic leukemia (AML), acute lymphocytic leukemia (ALL), mycosis fungoides, multiple myeloma, neuroblastoma, retinoblastoma, rhabdomyosarcoma, Ewing's sarcoma; breast, testicular, endometrial, ovarian, and lung cancers, and in conditioning regimens for bone marrow transplantation

Nononcologic: Prophylaxis of rejection for kidney, heart, liver, and bone marrow transplants, severe rheumatoid disorders, nephrotic syndrome, Wegener's granulomatosis, idiopathic pulmonary hemosideroses, myasthenia gravis, multiple sclerosis, systemic lupus erythematosus, lupus nephritis, autoimmune hemolytic anemia, idiopathic thrombocytic purpura (ITP), macroglobulinemia, and antibody-induced pure red cell aplasia

Mechanism of Action Interferes with the normal function of DNA by alkylation and cross-linking the strands of DNA, and by possible protein modification; cyclophosphamide also possesses potent immunosuppressive activity; note that cyclophosphamide must be metabolized to its active form in the liver (an alkylating agent)

Adverse Reactions

Cardiovascular: High-dose therapy may cause cardiac dysfunction manifested as congestive heart failure; cardiac necrosis or hemorrhagic myocarditis has occurred rarely, but is fatal; cyclophosphamide may also potentiate the cardiac toxicity of anthracyclines, tachycardia, facial flushing, cardiomegaly, cardiomyopathy, myocardial depression, sinus tachycardia

Central nervous system: Headache, dizziness, fatigue, psychosis

Dermatologic: Skin rash, skin hyperpigmentation (hyperpigmentation of palms and soles), transverse ridging of nails, hepatic toxicity, and dermatitis; allergic skin reactions, radiation recall dermatitis, cutaneous vasculitis

Alopecia: Frequent (occurs in 40% to 60% of patients), hair will regrow although it may be of a different color or texture; hair loss usually occurs 3 weeks after therapy

Endocrine & metabolic: Hypokalemia, ovotoxic, syndrome of inappropriate antidiuretic hormone has occurred with I.V. doses >50 mg/kg, hyperuricemia, nephrogenic diabetes insipidus

Fertility: May cause sterility; interferes with oogenesis and spermatogenesis; may be irreversible in some patients; gonadal suppression (amenorrhea)

Gastrointestinal: **Nausea and vomiting occur more frequently with larger doses, usually beginning 6-10 hours after administration; also seen are anorexia, diarrhea, stomatitis, mucositis,** pancreatitis, hemorrhagic colitis, feces discoloration (black)

Genitourinary: **Severe, potentially fatal acute hemorrhagic cystitis or urinary fibrosis,** believed to be a result of chemical irritation of the bladder by acrolein, a cyclophosphamide metabolite, occurs in 7% to 12% of patients and has been reported in up to 40% of patients in some series. Patients should be encouraged to drink plenty of fluids during therapy (most adults will require at least 2 L/day), void frequently, and avoid taking the drug at night. With large I.V. doses, I.V. hydration is usually recommended. The use of mesna and/or continuous bladder irrigation is rarely needed for doses <2 g/m².

Hematologic: **Thrombocytopenia and anemia are less common than leukopenia**

Onset: 7 days
Nadir: 10-14 days
Recovery: 21 days

Hepatic: **Jaundice,** acute liver failure, cholestasis

Local: Extravasation injury

Neuromuscular & skeletal: Rhabdomyolysis

Renal: Tubular necrosis (acute) has occurred, but usually resolves after the discontinuation of therapy; Fanconi syndrome, renal tubular acidosis type II

Respiratory: Interstitial pulmonary fibrosis with prolonged high dosage has occurred, rhinorrhea, sinus congestion, nasal stuffiness occurs when given in large I.V. doses, sneezing during or immediately after the infusion

Miscellaneous: Patients experience runny eyes, distortion; diaphoresis, anaphylaxis, aneuploidy induction

Signs and Symptoms of Overdose Agranulocytosis, azoospermia, AV block, colitis, erythema multiforme, granulocytopenia, hematuria, hemorrhagic cystitis, hyperglycemia, hyperpigmented hair, hypertension, hy-

peruricemia, hyponatremia, hypokalemia, leukopenia, Mees' lines, neutropenia, oligospermia, tachycardia

Pharmacodynamics/Kinetics

Absorption: Oral: Well absorbed

Distribution: V_d: 0.48-0.71 L/kg; crosses placenta; crosses into CSF (not in high enough concentrations to treat meningeal leukemia)

Protein binding: 10% to 56%

Metabolism: Hepatic to active metabolites acrolein, 4-aldophosphamide, 4-hydroperoxycyclophosphamide, and nor-nitrogen mustard

Bioavailability: >75%

Half-life elimination: 4-8 hours

Time to peak, serum: Oral: ~1 hour

Excretion: Urine (<30% as unchanged drug, 85% to 90% as metabolites)

Dosage

Refer to individual protocols

Patients who are heavily pretreated with cytotoxic radiation or chemotherapy, or who have compromised bone marrow function may require a 33% to 50% reduction in initial dose.

Children:
SLE: I.V.: 500-750 mg/m² every month; maximum dose: 1 g/m²
JRA/vasculitis: I.V.: 10 mg/kg every 2 weeks

Children and Adults:
Oral: 50-100 mg/m²/day as continuous therapy or 400-1000 mg/m² in divided doses over 4-5 days as intermittent therapy
I.V.:
Single doses: 400-1800 mg/m² (30-50 mg/kg) per treatment course (1-5 days) which can be repeated at 2-4 week intervals
Continuous daily doses: 60-120 mg/m² (1-2.5 mg/kg) per day
Autologous BMT: IVPB: 50 mg/kg/dose × 4 days or 60 mg/kg/dose for 2 days; total dose is usually divided over 2-4 days

Nephrotic syndrome: Oral: 2-3 mg/kg/day every day for up to 12 weeks when corticosteroids are unsuccessful

Dosing adjustment in renal impairment: A large fraction of cyclophosphamide is eliminated by hepatic metabolism
Some authors recommend no dose adjustment unless severe renal insufficiency (Cl_{cr} <20 mL/minute)
Cl_{cr} >10 mL/minute: Administer 100% of normal dose
Cl_{cr} <10 mL/minute: Administer 75% of normal dose

Hemodialysis: Moderately dialyzable (20% to 50%); administer dose posthemodialysis

CAPD effects: Unknown
CAVH effects: Unknown

Dosing adjustment in hepatic impairment: Some authors recommend dosage reductions (of up to 30%); however, the pharmacokinetics of cyclophosphamide are not significantly altered in the presence of hepatic insufficiency.

Stability Store intact vials of powder at room temperature of 15°C to 30°C (59°F to 86°F). Reconstitute vials with sterile water, normal saline, or 5% dextrose to a concentration of 20 mg/mL. Reconstituted solutions are stable for 24 hours at room temperature and 6 days under refrigeration at 2°C to 8°C (36°F to 46°F). Further dilutions in D₅W or NS are stable for 24 hours at room temperature and 6 days at refrigeration.

Monitoring Parameters CBC with differential and platelet count, BUN, UA, serum electrolytes, serum creatinine

Administration May be administered I.P., intrapleurally, IVPB, or continuous I.V. infusion; may also be administered slow IVP in doses ≤1 g. I.V. infusions may be administered over 1-24 hours
Doses >500 mg to approximately 2 g may be administered over 20-30 minutes
To minimize bladder toxicity, increase normal fluid intake during and for 1-2 days after cyclophosphamide dose. Most adult patients will require a fluid intake of at least 2 L/day. High-dose regimens should be accompanied by vigorous hydration with or without mesna therapy.
Tablets are not scored and should not be cut or crushed; should be administered during or after meals.

Contraindications Hypersensitivity to cyclophosphamide or any component of the formulation; pregnancy

Warnings Hazardous agent - use appropriate precautions for handling and disposal. Dosage adjustment needed for renal or hepatic failure.

Dosage Forms

Injection, powder for reconstitution (Cytoxan®): 500 mg, 1 g, 2 g [contains mannitol 75 mg per cyclophosphamide 100 mg]
Tablet (Cytoxan®): 25 mg, 50 mg

Overdosage/Treatment

Decontamination: Emesis within 30 minutes or lavage (within 1 hour)/activated charcoal

Supportive therapy: Hyperuricemia can be treated with alkalinization of urine along with allopurinol; cystitis (hemorrhagic) can be controlled with bladder irrigation of 5% to 10% formalin glutathione, 2-mercaptoethane sulfonate (30 mg/kg/day for 4 doses) may be uroprotective; additionally, bladder irrigation with prostaglandin F₂-alpha (carboprost tromethamine) has been used; bladder spasm can be controlled with oxybutynin chloride 2.5-5 mg orally 3 times/day. For extravasation, hyaluronidase or chondroitin sulfatase injected SubQ can be utilized; do not use warm packs. To prevent cyclophosphamide-induced antidiuresis, continuous infusion of furosemide (mean dose of 0.128 mg/kg/hour) may be useful. Amifostine (910 mg/m^2) pretreatment may be protective of drug-induced neutropenia, renal toxicity, or ototoxicity. Testosterone (100 mg I.M. every 15 days beginning 1 month before therapy) can prevent cyclophosphamide-induced azoospermia.

Enhancement of elimination: Multiple dosing of activated charcoal may be effective; hemodialysis may remove 36% of prodrug; moderately dialyzable (20% to 50%)

Antidote(s)
- Amifostine [ANTIDOTE]
- Thrombopoietin [ANTIDOTE]

Test Interactions Hyponatremia may develop due to syndrome of inappropriate antidiuretic hormone; ↑ uric acid (S)

Drug Interactions
Substrate of CYP2A6 (minor), 2B6 (major), 2C9 (minor), 2C19 (minor), 3A4 (major); **Inhibits** CYP3A4 (weak); **Induces** CYP2B6 (weak), 2C8 (weak), 2C9 (weak)

Allopurinol may cause increase in bone marrow depression and may result in significant elevations of cyclophosphamide cytotoxic metabolites.

Anesthetic agents: Cyclophosphamide reduces serum pseudocholinesterase concentrations and may prolong the neuromuscular blocking activity of succinylcholine; use with caution with halothane, nitrous oxide, and succinylcholine.

Chloramphenicol results in prolonged cyclophosphamide half-life to increase toxicity.

CYP2B6 inducers: May increase the levels/effects of acrolein (the active metabolite of cyclophosphamide). Example inducers include carbamazepine, nevirapine, phenobarbital, phenytoin, and rifampin.

CYP2B6 inhibitors: May decrease the levels/effects of acrolein (the active metabolite of cyclophosphamide). Example inhibitors include desipramine, paroxetine, and sertraline.

CYP3A4 inducers: CYP3A4 inducers may increase the levels/effects of acrolein (the active metabolite of cyclophosphamide). Example inducers include aminoglutethimide, carbamazepine, nafcillin, nevirapine, phenobarbital, phenytoin, and rifamycins.

CYP3A4 inhibitors: May decrease the levels/effects of acrolein (the active metabolite of cyclophosphamide). Example inhibitors include azole antifungals, ciprofloxacin, clarithromycin, diclofenac, doxycycline, erythromycin, imatinib, isoniazid, nefazodone, nicardipine, propofol, protease inhibitors, quinidine, and verapamil.

Digoxin: Cyclophosphamide may decrease digoxin serum levels.
Doxorubicin: Cyclophosphamide may enhance cardiac toxicity of anthracyclines.

Tetrahydrocannabinol results in enhanced immunosuppression in animal studies.

Thiazide diuretics: Leukopenia may be prolonged.

Pregnancy Risk Factor D
Pregnancy Implications Multiple anomalies (cleft palate, absent thumbs, dysmorphic facies, skeletal and CNS abnormalities noted); crosses the placenta

Lactation Enters breast milk/contraindicated
Nursing Implications Encourage adequate hydration and frequent voiding to help prevent cystitis (hemorrhagic)
Additional Information May be used in combination with mesna to prevent hemorrhagic cystitis. Rarely required for doses <1.5-2 g/m^2. Cardiac toxicity can occur at doses >2.4 g/m^2

Specific References
Elcombe CR, "Abstracts of the European Association of Poison Centres and Clinical Toxicologists XXVI International Congress," *Clin Toxicol*, 2006, 44:401-586.
Huang SH, Lee PY, and Niu CK, "Treatment of Pediatric Idiopathic Pulmonary Hemosiderosis with Low-Dose Cyclophosphamide," *Ann Pharmacother*, 2003, 37(11):1618-21.

CycloSERINE

CAS Number 68-41-7
U.S. Brand Names Seromycin®
Use Adjunctive treatment in pulmonary or extrapulmonary tuberculosis; treatment of acute urinary tract infections caused by *E. coli* or *Enterobacter* sp when less toxic conventional therapy has failed or is contraindicated
Unlabeled/Investigational Use Treatment of Gaucher's disease
Mechanism of Action Inhibits bacterial cell wall synthesis by competing with amino acid (D-alanine) for incorporation into the bacterial cell wall; bacteriostatic or bactericidal
Adverse Reactions
Cardiovascular: Cardiac arrhythmias, congestive heart failure at doses >1 g/day
Central nervous system: Dizziness, seizures, confusion, paranoia, psychosis, paresis, coma, drowsiness, headache, delirium, absence seizures, catatonia

Dermatologic: Rash, Stevens-Johnson syndrome
Endocrine & metabolic: Vitamin B$_{12}$ deficiency
Hematologic: Folate deficiency
Hepatic: Elevated liver enzymes
Neuromuscular & skeletal: Tremor, dysarthria, hyperreflexia
Miscellaneous: Pellagra

Admission Criteria/Prognosis Admit adult ingestions >2 g
Pharmacodynamics/Kinetics
Absorption: ~70% to 90%
Distribution: Widely to most body fluids and tissues including CSF, breast milk, bile, sputum, lymph tissue, lungs, and ascitic, pleural, and synovial fluids; crosses placenta
Half-life elimination: Normal renal function: 10 hours
Metabolism: Hepatic
Time to peak, serum: 3-4 hours
Excretion: Urine (60% to 70% as unchanged drug) within 72 hours; feces (small amounts); remainder metabolized

Dosage
Some of the neurotoxic effects may be relieved or prevented by the concomitant administration of pyridoxine
Tuberculosis: Oral:
Children: 10-20 mg/kg/day in 2 divided doses up to 1000 mg/day for 18-24 months
Adults: Initial: 250 mg every 12 hours for 14 days, then give 500 mg to 1 g/day in 2 divided doses for 18-24 months (maximum daily dose: 1 g)
Dosing interval in renal impairment:
Cl$_{cr}$ 10-50 mL/minute: Administer every 12-24 hours
Cl$_{cr}$ <10 mL/minute: Administer every 24 hours
Monitoring Parameters Periodic renal, hepatic, hematological tests, and plasma cycloserine concentrations
Contraindications Hypersensitivity to cycloserine or any component of the formulation
Warnings Epilepsy, depression, severe anxiety, psychosis, severe renal insufficiency, chronic alcoholism
Dosage Forms Capsule: 250 mg
Reference Range Toxicity is greatly increased at serum levels >30 mcg/mL; therapeutic cycloserine serum levels for *Mycobacterium* tuberculosis: 5-20 mcg/mL
Overdosage/Treatment
Supportive therapy: Neurotoxic effects can be prevented with use of pyridoxine (150-300 mg/day)
Enhanced elimination: Removed by dialysis
Test Interactions Possible assay interference with cyclosporine by HPLC
Drug Interactions Increased toxicity: Alcohol, isoniazid, ethionamide increase toxicity of cycloserine; cycloserine inhibits the hepatic metabolism of phenytoin
Pregnancy Risk Factor C
Lactation Enters breast milk/compatible

CycloSPORINE

Related Information
- Therapeutic Drugs Associated with Hallucinations
CAS Number 59865-13-3
U.S. Brand Names Gengraf™; Neoral®; Restasis™; Sandimmune®
Synonyms CsA; CyA; Cyclosporin A
Use
Prophylaxis of organ rejection in kidney, liver, and heart transplants, has been used with azathioprine and/or corticosteroids; severe, active rheumatoid arthritis (RA) not responsive to methotrexate alone; severe, recalcitrant plaque psoriasis in nonimmunocompromised adults unresponsive to or unable to tolerate other systemic therapy
Ophthalmic emulsion (Restasis™): Increase tear production when suppressed tear production is presumed to be due to keratoconjunctivitis sicca-associated ocular inflammation (in patients not already using topical anti-inflammatory drugs or punctal plugs)
Unlabeled/Investigational Use Short-term, high-dose cyclosporine as a modulator of multidrug resistance in cancer treatment; allogenic bone marrow transplants for prevention and treatment of graft-versus-host disease; also used in some cases of severe autoimmune disease (eg, SLE, myasthenia gravis) that are resistant to corticosteroids and other therapy; focal segmental glomerulosclerosis
Mechanism of Action Inhibition of production and release of interleukin II and inhibits interleukin II-induced activation of resting T lymphocytes
Adverse Reactions
Note: Adverse reactions reported with kidney, liver, and heart transplantation, unless otherwise noted. Although percentage is reported for specific condition, reaction may occur in anyone taking cyclosporine. [Reactions reported for rheumatoid arthritis (RA) are based on cyclosporine (modified) 2.5 mg/kg/day versus placebo.]
>10%:
Cardiovascular: Hypertension (13% to 53%; psoriasis 25% to 27%)

Central nervous system: Headache (2% to 15%; RA 17%, psoriasis 14% to 16%)

Dermatologic: Hirsutism (21% to 45%), hypertrichosis (RA 19%)

Endocrine & metabolic: Increased triglycerides (psoriasis 15%), female reproductive disorder (psoriasis 8% to 11%)

Gastrointestinal: Nausea (RA 23%), diarrhea (RA 12%), gum hyperplasia (4% to 16%), abdominal discomfort (RA 15%), dyspepsia (RA 12%)

Neuromuscular & skeletal: Tremor (12% to 55%)

Renal: Renal dysfunction/nephropathy (25% to 38%; RA 10%, psoriasis 21%), creatinine elevation ≥50% (RA 24%), increased creatinine (psoriasis 16% to 20%)

Respiratory: Upper respiratory infection (psoriasis 8% to 11%)

Miscellaneous: Infection (psoriasis 24% to 25%)

Kidney, liver, and heart transplant only (≤2% unless otherwise noted):

Cardiovascular: Flushes (<1% to 4%), myocardial infarction

Central nervous system: Convulsions (1% to 5%), anxiety, confusion, fever, lethargy

Dermatologic: Acne (1% to 6%), brittle fingernails, hair breaking, pruritus

Endocrine & metabolic: Gynecomastia (<1% to 4%), hyperglycemia

Gastrointestinal: Nausea (2% to 10%), vomiting (2% to 10%), diarrhea (3% to 8%), abdominal discomfort (<1% to 7%), cramps (0% to 4%), anorexia, constipation, gastritis, mouth sores, pancreatitis, swallowing difficulty, upper GI bleed, weight loss

Hematologic: Leukopenia (<1% to 6%), anemia, thrombocytopenia

Hepatic: Hepatotoxicity (<1% to 7%)

Neuromuscular & skeletal: Paresthesia (1% to 3%), joint pain, muscle pain, tingling, weakness

Ocular: Conjunctivitis, visual disturbance

Otic: Hearing loss, tinnitus

Renal: Hematuria

Respiratory: Sinusitis (<1% to 7%)

Miscellaneous: Lymphoma (<1% to 6%), allergic reactions, hiccups, night sweats

Rheumatoid arthritis only (1% to <3% unless otherwise noted):

Cardiovascular: Hypertension (8%), edema (5%), chest pain (4%), arrhythmia (2%), abnormal heart sounds, cardiac failure, myocardial infarction, peripheral ischemia

Central nervous system: Dizziness (8%), pain (6%), insomnia (4%), depression (3%), migraine (2%), anxiety, hypoesthesia, emotional lability, impaired concentration, malaise, nervousness, paranoia, somnolence, vertigo

Dermatologic: Purpura (3%), abnormal pigmentation, angioedema, cellulitis, dermatitis, dry skin, eczema, folliculitis, nail disorder, pruritus, skin disorder, urticaria

Endocrine & metabolic: Menstrual disorder (3%), breast fibroadenosis, breast pain, diabetes mellitus, goiter, hot flashes, hyperkalemia, hyperuricemia, hypoglycemia, libido increased/decreased

Gastrointestinal: Vomiting (9%), flatulence (5%), gingivitis (4%), gum hyperplasia (2%), constipation, dry mouth, dysphagia, enanthema, eructation, esophagitis, gastric ulcer, gastritis, gastroenteritis, gingival bleeding, glossitis, peptic ulcer, salivary gland enlargement, taste perversion, tongue disorder, tooth disorder, weight loss/gain

Genitourinary: Leukorrhea (1%), abnormal urine, micturition urgency, nocturia, polyuria, pyelonephritis, urinary incontinence, uterine hemorrhage

Hematologic: Anemia, leukopenia

Hepatic: Bilirubinemia

Neuromuscular & skeletal: Paresthesia (8%), tremor (8%), leg cramps/muscle contractions (2%), arthralgia, bone fracture, joint dislocation, myalgia, neuropathy, stiffness, synovial cyst, tendon disorder, weakness

Ocular: Abnormal vision, cataract, conjunctivitis, eye pain

Otic: Tinnitus, deafness, vestibular disorder

Renal: Increased BUN, hematuria, renal abscess

Respiratory: Cough (5%), dyspnea (5%), sinusitis (4%), abnormal chest sounds, bronchospasm, epistaxis

Miscellaneous: Infection (9%), abscess, allergy, bacterial infection, carcinoma, fungal infection, herpes simplex, herpes zoster, lymphadenopathy, moniliasis, diaphoresis increased, tonsillitis, viral infection

Psoriasis only (1% to <3% unless otherwise noted):

Cardiovascular: Chest pain, flushes

Central nervous system: Psychiatric events (4% to 5%), pain (3% to 4%), dizziness, fever, insomnia, nervousness, vertigo

Dermatologic: Hypertrichosis (5% to 7%), acne, dry skin, folliculitis, keratosis, pruritus, rash, skin malignancies

Endocrine & metabolic: Hot flashes

Gastrointestinal: Nausea (5% to 6%), diarrhea (5% to 6%), gum hyperplasia (4% to 6%), abdominal discomfort (3% to 6%),

dyspepsia (2% to 3%), abdominal distention, appetite increased, constipation, gingival bleeding

Genitourinary: Micturition increased

Hematologic: Bleeding disorder, clotting disorder, platelet disorder, red blood cell disorder

Hepatic: Hyperbilirubinemia

Neuromuscular & skeletal: Paresthesia (5% to 7%), arthralgia (1% to 6%)

Ocular: Abnormal vision

Respiratory: Bronchospasm (5%), cough (5%), dyspnea (5%), rhinitis (5%), respiratory infection

Miscellaneous: Flu-like symptoms (8% to 10%)

Postmarketing and/or case reports (any indication): Death (due to renal deterioration), mild hypomagnesemia, hyperkalemia, increased uric acid, gout, hyperbilirubinemia, increased cholesterol, encephalopathy, impaired consciousness, neurotoxicity

Ophthalmic emulsion (Restasis™): >10%: Ocular: Burning (17%)

1% to 10%: Ocular: Hyperemia (conjunctival 5%), eye pain, pruritus, stinging

Signs and Symptoms of Overdose Abdominal pain, cholestatic jaundice, colitis, coma, cortical blindness, deafness, delirium, dementia, diarrhea, dysgeusia, dysphoria, eclampsia, encephalopathy, facial flushing, fibrillation (atrial), gingival hyperplasia, gout, headache, hypercalcemia, hyperglycemia, hyperuricemia, hypertriglyceridemia, hypertrichosis, hypomagnesemia, hypertension, jaundice, leukopenia, lymphoma, malaise, mania, metabolic acidosis, myasthenia gravis (exacerbation or precipitation), myoclonus, renal dysfunction, seizures, sweating, thrombocytopenia, tubular necrosis, vomiting

Admission Criteria/Prognosis Admit any ingestion >150 mg/kg

Pharmacodynamics/Kinetics

Absorption:

Ophthalmic emulsion: Serum concentrations not detectable.

Oral:

Cyclosporine (non-modified): Erratic and incomplete; dependent on presence of food, bile acids, and GI motility; larger oral doses are needed in pediatrics due to shorter bowel length and limited intestinal absorption

Cyclosporine (modified): Erratic and incomplete; increased absorption, up to 30% when compared to cyclosporine (non-modified); less dependent on food, bile acids, or GI motility when compared to cyclosporine (non-modified)

Distribution: Widely in tissues and body fluids including the liver, pancreas, and lungs; crosses placenta; enters breast milk

V_{dss}: 4-6 L/kg in renal, liver, and marrow transplant recipients (slightly lower values in cardiac transplant patients; children <10 years have higher values)

Protein binding: 90% to 98% to lipoproteins

Metabolism: Extensively hepatic via CYP3A4; forms at least 25 metabolites; extensive first-pass effect following oral administration

Bioavailability: Oral:

Cyclosporine (non-modified): Dependent on patient population and transplant type (<10% in adult liver transplant patients and as high as 89% in renal transplant patients); bioavailability of Sandimmune® capsules and oral solution are equivalent; bioavailability of oral solution is ~30% of the I.V. solution

Children: 28% (range: 17% to 42%); gut dysfunction common in BMT patients and oral bioavailability is further reduced

Cyclosporine (modified): Bioavailability of Neoral® capsules and oral solution are equivalent:

Children: 43% (range: 30% to 68%)

Adults: 23% greater than with cyclosporine (non-modified) in renal transplant patients; 50% greater in liver transplant patients

Half-life elimination: Oral: May be prolonged in patients with hepatic impairment and shorter in pediatric patients due to the higher metabolism rate

Cyclosporine (non-modified): Biphasic: Alpha: 1.4 hours; Terminal: 19 hours (range: 10-27 hours)

Cyclosporine (modified): Biphasic: Terminal: 8.4 hours (range: 5-18 hours)

Time to peak, serum: Oral:

Cyclosporine (non-modified): 2-6 hours; some patients have a second peak at 5-6 hours

Cyclosporine (modified): Renal transplant: 1.5-2 hours

Excretion: Primarily feces; urine (6%, 0.1% as unchanged drug and metabolites)

Dosage

Note: Neoral® and Sandimmune® are not bioequivalent and cannot be used interchangeably

Children: Transplant: Refer to adult dosing; children may require, and are able to tolerate, larger doses than adults.

Adults:

Newly-transplanted patients: Adjunct therapy with corticosteroids is recommended. Initial dose should be given 4-12 hours prior to transplant or may be given postoperatively; adjust initial dose to achieve desired plasma concentration

Oral: Dose is dependent upon type of transplant and formulation:

Cyclosporine (modified):

Renal: 9 ± 3 mg/kg/day, divided twice daily

Liver: 8 ± 4 mg/kg/day, divided twice daily

Heart: 7 ± 3 mg/kg/day, divided twice daily

Cyclosporine (non-modified): Initial dose: 15 mg/kg/day as a single dose (range 14-18 mg/kg); lower doses of 10-14 mg/kg/day have been used for renal transplants. Continue initial dose daily for 1-2 weeks; taper by 5% per week to a maintenance dose of 5-10 mg/kg/day; some renal transplant patients may be dosed as low as 3 mg/kg/day

When using the non-modified formulation, cyclosporine levels may increase in liver transplant patients when the T-tube is closed; dose may need decreased

I.V.: Cyclosporine (non-modified): Initial dose: 5-6 mg/kg/day as a single dose ($^1/_3$ the oral dose), infused over 2-6 hours; use should be limited to patients unable to take capsules or oral solution; patients should be switched to an oral dosage form as soon as possible

Conversion to cyclosporine (modified) from cyclosporine (non-modified): Start with daily dose previously used and adjust to obtain preconversion cyclosporine trough concentration. Plasma concentrations should be monitored every 4-7 days and dose adjusted as necessary, until desired trough level is obtained. When transferring patients with previously poor absorption of cyclosporine (non-modified), monitor trough levels at least twice weekly (especially if initial dose exceeds 10 mg/kg/day); high plasma levels are likely to occur.

Rheumatoid arthritis: Oral: Cyclosporine (modified): Initial dose: 2.5 mg/kg/day, divided twice daily; salicylates, NSAIDs, and oral glucocorticoids may be continued (refer to Drug Interactions); dose may be increased by 0.5-0.75 mg/kg/day if insufficient response is seen after 8 weeks of treatment; additional dosage increases may be made again at 12 weeks (maximum dose: 4 mg/kg/day). Discontinue if no benefit is seen by 16 weeks of therapy.

Note: Increase the frequency of blood pressure monitoring after each alteration in dosage of cyclosporine. Cyclosporine dosage should be decreased by 25% to 50% in patients with no history of hypertension who develop sustained hypertension during therapy and, if hypertension persists, treatment with cyclosporine should be discontinued.

Psoriasis: Oral: Cyclosporine (modified): Initial dose: 2.5 mg/kg/day, divided twice daily; dose may be increased by 0.5 mg/kg/day if insufficient response is seen after 4 weeks of treatment. Additional dosage increases may be made every 2 weeks if needed (maximum dose: 4 mg/kg/day). Discontinue if no benefit is seen by 6 weeks of therapy. Once adequately controlled, the dose should be decreased to the lowest effective dose. Doses lower than 2.5 mg/kg/day may be effective. Treatment longer than 1 year is not recommended.

Note: Increase the frequency of blood pressure monitoring after each alteration in dosage of cyclosporine. Cyclosporine dosage should be decreased by 25% to 50% in patients with no history of hypertension who develop sustained hypertension during therapy and, if hypertension persists, treatment with cyclosporine should be discontinued.

Focal segmental glomerulosclerosis: Initial: 3 mg/kg/day divided every 12 hours

Autoimmune diseases: 1-3 mg/kg/day

Keratoconjunctivitis sicca: Ophthalmic: Children ≥ 16 years and Adults: Instill 1 drop in each eye every 12 hours

Dosage adjustment in renal impairment: For severe psoriasis:

Serum creatinine levels $\geq$25% above pretreatment levels: Take another sample within 2 weeks; if the level remains $\geq$25% above pretreatment levels, decrease dosage of cyclosporine (modified) by 25% to 50%. If two dosage adjustments do not reverse the increase in serum creatinine levels, treatment should be discontinued.

Serum creatinine levels $\geq$50% above pretreatment levels: Decrease cyclosporine dosage by 25% to 50%. If two dosage adjustments do not reverse the increase in serum creatinine levels, treatment should be discontinued.

Hemodialysis: Supplemental dose is not necessary.

Peritoneal dialysis: Supplemental dose is not necessary.

Dosage adjustment in hepatic impairment: Probably necessary; monitor levels closely

Stability Do **not** store oral solution in the refrigerator; use contents of oral solution within 2 months after opening; I.V. cyclosporine prepared in normal saline or D_5W is stable 6 hours in PVC or 24 hours in a glass container or PAB container or Excel® container; do not freeze

Monitoring Parameters

Monitor blood pressure and serum creatinine after any cyclosporine dosage changes or addition, modification, or deletion of other medications. Monitor plasma concentrations periodically.

Transplant patients: Cyclosporine trough levels, serum electrolytes, renal function, hepatic function, blood pressure, lipid profile

Psoriasis therapy: Baseline blood pressure, serum creatinine (2 levels each), BUN, CBC, serum magnesium, potassium, uric acid, lipid profile.

Biweekly monitoring of blood pressure, complete blood count, and levels of BUN, uric acid, potassium, lipids, and magnesium during the first 3 months of treatment for psoriasis. Monthly monitoring is recommended after this initial period. Also evaluate any atypical skin lesions prior to therapy. Increase the frequency of blood pressure monitoring after each alteration in dosage of cyclosporine. Cyclosporine dosage should be decreased by 25% to 50% in patients with no history of hypertension who develop sustained hypertension during therapy and, if hypertension persists, treatment with cyclosporine should be discontinued.

Rheumatoid arthritis: Baseline blood pressure, and serum creatinine (2 levels each); serum creatinine every 2 weeks for first 3 months, then monthly if patient is stable. Increase the frequency of blood pressure monitoring after each alteration in dosage of cyclosporine. Cyclosporine dosage should be decreased by 25% to 50% in patients with no history of hypertension who develop sustained hypertension during therapy and, if hypertension persists, treatment with cyclosporine should be discontinued.

Administration Oral solution: Do not administer liquid from plastic or styrofoam cup. May dilute Neoral® oral solution with orange juice or apple juice. May dilute Sandimmune® oral solution with milk, chocolate milk, or orange juice. Avoid changing diluents frequently. Mix thoroughly and drink at once. Use syringe provided to measure dose. Mix in a glass container and rinse container with more diluent to ensure total dose is taken. Do not rinse syringe before or after use (may cause dose variation).

I.V.: Following dilution, intravenous admixture should be administered over 2-6 hours. Discard solution after 24 hours. Anaphylaxis has been reported with I.V. use; reserve for patients who cannot take oral form. Patients should be under continuous observation for at least the first 30 minutes of the infusion, and should be monitored frequently thereafter. Maintain patent airway; other supportive measures and agents for treating anaphylaxis should be present when I.V. drug is given.

Ophthalmic emulsion: Prior to use, invert vial several times to obtain a uniform emulsion. Remove contact lenses prior to instillation of drops; may be reinserted 15 minutes after administration. May be used with artificial tears; allow 15 minute interval between products.

Contraindications Hypersensitivity to cyclosporine or any component of the formulation. Rheumatoid arthritis and psoriasis: Abnormal renal function, uncontrolled hypertension, malignancies. Concomitant treatment with PUVA or UVB therapy, methotrexate, other immunosuppressive agents, coal tar, or radiation therapy are also contraindications for use in patients with psoriasis. Ophthalmic emulsion is contraindicated in patients with active ocular infections.

Warnings

[U.S. Boxed Warning]: Use caution with other potentially nephrotoxic drugs (eg, acyclovir, aminoglycoside antibiotics, amphotericin B, ciprofloxacin). **[U.S. Boxed Warning]: Increased risk of lymphomas, other malignancies, infection. [U.S. Boxed Warning]: May cause hypertension.** Use caution when changing dosage forms; products are not equally interchangeable. Cyclosporine (modified) refers to the capsule dosage formulation of cyclosporine in an aqueous dispersion (previously referred to as "microemulsion"). **[U.S. Boxed Warning]: Cyclosporine (modified) has increased bioavailability as compared to cyclosporine (non-modified) and cannot be used interchangeably without close monitoring.** Monitor cyclosporine concentrations closely following the addition, modification, or deletion of other medications; live, attenuated vaccines may be less effective; use should be avoided.

Transplant patients: To be used initially with corticosteroids. May cause significant hyperkalemia and hyperuricemia. May cause seizures, particularly if used with high-dose corticosteroids. Encephalopathy has been reported, predisposing factors include hypertension, hypomagnesemia, hypocholesterolemia, high-dose corticosteroids, high cyclosporine serum concentration, and graft-versus-host disease; may be more common in patients with liver transplant. Make dose adjustments based on cyclosporine blood concentrations. **[U.S. Boxed Warning]: Adjustment of dose should only be made under the direct supervision of an experienced physician.** Anaphylaxis has been reported with I.V. use; reserve for patients who cannot take oral form.

Psoriasis: Patients should avoid excessive sun exposure; safety and efficacy in children <18 years of age have not been established. **[U.S. Boxed Warning]: Risk of skin cancer may be increased with a history of PUVA and possibly methotrexate or other immunosuppressants, UVB, coal tar, or radiation.**

Rheumatoid arthritis: Safety and efficacy for use in juvenile rheumatoid arthritis have not been established. If receiving other immunosuppressive agents, radiation or UV therapy, concurrent use of cyclosporine is not recommended.

Ophthalmic emulsion: Safety and efficacy have not been established in patients <16 years of age.

Products may contain corn oil, castor oil, ethanol, or propylene glycol; injection also contains Cremophor® EL (polyoxyethylated castor oil), which has been associated with rare anaphylactic reactions.

Dosage Forms

Capsule, soft gel, modified: 25 mg, 100 mg [contains castor oil, ethanol]
  Gengraf®: 25 mg, 100 mg [contains ethanol, castor oil, propylene glycol]
  Neoral®: 25 mg, 100 mg [contains dehydrated ethanol, corn oil, castor oil, propylene glycol]
Capsule, soft gel, non-modified (Sandimmune®): 25 mg, 100 mg [contains dehydrated ethanol, corn oil]
Emulsion, ophthalmic [preservative free, single-use vial] (Restasis®): 0.05% (0.4 mL) [contains glycerin, castor oil, polysorbate 80, carbomer 1342; 32 vials/box]
Injection, solution, non-modified (Sandimmune®): 50 mg/mL (5 mL) [contains Cremophor® EL (polyoxyethylated castor oil), ethanol]
Solution, oral, modified:
  Gengraf®: 100 mg/mL (50 mL) [contains castor oil, propylene glycol]
  Neoral®: 100 mg/mL (50 mL) [contains dehydrated ethanol, corn oil, castor oil, propylene glycol]
Solution, oral, non-modified (Sandimmune®): 100 mg/mL (50 mL) [contains olive oil, ethanol]

Reference Range Reference ranges are method dependent and specimen dependent; use the same analytical method consistently

Method-dependent and specimen-dependent: Trough levels should be obtained:
  Oral: 12-18 hours after dose (chronic usage)
  I.V.: 12 hours after dose **or** immediately prior to next dose

Therapeutic range: Not absolutely defined, dependent on organ transplanted, time after transplant, organ function and CsA toxicity:
  General range of 100-400 ng/mL
  Toxic level: Not well defined, nephrotoxicity may occur at any level

Overdosage/Treatment

Decontamination: Lavage (within 1 hour)/activated charcoal
Supportive therapy: Diazepam, lorazepam, phenytoin, or phenobarbital for seizure control; calcium channel blockers are preferred agent for treatment of hypertension (diltiazen or verapamil); azithromycin (500 mg/day for 1 day, then 250 mg/day for 4 days) or metronidazole (750 mg 3 times/day for 2 weeks) has been used to treat gingival hyperplasia; amlodipine (5 mg/day) in normotensive renal transplant recipients has resulted in decreased nephrotoxicity of cyclosporine. Cyclosporin-induced hypertension can be treated with labetalol or a dihydropyridine calcium antagonist.
Enhancement of elimination: Multiple dosing of activated charcoal can decrease half-life from 9 hours to under 3 hours (through enterohepatic recirculation of drug); hemodialysis is not useful (will remove ~3% of dose)

Diagnostic Procedures
- Cyclosporine, Blood

Test Interactions May falsely elevate specific whole blood, HPLC assay for cyclosporine if the sample is drawn from the same line through which the dose was administered (even with I.V. flush and/or the dose was administered hours before).

Drug Interactions

Substrate of CYP3A4 p-glycoprotein (major); **Inhibits** CYP2C9 p-glycoprotein (weak), 3A4 (moderate)
ACE inhibitors: May enhance nephrotoxic effects of cyclosporine.
Allopurinol: Increases cyclosporine concentrations by inhibiting cyclosporine metabolism.
Amiodarone: May increase cyclosporine concentrations by inhibiting cyclosporine metabolism.
Antibiotics: Concomitant use may potentiate renal dysfunction (seen with ciprofloxacin, gentamicin, tobramycin, vancomycin, trimethoprim and sulfamethoxazole); increased cyclosporine concentrations by inhibiting cyclosporine metabolism (seen with azithromycin, clarithromycin, erythromycin, and norfloxacin, quinupristin/dalfopristin); may decrease cyclosporine concentrations by inducing cyclosporine metabolism (seen with nafcillin, and rifampin); may decrease immunosuppressant effects (seen with ciprofloxacin); CNS disturbances, seizures (seen with imipenem).
Anticonvulsants: May decrease cyclosporine concentrations by inducing cyclosporine metabolism (seen with carbamazepine, phenobarbital, and phenytoin)
Antineoplastics: Concomitant use may potentiate renal dysfunction (seen with melphalan)
Antifungals: Concomitant use may potentiate renal dysfunction (seen with amphotericin B, ketoconazole); increase cyclosporine concentrations by inhibiting cyclosporine metabolism (seen with fluconazole, itraconazole, and ketoconazole)
Bosentan: Cyclosporine may increase the serum concentration of bosentan. Bosentan may decrease the serum concentration of cyclosporine. Concurrent use is contraindicated.

Bromocriptine: Increases cyclosporine concentrations by inhibiting cyclosporine metabolism
Calcium channel blockers (diltiazem, nicardipine, verapamil): Increase cyclosporine concentrations by inhibiting cyclosporine metabolism. Nifedipine has been reported to increase the risk of gingival hyperplasia.
Colchicine: May potentiate renal dysfunction; colchicine may increase cyclosporine concentrations by inhibiting metabolism. Cyclosporine may decrease the clearance of colchicine.
Corticosteroids: Systemic corticosteroids may increase the serum concentration of cyclosporine (reported with methylprednisolone). Cyclosporine may increase the serum concentration of systemic corticosteroids. Convulsions have been reported with high-dose methylprednisolone.
CYP3A4 inducers: CYP3A4 inducers may decrease the levels/effects of cyclosporine. Example inducers include aminoglutethimide, carbamazepine, nafcillin, nevirapine, phenobarbital, phenytoin, and rifamycins.
CYP3A4 inhibitors: May increase the levels/effects of cyclosporine. Example inhibitors include azole antifungals, clarithromycin, diclofenac, doxycycline, erythromycin, imatinib, isoniazid, nefazodone, nicardipine, propofol, protease inhibitors, quinidine, telithromycin, and verapamil.
CYP3A4 substrates: Cyclosporine may increase the levels/effects of CYP3A4 substrates. Example substrates include benzodiazepines, calcium channel blockers, cyclosporine, mirtazapine, nateglinide, nefazodone, sildenafil (and other PDE-5 inhibitors), tacrolimus, and venlafaxine. Selected benzodiazepines (midazolam and triazolam), cisapride, ergot alkaloids, selected HMG-CoA reductase inhibitors (lovastatin and simvastatin), and pimozide are generally contraindicated with strong CYP3A4 inhibitors.
Danazol: Increases cyclosporine concentrations by inhibiting cyclosporine metabolism
Digoxin: Decreased clearance and decreased volume of distribution of digoxin; severe digitalis toxicity has been observed.
Fibric acid derivatives: May increase the risk of renal dysfunction and may alter cyclosporine concentrations; monitor.
H_2 blockers: Concomitant use may potentiate renal dysfunction (seen with cimetidine, ranitidine).
HMG-CoA reductase inhibitors: Cyclosporine may increase levels/effects of HMG-CoA reductase inhibitors, resulting in myalgias, rhabdomyolysis, acute renal failure; dosage adjustments of HMG-CoA reductase inhibitors are recommended.
Imatinib: May increase cyclosporine serum concentrations by inhibiting cyclosporine metabolism.
Immunosuppressives: Concomitant use may potentiate renal dysfunction (seen with tacrolimus, muromonab-CD3).
Metoclopramide: Increases cyclosporine concentrations by inhibiting cyclosporine metabolism.
Methotrexate: Cyclosporine increases plasma levels of methotrexate and decreases plasma levels of its metabolite; monitor closely for signs of toxicity.
Minoxidil: Concomitant use may lead to severe hypertrichosis.
NSAIDs: Concomitant use may potentiate renal dysfunction, especially in dehydrated patients (seen with diclofenac, naproxen, sulindac). In addition, diclofenac plasma levels are doubled when given with cyclosporine; the lowest possible dose of diclofenac should be used. Monitor serum creatinine.
Octreotide: May decrease cyclosporine concentrations by inducing cyclosporine metabolism.
Oral contraceptives (hormonal): May increase serum levels of cyclosporine; monitor for signs of toxicity.
Orlistat: May decrease absorption of cyclosporine; avoid concomitant use.
Protease inhibitors: Formal interaction studies have not been done; protease inhibitors are known to induce CYP3A4; use caution when using cyclosporine with indinavir, nelfinavir, ritonavir, or saquinavir.
Rifabutin: Formal interaction studies have not been done; rifabutin is known to increase the metabolism of medications via CYP3A4.
Sirolimus: Cyclosporine may increase serum levels/effects; monitor. Concurrent therapy may increase the risk of HUS/TTP/TMA. Administer sirolimus 4 hours after cyclosporine to minimize the increase in sirolimus blood levels.
Sulfinpyrazone: May decrease cyclosporine levels by inducing cyclosporine metabolism; monitor.
Ticlopidine: May decrease cyclosporine concentrations by inducing cyclosporine metabolism.
Vaccines: Vaccination may be less effective; avoid use of live vaccines during therapy.
Voriconazole: Cyclosporine serum concentrations may be increased; monitor serum concentrations and renal function. Decrease cyclosporine dosage by 50% when initiating voriconazole.

Pregnancy Risk Factor C
Pregnancy Implications Cyclosporine crosses the placenta. Based on clinical use, premature births and low birth weight were consistently observed. Use only if the benefit to the mother outweighs the possible risks to the fetus.
Lactation Enters breast milk/not recommended

Nursing Implications Do not administer liquid from plastic or styrofoam cup; mixing with milk, chocolate milk, or orange juice preferably at room temperature, improves palatability; stir well and drink at once; do not allow to stand before drinking; rinse with more diluent to ensure that the total dose is taken; after use, dry outside of pipette; do not rinse with water or other cleaning agents; may cause inflamed gums

Additional Information
Cyclosporine (modified): Refers to the capsule dosage formulation of cyclosporine in an aqueous dispersion (previously referred to as "microemulsion"). Cyclosporine (modified) has increased bioavailability as compared to cyclosporine (non-modified) and cannot be used interchangeably without close monitoring.

Food interaction: Grapefruit juice increases absorption; unsupervised use should be avoided.

Herb/Nutraceutical interaction: Avoid St John's wort; as an enzyme inducer, it may increase the metabolism of and decrease plasma levels of cyclosporine; organ rejection and graft loss have been reported. Avoid cat's claw, echinacea (have immunostimulant properties).

Specific References
Akhlaghi F and Trull AK, "Distribution of Cyclosporin in Organ Transplant Recipients," Clin Pharmacokinet, 2002, 41(9):615-37.

Barone GW, Gurley BJ, Ketel BL, et al, "Drug Interaction Between St John's Wort and Cyclosporine," Ann Pharmacother, 2000, 34(9):1013-6.

Butch AW and Fukuchi AM, "Analytical Performance of the CEDIA® Cyclosporine PLUS Whole Blood Immunoassay," J Anal Toxicol, 2004, 28:204-10.

Caroli A, Fregonese D, Di Falco G, et al, "Aspergillus fumigatus Pneumonia During Cyclosporine Treatment for Ulcerative Colitis," Am J Gastroenterol, 2000, 95(10):3016-7.

Cohen E, Kramer MR, Maoz C, et al, "Cyclosporin Drug-Interaction-Induced Rhabdomyolysis: A Report of Two Cases in Lung Transplant Recipients," Transplantation, 2000, 70(1):119-22.

Colman E and Fossler M, "Reduction in Blood Cyclosporine Concentrations by Orlistat," N Engl J Med, 2000, 342(15):1141-2.

de Bono JS, Fraser JA, Lee F, et al, "Metastatic Extragonadal Seminoma Associated with Cardiac Transplantation," Ann Oncol, 2000, 11(6):749-52.

de Perrot M , Spiliopoulos A, Cottini S, et al, "Massive Cerebral Edema After I.V. Cyclosporin Overdose," Transplantation, 2000, 70(8):1259-60.

Dumont RJ and Ensom MH, "Methods for Clinical Monitoring of Cyclosporin in Transplant Patients," Clin Pharmacokinet, 2000, 38(5):427-47.

Filler G, Lepage N, Delisle B, et al, "Effect of Cyclosporine on Mycophenolic Acid Area Under the Concentration-Time Curve in Pediatric Kidney Transplant Recipients," Ther Drug Monit, 2001, 23(5):514-9.

Hakkaart-van Roijen L, Verboom P, Redekop WK, et al, "The Cost Effectiveness of Tapered Versus Abrupt Discontinuation of Oral Cyclosporin Microemulsion for the Treatment of Psoriasis," Pharmacoeconomics, 2001, 19(5 Pt 2):599-608.

Haug M 3rd and Wimberley SL, "Problems with the Automatic Switching of Generic Cyclosporine Oral Solution for the Innovator Product," Am J Health Syst Pharm, 2000, 57(14):1349-53.

Katz K, Curry S, Brooks D, et al, "Cyclosporine's Effect on Survival Time in a Rat Model of Acute Salicylate Toxicity," J Toxicol Clin Toxicol, 2002, 40(5):693.

Kirby B, Owen CM, Blewitt RW, et al, "Cutaneous T-Cell Lymphoma Developing in a Patient on Cyclosporin Therapy," J Am Acad Dermatol, 2002, 47(2 Suppl):S165-7.

Koide T, Yamada M, Takahashi T, et al, "Cyclosporine A-Associated Fatal Central Nervous System Angiopathy in a Bone Marrow Transplant Recipient: An Autopsy Case," Acta Neuropathol (Berl), 2000, 99(6):680-4.

Koshman SL, Lalonde LD, Burton I, et al, "Supratherapeutic Response to Ezetimibe Administered with Cyclosporine," Ann Pharmacother, 2005, 39(7):1561-5.

Kuiper RA, Malingré MM, Beijnen JH, et al, "Cyclosporine-Induced Anaphylaxis," Ann Pharmacother, 2000, 34(7-8):858-61.

Lee PC, Hung CJ, Lei HY, et al, "Suspected Acute Post-Transplant Neuropsychosis Due to Interaction of Morphine and Cyclosporin After a Renal Transplant," Anaesthesia, 2000, 55(8):827-8.

Leitner GC, Hiesmayr M, Hoecker P, et al, "Therapeutic Approaches in the Management of Oral Cyclosporine A Intoxication," Transplantation, 2003, 75(5):1764-5.

Lill J, Bauer LA, Horn JR, et al, "Cyclosporine-Drug Interactions and the Influence of Patient Age," Am J Health Syst Pharm, 2000, 57(17):1579-84.

LoVecchio FA and Goltz HR, "Atrial Fibrillation Following Acute Overdose with Oral Cyclosporin," Ann Pharmacother, 2000, 34(3):405.

Manadan AM, Sequeira W, and Block JA, "The Treatment of Psoriatic Arthritis," Am J Ther, 2006, 13(1):72-9.

Morris RG and Lam AK, "Cyclosporin Monitoring in Australasia: Survey of Laboratory Practices in 2000," Ther Drug Monit, 2002, 24(4):471-8.

Nicolas De Prado I, Miras Lopez M, Moran Sanchez S, et al, "Rhabdomyolysis Associated with Cerivastatin and Cyclosporine Combination Therapy," Med Clin (Barc), 2002, 118(18):716-7.

Oellerich M and Armstrong VW, "Two-Hour Cyclosporine Concentration Determination: An Appropriate Tool to Monitor Neoral Therapy?" Ther Drug Monit, 2002, 24(1):40-6.

Page RL 2nd, Ruscin JM, Fish D, et al, "Possible Interaction Between Intravenous Azithromycin and Oral Cyclosporine," Pharmacotherapy, 2001, 21(11):1436-43.

Pham CQ, Efros CB, and Berardi RR, "Cyclosporine for Severe Ulcerative Colitis," Ann Pharmacother, 2006, 40(1):96-101.

Pham PT, Peng A, Wilkinson AH, et al, "Cyclosporine and Tacrolimus-Associated Thrombotic Microangiopathy," Am J Kidney Dis, 2000, 36(4):844-50.

Qureshi ST and Smolinske S, "Cyclosporin Pharmacokinetics with Multidose Charcoal After a Ten-Fold Dosing Error," J Toxicol Clin Toxicol, 2003, 41(5):747.

Ramchandani M, Brown AM, Rippin JW, et al, "Labial Adenocarcinoma After Treatment with Cyclosporin A in a Patient with Panuveitis," Am J Ophthalmol, 2000, 130(1):127-8.

Ruschitzka F, Meier PJ, Turina M, et al, "Acute Heart Transplant Rejection Due to Saint John's Wort," Lancet, 2000, 355(9203):548-9.

Verdejo A, de Cos MA, and Zubimendi JA, "Drug Points: Probable Interaction Between Cyclosporin A and Low Dose Ticlopidine," BMJ, 2000, 320(7241):1037.

Walter SH, Bertz H, and Gerling J, "Bilateral Optic Neuropathy After Bone Marrow Transplantation and Cyclosporin A Therapy," Graefes Arch Clin Exp Ophthalmol, 2000, 238(6):472-6.

Cyproheptadine

CAS Number 129-03-3; 41354-29-4; 969-33-5
U.S. Brand Names Periactin® [DSC]
Synonyms Cyproheptadine Hydrochloride; Periactin
Use Perennial and seasonal allergic rhinitis and other allergic symptoms including urticaria
Unlabeled/Investigational Use Appetite stimulation, blepharospasm, cluster headaches, migraine headaches, Nelson's syndrome, pruritus, schizophrenia, spinal cord damage associated spasticity, and tardive dyskinesia
Mechanism of Action Direct serotonin antagonist with anticholinergic and antihistamine effects
Adverse Reactions
Cardiovascular: Hypotension, palpitations, tachycardia, sinus tachycardia, vasculitis
Central nervous system: **Slight to moderate drowsiness**, dizziness, fatigue, ataxia, euphoria, seizures, lethargy, hyperthermia, cognitive dysfunction, aggressive behavior
Dermatologic: Angioedema, urticaria, purpura, licheniform eruptions, exanthem
Endocrine & metabolic: Hyperprolactinemia, hypoprolactinemia
Gastrointestinal: Nausea, vomiting, diarrhea, weight gain
Genitourinary: Urinary retention, dysuria
Hepatic: Jaundice
Neuromuscular & skeletal: Paresthesia
Ocular: Diplopia, increased intraocular pressure, photosensitivity, mydriasis
Otic: Tinnitus
Respiratory: **Thickening of bronchial secretions**, bronchoconstriction
Miscellaneous: Systemic lupus erythematosus
Signs and Symptoms of Overdose Agitation, confusion, hallucinations, mydriasis, seizures, tachycardia
Pharmacodynamics/Kinetics
Absorption: Completely
Metabolism: Almost completely hepatic
Excretion: Urine (>50% primarily as metabolites); feces (~25%)
Dosage
Oral:
Children:
Allergic conditions: 0.25 mg/kg/day or 8 mg/m^2/day in 2-3 divided doses **or**
2-6 years: 2 mg every 8-12 hours (not to exceed 12 mg/day)
7-14 years: 4 mg every 8-12 hours (not to exceed 16 mg/day)
Migraine headaches: 4 mg 2-3 times/day
Children ≥12 years and Adults: Spasticity associated with spinal cord damage: 4 mg at bedtime; increase by a 4 mg dose every 3-4 days; average daily dose: 16 mg in divided doses; not to exceed 36 mg/day
Children >13 years and Adults: Appetite stimulation (anorexia nervosa): 2 mg 4 times/day; may be increased gradually over a 3-week period to 8 mg 4 times/day
Adults:
Allergic conditions: 4-20 mg/day divided every 8 hours (not to exceed 0.5 mg/kg/day)
Cluster headaches: 4 mg 4 times/day

Migraine headaches: 4-8 mg 3 times/day

Dosage adjustment in hepatic impairment: Reduce dosage in patients with significant hepatic dysfunction

Contraindications Hypersensitivity to cyproheptadine or any component of the formulation; narrow-angle glaucoma; bladder neck obstruction; acute asthmatic attack; stenosing peptic ulcer; GI tract obstruction; concurrent use of MAO inhibitors; avoid use in premature and term newborns due to potential association with SIDS

Warnings Do not use in neonates, safety and efficacy have not been established in children <2 years of age; symptomatic prostate hypertrophy; antihistamines are more likely to cause dizziness, excessive sedation, syncope, toxic confusion states, and hypotension in the elderly. In case reports, cyproheptadine has promoted weight gain in anorexic adults, though it has not been specifically studied in the elderly. All cases of weight loss or decreased appetite should be adequately assessed.

Dosage Forms

Syrup, as hydrochloride: 2 mg/5 mL (473 mL) [contains alcohol 5%; mint flavor]

Tablet, as hydrochloride: 4 mg

Reference Range Postmortem peripheral blood and urine concentrations following fatal overdose: 0.62 mg/L and 0.75 mg/L

Overdosage/Treatment

Referral and treatment of ingestions >3 times usual dose suggested

Decontamination: Avoid ipecac (except prehospital), charcoal recommended; lavage indicated if obtunded or within 1 hour of ingestion or evidence of gastric hypomotility

Supportive therapy: There is no routine specific treatment; severe life-threatening symptoms may be treated with physostigmine; hypotension is best treated with norepinephrine or phenylephrine; seizures should be treated with benzodiazepines; in absence of secondary complications (cardiac ischemia), sinus tachycardia does not require specific therapy; renal failure due to rhabdomyolysis, hemodialysis may be employed; sodium bicarbonate may be of some value in wide complex tachycardias.

Test Interactions ↑ serum amylase; ↓ serum prolactin; reduces hypoglycemia-induced growth hormone secretion; can cause false-positive screen for serum tricyclic antidepressant

Drug Interactions

Cyproheptadine may potentiate the effect of CNS depressants.

MAO inhibitors may cause hallucinations when taken with cyproheptadine.

Pregnancy Risk Factor B

Lactation Excretion in breast milk unknown/contraindicated

Additional Information Lowers serum prolactin levels; also has been used to treat serotonin syndrome induced by the combination of sertraline and isocarboxazid at a dose of 4 mg; can cause dependence

Specific References

Gunja N, Collins M, and Graudins A, "A Comparison of the Pharmacokinetics of Oral and Sublingual Cyproheptadine," *J Toxicol Clin Toxicol*, 2004, 42(1):79-83.

Meythaler JM, Roper JF, and Brunner RC, "Cyproheptadine for Intrathecal Baclofen Withdrawal," *Arch Phys Med Rehabil*, 2003, 84(5):638-42.

Yuan CM, Spandorfer PR, Miller SL, et al, "Evaluation of Tricyclic Antidepressant False Positivity in a Pediatric Case of Cyproheptadine (Periactin) Overdose," *Ther Drug Monit*, 2003, 25(3):299-304.

Cytarabine

CAS Number 147-94-4; 69-74-9

U.S. Brand Names Cytosar-U®

Synonyms Ara-C; Arabinosylcytosine; Cytarabine Hydrochloride; Cytosine Arabinosine Hydrochloride; NSC-63878

Use Cytarabine is one of the most active agents in leukemia; also active against lymphoma, meningeal leukemia, and meningeal lymphoma; has little use in the treatment of solid tumors

Mechanism of Action This is a sustained-release formulation of the active ingredient cytarabine, which acts through inhibition of DNA synthesis; cell cycle-specific for the S phase of cell division; cytosine gains entry into cells by a carrier process, and then must be converted to its active compound; cytosine acts as an analog and is incorporated into DNA; however, the primary action is inhibition of DNA polymerase resulting in decreased DNA synthesis and repair; degree of its cytotoxicity correlates linearly with its incorporation into DNA; therefore, incorporation into the DNA is responsible for drug activity and toxicity

Adverse Reactions

High-dose therapy toxicities: Cerebellar toxicity, keratoconjunctivitis (make sure the patient is on steroid eye drops during therapy), corneal keratitis, hyperbilirubinemia, pulmonary edema, pericarditis, and tamponade

Cardiovascular: Cardiomegaly, pericarditis, chest pain, vasculitis

Central nervous system: **Fever (>80%)**, leukoencephalopathy, dizziness, headache, somnolence, confusion, malaise, extrapyramidal reactions; has produced seizures when given I.T.; cerebellar syndrome (or cerebellar toxicity) in 8% of patients (fatal or permanent in 1%); manifested as ataxia, dysarthria, and dysdiadochokinesia; has been

reported to be dose-related at cumulative doses >30 g/m². This may or may not be reversible.

Dermatologic: **Rash**, skin freckling, itching, alopecia, cellulitis at injection site, palmar-plantar erythrodysesthesia, acral erythema, cutaneous vasculitis

Endocrine & metabolic: Parotid disorder

Gastrointestinal: **Nausea, vomiting, diarrhea, and mucositis which subside quickly after discontinuing the drug; GI effects may be more pronounced with divided I.V. bolus doses than with continuous infusion; oral/anal ulceration**; acute pancreatitis

   Emetic potential:

   ≤20 mg: Moderately low (10% to 30%)

   250 mg to 1 g: Moderately high (60% to 90%)

   >1 g: High (>90%)

Genitourinary: Urinary retention, hemorrhagic cystitis

Hematologic: **Myelosuppression; neutropenia and thrombocytopenia are severe, anemia may also occur**

   Onset: 4-7 days

   Nadir: 14-18 days

   Recovery: 21-28 days

Hepatic: **Hepatic dysfunction, mild jaundice and acute increase in transaminases can be produced**

Local: **Thrombophlebitis**, extravasation injury

Neuromuscular & skeletal: Myalgia, bone pain, neuropathy (peripheral), neuritis

Ocular: Photophobia, blurred vision

Respiratory: Syndrome of sudden respiratory distress progressing to pulmonary edema, pneumonia, hyposmia

Miscellaneous: Sepsis

Pharmacodynamics/Kinetics

Distribution: V_d: Total body water; widely and rapidly since it enters the cells readily; crosses blood-brain barrier with CSF levels of 40% to 50% of plasma level

Metabolism: Primarily hepatic; metabolized by deoxycytidine kinase and other nucleotide kinases to aracytidine triphosphate (active); about 86% to 96% of dose is metabolized to inactive uracil arabinoside

Half-life elimination: Initial: 7-20 minutes; Terminal: 0.5-2.6 hours

Excretion: Urine (~80% as metabolites) within 24-36 hours

Dosage

I.V. bolus, IVPB, and CIV doses of cytarabine are very different. Bolus doses are relatively well tolerated since the drug is rapidly metabolized; but are associated with greater neurotoxicity. Continuous infusion uniformly results in myelosuppression. Refer to individual protocols.

Children and Adults:

Remission induction:

   I.V.: 100-200 mg/m²/day for 5-10 days; a second course, beginning 2-4 weeks after the initial therapy, may be required in some patients.

   I.T.: 5-75 mg/m² every 2-7 days until CNS findings normalize; or age-based dosing:

      <1 year: 20 mg

      1-2 years: 30 mg

      2-3 years: 50 mg

      >3 years: 75 mg

Remission maintenance:

   I.V.: 70-200 mg/m²/day for 2-5 days at monthly intervals

   I.M., SubQ: 1-1.5 mg/kg single dose for maintenance at 1- to 4-week intervals

High-dose therapies:

Doses as high as 1-3 g/m² have been used for refractory or secondary leukemias or refractory non-Hodgkin's lymphoma.

Doses of 1-3 g/m² every 12 hours for up to 12 doses have been used

Bone marrow transplant: 1.5 g/m² continuous infusion over 48 hours

Hemodialysis: Supplemental dose is not necessary.

Peritoneal dialysis: Supplemental dose is not necessary.

Dosage adjustment in hepatic impairment: Dose may need to be adjusted since cytarabine is partially detoxified in the liver.

Stability Store intact vials of powder at room temperature 15°C to 30°C (59°F to 86°F). Reconstitute with SWI, D₅W or NS; reconstituted solutions are stable for up to 8 days at room temperature. Further dilution in D₅W or NS is stable for 8 days at room temperature (25°C).

Standard I.V. infusion dilution: Dose/250-1000 mL D₅W or NS.

Standard intrathecal dilutions: Dose/3-5 mL lactated Ringer's ± methotrexate (12 mg) ± hydrocortisone (15-50 mg); intrathecal solutions in 3-20 mL lactated Ringer's are stable for 7 days at room temperature (30°C); however, should be used within 24 hours due to sterility concerns

Note: Bacteriostatic diluent should not be used for the preparation of either high doses or intrathecal doses of cytarabine; may be used for I.M., SubQ, and low-dose (100-200 mg/m²) I.V. solution.

Monitoring Parameters Liver function tests, CBC with differential and platelet count, serum creatinine, BUN, serum uric acid

Administration

Can be administered I.M., I.V. infusion, I.T., or SubQ at a concentration not to exceed 100 mg/mL

I.V. may be administered either as a bolus, IVPB (high doses of >500 mg/m^2), or continuous intravenous infusion (doses of 100-200 mg/m^2)

I.V. doses of ≥1.5 g/m^2 may produce conjunctivitis which can be ameliorated with prophylactic use of corticosteroid (0.1% dexamethasone) eye drops. Dexamethasone eye drops should be administered at 1-2 drops every 6 hours during and for 2-7 days after cytarabine is done.

Contraindications Hypersensitivity to cytarabine or any component of the formulation

Warnings Hazardous agent - use appropriate precautions for handling and disposal. **[U.S. Boxed Warning]: Potent myelosuppressive agent;** use with caution in patients with prior bone marrow suppression; monitor for signs of febrile neutropenia. High-dose regimens are associated with CNS, gastrointestinal, ocular (prophylaxis with ophthalmic corticosteroid drops is recommended), and pulmonary toxicities. Use with caution in patients with impaired renal (high dose cytarabine) and hepatic function; may be at higher risk for CNS toxicities; dosage adjustments may be required. Tumor lysis syndrome and subsequent hyperuricemia may occur with high dose cytarabine; monitor, consider allopurinol and hydrate accordingly. Cytarabine syndrome is characterized by fever, myalgia, bone pain, chest pain, maculopapular rash, conjunctivitis, and malaise, and may occur 6-12 hours following administration; may be managed with corticosteroids. **[U.S. Boxed Warning]: Should be administered under the supervision of an experienced cancer chemotherapy physician.** Some products may contain benzyl alcohol; do not use products containing benzyl alcohol or products reconstituted with bacteriostatic diluent intrathecally or for high-dose cytarabine regimens.

Dosage Forms Injection, powder for reconstitution: 100 mg, 500 mg, 1 g, 2 g
Injection, solution: 20 mg/mL (5 mL, 25 mL, 50 mL); 100 mg/mL (20 mL)

Reference Range Cytotoxic plasma cytarabine range: 50-100 mg/L (0.2-0.4 mM/L)

Overdosage/Treatment Supportive therapy: High-dose methylprednisolone therapy (10 mg/kg) may be useful to treat cytarabine-induced ARDS. Additionally, compartment syndrome due to isolated extremity perfusion can be relieved with I.V. methylprednisolone (1 g). Keratoconjunctivitis can be avoided with prophylactic use of corticosteroid eye drops (1-2 drops of 0.1% dexamethasone ophthalmic solution in each eye) every 4-6 hours while awake for 1 week following high-dose cytarabine therapy; metoclopramide (2 mg/kg) before, 2,4, and 6 hours post-therapy can reduce vomiting by 70%

Drug Interactions

Digoxin: Cytarabine may decrease the levels/effects of digoxin (oral tablet).

Flucytosine: Cytarabine may decrease the therapeutic effect of flucytosine.

Pregnancy Risk Factor D

Pregnancy Implications Congenital limb abnormalities have been noted

Lactation Excretion in breast milk unknown/not recommended

Additional Information Supplied with diluent containing benzyl alcohol, which should not be used when preparing either high-dose or I.T. doses; patients with creatinine clearances <60 mL/minute may be particularly at risk for neurotoxicity

---

Dalteparin

U.S. Brand Names Fragmin®

Use Prevention of deep vein thrombosis which may lead to pulmonary embolism, in patients requiring abdominal surgery who are at risk for thromboembolism complications (eg, patients >40 years of age, obesity, patients with malignancy, history of deep vein thrombosis or pulmonary embolism, and surgical procedures requiring general anesthesia and lasting >30 minutes); prevention of DVT in patients undergoing hip-replacement surgery; patients immobile during an acute illness; acute treatment of unstable angina or non-Q-wave myocardial infarction; prevention of ischemic complications in patients on concurrent aspirin therapy

Active treatment of deep vein thrombosis

Mechanism of Action Low molecular weight heparin analog with a molecular weight of 4000-6000 daltons; the commercial product contains 3% to 15% heparin with a molecular weight <3000 daltons, 65% to 78% with a molecular weight of 3000-8000 daltons and 14% to 26% with a molecular weight >8000 daltons; while dalteparin has been shown to inhibit both factor Xa and factor IIa (thrombin), the antithrombotic effect of dalteparin is characterized by a higher ratio of antifactor Xa to antifactor IIa activity (ratio = 4)

Adverse Reactions

Cardiovascular: Edema

Central nervous system: Confusion, fever

Dermatologic: Ecchymosis, pruritus, alopecia

Hematologic: Hemorrhage, thrombocytopenia, erythema, hypochromic anemia, coagulopathy, hematoma

Gastrointestinal: Nausea

Local: Irritation, pain

Pharmacodynamics/Kinetics

Onset of action: 1-2 hours

Duration: >12 hours

Half-life elimination (route dependent): 2-5 hours

Time to peak, serum: 4 hours

Dosage

Adults: SubQ:

Abdominal surgery:

Low-to-moderate DVT risk: 2500 int. units 1-2 hours prior to surgery, then once daily for 5-10 days postoperatively

High DVT risk: 5000 int. units 1-2 hours prior to surgery and then once daily for 5-10 days postoperatively

Patients undergoing total hip surgery: **Note:** Three treatment options are currently available. Dose is given for 5-10 days, although up to 14 days of treatment have been tolerated in clinical trials:

Postoperative start:

Initial: 2500 int. units 4-8 hours* after surgery

Maintenance: 5000 int. units once daily; start at least 6 hours after postsurgical dose

Preoperative (starting day of surgery):

Initial: 2500 int. units within 2 hours before surgery

Adjustment: 2500 int. units 4-8 hours* after surgery

Maintenance: 5000 int. units once daily; start at least 6 hours after postsurgical dose

Preoperative (starting evening prior to surgery):

Initial: 5000 int. units 10-14 hours before surgery

Adjustment: 5000 int. units 4-8 hours* after surgery

Maintenance: 5000 int. units once daily, allowing 24 hours between doses.

*Dose may be delayed if hemostasis is not yet achieved.

Unstable angina or non-Q-wave myocardial infarction: 120 int. units/kg body weight (maximum dose: 10,000 int. units) every 12 hours for 5-8 days with concurrent aspirin therapy. Discontinue dalteparin once patient is clinically stable.

Immobility during acute illness: 5000 int. units once daily

Dosing adjustment in renal impairment: Half-life is increased in patients with chronic renal failure, use with caution, accumulation can be expected; specific dosage adjustments have not been recommended

Dosing adjustment in hepatic impairment: Use with caution in patients with hepatic insufficiency; specific dosage adjustments have not been recommended

Monitoring Parameters Periodic CBC including platelet count; stool occult blood tests; monitoring of PT and PTT is not necessary

Administration

For deep SubQ injection only. May be injected in a U-shape to the area surrounding the navel, the upper outer side of the thigh, or the upper outer quadrangle of the buttock. Apply pressure to injection site; do not massage. Use thumb and forefinger to lift a fold of skin when injecting dalteparin to the navel area or thigh. Insert needle at a 45- to 90-degree angle. The entire length of needle should be inserted. Do not expel air bubble from fixed-dose syringe prior to injection. Air bubble (and extra solution, if applicable) may be expelled from graduated syringes.

Administration once daily beginning prior to surgery and continuing 5-10 days after surgery prevents deep vein thrombosis in patients at risk for thromboembolic complications. For unstable angina or non-Q-wave myocardial infarction, dalteparin is administered every 12 hours until the patient is stable (5-8 days).

Contraindications Hypersensitivity to dalteparin or any component of the formulation; thrombocytopenia associated with a positive *in vitro* test for antiplatelet antibodies in the presence of dalteparin; hypersensitivity to heparin or pork products; patients with active major bleeding; patients with unstable angina or non-Q-wave MI undergoing regional anesthesia; not for I.M. or I.V. use

Warnings

[U.S. Boxed Warning]: Patients with recent or anticipated neuraxial anesthesia (epidural or spinal anesthesia) are at risk of spinal or epidural hematoma and subsequent paralysis. Consider risk versus benefit prior to neuraxial anesthesia. Risk is increased by concomitant agents which may alter hemostasis, as well as traumatic or repeated epidural or spinal puncture. Patient should be observed closely for bleeding if dalteparin is administered during or immediately following diagnostic lumbar puncture, epidural anesthesia, or spinal anesthesia.

Not to be used interchangeably (unit for unit) with heparin or any other low molecular weight heparins. Use with caution in patients with known hypersensitivity to methylparaben or propylparaben. Use with caution in patients with history of heparin-induced thrombocytopenia. Monitor platelet count closely. Rare thrombocytopenia may occur. Consider discontinuation of dalteparin in any patient developing significant thrombocytopenia. Monitor patient closely for signs or symptoms of bleeding. Certain patients are at increased risk of bleeding. Risk factors include bacterial endocarditis; congenital or acquired bleeding disorders; active ulcerative or angiodysplastic GI diseases; severe uncontrolled hypertension; hemorrhagic stroke; or use shortly after brain, spinal, or ophthalmology surgery; in patient treated concomitantly with platelet inhibitors; recent GI bleeding; thrombocytopenia or platelet defects; severe liver disease; hypertensive or diabetic retinopathy; or in patients undergoing invasive procedures.

Use with caution in patients with severe renal failure (has not been studied). Safety and efficacy in pediatric patients have not been established. Rare cases of thrombocytopenia with thrombosis have occurred. Multidose vials contain benzyl alcohol and should not be used in pregnant women. Heparin can cause hyperkalemia by affecting aldosterone. Similar reactions could occur with LMWHs. Monitor for hyperkalemia.

Dosage Forms

Injection, solution [multidose vial]: Antifactor Xa 10,000 int. units per 1 mL (9.5 mL) [contains benzyl alcohol]; antifactor Xa 25,000 units per 1 mL (3.8 mL) [contains benzyl alcohol]

Injection, solution [preservative free; prefilled syringe]: Antifactor Xa 2500 int. units per 0.2 mL (0.2 mL); antifactor Xa 5000 int. units per 0.2 mL (0.2 mL); antifactor Xa 7500 int. units per 0.3 mL (0.3 mL); antifactor Xa 10,000 int. units per 1 mL (1 mL)

Reference Range Therapeutic plasma anti-Xa levels (antifactor Xa): 0.1-0.6 units/mL (antithrombotic activity); activated partial thromboplastin time (APTT) is not considered useful for dalteparin monitoring

Overdosage/Treatment

Supportive therapy: Protamine can be used for severe bleeding upon withdrawal of heparin (1 mg of protamine for every 1 mg of dalteparin [100 units] by slow I.V. push up to 50 mg over 60 minutes). An additional 0.5 mg protamine per 100 int. units of dalteparin can be administered 2-4 hours after the initial dose if the PTT is till elevated. If serious bleeding occurs, give fresh frozen plasma in addition to protamine.

Enhancement of elimination: While hemodialysis is not beneficial, exchange transfusion has been used successfully in a neonate and plasma exchange has been used successfully in four older patients for thrombocytopenia

Antidote(s)
- Protamine Sulfate [ANTIDOTE]

Drug Interactions

Drugs which affect platelet function (eg, aspirin, NSAIDs, dipyridamole, ticlopidine, clopidogrel) may potentiate the risk of hemorrhage.
Thrombolytic agents increase the risk of hemorrhage.
Warfarin: Risk of bleeding may be increased during concurrent therapy. Dalteparin is commonly continued during the initiation of warfarin therapy to assure anticoagulation and to protect against possible transient hypercoagulability.

Pregnancy Risk Factor B

Pregnancy Implications Multiple-dose vials contain benzyl alcohol (avoid in pregnant women due to association with fetal syndrome in premature infants).

Lactation Excretion in breast milk unknown/use caution

Nursing Implications Not intended for I.M. administration

Additional Information Molecular weight: 5000; sulfur content: 11%

Specific References

Payne SM and Kovacs MJ, "Cutaneous Dalteparin Reactions Associated with Antibodies of Heparin-Induced Thrombocytopenia," *Ann Pharmacother*, 2003, 37(5):655-8.

Danaparoid

CAS Number 83513-48-8

U.S. Brand Names Orgaran® [DSC]

Synonyms Danaparoid Sodium

Use Prevention of postoperative deep vein thrombosis following elective hip replacement surgery

Unlabeled/Investigational Use Systemic anticoagulation for patients with heparin-induced thrombocytopenia: factor Xa inhibition is used to monitor degree of anticoagulation if necessary

Mechanism of Action A low molecular weight heparinoid with antifactor Xa activity and decreased platelet function effects (as compared with heparin)

Adverse Reactions

Cardiovascular: Peripheral edema, generalized edema
Central nervous system: Fever, insomnia, headache, dizziness
Dermatologic: Rash, pruritus
Gastrointestinal: Nausea, constipation, vomiting
Genitourinary: Urinary tract infections, urinary retention
Hematologic: Anemia, hemorrhage, hematoma, thrombocytopenia (7%)
Hepatic: Transient elevation of liver enzymes
Local: Injection site pain
Neuromuscular & skeletal: Joint disorder, weakness

Pharmacodynamics/Kinetics

Onset of action: Peak effect: SubQ: Maximum antifactor Xa and antithrombin (antifactor IIa) activities occur in 2-5 hours
Half-life elimination, plasma: Mean: Terminal: ~24 hours
Excretion: Primarily urine

Dosage

SubQ:
Children: Safety and effectiveness have not been established

Adults: 750 anti-Xa units (~55 mg) twice daily; beginning 1-4 hours before surgery and then not sooner than 2 hours after surgery and every 12 hours until the risk of DVT has diminished, the average duration of therapy is 7-10 days

Dosing adjustment in renal impairment: Adjustment may be necessary in elderly and patients with severe renal impairment; patients with serum creatinine levels ≥2.0 mg/dL should be carefully monitored

Monitoring Parameters Platelets, occult blood, and anti-Xa activity, if available; the monitoring of PT and/or PTT is not necessary

Administration

Administer by subcutaneous injection, **not** I.M. Have patient lie down and administer by deep SubQ injection using a fine needle (25- to 26-gauge). Rotate sites of injection.

Contraindications Hypersensitivity to danaparoid or thrombocytopenia associated with a positive *in vitro* test for antiplatelet antibodies in the presence of danaparoid; hypersensitivity to pork products or to sulfites (contains metabisulfite); patients with active major bleeding; severe hemorrhagic diathesis (hemophilia, idiopathic thrombocytopenic purpura); not for I.M. or I.V. use

Warnings

Patients with recent or anticipated neuraxial anesthesia (epidural or spinal anesthesia) are at risk of spinal or epidural hematoma and subsequent paralysis. Consider risk versus benefit prior to neuraxial anesthesia; risk is increased by concomitant agents which may alter hemostasis, as well as traumatic or repeated epidural or spinal puncture. Patient should be observed closely for bleeding if danaparoid is administered during or immediately following diagnostic lumbar puncture, epidural anesthesia, or spinal anesthesia.

Not to be used interchangeably (unit for unit) with heparin or any other low molecular weight heparins. Use with caution in patients with known hypersensitivity to methylparaben or propylparaben. Use with caution in patients with history of heparin-induced thrombocytopenia. Monitor patient closely for signs or symptoms of bleeding. Certain patients are at increased risk of bleeding. Risk factors include bacterial endocarditis; congenital or acquired bleeding disorders; active ulcerative or angiodysplastic GI diseases; severe uncontrolled hypertension; hemorrhagic stroke; use shortly after brain, spinal, or ophthalmology surgery; patient treated concomitantly with platelet inhibitors; recent GI bleeding; thrombocytopenia or platelet defects; severe liver disease; hypertensive or diabetic retinopathy; or patients undergoing invasive procedures. Use with caution in patients with severe renal failure (has not been studied). Safety and efficacy in pediatric patients have not been established. Heparin can cause hyperkalemia by affecting aldosterone. A similar reaction could occur with danaparoid. Monitor for hyperkalemia.

Dosage Forms

[CAN] = Canadian brand name
Injection, solution:
Orgaran® [CAN]: 750 anti-Xa units/0.6 mL (0.6 mL) [not available in the U.S.]

Reference Range After 3250 anti-Xa units given SubQ, peak plasma anti-Xa activity is ~0.4 anti-Xa unit/mL; anti-Xa activity >0.8 anti-Xa unit/mL may be associated with bleeding

Overdosage/Treatment Supportive therapy: Essentially the same treatment plan as with heparin; protamine sulfate is only partially effective in neutralizing danaparoid

Antidote(s)
- Protamine Sulfate [ANTIDOTE]

Drug Interactions Drugs which affect platelet function (eg, aspirin, NSAIDs, dipyridamole, ticlopidine, clopidogrel) may potentiate the risk of hemorrhage.
Thrombolytic agents increase the risk of hemorrhage.
Warfarin (and other oral anticoagulants) may increase the risk of bleeding with danaparoid.

Pregnancy Risk Factor B

Lactation Excretion in breast milk unknown/compatible

Danazol

CAS Number 17230-88-5

U.S. Brand Names Danocrine®

Use Treatment of endometriosis, fibrocystic breast disease, and hereditary angioedema; also used for refractory thrombocytopenic purpura in children

Unlabeled/Investigational Use Precocious puberty, gynecomastia, menorrhagia, idiopathic immune thrombocytopenia, lupus-associated thrombocytopenia, and autoimmune hemolytic anemia

Mechanism of Action Suppresses pituitary output of follicle-stimulating hormone and luteinizing hormone that causes regression and atrophy of normal and ectopic endometrial tissue; decreases rate of growth of abnormal breast tissue; reduces attacks associated with hereditary angioedema by increasing levels of C4 component of complement

Adverse Reactions

Cardiovascular: Hypertension, tachycardia, **edema**, sinus tachycardia
Central nervous system: Anxiety, depression, Guillain-Barré syndrome

Dermatologic: **Oily skin**, **acne**, **hirsutism**, photosensitivity, cystic acne, seborrheic dermatitis, alopecia, erythema multiforme, purpura, hypertrichosis, angioedema, urticaria, Stevens-Johnson syndrome, pruritus, exanthem

Endocrine & metabolic: **Amenorrhea, breakthrough bleeding, irregular menstrual periods, decreased breast size, fluid retention**, hyperglycemia, hot flashes, hypophosphatemia, hypoprolactinemia

Gastrointestinal: Pancreatitis, **weight gain**

Genitourinary: Monilial vaginitis, testicular atrophy, enlarged clitoris, cystitis

Hematologic: Thrombocytopenia, thrombocytosis, hypercalcemia, porphyrinogenic

Hepatic: Cholestatic jaundice, **hepatic impairment**, liver cancer

Neuromuscular & skeletal: Weakness, carpal tunnel syndrome, paresthesia

Otic: Hearing loss

Renal: Hematuria

Miscellaneous: **Voice deepening**, virilization, clitoral hypertrophy, hypoestrogenism, bleeding gums, benign intracranial hypertension, hypogonadism, peliosis of spleen and liver, systemic lupus erythematosus

Pharmacodynamics/Kinetics
Onset of action: Therapeutic: ~4 weeks
Metabolism: Extensively hepatic, primarily to 2-hydroxymethylethisterone
Half-life elimination: 4.5 hours (variable)
Time to peak, serum: Within 2 hours
Excretion: Urine

Dosage
Adults: Oral:
Female: Endometriosis: Initial: 200-400 mg/day in 2 divided doses for mild disease; individualize dosage. Usual maintenance dose: 800 mg/day in 2 divided doses to achieve amenorrhea and rapid response to painful symptoms. Continue therapy uninterrupted for 3-6 months (up to 9 months).
Female: Fibrocystic breast disease: Range: 100-400 mg/day in 2 divided doses
Male/Female: Hereditary angioedema: Initial: 200 mg 2-3 times/day; after favorable response, decrease the dosage by 50% or less at intervals of 1-3 months or longer if the frequency of attacks dictates. If an attack occurs, increase the dosage by up to 200 mg/day.

Monitoring Parameters
Signs and symptoms of intracranial hypertension (papilledema, headache, nausea, vomiting), lipoproteins, androgenic changes, hepatic function

Contraindications
Hypersensitivity to danazol or any component of the formulation; undiagnosed genital bleeding; pregnancy; breast-feeding; porphyria; markedly impaired hepatic, renal, or cardiac function

Warnings
Use with caution in patients with seizure disorders, migraine, or conditions influenced by edema. **[U.S. Boxed Warning]: Thromboembolism, thrombotic, and thrombophlebitic events have been reported (including life-threatening or fatal strokes). [U.S. Boxed Warning]: Peliosis hepatis and benign hepatic adenoma have been reported with long-term use** (may be complicated by acute intra-abdominal hemorrhage). **[U.S. Boxed Warning]: May cause benign intracranial hypertension (pseudotumor cerebri).** Breast cancer should be ruled out prior to treatment for fibrocystic breast disease. May increase risk of atherosclerosis and coronary artery disease due to decreased HDL and possible increase of LDL. May cause nonreversible androgenic effects. **[U.S. Boxed Warning]: Pregnancy must be ruled out prior to treatment.** Safety and efficacy in pediatric patients have not been established.

Dosage Forms
[DSC] = Discontinued product
Capsule: 50 mg, 100 mg, 200 mg
Danocrine®: 50 mg, 100 mg, 200 mg [DSC]

Reference Range
Oral dose of 400 mg results in a peak plasma level of 0.08 ng/mL

Overdosage/Treatment
Decontamination: Emesis with ipecac within 30 minutes or lavage within 1 hour; activated charcoal

Test Interactions
↑ serum glucagon; ↓ serum thyroxine levels, FSH, and LH

Drug Interactions
Inhibits CYP3A4 (weak)
Carbamazepine: Danazol may increase carbamazepine concentrations, requiring a decreased dosage of carbamazepine; monitor
Cyclosporine: Danazol may increase cyclosporine concentrations leading to increased toxicity; dosage of cyclosporine may need decreased; monitor
HMG-CoA reductase inhibitors: Concomitant use may lead to severe myopathy or rhabdomyolysis; effect seen with lovastatin
Hormonal contraceptives: Danazol also inhibits ovulation, possibly by acting at (and competing for) the same hormonal receptors; nonhormonal birth control methods are recommended during therapy.
Hypoglycemic agents: Danazol effects glucose metabolism, concurrent use may lead to hypoglycemia; monitor

Tacrolimus: Danazol may increase tacrolimus concentrations leading to increased toxicity; monitor
Warfarin: Increased anticoagulant effect; avoid concomitant use if possible

Pregnancy Risk Factor X

Pregnancy Implications Premature bone maturation, masculinization of urogenital sinus, clitoromegaly before 12th week of gestation in the female fetus; after the first trimester, clitoral hypertrophy would be primary effect in the female fetus

Lactation Enters breast milk/contraindicated

Nursing Implications Ensure patient is not pregnant before therapy

Dantrolene

Related Information
● Therapeutic Drugs Associated with Hallucinations
CAS Number 14663-23-1; 24868-20-0; 7261-97-4
U.S. Brand Names Dantrium®
Synonyms Dantrolene Sodium
Use Treatment of spasticity associated with spinal cord injury, stroke, cerebral palsy, or multiple sclerosis; treatment of malignant hyperthermia
Unlabeled/Investigational Use Neuroleptic malignant syndrome (NMS), considered possibly beneficial for fever and rigidity due to carbon monoxide, cocaine poisoning, alcohol withdrawal "ecstasy"
Mechanism of Action Acts directly on skeletal muscle by interfering with release of calcium ion from the sarcoplasmic reticulum; prevents or reduces the increase in myoplasmic calcium ion concentration that activates the acute catabolic processes associated with malignant hyperthermia

Adverse Reactions
Cardiovascular: Pleural effusion with pericarditis
Central nervous system: Convulsions, **drowsiness, dizziness, lightheadedness**, confusion, headache, **fatigue**, speech disturbances, slurred speech, **tiredness**, chills, fever, insomnia, nervousness, CNS depression, auditory and visual hallucinations
Dermatologic: **Rash**, urticaria, pruritus, exanthem
Gastrointestinal: **Diarrhea, nausea, vomiting**, severe constipation, anorexia, stomach cramps
Genitourinary: Urinary retention, crystalluria
Hepatic: Hepatitis
Neuromuscular & skeletal: **Weakness**
Ocular: Visual disturbances, diplopia
Otic: Ototoxicity, tinnitus
Renal: Hematuria
Respiratory: Apnea, respiratory depression, eosinophilic pneumonia
Miscellaneous: Lymphocytic lymphoma

Signs and Symptoms of Overdose
Crystalluria, disorientation, hematuria, hypotension, insomnia, jaundice, lethargy, lightheadedness, neutropenia, nocturia, pericarditis, respiratory depression, seizures

Pharmacodynamics/Kinetics
Absorption: Oral: Slow and incomplete
Metabolism: Hepatic
Half-life elimination: 8.7 hours
Excretion: Feces (45% to 50%); urine (25% as unchanged drug and metabolites)

Dosage
Spasticity: Oral:
Children: Initial: 0.5 mg/kg/dose twice daily, increase frequency to 3-4 times/day at 4- to 7-day intervals, then increase dose by 0.5 mg/kg to a maximum of 3 mg/kg/dose 2-4 times/day up to 400 mg/day
Adults: 25 mg/day to start, increase frequency to 2-4 times/day, then increase dose by 25 mg every 4-7 days to a maximum of 100 mg 2-4 times/day or 400 mg/day
Malignant hyperthermia: Children and Adults:
Oral: 4-8 mg/kg/day in 4 divided doses
Preoperative prophylaxis: Begin 1-2 days prior to surgery with last dose 3-4 hours prior to surgery
I.V.: 1 mg/kg; may repeat dose up to cumulative dose of 10 mg/kg (mean effective dose is 2.5 mg/kg), then switch to oral dose
Preoperative: 2.5 mg/kg ~1$^1/_4$ hours prior to anesthesia and infused over 1 hour with additional doses as needed and individualized

Stability
Reconstitute vial by adding 60 mL of sterile water for injection USP (**not bacteriostatic water for injection**); protect from light; use within 6 hours; avoid glass bottles for I.V. infusion

Monitoring Parameters
Motor performance should be monitored for therapeutic outcomes; nausea, vomiting, and liver function tests should be monitored for potential hepatotoxicity; intravenous administration requires cardiac monitor and blood pressure monitor

Administration
I.V.: Therapeutic or emergency dose can be administered with rapid continuous I.V. push. Follow-up doses should be administered over 2-3 minutes.

Contraindications
Active hepatic disease; should not be used where spasticity is used to maintain posture or balance

Warnings Use with caution in patients with impaired cardiac function or impaired pulmonary function. **[U.S. Boxed Warning]: Has potential for hepatotoxicity.** Overt hepatitis has been most frequently observed between the third and twelfth month of therapy. Hepatic injury appears to be greater in females and in patients >35 years of age.

Dosage Forms Capsule, as sodium: 25 mg, 50 mg, 100 mg
Dantrium®: 25 mg, 50 mg, 100 mg
Injection, powder for reconstitution, as sodium:
Dantrium®: 20 mg [contains mannitol 3 g]

Overdosage/Treatment
Decontamination: Lavage (within 1 hour)/activated charcoal; **do not** use ipecac
Supportive therapy: Hypotension can be treated with isotonic I.V. fluids with the patient placed in the Trendelenburg position; dopamine or norepinephrine can be given if hypotension is refractory to above therapy

Antidote(s)
● DOPamine [ANTIDOTE]
● Norepinephrine [ANTIDOTE]

Test Interactions ↑ serum AST, ALT, alkaline phosphatase, LDH, BUN, and total bilirubin

Drug Interactions
Substrate of CYP3A4 (major)
CYP3A4 inducers: CYP3A4 inducers may decrease the levels/effects of dantrolene. Example inducers include aminoglutethimide, carbamazepine, nafcillin, nevirapine, phenobarbital, phenytoin, and rifamycins.
CYP3A4 inhibitors: May increase the levels/effects of dantrolene. Example inhibitors include azole antifungals, clarithromycin, diclofenac, doxycycline, erythromycin, imatinib, isoniazid, nefazodone, nicardipine, propofol, protease inhibitors, quinidine, telithromycin, and verapamil.
Increased toxicity: Estrogens (hepatotoxicity), CNS depressants (sedation), MAO inhibitors, phenothiazines, clindamycin (increased neuromuscular blockade), verapamil (hyperkalemia and cardiac depression), warfarin, clofibrate, and tolbutamide

Pregnancy Risk Factor C

Lactation Excretion in breast milk unknown/not recommended

Nursing Implications 36 vials needed for adequate hyperthermia therapy; exercise caution at meals on the day of administration because difficulty swallowing and choking have been reported

Additional Information Routine I.V. prophylactic use of dantrolene for malignant hyperthermia is associated with multiple and frequent side effects and thus is **not** recommended

Specific References
Rusyniak DE and Sprague JE, "Toxin-Induced Hyperthermic Syndromes," *Med Clin North Am*, 2005, 89(6):1277-96 (review).

Dapsone

Related Information
● Therapeutic Drugs Associated with Hallucinations
CAS Number 80-08-0
U.S. Brand Names Aczone™
Synonyms Diaminodiphenylsulfone
Use Treatment of leprosy and dermatitis herpetiformis (infections caused by *Mycobacterium leprae*)
Prophylaxis of toxoplasmosis in severely immunocompromised patients; alternative agent for *Pneumocystis carinii* pneumonia prophylaxis (monotherapy) and treatment (in combination with trimethoprim); brown recluse spider bites

Mechanism of Action Dapsone is a sulfone antimicrobial; mechanism of action of the sulfones is similar to that of the sulfonamides. Sulfonamides are competitive antagonists of para-aminobenzoic acid (PABA) and prevent normal bacterial utilization of PABA for the synthesis of folic acid.

Adverse Reactions
Cardiovascular: Sinus tachycardia
Central nervous system: Insomnia, psychosis, dizziness, headache, visual hallucinations, axonopathy
Dermatologic: Exfoliative dermatitis, toxic epidermal necrolysis, erythema nodosum leprosum
Gastrointestinal: Nausea, vomiting
Hematologic: Hemolysis, methemoglobinemia, neutropenia, agranulocytosis, aplastic anemia, thrombocytosis, red blood cell aplasia, methemoglobinemia followed by hemolysis, pulmonary eosinophilia
Hepatic: Hepatitis, cholestatic jaundice
Neuromuscular & skeletal: Paresthesia, peripheral neuropathy
Ocular: Blurred vision
Otic: Ototoxicity, tinnitus
Miscellaneous: Mononucleosis-like syndrome

Signs and Symptoms of Overdose Aggressive behavior, coma (with large overdose), cyanosis, dyspnea, elevated bilirubin, elevated transaminases, erythema, erythema multiforme, hallucinations, hematuria, hemolysis with the appearance of Heinz bodies (common), hyperventilation, hypotension, insomnia, methemoglobinemia (common), nephrotic syndrome, oliguria, paresthesia (distal motor axonopathy),

photosensitivity, sulfhemoglobinemia and aplastic anemia (rare), tachycardia, toxic epidermal necrolysis, tubular necrosis, vomiting
Signs and symptoms can appear in a few minutes to within 24 hours following ingestion, with methemoglobinemia and CNS stimulation the most common.

Admission Criteria/Prognosis Any patient with change in mental status, cardiopulmonary complaints, or methemoglobin levels >30% should be admitted; asymptomatic patients with methemoglobin levels <30% may be considered for discharge after 6 hours of observation and if methemoglobin levels fall to <15%

Pharmacodynamics/Kinetics
Absorption:
Oral: Well absorbed
Topical: ~1% of the absorption of 100 mg tablet
Distribution: V_d: 1.5 L/kg; throughout total body water and present in all tissues, especially liver and kidney
Metabolism: Hepatic; forms metabolite
Half-life elimination: 30 hours (range: 10-50 hours)
Excretion: Urine (~85%)

Dosage
Oral:
Leprosy:
Children: 1-2 mg/kg/24 hours, up to a maximum of 100 mg/day
Adults: 50-100 mg/day for 3-10 years
Dermatitis herpetiformis: Adults: Start at 50 mg/day, increase to 300 mg/day, or higher to achieve full control, reduce dosage to minimum level as soon as possible
Pneumocystis carinii pneumonia (unlabeled use):
Prophylaxis:
Children >1 month: 2 mg/kg/day once daily (maximum dose: 100 mg/day) or 4 mg/kg/dose once weekly (maximum dose: 200 mg)
Adults: 100 mg/day
Treatment: Adults: 100 mg/day in combination with trimethoprim (15-20 mg/kg/day) for 21 days
Brown recluse spider bites: 100 mg twice daily for 14 days
Dosing adjustment in renal impairment: Necessary, but no specific guidelines are available

Stability Protect from light

Monitoring Parameters Monitor patient for signs of jaundice and hemolysis; CBC weekly for first month, monthly for 6 months, and semiannually thereafter

Administration Oral: May give with meals if GI upset occurs.
Topical: Apply to clean, dry skin; rub in completely. Wash hands after application.

Contraindications Hypersensitivity to dapsone or any component of the formulation

Warnings Use with caution in patients with severe anemia, G6PD, methemoglobin reductase or hemoglobin M deficiency; hypersensitivity to other sulfonamides; aplastic anemia, agranulocytosis and other severe blood dyscrasias have resulted in death; monitor carefully; treat severe anemia prior to therapy; serious dermatologic reactions (including toxic epidermal necrolysis) are rare but potential occurrences; sulfone reactions may also occur as potentially fatal hypersensitivity reactions; these, but not leprosy reactional states, require drug discontinuation; dapsone is carcinogenic in small animals. Safety and efficacy of topical dapsone has not been adequately evaluated in patient with G6PD deficiency or in patients <12 years of age.

Dosage Forms
Gel, topical (Aczone™): 5% (30 g)
Tablet: 25 mg, 100 mg

Reference Range Levels do not correlate with symptoms but may be used to confirm diagnosis; therapeutic concentrations: 0.5-5 mcg/mL; toxic effects can occur at levels >10 mcg/mL

Overdosage/Treatment
Decontamination: Emesis within 30 minutes, lavage (within 1 hour)/activated charcoal
Supportive therapy: Monitor methemoglobin, CBC, blood smear, platelets, urinalysis, liver function tests, and ABGs; hemolysis may require transfusion; methylene blue 1-2 mg/kg (up to 4 mg/kg) may be required for symptomatic patients or those with a methemoglobin >30%; methylene blue may precipitate hemolytic anemia in large doses, in patients with G6PD deficiency and in one case of dapsone overdose; cimetidine may decrease the rate of toxic metabolite although has not been tried in the overdose situation; cimetidine (400 mg 3 times/day) can lower methemoglobin levels by 25% in a nonoverdose setting
Enhanced elimination: Charcoal hemoperfusion may be useful (one case report) in patients who have clinical deterioration despite supportive care; hemodialysis has also been reported to decrease the half-life; plasma exchange has been utilized with varying degrees of success; multiple doses of activated charcoal enhance elimination and is considered treatment of choice and may be required for as long as 72 hours

Antidote(s)
- Methylene Blue [ANTIDOTE]

Drug Interactions **Substrate** of CYP2C8 (minor), 2C9 (major), 2C19 (minor), 2E1 (minor), 3A4 (major)

CYP2C9 Inducers may decrease the levels/effects of dapsone. Example inducers include carbamazepine, phenobarbital, phenytoin, rifampin, rifapentine, and secobarbital.

CYP2C9 Inhibitors may increase the levels/effects of dapsone. Example inhibitors include delavirdine, fluconazole, gemfibrozil, ketoconazole, nicardipine, NSAIDs, sulfonamides and tolbutamide.

CYP3A4 inducers: May decrease the levels/effects of dapsone. Example inducers include aminoglutethimide, carbamazepine, efavirenz, fosphenytoin, nafcillin, nevirapine, oxcarbazine, phenobarbital, phenytoin, primidone, and rifamycins.

CYP3A4 inhibitors: May increase the levels/effects of dapsone. Example inhibitors include azole antifungals, clarithromycin, diclofenac, doxycycline, erythromycin, imatinib, isoniazid, nefazodone, nicardipine, propofol, protease inhibitors, quinidine, telithromycin, and verapamil.

Didanosine: May decrease absorption of dapsone. Didanosine enteric coated capsules should not affect dapsone. Avoid other forms of didanosine.

Folic acid antagonists: May increase the risk of hematologic reactions of dapsone.

Probenecid: Decreases dapsone excretion.

Rifamycin derivatives: Increase metabolism of dapsone.

Trimethoprim: May increase toxic effects of both drugs.

Pregnancy Risk Factor C

Pregnancy Implications Does cross placenta but there have been cases with normal pregnancy outcomes with mothers taking dapsone; however, because it has the capacity to induce methemoglobinemia and hemolytic anemia, it has been suggested to limit its use in pregnancy; overdose in pregnancy has not been reported; secreted in milk with a few reports of neonatal hemolytic anemia

Lactation Enters breast milk/not recommended (AAP rates "compatible")

Additional Information Daspone accounts for about 42% of cases of acquired methemoglobinemia (with a mean peak methemoglobinemia of 7.6%)

Specific References

Ash-Bernal R, Wise R, and Wright SM. "Acquired Methemoglobinemia: A Retrospective Series of 138 Cases at 2 Teaching Hospitals," *Medicine*, 2004, 83(5):265-73.

Jha SH, Reddy JA, and Dave JK, "Dapsone-Induced Acute Pancreatitis," *Ann Pharmacother*, 2003, 37(10):1438-40.

Lee KB and Nashed TB, "Dapsone-Induced Sulfone Syndrome," *Ann Pharmacother*, 2003, 37(7-8):1044-6.

Shadnia S, Rahimi, M, Moeinsadat M, et al, "Acute Methemog lobinenia Following Attempted Suicide by Dapson," *Arch Med Res*, 2006, 37(3):410-4.

Talarico JF, Metro DG, "Presentation of Dapsone - Induced Methemoglobinemia in a Patient Status Post Small Bowel Transplant," *J. Clin. Anesth*, 2005, 17(7):568-570.

DAUNOrubicin Hydrochloride

CAS Number 20830-81-3; 23541-50-6

U.S. Brand Names Cerubidine®

Synonyms Daunomycin; DNR; NSC-82151; Rubidomycin Hydrochloride

Use Treatment of ANLL and myeloblastic leukemia; questionable results in neuroblastoma; has been used for advanced HIV-associated Kaposi's sarcoma (orphan drug status)

Mechanism of Action Inhibition of DNA and RNA synthesis, by intercalating between DNA base pairs and by steric obstruction; is not cell cycle-specific for the S phase of cell division; daunomycin is preferred over doxorubicin for the treatment of ANLL because of its dose-limiting toxicity (myelosuppression) is not of concern in the therapy of this disease; has less mucositis associated with its use

Adverse Reactions

Vesicant chemotherapy

Cardiovascular: Congestive heart failure; maximum lifetime dose: Refer to Warnings; pericarditis/myocarditis

Central nervous system: Chills

Dermatologic: **Alopecia (reversible)**, rash, pigmentation of nail beds, urticaria, hyperpigmentation, radiation recall dermatitis

Endocrine & metabolic: Hyperuricemia

Gastrointestinal: **Mild nausea or vomiting occurs in 50% of patients within the first 24 hours**; **stomatitis** may occur 3-7 days after administration, but is not as severe as that caused by doxorubicin; GI ulceration, diarrhea

Genitourinary: **Urine discoloration (red) for 1-2 days**

Hematologic:

Myelosuppressive: Dose-limiting toxicity, occurs in all patients; leukopenia is more significant than thrombocytopenia

WBC: Severe; Platelets: Severe; Onset (days): 7; Nadir (days): 14; Recovery (days): 21-28

Hepatic: Elevation of serum bilirubin, AST, and alkaline phosphatase

Local: Extravasation: Daunorubicin is a vesicant; infiltration can cause severe inflammation, tissue necrosis, and ulceration; if the drug is infiltrated, consult institutional policy, apply ice to the area, and elevate the limb

Miscellaneous: Fertility impairment

Pharmacodynamics/Kinetics

Distribution: Many body tissues, particularly the liver, kidneys, lung, spleen, and heart; not into CNS; crosses placenta; V_d: 40 L/kg

Metabolism: Primarily hepatic to daunorubicinol (active), then to inactive aglycones, conjugated sulfates, and glucuronides

Half-life elimination: Distribution: 2 minutes; Elimination: 14-20 hours; Terminal: 18.5 hours; Daunorubicinol plasma half-life: 24-48 hours

Excretion: Feces (40%); urine (~25% as unchanged drug and metabolites)

Dosage

I.V. (refer to individual protocols):

Children:

ALL combination therapy: Remission induction: 25-45 mg/m^2 on day 1 every week for 4 cycles **or** 30-45 mg/m^2/day for 3 days

AML combination therapy: Induction: I.V. continuous infusion: 30-60 mg/m^2/day on days 1-3 of cycle

Note: In children <2 years or <0.5 m^2, daunorubicin should be based on weight - mg/kg: 1 mg/kg per protocol with frequency dependent on regimen employed

Cumulative dose should not exceed 300 mg/m^2 in children >2 years; maximum cumulative doses for younger children are unknown.

Adults:

Range: 30-60 mg/m^2/day for 3-5 days, repeat dose in 3-4 weeks

AML: Single agent induction: 60 mg/m^2/day for 3 days; repeat every 3-4 weeks

AML: Combination therapy induction: 45 mg/m^2/day for 3 days of the first course of induction therapy; subsequent courses: Every day for 2 days

ALL combination therapy: 45 mg/m^2/day for 3 days

Cumulative dose should not exceed 400-600 mg/m^2

Dosing adjustment in renal impairment:

Cl_{cr} <10 mL/minute: Administer 75% of normal dose

S_{cr} >3 mg/dL: Administer 50% of normal dose

Dosing adjustment in hepatic impairment:

Serum bilirubin 1.2-3 mg/dL or AST 60-180 int. units: Reduce dose to 75%

Serum bilirubin 3.1-5 mg/dL or AST >180 int. units: Reduce dose to 50%

Serum bilirubin >5 mg/dL: Omit use

Stability Store intact vials at room temperature and protect from light. Dilute vials with 4 mL SWFI for a final concentration of 5 mg/mL; reconstituted solution is stable for 4 days at 15°C to 25°C. Further dilution in D$_5$W, LR, or NS is stable at room temperature (25°C) for up to 4 weeks if protected from light.

Monitoring Parameters CBC with differential and platelet count, liver function test, ECG, ventricular ejection fraction, renal function test

Administration

Not for I.M. or SubQ administration. Administer IVP over 1-5 minutes into the tubing of a rapidly infusing I.V. solution of D$_5$W or NS; daunorubicin has also been diluted in 100 mL of D$_5$W or NS and infused over 15-30 minutes.

Extravasation management: Apply ice immediately for 30-60 minutes; then alternate off/on every 15 minutes for 1 day. Topical cooling may be achieved using ice packs or cooling pad with circulating ice water. Cooling of site for 24 hours as tolerated by the patient. Elevate and rest extremity 24-48 hours, then resume normal activity as tolerated. Application of cold inhibits vesicant's cytotoxicity. Application of heat or sodium bicarbonate can be harmful and is contraindicated. If pain, erythema, and/or swelling persist beyond 48 hours, refer patient immediately to plastic surgeon for consultation and possible debridement.

Contraindications Hypersensitivity to daunorubicin or any component of the formulation; congestive heart failure or arrhythmias; previous therapy with high cumulative doses of daunorubicin and/or doxorubicin; pre-existing bone marrow suppression; pregnancy

Warnings

Hazardous agent - use appropriate precautions for handling and disposal. Use with caution in patients who have received radiation therapy; reduce dosage in patients who are receiving radiation therapy simultaneously.

[U.S. Boxed Warnings]: Use caution with renal impairment or in the presence of hepatic dysfunction; dosage reduction is recommended. Potent vesicant; if extravasation occurs, severe tissue damage leading to ulceration and necrosis, and pain may occur. For I.V. use only. Severe bone marrow suppression may occur.

[U.S. Boxed Warning]: May cause cumulative, dose-related myocardial toxicity (concurrent or delayed). Total cumulative dose should take into account previous or concomitant treatment with cardiotoxic agents or irradiation of chest.

Irreversible myocardial toxicity may occur as total dosage approaches:
550 mg/m^2 in adults
400 mg/m^2 in patients receiving chest radiation
300 mg/m^2 in children >2 years of age
[U.S. Boxed Warning]: Should be administered under the supervision of an experienced cancer chemotherapy physician].

Dosage Forms
Injection, powder for reconstitution: 20 mg, 50 mg
Cerubidine®: 20 mg
Injection, solution: 5 mg/mL (4 mL, 10 mL)

Overdosage/Treatment
Supportive therapy:
Extravasation management:
Apply ice immediately for 30-60 minutes; then alternate off/on every 15 minutes for one day
Topical cooling may be achieved using ice packs or cooling pad with circulating ice water; cooling of site for 24 hours as tolerated by the patient. Elevate and rest extremity 24-48 hours, then resume normal activity as tolerated. Application of cold inhibits vesicant's cytotoxicity.
Application of heat or sodium bicarbonate can be harmful and is contraindicated
If pain, erythema, and/or swelling persist beyond 48 hours, refer patient immediately to plastic surgeon for consultation and possible debridement
For extravasation, topical dimethyl sulfoxide (1.5 mL on site every 6-8 hours for 2 weeks) should be utilized; cardiomyopathy should be treated with salt restriction, diuretics and digitalis; allopurinol should be given to prevent urate nephropathy if massive cell lysis occurs

Test Interactions ↑ potassium (S), uric acid due to hyperuricemia secondary to cell lysis

Drug Interactions Patients may experience impaired immune response to vaccines; possible infection after administration of live vaccines in patients receiving immunosuppressants

Pregnancy Risk Factor D

Pregnancy Implications May cause fetal harm when administered to a pregnant woman. Animal studies have shown an increased incidence of fetal abnormalities.

Lactation Excretion in breast milk unknown/not recommended

Dehydroepiandrosterone

CAS Number 53-43-0

Use Not FDA approved: Has been used to boost the immune system, increase insulin sensitivity, improve symptoms in multiple sclerosis; as an antiobesity agent; for improvement of mood and memory in the elderly

Mechanism of Action An adrenal steroid and intermediate in testosterone and estradiol synthesis from cholesterol. It is secreted by the adrenal cortex primarily as a sulfate conjugate (DHEA-S).

Adverse Reactions
Dermatologic: Acne, hirsutism, alopecia
Hepatic: Transient hepatitis
Miscellaneous: Voice deepening (may be irreversible); may possibly increase development of breast, prostate, and ovarian cancer

Toxicodynamics/Kinetics Half-life: DHEA: 15-30 minutes; DHEA-S: 7-10 hours

Dosage
Oral:
Improvement of mood, energy, libido, and memory in the elderly: 30-90 mg/day for 4 weeks
Antiobesity: 1600 mg/day for 4 weeks
Increased insulin sensitivity in postmenopausal women: 50 mg daily for 3 weeks
Symptomatic improvement in systemic lupus erythematosus: 200 mg daily

Reference Range Average serum level of DHEA-S in men 25-34 years of age is ~6.44±2.29 μmol/L, falling to 1.15±0.5 μmol/L in men 75-84 years of age. Corresponding fall of DHEA levels is from 15.91±6.05 nmol/L to 5.36±1.69 nmol/L, respectively. The decline is relatively constant at ~2% per year. DHEA-S levels in young women are ~10% to 30% lower than in young men, but sex differences decline with age.

Overdosage/Treatment Decontamination: Oral: Emesis with syrup of ipecac within 30 minutes, or lavage within 1 hour; activated charcoal may be useful

Desipramine

Pronunciation (des IP ra meen)
Related Information
- Anticholinergic Effects of Common Psychotropics
- Antidepressant Agents
CAS Number 50-47-5; 58-28-6
U.S. Brand Names Norpramin®

Synonyms Desipramine Hydrochloride; Desmethylimipramine Hydrochloride

Use Treatment of depression

Unlabeled/Investigational Use Analgesic adjunct in chronic pain; peripheral neuropathies; substance-related disorders (eg, cocaine withdrawal); attention-deficit/hyperactivity disorder (ADHD); depression in children ≤12 years of age

Mechanism of Action Traditionally believed to increase the synaptic concentration of norepinephrine (and to a lesser extent, serotonin) in the central nervous system by inhibition of its reuptake by the presynaptic neuronal membrane. However, additional receptor effects have been found including desensitization of adenyl cyclase, down regulation of beta-adrenergic receptors, and down regulation of serotonin receptors.

Adverse Reactions
Cardiovascular: Cardiac arrhythmias, myocarditis, sinus tachycardia, tachycardia (supraventricular), torsade de pointes, exacerbation of Brugada syndrome
Central nervous system: **Drowsiness, dizziness, headache**, sedation, psychosis, confusion, excitation associated with falls, restlessness
Dermatologic: Photosensitivity, exfoliative dermatitis, acne, alopecia, angioedema, urticaria, purpura, pruritus, exanthem
Endocrine & metabolic: Syndrome of inappropriate antidiuretic hormone, gynecomastia
Gastrointestinal: **Constipation, increased appetite, unpleasant taste, nausea, weight gain, xerostomia**, vomiting, craving sweets, bowel ischemia, lingua villosa nigra
Genitourinary: Urinary retention
Hematologic: Blood dyscrasias
Hepatic: Hepatitis
Neuromuscular & skeletal: **Weakness**, clonus, myoclonus, paresthesia
Ocular: Blurred vision, diplopia, photophobia, increased intraocular pressure, mydriasis
Otic: Ototoxicity, tinnitus
Respiratory: Pulmonary edema
Miscellaneous: Hypersensitivity reactions

Signs and Symptoms of Overdose Symptoms include severe hypotension, agitation, confusion, hypo-/hyperthermia, hypotension (severe), urinary retention, CNS depression, coma, cyanosis, dry mucous membranes, cardiac arrhythmias, seizures, changes in ECG (particularly in QRS axis and width), transient visual hallucinations, stupor, and muscle rigidity.

Admission Criteria/Prognosis Admit any patient who is symptomatic (including sinus tachycardia) 6 hours postingestion; admit any pediatric ingestion >5 mg/kg

Pharmacodynamics/Kinetics
Onset of action: 1-3 weeks; Maximum antidepressant effect: >2 weeks
Absorption: Well absorbed
Metabolism: Hepatic
Half-life elimination: Adults: 7-60 hours
Time to peak, plasma: 4-6 hours
Excretion: Urine (70%)

Dosage
Oral (not recommended for use in children <12 years):
Adolescents: Initial: 25-50 mg/day; gradually increase to 100 mg/day in single or divided doses; maximum: 150 mg/day
Adults: Initial: 75 mg/day in divided doses; increase gradually to 150-200 mg/day in divided or single dose; maximum: 300 mg/day

Monitoring Parameters Monitor blood pressure and pulse rate prior to and during initial therapy evaluate mental status; monitor weight; ECG in older adults and those patients with cardiac disease; blood levels are useful for therapeutic monitoring

Contraindications Hypersensitivity to desipramine, drugs of similar chemical class, or any component of the formulation; use of MAO inhibitors within 14 days; use in a patient during the acute recovery phase of MI; concurrent use of thioridazine

Warnings
[U.S. Boxed Warning]: Antidepressants increase the risk of suicidal thinking and behavior in children and adolescents with major depressive disorder (MDD) and other depressive disorders; consider risk prior to prescribing. Closely monitor for clinical worsening, suicidality, or unusual changes in behavior; the child's family or caregiver should be instructed to closely observe the patient and communicate condition with healthcare provider. Such observation would generally include at least weekly face-to-face contact with patients or their family members or caregivers during the first 4 weeks of treatment, then every other week visits for the next 4 weeks, then at 12 weeks, and as clinically indicated beyond 12 weeks. Additional contact by telephone may be appropriate between face-to-face visits. Adults treated with antidepressants should be observed similarly for clinical worsening and suicidality, especially during the initial few months of a course of drug therapy, or at times of dose changes, either increases or decreases. A medication guide should be dispensed with each prescription. **Desipramine is FDA approved for the treatment of depression in adolescents.**

The possibility of a suicide attempt is inherent in major depression and may persist until remission occurs. Monitor for worsening of depression or suicidality, especially during initiation of therapy or with dose increases or decreases. Worsening depression and severe abrupt suicidality that are not part of the presenting symptoms may require discontinuation or modification of drug therapy. Use caution in high-risk patients during initiation of therapy. Prescriptions should be written for the smallest quantity consistent with good patient care. The patient's family or caregiver should be alerted to monitor patients for the emergence of suicidality and associated behaviors such as anxiety, agitation, panic attacks, insomnia, irritability, hostility, impulsivity, akathisia, hypomania, and mania; patients should be instructed to notify their healthcare provider if any of these symptoms or worsening depression occur.

May worsen psychosis in some patients or precipitate a shift to mania or hypomania in patients with bipolar disorder. Monotherapy in patients with bipolar disorder should be avoided. Patients presenting with depressive symptoms should be screened for bipolar disorder. **Desipramine is not FDA approved for the treatment of bipolar depression.**

May cause sedation, resulting in impaired performance of tasks requiring alertness (eg, operating machinery or driving). Sedative effects may be additive with other CNS depressants and/or ethanol. The degree of sedation is low-moderate relative to other antidepressants. May cause hyponatremia/SIADH. May increase the risks associated with electro-convulsive therapy. Consider discontinuing, when possible, prior to elective surgery. Therapy should not be abruptly discontinued in patients receiving high doses for prolonged periods.

May cause orthostatic hypotension (risk is moderate relative to other antidepressants) - use with caution in patients at risk of hypotension or in patients where transient hypotensive episodes would be poorly tolerated (cardiovascular disease or cerebrovascular disease). The degree of anticholinergic blockade produced by this agent is low relative to other cyclic antidepressants - however, caution should be used in patients with urinary retention, benign prostatic hyperplasia, narrow-angle glaucoma, xerostomia, visual problems, constipation, or a history of bowel obstruction.

Use with caution in patients with a history of cardiovascular disease (including previous MI, stroke, tachycardia, or conduction abnormalities). The risk conduction abnormalities with this agent is moderate relative to other antidepressants. Use caution in patients with a previous seizure disorder or condition predisposing to seizures such as brain damage, alcoholism, or concurrent therapy with other drugs which lower the seizure threshold. Use with caution in hyperthyroid patients or those receiving thyroid supplementation. Use with caution in patients with hepatic or renal dysfunction and in elderly patients.

Dosage Forms Tablet, as hydrochloride: 10 mg, 25 mg, 50 mg, 75 mg, 100 mg, 150 mg

Reference Range
Therapeutic: 150-300 ng/mL (SI: 560-1125 nmol/L)
Possible toxicity: >300 ng/mL (SI: >1070 nmol/L)
Toxic: >1000 ng/mL (SI: >3750 nmol/L)
In the postmortem state, anatomical site concentration differences (ie, postmortem redistribution) may occur.

Overdosage/Treatment
Decontamination: Lavage (within 2-3 hours)/activated charcoal; multiple dosing of activated charcoal is more effective

Treatment is supportive and symptom-directed. Initiate gastric decontamination (emesis is contraindicated) and ECG monitoring immediately; monitor for a minimum of 6 hours. Sodium bicarbonate is indicated when the QRS interval is ≥ 0.10 seconds or the QT_c is >0.42 seconds. Ventricular arrhythmias and ECG changes (eg, QRS widening) often respond with concurrent systemic alkalinization (sodium bicarbonate 0.5-2 mEq/kg I.V.). Arrhythmias unresponsive to phenytoin 15-20 mg/kg (adults) may respond to lidocaine 1 mg/kg I.V. followed by a titrated infusion. Physostigmine (1-2 mg slow I.V. for adults or 0.5 mg slow I.V. for children) may be indicated in reversing life-threatening cardiac arrhythmias. Seizures usually respond to diazepam I.V. boluses (5-10 mg for adults up to 30 mg or 0.25-0.4 mg/kg/dose for children up to 10 mg/dose). If seizures are unresponsive or recur, phenytoin or phenobarbital may be required. Dialysis and diuresis have not been proven beneficial.

Antidote(s)
• Sodium Bicarbonate [ANTIDOTE]

Test Interactions ↑ glucose

Drug Interactions
Substrate of CYP1A2 (minor), 2D6 (major); **Inhibits** CYP2A6 (moderate), 2B6 (moderate), 2D6 (moderate), 2E1 (weak), 3A4 (moderate)

α- and β-agonists: When combined with TCAs, may predispose patients to cardiac arrhythmias; may also enhance vasopressor effects; consider alternate therapy.

Altretamine: Concurrent use may cause orthostatic hypertension.

Amphetamines: TCAs may enhance the effect of amphetamines; monitor for adverse CV effects.

Anticholinergics: Combined use with TCAs may produce additive anticholinergic effects.

Barbiturates: May decrease the levels/effects of TCAs; monitor.

Bupropion: May increase the levels of tricyclic antidepressants; based on limited information; monitor response.

Carbamazepine: Tricyclic antidepressants may increase carbamazepine levels; monitor.

Cholestyramine and colestipol: May bind TCAs and reduce their absorption; monitor for altered response.

Clonidine: Abrupt discontinuation of clonidine may cause hypertensive crisis; amitriptyline may enhance the response.

CNS depressants: Sedative effects may be additive with TCAs; monitor for increased effect; includes benzodiazepines, barbiturates, antipsychotics, ethanol, and other sedative medications.

CYP2A6 substrates: Desipramine may increase the levels/effects of CYP2A6 substrates. Example substrates include dexmedetomidine and ifosfamide.

CYP2B6 substrates: Desipramine may increase the levels/effects of CYP2B6 substrates. Example substrates include bupropion, cyclophosphamide, irinotecan, ketamine, promethazine, propofol, and selegiline.

CYP2D6 inhibitors: May increase the levels/effects of desipramine. Example inhibitors include chlorpromazine, delavirdine, fluoxetine, miconazole, paroxetine, pergolide, quinidine, quinine, ritonavir, and ropinirole.

CYP2D6 substrates: Desipramine may increase the levels/effects of CYP2D6 substrates. Example substrates include amphetamines, selected beta-blockers, dextromethorphan, fluoxetine, lidocaine, mirtazapine, nefazodone, paroxetine, risperidone, ritonavir, thioridazine, tricyclic antidepressants, and venlafaxine. Concurrent use with thioridazine is contraindicated.

CYP2D6 prodrug substrates: Desipramine may decrease the levels/effects of CYP2D6 prodrug substrates. Example prodrug substrates include codeine, hydrocodone, oxycodone, and tramadol.

CYP3A4 substrates: Desipramine may increase the levels/effects of CYP3A4 substrates. Example substrates include benzodiazepines, calcium channel blockers, cyclosporine, mirtazapine, nateglinide, nefazodone, sildenafil (and other PDE-5 inhibitors), tacrolimus, and venlafaxine. Selected benzodiazepines (midazolam and triazolam), cisapride, ergot alkaloids, selected HMG-CoA reductase inhibitors (lovastatin and simvastatin), and pimozide are generally contraindicated with strong CYP3A4 inhibitors.

Epinephrine (and other direct alpha-agonists): Pressor response to I.V. epinephrine, norepinephrine, and phenylephrine may be enhanced in patients receiving TCAs. (**Note:** Effect is unlikely with epinephrine or levonordefrin dosages typically administered as infiltration in combination with local anesthetics.)

False neurotransmitters (eg, guanadrel, methyldopa): TCAs may diminish the antihypertensive effects of false neurotransmitters.

Fenfluramine: May increase tricyclic antidepressant levels/effects.

Hypoglycemic agents (including insulin): TCAs may enhance the hypoglycemic effects of tolazamide, chlorpropamide, or insulin; monitor for changes in blood glucose levels; reported with chlorpropamide, tolazamide, and insulin.

Levodopa: Tricyclic antidepressants may decrease the absorption (bioavailability) of levodopa; rare hypertensive episodes have also been attributed to this combination.

Linezolid: Hyperpyrexia, hypertension, tachycardia, confusion, seizures, and **deaths have been reported** with agents which inhibit MAO (serotonin syndrome); this combination should be avoided.

Lithium: Concurrent use with a TCA may increase the risk for neurotoxicity.

MAO inhibitors: Hyperpyrexia, hypertension, tachycardia, confusion, seizures, and **deaths have been reported** (serotonin syndrome); this combination should be avoided.

Methylphenidate: Metabolism of TCAs may be decreased.

Phenothiazines: Serum concentrations of some TCAs may be increased; in addition, TCAs may increase concentration of phenothiazines; monitor for altered clinical response.

Pramlintide: May increase the anticholinergic effects of TCAs.

QT_c-prolonging agents: Concurrent use of tricyclic agents with other drugs which may prolong QT_c interval may increase the risk of potentially fatal arrhythmias; includes type Ia and type III antiarrhythmics agents, selected quinolones (sparfloxacin, gatifloxacin, moxifloxacin, grepafloxacin), cisapride, and other agents.

Ritonavir: Combined use of high-dose tricyclic antidepressants with ritonavir may cause serotonin syndrome in HIV-positive patients; monitor.

Serotonin modulators, SSRIs, sibutramine: Concomitant use may increase serotonergic effects; concurrent use with sibutramine is contraindicated.

Sympathomimetics, indirect-acting: Tricyclic antidepressants may result in a decreased sensitivity to indirect-acting sympathomimetics; includes dopamine and ephedrine; also see interaction with epinephrine (and direct-acting sympathomimetics).

Terbinafine: May increase the levels/effects of TCAs; monitor.

Tramadol: Tramadol's risk of seizures may be increased with TCAs.

Valproic acid: May increase serum concentrations/adverse effects of some tricyclic antidepressants.

Warfarin (and other oral anticoagulants): TCAs may increase the anticoagulant effect in patients stabilized on warfarin; monitor INR.

Pregnancy Risk Factor C

Lactation Enters breast milk/not recommended (AAP rates "of concern")

Nursing Implications Monitor blood pressure and pulse rate prior to and during initial therapy; may increase appetite

Additional Information May unmask pheochromocytoma; nitroglycerin administration decreased survival time in a rodent model

Specific References

Amitai Y and Frischer H, "Excess Fatality from Desipramine in Children and Adolescents," *Clin Toxicol*, 2005, 43:631.

Amitai Y and Frischer H, "Excess Fatality from Desipramine and Dosage Recommendations," *J Toxicol Clin Toxicol*, 2003, 41(5):714.

Murphy PM and Wermuth ME, "Prolonged and Recurrent Cardiotoxicity from Desipramine Ingestion," *J Toxicol Clin Toxicol*, 2004, 42(5):737.

Seger DL, Hantsch C, Zavoral T, et al, "Variability of Recommendations for Serum Alkalinization in Tricyclic Antidepressant Overdose: A Survey of U.S. Poison Center Medical Directors," *J Toxicol Clin Toxicol*, 2003, 41(4):331-8.

Deslanoside

CAS Number 17598-65-1

Use Rapid digitalizing effect in emergency treatment of congestive heart failure, paroxysmal atrial tachycardia, fibrillation (atrial) and flutter

Adverse Reactions

Cardiovascular: Sinus bradycardia, AV block, S-A block, ectopic beats (atrial or nodal), arrhythmias (ventricular), bigemiry, trigeminy, atrial tachycardia with AV block, sinus tachycardia, tachycardia (supraventricular)

Central nervous system: Drowsiness, fatigue, neuralgia, dizziness, disorientation, chorea (extrapyramidal), visual hallucinations, paranoia, headache, extrapyramidal reactions

Endocrine & metabolic: Toxicity is enhanced by hypokalemia

Gastrointestinal: Vomiting, nausea, feeding intolerance, abdominal pain, diarrhea

Ocular: Blurred vision, halos, yellow or green vision, diplopia, photophobia, flashing lights

Signs and Symptoms of Overdose Arrhythmias, AV block, fibrillation (ventricular) or asystole, hyperkalemia, hypokalemia, hypotension, neuropathy (peripheral), tachycardia (ventricular), vision color changes (blue tinge; green tinge; red tinge; yellow tinge)

Toxicodynamics/Kinetics Half-life: 33 hours

Dosage I.M., I.V.:

Children:

Neonates, premature and full-term: 22 mcg divided into 2-3 doses every 3-4 hours

2 weeks to 3 years: 25 mcg/kg divided into 2-3 doses every 3-4 hours

>3 years: 22.5 mcg/kg divided into 2-3 doses every 3-4 hours

Children and Adults: Highly individualized

Adults: Loading dose: 1.2-1.6 mg in 2 divided doses over 24 hours

Reference Range

Therapeutic: 0.5-2.0 ng/mL (SI: 0.6-2.6 nmol/L); Adults: <0.5 ng/mL (SI: <0.6 nmol/L) probably indicates underdigitalization unless there are special circumstances

Toxic: >2.0 ng/mL (SI: >2.6 nmol/L)

Fatal: >3.5 ng/mL (>4.8 nmol/L)

Overdosage/Treatment

Decontamination: Lavage (within 1 hour)/activated charcoal; whole bowel irrigation may be useful

Supportive therapy: Antidote: Life-threatening digoxin toxicity is treated with Digibind®; phenytoin, magnesium, and lidocaine are useful for arrhythmias; atropine is useful for bradycardia; avoid quinidine, bretylium, or cardioversion

Enhancement of elimination: Multiple dosing of activated charcoal may be useful; hemodialysis/hemoperfusion is ineffective

Diagnostic Procedures

• Digoxin, Blood

Test Interactions Digibind® increases total serum digoxin level ~50-fold; digoxin-like immunoreactive substance (DLIS), which is an endogenous natriuretic substance, may cause false elevation

Pregnancy Risk Factor C

Dexamethasone

Related Information

• Corticosteroids

CAS Number 1177-87-3; 2265-64-7; 2392-39-4; 312-93-6; 3936-02-5; 50-02-2

U.S. Brand Names Decadron® Phosphate [DSC]; Decadron®; Dexamethasone Intensol®; DexPak® TaperPak®; Maxidex®

Synonyms Dexamethasone Sodium Phosphate

Use Systemically and locally for chronic inflammation, allergic, hematologic, neoplastic, and autoimmune diseases; may be used in management of cerebral edema, as a diagnostic agent, antiemetic; to prevent

neurologic sequelae in children with bacterial meningitis due to *Haemophilus influenzae* type b infections; no longer recommended for septic shock; used for thrombocytopenia in AIDS; may reduce peripheral edema due to docetaxel

Unlabeled/Investigational Use Dexamethasone suppression test: General indicator consistent with depression and/or suicide

Mechanism of Action Decreases inflammation by suppression of migration of polymorphonuclear leukocytes and reversal of increased capillary permeability; suppresses normal immune response. Dexamethasone's mechanism of antiemetic activity is unknown.

Adverse Reactions

Cardiovascular: Edema, hypertension, premature ventricular contraction, sinus bradycardia, arrhythmias (ventricular), QT prolongation, cardiomegaly, cardiomyopathy

Central nervous system: Headache, mania, dizziness, seizures, psychosis, pseudotumor cerebri, **insomnia**, CNS depression, depression, **nervousness**

Dermatologic: Acne, dermatitis, skin atrophy, hypertrichosis, acute generalized exanthematous pustulosis

Endocrine & metabolic: Pituitary-adrenal axis suppression, growth suppression, hyperthyroidism, glucose intolerance, hypokalemia, alkalosis, Cushing's syndrome, hyperglycemia, hypoprolactinemia

Gastrointestinal: Peptic ulcer, nausea, vomiting, pancreatitis, fecal discoloration (dark brown), **increased appetite, indigestion**

Hematologic: Eosinopenia, leukocytosis, leukemoid reaction, thrombocytopenia, porphyria

Neuromuscular & skeletal: Myalgia, osteoporosis, fractures, rhabdomyolysis, weakness

Ocular: Cataracts, ptosis, photophobia, diplopia, increased intraocular pressure, glaucoma, blindness

Renal: Proteinuria

Miscellaneous: Hiccups

Pharmacodynamics/Kinetics

Onset of action: Acetate: Prompt

Duration of metabolic effect: 72 hours; acetate is a long-acting repository preparation

Metabolism: Hepatic

Half-life elimination: Normal renal function: 1.8-3.5 hours; Biological half-life: 36-54 hours

Time to peak, serum: Oral: 1-2 hours; I.M.: ~8 hours

Excretion: Urine and feces

Dosage

Children:

Antiemetic (prior to chemotherapy): I.V. (should be given as sodium phosphate): 5-20 mg given 15-30 minutes before treatment

Anti-inflammatory immunosuppressant: Oral, I.M., I.V. (injections should be given as sodium phosphate): 0.08-0.3 mg/kg/day **or** 2.5-10 mg/m²/day in divided doses every 6-12 hours

Extubation or airway edema: Oral, I.M., I.V. (injections should be given as sodium phosphate): 0.5-2 mg/kg/day in divided doses every 6 hours beginning 24 hours prior to extubation and continuing for 4-6 doses afterwards

Cerebral edema: I.V. (should be given as sodium phosphate): Loading dose: 1-2 mg/kg/dose as a single dose; maintenance: 1-1.5 mg/kg/day (maximum: 16 mg/day) in divided doses every 4-6 hours for 5 days then taper for 5 days, then discontinue

Bacterial meningitis in infants and children >2 months: I.V. (should be given as sodium phosphate): 0.6 mg/kg/day in 4 divided doses every 6 hours for the first 4 days of antibiotic treatment; start dexamethasone at the time of the first dose of antibiotic

Physiologic replacement: Oral, I.M., I.V.: 0.03-0.15 mg/kg/day **or** 0.6-0.75 mg/m²/day in divided doses every 6-12 hours

Adults:

Antiemetic:

Prophylaxis: Oral, I.V.: 10-20 mg 15-30 minutes before treatment on each treatment day

Continuous infusion regimen: Oral or I.V.: 10 mg every 12 hours on each treatment day

Mildly emetogenic therapy: Oral, I.M., I.V.: 4 mg every 4-6 hours

Delayed nausea/vomiting: Oral: 4-10 mg 1-2 times/day for 2-4 days **or**

8 mg every 12 hours for 2 days; then

4 mg every 12 hours for 2 days **or**

20 mg 1 hour before chemotherapy; then

10 mg 12 hours after chemotherapy; then

8 mg every 12 hours for 4 doses; then

4 mg every 12 hours for 4 doses

Anti-inflammatory:

Oral, I.M., I.V. (injections should be given as sodium phosphate): 0.75-9 mg/day in divided doses every 6-12 hours

I.M. (as acetate): 8-16 mg; may repeat in 1-3 weeks

Intralesional (as acetate): 0.8-1.6 mg

Intra-articular/soft tissue (as acetate): 4-16 mg; may repeat in 1-3 weeks

Intra-articular, intralesional, or soft tissue (as sodium phosphate): 0.4-6 mg/day

Ophthalmic:

Ointment: Apply thin coating into conjunctival sac 3-4 times/day; gradually taper dose to discontinue

Suspension: Instill 2 drops into conjunctival sac every hour during the day and every other hour during the night; gradually reduce dose to every 3-4 hours, then to 3-4 times/day

Topical: Apply 1-4 times/day. Therapy should be discontinued when control is achieved; if no improvement is seen, reassessment of diagnosis may be necessary.

Chemotherapy: Oral, I.V.: 40 mg every day for 4 days, repeated every 4 weeks (VAD regimen)

Cerebral edema: I.V. 10 mg stat, 4 mg I.M./I.V. (should be given as sodium phosphate) every 6 hours until response is maximized, then switch to oral regimen, then taper off if appropriate; dosage may be reduced after 24 days and gradually discontinued over 5-7 days

Dexamethasone suppression test (depression indicator) or diagnosis for Cushing's syndrome (unlabeled uses): Oral: 1 mg at 11 PM, draw blood at 8 AM the following day for plasma cortisol determination

Physiological replacement: Oral, I.M., I.V. (should be given as sodium phosphate): 0.03-0.15 mg/kg/day **or** 0.6-0.75 mg/m^2/day in divided doses every 6-12 hours

Treatment of shock:

Addisonian crisis/shock (ie, adrenal insufficiency/responsive to steroid therapy): I.V. (given as sodium phosphate): 4-10 mg as a single dose, which may be repeated if necessary

Unresponsive shock (ie, unresponsive to steroid therapy): I.V. (given as sodium phosphate): 1-6 mg/kg as a single I.V. dose or up to 40 mg initially followed by repeat doses every 2-6 hours while shock persists

Hemodialysis: Supplemental dose is not necessary

Peritoneal dialysis: Supplemental dose is not necessary

Stability Injection solution: Store at room temperature; protect from light and freezing

Stability of injection of parenteral admixture at room temperature (25°C): 24 hours

Stability of injection of parenteral admixture at refrigeration temperature (4°C): 2 days; protect from light and freezing

Injection should be diluted in 50-100 mL NS or D$_5$W.

Monitoring Parameters Hemoglobin, occult blood loss, serum potassium, and glucose

Administration

Oral: Administer with meals to decrease GI upset.

I.M.: Acetate injection is **not** for I.V. use.

I.V.: Administer as a 5-10 minute bolus; rapid injection is associated with a high incidence of perianal discomfort.

Topical: For external use. Do not use on open wounds. Apply sparingly to occlusive dressings. Should not be used in the presence of open or weeping lesions.

Contraindications Hypersensitivity to dexamethasone or any component of the formulation; systemic fungal infections, cerebral malaria; ophthalmic use in viral (active ocular herpes simplex), fungal, or tuberculosis diseases of the eye

Warnings

Use with caution in patients with hypothyroidism, cirrhosis, hypertension, CHF, or thromboembolic disorders. Corticosteroids should be used with caution in patients with diabetes, glaucoma, cataracts, or tuberculosis; or patients at risk for osteoporosis. Use caution with GI diseases (diverticulitis, peptic ulcer, ulcerative colitis) due to perforation risk. Use caution following acute MI (corticosteroids have been associated with myocardial rupture). Use caution in renal and hepatic impairment. Because of the risk of adverse effects, systemic corticosteroids should be used cautiously in the elderly in the smallest possible effective dose for the shortest duration.

May cause suppression of hypothalamic-pituitary-adrenal (HPA) axis, particularly in younger children or in patients receiving high doses for prolonged periods. Symptoms of adrenocortical insufficiency in suppressed patients may result from rapid discontinuation/withdrawal; deficits in HPA response may persist for months following discontinuation and require supplementation during metabolic stress. Patients receiving ≥20 mg/day of prednisone (or equivalent) may be most susceptible. Particular care is required when patients are transferred from systemic corticosteroids to inhaled products due to possible adrenal insufficiency or exacerbation of underlying disease (an increase in allergic symptoms). Fatalities have occurred due to adrenal insufficiency in asthmatic patients during and after transfer from systemic corticosteroids to aerosol steroids; aerosol steroids do **not** provide the systemic steroid needed to treat patients having trauma, surgery, or infections. Dexamethasone does not provide adequate mineralocorticoid activity in adrenal insufficiency (may be employed as a single dose while cortisol assays are performed). The lowest possible dose should be used during treatment; discontinuation and/or dose reductions should be gradual.

Controlled clinical studies have shown that orally-inhaled and intranasal corticosteroids may cause a reduction in growth velocity in pediatric patients. (In studies of orally-inhaled corticosteroids, the mean reduction in growth velocity was ~1 cm per year [range 0.3-1.8 cm per year] and appears to be related to dose and duration of exposure). The growth of pediatric patients receiving inhaled corticosteroids, should be monitored routinely (eg, via stadiometry). To minimize the systemic effects of orally-inhaled and intranasal corticosteroids, each patient should be titrated to the lowest effective dose.

Acute myopathy has been reported with high dose corticosteroids, usually with use for neuromuscular transmission disorders; may involve ocular and/or respiratory muscles; monitor creatine kinase; recovery may be delayed. Corticosteroid use may cause psychiatric manifestations, including depression, euphoria, insomnia, mood swings, and personality changes. Pre-existing psychiatric conditions may be exacerbated by corticosteroid use.

May suppress the immune system; patients may be more susceptible to infection; use with caution in patients with systemic infections. Avoid exposure to chickenpox and measles.

Dosage Forms

[DSC] = Discontinued product

Elixir, as base: 0.5 mg/5 mL (240 mL)

Injection, solution, as sodium phosphate: 4 mg/mL (1 mL, 5 mL, 30 mL); 10 mg/mL (10 mL)

Injection, solution, as sodium phosphate [preservative free]: 10 mg/mL (1 mL)

Solution, ophthalmic, as sodium phosphate: 0.1% (5 mL)

Solution, oral: 0.5 mg/5 mL (500 mL)

Solution, oral concentrate:

Dexamethasone Intensol™: 1 mg/mL (30 mL) [contains alcohol 30%]

Suspension, ophthalmic:

Maxidex®: 0.1% (5 mL; 15 mL [DSC]) [contains benzalkonium chloride]

Tablet [scored]: 0.5 mg, 0.75 mg, 1 mg, 1.5 mg, 2 mg, 4 mg, 6 mg

DexPak® TaperPak®: 1.5 mg [51 tablets on taper dose card]

Reference Range Dexamethasone suppression test, overnight: 8 AM cortisol <6 mcg/100 mL (dexamethasone 1 mg)

Overdosage/Treatment

Decontamination: Emesis within 30 minutes or lavage (within 1 hour)/ activated charcoal; acute overdose does not require tapering of dose

Supportive therapy: Hiccups can be treated with metoclopramide (10 mg every 6 hours)

Test Interactions May result in false elevation of digoxin level (by RIA); >0.5 mg/day may interfere with TSH assay resulting in falsely low TSH levels

Drug Interactions

Substrate of CYP3A4 (minor); **Induces** CYP2A6 (weak), 2B6 (weak), 2C8 (weak), 2C9 (weak), 3A4 (weak)

Aminoglutethimide: May reduce the serum levels/effects of dexamethasone; likely via induction of microsomal isoenzymes.

Antacids: May increase the absorption of corticosteroids; separate administration by 2 hours.

Anticholinesterases: Concurrent use may lead to severe weakness in patients with myasthenia gravis.

Aprepitant: May increase the serum levels of corticosteroids; monitor.

Azole antifungals: May increase the serum levels of corticosteroids; monitor.

Barbiturates: May decrease the levels/effects of dexamethasone (systemic).

Bile acid sequestrants: May reduce the absorption of corticosteroids; separate administration by 2 hours.

Calcium channel blockers (nondihydropyridine): May increase the serum levels of corticosteroids; monitor.

Cyclosporine: Corticosteroids may increase the serum levels of cyclosporine. In addition, cyclosporine may increase levels of corticosteroids.

Estrogens: May increase the serum levels of corticosteroids; monitor.

Fluoroquinolones: Concurrent use may increase the risk of tendon rupture, particularly in elderly patients (overall incidence rare).

Isoniazid: Serum concentrations may be decreased by corticosteroids.

Macrolide antibiotics: May increase the levels/effects of dexamethasone (systemic).

Neuromuscular-blocking agents: Concurrent use with corticosteroids may increase the risk of myopathy.

Nonsteroidal anti-inflammatory drugs (NSAIDs): Concurrent use with corticosteroids may lead to an increased incidence of gastrointestinal adverse effects; use caution. NSAID (ophthalmic) may enhance the adverse/toxic effect of dexamethasone (ophthalmic).

Primidone: May decrease the levels/effects of dexamethasone (systemic); monitor.

Rifamycins: May decrease the levels/effects of dexamethasone (systemic); monitor.

Salicylates: Salicylates may increase the gastrointestinal adverse effects of corticosteroids.

Thalidomide: Concurrent use with corticosteroids may increase the risk of selected adverse effects (toxic epidermal necrolysis and DVT); use caution.

Vaccine (dead organism): Dexamethasone may decrease the effect of vaccines (dead organisms). In patients receiving high doses of systemic corticosteroids for ≥ 14 days, wait at least 1 month between discontinuing steroid therapy and administering immunization.

Vaccine (live organism): Dexamethasone may increase the risk of vaccinal infection. The use of live vaccines is contraindicated in immunosuppressed patients.

Pregnancy Risk Factor C

Pregnancy Implications Teratogenic effects have been observed in animal studies. Dexamethasone has been used in patients with premature labor (26-34 weeks gestation) to stimulate fetal lung maturation. Crosses the placenta; transient leukocytosis reported. Available evidence suggests safe use during pregnancy.

Lactation Enters breast milk/use caution

Nursing Implications Give oral formulation with meals to decrease gastritis; topical formation is for external use, do not use on open wounds; apply sparingly to occlusive dressings; should not be used in the presence of open or weeping lesions; **acetate injection is not for I.V. use**

Additional Information Not suitable for every-other-day dosing due to long duration of effect. Intravenous dexamethasone (2 mg I.V.) can impair ethyl alcohol's ability to stimulate sympathetic nerve discharge, and thus suppress alcohol-induced high blood pressure in the acute state. Nebulization of dexamethasone sodium phosphate (1.5 mg/kg up to 45 mg) may be as effective as oral prednisone in the emergency management of moderately severe asthma in children. Granisetron (3 mg I.V.) is effective when used with dexamethasone to prevent emesis due to chemotherapy.

Specific References

Bulloch B, Kabani A, and Tenenbein M, "Oral Dexamethasone for the Treatment of Pain in Children with Acute Pharyngitis: A Randomized, Double-Blind, Placebo-Controlled Trial," *Ann Emerg Med*, 2003, 41(5):601-8.

Cheng Y, Wong RS, Soo YO, et al, "Initial Treatment of Immune Thrombocytopenic Purpura with High-Dose Dexamethasone," *N Engl J Med*, 2003, 349(9):831-6.

Donaldson D, Poleski D, Knipple E, et al, "Intramuscular Versus Oral Dexamethasone for the Treatment of Moderate-to-Severe Croup: A Randomized, Double-blind Trial," *Acad Emerg Med*, 2003, 10(1):16-21.

Mitchell JC and Counselman FL, "A Taste Comparison of Three Different Liquid Steroid Preparations: Prednisone, Prednisolone, and Dexamethasone," *Acad Emerg Med*, 2003, 10(4):400-3.

Naumovski J, Bozinovska C, Kovkarova E, et al, "Single-Dose Dexamethasone-Induced Adrenocortical Suppression in an Intentional Self-Poisoning - Case Report," *J Toxicol Clin Toxicol*, 2003, 41(6):895.

Ng KH, "Chemotherapy-Induced Delayed Emesis: What Is the Role of 5-HT$_3$ Antagonists?" *J Pharm Technol*, 2003, 19:287-97.

Richardson PG, Sonneveld P, Schuster MW, et al, "Bortezomib or High-Dose Dexamethasone for Relapsed Multiple Myeloma," *N Engl J Med*, 2005, 16;352(24):2487-98.

Roy M, Bailey B, Amre DK, et al, "Dexamethasone for the Treatment of Sore Throat in Children with Suspected Infectious Mononucleosis: A Randomized, Double-Blind, Placebo-Controlled, Clinical Trial," *Arch Pediatr Adolesc Med*, 2004, 158(3):250-4.

Dexfenfluramine

CAS Number 3239-44-9; 3239-45-0

Synonyms Dexfenfluramine Hydrochloride; S5614

Use Management of obesity (initial body mass >30 kg/m^3 or >27 kg/m^3 with other risk factors such as hypertension, diabetes, or hyperlipidemia); given as an adjunct to dietary restriction; off the U.S. market as of September 15, 1997

Mechanism of Action Can cause elevation of serotonin in the brain which suppresses appetite for carbohydrates (but not protein-rich foods)

Adverse Reactions

Cardiovascular: Hypotension, primary pulmonary hypertension (18 cases per 1 million users per year), leukocytoclastic vasculitis

Central nervous system: Fatigue, **drowsiness**, **headache**, dizziness, **insomnia**, anxiety, depression (reactive), dysphoria, mania

Dermatologic: Urticaria, scleroderma

Endocrine & metabolic: Hyperprolactinemia

Gastrointestinal: **Abdominal discomfort, xerostomia,** nausea, vomiting, **diarrhea**

Hematologic: Porphyrinogenic

Neuromuscular & skeletal: **Weakness**

Renal: Polyuria

Pharmacodynamics/Kinetics

Peak serum levels: 2-4 hours

Metabolism: Hepatic to d-norfenfluramine (active metabolite)

Half-life:

18 hours (dexfenfluramine)

30 hours (d-norfenfluramine)

Dosage 15 mg 2 times/day with meals

Monitoring Parameters Monitor weight, eating habits, cardiopulmonary function including cardiac insufficiency, palpitations, exertional dyspnea, and/or chest pain; blood should also be monitored

Contraindications Hypersensitivity to dexfenfluramine or fenfluramine, glaucoma, pulmonary hypertension or use of monoamine oxidase inhibitors within 2 weeks of dexfenfluramine; children, pregnancy, or nursing women

Warnings Use with caution in patients with cardiac disease, renal or hepatic insufficiency, prophyria, drug abuse, psychiatric disorder, or organic causes for obesity

Dosage Forms Capsule, as hydrochloride: 15 mg

Reference Range After a 20 mg oral dose, peak serum level: ~16 mcg/L; peak serum metabolite d-norfenfluramine is 6 mcg/L

Overdosage/Treatment

Decontamination: **Do not** induce emesis; lavage (within 4 hours)/ activated charcoal

Supportive therapy: Treat hypotension with I.V. crystalloid solutions; vasopressors can be used for refractory cases; propranolol (1 mg/dose in adults or 0.01-0.1 mg/kg/dose in children over 10 minutes) or esmolol can be used to treat tachycardia; hyperpyrexia can be treated with external (passive) cooling

Test Interactions Can result in a positive urinary immunoassay for amphetamines, but will not confirm by gas chromatography/mass spectrometry

Drug Interactions Increased toxicity: Serotonin reuptake inhibitors and monoamine oxidase inhibitors may cause rigidity, hyperthermia, tremor, seizures, and delirium

Pregnancy Risk Factor C

Pregnancy Implications Spontaneous abortions in 1st trimester have been described

Additional Information On September 12, 1997, the FDA announced new summary information concerning abnormal echocardiogram findings in asymptomatic patients seen in five centers. These patients had been treated with fenfluramine or dexfenfluramine for up to 24 months, most often in combination with phentermine. Abnormal echocardiogram findings were reported in 92 of 291 subjects evaluated, including 80 reports of aortic regurgitation (mild or greater) and 23 reports of mitral regurgitation (moderate or greater). Those requiring further information can call 1-800-892-2718. Questions about returning products can be directed to 1-800-666-7248.

Specific References

Bryant SM, Lozada C, and Wahl M, "A Chinese Herbal Weight Loss Product Adulterated with Fenfluramine," *Ann Emerg Med*, 2005, 46(2):208.

Dextroamphetamine

Related Information

- Diethylpropion
- Fenproporex
- Phenmetrazine
- Therapeutic Drugs Associated with Hallucinations

CAS Number 51-63-8; 51-64-9; 7528-00-9

U.S. Brand Names Dexedrine®; Dextrostat®

Synonyms Dextroamphetamine Sulfate

Impairment Potential Yes

Use Narcolepsy; attention-deficit/hyperactivity disorder (ADHD)

Unlabeled/Investigational Use Exogenous obesity; depression; abnormal behavioral syndrome in children (minimal brain dysfunction)

Mechanism of Action Blocks reuptake of dopamine and norepinephrine from the synapse, thus increases the amount of circulating dopamine and norepinephrine in cerebral cortex to reticular activating system; inhibits the action of monoamine oxidase and causes catecholamines to be released

Adverse Reactions

Cardiovascular: Hypertension, tachycardia (ventricular), tachycardia, palpitations, **cardiac arrhythmias**, vasculitis, sinus tachycardia, tachycardia (supraventricular), arrhythmias (ventricular)

Central nervous system: **Insomnia**, headache, **nervousness**, dizziness, seizures, mania, may precipitate Tourette's syndrome, CNS depression, dysphonia, irritability, agitation, euphoria, hallucination, extrapyramidal reaction, movement disorders, depression, paranoia, sympathetic storm, fever, hyperthermia, **restlessness, false feeling of well being**

Dermatologic: Urticaria

Endocrine & metabolic: Growth suppression, respiratory alkalosis, increased serum thyroxine (hyperthyroidism)

Gastrointestinal: Anorexia, nausea, vomiting, diarrhea, abdominal cramps, metallic taste, xerostomia, bitter dysgeusia

Genitourinary: Impotence

Hematologic: Porphyria, porphyrinogenic

Neuromuscular & skeletal: Tremors, choreoathetoid movements, fasciculations, rhabdomyolysis

Renal: Myoglobinuria

Respiratory: Tachypnea

Pharmacodynamics/Kinetics

Onset of action: 1-1.5 hours

Distribution: V_d: Adults: 3.5-4.6 L/kg; distributes into CNS; mean CSF concentrations are 80% of plasma; enters breast milk

Metabolism: Hepatic via CYP monooxygenase and glucuronidation

Half-life elimination: Adults: 10-13 hours

Time to peak, serum: T_{max}: Immediate release: 3 hours; sustained release: 8 hours

Excretion: Urine (as unchanged drug and inactive metabolites)

Dosage

Oral:

Children:

Narcolepsy: 6-12 years: Initial: 5 mg/day; may increase at 5 mg increments in weekly intervals until side effects appear (maximum dose: 60 mg/day)

Attention-deficit/hyperactivity disorder (ADHD):

3-5 years: Initial: 2.5 mg/day given every morning; increase by 2.5 mg/day in weekly intervals until optimal response is obtained; usual range: 0.1-0.5 mg/kg/dose every morning with maximum of 40 mg/day

≥6 years: 5 mg once or twice daily; increase in increments of 5 mg/day at weekly intervals until optimal response is obtained; usual range: 0.1-0.5 mg/kg/dose every morning (5-20 mg/day) with maximum of 40 mg/day

Children >12 years and Adults:

Narcolepsy: Initial: 10 mg/day, may increase at 10 mg increments in weekly intervals until side effects appear; maximum: 60 mg/day

Exogenous obesity (unlabeled use): 5-30 mg/day in divided doses of 5-10 mg 30-60 minutes before meals

Stability Protect from light

Monitoring Parameters Growth in children and CNS activity in all

Administration

Do not crush sustained release drug product. Administer as single dose in morning or as divided doses with breakfast and lunch. Should be administered 30 minutes before meals and at least 6 hours before bedtime.

Contraindications Hypersensitivity or idiosyncrasy to dextroamphetamine or other sympathomimetic amines. Patients with advanced arteriosclerosis, symptomatic cardiovascular disease, moderate to severe hypertension (stage II or III), hyperthyroidism, glaucoma, agitated states, patients with a history of drug abuse, and during or within 14 days following MAO inhibitor therapy.

Warnings

[U.S. Boxed Warning]: **Dexamphetamine has been associated with serious cardiac cardiovascular events including sudden death in patients with pre-existing structural cardiac abnormalities or other serious heart problems.** Using CNS stimulant treatment at usual doses in children and adolescents with serious heart problems and structural cardiac abnormalities has been associated with sudden death. In adults, stimulant use has been associated with sudden deaths, stroke, and myocardial infarction. Stimulant products should be avoided in the patients with known serious structural cardiac abnormalities, cardiomyopathy, serious heart rhythm abnormalities, or other serious cardiac problems that could increase the risk of sudden death that these conditions alone carry. Caution should be used in patients with hypertension and other cardiovascular conditions that might be exacerbated by increases in blood pressure or heart rate. Use of stimulants can cause an increase in blood pressure (average 2-4 mm Hg) and increases in heart rate (average 3-6 bpm), although some patients may have larger than average increases.

Use with caution in patients with bipolar disorder, cardiovascular disease, diabetes, seizure disorders, insomnia, porphyria, hypertension (stage I), or history of substance abuse. May exacerbate symptoms of behavior and thought disorder in psychotic patients. Stimulants may unmask tics in individuals with coexisting Tourette's syndrome. Potential for drug dependency exists - avoid abrupt discontinuation in patients who have received for prolonged periods. [U.S. Boxed Warning]: **Use in weight reduction programs only when alternative therapy has been ineffective; due to high potential for abuse and/or nontherapeutic use should be prescribed/dispensed sparingly.** Products may contain tartrazine - use with caution in potentially sensitive individuals. Stimulant use in children has been associated with growth suppression. May cause visual disturbances.

Dosage Forms Capsule, sustained release, as sulfate: 5 mg, 10 mg, 15 mg

Dexedrine® Spansule®: 5 mg, 10 mg, 15 mg

Tablet, as sulfate: 5 mg, 10 mg

Dexedrine®: 5 mg [contains tartrazine]

Dextrostat®: 5 mg, 10 mg [contains tartrazine]

Reference Range Urinary amphetamine concentrations at steady state (30 mg/day) range from 1100-17,800 ng/mL

Overdosage/Treatment

Decontamination: Lavage (within 1 hour)/activated charcoal

Supportive therapy: Seizures can be treated with lorazepam, diazepam, phenytoin, or phenobarbital; ventricular arrhythmias should be treated with lidocaine

Enhancement of elimination: Hemodialysis may be useful; do not acidify urine

Test Interactions False-positive amphetamine assays may result from coadministration with ranitidine, phenylpropanolamine, brompheniramine, chlorpromazine, fluspiriline, or pipothiazine

Drug Interactions Substrate of CYP2D6 (major)

Acidifiers: Very large doses of potassium acid phosphate or ammonium chloride may increase the renal elimination of amphetamines due to urinary acidification, resulting in lower blood level and efficacy of amphetamines.

Alkalinizers: Large doses of sodium bicarbonate or other alkalinizers may increase renal tubular reabsorption (decreased elimination) and enhance the effect of amphetamine; includes potassium or sodium citrate and acetate.

Antipsychotics: Efficacy of amphetamines may be decreased by antipsychotics; in addition, amphetamines may induce an increase in psychotic symptoms in some patients.

CYP2D6 inhibitors: May increase the levels/effects of dextroamphetamine. Example inhibitors include chlorpromazine, delavirdine, fluoxetine, miconazole, paroxetine, pergolide, quinidine, quinine, ritonavir, and ropinirole.

Furazolidone: Amphetamines may induce hypertensive episodes in patients receiving furazolidone.

Guanethidine: Amphetamines inhibit the antihypertensive response to guanethidine; probably also may occur with guanadrel and other antihypertensives.

MAO inhibitors: Severe hypertensive episodes have occurred with amphetamine when used in patients receiving MAO inhibitors; concurrent use or use within 14 days is contraindicated.

Norepinephrine: Amphetamines enhance the pressor response to norepinephrine.

Sibutramine: Concurrent use of sibutramine and amphetamines may cause severe hypertension and tachycardia; use is contraindicated with SSRIs; amphetamines may increase the potential for serotonin syndrome when used concurrently with selective serotonin reuptake inhibitors (including fluoxetine, fluvoxamine, paroxetine, and sertraline).

Tricyclic antidepressants: Concurrent of amphetamines with TCAs may result in hypertension and CNS stimulation; avoid this combination.

Pregnancy Risk Factor C

Pregnancy Implications A case of bone deformity, tracheoesophageal fistula, and anal atresia has been noted in a fetus after first trimester use of lovastatin and dextroamphetamine.

Lactation Enters breast milk/contraindicated

Nursing Implications Last daily dose should be given 6 hours before retiring; do not crush sustained release drug product; dose should not be given in evening or at bedtime

Additional Information Illicit preparation may contain up to 24 g per spoon; 5 mg tablets contain tartrazine

Specific References

Klette KL, Kettle AR, and Jamerson MH, "Prevalence of Use Study for Amphetamine (AMP), Methamphetamine (MAMP), 3,4-Methylenedioxy-amphetamine (MDA), 3,4-Methylenedioxy-methamphetamine (MDMA), and 3,4-Methylenedioxy-ethylamphetamine (MDEA) in Military Entrance Processing Stations (MEPS) Specimens," *J Anal Toxicol*, 2006, 30:319-22.

Valtier S, McHugh KM and Cody JT, "Amphetamine Excretion Following Tablet and Gel Formulations of Dexedrine," *J Anal Toxicol*, 2006, 30:145.

Dextromethorphan

Related Information

● Therapeutic Drugs Associated with Hallucinations

CAS Number 125-69-9; 125-71-3; 6700-34-1

U.S. Brand Names Babee® Cof Syrup [OTC]; Benylin® Adult [OTC]; Benylin® Pediatric [OTC]; Creo-Terpin® [OTC]; Creomulsion® Cough [OTC]; Creomulsion® for Children [OTC]; Delsym® [OTC]; Dexalone® [OTC]; ElixSure™ Cough [OTC]; Hold® DM [OTC]; Pertussin® DM [OTC]; Robitussin® CoughGels™[OTC]; Robitussin® Honey Cough; Robitussin® Maximum Strength Cough [OTC]; Robitussin® Pediatric Cough [OTC]; Scot-Tussin DM® Cough Chasers [OTC]; Silphen DM® [OTC]; Simply Cough™ [OTC]; Vicks® 44® Cough Relief [OTC]

Impairment Potential Yes

Use Symptomatic relief of coughs caused by minor viral upper respiratory tract infections or inhaled irritants; most effective for a chronic nonproductive cough

Unlabeled/Investigational Use *N*-methyl-D-aspartate (NMDA) antagonist in cerebral injury

Mechanism of Action Chemical relative of morphine lacking narcotic properties; controls cough by depressing the medullary cough center; has virtually no analgesic activity; acts through the sigma receptor with little dependence effect

Adverse Reactions

Cardiovascular: Sinus tachycardia

Central nervous system: Drowsiness, dizziness, coma, auditory and visual hallucinations, insomnia, dystonia

Gastrointestinal: Nausea

Respiratory: Apnea, respiratory depression

Miscellaneous: Fixed drug eruption

Signs and Symptoms of Overdose Ataxia, coma, dystonic reaction, excitation, fever, hyperactivity, hypertension, hyperthermia, insomnia, miosis, respiratory depression, tachycardia, tremors

Pharmacodynamics/Kinetics

Onset of action: Antitussive: 15-30 minutes

Duration: ≤6 hours

Metabolism: In the liver to an active metabolite (dextrophan)

Half-life: 2-4 hours

Time to peak: 2.5 hours

Elimination: Principally in urine

Dosage

Oral:

Children:

2-5 years: 2.5-7.5 mg every 4-8 hours; extended release is 15 mg twice daily (maximum: 30 mg/24 hours)

6-12 years: 5-10 mg every 4 hours or 15 mg every 6-8 hours; extended release is 30 mg twice daily (maximum: 60 mg/24 hours)

Children >12 years and Adults: 10-30 mg every 4-8 hours or 30 mg every 6-8 hours; extended release is 60 mg twice daily (maximum: 120 mg/24 hours)

Contraindications Hypersensitivity to dextromethorphan or any component of the formulation

Dosage Forms

[DSC] = Discontinued product

Gelcap, as hydrobromide:

Dexalone®: 30 mg

Robitussin® CoughGels™: 15 mg [contains coconut oil]

Liquid, as hydrobromide:

Creo-Terpin®: 10 mg/15 mL (120 mL) [contains alcohol 25% and tartrazine]

Simply Cough®: 5 mg/5 mL (120 mL) [contains sodium benzoate; cherry berry flavor]

Vicks® 44® Cough Relief: 10 mg/5 mL (120 mL) [contains alcohol, sodium 10 mg/5 mL, sodium benzoate]

Liquid, oral, as hydrobromide [freezer pops] (PediaCare® Children's Medicated Freezer Pops Long Acting Cough): 7.5 mg/25 mL (8s) [alcohol free; contains sodium benzoate, berry flavor also contains benzyl alcohol; glacier grape™ and polar berry blue™ flavors]

Liquid, oral drops, as hydrobromide (PediaCare® Infants' Long-Acting Cough): 7.5 mg/0.8 mL (15 mL) [alcohol free, dye free; contains sodium benzoate; grape flavor]

Lozenge, as hydrobromide:

Hold® DM: 5 mg (10s) [cherry or original flavor]

Scot-Tussin DM® Cough Chasers: 5 mg (20s)

Strips, oral, as hydrobromide (Triaminic® Thin Strips™ Long Acting Cough): 7.5 mg [equivalent to dextromethorphan 5 mg; cherry flavor]

Suspension, extended release, as hydrobromide (Delsym®): 30 mg/5 mL (89 mL, 148 mL) [contains alcohol 0.26%, sodium 5 mg/5 mL; orange flavor]

Syrup, as hydrobromide:

Babee® Cof Syrup: 7.5 mg/5 mL (120 mL) [alcohol free, dye free; cherry flavor]

Benylin® Adult: 15 mg/5 mL (120 mL) [alcohol free, sugar free; contains sodium benzoate; raspberry flavor] [DSC]

Benylin® Pediatric: 7.5 mg/mL (120 mL) [alcohol free, sugar free; contains sodium benzoate; grape flavor] [DSC]

Creomulsion® Cough: 20 mg/15 mL (120 mL) [alcohol free; contains sodium benzoate]

Creomulsion® for Children: 5 mg/5 mL (120 mL) [alcohol free; contains sodium benzoate; cherry flavor]

ElixSure™ Cough: 7.5 mg/5 mL (120 mL) [cherry bubble gum flavor]

Robitussin® Honey Cough: 10 mg/5 mL (120 mL) [alcohol free; contains sodium benzoate]

Robitussin® Maximum Strength Cough: 15 mg/5 mL (120 mL, 240 mL) [contains alcohol, sodium benzoate]

Robitussin® Pediatric Cough: 7.5 mg/5 mL (120 mL) [alcohol free; contains sodium benzoate; fruit punch flavor]

Silphen DM®: 10 mg/5 mL (120 mL) [strawberry flavor]

Reference Range Serum level of 0.1 mcg/mL associated with coma

Overdosage/Treatment

Decontamination: Lavage (within 1 hour) is recommended for ingestions >10 mg/kg; activated charcoal is useful

Supportive therapy: Naloxone hydrochloride (0.4-2 mg I.V., SubQ, or through an endotracheal tube); a continuous infusion (at $^2/_3$ the response dose/hour) may be required; dystonic reactions can be treated with diphenhydramine (1 mg/kg up to 50 mg)

Antidote(s)

- Naloxone [ANTIDOTE]

Test Interactions Can result in a false-positive phencyclidine qualitative immunoassay screen

Drug Interactions Substrate of CYP2B6 (minor), 2C9 (minor), 2C19 (minor), 2D6 (major), 2E1 (minor), 3A4 (minor); **Inhibits** CYP2D6 (weak)

CYP2D6 inhibitors: May increase the levels/effects of dextromethorphan. Example inhibitors include chlorpromazine, delavirdine, fluoxetine, miconazole, paroxetine, pergolide, quinidine, quinine, ritonavir, and ropinirole.

MAO inhibitors: Dextromethorphan may increase effect/toxicity of MAO inhibitors.

Pregnancy Risk Factor C

Pregnancy Implications Dextromethorphan is teratogenic in chick embryos (neural crest/neural tube defects)

Nursing Implications Raise side rails, institute safety measures

Additional Information

Monitor for bromide poisoning.

According to the Drug Abuse Warning Network for 2004 (Dawn Report: Issue 32, 2006)

- An Estimated 12,584 Emergency Department visits involved pharmaceuticals containing dextromethorphan (DXM) which represented about 0.7% of all drug related ED visits.

- The rate of ED visits resulting from nonmedicinal use of DXM for those aged 12 to 20 years was 7.1 visits per 100,000 population compared with 2.6 visits or fewer per 100,000 for other age groups.

- ED patients aged 12 to 20 years accounted for nearly half (48%) of all the ED visits resulting from nonmedicinal use of DXM.

- Alcohol was implicated in over one third (36%) of ED visits involving nonmedicinal use of DXM for those aged 18 to 20 years and in 13% of visit for those age 12 to 17 years.

Specific References

Baker SD and Borys DJ, "A Possible Trend Suggesting Increased Abuse from Coricidin® Exposures Reported to the Texas Poison Network: Comparing 1998 to 1999," *Vet Hum Toxicol*, 2002, 44(3):169-71.

Betschart T, Rauber-Lüthy CH, Guirguis M, et al, "Dose Dependent Toxicity of Dextromethorphan Overdose," *J Toxicol Clin Toxicol*, 2000, 38(2):190.

Boland DM, Rein J, Lew EO, et al, "Fatal Cold Medication Intoxication in an Infant," *J Anal Toxicol*, 2004, 28:293.

Boyer EW, Mazzola J, and Hibberd PL, "Coricidin Abuse in Adolescent Females," *J Toxicol Clin Toxicol*, 2004, 42(5):761.

Budai B and Iskandar H, "Dextromethorphan Can Produce False Positive Phencyclidine Testing with HPLC," *Am J Emerg Med*, 2002, 20(1):61-2.

Burns MM and Law T, "Over-the-Counter Cough and Cold Preparations: At What Concentration Do They Produce a Positive Urine Toxicologic Screen?" *Acad Emerg Med*, 2001, 8(5):442.

Cochems A, Harding P, Johnson W, et al, "Dextromethorphan Concentrations in Wisconsin Drivers," *J Anal Toxicol*, 2006, 30:150.

Kirages TJ, Sule HP, and Mycyk MB, "Severe Manifestations of Coricidin Intoxication," *Am J Emerg Med*, 2003, 21(6):473-5.

Konrad D, Sobetzko D, Schmitt B, et al, "Insulin-Dependent Diabetes Mellitus Induced by the Antitussive Agent Dextromethorphan," *Diabetologia*, 2000, 43(2):261-2.

LoVecchio F, Pizon AF, O'Patry S, et al, "Accidental Dextromethorphan Ingestions in Children Less Than 5 Years Old," *Clin Toxicol (Phila)*, 2005, 43:659.

Price LH and Lebel J, "Dextromethorphan-Induced Psychosis," *Am J Psychiatry*, 2000, 157(2):304.

Roll D and Tispis G, "'Agent Lemon': A New Twist on Dextromethorphan Toxicity," *J Toxicol Clin Toxicol*, 2002, 40(5):655.

Diazepam

Related Information

- Seizures, Neonatal Guidelines
- Zopiclone

CAS Number 439-14-5

U.S. Brand Names Diastat® AcuDial™; Diastat®; Diazepam Intensol®; Valium®

Impairment Potential Yes. More than double-increased risk of involvement in injurious auto crash following ingestion of ≥20 mg diazepam in elderly drivers. Impairment can also occur at 10 mg doses in younger patients. Brief or extended period (up to 1 year) of use is consistent with driving impairment in the elderly; impairment is greatest in the first week of use. (Ray WA, Fought RL, and Decker MD, "Psychoactive Drugs and the Risk of Injurious Motor Vehicle Crashes in Elderly Drivers," *Am J Epidemiol*, 1992, 136(7):873-83.)

Use Management of anxiety disorders, ethanol withdrawal symptoms; skeletal muscle relaxant; treatment of convulsive disorders

Orphan drug: Viscous solution for rectal administration: Management of selected, refractory epilepsy patients on stable regimens of antiepileptic drugs (AEDs) requiring intermittent use of diazepam to control episodes of increased seizure activity

Unlabeled/Investigational Use Panic disorders; preoperative sedation, light anesthesia, amnesia

Mechanism of Action Depresses all levels of the CNS, including the limbic and reticular formation, probably through the increased action of gamma-aminobutyric acid (GABA), which is a major inhibitory neurotransmitter in the brain

Adverse Reactions

Cardiovascular: **Cardiac arrest, hypotension, bradycardia, cardiovascular collapse, tachycardia, chest pain**, syncope

Central nervous system: **Drowsiness, ataxia, amnesia, slurred speech, paradoxical excitement or rage, fatigue, lightheadedness, insomnia, memory impairment, headache, anxiety, depression**, confusion, nervousness, dizziness, akathisia, aggressive behavior

Dermatologic: **Rash**, dermatitis, exfoliative dermatitis, acne, angioedema, bullous eruptions, urticaria, purpura, pruritus, bullous skin disease/pemphigoid, exanthem, cutaneous vasculitis

Endocrine & metabolic: **Decreased libido**, menstrual irregularities, gynecomastia

Gastrointestinal: **Xerostomia, changes in salivation, constipation, nausea, vomiting, diarrhea, increased or decreased appetite**, weight gain or loss, xerostomia

Hematologic: Blood dyscrasias

Local: **Phlebitis, pain with injection**

Neuromuscular & skeletal: **Dysarthria**, rigidity, tremor, muscle cramps, reflex slowing, paresthesia

Ocular: **Blurred vision, diplopia**

Otic: Tinnitus

Respiratory: **Decrease in respiratory rate, apnea, laryngospasm**, nasal congestion, hyperventilation, pulmonary vasculitis

Miscellaneous: **Diaphoresis**, hiccups, physical and psychological dependence with prolonged use, fixed drug eruption, aneuploidy induction, acute atraumatic compartment syndrome

Signs and Symptoms of Overdose Ataxia, cognitive dysfunction, coma, confusion, dysarthria, dyspnea, eosinophilia, extrapyramidal reaction, gynecomastia, hiccups, hypoactive reflexes, hyporeflexia, hypotension, hypothermia, jaundice, memory loss, myoglobinuria, nystagmus, renal failure, respiratory depression, rhabdomyolysis, slurred speech, somnolence, thrombocytopenia

Pharmacodynamics/Kinetics

I.V.: Status epilepticus:
Onset of action: Almost immediate
Duration: 20-30 minutes

Absorption: Oral: 85% to 100%, more reliable than I.M.

Protein binding: 98%

Metabolism: Hepatic

Half-life elimination: Parent drug: Adults: 20-50 hours; increased half-life in neonates, elderly, and those with severe hepatic disorders; Active major metabolite (desmethyldiazepam): 50-100 hours; may be prolonged in neonates

Dosage

Oral absorption is more reliable than I.M.

Children:

Conscious sedation for procedures: Oral: 0.2-0.3 mg/kg (maximum: 10 mg) 45-60 minutes prior to procedure

Sedation/muscle relaxant/anxiety:
Oral: 0.12-0.8 mg/kg/day in divided doses every 6-8 hours
I.M., I.V.: 0.04-0.3 mg/kg/dose every 2-4 hours to a maximum of 0.6 mg/kg within an 8-hour period if needed

Status epilepticus:
Infants 30 days to 5 years: I.V.: 0.05-0.3 mg/kg/dose given over 2-3 minutes, every 15-30 minutes to a maximum total dose of 5 mg; repeat in 2-4 hours as needed **or** 0.2-0.5 mg/dose every 2-5 minutes to a maximum total dose of 5 mg

>5 years: I.V.: 0.05-0.3 mg/kg/dose given over 2-3 minutes every 15-30 minutes to a maximum total dose of 10 mg; repeat in 2-4 hours as needed **or** 1 mg/dose given over 2-3 minutes, every 2-5 minutes to a maximum total dose of 10 mg

Rectal: 0.5 mg/kg, then 0.25 mg/kg in 10 minutes if needed

Anticonvulsant (acute treatment): Rectal gel formulation:
Infants <6 months: Not recommended
Children <2 years: Safety and efficacy have not been studied
Children 2-5 years: 0.5 mg/kg
Children 6-11 years: 0.3 mg/kg
Children ≥12 years and Adults: 0.2 mg/kg
Note: Dosage should be rounded upward to the next available dose, 2.5, 5, 10, 15, and 20 mg/dose; dose may be repeated in 4-12 hours if needed; do not use more than 5 times per month or more than once every 5 days

Adolescents: Conscious sedation for procedures:
Oral: 10 mg
I.V.: 5 mg, may repeat with $^1/_2$ dose if needed

Adults:
Anxiety/sedation/skeletal muscle relaxant:
Oral: 2-10 mg 2-4 times/day
I.M., I.V.: 2-10 mg, may repeat in 3-4 hours if needed

Sedation in the ICU patient: I.V.: 0.03-0.1 mg/kg every 30 minutes to 6 hours

Status epilepticus: I.V.: 5-10 mg every 10-20 minutes, up to 30 mg in an 8-hour period; may repeat in 2-4 hours if necessary

Rapid tranquilization of agitated patient (administer every 30-60 minutes): Oral: 5-10 mg; average total dose for tranquilization: 20-60 mg

Elderly: Oral: Initial:
Anxiety: 1-2 mg 1-2 times/day; increase gradually as needed, rarely need to use >10 mg/day (watch for hypotension and excessive sedation)

Skeletal muscle relaxant: 2-5 mg 2-4 times/day

Hemodialysis: Not dialyzable (0% to 5%); supplemental dose is not necessary

Dosing adjustment in hepatic impairment: Reduce dose by 50% in cirrhosis and avoid in severe/acute liver disease

Monitoring Parameters Respiratory, cardiovascular, and mental status; check for orthostasis

Administration Intensol® should be diluted before use.

In children, do not exceed 1-2 mg/minute IVP; adults 5 mg/minute.

Rectal gel: Prior to administration, confirm that prescribed dose is visible and correct, and that the green "ready" band is visible. Patient should be positioned on side (facing person responsible for monitoring), with top leg bent forward. Insert rectal tip (lubricated) into rectum and push in plunger gently over 3 seconds. Remove tip of rectal syringe after 3 additional seconds. Buttocks should be held together for 3 seconds after removal. Dispose of syringe appropriately.

Contraindications Hypersensitivity to diazepam or any component of the formulation (cross-sensitivity with other benzodiazepines may exist); narrow-angle glaucoma; not for use in children <6 months of age (oral); pregnancy

Warnings

Diazepam has been associated with increasing the frequency of grand mal seizures. Withdrawal has also been associated with an increase in the seizure frequency. Use with caution with drugs which may decrease diazepam metabolism. Use with caution in elderly or debilitated patients, patients with hepatic disease (including alcoholics), or renal impairment. Active metabolites with extended half-lives may lead to delayed accumulation and adverse effects. Use with caution in patients with respiratory disease or impaired gag reflex.

Acute hypotension, muscle weakness, apnea, and cardiac arrest have occurred with parenteral administration. Acute effects may be more prevalent in patients receiving concurrent barbiturates, narcotics, or ethanol. Appropriate resuscitative equipment and qualified personnel should be available during administration and monitoring. Avoid use of the injection in patients with shock, coma, or acute ethanol intoxication. Intra-arterial injection or extravasation of the parenteral formulation should be avoided. Parenteral formulation contains propylene glycol, which has been associated with toxicity when administered in high dosages. Administration of rectal gel should only be performed by individuals trained to recognize characteristic seizure activity for which the product is indicated, and capable of monitoring response to determine need for additional medical intervention.

Causes CNS depression (dose-related) resulting in sedation, dizziness, confusion, or ataxia which may impair physical and mental capabilities. Patients must be cautioned about performing tasks which require mental alertness (eg, operating machinery or driving). Use with caution in patients receiving other CNS depressants or psychoactive agents. Effects with other sedative drugs or ethanol may be potentiated. The dosage of narcotics should be reduced by approximately 1/3 when diazepam is added. Benzodiazepines have been associated with falls and traumatic injury and should be used with extreme caution in patients who are at risk of these events (especially the elderly).

Use caution in patients with depression, particularly if suicidal risk may be present. Use with caution in patients with a history of drug dependence. Benzodiazepines have been associated with dependence and acute withdrawal symptoms on discontinuation or reduction in dose. Acute withdrawal, including seizures, may be precipitated in patients after administration of flumazenil to patients receiving long-term benzodiazepine therapy.

Diazepam has been associated with anterograde amnesia. Paradoxical reactions, including hyperactive or aggressive behavior, have been reported with benzodiazepines, particularly in adolescent/pediatric or psychiatric patients. Does not have analgesic, antidepressant, or antipsychotic properties.

Rectal gel: Safety and efficacy have not been established in children <2 years of age.

Oral: Safety and efficacy have not been established in children <6 months of age.

Injection: Safety and efficacy have not been established in children <30 days of age. Solution for injection may contain sodium benzoate, benzyl alcohol, or benzoic acid. Large amounts have been associated with "gasping syndrome" in neonates.

Dosage Forms

Gel, rectal:

Diastat®: Pediatric rectal tip [4.4 cm]: 5 mg/mL (2.5 mg, 5 mg) [contains ethyl alcohol 10%, sodium benzoate, benzyl alcohol 1.5%; twin pack]

Diastat® AcuDial™ delivery system:

10 mg: Pediatric/adult rectal tip [4.4 cm]: 5 mg/mL (delivers set doses of 5 mg, 7.5 mg, and 10 mg) [contains ethyl alcohol 10%, sodium benzoate, benzyl alcohol 1.5%; twin pack]

20 mg: Adult rectal tip [6 cm]: 5 mg/mL (delivers set doses of 10 mg, 12.5 mg, 15 mg, 17.5 mg, and 20 mg) [contains ethyl alcohol 10%, sodium benzoate, benzyl alcohol 1.5%; twin pack]

Injection, solution: 5 mg/mL (2 mL, 10 mL) [may contain benzyl alcohol, sodium benzoate, benzoic acid]

Solution, oral: 5 mg/5 mL (5 mL, 500 mL) [wintergreen-spice flavor]

Solution, oral concentrate:

Diazepam Intensol®: 5 mg/mL (30 mL)

Tablet: 2 mg, 5 mg, 10 mg

Valium®: 2 mg, 5 mg, 10 mg

Reference Range

Therapeutic:

Diazepam: 0.2-1.5 mcg/mL (SI: 0.7-5.3 µmol/L)

N-desmethyldiazepam (nordiazepam): 0.1-0.5 mcg/mL (SI: 0.35-1.8 µmol/L)

Urine drug screens can remain positive for 30 days

Overdosage/Treatment

Decontamination: Lavage (within 1 hour)/activated charcoal

Supportive therapy: Rarely is mechanical ventilation required; flumazenil has been shown to selectively block the binding of benzodiazepines to CNS receptors, resulting in a reversal of benzodiazepine-induced CNS depression and respiratory depression

Enhancement of elimination: Multiple dose activated charcoal may be effective

Antidote(s)

• Flumazenil [ANTIDOTE]

Test Interactions False-negative urinary glucose determination when using Clinistix® or Diastix®; may inhibit thyroxine binding; may increase plasma testosterone

Drug Interactions

Substrate of CYP1A2 (minor), 2B6 (minor), 2C9 (minor), 2C19 (major), 3A4 (major); **Inhibits** CYP2C19 (weak), 3A4 (weak)

Calcium channel blockers, nondihydropyridine (diltiazem, verapamil): May decrease the metabolism, via CYP isoenzymes, of diazepam.

Clozapine: Benzodiazepines may enhance the adverse/toxic effect of clozapine.

CNS depressants: Sedative effects and/or respiratory depression may be additive with CNS depressants; includes ethanol, barbiturates, narcotic analgesics, and other sedative agents; monitor for increased effect.

CYP2C19 inducers: May decrease the levels/effects of diazepam. Example inducers include aminoglutethimide, carbamazepine, phenytoin, and rifampin.

CYP2C19 inhibitors: May increase the levels/effects of diazepam. Example inhibitors include delavirdine, fluconazole, fluvoxamine, gemfibrozil, isoniazid, omeprazole, and ticlopidine.

CYP3A4 inducers: CYP3A4 inducers may decrease the levels/effects of diazepam. Example inducers include aminoglutethimide, carbamazepine, nafcillin, nevirapine, phenobarbital, phenytoin, and rifamycins.

CYP3A4 inhibitors: May increase the levels/effects of diazepam. Example inhibitors include azole antifungals, clarithromycin, diclofenac, doxycycline, erythromycin, imatinib, isoniazid, nefazodone, nicardipine, propofol, protease inhibitors, quinidine, telithromycin, and verapamil.

Levodopa: Therapeutic effects may be diminished in some patients following the addition of a benzodiazepine; limited/inconsistent data.

Oral contraceptives: May decrease the clearance of some benzodiazepines (those which undergo oxidative metabolism); monitor for increased benzodiazepine effect.

Theophylline: May partially antagonize some of the effects of benzodiazepines; monitor for decreased response; may require higher doses for sedation.

Pregnancy Risk Factor D

Pregnancy Implications Crosses the placenta. Oral clefts reported, however, more recent data does not support an association between drug and oral clefts; inguinal hernia, cardiac defects, spina bifida, dysmorphic facial features, skeletal defects, multiple other malformations reported; hypotonia and withdrawal symptoms reported following use near time of delivery

Lactation Enters breast milk/contraindicated (AAP rates "of concern")

Nursing Implications In children, do not exceed 1-2 mg/minute IVP; adults 5 mg/minute; provide safety measures (ie, side rails, night light, and call button); remove smoking materials from area; supervise ambulation; do not exceed 5 mg/minute IVP; provide safety measures

(ie, side rails, night light, and call button); remove smoking materials from area; supervise ambulation

Additional Information Benzyl alcohol toxicity can develop after administration of high-dose intravenous diazepam (2.4 mg/kg/hour in 36 hours) in children; oral absorption more reliable than I.M.; intra-arterial injection may cause tissue necrosis

Specific References

Bird SB, Gaspari RJ, Barnett KA, et al, "Diazepam Attenuates Acute Central Respiratory Depression from Acute Organophosphate Poisoning," Acad Emerg Med, 2003, 10:520b-21b.

de Jong LA, Verwey B, Essink G, et al, "Determination of the Benzodiazepine Plasma Concentrations in Suicidal Patients Using a Radioreceptor Assay," J Anal Toxicol, 2004, 28:587-92.

Dickson EW, Bird SB, Gaspari RJ, et al, "Diazepam Inhibits Organophosphate-Induced Central Respiratory Depression," Acad Emerg Med, 2003, 10(12): 1303-6.

Huffman JC and Stern TA, "The Use of Benzodiazepines in the Treatment of Chest Pain: A Review of the Literature," J Emerg Med, 2003, 25(4): 427-37.

Jones AW, Holmgren A, and Holmgren P, "High Concentrations of Diazepam and Nordiazepam in Blood of Impaired Drivers: Association with Age, Gender and Spectrum of Other Drugs Present," Forensic Sci Int, 2005, 146(1):1-7.

Marrs TC, "The Role of Diazepam in the Treatment of Nerve Agent Poisoning in a Civilian Population," Toxicol Rev, 2004, 23(3):145-57.

Marrs TC, "Diazepam in the Treatment of Organophosphorus Ester Pesticide Poisoning," Toxicol Rev, 2003, 22:(2):75-81.

Miner JR, Fringer R, Siegel T, et al, "Serial Bispectral Index Scores in Patients Undergoing Observation for Sedative Overdose in the Emergency Department," Am J Emerg Med. 2006, 24(1):53-7.

Murphy A and Wilbur K, "Phenytoin-Diazepam Interaction," Ann Pharmacother, 2003, 37(5):659-63.

Diazoxide

CAS Number 364-98-7

U.S. Brand Names Hyperstat®; Proglycem®

Use Oral: Hypoglycemia related to islet cell adenoma, carcinoma, hyperplasia, or adenomatosis, nesidioblastosis, leucine sensitivity, or extrapancreatic malignancy

I.V.: Emergency lowering of blood pressure

Mechanism of Action Inhibits insulin release from the pancreas; produces direct smooth muscle relaxation of the peripheral arterioles which results in decrease in blood pressure and reflex increase in heart rate and cardiac output

Adverse Reactions

Cardiovascular: Hypotension, cardiomyopathy, tachycardia, flushing, heart block, cardiomegaly, chest pain, sinus bradycardia, angina, myocardial depression, sinus tachycardia, vasodilation

Central nervous system: Dizziness, seizures, headache, **extrapyramidal reaction** and development of abnormal facies with chronic oral use

Dermatologic: Rash, hirsutism (long-term treatment), edema, cellulitis upon extravasation

Endocrine & metabolic: Hyperglycemia, ketoacidosis, labor (inhibition), hyperuricemia, sodium and water retention

Gastrointestinal: Nausea, vomiting, anorexia, constipation, pancreatitis, loss of taste perception

Hematologic: Leukopenia, thrombocytopenia, hemolysis

Local: Pain, burning, phlebitis upon extravasation

Neuromuscular & skeletal: Weakness

Ocular: Lacrimation, diplopia

Signs and Symptoms of Overdose Agranulocytosis, AV block, bradycardia, chest pain, congestive heart failure, dermatitis, diplopia, dysosmia, fever, galactorrhea, granulocytopenia, hematuria, hemiplegia, hyperglycemia, hyperthermia, hypertrichosis, hyperuricemia, hypotension, ketoacidosis, lacrimation, leukopenia, lichenoid eruptions, nephrotic syndrome, neutropenia

Pharmacodynamics/Kinetics

Onset of action: Hyperglycemic: Oral: ~1 hour

Peak effect: Hypotensive: I.V.: ~5 minutes

Duration: Hyperglycemic: Oral: Normal renal function: 8 hours; Hypotensive: I.V.: Usually 3-12 hours

Protein binding: 90%

Half-life elimination: Children: 9-24 hours; Adults: 20-36 hours; End-stage renal disease: >30 hours

Excretion: Urine (50% as unchanged drug)

Dosage

Hyperinsulinemic hypoglycemia: Oral:

Newborns and Infants: 8-15 mg/kg/day in divided doses every 8-12 hours

Children and Adults: 3-8 mg/kg/day in divided doses every 8-12 hours

Hypertension: I.V.: Children and Adults: 1-3 mg/kg (maximum: 150 mg in a single injection); repeat dose in 5-15 minutes until blood pressure adequately reduced; repeat administration every 4-24 hours monitoring blood pressure closely; do not use longer than 10 days

Stability Protect from light, heat, and freezing; avoid using darkened solutions; virtually insoluble in water

Monitoring Parameters Blood pressure, blood glucose, serum uric acid; intravenous administration requires cardiac monitor and blood pressure monitor

Administration
I.V. diazoxide is given undiluted by rapid I.V. injection over a period of 30 seconds or less, but may also be given by continuous infusion.

Contraindications Hypersensitivity to diazoxide, thiazides, or other sulfonamide derivatives; hypertension associated with aortic coarctation, arteriovenous shunts, pheochromocytoma, dissecting aortic aneurysm

Warnings Diabetes mellitus, renal or liver disease, coronary artery disease, or cerebral vascular insufficiency; patients may require a diuretic with repeated I.V. doses; use caution when reducing severely elevated blood pressure (use 150 mg minibolus only)

Dosage Forms
Capsule (Proglycem®): 50 mg [not available in the U.S.]
Injection, solution (Hyperstat®): 15 mg/mL (20 mL)
Suspension, oral (Proglycem®): 50 mg/mL (30 mL) [contains alcohol 7.25%; chocolate-mint flavor]

Reference Range Plasma level of 35 mg/L (152 μmol/L) produces a 25% reduction of mean arterial pressure

Overdosage/Treatment
Decontamination: Lavage (within 1 hour)/activated charcoal
Supportive therapy: Insulin for hyperglycemia, fluid, and electrolyte restoration; place patient in Trendelenburg position if hypotensive; isotonic saline and/or dopamine or norepinephrine can be used
Enhancement of elimination: Low recovery with dialysis

Test Interactions ↑ glucose, sodium (S), uric acid (S); false-negative insulin response to glucagon

Drug Interactions
Decreased effect: Diazoxide may increase phenytoin metabolism or free fraction
Increased toxicity:
Diuretics and hypotensive agents may potentiate diazoxide adverse effects
Diazoxide may decrease warfarin protein binding

Pregnancy Risk Factor C

Pregnancy Implications Can cause infantile alopecia along with neonatal hyperglycemia

Lactation Excretion in breast milk unknown

Nursing Implications I.V. diazoxide is given undiluted by rapid I.V. injection over a period of 30 seconds or less; shake suspension well before using; extravasation can be treated with warm compresses

Additional Information Patients may require a diuretic with repeated I.V. doses.

Dibenzepin

Pronunciation (dye BENZ e pin)

Related Information
- Amitriptyline
- Imipramine

CAS Number 315-80-0; 4498-32-2

Synonyms Dibenzepin Hydrochloride

Use Depression

Mechanism of Action A tricyclic antidepressant of the dibenzoepine group which selectively inhibits neuronal norepinephrine uptake

Adverse Reactions
Cardiovascular: Cardiac arrhythmias, cardiomyopathy, hypotension has been associated with falls, hypotension (orthostatic)
Central nervous system: **Drowsiness**, sedation, confusion, **dizziness**, psychosis, restlessness, fatigue, anxiety, nervousness, sleep disorders, seizures, delirium, hyperthermia, visual hallucinations
Dermatologic: Rash, photosensitivity
Endocrine & metabolic: Syndrome of inappropriate antidiuretic hormone
Gastrointestinal: **Nausea**, vomiting, **constipation, xerostomia**
Genitourinary: Urinary retention
Hematologic: Blood dyscrasias
Hepatic: Hepatitis, liver failure
Neuromuscular & skeletal: Clonus, myoclonus, weakness
Ocular: Blurred vision, photophobia, diplopia, increased intraocular pressure, mydriasis
Respiratory: Pulmonary edema may develop 45 hours postingestion
Miscellaneous: Hypersensitivity reactions, systemic lupus erythematosus

Signs and Symptoms of Overdose Agranulocytosis, alopecia, ataxia, cardiac arrhythmias, colitis, coma (mean duration: 6 hours), conduction defects, confusion, constipation, cyanosis, dementia, dental erosion, depression, disorientation, ejaculatory disturbances, eosinophilia, galactorrhea, granulocytopenia, hallucinations, hyperthyroidism, hypoglycemia, hyponatremia, hypotension, impotence, increased intraocular pressure, jaundice, lactation, leukopenia, mania, myasthenia gravis

(exacerbation or precipitation), myoclonus, neutropenia, nystagmus, ototoxicity, pulmonary edema (may develop 45 hours postingestion), QT prolongation, respiratory depression, seizure (usually within 3 hours of ingestion), QRS prolongation (with rightward terminal 40 millisecond frontal plane of QRS vector), tachycardia (sinus), tinnitus

Admission Criteria/Prognosis Admit any adult ingestion >1 g

Pharmacodynamics/Kinetics
Metabolism: Hepatic demethylation to an active metabolite
Half-life: 5 hours

Dosage
Oral: 240-480 mg/day; maximum daily dose: 720 mg
I.M., I.V.: 360 mg/day

Overdosage/Treatment
Decontamination: **Do not** induce emesis; lavage is effective if performed within 90 minutes/activated charcoal; multiple dosing of activated charcoal would be expected to be useful
Supportive therapy: Following initiation of essential overdose management, toxic symptoms should be treated. Ventricular arrhythmias and ventricular conduction defects often respond to phenytoin 15-20 mg/kg (adults) with concurrent systemic alkalinization (sodium bicarbonate 0.5-2 mEq/kg I.V.). Titrate to a serum pH of 7.45-7.55. Arrhythmias unresponsive to this therapy may respond to lidocaine 1 mg/kg I.V. followed by a titrated infusion. Physostigmine (1-2 mg I.V. slowly for adults or 0.5 mg I.V. slowly for children) may be indicated for seizures or movement disorders but only as **a last resort**. Propranolol may also be utilized for supraventricular arrhythmias (rate: >160) at 1 mg/minute to a maximum of 5 mg in adults; pediatric dosage of 0.1 mg/kg/dose to 1 mg I.V.. Seizures usually respond to lorazepam or diazepam I.V. boluses (5-10 mg for adults up to 30 mg or 0.25-0.4 mg/kg/dose for children up to 10 mg/dose). If seizures are unresponsive or recur, phenytoin or phenobarbital may be required. Patients must be monitored for at least 24 hours if any signs or symptoms are exhibited. Dobutamine is preferred over dopamine for hypotension; glucagon (10 mg I.V.) can be given to treat hypotension. Flumazenil is contraindicated; magnesium has potentiated adverse cardiac effects (ie, asystole, decreased left ventricular pressure) in an animal model.

Additional Information Lethal dose: 35 mg/kg

Dibucaine

CAS Number 61-12-1; 85-79-0

U.S. Brand Names Nupercainal® [OTC]

Use Fast, temporary relief of pain and itching due to hemorrhoids, minor burns, other minor skin conditions

Mechanism of Action Blocks both initiation and conduction of nerve impulses by decreasing the neuronal membrane's permeability to sodium ions, which results in inhibition of depolarization with resultant blockade of conduction; it is an amide anesthetic, one of the most potent and long-acting and more vasodilatory properties; quinolone derivative

Adverse Reactions
Cardiovascular: Edema, fibrillation (atrial), AV block, sinus bradycardia
Dermatologic: Urticaria, cutaneous lesions
Gastrointestinal: Nausea, vomiting
Local: Burning, tenderness, irritation, inflammation, contact dermatitis, pruritus
Otic: Ototoxicity, tinnitus

Signs and Symptoms of Overdose Acidosis, ARDS, ataxia, bradycardia, coma, CNS depression, cough, cyanosis, flutter (atrial), hypotension, lethargy, ototoxicity, tinnitus, respiratory depression, seizures, ventricular arrhythmias, vomiting

Pharmacodynamics/Kinetics
Onset of action: ~15 minutes
Duration: 2-4 hours
Absorption: Poor through intact skin; well absorbed through mucous membranes and excoriated skin

Dosage
Children and Adults:
Rectal: Hemorrhoids: Insert ointment into rectum using a rectal applicator; administer each morning, evening, and after each bowel movement
Topical: Apply gently to the affected areas; no more than 30 g for adults or 7.5 g for children should be used in any 24-hour period

Stability Darkens on light exposure

Contraindications Hypersensitivity to amide-type anesthetics, ophthalmic use

Dosage Forms
Ointment: 1% (30 g, 454 g)
Nupercainal®: 1% (30 g, 60g) [contains sodium bisulfite]

Reference Range Plasma level of 71 ng/mL associated with seizures

Overdosage/Treatment
Decontamination: Lavage (within 1 hour)/activated charcoal
Supportive therapy: Treat seizures with lorazepam or diazepam; recurring seizures may require phenytoin or phenobarbital; sodium bicarbonate (1-2 mEq/kg) for treatment of acidosis; **do not** use lidocaine in order to treat ventricular arrhythmias; bretylium may be particularly effective;

although no cases exist for development of methemoglobin, amide anesthetics may cause this entity

Enhancement of elimination: Forced diuresis and hemodialysis may be beneficial

Drug Interactions No data reported

Pregnancy Risk Factor C

Nursing Implications Do not use near the eyes or over denuded surfaces or blistered areas

Additional Information Fatal oral dose: 0.8 mg/kg.

Formerly marketed as Percaine; not available in the U.S. as an injectable. Child-resistant packaging was ordered by the U.S. Consumer Product Safety Commission for products containing more than 0.5 mg dibucaine. Dibucaine is 10 and 20 times more toxic than lidocaine and procaine, respectively.

Diclofenac

Related Information

- Nonsteroidal Anti-inflammatory Drugs

CAS Number 15307-79-6

U.S. Brand Names Cataflam®; Solaraze™; Voltaren Ophthalmic®; Voltaren®-XR; Voltaren®

Synonyms Diclofenac Potassium; Diclofenac Sodium

Use Acute and chronic treatment of rheumatoid arthritis, ankylosing spondylitis, and osteoarthritis; ophthalmic solution for postoperative inflammation after cataract extraction

Juvenile rheumatoid arthritis, gout, dysmenorrhea, biliary and renal colic, fever, and pain relief

Mechanism of Action Inhibits prostaglandin synthesis by decreasing the activity of the enzyme, cyclooxygenase, which results in decreased formation of prostaglandin precursors. Mechanism of action for the treatment of AK has not been established.

Adverse Reactions

Cardiovascular: Circulatory collapse, vasculitis

Central nervous system: Headache, dizziness, aseptic meningitis, psychosis, cognitive dysfunction, coma, seizures

Dermatologic: **Rash**, pruritus, bullous lesions, exfoliative dermatitis, erythema multiforme, alopecia, angioedema, toxic epidermal necrolysis, urticaria, purpura, Stevens-Johnson syndrome, photosensitivity, psoriasis, exanthem, scalded skin syndrome

Endocrine & metabolic: Hyperkalemia, anion gap metabolic acidosis, fluid retention, erythema nodosum

Gastrointestinal: **Abdominal cramps, heartburn, indigestion, nausea**, vomiting, GI bleeding, GI ulceration, constipation, diarrhea, dyspepsia, cecal diaphragm/intestinal stricture, diaphragm disease, aphthous stomatitis, xerostomia

Hematologic: Leukopenia, neutropenia, agranulocytosis, granulocytopenia; aplastic anemia (rare), platelet inhibition, thrombocytopenia, hemolytic anemia, immune hemolytic anemia

Hepatic: Elevated transaminases, hepatitis (fulminant), hepatic necrosis

Neuromuscular & skeletal: Clonus, myoclonus, paresthesia

Otic: Ototoxicity, tinnitus

Renal: Renal failure (acute), albuminuria, nephrotic syndrome, chronic renal failure

Respiratory: Wheezing, respiratory depression

Miscellaneous: Hypersensitivity, systemic lupus erythematosus (SLE)

Signs and Symptoms of Overdose Coagulopathy, cognitive dysfunction, drowsiness, GI bleeding, GI upset, lichenoid eruptions, nausea, nephrotic syndrome, ototoxicity, tinnitus, vomiting, wheezing. Severe poisoning can manifest with coma, hypotension, renal and/or hepatic failure, respiratory depression, and seizures.

Pharmacodynamics/Kinetics

Onset of action: Cataflam® is more rapid than sodium salt (Voltaren®) because it dissolves in the stomach instead of the duodenum

Absorption: Topical gel: 10%

Protein binding: 99% to albumin

Metabolism: Hepatic to several metabolites

Half-life elimination: 2 hours

Time to peak, serum: Cataflam®: ~1 hour; Voltaren®: ~2 hours

Excretion: Urine (65%); feces (35%)

Dosage

Adults:

Oral:

Analgesia (Cataflam®): Starting dose: 50 mg 3 times/day

Rheumatoid arthritis: 150-200 mg/day in 2-4 divided doses

Osteoarthritis: 100-150 mg/day in 2-3 divided doses

Ankylosing spondylitis: 100-125 mg/day in 4-5 divided doses

Ophthalmic: Instill 1 drop into affected eye 4 times/day beginning 24 hours after cataract surgery and continuing for 2 weeks

Monitoring Parameters Monitor CBC, liver enzymes; monitor urine output and BUN/serum creatinine; occult blood loss, hemoglobin, hematocrit

Administration

Oral: Do not crush tablets. Administer with food or milk to avoid gastric distress. Take with full glass of water to enhance absorption.

Ophthalmic: Wait at least 5 minutes before administering other types of eye drops.

Topical gel: Cover lesion with gel and smooth into skin gently. Do not cover lesion with occlusive dressings or apply sunscreens, cosmetics, or other medications to affected area.

Contraindications Hypersensitivity to diclofenac, aspirin, other NSAIDs, or any component of the formulation; perioperative pain in the setting of coronary artery bypass surgery (CABG); pregnancy (3rd trimester)

Warnings [U.S. Boxed Warning]: NSAIDs are associated with an increased risk of adverse cardiovascular events, including MI, stroke, and new onset or worsening of pre-existing hypertension. Risk may be increased with duration of use or pre-existing cardiovascular risk factors or disease. Carefully evaluate individual cardiovascular risk profiles prior to prescribing. Use caution with fluid retention, CHF, or hypertension.

Use of NSAIDs can compromise existing renal function. Renal toxicity can occur in patient with impaired renal function, dehydration, heart failure, liver dysfunction, those taking diuretics and ACEI, and the elderly. Rehydrate patient before starting therapy. Monitor renal function closely. Not recommended for use in patients with advanced renal disease.

[U.S. Boxed Warning]: NSAIDs may increase risk of gastrointestinal irritation, ulceration, bleeding, and perforation. These events may occur at any time during therapy and without warning. Use caution with a history of GI disease (bleeding or ulcers), concurrent therapy with aspirin, anticoagulants and/or corticosteroids, smoking, use of alcohol, the elderly or debilitated patients.

Use the lowest effective dose for the shortest duration of time, consistent with individual patient goals, to reduce risk of cardiovascular or GI adverse events. Alternate therapies should be considered for patients at high risk.

NSAIDs may cause serious skin adverse events including exfoliative dermatitis, Stevens-Johnson syndrome (SJS), and toxic epidermal necrolysis (TEN). Anaphylactoid reactions may occur, even without prior exposure; patients with "aspirin triad" (bronchial asthma, aspirin intolerance, rhinitis) may be at increased risk. Do not use in patients who experience bronchospasm, asthma, rhinitis, or urticaria with NSAID or aspirin therapy.

Use with caution in patients with decreased hepatic function. Closely monitor patients with any abnormal LFT. Severe hepatic reactions (eg, fulminant hepatitis, liver failure) have occurred with NSAID use, rarely; discontinue if signs or symptoms of liver disease develop, or if systemic manifestations occur.

The elderly are at increased risk for adverse effects (especially peptic ulceration, CNS effects, renal toxicity) from NSAIDs even at low doses.

Withhold for at least 4-6 half-lives prior to surgical or dental procedures.

Topical gel should not be applied to the eyes, open wounds, infected areas, or to exfoliative dermatitis. Monitor patients for 1 year following application of ophthalmic drops for corneal refractive procedures. Patients using ophthalmic drops should not wear soft contact lenses. Ophthalmic drops may slow/delay healing or prolong bleeding time following surgery.

Dosage Forms

[DSC] = Discontinued product

Gel, as sodium:

Solaraze®: 30 mg/g (50 g)

Solution, ophthalmic, as sodium:

Voltaren Ophthalmic®: 0.1% (2.5 mL, 5 mL)

Tablet, as potassium: 50 mg

Cataflam®: 50 mg

Tablet, delayed release, enteric coated, as sodium: 50 mg, 75 mg

Voltaren®: 25 mg [DSC], 50 mg [DSC], 75 mg

Tablet, extended release, as sodium: 100 mg

Voltaren®-XR: 100 mg

Reference Range Peak plasma diclofenac level after a 50 mg dose: ~735 ng/mL

Overdosage/Treatment

Decontamination: Ipecac within 30 minutes or lavage (within 1 hour)/activated charcoal

Supportive therapy: Hypotension/dehydration can be managed with I.V. fluid therapy; acidosis should be treated with I.V. sodium bicarbonate; seizures with benzodiazepines; antacids, blood products are indicated, as appropriate, for hemorrhage; famotidine (40 mg 2 times/day) can decrease incidence of gastric or duodenal ulcers in patients receiving long-term therapy of this drug

Enhancement of elimination: Dialysis or perfusion is indicated for secondary complications, acidosis, or renal failure and not toxin removal alone; multiple dosing of activated charcoal may be useful

Test Interactions ↑ bleeding time; causes falsely increased free thyroxine level

Drug Interactions **Substrate** (minor) of CYP1A2, 2B6, 2C8, 2C9, 2C19, 2D6, 3A4; **Inhibits** CYP1A2 (moderate), 2C9 (weak), 2E1 (weak), 3A4 (strong)

ACE inhibitors: Antihypertensive effects may be decreased by concurrent therapy with NSAIDs; monitor blood pressure

Angiotensin II antagonists: Antihypertensive effects may be decreased by concurrent therapy with NSAIDs; monitor blood pressure

Anticoagulants (warfarin, heparin, LMWHs) in combination with NSAIDs can cause increased risk of bleeding.

Antiplatelet drugs (ticlopidine, clopidogrel, aspirin, abciximab, dipyridamole, eptifibatide, tirofiban) can cause an increased risk of bleeding.

Beta-blockers: NSAIDs may decrease the antihypertensive effect of beta-blockers. Monitor.

Cholestyramine (and other bile acid sequestrants): May decrease the absorption of NSAIDs. Separate by at least 2 hours.

Corticosteroids may increase the risk of GI ulceration; avoid concurrent use.

Cyclosporine: NSAIDs may increase serum creatinine, potassium, blood pressure, and cyclosporine levels; monitor cyclosporine levels and renal function carefully.

CYP1A2 substrates: Diclofenac may increase the levels/effects of CYP1A2 substrates. Example substrates include aminophylline, fluvoxamine, mexiletine, mirtazapine, ropinirole, theophylline, and trifluoperazine.

CYP3A4 substrates: Diclofenac may increase the levels/effects of CYP3A4 substrates. Example substrates include benzodiazepines, calcium channel blockers, mirtazapine, nateglinide, nefazodone, tacrolimus, and venlafaxine. Selected benzodiazepines (midazolam and triazolam), cisapride, ergot alkaloids, selected HMG-CoA reductase inhibitors (lovastatin and simvastatin), and pimozide are generally contraindicated with strong CYP3A4 inhibitors.

Gentamicin and amikacin serum concentrations are increased by indomethacin in premature infants. Results may apply to other aminoglycosides and NSAIDs.

Hydralazine's antihypertensive effect is decreased; avoid concurrent use.

Lithium levels can be increased; avoid concurrent use if possible or monitor lithium levels and adjust dose. Sulindac may have the least effect. When NSAID is stopped, lithium will need adjustment again.

Loop diuretics efficacy (diuretic and antihypertensive effect) is reduced. Indomethacin reduces this efficacy, however, it may be anticipated with any NSAID.

Methotrexate: Severe bone marrow suppression, aplastic anemia, and GI toxicity have been reported with concomitant NSAID therapy. Avoid use during moderate or high-dose methotrexate (increased and prolonged methotrexate levels). NSAID use during low-dose treatment of rheumatoid arthritis has not been fully evaluated; extreme caution is warranted.

Thiazides antihypertensive effects are decreased; avoid concurrent use.

Verapamil plasma concentration is decreased by diclofenac; avoid concurrent use.

Warfarin's INRs may be increased by piroxicam. Other NSAIDs may have the same effect depending on dose and duration. Monitor INR closely. Use the lowest dose of NSAIDs possible and for the briefest duration.

Pregnancy Risk Factor B (topical); C (oral)/D (3rd trimester)

Pregnancy Implications Closure of the ductus arteriosus in a fetus following *in utero* exposure

Lactation Excretion in breast milk unknown/not recommended

Additional Information Misoprostol (200 mcg) can prevent diclofenac-induced gastric ulcers (**not** duodenal ulcers)

Specific References

Schechner V, Hershcovici T, and Beigel Y, "Rhabdomyolysis Due to Combined Therapy with Cerivastatin and Diclofenac," *J Pharm Technol*, 2003(19):219-21.

Dicumarol

Pronunciation (dye KOO ma role)

Related Information

- Warfarin

CAS Number 66-76-2

Synonyms Bishydroxycoumarin

Use Prophylaxis and treatment of thromboembolic disorders

Mechanism of Action Depression of factors VII, IX, X, and II (sequential) - a hydroxycoumarin

Adverse Reactions

More likely to have gastrointestinal side effects than warfarin

Cardiovascular: Circulatory collapse, pericardial effusion/pericarditis

Central nervous system: Fever, intracranial hemorrhage

Dermatologic: Skin lesions, skin necrosis, alopecia, angioedema, bullous skin disease, urticaria, purpura, pruritus, exanthem

Gastrointestinal: Anorexia, nausea, vomiting, diarrhea, pancreatitis, hemorrhagic pancreatitis

Genitourinary: Priapism

Hematologic: Hemorrhage, ocular hemorrhage, bleeding gums, coagulopathy

Hepatic: Elevated prothrombin time

Renal: Renal tubular necrosis

Respiratory: Hemoptysis, alveolar hemorrhage, pulmonary hemorrhage

Miscellaneous: Feces discoloration (black), feces discoloration (light brown), feces discoloration (pink), feces discoloration (red)

Pharmacodynamics/Kinetics

Duration of action: 5-6 days

Absorption: Oral: Well (but unpredictably) absorbed - affected by food

Protein binding: 97%

Metabolism: In the liver

Half-life: Plasma: 1-2 days

Time to peak serum concentration: 1-9 hours

Elimination: In urine

Dosage Adults: Oral: 25-200 mg/day based on prothrombin time (PT) determinations

Stability Insoluble in water or alcohol

Contraindications Severe liver or kidney disease; open wounds; uncontrolled bleeding; hypersensitivity to dicumarol or any component

Warnings Concomitant use with vitamin K may decrease anticoagulant effect; monitor carefully; concomitant use with ethacrynic acid, indomethacin, mefenamic acid, phenylbutazone, or aspirin increases warfarin's anticoagulant effect and may cause severe GI bleeding; the plasma half-life of dicumarol is 1-2 days and its duration of action is 2-10 days; as this is considerably longer than warfarin, prescribers should be aware of this difference; peak levels should be expected 1-2 weeks after dose adjustment

Dosage Forms Tablet: 25 mg

Reference Range

Normal: 20-30 mcg/mL

Toxic: >70 mcg/mL

Overdosage/Treatment

Decontamination: Activated charcoal should be given; lavage can be performed within 1 hour of ingestion

Supportive therapy: Vitamin K_1 should be given in doses as outlined in phytonadione; monitor PT and INR till normalization

Enhancement of elimination: Multiple dosing of activated charcoal or cholestyramine may be useful

Antidote(s)

- Cholestyramine Resin [ANTIDOTE]
- Phytonadione [ANTIDOTE]

Diagnostic Procedures

- Bishydroxycoumarin, Blood

Drug Interactions May accentuate toxicities of oral hypoglycemics and anticonvulsants. The following will decrease prothrombin time - antacids, antihistamines, phenobarbital, carbamazepine, cholestyramine, meprobamate, glutethimide, ethchlorvynol, oral contraceptives, ranitidine, chloral hydrate, diuretics. Increased prothrombin time due to allopurinol, amiodarone, cimetidine, clofibrate, dextran, diazoxide, diflunisal, diuretics, disulfiram, fenoprofen, ibuprofen, indomethacin, influenza virus vaccine, methyldopa, methylphenidate, MAO inhibitors, naproxen, nortriptyline, phenytoin, propylthiouracil, salicylates, quinidine, quinine, ranitidine, tolbutamide, thyroid drugs, sulindac, co-trimoxazole

Pregnancy Risk Factor D

Additional Information TLV-TWA: 0.1 mg/m^3; IDLH: 200 mg/m^3

Dicyclomine

Pronunciation (dye SYE kloe meen)

CAS Number 67-92-5; 77-19-0

U.S. Brand Names Bentyl®

Synonyms Dicyclomine Hydrochloride; Dicycloverine Hydrochloride

Use Treatment of functional disturbances of GI motility such as irritable bowel syndrome

Unlabeled/Investigational Use Urinary incontinence

Mechanism of Action Blocks the action of acetylcholine at parasympathetic sites in smooth muscle, secretory glands and the CNS

Adverse Reactions

Cardiovascular: Hypotension (orthostatic), tachycardia, palpitations, thrombosis with I.V. administration, cardiomegaly, cardiomyopathy

Central nervous system: Confusion, drowsiness, headache, lightheadedness, memory disturbance, loss of short-term memory, tiredness, seizures, coma, nervousness, excitement, insomnia, dizziness, delirium, psychosis

Dermatologic: **Dry skin**, rash, urticaria, pruritus

Endocrine & metabolic: Decreased flow of breast milk

Gastrointestinal: **Constipation, xerostomia and dry throat**, dysphagia, bloated feeling, nausea, vomiting, loss of taste perception

Genitourinary: Dysuria, urinary retention

Local: **Injection site reactions**

Neuromuscular & skeletal: Muscular hypotonia, weakness

Ocular: Blurred vision, intraocular pain (increased), sensitivity to light (increased)

Respiratory: **Dry nose**, asphyxia, respiratory distress, apnea (in neonates)

Miscellaneous: **Diaphoresis (decreased)**

Signs and Symptoms of Overdose Dry mouth, hypertension, hyperthermia, ileus, mydriasis, tachycardia, urinary retention

Pharmacodynamics/Kinetics

Onset of action: 1-2 hours

Duration: ≤ 4 hours

Absorption: Oral: Well absorbed

Metabolism: Extensive

Half-life elimination: Initial: 1.8 hours; Terminal: 9-10 hours

Excretion: Urine (small amounts as unchanged drug)

Dosage

Oral:

Infants >6 months: 5 mg/dose 3-4 times/day

Children: 10 mg/dose 3-4 times/day

Urinary incontinence: 8 mg/kg/day in 3 divided doses

Adults: Begin with 80 mg/day in 4 equally divided doses, then increase up to 160 mg/day

Urinary incontinence: 60-100 mg/day

I.M. **(should not be used I.V.)**: Adults: 80 mg/day in 4 divided doses (20 mg/dose)

Monitoring Parameters Pulse, anticholinergic effect, urinary output, GI symptoms

Administration Do not administer I.V.

Contraindications Hypersensitivity to any anticholinergic drug; narrow-angle glaucoma; myasthenia gravis; should not be used in infants <6 months of age

Warnings Use with caution in patients with hepatic or renal disease, ulcerative colitis, hyperthyroidism, cardiovascular disease, hypertension, tachycardia, GI obstruction, obstruction of the urinary tract. The elderly are at increased risk for anticholinergic effects, confusion, and hallucinations.

Dosage Forms Capsule, as hydrochloride: 10 mg

Injection, solution, as hydrochloride: 10 mg/mL (2 mL)

Syrup, as hydrochloride: 10 mg/5 mL (480 mL)

Tablet, as hydrochloride: 20 mg

Overdosage/Treatment

Decontamination: Lavage (within 1 hour)/activated charcoal

Supportive therapy: Physostigmine should be reserved for life-threatening anticholinergic effects; tachyarrhythmias can respond to physostigmine or I.V. beta-adrenergic blockers; agitation can be treated with benzodiazepines

Drug Interactions Decreased effect: Phenothiazines, anti-Parkinson's drugs, haloperidol, sustained release dosage forms; decreased effect with antacids

Increased toxicity: Anticholinergics, amantadine, narcotic analgesics, type I antiarrhythmics, antihistamines, phenothiazines, TCAs

Pregnancy Risk Factor B

Pregnancy Implications No increase in fetal abnormalities in mothers taking 40 mg/day during first trimester

Lactation Enters breast milk/contraindicated

Nursing Implications Raise bed rails, institute safety measures

---

Didanosine

CAS Number 69655-05-6

U.S. Brand Names Videx® EC; Videx®

Synonyms ddI; Dideoxyinosine

Use Treatment of HIV infection; always to be used in combination with at least two other antiretroviral agents

Mechanism of Action Didanosine, a purine nucleoside (adenosine) analog and the deamination product of dideoxyadenosine (ddA), inhibits HIV replication *in vitro* in both T cells and monocytes. Didanosine is converted within the cell to the mono-, di-, and triphosphates of ddA. These ddA triphosphates act as substrate and inhibitor of HIV reverse transcriptase substrate and inhibitor of HIV reverse transcriptase, thereby blocking viral DNA synthesis and suppressing HIV replication.

Adverse Reactions

Cardiovascular: Heart failure, cardiomyopathy, cardiomegaly, QT prolongation, vasodilation

Central nervous system: **Headache, anxiety, irritability, restlessness, insomnia**, malaise, CNS depression, cranial nerve palsies, fever, mania

Dermatologic: Rash, pruritus, erythema, eczema, alopecia, cutaneous vasculitis

Endocrine & metabolic: Hypokalemia, hyperuricemia (dose related), hypomagnesemia, hypocalcemia, hyperlactatemia (symptomatic)

Gastrointestinal: **Diarrhea**, **nausea**, dyspepsia, vomiting, anorexia, stomatitis, **pancreatitis**, **abdominal pain**

Hematologic: Thrombocytopenia

Hepatic: Elevated liver enzymes, hepatic failure, hepatitis (fulminant)

Neuromuscular & skeletal: **Paresthesia, peripheral neuropathy**, weakness

Ocular: Retinal depigmentation, photophobia, diplopia, amblyopia, blindness

Otic: Deafness

Respiratory: Cough, apnea, dyspnea, rhinitis

Signs and Symptoms of Overdose Fanconi syndrome, myalgia; peripheral neuropathy can occur at doses >20 mg/kg/day

Pharmacodynamics/Kinetics

Absorption: Subject to degradation by acidic pH of stomach; some formulations are buffered to resist acidic pH; $\leq 50\%$ reduction in peak plasma concentration is observed in presence of food. Delayed release capsules contain enteric-coated beadlets which dissolve in the small intestine.

Distribution: V_d: Children: 35.6 L/m²; Adults: 1.08 L/kg

Protein binding: <5%

Metabolism: Has not been evaluated in humans; studies conducted in dogs show extensive metabolism with allantoin, hypoxanthine, xanthine, and uric acid being the major metabolites found in urine

Bioavailability: 42%

Half-life elimination:

Children and Adolescents: 0.8 hour

Adults: Normal renal function: 1.5 hours; active metabolite, ddATP, has an intracellular half-life >12 hours *in vitro*; Renal impairment: 2.5-5 hours

Time to peak: Buffered tablets: 0.67 hours; Delayed release capsules: 2 hours

Excretion: Urine (~55% as unchanged drug)

Clearance: Total body: Averages 800 mL/minute

Dosage Treatment of HIV infection: Oral (administer on an empty stomach):

Children:

2 weeks to 8 months: 100 mg/m² twice daily; 50 mg/m² may be considered in infants 2 weeks to 4 months

>8 months: 120 mg/m² twice daily; dosing range: 90-150 mg/m² twice daily; patients with CNS disease may require higher dose

Note: At least 2 tablets per dose should be administered for adequate buffering and absorption; tablets should be chewed or dispersed (in 1 ounce of water).

Adolescents and Adults: Dosing based on patient weight:

Note: Preferred dosing frequency is twice daily for didanosine tablets/oral solution

Chewable tablets, powder for oral solution:

<60 kg: 125 mg twice daily or 250 mg once daily

≥ 60 kg: 200 mg twice daily or 400 mg once daily

Note: Adults should receive 2-4 tablets per dose for adequate buffering and absorption; tablets should be chewed or dispersed

Delayed release capsule (Videx® EC):

<60 kg: 250 mg once daily

≥ 60 kg: 400 mg once daily

Dosing adjustment with tenofovir (didanosine tablets or delayed release capsules; based on tenofovir product labeling):

<60 kg: 200 mg once daily

≥ 60 kg: 250 mg once daily

Dosage adjustment in renal impairment: Dosing based on patient weight, creatinine clearance, and dosage form: See table.

Recommended Dose (mg) of Didanosine by Body Weight				
Creatinine Clearance (mL/min)	≥ 60 kg		<60 kg	
	Tablet[1] (mg)	Delayed Release Capsule (mg)	Tablet[1] (mg)	Delayed Release Capsule (mg)
≥ 60	400 qd or 200 bid	400 qd	250 qd or 125 bid	250 qd
30-59	200 qd or 100 bid	200 qd	150 qd or 75 bid	125 qd
10-29	150 qd	125 qd	100 qd	125 qd
<10	100 qd	125 qd	75 qd	See footnote 2.

[1]Chewable/dispersible buffered tablet; 2 tablets must be taken with each dose; different strengths of tablets may be combined to yield the recommended dose.

[2]Not suitable for use in patients <60 kg with Cl_{cr} <10 mL/minute; use alternate formulation.

Patients requiring hemodialysis or CAPD: Dose per Cl_{cr} <10 mL/minute

Hemodialysis: Removed by hemodialysis (40% to 60%)

Dosing adjustment in hepatic impairment: Should be considered; monitor for toxicity

Elderly patients have a higher frequency of pancreatitis (10% versus 5% in younger patients); monitor renal function and dose accordingly

Monitoring Parameters Serum potassium, uric acid, creatinine; hemoglobin, CBC with neutrophil and platelet count, CD4 cells; viral load; liver function tests, amylase; weight gain; perform dilated retinal exam every 6 months

Administration

Videx® EC: Take on an empty stomach; administer at least 1 hour before or 2 hours after eating.

Chewable/dispersible buffered tablets: The 200 mg tablet should only be used in once-daily dosing. At least 2 tablets, but no more than 4 tablets, should be taken together to allow adequate buffering. Tablets may be chewed or dispersed prior to consumption. To disperse, dissolve in 1 oz water, stir until uniform dispersion is formed, and drink immediately. May also add 1 oz of clear apple juice to initial dispersion if additional flavor is needed. The apple juice dilution is stable for 1 hour at room temperature. Do not mix with other juices.

Pediatric powder for oral solution: Prior to dispensing, the powder should be mixed with purified water USP to an initial concentration of 20 mg/mL and then further diluted with an appropriate antacid suspension to a final mixture of 10 mg/mL. Shake well prior to use.

Contraindications Hypersensitivity to didanosine or any component of the formulation

Warnings

[U.S. Boxed Warning]: Pancreatitis (sometimes fatal) has been reported; incidence is dose related. Risk factors for developing pancreatitis include a previous history of the condition, concurrent cytomegalovirus or *Mycobacterium avium-intracellulare* infection, and concomitant use of stavudine, pentamidine, or co-trimoxazole. Discontinue didanosine if clinical signs of pancreatitis occur. **[U.S. Boxed Warning]: Lactic acidosis, symptomatic hyperlactatemia, and severe hepatomegaly with steatosis (sometimes fatal) have occurred with antiretroviral nucleoside analogues, including didanosine.** Hepatotoxicity may occur even in the absence of marked transaminase elevations; suspend therapy in any patient developing clinical/laboratory findings which suggest hepatotoxicity. Pregnant women may be at increased risk of lactic acidosis and liver damage.

Peripheral neuropathy occurs in ~20% of patients receiving the drug. Retinal changes (including retinal depigmentation) and optic neuritis have been reported in adults and children using didanosine. Patients should undergo retinal examination every 6-12 months. Use with caution in patients with decreased renal or hepatic function, phenylketonuria, sodium-restricted diets, or with edema, CHF, or hyperuricemia. Twice-daily dosing is the preferred dosing frequency for didanosine tablets. Didanosine delayed release capsules are indicated for once-daily use.

Dosage Forms Capsule, delayed release: 200 mg, 250 mg, 400 mg
Videx® EC: 125 mg, 200 mg, 250 mg, 400 mg
Powder for oral solution, pediatric:
Videx®: 2 g, 4 g [makes 10 mg/mL solution after final mixing]
Tablet, buffered, chewable/dispersible:
Videx®: 25 mg, 50 mg, 100 mg, 150 mg, 200 mg [all strengths contain phenylalanine 36.5 mg/tablet; orange flavor] [DSC]

Reference Range Peak plasma level of 1-29 μmol/L following oral dose of 0.8-33 mg/kg

Overdosage/Treatment

Decontamination: Lavage (within 1 hour)/activated charcoal

Enhancement of elimination: Multiple dosing of activated charcoal may be effective; hemodialysis may be effective in removing approximately 20% of dose

Test Interactions ↑ serum triglycerides, uric acid; ↓ serum calcium, potassium, magnesium

Drug Interactions Drugs whose absorption depends on the level of acidity in the stomach (such as ketoconazole, itraconazole, and dapsone) should be administered at least 2 hours prior to the buffered formulations of didanosine (not affected by delayed release capsules)

Decreased effect: Buffered formulations of didanosine (tablets, pediatric oral solution) may decrease absorption of quinolones or tetracyclines, separate dosing by 2 hours; didanosine should be held during PCP treatment with pentamidine; didanosine may decrease levels of indinavir.

Increased toxicity: Concomitant administration of other drugs (including hydroxyurea) which have the potential to cause peripheral neuropathy or pancreatitis may increase the risk of these toxicities.

Allopurinol: May increase didanosine concentration; avoid concurrent use.

Antacids: Concomitant use with buffered tablet or pediatric didanosine solution may potentiate adverse effects of aluminum- or magnesium-containing antacids.

Ganciclovir: May increase didanosine concentration; monitor.

Hydroxyurea: May precipitate didanosine-induced pancreatitis if added to therapy; concomitant use is not recommended.

Methadone: May decrease didanosine concentration; monitor.

Ribavirin: Coadministration may increase exposure to didanosine and/or its active metabolite, increasing the risk of hepatic decompensation or other signs of mitochondrial toxicity, including pancreatitis, lactic acidosis, and peripheral neuropathy. Coadministration of ribavirin with didanosine should be undertaken with caution, and patients should be monitored closely for didanosine-related toxicities; suspend therapy if signs or symptoms of toxicity are noted.

Tenofovir: Coadministration may increase exposure to didanosine and/or its active metabolite increasing the risk or severity of didanosine toxicities, including pancreatitis, hyperglycemia, lactic acidosis, and peripheral neuropathy. Some patients have experienced reduced CD4 cell counts and/or decreased virologic response. Coadministration of tenofovir with didanosine should be undertaken with caution, and patients should be monitored closely for didanosine-related toxicities; specific dosing adjustment is recommended; suspend therapy if signs or symptoms of toxicity are noted.

Pregnancy Risk Factor B

Pregnancy Implications Cases of fatal and nonfatal lactic acidosis, with or without pancreatitis, have been reported in pregnant women. It is not known if pregnancy itself potentiates this known side effect; however, pregnant women may be at increased risk of lactic acidosis and liver damage. Hepatic enzymes and electrolytes should be monitored frequently during the 3rd trimester of pregnancy. Use during pregnancy only if the potential benefit to the mother outweighs the potential risk of this complication. Phase I/II studies have shown limited placental transfer. Health professionals are encouraged to contact the antiretroviral pregnancy registry to monitor outcomes of pregnant women exposed to antiretroviral medications (1-800-258-4263).

Lactation Excretion in breast milk unknown/contraindicated

Nursing Implications Administer liquified powder immediately after dissolving; avoid creating dust if powder spilled, use wet mop or damp sponge

Additional Information Each chewable tablet contains 36.5 mg phenylalanine and 8.6 mEq magnesium. Sodium content of buffered tablets: 264.5 mg (11.5 mEq).

Specific References

Kirian MA, Higginson RT, and Fulco PP, "Acute Onset of Pancreatitis with Concomitant Use of Tenofovir and Didanosine," *Ann Pharmacother*, 2004, 38(10):1660-3.

Diethylcarbamazine

CAS Number 1642-54-2; 90-89-1

Use An antihelmintic agent used to treat *Wuchereria bancrofti*, *Brugia malayi*, *Brugia timori*, or *Onchocerca volvulus*; has been used to treat dog heartworm

Mechanism of Action Antifilarial agent which kills parasite in adult stage (a piperazine derivative)

Adverse Reactions

Cardiovascular: Hypotension, tachycardia

Central nervous system: Dizziness, headache, fever

Dermatologic: Pruritus

Endocrine & metabolic: Abortifacient

Gastrointestinal: Vomiting, nausea

Neuromuscular & skeletal: Arthralgia

Ocular: Eye discomfort (optic neuritis)

Renal: Proteinuria

Miscellaneous: Hypersensitivity due to microfilariae death (Mazzotti reaction) which can occur within 2 hours; lymphadenopathy

Signs and Symptoms of Overdose Abdominal cramping, anorexia, dizziness, nausea, vomiting (>1 g)

Admission Criteria/Prognosis Consider admitting hypersensitivity reactions (especially due onchocerciasis) or ingestions >1 g

Toxicodynamics/Kinetics

Metabolism: N-oxide metabolites

Half-life: 9-13 hours; 15 hours in renal failure

Elimination: Renal

Dosage

Bancroftian filariasis: 6 mg/kg/day in 3 divided doses for 12 days

Brugian filariasis: 3-6 mg/kg/day in 3 divided doses for 6-12 days

In order to decrease severity of hypersensitivity reactions, initial dosage of 1 mg/kg/day can be increased to 6 mg/kg/day over 3 days; a corticosteroid agent can be added

Prophylaxis of Bancroftian/Malayan filariasis: 50 mg/month

Prophylaxis of loiasis: 4-5 mg/kg for 3 successive days each month

Onchocerciasis: 0.5-1 mg/kg for first 1-2 days, then 2 mg/kg twice daily for next 5-7 days

Reference Range Dose of 0.5 mg/kg can result in a peak plasma diethylcarbamazine citrate concentration of 100-150 ng/mL

Overdosage/Treatment

Decontamination: Oral: Lavage ingestions >10 mg/kg/activated charcoal

Supportive therapy: Betamethasone can be used to treat hypersensitivity reactions during onchocerciasis treatment; antihistamines are of no value, although antipyretic or analgesic agents may be useful

Enhanced elimination: Avoid alkalinization of urine if possible due to prolongation of serum half-life; multiple dosing of activated charcoal may be useful

Pregnancy Implications Uterine hypermotility (due to prostaglandin synthesis) may occur

Additional Information Encephalitis due to *Loa loa* infection may worsen during initial treatment with diethylcarbamazine citrate; use of corticosteroids may be useful for such treatment

Diethylpropion

CAS Number 134-80-5; 90-84-6
U.S. Brand Names Tenuate® Dospan®; Tenuate®
Synonyms Amfepramone; Diethylpropion Hydrochloride
Use Short-term adjunct in exogenous obesity
Unlabeled/Investigational Use Migraine
Mechanism of Action Diethylpropion is used as an anorexiant agent possessing pharmacological and chemical properties similar to those of amphetamines. The mechanism of action of diethylpropion in reducing appetite appears to be secondary to CNS effects, specifically stimulation of the hypothalamus to release catecholamines into the central nervous system; anorexiant effects are mediated via norepinephrine and dopamine metabolism. An increase in physical activity and metabolic effects (inhibition of lipogenesis and enhancement of lipolysis) may also contribute to weight loss.
Adverse Reactions
Cardiovascular: **Hypertension**, tachycardia, arrhythmias
Central nervous system: **Euphoria, nervousness, insomnia**, confusion, headache, psychosis, paranoid psychosis, auditory hallucinations, CNS depression, paranoia
Dermatologic: Alopecia, urticaria, ecchymosis
Endocrine & metabolic: Changes in libido, gynecomastia
Gastrointestinal: Nausea, vomiting, restlessness, constipation, diarrhea, abdominal cramps, metallic taste
Genitourinary: Dysuria, impotence
Hematologic: Blood dyscrasias, agranulocytosis, leukopenia
Neuromuscular & skeletal: Tremor, myalgia
Ocular: Blurred vision, mydriasis
Renal: Polyuria
Respiratory: Dyspnea
Miscellaneous: Diaphoresis (increased)
Pharmacodynamics/Kinetics
Onset of action: 1 hour
Duration: 12-24 hours
Dosage Adults: Oral:
Tablet: 25 mg 3 times/day before meals or food
Tablet, controlled release: 75 mg at midmorning
Monitoring Parameters Monitor CNS
Administration Do not crush 75 mg controlled release tablet. Dose should not be given in evening or at bedtime. Take tablets 1 hour before meals. Take controlled release tablet at midmorning.
Contraindications Hypersensitivity or idiosyncrasy to sympathomimetic amines. Patients with advanced arteriosclerosis, symptomatic cardiovascular disease, moderate to severe hypertension (stage II or III), hyperthyroidism, glaucoma, agitated states, patients with a history of drug abuse, and during or within 14 days following MAO inhibitor therapy. Concurrent use with other anorectic agents; stimulant medications are contraindicated for use in children with attention-deficit/hyperactivity disorders and concomitant Tourette's syndrome or tics.
Warnings
Use with caution in patients with bipolar disorder, diabetes mellitus, cardiovascular disease, seizure disorders, insomnia, porphyria, or mild hypertension (stage I). May exacerbate symptoms of behavior and thought disorder in psychotic patients. Stimulants may unmask tics in individuals with coexisting Tourette's syndrome. Potential for drug dependency exists - avoid abrupt discontinuation in patients who have received for prolonged periods. Stimulant use in children has been associated with growth suppression. Not recommended for use in patients <12 years of age.
Serious, potentially life-threatening toxicities may occur when thyroid hormones (at dosages above usual daily hormonal requirements) are used in combination with sympathomimetic amines to induce weight loss. Treatment of obesity is not an approved use for thyroid hormone.
Dosage Forms Tablet, as hydrochloride (Tenuate®): 25 mg
Tablet, controlled release, as hydrochloride (Tenuate® Dospan®): 75 mg
Overdosage/Treatment
Decontamination: **Do not** induce emesis; lavage (within 4 hours)/ activated charcoal
Supportive therapy: Treat hypotension with I.V. crystalloid solutions; vasopressors can be used for refractory cases; propranolol (1 mg/dose in adults or 0.01-0.1 mg/kg/dose in children over 10 minutes) or esmolol can be used to treat tachycardia; hyperpyrexia can be treated with external (passive) cooling

Drug Interactions Anorectic agents: Concurrent use with other anorectic agents may cause serious cardiac problems and is contraindicated.
Furazolidone: May induce a hypertensive episode in patients receiving furazolidone.
Guanethidine: Diethylpropion may inhibit the antihypertensive response to guanethidine; probably also may occur with guanadrel.
MAO inhibitors: Severe hypertensive episodes have occurred with amphetamine when used in patients receiving MAO inhibitors; concurrent use or use within 14 days is contraindicated.
Norepinephrine: Diethylpropion may enhance the pressor response to norepinephrine.
Sibutramine: Concurrent use of sibutramine and diethylpropion may cause severe hypertension and tachycardia; use is contraindicated.
Tricyclic antidepressants: Concurrent use with tricyclic antidepressants may result in hypertension and CNS stimulation; avoid this combination.
Pregnancy Risk Factor B
Lactation Enters breast milk/not recommended
Nursing Implications Do not crush 75 mg controlled release tablets; dose should not be given in evening or at bedtime

Diethylstilbestrol

Pronunciation (dye eth il stil BES trole)
CAS Number 130-80-3; 56-53-1
Synonyms DES; Diethylstilbestrol Diphosphate Sodium; Stilbestrol
Use Palliative treatment of inoperable metastatic prostatic carcinoma and postmenopausal inoperable, progressing breast cancer
Mechanism of Action Competes with estrogenic and androgenic compounds for binding onto tumor cells and thereby inhibits their effects on tumor growth
Adverse Reactions
Cardiovascular: Hypertension, thromboembolism, myocardial infarction, **peripheral edema**, edema, angina
Central nervous system: Headache, CNS depression, dizziness, anxiety, stroke
Dermatologic: Rash, chloasma, melasma, bullous lesions, hypertrichosis, exfoliative dermatitis, angioedema, urticaria, purpura, pruritus, acanthosis nigricans, exanthem
Endocrine & metabolic: Gynecomastia, amenorrhea, **breast tenderness, enlargement of breasts (female & male)**, alterations in frequency and flow of menses, decreased glucose tolerance, decreased libido in males, increased libido in females
Gastrointestinal: **Nausea, anorexia, bloating**, vomiting, diarrhea, GI distress, pancreatitis
Hematologic: Thrombocytopenia, hemolytic anemia, pancytopenia, hypercalcemia, porphyrinogenic
Hepatic: Cholestatic jaundice, increased triglycerides and LDL
Ocular: Intolerance to contact lenses
Miscellaneous: Breast tumors, breast cancer, susceptibility to *Candida* infection (increased), risk of pre-eclampsia (increased), systemic lupus erythematosus
Signs and Symptoms of Overdose Chest pain, depression, dysuria, ectopic pregnancy, gynecomastia, hirsutism, hyperactivity, hyperprolactinemia, hypocalcemia, nausea
Pharmacodynamics/Kinetics
Metabolism: Hepatic
Excretion: Urine and feces
Dosage Adults:
Male:
Prostate carcinoma: Oral: 1-3 mg/day
Diphosphate: Inoperable progressing prostate cancer:
Oral: 50 mg 3 times/day; increase up to 200 mg or more 3 times/ day; maximum daily dose: 1 g
I.V.: Give 0.5 g, dissolved in 250 mL of saline or D_5W, administer slowly the first 10-15 minutes then adjust rate so that the entire amount is given in 1 hour; repeat for ≥5 days depending on patient response, then repeat 0.25-0.5 g 1-2 times for 1 week or change to oral therapy
Female: Postmenopausal inoperable, progressing breast carcinoma: Oral: 15 mg/day
Stability Intravenous solution should be stored at room temperature and away from direct light; solution is stable for 3 days as long as cloudiness or precipitation has not occurred
Monitoring Parameters Mammography should be performed in all women prior to starting estrogen therapy and then annually; blood pressure, Pap smear annually
Administration I.V. infusion: Dilute 0.5-1 g in 250-500 mL D_5W or NS; give 1-2 mL/minute for 10-15 minutes, then infuse remaining solution over 1 hour
Contraindications Undiagnosed vaginal bleeding; breast cancer except in select patients with metastatic disease; pregnancy
Warnings Use with caution in patients with a history of thromboembolism, stroke, myocardial infarction (especially >40 years of age who smoke), liver tumor, hypertension, cardiac, renal, or hepatic insufficiency; estro-

gens have been reported to increase the risk of endometrial carcinoma; do not use estrogens during pregnancy

Dosage Forms Injection, as diphosphate sodium (Stilphostrol®): 0.25 g (5 mL)
Tablet (Honvol®): 0.1 mg, 0.5 mg, 1 mg

Overdosage/Treatment
Decontamination: Emesis within 30 minutes or lavage within 1 hour; activated charcoal
Enhancement of elimination: Due to enterohepatic recirculation of drug, multiple dosing of activated charcoal may be effective

Test Interactions ↓ antithrombin III; ↓ serum folate concentration; ↑ prothrombin and factors VII, VIII, IX, X; ↑ platelet aggregability; ↑ thyroid binding globulin; ↑ total thyroid hormone (T_4); ↑ serum triglycerides/phospholipids; ↑ prolactin

Drug Interactions Decreased effect of oral anticoagulants
Increased effect of corticosteroids, succinylcholine, TCAs
Decreased DES levels: Barbiturates, phenytoin, rifampin

Pregnancy Risk Factor X

Nursing Implications Note potency difference between DES base and DES diphosphonate

Additional Information Neoplasms associated with diethylstilbestrol use include renal, hepatic, angiosarcoma, breast, and clear-cell adenocarcinoma of the genital tract in women exposed to diethylstilbestrol *in utero*. The benefits of postmenopausal estrogen therapy may be substantial for some women. Diethylstilbestrol is not the drug of choice for vasomotor symptoms, to prevent bone loss, or to treat vaginal atrophy or urinary incontinence secondary to estrogen deficiency. Diethylstilbestrol does have a role in the treatment of inoperable, progressive prostatic carcinoma and inoperable, progressive breast cancer in select men and women. Risk of developing vaginal or cervical adenocarcinoma is 3 times greater with *in utero* exposure during first trimester as compared with fetal exposure after 13 weeks. *In utero* exposure to diethylstilbestrol does not appear to affect fertility or sexual function in males.

Diethyltoluamide

CAS Number 134-62-3

U.S. Brand Names OFF®

Synonyms 3-Methyl-N,N-Diethylbenzamide; Benzamide; DEET; Diethylamide; M-delphene; M-det; M-deta; M-Toluamide; M-Toluic Acid Diethylamide; Metadelphene; MGK Diethyltoluamide; N,N-Diethyl-3-Methyl-Diethyl-M-Toluamide; N,N-Diethyl-M-Toluamide; N,N-Diethyl-M-Toluic Acid

Commonly Found In Some formulations use as vehicles ethyl and isopropyl alcohols and freon, which may contribute significantly to toxicity

Use Insect repellent against mosquitoes, ticks, fleas, leeches, blackflies; used since 1957

Adverse Reactions
Cardiovascular: Hypotension, bradycardia, Reye's syndrome, sinus bradycardia
Central nervous system: Psychosis, seizures, coma, drowsiness, headache, mania, slurred speech, ataxia
Dermatologic: Urticaria, skin necrosis, bullous eruption
Gastrointestinal: Nausea, vomiting
Hepatic: Hepatic necrosis, steatosis
Neuromuscular & skeletal: Tremors, myoclonus, athetosis, hypertonicity
Miscellaneous: Anaphylactic shock

Signs and Symptoms of Overdose Coma and seizures may occur rapidly within 30-60 minutes after ingestion.
Abdominal pain, acute psychosis, anaphylactic shock, ataxia, bradycardia, bullous eruption/skin necrosis, burning sensation (eyes, lips, tongue, mouth), cerebral edema, clonic jerking, coma, confusion, contact rash, hypertonicity, hypotension, nausea, renal damage, seizures, skin irritation, toxic hepatitis, urticaria, vomiting

Toxicodynamics/Kinetics
Onset of action: Oral: Rapid
Absorption: Oral: Rapid. Topical: Within 6 hours
Distribution: Skin and fatty tissues retain DEET and its metabolites for 1-2 months after topical application and may act as reservoirs for DEET
Metabolism: Occurs in the liver by oxidative enzymes
Peak plasma concentration: 1 hour

Monitoring Parameters Monitor for renal and hepatic dysfunction with chronic oral and dermal exposures; consider CT and LP to rule out other causes for neurologic effects; sterile CSF pleocytosis, usually with lymphocytic predominance, has been associated with DEET
Significant and severe toxicity has occurred following both dermal and oral exposures to large amounts of DEET

Reference Range DEET serum level 8 hours after dermal application: 0.3 mg/dL (0.016 mM/L) in asymptomatic patient; serum concentration of DEET of 63 mg/L associated with hypotension, lethargy, and ECG changes (S-T abnormalities); serum DEET level of 168 mg/L to 239 mg/L associated with fatality

Overdosage/Treatment
Decontamination: **Oral**: Syrup of ipecac/emesis is contraindicated following oral ingestions due to rapid onset of coma and seizures; cautious gastric lavage (within 1 hour) followed by activated charcoal. **Dermal**: Topical corticosteroid or oral antihistamines can be used for dermal reaction.
Supportive therapy: Diazepam or lorazepam for seizures; phenobarbital for recurrent seizures. For dermal exposures, wash twice with copious amounts of soap and water, preferably using alcohol-detergent solutions such as "green soap". If irritation or pain persists after washing, consult physician to examine affected area. For eye exposure, irrigate with copious amounts of tepid water for at least 15 minutes. Patients should seek medical advice if irritation, pain, swelling, lacrimation, or photophobia persists.
Enhancement of elimination: Lipid based hemodialysis may be helpful, although there is no data on this modality.

Additional Information Severe toxicity occurred in a child 1 year of age following oral ingestion of 25 mL of 50% DEET. Severe toxicity and death occurred following oral ingestion of 50 mL of 100% DEET in adolescents or adults. Extensive daily dermal applications of 10% to 15% solutions for 2 days to 3 months have resulted in encephalopathy in children.
National DEET Registry (Pegus Research, Inc), Salt Lake City, UT, (800)-949-0089

Specific References
Cherstniakova SA, Garcia GE, Strong J, et al, "Rapid Determination of N,N-Diethyl-m-Toluamide and Permethrin in Human Plasma by Gas Chromatography-Mass Spectrometry and Pyridostigmine Bromide by High-Performance Liquid Chromatography," *J Anal Toxicol*, 2006, 30:21-30.
Sudakin DL and Trevathan WR, "DEET: A Review and Update of Safety and Risk in the General Population," *J Toxicol Clin Toxicol*, 2003, 41(6):831-9.

Diflunisal

Pronunciation (dye FLOO ni sal)

Related Information
• Nonsteroidal Anti-inflammatory Drugs

CAS Number 22494-42-4

U.S. Brand Names Dolobid®

Use Management of inflammatory disorders usually including rheumatoid arthritis and osteoarthritis; can be used as an analgesic for treatment of mild to moderate pain. Difluorophenyl derivative of salicyclic acid.

Mechanism of Action Inhibits prostaglandin synthesis by decreasing the activity of the enzyme, cyclooxygenase, which results in decreased formation of prostaglandin precursors

Adverse Reactions
Cardiovascular: Tachycardia, palpitations, sinus tachycardia, vasculitis
Central nervous system: Dizziness, somnolence, insomnia, **headache**
Dermatologic: Rash, pruritus, Stevens-Johnson syndrome, toxic epidermal necrolysis, exfoliative dermatitis, alopecia, angioedema, bullous skin disease, urticaria, purpura, onycholysis, licheniform eruptions, exanthem
Endocrine & metabolic: **Fluid retention**
Gastrointestinal: Nausea, dyspepsia, GI pain, diarrhea, vomiting, constipation, flatulence, GI bleeding/perforation, aphthous stomatitis, xerostomia
Genitourinary: Dysuria
Hepatic: Intrahepatic cholestasis
Neuromuscular & skeletal: Paresthesia
Otic: Tinnitus (rare)
Renal: Interstitial nephritis, hematuria, albuminuria
Respiratory: Tachypnea, eosinophilic pneumonitis, pulmonary vasculitis
Miscellaneous: Hypersensitivity reactions, diaphoresis, fixed drug eruption

Signs and Symptoms of Overdose Chills, cholestatic jaundice, coagulopathy, coma, confusion, depression, dermatitis, drowsiness, eosinophilia, erythema multiforme, fever, gastritis, GI bleeding, hematuria, hyperthermia, hyperventilation, insomnia, lightheadedness, malaise, myalgia, nausea, nephritis, nephrotic syndrome, neutropenia, ototoxicity, photosensitivity, stomatitis, stupor, tachycardia, thrombocytopenia, tinnitus, toxic epidermal necrolysis, vomiting, wheezing

Pharmacodynamics/Kinetics
Onset of action: Analgesic: ~1 hour; maximal effect: 2-3 hours
Duration: 8-12 hours
Absorption: Well absorbed
Protein binding: >99%
Distribution: Enters breast milk
Metabolism: Extensively hepatic; metabolic pathways are saturable
Half-life elimination: 8-12 hours; prolonged with renal impairment
Time to peak, serum: 2-3 hours
Excretion: Urine (~3% as unchanged drug, 90% as glucuronide conjugates) within 72-96 hours

Dosage

Adults: Oral:

Pain: Initial: 500-1000 mg followed by 250-500 mg every 8-12 hours; maximum daily dose: 1.5 g

Inflammatory condition: 500-1000 mg/day in 2 divided doses; maximum daily dose: 1.5 g

Dosing adjustment in renal impairment: Cl_{cr} <50 mL/minute: Administer 50% of normal dose

Administration

Tablet should be swallowed whole; do not crush or chew.

Contraindications Hypersensitivity to diflunisal, aspirin, other NSAIDs, or any component of the formulation; perioperative pain in the setting of coronary artery bypass surgery (CABG); pregnancy (3rd trimester)

Warnings [U.S. Boxed Warning]: NSAIDs are associated with an increased risk of adverse cardiovascular events, including MI, stroke, and new onset or worsening of pre-existing hypertension. Risk may be increased with duration of use or pre-existing cardiovascular risk-factors or disease. Carefully evaluate individual cardiovascular risk profiles prior to prescribing. Use caution with fluid retention, CHF, or hypertension.

[U.S. Boxed Warning]: NSAIDs may increase risk of gastrointestinal irritation, ulceration, bleeding, and perforation. These events may occur at any time during therapy and without warning. Use caution with a history of GI disease (bleeding or ulcers), concurrent therapy with aspirin, anticoagulants and/or corticosteroids, smoking, use of alcohol, the elderly or debilitated patients.

Use of NSAIDs can compromise existing renal function. Renal toxicity can occur in patient with impaired renal function, dehydration, heart failure, liver dysfunction, those taking diuretics and ACEI and the elderly. Rehydrate patient before starting therapy. Monitor renal function closely. Diflunisal is not recommended for patients with advanced renal disease.

Use the lowest effective dose for the shortest duration of time, consistent with individual patient goals, to reduce risk of cardiovascular or GI adverse events. Alternate therapies should be considered for patients at high risk.

NSAIDs may cause serious skin adverse events including exfoliative dermatitis, Stevens-Johnson syndrome (SJS), and toxic epidermal necrolysis (TEN). Anaphylactoid reactions may occur, even without prior exposure; patients with "aspirin triad" (bronchial asthma, aspirin intolerance, rhinitis) may be at increased risk. Do not use in patients who experience bronchospasm, asthma, rhinitis, or urticaria with NSAID or aspirin therapy.

A hypersensitivity syndrome has been reported; monitor for constitutional symptoms and cutaneous findings; other organ dysfunction may be involved.

Use with caution in patients with decreased hepatic function. Closely monitor patients with any abnormal LFT. Severe hepatic reactions (eg, fulminant hepatitis, liver failure) have occurred with NSAID use, rarely; discontinue if signs or symptoms of liver disease develop, or if systemic manifestations occur.

Diflunisal is a derivative of acetylsalicylic acid and therefore may be associated with Reye's syndrome. Withhold for at least 4-6 half-lives prior to surgical or dental procedures. Safety and efficacy have not been established in children <12 years of age.

Dosage Forms

[DSC] = Discontinued product

Tablet: 500 mg

Dolobid®: 250 mg, 500 mg [DSC]

Overdosage/Treatment

Decontamination: Lavage/activated charcoal

Supportive therapy: Management of a nonsteroidal anti-inflammatory agent (NSAID) intoxication is primarily supportive and symptomatic. Fluid therapy is commonly effective in managing the hypotension that may occur following an acute NSAID overdose, except when this is due to an acute blood loss.

Enhancement of elimination: NSAID: Forced diuresis/hemodialysis are of no benefit

Test Interactions ↑ prothrombin time; ↓ uric acid (S); may cross-react with some salicylate assays

Drug Interactions

ACE inhibitors: Antihypertensive effects may be decreased by concurrent therapy with NSAIDs; monitor blood pressure.

Aminoglycosides: NSAIDs may decrease the excretion of aminoglycosides.

Angiotensin II antagonists: Antihypertensive effects may be decreased by concurrent therapy with NSAIDs; monitor blood pressure.

Anticoagulants (warfarin, heparin, LMWHs) in combination with NSAIDs can cause increased risk of bleeding.

Antiplatelet agents (ticlopidine, clopidogrel, aspirin, abciximab, dipyridamole, eptifibatide, tirofiban) can cause an increased risk of bleeding.

Beta-blockers: NSAIDs may diminish the antihypertensive effects of beta blockers.

Bisphosphonates: NSAIDs may increase the risk of gastrointestinal ulceration.

Cholestyramine (and other bile acid sequestrants): May decrease the absorption of NSAIDs. Separate by at least 2 hours.

Corticosteroids may increase the risk of GI ulceration; avoid concurrent use.

Cyclosporine: NSAIDs may increase serum creatinine, potassium, blood pressure, and cyclosporine levels; monitor cyclosporine levels and renal function carefully.

Hydralazine's antihypertensive effect is decreased; avoid concurrent use.

Lithium levels can be increased; avoid concurrent use if possible or monitor lithium levels and adjust dose.

Sulindac may have the least effect. When NSAID is stopped, lithium will need adjustment again.

Loop diuretics efficacy (diuretic and antihypertensive effect) is reduced. Indomethacin reduces this efficacy, however, it may be anticipated with any NSAID.

Methotrexate: Severe bone marrow suppression, aplastic anemia, and GI toxicity have been reported with concomitant NSAID therapy. Avoid use during moderate or high-dose methotrexate (increased and prolonged methotrexate levels). NSAID use during low-dose treatment of rheumatoid arthritis has not been fully evaluated; extreme caution is warranted.

Pemetrexed: NSAIDs may decrease the excretion of pemetrexed. Patients with Cl_{cr} 45-79 mL/minute should avoid long acting NSAIDs for 5 days before and 2 days after pemetrexed treatment.

Thiazides antihypertensive effects are decreased; avoid concurrent use.

Treprostinil: May enhance the risk of bleeding with concurrent use.

Vancomycin: NSAID's may decrease the excretion of vancomycin.

Pregnancy Risk Factor C (1st and 2nd trimesters); D (3rd trimester)

Pregnancy Implications C (first and second trimester); D (third trimester)

Lactation Enters breast milk/not recommended

Additional Information Fewer GI and antiplatelet effects as opposed to salicyclate

Specific References

Proudfoot AT, Krenzelok EP, Vale JA, et al, "AACT/EAPCCT Position Paper on Urine Alkalinization," *J Toxicol Clin Toxicol*, 2004, 42(1):1-26.

Digitoxin

Related Information

- Ouabain

CAS Number 71-63-6

Synonyms Crystodigin

Use Congestive heart failure, fibrillation (atrial), flutter (atrial), paroxysmal atrial tachycardia, and cardiogenic shock

Mechanism of Action Indirect effect through vagal stimulation. Most clinically important actions of digitalis on the S-A and AV nodes are mediated through the autonomic nervous system. Digitalis increases efferent vagal impulses, reflexly reduces sympathetic tone, and decreases the sinus rate. In a normal heart, the augmented vagal activity decreases the rate of generation of impulses in the S-A node. A decrease in sinus rate may not occur, but the maximum heart rate achieved during exercise is diminished. When the sinus rate is increased due to heart failure, digitalis has prominent negative chronotropic effects.

Adverse Reactions

Cardiovascular: Sinus bradycardia, AV block, S-A block, ectopic beats (atrial or nodal), arrhythmias (ventricular), bigeminy, trigeminy, tachycardia (atrial) with AV block, superior mesenteric artery thrombosis, QRS prolongation, sinus tachycardia, tachycardia (supraventricular), bidirectional ventricular tachycardia

Central nervous system: Drowsiness, fatigue, drowsiness, disorientation, dizziness, visual hallucinations, headache, psychosis

Dermatologic: Stevens-Johnson syndrome, exanthem

Endocrine & metabolic: Hyperkalemia with acute toxicity

Gastrointestinal: Vomiting, nausea, feeding intolerance, anorexia, abdominal pain, diarrhea, feces discoloration (black), colonic ischemia

Hematologic: Thrombocytopenia

Neuromuscular & skeletal: Neuralgia

Ocular: Blurred vision, halos, yellow or green vision, diplopia, photophobia, flashing lights, decreased visual acuity

Signs and Symptoms of Overdose Arrhythmias, asystole, AV block, bowel ischemia, delirium, depression, fibrillation (ventricular), gynecomastia, hyperkalemia, hypotension, neuropathy (peripheral), ototoxicity, photophobia, tachycardia (ventricular), tachycardia (ventricular, bidirectional), tinnitus, tremor, vision color changes (blue tinge; green tinge; orange tinge; red tinge; yellow tinge)

Pharmacodynamics/Kinetics

Absorption: 90% to 100%

Distribution: V_d: 7 L/kg

Protein binding: 90% to 97%

Metabolism: Hepatic (50% to 70%)

Half-life elimination: 7-8 days

Time to peak: 8-12 hours

Excretion: Urine and feces (30% to 50% as unchanged drug)

Dosage Oral:

Children: Doses are very individualized; **when recommended**, digitalizing dose is as follows:

<1 year: 0.045 mg/kg

1-2 years: 0.04 mg/kg

>2 years: 0.03 mg/kg which is equivalent to 0.75 mg/m^2

Maintenance: Approximately $^1/_{10}$ of the digitalizing dose

Adults:

Rapid loading dose: Initial: 0.6 mg followed by 0.4 mg and then 0.2 mg at intervals of 4-6 hours

Slow loading dose: 0.2 mg twice daily for a period of 4 days followed by a maintenance dose

Maintenance: 0.05-0.3 mg/day

Most common dose: 0.15 mg/day

Dosing adjustment in renal impairment: Cl_{cr} <10 mL/minute: Administer 50% to 75% of normal dose.

Hemodialysis: Not dialyzable (0% to 5%)

Dosing adjustment in hepatic impairment: Dosage reduction is necessary in severe liver disease.

Stability Insoluble in water

Monitoring Parameters Monitor blood pressure and ECG closely

Contraindications Hypersensitivity to digitoxin or any component (rare); digitalis toxicity; beriberi heart disease; AV block; idiopathic hypertrophic subaortic stenosis; constrictive pericarditis; ventricular fibrillation; ventricular tachycardia

Warnings Use with caution in patients with hypoxia, hypothyroidism, or acute myocarditis. Do not use to treat obesity. Patients with incomplete AV block (Stokes-Adams attack) may progress to complete block with digitalis drug administration. Use with caution in patients with acute myocardial infarction, severe pulmonary disease, idiopathic hypertrophic subaortic stenosis, Wolff-Parkinson-White syndrome, sick sinus syndrome (bradyarrhythmias), amyloid heart disease, and constrictive cardiomyopathies. Adjust dose with renal or hepatic impairment and aged patients. Elderly may develop exaggerated serum/tissue concentrations due to decreased lean body mass, total body water, and age-related reduction in renal/hepatic function. Exercise will reduce serum concentrations of digoxin due to increased skeletal muscle uptake.

Dosage Forms Tablet: 0.1 mg, 0.2 mg

Reference Range

Therapeutic: 18-22 ng/mL (23-28 nmol/L)

Toxic: >25 ng/mL (>32 nmol/L)

Overdosage/Treatment

Decontamination: Lavage (within 1 hour)/activated charcoal

Supportive therapy: Antidote: Life-threatening digoxin toxicity is treated with Digibind®; ventricular pacing should be reserved for those patients not responding to Digibind®; torsade de pointes can be treated with magnesium sulfate and overdrive pacing (try to avoid isoproterenol)

Enhancement of elimination: Since enterohepatic recirculation accounts for a low percentage of digitoxin metabolism (6.6%/day), cholestyramine or multiple dosing of activated charcoal would have virtually no effect on decreasing half-life; not dialyzable (0% to 5%); although hemodialysis is not useful, charcoal hemoperfusion (clearance ~30 mL/minute) can increase total body clearance of the drug 8-20 times (14% of drug removed during 4 hours)

Antidote(s)

● Cholestyramine Resin [ANTIDOTE]

● Digoxin Immune Fab [ANTIDOTE]

Diagnostic Procedures

● Digitoxin, Blood

Test Interactions Digibind® increases serum digitoxin level tenfold; digitoxin may interfere with a urinary 17-hydroxycorticosteroid assay; digoxin-like immunoreactive substance (DLIS), an endogenous natriuretic substance, may cause false elevation

Drug Interactions **Substrate** of CYP3A4 (major)

Amiloride may reduce the inotropic response to digitoxin.

Amiodarone reduces renal and nonrenal clearance of digitoxin and may have additive effects on heart rate.

Beta-blocking agents (propranolol) may have additive effects on heart rate.

Calcium preparations: Rare cases of acute digitalis glycoside toxicity have been associated with parental calcium (bolus) administration.

Cholestyramine, colestipol, kaolin-pectin may reduce digitoxin absorption.

CYP3A4 inducers: CYP3A4 inducers may decrease the levels/effects of digitoxin. Example inducers include aminoglutethimide, carbamazepine, nafcillin, nevirapine, phenobarbital, phenytoin, and rifamycins.

CYP3A4 inhibitors: May increase the levels/effects of digitoxin. Example inhibitors include azole antifungals, clarithromycin, diclofenac, doxycycline, erythromycin, imatinib, isoniazid, nefazodone, nicardipine, propofol, protease inhibitors, quinidine, telithromycin, and verapamil.

Levothyroxine (and other thyroid supplements) may decrease digitoxin blood levels.

Moricizine may increase the toxicity of digitalis glycosides (mechanism undefined).

Propafenone increases digoxin blood levels. Effects may also occur with digitoxin. Monitor closely.

Propylthiouracil and methimazole may increase digitoxin blood levels by reducing thyroid hormone.

Quinidine increases digitoxin blood levels substantially; monitor blood levels/effect closely. Other related agents (hydroxychloroquine, quinine) should be used with caution.

Verapamil, diltiazem, bepridil, and nitrendipine increase digoxin concentrations, and may have similar effect on digitoxin. Other calcium channel blocking agents do not appear to share this effect.

Drugs which cause hypokalemia (thiazide and loop diuretics, amphotericin B): Hypokalemia may potentiate toxicity of digitalis glycosides.

These medications have been associated with reduced blood levels of digitalis glycosides which appear to be of limited clinical significance: Aminoglutethimide, antacids (magnesium- and aluminum-containing), sucralfate, sulfasalazine, ticlopidine.

These medications have been associated with increased digitalis glycoside blood levels which appear to be of limited clinical significance: Famciclovir, flecainide, ibuprofen, itraconazole, cimetidine, famotidine, fluoxetine, nefazodone, omeprazole, ranitidine, trimethoprim.

Pregnancy Risk Factor C

Nursing Implications Check apical pulse before administering

Additional Information Not available in U.S.

Digoxin

Related Information

● Ouabain

● Therapeutic Drugs Associated with Hallucinations

CAS Number 20830-75-5

U.S. Brand Names Digitek®; Lanoxicaps®; Lanoxin®

Use Treatment of congestive heart failure; slows the ventricular rate in tachyarrhythmias such as fibrillation (atrial), flutter (atrial), tachycardia (ventricular), paroxysmal atrial tachycardia, cardiogenic shock

Mechanism of Action Increases the influx of calcium ions, from extracellular to intracellular cytoplasm by inhibition of sodium and potassium ion movement across the myocardial membranes; this increase in calcium ions results in a potentiation of the activity of the contractile heart muscle fibers and an increase in the force of myocardial contraction (positive inotropic effect); inhibits adenosine triphosphatase (ATPase); decreases conduction through the S-A and AV nodes

Adverse Reactions

Cardiovascular: Sinus bradycardia, AV block, S-A block, ectopic beats (atrial or nodal), tachycardia (ventricular), arrhythmias (ventricular), bigeminy, trigeminy, tachycardia (atrial) with AV block, superior mesenteric artery thrombosis, QRS prolongation, sinus tachycardia, tachycardia (supraventricular), vasculitis, tachycardia (ventricular, bidirectional)

Central nervous system: Drowsiness, fatigue, disorientation, dizziness, auditory and visual hallucinations, paranoia, headache, psychosis, cerebral arteritis, extrapyramidal reaction

Dermatologic: Stevens-Johnson syndrome, bullous skin disease, urticaria, purpura, pruritus, psoriasis, exanthem

Endocrine & metabolic: Toxicity is enhanced by hypokalemia

Gastrointestinal: Vomiting, nausea, feeding intolerance, anorexia, abdominal pain, diarrhea, fecal discoloration (black), colonic ischemia, esophagitis

Hematologic: Thrombocytopenia

Neuromuscular & skeletal: Neuralgia, chorea (extrapyramidal)

Ocular: Blurred vision, halos, yellow or green vision, diplopia, photophobia, flashing lights, decreased visual acuity, color vision abnormalities

Signs and Symptoms of Overdose AV block, arrhythmias, bowel ischemia, delirium, dementia, depression, dysphagia, fibrillation (ventricular) or asystole, gynecomastia, heart block, hyperkalemia, hypokalemia, hypotension, impotence, neuropathy (peripheral), night terrors, ototoxicity, photophobia, seizures, tachycardia (ventricular, bidirectional), tinnitus, tremors, vision color changes (blue tinge; green tinge; orange tinge; red tinge)

Pharmacodynamics/Kinetics

Onset of action: Oral: 1-2 hours; I.V.: 5-30 minutes

Peak effect: Oral: 2-8 hours; I.V.: 1-4 hours

Duration: Adults: 3-4 days both forms

Absorption: By passive nonsaturable diffusion in the upper small intestine; food may delay, but does not affect extent of absorption

Distribution:

Normal renal function: 6-7 L/kg

V_d: Extensive to peripheral tissues, with a distinct distribution phase which lasts 6-8 hours; concentrates in heart, liver, kidney, skeletal muscle, and intestines. Heart/serum concentration is 70:1. Pharmacologic effects are delayed and do not correlate well with serum concentrations during distribution phase.

Hyperthyroidism: Increased V_d

Hyperkalemia, hyponatremia: Decreased digoxin distribution to heart and muscle

Hypokalemia: Increased digoxin distribution to heart and muscles

Concomitant quinidine therapy: Decreased V_d

Chronic renal failure: 4-6 L/kg

Decreased sodium/potassium ATPase activity - decreased tissue binding
Neonates, full-term: 7.5-10 L/kg
Children: 16 L/kg
Adults: 7 L/kg, decreased with renal disease
Protein binding: 30%; in uremic patients, digoxin is displaced from plasma protein binding sites
Metabolism: Via sequential sugar hydrolysis in the stomach or by reduction of lactone ring by intestinal bacteria (in ~10% of population, gut bacteria may metabolize up to 40% of digoxin dose); metabolites may contribute to therapeutic and toxic effects of digoxin; metabolism is reduced with CHF
Bioavailability: Oral (formulation dependent): Elixir: 75% to 85%; Tablet: 70% to 80%
Half-life elimination (age, renal and cardiac function dependent):
Neonates: Premature: 61-170 hours; Full-term: 35-45 hours
Infants: 18-25 hours
Children: 35 hours
Adults: 38-48 hours
Adults, anephric: 4-6 days
Half-life elimination: Parent drug: 38 hours; Metabolites: Digoxigenin: 4 hours; Monodigitoxoside: 3-12 hours
Time to peak, serum: Oral: ~1 hour
Excretion: Urine (50% to 70% as unchanged drug)

Toxicodynamics/Kinetics
Onset of action: Oral: 1-2 hours; I.V.: 5-30 minutes;
Peak effect: Oral: 2-8 hours; I.V.: 1-4 hours
Duration: Adults: 3-4 days
Distribution: Minimal to body fat; high concentrations in myocardium, skeletal muscle, and kidney; crosses blood-brain barrier
V_d: Neonates, premature: 4.5 L/kg; Neonates, full-term: 7.5-10 L/kg; Children: 16 L/kg; Adults: 7 L/kg; decreased V_d with renal disease
Protein binding: 23%
Metabolism: Small amount in the liver and gut by bacteria
Bioavailability: Dependent upon formulation, elixir: 70% to 85%, tablets: 60% to 80%, capsules: 90% to 100%
Half-life: Dependent upon age, renal and cardiac function: Premature: 61-170 hours; Neonates, full-term: 35-45 hours; Infants: 18-25 hours; Children: 35 hours; Adults: 38-48 hours; Anephric: >4.5 days
Elimination: 50% to 70% excreted unchanged in urine; ~7% of the drug is normally excreted in 4 hours in a healthy person

Dosage When changing from oral (tablets or liquid) or I.M. to I.V. therapy, dosage should be reduced by 20% to 25%. See table.

Dosage Recommendations for Digoxin*

Age	Total Digitalizing Dose† (mcg/kg)		Daily Maintenance Dose‡ (mcg/kg)	
	P.O.	I.V. or I.M.	P.O.	I.V. or I.M.
Preterm infant	20-30	15-25	5-7.5	4-6
Full term infant	25-35	20-30	6-10	5-8
1 mo-2 y	35-60	30-50	10-15	7.5-12
2-5 y	30-40	25-35	7.5-10	6-9
5-10 y	20-35	15-30	5-10	4-8
>10 y	10-15	8-12	2.5-5	2-3
Adult	0.75-1.5 mg	0.5-1 mg	0.125-0.5 mg	0.1-0.4 mg

*Based on lean body weight and normal renal function for age. Decrease dose in patients with decreased renal function.
†Give one-half of the total digitalizing dose (TDD) in the initial dose, then give one-quarter of the TDD in each of two subsequent doses at 8- to 12-hour intervals. Obtain EKG 6 hours after each dose to assess potential toxicity.
‡Divided every 12 hours in infants and children <10 years of age. Given once daily to children >10 years and adults.

Dosing adjustment/interval in renal impairment:
Cl_{cr} 10-50 mL/minute: Administer 25% to 75% of dose or every 36 hours
Cl_{cr} <10 mL/minute: Administer 10% to 25% of dose or every 48 hours
Reduce loading dose by 50% in ESRD
Stability Protect elixir and injection from light; solution compatibility: D_5W, $D_{10}W$, NS, sterile water for injection (when diluted fourfold or greater)
Monitoring Parameters When to draw serum digoxin concentrations: Digoxin serum concentrations are monitored because digoxin possesses a narrow therapeutic serum range; the therapeutic endpoint is difficult to quantify and digoxin toxicity may be life-threatening. Digoxin serum levels should be drawn **at least 4 hours after an intravenous dose** and **at least 6 hours after an oral dose (optimally 12-24 hours after a dose).**
Initiation of therapy:

If a loading dose is given: Digoxin serum concentration may be drawn within 12-24 hours after the initial loading dose administration. Levels drawn this early may confirm the relationship of digoxin plasma levels and response but are of little value in determining maintenance doses.
If a loading dose is not given: Digoxin serum concentration should be obtained after 3-5 days of therapy
Maintenance therapy:
Trough concentrations should be followed just prior to the next dose or at a minimum of 4 hours after an I.V. dose and at least 6 hours after an oral dose
Digoxin serum concentrations should be obtained within 5-7 days (approximate time to steady-state) after any dosage changes. Continue to obtain digoxin serum concentrations 7-14 days after any change in maintenance dose. **Note:** In patients with end-stage renal disease, it may take 15-20 days to reach steady-state.
Additionally, patients who are receiving potassium-depleting medications such as diuretics, should be monitored for potassium, magnesium, and calcium levels
Digoxin serum concentrations should be obtained whenever any of the following conditions occur:
Questionable patient compliance or to evaluate clinical deterioration following an initial good response
Changing renal function
Suspected digoxin toxicity
Initiation or discontinuation of therapy with drugs (amiodarone, quinidine, verapamil) which potentially interact with digoxin; if quinidine therapy is started; digoxin levels should be drawn within the first 24 hours after starting quinidine therapy, then 7-14 days later or empirically skip one day's digoxin dose and decrease the daily dose by 50%
Any disease changes (hypothyroidism)
Heart rate and rhythm should be monitored along with periodic ECGs to assess both desired effects and signs of toxicity
Follow closely (especially in patients receiving diuretics or amphotericin) for decreased serum potassium and magnesium or increased calcium, all of which predispose to digoxin toxicity
Assess renal function
Be aware of drug interactions
Administration
I.M.: Inject no more than 2 mL per injection site. May cause intense pain.
I.V.: May be administered undiluted or diluted fourfold in D_5W, NS, or SWFI for direct injection. Less than fourfold dilution may permit drug precipitation. Inject slowly 1-5 minutes for undiluted form.
Contraindications Hypersensitivity to digoxin or any component of the formulation; hypersensitivity to cardiac glycosides (another may be tried); history of toxicity; ventricular tachycardia or fibrillation; idiopathic hypertrophic subaortic stenosis; constrictive pericarditis; amyloid disease; second- or third-degree heart block (except in patients with a functioning artificial pacemaker); Wolff-Parkinson-White syndrome and atrial fibrillation concurrently
Warnings Withdrawal in CHF patients may lead to recurrence of CHF symptoms. Some arrhythmias that digoxin is used to treat may be exacerbated in digoxin toxicity. Sinus nodal disease may be worsened. Adjust doses in renal impairment and when verapamil, quinidine or amiodarone are added to a patient on digoxin. Correct hypokalemia and hypomagnesemia before initiating therapy. Calcium, especially when administered rapidly I.V., can produce serious arrhythmias. Atrial arrhythmias associated with hypermetabolic states are very difficult to treat. Rate control in atrial fibrillation may be better in a sedentary patient than an active one. Use with caution in acute MI (within 6 months). Serum concentration monitoring should be done before the next dose (patient can hold AM dose for blood test) for an accurate assessment. Reduce or hold dose 1-2 days before elective electrical cardioversion.
Dosage Forms Capsule:
Lanoxicaps®: 100 mcg, 200 mcg [contains ethyl alcohol]
Injection, solution: 250 mcg/mL (1 mL, 2 mL)
Lanoxin®: 250 mcg/mL (2 mL) [contains alcohol 10% and propylene glycol 40%]
Injection, solution [pediatric]: 100 mcg/mL (1 mL)
Solution, oral: 50 mcg/mL (2.5 mL, 5 mL, 60 mL)
Tablet: 125 mcg, 250 mcg
Digitek®, Lanoxin®: 125 mcg, 250 mcg
Reference Range
Therapeutic: 0.5-2.0 ng/mL (SI: 0.6-2.6 nmol/L); Adults: <0.5 ng/mL (SI: <0.6 nmol/L) probably indicates underdigitalization unless there are special circumstances
Toxic: >2.0 ng/mL (SI: >2.6 nmol/L); fatalities associated with levels >3.5 ng/mL (>4.8 nmol/L)
In the postmortem state, anatomical site concentration differences (ie, postmortem redistribution) may occur.
Overdosage/Treatment
Decontamination: Lavage (within 1 hour)/activated charcoal; whole bowel irrigation may be useful

Supportive therapy: Antidote: Life-threatening digoxin toxicity is treated with Digibind®; phenytoin, magnesium, and lidocaine are useful for cardiac arrhythmias; atropine is useful for bradycardia; avoid quinidine, bretylium, or cardioversion; ventricular pacing should be reserved for patients not responding to Digibind®; delirium can also respond to Digibind®; torsade de pointes can be treated with magnesium sulfate and overdrive pacing (try to avoid isoproterenol)

Enhancement of elimination: Multiple dosing of activated charcoal may be useful but is usually not required if Digibind® is used; exchange transfusion is of no benefit; hemodialysis/hemoperfusion is ineffective; not dialyzable (0% to 5%); multiple doses of cholestyramine (4 g every 4 hours for four doses) can help enhance elimination

Antidote(s)
- Cholestyramine Resin [ANTIDOTE]
- Digoxin Immune Fab [ANTIDOTE]

Diagnostic Procedures
- Digoxin, Blood

Test Interactions Digibind® increases total serum digoxin level ~50-fold; digoxin-like immunoreactive substance (DLIS), an endogenous natriuretic substance, may cause false elevation

Drug Interactions Substrate of CYP3A4 (minor)

Amiloride may reduce the inotropic response to digoxin.

Amiodarone reduces renal and nonrenal clearance of digoxin and may have additive effects on heart rate. Reduce digoxin dose by 50% with start of amiodarone.

Benzodiazepines (alprazolam, diazepam) have been associated with isolated reports of digoxin toxicity.

Beta-blocking agents (propranolol) may have additive effects on heart rate.

Calcium preparations: Rare cases of acute digoxin toxicity have been associated with parenteral calcium (bolus) administration.

Carvedilol may increase digoxin blood levels in addition to potentiating its effects on heart rate.

Cholestyramine, colestipol, kaolin-pectin may reduce digoxin absorption. Separate administration.

Cyclosporine may increase digoxin levels, possibly due to reduced renal clearance.

Erythromycin, clarithromycin, and tetracyclines may increase digoxin (not capsule form) blood levels in a subset of patients.

Indomethacin has been associated with isolated reports of increased digoxin blood levels/toxicity.

Itraconazole may increase digoxin blood levels in some patients; monitor.

Levothyroxine (and other thyroid supplements) may decrease digoxin blood levels.

Metoclopramide may reduce the absorption of digoxin tablets.

Moricizine may increase the toxicity of digoxin (mechanism undefined).

Penicillamine has been associated with reductions in digoxin blood levels

Propafenone increases digoxin blood levels. Effects are highly variable; monitor closely.

Propylthiouracil (and methimazole) may increase digoxin blood levels by reducing thyroid hormone.

Quinidine increases digoxin blood levels substantially. Effect is variable (33% to 50%). Monitor digoxin blood levels/effect closely. Reduce digoxin dose by 50% with start of quinidine. Other related agents (hydroxychloroquine, quinine) should be used with caution.

Spironolactone may interfere with some digoxin assays, but may also increase blood levels directly. However, spironolactone may attenuate the inotropic effect of digoxin. Monitor effects of digoxin closely.

Succinylcholine administration to patients on digoxin has been associated with an increased risk of arrhythmias.

Verapamil diltiazem, bepridil, and nitrendipine increased serum digoxin concentrations. Other calcium channel blocking agents do not appear to share this effect. Reduce digoxin's dose with the start of verapamil.

Drugs which cause hypokalemia (thiazide and loop diuretics, amphotericin B): Hypokalemia may potentiate digoxin toxicity.

These medications have been associated with reduced digoxin blood levels which appear to be of limited clinical significance: Aminoglutethimide, aminosalicylic acid, aluminum-containing antacids, sucralfate, sulfasalazine, neomycin, ticlopidine.

These medications have been associated with increased digoxin blood levels which appear to be of limited clinical significance: Famciclovir, flecainide, ibuprofen, fluoxetine, nefazodone, cimetidine, famotidine, ranitidine, omeprazole, trimethoprim.

Pregnancy Risk Factor C

Pregnancy Implications Crosses the placenta

Lactation Enters breast milk (small amounts)/compatible

Nursing Implications Check apical pulse before administering

Additional Information Lethal dose: Children: 4 mg; Adults: 10 mg; Toxic dose: Oral: 2 mg

Death rate approaches 50% when serum digoxin levels are >6 ng/mL; digoxin-specific antibodies have reversed thrombocytopenia caused by digoxin;

Mean total hospital cost of digoxin toxicity is $4,087.05 ± 2,659.76; mean length of stay: 3.3 ± 1.2 days

Herbs with digoxin-like substances or effects: *Adonis vernalis*, *Apocynum androsaemifolium*, *Apocynum canabinum*, *Asclepias tuberosa*, *Convallaria majalis*, *Cystisus scoparius*, *Digitalis lanata*, *Digitalis purpura*, *Elutherococcus senticosus*, *Kyushin*, *Leonurus cardica*, *Scilla maritima*, *Scrophularia nodosa*, *Strophantus kombe*, *Uzarae radix*, *Crategus* (sp) berries

Specific References

Aaron CK and Stiles P, "Factitious Digoxin Toxicity from Interference with an Automated Immunoassay," *J Toxicol Clin Toxicol*, 2003, 41(5):678.

Bateman DN, "Digoxin-Specific Antibody Fragments: How Much and When?" *Toxicol Rev*, 2004, 23(3):135-43.

Bottei EM, Moreland JG, Gottsch SG, et al, "Accidental Overdose of Digoxin in a 9-Minute-Old Neonate," *J Toxicol Clin Toxicol*, 2004, 42(5):729.

Delacretaz E, "Clinical Practice: Supraventricular Tachycardia," *N Engl J Med*, 2006, 354(10):1039-51 (review).

El-Desoky ES, AL-Ghamdi HA, Halaby FH, et al, "Therapeutic Monitoring of Digoxin and Antiepileptic Drugs in Egypt and Saudi Arabia," *Ther Drug Monit*, 2003, 25(2):211-4.

El-Desoky ES, Madabushi R, Amry Sel-D, et al, "Application of Two-point Assay of Digoxin Serum Concentration in Studying Population Pharmacokinetics in Egyptian Pediatric Patients with Heart Failure: Does It Make Sense?" *Am J Ther*, 2005, 12(4):320-7.

Eisenberg J, "Chronic Digoxin Intoxication and Hypokalemia," *J Toxicol Clin Toxicol*, 2004, 42(5):738.

Eyal D, Molczan KA, and Carroll LS, "Digoxin Toxicity: Pediatric Survival After Asystolic Arrest," *Clin Toxicol (Phila)*, 2005, 43(1):51-4.

Hack JB, Woody JH, Brewer K, et al, "Pilot Study: Use of Calcium Chloride to Treat Hyperkalemia Due to Acute Digoxin Toxicity in a Swine Model," *J Toxicol Clin Toxicol*, 2003, 41(5):696.

Heinrich K, Prendergast HM, and Erickson T, "Chronic Digoxin Toxicity and Significantly Elevated BNP Levels in the Presence of Mild Heart Failure," *Am J Emerg Med*, 2005, 23(4):561-2.

Lien WC, Huang CH, and Chen WJ, "Bidirectional Ventricular Tachycardia Resulting from Digoxin and Amiodarone Treatment of Rapid Atrial Fibrillation," *Am J Emerg Med*, 2004, 22(3):235-6.

Matsumoto K, Ueno K, Nakabayashi T, et al, "Amiodarone Interaction Time Differences with Warfarin and Digoxin," *J Pharm Technol*, 2003, 19:83-90.

Offhaus JM and Judge BS, " Massive Unintentional Digoxin Ingestion Successfully Managed Without the Use of Activated Charcoal or Digoxin-Specific Antibody Fragments," *Clin Toxicol (Phila)*. 2005, 43:650.

Robert R, Frat JP, Veinstein A, et al, "Protective Effect of Medication Bezoar After a Massive Beta-Blocker, Digoxin, and Amitriptyline Poisoning," *Clin Toxicol*, 2005, 43(5):381-2.

Somberg JC and Molnar J, "The Pharmacologic Treatment of Heart Failure," *Am J Ther*, 2004, 11(6):480-8.

Tzimenatos L and Bond GR, "65 Cases of Severe Injury or Death in Children Resulting from Unintentional Therapeutic Error in a Health Care Facility," *Clin Toxicol (Phila)*, 2005, 43:651.

Diltiazem

Related Information
- Calcium Channel Blockers

CAS Number 33286-22-5; 42399-41-7

U.S. Brand Names Cardizem® CD; Cardizem® LA; Cardizem® SR; Cardizem®; Cartia XT™; Dilacor® XR; Diltia XT®; Taztia XT™; Tiazac®

Synonyms Diltiazem Hydrochloride

Use

Oral: Essential hypertension; chronic stable angina or angina from coronary artery spasm

Injection: Atrial fibrillation or atrial flutter; paroxysmal supraventricular tachycardia (PSVT)

Unlabeled/Investigational Use Investigational: Therapy of Duchenne muscular dystrophy

Mechanism of Action A benzothiazepine calcium channel blocker which inhibits calcium ion from entering the "slow channels" or select voltage-sensitive areas of vascular smooth muscle and myocardium during depolarization, producing a relaxation of coronary vascular smooth muscle and coronary vasodilation; increases myocardial oxygen delivery in patients with vasospastic angina

Adverse Reactions

Cardiovascular: Edema* (2% to 15%), AV block, pain, bradycardia, hypotension, vasodilation, extrasystoles, flushing, palpitations, angina, arrhythmia, bundle branch block, congestive heart failure, ECG abnormalities, ventricular extrasystoles, asystole

Central nervous system: Headache* (5% to 12%), dizziness, nervousness, amnesia, depression, abnormal dreams, hallucinations, insomnia, pain, personality change, extrapyramidal symptoms

Dermatologic: Rash, bruising, petechiae, photosensitivity, pruritus, alopecia, angioedema, erythema multiforme, exfoliative dermatitis, purpura, Stevens-Johnson syndrome, toxic epidermal necrolysis

Endocrine & metabolic: Gout, gynecomastia, hyperglycemia, hyperuricemia

Gastrointestinal: Dyspepsia, constipation, vomiting, diarrhea, anorexia, dry mouth, dysgeusia, nausea, weight gain, gingival hyperplasia

Genitourinary: Crystalluria, impotence, nocturia

Hematologic: Bleeding time increased, hemolytic anemia, leukopenia, thrombocytopenia

Hepatic: Alkaline phosphatase increased, LDH increased, SGOT increased, SGPT increased

Local: Injection site reactions: Burning, itching

Neuromuscular & skeletal: Weakness, myalgia, CPK elevated, gait abnormality, muscle cramps, neck rigidity, paresthesia, tremor

Ocular: Amblyopia, retinopathy

Otic: Tinnitus

Renal: Albuminuria, polyuria

Respiratory: Rhinitis, pharyngitis, dyspnea, bronchitis, sinus congestion, epistaxis

Miscellaneous: Allergic reaction

*Represents range for various dosage forms

Signs and Symptoms of Overdose Asystole, AV block, bradycardia, congestive heart failure, constipation, erythema multiforme, gingival hyperplasia, gynecomastia, hyperglycemia, hypotension, hypothermia, mania, myopathy, purpura, toxic epidermal necrolysis

Pharmacodynamics/Kinetics

Onset of action: Oral: Immediate release tablet: 30-60 minutes

Absorption: 70% to 80%

Distribution: V_d: 3-13 L/kg; enters breast milk

Protein binding: 70% to 80%

Metabolism: Hepatic; extensive first-pass effect; following single I.V. injection, plasma concentrations of N-monodesmethyldiltiazem and desacetyldiltiazem are typically undetectable; however, these metabolites accumulate to detectable concentrations following 24-hour constant rate infusion. N-monodesmethyldiltiazem appears to have 20% of the potency of diltiazem; desacetyldiltiazem is about 25% to 50% as potent as the parent compound.

Bioavailability: Oral: ~40%

Half-life elimination: Immediate release tablet: 3-4.5 hours, may be prolonged with renal impairment

Time to peak, serum: Immediate release tablet: 2-4 hours

Excretion: Urine and feces (primarily as metabolites)

Dosage Adults:

Oral:

Angina:

Capsule, extended release (Cardizem® CD, Cartia XT™, Dilacor XR®, Diltia XT™, Tiazac®): Initial: 120-180 mg once daily (maximum dose: 480 mg/day)

Tablet, extended release (Cardizem® LA): 180 mg once daily; may increase at 7- to 14-day intervals (maximum recommended dose: 360 mg/day)

Tablet, immediate release (Cardizem®): Usual starting dose: 30 mg 4 times/day; usual range: 180-360 mg/day

Hypertension:

Capsule, extended release (Cardizem® CD, Cartia XT™, Dilacor XR®, Diltia XT™, Tiazac®): Initial: 180-240 mg once daily; dose adjustment may be made after 14 days; usual dose range (JNC 7): 180-420 mg/day; Tiazac®: usual dose range: 120-540 mg/day

Capsule, sustained release (Cardizem® SR): Initial: 60-120 mg twice daily; dose adjustment may be made after 14 days; usual range: 240-360 mg/day

Tablet, extended release (Cardizem® LA): Initial: 180-240 mg once daily; dose adjustment may be made after 14 days; usual dose range (JNC 7): 120-540 mg/day

Note: Elderly: Patients ≥60 years may respond to a lower initial dose (ie, 120 mg once daily using extended release capsule)

I.V.: Atrial fibrillation, atrial flutter, PSVT:

Initial bolus dose: 0.25 mg/kg actual body weight over 2 minutes (average adult dose: 20 mg)

Repeat bolus dose (may be administered after 15 minutes if the response is inadequate.): 0.35 mg/kg actual body weight over 2 minutes (average adult dose: 25 mg)

Continuous infusion (requires an infusion pump; infusions >24 hours or infusion rates >15 mg/hour are not recommended): Initial infusion rate of 10 mg/hour; rate may be increased in 5 mg/hour increments up to 15 mg/hour as needed; some patients may respond to an initial rate of 5 mg/hour.

If diltiazem injection is administered by continuous infusion for >24 hours, the possibility of decreased diltiazem clearance, prolonged elimination half-life, and increased diltiazem and/or diltiazem metabolite plasma concentrations should be considered.

Conversion from I.V. diltiazem to oral diltiazem: Start oral approximately 3 hours after bolus dose.

Oral dose (mg/day) is approximately equal to [rate (mg/hour) × 3 + 3] × 10.

3 mg/hour = 120 mg/day

5 mg/hour = 180 mg/day

7 mg/hour = 240 mg/day

11 mg/hour = 360 mg/day

Dosing comments in renal/hepatic impairment: Use with caution as extensively metabolized by the liver and excreted in the kidneys and bile.

Dialysis: Not removed by hemo- or peritoneal dialysis; supplemental dose is not necessary.

Monitoring Parameters Liver function tests, blood pressure, ECG

Administration

Oral: Do not crush long acting dosage forms.

Tiazac®: Capsules may be opened and sprinkled on a spoonful of applesauce. Applesauce should be swallowed without chewing, followed by drinking a glass of water.

I.V.: Bolus doses given over 2 minutes with continuous ECG and blood pressure monitoring. Continuous infusion should be via infusion pump.

Contraindications Hypersensitivity to diltiazem or any component of the formulation; sick sinus syndrome; second- or third-degree AV block (except in patients with a functioning artificial pacemaker); hypotension (systolic <90 mm Hg); acute MI and pulmonary congestion

Warnings Concomitant use with beta-blockers or digoxin can result in conduction disturbances. Avoid concurrent I.V. use of diltiazem and a beta-blocker. Use caution in left ventricular dysfunction (can exacerbate condition). Symptomatic hypotension can occur. Use with caution in hepatic or renal dysfunction.

Dosage Forms [DSC] = Discontinued product

Capsule, extended release, as hydrochloride [once-daily dosing]: 120 mg, 180 mg, 240 mg, 300 mg

Cardizem® CD: 120 mg, 180 mg, 240 mg, 300 mg, 360 mg

Cartia XT™: 120 mg, 180 mg, 240 mg, 300 mg

Dilacor® XR, Diltia XT®: 120 mg, 180 mg, 240 mg

Taztia XT™: 120 mg, 180 mg, 240 mg, 300 mg, 360 mg

Tiazac®: 120 mg, 180 mg, 240 mg, 300 mg, 360 mg, 420 mg

Capsule, sustained release, as hydrochloride [twice-daily dosing] (Cardizem® SR [DSC]): 60 mg, 90 mg, 120 mg

Injection, solution, as hydrochloride: 5 mg/mL (5 mL, 10 mL, 25 mL)

Injection, powder for reconstitution, as hydrochloride (Cardizem®): 25 mg

Tablet, as hydrochloride (Cardizem®): 30 mg, 60 mg, 90 mg, 120 mg

Tablet, extended release, as hydrochloride (Cardizem® LA): 120 mg, 180 mg, 240 mg, 300 mg, 360 mg, 420 mg

Reference Range Zero order kinetics are noted with massive ingestion relating to plasma levels >2000 ng/mL; therapeutic serum diltiazem levels: 50-200 ng/mL; peak plasma diltiazem and desacetyldiltiazem plasma levels following a 14.94 g (150 mg/kg) diltiazem overdose were 7044 ng/mL and 1837.55 ng/mL, respectively; this was associated with cardiogenic shock and asystole

Overdosage/Treatment

Multiple doses may be necessary with SR products. Whole bowel irrigation may be used; monitor bowel sounds and blood pressure.

Decontamination: Lavage (within 1 hour)/activated charcoal is useful; ipecac-induced emesis can hypothetically worsen calcium antagonist toxicity, since it can produce vagal stimulation. The potential for seizures precipitously following acute ingestion of large doses of a calcium antagonist may also contraindicate the use of ipecac.

Supportive therapy: Supportive and symptomatic treatment, including I.V. fluids and Trendelenburg positioning, should be initiated as intoxication may cause hypotension. Intra-aortic balloon pump may be useful. Calcium (calcium chloride I.V. 1-3 g in adults or 10-30 mg/kg in children over 5-10 minutes with repeats as needed) has been used as a treatment for acute intoxications, it should be reserved for those cases where definite signs of myocardial depression are evident and as a second line therapy for refractory hypotension following use of vasopressors. Hyperinsulinemic therapy with 0.5-1.0 unit I.V. insulin bolus with an infusion of 0.2-1 unit/kg/hour plus a glucose bolus of 25 g I.V. and dextrose infusion to maintain a serum glucose >100 mg/dL may reverse cardiogenic shock due to calcium blockers. Diltiazem may be particularly unresponsive to calcium; heart block may respond to isoproterenol, glucagon, atropine and/or calcium, although a temporary pacemaker may be required. Hypotension can be treated with norepinephrine, dopamine, or amrinone; use diazepam or lorazepam for seizures. Glucagon may increase myocardial contractility.

Enhancement of elimination: Multiple dosing of activated charcoal may not be effective; charcoal hemoperfusion may not be effective; following $3^1/_2$ hours of charcoal hemoperfusion, diltiazem levels fell from 1100 ng/mL to 375 ng/mL in one case; thus, therapeutic effectiveness of this modality is questionable. Albumin dialysis using molecular adsorbents recirculating system (MARS®) may assist in improving hemodynamic status.

Vasopressin (20 IU bolus I.V. titrated by blood pressure to 4 to 5 IU/hour infusion) can increase systemic vascular resistance and cardiac output.

Antidote(s)

- Glucagon [ANTIDOTE]

Drug Interactions **Substrate** of CYP2C9 p-glycoprotein (minor), 2D6 (minor), 3A4 p-glycoprotein (major); **Inhibits** CYP2C9 p-glycoprotein (weak), 2D6 (weak), 3A4 p-glycprotein (moderate)

Alfentanil's plasma concentration is increased. Fentanyl and sufentanil may be affected similarly.

Amiodarone use may lead to bradycardia, other conduction delays, and decreased cardiac output; monitor closely if using together.

Azole antifungals may inhibit the calcium channel blocker's metabolism; avoid this combination. Try an antifungal like terbinafine (if appropriate) or monitor closely for altered effect of the calcium channel blocker.

Benzodiazepines (midazolam, triazolam) plasma concentrations are increased by diltiazem; monitor for prolonged CNS depression.

Beta-blockers may have increased pharmacodynamic interactions with diltiazem (see Warnings/Precautions).

Buspirone: Diltiazem may increase serum levels of buspirone; monitor.

Calcium may reduce the calcium channel blocker's effects, particularly hypotension.

Carbamazepine's serum concentration is increased and toxicity may result; avoid this combination.

Cimetidine reduced diltiazem's metabolism; consider an alternative H$_2$ antagonist.

Cyclosporine's serum concentrations are increased by diltiazem; avoid the combination. Use another calcium channel blocker or monitor cyclosporine trough levels and renal function closely.

CYP3A4 inducers: CYP3A4 inducers may decrease the levels/effects of diltiazem. Example inducers include aminoglutethimide, carbamazepine, nafcillin, nevirapine, phenobarbital, phenytoin, and rifamycins.

CYP3A4 inhibitors: May increase the levels/effects of diltiazem. Example inhibitors include azole antifungals, clarithromycin, diclofenac, doxycycline, erythromycin, imatinib, isoniazid, nefazodone, nicardipine, propofol, protease inhibitors, quinidine, telithromycin, and verapamil.

CYP3A4 substrates: Diltiazem may increase the levels/effects of CYP3A4 substrates. Example substrates include benzodiazepines, calcium channel blockers, cyclosporine, mirtazapine, nateglinide, nefazodone, sildenafil (and other PDE-5 inhibitors), tacrolimus, and venlafaxine. Selected benzodiazepines (midazolam and triazolam), cisapride, ergot alkaloids, selected HMG-CoA reductase inhibitors (lovastatin and simvastatin), and pimozide are generally contraindicated with strong CYP3A4 inhibitors.

Digoxin's serum concentration can be increased in some patients; monitor for increased effects of digoxin.

HMG-CoA reductase inhibitors (atorvastatin, lovastatin, simvastatin): Serum concentration will likely be increased; consider pravastatin/fluvastatin or a second generation dihydropyridine calcium channel blocker as an alternative.

Lithium neurotoxicity may result when diltiazem is added; monitor lithium levels.

Moricizine's serum concentration is increased; monitor clinical response closely.

Nafcillin decreases plasma concentration of diltiazem; avoid this combination.

Nitroprusside's dose required reduction in patients started on diltiazem; monitor blood pressure.

Protease inhibitor like amprenavir and ritonavir may increase diltiazem's serum concentration.

Quinidine: Diltiazem may increase serum levels of quinidine. Dosage adjustment may be required.

Rifampin increases the metabolism of calcium channel blockers; adjust the dose of the calcium channel blocker to maintain efficacy or consider an alternative to rifampin.

Sildenafil, tadalafil, vardenafil: Blood pressure-lowering effects may be additive; use caution.

Tacrolimus's serum concentrations are increased by diltiazem; avoid the combination. Use another calcium channel blocker or monitor tacrolimus trough levels and renal function closely.

Pregnancy Risk Factor C

Pregnancy Implications Teratogenic and embryotoxic effects have been demonstrated in small animals

Lactation Enters breast milk/not recommended (AAP considers "compatible")

Nursing Implications Do not crush sustained release capsules

Additional Information Toxic dose: Children: 6 mg/kg. Adults: 2 g

Response to atropine may not be observed until after I.V. calcium administration; erythema may precede elevation of liver function tests by 3-5 days; most effective for treating hypertension in African-Americans Formula for I.V. to Oral diltiazem conversion: Daily diltiazem oral dose = [(mg/hour infusion rate) × 3 + 3] × 10. Discontinue the continuous infusion ~4 hours after the first dose of Cardizem® CD.

Specific References

Cantrell FL, Clark RF, and Manoguerra AS, "Determining Triage Guidelines for Unintentional Overdoses with Calcium Channel Antagonists," *Clin Toxicol (Phila)*, 2005, 43(7):849-53 (review).

Cantrell FL and Williams SR, "Fatal Unintentional Overdose of Diltiazem with Antemortem and Postmortem Values," *Clin Toxicol*, 2005, 43(6):587-8.

Chobanian AV, Bakris GL, Black HR, et al, "The Seventh Report of the Joint National Committee on Prevention, Detection, Evaluation, and Treatment of High Blood Pressure: The JNC 7 Report," *JAMA*, 2003, 289(19):2560-71.

DeWitt CR and Waksman JC. "Pharmacology, Pathophysiology and Management of Calcium Channel Blocker and Beta-Blocker Toxicity," *Toxicol Rev*, 2004, 23(4):223-38.

Megarbane B, Karyo S, and Baud FJ, "The Role of Insulin and Glucose (Hyperinsulinaemia/Euglycaemia) Therapy in Acute Calcium Channel Antagonist and Beta-Blocker Poisoning," *Toxicol Rev*, 2004, 23(4): 215-22.

Moriya F and Hashimoto Y, "Redistribution of Diltiazem in the Early Postmortem Period," *J Anal Toxicol*, 2004, 28:269-75.

Olson KR, Erdman AR, Woolf AD, et al, "Calcium Channel Blocker Ingestion: An Evidence-Based Consensus Guideline for Out-of-Hospital Management," *Clin Toxicol (Phila)*, 2005, 43(7):797-822.

Pichon N, Francois B, Clavel M, et al, "Albumin Dialysis: A New Therapeutic Alternative for Severe Diltiazem Intoxication," *Clin Toxicol*, 2006, 44:195-6.

Punukollu G, Gowda RM, Khan IA, et al, "Delayed Presentation of Calcium Channel Antagonist Overdose," *Am J Ther*, 2003, 10(2):132-4.

Satar S, Acikalin A, and Akpinar O, "Unusual Electrocardiographic Changes with Propranolol and Diltiazem Overdosage: A Case Report," *Am J Ther*, 2003, 10(4):299-302.

Shepherd G and Klein-Schwartz W, "High-Dose Insulin Therapy for Calcium-Channel Blocker Overdose," *Ann Pharmacother*, 2005, 39(5):923-30.

Wills BK, Liu J, Montana R, et al, "3° AV Block from Diltiazem XR Ingestion in a Nine-Month-Old," *Clin Toxicol (Phila)*. 2005, 43:652.

DimenhyDRINATE

Related Information

- Therapeutic Drugs Associated with Hallucinations

CAS Number 523-87-5

U.S. Brand Names Dramamine® [OTC]; Hydrate® [DSC]; TripTone® [OTC]

Impairment Potential Yes

Use Treatment and prevention of nausea, dizziness, and vomiting associated with motion sickness

Treatment of Meniere's disease

Mechanism of Action Competes with histamine for H$_1$-receptor sites on effector cells in the GI tract, blood vessels, and respiratory tract; blocks chemoreceptor trigger zone, diminishes vestibular stimulation and depresses labyrinthine function through its central anticholinergic activity

Adverse Reactions

Cardiovascular: Hypotension, sinus tachycardia

Central nervous system: **Drowsiness**, paradoxical CNS stimulation, dizziness, auditory and visual hallucinations, headache, ataxia

Gastrointestinal: Anorexia, dry mucous membranes

Genitourinary: Urinary frequency

Hematologic: Porphyria

Local: Pain at the injection site

Ocular: Blurred vision, affects color/night vision

Otic: Ototoxicity, tinnitus

Respiratory: **Thickening of bronchial secretions**

Signs and Symptoms of Overdose Toxicity may resemble atropine overdosage; CNS depression or CNS stimulation, mydriasis; dry mucous membranes

Pharmacodynamics/Kinetics

Onset of action: Oral: ~15-30 minutes

Duration: ~4-6 hours

Absorption: Oral: Well absorbed

Distribution: Wide throughout body

Metabolism: Extensive in the liver

Elimination: Renal

Dosage

Children:

Oral:

2-5 years: 12.5-25 mg every 6-8 hours, maximum: 75 mg/day

6-12 years: 25-50 mg every 6-8 hours, maximum: 150 mg/day

I.M.: 1.25 mg/kg or 37.5 mg/m^2 4 times/day, not to exceed 300 mg/day

Adults: Oral, I.M., I.V.: 50-100 mg every 4-6 hours, not to exceed 400 mg/day

Contraindications Hypersensitivity to dimenhydrate or any component

Warnings

Causes sedation, caution must be used in performing tasks which require alertness (eg, operating machinery or driving). Sedative effects of CNS depressants or ethanol are potentiated. Use with caution in patients with angle-closure glaucoma, pyloroduodenal obstruction (including stenotic peptic ulcer), urinary tract obstruction (including bladder neck obstruction and symptomatic prostatic hyperplasia), hyperthyroidism, increased intraocular pressure, and cardiovascular disease (including hypertension and tachycardia). May cause paradoxical excitation in pediatric patients, and can result in hallucinations, coma, and death in overdose.

Note: Parenteral formulations (not available in the U.S.) intended for I.V. and I.M. use are distinct and should not be confused. The I.M. formulation can be used for I.V. administration only after dilution.

Dosage Forms
[CAN] = Canadian brand name
Caplet (TripTone®): 50 mg [DSC]
Capsule, softgel (Gravol®) [CAN]: 50 mg [not available in the U.S.]
Capsule, long-acting (Gravol® L/A) [CAN]: 75 mg, 100 mg [not available in the U.S.]
Injection, solution:
  Gravol® I.M. [CAN]: 50 mg/mL (1 mL, 5 mL) [not available in the U.S.]
  Gravol® I.V. [CAN]: 10 mg/mL (5 mL) [not available in the U.S.]
Solution, oral (Gravol® [CAN], Children's Motion Sickness [CAN]): 3 mg/mL (75 mL) [not available in the U.S.]
Suppository, rectal (Gravol® [CAN], Sab-Dimenhydrinate [CAN]): 75 mg, 100 mg [not available in the U.S.]
Tablet:
  Dinate® [CAN], Jamp® Travel Tablet [CAN], Nauseatol® [CAN]: 50 mg
  Dramamine®: 50 mg
  Gravol® Filmkote Jr [CAN]: 25 mg [not available in the U.S.]
  Gravol® Filmkote [CAN]: 50 mg [not available in the U.S.]
Tablet, chewable:
  Dramamine®: 50 mg [contains phenylalanine 1.5 mg/tablet and tartrazine; orange flavor]
  Gravol® Chewable for Children [CAN]: 25 mg [not available in the U.S.]
  Gravol® Chewable for Adults [CAN]: 50 mg [not available in the U.S.]

Overdosage/Treatment Supportive therapy: There is no specific treatment for an antihistamine overdose; however, most of its clinical toxicity is due to anticholinergic effects. Anticholinesterase inhibitors may be useful by reducing acetylcholinesterase. Anticholinesterase inhibitors include physostigmine, neostigmine, pyridostigmine, and edrophonium. For anticholinergic overdose with severe life-threatening symptoms, physostigmine 1-2 mg (0.5 or 0.02 mg/kg for children) I.V., slowly may be given to reverse these effects.

Drug Interactions
Increased effect/toxicity with CNS depressants, anticholinergics, TCAs, MAO inhibitors
Increased toxicity of antibiotics, especially aminoglycosides (ototoxicity)

Pregnancy Risk Factor B

Pregnancy Implications Crosses placenta; possible oxytocic effect on the uterus at term

Nursing Implications I.V. injection must be diluted to 10 mL with NS and given at 25 mg/minute

Additional Information Dramamine® II contains meclizine

Dimethyl Sulfoxide

Pronunciation (dye meth il sul FOKS ide)
CAS Number 67-68-5
U.S. Brand Names Rimso®-50
Synonyms DMSO
Use Industrial solvent; only approved by FDA for treatment of interstitial cystitis; may be a vehicle for other agents; extravasation of chemotherapy agents
Unlabeled/Investigational Use I.V. use (dose 1 mg/kg) to reduce intracranial pressure in trauma patients; also being studied for its free radical scavenging properties, stress-induced gastric ulcers, and tissue protectant

Adverse Reactions
Cardiovascular: Sinus tachycardia
Gastrointestinal: **Garlic-like breath**

Signs and Symptoms of Overdose
Symptoms are rarely reported.
Agitation, altered taste, diarrhea, dizziness, dysosmia, facial flushing, garlic-onion odor of breath, headache, hemoglobinuria, hypernatremia, mild elevation of liver function tests, photophobia, possible hemolysis when given I.V., pruritus, vasodilation, tachycardia, urine discoloration (red), possible encephalopathy (rare), vomiting

Toxicodynamics/Kinetics
Absorption: Well absorbed from all routes
Distribution: Rapid
Metabolism: Oxidized to dimethylsulfone and reduced to dimethylsulfide
Half-life: Parent drug: 11-14 hours; dimethylsulfone: 60-70 hours
Time to peak: Dermal: 4-8 hours
Elimination: Most DMS0 and metabolites excreted in urine

Dosage
Topical: 1.5 mL of a 90% solution every 6 hours for 2 weeks can be used to treat extravasation of anthracycline chemotherapeutic agents or mitomycin
One protocol that is effective for prevention of soft tissue injury due to extravasation of vesicant cytotoxic drugs (excluding vinca alkaloids): Topical application of 4 drops/10 cm^2 of skin surface of 99% DMSO over an area twice affected and left to air dry without dressings. Repeat every 8 hours for 1 week. Apply local cooling every 8 hours for 3 days.

Monitoring Parameters May be analyzed but levels are not helpful
Administration Not for I.V. or I.M. use
Dosage Forms Solution, intravesical: 50% [500 mg/mL] (50 mL)
Reference Range Dermal dose of 1 g/kg resulted in peak serum dimethyl sulfoxide level of 504-506 mg/L and peak dimethyl sulfone serum level of 333-514 mg/L; oral dose of 1 g/kg resulted in peak serum dimethyl sulfoxide levels of 1029-3380 mg/L and peak dimethyl sulfone level of 263-596 mg/L

Overdosage/Treatment
Decontamination: Emesis within 30 minutes, lavage (within 1 hour)/ activated charcoal with sorbitol
Supportive therapy: Evaluate and monitor liver function, renal function, hemoglobin, and platelet count. Prevention of soft tissue injury due to extravasation of vesicant cytotoxic drugs (excluding vinca alkaloids): See protocol in Usual Dosage
Enhancement of elimination: No data; multiple dosing with activated charcoal may be effective; dialysis does not appear to be effective

Drug Interactions Inhibits CYP2C9 (weak), 2C19 (weak)
Increased toxicity with sulindac
Pregnancy Risk Factor C
Pregnancy Implications Unknown risk; appears to be teratogenic in animals
Lactation Excretion in breast milk unknown
Additional Information Symptoms from DMS0 exposure may be due to other substances carried into the body; it may carry water soluble drugs and provide a dermal reservoir for sustained effect

Specific References
Topacoglu H, Karcioglu O, Ozsarac M, et al, "Massive Intracranial Hemorrhage Associated with the Ingestion of Dimethyl Sulfoxide," *Vet Hum Toxicol*, 2004, 46(3):138-40.

DiphenhydrAMINE

Related Information
- Anticholinergic Effects of Common Psychotropics
- Therapeutic Drugs Associated with Hallucinations

CAS Number 147-24-0

U.S. Brand Names Aler-Cap [OTC]; Aler-Dryl [OTC]; Aler-Tab [OTC]; AllerMax® [OTC]; Altaryl [OTC]; Banophen® Anti-Itch [OTC]; Banophen® [OTC]; Benadryl® Allergy [OTC]; Benadryl® Children's Allergy Fastmelt® [OTC]; Benadryl® Children's Allergy [OTC]; Benadryl® Dye-Free Allergy [OTC]; Benadryl® Injection; Benadryl® Itch Stopping Extra Strength [OTC]; Benadryl® Itch Stopping [OTC]; Compoz® Nighttime Sleep Aid [OTC]; Dermamycin® [OTC]; Dermarest® Plus [OTC]; Dermarest® Insect Bite [OTC]; Diphenhist [OTC]; Diphen® AF [OTC]; Diphen® [OTC]; Dytan™; Genahist® [OTC]; Hydramine® [OTC]; Nytol® Quick Caps [OTC]; Nytol® Quick Gels [OTC]; Q-Dryl [OTC]; Quenalin [OTC]; Siladryl® Allergy [OTC]; Siladryl® DAS [OTC]; Silphen® [OTC]; Simply Sleep® [OTC]; Sleep-ettes D [OTC]; Sleepinal® [OTC]; Sominex® Maximum Strength [OTC]; Sominex® [OTC]; Triaminic® Thin Strips™ Cough and Runny Nose [OTC]; Twilite® [OTC]; Unisom® Maximum Strength SleepGels® [OTC]

Synonyms Diphenhydramine Citrate; Diphenhydramine Hydrochloride; Diphenhydramine Tannate

Impairment Potential Yes. Doses >50 mg or serum levels >50 ng/mL are consistent with impairment (Gengo FM and Manning C, "A Review of the Effects of Antihistamines on Mental Processes Related to Automobile Driving," *J Allergy Clin Immunol*, 1990, 86(2): 1034-9.)

Use Reversal of toxin-induced extrapyramidal reactions or serum sickness secondary to antivenin; antitussive; antimotion sickness; sleep-aid; useful in anaphylaxis and allergy treatment

Mechanism of Action Competes with histamine for H_1-receptor sites on effector cells in the gastrointestinal tract, blood vessels, and respiratory tract; anticholinergic and sedative effects are also seen

Adverse Reactions
Cardiovascular: Hypotension, palpitations, prolonged QT interval, QRS prolongation, sinus tachycardia, vasculitis
Central nervous system: **Slight to moderate drowsiness**, sedation, disorientation, dizziness, paradoxical excitement, extrapyramidal symptoms, fatigue, insomnia, visual hallucinations, acute dystonia, fever, hyperthermia, seizures, ataxia
Dermatologic: Angioedema, toxic epidermal necrolysis, urticaria, purpura, pruritus, exanthem, photoallergic reaction, cutaneous vasculitis
Gastrointestinal: Nausea, vomiting, dry mucous membranes, xerostomia
Genitourinary: Urinary retention, impotence, urinary incontinence

Hematologic: Porphyria

Neuromuscular & skeletal: Tremors, trismus

Ocular: Blurred vision, mydriasis, nystagmus (vertical/horizontal), color vision abnormalities

Respiratory: **Thickening of bronchial secretions**, bronchospasm

Miscellaneous: Dental erosion, fixed drug eruption

Signs and Symptoms of Overdose Overdose may result in death in infants and children. Catatonic stupor (15%), coma, CNS stimulation or depression, delirium, mydriasis, nystagmus, rhabdomyolysis, seizures, tachycardia, toxic psychosis

Admission Criteria/Prognosis Any symptomatic patient with ECG abnormalities or ingestions over 10 mg/kg should be considered for admission

Pharmacodynamics/Kinetics

Onset of action: Maximum sedative effect: 1-3 hours

Duration: 4-7 hours

Protein binding: 78%

Metabolism: Extensively hepatic; smaller degrees in pulmonary and renal systems; significant first-pass effect

Bioavailability: Oral: 40% to 60%

Half-life elimination: 2-8 hours; Elderly: 13.5 hours

Time to peak, serum: 2-4 hours

Excretion: Urine (as unchanged drug)

Dosage Children: Oral, I.M., I.V.: 5 mg/kg/day or 150 mg/m^2/day in divided doses every 6-8 hours, not to exceed 300 mg/day

Adults:

Oral: 25-50 mg every 4-6 hours

I.M., I.V.: 10-50 mg in a single dose every 2-4 hours, not to exceed 400 mg/day

Fatal dose: 25 mg/kg

Stability Protect from light

Monitoring Parameters Relief of symptoms, mental alertness

Contraindications Hypersensitivity to diphenhydramine or any component of the formulation; acute asthma; not for use in neonates

Warnings Causes sedation, caution must be used in performing tasks which require alertness (eg, operating machinery or driving). Sedative effects of CNS depressants or ethanol are potentiated. Use with caution in patients with angle-closure glaucoma, pyloroduodenal obstruction (including stenotic peptic ulcer), urinary tract obstruction (including bladder neck obstruction and symptomatic prostatic hyperplasia), hyperthyroidism, increased intraocular pressure, and cardiovascular disease (including hypertension and tachycardia). Diphenhydramine has high sedative and anticholinergic properties, so it may not be considered the antihistamine of choice for prolonged use in the elderly. May cause paradoxical excitation in pediatric patients, and can result in hallucinations, coma, and death in overdose. Some preparations contain sodium bisulfite; syrup formulations may contain alcohol. Some preparations contain soy protein; patients with soy protein or peanut allergies should avoid.

Dosage Forms Caplet, as hydrochloride: 25 mg, 50 mg

Aler-Dryl, AllerMax®, Compoz® Nighttime Sleep Aid, Sleep-ettes D, Sominex® Maximum Strength, Twilite®: 50 mg

Simply Sleep®, Nytol® Quick Caps: 25 mg

Capsule, as hydrochloride: 25 mg, 50 mg

Aler-Cap, Banophen®, Benadryl® Allergy, Diphen®, Diphenhist, Genahist®, Q-Dryl: 25 mg

Sleepinal®: 50 mg

Capsule, softgel, as hydrochloride: 50 mg

Benadryl® Dye-Free Allergy: 25 mg [dye-free]

Compoz® Nighttime Sleep Aid, Nytol® Quick Gels, Sleepinal®, Unisom® Maximum Strength SleepGels®: 50 mg

Captab, as hydrochloride (Diphenhist®): 25 mg

Cream, as hydrochloride: 2% (30 g) [contains zinc acetate 0.1%]

Banophen® Anti-Itch: 2% (30 g) [contains zinc acetate 0.1%]

Benadryl® Itch Stopping: 1% (30 g) [contains zinc acetate 0.1%]

Benadryl® Itch Stopping Extra Strength: 2% (30 g) [contains zinc acetate 0.1%]

Diphenhist®: 2% (30 g) [contains zinc acetate 0.1%]

Elixir, as hydrochloride:

Altaryl: 12.5 mg/5 mL (120 mL, 480 mL, 3840 mL) [cherry flavor]

Banophen®: 12.5 mg/5 mL (120 mL)

Diphen AF: 12.5 mg/5 mL (120 mL, 240 mL, 480 mL) [alcohol free; cherry flavor]

Q-Dryl: 12.5 mg/5 mL (480 mL) [alcohol free]

Gel, topical, as hydrochloride:

Benadryl® Itch Stopping Extra Strength: 2% (120 mL)

Dermarest® Plus: 2% (28 g, 42 g) [contains menthol 1%]

Injection, solution, as hydrochloride: 50 mg/mL (1 mL)

Benadryl®: 50 mg/mL (1 mL, 10 mL)

Liquid, as hydrochloride:

AllerMax®: 12.5 mg/5 mL (120 mL)

Benadryl® Allergy: 12.5 mg/5 mL (120 mL, 240 mL) [alcohol free; contains sodium benzoate; cherry flavor]

Benadryl® Dye-Free Allergy: 12.5 mg/5 mL (120 mL) [alcohol free, dye free, sugar free; contains sodium benzoate; bubble gum flavor]

Genahist®: 12.5 mg/5 mL (120 mL) [alcohol free, sugar free; contains sodium benzoate; cherry flavor]

Hydramine®: 12.5 mg/5 mL (120 mL, 480 mL) [alcohol free]

Q-Dryl: 12.5 mg/5 mL (120 mL) [alcohol free; cherry flavor]

Quenalin: 12.5 mg/5 mL (120 mL) [fruit flavor]

Siladryl® Allergy: 12.5 mg/5 mL (120 mL, 240 mL, 480 mL) [alcohol free, sugar free; black cherry flavor]

Siladryl® DAS: 12.5 mg/5 mL (120 mL) [alcohol free, dye free, sugar free; black cherry flavor]

Liquid, topical, as hydrochloride [stick] (Benadryl® Itch Stopping Extra Strength): 2% (14 mL) [contains zinc acetate 0.1% and alcohol]

Solution, oral, as hydrochloride:

Banophen®: 12.5 mg/5mL (480 mL) [sugar free]

Diphenhist: 12.5 mg/5 mL (120 mL, 480 mL) [alcohol free; contains sodium benzoate]

Solution, topical, as hydrochloride [spray]:

Benadryl® Itch Stopping Extra Strength: 2% (60 mL) [contains zinc acetate 0.1% and alcohol]

Dermamycin®, Dermarest® Insect Bite: 2% (60 mL) [contains menthol 1%]

Strips, oral, as hydrochloride (Triaminic® Thin Strips™ Cough and Runny Nose): 12. 5 mg (16s) [grape flavor]

Suspension, as tannate: 25 mg/5 mL (120 mL)

Dytan™: 25 mg/5 mL (120 mL) [strawberry flavor]

Syrup, as hydrochloride (Silphen® Cough): 12.5 mg/5 mL (120 mL, 240 mL, 480 mL) [contains alcohol; 5%; strawberry flavor]

Tablet, as hydrochloride: 25 mg, 50 mg

Aler-Tab, Benadryl® Allergy, Genahist®, Sleepinal®, Sominex®: 25 mg

Tablet, chewable, as hydrochloride (Benadryl® Children's Allergy): 12.5 mg [contains phenylalanine 4.2 mg/tablet; grape flavor]

Tablet, chewable, as tannate (Dytan™): 25 mg [contains phenylalanine; strawberry flavor]

Tablet, orally disintegrating, as citrate (Benadryl® Children's Allergy Fastmelt®): 19 mg [equivalent to diphenhydramine hydrochloride 12.5 mg; contains phenylalanine 4.5 mg/tablet and soy protein isolate; cherry flavor]

Reference Range

Therapeutic: Serum: Antihistamine 30-50 ng/mL (117.5-195.8 nmol/L); Sedative: 50-300 ng/mL (195.8-1174.9 nmol/L)

Toxic: Diphenhydramine level of 12.8 mg/L has been associated with fatality

In the postmortem state, anatomical site concentration differences (ie, postmortem redistribution) may occur.

Overdosage/Treatment

Decontamination: Lavage (within 1 hour) with ingestions over 5 mg/kg in pediatrics or over 150 mg in adults; activated charcoal can be most useful; **do not** use a cathartic if diarrhea is present

Supportive therapy: Propranolol or esmolol can be used for tachyarrhythmias (avoid quinidine or disopyramide in that conduction disturbances can occur); benzodiazepine can be utilized for seizures; if anticholinergic findings are present with the seizures (or if coma or delirium is present) a trial of physostigmine may be useful; wide complex QRS conduction defects may respond to I.V. sodium bicarbonate; seizures have responded to sodium bicarbonate in a rodent model. Initiate cooling technique if core body temperature is >104 °F (40 °C).

Enhanced elimination: Dialysis/hemoperfusion is not useful; charcoal hemoperfusion with in-line hemodialysis and regional citrate anticoagulation may be beneficial in patients with cardiac abnormalities

Antidote(s)

- Physostigmine [ANTIDOTE]

Test Interactions May suppress wheal and flare reaction to skin test antigens; false-positive methadone or opiate enzyme immunoassay may result with diphenhydramine or doxylamine; may cause false-positive urinary assay for propoxyphene on EMIT II immunoassay. May cause false-positive phencyclidine on fluorescence polarization urinary immunoassay.

Drug Interactions Inhibits CYP2D6 (moderate)

Amantadine, rimantadine: Central and/or peripheral anticholinergic syndrome can occur when administered with amantadine or rimantadine

Anticholinergic agents: Central and/or peripheral anticholinergic syndrome can occur when administered with narcotic analgesics, phenothiazines and other antipsychotics (especially with high anticholinergic activity), tricyclic antidepressants, quinidine and some other antiarrhythmics, and antihistamines

Atenolol: Drugs with high anticholinergic activity may increase the bioavailability of atenolol (and possibly other beta-blockers); monitor for increased effect

Cholinergic agents: Drugs with high anticholinergic activity may antagonize the therapeutic effect of cholinergic agents; includes donepezil, rivastigmine, and tacrine

CNS depressants: Sedative effects may be additive with CNS depressants; includes ethanol, benzodiazepines, barbiturates, narcotic analgesics, and other sedative agents; monitor for increased effect

CYP2D6 substrates: Diphenhydramine may increase the levels/effects of CYP2D6 substrates. Example substrates include amphetamines, selected beta-blockers, dextromethorphan, fluoxetine, lidocaine, mirtazapine, nefazodone, paroxetine, risperidone, ritonavir, thioridazine, tricyclic antidepressants, and venlafaxine.

CYP2D6 prodrug substrates: Diphenhydramine may decrease the levels/effects of CYP2D6 prodrug substrates. Example prodrug substrates include codeine, hydrocodone, oxycodone, and tramadol.

Digoxin: Drugs with high anticholinergic activity may decrease gastric degradation and increase the amount of digoxin absorbed by delaying gastric emptying

Ethanol: Syrup should not be given to patients taking drugs that can cause disulfiram reactions (ie, metronidazole, chlorpropamide) due to high alcohol content

Levodopa: Drugs with high anticholinergic activity may increase gastric degradation and decrease the amount of levodopa absorbed by delaying gastric emptying

Neuroleptics: Drugs with high anticholinergic activity may antagonize the therapeutic effects of neuroleptics

Pregnancy Risk Factor B

Pregnancy Implications Crosses placenta; use with temazepam can cause profound fetal CNS depression

Lactation Enters breast milk/contraindicated

Nursing Implications I.V. must be given slowly

Additional Information Has antinauseant and topical anesthetic properties; false-positive results with methadone or opiate enzyme immunoassay may occur with diphenhydramine or doxylamine; liquid preparations may also contain significant amounts of alcohol; topical administration on infants and small children has lead to severe systemic toxicity, particularly in presence of varicella infection

Specific References

Bird SB, Gaspari RJ, Lee WJ, et al, "Diphenhydramine As a Protective Agent in a Rat Model of Acute, Lethal Organophosphate Poisoning," *Acad Emerg Med*, 2002, 9(12):1369-72.

Bird SB, Gaspari RJ, Lee WJ, et al, "Diphenhydramine As a Protective Agent in Severe Organophosphate Poisoning," *Acad Emerg Med*, 2002, 9(5):357-8.

Christensen RC, "Screening for Anticholinergic Abuse in Patients with Chronic Mental Illness," *Am J Emerg Med*, 2003, 21(6):508.

Dawson A, "Diphenhydramine-Associated Wide Complex Dysrhythmia," *Am J Emerg Med*, 2004, 22(6):496.

Foresto CM, Caraccio TR, and McFee RL, "Atypical Presentation Including Decerebrate Posturing from Diphenhydramine (DPH) Toxicity in a 23-Year-Old," *J Toxicol Clin Toxicol*, 2003, 41(5):670.

Goklaney A, Mullins ME, Halcomb SE, et al, "Pharmacokinetic Effects of Co-Ingested Diphenhydramine or Oxycodone on Simulated Acetaminophen Overdose," *Acad Emerg Med*, 2003, 10:510a.

Haas CE, Magram Y, and Mishra A, "Rhabdomyolysis and Acute Renal Failure Following an Ethanol and Diphenhydramine Overdose," *Ann Pharmacother*, 2003, 37(4):538-42.

Kearney TE, Hiatt PH, Machado L, et al, "Validating Send-In Guidelines: Factors Influencing Triage Decisions for Pediatric Diphenhydramine Ingestions," *J Toxicol Clin Toxicol*, 2004, 42(5):815-6.

Khosla U, Ruel KS, and Hunt DP, "Antihistamine-Induced Rhabdomyolysis," *South Med J*, 2003, 96(10):1023-6.

Marinetti L, Lehman L, Casto B, et al, "Over-the-Counter Cold Medications - Postmortem Findings in Infants and Relationship to Cause of Death," *J Anal Toxicol*, 2005, 29:738-43.

Mason A, Winecker R, and Ropero-Miller J, "Chemical Restraint of an Infant Using Diphenhydramine Associated with a Fatality," *J Anal Toxicol*, 2003, 27:193.

Richardson WH 3rd, Williams SR, and Carstairs SD, "A Picturesque Reversal of Antimuscarinic Delirium," *J Emerg Med*, 2004, 26(4):463.

Scharman EJ, Erdman AR, Wax PM, et al, "Diphenhydramine and Dimenhydrinate Poisoning: An Evidence-Based Consensus Guideline for Out-of-Hospital Management," *Clin Toxicol*, 2006, 44(3):205-23.

Schneir AB, Munday S, Ly BT, et al, "Diphenhydramine-Induced Wide Complex Tachycardia Shown by Exercise Treadmill Testing Not to Be Entirely Rate Related," *J Toxicol Clin Toxicol*, 2003, 41(5):656.

Sharma AN, Hexdall AH, Chang EK, et al, "Diphenhydramine-Induced Wide Complex Dysrhythmia Responds to Treatment with Sodium Bicarbonate," *Am J Emerg Med*, 2003, 21(3):212-5.

Stojanovski SD, Robinson RF, Baker DS, et al, "Relationship Between Reported Single Acute Dose of Diphenhydramine Hydrochloride Exposures in Children ≤6 Years of Age and Clinical Outcomes," *Clin Toxicol (Phila)*, 2005, 43:659.

Stucka KR, Mycyk MB, Leikin JB, et al, "Rhabdomyolysis Associated with Unintentional Antihistamine Overdose in a Child," *Pediatr Emerg Care*, 2003, 19(2):25-6.

Diphenoxylate and Atropine

CAS Number 3810-80-8; 915-30-0

U.S. Brand Names Lomocot®; Lomotil®; Lonox®

Synonyms Atropine and Diphenoxylate

Use Treatment of diarrhea with nonbacterial causes

Mechanism of Action Diphenoxylate inhibits excessive gastrointestinal motility and gastrointestinal propulsion (an analogue of meperidine); commercial preparations contain a subtherapeutic amount of atropine to discourage abuse

Adverse Reactions

Effects of atropine are noted first followed by diphenoxylate

Cardiovascular: Tachycardia, flushing, sinus tachycardia

Central nervous system: Sedation, dizziness, headache, hyperthermia, euphoria, drowsiness, irritability, seizures, coma, hallucination, hyperexcitability, ataxia

Dermatologic: Pruritus, rash

Gastrointestinal: Nausea, vomiting, abdominal pain, abdominal discomfort, paralytic ileus, pancreatitis, xerostomia, anorexia, constipation

Genitourinary: Urinary retention

Neuromuscular & skeletal: Weakness

Ocular: Blurred vision

Respiratory: Apnea, respiratory depression (young children may be at greater risk)

Miscellaneous: Physical and psychological dependence with prolonged use

Signs and Symptoms of Overdose Paralytic ileus

Admission Criteria/Prognosis Admit any significant pediatric ingestion due to delayed symptom progression of toxicity.

Pharmacodynamics/Kinetics

Atropine: See Atropine monograph.

Diphenoxylate:

Onset of action: Antidiarrheal: 45-60 minutes

Duration: Antidiarrheal: 3-4 hours

Absorption: Well absorbed

Metabolism: Extensively hepatic via ester hydrolysis to diphenoxylic acid (active)

Half-life elimination: Diphenoxylate: 2.5 hours; Diphenoxylic acid: 12-14 hours

Time to peak, serum: 2 hours

Excretion: Primarily feces (49% as unchanged drug and metabolites); urine (~14%, <1% as unchanged drug)

Dosage

Use with caution in young children due to variable responses; if there is no response within 48 hours, the drug is unlikely to be effective and should be discontinued.

Oral:

Children 2-12 years: 0.3-0.4 mg/kg/day of diphenoxylate in 2-4 divided doses

Adults: 15-20 mg/day of diphenoxylate in 3-4 divided doses

Monitoring Parameters Watch for signs of atropinism (dryness of skin and mucous membranes, tachycardia, thirst, flushing); monitor number and consistency of stools; observe for signs of toxicity, fluid and electrolyte loss, hypotension, and respiratory depression

Administration If there is no response within 48 hours of continuous therapy, this medication is unlikely to be effective and should be discontinued; if chronic diarrhea is not improved symptomatically within 10 days at maximum dosage, control is unlikely with further use. Use of the liquid preparation is recommended in children <13 years of age; use plastic dropper provided when measuring liquid.

Contraindications Hypersensitivity to diphenoxylate, atropine, or any component of the formulation; obstructive jaundice; diarrhea associated with pseudomembranous enterocolitis or enterotoxin-producing bacteria; not for use in children <2 years of age

Warnings

Use in conjunction with fluid and electrolyte therapy when appropriate. In case of severe dehydration or electrolyte imbalance, withhold diphenoxylate/atropine treatment until corrective therapy has been initiated. Inhibiting peristalsis may lead to fluid retention in the intestine aggravating dehydration and electrolyte imbalance. Reduction of intestinal motility may be deleterious in diarrhea resulting from *Shigella*, *Salmonella*, toxigenic strains of *E. coli*, and pseudomembranous enterocolitis associated with broad-spectrum antibiotics; use is not recommended.

Use with caution in children. Younger children may be predisposed to toxicity; signs of atropinism may occur even at recommended doses, especially in patients with Down syndrome. Overdose in children may result in severe respiratory depression, coma, and possibly permanent brain damage.

Use caution with acute ulcerative colitis, hepatic or renal dysfunction. If there is no response with 48 hours, this medication is unlikely to be effective and should be discontinued; if chronic diarrhea is not improved symptomatically within 10 days at maximum dosage, control is unlikely with further use. Physical and psychological dependence have been reported with higher than recommended dosing.

Dosage Forms

Solution, oral: Diphenoxylate hydrochloride 2.5 mg and atropine sulfate 0.025 mg per 5 mL (5 mL, 10 mL, 60 mL)

Lomotil®: Diphenoxylate hydrochloride 2.5 mg and atropine sulfate 0.025 mg per 5 mL (60 mL) [contains alcohol 15%; cherry flavor]

Tablet: Diphenoxylate hydrochloride 2.5 mg and atropine sulfate 0.025 mg

Lomotil®, Lonox®: Diphenoxylate hydrochloride 2.5 mg and atropine sulfate 0.025 mg

Reference Range Peak plasma level after 5 mg of diphenoxylate: 0.01 mg/L of diphenoxylate and 0.04 mg/L of difenoxine

Overdosage/Treatment

Decontamination: Lavage (within 3 hours)/activated charcoal

Supportive therapy: Naloxone for respiratory/central nervous system depression

Enhanced elimination: Due to delayed drug absorption and enterohepatic recirculation, multiple dosing of activated charcoal may be useful

Antidote(s)

- Naloxone [ANTIDOTE]

Drug Interactions Pramlintide: Pramlintide may enhance the anticholinergic effect of anticholinergics; additive effects on reduced GI motility may occur.

Pregnancy Risk Factor C

Pregnancy Implications Neonatal respiratory depression/withdrawal can occur

Lactation Enters breast milk/use caution

Dipyridamole

CAS Number 58-32-2

U.S. Brand Names Persantine®

Use Maintain patency after surgical grafting procedures including coronary artery bypass; with warfarin to decrease thrombosis in patients after artificial heart valve replacement; for chronic management of angina pectoris; with aspirin to prevent coronary artery thrombosis; in combination with aspirin or warfarin to prevent other thromboembolic disorders

Mechanism of Action Inhibits the activity of adenosine deaminase and phosphodiesterase, which causes an accumulation of adenosine, adenine nucleotides, and cyclic AMP; these mediators then inhibit platelet aggregation and may cause vasodilation; may also stimulate release of prostacyclin or PGD_2

Adverse Reactions

Cardiovascular: **Exacerbation of angina pectoris**, vasodilation, flushing, angina, pericardial effusion/pericarditis, sinus bradycardia, vasodilation, syncope

Central nervous system: **Dizziness**, headache (dose related)

Dermatologic: Rash, pruritus, angioedema

Gastrointestinal: Abdominal distress, nausea, vomiting, hemorrhoids, salty taste

Neuromuscular & skeletal: Weakness

Respiratory: Asthma, pulmonary edema, hyposmia

Signs and Symptoms of Overdose Bradycardia, chest pain, cholelithiasis, coagulopathy, hypotension, myalgia, metallic taste, peripheral vasodilation, wheezing

Pharmacodynamics/Kinetics

Absorption: Readily, but variable

Distribution: Adults: V_d: 2-3 L/kg

Protein binding: 91% to 99%

Metabolism: Hepatic

Half-life elimination: Terminal: 10-12 hours

Time to peak, serum: 2-2.5 hours

Excretion: Feces (as glucuronide conjugates and unchanged drug)

Dosage Oral:

Children: 4-10 mg/kg/day in 3 divided doses

Doses of 4-10 mg/kg/day have been used investigationally to treat albuminuria in pediatric renal disease

Adults: 75-400 mg/day in 3-4 divided doses

I.V.: 0.14 mg/kg/minute for 4 minutes; maximum dose: 60 mg

Stability Insoluble in water

Monitoring Parameters Blood pressure, heart rate

Administration

I.V.: Infuse diluted solution over 4 minutes; following dipyridamole infusion, inject thallium-201 within 5 minutes. **Note:** Aminophylline should be available for urgent/emergent use; dosing of 50-100 mg (range: 50-250 mg) IVP over 30-60 seconds.

Tablet: Administer with water 1 hour before meals.

Contraindications Hypersensitivity to dipyridamole or any component of the formulation

Warnings Use caution in patients with hypotension and severe cardiac disease. Use caution in patients on other antiplatelet agents or anticoagulation. Severe adverse reactions have occurred rarely with I.V. administration. Use the I.V. form with caution in patients with bronchos-

pastic disease or unstable angina. Have aminophylline ready in case of urgency or emergency with I.V. use. Safety and efficacy in children <12 years of age have not been established.

Dosage Forms Injection, solution: 5 mg/mL (2 mL, 10 mL)

Tablet: 25 mg, 50 mg, 75 mg

Persantine®: 25 mg, 50 mg, 75 mg

Reference Range 300 mg oral dose associated with a serum dipyridamole level of 2.9 mcg/mL

Overdosage/Treatment

Decontamination: Ipecac within 30 minutes or lavage (within 1 hour)/ activated charcoal

Supportive therapy: Fluids and vasopressors may be helpful although hypotension is often transient; coronary vasodilation may be reversed by aminophylline

Enhancement of elimination: Multiple dose of activated charcoal may be useful; dialysis unlikely to help because highly protein bound

Test Interactions May result in falsely elevated lipoprotein

Drug Interactions Adenosine: Blood levels and pharmacologic effects of adenosine are increased; consider reduced doses of adenosine.

Cholinesterase inhibitors: May counteract effect of cholinesterase inhibitor and may aggravate myasthenia gravis.

Xanthine derivatives (eg, theophylline): May reduce the pharmacologic effects of dipyridamole; hold theophylline preparations for 36-48 hours before dipyridamole facilitated stress test.

Pregnancy Risk Factor B

Pregnancy Implications Small amounts cross placenta

Lactation Enters breast milk/use caution

Nursing Implications Dilute I.V. dipyridamole in at least a 1:2 ratio with D_5W

Additional Information Dipyridamole may also be given 2 days prior to open heart surgery to prevent platelet activation by extracorporeal bypass pump; doses of 4-10 mg/kg/day have been used investigationally to treat albuminuria in pediatric renal disease

---

Dirithromycin

CAS Number 62013-04-1

U.S. Brand Names Dynabac®

Use Not yet FDA-approved for community-acquired pneumonia, pharyngitis/tonsillitis, bronchitis, skin and skin structure infections

Mechanism of Action Macrolide antibiotic similar to erythromycin, dirithromycin; inhibits RNA-dependent protein synthesis by binding to 50-S subunit of ribosomes

Adverse Reactions

Central nervous system: Headache, dizziness

Dermatologic: Urticaria

Gastrointestinal: Abdominal pain, diarrhea, nausea, dyspepsia, flatulence

Neuromuscular & skeletal: Weakness

Respiratory: Rhinitis

Pharmacodynamics/Kinetics

Absorption: Rapid

Distribution: V_d: 800 L; rapidly and widely (higher levels in tissues than plasma)

Protein binding: 14% to 30%

Metabolism: Hydrolyzed to erythromycylamine

Bioavailability: 10%

Half-life elimination: 8 hours (range: 2-36 hours)

Time to peak: 4 hours

Excretion: Feces (81% to 97%)

Dosage 500 mg/day

Monitoring Parameters Temperature, CBC

Administration Administer with food or within an hour following a meal. Do not alter (chew or crush) enteric coated dosage form.

Contraindications Hypersensitivity to any macrolide or component of dirithromycin; use with pimozide

Warnings Pseudomembranous colitis has been reported and should be considered in patients presenting with diarrhea subsequent to therapy with dirithromycin.

Dosage Forms

[DSC] = Discontinued product

Tablet, enteric coated: 250 mg [DSC]

Reference Range After a 500 mg oral dose, peak plasma level was 0.5 mg/L

Overdosage/Treatment

Decontamination: Lavage (within 1 hour)/activated charcoal

Supportive therapy: Acute gastrointestinal irritation can be treated with milk or bismuth subsalicylate; lidocaine can be used for ventricular arrhythmias

Elimination: Hemodialysis is not effective

Drug Interactions Substrate of CYP3A4 (minor)

Increased effect: Absorption of dirithromycin is slightly enhanced with concomitant antacids and H_2 antagonists; dirithromycin may, like erythromycin, increase the effect of alfentanil, anticoagulants, bromocriptine, carbamazepine, cyclosporine, digoxin, disopyramide, ergots, methylprednisolone, cisapride.

Increased toxicity: Avoid use with pimozide (due to risk of significant cardiotoxicity) and triazolam.

Note: Interactions with nonsedating antihistamines (eg, astemizole), cisapride, and theophylline are not known to occur; however, caution is advised with coadministration.

Pregnancy Risk Factor C

Pregnancy Implications Animal studies indicate the use of dirithromycin during pregnancy should be avoided if possible.

Lactation Excretion in breast milk unknown/use caution

Additional Information Effective against gram-positive organisms (*Legionella*, *Helicobacter pylori*, and *Chlamydia trachomatis*)

Disopyramide

Related Information
- Therapeutic Drugs Associated with Hallucinations

CAS Number 22059-60-5; 3737-09-5

U.S. Brand Names Norpace® CR; Norpace®

Synonyms Disopyramide Phosphate

Use Suppression and prevention of unifocal and multifocal premature, ventricular premature complexes, coupled tachycardia (ventricular); also effective in the conversion of fibrillation (atrial), flutter (atrial), and paroxysmal atrial tachycardia to normal sinus rhythm and prevention of the reoccurrence of these arrhythmias after conversion by other methods

Unlabeled/Investigational Use Hypertrophic obstructive cardiomyopathy (HOCM)

Mechanism of Action Class IA antiarrhythmic: Decreases myocardial excitability and conduction velocity; reduces disparity in refractory between normal and infarcted myocardium; possesses anticholinergic, peripheral vasoconstrictive, and negative inotropic effects

Adverse Reactions

Cardiovascular: Congestive heart failure, edema, chest pain, syncope and hypotension; conduction disturbances including AV block, QRS prolongation, QT prolongation, fibrillation (atrial), flutter (atrial), sinus bradycardia, angina, myocardial depression, tachycardia (supraventricular), arrhythmias (ventricular)

Central nervous system: Fatigue, malaise, nervousness, acute psychosis, CNS depression, dizziness, headache, auditory and visual hallucinations, psychosis

Dermatologic: Generalized rashes

Endocrine & metabolic: Hypoglycemia, may initiate contractions of pregnant uterus, hyperkalemia may enhance toxicities, hyperinsulinemia, elevation of cholesterol and triglycerides

Gastrointestinal: Constipation, nausea, vomiting, diarrhea, GI pain, gas, anorexia, xerostomia, decreased bowel sounds, weight gain, dry throat

Genitourinary: **Urinary retention/hesitancy**, impotence

Hematologic: Granulocytopenia

Hepatic: Hepatic cholestasis, liver enzymes (elevated)

Neuromuscular & skeletal: Paresthesia, weakness

Ocular: Blurred vision, photophobia, diplopia, mydriasis, acute angle-closure glaucoma, dry eyes

Respiratory: Dyspnea, dry nose

Miscellaneous: Anaphylactic shock

Signs and Symptoms of Overdose Agranulocytosis, anticholinergic effects, apnea, asystole, AV block, bradycardia, cardiac arrhythmias, cardiac conduction disturbances, coma, congestive heart failure, drowsiness, granulocytopenia, heart block, hypoglycemia, hypotension, impotence, increased intraocular pressure, jaundice, leukopenia, loss of consciousness, mydriasis, neutropenia, paroxysmal tachycardia (ventricular), photosensitivity, QRS prolongation, QT prolongation, respiratory arrest, seizures, slurred speech, torsade de pointes, urine discoloration (milky)

Pharmacodynamics/Kinetics

Onset of action: 0.5-3.5 hours

Duration: 1.5-8.5 hours

Absorption: 60% to 83%

Protein binding (concentration dependent): 20% to 60%

Metabolism: Hepatic to inactive metabolites

Half-life elimination: Adults: 4-10 hours; prolonged with hepatic or renal impairment

Excretion: Urine (40% to 60% as unchanged drug); feces (10% to 15%)

Dosage Oral:

Children:

<1 year: 10-30 mg/kg/24 hours in 4 divided doses

1-4 years: 10-20 mg/kg/24 hours in 4 divided doses

4-12 years: 10-15 mg/kg/24 hours in 4 divided doses

12-18 years: 6-15 mg/kg/24 hours in 4 divided doses

Note: 600 mg ingestion in a child can be fatal

Adults:

<50 kg: 100 mg every 6 hours or 200 mg every 12 hours (controlled release)

>50 kg: 150 mg every 6 hours or 300 mg every 12 hours (controlled release); if no response, may increase to 200 mg every 6 hours; maximum dose required for patients with severe refractory tachycardia (ventricular) is 400 mg every 6 hours

Dosing adjustment in renal impairment: 100 mg (nonsustained release) given at the following intervals, based on creatinine clearance (mL/minute):

Cl_{cr} 30-40 mL/minute: Administer every 8 hours

Cl_{cr} 15-30 mL/minute: Administer every 12 hours

Cl_{cr} <15 mL/minute: Administer every 24 hours

or alter the dose as follows:

Cl_{cr} 30-<40 mL/minute: Reduce dose 50%

Cl_{cr} 15-30 mL/minute: Reduce dose 75%

Dosing interval in hepatic impairment: 100 mg every 6 hours or 200 mg every 12 hours (controlled release)

Monitoring Parameters ECG, blood pressure, urinary retention, CNS anticholinergic effects (confusion, agitation, hallucinations, etc)

Administration Do not break or chew controlled release capsules. Administer around-the-clock to Administer around-the-clock rather than 4 times/day (ie, 12-6-12-6, not 9-1-5-9) to promote less variation in peak and trough serum levels

Contraindications Hypersensitivity to disopyramide or any component of the formulation; cardiogenic shock; pre-existing second- or third-degree heart block (except in patients with a functioning artificial pacemaker); congenital QT syndrome; sick sinus syndrome

Warnings Monitor and adjust dose to prevent QT_c prolongation. Avoid concurrent use with other medications that prolong QT interval or decrease myocardial contractility. Correct hypokalemia before initiating therapy; may worsen toxicity. Watch for proarrhythmic effects. **[U.S. Boxed Warning]: In the Cardiac Arrhythmia Suppression Trial (CAST), recent (>6 days but <2 years ago) myocardial infarction patients with asymptomatic, nonlife-threatening ventricular arrhythmias did not benefit and may have been harmed by attempts to suppress the arrhythmia with flecainide or encainide. An increased mortality or nonfatal cardiac arrest rate (7.7%) was seen in the active treatment group compared with patients in the placebo group (3%). The applicability of the CAST results to other populations is unknown. Antiarrhythmic agents should be reserved for patients with life-threatening ventricular arrhythmias.** May precipitate or exacerbate CHF. Due to significant anticholinergic effects, do not use in patients with urinary retention, BPH, glaucoma, or myasthenia gravis. Reduce dosage in renal or hepatic impairment. The extended release form is not recommended for Cl_{cr} <40 mL/minute. In patients with atrial fibrillation or flutter, block the AV node before initiating. Use caution in Wolff-Parkinson-White syndrome or bundle branch block. Monitor closely for hypotension during the initiation of therapy.

Dosage Forms Capsule (Norpace®): 100 mg, 150 mg

Capsule, controlled release (Norpace® CR): 100 mg, 150 mg

Reference Range

Therapeutic:

Atrial arrhythmias: 2.8-3.2 mcg/mL (SI: 8.3-9.4 μmol/L)

Ventricular arrhythmias: 3.3-7.5 mcg/mL (SI: 9.7-22.0 μmol/L)

Toxic: >7.0 mcg/mL (SI: >20.7 μmol/L)

Fatal: Levels >16.0 mcg/mL

Overdosage/Treatment

Decontamination: Lavage (within 1 hour)/activated charcoal

Supportive therapy: Phenytoin and lidocaine are useful for ventricular arrhythmia; isoproterenol is useful to reverse cardiac depressant effects. Resuscitative effort may need to be prolonged. Calcium chloride may be useful for electromechanical disassociation.

Enhancement of elimination: Forced diuresis, charcoal hemoperfusion is effective; multiple dosing of activated charcoal may be effective; since plasma protein decreases as disopyramide levels rise, hemodialysis may be useful in enhancing elimination (clearance of 123 mL/minute with 40% of drug removed during 4 hours of hemodialysis)

Test Interactions ↓ glucose; disopyramide can cross react with methadone urinary immunoassay tests

Drug Interactions Substrate of CYP3A4 (major)

Beta-blockers may cause additive/excessive negative inotropic activity.

CYP3A4 inducers: CYP3A4 inducers may decrease the levels/effects of disopyramide. Example inducers include aminoglutethimide, carbamazepine, nafcillin, nevirapine, phenobarbital, phenytoin, and rifamycins.

CYP3A4 inhibitors: May increase the levels/effects of disopyramide. Example inhibitors include azole antifungals, clarithromycin, diclofenac, doxycycline, erythromycin, imatinib, isoniazid, nefazodone, nicardipine, propofol, protease inhibitors, quinidine, telithromycin, and verapamil.

Erythromycin and clarithromycin increase disopyramide blood levels; may cause QRS widening and/or QT interval prolongation.

Procainamide, quinidine, propafenone, or flecainide can cause increased/excessive negative inotropic effects or prolonged conduction.

Drugs which may prolong the QT interval (amiodarone, amitriptyline, bepridil, cisapride, disopyramide, erythromycin, haloperidol, imipramine, pimozide, quinidine, sotalol, and thioridazine) may be additive with disopyramide; use with caution.

Sparfloxacin, gatifloxacin, and moxifloxacin may result in additional prolongation of the QT interval; concurrent use is contraindicated.

Pregnancy Risk Factor C

Pregnancy Implications May cause uterine contractions

Lactation Enters breast milk/compatible

Disulfiram

Related Information
- Drugs Used in Addiction Treatment
- Therapeutic Drugs Associated with Hallucinations

CAS Number 97-77-8

U.S. Brand Names Antabuse®

Use Management of chronic alcoholics; also used to treat allergic nickel dermatitis and can enhance the elimination of nickel

Mechanism of Action Disulfiram is a thiuram derivative which interferes with aldehyde dehydrogenase. When taken concomitantly with alcohol, there is an increase in serum acetaldehyde levels. High acetaldehyde causes uncomfortable symptoms, including flushing, nausea, thirst, palpitations, chest pain, dizziness, and hypotension. This reaction is the basis for disulfiram use in postwithdrawal long-term care of alcoholism. May also boost the immune function in HIV patients.

Adverse Reactions

Alcohol-disulfiram reaction:

Cardiovascular: Flushing, cardiovascular collapse, myocardial infarction, chest pain, angina, vasodilation, Reye's-like syndrome

Central nervous system: **Drowsiness**, dizziness, seizures, death, auditory and visual hallucinations, psychosis, headache, paranoia, gustatory hallucinations, parkinsonism, catatonia, extrapyramidal reactions, axonopathy

Dermatologic: Systemic contact dermatitis, nickel dermatitis recall

Gastrointestinal: Nausea, vomiting, metallic taste

Hematologic: Methemoglobin (as high as 52.8% has been described in a disulfiram ethanol reaction)

Hepatic: Hepatitis

Ocular: Retrobulbar neuritis, blepharospasm

Respiratory: Dyspnea

Miscellaneous: Diaphoresis

Signs and Symptoms of Overdose Symptoms develop within 12 hours; Ataxia, blindness, dementia, depression, dysphoria, eczema, facial flushing, garlic-like breath, impotence, mania, memory loss, metallic taste, nystagmus, paresthesia, ptosis, rotten egg breath, seizures, syncope, thrombocytopenia

Pharmacodynamics/Kinetics

Onset of action: Full effect: 12 hours

Duration: ~1-2 weeks after last dose

Absorption: Rapid

Metabolism: To diethylthiocarbamate

Protein binding: 96%

Excretion: Feces and exhaled gases (as metabolites)

Dosage Adults: Oral: Maximum daily dose: 500 mg/day in a single dose for 1-2 weeks; average maintenance dose: 250 mg/day; range: 125-500 mg; duration of therapy is to continue until the patient is fully recovered socially and a basis for permanent self control has been established; maintenance therapy may be required for months or even years

Monitoring Parameters Hypokalemia; liver function tests at baseline and after 10-14 days of treatment; CBC, serum chemistries, liver function tests should be monitored during therapy

Administration Administration of any medications containing alcohol, including topicals, is contraindicated. Do not administer disulfiram if ethanol has been consumed within the prior 12 hours.

Contraindications Hypersensitivity to disulfiram and related compounds or any component of the formulation; patients receiving or using ethanol, metronidazole, paraldehyde, or ethanol-containing preparations like cough syrup or tonics; psychosis; severe myocardial disease and coronary occlusion

Warnings Use with caution in patients with diabetes, hypothyroidism, seizure disorders, nephritis (acute or chronic), hepatic cirrhosis or insufficiency. **[U.S. Boxed Warning]: Should never be administered to a patient when he/she is in a state of ethanol intoxication, or without his/her knowledge.** Patient must receive appropriate counseling, including information on "disguised" forms of ethanol (tonics, mouthwashes, etc) and the duration of the drug's activity (up to 14 days). Severe (sometimes fatal) hepatitis and/or hepatic failure have been associated with disulfiram. May occur in patients with or without prior history of abnormal hepatic function.

Dosage Forms Tablet: 250 mg

Reference Range Peak blood disulfiram level after a 500 mg dose: 0.38 mg/L; peak DDC level is ~1.2 mg/L; peak carbon disulfide level is 14 mg/L; concomitant ethanol levels >0.12 g/dL associated with unconsciousness when ethanol is used with disulfiram

Overdosage/Treatment To prevent absorption, lavage (up to 10 hours postingestion) and activated charcoal should be given; management of

disulfiram reaction: Institute support measures to restore blood pressure (pressors and fluids); antihistamines are useful to treat flushing; monitor for hypokalemia; metoclopramide or prochlorperazine can be used for vomiting; dopamine is not useful to treat disulfiram-ethanol induced hypotension; norepinephrine is the preferred agent; use of 4-methylpyrazole (7-10 mg/kg) or ascorbic acid (1 g I.V.) is investigational and not well documented in treating disulfiram-ethanol reaction; multiple dosing of activated charcoal may be useful in disulfiram overdose

Antidote(s)
- Norepinephrine [ANTIDOTE]

Test Interactions ↑ cholesterol (S), acetone levels; ↓ catecholamines (U)

Drug Interactions

Substrate (minor) of CYP1A2, 2A6, 2B6, 2D6, 2E1, 3A4; **Inhibits** CYP1A2 (weak), 2A6 (weak), 2B6 (weak), 2C9 (weak), 2D6 (weak), 2E1 (strong), 3A4 (weak)

Benzodiazepines: Disulfiram may increase serum concentrations of benzodiazepines; includes only benzodiazepines which undergo oxidative metabolism (all but oxazepam, lorazepam, temazepam).

Cocaine: Disulfiram may increase serum concentrations of cocaine; avoid concurrent use.

Co-trimoxazole: Intravenous trimethoprim-sulfamethoxazole contains 10% ethanol as a solubilizing agent and may interact with disulfiram; monitor for disulfiram reaction.

CYP2E1 substrates: Disulfiram may increase the levels/effects of CYP2E1 substrates. Example substrates include inhalational anesthetics, theophylline, and trimethadione.

Diphenhydramine: Syrup contains ethanol, avoid use of syrup; monitor for disulfiram reaction.

Ethanol: Disulfiram results in severe ethanol intolerance (disulfiram reaction) secondary to disulfiram's ability to inhibit aldehyde dehydrogenase; this combination should be avoided. Pharmaceutical products should be evaluated for possible inclusion of ethanol (eg, elixirs).

Isoniazid: Concurrent use with disulfiram may result in adverse CNS effects; this combination should be avoided.

MAO inhibitors: Concurrent use with disulfiram may result in adverse CNS effects; this combination should be avoided.

Metronidazole: Concurrent use with disulfiram may result in adverse CNS effects; this combination should be avoided.

Omeprazole: May cause CNS adverse effects (limited documentation); monitor.

Phenytoin: Disulfiram may increase theophylline serum concentrations; toxicity may occur.

Theophylline: Disulfiram may increase theophylline serum concentrations; toxicity may occur.

Tricyclic antidepressants: Disulfiram may increase adverse CNS effects; monitor for acute changes in mental status.

Warfarin: Disulfiram inhibits the metabolism of warfarin resulting in an increased hypoprothrombinemic response; avoid when possible or monitor INR closely and adjust warfarin dosage.

Pregnancy Risk Factor C

Pregnancy Implications Increased incidence of clubfoot, limb reduction, vertebral fusion have been reported

Lactation Excretion in breast milk unknown

Nursing Implications Administration of any medications containing alcohol including topicals is contraindicated

Docetaxel

Related Information
- Paclitaxel

CAS Number 114977-28-5; 148408-66-6

U.S. Brand Names Taxotere®

Synonyms NSC-628503; RP-6976

Use Treatment of locally-advanced or metastatic breast cancer, after failure of prior chemotherapy; treatment of locally-advanced or metastatic nonsmall cell lung cancer (NSCLC) after failure of prior platinum-based chemotherapy; in combination with cisplatin in treatment of patients who have not previously received chemotherapy for unresected NSCLC

Unlabeled/Investigational Use: Treatment of pancreatic, head and neck, and ovarian cancers, soft tissue sarcoma, and melanoma

Mechanism of Action Semisynthetic agent prepared from a noncytotoxic precursor which is extracted from the needles of the European Yew *Taxus baccata*. Docetaxel differs structurally from the prototype taxoid, paclitaxel, by substitutions at the C-10 and C-5 positions. It is an antimicrotubule agent, but exhibits a unique mechanism of action. Unlike other antimicrotubule agents that induce microtubule disassembly (eg, vinca alkaloids and colchicine), docetaxel promotes the assembly of microtubules from tubulin dimers, and inhibits the depolymerization of tubulin which leads to bundles of microtubules in the cell.

Adverse Reactions

Note: Frequencies cited for nonsmall cell lung cancer and breast cancer treatment. Exact frequency may vary based on tumor type, prior treatment, premedication, and dosage of docetaxel.

Cardiovascular: **Fluid retention, including peripheral edema, pleural effusions, and ascites (33% to 47%)**; may be more common at cumulative doses ≥ 400 mg/m^2 (up to 64% in breast cancer patients with dexamethasone premedication); hypotension, arrhythmias, atrial fibrillation, MI

Central nervous system: Confusion, loss of consciousness (transient), seizures

Dermatologic: **Alopecia (56% to 76%); nail disorder (11% to 31%, banding, onycholysis, hypo- or hyperpigmentation)**, rash, skin eruptions, erythema multiforme, radiation recall, Stevens-Johnson syndrome

Endocrine & metabolic: Dehydration

Gastrointestinal: **Mucositis/stomatitis (26% to 42%, severe in 6% to 7%)**, may be dose-limiting (premedication may reduce frequency and severity); **nausea and vomiting (40% to 80%, severe in 1% to 5%); diarrhea (33% to 43%)**, taste perversion, gastrointestinal hemorrhage, gastrointestinal obstruction, gastrointestinal perforation, ileus, ischemic colitis, neutropenic enterocolitis

Hematologic: **Myelosuppression, neutropenia (75% to 85%), thrombocytopenia, anemia**
Onset: 4-7 days
Nadir: 5-9 days
Recovery: 21 days

Hepatic: **Transaminase levels increased**, bilirubin increased, hepatitis

Neuromuscular & skeletal: **Neurosensory changes (paresthesia, dysesthesia, pain) noted in 23% to 49% (severe in up to 6%). Motor neuropathy, including weakness**, noted in as many as 16% of lung cancer patients (severe in up to 5%); **myalgia (3% to 21%)**, arthralgia. Neuropathy may be more common at higher cumulative docetaxel dosages or with prior cisplatin therapy.

Ocular: Lacrimal duct obstruction, visual disturbances

Respiratory: Acute respiratory distress syndrome (ARDS), interstitial pneumonia, pulmonary edema, pulmonary embolism, pulmonary fibrosis

Miscellaneous: **Hypersensitivity reactions (6% to 13%; angioedema, rash, flushing, fever, hypotension)**; frequency substantially reduced by premedication with dexamethasone starting one day prior to docetaxel administration; infusion site reactions

Pharmacodynamics/Kinetics
Administered by I.V. infusion and exhibits linear pharmacokinetics at the recommended dosage range

Distribution: V_d: 12-16 L/kg. Exhibits a triphasic decline in plasma concentrations. Initial rapid decline represents distribution to the peripheral compartment and the terminal phase reflects a relatively slow efflux of docetaxel from the peripheral compartment. Mean steady state: 36.6-95.6 L/m^2, indicating extensive extravascular distribution and/or tissue binding. Mean steady state volume of distribution is 113 liters.

Protein binding: 94% mainly to alpha$_1$-acid glycoprotein, albumin, and lipoproteins

Metabolism: Oxidative metabolism by the liver; isoenzymes of cytochrome P450 (CYA3A) are involved in metabolism

Half-life: α, β, and γ phases: 4 minutes, 36 minutes, and 11.1 hours, respectively

Elimination: Following oxidative metabolism, docetaxel is eliminated in both urine (6%) and feces (75%) with approximately 80% eliminated in the first 48 hours

Mean values for total body clearance: 21 L/hour/m^2

Dosage
Adults: I.V. infusion: Refer to individual protocols:
Breast cancer (locally-advanced or metastatic): 60-100 mg/m^2 over 1 hour every 3 weeks; patients initially started at 60 mg/m^2 who do not develop toxicity may tolerate higher doses

Nonsmall-cell lung cancer: I.V.: 75 mg/m^2 over 1 hour every 3 weeks

Dosing adjustment for toxicity:
Note: Toxicity includes febrile neutropenia, neutrophils ≤ 500/mm^3 for >1 week, severe or cumulative cutaneous reactions; in nonsmall cell lung cancer, this may also include other grade 3/4 nonhematologic toxicities.

Breast cancer: Patients dosed initially at 100 mg/m^2; reduce dose to 75 mg/m^2; **Note:** If the patient continues to experience these adverse reactions, the dosage should be reduced to 55 mg/m^2 or therapy should be discontinued

Nonsmall cell lung cancer:
Monotherapy: Patients dosed initially at 75 mg/m^2 should have dose held until toxicity is resolved, then resume at 55 mg/m^2; discontinue patients who develop $\geq$ grade 3 peripheral neuropathy.
Combination therapy: Patients dosed initially at 75 mg/m^2, in combination with cisplatin, should have the docetaxel dosage reduced to 65 mg/m^2 in subsequent cycles; if further adjustment is required, dosage may be reduced to 50 mg/m^2

Dosing adjustment in hepatic impairment: Total bilirubin $\geq$ the upper limit of normal (ULN), or AST/ALT >1.5 times the ULN concomitant with alkaline phosphatase >2.5 times the ULN: Docetaxel **should not be administered**.

Stability
Store intact vials at 2°C to 25°C (36°F to 77°F) and protect from light. Intact vials of solution should be further diluted with 13% (w/w) ethanol/water to a final concentration of 10 mg/mL. Do not shake. Initial diluted solution is stable for 8 hours at room temperature or under refrigeration.

Docetaxel dose should be further diluted with 0.9% sodium chloride or 5% dextrose in water to a final concentration of 0.3-0.9 mg/mL and must be prepared in a glass bottle, polypropylene, or polyolefin plastic bag to prevent leaching of plasticizers.

Non-PVC tubing **must** be used. Diluted solutions are stable for up to 4 weeks at room temperature 15°C to 25°C (59°F to 77°F) in polyolefin containers. (Thiesen J and Kramer I, *Pharm World Sci*, 1999, 21(3): 137-41.)

Although the stability of some antineoplastic agents may be long, it is probably considered good pharmaceutical practice to allow a maximum expiration dating of 24 hours due to possible sterility concerns. The manufacturer recommends using within 4 hours.

Monitoring Parameters
Monitor for hypersensitivity reactions and fluid retention

Administration
Anaphylactoid-like reactions have been reported: Premedication with dexamethasone (4-8 mg orally twice daily for 3 or 5 days starting 1 day prior to administration of docetaxel).

Administer I.V. infusion over 1-hour through nonsorbing (nonpolyvinylchloride) tubing; in-line filter is not necessary. When administered as sequential infusions, taxane derivatives should be administered before platinum derivatives (cisplatin, carboplatin) to limit myelosuppression and to enhance efficacy.

Contraindications
Hypersensitivity to docetaxel or any component of the formulation; prior hypersensitivity to medications containing polysorbate 80; pre-existing bone marrow suppression (neutrophils <1500 cells/mm^3); pregnancy

Warnings
Hazardous agent – use appropriate precautions for handling and disposal.

[U.S. Boxed Warnings]: Use caution in hepatic disease; avoid use in patients with bilirubin exceeding upper limit of normal (ULN) or AST and/or ALT >1.5 times ULN in conjunction with alkaline phosphatase >2.5 times ULN; patients with abnormal liver function are at increased risk of treatment-related adverse events. Severe hypersensitivity reactions characterized by hypotension, bronchospasms, anaphylaxis, or minor reactions characterized by generalized rash/erythema may occur. Fluid retention syndrome characterized by pleural effusions, ascites, edema, and weight gain (2-15 kg) has also been reported. The incidence and severity of the syndrome increase sharply at cumulative doses ≥ 400 mg/m^2. Patients should be premedicated with a corticosteroid to prevent hypersensitivity reactions and fluid retention; severity is reduced with dexamethasone premedication starting one day prior to docetaxel administration.

Neutropenia is the dose-limiting toxicity; however, this rarely results in treatment delays and prophylactic colony stimulating factors have not been routinely used. **[U.S. Boxed Warning]: Patients with abnormal liver function, those receiving higher doses and patients with non-small cell lung cancer and a history of prior treatment with platinum derivatives who receive docetaxel doses higher than 100 mg/m^2 are at higher risk for treatment-related mortality.** Patients with increased liver function tests experienced more episodes of neutropenia with a greater number of severe infections. **[U.S. Boxed Warning]: Patients with an absolute neutrophil count <1500 cells/mm^3 should not receive docetaxel.** When administered as sequential infusions, taxane derivatives (docetaxel, paclitaxel) should be administered before platinum derivatives (carboplatin, cisplatin) to limit myelosuppression and to enhance efficacy.

Cutaneous reactions including erythema and desquamation have been reported; may require dose reduction. Dosage adjustment is recommended with severe neurosensory symptoms (paresthesia, dysesthesia, pain). **[U.S. Boxed Warning]: Should be administered under the supervision of an experienced cancer chemotherapy physician.** Safety and efficacy in children <16 years of age have not been established.

Dosage Forms
Injection, solution [concentrate]:
Taxotere®: 20 mg/0.5 mL (0.5 mL, 2 mL) [contains Polysorbate 80®; diluent contains ethanol 13%]

Overdosage/Treatment
Supportive therapy: Extravasation of docetaxel does not usually cause significant injury. Hypersensitivity reactions should be treated with standard therapy.

Drug Interactions
Substrate of CYP3A4 (major); **Inhibits** CYP3A4 (weak)

Antifungal agents (imidazole): Imidazole antifungal agents may decrease the metabolism (via CYP isoenzymes) of docetaxel; avoid concurrent use.

Carboplatin, cisplatin (platinum derivatives): When administered as sequential infusions, taxane derivatives should be administered before platinum derivatives to limit myelosuppression.

CYP3A4 inducers: CYP3A4 inducers may decrease the levels/effects of docetaxel. Example inducers include aminoglutethimide, carbamazepine, nafcillin, nevirapine, phenobarbital, phenytoin, and rifamycins.

CYP3A4 inhibitors: May increase the levels/effects of docetaxel. Example inhibitors include azole antifungals, clarithromycin, diclofenac, doxycycline, erythromycin, imatinib, isoniazid, nefazodone, nicardipine, propofol, protease inhibitors, quinidine, telithromycin, and verapamil.

Pregnancy Risk Factor D

Pregnancy Implications Animal studies have demonstrated embryotoxicity, fetal toxicity, and maternal toxicity. There are no adequate and well-controlled studies in pregnant women; however, fetal harm may occur. Women of childbearing potential should avoid becoming pregnant. A pregnancy registry is available for all cancers diagnosed during pregnancy at Cooper Health (856-757-7876).

Lactation Excretion in breast milk unknown/contraindicated

Additional Information St John's wort may decrease docetaxel levels.

Specific References

Behrens RJ, Gulley JL, and Dahut WL, "Pulmonary Toxicity During Prostate Cancer Treatment with Docetaxel and Thalidomide," *Am J Ther*, 2003, 10(3):228-32.

Docusate

CAS Number 128-49-4; 577-11-7; 7491-09-0

U.S. Brand Names Colace® [OTC]; D-S-S® [OTC]; Diocto® [OTC]; Docusoft-S™ [OTC]; DOS® [OTC]; ex-lax® Stool Softener [OTC]; Fleet® Sof-Lax® [OTC]; Genasoft® [OTC]; Phillips'® Stool Softener Laxative [OTC]; Surfak® [OTC]

Synonyms Dioctyl Calcium Sulfosuccinate; Dioctyl Sodium Sulfosuccinate; Docusate Calcium; Docusate Potassium; Docusate Sodium; DOSS; DSS

Use Stool softener in patients who should avoid straining during defecation and constipation associated with hard, dry stools

Unlabeled/Investigational Use Ceruminolytic

Mechanism of Action An emollient laxative which reduces surface tension of the oil-water interface of the stool resulting in enhanced incorporation of water and fat allowing for stool softening; also promotes intestinal secretion of potassium, water, sodium, and chloride

Adverse Reactions Gastrointestinal: Intestinal obstruction, diarrhea, abdominal cramping, throat irritation

Signs and Symptoms of Overdose Abdominal cramps, diarrhea, fluid loss, hypokalemia, hypomagnesemia, nausea, vomiting

Pharmacodynamics/Kinetics

Onset of action: 12-72 hours

Excretion: Feces

Dosage Docusate salts are interchangeable; the amount of sodium or calcium per dosage unit is clinically insignificant

Infants and Children <3 years: Oral: 10-40 mg/day in 1-4 divided doses

Children: Oral:

3-6 years: 20-60 mg/day in 1-4 divided doses

6-12 years: 40-150 mg/day in 1-4 divided doses

Adolescents and Adults: Oral: 50-500 mg/day in 1-4 divided doses

Older Children and Adults: Rectal: Add 50-100 mg of docusate liquid to enema fluid (saline or water); administer as retention or flushing enema

Ceruminolytic (unlabeled use): Intra-aural: Administer 1 mL of docusate sodium in 2 mL syringes; if no clearance in 15 minutes, irrigate with 50-100 mL normal saline (this method is 80% effective)

Stability

Store intact vials at 2°C to 25°C (36°F to 77°F) and protect from light. Intact vials of solution should be further diluted with 13% (w/w) ethanol/water to a final concentration of 10 mg/mL. Do not shake. Initial diluted solution is stable for 8 hours at room temperature or under refrigeration.

Docetaxel dose should be further diluted with 0.9% sodium chloride or 5% dextrose in water to a final concentration of 0.3-0.9 mg/mL and must be prepared in a glass bottle, polypropylene, or polyolefin plastic bag to prevent leaching of plasticizers.

Non-PVC tubing **must** be used. Diluted solutions are stable for up to 4 weeks at room temperature 15°C to 25°C (59°F to 77°F) in polyolefin containers. (Thiesen J and Kramer I, *Pharm World Sci*, 1999, 21(3):137-41.)

Although the stability of some antineoplastic agents may be long, it is probably considered good pharmaceutical practice to allow a maximum expiration dating of 24 hours due to possible sterility concerns. The manufacturer recommends using within 4 hours.

Administration Anaphylactoid-like reactions have been reported: Premedication with dexamethasone (8 mg orally twice daily for 3 or 5 days starting 1 day prior to administration of docetaxel).

Administer I.V. infusion over 1-hour. When administered as sequential infusions, taxane derivatives should be administered before platinum derivatives (cisplatin, carboplatin) to limit myelosuppression and to enhance efficacy.

Contraindications Hypersensitivity to docusate or any component of the formulation; concomitant use of mineral oil; intestinal obstruction, acute abdominal pain, nausea, or vomiting

Warnings Prolonged, frequent or excessive use may result in dependence or electrolyte imbalance

Dosage Forms Capsule, as calcium (Surfak®): 240 mg

Capsule, as sodium: 100 mg, 250 mg

Colace®: 50 mg [contains sodium 3 mg], 100 mg [contains sodium 5 mg]

Docusoft-S™: 100 mg [contains sodium 5 mg]

DOK™, Genasoft®: 100 mg

DOS®, D-S-S®: 100 mg, 250 mg

Dulcolax® Stool Softener: 100 mg [contains sodium 5 mg]

Phillips'® Stool Softener Laxative: 100 mg [contains sodium 5.2 mg]

Enema, rectal, as sodium (Enemeez®): 283 mg/5 mL 5 mL

Gelcap, as sodium (Fleet® Sof-Lax®): 100 mg

Liquid, as sodium: 150 mg/15 mL (480 mL)

Colace®: 150 mg/15 mL (30 mL) [contains sodium 1 mg/mL]

Diocto®: 150 mg/15 mL (480 mL) [vanilla flavor]

Silace: 150 mg/15 mL (480 mL) [lemon-vanilla flavor]

Syrup, as sodium: 60 mg/15 mL (480 mL)

Colace®, Diocto®: 60 mg/15 mL (480 mL) [alcohol free, sugar free; contains sodium 36 mg/5 mL]

Silace: 20 mg/5 mL (480 mL) [peppermint flavor]

Overdosage/Treatment

Decontamination: Lavage (within 1 hour)/activated charcoal without a cathartic

Supportive therapy: I.V. fluid and electrolyte replacement; restrict solid food

Test Interactions ↑ transaminases; ↓ potassium (S), chloride (S)

Pregnancy Risk Factor C

Pregnancy Implications Can cause hypomagnesemia in the neonate; no evidence for congenital malformations

Lactation Excretion in breast milk unknown/compatible

Nursing Implications Docusate liquid should be given with milk, fruit juice, or infant formula to mask the bitter taste

Additional Information Docusate sodium 5-10 mg/mL liquid instilled in the ear as a ceruminolytic produces substantial ear wax disintegration within 15 minutes and complete disintegration after 24 hours. A safe agent to be used in elderly; some evidence that doses <200 mg are ineffective; stool softeners are unnecessary if stool is well hydrated or "mushy" and soft; shown to be ineffective used long-term.

Dofetilide

U.S. Brand Names Tikosyn™

Use Prevention and treatment of fibrillation (atrial), flutter (atrial), paroxysmal tachycardia (ventricular), tachycardia (ventricular), fibrillation (ventricular); used in conjunction with implantable defibrillator

Mechanism of Action Selective class III antiarrhythmic agent (investigational agent undergoing phase III trials in U.S.); more potent than sotalol, it causes selective blockade of potassium channels in the myocardium that prolongs ventricular refractoriness

Adverse Reactions Cardiovascular: Prolongs QT intervals on ECG (dose dependent), possible increase in incidence of torsade de pointes (4% to 8%), sinus bradycardia

Pharmacodynamics/Kinetics

Absorption: >90%

Distribution: V_d: 3 L/kg

Protein binding: 60% to 70%

Metabolism: Hepatic via CYP3A4, but low affinity for it; metabolites formed by N-dealkylation and N-oxidation

Bioavailability: >90%

Half-life elimination: 10 hours

Time to peak: Fasting: 2-3 hours

Excretion: Urine (80%, 80% as unchanged drug, 20% as inactive or minimally active metabolites); renal elimination consists of glomerular filtration and active tubular secretion via cationic transport system

Dosage Oral: 0.25-1 mg twice daily in patients with sustained tachycardia (ventricular) (lower dose in patients with renal insufficiency)

I.V.:

Supraventricular tachycardia: 1-10 mcg/kg over 15 minutes followed by 0.12-0.5 mcg/kg maintenance infusion

Ventricular arrhythmia: 1.5-15 mcg/kg

Monitoring Parameters ECG monitoring with attention to QT_c and occurrence of ventricular arrhythmias, baseline serum creatinine and changes in serum creatinine. Check serum potassium and magnesium levels if on medications where these electrolyte disturbances can occur, or if patient has a history of hypokalemia or hypomagnesemia. QT or QT_c must be monitored at specific times prior to the first dose and during the first 3 days of therapy. Thereafter, QT or QT_c and creatinine clearance must be evaluated at 3-month intervals.

Administration Do not open capsules.

Contraindications Hypersensitivity to dofetilide or any component of the formulation; patients with congenital or acquired long QT syndromes; do not use if a baseline QT interval or QT_c is >440 msec (500 msec in patients with ventricular conduction abnormalities); severe renal impairment (estimated Cl_{cr} <20 mL/minute); concurrent use with verapamil, cimetidine, hydrochlorothiazide (alone or in combinations), trimethoprim (alone or in combination with sulfamethoxazole), itraconazole, ketoconazole, prochlorperazine, or megestrol; baseline heart rate <50 beats/ minute; other drugs that prolong QT intervals (phenothiazines, cisapride, bepridil, tricyclic antidepressants, sparfloxacin, gatifloxacin, moxifloxacin; hypokalemia or hypomagnesemia; concurrent amiodarone, clarithromycin, or erythromycin

Warnings

[U.S. Boxed Warning]: Must be initiated (or reinitiated) in a setting with continuous monitoring and staff familiar with the recognition and treatment of life-threatening arrhythmias. Patients must be monitored with continuous ECG for a minimum of 3 days, or for a minimum of 12 hours after electrical or pharmacological cardioversion to normal sinus rhythm, whichever is greater. Patients should be readmitted for continuous monitoring if dosage is later increased.

Reserve for patients who are highly symptomatic with atrial fibrillation/ atrial flutter; torsade de pointes significantly increases with doses >500 mcg twice daily; hold class I or class III antiarrhythmics for at least three half-lives prior to starting dofetilide; use in patients on amiodarone therapy only if serum amiodarone level is <0.3 mg/L or if amiodarone was stopped for >3 months previously; correct hypokalemia or hypomagnesemia before initiating dofetilide and maintain within normal limits during treatment. Risk of hypokalemia and/or hypomagnesemia may be increased by potassium-depleting diuretics, increasing the risk of torsade de pointes. Concurrent use with other drugs known to prolong QT_c interval is not recommended.

Patients with sick sinus syndrome or with second or third-degree heart block should not receive dofetilide unless a functional pacemaker is in place. Defibrillation threshold is reduced in patients with ventricular tachycardia or ventricular fibrillation undergoing implantation of a cardioverter-defibrillator device. Safety and efficacy in children (<18 years old) have not been established. Use with caution in renal impairment; not recommended in patients receiving drugs which may compete for renal secretion via cationic transport. Use with caution in patients with severe hepatic impairment.

Dosage Forms Capsule: 125 mcg, 250 mcg, 500 mcg

Overdosage/Treatment

Decontamination: Lavage (within 1 hour)/activated charcoal (for oral ingestion)

Supportive therapy: No human overdose experience since this agent inhibits intracellular potassium transport, agents such as glucose/insulin and hyperventilation may assist in creasing intracellular potassium concentrations; need to monitor for hypokalemia and torsade de pointes

Enhancement of elimination: Multiple dosing of activated charcoal may be effective

Drug Interactions **Substrate** of CYP3A4 (minor)

If dofetilide needs to be discontinued to allow dosing of other potentially interacting drug(s) (see below), a washout period of at least 2 days is needed before starting the other drug(s).

Cimetidine, a cation transport system inhibitor, inhibits dofetilide's elimination and can cause a 58% increase in dofetilide's plasma levels; concomitant use is contraindicated.

Diuretics and other drugs (aminoglycosides) which deplete potassium or magnesium may increase dofetilide toxicity (torsade de pointes). Concurrent use of hydrochlorothiazide is contraindicated.

Hydrochlorothiazide: May enhance the QT_c-prolonging effect of dofetilide. May increase serum concentration of dofetilide. Concurrent use is contraindicated.

Itraconazole: May decrease the metabolism of dofetilide. Concurrent use is contraindicated.

Ketoconazole increases dofetilide's C_{max} (53% males, 97% females) and the AUC (41% males, 69% females) when used concurrently; concomitant use is contraindicated.

QT_c-prolonging agents (including bepridil, cisapride, clarithromycin, erythromycin, tricyclic antidepressants, phenothiazines, sparfloxacin, gatifloxacin, moxifloxacin): Use is contraindicated.

Renal cationic transport inhibitors (including triamterene, metformin, amiloride, prochlorperazine, megestrol) may increase dofetilide levels; coadminister with caution.

Trimethoprim (alone or in combination with sulfamethoxazole) increases dofetilide's C_{max} (103%) and AUC (93%); concomitant use is contraindicated.

Verapamil causes an increase in dofetilide's peak plasma levels by 42%. In the supraventricular arrhythmia and a higher incidence of torsade de pointes was seen in patients on verapamil; concomitant use is contraindicated.

Pregnancy Risk Factor C

Pregnancy Implications Dofetilide has been shown to adversely affect *in utero* growth, organogenesis, and survival of rats and mice. There are no adequate and well controlled studies in pregnant women. Dofetilide should be used with extreme caution in pregnant women and in women of childbearing age only when the benefit to the patient unequivocally justifies the potential risk to the fetus.

Lactation Excretion in breast milk unknown/not recommended

Additional Information Increases myocardial refractoriness; peak onset of torsade de pointes is within 1 hour of I.V. use and within 2 hours of oral use

Donepezil

U.S. Brand Names Aricept®

Synonyms E2020

Use Treatment of mild to moderate dementia of the Alzheimer's type

Unlabeled/Investigational Use Attention-deficit/hyperactivity disorder (ADHD), behavioral syndromes in dementia

Mechanism of Action Alzheimer's disease is characterized by cholinergic deficiency in the cortex and basal forebrain, which contributes to cognitive deficits. Donepezil reversibly and noncompetitively inhibits centrally-active acetylcholinesterase, the enzyme responsible for hydrolysis of acetylcholine. This appears to result in increased concentrations of acetylcholine available for synaptic transmission in the central nervous system.

Adverse Reactions

Cardiovascular: Syncope, chest pain

Central nervous system: **Headache**, fatigue, insomnia, dizziness, depression, abnormal dreams, somnolence, seizures, paranoia

Dermatologic: Bruising

Gastrointestinal: **Nausea, diarrhea**, anorexia, vomiting, weight loss

Genitourinary: Urinary incontinence

Neuromuscular & skeletal: Muscle cramps, arthritis, body pain

Renal: Polyuria

Pharmacodynamics/Kinetics

Absorption: Well absorbed

Protein binding: 96%, primarily to albumin (75%) and α_1-acid glycoprotein (21%)

Metabolism: Extensively to four major metabolites (two are active) via CYP2D6 and 3A4; undergoes glucuronidation

Bioavailability: 100%

Half-life elimination: 70 hours; time to steady-state: 15 days

Time to peak, plasma: 3-4 hours

Excretion: Urine 57% (17% as unchanged drug); feces 15%

Dosage Oral:

Children: ADHD (unlabeled use): 5 mg/day

Adults: Dementia of Alzheimer's type: Initial: 5 mg/day at bedtime; may increase to 10 mg/day at bedtime after 4-6 weeks

Monitoring Parameters Behavior, mood, bowel function

Administration Aricept® ODT: Allow tablet to dissolve completely on tongue and follow with water.

Contraindications Hypersensitivity to donepezil, piperidine derivatives, or any component of the formulation

Warnings Cholinesterase inhibitors may have vagotonic effects which may cause bradycardia and/or heart block with or without a history of cardiac disease; syncopal episodes have been associated with donepezil. Use with caution with sick sinus syndrome or other supraventricular cardiac conduction abnormalities, with seizures, COPD, or asthma. Use with caution in patients at risk of ulcer disease (ie, previous history or NSAID use), or in patients with bladder outlet obstruction. May cause diarrhea, nausea, and/or vomiting, which may be dose-related.

Dosage Forms Tablet, as hydrochloride (Aricept®): 5 mg, 10 mg

Tablet, orally disintegrating, as hydrochloride (Aricept® ODT): 5 mg, 10 mg

Reference Range Following a 5 mg oral dosing regimen, steady-state plasma donepezil concentration is ~30 ng/mL

Overdosage/Treatment

Decontamination: Lavage within 1 hour/activated charcoal

Supportive therapy: Atropine can be used to treat bradycardia

Drug Interactions **Substrate** (minor) of CYP2D6, 3A4

Anticholinergic agents: Effects of donepezil may be inhibited by anticholinergic agents (benztropine)

Antipsychotic agents: Acetylcholinesterase inhibitors (central) may increase the risk of antipsychotic-related extrapyramidal symptoms; monitor.

Cholinergic agents: A synergistic effect may be seen with concurrent administration of succinylcholine or cholinergic agonists (bethanechol); excessive cholinergic stimulation and toxicity may occur; use caution.

Cocaine may prolong or potentiate cocaine activity.

Pregnancy Risk Factor C

Pregnancy Implications Teratogenic effects were not observed in animal studies. There are no adequate and well-controlled studies in pregnant women.

Lactation Excretion in breast milk unknown/not recommended

Specific References

Bynum N, Poklis J, Garside D, et al, "Postmortem Donepezil and Memantine Concentrations," *J Anal Toxicol*, 2006, 30:153-4.

Kondoh T, Amamoto N, Doi T, et al, "Dramatic Improvement in Down Syndrome-Associated Cognitive Impairment with Donepezil," *Ann Pharmacother*, 2005, 39(3):563-6.

Lintemoot J, Anderson D, and Urizar B, "Donepezil (Aricept®): An Incidental Finding in Eleven Postmortem Cases," *J Anal Toxicol*, 2006, 30:133.

Dornase Alfa

U.S. Brand Names Pulmozyme®

Synonyms DNase; Recombinant Human Deoxyribonuclease

Use Management of cystic fibrosis patients to reduce the frequency of respiratory infections that require parenteral antibiotics, and to improve pulmonary function

Unlabeled/Investigational Use Treatment of chronic bronchitis

Mechanism of Action The hallmark of cystic fibrosis lung disease is the presence of abundant, purulent airway secretions composed primarily of highly polymerized DNA. The principal source of this DNA is the nuclei of degenerating neutrophils, which is present in large concentrations in infected lung secretions. The presence of this DNA produces a viscous mucous that may contribute to the decreased mucociliary transport and persistent infections that are commonly seen in this population. Dornase alfa is a deoxyribonuclease (DNA) enzyme produced by recombinant gene technology. Dornase selectively cleaves DNA, thus reducing mucous viscosity and, as a result, airflow in the lung is improved and the risk of bacterial infection may be decreased. Pulmonary function improves after 3 days of use.

Adverse Reactions

Cardiovascular: **Chest pain**, angina

Dermatologic: **Rash**

Ocular: Conjunctivitis

Respiratory: Cough, dyspnea, **pharyngitis**, laryngitis, hoarse throat, wheezing, rhinitis, hemoptysis

Miscellaneous: **Voice alteration** (most noted in female patients)

Pharmacodynamics/Kinetics

Onset of action: Nebulization: Enzyme levels are measured in sputum in ~15 minutes

Duration: Rapidly declines

Dosage Children >5 years and Adults: Inhalation: 2.5 mg once daily through selected nebulizers in conjunction with a Pulmo-Aide® or a Pari-Proneb® compressor

Stability Must be stored in the refrigerator at 2°C to 8°C (36°F to 46°F) and protected from strong light; should not be exposed to room temperature for a total of 24 hours

Administration Nebulization: Should not be diluted or mixed with any other drugs in the nebulizer, this may inactivate the drug

Contraindications Hypersensitivity to dornase alfa, Chinese hamster ovary cell products (eg, epoetin alfa), or any component of the formulation

Warnings No clinical trials have been conducted to demonstrate safety and effectiveness of dornase in patients with pulmonary function <40% of normal or in patients for longer treatment periods >12 months; no data exists regarding safety during lactation

Dosage Forms Solution for nebulization: 1 mg/mL (2.5 mL)

Overdosage/Treatment Supportive therapy: 100% humidified oxygen; beta agonist bronchodilation for wheezing

Drug Interactions Dornase alfa can be effectively and safely used in conjunction with standard CF therapies including oral, inhaled, and parenteral antibiotics, bronchodilators, enzyme supplements, vitamins, oral and inhaled corticosteroids, and analgesics. No formal drug interaction studies have been performed.

Pregnancy Risk Factor B

Lactation Excretion in breast milk unknown

Nursing Implications Should not be diluted or mixed with any other drugs in the nebulizer, this may inactivate the drug

Doxazosin

CAS Number 74191-85-8; 77883-43-3

U.S. Brand Names Cardura®

Synonyms Doxazosin Mesylate

Use Alpha-blocking agent for treatment of hypertension; treatment of benign prostatic hyperplasia (BPH)

Mechanism of Action Doxazosin is a long-acting selective inhibitor of postjunctional α_1-adrenoceptors as demonstrated in isolated animal tissues and anesthetized healthy animals. Doxazosin is a water soluble quinazoline analogue of prazosin, and on a weight-for-weight basis is approximately half as potent as prazosin in postsynaptic α_1-adrenoceptor inhibition in animals and man. Inhibition of these α_1-adrenergic receptors in the peripheral vasculature prevents vasoconstriction from adrenergic stimulation; therefore, allowing vasodilation and a reduction in blood pressure. Because of doxazosin's and similar α_1-adrenergic blockers specificity, they preserve feedback control of transmitter norepinephrine release and, therefore, cause minimal reflex activation.

Adverse Reactions

Cardiovascular: Palpitations, arrhythmia, orthostatic hypotension (dose-related), hypotension, tachycardia, edema, chest pain, syncope, flushing, angina, bradycardia, myocardial infarction, pallor, peripheral ischemia

Central nervous system: **Dizziness, headache**, vertigo, nervousness, somnolence, anxiety, depression, ataxia, abnormal thinking, agitation, amnesia, confusion, depersonalization, emotional lability, fever, hyp-oesthesia, impaired concentration, migraine, paranoia, paresis, stroke, fatigue, insomnia

Dermatologic: Alopecia, xerosis, urticaria, purpura, pruritus, licheniform eruptions, exanthem, rash, eczema,

Endocrine & metabolic: Decreased libido, sexual dysfunction, breast pain, gout, hot flashes, hypokalemia, gynecomastia, lymphadenopathy, impotence

Gastrointestinal: Nausea, vomiting, xerostomia, diarrhea, constipation, abdominal discomfort, flatulence, anorexia, fecal incontinence, gastroenteritis, taste perversion, weight gain, weight loss, dyspepsia

Genitourinary: Incontinence, polyuria, priapism, enuresis, micturition abnormality, nocturia, urinary tract infection

Hematologic: Leukopenia, thrombocytopenia

Hepatic: Cholestasis, hepatitis

Neuromuscular & skeletal: Back pain; paresthesia, movement disorder, hypertonia, weakness, myalgia, muscle cramps, rigors, twitching, cataplexy, arthritis

Ocular: Abnormal vision, conjunctivitis, abnormal lacrimation, photophobia

Otic: Tinnitus, earache, parosmia

Renal: Renal calculus, hematuria

Respiratory: Rhinitis, dyspnea, sinusitis, epistaxis, bronchospasm, coughing, pharyngitis

Miscellaneous: Systemic lupus erythematosus, flu-like syndrome, diaphoresis, infection, thirst, allergic reaction

Signs and Symptoms of Overdose Drowsiness, lightheadedness, severe hypotension, tachycardia

Pharmacodynamics/Kinetics

Not significantly affected by increased age

Duration: >24 hours

Protein binding: Extended release: 98%

Metabolism: Extensively hepatic to active metabolites; primarily via CYP3A4; secondary pathways involve CYP2D6 and 2C19

Bioavailability: Extended release relative to immediate release: 54% to 59%

Half-life elimination: 15-22 hours

Time to peak, serum: Immediate release: 2-3 hours; extended release: 8-9 hours

Excretion: Feces (63% primarily as metabolites); urine (9%)

Dosage Oral:

Adults: 1 mg once daily in morning or evening; may be increased to 2 mg once daily. Thereafter titrate upwards, if needed, over several weeks, balancing therapeutic benefit with doxazosin-induced postural hypotension

Hypertension: Maximum dose: 16 mg/day

BPH: Goal: 4-8 mg/day; maximum dose: 8 mg/day

Elderly: Initial: 0.5 mg once daily

Monitoring Parameters Blood pressure, standing and sitting/supine

Administration Cardura® XL: Tablets should be swallowed whole; do not crush, chew, or divide.

Contraindications Hypersensitivity to quinazolines (prazosin, terazosin), doxazosin, or any component of the formulation

Warnings

Can cause significant orthostatic hypotension and syncope, especially with first dose; anticipate a similar effect if therapy is interrupted for a few days, if dosage is rapidly increased, or if another antihypertensive drug (particularly vasodilators) or a PDE5 inhibitor is introduced. Patients should be cautioned about performing hazardous tasks when starting new therapy or adjusting dosage upward. Prostate cancer should be ruled out before starting for BPH. Use with caution in mild to moderate hepatic impairment; not recommended in severe dysfunction. Intraoperative floppy iris syndrome has been observed in cataract surgery patients who were on or were previously treated with alpha1 blockers. Causality has not been established and there appears to be no benefit in discontinuing alpha blocker therapy prior to surgery. Safety and efficacy in children have not been established.

The extended release formulation consists of drug within a nondeformable matrix; following drug release/absorption, the matrix/shell is expelled in the stool. The use of nondeformable products in patients with known stricture/narrowing of the GI tract has been associated with symptoms of obstruction. Use caution in patients with increased GI retention (eg, chronic constipation) as doxazosin exposure may be increased. Extended release formulation is not approved for the treatment of hypertension.

Dosage Forms Tablet: 1 mg, 2 mg, 4 mg, 8 mg

Cardura®: 1 mg, 2 mg, 4 mg, 8 mg

Tablet, extended release:

Cardura® XL: 4 mg, 8 mg

Reference Range 8 mg dose is associated with a serum level of 60 ng/mL

Overdosage/Treatment

Decontamination: Lavage (within 1 hour)/activated charcoal

Supportive therapy: Treatment is supportive with fluids; use only pure alpha-adrenergic pressors for hypotension (norepinephrine, phenylephrine); dobutamine may also be helpful

Enhancement of elimination: Multiple dose of activated charcoal may be effective; not removed by dialysis

Antidote(s)
- DOBUTamine [ANTIDOTE]

Drug Interactions ACE inhibitors: Hypotensive effect (particularly orthostasis) may be increased.

Beta-blockers: Hypotensive effect may be increased.

Calcium channel blockers: Hypotensive effect may be increased.

Phosphodiesterase-5 (PDE5) inhibitors (eg, sildenafil, tadalafil, vardenafil): Blood pressure-lowering effects are additive. Use with caution and monitor.

Pregnancy Risk Factor C

Pregnancy Implications Some studies demonstrated embryolethality resulting from doxazosin exposure during organogenesis. Delayed postnatal development was also noted. There are no adequate and well-controlled studies in pregnant women. Use only if benefit outweighs risk.

Lactation Excretion in breast milk unknown/not recommended

Nursing Implications Syncope may occur (usually within 90 minutes of the initial dose)

Specific References

McConnell JD, Roehrborn CG, Bautista OM, et al, "The Long-Term Effect of Doxazosin, Finasteride, and Combination Therapy on the Clinical Progression of Benign Prostatic Hyperplasia: Medical Therapy of Prostatic Symptoms (MTOPS) Research Group," *N Engl J Med*, 2003, 349(25):2387-98.

Doxepin

Related Information
- Anticholinergic Effects of Common Psychotropics
- Antidepressant Agents
- Therapeutic Drugs Associated with Hallucinations

CAS Number 1229-29-4; 1668-19-5; 25127-31-5; 4698-39-9

U.S. Brand Names Prudoxin™; Sinequan®; Zonalon®

Synonyms Doxepin Hydrochloride

Impairment Potential Yes. Single oral dose of 25 mg can prolong choice reaction time. (Stromberg C, Seppala T, and Mattila MJ, "Acute Effects of Maprotiline, Doxepin, and Zimeldine with Alcohol in Healthy Volunteers," *Arch Int Pharmacodyn Ther*, 1988, 291:217-28.)

Use

Oral: Depression

Topical: Short-term (<8 days) management of moderate pruritus in adults with atopic dermatitis or lichen simplex chronicus

Unlabeled/Investigational Use Analgesic for certain chronic and neuropathic pain; anxiety

Mechanism of Action Increases the synaptic concentration of serotonin and/or norepinephrine in the central nervous system by inhibition of their reuptake by the presynaptic neuronal membrane; also an H_2-receptor antagonist

Adverse Reactions

Oral: Frequency not defined.

Cardiovascular: Hypotension, hypertension, tachycardia

Central nervous system: Drowsiness, dizziness, headache, disorientation, ataxia, confusion, seizure

Dermatologic: Alopecia, photosensitivity, rash, pruritus

Endocrine & metabolic: Breast enlargement, galactorrhea, SIADH, increase or decrease in blood sugar, increased or decreased libido

Gastrointestinal: Xerostomia, constipation, vomiting, indigestion, anorexia, aphthous stomatitis, nausea, unpleasant taste, weight gain, diarrhea, trouble with gums, decreased lower esophageal sphincter tone may cause GE reflux

Genitourinary: Urinary retention, testicular edema

Hematologic: Agranulocytosis, leukopenia, eosinophilia, thrombocytopenia, purpura

Neuromuscular & skeletal: Weakness, tremors, numbness, paresthesia, extrapyramidal symptoms, tardive dyskinesia

Ocular: Blurred vision

Otic: Tinnitus

Miscellaneous: Diaphoresis (excessive), allergic reactions

Topical:

Cardiovascular: Edema

Central nervous system: **Drowsiness (22%)**, anxiety, dizziness, emotional changes

Dermatologic: **Stinging/burning (23%)**, contact dermatitis

Gastrointestinal: **Xerostomia**, taste alteration, tongue numbness

Signs and Symptoms of Overdose Ataxia, confusion, cyanosis, dental erosion, ejaculatory disturbances, extrapyramidal reaction, galactorrhea, gynecomastia, hallucinations, hypoglycemia, myoglobinuria, hypotension, hypothermia, nystagmus, photosensitivity, priapism, QT prolongation, respiratory depression, rhabdomyolysis, seizures, tachycardia, urinary retention

Pharmacodynamics/Kinetics

Onset of action: Peak effect: Antidepressant: Usually >2 weeks; Anxiolytic: may occur sooner

Absorption: Following topical application, plasma levels may be similar to those achieved with oral administration

Distribution: Crosses placenta; enters breast milk

Protein binding: 80% to 85%

Metabolism: Hepatic; metabolites include desmethyldoxepin (active)

Half-life elimination: Adults: 6-8 hours

Excretion: Urine

Dosage Oral (entire daily dose may be given at bedtime): Depression or anxiety (unlabeled use):

Children: 1-3 mg/kg/day in single or divided doses

Adolescents: Initial: 25-50 mg/day in single or divided doses; gradually increase to 100 mg/day

Adults: Initial: 30-150 mg/day at bedtime or in 2-3 divided doses; may gradually increase up to 300 mg/day; single dose should not exceed 150 mg; select patients may respond to 25-50 mg/day

Elderly: Use a lower dose and adjust gradually

Dosing adjustment in hepatic impairment: Use a lower dose and adjust gradually

Topical: Pruritus: Adults and Elderly: Apply a thin film 4 times/day with at least 3- to 4-hour interval between applications; not recommended for use >8 days. **Note:** Low-dose (25-50 mg) oral administration has also been used to treat pruritus, but systemic effects are increased.

Stability Protect from light

Monitoring Parameters Monitor blood pressure and pulse rate prior to and during initial therapy; monitor mental status, weight; ECG in older adults; adverse effects may be increased if topical formulation is applied to >10% of body surface area

Administration Oral: Do not mix oral concentrate with carbonated beverages (physically incompatible).

Topical: Apply thin film to affected area; use of occlusive dressings is not recommended.

Contraindications Hypersensitivity to doxepin, drugs from similar chemical class, or any component of the formulation; narrow-angle glaucoma; urinary retention; use of MAO inhibitors within 14 days; use in a patient during acute recovery phase of MI

Warnings

[U.S. Boxed Warning]: Antidepressants increase the risk of suicidal thinking and behavior in children and adolescents with major depressive disorder (MDD) and other depressive disorders; consider risk prior to prescribing. Closely monitor for clinical worsening, suicidality, or unusual changes in behavior; the child's family or caregiver should be instructed to closely observe the patient and communicate condition with healthcare provider. Such observation would generally include at least weekly face-to-face contact with patients or their family members or caregivers during the first 4 weeks of treatment, then every other week visits for the next 4 weeks, then at 12 weeks, and as clinically indicated beyond 12 weeks. Additional contact by telephone may be appropriate between face-to-face visits. Adults treated with antidepressants should be observed similarly for clinical worsening and suicidality, especially during the initial few months of a course of drug therapy, or at times of dose changes, either increases or decreases. A medication guide should be dispensed with each prescription. **Doxepin is approved for treatment of depression in adolescents.**

The possibility of a suicide attempt is inherent in major depression and may persist until remission occurs. Monitor for worsening of depression or suicidality, especially during initiation of therapy or with dose increases or decreases. Worsening depression and severe abrupt suicidality that are not part of the presenting symptoms may require discontinuation or modification of drug therapy. Use caution in high-risk patients during initiation of therapy. Prescriptions should be written for the smallest quantity consistent with good patient care. The patient's family or caregiver should be alerted to monitor patients for the emergence of suicidality and associated behaviors such as anxiety, agitation, panic attacks, insomnia, irritability, hostility, impulsivity, akathisia, hypomania, and mania; patients should be instructed to notify their healthcare provider if any of these symptoms or worsening depression occur.

May worsen psychosis in some patients or precipitate a shift to mania or hypomania in patients with bipolar disorder. Monotherapy in patients with bipolar disorder should be avoided. Patients presenting with depressive symptoms should be screened for bipolar disorder. **Doxepin is not FDA approved for the treatment of bipolar depression.**

Often causes sedation, which may result in impaired performance of tasks requiring alertness (eg, operating machinery or driving). Sedative effects may be additive with other CNS depressants and/or ethanol. The degree of sedation is very high relative to other antidepressants. May increase the risks associated with electroconvulsive therapy. Consider discontinuing, when possible, prior to elective surgery. Therapy should not be abruptly discontinued in patients receiving high doses for prolonged periods.

May cause orthostatic hypotension (risk is moderate relative to other antidepressants) - use with caution in patients at risk of hypotension or in patients where transient hypotensive episodes would be poorly tolerated (cardiovascular disease or cerebrovascular disease). The degree of anticholinergic blockade produced by this agent is high relative to other cyclic antidepressants - use caution in patients with benign prostatic hyperplasia, xerostomia, visual problems, constipation, or history of bowel obstruction.

Use with caution in patients with a history of cardiovascular disease (including previous MI, stroke, tachycardia, or conduction abnormalities). The risk conduction abnormalities with this agent is moderate relative to other antidepressants. Use caution in patients with a previous seizure disorder or condition predisposing to seizures such as brain damage, alcoholism, or concurrent therapy with other drugs which lower the seizure threshold. Use with caution in hyperthyroid patients or those receiving thyroid supplementation. Use with caution in patients with hepatic or renal dysfunction and in elderly patients. Cream formulation is for external use only (not for ophthalmic, vaginal, or oral use). Do not use occlusive dressings. Use for >8 days may increase risk of contact sensitization. Doxepin is significantly absorbed following topical administration; plasma levels may be similar to those achieved with oral administration.

Dosage Forms [DSC] = Discontinued product
Capsule, as hydrochloride: 10 mg, 25 mg, 50 mg, 75 mg, 100 mg, 150 mg
  Sinequan®: 10 mg, 25 mg, 50 mg, 75 mg, 100 mg, 150 mg [DSC]
Cream, as hydrochloride:
  Prudoxin™: 5% (45 g) [contains benzyl alcohol]
  Zonalon®: 5% (30 g, 45 g) [contains benzyl alcohol]
Solution, oral concentrate, as hydrochloride (Sinequan®): 10 mg/mL (120 mL)
  Sinequan®: 10 mg/mL (120 mL) [DSC]

Reference Range
Therapeutic: 110-250 ng/mL
Toxic: >500 ng/mL
In the postmortem state, anatomical site concentration differences (ie, postmortem redistribution) may occur.

Overdosage/Treatment
Decontamination: Lavage (within 1 hour)/activated charcoal; multiple dosing of activated charcoal may be effective
Supportive therapy: Following initiation of essential overdose management, toxic symptoms should be treated. Ventricular arrhythmias often respond to systemic alkalinization (sodium bicarbonate 0.5-2 mEq/kg I.V.). Arrhythmias unresponsive to this therapy may respond to lidocaine 1 mg/kg I.V. followed by a titrated infusion. Seizures usually respond to diazepam or lorazepam I.V. boluses. If seizures are unresponsive or recur, phenobarbital may be required. Quinidine, disopyramide, and procainamide are contraindicated. Hemoperfusion or hemodialysis is generally not of benefit. Hypotension can respond to crystalloid infusion; norepinephrine or dopamine can be used as a second line agent.

Antidote(s)
• Sodium Bicarbonate [ANTIDOTE]

Test Interactions ↑ glucose, catecholamine

Drug Interactions Substrate (major) of CYP1A2, 2D6, 3A4
Altretamine: Concurrent use may cause orthostatic hypertension.
Amphetamines: TCAs may enhance the effect of amphetamines; monitor for adverse CV effects.
Anticholinergics: Combined use with TCAs may produce additive anticholinergic effects
Antihypertensives: TCAs may inhibit the antihypertensive response to bethanidine, clonidine, debrisoquin, guanadrel, guanethidine, guanabenz, guanfacine; monitor BP; consider alternate antihypertensive agent.
Beta-agonists (nonselective): When combined with TCAs may predispose patients to cardiac arrhythmias.
Bupropion: May increase the levels of tricyclic antidepressants; based on limited information; monitor response.
Carbamazepine: Tricyclic antidepressants may increase carbamazepine levels; monitor.
Cholestyramine and colestipol: May bind TCAs and reduce their absorption; monitor for altered response.
Clonidine: Abrupt discontinuation of clonidine may cause hypertensive crisis, amitriptyline may enhance the response.
CNS depressants: Sedative effects may be additive with TCAs; monitor for increased effect; includes benzodiazepines, barbiturates, antipsychotics, ethanol and other sedative medications.
CYP1A2 inducers: May decrease the levels/effects of doxepin. Example inducers include aminoglutethimide, carbamazepine, phenobarbital, and rifampin.
CYP1A2 inhibitors: May increase the levels/effects of doxepin. Example inhibitors include ciprofloxacin, fluvoxamine, ketoconazole, norfloxacin, ofloxacin, and rofecoxib.
CYP2D6 inhibitors: May increase the levels/effects of doxepin. Example inhibitors include chlorpromazine, delavirdine, fluoxetine, miconazole, paroxetine, pergolide, quinidine, quinine, ritonavir, and ropinirole.

CYP3A4 inducers: CYP3A4 inducers may decrease the levels/effects of doxepin. Example inducers include aminoglutethimide, carbamazepine, nafcillin, nevirapine, phenobarbital, phenytoin, and rifamycins.
CYP3A4 inhibitors: May increase the levels/effects of doxepin. Example inhibitors include azole antifungals, clarithromycin, diclofenac, doxycycline, erythromycin, imatinib, isoniazid, nefazodone, nicardipine, propofol, protease inhibitors, quinidine, telithromycin, and verapamil.
Epinephrine (and other direct alpha-agonists): Pressor response to I.V. epinephrine, norepinephrine, and phenylephrine may be enhanced in patients receiving TCAs. (**Note:** Effect is unlikely with epinephrine or levonordefrin dosages typically administered as infiltration in combination with local anesthetics.)
Fenfluramine: May increase tricyclic antidepressant levels/effects.
Hypoglycemic agents (including insulin): TCAs may enhance the hypoglycemic effects of tolazamide, chlorpropamide, or insulin; monitor for changes in blood glucose levels; reported with chlorpropamide, tolazamide, and insulin.
Levodopa: Tricyclic antidepressants may decrease the absorption (bioavailability) of levodopa; rare hypertensive episodes have also been attributed to this combination.
Linezolid: Hyperpyrexia, hypertension, tachycardia, confusion, seizures, and **deaths have been reported** with agents which inhibit MAO (serotonin syndrome); this combination should be avoided.
Lithium: Concurrent use with a TCA may increase the risk for neurotoxicity.
MAO inhibitors: Hyperpyrexia, hypertension, tachycardia, confusion, seizures, and **deaths have been reported** (serotonin syndrome); this combination is contraindicated.
Methylphenidate: Metabolism of TCAs may be decreased.
Phenothiazines: Serum concentrations of some TCAs may be increased; in addition, TCAs may increase concentration of phenothiazines; monitor for altered clinical response.
QTc-prolonging agents: Concurrent use of tricyclic agents with other drugs which may prolong QTc interval may increase the risk of potentially fatal arrhythmias; includes type Ia and type III antiarrhythmics agents, selected quinolones (sparfloxacin, gatifloxacin, moxifloxacin, grepafloxacin), cisapride, and other agents.
Ritonavir: Combined use of high-dose tricyclic antidepressants with ritonavir may cause serotonin syndrome in HIV-positive patients; monitor.
Sucralfate: Absorption of tricyclic antidepressants may be reduced with coadministration.
Sympathomimetics, indirect-acting: Tricyclic antidepressants may result in a decreased sensitivity to indirect-acting sympathomimetics; includes dopamine and ephedrine; also see interaction with epinephrine (and direct-acting sympathomimetics).
Tramadol: Tramadol's risk of seizures may be increased with TCAs.
Valproic acid: May increase serum concentrations/adverse effects of some tricyclic antidepressants.
Warfarin (and other oral anticoagulants): TCAs may increase the anticoagulant effect in patients stabilized on warfarin; monitor INR.

Pregnancy Risk Factor B (cream); C (all other forms)
Pregnancy Implications Teratogenic effects were not observed in animal studies; however, there are no adequate and well-controlled studies in pregnant women. Use during pregnancy only if clearly needed.
Lactation Enters breast milk/not recommended (AAP rates "of concern")
Additional Information Entire daily dose may be given at bedtime; avoid unnecessary exposure to sunlight; found in a 5% concentration in Zonalon® topical cream for pruritus; toxic reactions can occur due to percutaneous absorption
Specific References
Martínez MA, Sánchez de la Torre C, and Almarza E, "A Comparative Solid-Phase Extraction Study for the Simultaneous Determination of Fluvoxamine, Mianserin, Doxepin, Citalopram, Paroxetine, and Etoperidone in Whole Blood by Capillary Gas-Liquid Chromatography with Nitrogen-Phosphorus Detection," *J Anal Toxicol*, 2004, 28(4):174-80.
Wammack R, Remzi M, Seitz C, et al, "Efficacy of Oral Doxepin and Piroxicam Treatment for Interstitial Cystitis," *Eur Urol*, 41(6):596-600.

DOXOrubicin

Related Information
• DAUNOrubicin Hydrochloride
CAS Number 23214-92-8; 25316-40-9
U.S. Brand Names Adriamycin PFS®; Adriamycin RDF®; Rubex®
Synonyms ADR (error-prone abbreviation); Adria; Doxorubicin Hydrochloride; Hydroxydaunomycin Hydrochloride; Hydroxyldaunorubicin Hydrochloride; NSC-123127
Use Leukemias, lymphomas, multiple myeloma, osseous and nonosseous sarcomas, mesotheliomas, germ cell tumors of the ovary or testis, and carcinomas of the head and neck, thyroid, lung, breast, stomach,

pancreas, liver, ovary, bladder, prostate, and uterus; neuroblastoma, osteosarcoma

Mechanism of Action Inhibition of DNA and RNA synthesis by intercalation between DNA base pairs by inhibition of topoisomerase II and by steric obstruction. Doxorubicin intercalates at points of local uncoiling of the double helix. Although the exact mechanism is unclear, it appears that direct binding to DNA (intercalation) and inhibition of DNA repair (topoisomerase II inhibition) result in blockade of DNA and RNA synthesis and fragmentation of DNA. Doxorubicin is also a powerful iron chelator; the iron-doxorubicin complex can bind DNA and cell membranes and produce free radicals that immediately cleave the DNA and cell membranes.

Adverse Reactions Cardiovascular: Myocarditis, myocardial infection, pericarditis, transient ECG abnormalities (supraventricular tachycardia, S-T wave changes, atrial or ventricular extrasystoles); generally asymptomatic and self-limiting. Congestive heart failure, dose-related, may be delayed for 7-8 years after treatment. Cumulative dose, mediastinal/pericardial radiation therapy, cardiovascular disease, age, and use of cyclophosphamide (or other cardiotoxic agents) all increase the risk.

Recommended maximum cumulative doses:
No risk factors: 550 mg/m^2
Concurrent radiation: 450 mg/m^2
Note: Regardless of cumulative dose, if the left ventricular ejection fraction is <30% to 40%, the drug is usually not given.
Dermatologic: **Alopecia, radiation recall**, skin "flare" at injection site; discoloration of saliva, sweat, or tears; skin rash, pigmentation of nail beds, nail banding, onycholysis, urticaria
Endocrine & metabolic: Hyperuricemia, infertility, sterility
Gastrointestinal: **Nausea, vomiting, stomatitis, GI ulceration, anorexia, diarrhea**
Genitourinary: **Discoloration of urine, mild dysuria, urinary frequency, hematuria, bladder spasms, cystitis following bladder instillation**
Hematologic: **Myelosuppression, primarily leukopenia (75%); thrombocytopenia and anemia** (onset: 7 days, nadir: 10-14 days, recovery: 21-28 days)
Hepatic: Hepatitis, elevations of bilirubin and transaminases
Miscellaneous: Systemic hypersensitivity (including urticaria, pruritus, angioedema, dysphagia, and dyspnea)

Signs and Symptoms of Overdose Dysuria, hematuria, hyperuricemia, lacrimation, leukopenia or neutropenia (agranulocytosis, granulocytopenia), Mees' lines, myocardial depression, onycholysis, tongue discoloration

Admission Criteria/Prognosis May discharge asymptomatic patients after 8 hours of observation

Pharmacodynamics/Kinetics
Absorption: Oral: Poor (<50%)
Distribution: V$_d$: 25 L/kg; to many body tissues, particularly liver, spleen, kidney, lung, heart; does not distribute into the CNS; crosses placenta
Protein binding, plasma: 70%
Metabolism: Primarily hepatic to doxorubicinol (active), then to inactive aglycones, conjugated sulfates, and glucuronides
Half-life elimination:
Distribution: 10 minutes
Elimination: Doxorubicin: 1-3 hours; Metabolites: 3-3.5 hours
Terminal: 17-30 hours
Male: 54 hours; Female: 35 hours
Excretion: Feces (~40% to 50% as unchanged drug); urine (~3% to 10% as metabolites, 1% doxorubicinol, <1% Adriamycin aglycones, and unchanged drug)
Clearance: Male: 113 L/hour; Female: 44 L/hour

Dosage Refer to individual protocols. I.V.:
Children:
35-75 mg/m^2 as a single dose, repeat every 21 days **or**
20-30 mg/m^2 once weekly **or**
60-90 mg/m^2 given as a continuous infusion over 96 hours every 3-4 weeks
Adults: Usual or typical dose: 60-75 mg/m^2 as a single dose, repeat every 21 days **or** other dosage regimens like 20-30 mg/m^2/day for 2-3 days, repeat in 4 weeks **or** 20 mg/m^2 once weekly
The lower dose regimen should be given to patients with decreased bone marrow reserve, prior therapy or marrow infiltration with malignant cells
Dosing adjustment in renal impairment:
Mild to moderate renal failure: Adjustment is not required
Cl$_{cr}$ <10 mL/minute: Administer 75% of normal dose
Hemodialysis: Supplemental dose is not necessary
Dosing adjustment in hepatic impairment:
Bilirubin 1.2-3 mg/dL: Administer 50% of dose
Bilirubin 3.1-5 mg/dL: Administer 25% of dose
Bilirubin >5 mg/dL: Do not administer drug

Stability Protect from light, must be dispensed in an amber bag; store powder vials at room temperature, refrigerate liquid vials; reconstituted powder vials stable for 24 hours at room temperature and 48 hours if refrigerated; unstable in solutions with a pH <3 or >7. **Incompatible** with heparin, fluorouracil, aminophylline, cephalothin, methotrexate, dexamethasone, diazepam, hydrocortisone, furosemide. Y-site is **compatible** with doxorubicin, vincristine, cyclophosphamide, dacarbazine, bleomycin, vinblastine.

Monitoring Parameters CBC with differential and platelet count, cardiac and liver function tests

Administration
Administer I.V. push over 1-2 minutes or IVPB. Continuous infusions may be administered via central line. **Avoid extravasation**, associated with severe ulceration and soft tissue necrosis. Flush with 5-10 mL of I.V. solution before and after drug administration. Incompatible with heparin. Monitor for local erythematous streaking along vein and/or facial flushing (may indicate rapid infusion rate).
Extravasation management: Apply ice immediately for 30-60 minutes; then alternate off/on every 15 minutes for 1 day. Topical cooling may be achieved using ice packs or cooling pad with circulating ice water. Cooling of site for 24 hours as tolerated by the patient. Elevate and rest extremity 24-48 hours, then resume normal activity as tolerated. Application of cold inhibits vesicant's cytotoxicity. **Application of heat or sodium bicarbonate can be harmful and is contraindicated.** If pain, erythema, and/or swelling persist beyond 48 hours, refer patient immediately to plastic surgeon for consultation and possible debridement.

Contraindications Hypersensitivity to doxorubicin or any component of the formulation; congestive heart failure or arrhythmias; previous therapy with high cumulative doses of doxorubicin and/or daunorubicin; pre-existing bone marrow suppression; pregnancy

Warnings Hazardous agent - use appropriate precautions for handling and disposal. Use with caution in patients who have received radiation therapy or in the presence of hepatobiliary dysfunction; reduce dosage in patients who are receiving radiation therapy simultaneously. Administration of live vaccines to immunosuppressed patients may be hazardous. Total dose should not exceed 550 mg/m^2 or 450 mg/m^2 in patients with previous or concomitant treatment with daunorubicin, cyclophosphamide, or irradiation of the cardiac region. **[U.S. Boxed Warning]: Irreversible myocardial toxicity may occur** as total dosage approaches 550 mg/m^2. A baseline cardiac evaluation (ECG, LVEF, +/- ECHO) is recommended, especially in patients with risk factors for increased cardiac toxicity and in pediatric patients. Pediatric patients are at increased risk for delayed cardiotoxicity. **[U.S. Boxed Warnings]: Reduce dose in patients with impaired hepatic function; severe myelosuppression is also possible. Secondary acute myelogenous leukemia may occur following treatment.**
[U.S. Boxed Warnings]: I.V. use only. Doxorubicin is a potent vesicant; if extravasation occurs, severe tissue damage leading to ulceration and necrosis, and pain may occur. Should be administered under the supervision of an experienced cancer chemotherapy physician.

Dosage Forms
Injection, powder for reconstitution, as hydrochloride: 10 mg, 20 mg, 50 mg [contains lactose]
Adriamycin RDF®: 10 mg, 20 mg, 50 mg, 150 mg [contains lactose; rapid dissolution formula]
Rubex®: 50 mg, 100 mg [contains lactose]
Injection, solution, as hydrochloride [preservative free]: 2 mg/mL (5 mL, 10 mL, 25 mL, 100 mL)
Adriamycin PFS® [preservative free]: 2 mg/mL (5 mL, 10 mL, 25 mL, 37.5 mL, 100 mL)

Reference Range No relationship between serum level and cytotoxicity; mean plasma doxorubicin level following 10-15 mg/m^2/day for 5 days of doxorubicin was 7.8-90 ng/mL

Overdosage/Treatment
Supportive therapy: Prophylactically, dexrazoxane (Zinecard®) (10 times the dose of doxorubicin 30 minutes prior to doxorubicin treatment) may reduce cardiotoxicity of doxorubicin; topical DMSO (1.5 mL of a 50% solution every 6 hours for 2 weeks) with cold compresses can be used to treat extravasation. Levocarnitine daily 2-3 days before and 2 days after (1 g 3 times with 1 g I.V. on day of therapy doxorubicin treatment) may decrease cardiotoxicity; topical dimethylsulfoxide or local hydrocortisone (100 mg/2 mL) injections with cold compresses can be used to treat extravasation injury
Enhancement of elimination: While hemodialysis is not useful, Amberlite hemoperfusion may be effective if initiated within 1 hour of administration

Antidote(s)
● Dexrazoxane [ANTIDOTE]
● Levocarnitine [ANTIDOTE]

Drug Interactions Substrate (major) of CYP2D6, 3A4; **Inhibits** CYP2B6 (moderate), 2D6 (weak), 3A4 (weak)
Allopurinol may enhance the antitumor activity of doxorubicin (animal data only).
Cyclophosphamide enhances the cardiac toxicity of doxorubicin by producing additional myocardial cell damage.

267

Cyclosporine may decrease clearance of parent and metabolite and may induce coma or seizures and enhance hematologic toxicity.

CYP2B6 substrates: Doxorubicin may increase the levels/effects of CYP2B6 substrates. Example substrates include bupropion, promethazine, propofol, selegiline, and sertraline.

CYP2D6 inhibitors: May increase the levels/effects of doxorubicin. Example inhibitors include chlorpromazine, delavirdine, fluoxetine, miconazole, paroxetine, pergolide, quinidine, quinine, ritonavir, and ropinirole.

CYP3A4 inducers: CYP3A4 inducers may decrease the levels/effects of doxorubicin. Example inducers include aminoglutethimide, carbamazepine, nafcillin, nevirapine, phenobarbital, phenytoin, and rifamycins.

CYP3A4 inhibitors: May increase the levels/effects of doxorubicin. Example inhibitors include azole antifungals, clarithromycin, diclofenac, doxycycline, erythromycin, imatinib, isoniazid, nefazodone, nicardipine, propofol, protease inhibitors, quinidine, telithromycin, and verapamil.

Digoxin: Doxorubicin may decrease plasma levels and effectiveness of digoxin.

Mercaptopurine increases toxicities.

Paclitaxel reduces doxorubicin clearance and increases toxicity if administered prior to doxorubicin.

Phenobarbital increases elimination (decreases effect) of doxorubicin.

Phenytoin: Doxorubicin may decrease plasma levels and effectiveness of phenytoin.

Progesterone: High doses of progesterone enhance toxicity (neutropenia and thrombocytopenia).

Streptozocin greatly enhances leukopenia and thrombocytopenia.

Verapamil alters the cellular distribution of doxorubicin and may result in increased cell toxicity by inhibition of the P-glycoprotein pump. Based on mouse studies, cardiotoxicity may be enhanced by verapamil.

Zidovudine: Doxorubicin may decrease the antiviral activity of zidovudine.

Pregnancy Risk Factor D

Pregnancy Implications Advise patients to avoid becoming pregnant (females) and to avoid causing pregnancy (males).

Lactation Enters breast milk/contraindicated

Nursing Implications Local erythematous streaking along the vein and/or facial flushing may indicate too rapid a rate of administration; avoid extravasation, drug is a vesicant; if extravasation occurs, apply ice

Additional Information Cutaneous squamous cell carcinoma (Marjolin's ulcer) has been associated at the site of doxorubicin extravasation 10 years after drug administration

Myelosuppressive effects: **WBC**: Moderate. **Platelets**: Moderate. Onset (days): 7. Nadir (days): 10-14. Recovery (days): 21-28

Doxycycline

CAS Number 10592-13-9; 17086-28-1; 24390-14-5; 564-25-0; 83038-87-3

U.S. Brand Names Adoxa™; Doryx®; Doxy-100®; Monodox®; Oracea™; Periostat®; Vibra-Tabs®; Vibramycin®

Synonyms Doxycycline Calcium; Doxycycline Hyclate; Doxycycline Monohydrate

Use Principally in the treatment of infections caused by susceptible *Rickettsia*, *Chlamydia*, and *Mycoplasma*; alternative to mefloquine for malaria prophylaxis; treatment for syphilis, uncomplicated *Neisseria gonorrhoeae*, *Listeria*, *Actinomyces israelii*, and *Clostridium* infections in penicillin-allergic patients; used for community-acquired pneumonia and other common infections due to susceptible organisms; anthrax due to *Bacillus anthracis*, including inhalational anthrax (postexposure); treatment of infections caused by uncommon susceptible gram-negative and gram-positive organisms including *Borrelia recurrentis*, *Ureaplasma urealyticum*, *Haemophilus ducreyi*, *Yersinia pestis*, *Francisella tularensis*, *Vibrio cholerae*, *Campylobacter fetus*, *Brucella* spp, *Bartonella bacilliformis*, and *Calymmatobacterium granulomatis*; treatment of inflammatory lesions associated with rosacea

Unlabeled/Investigational Use Sclerosing agent for pleural effusion injection; vancomycin-resistant enterococci (VRE)

Mechanism of Action Inhibits protein synthesis by binding with the 30S and possibly the 50S ribosomal subunit(s) of susceptible bacteria; may also cause alterations in the cytoplasmic membrane

Adverse Reactions

Cardiovascular: Vasculitis

Central nervous system: Increased intracranial pressure, bulging fontanels in infants, headache

Dermatologic: Rash, photosensitivity, hyperpigmentation, toxic pustuloderma, Stevens-Johnson syndrome, exfoliative dermatitis, erythema multiforme, angioedema, toxic epidermal necrolysis, urticaria, purpura, psoriasis, yellow fingernail, exanthem

Endocrine & metabolic: Parotitis, black thyroid

Gastrointestinal: Nausea, diarrhea, esophagitis and esophageal ulceration with the hyclate salt formulation; vomiting

Hematologic: Neutropenia, eosinophilia, porphyria

Hepatic: Hepatotoxicity

Local: Phlebitis (I.V. administration)

Neuromuscular & skeletal: Paresthesia

Renal: Polyuria, Fanconi-like reaction (albuminuria, hypokalemia, acidosis) with outdated drug

Respiratory: Hyposmia

Miscellaneous: May cause **discoloration of teeth in children**, hiccups, systemic lupus erythematosus, fixed drug eruption

Signs and Symptoms of Overdose Leukopenia or neutropenia (agranulocytosis, granulocytopenia); photosensitivity, hypokalemia, flatulence

Pharmacodynamics/Kinetics

Absorption: Oral: Almost complete; reduced by food or milk by 20%

Distribution: Widely into body tissues and fluids including synovial, pleural, prostatic, seminal fluids, and bronchial secretions; saliva, aqueous humor, and CSF penetration is poor; readily crosses placenta; enters breast milk

Protein binding: 90%

Metabolism: Not hepatic; partially inactivated in GI tract by chelate formation

Half-life elimination: 12-15 hours (usually increases to 22-24 hours with multiple doses); End-stage renal disease: 18-25 hours

Time to peak, serum: 1.5-4 hours

Excretion: Feces (30%); urine (23%)

Dosage Children:

Anthrax: Doxycycline should be used in children if antibiotic susceptibility testing, exhaustion of drug supplies, or allergic reaction preclude use of penicillin or ciprofloxacin. For treatment, the consensus recommendation does not include a loading dose for doxycycline.

Inhalational (postexposure prophylaxis) (*MMWR*, 2001, 50:889-893): Oral, I.V. (use oral route when possible):

≤8 years: 2.2 mg/kg every 12 hours for 60 days

>8 years and ≤45 kg: 2.2 mg/kg every 12 hours for 60 days

>8 years and >45 kg: 100 mg every 12 hours for 60 days

Cutaneous (treatment): Oral: See dosing for "Inhalational (post-exposure prophylaxis)"

Note: In the presence of systemic involvement, extensive edema, and/or lesions on head/neck, doxycycline should initially be administered I.V.

Inhalational/gastrointestinal/oropharyngeal (treatment): I.V.: Refer to dosing for inhalational anthrax (postexposure prophylaxis); switch to oral therapy when clinically appropriate; refer to Adults dosing for "Note" on combined therapy and duration

Children ≥8 years (<45 kg): Susceptible infections: Oral, I.V.: 2-5 mg/kg/day in 1-2 divided doses, not to exceed 200 mg/day

Children >8 years (>45 kg) and Adults: Susceptible infections: Oral, I.V.: 100-200 mg/day in 1-2 divided doses

Acute gonococcal infection (PID) in combination with another antibiotic: 100 mg every 12 hours until improved, followed by 100 mg orally twice daily to complete 14 days

Community-acquired pneumonia: 100 mg twice daily

Lyme disease: Oral: 100 mg twice daily for 14-21 days

Early syphilis: 200 mg/day in divided doses for 14 days

Late syphilis: 200 mg/day in divided doses for 28 days

Uncomplicated chlamydial infections: 100 mg twice daily for ≥7 days

Endometritis, salpingitis, parametritis, or peritonitis: I.V. twice daily with cefoxitin 2 g every 6 hours for 4 days and for ≥48 hours after patient improves; then continue with oral therapy 100 mg twice daily to complete a 10- to 14-day course of therapy

Sclerosing agent for pleural effusion injection (unlabeled use): 500 mg as a single dose in 30-50 mL of NS or SWI

Periodontitis: Oral (Periostat®): 20 mg twice daily as an adjunct following scaling and root planing; may be administered for up to 9 months. Safety beyond 12 months of treatment and efficacy beyond 9 months of treatment have not been established.

Adults:

Anthrax:

Inhalational (postexposure prophylaxis): Oral, I.V. (use oral route when possible): 100 mg every 12 hours for 60 days (*MMWR*, 2001, 50:889-93); **Note:** Preliminary recommendation, FDA review and update is anticipated.

Cutaneous (treatment): Oral: 100 mg every 12 hours for 60 days. **Note:** In the presence of systemic involvement, extensive edema, lesions on head/neck, refer to I.V. dosing for treatment of inhalational/gastrointestinal/oropharyngeal anthrax

Inhalational/gastrointestinal/oropharyngeal (treatment): I.V.: Initial: 100 mg every 12 hours; switch to oral therapy when clinically appropriate; some recommend initial loading dose of 200 mg, followed by 100 mg every 8-12 hours (*JAMA*, 1997, 278:399-411). **Note:** Initial treatment should include two or more agents predicted to be effective (per CDC recommendations). Agents suggested for use in conjunction with doxycycline or ciprofloxacin include rifampin, vancomycin, imipenem, penicillin, ampicillin, chloramphenicol, clindamycin, and clarithromycin. May switch to oral antimicrobial therapy when clinically appropriate. Continue combined therapy for 60 days

Rosacea: (Oracea™): Oral: 40 mg once daily in the morning

Dosing adjustment in renal impairment: No adjustment necessary

Dialysis: Not dialyzable; 0% to 5% by hemo- and peritoneal methods or by continuous arteriovenous or venovenous hemofiltration: No supplemental dosage necessary

Stability Tetracyclines form toxic products when outdated or when exposed to light, heat, or humidity; reconstituted solution is stable for 72 hours (refrigerated); for I.V. infusion in NS or D₅W solution, complete infusion should be completed within 12 hours; discard remaining solution

Monitoring Parameters Periodic monitoring of renal, hepatic, and hematologic function tests

Administration Oral: Administer with adequate fluid to reduce risk of esophageal irritation and ulceration; may administer with meals to decrease GI upset

Doryx®: Capsules may be opened and contents sprinkled on applesauce. Applesauce should be swallowed immediately; do not chew. Follow with 8 ounces of water. Applesauce should not be hot and should be soft enough to swallow without chewing.

I.V.: Infuse I.V. doxycycline over 1-4 hours

Contraindications Hypersensitivity to doxycycline, tetracycline or any component of the formulation; children <8 years of age, except in treatment of anthrax (including inhalational anthrax postexposure prophylaxis); severe hepatic dysfunction; pregnancy

Warnings

Do not use during pregnancy - use of tetracyclines during tooth development may cause permanent discoloration of the teeth and enamel hypoplasia; prolonged use may result in superinfection, including oral or vaginal candidiasis; photosensitivity reaction may occur with this drug; avoid prolonged exposure to sunlight or tanning equipment. Anti-anabolic effects of tetracyclines can increase BUN leading to significant renal dysfunction and hepatotoxicity in patients with preexisting renal impairment. Autoimmune syndromes have been reported; if symptomatic conduct LFT and discontinue drug. Tetracyclines have been associated with pseudotumor cerebri. Avoid in children ≤8 years of age.

Additional specific warnings: Periostat®: Effectiveness has not been established in patients with coexistent oral candidiasis; use with caution in patients with a history or predisposition to oral candidiasis. Oracea™: Should not be used for the treatment or prophylaxis of bacterial infections, since the lower dose of drug per capsule may be sub-efficacious and promote resistance.

Dosage Forms [DSC] = Discontinued product

Capsule, as hyclate: 50 mg, 100 mg
Vibramycin®: 100 mg
Capsule, as monohydrate (Monodox®): 50 mg, 100 mg
Capsule, coated pellets, as hyclate (Doryx®): 75 mg, 100 mg [DSC]
Capsule, variable release (Oracea™): 40 mg [30 mg (immediate-release) and 10 mg (delayed-release)]
Injection, powder for reconstitution, as hyclate (Doxy-100®): 100 mg
Powder for oral suspension, as monohydrate (Vibramycin®): 25 mg/5 mL (60 mL) [raspberry flavor]
Syrup, as calcium (Vibramycin®): 50 mg/5 mL (480 mL) [contains sodium metabisulfite; raspberry-apple flavor]
Tablet, as hyclate: 100 mg
Periostat®: 20 mg
Vibra-Tabs®: 100 mg
Tablet, as monohydrate:
Adoxa™: 50 mg, 75 mg, 100 mg
Adoxa® Pak™ 1/75 [unit-dose pack]: 75 mg (31s)
Adoxa® Pak™ 1/100 [unit-dose pack]: 100 mg (31s)
Adoxa® Pak™ 1/150 [unit-dose pack]: 150 mg (30s)
Adoxa® Pak™ 2/100 [unit-dose pack]: 100 mg (60s)
Tablet, delayed-release coated pellets, as hyclate (Doryx®): 75 mg [contains sodium 4.5 mg (0.196 mEq)], 100 mg [contains sodium 6 mg (0.261 mEq)]

Reference Range Peak plasma level of 3 mg/L (6.5 µmol/L) following a 200 mg dose

Overdosage/Treatment

Decontamination: Lavage (within 1 hour)/activated charcoal; dilute with milk or water to avoid corrosive gastrointestinal effects

Supportive therapy: Antacids effective for gastrointestinal irritation

Enhancement of elimination: Multiple dosing of activated charcoal may be effective; can increase fecal elimination by binding to doxycycline after intestinal secretion; not dialyzable

Test Interactions False-negative urine glucose using Clinistix®, Tes-Tape®

Drug Interactions **Substrate** of CYP3A4 (major); **Inhibits** CYP3A4 (moderate)

Antacids (containing aluminum, calcium, or magnesium): Decreased absorption of tetracyclines

Anticoagulants: Tetracyclines may decrease plasma thrombin activity; monitor

Barbiturates: Decreased half-life of doxycycline

Carbamazepine: Decreased half-life of doxycycline

CYP3A4 inducers: CYP3A4 inducers may decrease the levels/effects of doxycycline. Example inducers include aminoglutethimide, carbamazepine, nafcillin, nevirapine, phenobarbital, phenytoin, and rifamycins.

CYP3A4 substrates: Doxycycline may increase the levels/effects of CYP3A4 substrates. Example substrates include benzodiazepines, calcium channel blockers, mirtazapine, nateglinide, nefazodone, tacrolimus, and venlafaxine. Selected benzodiazepines (midazolam and triazolam), cisapride, ergot alkaloids, selected HMG-CoA reductase inhibitors (lovastatin and simvastatin), and pimozide are generally contraindicated with strong CYP3A4 inhibitors.

Iron-containing products: Decreased absorption of tetracyclines

Methoxyflurane: Concomitant use may cause fatal renal toxicity.

Oral contraceptives: Anecdotal reports suggesting decreased contraceptive efficacy with tetracyclines have been refuted by more rigorous scientific and clinical data.

Phenytoin: Decreased half-life of doxycycline

Pregnancy Risk Factor D

Pregnancy Implications Exposure during the last half or pregnancy causes permanent yellow-gray-brown discoloration of the teeth. Tetracyclines also form a complex in bone forming tissue, leading to a decreased fibula growth rate when given to premature infants. According to the FDA, the Teratogen Information System concluded that therapeutic doses during pregnancy are unlikely to produce substantial teratogenic risk, but data are insufficient to say that there is no risk. In general, reports of exposure have been limited to short durations of therapy in the first trimester. When considering treatment for life-threatening infection and/or prolonged duration of therapy (such as in anthrax), the potential risk to the fetus must be balanced against the severity of the potential illness.

Lactation Enters breast milk/not recommended

Nursing Implications Infuse I.V. doxycycline over 1 hour

Additional Information

Not as antianabolic as other tetracyclines.

If liquid doxycycline is unavailable for the treatment of anthrax, emergency doses may be prepared for children using the tablets.

Crush one 100 mg tablet and grind into a fine powder. Mix with 4 teaspoons of food or drink (lowfat milk, chocolate milk, chocolate pudding, or apple juice). Appropriate dose may be taken from this mixture. Mixture may be stored for up to 24 hours. Dairy mixtures should be refrigerated; apple juice may be stored at room temperature

U.S. Food and Drug Administration, Center for Drug Evaluation and Research, "How to Prepare Emergency Dosages of Doxycycline at Home for Infants and Children," April 25, 2003, viewable at http://www.fda.gov/cder/drug/infopage/penG_doxy/doxycyclinePeds.htm, last accessed May 8, 2003.

Doxylamine

CAS Number 562-10-7

U.S. Brand Names Good Sense Sleep Aid [OTC]; Unisom® SleepTabs® [OTC]

Synonyms Doxylamine Succinate

Use Sleep aid; antihistamine for hypersensitivity reactions and antiemetic

Mechanism of Action Competes with histamine at H₁-receptor sites on effector cells in blood vessels, central nervous system, GI tract, striated muscle, and respiratory tract

Adverse Reactions

Cardiovascular: Tachycardia

Central nervous system: Sedation, paradoxical stimulation in children, hyperthermia

Gastrointestinal: Dry mucous membranes, constipation, nausea, vomiting, pancreatitis

Genitourinary: Urinary retention

Neuromuscular & skeletal: Tremors

Ocular: Blurred vision, mydriasis

Signs and Symptoms of Overdose Overdose may result in death; cardiopulmonary arrest, catatonic psychosis, CNS depression or stimulation, elevated CPK, mydriasis, seizures, rhabdomyolysis, tachycardia

Admission Criteria/Prognosis Any symptomatic patient and/or elevated CPK

Pharmacodynamics/Kinetics

Onset of effect: 30 minutes

Duration: 4-6 hours

Absorption: Well absorbed

Distribution: V_d: 2.5 L/kg

Metabolism: Via multiple metabolic pathways including N-demethylation, oxidation, hydroxylation, N-acetylation to metabolites including nordoxylamine, dinordoxylamine

Half-life elimination: 10-12 hours

Excretion: Urine (primarily as metabolites)

Dosage Oral: Children >12 years and adults: 25 mg at bedtime

Administration

Main dose should be taken at bedtime to provide relief in the early morning hours.

Contraindications Hypersensitivity to doxylamine or any component of the formulation

Warnings May cause drowsiness; patient should avoid tasks requiring alertness (eg, driving, operating machinery) until effects are known. Sedative effects of CNS depressants or ethanol are potentiated. Use with caution in patients with angle-closure glaucoma, pyloroduodenal obstruction (including stenotic peptic ulcer), urinary tract obstruction (including bladder neck obstruction and symptomatic prostatic hyperplasia), hyperthyroidism, increased intraocular pressure, and cardiovascular disease (including hypertension and tachycardia). If sleeplessness persists for >2 weeks, medical evaluation should occur. Safety and efficacy not established in children <12 years of age.

Dosage Forms Tablet, a succinate:
Good Sense Sleep Aid, Unisom® SleepTabs®: 25 mg

Reference Range
Therapeutic: Not established; nonintoxicated postmortem blood concentrations range from 0.05-0.8 mg/L
Toxic: Fatalities reported with concentrations of 0.7, 12.0, and 17.0 mg/L in blood, postmortem blood, and urine, respectively
Retrospective review has found no correlation between concentrations and toxic effects in intoxicated patients.
In the postmortem state, anatomical site concentration differences (ie, postmortem redistribution) may occur.

Overdosage/Treatment
Decontamination: Lavage (within 1 hour)/activated charcoal can be most useful; **do not** use a cathartic if diarrhea is present
Supportive therapy: Propranolol or esmolol can be used for tachyarrhythmias (avoid quinidine or disopyramide in that conduction disturbances can occur); benzodiazepine can be utilized for seizures; if anticholinergic findings are present with the seizures (or if coma is present) a trial of physostigmine may be useful; wide complex QRS conduction defects may respond to sodium bicarbonate; seizures have responded to sodium bicarbonate in a rodent model
Enhanced elimination: Dialysis/hemoperfusion is not useful

Test Interactions May suppress wheal and flare reactions to skin test antigens; false-positive results with methadone or opiate enzyme immunoassay may occur with diphenhydramine or doxylamine

Drug Interactions
Anticholinergic agents: Central and/or peripheral anticholinergic syndrome can occur when administered with narcotic analgesics, phenothiazines and other antipsychotics (especially with high anticholinergic activity), tricyclic antidepressants, quinidine and some other antiarrhythmics, and antihistamines.
Cholinergic agents: Drugs with high anticholinergic activity may antagonize the therapeutic effect of cholinergic agents; includes donepezil, rivastigmine, and tacrine.
CNS depressants: Sedative effects may be additive with CNS depressants; includes ethanol, benzodiazepines, barbiturates, narcotic analgesics, and other sedative agents; monitor for increased effect.

Pregnancy Risk Factor B

Pregnancy Implications Doxylamine has been approved for used in pregnancy-associated nausea and vomiting.

Lactation Excretion in breast milk unknown

Additional Information Found in many OTC cough/cold preparations

Specific References
Khosla U, Ruel KS, and Hunt DP, "Antihistamine-Induced Rhabdomyolysis," *South Med J*, 2003, 96(10):1023-6.

Droperidol

CAS Number 548-72-3
U.S. Brand Names Inapsine®
Synonyms Dehydrobenzperidol
Impairment Potential Yes
Use Antiemetic in surgical and diagnostic procedures; preoperative medication in patients when other treatments are ineffective or inappropriate
Mechanism of Action Alters the action of dopamine in the CNS, at subcortical levels, to produce sedation; it is a butyrophenone with phenothiazine-like properties

Adverse Reactions
ECG changes and retinal pigmentation are more common than with chlorpromazine. Relative to other neuroleptics, droperidol has a low potency of cholinergic blockade.
Cardiovascular: **QT_c** prolongation (dose dependent), hypotension (especially orthostatic), tachycardia, abnormal T waves with prolonged ventricular repolarization, arrhythmia, torsade de pointes, ventricular tachycardia
Central nervous system: **Restlessness, anxiety, extrapyramidal symptoms, dystonic reactions, pseudoparkinsonian signs and symptoms, tardive dyskinesia, seizures, altered central temperature regulation, akathisia,** hallucinations, sedation, drowsiness, neuroleptic malignant syndrome, tardive dystonia

Dermatologic: Alopecia, contact dermatitis, hyperpigmentation, photosensitivity (rare), pruritus, rash
Endocrine & metabolic: **Swelling of breasts,** amenorrhea, galactorrhea, gynecomastia, sexual dysfunction
Gastrointestinal: **Weight gain, constipation,** nausea, vomiting, adynamic ileus, xerostomia
Genitourinary: Dysuria, overflow incontinence, priapism, urinary retention
Hematologic: Agranulocytosis, leukopenia (usually with large doses for prolonged periods)
Hepatic: Cholestatic jaundice, obstructive jaundice
Ocular: Decreased visual acuity, blurred vision, retinal pigmentation
Respiratory: Laryngospasm, respiratory depression
Miscellaneous: Heat stroke

Signs and Symptoms of Overdose Cardiac conduction disturbances can occur if daily intravenous dose exceeds 50 mg. Chills, coma, extrapyramidal reaction, hallucinations, hypotension, myasthenia gravis (exacerbation or precipitation), neuroleptic malignant syndrome, Parkinson's-like symptoms, tachycardia, wheezing

Pharmacodynamics/Kinetics
Onset of action: Peak effect: Parenteral: ~30 minutes
Duration: Parenteral: 2-4 hours, may extend to 12 hours
Absorption: I.M.: Rapid
Distribution: Crosses blood-brain barrier and placenta
V_d: Children: ~0.25-0.9 L/kg; Adults: ~2 L/kg
Protein binding: Extensive
Metabolism: Hepatic, to *p*-fluorophenylacetic acid, benzimidazolone, *p*-hydroxypiperidine
Half-life elimination: Adults: 2.3 hours
Excretion: Urine (75%, <1% as unchanged drug); feces (22%, 11% to 50% as unchanged drug)

Dosage
Titrate carefully to desired effect
Children 2-12 years: Nausea and vomiting: I.M., I.V.: 0.05-0.06 mg/kg (maximum initial dose: 0.1 mg/kg); additional doses may be repeated to achieve effect; administer additional doses with caution
Adults: Nausea and vomiting: I.M., I.V.: Initial: 2.5 mg; additional doses of 1.25 mg may be administered to achieve desired effect; administer additional doses with caution

Stability Stability of parenteral admixture at room temperature (25°C): 24 hours

Monitoring Parameters To identify QT prolongation, a 12-lead ECG prior to use is recommended; continued ECG monitoring for 2-3 hours following administration is recommended. Vital signs; lipid profile, fasting blood glucose/Hgb A$_{1c}$, serum magnesium and potassium; BMI; mental status, abnormal involuntary movement scale (AIMS); observe for dystonias, extrapyramidal side effects, and temperature changes

Administration Administer I.M. or I.V.; I.V. should be administered slow IVP (over 2-5 minutes) or IVPB; ECG monitoring for 2-3 hours after administration is recommended

Contraindications Hypersensitivity to droperidol or any component of the formulation; known or suspected QT prolongation, including congenital long QT syndrome (prolonged QT$_c$ is defined as >440 msec in males or >450 msec in females)

Warnings
May alter cardiac conduction. **[U.S. Boxed Warning]: Cases of QT prolongation and torsade de pointes, including some fatal cases, have been reported.** Use extreme caution in patients with bradycardia (<50 bpm), cardiac disease, concurrent MAOI therapy, Class I and Class III antiarrhythmics or other drugs known to prolong QT interval, and electrolyte disturbances (hypokalemia or hypomagnesemia), including concomitant drugs which may alter electrolytes (diuretics).
Use with caution in patients with seizures, bone marrow suppression, or severe liver disease. May be sedating, use with caution in disorders where CNS depression is a feature. Caution in patients with hemodynamic instability, predisposition to seizures, subcortical brain damage, renal or respiratory disease. Esophageal dysmotility and aspiration have been associated with antipsychotic use - use with caution in patients at risk of pneumonia (ie, Alzheimer's disease). Caution in breast cancer or other prolactin-dependent tumors (may elevate prolactin levels). May alter temperature regulation or mask toxicity of other drugs due to antiemetic effects. May cause orthostatic hypotension - use with caution in patients at risk of this effect or those who would tolerate transient hypotensive episodes (cerebrovascular disease, cardiovascular disease, or other medications which may predispose). Significant hypotension may occur; injection contains benzyl alcohol; injection also contains sulfites which may cause allergic reaction.
May cause anticholinergic effects (confusion, agitation, constipation, xerostomia, blurred vision, urinary retention). Therefore, they should be used with caution in patients with decreased gastrointestinal motility, urinary retention, BPH, xerostomia, or visual problems. Conditions which also may be exacerbated by cholinergic blockade include narrow-angle glaucoma (screening is recommended) and worsening of myasthenia gravis. Relative to other neuroleptics, droperidol has a low potency of cholinergic blockade.

May cause extrapyramidal symptoms, including pseudoparkinsonism, acute dystonic reactions, akathisia, and tardive dyskinesia (risk of these reactions is high relative to other neuroleptics). May be associated with neuroleptic malignant syndrome (NMS) or pigmentary retinopathy. Safety in children <6 months of age has not been established.

Dosage Forms Injection, solution: 2.5 mg/mL (1 mL, 2 mL)

Overdosage/Treatment

Decontamination: Lavage (within 1 hour)/activated charcoal

Supportive therapy: Following initiation of essential overdose management, toxic symptom treatment and supportive treatment should be initiated. Hypotension usually responds to I.V. fluids or Trendelenburg positioning. If unresponsive to these measures, the use of a parenteral inotrope may be required (eg, norepinephrine 0.1-0.2 mcg/kg/minute titrated to response). Seizures commonly respond to lorazepam or diazepam (I.V. 5-10 mg bolus in adults every 15 minutes if needed up to a total of 30 mg; I.V. 0.25-0.4 mg/kg/dose up to a total of 10 mg in children) or to phenytoin or phenobarbital. Also critical cardiac arrhythmias often respond to I.V. phenytoin (15 mg/kg up to 1 g), while other antiarrhythmics can be used. Neuroleptics often cause extrapyramidal reaction (eg, dystonic reactions) requiring management with diphenhydramine 1-2 mg/kg (adults) up to a maximum of 50 mg I.M. or I.V. slow push followed by a maintenance dose for 48-72 hours. When these reactions are unresponsive to diphenhydramine, benztropine mesylate I.V. 1-2 mg (adults) may be effective. These agents are generally effective within 2-5 minutes.

Drug Interactions Acetylcholinesterase inhibitors (central): May increase the risk of antipsychotic-related extrapyramidal symptoms; monitor.

CNS depressants: Sedative effects may be additive with other CNS depressants; monitor for increased effect; includes benzodiazepines, barbiturates, antipsychotics, ethanol, opiates, and other sedative medications

Cyclobenzaprine: Droperidol and cyclobenzaprine may have an additive effect on prolonging the QT interval; based on limited documentation; monitor

Inhalation anesthetics: Droperidol in combination with certain forms of induction anesthesia may produce peripheral vasodilitation and hypotension

Metoclopramide: May increase extrapyramidal symptoms (EPS) or risk.

Potassium- or magnesium-depleting agents: May increase the risk of serious arrhythmias with droperidol; includes many diuretics, aminoglycosides, cyclosporine, supraphysiologic doses of corticosteroids with mineralocorticoid effects, laxatives, and amphotericin B; monitor serum potassium and magnesium levels closely.

Propofol: An increased incidence of postoperative nausea and vomiting have been reported following coadministration

QT_c-prolonging agents: May result in additive effects on cardiac conduction, potentially resulting in malignant or lethal arrhythmias; concurrent use is contraindicated. Includes cisapride, Class I and Class III antiarrhythmics (amiodarone, dofetilide, procainamide, quinidine, sotalol), pimozide, some quinolone antibiotics (moxifloxacin, sparfloxacin, gatifloxacin), tricyclic antidepressants, and some phenothiazines (mesoridazine, thioridazine).

Pregnancy Risk Factor C

Pregnancy Implications Crosses the placenta

Lactation Excretion in breast milk unknown

Additional Information

Butyrophenone derivative that produces tranquilization, sedation, and an antiemetic effect; does not possess analgesic effects; has little or no amnesic properties.

May cause hypotension and reflex tachycardia. This is more pronounced when the drug is given intravenously. Warnings concerning QT prolongation have altered recommendations concerning perioperative use and monitoring. Baseline 12-lead ECG screening is recommended, and continued ECG monitoring for 2-3 hours postadministration is advised. Use should be limited to patients in whom alternatives are unacceptable.

Duloxetine

Pronunciation (doo LOX e teen)

CAS Number 136434-34-9

U.S. Brand Names Cymbalta®

Synonyms (+)-(S)-N-Methyl-γ-(1-naphthyloxy)-2-thiophenepropylamine Hydrochloride; Duloxetine Hydrochloride; LY248686

Use Treatment of major depressive disorder; management of pain associated with diabetic neuropathy

Unlabeled/Investigational Use Treatment of stress incontinence; management of chronic pain syndromes; management of fibromyalgia

Mechanism of Action Duloxetine is a potent inhibitor of neuronal serotonin and norepinephrine reuptake and a weak inhibitor of dopamine reuptake. Duloxetine has no significant activity for muscarinic cholinergic, H_1-histaminergic, or alpha$_2$-adrenergic receptors. Duloxetine does not possess MAO-inhibitory activity.

Adverse Reactions

>10%:

Central nervous system: Somnolence (7% to 15%), dizziness (6% to 14%), headache (13%), insomnia (8% to 11%%)

Gastrointestinal: Nausea (14% to 22% - usually subsides within 1-2 weeks), xerostomia (5% to 15%), diarrhea (8% to 13%), constipation (5% to 11%)

1% to 10%:

Cardiovascular: Palpitations (1%)

Central nervous system: Fatigue (2% to 10%), anxiety (3%), fever (1% to 2%), hypoesthesia (1%), irritability (1%), lethargy (1%), nervousness (1%), nightmares (1%), restlessness (1%), sleep disorder (1%), vertigo (1%), yawning (1%)

Dermatologic: Hyperhydrosis (6%), pruritus (1%), rash (1%)

Endocrine & metabolic: Libido decreased (3% to 6%), orgasm abnormality (3% to 4%), hot flushes (2%), anorgasmia (1%), hypoglycemia (1%)

Gastrointestinal: Appetite decreased (3% to 8%), vomiting (5% to 6%), dyspepsia (4%), loose stools (2% to 3%), weight loss (1% to 2%), gastritis (1%)

Genitourinary: Erectile dysfunction (1% to 4%), ejaculation delayed (3%), ejaculatory dysfunction (3%), pollakiuria (1% to 3%), dysuria (1%), urinary symptoms (hesitancy, obstructive symptoms; 1%)

Hepatic: Transaminases increased transiently: Occasionally associated with hyperbilirubinemia and/or increased alkaline phosphatase (1%)

Neuromuscular & skeletal: Muscle cramp (4% to 5%), weakness (2% to 4%), myalgia (1% to 3%), tremor (1% to 3%), muscle tightness (1%), muscle twitching (1%), rigors (1%)

Ocular: Blurred vision (4%), mydriasis

Respiratory: Nasopharyngitis (7% to 9%), cough (3% to 6%), pharyngolaryngeal pain (1% to 3%)

Miscellaneous: Diaphoresis increased (6%), night sweats (1%)

<1%: Abdominal pain, acne, agitation, alopecia, anemia, aphthous stomatitis, ataxia, atrial fibrillation, bloody stools, bruxism, bundle branch block, CHF, cholesterol increased, colitis, dehydration, diplopia, disorientation, diverticulitis, dysarthria, dyslipidemia, dysphagia, ecchymosis, eczema, edema (peripheral), eructation, erythema, esophageal stenosis, facial edema, flu-like syndrome, gastric emptying impaired, gastric irritation, gastric ulcer, gingivitis, glaucoma, hepatic steatosis, hypercholesterolemia, hyperlipidemia, hypertensive crisis, hypertriglyceridemia, irritable bowel syndrome, keroconjunctivitis sicca, leukopenia, lymphadenopathy, macular degeneration, maculopathy, malaise, mania, melena, MI, micturation urgency, mood swings, muscle weakness, nephropathy, nocturia, oropharyngeal edema, phlebitis, photopsia, photosensitivity, retinal detachment, seizure, stomatitis, suicide, tachycardia, thirst, thrombocytopenia, urinary retention, visual disturbance, weight increased; withdrawal syndrome (including headache, dizziness, nightmares, irritability, paresthesia, and/or vomiting)

Postmarketing and/or case reports: Anaphylactic reaction, angioneurotic edema, bilirubin increased, hepatitis, hyponatremia, jaundice, orthostatic hypotension, Stevens-Johnson syndrome, syncope, urticaria

Pharmacodynamics/Kinetics

Absorption: Well absorbed, 3-hour delay in absorption after ingestion

Distribution: 1640 L

Protein binding: >90%

Metabolism: Hepatic, via CYP1A2 and CYP2D6; forms multiple metabolites (inactive)

Half-life elimination: 12 hours (range 8-17 hours)

Time to peak: 6 hours

Excretion: As metabolites; urine (70%), feces (20%); total body clearance: 114 L/hour

Bioavailability: <70% (oral)

Dosage Oral:

Adults:

Treatment of major depressive disorder: Initial: 40-60 mg/day; dose may be divided (ie, 20 or 30 mg twice daily) or given as a single daily dose of 60 mg; maximum dose: 60 mg/day

Management of diabetic neuropathy: 60 mg once daily; lower initial doses may be considered in patients where tolerability is a concern and/or renal impairment is present

Management of chronic pain syndromes (unlabeled use): 60 mg once daily

Management of fibromyalgia (unlabeled use): 60 mg twice daily

Management of stress incontinence (unlabeled use): 40 mg twice daily

Elderly:

Treatment of major depressive disorder: Initial dose: 20 mg 1-2 times/day; increase to 40-60 mg/day as a single daily dose or in divided doses

Other indications: Refer to Adults dosing

Dosage adjustment in renal impairment: Not recommended for use in Cl_{cr} <30 mL/minute or ESRD; in mild-moderate impairment, lower initial doses may be considered with titration guided by response and tolerability

Dosage adjustment in hepatic impairment: Not recommended for use in hepatic impairment

Stability Store at 25°C (77°F), excursions permitted to 15°C to 30°C (59°F to 86°F)

Monitoring Parameters Blood pressure should be regularly monitored, especially in patients with a high baseline blood pressure; mental status for depression, suicidal ideation (especially at the beginning of therapy or when doses are increased or decreased), anxiety, social functioning, mania, panic attacks

Administration Capsule should be swallowed whole; do not break open or crush.

Contraindications Hypersensitivity to duloxetine or any component of the formulation; concomitant use or within 2 weeks of MAO inhibitors; uncontrolled narrow angle glaucoma

Warnings *Major psychiatric warnings:*
- Antidepressants increase the risk of suicidal thinking and behavior in children and adolescents with major depressive disorder (MDD) and other depressive disorders; consider risk prior to prescribing. Closely monitor for clinical worsening, suicidality, or unusual changes in behavior; the child's family or caregiver should be instructed to closely observe the patient and communicate condition with healthcare provider. A medication guide concerning the use of antidepressants in children and teenagers should be dispensed with each prescription. **Duloxetine is not FDA approved for use in children.**
- The possibility of a suicide attempt is inherent in major depression and may persist until remission occurs. Patients treated with antidepressants should be observed for clinical worsening and suicidality, especially during the initial few months of a course of drug therapy, or at times of dose changes, either increases or decreases. Worsening depression and severe abrupt suicidality that are not part of the presenting symptoms may require discontinuation or modification of drug therapy. Use caution in high-risk patients during initiation of therapy.
- Prescriptions should be written for the smallest quantity consistent with good patient care. The patient's family or caregiver should be alerted to monitor patients for the emergence of suicidality and associated behaviors such as anxiety, agitation, panic attacks, insomnia, irritability, hostility, impulsivity, akathisia, hypomania, and mania; patients should be instructed to notify their healthcare provider if any of these symptoms or worsening depression or psychosis occur.
- May worsen psychosis in some patients or precipitate a shift to mania or hypomania in patients with bipolar disorder. Monotherapy in patients with bipolar disorder should be avoided. Patients presenting with depressive symptoms should be screened for bipolar disorder. **Duloxetine is not FDA approved for the treatment of bipolar depression.**

Key adverse effects:
- CNS depression: Has a low potential to impair cognitive or motor performance; caution operating hazardous machinery or driving.
- SIADH and hyponatremia: Has been associated with the development of SIADH; hyponatremia has been reported rarely, predominately in the elderly
- Urinary hesitancy: May cause increased urinary resistance; advise patient to report symptoms of urinary hesitation/difficulty.

Concurrent disease:
- Hepatic impairment and/or ethanol use: May cause hepatotoxicity; avoid use in patients with substantial alcohol intake, evidence of chronic liver disease, or hepatic impairment.
- Narrow-angle glaucoma: Associated with an increased risk of mydriasis in patients with controlled narrow-angle glaucoma.
- Renal impairment: Use with caution; clearance is decreased and plasma concentrations are increased; not recommended for use when $Cl_{cr} < 30$ mL/minute or ESRD.
- Sexual dysfunction: May cause or exacerbate sexual dysfunction.
- Seizure disorders: Use caution with a previous seizure disorder or condition predisposing to seizures such as brain damage or alcoholism.

Concurrent drug therapy:
- Agents which lower seizure threshold: Concurrent therapy with other drugs which lower the seizure threshold.
- CNS depressants: Use caution with concomitant therapy.
- MAO inhibitors: Potential for severe reaction when used with MAO inhibitors; autonomic instability, coma, death, delirium, diaphoresis, hyperthermia, mental status changes/agitation, muscular rigidity, myoclonus, neuroleptic malignant syndrome features, and seizures may occur.

Can increase serum half-life and concentration of desipramine

Special notes:
- Electroconvulsive therapy: May increase the risks associated with electroconvulsive therapy; consider discontinuing, when possible, prior to ECT treatment.
- Withdrawal syndrome: May cause dysphoric mood, irritability, agitation, dizziness, sensory disturbances, anxiety, confusion, headache, lethargy, emotional lability, insomnia, hypomania, tinnitus, and seizures. Upon discontinuation of duloxetine therapy, gradually taper dose. If intolerable symptoms occur following a decrease in dosage or upon discontinuation of therapy, then resuming the previous dose with a more gradual taper should be considered.

Dosage Forms Capsule: 20 mg, 30 mg, 60 mg [contains enteric coated pellets]

Reference Range Peak plasma duloxetine and desmethyl metabolite level following a 20 mg oral dose is approximately 13 ng/mL and <2 ng/mL, respectively

Overdosage/Treatment
Decontamination: Lavage (within 3 hours) or administer oral activated charcoal for adult ingestions >1.5 g
Supportive: Monitor for serotonin syndrome; care is supportive

Drug Interactions **Substrate** (major) of CYP1A2, 2D6; **inhibits** CYP2D6 (moderate)
Buspirone: Concurrent use of duloxetine with buspirone may cause serotonin syndrome; avoid concurrent use.
CYP1A2 inducers: May decrease the levels/effects of duloxetine. Example inducers include aminoglutethimide, carbamazepine, phenobarbital, and rifampin.
CYP1A2 inhibitors: May increase the levels/effects of duloxetine. Example inhibitors include ciprofloxacin, fluvoxamine, ketoconazole, norfloxacin, ofloxacin, and rofecoxib.
CYP2D6 inhibitors: May increase the levels/effects of duloxetine. Example inhibitors include chlorpromazine, delavirdine, fluoxetine, miconazole, paroxetine, pergolide, quinidine, quinine, ritonavir, and ropinirole.
Desipramine: Duloxetine may increase desipramine levels.
Linezolid: Hyperpyrexia, hypertension, tachycardia, confusion, seizures, and deaths have been reported with agents which inhibit MAO (serotonin syndrome); this combination should be avoided.
MAO inhibitors: Hyperpyrexia, hypertension, tachycardia, confusion, seizures, and deaths have been reported with MAO inhibitors (serotonin syndrome); this combination is contraindicated. Wait 5 days after discontinuation of duloxetine before initiating therapy with a MAO inhibitor.
Meperidine: Combined use theoretically may increase the risk of serotonin syndrome.
Moclobemide: Concurrent use of duloxetine with moclobemide may cause serotonin syndrome; avoid concurrent use.
Nefazodone: Concurrent use of duloxetine with nefazodone may cause serotonin syndrome.
Selegiline: Concurrent use with SSRIs has been reported to cause serotonin syndrome; as an MAO type B inhibitor, the risk of serotonin syndrome may be less than with nonselective MAO inhibitors, and reports indicate that this combination has been well tolerated in Parkinson's patients.
SSRIs: Concurrent use with serotonin reuptake inhibitors may increase the risk of serotonin syndrome.
Sibutramine: May increase the risk of serotonin syndrome with SNRIs.
Sumatriptan (and other serotonin agonists): Concurrent use may result in toxicity; weakness, hyper-reflexia, and incoordination have been observed with sumatriptan and SSRIs (and/or SNRIs). In addition, concurrent use may theoretically increase the risk of serotonin syndrome; includes almotriptan, sumatriptan, naratriptan, rizatriptan, and zolmitriptan.
Thioridazine: Duloxetine may increase serum concentrations of thioridazine, which has been associated with the development of malignant ventricular arrhythmias; use caution
Tramadol: Concurrent use of duloxetine with tramadol may cause serotonin syndrome; avoid concurrent use.
Trazodone: Concurrent use of duloxetine with trazodone may cause serotonin syndrome.
Tricyclic antidepressants: Serum levels/effects may be increased by duloxetine; use caution
Venlafaxine: Combined use with duloxetine may increase the risk of serotonin syndrome.

Pregnancy Risk Factor C
Nonteratogenic effects including respiratory distress, cyanosis, apnea, seizures, temperature instability, feeding difficulty, vomiting, hypoglycemia, hypo- or hypertonia, hyper-reflexia, jitteriness, irritability, constant crying, and tremor have been reported in the neonate immediately following delivery after exposure late in the third trimester. Adverse effects may be due to toxic effects of SNRI or drug discontinuation. There are no adequate and well-controlled studies in pregnant women. Use during pregnancy only if the potential benefit to the mother outweighs the possible risk to the fetus. If treatment during pregnancy is required, consider tapering therapy during the third trimester.

Pregnancy Implications Decreased fetal weight and behavioral effects have been reported in animal studies. Nonteratogenic effects including respiratory distress, cyanosis, apnea, seizures, temperature instability, feeding difficulty, vomiting, hypoglycemia, hypo- or hypertonia, hyper-reflexia, jitteriness, irritability, constant crying, and tremor have been reported in the neonate immediately following delivery after exposure late in the third trimester. Adverse effects may be due to toxic effects of SNRI or drug discontinuation. There are no adequate and well-controlled studies in pregnant women. Use during pregnancy only if the potential benefit to the mother outweighs the possible risk to the fetus. If treatment during pregnancy is required, consider tapering therapy during the third trimester.

Lactation Enters breast milk/not recommended

Edrophonium

Specific References
Cruz MP, Gonzales ME, Jacobs J, et al, "Duloxetine HCl (Cymbalta) for the Treatment of Depression, Neuropathic Pain, Fibromyalgia, and Stress Urinary Incontinence," *P&T*, 2006, 31(2):84-97.

CAS Number 116-38-1; 312-42-1
U.S. Brand Names Enlon®; Reversol®
Synonyms Edrophonium Chloride
Use Diagnosis of myasthenia gravis; differentiation of cholinergic crises from myasthenia crises; reversal of nondepolarizing neuromuscular blockers; adjunct treatment of respiratory depression caused by curare overdose
Mechanism of Action Inhibits destruction of acetylcholine by acetylcholinesterase which facilitates transmission of impulses across myoneural junction
Adverse Reactions
Cardiovascular: Arrhythmias, hypotension, bradyarrhythmias, ventricular asystole (after a dose of 10 mg), chest pain, flutter (atrial), sinus bradycardia, angina
Central nervous system: Convulsions, seizures
Gastrointestinal: **Nausea**, **vomiting**, abdominal pain, **diarrhea**, **excessive salivation**, **stomach cramps**
Genitourinary: Urinary frequency
Neuromuscular & skeletal: Weakness, muscle cramps
Ocular: Diplopia, photophobia, miosis, blurred vision
Respiratory: Laryngospasm, wheezing, respiratory paralysis, tachypnea
Miscellaneous: **Diaphoresis**, increased secretions
Signs and Symptoms of Overdose Bronchospasm, fibrillation (atrial), hypotension, miosis, muscle weakness, nausea, respiratory paralysis, seizures, vomiting, wheezing
Pharmacodynamics/Kinetics
Onset of action: I.M.: 2-10 minutes; I.V.: 30-60 seconds
Duration: I.M.: 5-30 minutes: I.V.: 10 minutes
Distribution: V_d: Adults: 1.1 L/kg
Half-life elimination: Adults: 1.2-2.4 hours; Anephric patients: 2.4-4.4 hours
Excretion: Adults: Primarily urine (67%)
Dosage
Usually administered I.V., however, if not possible, I.M. or SubQ may be used:
Infants:
I.M.: 0.5-1 mg
I.V.: Initial: 0.1 mg, followed by 0.4 mg if no response; total dose = 0.5 mg
Children:
Diagnosis: Initial: 0.04 mg/kg over 1 minute followed by 0.16 mg/kg if no response, to a maximum total dose of 5 mg for children <34 kg, or 10 mg for children >34 kg **or**
Alternative dosing (manufacturer's recommendation):
≤34 kg: 1 mg; if no response after 45 seconds, repeat dosage in 1 mg increments every 30-45 seconds, up to a total of 5 mg
>34 kg: 2 mg; if no response after 45 seconds, repeat dosage in 1 mg increments every 30-45 seconds, up to a total of 10 mg
I.M.:
<34 kg: 1 mg
>34 kg: 5 mg
Titration of oral anticholinesterase therapy: 0.04 mg/kg once given 1 hour after oral intake of the drug being used in treatment; if strength improves, an increase in neostigmine or pyridostigmine dose is indicated
Adults:
Diagnosis:
I.V.: 2 mg test dose administered over 15-30 seconds; 8 mg given 45 seconds later if no response is seen; test dose may be repeated after 30 minutes
I.M.: Initial: 10 mg; if no cholinergic reaction occurs, administer 2 mg 30 minutes later to rule out false-negative reaction
Titration of oral anticholinesterase therapy: 1-2 mg given 1 hour after oral dose of anticholinesterase; if strength improves, an increase in neostigmine or pyridostigmine dose is indicated
Reversal of nondepolarizing neuromuscular blocking agents (neostigmine with atropine usually preferred): I.V.: 10 mg over 30-45 seconds; may repeat every 5-10 minutes up to 40 mg
Termination of paroxysmal atrial tachycardia: I.V. rapid injection: 5-10 mg
Differentiation of cholinergic from myasthenic crisis: I.V.: 1 mg; may repeat after 1 minute. **Note:** Intubation and controlled ventilation may be required if patient has cholinergic crisis
Dosing adjustment in renal impairment: Dose may need to be reduced in patients with chronic renal failure
Monitoring Parameters Pre- and postinjection strength (cranial musculature is most useful); heart rate, respiratory rate, blood pressure
Administration Edrophonium is administered by direct I.V. injection; see Dosage
Contraindications Hypersensitivity to edrophonium, sulfites, or any component of the formulation; GI or GU obstruction
Warnings Use with caution in patients with bronchial asthma and those receiving a cardiac glycoside; atropine sulfate should always be readily available as an antagonist. Overdosage can cause cholinergic crisis which may be fatal. I.V. atropine should be readily available for treatment of cholinergic reactions.
Dosage Forms Injection, solution, as chloride:
Enlon®: 10 mg/mL (15 mL) [contains sodium sulfite]
Reversol®: 10 mg/mL (10 mL) [contains sodium sulfite]
Reference Range Dose of 0.5 mcg/kg gives mean plasma concentration of 7.82 nmol/mL and will probably decrease cholinesterase levels by >80%
Overdosage/Treatment Supportive therapy: For muscarinic symptoms, the antidote is atropine 0.4-0.5 mg I.V. repeated every 3-10 minutes (initial doses as high as 1.2 mg have been administered). Skeletal muscle effects of edrophonium are not alleviated by atropine. Pralidoxime (2-PAM) may be needed to reverse severe muscle asthenia or paralysis; although, since edrophonium is such a short-acting drug, 2-PAM use is usually not necessary.
Antidote(s)
- Atropine [ANTIDOTE]
- Pralidoxime [ANTIDOTE]

Test Interactions ↑ aminotransferases (ALT, AST) (S), amylase (S)
Drug Interactions Decreased effect: Atropine, nondepolarizing muscle relaxants, procainamide, quinidine
Increased effect: Succinylcholine, digoxin, I.V. acetazolamide, neostigmine, physostigmine
Pregnancy Risk Factor C
Lactation Excretion in breast milk unknown
Nursing Implications Atropine sulfate should be available at bedside
Additional Information Overdosage can cause cholinergic crisis which may be fatal. Atropine should be readily available for treatment of cholinergic reactions. Pralidoxime may reverse muscle asthenia.

Eflornithine

CAS Number 96020-91-6
U.S. Brand Names Vaniqa™
Synonyms DFMO; Eflornithine Hydrochloride
Use
Cream: Females ≥12 years: Reduce unwanted hair from face and adjacent areas under the chin
Orphan status: Injection: Treatment of meningoencephalitic stage of *Trypanosoma brucei gambiense* infection (sleeping sickness) *P. carinii* infection, cryptosporidiosis infections in HIV-infected patients
Mechanism of Action Eflornithine exerts antitumor and antiprotozoal effects through specific, irreversible ("suicide") inhibition of the enzyme ornithine decarboxylase (ODC). ODC is the rate-limiting enzyme in the biosynthesis of putrescine, spermine, and spermidine, the major polyamines in nucleated cells. Polyamines are necessary for the synthesis of DNA, RNA, and proteins and are, therefore, necessary for cell growth and differentiation. Although many microorganisms and higher plants are able to produce polyamines from alternate biochemical pathways, all mammalian cells depend on ornithine decarboxylase to produce polyamines. Eflornithine inhibits ODC and rapidly depletes animal cells of putrescine and spermidine; the concentration of spermine remains the same or may even increase. Rapidly dividing cells appear to be most susceptible to the effects of eflornithine.
Adverse Reactions
Central nervous system: Convulsions
Dermatologic: Alopecia
Gastrointestinal: Diarrhea, vomiting
Hematologic: **Anemia**, **leukopenia**, **thrombocytopenia**
Otic: Hearing impairment, deafness
Signs and Symptoms of Overdose In mice and rats CNS depression, seizures and death have occurred. Human overdose cases have not been published. Leukopenia, neutropenia, agranulocytosis, granulocytopenia
Pharmacodynamics/Kinetics
Absorption: Topical: <1%
Half-life elimination: I.V.: 3-3.5 hours; Topical: 8 hours
Excretion: Primarily urine (as unchanged drug)
Dosage
Children ≥12 years and Adults: Females: Topical: Apply thin layer of cream to affected areas of face and adjacent chin twice daily, at least 8 hours apart
Adults: I.V. infusion: 100 mg/kg/dose given every 6 hours (over at least 45 minutes) for 14 days
Dosing adjustment in renal impairment: Injection: Dose should be adjusted although no specific guidelines are available
Monitoring Parameters CBC with platelet counts

Administration

I.V.: Administred I.V. only; infuse over 45 minutes. Not for I.M. administration.

Cream: Apply thin layer of eflornithine cream to affected areas of face and adjacent chin area twice daily, at least 8 hours apart. Rub in thoroughly. Hair removal techniques must still be continued; wait at least 5 minutes after removing hair to apply cream. Do not wash affected area for at least 8 hours following application.

Contraindications Hypersensitivity to eflornithine or any component of the formulation

Warnings Injection: For I.V. use only; not for I.M. administration. Must be diluted before use; frequent monitoring for myelosuppression should be done; use with caution in patients with a history of seizures and in patients with renal impairment; serial audiograms should be obtained; due to the potential for relapse, patients should be followed up for at least 24 months

Cream: For topical use by females only; discontinue if hypersensitivity occurs; safety and efficacy in children <12 years has not been studied

Dosage Forms

Cream, topical, as hydrochloride: 13.9% (30 g)

Injection, solution, as hydrochloride: 200 mg/mL (100 mL) [orphan drug status]

Overdosage/Treatment

Decontamination: Activated charcoal

Supportive therapy: General poison management; no known antidote

Test Interactions ↑ BUN; ↓ RBC, WBC, platelets

Drug Interactions Cream: Possible interactions with other topical products have not been studied.

Pregnancy Risk Factor C

Pregnancy Implications There are no adequate and well-controlled studies of topical eflornithine cream in pregnant women. The potential benefits to the mother versus the possible risks to the fetus should be considered prior to use.

Lactation Excretion in breast milk unknown/use caution

Nursing Implications Must be diluted before use and used within 24 hours of preparation

---

Enalapril

Related Information
- Angiotensin Agents

CAS Number 75847-73-3; 76095-16-4

U.S. Brand Names Vasotec®

Synonyms Enalapril Maleate; Enalaprilat

Use Management of mild to severe hypertension; treatment of congestive heart failure, left ventricular dysfunction after myocardial infarction

Unlabeled/Investigational Use Unlabeled: Hypertensive crisis, diabetic nephropathy, rheumatoid arthritis, diagnosis of anatomic renal artery stenosis, hypertension secondary to scleroderma renal crisis, diagnosis of aldosteronism, idiopathic edema, Bartter's syndrome, postmyocardial infarction for prevention of ventricular failure

Investigational: Severe congestive heart failure in infants, neonatal hypertension, acute pulmonary edema

Mechanism of Action Competitive inhibitor of angiotensin-converting enzyme (ACE); prevents conversion of angiotensin I to angiotensin II, a potent vasoconstrictor; results in lower levels of angiotensin II which causes an increase in plasma renin activity and a reduction in aldosterone secretion

Adverse Reactions

Cardiovascular: Hypotension, chest pain, syncope, bradycardia, sinus bradycardia, angina, vasodilation, vasculitis

Central nervous system: Fatigue, psychosis, insomnia, dizziness, headache

Dermatologic: Rash, pemphigus, angioedema (0.68%), toxic pustuloderma, toxic epidermal necrolysis, exfoliative dermatitis, erythema multiforme, alopecia, urticaria, purpura, Stevens-Johnson syndrome, photosensitivity, pruritus, licheniform eruptions, exanthem, scalded mouth syndrome, Henoch-Schönlein purpura, cutaneous vasculitis

Endocrine & metabolic: Hypoglycemia, gynecomastia, hyperkalemia, syndrome of inappropriate antidiuretic hormone secretion

Gastrointestinal: Nausea, dyspepsia, diarrhea, pancreatitis, loss of taste perception (less than with captopril), metallic taste, salty taste

Genitourinary: Impotence

Hematologic: Leukopenia/neutropenia (agranulocytosis, granulocytopenia), anemia, pancytopenia

Neuromuscular & skeletal: Muscle cramps

Otic: Decreased hearing acuity

Renal: Deterioration in renal function, proteinuria, diuresis, renal vasculitis

Respiratory: Cough, hyposmia

Miscellaneous: Systemic lupus erythematosus

Signs and Symptoms of Overdose Hypotension is usually not severe in overdose patients and manifests itself within 1 hour with a maximal effect at 4 hours. Azotemia, bradycardia, coagulopathy deafness, depression, eosinophilia, hypoglycemia, insomnia, pemphigus, ototoxicity, thrombocytopenia, tinnitus

Pharmacodynamics/Kinetics

Onset of action: Oral: ~1 hour

Duration: Oral: 12-24 hours

Absorption: Oral: 55% to 75%

Protein binding: 50% to 60%

Metabolism: Prodrug, undergoes hepatic biotransformation to enalaprilat

Half-life elimination:
Enalapril: Adults: Healthy: 2 hours; Congestive heart failure: 3.4-5.8 hours
Enalaprilat: Infants 6 weeks to 8 months old: 6-10 hours; Adults: 35-38 hours

Time to peak, serum: Oral: Enalapril: 0.5-1.5 hours; Enalaprilat (active): 3-4.5 hours

Excretion: Urine (60% to 80%); some feces

Dosage

Use lower listed initial dose in patients with hyponatremia, hypovolemia, severe congestive heart failure, decreased renal function, or in those receiving diuretics.

Oral: **Enalapril:** Children 1 month to 16 years: Hypertension: Initial: 0.08 mg/kg (up to 5 mg) once daily; adjust dosage based on patient response; doses >0.58 mg/kg (40 mg) have not been evaluated in pediatric patients

Investigational: Congestive heart failure: Initial oral doses of **enalapril**: 0.1 mg/kg/day increasing as needed over 2 weeks to 0.5 mg/kg/day have been used in infants

Investigational: Neonatal hypertension: I.V. doses of **enalaprilat**: 5-10 mcg/kg/dose administered every 8-24 hours have been used; monitor patients carefully; select patients may require higher doses

Adults:

Oral: **Enalapril:**
Hypertension: 2.5-5 mg/day then increase as required; usual dose range (JNC 7): 2.5-40 mg/day in 1-2 divided doses. **Note:** Initiate with 2.5 mg if patient is taking a diuretic which cannot be discontinued. May add a diuretic if blood pressure cannot be controlled with enalapril alone.

Heart failure: As standard therapy alone or with diuretics, beta-blockers, and digoxin, initiate with 2.5 mg once or twice daily (usual range: 5-20 mg/day in 2 divided doses; target: 40 mg)

Asymptomatic left ventricular dysfunction: 2.5 mg twice daily, titrated as tolerated to 20 mg/day

I.V.: **Enalaprilat:**
Hypertension: 1.25 mg/dose, given over 5 minutes every 6 hours; doses as high as 5 mg/dose every 6 hours have been tolerated for up to 36 hours. **Note:** If patients are concomitantly receiving diuretic therapy, begin with 0.625 mg I.V. over 5 minutes; if the effect is not adequate after 1 hour, repeat the dose and administer 1.25 mg at 6-hour intervals thereafter; if adequate, administer 0.625 mg I.V. every 6 hours.

Heart failure: Avoid I.V. administration in patients with unstable heart failure or those suffering acute myocardial infarction.

Conversion from I.V. to oral therapy if not concurrently on diuretics: 5 mg once daily; subsequent titration as needed; if concurrently receiving diuretics and responding to 0.625 mg I.V. every 6 hours, initiate with 2.5 mg/day.

Dosing adjustment in renal impairment:
Oral: Enalapril:
Cl_{cr} 30-80 mL/minute: Administer 5 mg/day titrated upwards to maximum of 40 mg.
Cl_{cr} <30 mL/minute: Administer 2.5 mg day; titrated upward until blood pressure is controlled.
For heart failure patients with sodium <130 mEq/L or serum creatinine >1.6 mg/dL, initiate dosage with 2.5 mg/day, increasing to twice daily as needed. Increase further in increments of 2.5 mg/dose at >4-day intervals to a maximum daily dose of 40 mg.

I.V.: Enalaprilat:
Cl_{cr} >30 mL/minute: Initiate with 1.25 mg every 6 hours and increase dose based on response.
Cl_{cr} <30 mL/minute: Initiate with 0.625 mg every 6 hours and increase dose based on response.

Hemodialysis: Moderately dialyzable (20% to 50%); administer dose postdialysis (eg, 0.625 mg I.V. every 6 hours) or administer 20% to 25% supplemental dose following dialysis; Clearance: 62 mL/minute.

Peritoneal dialysis: Supplemental dose is not necessary, although some removal of drug occurs.

Dosing adjustment in hepatic impairment: Hydrolysis of enalapril to enalaprilat may be delayed and/or impaired in patients with severe hepatic impairment, but the pharmacodynamic effects of the drug do not appear to be significantly altered; no dosage adjustment.

Stability Solutions for I.V. infusion mixed in NS or D_5W, are stable for 24 hours at room temperature

Monitoring Parameters Blood pressure, renal function, WBC, serum potassium; blood pressure monitor required during intravenous administration

Administration Administer direct IVP over at least 5 minutes or dilute up to 50 mL and infuse; discontinue diuretic, if possible, for 2-3 days before beginning enalapril therapy

Contraindications Hypersensitivity to enalapril or enalaprilat; angioedema related to previous treatment with an ACE inhibitor; patients with idiopathic or hereditary angioedema; bilateral renal artery stenosis; pregnancy (2nd and 3rd trimesters)

Warnings

Anaphylactic reactions can occur. Angioedema can occur at any time during treatment (especially following first dose). It may involve head and neck (potentially affecting the airway) or the intestine (presenting with abdominal pain). Prolonged monitoring may be required especially if tongue, glottis, or larynx are involved as they are associated with airway obstruction. Those with a history of airway surgery in this situation have a higher risk. Careful blood pressure monitoring with first dose (hypotension can occur especially in volume-depleted patients).

[U.S. Boxed Warning]: Based on human data, ACEIs can cause injury and death to the developing fetus when used in the second and third trimesters. ACEIs should be discontinued as soon as possible once pregnancy is detected. Dosage adjustment needed in renal impairment. Use with caution in hypovolemia; collagen vascular diseases; valvular stenosis (particularly aortic stenosis); hyperkalemia; or before, during, or immediately after anesthesia. Avoid rapid dosage escalation which may lead to renal insufficiency.

Rare toxicities associated with ACE inhibitors include cholestatic jaundice (which may progress to hepatic necrosis) and neutropenia/agranulocytosis with myeloid hyperplasia. Hypersensitivity reactions may be seen during hemodialysis with high-flux dialysis membranes (eg, AN69). Hyperkalemia may rarely occur. If patient has renal impairment then a baseline WBC with differential and serum creatinine should be evaluated and monitored closely during the first 3 months of therapy. Use with caution in unilateral renal artery stenosis and pre-existing renal insufficiency.

Dosage Forms

Injection, solution, as enalaprilat: 1.25 mg/mL (1 mL, 2 mL) [contains benzyl alcohol]

Tablet, as maleate (Vasotec®): 2.5 mg, 5 mg, 10 mg, 20 mg

Reference Range Enalaprilat plasma level of 40 mcg/L (104 mM/L) can produce a mean blood pressure reduction of 12 mm Hg

Overdosage/Treatment

Decontamination: Ipecac (within 30 minutes)/lavage (within 1 hour)/activated charcoal

Supportive therapy: Following initiation of essential overdose management, toxic symptom treatment and supportive treatment should be initiated. Hypotension usually responds to I.V. normal saline or Trendelenburg positioning. If unresponsive to these measures, the use of a parenteral inotrope may be required (eg, norepinephrine 0.1-0.2 mcg/kg/minute titrated to response). Seizures commonly respond to lorazepam or diazepam (I.V. 5-10 mg bolus in adults every 15 minutes if needed up to a total of 30 mg; I.V. 0.25-0.4 mg/kg/dose up to a total of 10 mg in children) or to phenytoin or phenobarbital. Naloxone may antagonize hypotensive effects. Inhaled sodium cromoglycate (total dose: 40 mg/day) can decrease ACE-inhibitor cough by 50%. Picotamide (600 mg twice daily) can also decrease ACE-inhibitor cough. In Great Britain, I.V. use of angiotensin II at a dose of 22 ng/kg/minute has been shown to result in elevation of blood pressure and cardiac output in an enalapril overdose. For refractory hypotension, angiotensin amide infusion may be attempted.

Enhanced elimination: Multiple dosing of activated charcoal may be effective

Test Interactions ↑ BUN, creatinine, potassium; positive Coombs' [direct]; ↓ cholesterol (S); may cause false-positive urine acetone determinations using sodium nitroprusside reagent

Drug Interactions Substrate of CYP3A4 (major)

α_1 blockers: Hypotensive effect increased.

Aspirin: The effects of ACE inhibitors may be blunted by aspirin administration, particularly at higher dosages (see Cardiovascular Considerations) and/or increase adverse renal effects.

CYP3A4 inducers: CYP3A4 inducers may decrease the levels/effects of enalapril. Example inducers include aminoglutethimide, carbamazepine, nafcillin, nevirapine, phenobarbital, phenytoin, and rifamycins.

Diuretics: Hypovolemia due to diuretics may precipitate acute hypotensive events or acute renal failure.

Insulin: Risk of hypoglycemia may be increased.

Lithium: Risk of lithium toxicity may be increased; monitor lithium levels, especially in the first 4 weeks of therapy.

Mercaptopurine: Risk of neutropenia may be increased.

NSAIDs: May attenuate hypertensive efficacy; effect has been seen with captopril and may occur with other ACE inhibitors; monitor blood pressure. May increase risk of renal adverse effects.

Potassium-sparing diuretics (amiloride, spironolactone, triamterene): Increased risk of hyperkalemia.

Potassium supplements may increase the risk of hyperkalemia.

Trimethoprim (high dose) may increase the risk of hyperkalemia.

Pregnancy Risk Factor C (1st trimester)/D (2nd and 3rd trimesters)

Pregnancy Implications Decreased placental blood flow, low birth weight, fetal hypotension, preterm delivery, and fetal death have been noted with the use of some ACE inhibitors (ACEIs) in animal studies. Neonatal hypotension, skull hypoplasia, anuria, renal failure, oligohydramnios (associated with fetal limb contractures, craniofacial deformities, hypoplastic lung development), prematurity, intrauterine growth retardation, and patent ductus arteriosus have been reported with the use of ACEIs, primarily in the 2nd and 3rd trimesters. The risk of neonatal toxicity has been considered less when ACEIs have been used in the 1st trimester; however, major congenital malformations have been reported. The cardiovascular and/or central nervous systems are most commonly affected. Unless alternative agents are not appropriate, ACEIs should be discontinued as soon as possible once pregnancy is detected.

Lactation Enters breast milk/not recommended (AAP rates "compatible")

Nursing Implications May cause depression in some patients; discontinue if angioedema of the face, extremities, lips, tongue, or glottis occurs

Additional Information Severe hypotension may occur in patients who are sodium and/or volume depleted. Initiate lower doses and monitor closely when starting therapy in these patients. Reduces albuminuria in sickle cell anemia by up to 70%

Angioedema is more likely to occur in black patients, those older than 65 years, and those with a history of drug rash or seasonal allergies.

Specific References

Chobanian AV, Bakris GL, Black HR, et al, "The Seventh Report of the Joint National Committee on Prevention, Detection, Evaluation, and Treatment of High Blood Pressure: The JNC 7 Report," *JAMA*, 2003, 289(19):2560-71.

Cooper W, Hernandez-Diaz S, Arbogast P, et al, "Major Congenital Malformations After First Trimester Exposure to ACE Inhibitors," *N Engl J Med*, 2006, 354:2443-51.

Kostis JB, Kim HJ, Rusnak J, et al, "Incidence and Characteristics of Angioedema Associated with Enalapril," *Arch Intern Med*, 2005, 165(14):1637-42.

Mastrobattista J, "Angiontensin-Converting Enzyme Inhibitors in Pregnancy," *Semin Perinatol*, 1997, 21(2):124-34.

Quan A, "Fetopathy Associated with Exposure to Angiotensin-Converting Enzyme Inhibitors and Angiontensin Receptor Antagonists," *Early Hum Dev*, 2006, 82(1):23-8.

Enfuvirtide

U.S. Brand Names Fuzeon™

Synonyms T-20

Use Treatment of HIV-1 infection in combination with other antiretroviral agents in treatment-experienced patients with evidence of HIV-1 replication despite ongoing antiretroviral therapy

Mechanism of Action Binds to the first heptad-repeat (HR1) in the gp41 subunit of the viral envelope glycoprotein. Inhibits the fusion of HIV-1 virus with CD4 cells by blocking the conformational change in gp41 required for membrane fusion and entry into CD4 cells

Adverse Reactions

Central nervous system: **Insomnia**, depression, anxiety, Guillain-Barré syndrome

Dermatologic: Pruritus

Endocrine & metabolic: Weight loss, anorexia, hyperglycemia

Gastrointestinal: Triglycerides increased, appetite decreased, constipation, abdominal pain, pancreatitis, taste disturbance, serum amylase increased

Hematologic: Eosinophilia, anemia, thrombocytopenia, neutropenia

Hepatic: Serum transaminases increased

Local: **Injection site reactions (98%; may include pain, erythema, induration, pruritus, ecchymosis, nodule or cyst formation)**, injection site infection

Neuromuscular & skeletal: Neuropathy, weakness, myalgia

Ocular: Conjunctivitis

Renal: Renal insufficiency, renal failure

Respiratory: Cough, pneumonia (4.7 events per 100 patient years vs 0.61 events per 100 patient years in control group), sinusitis

Miscellaneous: Infections, flu-like symptoms, lymphadenopathy, hypersensitivity reactions (symptoms may include rash, fever, nausea, vomiting, hypotension, and hepatic transaminases increased), worsening of abacavir hypersensitivity, sixth nerve palsy

Pharmacodynamics/Kinetics

Distribution: V_d: 5.5 L

Protein binding: 92%

Metabolism: Proteolytic hydrolysis (CYP isoenzymes do not appear to contribute to metabolism); clearance: 24.8 mL/hour/kg

Half-life elimination: 3.8 hours

Time to peak: 8 hours

Dosage

SubQ:

Children ≥6 years: 2 mg/kg twice daily (maximum dose: 90 mg twice daily)

Adults: 90 mg twice daily

Dosage adjustment in renal impairment: No dosage adjustment required

Stability Store powder at 25°C (77°F); excursions permitted to 15°C to 30°C (59 to 86°F). Reconstitute with 1.1 mL SWFI; tap vial for 10 seconds and roll gently to ensure contact with diluent; then allow to stand until solution is completed; may require up to 45 minutes to form solution. Reconstituted solutions should be refrigerated and must be used within 24 hours.

Administration Inject subcutaneously into upper arm, abdomen, or anterior thigh. Do not inject into moles, scar tissue, bruises, or the navel. Rotate injection site, give injections at a site different from the preceding injection site; do not inject into any site where an injection site reaction is evident.

Contraindications Hypersensitivity to enfuvirtide or any component of the formulation

Warnings Monitor closely for signs/symptoms of pneumonia; associated with an increased incidence during clinical trials, particularly in patients with a low CD4 cell count, high initial viral load, I.V. drug use, smoking, or a history of lung disease. May cause hypersensitivity reactions (symptoms may include rash, fever, nausea, vomiting, hypotension, and elevated transaminases). In addition, local injection site reactions may occur. An inflammatory response to indolent or residual opportunistic infections (immune reconstitution syndrome) has occurred with antiretroviral therapy; further investigation is warranted. Safety and efficacy have not been established in children <6 years of age.

Dosage Forms Injection, powder for reconstitution [preservative free]:

Fuzeon®: 108 mg [90 mg/mL following reconstitution; available in convenience kit of 60 vials, SWFI, syringes, alcohol wipes, patient instructions]

Drug Interactions No interactions have been identified which would require alteration of other antiretroviral drugs.

Pregnancy Risk Factor B

Pregnancy Implications An antiretroviral registry has been established to monitor maternal and fetal outcomes in women receiving antiretroviral drugs. Physicians are encouraged to register patients at 1-800-258-4263.

Lactation Excretion in breast milk unknown/contraindicated

Enoxacin

Related Information

• Therapeutic Drugs Associated with Hallucinations

CAS Number 74011-58-8

Use Complicated and uncomplicated urinary tract infections caused by susceptible gram-negative and gram-positive bacteria

Mechanism of Action Enoxacin exerts its antibacterial activity, as do other quinoline-azaquinolone antibiotics, by inhibition of bacterial DNA gyrase

Adverse Reactions

Central nervous system: Restlessness, dizziness, confusion, seizures, headache, CNS depression, visual hallucinations, depression

Dermatologic: Rash, photosensitivity, urticaria, exanthem, photoallergic reaction

Gastrointestinal: Nausea, diarrhea, vomiting, GI bleeding, feces discoloration (white/speckling)

Hematologic: Anemia

Hepatic: Elevated liver enzymes

Neuromuscular & skeletal: Tremors, arthralgia

Ocular: Phototoxic

Renal: Renal failure (acute), elevation of serum creatinine and BUN

Toxicodynamics/Kinetics

Absorption: 98%

Distribution: Penetrates well into tissues and body secretions

Bioavailability: Essentially the bioavailability as I.V. administration; administration with food does not affect bioavailability

Half-life: 3-6 hours (average)

Elimination: Primarily excreted in urine; however, significant drug concentrations are achieved in feces

Dosage Adults: Oral: 400 mg twice daily

Dosing adjustment in renal impairment: Cl_cr <50 mL/minute: Administer 50% of dose

Reference Range Peak plasma level: 3 mg/L after a 750 mg oral dose

Overdosage/Treatment

Decontamination: Lavage (within 1 hour)/activated charcoal

Enhancement of elimination: Multiple dosing of activated charcoal may be effective

Pregnancy Risk Factor C

Enoxaparin

CAS Number 74011-58-8
U.S. Brand Names Lovenox®
Synonyms Enoxaparin Sodium

Use

DVT Treatment (acute): Inpatient treatment (patients with and without pulmonary embolism) and outpatient treatment (patients without pulmonary embolism)

DVT prophylaxis: Following hip or knee replacement surgery, abdominal surgery, or in medical patients with severely-restricted mobility during acute illness in patients at risk of thromboembolic complications

Note: High-risk patients include those with one or more of the following risk factors: >40 years of age, obesity, general anesthesia lasting >30 minutes, malignancy, history of deep vein thrombosis or pulmonary embolism

Unstable angina and non-Q-wave myocardial infarction (to prevent ischemic complications)

Unlabeled/Investigational Use Prophylaxis and treatment of thromboembolism in children

Mechanism of Action Inhibits thrombin

Adverse Reactions

Cardiovascular: Edema

Central nervous system: Confusion, fever, intracranial bleed

Dermatologic: Ecchymosis, erythema, skin necrosis, eczematous plaques, itchy erythematous patches, pruritus, urticaria, vesicobullous rash, purpura, skin necrosis

Endocrine & metabolic: Hyperlipidemia, hypertriglyceridemia

Gastrointestinal: Nausea, diarrhea

Hematologic: Hemorrhage, thrombocytopenia, hypochromic anemia, coagulopathy, thrombocytosis, hematoma, spontaneous splenic rupture

Hepatic: Increased ALT/AST

Local: Local irritation, pain

Neuromuscular & skeletal: Erythromelalgia

Miscellaneous: Allergic reaction, anaphylactoid reaction, retroperitoneal bleed

Spinal or epidural hematomas can occur following neuraxial anesthesia or spinal puncture, resulting in paralysis. Risk is increased in patients with indwelling epidural catheters or concomitant use of other drugs affecting hemostasis. Prosthetic valve thrombosis, including fatal cases, has been reported in pregnant women receiving enoxaparin as thromboprophylaxis. Thrombocytopenia with thrombosis: Cases of heparin-induced thrombocytopenia (some complicated by organ infarction, limb ischemia, or death) have been reported.

Pharmacodynamics/Kinetics

Onset of action: Peak effect: SubQ: Antifactor Xa and antithrombin (antifactor IIa): 3-5 hours

Duration: 40 mg dose: Antifactor Xa activity: ~12 hours

Metabolism: Hepatic, to lower molecular weight fragments (little activity)

Protein binding: Does not bind to heparin binding proteins

Half-life elimination, plasma: 2-4 times longer than standard heparin, independent of dose; based on anti-Xa activity: 4.5-7 hours

Excretion: Urine (40% of dose; 10% as active fragments)

Dosage

SubQ:

Infants and Children (unlabeled use):

Infants <2 months: Initial:
Prophylaxis: 0.75 mg/kg every 12 hours
Treatment: 1.5 mg/kg every 12 hours

Infants >2 months and Children ≤18 years: Initial:
Prophylaxis: 0.5 mg/kg every 12 hours
Treatment: 1 mg/kg every 12 hours

Adults:

DVT prophylaxis:

Hip replacement surgery:

Twice-daily dosing: 30 mg twice daily, with initial dose within 12-24 hours after surgery, and every 12 hours until risk of DVT has diminished or the patient is adequately anticoagulated on warfarin.

Once-daily dosing: 40 mg once daily, with initial dose within 9-15 hours before surgery, and daily until risk of DVT has diminished or the patient is adequately anticoagulated on warfarin.

Knee replacement surgery: 30 mg twice daily, with initial dose within 12-24 hours after surgery, and every 12 hours until risk of DVT has diminished (usually 7-10 days).

Abdominal surgery: 40 mg once daily, with initial dose given 2 hours prior to surgery; continue until risk of DVT has diminished (usual 7-10 days).

Medical patients with severely-restricted mobility during acute illness: 40 mg once daily; continue until risk of DVT has diminished

DVT treatment (acute): **Note:** Start warfarin within 72 hours and continue enoxaparin until INR is between 2.0 and 3.0 (usually 7 days).

Inpatient treatment (with or without pulmonary embolism): 1 mg/kg/dose every 12 hours or 1.5 mg/kg once daily.

Outpatient treatment (without pulmonary embolism): 1 mg/kg/dose every 12 hours.

Unstable angina or non-Q-wave MI: 1 mg/kg twice daily in conjunction with oral aspirin therapy (100-325 mg once daily); continue until clinical stabilization (a minimum of at least 2 days)

Elderly: Increased incidence of bleeding with doses of 1.5 mg/kg/day or 1 mg/kg every 12 hours; injection-associated bleeding and serious adverse reactions are also increased in the elderly. Careful attention should be paid to elderly patients <45 kg.

Dosing adjustment in renal impairment: SubQ:

$Cl_{cr} \geq 30$ mL/minute: No specific adjustment recommended (per manufacturer); monitor closely for bleeding

$Cl_{cr} < 30$ mL/minute:

DVT prophylaxis in abdominal surgery, hip replacement, knee replacement, or in medical patients during acute illness: 30 mg once daily

DVT treatment (inpatient or outpatient treatment in conjunction with warfarin): 1 mg/kg once daily

Unstable angina, non-Q-wave MI (with ASA): 1 mg/kg once daily

Dialysis: Enoxaparin has not been FDA approved for use in dialysis patients. It's elimination is primarily via the renal route. Serious bleeding complications have been reported with use in patients who are dialysis dependent or have severe renal failure. LMWH administration at fixed doses without monitoring has greater unpredictable anticoagulant effects in patients with chronic kidney disease. If used, dosages should be reduced and anti-Xa activity frequently monitored, as accumulation may occur over days. Many clinicians would not use enoxaparin in this population especially without timely anti-Xa activity assay results.

Hemodialysis: Supplemental dose is not necessary.

Peritoneal dialysis: Significant drug removal is unlikely based on physiochemical characteristics.

Stability Incompatible with gentamicin

Monitoring Parameters Platelets, occult blood, and anti-Xa activity, if available; the monitoring of PT and/or PTT is not necessary

Administration Should be administered by deep SubQ injection to the left or right anterolateral and left or right posterolateral abdominal wall. To avoid loss of drug from the 30 mg and 40 mg syringes, do not expel the air bubble from the syringe prior to injection. In order to minimize bruising, do not rub injection site. An automatic injector (Lovenox EasyInjector™) is available with the 30 mg and 40 mg syringes to aid the patient with self-injections. **Note:** Enoxaparin is available in 100 mg/mL and 150 mg/mL concentrations.

Contraindications Hypersensitivity to enoxaparin, heparin, or any component of the formulation; thrombocytopenia associated with a positive *in vitro* test for antiplatelet antibodies in the presence of enoxaparin; hypersensitivity to pork products; active major bleeding; not for I.M. or I.V. use

Warnings

[U.S. Boxed Warning]: Patients with recent or anticipated neuraxial anesthesia (epidural or spinal anesthesia) are at risk of spinal or epidural hematoma and subsequent paralysis. Consider risk versus benefit prior to neuraxial anesthesia; risk is increased by concomitant agents which may alter hemostasis, as well as traumatic or repeated epidural or spinal puncture. Patient should be observed closely for bleeding if enoxaparin is administered during or immediately following diagnostic lumbar puncture, epidural anesthesia, or spinal anesthesia.

Do not administer intramuscularly. Not recommended for thromboprophylaxis in patients with prosthetic heart valves (especially pregnant women). Not to be used interchangeably (unit for unit) with heparin or any other low molecular weight heparins. Use caution in patients with history of heparin-induced thrombocytopenia. Monitor patient closely for signs or symptoms of bleeding. Certain patients are at increased risk of bleeding. Risk factors include bacterial endocarditis; congenital or acquired bleeding disorders; active ulcerative or angiodysplastic GI diseases; severe uncontrolled hypertension; hemorrhagic stroke; use shortly after brain, spinal, or ophthalmology surgery; patients treated concomitantly with platelet inhibitors; recent GI bleeding; thrombocytopenia or platelet defects; severe liver disease; hypertensive or diabetic retinopathy; or in patients undergoing invasive procedures. Monitor platelet count closely. Rare cases of thrombocytopenia have occurred. Manufacturer recommends discontinuation of therapy if platelets are <100,000/mm^3. Risk of bleeding may be increased in women <45 kg and in men <57 kg. Use caution in patients with renal failure; dosage adjustment needed if $Cl_{cr} < 30$ mL/minute. Safety and efficacy in pediatric patients have not been established. Use with caution in the elderly (delayed elimination may occur). Heparin can cause hyperkalemia by affecting aldosterone. Similar reactions could occur with LMWHs. Monitor for hyperkalemia. Multiple-dose vials contain benzyl alcohol (use caution in pregnant women).

Dosage Forms

Injection, solution, as sodium [graduated prefilled syringe; preservative free]: 60 mg/0.6 mL (0.6 mL); 80 mg/0.8 mL (0.8 mL); 100 mg/mL (1 mL); 120 mg/0.8 mL (0.8 mL); 150 mg/mL (1 mL)

Injection, solution, as sodium [multidose vial]: 100 mg/mL (3 mL) [contains benzyl alcohol]

Injection, solution, as sodium [prefilled syringe; preservative free]: 30 mg/0.3 mL (0.3 mL); 40 mg/0.4 mL (0.4 mL)

Reference Range Risk of bleeding increases when antifactor Xa levels exceed 0.4 unit/mL

Overdosage/Treatment

Supportive therapy: In the event of a serious bleeding episode in a patient receiving enoxaparin therapy, protamine may be used. The recommended dose of protamine can be found in the following table. It is important to realize that protamine will neutralize a maximum of 60% to 70% of enoxaparin. If serious bleeding occurs, protamine should be used in conjunction with FFP. An additional 0.5 mg protamine per 1 mg enoxaparin can be administered 2-4 hours after the initial dose if PTT is still elevated at this time.

Enhancement of elimination: While hemodialysis is not beneficial, exchange transfusion has been used successfully in a neonate and plasma exchange has been used successfully in four older patients for thrombocytopenia. See table.

Recommended Protamine Dosing

<8 Hours Since Last Dose	8-12 Hours Since Last Dose	>12 Hours Since Last Dose
1 mg protamine per 1 mg enoxaparin	0.5 mg protamine per 1 mg enoxaparin	No recommended dose: protamine probably not of value at this time

Antidote(s)

- Protamine Sulfate [ANTIDOTE]

Drug Interactions

Drugs which affect platelet function (eg, aspirin, NSAIDs, dipyridamole, ticlopidine, clopidogrel) may potentiate the risk of hemorrhage.

Thrombolytic agents increase the risk of hemorrhage.

Warfarin: Risk of bleeding may be increased during concurrent therapy. Enoxaparin is commonly continued during the initiation of warfarin therapy to assure anticoagulation and to protect against possible transient hypercoagulability.

Pregnancy Risk Factor B

Pregnancy Implications There are no adequate and well-controlled studies using enoxaparin in pregnant women. Animal studies have not shown teratogenic or fetotoxic effects. Postmarketing reports include congenital abnormalities (cause and effect not established) and also fetal death when used in pregnant women. In addition, prosthetic valve thrombosis, including fatal cases, has been reported in pregnant women receiving enoxaparin as thromboprophylaxis. Multiple-dose vials contain benzyl alcohol; use caution in pregnant women.

Lactation Excretion in breast milk unknown/use caution

Additional Information ~$^1/_2$ the weight of heparin with 20% of the activity

Specific References

Argenti D, Hoppensteadt D, Heald D, et al, "Pharmacokinetics of Enoxaparin in Patients Undergoing Percutaneous Coronary Intervention with and without Glycoprotein IIb/IIIa Therapy," *Am J Ther*, 2003, 10(4):241-6.

Gosselin RC, King JH, Janatpour KA, et al, "Variability of Plasma Anti-Xa Activities with Different Lots of Enoxaparin," *Ann Pharmacother*, 2004, 38(4):563-8. Epub 2004 Feb 24.

Shapiro NI, Spear J, Sheehy S, et al, "Barriers to the Use of Outpatient Enoxaparin Therapy in Patients with Deep Venous Thrombosis," *Am J Emerg Med*, 2005, 23(1):30-4.

Ephedrine

Related Information

- Ephedra
- Therapeutic Drugs Associated with Hallucinations

CAS Number 134-72-5; 299-42-3; 50906-05-3

U.S. Brand Names Pretz-D® [OTC]

Synonyms Ephedrine Sulfate

Impairment Potential Yes

Use Bronchial asthma; nasal congestion; acute wheezing; acute hypotensive states

Mechanism of Action Releases tissue stores of epinephrine and thereby produces an alpha- and beta-adrenergic stimulation

Adverse Reactions

Cardiovascular: Hypertension, cardiomyopathy, cardiomegaly, sinus tachycardia

Central nervous system: **CNS-stimulating effects, nervousness, anxiety, fear,** psychosis, **tension, agitation, excitation, restlessness, irritability, insomnia,** auditory and visual hallucinations, vasculitis, mania, paranoia, psychosis, sympathetic storm, **apprehension, hyperactivity**

Endocrine & metabolic: Hypokalemia

Gastrointestinal: Nausea, anorexia

Neuromuscular & skeletal: Tremors, weakness

Signs and Symptoms of Overdose CNS depression, depression, dry skin, dysrhythmias, insomnia, mydriasis, respiratory alkalosis, respiratory depression, seizures, vomiting

Pharmacodynamics/Kinetics

Onset of action: Oral: Bronchodilation: 0.25-1 hour

Duration: Oral: 3-6 hours

Distribution: Crosses placenta; enters breast milk

Metabolism: Minimally hepatic

Half-life elimination: 2.5-3.6 hours

Excretion: Urine (60% to 77% as unchanged drug) within 24 hours

Dosage

Children:

Oral, SubQ: 3 mg/kg/day or 25-100 mg/m^2/day in 4-6 divided doses every 4-6 hours

I.M., slow I.V. push: 0.2-0.3 mg/kg/dose every 4-6 hours

Adults:

Oral: 25-50 mg every 3-4 hours as needed

I.M., SubQ: 25-50 mg, parenteral adult dose should not exceed 150 mg in 24 hours

I.V.: 5-25 mg/dose slow I.V. push repeated after 5-10 minutes as needed, then every 3-4 hours not to exceed 150 mg/24 hours

Nasal spray:

Children 6-12 years: 1-2 sprays into each nostril, not more frequently than every 4 hours

Children ≥12 years and Adults: 2-3 sprays into each nostril, not more frequently than every 4 hours

Stability Protect all dosage forms from light

Monitoring Parameters Blood pressure, pulse, urinary output, mental status; cardiac monitor and blood pressure monitor required

Contraindications Hypersensitivity to ephedrine or any component of the formulation; cardiac arrhythmias; angle-closure glaucoma; concurrent use of other sympathomimetic agents

Warnings Blood volume depletion should be corrected before ephedrine therapy is instituted; use caution in patients with unstable vasomotor symptoms, diabetes, hyperthyroidism, prostatic hyperplasia, or a history of seizures; also use caution in the elderly and those patients with cardiovascular disorders such as coronary artery disease, arrhythmias, and hypertension. Ephedrine may cause hypertension resulting in intracranial hemorrhage. Long-term use may cause anxiety and symptoms of paranoid schizophrenia. Avoid as a bronchodilator; generally not used as a bronchodilator since new beta$_2$ agents are less toxic. Use with caution in the elderly, since it crosses the blood-brain barrier and may cause confusion.

Dosage Forms

Capsule, as sulfate: 25 mg

Injection, solution, as sulfate: 50 mg/mL (1 mL, 10 mL)

Solution, intranasal spray, as sulfate (Pretz-D®): 0.25% (50 mL)

Reference Range Postmortem blood level of 11 mg/L associated with a fatal ephedrine overdose; therapeutic serum level: 0.04-0.08 mcg/mL

Overdosage/Treatment

Decontamination: Lavage (within 1 hour)/activated charcoal

Supportive therapy: There is no specific antidote for ephedrine intoxication and the bulk of the treatment is supportive. Hyperactivity and agitation usually respond to reduced sensory input, however with extreme agitation haloperidol (2-5 mg I.M. for adults) may be required. Hyperthermia is best treated with external cooling measures, or when severe or unresponsive, muscle paralysis with pancuronium may be needed. Hypertension is usually transient and generally does not require treatment unless severe. For diastolic blood pressures >110 mm Hg, a nitroprusside infusion should be initiated. Seizures usually respond to diazepam or lorazepam I.V. and/or phenytoin maintenance regimens.

Drug Interactions

Alpha- and beta-adrenergic-blocking agents decrease ephedrine vasopressor effects.

Cardiac glycosides or general anesthetics may increase cardiac stimulation.

MAO inhibitors or atropine may increase blood pressure

Sympathomimetic agents: Additive cardiostimulation with other sympathomimetic agents.

Theophylline may lead to cardiostimulation.

Pregnancy Risk Factor C

Pregnancy Implications Crosses the placenta; fetal tachycardia can occur

Lactation Enters breast milk/not recommended

Nursing Implications Protect from light; do not administer unless solution is clear

Additional Information Ephedrine is a precursor in the illicit manufacture of methamphetamine; ephedrine is extracted by dissolving ephedrine tablets in water or alcohol (50,000 tablets can result in 1 kg of ephedrine); conversion to methamphetamine occurs at a rate of 50% to 70% of the weight of ephedrine; ephedrine is synthesized by the reductive condensation of L-1-phenyl-1-acetylcarbinol with methylamine. See table.

Ephedrine products are marketed under a variety of packaging gimmicks and names. The following products are marketed as natural versions of illegal drugs:		
Cloud 9	Herbal Ecstasy	Ritual Spirit
Fat Burner	Herbal × GWM	Thermoslim
Herbal Bliss		

Truck stop ephedrine products include the following:		
357 Magnum	Heads Up	Mini-Thins
Efedrin	Max Alert	Thin-Edrine
GoPower	Maxephedrine	Turbo Tabs

Many products contain a form of ephedrine called ma huang, with ephedrine concentrations as much as 16 times higher than the naturally occurring levels.		
AM Trim and Firm	Herbal Fuel	Super Day Trim
Blasting Caps	Kickers Instant Energy Caplets	Summit Select
Chi Powder	Mega Ripped	Super Fat Burners
Cybergenics	New Zest	Smart Body
Dextrate	New Zest Plus	Thermo Diet
Diet Max	Now	Thermo Slim
Diet Max LiquidGels	Nura One	Thermogenics
Diet Now	Performance Energy	Thermojetics
Diet Pep	Power Trim	Thinline III
Ephedra 850	Pro Ripped	Trim Time Tea
Excell Energy	Ripped Fuel Tea	Ultra Diet Prep
Excell Ultra High Energy Performance	Quick Shot Energel	Up Your Gas
Formula One		

Specific References

Jackson GF and Dunn WA, "An Analysis of Drug Findings in Drug-Facilitated Sexual Assault Cases," *J Anal Toxicol*, 2003, 27(3):179.

Manno BR and Colon MA, "Ephedrine Toxicity and Psychiatric Consequences: Case Reports and Literature Review," *J Anal Toxicol*, 2004, 28:290-1.

Kaye AD, Hoover JM, Baber SR, et al, "Influence of Ephedrine and the Role of Alpha Subtype Adrenoreceptors in the Vascular Bed of the Cat Lung," *Am J Ther*, 2006, 13(1):12-7.

Palmer ME, Haller C, McKinney PE, et al, "Adverse Events Associated with Dietary Supplements: An Observational Study," *Lancet*, 2003, 361(9352):101-6.

Schier JG, Traub SJ, Hoffman RS, et al, "Ephedrine-Induced Cardiac Ischemia: Exposure Confirmed with a Serum Level," *J Toxicol Clin Toxicol*, 2003, 41(6):849-53.

Sharma AN and Olmedo R, "Ephedrine-Induced Tourette Syndrome," *J Toxicol Clin Toxicol*, 2003, 41(5):668.

Shekelle PG, Hardy ML, Morton SC, et al, "Efficacy and Safety of Ephedra and Ephedrine for Weight Loss and Athletic Performance: A Meta-Analysis," *JAMA*, 2003, 289(12):1537-45.

Tseng YL, Hsu HR, Kuo FH, et al, "Ephedrines in Over-the-Counter Cold Medicines and Urine Specimens Collected During Sport Competitions," *J Anal Toxicol*, 2003, 27(6):359-65.

Vasiliades J and Colonna K, "Determination of Ephedrine/Pseudoephedrine in Over-the-Counter Medications by Gas Chromatography," *J Anal Toxicol*, 2006, 30:128.

Wilson M, Friel P, Gordon AM, et al, "Driving Under the Influence of Ephedrine," *J Anal Toxicol*, 2004, 28:281-2.

Epoetin Alfa

Related Information

● Therapeutic Drugs Associated with Hallucinations

CAS Number 113427-24-0; 122312-54-3

U.S. Brand Names Epogen®; Procrit®

Synonyms rHuEPO-α; EPO; Erythropoietin; NSC-724223

Use

Treatment of anemia related to zidovudine therapy in HIV-infected patients; in patients when the endogenous erythropoietin level is ≤500 mU/mL and the dose of zidovudine is ≤4200 mg/week

Treatment of anemia associated with chronic renal failure (CRF) including dialysis (end-stage renal disease, ESRD) and nondialysis patients. Prior to therapy, serum ferritin should be >100 ng/dL and transferrin saturation (serum iron/iron binding capacity × 100) of 20% to 30%; nondialysis patients should have a hematocrit <30%

Treatment of anemia in cancer patients on chemotherapy; in patients with nonmyeloid malignancies where anemia is caused by the effect of the concomitantly administered chemotherapy; to decrease the need for transfusions in patients who will be receiving chemotherapy for a minimum of 2 months

Reduction of allogeneic blood transfusion in surgery patients (with hemoglobin >10 g/dL up to 13 g/dL) scheduled to undergo elective, noncardiac, nonvascular surgery

Unlabeled/Investigational Use Anemia associated with rheumatic disease; hypogenerative anemia of Rh hemolytic disease; sickle cell anemia; acute renal failure; Gaucher's disease; Castleman's disease; paroxysmal nocturnal hemoglobinuria; anemia of critical illness (limited documentation); anemia of prematurity

Mechanism of Action A glycosylated protein hormone which induces erythropoiesis by stimulating the division and differentiation of committed erythroid progenitor cells; induces the release of reticulocytes from the bone marrow into the bloodstream, where they mature to erythrocytes. There is a dose response relationship with this effect. This results in an increase in reticulocyte counts followed by a rise in hematocrit and hemoglobin levels. Studies in lab animals suggest that epoetin may have an effect on megakaryoblast development, and increased platelet counts have been noted in dialysis patients receiving epoetin.

Adverse Reactions

Cardiovascular: **Hypertension**, edema, chest pain, CVA/TIA, MI, thrombosis

Central nervous system: **Headache, fever**, fatigue, seizures

Dermatologic: Rash

Endocrine & metabolic: Hyperkalemia

Gastrointestinal: **Nausea**, vomiting, diarrhea

Neuromuscular & skeletal: **Arthralgia**, asthenia

Miscellaneous: Flu-like syndrome, hypersensitivity reactions

Signs and Symptoms of Overdose Coagulopathy, conjunctivitis, erythrocytosis, hallucinations, polycythemia

Pharmacodynamics/Kinetics

Onset of action: Several days

Peak effect: 2-3 weeks

Distribution: V_d: 9 L; rapid in the plasma compartment; concentrated in liver, kidneys, and bone marrow

Metabolism: Some degradation does occur

Bioavailability: SubQ: ~21% to 31%; intraperitoneal epoetin: 3% (a few patients)

Half-life elimination: Cancer: SubQ: 16-67 hours; Chronic renal failure: 4-13 hours

Time to peak, serum: Chronic renal failure: 5-13 hours

Excretion: Feces (majority); urine (small amounts, 10% unchanged in normal volunteers)

Dosage Chronic renal failure patients: I.V., SubQ:

Children: Initial dose: 50 units/kg 3 times/week

Adults: Initial dose: 50-100 units/kg 3 times/week

Reduce dose when

1) hematocrit approaches 36% **or**

2) when hematocrit increases >4 points in any 2-week period

Increase dose if hematocrit does not increase by 5-6 points after 8 weeks of therapy and hematocrit is below suggested target range

Suggested target hematocrit range: 30% to 36%

Maintenance dose: Individualize to target range

Dialysis patients: Median dose:

Children: 167 units/kg/week **or** 76 units/kg 2-3 times/week

Adults: 75 units/kg 3 times/week

Nondialysis patients:

Children: Dosing range: 50-250 units/kg 1-3 times/week

Adults: Median dose: 75-150 units/kg

Zidovudine-treated, HIV-infected patients (patients with erythropoietin levels >500 mU/mL are unlikely to respond): I.V., SubQ:

Children: Initial dose: Reported dosing range: 50-400 units/kg 2-3 times/week

Adults: 100 units/kg 3 times/week for 8 weeks

Increase dose by 50-100 units/kg 3 times/week if response is not satisfactory in terms of reducing transfusion requirements or increasing hematocrit after 8 weeks of therapy

Evaluate response every 4-8 weeks thereafter and adjust the dose accordingly by 50-100 units/kg increments 3 times/week

If patients have not responded satisfactorily to a 300 unit/kg dose 3 times/week, it is unlikely that they will respond to higher doses

Stop dose if hematocrit exceeds 40% and resume treatment at a 25% dose reduction when hematocrit drops to 36%

Cancer patients on chemotherapy: Treatment of patients with erythropoietin levels >200 mU/mL is **not recommended**

Children: I.V.: 600 units/kg once weekly (maximum: 40,000 units)

Adults: SubQ: Initial dose: 150 units/kg 3 times/week or 40,000 units once weekly; commonly used doses range from 10,000 units 3 times/week to 40,000-60,000 units once weekly.

Dose adjustment: If response is not satisfactory in terms of reducing transfusion requirement or increasing hematocrit after 8 weeks of therapy, the dose may be increased up to 300 units/kg 3 times/week.

If patients do not respond, it is unlikely that they will respond to higher doses.

If hematocrit exceeds 40%, hold the dose until it falls to 36% and reduce the dose by 25% when treatment is resumed.

Surgery patients: Prior to initiating treatment, obtain a hemoglobin to establish that is >10 mg/dL or ≤13 mg/dL: Adults: SubQ: Initial dose: 300 units/kg/day for 10 days before surgery, on the day of surgery, and for 4 days after surgery

Alternative dose: 600 units/kg in once weekly doses (21, 14, and 7 days before surgery) plus a fourth dose on the day of surgery

Anemia of critical illness (unlabeled use): Adults: SubQ: 40,000 units once weekly

Anemia of prematurity (unlabeled use): Infants: I.V., SubQ: Dosing range: 500-1250 units/kg/week; commonly used dose: 250 units/kg 3 times/week; supplement with oral iron therapy 3-8 mg/kg/day

Dosage adjustment in renal impairment:

Dialysis patient: Usually administered as I.V. bolus 3 times/week. While administration is independent of the dialysis procedure, it may be administered into the venous line at the end of the dialysis procedure to obviate the need for additional venous access.

Chronic renal failure patients not on dialysis: May be given either as an I.V. or SubQ injection.

Hemodialysis: Supplemental dose is not necessary.

Peritoneal dialysis: Supplemental dose is not necessary.

Monitoring Parameters Blood pressure; hematocrit/hemoglobin, CBC with differential and platelets, transferring saturation and ferritin

Suggested tests to be monitored and their frequency: See table.

Test	Initial Phase Frequency	Maintenance Phase Frequency
Hematocrit/hemoglobin	2 ×/week	2-4 ×/month
Blood pressure	3 ×/week	3 ×/week
Serum ferritin	Monthly	Quarterly
Transferrin saturation	Monthly	Quarterly
Serum chemistries including CBC with differential, creatinine, blood urea nitrogen, potassium, phosphorous	Regularly per routine	Regularly per routine

Hematocrit should be determined twice weekly until stabilization within the target range (30% to 36%), and twice weekly for at least 2-6 weeks after a dose increase.

Administration Patients with CRF on dialysis: May be administered I.V. bolus into the venous line after dialysis.

Patients with CRF not on dialysis: May be administered I.V. or SubQ

Contraindications Hypersensitivity to erythropoietin, albumin (human) or mammalian cell-derived products, or any component of the formulation; uncontrolled hypertension

Warnings

Use caution with history of seizures or hypertension; blood pressure should be controlled prior to start of therapy and monitored closely throughout treatment. Excessive rate of rise of hematocrit may be possibly associated with the exacerbation of hypertension or seizures; decrease the epoetin dose if the hemoglobin increase exceeds 1 g/dL in any 2-week period. Use caution in patients at risk for thrombosis or with history of cardiovascular disease. Increased mortality has been observed when aggressive dosing is used in CHF or anginal patients undergoing hemodialysis. Multidose vials contain benzyl alcohol; do not use in premature infants.

Pure red cell aplasia (PRCA) with neutralizing antibodies to erythropoietin has been reported in patients treated with recombinant products; may occur more in patients with CRF. Patients should be evaluated for any loss of effect to therapy and treatment discontinued with evidence of PRCA. Response to therapy may be limited by multiple factors; refer to Additional Information for details.

Prior to and during therapy, iron stores must be evaluated; iron supplementation should be given during therapy. Use caution with porphyria, exacerbation of porphyria has been reported in patients with chronic renal failure. Not recommended for acute correction of severe anemia or as a substitute for transfusion. Safety and efficacy in children <1 month of age have not been established.

Dosage Forms Injection, solution [preservative free]: 2000 units/mL (1 mL); 3000 units/mL (1 mL); 4000 units/mL (1 mL); 10,000 units/mL (1 mL); 40,000 units/mL (1 mL) [contains human albumin]

Injection, solution [with preservative]: 10,000 units/mL (2 mL); 20,000 units/mL (1 mL) [contains human albumin and benzyl alcohol]

Reference Range

Guidelines should be based on the following figure or published literature

Guidelines for estimating appropriateness of endogenous EPO levels for varying levels of anemia via the EIA assay method: See figure. The reference range for erythropoietin in serum, for subjects with normal hemoglobin and hematocrit, is 4.1-22.2 mU/mL by the EIA method. Erythropoietin levels are typically inversely related to hemoglobin (and hematocrit) levels in anemias not attributed to impaired erythropoietin production.

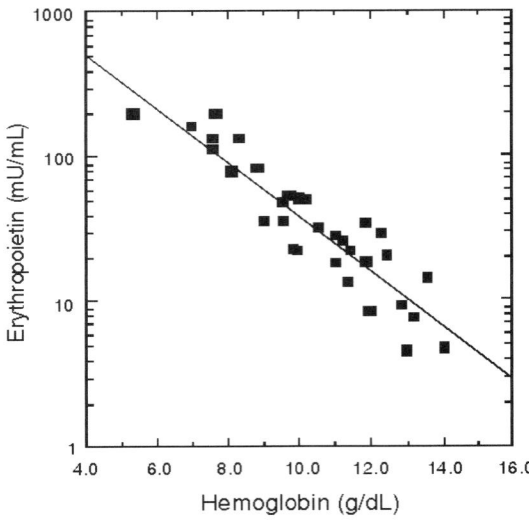

Zidovudine-treated HIV patients: Available evidence indicates patients with endogenous serum erythropoietin levels >500 mU/mL are unlikely to respond

Cancer chemotherapy patients: Treatment of patients with endogenous serum erythropoietin levels >200 mU/mL is not recommended

Overdosage/Treatment Supportive therapy: Adequate airway and other supportive measures and agents for treating anaphylaxis should be present when I.V. drug is given; venesection can successfully reduce blood pressure if hypertension does **not** respond to antihypertensive agents in the setting of erythropoietin overdosage

Pregnancy Risk Factor C

Pregnancy Implications Epoetin alfa has been shown to have adverse effects in animal studies. Studies suggest that rHuEPO-α does not cross the human placenta. Based on case reports, treatment with rHuEPO-α may be an option in pregnant women with ESRD on dialysis. Amenorrheic premenopausal women should be cautioned that menstruation may resume following treatment with rHuEPO-α and contraception should be considered if pregnancy is to be avoided.

Lactation Excretion in breast milk unknown/use caution

Additional Information

May require supplemental iron to keep ferritin levels >100 ng/dL; frequently used by athletes for "blood doping"; response to erythropoietin of metastatic renal cell carcinoma has been reported; high ratio of soluble transferrin to ferritin may be indicative of exogenous erythropoietin use

Due to the delayed onset of erythropoiesis (7-10 days to ↑ reticulocyte count; 2-6 weeks to ↑ hemoglobin), erythropoietin is of no value in the acute treatment of anemia. Emergency/stat orders for erythropoietin are inappropriate.

Professional Services:

Amgen (Epogen®): 1-800-772-6436

Ortho Biotech (Procrit®): 1-800-325-7504

Reimbursement Assistance:

Amgen: 1-800-272-9376

Ortho Biotech: 1-800-553-3851

Factors Limiting Response to Epoetin Alfa

Factor	Mechanism
Iron deficiency	Limits hemoglobin synthesis
Blood loss/hemolysis	Counteracts epoetin alfa-stimulated erythropoiesis
Infection/inflammation	Inhibits iron transfer from storage to bone marrow
	Suppresses erythropoiesis through activated macrophages
Aluminum overload	Inhibits iron incorporation into heme protein
Bone marrow replacement Hyperparathyroidism Metastatic, neoplastic	Limits bone marrow volume
Folic acid/vitamin B$_{12}$ deficiency	Limits hemoglobin synthesis
Patient compliance	Self-administered epoetin alfa or iron therapy

Specific References

Czogala J and Goniewicz ML, "The Complex Analytical Method for Assessment of Passive Smokers' Exposure to Carbon Monoxide," *J Anal Toxicol*, 2005, 29(8):830-4.

Juul SE and Christensen RD, "Absorption of Enteral Recombinant Human Erythropoietin by Neonates," *Ann Pharmacother*, 2003, 37(6):782-6.

Pajoumand M, Erstad BL, and Camamo JM, "Use of Epoetin Alfa in Critically Ill Patients," *Ann Pharmacother*, 2004, 38(4):641-8. Epub 2004 Feb 13.

Varlet-Marie E, Gaudard A, Audran M, et al, "Pharmacokinetics/Pharmacodynamics of Recombinant Human Erythropoietins in Doping Control," *Sports Med*, 2003, 33(4):301-15.

Eptifibatide

U.S. Brand Names Integrilin®

Synonyms Intrifiban

Use Treatment of patients with acute coronary syndrome (UA/NQMI), including patients who are to be managed medically and those undergoing percutaneous coronary intervention (PCI including PTCA; intracoronary stenting)

Mechanism of Action Eptifibatide is a synthetic cyclic heptapeptide which blocks the platelet glycoprotein IIb/IIIa receptor, the binding site for fibrinogen, von Willebrand factor, and other ligands. Inhibition of binding at this final common receptor reversibly blocks platelet aggregation and prevents thrombosis.

Adverse Reactions

Bleeding is the major drug-related adverse effect. Major bleeding was reported in 4.4% to 10.5%, minor bleeding was reported in 10.5% to 14.2%, requirement for transfusion was reported in 5.5% to 12.8%.

Cardiovascular: Hypotension

Central nervous system: Intracranial hemorrhage

Hematologic: Acute profound thrombocytopenia, fatal bleeding events

Local: Injection site reaction

Neuromuscular & skeletal: Back pain

Miscellaneous: Anaphylaxis

Pharmacodynamics/Kinetics

Onset of action: Within 1 hour

Duration: Platelet function restored ~4 hours following discontinuation

Protein binding: ~25%

Half-life elimination: 2.5 hours

Excretion: Primarily urine (as eptifibatide and metabolites); significant renal impairment may alter disposition of this compound

Clearance: Total body: 55-58 mL/kg/hour; Renal: ~50% of total in healthy subjects

Dosage

I.V.: Adults:

Acute coronary syndrome: Bolus of 180 mcg/kg (maximum: 22.6 mg) over 1-2 minutes, begun as soon as possible following diagnosis, followed by a continuous infusion of 2 mcg/kg/minute (maximum: 15 mg/hour) until hospital discharge or initiation of CABG surgery, up to 72 hours. Concurrent aspirin (160-325 mg initially and daily thereafter) and heparin therapy (target aPTT 50-70 seconds) are recommended.

Percutaneous coronary intervention (PCI) with or without stenting: Bolus of 180 mcg/kg (maximum: 22.6 mg) administered immediately before the initiation of PCI, followed by a continuous infusion of 2 mcg/kg/minute (maximum: 15 mg/hour). A second 180 mcg/kg bolus (maximum: 22.6 mg) should be administered 10 minutes after the first bolus. Infusion should be continued until hospital discharge or for up to 18-24 hours, whichever comes first; minimum of 12 hours of infusion is recommended. Concurrent aspirin (160-325 mg 1-24 hours before PCI and daily thereafter) and heparin therapy (ACT 200-300 seconds during PCI) are recommended. Heparin infusion after PCI is discouraged. In patients who undergo coronary artery bypass graft surgery, discontinue infusion prior to surgery.

Dosing adjustment in renal impairment: Dialysis is a contraindication to use.

Acute coronary syndrome: Cl$_{cr}$ <50 mL/minute or S$_{cr}$ >2 mg/dL: Use 180 mcg/kg bolus (maximum: 22.6 mg) and 1 mcg/kg/minute infusion (maximum: 7.5 mg/hour)

Percutaneous coronary intervention (PCI) with or without stenting: Cl$_{cr}$ <50 mL/minute or S$_{cr}$ >2 mg/dL: Use 180 mcg/kg bolus (maximum: 22.6 mg) administered immediately before the initiation of PCI and followed by a continuous infusion of 1 mcg/kg/minute (maximum: 7.5 mg/hour). A second 180 mcg/kg (maximum: 22.6 mg) bolus should be administered 10 minutes after the first bolus.

Stability Vials should be stored refrigerated at 2°C to 8°C (36°F to 46°F). Protect from light until administration. Do not use beyond the expiration date. Discard any unused portion left in the vial.

Monitoring Parameters Coagulation parameters, signs/symptoms of excessive bleeding. Laboratory tests at baseline and monitoring during therapy: hematocrit and hemoglobin, platelet count, serum creatinine, PT/

aPTT (maintain aPTT between 50-70 seconds unless PCI is to be performed), and ACT with PCI (maintain ACT between 200-300 seconds during PCI).

Administration Visually inspect for discoloration or particulate matter prior to administration

The bolus dose should be withdrawn from the 10 mL vial into a syringe and administered by I.V. push over 1-2 minutes

Begin continuous infusion immediately following bolus administration, administered directly from the 100 mL vial

The 100 mL vial should be spiked with a vented infusion set

Contraindications Hypersensitivity to eptifibatide or any component of the product; active abnormal bleeding or a history of bleeding diathesis within the previous 30 days; history of CVA within 30 days or a history of hemorrhagic stroke; severe hypertension (systolic blood pressure >200 mm Hg or diastolic blood pressure >110 mm Hg) not adequately controlled on antihypertensive therapy; major surgery within the preceding 6 weeks; current or planned administration of another parenteral GP IIb/IIIa inhibitor; thrombocytopenia; dependency on renal dialysis

Warnings Bleeding is the most common complication. Most major bleeding occurs at the arterial access site where the cardiac catheterization was done. When bleeding can not be controlled with pressure, discontinue infusion and heparin. Use caution in patients with hemorrhagic retinopathy or with other drugs that affect hemostasis. Concurrent use with thrombolytics has not been established as safe. Minimize other procedures including arterial and venous punctures, I.M. injections, nasogastric tubes, etc. Sheath should not be removed unless the aPTT <45 sec or the ACT <150 sec. Use caution in renal dysfunction (estimated Cl$_{cr}$ <50 mL/minute); dosage adjustment required. Safety and efficacy in pediatric patients have not been determined.

Dosage Forms Injection, solution: 0.75 mg/mL (100 mL); 2 mg/mL (10 mL, 100 mL)

Overdosage/Treatment Supportive therapy: Essentially no overdose experience; anaphylaxis may be treated with standard treatment; discontinue heparin; use pressure techniques if bleeding develops; consider platelet transfusion for patients with serious, uncontrolled bleeding and if bleeding time is >10 minutes

Drug Interactions

Cephalosporins which contain the MTT side chain may theoretically increase the risk of hemorrhage.

Drotrecogin alfa: Antiplatelet agents (eg, eptifibatide) may enhance the adverse/toxic effect of drotrecogin alfa; bleeding may occur.

Drugs which affect platelet function (eg, aspirin, NSAIDs, dipyridamole, ticlopidine, clopidogrel) may potentiate the risk of hemorrhage; use with caution.

Heparin and aspirin: Use with aspirin and heparin may increase bleeding over aspirin and heparin alone. However, aspirin and heparin were used concurrently in the majority of patients in the major clinical studies of eptifibatide.

Thrombolytic agents theoretically may increase the risk of hemorrhage; use with caution.

Warfarin and oral anticoagulants: Risk of bleeding may be increased during concurrent therapy.

Other IIb/IIIa antagonists: Avoid concomitant use of other glycoprotein IIb/IIIa antagonists (see Contraindications).

Pregnancy Risk Factor B

Pregnancy Implications Teratogenic effects were not observed in animal studies

Lactation Excretion in breast milk unknown/use caution

Nursing Implications

Do not shake the vial; maintain bleeding precautions, avoid unnecessary arterial and venous punctures, use saline or heparin lock for blood drawing, assess sheath insertion site and distal pulses of affected leg every 15 minutes for the first hour and then every 1 hour for the next 6 hours. Arterial access site care is important to prevent bleeding. Care should be taken when attempting vascular access that only the anterior wall of the femoral artery is punctured, avoiding a Seldinger (through and through) technique for obtaining sheath access. Femoral vein sheath placement should be avoided unless needed. While the vascular sheath is in place, patients should be maintained on complete bedrest with the head of the bed at a 30° angle and the affected limb restrained in a straight position.

Observe patient for mental status changes, hemorrhage, assess nose and mouth mucous membranes, puncture sites for oozing, ecchymosis and hematoma formation, and examine urine, stool and emesis for presence of occult or frank blood; gentle care should be provided when removing dressings.

Ergotamine

CAS Number 379-79-3
U.S. Brand Names Ergomar®
Synonyms Ergotamine Tartrate
Use Abort or prevent vascular headaches, such as migraine, migraine variants, or so-called "histaminic cephalalgia"

Mechanism of Action Ergot alkaloid alpha-adrenergic blocker directly stimulates vascular smooth muscle to vasoconstrict peripheral and cerebral vessels; may also have antagonist effects on serotonin

Adverse Reactions

Cardiovascular: Absence of pulse, bradycardia, cardiac valvular fibrosis, cyanosis, edema, ECG changes, hypertension, ischemia, precordial distress and pain, tachycardia, vasospasm

Central nervous system: Vertigo

Dermatologic: Gangrene, itching

Gastrointestinal: Anal or rectal ulcer (with overuse of suppository), nausea, vomiting

Genitourinary: Retroperitoneal fibrosis

Neuromuscular & skeletal: Muscle pain, numbness, paresthesias, weakness

Respiratory: Pleuropulmonary fibrosis

Miscellaneous: Cold extremities

Signs and Symptoms of Overdose Asthenia, bradycardia, chest pain, colitis, drowsiness, hypertension, hypotension, impaired mental function, myalgia, nausea, nystagmus, seizures, shock and death, unconsciousness, vasospastic effects, vision color changes (red tinge), vomiting

Pharmacodynamics/Kinetics

Absorption: Oral: Erratic; enhanced by caffeine coadministration

Metabolism: Extensively hepatic

Time to peak, serum: 0.5-3 hours

Half-life elimination: 2 hours

Excretion: Feces (90% as metabolites)

Dosage

Oral (Cafergot®, Wigraine®): 2 tablets at onset of attack; then 1 tablet every 30 minutes as needed; maximum: 6 tablets per attack; do not exceed 10 tablets/week.

Sublingual (Ergomar®): 1 tablet under tongue at first sign, then 1 tablet every 30 minutes if needed; maximum dose: 3 tablets/24 hours, 5 tablets/week

Rectal (Cafergot®): 1 suppository rectally at first sign of an attack; follow with second dose after 1 hour, if needed; maximum: 2 per attack; do not exceed 5/week.

Administration

Do not crush sublingual tablets.

Contraindications Hypersensitivity to ergotamine or any component of the formulation; peripheral vascular disease; hepatic or renal disease; coronary artery disease; hypertension; sepsis; ergot alkaloids are contraindicated with strong inhibitors of CYP3A4 (includes protease inhibitors, azole antifungals, and some macrolide antibiotics); pregnancy

Warnings

Avoid prolonged administration or excessive dosage because of the danger of ergotism (intense vasoconstriction), gangrene, cardiac valvular fibrosis, retroperitoneal and/or pleuropulmonary fibrosis. Patients who take ergotamine for extended periods of time may experience withdrawal symptoms and rebound headache when ergotamine is discontinued. May be harmful due to reduction in cerebral blood flow; may precipitate angina, myocardial infarction, or aggravate intermittent claudication; therefore, not considered a drug of choice in the elderly.

[U.S. Boxed Warning]: Concomitant use with medications considered to be "strong" CYP3A4 inhibitors has been associated with acute ergot toxicity; use caution with inhibitors of CYP3A4 enzymes.

Dosage Forms Tablet, sublingual: Ergotamine tartrate 2 mg

Reference Range Serum levels >1.8 ng/mL are toxic

Overdosage/Treatment

Decontamination: Gastric lavage within 1 hour or induction of emesis within 30 minutes, activated charcoal; keep extremities warm; consider gastric decontamination for ingestions >1 mg/kg

Supportive therapy: Treatment is symptomatic with captopril, nifedipine, prazosin, vasodilators (nitroprusside) or nitroglycerin for hypertension. Intra-arterial bolus of phentolamine (5-25 mg) or tolazoline (25-100 mg) followed by infusions are effective for arterial vasodilitation. Aspirin (325 mg) should be used for antiplatelet effect. Prostaglandins (alprostadil at doses of 1-20 ng/kg/minute or epoprostenol at 20 ng/kg/minute) are also effective treatment. Diazepam can be utilized for seizures. Heparin can be used for hypercoagulable state; titrate to a PTT of 70-90 seconds. Hyperbaric oxygen can be used to treat peripheral ischemia. Cyproheptadine (4 mg 3 times/day orally) can be used to reverse ergot-induced vasoconstriction.

Enhancement of elimination: Multiple dosing of activated charcoal may be effective.

Drug Interactions

Substrate of CYP3A4 (major); **Inhibits** CYP3A4 (weak)

Antifungals, azole derivatives (itraconazole, ketoconazole) increase levels of ergot alkaloids by inhibiting CYP3A4 metabolism, resulting in toxicity; concomitant use is contraindicated.

Antipsychotics: May diminish the effects of ergotamine (due to dopamine antagonism); these combinations should generally be avoided.

Beta blockers: Severe peripheral vasoconstriction has been reported with concomitant use of beta blockers and ergot derivatives; monitor.

CYP3A4 inhibitors: May increase the levels/effects of ergotamine. Example inhibitors include azole antifungals, clarithromycin, diclofenac, doxycycline, erythromycin, imatinib, isoniazid, nefazodone, nicardipine, propofol, protease inhibitors, quinidine, telithromycin, and verapamil. Ergot alkaloids are contraindicated with potent CYP3A4 inhibitors.

Macrolide antibiotics: Erythromycin, clarithromycin, and troleandomycin may increase levels of ergot alkaloids by inhibiting CYP3A4 metabolism, resulting in toxicity (ischemia, vasospasm); concomitant use is contraindicated.

MAO inhibitors: The serotonergic effects of ergot derivatives may be increased by MAO inhibitors. Monitor for signs and symptoms of serotonin syndrome.

Metoclopramide: May diminish the effects of ergotamine (due to dopamine antagonism); concurrent therapy should generally be avoided.

Protease inhibitors (ritonavir, amprenavir, atazanavir, indinavir, nelfinavir, and saquinavir) increase blood levels of ergot alkaloids by inhibiting CYP3A4 metabolism, acute ergot toxicity has been reported; concomitant use is contraindicated.

Sibutramine: May cause serotonin syndrome; concurrent use with ergot alkaloids is contraindicated.

Serotonin agonists: Concurrent use with ergotamine may increase the risk of serotonin syndrome (includes buspirone, SSRIs, TCAs, nefazodone, sumatriptan, and trazodone).

Sumatriptan and other serotonin 5-HT$_1$ receptor agonists: Prolong vasospastic reactions; do not use sumatriptan or ergot-containing drugs within 24 hours of each other.

Vasoconstrictors: Concomitant use of some ergot derivatives and peripheral vasoconstrictors may cause synergistic elevation of blood pressure; use is contraindicated.

Pregnancy Risk Factor X

Pregnancy Implications May cause prolonged constriction of the uterine vessels and/or increased myometrial tone leading to reduced placental blood flow. This has contributed to fetal growth retardation in animals. Ergotamine also has oxytocic effects.

Lactation Enters breast milk/not recommended

Nursing Implications Do not crush sublingual drug product

Erythromycin

Related Information
- Clarithromycin

CAS Number 114-07-8; 134-36-1; 23067-13-2; 304-63-2; 3521-62-8; 3847-29-8; 41342-53-4; 643-22-1; 96128-89-1

U.S. Brand Names A/T/S®; Akne-Mycin®; E.E.S.®; Emgel®; Ery-Tab®; Erycette®; Eryc®; Eryderm®; Erygel®; EryPed®; Erythra-Derm™; Erythrocin®; PCE®; Romycin®; Staticin®; T-Stat®; Theramycin Z®

Synonyms Erythromycin Base; Erythromycin Estolate; Erythromycin Ethylsuccinate; Erythromycin Gluceptate; Erythromycin Lactobionate; Erythromycin Stearate

Use
Systemic: Treatment of susceptible bacterial infections including *S. pyogenes*, some *S. pneumoniae*, some *S. aureus*, *M. pneumoniae*, *Legionella pneumophila*, diphtheria, pertussis, chancroid, *Chlamydia*, erythrasma, *N. gonorrhoeae*, *E. histolytica*, syphilis and nongonococcal urethritis, and *Campylobacter* gastroenteritis; used in conjunction with neomycin for decontaminating the bowel

Ophthalmic: Treatment of superficial eye infections involving the conjunctiva or cornea; neonatal ophthalmia

Topical: Treatment of acne vulgaris

Unlabeled/Investigational Use Systemic: Treatment of gastroparesis

Mechanism of Action Inhibits RNA-dependent protein synthesis at the chain elongation step; binds to the 50S ribosomal subunit resulting in blockage of transpeptidation

Adverse Reactions
Cardiovascular: Ventricular arrhythmias, QT$_c$ prolongation, torsade de pointes (rare), ventricular tachycardia (rare)

Central nervous system: Headache, pain, fever, seizures

Dermatitis: Rash, erythema, desquamation, dryness, pruritus

Gastrointestinal: Abdominal pain, cramping, nausea, oral candidiasis, vomiting, diarrhea, dyspepsia, flatulence, anorexia, pseudomembranous colitis, hypertrophic pyloric stenosis (including cases in infants or IHPS), pancreatitis

Hematologic: Eosinophilia

Hepatic: Cholestatic jaundice (most common with estolate), elevated liver function tests

Local: Phlebitis at the injection site, thrombophlebitis

Neuromuscular & skeletal: Weakness

Respiratory: Dyspnea, cough

Miscellaneous: Hypersensitivity reactions, allergic reactions

Admission Criteria/Prognosis Admit ingestions >5 g

Pharmacodynamics/Kinetics
Absorption: Oral: Variable but better with salt forms than with base form; 18% to 45%; ethylsuccinate may be better absorbed with food

Distribution: Crosses placenta; enters breast milk

Relative diffusion from blood into CSF: Minimal even with inflammation

CSF: blood level ratio: Normal meninges: 1% to 12%; Inflamed meninges: 7% to 25%

Protein binding: 75% to 90%

Metabolism: Hepatic via demethylation

Half-life elimination: Peak: 1.5-2 hours; End-stage renal disease: 5-6 hours

Time to peak, serum: Base: 4 hours; Ethylsuccinate: 0.5-2.5 hours; delayed with food due to differences in absorption

Excretion: Primarily feces; urine (2% to 15% as unchanged drug)

Dosage Neonates: Ophthalmic: Prophylaxis of neonatal gonococcal or chlamydial conjunctivitis: 0.5-1 cm ribbon of ointment should be instilled into each conjunctival sac

Infants and Children:

Usual dosage range:

Oral: (**Note:** Due to differences in absorption, 400 mg erythromycin ethylsuccinate produces the same serum levels as 250 mg erythromycin base, sterate or estolate)

Base: 30-50 mg/kg/day in 2-4 divided doses; do not exceed 2 g/day

Estolate: 30-50 mg/kg/day in 2-4 divided doses; do not exceed 2 g/day

Ethylsuccinate: 30-50 mg/kg/day in 2-4 divided doses; do not exceed 3.2 g/day

Stearate: 30-50 mg/kg/day in 2-4 divided doses; do not exceed 2 g/day

I.V.: Lactobionate: 15-50 mg/kg/day divided every 6 hours, not to exceed 4 g/day

Indication-specific dosing: Oral:

Acne vulgaris (unlabeled use): Adolescents: 250-1500 mg/day in 2 divided doses; therapy may be continued for 4-6 weeks at lowest possible dose

Pharyngitis: 40 mg/kg/day in 2 doses; maximum: 1600 mg/day; short-course therapy for 5 days may be considered

Pertussis (CDC guidelines): 40-50 mg/kg/day in 4 divided doses for 14 days; maximum 2 g/day (not preferred agent for infants <1 month)

Preop bowel preparation: 20 mg/kg erythromycin base at 1, 2, and 11 PM on the day before surgery combined with mechanical cleansing of the large intestine and oral neomycin

Children and Adults:

Ophthalmic: Instill $^1/_2$" (1.25 cm) 2-6 times/day depending on the severity of the infection

Topical: Apply over the affected area twice daily after the skin has been thoroughly washed and patted dry

Adults:

Usual dosage range:

Oral:

Base: 250-500 mg every 6-12 hours

Ethylsuccinate: 400-800 mg every 6-12 hours

I.V. (lactobionate): 15-20 mg/kg/day divided every 6 hours or 500 mg to 1 g every 6 hours, or given as a continuous infusion over 24 hours (maximum: 4 g/24 hours)

Indication-specific dosing:

Cervicitis: Oral: 500 mg 4 times/day for 7 days

Chancroid (unlabeled use; not a preferred agent): Oral: 500 mg 4 times/day for 7 days

Community-acquired pneumonia, bronchitis: Oral, I.V.: 500-1000 mg 4 times/day for 10-14 days. If *Legionella* is suspected/confirmed, 750-1000 mg 4 times/day for 21 days or more may be recommended. **Note:** Other macrolides and/or fluoroquinolones may be preferred and better tolerated.

Lymphogranuloma venereum: Oral: 500 mg 4 times/day for 21 days

Nongonococcal urethritis (recurrent): Oral: CDC Guidelines for the Treatment of Sexually Transmitted Diseases recommendation: Metronidazole (2 g as a single dose) plus 7 days of erythromycin base (500 mg 4 times/day) or erythromycin ethylsuccinate (800 mg 4 times/day)

Pertussis (CDC guidelines): 500 mg every 6 hours for 14 days

Preop bowel preparation (unlabeled use): Oral: 1 g erythromycin base at 1, 2, and 11 PM on the day before surgery combined with mechanical cleansing of the large intestine and oral neomycin

Gastrointestinal prokinetic (unlabeled use): Oral: Erythromycin has been used as a prokinetic agent to improve gastric emptying time and intestinal motility. In adults, 200 mg was infused I.V. initially followed by 250 mg orally 3 times/day 30 minutes before meals. Lower dosages have been used in some trials.

Dosage adjustment in renal impairment: Dialysis: Slightly dialyzable (5% to 20%); no supplemental dosage necessary in hemo- or peritoneal dialysis or in continuous arteriovenous or venovenous hemofiltration

Stability Erythromycin lactobionate should be reconstituted with sterile water for injection without preservatives to avoid gel formation; the reconstituted solution is stable for 2 weeks when refrigerated or 24 hours at room temperature. Erythromycin I.V. infusion solution is stable at pH 6-8. Do not use D$_5$W as a diluent unless sodium bicarbonate is added to solution.

Monitoring Parameters Liver function tests

Administration Oral: Do not crush enteric coated drug product. GI upset, including diarrhea, is common. May be administered with food to decrease GI upset. Do not give with milk or acidic beverages.

I.V.: Infuse 1 g over 20-60 minutes. I.V. infusion may be very irritating to the vein. If phlebitis/pain occurs with used dilution, consider diluting further (eg, 1:5) if fluid status of the patient will tolerate, or consider administering in larger available vein. The addition of lidocaine or bicarbonate does not decrease the irritation of erythromycin infusions.

Ophthalmic: Avoid contact of tip of ophthalmic ointment tube with affected eye

Contraindications Hypersensitivity to erythromycin or any component of the formulation

Systemic: Pre-existing liver disease (erythromycin estolate); concomitant use with ergot derivatives, pimozide, or cisapride

Warnings Systemic: Use caution with hepatic impairment with or without jaundice has occurred, it may be accompanied by malaise, nausea, vomiting, abdominal colic, and fever; discontinue use if these occur; avoid using erythromycin lactobionate in neonates since formulations may contain benzyl alcohol which is associated with toxicity in neonates; observe for superinfections. Use in infants has been associated with infantile hypertrophic pyloric stenosis (IHPS). Macrolides have been associated with rare QT prolongation and ventricular arrhythmias, including torsade de pointes. Elderly may be at increased risk of adverse events, including hearing loss and/or torsade de pointes when dosage ≥ 4 g/day, particularly if concurrent renal/hepatic impairment.

Dosage Forms

[DSC] = Discontinued product; [CAN] = Canadian brand name

Capsule, delayed release, enteric-coated pellets, as base (Eryc®): 250 mg

Gel, topical: 2% (30 g, 60 g)

A/T/S®: 2% (30 g) [contains alcohol 92%]

Erygel®: 2% (30 g, 60 g) [contains alcohol 92%]

Granules for oral suspension, as ethylsuccinate (E.E.S.®): 200 mg/5 mL (100 mL, 200 mL) [cherry flavor]

Injection, powder for reconstitution, as lactobionate (Erythrocin®): 500 mg, 1 g

Ointment, ophthalmic: 0.5% [5 mg/g] (1 g, 3.5 g)

Romycin®: 0.5% [5 mg/g] (3.5 g)

Ointment, topical (Akne-Mycin®): 2% (25 g)

Powder for oral suspension, as ethylsuccinate (EryPed®): 200 mg/5 mL (100 mL, 200 mL) [fruit flavor]; 400 mg/5 mL (100 mL, 200 mL) [banana flavor]

Powder for oral suspension, as ethylsuccinate [drops] (EryPed®): 100 mg/2.5 mL (50 mL) [fruit flavor]

Solution, topical: 2% (60 mL)

A/T/S®: 2% (60 mL) [contains alcohol 66%]

Eryderm®, T-Stat® [DSC], Theramycin Z®: 2% (60 mL) [contain alcohol]

Sans Acne® [CAN]: 2% (60 mL) [contains ethyl alcohol 44%; not available in U.S.]

Staticin®: 1.5% (60 mL) [DSC]

Suspension, oral, as estolate: 125 mg/5 mL (480 mL); 250 mg/5 mL (480 mL)

Suspension, oral, as ethylsuccinate: 200 mg/5 mL (480 mL); 400 mg/5 mL (480 mL)

E.E.S.®: 200 mg/5 mL (100 mL, 480 mL) [fruit flavor]; 400 mg/5 mL (100 mL, 480 mL) [orange flavor]

Swab (T-Stat® [DSC]): 2% (60s)

Tablet, chewable, as ethylsuccinate (EryPed®): 200 mg [fruit flavor] [DSC]

Tablet, delayed release, enteric coated, as base (Ery-Tab®): 250 mg, 333 mg, 500 mg

Tablet, as base: 250 mg, 500 mg

Tablet, as ethylsuccinate (E.E.S.®): 400 mg

Tablet, as stearate: 250 mg

Erythrocin®: 250 mg, 500 mg

Tablet [polymer-coated particles], as base (PCE®): 333 mg, 500 mg

Reference Range Peak plasma level after 500 mg dose: 2-20 mg/L

Overdosage/Treatment

Decontamination: Lavage (within 1 hour)/activated charcoal

Supportive therapy: Acute gastrointestinal irritation can be treated with milk or bismuth subsalicylate; QT prolongation, hypotension, or ventricular arrhythmias can be treated with sodium bicarbonate; lidocaine can be useful for ventricular tachycardia; magnesium sulfate can be useful in treating torsade de pointes

Enhanced elimination: Slightly dialyzable

Test Interactions False-positive urinary catecholamines and 17-hydroxycorticosteroids; estolate salt may result in false-positive elevation of serum AST when assayed colorimetrically

Drug Interactions

Substrate of CYP2B6 (minor), 3A4 (major); **Inhibits** CYP1A2 (weak), 3A4 (moderate)

Alfentanil (and possibly other narcotic analgesics): Serum levels may be increased by erythromycin; monitor for increased effect.

Antipsychotic agents (particularly mesoridazine and thioridazine): Risk of QT_c prolongation and malignant arrhythmias may be increased.

Benzodiazepines (those metabolized by CYP3A4, including alprazolam and triazolam): Serum levels may be increased by erythromycin; somnolence and confusion have been reported.

Bromocriptine: Serum levels may be increased by erythromycin; monitor for increased effect.

Buspirone: Serum levels may be increased by erythromycin; monitor.

Calcium channel blockers (felodipine, verapamil, and potentially others metabolized by CYP3A4): Serum levels may be increased by erythromycin; monitor.

Carbamazepine: Serum levels may be increased by erythromycin; monitor.

Cilostazol: Serum levels may be increased by erythromycin.

Cisapride: Serum levels may be increased by erythromycin; serious arrhythmias have occurred; concurrent use contraindicated.

Clindamycin (and lincomycin): Use with erythromycin may result in pharmacologic antagonism; manufacturer recommends avoiding this combination.

Clozapine: Serum levels may be increased by erythromycin; monitor.

Colchicine: serum levels/toxicity may be increased by erythromycin; monitor. Avoid use, if possible.

Cyclosporine: Serum levels may be increased by erythromycin; monitor serum levels.

CYP3A4 inducers: CYP3A4 inducers may decrease the levels/effects of erythromycin. Example inducers include aminoglutethimide, carbamazepine, nafcillin, nevirapine, phenobarbital, phenytoin, and rifamycins.

CYP3A4 inhibitors: May increase the levels/effects of erythromycin. Example inhibitors include azole antifungals, clarithromycin, diclofenac, doxycycline, imatinib, isoniazid, nefazodone, nicardipine, propofol, protease inhibitors, quinidine, telithromycin, and verapamil.

CYP3A4 substrates: Erythromycin may increase the levels/effects of CYP3A4 substrates. Example substrates include benzodiazepines, calcium channel blockers, cyclosporine, mirtazapine, nateglinide, nefazodone, sildenafil (and other PDE-5 inhibitors), tacrolimus, and venlafaxine. Selected benzodiazepines (midazolam and triazolam), cisapride, ergot alkaloids, selected HMG-CoA reductase inhibitors (lovastatin and simvastatin), and pimozide are generally contraindicated with strong CYP3A4 inhibitors.

Delavirdine: Serum levels of erythromycin may be increased; also, serum levels of delavirdine may increased by erythromycin (low risk); monitor.

Digoxin: Serum levels may be increased by erythromycin; monitor digoxin levels.

Disopyramide: Serum levels may be increased by erythromycin; in addition, QT_c prolongation and risk of malignant arrhythmia may be increased; avoid combination.

Ergot alkaloids: Concurrent use may lead to acute ergot toxicity (severe peripheral vasospasm and dysesthesia).

HMG-CoA reductase inhibitors (atorvastatin, lovastatin, and simvastatin); Erythromycin may increase serum levels of "statins" metabolized by CYP3A4, increasing the risk of myopathy/rhabdomyolysis (does not include fluvastatin and pravastatin). Switch to pravastatin/fluvastatin or suspend treatment during course of erythromycin therapy.

Loratadine: Serum levels may be increased by erythromycin; monitor.

Methylprednisolone: Serum levels may be increased by erythromycin; monitor.

Neuromuscular-blocking agents: May be potentiated by erythromycin (case reports).

Phenytoin: Serum levels may be increased by erythromycin; other evidence suggested phenytoin levels may be decreased in some patients; monitor.

Pimozide: Serum levels may be increased, leading to malignant arrhythmias; concomitant use is contraindicated.

Protease inhibitors (amprenavir, nelfinavir, and ritonavir): May increase serum levels of erythromycin.

QT_c-prolonging agents: Concomitant use may increase the risk of malignant arrhythmias.

Quinidine: Serum levels may be increased by erythromycin; in addition, the risk of QT_c prolongation and malignant arrhythmias may be increased during concurrent use.

Quinolone antibiotics (sparfloxacin, gatifloxacin, and moxifloxacin): Concurrent use may increase the risk of malignant arrhythmias.

Rifabutin: Serum levels may be increased by erythromycin; monitor.

Sildenafil, tadalafil, vardenafil: Serum concentration may be substantially increased by erythromycin. Do not exceed single sildenafil doses of 25 mg in 48 hours, a single tadalafil dose of 10 mg in 72 hours, or a single vardenafil dose of 2.5 mg in 24 hours.

Tacrolimus: Serum levels may be increased by erythromycin; monitor serum concentration.

Theophylline: Serum levels may be increased by erythromycin; monitor.

Valproic acid (and derivatives): Serum levels may be increased by erythromycin; monitor.

Vinblastine (and vincristine): Serum levels may be increased by erythromycin.

Warfarin: Effects may be potentiated; monitor INR closely and adjust warfarin dose as needed or choose another antibiotic.

Zafirlukast: Serum levels may be decreased by erythromycin; monitor.

Zopiclone: Serum levels may be increased by erythromycin; monitor.

Pregnancy Risk Factor B

Pregnancy Implications Crosses the placenta; avoid erythromycin estolate in that elevated serum aspartate aminotransferase can occur in 14% of patients (not a false-positive)

Lactation Enters breast milk/use caution (AAP considers "compatible")

Nursing Implications Gastrointestinal upset, including diarrhea, is common; can give with food to decrease gastritis; some formulations may contain benzyl alcohol as a preservative; use with extreme care in neonates

Additional Information Sodium content of oral suspension (ethylsuccinate) 200 mg/5 mL: 29 mg (1.3 mEq); sodium content of base Filmtab® 250 mg: 70 mg (3 mEq)

Specific References

Cvetanovic I, Ranade V, Lin C, et al, "The Differential Antibacterial and Gastrointestinal Effects of Erythromycin and Its Chiral Isolates," *Am J Ther*, 2006, 13(1):48-56.

Rosenman MB, Mahon BE, Downs SM, et al, "Oral Erythromycin Prophylaxis vs Watchful Waiting in Caring for Newborns Exposed to *Chlamydia trachomatis*," *Arch Pediatr Adolesc Med*, 2003, 157(6): 565-71.

Tenenbein MS and Tenenbein M, "Acute Pancreatitis Following an Overdose of Erythromycin," *J Toxicol Clin Toxicol*, 2004, 42(5):717.

Escitalopram

Pronunciation (es sye TAL oh pram)

Related Information
- Antidepressant Agents
- Citalopram

CAS Number 128196-01-0; 219861-08-2

U.S. Brand Names Lexapro®

Synonyms Escitalopram Oxalate; Lu-26-054; S-Citalopram

Use Treatment of major depressive disorder; generalized anxiety disorders (GAD)

Mechanism of Action Escitalopram is the S-enantiomer of the racemic derivative (bicyclic) citalopram, which selectively inhibits the reuptake of serotonin with little to no effect on norepinephrine or dopamine reuptake. It has no or very low affinity for 5-HT$_{1-7}$, alpha- and beta-adrenergic, D$_{1-5}$, H$_{1-3}$, M$_{1-5}$, and benzodiazepine receptors. Escitalopram does not bind or has low affinity for Na$^+$, K$^+$, Cl$^-$, and Ca^{++} ion channels.

Adverse Reactions

>10%:

Central nervous system: Headache (24%), somnolence (6% to 13%), insomnia (9% to 12%)

Gastrointestinal: Nausea (15%)

Genitourinary: Ejaculation disorder (9% to 14%)

1% to 10%:

Cardiovascular: Chest pain, hypertension, palpitation

Central nervous system: Dizziness (5%), fatigue (5% to 8%), dreaming abnormal, concentration impaired, fever, irritability, lethargy, lightheadedness, migraine, vertigo, yawning

Dermatologic: Rash

Endocrine & metabolic: Libido decreased (3% to 7%), anorgasmia (2% to 6%), hot flashes, menstrual cramps, menstrual disorder

Gastrointestinal: Diarrhea (8%), xerostomia (6% to 9%), appetite decreased (3%), constipation (3% to 5%), indigestion (3%), abdominal pain (2%), abdominal cramps, appetite increased, flatulence, gastroenteritis, gastroesophageal reflux, heartburn, toothache, vomiting, weight gain/loss

Genitourinary: Impotence (3%), urinary tract infection, urinary frequency

Neuromuscular & skeletal: Arthralgia, limb pain, muscle cramp, myalgia, neck/shoulder pain, paresthesia, tremor

Ocular: Blurred vision

Otic: Earache, tinnitus

Respiratory: Rhinitis (5%), sinusitis (3%), bronchitis, cough, nasal or sinus congestion, sinus headache

Miscellaneous: Diaphoresis (4% to 5%), flu-like syndrome (5%), allergy

<1%: Abdominal discomfort, acne, agitation, alopecia, amnesia, anaphylaxis, anemia, anxiety attack, apathy, arthritis, arthropathy, asthma, auditory hallucination, back discomfort, belching, bilirubin increased, bloating, bradycardia, bruise, bruxism, carbohydrate craving, carpal tunnel syndrome, chest tightness, chills, confusion, conjunctivitis, crying abnormal, depersonalization, depression aggravated, depression, dermatitis, dry eyes, dry skin, dysequilibrium, dyspepsia, dysuria, ECG abnormal, eczema, edema, emotional lability, excitability, eye infection, eye irritation, faintness, feeling unreal, flushing, folliculitis, forgetfulness, furunculosis, gagging, gastritis, gout, hematoma, hemorrhoids, hyper-cholesterolemia, hyperglycemia, hyper-reflexia, jaw pain, jaw stiffness,

jitteriness, joint stiffness, kidney stone, laryngitis, leg pain, lipoma, malaise, menorrhagia, muscle contractions (involuntary), muscle stiffness, muscle weakness, muscular tone increased, nervousness, nosebleed, panic reaction, pelvic inflammation, pneumonia, pruritus, pupils dilated, restless legs, restlessness aggravated, shaking, shortness of breath, spotting between menses, stool frequency increased, suicidal tendency, suicide attempt, syncope, tachycardia, taste alteration, tics, tracheitis, tremulousness nervous, twitching, urinary frequency, varicose vein, vision abnormal, visual disturbance, weakness

Postmarketing and/or case reports: Acute renal failure, aggression, akathisia, allergic reaction, angioedema, atrial fibrillation, choreoathetosis, delirium, dyskinesia, ecchymosis, epidermal necrolysis, erythema multiforme, grand mal seizure, hallucination, hemolytic anemia, hepatic necrosis, hepatitis, nystagmus, pancreatitis, priapism, prolactinemia, prothrombin decreased, pulmonary embolism, QT prolonged, rhabdomyolysis, serotonin syndrome, SIADH, spontaneous abortion, thrombocytopenia, thrombosis, torsade de pointes, ventricular arrhythmia, withdrawal syndrome

Signs and Symptoms of Overdose Seizure, QT prolongation, serotonin syndrome, drowsiness, agitation, fever, clonus

Pharmacodynamics/Kinetics

Protein binding: 56% to plasma proteins

Metabolism: Hepatic via CYP2C19 and 3A4 to an active metabolite, S-desmethylcitalopram (S-DCT; 1/7 the activity); S-DCT is metabolized to S-didesmethylcitalopram (S-DDCT; active; 1/27 the activity) via CYP2D6

Volume of distribution: 12-26 L/kg

Half-life elimination: Escitalopram: 27-32 hours; S-desmethylcitalopram: 59 hours

Time to peak: Escitalopram: 5±1.5 hours; S-desmethylcitalopram: 14 hours

Excretion: Urine (Escitalopram: 8%; S-DCT: 10%)

Clearance: Total body: 37-40 L/hour; Renal: Escitalopram: 2.7 L/hour; S-desmethylcitalopram: 6.9 L/hour

Dosage Oral:

Adults: Depression, GAD: Initial: 10 mg/day; dose may be increased to 20 mg/day after at least 1 week

Elderly: 10 mg/day; bioavailability and half-life are increased by 50% in the elderly

Dosage adjustment in renal impairment:

Mild to moderate impairment: No dosage adjustment needed

Severe impairment: Cl$_{cr}$ <20 mL/minute: Use caution

Dosage adjustment in hepatic impairment: 10 mg/day

Stability Store at 25°C (77°F).

Monitoring Parameters Mental status for depression, suicidal ideation (especially at the beginning of therapy or when doses are increased or decreased), anxiety, social functioning, mania, panic attacks; akathisia

Administration Administer once daily (morning or evening), with or without food.

Contraindications Hypersensitivity to escitalopram, citalopram, or any component of the formulation; concomitant use or within 2 weeks of MAO inhibitors

Warnings

Major psychiatric warnings:

- **[U.S. Boxed Warning]: Antidepressants increase the risk of suicidal thinking and behavior in children and adolescents with major depressive disorder (MDD) and other depressive disorders;** consider risk prior to prescribing. Closely monitor for clinical worsening, suicidality, or unusual changes in behavior; the child's family or caregiver should be instructed to closely observe the patient and communicate condition with healthcare provider. A medication guide concerning the use of antidepressants in children and teenagers should be dispensed with each prescription. **Escitalopram is not FDA approved for use in children.**

- The possibility of a suicide attempt is inherent in major depression and may persist until remission occurs. Patients treated with antidepressants should be observed for clinical worsening and suicidality, especially during the initial few months of a course of drug therapy, or at times of dose changes, either increases or decreases. Worsening depression and severe abrupt suicidality that are not part of the presenting symptoms may require discontinuation or modification of drug therapy. Use caution in high-risk patients during initiation of therapy.

- Prescriptions should be written for the smallest quantity consistent with good patient care. The patient's family or caregiver should be alerted to monitor patients for the emergence of suicidality and associated behaviors such as anxiety, agitation, panic attacks, insomnia, irritability, hostility, impulsivity, akathisia, hypomania, and mania; patients should be instructed to notify their healthcare provider if any of these symptoms or worsening depression or psychosis occur.

- May worsen psychosis in some patients or precipitate a shift to mania or hypomania in patients with bipolar disorder. Monotherapy in patients with bipolar disorder should be avoided. Patients presenting with depressive symptoms should be screened for bipolar disorder.

Escitalopram is not FDA approved for the treatment of bipolar depression.

Key adverse effects:
- Anticholinergic effects: Relatively devoid of these side effects.
- CNS depression: Has a low potential to impair cognitive or motor performance; caution operating hazardous machinery or driving.
- SIADH and hyponatremia: Has been associated with the development of SIADH; hyponatremia has been reported rarely, predominately in the elderly

Concurrent disease:
- Hepatic impairment: Use caution; clearance is decreased and plasma concentrations are increased; a lower dosage may be needed.
- Platelet aggregation: May impair platelet aggregation, resulting in bleeding.
- Renal impairment: Use caution; clearance is decreased and plasma concentrations are increased; a lower dosage may be needed.
- Seizure disorders: Use caution with a previous seizure disorder or condition predisposing to seizures such as brain damage or alcoholism.
- Sexual dysfunction: May cause or exacerbate sexual dysfunction.

Concurrent drug therapy:
- Agents which lower seizure threshold: Concurrent therapy with other drugs which lower the seizure threshold.
- Anticoagulants/Antiplatelets: Use caution with concomitant use of NSAIDs, ASA, or other drugs that affect coagulation; the risk of bleeding is potentiated.
- CNS depressants: Use caution with concomitant therapy.
- MAO inhibitors: Potential for severe reaction when used with MAO inhibitors; autonomic instability, coma, death, delirium, diaphoresis, hyperthermia, mental status changes/agitation, muscular rigidity, myoclonus, neuroleptic malignant syndrome features, and seizures may occur.

Special populations:
- Elderly: Use caution in elderly patients.
- Pregnancy: Use caution in pregnant patients; high doses of citalopram have been associated with teratogenicity in animals.

Special notes:
- Electroconvulsive therapy: May increase the risks associated with electroconvulsive therapy; consider discontinuing, when possible, prior to ECT treatment.
- Withdrawal syndrome: May cause dysphoric mood, irritability, agitation, dizziness, sensory disturbances, anxiety, confusion, headache, lethargy, emotional lability, insomnia, hypomania, tinnitus, and seizures. Upon discontinuation of escitalopram therapy, gradually taper dose. If intolerable symptoms occur following a decrease in dosage or upon discontinuation of therapy, then resuming the previous dose with a more gradual taper should be considered.

Dosage Forms
Solution, oral: 1 mg/mL (240 mL) [peppermint flavor]
Tablet: 5 mg, 10 mg, 20 mg
   Note: Cipralex® [CAN] is available only in 10 mg and 20 mg strengths.
Reference Range Daily dose of 10 mg achieves steady state escitalopram plasma levels of 20-125 nmol/L

Overdosage/Treatment
Decontamination: Lavage/activated charcoal
Treatment should be symptom-directed and supportive. Hypertension can be treated with nitroprusside. Seizures can be treated with benzodiazepine or phenobarbital.

Drug Interactions   Substrate (major) of CYP2C19, 3A4; **Inhibits** CYP2D6 (weak)
Aspirin: Concomitant use of escitalopram and NSAIDs, aspirin, or other drugs affecting coagulation has been associated with an increased risk of bleeding; monitor.
Buspirone: Concurrent use of citalopram with buspirone may cause serotonin syndrome; avoid concurrent use.
Cimetidine: May inhibit the metabolism of citalopram.
CYP2C19 inducers: May decrease the levels/effects of escitalopram. Example inducers include aminoglutethimide, carbamazepine, phenytoin, and rifampin.
CYP2C19 inhibitors: May increase the levels/effects of escitalopram. Example inhibitors include delavirdine, fluconazole, fluvoxamine, gemfibrozil, isoniazid, omeprazole, and ticlopidine.
CYP3A4 inducers: CYP3A4 inducers may decrease the levels/effects of escitalopram. Example inducers include aminoglutethimide, carbamazepine, nafcillin, nevirapine, phenobarbital, phenytoin, and rifampicins.
CYP3A4 inhibitors: May increase the levels/effects of escitalopram. Example inhibitors include azole antifungals, clarithromycin, diclofenac, doxycycline, erythromycin, imatinib, isoniazid, nefazodone, nicardipine, propofol, protease inhibitors, quinidine, telithromycin, and verapamil.
Desipramine: Escitalopram may increase desipramine levels.
Linezolid: Hyperpyrexia, hypertension, tachycardia, confusion, seizures, and deaths have been reported with agents which inhibit MAO (serotonin syndrome); this combination should be avoided.

MAO inhibitors: Hyperpyrexia, hypertension, tachycardia, confusion, seizures, and deaths have been reported with MAO inhibitors (serotonin syndrome); this combination should be avoided.
Meperidine: Combined use theoretically may increase the risk of serotonin syndrome.
Metoprolol: Escitalopram may increase plasma levels of metoprolol; monitor for increased effect.
Moclobemide: Concurrent use of citalopram with moclobemide may cause serotonin syndrome; avoid concurrent use.
Nefazodone: Concurrent use of citalopram with nefazodone may cause serotonin syndrome.
NSAIDs: Concomitant use of escitalopram and NSAIDs, aspirin, or other drugs affecting coagulation has been associated with an increased risk of bleeding; monitor.
Selegiline: Concurrent use with citalopram has been reported to cause serotonin syndrome; as an MAO type B inhibitor, the risk of serotonin syndrome may be less than with nonselective MAO inhibitors, and reports indicate that this combination has been well tolerated in Parkinson's patients.
SSRIs: Concurrent use with other reuptake inhibitors may increase the risk of serotonin syndrome.
Sibutramine: May increase the risk of serotonin syndrome with SSRIs.
Sumatriptan (and other serotonin agonists): Concurrent use may result in toxicity; weakness, hyper-reflexia, and incoordination have been observed with sumatriptan and SSRIs. In addition, concurrent use may theoretically increase the risk of serotonin syndrome; includes sumatriptan, naratriptan, rizatriptan, and zolmitriptan.
Tramadol: Concurrent use of citalopram with tramadol may cause serotonin syndrome; avoid concurrent use.
Trazodone: Concurrent use of citalopram with trazodone may cause serotonin syndrome.
Venlafaxine: Combined use with citalopram may increase the risk of serotonin syndrome.
Warfarin: Use with caution; may increase risk of bleeding.

Pregnancy Risk Factor C
Teratogenic effects have been reported in animal studies. Nonteratogenic effects including respiratory distress, cyanosis, apnea, seizures, temperature instability, feeding difficulty, vomiting, hypoglycemia, hypo- or hypertonia, hyper-reflexia, jitteriness, irritability, constant crying, and tremor have been reported in the neonate immediately following delivery after exposure late in the third trimester. Adverse effects may be due to toxic effects of SSRI or drug discontinuation. In some cases, may present clinically as serotonin syndrome. There are no adequate and well-controlled studies in pregnant women. Use during pregnancy only if the potential benefit to the mother outweighs the possible risk to the fetus. If treatment during pregnancy is required, consider tapering therapy during the third trimester.

Pregnancy Implications Teratogenic effects have been reported in animal studies. Nonteratogenic effects including respiratory distress, cyanosis, apnea, seizures, temperature instability, feeding difficulty, vomiting, hypoglycemia, hypo- or hypertonia, hyper-reflexia, jitteriness, irritability, constant crying, and tremor have been reported in the neonate immediately following delivery after exposure late in the third trimester. Adverse effects may be due to toxic effects of SSRI or drug discontinuation. In some cases, may present clinically as serotonin syndrome. There are no adequate and well-controlled studies in pregnant women. Use during pregnancy only if the potential benefit to the mother outweighs the possible risk to the fetus. If treatment during pregnancy is required, consider tapering therapy during the third trimester.

Lactation Enters breast milk/not recommended

Additional Information The tablet and oral solution dosage forms are bioequivalent. Clinically, escitalopram 20 mg is equipotent to citalopram 40 mg. Do not coadminister with citalopram.

Specific References
Barnett AK, Brush DE, and Schroeder W, "The Pharmacology and Toxicology of Escitalopram," *Int J Med Toxicol*, 2003, 6(3):14.
Bernard L, Stern R, Lew D, et al, "Serotonin Syndrome After Concomitant Treatment with Linezolid and Citalopram," *Clin Infect Dis*, 2003, 36(9):1197.
Mahlberg R, Kunz D, Sasse J, et al, "Serotonin Syndrome with Tramadol and Citalopram," *Am J Psychiatry*, 2004, 161(6):1129.
Mokhlesi B, Leikin JB, Murray P, et al, "Adult Toxicology in Critical Care: Part II: Specific Poisonings," *Chest*, 2003, 123(3):897-922.
Pass SE and Simpson RW, "Discontinuation and Reinstitution of Medications During the Perioperative Period," *Am J Health Syst Pharm*, 2004, 61(9):899-912.
Tahir N, "Serotonin Syndrome as a Consequence of Drug-Resistant Infections: An Interaction Between Linezolid and Citalopram, *J Am Med Dir Assoc*, 2004, 5(2):111-3.

Esmolol

Related Information
- Selected Properties of Beta-Adrenergic Blocking Drugs

CAS Number 103598-03-4; 81161-17-3; 84057-94-3

U.S. Brand Names Brevibloc®

Synonyms Esmolol Hydrochloride

Use Treatment of tachycardia (ventricular), fibrillation (atrial)/flutter (primarily to control ventricular rate), and hypertension (especially perioperatively); may be effective for thyrotoxic crisis; has been used to treat tachycardia due to neonatal tetanus

Unlabeled/Investigational Use In children, for SVT and postoperative hypertension

Mechanism of Action Class II antiarrhythmic: Competitively blocks response to beta$_1$ stimulation with little or no effect of beta$_2$ receptors except at high doses, no intrinsic sympathomimetic activity, no membrane stabilizing activity

Adverse Reactions

Cardiovascular: **Hypotension (especially with doses >200 mcg/kg/minute)**, bradycardia, exacerbation of Raynaud's phenomenon, sinus bradycardia, QRS prolongation

Central nervous system: Dizziness, somnolence, confusion, drowsiness, CNS depression, headache, seizures

Gastrointestinal: Nausea, vomiting, dyspepsia, constipation

Local: Phlebitis (at concentrations >20 mg/mL), skin necrosis after extravasation

Otic: Ototoxicity, tinnitus

Respiratory: Bronchoconstriction (less than propranolol, but more likely with higher doses), bronchospasm

Miscellaneous: Other adverse reactions similar to other beta-blockers may occur, **diaphoresis**

Signs and Symptoms of Overdose Abdominal pain, ataxia, AV block, depression, dizziness, dose-related hypotension, dry mouth, dyspnea, headache, heart block, hypoglycemia, lightheadedness, wheezing

Pharmacodynamics/Kinetics

Onset of action: Beta-blockade: I.V.: 2-10 minutes (quickest when loading doses are administered)

Duration of hemodynamic effects: 10-30 minutes; prolonged following higher cumulative doses, extended duration of use

Protein binding: 55%

Metabolism: In blood by red blood cell esterases

Half-life elimination: Adults: 9 minutes; elimination of metabolite decreases with end stage renal disease

Excretion: Urine (~69% as metabolites, 2% unchanged drug)

Dosage

I.V. (Must be adjusted to individual response and tolerance):

Children: An extremely limited amount of information regarding esmolol use in pediatric patients is currently available. Some centers have utilized doses of 100-500 mcg/kg given over 1 minute for control of tachycardia (ventricular)s. Loading doses of 500 mcg/kg/minute over 1 minute with maximal doses of 50-250 mcg/kg/minute (mean 173) have been used in addition to nitroprusside in a small number of patients (7 patients, 7-19 years of age, median 13 years) to treat postoperative hypertension after coarctation of aorta repair.

Adults: Loading dose: 500 mcg/kg over 1 minute; follow with a 50 mcg/kg/minute infusion for 4 minutes; if response is inadequate, rebolus with another 500 mcg/kg loading dose over 1 minute, and increase the maintenance infusion to 100 mcg/kg/minute. Repeat this process until a therapeutic effect has been achieved or to a maximum recommended maintenance dose of 200 mcg/kg/minute. Usual dosage range: 50-200 mcg/kg/minute with average dose of 100 mcg/kg/minute.

Monitoring Parameters Blood pressure, heart rate, MAP, ECG, respiratory rate, I.V. site; cardiac monitor and blood pressure monitor required

Administration Infusions must be administered with an infusion pump. The concentrate (250 mg/mL ampul) is **not** for direct I.V. injection, but rather must first be diluted to a final concentration of 10 mg/mL (ie, 2.5 g in 250 mL or 5 g in 500 mL). Concentrations >10 mg/mL or infusion into small veins or through a butterfly catheter should be avoided (can cause thrombophlebitis). Decrease or discontinue infusion if hypotension or congestive heart failure occur. Medication port of premixed bags should be used to withdraw only the initial bolus, if necessary (not to be used for withdrawal of additional bolus doses).

Contraindications Hypersensitivity to esmolol or any component of the formulation; sinus bradycardia; heart block greater than first degree (except in patients with a functioning artificial pacemaker); cardiogenic shock; bronchial asthma (relative); uncompensated cardiac failure; hypotension; pregnancy (2nd and 3rd trimesters)

Warnings Hypotension is common; patients need close blood pressure monitoring. Administer cautiously in compensated heart failure and monitor for a worsening of the condition. Use caution in patients with PVD (can aggravate arterial insufficiency). Use caution with concurrent use of beta-blockers and either verapamil or diltiazem; bradycardia or heart block can occur. Avoid concurrent I.V. use of both agents. Use beta-blockers cautiously in patients with bronchospastic disease; monitor

pulmonary status closely. Use cautiously in diabetics because it can mask prominent hypoglycemic symptoms. Can mask signs of thyrotoxicosis. Can cause fetal bradycardia when administered in the 3rd trimester of pregnancy or at delivery. Use caution in patients with renal dysfunction (active metabolite retained). Do not use in the treatment of hypertension associated with vasoconstriction related to hypothermia. Concentrations >10 mg/mL or infusion into small veins or through a butterfly catheter should be avoided (can cause thrombophlebitis). Extravasation can lead to skin necrosis and sloughing.

Dosage Forms Infusion [premixed in sodium chloride; preservative free]:
Brevibloc®: 2000 mg (100 mL) [20 mg/mL; double strength]; 2500 mg (250 mL) [10 mg/mL]

Injection, solution, as hydrochloride: 10 mg/mL (10 mL) [premixed in sodium chloride]
Brevibloc®: 10 mg/mL (10 mL) [alcohol free; premixed in sodium chloride]; 20 mg/mL (5 mL, 100 mL) [alcohol free; double strength; premixed in sodium chloride]; 250 mg/mL (10 mL) [contains alcohol 25%, propylene glycol 25%; concentrate]

Reference Range Therapeutic: 1.0-1.5 mg/L (3.4-5.1 μmol/L); note that arterial esmolol levels are sevenfold higher than venous levels

Overdosage/Treatment Supportive therapy: Usually discontinuation of the infusion will result in resolution of adverse effects within 30 minutes; hypotension can be treated with crystalloid infusion; beta agonist agents or aminophylline can be used for bronchoconstriction

Drug Interactions

Acetylcholinesterase Inhibitors: May enhance the bradycardic effect of beta-blockers.

Alpha/beta agonists (direct acting): Beta blockers may enhance the vasopressor effect of alpha/beta agonists (direct-acting). Epinephrine used as a local anesthetic for dental procedures will not likely cause clinically-relevant problems.

α_1-blockers: Beta blockers may enhance the orthostatic effect of α_1 blockers. The risk associated with ophthalmic products is probably less than systemic products.

α_2 agonists: Beta blockers may enhance the rebound hypertensive effect of α_2 agonists. This effect can occur when the α_2 agonist is abruptly withdrawn.

Amiodarone: May enhance the bradycardic effect of beta-blockers. Possibly to the point of cardiac arrest. Consider therapy modification.

β_2 agonists: May diminish the bradycardic effect of beta-blockers (β_1 selective); of concern with high doses of some beta-blockers.

Calcium channel blockers (nondihydropyridine): May enhance the hypotensive effect of beta-blockers. Bradycardia and signs of heart failure have also been reported.

Cardiac glycosides: Beta-blockers may enhance the bradycardic effect of cardiac glycosides.

Disopyramide: May enhance the bradycardic effect of beta-blockers. Use caution if coadministering disopyramide and a beta-blocker (especially if both are I.V.).

Insulin preparations: Beta-blockers may mask the hypoglycemic effect of insulin preparations.

NSAIDs: May diminish the antihypertensive effect of beta-blockers.

Sulfonylureas: Beta-blockers may enhance the hypoglycemic effect of sulfonylureas. Cardioselective beta-blockers (eg, esmolol) may be safer than nonselective beta-blockers. All beta-blockers appear to mask tachycardia as an initial symptom of hypoglycemia.

Pregnancy Risk Factor C (manufacturer); D (2nd and 3rd trimesters - expert analysis)

Pregnancy Implications Teratogenic effects are not noted in animal studies. Fetal bradycardia can occur when administered in the 3rd trimester of pregnancy or at delivery.

Lactation Excretion in breast milk unknown/use with caution

Additional Information 1.3 g overdose of esmolol associated with asystole and seizures; propylene glycol level in this case was 4 mg/dL (note that the more concentrated solution contains 25% propylene glycol)

Esomeprazole

Pronunciation (es oh ME pray zol)

U.S. Brand Names Nexium®

Synonyms Esomeprazole Magnesium

Use

Oral: Short-term (4-8 weeks) treatment of erosive esophagitis; maintaining symptom resolution and healing of erosive esophagitis; treatment of symptomatic gastroesophageal reflux disease (GERD); as part of a multidrug regimen for Helicobacter pylori eradication in patients with duodenal ulcer disease (active or history of within the past 5 years); prevention of gastric ulcers in patients at risk (age ≥60 years and/or history of gastric ulcer) associated with continuous NSAID therapy

I.V.: Short-term (≤10 weeks) treatment of gastroesophageal reflux disease (GERD) when oral therapy is not possible or appropriate

Mechanism of Action Proton pump inhibitor suppresses gastric acid secretion by inhibition of the H$^+$/K$^+$-ATPase in the gastric parietal cell

Adverse Reactions

Unless otherwise specified, percentages represent adverse reactions identified in clinical trials evaluating the intravenous formulation.

>10%: Central nervous system: Headache (I.V. 11%; oral 4% to 8%)

1% to 10%:

Central nervous system: Dizziness (3%)

Dermatologic: Pruritus ($\leq$1%)

Gastrointestinal: Flatulence (10%), nausea (2% to 6%), abdominal pain (6%; oral 3% to 4%), diarrhea (4%), xerostomia (2% to 4%), dyspepsia (<1% to 6%), constipation (3%)

Local: Injection site reaction (2%)

Respiratory: Sinusitis ($\leq$2%), respiratory infection (1%)

<1% (Limited to important or life-threatening): Albuminuria, alkaline phosphatase increased, allergic reactions, anemia, angioedema, arthritis exacerbation, arthropathy, asthenia, asthma exacerbation, Barrett's esophagus, benign polyps/nodules, bilirubinemia, cervical lymphadenopathy, chest pain, confusion, creatinine increased, cystitis, depression exacerbation, dermatitis, duodenitis, dysmenorrhea, dysphagia, dyspnea, epigastric pain, epistaxis, esophageal stricture, esophageal ulceration, esophageal varices, esophagitis, facial edema, fever, fibromyalgia syndrome, flu-like syndrome, flushing, fungal infection, gastric ulcer, gastritis, gastroenteritis, genital moniliasis, GI dysplasia, GI hemorrhage, glycosuria, goiter, hematuria, hepatic enzymes increased, hernia, hot flushes, hypertension, hypertonia, hyperuricemia, hypochromic anemia, hypoesthesia, hyponatremia, larynx edema, leukocytosis, leukopenia, maculopapular rash, migraine, pain, paresthesia, parosmia, peripheral edema, polymyalgia rheumatica, polyuria, pruritus ani, rash, rigors, serum gastrin increased, substernal chest pain, tachycardia, thrombocytopenia, thyroid stimulating hormone increased, tinnitus, tongue edema, total bilirubin increased, tremor, ulcerative stomatitis, urticaria, vaginitis, vertigo, vision change, vitamin B_{12} deficiency, vomiting

Postmarketing and/or case reports: Agranulocytosis, alopecia, anaphylaxis, anaphylactic shock, blurred vision, depression, erythema multiforme, hepatitis, jaundice, myalgia, pancreatitis, pancytopenia, Stevens-Johnson syndrome, toxic epidermal necrolysis

Pharmacodynamics/Kinetics

Distribution: V_{dss}: 16 L

Protein binding: 97%

Metabolism: Hepatic via CYP2C19 and 3A4 enzymes to hydroxy, desmethyl, and sulfone metabolites (all inactive)

Bioavailability: 90% with repeat dosing

Half-life elimination: 1-1.5 hours

Time to peak: 1.5 hours

Excretion: Urine (80%); feces (20%)

Dosage Note: Delayed-release capsules should be swallowed whole and taken at least 1 hour before eating

Adolescents 12-17 years: Oral: GERD: 20-40 mg once daily for up to 8 weeks

Adults:

Oral:

Erosive esophagitis (healing): Initial: 20-40 mg once daily for 4-8 weeks; if incomplete healing, may continue for an additional 4-8 weeks; maintenance: 20 mg once daily

Symptomatic GERD: 20 mg once daily for 4 weeks; may continue an additional 4 weeks if symptoms persist

Helicobacter pylori eradication: 40 mg once daily for 10 days; requires combination therapy

Prevention of NSAID-induced gastric ulcers: 20-40 mg once daily for up to 6 months

I.V.: GERD: 20 mg or 40 mg once daily for $\leq$10 days; change to oral therapy as soon as appropriate

Elderly: No dosage adjustment needed

Dosage adjustment in renal impairment: No dosage adjustment needed

Dosage adjustment in hepatic impairment:

Mild-to-moderate hepatic impairment (Child-Pugh Class A or B): No dosage adjustment needed

Severe hepatic impairment (Child-Pugh Class C): Dose should not exceed 20 mg/day

Stability

Capsule: Store at 15°C to 30°C (59°F to 86°F); keep container tightly closed

Powder for injection: Store at 15°C to 30°C (59°F to 86°F); protect from light.

For I.V. injection: Reconstitute powder with 5 mL NS.

For I.V. infusion: Initially reconstitute powder with 5 mL of NS, LR, or D_5W, then further dilute to a final volume of 50 mL.

Following reconstitution, solution for injection prepared in NS, and solution for infusion prepared in NS or LR should be used within 12 hours. Following reconstitution, solution for infusion prepared in D_5W should be used within 6 hours. Refrigeration is not required following reconstitution.

Monitoring Parameters Susceptibility testing recommended in patients who fail *H. pylori* eradication regimen (esomeprazole, clarithromycin, and amoxicillin)

Administration

Oral: Capsule should be swallowed whole and taken at least 1 hour before eating (best if taken before breakfast). For patients with difficulty swallowing, open capsule and mix contents with 1 tablespoon of applesauce. Swallow immediately; mixture should not be chewed or warmed. The mixture should not be stored for future use.

I.V.: May be administered by injection ($\geq$3 minutes) or infusion (10-30 minutes). Flush line prior to and after administration with NS, LR, or D_5W.

Nasogastric tube: Open capsule and place intact granules into a 60 mL syringe; mix with 50 mL of water. Replace plunger and shake vigorously for 15 seconds. Ensure that no granules remain in syringe tip. Do not administer if pellets dissolve or disintegrate. After administration, flush nasogastric tube with additional water. Use suspension immediately after preparation.

Contraindications Hypersensitivity to esomeprazole, substituted benzimidazoles (ie, lansoprazole, omeprazole, pantoprazole, rabeprazole), or any component of the formulation

Warnings Relief of symptoms does not preclude the presence of a gastric malignancy. Atrophic gastritis (by biopsy) has been noted with long-term omeprazole therapy; this may also occur with esomeprazole. No reports of enterochromaffin-like (ECL) cell carcinoids, dysplasia, or neoplasia has occurred. No reports of enterochromaffin-like (ECL) cell carcinoids, dysplasia, or neoplasia has occurred. Safety and efficacy in children <12 years of age have not been established.

Dosage Forms Capsule, delayed release:

Nexium®: 20 mg, 40 mg

Injection, powder for reconstitution:

Nexium®: 20 mg, 40 mg [contains edetate sodium]

Drug Interactions

Substrate of CYP2C19 (major), 3A4 (minor); **Inhibits** CYP2C19 (moderate)

Benzodiazepines metabolized by oxidation (eg, diazepam, midazolam, triazolam): Esomeprazole and omeprazole may increase levels of benzodiazepines metabolized by oxidation.

Carbamazepine: Esomeprazole and omeprazole may increase carbamazepine levels. Carbamazepine may decrease the effects of esomeprazole.

CYP2C19 inducers: May decrease the levels/effects of esomeprazole. Example inducers include aminoglutethimide, carbamazepine, phenytoin, and rifampin.

CYP2C19 substrates: Esomeprazole may increase the levels/effects of CYP2C19 substrates. Example substrates include citalopram, diazepam, methsuximide, phenytoin, propranolol, and sertraline.

HMG-CoA reductase inhibitors: Esomeprazole may increase the levels/effects; monitor.

Iron salts: Esomeprazole may decrease the absorption of orally-administered iron salts.

Itraconazole and ketoconazole: Proton pump inhibitors may decrease the absorption of itraconazole and ketoconazole.

Protease inhibitors: Proton pump inhibitors may decrease absorption of some protease inhibitors (atazanavir and indinavir).

Pregnancy Risk Factor B

Pregnancy Implications Teratogenic effects were not observed in animal studies. However, there are no adequate and well-controlled studies in pregnant women. Congenital abnormalities have been reported sporadically following omeprazole use during pregnancy.

Lactation Excretion in breast milk unknown/not recommended

Additional Information Esomeprazole is the S-isomer of omeprazole.

Specific References

Li X-Q, Anderson TB, Ahlstrom M, et al, "Comparison of Inhibitory Effects of the Proton Pump-Inhibiting Drugs Omeprazole, Esomeprazole, Lansoprazole, Pantoprazole, and Rabeprazole on Human Cytochrome P450 Activities," *Drug Metab Disp*, 2004, 32(8):821-7.

Estazolam

CAS Number 29975-16-4

U.S. Brand Names ProSom®

Impairment Potential Yes

Use Short-term management of insomnia

Mechanism of Action Has not been fully elucidated in humans; the most promising hypothesis involves GABA transmission. GABA is a major inhibitory transmitter in the CNS. Benzodiazepines may exert their pharmacologic effect through potentiation of the inhibitory activity of GABA. Specific benzodiazepine receptors have been identified in the rat brain located in proximity to dense areas of GABA receptors, primarily in the frontal and occipital cortex. Benzodiazepines do not alter the synthesis, release, reuptake, or enzymatic degradation of GABA.

Adverse Reactions

Cardiovascular: Syncope

Central nervous system: **Somnolence** (42%), agitation (4%), amnesia (4%), apathy (4%), emotional lability (4%), hostility seizures (4%), sleep disorder (4%), stupor (4%), ataxia (4%), anxiety (1%), "hangover effect" (3%), abnormal thinking (2%), hypokinesia (8%), neuritis (4%)

Dermatologic: Urticaria, acne, dry skin, photosensitivity, xerosis, purpura, pruritus

Endocrine & metabolic: Decreased libido, gynecomastia

Gastrointestinal: Dyspepsia, increased or decreased appetite, flatulence, gastritis, enterocolitis, melena, mouth ulcerations, xerostomia

Genitourinary: Urinary incontinence, nocturia

Hematologic: Agranulocytosis

Hepatic: Elevated AST

Neuromuscular & skeletal: **Weakness** (11%), twitching (4%), decreased reflexes (4%), paresthesia

Renal: Hematuria, oliguria

Respiratory: Cold symptoms, pharyngitis, asthma, cough, dyspnea, rhinitis, epistaxis, laryngitis

Signs and Symptoms of Overdose Confusion, coma, diminished reflexes, mydriasis, respiratory depression, somnolence

Admission Criteria/Prognosis Admit any patient with CNS depression or ingestions >3 mg

Pharmacodynamics/Kinetics

Onset of action: ~1 hour

Duration: Variable

Metabolism: Extensively hepatic

Half-life elimination: 10-24 hours (no significant changes in elderly)

Time to peak, serum: 0.5-1.6 hours

Excretion: Urine (<5% as unchanged drug)

Dosage Adults: Oral: 1 mg at bedtime, some patients may require 2 mg; start at doses of 0.5 mg in debilitated or small elderly patients

Dosing adjustment in hepatic impairment: May be necessary

Monitoring Parameters Respiratory and cardiovascular status

Contraindications Hypersensitivity to estazolam or any component of the formulation (cross-sensitivity with other benzodiazepines may exist); pregnancy

Note: Manufacturer states concurrent therapy with itraconazole or ketoconazole is contraindicated.

Warnings

As a hypnotic, should be used only after evaluation of potential causes of sleep disturbance. Failure of sleep disturbance to resolve after 7-10 days may indicate psychiatric or medical illness. Use is not recommended in patients with depressive disorders or psychoses. Avoid use in patients with sleep apnea. Use with caution in patients receiving concurrent CYP3A4 inhibitors, particularly when these agents are added to therapy. Use with caution in elderly or debilitated patients, patients with hepatic disease (including alcoholics), renal impairment, respiratory disease, impaired gag reflex, or obese patients.

Causes CNS depression (dose related) which may impair physical and mental capabilities. Use with caution in patients receiving other CNS depressants or psychoactive agents. Benzodiazepines have been associated with falls and traumatic injury and should be used with extreme caution in patients who are at risk of these events (especially the elderly). May cause physical or psychological dependence - use with caution in patients with a history of drug dependence.

Benzodiazepines have been associated with anterograde amnesia. Paradoxical reactions, including hyperactive or aggressive behavior, have been reported with benzodiazepines, particularly in adolescent/pediatric or psychiatric patients. Does not have analgesic, antidepressant, or antipsychotic properties.

Dosage Forms Tablet: 1 mg, 2 mg

Overdosage/Treatment

Decontamination: Lavage (within 1 hour)/activated charcoal

Supportive therapy: Treatment for benzodiazepine overdose is supportive; rarely is mechanical ventilation required. Flumazenil (Romazicon™) has been shown to selectively block the binding of benzodiazepines to CNS receptors, resulting in a reversal of benzodiazepine-induced CNS depression. Do not use in concomitant tricyclic ingestion; treat hypotension with isotonic crystalloids, place in Trendelenburg position or give dopamine or norepinephrine.

Enhancement of elimination: Multiple dose of activated charcoal may enhance elimination

Antidote(s)

● Flumazenil [ANTIDOTE]

Test Interactions Visine®, Drano®, and bleach may result in false-negative urine tests

Drug Interactions

Substrate of CYP3A4 (minor)

CNS depressants: Sedative effects and/or respiratory depression may be additive with CNS depressants; includes ethanol, barbiturates, narcotic analgesics, and other sedative agents; monitor for increased effect.

Itraconazole, ketoconazole: Concurrent use is contraindicated (per manufacturer); however, estazolam is a minor CYP3A4 substrate and an effect has not been documented in clinical studies.

Levodopa: Therapeutic effects may be diminished in some patients following the addition of a benzodiazepine; limited/inconsistent data.

Oral contraceptives: May decrease the clearance of some benzodiazepines (those which undergo oxidative metabolism); monitor for increased benzodiazepine effect.

Theophylline: May partially antagonize some of the effects of benzodiazepines; monitor for decreased response; may require higher doses for sedation.

Pregnancy Risk Factor X

Pregnancy Implications Suggested to be teratogenic in animal and human data; can precipitate neonatal respiratory depression when given during delivery

Lactation Enters breast milk/contraindicated

Nursing Implications Provide safety measures (ie, side rails, night light, and call button); remove smoking materials from area; supervise ambulation; avoid abrupt discontinuance in patients with prolonged therapy or seizure disorders

---

Estrogens, Conjugated

U.S. Brand Names Premarin®

Synonyms C.E.S.; CEE; Estrogenic Substances, Conjugated

Use Treatment of moderate to severe vasomotor symptoms associated with menopause; treatment of vulvar and vaginal atrophy; hypoestrogenism (due to hypogonadism, castration, or primary ovarian failure); prostatic cancer (palliation); breast cancer (palliation); osteoporosis (prophylaxis, postmenopausal women at significant risk only); abnormal uterine bleeding

Unlabeled/Investigational Use Uremic bleeding

Mechanism of Action Conjugated estrogens contain a mixture of estrone sulfate, equilin sulfate, 17 alpha-dihydroequilin, 17 alpha-estradiol and 17 beta-dihydroequilin. Estrogens are responsible for the development and maintenance of the female reproductive system and secondary sexual characteristics. Estradiol is the principle intracellular human estrogen and is more potent than estrone and estriol at the receptor level; it is the primary estrogen secreted prior to menopause. Following menopause, estrone and estrone sulfate are more highly produced. Estrogens modulate the pituitary secretion of gonadotropins, luteinizing hormone, and follicle-stimulating hormone through a negative feedback system; estrogen replacement reduces elevated levels of these hormones in postmenopausal women.

Adverse Reactions

Cardiovascular: Edema, hypertension, venous thromboembolism, myocardial infarction, stroke

Central nervous system: Dizziness, **headache (26% to 32%)**, mental depression, migraine, epilepsy exacerbation, irritability, mood disturbances, nervousness

Dermatologic: Chloasma, erythema multiforme, erythema nodosum, hemorrhagic eruption, hirsutism, loss of scalp hair, melasma, angioedema, pruritus, rash, urticaria

Endocrine & metabolic: Breast cancer, breast enlargement, breast tenderness, changes in libido, increased thyroid-binding globulin, increased total thyroid hormone (T_4), increased serum triglycerides/phospholipids, increased HDL-cholesterol, decreased LDL-cholesterol, impaired glucose tolerance, hypercalcemia, hypocalcemia

Gastrointestinal: Abdominal cramps, bloating, cholecystitis, cholelithiasis, gallbladder disease, nausea, pancreatitis, vomiting, weight gain/loss

Genitourinary: Alterations in frequency and flow of menses, changes in cervical secretions, endometrial cancer, increased size of uterine leiomyomata, vaginal candidiasis, endometrial hyperplasia

Hematologic: Aggravation of porphyria, decreased antithrombin III and antifactor Xa, increased levels of fibrinogen, increased platelet aggregability and platelet count; increased prothrombin and factors VII, VIII, IX, X

Hepatic: Cholestatic jaundice, hepatic hemangiomas enlarged

Local: Thrombophlebitis

Neuromuscular & skeletal: Chorea, arthralgias, leg cramps

Ocular: Intolerance to contact lenses, steepening of corneal curvature, retinal vascular thrombosis

Respiratory: Pulmonary thromboembolism, asthma exacerbation

Miscellaneous: Carbohydrate intolerance, anaphylactoid/anaphylactic reactions

Signs and Symptoms of Overdose Depression, dizziness, ectopic pregnancy, fluid retention, gynecomastia, hypophosphatemia, impotence, jaundice, sexual dysfunction, thrombophlebitis

Pharmacodynamics/Kinetics

Absorption: Well absorbed

Metabolism: Hepatic via CYP3A4; estradiol is converted to estrone and estriol; also undergoes enterohepatic recirculation; estrone sulfite is the main metabolite in postmenopausal women

Excretion: Urine (primarily estriol, also as estradiol, estrone, and conjugates)

Dosage Adults:

Male: Androgen-dependent prostate cancer: Oral: 1.25-2.5 mg 3 times/day

Female:

Prevention of osteoporosis in postmenopausal women: Oral: Initial: 0.3 mg/day cyclically* or daily, depending on medical assessment of patient. Dose may be adjusted based on bone mineral density and clinical response. The lowest effective dose should be used.

Moderate to severe vasomotor symptoms associated with menopause: Oral: Initial: 0.3 mg/day, cyclically* or daily, depending on medical assessment of patient. The lowest dose that will control symptoms should be used. Medication should be discontinued as soon as possible.

Vulvar and vaginal atrophy:

Oral: Initial: 0.3 mg/day; the lowest dose that will control symptoms should be used. May be given cyclically* or daily, depending on medical assessment of patient. Medication should be discontinued as soon as possible.

Vaginal cream: Intravaginal: $^1/_2$ to 2 g/day given cyclically*

Abnormal uterine bleeding:

Acute/heavy bleeding:

Oral (unlabeled route): 1.25 mg, may repeat every 4 hours for 24 hours, followed by 1.25 mg once daily for 7-10 days

I.V.: 25 mg, may repeat in 6-12 hours if needed

Note: Oral/I.V.: Treatment should be followed by a low-dose oral contraceptive; medroxyprogesterone acetate along with or following estrogen therapy can also be given

Nonacute/lesser bleeding: Oral (unlabeled route): 1.25 mg once daily for 7-10 days

Female hypogonadism: Oral: 0.3-0.625 mg/day given cyclically*; dose may be titrated in 6- to 12-month intervals; progestin treatment should be added to maintain bone mineral density once skeletal maturity is achieved.

Female castration, primary ovarian failure: Oral: 1.25 mg/day given cyclically*; adjust according to severity of symptoms and patient response. For maintenance, adjust to the lowest effective dose.

***Cyclic administration:** Either 3 weeks on, 1 week off **or** 25 days on, 5 days off

Male and Female:

Breast cancer palliation, metastatic disease in selected patients: Oral: 10 mg 3 times/day for at least 3 months

Uremic bleeding (unlabeled use): I.V.: 0.6 mg/kg/day for 5 days

Elderly: Refer to Adults dosing; a higher incidence of stroke and invasive breast cancer was observed in women >75 years in a WHI substudy.

Stability

Injection: Refrigerate at 2°C to 8°C (36°F to 46°F) prior to reconstitution. Reconstitute using provided diluent; do not shake violently. Following reconstitution, solution is stable for 60 days under refrigeration.

Compatible with normal saline, dextrose

Incompatible with ascorbic acid

Tablets, vaginal cream: Store at room temperature (25°C)

Monitoring Parameters Yearly physical examination that includes blood pressure and Papanicolaou smear, breast exam, mammogram. Monitor for signs of endometrial cancer in female patients with uterus. Adequate diagnostic measures, including endometrial sampling, if indicated, should be performed to rule out malignancy in all cases of undiagnosed abnormal vaginal bleeding.

Menopausal symptoms: Assess need for therapy at 3- to 6-month intervals

Prevention of osteoporosis: Bone density measurement

Administration Injection: May also be administered intramuscularly; when administered I.V., drug should be administered slowly to avoid the occurrence of a flushing reaction

Oral tablet, vaginal cream: Administer at bedtime to minimize adverse effects.

Contraindications Hypersensitivity to estrogens or any component of the formulation; undiagnosed abnormal vaginal bleeding; history of or current thrombophlebitis or venous thromboembolic disorders (including DVT, PE); active or recent (within 1 year) arterial thromboembolic disease (eg, stroke, MI); carcinoma of the breast (except in appropriately selected patients being treated for metastatic disease); estrogen-dependent tumor; hepatic dysfunction or disease; pregnancy

Warnings

Cardiovascular-related considerations: **[U.S. Boxed Warning]: Estrogens with or without progestin should not be used to prevent coronary heart disease.** Use caution with cardiovascular disease or dysfunction. May increase the risks of hypertension, myocardial infarction (MI), stroke, pulmonary emboli (PE), and deep vein thrombosis; incidence of these effects was shown to be significantly increased in postmenopausal women using conjugated equine estrogens (CEE) in combination with medroxyprogesterone acetate (MPA). Nonfatal MI, PE, and thrombophlebitis have also been reported in males taking high doses of CEE (eg, for prostate cancer). Estrogen compounds are generally associated with lipid effects such as increased HDL-cholesterol and decreased LDL-cholesterol. Triglycerides may also be in-creased; use with caution in patients with familial defects of lipoprotein metabolism. Whenever possible, estrogens should be discontinued at least 4 weeks prior to and for 2 weeks following elective surgery associated with an increased risk of thromboembolism or during periods of prolonged immobilization.

Neurological considerations: **[U.S. Boxed Warning]: The risk of dementia may be increased in postmenopausal women;** increased incidence was observed in women ≥65 years of age taking CEE alone or in combination with MPA.

Cancer-related considerations: **[U.S. Boxed Warning]: Unopposed estrogens may increase the risk of endometrial carcinoma in postmenopausal women.** Estrogens may exacerbate endometriosis. Malignant transformation of residual endometrial implants has been reported posthysterectomy with estrogen only therapy. Consider adding a progestin in women with residual endometriosis posthysterectomy. Estrogens may increase the risk of breast cancer. An increased risk of invasive breast cancer was observed in postmenopausal women using CEE in combination with MPA; a smaller increase in risk was seen with estrogen therapy alone in observational studies. An increase in abnormal mammograms has also been reported with estrogen and progestin therapy. Estrogen use may lead to severe hypercalcemia in patients with breast cancer and bone metastases; discontinue estrogen if hypercalcemia occurs.

Estrogens may cause retinal vascular thrombosis; discontinue permanently if papilledema or retinal vascular lesions are observed on examination. Use with caution in patients with diseases which may be exacerbated by fluid retention, including asthma, epilepsy, migraine, diabetes or renal dysfunction. Use with caution in patients with a history of severe hypocalcemia, SLE, hepatic hemangiomas, porphyria, endometriosis, and gallbladder disease. Use caution with history of cholestatic jaundice associated with past estrogen use or pregnancy. Safety and efficacy in pediatric patients have not been established. Prior to puberty, estrogens may cause premature closure of the epiphyses, premature breast development in girls or gynecomastia in boys. Vaginal bleeding and vaginal cornification may also be induced in girls.

Before prescribing estrogen therapy to postmenopausal women, the risks and benefits must be weighed for each patient. Women should be informed of these risks and benefits, as well as possible effects of progestin when added to estrogen therapy. Estrogens with or without progestin should be used for shortest duration possible consistent with treatment goals. Conduct periodic risk:benefit assessments.

When used solely for prevention of osteoporosis in women at significant risk, nonestrogen treatment options should be considered. When used solely for the treatment of vulvar and vaginal atrophy, topical vaginal products should be considered. Use caution applying topical products to severely atrophic vaginal mucosa.

Dosage Forms Cream, vaginal: 0.625 mg/g (42.5 g)

Injection, powder for reconstitution: 25 mg [contains lactose 200 mg; diluent contains benzyl alcohol]

Tablet: 0.3 mg, 0.45 mg, 0.625 mg, 0.9 mg, 1.25 mg

Reference Range

Children: <10 mcg/24 hours (SI: <35 µmol/day) (values at Mayo Medical Laboratories)

Adults:

Male: 15-40 mcg/24 hours (SI: 52-139 µmol/day)

Female:

Menstruating: 15-80 mcg/24 hours (SI: 52-277 µmol/day)

Postmenopausal: <20 mcg/24 hours (SI: <69 µmol/day)

Overdosage/Treatment

Decontamination: Emesis within 30 minutes or lavage within 1 hour; activated charcoal

Enhancement of elimination: Due to enterohepatic recirculation of drug, multiple dosing of activated charcoal may be effective

Test Interactions Pathologist should be advised of estrogen/progesterone therapy when specimens are submitted. Reduced response to metyrapone test.

Drug Interactions

Based on estradiol and estrone: **Substrate** of CYP1A2 (major), 2A6 (minor), 2B6 (minor), 2C9 (minor), 2C19 (minor), 2D6 (minor), 2E1 (minor), 3A4 (major); **Inhibits** CYP1A2 (weak), 2C8 (weak); **Induces** CYP3A4 (weak)

Anticoagulants: Increase potential for thromboembolic events

Cyclosporine: Estrogen derivatives may enhance the hepatotoxic effect of cyclosporine. Estrogen derivatives may increase the serum concentration of cyclosporine.

CYP1A2 inducers: May decrease the levels/effects of estrogens. Example inducers include aminoglutethimide, carbamazepine, phenobarbital, and rifampin.

CYP3A4 inducers: CYP3A4 inducers may decrease the levels/effects of estrogens. Example inducers include aminoglutethimide, carbamazepine, nafcillin, nevirapine, phenobarbital, phenytoin, and rifamycins.

Thyroid products: Estrogen derivatives may diminish the therapeutic effect of thyroid products; monitor.

Pregnancy Risk Factor X

Pregnancy Implications Increased risk of fetal reproductive tract disorders and other birth defects; do not use during pregnancy

Lactation Enters breast milk/use caution

Nursing Implications May also be administered intramuscularly; give at bedtime to minimize occurrence of adverse effects; when administered I.V., drug should be administered slowly to avoid the occurrence of a flushing reaction

Additional Information

The use of estrogens for the prevention of other chronic diseases, as well as their potential negative effects on women's health, has been debated. Data published from the Women's Health Initiative (WHI) has provided some additional insight on this controversial topic. In the WHI, one arm of the study compared postmenopausal women with an intact uterus using CEE 0.625 mg in combination with MPA 2.5 mg daily, versus placebo. This arm of the study was stopped in 2002. In March, 2004, it was announced that the arm of the study comparing placebo to CEE alone in postmenopausal women without a uterus was ended.

Based on preliminary findings, the FDA has requested labeling changes be made to estrogen products used in postmenopausal women. The updates include information from the Women's Health Initiative Memory Study (WHIMS) as well as information collected from the completed CEE/MPA arm of the WHI study. Complete analysis of the WHI data is forthcoming, and will include all information collected through February, 2004.

Specific References

Roy PM and Gras E, "Images in Clinical Medicine: Cerebral Venous Thrombosis," *N Engl J Med*, 2003, 349(18):1730.

U.S. Food and Drug Administration, Department of Health and Human Services, "FDA Approves New Labels for Estrogen and Estrogen with Progestin Therapies for Postmenopausal Women Following Review of Women's Health Initiative Data," January 8, 2003, viewable at http://www.fda.gov/medwatch/SAFETY/2003/safety03.htm#prempr, last accessed January 9, 2003.

Estrogens (Esterified)

U.S. Brand Names Menest®

Synonyms Esterified Estrogens

Use Treatment of moderate to severe vasomotor symptoms associated with menopause; treatment of vulvar and vaginal atrophy; hypoestrogenism (due to hypogonadism, castration, or primary ovarian failure); prostatic cancer (palliation); breast cancer (palliation); osteoporosis (prophylaxis, in women at significant risk only)

Mechanism of Action All estrogens, including esterified estrogens, act in a similar manner. Estrogens exert their primary effects on the interphase DNA-protein complex (chromatin) by binding to a receptor (usually located in the cytoplasm of a target cell) and initiating translocation of the hormone-receptor complex to the nucleus. The specificity of estrogen action depends upon the presence and concentration of estrogen targets, which are defined as tissues containing a high concentration of estrogen receptors.

Adverse Reactions

Cardiovascular: Edema, hypertension, venous thromboembolism

Central nervous system: Dizziness, headache, mental depression, migraine

Dermatologic: Chloasma, erythema multiforme, erythema nodosum, hemorrhagic eruption, hirsutism, loss of scalp hair, melasma

Endocrine & metabolic: Breast enlargement, breast tenderness, changes in libido, increased thyroid-binding globulin, increased total thyroid hormone (T_4), increased serum triglycerides/phospholipids, increased HDL cholesterol, decreased LDL cholesterol, impaired glucose tolerance, hypercalcemia

Gastrointestinal: Abdominal cramps, bloating, cholecystitis, cholelithiasis, gallbladder disease, nausea, pancreatitis, vomiting, weight gain/loss

Genitourinary: Alterations in frequency and flow of menses, changes in cervical secretions, endometrial cancer, increased size of uterine leiomyomata, vaginal candidiasis

Hematologic: Aggravation of porphyria, decreased antithrombin III and antifactor Xa, increased levels of fibrinogen, increased platelet aggregability and platelet count; increased prothrombin and factors VII, VIII, IX, X

Hepatic: Cholestatic jaundice

Neuromuscular & skeletal: Chorea

Ocular: Intolerance to contact lenses, steepening of corneal curvature

Respiratory: Pulmonary thromboembolism

Miscellaneous: Carbohydrate intolerance

Signs and Symptoms of Overdose Toxicity is unlikely following single exposures of excessive doses. Fluid retention, gynecomastia, hypophosphatemia, impotence, jaundice, migraine headache (exacerbation), sexual dysfunction, thrombophlebitis

Pharmacodynamics/Kinetics

Absorption: Readily

Metabolism: Rapidly hepatic to estrone sulfate, conjugated and unconjugated metabolites; first-pass effect

Excretion: Urine (as unchanged drug and as glucuronide and sulfate conjugates)

Dosage

Oral: Adults:

Prostate cancer (palliation): 1.25-2.5 mg 3 times/day

Female hypogonadism: 2.5-7.5 mg of estrogen daily for 20 days followed by a 10-day rest period. Administer cyclically (3 weeks on and 1 week off). If bleeding does not occur by the end of the 10-day period, repeat the same dosing schedule; the number of courses is dependent upon the responsiveness of the endometrium. If bleeding occurs before the end of the 10-day period, begin an estrogen-progestin cyclic regimen of 2.5-7.5 mg esterified estrogens daily for 20 days. During the last 5 days of estrogen therapy, give an oral progestin. If bleeding occurs before regimen is concluded, discontinue therapy and resume on the fifth day of bleeding.

Moderate to severe vasomotor symptoms associated with menopause: 1.25 mg/day administered cyclically (3 weeks on and 1 week off). If patient has not menstruated within the last 2 months or more, cyclic administration is started arbitrary. If the patient is menstruating, cyclical administration is started on day 5 of the bleeding. For short-term use only and should be discontinued as soon as possible. Re-evaluate at 3- to 6-month intervals for tapering or discontinuation of therapy.

Atopic vaginitis and kraurosis vulvae: 0.3 to $\geq$ 1.25 mg/day, depending on the tissue response of the individual patient. Administer cyclically. For short-term use only and should be discontinued as soon as possible. Re-evaluate at 3- to 6-month intervals for tapering or discontinuation of therapy.

Breast cancer (palliation): 10 mg 3 times/day for at least 3 months

Osteoporosis in postmenopausal women: Initial: 0.3 mg/day and increase to a maximum daily dose of 1.25 mg/day; initiate therapy as soon as possible after menopause; cyclically or daily, depending on medical assessment of patient. Monitor patients with an intact uterus for signs of endometrial cancer; rule out malignancy if unexplained vaginal bleeding occurs

Female castration and primary ovarian failure: 1.25 mg/day, cyclically. Adjust dosage upward or downward, according to the severity of symptoms and patient response. For maintenance, adjust dosage to lowest level that will provide effective control.

Elderly: Refer to Adults dosing. A higher incidence of stroke and invasive breast cancer were observed in women >75 years in a Women's Health Initiative (WHI) substudy using conjugated equine estrogen.

Dosing adjustment in hepatic impairment:

Mild to moderate liver impairment: Dosage reduction of estrogens is recommended

Severe liver impairment: **Not recommended**

Monitoring Parameters

Yearly physical examination that includes blood pressure and Papanicolaou smear, breast exam, mammogram. Monitor for signs of endometrial cancer in female patients with uterus. Adequate diagnostic measures, including endometrial sampling, if indicated, should be performed to rule out malignancy in all cases of undiagnosed abnormal vaginal bleeding.

Menopausal symptoms: Assess need for therapy at 3- to 6-month intervals

Prevention of osteoporosis: Bone density measurement

Contraindications Hypersensitivity to estrogens or any component of the formulation; undiagnosed abnormal vaginal bleeding; history of or current thrombophlebitis or venous thromboembolic disorders (including DVT, PE); active or recent (within 1 year) arterial thromboembolic disease (eg, stroke, MI); carcinoma of the breast, except in appropriately selected patients being treated for metastatic disease; estrogen-dependent tumor; hepatic dysfunction or disease; pregnancy

Warnings

Cardiovascular-related considerations: **[U.S. Boxed Warning]: Estrogens with or without progestin should not be used to prevent coronary heart disease.** Use caution with cardiovascular disease or dysfunction. May increase the risks of hypertension, myocardial infarction (MI), stroke, pulmonary emboli (PE), and deep vein thrombosis; incidence of these effects was shown to be significantly increased in postmenopausal women using conjugated equine estrogens (CEE) in combination with medroxyprogesterone acetate (MPA). Nonfatal MI, PE, and thrombophlebitis have also been reported in males taking high doses of CEE (eg, for prostate cancer). Estrogen compounds are generally associated with lipid effects such as increased HDL-cholesterol and decreased LDL-cholesterol. Triglycerides may also be increased; use with caution in patients with familial defects of lipoprotein metabolism. Whenever possible, estrogens should be discontinued at least 4 weeks prior to and for 2 weeks following elective surgery associated with an increased risk of thromboembolism or during periods of prolonged immobilization.

Neurological considerations: **[U.S. Boxed Warning]: The risk of dementia may be increased in postmenopausal women;** increased incidence was observed in women ≥65 years of age taking CEE alone or in combination with MPA.

Cancer-related considerations: **[U.S. Boxed Warning]: Unopposed estrogens may increase the risk of endometrial carcinoma in postmenopausal women.** Estrogens may exacerbate endometriosis. Malignant transformation of residual endometrial implants has been reported post-hysterectomy with estrogen only therapy. Consider adding a progestin in women with residual endometriosis post-hysterectomy. Estrogens may increase the risk of breast cancer. An increased risk of invasive breast cancer was observed in postmenopausal women using CEE in combination with MPA; a smaller increase in risk was seen with estrogen therapy alone in observational studies. An increase in abnormal mammograms has also been reported with estrogen and progestin therapy. Estrogen use may lead to severe hypercalcemia in patients with breast cancer and bone metastases; discontinue estrogen if hypercalcemia occurs.

Estrogens may cause retinal vascular thrombosis; discontinue permanently if papilledema or retinal vascular lesions are observed on examination. Use with caution in patients with diseases which may be exacerbated by fluid retention, including asthma, epilepsy, migraine, diabetes or renal dysfunction. Use with caution in patients with a history of severe hypocalcemia, SLE, hepatic hemangiomas, porphyria, endometriosis, and gallbladder disease. Use caution with history of cholestatic jaundice associated with past estrogen use or pregnancy. Safety and efficacy in pediatric patients have not been established. Prior to puberty, estrogens may cause premature closure of the epiphyses, premature breast development in girls or gynecomastia in boys. Vaginal bleeding and vaginal cornification may also be induced in girls.

Before prescribing estrogen therapy to postmenopausal women, the risks and benefits must be weighed for each patient. Women should be informed of these risks and benefits, as well as possible effects of progestin when added to estrogen therapy. Estrogens with or without progestin should be used for shortest duration possible consistent with treatment goals. Conduct periodic risk:benefit assessments.

When used solely for prevention of osteoporosis in women at significant risk, nonestrogen treatment options should be considered. When used solely for the treatment of vulvar and vaginal atrophy, topical vaginal products should be considered.

Dosage Forms Tablet: 0.3 mg, 0.625 mg, 1.25 mg, 2.5 mg

Reference Range
Children: <10 mcg/24 hours (SI: <35 µmol/day) (values at Mayo Medical Laboratories)
Adults:
Male: 15-40 mcg/24 hours (SI: 52-139 µmol/day)
Female:
Menstruating: 15-80 mcg/24 hours (SI: 52-277 µmol/day)
Postmenopausal: <20 mcg/24 hours (SI: <69 µmol/day)

Overdosage/Treatment Toxicity is unlikely following single exposures of excessive doses, any treatment following emesis and charcoal administration should be supportive and symptomatic. Effects noted after large doses include headache, nausea, and vomiting. Bleeding may occur in females.

Test Interactions Pathologist should be advised of estrogen/progesterone therapy when specimens are submitted. Reduced response to metyrapone test.

Drug Interactions
Based on estrone: **Substrate** of CYP1A2 (major), 2B6 (minor), 2C9 (minor), 2E1 (minor), 3A4 (major)
Anticoagulants: Increases potential for thromboembolic events with anticoagulants
Corticosteroids: Estrogens may enhance the effects of hydrocortisone and prednisone.
Cyclosporine: Estrogen derivatives may enhance the hepatotoxic effect of cyclosporine. Estrogen derivatives may increase the serum concentration of cyclosporine.
CYP1A2 inducers: May decrease the levels/effects of estrogens. Example inducers include aminoglutethimide, carbamazepine, phenobarbital, and rifampin.
CYP3A4 inducers: CYP3A4 inducers may decrease the levels/effects of estrogens. Example inducers include aminoglutethimide, carbamazepine, nafcillin, nevirapine, phenobarbital, phenytoin, and rifamycins.
Thyroid products: Estrogen derivatives may diminish the therapeutic effect of thyroid products; monitor.

Pregnancy Risk Factor X
Pregnancy Implications Increased risk of fetal reproductive tract disorders and other birth defects; do not use during pregnancy
Lactation Enters breast milk/use caution
Additional Information
The use of estrogens for the prevention of other chronic diseases, as well as their potential negative effects on women's health, has been debated. Data published from the Women's Health Initiative (WHI) has provided

some additional insight on this controversial topic. In the WHI, one arm of the study compared postmenopausal women with an intact uterus using CEE 0.625 mg in combination with MPA 2.5 mg daily, versus placebo. This arm of the study was stopped in 2002. In March, 2004, it was announced that the arm of the study comparing placebo to CEE alone in postmenopausal women without a uterus was ended.

Based on preliminary findings, the FDA has requested labeling changes be made to estrogen products used in postmenopausal women. The updates include information from the Women's Health Initiative Memory Study (WHIMS) as well as information collected from the completed CEE/MPA arm of the WHI study. Complete analysis of the WHI data is forthcoming, and will include all information collected through February, 2004.

Ethacrynic Acid

CAS Number 58-54-8
U.S. Brand Names Edecrin®
Synonyms Ethacrynate Sodium
Use Management of edema secondary to congestive heart failure; hepatic or renal disease, hypertension
Mechanism of Action Inhibits reabsorption of sodium and chloride in the ascending loop of Henle and distal renal tubule, interfering with the chloride-binding cotransport system, thus causing increased excretion of water, sodium, chloride, magnesium, and calcium
Adverse Reactions
Cardiovascular: Hypotension, diuresis
Dermatologic: Rash
Endocrine & metabolic: Fluid and electrolyte imbalances (fluid depletion, hypokalemia, hyponatremia, hyperglycemia), hyperuricemia
Gastrointestinal: GI irritation, **diarrhea**, GI bleeding (especially when used with warfarin); feces discoloration (black)
Hematologic: Thrombocytopenia, leukopenia, neutropenia, agranulocytosis, granulocytopenia
Hepatic: Abnormal liver function tests
Otic: Ototoxicity, tinnitus, deafness
Renal: Renal injury
Signs and Symptoms of Overdose Agranulocytosis, dizziness, dysosmia, gout, granulocytopenia, hyperglycemia, hyperuricemia, hypocalcemia, hypoglycemia, hypokalemia, hypomagnesemia, hyponatremia, hypotension, leukopenia, myasthenia gravis (exacerbation or precipitation), thrombocytopenia, neutropenia, nocturia, nystagmus, pancreatitis
Pharmacodynamics/Kinetics
Onset of action: Diuresis: Oral: ~30 minutes; I.V.: 5 minutes
Peak effect: Oral: 2 hours; I.V.: 30 minutes
Duration: Oral: 12 hours; I.V.: 2 hours
Absorption: Oral: Rapid
Protein binding: >90%
Metabolism: Hepatic (35% to 40%) to active cysteine conjugate
Half-life elimination: Normal renal function: 2-4 hours
Excretion: Feces and urine (30% to 60% as unchanged drug)
Dosage
Children:
Oral: 25 mg/day to start, increase by 25 mg/day at intervals of 2-3 days as needed, to a maximum of 3 mg/kg/day
I.V.: 1 mg/kg/dose, (maximum: 50 mg/dose); repeat doses not recommended
Adults:
Oral: 50-100 mg/day in 1-2 divided doses; may increase in increments of 25-50 mg at intervals of several days to a maximum of 400 mg/24 hours
I.V.: 0.5-1 mg/kg/dose (maximum: 100 mg/dose); repeat doses not recommended
Dosing adjustment/comments in renal impairment: Cl_{cr} <10 mL/minute: Avoid use
Monitoring Parameters Blood pressure, renal function, serum electrolytes, and fluid status closely, including weight and I & O daily; hearing
Administration Injection should **not** be given SubQ or I.M. due to local pain and irritation; single I.V. doses should not exceed 100 mg; if a second dose is needed, use a new injection site to avoid possible thrombophlebitis
Contraindications Hypersensitivity to ethacrynic acid or any component of the formulation; anuria; history of severe watery diarrhea caused by this product; infants
Warnings Adjust dose to avoid dehydration. In cirrhosis, avoid electrolyte and acid/base imbalances that might lead to hepatic encephalopathy. Ototoxicity is associated with rapid I.V. administration, renal impairment, excessive doses, and concurrent use of other ototoxins. Has been associated with a higher incidence of ototoxicity than other loop diuretics. Hypersensitivity reactions can rarely occur, however, ethacrynic acid has no cross-reactivity to sulfonamides or sulfonylureas. Monitor fluid status and renal function in an attempt to prevent oliguria, azotemia, and reversible increases in BUN and creatinine. Close medical supervision of aggressive diuresis required. Watch for and correct electrolyte disturbances. Coadministration of antihypertensives may increase the risk of

hypotension. Increased risk of gastric hemorrhage associated with corticosteroid therapy.

Dosage Forms
Injection, powder for reconstitution, as ethacrynate sodium: 50 mg
Tablet: 25 mg

Overdosage/Treatment
Decontamination: Activated charcoal for gastric decontamination
Supportive therapy: I.V. hydration with 0.9% saline; replace electrolyte deficiency

Drug Interactions
ACE inhibitors: Hypotensive effects and/or renal effects are potentiated by hypovolemia.
Antidiabetic agents: Glucose tolerance may be decreased.
Antihypertensive agents: Hypotensive effects may be enhanced.
Cephaloridine or cephalexin: Nephrotoxicity may occur.
Cholestyramine or colestipol may reduce bioavailability of ethacrynic acid.
Clofibrate: Protein binding may be altered in hypoalbuminemic patients receiving ethacrynic acid, potentially increasing toxicity.
Digoxin: Ethacrynic acid-induced hypokalemia may predispose to digoxin toxicity; monitor potassium.
Indomethacin (and other NSAIDs) may reduce natriuretic and hypotensive effects of diuretics.
Lithium: Renal clearance may be reduced. Isolated reports of lithium toxicity have occurred; monitor lithium levels.
NSAIDs: Risk of renal impairment may increase when used in conjunction with diuretics.
Ototoxic drugs (aminoglycosides, cis-platinum): Concomitant use of ethacrynic acid may increase risk of ototoxicity, especially in patients with renal dysfunction.
Peripheral adrenergic-blocking drugs or ganglionic blockers: Effects may be increased.
Salicylates (high-dose) with diuretics may predispose patients to salicylate toxicity due to reduced renal excretion or alter renal function.
Thiazides: Synergistic diuretic effects occur.

Pregnancy Risk Factor B
Pregnancy Implications No data available. Generally, use of diuretics during pregnancy is avoided due to risk of decreased placental perfusion.
Lactation Contraindicated
Nursing Implications Tissue irritant; not to be administered I.M. or SubQ; dilute injection with 50 mL dextrose 5% or normal saline (1 mg/mL concentration resulting); may be injected without further dilution over a period of several minutes or infused over 20-30 minutes
Monitor blood pressure, serum electrolytes, renal function, hearing
Additional Information Injection contains thimerosal
Specific References
Wall GC, Bigner D, and Craig S, "Ethacrynic Acid and the Sulfa-Sensitive Patient," *Arch Intern Med*, 2003, 163(1):116-7.

Ethambutol

Related Information
• Therapeutic Drugs Associated with Hallucinations
CAS Number 1070-11-7
U.S. Brand Names Myambutol®
Synonyms Ethambutol Hydrochloride
Use Treatment of tuberculosis and other mycobacterial diseases in conjunction with other antituberculosis agents
Mechanism of Action Suppresses mycobacteria multiplication by interfering with RNA synthesis
Adverse Reactions
Cardiovascular: Myocarditis, pericarditis
Central nervous system: Headache, confusion, disorientation, malaise, mental confusion, fever, dizziness, hallucinations
Dermatologic: Rash, pruritus, dermatitis, exfoliative dermatitis
Endocrine & metabolic: Acute gout or hyperuricemia
Gastrointestinal: Abdominal pain, anorexia, nausea, vomiting
Hematologic: Leukopenia, thrombocytopenia, eosinophilia, neutropenia, lymphadenopathy
Hepatic: Abnormal LFTs, hepatotoxicity (possibly related to concurrent therapy), hepatitis
Neuromuscular & skeletal: Peripheral neuritis, arthralgia
Ocular: Optic neuritis; symptoms may include decreased acuity, scotoma, color blindness, or visual defects (usually reversible with discontinuation, irreversible blindness has been described)
Renal: Nephritis
Respiratory: Infiltrates (with or without eosinophilia), pneumonitis
Miscellaneous: Anaphylaxis, anaphylactoid reaction; hypersensitivity syndrome (rash, eosinophilia, and organ-specific inflammation)
Signs and Symptoms of Overdose Alopecia, anorexia, arthralgia, blindness, disorientation, eosinophilia, fever, hallucinations, hyperuricemia, jaundice, mental confusion, nausea, neuropathy (peripheral), neutropenia, numbness of the extremities, optic neuropathy, purpura, toxic epidermal necrolysis, visual changes, vomiting

Admission Criteria/Prognosis Admit any patient with CNS abnormalities or ingestions >8 g in adults
Pharmacodynamics/Kinetics
Absorption: ~80%
Distribution: Widely throughout body; concentrated in kidneys, lungs, saliva, and red blood cells
Relative diffusion from blood into CSF: Adequate with or without inflammation (exceeds usual MICs)
CSF:blood level ratio: Normal meninges: 0%; Inflamed meninges: 25%
Protein binding: 20% to 30%
Metabolism: Hepatic (20%) to inactive metabolite
Half-life elimination: 2.5-3.6 hours; End-stage renal disease: 7-15 hours
Time to peak, serum: 2-4 hours
Excretion: Urine (~50%) and feces (20%) as unchanged drug
Dosage
Oral:
Ethambutol is generally not recommended in children whose visual acuity cannot be monitored. However, ethambutol should be considered for all children with organisms resistant to other drugs, when susceptibility to ethambutol has been demonstrated, or susceptibility is likely.
Note: A four-drug regimen (isoniazid, rifampin, pyrazinamide, and either streptomycin or ethambutol) is preferred for the initial, empiric treatment of TB. When the drug susceptibility results are available, the regimen should be altered as appropriate.
Children and Adults:
Daily therapy: 15-25 mg/kg/day (maximum: 2.5 g/day)
Directly observed therapy (DOT): Twice weekly: 50 mg/kg (maximum: 2.5 g)
DOT: 3 times/week: 25-30 mg/kg (maximum: 2.5 g)
Adults: Treatment of disseminated *Mycobacterium avium* complex (MAC) in patients with advanced HIV infection: 15 mg/kg ethambutol in combination with azithromycin 600 mg daily
Dosing interval in renal impairment:
Cl$_{cr}$ 10-50 mL/minute: Administer every 24-36 hours
Cl$_{cr}$ <10 mL/minute: Administer every 48 hours
Hemodialysis: Slightly dialyzable (5% to 20%); Administer dose postdialysis
Peritoneal dialysis: Dose for Cl$_{cr}$ <10 mL/minute
Continuous arteriovenous or venovenous hemofiltration: Administer every 24-36 hours
Monitoring Parameters Baseline and periodic (monthly) visual testing (each eye individually, as well as both eyes tested together) in patients receiving >15 mg/kg/day; baseline and periodic renal, hepatic, and hematopoietic tests
Contraindications Hypersensitivity to ethambutol or any component of the formulation; optic neuritis; use in children, unconscious patients, or any other patient who may be unable to discern and report visual changes
Warnings May cause optic neuritis, resulting in decreased visual acuity or other vision changes. Discontinue promptly in patients with changes in vision, color blindness, or visual defects (effects normally reversible, but reversal may require up to a year). Use only in children whose visual acuity can accurately be determined and monitored (not recommended for use in children <13 years of age unless the benefit outweighs the risk). Dosage modification is required in patients with renal insufficiency. Hepatic toxicity has been reported, possibly due to concurrent therapy.
Dosage Forms Tablet, as hydrochloride: 100 mg, 400 mg
Reference Range Peak plasma ethambutol level after a dose of 25 mg/kg: ~5 mcg/mL
Overdosage/Treatment
Decontamination: Activated charcoal/lavage within 1 hour
Supportive therapy: Replace potassium/sodium losses
Enhancement of elimination: Slightly dialyzable (5% to 20%) and possibly effective
Test Interactions ↑ uric acid (S)
Drug Interactions Decreased absorption with aluminum hydroxide. Avoid concurrent administration of aluminum-containing antacids for at least 4 hours following ethambutol.
Pregnancy Risk Factor B
Pregnancy Implications There are no adequate and well-controlled studies in pregnant women; teratogenic effects have been seen in animals. Ethambutol has been used safely during pregnancy.
Lactation Enters breast milk/use caution (AAP considers "compatible")
Additional Information Incidence of optic neuropathy increases significantly with dosages above 15 mg/kg/day but may be idiosyncratic

---

Ethchlorvynol

Related Information
• Therapeutic Drugs Associated with Hallucinations
CAS Number 113-18-8
Impairment Potential Yes
Use Short-term management of insomnia
Mechanism of Action A chlorinated acetylenic carbinol which causes nonspecific depression of the reticular activating system

Adverse Reactions

Cardiovascular: Bradycardia, sinus bradycardia

Central nervous system: Facial numbness, residual sedation, headache, **dizziness**, psychosis, nervousness, excitation, clumsiness, confusion, drowsiness (daytime), visual hallucinations, slurred speech, retrograde amnesia, gustatory hallucinations

Dermatologic: Rash

Gastrointestinal: **Nausea, indigestion, stomach pain, unpleasant aftertaste**, vomiting

Genitourinary: Urinary retention

Hematologic: Thrombocytopenia, porphyria, pancytopenia

Hepatic: Jaundice

Neuromuscular & skeletal: **Weakness**, trembling

Ocular: **Blurred vision**, diplopia, mydriasis, nystagmus

Renal: Myoglobinuria

Respiratory: Dyspnea

Miscellaneous: **Unpleasant aftertaste** (mint-like)

Signs and Symptoms of Overdose Ataxia, bradycardia, bullous skin lesions, cough, hypotension, hypothermia, myopathy, numbness, pleural effusion, prolonged coma lasting over 100 hours, pulmonary edema, respiratory depression, rhabdomyolysis

Pharmacodynamics/Kinetics

Onset of action: 15-60 minutes

Duration: 5 hours

Absorption: Rapidly

Metabolism: Hepatic

Half-life elimination: 10-20 hours

Time to peak, serum: 2 hours

Excretion: Urine

Dosage Adults: Oral: 500-1000 mg at bedtime

Dosing adjustment in renal impairment: $Cl_{cr} < 50$ mL/minute: Avoid use

Monitoring Parameters Cardiac and respiratory function and abuse potential

Contraindications Hypersensitivity to ethchlorvynol or any component of the formulation; porphyria

Warnings Administer with caution to depressed or suicidal patients or to patients with a history of drug abuse; intoxication symptoms may appear with prolonged daily doses of as little as 1 g; withdrawal symptoms may be seen upon abrupt discontinuation; use with caution in the elderly and in patients with hepatic or renal dysfunction; use with caution in patients who have a history of paradoxical restlessness to barbiturates or alcohol; some products may contain tartrazine

Dosage Forms Capsule: 200 mg, 500 mg, 750 mg

Reference Range

Therapeutic: 2-8 mcg/mL

Toxic: >20 mcg/mL

Overdosage/Treatment

Decontamination: Lavage (within 1 hour)/activated charcoal

Supportive therapy: Hypotension can be treated with isotonic saline infusion (10-20 mL/kg), and/or dopamine or norepinephrine

Enhancement of elimination: Multiple dosing of activated charcoal is effective for ingestions >10 g (or over 100 mg/kg); or for prolonged coma; hemodialysis (or preferably hemoperfusion) should be initiated; consider hemodialysis/hemoperfusion if ethchlorvynol serum levels are >10 mcg/mL; monitor for rebound effect with redistribution of drug from fat storage; thus prolonged or repeated hemoperfusion may be needed; ~17% to 23% of the drug can be removed during 4 hours of hemodialysis or hemoperfusion

Antidote(s)

- DOPamine [ANTIDOTE]
- Norepinephrine [ANTIDOTE]

Drug Interactions

CNS depressants: Sedative effects may be additive with other CNS depressants; monitor for increased effect; includes benzodiazepines, barbiturates, antipsychotics, ethanol, and other sedative medications

Warfarin: May inhibit the hypoprothrombinemic response to warfarin via an unknown mechanism; monitor for altered anticoagulant effect or consider using a benzodiazepine

Pregnancy Risk Factor C

Nursing Implications Raise bed rails, institute safety measures, assist with ambulation

Ethionamide

CAS Number 536-33-4

U.S. Brand Names Trecator®-SC

Use In conjunction with other antituberculosis agents in the treatment of tuberculosis and other mycobacterial diseases

Mechanism of Action Inhibits peptide synthesis

Adverse Reactions

Cardiovascular: Postural hypotension

Central nervous system: Drowsiness, psychosis, dizziness, seizures, headache, peripheral neuritis (sensory neuropathy)

Dermatologic: Rash

Endocrine & metabolic: Hypoglycemia, goiter, gynecomastia

Gastrointestinal: **Nausea, vomiting**, abdominal pain, diarrhea, **anorexia**, metallic taste, stomatitis

Hematologic: Thrombocytopenia, porphyria

Hepatic: Hepatitis

Ocular: Optic neuritis, photophobia, diplopia

Signs and Symptoms of Overdose Anorexia, arthralgia, extensor plantar response, hypoglycemia, impotence, neuropathy (peripheral), paresthesias, personality changes, stomatitis, vision color changes (increased color perception)

Pharmacodynamics/Kinetics

Absorption: Rapid, complete

Distribution: Crosses placenta; V_d: 93.5 L

Protein binding: ~30%

Metabolism: Extensively hepatic to active and inactive metabolites

Bioavailability: 80%

Half-life elimination: 2-3 hours

Time to peak, serum: 1 hour

Excretion: Urine (<1% as unchanged drug; as active and inactive metabolites)

Dosage

Oral:

Children: 15-20 mg/kg/day in 2 divided doses, not to exceed 1 g/day

Adults: 500-1000 mg/day in 1-3 divided doses

Dosing adjustment in renal impairment: $Cl_{cr} < 50$ mL/minute: Administer 50% of dose

Monitoring Parameters Initial and periodic serum ALT and AST

Administration

Neurotoxic effects may be relieved by the administration of pyridoxine (6-100 mg daily, lower doses are more common). May be taken with or without meals. Gastrointestinal adverse effects may be decreased by administration at bedtime, decreased dose, or giving antiemetics.

Contraindications Hypersensitivity to ethionamide or any component of the formulation; severe hepatic impairment

Warnings Use with caution in patients with diabetes mellitus; use with caution in patients receiving cycloserine or isoniazid. Use caution when switching patients from the sugar-coated tablet formulation (Trecator®-SC) to film-coated tablet (Trecator®); the dosage may need retitrated in order to avoid intolerance.

Dosage Forms Tablet: 250 mg

Reference Range Peak serum concentration: 2 mcg/mL after an oral dose of 250 mg

Overdosage/Treatment

Decontamination: Charcoal/lavage within 1 hour as indicated

Supportive therapy: Neurologic symptoms may resolve with pyridoxine or nicotinamide therapy

Test Interactions ↓ thyroxine (S)

Pregnancy Risk Factor C

Pregnancy Implications Crosses the placenta

Lactation Excretion in breast milk unknown/use caution

Ethosuximide

Related Information

- Therapeutic Drugs Associated with Hallucinations

CAS Number 77-67-8

U.S. Brand Names Zarontin®

Impairment Potential Yes

Use Management of absence (petit mal) seizures, myoclonic seizures, and akinetic epilepsy

Mechanism of Action Increases the seizure threshold and suppresses paroxysmal spike-and-wave pattern in absence seizures; depresses nerve transmission in the motor cortex

Adverse Reactions

Cardiovascular: Raynaud's phenomenon

Central nervous system: **Sedation, dizziness, drowsiness, euphoria**, visual hallucinations, **insomnia**, psychosis (especially in pediatric patients), **agitation, behavioral changes**, parkinsonism, **headache, ataxia, lethargy, hallucinations**

Dermatologic: Rashes, **Stevens-Johnson syndrome**, hypertrichosis, alopecia, urticaria, scleroderma, pruritus, exanthem

Gastrointestinal: **Nausea, vomiting, anorexia** (dose related), **abdominal pain** (epigastric), **weight loss**, gingival hyperplasia

Hematologic: Leukopenia, aplastic anemia, thrombocytopenia

Hepatic: Liver enzyme elevation

Ocular: Photophobia, diplopia

Miscellaneous: **Hiccups, systemic lupus erythematosus**

Signs and Symptoms of Overdose Agranulocytosis, granulocytopenia, insomnia myasthenia gravis (exacerbation or precipitation), neutropenia

Acute overdosage can cause ataxia, CNS depression, coma, hypotension, stupor

Chronic overdose can cause albuminuria, confusion, dementia, erythema multiforme, extrapyramidal reaction, hematuria, hepatic dysfunction, leukopenia, skin rash

Pharmacodynamics/Kinetics

Distribution: Adults: V_d: 0.62-0.72 L/kg

Metabolism: Hepatic (~80% to 3 inactive metabolites)

Half-life elimination, serum: Children: 30 hours; Adults: 50-60 hours

Time to peak, serum: Capsule: ~2-4 hours; Syrup: <2-4 hours

Excretion: Urine, slowly (50% as metabolites, 10% to 20% as unchanged drug); feces (small amounts)

Dosage

Oral:

Children 3-6 years: Initial: 250 mg/day (or 15 mg/kg/day) in 2 divided doses; increase every 4-7 days; usual maintenance dose: 15-40 mg/kg/day in 2 divided doses

Children >6 years and Adults: Initial: 250 mg twice daily; increase by 250 mg as needed every 4-7 days up to 1.5 g/day in 2 divided doses; usual maintenance dose: 20-40 mg/kg/day in 2 divided doses

Monitoring Parameters Seizure frequency, trough serum concentrations; CBC, platelets, liver enzymes, urinalysis

Administration Administer with food or milk to avoid GI upset

Contraindications Hypersensitivity to succinimides or any component of the formulation

Warnings Use with caution in patients with hepatic or renal disease; abrupt withdrawal of the drug may precipitate absence status; ethosuximide may increase tonic-clonic seizures in patients with mixed seizure disorders; ethosuximide must be used in combination with other anticonvulsants in patients with both absence and tonic-clonic seizures. Succinimides have been associated with severe blood dyscrasias and cases of systemic lupus erythematosus. Consider evaluation of blood counts in patients with signs/symptoms of infection. Safety and efficacy in patients <3 years of age have not been established.

Dosage Forms Capsule: 250 mg

Syrup: 250 mg/5 mL (473 mL) [contains sodium benzoate; raspberry flavor]

Reference Range

Therapeutic: 40-100 mcg/mL (SI: 280-710 µmol/L)

Toxic: >100 mcg/mL (SI: >710 µmol/L); at steady-state, each 1 mg/kg will result in a serum rise of 2 mcg/mL

Overdosage/Treatment

Decontamination: Lavage (within 1 hour)/activated charcoal

Supportive therapy: Treatment is supportive; benzodiazepine (diazepam or lorazepam) for seizures

Enhanced elimination: Hemoperfusion and hemodialysis may be useful; hemodialysis has an extraction efficiency of 61% to 100%; forced diuresis is not useful; multiple dosing of activated charcoal may be useful; hemodialyzer clearance is ~140 mL/minute

Test Interactions ↑ alkaline phosphatase (S); positive Coombs' [direct]; ↓ calcium (S)

Drug Interactions Substrate of CYP3A4 (major)

CNS depressants: Sedative effects and/or respiratory depression may be additive with CNS depressants; includes ethanol, benzodiazepines, barbiturates, narcotic analgesics, and other sedative agents; monitor for increased effect

CYP3A4 inducers: CYP3A4 inducers may decrease the levels/effects of ethosuximide. Example inducers include aminoglutethimide, carbamazepine, nafcillin, nevirapine, phenobarbital, phenytoin, and rifamycins.

CYP3A4 inhibitors: May increase the levels/effects of ethosuximide. Example inhibitors include azole antifungals, clarithromycin, diclofenac, doxycycline, erythromycin, imatinib, isoniazid, nefazodone, nicardipine, propofol, protease inhibitors, quinidine, telithromycin, and verapamil.

Isoniazid: May inhibit hepatic metabolism of ethosuximide with a resultant increase in ethosuximide serum concentrations

Phenytoin: Ethosuximide may elevate phenytoin levels; phenytoin may decrease ethosuximide levels (see enzyme inducers)

Valproic acid: Has been reported to both increase and decrease ethosuximide levels

Pregnancy Risk Factor C

Pregnancy Implications Low teratogenicity in mice

Lactation Enters breast milk/compatible

Nursing Implications Observe patient for excess sedation

Additional Information Considered to be drug of choice for simple absence seizures

Ethotoin

Pronunciation (ETH oh toyn)

CAS Number 86-35-1

U.S. Brand Names Peganone®

Synonyms Ethylphenylhydantoin

Use Generalized tonic-clonic or complex-partial seizures

Mechanism of Action Exerts an anticonvulsant effect without causing general central nervous system depression. The mechanism of action is believed to be similar to that of phenytoin which appears to stabilize the normal seizure threshold and to prevent the spread of seizure activity rather than to abolish the primary focus of seizure discharges. Ethotoin is effective in protecting against electroshock seizures and, to a lesser extent, against pentylenetetrazol-induced seizures in laboratory animals.

Adverse Reactions

Frequency not defined.

Cardiovascular: Arrhythmias, ataxia, cardiovascular collapse, venous irritation and pain

Central nervous system: Psychiatric changes, slurred speech, trembling, dizziness, drowsiness, headache, insomnia

Dermatologic: Skin rash, Stevens-Johnson syndrome

Gastrointestinal: Constipation, nausea, vomiting, gingival hyperplasia, anorexia, weight loss

Hematologic: Leukopenia, blood dyscrasias

Hepatic: Hepatitis

Local: Thrombophlebitis

Neuromuscular & skeletal: Paresthesia, peripheral neuropathy

Ocular: Nystagmus

Renal: Serum creatinine increased

Miscellaneous: Lymphadenopathy, SLE-like syndrome

Signs and Symptoms of Overdose Anemia (megaloblastic), ataxia, bradycardia, coma, diplopia, gingival hyperplasia, hypotension, insomnia, numbness

Toxicodynamics/Kinetics

Absorption: Rapidly although the extent of oral absorption is unknown

Metabolism: Exhibits saturable metabolism relative to the formation of N-diethyl and p-hydroxylethotoin which are the major metabolites

Half-life: 3-9 hours with low plasma levels (<8 mcg/mL); average: ~5 hours; above this concentration, the half-life may be prolonged because of the nonlinear kinetics

Dosage

Oral:

Children: 30-60 mg/kg/day or 250 mg twice daily, may be increased up to 2-3 g/day

Adults: 250 mg 4 times/day after meals, may be increased up to 3 g/day in divided doses 4 times/day

Contraindications Hypersensitivity to ethotoin or any component of the formulation; hepatic abnormalities; hematologic disorders; pregnancy; breast-feeding

Warnings Avoid abrupt withdrawal (can precipitate status epilepticus); hypersensitivity reactions may occur

Dosage Forms Tablet: 250 mg

Reference Range Although the therapeutic range is poorly documented, most reports indicate that therapeutic plasma concentrations fall between 15-50 mcg/mL

Overdosage/Treatment

Decontamination: Lavage (within 1 hour)/activated charcoal

Supportive: Bradycardia may be treated with atropine; benzodiazepine or phenobarbital for seizures

Enhancement of elimination: Multiple dosing of activated charcoal may be useful

Test Interactions ↑ alkaline phosphatase (S); ↓ calcium (S)

Drug Interactions Inhibits CYP2C19 (weak)

Pregnancy Risk Factor D

Pregnancy Implications Maternal ingestion of antiepileptic agents has been associated with neonatal coagulation defects/bleeding usually within 24 hours of birth.

Lactation Enters breast milk/not recommended

Ethyl Alcohol

Related Information

● Substance-Related Disorders

CAS Number 64-17-5

UN Number 1170

Impairment Potential Yes. Blood ethanol >0.03% may cause driving impairment. Most studies report significant impairment (particularly eye movement, glare resistance, visual perception, and reaction time) at blood ethanol levels of 0.05%; and 94% of studies report impairment at 0.08%. At blood ethanol levels of ~0.02%, the ability to divide attention between two or more visual stimuli is impaired. At blood ethanol levels between 0.08% and 0.10%, the relative risk of a fatal single-vehicle crash varies between 11% (for drivers 35 years of age and older) and 52% (for male drivers 16-20 years of age). See figure.

Comparison of Various Categories of Alcohol-Related Effects as Function of Blood Alcohol Concentrations

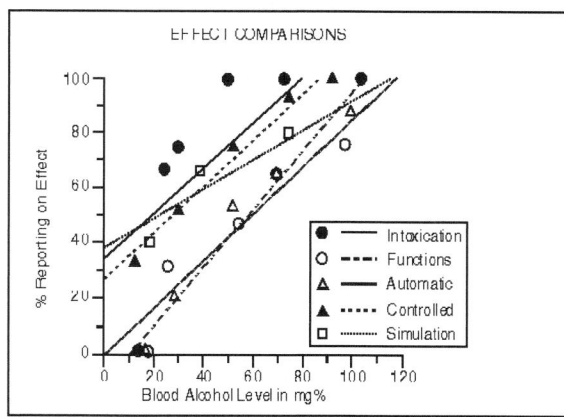

From Brain Information Service, Brain Research Institute, University of California, Los Angeles, CA 90024-1746.

Use Topical anti-infective; pharmaceutical aid; as an antidote for ethylene glycol overdose; as antidote for methanol overdose; may also be useful in propylene glycol. See Alcohol, Ethyl [ANTIDOTE]

Mechanism of Action Central nervous system depressant

Adverse Reactions

Cardiovascular: Tachycardia, hypertension, fibrillation (atrial), flutter (atrial), cardiomegaly, angina, chest pain, congestive heart failure, sinus tachycardia, tachycardia (supraventricular), arrhythmias (ventricular), vasodilation

Central nervous system: Ataxia, dementia, Wernicke-Korsakoff syndrome, amnesia, paranoia, hyperthermia, aggressive behavior, leukoencephalopathy

Gastrointestinal: Nausea, diarrhea, abdominal pain, dyspepsia, vomiting, GI hemorrhage, anorexia, pancreatitis, decreased esophageal sphincter tone

Hematologic: Porphyria, megaloblastic anemia

Hepatic: Hepatic cirrhosis, fatty degeneration of liver, hepatic steatosis, impaired gluconeogenesis, aminotransferase level elevation (asymptomatic)

Neuromuscular & skeletal: Dysarthria, neuropathy (peripheral), osteoporosis

Ocular: Visual evoked potential abnormalities

Miscellaneous: Impaired judgment, hiccups, breast cancer, acute atraumatic compartment syndrome; see Impairment Potential

Signs and Symptoms of Overdose Acetone breath, acidosis, apnea, atrial tachycardia, cardiomyopathy, chorea (extrapyramidal), CNS depression, dementia, depression, diplopia, dysphagia, encephalopathy, fever, gynecomastia, hyperuricemia, hyperventilation, hypocalcemia, hypoglycemia (3.4%), hypokalemia, hypomagnesemia, hyponatremia, hypophosphatemia, hyporeflexia, hypotension, hypothermia, impotence, leukocytosis, lymphopenia, mydriasis, myocardial depression, myoclonus, myoglobinuria, myopathy, numbness, nystagmus, optic neuropathy, ototoxicity, paresthesia, porphyria, rhabdomyolysis, respiratory depression, sedation, seizures, tremors, thrombocytopenia, tinnitus

Admission Criteria/Prognosis Any pediatric patient with electrolyte or acid-base disturbance or ingestion of >60 mL of cosmetic fragrances should be admitted

Toxicodynamics/Kinetics

Distribution: V_d: 0.6 L/kg

Metabolism: Hepatic to acetaldehyde by alcohol dehydrogenase at a rate of 10-30 mg/dL/hour

Dosage I.V. doses of 100-125 mg/kg/hour to maintain blood levels of 100 mg/dL are recommended after a loading dose of 0.6 g/kg; maximum dose: 400 mL of a 5% solution within 1 hour

Administration Caution must be taken to avoid extravasation; administer only by slow I.V. infusion

Reference Range Levels >100 mg/dL can cause nausea and vomiting; levels >300 mg/dL can be associated with coma and fatalities

Overdosage/Treatment

Decontamination: Lavage within 2 hours/activated charcoal

Supportive therapy: Flumazenil (2-5 mg) or naloxone may alleviate respiratory depression but not CNS depression, there is conflicting data regarding these two agents; crystalloid infusion for hypotension (will not increase ethanol clearance); monitor glucose; thiamine (50-100 mg) should also be given; monitor magnesium level; for rate control of atrial fibrillation, digoxin or I.V. diltiazem can be used; lorazepam (2 mg I.V.) can prevent recurrent seizures due to ethanol

Enhancement of elimination: Hemodialysis removes 50% to 100%; clearance of ethanol through hemodialysis is ~300-400 mL/minute with an ethanol removal rate of 280 mg/minute

Antidote(s)

- Alcohol, Ethyl [ANTIDOTE]
- Flumazenil [ANTIDOTE]

Diagnostic Procedures

- Alcohol, Semiquantitative, Urine
- Alcohol, Serum

Test Interactions ↑ ammonia (B), creatine phosphokinase (CPK) (S), serum osmolarity gap increases an average of 20 mOsm for every 100 mg/dL of ethanol; ↓ glucose, magnesium

Pregnancy Risk Factor D/X (prolonged use or high doses at term)

Pregnancy Implications Causes fetal alcohol syndrome, facial dysmorphias, growth retardation

Additional Information

Energy content of ethanol: 7.1 kcal (29.7 kg) per g

Highest serum level recorded with full recovery: 1510 mg/dL (327.8 mM/L) in an adult; in an adolescent it is 757 mg/dL; children who ingest a significant amount of alcohol should be monitored hourly for up to 6 hours; elevated serum lactate and lactate dehydrogenase levels may interfere with enzymatic ethanol assays; intravenous dexamethasone (2 mg I.V.) can impair ethyl alcohol's ability to stimulate sympathetic nerve discharge and thus suppress alcohol-induced high blood pressure in the acute state

Moderate drinking is defined as not more than 2 drinks (28 g) of ethanol daily in men and only 1 drink (14 g) daily in women. Corpus callosum atrophy can occur in the brain with chronic ethyl alcohol intake; daily ingestion of 40-60 g of ethanol in men and 20 g of ethanol in women can significantly increase the incidence of cirrhosis in individuals who are well nourished.

While the reduced risk for coronary heart disease by ethanol appears to be related to elevation of high density lipoprotein (HDL cholesterol) levels, the maximal benefit appears to be at the amount of one drink daily. Hepatic toxicity can occur at lower ethanol amounts in women as opposed to men. Serum selenium levels are significantly lower (24 ng/mL versus 39 ng/mL in control patients) in chronic alcohol abuse patients.

Odor threshold: 10 ppm; TLV-TWA: 1000 ppm.

Ethanol Content	
Beverages	**Percent Ethanol**
7-Up (diet)	0.077
7-Up (diet cherry)	0.017
Ale	5-8
Beer	4-6
Bourbon	40-50
Brandy	35-40
Calistoga Lemon Flavor	0.096
Calistoga Lime Flavor	0.084
Cognac	40-41
Coca-Cola (Caffeine-free, diet)	0.005
Coca-Cola	0.004
Distilled liquors	22-50
Dr. Pepper (diet)	0.024
Fruit Punch (Hawaiian Punch orange creme)	0.040
Fruit Punch (Tropicana)	0.096
Fruit Punch (Veryfine papaya)	0.058
Gin	40-47
Ginger ale (Canada Dry)	0.065
Lemonade (Elliott's)	0.037
Light beer	2.5-3.5
Mountain Dew	0.024
Peppermint Schnapps	20-30
Root beer (A&W)	0.004
Rum	40-41
Scotch	40-50
Second Wind (sports drink)	0.025
Slice (lemon-lime)	0.056
Sprite (diet)	0.054
Tea (Elliott's Brewed Ice)	0.017
Tequila	40-46
Vodka	40-41
Whiskey	40-45
Wine	10-18
Nonmedicinal	
Cements	7-30
Colognes and perfumes	40-60

Table (Continued)	
Beverages	**Percent Ethanol**
Gasohol	10
Glass cleaners	10
Hair tonics	25-65
Liquid hand-washing detergent	1-10
Paint stripper	25
Medicinal (Oral)	
Cough/cold preparations	3-25
Geritol®	12
Homeopathic/herbal medicine	Varies
Mouthwashes	14-27
Vitameatavegamin	23

Mid-Year 2000 Emergency Department Drug Abuse Warning Network (DAWN) data: Mentions of alcohol-in-combination occurred in 33% (97,143) of Emergency Department drug episodes in the first half of 2000. Mentions of alcohol-in-combination remained stable between the first half of 1999 and the first half of 2000.
See figure.

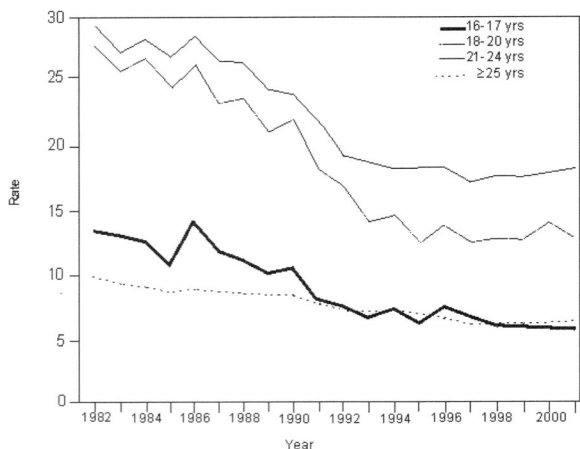

Rate* of Drinking Drivers in Fatal Alcohol-Related Crashes, by Age Group
Fatality Analysis Reporting System, United States, 1982-2001†

*Per 100,000 population
†Because of the unavailability of census data, crash rates for 2001 were calculated by using 2000 population estimates.

Specific References

Burnhill Jr. MT, Herbert D, Wells Jr. DJ, "Comparison of Hospital Laboratory Serum Alcohol Levels Obtained by an Enzymatic Method with Whole Blood Levels Forensically Determined by Gas Chromatography," *J Anal Tox*, 2007, 31:23-30.

Centers for Disease Control and Prevention (CDC), "Alcohol Consumption Among Women Who Are Pregnant or Who Might Become Pregnant–United States, 2002," *MMWR Morb Mortal Wkly Rep*, 2004, 53(50):1178-81.

Chan GM, Su M, Donnelly JG, et al, "Serum Homocysteine Levels Do Not Correlate with Severity of Alcohol Withdrawal," *J Toxicol Clin Toxicol*, 2003, 41(5):745.

Collison IB, "Elevated Postmortem Ethanol Concentrations in an Insulin-Dependent Diabetic," *J Anal Toxicol*, 2005, 29:762-4.

Cukor JM, Rose RB, Fleming JK, et al, "Relationship Between Traumatic Injury, Alcohol Consumption, and Previous Emergency Department Visits: Opportunity for Early Screening and Intervention?" *SAEM Annual Meeting Abstracts*, 2004, 544.

Edwards RP, Flammia DD, Pearson JM, et al, "Driving Under the Influence of Drugs (DUID) Cases in Virginia for 2001," *J Anal Toxicol*, 2003, 27(3):188.

Gaetz A, Miner JR, Biros M, et al, "Breath Alcohol Concentration, Bispectral Index, and a Standardized Scale as Predictors of Observation Time for Intoxicated Patients," *SAEM Annual Meeting Abstracts*, 2004, 468-9.

Gentilello LM, "Alcohol Interventions in Trauma Centers: The Opportunity and the Challenge," *J Trauma*, 2006, 59(3 Suppl):S18-20.

Gowda RM, Khan IA, Vasavada BC, et al, "Alcohol-Triggered Acute Myocardial Infarction," *Am J Ther*, 2003, 10(1):71-2.

Haas CE, Magram Y, and Mishra A, "Rhabdomyolysis and Acute Renal Failure Following an Ethanol and Diphenhydramine Overdose," *Ann Pharmacother*, 2003, 37(4):538-42.

Helander A and Beck O, "Ethyl Sulfate: A Metabolite of Ethanol in Humans and a Potential Biomarker of Acute Alcohol Intake," *J Anal Toxicol*, 2005, 29(5):270-4.

Hochman S, Hung O, and Shih RD, "Methods of Determining Sobriety in Evaluating Alcohol-Intoxicated Patients," *Ann Emerg Med*, 2003, 42(4):S21.

Holstege CP, Ferguson JD, Wolf CE, et al, "Analysis of Moonshine for Contaminants," *J Toxicol Clin Toxicol*, 2004, 42(5):597-601.

Honey D, Caylor C, Luthi R, et al, "Comparative Alcohol Concentrations in Blood and Vitreous Fluid with Illustrative Case Studies," *J Anal Toxicol*, 2005, 29(5):365-9.

Hungerford DW, Williams JM, Furbee PM, et al, "Feasibility of Screening and Intervention for Alcohol Problems Among Young Adults in the ED," *Am J Emerg Med*, 2003, 21(1):14-22.

Jivcu C, Lotfipour S, Winn D, et al, "The Role of Alcohol in Traffic Collisions Involving Older Drivers in Orange County, California," *SAEM Annual Meeting Abstracts*, 2004, 544.

Johnson RD, Lewis RJ, Canfield DV, et al, "Ethanol Origin in Postmortem Urine: The LC/MS Determination of Serotonin Metabolites," *J Anal Toxicol*, 2004, 28:297.

Jones AW, "Time-Adjusted Urine/Blood Ratios of Ethanol in Drinking Drivers," *J Anal Toxicol*, 2003, 27(3):167-8.

Kancler J, "Static Headspace Analysis of Alcohol and Common Abused Inhalants in Blood Using Dual-Column Gas Chromatography," *J Anal Toxicol*, 2004, 28:290.

Karlovsek MZ and Balazic J, "Evaluation of the Post-Rotational Nystagmus Test (PRN) in Determining Alcohol Intoxication," *J Anal Toxicol*, 2005, 29(5):390-3.

Leman P, Greene SL, Kerins M, et al, "The Effect of Alcohol Co-Ingestion on Patient Behaviour in Acute Drug Overdose," *J Toxicol Clin Toxicol*, 2003, 41(5):743.

Martinez S, Enriquez P, and Kerrigan S, "Drug-Impaired Driving in New Mexico: A Six-Year Retrospective Study," *J Anal Toxicol*, 2003, 27(3): 180-1.

Mello MJ, Nirenberg TD, Longabaugh R, et al, "Emergency Department Brief Motivational Interventions for Alcohol with Motor Vehicle Crash Patients," *Ann Emerg Med*, 2005, 45(6):620-5.

Miner JR, McCoy C, and Biros M, "A Standardized Intoxication Scale vs Breath Ethanol Level as a Predictor of Observation Time in the Emergency Department," *Acad Emerg Med*, 2003, 10:520.

Morris-Kukoski CL, Jagerdeo E, Schaff JE, et al, "Ethanol Analysis from Biological Samples by Dual Arm Robotic Autosampler," *J Anal Toxicol*, 2006, 30:131.

Mozayani A, Schrode P, Carter J, et al, "A Multiple Drug Fatality Involving MK-801 (Dizocilpine), A Mimic of Phencyclidine," *Forensic Sci Int*, 2003, 133(1-2):113-7.

Mukamal KJ, Conigrave KM, Mittleman MA, et al, "Roles of Drinking Pattern and Type of Alcohol Consumed in Coronary Heart Disease in Men," *N Engl J Med*, 2003, 348(2):109-18.

O'Connor AD, Rusyniak DE, and Bruno A., "Cerebrovascular and Cardiovascular Complications of Alcohol and Sympathomimetic Drug Abuse, *Med Clin North Am*, 2005, 89(6):1343-58 (review).

Olsen T and Hearn WL, "Stability of Ethanol in Postmortem Blood and Vitreous Humor in Long-Term Refrigerated Storage," *J Anal Toxicol*, 2003, 27:517-9.

Pedersen-Bjergaard U, Reubsaet JL, Nielsen SL, et al, "Psychoactive Drugs, Alcohol, and Severe Hypoglycemia in Insulin-Treated Diabetes: Analysis of 141 Cases," *Am J Med*, 2005, 118(3):307-10.

Pemberton ML and Logan BK, "Driver Behavior, Responses and Performance with Blood Alcohol Concentration (BAC) Greater than 0.30 g/100 mL," *J Anal Toxicol*, 2004, 28:291.

Pittler MH, Verster JC, and Ernst E, "Interventions for Preventing or Treating Alcohol Hangover: Systematic Review of Randomised Controlled Trials," *BMJ*, 2006, 331(7531):1515-8 (review).

Ratzan RM, "Ethanol and Embrace: Emergency Medicine and the Health Care Giver-Patient Relationship Revisited," *J Emerg Med*, 2003, 24(3):335-9.

Readie J, Hung OL, Hochman S, et al, "Determining Alcohol Elimination Rates in Chronic Alcoholics Presenting to the ED," *Clin Toxicol (Phila)*, 2005, 43:775.

Saitz R, Horton NJ, and Samet JH, "Alcohol and Medication Interactions in Primary Care Patients: Common and Unrecognized," *Am J Med*, 2003, 114(5):407-10.

Schwilke EW, dos Santos IS, and Logan BK, "Changes in Patterns of Drug and Alcohol Use in Fatally Injured Drivers in Washington State," *J Anal Toxicol*, 2004, 28:280.

Sezhian N, Rimal D, and Suresh G, "Isolated Intraperitoneal Bladder Rupture Following Minor Trauma After Alcohol Ingestion," *South Med J*, 2005, 98(5):573-4.

Stampfer MJ, Kang JH, Chen J, et al, "Effects of Moderate Alcohol Consumption on Cognitive Function in Women," *N Engl J Med*, 2005, 352(3):245-53.

Umberger LB, Tobin J, and Jufer RA, "*In vitro* Production of an Unusually High Ethanol Concentration in a Postmortem Blood Specimen," *J Anal Toxicol*, 2003, 27(3):185.

Wansink B and van Ittersum K, "Shape of Glass and Amount of Alcohol Poured: Comparative Study of Effect of Practice and Concentration," *BMJ*, 2006, 331(7531):1512-4.

Williams E, Fasano C, Bryant E, et al, "Effect of Ethanol and Glasgow Coma Scale Score on the Sensitivity of the History and Physical Examination in Detecting Acute Pelvic Trauma," *Ann Emerg Med*, 2003, 42(4):S98.

Zehtabchi S, Sinert R, Baron BJ, et al, "Does Ethanol Intoxication Explain the Acidosis Commonly Seen in Minor Trauma Patients?" *Acad Emerg Med*, 2004, 11(5):471.

Zehtabchi S, Sinert R, Baron BJ, et al, "Does Ethanol Explain the Acidosis Commonly Seen in Ethanol-Intoxicated Patients?" *Clin Toxicol (Phila)*, 2005, 43(3):161-6.

Ethyl Chloride

Pronunciation (ETH il KLOR ide)
CAS Number 75-00-3
UN Number 1037
U.S. Brand Names Gebauer's Ethyl Chloride®
Synonyms Chloroethane
Use
Medical: Local anesthetic in minor operative procedures and to relieve pain caused by insect stings and burns and irritation caused by myofascial and visceral pain syndromes
Industrial: Currently primarily utilized in the production of tetraethyl lead and ethyl cellulose; also used as a solvent and refrigerant
Mechanism of Action Results in tissue hypothermia (-10°C) when used topically
Adverse Reactions Gastrointestinal: Mucous membrane irritation, excessive salivation
Signs and Symptoms of Overdose Coma, laryngospasm, respiratory and cardiac arrest when taken systemically. Abdominal cramps, ataxia, chemical frostbite, coma, contact dermatitis, cyanosis, hepatomegaly, nausea, nystagmus, ocular irritation (at 40,000 ppm), unconsciousness, visual hallucinations, vomiting. Prolonged spraying may cause frostbite.
Toxicodynamics/Kinetics
Absorption: Readily through lungs; pulmonary route (82% retention); not absorbed dermally
Half-life: 1-3 minutes (when taken systemically)
Elimination: Through lungs
Dosage Dosage varies with use
Stability Refrigerate; store in airtight containers preferably hermetically sealed at a temperature not exceeding 15°C; protect from light
Administration Spray for a few seconds to the point of frost formation when the tissue becomes white; avoid prolonged spraying of skin beyond this point; avoid broken skin or mucous membranes
Dosage Forms Aerosol: 100% (103 mL) [available as a fine-point or medium spray]
Reference Range Serum ethyl chloride level of 200 mg/L associated with fatality following recreational use; postmortem ethyl chloride blood and urine levels of 423 mg/L and 35 mg/L, respectively, associated with fatality
Overdosage/Treatment Decontamination: **Dermal**: Irrigate exposed areas with soap and water; **Inhalation**: Administer 100% humidified oxygen
Pregnancy Risk Factor C
Additional Information
Spray for a few seconds to the point of frost formation when the tissue becomes white; avoid prolonged spraying of skin beyond this point. Essentially acts as a general anesthetic at air concentrations >30,000 ppm by means of interference of calcium-mediated channels in neurons.
Highly flammable; air concentrations >5% may be explosive.
Ambient air levels of 40,000 ppm can be fatal. IDLH: 20,000 ppm

Ethyl Loflazepate

CAS Number 29177-84-2
U.S. Brand Names Meilax; Victan
Synonyms Dichlorotetrafluoroethane and Ethyl Chloride
Use Short-term treatment of anxiety disorders
Mechanism of Action Binds to stereospecific benzodiazepine receptors on the postsynaptic GABA neuron at several sites within the central nervous system, including the limbic system, reticular formation. Enhancement of the inhibitory effect of GABA on neuronal excitability results by increased neuronal membrane permeability to chloride ions. This shift in chloride ions results in hyperpolarization (a less excitable state) and stabilization.

Adverse Reactions
Frequency not defined.
Cardiovascular: Hypotension
Central nervous system: Drowsiness, ataxia, amnesia, slurred speech, paradoxical excitement or rage, fatigue, insomnia, memory impairment, headache, anxiety, depression, vertigo, confusion
Dermatologic: Rash
Endocrine & metabolic: Changes in libido
Gastrointestinal: Changes in salivation, constipation, nausea
Genitourinary: Incontinence, urinary retention
Hepatic: Jaundice
Local: Phlebitis, pain with injection
Neuromuscular & skeletal: Dysarthria, tremor
Ocular: Blurred vision, diplopia
Respiratory: Decrease in respiratory rate, apnea
Pharmacodynamics/Kinetics
Metabolism: Hepatic to active metabolites
Half-life: 75-80 hours
Protein binding: Metabolites (99%)
Dosage Oral: 1-4 mg/day in single or divided doses
Dosage Forms Aerosol: Ethyl chloride 25% and dichlorotetrafluoroethane 75% (148 mL)
Reference Range Peak ethyl loflazepate serum concentrations after 4 mg dose is about 200 ng/mL
Overdosage/Treatment
Decontamination: Lavage (within 1 hour)/activated charcoal
Supportive therapy: Rarely is mechanical ventilation required; flumazenil has been shown to selectively block the binding of benzodiazepines to CNS receptors, resulting in a reversal of benzodiazepine-induced CNS depression and respiratory depression
Enhancement of elimination: Multiple dose activated charcoal may be effective
Pregnancy Risk Factor C
Specific References
Kamijo Y, Hayaski I, Nishikawa T, et al, "Pharmacokinetics of the Active Metabolites of Ethyl Loflazepate in Elderly Patients Who Died of Asphyxia Associated with Benzodiazepine-Related Toxicity," *J Anal Toxicol*, 2005, 29:140-4.

Etidronate Disodium

CAS Number 2809-21-4; 7414-83-7
U.S. Brand Names Didronel®
Synonyms EHDP; Sodium Etidronate
Use Symptomatic treatment of Paget's disease and heterotopic ossification due to spinal cord injury or after total hip replacement, hypercalcemia associated with malignancy
Postmenopausal osteoporosis
Mechanism of Action Decreases bone resorption by inhibiting osteocystic osteolysis; decreases mineral release and matrix or collagen breakdown in bone
Adverse Reactions
Endocrine & metabolic: Hyperphosphatemia, hypocalcemia, pseudogout
Gastrointestinal: Diarrhea, nausea, vomiting, altered taste
Hematologic: Occult blood in stools
Neuromuscular & skeletal: Risk of fractures (increased), microfractures, bone pain (increased), dose-related osteomalacia
Renal: Nephrotoxicity
Miscellaneous: Hypersensitivity reactions
Signs and Symptoms of Overdose Diarrhea, hypocalcemia, nausea
Pharmacodynamics/Kinetics
Onset of action:
Paget's disease: May be observed after 1 month of treatment; initially observed as a reduction in urinary hydroxyproline
Hypercalcemia: Reductions in urinary calcium excretion which accompany reductions in bone resorption; may become apparent after 24 hours
Duration of action: Cleared from blood in 6 hours
Absorption: Dependent upon dose administered; decreased oral absorption with calcium-rich foods
Distribution: ~$\frac{1}{2}$ absorbed dose is chemically absorbed to bone, presumably upon hydroxyapatite crystals, in areas of elevated osteogenesis
Metabolism: Not metabolized
Half-life: 5-7 hours in plasma; 90 days in bone
Elimination: Excreted as unchanged drug primarily in the urine with unabsorbed drug being eliminated in the feces
Onset of therapeutic effects: Within 1-3 months of therapy
Duration: 12 months without continuous therapy
Dosage
Adults:
Paget's disease: Oral: 5 mg/kg/day given every day for no more than 6 months; may give 10 mg/kg/day for up to 3 months; daily dose may be divided if adverse gastrointestinal effects occur

Heterotopic ossification with spinal cord injury: 20 mg/kg/day for 2 weeks, then 10 mg/kg/day for 10 weeks (this dosage has been used in children, however, treatment >1 year has been associated with a rachitic syndrome)

Hypercalcemia associated with malignancy:
  I.V. (dilute dose in at least 250 mL NS): 7.5 mg/kg/day for 3 days; there should be at least 7 days between courses of treatment
  Oral: Start 20 mg/kg/day on the last day of infusion and continue for 30-90 days

Dosing adjustment in renal impairment:
  S_{cr} 2.5-5 mg/dL: Use with caution
  S_{cr} >5 mg/dL: Do not use

Stability Dilute I.V. dose in at least 250 mL NS; stable for 48 hours at room temperature or refrigerated

Monitoring Parameters Serum calcium and phosphorous; serum creatinine and BUN

Administration
  I.V. doses should be diluted in at least 250 mL normal saline.

Contraindications Hypersensitivity to bisphosphonates or any component of the formulation; overt osteomalacia

Warnings

Ensure adequate calcium and vitamin D intake. Etidronate may retard mineralization of bone; treatment may need delayed or interrupted until callus is present. Use caution in patients with renal impairment. Use caution with enterocolitis; diarrhea has been reported at high doses and therapy may need to be withheld.

Bisphosphonate therapy has been associated with osteonecrosis, primarily of the jaw; this has been observed mostly in cancer patients, but also in patients with postmenopausal osteoporosis and other diagnoses. Risk factors include a diagnosis of cancer, with concomitant chemotherapy, radiotherapy or corticosteroids; anemia, coagulopathy, infection or pre-existing dental disease. Symptoms included nonhealing extraction socket or an exposed jawbone. There are no data addressing whether discontinuation of therapy reduces the risk of developing osteonecrosis. However, as a precautionary measure, dental exams and preventative dentistry should be performed prior to placing patients with risk factors on chronic bisphosphonate therapy. Invasive dental procedures should be avoided during treatment.

Infrequently, severe (and occasionally debilitating) bone, joint, and/or muscle pain have been reported during bisphosphonate treatment. The onset of pain ranged from a single day to several months. Symptoms usually resolve upon discontinuation. Some patients experienced recurrence when rechallenged with same drug or another bisphosphonate; avoid use in patients with a history of these symptoms in association with bisphosphonate therapy.

Safety and efficacy in pediatric patients have not been established.

Dosage Forms Tablet: 200 mg, 400 mg

Reference Range Calcium (total): Adults: 9.0-11.0 mg/dL

Overdosage/Treatment Supportive therapy: I.V. hydration; monitor urine flow and calcium and phosphorus level

Drug Interactions

Aminoglycosides: May lower serum calcium levels with prolonged administration. Concomitant use may have an additive hypocalcemic effect.

Antacids: May decrease the absorption of bisphosphonate derivatives; should be administered at a different time of the day. Antacids containing aluminum, calcium, or magnesium are of specific concern.

Calcium salts: May decrease the absorption of bisphosphonate derivatives. Separate oral dosing in order to minimize risk of interaction.

Iron salts: May decrease the absorption of bisphosphonate derivatives. Only oral iron salts and oral bisphosphonates are of concern.

Magnesium salts: May decrease the absorption of bisphosphonate derivatives. Only oral magnesium salts and oral bisphosphonates are of concern.

Nonsteroidal anti-inflammatory drugs (NSAIDs): May enhance the gastrointestinal adverse/toxic effects (increased incidence of GI ulcers) of bisphosphonate derivatives.

Phosphate supplements: Bisphosphonate derivatives may enhance the hypocalcemic effect of phosphate supplements.

Pregnancy Risk Factor B (oral); C (parenteral)

Pregnancy Implications Teratogenic effects have been reported in some but not all animal studies. There are no adequate and well-controlled studies in pregnant women. Bisphosphonates are incorporated into the bone matrix and gradually released over time. Theoretically, there may be a risk of fetal harm when pregnancy follows the completion of therapy. Based on limited case reports with pamidronate, serum calcium levels in the newborn may be altered if administered during pregnancy.

Lactation Excretion in breast milk unknown/use caution

Nursing Implications Dilute I.V. dose in at least 250 mL NS, ensure adequate hydration; dosage modification required in renal insufficiency

Specific References
French AE, Kaplan N, Lishner M, et al, "Taking Bisphosphonates During Pregnancy," *Can Fam Physician*, 2003, 49:1281-2.

Etodolac

Related Information
● Nonsteroidal Anti-inflammatory Drugs

CAS Number 41340-25-4

U.S. Brand Names Lodine® XL; Lodine®

Synonyms Etodolic Acid

Use Acute and long-term use in the management of signs and symptoms of osteoarthritis and management of pain; rheumatoid arthritis; juvenile rheumatoid arthritis

Mechanism of Action Inhibits prostaglandin synthesis by decreasing the activity of the enzyme, cyclooxygenase, which results in decreased formation of prostaglandin precursors

Adverse Reactions

Cardiovascular: Circulatory collapse

Central nervous system: **Dizziness**, headache, aseptic meningitis, psychosis, cognitive dysfunction, coma, seizures

Dermatologic: **Rash**, pruritus, hypersensitivity vasculitis, exfoliative dermatitis, alopecia, angioedema, urticaria, Stevens-Johnson syndrome, photosensitivity, exanthem, cutaneous vasculitis

Endocrine & metabolic: Hyperkalemia, anion gap metabolic acidosis, fluid retention, gynecomastia

Gastrointestinal: **Abdominal cramps, heartburn, indigestion, nausea**, vomiting, GI bleeding, GI ulceration, constipation, diarrhea, dyspepsia, xerostomia, colitis

Hematologic: Leukopenia, neutropenia, agranulocytosis, granulocytopenia, aplastic anemia (rare), platelet inhibition, hepatic necrosis

Hepatic: Elevated transaminases, hepatitis (fulminant)

Neuromuscular & skeletal: Paresthesia

Otic: Ototoxicity; tinnitus, deafness

Renal: Renal failure (acute), nephrotic syndrome, chronic renal failure, albuminuria

Respiratory: Wheezing, respiratory depression, rhinitis

Miscellaneous: Hypersensitivity

Signs and Symptoms of Overdose Cognitive dysfunction, conjunctivitis, drowsiness, dysuria, flatulence, gastritis, GI bleeding, hematuria, nausea, nephrotic syndrome, ototoxicity, tinnitus, wheezing, vomiting

Severe poisoning can manifest with coma, hypotension, leukocytosis, renal failure and/or hepatic failure, respiratory depression, seizures

Pharmacodynamics/Kinetics

Onset of action: Analgesic: 2-4 hours; Maximum anti-inflammatory effect: A few days

Absorption: ≥80%

Distribution: V_d:
  Immediate release: Adults:0.4 L/kg
  Extended release: Adults: 0.57 L/kg; Children (6-16 years): 0.08 L/kg

Protein binding: ≥99%, primarily albumin

Metabolism: Hepatic

Half-life elimination: Terminal: Adults: 5-8 hours
  Extended release: Children (6-16 years): 12 hours

Time to peak, serum:
  Immediate release: Adults: 1-2 hours
  Extended release: Extended release: 5-7 hours, increased 1.4-3.8 hours with food

Excretion: Urine 73% (1% unchanged); feces 16%

Dosage

Single dose of 76-100 mg is comparable to the analgesic effect of aspirin 650 mg; in patients ≥65 years, no substantial differences in the pharmacokinetics or side-effects profile were seen compared with the general population

Children 6-16 years: Oral: Juvenile rheumatoid arthritis (Lodine® XL):
  20-30 kg: 400 mg once daily
  31-45 kg: 600 mg once daily
  46-60 kg: 800 mg once daily
  >60 kg: 1000 mg once daily

Adults: Oral:
  Acute pain: 200-400 mg every 6-8 hours, as needed, not to exceed total daily doses of 1200 mg; for patients weighing <60 kg, total daily dose should not exceed 20 mg/kg/day

  Rheumatoid arthritis, osteoarthritis: Initial: 600-1200 mg/day given in divided doses: 400 mg 2 times/day; 300 mg 2 or 3 times/day; 500 mg 2 times/day; total daily dose should not exceed 1200 mg; for patients weighing <60 kg, total daily dose should not exceed 20 mg/kg/day
    Lodine® XL: 400-1000 mg once daily

Elderly: Refer to adult dosing; in patients ≥65 years, no dosage adjustment required based on pharmacokinetics. The elderly are more sensitive to antiprostaglandin effects and may need dosage adjustments.

Monitoring Parameters Monitor CBC, liver enzymes; in patients receiving diuretics, monitor urine output and BUN/serum creatinine

Contraindications Hypersensitivity to etodolac, aspirin, other NSAIDs, or any component of the formulation; perioperative pain in the setting of coronary artery bypass surgery (CABG); pregnancy

Warnings [U.S. Boxed Warning]: NSAIDs are associated with an increased risk of adverse cardiovascular events, including MI, stroke, and new onset or worsening of pre-existing hypertension. Risk may be increased with duration of use or pre-existing cardiovascular risk-factors or disease. Carefully evaluate individual cardiovascular risk profiles prior to prescribing. Use caution with fluid retention, CHF, or hypertension.

[U.S. Boxed Warning]: NSAIDs may increase risk of gastrointestinal irritation, ulceration, bleeding, and perforation. These events may occur at any time during therapy and without warning. Use caution with a history of GI disease (bleeding or ulcers), concurrent therapy with aspirin, anticoagulants and/or corticosteroids, smoking, use of alcohol, the elderly or debilitated patients.

Use of NSAIDs can compromise existing renal function. Renal toxicity can occur in patient with impaired renal function, dehydration, heart failure, liver dysfunction, those taking diuretics and ACE inhibitors and the elderly. Rehydrate patient before starting therapy. Monitor renal function closely. Etodolac is not recommended for patients with advanced renal disease.

Use the lowest effective dose for the shortest duration of time, consistent with individual patient goals, to reduce risk of cardiovascular or GI adverse events. Alternate therapies should be considered for patients at high risk.

NSAIDs may cause serious skin adverse events including exfoliative dermatitis, Stevens-Johnson syndrome (SJS), and toxic epidermal necrolysis (TEN). Anaphylactoid reactions may occur, even without prior exposure; patients with "aspirin triad" (bronchial asthma, aspirin intolerance, rhinitis) may be at increased risk. Do not use in patients who experience bronchospasm, asthma, rhinitis, or urticaria with NSAID or aspirin therapy.

Use with caution in patients with decreased hepatic function. Closely monitor patients with any abnormal LFT. Severe hepatic reactions (eg, fulminant hepatitis, liver failure) have occurred with NSAID use, rarely; discontinue if signs or symptoms of liver disease develop, or if systemic manifestations occur. The elderly are at increased risk for adverse effects (especially peptic ulceration, CNS effects, renal toxicity) from NSAIDs even at low doses.

Withhold for at least 4-6 half-lives prior to surgical or dental procedures.

Use of extended release product consisting of a nondeformable matrix should be avoided in patients with stricture/narrowing of the GI tract; symptoms of obstruction have been associated with nondeformable products.

Dosage Forms [DSC] = Discontinued product
Capsule: 200 mg, 300 mg
  Lodine®: 200 mg, 300 mg [DSC]
Tablet: 400 mg, 500 mg
Tablet, extended release (Lodine® XL): 400 mg, 500 mg [DSC]

Reference Range After a 200 mg oral dose, peak plasma levels are ~12-16 mg/L; after a 400 mg oral dose, peak plasma level is ~21 mg/L

Overdosage/Treatment
Decontamination: Ipecac within 30 minutes or lavage (within 1 hour)/activated charcoal

Supportive therapy: Hypotension/dehydration can be managed with I.V. fluid therapy; acidosis should be treated with bicarbonates, seizures with benzodiazepines; antacids, blood products are indicated, as appropriate, for hemorrhage

Enhancement of elimination: Dialysis or perfusion is indicated for secondary complications, acidosis, or renal failure and not toxin removal alone; multiple dosing of activated charcoal may be useful

Test Interactions False-positive for urinary bilirubin and ketone

Drug Interactions ACE inhibitors: Antihypertensive effects may be decreased by concurrent therapy with NSAIDs; monitor blood pressure.

Aminoglycosides: NSAIDs may decrease the excretion of aminoglycosides.

Angiotensin II antagonists: Antihypertensive effects may be decreased by concurrent therapy with NSAIDs; monitor blood pressure.

Anticoagulants (warfarin, heparin, LMWHs) in combination with NSAIDs can cause increased risk of bleeding.

Antiplatelet agents (ticlopidine, clopidogrel, aspirin, abciximab, dipyridamole, eptifibatide, tirofiban) can cause an increased risk of bleeding.

Beta-blockers: NSAIDs may diminish the antihypertensive effects of beta-blockers.

Bisphosphonates: NSAIDs may increase the risk of gastrointestinal ulceration.

Cholestyramine and colestipol reduce the bioavailability of some NSAIDs; separate administration times.

Corticosteroids may increase the risk of GI ulceration; avoid concurrent use.

Cyclosporine: NSAIDs may increase serum creatinine, potassium, blood pressure, and cyclosporine levels; monitor cyclosporine levels and renal function carefully.

Hydralazine's antihypertensive effect is decreased; avoid concurrent use.

Lithium levels can be increased; avoid concurrent use if possible or monitor lithium levels and adjust dose. Sulindac may have the least effect. When NSAID is stopped, lithium will need adjustment again.

Loop diuretics efficacy (diuretic and antihypertensive effect) is reduced. Indomethacin reduces this efficacy, however, it may be anticipated with any NSAID.

Methotrexate: Severe bone marrow suppression, aplastic anemia, and GI toxicity have been reported with concomitant NSAID therapy. Avoid use during moderate or high-dose methotrexate (increased and prolonged methotrexate levels). NSAID use during low-dose treatment of rheumatoid arthritis has not been fully evaluated; extreme caution is warranted.

Pemetrexed: NSAIDs may decrease the excretion of pemetrexed. Patients with Cl$_{cr}$ 45-79 mL/minute should avoid short acting NSAIDs for 2 days before and 2 days after pemetrexed treatment.

Thiazides antihypertensive effects are decreased; avoid concurrent use.

Treprostinil: May enhance the risk of bleeding with concurrent use.

Vancomycin: NSAIDs may decrease the excretion of vancomycin. Avoid concurrent use.

Verapamil plasma concentration is decreased by some NSAIDs; avoid concurrent use.

Pregnancy Risk Factor C/D (3rd trimester)
Lactation Excretion in breast milk unknown/not recommended
Nursing Implications Do not crush tablets

Etoposide

CAS Number 33419-42-0
U.S. Brand Names Toposar®; VePesid®
Synonyms Epipodophyllotoxin; VP-16-213; VP-16
Use Treatment of refractory testicular tumors; treatment of small cell lung cancer
Unlabeled/Investigational Use Treatment of lymphomas, acute non-lymphocytic leukemia (ANLL); lung, bladder, and prostate carcinoma; hepatoma, rhabdomyosarcoma, uterine carcinoma, neuroblastoma, mycosis fungoides, Kaposi's sarcoma, histiocytosis, gestational trophoblastic disease, Ewing's sarcoma, Wilms' tumor, brain tumors
Mechanism of Action Inhibits mitotic activity; inhibits cells from entering prophase; inhibits DNA synthesis. Initially thought to be mitotic inhibitors similar to podophyllotoxin, but actually have no effect on microtubule assembly. However, later shown to induce DNA strand breakage and inhibition of topoisomerase II (an enzyme which breaks and repairs DNA); etoposide acts in late S or early G2 phases.
Adverse Reactions
Cardiovascular: Tachycardia
  Hypotension: Related to drug infusion time; may be related to vehicle used in the I.V. preparation (polysorbate 80 plus polyethylene glycol). Best to administer the drug over 1 hour.
Central nervous system: Unusual tiredness, neurotoxicity, somnolence, fever, headache, dystonia
Dermatologic: **Alopecia** (reversible 66%), radiation recall dermatitis, rash, urticaria, Stevens-Johnson syndrome, onycholysis, toxic epidermal necrolysis
Endocrine & metabolic: Syndrome of inappropriate antidiuretic hormone secretion
Gastrointestinal: **Emetic potential:** Moderately low (10% to 30%); occasional **diarrhea** and **infrequent nausea and vomiting** at standard doses; **severe mucositis** occurs with high (BMT) doses; **anorexia** (10% to 13%); stomatitis, abdominal pain, hepatitic dysfunction, paralytic ileus
Hematologic:
  Myelosuppressive: Principal dose-limiting toxicity of VP-16. White blood cell count nadir is 5-15 days after administration and is more frequent than thrombocytopenia. Recovery is usually within 24-28 days and cumulative toxicity has not been noted with VP-16 as a single agent. No difference in toxicity is seen when VP-16 is administered over a 24-hour period or over 2 hours on 5 consecutive days.
    WBC: Mild to severe
    Platelets: Mild
    Onset (days): 10
    Nadir (days): 14-16
    Recovery (days): 21-28
    Hepatic: Toxic hepatitis (with high-dose therapy); hepatic necrosis at doses >600 mg/m^2
    Local: **Irritant chemotherapy**, thrombophlebitis has been reported (0.7% to 2%), extravasation injury
    Neuromuscular & skeletal: Neuropathy (peripheral) 1% to 2%
    Respiratory: Dyspnea, bronchospasm, apnea, pulmonary interstitial fibrosis
    Miscellaneous: Hiccups
      Hypersensitivity: Reports of flushing or bronchospasm, which, in one report, did not recur if patients were pretreated with corticosteroids and antihistamines
Admission Criteria/Prognosis Admit any symptomatic patient

Pharmacodynamics/Kinetics

Absorption: Oral: 25% to 75%; significant inter- and intrapatient variation

Distribution: Average V_d: 7-17 L/m^2; poor penetration across the blood-brain barrier; CSF concentrations <10% of plasma concentrations

Protein binding: 94% to 97%

Metabolism: Hepatic to hydroxy acid and cislactone metabolites

Bioavailability: Oral: ~50% (range 25% to 75%)

Half-life elimination: Terminal: 4-11 hours; Children: Normal renal/hepatic function: 6-8 hours

Time to peak, serum: Oral: 1-1.5 hours

Excretion:

Children: Urine (≤55% as unchanged drug)

Adults: Urine (42% to 67%; 8% to 35% as unchanged drug) within 24 hours; feces (up to 44%)

Dosage Refer to individual protocols

Oral: Twice the I.V. dose rounded to the nearest 50 mg given once daily if total dose ≤400 mg or in divided doses if >400 mg

Children: I.V.: 60-120 mg/m^2/day for 3-5 days every 3-6 weeks

AML:

Remission induction: 150 mg/m^2/day for 2-3 days for 2-3 cycles

Intensification or consolidation: 250 mg/m^2/day for 3 days, courses 2-5

Conditioning regimen for allogeneic BMT: 60 mg/kg/dose as a single dose

Adults:

Small cell lung cancer:

I.V.: 35 mg/m^2/day for 4 days or 50 mg/m^2/day for 5 days every 3-4 weeks total dose ≤400 mg/day or in divided doses if >400 mg/day

IVPB: 200-250 mg/m^2 repeated every 7 weeks

Continuous intravenous infusion: 500 mg/m^2 over 24 hours every 3 weeks

Testicular cancer:

IVPB: 50-100 mg/m^2/day for 5 days repeated every 3-4 weeks

I.V.: 100 mg/m^2 every other day for 3 doses repeated every 3-4 weeks

BMT/relapsed leukemia: I.V.: 2.4-3.5 g/m^2 or 25-70 mg/kg administered over 4-36 hours

Dosage adjustment in renal impairment:

Cl_{cr} 10-50 mL/minute: Administer 75% of normal dose

Cl_{cr} <10 mL minute: Administer 50% of normal dose

Hemodialysis effects: Supplemental dose is not necessary

CAPD effects: Unknown

CAVH effects: Unknown

Dosage adjustment in hepatic impairment:

Bilirubin 1.5-3 mg/dL or AST 60-180 units: Reduce dose by 50%

Bilirubin >3 mg/dL or AST >180 units: Reduce by 75%

Stability

Store intact vials of injection at room temperature and protected from light; injection solution contains polyethylene glycol vehicle with absolute alcohol; store oral capsules under refrigeration

VP-16 should be further diluted in D_5W or NS for administration; diluted solutions have concentration-dependent stability: More concentrated solutions have shorter stability times

At room temperature in D_5W or NS in polyvinyl chloride, the concentration is stable as follows: 0.2 mg/mL: 96 hours; 0.4 mg/mL: 48 hours; 0.6 mg/mL: 8 hours; 1 mg/mL: 2 hours; 2 mg/mL: 1 hour; 20 mg/mL (undiluted): 24 hours

Y-site compatible with carboplatin, cytarabine, mesna, daunorubicin

Standard I.V. dilution:

Lower dose regimens (<1 g/dose):

Doses may be diluted in 100-1000 mL of D_5W or NS

If the concentration is less than or equal to 0.6 mg/mL, the bag should be mixed with the appropriate expiration dating

If the concentration is >0.6 mg/mL, the concentration is highly unstable and a syringe of undiluted etoposide accompanied with the appropriate volume of diluent will be sent to the nursing unit to be mixed at the bedside just prior to administration.

High-dose regimens (>1g/dose):

Total dose should be drawn into an empty viaflex container and the appropriate amount of diluent (for a final concentration of 1 mg/mL) will be sent

Use the **2-Channel Pump Method**: Instill all of the etoposide dose into one viaflex container (concentration = 20 mg/mL). Infuse this into one channel (Baxter Flow-Guard 6300 Dual Channel Volumetric Infusion Pump - or any 2-channel infusion pump that does not require a "hard" plastic cassette). Infuse the indicated diluent (ie, D_5W or NS) at a rate of at least 20 times the infusion rate of the etoposide to simulate a 1 mg/mL concentration in the line. The etoposide should be Y-sited into the port most proximal to the patient. A 0.22 micron filter should be attached to the line after the Y-site and before entry into the patient.

Monitoring Parameters CBC with differential, platelet count, and hemoglobin, vital signs (blood pressure), bilirubin, and renal function tests

Administration

Administer lower doses IVPB over at least 30 minutes to minimize the risk of hypotensive reactions.

Administer high-doses (>1 g/dose) via the 2-channel pump method.

An in-line 0.22 micron filter should be attached to **all** etoposide infusions due to the high potential for precipitation

Contraindications Hypersensitivity to etoposide or any component of the formulation; pregnancy

Warnings Hazardous agent – use appropriate precautions for handling and disposal. **[U.S. Boxed Warning]: Severe myelosuppression with resulting infection or bleeding may occur.** Treatment should be withheld for platelets <50,000/mm^3 or absolute neutrophil count (ANC) <500/mm^3. May cause anaphylactic reaction manifested by chills, fever, tachycardia, bronchospasm, dyspnea, and hypotension. In children, the use of concentrations higher than recommended were associated with higher rates of anaphylactic-like reactions. Infusion should be interrupted and medications for the treatment of anaphylaxis should be available for immediate use. Must be diluted; do not give I.V. push, infuse over at least 30-60 minutes; hypotension is associated with rapid infusion. Dosage should be adjusted in patients with hepatic or renal impairment. **[U.S. Boxed Warning]: Should be administered under the supervision of an experienced cancer chemotherapy physician.** Injectable formula contains polysorbate 80; do not use in premature infants. May contain benzyl alcohol; do not use in newborn infants. Safety and efficacy in children have not been established.

Dosage Forms Capsule, softgel:

VePesid®: 50 mg

Injection, solution: 20 mg/mL (5 mL, 25 mL, 50 mL)

Toposar®: 20 mg/mL (5 mL, 25 mL, 50 mL) [contains alcohol 33% and polysorbate 80]

Reference Range 5 minutes following intravenous infusion of 100 mg/m^2 over 30-60 minutes, plasma etoposide level of 21 mg/L was obtained

Overdosage/Treatment

Decontamination: Oral: Emesis within 30 minutes or lavage within 2 hours of ingestion; activated charcoal

Supportive therapy: Hypotension usually responds to discontinuation of drug to I.V. fluids and diphenhydramine; bronchospasm and dystonia also respond to diphenhydramine; recombinant human erythropoietin (150-300 units/kg subcutaneously 3 times weekly) may be used to treat anemia along with red blood cell transfusions; granulocyte-macrophage colony stimulating factor or granulocyte colony stimulating factor can be used to treat bone marrow infection; diphenhydramine (1 mg/kg up to 50 mg I.V.) or benztropine (1-2 mg/kg I.V.) can be used to treat dystonia; **extravasation treatment**: Inject 150-900 units of hyaluronidase SubQ clockwise into the infiltrated area using a 25-gauge needle; change the needle with each injection; apply heat immediately for 1 hour, repeat 4 times/day for 3-5 days; **application of cold or hydrocortisone is contraindicated**

Antidote(s)

- Thrombopoietin [ANTIDOTE]

Drug Interactions Substrate of CYP1A2 (minor), 2E1 (minor), 3A4 (major); **Inhibits** CYP2C9 (weak), 3A4 (weak)

Barbiturates: May increase metabolism/decrease the effects of etoposide; monitor.

Cyclosporine: May decrease the metabolism/increase the levels of etoposide; consider reducing the dose of etoposide by 50% if the patient is receiving, or has recently received, cyclosporine. Monitor for increased toxic effects of etoposide if cyclosporine is initiated, the dose is increased, or it has been recently discontinued.

CYP3A4 inducers: CYP3A4 inducers may decrease the levels/effects of etoposide. Example inducers include aminoglutethimide, carbamazepine, nafcillin, nevirapine, phenobarbital, phenytoin, and rifamycins.

CYP3A4 inhibitors: May increase the levels/effects of etoposide. Example inhibitors include azole antifungals, clarithromycin, diclofenac, doxycycline, erythromycin, imatinib, isoniazid, nefazodone, nicardipine, propofol, protease inhibitors, quinidine, telithromycin, and verapamil.

Phenytoin: May increase metabolism/decrease effects of etoposide; monitor.

Warfarin may elevate prothrombin time with concurrent use.

Pregnancy Risk Factor D

Pregnancy Implications Fetotoxic and teratogenic in rats

Lactation Enters breast milk/contraindicated

Nursing Implications If necessary, the injection may be used for oral administration; mix with orange juice, apple juice, or lemonade to a concentration of 0.4 mg/mL or less, and use within a 3-hour period

Additional Information Derived from the May Apple plant

Famciclovir

Related Information
- Acyclovir

CAS Number 104227-87-4

U.S. Brand Names Famvir®

Use Management of acute herpes zoster (shingles); treatment of recurrent herpes simplex (genital herpes) in immunocompetent patients

Mechanism of Action After undergoing rapid biotransformation to the active compound, penciclovir, famciclovir is phosphorylated by viral thymidine kinase in HSV-1, HSV-2, and VZV-infected cells to a monophosphate form; this is then converted to penciclovir triphosphate and competes with deoxyguanosine triphosphate to inhibit HSV-2 polymerase (ie, herpes viral DNA synthesis/replication is selectively inhibited)

Adverse Reactions

Central nervous system: **Headache**, fatigue, fever, dizziness, somnolence

Dermatologic: Pruritus

Gastrointestinal: **Nausea**, diarrhea, vomiting, constipation, anorexia, abdominal pain, pancreatitis

Neuromuscular & skeletal: Rigors, paresthesia

Pharmacodynamics/Kinetics

Absorption: Food decreases maximum peak concentration and delays time to peak; AUC remains the same

Distribution: V_{dss}: 0.91-1.25 L/kg

Protein binding: $\leq 20\%$

Metabolism: Rapidly deacetylated and oxidized to penciclovir; not via CYP

Bioavailability: 69% to 85%

Half-life elimination: Penciclovir: 2-3 hours (10, 20, and 7 hours in HSV-1, HSV-2, and VZV-infected cells, respectively); prolonged with renal impairment

Time to peak: 0.9 hours; C_{max} and T_{max} are decreased and prolonged with noncompensated hepatic impairment

Excretion: Urine (73% primarily as penciclovir); feces (27%)

Dosage Herpes zoster: Adults: Oral: 500 mg every 8 hours for 7 days

First episode genital herpes simplex: 750 mg every 8 hours for 5 days

Dosing interval in renal impairment:

$Cl_{cr} \geq 60$ mL/minute: Administer 500 mg every 8 hours

Cl_{cr} 40-59 mL/minute: Administer 500 mg every 12 hours

Cl_{cr} 20-39 mL/minute: Administer 500 mg every 24 hours

$Cl_{cr} < 20$ mL/minute: Unknown

Monitoring Parameters Periodic CBC during long-term therapy

Contraindications Hypersensitivity to famciclovir, penciclovir, or any component of the formulation

Warnings Has not been established for use in initial episodes of genital herpes, patients with ophthalmic or disseminated zoster, or in immunocompromised patients with herpes zoster. Dosage adjustment is required in patients with renal insufficiency. Tablets contain lactose; do not use with galactose intolerance, severe lactase deficiency, or glucose-galactose malabsorption syndromes. Safety and efficacy have not been established in children <18 years of age.

Dosage Forms Tablet: 125 mg, 250 mg, 500 mg [contains lactose]

Reference Range Peak serum penciclovir levels after a 250 mg oral dose range from 1.6-1.9 mcg/mL; after a 500 mg dose, peak serum penciclovir levels are ~3.5 mcg/mL; peak serum penciclovir level after a 10 mg/kg I.V. dose is ~12 mcg/mL

Overdosage/Treatment

Decontamination: Ipecac within 30 minutes or lavage (within 1 hour)/activated charcoal

Supportive therapy: Renal toxicity and crystalluria can be managed with I.V. fluid hydration

Enhancement of elimination: Multiple dosing of activated charcoal may be effective; while no studies have been performed, hemodialysis would appear to be an effective modality for drug removal; hemodialysis can remove as much as 76% of the drug within 4 hours

Pregnancy Risk Factor B

Pregnancy Implications Use only if the benefit to the patient clearly exceeds the potential risk to the fetus; due to potential for excretion of famciclovir in breast milk and for its associated tumorigenicity, discontinue nursing or discontinue the drug during lactation

Lactation Excretion in breast milk unknown/use caution

Additional Information Most effective if therapy is initiated within 72 hours of initial lesion; currently also being studied for chronic hepatitis B infections

Famotidine

CAS Number 76824-35-6

U.S. Brand Names Pepcid® AC [OTC]; Pepcid®

Use Therapy and treatment of duodenal ulcer, gastric ulcer, control gastric pH in critically-ill patients, symptomatic relief in gastritis, gastroesophageal reflux, active benign ulcer, and pathological hypersecretory conditions

OTC labeling: Relief of heartburn, acid indigestion, and sour stomach

Unlabeled/Investigational Use Part of a multidrug regimen for *H. pylori* eradication to reduce the risk of duodenal ulcer recurrence

Mechanism of Action Competitive inhibition of histamine at H_2-receptors of the gastric parietal cells, which inhibits gastric acid secretion

Adverse Reactions

Note: Agitation and vomiting have been reported in up to 14% of pediatric patients <1 year of age.

Cardiovascular: Arrhythmia, bradycardia, hypertension, palpitations, tachycardia

Central nervous system: Dizziness, headache, drowsiness, fatigue, fever, insomnia, psychiatric disturbances, seizures

Dermatologic: Acne, dry skin, pruritus, rash, urticaria

Gastrointestinal: Constipation, diarrhea, abdominal discomfort, anorexia, belching, flatulence

Hematologic: Agranulocytosis, neutropenia, thrombocytopenia

Hepatic: AST/ALT increased, jaundice

Neuromuscular & skeletal: Paresthesia, weakness

Renal: BUN/creatinine increased, proteinuria

Respiratory: Bronchospasm

Miscellaneous: Allergic reaction, anaphylaxis

Signs and Symptoms of Overdose Abdominal pain, AV block, CNS depression, confusion, depression, dry skin, hypotension, impotence, insomnia, neutropenia, seizures, tachycardia, vomiting

Pharmacodynamics/Kinetics

Onset of action: GI: Oral: Within 1-3 hour

Duration: 10-12 hours

Protein binding: 15% to 20%

Bioavailability: Oral: 40% to 50%

Half-life elimination: Injection, oral suspension, tablet: 2.5-3.5 hours; prolonged with renal impairment; Oliguria: 20 hours

Time to peak, serum: Oral: ~1-3 hours

Excretion: Urine (as unchanged drug)

Dosage

Children: Treatment duration and dose should be individualized

Peptic ulcer: 1-16 years:

Oral: 0.5 mg/kg/day at bedtime or divided twice daily (maximum dose: 40 mg/day); doses of up to 1 mg/kg/day have been used in clinical studies

I.V.: 0.25 mg/kg every 12 hours (maximum dose: 40 mg/day); doses of up to 0.5 mg/kg have been used in clinical studies

GERD: Oral:

<3 months: 0.5 mg/kg once daily

3-12 months: 0.5 mg/kg twice daily

1-16 years: 1 mg/kg/day divided twice daily (maximum dose: 40 mg twice daily); doses of up to 2 mg/kg/day have been used in clinical studies

Children ≥ 12 years and Adults: Heartburn, indigestion, sour stomach:

OTC labeling: Oral: 10-20 mg every 12 hours; dose may be taken 15-60 minutes before eating foods known to cause heartburn

Adults:

Duodenal ulcer: Oral: Acute therapy: 40 mg/day at bedtime for 4-8 weeks; maintenance therapy: 20 mg/day at bedtime

Helicobacter pylori eradication (unlabeled use): 40 mg once daily; requires combination therapy with antibiotics

Gastric ulcer: Oral: Acute therapy: 40 mg/day at bedtime

Hypersecretory conditions: Oral: Initial: 20 mg every 6 hours, may increase in increments up to 160 mg every 6 hours

GERD: Oral: 20 mg twice daily for 6 weeks

Esophagitis and accompanying symptoms due to GERD: Oral: 20 mg or 40 mg twice daily for up to 12 weeks

Patients unable to take oral medication: I.V.: 20 mg every 12 hours

Dosing adjustment in renal impairment: $Cl_{cr} < 50$ mL/minute: Manufacturer recommendation: Administer 50% of dose **or** increase the dosing interval to every 36-48 hours (to limit potential CNS adverse effects).

Monitoring Parameters ECG, CBC, electrolytes

Administration I.V. push: Inject over at least 2 minutes

Solution for infusion: Administer over 15-30 minutes

Contraindications Hypersensitivity to famotidine, other H_2 antagonists, or any component of the formulation

Warnings

Modify dose in patients with renal impairment; chewable tablets contain phenylalanine; multidose vials contain benzyl alcohol

OTC labeling: When used for self-medication, patients should be instructed not to use if they have difficulty swallowing, have vomiting with blood, or bloody or black stools. Not for use with other acid reducers.

Dosage Forms [DSC] = Discontinued product

Gelcap:

Pepcid® AC: 10 mg

Infusion [premixed in NS]: 20 mg (50 mL)

Pepcid®: 20 mg (50 mL)

Injection, solution: 10 mg/mL (4 mL, 20 mL)

Pepcid®: 10 mg/mL (20 mL) [contains benzyl alcohol]

Injection, solution [preservative free]: 10 mg/mL (2 mL)

Pepcid®: 10 mg/mL (2 mL)

Powder for oral suspension:

Pepcid®: 40 mg/5 mL (50 mL) [contains sodium benzoate; cherry-banana-mint flavor]

Tablet: 10 mg [OTC], 20 mg, 40 mg

Pepcid®: 20 mg, 40 mg

Pepcid® AC: 10 mg, 20 mg

Tablet, chewable:

Pepcid® AC: 10 mg [contains phenylalanine 1.4 mg/tablet; mint flavor]

Reference Range Serum level of 13 ng/mL will produce 50% inhibition of gastric acid secretion

Overdosage/Treatment

Decontamination: Lavage (within 1 hour)/activated charcoal

Supportive therapy: Treatment is primarily symptomatic and supportive

Enhancement of elimination: Hemodialysis may be useful (four- to sixfold increase in clearance)

Drug Interactions

Cefpodoxime: Histamine H$_2$ antagonists may decrease the absorption of cefpodoxime; separate oral doses by at least 2 hours. Risk: Moderate

Cefuroxime: Histamine H$_2$ antagonists may decrease the absorption of cefuroxime; separate oral doses by at least 2 hours. Risk: Moderate

Cyclosporine: Histamine H$_2$ antagonists may increase the serum concentration of cyclosporine; monitor

Delavirdine: Delavirdine's absorption is decreased; avoid concurrent use with H$_2$ antagonists

Itraconazole: Histamine H$_2$ antagonists may decrease the absorption of itraconazole; monitor

Ketoconazole: Histamine H$_2$ antagonists may decrease the absorption of ketoconazole; monitor

Pregnancy Risk Factor B

Pregnancy Implications Crosses the placenta; insufficient data concerning effects on the fetus

Lactation Enters breast milk/not recommended

Additional Information The expensive parenteral route should only be used when a patient is unable to take oral medication. Less antiandrogenic than cimetidine.

Felodipine

Related Information

• Calcium Channel Blockers

CAS Number 72509-76-3; 86189-69-7

U.S. Brand Names Plendil®

Use Treatment of hypertension, congestive heart failure

Mechanism of Action Dihydropyridine calcium channel blocking agent similar to nifedipine; predominantly vasodilatory actions

Adverse Reactions

Cardiovascular: **Peripheral edema**, flushing, tachycardia, sinus bradycardia, angina, chest pain, QRS prolongation, sinus tachycardia

Central nervous system: Headache, dizziness, insomnia, night terrors, CNS depression, depression

Dermatologic: Urticaria, eczema, purpura, pruritus, exanthem

Gastrointestinal: Vomiting, xerostomia, flatulence, gingival hyperplasia, constipation

Neuromuscular & skeletal: Weakness, paresthesia, exacerbation of myasthenia gravis in elderly

Respiratory: Cough, hyposmia

Signs and Symptoms of Overdose Bradycardia, hypotension

Pharmacodynamics/Kinetics

Onset of action: Antihypertensive: 2-5 hours

Duration of antihypertensive effect: 24 hours

Absorption: 100%; Absolute: 20% due to first-pass effect

Protein binding: >99%

Metabolism: Hepatic; CYP3A4 substrate (major); extensive first-pass effect

Half-life elimination: Immediate release: 11-16 hours

Excretion: Urine (70% as metabolites); feces 10%

Dosage

Adults: Oral: 2.5-10 mg once daily; usual initial dose: 5 mg; increase by 5 mg at 2-week intervals, as needed; maximum: 10 mg

Usual dose range (JNC 7) for hypertension: 2.5-20 mg once daily

Elderly: Begin with 2.5 mg/day

Dosing adjustment/comments in hepatic impairment: May require lower dosages (initial: 2.5 mg/day); monitor blood pressure

Administration Do not crush or chew extended release tablets; swallow whole.

Contraindications Hypersensitivity to felodipine, any component of the formulation, or other calcium channel blocker

Warnings Watch for hypotension and syncope (can rarely occur). Reflex tachycardia may occur. Use caution in patients with heart failure particularly with concurrent beta-blocker use. Elderly patients and patients with hepatic impairment should start off with a lower dose. Peripheral edema is the most common side effect (occurs within 2-3 weeks of starting therapy). Use caution in hepatic impairment. Safety and efficacy in children have not been established. Dosage titration should occur after 14 days on a given dose.

Dosage Forms Tablet, extended release: 2.5 mg, 5 mg, 10 mg

Reference Range Therapeutic plasma level: 5-10 nmol/L; toxic: >30 nmol/L

Overdosage/Treatment

Decontamination: Ipecac-induced emesis can hypothetically worsen calcium antagonist toxicity, since it can produce vagal stimulation. The potential for seizures precipitously following acute ingestion of large doses of a calcium antagonist may also contraindicate the use of ipecac. Lavage (within 1 hour)/activated charcoal is useful. Whole bowel irrigation for sustained release preparations.

Supportive therapy: I.V. fluids and Trendelenburg positioning should be initiated as intoxication may cause hypotension. Calcium (calcium chloride I.V. 1-3 g in adults or 10-30 mg/kg in children over 5-10 minutes with repeats as needed) has been used as an "antidote" for acute intoxications and is the second line therapy for shock next to traditional vasopressors. Heart block may respond to isoproterenol, glucagon, atropine and/or calcium, although a temporary pacemaker may be required. Inamrinone or dopamine may be required for hypotension and is the first-line treatment for shock. Glucagon may increase myocardial contractility.

Enhancement of elimination: Multiple dosing of activated charcoal is useful; ~9% of the parent drug can be removed by hemodialysis

Test Interactions May cause increased serum alkaline phosphatase, serum calcium, serum creatinine, serum gamma glutamyl transferase, serum norepinephrine, renin

Drug Interactions

Substrate of CYP3A4 (major); **Inhibits** CYP2C8 (moderate), 2C9 (weak), 2D6 (weak), 3A4 (weak)

Azole antifungals may inhibit calcium channel blocker's metabolism; avoid this combination. Try an antifungal like terbinafine (if appropriate) or monitor closely for altered effect of the calcium channel blocker.

Beta-blockers may have increased pharmacokinetic or pharmacodynamic interactions with felodipine.

Calcium may reduce the calcium channel blocker's effects, particularly hypotension.

Carbamazepine significantly reduces felodipine's bioavailability; avoid this combination.

Cimetidine may inhibit felodipine metabolism (AUC increased by 50%); use caution and monitor for potential hypotension.

Cyclosporine increases felodipine's serum concentration; avoid the combination or reduce dose of felodipine and monitor blood pressure.

CYP2C8 Substrates: Felodipine may increase the levels/effects of CYP2C8 substrates. Example substrates include amiodarone, paclitaxel, pioglitazone, repaglinide, and rosiglitazone.

CYP3A4 inducers: CYP3A4 inducers may decrease the levels/effects of felodipine. Example inducers include aminoglutethimide, carbamazepine, nafcillin, nevirapine, phenobarbital, phenytoin, and rifamycins.

CYP3A4 inhibitors: May increase the levels/effects of felodipine. Example inhibitors include azole antifungals, clarithromycin, diclofenac, doxycycline, erythromycin, imatinib, isoniazid, nefazodone, nicardipine, propofol, protease inhibitors, quinidine, telithromycin, and verapamil.

Erythromycin decreases felodipine's metabolism; coadministration results in a twofold increase in the AUC and half-life of felodipine; monitor for hypotension.

Nafcillin decreases plasma concentration of felodipine; avoid this combination.

Rifampin increases the metabolism of the calcium channel blocker; adjust the dose of the calcium channel blocker to maintain efficacy.

Sildenafil, tadalafil, vardenafil: Blood pressure-lowering effects may be additive; use caution.

Tacrolimus: Felodipine may increase tacrolimus serum levels; monitor.

Pregnancy Risk Factor C

Pregnancy Implications Potentially, calcium channel blockers may prolong labor. There are no adequate or well-controlled studies in pregnant women.

Lactation Excretion in breast milk unknown/not recommended

Additional Information Do not crush or chew pills; increased bioavailability when taken with grapefruit juice

Specific References

Chobanian AV, Bakris GL, Black HR, et al, "The Seventh Report of the Joint National Committee on Prevention, Detection, Evaluation, and Treatment of High Blood Pressure: The JNC 7 Report," *JAMA*, 2003, 289(19):2560-71.

Femoxetine

CAS Number 59859-58-4

Unlabeled/Investigational Use Antidepressant, narcolepsy, tension headache

Mechanism of Action A phenylpiperidine derivative which selectively inhibits reuptake of serotonin

Adverse Reactions

Cardiovascular: Palpitations

Central nervous system: Nervousness, anxiety, insomnia, dizziness, headache

Dermatologic: Urticaria
Gastrointestinal: Nausea, xerostomia, constipation
Genitourinary: Dysuria
Hepatic: Hepatitis
Neuromuscular & skeletal: Tremor
Respiratory: Nasal congestion
Miscellaneous: Diaphoresis

Toxicodynamics/Kinetics
Metabolism: Hepatic to active (norfemoxetine) and inactive metabolites
Bioavailability: 5% to 10%
Half-life: ~20 hours (norfemoxetine half-life: 4-19 hours)
Elimination: Primarily renal (54% to 81%). Total body clearance: 8-50 L/hour/kg; Feces (6% to 11%)

Dosage
Depression: 300-600 mg in 3 divided doses; start at the lower dose
Narcolepsy: 300 mg twice daily
Tension headache: 100 mg 4 times/day
Dosing adjustment in hepatic impairment: Reduce initial dose to 100 mg/day

Reference Range Peak serum levels following a 500-600 mg dose: 120 ng/mL

Overdosage/Treatment
Decontamination: Lavage (within 1 hour)/activated charcoal. Consider gastric decontamination for ingestions >1 g.
Supportive therapy: Toxic symptoms should be treated supportively. Diazepam I.V. boluses (5-10 mg for adults up to 30 mg or 0.25-0.4 mg/kg/dose for children up to 10 mg/dose). If seizures are unresponsive or recur, phenytoin or phenobarbital may be required.
Enhancement of elimination: Multiple dosing of activated charcoal may not be useful; hemodialysis does not appear to be useful

Additional Information Does not appear to be as effective as propranolol for migraine prophylaxis

Fenoldopam

CAS Number 67227-56-9; 67227-57-0
U.S. Brand Names Corlopam®
Synonyms Fenoldopam Mesylate
Use Treatment of severe hypertension (up to 48 hours in adults), including in patients with renal compromise; short-term (up to 4 hours) blood pressure reduction in pediatric patients
Mechanism of Action A selective dopamine agonist (D_1-receptors) with vasodilatory properties; 6 times as potent as dopamine in producing vasodilatation

Adverse Reactions
Cardiovascular: Fibrillation (atrial), hypotension, edema, tachycardia, facial flushing, asymptomatic T wave flattening on ECG, flutter (atrial), chest pain, angina
Central nervous system: Headache, dizziness
Gastrointestinal: Nausea, vomiting, diarrhea
Ocular: Increased intraocular pressure

Pharmacodynamics/Kinetics
Onset of action: I.V.: 10 minutes
Duration: I.V.: 1 hour
Distribution: V_d: 0.6 L/kg
Half-life elimination: I.V.: Children: 3-5 minutes; Adults: ~5 minutes
Metabolism: Hepatic via methylation, glucuronidation, and sulfation; the 8-sulfate metabolite may have some activity; extensive first-pass effect
Excretion: Urine (90%); feces (10%)

Dosage I.V.: Hypertension, severe:
Children: Initial: 0.2 mcg/kg/minute; may be increased to dosages of 0.3-0.5 mcg/kg/minute every 20-30 minutes (maximum dose: 0.8 mcg/kg/minute); limited to short-term (4 hours) use
Adults: Initial: 0.1-0.3 mcg/kg/minute (lower initial doses may be associated with less reflex tachycardia); may be increased in increments of 0.05-0.1 mcg/kg/minute every 15 minutes until target blood pressure is reached; the maximal infusion rate reported in clinical studies was 1.6 mcg/kg/minute
Dosing adjustment in renal impairment: None required
Dosing adjustment in hepatic impairment: None published
Monitoring Parameters Blood pressure, heart rate, ECG, renal/hepatic function tests
Administration For I.V. infusion using an infusion pump.
Contraindications Hypersensitivity of fenoldopam or any component of the formulation
Warnings Use caution in patients with glaucoma or intraocular hypertension. A dose-related tachycardia can occur, especially at infusion rates >0.1 mcg/kg/minute. Use caution in angina patients (can increase myocardial oxygen demand with tachycardia). Close monitoring of blood pressure is necessary (hypotension can occur). Monitor for hypokalemia at intervals of 6 hours during infusion. For continuous infusion only (no bolus doses). The effects of hemodialysis on the pharmacokinetics of fenoldopam have not been evaluated. Use caution with increased intracranial pressure. Contains sulfites; may cause allergic reaction in susceptible individuals.
Dosage Forms Injection, solution: 10 mg/mL (1 mL, 2 mL) [contains sodium metabisulfite and propylene glycol]
Reference Range Mean plasma fenoldopam levels after a 2 hour infusion (at 0.5 mcg/kg/minute) and a 100 mg dose is approximately 13 ng/mL and 50 ng/mL
Overdosage/Treatment Supportive: I.V.: Usually discontinuing medication will often return blood pressure to baseline levels within 1 hour
Drug Interactions Concurrent acetaminophen may increase fenoldopam levels (30% to 70%).
Beta-blockers increase the risk of hypotension. Avoid concurrent use; if used concurrently, close monitoring is recommended.
Pregnancy Risk Factor B
Pregnancy Implications Fetal harm was not observed in animal studies; however, safety and efficacy have not been established for use during pregnancy. Use during pregnancy only if clearly needed. Fetal heart rate monitoring is recommended.
Lactation Excretion in breast milk unknown/use caution
Specific References
Devlin JW, Seta ML, Kanji S, et al, "Fenoldopam Versus Nitroprusside for the Treatment of Hypertensive Emergency," *Ann Pharmacother*, 2004, 38(5):755-59.
Stone GW, McCullough PA, Tumlin JA, et al, "Fenoldopam Mesylate for the Prevention of Contrast-Induced Nephropathy: A Randomized Controlled Trial," *JAMA*, 2003, 290(17):2284-91.

Fenoprofen

Related Information
• Nonsteroidal Anti-inflammatory Drugs
CAS Number 53746-45-5
U.S. Brand Names Nalfon®
Synonyms Fenoprofen Calcium
Use Symptomatic treatment of acute and chronic rheumatoid arthritis and osteoarthritis; relief of mild to moderate pain
Mechanism of Action Inhibits prostaglandin synthesis by decreasing the activity of the enzyme, cyclooxygenase, which results in decreased formation of prostaglandin precursors; propionic acid derivative (like ibuprofen)

Adverse Reactions
Cardiovascular: Circulatory collapse, sinus tachycardia
Central nervous system: **Dizziness**, headache, aseptic meningitis, psychosis, cognitive dysfunction, coma, seizures
Dermatologic: **Rash**, pruritus, toxic epidermal necrolysis, exfoliative dermatitis, acne, alopecia, angioedema, urticaria, purpura, exanthem
Endocrine & metabolic: Hyperkalemia, anion gap metabolic acidosis, fluid retention
Gastrointestinal: **Abdominal cramps, heartburn, indigestion, nausea**, vomiting, GI bleeding, GI ulceration, constipation, diarrhea, dyspepsia, feces discoloration (black), aphthous stomatitis, xerostomia, stomatitis
Hematologic: Leukopenia, neutropenia, agranulocytosis, granulocytopenia; aplastic anemia (rare), platelet inhibition, red blood cell aplasia
Hepatic: Elevated transaminases, hepatitis (fulminant)
Ocular: Diplopia
Otic: Ototoxicity, tinnitus
Renal: Renal failure (acute), nephrotic syndrome, chronic renal failure, albuminuria, glomerulosclerosis
Respiratory: Wheezing, respiratory depression
Miscellaneous: Hypersensitivity
Signs and Symptoms of Overdose Azotemia, coagulopathy, cognitive dysfunction, drowsiness, erythema multiforme, gastritis, GI bleeding, nausea, nephrotic syndrome, ototoxicity, tinnitus, vomiting, wheezing
Severe poisoning can manifest with agranulocytosis, coma, granulocytopenia, hypotension, hypothermia, leukopenia, neutropenia, renal failure and/or hepatic failure, respiratory depression, seizures, tachycardia
Pharmacodynamics/Kinetics
Onset of action: A few days
Absorption: Rapid, 80%
Distribution: Does not cross the placenta
Protein binding: 99%
Metabolism: Extensively hepatic
Half-life elimination: 2.5-3 hours
Time to peak, serum: ~2 hours
Excretion: Urine (2% to 5% as unchanged drug); feces (small amounts)
Dosage
Adults: Oral:
Rheumatoid arthritis: 300-600 mg 3-4 times/day up to 3.2 g/day
Mild to moderate pain: 200 mg every 4-6 hours as needed
Monitoring Parameters Monitor CBC, liver enzymes; monitor urine output and BUN/serum creatinine in patients receiving diuretics
Administration
Do not crush tablets. Swallow whole with a full glass of water. Take with food to minimize stomach upset.

Contraindications Hypersensitivity to fenoprofen, aspirin, or other NSAIDs, or any component of the formulation; perioperative pain in the setting of coronary artery bypass surgery (CABG); significant renal dysfunction; pregnancy (3rd trimester)

Warnings [U.S. Boxed Warning]: NSAIDs are associated with an increased risk of adverse cardiovascular events, including MI, stroke, and new onset or worsening of pre-existing hypertension. Risk may be increased with duration of use or pre-existing cardiovascular risk-factors or disease. Carefully evaluate individual cardiovascular risk profiles prior to prescribing. Use caution with fluid retention, CHF, or hypertension.

Use of NSAIDs can compromise existing renal function. Renal toxicity can occur in patient with impaired renal function, dehydration, heart failure, liver dysfunction, those taking diuretics and ACEI, and the elderly. Rehydrate patient before starting therapy. Monitor renal function closely. Not recommended for use in patients with advanced renal disease.

[U.S. Boxed Warning]: NSAIDs may increase risk of gastrointestinal irritation, ulceration, bleeding, and perforation. These events may occur at any time during therapy and without warning. Use caution with a history of GI disease (bleeding or ulcers), concurrent therapy with aspirin, anticoagulants and/or corticosteroids, smoking, use of alcohol, the elderly or debilitated patients.

Use the lowest effective dose for the shortest duration of time, consistent with individual patient goals, to reduce risk of cardiovascular or GI adverse events. Alternate therapies should be considered for patients at high risk.

NSAIDs may cause serious skin adverse events including exfoliative dermatitis, Stevens-Johnson syndrome (SJS), and toxic epidermal necrolysis (TEN). Anaphylactoid reactions may occur, even without prior exposure; patients with "aspirin triad" (bronchial asthma, aspirin intolerance, rhinitis) may be at increased risk. Do not use in patients who experience bronchospasm, asthma, rhinitis, or urticaria with NSAID or aspirin therapy.

Use with caution in patients with decreased hepatic function. Closely monitor patients with any abnormal LFT. Severe hepatic reactions (eg, fulminant hepatitis, liver failure) have occurred with NSAID use, rarely; discontinue if signs or symptoms of liver disease develop, or if systemic manifestations occur.

The elderly are at increased risk for adverse effects (especially peptic ulceration, CNS effects, renal toxicity) from NSAIDs even at low doses.

Withhold for at least 4-6 half-lives prior to surgical or dental procedures. Safety and efficacy have not been established in children <18 years of age.

Dosage Forms
Capsule, as calcium (Nalfon®): 200 mg, 300 mg
Tablet, as calcium: 600 mg

Reference Range Therapeutic: 20-65 mcg/mL (SI: 82-268 μmol/L), not readily available

Overdosage/Treatment
Decontamination: Ipecac within 30 minutes or lavage (within 1 hour)/activated charcoal
Supportive therapy: Hypotension/dehydration can be managed with I.V. fluid therapy; acidosis should be treated with bicarbonates, seizures with benzodiazepines; antacids, blood products are indicated, as appropriate, for hemorrhage
Enhancement of elimination: Dialysis or hemoperfusion is indicated for secondary complications, acidosis, or renal failure and not toxin removal alone; multiple dosing of activated charcoal may be useful

Diagnostic Procedures
- Electrolytes, Blood
- Electrolytes, Urine
- Urinalysis

Test Interactions ↑ chloride (S), sodium (S); may yield false-positive for benzodiazepine and barbiturate assay

Drug Interactions ACE inhibitors: Antihypertensive effects may be decreased by concurrent therapy with NSAIDs; monitor blood pressure.
Angiotensin II antagonists: Antihypertensive effects may be decreased by concurrent therapy with NSAIDs; monitor blood pressure.
Anticoagulants (warfarin, heparin, LMWHs) in combination with NSAIDs can cause increased risk of bleeding.
Antiplatelet drugs (ticlopidine, clopidogrel, aspirin, abciximab, dipyridamole, eptifibatide, tirofiban) can cause an increased risk of bleeding.
Beta-blockers: NSAIDs may decrease the antihypertensive effect of beta-blockers. Monitor.
Cholestyramine (and other bile acid sequestrants): May decrease the absorption of NSAIDs. Separate by at least 2 hours.
Corticosteroids may increase the risk of GI ulceration; avoid concurrent use.
Cyclosporine: NSAIDs may increase serum creatinine, potassium, blood pressure, and cyclosporine levels; monitor cyclosporine levels and renal function carefully.
Gentamicin and amikacin serum concentrations are increased by indomethacin in premature infants. Results may apply to other aminoglycosides and NSAIDs.
Hydralazine's antihypertensive effect is decreased; avoid concurrent use.

Lithium levels can be increased; avoid concurrent use if possible or monitor lithium levels and adjust dose. Sulindac may have the least effect. When NSAID is stopped, lithium will need adjustment again.
Loop diuretics efficacy (diuretic and antihypertensive effect) is reduced. Indomethacin reduces this efficacy, however, it may be anticipated with any NSAID.
Methotrexate: Severe bone marrow suppression, aplastic anemia, and GI toxicity have been reported with concomitant NSAID therapy. Avoid use during moderate or high-dose methotrexate (increased and prolonged methotrexate levels). NSAID use during low-dose treatment of rheumatoid arthritis has not been fully evaluated; extreme caution is warranted.
Thiazide efficacy (diuretic and antihypertensive effect) may be reduced. Indomethacin may reduce this efficacy and it may be anticipated with any NSAID.
Verapamil plasma concentration is decreased by diclofenac; avoid concurrent use.
Warfarin's INRs may be increased by piroxicam. Other NSAIDs may have the same effect depending on dose and duration. Monitor INR closely. Use the lowest dose of NSAIDs possible and for the briefest duration.

Pregnancy Risk Factor B/D (3rd trimester)
Pregnancy Implications Does not cross the placenta
Lactation Enters breast milk/not recommended
Additional Information Generally nontoxic ingestions

Fenproporex

CAS Number 15686-61-0; 18305-29-8
Unlabeled/Investigational Use Anorectic agent (not FDA approved in U.S.)
Mechanism of Action Stimulant effects
Adverse Reactions
Cardiovascular: Palpitations, tachycardia
Central nervous system: Anxiety, headache, sleep disturbances
Gastrointestinal: Xerostomia
Toxicodynamics/Kinetics
Metabolism: Metabolized to amphetamine (both enantiomers)
Peak urine levels of amphetamine: 6-20 hours postdose
Elimination: Renal
Dosage Oral: 10-25 mg/day in divided doses before meals; long-acting preparation can be given at a dose of 20 mg before breakfast
Overdosage/Treatment
Decontamination: Lavage (within 1 hour)/activated charcoal
Supportive therapy: Seizures can be treated with lorazepam, diazepam, phenytoin, or phenobarbital; ventricular arrhythmias should be treated with lidocaine
Additional Information Will cause a positive urine amphetamine screen for up to 119 hours postdose (level of detection >5 ng/mL). Maximal urinary amphetamine concentration after one 10 mg dose: ~2099 ng/mL. Available in Mexico (since 1972), Costa Rica, Spain, El Salvador, Panama, France, and Germany.

Fentanyl

Related Information
- Carfentanil Citrate
CAS Number 437-38-7; 990-73-8
U.S. Brand Names Actiq®; Duragesic®; Ionsys™; Sublimaze®
Synonyms Fentanyl Citrate; Fentanyl Hydrocholoride
Impairment Potential Yes
Use Sedation, relief of pain, preoperative medication, adjunct to general or regional anesthesia, management of chronic pain (transdermal product) Actiq® is indicated only for management of breakthrough cancer pain in patients who are tolerant to and currently receiving opioid therapy for persistent cancer pain.
Mechanism of Action Binds with stereospecific receptors at many sites within the CNS, increases pain threshold, alters pain reception, inhibits ascending pain pathways
Adverse Reactions
Cardiovascular: **Hypotension, bradycardia**, sinus bradycardia, angina, sinus tachycardia
Central nervous system: **CNS depression**, agitation, **drowsiness**, dizziness, **sedation**, electroencephalogram abnormalities, amnesia, paranoia
Dermatologic: Erythema, pruritus, urticaria, exanthem
Endocrine & metabolic: ADH release
Gastrointestinal: **Nausea**, dyspepsia, **vomiting**, **constipation**, biliary tract spasm, xerostomia, dysphagia (following intrathecal administration)
Genitourinary: Urinary tract spasm
Local: Transdermal system: Edema, erythema, pruritus
Neuromuscular & skeletal: Skeletal and thoracic muscle rigidity especially following rapid I.V. administration; dyskinesias; paresthesia
Ocular: Miosis

Respiratory: Apnea, **respiratory depression**, laryngospasm

Miscellaneous: Physical and psychological dependence with prolonged use; chest wall rigidity can occur in neonates

Signs and Symptoms of Overdose Apnea, chest pain, coma, confusion, depression, dyspnea, exfoliative dermatitis, flatulence, hiccups, hypertension, hypertonia, hypotension, laryngospasm, pseudotumor cerebri, respiratory depression (especially with doses >200 mcg), seizures

Pharmacodynamics/Kinetics

Onset of action: Analgesic: I.M.: 7-15 minutes; I.V.: Almost immediate; Transmucosal: 5-15 minutes

Peak effect: Transmucosal: Analgesic: 20-30 minutes

Duration: I.M.: 1-2 hours; I.V.: 0.5-1 hour; Transmucosal: Related to blood level; respiratory depressant effect may last longer than analgesic effect

Absorption:

Transmucosal: Rapid, ~25% from the buccal mucosa; 75% swallowed with saliva and slowly absorbed from GI tract

Iontophoretic transdermal system (Ionsys™): Fentanyl levels continue to rise for 5 minutes after the completion of each 10-minute dose

Distribution: Highly lipophilic, redistributes into muscle and fat

Metabolism: Hepatic, primarily via CYP3A4

Bioavailability: Transmucosal: ~50% (range: 36% to 71%)

Half-life elimination: 2-4 hours

Iontophoretic transdermal system (Ionsys™): 11 hours

Transdermal patch: 17 hours (half-life is influenced by absorption rate)

Transmucosal: 6.6 hours (range: 5-15 hours)

Time to peak: Transdermal patch: 24-72 hours

Excretion: Urine (primarily as metabolites, 10% as unchanged drug)

Dosage

Note: These are guidelines and do not represent the maximum doses that may be required in all patients. Doses should be titrated to pain relief/prevention. Monitor vital signs routinely. Single I.M. doses have a duration of 1-2 hours, single I.V. doses last 0.5-1 hour.

Children 1-12 years:

Sedation for minor procedures/analgesia: I.M., I.V.: 1-2 mcg/kg/dose; may repeat at 30- to 60-minute intervals.

Note: Children 18-36 months of age may require 2-3 mcg/kg/dose

Continuous sedation/analgesia: Initial I.V. bolus: 1-2 mcg/kg then 1 mcg/kg/hour; titrate upward; usual: 1-3 mcg/kg/hour

Pain control: Transdermal (limited to children >2 years who are opioid tolerant): Initial dose: 25 mcg/hour system (higher doses have been used based on equianalgesic conversion); change patch every 72 hours

Children >12 years and Adults:

Sedation for minor procedures/analgesia: I.M., I.V.: 0.5-1 mcg/kg/dose; higher doses are used for major procedures

Pain control: Transdermal: Initial: 25 mcg/hour system; if currently receiving opiates, convert to fentanyl equivalent and administer equianalgesic dosage titrated to minimize the adverse effects and provide analgesia. Change patch every 72 hours. To convert patients from oral or parenteral opioids to Duragesic®, the previous 24-hour analgesic requirement should be calculated. This analgesic requirement should be converted to the equianalgesic oral morphine dose.

Adults:

Premedication: I.M., slow I.V.: 50-100 mcg/dose 30-60 minutes prior to surgery

Adjunct to regional anesthesia: I.M., slow I.V.: 50-100 mcg/dose; if I.V. used, give over 1-2 minutes

Severe pain: I.M.: 50-100 mcg/dose every 1-2 hours as needed; patients with prior opiate exposure may tolerate higher initial doses

Adjunct to general anesthesia: Slow I.V.:

Low dose: Initial: 2 mcg/kg/dose; Maintenance: Additional doses infrequently needed

Moderate dose: Initial: 2-20 mcg/kg/dose; Maintenance: 25-100 mcg/dose may be given slow I.V. or I.M. as needed

High dose: Initial: 20-50 mcg/kg/dose; Maintenance: 25 mcg to one-half the initial loading dose may be given as needed

General anesthesia without additional anesthetic agents: Slow I.V.: 50-100 mcg/kg with O₂ and skeletal muscle relaxant

Mechanically-ventilated patients (based on 70 kg patient): Slow I.V.: 0.35-1.5 mcg/kg every 30-60 minutes as needed; infusion: 0.7-10 mcg/kg/hour

Patient-controlled analgesia (PCA): I.V.: Usual concentration: 50 mcg/mL

Demand dose: Usual: 10 mcg; range: 10-50 mcg

Lockout interval: 5-8 minutes

Iontophoretic transdermal system: 40 mcg per activation on-demand (maximum: 6 doses/hour). Note: Patient's pain should be controlled prior to initiating system. Instruct patient how to operate system. Only the patient should initiate system. Each system operates for 24 hours or until 80 doses have been administered, whichever comes first.

Breakthrough cancer pain: Adults: Transmucosal: Actiq® dosing should be individually titrated to provide adequate analgesia with minimal side effects. It is indicated only for management of breakthrough cancer pain in patients who are tolerant to and currently receiving opioid therapy for persistent cancer pain. An initial starting dose of 200 mcg should be used for the treatment of breakthrough cancer pain. Patients should be monitored closely in order to determine the proper dose. If redosing for the same episode is necessary, the second dose may be started 15 minutes after completion of the first dose. Dosing should be titrated so that the patient's pain can be treated with one single dose. Generally, 1-2 days is required to determine the proper dose of analgesia with limited side effects. Once the dose has been determined, consumption should be limited to 4 units/day or less. Patients needing more than 4 units/day should have the dose of their long-term opioid re-evaluated. If signs of excessive opioid effects occur before a dose is complete, the unit should be removed from the patient's mouth immediately, and subsequent doses decreased.

See tables.

Equianalgesic Doses of Opioid Agonists

Drug	Equianalgesic Dose (mg)	
	I.M.	P.O.
Codeine	75	130
Hydromorphone	1.5	7.5
Levorphanol	2 (acute)	4 (acute)
Meperidine	75	300
Methadone	10 (acute)	20 (acute)
Morphine	10	30
Oxycodone	—	20
Oxymorphone	1	10 (PR)

From "Principles of Analgesic Use," *Am Pain Soc*, 1999.

Corresponding Doses of Oral/Intramuscular Morphine and Duragesic™

P.O. 24-Hour Morphine (mg/d)	I.M. 24-Hour Morphine (mg/d)	Duragesic™ Dose (mcg/h)
45-134	8-22	25
135-224	28-37	50
225-314	38-52	75
315-404	53-67	100
405-494	68-82	125
495-584	83-97	150
585-674	98-112	175
675-764	113-127	200
765-854	128-142	225
855-944	143-157	250
945-1034	158-172	275
1035-1124	173-187	300

Product information, Duragesic™ — Janssen Pharmaceutica, January, 1991.

The dosage should not be titrated more frequently than every 3 days after the initial dose or every 6 days thereafter. The majority of patients are controlled on every 72-hour administration, however, a small number of patients require every 48-hour administration.

Elderly >65 years: Transmucosal: Actiq®: Dose should be reduced to 2.5-5 mcg/kg; elderly have been found to be twice as sensitive as younger patients to the effects of fentanyl. Patients in this age group generally require smaller doses of Actiq® than younger patients

Dosing adjustment in hepatic impairment: Actiq®: Although fentanyl kinetics may be altered in hepatic disease, Actiq® can be used successfully in the management of breakthrough cancer pain. Doses should be titrated to reach clinical effect with careful monitoring of patients with severe hepatic disease.

Stability

Protect from light; **incompatible** when mixed in the same syringe with pentobarbital; **incompatible** with thiopental sodium and methohexital sodium

Transmucosal: Store at controlled room temperature of 15°C to 30°C (59°F to 86°F)

Monitoring Parameters Respiratory and cardiovascular status, blood pressure, heart rate

Administration

I.V.: Muscular rigidity may occur with rapid I.V. administration. During prolonged administration, dosage requirements may decrease.

Transdermal: Apply to nonirritated and nonirradiated skin, such as chest, back, flank, or upper arm. Upper back is preferred location in children. Do not shave skin; hair at application site should be clipped. Prior to application, clean site with clear water and allow to dry completely. Do not cut patch. Apply patch immediately after removing from package. Firmly press in place and hold for 30 seconds. Change patch every 72 hours. Keep transdermal product (both used and unused) out of the reach of children. Do **not** use soap, alcohol, or other solvents to remove transdermal gel if it accidentally touches skin, as they may increase transdermal absorption; use copious amounts of water. Avoid exposing application site to external heat sources (eg, heating pad, electric blanket, heat lamp, hot tub).

Transmucosal: Foil overwrap should be removed just prior to administration. Once removed, patient should place the unit in mouth and allow it to dissolve. Do **not** chew. Actiq® units may be occasionally moved from one side of the mouth to the other. The unit should be consumed over a period of 15 minutes. Unit should be removed after it is consumed or if patient has achieved an adequate response and/or shows signs of respiratory depression. For patients who have received transmucosal product within 6-12 hours, it is recommended that if other narcotics are required, they should be used at starting doses $^1/_4$ to $^1/_3$ those usually recommended.

Contraindications

Hypersensitivity to fentanyl or any component of the formulation; increased intracranial pressure; severe respiratory disease or depression including acute asthma (unless patient is mechanically ventilated); paralytic ileus; severe liver or renal insufficiency; pregnancy (prolonged use or high doses near term)

Iontophoretic transdermal system (Ionsys™): Hypersensitivity to fentanyl, cetylpyridinium chloride (eg, Cepacol®) or any component of Ionsys™ system

Transmucosal lozenges (Actiq®) or transdermal patches (eg, Duragesic®) must not be used in patients who are not opioid tolerant. Patients are considered opioid-tolerant if they are taking at least 60 mg morphine/day, 30 mg oral oxycodone/day, 8 mg oral hydromorphone/day, 25 mcg transdermal fentanyl/hour, or an equivalent dose of another opioid for ≥1 week. Transdermal patches are not for use in acute pain, mild pain, intermittent pain, or postoperative pain management.

Warnings

An opioid-containing analgesic regimen should be tailored to each patient's needs and based upon the type of pain being treated (acute versus chronic), the route of administration, degree of tolerance for opioids (naive versus chronic user), age, weight, and medical condition. The optimal analgesic dose varies widely among patients. Doses should be titrated to pain relief/prevention. When using with other CNS depressants, reduce dose of one or both agents. Fentanyl shares the toxic potentials of opiate agonists, and precautions of opiate agonist therapy should be observed; use with caution in patients with bradycardia; rapid I.V. infusion may result in skeletal muscle and chest wall rigidity leading to respiratory distress and/or apnea, bronchoconstriction, laryngospasm; inject slowly over 3-5 minutes. Tolerance or drug dependence may result from extended use. Use caution in patients with a history of drug dependence or abuse. The elderly may be particularly susceptible to the CNS depressant and constipating effects of narcotics. Use extreme caution in patients with COPD or other chronic respiratory conditions. Use caution with head injuries, hepatic or renal dysfunction.

Actiq®: **[U.S. Boxed Warning]: Should be used only for the care of cancer patients and is intended for use by specialists who are knowledgeable in treating cancer pain.** For patients who have received transmucosal product within 6-12 hours, it is recommended that if other narcotics are required, they should be used at starting doses 1/4 to 1/3 those usually recommended. **[U.S. Boxed Warning]:Actiq® preparations contain an amount of medication that can be fatal to children.** Keep all units out of the reach of children and discard any open units properly. Patients and caregivers should be counseled on the dangers to children including the risk of exposure to partially-consumed units. Safety and efficacy have not been established in children <16 years of age.

Transdermal patches (eg, Duragesic®): **[U.S. Boxed Warning]: Serious or life-threatening hypoventilation may occur, even in opioid-tolerant patients.** Serum fentanyl concentrations may increase approximately one-third for patients with a body temperature of 40°C secondary to a temperature-dependent increase in fentanyl release from the patch and increased skin permeability. Avoid exposure of application site to direct external heat sources. Patients who experience adverse reactions should be monitored for at least 24 hours after removal of the patch. Transdermal patch does not contain any metal-based compounds; the printed ink used to indicate strength on the outer surface of the patch does contain titanium dioxide but the amount is minimal; adverse events have not been reported while wearing during an MRI. **[U.S. Boxed Warning]: Safety and efficacy of transdermal patch have been limited to children ≥2 years of age who are opioid tolerant.**

Iontophoretic transdermal system (Ionsys™): **[U.S. Boxed Warning]: Should only be used for the treatment of hospitalized patients. To avoid overdose, the patient should be the only one to activate the**

system. **Unintended exposure to fentanyl hydrogel could lead to absorption of fatal dose; hydrogel should not come in contact with fingers or mouth.** Should be used only in patients who are able to understand and follow instructions to operate the system. The error detection circuit uses a series of audible signals to alert the patient when a dose is not being delivered; use caution in patients who have high frequency hearing impairment. Ionsys™ contains metal parts; remove prior to MRI procedure, cardioversion, or defibrillation. May interfere with radiographic image or CAT scan as system contains radiopaque components. Patients on chronic opioids or with a history of opioid abuse may require higher analgesic doses than Ionsys™ is able to provide. Prior to patient's hospital discharge, the system must be removed and disposed of in accordance with State and Federal regulations for a C-II substance. **[U.S. Boxed Warning]: Even if all 80 doses are used, a significant amount of fentanyl remains in the iontophoretic transdermal system and requires proper removal and disposal to avoid misuse, abuse, or diversion.** Safety and efficacy of iontophoretic transdermal system have not been established in children <18 years of age.

Dosage Forms

Infusion [premixed in NS]: 0.05 mg (10 mL); 1 mg (100 mL); 1.25 mg (250 mL); 2 mg (100 mL); 2.5 mg (250 mL)

Injection, solution, as citrate [preservative free]: 0.05 mg/mL (2 mL, 5 mL, 10 mL, 20 mL, 30 mL, 50 mL)

   Sublimaze®: 0.05 mg/mL (2 mL, 5 mL, 10 mL, 20 mL)

Lozenge, oral transmucosal, as citrate:

   Actiq®: 200 mcg, 400 mcg, 600 mcg, 800 mcg, 1200 mcg, 1600 mcg [mounted on a plastic radiopaque handle; contains sugar 2 g/unit; raspberry flavor]

Transdermal patch: 25 mcg/hour [6.25 cm^2] (5s); 50 mcg/hour [12.5 cm^2] (5s); 75 mcg/hour [18.75 cm^2]; 100 mcg/hour [25 cm^2] (5s)

   Duragesic®: 12 [delivers 12.5 mcg/hour; 5 cm^2; contains alcohol 0.1 mL/10 cm^2] (5s); 25 [delivers 25 mcg/hour; 10 cm^2; contains alcohol 0.1 mL/10 cm^2] (5s); 50 [delivers 50 mcg/hour; 20 cm^2; contains alcohol 0.1 mL/10 cm^2] (5s); 75 [delivers 75 mcg/hour; 30 cm^2; contains alcohol 0.1 mL/10 cm^2]; 100 [delivers 100 mcg/hour; 40 cm^2; contains alcohol 0.1 mL/10 cm^2] (5s)

Transdermal iontophoretic system:

   Ionsys™: Fentanyl hydrochloride 40 mcg/dose [80 doses/patch; contains 3-volt lithium battery]

Reference Range

Therapeutic: 2-200 mcg/L; opioid naive patients may exhibit CNS toxicity at serum fentanyl >3 mcg/L.

Serum level of 17.7 mcg/L has been correlated with fatality. Postmortem redistribution of drug may occur.

Overdosage/Treatment

Decontamination: Lavage (within 1 hour)/activated charcoal for oral ingestion

Supportive therapy: Naloxone in large doses and/or a continuous infusion may be necessary; laryngospasm and masseter muscle spasm also respond to naloxone; inhaled beta adrenergic agents can be used to treat fentanyl-induced coughing; seizures can be treated with diazepam or thiopental

Enhancement of elimination: Not dialyzable

Antidote(s)

- Nalmefene [ANTIDOTE]
- Naloxone [ANTIDOTE]

Drug Interactions **Substrate** of CYP3A4 (major); **Inhibits** CYP3A4 (weak)

Antipsychotic agents (phenothiazines): May enhance the hypotensive effect of analgesics (narcotic).

CNS depressants: Increased sedation with CNS depressants.;

CYP3A4 inhibitors: May increase the levels/effects of fentanyl. Potentially fatal respiratory depression may occur when a potent inhibitor is used in a patient receiving chronic fentanyl (eg, transdermal patch). Example inhibitors include azole antifungals, clarithromycin, diclofenac, doxycycline, erythromycin, imatinib, isoniazid, nefazodone, nicardipine, propofol, protease inhibitors, quinidine, telithromycin, and verapamil.

MAO inhibitors: Not recommended to use Actiq® within 14 days. Severe and unpredictable potentiation by MAO inhibitors has been reported with opioid analgesics.

Pegvisomant: Analgesics (narcotic) may diminish the therapeutic effect of pegvisomant.

Protease inhibitors: May decrease the metabolism, via CYP isoenzymes, of fentanyl.

Selective serotonin reuptake inhibitors (SSRIs): Analgesics (narcotic) may enhance the serotonergic effect of SSRIs. This may cause serotonin syndrome.

Sibutramine: Fentanyl may enhance the serotonergic effect of sibutramine.

Pregnancy Risk Factor B/D (prolonged use or high doses at term)

Pregnancy Implications Fentanyl crosses the placenta and has been used safely during labor. Chronic use during pregnancy has shown detectable serum levels in the newborn with mild opioid withdrawal (case report).

Lactation Enters breast milk/not recommended (AAP rates "compatible")

Additional Information Lethal dose: Adults: I.V.: 1 mg

Specific References

Barrueto F Jr, Howland MA, Hoffman RS, et al, "The Fentanyl Tea Bag," *Vet Hum Toxicol*, 2004, 46(1):30-1.

Coon TP, Miller M, Kaylor D, et al, "Rectal Insertion of Fentanyl Patches: A New Route of Toxicity," *Ann Emerg Med*, 2005, 46(5):473.

Day J, Slawson M, Lugo RA, et al, "Analysis of Fentanyl and Norfentanyl in Human Plasma by Liquid Chromatography-Tandem Mass Spectrometry Using Electrospray Ionization," *J Anal Toxicol*, 2003, 27:513-6.

Dominguez KD, Lomako DM, Katz RW, et al, "Opioid Withdrawal in Critically Ill Neonates," *Ann Pharmacother*, 2003, 37(4):473-7.

Frakes MA, Lord WR, Kociszewski C, et al, "Efficacy of Fentanyl Analgesia for Trauma in Critical Care Transport," *Am J Emerg Med*, 2006, 24:286-9.

Galinski M, Dolveck F, Borron SW, et al, "A Randomized, Double-Blind Study Comparing Morphine with Fentanyl in Prehospital Analgesia," *Am J Emerg Med*, 2005, 23(2):114-9.

Han PK, Arnold R, Bond G, et al, "Myoclonus Secondary to Withdrawal from Transdermal Fentanyl: Case Report and Literature Review," *J Pain Symptom Manage*, 2002, 23(1):66-72.

Hughes AA, Dart RC, and Bailey JE, "Lick or Stick: The Common Routes of the Misuse and Abuse of Fentanyl," *Clin Toxicol (Phila)*, 2005, 43:668.

Jin M, Gock SB, Jannetoo PJ, et al, "Pharmacogenomics as Molecular Autopsy for Forensic Toxicology: Genotyping Cytochrome P450 3A4*1B and 3A5*3 for 25 Fentanyl Cases," *J Anal Toxicol*, 2005, 29:590-606.

Kaye AD, Hoover JM, Ibrahim IN, et al, "Analysis of the Effects of Fentanyl in the Feline Pulmonary Vascular Bed." *Am J Therapeutics*, 2006, 13:478-84.

Kuhlman JJ Jr, McCaulley R, Valouch TJ, et al, "Fentanyl Use, Misuse, and Abuse: A Summary of 23 Postmortem Cases," *J Anal Toxicol*, 2003, 27:499-512.

Miller MA, Kaylor DW, Jones-Spangle K, et al, "Rectal Overdose with Fentanyl Patches; A Case Report," *Clin Toxicol (Phila)*, 2005, 43:666.

Pizon AF and Brooks DE, "Fentanyl Patch Abuse: Naloxone Complications and Extracorporeal Membrane Oxygenation Rescue," *Vet Hum Toxicol*, 2004, 46(5):256-7.

Poklis A and Backer R, "Urine Concentrations of Fentanyl and Norfentanyl During Application of Duragesic® Transdermal Patches," *J Anal Toxicol*, 2004, 28(6):422-5.

Tharp AM, Winecker RE, and Winston DC, "Fatal Intravenous Fentanyl Abuse: Four Cases Involving Extraction of Fentanyl from Transdermal Patches," *Am J Forensic Med Pathol*, 2004, 25(2):178-81.

Viscusi ER, Reynolds L, Chung F, et al, "Patient-Controlled Transdermal Fentanyl Hydrochloride vs Intravenous Morphine Pump for Postoperative Pain: A Randomized Controlled Trial," *JAMA*, 2004, 291(11): 1333-41.

Fexofenadine

CAS Number 138452-21-8

U.S. Brand Names Allegra®

Synonyms Fexofenadine Hydrochloride

Impairment Potential None documented at 60 mg dose; impairment may occur at double the therapeutic dose

Use Relief of symptoms associated with seasonal allergic rhinitis; treatment of chronic idiopathic urticaria

Mechanism of Action Fexofenadine is an active metabolite of terfenadine and like terfenadine it competes with histamine for H_1-receptor sites on effector cells in the gastrointestinal tract, blood vessels, and respiratory tract; it appears that fexofenadine does not cross the blood brain barrier to any appreciable degree, resulting in a greatly reduced potential for sedation

Adverse Reactions

Central nervous system: **Headache** (with once-daily dosing) fever, dizziness, pain, drowsiness, fatigue, insomnia, nervousness, sleep disorders

Endocrine & metabolic: Dysmenorrhea

Gastrointestinal: Nausea, dyspepsia

Neuromuscular & skeletal: Back pain

Otic: Otitis media

Respiratory: Cough, upper respiratory tract infection, sinusitis

Miscellaneous: Viral infection, hypersensitivity reactions (anaphylaxis, angioedema, dyspnea, flushing, pruritus, rash, urticaria), paroniria

Pharmacodynamics/Kinetics

Onset of action: 60 minutes

Duration: Antihistaminic effect: $\geq$12 hours

Protein binding: 60% to 70%, primarily albumin and alpha$_1$-acid glycoprotein

Metabolism: Minimal ($\sim$5%)

Half-life elimination: 14.4 hours

Time to peak, serum: $\sim$2.6 hours

Excretion: Feces ($\sim$80%) and urine ($\sim$11%) as unchanged drug

Dosage Oral:

Children 6-11 years: 30 mg twice daily

Children $\geq$12 years and Adults:

Seasonal allergic rhinitis: 60 mg twice daily **or** 180 mg once daily

Chronic idiopathic urticaria: 60 mg twice daily

Dosing adjustment in renal impairment: Cl_{cr} <80 mL/minute:

Children 6-11 years: Initial: 30 mg once daily

Children $\geq$12 years and Adults: Initial: 60 mg once daily

Stability Store capsules at controlled room temperature of 20°C to 25°C (68°F to 77°F). Protect from excessive moisture.

Monitoring Parameters Relief of symptoms

Administration Administer with water.

Contraindications Hypersensitivity to fexofenadine or any component of the formulation

Warnings Safety and effectiveness in children <6 years of age have not been established.

Dosage Forms Tablet, as hydrochloride: 30 mg, 60 mg, 180 mg

Overdosage/Treatment

Decontamination: Lavage within 1 hour/activated charcoal

Enhancement of elimination: Hemodialysis removes <2% of dose

Drug Interactions Substrate of CYP3A4 (minor); **Inhibits** CYP2D6 (weak)

Antacids (containing aluminum or magnesium): AUC of fexofenadine was decreased by 41% and C_{max} by 43% with concomitant administration; separate administration is recommended.

Erythromycin: Levels of fexofenadine are increased (82% higher); not associated with increased adverse effects and no difference in QT_c intervals.

Ketoconazole: Levels of fexofenadine are increased (135% higher); not associated with increased adverse effects and no difference in QT_c intervals.

Pregnancy Risk Factor C

Pregnancy Implications There are no adequate and well-controlled studies in pregnant women; use during pregnancy only if potential benefit to mother outweighs possible risk to fetus.

Lactation Excretion in breast milk unknown/use caution (AAP rates "compatible")

Finasteride

CAS Number 98319-26-7

U.S. Brand Names Propecia®; Proscar®

Use Early data indicate that finasteride is useful in the treatment of symptomatic benign prostatic hyperplasia (BPH)

Unlabeled/Investigational Use Adjuvant monotherapy after radical prostatectomy in the treatment of prostatic cancer; female hirsutism

Mechanism of Action

Finasteride is a 4-azo analog of testosterone and is a competitive inhibitor of both tissue and hepatic 5-alpha reductase. This results in inhibition of the conversion of testosterone to dihydrotestosterone; markedly suppresses serum dihydrotestosterone levels; dependent on dose and duration, serum testosterone concentrations may or may not increase. Testosterone-dependent processes such as fertility, muscle strength, potency, and libido are not affected by finasteride.

In addition to hydrotestosterone levels, androstenediol and androsterone glucuronide are also suppressed, indicating inhibition of the formation of both unconjugated and conjugated 5-alpha reduced androgens

Adverse Reactions

Endocrine & metabolic: Decreased libido, breast tenderness, breast enlargement

Genitourinary: <4% incidence of erectile dysfunction, decreased volume of ejaculate, testicular pain

Miscellaneous: Hypersensitivity (pruritus, urticaria, swelling of face/lips), breast cancer (males)

Admission Criteria/Prognosis Asymptomatic patients may be managed as out patients

Pharmacodynamics/Kinetics

Onset of action: 3-6 months of ongoing therapy

Duration:

After a single oral dose as small as 0.5 mg: 65% depression of plasma dihydrotestosterone levels persists 5-7 days

After 6 months of treatment with 5 mg/day: Circulating dihydrotestosterone levels are reduced to castrate levels without significant effects on circulating testosterone; levels return to normal within 14 days of discontinuation of treatment

Distribution: V_{dss}: 76 L

Protein binding: 90%

Metabolism: Hepatic via CYP3A4; two active metabolites (<20% activity of finasteride)

Bioavailability: Mean: 63%

Half-life elimination, serum: Elderly: 8 hours; Adults: 6 hours (3-16)

Time to peak, serum: 2-6 hours

Excretion: Feces (57%) and urine (39%) as metabolites

Dosage

Adults: Male: Benign prostatic hyperplasia: Oral: 5 mg/day as a single dose; clinical responses occur within 12 weeks to 6 months of initiation of therapy; long-term administration is recommended for maximal response

Dosing adjustment in renal impairment: No dosage adjustment is necessary

Monitoring Parameters Objective and subjective signs of relief of benign prostatic hyperplasia, including improvement in urinary flow, reduction in symptoms of urgency, and relief of difficulty in micturition

Administration Administration with food may delay the rate and reduce the extent of oral absorption. Childbearing age women should not touch or handle this medication.

Contraindications Hypersensitivity to finasteride or any component of the formulation; pregnancy; not for use in children

Warnings Hazardous agent - use appropriate precautions for handling and disposal. A minimum of 6 months of treatment may be necessary to determine whether an individual will respond to finasteride. Use with caution in those patients with hepatic dysfunction. Carefully monitor patients with a large residual urinary volume or severely diminished urinary flow for obstructive uropathy. These patients may not be candidates for finasteride therapy.

Dosage Forms Tablet: 5 mg

Propecia®: 1 mg

Proscar®: 5 mg

Reference Range Peak plasma level: 1-2 hours; peak plasma finasteride concentration after a 100 mg dose is ~835.5 ($\pm$199) mcg/L

Overdosage/Treatment Decontamination: Emesis within 30 minutes or lavage within 2 hours of ingestion; activated charcoal may be given; decontamination should be aggressive in a pregnant female

Test Interactions Finasteride does not influence plasma FSH, LH, cortisol, or estradiol levels; increases plasma testosterone levels; decreases plasma dihydrotestosterone and prostate specific antigen levels; no clinically significant effects on serum lipids

Drug Interactions Substrate of CYP3A4 (minor)

Pregnancy Risk Factor X

Pregnancy Implications Abnormalities of external male genitalia were reported in animal studies. Pregnant women are advised to avoid contact with crushed or broken tablets.

Lactation Excretion in breast milk unknown/contraindicated

Nursing Implications Administration with food may delay the rate and reduce the extent of oral absorption

Additional Information May be useful in men with moderately symptomatic BPH who either refuse prostatectomy or are poor surgical candidates. The risk/benefit ratio and cost must be explained to the patient. Currently, there is no way to predict which men will respond to finasteride. The Washington Poison Control Center (206) 526-2121 can be contacted regarding toxicities of the Finasteride Study.

Flecainide

Related Information

● Lorcainide

CAS Number 54143-55-4

U.S. Brand Names Tambocor™

Synonyms Flecainide Acetate

Use Prevention and suppression of documented life-threatening ventricular arrhythmias (ie, sustained tachycardia (ventricular)); controlling symptomatic, disabling tachycardia (ventricular) in patients without structural heart disease (class I agent)

Mechanism of Action Class IC antiarrhythmic; slows conduction in cardiac tissue by altering transport of ions across cell membranes; causes slight prolongation of refractory periods; decreases the rate of rise of the action potential without affecting its duration; increases electrical stimulation threshold of ventricle, His-Purkinje system; possesses local anesthetic and moderate negative inotropic effects

Adverse Reactions

Cardiovascular: Bradycardia, heart block, P-R prolongation, QRS prolongation, QT_c interval prolongation is minimal; worsening arrhythmias (ventricular), congestive heart failure, palpitations, chest pain, edema, cardiac arrest, hypotension, syncope, sinus bradycardia, angina, myocardial depression, sinus tachycardia, tachycardia (supraventricular), atrial flutter, exacerbation of Brugada syndrome

Central nervous system: **Dizziness**, fatigue, nervousness, hypoesthesia, seizures, psychosis, visual hallucinations, headache

Dermatologic: Rashes

Gastrointestinal: Nausea, metallic taste, vomiting

Hematologic: Blood dyscrasias

Hepatic: Possible hepatic dysfunction

Neuromuscular & skeletal: Tremors, dysarthria, paresthesia

Ocular: **Visual disturbances**, blurred vision, photophobia, diplopia

Respiratory: **Dyspnea**

Miscellaneous: Systemic lupus-like syndrome

Signs and Symptoms of Overdose Arthralgia, AV block, blurred vision, conduction disturbances, congestive heart failure, heart block, hypotension and death, impotence, increased T-wave amplitude, neutropenia, primary arrhythmia has been noted, P-R prolongation, polymorphous or wide-complex ventricular tachycardia (although wide-complex supraventricular arrhythmias can occur), QRS prolongation, QT prolongation, syncope, reduced heart rate and myocardial contractility, tachycardia (ventricular)

Pharmacodynamics/Kinetics

Absorption: Oral: Rapid

Distribution: Adults: V_d: 5-13.4 L/kg

Protein binding: Alpha$_1$ glycoprotein: 40% to 50%

Metabolism: Hepatic

Bioavailability: 85% to 90%

Half-life elimination: Infants: 11-12 hours; Children: 8 hours; Adults: 7-22 hours, increased with congestive heart failure or renal dysfunction; End-stage renal disease: 19-26 hours

Time to peak, serum: ~1.5-3 hours

Excretion: Urine (80% to 90%, 10% to 50% as unchanged drug and metabolites)

Dosage

Oral:

Children: Initial: 3 mg/kg/day in 3 divided doses; usual 3-6 mg/kg/day in 3 divided doses; up to 11 mg/kg/day for uncontrolled patients with subtherapeutic levels

Adults: Initial: 100 mg every 12 hours, increase by 100 mg/day (given in 2 doses/day) every 4 days to maximum of 400 mg/day; for patients receiving 400 mg/day who are not controlled and have trough concentrations <0.6 mcg/mL, dosage may be increased to 600 mg/day

Children and Adults:

Dosing adjustment in severe renal impairment: Cl_{cr} <10 mL/minute: Decrease usual dose by 25% to 50%

Dosing adjustment/comments in hepatic impairment: Monitoring of plasma levels is recommended because of significantly increased half-life

Monitoring Parameters ECG, blood pressure, pulse, periodic serum concentrations, especially in patients with renal or hepatic impairment

Administration Administer around-the-clock to promote less variation in peak and trough serum levels

Contraindications Hypersensitivity to flecainide or any component of the formulation; pre-existing second- or third-degree AV block or with right bundle branch block when associated with a left hemiblock (bifascicular block) (except in patients with a functioning artificial pacemaker); cardiogenic shock; coronary artery disease (based on CAST study results); concurrent use of ritonavir or amprenavir

Warnings [U.S. Boxed Warning]: In the Cardiac Arrhythmia Suppression Trial (CAST), recent (>6 days but <2 years ago) myocardial infarction patients with asymptomatic, nonlife-threatening ventricular arrhythmias did not benefit and may have been harmed by attempts to suppress the arrhythmia with flecainide or encainide. An increased mortality or nonfatal cardiac arrest rate (7.7%) was seen in the active treatment group compared with patients in the placebo group (3%). The applicability of the CAST results to other populations is unknown. The risks of class 1C agents and the lack of improved survival make use in patients without life-threatening arrhythmias generally unacceptable. Not recommended for patients with chronic atrial fibrillation; may have proarrhythmic effects. When treating atrial flutter, 1:1 atrioventricular conduction may occur; pre-emptive negative chronotropic therapy (eg, digoxin, beta-blockers) may lower the risk. Pre-existing hypokalemia or hyperkalemia should be corrected before initiation (can alter drug's effect). A worsening or new arrhythmia may occur (proarrhythmic effect). Use caution in heart failure (may precipitate or exacerbate CHF). Dose-related increases in PR, QRS, and QT intervals occur. Use with caution in sick sinus syndrome or with permanent pacemakers or temporary pacing wires (can increase endocardial pacing thresholds). Cautious use in significant hepatic impairment.

Dosage Forms Tablet, as acetate: 50 mg, 100 mg, 150 mg

Reference Range

Therapeutic: 0.2-1.0 mcg/mL (SI: 0.4-2.0 μmol/L)

Fatal: 21.3 mcg/mL associated with fatality

Postmortem flecainide blood concentration was 6.87 mcg/mL following pediatric overdose.

Overdosage/Treatment

Decontamination: Lavage (within 1 hour)/activated charcoal

Supportive therapy: Monitoring; flecainide-induced tachycardia (ventricular) should be treated with ventricular pacing, antiarrhythmic drugs and/or cardioversion; however, it is commonly refractory to these measures; isoproterenol can be used for bradyarrhythmias; sodium bicarbonate (1-2 mEq/kg) can be given for ventricular conduction delays; sotalol can be used to treat flecainide-induced atrial flutter; peripheral cardiopulmonary bypass support can assist in hemodynamic support for improvement of drug clearance and allows time for redistribution

Enhancement of elimination: Multiple dosing of activated charcoal or charcoal hemoperfusion may be helpful; do not alkalinize the urine

Drug Interactions **Substrate** of CYP1A2 (minor), 2D6 (major); **Inhibits** CYP2D6 (weak)

Amiodarone increases in flecainide plasma levels; consider reducing flecainide dose by 25% to 33% with concurrent use.

Amprenavir and ritonavir may increase cardiotoxicity of flecainide (decrease metabolism).

Cimetidine may decrease flecainide's metabolism; monitor cardiac status or use an alternative H_2 antagonist.

CYP2D6 inhibitors: May increase the levels/effects of flecainide. Example inhibitors include chlorpromazine, delavirdine, fluoxetine, miconazole, paroxetine, pergolide, quinidine, quinine, ritonavir, and ropinirole.

Digoxin's serum concentration may increase slightly.

Propranolol (and possibly other beta-blockers) increases flecainide blood levels, and propranolol blood levels are increased with concurrent use; monitor for excessive negative inotropic effects.

Quinidine may decrease flecainide's metabolism; monitor cardiac status.

Urinary alkalinizers (antacids, sodium bicarbonate, acetazolamide) may increase flecainide blood levels.

Pregnancy Risk Factor C

Pregnancy Implications Can cause transient neonatal conjugated hyperbilirubinemia

Lactation Enters breast milk/compatible

Additional Information Based on adverse outcomes noted with flecainide in the CAST trial, the FDA recommends that use of flecainide be limited to patients with life-threatening ventricular arrhythmias; case fatality rate in overdose setting is 8%

Specific References

Benijts T, Borrey D, Lambert WE, et al, "Analysis of Flecainide and Two Metabolites in Biological Specimens of HPLC: Application to a Fatal Intoxication," *J Anal Toxicol*, 2003, 27(1):47-52.

Bottema C, Bilden EF, and Bangh S, "Pediatric Fatality Following Accidental Flecainide Ingestion," *Clin Toxicol*, 2005, 43:633.

Resiere D, Megarbane B, Guerrier G, et al, "Prognositc Factors and Toxicokinetic-Toxicodynamic Relationships in Flecainide Poisonings," *Clin Toxicol (Phila)*, 2005, 43:731.

Wood DM, Angel T, Dargan PI, et al, "Flecainide Toxicity: A Case Report with Toxicokinetic Data," *Br J Clin Pharmacol*, 2003, 55:431-2.

Fleroxacin

CAS Number 79660-72-3

Unlabeled/Investigational Use Urinary tract infections, sexually transmitted diseases, skin/soft tissue infections, bone and joint infections, respiratory tract infections, chancroid, bacterial diarrhea, typhoid fever, effective against Enterobacteriaceae, *Acetobacter*, *Haemophilus*, *Neisseria*, *Moraxella*

Mechanism of Action Fluoroquinolone which inhibits bacterial DNA gyrase and thus has bactericidal activity

Adverse Reactions

Cardiovascular: Flushing

Central nervous system: Insomnia, headache, dizziness, night terrors, lethargy

Dermatologic: Photosensitivity, pruritus

Gastrointestinal: Nausea, vomiting, diarrhea, flatulence, xerostomia

Hematologic: Eosinophilia

Toxicodynamics/Kinetics

Distribution: V_d: 1.3-1.8 L/kg

Protein binding: 30%

Metabolism: Hepatic N-demethylation and N-oxidation to N-desmethyl-fleroxacin (active metabolite) and to fleroxacin-N-oxide (inactive)

Bioavailability: 96% to 100%

Half-life: 8.9-10.3 hours

Elimination: Urine

Dosage

Oral:

Uncomplicated urinary tract infection: 200 mg/day for 10 days

Complicated urinary tract infection: 400 mg/day for 10 days

Uncomplicated cervical or urethral gonorrhea: Single 400 mg dose

Bronchitis: 400 mg once daily

Skin/soft tissue infection: 400 mg/day

Typhoid fever: 400 mg/day for 7 days

I.V.: Urinary tract infection: 400 mg

Reference Range After an 800 mg oral dose, peak serum fleroxacin levels range from 7-15.6 mcg/mL; therapeutic serum levels: 1-4 mcg/mL

Overdosage/Treatment

Decontamination: Lavage (within 1 hour)/activated charcoal

Supportive therapy: Do **not** use flumazenil; diazepam, phenobarbital; phenytoin can be used for seizures

Enhancement of elimination: Multiple dosing of activated charcoal may be effective

Additional Information Less effective than other quinolones against *Streptococcus pneumoniae*, or *Pseudomonas aeruginosa*

Floxuridine

Related Information

● Fluorouracil

CAS Number 50-91-9

U.S. Brand Names FUDR®

Synonyms 5-FUDR; Fluorodeoxyuridine; FUDR; NSC-27640

Use Antineoplastic agent usually used to treat hepatic metastasis from gastrointestinal carcinoma or other solid neoplasms.

Mechanism of Action Mechanism of action and pharmacokinetics are very similar to fluorouracil; floxuridine is the deoxyribonucleotide of fluorouracil. Floxuridine is a fluorinated pyrimidine antagonist which inhibits DNA and RNA synthesis and methylation of deoxyuridylic acid to thymidylic acid.

Adverse Reactions

Dermatologic: Alopecia, photosensitivity, hyperpigmentation of the skin, localized erythema, dermatitis

Gastrointestinal: **Stomatitis, diarrhea**; may be dose-limiting; anorexia, nausea, vomiting

Hematologic: **Myelosuppression**, may be dose-limiting; **leukopenia, thrombocytopenia, anemia**

Onset: 4-7 days

Nadir: 5-9 days

Recovery: 21 days

Hepatic: Biliary sclerosis, cholecystitis, jaundice, intrahepatic abscess

Pharmacodynamics/Kinetics

Metabolism: Hepatic; Active metabolites: Floxuridine monophosphate (FUDR-MP) and fluorouracil; Inactive metabolites: Urea, CO_2, α-fluoro-β-alanine, α-fluoro-β-guanidopropionic acid, α-fluoro-β-ureidopropionic acid, and dihydrofluorouracil

Excretion: Urine: Fluorouracil, urea, α-fluoro-β-alanine, α-fluoro-β-guanidopropionic acid, α-fluoro-β-ureidopropionic acid, and dihydrofluorouracil; exhaled gases (CO_2)

Dosage

Intra-arterial through infusion pump: 0.1-0.6 mg/kg/day. Ranitidine (150 mg twice daily) and heparin (10,000 units/50 mL of solution added to floxuridine infusate) are usually given concomitantly. Dose is usually given for 1-6 weeks.

Meningeal neoplasia: Intraventricular: 4-16 mg

Solid tumors: I.V.: 0.5-1 mg/kg/day for 6-15 days by continuous infusion. May be administered with thymidine (30 mg/kg/day) to decrease toxicity. Bolus infusions of 30 mg/kg/day every other day for up to 11 days or until toxicity occurs have also been used to treat solid tumors.

Monitoring Parameters WBC and platelet counts. If WBC falls below $3500/mm^3$ or platelet count falls below $100,000/mm^3$, treatment should be stopped.

Administration Continuous intra-arterial or I.V. infusion (unlabeled use)

Contraindications Hypersensitivity to floxuridine, fluorouracil, or any component of the formulation; pregnancy

Warnings Hazardous agent – use appropriate precautions for handling and disposal. Use caution in impaired kidney or liver function. Discontinue if intractable vomiting, diarrhea, precipitous fall in leukocyte or platelet counts, myocardial ischemia, hemorrhage, gastrointestinal ulcer, or stomatitis occur. Use with caution in patients with poor nutritional status; depressed (leukocyte count $<5000/mm^3$ or platelet count $<100,000/mm^3$) bone marrow function; potentially serious infections. Use with caution in patients who have had high-dose pelvic radiation or previous use of alkylating agents. Use of floxuridine with pentostatin has been associated with a high incidence of fatal pulmonary toxicity; this combination is not recommended. **[U.S. Boxed Warnings]: Should be administered under the supervision of an experienced cancer chemotherapy physician. Patients should be hospitalized for initiation of the first course of therapy due to the risk for severe toxic reactions.**

Dosage Forms Injection, powder for reconstitution: 500 mg

Overdosage/Treatment

Decontamination: Emesis within 30 minutes or lavage (within 1 hour)/activated charcoal for oral ingestion

Supportive therapy: Allopurinol (300 mg 3 times/day) may be useful in decreasing toxicity; for treatment of acute encephalopathy, dexamethasone (10 mg every 6 hours I.V.) and thiamine may expedite neurologic recovery. High dose prednisone can be used to treat interstitial pneumonitis.

Enhancement of elimination: Forced diuresis or hemodialysis may enhance elimination

Drug Interactions Patients may experience impaired immune response to vaccines

Possible infection after administration of live vaccines in patients receiving immunosuppressants

Pregnancy Risk Factor D

Lactation Excretion in breast milk unknown/contraindicated

Fluconazole

CAS Number 86386-73-4
U.S. Brand Names Diflucan®
Use
  Treatment of oral or vaginal candidiasis unresponsive to nystatin or clotrimazole; nonlife-threatening *Candida* infections (eg, cystitis, esophagitis); treatment of hepatosplenic candidiasis; treatment of other *Candida* infections in persons unable to tolerate amphotericin B; treatment of cryptococcal infections; secondary prophylaxis for cryptococcal meningitis in persons with AIDS; antifungal prophylaxis in allogeneic bone marrow transplant recipients
  Oral fluconazole should be used in persons able to tolerate oral medications; parenteral fluconazole should be reserved for patients who are both unable to take oral medications and are unable to tolerate amphotericin B (eg, due to hypersensitivity or renal insufficiency)

Mechanism of Action Interferes with cytochrome P450 activity, decreasing ergosterol synthesis (principal sterol in fungal cell membrane) and inhibiting cell membrane formation

Adverse Reactions
  Cardiovascular: Pallor, torsade de pointes
  Central nervous system: Dizziness, seizures, headache
  Dermatologic: Skin rash, exfoliative dermatitis, alopecia, urticaria, erythema multiforme, angioedema, bullous skin disease, toxic epidermal necrolysis, purpura, Stevens-Johnson syndrome, pruritus, exanthem
  Endocrine & metabolic: Hypokalemia, amenorrhea
  Gastrointestinal: Nausea, abdominal pain, vomiting, diarrhea
  Hematologic: Thrombocytopenia
  Hepatic: Elevation of AST, ALT, or alkaline phosphatase; hepatic necrosis, aminotransferase level elevation (asymptomatic)
  Neuromuscular & skeletal: Paresthesia
  Renal: Renal failure
  Miscellaneous: Fixed drug eruption

Signs and Symptoms of Overdose Convulsions, hepatic failure, hepatitis, hypokalemia, nausea, vomiting

Pharmacodynamics/Kinetics
  Distribution: Widely throughout body with good penetration into CSF, eye, peritoneal fluid, sputum, skin, and urine
    Relative diffusion blood into CSF: Adequate with or without inflammation (exceeds usual MICs)
    CSF: blood level ratio: Normal meninges: 70% to 80%; Inflamed meninges: >70% to 80%
  Protein binding, plasma: 11% to 12%
  Bioavailability: Oral: >90%
  Half-life elimination: Normal renal function: ~30 hours
  Time to peak, serum: Oral: 1-2 hours
  Excretion: Urine (80% as unchanged drug)

Dosage The daily dose of fluconazole is the same for oral and I.V. administration
  Usual dosage ranges:
  Neonates: First 2 weeks of life, especially premature neonates: Same dose as older children every 72 hours
  Children: Loading dose: 6-12 mg/kg; maintenance: 3-12 mg/kg/day; duration and dosage depends on severity of infection
  Adults: 200-400 mg/day; duration and dosage depends on severity of infection
  Indication-specific dosing:
  Children:
  Candidiasis:
  Oropharyngeal: Loading dose: 6 mg/kg; maintenance: 3 mg/kg/day for 2 weeks
  Esophageal: Loading dose: 6 mg/kg; maintenance: 3-12 mg/kg/day for 21 days and at least 2 weeks following resolution of symptoms
  Systemic infection: 6 mg/kg every 12 hours for 28 days
  Meningitis, cryptococcal: Loading dose: 12 mg/kg; maintenance: 6-12 mg/kg/day for 10-12 weeks following negative CSF culture; relapse suppression: 6 mg/kg/day
  Adults:
  Candidiasis:
  Candidemia, primary therapy, non-neutropenic: 400-800 mg/day for 14 days after last positive blood culture and resolution of signs/symptoms
  Alternate therapy: 800 mg/day with amphotericin B for 4-7 days followed by 800 mg/day for 14 days after last positive blood culture and resolution of signs/symptoms
  Candidemia, secondary, neutropenic: 6-12 mg/kg/day for 14 days after last positive blood culture and resolution of signs/symptoms
  Chronic, disseminated: 6 mg/kg/day for 3-6 months
  Oropharyngeal (long-term suppression): 200 mg/day; chronic therapy is recommended in immunocompromised patients with history of oropharyngeal candidiasis (OPC)
  Osteomyelitis: 6 mg/kg/day for 6-12 months
  Esophageal: 200 mg on day 1, then 100-200 mg/day for 2-3 weeks after clinical improvement

Prophylaxis in bone marrow transplant: 400 mg/day; begin 3 days before onset of neutropenia and continue for 7 days after neutrophils >1000 cells/mm^3
  Urinary: 200 mg/day for 1-2 weeks
  Vaginal: 150 mg as a single dose
  Coccidiomycosis: 400 mg/day; doses of 800-1000 mg/day have been used for meningeal disease; usual duration of therapy ranges from 3-6 months for primary uncomplicated infections and up to 1 year for pulmonary (chronic and diffuse) infection
  Endocarditis, prosthetic valve, early: 6-12 mg/kg/day for 6 weeks after valve replacement
  Endophthalmitis: 6-12 mg/kg/day or 400-800 mg/day for 6-12 weeks after surgical intervention. Note: C. krusei and C. galbrata infection acquired exogenously should be treated with voriconazole.
  Meningitis, cryptococcal: 400-800 mg/day for 10-12 weeks or with flucytosine 100-150 mg/day for 6 weeks; maintenance: 200-400 mg/day
  Pneumonia, cryptococcal (mild-to-moderate): 200-400 mg/day for 6-12 months (life-long in HIV-positive patients)
  Dosing adjustment/interval in renal impairment:
    No adjustment for vaginal candidiasis single-dose therapy
    For multiple dosing, administer usual load then adjust daily doses
    Cl$_{cr}$ ≤50 mL/minute (no dialysis): Administer 50% of recommended dose or administer every 48 hours.
  Hemodialysis: 50% is removed by hemodialysis; administer 100% of daily dose (according to indication) after each dialysis treatment.
  Continuous arteriovenous or venovenous hemodiafiltration effects: Dose as for Cl$_{cr}$ 10-50 mL/minute

Stability Parenteral admixture at room temperature (25°C): Manufacturer expiration dating; do not refrigerate

Monitoring Parameters Periodic liver function tests (AST, ALT, alkaline phosphatase) and renal function tests, potassium

Administration
  Parenteral fluconazole must be administered by I.V. infusion over approximately 1-2 hours; do not exceed 200 mg/hour when giving I.V. infusion

Contraindications Hypersensitivity to fluconazole, other azoles, or any component of the formulation; concomitant administration with cisapride

Warnings Should be used with caution in patients with renal and hepatic dysfunction or previous hepatotoxicity from other azole derivatives. Patients who develop abnormal liver function tests during fluconazole therapy should be monitored closely and discontinued if symptoms consistent with liver disease develop. Use caution in patients at risk of proarrhythmias.

Dosage Forms
  Infusion [premixed in sodium chloride]: 2 mg/mL (100 mL, 200 mL)
    Diflucan® [premixed in sodium chloride or dextrose] 2 mg/mL (100 mL, 200 mL)
  Powder for oral suspension (Diflucan®): 10 mg/mL (35 mL); 40 mg/mL (35 mL) [contains sodium benzoate; orange flavor]
  Tablet (Diflucan®): 50 mg, 100 mg, 150 mg, 200 mg

Reference Range Serum fluconazole trough levels >80 mcg/mL may be associated with seizures.

Overdosage/Treatment Enhancement of elimination: 3-hour hemodialysis will remove 50% (unlikely to require this procedure)

Drug Interactions
  Inhibits CYP1A2 (weak), 2C9 (strong), 2C19 (strong), 3A4 (moderate)
  Benzodiazepines (metabolized by oxidation, eg, alprazolam, triazolam, midazolam, diazepam) serum concentrations are increased by fluconazole which may cause increased CNS sedation. Consider a benzodiazepine not metabolized by CYP3A4 or another antifungal.
  Caffeine's metabolism is decreased; monitor for tachycardia, nervousness, and anxiety.
  Calcium channel blockers may have increased serum concentrations; consider another agent instead of a calcium channel blocker, another antifungal, or reduce the dose of the calcium channel blocker. Monitor blood pressure.
  Cisapride's serum concentration is increased which may lead to malignant arrhythmias; concurrent use is contraindicated.
  Cyclosporine's serum concentration is increased; monitor cyclosporine's serum concentration and renal function.
  CYP2C9 Substrates: Fluconazole may increase the levels/effects of CYP2C9 substrates. Example substrates include bosentan, dapsone, fluoxetine, glimepiride, glipizide, losartan, montelukast, nateglinide, paclitaxel, phenytoin, warfarin, and zafirlukast.
  CYP2C19 substrates: Fluconazole may increase the levels/effects of CYP2C19 substrates. Example substrates include citalopram, diazepam, methsuximide, phenytoin, propranolol, and sertraline.
  CYP3A4 substrates: Fluconazole may increase the levels/effects of CYP3A4 substrates. Example substrates include benzodiazepines, calcium channel blockers, cyclosporine, mirtazapine, nateglinide, nefazodone, sildenafil (and other PDE-5 inhibitors), tacrolimus, and venlafaxine. Selected benzodiazepines (midazolam and triazolam), cisapride, ergot alkaloids, selected HMG-CoA reductase inhibitors

(lovastatin and simvastatin), and pimozide are generally contraindicated with strong CYP3A4 inhibitors.

HMG-CoA reductase inhibitors (except pravastatin and fluvastatin) have increased serum concentrations; switch to pravastatin/fluvastatin or monitor for development of myopathy.

Losartan's active metabolite is reduced in concentration; consider another antihypertensive agent unaffected by the azole antifungals, another antifungal, or monitor blood pressure closely.

Phenytoin's serum concentration is increased; monitor phenytoin levels and adjust dose as needed.

Rifampin decreases fluconazole's serum concentration; monitor infection status.

Tacrolimus's serum concentration is increased; monitor tacrolimus's serum concentration and renal function.

Warfarin's effects are increased; monitor INR and adjust warfarin's dose as needed.

Pregnancy Risk Factor C

Pregnancy Implications When used in high doses, fluconazole is teratogenic in animal studies. Following exposure during the first trimester, case reports have noted similar malformations in humans when used in higher doses (400 mg/day) over extended periods of time. Use of lower doses (150 mg as a single dose or 200 mg/day) may have less risk; however, additional data is needed. Use during pregnancy only if the potential benefit to the mother outweighs any potential risk to the fetus.

Lactation Enters breast/not recommended (AAP rates "compatible")

Nursing Implications Monitor renal function as dosage adjustments are required with significant changes in renal function

Additional Information Expensive oral alternative to I.V. amphotericin B infusions; in some clinical studies it has been as effective as amphotericin B, but is less likely to cause serious adverse reactions; represents a significant advancement in the treatment of systemic cryptococcosis, including meningitis

Flunitrazepam

Related Information
- Clonazepam
- Nitrazepam

CAS Number 1622-62-4

Synonyms RO5-4200

Impairment Potential Yes. Serum flunitrazepam levels >0.01 mg/L are associated with driving impairment

Use Not marketed in United States, but is encountered in the U.S. as a drug of abuse; used for insomnia and sedation (short-term therapy) and anesthesia induction or supplementation in Europe

Mechanism of Action Intermediate to long-acting benzodiazepine, this agent facilitates the gamma-aminobutyric acid-mediated neuroreceptors

Adverse Reactions
Cardiovascular: Tachycardia, myocardial depression, hypotension, shock, congestive heart failure, sinus tachycardia

Central nervous system: Lethargy, dizziness, ataxia, headache, night terrors, amnesia (anterograde), cognitive dysfunction

Gastrointestinal: Nausea, diarrhea

Hematologic: Porphyria

Neuromuscular & skeletal: Tremor

Respiratory: Cough, apnea

Miscellaneous: Hiccups

Signs and Symptoms of Overdose Apnea, ataxia, coma, hypotension

Pharmacodynamics/Kinetics
Onset: 20 minutes

Peak sedation: 1-2 hours

Duration of sedation: 8-12 hours

Absorption: Food can reduce absorption by 50%

Distribution: V_d: 3.4-5.5 L/kg

Protein binding: 80% to 90%

Metabolism: Hepatic to 7-aminoflunitrazepam and other metabolites

Bioavailability: 80% to 90%

Half-life: 19-22 hours

Elimination: Renal

Dosage
Anesthesia induction: I.V.: 0.015-0.03 mg/kg slowly over 30-60 seconds

Premedication for anesthesia: I.M.: 0.015-0.03 mg/kg slowly over 30-60 seconds

Anesthesia maintenance: I.V.: 0.2-0.5 mg (0.005-0.01 mg/kg) 2-3 hours after anesthesia induction

Insomnia: Oral: 0.5-2 mg nightly; in elderly, 0.5 mg dose should be initiated

Monitoring Parameters Blood pressure, heart rate, arterial blood gas

Contraindications Hypersensitivity to flunitrazepam, nitrazepam, or clonazepam

Warnings Use with caution in patients with porphyria, myasthenia gravis, cardiovascular disease, or hepatic/renal insufficiency; reduce dosage in elderly; dependence may occur

Dosage Forms Injection: 2 mg/mL

Tablet: 0.5 mg, 1 mg, 2 mg

Reference Range

Peak plasma levels after a 2 mg oral dose: 10-15 ng/mL

Urinary benzodiazepine micro-plate enzyme immunoassay can detect flunitrazepam and its metabolites up to 21 days after drug administration

Overdosage/Treatment

Decontamination: Lavage (within 1 hour)/activated charcoal

Supportive therapy: Flumazenil has been shown to selectively block the binding of benzodiazepines to CNS receptors, resulting in a reversal of benzodiazepine-induced CNS depression and apnea; sedation also has been reversed with administration of aminophylline at a low-dose of 2 mg/kg I.V.

Enhancement of elimination: Multiple dose of activated charcoal may be effective

Antidote(s)
- Flumazenil [ANTIDOTE]

Test Interactions Urinary diazepam levels >1000 mcg/L may cross-react with flunitrazepam ELISA immunoassays.

Drug Interactions Enhances sedative effects of ethanol and general anaesthesias; with succinylcholine, increased intraovular pressure can occur; theophylline antagonizes sedative effects

Pregnancy Risk Factor D

Pregnancy Implications Can cross the placenta (no congenital malformations described) and accumulate in the fetus

Additional Information

About 10 times as potent as diazepam; insoluble in water; a growing drug of abuse in Europe and in the U.S. due to its euphoric producing qualities and low street price ($1-$3/tablet); usually several tablets are required for a euphoric effect; oral dose of 28 mg associated with fatality; psychomotor effects may last for 12 hours postdose; often abused in combination with heroin, ethanol, cocaine, or methamphetamine; not detectable on urine assays by EMIT for most benzodiazepine tests.

Hoffman-LaRoche can assist in analyzing urine specimens (1-800-608-6540) with a turnaround time of 1 week. General phone number for information (1-800-720-1076).

Urinary immunoassay for flunitrazepam may remain positive for up to 1 week (using an ELISA assay).

Specific References

Lin DL, Yin RM, Chen CH, et al, "Performance Characteristics of 7-Aminoflunitrazepam Specific Enzyme-Linked Immunosorbent Assays," *J Anal Toxicol*, 2005, 29:718-23.

Mayer BA, Heller TA, and Schroedter DE, "Detection of Club Drugs and Drugs Associated with Drug-Facilitated Sexual Assault in Human Urine by Immunoassay," *J Anal Toxicol*, 2003, 27(3):183-4.

McKinnon A, Humphreys I, and Scott-Ham M, "Flunitrazepam in Doping and Robbery Cases in the U.K.," *J Anal Toxicol*, 2006, 30:149.

Testorf MF, Kronstrand R, Svensson SP, et al, "Characterization of [^{3}H]-Flunitrazepam Binding to Melanin," *J Anal Toxicol*, 2003, 27(3):188-9.

Fluoride

CAS Number 7681-49-4

UN Number 1690

U.S. Brand Names ACT® [OTC]; Fluor-A-Day [OTC]; Fluorigard® [OTC]; Fluorinse®; Flura-Drops®; Flura-Loz®; Gel-Kam® Rinse; Gel-Kam® [OTC]; Lozi-Flur™; Luride® Lozi-Tab®; Luride®; NeutraCare®; NeutraGard® [OTC]; Pediaflor®; Pharmaflur 1.1; Pharmaflur®; Phos-Flur® Rinse [OTC]; Phos-Flur®; PreviDent® 5000 Plus™; PreviDent®; Stan-gard®; Stop®; Thera-Flur-N®

Synonyms Acidulated Phosphate Fluoride; Sodium Fluoride; Stannous Fluoride

Use Prevention of dental caries

Mechanism of Action Derived from hydrofluoric acid, reduces acid production by dental bacteria; increases tooth resistance to acid dissolution

Adverse Reactions
Cardiovascular: Arrhythmias (ventricular)

Dermatologic: Rash

Gastrointestinal: GI upset, nausea, feces discoloration (black), vomiting, stomach cramps

Neuromuscular & skeletal: Tremors, paresthesia, fasciculations

Respiratory: Asthma

Miscellaneous: Products containing stannous fluoride may stain the teeth; ulceration of mucous membranes

Signs and Symptoms of Overdose Abdominal pain, apnea, delirium, diarrhea, epigastric pain, esophageal stricture, fibrillation (ventricular), GI hemorrhage, hematuria, hyperkalemia, hypocalcemia, hypomagnesemia, hypotension, hypothyroidism, mydriasis, nausea, osteomalacia, respiratory paralysis, seizures, slurred speech, tetany, tremors, urine discoloration (milky), vomiting

Pharmacodynamics/Kinetics

Absorption: Oral: Rapid and complete; sodium fluoride; other soluble fluoride salts; calcium, iron, or magnesium may delay absorption

Distribution: 50% of fluoride is deposited in teeth and bone after ingestion; topical application works superficially on enamel and plaque; crosses placenta; enters breast milk

Excretion: Urine and feces

Dosage Oral:

Recommended daily fluoride supplement (2.2 mg of sodium fluoride is equivalent to 1 mg of fluoride ion): See table.

Fluoride Ion	
Fluoride Content of Drinking Water	**Daily Dose, Oral (mg)**
<0.3 ppm	
Birth - 6 mo	0
6 mo - 3 y	0.25
3-6 y	0.5
6 y	1.0
0.3-0.7 ppm	
Birth - 6 mo	0
6 mo - 3 y	0.125
3-6 y	0.25
6 y	0.5

Dental rinse or gel:

Children 6-12 years: 5-10 mL rinse or apply to teeth and spit daily after brushing

Adults: 10 mL rinse or apply to teeth and spit daily after brushing

Stability Store in tight plastic containers (not glass)

Contraindications Hypersensitivity to fluoride, tartrazine, or any component of the formulation; when fluoride content of drinking water exceeds 0.7 ppm; low sodium or sodium-free diets; do not use 1 mg tablets in children <3 years of age or when drinking water fluoride content is ≥0.3 ppm; do not use 1 mg/5 mL rinse (as supplement) in children <6 years of age

Warnings Prolonged ingestion with excessive doses may result in dental fluorosis and osseous changes; do **not** exceed recommended dosage; some products contain tartrazine

Dosage Forms [DSC] = Discontinued product

Cream, oral, as sodium [toothpaste]: 1.1% (51 g) [fluoride 2.5 mg/dose]
Denta 5000 Plus: 1.1% (51g) [fluoride 2.5 mg/dose; spearmint flavor]
EtheDent™: 1.1% (51g) [fluoride 2.5 mg/dose]

Gel-drops, as sodium fluoride (Thera-Flur-N®): 1.1% (24 mL) [fluoride 0.5%; neutral pH; no artificial color or flavor]

Gel, topical, as acidulated phosphate fluoride (Phos-Flur®): 1.1% (60 g) [fluoride 0.5%; cherry and mint flavors]

Gel, topical, as sodium fluoride: 1.1% (56 g) [fluoride 2 mg/dose]
DentaGel, EtheDent™: 1.1% (56 g) [fluoride 2 mg/dose; fresh mint flavor]
NeutraCare®: 1.1% (60 g) [neutral pH; grape and mint flavors]
NeutraGard® Advanced: 1.1% (60 g) [cinnamon and mint flavors]
PreviDent®: 1.1% (60 g) [fluoride 2 mg/dose; berry, cherry, and mint flavors]

Gel, topical, as stannous fluoride:
Gel-Kam®: 0.4% (129 g) [bubble gum, cinnamon, fruit/berry, and mint flavors]
Just for Kids™: 0.4% (122 g) [bubble gum, fruit punch, and grapey grape flavors]
Omnii Gel™: 0.4% (122 g) [cinnamon, grape, natural, mint, and raspberry flavors]
StanGard®: 0.4% (122 g) [bubble gum, cherry, mint, and raspberry flavors]

Stop®: 0.4% (120 g) [bubble gum, cinnamon, grape, and mint flavors]
Lozenge, as sodium (Lozi-Flur™): 2.21 mg [fluoride 1 mg; cherry flavor]
Paste, oral, as sodium [toothpaste] (ControlRx®): 1.1% (56 g) [vanilla mint flavor]

Solution, oral drops, as sodium: 1.1 mg/mL (50 mL) [fluoride 0.5 mg/mL]
Flura-Drops®: 0.55 mg/drop (24 mL) [fluoride 0.25 mg/drop; dye free, sugar free]
Luride®: 1.1 mg/mL (50 mL) [fluoride 0.5 mg/mL; sugar free]
Pediaflor®: 1.1 mg/mL (50 mL) [fluoride 0.5 mg/mL; contains alcohol <0.5%; sugar free; cherry flavor] [DSC]

Solution, oral rinse, as sodium:
ACT®: 0.05% (530 mL) [fluoride 0.02%; bubble gum, cinnamon (contains tartrazine), and mint flavors]
ACT® Plus: 0.05% (530 mL) [fluoride 0.02%; alcohol free; icy cool mint flavor]
ACT® x2™: 0.5% (530 mL) [fluoride 0.02%; contains alcohol 11%; icy cool mint and spearmint flavors]
CaviRinse™: 0.2% (240 mL) [mint flavor]

Fluorigard®: 0.05% (480 mL) [alcohol free, sugar free; contains sodium benzoate and tartrazine; mint flavor]
Fluorinse®: 0.2% (480 mL) [alcohol free; cinnamon and mint flavors]
NeutraGard®: 0.05% (480 mL) [neutral pH; mint and tropical blast flavors]
NeutraGard® Plus: 0.2% (480 mL) [neutral pH; mint and tropical blast flavors]
Phos-Flur®: 0.44% (500 mL) [bubble gum, cherry, grape, and mint flavors]
PreviDent®: 0.2% (250 mL) [contains alcohol; mint flavor]

Solution, oral rinse concentrate, as stannous fluoride:
Gel-Kam®: 0.63% (300 mL) [fluoride 0.1%/dose; cinnamon and mint flavors]
PerioMed™: 0.63% (284 mL) [fluoride 7 mg/30 mL; alcohol free; cinnamon, mint and tropical fruit flavors]
StanGard® Perio: 0.63% (284 mL) [mint flavor]

Tablet, chewable, as sodium: 0.5 mg [fluoride 0.25 mg]; 1.1 mg [fluoride 0.5 mg]; 2.2 mg [fluoride 1 mg]
EtheDent™:
0.55 mg [fluoride 0.25 mg; sugar free; contains aspartame; vanilla flavor]
1.1 mg [fluoride 0.5 mg; sugar free; contains aspartame; grape flavor]
2.2 mg [fluoride 1 mg; sugar free; contains aspartame; cherry flavor]
Fluor-A-Day:
0.56 mg [fluoride 0.25 mg; raspberry flavor]
1.1 mg [fluoride 0.5 mg; raspberry flavor]
2.21 mg [fluoride 1 mg; raspberry flavor]
Luride® Lozi-Tab®:
0.55 mg [fluoride 0.25 mg; sugar free; vanilla flavor]
1.1 mg [fluoride 0.5 mg; sugar free; grape flavor]
2.2 mg [fluoride 1 mg; sugar free; cherry flavor]
Pharmaflur®: 2.2 mg [fluoride 1 mg; dye free, sugar free; cherry flavor]
Pharmaflur 1.1: 1.1 mg [fluoride 0.5 mg; dye free, sugar free; grape flavor]

Reference Range Normal serum level of fluoride: 1.9-7.6 mcg/dL (SI: 1-4 μmol/L); toxic serum fluoride level: >28.5 mcg/dL (SI: >15 μmol/L); toxic urine fluoride level is >10 mg/L

Overdosage/Treatment

Decontamination: Lavage (within 1 hour) with 10% calcium gluconate; if <8 mg/kg is ingested, dilute with milk; do **not** induce emesis; do **not** administer sodium bicarbonate; magnesium based cathartics are preferred; calcium binds to fluoride to decrease the absorption

Supportive therapy: Calcium gluconate to reduce tetanic contractures; quinidine may be particularly effective for treatment of ventricular arrhythmias; monitor magnesium

Enhancement of elimination: Hemodialysis can be utilized; hemodialysis can remove over 80% of body stores of fluoride within 4 hours

Antidote(s)
● Calcium Gluconate [ANTIDOTE]

Test Interactions ↑ potassium; ↓ calcium

Drug Interactions Decreased effect/absorption with magnesium-, aluminum-, and calcium-containing products

Pregnancy Risk Factor C

Pregnancy Implications Crosses placenta

Nursing Implications Avoid giving with milk or dairy products

Additional Information

Fatal oral dose: 5-10 g

Odorless; not flammable; seafood can contain large amounts of fluoride (up to 28 mg/kg); tea can contain 0.5 mg/cup

PEL-TWA: 2.5 mg/m³; IDLH: 500 mg/m³

Total daily intake of fluoride: 2.1-2.4 mg (diet) and 2.8-5.9 mg (water)

In pediatrics, the therapeutic fluoride dosage is 0.05-0.07 mg/kg/day; fluorosis can develop at daily fluoride doses exceeding 0.1 mg/kg; fluoride supplementation should occur at age 6 months at a dose of 0.25 mg/day if their formulas or water contains <0.3 mg/L (0.3 ppm); this increases to daily supplementation of 0.5 mg at age 3 years and 1 mg at 6 years. Children >3 years of age require 0.25 mg/day of fluoride (0.5 mg/day at 6 years) if water fluoride ion level is 0.3-0.6 mg/L (0.3-0.6 ppm); fluoride levels in drinking water >0.6 mg/L (0.6 ppm) require no supplementation. Most fluoridated toothpastes contain ~1000 ppm of fluoride; thus, the daily dose of fluoride by brushing teeth is 0.134 mg from brushing once daily and 0.268 mg brushing twice daily. 53% of U.S. population drinks artificially fluoridated water at an optimal level of 1 mg/L (maximum allowable level 4 mg/L); carbonated beverages contain ~0.74 ppm of fluoride while tea contains ~2.6 ppm. Patients with skeletal fluorosis may exhibit lower serum testosterone levels

Specific References

Buzalaf MA, Caroselli EE, de Carvalho JG, et al, "Bone Surface and Whole Bone as Biomarkers for Acute Fluoride Exposure" *J Anal Toxicol*, 2005, 29(8):810-3.

Buzalaf MA, Caroselli EE, de Oliveira RC, et al, "Nail and Bone Surface as Biomarkers for Acute Fluoride Exposure in Rats," *J Anal Toxicol*, 2004, 28:249-52.

Chu J, Bania TC, Su M, et al, "The Effect of Amiodarone on Fluoride-Induced Ventricular Tachycardia," *Clin Toxicol (Phila)*, 2005, 43:729.

Chu J, Su M, Bania TC, et al, "The Effect of Amiodarone on Survival in a Murine Model of Fluoride Toxicity," *J Toxicol Clin Toxicol*, 2003, 41(5):749.

Kao WF, Deng JF, Chiang SC, et al, "A Simple, Safe, and Efficient Way to Treat Severe Fluoride Poisoning - Oral Calcium or Magnesium," *J Toxicol Clin Toxicol*, 2004, 42(1):33-40.

Proudfoot AT, Krenzelok EP, Vale JA, et al, "AACT/EAPCCT Position Paper on Urine Alkalinization," *J Toxicol Clin Toxicol*, 2004, 42(1):1-26.

Fluorouracil

Related Information
- Floxuridine

CAS Number 51-21-8

U.S. Brand Names Adrucil®; Carac™; Efudex®; Fluoroplex®

Synonyms 5-Fluorouracil; 5-FU; FU

Use Treatment of carcinomas of the breast, colon, head and neck, pancreas, rectum, or stomach; topically for the management of actinic or solar keratoses and superficial basal cell carcinomas

Mechanism of Action A pyrimidine antimetabolite that interferes with DNA synthesis by blocking the methylation of deoxyuridylic acid; fluorouracil inhibits thymidylate synthetase (TS), or is incorporated into RNA. The reduced folate cofactor is required for tight binding to occur between the 5-FdUMP and TS.

Adverse Reactions

Toxicity depends on route and duration of treatment

I.V.:
Cardiovascular: Angina, myocardial ischemia, nail changes

Central nervous system: Acute cerebellar syndrome, confusion, disorientation, euphoria, headache, nystagmus

Dermatologic: Alopecia, dermatitis, dry skin, fissuring, palmar-plantar erythrodysesthesia syndrome, pruritic maculopapular rash, photosensitivity, vein pigmentations

Gastrointestinal: Anorexia, bleeding, diarrhea, esophagopharyngitis, nausea, sloughing, stomatitis, ulceration, vomiting

Hematologic: Agranulocytosis, anemia, leukopenia, pancytopenia, thrombocytopenia

Myelosuppression:

Onset: 7-10 days

Nadir: 9-14 days

Recovery: 21-28 days

Local: Thrombophlebitis

Ocular: Lacrimation, lacrimal duct stenosis, photophobia, visual changes

Respiratory: Epistaxis

Miscellaneous: Anaphylaxis, generalized allergic reactions, loss of nails

Topical: Note: Systemic toxicity normally associated with parenteral administration (including neutropenia, neurotoxicity, and gastrointestinal toxicity) has been associated with topical use particularly in patients with a genetic deficiency of dihydropyrimidine dehydrogenase (DPD).

Central nervous system: Headache, telangiectasia

Dermatologic: Photosensitivity, pruritus, rash, scarring

Hematologic: Leukocytosis

Local: Allergic contact dermatitis, burning, crusting, dryness, edema, erosion, erythema, hyperpigmentation, irritation, pain, soreness, ulceration

Ocular: Eye irritation (burning, watering, sensitivity, stinging, itching)

Miscellaneous: Birth defects, miscarriage

Signs and Symptoms of Overdose Acrodynia, alopecia, bullous skin disease/pemphigoid, cardiogenic shock, coagulopathy, coma, dermatitis, drowsiness, encephalopathy, hypercalcemia, hyperkeratosis, hypotonia, lacrimation, myocarditis, neutropenia, pemphigus, photosensitivity

Pharmacodynamics/Kinetics

Duration: ~3 weeks

Distribution: V_d: ~22% of total body water; penetrates extracellular fluid, CSF, and third space fluids (eg, pleural effusions and ascitic fluid)

Metabolism: Hepatic (90%); via a dehydrogenase enzyme; FU must be metabolized to be active

Bioavailability: <75%, erratic and undependable

Half-life elimination: Biphasic: Initial: 6-20 minutes; two metabolites, FdUMP and FUTP, have prolonged half-lives depending on the type of tissue

Excretion: Lung (large amounts as CO_2); urine (5% as unchanged drug) in 6 hours

Dosage Adults:

Refer to individual protocols:

I.V. bolus: 500-600 mg/m² every 3-4 hours **or** 425 mg/m² on days 1-5 every 4 weeks

Continuous I.V. infusion: 1000 mg/m²/day for 4-5 days every 3-4 weeks **or**

2300-2600 mg/m² on day 1 every week **or**

300-400 mg/m²/day **or**

225 mg/m²/day for 5-8 weeks (with radiation therapy)

Actinic keratoses: Topical:

Carac™: Apply thin film to lesions once daily for up to 4 weeks, as tolerated

Efudex®: Apply to lesions twice daily for 2-4 weeks; complete healing may not be evident for 1-2 months following treatment

Fluoroplex®: Apply to lesions twice daily for 2-6 weeks

Basal cell carcinoma: Topical: Efudex®: Apply to affected lesions twice daily for 3-6 weeks; treatment may be continued for up to 10-12 weeks

Dosage adjustment for renal impairment: Hemodialysis: Administer dose following hemodialysis.

Dosage adjustment for hepatic impairment: Bilirubin >5 mg/dL: Omit use.

Stability Injection: Store intact vials at room temperature and protect from light; slight discoloration does not usually denote decomposition. If exposed to cold, a precipitate may form; **gentle** heating to 60°C will dissolve the precipitate without impairing the potency; solutions in 50-1000 mL NS or D_5W, or undiluted solutions in syringes are stable for 72 hours at room temperature.

Topical: Store at controlled room temperature.

Monitoring Parameters CBC with differential and platelet count, renal function tests, liver function tests

Administration

I.V.: I.V. bolus as a slow push or short (5-15 minutes) bolus infusion, or as a continuous infusion. I.V. formulation may be given orally mixed in water, grape juice, or carbonated beverage. It is generally best to drink undiluted solution, then rinse the mouth. CocaCola® has been recommended as the "best chaser" for oral fluorouracil.

Topical: Apply 10 minutes after washing, rinsing, and drying the affected area. Apply using fingertip (wash hands immediately after application) or nonmetal applicator. Avoid eyes, nostrils, and mouth. Do not cover area with an occlusive dressing.

Contraindications Hypersensitivity to fluorouracil or any component of the formulation; dihydropyrimidine dehydrogenase (DPD) enzyme deficiency; pregnancy

Warnings

Hazardous agent – use appropriate precautions for handling and disposal. Use with caution in patients with impaired kidney or liver function. The drug should be discontinued if intractable vomiting or diarrhea, precipitous falls in leukocyte or platelet counts, stomatitis, hemorrhage, or myocardial ischemia occurs. Use with caution in patients who have had high-dose pelvic radiation or previous use of alkylating agents. Palmar-plantar erythrodysesthesia (hand-foot) syndrome has been associated with use. Safety and efficacy have not been established in pediatric patients.

Administration to patients with a genetic deficiency of dihydropyrimidine dehydrogenase (DPD) has been associated with diarrhea, neutropenia, and neurotoxicity. Systemic toxicity normally associated with parenteral administration has also been associated with topical use, particularly in patients with DPD. Discontinue if symptoms of DPD occur. **[U.S. Boxed Warning]: Should be administered under the supervision of an experienced cancer chemotherapy physician.**

Avoid topical application to mucous membranes due to potential for local inflammation and ulceration. The use of occlusive dressings with topical preparations may increase the severity of inflammation in nearby skin areas. Avoid exposure to ultraviolet rays during and immediately following therapy.

Dosage Forms Cream, topical:

Carac™: 0.5% (30 g)

Efudex®: 5% (25 g, 40 g)

Fluoroplex®: 1% (30 g) [contains benzyl alcohol]

Injection, solution: 50 mg/mL (10 mL, 20 mL, 50 mL, 100 mL)

Adrucil®: 50 mg/mL (10 mL, 50 mL, 100 mL)

Solution, topical (Efudex®): 2% (10 mL); 5% (10 mL)

Reference Range Plasma 5-FU level of 3.37×10^{-6}M with dose of 1.25 g/m²/day

Overdosage/Treatment

Decontamination: Emesis within 30 minutes or lavage (within 1 hour)/activated charcoal for oral ingestion

Supportive therapy: Allopurinol (300 mg 3 times/day) may be useful in decreasing toxicity; for treatment of acute encephalopathy, dexamethasone (10 mg every 6 hours I.V.) and thiamine may expedite neurologic recovery; palmar-plantar erythrodysesthesia syndrome can be treated with pyroxidine 50-150 mg daily; hyperammonemia dissipates upon 5-FU removal.

Enhancement of elimination: Forced diuresis or hemodialysis may enhance elimination

Antidote(s)
- Thrombopoietin [ANTIDOTE]

Test Interactions Fecal discoloration; may elevate total thyroxine level

Drug Interactions Warfarin: May increase aPTT and bleeding time; monitor

Pregnancy Risk Factor D (injection); X (topical)

Pregnancy Implications There are no adequate and well-controlled studies in pregnant women, however, fetal defects and miscarriages have been reported following use of topical and intravenous products. Use is contraindicated during pregnancy.

Lactation Excretion in breast milk unknown/not recommended

Nursing Implications Warm to body temperature before using; after vial has been entered, any unused portion should be discarded within 1 hour; wash hands immediately after topical application of the 5% cream; I.V. formulation may be given orally mixed in water, grape juice, or carbonated beverage

Additional Information May be permeable to PVC gloves as opposed to latex gloves; risk factors for developing fluorouracil-induced mucositis include low salivary flow and neutrophil level <4000 cells/m^3

Specific References
Weng T, Shih FF, and Chen WJ, "Unusual Causes of Hyperammonemia in the ED," *Am J Emerg Med*, 2004, 22:105-7.

Fluoxetine

Related Information
- Anticholinergic Effects of Common Psychotropics
- Antidepressant Agents
- Citalopram

CAS Number 54910-89-3

U.S. Brand Names Prozac® Weekly™; Prozac®; Sarafem™

Synonyms Fluoxetine Hydrochloride

Use Treatment of major depressive disorder; treatment of binge-eating and vomiting in patients with moderate-to-severe bulimia nervosa; obsessive-compulsive disorder (OCD); premenstrual dysphoric disorder (PMDD); panic disorder with or without agoraphobia

Unlabeled/Investigational Use Selective mutism

Mechanism of Action Inhibits CNS neuron serotonin uptake; minimal or no effect on reuptake of norepinephrine or dopamine; does not significantly bind to alpha-adrenergic, histamine, or cholinergic receptors; may therefore be useful in patients at risk from sedation, hypotension, and anticholinergic effects of tricyclic antidepressants

Adverse Reactions
Predominant adverse effects are CNS and GI

Cardiovascular: Vasodilation, palpitations, hypertension, angina, arrhythmia, congestive heart failure, edema, heart arrest, hypotension, myocardial infarction, postural hypotension, QT prolongation, syncope, tachycardia, vasculitis, ventricular tachycardia (including torsade de pointes)

Central nervous system: Amnesia, **anxiety**, confusion, drowsiness, **headache**, emotional lability, sleep disorder, dizziness, agitation, yawning, pain, fever, abnormal dreams, chills, confusion, euphoria, **insomnia**, extrapyramidal reactions (rare), hallucinations, hostility, malaise, migraine, neuroleptic malignant syndrome, **nervousness**, serotonin syndrome, suicidal ideation, fever

Dermatologic: Rash, pruritus, cutaneous vasculitis, acne, alopecia, bruising, ecchymosis, erythema nodosum, exfoliative dermatitis, photosensitivity reaction, Stevens-Johnson syndrome

Systemic events, possibly related to vasculitis (including lupus-like syndrome), have occurred rarely in patients with rash; may include lung, kidney, and/or hepatic involvement. Death has been reported.

Endocrine & metabolic: Syndrome of inappropriate ADH secretion, hypoglycemia, hyponatremia (elderly or volume-depleted patients), dehydration, gout, hypercholesterolemia, hyperprolactinemia, hypokalemia, hypothyroidism

Gastrointestinal: **Nausea, diarrhea, xerostomia, anorexia**, dyspepsia, increased appetite, constipation, vomiting, flatulence, weight gain/loss, abdominal pain, dyspepsia, aphthous stomatitis, colitis, dysphagia, esophagitis, gastritis, glossitis, gynecomastia, pancreatitis, taste perversion

Genitourinary: Sexual dysfunction, urinary frequency, amenorrhea, priapism

Hematologic: Anemia, hemorrhage, immune-related hemolytic anemia, pancytopenia, thrombocytopenia, thrombocytopenic purpura

Hepatic: Cholelithiasis, cholestatic jaundice, hepatic failure/necrosis, liver function test abnormalities

Neuromuscular & skeletal: **Weakness, tremor**, arthritis, bone pain, bursitis, dyskinesia, leg cramps

Ocular: Abnormal vision, aggravation of glaucoma, cataract, optic neuritis

Otic: Tinnitus

Renal: Albuminuria, kidney failure

Respiratory: Pharyngitis, asthma, eosinophilic pneumonia, epistaxis, hyperventilation, laryngospasm, pulmonary embolism, pulmonary hypertension

Miscellaneous: Diaphoresis, flu syndrome, infection, abnormal thinking, allergies, anaphylactoid reactions, hiccups, lupus-like syndrome, misuse/abuse

Signs and Symptoms of Overdose Agitation, AV block, bradycardia, cognitive dysfunction, cystitis, delirium, depression, drowsiness, eosinophilia, extrapyramidal reaction, generalized seizures, gout, hallucinations, hirsutism, hypoglycemia, hypokalemia, hypomania, hyponatremia, insomnia, leukocytosis, lightheadedness, mania, myoclonus, myoglobinuria, nausea, nystagmus, QT prolongation, rhabdomyolysis, spontaneous vomiting, tachycardia (ventricular), vasculitis

Pharmacodynamics/Kinetics
Absorption: Well absorbed; delayed 1-2 hours with weekly formulation
Protein binding: 95%
Metabolism: Hepatic to norfluoxetine (activity equal to fluoxetine)
Half-life elimination: Adults:
    Parent drug: 1-3 days (acute), 4-6 days (chronic), 7.6 days (cirrhosis)
    Metabolite (norfluoxetine): 9.3 days (range: 4-16 days), 12 days (cirrhosis)
Time to peak: 6-8 hours
Excretion: Urine (10% as norfluoxetine, 2.5% to 5% as fluoxetine)
Note: Weekly formulation results in greater fluctuations between peak and trough concentrations of fluoxetine and norfluoxetine compared to once-daily dosing (24% daily/164% weekly; 17% daily/43% weekly, respectively). Trough concentrations are 76% lower for fluoxetine and 47% lower for norfluoxetine than the concentrations maintained by 20 mg once-daily dosing. Steady-state fluoxetine concentrations are ~50% lower following the once-weekly regimen compared to 20 mg once daily. Average steady-state concentrations of once-daily dosing were highest in children ages 6 to <13 (fluoxetine 171 ng/mL; norfluoxetine 195 ng/mL), followed by adolescents ages 13 to <18 (fluoxetine 86 ng/mL; norfluoxetine 113 ng/mL); concentrations were considered to be within the ranges reported in adults (fluoxetine 91-302 ng/mL; norfluoxetine 72-258 ng/mL).

Dosage
Oral:
Children:
    Depression: 8-18 years: 10-20 mg/day; lower-weight children can be started at 10 mg/day, may increase to 20 mg/day after 1 week if needed
    OCD: 7-18 years: Initial: 10 mg/day; in adolescents and higher-weight children, dose may be increased to 20 mg/day after 2 weeks. Range: 10-60 mg/day
    Selective mutism (unlabeled use):
        <5 years: No dosing information available
        5-18 years: Initial: 5-10 mg/day; titrate upwards as needed (usual maximum dose: 60 mg/day)
Adults: 20 mg/day in the morning; may increase after several weeks by 20 mg/day increments; maximum: 80 mg/day; doses >20 mg may be given once daily or divided twice daily. **Note:** Lower doses of 5-10 mg/day have been used for initial treatment.
    Usual dosage range:
        Bulimia nervosa: 60-80 mg/day
        Depression: 20-40 mg/day; patients maintained on Prozac® 20 mg/day may be changed to Prozac® Weekly™ 90 mg/week, starting dose 7 days after the last 20 mg/day dose
        OCD: 40-80 mg/day
        Panic disorder: Initial: 10 mg/day; after 1 week, increase to 20 mg/day; may increase after several weeks; doses >60 mg/day have not been evaluated
        PMDD (Sarafem™): 20 mg/day continuously, **or** 20 mg/day starting 14 days prior to menstruation and through first full day of menses (repeat with each cycle)
Elderly: Depression: Some patients may require an initial dose of 10 mg/day with dosage increases of 10 and 20 mg every several weeks as tolerated; should not be taken at night unless patient experiences sedation

Dosing adjustment in renal impairment:
Single dose studies: Pharmacokinetics of fluoxetine and norfluoxetine were similar among subjects with all levels of impaired renal function, including anephric patients on chronic hemodialysis
Chronic administration: Additional accumulation of fluoxetine or norfluoxetine may occur in patients with severely impaired renal function
Hemodialysis: Not removed by hemodialysis; use of lower dose or less frequent dosing is not usually necessary

Dosing adjustment in hepatic impairment: Elimination half-life of fluoxetine is prolonged in patients with hepatic impairment; a lower or less frequent dose of fluoxetine should be used in these patients
    Cirrhosis patients: Administer a lower dose or less frequent dosing interval
    Compensated cirrhosis without ascites: Administer 50% of normal dose

Monitoring Parameters Mental status for depression, suicidal ideation, anxiety, social functioning, mania, panic attacks; akathisia, sleep

Contraindications Hypersensitivity to fluoxetine or any component of the formulation; patients currently receiving MAO inhibitors, pimozide, or thioridazine
    Note: MAO inhibitor therapy must be stopped for 14 days before fluoxetine is initiated. Treatment with MAO inhibitors, thioridazine, or mesoridazine should not be initiated until 5 weeks after the discontinuation of fluoxetine.

Warnings

Major psychiatric warnings:

- **[U.S. Boxed Warning]: Antidepressants increase the risk of suicidal thinking and behavior in children and adolescents with major depressive disorder (MDD) and other depressive disorders;** consider risk prior to prescribing. Closely monitor for clinical worsening, suicidality, or unusual changes in behavior; the child's family or caregiver should be instructed to closely observe the patient and communicate condition with healthcare provider. A medication guide concerning the use of antidepressants in children and teenagers should be dispensed with each prescription. **Fluoxetine is FDA approved for the treatment of OCD in children ≥7 years of age and MDD in children ≥8 years of age.**
- The possibility of a suicide attempt is inherent in major depression and may persist until remission occurs. Patients treated with antidepressants should be observed for clinical worsening and suicidality, especially during the initial few months of a course of drug therapy, or at times of dose changes, either increases or decreases. Worsening depression and severe abrupt suicidality that are not part of the presenting symptoms may require discontinuation or modification of drug therapy. Use caution in high-risk patients during initiation of therapy.
- Prescriptions should be written for the smallest quantity consistent with good patient care. The patient's family or caregiver should be alerted to monitor patients for the emergence of suicidality and associated behaviors such as anxiety, agitation, panic attacks, insomnia, irritability, hostility, impulsivity, akathisia, hypomania, and mania; patients should be instructed to notify their healthcare provider if any of these symptoms or worsening depression or psychosis occur.
- May worsen psychosis in some patients or precipitate a shift to mania or hypomania in patients with bipolar disorder. Monotherapy in patients with bipolar disorder should be avoided. Patients presenting with depressive symptoms should be screened for bipolar disorder. **Fluoxetine is not FDA approved for the treatment of bipolar depression.** Safety and efficacy in children <8 years of age (major depressive disorder) and <7 years of age (OCD) have not been established.

Key adverse effects:

- Allergic events and rash: Fluoxetine use has been associated with occurrences of significant rash and allergic events, including vasculitis, lupus-like syndrome, laryngospasm, anaphylactoid reactions, and pulmonary inflammatory disease. Discontinue if underlying cause of rash cannot be identified.
- Anticholinergic effects: Relatively devoid of these side effects
- CNS depression: Has a low potential to impair cognitive or motor performance; caution operating hazardous machinery or driving.
- CNS effects: May cause insomnia, anxiety, nervousness or anorexia.
- SIADH and hyponatremia: Has been associated with the development of SIADH; hyponatremia has been reported rarely, predominately in the elderly.

Concurrent disease:

- Diabetes: May alter glycemic control in patients with diabetes.
- Hepatic impairment: Use caution; clearance is decreased and plasma concentrations are increased; a lower dosage may be needed.
- Platelet aggregation: May impair platelet aggregation, resulting in bleeding.
- Renal impairment: Use caution; clearance is decreased and plasma concentrations are increased; a lower dosage may be needed.
- Seizure disorders: Use caution with a previous seizure disorder or condition predisposing to seizures such as brain damage or alcoholism.
- Sexual dysfunction: May cause or exacerbate sexual dysfunction.
- Weight loss: May cause weight loss. Use caution in patients where weight loss is undesirable.

Concurrent drug therapy:

- Agents which lower seizure threshold: Use caution with concurrent therapy.
- Anticoagulants/Antiplatelets: Use caution with concomitant use of NSAIDs, ASA, or other drugs that affect coagulation; the risk of bleeding is potentiated.
- Cardiovascular: Use caution with history of MI or unstable heasrt disease; use in these patients is limited
- CNS depressants: Use caution with concomitant therapy.
- MAO inhibitors: Potential for severe reaction when used with MAO inhibitors; autonomic instability, coma, death, delirium, diaphoresis, hyperthermia, mental status changes/agitation, muscular rigidity, myoclonus, neuroleptic malignant syndrome features, and seizures may occur.
- Thioridazine: Fluoxetine may elevate plasma levels of thioridazine; increasing risk of QTc interval prolongation; this may lead to serious ventricular arrhythmias such as torsade de pointes-type arrhythmias and sudden death. **Concurrent use is contraindicated.**

Special populations:

- Elderly: Use caution in elderly patients.

Special notes:

- Electroconvulsive therapy: May increase the risks associated with electroconvulsive therapy; consider discontinuing, when possible, prior to ECT treatment.
- Long half-life: Due to the long half-life of fluoxetine and its metabolites, the effects and interactions noted may persist for prolonged periods following discontinuation.
- Withdrawal syndrome: May cause dysphoric mood, irritability, agitation, dizziness, sensory disturbances, anxiety, confusion, headache, lethargy, emotional lability, insomnia, hypomania, tinnitus, and seizures. Upon discontinuation of fluoxetine therapy, gradually taper dose. If intolerable symptoms occur following a decrease in dosage or upon discontinuation of therapy, then resuming the previous dose with a more gradual taper should be considered.

Dosage Forms [DSC] = Discontinued product

Capsule, as hydrochloride: 10 mg, 20 mg, 40 mg
  Prozac®: 10 mg, 20 mg, 40 mg
  Sarafem®: 10 mg, 20 mg
Capsule, delayed release, as hydrochloride (Prozac® Weekly™): 90 mg
Solution, oral, as hydrochloride (Prozac®): 20 mg/5 mL (120 mL) [contains alcohol 0.23% and benzoic acid; mint flavor]
Tablet, as hydrochloride: 10 mg, 20 mg
  Prozac® [scored]: 10 mg [DSC]

Reference Range

Therapeutic:
Fluoxetine: 100-800 ng/mL (SI: 289-2314 nmol/L); serum level of 1956 ng/mL (norfluoxetine level of 416 ng/mL) associated with seizure
Norfluoxetine: 100-600 ng/mL (SI: 289-1735 nmol/L)
In the postmortem state, anatomical site concentration differences (ie, postmortem redistribution) may occur.
Postmortem blood fluoxetine level of 0.63 mg/L may indicate that this drug was the cause of death.

Overdosage/Treatment

Decontamination: Lavage (within 1 hour)/activated charcoal
Supportive therapy: Toxic symptoms should be treated. Seizures usually respond to lorazepam or diazepam I.V. boluses (5-10 mg for adults up to 30 mg or 0.25-0.4 mg/kg/dose for children up to 10 mg/dose). If seizures are unresponsive or recur, phenytoin or phenobarbital may be required. Amantadine (100-200 mg 2 times/day) has been used successfully in treating sexual dysfunction; sildenafil (50-100 mg) can be used to treat sexual dysfunction; bruxism can be treated with buspirone (5 mg at night)
Enhancement of elimination: Multiple dosing of activated charcoal may not be useful; hemodialysis does not appear to be useful

Test Interactions Increases albumin in urine; fluoxetine can interfere with bupropion quantitation by HPLC analysis in plasma or serum

Drug Interactions Substrate of CYP1A2 (minor), 2B6 (minor), 2C9 (major), 2C19 (minor), 2D6 (major), 2E1 (minor), 3A4 (minor); **Inhibits** CYP1A2 (moderate), 2B6 (weak), 2C9 (weak), 2C19 (moderate), 2D6 (strong), 3A4 (weak)

Amphetamines: SSRIs may increase the sensitivity to amphetamines, and amphetamines may increase the risk of serotonin syndrome.

Benzodiazepines: Fluoxetine may inhibit the metabolism of alprazolam and diazepam resulting in elevated serum levels; monitor for increased sedation and psychomotor impairment.

Beta-blockers: Fluoxetine may inhibit the metabolism of metoprolol and propranolol resulting in cardiac toxicity; monitor for bradycardia, hypotension, and heart failure if combination is used; not established for all beta-blockers (unlikely with atenolol or nadolol due to renal elimination).

Buspirone: Fluoxetine inhibits the reuptake of serotonin; combined use with a serotonin agonist (buspirone) may cause serotonin syndrome.

Carbamazepine: Fluoxetine may inhibit the metabolism of carbamazepine resulting in increased carbamazepine levels and toxicity; monitor for altered carbamazepine response.

Carvedilol: Serum concentrations may be increased; monitor carefully for increased carvedilol effect (hypotension and bradycardia).

Clozapine: Fluoxetine may increase serum levels of clozapine; levels may increase by 76%; monitor for increased effect/toxicity.

Cyclosporine: Fluoxetine may increase serum levels of cyclosporine (and possibly tacrolimus); monitor.

CYP1A2 substrates: Fluoxetine may increase the levels/effects of CYP1A2 substrates. Example substrates include aminophylline, fluvoxamine, mexiletine, mirtazapine, ropinirole, theophylline, and trifluoperazine.

CYP2C9 inducers: May decrease the levels/effects of fluoxetine. Example inducers include carbamazepine, phenobarbital, phenytoin, rifampin, rifapentine, and secobarbital.

CYP2C9 Inhibitors may increase the levels/effects of fluoxetine. Example inhibitors include delavirdine, fluconazole, gemfibrozil, ketoconazole, nicardipine, NSAIDs, sulfonamides and tolbutamide.

CYP2C19 substrates: Fluoxetine may increase the levels/effects of CYP2C19 substrates. Example substrates include citalopram, diazepam, methsuximide, phenytoin, propranolol, and sertraline.

CYP2D6 inhibitors: May increase the levels/effects of fluoxetine. Example inhibitors include chlorpromazine, delavirdine, miconazole, paroxetine, pergolide, quinidine, quinine, ritonavir, and ropinirole.

CYP2D6 substrates: Fluoxetine may increase the levels/effects of CYP2D6 substrates. Example substrates include amphetamines, selected beta-blockers, dextromethorphan, lidocaine, mirtazapine, nefazodone, paroxetine, risperidone, ritonavir, thioridazine, tricyclic antidepressants, and venlafaxine.

CYP2D6 prodrug substrates: Fluoxetine may decrease the levels/effects of CYP2D6 prodrug substrates. Example prodrug substrates include codeine, hydrocodone, oxycodone, and tramadol.

Cyproheptadine: May inhibit the effects of serotonin reuptake inhibitors (fluoxetine); monitor for altered antidepressant response; cyproheptadine acts as a serotonin agonist.

Dextromethorphan: Fluoxetine inhibits the metabolism of dextromethorphan; visual hallucinations occurred in a patient receiving this combination; monitor for serotonin syndrome.

Digoxin: Fluoxetine may increase serum levels of digoxin; monitor.

Haloperidol: Fluoxetine may inhibit the metabolism of haloperidol and cause extrapyramidal symptoms (EPS); monitor patients for EPS if combination is utilized.

HMG-CoA reductase inhibitors: Fluoxetine may inhibit the metabolism of lovastatin and simvastatin resulting in myositis and rhabdomyolysis; these combinations are best avoided.

Lithium: Reports of both increased and decreased lithium levels when used concomitantly with fluoxetine. Patients receiving fluoxetine and lithium have developed neurotoxicity. If combination is used; monitor lithium levels and for neurotoxicity.

Loop diuretics: Fluoxetine may cause hyponatremia; additive hyponatremic effects may be seen with combined use of a loop diuretic (bumetanide, furosemide, torsemide); monitor for hyponatremia.

MAO inhibitors: Combined use of fluoxetine with nonselective MAOIs (ie, isocarboxazid, phenelzine) is contraindicated; fatal reactions have been reported; wait 5 weeks after stopping fluoxetine before starting an MAO inhibitor and 2 weeks after stopping an MAO inhibitor before starting fluoxetine.

Meperidine: Combined use with fluoxetine theoretically may increase the risk of serotonin syndrome.

Nefazodone: May increase the risk of serotonin syndrome with SSRIs; monitor.

NSAIDs: Concomitant use of fluoxetine and NSAIDs, aspirin, or other drugs affecting coagulation has been associated with an increased risk of bleeding; monitor.

Phenytoin: Fluoxetine inhibits the metabolism of phenytoin and may result in phenytoin toxicity; monitor for phenytoin toxicity (ataxia, confusion, dizziness, nystagmus, involuntary muscle movement).

Pimozide: Due to potential QT_c interval prolongation, concomitant use is contraindicated.

Propafenone: Serum concentrations and/or toxicity may be increased by fluoxetine; avoid concurrent administration.

Ritonavir: Combined use of fluoxetine with ritonavir may cause serotonin syndrome in HIV-positive patients; monitor.

Selegiline: Fluoxetine has been reported to cause mania or hypertension when combined with selegiline; this combination is best avoided. Concurrent use with SSRIs has also been reported to cause serotonin syndrome. As a MAO type B inhibitor, the risk of serotonin syndrome may be less than with nonselective MAO inhibitors.

Sibutramine: May increase the risk of serotonin syndrome with SSRIs; avoid coadministration.

SSRIs: Fluoxetine inhibits the reuptake of serotonin; combined use with other drugs which inhibit the reuptake may cause serotonin syndrome.

Sumatriptan (and other serotonin agonists): Concurrent use may result in toxicity; weakness, hyper-reflexia, and incoordination have been observed with sumatriptan and SSRIs. In addition, concurrent use may theoretically increase the risk of serotonin syndrome; includes sumatriptan, naratriptan, rizatriptan, and zolmitriptan.

Sympathomimetics: May increase the risk of serotonin syndrome with SSRIs.

Thioridazine: Fluoxetine may inhibit the metabolism of thioridazine, resulting in increased plasma levels and increasing the risk of QT_c interval prolongation. This may lead to serious ventricular arrhythmias, such as torsade de pointes-type arrhythmias and sudden death. Do not use together. Wait at least 5 weeks after discontinuing fluoxetine prior to starting thioridazine.

Tramadol: Fluoxetine combined with tramadol (serotonergic effects) may cause serotonin syndrome; monitor.

Trazodone: Fluoxetine may inhibit the metabolism of trazodone resulting in increased toxicity; monitor.

Tricyclic antidepressants: Fluoxetine inhibits the metabolism of tricyclic antidepressants (amitriptyline, desipramine, imipramine, nortriptyline) resulting is elevated serum levels; if combination is warranted, a low dose of TCA (10-25 mg/day) should be utilized.

Tryptophan: Fluoxetine inhibits the reuptake of serotonin; combination with tryptophan, a serotonin precursor, may cause agitation and restlessness; this combination is best avoided.

Valproic acid: Fluoxetine may increase serum levels of valproic acid; monitor.

Venlafaxine: Fluoxetine may increase the risk of serotonin syndrome.

Warfarin: Fluoxetine may alter the hypoprothrombinemic response to warfarin; monitor.

Pregnancy Risk Factor C
Pregnancy Implications Fluoxetine crosses the placenta
Lactation Enters breast milk/not recommended (AAP rates "of concern")
Nursing Implications Offer patient sugarless hard candy for dry mouth
Additional Information

ECG may reveal S-T segment depression; not shown to be teratogenic in rodents; 15-60 mg/day, buspirone and cyproheptadine, may be useful in treatment of sexual dysfunction during treatment with a selective serotonin reuptake inhibitor.

Weekly capsules are a delayed release formulation containing enteric-coated pellets of fluoxetine hydrochloride, equivalent to 90 mg fluoxetine. Therapeutic equivalence of weekly formulation with daily formulation for delaying time to relapse has not been established.

Specific References

Baker SD and Morgan DL, "Fluoxetine Exposures: Are They Safe for Children?" *Am J Emerg Med*, 2004, 22(3):211-3.

Bogdanovic Z, Nalamati JR, Kilcullen JK, et al, "Antidepressant-Induced Adverse Reactions in a Patient with Hemorrhagic Stroke," *Ann Pharmacother*, 2005, 39(10):1755-7.

Boyer EW and Shannon M, "The Serotonin Syndrome," *N Engl J Med*, 2005, 352(11):1112-20 (review).

Charlier C, Broly F, Lhermitte M, et al, "Polymorphisms in the CYP 2D6 Gene: Association with Plasma Concentrations of Fluoxetine and Paroxetine," *Ther Drug Monit*, 2003, 25(6):738-42.

Compton R, Spiller HA, and Bosse GM, "Fatal Fluoxetine Ingestion with Postmortem Blood Concentrations," *Clin Toxicol (Phila)*, 2005, 43(4):277-9.

Hemels ME, Einarson A, Koren G, et al, "Antidepressant Use During Pregnancy and the Rates of Spontaneous Abortions: A Meta-Analysis," *Ann Pharmacother*, 2005, 39(5):803-9.

Kim SS, "Role of Fluoxetine in Anorexia Nervosa," *Ann Pharmacother*, 2003, 37(6):890-2.

Nykamp DL, Blackmon CL, Schmidt PE, et al, "QTc Prolongation Associated with Combination Therapy of Levofloxacin, Imipramine, and Fluoxetine," *Ann Pharmacother*, 2005, 39(3):543-6.

Prybys KM, "Deadly Drug Interactions in Emergency Medicine," *Emerg Med Clin N Am*, 2004, 22:845-63.

Ramagiri, S, Skukla SK, Sai Prakash PK, "Stability Study of Fluoxetine in Formaline - Fixed Liver Tissue," *J Anal Tox*, 2006, 30:692-696.

Serebruany VL, "Selective Serotonin Reuptake Inhibitors and Increased Bleeding Risk: Are We Missing Something?" *Am J Med*, 2006, 119(2):113-6 (review).

Sullivan PW, Valuck R, Brixner DI, et al, "Managed Care's Response to a Pharmacoeconomic Model of Serotonin Reuptake Inhibitors," *P&T*, 2005 30(3):178-82.

Thompson DS, Kirshner MA, Klug TL, et al, "A Preliminary Study of the Effect of Fluoxetine Treatment on the 2:16-α-Hydroxyestrone Ratio in Young Women," *Ther Drug Monit*, 2003, 25(1):125-8.

Fluphenazine

Related Information
- Anticholinergic Effects of Common Psychotropics
- Antipsychotic Agents

CAS Number 146-56-5; 2746-81-8; 69-23-8
U.S. Brand Names Prolixin Decanoate®; Prolixin® [DSC]
Synonyms Fluphenazine Decanoate
Use Management of manifestations of psychotic disorders and schizophrenia; depot formulation may offer improved outcome in individuals with psychosis who are nonadherent with oral antipsychotics
Unlabeled/Investigational Use Pervasive developmental disorder
Mechanism of Action Blocks postsynaptic mesolimbic dopaminergic receptors in the brain; exhibits a strong alpha-adrenergic blocking effect and depresses the release of hypothalamic and hypophyseal hormones
Adverse Reactions

Cardiovascular: **Hypotension (especially orthostatic)**, tachycardia, **cardiac arrhythmias**, abnormal T waves with prolonged ventricular repolarization, sinus tachycardia, **hypotension**

Central nervous system: Sedation, drowsiness, fever, restlessness, anxiety, extrapyramidal reactions, **dystonic reactions**, **pseudoparkinsonian signs and symptoms**, **tardive dyskinesia**, neuroleptic malignant syndrome, seizures, altered central temperature regulation, gustatory hallucinations, **akathisia**, **dizziness**

Dermatologic: Hyperpigmentation, pruritus, rash, contact dermatitis, photosensitivity (rare), exfoliative dermatitis, angioedema, toxic epidermal necrolysis, urticaria, purpura, exanthem

Endocrine & metabolic: Amenorrhea, galactorrhea, gynecomastia, syndrome of inappropriate antidiuretic hormone, sexual dysfunction

Gastrointestinal: **Constipation**, adynamic ileus, GI upset, xerostomia (problem for denture user), nausea, vomiting, weight gain

Genitourinary: Urinary retention, overflow incontinence, priapism

Hematologic: Leukopenia/neutropenia (agranulocytosis, granulocytopenia) usually inpatients with large doses for prolonged periods

Hepatic: Cholestatic jaundice, cholestasis

Ocular: Blurred vision, photophobia, diplopia, **retinal pigmentation**, pigmentary deposits in the lens and cornea, bilateral maculopathy

Respiratory: **Nasal congestion**

Miscellaneous: Systemic lupus erythematosus, **diaphoresis**

Signs and Symptoms of Overdose Deep sleep, depression, dystonic reactions, ejaculatory disturbances, extrapyramidal reaction, gynecomastia, enuresis, hyperthermia, hypotension or hypertension, hyponatremia, hypothermia, lactation, neuroleptic malignant syndrome, Parkinson's-like symptoms, photosensitivity, respiratory failure, seizures, QT prolongation, urine discoloration (pink; red; red-brown) vision color changes (brown tinge; yellow tinge)

Pharmacodynamics/Kinetics

Onset of action: I.M., SubQ (derivative dependent): Hydrochloride salt: ~1 hour

Peak effect: Neuroleptic: Decanoate: 48-96 hours

Duration: Hydrochloride salt: 6-8 hours; Decanoate: 24-72 hours

Absorption: Oral: Erratic and variable

Distribution: Crosses placenta; enters breast milk

Protein binding: 91% and 99%

Metabolism: Hepatic

Half-life elimination (derivative dependent): Hydrochloride: 33 hours; Decanoate: 163-232 hours

Excretion: Urine (as metabolites)

Dosage

Children: Oral: Childhood-onset pervasive developmental disorder (unlabeled use): 0.04 mg/kg/day

Adults: Psychoses:

Oral: 0.5-10 mg/day in divided doses at 6- to 8-hour intervals; some patients may require up to 40 mg/day

I.M.: 2.5-10 mg/day in divided doses at 6- to 8-hour intervals (parenteral dose is $^1/_3$ to $^1/_2$ the oral dose for the hydrochloride salts)

I.M. (decanoate): 12.5 mg every 2 weeks

Conversion from hydrochloride to decanoate I.M. 0.5 mL (12.5 mg) decanoate every 3 weeks is approximately equivalent to 10 mg hydrochloride/day

I.M. (enanthate): 12.5-25 mg every 2 weeks

Hemodialysis: Not dialyzable (0% to 5%)

Monitoring Parameters Vital signs; lipid profile, fasting blood glucose/Hgb A_{1c}; BMI; mental status, abnormal involuntary movement scale (AIMS), extrapyramidal symptoms (EPS)

Administration Avoid contact of oral solution or injection with skin (contact dermatitis). Oral liquid should be diluted in the following **only**: Water, saline, homogenized milk, carbonated orange beverages, pineapple, apricot, prune, orange, tomato, and grapefruit juices. Do **not** dilute in beverages containing caffeine, tannics, or pectinate. Watch for hypotension when administering I.M.

Contraindications Hypersensitivity to fluphenazine or any component of the formulation (cross-reactivity between phenothiazines may occur); severe CNS depression; coma; subcortical brain damage; blood dyscrasias; hepatic disease

Warnings

May be sedating, use with caution in disorders where CNS depression is a feature. Use with caution in Parkinson's disease. Caution in patients with hemodynamic instability; bone marrow suppression; predisposition to seizures; severe cardiac, renal, or respiratory disease. Esophageal dysmotility and aspiration have been associated with antipsychotic use - use with caution in patients at risk of pneumonia (ie, Alzheimer's disease). Caution in breast cancer or other prolactin-dependent tumors (may elevate prolactin levels). May alter temperature regulation or mask toxicity of other drugs due to antiemetic effects. May alter cardiac conduction; life-threatening arrhythmias have occurred with therapeutic doses of phenothiazines. Hypotension may occur, particularly with I.M. administration. May cause orthostatic hypotension - use with caution in patients at risk of this effect or those who would tolerate transient hypotensive episodes (cerebrovascular disease, cardiovascular disease, or other medications which may predispose). Adverse effects of depot injections may be prolonged.

Phenothiazines may cause anticholinergic effects (confusion, agitation, constipation, xerostomia, blurred vision, urinary retention). Therefore, they should be used with caution in patients with decreased gastrointestinal motility, urinary retention, BPH, xerostomia, or visual pro-

blems. Conditions which also may be exacerbated by cholinergic blockade include narrow-angle glaucoma (screening is recommended) and worsening of myasthenia gravis. Relative to other antipsychotics, fluphenazine has a low potency of cholinergic blockade.

May cause extrapyramidal symptoms, including pseudoparkinsonism, acute dystonic reactions, akathisia and tardive dyskinesia (risk of these reactions is high relative to other antipsychotics). May be associated with neuroleptic malignant syndrome (NMS) or pigmentary retinopathy.

Dosage Forms [DSC] = Discontinued product

Elixir, as hydrochloride (Prolixin®): 2.5 mg/5 mL (60 mL) [contains alcohol 14% and sodium benzoate] [DSC]

Injection, oil, as decanoate: 25 mg/mL (5 mL) [may contain benzyl alcohol, sesame oil]

Prolixin Decanoate®: 25 mg/mL (5 mL) [contains benzyl alcohol, sesame oil]

Injection, solution, as hydrochloride (Prolixin® [DSC]): 2.5 mg/mL (10 mL)

Solution, oral concentrate, as hydrochloride (Prolixin®): 5 mg/mL (120 mL) [contains alcohol 14%] [DSC]

Tablet, as hydrochloride: 1 mg, 2.5 mg, 5 mg, 10 mg

Prolixin®: 1 mg, 2.5 mg, 5 mg [contains tartrazine], 10 mg [DSC]

Reference Range Therapeutic: 5-20 ng/mL (SI: 10-40 nmol/L)

Overdosage/Treatment

Decontamination: Lavage (within 1 hour)/activated charcoal

Supportive therapy: Toxic symptom treatment and supportive treatment should be initiated. Hypotension usually responds to I.V. fluids or Trendelenburg positioning. If unresponsive to these measures, the use of a parenteral inotrope may be required (eg, norepinephrine 0.1-0.2 mcg/kg/minute titrated to response). Seizures commonly respond to lorazepam or diazepam (I.V. 5-10 mg bolus in adults every 15 minutes if needed up to a total of 30 mg; I.V. 0.25-0.4 mg/kg/dose up to a total of 10 mg in children) or to phenytoin or phenobarbital. Also critical cardiac arrhythmias often respond to I.V. phenytoin (15 mg/kg up to 1 g), while other antiarrhythmics can be used. Neuroleptics often cause extrapyramidal reaction (eg, dystonic reactions) requiring management with diphenhydramine 1-2 mg/kg (adults) up to a maximum of 50 mg I.M. or I.V. slow push followed by a maintenance dose for 48-72 hours. When these reactions are unresponsive to diphenhydramine, benztropine mesylate I.V. 1-2 mg (adults) may be effective. These agents are generally effective within 2-5 minutes. Ventricular arrhythmias often respond to quinidine or phenytoin; avoid quinidine or procainamide. Blepharospasm can be treated with clozapine (125-200 mg/day).

Enhancement of elimination: Multiple dosing of activated charcoal may be useful; not dialyzable (0% to 5%)

Test Interactions ↑ cholesterol (S), glucose; ↓ uric acid (S)

Drug Interactions Substrate of CYP2D6 (major); **Inhibits** CYP1A2 (weak), 2C9 (weak), 2D6 (weak), 2E1 (weak)

Acetylcholinesterase inhibitors (central): May increase the risk of antipsychotic-related extrapyramidal symptoms; monitor.

Aluminum salts: May decrease the absorption of phenothiazines; monitor

Amphetamines: Efficacy may be diminished by antipsychotics; in addition, amphetamines may increase psychotic symptoms. Avoid concurrent use

Anticholinergics: May inhibit the therapeutic response to phenothiazines and excess anticholinergic effects may occur; includes benztropine, trihexyphenidyl, biperiden, and drugs with significant anticholinergic activity (TCAs, antihistamines, disopyramide)

Antihypertensives: Concurrent use of phenothiazines with an antihypertensive may produce additive hypotensive effects (particularly orthostasis)

Bromocriptine: Phenothiazines inhibit the ability of bromocriptine to lower serum prolactin concentrations

CNS depressants: Sedative effects may be additive with phenothiazines; monitor for increased effect; includes barbiturates, benzodiazepines, narcotic analgesics, ethanol, and other sedative agents

CYP2D6 inhibitors: May increase the levels/effects of fluphenazine. Example inhibitors include chlorpromazine, delavirdine, fluoxetine, miconazole, paroxetine, pergolide, quinidine, quinine, ritonavir, and ropinirole.

Epinephrine: Chlorpromazine (and possibly other low potency antipsychotics) may diminish the pressor effects of epinephrine

Guanethidine and guanadrel: Antihypertensive effects may be inhibited by phenothiazines

Levodopa: Phenothiazines may inhibit the antiparkinsonian effect of levodopa; avoid this combination

Lithium: Phenothiazines may produce neurotoxicity with lithium; this is a rare effect

Metoclopramide: May increase extrapyramidal symptoms (EPS) or risk.

Phenytoin: May reduce serum levels of phenothiazines; phenothiazines may increase phenytoin serum levels

Propranolol: Serum concentrations of phenothiazines may be increased; propranolol also increases phenothiazine concentrations

Polypeptide antibiotics: Rare cases of respiratory paralysis have been reported with concurrent use of phenothiazines

QT$_c$-prolonging agents: Effects on QT$_c$ interval may be additive with phenothiazines, increasing the risk of malignant arrhythmias; includes type Ia antiarrhythmics, TCAs, and some quinolone antibiotics (sparfloxacin, moxifloxacin and gatifloxacin)

Sulfadoxine-pyrimethamine: May increase phenothiazine concentrations

Tricyclic antidepressants: Concurrent use may produce increased toxicity or altered therapeutic response

Trazodone: Phenothiazines and trazodone may produce additive hypotensive effects

Valproic acid: Serum levels may be increased by phenothiazines

Pregnancy Risk Factor C

Pregnancy Implications Extrapyramidal reaction may develop in neonates from maternally-administered drug; crosses the placenta

Lactation Enters breast milk/not recommended

Nursing Implications Dilute oral concentrate solution in juice before administration; avoid contact of oral solution or injection with skin (contact dermatitis); watch for hypotension when administering I.M. or I.V.

Additional Information Oral liquid to be diluted in the following **only**: water, saline, 7-UP®, homogenized milk, carbonated orange beverages, pineapple, apricot, prune, orange, V8® juice, tomato, and grapefruit juices. Benztropine can be used to treat nausea/vomiting.

Flurazepam

CAS Number 1172-18-5; 17617-23-1

U.S. Brand Names Dalmane®

Synonyms Flurazepam Hydrochloride

Impairment Potential Yes. A 15 mg ingestion of flurazepam at bedtime has been demonstrated to result in driving impairment the next morning. A brief or extended period (up to 1 year) of use is consistent with driving impairment in the elderly; impairment is greatest in the first week of use. (Betts TA and Birtle J, "Effect of Two Hypnotic Drugs on Actual Driving Performances Next Morning," Br Med J, 1982, 285(6345):852.)

Use Short-term treatment of insomnia

Mechanism of Action Depresses all levels of the CNS, including the limbic and reticular formation, probably through the increased action of gamma-aminobutyric acid (GABA), which is a major inhibitory neurotransmitter in the brain

Adverse Reactions

Cardiovascular: Tachycardia

Central nervous system: **Drowsiness, ataxia, lightheadedness, dizziness, slurred speech**, euphoria, headache, mental depression, hallucinations, insomnia, convulsions, paranoid symptoms, confusion, dystonic reactions

Dermatologic: Urticaria, purpura, pruritus, exanthem

Endocrine & metabolic: Changes in libido

Gastrointestinal: Nausea, xerostomia, vomiting, diarrhea, constipation, abdominal cramps

Hematologic: Thrombocytopenia, anemia, leukopenia, neutropenia, agranulocytosis

Hepatic: Liver dysfunction

Local: Phlebitis

Neuromuscular & skeletal: Paresthesia, muscle spasm, trembling

Ocular: Blurred vision, photophobia

Miscellaneous: Allergic reaction, drug dependence, diaphoresis (excessive)

Signs and Symptoms of Overdose Adult respiratory distress syndrome, apnea, asterixis, ataxia, coma, drowsiness, hyperactivity, hypoactive reflexes, hyporeflexia, hypotension, metallic taste, mydriasis, nystagmus, respiratory depression, unsteady gait

Pharmacodynamics/Kinetics

Onset of action: Hypnotic: 15-20 minutes

Peak effect: 3-6 hours

Duration: 7-8 hours

Metabolism: Hepatic to N-desalkylflurazepam (active)

Half-life elimination: Desalkylflurazepam:

Adults: Single dose: 74-90 hours; Multiple doses: 111-113 hours

Elderly (61-85 years): Single dose: 120-160 hours; Multiple doses: 126-158 hours

Dosage

Oral:

Children:

≤15 years: Dose not established

>15 years: 15 mg at bedtime

Adults: 15-30 mg at bedtime

Elderly: Oral: 15 mg at bedtime; avoid use if possible

Stability Store in light-resistant containers

Monitoring Parameters Respiratory and cardiovascular status

Administration Give 30 minutes to 1 hour before bedtime on an empty stomach with full glass of water. May be taken with food if GI distress occurs.

Contraindications Hypersensitivity to flurazepam or any component of the formulation (cross-sensitivity with other benzodiazepines may exist); narrow-angle glaucoma; pregnancy

Warnings

Use with caution in elderly or debilitated patients, patients with hepatic disease (including alcoholics), or renal impairment. Active metabolites with extended half-lives may lead to delayed accumulation and adverse effects. Use with caution in patients with respiratory disease, or impaired gag reflex. Avoid use in patients with sleep apnea.

Causes CNS depression (dose-related) resulting in sedation, dizziness, confusion, or ataxia which may impair physical and mental capabilities. Patients must be cautioned about performing tasks which require mental alertness (eg, operating machinery or driving). Use with caution in patients receiving other CNS depressants or psychoactive agents. Effects with other sedative drugs or ethanol may be potentiated. Benzodiazepines have been associated with falls and traumatic injury and should be used with extreme caution in patients who are at risk of these events (especially the elderly).

Use caution in patients with depression, particularly if suicidal risk may be present. Use with caution in patients with a history of drug dependence. Benzodiazepines have been associated with dependence and acute withdrawal symptoms on discontinuation or reduction in dose (may occur after as little as 10 days of use). Acute withdrawal, including seizures, may be precipitated in patients after administration of flumazenil to patients receiving long-term benzodiazepine therapy.

As a hypnotic, should be used only after evaluation of potential causes of sleep disturbance. Failure of sleep disturbance to resolve after 7-10 days may indicate psychiatric or medical illness. A worsening of insomnia or the emergence of new abnormalities of thought or behavior may represent unrecognized psychiatric or medical illness and requires immediate and careful evaluation.

Benzodiazepines have been associated with anterograde amnesia. Paradoxical reactions, including hyperactive or aggressive behavior have been reported with benzodiazepines, particularly in adolescent/pediatric or psychiatric patients. Does not have analgesic, antidepressant, or antipsychotic properties.

Dosage Forms Capsule, as hydrochloride: 15 mg, 30 mg

Reference Range

Therapeutic: 0-4 ng/mL (SI: 0-9 nmol/L)

Metabolite N-desalkylflurazepam: 20-110 ng/mL (SI: 43-240 nmol/L)

Toxic: 2000 ng/mL (SI: 4300 nmol/L)

Overdosage/Treatment

Decontamination: Lavage (within 1 hour)/activated charcoal

Supportive therapy: Treatment for benzodiazepine overdose is supportive. Rarely is mechanical ventilation required. Flumazenil has been shown to selectively block the binding of benzodiazepines to CNS receptors, resulting in a reversal of benzodiazepine-induced CNS depression. Hypotension can be treated with isotonic I.V. fluids with placement in Trendelenburg position; dopamine and norepinephrine can be used.

Enhancement of elimination: Forced diuresis or hemodialysis is not useful; multiple dosing of activated charcoal may be useful

Drug Interactions Substrate of CYP3A4 (major); **Inhibits** CYP2E1 (weak)

CNS depressants: Sedative effects and/or respiratory depression may be additive with CNS depressants; includes ethanol, barbiturates, narcotic analgesics, and other sedative agents; monitor for increased effect

CYP3A4 inducers: CYP3A4 inducers may decrease the levels/effects of flurazepam. Example inducers include aminoglutethimide, carbamazepine, nafcillin, nevirapine, phenobarbital, phenytoin, and rifamycins.

CYP3A4 inhibitors: May increase the levels/effects of flurazepam. Example inhibitors include azole antifungals, clarithromycin, diclofenac, doxycycline, erythromycin, imatinib, isoniazid, nefazodone, nicardipine, propofol, protease inhibitors, quinidine, telithromycin, and verapamil.

Levodopa: Therapeutic effects may be diminished in some patients following the addition of a benzodiazepine; limited/inconsistent data

Oral contraceptives: May decrease the clearance of some benzodiazepines (those which undergo oxidative metabolism); monitor for increased benzodiazepine effect

Theophylline: May partially antagonize some of the effects of benzodiazepines; monitor for decreased response; may require higher doses for sedation

Pregnancy Risk Factor X

Lactation Excretion in breast milk unknown/not recommended

Nursing Implications Provide safety measures (ie, side rails, night light, and call button); remove smoking materials from area; supervise ambulation; avoid abrupt discontinuance in patients with prolonged therapy or seizure disorders

Flurbiprofen

Related Information

- Ibuprofen
- Nonsteroidal Anti-inflammatory Drugs

CAS Number 5104-49-4

U.S. Brand Names Ansaid®; Ocufen®

Synonyms Flurbiprofen Sodium

Use
Oral: Treatment of rheumatoid arthritis and osteoarthritis
Ophthalmic: Inhibition of intraoperative miosis

Mechanism of Action Propionic acid derivative (like ibuprofen); inhibits prostaglandin synthesis by decreasing the activity of the enzyme, cyclooxygenase, which results in decreased formation of prostaglandin precursors

Adverse Reactions
Ophthalmic: Frequency not defined: Ocular: Slowing of corneal wound healing, mild ocular stinging, itching and burning, ocular irritation, fibrosis, miosis, mydriasis, bleeding tendency increased

Oral:
Cardiovascular: Edema, cerebrovascular ischemia, CHF, hypertension, vasodilation

Central nervous system: Amnesia, anxiety, depression, dizziness, headache, insomnia, malaise, nervousness, somnolence, confusion, fever

Dermatologic: Rash, angioedema, bruising, eczema, exfoliative dermatitis, photosensitivity, pruritus, purpura, toxic epidermal necrolysis, urticaria

Endocrine & metabolic: Hyperuricemia

Gastrointestinal: Abdominal pain, constipation, diarrhea, dyspepsia, flatulence, GI bleeding, nausea, vomiting, weight changes, gastric/peptic ulcer, stomatitis

Hematologic: Anemia, eosinophilia, hematocrit decreased, hemoglobin decreased, leukopenia, thrombocytopenia

Hepatic: Liver enzymes elevated, hepatitis, jaundice

Neuromuscular & skeletal: Reflexes increased, tremor, vertigo, weakness, paresthesia

Ocular: Vision changes

Otic: Tinnitus

Renal: Hematuria, interstitial nephritis, renal failure

Respiratory: Rhinitis, asthma, epistaxis

Miscellaneous: Anaphylactic reaction, parosmia

Signs and Symptoms of Overdose Cognitive dysfunction, drowsiness, gastritis, GI bleeding, nausea, nephrotic syndrome, ototoxicity, tinnitus, vomiting, wheezing. Severe poisoning can manifest with coma, renal and/or hepatic failure, hypotension, seizures, and respiratory depression.

Pharmacodynamics/Kinetics
Onset of action: ~1-2 hours
Distribution: V_d: 0.12 L/kg
Protein binding: 99%, primarily albumin
Metabolism: Hepatic via CYP2C9; forms metabolites such as 4-hydroxyflurbiprofen (inactive)
Half-life elimination: 5.7 hours
Time to peak: 1.5 hours
Excretion: Urine (primarily as metabolites)

Dosage
Oral: Rheumatoid arthritis and osteoarthritis: 200-300 mg/day in 2-, 3-, or 4 divided doses; do not administer more than 100 mg for any single dose; maximum: 300 mg/day

Ophthalmic: Instill 1 drop every 30 minutes, beginning 2 hours prior to surgery (total of 4 drops in each affected eye)

Administration
Tablet: Take with a full glass of water.

Contraindications Hypersensitivity to flurbiprofen, aspirin, other NSAIDs, or any component of the formulation; perioperative pain in the setting of coronary artery bypass surgery (CABG); dendritic keratitis; pregnancy (3rd trimester)

Warnings [U.S. Boxed Warning]: NSAIDs are associated with an increased risk of adverse cardiovascular events, including MI, stroke, and new onset or worsening of pre-existing hypertension. Risk may be increased with duration of use or pre-existing cardiovascular risk-factors or disease. Carefully evaluate individual cardiovascular risk profiles prior to prescribing. Use caution with fluid retention, CHF, or hypertension.

Use of NSAIDs can compromise existing renal function. Renal toxicity can occur in patient with impaired renal function, dehydration, heart failure, liver dysfunction, those taking diuretics and ACEI, and the elderly. Rehydrate patient before starting therapy. Monitor renal function closely. Not recommended for use in patients with advanced renal disease.

[U.S. Boxed Warning]: NSAIDs may increase risk of gastrointestinal irritation, ulceration, bleeding, and perforation. These events may occur at any time during therapy and without warning. Use caution with a history of GI disease (bleeding or ulcers), concurrent therapy with aspirin, anticoagulants and/or corticosteroids, smoking, use of alcohol, the elderly or debilitated patients.

Use the lowest effective dose for the shortest duration of time, consistent with individual patient goals, to reduce risk of cardiovascular or GI adverse events. Alternate therapies should be considered for patients at high risk.

NSAIDs may cause serious skin adverse events including exfoliative dermatitis, Stevens-Johnson syndrome (SJS), and toxic epidermal necrolysis (TEN). Anaphylactoid reactions may occur, even without

prior exposure; patients with "aspirin triad" (bronchial asthma, aspirin intolerance, rhinitis) may be at increased risk. Do not use in patients who experience bronchospasm, asthma, rhinitis, or urticaria with NSAID or aspirin therapy.

Use with caution in patients with decreased hepatic function. Closely monitor patients with any abnormal LFT. Severe hepatic reactions (eg, fulminant hepatitis, liver failure) have occurred with NSAID use, rarely; discontinue if signs or symptoms of liver disease develop, or if systemic manifestations occur.

The elderly are at increased risk for adverse effects (especially peptic ulceration, CNS effects, renal toxicity) from NSAIDs even at low doses.

Withhold for at least 4-6 half-lives prior to surgical or dental procedures. Safety and efficacy have not been established in children <18 years of age.

Dosage Forms
[DSC] = Discontinued product
Solution, ophthalmic, as sodium (Ocufen®): 0.03% (2.5 mL) [contains thimerosal]
Tablet: 50 mg, 100 mg
Ansaid®: 50 mg, 100 mg [DSC]

Reference Range
Mean steady-state levels: ~6 mg/mL (not age-dependent)
Peak serum flurbiprofen levels after a single 50 mg dose: ~8-9.4 mg/L

Overdosage/Treatment
Decontamination: Ipecac within 30 minutes or lavage (within 1 hour)/activated charcoal

Supportive therapy: Hypotension/dehydration can be managed with I.V. fluid therapy; acidosis should be treated with bicarbonates, seizures with benzodiazepines; antacids, blood products are indicated, as appropriate, for hemorrhage

Enhancement of elimination: Dialysis or perfusion is indicated for secondary complications, acidosis, or renal failure and not toxin removal alone; multiple dosing of activated charcoal may be effective

Drug Interactions
Substrate of CYP2C9 (minor); **Inhibits** CYP2C9 (strong)
ACE inhibitors: Antihypertensive effects may be decreased by concurrent therapy with NSAIDs; monitor blood pressure.

Angiotensin II antagonists: Antihypertensive effects may be decreased by concurrent therapy with NSAIDs; monitor blood pressure.

Anticoagulants (warfarin, heparin, LMWHs) in combination with NSAIDs can cause increased risk of bleeding.

Antiplatelet drugs (ticlopidine, clopidogrel, aspirin, abciximab, dipyridamole, eptifibatide, tirofiban) can cause an increased risk of bleeding.

Beta-blockers: NSAIDs may decrease the antihypertensive effect of beta-blockers. Monitor.

Cholestyramine (and other bile acid sequestrants): May decrease the absorption of NSAIDs. Separate by at least 2 hours.

Corticosteroids may increase the risk of GI ulceration; avoid concurrent use.

Cyclosporine: NSAIDs may increase serum creatinine, potassium, blood pressure, and cyclosporine levels; monitor cyclosporine levels and renal function carefully.

CYP2C9 Substrates: Flurbiprofen may increase the levels/effects of CYP2C9 substrates. Example substrates include bosentan, dapsone, fluoxetine, glimepiride, glipizide, losartan, montelukast, nateglinide, paclitaxel, phenytoin, warfarin, and zafirlukast.

Gentamicin and amikacin serum concentrations are increased by indomethacin in premature infants. Results may apply to other aminoglycosides and NSAIDs.

Hydralazine's antihypertensive effect is decreased; avoid concurrent use.

Lithium levels can be increased; avoid concurrent use if possible or monitor lithium levels and adjust dose. Sulindac may have the least effect. When NSAID is stopped, lithium will need adjustment again.

Loop diuretics efficacy (diuretic and antihypertensive effect) is reduced. Indomethacin reduces this efficacy, however, it may be anticipated with any NSAID.

Methotrexate: Severe bone marrow suppression, aplastic anemia, and GI toxicity have been reported with concomitant NSAID therapy. Avoid use during moderate or high-dose methotrexate (increased and prolonged methotrexate levels). NSAID use during low-dose treatment of rheumatoid arthritis has not been fully evaluated; extreme caution is warranted.

Thiazides antihypertensive effects are decreased; avoid concurrent use.

Warfarin's INRs may be increased by piroxicam. Other NSAIDs may have the same effect depending on dose and duration. Monitor INR closely. Use the lowest dose of NSAIDs possible and for the briefest duration.

Verapamil plasma concentration is decreased by some NSAIDs; avoid concurrent use.

Pregnancy Risk Factor C/D (3rd trimester)

Pregnancy Implications Teratogenic effects were not observed in animal studies, however, adequate and well-controlled studies have not been conducted in pregnant women. Exposure late in pregnancy may lead to premature closure of the ductus arteriosus.

Lactation Enters breast milk/not recommended

Nursing Implications Care should be taken to avoid contamination of the solution container tip

Flutamide

CAS Number 13311-84-7

U.S. Brand Names Eulexin®

Synonyms 4'-Nitro-3'-Trifluoromethylisobutyrantide; Niftolid; NSC-147834; SCH 13521

Use Treatment of metastatic prostatic carcinoma in combination therapy with LHRH agonist analogues

Unlabeled/Investigational Use Female hirsutism

Mechanism of Action Nonsteroidal antiandrogen with properties which block the action of dihydrotestosterone on the prostatic tissue and testes

Adverse Reactions

Cardiovascular: Hypertension, edema, myocardial infarction

Central nervous system: Drowsiness, confusion, depression, anxiety, nervousness, headache, dizziness, insomnia

Dermatologic: Pruritus, ecchymosis, photosensitivity

Endocrine & metabolic: **Gynecomastia, hot flashes, breast tenderness, galactorrhea; impotence; decreased libido; tumor flare**

Gastrointestinal: **Nausea, vomiting,** anorexia, increased appetite, constipation, indigestion, upset stomach; diarrhea

Genitourinary: Discoloration of urine (yellow)

Hematologic: Anemia, leukopenia, thrombocytopenia, hepatitis, hepatic failure, jaundice, sulfhemoglobinemia

Hepatic: **Increased AST (SGOT) and LDH levels, transient, mild**

Local: Thrombophlebitis

Neuromuscular & skeletal: Weakness

Respiratory: Pulmonary embolism

Miscellaneous: Herpes zoster

Signs and Symptoms of Overdose Apnea, ataxia, hypoactivity, lacrimation, lethargy, methemoglobinemia (up to 16.2% has been described), vomiting

Pharmacodynamics/Kinetics

Absorption: Oral: Rapid and complete

Protein binding: Parent drug: 94% to 96%; 2-hydroxyflutamide: 92% to 94%

Metabolism: Extensively hepatic to more than 10 metabolites, primarily 2-hydroxyflutamide (active)

Half-life elimination: 5-6 hours (2-hydroxyflutamide)

Excretion: Primarily urine (as metabolites)

Dosage

Oral: Adults:

Prostatic carcinoma: 250 mg 3 times/day **or** 1.5 g once daily

Female hirsutism: 250 mg daily

Monitoring Parameters Serum transaminase levels should be measured prior to starting treatment and should be repeated monthly for the first 4 months of therapy, and periodically thereafter. LFTs should be checked at the first sign or symptom of liver dysfunction (eg, nausea, vomiting, abdominal pain, fatigue, anorexia, flu-like symptoms, hyperbilirubinuria, jaundice, or right upper quadrant tenderness). Other parameters include tumor reduction, testosterone/estrogen, and phosphatase serum levels.

Administration Usually administered orally in 3 divided doses; contents of capsule may be opened and mixed with applesauce, pudding, or other soft foods; mixing with a beverage is not recommended

Contraindications Hypersensitivity to flutamide or any component of the formulation; severe hepatic impairment; pregnancy

Warnings

[U.S. Boxed Warning]: Hospitalization and, rarely, death due to liver failure has been reported in patients taking flutamide. Elevated serum transaminase levels, jaundice, hepatic encephalopathy, and acute hepatic failure have been reported. Product labeling states flutamide is not for use in women, particularly for nonlife-threatening conditions. In some patients, the toxicity reverses after discontinuation of therapy. About 50% of the cases occur within the first 3 months of treatment. Serum transaminase levels should be measured prior to starting treatment, monthly for 4 months, and periodically thereafter. Liver function tests should be obtained at the first suggestion of liver dysfunction (nausea, vomiting, abdominal pain, fatigue, anorexia, "flu-like" symptoms, hyperbilirubinuria, jaundice, or right upper quadrant tenderness). Flutamide should be immediately discontinued any time a patient has jaundice, and/or an ALT level greater than twice the upper limit of normal. Flutamide should not be used in patients whose ALT values are greater than twice the upper limit of normal.

Patients with glucose-6 phosphate dehydrogenase deficiency or hemoglobin M disease or smokers are at risk of toxicities associated with aniline exposure, including methemoglobinemia, hemolytic anemia, and cholestatic jaundice. Monitor methemoglobin levels.

Dosage Forms Capsule: 125 mg

Reference Range At steady-state; plasma 2-hydroxyflutamide levels range from 1556-2284 ng/mL

Overdosage/Treatment

Decontamination: Emesis within 30 minutes or lavage (within 1 hour)/ activated charcoal

Supportive therapy: Treat symptomatic methemoglobinemia with methylene blue

Enhancement of elimination: Multiple dosing of activated charcoal may be beneficial; hemodialysis is not expect to be of benefit

Drug Interactions Substrate (major) of CYP1A2, 3A4; **Inhibits** CYP1A2 (weak)

CYP1A2 inducers: May decrease the levels/effects of flutamide. Example inducers include aminoglutethimide, carbamazepine, phenobarbital, and rifampin.

CYP1A2 inhibitors: May increase the levels/effects of flutamide. Example inhibitors include ciprofloxacin, fluvoxamine, ketoconazole, lomefloxacin, ofloxacin, and rofecoxib.

CYP3A4 inducers: CYP3A4 inducers may decrease the levels/effects of flutamide. Example inducers include aminoglutethimide, carbamazepine, nafcillin, nevirapine, phenobarbital, phenytoin, and rifamycins.

CYP3A4 inhibitors: May increase the levels/effects of flutamide. Example inhibitors include azole antifungals, clarithromycin, diclofenac, doxycycline, erythromycin, imatinib, isoniazid, nefazodone, nicardipine, propofol, protease inhibitors, quinidine, telithromycin, and verapamil.

Warfarin: Warfarin effects may be increased

Pregnancy Risk Factor D

Lactation Excretion in breast milk unknown/not recommended

Additional Information Diarrhea may occur due to lactose intolerance; plasma testosterone and estradiol levels may be elevated

Fluvastatin

CAS Number 93957-54-1; 93957-55-2

U.S. Brand Names Lescol® XL; Lescol®

Use

To be used as a component of multiple risk factor intervention in patients at risk for atherosclerosis vascular disease due to hypercholesterolemia

Adjunct to dietary therapy to reduce elevated total cholesterol (total-C), LDL-C, triglyceride, and apolipoprotein B (apo-B) levels and to increase HDL-C in primary hypercholesterolemia and mixed dyslipidemia (Fredrickson types IIa and IIb); to slow the progression of coronary atherosclerosis in patients with coronary heart disease; reduce risk of coronary revascularization procedures in patients with coronary heart disease

Mechanism of Action HMG-CoA reductase inhibitor, the enzyme responsible for cholesterol synthesis

Adverse Reactions

Cardiovascular: Vasculitis

Central nervous system: Headache, insomnia

Dermatologic: Rash, erythema multiforme, alopecia, angioedema, toxic epidermal necrolysis, xerosis, urticaria, purpura, Stevens-Johnson syndrome, photosensitivity, pruritus

Endocrine & metabolic: Gynecomastia

Gastrointestinal: Dyspepsia, diarrhea, nausea

Hepatic: Hepatotoxicity

Neuromuscular & skeletal: Paresthesia

Respiratory: Adult respiratory distress syndrome

Miscellaneous: Systemic lupus erythematosus

Pharmacodynamics/Kinetics

Onset: Peak effect: Maximal LDL-C reductions achieved within 4 weeks

Distribution: V_d: 0.35 L/kg

Protein binding: >98%

Metabolism: To inactive and active metabolites (oxidative metabolism via CYP2C9 [75%], 2C8 [~5%], and 3A4 [~20%] isoenzymes); active forms do not circulate systemically; extensive (saturable) first-pass hepatic extraction

Bioavailability: Absolute: Capsule: 24%; Extended release tablet: 29%

Half-life elimination: Capsule: <3 hours; Extended release tablet: 9 hours

Time to peak: Capsule: 1 hour; Extended release tablet: 3 hours

Excretion: Feces (90%): urine (5%)

Dosage Adults: Oral:

Patients requiring ≥25% decrease in LDL-C: 40 mg capsule or 80 mg extended release tablet once daily in the evening; may also use 40 mg capsule twice daily

Patients requiring <25% decrease in LDL-C: 20 mg capsule once daily in the evening

Note: Dosing range: 20-80 mg/day; adjust dose based on response to therapy; maximum response occurs within 4-6 weeks

Dosage adjustment in renal impairment: Less than 6% excreted renally; no dosage adjustment needed with mild to moderate renal impairment; use with caution in severe impairment

Dosage adjustment in hepatic impairment: Levels may accumulate in patients with liver disease (increased AUC and C_{max}); use caution with severe hepatic impairment or heavy ethanol ingestion; contraindicated in active liver disease or unexplained transaminase elevations; decrease dose and monitor effects carefully in patients with hepatic insufficiency

Elderly: No dosage adjustment necessary based on age

Monitoring Parameters Obtain baseline LFTs and total cholesterol profile; repeat tests at 12 weeks after initiation of therapy or elevation in dose, and periodically thereafter. Monitor LDL-C at intervals no less than 4 weeks.

Administration Patient should be placed on a standard cholesterol-lowering diet before and during treatment; fluvastatin may be taken without regard to meals; adjust dosage as needed in response to periodic lipid determinations during the first 4 weeks after a dosage change; lipid-lowering effects are additive when fluvastatin is combined with a bile-acid binding resin or niacin, however, it must be administered at least 2 hours following these drugs. Do not break, chew, or crush extended release tablets; do not open capsules.

Contraindications Hypersensitivity to fluvastatin or any component of the formulation; active liver disease; unexplained persistent elevations of serum transaminases; pregnancy; breast-feeding

Warnings Secondary causes of hyperlipidemia should be ruled out prior to therapy. Liver function must be monitored by periodic laboratory assessment. Rhabdomyolysis with acute renal failure has occurred with fluvastatin and other HMG-CoA reductase inhibitors. Risk may be increased with concurrent use of other drugs which may cause rhabdomyolysis (including gemfibrozil, fibric acid derivatives, or niacin at doses ≥ 1 g/day). Temporarily discontinue in any patient experiencing markedly elevated CPK levels, myopathy, or an acute/serious condition predisposing to renal failure secondary to rhabdomyolysis. Use caution in patients with previous liver disease or heavy ethanol use. Use caution in patients with concurrent medications or conditions which reduce steroidogenesis. Efficacy and safety in children <10 years of age have not been established.

Dosage Forms Capsule (Lescol®): 20 mg, 40 mg
Tablet, extended release (Lescol® XL): 80 mg

Reference Range Peak plasma fluvastatin level after a 10 mg oral dose: ~23 ng/mL

Overdosage/Treatment Decontamination: Lavage (within 1 hour)/cholestyramine can inhibit absorption

Drug Interactions Substrate of CYP2C9 (major), 2C8 (minor), 2D6 (minor), 3A4 (minor); **Inhibits** CYP1A2 (weak), 2C8 (weak), 2C9 (moderate), 2D6 (weak), 3A4 (weak)

Cholestyramine: Cholestyramine may decrease the absorption of fluvastatin. Separate administration times by at least 4 hours. Cholestyramine may increase the therapeutic effects of fluvastatin.

CYP2C9 inhibitors: May increase the levels/effects of fluvastatin. Example inhibitors include delavirdine, fluconazole, gemfibrozil, ketoconazole, nicardipine, NSAIDs, sulfonamides, and tolbutamide.

CYP2C9 substrates: Fluvastatin may increase levels/effects of CYP2C9 substrates. Example substrates include bosentan, dapsone, fluoxetine, glimepiride, glipizide, losartan, montelukast, nateglinide, paclitaxel, phenytoin, warfarin, and zafirlukast.

Fibric acid derivatives: May increase the risk of myopathy and rhabdomyolysis.

Fluconazole: May increase the levels/effects of fluvastatin; monitor.

Glyburide: C_{max} and AUC of both fluvastatin and glyburide may increase; half-life of glyburide may also increase; monitor

Omeprazole: Omeprazole may increase serum concentrations of fluvastatin

Phenytoin: C_{max} and AUC of both phenytoin and fluvastatin may be increased when given together; monitor phenytoin when fluvastatin is initiated, modified, or discontinued

Rifamycin derivatives: May decrease serum concentrations of fluvastatin

Warfarin: Fluvastatin may increase hypoprothrombinemic effects of warfarin; monitor INR closely when fluvastatin is initiated, modified, or discontinued

Pregnancy Risk Factor X

Pregnancy Implications Animal studies have shown delays in fetal skeletal development and fetal, neonatal, and maternal mortality. Congenital anomalies following use of other HMG-CoA reductase inhibitors in humans have been reported (rare). Use in women of childbearing potential only if they are highly unlikely to conceive; discontinue if pregnancy occurs.

Lactation Enters breast milk/contraindicated

Additional Information Food can increase absorption.

Specific References

Holdaas H, Fellström B, Jardine AG, et al, "Effect of Fluvastatin on Cardiac Outcomes in Renal Transplant Recipients: A Multicentre, Randomised, Placebo-Controlled Trial," *Lancet*, 2003, 361(9374): 2024-31.

Fluvoxamine

Related Information
- Antidepressant Agents

Synonyms Luvox

Use Treatment of obsessive-compulsive disorder (OCD) in children ≥ 8 years of age and adults

Treatment of major depression; panic disorder; anxiety disorders in children

Mechanism of Action Serotonin reuptake inhibitor

Adverse Reactions

Cardiovascular: Syncope, Raynaud's phenomenon, sinus bradycardia, sinus tachycardia

Central nervous system: Somnolence, headache, agitation, insomnia, dizziness, psychosis, hypokinesia, akathisia, electroencephalogram abnormalities, extrapyramidal reactions

Dermatologic: Toxic epidermal necrolysis, photosensitivity, alopecia, ecchymosis, Stevens-Johnson syndrome, angioedema, urticaria, exanthem

Endocrine & metabolic: Sexual dysfunction (delayed orgasm), syndrome of inappropriate antidiuretic hormone, hyponatremia due to SIADH, anorgasmia; nephrogenic diabetes insipidus

Gastrointestinal: Xerostomia, **nausea**, vomiting, constipation

Hepatic: Elevated liver function test results

Neuromuscular & skeletal: Tremor, weakness

Ocular: Aggravation of glaucoma

Respiratory: Epistaxis

Signs and Symptoms of Overdose Amenorrhea, bradycardia, coma, death, depression, elevated liver function tests, hypotension, insomnia, mania, seizures, tachycardia, toxic epidermal necrolysis, syndrome of inappropriate antidiuretic hormone (SIADH)

Pharmacodynamics/Kinetics

Absorption: Steady-state plasma concentrations have been noted to be 2-3 times higher in children than those in adolescents; female children demonstrated a significantly higher AUC than males

Distribution: V_d: ~25 L/kg

Protein binding: ~80%, primarily to albumin

Metabolism: Hepatic

Bioavailability: 53%; not significantly affected by food

Half-life elimination: ~15 hours

Time to peak, plasma: 3-8 hours

Excretion: Urine

Dosage

Oral: **Note:** When total daily dose exceeds 50 mg, the dose should be given in 2 divided doses:

Children 8-17 years: Initial: 25 mg at bedtime; adjust in 25 mg increments at 4- to 7-day intervals, as tolerated, to maximum therapeutic benefit: Range: 50-200 mg/day

Maximum: Children: 8-11 years: 200 mg/day, adolescents: 300 mg/day; lower doses may be effective in female versus male patients

Adults: Initial: 50 mg at bedtime; adjust in 50 mg increments at 4- to 7-day intervals; usual dose range: 100-300 mg/day; divide total daily dose into 2 doses; administer larger portion at bedtime

Elderly: Reduce dose, titrate slowly

Dosage adjustment in hepatic impairment: Reduce dose, titrate slowly

Monitoring Parameters Mental status for depression, suicidal ideation, anxiety, social functioning, mania, panic attacks; akathisia, weight gain or loss, nutritional intake, sleep

Contraindications Hypersensitivity to fluvoxamine or any component of the formulation; concurrent use with alosetron, pimozide, thioridazine, tizanidine, mesoridazine, or cisapride; use of MAO inhibitors within 14 days

Warnings

Major psychiatric warnings:

- [U.S. Boxed Warning]: **Antidepressants increase the risk of suicidal thinking and behavior in children and adolescents with major depressive disorder (MDD) and other depressive disorders;** consider risk prior to prescribing. Closely monitor for clinical worsening, suicidality, or unusual changes in behavior; the child's family or caregiver should be instructed to closely observe the patient and communicate condition with healthcare provider. A medication guide concerning the use of antidepressants in children and teenagers should be dispensed with each prescription. **Fluvoxamine is not FDA approved for use in children.**

- The possibility of a suicide attempt is inherent in major depression and may persist until remission occurs. Patients treated with antidepressants should be observed for clinical worsening and suicidality, especially during the initial few months of a course of drug therapy, or at times of dose changes, either increases or decreases. Worsening depression and severe abrupt suicidality that are not part of the presenting symptoms may require discontinuation or modification of drug therapy. Use caution in high-risk patients during initiation of therapy.

• Prescriptions should be written for the smallest quantity consistent with good patient care. The patient's family or caregiver should be alerted to monitor patients for the emergence of suicidality and associated behaviors such as anxiety, agitation, panic attacks, insomnia, irritability, hostility, impulsivity, akathisia, hypomania, and mania; patients should be instructed to notify their healthcare provider if any of these symptoms or worsening depression or psychosis occur.

• May worsen psychosis in some patients or precipitate a shift to mania or hypomania in patients with bipolar disorder. Monotherapy in patients with bipolar disorder should be avoided. Patients presenting with depressive symptoms should be screened for bipolar disorder. **Fluvoxamine is not FDA approved for the treatment of bipolar depression.**

Key adverse effects:
• Anticholinergic effects: Relatively devoid of these side effects
• CNS depression: Has a low potential to impair cognitive or motor performance; caution operating hazardous machinery or driving.
• SIADH and hyponatremia: Has been associated with the development of SIADH; hyponatremia has been reported rarely, predominately in the elderly

Concurrent disease:
• Cardiovascular disease: Use caution in patients with cardiovascular disease; fluvoxamine has not been systemically evaluated in patients with a recent history of MI or unstable heart disease.
• Hepatic impairment: Use caution; clearance is decreased and plasma concentrations are increased; a lower dosage may be needed.
• Platelet aggregation: May impair platelet aggregation, resulting in bleeding.
• Renal impairment: Use caution; clearance is decreased and plasma concentrations are increased; a lower dosage may be needed.
• Seizure disorders: Use caution with a previous seizure disorder or condition predisposing to seizures such as brain damage or alcoholism.
• Sexual dysfunction: May cause or exacerbate sexual dysfunction.

Concurrent drug therapy:
• Agents which lower seizure threshold: Concurrent therapy with other drugs which lower the seizure threshold.
• Anticoagulants/Antiplatelets: Use caution with concomitant use of NSAIDs, ASA, or other drugs that affect coagulation; the risk of bleeding is potentiated.
• CNS depressants: Use caution with concomitant therapy.
• MAO inhibitors: Potential for severe reaction when used with MAO inhibitors; autonomic instability, coma, death, delirium, diaphoresis, hyperthermia, mental status changes/agitation, muscular rigidity, myoclonus, neuroleptic malignant syndrome features, and seizures may occur.

Special populations:
• Elderly: Use caution in elderly patients.

Special notes:
• Electroconvulsive therapy: May increase the risks associated with electroconvulsive therapy; consider discontinuing, when possible, prior to ECT treatment.
• Withdrawal syndrome: May cause dysphoric mood, irritability, agitation, dizziness, sensory disturbances, anxiety, confusion, headache, lethargy, emotional lability, insomnia, hypomania, tinnitus, and seizures. Upon discontinuation of fluvoxamine therapy, gradually taper dose. If intolerable symptoms occur following a decrease in dosage or upon discontinuation of therapy, then resuming the previous dose with a more gradual taper should be considered.

Dosage Forms Tablet: 25 mg, 50 mg, 100 mg

Overdosage/Treatment
Decontamination: Lavage (within 1 hour)/activated charcoal
Supportive therapy: Mianserin (15 mg at night) has been used to treat fluvoxamine-induced akathisia; akathisia can be treated with propranolol (60-120 mg/day) and trihexiphenidyl (2 mg/day)
Enhancement of elimination: Multiple dose activated charcoal may be useful

Drug Interactions
Substrate (major) of CYP1A2, 2D6; **Inhibits** CYP1A2 (strong), 2B6 (weak), 2C9 (weak), 2C19 (strong), 2D6 (weak), 3A4 (weak)
Alosetron: Serum concentrations may be increased by fluvoxamine; concurrent use is not recommended.
Amphetamines: SSRIs may increase the sensitivity to amphetamines, and amphetamines may increase the risk of serotonin syndrome
Benzodiazepines: Fluvoxamine may inhibit the metabolism of alprazolam, diazepam, and triazolam resulting in elevated serum levels; monitor for increased sedation and psychomotor impairment
Beta-blockers: Fluvoxamine may inhibit the metabolism of metoprolol and propranolol resulting in cardiac toxicity; monitor for bradycardia, hypotension, and heart failure if combination is used; not established for all beta-blockers (unlikely with atenolol or nadolol due to renal elimination)

Buspirone: Fluvoxamine inhibits the reuptake of serotonin; combined use with a serotonin agonist (buspirone) may cause serotonin syndrome; fluvoxamine may also increase serum concentrations of buspirone
Carbamazepine: Fluvoxamine may inhibit the metabolism of carbamazepine resulting in increased carbamazepine levels and toxicity; monitor for altered carbamazepine response
Carvedilol: Serum concentrations may be increased; monitor carefully for increased carvedilol effect (hypotension and bradycardia)
Cisapride: Concurrent use is contraindicated
Clozapine: Fluvoxamine inhibits the metabolism of clozapine; adjust clozapine dosage downward or use an alternative SSRI
CYP1A2 inducers: May decrease the levels/effects of fluvoxamine. Example inducers include aminoglutethimide, carbamazepine, phenobarbital, and rifampin.
CYP1A2 inhibitors: May increase the levels/effects of fluvoxamine. Example inhibitors include ciprofloxacin, ketoconazole, norfloxacin, ofloxacin, and rofecoxib.
CYP1A2 substrates: Fluvoxamine may increase the levels/effects of CYP1A2 substrates. Example substrates include aminophylline, mexiletine, mirtazapine, ropinirole, theophylline, and trifluoperazine.
CYP2C19 substrates: Fluvoxamine may increase the levels/effects of CYP2C19 substrates. Example substrates include citalopram, diazepam, methsuximide, phenytoin, propranolol, and sertraline.
CYP2D6 inhibitors: May increase the levels/effects of fluvoxamine. Example inhibitors include chlorpromazine, delavirdine, fluoxetine, miconazole, paroxetine, pergolide, quinidine, quinine, ritonavir, and ropinirole.
Cyproheptadine: May inhibit the effects of serotonin reuptake inhibitors (fluvoxamine); monitor for altered antidepressant response; cyproheptadine acts as a serotonin agonist
Dextromethorphan: Fluvoxamine inhibits the metabolism of dextromethorphan; visual hallucinations occurred in a patient receiving this combination; monitor for serotonin syndrome
Haloperidol: Fluvoxamine may inhibit the metabolism of haloperidol and cause extrapyramidal symptoms (EPS); monitor patients for EPS if combination is utilized
HMG-CoA reductase inhibitors: Fluvoxamine may inhibit the metabolism of lovastatin and simvastatin resulting in myositis and rhabdomyolysis; these combinations are best avoided
Lithium: Patients receiving SSRIs and lithium have developed neurotoxicity; if combination is used, monitor for neurotoxicity
Loop diuretics: Fluvoxamine may cause hyponatremia; additive hyponatremic effects may be seen with combined use of a loop diuretic (bumetanide, furosemide, torsemide); monitor for hyponatremia
MAO inhibitors: Fluvoxamine should not be used with nonselective MAO inhibitors (isocarboxazid, phenelzine); fatal reactions have been reported; this combination should be avoided
Meperidine: Combined use with fluvoxamine theoretically may increase the risk of serotonin syndrome
Methadone: Fluvoxamine may increase serum concentrations of methadone; monitor for increased effect
Mexiletine: Clearance of mexiletine was reduced by 38% following coadministration with fluvoxamine. If used concurrently, mexiletine levels should be monitored.
Nefazodone: May increase the risk of serotonin syndrome with SSRIs
NSAIDs: Concomitant use of fluvoxamine and NSAIDs, aspirin, or other drugs affecting coagulation has been associated with an increased risk of bleeding; monitor.
Pimozide: Concurrent use is contraindicated
Phenothiazines: Fluvoxamine may inhibit metabolism of phenothiazines; **concurrent use of agents associated with QT prolongation (thioridazine, mesoridazine) is contraindicated**
Phenytoin: Fluvoxamine inhibits the metabolism of phenytoin and may result in phenytoin toxicity; monitor for phenytoin toxicity (ataxia, confusion, dizziness, nystagmus, involuntary muscle movement)
Propafenone: Serum concentrations and/or toxicity may be increased by fluoxetine; avoid concurrent administration
Quinidine: Serum concentrations may be increased with fluvoxamine; avoid concurrent use
Ritonavir: Combined use of fluvoxamine with ritonavir may cause serotonin syndrome in HIV-positive patients; monitor
Selegiline: SSRIs have been reported to cause mania or hypertension when combined with selegiline; this combination is best avoided. In addition, use with some SSRIs has been reported to cause serotonin syndrome. As an MAO type B inhibitor, the risk of serotonin syndrome may be less than with nonselective MAO inhibitors.
Serotonin reuptake inhibitors: Combined use with other drugs which inhibit the reuptake may cause serotonin syndrome; monitor patient for altered response with nefazodone; avoid sibutramine combination
Sibutramine: May increase the risk of serotonin syndrome with SSRIs
Sumatriptan (and other serotonin agonists): Concurrent use may result in toxicity; weakness, hyper-reflexia, and incoordination have been observed with sumatriptan and SSRIs. In addition, concurrent use

may theoretically increase the risk of serotonin syndrome; includes sumatriptan, naratriptan, rizatriptan, and zolmitriptan.

Sympathomimetics: May increase the risk of serotonin syndrome with SSRIs

Tacrine: Fluvoxamine inhibits the metabolism of tacrine; use alternative SSRI

Tacrolimus: Fluvoxamine may inhibit the metabolism of tacrolimus; monitor for adverse effects; consider an alternative SSRI

Theophylline: Fluvoxamine inhibits the metabolism of theophylline; monitor for theophylline toxicity or use alternative SSRI

Tizanidine: Serum concentrations may be increased by fluvoxamine; concurrent use is not recommended.

Tramadol: Fluvoxamine combined with tramadol (serotonergic effects) may cause serotonin syndrome; monitor

Trazodone: Fluvoxamine may inhibit the metabolism of trazodone resulting in increased toxicity; monitor

Tricyclic antidepressants Fluvoxamine inhibits the metabolism of tricyclic antidepressants (amitriptyline, desipramine, imipramine, nortriptyline) resulting is elevated serum levels; if combination is warranted, a low dose of TCA (10-25 mg/day) should be utilized

Tryptophan: Fluvoxamine inhibits the reuptake of serotonin; combination with tryptophan, a serotonin precursor, may cause agitation and restlessness; this combination is best avoided

Venlafaxine: Combined use with fluvoxamine may increase the risk of serotonin syndrome

Warfarin: Fluvoxamine may alter the hypoprothrombinemic response to warfarin; monitor

Pregnancy Risk Factor C

Pregnancy Implications Nonteratogenic effects including respiratory distress, cyanosis, apnea, seizures, temperature instability, feeding difficulty, vomiting, hypoglycemia, hypo- or hypertonia, hyper-reflexia, jitteriness, irritability, constant crying, and tremor have been reported in the neonate immediately following delivery after exposure to other SSRIs late in the third trimester. Adverse effects may be due to toxic effects of SSRI or drug discontinuation. In some cases, may present clinically as serotonin syndrome. There are no adequate and well-controlled studies in pregnant women. Use during pregnancy only if the potential benefit to the mother outweighs the possible risk to the fetus. If treatment during pregnancy is required, consider tapering therapy during the third trimester.

Lactation Enters breast milk/not recommended (AAP rates "of concern")

Additional Information Rate of serotonin syndrome-like symptoms: ~0.04-0.006/100 treatment days

Specific References

Karunatilake H and Buckley NA, "Serotonin Syndrome Induced by Fluvoxamine and Oxycodone," *Ann Pharmacother*, 2006, 40(1):155-7.

Martínez MA, Sánchez de la Torre C, and Almarza E, "A Comparative Solid-Phase Extraction Study for the Simultaneous Determination of Fluvoxamine, Mianserin, Doxepin, Citalopram, Paroxetine, and Etoperidone in Whole Blood by Capillary Gas-Liquid Chromatography with Nitrogen-Phosphorus Detection," *J Anal Toxicol*, 2004, 28(4):174-80.

Foscarnet

CAS Number 34156-56-4; 63585-09-1

U.S. Brand Names Foscavir®

Synonyms PFA; Phosphonoformate; Phosphonoformic Acid

Use Treatment of herpes virus infections suspected to be caused by acyclovir-resistant (HSV, VZV) or ganciclovir-resistant (CMV) strains; this occurs almost exclusively in immunocompromised persons (eg, with advanced AIDS) who have received prolonged treatment for a herpes virus infection

Treatment of CMV retinitis in persons with AIDS

Unlabeled/Investigational Use Other CMV infections (eg, colitis, esophagitis, neurological disease)

Mechanism of Action Pyrophosphate analogue which acts as a noncompetitive inhibitor of many viral RNA and DNA polymerases as well as HIV reverse transcriptase. Inhibitory effects occur at concentrations which do not affect host cellular DNA polymerases; however, some human cell growth suppression has been observed with high *in vitro* concentrations. Similar to ganciclovir, foscarnet is a virostatic agent. Foscarnet does not require activation by thymidine kinase.

Adverse Reactions

Cardiovascular: Cardiomyopathy, fibrillation (atrial), flutter (atrial), sinus bradycardia, cardiomegaly, palpitations

Central nervous system: Fatigue, **fever, headache, seizures**, hallucinations, electroencephalogram abnormalities, amnesia

Dermatologic: Alopecia, xerosis, urticaria, psoriasis, exanthem, toxic epidermal necrolysis

Endocrine & metabolic: Hypocalcemia, hypomagnesemia, hypokalemia, change in serum phosphorus, hypophosphatemia, hypercalcemia, nephrogenic diabetes insipidus

Gastrointestinal: **Nausea, diarrhea**, dyspepsia, **vomiting**

Genitourinary: Genital ulcers

Hematologic: **Anemia**, decreases in hemoglobin and hematocrit

Hepatic: Elevated liver enzymes

Local: Thrombophlebitis

Neuromuscular & skeletal: Paresthesia

Renal: **Abnormal renal function** including renal failure, albuminuria, acidosis (renal tubular), renal tubular necrosis; **decreased creatinine clearance** at continuous dosing of 130-230 mg/kg/day,

Respiratory: Rhinitis

Miscellaneous: Penile ulceration (at 7-24 days), nephrogenic diabetes insipidus, lymphadenopathy, fixed drug eruption

Signs and Symptoms of Overdose Cough, dementia, depression, dry mouth, dysphagia, dysuria, hypercalcemia, hypocalcemia, hypokalemia, hypomagnesemia, hyponatremia, hypophosphatemia, leg cramps, leukocytosis, lymphopenia, malaise, meningitis, myalgia, nocturia, perioral or limb paresthesias, renal dysfunction, seizures, thrombocytopenia, wheezing

Pharmacodynamics/Kinetics

Distribution: Up to 28% of cumulative I.V. dose may be deposited in bone

Metabolism: Biotransformation does not occur

Half-life elimination: ~3 hours

Excretion: Urine ($\leq$28% as unchanged drug)

Dosage

CMV retinitis: I.V.:

Induction treatment: 60 mg/kg/dose every 8 hours **or** 100 mg/kg every 12 hours for 14-21 days

Maintenance therapy: 90-120 mg/kg/day as a single infusion

Acyclovir-resistant HSV induction treatment: I.V.: 40 mg/kg/dose every 8-12 hours for 14-21 days

Dosage adjustment in renal impairment:

Induction and maintenance dosing schedules based on creatinine clearance (mL/kg/minute): See tables.

Maintenance Dosing of Foscarnet in Patients with Abnormal Renal Function

Cl_{cr} (mL/min/kg)	CMV Equivalent to 90 mg/kg q24h	CMV Equivalent to 120 mg/kg q24h
<0.4	Not recommended	Not recommended
$\geq$0.4-0.5	50 mg/kg every 48 hours	65 mg/kg every 48 hours
>0.5-0.6	60 mg/kg every 48 hours	80 mg/kg every 48 hours
>0.6-0.8	80 mg/kg every 48 hours	105 mg/kg every 48 hours
>0.8-1.0	50 mg/kg every 24 hours	65 mg/kg every 24 hours
>1.0-1.4	70 mg/kg every 24 hours	90 mg/kg every 24 hours
>1.4	90 mg/kg every 24 hours	120 mg/kg every 24 hours

Hemodialysis:

Foscarnet is highly removed by hemodialysis (30% in 4 hours HD) Doses of 50 mg/kg/dose posthemodialysis have been found to produce similar serum concentrations as doses of 90 mg/kg twice daily in patients with normal renal function

Doses of 60-90 mg/kg/dose loading dose (posthemodialysis) followed by 45 mg/kg/dose posthemodialysis (3 times/week) with the monitoring of weekly plasma concentrations to maintain peak plasma concentrations in the range of 400-800 µMolar has been recommended by some clinicians

Continuous arteriovenous or venovenous hemodiafiltration effects: Dose as for Cl_{cr} 10-50 mL/minute

Stability Do not admix or run with other drugs, multiple incompatibilities

Monitoring Parameters Serum creatinine, calcium, phosphorus, potassium, magnesium; hemoglobin

Administration Administer diluted to 12 mg/mL through a peripheral line; may be administered undiluted through a central line; infuse over 1 hour

Contraindications Hypersensitivity to foscarnet or any component of the formulation; Cl_{cr} <0.4 mL/minute/kg during therapy

Warnings

Hazardous agent – use appropriate precautions for handling and disposal. **[U.S. Boxed Warning]: Indicated only for immunocompromised patients with CMV retinitis and mucocutaneous acyclovir-resistant HSV infection.[U.S. Boxed Warning]: Renal impairment occurs to some degree in the majority of patients treated with foscarnet;** renal impairment may occur at any time and is usually reversible within 1 week following dose adjustment or discontinuation of therapy, however, several patients have died with renal failure within 4 weeks of stopping foscarnet; therefore, renal function should be closely monitored. To reduce the risk of nephrotoxicity and the potential to administer a relative overdose, always calculate the Cl_{cr} even if serum creatinine is within the normal range. Adequate hydration

Induction Dosing of Foscarnet in Patients with Abnormal Renal Function

Clcr (mL/min/kg)	HSV Equivalent to 40 mg/kg q12h	HSV Equivalent to 40 mg/kg q8h	CMV Equivalent to 60 mg/kg q8h	CMV Equivalent to 90 mg/kg q12h
<0.4	Not recommended	Not recommended	Not recommended	Not recommended
≥0.4-0.5	20 mg/kg every 24 hours	35 mg/kg every 24 hours	50 mg/kg every 24 hours	50 mg/kg every 24 hours
>0.5-0.6	25 mg/kg every 24 hours	40 mg/kg every 24 hours	60 mg/kg every 24 hours	60 mg/kg every 24 hours
>0.6-0.8	35 mg/kg every 24 hours	25 mg/kg every 12 hours	40 mg/kg every 12 hours	80 mg/kg every 24 hours
>0.8-1.0	20 mg/kg every 12 hours	35 mg/kg every 12 hours	50 mg/kg every 12 hours	50 mg/kg every 12 hours
>1.0-1.4	30 mg/kg every 12 hours	30 mg/kg every 8 hours	45 mg/kg every 8 hours	70 mg/kg every 12 hours
>1.4	40 mg/kg every 12 hours	40 mg/kg every 8 hours	60 mg/kg every 8 hours	90 mg/kg every 12 hours

may reduce the risk of nephrotoxicity; the manufacturer makes specific recommendations regarding this (see Administration).

Imbalance of serum electrolytes or minerals occurs in at least 15% of patients (hypocalcemia, low ionized calcium, hypophosphatemia, hypomagnesemia, or hypokalemia). Patients with low ionized calcium may experience perioral tingling, numbness, paresthesias, tetany, and seizures. Correct electrolytes before initiating therapy; use caution in patients who have any underlying electrolyte imbalances, those with neurologic or cardiac abnormalities and those receiving medications that are influenced by calcium levels. Use caution when administering other medications that cause electrolyte imbalances. Patients who experience signs or symptoms of an electrolyte imbalance should be assessed immediately. **[U.S. Boxed Warning]: Seizures related to plasma electrolyte/mineral imbalance may occur;** incidence has been reported in up to 10% of AIDS patients. Risk factors for seizures include impaired baseline renal function and low total serum calcium. Some patients who have experienced seizures have been able to continue or resume foscarnet treatment after their mineral or electrolyte abnormality has been corrected, their underlying disease state treated, or their dose decreased. May cause anemia and granulocytopenia. Foscarnet has been shown to be mutagenic in animal studies. Foscarnet is deposited in teeth and bone of young, growing animals; it has adversely affected tooth enamel development in rats. Safety and efficacy in children have not been established.

Dosage Forms
Injection, solution: 24 mg/mL (250 mL, 500 mL)
Foscavir®: 24 mg/mL (500 mL)

Reference Range Therapeutic for CMV: 150 mcg/mL

Overdosage/Treatment
Supportive therapy: I.V. calcium salts for hypocalcemia; I.V. hydration is essential
Enhancement of elimination: Hemodialysis may be useful to aid in removal of the drug, although this has not been formally studied

Drug Interactions
Ciprofloxacin: May enhance the neuroexcitatory and/or seizure-potentiating effect of foscarnet.
Nephrotoxic drugs (amphotericin B, I.V. pentamidine, aminoglycosides, etc): Should be avoided, if possible, to minimize additive renal risk with foscarnet.
QTc-prolonging agents: May enhance the adverse/toxic effect of other QTc-prolonging agents such as foscarnet. Any electrolyte abnormalities caused by foscarnet may exacerbate the situation.
Pentamidine: Increases risk of severe hypocalcemia.
Ritonavir, saquinavir: Increased risk of renal impairment has been associated with concurrent use with foscarnet.
Thioridazine: Foscarnet may enhance the QTc-prolonging effect of thioridazine.
Zalcitabine: Foscarnet may enhance the neurotoxic (peripheral) effect of zalcitabine.

Pregnancy Risk Factor C

Pregnancy Implications Associated with an increase in skeletal anomalies in animal studies. There are no adequate and well controlled studies in pregnant women. A single case report of use during the third trimester with normal infant outcome was observed. Monitoring of amniotic fluid volumes by ultrasound is recommended weekly after 20 weeks of gestation to detect oligohydramnios.

Lactation Excretion in breast milk unknown/contraindicated

Nursing Implications Provide adequate hydration with I.V. normal saline prior to and during treatment to minimize nephrotoxicity

Fosfomycin

CAS Number 23155-02-4; 78964-85-9
U.S. Brand Names Monurol™
Synonyms Fosfomycin Tromethamine
Use Antibiotic for uncomplicated urinary tract infections
Unlabeled/Investigational Use Multiple doses have been investigated for complicated urinary tract infections in men
Mechanism of Action A phosphoric acid derivative, fosfomycin inhibits bacterial wall synthesis and thus is bactericidal
Adverse Reactions
Central nervous system: **Headache** (10.3%)
Gastrointestinal: **Diarrhea** 10.4% (diarrhea is dose related); anorexia
Hematologic: Eosinophilia
Miscellaneous: Anaphylaxis
Signs and Symptoms of Overdose Not documented in humans; animal studies at doses of 5 g/kg demonstrated little toxicity (outside of watery diarrhea)
Pharmacodynamics/Kinetics
Absorption: Well absorbed
Distribution: V_d: 2 L/kg; high concentrations in urine; well into other tissues; crosses maximally into CSF with inflamed meninges
Protein binding: <3%
Bioavailability: 34% to 58%
Half-life elimination: 4-8 hours; Cl_{cr} <10 mL/minute: 50 hours
Time to peak, serum: 2 hours
Excretion: Urine (as unchanged drug); high urinary levels (100 mcg/mL) persist for >48 hours
Dosage Oral:
Infants <1 year: 1 g single dose
Children: 2 g single dose
Adults: 3 g single dose
Doses should be taken on an empty stomach as food can impair its absorption; use in children <12 years of age has not been established
Monitoring Parameters Signs and symptoms of urinary tract infection
Administration Always mix with water before ingesting; do not administer in its dry form; pour contents of envelope into 90-120 mL of water (not hot), stir to dissolve and take immediately
Dosage Forms Powder, as tromethamine: 3 g
Reference Range Peak serum fosfomycin level ranges from 22-43 mcg/mL after a 50 mg/kg oral dose; therapeutic range: 8-32 mcg/mL
Overdosage/Treatment
Decontamination: Oral: Ipecac within 30 minutes or lavage within 1 hour/activated charcoal
Supportive therapy: Crystalloid I.V. fluids to replace watery diarrhea
Enhanced elimination: Hemodialysis can enhance fosfomycin elimination
Drug Interactions
Antacids or calcium salts may cause precipitate formation and decrease fosfomycin absorption
Metoclopramide: Increased gastrointestinal motility may lower fosfomycin tromethamine serum concentrations and urinary excretion. This drug interaction possibly could be extrapolated to other medications which increase gastrointestinal motility.

Pregnancy Risk Factor B

Lactation Enters breast milk/not recommended

Additional Information Cross resistance with other antibiotics does not appear to occur.

Fosinopril

Related Information
- Angiotensin Agents

CAS Number 88889-14-9; 97825-24-6

U.S. Brand Names Monopril®

Synonyms Fosinopril Sodium

Use Treatment of hypertension, either alone or in combination with other antihypertensive agents; treatment of congestive heart failure, left ventricular dysfunction after myocardial infarction

Mechanism of Action Competitive inhibition of angiotensin I being converted to angiotensin II, a potent vasoconstrictor, through the angiotensin I-converting enzyme (ACE) activity, with resultant lower levels of angiotensin II which causes an increase in plasma renin activity and a reduction in aldosterone secretion

Adverse Reactions
Cardiovascular: Hypotension (orthostatic), vasodilation, vasculitis

Central nervous system: Headache, fatigue, dizziness, syncope, vertigo, insomnia

Dermatologic: Angioedema, rash, scleroderma, exfoliative dermatitis, urticaria, photosensitivity, pemphigus

Endocrine & metabolic: Hypoglycemia, hyperkalemia, sexual dysfunction

Gastrointestinal: Diarrhea, nausea, vomiting, loss of taste perception, xerostomia

Genitourinary: Impotence

Hematologic: Neutropenia, agranulocytosis, anemia

Neuromuscular & skeletal: Muscle cramps, eosinophilic fasciitis, paresthesia

Renal: Deterioration in renal function, proteinuria

Respiratory: Cough

Pharmacodynamics/Kinetics
Onset of action: 1 hour

Duration: 24 hours

Absorption: 36%

Protein binding: 95%

Metabolism: Prodrug, hydrolyzed to its active metabolite fosinoprilat by intestinal wall and hepatic esterases

Bioavailability: 36%

Half-life elimination, serum (fosinoprilat): 12 hours

Time to peak, serum: ~3 hours

Excretion: Urine and feces (as fosinoprilat and other metabolites in roughly equal proportions, 45% to 50%)

Dosage
Oral:

Children >50 kg: Hypertension: Initial: 5-10 mg once daily

Adults:

Hypertension: Initial: 10 mg/day; most patients are maintained on 20-40 mg/day. May need to divide the dose into two if trough effect is inadequate; discontinue the diuretic, if possible 2-3 days before initiation of therapy; resume diuretic therapy carefully, if needed.

Heart failure: Initial: 10 mg/day (5 mg if renal dysfunction present) and increase, as needed, to a maximum of 40 mg once daily over several weeks; usual dose: 20-40 mg/day. If hypotension, orthostasis, or azotemia occur during titration, consider decreasing concomitant diuretic dose, if any.

Dosing adjustment/comments in renal impairment: None needed since hepatobiliary elimination compensates adequately diminished renal elimination.

Hemodialysis: Moderately dialyzable (20% to 50%)

Monitoring Parameters Blood pressure (supervise for at least 2 hours after the initial dose or any increase for significant orthostasis); serum potassium, creatinine, BUN, WBC

Contraindications Hypersensitivity to fosinopril or any component of the formulation; angioedema related to previous treatment with an ACE inhibitor; idiopathic or hereditary angioedema; bilateral renal artery stenosis; pregnancy (2nd and 3rd trimesters)

Warnings Anaphylactic reactions can occur. Angioedema can occur at any time during treatment (especially following first dose). It may involve head and neck (potentially affecting the airway) or the intestine (presenting with abdominal pain). Prolonged monitoring may be required especially if tongue, glottis, or larynx are involved as they are associated with airway obstruction. Those with a history of airway surgery in this situation have a higher risk. Careful blood pressure monitoring (hypotension can occur especially in volume-depleted patients). **[U.S. Boxed Warning]: Based on human data, ACEIs can cause injury and death to the developing fetus when used in the second and third trimesters. ACEIs should be discontinued as soon as possible**

once pregnancy is detected. Dosage adjustment needed in severe renal impairment (Cl_{cr} <10 mL/minute). Use with caution in hypovolemia; collagen vascular diseases; valvular stenosis (particularly aortic stenosis); hyperkalemia; or before, during, or immediately after anesthesia. Avoid rapid dosage escalation which may lead to renal insufficiency. Rare toxicities associated with ACE inhibitors include cholestatic jaundice (which may progress to hepatic necrosis) and neutropenia/agranulocytosis with myeloid hyperplasia. Hypersensitivity reactions may be seen during hemodialysis with high-flux dialysis membranes (eg, AN69). Hyperkalemia may rarely occur. If patient has renal impairment, then a baseline WBC with differential and serum creatinine should be evaluated and monitored closely during initial therapy. Use with caution in unilateral renal artery stenosis and pre-existing renal insufficiency.

Dosage Forms Tablet, as sodium: 10 mg, 20 mg, 40 mg

Monopril®: 10 mg, 20 mg, 40 mg

Reference Range Peak serum fosinoprilat level after a 40 mg dose: ~600 ng/mL

Overdosage/Treatment
Decontamination: Lavage (within 1 hour)/activated charcoal

Supportive therapy: Following initiation of essential overdose management, toxic symptom treatment and supportive treatment should be initiated. Hypotension usually responds to I.V. fluids or Trendelenburg positioning. If unresponsive to these measures, the use of a parenteral inotrope may be required (eg, norepinephrine 0.1-0.2 mcg/kg/minute titrated to response). Seizures commonly respond to diazepam (I.V. 5-10 mg bolus in adults every 15 minutes if needed up to a total of 30 mg; I.V. 0.25-0.4 mg/kg/dose up to a total of 10 mg in children) or to phenytoin or phenobarbital. Naloxone has been shown to antagonize hypotensive effects of captopril, but routine use in an overdose situation due to this agent is uncertain. For refractory hypotension, angiotensin amide infusion may be attempted.

Enhancement of elimination: Multiple dosing of activated charcoal may be effective; hemodialysis is not effective

Test Interactions Positive Coombs' [direct]; may cause false-positive urine acetone determinations using sodium nitroprusside reagent; may cause a falsely low serum digoxin level (with Digi-Tab® RIA kit)

Drug Interactions α_1 blockers: Hypotensive effect increased.

Antacids (aluminum hydroxide, magnesium hydroxide and simethicone): Absorption of fosinopril impaired; separate dose by 2 hours.

Aspirin: The effects of ACE inhibitors may be blunted by aspirin administration, particularly at higher dosages (see Cardiovascular Considerations) and/or increase adverse renal effects.

Diuretics: Hypovolemia due to diuretics may precipitate acute hypotensive events or acute renal failure.

Insulin: Risk of hypoglycemia may be increased.

Lithium: Risk of lithium toxicity may be increased; monitor lithium levels, especially the first 4 weeks of therapy.

Mercaptopurine: Risk of neutropenia may be increased.

NSAIDs: May attenuate hypertensive efficacy; effect has been seen with captopril and may occur with other ACE inhibitors; monitor blood pressure. May increase risk of adverse renal effects.

Potassium-sparing diuretics (amiloride, spironolactone, triamterene): Increased risk of hyperkalemia.

Potassium supplements may increase the risk of hyperkalemia.

Trimethoprim (high dose) may increase the risk of hyperkalemia.

Pregnancy Risk Factor C (1st trimester)/D (2nd and 3rd trimesters)

Pregnancy Implications Decreased placental blood flow, low birth weight, fetal hypotension, preterm delivery, and fetal death have been noted with the use of some ACE inhibitors (ACEIs) in animal studies. Neonatal hypotension, skull hypoplasia, anuria, renal failure, oligohydramnios (associated with fetal limb contractures, craniofacial deformities, hypoplastic lung development), prematurity, intrauterine growth retardation, and patent ductus arteriosus have been reported with the use of ACEIs, primarily in the 2nd and 3rd trimesters. The risk of neonatal toxicity has been considered less when ACEIs have been used in the 1st trimester; however, major congenital malformations have been reported. The cardiovascular and/or central nervous systems are most commonly affected. Unless alternative agents are not appropriate, ACEIs should be discontinued as soon as possible once pregnancy is detected.

Lactation Enters breast milk/not recommended

Nursing Implications May cause depression in some patients; discontinue if angioedema of the face, extremities, lips, tongue, or glottis occurs; watch for hypotensive effects within 1-3 hours of first dose or new higher dose

Additional Information
Some patients may have a decreased hypotensive effect between 12-16 hours; consider dividing total daily dose into 2 doses 12 hours apart. If receiving a diuretic, the potential for first-dose hypotension is increased. To decrease this potential, stop the diuretic for 2-3 days prior to initiating fosinopril, if possible. Continue the diuretic if needed to control blood pressure.

Due to frequent decreases in glomerular filtration (also creatinine clearance) with aging, elderly patients may have exaggerated responses to ACE inhibitors; differences in clinical response due to hepatic changes are not observed. ACE inhibitors may be preferred agents in elderly patients with congestive heart failure and diabetes mellitus. Diabetic proteinuria is reduced and insulin sensitivity is enhanced. In general, the side effect profile is favorable in elderly and causes little or no CNS confusion; use lowest dose recommendations initially. Pediatric ingestion of 15 mg/kg is survivable with supportive therapy. Should not take a potassium salt supplement without the advice of healthcare provider.

Specific References

Cooper W, Hernandez-Diaz S, Arbogast P, et al, "Major Congenital Malformations After First Trimester Exposure to ACE Inhibitors," *N Engl J Med*, 2006, 354:2443-51.

Graham MR, Allcock NM, and Lindsey CC, "Maintenance of Goal Blood Pressure Following Conversion from Lisinopril to Fosinopril," *J Pharm Technol*, 2003, 19:266-70.

Mastrobattista J, "Angiotensin-Converting Enzyme Inhibitors in Pregnancy," *Semin Perinatol*, 1997, 21(2):124-34.

Quan A, "Fetopathy Associated with Exposure to Angiotensin-Converting Enzyme Inhibitors and Angiontensin Receptor Antagonists," *Early Hum Dev*, 2006, 82(1):23-8.

Fosphenytoin

U.S. Brand Names Cerebyx®
Synonyms Fosphenytoin Sodium
Use Management of generalized tonic-clonic (grand mal), simple partial and complex partial seizures; prevention of seizures following head trauma/neurosurgery; ventricular arrhythmias, including those associated with digitalis intoxication; beneficial effects in the treatment of migraine or trigeminal neuralgia in some patients; usually used in short-term seizure management
Mechanism of Action Diphosphate ester salt of phenytoin which acts as a water soluble prodrug of phenytoin; after administration, plasma esterases convert to phenytoin as the active moiety

Adverse Reactions

Cardiovascular: Sinus bradycardia, facial edema
Central nervous system: Slurred speech, dizziness, drowsiness, fever, visual hallucinations
Dermatologic: Rash, exfoliative dermatitis, erythema multiforme, acne
Endocrine & metabolic: Folic acid depletion, hyperglycemia, reduced plasma testosterone, gynecomastia
Gastrointestinal: Nausea, vomiting, gingival hyperplasia
Genitourinary: Priapism
Hematologic: Neutropenia, thrombocytopenia, anemia (megaloblastic)
Local: Pain on injection
Neuromuscular & skeletal: **Sensory paresthesia** (up to 30% of patients on long-term treatment), choreoathetosis, osteomalacia
Ocular: Nystagmus, blurred vision, diplopia
Renal: Nephrotic syndrome
Miscellaneous: Due to the fact that fosphenytoin is water soluble and has a lower pH (8.8) than phenytoin (12), necrosis or irritation at injection site is reduced, systemic lupus erythematosus (SLE), lymphadenopathy
Signs and Symptoms of Overdose Agranulocytosis, chorea (extrapyramidal), coma, confusion, drowsiness, encephalopathy, fever, gingival hyperplasia, granulocytopenia, gynecomastia, hyperthermia, hyperglycemia, hyperreflexia, hypotension, hypothermia, leukopenia, mydriasis, myoclonus, myoglobinuria, nausea, nephrotic syndrome, neutropenia, ophthalmoplegia, respiratory depression, slurred speech, tremors, unsteady gait

Pharmacodynamics/Kinetics

Also refer to Phenytoin monograph for additional information.
Protein binding: Fosphenytoin: 95% to 99% to albumin; can displace phenytoin and increase free fraction (up to 30% unbound) during the period required for conversion of fosphenytoin to phenytoin
Metabolism: Fosphenytoin is rapidly converted via hydrolysis to phenytoin; phenytoin is metabolized in the liver and forms metabolites
Bioavailability: I.M.: Fosphenytoin: 100%
Half-life elimination:
 Fosphenytoin: 15 minutes
 Phenytoin: Variable (mean: 12-29 hours); kinetics of phenytoin are saturable
Time to peak: Conversion to phenytoin: Following I.V. administration (maximum rate of administration): 15 minutes; following I.M. administration, peak phenytoin levels are reached in 3 hours
Excretion: Phenytoin: Urine (as inactive metabolites)

Dosage

I.M.: Up to 450 mg has been used in adults
I.V.: 14-17 mg/kg (suggested); doses up to 3000 mg (38 mg/kg) have been used. Rates as high as 150-218 mg/minute have been administered. Usual infusion time: ~30 minutes

Monitoring Parameters Blood pressure, vital signs (with I.V. use), plasma level monitoring, CBC, liver function tests
Administration
I.M.: May be administered as a single daily dose using either 1 or 2 injection sites.
I.V.: Rates of infusion:
 Children: 1-3 mg PE/kg/minute
 Adults: Should not exceed 150 mg PE/minute
Contraindications Hypersensitivity to phenytoin, other hydantoins, or any component of the formulation; patients with sinus bradycardia, sinoatrial block, second- and third-degree AV block, or Adams-Stokes syndrome; occurrence of rash during treatment (should not be resumed if rash is exfoliative, purpuric, or bullous); treatment of absence seizures
Warnings Doses of fosphenytoin are expressed as their phenytoin sodium equivalent (PE). Antiepileptic drugs should not be abruptly discontinued. Hypotension may occur, especially after I.V. administration at high doses and high rates of administration. Administration of phenytoin has been associated with atrial and ventricular conduction depression and ventricular fibrillation. Careful cardiac monitoring is needed when administering I.V. loading doses of fosphenytoin. Acute hepatotoxicity associated with a hypersensitivity syndrome characterized by fever, skin eruptions, and lymphadenopathy has been reported to occur within the first 2 months of treatment. Discontinue if skin rash or lymphadenopathy occurs. Use with caution in patients with hypotension, severe myocardial insufficiency, diabetes mellitus, porphyria, hypoalbuminemia, hypothyroidism, fever, or hepatic or renal dysfunction.
Dosage Forms Injection, solution, as sodium: 75 mg/mL [equivalent to phenytoin sodium 50 mg/mL] (2 mL, 10 mL)

Reference Range

Therapeutic: 10-20 mcg/mL (SI: 40-79 μmol/L); toxicity is measured clinically, and some patients require levels outside the suggested therapeutic range
Toxic: 30-50 mcg/mL (SI: 120-200 μmol/L)
Lethal: >100 mcg/mL (SI: >400 μmol/L)
Manifestations of toxicity:
Nystagmus: 20 mcg/mL (SI: 79 μmol/L)
Ataxia: 30 mcg/mL (SI: 118.9 μmol/L)
Decreased mental status: 40 mcg/mL (SI: 159 μmol/L)
Coma: 50 mcg/mL (SI: 200 μmol/L)
Peak serum phenytoin level after a 375 mg I.M. fosphenytoin dose in healthy males: 5.7 mcg/mL
Peak serum fosphenytoin levels and phenytoin levels after a 1.2 g infusion (I.V.) in healthy subjects over 30 minutes were 129 mcg/mL and 17.2 mcg/mL, respectively

Overdosage/Treatment

Supportive therapy: Treatment is supportive for hypotension; treat with I.V. fluids and place patient in Trendelenburg position; seizures may be controlled with lorazepam or diazepam 5-10 mg (0.25-0.4 mg/kg in children); I.V. albumin (25 g every 6 hours has been used to increase bound fraction of drug)
Enhancement of elimination: Multiple dosing of activated charcoal may be effective; peritoneal dialysis, diuresis, hemodialysis, hemoperfusion, and plasmapheresis are of little value; 4 hours of continuous venovenous hemofiltration can enhance elimination

Diagnostic Procedures

• Phenytoin, Blood

Test Interactions ↑ glucose, alkaline phosphatase (S); ↓ thyroxine (S), calcium (S); serum sodium increases in overdose setting
Drug Interactions
As phenytoin: **Substrate** of CYP2C9 (major), 2C19 (major), 3A4 (minor); **Induces** CYP2B6 (strong), 2C8 (strong), 2C9 (strong), 2C19 (strong), 3A4 (strong)
Acetaminophen: Phenytoin may enhance the hepatotoxic potential of acetaminophen overdoses
Acetazolamide: Concurrent use with phenytoin may result in an increased risk of osteomalacia
Acyclovir: May decrease phenytoin serum levels; limited documentation; monitor
Allopurinol: May increase phenytoin serum concentrations; monitor
Antiarrhythmics: Phenytoin may increase the metabolism of antiarrhythmics, decreasing their clinical effect; includes disopyramide, propafenone, and quinidine; amiodarone also may increase phenytoin concentrations (see CYP inhibitors)
Anticonvulsants: Phenytoin may increase the metabolism of anticonvulsants; includes barbiturates, carbamazepine, ethosuximide, felbamate, lamotrigine, tiagabine, topiramate, and zonisamide; does not appear to affect gabapentin or levetiracetam; felbamate and gabapentin may increase phenytoin levels; monitor
Antineoplastics: Several chemotherapeutic agents have been associated with a decrease in serum phenytoin levels; includes cisplatin, bleomycin, carmustine, methotrexate, and vinblastine; monitor phenytoin serum levels. Limited evidence also suggest that enzyme-inducing

anticonvulsant therapy may reduce the effectiveness of some che-motherapy regimens (specifically in ALL). Teniposide and methotrexate may be cleared more rapidly in these patients.

Antipsychotics: Phenytoin may enhance the metabolism (decrease the efficacy) of antipsychotics; monitor for altered response; dose adjust-ment may be needed; also see note on clozapine

Benzodiazepines: Phenytoin may decrease the serum concentrations of some benzodiazepines; monitor for decreased benzodiazepine effect

Beta-blockers: Metabolism of beta-blockers may be increased and clinical effect decreased; atenolol and nadolol are unlikely to interact given their renal elimination

Calcium channel blockers: Phenytoin may enhance the metabolism of calcium channel blockers, decreasing their clinical effect; calcium channel blockers (diltiazem, nifedipine) have been reported to increase phenytoin levels (case report); monitor

Capecitabine: May increase the serum concentrations of phenytoin; monitor

Chloramphenicol: Phenytoin may increase the metabolism of chloram-phenicol and chloramphenicol may inhibit phenytoin metabolism; monitor for altered response

Cimetidine: May increase the serum concentrations of phenytoin; monitor.

Ciprofloxacin: Case reports indicate ciprofloxacin may increase or decrease serum phenytoin concentrations; monitor

Clozapine: May decrease phenytoin serum concentrations; monitor

CNS depressants: Sedative effects may be additive with other CNS depressants; monitor for increased effect; includes ethanol, barbitu-rates, sedatives, antidepressants, narcotic analgesics, and benzodia-zepines

Corticosteroids: Phenytoin may increase the metabolism of corticoster-oids, decreasing their clinical effect; also see dexamethasone

Cyclosporine and tacrolimus: Levels may be decreased by phenytoin; monitor

CYP2B6 substrates: Phenytoin may decrease the levels/effects of CYP2B6 substrates. Example substrates include bupropion, efavirenz, promethazine, selegiline, and sertraline.

CYP2C9 inducers: May decrease the levels/effects of phenytoin. Exam-ple inducers include carbamazepine, phenobarbital, rifampin, rifapen-tine, and secobarbital.

CYP2C9 Inhibitors may increase the levels/effects of phenytoin. Example inhibitors include delavirdine, fluconazole, gemfibrozil, ketoconazole, nicardipine, NSAIDs, sulfonamides and tolbutamide.

CYP2C8 Substrates: Phenytoin may decrease the levels/effects of CYP2C8 substrates. Example substrates include amiodarone, pacli-taxel, pioglitazone, repaglinide, and rosiglitazone.

CYP2C9 Substrates: Phenytoin may decrease the levels/effects of CYP2C9 substrates. Example substrates include bosentan, cele-coxib, dapsone, fluoxetine, glimepiride, glipizide, losartan, montelukast, nateglinide, paclitaxel, sulfonamides, trimethoprim, warfarin, and zafir-lukast.

CYP2C19 inducers: May decrease the levels/effects of phenytoin. Example inducers include aminoglutethimide, carbamazepine, pheny-toin, and rifampin.

CYP2C19 inhibitors: May increase the levels/effects of phenytoin. Example inhibitors include delavirdine, fluconazole, fluvoxamine, gemfi-brozil, isoniazid, omeprazole, and ticlopidine.

CYP2C19 substrates: Phenytoin may decrease the levels/effects of CYP2C19 substrates. Example substrates include citalopram, diaze-pam, methsuximide, phenytoin, propranolol, proton pump inhibitors, sertraline, and voriconazole

CYP3A4 substrates: Phenytoin may decrease the levels/effects of CYP3A4 substrates. Example substrates include benzodiazepines, calcium channel blockers, clarithromycin, cyclosporine, erythromycin, estrogens, mirtazapine, nateglinide, nefazodone, nevirapine, protease inhibitors, tacrolimus, and venlafaxine

Dexamethasone: May decrease serum phenytoin due to increased metabolism; monitor

Digoxin: Effects and/or levels of digitalis glycosides may be decreased by phenytoin

Disulfiram: May increase serum phenytoin concentrations; monitor

Dopamine: Phenytoin (I.V.) may increase the effect of dopamine (enhanced hypotension)

Doxycycline: Phenytoin may enhance the metabolism of doxycycline, decreasing its clinical effect; higher dosages may be required

Estrogens: Phenytoin may increase the metabolism of estrogens, decreasing their clinical effect; monitor

Folic acid: Replacement of folic acid has been reported to increase the metabolism of phenytoin, decreasing its serum concentrations and/or increasing seizures

HMG-CoA reductase inhibitors: Phenytoin may increase the metabolism of these agents, reducing their clinical effect; monitor

Itraconazole: Phenytoin may decrease the effect of itraconazole

Levodopa: Phenytoin may inhibit the anti-Parkinson effect of levodopa

Lithium: Concurrent use of phenytoin and lithium has resulted in lithium intoxication

Methadone: Phenytoin may enhance the metabolism of methadone resulting in methadone withdrawal

Methylphenidate: May increase serum phenytoin concentrations; monitor

Metronidazole: May increase the serum concentrations of phenytoin; monitor.

Neuromuscular-blocking agents: Duration of effect may be decreased by phenytoin

Omeprazole: May increase serum phenytoin concentrations; monitor

Oral contraceptives: Phenytoin may enhance the metabolism of oral contraceptives, decreasing their clinical effect; an alternative method of contraception should be considered

Primidone: Phenytoin enhances the conversion of primidone to pheno-barbital resulting in elevated phenobarbital serum concentrations

Quetiapine: Serum concentrations may be substantially reduced by phenytoin, potentially resulting in a loss of efficacy; limited documenta-tion; monitor

SSRIs: May increase phenytoin serum concentrations; fluoxetine and fluvoxamine are known to inhibit metabolism via CYP enzymes; sertraline and paroxetine have also been shown to increase concentra-tions in some patients; monitor

Theophylline: Phenytoin may increase metabolism of theophylline deri-vatives and decrease their clinical effect; theophylline may also increase phenytoin concentrations

Thyroid hormones (including levothyroxine): Phenytoin may alter the metabolism of thyroid hormones, reducing its effect; there is limited documentation of this interaction, but monitoring should be considered

Ticlopidine: May increase serum phenytoin concentrations and/or toxicity; monitor

Tricyclic antidepressants: Phenytoin may increase metabolism of tricyclic antidepressants and decrease their clinical effect; sedative effects may be additive; tricyclics may also increase phenytoin concentrations

Topiramate: Phenytoin may decrease serum levels of topiramate; topiramate may increase the effect of phenytoin

Trazodone: Serum levels of phenytoin may be increased; limited documentation; monitor

Trimethoprim: May increase serum phenytoin concentrations; monitor

Valproic acid (and sulfisoxazole): May displace phenytoin from binding sites; valproic acid may increase, decrease, or have no effect on phenytoin serum concentrations

Vigabatrin: May reduce phenytoin serum concentrations; monitor

Warfarin: Phenytoin transiently increased the hypothrombinemia re-sponse to warfarin initially; this is followed by an inhibition of the hypoprothrombinemic response

Pregnancy Risk Factor D

Pregnancy Implications Crosses placenta with fetal serum concentra-tions equal to those of mother; eye, cardiac, cleft palate, and skeletal malformations have been noted; fetal hydantoin syndrome associated with maternal ingestion of 100-800 mg/kg during 1st trimester

Lactation Excretion in breast milk unknown/not recommended

Additional Information Infusion of 71 mg/kg in an infant resulted in cardiac arrest.

Fosphenytoin 1.5 mg is approximately equivalent to 1 mg phenytoin; equimolar fosphenytoin dose is 375 mg (75 mg/mL solution) to phenytoin 250 mg (50 mg/mL)

Water solubility: 142 mg/mL at pH of 9

Compatible with all diluents and does not require propylene glycol or ethanol for solubility; no drug interaction noted with diazepam; since there is no precipitation problem with fosphenytoin, no I.V. filter is required; antiarrhythmic effects may be similar to phenytoin; parenteral product contains no propylene sterol; this should allow for rapid intravenous bolus dosing without cardiovascular complications; formaldehyde production is not expected to be clinically consequential (~200 mg) if used for 1 week

Furosemide

CAS Number 54-31-9

U.S. Brand Names Lasix®

Synonyms Frusemide

Use Management of edema associated with congestive heart failure and hepatic or renal disease; used alone or in combination with antihyperten-sives in treatment of hypertension

Mechanism of Action Inhibits reabsorption of sodium and chloride in the ascending loop of Henle and distal renal tubule, interfering with the chloride-binding cotransport system, thus causing increased excretion of water, sodium, chloride, magnesium, and calcium

Adverse Reactions

Cardiovascular: Sinus bradycardia, tachycardia (supraventricular), vaso-dilation, **orthostatic hypotension**

Central nervous system: **Dizziness**, headache, fever, gustatory hallucinations

Dermatologic: Urticaria, Stevens-Johnson syndrome, exfoliative dermatitis, photosensitivity, lichenoid eruptions, erythema multiforme, purpura, bullous pemphigoid, acute generalized exanthematous pustulosis, pruritus, erythema nodosum, exanthem, pseudoporphyria cutanea tarda, cutaneous vasculitis

Endocrine & metabolic: Hypokalemia, hypomagnesemia, hypercalcemia, hyponatremia, hypochloremia, alkalosis, hypocalcemia, hyperglycemia, dehydration, hyperuricemia

Gastrointestinal: Pancreatitis, nausea, oral solutions may cause diarrhea due to sorbitol content, sweet dysgeusia, xerostomia

Genitourinary: Nocturia, urinary incontinence

Hematologic: Leukopenia/neutropenia (agranulocytosis, granulocytopenia), anemia, thrombocytopenia, eosinophilia

Neuromuscular & skeletal: Myasthenia gravis (exacerbation or precipitation of), paresthesia

Ocular: Phototoxic, xanthopsia

Otic: Potential ototoxicity, deafness, tinnitus

Renal: Nephrocalcinosis, proteinuria, interstitial nephritis, hypercalciuria, diuresis, prerenal azotemia, renal vasculitis

Miscellaneous: Systemic lupus erythematosus (SLE)

Signs and Symptoms of Overdose Periarteritis nodosa, photophobia, vision color changes (yellow tinge)

Pharmacodynamics/Kinetics
Onset of action: Diuresis: Oral: 30-60 minutes; I.M.: 30 minutes; I.V.: ~5 minutes
 Peak effect: Oral: 1-2 hours
Duration: Oral: 6-8 hours; I.V.: 2 hours
Absorption: Oral: 60% to 67%
Protein binding: >98%
Metabolism: Minimally hepatic
Half-life elimination: Normal renal function: 0.5-1.1 hours; End-stage renal disease: 9 hours
Excretion: Urine (Oral: 50%, I.V.: 80%) within 24 hours; feces (as unchanged drug); nonrenal clearance prolonged in renal impairment

Dosage
Infants and Children:
 Oral: 1-2 mg/kg/dose increased in increments of 1 mg/kg/dose with each succeeding dose until a satisfactory effect is achieved to a maximum of 6 mg/kg/dose no more frequently than 6 hours.
 I.M., I.V.: 1 mg/kg/dose, increasing by each succeeding dose at 1 mg/kg/dose at intervals of 6-12 hours until a satisfactory response up to 6 mg/kg/dose.
Adults:
 Oral: 20-80 mg/dose initially increased in increments of 20-40 mg/dose at intervals of 6-8 hours; usual maintenance dose interval is twice daily or every day; may be titrated up to 600 mg/day with severe edematous states.
  Hypertension (JNC 7): 20-80 mg/day in 2 divided doses
 I.M., I.V.: 20-40 mg/dose, may be repeated in 1-2 hours as needed and increased by 20 mg/dose until the desired effect has been obtained. Usual dosing interval: 6-12 hours; for acute pulmonary edema, the usual dose is 40 mg I.V. over 1-2 minutes. If not adequate, may increase dose to 80 mg.
 Continuous I.V. infusion: Initial I.V. bolus dose of 0.1 mg/kg followed by continuous I.V. infusion doses of 0.1 mg/kg/hour doubled every 2 hours to a maximum of 0.4 mg/kg/hour if urine output is <1 mL/kg/hour have been found to be effective and result in a lower daily requirement of furosemide than with intermittent dosing. Other studies have used a rate of ≤4 mg/minute as a continuous I.V. infusion.
Elderly: Oral, I.M., I.V.: Initial: 20 mg/day; increase slowly to desired response.
Refractory heart failure: Oral, I.V.: Doses up to 8 g/day have been used.
Dosing adjustment/comments in renal impairment: Acute renal failure: High doses (up to 1-3 g/day - oral/I.V.) have been used to initiate desired response; avoid use in oliguric states.
Dialysis: Not removed by hemo- or peritoneal dialysis; supplemental dose is not necessary.
Dosing adjustment/comments in hepatic disease: Diminished natriuretic effect with increased sensitivity to hypokalemia and volume depletion in cirrhosis; monitor effects, particularly with high doses.

Monitoring Parameters Monitor weight and I & O daily; blood pressure, serum electrolytes, renal function; in high doses, monitor hearing

Administration Replace parenteral therapy with oral therapy as soon as possible. I.V. injections should be given slowly may be administered undiluted direct I.V. at a maximum rate of 0.5 mg/kg/minute for doses <120 mg and 4 mg/minute for doses >120 mg; maximum rate of administration for IVPB or infusion: 4 mg/minute. For continuous infusion furosemide in patients with severely-impaired renal function, do not exceed 4 mg/minute.

Contraindications Hypersensitivity to furosemide, any component, or sulfonylureas; anuria; patients with hepatic coma or in states of severe electrolyte depletion until the condition improves or is corrected

Warnings
Adjust dose to avoid dehydration. In cirrhosis, avoid electrolyte and acid/base imbalances that might lead to hepatic encephalopathy. Ototoxicity is associated with rapid I.V. administration, renal impairment, excessive doses, and concurrent use of other ototoxins. Hypersensitivity reactions can rarely occur. Monitor fluid status and renal function in an attempt to prevent oliguria, azotemia, and reversible increases in BUN and creatinine. Close medical supervision of aggressive diuresis required. Monitor closely for electrolyte imbalances particularly hypokalemia. Watch for and correct electrolyte disturbances. Coadministration of antihypertensives may increase the risk of hypotension. Avoid use of medications in which the toxicity is enhanced by hypokalemia (including quinolones with QT prolongation).

Chemical similarities are present among sulfonamides, sulfonylureas, carbonic anhydrase inhibitors, thiazides, and loop diuretics (except ethacrynic acid). Use in patients with sulfonylurea allergy is specifically contraindicated in product labeling, however, a risk of cross-reaction exists in patients with allergy to any of these compounds; avoid use when previous reaction has been severe.

Dosage Forms
Injection, solution: 10 mg/mL (2 mL, 4 mL, 8 mL, 10 mL)
Solution, oral: 10 mg/mL (60 mL, 120 mL) [orange flavor]; 40 mg/5 mL (5 mL, 500 mL) [pineapple-peach flavor]
Tablet (Lasix®): 20 mg, 40 mg, 80 mg

Reference Range
Therapeutic: 1-2 mcg/mL (SI: 3-6 μmol/L)
Toxic: >50 mcg/mL may be associated with toxicity

Overdosage/Treatment
Decontamination: Activated charcoal
Supportive therapy: I.V. hydration with 0.9% saline and electrolyte replacement

Test Interactions ↑ ammonia (B), amylase (S), glucose, uric acid (S); ↓ calcium (S), chloride (S), magnesium, sodium (S). I.V. furosemide (>80 mg/day) causes a falsely increased free thyroxine level

Drug Interactions ACE inhibitors: Hypotensive effects and/or renal effects are potentiated by hypovolemia.
Antidiabetic agents: Glucose tolerance may be decreased.
Antihypertensive agents: Hypotensive effects may be enhanced.
Cephaloridine or cephalexin: Nephrotoxicity may occur.
Cholestyramine or colestipol may reduce bioavailability of furosemide.
Digoxin: Furosemide-induced hypokalemia may predispose to digoxin toxicity. Monitor potassium.
Fibric acid derivatives: Blood levels of furosemide and fibric acid derivatives (ie, clofibrate and fenofibrate) may be increased during concurrent dosing (particularly in hypoalbuminemia). Limited documentation; monitor for increased effect/toxicity.
Indomethacin (and other NSAIDs) may reduce natriuretic and hypotensive effects of furosemide.
Lithium: Renal clearance may be reduced. Isolated reports of lithium toxicity have occurred; monitor lithium levels.
Metformin may decrease furosemide concentrations.
Metformin blood levels may be increased by furosemide.
NSAIDs: Risk of renal impairment may increase when used in conjunction with furosemide.
Ototoxic drugs (aminoglycosides, cis-platinum): Concomitant use of furosemide may increase risk of ototoxicity, especially in patients with renal dysfunction.
Peripheral adrenergic-blocking drugs or ganglionic blockers: Effects may be increased.
Phenobarbital or phenytoin may reduce diuretic response to furosemide.
Salicylates (high-dose) with furosemide may predispose patients to salicylate toxicity due to reduced renal excretion or alter renal function.
Succinylcholine: Action may be potentiated by furosemide.
Sucralfate may limit absorption of furosemide, effects may be significantly decreased; separate oral administration by 2 hours.
Thiazides: Synergistic diuretic effects occur.
Tubocurarine: The skeletal muscle-relaxing effect may be attenuated by furosemide.

Pregnancy Risk Factor C

Pregnancy Implications Neonatal hyponatremia/hyperuricemia can occur; possible increase in incidence of patent ductus arteriolysis

Lactation Enters breast milk/use caution

Additional Information Increased diuretic response in patients with cystic fibrosis; can cause elevation of parathyroid hormone; 40 mg furosemide is equivalent to 1 mg of bumetanide, 12 mg of piretanide, and 10-20 mg of torsemide; sodium content of 1 mL (injection): 0.162 mEq. Incidence of cochleotoxicity is 0% to 6%; aminoglycosides are ototoxic synergistic.

Specific References

Chobanian AV, Bakris GL, Black HR, et al, "The Seventh Report of the Joint National Committee on Prevention, Detection, Evaluation, and Treatment of High Blood Pressure: The JNC 7 Report," *JAMA*, 2003, 289(19):2560-71.

Juang P, Page RL 2nd, and Zolty R, "Probable Loop Diuretic-Induced Pancreatitis in a Sulfonamide-allergic Patient," *Ann Pharmacother*, 2006, 40(1):128-34.

Margalho C, de Boer D, Gallardo E, et al, "Determination of Furosemide in Whole Blood Using SPE and GC-EI-MS," *J Anal Toxicol*, 2005, 29(5):309-13.

Niven AS and Argyros G, "Alternate Treatments in Asthma," *Chest*, 2003, 123(4):1254-65.

Somberg JC and Molnar J, "The Pharmacologic Treatment of Heart Failure," *Am J Ther*, 2004, 11(6):480-8.

Verma AK, da Silva JH, and Kuhl DR, "Diuretic Effects of Subcutaneous Furosemide in Human Volunteers: A Randomized Pilot Study," *Ann Pharmacother*, 2004, 38(4):544-9. Epub 2004 Feb 24.

Gabapentin

CAS Number 60142-96-3

U.S. Brand Names Neurontin®

Use Partial or secondary generalized seizures; possibly useful for pain relief due to reflex sympathetic dystrophy. Used to treat adverse effects of ciguatera fish exposure and paclitaxel toxicity.

Unlabeled/Investigational Use Social phobia; chronic pain

Mechanism of Action Structural analog to gamma amino butyric acid (GABA). Binds to gabapentin receptors in hippocampus. No effect on GABA system.

Adverse Reactions

Cardiovascular: Vasodilation

Central nervous system: **Dizziness, somnolence, fatigue, ataxia**, drowsiness, psychosis, slurred speech, stuttering, polyneuropathy, aggressive behavior

Dermatologic: Eczema, Stevens-Johnson syndrome, alopecia

Endocrine & metabolic: Sexual dysfunction

Gastrointestinal: Nausea, vomiting, xerostomia, weight gain (average of 6.9 kg)

Genitourinary: Impotence, anorgasmia

Neuromuscular & skeletal: Tremors, choreoathetosis, asterixis

Ocular: Nystagmus, reversible visual field constriction

Respiratory: Cough, rhinitis

Pharmacodynamics/Kinetics

Absorption: 50% to 60% from proximal small bowel by L-amino transport system

Distribution: V_d: 0.6-0.8 L/kg

Protein binding: <3%

Bioavailability: Inversely proportional to dose due to saturable absorption:

900 mg/day: 60%

1200 mg/day: 47%

2400 mg/day: 34%

3600 mg/day: 33%

4800 mg/day: 27%

Half-life elimination: 5-7 hours; anuria 132 hours; during dialysis 3.8 hours

Excretion: Proportional to renal function; urine (as unchanged drug)

Dosage

If gabapentin is discontinued or if another anticonvulsant is added to therapy, it should be done slowly over a minimum of 1 week

Children >12 years and Adults: Oral:

Initial: 300 mg on day 1 (at bedtime to minimize sedation), then 300 mg twice daily on day 2, and then 300 mg 3 times/day on day 3

Total daily dosage range: 900-1800 mg/day administered in 3 divided doses at 8-hour intervals

Pain: 300-1800 mg/day given in 3 divided doses has been the most common dosage range

Dosing adjustment in renal impairment:

Cl_{cr} >60 mL/minute: Administer 1200 mg/day

Cl_{cr} 30-60 mL/minute: Administer 600 mg/day

Cl_{cr} 15-30 mL/minute: Administer 300 mg/day

Cl_{cr} <15 mL/minute: Administer 150 mg/day

Hemodialysis: 200-300 mg after each 4-hour dialysis following a loading dose of 300-400 mg

Monitoring Parameters Monitor serum levels of concomitant anticonvulsant therapy

Administration Administer first dose on first day at bedtime to avoid somnolence and dizziness. Dosage must be adjusted for renal function; when given 3 times daily, the maximum time between doses should not exceed 12 hours.

Contraindications Hypersensitivity to gabapentin or any component of the formulation

Warnings Avoid abrupt withdrawal, may precipitate seizures; use cautiously in patients with severe renal dysfunction; male rat studies demonstrated an association with pancreatic adenocarcinoma (clinical implication unknown). May cause CNS depression, which may impair physical or mental abilities. Patients must be cautioned about performing tasks which require mental alertness (eg, operating machinery or driving). Effects with other sedative drugs or ethanol may be potentiated. Pediatric patients (3-12 years of age) have shown increased incidence of CNS-related adverse effects, including emotional lability, hostility, thought disorder, and hyperkinesia. Safety and efficacy in children <3 years of age have not been established.

Dosage Forms

Capsule (Neurontin®): 100 mg, 300 mg, 400 mg

Solution, oral (Neurontin®): 250 mg/5 mL (480 mL) [cool strawberry anise flavor]

Tablet: 100 mg, 300 mg, 400 mg

Neurontin®: 600 mg, 800 mg

Reference Range Peak plasma level: 2 mcg/mL 1.5-3 hours after a 200 mg dose; serum gabapentin concentration of 104.5 u/mL associated with coma, respiratory depression requiring mechanical ventilation, and hypotension.

Overdosage/Treatment

Decontamination: Lavage (within 1 hour)/activated charcoal

Supportive therapy: In one case report flumazenil has reversed gabapentin-induced coma

Enhancement of elimination: Multiple dosing of activated charcoal may be useful; hemodialysis will be useful; see Dosage

Drug Interactions CNS depressants: Sedative effects may be additive with CNS depressants; includes ethanol, barbiturates, narcotic analgesics, and other sedative agents. Monitor for increased effect.

Pregnancy Risk Factor C

Pregnancy Implications No teratogenicity

Lactation Enters breast milk/use caution

Additional Information Not effective for absence seizures; benign pancreatic tumors noted in rodents administered high doses, ingestion of 48.9 g resulted in minimal symptoms; gabapentin levels 5 times over therapeutic limit result in minimal clinical effects; proposed use for amyotrophic lateral sclerosis

Specific References

Bekkelund SI, Lilleng H, and tonseth S, "Gabapentin May Cause Reversible Visual Field Constriction," *BMJ*, 2006, 332:1193..

Butler TC, Rosen RM, Wallace AL, et al, "Flumazenil and Dialysis for Gabapentin-Induced Coma," *Ann Pharmacother*, 2003, 37(1):74-6.

Faulkner MA, Bertoni JM, and Lenz TL, "Gabapentin for the Treatment of Tremor," *Ann Pharmacother*, 2003, 37(2):282-6.

Gatti G, Ferrari AR, Guerrini R, et al, "Plasma Gabapentin Concentrations in Children with Epilepsy: Influence of Age, Relationship with Dosage, and Preliminary Observations on Correlation with Clinical Response," *Ther Drug Monit*, 2003, 25(1):54-60.

Gonyeau MJ, Rooney CA, "Should Gabapertin Be Dose Adjusted: What are the Clinical Consequences?," *J Pharm Technol*, 2007, 23:30-4.

Klein-Schwartz W, Shepherd JG, Gorman S, et al, "Characterization of Gabapentin Overdose Using a Poison Center Case Series," *J Toxicol Clin Toxicol*, 2003, 41(1):11-5.

Lindberger M, Luhr O, Johannessen SI, et al, "Serum Concentrations and Effects of Gabapentin and Vigabatrin: Observations from a Dose Titration Study," *Ther Drug Monit*, 2003, 25(4):457-62.

Malek-Ahmadi P, "Gabapentin and Post-Traumatic Stress Disorder," *Ann Pharmacother*, 2003, 37(5):664-6.

Pina MA and Modrego PJ, "Dystonia Induced by Babapentin," *Ann Pharmacother*, 2005, 39(2):380-2.

Rodrigues JP, Edwards DJ, Walters SE, et al, "Gabapentin Can Improve Postural Stability and Quality of Life in Primary Orthostatic Tremor," *Mov Disord*, 2005, 20(7):865-70.

Stacey B, Parsons B, Huang S, et al, "Gabapentin and Improved Health Status in Elderly Patients with Postherpetic Neuralgia: A Pooled Analysis of Three Clinical Studies," *P&T*, 2004, 29(10):646-50.

Wogoman H, Bultman S, Smith R, et al, "Increased Incidence of Gabapentin and Baclofen in Postmortem Casework, Both Alone and in Combination with Other Drugs," *J Anal Toxicol*, 2004, 28:301.

Gallium Nitrate

CAS Number 13494-90-1; 135886-70-3

U.S. Brand Names Ganite™

Synonyms NSC-15200

Use Treatment of hypercalcemia

Mechanism of Action Gallium is a naturally occurring group IIIa heavy metal. It is the second metal, in addition to salts of platinum (group VIII metal), which has demonstrated significant clinical antitumor activity. The mechanism of hypocalcemia induced by gallium is primarily via inhibition of bone resorption with associated reduction in urinary calcium excretion. Gallium has increased the calcium content of newly mineralized bone following short-term treatment *in vitro*, and this effect combined with its ability to inhibit bone resorption has suggested the use of gallium for other disorders associated with increased bone loss. Gallium has produced significant decreases in urinary excretion of calcium and hydroxyproline in patients with solitary or multiple lytic bone metastases, and may be useful for preventing pathologic conditions in these patients.

Adverse Reactions
Not all frequencies defined.
Cardiovascular: Hypotension, tachycardia, edema of lower extremities
Central nervous system: Lethargy, confusion, dreams, hallucinations, hypothermia, fever
Dermatologic: Rash
Endocrine & metabolic: **Hypophosphatemia** (>50%, usually asymptomatic); hypocalcemia; mild respiratory alkalosis with hyperchloremia
Gastrointestinal: **Nausea** (14%, generally mild), vomiting, diarrhea, constipation
Hematologic: Anemia, leukopenia
Neuromuscular & skeletal: Paresthesia
Renal: **Nephrotoxicity** (>10%, generally reversible and reported to be minimized with adequate hydration and urine output)
Respiratory: Dyspnea, rales, rhonchi, pleural effusion, pulmonary infiltrates. **Note:** Toxicities reported with doses higher than those used to treat hypercalcemia (ie, in trials evaluating anticancer effect): Optic neuritis, tinnitus, hearing acuity decreased, metallic taste, hypomagnesemia, encephalopathy

Pharmacodynamics/Kinetics
Onset of calcium lowering: Seen within 24-48 hours of beginning therapy, with normocalcemia achieved within 4-7 days of beginning therapy
Bioavailability: Oral: 5%
Distribution: Tissue concentrations were determined postmortem in one patient and concentrations were higher in liver and kidney than in lung, skin, muscle, heart, and cervix tumor; in dogs, tissue gallium concentrations were higher in renal cortex, bone, bone marrow, small intestine, and liver than in skeletal muscle and brain
Half-life elimination: Alpha: 1.25 hours; Beta: ~24 hours
Elimination half-life varies with method of administration (72-115 hours with prolonged intravenous infusion versus 24 hours with bolus administration); long elimination half-life may be related to slow release from tissue such as bone
Excretion: Primarily renal with no prior metabolism in the liver or kidney

Dosage
I.V.: Adults: 200 mg/m²/day for 5 days; duration may be shortened during a course if normocalcemia is achieved. If hypercalcemia is mild and with very few symptoms, 100 mg/m²/day may be used.
Dosage adjustment in renal impairment:
Serum creatinine >2.5 mg/dL: Contraindicated
Serum creatinine 2 to <2.5 mg/dL: No guidelines exist; frequent monitoring is recommended

Monitoring Parameters Renal function, serum calcium (daily), serum phosphorus (twice weekly)

Administration
I.V. infusion over 30 minutes to 24 hours

Contraindications Hypersensitivity to gallium nitrate or any component of the formulation; severe renal dysfunction (creatinine >2.5 mg/dL)

Warnings Hazardous agent - use appropriate precautions for handling and disposal. **[U.S. Boxed Warning]: Use caution with renal impairment or when administering other nephrotoxic drugs (eg, aminoglycosides, amphotericin B);** consider discontinuing gallium nitrate during treatment with nephrotoxic drugs. Maintain adequate hydration. Safety and efficacy in pediatric patients have not been established.

Dosage Forms Injection, solution [preservative free]: 25 mg/mL (20 mL)

Reference Range Steady-state gallium serum levels: Generally obtained within 2 days following initiation of continuous I.V. infusions of gallium nitrate

Overdosage/Treatment Supportive therapy: Give calcium chloride for hypocalcemia

Drug Interactions
Cyclophosphamide: Concurrent use of low dose gallium nitrate has been associated with dyspnea, stomatitis, asthenia, and rarely interstitial pneumonitis.
Nephrotoxic drugs (eg, aminoglycosides, amphotericin B): Concurrent use with gallium nitrate may increase nephrotoxic effects.

Pregnancy Risk Factor C

Pregnancy Implications Reproduction studies have not been conducted

Lactation Excretion in breast milk unknown/not recommended

Nursing Implications Patients should have adequate I.V. hydration, serum creatinine levels should be monitored during gallium nitrate therapy

Additional Information Has shown to be more effective in lowering serum calcium levels in patients with cancer-related hypercalcemia than calcitonin; due to the potential for drug-induced renal dysfunction, patients receiving gallium nitrate should be adequately hydrated to minimize risk

Gallopamil

Related Information
● Calcium Channel Blockers
CAS Number 16662-47-8
Use Angina, hypertension
Mechanism of Action Second generation calcium antagonist with actions very similar to verapamil, but ~8 times as potent
Adverse Reactions
Cardiovascular: Bradycardia, palpitations, edema, flushing, sinus bradycardia, angina, chest pain
Central nervous system: Headache, drowsiness, dizziness
Gastrointestinal: Constipation
Hepatic: Cholestatic jaundice
Signs and Symptoms of Overdose Atrioventricular dissociations
Pharmacodynamics/Kinetics
Peak serum level: 1-2 hours; sustained release: 4 hours
Distribution: ≈2 L/kg
Metabolism: Hepatic
Protein binding: 93%
Half-life: 4-8 hours; cirrhotic patients: 5-20 hours
Bioavailability: 25%
Dosage
Angina:
Oral: 50-75 mg 3 times/day
I.V. bolus: 0.03 mg/kg
I.V. infusion: 0.02 mg/kg/hour; can titrate up to 0.03 mg/kg/hour after 2 days
Hypertension: Oral: 50 mg 2-3 times/day; reduce dose by 50% to 75% in liver disease
Paroxysmal supraventricular tachycardia: I.V.: 0.03-0.05 mg/kg bolus
Contraindications Hypersensitivity to gallopamil, second/third degree atrioventricular block, Wolff-Parkinson-White syndrome, hypotension, cardiogenic shock
Warnings Use with caution in patients hypersensitive to verapamil, patients with bradycardia, heart failure, aortic stenosis, liver disease, patients taking calcium supplements or beta-blocking agents
Reference Range Mean serum level 2 hours after a 50 mg dose: ~40 ng/mL
Overdosage/Treatment
Decontamination: Ipecac-induced emesis can hypothetically worsen calcium antagonist toxicity, since it can produce vagal stimulation. The potential for seizures precipitously following acute ingestion of large doses of a calcium antagonist may also contraindicate the use of ipecac. Lavage (within 1 hour)/activated charcoal; whole bowel irrigation may be effective for sustained release preparations
Supportive therapy: Supportive and symptomatic treatment, including I.V. fluids and Trendelenburg positioning, should be initiated as intoxication may cause hypotension. Although calcium (calcium chloride I.V. 1-3 g in adults or 10-30 kg in children over 5-10 minutes with repeats as needed) has been used as an "antidote" for acute intoxications, although inamrinone or dopamine may be needed for hypotension and are first line agents for treatment of shock. Heart block may respond to isoproterenol, glucagon, atropine and/or calcium, although a temporary pacemaker may be required; sodium bicarbonate should be given for acidosis. Glucagon may increase myocardial contractility. In an animal model, the therapy of hyperinsulinemia with euglycemia allowed for larger increases in myocardial contractility than calcium chloride, epinephrine, and glucagon.
Enhancement of elimination: Multiple dosing of activated charcoal may be effective; not dialyzable (0% to 5%)
Drug Interactions Enhances hypotensive effects of monoxidine; can increase anti-ischemic effect of isosorbide mononitrate

Galsulfase

Pronunciation (gal SUL fase)
U.S. Brand Names Naglazyme™
Synonyms Recombinant N-Acetylgalactosamine 4-Sulfatase; rhASB
Use Replacement therapy in mucopolysaccharidosis VI (MPS VI; Maroteaux-Lamy syndrome) for improvement of walking and stair-climbing capacity
Mechanism of Action Galsulfase is a recombinant form of N-acetylgalactosamine 4-sulfatase, produced in Chinese hamster cells. A deficiency of this enzyme leads to accumulation of the glycosaminoglycan dermatan sulfate in various tissues, causing progressive disease which includes decreased growth, skeletal deformities, upper airway obstruction, clouding of the cornea, heart disease, and coarse facial features. Replacement of this enzyme has been shown to improve mobility and physical function (measured by walking and stair-climbing).
Adverse Reactions
Note: Percentages reported are from a placebo-controlled study (39 patients, 19 on galsulfase); also included are adverse effects noted during other clinical studies.

Cardiovascular: Chest pain (16%), facial edema (11%), hypertension (11%)

Central nervous system: Pain (26%), malaise (11%), fever, headache

Gastrointestinal: Abdominal pain (53%), gastroenteritis (11%), diarrhea, vomiting

Neuromuscular & skeletal: Rigors (21%), areflexia (11%), arthralgia

Ocular: Conjunctivitis (21%), corneal opacification increased (11%)

Otic: ear pain (42%), otitis media

Respiratory: dyspnea (21%), pharyngitis (16%), nasal congestion (11%), cough, upper respiratory tract infections

Miscellaneous: Antigalsulfase antibodies (98%), umbilical hernia (11%)

Infusion-related reactions: angioedema, apnea, bronchospasm, chills, facial and neck urticaria, hypotension, rash, respiratory distress

Pharmacodynamics/Kinetics Half-life elimination: Week 1: Median 9 hours (range: 6-21 hours); Week 24: Median 26 hours (range: 8-40 hours)

Dosage MPS VI: Children >5 years: I.V.: 1 mg/kg once weekly

Stability

Prior to use, store vials under refrigeration at 2°C to 8°C (36°F to 46°F). Do not freeze or shake. Allow vials to reach room temperature prior to dilution. Do not keep at room temperature >24 hours. Do not heat or microwave vials.

After calculating dose, round to the nearest whole vial to prepare infusion (do not use partial vials). Dilute in NS to a final volume of 250 mL (including volume of galsulfase). Slowly add galsulfase to infusion bag (compatibility in glass containers has not been studied). Gently rotate to distribute. Do not shake or agitate, do not use filter needle. In patients <20 kg or in those who are susceptible to volume overload, dose may be diluted into 100 mL NS.

Following dilution, use immediately. May store under refrigeration if used within 48 hours from the time of preparation to the completion of infusion. Do not store solution for infusion at room temperature.

Monitoring Parameters In clinical studies, tests of mobility and physical function were monitored at baseline and every 6 weeks.

Administration Administer using infusion pump and PVC infusion set with in-line low protein binding 0.2 micrometer filter. Pretreatment with antihistamines with or without antipyretics is recommended 30-60 minutes prior to infusion. Infuse a 250 mL solution at 6 mL/hour for the first hour. If well-tolerated, increase to 80 mL/hour for the remaining 3 hours. Doses prepared in 100 mL should also be infused over at least 4 hours. In case of infusion-related reactions, decrease infusion rate or temporarily discontinue. Infusion time can be extended up to 20 hours if infusion reactions occur. Discontinue immediately if severe reaction occurs. Patients requiring supplemental oxygen or CPAP during sleep should have these treatments readily available in case of infusion-related or antihistamine-induced reaction.

Contraindications None known

Warnings Patients should be premedicated with antihistamines and/or antipyretics prior to infusion. Infusion-related reactions have been reported as late as week 55 of treatment. Evaluate airway prior to therapy (due to possible effects of antihistamine use). Consider delaying treatment in patients with an acute febrile or respiratory illness. Excess agitation of solution prior to or after dilution may denature galsulfase rendering it inactive. Studies did not include patients <5 years of age or >29 years.

Dosage Forms Injection, solution [preservative free]: 5 mg/5 mL (5 mL)

Overdosage/Treatment Supportive therapy: Treat symptomatically; Bronchospasm can be treated with beta-adrenergic agents

Pregnancy Risk Factor B

Pregnancy Implications Fetal harm was not reported in animal studies. There are no studies in pregnant women. Pregnant women are encouraged to enroll in the Clinical Surveillance Program.

Lactation Excretion in breast milk unknown/use caution

Additional Information A Clinical Surveillance Program has been created to monitor therapeutic response, progression of disease, and adverse effects during long-term treatment; patients should be encouraged to register (866-906-6100).

Gamma Hydroxybutyric Acid

Related Information

• Highlights of Recent Reports (2006) on Substance Abuse and Mental Health

CAS Number 502-85-2

U.S. Brand Names Xyrem® (Schedule 111 drug)

Synonyms 4-Hydroxybutyrate; Gamma Hydroxybutyric Acid; GHB; Sodium 4-Hydroxybutyrate

Impairment Potential Yes. Ingestion of >100 mg/kg, urinary gamma/hydroxybutyrate level >2000 mg/L, or blood GHB level >26 mg/L is consistent with driving impairment. (Stephens BG and Baselt RC, "Driving Under the Influence of GHB?" *J Anal Toxicol*, 1994, 18(6): 357-8.) (Couper FJ and Logan BK, "Driving Under the Influence of GHB," *J Anal Toxicol*, 2001, 25:365.)

Use Treatment of cataplexy and daytime sleepiness in patients with narcolepsy

Unlabeled/Investigational Use Narcolepsy; anesthetic agent

Mechanism of Action Central nervous system depressant which has anesthetic action; possible role as a neurotransmitter particularly in the substantia nigra influencing dopamine release

Adverse Reactions

Cardiovascular: Bradycardia, hypertension, hypotension, atrial fibrillation, nonsustained ventricular tachycardia, QT prolongation

Central nervous system: Confusion, seizures, coma (1-2 hours duration), dizziness, relaxation, euphoria, amnesia, hypotonia (dose related), ataxia, extrapyramidal reaction

Gastrointestinal: Fecal incontinence, excessive salivation

Genitourinary: Urinary incontinence

Hematologic: Porphyria

Neuromuscular & skeletal: Tremors

Ocular: Nystagmus

Respiratory: Apnea, respiratory depression

Signs and Symptoms of Overdose (usually over 20 mg/kg): Coma, somnolence, dizziness, hypotonia, apnea, spontaneous emsis, seizures.

Pharmacodynamics/Kinetics

Onset: IV: 2–15 min

Oral: 15–30 min

Absorption: Rapid

Distribution: 190-384 mL/kg

Protein binding: <1%

Metabolism: Primarily via the Krebs cycle to form water and carbon dioxide; secondarily via beta oxidation; significant first-pass effect; no active metabolites; metabolic pathways are saturable

Bioavailability: 25%

Half-life elimination: 30-60 minutes

Time to peak: 30-75 minutes

Excretion: Primarily pulmonary (as carbon dioxide); urine (<5% unchanged drug)

Dosage

Analgesia/amnesia and hypotonia: 10-20 mg

General anesthesia coma, bradycardia: 50 mg/kg

Intoxicating dose: 15 mg/kg

Monitoring Parameters Respiratory status, ECG

Administration Take on an empty stomach; separate last meal (or food) and first dose by several hours; try to take at similar time each day. Doses should be administered while patient is sitting up in bed. Both doses should be prepared prior to bedtime. The first dose is taken at bedtime and the second dose is taken 2.5-4 hours later; an alarm clock may need to be set for the second dose. After taking the dose, patient is to lie down and remain in bed.

Contraindications Hypersensitivity to sodium oxybate or any component of the formulation; ethanol and other CNS depressants; semialdehyde dehydrogenase deficiency

Warnings

[U.S. Boxed Warning]: Sodium oxybate is a CNS depressant with abuse potential; it should not be used with ethanol or other CNS depressants. Seizures, respiratory depression, decreases in level of consciousness, coma, and death have been reported when used for nonprescription purposes. Due to the rapid onset of CNS depressant effects, doses should be administered only at bedtime and while the patient is sitting up in bed. May impair respiratory drive; use caution with compromised respiratory function. Most patients (~80%) in clinical trials were also treated with stimulants; therefore, an independent assessment of the effects of sodium oxybate is lacking. May cause confusion, psychosis, paranoia, hallucinations, agitation, and depression; use caution with history of depression or suicide attempt. May cause sleepwalking, urinary, and/or fecal incontinence. Use caution with hepatic dysfunction. Contains significant amounts of sodium; use caution with heart failure, hypertension, or compromised renal function.

Patients should be instructed not to engage in hazardous activities requiring mental alertness for at least 6 hours after taking this medication and that CNS effects may carryover to the next day. Tolerance to sodium oxybate, or withdrawal following its discontinuation, have not been clearly defined in controlled clinical trials, but have been reported at larger doses used for illicit purposes. Safety and efficacy have not been established in patients <16 years of age.

[U.S. Boxed Warning]: Sodium oxybate oral solution will be available only to prescribers enrolled in the Xyrem® Patient Success Program® and dispensed to the patient through the designated centralized pharmacy (1-866-997-3688).

Dosage Forms Solution, oral: 500 mg/mL (180 mL) [supplied in a kit containing two dosing cups and measuring device]

Reference Range 4-butyrolactone plasma levels >2.5 mM/L are associated with coma; oral doses (in mg/kg) approximate plasma levels (in mcg/mL); following an oral dose of 100 mg, peak urinary GHB concentrations are approximately 1100 mg/L; urinary levels are undetectable in 12 hours. Postmortem gamma-hydroxybutyric acid levels following a gamma-butyrolactone (GBL) overdose were reported as: Heart blood: 583 mg/L; vitreous: 652 mg/L; and urine: 2927 mg/L. Postmortem urine and blood levels of a 1,4-butanediol overdose fatality were 146 mcg/mL and 7.6 mcg/mL, respectively. Corresponding urine and blood GHB levels were 6171 mcg/mL and 280 mcg/mL. Urinary GHB level >5 mg/L is reflective of GHB ingestion.

Overdosage/Treatment

Decontamination: Lavage (within 1 hour)/activated charcoal; **do not** induce emesis

Supportive therapy: Atropine can be utilized for bradycardia; naloxone or flumazenil has been effective in reversing the effect in animals, however, human experience is disappointing; pentobarbital (2.5-5 mg/kg I.V. infused over 30 minutes) can be used to treat GHB withdrawal. Supportive therapy (with possible mechanical ventilation) is the mainstay of therapy. Symptoms usually resolve in ~8 hours. Physostigmine (0.5-2 mg I.V.) has been used successfully to reverse coma.

Enhancement of elimination: Multiple dosing of charcoal may be effective

Antidote(s)

● Physostigmine [ANTIDOTE]

Test Interactions Increases growth hormone and prolactin levels as little as a 3 g dose; sodium salt can cause hypernatremia; hypokalemia has also been reported

Drug Interactions CNS depressants: CNS depressant effects are potentiated; concomitant use with sodium oxybate is contraindicated.

Pregnancy Risk Factor B

Pregnancy Implications Has been used as an obstetric anesthetic agent; while GHB crosses the placenta, no fetal effects are known; can increase uterine contractions

Lactation Excretion in breast milk unknown/use caution

Additional Information

Lethal dose: ~4 g; Minimal lethal dose of 1,4-butanediol: Oral: 5.4 g

Recalled by the FDA in November 1990; found in certain ripe fruits such as guava; can be synthesized by titrating gamma butyryl lactone with sodium hydroxide to a pH of 6-7; withdrawal symptoms (insomnia, anxiety, tremors) may last 3-12 days; more commonly sold as a liquid form in its sodium salt form dissolved in ethanol or water. GHB can increase plasma growth hormone levels up to 40 ng/mL.

Osmolality gap determination formula: (GHB) mg/L divided by MW of GHB = (104) = calculated osmolality in mOsm/L.

Sources for GHB analysis include: Kathleen Andrews, DEA Western Laboratory, 390 Main Street, Room #700, San Francisco, CA 94105, (415) 744-7051 ext 33; Adrian Krawczeniuk, DEA Northeast Laboratory, 99 Tenth Avenue, Suite 721, New York, NY 10011, (212) 620-3684; Peter K Poole, DEA North Central Laboratory, 536 South Clark Street, Room 8, Chicago IL 60605, (312) 353-3640 ext 1601

GHB cases can be reported to the DEA through: Office of Diversion Control, Drug and Chemical Evaluation Section, Drug Enforcement Administration, Washington, DC 20537, (202) 307-7183.

GHB tolerance can occur with ingestion over 20 grams per day for over 1.5 years. Sings of withdrawal include disorientation, tremors, hallucinations, tachycardia, hypertension and nystagmus. Seizures and fever do not occur. Benzodiazepines are the mainstay of therapy.

Specific References

Anderson IB, Kim SY, Dyer JE, et al, "Trends in Gamma-Hydroxybutyrate (GHB) and Related Drug Intoxication: 1999 to 2003," *Ann Emerg Med*, 2006, 47(2):177-83.

Bania TC, Chu J, Ashar T, et al, "Severe Gamma-Hyroxybutyric Acid Withdrawal in an Animal Model," *Acad Emerg Med*, 2003, 10:518b-19b.

Bania TC, Chu J, and O'Neill M, "Effect of Haloperidol on Gamma-Hydroxybutyrate (GHB) Withdrawal in an Animal Model," *SAEM Annual Meeting Abstracts*, 2004, 470.

Bania TC, Chu J, and O'Neill M, "Optimal Dosing Regimen to Produce Gamma-Hydroxybutyrate (GHB) Withdrawal in an Animal Model," *SAEM Annual Meeting Abstracts*, 2004, 470-1.

Bania TC, Chu J, O'Neil M, et al, "Effects of Physostigmine Following Cessation of Chronic GHB Administration in Mice," *Acad Emerg Med*, 2003, 10:518.

Brenneisen R, Elsohly MA, Murphy TP, et al, "Pharmacokinetics and Excretion of Gamma-hydroxybutyrate (GHB) in Healthy Subjects," *J Anal Toxicol*, 2004, 28(8):625-30.

Brown JJ and Nanayakkara CS, "Acetone-Free Nail Polish Removers: Are They Safe?" *Clin Toxicol (Phila)*, 2005, 43(4):297-9.

Carai MA, Colombo G, and Gessa GL, "Resuscitative Effect of a Gamma-aminobutyric Acid B Receptor Antagonist on Gamma-hydroxybutyric Acid Mortality in Mice," *Ann Emerg Med*, 2005, 45(6):614-9.

Chen M, Andrenyak DM, Moody DE, et al, "Stability of Plasma Gamma-Hydroxybutyrate Determined by Gas Chromatography-Positive Ion Chemical Ionization-Mass Spectrometry," *J Anal Toxicol*, 2003, 27:445-8.

Couper FJ and Logan BK, "Addicted to Driving Under the Influence - A GHB/GBL Case Report," *J Anal Toxicol*, 2004, 28(6):512-5.

Couper FJ, Thatcher JE, and Logan BK, "Suspected GHB Overdoses in the Emergency Department," *J Anal Toxicol*, 2004, 28(6):481-4.

Crookes CE, Faulds MC, Forrest AR, et al, "A Reference Range for Endogenous Gamma-hydroxybutyrate in Urine by Gas Chromatography-mass Spectrometry," *J Anal Toxicol*, 2004, 28(8):644-9.

Elliott SP, "Further Evidence for the Presence of GHB in Postmortem Biological Fluid: Implications for the Interpretation of Findings," *J Anal Toxicol*, 2004, 28(1):20-6.

Goulle JP, Cheze M, and Pepin G, "Determination of Endogenous Levels of GHB in Human Hair: Are There Possibilities for the Identification of GHB Administration Through Hair Analysis in Cases of Drug-Facilitated Sexual Assault?" *J Anal Toxicol*, 2003, 27(8):574-80.

Haller C, Thai D, and Benowitz N, "Cardiovascular Responses to GHB and Ethanol in Human Subjects," *J Toxicol Clin Toxicol*, 2004, 42(5):761-2.

Haller C, Thai D, Manktelow TC, et al, "Cognitive and Mood Effects of GHB and Ethanol in Humans," *J Toxicol Clin Toxicol*, 2004, 42(5):762.

Haroz R and Greenberg MI, "Emerging Drugs of Abuse," *Med Clin North Am*, 2005, 89(6):1259-76 (review).

Karas RP, Jagerdeo E, Deakin AL, et al, "Quantitative Analysis of Gamma-Hydroxy-Butyrate (GHB) in Urine by Direct Analysis in Real Time (DART™) Time-of-Flight Mass Spectrometry (TOF-MS)," *J Anal Toxicol*, 2006, 30:140.

Kintz P, Villain M, Pelissier AL, et al, "Unusually High Concentrations in a Fatal GHB Case," *J Anal Toxicol*, 2005, 29:582-5.

Larson SJ, Putnam EA, Schwarke CM, Pershouse MA, "Potential Surrogate Markers for Gamma-Hydroxybutyrate Administration May Extend the Detection Window from 12 to 48 Hours" *J Anal Tox*, 2007, 31:15-22.

LeBeau MA, Montgomery MA, Morris-Kukoski C, et al, "A Comprehensive Study on the Variations in Urinary Concentrations of Endogenous Gamma-Hydroxybutyrate (GHB)," *J Anal Toxicol*, 2006, 30:98-105.

Liechti ME and Kupferschmidt H, "Gamma-Hydroxybutyrate (GHB) and Gamma-Butyrolactone (GBL) Poisoning," *J Toxicol Clin Toxicol*, 2004, 42(5):758-9.

Marinetti LJ and Commissaris RL, "The Pharmacological Characterization of Gamma Valerolactone (GVL) in Rats as Compared to Gamma Hydroxybutyric Acid (GHB), Gamma Butyrolactone (GBL), and Ethanol (EtOH)," *J Anal Toxicol*, 2003, 27(3):189.

Marinetti LJ, Isenschmid DS, Hepler BR, et al, "Analysis of GHB and 4-Methyl-GHB in Postmortem Matrices After Long-Term Storage," *J Anal Toxicol*, 2005, 29:41-7.

Mazarr-Proo S and Kerrigan S,, "Distribution of GHB in Tissues and Fluids Following a Fatal Overdose," *J Anal Toxicol*, 2005, 29(5):398-400.

Meyers JE and Almirall JR, "A Study of the Effectiveness of Commercially Available Drink Test Coasters for the Detection of "Date Rape" Drugs in Beverages," *J Anal Toxicol*, 2004, 28(8):685-8.

Morris-Kukoski CL, "Gamma-Hydroxybutyrate: Bridging the Clinical-analytical Gap," *Toxicol Rev*, 2004, 23(1):33-43 (review).

Palmer RB, "Gamma-butyrolactone and 1,4-butanediol: Abused Analogues of Gamma-Hydroxybutyrate," *Toxicol Rev*, 2004, 23(1):21-31 (review).

Quang LS, Amer A, and Maher TJ, "Orexin-A Attenuates GBL/GHB Toxicity in Rodent Overdose," *J Toxicol Clin Toxicol*, 2004, 42(5):741.

Quang LS, Carai MA, Atzeri S, et al, "Audiogenic Withdrawal Seizures from GHB and 1,4-Butanediol (1,4-BD) in Sardinian Alcohol-Preferring (SP) Rats," *Clin Toxicol (Phila)*, 2005, 43:692.

Quang LS, Carai MA, Atzeri S, et al, "Role of the GABA$_B$ Receptor in Audiogenic Withdrawal Seizures from 1,4-Butanediol (1,4-BD) in Sardinian Alcohol-Preferring (SP) Rats," *Clin Toxicol (Phila)*, 2005, 43:691.

Quang LS, Gupta M, Maher TJ, et al, "4,5-DHHA is a Biomarker for 1,4-BD and GBL in Murine Overdose," *J Toxicol Clin Toxicol*, 2004, 42(5):754-5.

Quang LS, Gupta M, Maher TJ, et al, "4,5-DHHA is a Biomarker for GHB in GHB Mutant Mice," *J Toxicol Clin Toxicol*, 2004, 42(5):755.

Quang LS, Sadasivan S, Maher TJ, et al, "Neuroprotective Effect of GHB, GBL, and 1,4-BD on Rat Focal Cerebral Ischemia by Permanent Middle Cerebral Artery Occlusion (MCAO)," *J Toxicol Clin Toxicol*, 2003, 41(5):750.

Quang LS, Vo T, Maher TJ, et al, "A Dose-Response Evaluation of the GHB Precursor, Tetrahydrofuran," *J Toxicol Clin Toxicol*, 2003, 41(5):692.

Saudan C, Augsburger M, Kintz P, et al, "Detection of Exogenous GHB in Blood by Gas Chromatography-Combustion-Isotope Ratio Mass Spectrometry: Implications in Postmortem Toxicology," *J Anal Toxicol*, 2005, 29(9):777-81.

Shah PP, Bohlke M, Quang LS, et al, "Determination of Gamma Hydroxy Butyrate in Striatal Dialysates of Rats Treated with 1,4-Butanediol," *J Toxicol Clin Toxicol*, 2003, 41(5):693.

Snead OC 3rd and Gibson KM, "Gamma-Hydroxybutyric Acid," *N Engl J Med*, 2005, 352(26):2721-32 (review).

Sporer KA, Chin RL, Dyer JE, et al, "Gamma-Hydroxybutyrate Serum Levels and Clinical Syndrome After Severe Overdose," *Ann Emerg Med*, 2003, 42(1):3-8.

Stolbach A, Chu J, Lee DC, et al, "Repetitive Naloxone Dosing Does Not Reverse Gamma-Butyrolactone (GBL) Sedation in a Rat Model of Severe Intoxication," *J Toxicol Clin Toxicol*, 2004, 42(5):735-6.

Suchard JR and Attai S, "GHB-Associated Ventricular Tachycardia and QT Prolongation," *J Toxicol Clin Toxicol*, 2003, 41(5):645.

Tarabar AF and Nelson LS, "The Gamma-Hydroxybutyrate Withdrawal Syndrome," *Toxicol Rev*, 2004, 23(1):45-9 (review).

Thai D, Haller C, Jacob III P, et al, "Pharmacokinetic Interactions of GHB and Ethanol in Humans," *J Toxicol Clin Toxicol*, 2004, 42(5):760.

U.S. Xyrem® Multi-Center Study Group, "The Abrupt Cessation of Therapeutically Administered Sodium Oxybate (GHB) Does Not Cause Withdrawal Symptoms," *J Toxicol Clin Toxicol*, 2003, 41(2):131-5.

Van Sassenbroeck DK, De Paepe P, Belpaire FM, "Characterization of the Pharmacokinetic and Pharmacodynamic Interaction Between Gamma-Hydroxybutyrate and Ethanol in the Rat," *Toxicol Sci*, 2003, 73(2):270-8.

Vasiliades J and Ford K, "Simple, Rapid, Sensitive, Direct Method for the Identification and Quantitation of Gammahydroxybutyric Acid (GHB) in Urine," *J Anal Toxicol*, 2003, 27(3):178.

Wiegand TJ, Zvosec DL, and Smith SW, "Use of Propofol for Severe GHB Withdrawal: Two Cases," *Clin Toxicol (Phila)*, 2005, 43:665.

Wong CG, Chan KF, Gibson KM, et al, "Gamma-Hydroxybutyric Acid: Neurobiology and Toxicology of a Recreational Drug," *Toxicol Rev*, 2004, 23(1):3-20 (review).

Yambo CM, McFee RB, Caraccio TR, et al, "The Case of Inkjet Cleaner 'Hurricaine' - Another GHB Recipe," *J Toxicol Clin Toxicol*, 2004, 46(6):329-30.

Yeatman DT and Reid K, "A Study of Urinary Endogenous Gamma-Hydroxybutyrate (GHB) Levels," *J Anal Toxicol*, 2003, 27(1):40-2.

Zvosec D and Smith SW, "Gamma-Hydroxybutyrate Addiction and Withdrawal: From the Gamma Hydroxybutyrate Addiction Study," *Ann Emerg Med*, 2004, 44:S91.

Zvosec DL, Smith SW, and Litonjua MR, "Physostigmine for Gamma Hydroxybutyrate Coma: Lack of Efficacy and Adverse Events in 5 Patients," *Clin Toxicol (Phila)*, 2005, 43:674.

Zvosec DL, Smith SW, Porrata T, et al, "Gamma Hydroxybutyrate-Related Fatalities: 146 Deaths," *Clin Toxicol (Phila)*, 2005, 43:665.

Ganciclovir

CAS Number 107910-75-8; 82410-32-0

U.S. Brand Names Cytovene®; Vitrasert®

Synonyms DHPG Sodium; GCV Sodium; Nordeoxyguanosine

Use

Parenteral: Treatment of CMV retinitis in immunocompromised individuals, including patients with acquired immunodeficiency syndrome; prophylaxis of CMV infection in transplant patients

Oral: Alternative to the I.V. formulation for maintenance treatment of CMV retinitis in immunocompromised patients, including patients with AIDS, in whom retinitis is stable following appropriate induction therapy and for whom the risk of more rapid progression is balanced by the benefit associated with avoiding daily I.V. infusions.

Implant: Treatment of CMV retinitis

Unlabeled/Investigational Use May be given in combination with foscarnet in patients who relapse after monotherapy with either drug;

Mechanism of Action Ganciclovir is phosphorylated to a substrate which competitively inhibits the binding of deoxyguanosine triphosphate to DNA polymerase resulting in inhibition of viral DNA synthesis

Adverse Reactions

Cardiovascular: Edema, cardiac arrhythmias, hypertension, tachycardia (ventricular), sinus tachycardia, arrhythmias (ventricular), vasodilation

Central nervous system: **Headache**, seizures, confusion, nervousness, dizziness, psychosis, hallucinations, coma, fever, encephalopathy, malaise, amnesia, mania, hyperthermia

Dermatologic: Rash, alopecia, purpura, pruritus, exanthem, vitiligo

Endocrine & metabolic: Hypoglycemia, hypercalcemia

Gastrointestinal: Nausea, vomiting, diarrhea, anorexia

Hematologic: **Reversible neutropenia, granulocytopenia, thrombocytopenia**, leukopenia, anemia, eosinophilia

Hepatic: Elevated liver function tests

Local: Phlebitis

Neuromuscular & skeletal: Myalgia, trismus, paresthesia

Ocular: Retinal detachment

Renal: Hematuria, elevated BUN/serum creatinine

Respiratory: Dyspnea

Signs and Symptoms of Overdose Bone marrow depression, hematuria, hypoglycemia, leukopenia or neutropenia (agranulocytosis, granulocytopenia), myalgia, and tachycardia (ventricular)

Pharmacodynamics/Kinetics

Distribution: V_d: 15.26 L/1.73 m²; widely to all tissues including CSF and ocular tissue

Protein binding: 1% to 2%

Bioavailability: Oral: Fasting: 5%; Following food: 6% to 9%; Following fatty meal: 28% to 31%

Half-life elimination: 1.7-5.8 hours; prolonged with renal impairment; End-stage renal disease: 5-28 hours

Excretion: Urine (80% to 99% as unchanged drug)

Dosage CMV retinitis: Slow I.V. infusion (dosing is based on total body weight):

Children >3 months and Adults:

Induction therapy: 5 mg/kg/dose every 12 hours for 14-21 days followed by maintenance therapy

Maintenance therapy: 5 mg/kg/day as a single daily dose for 7 days/ week or 6 mg/kg/day for 5 days/week

CMV retinitis: Oral: 1000 mg 3 times/day with food **or** 500 mg 6 times/day with food

Prevention of CMV disease in patients with advanced HIV infection and normal renal function: Oral: 1000 mg 3 times/day with food

Prevention of CMV disease in transplant patients: Same initial and maintenance dose as CMV retinitis except duration of initial course is 7-14 days, duration of maintenance therapy is dependent on clinical condition and degree of immunosuppression

Intravitreal implant: One implant for 5- to 8-month period; following depletion of ganciclovir, as evidenced by progression of retinitis, implant may be removed and replaced

Elderly: Refer to adult dosing; in general, dose selection should be cautious, reflecting greater frequency of organ impairment

Dosing adjustment in renal impairment:

I.V. (Induction):

Cl_{cr} 50-69 mL/minute: Administer 2.5 mg/kg/dose every 12 hours

Cl_{cr} 25-49 mL/minute: Administer 2.5 mg/kg/dose every 24 hours

Cl_{cr} 10-24 mL/minute: Administer 1.25 mg/kg/dose every 24 hours

Cl_{cr} <10 mL/minute: Administer 1.25 mg/kg/dose 3 times/week following hemodialysis

I.V. (Maintenance):

Cl_{cr} 50-69 mL/minute: Administer 2.5 mg/kg/dose every 24 hours

Cl_{cr} 25-49 mL/minute: Administer 1.25 mg/kg/dose every 24 hours

Cl_{cr} 10-24 mL/minute: Administer 0.625 mg/kg/dose every 24 hours

Cl_{cr} <10 mL/minute: Administer 0.625 mg/kg/dose 3 times/week following hemodialysis

Oral:

Cl_{cr} 50-69 mL/minute: Administer 1500 mg/day or 500 mg 3 times/ day

Cl_{cr} 25-49 mL/minute: Administer 1000 mg/day or 500 mg twice daily

Cl_{cr} 10-24 mL/minute: Administer 500 mg/day

Cl_{cr} <10 mL/minute: Administer 500 mg 3 times/week following hemodialysis

Hemodialysis effects: Dialyzable (50%) following hemodialysis; administer dose postdialysis. During peritoneal dialysis, dose as for Cl_{cr} <10 mL/minute. During continuous arteriovenous or venovenous hemofiltration, administer 2.5 mg/kg/dose every 24 hours.

Stability Reconstituted solution is stable for 12 hours at room temperature; **do not refrigerate**; reconstitute with sterile water **not** bacteriostatic water because parabens may cause precipitation

Monitoring Parameters CBC with differential and platelet count, serum creatinine, ophthalmologic exams

Administration Administer by slow I.V. infusion over at least 1 hour at a final concentration for administration not to exceed 10 mg/mL

Contraindications Hypersensitivity to ganciclovir, acyclovir, or any component of the formulation; absolute neutrophil count <500/mm³; platelet count <25,000/mm³

Warnings Hazardous agent – use appropriate precautions for handling and disposal. **[U.S. Boxed Warning]: Granulocytopenia, anemia, and thrombocytopenia may occur.** Dosage adjustment or interruption of ganciclovir therapy may be necessary in patients with neutropenia and/or thrombocytopenia and patients with impaired renal function. Use with extreme caution in children since long-term safety has not been determined and **[U.S. Boxed Warning]: Animal studies have demonstrated carcinogenic and teratogenic effects, and inhibition of spermatogenesis;** contraceptive precautions for female and male patients need to be followed during and for at least 90 days after therapy with the drug; take care to administer only into veins with good blood flow. **[U.S. Boxed Warning]: Indicated only for treatment of CMV retinitis in the immunocompromised patient and CMV prevention in transplant patients at risk.**

Dosage Forms [DSC] = Discontinued product

Capsule: 250 mg, 500 mg

Cytovene®: 250 mg, 500 mg [DSC]

Implant, intravitreal (Vitrasert®): 4.5 mg [released gradually over 5-8 months]

Injection, powder for reconstitution, as sodium (Cytovene®): 500 mg

Reference Range Peak steady state serum level of 5 mg/kg/dose: 15 mcg/mL (44.5 μmol/L)

Overdosage/Treatment

Decontamination: Emesis within 30 minutes or lavage (within 1 hour)/ activated charcoal

Supportive therapy: Colony-stimulating factor may decrease hematologic toxicity

Enhancement of elimination: Multiple dosing may be effective; hemodialysis may be effective (40% to 50% removed by a 4-hour hemodialysis)

Test Interactions May increase serum alkaline phosphatase and serum bilirubin

Drug Interactions

Decreased effect: Didanosine: A decrease in steady-state ganciclovir AUC may occur

Increased toxicity:

Immunosuppressive agents may increase cytotoxicity of ganciclovir

Imipenem/cilastatin may increase seizure potential

Zidovudine: Oral ganciclovir increased the AUC of zidovudine, although zidovudine decreases steady state levels of ganciclovir. Since both drugs have the potential to cause neutropenia and anemia, some patients may not tolerate concomitant therapy with these drugs at full dosage.

Probenecid: The renal clearance of ganciclovir is decreased in the presence of probenecid

Didanosine levels are increased with concurrent ganciclovir

Other nephrotoxic drugs (eg, amphotericin and cyclosporine) may have additive nephrotoxicity with ganciclovir

Pregnancy Risk Factor C

Pregnancy Implications Animal studies reveal growth retardation, cleft palate, microphthalmia, hydrocephaly

Lactation Excretion in breast milk unknown/contraindicated

Nursing Implications Must be prepared in vertical flow hood; use chemotherapy precautions during administration; discard appropriately

Additional Information Sodium content of 500 mg vial: 46 mg

Questions about this drug can be directed to the Ganciclovir Study Center (301) 497-9888 or Syntex Laboratories (415) 496-3648

Gemfibrozil

CAS Number 25812-30-0

U.S. Brand Names Lopid®

Synonyms CI-719

Use Treatment of hypertriglyceridemia in types IV and V hyperlipidemia for patients who are at greater risk for pancreatitis and who have not responded to dietary intervention

Mechanism of Action Exact mechanism of action unknown, however, several theories exist regarding the VLDL effect; it can inhibit lipolysis and decrease subsequent hepatic fatty acid uptake as well as inhibit hepatic secretion of VLDL; together these actions decrease serum VLDL levels; increases HDL cholesterol; the mechanism behind HDL elevation is currently unknown

Adverse Reactions

Cardiovascular: Exacerbation of Raynaud's phenomenon, vasculitis

Central nervous system: Dizziness, drowsiness, somnolence, frontal headache, CNS depression

Dermatologic: Exacerbation of psoriasis, hypertrichosis, exfoliative dermatitis, erythema multiforme, alopecia, angioedema, xerosis, urticaria, pruritus, acanthosis nigricans, licheniform eruptions, exanthem

Gastrointestinal: **Abdominal pain, dyspepsia**, nausea, vomiting, diarrhea, constipation, flatulence, xerostomia

Genitourinary: Impotence

Hepatic: Cholelithiasis, cholecystitis

Neuromuscular & skeletal: Paresthesia, polymyositis (dermatomyositis), rhabdomyolysis

Ocular: Blurred vision

Renal: Myoglobinuria

Miscellaneous: Systemic lupus erythematosus

Pharmacodynamics/Kinetics

Onset of action: May require several days

Absorption: Well absorbed

Protein binding: 99%

Metabolism: Hepatic via oxidation to two inactive metabolites; undergoes enterohepatic recycling

Half-life elimination: 1.4 hours

Time to peak, serum: 1-2 hours

Excretion: Urine (70% primarily as conjugated drug); feces (6%)

Dosage

Adults: Oral: 1200 mg/day in 2 divided doses, 30 minutes before breakfast and dinner

Hemodialysis: Not removed by hemodialysis; supplemental dose is not necessary

Monitoring Parameters Serum cholesterol, LFTs

Contraindications Hypersensitivity to gemfibrozil or any component of the formulation; significant hepatic or renal dysfunction; primary biliary cirrhosis; pre-existing gallbladder disease

Warnings Possible increased risk of malignancy and cholelithiasis. No evidence of cardiovascular mortality benefit. Anemia and leukopenia have been reported. Elevations in serum transaminases can be seen. Discontinue if lipid response not seen. Be careful in patient selection; this is not a first- or second-line choice. Other agents may be more suitable. Adjustments in warfarin therapy may be required with concurrent use. Use caution when combining gemfibrozil with HMG-CoA reductase inhibitors (may lead to myopathy, rhabdomyolysis). Renal function

deterioration has been seen when used in patients with a serum creatinine >2.0 mg/dL. Safety and efficacy in pediatric patients have not been established.

Dosage Forms Tablet: 600 mg

Overdosage/Treatment

Decontamination: Emesis within 30 minutes or lavage (within 1 hour)/activated charcoal

Enhancement of elimination: Multiple dosing of activated charcoal may increase clearance

Test Interactions Possible false positive urinary assay for cannabinoids utilizing the OnTrak TesTcup method (Roche Diagnostic Systems, Inc)

Drug Interactions Substrate of CYP3A4 (minor); **Inhibits** CYP1A2 (moderate), 2C8 (strong), 2C9 (strong), 2C19 (strong)

Bexarotene's serum concentration is significantly increased; avoid concurrent use.

Chlorpropamide: May increase risk of hypoglycemia.

Cyclosporine's blood levels may be reduced; monitor cyclosporine levels and renal function.

CYP1A2 substrates: Gemfibrozil may increase the levels/effects of CYP1A2 substrates. Example substrates include aminophylline, fluvoxamine, mexiletine, mirtazapine, ropinirole, theophylline, and trifluoperazine.

CYP2C8 substrates: Gemfibrozil may increase the levels/effects of CYP2C8 substrates. Example substrates include amiodarone, paclitaxel, pioglitazone, repaglinide, and rosiglitazone.

CYP2C9 substrates: Gemfibrozil may increase the levels/effects of CYP2C9 substrates. Example substrates include bosentan, dapsone, fluoxetine, glimepiride, glipizide, losartan, montelukast, nateglinide, paclitaxel, phenytoin, warfarin, and zafirlukast.

CYP2C19 substrates: Gemfibrozil may increase the levels/effects of CYP2C19 substrates. Example substrates include citalopram, diazepam, methsuximide, phenytoin, propranolol, and sertraline.

Furosemide: Increased blood levels of both in hypoalbuminemia.

Glyburide (and possibly other sulfonylureas): The hypoglycemic effects may be increased.

HMG-CoA reductase inhibitors (atorvastatin, fluvastatin, lovastatin, pravastatin, simvastatin) may increase the risk of myopathy and rhabdomyolysis. The manufacturer warns against the concurrent use of lovastatin (if unavoidable, limit lovastatin to <20 mg/day). Combination therapy with statins has been used in some patients with resistant hyperlipidemias (with great caution).

Repaglinide: Gemfibrozil may increase the serum concentration of repaglinide (prolonged, severe hypoglycemia has been reported). The addition of itraconazole may augment the effects of gemfibrozil on repaglinide. Consider alternative therapy.

Rifampin: Decreased gemfibrozil blood levels.

Warfarin: Hypoprothrombinemic response increased; monitor INRs closely when gemfibrozil is initiated or discontinued.

Pregnancy Risk Factor C

Lactation Excretion in breast milk unknown/contraindicated

Specific References

Layne RD, Sehbai AS, and Stark LJ, "Rhabdomyolysis and Renal Failure Associated with Gemfibrozil Monotherapy," *Ann Pharmacother*, 2004, 38(2):232-4.

Gentamicin

Related Information

● Therapeutic Drugs Associated with Hallucinations

CAS Number 1405-41-0

U.S. Brand Names Garamycin® [DSC]; Genoptic®; Gentacidin®; Gentak®

Synonyms Gentamicin Sulfate

Use Treatment of susceptible bacterial infections, normally gram-negative organisms including *Pseudomonas*, *Proteus*, *Serratia*, and gram-positive *Staphylococcus*; treatment of bone infections, respiratory tract infections, skin and soft tissue infections, as well as abdominal and urinary tract infections, endocarditis, and septicemia; used topically to treat superficial infections of the skin or ophthalmic infections caused by susceptible bacteria; prevention of bacterial endocarditis prior to dental or surgical procedures

Mechanism of Action Interferes with bacterial protein synthesis by binding to 30S and 50S ribosomal subunits resulting in a defective bacterial cell membrane

Adverse Reactions

Cardiovascular: Vasoconstriction, congestive heart failure, myocardial depression

Central nervous system: Psychosis, **dizziness**, hallucinations, anxiety, **ataxia**, arachnoiditis

Dermatologic: Rash, systemic contact dermatitis, immunologic contact urticaria, toxic pustuloderma, acute generalized exanthematous pustulosis

Endocrine & metabolic: Hypomagnesemia

Hematologic: Granulocytopenia

Hepatic: Elevation of AST and ALT

Local: Thrombophlebitis

Neuromuscular & skeletal: Neuromuscular blockade, **gait instability**

Ocular: Nystagmus

Otic: **Ototoxicity** (auditory and vestibular), tinnitus (peak >12-15 mcg/mL and high trough levels)

Renal: **Nephrotoxicity** (high trough levels) with albuminuria, reduction in glomerular filtration rate, elevated serum creatinine, decrease in urine specific gravity, casts in urine and possible electrolyte wasting, **decreased creatinine clearance**

Signs and Symptoms of Overdose Deafness, eczema, Fanconi syndrome, hypokalemia, hypomagnesemia, leukopenia or neutropenia (agranulocytosis, granulocytopenia), myasthenia gravis (exacerbation or precipitation), pseudotumor cerebri, seizures thrombocytopenia, tubular necrosis

Pharmacodynamics/Kinetics

Absorption:

Intramuscular: Rapid and complete

Oral: None

Distribution: Primarily into extracellular fluid (highly hydrophilic); crosses placenta and excreted in breast milk; high concentration in the renal cortex; minimal penetration to ocular tissues via I.V. route

V_d: Increased by edema, ascites, fluid overload; decreased with dehydration

Neonates: 0.4-0.6 L/kg

Children: 0.3-0.35 L/kg

Adults: 0.2-0.3 L/kg

Relative diffusion from blood into CSF: Minimal even with inflammation

CSF: blood level ratio: Normal meninges: Nil; Inflamed meninges: 10% to 30%

Protein binding: <30%

Half-life elimination:

Infants: <1 week: 3-11.5 hours; 1 week to 6 months: 3-3.5 hours

Adults: 1.5-3 hours; End-stage renal disease: 36-70 hours

Time to peak, serum: I.M.: 30-90 minutes; I.V.: 30 minutes after 30-minute infusion

Excretion: Urine (as unchanged drug)

Clearance: Directly related to renal function

Dosage Individualization is critical because of the low therapeutic index

Use of ideal body weight (IBW) for determining the mg/kg/dose appears to be more accurate than dosing on the basis of total body weight (TBW).

In morbid obesity, dosage requirement may best be estimated using a dosing weight of IBW + 0.4 (TBW - IBW)

Initial and periodic peak and trough plasma drug levels should be determined, particularly in critically-ill patients with serious infections or in disease states known to significantly alter aminoglycoside pharmacokinetics (eg, cystic fibrosis, burns, or major surgery)

Newborns: Intrathecal: 1 mg every day

Infants >3 months: Intrathecal: 1-2 mg/day

Infants and Children <5 years: I.M., I.V.: 2.5 mg/kg/dose every 8 hours*

Cystic fibrosis: 2.5 mg/kg/dose every 6 hours

Children >5 years: I.M., I.V.: 1.5-2.5 mg/kg/dose every 8 hours*

Prevention of bacterial endocarditis: Dental, oral, upper respiratory procedures, GI/GU procedures: 2 mg/kg with ampicillin (50 mg/kg) 30 minutes prior to procedure

*Some patients may require larger or more frequent doses (eg, every 6 hours) if serum levels document the need (ie, cystic fibrosis or febrile granulocytopenic patients)

Adults: I.M., I.V.:

Severe life-threatening infections: 2-2.5 mg/kg/dose

Urinary tract infections: 1.5 mg/kg/dose

Synergy (for gram-positive infections): 1 mg/kg/dose

Prevention of bacterial endocarditis:

Dental, oral, or upper respiratory procedures: 1.5 mg/kg not to exceed 80 mg with ampicillin (1-2 g) 30 minutes prior to procedure

GI/GU surgery: 1.5 mg/kg not to exceed 80 mg with ampicillin (2 g) 30 minutes prior to procedure

Some clinicians suggest a daily dose of 4-7 mg/kg for all patients with normal renal function. This dose is at least as efficacious with similar, if not less, toxicity than conventional dosing.

Children and Adults:

Intrathecal: 4-8 mg/day

Ophthalmic:

Ointment: Instill $^1/_2$" (1.25 cm) 2-3 times/day to every 3-4 hours

Solution: Instill 1-2 drops every 2-4 hours, up to 2 drops every hour for severe infections

Topical: Apply 3-4 times/day to affected area

Dosing interval in renal impairment:

Cl_{cr} ≥60 mL/minute: Administer every 8 hours

Cl_{cr} 40-60 mL/minute: Administer every 12 hours

Cl_{cr} 20-40 mL/minute: Administer every 24 hours

Cl_{cr} <20 mL/minute: Loading dose, then monitor levels

Hemodialysis: Dialyzable; removal by hemodialysis: 30% removal of aminoglycosides occurs during 4 hours of HD; administer dose after dialysis and follow levels

Removal by continuous ambulatory peritoneal dialysis (CAPD):

Administration via CAPD fluid:

Gram-negative infection: 4-8 mg/L (4-8 mcg/mL) of CAPD fluid

Gram-positive infection (ie, synergy): 3-4 mg/L (3-4 mcg/mL) of CAPD fluid

Administration via I.V., I.M. route during CAPD: Dose as for Cl_{cr} <10 mL/minute and follow levels

Removal via continuous arteriovenous or venovenous hemofiltration: Dose as for Cl_{cr} 10-40 mL/minute and follow levels

Dosing adjustment/comments in hepatic disease: Monitor plasma concentrations

Stability I.V. infusion solutions mixed in NS or D_5W solution are stable for 24 hours at room temperature; **incompatible** with penicillins

Monitoring Parameters Urinalysis, urine output, BUN, serum creatinine; hearing should be tested before, during, and after treatment; particularly in those at risk for ototoxicity or who will be receiving prolonged therapy (>2 weeks)

Administration Administer by I.V. slow intermittent infusion over 30 minutes; final concentration for administration should not exceed 10 mg/mL

Contraindications Hypersensitivity to gentamicin or other aminoglycosides

Warnings

[U.S. Boxed Warning]: Aminoglycosides may cause neurotoxicity and/or nephrotoxicity; usual risk factors include pre-existing renal impairment, concomitant neuro-/nephrotoxic medications, advanced age and dehydration. Ototoxicity may be directly proportional to the amount of drug given and the duration of treatment; tinnitus or vertigo are indications of vestibular injury and impending hearing loss; renal damage is usually reversible

Not intended for long-term therapy due to toxic hazards associated with extended administration; use caution in pre-existing renal insufficiency, vestibular or cochlear impairment, myasthenia gravis, hypocalcemia, conditions which depress neuromuscular transmission. Dosage modification required in patients with impaired renal function

Dosage Forms [DSC] = Discontinued product

Cream, topical, as sulfate: 0.1% (15 g, 30 g)

Infusion, as sulfate [premixed in NS]: 40 mg (50 mL); 60 mg (50 mL, 100 mL); 70 mg (50 mL); 80 mg (50 mL, 100 mL); 90 mg (100 mL); 100 mg (50 mL, 100 mL); 120 mg (100 mL)

Injection, solution, as sulfate [ADD-Vantage® vial]: 10 mg/mL (6 mL, 8 mL, 10 mL)

Injection, solution, as sulfate: 40 mg/mL (2 mL, 20 mL) [may contain sodium metabisulfite]

Injection, solution, pediatric, as sulfate: 10 mg/mL (2 mL) [may contain sodium metabisulfite]

Injection, solution, pediatric, as sulfate [preservative free]: 10 mg/mL (2 mL)

Ointment, ophthalmic, as sulfate (Gentak®): 0.3% [3 mg/g] (3.5 g)

Ointment, topical, as sulfate: 0.1% (15 g, 30 g)

Solution, ophthalmic, as sulfate: 0.3% (5 mL, 15 mL) [contains benzalkonium chloride]

Genoptic®: 0.3% (1 mL) [contains benzalkonium chloride] [DSC]

Gentak®: 0.3% (5 mL; 15 mL [DSC]) [contains benzalkonium chloride]

Reference Range

Therapeutic: Peak: 4-8 mcg/mL (SI: 8-17 µmol/L); Trough: <2 mcg/mL (SI: <4 µmol/L) (depends in part on the minimal inhibitory concentration of drug against organism being treated)

Toxic: Peak: >10 mcg/mL (SI: >21 µmol/L); Trough: >2 mcg/mL (SI: >4 µmol/L)

Overdosage/Treatment

Supportive therapy: 14 day-therapy with aspirin (1 g 3 times/day) may provide antioxidant protection against ototoxicity

Enhancement of elimination: While hemodialysis is of questionable benefit in those patients with normal renal function, it should be performed in patients with renal insufficiency; the addition of ticarcillin (2-5 g I.V. every 4-6 hours until gentamicin serum levels are <0.2 mcg/mL) may complex with gentamicin and decrease the half-life of gentamicin by enhancing renal excretion

Test Interactions ↑ protein, BUN, AST, GPT, alkaline phosphatase, creatinine (S); ↓ magnesium, potassium, sodium, calcium; the presence of this drug may result in decreased reactivity of urinary leukocyte esterase

Drug Interactions Increased toxicity:

Aminoglycosides may potentiate the effects of neuromuscular-blocking agents.

Penicillins, cephalosporins, amphotericin B, loop diuretics may increase nephrotoxic potential

Decreased effect: Gentamicin's efficacy reduced when given concurrently with carbenicillin, ticarcillin, or piperacillin to patients with severe renal impairment (inactivation). Separate administration.

Pregnancy Risk Factor C
Pregnancy Implications Crosses the placenta
Lactation Enters breast milk (small amounts)/use caution (AAP rates "compatible")
Nursing Implications Slower absorption and lower peak concentrations probably due to poor circulation in the atrophic muscle, may occur following I.M. injection in paralyzed patients (suggest I.V. route); aminoglycoside levels measured in blood taken from Silastic® central catheters can sometimes give falsely high readings (draw via separate lumen or peripheral site if possible, otherwise flush very well). Monitor serum creatinine and urine output; obtain drug levels after the third dose unless otherwise directed (eg, suspected toxicity or renal dysfunction). Peak levels are drawn 30 minutes after the end of a 30-minute infusion or 60 minutes following I.M. injection; trough levels are drawn within 30 minutes before the next dose. Separate administration of extended-spectrum penicillins (eg, carbenicillin, ticarcillin, piperacillin) from gentamicin in patients with severe renal impairment; gentamicin's efficacy may be reduced if given concurrently. Hearing should be tested before, during, and after treatment in patients at risk for ototoxicity.

Additional Information Incidence of cochlear toxicity: 10% to 16%; vestibular toxicity: 5% to 15%; nephrotoxicity: 10% to 35%; ototoxicity may be related to hypovolemia, hepatic disease, and critical illness. Additionally, limiting the total dose to <2 g while limiting the duration of therapy to <10 days may limit ototoxicity, although appears idiosyncratic occurring with first dose. Nephrotoxicity is **not** related to ototoxicity.

Incidence of cochleotoxicity is ~10% to 63% with loop diuretics and noise exposure being ototoxic synergistic. Inhaled tobramycin appears to exhibit minimal ototoxic effects. There may be a genetic basis (in the mitochondrial 12 S ribosomal RNA gene) for ototoxicity in 17% to 33% of cases. Suggested evaluation for ototoxicity with aminoglycoside treatment includes:

- baseline audiometric evaluation (tonal air conduction thresholds from 250-20,000 Hz)
- monitoring during aminoglycoside treatment (to a tonal-air conduction threshold at frequency >8000 Hz)
- follow-up audiometric assessment (tonal air conduction thresholds at frequencies >8000 Hz) until the threshold stabilizes

Specific References

Baciewicz AM, Sokos DR, and Cowan RI, "Aminoglycoside-Associated Nephrotoxicity in the Elderly," *Ann Pharmacother*, 2003, 37(2):182-6.

Bailey DN and Briggs JR, "Gentamicin and Tobramycin Binding to Human Serum In Vitro," *J Anal Toxicol*, 2004, 28:187-95.

Bartal C, Danon A, Schlaeffer F, et al, "Pharmacokinetic Dosing of Aminoglycosides: A Controlled Trial," *Am J Med*, 2003, 114(3):194-8.

Dager WE and King JH, "Aminoglycosides in Intermittent Hemodialysis: Pharmacokinetics with Individual Dosing," *Ann Pharmacother*, 2006, 40(1):9-14.

Kirkpatrick CM, Duffull SB, Begg EJ, et al, "The Use of a Change in Gentamicin Clearance as an Early Predictor of Gentamicin-Induced Nephrotoxicity," *Ther Drug Monit*, 2003, 25(5):623-30.

Sha SH, Qiu JH, and Schacht J, "Aspirin to Prevent Gentamicin-Induced Hearing Loss," *N Engl J Med*, 2006, 354(17):1856-7.

Winston L and Benowitz N, "Once-Daily Dosing of Aminoglycosides: How Much Monitoring is Truly Required?," *Am J Med*, 2003, 114(3):239-40.

Glimepiride

CAS Number 93479-97-1
U.S. Brand Names Amaryl®
Use Management of type 2 diabetes mellitus (noninsulin dependent, NIDDM) as an adjunct to diet and exercise to lower blood glucose or in combination with metformin; use in combination with insulin to lower blood glucose in patients whose hyperglycemia cannot be controlled by diet and exercise in conjunction with an oral hypoglycemic agent
Mechanism of Action Stimulates insulin release from the pancreatic beta cells; reduces glucose output from the liver; insulin sensitivity is increased at peripheral target sites by affecting insulin receptor binding or coupling mechanisms (especially in adipose tissue). It is structurally similar to glyburide.

Adverse Reactions
Central nervous system: Dizziness, **headache**
Endocrine & metabolic: Hypoglycemia
Gastrointestinal: Nausea
Neuromuscular & skeletal: Weakness
Rare but important or life-threatening: Agranulocytosis, anorexia, aplastic anemia, cholestatic jaundice, constipation, diarrhea, disulfiram-like reaction, diuretic effect, edema, epigastric fullness, gastrointestinal pain, erythema, heartburn, hemolytic anemia, hepatitis, hypoglycemia, hyponatremia, leukopenia, liver function tests abnormal, nausea, pancytopenia, photosensitivity, porphyria cutanea tarda, pruritus, rash (morbilliform or maculopapular), SIADH, thrombocytopenia, urticaria, vasculitis (allergic), visual accommodation changes (early treatment), vomiting

Signs and Symptoms of Overdose Low blood sugar, tingling of lips and tongue, nausea, yawning, confusion, agitation, tachycardia, sweating, convulsions, stupor, and coma.

Admission Criteria/Prognosis Admit all intentional adult overdoses. Pediatric patients should be observed in a medical setting through an overnight sleep cycle (and for a minimum of 8 hours). No intravenous glucose or dextrose should be given prophylactically. Asymptomatic pediatric patients should have a blood glucose determination at 3-6 hours postingestion or immediately when symptoms (hunger, irritability, lethargy, tremulousness, tachycardia, diaphoresis, or seizures) develop. Any borderline blood glucose reading (about 70 mg/dL) are repeated in one hour. Consider regular 2- to 3-hour interval blood glucose measurements during sleep. If no hypoglycemic events occur and prebreakfast blood glucose levels are normal, pediatric patients can be monitored by parental observation at home.

Pharmacodynamics/Kinetics
Onset of action: Peak effect: Blood glucose reductions: 2-3 hours
Duration: 24 hours
Absorption: 100%; delayed when given with food
Distribution: V_d: 8.8 L
Protein binding: >99.5%
Metabolism: Hepatic oxidation via CYP2C9 to M1 metabolite (~33% activity of parent compound); further oxidative metabolism to inactive M2 metabolite
Half-life elimination: 5-9 hours
Time to peak, plasma: 2-3 hours
Excretion: Urine (60%, 80% to 90% M1 and M2); feces (40%, 70% M1 and M2)

Dosage
Oral (allow several days between dose titrations):
Adults: Initial: 1-2 mg once daily, administered with breakfast or the first main meal; usual maintenance dose: 1-4 mg once daily; after a dose of 2 mg once daily, increase in increments of 2 mg at 1- to 2-week intervals based upon the patient's blood glucose response to a maximum of 8 mg once daily
Combination with insulin therapy (fasting glucose level for instituting combination therapy is in the range of >150 mg/dL in plasma or serum depending on the patient): initial recommended dose: 8 mg once daily with the first main meal
After starting with low-dose insulin, upward adjustments of insulin can be done approximately weekly as guided by frequent measurements of fasting blood glucose. Once stable, combination-therapy patients should monitor their capillary blood glucose on an ongoing basis, preferably daily.
Dosing adjustment/comments in renal impairment: Cl_{cr} <22 mL/minute: Initial starting dose should be 1 mg and dosage increments should be based on fasting blood glucose levels
Dosing adjustment in hepatic impairment: No data available
Elderly: Initial: 1 mg/day; dose titration and maintenance dosing should be conservative to avoid hypoglycemia
Monitoring Parameters Urine for glucose and ketones; monitor for signs and symptoms of hypoglycemia (fatigue, excessive hunger, profuse sweating, numbness of extremities), fasting blood glucose, hemoglobin A_{1c}, fructosamine
Administration May be administered with a meal/food
Contraindications Hypersensitivity to glimepiride, any component of the formulation, or sulfonamides; diabetic ketoacidosis (with or without coma)
Warnings
All sulfonylurea drugs are capable of producing severe hypoglycemia. Hypoglycemia is more likely to occur when caloric intake is deficient, after severe or prolonged exercise, when ethanol is ingested, or when more than one glucose-lowering drug is used.
Chemical similarities are present among sulfonamides, sulfonylureas, carbonic anhydrase inhibitors, thiazides, and loop diuretics (except ethacrynic acid). Use in patients with sulfonamide allergy is specifically contraindicated in product labeling, however, a risk of cross-reaction exists in patients with allergy to any of these compounds; avoid use when previous reaction has been severe.
Product labeling states oral hypoglycemic drugs may be associated with an increased cardiovascular mortality as compared to treatment with diet alone or diet plus insulin. Data to support this association are limited, and several studies, including a large prospective trial (UKPDS) have not supported an association. Safety and efficacy in pediatric patients have not been established.
Dosage Forms Tablet: 1 mg, 2 mg, 4 mg
Reference Range Mean peak serum glimepiride concentrations after single dose of 4 mg and 8 mg were 352 ng/mL and 591 ng/mL, respectively
Overdosage/Treatment
Intoxication with sulfonylureas can cause hypoglycemia and are best managed with glucose administration (oral for milder hypoglycemia or by injection in more severe forms). Patients should be monitored for a minimum of 24-48 hours after ingestion.
Decontamination: Lavage/activated charcoal

Supportive therapy: Glucose (25 g I.V.) is mainstay of therapy; glucagon (1-5 mg I.V., I.M., or SubQ) (0.03-0.1 mg/kg in pediatrics) will have limited benefit; diazoxide is a third-line agent (3-8 mg/kg/24 hours); octreotide (50 mcg SubQ every 12 hours) may be helpful in sulfonylurea overdose

For pediatric patients with profound sulfonylurea-induced hypoglycemia: Give 0.5 g of dextrose per kg of body weight (5 mL/kg of 10% dextrose concentration of intravenous fluid, 2 mL/kg of D_{25} or 1 mL/kg of D_{50}).

Drug Interactions Substrate of CYP2C9 (major)

Beta blockers: Beta blockers may enhance the effects of sulfonylureas.

Chloramphenicol: Chloramphenicol may increase the effects of sulfonylureas.

Cimetidine: Cimetidine may increase the effects of glimepiride.

Cyclosporine: Sulfonylureas may increase the levels of cyclosporine.

CYP2C9 inducers: May decrease the levels/effects of glimepiride. Example inducers include carbamazepine, phenobarbital, phenytoin, rifampin, rifapentine, and secobarbital.

CYP2C9 inhibitors: May increase the levels/effects of glimepiride. Example inhibitors include delavirdine, fluconazole, gemfibrozil, ketoconazole, nicardipine, NSAIDs, sulfonamides, and tolbutamide.

Ethanol: Sulfonylureas may induce a disulfiram-like reaction.

Fibric acid derivatives: May increase the hypoglycemic effects of sulfonylureas; monitor.

Fluconazole: Fluconazole may increase the levels of sulfonylureas.

Hyperglycemia-producing agents: Certain drugs tend to produce hyperglycemia and may lead to loss of control. These drugs include the thiazides and other diuretics, corticosteroids, phenothiazines, thyroid products, estrogens, oral contraceptives, phenytoin, nicotinic acid, sympathomimetics, and isoniazid.

Pegvisomant: Pegvisomant may increase the effects of sulfonylureas.

Rifampin: Rifampin may decrease the effects of sulfonylureas.

Salicylates: Salicylates may increase the effects of sulfonylureas.

Sulfonamides: Sulfonamides may increase the effects of sulfonylureas.

Tricyclic antidepressants: TCAs may increase the effects of sulfonylureas.

Pregnancy Risk Factor C

Pregnancy Implications Animal studies did not show any direct drug relationship with congenital malformations. Primary adverse effects are associated with maternal hypoglycemia. Abnormal blood glucose levels are associated with a higher incidence of congenital abnormalities. Insulin is the drug of choice for the control of diabetes mellitus during pregnancy.

Lactation Excretion in breast milk unknown/contraindicated

Additional Information Oral aloe, bitter melon (karela), eucalyptus, fenugreek, and ginseng may increase the effects of glimepiride.

Caution with ethanol, chromium, garlic, gymnema (may cause hypoglycemia)

Specific References

Calello D, Kelly A, and Osterhoudt KC, "Case Files of the Medical Toxicology Fellowship Training Program at the Childrens Hospital of Philadelphia: A Pediatric Exploratory Sulfonylurea Ingestion," *J Med Toxicol*, 2006, 2(1):19-26.

Johnson KK, Green DL, Rife JP, et al, "Sulfonamide Cross-Reactivity: Fact or Fiction?" *Ann Pharmacother*, 2005, 39(2):290-301.

GlipiZIDE

CAS Number 29094-61-9

U.S. Brand Names Glucotrol® XL; Glucotrol®

Synonyms Glydiazinamide

Use Management of type 2 diabetes mellitus (noninsulin dependent, NIDDM)

Mechanism of Action Sulfonylurea which stimulates insulin release from the pancreatic beta cells; reduces glucose output from the liver; insulin sensitivity is increased at peripheral target sites

Adverse Reactions

Frequency not defined.

Cardiovascular: Edema, syncope

Central nervous system: Anxiety, depression, dizziness, headache, insomnia, nervousness

Dermatologic: Rash, urticaria, photosensitivity, pruritus

Endocrine & metabolic: Hypoglycemia, hyponatremia, SIADH (rare)

Gastrointestinal: Anorexia, nausea, vomiting, diarrhea, epigastric fullness, constipation, heartburn, flatulence

Hematologic: Blood dyscrasias, aplastic anemia, hemolytic anemia, bone marrow suppression, thrombocytopenia, agranulocytosis

Hepatic: Cholestatic jaundice, hepatic porphyria

Neuromuscular & skeletal: Arthralgia, leg cramps, myalgia, tremor

Ocular: Blurred vision

Renal: Diuretic effect (minor)

Miscellaneous: Diaphoresis, disulfiram-type reaction

Postmarketing and/or case reports: Abdominal pain

Admission Criteria/Prognosis Admit all intentional adult overdoses. Pediatric patients should be observed in a medical setting through an overnight sleep cycle (and for a minimum of 8 hours). No intravenous

glucose or dextrose should be given prophylactically. Asymptomatic pediatric patients should have a blood glucose determination at 3-6 hours postingestion or immediately when symptoms (hunger, irritability, lethargy, tremulousness, tachycardia, diaphoresis, or seizures) develop. Any borderline blood glucose reading (about 70 mg/dL) are repeated in one hour. Consider regular 2- to 3-hour interval blood glucose measurements during sleep. If no hypoglycemic events occur and prebreakfast blood glucose levels are normal, pediatric patients can be monitored by parental observation at home.

Pharmacodynamics/Kinetics

Onset of action: Peak effect: Blood glucose reductions: 1.5-2 hours

Duration: 12-24 hours

Absorption: Delayed with food

Protein binding: 92% to 99%

Metabolism: Hepatic with metabolites

Half-life elimination: 2-4 hours

Excretion: Urine (60% to 80%, 91% to 97% as metabolites); feces (11%)

Dosage

Oral (allow several days between dose titrations): Adults: Initial: 5 mg/day; adjust dosage at 2.5-5 mg daily increments as determined by blood glucose response at intervals of several days.

Immediate release tablet: Maximum recommended once-daily dose: 15 mg; maximum recommended total daily dose: 40 mg

Extended release tablet (Glucotrol® XL): Maximum recommended dose: 20 mg

When transferring from insulin to glipizide:

Current insulin requirement ≤20 units: Discontinue insulin and initiate glipizide at usual dose

Current insulin requirement >20 units: Decrease insulin by 50% and initiate glipizide at usual dose; gradually decrease insulin dose based on patient response. Several days should elapse between dosage changes.

Elderly: Initial: 2.5 mg/day; increase by 2.5-5 mg/day at 1- to 2-week intervals

Dosing adjustment/comments in renal impairment: Cl_{cr} <10 mL/minute: Some investigators recommend not using

Dosing adjustment in hepatic impairment: Initial dosage should be 2.5 mg/day

Monitoring Parameters Urine for glucose and ketones; monitor for signs and symptoms of hypoglycemia (fatigue, excessive hunger, profuse sweating, numbness of extremities), fasting blood glucose, hemoglobin A_{1c}, fructosamine

Administration Administer immediate release tablets 30 minutes before a meal to achieve greatest reduction in postprandial hyperglycemia. Extended release tablets should be given with breakfast. Patients who are NPO may need to have their dose held to avoid hypoglycemia.

Contraindications Hypersensitivity to glipizide or any component of the formulation, other sulfonamides; type 1 diabetes mellitus (insulin dependent, IDDM)

Warnings

Use with caution in patients with severe hepatic disease.

Chemical similarities are present among sulfonamides, sulfonylureas, carbonic anhydrase inhibitors, thiazides, and loop diuretics (except ethacrynic acid). Use in patients with sulfonamide allergy is specifically contraindicated in product labeling, however, a risk of cross-reaction exists in patients with allergy to any of these compounds; avoid use when previous reaction has been severe.

The extended release formulation consists of drug within a nondeformable matrix; following drug release/absorption, the matrix/shell is expelled in the stool. The use of nondeformable products in patients with known stricture/narrowing of the GI tract has been associated with symptoms of obstruction. Avoid use of extended release tablets (Glucotrol® XL) in patients with severe gastrointestinal narrowing or esophageal dysmotility.

Product labeling states oral hypoglycemic drugs may be associated with an increased cardiovascular mortality as compared to treatment with diet alone or diet plus insulin. Data to support this association are limited, and several studies, including a large prospective trial (UKPDS) have not supported an association.

Dosage Forms Tablet (Glucotrol®): 5 mg, 10 mg

Tablet, extended release: 5 mg, 10 mg

Glucotrol® XL: 2.5 mg, 5 mg, 10 mg

Reference Range Glucose: Adults: 80-140 mg/dL; Elderly: 100-180 mg/dL

Overdosage/Treatment

Decontamination: Lavage (within 1 hour)/activated charcoal

Supportive therapy: Glucose (25 g I.V.) is mainstay of therapy; glucagon (1-5 mg I.V., I.M., or SubQ) (0.03-0.1 mg/kg in pediatrics) will have limited benefit; diazoxide is a third-line agent (3-8 mg/kg/24 hours); octreotide (50 mcg SubQ every 12 hours) may be helpful in sulfonylurea overdose

For pediatric patients with profound sulfonylurea-induced hypoglycemia: Give 0.5 g of dextrose per kg of body weight (5 mL/kg of 10% dextrose concentration of intravenous fluid, 2 mL/kg of D_{25} or 1 mL/kg of D_{50}).

Enhancement of elimination: Multiple dosing of activated charcoal may be more effective for this agent than for other oral hypoglycemics due to enterohepatic recirculation of glipizide; peritoneal dialysis has been used with some success, but is not recommended as a routine procedure; urine alkalinization is also useful

Antidote(s)
- Dextrose [ANTIDOTE]
- Glucagon [ANTIDOTE]
- Octreotide [ANTIDOTE]

Diagnostic Procedures
- Electrolytes, Blood
- Glucose, Random

Drug Interactions Substrate of 2C8/9 (major)

Anabolic steroids may increase hypoglycemic effect; monitor blood glucose.

ACE inhibitors may increase hypoglycemic effect; monitor blood glucose.

Beta-blockers decrease hypoglycemic effect, mask most hypoglycemic symptoms, decrease glycogenolysis; avoid use in diabetics with frequent hypoglycemic episodes.

Cholestyramine decreases glipizide's absorption; separate administration times.

Corticosteroids cause hyperglycemia; adjustment of hypoglycemic agent may be necessary.

Cyclosporine serum concentration is increased; monitor cyclosporine levels and renal function.

CYP2C8/9 inducers: May decrease the levels/effects of glipizide. Example inducers include carbamazepine, phenobarbital, phenytoin, rifampin, rifapentine, and secobarbital.

CYP2C8/9 inhibitors: May increase the levels/effects of glipizide. Example inhibitors include delavirdine, fluconazole, gemfibrozil, ketoconazole, nicardipine, NSAIDs, pioglitazone, and sulfonamides.

Ethanol (large amounts) decreases hypoglycemic effect; avoid concurrent use; rare disulfiram reaction.

H$_2$ antagonists, antacids, oral sodium bicarbonate may increase the hypoglycemic effect; monitor glucose response.

Rifampin may decrease hypoglycemic effects of glipizide; monitor blood glucose.

Tacrolimus serum concentrations may be increased; monitor tacrolimus serum concentrations and renal function.

Pregnancy Risk Factor C

Pregnancy Implications Crosses the placenta. Abnormal blood glucose levels are associated with a higher incidence of congenital abnormalities. Insulin is the drug of choice for the control of diabetes mellitus during pregnancy. If glipizide is used during pregnancy, discontinue and change to insulin at least 1 month prior to delivery to decrease prolonged hypoglycemia in the neonate.

Lactation Excretion in breast milk unknown/not recommended

Nursing Implications Monitor for signs and symptoms of hypoglycemia; patients who are anorexic or NPO, may need to have their dose held to avoid hypoglycemia

Additional Information Exhibits more diuretic action than chlorpropamide

Food: A delayed release of insulin may occur if glipizide is taken with food. Immediate release tablets should be administered 30 minutes before meals to avoid erratic absorption.

Specific References

Calello D, Kelly A, and Osterhoudt KC, "Case Files of the Medical Toxicology Fellowship Training Program at the Childrens Hospital of Philadelphia: A Pediatric Exploratory Sulfonylurea Ingestion," *J Med Toxicol* , 2006, 2(1):19-26.

DeWitt C, Waksman J, and Heard K, "Insulin and C-Peptide in Sulfonylurea-Induced Hypoglycemia," *J Toxicol Clin Toxicol*, 2004, 42(5):796.

Johnson KK, Green DL, Rife JP, et al, "Sulfonamide Cross-Reactivity: Fact or Fiction?" *Ann Pharmacother*, 2005, 39(2):290-301.

Glutamine

Pronunciation (GLOO ta meen)

U.S. Brand Names Enterex® Glutapak-10® [OTC]; NutreStore™; Resource® GlutaSolve® [OTC]; Sympt-X G.I. [OTC]; Sympt-X [OTC]

Synonyms Gln; L-Glutamine

Use Treatment of short bowel syndrome when used in combination with nutritional support and growth hormone therapy; a medical food used to promote GI tract healing and nutritional supplementation with GI disorders, HIV/AIDS, cancer, and other critical illnesses

Mechanism of Action Glutamine regulates gastrointestinal cell growth, function, and regeneration. Considered a "conditionally essential" amino acid during metabolic stress and injury.

Adverse Reactions

Frequency not defined.

Cardiovascular: Facial edema, peripheral edema

Central nervous system: Dizziness, fever, headache, pain

Dermatologic: Pruritus, rash

Gastrointestinal: Abdominal pain, flatulence, nausea, pancreatitis, tenesmus, vomiting

Neuromuscular & skeletal: Arthralgia, back pain, hypoesthesia

Otic: Ear or hearing symptoms

Respiratory: Rhinitis

Miscellaneous: Flu-like syndrome, infection, sepsis

Pharmacodynamics/Kinetics

As reported in healthy adults; parameters may vary following oral administration in patients with short bowel syndrome.

Distribution: I.V.: V$_d$: 200 mL/kg

Metabolism: Via splanchnic tissue, lymphocytes, kidney, and liver to glutamate and ammonia

Half-life elimination: I.V.: 1 hour

Dosage

Oral: Adults:

Nutritional supplement (Enterex® Glutapak-10®, Resource® GlutaSolve®, Sympt-X, Sympt-X G.I.): Average dose: 10 g 3 times/day; dosing range: 5-30 g/day

Short bowel syndrome (NutreStore™): 30 g/day administered as 5 g 6 times/day (every 2-3 hours while awake) for up to 16 weeks; to be used in combination with growth hormone and nutritional support

Stability Store at controlled room temperature.

Monitoring Parameters BUN; body weight, nutritional status

Administration

Enterex® Glutapak-10®: Prior to use, mix with clear liquids or semi-solid food. If administering via feeding tube, mix each 10 g packet with ≥60 mL water. Use immediately after preparation. May also be added directly to enteral formula if used within 24 hours.

Resource® GlutaSolve®: Mix each 15 g packet with 120-240 mL of water. May also be mixed in hot or cold beverages, applesauce, or pudding. If administering via feeding tube, mix with 60-120 mL water. Use immediately after preparation.

NutreStore™: Mix each packet (5 g) with ~240 mL of water prior to administration. May be given with meals or snacks

Sympt-X, Sympt-X G.I.: Mix dose with 6-8 ounces of juice or another beverage, may also be mixed with applesauce or pudding. Administer with meals. If administering via feeding tube, mix with ≥60 mL water; do not add directly to feeding bag. Use immediately after preparation.

Warnings Use caution with hepatic or renal impairment. NutreStore™ should be used with nutritional support based on individual patient requirements. Medical foods are intended to be used under the direction of a healthcare provider.

Dosage Forms Powder for oral solution:

Enterex® Glutapak-10®: 10 g/packet (50s)

NutreStore™: 5 g/packet

Resource® GlutaSolve®: 15 g/packet (56s)

Sympt-X, Sympt-X G.I.: 10 g/packet (60s)

Pregnancy Risk Factor C

Pregnancy Implications Reproduction studies have not been conducted.

Lactation Excretion in breast milk unknown/use caution

Glutethimide

Pronunciation (gloo TETH i mide)

Related Information
- Toxins Which Should Be Lavaged with Solutions Other Than Water

CAS Number 77-21-4

Impairment Potential

Yes. Blood glutethimide level >5 mg/L is associated with intoxication. (Chazan JA and Garella S, "Glutethimide Intoxication: A Prospective Study of 70 Patients Treated Conservatively Without Hemodialysis," *Arch Intern Med*, 1971, 128(2):215-9.)

Use Short-term treatment of insomnia; introduced in 1954

Mechanism of Action Central nervous system depressant with hypnotic action of phenobarbital and antimuscarinic effects

Adverse Reactions

Cardiovascular: Bradycardia, hypotension, sinus bradycardia

Central nervous system: **Daytime drowsiness**, convulsions, confusion, slurred speech, dizziness, headache, prolonged coma, fever, ataxia, hypothermia, axonopathy

Dermatologic: Skin rash; bullous eruptions

Endocrine & metabolic: Hypocalcemia (with chronic use)

Gastrointestinal: Nausea, vomiting, ileus

Genitourinary: Urinary retention

Hematologic: Blood dyscrasias, methemoglobinemia, thrombocytopenia, leukopenia (with chronic use), porphyrinogenic

Neuromuscular & skeletal: Muscle spasm, rhabdomyolysis, peripheral neuropathy

Ocular: Nystagmus, mydriasis, diplopia, papilledema

Respiratory: Apnea, respiratory depression, pulmonary edema

Signs and Symptoms of Overdose Anemia (megaloblastic), apnea, bezoars, dry skin, hypocalcemia, hyporeflexia, hypothermia, leukopenia or neutropenia (agranulocytosis, granulocytopenia)

Admission Criteria/Prognosis
Admit any patient with central nervous system depression, or adult ingestion >3 g.

Toxicodynamics/Kinetics
Protein binding: 50%
Metabolism: Hepatic to an active metabolite (4-hydroxy-2-ethyl-2-phenylglutarimide); significant enterohepatic recirculation
Half-life: 5-22 hours
Elimination: ~20% of the drug is normally excreted in 4 hours in a healthy person

Dosage Oral:
Adults: 250-500 mg at bedtime, dose may be repeated but not less than 4 hours before intended awakening; maximum: 1 g/day
Elderly/debilitated patients: Total daily dose should not exceed 500 mg

Contraindications Hypersensitivity to glutethimide; porphyria

Dosage Forms Tablet: 250 mg

Reference Range
Therapeutic: 2-6 mcg/mL
Toxic: >10 mcg/mL; fatalities have occurred with serum levels between 10-100 mcg/mL (average, 50 mcg/mL)

Overdosage/Treatment
Decontamination: Aggressively lavage within 1 hour (with water or castor oil in a 1:1 mixture)/activated charcoal (1 g for every 50 g of ingested drug)
Supportive therapy: Avoid overhydration, anticholinergic
Enhancement of elimination: Multiple dosing of activated charcoal is effective; hemoperfusion is effective in removing metabolite and is preferred over hemodialysis (which is only about half as effective as charcoal hemoperfusion in removing glutethimide); considerations for extracorporeal removal of drug include ingestions >10 g (or a serum level >6 mcg/mL), prolonged coma, flat line on EEG, or progressive systemic deterioration; do not alkalinize the urine; hemoperfusion clearance ranges from 60-250 mL/minute with 32% fractional removal of drug during 4 hours

Drug Interactions Decreased effect of anticoagulants

Pregnancy Risk Factor C

Pregnancy Implications Neonatal respiratory depression/apnea have been noted as have neonatal withdrawal from chronic maternal use

Additional Information Lethal dose: 10 g. Overdose symptoms occur at 3 g ingestion. Often ingested with acetaminophen and codeine ("Fours and Doors") Not available in U.S.

GlyBURIDE

CAS Number 10238-21-8
U.S. Brand Names Diaβeta®; Glynase® PresTab®; Micronase®
Synonyms Diabeta; Glibenclamide; Glybenclamide; Glybenzcyclamide
Use Management of noninsulin-dependent diabetes mellitus (type II)
Unlabeled/Investigational Use Alternative to insulin in women for the treatment of gestational diabetes (11-33 weeks gestation)
Mechanism of Action A sulfonylurea which stimulates insulin release from the pancreatic beta cells; reduces glucose output from the liver; insulin sensitivity is increased at peripheral target sites

Adverse Reactions
Cardiovascular: Sinus tachycardia, tachycardia (supraventricular), vasculitis
Central nervous system: **Headache**, ataxia, **dizziness**
Dermatologic: Pruritus, rash, photosensitivity, hives, bullous skin disease, purpura, psoriasis, photoallergy, exanthem
Endocrine & metabolic: Hypoglycemia (12-72 hours), syndrome of inappropriate antidiuretic hormone effect, hyperinsulinemia, exanthem
Gastrointestinal: **Nausea**, **epigastric fullness**, abdominal pain, **heartburn, constipation, diarrhea, anorexia**
Genitourinary: Nocturia
Hematologic: Thrombocytopenia, hemolysis, aplastic anemia, leukopenia, neutropenia, agranulocytosis, granulocytopenia, bone marrow suppression
Hepatic: Cholestatic jaundice, granulomatous hepatitis, intrahepatic cholestasis, jaundice
Neuromuscular & skeletal: Arthralgia, paresthesia
Ocular: Myopia, optic atrophy (infant), diplopia

Signs and Symptoms of Overdose Coagulopathy, diuresis, enuresis, eosinophilia, exfoliative dermatitis, hypoglycemia, hyponatremia, leukopenia or neutropenia (agranulocytosis, granulocytopenia), nocturia, photosensitivity

Admission Criteria/Prognosis Admit all intentional adult overdoses. Pediatric patients should be observed in a medical setting through an overnight sleep cycle (and for a minimum of 8 hours). No intravenous glucose or dextrose should be given prophylactically. Asymptomatic pediatric patients should have a blood glucose determination at 3-6 hours postingestion or immediately when symptoms (hunger, irritability,

lethargy, tremulousness, tachycardia, diaphoresis, or seizures) develop. Any borderline blood glucose reading (about 70 mg/dL) are repeated in one hour. Consider regular 2- to 3-hour interval blood glucose measurements during sleep. If no hypoglycemic events occur and prebreakfast blood glucose levels are normal, pediatric patients can be monitored by parental observation at home.

Pharmacodynamics/Kinetics
Onset of action: Serum insulin levels begin to increase 15-60 minutes after a single dose
Duration: ≤24 hours
Protein binding, plasma: >99%
Metabolism: To one moderately active and several inactive metabolites
Half-life elimination: 5-16 hours; may be prolonged with renal or hepatic impairment
Time to peak, serum: Adults: 2-4 hours
Excretion: Feces (50%) and urine (50%) as metabolites

Dosage Oral:
Adults: 1.25-5 mg to start then increase at weekly intervals to 1.25-20 mg maintenance dose/day divided in 1-2 doses
Elderly: Initial: 1.25-2.5 mg/day, increase by 1.25-2.5 mg/day every 1-3 weeks
PresTab™: Initial: 0.75-3 mg/day, increase by 1.5 mg/day in weekly intervals, maximum: 12 mg/day
Dosing adjustment/comments in renal impairment:
Cl_{cr} 10-50 mL/minute: Use conservative initial and maintenance doses
Cl_{cr} <10 mL/minute: Avoid use
Dosing adjustment in hepatic impairment: Use conservative initial and maintenance doses and avoid use in severe disease

Monitoring Parameters Signs and symptoms of hypoglycemia, fasting blood glucose, hemoglobin A_{1c}

Administration Administer with meals at the same time each day. Patients who are anorexic or NPO may need to have their dose held to avoid hypoglycemia.

Contraindications Hypersensitivity to glyburide, any component of the formulation, or other sulfonamides; type 1 diabetes mellitus (insulin dependent, IDDM), diabetic ketoacidosis with or without coma

Warnings
Elderly: Rapid and prolonged hypoglycemia (>12 hours) despite hypertonic glucose injections have been reported; age and hepatic and renal impairment are independent risk factors for hypoglycemia; dosage titration should be made at weekly intervals. Use with caution in patients with renal and hepatic impairment, malnourished or debilitated conditions, or adrenal or pituitary insufficiency.
Chemical similarities are present among sulfonamides, sulfonylureas, carbonic anhydrase inhibitors, thiazides, and loop diuretics (except ethacrynic acid). Use in patients with sulfonamide allergy is specifically contraindicated in product labeling, however, a risk of cross-reaction exists in patients with allergy to any of these compounds; avoid use when previous reaction has been severe.
Product labeling states oral hypoglycemic drugs may be associated with an increased cardiovascular mortality as compared to treatment with diet alone or diet plus insulin. Data to support this association are limited, and several studies, including a large prospective trial (UKPDS) have not supported an association.

Dosage Forms [DSC] = Discontinued product
Tablet (Diaβeta®, Micronase®): 1.25 mg, 2.5 mg, 5 mg
Tablet, micronized: 1.5 mg, 3 mg, 6 mg
Glynase® PresTab®: 1.5 mg [DSC], 3 mg, 6 mg

Reference Range Normal fasting glucose: Adults: 80-140 mg/dL; Elderly: 100-180 mg/dL
Therapeutic glyburide level: 40-50 ng/mL

Overdosage/Treatment
Decontamination: Lavage (within 1 hour)/activated charcoal
Supportive therapy: Glucose (25 g I.V.) is mainstay of therapy; glucagon (1-5 mg I.V., I.M., or SubQ) (0.03-0.1 mg/kg in pediatrics) will have limited benefit; diazoxide is a third-line agent (3-8 mg/kg/24 hours); octreotide (50 mcg SubQ every 12 hours) may be helpful in sulfonylurea overdose
For pediatric patients with profound sulfonylurea-induced hypoglycemia: Give 0.5 g of dextrose per kg of body weight (5 mL/kg of 10% dextrose concentration of intravenous fluid, 2 mL/kg of D_{25} or 1 mL/kg of D_{50}).
Enhancement of elimination: Multiple dosing of activated charcoal may be effective; peritoneal dialysis has been used with some success, but is not recommended as a routine procedure; urine alkalinization is also useful

Antidote(s)
- Dextrose [ANTIDOTE]
- Glucagon [ANTIDOTE]
- Octreotide [ANTIDOTE]

Diagnostic Procedures
- Electrolytes, Blood
- Glucose, Random

Drug Interactions **Inhibits** CYP2C8 (weak), 3A4 (weak)
Decreased effect: Thiazides may decrease effectiveness of glyburide

Increased effect: Possible interaction between glyburide and fluoroquinolone antibiotics has been reported resulting in a potentiation of hypoglycemic action of glyburide

Increased toxicity:

Since this agent is highly protein bound, the toxic potential is increased when given concomitantly with other highly protein bound drugs (ie, phenylbutazone, oral anticoagulants, hydantoins, salicylates, NSAIDs, beta-blockers, sulfonamides) - increase hypoglycemic effect

Ethanol increases disulfiram reactions

Phenylbutazone can increase hypoglycemic effects

Certain drugs tend to produce hyperglycemia and may lead to loss of control (ie, thiazides and other diuretics, corticosteroids, phenothiazines, thyroid products, estrogens, oral contraceptives, phenytoin, nicotinic acid, sympathomimetics, calcium channel blocking drugs, and isoniazid)

Possible interactions between glyburide and coumarin derivatives have been reported that may either potentiate or weaken the effects of coumarin derivatives

Pregnancy Risk Factor C

Pregnancy Implications Crosses the placenta. Hypoglycemia; ear defects reported; other malformations reported but may have been secondary to poor maternal glucose control/diabetes. Insulin is the drug of choice for the control of diabetes mellitus during pregnancy.

Lactation Does not enter breast milk/ use caution

Nursing Implications Monitor for signs and symptoms of hypoglycemia; patients who are anorexic or NPO, may need to have their dose held to avoid hypoglycemia

Additional Information More diuretic effect than chlorpropamide; glyburide-microsed dust may cause hypoglycemia by inhalation

Specific References

Alsop JA and Welch RA, "Incidence of Grandparent's Oral Hypoglycemic Medications as a Source of Pediatric Ingestions," *J Toxicol Clin Toxicol*, 2003, 41(5):649.

Calello D, Kelly A, and Osterhoudt KC, "Case Files of the Medical Toxicology Fellowship Training Program at the Childrens Hospital of Philadelphia: A Pediatric Exploratory Sulfonylurea Ingestion," *J Med Toxicol*, 2006, 2(1):19-26.

Chin RL, "Oral Hypoglycemics Sold as Valium on the Streets: A Case Report," *Ann Emerg Med*, 2004, 44(5):552.

Johnson KK, Green DL, Rife JP, et al, "Sulfonamide Cross-Reactivity: Fact or Fiction?" *Ann Pharmacother*, 2005, 39(2):290-301.

Kent DA, Main BA, and Friesen MS, "Use of Octreotide in Sulfonylurea Poisoning in a Child," *J Toxicol Clin Toxicol*, 2003, 41(5):669.

Roberge R, Comment on "Refractory Hypoglycemia from Ciprofloxacin and Glyburide Interaction," *Clin Toxicol (Phila)*, 2005, 43(3):213-4.

Glycerin

CAS Number 56-81-5

U.S. Brand Names Bausch & Lomb® Computer Eye Drops [OTC]; Fleet® Babylax® [OTC]; Fleet® Glycerin Suppositories Maximum Strength [OTC]; Fleet® Glycerin Suppositories [OTC]; Fleet® Liquid Glycerin Suppositories [OTC]; Osmoglyn®; Sani-Supp® [OTC]

Synonyms Glycerol

Use Constipation; reduction of intraocular pressure; reduction of corneal edema; glycerin has been administered orally to reduce intracranial pressure

Mechanism of Action Osmotic dehydrating agent which increases osmotic pressure; draws fluid into colon and thus stimulates evacuation

Adverse Reactions

Cardiovascular: Arrhythmias

Central nervous system: **Headache**, dizziness, confusion, amnesia, pain

Endocrine & metabolic: Polydipsia, hyperglycemia

Gastrointestinal: **Vomiting**, diarrhea, nausea, tenesmus, xerostomia

Hematologic: Hemolytic anemia

Local: Rectal irritation, burning, cramping pain

Otic: Temporary hearing loss

Renal: Renal failure secondary to hemolysis, proteinuria

Miscellaneous: Thirst

Pharmacodynamics/Kinetics

Onset of action:

Decrease in intraocular pressure: Oral: 10-30 minutes

Reduction of intracranial pressure: Oral: 10-60 minutes

Constipation: Suppository: 15-30 minutes

Peak effect:

Decrease in intraocular pressure: Oral: 60-90 minutes

Reduction of intracranial pressure: Oral: 60-90 minutes

Duration:

Decrease in intraocular pressure: Oral: 4-8 hours

Reduction of intracranial pressure: Oral: ~2-3 hours

Absorption: Oral: Well absorbed; Rectal: Poorly absorbed

Half-life elimination, serum: 30-45 minutes

Dosage Constipation: Rectal:

Neonates: 0.5 mL/kg/dose

Children <6 years: 1 infant suppository 1-2 times/day as needed or 2-5 mL as an enema

Children >6 years and Adults: 1 adult suppository 1-2 times/day as needed or 5-15 mL as an enema

Children and Adults:

Oral: Maximum daily dose: 120 mg

Reduction of intraocular pressure: 1-1.8 g/kg 1-1$^1/_2$ hours preoperatively; additional doses may be administered at 5-hour intervals

Reduction of intracranial pressure: 1.5 g/kg/day divided every 4 hours; 1 g/kg/dose every 6 hours has also been used

Ophthalmic solution: Reduction of corneal edema: Instill 1-2 drops in eye(s) prior to examination OR for lubricant effect, instill 1-2 drops in eye(s) every 3-4 hours

Stability Refrigerate suppositories; protect from heat; freezing should be avoided

Ophthalmic: Keep bottle tightly closed; store at room temperature; discard 6 months after dropper is first placed in the solution

Administration Oral: Orange or lemon juice may be added to unflavored 50% oral solution; pour solution over crushed ice and drink through a straw to improve palatability; headache can be minimized by having the patient lie down during and after administration

Rectal: Inset suppository high in the rectum and retain 15 minutes

Dosage Forms [DSC] = Discontinued product

Solution, ophthalmic, sterile (Bausch & Lomb® Computer Eye Drops): 1% (15 mL) [contains benzalkonium chloride]

Solution, oral (Osmoglyn®): 50% (220 mL) [lime flavor] [DSC]

Solution, rectal:

Fleet® Babylax®: 2.3 g/2.3 mL (4 mL) [6 units per box]

Fleet® Liquid Glycerin Suppositories: 5.6 g/5.5 mL (7.5 mL) [4 units per box]

Suppository, rectal: 82.5% (12s, 25s) [pediatric size]; 82.5% (12s, 24s, 25s, 50s, 100s) [adult size]

Colace® Adult/Children: 2.1 g (12s, 24s, 48s, 100s)

Colace® Infant/Children: 1.2 g (12s, 24s)

Fleet® Glycerin Suppositories: 1 g (12s) [pediatric size]; 2g (12s, 24s, 50s) [adult size]

Fleet® Glycerin Suppositories Maximum Strength: 3g (18s) [adult size]

Sani-Supp®: 82.5% (10s, 25s) [pediatric size]; 82.5% (10s, 25s, 50s) [adult size]

Reference Range 1-1.3 g/kg oral dose results in plasma glycerin levels of 1.45 mg/mL

Overdosage/Treatment

Decontamination: **Oral**: Lavage (within 1 hour)/activated charcoal. **Ocular**: Irrigate with copious amounts of saline

Supportive therapy: Monitor serum electrolytes; replace fluids and electrolytes

Pregnancy Risk Factor C

Nursing Implications Apply topical anesthetic before instilling ophthalmic drops. Use caution during insertion of suppository to avoid intestinal perforation, especially in neonates; suppository needs to melt to provide laxative effect; primary use of glycerin in the elderly is as a laxative, although it is not recommended as a first-line treatment.

Gold Compounds

CAS Number 7440-57-5

Synonyms Auranofin; Aurothioglucose; Gold Sodium Thiomalate; Sodium Aurothiomalate

Use Metallic use in dentistry; food coloring agent; auric drug used for treatment of progressive rheumatoid arthritis; adjunctive treatment in adult and juvenile active rheumatoid arthritis; alternative or adjunct in treatment of pemphigus; psoriatic patients who do not respond to NSAIDs

Mechanism of Action May inhibit phagocytosis and lysosomal enzyme

Adverse Reactions

Cardiovascular: Flushing, sinus tachycardia, arrhythmias (ventricular), vasculitis

Central nervous system: Gustatory hallucinations, axonopathy

Dermatologic: Pruritus, hypersensitivity, alopecia, dermal eruption, rash, photosensitivity/phototoxicity, toxic epidermal necrolysis, exfoliative dermatitis, erythema, pemphigus, chrysiasis (total dose ~1 g), pityriasis rosea-like reaction, discoid eczema, erythema annulare centri fugum, acne, angioedema, xerosis, urticaria, purpura, erythema nodosum, exanthem, cutaneous vasculitis

Endocrine & metabolic: Gynecomastia

Gastrointestinal: Nausea, vomiting, diarrhea, gingivitis, loss of taste perception, aphthous stomatitis

Hematologic: Thrombocytopenia, eosinophilia, leukopenia, anemia, red blood cell aplasia

Hepatic: Cholestatic jaundice, hepatitis, hepatic necrosis in overdose situation, cholestatic hepatitis

Neuromuscular & skeletal: Paresthesia

Ocular: Corneal crystalline deposits that usually do not affect vision, iritis

Renal: Proteinuria (17%), tubular necrosis (acute), interstitial nephritis (oral gold is less nephrotoxic than parenteral gold administration), glomerulonephritis, nephrotic syndrome (2.6% to 5.3%)

Respiratory: Wheezing, cough, interstitial lung disease, bronchiolitis obliterans, interstitial pulmonary fibrosis, eosinophilic pneumonia

Miscellaneous: Drug-induced SLE, fixed drug eruption, elevated antineutrophilic cytoplasmic antibodies (ANCA)

Signs and Symptoms of Overdose Agranulocytosis, bleeding, blood dyscrasias, cataract, crystalluria, dementia, dysosmia, eosinophilia, feces discoloration (yellow-green), granulocytopenia, hematuria, leukopenia, lichenoid eruptions, metallic taste, pancreatitis, pemphigus, periarteritis nodosa, photosensitivity, nephrotic syndrome, neutropenia, nystagmus, toxic epidermal necrolysis, ventricular tachycardia, wheezing

Pharmacodynamics/Kinetics

Distribution: V_d: 0.1 L/kg

Protein binding: 95%

Half-life: 5-16 days

Elimination: Normal urinary excretion is 0.1-1 mg/day; 10% to 40% excreted by feces

Dosage

Auranofin: Oral:

Children: Initial: 0.1 mg/kg/day divided daily; usual maintenance: 0.15 mg/kg/day in 1-2 divided doses; maximum: 0.2 mg/kg/day in 1-2 divided doses

Adults: 6 mg/day in 1-2 divided doses; after 3 months may be increased to 9 mg/day in 3 divided doses; if still no response after 3 months at 9 mg/day, discontinue drug

Aurothioglucose: I.M.: Doses should initially be given at weekly intervals

Children 6-12 years: Initial: 0.25 mg/kg/dose first week; increment at 0.25 mg/kg/dose increasing with each weekly dose; maintenance: 0.75-1 mg/kg/dose weekly not to exceed 25 mg/dose to a total of 20 doses, then every 2-4 weeks

Adults: 10 mg first week; 25 mg second and third week; then 50 mg/week until 800 mg to 1 g cumulative dose has been given; if improvement occurs without adverse reactions, give 25-50 mg every 2-3 weeks, then every 3-4 weeks

Gold sodium thiomalate: I.M.:

Children: Initial: Test dose of 10 mg is recommended, followed by 1 mg/kg/week for 20 weeks; maintenance: 1 mg/kg/dose at 2- to 4-week intervals thereafter for as long as therapy is clinically beneficial and toxicity does not develop. Administration for 2-4 months is usually required before clinical improvement is observed.

Adults: 10 mg first week; 25 mg second week; then 25-50 mg/week until 1 g cumulative dose has been given; if improvement occurs without adverse reactions, give 25-50 mg every 2-3 weeks for 2-20 weeks, then every 3-4 weeks indefinitely

Monitoring Parameters CBC, liver function tests, renal function

Dosage Forms Capsule (Auranofin [Ridaura®]): 3 mg [gold 29%]

Injection (Gold Sodium Thiomalate [Myochrysine® Injection]): 25 mg/mL (1 mL); 50 mg/mL (1 mL, 10 mL)

Suspension, sterile (Aurothioglucose [Solganal®]): 50 mg/mL [gold 50%] (10 mL)

Reference Range

Gold: Normal: 0-0.1 mcg/mL (SI: 0-0.0064 μmol/L); Therapeutic: 1-3 mcg/mL (SI: 0.06-0.18 μmol/L)

Urine: <0.1 mcg/24 hours

Peak serum gold levels after a 50 mg injection: 6-8 mg/L; after a 450 mg I.M. injection: 29.7 mg/L

Overdosage/Treatment

Decontamination: Emesis within 30 minutes or lavage (within 1 hour)/activated charcoal

Supportive therapy: For thrombocytopenia refractory to chelation therapy, cyclophosphamide (100 mg/day for 6 months or until platelet count was >100,000 with subsequent reduction of dose to 75 mg/day) can be utilized; high-dose I.V. N-acetylcysteine may be useful to treat hematologic toxicity due to gold (2-9 g in 100 mL of $D_5^{1}/_2NS$ over 2-6 hours, total dose: 13-153 g); chrysiasis can be treated with corticosteroids (systemically) and topical 2% solution of hydroquinone; gold-induced pulmonary disease should be treated with prednisone (30-60 mg/day); agranulocytosis can be treated with SubQ granulocyte-colony stimulating factor (5 mcg/kg/day)

Enhancement of elimination: Chelation with BAL (dimercaprol) or D-penicillamine (250 mg 4 times/day for 11 days) can increase elimination; hemodialysis is not useful

Antidote(s)
- Dimercaprol [ANTIDOTE]
- Penicillamine [ANTIDOTE]

Diagnostic Procedures
- Gold Level

Pregnancy Risk Factor C

Pregnancy Implications Teratogenic in animals; not proven to be teratogenic in humans; not compatible for breast-feeding since it is excreted in breast milk

Additional Information Mean cumulative dose of gold for gold-induced thrombocytopenia is 840 mg. HLA-DR3 positive individuals exhibit an 8.9 times increased risk of thrombocytopenia and a 32 times increased risk of proteinuria

Granisetron

CAS Number 109889-09-0

U.S. Brand Names Kytril®

Synonyms BRL 43694

Use

Prophylaxis of chemotherapy-related emesis; prophylaxis of nausea and vomiting associated with radiation therapy, including total body irradiation and fractionated abdominal radiation; prophylaxis of postoperative nausea and vomiting (PONV)

Generally **not** recommended for treatment of existing chemotherapy-induced emesis (CIE) or for prophylaxis of nausea from agents with a low emetogenic potential.

Mechanism of Action Selective 5-HT$_3$ receptor antagonist, blocking serotonin, both peripherally on vagal nerve terminals and centrally in the chemoreceptor trigger zone

Adverse Reactions

Cardiovascular: Transient blood pressure changes

Central nervous system: Agitation, **headache**, fever, insomnia, somnolence, extrapyramidal reactions

Endocrine & metabolic: Hot flashes

Gastrointestinal: Constipation, diarrhea, pancreatitis

Hepatic: Liver enzyme elevations

Neuromuscular & skeletal: Weakness

Signs and Symptoms of Overdose Myalgia, somnolence

Pharmacodynamics/Kinetics

Duration: Generally up to 24 hours

Absorption: Tablets and oral solution are bioequivalent

Distribution: V_d: 2-4 L/kg; widely throughout body

Protein binding: 65%

Metabolism: Hepatic via N-demethylation, oxidation, and conjugation; some metabolites may have 5-HT$_3$ antagonist activity

Half-life elimination: Terminal: 5-9 hours

Excretion: Urine (12% as unchanged drug, 48% to 49% as metabolites); feces (34% to 38% as metabolites)

Dosage

Oral: Adults:

Prophylaxis of chemotherapy-related emesis: 2 mg once daily up to 1 hour before chemotherapy or 1 mg twice daily; the first 1 mg dose should be given up to 1 hour before chemotherapy.

Prophylaxis of radiation therapy-associated emesis: 2 mg once daily given 1 hour before radiation therapy.

I.V.:

Children ≥2 years and Adults: Prophylaxis of chemotherapy-related emesis:

Within U.S.: 10 mcg/kg/dose (or 1 mg/dose) administered IVPB over 5 minutes given within 30 minutes of chemotherapy: for some drugs (eg, carboplatin, cyclophosphamide) with a later onset of emetic action, 10 mcg/kg every 12 hours may be necessary.

Outside U.S.: 40 mcg/kg/dose (or 3 mg/dose); maximum: 9 mg/24 hours

Breakthrough: Repeat the dose 2-3 times within the first 24 hours as necessary **(not based on controlled trials, or generally recommended)**

Adults: PONV:

Prevention: 1 mg given undiluted over 30 seconds; administer before induction of anesthesia or before reversal of anesthesia

Treatment: 1 mg given undiluted over 30 seconds

Dosing interval in renal impairment: No dosage adjustment required.

Dosing interval in hepatic impairment: Kinetic studies in patients with hepatic impairment showed that total clearance was approximately halved, however, standard doses were very well tolerated

Monitoring Parameters Liver function tests

Administration Oral: Doses should be given up to 1 hour prior to initiation of chemotherapy/radiation

I.V.: Administer as rapid (30 second) I.V. push or a short (5-10 minutes) infusion

For prevention of PONV, administer before induction of anesthesia or before reversal of anesthesia.

For PONV, administer undiluted over 30 seconds.

Contraindications Previous hypersensitivity to granisetron, other 5-HT$_3$ receptor antagonists, or any component of the formulation

Warnings

Chemotherapy-related emesis: **Granisetron should be used on a scheduled basis, not on an "as needed" (PRN) basis**, since data support the use of this drug in the prevention of nausea and vomiting and not in the rescue of nausea and vomiting. Granisetron should be used only in the first 24-48 hours of receiving chemotherapy or radiation. Data do not support any increased efficacy of granisetron in delayed nausea and vomiting. May be prescribed for patients who are refractory to or have severe adverse reactions to standard antiemetic therapy or young patients (ie, <45 years of age who are more likely to develop extrapyramidal symptoms to high-dose metoclopramide) who are to receive highly emetogenic chemotherapeutic agents. Should not be prescribed for chemotherapeutic agents with a low emetogenic potential (eg, bleomycin, busulfan, etoposide, 5-fluorouracil, vinblastine, vincristine).

Routine prophylaxis for PONV is not recommended. In patients where nausea and vomiting must be avoided postoperatively, administer to all patients even when expected incidence of nausea and vomiting is low. Use caution following abdominal surgery or in chemotherapy-induced nausea and vomiting; may mask progressive ileus or gastric distention. Use caution in patients with liver disease or in pregnancy. Safety and efficacy in children <2 years of age have not been established. Injection contains benzyl alcohol (1 mg/mL) and should not be used in neonates.

Dosage Forms Injection, solution: 1 mg/mL (1 mL, 4 mL) [contains benzyl alcohol]

Injection, solution [preservative free]: 0.1 mg/mL (1 mL)

Solution, oral: 2 mg/10 mL (30 mL) [contains sodium benzoate; orange flavor]

Tablet: 1 mg

Reference Range Peak serum levels: 11-124 ng/mL following a 40 mcg/kg dose

Overdosage/Treatment

Decontamination: Lavage (within 1 hour)/activated charcoal

Enhancement of elimination: Multiple dosing of activated charcoal may be effective

Drug Interactions Substrate of CYP3A4 (minor)

Apomorphine: Due to reports of profound hypotension during concomitant therapy with other 5-HT3 antagonists, the manufacturer of apomorphine contraindicates its use with granisetron.

Pregnancy Risk Factor B

Pregnancy Implications There are no adequate or well-controlled studies in pregnant women. Teratogenic effects were not observed in animal studies. Injection (1 mg/mL strength) contains benzyl alcohol which may cross the placenta. Use only if benefit exceeds the risk.

Lactation Excretion in breast milk unknown/use caution

Nursing Implications Doses should be given at least 15 minutes prior to initiation of chemotherapy

Additional Information Granisetron (10 mcg/kg I.V.) can decrease nausea and emesis associated with activated charcoal/sorbitol administration; granisetron (3 mg I.V.) is effective when used with dexamethasone to prevent emesis due to chemotherapy

Griseofulvin

Related Information

• Therapeutic Drugs Associated with Hallucinations

CAS Number 126-07-8

U.S. Brand Names Fulvicin-U/F®; Fulvicin® P/G; Grifulvin® V; Gris-PEG®

Synonyms Griseofulvin Microsize; Griseofulvin Ultramicrosize

Use Treatment of susceptible tinea infections of the skin, hair, and nails

Mechanism of Action Inhibits fungal cell mitosis at metaphase; binds to human keratin making it resistant to fungal invasion

Adverse Reactions

Central nervous system: Headache, fatigue, dizziness, insomnia, mental confusion

Dermatologic: Rash (most common), urticaria (most common), photosensitivity, erythema multiforme, angioneurotic edema (rare)

Gastrointestinal: Nausea, vomiting, epigastric distress, diarrhea, GI bleeding

Genitourinary: Menstrual irregularities (rare)

Hematologic: Leukopenia, granulocytopenia

Neuromuscular & skeletal: Paresthesia (rare)

Renal: Hepatotoxicity, proteinuria, nephrosis

Miscellaneous: Oral thrush, drug-induced lupus-like syndrome (rare)

Signs and Symptoms of Overdose Cholestatic jaundice, depression, erythema multiforme, leukopenia or neutropenia (agranulocytosis, granulocytopenia), insomnia, photosensitivity, toxic epidermal necrolysis, vision color changes (green tinge); porphyrinogenic

Pharmacodynamics/Kinetics

Absorption: Ultramicrosize griseofulvin absorption is almost complete; absorption of microsize griseofulvin is variable (25% to 70% of an oral dose); enhanced by ingestion of a fatty meal (GI absorption of ultramicrosize is ~1.5 times that of microsize)

Distribution: Crosses placenta

Metabolism: Extensively hepatic

Half-life elimination: 9-22 hours

Excretion: Urine (<1% as unchanged drug); feces; perspiration

Dosage

Oral:

Children >2 years:

Microsize: 10-20 mg/kg/day in single or 2 divided doses

Ultramicrosize: >2 years: 5-10 mg/kg/day in single or 2 divided doses

Adults:

Microsize: 500-1000 mg/day in single or divided doses

Ultramicrosize: 330-375 mg/day in single or divided doses; doses up to 750 mg/day have been used for infections more difficult to eradicate such as tinea unguium

Duration of therapy depends on the site of infection:

Tinea corporis: 2-4 weeks

Tinea capitis: 4-6 weeks or longer

Tinea pedis: 4-8 weeks

Tinea unguium: 3-6 months or longer

Monitoring Parameters Periodic renal, hepatic, and hematopoietic function tests

Administration Oral: Administer with a fatty meal (peanuts or ice cream) to increase absorption, or with food or milk to avoid GI upset

Contraindications Hypersensitivity to griseofulvin or any component of the formulation; severe liver disease; porphyria (interferes with porphyrin metabolism)

Warnings Safe use in children ≤2 years of age has not been established; during long-term therapy, periodic assessment of hepatic, renal, and hematopoietic functions should be performed; may cause fetal harm when administered to pregnant women; avoid exposure to intense sunlight to prevent photosensitivity reactions; hypersensitivity cross reaction between penicillins and griseofulvin is possible

Dosage Forms

Suspension, oral, microsize (Grifulvin® V): 125 mg/5 mL (120 mL) [contains alcohol 0.2%]

Tablet, microsize (Grifulvin® V): 500 mg

Tablet, ultramicrosize: 125 mg, 250 mg, 330 mg

Gris-PEG®: 125 mg, 250 mg

Reference Range Peak plasma griseofulvin level of 1 mcg/mL after a 500 mg dose

Overdosage/Treatment

Decontamination: Lavage (within 1 hour)/activated charcoal

Supportive therapy: For treatment of lingua villosa nigra, discontinue causative agent. Clean the tongue with a toothbrush and rinse mouth with a half-strength solution of hydrogen peroxide or 10% carbamide peroxide. Symptoms should subside in a few days.

Enhancement of elimination: Multiple dosing of activated charcoal may be effective

Test Interactions False-positive urinary VMA levels

Drug Interactions Induces CYP1A2 (weak), 2C8 (weak), 2C9 (weak), 3A4 (weak)

Decreased effect:

Barbiturates may decrease levels of griseofulvin

Decreased warfarin, cyclosporine, and salicylate activity with griseofulvin

Griseofulvin decreases oral contraceptive effectiveness

Increased toxicity: With ethanol, may cause tachycardia and flushing

Pregnancy Risk Factor C

Lactation Excretion in breast milk unknown

Additional Information Microsize: Fulvicin-U/F®, Grifulvin® V, Grisactin®: 66% effective for treating pediatric tinea capitus

Ultramicrosize: Fulvicin® P/G, Grisactin® Ultra, Gris-PEG®; gastrointestinal absorption of ultramicrosize is ~1.5 times that of microsize

Specific References

Colton RL, Amir J, Mimouni M, et al, "Serum Sickness-Like Reaction Associated with Griseofulvin," *Ann Pharmacother*, 2004, 38(4):609-11. Epub 2004 Feb 24.

Guaifenesin

CAS Number 93-14-1

U.S. Brand Names Allfen Jr; Amibid LA [DSC]; Diabetic Tussin® EX [OTC]; Ganidin NR; Guiatuss™ [OTC]; Humibid® LA [DSC]; Humibid® Pediatric [DSC]; Iophen NR; Liquibid® 1200 [DSC]; Liquibid® [DSC]; Mucinex® [OTC]; Naldecon Senior EX® [OTC]; Organ-1 NR; Organidin® NR; Phanasin [OTC]; Phanasin® Diabetic Choice [OTC]; Q-Tussin [OTC]; Respa-GF® [DSC]; Robitussin® [OTC]; Scot-Tussin® Expectorant [OTC]; Siltussin DAS [OTC]; Siltussin SA [OTC]; Touro Ex® [DSC]; Tussin [OTC]

Synonyms GG; Glyceryl Guaiacolate

Use Help loosen phlegm and thin bronchial secretions to make coughs more productive

Mechanism of Action Thought to act as an expectorant by irritating the gastric mucosa and stimulating respiratory tract secretions, thereby increasing respiratory fluid volumes and decreasing phlegm viscosity

Adverse Reactions

Frequency not defined.

Central nervous system: Dizziness, drowsiness, headache

Dermatologic: Rash

Endocrine & metabolic: Uric acid levels decreased

Gastrointestinal: Nausea, vomiting, stomach pain

Renal: Kidney stone formation (with consumption of large quantities)

Signs and Symptoms of Overdose Coma, lethargy, nausea, respiratory depression, vomiting

Pharmacodynamics/Kinetics
Absorption: Well absorbed
Half-life elimination: ~1 hour
Excretion: Urine (as unchanged drug and metabolites)

Dosage
Oral:
Children:
6 months to 2 years: 25-50 mg every 4 hours, not to exceed 300 mg/day
2-5 years: 50-100 mg every 4 hours, not to exceed 600 mg/day
6-11 years: 100-200 mg every 4 hours, not to exceed 1.2 g/day
Children >12 years and Adults: 200-400 mg every 4 hours to a maximum of 2.4 g/day
Extended release tablet: 600-1200 mg every 12 hours, not to exceed 2.4 g/day

Monitoring Parameters Cough, sputum consistency and volume

Administration Do not crush, chew, or break extended release tablets; administer with a full glass of water

Contraindications Hypersensitivity to guaifenesin or any component of the formulation

Warnings Not for persistent cough such as occurs with smoking, asthma, chronic bronchitis, or emphysema or cough accompanied by excessive secretions. When used for self-medication (OTC), contact healthcare provider if needed for >7 days or for a cough with a fever, rash, or persistent headache.

Dosage Forms [DSC] = Discontinued product
Liquid: 100 mg/5 mL (120 mL, 480 mL)
Diabetic Tussin EX®: 100 mg/5 mL (120 mL) [alcohol free, sugar free, dye free; contains phenylalanine 8.4 mg/5 mL]
Ganidin NR: 100 mg/5 mL (480 mL) [raspberry flavor]
Iophen NR: 100 mg/5 mL (480 mL)
Organidin® NR: 100 mg/5 mL (480 mL) [contains sodium benzoate; raspberry flavor]
Q-Tussin: 100 mg/5 mL (120 mL, 240 mL, 480 mL, 3840 mL) [alcohol free; cherry flavor]
Siltussin DAS: 100 mg/5 mL (120 mL) [alcohol free, dye free, sugar free; strawberry flavor]
Syrup: 100 mg/5 mL (120 mL, 480 mL)
Guiatuss™: 100 mg/5 mL (120 mL, 480 mL) [alcohol free; fruit-mint flavor]
Phanasin®: 100 mg/5 mL (120 mL, 240 mL) [alcohol free, sugar free; mint flavor]
Phanasin® Diabetic Choice: 100 mg/5 mL (120 mL) [alcohol free, sugar free; mint flavor]
Robitussin®: 100 mg/5 mL (5 mL, 10 mL, 15 mL, 30 mL, 120 mL, 240 mL, 480 mL) [alcohol free; contains sodium benzoate]
Scot-Tussin® Expectorant: 100 mg/5 mL (120 mL) [alcohol free, dye free, sugar free; contains benzoic acid; grape flavor]
Siltussin SA: 100 mg/5 mL (120 mL, 240 mL, 480 mL) [alcohol free, sugar free; strawberry flavor]
Tussin: 100 mg/5 mL (120 mL, 240 mL)
Vicks® Casero™: 100 mg/6.25 mL (120 mL, 480 mL) [contains phenylalanine 5.5 mg/12.5 mL, sodium 32 mg/12.5 mL, and sodium benzoate; honey menthol flavor]
Syrup, oral drops (Phanasin®): 50 mg/mL (50 mL) [alcohol free, sugar free; fruit flavor]
Tablet: 200 mg
Allfen Jr: 400 mg [dye free]
Humibid® e: 400 mg [DSC]
Organ-1 NR, Organidin® NR: 200 mg
XPECT™: 400 mg
Tablet, extended release:
Humibid® Maximum Strength: 1200 mg
Mucinex®: 600 mg

Reference Range 600 mg oral dose results in a peak guaifenesin blood level of 1.4 mg/L

Overdosage/Treatment
Decontamination: Lavage (within 1 hour)/activated charcoal
Enhancement of elimination: Multiple dosing of activated charcoal may be effective

Test Interactions Possible color interference with determination of 5-HIAA and VMA; ↓ serum uric acid (uricosuric)

Pregnancy Risk Factor C

Lactation Excretion in breast milk unknown/use caution

Guanabenz

CAS Number 23256-50-0; 5051-62-7
U.S. Brand Names Wytensin® [DSC]
Synonyms Guanabenz Acetate
Impairment Potential Yes
Use Management of mild to moderate hypertension

Mechanism of Action Stimulates alpha$_2$-adrenoreceptors in the brain stem, thus activating an inhibitory neuron, resulting in reduced sympathetic outflow, producing a decrease in vasomotor tone and heart rate

Adverse Reactions
Cardiovascular: Bradycardia, chest pain, sinus bradycardia, angina, palpitations, vasodilation
Central nervous system: **Drowsiness, dizziness**, hypothermia, headache
Gastrointestinal: Nausea, **xerostomia**
Neuromuscular & skeletal: **Weakness**
Ocular: Miosis

Signs and Symptoms of Overdose Apnea, bradycardia, CNS depression, depression, diarrhea, drowsiness, dyspnea, gynecomastia, hyperglycemia, hypoglycemia, hypotension, hypothermia, impotence, miosis, myalgia

Pharmacodynamics/Kinetics
Onset of action: Antihypertensive effects occur within 60 minutes
Duration: 12 hours
Absorption: Oral: ~75% from gastrointestinal tract
Distribution: V$_d$: 7.4-17 L/kg; widely distributed into body
Protein binding: 90%
Metabolism: Extensive
Bioavailability: Very low because of extensive first-pass metabolism
Half-life: 7-10 hours
Time to peak serum concentration: 2-5 hours
Elimination: <1% excreted as unchanged drug in urine

Dosage
Adults: Oral: Initial: 4 mg twice daily, increase in increments of 4-8 mg/day every 1-2 weeks to a maximum of 32 mg twice daily
Dosing adjustment in hepatic impairment: Probably necessary

Stability Protect from light

Monitoring Parameters Blood pressure, standing and sitting/supine

Contraindications Hypersensitivity to guanabenz or any component of the formulation

Warnings Use with caution in severe hepatic or renal failure. Avoid in pregnancy and breast-feeding. Safety and efficacy for use in children <12 years of age have not been demonstrated. Use with caution in patients with severe coronary insufficiency, recent MI or cerebrovascular disease. Abrupt discontinuation can result in rebound hypertension. Avoid use in CNS disease, elderly or with other CNS depressants (can cause sedation and drowsiness alone). May cause significant orthostasis.

Dosage Forms Tablet: 4 mg, 8 mg

Overdosage/Treatment
Decontamination: Ipecac within 30 minutes or lavage (within 1 hour)/activated charcoal
Supportive therapy: Hypotension usually responds to I.V. fluids or Trendelenburg positioning. If unresponsive to these measures, the use of a parenteral vasoconstrictor may be required (eg, norepinephrine 0.1-0.2 mcg/kg/minute titrated to response). Naloxone may be utilized in treating the hypotension, CNS depression, and/or apnea and should be given I.V. 0.4-2 mg, with repeats as needed. Atropine 15 mcg/kg I.V. or I.M. may be needed for symptomatic bradycardia.
Enhancement of elimination: Multiple dosing of activated charcoal would not be useful; hemodialysis is not useful

Test Interactions ↑ sodium (S)

Drug Interactions Substrate of CYP1A2 (major)
CYP1A2 inducers: May decrease the levels/effects of guanabenz. Example inducers include aminoglutethimide, carbamazepine, phenobarbital, and rifampin.
CYP1A2 inhibitors: May increase the levels/effects of guanabenz. Example inhibitors include ciprofloxacin, fluvoxamine, ketoconazole, norfloxacin, ofloxacin, and rofecoxib.
Hypoglycemic symptoms may be reduced. Educate patient about decreased signs and symptoms of hypoglycemia or avoid use in patients with frequent episodes of hypoglycemia.
Nitroprusside and guanabenz have additive hypotensive effects.
Noncardioselective beta-blockers (nadolol, propranolol, timolol) may exacerbate rebound hypertension when guanabenz is withdrawn. The beta-blocker should be withdrawn first. The gradual withdrawal of guanabenz or a cardioselective beta-blocker could be substituted.
TCAs decrease the hypotensive effect of guanabenz.

Pregnancy Risk Factor C

Additional Information Guanabenz is considered an alternate to clonidine; it causes less sodium retention than clonidine or methyldopa.

Guanadrel

CAS Number 22195-34-2; 40580-59-4
U.S. Brand Names Hylorel®
Synonyms Guanadrel Sulfate
Impairment Potential Yes
Use Step 2 agent in stepped-care treatment of hypertension, usually with a diuretic

Mechanism of Action Acts as a false neurotransmitter that blocks the adrenergic actions of norepinephrine; it displaces norepinephrine form its presynaptic storage granules and thus exposes it to degradation; it thereby produces a reduction in total peripheral resistance and therefore blood pressure

Adverse Reactions

Cardiovascular: Hypotension (orthostatic), **palpitations, chest pain**, angina, **peripheral edema**

Central nervous system: **Fatigue**, dizziness, **headache, faintness, drowsiness, confusion**

Gastrointestinal: Diarrhea, **increased bowel movements, constipation, gas pain, anorexia, weight gain or loss**

Genitourinary: **Ejaculatory disturbances, nocturia**

Neuromuscular & skeletal: Weakness, **paresthesia, aching limbs, leg cramps, backache, arthralgia**

Ocular: Blurred vision, **visual disturbances**

Renal: **Polyuria**

Respiratory: **Dyspnea, coughing**

Signs and Symptoms of Overdose Blurred vision, ejaculatory disturbances, dizziness, hypotension, nausea, nocturia, vomiting

Pharmacodynamics/Kinetics

Onset of action: Peak effect: 4-6 hours

Duration: 4-14 hours

Absorption: Rapid

Half-life elimination, serum: Biphasic: Initial: 1-4 hours; Terminal: 5-45 hours

Time to peak, serum: 1.5-2 hours

Dosage Adults: Oral: Initial: 10 mg/day (5 mg twice daily); adjust dosage until blood pressure is controlled, usual dosage: 20-75 mg/day, given twice daily

Dosing in renal impairment:

Cl_{cr} 10-50 mL/minute: Administer every 12-24 hours

Cl_{cr} <10 mL/minute: Administer every 24-48 hours

Monitoring Parameters Blood pressure, standing and sitting/supine

Contraindications Hypersensitivity to guanadrel or any component of the formulation; known or suspected pheochromocytoma; concurrent use or within 1 week of any MAO inhibitor; exacerbation of CHF

Warnings Orthostatic hypotension is common. Avoid using other drugs that cause orthostatic hypotension (alpha-blocking agents or reserpine). Discontinue 48-72 hours before elective surgery (reduces potential for vascular collapse). If emergency surgery required, notify anesthesiologist of the drug regimen. Avoid using tricyclic antidepressants and indirect-acting sympathomimetics (can reverse the blood pressure lowering effects). Use cautiously in asthma (may aggravate condition), CHF (sodium and water retention), and PUD (may aggravate condition). Safety and efficacy have not been established in pediatric patients. Dosage adjustment required with renal dysfunction.

Dosage Forms Tablet, as sulfate: 10 mg, 25 mg

Overdosage/Treatment

Decontamination: Ipecac within 30 minutes or lavage (within 1 hour)/ activated charcoal

Supportive therapy: Hypotension usually responds to I.V. fluids or Trendelenburg positioning. If unresponsive to these measures, the use of a parenteral vasoconstrictor may be required (eg, dopamine 2-5 mcg/kg/minute titrated to 10 mcg/kg/minute). Naloxone may be utilized in treating hypotension, CNS depression, and/or apnea and should be given I.V. 0.4-2 mg, with repeats as needed. Atropine 15 mcg/kg I.V. or I.M. may be needed for symptomatic bradycardia.

Enhancement of elimination: Multiple dosing of activated charcoal may be effective

Test Interactions ↑ sodium (S)

Drug Interactions TCAs decrease hypotensive effect of guanadrel.

Increased toxicity of direct-acting amines (epinephrine, norepinephrine) by guanadrel; the hypotensive effect of guanadrel may be potentiated. Increased effect of beta-blockers, vasodilators.

Phenothiazines may inhibit the antihypertensive response to guanadrel; consider an alternative antihypertensive with different mechanism of action.

Amphetamines, related sympathomimetics, and methylphenidate decrease the antihypertensive response to guanadrel; consider an alternative antihypertensive with different mechanism of action. Reassess the need for amphetamine, related sympathomimetic, or methylphenidate; consider alternatives.

Ephedrine may inhibit the antihypertensive response to guanadrel; consider an alternative antihypertensive with different mechanism of action. Reassess the need for ephedrine.

Norepinephrine/phenylephrine have exaggerated pressor response; monitor blood pressure closely.

MAO inhibitors may cause severe hypertension; give at least 1 week apart.

Pregnancy Risk Factor B

Pregnancy Implications Crosses the placenta

Nursing Implications Tablet may be crushed; assist patient with rising and ambulation

Additional Information Considered an alternative to guanethidine

Guanethidine

CAS Number 55-65-2; 645-43-2

Synonyms Guanethidine Monosulfate

Impairment Potential Yes

Use Treatment of moderate to severe hypertension; also useful in treating vasopressin extravasation

Mechanism of Action Acts as a false neurotransmitter that blocks the adrenergic actions of norepinephrine; it displaces norepinephrine from its presynaptic storage granules and thus exposes it to degradation; it thereby produces a reduction in total peripheral resistance and therefore blood pressure

Adverse Reactions

Cardiovascular: **Palpitations, chest pain**, hypotension (orthostatic), vasculitis, hypertension in patients with pheochromocytoma, AV block, sinus bradycardia, angina, vasodilation, **peripheral edema**

Central nervous system: **Fatigue**, dizziness, **drowsiness, faintness, headache, confusion**

Dermatologic: Cutaneous vasculitis

Endocrine & metabolic: Parotitis, hypoglycemia

Gastrointestinal: Diarrhea, **increased bowel movements, gas pain, constipation, anorexia, weight gain or loss**

Genitourinary: **Ejaculatory disturbances, nocturia, impotence**

Neuromuscular & skeletal: Weakness, **paresthesia, aching limbs, leg cramps, backache, arthralgia**

Ocular: Blurred vision, diplopia, **visual disturbances**

Renal: **Polyuria**, renal vasculitis

Respiratory: **Dyspnea, coughing**

Signs and Symptoms of Overdose Blurred vision, dizziness, ejaculatory disturbances, hypotension, impotence, nausea, nocturia, periarteritis nodosa, ptosis, syncope, vomiting

Pharmacodynamics/Kinetics

Onset of action: 0.5-2 hours

Peak effect: Antihypertensive: 6-8 hours

Duration: 24-48 hours

Absorption: Irregular (3% to 55%)

Half-life elimination, serum: 5-10 days

Dosage Oral:

Children: Initial: 0.2 mg/kg/day, increase by 0.2 mg/kg/day at 7- to 10-day intervals to a maximum of 3 mg/kg/day

Adults:

Ambulatory patients: Initial: 10 mg/day, increase at 5- to 7-day intervals to a maximum of 25-50 mg/day

Hospitalized patients: Initial: 25-50 mg/day, increase by 25-50 mg/day or every other day to desired therapeutic response

Vasopressin extravasation: 10 mg in 0.9% saline (10 mL) with 1000 units of heparin either through offending I.V. cannulas or through multiple SubQ injections after removal of catheter; apply ice to affected area

Dosing interval in renal impairment: Cl_{cr} <10 mL/minute: Administer every 24-36 hours

Monitoring Parameters Blood pressure, standing and sitting/supine

Contraindications Hypersensitivity to guanethidine or any component of the formulation; known or suspected pheochromocytoma; concurrent use or within 1 week of any MAO inhibitor; exacerbation of CHF (unrelated to HTN)

Warnings Orthostatic hypotension is common. Avoid using other drugs that cause orthostatic hypotension (alpha-blocking agents or reserpine). Discontinue 2 weeks before elective surgery (reduces potential for vascular collapse). If emergency surgery required, notify anesthesiologist of the drug regimen. Fever reduces dosage requirements. Avoid using tricyclic antidepressants and indirect-acting sympathomimetics (can reverse the blood pressure lowering effects). Use cautiously in asthma (may aggravate condition), CHF (sodium and water retention), renal dysfunction (can worsen renal function), recent MI, cerebrovascular disease with encephalopathy, and PUD (may aggravate condition). Safety and efficacy have not been established in pediatric patients. Dosage adjustment required with severe renal dysfunction.

Dosage Forms Tablet, as monosulfate: 10 mg, 25 mg

Reference Range Adrenergic blockade at plasma concentrations of 8 ng/mL

Overdosage/Treatment Supportive therapy: Hypotension usually responds to I.V. fluids or Trendelenburg positioning. If unresponsive to these measures, the use of a parenteral vasoconstrictor may be required (eg, dopamine at 2-5 mcg/kg/minute titrated to 10 mcg/kg/minute). Treatment is primarily supportive and symptomatic; overdose symptoms usually last for 72 hours.

Test Interactions ↑ sodium (S); ↓ catecholamines (U)

Drug Interactions TCAs decrease hypotensive effect of guanethidine.

Phenothiazines may inhibit the antihypertensive response to guanethidine consider an alternative antihypertensive with different mechanism of action.

Amphetamines, related sympathomimetics, and methylphenidate decrease the antihypertensive response to guanethidine; consider an alternative antihypertensive with different mechanism of action. Reassess the need for amphetamine, related sympathomimetic, or methylphenidate; consider alternatives.

Ephedrine may inhibit the antihypertensive response to guanethidine; consider an alternative antihypertensive with different mechanism of action. Reassess the need for ephedrine.

Norepinephrine/phenylephrine have exaggerated pressor response; monitor blood pressure closely.

Oral contraceptives may decrease hypotensive effect; avoid concurrent use.

Minoxidil may cause severe orthostatic hypotension; avoid concurrent use. Enflurane may cause hypotension; avoid concurrent use.

Pregnancy Risk Factor C
Nursing Implications Tablet may be crushed

Guanfacine

CAS Number 29110-47-2
U.S. Brand Names Tenex®
Synonyms Guanfacine Hydrochloride
Use Management of hypertension
Unlabeled/Investigational Use ADHD, tic disorder, aggression
Mechanism of Action False neurotransmitter (alpha$_2$-adrenoceptor agonist) that blocks the adrenergic actions of norepinephrine; displaces norepinephrine form its presynaptic storage granules and thus exposes it to degradation and, thereby, produces a reduction in total peripheral resistance and, therefore, blood pressure; structurally related to guanabenz, methyldopa, and clonidine
Adverse Reactions

Cardiovascular: Bradycardia, chest pain, edema, hypotension, orthostasis, palpitations, rebound hypertension, syncope

Central nervous system: Agitation, amnesia, confusion, depression, **dizziness, headache**, fatigue, insomnia, malaise, nervousness, **somnolence**, vertigo

Dermatologic: Alopecia, dermatitis, exfoliative dermatitis, pruritus, rash

Endocrine & metabolic: Impotence

Gastrointestinal: **Xerostomia, constipation**, dysphagia

Genitourinary: Urinary incontinence

Neuromuscular & skeletal: Hypokinesia, leg cramps, paresthesia

Ocular: Blurred vision

Otic: Tinnitus

Respiratory: Dyspnea

Miscellaneous: Diaphoresis

Note: Mania and aggressive behavior have been reported in pediatric patients with ADHD who received guanfacine.

Signs and Symptoms of Overdose Apnea, bradycardia (within 2 hours of ingestion), CNS depression, dermatitis, diarrhea, drowsiness, dysphagia, hypomagnesemia, hypotension (4-8 hours postingestion), hypothermia, impotence, insomnia, leg cramps, myalgia. Paradoxical hypertension can occur.

Admission Criteria/Prognosis Admit ingestions >3 mg in children or 30 mg in adults

Pharmacodynamics/Kinetics

Onset of action: Peak effect: 8-11 hours

Duration: 24 hours following single dose

Half-life elimination, serum: 17 hours

Time to peak, serum: 1-4 hours

Dosage

Adults: Oral: Hypertension: 1 mg usually at bedtime, may increase if needed at 3- to 4-week intervals; usual dose range (JNC 7): 0.5-2 mg once daily

Monitoring Parameters Blood pressure, standing and sitting/supine, ECG

Contraindications Hypersensitivity to guanfacine or any component of the formulation

Warnings Use caution with severe coronary insufficiency, recent MI, cerebrovascular disease, or chronic renal or hepatic disease. Abrupt discontinuation can result in nervousness, anxiety and rarely, rebound hypertension (occurs 2-4 days after withdrawal). Avoid use in CNS disease, elderly, or with other CNS depressants (can cause sedation and drowsiness alone). Caution in diabetes; may mask signs of hypoglycemia. Safety and efficacy in children <12 years of age have not been demonstrated. May cause orthostasis.

Dosage Forms Tablet: 1 mg, 2 mg

Reference Range Adult therapeutic effect at serum levels of 1.5-2.0 ng/mL

Overdosage/Treatment

Decontamination: Lavage (within 1 hour)/activated charcoal

Supportive therapy: Hypotension usually responds to I.V. fluids or Trendelenburg positioning. If unresponsive to these measures, the use of a parenteral vasoconstrictor may be required (eg, norepinephrine 0.1-0.2 mcg/kg/minute titrated to response). Naloxone may be utilized in treating the hypotension, CNS depression and/or apnea and should be given I.V. 0.4-2 mg, with repeats as needed. Atropine 15 mcg/kg I.V. or I.M. may be needed for symptomatic bradycardia.

Enhancement of elimination: Hemodialysis is not useful due to its large volume of distribution.

Antidote(s)

● Naloxone [ANTIDOTE]

Test Interactions ↑ cholesterol, sodium (S), triglycerides, AST, GPT

Drug Interactions

Nitroprusside and guanfacine have additive hypotensive effects.

Noncardioselective beta-blockers (nadolol, propranolol, timolol) may exacerbate rebound hypertension when guanfacine is withdrawn. The beta-blocker should be withdrawn first. The gradual withdrawal of guanfacine or a cardioselective beta-blocker could be substituted.

TCAs decrease the hypotensive effect of guanfacine.

Pregnancy Risk Factor B

Nursing Implications Tablet may be crushed; assist patient with rising and ambulation

Additional Information Usually given with a thiazide diuretic

Specific References

Chobanian AV, Bakris GL, Black HR, et al, "The Seventh Report of the Joint National Committee on Prevention, Detection, Evaluation, and Treatment of High Blood Pressure: The JNC 7 Report," *JAMA*, 2003, 289(19):2560-71.

Guanidine

Pronunciation (GWAHN i deen)
CAS Number 113-00-8; 50-01-1
Synonyms Guanidine Hydrochloride
Use Reduction of symptoms of muscle weakness associated with the myasthenic syndrome of Eaton-Lambert, not for myasthenia gravis; has been used in botulism (type B) to reverse neuromuscular blockade with disappointing results
Adverse Reactions

Cardiovascular: Bradycardia, AV block, chest pain, sinus bradycardia, angina

Central nervous system: Headache, seizures, dysphoria, drowsiness, ataxia

Endocrine & metabolic: Hypoglycemia

Gastrointestinal: **Diarrhea, nausea**, abdominal pain, **stomach cramps**

Genitourinary: Urge to urinate

Hematologic: Aplastic anemia

Local: Thrombophlebitis

Neuromuscular & skeletal: Muscle spasm, tremors, weakness

Ocular: Lacrimation, miosis, diplopia

Respiratory: Increased bronchial secretions, respiratory paralysis, laryngospasm

Miscellaneous: **Diaphoresis and mouth watering (increased)**, hypersensitivity, hyper-reactive cholinergic responses

Dosage Adults: Oral: Initial: 10-15 mg/kg/day in 3-4 divided doses, gradually increase to 40 mg/kg/day

Dosage Forms Tablet, as hydrochloride: 125 mg

Overdosage/Treatment

Decontamination: Lavage (within 1 hour)/activated charcoal

Supportive therapy: Treat symptomatic bradycardia with atropine

Test Interactions ↑ creatinine; ↓ glucose

Additional Information Primary effect on botulism is on improvement in ocular muscles; little effect on respiratory function

Haloperidol

Related Information

● Anticholinergic Effects of Common Psychotropics

● Antipsychotic Agents

CAS Number 52-86-8; 74050-97-8

U.S. Brand Names Haldol® Decanoate; Haldol®

Synonyms Haloperidol Decanoate; Haloperidol Lactate

Impairment Potential Yes

Use Management of schizophrenia; control of tics and vocal utterances of Tourette's disorder in children and adults; severe behavioral problems in children

Unlabeled/Investigational Use Treatment of psychosis; may be used for the emergency sedation of severely-agitated or delirious patients; adjunctive treatment of ethanol dependence; antiemetic

Mechanism of Action Competitive blockade of postsynaptic dopamine receptors in the mesolimbic dopaminergic system; depresses cerebral cortex and hypothalamus; exhibits a strong alpha-adrenergic and anticholinergic-blocking activity

Adverse Reactions

Sedation and anticholinergic effects are more pronounced than extrapyramidal effects; ECG changes, retinal pigmentation are more common than with chlorpromazine; concomitant therapy with perazine can cause agranulocytosis and hepatotoxicity

Cardiovascular: Hypotension (especially orthostatic hypotension), tachycardia, cardiac arrhythmias, abnormal T waves with prolonged ventricular repolarization, sinus bradycardia, sinus tachycardia, arrhythmias (ventricular), torsade de pointes (case-control study ~4%)

Central nervous system: Sedation, drowsiness, **restlessness, anxiety, extrapyramidal reactions, dystonic reactions, pseudoparkinsonian signs and symptoms, tardive dyskinesia, neuroleptic malignant syndrome, seizures, altered central temperature regulation,** electroencephalogram abnormalities, memory disturbance, **akathisia**

Dermatologic: Hyperpigmentation, pruritus, rash, contact dermatitis, photosensitivity (rare), alopecia, exfoliative dermatitis, acne, urticaria, purpura, exanthem

Endocrine & metabolic: Amenorrhea, galactorrhea, gynecomastia, syndrome of inappropriate antidiuretic hormone, sexual dysfunction, **edema of the breasts**

Gastrointestinal: **Constipation**, adynamic ileus, dyspepsia, GI upset, xerostomia (problem for denture user), **weight gain**

Genitourinary: Urinary retention, overflow incontinence, priapism

Hematologic: Leukopenia/neutropenia (agranulocytosis, granulocytopenia) (usually inpatients with large doses for prolonged periods), thrombocytopenia

Hepatic: Cholestatic jaundice

Neuromuscular & skeletal: Trismus, rhabdomyolysis, Meige syndrome

Ocular: **Blurred vision**, retinal pigmentation, decreased visual acuity (may be irreversible)

Renal: Myoglobinuria

Miscellaneous: Bruxism, systemic lupus erythematosus

Signs and Symptoms of Overdose Agitation, alopecia, arrhythmias, bradycardia, chorea (extrapyramidal), confusion, deep sleep, dementia, disorientation, dry mouth, dysphagia, dystonic reactions, ejaculatory disturbances, extrapyramidal reaction, fever, gynecomastia, hyperglycemia, hyperprolactinemia, hyperreflexia, hyperthermia, hypoglycemia, hypokalemia, hypopigmented hair, hypothermia, impotence, lactation, memory loss, neuroleptic malignant syndrome, myasthenia gravis (exacerbation or precipitation), Parkinson's-like symptoms, ptosis, pulmonary edema, QT prolongation, urine discoloration (pink; red; red-brown). Cardiac conduction abnormalities can occur if daily I.V. dose exceeds 50 mg

Pharmacodynamics/Kinetics

Onset of action: Sedation: I.V.: ~1 hour

Duration: Decanoate: ~3 weeks

Distribution: Crosses placenta; enters breast milk

Protein binding: 90%

Metabolism: Hepatic to inactive compounds

Bioavailability: Oral: 60%

Half-life elimination: 20 hours

Time to peak, serum: 20 minutes

Excretion: Urine (33% to 40% as metabolites) within 5 days; feces (15%)

Dosage Children: 3-12 years (15-40 kg): Oral:

Initial: 0.05 mg/kg/day or 0.25-0.5 mg/day given in 2-3 divided doses; increase by 0.25-0.5 mg every 5-7 days; maximum: 0.15 mg/kg/day

Usual maintenance:

Agitation or hyperkinesia: 0.01-0.03 mg/kg/day once daily

Nonpsychotic disorders: 0.05-0.075 mg/kg/day in 2-3 divided doses

Psychotic disorders: 0.05-0.15 mg/kg/day in 2-3 divided doses

Children 6-12 years: Sedation/psychotic disorders: I.M. (as lactate): 1-3 mg/dose every 4-8 hours to a maximum of 0.15 mg/kg/day; change over to oral therapy as soon as able

Adults:

Psychosis:

Oral: 0.5-5 mg 2-3 times/day; usual maximum: 30 mg/day

I.M. (as lactate): 2-5 mg every 4-8 hours as needed

I.M. (as decanoate): Initial: 10-20 times the daily oral dose administered at 4-week intervals

Maintenance dose: 10-15 times initial oral dose; used to stabilize psychiatric symptoms

Delirium in the intensive care unit (unlabeled use, unlabeled route):

I.V.: 2-10 mg; may repeat bolus doses every 20-30 minutes until calm achieved then administer 25% of the maximum dose every 6 hours; monitor ECG and QT$_c$ interval

Intermittent I.V.: 0.03-0.15 mg/kg every 30 minutes to 6 hours

Oral: Agitation: 5-10 mg

Continuous intravenous infusion (100 mg/100 mL D$_5$W): Rates of 3-25 mg/hour have been used

Rapid tranquilization of severely-agitated patient (unlabeled use): Administer every 30-60 minutes:

Oral: 5-10 mg

I.M.: 5 mg

Average total dose (oral or I.M.) for tranquilization: 10-20 mg

Elderly: Initial: Oral: 0.25-0.5 mg 1-2 times/day; increase dose at 4- to 7-day intervals by 0.25-0.5 mg/day; increase dosing intervals (twice daily, 3 times/day, etc) as necessary to control response or side effects

Hemodialysis/peritoneal dialysis: Supplemental dose is not necessary

Stability Protect oral dosage forms from light; insoluble in water

Monitoring Parameters Vital signs; lipid profile, fasting blood glucose/Hgb A$_{1c}$; BMI; mental status, abnormal involuntary movement scale (AIMS), extrapyramidal symptoms (EPS)

Administration The decanoate injectable formulation should be administered I.M. only, **do not administer decanoate I.V.** Dilute the oral concentrate with water or juice before administration. Avoid skin contact with oral suspension or solution; may cause contact dermatitis.

Contraindications Hypersensitivity to haloperidol or any component of the formulation; Parkinson's disease; severe CNS depression; bone marrow suppression; severe cardiac or hepatic disease; coma

Warnings

Hypotension may occur, particularly with parenteral administration. Decanoate form should never be administered I.V. Avoid in thyrotoxicosis. May be sedating, use with caution in disorders where CNS depression is a feature. Caution in patients with hemodynamic instability, predisposition to seizures, subcortical brain damage, renal or respiratory disease. Esophageal dysmotility and aspiration have been associated with antipsychotic use - use with caution in patients at risk of pneumonia (ie, Alzheimer's disease). Caution in breast cancer or other prolactin-dependent tumors (may elevate prolactin levels). May alter temperature regulation or mask toxicity of other drugs due to antiemetic effects. May alter cardiac conduction - life-threatening arrhythmias have occurred with therapeutic doses of antipsychotics. Adverse effects of decanoate may be prolonged. May cause orthostatic hypotension - use with caution in patients at risk of this effect or those who would tolerate transient hypotensive episodes (cerebrovascular disease, cardiovascular disease, or other medications which may predispose). Some tablets contain tartrazine.

May cause anticholinergic effects (confusion, agitation, constipation, xerostomia, blurred vision, urinary retention). Therefore, they should be used with caution in patients with decreased gastrointestinal motility, urinary retention, BPH, xerostomia, or visual problems. Conditions which also may be exacerbated by cholinergic blockade include narrow-angle glaucoma (screening is recommended) and worsening of myasthenia gravis. Relative to other neuroleptics, haloperidol has a low potency of cholinergic blockade.

May cause extrapyramidal symptoms, including pseudoparkinsonism, acute dystonic reactions, akathisia, and tardive dyskinesia (risk of these reactions is high relative to other neuroleptics). May be associated with neuroleptic malignant syndrome (NMS) or pigmentary retinopathy.

Dosage Forms [DSC] = Discontinued product

Note: Strength expressed as base.

Injection, oil, as decanoate: 50 mg/mL (1 mL, 5 mL); 100 mg/mL (1 mL, 5 mL)

Haldol® Decanoate: 50 mg/mL (1 mL; 5 mL [DSC]); 100 mg/mL (1 mL; 5 mL [DSC]) [contains benzyl alcohol, sesame oil]

Injection, solution, as lactate: 5 mg/mL (1 mL, 10 mL)

Haldol®: 5 mg/mL (1 mL)

Solution, oral concentrate, as lactate: 2 mg/mL (15 mL, 120 mL)

Tablet: 0.5 mg, 1 mg, 2 mg, 5 mg, 10 mg, 20 mg

Reference Range

Therapeutic: 5-15 ng/mL (SI: 10-30 nmol/L) (psychotic disorders - less for Tourette's and mania)

Toxic: >28 ng/mL (SI: >56 nmol/L)

Overdosage/Treatment

Decontamination: Lavage (within 1 hour)/activated charcoal

Supportive therapy: Hypotension usually responds to I.V. fluids or Trendelenburg positioning. If unresponsive to these measures, the use of a parenteral inotrope may be required (eg, norepinephrine 0.1-0.2 mcg/kg/minute titrated to response). Seizures commonly respond to lorazepam or diazepam (I.V. 5-10 mg bolus in adults every 15 minutes if needed up to a total of 30 mg; I.V. 0.25-0.4 mg/kg/dose up to a total of 10 mg in children) or to phenytoin or phenobarbital. Also critical cardiac arrhythmias often respond to I.V. phenytoin (15 mg/kg up to 1 g), while other antiarrhythmics (ie, lidocaine) can be used. Neuroleptics often cause extrapyramidal reaction (eg, dystonic reactions) requiring management with diphenhydramine 1-2 mg/kg (adults) up to a maximum of 50 mg I.M. or I.V. slow push followed by a maintenance dose for 48-72 hours. When these reactions are unresponsive to diphenhydramine, benztropine mesylate I.V. 1-2 mg (adults) may be effective. These agents are generally effective within 2-5 minutes. Propranolol can be used to treat haloperidol-related nocturnal bruxism.

Enhancement of elimination: Multiple dosing of activated charcoal would not be expected to be useful

Test Interactions ↓ cholesterol (S)

Drug Interactions Substrate of CYP1A2 (minor), 2D6 (major), 3A4 (major); **Inhibits** CYP2D6 (moderate), 3A4 (moderate)

Acetylcholinesterase inhibitors (central): May increase the risk of antipsychotic-related extrapyramidal symptoms; monitor.

Anticholinergics: May inhibit the therapeutic response to haloperidol and excess anticholinergic effects may occur; tardive dyskinesias have also been reported; includes benztropine and trihexyphenidyl

Antihypertensives: Concurrent use of haloperidol with an antihypertensive may produce additive hypotensive effects (particularly orthostasis)

Bromocriptine: Antipsychotics inhibit the ability of bromocriptine to lower serum prolactin concentrations

Chloroquine: Serum concentrations of haloperidol may be increased by chloroquine

CNS depressants: Sedative effects may be additive; monitor for increased effect; includes barbiturates, benzodiazepines, narcotic analgesics, ethanol and other sedative agents

CYP2D6 inhibitors: May increase the levels/effects of haloperidol. Example inhibitors include chlorpromazine, delavirdine, fluoxetine, miconazole, paroxetine, pergolide, quinidine, quinine, ritonavir, and ropinirole.

CYP2D6 substrates: Haloperidol may increase the levels/effects of CYP2D6 substrates. Example substrates include amphetamines, selected beta-blockers, dextromethorphan, fluoxetine, lidocaine, mirtazapine, nefazodone, paroxetine, risperidone, ritonavir, thioridazine, tricyclic antidepressants, and venlafaxine.

CYP2D6 prodrug substrates: Haloperidol may decrease the levels/effects of CYP2D6 prodrug substrates. Example prodrug substrates include codeine, hydrocodone, oxycodone, and tramadol.

CYP3A4 inducers: CYP3A4 inducers may decrease the levels/effects of haloperidol. Example inducers include aminoglutethimide, carbamazepine, nafcillin, nevirapine, phenobarbital, phenytoin, and rifamycins.

CYP3A4 inhibitors: May increase the levels/effects of haloperidol. Example inhibitors include azole antifungals, clarithromycin, diclofenac, doxycycline, erythromycin, imatinib, isoniazid, nefazodone, nicardipine, propofol, protease inhibitors, quinidine, telithromycin, and verapamil.

CYP3A4 substrates: Haloperidol may increase the levels/effects of CYP3A4 substrates. Example substrates include benzodiazepines, calcium channel blockers, cyclosporine, mirtazapine, nateglinide, nefazodone, sildenafil (and other PDE-5 inhibitors), tacrolimus, and venlafaxine. Selected benzodiazepines (midazolam and triazolam), cisapride, ergot alkaloids, selected HMG-CoA reductase inhibitors (lovastatin and simvastatin), and pimozide are generally contraindicated with strong CYP3A4 inhibitors.

Indomethacin: Haloperidol in combination with indomethacin may result in drowsiness, tiredness, and confusion; monitor for adverse effects

Inhalation anesthetics: Haloperidol in combination with certain forms of induction anesthesia may produce peripheral vasodilitation and hypotension

Levodopa: Haloperidol may inhibit the antiparkinsonian effect of levodopa; avoid this combination

Lithium: Haloperidol may produce neurotoxicity with lithium; this is a rare effect

Methyldopa: Effect of haloperidol may be altered; enhanced effects, as well as reduced efficacy have been reported

Metoclopramide: May increase extrapyramidal symptoms (EPS) or risk.

Nefazodone: Haloperidol and nefazodone may produce additive CNS toxicity, including sedation

Propranolol: Serum concentrations of haloperidol may be increased

Quinidine: May increase haloperidol concentrations; monitor for EPS and/or QT_c prolongation

SSRIs: Fluoxetine, fluvoxamine, and paroxetine may inhibit the metabolism of haloperidol resulting in EPS; monitor for EPS

Sulfadoxine-pyrimethamine: May increase fluphenazine concentrations

Tricyclic antidepressants: Concurrent use may produce increased toxicity or altered therapeutic response

Trazodone: Haloperidol and trazodone may produce additive hypotensive effects

Pregnancy Risk Factor C

Pregnancy Implications Decline in developmental scores may be seen in nursing infants

Lactation Enters breast milk/not recommended (AAP rates "of concern")

Nursing Implications Observe for extrapyramidal effects

Additional Information 5 mg of haloperidol (I.V.) followed by a bolus of 1 L of normal saline has been used to treat migraine headaches; may be used for the emergency sedation of severely psychotic agitated patients (5 mg I.M. With 2 mg of lorazepam I.M.); hyperprolactinemia can develop during the first week of haloperidol therapy

Specific References

Hassaballa HA and Balk RA, "Torsade de Pointes Associated with the Administration of Intravenous Haloperidol," *Am J Ther*, 2003, 10(1):58-60.

Jhee SS, Zarotsky V, Mohaupt SM, et al, "Delayed Onset of Oculogyric Crisis and Torticollis with Intramuscular Haloperidol," *Ann Pharmacother*, 2003, 37(10):1434-7.

Kipps CM, Fung VS, Grattan-Smith P, et al, "Movement Disorder Emergencies," *Mov Disord*, 2005, 20(3):322-34.

Yasui-Furukori N, Furukori H, Saito M, et al, "Poor Reliability of Therapeutic Drug Monitoring Data for Haloperidol and Bromperidol Using Enzyme Immunoassay," *Ther Drug Monit*, 2003, 25(6):709-14.

Heparin

CAS Number 37270-89-6; 9005-49-6; 9041-08-1

U.S. Brand Names Hep-Lock®

Synonyms Heparin Calcium; Heparin Lock Flush; Heparin Sodium

Use Prophylaxis and treatment of thromboembolic disorders

Unlabeled/Investigational Use Acute MI – combination regimen of heparin (unlabeled dose), tenecteplase (half dose), and abciximab (full dose)

Mechanism of Action Potentiates the action of antithrombin III and thereby inactivates thrombin (as well as activated coagulation factors IX, X, XI, XII, and plasmin) and prevents the conversion of fibrinogen to fibrin; heparin also stimulates release of lipoprotein lipase (lipoprotein lipase hydrolyzes triglycerides to glycerol and free fatty acids)

Adverse Reactions

Cardiovascular: Cardiac tamponade, pericardial effusion/pericarditis, vasoconstriction, vasculitis

Central nervous system: Fever, headache, chills, hallucinations, amnesia, transient global amnesia (TGA), intracranial hemorrhage

Dermatologic: Urticaria, pruritus, eczema, alopecia, skin necrosis, purpura, unexplained bruising, angioedema, toxic epidermal necrolysis, cutaneous vasculitis, exanthem

Endocrine & metabolic: Hyperkalemia with prolonged therapy from hypoaldosteronism, nephrogenic diabetes insipidus

Gastrointestinal: Nausea, vomiting, fecal discoloration (black), fecal discoloration (pink), fecal discoloration (red), **constipation, vomiting of blood**

Genitourinary: Priapism, urine discoloration (orange), urine discoloration (red)

Hematologic: **Hemorrhage** (risk is threefold with APTT between 2-2.9 times control and eightfold when APTT is over 3 times control); thrombocytopenia; incidence of thrombocytopenia is greater with bovine than porcine heparin preparations; begins 1 week after therapy ocular hemorrhage, coagulopathy, eosinophilia, spontaneous splenic rupture

Hepatic: Elevated liver enzymes

Local: Irritation, ulceration, cutaneous necrosis have been rarely reported with deep SubQ injections, extravasation injury

Neuromuscular & skeletal: Osteoporosis with doses >15,000 units/day or therapy of over 5 months

Ocular: Conjunctivitis

Renal: Hematuria

Miscellaneous: Bleeding from gums, fixed drug eruption, anaphylaxis (0.2%)

Pharmacodynamics/Kinetics

Onset of action: Anticoagulation: I.V.: Immediate; SubQ: ~20-30 minutes

Absorption: Oral, rectal, I.M.: Erratic at best from all these routes of administration; SubQ absorption is also erratic, but considered acceptable for prophylactic use

Distribution: Does not cross placenta; does not enter breast milk

Metabolism: Hepatic; may be partially metabolized in the reticuloendothelial system

Half-life elimination: Mean: 1.5 hours; Range: 1-2 hours; affected by obesity, renal function, hepatic function, malignancy, presence of pulmonary embolism, and infections

Excretion: Urine (small amounts as unchanged drug)

Dosage

Children:

Intermittent I.V.: Initial: 50-100 units/kg, then 50-100 units/kg every 4 hours

I.V. infusion: Initial: 50 units/kg, then 15-25 units/kg/hour; increase dose by 2-4 units/kg/hour every 6-8 hours as required

Adults:

Prophylaxis (low-dose heparin): SubQ: 5000 units every 8-12 hours

Intermittent I.V.: Initial: 10,000 units, then 50-70 units/kg (5000-10,000 units) every 4-6 hours

I.V. infusion (weight-based dosing per institutional nomogram recommended):

Acute coronary syndromes: MI: Fibrinolytic therapy:

Alteplase or reteplase with first or second bolus: Concurrent bolus of 60 units/kg (maximum: 4000 units), then 12 units/kg/hour (maximum: 1000 units/hour) as continuous infusion. Check aPTT every 4-6 hours; adjust to target of 1.5-2 times the upper limit of control (50-70 seconds in clinical trials); usual range 10-30 units/kg/hour. Duration of heparin therapy depends on concurrent therapy and the specific patient risks for systemic or venous thromboembolism.

Streptokinase: Heparin use optional depending on concurrent therapy and specific patient risks for systemic or venous thromboembolism (anterior MI, CHF, previous embolus, atrial fibrillation, LV thrombus): If heparin is administered, start when aPTT <2 times the upper limit of control; do not use a bolus, but initiate infusion adjusted to a target aPTT of 1.5-2 times the upper limit of control (50-70 seconds in clinical trials). If heparin is not administered by infusion, 7500-12,500 units SubQ every 12 hours (when aPTT <2 times the upper limit of control) is recommended.

Percutaneous coronary intervention: Heparin bolus and infusion may be administered to an activated clotting time (ACT) of 300-350 seconds if no concurrent GPIIb/IIIa receptor antagonist is administered or 200-250 seconds if a GPIIb/IIIa receptor antagonist is administered.

Treatment of unstable angina (high-risk and some intermediate-risk patients): Initial bolus of 60-70 units/kg (maximum: 5000 units), followed by an initial infusion of 12-15 units/kg/hour (maximum: 1000 units/hour). The American College of Chest Physicians consensus conference has recommended dosage adjustments to correspond to a therapeutic range equivalent to heparin levels of 0.3-0.7 units/mL by antifactor Xa determinations, which correlates with aPTT values between 60 and 80 seconds

Treatment of venous thromboembolism (DVT/PE): 80 units/kg I.V. push followed by continuous infusion of 18 units/kg/hour

Line flushing: When using daily flushes of heparin to maintain patency of single and double lumen central catheters, 10 units/mL is commonly used for younger infants (eg, <10 kg) while 100 units/mL is used for older infants, children, and adults. Capped PVC catheters and peripheral heparin locks require flushing more frequently (eg, every 6-8 hours). Volume of heparin flush is usually similar to volume of catheter (or slightly greater). Additional flushes should be given when stagnant blood is observed in catheter, after catheter is used for drug or blood administration, and after blood withdrawal from catheter.

Addition of heparin (0.5-3 unit/mL) to peripheral and central parenteral nutrition has not been shown to decrease catheter-related thrombosis. The final concentration of heparin used for TPN solutions may need to be decreased to 0.5 units/mL in small infants receiving larger amounts of volume in order to avoid approaching therapeutic amounts. Arterial lines are heparinized with a final concentration of 1 unit/mL.

Using a standard heparin solution (25,000 units/500 mL D$_5$W), the following infusion rates can be used to achieve the listed doses.
For a dose of:
    400 units/hour: Infuse at 8 mL/hour
    500 units/hour: Infuse at 10 mL/hour
    600 units/hour: Infuse at 12 mL/hour
    700 units/hour: Infuse at 14 mL/hour
    800 units/hour: Infuse at 16 mL/hour
    900 units/hour: Infuse at 18 mL/hour
    1000 units/hour: Infuse at 20 mL/hour
    1100 units/hour: Infuse at 22 mL/hour
    1200 units/hour: Infuse at 24 mL/hour
    1300 units/hour: Infuse at 26 mL/hour
    1400 units/hour: Infuse at 28 mL/hour
    1500 units/hour: Infuse at 30 mL/hour
    1600 units/hour: Infuse at 32 mL/hour
    1700 units/hour: Infuse at 34 mL/hour
    1800 units/hour: Infuse at 36 mL/hour
    1900 units/hour: Infuse at 38 mL/hour
    2000 units/hour: Infuse at 40 mL/hour

Dosing adjustments in the elderly: Patients >60 years of age may have higher serum levels and clinical response (longer aPTTs) as compared to younger patients receiving similar dosages; lower dosages may be required

Stability Stable at room temperature; protect from freezing

Monitoring Parameters

Platelet counts, aPTT, hemoglobin, hematocrit, signs of bleeding

For intermittent I.V. injections, aPTT is measured 3.5-4 hours after I.V. injection

Note: Continuous I.V. infusion is preferred over I.V. intermittent injections. For full-dose heparin (ie, nonlow-dose), the dose should be titrated according to aPTT results. For anticoagulation, an aPTT 1.5-2.5 times normal is usually desired. Because of variation among hospitals in the control aPTT values, nomograms should be established at each institution, designed to achieve aPTT values in the target range (eg, for a control aPTT of 30 seconds, the target range [1.5-2.5 times control] would be 45-75 seconds). Measurements should be made prior to heparin therapy, 6 hours after initiation, and 6 hours after any dosage change, and should be used to adjust the heparin infusion until the aPTT exhibits a therapeutic level. When two consecutive aPTT values are therapeutic, the measurements may be made every 24 hours, and if necessary, dose adjustment carried out. In addition, a significant change in the patient's clinical condition (eg, recurrent ischemia, bleeding, hypotension) should prompt an immediate aPTT determination, followed by dose adjustment if necessary. Increase or decrease infusion by 2-4 units/kg/hour dependent upon aPTT.

Heparin infusion dose adjustment:
    aPTT >3x control: Decrease infusion rate 50%
    aPTT 2-3x control: Decrease infusion rate 25%
    aPTT 1.5-2x control: No change
    aPTT <1.5x control: Increase rate of infusion 25%; max 2500 units/hour

Administration

Do not administer I.M. due to pain, irritation, and hematoma formation; central venous catheters must be flushed with heparin solution when newly inserted, daily (at the time of tubing change), after blood withdrawal or transfusion, and after an intermittent infusion through an injectable cap. A volume of at least 10 mL of blood should be removed and discarded from a heparinized line before blood samples are sent for coagulation testing.

Using a standard heparin solution (25,000 units/500 mL D$_5$W), the following infusion rates can be used to achieve the listed doses.
For a dose of:
    400 units/hour: Infuse at 8 mL/hour
    500 units/hour: Infuse at 10 mL/hour
    600 units/hour: Infuse at 12 mL/hour
    700 units/hour: Infuse at 14 mL/hour
    800 units/hour: Infuse at 16 mL/hour
    900 units/hour: Infuse at 18 mL/hour
    1000 units/hour: Infuse at 20 mL/hour
    1100 units/hour: Infuse at 22 mL/hour
    1200 units/hour: Infuse at 24 mL/hour
    1300 units/hour: Infuse at 26 mL/hour
    1400 units/hour: Infuse at 28 mL/hour
    1500 units/hour: Infuse at 30 mL/hour
    1600 units/hour: Infuse at 32 mL/hour
    1700 units/hour: Infuse at 34 mL/hour
    1800 units/hour: Infuse at 36 mL/hour
    1900 units/hour: Infuse at 38 mL/hour
    2000 units/hour: Infuse at 40 mL/hour

Contraindications Hypersensitivity to heparin or any component of the formulation; severe thrombocytopenia; uncontrolled active bleeding except when due to DIC; suspected intracranial hemorrhage; not for I.M. use; not for use when appropriate monitoring parameters cannot be obtained

Warnings

Use cautiously in patients with a documented hypersensitivity reaction and only in life-threatening situations. Hemorrhage is the most common complication. Monitor for signs and symptoms of bleeding. Certain patients are at increased risk of bleeding. Risk factors include bacterial endocarditis; congenital or acquired bleeding disorders; active ulcerative or angiodysplastic GI diseases; severe uncontrolled hypertension; hemorrhagic stroke; or use shortly after brain, spinal, or ophthalmology surgery; patient treated concomitantly with platelet inhibitors; conditions associated with increased bleeding tendencies (hemophilia, vascular purpura); recent GI bleeding; thrombocytopenia or platelet defects; severe liver disease; hypertensive or diabetic retinopathy; or in patients undergoing invasive procedures. A higher incidence of bleeding has been reported in patients >60 years of age, particularly women. They are also more sensitive to the dose.

Patients who develop thrombocytopenia on heparin may be at risk of developing a new thrombus ("White-clot syndrome"). Hypersensitivity reactions can occur. Osteoporosis can occur following long-term use (>6 months). Monitor for hyperkalemia. Discontinue therapy and consider alternatives if platelets are <100,000/mm^3. Patients >60 years of age may require lower doses of heparin.

Some preparations contain benzyl alcohol as a preservative. In neonates, large amounts of benzyl alcohol (>100 mg/kg/day) have been associated with fatal toxicity (gasping syndrome). The use of preservative-free heparin is, therefore, recommended in neonates. Some preparations contain sulfite which may cause allergic reactions.

Heparin does not possess fibrinolytic activity and, therefore, cannot lyse established thrombi; discontinue heparin if hemorrhage occurs; severe hemorrhage or overdosage may require protamine

Dosage Forms [DSC] = Discontinued product

Infusion, as sodium [premixed in NaCl 0.45%; porcine intestinal mucosa source]: 12,500 units (250 mL); 25,000 units (250 mL, 500 mL)

Infusion, as sodium [preservative free; premixed in D$_5$W; porcine intestinal mucosa source]: 10,000 units (100 mL) [contains sodium metabisulfite]; 12,500 units (250 mL) [contains sodium metabisulfite]; 20,000 units (500 mL) [contains sodium metabisulfite]; 25,000 units (250 mL, 500 mL) [contains sodium metabisulfite]

Infusion, as sodium [preservative free; premixed in NaCl 0.9%; porcine intestinal mucosa source]: 1000 units (500 mL); 2000 units (1000 mL)

Injection, solution, as sodium [lock flush preparation; porcine intestinal mucosa source; multidose vial]: 10 units/mL (1 mL, 10 mL, 30 mL) [contains parabens]; 100 units/mL (1 mL, 5 mL) [contains parabens]

Injection, solution, as sodium [lock flush preparation; porcine intestinal mucosa source; multidose vial]: 10 units/mL (10 mL, 30 mL); 100 units/mL (10 mL, 30 mL) [contains benzyl alcohol]

  Hep-Lock®: 10 units/mL (1 mL, 2 mL, 10 mL, 30 mL); 100 units/mL (1 mL, 2 mL, 10 mL, 30 mL) [contains benzyl alcohol]

Injection, solution, as sodium [lock flush preparation; porcine intestinal mucosa source; prefilled syringe]: 10 units/mL (1 mL, 2 mL, 3 mL, 5 mL); 100 units/mL (1 mL, 2 mL, 3 mL, 5 mL) [contains benzyl alcohol]

Injection, solution, as sodium [preservative free; lock flush preparation; porcine intestinal mucosa source; prefilled syringe]: 100 units/mL (5 mL)

Injection, solution, as sodium [preservative free; lock flush preparation; porcine intestinal mucosa source; vial]:

  HepFlush®-10: 10 units/mL (10 mL)

Hep-Lock U/P: 10 units/mL (1 mL); 100 units/mL (1 mL)

Injection, solution, as sodium [porcine intestinal mucosa source; multi-dose vial]: 1000 units/mL (1 mL, 10 mL, 30 mL) [contains benzyl alcohol]; 1000 units/mL (1 mL, 10 mL, 30 mL) [contains methylparabens]; 5000 units/mL (1 mL, 10 mL) [contains benzyl alcohol]; 5000 units/mL (1 mL) [contains methylparabens]; 10,000 units/mL (1 mL, 4 mL) [contains benzyl alcohol]; 10,000 units/mL (1 mL, 5 mL) [contains methylparabens]; 20,000 units/mL (1 mL) [contains methylparabens]

Injection, solution, as sodium [porcine intestinal mucosa source; prefilled syringe]: 5000 units/mL (1 mL) [contains benzyl alcohol]

Injection, solution, as sodium [preservative free; porcine intestinal mucosa source; prefilled syringe]: 10,000 units/mL (0.5 mL)

Injection, solution, as sodium [preservative free; porcine intestinal mucosa source; vial]: 1000 units/mL (2 mL); 2000 units/mL (5 mL); 2500 units/mL (10 mL)

Reference Range Therapeutic: 0.3-0.5 units/mL

Overdosage/Treatment

Supportive therapy: Protamine can be used for severe bleeding upon withdrawal of heparin (1 mg of protamine for every 80-100 units of heparin by slow I.V. push); Effect on PTT can be seen within 15 minutes recombinant hirudin lepirudin or argatroban (both direct thrombin inhibitors) have been used successfully in treating heparin-induced thrombocytopenia. Danaparoid sodium or recombinant hirudin can be given if heparin-induced thrombocytopenia develops. Heparin should be discontinued once the clinical diagnosis is made. Do not wait for confirmatory test results (platelet aggregometry assay or enzyme-linked immunosorbent assay for heparin-induced thrombocytopenia IgG antibody). Do not start warfarin until thrombotic event is controlled and thrombocytopenia has resolved. Oral fludrocortisone (0.1 mg/day) can help resolve heparin-induced hyperkalemia.

Enhancement of elimination: While hemodialysis is not beneficial, exchange transfusion has been used successfully in a neonate and plasma exchange has been used successfully in four older patients for thrombocytopenia

Antidote(s)

- Protamine Sulfate [ANTIDOTE]

Test Interactions Increases thyroxine (S) (false elevation with competitive protein binding methods), PT, PTT, bleeding time; interferes with calcium assay techniques leading to false depression of calcium. Note that serum electrolyte assays obtained through heparin-based cannulas may result in factitious hyperkalemia and/or hypernatremia. Heparin may cause falsely elevated free thyroxine levels when measured by direct equilibrium dialysis method; I.V. heparin may produce a fivefold increase in free thyroxine

Drug Interactions Cephalosporins which contain the MTT side chain may increase the risk of hemorrhage.

Drugs which affect platelet function (eg, aspirin, NSAIDs, dipyridamole, ticlopidine, clopidogrel, IIb/IIIa antagonists) may potentiate the risk of hemorrhage.

Nitroglycerin (I.V.) may decrease heparin's anticoagulant effect. This interaction has not been validated in some studies, and may only occur at high nitroglycerin dosages.

Penicillins (parenteral) may prolong bleeding time via inhibition of platelet aggregation, potentially increasing the risk of hemorrhage.

Thrombolytic agents increase the risk of hemorrhage.

Warfarin: Risk of bleeding may be increased during concurrent therapy. Heparin is commonly continued during the initiation of warfarin therapy to assure anticoagulation and to protect against possible transient hypercoagulability.

Other drugs reported to increase heparin's anticoagulant effect include antihistamines, tetracycline, quinine, nicotine, and cardiac glycosides (digoxin).

Pregnancy Risk Factor C

Pregnancy Implications Does not cross placenta; while maternal thrombocytopenia and bleeding must be monitored, no congenital defects have been documented; heparin is probably safer than warfarin during pregnancy

Lactation Does not enter breast milk/compatible

Nursing Implications Do not administer I.M. due to pain, irritation, and hematoma formation

Additional Information Low molecular weight heparin agents carry a lower risk of thrombocytopenia; thrombocytopenia is more likely to occur with unfractionated heparin than low molecular weight heparin; thrombocytopenia can occur in patients given heparin with lupus anticoagulant; a value of 300-500 seconds (with control of 150-180 seconds) of activated clotting time is an appropriate target during heparin therapy. When patients present with thrombocytopenia and thrombosis up to 3 weeks after exposure to heparin, delayed-onset heparin-induced thrombocytopenia should be suspected.

A 50% or greater fall in the platelet count from the postoperative peak is a sensitive definition indicating possible heparin-induced thrombocytopenia that is associated with an increased risk of thrombosis.

Specific References

Dager WE and White RH, "Argatroban for Heparin-Induced Thrombocytopenia in Hepato-Renal Failure and CVVHD," *Ann Pharmacother*, 2003, 37(9):1232-6.

Hernandez MA, Holanda MS, Tejerina EE, et al, "Methanol Poisoning and Heparin: A Dangerous Couple?" *Am J Emer Med*, 2004, 22(7):620-1.

Howell MD and Powers RD, "Utility of Thrombocytopenia as a Marker for Heparin Allergy in Adult ED Patients," *Am J Emer Med*, 2006, 24: 268-70.

Klerk CP, Smorenburg SM, and Buller HR, "Thrombosis Prophylaxis in Patient Populations with A Central Venous Catheter: A Systematic Review," *Arch Intern Med*, 2003, 163(16):1913-21.

Levine RL, Hursting MJ, Drexler A, et al, "Heparin-induced Thrombocytopenia in the Emergency Department," *Ann Emerg Med*, 2004, 44(5): 511-5.

Mathis AS, Davé N, Shah NK, et al, "Bleeding and Thrombosis in High-Risk Renal Transplantation Candidates Using Heparin," *Ann Pharmacother*, 2004, 38(4):537-43. Epub 2004 Feb 06.

Nguyen TN, Gal P, Ransom JL, et al, "Lepirudin Use in a Neonate with Heparin-Induced Thrombocytopenia," *Ann Pharmacother*, 2003, 37(2): 229-33.

Norman NE, Sneed AM, Brown C, et al, "Heparin-Induced Hyponatremia," *Ann Pharmacother*, 2004, 38(3):404-7.

Rice L, "Heparin-induced Thrombocytopenia: Myths and Misconceptions (That will Cause Trouble For You and Your Patient)," *Arch Intern Med*, 2004, 164(18):1961-4 (review).

Schwiesow SJ, Wessell AM, and Steyer TE, "Use of a Modified Dosing Weight for Heparin Therapy in a Morbidly Obese Patient," *Ann Pharmacother*, 2005, 39(4):753-6.

Tang IY, Cox DS, Patel K, et al, "Argatroban and Renal Replacement Therapy in Patients with Heparin-induced Thrombocytopenia," *Ann Pharmacother*, 2005, 39(2):231-6.

Verme-Gibboney CN and Hursting MJ, "Argatroban Dosing in Patients with Heparin-Induced Thrombocytopenia," *Ann Pharmacother*, 2003, 37(7-8):970-5.

Warkentin TE, "Heparin-Induced Thrombocytopenia, Part 2: Clinical Course and Treatment," *J Crit Illness*, 2005, 20(2):36-43.

Warkentin TE, Roberts RS, Hirsh J, et al, "An Improved Definition of Immune Heparin-Induced Thrombocytopenia in Postoperative Orthopedic Patients," *Arch Intern Med*, 2003, 163(20):2518-24.

Yalamanchili K, Sukhija R, Sinha N, et al, "Efficacy of Unfractionated Heparin for Thromboembolism Prophylaxis in Medical Patients," *Am J Ther*, 2005, 12(4):293-9.

Heroin

Related Information

- Highlights of Recent Reports (2006) on Substance Abuse and Mental Health
- Morphine Sulfate

CAS Number 1502-95-0; 561-27-3

Synonyms Acetomorphine; Diacetylmorphine; Diamorphine Hydrochloride; Heroin Hydrochloride

Impairment Potential Yes. Urine 6-acetylmorphine levels >10 ng/mL are consistent with recent use. (Jones AW, "Heroin Use by Motorists in Sweden Confirmed by Analysis of 6-Acetylmorphine in Urine," *J Anal Toxicol*, 2001, 25:353-5.)

Use Most commonly a drug of abuse in the United States; used as an analgesic agent or cough suppressant in Britain

Mechanism of Action Acetylated morphine derivative with CNS depressant effects

Adverse Reactions

Cardiovascular: Hypotension, congestive heart failure, vasculitis

Central nervous system: Lethargy, coma, euphoria, hallucinations, CNS depression, depression, paranoia, aggressive behavior, leukoencephalopathy, progressive spongiform leukoencephalopathy

Dermatologic: Pemphigus, acne, angioedema, toxic epidermal necrolysis, purpura, photosensitivity, pruritus, acanthosis nigricans, exanthem

Gastrointestinal: Constipation, xerostomia, nausea, vomiting, Ogilvie's syndrome, decreased esophageal sphincter tone

Genitourinary: Urinary retention, priapism

Hematologic: Thrombocytopenia,

Neuromuscular & skeletal: Myoclonus, rhabdomyolysis

Ocular: Miosis, photophobia

Renal: Renal failure, proteinuria

Respiratory: Apnea, respiratory depression, bronchospasm (upon nasal insufflation), pulmonary edema, aspiration, asthma, acute respiratory distress syndrome, eosinophilic pneumonia, bronchiectasis

Miscellaneous: Fixed drug eruption, acute atraumatic compartment syndrome

Signs and Symptoms of Overdose Amenorrhea, constipation, delirium, disorientation, dry mouth, dysphoria, encephalopathy, extrapyramidal reaction, hypothermia, impotence, myocardial depression, myopathy, nephrotic syndrome, pemphigus, photophobia, tongue discoloration

Admission Criteria/Prognosis

Ongoing respiratory depression after 4 hours postexposure should be admitted for 24-48 hours in the hospital; admit any hypoxemic patient (these patients are at risk for development of noncardiogenic pulmonary edema)

Patients with presumed opioid overdose can be safely discharged 1 hour after naloxone administration if they - 1) can mobilize as usual; 2) have oxygen saturation on room air of >92%; 3) have a respiratory rate >10 breaths per minute and <20 breaths per minute; 4) have a temperature of >35.0°C and <37.5°C; 5) have a heart rate >50 beats per minute, and <100 beats per minute; and 6) have a Glasgow Coma Scale score of 15.

Pharmacodynamics/Kinetics

Peak plasma level: 10 minutes after I.M. absorption

Distribution: V_d: 25 L/kg

Protein binding: 40%

Metabolism: Deacetylation to 6-acetylmorphine and then to morphine in the liver (both active metabolites)

Half-life: 3-20 minutes

Elimination: Urine (as morphine glucuronides); total clearance: 31 mL/kg/minute

Dosage Analgesia (in Europe):

Oral: 5-10 mg

I.M., SubQ: 5 mg (usually I.V. dose)

As a drug of abuse:

Nasal insufflation, I.V., SubQ: Up to 200 mg; usual dose: ~2 mg

Contraindications Hypersensitivity to morphine or diamorphine, acute respiratory depression

Warnings May provoke hypertension and tachycardia in patients with pheochromocytoma; use with caution in renal/liver insufficiency, diarrhea associated with antibiotics; pulmonary disease, gallbladder disease, hypothyroidism, inflammatory bowel disease, prostatic hypertrophy, increased intracranial pressure

Reference Range

Heroin doses of 150-200 mg can produce plasma morphine levels of 300 ng/mL; analgesic level: 20-65 ng/mL

Screening cutoffs for 6-Monoacetyl Morphine

- Urine - 10 ng/ml
- Hair 200 pg/mg
- Oral Fluid 4 ng/ml
- Sweat 25 ng/patch

Overdosage/Treatment

Decontamination: Oral: Activated charcoal; for asymptomatic body packers, whole bowel irrigation with polyethylene glycol (PEG) solution is recommended

Supportive therapy: Antidote of choice is naloxone (bolus: 0.4-2 mg I.V.); a continuous infusion may be required, especially in the management of a body stuffer/packer

Antidote(s)

- Nalmefene [ANTIDOTE]
- Naloxone [ANTIDOTE]

Diagnostic Procedures

- Morphine, Urine

Drug Interactions Subcutaneous absorption may be delayed when coadministered with cocaine

Pregnancy Risk Factor B; D (if used for prolonged periods or near term)

Pregnancy Implications Associated with increased incidence of congenital abnormalities; higher rates of neonatal jaundice (due to accelerated liver maturity), lower birth rates, and perinatal mortality have been reported; narcotic withdrawal (incidence of 85% usually appearing within 48 hours) with associated elevated neonatal serum magnesium levels must be monitored; withdrawal is related to dose and length of exposure

Additional Information Use and purity has been increasing; purity ranges from 3% to 30%; often combined with cocaine ("speedball") or phenobarbital/methaqualone ("karachi"); annual prevalence according to 1991 NIDA survey in U.S. population is ~0.3%.

It appears that older users are more likely to inject while younger users are more likely to snort or smoke. Dark (Mexican) heroin is usually less potent than white (Asian) heroin. Urine drug screen will remain positive for ~40 hours; adulterants include talc, cornstarch, quinine, lead, mannitol, sodium bicarbonate, and lidocaine. Delayed encephalopathy (after 4 days) can occur.

Heroin-associated renal disease has been declining since 1990 in New York City and Miami, Florida. With the average purity of New York street heroin increasing, this has led to the speculation that it was the impurities associated with heroin injection that led to the development of heroin-associated renal disease.

Wound botulism has been associated with black tar heroin use (through skin popping)

Thallium contaminated heroin has been documented in France

Behavioral and psychological effects of 12 mg intranasal heroin are equivalent to 6 mg intramuscular heroin. See table.

Celebrities in Whom Heroin Was Involved in Their Deaths

Matthew Ansara (Barbara Eden's son)
Chet Baker (Jazz musician)
Francisco Javier Barrios (Baseball Pitcher)
Jean-Michel Basquiat (Graffiti artist)
John Belushi (Comedian/actor)
Mike Bloomfield (Guitarist)
Tommy Bolin (Guitarist - Deep Purple)
Graham Bond (Musician)
Lenny Bruce (Comedian)
Tim Buckley (Guitarist, composer)
John Coltrane (Tenor saxophonist)
Raphael de Rothschild (Banking heir)
Chris Farley (Comedian)
Trevor Goddard (Actor)
Rodney Harvey (Actor)
Mitch Hedberg (Comedian)
Billie Holiday (Jazz singer)
Shannon Hoon (Singer - Blind Melon)
Janis Joplin (Rock/blues singer)
"Big Daddy" Lipscombe (Football star)
Frankie Lymon (Singer)
Phil Lynott (Guitarist - Thin Lizzy)
James D McElroy (Baseball Pitcher)
Robbie McIntosh (Drummer - Average White Band)
Johnathan Melvoin (Keyboard - Smashing Pumpkins)
Pamela Morrison (Widow of Jim Morrison - Lead singer of the Doors)
Gram Parsons (Guitarist - Byrds and Flying Burrito Brothers)
Kristine Pfaff (Bassist - Hole)
River Phoenix (Actor)
Robert Quine (Guitarist)
Oscar Scaggs (Son of singer Boz Scaggs)
Eddy Shaver (Country-rock guitarist)
Hillel Slovek (Red Hot Chili Peppers)
Eric Vaughn Show (Baseball Pitcher - San Diego Padres)
Daride Sorrenti (Fashion photographer)
Layne Staley (Frontman - Alice in Chains)
Mark Tuinei (Football player)
Sid Vicious (Bassist - Sex Pistols)
Danny Whitten (Guitarist - Crazy Horse)
Andrew Wood (Band member - Mother Love Bone)
Primary source: Caro M, "Heroin Leaves FreshTrack in Entertainment World," *Chicago Tribune*, July 14, 1996, 1-6.

Injection of "black tar" heroin (which has been the predominant form of heroin in the western United States during the 1990s) either intramuscularly or subcutaneously is the primary risk factor for development of wound botulism (46 cases in California from 1988 to 1995).

Combining lemon juice to solubilize heroin can reduce its pH to 2.8 and predispose the user to *Candida* septicemia.

Seven times as toxic as morphine; average yearly mortality rate among heroin injectors is 2%

- Heroin/morphine mentions increased 22% from the first half of 1999 (38,565 mentions) to the first half of 2000 (47,008).
- From the first half of 1999 to the first half of 2000, heroin/morphine mentions increased:

U.S. retail price per pure gram: About $1,000. Opium production in certain countries in 2000: Afghanistan: 3276 tons; Myanmar: 1087 tons; Laos: 167 tons; Columbia: 88 tons; Mexico: 21 tons; Pakistan: 8 tons; Thailand: 6 tons; Vietnam: 2 tons. U.S. spending on illicit heroin in 2000: About 12 billion dollars. Recovery rate from addiction is 40% to 50%; 33% of all drug users in the U.S. are addicted to heroin (1999 data).

According to the Drug Abuse warning Network in 2004:

- Heroin was involved in an estimated 162,137 Emergency Department (ED) Visits
- Heroin and alcohol combination was involved in an estimated 14,669 ED visits
- Heroin was involved in about 2% of visits involving suicide attempts and in 30% of visits seeking detox in ED.
- Peak age of ED visit for heroin abuse was 25 to 29 years.

U.S. retail price per pure gram: About $1,000. Opium production in certain countries in 2000: Afghanistan: 3276 tons; Myanmar: 1087 tons; Laos: 167 tons; Columbia: 88 tons; Mexico: 21 tons; Pakistan: 8 tons; Thailand: 6 tons; Vietnam: 2 tons. U.S. spending on illicit heroin in 2000: About 12 billion dollars. Recovery rate from addiction is 40% to 50%; 33% of all drug users in the U.S. are addicted to heroin (1999 data).

Specific References

Beck O and Böttcher M, "Paradoxical Results in Urine Drug Testing for 6-Acetylmorphine and Total Opiates: Implications for Best Analytical Strategy," *J Anal Toxicol*, 2006, 30:73-9.

Centers for Disease Control and Prevention (CDC), "Atypical Reactions Associated with Heroin Use - Five States, January-April 2005," *MMWR Morb Mortal Wkly Rep*, 2005, 54(32):793-6.

Centers for Disease Control and Prevention (CDC), "Unintentional Deaths from Drug Poisoning by Urbanization of Area—New Mexico, 1994-2003," *MMWR Morb Mortal Wkly Rep*, 2005, 54(35):870-3.

Charles BK, Day JE, Rollins DE, et al, "Opiate Recidivism in a Drug-Treatment Program: Comparison of Hair and Urine Data," *J Anal Toxicol*, 2003, 27:412-9.

Cibull DL, Lyons TP, and Sartori DA, "Positive Pressure Solid-Phase Extraction and GC-MS Analysis of 6-Monoacetylmorphine in Urine for Production Forensicc Drug Testing Labs," *J Anal Toxicol*, 2006, 30:130.

Cingolani M, Scavella S, Mencarelli R, et al, "Simultaneous Detection and Quantitation of Morphine, 6-Acetylmorphine, and Cocaine in Toenails: Comparison with Hair Analysis," *J Anal Toxicol*, 2004, 28(2):128-31.

Clarke J, Blum K, Newland G, et al, "Identification of Polydrug Use by Bilateral (Paired) Oral Fluid Specimen Collection," *J Anal Toxicol*, 2006, 30:145.

Collins ED, Kleber HD, Whittington RA, et al, "Anesthesia-Assisted vs Buprenorphine- or Clonidine-Assisted Heroin Detoxification and Naltrexone Induction: A Randomized Trial," *JAMA*, 2005, 294(8):903-13.

Colombage SM, "Laryngeal Obstruction by Heroin Packets," *Am J Forensic Med Pathol*, 2003, 24(2):153-4.

Fajemirokun-Odudeyi O, Sinha C, Tutty S, et al, "Pregnancy Outcome in Women Who Use Opiates," *Eur J Obstet Gynecol Reprod Biol*, 2005 Sep 30 (Epub ahead of print)

Gill AC, Oei J, Lewis NL, et al, "Strabismus in Infants of Opiate-Dependent Mothers," *Acta Paediatr*, 2003, 92(3):379-85.

Gupta R and Haydock T, "Severe Hypercapnia Caused by Acute Heroin Overdose," *Ann Emerg Med*, 2004, 43(5):665-6.

Hoffman RS, Burkhart K, Chan G, et al, "Multistate Outbreak of Clenbuterol Contaminated Heroin and Cocaine," *Clin Toxicol (Phila)*, 2005, 43:683.

Holler JM, Bosy TZ, Klette KL, et al, "Comparison of the Microgenics CEDIA® Heroin Metaboite (6-AM) and the Roche Abuscreen® ONLINE Opiate Immunoassays for the Detection of Heroin Use in Forensic Urine Samples," *J Anal Toxicol*, 2004, 28(6):489-93.

Jenkins AJ, Lavins ES, and Snyder A, "Evaluation of the Cedia Heroin Metabolite (6-AM) Immunoassay with Urine Specimens from A Criminal Justice Drug-Testing Program," *J Anal Toxicol*, 2005, 29(3):201-4.

Johnson K, Gerada C, and Greenough A, "Treatment of Neonatal Abstinence Syndrome," *Arch Dis Child Fetal Neonatal Ed*, 2003, 88(1):F2-5 (review).

Jordan MT, Bryant SM, Aks SE, et al, "Outcome of Heroin Body Stuffers: A Case Series," *J Toxicol Clin Toxicol*, 2003, 41(5):654.

Klous MG, Lee WC, Hillebrand MJ, et al, "Analysis of Diacetylmorphine, Caffeine, and Degradation Products After Volatilization of Pharmaceutical Heroin for Inhalation," *J Anal Toxicol*, 2006, 30:6-13.

Klous MG, Rook EJ, Hillebrand MJ, et al, "Deuterodiacetylmorphine as a Marker for Use of Illicit Heroin by Addicts in a Heroin-Assisted Treatment Program," *J Anal Toxicol*, 2005, 29:564-5.

Lavins ES, Snyder A, and Jenkins AJ, "Evaluation of the Cedia® 6-Acetylmorphine Immunoassay with Urine Specimens from a Criminal Justice Drug Testing Program," *J Anal Toxicol*, 2004, 28:296.

Liao KF, Peg CY, Lai SW, et al, "Descriptive Epidemiology of Hepatitis C Virus Among Male Heroin Abusers in Taiwan," *So Med J*, 2006, 99:348-51.

Long H, Deore K, Hoffman RS, et al, "A Fatal Case of Spongiform Leukoencephalopathy Linked to "Chasing the Dragon"," *J Toxicol Clin Toxicol*, 2003, 41(6):887-91.

Mabry B, Greller HA, and Nelson LS, "Patterns of Heroin Overdose-Induced Pulmonary Edema," *Am J Emerg Med*, 2004, 22(4):316.

Martin TG and Mount C, "Emergency Department Clinical Course of Opiate Overdoses," *J Toxicol Clin Toxicol*, 2003, 41(5):751.

Mell HK and Sztajnkrycer MD, "Clinical Images in Medical Toxicology: Heroin Overdose with Noncardiogenic Pulmonary Edema," *Clin Toxicol*, 2006, 44:399.

Mirakbari SM, Innes GD, Christenson J, et al, "Do Co-Intoxicants Increase Adverse Event Rates in the First 24 Hours in Patients Resuscitated from Acute Opioid Overdose?" *J Toxicol Clin Toxicol*, 2003, 41(7):947-53.

Musshoff F, Lachenmeier K, Wollersen H, et al, "Opiate Concentrations in Hair from Subjects in a Controlled Heroin-Maintenance Program and from Opiate-Associated Fatalities," *J Anal Toxicol*, 2005, 29(5):345-52.

Osselton M and Robinson S, "Analysis of 6-Monoacetyl Morphine, Morphine, Codeine, and Dihydrocodeine in Oral Fluid Collected from a Population of Drug Users," *J Anal Toxicol*, 2003, 27:195.

Patterson S and Cordero R, "Comparison of the Various Opiate Alkaloid Contaminants and Their Metabolites Found in Illicit Heroin with 6-Monoacetyl Morphine as Indicators of Heroin Ingestion," *J Anal Toxicol*, 2006, 30:267-73.

Pearson J and Saady J, "Utility of Vitreous Humor in Investigations of Heroin-Related Deaths," *J Anal Toxicol*, 2003, 27:199.

Seiter W, Robinson R, Porter T, et al, "Opiate Prevalence in Oral Fluid," *J Anal Toxicol*, 2004, 28:302.

Sterrett C, Brownfield J, Korn CS, et al, "Patterns of Presentation in Heroin Overdose Resulting in Pulmonary Edema," *Am J Emerg Med*, 2003, 21(1):32-4.

Traub SJ, Hoffman RS, and Nelson LS, "Pediatric Body-Packing: A 12-Year-Old 'Mule'," *J Toxicol Clin Toxicol*, 2002, 40(5):614.

Traub SJ, Hoffman RS, and Nelson LS, et al, "Body Packing - The Internal Concealment of Illicit Drugs," *N Engl J Med*, 2003, 349(26):2519-26.

von Euler M, Villen T, Svensson JO, et al, "Interpretation of the Presence of 6-Monoacetylmorphine in the Absence of Morphine-3-Glucuronide in Urine Samples: Evidence of Heroin Abuse," *Ther Drug Monit*, 2003, 25(5):645-8.

Wang SM, Sung UW, Lin CC, et al, "Distribution Characteristics of Opiates in Urine and Hair Specimens Collected from Alleged Heroin-Users in Northern Taiwan," *J Anal Toxicol*, 2006, 30:132.

Wills B, Aks S, Mazor S, et al, "Delayed Passage of Heroin Packets by a Body Stuffer," *J Toxicol Clin Toxicol*, 2004, 42(5):758.

Wyman J and Bultman S, "Postmortem Distribution of Heroin Metabolites in Femoral Blood, Liver, Cerebrospinal Fluid, and Vitreous Humor," *J Anal Toxicol*, 2004, 28:260-3.

Yegles M, "Pitfalls in Hair Analysis: Cosmetic Treatment," *Annale de Toxicologie Analytique*, 2005, 17(4):275-8.

Hexachlorophene

CAS Number 70-30-4
UN Number 2875
U.S. Brand Names pHisoHex®
Use Surgical scrub and as a bacteriostatic skin cleanser; control an outbreak of gram-positive infection when other procedures have been unsuccessful
Mechanism of Action Bacteriostatic polychlorinated biphenyl which inhibits membrane-bound enzymes and disrupts the cell membrane
Adverse Reactions
Cardiovascular: Hypotension, bradycardia, sinus bradycardia, cerebral edema
Central nervous system: Convulsions, irritability, fever, pseudotumor cerebri, vascular encephalopathy, dementia, confusion, drowsiness, coma, myelinopathy, leukoencephalopathy
Dermatologic: Dermatitis, erythema, dry skin, photosensitivity
Gastrointestinal: Anorexia, nausea, vomiting, diarrhea
Ocular: Optic neuropathy, blindness, diplopia
Respiratory: Wheezing upon exposure to hexachlorophene powder; respiratory failure, respiratory arrest
Admission Criteria/Prognosis Admit any patient with nervous system or cardiac toxicity or ingestions >20 mg/kg
Pharmacodynamics/Kinetics
Absorption: Percutaneously through inflamed, excoriated, and intact skin
Distribution: Crosses placenta
Half-life elimination: Infants: 6.1-44.2 hours
Dosage Children and Adults: Topical: Apply 5 mL cleanser and water to area to be cleansed; lather and rinse thoroughly under running water
Stability Store in nonmetallic container (**incompatible** with many metals)
Contraindications Hypersensitivity to halogenated phenol derivatives or hexachlorophene; use in premature infants; use on burned or denuded skin; occlusive dressing; application to mucous membranes
Warnings Discontinue use if signs of cerebral irritability occur; exposure of preterm infants or patients with extensive burns has been associated with apnea, convulsions, agitation and coma; do not use for bathing infants, premature infants are particularly susceptible to hexachlorophene topical absorption
Dosage Forms Liquid, topical: 3% (150 mL, 500 mL, 3840 mL)
Reference Range Lethal oral dose: 2-10 g; Death in a child associated with a serum hexachlorophene level of 0.78 mcg/mL
Overdosage/Treatment
Decontamination: **Oral:** Lavage (within 4 hours) >10 mg/kg; activated charcoal may not be useful. **Dermal:** Vigorous irrigation with soap and water; olive oil or castor oil can dissolve hexachlorophene and also be utilized
Enhancement of elimination: Peritoneal dialysis is not useful
Drug Interactions No data reported
Pregnancy Risk Factor C
Pregnancy Implications Crosses the placenta; spongiform encephalopathy in low birth weight infants
Nursing Implications Do not use for bathing infants; premature infants are particularly susceptible to hexachlorophene topical absorption
Additional Information In cosmetics, usually not at a concentration >0.1%

Hirudin

Unlabeled/Investigational Use Thrombolysis in acute myocardial infarction to prevent reocclusion

Mechanism of Action Derived from the leech (*Hirudo medicinalis*), hirudin is a specific thrombin inhibitor; inhibits conversion of fibrinogen to fibrin

Adverse Reactions Hematologic: Bleeding, hemorrhage, disseminated intravascular coagulation

Toxicodynamics/Kinetics

Absorption: SubQ: 36%

Distribution: V_d: 0.2 L/kg

Half-life: I.V.: 0.6-1.6 hours; SubQ: 0.6-3 hours

Elimination: Renal

Dosage I.V.:

Bolus: 0.1-0.4 mg/kg

Infusion: 0.06-0.15 mg/kg/hour

Monitoring Parameters Activated PTT, CBC

Overdosage/Treatment

Supportive therapy: Monitor APTT; bleeding is dose related; treat hemorrhage with local therapy; prothrombin complex concentrate can aid in decreasing bleeding

Enhanced elimination: Hemodiafiltration using a high-flux capillary dialyzer can assist in enhancing hirudin elimination

Additional Information Not available in U.S.

1 mcg of hirudin inhibits ~10 units of human thrombin. Risk of bleeding increases with bolus >0.6 mg/kg and infusion >0.2 mg/kg.

Histoplasmin

Pronunciation (hiss toe PLAZ min)

CAS Number 9008-05-3

U.S. Brand Names Histolyn-CYL®

Synonyms Histoplasmosis Skin Test Antigen

Use Diagnosing histoplasmosis; to assess cell-mediated immunity

Mechanism of Action In persons that have become sensitized to histoplasmin fungus, intradermal administration of histoplasmin skin test antigen evokes a delayed hypersensitivity reaction at the site of administration, if the T-cell immune system is intact

Adverse Reactions Local: Vesiculation, ulceration, or necrosis at site of administration

Signs and Symptoms of Overdose Excessive dosage may result in severe erythema and induration, followed by necrosis and ulceration which may last for several weeks.

Dosage Adults: Intradermally: 0.1 mL of 1:100 dilution into volar surface of forearm; induration of ≥5 mm in diameter indicates a positive reaction

Stability Store in refrigerator (2°C to 8°C)

Administration Use a $^3/_8$" to $^1/_2$" 26- or 27-gauge needle

Contraindications Known hypersensitivity to phenol or polysorbate 80

Warnings Epinephrine should be available for immediate treatment of anaphylactic reaction; use with caution in patients with coccidioidal erythema nodosum; a dilution of 1:10,000 should be used for the initial skin test; resuscitative equipment and drugs should be available

Dosage Forms Injection: 1:100 (0.1 mL, 1.3 mL)

Overdosage/Treatment Treatment is dilution of site of exposure

Drug Interactions Any live virus vaccine, corticosteroids, immunosuppressive agents may inhibit the immune response to the skin test

Pregnancy Risk Factor C

Nursing Implications Examine reaction site at 24-48 hours for cell-mediated immunity and 48-72 hours for histoplasmosis; use a $^3/_8$" to $^1/_2$" 26- or 27-gauge needle

Additional Information Some formulations may contain phenol.

Histrelin

Pronunciation (his TREL in)

U.S. Brand Names Vantas™

Synonyms GnRH Agonist; Histrelin Acetate; LH-RH Agonist

Use Palliative treatment of advanced prostate cancer

Mechanism of Action Potent inhibitor of gonadotropin secretion; continuous administration results in, after an initiation phase, the suppression of luteinizing hormone (LH), follicle-stimulating hormone (FSH), and a subsequent decrease in testosterone.

Adverse Reactions

>10%: Endocrine & metabolic: Expected pharmacological consequence of testosterone suppression: Hot flashes (66%)

2% to 10%:

Central nervous system: Fatigue (10%), headache (3%), insomnia (3%)

Endocrine & metabolic: Expected pharmacological consequences of testosterone suppression: Gynecomastia (4%), sexual dysfunction (4%), libido decreased (2%)

Gastrointestinal: Constipation (4%), weight gain (2%)

Genitourinary: Expected pharmacological consequence of testosterone suppression: Testicular atrophy (5%)

Local: Implant site reaction (6%)

Renal: Renal impairment (5%)

<2%: Abdominal discomfort, alopecia, anemia, appetite increased, arthralgia, AST increased, back pain, bone density decreased, bone pain, breast pain, breast tenderness, contusion, craving food, creatinine increased, depression, diaphoresis, dizziness, dyspnea (exertional), dysuria, feeling cold, fluid retention, genital pruritus, hematuria, hypercalcemia, hypercholesterolemia, hyperglycemia, irritability, LDH increased, lethargy, liver disorder, malaise, muscle twitching, nausea, neck pain, palpitation, peripheral edema, prostatic acid phosphatase increased, renal calculi, renal failure, stent occlusion, testosterone increased, tremor, urinary frequency, urinary retention, ventricular asystoles, weight loss

Pharmacodynamics/Kinetics

Onset: Chemical castration: 14 days

Duration: 1 year

Distribution: V_d: ~58 L

Protein binding: 70% ± 9%

Metabolism: Hepatic via C-terminal dealkylation and hydrolysis

Bioavailability: 92%

Half-life elimination: Terminal: ~4 hours

Time to peak, serum: 12 hours

Dosage SubQ:

Adults: 50 mg implant surgically inserted every 12 months

Elderly: See Adults dosing

Dosage adjustment in renal impairment: Cl_{cr}: 15-60 mL/minute: Adjustment not needed

Stability Vantas™: Upon delivery, separate contents of implant carton. Store implant under refrigeration at 2°C to 8°C (36°F to 46°F), wrapped in the amber pouch for protection from light; do not freeze. The implantation kit does not require refrigeration.

Monitoring Parameters LH and FSH levels, serum testosterone levels, prostate specific antigen (PSA), bone mineral density; weakness, paresthesias, and urinary tract obstruction (especially during first few weeks of therapy)

Administration SubQ: The implant must be removed from within the glass vial prior to implantation. Surgical implantation into the inner portion of the upper arm requires the use of the implantation device provided. Use the patient's nondominant arm for placement. Removal must occur after 12 months; a replacement implant may be required.

Contraindications Hypersensitivity to histrelin acetate, GnRH, GnRH-agonist analogs, or any component of the formulation; children; females

Warnings Transient increases in testosterone serum levels occur during the first week of use. Worsening symptoms such as bone pain, neuropathy, ureteral or bladder outlet obstruction, and spinal cord compression have been reported. Spinal cord compression and ureteral obstruction may contribute to paralysis; close attention should be given during the first few weeks of therapy to both patients having metastatic vertebral lesions and/or urinary tract obstructions, and to any patients reporting weakness, paresthesias or poor urine output. Safety and efficacy have not been established in patients with hepatic dysfunction.

Dosage Forms Implant: 50 mg [released over 12 months; packaged with implantation kit]

Reference Range

Testosterone level: Expected to rise during the first few days and decline to below initiation level by week 2 before reaching ≤50 ng/dL (castrate level)

PSA: Expected to decrease to normal levels after 6 months of therapy

Note: Lack of response (testosterone and PSA decreases) should prompt suspicion that the implant has been expelled.

Test Interactions Results of diagnostic test of pituitary gonadotropic and gonadal functions may be affected during and after therapy

Drug Interactions Not studied

Pregnancy Risk Factor X

Pregnancy Implications Fetal harm and an increase in fetal mortalities have been noted in animal studies. Histrelin is contraindicated for use in females.

Lactation Excretion in breast milk unknown/contraindicated

HydrALAZINE

CAS Number 304-20-1; 86-54-5

Synonyms Apresoline [DSC]; Hydralazine Hydrochloride

Use Management of moderate to severe hypertension, congestive heart failure, hypertension secondary to pre-eclampsia/eclampsia; treatment of primary pulmonary hypertension

Mechanism of Action Direct vasodilation of arterioles (with little effect on veins) with decreased systemic resistance

Adverse Reactions

Cardiovascular: **Palpitations**, **flushing**, **tachycardia**, edema, myocardial ischemia, pericardial effusion/pericarditis, pulmonary hypertension, sinus tachycardia, vasodilation, **angina pectoris**, vasculitis

Central nervous system: Malaise, dizziness, fever, **headache**, depression, CNS depression, axonopathy

Dermatologic: Rash, pruritus, neutrophilic dermatosis (Sweet's syndrome), Stevens-Johnson syndrome, angioedema, bullous skin disease, urticaria, purpura, photosensitivity, erythema nodosum, exanthem, cutaneous vasculitis

Endocrine & metabolic: Nephrogenic diabetes insipidus

Gastrointestinal: **Anorexia, nausea, vomiting, diarrhea**, feces discoloration (black), loss of taste perception

Hepatic: Granulomatous hepatitis

Neuromuscular & skeletal: Arthralgia, peripheral neuritis, paresthesia, weakness

Ocular: Lacrimation, blurred vision, eyelid edema

Renal: Glomerulonephritis, renal vasculitis

Respiratory: Asthma, eosinophilic pneumonia, pulmonary vasculitis

Miscellaneous: Positive ANA, positive LE cells, systemic lupus erythematosus, fixed drug eruption, elevated antineutrophilic cytoplasmic antibodies (ANCA)

Signs and Symptoms of Overdose Agranulocytosis, arrhythmias, cholestatic jaundice, erythema multiforme, granulocytopenia, hyperthermia, hypokalemia, hypotension, impotence, lacrimation, lactic acidosis, leukopenia, neuropathy (peripheral), neutropenia, shock, tachycardia, thrombocytopenia, wheezing

Pharmacodynamics/Kinetics

Onset of action: Oral: 20-30 minutes; I.V.: 5-20 minutes

Duration: Oral: Up to 8 hours; I.V.: 1-4 hours; **Note:** May vary depending on acetylator status of patient

Distribution: Crosses placenta; enters breast milk

Protein binding: 85% to 90%

Metabolism: Hepatically acetylated; extensive first-pass effect (oral)

Bioavailability: 30% to 50%; increased with food

Half-life elimination: Normal renal function: 2-8 hours; End-stage renal disease: 7-16 hours

Excretion: Urine (14% as unchanged drug)

Dosage

Children:

Oral: Initial: 0.75-1 mg/kg/day in 2-4 divided doses; increase over 3-4 weeks to maximum of 7.5 mg/kg/day in 2-4 divided doses; maximum daily dose: 200 mg/day

I.M., I.V.: 0.1-0.2 mg/kg/dose (not to exceed 20 mg) every 4-6 hours as needed, up to 1.7-3.5 mg/kg/day in 4-6 divided doses

Adults:

Oral: Hypertension:

Initial dose: 10 mg 4 times/day for first 2-4 days; increase to 25 mg 4 times/day for the balance of the first week

Increase by 10-25 mg/dose gradually to 50 mg 4 times/day (maximum: 300 mg/day); usual dose range (JNC 7): 25-100 mg/day in 2 divided doses

Oral: Congestive heart failure:

Initial dose: 10-25 mg 3-4 times/day

Adjustment: Dosage must be adjusted based on individual response

Target dose: 225-300 mg/day; use in combination with isosorbide dinitrate

I.M., I.V.:

Hypertension: Initial: 10-20 mg/dose every 4-6 hours as needed, may increase to 40 mg/dose; change to oral therapy as soon as possible.

Pre-eclampsia/eclampsia: 5 mg/dose then 5-10 mg every 20-30 minutes as needed.

Elderly: Oral: Initial: 10 mg 2-3 times/day; increase by 10-25 mg/day every 2-5 days.

Dosing interval in renal impairment:

Cl_{cr} 10-50 mL/minute: Administer every 8 hours.

Cl_{cr} <10 mL/minute: Administer every 8-16 hours in fast acetylators and every 12-24 hours in slow acetylators.

Hemodialysis: Supplemental dose is not necessary.

Peritoneal dialysis: Supplemental dose is not necessary.

Stability Changes color after contact with a metal filter; do not store intact ampuls in refrigerator

Monitoring Parameters Blood pressure (monitor closely with I.V. use), standing and sitting/supine, heart rate, ANA titer

Administration Inject over 1 minute. Hypotensive effect may be delayed and unpredictable in some patients.

Contraindications Hypersensitivity to hydralazine or any component of the formulation; mitral valve rheumatic heart disease

Warnings May cause a drug-induced lupus-like syndrome (more likely on larger doses, longer duration). Adjust dose in severe renal dysfunction. Use with caution in CAD (increase in tachycardia may increase myocardial oxygen demand). Use with caution in pulmonary hypertension (may cause hypotension). Patients may be poorly compliant because of frequent dosing.

Monitor blood pressure closely following I.V. administration. Response may be delayed and unpredictable in some patients. Titrate cautiously to response. Hydralazine-induced fluid and sodium retention may require addition or increased dosage of a diuretics.

Dosage Forms Injection, solution, as hydrochloride: 20 mg/mL (1 mL)

Tablet, as hydrochloride: 10 mg, 25 mg, 50 mg, 100 mg

Overdosage/Treatment

Decontamination: Ipecac (within 30 minutes)/lavage (within 1 hour)/activated charcoal

Supportive therapy: Hypotension usually responds to I.V. fluids or Trendelenburg positioning. If unresponsive to these measures, the use of a parenteral vasoconstrictor may be required (eg, norepinephrine 0.1-0.2 mcg/kg/minute titrated to response). Treatment is primarily supportive and symptomatic. Verapamil, esmolol, or propranolol may be used to treat tachycardia. Polyneuropathy may respond to pyridoxine.

Enhancement of elimination: Multiple dosing of activated charcoal may be useful

Test Interactions ↑ calcium (S)

Drug Interactions Inhibits CYP3A4 (weak)

Beta-blockers (metoprolol, propranolol) serum concentrations and pharmacologic effects may be increased. Monitor cardiovascular status.

Propranolol increases hydralazine's serum concentrations. Acebutolol, atenolol, and nadolol (low hepatic clearance or no first-pass metabolism) are unlikely to be affected.

NSAIDs may decrease the hemodynamic effects of hydralazine; avoid use if possible or closely monitor cardiovascular status.

Pregnancy Risk Factor C

Pregnancy Implications Crosses the placenta. One report of fetal arrhythmia; transient neonatal thrombocytopenia and fetal distress reported following late 3rd trimester use. A large amount of clinical experience with the use of this drug for management of hypertension during pregnancy is available. Available evidence suggests safe use during pregnancy.

Lactation Enters breast milk/compatible

Nursing Implications Monitor blood pressure closely with I.V. use; dextrose solutions suggested

Additional Information Slow acetylators, patients with decreased renal function and patients receiving >200 mg/day (chronically) are at higher risk for systemic lupus erythematosus (SLE). Usually administered with diuretic and a beta-blocker to counteract side effects of sodium and water retention and reflex tachycardia although the beta-blocker may not be necessary in the elderly; odorless, bitter-tasting powder.

Specific References

Chobanian AV, Bakris GL, Black HR, et al, "The Seventh Report of the Joint National Committee on Prevention, Detection, Evaluation, and Treatment of High Blood Pressure: The JNC 7 Report," *JAMA*, 2003, 289(19):2560-71.

Finks SW, Finks AC, and Self TH, "Hydralazine-Induced Lupus: Maintaining Vigilance with Increased Use in Patients with Heart Failure," *So Med J*, 2006, 99(1):18-25.

Hydrochlorothiazide

CAS Number 58-93-5

U.S. Brand Names Aquazide® H; Microzide™; Oretic®

Synonyms HCTZ (error-prone abbreviation)

Use Management of mild to moderate hypertension; treatment of edema in congestive heart failure and nephrotic syndrome

Unlabeled/Investigational Use Treatment of lithium-induced diabetes insipidus

Mechanism of Action Inhibits sodium reabsorption in the distal tubules causing increased excretion of sodium and water as well as potassium and hydrogen ions; at high doses may inhibit carbonic anhydrase

Adverse Reactions

Cardiovascular: Myocarditis (hypersensitivity), postural hypotension

Central nervous system: Drowsiness, hyperthermia, fever

Dermatologic: Photosensitivity, exfoliative dermatitis, erythema multiforme, bullous skin disease, toxic epidermal necrolysis, urticaria, purpura, pruritus, licheniform eruptions, exanthem, photoallergic reaction

Endocrine & metabolic: Hypokalemia, hypercalcemia, hyperglycemia, hypochloremic metabolic alkalosis, hyperlipidemia, hyperuricemia, syndrome of inappropriate antidiuretic hormone, hypophosphatemia, hyponatremia, hypomagnesemia

Gastrointestinal: Nausea, vomiting, anorexia, loss of taste perception, xerostomia, pancreatitis

Hematologic: Aplastic anemia, hemolysis, leukopenia, neutropenia, agranulocytosis, granulocytopenia, thrombocytopenia

Hepatic: Hepatitis, intrahepatic cholestasis

Neuromuscular & skeletal: Paresthesia, weakness

Ocular: Acute angle-closure glaucoma, color vision abnormalities, phototoxic

Renal: Polyuria, prerenal azotemia

Miscellaneous: Systemic lupus erythematosus, fixed drug eruption, zinc depletion

Signs and Symptoms of Overdose Agranulocytosis, AV block, cystitis, diabetes insipidus, diuresis, fever, granulocytopenia, hypercalcemia, hyperglycemia, hyperperistalsis, hyperuricemia, hypokalemia, hyponatremia, impotence, leukopenia, myalgia, myasthenia gravis (exacerbation or precipitation), myocarditis, neutropenia, nocturia, pancreatitis, photosensitivity, vision color changes (yellow tinge)

Pharmacodynamics/Kinetics
Onset of action: Diuresis: ~2 hours
  Peak effect: 4-6 hours
Duration: 6-12 hours
Absorption: ~50% to 80%
Distribution: 3.6-7.8 L/kg
Protein binding: 68%
Metabolism: Not metabolized
Bioavailability: 50% to 80%
Half-life elimination: 5.6-14.8 hours
Time to peak: 1-2.5 hours
Excretion: Urine (as unchanged drug)

Dosage Oral (effect of drug may be decreased when used every day):
Children (in pediatric patients, chlorothiazide may be preferred over hydrochlorothiazide as there are more dosage formulations [eg, suspension] available):
  <6 months: 2-3 mg/kg/day in 2 divided doses
  >6 months: 2 mg/kg/day in 2 divided doses
Adults:
  Edema: 25-100 mg/day in 1-2 doses; maximum: 200 mg/day
  Hypertension: 12.5-50 mg/day; minimal increase in response and more electrolyte disturbances are seen with doses >50 mg/day
Elderly: 12.5-25 mg once daily
Dosing adjustment/comments in renal impairment: Cl_{cr} 25-50 mL/minute: Not effective

Monitoring Parameters Assess weight, I & O reports daily to determine fluid loss; blood pressure, serum electrolytes, BUN, creatinine

Administration May be taken with food or milk. Take early in day to avoid nocturia. Take the last dose of multiple doses no later than 6 PM unless instructed otherwise.

Contraindications Hypersensitivity to hydrochlorothiazide or any component of the formulation, thiazides, or sulfonamide-derived drugs; anuria; renal decompensation; pregnancy

Warnings
Avoid in severe renal disease (ineffective). Electrolyte disturbances (hypokalemia, hypochloremic alkalosis, hyponatremia) can occur. Use with caution in severe hepatic dysfunction; hepatic encephalopathy can be caused by electrolyte disturbances. Gout can be precipitate in certain patients with a history of gout, a familial predisposition to gout, or chronic renal failure. Cautious use in diabetics; may see a change in glucose control. Hypersensitivity reactions can occur. Can cause SLE exacerbation or activation. Use with caution in patients with moderate or high cholesterol concentrations. Photosensitization may occur. Correct hypokalemia before initiating therapy.
Chemical similarities are present among sulfonamides, sulfonylureas, carbonic anhydrase inhibitors, thiazides, and loop diuretics (except ethacrynic acid). Use in patients with sulfonamide allergy is specifically contraindicated in product labeling, however, a risk of cross-reaction exists in patients with allergy to any of these compounds; avoid use when previous reaction has been severe.

Dosage Forms Capsule (Microzide™): 12.5 mg
Tablet: 25 mg, 50 mg

Reference Range Serum level of 2 mcg/mL associated with peak diuretic effect

Overdosage/Treatment
Decontamination: Activated charcoal
Supportive therapy: I.V. hydration with 0.9% saline with electrolyte replacement; diuresis is usually short-lived
Enhancement of elimination: Hemodialysis may be effective

Test Interactions ↑ creatine phosphokinase (S), ammonia (B), amylase (S), calcium (S), cholesterol (S), glucose, acid (S); ↓ chloride (S), magnesium, potassium (S), sodium (S); hydrochlorothiazide may cause false increase in acetaminophen assay by HPLC

Drug Interactions ACE inhibitors: Increased hypotension if aggressively diuresed with a thiazide diuretic.
Beta-blockers increase hyperglycemic effects in type 2 diabetes mellitus (noninsulin dependent, NIDDM)
Cholestyramine: Hydrochlorothiazide absorption may be decreased.
Colestipol: Hydrochlorothiazide absorption may be decreased.
Cyclosporine and thiazides can increase the risk of gout or renal toxicity; avoid concurrent use.
Digoxin toxicity can be exacerbated if a thiazide induces hypokalemia or hypomagnesemia.
Lithium toxicity can occur by reducing renal excretion of lithium; monitor lithium concentration and adjust as needed.
Neuromuscular blocking agents can prolong blockade; monitor serum potassium and neuromuscular status.
NSAIDs can decrease the efficacy of thiazides reducing the diuretic and antihypertensive effects.

Pregnancy Risk Factor B (manufacturer); D (expert analysis)

Pregnancy Implications Although there are no adequate and well-controlled studies using hydrochlorothiazide in pregnancy, thiazide diuretics may cause an increased risk of congenital defects. Hypoglycemia, hypokalemia, hyponatremia, jaundice, and thrombocytopenia are also reported as possible complications to the fetus or newborn.

Lactation Enters breast milk/use caution (AAP rates "compatible")

Additional Information Inhibits insulin secretion/vitamin D synthesis

Specific References
Odvina CV, Mason RP, and Pak CC, "Prevention of Thiazide-Induced Hypokalemia Without Magnesium Depletion by Potassium-Magnesium-Citrate," *Am J Ther*, 2006, 13:101-8.
Schoofs MW, van der Klift M, Hofman A, et al, "Thiazide Diuretics and the Risk for Hip Fracture," *Ann Intern Med*, 2003, 139(6):476-82.

Hydrocodone and Acetaminophen

U.S. Brand Names Anexsia®; Bancap HC®; Ceta-Plus®; Co-Gesic®; hycet™; Lorcet® 10/650; Lorcet® Plus; Lorcet®-HD; Lortab®; Margesic® H; Maxidone™; Norco®; Stagesic®; Vicodin® ES; Vicodin® HP; Vicodin®; Zydone®

Synonyms Acetaminophen and Hydrocodone

Use Relief of moderate to severe pain; antitussive (hydrocodone)

Mechanism of Action Hydrocodone, as with other narcotic (opiate) analgesics, blocks pain perception in the cerebral cortex by binding to specific receptor molecules (opiate receptors) within the neuronal membranes of synapses. This binding results in a decreased synaptic chemical transmission throughout the CNS thus inhibiting the flow of pain sensations into the higher centers. Mu and kappa are the two subtypes of the opiate receptor which hydrocodone binds to cause analgesia.
Acetaminophen inhibits the synthesis of prostaglandins in the CNS and peripherally blocks pain impulse generation; produces antipyresis from inhibition of hypothalamic heat-regulating center.

Adverse Reactions
Cardiovascular: Hypotension, bradycardia, hypertension
Central nervous system: Lightheadedness, dizziness, sedation, drowsiness, fatigue, confusion, hallucinations
Gastrointestinal: Nausea, vomiting, xerostomia, anorexia, biliary tract spasm
Genitourinary: Decreased urination
Neuromuscular & skeletal: Weakness
Ocular: Diplopia, miosis
Respiratory: Dyspnea
Miscellaneous: Histamine release, physical and psychological dependence with prolonged use

Signs and Symptoms of Overdose Blood dyscrasias, hepatic necrosis, respiratory depression

Pharmacodynamics/Kinetics
Acetaminophen: See Acetaminophen monograph.
Hydrocodone:
Onset of action: Narcotic analgesic: 10-20 minutes
Duration: 4-8 hours
Distribution: Crosses placenta
Metabolism: Hepatic; O-demethylation; N-demethylation and 6-ketosteroid reduction
Half-life elimination: 3.3-4.4 hours
Excretion: Urine

Dosage
Oral (doses should be titrated to appropriate analgesic effect); for children ≥12 years of age and adults, the dosage of acetaminophen should be limited to ≤4 g/day (and possibly less in patients with hepatic impairment or ethanol use)
Children:
  Antitussive (hydrocodone): 0.6 mg/kg/day in 3-4 divided doses; even though dosing by hydrocodone, make sure to keep within age-specific acetaminophen doses as well
    A single dose should not exceed 10 mg in children >12 years, 5 mg in children 2-12 years, and 1.25 mg in children <2 years of age
  Analgesic (acetaminophen): Refer to Acetaminophen
Adults: Analgesic: 1-2 tablets or capsules every 4-6 hours or 5-10 mL solution every 4-6 hours as needed for pain; do not exceed 4 g/day of acetaminophen
  Hydrocodone 2.5-5 mg and acetaminophen 400-500 mg; maximum: 8 tablets/capsules per day
  Hydrocodone 7.5 mg and acetaminophen: 400-650 mg; maximum: 6 tablets/capsules per day
  Hydrocodone 2.5 mg and acetaminophen: 167 mg/5 mL (elixir/solution); maximum: 6 Tbsp/day
  Hydrocodone 7.5 mg and acetaminophen 750 mg; maximum: 5 tablets/capsules per day
  Hydrocodone 10 mg and acetaminophen: 350-660 mg; maximum: 6 tablets/day per product labeling
  Do not exceed 4 g/day of acetaminophen

Monitoring Parameters Pain relief, respiratory and mental status, blood pressure

Contraindications Hypersensitivity to hydrocodone, acetaminophen, or any component of the formulation; CNS depression; severe respiratory depression

Warnings

Use with caution in patients with hypersensitivity reactions to other phenanthrene derivative opioid agonists (morphine, hydromorphone, levorphanol, oxycodone, oxymorphone); tolerance or drug dependence may result from extended use.

Respiratory depressant effects may be increased with head injuries. Use caution with acute abdominal conditions; clinical course may be obscured. Use caution with thyroid dysfunction, prostatic hyperplasia, hepatic or renal disease, and in the elderly. Causes sedation; caution must be used in performing tasks which require alertness (eg, operating machinery or driving).

Limit acetaminophen to <4 g/day. May cause severe hepatic toxicity in acute overdose; in addition, chronic daily dosing in adults has resulted in liver damage in some patients. Use with caution in patients with alcoholic liver disease; consuming ≥3 alcoholic drinks/day may increase the risk of liver damage. Use with caution in patients with known G6PD deficiency.

Dosage Forms Capsule:

Bancap HC®, Ceta-Plus®, Margesic® H, Stagesic®: Hydrocodone bitartrate 5 mg and acetaminophen 500 mg

Elixir: Hydrocodone bitartrate 7.5 mg and acetaminophen 500 mg per 15 mL (480 mL)

Lortab®: Hydrocodone bitartrate 7.5 mg and acetaminophen 500 mg per 15 mL (480 mL) [contains alcohol 7%; tropical fruit punch flavor]

Solution, oral:

hycet™: Hydrocodone bitartrate 7.5 mg and acetaminophen 325 mg per 15 mL (480 mL) [contains alcohol 7%; tropical fruit punch flavor]

Tablet:

Hydrocodone bitartrate 2.5 mg and acetaminophen 500 mg
Hydrocodone bitartrate 5 mg and acetaminophen 325 mg
Hydrocodone bitartrate 5 mg and acetaminophen 500 mg
Hydrocodone bitartrate 7.5 mg and acetaminophen 325 mg
Hydrocodone bitartrate 7.5 mg and acetaminophen 500 mg
Hydrocodone bitartrate 7.5 mg and acetaminophen 650 mg
Hydrocodone bitartrate 7.5 mg and acetaminophen 750 mg
Hydrocodone bitartrate 10 mg and acetaminophen 325 mg
Hydrocodone bitartrate 10 mg and acetaminophen 500 mg
Hydrocodone bitartrate 10 mg and acetaminophen 650 mg
Hydrocodone bitartrate 10 mg and acetaminophen 660 mg

Anexsia®:

5/500: Hydrocodone bitartrate 5 mg and acetaminophen 500 mg [DSC]

7.5/650: Hydrocodone bitartrate 7.5 mg and acetaminophen 650 mg

Co-Gesic® 5/500: Hydrocodone bitartrate 5 mg and acetaminophen 500 mg

Lorcet® 10/650: Hydrocodone bitartrate 10 mg and acetaminophen 650 mg

Lorcet® Plus: Hydrocodone bitartrate 7.5 mg and acetaminophen 650 mg

Lortab®:

2.5/500: Hydrocodone bitartrate 2.5 mg and acetaminophen 500 mg
5/500: Hydrocodone bitartrate 5 mg and acetaminophen 500 mg
7.5/500: Hydrocodone bitartrate 7.5 mg and acetaminophen 500 mg
10/500: Hydrocodone bitartrate 10 mg and acetaminophen 500 mg

Maxidone™: Hydrocodone bitartrate 10 mg and acetaminophen 750 mg

Norco®:

Hydrocodone bitartrate 5 mg and acetaminophen 325 mg
Hydrocodone bitartrate 7.5 mg and acetaminophen 325 mg
Hydrocodone bitartrate 10 mg and acetaminophen 325 mg

Vicodin®: Hydrocodone bitartrate 5 mg and acetaminophen 500 mg

Vicodin® ES: Hydrocodone bitartrate 7.5 mg and acetaminophen 750 mg

Vicodin® HP: Hydrocodone bitartrate 10 mg and acetaminophen 660 mg

Zydone®:

Hydrocodone bitartrate 5 mg and acetaminophen 400 mg
Hydrocodone bitartrate 7.5 mg and acetaminophen 400 mg
Hydrocodone bitartrate 10 mg and acetaminophen 400 mg

Overdosage/Treatment

Treatment consists of acetylcysteine 140 mg/kg orally (loading) followed by 70 mg/kg every 4 hours for 17 doses; therapy should be initiated based upon laboratory analysis suggesting a high probability for hepatotoxic potential or I.V Prescott Protocol. See Acetaminophen. Naloxone, 2 mg I.V. With repeat administration as necessary up to a total of 10 mg, can also be used to reverse toxic effects of the opiate.

Decontamination: Oral: Activated charcoal is effective at binding certain chemicals, and this is especially true for acetaminophen.

Drug Interactions Hydrocodone: **Substrate** of CYP2D6 (major)

Acetaminophen: **Substrate** (minor) of CYP1A2, 2A6, 2C9, 2D6, 2E1, 3A4; **Inhibits** CYP3A4 (weak)

Acetaminophen component: Refer to Acetaminophen monograph.

Hydrocodone component:

CYP2D6 inhibitors may decrease the effects of hydrocodone. Example inhibitors include chlorpromazine, delavirdine, fluoxetine, miconazole, paroxetine, pergolide, quinidine, quinine, ritonavir, and ropinirole.

CNS depressants (including antianxiety agents, antihistamines, antipsychotics, narcotics): CNS depression is additive; dose adjustment may be needed

MAO inhibitors: May see increased effects of MAO inhibitor and hydrocodone.

Tricyclic antidepressants (TCAs): May see increased effects of TCA and hydrocodone.

Pregnancy Risk Factor C

Pregnancy Implications Animal reproduction studies have not been conducted with this combination product. Opioid analgesics are considered FDA risk category D if used for prolonged periods or in large doses near term. Withdrawal symptoms may be observed in babies born to mothers taking opioids regularly during pregnancy. Respiratory depression may be observed in the newborn if opioids are given close to delivery.

Lactation Excretion in breast milk unknown/contraindicated

Nursing Implications Observe patient for excessive sedation, respiratory depression

Additional Information Acetaminophen dosing for pediatric patients: 10-15 mg/kg/dose **or alternatively,**

Up to 3 months: 40 mg
4-11 months: 80 mg
1-2 years: 120 mg
2-3 years: 160 mg
4-5 years: 240 mg
6-8 years: 320 mg
9-10 years: 400 mg
11 years: 480 mg

Mid-Year 2000 Emergency Department Drug Abuse Warning Network (DAWN) data:

A comparison of the first half of 1999 and the first half of 2000 revealed significant increases in mentions of hydrocodone (51% from 6341 to 9549).

Specific References

Miller NS and Greenfeld A, "Patient Characteristics and Risks Factors for Development of Dependence on Hydrocodone and Oxycodone," *Am J Ther*, 2004, 11(1):26-32.

Mycyk MB, Tudor BC, and DiMaano JQ, "ED Visits and Hospitalizations Are Increasing Among Young Adults Abusing Oral Narcotics," *Clin Toxicol (Phila)*, 2005, 43:668.

Hydrocortisone

Related Information

● Corticosteroids

CAS Number 125-04-2; 13609-67-1; 2203-97-6; 50-03-3; 50-23-7; 508-99-6; 57524-89-7; 6000-74-4; 83784-20-7

U.S. Brand Names A-hydroCort®; Anucort-HC®; Anusol-HC®; Anusol® HC-1 [OTC]; Aquanil™ HC [OTC]; CaldeCORT® [OTC]; Cetacort®; Colocort™; CortaGel® Maximum Strength [OTC]; Cortaid® Intensive Therapy [OTC]; Cortaid® Maximum Strength [OTC]; Cortaid® Sensitive Skin with Aloe [OTC]; Cortef®; Corticool® [OTC]; Cortifoam®; Cortizone® 10 Quick Shot [OTC]; Cortizone® for Kids [OTC]; Cortizone®-10 Maximum Strength [OTC]; Cortizone®-10 Plus Maximum Strength [OTC]; Cortizone®-5 [OTC]; Dermarest Dricort® [OTC]; Dermtex® HC [OTC]; EarSol® HC; Hemril-HC®; Hydrocortone® Phosphate; Hydrocortone® [DSC]; Hytone®; LactiCare-HC®; Locoid Lipocream®; Locoid®; Nupercainal® Hydrocortisone Cream [OTC]; Nutracort®; Pandel®; Post Peel Healing Balm [OTC]; Preparation H® Hydrocortisone [OTC]; Proctocort®; ProctoCream® HC; Proctosol-HC®; Sarnol®-HC [OTC]; Solu-Cortef®; Summer's Eve® SpecialCare™ Medicated Anti-Itch Cream [OTC]; Texacort®; Theracort® [OTC]; Westcort®

Synonyms A-hydroCort; Compound F; Cortisol; Hemorrhoidal HC; Hydrocortisone Acetate; Hydrocortisone Butyrate; Hydrocortisone Probutate; Hydrocortisone Sodium Succinate; Hydrocortisone Valerate

Use Management of adrenocortical insufficiency; relief of inflammation of corticosteroid-responsive dermatoses (low and medium potency topical corticosteroid); adjunctive treatment of ulcerative colitis

Mechanism of Action Decreases inflammation by suppression of migration of polymorphonuclear leukocytes and reversal of increased capillary permeability

Adverse Reactions

Systemic:

Cardiovascular: Hypotension, edema

Central nervous system: **Insomnia, nervousness**, euphoria, headache, delirium, hallucinations, seizures, mood swings

Dermatologic: Hirsutism, acne, dermatitis, skin atrophy, bruising, hyperpigmentation

Endocrine & metabolic: Diabetes mellitus, hypokalemia, hyperglycemia, Cushing's syndrome, sodium and water retention, bone growth suppression, amenorrhea

Gastrointestinal: **Increased appetite, indigestion**, peptic ulcer, abdominal distention, ulcerative esophagitis, pancreatitis

Neuromuscular & skeletal: Arthralgia, muscle wasting

Ocular: Cataracts

Respiratory: Epistaxis

Miscellaneous: Hypersensitivity reactions, immunosuppression

Topical:

Dermatologic: **Eczema**, pruritus, stinging, dry skin, allergic contact dermatitis, hypopigmentation, striae dermal atrophy, folliculitis

Endocrine & metabolic: HPA axis suppression, hyperglycemia, hypokalemia

Local: Burning

Signs and Symptoms of Overdose Cushingoid appearance, muscle weakness, osteoporosis (with systemic long-term use only). When consumed in excessive quantities for prolonged periods, systemic hypercorticism and adrenal suppression may occur. In those cases, discontinuation and withdrawal of the corticosteroid should be done judiciously.

Pharmacodynamics/Kinetics

Onset of action:

Hydrocortisone acetate: Slow

Hydrocortisone sodium succinate (water soluble): Rapid

Duration: Hydrocortisone acetate: Long

Absorption: Rapid by all routes, except rectally

Metabolism: Hepatic

Half-life elimination: Biologic: 8-12 hours

Excretion: Urine (primarily as 17-hydroxysteroids and 17-ketosteroids)

Dosage

Dose should be based on severity of disease and patient response

Acute adrenal insufficiency: I.M., I.V.:

Infants and young Children: Succinate: 1-2 mg/kg/dose bolus, then 25-150 mg/day in divided doses every 6-8 hours

Older Children: Succinate: 1-2 mg/kg bolus then 150-250 mg/day in divided doses every 6-8 hours

Adults: Succinate: 100 mg I.V. bolus, then 300 mg/day in divided doses every 8 hours or as a continuous infusion for 48 hours; once patient is stable change to oral, 50 mg every 8 hours for 6 doses, then taper to 30-50 mg/day in divided doses

Chronic adrenal corticoid insufficiency: Adults: Oral: 20-30 mg/day

Anti-inflammatory or immunosuppressive:

Infants and Children:

Oral: 2.5-10 mg/kg/day **or** 75-300 mg/m²/day every 6-8 hours

I.M., I.V.: Succinate: 1-5 mg/kg/day **or** 30-150 mg/m²/day divided every 12-24 hours

Adolescents and Adults: Oral, I.M., I.V.: Succinate: 15-240 mg every 12 hours

Congenital adrenal hyperplasia: Oral: Initial: 10-20 mg/m²/day in 3 divided doses; a variety of dosing schedules have been used. **Note:** Inconsistencies have occurred with liquid formulations; tablets may provide more reliable levels. Doses must be individualized by monitoring growth, bone age, and hormonal levels. Mineralocorticoid and sodium supplementation may be required based upon electrolyte regulation and plasma renin activity.

Physiologic replacement: Children:

Oral: 0.5-0.75 mg/kg/day **or** 20-25 mg/m²/day every 8 hours

I.M.: Succinate: 0.25-0.35 mg/kg/day **or** 12-15 mg/m²/day once daily

Shock: I.M., I.V.: Succinate:

Children: Initial: 50 mg/kg, then repeated in 4 hours and/or every 24 hours as needed

Adolescents and Adults: 500 mg to 2 g every 2-6 hours

Status asthmaticus: Children and Adults: I.V.: Succinate: 1-2 mg/kg/dose every 6 hours for 24 hours, then maintenance of 0.5-1 mg/kg every 6 hours

Adults:

Rheumatic diseases:

Intralesional, intra-articular, soft tissue injection: Acetate:

Large joints: 25 mg (up to 37.5 mg)

Small joints: 10-25 mg

Tendon sheaths: 5-12.5 mg

Soft tissue infiltration: 25-50 mg (up to 75 mg)

Bursae: 25-37.5 mg

Ganglia: 12.5-25 mg

Stress dosing (surgery) in patients known to be adrenally-suppressed or on chronic systemic steroids: I.V.:

Minor stress (ie, inguinal herniorrhaphy): 25 mg/day for 1 day

Moderate stress (ie, joint replacement, cholecystectomy): 50-75 mg/day (25 mg every 8-12 hours) for 1-2 days

Major stress (pancreatoduodenectomy, esophagogastrectomy, cardiac surgery): 100-150 mg/day (50 mg every 8-12 hours) for 2-3 days

Dermatosis: Children >2 years and Adults: Topical: Apply to affected area 2-4 times/day (Buteprate: Apply once or twice daily). Therapy should be discontinued when control is achieved; if no improvement is seen, reassessment of diagnosis may be necessary.

Ulcerative colitis: Adults: Rectal: 10-100 mg 1-2 times/day for 2-3 weeks

Stability Hydrocortisone sodium phosphate and hydrocortisone sodium succinate are clear, light yellow solutions which are heat labile

After initial reconstitution, hydrocortisone sodium succinate solutions are stable for 3 days at room temperature and refrigeration if protected from light

Stability of parenteral admixture (Solu-Cortef®) at room temperature (25°C) and at refrigeration temperature (4°C) is concentration dependent

Minimum volume: Concentration should not exceed 1 mg/mL

Stability of concentration ≤1 mg/mL: 24 hours

Stability of concentration >1 mg/mL to <25 mg/mL: Unpredictable, 4-6 hours

Stability of concentration ≥25 mg/mL: 3 days

Standard diluent (Solu-Cortef®): 50 mg/50 mL D₅W; 100 mg/100 mL D₅W

Comments: Should be administered in a 0.1-1 mg/mL concentration due to stability problems

Monitoring Parameters Blood pressure, weight, serum glucose, and electrolytes

Administration Oral: Administer with food or milk to decrease GI upset

Parenteral: Hydrocortisone sodium succinate may be administered by I.M. or I.V. routes

I.V. bolus: Dilute to 50 mg/mL and give over 30 seconds to several minutes (depending on the dose)

I.V. intermittent infusion: Dilute to 1 mg/mL and give over 20-30 minutes

Topical: Apply a thin film to clean, dry skin and rub in gently

Contraindications Hypersensitivity to hydrocortisone or any component of the formulation; serious infections, except septic shock or tuberculous meningitis; viral, fungal, or tubercular skin lesions

Warnings

Use with caution in patients with hyperthyroidism, cirrhosis, nonspecific ulcerative colitis, hypertension, osteoporosis, thromboembolic tendencies, CHF, convulsive disorders, myasthenia gravis, thrombophlebitis, peptic ulcer, diabetes, glaucoma, cataracts, or tuberculosis. Use caution in hepatic impairment.

May cause HPA axis suppression. Acute adrenal insufficiency may occur with abrupt withdrawal after long-term therapy or with stress; young pediatric patients may be more susceptible to adrenal axis suppression from topical therapy. Avoid use of topical preparations with occlusive dressings or on weeping or exudative lesions.

Because of the risk of adverse effects, systemic corticosteroids should be used cautiously in the elderly, in the smallest possible dose, and for the shortest possible time

Dosage Forms [DSC] = Discontinued product

Aerosol, rectal, as acetate (Cortifoam®): 10% (15 g) [90 mg/applicator]

Cream, rectal, as acetate (Nupercainal® Hydrocortisone Cream): 1% (30 g) [strength expressed as base]

Cream, rectal, as base:

Cortizone®-10: 1% (30 g) [contains aloe]

Preparation H® Hydrocortisone: 1% (27 g)

Cream, topical, as acetate: 0.5% (9 g, 30 g, 60 g) [available with aloe]; 1% (30 g, 454 g) [available with aloe]

Cream, topical, as base: 0.5% (30 g); 1% (1.5 g, 30 g, 114 g, 454 g); 2.5% (20 g, 30 g, 454 g)

Anusol-HC®: 2.5% (30 g) [contains benzyl alcohol]

Caldecort®: 1% (30 g) [contains aloe vera gel]

Cortaid® Intensive Therapy: 1% (60 g)

Cortaid® Maximum Strength: 1% (15 g, 30 g, 40 g, 60 g) [contains aloe vera gel and benzyl alcohol]

Cortaid® Sensitive Skin: 0.5% (15 g) [contains aloe vera gel]

Cortizone®-10 Maximum Strength: 1% (15 g, 30 g, 60 g) [contains aloe]

Cortizone®-10 Plus Maximum Strength: 1% (30 g, 60 g) [contains vitamins A, D, E and aloe]

Dermarest® Dricort®: 1% (15 g, 30 g)

HydroZone Plus, Proctocort®, Procto-Pak™: 1% (30 g)

Hytone®: 2.5% (30 g, 60 g)

IvySoothe®: 1% (30 g) [contains aloe]

Post Peel Healing Balm: 1% (23 g)

ProctoCream® HC: 2.5% (30 g) [contains benzyl alcohol]

Procto-Kit™: 1% (30 g) [packaged with applicator tips and finger cots]; 2.5% (30 g) [packaged with applicator tips and finger cots]

Proctosol-HC®, Proctozone-HC™: 2.5% (30 g)

Summer's Eve® SpecialCare™ Medicated Anti-Itch Cream: 1% (30 g)

Cream, topical, as butyrate (Locoid®, Locoid Lipocream®): 0.1% (15 g, 45 g)

Cream, topical, as probutate (Pandel®): 0.1% (15 g, 45 g, 80 g)

Cream, topical, as valerate (Westcort®): 0.2% (15 g, 45 g, 60 g)

Gel, topical, as base (Corticool®): 1% (45 g)

Injection, powder for reconstitution, as sodium succinate (Solu-Cortef®): 100 mg, 250 mg, 500 mg, 1 g [diluent contains benzyl alcohol; strength expressed as base]

Lotion, topical, as base: 1% (120 mL); 2.5% (60 mL)
  Aquanil™ HC: 1% (120 mL)
  Beta-HC®, Cetacort®, Sarnol®-HC: 1% (60 mL)
  HydroZone Plus: 1% (120 mL)
  Hytone®: 2.5% (60 mL)
  Nutracort®: 1% (60 mL, 120 mL); 2.5% (60 mL, 120 mL)

Ointment, topical, as acetate: 1% (30 g) [strength expressed as base; available with aloe]
  Anusol® HC-1: 1% (21 g) [strength expressed as base]
  Cortaid® Maximum Strength: 1% (15 g, 30 g) [strength expressed as base]

Ointment, topical, as base: 0.5% (30 g); 1% (30 g, 454 g); 2.5% (20 g, 30 g, 454 g)
  Cortizone®-10 Maximum Strength: 1% (30 g, 60 g)
  Hytone®: 2.5% (30 g) [DSC]

Ointment, topical, as butyrate (Locoid®): 0.1% (15 g, 45 g)

Ointment, topical, as valerate (Westcort®): 0.2% (15 g, 45 g, 60 g)

Solution, otic, as base (EarSol® HC): 1% (30 mL) [contains alcohol 44%, benzyl benzoate, yerba santa]

Solution, topical, as base (Texacort®): 2.5% (30 mL) [contains alcohol]

Solution, topical, as butyrate (Locoid®): 0.1% (20 mL, 60 mL) [contains alcohol 50%]

Solution, topical spray, as base:
  Cortaid® Intensive Therapy: 1% (60 mL) [contains alcohol]
  Cortizone®-10 Quick Shot: 1% (44 mL) [contains benzyl alcohol]
  Dermtex® HC: 1% (52 mL) [contains menthol 1%]

Suppository, rectal, as acetate: 25 mg (12s, 24s, 100s)
  Anucort-HC®, Tucks® Anti-Itch: 25 mg (12s, 24s, 100s) [strength expressed as base; Anucort-HC® renamed Tucks® Anti-Itch]
  Anusol-HC®, Proctosol-HC®: 25 mg (12s, 24s)
  Encort™: 30 mg (12s)
  Hemril®-30, Proctocort®, Proctosert: 30 mg (12s, 24s)

Suspension, rectal, as base: 100 mg/60 mL (7s)
  Colocort®: 100 mg/60 mL (1s, 7s)

Tablet, as base: 20 mg
  Cortef®: 5 mg, 10 mg, 20 mg

Reference Range Therapeutic: AM: 5-25 mcg/dL (SI: 138-690 nmol/L), PM: 2-9 mcg/dL (SI: 55-248 nmol/L) depending on test, assay

Overdosage/Treatment Decontamination: Emesis or lavage within 1 hour; activated charcoal or cholestyramine (4 g) can decrease absorption

Test Interactions >100 mg/day may interfere with the TSH assay resulting in falsely low TSH levels

Drug Interactions Substrate of CYP3A4 (minor); **Induces** CYP3A4 (weak)
  Decreased effect:
    Insulin decreases hypoglycemic effect
    Phenytoin, phenobarbital, ephedrine, and rifampin increase metabolism of hydrocortisone and decrease steroid blood level
  Increased toxicity:
    Oral anticoagulants change prothrombin time
    Potassium-depleting diuretics increase risk of hypokalemia
    Cardiac glucosides increase risk of arrhythmias or digitalis toxicity secondary to hypokalemia

Pregnancy Risk Factor C

Pregnancy Implications No adequate studies in pregnant women. Corticosteroid use has been associated with cleft palate, neonatal adrenal suppression, low birth weight, and cataracts in the infant; including cases associated with topical administration. Use only if potential benefit to the mother exceeds the potential risk to the fetus. Avoid high doses or prolonged use.

Lactation Excretion in breast milk unknown/use caution

Additional Information Sodium content of 1 g (sodium succinate injection): 47.5 mg (2.07 mEq)
  Hydrocortisone base topical cream, lotion, and ointments in concentrations of 0.25%, 0.5%, and 1% may be OTC or prescription depending on the product labeling
  Food reduces absorption

Specific References
Odeh M, Lavy A, and Stermer E, "Hydrocortisone-Induced Convulsions," J Toxicol Clin Toxicol, 2003, 41(7):995-7.

Hydrogen Peroxide

CAS Number 7722-84-1

UN Number 2015

Synonyms H_2O_2; Hydrogen Dioxide; Peroxide

Commonly Includes Bleaching textiles, antiseptics, hair bleaching agents, loosens ear cerumen, recent intravenous use by AIDS patients to "cleanse blood." Household concentrations: 3%; industrial concentrations: 35%.

Use Cleanse wounds, suppurating ulcers, and local infections; used in the treatment of inflammatory conditions of the external auditory canal and as a mouthwash or gargle

Mechanism of Action Antiseptic oxidant that slowly releases oxygen and water upon contact with serum or tissue catalase; potent oxidizing agent

Adverse Reactions
  Cardiovascular: Gas embolism, angina
  Dermatologic: Bleaching effect on hair
  Gastrointestinal: Rupture of the colon, proctitis, abdominal pain, ulcerative colitis, small bowel perforation, GI bleeding
  Hematologic: Hemolysis
  Local: Irritation of the buccal mucous membrane
  Respiratory: Interstitial lung disease
  Renal: Myoglobinuria, renal failure

Signs and Symptoms of Overdose Abdominal pain, chest pain, colitis, coma, dyspnea, gastric distention, gingival ulceration, metabolic acidosis, oropharyngeal burns, seizures (35% hydrogen peroxide), vomiting. Inhalation can cause cough and interstitial lung disease. Ocular exposure causes corneal ulceration, irritation, and lacrimation. Systemic embolization can produce cardiac arrest.

Admission Criteria/Prognosis Asymptomatic patients 6 hours post-exposure may be released; any patient with cardiopulmonary complaint should be admitted for 24-72 hours observation. Admit any pediatric ingestion of >10% concentration of hydrogen peroxide.

Pharmacodynamics/Kinetics Duration of action: Only while bubbling action occurs

Dosage Children and Adults:
  Mouthwash or gargle: Dilute the 3% solution with an equal volume of water; swish around in the mouth over the affected area for at least 1 minute and then expel; use up to 4 times/day (after meals and at bedtime)
  Topical: 1.5% to 3% solution for cleansing wounds

Stability Keep tightly covered; decomposition is accelerated by metals and metallic salts; protect from heat and light

Monitoring Parameters CBC, renal status, x-rays

Contraindications Should not be used in abscesses

Warnings Repeat use as a mouthwash or gargle may produce irritation of the buccal mucous membrane or "hairy tongue"; bandages should not be applied too quickly after its use; 10% and 30% solutions must be diluted prior to use

Dosage Forms Gel, oral: 1.5% (15 g)
  Solution:
    Concentrate: 30.5% (480 mL)
    Topical: 3% (120 mL, 480 mL)

Overdosage/Treatment
  Decontamination: Dilute with water; use nasogastric tube for gastric decompression or removal of hydrogen peroxide
  Supportive therapy: Hyperbaric oxygen advocated for reducing size of gas emboli; cerebral gas embolism can be treated with hyperbaric oxygen (3 ATA); avoid use of the Trendelenburg positioning in that it may trap air in the right ventricle; endoscopy and abdominal x-rays should be obtained within 48 hours if ingested hydrogen peroxide concentration exceeds 10% to examine local mucosal burns and abdominal distention; seizures can be treated with benzodiazepines

Additional Information Clear, colorless fluid; bitter acid taste. Intravenous use is associated with hemolytic anemia and subsequent renal failure. 1 mL of 3% hydrogen peroxide liberates 10 mL of oxygen. TLV-TWA: 1 ppm; IDLH: 75 ppm; PEL-TWA: 1 ppm

Specific References
Sansone J, Vidal N, Bigliardi R, et al, "Unintentional Ingestion of 60% Hydrogen Peroxide by a Six-Year-Old Child," J Toxicol Clin Toxicol, 2004, 42(2):197-9.

Sudakin DL, "Biopesticides," Toxicol Rev, 2003, 22(2):83-90.

Watt BE, Proudfoot AT, and Vale JA, "Hydrogen Peroxide Poisoning," Toxicol Rev, 2004, 23(1):51-7 (review).

Yegles M, "Pitfalls in Hair Analysis: Cosmetic Treatment," Annale de Toxicologie Analytique, 2005, 17(4):275-8.

Hydromorphone

CAS Number 466-99-9; 71-68-1
U.S. Brand Names Dilaudid-HP®; Dilaudid®
Synonyms Dihydromorphinone; Hydromorphone Hydrochloride
Impairment Potential Yes
Use Management of moderate to severe pain
Unlabeled/Investigational Use Antitussive
Mechanism of Action Binds to opiate receptors in the CNS, causing inhibition of ascending pain pathways, altering the perception of and response to pain; causes cough supression by direct central action in the medulla; produces generalized CNS depression

Adverse Reactions
Cardiovascular: **Palpitations**, **hypotension**, bradycardia, **peripheral vasodilation**, sinus bradycardia
Central nervous system: CNS depression, agitation, increased intracranial pressure, **drowsiness, dizziness**, sedation, **lightheadedness**
Dermatologic: Pruritus, systemic contact dermatitis
Endocrine & metabolic: Antidiuretic hormone release
Gastrointestinal: Nausea, vomiting, constipation, biliary tract spasm, **anorexia**
Genitourinary: Urinary tract spasm
Ocular: Miosis
Respiratory: Apnea, respiratory depression
Miscellaneous: Physical and psychological dependence, histamine release, Myoclonus

Signs and Symptoms of Overdose Apnea, bradycardia, confusion, coma, flaccidity, hypotension, myasthenia gravis (exacerbation or precipitation), respiratory depression, syndrome of inappropriate antidiuretic hormone (SIADH).

Pharmacodynamics/Kinetics
Onset of action: Analgesic: Immediate release formulations:
  Oral: 15-30 minutes
  Peak effect: Oral: 30-60 minutes
Duration: Immediate release formulations: 4-5 hours
Absorption: I.M.: Variable and delayed
Distribution: V_d: 4 L/kg
Protein binding: ~8% to 19%
Metabolism: Hepatic via glucuronidation; to inactive metabolites
Bioavailability: 62%
Half-life elimination: Immediate release formulations: 1-3 hours
Excretion: Urine (primarily as glucuronide conjugates)

Dosage
Acute pain (moderate to severe): **Note:** These are guidelines and do not represent the maximum doses that may be required in all patients. Doses should be titrated to pain relief/prevention.
Young Children ≥6 months and <50 kg:
  Oral: 0.03-0.08 mg/kg/dose every 3-4 hours as needed
  I.V.: 0.015 mg/kg/dose every 3-6 hours as needed
Older Children >50 kg and Adults:
  Oral: Initial: Opiate-naive: 2-4 mg every 3-4 hours as needed; patients with prior opiate exposure may require higher initial doses; usual dosage range: 2-8 mg every 3-4 hours as needed
  I.V.: Initial: Opiate-naive: 0.2-0.6 mg every 2-3 hours as needed; patients with prior opiate exposure may tolerate higher initial doses
    Note: More frequent dosing may be needed.
    Mechanically-ventilated patients (based on 70 kg patient): 0.7-2 mg every 1-2 hours as needed; infusion (based on 70 kg patient): 0.5-1 mg/hour
  Patient-controlled analgesia (PCA): (Opiate-naive: Consider lower end of dosing range)
    Usual concentration: 0.2 mg/mL
    Demand dose: Usual: 0.1-0.2 mg; range: 0.05-0.5 mg
    Lockout interval: 5-15 minutes
    4-hour limit: 4-6 mg
  Epidural:
    Bolus dose: 1-1.5 mg
    Infusion concentration: 0.05-0.075 mg/mL
    Infusion rate: 0.04-0.4 mg/hour
    Demand dose: 0.15 mg
    Lockout interval: 30 minutes
  I.M., SubQ: **Note:** I.M. use may result in variable absorption and a lag time to peak effect.
    Initial: Opiate-naive: 0.8-1 mg every 4-6 hours as needed; patients with prior opiate exposure may require higher initial doses; usual dosage range: 1-2 mg every 3-6 hours as needed
  Rectal: 3 mg every 4-8 hours as needed
Chronic pain: Patients taking opioids chronically may become tolerant and require doses higher than the usual dosage range to maintain the desired effect. Tolerance can be managed by appropriate dose titration. There is no optimal or maximal dose for hydromorphone in chronic pain.

The appropriate dose is one that relieves pain throughout its dosing interval without causing unmanageable side effects.
  Adults: Oral, controlled release formulation (Hydromorph Contin®, not available in U.S.): 3-30 mg every 12 hours. **Note:** A patient's hydromorphone requirement should be established using prompt release formulations; conversion to long acting products may be considered when chronic, continuous treatment is required. Higher dosages should be reserved for use only in opioid-tolerant patients.
Antitussive: Oral:
  Children 6-12 years: 0.5 mg every 3-4 hours as needed
  Children >12 years and Adults: 1 mg every 3-4 hours as needed
Dosing adjustment in hepatic impairment: Should be considered
Stability Protect tablets from light; do not store intact ampuls in refrigerator; a slightly yellowish discoloration has not been associated with a loss of potency; I.V. is **incompatible** when mixed with minocycline, prochlorperazine, sodium bicarbonate, tetracycline, thiopental, dexamethasone
Monitoring Parameters Pain relief, respiratory and mental status, blood pressure
Administration Parenteral: May be given SubQ or I.M.; vial stopper contains latex
  I.V.: For IVP, must be given slowly over 2-3 minutes (rapid IVP has been associated with an increase in side effects, especially respiratory depression and hypotension)
  Oral: Hydromorph Contin®: Capsule should be swallowed whole; do not crush or chew; contents may be sprinkled on soft food and swallowed
Contraindications Hypersensitivity to hydromorphone, any component of the formulation; acute or severe asthma, severe respiratory depression (in absence of resuscitative equipment or ventilatory support); severe CNS depression; pregnancy (prolonged use or high doses at term); obstetrical analgesia
Warnings Hydromorphone shares toxic potential of opiate agonists, including CNS depression and respiratory depression. Precautions associated with opiate agonist therapy should be observed. Critical respiratory depression may occur, even at therapeutic dosages, particularly in elderly or debilitated patients or in patients with pre-existing respiratory compromise (hypoxia and/or hypercapnia). Use caution in COPD or other obstructive pulmonary disease. Use with caution in patients with hypersensitivity to other phenanthrene opiates, biliary tract disease, acute pancreatitis, adrenocortical insufficiency, hypothyroidism, acute alcoholism, toxic psychoses, or severe liver or renal failure. Use extreme caution in patients with head injury, intracranial lesions, or elevated intracranial pressure; exaggerated elevation of ICP may occur (in addition, hydromorphone may complicate neurologic evaluation due to pupillary dilation and CNS depressant effects). Use with caution in patients with depleted blood volume or drugs which may exaggerate hypotensive effects (including phenothiazines or general anesthetics).

[U.S. Boxed Warning]: Hydromorphone has a high potential for abuse. Those at risk for opioid abuse include patients with a history of substance abuse or mental illness. Tolerance or drug dependence may result from extended use; however, concerns for abuse should not prevent effective management of pain. In general, abrupt discontinuation of therapy in dependent patients should be avoided.

An opioid-containing analgesic regimen should be tailored to each patient's needs and based upon the type of pain being treated (acute versus chronic), the route of administration, degree of tolerance for opioids (naive versus chronic user), age, weight, and medical condition. The optimal analgesic dose varies widely among patients. Doses should be titrated to pain relief/prevention. I.M. use may result in variable absorption and a lag time to peak effect.

Dosage form-specific warnings:
  [U.S. Boxed Warning]: Dilaudid-HP®: Extreme caution should be taken to avoid confusing the highly-concentrated (Dilaudid-HP®) injection with the less-concentrated (Dilaudid®) injectable product. Dilaudid-HP® should only be used in patients who are opioid-tolerant.
  Controlled release: Capsules should only be used when continuous analgesia is required over an extended period of time. Controlled release products are not to be used on an "as needed" (PRN) basis.
  Some dosage forms contain trace amounts of sodium metabisulfite which may cause allergic reactions in susceptible individuals.
Dosage Forms [CAN] = Canadian brand name
Capsule, controlled release (Hydromorph Contin®) [CAN]: 3 mg, 6 mg, 12 mg, 18 mg, 24 mg, 30 mg [not available in U.S.]
Injection, powder for reconstitution, as hydrochloride (Dilaudid-HP®): 250 mg
Injection, solution, as hydrochloride: 1 mg/mL (1 mL); 2 mg/mL (1 mL, 20 mL); 4 mg/mL (1 mL); 10 mg/mL (1 mL, 5 mL, 10 mL)
  Dilaudid®: 1 mg/mL (1 mL); 2 mg/mL (1 mL, 20 mL) [20 mL size contains edetate sodium; vial stopper contains latex]; 4 mg/mL (1 mL)
  Dilaudid-HP®: 10 mg/mL (1 mL, 5 mL, 50 mL)
Liquid, oral, as hydrochloride (Dilaudid®): 1 mg/mL (480 mL) [may contain trace amounts of sodium bisulfite]

Suppository, rectal, as hydrochloride (Dilaudid®): 3 mg (6s)

Tablet, as hydrochloride (Dilaudid®): 2 mg, 4 mg, 8 mg (8 mg tablets may contain trace amounts of sodium bisulfite)

Reference Range Serum therapeutic (pain control): 0.001-0.032 mg/L; fatalities due to hydromorphone can occur at postmortem levels (blood) over 51 ng/mL

Overdosage/Treatment

Decontamination: Lavage (within 1 hour)/activated charcoal

Supportive therapy: Naloxone hydrochloride (0.4-2 mg I.V., SubQ, or through an endotracheal tube); a continuous infusion (at $^2/_3$ the response dose/hour) may be required

Antidote(s)

- Nalmefene [ANTIDOTE]
- Naloxone [ANTIDOTE]

Test Interactions ↑ aminotransferases (ALT, AST) (S)

Drug Interactions Ammonium chloride: May decrease the levels/effects of hydromorphone.

CNS depressants: Effects with hydromorphone may be additive.

General anesthetics: May enhance the hypotensive and CNS depressant effects of hydromorphone.

Pegvisomant: Analgesics (narcotic) may diminish the therapeutic effect of pegvisomant; increased pegvisomant doses may be needed.

Phenothiazines: May enhance the hypotensive and CNS depressant effects of hydromorphone.

Selective serotonin reuptake inhibitors (SSRIs): Serotonergic effects may be additive, leading to serotonin syndrome.

Pregnancy Risk Factor B/D (prolonged use or high doses at term)

Pregnancy Implications Crosses the placenta

Lactation Excretion in breast milk unknown/not recommended

Nursing Implications Observe patient for oversedation, respiratory depression, implement safety measures

Additional Information Equianalgesic doses: Morphine 10 mg I.M. = hydromorphone 1.5 mg I.M.; no cough suppressant effects

Specific References

Caplan YH, Cone EJ, Heit HA, et al, "Detection of Hydromorphone in Chronic Pain Patients with Correspondingly High Concentrations of Morphine in Urine," *J Anal Toxicol*, 2006, 30:149.

Patel S, Rosham VR, Lee KC, Cheung RJ et al, "A Myoclonic Reaction with Low-Dose Hydromorphone," *Ann Pharmacol*, 40(11):2068-2070.

Poklis A and Levine B, "A Fatal Therapeutic Misadventure: Mismanagement of Pain with Excessive Over Prescribing of Opiate Drugs," *J Anal Toxicol*, 2006, 30:152-3.

Wallage HR and Palmentire JP, "Hydromorphone-Related Fatalities in Ontario," *J Anal Toxicol*, 2006, 30:2002-9.

Yazzie J, Mazarr-Proo S, and Kerrigan S, "Analysis of Keto Opioids Using Solid-Phase Extraction and Gas Chromatography-Mass Spectrometry," *J Anal Toxicol*, 2004, 28:298.

Hydroquinone

CAS Number 123-31-9

UN Number 2662

U.S. Brand Names Alphaquin HP; Alustra™; Claripel™; Eldopaque Forte®; Eldopaque® [OTC]; Eldoquin Forte®; Eldoquin® [OTC]; EpiQuin™ Micro; Esoterica® Regular [OTC]; Glyquin®; Lustra-AF™; Lustra®; Melanex®; Melpaque HP®; Melquin HP®; Melquin-3®; NeoStrata AHA [OTC]; Nuquin HP®; Palmer's® Skin Success Fade Cream™ [OTC]; Solaquin Forte®; Solaquin® [OTC]

Synonyms Hydroquinol; Quinol

Use Gradual bleaching of hyperpigmented skin conditions

Mechanism of Action Produces reversible depigmentation of the skin by suppression of melanocyte metabolic processes, in particular the inhibition of the enzymatic oxidation of tyrosine to DOPA (3,4-dihydroxyphenylalanine); sun exposure reverses this effect and will cause repigmentation.

Adverse Reactions

Central nervous system: Dizziness, headache, delirium

Dermatologic: Dermatitis, dry skin, erythema, stinging, inflammatory reaction, sensitization, leukoderma, hair discoloration (red), nail discoloration (brown), hypopigmentation

Genitourinary: Discoloration of urine (black) after 12 g ingestion

Hematologic: Methemoglobinemia, hemolysis

Local: Irritation

Ocular: Keratitis, corneal ulceration

Admission Criteria/Prognosis Admit any oral ingestion >1 g

Pharmacodynamics/Kinetics Onset and duration of depigmentation produced by hydroquinone varies among individuals

Dosage Children >12 years and Adults: Topical: Apply thin layer and rub in twice daily

Administration For external use only; avoid contact with eyes

Contraindications Hypersensitivity to hydroquinone or any component of the formulation; sunburn, depilatory usage

Warnings Limit application to area no larger than face and neck or hands and arms

Dosage Forms

Cream, topical: 4% (30 g) [may contain sodium metabisulfite]

Alphaquin HP®: 4% (30 g, 60 g)

Eldoquin®: 2% (15 g, 30 g)

Eldoquin Forte®: 4% (30 g) [contains sodium metabisulfite]

EpiQuin™ Micro: 4% (30 g) [contains benzyl alcohol and sodium metabisulfite]

Esoterica® Regular: 2% (85 g) [contains sodium bisulfite]

Lustra®: 4% (30 g) [contains sodium metabisulfite]

Melquin HP®: 4% (15 g, 30 g) [contains sodium metabisulfite]

Cream, topical [with sunscreen]: 4% (30 g) [may contain sodium metabisulfite]

Claripel™: 4% (30 g, 45 g) [contains sodium metabisulfite]

Dermarest® Skin Correcting Cream Plus: 2% (85 g) [contains aloe vera, sodium bisulfite]

Eldopaque®: 2% (15 g, 30 g)

Eldopaque Forte®: 4% (30 g) [contains sodium metabisulfite]

Glyquin®: 4% (30 g)

Glyquin-XM™: 4% (30 g)

Lustra-AF™: 4% (30 g, 60 g) [contains sodium metabisulfite]

Melpaque HP®: 4% (15 g, 30 g) [contains sodium metabisulfite; sunblocking cream base]

Nuquin HP®: 4% (15 g, 30 g, 60 g) [contains sodium metabisulfite]

Palmer's® Skin Success Eventone® Fade Cream: 2% (81 g, 132 g) [contains sodium sulfite; available in regular, oily skin, and dry skin formulas]

Solaquin®: 2% (30 g)

Solaquin Forte®: 4% (30 g) [contains sodium metabisulfite]

Gel, topical (NeoStrata® AHA): 2% (45 g) [contains glycolic acid 10%, sodium bisulfite, and sodium sulfite]

Gel, topical [with sunscreen]: 4% (30 g)

Nuquin HP®: 4% (15 g, 30 g) [contains sodium bisulfite]

Solaquin Forte®: 4% (30 g) [contains sodium metabisulfite]

Solution, topical (Melanex®, Melquin-3®): 3% (30 mL) [contains alcohol]

Reference Range Acute GI symptoms associated with serum hydroquinone levels >0.1 mcg/mL

Overdosage/Treatment Decontamination: **Oral**: Dilute with milk or water; lavage (within 1 hour)/activated charcoal **Dermal**: Wash with soap and water. **Ocular**: Irrigate with copious amounts of saline

Test Interactions May result in positive urinary test for phenol

Drug Interactions No data reported

Pregnancy Risk Factor C

Lactation Excretion in breast milk unknown

Additional Information Lethal oral dose: Adults: 5 g

Specific gravity: 1.332; vapor density: 3.81; has a sweet taste

Hydroxychloroquine

Related Information

- Chloroquine

CAS Number 118-42-3; 747-36-4

U.S. Brand Names Plaquenil®

Synonyms Hydroxychloroquine Sulfate

Use Suppresses and treats acute attacks of malaria; treatment of systemic lupus erythematosus and rheumatoid arthritis

Unlabeled/Investigational Use Porphyria cutanea tarda, polymorphous light eruptions; nonbronchodilating antiasthmatic drug with potential steroid sparing effects due to immunomodulation

Mechanism of Action Interferes with digestive vacuole function within sensitive malarial parasites by increasing the pH and interfering with lysosomal degradation of hemoglobin; inhibits locomotion of neutrophils and chemotaxis of eosinophils; impairs complement-dependent antigen-antibody reactions

Adverse Reactions

Cardiovascular: Hypotension, arrhythmia (ventricular), torsade de pointes, bradycardia, sinus bradycardia

Central nervous system: Insomnia, nervousness, night terrors, psychosis, **headache**, confusion, agitation, seizures, dizziness, ataxia, global amnesia, extrapyramidal reactions

Dermatologic: Lichenoid dermatitis, exfoliative dermatitis, bleaching of the hair, hypopigmented hair, **pruritus**, phototoxicity, pustulosis

Endocrine & metabolic: Hypokalemia, hypoglycemia

Gastrointestinal: GI irritation, anorexia, **nausea, vomiting, diarrhea**, dysgeusia, **loss of appetite**, **stomach cramps**

Hematologic: Bone marrow suppression, hemolysis, thrombocytopenia, leukopenia, neutropenia, agranulocytosis, granulocytopenia, aplastic anemia, porphyria, porphyrinogenic

Neuromuscular & skeletal: Weakness

Ocular: Visual field defects, vision color changes (blue tinge); vision color changes (green tinge); vision color changes (yellow tinge); photophobia, blindness, diplopia, retinitis, retinopathy threshold dose is 7.8 mg/kg/day (less ocular toxicity than chloroquine), **ciliary muscle dysfunction**

Otic: Hearing loss

Signs and Symptoms of Overdose Lymphocytosis

Admission Criteria/Prognosis Admit any symptomatic patient, or ingestion >10 mg/kg; asymptomatic patients should be observed on an ECG monitor for 8 hours.

Pharmacodynamics/Kinetics

Onset of action: Rheumatic disease: May require 4-6 weeks to respond

Absorption: Complete

Protein binding: 55%

Metabolism: Hepatic

Half-life elimination: 32-50 days

Time to peak: Rheumatic disease: Several months

Excretion: Urine (as metabolites and unchanged drug); may be enhanced by urinary acidification

Dosage

Oral:

Children:

Chemoprophylaxis of malaria: 5 mg/kg (base) once weekly; should not exceed the recommended adult dose; begin 2 weeks before exposure; continue for 4-6 weeks after leaving endemic area

Acute attack: 10 mg/kg (base) initial dose; followed by 5 mg/kg in 6 hours on day 1; 5 mg/kg in 1 dose on day 2 and on day 3

JRA or SLE: 3-5 mg/kg/day divided 1-2 times/day to a maximum of 400 mg/day; not to exceed 7 mg/kg/day

Adults:

Chemoprophylaxis of malaria: 2 tablets/week on same day each week; begin 2 weeks before exposure; continue for 4-6 weeks after leaving endemic area

Acute attack: 4 tablets first dose day 1; 2 tablets in 6 hours day 1; 2 tablets in 1 dose day 2; and 2 tablets in 1 dose on day 3

Rheumatoid arthritis: 2-3 tablets/day to start taken with food or milk; increase dose until optimum response level is reached; usually after 4-12 weeks dose should be reduced by $1/_2$ and a maintenance dose of 1-2 tablets/day given

Lupus erythematosus: 2 tablets every day or twice daily for several weeks depending on response; 1-2 tablets/day for prolonged maintenance therapy

Asthma: 300-600 mg/day up to 3 years

To limit incidence of retinopathy, do not give more than 400 mg/day

Monitoring Parameters Ophthalmologic exam, CBC

Administration Administer with food or milk

Contraindications Hypersensitivity to hydroxychloroquine, 4-aminoquinoline derivatives, or any component of the formulation; retinal or visual field changes attributable to 4-aminoquinolines

Warnings Use with caution in patients with hepatic disease, G6PD deficiency, psoriasis, and porphyria; long-term use in children is not recommended; perform baseline and periodic (6 months) ophthalmologic examinations; test periodically for muscle weakness. **[U.S. Boxed Warning]: Should be prescribed by physicians familiar with its use.**

Dosage Forms Tablet, as sulfate: 200 mg [equivalent to 155 mg base]

Reference Range Peak serum level of 427 ng/mL after an oral dose of 200 mg (155 mg base); plasma level after ingestion of 20 g, with severe symptoms, was reported as 9.9 mg/L (29.4 µmol/L)

Overdosage/Treatment

Decontamination: Lavage (within 1 hour)/activated charcoal

Supportive therapy: Electrolyte balance should be monitored and treated, especially when refractory arrhythmias develop. Sodium bicarbonate 1-2 mEq/kg I.V. (or 0.5-1 mEq/kg in children) may decrease conduction defects. Phenytoin or lidocaine are often effective at controlling drug-induced arrhythmias, while phenytoin is preferred due to its beneficial effects on AV conduction velocity. Diazepam should also be administered to treat cardiac toxicity. Epinephrine is useful in treating hypotension or cardiac dysrhythmias. Monitor for hypokalemia and replace potassium as necessary. Treatment is similar to that of chloroquine toxicity. Torsade de pointes can be treated with magnesium sulfate or overdrive pacemaker. Avoid class I antiarrhythmic agents; avoid administration of thiopentone.

Enhancement of elimination: Multiple dosing of activated charcoal is effective; exchange transfusion can be utilized to remove toxic metabolites; hemodialysis or charcoal hemoperfusion have little effect; slightly dialyzable (5% to 20%). Plasmapheresis is not useful.

Drug Interactions Chloroquine and other 4-aminoquinolones may be decreased due to GI binding with kaolin or magnesium trisilicate

Increased effect: Cimetidine increases levels of chloroquine and probably other 4-aminoquinolones

Pregnancy Risk Factor C

Pregnancy Implications No evidence of teratogenesis

Lactation Enters breast milk/compatible

Nursing Implications Periodic blood counts and eye examinations are recommended when patient is on chronic therapy; give with food or milk

Specific References

Audi J, Schwartz M, Morgan B, et al, "Acute Hydroxychloroquine Ingestion Treated with Intravenous Diazepam - Case Report and Literature Review," *J Toxicol Clin Toxicol*, 2004, 42(5):721.

Carmichael SJ, Charles B, and Tett SE, "Population Pharmacokinetics of Hydroxychloroquine in Patients with Rheumatoid Arthritis," *Ther Drug Monit*, 2003, 25(6):671-81.

Chen CY, Wang FL, and Lin CC, "Chronic Hydroxychloroquine Use Associated with QT Prolongation and Refractory Ventricular Arrhythmia," *Clin Toxicol*, 2006, 44:173-5.

Singer P and Jones G, "Fatalities Involving Hydroxychloroquine: Chronic Accumulation?" *J Anal Toxicol*, 2003, 27(3):194.

Hydroxyurea

CAS Number 127-07-1

U.S. Brand Names Droxia™; Hydrea®; Mylocel™

Synonyms Hydroxycarbamide

Use Treatment of melanoma, refractory chronic myelocytic leukemia (CML), relapsed and refractory metastatic ovarian cancer; radiosensitizing agent in the treatment of squamous cell head and neck cancer (excluding lip cancer); adjunct in the management of sickle cell patients who have had at least three painful crises in the previous 12 months (to reduce frequency of these crises and the need for blood transfusions)

Unlabeled/Investigational Use Treatment of HIV; treatment of psoriasis, treatment of hematologic conditions such as essential thrombocythemia, polycythemia vera, hypereosinophilia, and hyperleukocytosis due to acute leukemia; treatment of uterine, cervix and nonsmall cell lung cancers; radiosensitizing agent in the treatment of primary brain tumors; has shown activity against renal cell cancer and prostate cancer

Mechanism of Action Interferes with synthesis of DNA, during the S phase of cell division, without interfering with RNA synthesis; inhibits ribonucleoside diphosphate reductase, preventing conversion of ribonucleotides to deoxyribonucleotides; cell-cycle specific for the S phase and may hold other cells in the G_1 phase of the cell cycle.

Adverse Reactions

Central nervous system: Drowsiness (with high doses), hallucinations, headache, neurotoxicity, seizures

Dermatologic: Erythema of the hands and face, maculopapular rash, pruritus or dry skin, skin cancer, alopecia is rare. Hyperpigmentation with radiation exposure.

Endocrine & metabolic: Hyperuricemia

Gastrointestinal: Mild nausea and vomiting may occur, as well as diarrhea, constipation, stomatitis, anorexia, pancreatitis

Emetic potential: Low

Hematologic: Myelosuppression (primarily leukopenia); Dose-limiting toxicity, causes a rapid drop in leukocyte count (seen in 4-5 days in nonhematologic malignancy and more rapidly in leukemia); thrombocytopenia and anemia occur less often; reversal of WBC count occurs rapidly, but the platelet count may take 7-10 days to recover

Onset: 24-48 hours; Nadir: 10 days; Recovery: 7 days after stopping drug

Hepatic: Elevation of hepatic enzymes, hepatotoxicity

Neuromuscular & skeletal: Peripheral neuropathy

Renal: Increased creatinine and BUN due to impairment of renal tubular function

Respiratory: Acute diffuse pulmonary infiltrates (rare)

Miscellaneous: Nail banding

Pharmacodynamics/Kinetics

Absorption: Readily (≥80%)

Distribution: Readily crosses blood-brain barrier; distributes into intestine, brain, lung, kidney tissues, effusions, and ascites

Metabolism: 60% via hepatic and GI tract

Half-life elimination: 3-4 hours

Time to peak: 1-4 hours

Excretion: Urine (80%, 50% as unchanged drug, 30% as urea); exhaled gases (as CO_2)

Dosage

Oral (refer to individual protocols): All dosage should be based on ideal or actual body weight, whichever is less:

Children:

No FDA-approved dosage regimens have been established; dosages of 1500-3000 mg/m² as a single dose in combination with other agents every 4-6 weeks have been used in the treatment of pediatric astrocytoma, medulloblastoma, and primitive neuroectodermal tumors

CML: Initial: 10-20 mg/kg/day once daily; adjust dose according to hematologic response

Adults: Dose should always be titrated to patient response and WBC counts; usual oral doses range from 10-30 mg/kg/day or 500-3000 mg/day; if WBC count falls to <2500 cells/mm³, or the platelet count to <100,000/mm³, therapy should be stopped for at least 3 days and resumed when values rise toward normal

Solid tumors:

Intermittent therapy: 80 mg/kg as a single dose every third day

Continuous therapy: 20-30 mg/kg/day given as a single dose/day

Concomitant therapy with irradiation: 80 mg/kg as a single dose every third day starting at least 7 days before initiation of irradiation

Resistant chronic myelocytic leukemia: Continuous therapy: 20-30 mg/kg as a single daily dose

HIV (unlabeled use; in combination with antiretroviral agents): 1000-1500 mg daily in a single dose or divided doses

Psoriasis (unlabeled use): 1000-1500 mg/day in a single dose or divided doses

Sickle cell anemia (moderate/severe disease): Initial: 15 mg/kg/day, increased by 5 mg/kg every 12 weeks if blood counts are in an acceptable range until the maximum tolerated dose of 35 mg/kg/day is achieved or the dose that does not produce toxic effects

Acceptable range:
Neutrophils $\geq$2500 cells/mm^3
Platelets $\geq$95,000/mm^3
Hemoglobin >5.3 g/dL, and
Reticulocytes $\geq$95,000/mm^3 if the hemoglobin concentration is <9 g/dL

Toxic range:
Neutrophils <2000 cells/mm^3
Platelets <80,000/mm^3
Hemoglobin <4.5 g/dL
Reticulocytes <80,000/mm^3 if the hemoglobin concentration is <9 g/dL

Monitor for toxicity every 2 weeks; if toxicity occurs, stop treatment until the bone marrow recovers; restart at 2.5 mg/kg/day less than the dose at which toxicity occurs; if no toxicity occurs over the next 12 weeks, then the subsequent dose should be increased by 2.5 mg/kg/day; reduced dosage of hydroxyurea alternating with erythropoietin may decrease myelotoxicity and increase levels of fetal hemoglobin in patients who have not been helped by hydroxyurea alone

Dosing adjustment in renal impairment:
Sickle cell anemia: Cl$_{cr}$ <60 mL/minute or ESRD: Reduce initial dose to 7.5 mg/kg; titrate to response/avoidance of toxicity (refer to usual dosing)
Other indications:
Cl$_{cr}$ 10-50 mL/minute: Administer 50% of normal dose
Cl$_{cr}$ <10 mL/minute: Administer 20% of normal dose
Hemodialysis: Supplemental dose is not necessary. Hydroxyurea is a low molecular weight compound with high aqueous solubility that may be freely dialyzable, however, clinical studies confirming this hypothesis have not been performed; peak serum concentrations are reached within 2 hours after oral administration and by 24 hours, the concentration in the serum is zero
CAPD effects: Unknown
CAVH effects: Dose for GFR 10-50 mL/minute

Stability Store capsules at room temperature; capsules may be opened and emptied into water (will not dissolve completely)

Monitoring Parameters CBC with differential, platelets, hemoglobin, renal function and liver function tests, serum uric acid

Administration Capsules may be opened and emptied into water (will not dissolve completely); observe proper handling procedures

Contraindications Hypersensitivity to hydroxyurea or any component of the formulation; severe anemia; severe bone marrow suppression; WBC <2500/mm^3 or platelet count <100,000/mm^3; pregnancy

Warnings Hazardous agent – use appropriate precautions for handling and disposal. Patients with a history of prior cytotoxic chemotherapy and radiation therapy are more likely to experience bone marrow depression. Patients with a history of radiation therapy are also at risk for exacerbation of post irradiation erythema. Megaloblastic erythropoiesis may be seen early in hydroxyurea treatment; plasma iron clearance may be delayed and the rate of utilization of iron by erythrocytes may be delayed. HIV-infected patients treated with hydroxyurea and didanosine (with or without stavudine) are at higher risk for pancreatitis, hepatotoxicity, hepatic failure, and severe peripheral neuropathy. **[U.S. Boxed Warning]: Hydroxyurea is mutagenic and clastogenic. Treatment of myeloproliferative disorders (polycythemia vera and thrombocythemia) with long-term hydroxyurea is associated with secondary leukemia**; it is unknown if this is drug-related or disease-related. Cutaneous vasculitic toxicities (vasculitic ulceration and gangrene) have been reported with hydroxyurea treatment, most often in patients with a history of or receiving concurrent interferon therapy; discontinue hydroxyurea and consider alternate cytoreductive therapy if cutaneous vasculitic toxicity develops. Use caution with renal dysfunction; may require dose reductions. Safety and efficacy in children have not been established. **[U.S. Boxed Warning]: Should be administered under the supervision of a physician experienced in cancer chemotherapy or in the treatment of sickle cell anemia.**

Dosage Forms Capsule: 500 mg
Droxia®: 200 mg, 300 mg, 400 mg
Hydrea®: 500 mg
Tablet (Mylocel™): 1000 mg

Overdosage/Treatment
Supportive therapy: Leg ulcers can be treated with a single application of Apligraf.
Decontamination: Lavage (within 1 hour)/activated charcoal

Enhancement of elimination: Multiple dosing of activated charcoal may be useful

Test Interactions ↑ uric acid, BUN, creatinine

Drug Interactions Didanosine: Hydroxyurea may increase risk of didanosine-induced pancreatitis, hepatotoxicity, or neuropathy; concomitant use is not recommended

Pregnancy Risk Factor D

Pregnancy Implications Hydroxyurea is teratogenic and fetotoxic in animals; data on use during human pregnancy is limited. Effective contraception is recommended in women of childbearing potential.

Lactation Enters breast milk/contraindicated

Additional Information Handle urine from patients taking hydroxyurea with care. Myelosuppressive effects: **WBC**: Moderate. **Platelets**: Moderate. Onset (days): 7. Nadir (days): 10. Recovery (days): 21

Specific References
Seki JT, Al-Omar HM, Amato D, et al, "Acute Tumor Lysis Syndrome Secondary to Hydroxyurea in Acute Myeloid Leukemia," *Ann Pharmacother*, 2003, 37(5):675-8.

HydrOXYzine

Related Information
• Cetirizine

CAS Number 10246-75-0; 2192-20-3; 68-88-2

U.S. Brand Names Atarax®; Vistaril®

Synonyms Hydroxyzine Hydrochloride; Hydroxyzine Pamoate

Impairment Potential Yes. Impairment occurs (over about a 6-hour period) at doses of 25 mg. (Gengo FM and Manning C, "A Review of the Effects of Antihistamines on Mental Processes Related to Automobile Driving," *J Allergy Clin Immunol*, 1990 86(2):1034-9.)

Use Treatment of anxiety, as a preoperative sedative, an antipruritic

Unlabeled/Investigational Use Antiemetic; ethanol withdrawal symptoms

Mechanism of Action A piperazine compound which competes with histamine for H$_1$-receptor sites on effector cells in the gastrointestinal tract, blood vessels, and respiratory tract

Adverse Reactions
Cardiovascular: Palpitations, hypotension, sinus bradycardia, sinus tachycardia
Central nervous system: **Slight to moderate drowsiness**, headache, fatigue, nervousness, dizziness, CNS depression, sedation, paradoxical excitement, insomnia, fever, hyperthermia, ataxia
Dermatologic: Photosensitivity, rash, angioedema, fixed drug eruption, erythema multiforme, urticaria, purpura, exanthem
Gastrointestinal: Increased appetite, increased weight, nausea, diarrhea, abdominal pain, xerostomia
Genitourinary: Urinary retention
Hematologic: Hemolysis (I.V. administration), porphyrinogenic
Hepatic: Hepatitis
Neuromuscular & skeletal: Arthralgia, myalgia, tremors, paresthesia, rhabdomyolysis
Ocular: Blurred vision
Respiratory: **Thickening of bronchial secretions**, bronchospasm, pharyngitis, epistaxis

Signs and Symptoms of Overdose Depression, hypotension, impotence, insomnia, myalgia, seizures, sedation

Admission Criteria/Prognosis Observe ingestions for 12 hours; admit ingestions >300 mg

Pharmacodynamics/Kinetics
Onset of action: 15-30 minutes
Duration: 4-6 hours
Absorption: Oral: Rapid
Metabolism: Exact fate unknown
Half-life elimination: 3-7 hours
Time to peak: ~2 hours

Dosage
Children:
Oral: 0.6 mg/kg/dose every 6 hours
I.M.: 0.5-1 mg/kg/dose every 4-6 hours as needed
Adults:
Antiemetic: I.M.: 25-100 mg/dose every 4-6 hours as needed
Anxiety: Oral: 25-100 mg 4 times/day; maximum dose: 600 mg/day
Preoperative sedation:
Oral: 50-100 mg
I.M.: 25-100 mg
Management of pruritus: Oral: 25 mg 3-4 times/day

Dosing interval in hepatic impairment: Change dosing interval to every 24 hours in patients with primary biliary cirrhosis

Stability Protect from light; I.V. is **incompatible** when mixed with aminophylline, amobarbital, chloramphenicol, dimenhydrinate, heparin, penicillin G, pentobarbital, phenobarbital, phenytoin, ranitidine, sulfisoxazole, thioridazine, vitamin B complex with C

Monitoring Parameters Relief of symptoms, mental status, blood pressure

Administration

Do not administer SubQ or intra-arterially.

I.M.: For administration in children, injections should be made into the midlateral muscles of the thigh.

I.V.: Not generally recommended; may be given as a short (30-60 minute) infusion.

Contraindications Hypersensitivity to hydroxyzine or any component of the formulation; early pregnancy

Warnings

Causes sedation, caution must be used in performing tasks which require alertness (eg, operating machinery or driving). Sedative effects of CNS depressants or ethanol are potentiated. SubQ and intra-arterial administration are not recommended since thrombosis and digital gangrene can occur; should be used with caution in patients with narrow-angle glaucoma, prostatic hyperplasia, and bladder neck obstruction; should also be used with caution in patients with asthma or COPD.

Anticholinergic effects are not well tolerated in the elderly. Hydroxyzine may be useful as a short-term antipruritic, but it is not recommended for use as a sedative or anxiolytic in the elderly.

Dosage Forms

Capsule, as pamoate: 25 mg, 50 mg, 100 mg
Vistaril®: 25 mg, 50 mg

Injection, solution, as hydrochloride: 25 mg/mL (1 mL); 50 mg/mL (1 mL, 2 mL, 10 mL)

Suspension, oral, as pamoate:
Vistaril®: 25 mg/5 mL (120 mL, 480 mL) [lemon flavor]

Syrup, as hydrochloride: 10 mg/5 mL (120 mL, 480 mL)

Tablet, as hydrochloride: 10 mg, 25 mg, 50 mg

Reference Range Plasma hydroxyzine level of 5.6-41.8 mcg/dL (13.2-102.0 nmol/L) therapeutic for pruritus in children; peak plasma level is 73 mcg/L after 0.7 mg/kg dose in adults

Overdosage/Treatment

Decontamination: Lavage (within 1 hour)/activated charcoal

Supportive therapy: Physostigmine should be utilized in severe life-threatening anticholinergic crisis; norepinephrine or metaraminol are the vasopressors of choice; epinephrine is **not** useful

Enhancement of elimination: Multiple dosing of activated charcoal may be effective

Test Interactions Can suppress wheal and flare of antigen skin testing for 4 days

Drug Interactions Inhibits CYP2D6 (weak)

Acetylcholinesterase Inhibitors (Central): May diminish the anticholinergic of hydroxyzine. If the anticholinergic effect is a side effect of the agent, as is the case with hydroxyzine, the result may be beneficial.

Anticholinergic agents: Central and/or peripheral anticholinergic syndrome can occur when administered with narcotic analgesics, phenothiazines and other antipsychotics (especially with high anticholinergic activity), tricyclic antidepressants, quinidine and some other antiarrhythmics, and antihistamines

CNS depressants: Sedative effects of hydroxyzine may be additive with CNS depressants; includes ethanol, benzodiazepines, barbiturates, narcotic analgesics, and other sedative agents; monitor for increased effect

Pramlintide: May enhance the GI-related anticholinergic effect of hydroxyzine.

Pregnancy Risk Factor C

Pregnancy Implications Neonatal withdrawal syndrome may occur

Lactation Enters breast milk/contraindicated

Nursing Implications Extravasation can result in sterile abscess and marked tissue induration; provide safety measures (ie, side rails, night light, and call button); remove smoking materials from area; supervise ambulation

Additional Information Estimated lethal dose: 25-250 mg/kg

Hydroxyzine hydrochloride: Atarax®, Vistaril® injection

Hydroxyzine pamoate: Vistaril® capsule and suspension

Hyoscyamine

CAS Number 101-31-5; 620-61-1; 6835-16-1

U.S. Brand Names Anaspaz®; Cystospaz-M®; Cystospaz®; Hyosine; Levbid®; Levsin/SL®; Levsinex®; Levsin®; NuLev™; Spacol T/S; Spacol; Symax SL; Symax SR

Synonyms l-Hyoscyamine Sulfate; Hyoscyamine Sulfate

Use

Oral: Adjunctive therapy for peptic ulcers, irritable bowel, neurogenic bladder/bowel; treatment of infant colic, GI tract disorders caused by spasm; to reduce rigidity, tremors, sialorrhea, and hyperhidrosis associated with parkinsonism; as a drying agent in acute rhinitis

Injection: Preoperative antimuscarinic to reduce secretions and block cardiac vagal inhibitory reflexes; to improve radiologic visibility of the kidneys; symptomatic relief of biliary and renal colic; reduce GI motility to facilitate diagnostic procedures (ie, endoscopy, hypotonic duodenography); reduce pain and hypersecretion in pancreatitis, certain cases of partial heart block associated with vagal activity; reversal of neuromuscular blockade

Mechanism of Action Blocks the action of acetylcholine at parasympathetic sites in smooth muscle, secretory glands and the CNS; increases cardiac output, dries secretions, antagonizes histamine and serotonin, antimuscarinic agent; found in the plant *Hyoscyamus niger*

Adverse Reactions

Cardiovascular: Tachycardia, palpitations, hypotension (orthostatic), sinus tachycardia, tachycardia (supraventricular)

Central nervous system: Fatigue, delirium, restlessness, headache, lightheadedness, anxiety, memory disturbance, ataxia, mania, paranoia, psychosis

Dermatologic: **Dry skin**, hot skin; photosensitivity, skin rash, urticaria

Gastrointestinal: Impaired gastrointestinal motility, constipation, dysphagia, **xerostomia and dry throat**, loss of taste perception, impotence, urinary retention

Genitourinary: Dysuria

Local: **Irritation at injection site**

Neuromuscular & skeletal: Tremors

Ocular: Mydriasis, blurred vision, increased intraocular pressure

Respiratory: **Dry nose**

Miscellaneous: **Diaphoresis (decreased)**

Signs and Symptoms of Overdose Ataxia, blurred vision, coma, dilated unreactive pupils, diminished or absent bowel sounds, dryness of mucous membranes, dysphagia, facial flushing, foul breath, hallucinations (lilliputian), hypertension, hyperthermia, ileus, impotence, increased intraocular pressure, increased respiratory rate, lightheadedness, memory loss, myoglobinuria, photophobia, rhabdomyolysis, seizures, tachycardia, urinary retention

Pharmacodynamics/Kinetics

Onset of action: 2-3 minutes

Duration: 4-6 hours

Absorption: Well absorbed

Distribution: Crosses placenta; small amounts enter breast milk

Protein binding: 50%

Metabolism: Hepatic

Half-life elimination: 3-5 hours

Excretion: Urine

Dosage

Oral: Children: Gastrointestinal disorders: Dose as listed, based on age and weight (kg) using 0.125 mg/mL drops; repeat dose every 4 hours as needed:
Children <2 years:
3.4 kg: 4 drops; maximum: 24 drops/24 hours
5 kg: 5 drops; maximum: 30 drops/24 hours
7 kg: 6 drops; maximum: 36 drops/24 hours
10 kg: 8 drops; maximum: 48 drops/24 hours

Oral, S.L.:
Children 2-12 years: Gastrointestinal disorders: Dose as listed, based on age and weight (kg); repeat dose every 4 hours as needed:
10 kg: 0.031-0.033 mg; maximum: 0.75 mg/24 hours
20 kg: 0.0625 mg; maximum: 0.75 mg/24 hours
40 kg: 0.0938 mg; maximum: 0.75 mg/24 hours
50 kg: 0.125 mg; maximum: 0.75 mg/24 hours

Children >12 years and Adults: Gastrointestinal disorders: 0.125-0.25 mg every 4 hours or as needed (before meals or food); maximum: 1.5 mg/24 hours
Cystospaz®: 0.15-0.3 mg up to 4 times/day

Oral (timed release): Children >12 years and Adults: Gastrointestinal disorders: 0.375-0.75 mg every 12 hours; maximum: 1.5 mg/24 hours

I.M., I.V., SubQ: Children >12 years and Adults: Gastrointestinal disorders: 0.25-0.5 mg; may repeat as needed up to 4 times/day, at 4-hour intervals

I.V.: Children >2 year and Adults: I.V.: Preanesthesia: 5 mcg/kg given 30-60 minutes prior to induction of anesthesia or at the time preoperative narcotics or sedatives are administered

I.V.: Adults: Diagnostic procedures: 0.25-0.5 mg given 5-10 minutes prior to procedure

To reduce drug-induced bradycardia during surgery: 0.125 mg; repeat as needed

To reverse neuromuscular blockade: 0.2 mg for every 1 mg neostigmine (or the physostigmine/pyridostigmine equivalent)

Stability Insoluble in ether; soluble in water

Administration

Oral: Tablets should be administered before meals or food.

Levbid®: Tablets are scored and may be broken in half for dose titration; do not crush or chew.

Levsin/SL®: Tablets may be used sublingually, chewed, or swallowed whole.

NuLev™: Tablet is placed on tongue and allowed to disintegrate before swallowing; may take with or without water.

Symax SL: Tablets may be used sublingually or swallowed whole.

I.M.: May be administered without dilution.

Inject over at least 1 minute. May be administered without dilution.

Contraindications Hypersensitivity to belladonna alkaloids or any component of the formulation; glaucoma; obstructive uropathy; myasthenia gravis; obstructive GI tract disease, paralytic ileus, intestinal atony of elderly or debilitated patients, severe ulcerative colitis, toxic megacolon complicating ulcerative colitis; unstable cardiovascular status in acute hemorrhage, myocardial ischemia

Warnings Heat prostration may occur in hot weather. Diarrhea may be a sign of incomplete intestinal obstruction, treatment should be discontinued if this occurs. May produce side effects as seen with other anticholinergic medications including drowsiness, dizziness, blurred vision, or psychosis. Children and the elderly may be more susceptible to these effects. Use with caution in children with spastic paralysis. Use with caution in patients with autonomic neuropathy, coronary heart disease, CHF, cardiac arrhythmias, prostatic hyperplasia, hyperthyroidism, hypertension, chronic lung disease, renal disease, and hiatal hernia associated with reflux esophagitis. Use with caution in the elderly, may precipitate undiagnosed glaucoma and/or severely impair memory function (especially in those patients with previous memory problems).
NuLev™: Contains phenylalanine

Dosage Forms [DSC] = Discontinued product
Capsule, timed release, as sulfate (Cystospaz-M® [DSC], Levsinex®): 0.375 mg
Elixir, as sulfate: 0.125 mg/5 mL (480 mL)
 Hyosine: 0.125 mg/5 mL (480 mL) [contains alcohol 20% and sodium benzoate; orange flavor]
 Levsin®: 0.125 mg/5 mL (480 mL) [contains alcohol 20%; orange flavor]
Injection, solution, as sulfate (Levsin®): 0.5 mg/mL (1 mL)
Liquid, as sulfate (Spacol [DSC]): 0.125 mg/5 mL (120 mL) [sugar free, alcohol free, simethicone based, bubble gum flavor]
Solution, oral drops, as sulfate: 0.125 mg/mL (15 mL)
 Hyosine: 0.125 mg/mL (15 mL) [contains alcohol 5% and sodium benzoate; orange flavor]
 Levsin®: 0.125 mg/mL (15 mL) [contains alcohol 5%; orange flavor]
Tablet (Cystospaz®): 0.15 mg
Tablet, as sulfate (Anaspaz®, Levsin®, Spacol [DSC]): 0.125 mg
Tablet, extended release, as sulfate (Levbid®, Symax SR, Spacol T/S [DSC]): 0.375 mg
Tablet, orally disintegrating, as sulfate (NuLev™): 0.125 mg [contains phenylalanine 1.7 mg/tablet, mint flavor]
Tablet, sublingual, as sulfate: 0.125 mg
 Levsin/SL®: 0.125 mg [peppermint flavor]
 Symax SL: 0.125 mg

Overdosage/Treatment
Decontamination: Lavage (within 1 hour)/activated charcoal; **do not** induce emesis
Supportive therapy: Physostigmine should be used as a last resort for life-threatening seizures, arrhythmias, or hypertension that is refractory to standard supportive therapy; rhabdomyolysis can be treated with alkaline diuresis and mannitol; esmolol can be used for tachyarrhythmias; bethanechol (5-10 mg 3 times/day) can be given for peripheral anticholinergic signs
Enhancement of elimination: Multiple dosing of activated charcoal may be effective

Antidote(s)
- Mannitol [ANTIDOTE]
- Physostigmine [ANTIDOTE]

Drug Interactions Amantadine: Additive adverse effects may occur due to cholinergic blockade.
Antacids: Antacids may decrease absorption of hyoscyamine; administer hyoscyamine before meals and give antacids after meals.
Antihistamines: Additive adverse effects may occur with some antihistamines due to cholinergic blockade.
Antimuscarinics: Additive adverse effects may occur due to cholinergic blockade.
Haloperidol: Additive adverse effects may occur due to cholinergic blockade.
MAO inhibitors: Additive adverse effects may occur due to cholinergic blockade.
Phenothiazines: Additive adverse effects may occur due to cholinergic blockade.
Tricyclic antidepressants: Additive adverse effects may occur due to cholinergic blockade.

Pregnancy Risk Factor C
Pregnancy Implications Crosses the placenta, effects to the fetus not known; use during pregnancy only if clearly needed
Lactation Enters breast milk/not recommended
Nursing Implications Observe for tachycardia if the patient has cardiac problems.

Ibuprofen

Related Information
- Flurbiprofen
- Nonsteroidal Anti-inflammatory Drugs

CAS Number 15687-27-1

U.S. Brand Names Advil® Children's [OTC]; Advil® Infants' [OTC]; Advil® Junior [OTC]; Advil® Migraine [OTC]; Advil® [OTC]; ElixSure™ IB [OTC] ; Genpril® [OTC]; I-Prin [OTC]; Ibu-200 [OTC]; Midol® Cramp and Body Aches [OTC]; Motrin® Children's [OTC]; Motrin® IB [OTC]; Motrin® Infants' [OTC]; Motrin® Junior Strength [OTC]; Motrin®; NeoProfen®; Proprinal [OTC]; Ultraprin [OTC]

Synonyms p-Isobutylhydratropic Acid; Ibuprofen Lysine

Use
Oral: Inflammatory diseases and rheumatoid disorders including juvenile rheumatoid arthritis, mild-to-moderate pain, fever, dysmenorrhea
Injection: Ibuprofen lysine is for use in premature infants weighing between 500-1500 g and who are ≤ 32 weeks gestational age (GA) to induce closure of a clinically-significant patent ductus arteriosus (PDA) when usual treatments are ineffective
Cystic fibrosis, gout, ankylosing spondylitis, acute migraine headache

Mechanism of Action Inhibits prostaglandin synthesis by decreasing the activity of the enzyme, cyclooxygenase, which results in decreased formation of prostaglandin precursors

Adverse Reactions
Cardiovascular: Circulatory collapse, arrhythmias (ventricular), vasculitis
Central nervous system: **Dizziness, fatigue**, headache, aseptic meningitis, psychosis, cognitive dysfunction, coma, seizures
Dermatologic: **Rash, urticaria**, pruritus, Stevens-Johnson syndrome, erythema multiforme, angioedema, toxic epidermal necrolysis, onycholysis, psoriasis, erythema nodosum, exanthem, photoallergic reaction, lichen planus, cutaneous vasculitis
Endocrine & metabolic: Hyperkalemia, anion gap metabolic acidosis, fluid retention, gynecomastia
Gastrointestinal: **Abdominal cramps, heartburn, indigestion, nausea**, vomiting, GI bleeding, GI ulceration, constipation, diarrhea, dyspepsia, fecal discoloration (black), vanishing bile duct syndrome, esophagitis, aphthous stomatitis, xerostomia, stomatitis
Hematologic: Leukopenia, neutropenia, agranulocytosis, granulocytopenia; aplastic anemia (rare), platelet inhibition, hemolytic anemia (Coombs' positive)
Hepatic: Elevated transaminases, hepatitis (fulminant), aminotransferase level elevation (asymptomatic)
Neuromuscular & skeletal: Paresthesia
Ocular: Diplopia, vortex keratopathy, amblyopia, color vision abnormalities
Otic: Ototoxicity, tinnitus
Renal: Renal failure (acute), nephrotic syndrome, chronic renal failure, albuminuria
Respiratory: Wheezing, respiratory depression, aspiration
Miscellaneous: Hypersensitivity, systemic lupus erythematosus (SLE), fixed drug eruption

Signs and Symptoms of Overdose Azotemia, coagulopathy, cognitive dysfunction, depression, drowsiness, flatulence, GI bleeding, hyperthermia, gastritis, hypoglycemia, hyponatremia, leukocytosis, lightheadedness, mental confusion, nausea, nephrotic syndrome, ototoxicity, photosensitivity, purpura, vomiting, thrombocytopenia, tinnitus, wheezing Severe poisoning can manifest with apnea, coma, hepatic failure, hypotension, hypothermia, metabolic acidosis, nystagmus, respiratory depression, and seizures. More significant exposures have been associated with ingestions >400 mg/kg. Alopecia, feces discoloration (tarry), fever, hypocalcemia, hypophosphatemia, hypomagnesemia, urine discoloration (red; red-purple). Acute renal papillary necrosis and renal failure at ingestions >6 g.

Admission Criteria/Prognosis Admit any patient with acidosis, symptoms occurring over 4 hours postingestion, or ingestions >400 mg/kg

Pharmacodynamics/Kinetics
Onset of action: Analgesic: 30-60 minutes; Anti-inflammatory: ≤ 7 days
 Peak effect: 1-2 weeks
Duration: 4-6 hours
Absorption: Oral: Rapid (85%)
Distribution: Premature infants with ductal closure (highly variable between studies):
 Day 3: 145-349 mL/kg
 Day 5: 72-222 mL/kg
Protein binding: 90% to 99%
Metabolism: Hepatic via oxidation
Half-life elimination:
 Premature infants (highly variable between studies):
  Day 3: 35-51 hours
  Day 5: 20-33 hours
 Children 3 months to 10 years: 1.6 ± 0.7 hours
 Adults: 2-4 hours; End-stage renal disease: Unchanged
Time to peak: ~1-2 hours
Excretion: Urine (1% as free drug); some feces

Dosage
I.V.: Infants between 500-1500 g and ≤ 32 weeks GA: Patent ductus arteriosus: Initial dose: Ibuprofen 10 mg/kg, followed by two doses of 5 mg/kg at 24 and 48 hours. Dose should be based on birth weight.
Oral:
Children:

Antipyretic: 6 months to 12 years: Temperature <102.5°F (39°C): 5 mg/kg/dose; temperature >102.5°F: 10 mg/kg/dose given every 6-8 hours (maximum daily dose: 40 mg/kg/day)

Juvenile rheumatoid arthritis: 30-50 mg/kg/24 hours divided every 8 hours; start at lower end of dosing range and titrate upward (maximum: 2.4 g/day)

Analgesic: 4-10 mg/kg/dose every 6-8 hours

Cystic fibrosis (unlabeled use): Chronic (>4 years) twice daily dosing adjusted to maintain serum levels of 50-100 mcg/mL has been associated with slowing of disease progression in younger patients with mild lung disease

OTC labeling (analgesic, antipyretic):

Children 6 months to 11 years: See table; use of weight to select dose is preferred; doses may be repeated every 6-8 hours (maximum: 4 doses/day)

Children ≥12 years: 200 mg every 4-6 hours as needed (maximum: 1200 mg/24 hours)

Ibuprofen Dosing

Weight (lbs)	Age	Dosage (mg)
12-17	6-11 mo	50
18-23	12-23 mo	75
24-35	2-3 y	100
36-47	4-5 y	150
48-59	6-8 y	200
60-71	9-10 y	250
72-95	11 y	300

Adults:

Inflammatory disease: 400-800 mg/dose 3-4 times/day (maximum dose: 3.2 g/day)

Analgesia/pain/fever/dysmenorrhea: 200-400 mg/dose every 4-6 hours (maximum daily dose: 1.2 g, unless directed by physician)

OTC labeling (analgesic, antipyretic): 200 mg every 4-6 hours as needed (maximum: 1200 mg/24 hours)

Dosing adjustment/comments in severe hepatic impairment: Avoid use

Monitoring Parameters CBC; occult blood loss and periodic liver function tests; monitor response (pain, range of motion, grip strength, mobility, ADL function), inflammation; observe for weight gain, edema; monitor renal function (urine output, serum BUN and creatinine); observe for bleeding, bruising; evaluate gastrointestinal effects (abdominal pain, bleeding, dyspepsia); mental confusion, disorientation; with long-term therapy, periodic ophthalmic exams

Administration

Oral: Administer with food

I.V.: For I.V. administration only; administration via umbilical line has not been evaluated. Infuse over 15 minutes through port closest to insertion site. Avoid extravasation. Do not administer simultaneously via same line with TPN. If needed, interrupt TPN for 15 minutes prior to and after ibuprofen administration, keeping line open with dextrose or saline.

Contraindications

Hypersensitivity to ibuprofen, aspirin, other NSAIDs, or any component of the formulation; perioperative pain in the setting of coronary artery bypass surgery (CABG); pregnancy (3rd trimester)

Ibuprofen lysine is contraindicated in preterm infants with untreated proven or suspected infection; congenital heart disease where patency of the PDA is necessary for pulmonary or systemic blood flow; bleeding (especially with active intracranial hemorrhage or GI bleed); thrombocytopenia; coagulation defects; proven or suspected necrotizing enterocolitis (NEC); significant renal dysfunction

Warnings [U.S. Boxed Warning]: NSAIDs are associated with an increased risk of adverse cardiovascular events, including MI, stroke, and new onset or worsening of pre-existing hypertension. Risk may be increased with duration of use or pre-existing cardiovascular risk-factors or disease. Carefully evaluate individual cardiovascular risk profiles prior to prescribing. Use caution with fluid retention, CHF or hypertension.

Use of NSAIDs can compromise existing renal function. Renal toxicity can occur in patient with impaired renal function, dehydration, heart failure, liver dysfunction, those taking diuretics and ACEI and the elderly. Rehydrate patient before starting therapy. Monitor renal function closely. Ibuprofen is not recommended for patients with advanced renal disease.

NSAIDs may increase risk of gastrointestinal irritation, ulceration, bleeding, and perforation. These events may occur at any time during therapy and without warning. Use caution with a history of GI disease (bleeding or ulcers), concurrent therapy with aspirin, anticoagulants and/or corticosteroids, smoking, use of alcohol, the elderly or debilitated patients.

Use the lowest effective dose for the shortest duration of time, consistent with individual patient goals, to reduce risk of cardiovascular or GI adverse events. Alternate therapies should be considered for patients at high risk.

NSAIDs may cause serious skin adverse events including exfoliative dermatitis, Stevens-Johnson syndrome (SJS) and toxic epidermal necrolysis (TEN). Anaphylactoid reactions may occur, even without prior exposure; patients with "aspirin triad" (bronchial asthma, aspirin intolerance, rhinitis) may be at increased risk. Do not use in patients who experience bronchospasm, asthma, rhinitis, or urticaria with NSAID or aspirin therapy.

Use with caution in patients with decreased hepatic function. Closely monitor patients with any abnormal LFT. Severe hepatic reactions (eg, fulminant hepatitis, liver failure) have occurred with NSAID use, rarely; discontinue if signs or symptoms of liver disease develop, or if systemic manifestations occur.

The elderly are at increased risk for adverse effects (especially peptic ulceration, CNS effects, renal toxicity) from NSAIDs even at low doses.

Withhold for at least 4-6 half-lives prior to surgical or dental procedures.

Injection: Hold second or third doses if urinary output is <0.6 mL/kg/hour. May alter signs of infection. May inhibit platelet aggregation; monitor for signs of bleeding. May displace bilirubin; use caution when total bilirubin is elevated. Long-term evaluations of neurodevelopment, growth, or diseases associated with prematurity following treatment have not been conducted. A second course of treatment, alternative pharmacologic therapy or surgery may be needed if the ductus arteriosus fails to close or reopens following the initial course of therapy.

OTC labeling: Prior to self-medication, patients should contact health care provider if they have had recurring stomach pain or upset, ulcers, bleeding problems, high blood pressure, heart or kidney disease, other serious medical problems, are currently taking a diuretic, or are ≥60 years of age. Recommended dosages should not be exceeded, due to an increased risk of GI bleeding. Consuming ≥3 alcoholic beverages/day or taking longer than recommended may increase the risk of GI bleeding. When used for self-medication, patients should contact healthcare provider if used for fever lasting >3 days or for pain lasting >10 days in adults or >3 days in children. In children with a sore throat, do not use for >2 days or administer to children <3 years of age unless instructed by healthcare provider. Consult healthcare provider when sore throat pain is severe, persistent, or accompanied by fever, headache, nausea, and/or vomiting. Notify healthcare provider of worsening stomach pain, feeling faint, vomiting of blood or bloody black stools.

Dosage Forms

Caplet: 200 mg [OTC]

Advil®: 200 mg [contains sodium benzoate]

Ibu-200, Motrin® IB: 200 mg

Motrin® Junior Strength: 100 mg

Capsule, liqui-gel:

Advil®: 200 mg

Advil® Migraine: 200 mg [solubilized ibuprofen; contains potassium 20 mg]

Gelcap:

Advil®: 200 mg [contains coconut oil]

Injection, solution, as lysine [preservative free]:

NeoProfen®: 17.1 mg/mL (2 mL) [equivalent to ibuprofen 10 mg/mL]

Suspension, oral: 100 mg/5 mL (5 mL, 120 mL, 480 mL)

Advil® Children's: 100 mg/5 mL (60 mL, 120 mL) [contains sodium benzoate; blue raspberry, fruit, and grape flavors]

ElixSure™ IB: 100 mg/5 mL (120 mL) [berry flavor]

Motrin® Children's: 100 mg/5 mL (60 mL, 120 mL) [contains sodium benzoate; berry, dye free berry, bubble gum, and grape flavors]

Suspension, oral drops: 40 mg/mL (15 mL)

Advil® Infants': 40 mg/mL (15 mL) [contains sodium benzoate; fruit and grape flavors]

Motrin® Infants': 40 mg/mL (15 mL, 30 mL) [contains sodium benzoate; berry and dye-free berry flavors]

Tablet: 200 mg [OTC], 400 mg, 600 mg, 800 mg

Advil®: 200 mg [contains sodium benzoate]

Advil® Junior: 100 mg [contains sodium benzoate; coated tablets]

Genpril®, I-Prin, Midol® Cramp and Body Aches, Motrin® IB, Proprinal, Ultraprin: 200 mg

Motrin®: 400 mg, 600 mg, 800 mg

Tablet, chewable:

Advil® Children's: 50 mg [contains phenylalanine 2.1 mg; grape flavors]

Advil® Junior: 100 mg [contains phenylalanine 4.2 mg; grape flavors]

Motrin® Children's: 50 mg [contains phenylalanine 1.4 mg; grape and orange flavor]

Motrin® Junior Strength: 100 mg [contains phenylalanine 2.1 mg; grape and orange flavors]

Reference Range Plasma concentrations >200 mcg/mL (971 μmol/L) may be associated with severe toxicity; serum levels are not readily available, thus not recommended routinely; antipyretic effect can occur at plasma concentrations of 10 mcg/mL (48 μmol/L)

Overdosage/Treatment

Decontamination: Ipecac within 30 minutes or lavage (within 1 hour)/ activated charcoal at ingestions >200 mg/kg; whole bowel irrigation is effective but usually not required

Supportive therapy: Hypotension/dehydration can be managed with I.V. fluid therapy; acidosis should be treated with bicarbonates, seizures with benzodiazepines; antacids, blood products are indicated, as appropriate, for hemorrhage; famotidine (40 mg 2 times/day) can decrease incidence of gastric or duodenal ulcers in patients receiving long-term therapy of this drug. Monitor renal function with ingestions >6 g.

Enhancement of elimination: Dialysis or perfusion is indicated for secondary complications, acidosis, or renal failure and not toxin removal alone; multiple dosing of activated charcoal may be effective.

Diagnostic Procedures

- Anion Gap, Blood
- Stool Culture
- Urinalysis

Test Interactions ↑ chloride (S), sodium (S); may cause false-positive on benzodiazepine assay

Drug Interactions **Substrate** (minor) of CYP2C9, 2C19; **Inhibits** CYP2C9 (strong)

ACE inhibitors: Antihypertensive effects may be decreased by concurrent therapy with NSAIDs; monitor blood pressure.

Aminoglycosides: NSAIDs may decrease the excretion of aminoglycosides; this is of particular concern in preterm infants.

Angiotensin II antagonists: Antihypertensive effects may be decreased by concurrent therapy with NSAIDs; monitor blood pressure.

Anticoagulants (warfarin, heparin, LMWHs) in combination with NSAIDs can cause increased risk of bleeding.

Antiplatelet drugs (ticlopidine, clopidogrel, aspirin, abciximab, dipyridamole, eptifibatide, tirofiban) can cause an increased risk of bleeding.

Aspirin: Ibuprofen and other COX-1 inhibitors may reduce the cardioprotective effects of aspirin. Avoid giving prior to aspirin therapy or on a regular basis in patients with CAD.

Beta-blockers: NSAIDs may decrease the antihypertensive effect of beta-blockers. Monitor.

Bisphosphonate derivatives: NSAIDs may enhance the adverse/toxic effect of bisphosphonate derivatives. An increased incidence of gastrointestinal ulceration is of concern.

Cholestyramine (and other bile acid sequestrants): May decrease the absorption of NSAIDs. Separate by at least 2 hours.

Corticosteroids: May increase the risk of GI ulceration; avoid concurrent use

Cyclosporine: NSAIDs may increase serum creatinine, potassium, blood pressure, and cyclosporine levels; monitor cyclosporine levels and renal function carefully.

CYP2C9 Substrates: Ibuprofen may increase the levels/effects of CYP2C9 substrates. Example substrates include bosentan, dapsone, fluoxetine, glimepiride, glipizide, losartan, montelukast, nateglinide, paclitaxel, phenytoin, warfarin, and zafirlukast.

Hydralazine's antihypertensive effect is decreased; avoid concurrent use

Lithium levels can be increased; avoid concurrent use if possible or monitor lithium levels and adjust dose. Sulindac may have the least effect. When NSAID is stopped, lithium will need adjustment again.

Loop diuretics efficacy (diuretic and antihypertensive effect) is reduced. Indomethacin reduces this efficacy, however, it may be anticipated with any NSAID.

Methotrexate: Severe bone marrow suppression, aplastic anemia, and GI toxicity have been reported with concomitant NSAID therapy. Avoid use during moderate or high-dose methotrexate (increased and prolonged methotrexate levels). NSAID use during low-dose treatment of rheumatoid arthritis has not been fully evaluated; extreme caution is warranted

Pemetrexed: NSAIDs may decrease the excretion of pemetrexed.

Probenecid: Probenecid may increase the serum concentration of NSAIDs.

Vancomycin: NSAIDs may decrease the excretion of vancomycin; this is of particular concern in preterm infants.

Warfarin's INRs may be increased by piroxicam. Other NSAIDs may have the same effect depending on dose and duration. Monitor INR closely. Use the lowest dose of NSAIDs possible and for the briefest duration. May alter the anticoagulant effects of warfarin; concurrent use with other antiplatelet agents or anticoagulants may increase risk of bleeding.

Pregnancy Risk Factor B/D (3rd trimester)

Lactation Enters breast milk/use caution (AAP rates "compatible")

Additional Information Largest ibuprofen ingestion reported was 72 g in an adult; while hyperkalemia, metabolic acidosis, and rhabdomyolysis was noted, the patient did well with supportive therapy and did not require dialysis

Specific References

Bell EC, Ravis WR, Lloyd KB, Stokes TJ, "Effects of St. John's Wort Supplementation on Ibuprofen" *Pharmacokinetics.*

Bernstein AL and Werlin A, "Pseudodementia Associated with Use of Ibuprofen," *Ann Pharmacother*, 2003, 37(1):80-2.

Clarke SF, Arepalli N, Armstrong C, et al, "Duodenal Perforation After Ibuprofen Overdose," *J Toxicol Clin Toxicol*, 2004, 42(7):983-5.

Desai PR and Sriskandan S, "Hypothermia in a Child Secondary to Ibuprofen," *Arch Dis Child*, 2003, 88(1):87-8.

Eldridge DL and holstege CP, "Massive Ibuprofen Overdose Associated with Electrocardiographic Changes," *Clin Toxicol (Phila)*, 2005, 43:739.

Fosnocht DE, Swanson ER, Donaldson GW, et al, "Pain Medication Use Before ED Arrival," *Am J Emerg Med*, 2003, 21(5):435-7.

Gamulescu MA, Schalke B, Schuierer G, et al, "Optic Neuritis with Visual Field Defect – Possible Ibuprofen-related Toxicity," *Ann Pharmacother*, 2006, 40(3):571-3.

Goddard J, Strachan FE, and Bateman DN, "Urinary Sodium and Potassium Excretion as Measures of Ibuprofen Nephrotoxicity," *J Toxicol Clin Toxicol*, 2003, 41(5):747.

Goldenberg NA, Jacobson L, and Manco-Johnson MJ, "Brief Communication: Duration of Platelet Dysfunction After a 7-day Course of Ibuprofen," *Ann Intern Med*, 2005, 5;142(7):506-9.

Kearney TE, Van Bebber SL, Olson KR, et al, "Validating Send-In Guidelines: Factors Influencing Triage Decisions for Pediatric Ibuprofen Ingestions," *J Toxicol Clin Toxicol*, 2004, 42(5):815.

Lipworth L, Friis S, Blot WJ, et al, "A Population-based Cohort Study of Mortality Among Users of Ibuprofen in Denmark," *Am J Ther*, 2004, 11(3):156-63.

Miksa IR, Cummings MR, and Poppenga RH, "Multi-Residue Determination of Anti-Inflammatory Analgesics in Sera by Liquid Chromatography-Mass Spectrometry," *J Anal Toxicol*, 2005, 29:95-104.

Nguyen HT and Juurlink DN, "Recurrent Ibuprofen-Induced Aseptic Meningitis," *Ann Pharmacother*, 2004, 38(3):408-10.

Re VL 3rd and Gluckman SJ, "Eosinophilic Meningitis," *Am J Med*, 2003, 114(3):217-23.

Smolinske SC and Kaufmann M, "Consumer Perception of Household Hazardous Materials," *Clin Toxicol (Phila)*, 2005, 43:706.

Ibutilide

U.S. Brand Names Corvert®

Synonyms Ibutilide Fumarate

Use Rapid conversion of atrial fibrillation or flutter of recent (<90 days) onset to sinus rhythm

Mechanism of Action A class III antiarrhythmic agent which prolongs action potential in atrium and ventricular myocytes; slow inward sodium current is activated and thus atrial and ventricular action potential refractoriness and duration are prolonged

Adverse Reactions

Cardiovascular: **Torsade de pointes** (1.7%), tachycardia (ventricular) (7.5%), hypotension (orthostatic), syncope, bundle branch block, premature ventricular contractions, atrioventricular block (1.7%), congestive heart failure, myocardial depression, sinus arrest

Central nervous system: Headache

Gastrointestinal: Nausea (2%)

Renal: Renal failure

Signs and Symptoms of Overdose Third degree AV block, torsade de pointes, ventricular ectopy

Pharmacodynamics/Kinetics

Onset of action: ~90 minutes after start of infusion ($^1/_2$ of conversions to sinus rhythm occur during infusion)

Distribution: V_d: 11 L/kg

Protein binding: 40%

Metabolism: Extensively hepatic; oxidation

Half-life elimination: 2-12 hours (average: 6 hours)

Excretion: Urine (82%, 7% as unchanged drug and metabolites); feces (19%)

Dosage

Acute conversion of atrial fibrillation and flutter:

Weight <60 kg: 0.01 mg/kg

Weight >60 kg: 0.1 mg/kg

A second dose may be given 10 minutes after the first infusion if arrhythmia persists

Monitoring Parameters Observe patient with continuous ECG monitoring for at least 4 hours following infusion or until QT_c has returned to baseline; skilled personnel and proper equipment should be available during administration of ibutilide and subsequent monitoring of the patient

Administration May be administered undiluted or diluted in 50 mL diluent (0.9% NS or D_5W); infuse over 10 minutes

Contraindications Hypersensitivity to ibutilide or any component of the formulation; QT_c >440 msec

Warnings [U.S. Boxed Warning]: Potentially fatal arrhythmias (eg, polymorphic ventricular tachycardia) can occur with ibutilide, usually in association with torsade de pointes (QT prolongation).

Studies indicate a 1.7% incidence of arrhythmias in treated patients. The drug should be given in a setting of continuous ECG monitoring and by personnel trained in treating arrhythmias particularly polymorphic ventricular tachycardia. **[U.S. Boxed Warning]: Patients with chronic atrial fibrillation may not be the best candidates for ibutilide since they often revert after conversion and the risks of treatment may not be justified when compared to alternative management.** Dosing adjustments are not required in patients with renal or hepatic dysfunction since a maximum of only two 10-minute infusions are utilized. Drug distribution, rather than administration, are the primary mechanisms responsible for termination of the pharmacologic effect. Use caution in elderly patients. Safety and efficacy in children have not been established. Avoid any drug that can prolong QT interval. Correct hyperkalemia and hypomagnesemia before using. Monitor for heart block.

Dosage Forms Injection, solution, as fumarate: 0.1 mg/mL (10 mL)

Reference Range Peak serum levels after infusion of 0.01 mg/kg: ~10 ng/mL

Overdosage/Treatment Supportive therapy: Polymorphic ventricular tachycardia should be treated with discontinuation of drug, monitoring of potassium and magnesium and correction of electrolyte abnormalities, overdrive pacing, electrical cardioversion, or magnesium sulfate; monitor ECG for at least 4 hours postinfusion

Drug Interactions Antiarrhythmics: Class Ia antiarrhythmic drugs (disopyramide, quinidine, and procainamide) and other class III drugs such as amiodarone and sotalol, should not be given concomitantly with ibutilide due to their potential to prolong refractoriness.

Other drugs which may prolong QT interval: Phenothiazines, tricyclic and tetracyclic antidepressants, and cisapride, sparfloxacin, gatifloxacin, moxifloxacin, erythromycin may increase risk of toxicity; avoid concurrent use.

Digoxin: Signs of digoxin toxicity may be masked when coadministered with ibutilide.

Pregnancy Risk Factor C

Pregnancy Implications Teratogenic in rodents (adactyly, cleft palate, scoliosis)

Lactation Enters breast milk/contraindicated

Additional Information Overall efficacy rate is 43% to 58% (conversion rate of atrial fibrillation ranges from 30% to 51% while conversion rate for atrial flutter ranges from 55% to 76%); termination rate is higher with recent onset of arrhythmia (<30 days); mean time to conversion is 13-21 minutes; patients with atrial arrhythmias over 2- to 3- day duration should be anticoagulated before conversion. Torsade de pointes usually occurs within 30 minutes of infusion but recurrent polymorphic ventricular tachycardia may occur as long as 3 hours postinfusion. Patients with congestive heart failure, bradycardia, prolonged QT interval or hypokalemia are at risk for torsade de pointes.

Specific References

Gowda RM, Khan IA, Punukollu G, et al, "Use of Ibutilide for Cardioversion of Recent-Onset Atrial Fibrillation and Flutter in Elderly," *Am J Ther*, 2004, 11(2):95-7.

Gowda RM, Punukollu G, Khan IA, et al, "Ibutilide for Pharmacological Cardioversion of Atrial Fibrillation and Flutter: Impact of Race on Efficacy and Safety," *Am J Ther*, 2003, 10(4):259-63.

Ifosfamide

CAS Number 3778-73-2

U.S. Brand Names Ifex®

Synonyms Isophosphamide; NSC-109724; Z4942

Use Treatment of lung cancer, Hodgkin's and non-Hodgkin's lymphoma, breast cancer, acute and chronic lymphocytic leukemias, ovarian cancer, sarcomas, pancreatic and gastric carcinomas

Orphan drug: Treatment of testicular cancer

Mechanism of Action Causes cross-linking of strands of DNA by binding with nucleic acids and other intracellular structures; inhibits protein synthesis and DNA synthesis

Adverse Reactions

Cardiovascular: Cardiotoxicity

Central nervous system: Somnolence, confusion, hallucinations in 12% and coma (rare) have occurred and are usually reversible; usually occur with higher doses or in patients with reduced renal function; depressive psychoses, polyneuropathy

Dermatologic: Alopecia occurs in 50% to 83% of patients 2-4 weeks after initiation of therapy; may be as high as 100% in combination therapy; phlebitis, dermatitis, nail ridging, skin hyperpigmentation, impaired wound healing

Endocrine & metabolic: SIADH, metabolic acidosis

Gastrointestinal: Nausea and vomiting in 58% of patients is dose and schedule related (more common with higher doses and after bolus regimens); nausea and vomiting can persist up to 3 days after therapy; also anorexia, diarrhea, constipation, transient increase in liver function test results and stomatitis noted, pancreatitis

Emetic potential: Moderate (58%)

Time course of nausea/vomiting: Onset: 2-3 hours; Duration: 12-72 hours

Genitourinary: Hemorrhagic cystitis has been frequently associated with the use of ifosfamide. A urinalysis prior to each dose should be obtained. **Ifosfamide should never be administered without a uroprotective agent (mesna).** Hematuria has been reported in 6% to 92% of patients.

Hematologic: Myelosuppression: Less of a problem than with cyclophosphamide if used alone. Leukopenia is mild to moderate, thrombocytopenia and anemia are rare. However, myelosuppression can be severe when used with other chemotherapeutic agents or with high-dose therapy. Be cautious with patients with compromised bone marrow reserve. Methemoglobinemia.

WBC: Moderate; Platelets: Mild; Onset (days): 7; Nadir (days): 10-14

Hepatic: Elevated liver enzymes

Renal: Fanconi-like syndrome; renal toxicity occurs in 6% of patients and is manifested as an increase in BUN or serum creatinine and is most likely related to tubular damage. Renal toxicity, including ARF, may occur more frequently with high-dose ifosfamide. Metabolic acidosis may occur in up to 31% of patients.

Respiratory: Nasal congestion, pulmonary fibrosis, pulmonary toxicity

Miscellaneous: Immunosuppression, sterility, possible secondary malignancy, allergic reactions

Signs and Symptoms of Overdose Symptoms of overdose include alopecia, diarrhea, myelosuppression, nausea, vomiting. Direct extension of the drug's pharmacologic effect: Myocardial depression at doses >15 g/m²

Pharmacodynamics/Kinetics

Pharmacokinetics are dose dependent

Distribution: V_d: 5.7-49 L; does penetrate CNS, but not in therapeutic levels

Protein binding: Negligible

Metabolism: Hepatic to active metabolites phosphoramide mustard, acrolein, and inactive dichloroethylated and carboxy metabolites; acrolein is the agent implicated in development of hemorrhagic cystitis

Bioavailability: Estimated at 100%

Half-life elimination: Beta: High dose: 11-15 hours (3800-5000 mg/m²); Lower dose: 4-7 hours (1800 mg/m²)

Time to peak, plasma: Oral: Within 1 hour

Excretion: Urine (15% to 50% as unchanged drug, 41% as metabolites)

Dosage Refer to individual protocols. To prevent bladder toxicity, ifosfamide should be given with the urinary protector mesna and hydration of at least 2 L of oral or I.V. fluid per day. I.V.:

Children:

1200-1800 mg/m²/day for 3-5 days every 21-28 days **or**

5 g/m² once every 21-28 days **or**

3 g/m²/day for 2 days every 21-28 days

Adults:

50 mg/kg/day or 700-2000 mg/m² for 5 days every 3-4 weeks

Alternatives: 2400 mg/m²/day for 3 days or 5000 mg/m² as a single dose every 3-4 weeks

Dosing adjustment in renal impairment:

S_{cr} 2.1-3.0 mg/dL: Reduce dose by 25% to 50%

S_{cr} >3.0 mg/dL: Withhold drug

Dosing adjustment in hepatic impairment: Although no specific guidelines are available, it is possible that adjusted doses are indicated in hepatic disease. Falkson G, et al (*Invest New Drugs*, 1992, 10:337-43) recommended the following dosage adjustments:

AST >300 or bilirubin >3.0 mg/dL: Decrease ifosfamide dose by 75%

Stability Store intact vials at room temperature. Dilute powder with SWI or NS to a concentration of 50 mg/mL. Further dilution in 50-1000 mL D_5W or NS is recommended for I.V. infusion. Reconstituted solutions may be stored under refrigeration for up to 21 days. Solutions diluted for administration are stable for 7 days at room temperature and for 6 weeks under refrigeration.

Monitoring Parameters CBC with differential, hemoglobin, and platelet count, urine output, urinalysis, liver function, and renal function tests

Administration Administer slow I.V. push, IVPB over 30 minutes to several hours or continuous I.V. over 5 days

Contraindications Hypersensitivity to ifosfamide or any component of the formulation; patients with severely depressed bone marrow function; pregnancy

Warnings Hazardous agent – use appropriate precautions for handling and disposal. **[U.S. Boxed Warning]: Urotoxic side effects, primarily hemorrhagic cystitis, may occur.** Hydration and/or mesna administration will protect against hemorrhagic cystitis. **[U.S. Boxed Warning]: Severe bone marrow suppression may occur. May cause CNS toxicity, including confusion and coma;** reversible upon discontinuation of treatment. Use with caution in patients with impaired renal function or those with compromised bone marrow reserve. May interfere with wound healing. **[U.S. Boxed Warning]: Should be administered under the supervision of an experienced cancer chemotherapy physician.** Safety and efficacy in children have not been established.

Dosage Forms

Injection, powder for reconstitution: 1 g

Ifex®: 1 g, 3 g

Overdosage/Treatment Supportive therapy: Ifosfamide neurotoxicity has been successfully treated with methylene blue (1-2 mg/kg in children or 50 mg in 1% aqueous solution administered over 5 minutes in adults). Adequate hydration is also suggested. Congestive heart failure can be treated with diuretics, inotropic and vasodilator agents.

Antidote(s)

- Methylene Blue [ANTIDOTE]

Drug Interactions Substrate of CYP2A6 (minor), 2B6 (minor), 2C8 (minor), 2C9 (minor), 2C19 (minor), 3A4 (major); **Inhibits** CYP3A4 (weak); **Induces** CYP2C8 (weak), 2C9 (weak)

CYP3A4 inducers: CYP3A4 inducers may increase the levels/effects of acrolein (the active metabolite of ifosfamide). Example inducers include aminoglutethimide, carbamazepine, nafcillin, nevirapine, phenobarbital, phenytoin, and rifamycins.

CYP3A4 inhibitors: May decrease the levels/effects of acrolein (the active metabolite of ifosfamide). Example inhibitors include azole antifungals, clarithromycin, diclofenac, doxycycline, erythromycin, imatinib, isoniazid, nefazodone, nicardipine, propofol, protease inhibitors, quinidine, telithromycin, and verapamil.

Pregnancy Risk Factor D

Lactation Enters breast milk/contraindicated

Nursing Implications Mesna to be used concomitantly for prophylaxis against hemorrhagic cystitis

Additional Information Development of ifosfamide neurotoxicity appears to be related to low serum albumin (<3 g/dL), dehydration, extremes of age, renal dysfunction, and previous therapy with cis-platinum. Encephalopathy occurs in 9% of patients receiving doses of 5 g/m².

Specific References

Kilickap S, Cakar M, Onal IK, et al, "Nonconvulsive Status Epilepticus Due to Ifosfamide," *Ann Pharmacother*, 2006, 40(2):332-5.

Imipenem and Cilastatin

Related Information

- Meropenem

CAS Number 64221-86-9; 74431-23-5; 81129-83-1; 82009-34-5

U.S. Brand Names Primaxin®

Synonyms Imipemide

Use Treatment of documented multidrug-resistant gram-negative infection due to organisms proven or suspected to be susceptible to imipenem/cilastatin; treatment of multiple organism infection in which other agents have an insufficient spectrum of activity or are contraindicated due to toxic potential; imipenem is usually given with a dehydropeptidase I inhibitor cilastatin sodium which inhibits renal breakdown of imipenem

Mechanism of Action Inhibits bacterial cell wall synthesis by binding to one or more of the penicillin binding proteins (PBPs); which in turn inhibits the final transpeptidation step of peptidoglycan synthesis in bacterial cell walls, thus inhibiting cell wall biosynthesis. Bacteria eventually lyse due to ongoing activity of cell wall autolytic enzymes (autolysins and murein hydrolases) while cell wall assembly is arrested.

Adverse Reactions

Cardiovascular: Hypotension, palpitations, tachycardia, sinus tachycardia

Central nervous system: Seizures, dizziness, confusion

Dermatologic: Rash, pruritus, urticaria

Gastrointestinal: Nausea, diarrhea, vomiting, pseudomembranous colitis, dental staining

Hematologic: Neutropenia, eosinophilia, thrombocytosis, aplastic anemia, leukopenia

Hepatic: Hepatotoxicity

Local: Phlebitis, pain at injection site

Neuromuscular & skeletal: Myasthenia gravis may worsen

Miscellaneous: Emergence of resistant strains of *P. aeruginosa*, anaphylactic reaction

Signs and Symptoms of Overdose Myasthenia gravis (exacerbation or precipitation), seizures, tremors

Pharmacodynamics/Kinetics

Absorption: I.M.: Imipenem: 60% to 75%; cilastatin: 95% to 100%

Distribution: Rapidly and widely to most tissues and fluids including sputum, pleural fluid, peritoneal fluid, interstitial fluid, bile, aqueous humor, reproductive organs, and bone; highest concentrations in pleural fluid, interstitial fluid, peritoneal fluid, and reproductive organs; low concentrations in CSF; crosses placenta; enters breast milk

Protein binding: Imipenem: 20%; cilastatin: 40%

Metabolism: Renally by dehydropeptidase; activity is blocked by cilastatin; cilastatin is partially metabolized renally

Half-life elimination: I.V.: Both drugs: 60 minutes; prolonged with renal impairment; I.M.: Imipenem: 2-3 hours

Time to peak: I.M.: 3.5 hours

Excretion: Both drugs: Urine (~70% as unchanged drug)

Dosage

I.V. infusion (dosage recommendation based on imipenem component):

Children: 25 mg/kg every 6 hours

Adults: 1-4 g/day not to exceed 50 mg/kg/day; reduce dose in renal failure; usually given twice daily

Stability Stable for 10 hours at room temperature following reconstitution with 100 mL of 0.9% sodium chloride injection; up to 48 hours when refrigerated at 5°C. If reconstituted with 5% or 10% dextrose injection, 5% dextrose and sodium bicarbonate, 5% dextrose and 0.9% sodium chloride, is stable for 4 hours at room temperature and 24 hours when refrigerated.

Monitoring Parameters Periodic renal, hepatic, and hematologic function tests; monitor for signs of anaphylaxis during first dose

Administration

I.M.: **Note:** I.M. administration is not intended for severe or life-threatening infections (eg, septicemia, endocarditis, shock). Administer by deep injection into a large muscle (gluteal or lateral thigh). **Only the I.M. formulation can be used for I.M. administration.**

I.V.: Do not administer I.V. push. Infuse doses ≤500 mg over 20-30 minutes; infuse doses ≥750 mg over 40-60 minutes. **Only the I.V. formulation can be used for I.V. administration.**

Contraindications Hypersensitivity to imipenem/cilastatin or any component of the formulation

Warnings Dosage adjustment required in patients with impaired renal function; elderly patients often require lower doses (adjust carefully to renal function); Prolonged use may result in superinfection, including pseudomembranous colitis. Has been associated with CNS adverse effects, including confusional states and seizures; use with caution in patients with a history of seizures or hypersensitivity to beta-lactams (including penicillins and cephalosporins); patients with impaired renal function are at increased risk of seizures if not properly dose adjusted. Not recommended in pediatric CNS infections due to seizure potential. Serious hypersensitivity reactions, including anaphylaxis, have been reported (some without a history of previous allergic reactions to beta-lactams). Doses for I.M. administration are mixed with lidocaine, consult information on lidocaine for associated warnings/precautions. Two different imipenem/cilastatin products are available; due to differences in formulation, the I.V. and I.M. preparations **cannot** be interchanged. Safety and efficacy of I.M. administration in children <12 years have not been established.

Dosage Forms

Injection, powder for reconstitution [I.M.]: Imipenem 500 mg and cilastatin 500 mg [contains sodium 32 mg (1.4 mEq)]

Injection, powder for reconstitution [I.V.]: Imipenem 250 mg and cilastatin 250 mg [contains sodium 18.8 mg (0.8 mEq)]; imipenem 500 mg and cilastatin 500 mg [contains sodium 37.5 mg (1.6 mEq)]

Reference Range Peak plasma imipenem concentration following a 500 mg I.V. dose of imipenem/cilastatin: ~40-50 mcg/mL

Overdosage/Treatment

Supportive therapy: Diazepam or phenytoin may be useful for treatment of seizures; fentanyl (100 mcg in adults) has been used with diazepam (5 mg) to treat tremors and seizures

Enhancement of elimination: Hemodialysis is particularly useful to increase clearance of imipenem and cilastatin; ~73% of imipenem and 82% of cilastatin are cleared by a 4-hour dialysis; peritoneal dialysis is not useful in enhancing elimination

Test Interactions Interferes with urinary glucose determination using Clinitest®; can cause false elevations of amylase and lipase

Drug Interactions

Cyclosporine: May increase neurotoxicity of imipenem; conversely, imipenem may increase the serum levels/effects of cyclosporine; monitor.

Ganciclovir: May increase the risk of seizures; concomitant use not recommended.

Typhoid vaccine: Concomitant antibiotics may decrease the effectiveness of live, attenuated Ty21a typhoid vaccine; delay vaccination for >24 hours after administration of antibiotic.

Uricosuric agents: May increase the levels/effects imipenem; monitor.

Valproic acid: Imipenem may decrease valproic acid concentrations to subtherapeutic levels; monitor.

Pregnancy Risk Factor C

Pregnancy Implications Teratogenic effects were not observed in animal studies; however, maternal toxicity was noted. There are no well-controlled or adequate studies in pregnant women. Use during pregnancy only if the potential benefits outweigh the potential risks to mother and fetus.

Lactation Excretion in breast milk unknown/use caution

Nursing Implications Not for direct infusion; vial contents must be transferred to 100 mL of infusion solution; final concentration should not exceed 5 mg/mL; infuse over 30-60 minutes; watch for seizures; do not mix with or physically add to other antibiotics; however, may administer concomitantly

Additional Information

Seizure frequency is ~1.5% to 2% and usually occurs ~7 days after initiation of therapy; risk factors include brain lesions, epilepsy or previous seizure disorder, and renal insufficiency; the mechanism of action for seizures may be due to binding of imipenem to gamma-aminobutyric acid (GABA) receptors in the central nervous system

Sodium content of 1 g injection: I.M.: 64.4 mg (2.8 mEq); I.V.: 73.6 mg (3.2 mEq)

Imipramine

Related Information

- Anticholinergic Effects of Common Psychotropics
- Antidepressant Agents
- Dibenzepin
- Therapeutic Drugs Associated with Hallucinations

CAS Number 10075-24-8; 113-52-0; 50-49-7

U.S. Brand Names Tofranil-PM®; Tofranil®

Synonyms Imipramine Hydrochloride; Imipramine Pamoate

Use Treatment of various forms of depression, often in conjunction with psychotherapy; enuresis in children

Unlabeled/Investigational Use Analgesic for certain chronic and neuropathic pain; panic disorder; attention-deficit/hyperactivity disorder (ADHD)

Mechanism of Action Increases the synaptic concentration of serotonin, norepinephrine, and/or dopamine in the central nervous system by inhibition of their reuptake by the presynaptic neuronal membrane; peripheral alpha-receptor blockade may be the cause of hypotension (orthostatic).

Adverse Reactions

Cardiovascular: Cardiac arrhythmias, cardiomyopathy; hypotension has been associated with falls; hypotension (orthostatic), cardiomegaly, myocarditis, tachycardia (supraventricular), torsade de pointes, vasoconstriction, vasculitis, exacerbation of Brugada syndrome

Central nervous system: **Drowsiness**, **headache**, sedation, confusion, **dizziness**, psychosis, restlessness, fatigue, anxiety, nervousness, sleep disorders, seizures, delirium, hyperthermia, visual hallucinations, paranoia, extrapyramidal reactions

Dermatologic: Rash, photosensitivity, exfoliative dermatitis, angioedema, urticaria, purpura, pruritus, bullous eruptions, licheniform eruptions, exanthem, photoallergic reaction

Endocrine & metabolic: Syndrome of inappropriate antidiuretic hormone, gynecomastia

Gastrointestinal: **Nausea**, vomiting, **constipation, xerostomia**, Ogilvie's syndrome, **increased appetite, weight gain, unpleasant taste**, stomatitis, lingua villosa nigra

Genitourinary: **Urinary retention**

Hematologic: Blood dyscrasias

Hepatic: Hepatitis, liver failure, liver necrosis, cholestasis

Neuromuscular & skeletal: Clonus, myoclonus, **weakness**, paresthesia

Ocular: Blurred vision, photophobia, diplopia, intraocular pressure (increased), mydriasis

Respiratory: Pulmonary edema, eosinophilic pneumonia

Miscellaneous: Hypersensitivity reactions, systemic lupus erythematosus (SLE), fixed drug eruption

Signs and Symptoms of Overdose Agranulocytosis, alopecia, ataxia, cardiac arrhythmias, colitis, coma (mean duration: 6 hours), conduction defects, confusion, constipation, cyanosis, dementia, dental erosion, depression, disorientation, ejaculatory disturbances, eosinophilia, galactorrhea, granulocytopenia, hallucinations, hyperthyroidism, hypoglycemia, hyponatremia, hypotension, impotence, increased intraocular pressure, jaundice, lactation, leukopenia, mania, myasthenia gravis (exacerbation or precipitation), myoclonus, neutropenia, nystagmus, ototoxicity, pulmonary edema, QT prolongation, respiratory depression, seizures (within 3 hours of ingestion), tachycardia (sinus), tinnitus; QRS prolongation (with rightward terminal 40 millisecond frontal plane of QRS vector)

Admission Criteria/Prognosis Admit any symptomatic patient (including persistent tachycardia) following 6 hours of ER observation; admit any pediatric ingestion >5 mg/kg

Pharmacodynamics/Kinetics

Onset of action: Peak antidepressant effect: Usually after ≥2 weeks

Absorption: Well absorbed

Distribution: Crosses placenta

Metabolism: Hepatic via CYP to desipramine (active) and other metabolites; significant first-pass effect

Half-life elimination: 6-18 hours

Excretion: Urine (as metabolites)

Dosage Maximum antidepressant effect may not be seen for 2 or more weeks after initiation of therapy

Children: Oral:

Depression: 1.5 mg/kg/day with dosage increments of 1 mg/kg every 3-4 days to a maximum dose of 5 mg/kg/day in 1-4 divided doses; monitor carefully especially with doses ≥3.5 mg/kg/day

Enuresis: ≥6 years: Initial: 10-25 mg at bedtime, if inadequate response still seen after 1 week of therapy, increase by 25 mg/day; dose should not exceed 2.5 mg/kg/day or 50 mg at bedtime if 6-12 years of age or 75 mg at bedtime if ≥12 years of age

Adjunct in the treatment of cancer pain: Initial: 0.2-0.4 mg/kg at bedtime; dose may be increased by 50% every 2-3 days up to 1-3 mg/kg/dose at bedtime

Adolescents: Oral: Initial: 25-50 mg/day; increase gradually; maximum: 100 mg/day in single or divided doses

Adults:

Oral: Initial: 25 mg 3-4 times/day, increase dose gradually, total dose may be given at bedtime; maximum: 300 mg/day

I.M.: Initial: Up to 100 mg/day in divided doses; change to oral as soon as possible

Stability Solutions stable at a pH of 4-5; turns yellowish or reddish on exposure to light. Slight discoloration does not affect potency; marked discoloration is associated with loss of potency. Capsules stable for 3 years following date of manufacture.

Monitoring Parameters Monitor blood pressure and pulse rate prior to and during initial therapy; ECG in older adults; evaluate mental status; blood levels are useful for therapeutic monitoring

Contraindications Hypersensitivity to imipramine (cross-reactivity with other dibenzodiazepines may occur) or any component of the formulation; concurrent use of MAO inhibitors (within 14 days); in a patient during acute recovery phase of MI; pregnancy

Warnings[U.S. Boxed Warning]: Antidepressants increase the risk of suicidal thinking and behavior in children and adolescents with major depressive disorder (MDD) and other depressive disorders; consider risk prior to prescribing. Closely monitor for clinical worsening, suicidality, or unusual changes in behavior; the child's family or caregiver should be instructed to closely observe the patient and communicate condition with healthcare provider. Such observation would generally include at least weekly face-to-face contact with patients or their family members or caregivers during the first 4 weeks of treatment, then every other week visits for the next 4 weeks, then at 12 weeks, and as clinically indicated beyond 12 weeks. Additional contact by telephone may be appropriate between face-to-face visits. Adults treated with antidepressants should be observed similarly for clinical worsening and suicidality, especially during the initial few months of a course of drug therapy, or at times of dose changes, either increases or decreases. A medication guide should be dispensed with each prescription. **Imipramine is FDA approved for the treatment of nocturnal enuresis in children ≥6 years of age.**

The possibility of a suicide attempt is inherent in major depression and may persist until remission occurs. Monitor for worsening of depression or suicidality, especially during initiation of therapy or with dose increases or decreases. Worsening depression and severe abrupt suicidality that are not part of the presenting symptoms may require discontinuation or modification of drug therapy. Use caution in high-risk patients during initiation of therapy. Prescriptions should be written for the smallest quantity consistent with good patient care. The patient's family or caregiver should be alerted to monitor patients for the emergence of suicidality and associated behaviors such as anxiety, agitation, panic attacks, insomnia, irritability, hostility, impulsivity, akathisia, hypomania, and mania; patients should be instructed to notify their healthcare provider if any of these symptoms or worsening depression occur. May worsen psychosis in some patients or precipitate a shift to mania or hypomania in patients with bipolar disorder. Monotherapy in patients with bipolar disorder should be avoided. Patients presenting with depressive symptoms should be screened for bipolar disorder. **Imipramine is not FDA approved for the treatment of bipolar depression.**

May cause sedation, resulting in impaired performance of tasks requiring alertness (eg, operating machinery or driving). Sedative effects may be additive with other CNS depressants and/or ethanol. The degree of sedation is high relative to other antidepressants. May increase the risks associated with electroconvulsive therapy. Consider discontinuing, when possible, prior to elective surgery. Therapy should not be abruptly discontinued in patients receiving high doses for prolonged periods.

May cause orthostatic hypotension (risk is very high relative to other antidepressants) - use with caution in patients at risk of hypotension or in patients where transient hypotensive episodes would be poorly tolerated (cardiovascular disease or cerebrovascular disease). The degree of anticholinergic blockade produced by this agent is high relative to other cyclic antidepressants - use caution in patients with urinary retention, benign prostatic hyperplasia, narrow-angle glaucoma, xerostomia, visual problems, constipation, or history of bowel obstruction.

Use with caution in patients with a history of cardiovascular disease (including previous MI, stroke, tachycardia, or conduction abnormalities). The risk of conduction abnormalities with this agent is high relative to other antidepressants. ECG monitoring is recommended if high dosages are used. Use caution in patients with a previous seizure disorder or condition predisposing to seizures such as brain damage, alcoholism, or concurrent therapy with other drugs which lower the seizure threshold. Use with caution in hyperthyroid patients or those receiving thyroid supplementation. Use with caution in patients with hepatic or renal dysfunction and in elderly patients. Has been associated with photosensitization.

Dosage Forms

Capsule, as pamoate (Tofranil-PM®): 75 mg, 100 mg, 125 mg, 150 mg

Tablet, as hydrochloride (Tofranil®): 10 mg, 25 mg, 50 mg [generic tablets may contain sodium benzoate]

Reference Range

Therapeutic:

Imipramine and desipramine 150-250 ng/mL (SI: 530-890 nmol/L)

Desipramine 150-300 ng/mL (SI: 560-1125 nmol/L)

Metabolism may be impaired in elderly patients; toxic: >300 ng/mL (SI: >1070 nmol/L); serious symptoms are associated with levels >1000 ng/mL (SI: >3566 nmol/L)

In the postmortem state, anatomical site concentration differences (ie, postmortem redistribution) may occur.

Overdosage/Treatment

Decontamination: **Do not** induce emesis; lavage within 2-3 hours/ activated charcoal; multiple dosing of activated charcoal would be expected to be useful

Supportive therapy: Following initiation of essential overdose management, toxic symptoms should be treated. Ventricular arrhythmias and ventricular conduction defects often respond to concurrent systemic alkalinization (sodium bicarbonate 0.5-2 mEq/kg I.V.). Titrate to a serum pH of 7.45-7.55. Arrhythmias unresponsive to this therapy may respond to lidocaine 1 mg/kg I.V. followed by a titrated infusion. Phenytoin is also useful in treating ventricular dysrhythmias (15 mg/kg up to 1 g I.V.). Physostigmine (1-2 mg I.V. slowly for adults or 0.5 mg I.V. slowly for children) may be indicated for seizures or movement disorders but only as **a last resort**. Propranolol may also be utilized for supraventricular arrhythmias (rate: >160) at 1 mg/minute to a maximum of 5 mg in adults; pediatric dosage of 0.1 mg/kg/dose to 1 mg I.V.. Seizures usually respond to lorazepam or diazepam I.V. boluses (5-10 mg for adults up to 30 mg or 0.25-0.4 mg/kg/dose for children up to 10 mg/ dose). If seizures are unresponsive or recur, phenytoin or phenobarbital may be required. Patients must be monitored for at least 24 hours if any signs or symptoms are exhibited. Dobutamine is preferred over dopamine for hypotension, although there is conflicting animal data. Norepinephrine appears effective in treating hypotension; glucagon (10 mg I.V.) can be given to treat hypotension. Flumazenil is contraindicated; magnesium has potentiated adverse cardiac effects (ie, asystole, decreased left ventricular pressure) in an animal model, although it was used successfully in treating refractory ventricular fibrillation at a dose of 20 nmol I.V. (a total of 2 doses). For treatment of lingua villosa nigra, discontinue causative agent. Clean the tongue with a toothbrush and rinse mouth with a half-strength solution of hydrogen peroxide or 10% carbamide peroxide. Oral symptoms should subside in a few days.

TCA ovine antibody fragments (TCA Fab, Protherics Inc) have been developed and used investigationally at a dose of 1-2 g over 30 minutes I.V.; if QRS was >100 msec or terminal deflection of QRS in lead aVR was >3 mm, a second dose (2 g over 30 min or 4 g over 1 hour) was given. If no response, a third infusion (4 g over 60 minutes or 8 g over 2 hours) was given.

Antidote(s)

• Sodium Bicarbonate [ANTIDOTE]

Test Interactions Increases glucose, increases plasma norepinephrine levels and plasma epinephrine levels threefold to fivefold; EMIT assays may be false-positive in the presence of diphenhydramine, thioridazine, chlorpromazine, alimenazine, carbamazepine, cyclobenzaprine, or perphenazine

Drug Interactions Substrate of CYP1A2 (minor), 2B6 (minor), 2C19 (major), 2D6 (major), 3A4 (minor); **Inhibits** CYP1A2 (weak), 2C19 (weak), 2D6 (moderate), 2E1 (weak)

Altretamine: Concurrent use may cause orthostatic hypertension

Amphetamines: TCAs may enhance the effect of amphetamines; monitor for adverse CV effects

Anticholinergics: Combined use with TCAs may produce additive anticholinergic effects

Antihypertensives: TCAs may inhibit the antihypertensive response to bethanidine, clonidine, debrisoquin, guanadrel, guanethidine, guanabenz, guanfacine; monitor BP; consider alternate antihypertensive agent

Beta-agonists: When combined with TCAs may predispose patients to cardiac arrhythmias

Bupropion: May increase the levels of tricyclic antidepressants; based on limited information; monitor response

Carbamazepine: Tricyclic antidepressants may increase carbamazepine levels; monitor

Cholestyramine and colestipol: May bind TCAs and reduce their absorption; monitor for altered response

Clonidine: Abrupt discontinuation of clonidine may cause hypertensive crisis, amitriptyline may enhance the response

CNS depressants: Amitriptyline may be additive with or may potentiate sedation; sedative effects may be additive with TCAs; monitor for increased effect; includes benzodiazepines, barbiturates, antipsychotics, ethanol, and other sedative medications

CYP2C19 inducers: May decrease the levels/effects of imipramine. Example inducers include aminoglutethimide, carbamazepine, phenytoin, and rifampin.

CYP2C19 inhibitors: May increase the levels/effects of imipramine. Example inhibitors include delavirdine, fluconazole, fluvoxamine, gemfibrozil, isoniazid, omeprazole, and ticlopidine.

CYP2D6 inhibitors: May increase the levels/effects of imipramine. Example inhibitors include chlorpromazine, delavirdine, fluoxetine, miconazole, paroxetine, pergolide, quinidine, quinine, ritonavir, and ropinirole.

Epinephrine (and other direct alpha-agonists): The pressor response to I.V. epinephrine, norepinephrine, and phenylephrine may be enhanced in patients receiving TCAs; this combination is best avoided

Fenfluramine: May increase tricyclic antidepressant levels/effects

Hypoglycemic agents (including insulin): TCAs may enhance the hypoglycemic effects of tolazamide, chlorpropamide, or insulin; monitor for changes in blood glucose levels; reported with chlorpropamide, tolazamide, and insulin

Levodopa: Tricyclic antidepressants may decrease the absorption (bioavailability) of levodopa; rare hypertensive episodes have also been attributed to this combination

Linezolid: Hyperpyrexia, hypertension, tachycardia, confusion, seizures, and **deaths have been reported** with agents which inhibit MAO (serotonin syndrome); this combination should be avoided

Lithium: Concurrent use with a TCA may increase the risk for neurotoxicity

MAO inhibitors: Hyperpyrexia, hypertension, tachycardia, confusion, seizures, and **deaths have been reported** (serotonin syndrome); this combination should be avoided

Methylphenidate: Metabolism of TCAs may be decreased

Phenothiazines: Serum concentrations of some TCAs may be increased; in addition, TCAs may increase concentration of phenothiazines; monitor for altered clinical response

QT_c-prolonging agents: Concurrent use of tricyclic agents with other drugs which may prolong QT_c interval may increase the risk of potentially fatal arrhythmias; includes type Ia and type III antiarrhythmics agents, selected quinolones (sparfloxacin, gatifloxacin, moxifloxacin, grepafloxacin), cisapride, and other agents

Ritonavir: Combined use of high-dose tricyclic antidepressants with ritonavir may cause serotonin syndrome in HIV-positive patients; monitor

Sucralfate: Absorption of tricyclic antidepressants may be reduced with coadministration

Sympathomimetics, indirect-acting: Tricyclic antidepressants may result in a decreased sensitivity to indirect-acting sympathomimetics; includes dopamine and ephedrine; also see interaction with epinephrine (and direct-acting sympathomimetics)

Tramadol: Tramadol's risk of seizures may be increased with TCAs

Valproic acid: May increase serum concentrations/adverse effects of some tricyclic antidepressants

Warfarin (and other oral anticoagulants): TCAs may increase the anticoagulant effect in patients stabilized on warfarin; monitor INR

Pregnancy Risk Factor D

Pregnancy Implications Has been known to cause neonatal withdrawal consisting of tachypnea, restlessness, and insomnia; crosses the placenta

Lactation Enters breast milk/not recommended (AAP rates "of concern")

Nursing Implications May increase appetite

Additional Information Imipramine hydrochloride: Tofranil®, Janimine® Imipramine Pamoate: Tofranil-PM®; monoclonal anti-imipramine antibodies are investigational

Hypericum extract ZE, 250 mg twice daily, appears to be as effective as imipramine, 75 mg twice daily, for treatment of mild to moderate depression for 6 weeks.

Specific References

Heard K, Dart RC, Bogdan G, et al, "A Preliminary Study of Tricyclic Antidepressant (TCA) Ovine FAB for TCA Toxicity," *J Toxicol Clin Toxicol*, 2006, 44:275-81.

Nykamp DL, Blackmon CL, Schmidt PE, et al, "QTc Prolongation Associated with Combination Therapy of Levofloxacin, Imipramine, and Fluoxetine," *Ann Pharmacother*. 2005, 39(3):543-6.

Inamrinone

CAS Number 60719-84-8

Synonyms Amrinone Lactate

Use Treatment of low cardiac output states (sepsis, congestive heart failure); adjunctive therapy of pulmonary hypertension; normally prescribed for patients who have not responded well to therapy with digitalis, diuretics, and vasodilators; effective for calcium channel blocker toxicity

Mechanism of Action Inhibits myocardial cyclic adenosine monophosphate (cAMP) phosphodiesterase activity and increases cellular levels of cAMP resulting in a positive inotropic effect; also possesses systemic and pulmonary vasodilator effects

Adverse Reactions

Cardiovascular: Hypotension, ventricular and arrhythmias (supraventricular); may be related to infusion rate, angina, tachycardia (sinus); tachycardia (supraventricular)

Central nervous system: Headache, fever, mania

Dermatologic: Yellow fingernail discoloration

Endocrine & metabolic: Nephrogenic diabetes insipidus

Gastrointestinal: Nausea, vomiting, abdominal pain, anorexia, hypogeusia, splenomegaly, stomatitis, altered taste

Hematologic: Thrombocytopenia

Hepatic: Hepatotoxicity: Discontinue inamrinone if significant elevation in liver enzymes (serum lactic dehydrogenase or glutamic oxaloacetic transaminase) with symptoms of idiosyncratic hypersensitivity reaction (eg, eosinophilia) occurs

Neuromuscular & skeletal: Myalgia

Renal: Diuresis

Respiratory: Hyposmia

Signs and Symptoms of Overdose
Chest pain, diabetes insipidus, hyperthermia, hypotension, lightheadedness, myalgia, tachycardia

Pharmacodynamics/Kinetics

Onset of action: I.V.: 2-5 minutes

  Peak effect: ~10 minutes

Duration (dose dependent): Low dose: ~30 minutes; Higher doses: ~2 hours

Half-life elimination, serum: Adults: Healthy volunteers: 3.6 hours, Congestive heart failure: 5.8 hours

Dosage

Dosage is based on clinical response. **Note:** Dose should not exceed 10 mg/kg/24 hours

Neonates: 0.75 mg/kg I.V. bolus over 2-3 minutes followed by maintenance infusion 3-5 mcg/kg/minute; I.V. bolus may need to be repeated in 30 minutes

Children and Adults: 0.75 mg/kg I.V. bolus over 2-3 minutes followed by maintenance infusion 5-10 mcg/kg/minute; I.V. bolus may need to be repeated in 30 minutes

Dosing adjustment in renal failure: Cl_{cr} <10 mL/minute: Administer 50% to 75% of dose

Stability
May be administered undiluted for I.V. bolus doses. For continuous infusion: Dilute with 0.45% or 0.9% sodium chloride to final concentration of 1-3 mg/mL; use within 24 hours; do not directly dilute with dextrose-containing solutions, chemical interaction occurs; may be administered I.V. into running dextrose infusions. Furosemide forms a precipitate when injected in I.V. lines containing amrinone.

Monitoring Parameters
Cardiac index, stroke volume, systemic vascular resistance, and pulmonary vascular resistance (if Swan-Ganz catheter available); CVP, SBP, DBP, heart rate; platelet count, CBC, liver function and renal function tests

Administration
Should be administered solely via an I.V. pump

Contraindications
Hypersensitivity to inamrinone, any component of the formulation, or bisulfites (contains sodium metabisulfite); patients with severe aortic or pulmonic valvular disease

Warnings
Due to a slight effect on AV conduction, may increase ventricular response rate in atrial fibrillation/atrial flutter; prior treatment with digoxin is recommended. Monitor liver function. Discontinue therapy if alteration in LFTs and clinical symptoms of hepatotoxicity occur. Observe for arrhythmias in this very high-risk patient population. Not recommended in acute MI treatment. Monitor fluid status closely; patients may require adjustment of diuretic and electrolyte replacement therapy. Can cause thrombocytopenia (dose dependent). Correct hypokalemia before initiating therapy. Increase risk of hospitalization and death with long-term therapy.

Dosage Forms
Injection, solution, as lactate: 5 mg/mL (20 mL) [contains sodium metabisulfite]

Reference Range
Therapeutic range: 2-7 mcg/mL (serum) serum level of 75.9 mcg/mL correlated with dose of 180-198 mcg/kg/minute refractory hypotension and death

Overdosage/Treatment
Supportive therapy: There is no specific antidote for inamrinone intoxication. Overdosage with inamrinone has caused severe hypotension by vasodilation; if this occurs, general measures for circulatory support should be taken (isotonic saline, dopamine)

Test Interactions
↓ potassium

Drug Interactions
Furosemide: A precipitate forms on admixture with inamrinone.

Diuretics may cause significant hypovolemia and decrease filling pressure.

Digitalis: Inotropic effects are additive.

Pregnancy Risk Factor
C

Nursing Implications
Patients should be carefully monitored for hemodynamic response (hypotension) and potential adverse effects (ie, thrombocytopenia, hepatitis, and GI effects)

Additional Information
To avoid confusion with amiodarone, the generic name "amrinone" was changed to "inamrinone" in July, 2000. Normally prescribed for patients who have not responded well to therapy with digitalis, diuretics, and vasodilators

Indapamide

CAS Number 26807-65-8

U.S. Brand Names Lozol®

Use Hypertension; edema due to congestive heart failure, renal calculi due to hypercalciuria, Raynaud's disease

Mechanism of Action Similar diuretic action as with thiazide diuretics with additional action on blood vessels resulting in decreased peripheral vascular resistance (possibly due to a calcium channel blocking effect)

Adverse Reactions

Cardiovascular: Hypotension (orthostatic), palpitations, vasculitis

Central nervous system: Vertigo, headache

Dermatologic: Hives, pruritus, epidermal necrolysis, erythema multiforme, angioedema, Stevens-Johnson syndrome, exanthem

Endocrine & metabolic: **Hypokalemia** (12% on 2.5 mg/day, 27% on 5 mg/day), uric acid levels (increased), hypochloremia, hyponatremia (rare), toxic epidermal necrolysis, hypercalcemia

Gastrointestinal: Nausea, vomiting, constipation, anorexia, xerostomia, pancreatitis

Genitourinary: Nocturia, impotence

Hepatic: Hepatotoxicity (cirrhosis)

Neuromuscular & skeletal: Paresthesias

Renal: Azotemia, interstitial nephritis

Respiratory: Rhinorrhea

Miscellaneous: Fixed drug eruption

Pharmacodynamics/Kinetics

Onset of action: 1-2 hours

Duration: ≤36 hours

Absorption: Complete

Protein binding, plasma: 71% to 79%

Metabolism: Extensively hepatic

Half-life elimination: 14-18 hours

Time to peak: 2-2.5 hours

Excretion: Urine (~60%) within 48 hours; feces (~16% to 23%)

Dosage
Oral: 2.5-5 mg once daily

Monitoring Parameters
Blood pressure (both standing and sitting/supine), serum electrolytes, renal function, assess weight, I & O reports daily to determine fluid loss

Administration
May be taken with food or milk. Administer early in day to avoid nocturia. Administer the last dose of multiple doses no later than 6 PM unless instructed otherwise.

Contraindications
Hypersensitivity to indapamide or any component of the formulation, thiazides, or sulfonamide-derived drugs; anuria; renal decompensation; pregnancy (based on expert analysis)

Warnings
Use with caution in severe renal disease. Electrolyte disturbances (hypokalemia, hypochloremic alkalosis, hyponatremia) can occur. Use with caution in severe hepatic dysfunction; hepatic encephalopathy can be caused by electrolyte disturbances. Gout can be precipitate in certain patients with a history of gout, a familial predisposition to gout, or chronic renal failure. Cautious use in diabetics; may see a change in glucose control. I.V. use is generally not recommended (but is available). Hypersensitivity reactions can occur. Can cause SLE exacerbation or activation. Use with caution in patients with moderate or high cholesterol concentrations. Photosensitization may occur. Correct hypokalemia before initiating therapy.

Chemical similarities are present among sulfonamides, sulfonylureas, carbonic anhydrase inhibitors, thiazides, and loop diuretics (except ethacrynic acid). Use in patients with thiazide or sulfonamide allergy is specifically contraindicated in product labeling, however, a risk of cross-reaction exists in patients with allergy to any of these compounds; avoid use when previous reaction has been severe.

Dosage Forms

Tablet: 1.25 mg, 2.5 mg

  Lozol®: 1.25 mg

Reference Range
After a 5 mg oral dose, peak serum indapamide levels of 221 ng/mL are achieved (after 3 hours)

Overdosage/Treatment

Decontamination: Activated charcoal

Supportive therapy: I.V. hydration with 0.9% saline and electrolyte replacement

Enhancement of elimination: Hemodialysis may be effective; not dialyzable

Drug Interactions

ACE inhibitors: Increased hypotension if aggressively diuresed with a thiazide diuretic.

Beta-blockers increase hyperglycemic effects in type 2 diabetes mellitus (noninsulin dependent, NIDDM)

Cyclosporine and thiazides can increase the risk of gout or renal toxicity; avoid concurrent use.

Digoxin toxicity can be exacerbated if a thiazide induces hypokalemia or hypomagnesemia.

Lithium toxicity can occur by reducing renal excretion of lithium; monitor lithium concentration and adjust as needed.

Neuromuscular blocking agents can prolong blockade; monitor serum potassium and neuromuscular status.

NSAIDs can decrease the efficacy of thiazides reducing the diuretic and antihypertensive effects.

Pregnancy Risk Factor B (manufacturer); D (expert analysis)

Lactation Excretion in breast milk unknown

Indinavir

U.S. Brand Names Crixivan®

Synonyms Indinavir Sulfate

Use Treatment of HIV infection; should always be used as part of a multidrug regimen (at least three antiretroviral agents)

Mechanism of Action Indinavir is a human immunodeficiency virus protease inhibitor, binding to the protease activity site and inhibiting the activity of this enzyme. HIV protease is an enzyme required for the cleavage of viral polyprotein precursors into individual functional proteins found in infectious HIV. Inhibition prevents cleavage of these polyproteins resulting in the formation of immature noninfectious viral particles.

Adverse Reactions

Protease inhibitors cause dyslipidemia which includes elevated cholesterol and triglycerides and a redistribution of body fat centrally to cause "protease paunch", buffalo hump, facial atrophy, and breast enlargement. These agents also cause hyperglycemia (exacerbation or new-onset diabetes).

Cardiovascular: Myocardial infarction

Central nervous system: Headache, insomnia, malaise, dizziness, somnolence, depression, fever

Dermatologic: Urticaria, alopecia, erythema multiforme, Stevens-Johnson syndrome

Endocrine & metabolic: Increased serum cholesterol, hyperglycemia, new-onset diabetes

Gastrointestinal: **Nausea**, abdominal pain, diarrhea/vomiting, taste perversion, anorexia, pancreatitis

Genitourinary: Leukocyturia (severe and asymptomatic)

Hematologic: Decreased hemoglobin

Hepatic: **Hyperbilirubinemia (14%)**, hepatic failure, hepatitis

Neuromuscular & skeletal: Weakness, flank pain

Ocular: Photophobia

Renal: **Nephrolithiasis/urolithiasis (29%, pediatric patients; 12%, adult patients)**, hematuria, acute renal failure, crystalluria, pyelonephritis, interstitial nephritis (with medullary calcification and cortical atrophy)

Miscellaneous: Anaphylactoid reactions

Signs and Symptoms of Overdose Dizziness, drowsiness, nausea, paresthesias

Admission Criteria/Prognosis Admit any ingestion >5 g.

Pharmacodynamics/Kinetics

Absorption: Administration with a high fat, high calorie diet resulted in a reduction in AUC and in maximum serum concentration (77% and 84% respectively); lighter meal resulted in little or no change in these parameters.

Protein binding, plasma: 60%

Metabolism: Hepatic via CYP3A4; seven metabolites of indinavir identified

Bioavailability: Good

Half-life elimination: 1.8 ± 0.4 hour

Time to peak: 0.8 ± 0.3 hour

Excretion: Urine and feces

Dosage

Children 4-15 years (investigational): 500 mg/m² every 8 hours

Adults: Oral:

Unboosted regimen: 800 mg every 8 hours

Ritonavir-boosted regimens:

Ritonavir 100-200 mg twice daily plus indinavir 800 mg twice daily **or** Ritonavir 400 mg twice daily plus indinavir 400 mg twice daily

Dosage adjustments for indinavir when administered in combination therapy:

Delavirdine, itraconazole, or ketoconazole: Reduce indinavir dose to 600 mg every 8 hours

Efavirenz: Increase indinavir dose to 1000 mg every 8 hours

Lopinavir and ritonavir (Kaletra™): Indinavir 600 mg twice daily

Nelfinavir: Increase indinavir dose to 1200 mg twice daily

Nevirapine: Increase indinavir dose to 1000 mg every 8 hours

Rifabutin: Reduce rifabutin to 1/2 the standard dose plus increase indinavir to 1000 mg every 8 hours

Dosage adjustment in hepatic impairment: Mild-moderate impairment due to cirrhosis: 600 mg every 8 hours or with ketoconazole coadministration

Monitoring Parameters Monitor viral load, CD4 count, triglycerides, cholesterol, glucose, liver function tests, CBC, urinalysis (severe leukocyturia should be monitored frequently).

Administration Drink at least 48 oz of water daily. Administer with water, 1 hour before or 2 hours after a meal. Administer around-the-clock to avoid significant fluctuation in serum levels. May be taken with food when administered in combination with ritonavir.

Contraindications Hypersensitivity to indinavir or any component of the formulation; concurrent use of amiodarone, cisapride, triazolam, midazolam, pimozide, or ergot alkaloids

Warnings Because indinavir may cause nephrolithiasis/urolithiasis the drug should be discontinued if signs and symptoms occur; risk is substantially higher in pediatric patients versus adults. Adequate hydration is recommended. May cause tubulointerstitial nephritis (rare); severe asymptomatic leukocyturia may warrant evaluation. Indinavir should not be administered concurrently with lovastatin or simvastatin (caution with atorvastatin and cerivastatin) because of competition for metabolism of these drugs through the CYP3A4 system, and potential serious or life-threatening events. Use caution with other drugs metabolized by this enzyme (particular caution with phosphodiesterase-5 inhibitors, including sildenafil). Avoid concurrent use of St John's wort (may lead to loss of virologic response and/or resistance). Patients with hepatic insufficiency due to cirrhosis should have dose reduction. Warn patients about fat redistribution that can occur. Indinavir has been associated with hemolytic anemia (discontinue if diagnosed), hepatitis, and hyperglycemia (exacerbation or new-onset diabetes). Treatment may result in immune reconstitution syndrome (acute inflammatory response to indolent or residual opportunistic infections). Use caution in patients with hemophilia; spontaneous bleeding has been reported.

Dosage Forms Capsule: 100 mg, 200 mg, 333 mg, 400 mg

Reference Range Therapeutic drug concentration (serum) is 251-12,617 nmol

Overdosage/Treatment

Decontamination: Lavage any ingestion >3 g in adults within 1 hour; activated charcoal should be given.

Supportive therapy: Aggressively hydrate (200 mL/hour normal saline in adults) to prevent nephrolithiasis.

Drug Interactions Substrate of CYP2D6 (minor), 3A4 (major); **Inhibits** CYP2C9 (weak), 2C19 (weak), 2D6 (weak), 3A4 (strong)

Amiodarone: Serum levels/toxicity may be increased by indinavir; serious and/or life-threatening reactions may occur; concurrent use is contraindicated.

Anticonvulsants: Phenobarbital, and carbamazepine may decrease serum levels and consequently effectiveness of indinavir.

Benzodiazepines: An increase in midazolam and triazolam serum levels may occur resulting in significant oversedation when administered with indinavir. Concurrent use is contraindicated. Use caution with other benzodiazepines.

Calcium channel blockers: Indinavir may increase the serum concentrations of calcium channel blockers.

Cisapride: Indinavir inhibits the metabolism of cisapride and should not be administered concurrently due to risk of life-threatening cardiac arrhythmias.

CYP3A4 inducers: CYP3A4 inducers may decrease the levels/effects of indinavir. Example inducers include aminoglutethimide, carbamazepine, nafcillin, nevirapine, phenobarbital, phenytoin, and rifamycins. Dosage adjustment may be recommended; see individual agents.

CYP3A4 inhibitors: May increase the levels/effects of indinavir. Example inhibitors include azole antifungals, clarithromycin, diclofenac, doxycycline, erythromycin, imatinib, isoniazid, nefazodone, nicardipine, propofol, protease inhibitors, quinidine, telithromycin, and verapamil.

CYP3A4 substrates: Indinavir may increase the levels/effects of CYP3A4 substrates. Example substrates include benzodiazepines, calcium channel blockers, mirtazapine, nateglinide, nefazodone, and tacrolimus. Selected benzodiazepines (midazolam and triazolam), cisapride, ergot alkaloids, selected HMG-CoA reductase inhibitors (lovastatin and simvastatin), and pimozide are generally contraindicated with strong CYP3A4 inhibitors.

Didanosine: Separate administration of indinavir from buffered formulations by at least 1 hour.

Ergot alkaloids: Serum levels/toxicity may be increased by indinavir; serious and/or life-threatening reactions may occur; concurrent use is contraindicated.

HMG-CoA reductase inhibitors: Indinavir may increase levels of HMG-CoA reductase inhibitors, increasing the risk of myopathy. Lovastatin and simvastatin should not be coadministered with indinavir (per manufacturer). Atorvastatin may be used with careful monitoring, in the lowest dose possible. Fluvastatin and pravastatin may have lowest risk.

Immunosuppressants: Indinavir may increase the serum levels of cyclosporine, sirolimus or tacrolimus.

Itraconazole or ketoconazole: May increase the serum concentrations of indinavir. Dosage adjustment of indinavir is recommended.

Non-nucleoside reverse transcriptase inhibitors: When used with delavirdine, serum levels of indinavir are increased. The serum concentrations of indinavir may be decreased by efavirenz or nevirapine. Dosage adjustment of indinavir may be required for these combinations.

Phosphodiesterase-5 (PDE-5) inhibitors (sildenafil, tadalafil, vardenafil): Serum concentrations/effects may be substantially increased by indinavir. Dosage restriction/limitation is recommended.

Pimozide: Serum levels/toxicity may be increased by indinavir; serious and/or life-threatening reactions may occur; concurrent use is contraindicated.

Protease inhibitors: Serum levels of both nelfinavir and indinavir are increased with concurrent use. Serum concentrations of indinavir may be increased by ritonavir. Serum levels of ritonavir and saquinavir may be increased. Dosage adjustments of both agents may be required during concurrent therapy. Concurrent use of atazanavir may increase the risk of hyperbilirubinemia.

Quinidine: Serum levels/toxicity may be increased by indinavir; serious and/or life-threatening reactions may occur; concurrent use is contraindicated.

Rifabutin: A 200% increase in rifabutin plasma AUC has been observed when coadministered with indinavir. Rifabutin may decrease the serum concentrations of indinavir. Dosage adjustment of both agents required.

Rifampin: Rifampin decreases indinavir's serum concentrations; loss of virologic response and resistance may occur; the two drugs should not be administered together.

St John's wort (*Hypericum perforatum*): Appears to induce CYP3A enzymes and may lead to reduction in trough serum concentrations, which may lead to treatment failures. Alternatively, changes may involve P-glycoprotein. The two drugs should not be used together.

Venlafaxine: May decrease indinavir levels/effects; use caution.

Pregnancy Risk Factor C

Pregnancy Implications Safety and pharmacokinetic studies are currently underway in pregnant women; hyperbilirubinemia may be exacerbated in neonates. Pregnancy and protease inhibitors are both associated with an increased risk of hyperglycemia. Glucose levels should be closely monitored. Healthcare professionals are encouraged to contact the antiretroviral pregnancy registry to monitor outcomes of pregnant women exposed to antiretroviral medications (1-800-258-4263).

Lactation Enters breast milk/contraindicated

Nursing Implications Administer around-the-clock to avoid significant fluctuation in serum levels; administer with plenty of water

Specific References

Huitema AD, Kuiper RA, Meenhorst PL, et al, "Photophobia in a Patient with High Indinavir Plasma Concentrations," *Ther Drug Monit*, 2003, 25(6):735-7.

Indomethacin

Related Information
- Nonsteroidal Anti-inflammatory Drugs
- Therapeutic Drugs Associated with Hallucinations

CAS Number 53-86-1 (Base); 74252-25-8 (Sodium)

U.S. Brand Names Indocin® I.V.; Indocin® SR; Indocin®

Synonyms Indometacin; Indomethacin Sodium Trihydrate

Use Management of inflammatory diseases and rheumatoid disorders; moderate pain; acute gouty arthritis, acute bursitis/tendonitis, moderate to severe osteoarthritis, rheumatoid arthritis, ankylosing spondylitis; I.V. form used as alternative to surgery for closure of patent ductus arteriosus in neonates

Mechanism of Action Inhibits prostaglandin synthesis by decreasing the activity of the enzyme, cyclooxygenase, which results in decreased formation of prostaglandin precursors

Adverse Reactions

Cardiovascular: Tachycardia

Central nervous system: Arrhythmias, aseptic meningitis, confusion, depression, dizziness, drowsiness, fatigue, hallucinations, **headache**, hypertension, malaise, psychic disturbances, psychosis, shock, somnolence, vertigo

Dermatologic: Angioedema, erythema multiforme, exfoliative dermatitis, itching, rash, Stevens-Johnson syndrome, toxic epidermal necrolysis, urticaria

Endocrine & metabolic: Hot flashes, hyperkalemia, dilutional hyponatremia (I.V.), hypoglycemia (I.V.), polydipsia

Gastrointestinal: Abdominal pain, abdominal cramps, abdominal distress, anorexia, constipation, diarrhea, dyspepsia, epigastric pain, flatulence, gastritis, GI bleeding, GI ulceration, heartburn, indigestion, perforation, proctitis, nausea, stomatitis

Genitourinary: Cystitis

Hematologic: Agranulocytosis, anemia, bone marrow suppression, hemolytic anemia, inhibition of platelet aggregation, leukopenia, thrombocytopenia

Hepatic: Cholestatic jaundice, hepatitis (including fatal cases)

Ocular: Blurred vision, conjunctivitis, corneal opacities, dry eyes, retinal/macular disturbances, toxic amblyopia

Otic: Decreased hearing, tinnitus

Neuromuscular & skeletal: Peripheral neuropathy

Renal: Interstitial nephritis, nephrotic syndrome, oliguria, polyuria, renal failure

Respiratory: Acute respiratory distress, allergic rhinitis, asthma, bronchospasm, CHF, dyspnea, epistaxis

Miscellaneous: Anaphylaxis, hypersensitivity reactions

Signs and Symptoms of Overdose Azotemia, cholestatic jaundice, coagulopathy, colitis, corneal microdeposits, dementia, drowsiness, esophageal ulceration, gastrointestinal upset, GI bleeding, hematuria, hypoglycemia, hyponatremia, impotence, nausea, ototoxicity, photosensitivity, pseudotumor cerebri, syndrome of inappropriate antidiuretic hormone (SIADH), tinnitus, vomiting, wheezing

Severe poisoning can manifest with blindness, blurred vision, coma, feces discoloration (green), hyperglycemia, hypotension, renal and/or hepatic failure, respiratory depression, seizures, thrombocytopenia, urine discoloration (green)

Pharmacodynamics/Kinetics

Onset of action: ~30 minutes

Duration: 4-6 hours

Absorption: Prompt and extensive

Distribution: V_d: 0.34-1.57 L/kg; crosses blood brain barrier and placenta; enters breast milk

Protein binding: 99%

Metabolism: Hepatic; significant enterohepatic recirculation

Bioavailability: 100%

Half-life elimination: 4.5 hours; prolonged in neonates

Time to peak: Oral: 2 hours

Excretion: Urine (60%, primarily as glucuronide conjugates); feces (33%, primarily as metabolites)

Dosage

Patent ductus arteriosus:

Neonates: I.V.: Initial: 0.2 mg/kg, followed by 2 doses depending on postnatal age (PNA):

PNA **at time of first dose** <48 hours: 0.1 mg/kg at 12- to 24-hour intervals

PNA **at time of first dose** 2-7 days: 0.2 mg/kg at 12- to 24-hour intervals

PNA **at time of first dose** >7 days: 0.25 mg/kg at 12- to 24-hour intervals

In general, may use 12-hour dosing interval if urine output >1 mL/kg/hour after prior dose; use 24-hour dosing interval if urine output is <1 mL/kg/hour but >0.6 mL/kg/hour; doses should be withheld if patient has oliguria (urine output <0.6 mL/kg/hour) or anuria

Inflammatory/rheumatoid disorders: Oral:

Children: 1-2 mg/kg/day in 2-4 divided doses; maximum dose: 4 mg/kg/day; not to exceed 150-200 mg/day

Adults: 25-50 mg/dose 2-3 times/day; maximum dose: 200 mg/day; extended release capsule should be given on a 1-2 times/day schedule

Stability Protect from light; not stable in alkaline solution; reconstitute just prior to administration; discard any unused portion; do not use preservative containing diluents for reconstitution

Monitoring Parameters Monitor response (pain, range of motion, grip strength, mobility, ADL function), inflammation; observe for weight gain, edema; monitor renal function (serum creatinine, BUN); observe for bleeding, bruising; evaluate gastrointestinal effects (abdominal pain, bleeding, dyspepsia); mental confusion, disorientation, CBC, liver function tests

Administration

Oral: Administer with food, milk, or antacids to decrease GI adverse effects; extended release capsules must be swallowed whole, do not crush

I.V.: Administer over 20-30 minutes at a concentration of 0.5-1 mg/mL in preservative-free sterile water for injection or normal saline. Reconstitute I.V. formulation just prior to administration; discard any unused portion; avoid I.V. bolus administration or infusion via an umbilical catheter into vessels near the superior mesenteric artery as these may cause vasoconstriction and can compromise blood flow to the intestines. Do not administer intra-arterially.

Contraindications Hypersensitivity to indomethacin, aspirin, other NSAIDs, or any component of the formulation; perioperative pain in the setting of coronary artery bypass surgery (CABG); pregnancy (3rd trimester)

Neonates: Necrotizing enterocolitis, impaired renal function, active bleeding, thrombocytopenia, coagulation defects, untreated infection

Warnings [U.S. Boxed Warning]: NSAIDs are associated with an increased risk of adverse cardiovascular events, including MI, stroke, and new onset or worsening of pre-existing hypertension. Risk may be increased with duration of use or pre-existing cardiovascular risk-factors or disease. Carefully evaluate individual cardiovascular risk profiles prior to prescribing. Use caution with fluid retention, CHF or hypertension.

Use of NSAIDs can compromise existing renal function. Renal toxicity can occur in patient with impaired renal function, dehydration, heart failure, liver dysfunction, those taking diuretics and ACEI and the elderly. Rehydrate patient before starting therapy. Monitor renal function closely. Indomethacin is not recommended for patients with advanced renal disease.

[U.S. Boxed Warning]: NSAIDs may increase risk of gastrointestinal irritation, ulceration, bleeding, and perforation. These events may occur at any time during therapy and without warning. Use caution with a history of GI disease (bleeding or ulcers), concurrent therapy with aspirin, anticoagulants and/or corticosteroids, smoking, use of alcohol, the elderly or debilitated patients.

Use the lowest effective dose for the shortest duration of time, consistent with individual patient goals, to reduce risk of cardiovascular or GI adverse events. Alternate therapies should be considered for patients at high risk.

NSAIDs may cause serious skin adverse events including exfoliative dermatitis, Stevens-Johnson syndrome (SJS) and toxic epidermal necrolysis (TEN). Anaphylactoid reactions may occur, even without prior exposure; patients with "aspirin triad" (bronchial asthma, aspirin intolerance, rhinitis) may be at increased risk. Do not use in patients who experience bronchospasm, asthma, rhinitis, or urticaria with NSAID or aspirin therapy.

Use with caution in patients with decreased hepatic function. Closely monitor patients with any abnormal LFT. Severe hepatic reactions (eg, fulminant hepatitis, liver failure) have occurred with NSAID use, rarely; discontinue if signs or symptoms of liver disease develop, or if systemic manifestations occur.

Withhold for at least 4-6 half-lives prior to surgical or dental procedures.

Dosage Forms
Capsule (Indocin®): 25 mg, 50 mg
Capsule, sustained release (Indocin® SR): 75 mg
Injection, powder for reconstitution, as sodium trihydrate (Indocin® I.V.): 1 mg
Suspension, oral (Indocin®): 25 mg/5 mL (237 mL) [contains alcohol 1%; pineapple-coconut-mint flavor]

Reference Range Therapeutic: 0.3-3.0 mg/L (0.8-8.0 µmol/L)
Overdosage/Treatment
Decontamination: Ipecac within 30 minutes or lavage (within 4 hours) for ingestions >10 mg/kg; activated charcoal can be utilized
Supportive therapy: Hypotension/dehydration can be managed with I.V. fluid therapy; dopamine is vasopressor of choice; acidosis should be treated with bicarbonates, seizures with benzodiazepines; antacids, blood products are indicated, as appropriate, for hemorrhage; famotidine (40 mg 2 times/day) can decrease incidence of gastric or duodenal ulcers in patients receiving long-term therapy of this drug
Enhancement of elimination: Multiple doses of activated charcoal; dialysis or perfusion is indicated for secondary complications, acidosis, or renal failure and not toxin removal alone

Test Interactions Positive Coombs' [direct]
Drug Interactions Substrate (minor) of CYP2C9, 2C19; **Inhibits** CYP2C9 (strong), 2C19 (weak)
ACE inhibitors: Antihypertensive effects may be decreased by concurrent therapy with NSAIDs; monitor blood pressure.
Aminoglycosides: NSAIDs may decrease the excretion of aminoglycosides.
Angiotensin II antagonists: Antihypertensive effects may be decreased by concurrent therapy with NSAIDs; monitor blood pressure.
Anticoagulants (warfarin, heparin, LMWHs) in combination with NSAIDs can cause increased risk of bleeding.
Antiplatelet drugs (ticlopidine, clopidogrel, aspirin, abciximab, dipyridamole, eptifibatide, tirofiban) can cause an increased risk of bleeding.
Beta-blockers: NSAIDs may diminish the antihypertensive effects of beta blockers.
Bisphosphonates: NSAIDs may increase the risk of gastrointestinal ulceration.
Cholestyramine (and other bile acid sequestrants): May decrease the absorption of NSAIDs. Separate by at least 2 hours.
Corticosteroids may increase the risk of GI ulceration; avoid concurrent use.
Cyclosporine: NSAIDs may increase serum creatinine, potassium, blood pressure, and cyclosporine levels; monitor cyclosporine levels and renal function carefully.
CYP2C9 Substrates: Indomethacin may increase the levels/effects of CYP2C9 substrates. Example substrates include bosentan, dapsone, fluoxetine, glimepiride, glipizide, losartan, montelukast, nateglinide, paclitaxel, phenytoin, warfarin, and zafirlukast.
Gentamicin and amikacin serum concentrations are increased by indomethacin in premature infants. Results may apply to other aminoglycosides and NSAIDs.
Hydralazine's antihypertensive effect is decreased; avoid concurrent use.
Lithium levels can be increased; avoid concurrent use if possible or monitor lithium levels and adjust dose. Sulindac may have the least effect. When NSAID is stopped, lithium will need adjustment again.
Loop diuretics efficacy (diuretic and antihypertensive effect) is reduced. Indomethacin reduces this efficacy, however, it may be anticipated with any NSAID.

Methotrexate: Severe bone marrow suppression, aplastic anemia, and GI toxicity have been reported with concomitant NSAID therapy. Avoid use during moderate or high-dose methotrexate (increased and prolonged methotrexate levels). NSAID use during low-dose treatment of rheumatoid arthritis has not been fully evaluated; extreme caution is warranted.
Pemetrexed: NSAIDs may decrease the excretion of pemetrexed. Patients with Cl$_{cr}$ 45-79 mL/minute should avoid short acting NSAIDs for 2 days before and 2 days after pemetrexed treatment.
Thiazides antihypertensive effects are decreased; avoid concurrent use.
Tiludronate: Indomethacin may increase serum concentration of tiludronate.
Treprostinil: May enhance the risk of bleeding with concurrent use.
Vancomycin: NSAIDs may decrease the excretion of vancomycin.
Pregnancy Risk Factor B/D (3rd trimester)
Pregnancy Implications May have adverse effects on fetus; crosses the placenta; anhydramnios without adverse fetal effects has been associated with 100 mg/day ingestion; renal failure, metabolic acidosis, patent ductus arteriosus and tricuspid regurgitation in neonates can follow in utero exposure; dramatic increase in the incidence of indomethacin-induced ductal constriction occurs at 31 weeks gestation
Lactation Enters breast milk/use caution (AAP rates "compatible")
Nursing Implications Reconstitute just prior to administration; discard any unused portion; inject I.V. over 5-10 seconds; extended release capsules must be swallowed intact
Additional Information May affect platelet and renal function in neonates; misoprostol (200 mcg) can reverse indomethacin-induced renal dysfunction in patients with stable alcoholic cirrhosis

Insulin Lispro

CAS Number 133107-64-9
U.S. Brand Names Humalog®
Synonyms Lispro Insulin
Use Treatment of insulin-dependent diabetes mellitus, also noninsulin-dependent diabetes mellitus unresponsive to treatment with diet and/or oral hypoglycemics; to assure proper utilization of glucose and reduce glucosuria in nondiabetic patients receiving parenteral nutrition whose glucosuria cannot be adequately controlled with infusion rate adjustments or those who require assistance in achieving optimal caloric intakes; used to treat hyperkalemia
Mechanism of Action Equipotent to regular insulin, insulin lispro is a human insulin analog which is more rapidly adsorbed
Pharmacodynamics/Kinetics
Onset of action: 0.2-0.5 hours
Duration: 3-4 hours
Distribution: 0.26-0.36 L/kg
Bioavailability: 55% to 77%
Time to peak: 30-90 minutes
Excretion: Urine
Dosage 100 units/mL
Monitoring Parameters Urine sugar and acetone, serum glucose, electrolytes
Administration Insulin lispro (Humalog®): SubQ administration: May be administered within 15 minutes before or immediately after a meal. Cold injections should be avoided. SubQ administration is usually made into the thighs, arms, buttocks, or abdomen, with sites rotated. Can be infused SubQ by external insulin pump; however, when used in an external pump, should not be diluted or mixed with other insulins.
Note: May be mixed in the same syringe as Humulin® N or Humulin® U, but Humalog® should be drawn into the syringe first.
Contraindications Hypersensitivity to any component of the formulation
Warnings In type 1 diabetes mellitus (insulin dependent, IDDM), insulin lispro (Humalog®) and insulin glulisine (Apidra™) should be used in combination with a long-acting insulin. However, in type 2 diabetes mellitus (noninsulin dependent, NIDDM), insulin lispro (Humalog®) may be used without a long-acting insulin when used in combination with a sulfonylurea.
Dosage Forms Injection, solution (Humalog®): 100 units/mL (3 mL) [prefilled cartridge or prefilled disposable pen]; (10 mL) [vial]
Reference Range Peak serum insulin level of 4.1 ng/mL obtained 1 hour after subcutaneous injection of 10 units of insulin lispro
Overdosage/Treatment
Decontamination: Excision of tissue near insulin injection site can be performed
Supportive therapy: 50 mL D$_{50}$W given I.V.; if no I.V. is available, glucagon 0.5-1 mg SubQ or I.M.; give 300 g of carbohydrates orally when patient awakens; insulin-induced peripheral and sacral edema has been successfully treated with oral ephedrine (15 mg every 8 hours); for most insulin overdoses, anticipate a need of 400-600 mg of glucose/kg/hour; continuous infusions of glucose with concentrations exceeding 20% should be given by central venous line

Drug Interactions Refer to Insulin Preparations - Regular

Pregnancy Risk Factor B

Pregnancy Implications Does not cross the placenta. Insulin is the drug of choice for control of diabetes mellitus during pregnancy.

Lactation Excretion in breast milk unknown/compatible

Additional Information Less late hypoglycemia and better postprandial glucose control than with regular insulin. NPH insulin should be added to insulin lispro at any meal when the next insulin injection is due no sooner than 3-4 hours later. Insulin lispro costs ~30% more than regular human insulin.

Insulin Preparations

Related Information

- Donor Victims of Poisoning in Whom Transplantation of Organs Occurred
- Insulin Lispro

CAS Number 11061-68-0; 11070-73-8; 11091-62-6; 12584-58-6; 51798-72-2; 53027-39-7; 68859-20-1; 8049-62-5; 8063-29-4; 9004-10-8; 9004-12-0; 9004-21-1

U.S. Brand Names Apidra™; Humalog® Mix 75/25™; Humalog®; Humulin® 50/50; Humulin® 70/30; Humulin® L; Humulin® N; Humulin® R (Concentrated) U-500; Humulin® R; Humulin® U; Lantus®; Lente® Iletin® II [DSC]; Novolin® 70/30; Novolin® L [DSC]; Novolin® N; Novolin® R; NovoLog® Mix 70/30; NovoLog®; NPH Iletin® II; Regular Iletin® II; Velosulin® BR (Buffered) [DSC]

Use Treatment of type 1 diabetes mellitus (insulin dependent, IDDM); type 2 diabetes mellitus (noninsulin dependent, NIDDM) unresponsive to treatment with diet and/or oral hypoglycemics; adjunct to parenteral nutrition

Unlabeled/Investigational Use Hyperkalemia (regular insulin only; use with glucose to shift potassium into cells to lower serum potassium levels); therapy of severe calcium channel blocker poisoning

Mechanism of Action Replacement therapy for persons unable to produce the hormone naturally or in insufficient amounts to maintain glycemic control

Adverse Reactions

Primarily symptoms of hypoglycemia

Cardiovascular: Palpitations, tachycardia, pallor, sinus tachycardia, vasodilation, vasculitis

Central nervous system: Fatigue, tingling of fingers, mental confusion, loss of consciousness, headache, hypothermia

Dermatologic: Urticaria, angioedema, bullous skin disease, purpura, exanthem

Endocrine & metabolic: Hypoglycemia, hypokalemia, parotitis, insulin antibody formation

Gastrointestinal: Hunger, nausea, numbness of mouth, loss of taste perception

Local: Itching, redness, edema, stinging, or warmth at injection site; atrophy or hypertrophy of SubQ fat tissue

Neuromuscular & skeletal: Tremors, fasciculations, weakness

Ocular: Transient presbyopia or blurred vision, nystagmus

Miscellaneous: Anaphylactoid reactions, diaphoresis, hiccups

Signs and Symptoms of Overdose Apnea, ataxia, coma, dysarthria, hepatomegaly, hyperglycemia, hypoglycemia, hypokalemia, hypothermia, mydriasis, noncardiogenic pulmonary edema, numbness, nystagmus, parotid pain, periarteritis nodosa, seizures

Admission Criteria/Prognosis Admit any patient who has taken a massive insulin overdose or any child in whom insulin was given without any indication.

Toxicodynamics/Kinetics

Onset of action and duration: Biosynthetic NPH human insulin shows a more rapid onset and shorter duration of action than corresponding porcine insulins; human insulin and purified porcine regular insulin are similarly efficacious following SubQ administration. The duration of action of highly purified porcine insulins is shorter than that of conventional insulin equivalents. Duration depends on type of preparation and route of administration as well as patient-related variables. In general, the larger the dose of insulin, the longer the duration of activity.

Absorption: Biosynthetic regular human insulin is absorbed from the SubQ injection site more rapidly than insulins of animal origin (60-90 minutes peak vs 120-150 minutes peak respectively) and lowers the initial blood glucose much faster. Human Ultralente® insulin is absorbed about twice as quickly as its bovine equivalent, and bioavailability is also improved. Human Lente® insulin preparations are also absorbed more quickly than their animal equivalents. Insulin glargine (Lantus®) is designed to form microprecipitates when injected subcutaneously. Small amounts of insulin glargine are then released over a 24-hour period, with no pronounced peak. Insulin glargine (Lantus®) for the treatment of type 1 diabetes (insulin dependent, IDDM) and type 2 diabetes mellitus (noninsulin dependent, NIDDM) in patients who require basal (long-acting) insulin.

Bioavailability: Medium-acting SubQ Lente®-type human insulins did not differ from the corresponding porcine insulins

Insulin aspart (NovoLog®):
Onset: 0.17-0.33 hours; Peak effect: 1-3 hours; Duration: 3-5 hours

Lispro (Humalog®):
Onset: 0.25 hours; Peak effect: 0.5-1.5 hours; Duration: 6-8 hours

Insulin, regular (Novolin® R):
Onset: 0.5-1 hours; Peak effect: 2-3 hours; Duration: 8-12 hours

Isophane insulin suspension (NPH) (Novolin® N):
Onset: 1-1.5 hours; Peak effect: 4-12 hours; Duration: 24 hours

Insulin zinc suspension (Lente®):
Onset: 1-2.5 hours; Peak effect: 8-12 hours; Duration: 18-24 hours

Isophane insulin suspension and regular insulin injection (Novolin® 70/30):
Onset: 0.5 hours; Peak effect: 2-12 hours; Duration: 24 hours

Extended insulin zinc suspension (Ultralente®):
Onset: 4-8 hours; Peak effect: 16-18 hours; Duration: >36 hours

Insulin glargine (Lantus®):
Duration: 24 hours

Dosage

Dose requires continuous medical supervision; may administer I.V. (regular), I.M., or SubQ; regular insulin may also be administered I.V.

Diabetes mellitus: The number and size of daily doses, time of administration, and diet and exercise require continuous medical supervision. In addition, specific formulations may require distinct administration procedures (see Administration).

Children and Adults: 0.5-1 unit/kg/day in divided doses

Adolescents (growth spurts): 0.8-1.2 units/kg/day in divided doses

Adjust dose to maintain premeal and bedtime blood glucose of 80-140 mg/dL (children <5 years: 100-200 mg/dL)

Insulin glargine (Lantus®): SubQ:

Type 2 diabetes (patient not already on insulin): 10 units once daily, adjusted according to patient response (range in clinical study 2-100 units/day)

Patients already receiving insulin: In clinical studies, when changing to insulin glargine from once-daily NPH or Ultralente® insulin, the initial dose was not changed; when changing from twice-daily NPH to once-daily insulin glargine, the total daily dose was reduced by 20% and adjusted according to patient response

Hyperkalemia (unlabeled use): Administer dextrose at 0.5-1 mL/kg and regular insulin 1 unit for every 4-5 g dextrose given

Diabetic ketoacidosis: Children and Adults: Regular insulin: I.V. loading dose: 0.1 unit/kg, then maintenance continuous infusion: 0.1 unit/kg/hour (range: 0.05-0.2 units/kg/hour depending upon the rate of decrease of serum glucose - too rapid decrease of serum glucose may lead to cerebral edema).

Optimum rate of decrease (serum glucose): 80-100 mg/dL/hour

Note: Newly-diagnosed patients with IDDM presenting in DKA and patients with blood sugars <800 mg/dL may be relatively "sensitive" to insulin and should receive loading and initial maintenance doses approximately $^1/_2$ of those indicated above.

Dosing adjustment in renal impairment (regular): Insulin requirements are reduced due to changes in insulin clearance or metabolism

Cl_{cr} 10-50 mL/minute: Administer at 75% of normal dose

Cl_{cr} <10 mL/minute: Administer at 25% to 50% of normal dose and monitor glucose closely

Hemodialysis: Because of a large molecular weight (6000 daltons), insulin is not significantly removed by either peritoneal or hemodialysis Supplemental dose is not necessary

Peritoneal dialysis: Supplemental dose is not necessary

Continuous arteriovenous or venovenous hemofiltration effects: Supplemental dose is not necessary

Monitoring Parameters Urine sugar and acetone, serum glucose, electrolytes, Hb A_{1c}, lipid profile

Administration

SubQ administration: Cold injections should be avoided. SubQ administration is usually made into the thighs, arms, buttocks, or abdomen, with sites rotated. When mixing regular insulin with other preparations of insulin, regular insulin should be drawn into syringe first. Buffered insulin (Velosulin® BR) should not be mixed with any other form of insulin.

Insulin lispro (Humalog®): May be administered within 15 minutes before or immediately after a meal.

Insulin aspart (NovoLog®): Should be administered immediately before a meal (within 5-10 minutes of the start of a meal). Can be infused SubQ by external insulin pump; do not dilute or mix with other insulins when used in an external pump for SubQ infusion; should replace insulin in reservoir every 48 hours.

Human regular insulin: Should be administered within 30-60 minutes before a meal.

Intermediate-acting insulins (such as NPH): May be administered 1-2 times/day.

Long-acting insulins (such as Ultralente®, Lantus®): May be administered once daily.

Insulin glargine (Lantus®): Should be administered once daily, at any time of day, but should be administered at the same time each day. Cannot be diluted or mixed with any other insulin or solution.

Regular insulin may be administered by SubQ, I.M., or I.V. routes
I.V. administration (requires use of an infusion pump): **Only regular insulin** may be administered I.V.
I.V. infusions: To minimize adsorption problems to I.V. solution bag:
If new tubing is **not** needed: Wait a minimum of 30 minutes between the preparation of the solution and the initiation of the infusion
If new tubing is needed: After receiving the insulin drip solution, the administration set should be attached to the I.V. container and the line should be flushed with the insulin solution. The nurse should then wait 30 minutes, then flush the line again with the insulin solution prior to initiating the infusion
If insulin is required prior to the availability of the insulin drip, regular insulin should be administered by I.V. push injection
Because of adsorption, the actual amount of insulin being administered could be substantially less than the apparent amount. Therefore, adjustment of the insulin drip rate should be based on effect and not solely on the apparent insulin dose. Furthermore, the apparent dose should not be used as the basis for determining the subsequent insulin dose upon discontinuing the insulin drip. Dose requires continuous medical supervision.

To be ordered as units/hour
Example: Standard diluent of regular insulin only: 100 units/100 mL NS (can be administered as a more diluted solution, ie, 100 units/250 mL NS)
Insulin rate of infusion (100 units regular/100 mL NS)
1 unit/hour: 1 mL/hour
2 units/hour: 2 mL/hour
3 units/hour: 3 mL/hour
4 units/hour: 4 mL/hour
5 units/hour: 5 mL/hour, etc

Reference Range
Therapeutic, serum insulin (fasting): 5-20 µIU/mL (SI: 35-145 pmol/L)
Glucose: Newborns: 20-80 mg/dL; Adults: 60-115 mg/dL; Elderly: 100-180 mg/dL
Peptide fragments are low (<0.5 ng/mL) in cases of exogenous insulin administration but high in insulinoma or sulfonylurea ingestion
Plasma insulin levels which are very high (>10,000 pmol/L), consistent with exogenous administration

Overdosage/Treatment
Decontamination: Excision of tissue near insulin injection site can be performed
Supportive therapy: 50 mL $D_{50}W$ given I.V.; if no I.V. is available, glucagon 0.5-1 mg SubQ or I.M.; give 300 g of carbohydrates orally when patient awakens; insulin-induced peripheral and sacral edema has been successfully treated with oral ephedrine (15 mg every 8 hours); for most insulin overdoses, anticipate a need of 400-600 mg of glucose/kg/hour; continuous infusions of glucose with concentrations exceeding 20% should be given by central venous line

Antidote(s)
- Dextrose [ANTIDOTE]
- Glucagon [ANTIDOTE]

Nursing Implications Patients using human insulin may be less likely to recognize hypoglycemia than if they use pork insulin; patients on pork insulin that have low blood sugar exhibit hunger and sweating; regular insulin is the only form for I.V. use; patients who are unable to accurately draw up their dose will need assistance such as prefilled syringes

Additional Information The term "purified" refers to insulin preparations containing no more than 10 ppm proinsulin (purified and human insulins are less immunogenic). Insulin abuse can be identified by presence of anti-insulin antibodies or decreased plasma C-peptide concentration; aspirin may be useful in alleviating hypersensitivity reactions; gas gangrene may occur secondary to SubQ insulin injection; buffering agent in Velosulin® BR may alter the activity of other insulin products

Specific References
Brvar M, Mozina M, and Bunc M, "Poisoning with Insulin Glargine," *Clin Toxicol (Phila)*, 2005, 43(3):219-20.
Deakin A, Montgomery M, and LeBeau M, "ELISA Screen for Human Insulin and Insulin Analogs in Serum<" *J Anal Toxicol*, 2006, 30:130.
Holger JS, Engebretsen KM, Fritzlar SJ, et al, "Insulin Versus Vasopressin and Epinephrine to Treat Beta-Blocker Toxicity," *Clin Toxicol (Phila)*, 2005, 43:729.
Shepherd G and Klein-Schwartz W, "High-Dose Insulin Therapy for Calcium Channel Blocker Overdose," *Ann Pharmacother*, 2005, 39:923-30.
Van den Berghe G, Wilmer A, Hermans G, et al, "Intensive Insulin Therapy in the Medical ICU," *N Engl J Med*. 2006, 2;354(5):449-61.

Interferon Alfa-2a

CAS Number 76543-88-9
U.S. Brand Names Roferon-A®
Synonyms IFLrA; rIFN-A
Use Patients >18 years of age: Hairy cell leukemia, AIDS-related Kaposi's sarcoma, chronic hepatitis C

Children and Adults: Chronic myelogenous leukemia (CML), Philadelphia chromosome positive, within 1 year of diagnosis (limited experience in children)

Unlabeled/Investigational Use Adjuvant therapy for malignant melanoma, AIDS-related thrombocytopenia, cutaneous ulcerations of Behüïet's disease, brain tumors, metastatic ileal carcinoid tumors, cervical and colorectal cancers, genital warts, idiopathic mixed cryoglobulinemia, hemangioma, hepatitis D, hepatocellular carcinoma, idiopathic hypereosinophilic syndrome, mycosis fungoides, Sézary syndrome, low-grade non-Hodgkin's lymphoma, macular degeneration, multiple myeloma, renal cell carcinoma, basal and squamous cell skin cancer, essential thrombocythemia, cutaneous T-cell lymphoma

Mechanism of Action Following activation, multiple effects can be detected including induction of gene transcription. Inhibits cellular growth, alters the state of cellular differentiation, interferes with oncogene expression, alters cell surface antigen expression, increases phagocytic activity of macrophages, and augments cytotoxicity of lymphocytes for target cells

Adverse Reactions
Flu-like symptoms (fever, fatigue/malaise, myalgia, chills, headache, arthralgia, rigors) begin ~2-6 hours after the dose is given and may persist as long as 24 hours; usually patient can build up a tolerance to side effects
Cardiovascular: Tachycardia, cardiac arrhythmias, hypotension, edema, chest pain, cardiomegaly, cardiomyopathy, angina, congestive heart failure, myocardial depression, sinus tachycardia, acrocyanosis
Central nervous system: **Fatigue/malaise, dizziness**, CNS depression, confusion, sensory neuropathy, psychiatric effects, headache, EEG abnormalities, **chills**, abducent nerve paralysis, psychosis, **fever**
Dermatologic: **Alopecia, rash**, lichen planus, vitiligo
Endocrine & metabolic: Increased uric acid level, Graves' disease, thyroid dysfunction, autoimmune thyroiditis
Gastrointestinal: Anorexia, **xerostomia, nausea, vomiting, diarrhea, abdominal cramps, weight loss**, change in taste, **metallic taste**
Genitourinary: Impotence
Hematologic: **Leukopenia** (mainly neutropenia), **anemia, thrombocytopenia**; **decreased hemoglobin, hematocrit, platelets**; neutralizing antibodies
Hepatic: Elevation of ALT and AST
Neuromuscular & skeletal: **Rigors**, myasthenia gravis, chorea, **arthralgia**, myopathy
Ocular: Blurred vision
Renal: Proteinuria, creatinine/BUN (elevated)
Respiratory: Coughing, nasal congestion, pneumonitis, pneumonia
Miscellaneous: **Diaphoresis**, subacute thyroiditis, psoriatic arthritis, systemic lupus erythematosus-like syndrome, herpes labialis

Signs and Symptoms of Overdose Agranulocytosis, AV block, coma, encephalopathy, granulocytopenia, hyperglycemia, impotence, leukopenia, mania, Mees' lines, neutropenia

Pharmacodynamics/Kinetics
Absorption: Filtered and absorbed at the renal tubule
Distribution: V_d: 0.223-0.748 L/kg
Metabolism: Primarily renal; filtered through glomeruli and undergoes rapid proteolytic degradation during tubular reabsorption
Bioavailability: I.M.: 83%; SubQ: 90%
Half-life elimination: I.V.: 3.7-8.5 hours (mean ~5 hours)
Time to peak, serum: I.M., SubQ: ~6-8 hours

Dosage Refer to individual protocols
Children (limited data):
Chronic myelogenous leukemia (CML): I.M.: 2.5-5 million units/m²/day; **Note:** In juveniles, higher dosages (30 million units/m²/day) have been associated with severe adverse events, including death
Adults:
Hairy cell leukemia: SubQ, I.M.: 3 million units/day for 16-24 weeks, then 3 million units 3 times/week for up to 6-24 months
Chronic myelogenous leukemia (CML): SubQ, I.M.: 9 million units/day, continue treatment until disease progression
AIDS-related Kaposi's sarcoma: SubQ, I.M.: 36 million units/day for 10-12 weeks, then 36 million units 3 times/week; to minimize adverse reactions, can use escalating dose (3-, 9-, then 18 million units each day for 3 days, then 36 million units daily thereafter)
Hepatitis C: SubQ, I.M.: 3 million units 3 times/week for 12 months

Dosage adjustment in renal impairment: Not removed by hemodialysis
Stability Refrigerate (2°C to 8°C/36°F to 46°F); do not freeze; do not shake. Reconstitute vial with the diluent provided, or SWFI, NS, or D_5W; concentrations ≥3×10⁶ units/mL are hypertonic. After reconstitution, the solution is stable for 24 hours at room temperature and for 1 month when refrigerated.
Monitoring Parameters Chronic hepatitis C: Monitor ALT and HCV-RNA to assess response (particularly in first 3 months of therapy)
CML/hairy cell leukemia: Hematologic monitoring should be performed monthly
Administration SubQ administration is suggested for those who are at risk for bleeding or are thrombocytopenic; rotate SubQ injection site; patient should be well hydrated

Contraindications Hypersensitivity to alfa interferon, benzyl alcohol, or any component of the formulation; autoimmune hepatitis; hepatic decompensation (Child-Pugh class B or C)

Warnings Use caution in patients with a history of depression. May cause severe psychiatric adverse events (psychosis, mania, depression, suicidal behavior/ideation) in patients with and without previous psychiatric symptoms; careful neuropsychiatric monitoring is required during therapy. Use with caution in patients with seizure disorders, brain metastases, or compromised CNS function. Higher doses in the elderly or in malignancies other than hairy cell leukemia may result in severe obtundation.

Use caution in patients with autoimmune diseases; development or exacerbation of autoimmune diseases has been reported. Use caution in patients with pre-existing cardiac disease (ischemic or thromboembolic), arrhythmias, renal impairment (Cl_{cr} <50 mL/minute), mild hepatic impairment, or myelosuppression. Also use caution in patients receiving therapeutic immunosuppression. May cause thyroid dysfunction or hyperglycemia, use caution in patients with diabetes or pre-existing thyroid disease. Pulmonary dysfunction may be induced or aggravated by interferon alpha; discontinue if persistent unexplained pulmonary infiltrates are noted. Gastrointestinal ischemia, ulcerative colitis and hemorrhage have been associated rarely with alpha interferons; some cases are severe and life-threatening. Ophthalmologic disorders (including retinal hemorrhages, cotton wool spots, and retinal artery or vein obstruction) have occurred in patients receiving alpha interferons; close monitoring is warranted.

[U.S. Boxed Warning]: Treatment should be discontinued in patients with worsening or persistently severe signs/symptoms of autoimmune, infectious, ischemic, or neuropsychiatric disorders (including depression and/or suicidal thoughts/behavior). Discontinue treatment if neutrophils <0.5×10^9/L or platelets <25×10^9/L. **Due to differences in dosage, patients should not change brands of interferons.** Injection solution contains benzyl alcohol; do not use in neonates or infants. Safety and efficacy in children <18 years of age have not been established.

Dosage Forms Injection, solution [single-dose prefilled syringe; SubQ use only]: 3 million units/0.5 mL (0.5 mL); 6 million units/0.5 mL (0.5 mL); 9 million units/0.5 mL (0.5 mL) [contains benzyl alcohol]

Reference Range
Peak serum concentration following an I.V. dose of 36 million units: 10,400-17,470 pg/mL

Overdosage/Treatment
Supportive therapy: Indomethacin or acetaminophen can be given for fever; avoid glucocorticoids; I.V. crystalloid therapy is usually adequate to treat hypotension
Enhancement of elimination: Hemodialysis is not useful

Test Interactions Increases norepinephrine plasma levels

Drug Interactions Inhibits CYP1A2 (weak)

Note: May exacerbate the toxicity of other agents with respect to CNS, myelotoxicity, or cardiotoxicity.

ACE inhibitors: Interferons may increase the adverse/toxic effects of ACE inhibitors, specifically the development of granulocytopenia. Risk: Monitor

Clozapine: A case report of agranulocytosis with concurrent use.

Erythropoietin: Case reports of decreased hematopoietic effect

Melphalan: Interferon alpha may decrease the serum concentrations of melphalan; this may or may not decrease the potential toxicity of melphalan. Risk: Monitor

Prednisone: Prednisone may decrease the therapeutic effects of interferon alpha. Risk: Moderate

Ribavirin: Concurrent therapy may increase the risk of hemolytic anemia.

Theophylline: Interferon alpha may decrease the P450 isoenzyme metabolism of theophylline. Risk: Moderate

Warfarin: Interferons may increase the anticoagulant effects of warfarin. Risk: Monitor

Zidovudine: Interferons may decrease the metabolism of zidovudine. Risk: Monitor

Pregnancy Risk Factor C

Pregnancy Implications Safety and efficacy for use during pregnancy have not been established. Interferon alpha has been shown to decrease serum estradiol and progesterone levels in humans. Menstrual irregularities and abortion have been reported in animals. Effective contraception is recommended during treatment.

Lactation Enters breast milk/contraindicated (AAP rates "compatible")

Nursing Implications Flu-like syndrome (fever, chills) occurs in the majority of patients 2-6 hours after a dose; use acetaminophen to prevent or partially alleviate headache and fever

Additional Information Indications and dosage regimens are specific for a particular brand of interferon; other brands of interferon (ie, Intron® A) have different indications and dosage guidelines; do not change brands of interferon as changes in dosage may result. Women with hepatitis C should be instructed that there is a theoretical risk the virus may be transmitted in breast milk. HIV-infected mothers are discouraged from breast-feeding to decrease potential transmission of HIV.

Specific References
Solomon T, Dung NM, Wills B, et al, "Interferon Alfa-2a in Japanese Encephalitis: A Randomised Double-Blind Placebo-Controlled Trial," *Lancet*, 2003, 361(9360):821-6.

Interferon Alfa-2b

CAS Number 99210-65-8
U.S. Brand Names Intron® A
Synonyms INF-alpha 2; rLFN-α2; α-2-interferon
Use
Patients ≥1 year of age: Chronic hepatitis B
Patients ≥18 years of age: Condyloma acuminata, chronic hepatitis C, hairy cell leukemia, malignant melanoma, AIDS-related Kaposi's sarcoma, follicular non-Hodgkin's lymphoma

Unlabeled/Investigational Use AIDS-related thrombocytopenia, cutaneous ulcerations of Behûlet's disease, carcinoid syndrome, cervical cancer, lymphomatoid granulomatosis, genital herpes, hepatitis D, chronic myelogenous leukemia (CML), non-Hodgkin's lymphomas (other than follicular lymphoma, see approved use), polycythemia vera, medullary thyroid carcinoma, multiple myeloma, renal cell carcinoma, basal and squamous cell skin cancers, essential thrombocytopenia, thrombocytopenic purpura
Investigational: West Nile virus

Mechanism of Action Following activation, multiple effects can be detected including induction of gene transcription. Inhibits cellular growth, alters the state of cellular differentiation, interferes with oncogene expression, alters cell surface antigen expression, increases phagocytic activity of macrophages, and augments cytotoxicity of lymphocytes for target cells

Adverse Reactions
Flu-like symptoms (fever, fatigue/malaise, myalgia, chills, headache, arthralgia, rigors) begin ~2-6 hours after the dose is given and may persist as long as 24 hours; usually patient can build up a tolerance to side effects
Cardiovascular: Tachycardia, cardiac arrhythmias, hypotension, edema, chest pain, Raynaud's disease, cardiomyopathy, cardiomegaly, angina, congestive heart failure, myocardial infarction, sinus tachycardia
Central nervous system: **Fatigue/malaise, dizziness,** CNS depression, confusion, sensory neuropathy, psychiatric effects, **fever,** headache, EEG abnormalities, **chills,** psychosis, hallucinations
Dermatologic: Partial alopecia, **rash,** purpura, skin necrosis
Endocrine & metabolic: Increased uric acid level, thyroid dysfunction, impaired spermatogenesis, thyroiditis
Gastrointestinal: **Anorexia, xerostomia, nausea, vomiting, diarrhea, abdominal cramps, weight loss,** change in taste, **metallic taste,** pancreatitis
Hematologic: **Leukopenia** (mainly neutropenia), agranulocytosis, **anemia,** thrombocytopenic purpura, **thrombocytopenia; decreased hemoglobin, hematocrit, platelets;** neutralizing antibodies, hemolytic anemia
Hepatic: Elevation of ALT and AST, primary biliary cirrhosis, hepatotoxic reaction
Local: Injection site alopecia
Neuromuscular & skeletal: Myalgia, **arthralgia, rigors,** myasthenia gravis, polymyositis (dermatomyositis), poliomyositis, rhabdomyolysis
Ocular: Blurred vision
Renal: Proteinuria, elevated creatinine/BUN, glomerulonephritis, nephrotic syndrome, renal failure
Respiratory: Coughing, nasal congestion, exacerbation of asthma
Miscellaneous: **Diaphoresis,** digital necrosis, Sjögren's syndrome, psoriatic arthritis, lupus erythematosus

Signs and Symptoms of Overdose Agranulocytosis, AV block, encephalopathy, granulocytopenia, hyperglycemia, leukopenia, lymphopenia, Mees' lines, neutropenia

Pharmacodynamics/Kinetics
Distribution: V_d: 31 L; but has been noted to be much greater (370-720 L) in leukemia patients receiving continuous infusion IFN; IFN does not penetrate the CSF
Metabolism: Primarily renal
Bioavailability: I.M.: 83%; SubQ: 90%
Half-life elimination: I.M., I.V.: 2 hours; SubQ: 3 hours
Time to peak, serum: I.M., SubQ: ~3-12 hours

Dosage
Refer to individual protocols
Children 1-17 years: Chronic hepatitis B: SubQ: 3 million units/m² 3 times/week for 1 week; then 6 million units/m² 3 times/week; maximum: 10 million units 3 times/week; total duration of therapy 16-24 weeks
Adults:
Hairy cell leukemia: I.M., SubQ: 2 million units/m² 3 times/week for 2-6 months
Lymphoma (follicular): SubQ: 5 million units 3 times/week for up to 18 months

Malignant melanoma: 20 million units/m^2 I.V. for 5 consecutive days per week for 4 weeks, then 10 million units/m^2 SubQ 3 times/week for 48 weeks

AIDS-related Kaposi's sarcoma: I.M., SubQ: 30 million units/m^2 3 times/week

Chronic hepatitis B: I.M., SubQ: 5 million units/day or 10 million units 3 times/week for 16 weeks

Chronic hepatitis C: I.M., SubQ: 3 million units 3 times/week for 16 weeks. In patients with normalization of ALT at 16 weeks, continue treatment for 18-24 months; consider discontinuation if normalization does not occur at 16 weeks. **Note:** May be used in combination therapy with ribavirin in previously untreated patients or in patients who relapse following alpha interferon therapy; refer to Interferon Alfa-2b and Ribavirin Combination Pack monograph.

Condyloma acuminata: Intralesionally: 1 million units/lesion (maximum: 5 lesions/treatment) 3 times/week (on alternate days) for 3 weeks. Use 1 million unit per 0.1 mL concentration.

Dosage adjustment in renal impairment: Not removed by peritoneal or hemodialysis

Dosage adjustment for toxicity: Manufacturer-recommended adjustments, listed according to indication:

Follicular lymphoma:
Severe toxicity (neutrophils <1000 cells/mm^3 or platelets <50,000 cells/mm^3): Reduce dose by 50% or temporarily discontinue
AST/ALT >5 times ULN: Permanently discontinue

Hairy cell leukemia:
Severe toxicity: Reduce dose by 50% or temporarily discontinue; permanently discontinue if persistent or recurrent severe toxicity is noted

Hepatitis B or C:
WBC <1500 cells/mm^3, granulocytes <750 cells/mm^3, or platelet count <50,000 cells/mm^3: Reduce dose by 50%
WBC <1000 cells/mm^3, granulocytes <500 cells/mm^3, or platelet count <25,000 cells/mm^3: Permanently discontinue

Kaposi sarcoma: Severe toxicity: Reduce dose by 50% or temporarily discontinue

Malignant melanoma:
Severe toxicity (neutrophils <500 cells/mm^3 or AST/ALT >5 times ULN): Reduce dose by 50% or temporarily discontinue
Neutrophils <250 cells/mm^3 or AST/ALT >10 times ULN: Permanently discontinue

See table.

Effects of Interferon Alpha-2b on Cell Counts

Granulocyte Count	Platelet Count	Interferon 2b dose
<750/mm^3	<50,000/mm^3	Decrease by 50%
<500/mm^3	<30,000/mm^3	Interrupt

When platelet/granulocyte count returns to normal, reinstitute therapy

Monitoring Parameters Baseline chest x-ray, ECG, CBC with differential, liver function tests, electrolytes, thyroid function tests, platelets, weight; patients with pre-existing cardiac abnormalities, or in advanced stages of cancer should have ECGs taken before and during treatment.

Administration Injection: Do not use 3-, 5-, 18-, and 25 million unit strengths intralesionally, solutions are hypertonic; 50 million unit strength is not for use in condylomata, hairy cell leukemia, or chronic hepatitis. Patients with platelet count <50,000/mm^3 should receive doses SubQ, not I.M.

Oral: Capsules should not be crushed, chewed, or opened.

Contraindications Hypersensitivity to interferon alfa or any component of the formulation; decompensated liver disease; autoimmune hepatitis; history of autoimmune disease; immunosuppressed transplant patients

Warnings
Suicidal ideation or attempts may occur more frequently in pediatric patients when compared to adults. May cause severe psychiatric adverse events (psychosis, mania, depression, suicidal behavior/ideation) in patients with and without previous psychiatric symptoms, avoid use in severe psychiatric disorders or in patients with a history of depression; careful neuropsychiatric monitoring is required during therapy. Use with caution in patients with a history of seizures, brain metastases, multiple sclerosis, cardiac disease (ischemic or thromboembolic), arrhythmias, myelosuppression, hepatic impairment, or renal dysfunction (use is not recommended if Cl$_{cr}$<50 mL/minute). Use caution in patients with a history of pulmonary disease, coagulopathy, thyroid disease (monitor thyroid function), hypertension, or diabetes mellitus (particularly if prone to DKA). Caution in patients receiving drugs that may cause lactic acidosis (eg, nucleoside analogues).

Avoid use in patients with autoimmune disorders; worsening of psoriasis and/or development of autoimmune disorders has been associated with alpha interferons. Higher doses in elderly patients, or diseases other than hairy cell leukemia, may result in increased CNS toxicity. **[U.S.**

Boxed Warning]: Treatment should be discontinued in patients who develop severe pulmonary symptoms with chest x-ray changes, autoimmune disorders, worsening of hepatic function, psychiatric symptoms (including depression and/or suicidal thoughts/behaviors), ischemic and/or infectious disorders. Ophthalmologic disorders (including retinal hemorrhages, cotton wool spots and retinal artery or vein obstruction) have occurred in patients receiving alpha interferons. Hypertriglyceridemia has been reported (discontinue if severe).

Safety and efficacy in children <1 year of age have not been established. Do not treat patients with visceral AIDS-related Kaposi's sarcoma associated with rapidly-progressing or life-threatening disease. A transient increase in SGOT (>2x baseline) is common in patients treated with interferon alfa-2b for chronic hepatitis. Therapy generally may continue, however, functional indicators (albumin, prothrombin time, bilirubin) should be monitored at 2-week intervals. **Due to differences in dosage, patients should not change brands of interferons without the prescribers knowledge.**

Intron® A may cause bone marrow suppression, including very rarely, aplastic anemia. Hemolytic anemia (hemoglobin <10 g/dL) was observed in up to 10% of treated patients in clinical trials when combined with ribavirin; anemia occurred within 1-2 weeks of initiation of therapy.

Dosage Forms
Injection, powder for reconstitution: 10 million units; 18 million units; 50 million units [contains human albumin]
Injection, solution [multidose prefilled pen]:
Delivers 3 million units/0.2 mL (1.5 mL) [delivers 6 doses; 18 million units]
Delivers 5 million units/0.2 mL (1.5 mL) [delivers 6 doses; 30 million units]
Delivers 10 million units/0.2 mL (1.5 mL) [delivers 6 doses; 60 million units]
Injection, solution [multidose vial]: 6 million units/mL (3 mL); 10 million units/mL (2.5 mL)
Injection, solution [single-dose vial]: 10 million units/ mL (1 mL)
See also Interferon Alfa-2b and Ribavirin Combination Pack monograph.

Reference Range Peak serum level after I.V. infusion of 10 million units: 546 units/mL

Overdosage/Treatment
Supportive therapy: Indomethacin or acetaminophen can be given for fever; avoid glucocorticoids
Enhancement of elimination: Hemodialysis is not useful

Drug Interactions
Inhibits CYP1A2 (weak)
ACE inhibitors: Interferons may increase the adverse/toxic effects of ACE inhibitors, specifically the development of granulocytopenia; monitor.
Clozapine: A case report of agranulocytosis with concurrent use.
Erythropoietin: Case reports of decreased hematopoietic effect.
Melphalan: Interferon alfa may decrease the serum concentrations of melphalan; this may or may not decrease the potential toxicity of melphalan; monitor.
Prednisone: Prednisone may decrease the therapeutic effects of interferon alfa. Risk: Moderate
Ribavirin: Concurrent therapy may increase the risk of hemolytic anemia.
Theophylline: Interferon alfa may decrease the P450 isoenzyme metabolism of theophylline. Risk: Moderate
Warfarin: Interferons may increase the anticoagulant effects of warfarin; monitor.
Zidovudine: Interferons may decrease the metabolism of zidovudine; monitor.

Pregnancy Risk Factor C

Pregnancy Implications Safety and efficacy for use during pregnancy have not been established. Interferon alpha has been shown to decrease serum estradiol and progesterone levels in humans. Menstrual irregularities and abortion have been reported in animals. Effective contraception is recommended during treatment.

Lactation Enters breast milk/not recommended (AAP rates "compatible")

Nursing Implications Use acetaminophen to prevent or partially alleviate headache and fever; do not use 3, 5, and 25 million unit strengths intralesionally, solutions are hypertonic; 50 million unit strength is not for use in condylomata

Additional Information Induction of insulin antibodies may result
Myelosuppressive effects: **WBC**: Mild. **Platelets**: Mild. Onset (days): 7-10. Nadir (days): 14. Recovery (days): 21

Interferon Alfa-n3

Pronunciation (in ter FEER on AL fa en three)
U.S. Brand Names Alferon® N
Use FDA approved: Condylomata acuminata, intralesional treatment of refractory or recurring genital or venereal warts; useful in patients who do not respond or are not candidates for usual treatments; indications and dosage regimens are specific for a particular brand of interferon

Mechanism of Action Alpha interferons are a family of proteins, produced by nucleated cells, that have antiviral, antiproliferative, and immune-regulating activity. There are 16 known subtypes of alpha interferons. Interferons interact with cells through high affinity cell surface receptors. Following activation, multiple effects can be detected including induction of gene transcription. Inhibits cellular growth, alters the state of cellular differentiation, interferes with oncogene expression, alters cell surface antigen expression, increases phagocytic activity of macrophages, and augments cytotoxicity of lymphocytes for target cells.

Adverse Reactions

Cardiovascular: Tachycardia, cardiac arrhythmias, chest pain, hypotension, SVT, edema, cardiomyopathy, cardiomegaly, angina, congestive heart failure, myocardial depression, sinus tachycardia

Central nervous system: **Dizziness, tiredness, fatigue, malaise, fever, chills**, lightheadedness, confusion, CNS depression, sensory neuropathy, psychiatric effects, EEG abnormalities, neurotoxicity, psychosis

Dermatologic: **Skin rash**, dry skin, alopecia

Endocrine & metabolic: Increased uric acid level

Gastrointestinal: **Nausea, anorexia, vomiting, xerostomia, diarrhea, abdominal cramps, weight loss, metallic tastes**, stomatitis

Hematologic: Mildly myelosuppressive and well tolerated if used without adjunct antineoplastic agents; **thrombocytosis** has been reported, **leukopenia** (mainly neutropenia), **anemia, thrombocytopenia, decreased hemoglobin, hematocrit, platelets**

Hepatic: Hepatotoxicity; hepatic transaminase, elevation of ALT and AST

Local: Sensitivity to injection

Neuromuscular & skeletal: **Rigors, arthralgia**, leg cramps, paresthesia

Ocular: Blurred vision

Renal: Creatinine/BUN (elevated), albuminuria

Respiratory: Cough, nasal congestion, dyspnea

Miscellaneous: **Flu-like syndrome**, neutralizing antibodies; usually patient can build up a tolerance to side effects, **diaphoresis**

Signs and Symptoms of Overdose Agranulocytosis, coagulopathy, encephalopathy, granulocytopenia, hyperglycemia, leukopenia, lightheadedness, neutropenia, syndrome of inappropriate antidiuretic hormone (SIADH)

Toxicodynamics/Kinetics Elimination: Renal

Dosage Adults: Inject 250,000 units (0.05 mL) in each wart twice weekly for a maximum of 8 weeks; therapy should not be repeated for at least 3 months after the initial 8-week course of therapy

Stability Store solution at 2°C to 8°C (36°F to 46°F); do not freeze or shake solution

Administration Inject into base of wart with a small 30-gauge needle

Contraindications Hypersensitivity to alpha interferon or any component of the formulation; anaphylactic sensitivity to mouse immunoglobulin, egg protein, or neomycin

Warnings Use with caution in patients with pre-existing cardiac disease, including unstable angina, uncontrolled CHF, or arrhythmias; severe pulmonary disease; diabetes with ketoacidosis; coagulation disorders (such as thrombophlebitis, pulmonary embolism, hemophilia); severe myelosuppression; or seizure disorder. **Due to differences in dosage, patients should not change brands of interferons.** Safety and efficacy in patients <18 years of age have not been not established.

Dosage Forms Injection, solution: 5 million int. units (1 mL) [contains albumin]

Overdosage/Treatment

Supportive therapy: Indomethacin or acetaminophen can be given for fever; avoid glucocorticoids

Enhancement of elimination: Hemodialysis is not useful

Drug Interactions

ACE inhibitors: Interferons may increase the adverse/toxic effects of ACE inhibitors, specifically the development of granulocytopenia. Risk: Monitor

Clozapine: A case report of agranulocytosis with concurrent use.

Erythropoietin: Case reports of decreased hematopoietic effect

Melphalan: Interferon alpha may decrease the serum concentrations of melphalan; this may or may not decrease the potential toxicity of melphalan. Risk: Monitor

Prednisone: Prednisone may decrease the therapeutic effects of Interferon alpha. Risk: Moderate

Theophylline: Interferon alpha may decrease the P450 isoenzyme metabolism of theophylline. Risk: Moderate

Warfarin: Interferons may increase the anticoagulant effects of warfarin. Risk: Monitor

Zidovudine: Interferons may decrease the metabolism of zidovudine. Risk: Monitor

Pregnancy Risk Factor C

Pregnancy Implications Safety and efficacy for use during pregnancy have not been established. Interferon alpha has been shown to decrease serum estradiol and progesterone levels in humans. Menstrual irregularities and abortion have been reported in animals. Effective contraception is recommended during treatment.

Lactation Excretion in breast milk unknown/not recommended

Nursing Implications Inject into base of wart with a small 30-gauge needle

Interferon Beta-1a

CAS Number 145258-61-3

U.S. Brand Names Avonex®; Rebif®

Synonyms rIFN beta-1a

Use Treatment of relapsing forms of multiple sclerosis (MS)

Mechanism of Action Interferon beta differs from naturally occurring human protein by a single amino acid substitution and the lack of carbohydrate side chains; alters the expression and response to surface antigens and can enhance immune cell activities. Properties of interferon beta that modify biologic responses are mediated by cell surface receptor interactions; mechanism in the treatment of MS is unknown.

Adverse Reactions

Cardiovascular: Chest pain, vasodilation, cardiomyopathy, CHF

Central nervous system: **Headache** (Avonex® 58%; Rebif® 65% to 70%), **fatigue** (Rebif® 33% to 41%), **fever** (Avonex® 20%; Rebif® 25% to 28%), convulsions, malaise, migraine, somnolence **pain** (Avonex® 23%), **chills** (Avonex® 19%), **depression** (Avonex® 18%), **dizziness** (Avonex® 14%), psychiatric disorders (new or worsening)

Dermatologic: Alopecia, rash

Endocrine & metabolic: Thyroid disorder, menorrhagia, metrorrhagia

Gastrointestinal: **Nausea** (Avonex® 23%), **abdominal pain** (Avonex® 8%; Rebif® 20% to 22%), toothache, xerostomia

Genitourinary: **Urinary tract infection** (Avonex® 17%), micturition frequency, urinary incontinence

Hematologic: **Leukopenia** (Rebif® 28% to 36%), anemia, thrombocytopenia, idiopathic thrombocytopenia, pancytopenia

Hepatic: **ALT increased** (Rebif® 20% to 27%), **AST increased** (Rebif® 10% to 17%), bilirubinemia, hepatic function abnormal, autoimmune hepatitis, hepatitis

Local: **Injection site reaction** (Avonex® 3%; Rebif® 89% to 92%)

Neuromuscular & skeletal: **Myalgia** (Avonex® 29%; Rebif® 25%), **back pain** (Rebif® 23% to 25%), **weakness** (Avonex® 24%), **skeletal pain** (Rebif® 10% to 15%), **rigors** (Rebif® 6% to 13%), arthralgia, coordination abnormal, hypertonia

Ocular: **Vision abnormal** (Rebif® 7% to 13%), eye disorder, xerophthalmia

Respiratory: **Sinusitis** (Avonex® 14%), **upper respiratory tract infection** (Avonex® 14%), bronchitis

Miscellaneous: **Flu-like symptoms** (Avonex® 49%; Rebif® 56% to 59%), **neutralizing antibodies** (significance not known; Avonex® 5%; Rebif® 24%), **lymphadenopathy** (Rebif® 11% to 12%), infection, anaphylaxis

Signs and Symptoms of Overdose CNS depression, flu-like symptoms, myelosuppression, obtundation

Pharmacodynamics/Kinetics

Limited data due to small doses used

Half-life elimination: Avonex®: 10 hours; Rebif®: 69 hours

Time to peak, serum: Avonex® (I.M.): 3-15 hours; Rebif® (SubQ): 16 hours

Dosage Adults:

I.M. (Avonex®): 30 mcg once weekly

SubQ (Rebif®): Initial: 8.8 mcg 3 times/week, increasing over a 4-week period to the recommended dose of 44 mcg 3 times/week; doses should be separated by at least 48 hours

Dosage adjustment in hepatic impairment: Rebif®: If liver function tests increase or in case of leukopenia: Decrease dose 20% to 50% until toxicity resolves.

Monitoring Parameters Monitor for signs and symptoms of thyroid abnormalities, hematologic suppression, liver functions tests, symptoms of autoimmune disorders

Avonex®: Frequency of monitoring for patients receiving Avonex® has not been specifically defined; in clinical trials, monitoring was at 6-month intervals.

Rebif®: CBC and liver function testing at 1-, 3-, and 6 months, then periodically thereafter. Thyroid function every 6 months (in patients with pre-existing abnormalities and/or clinical indications)

Administration Avonex®: Must be administered by I.M. injection

Rebif®: Administer SubQ at the same time of day on the same 3 days each week (ie, late afternoon/evening Mon, Wed, Fri)

Contraindications Hypersensitivity to natural or recombinant interferons, human albumin, or any other component of the formulation

Warnings Interferons have been associated with severe psychiatric adverse events (psychosis, mania, depression, suicidal behavior/ideation) in patients with and without previous psychiatric symptoms, avoid use in severe psychiatric disorders and use caution in patients with a history of depression; patients exhibiting depressive symptoms should be closely monitored and discontinuation of therapy should be considered.

Allergic reactions, including anaphylaxis, have been reported. Caution should be used in patients with hepatic impairment or in those who abuse alcohol. Rare cases of severe hepatic injury, including hepatic failure, have been reported in patients receiving interferon beta-1a; risk may be increased by ethanol use or concurrent therapy with hepatotoxic drugs. Treatment should be suspended if jaundice or symptoms of hepatic dysfunction occur. Some reports indicate symptoms began after

1-6 months of treatment. Hematologic effects, including pancytopenia (rare) and thrombocytopenia, have been reported. Associated with a high incidence of flu-like adverse effects; use of analgesics and/or antipyretics on treatment days may be helpful. Use caution in patients with pre-existing cardiovascular disease, pulmonary disease, seizure disorders, myelosuppression, or renal impairment. Some formulations contain albumin, which may carry a remote risk of transmitting Creutzfeldt-Jakob or other viral diseases. Safety and efficacy in patients <18 years of age have not been established.

Dosage Forms Combination package [preservative free] (Rebif® Titration Pack):

Injection, solution: 8.8 mcg/0.2 mL (0.2 mL) [6 prefilled syringes; contains albumin]

Injection, solution: 22 mcg/0.5 mL (0.5 mL) [6 prefilled syringes; contains albumin]

Injection, powder for reconstitution (Avonex®): 33 mcg [6.6 million units; provides 30 mcg/mL following reconstitution] [contains albumin; packaged with SWFI, alcohol wipes, and access pin and needle]

Injection, solution (Avonex®): 30 mcg/0.5 mL (0.5 mL) [albumin free; prefilled syringe; syringe cap contains latex; packaged with alcohol wipes, gauze pad, and adhesive bandages]

Injection, solution [preservative free] (Rebif®): 22 mcg/0.5 mL (0.5 mL) [prefilled syringe; contains albumin]; 44 mcg/0.5 mL (0.5 mL) [prefilled syringe; contains albumin]

Reference Range Mean serum interferon beta-1a levels during therapy range from 76.8 int. unit/mL to 94.8 int. unit/mL

Overdosage/Treatment Treatment is supportive

Drug Interactions

ACE inhibitors: Interferons may increase the adverse/toxic effects of ACE inhibitors, specifically the development of granulocytopenia; monitor.

Hepatotoxic drugs: May increase the risk of hepatic injury in patients receiving interferon beta-1a.

Warfarin: Interferons may increase the anticoagulant effects of warfarin; monitor.

Zidovudine: Interferons may decrease the metabolism of zidovudine; monitor.

Pregnancy Risk Factor C

Pregnancy Implications There are no adequate and well-controlled studies in pregnant women. Consideration should be given to discontinue treatment if a woman becomes pregnant, or plans to become pregnant during therapy. A dose-related abortifacient activity was reported in Rhesus monkeys. Healthcare providers are encouraged to register pregnant women receiving Rebif® during pregnancy online at www.rebifpregnancyregistry.com or by telephone at MS LifeLines 1-877-44-REBIF. A registry has been established for women who become pregnant while receiving Avonex®. Women may be enrolled in the registry by calling 1-800-456-2255.

Lactation Excretion in breast milk unknown/not recommended

Nursing Implications Suicidal ideations, and the risk of abortion; flu-like symptoms such as chills, fever, malaise, diaphoresis, and myalgia are common

Specific References

Falcone NP, Nappo A, and Neuteboom B, "Interferon Beta-1a Overdose in a Multiple Sclerosis Patient," *Ann Pharmacother*, 2005, 39(11): 1950-2.

Interferon Beta-1b

CAS Number 9008-11-1

U.S. Brand Names Betaseron®

Synonyms rIFN beta-1b

Use Treatment of relapsing forms of multiple sclerosis (MS)

Mechanism of Action Interferon beta-1b differs from naturally occurring human protein by a single amino acid substitution and the lack of carbohydrate side chains; alters the expression and response to surface antigens and can enhance immune cell activities. Properties of interferon beta-1b that modify biologic responses are mediated by cell surface receptor interactions; mechanism in the treatment of MS is unknown.

Adverse Reactions

Note: Flu-like symptoms (including at least two of the following - headache, fever, chills, malaise, diaphoresis, and myalgias) are reported in the majority of patients (60%) and decrease over time (average duration ~1 week).

Cardiovascular: **Peripheral edema, chest pain**, palpitation, vasodilation, hypertension, tachycardia, peripheral vascular disorder, arrhythmia, cardiac arrest, cardiomegaly, cerebral hemorrhage, heart failure, MI, pericardial effusion, shock, syncope, DVT, capillary leak syndrome

Central nervous system: **Headache (57%), fever (36%), pain (51%), chills (25%), dizziness (24%), insomnia (24%), anxiety,** malaise, nervousness, coma, delirium, hallucinations, hypothermia, manic reaction, psychosis, ataxia, confusion, convulsion, depersonalization, emotional lability

Dermatologic: **Rash (24%), skin disorder,** alopecia, erythema nodosum, exfoliative dermatitis, skin necrosis, photosensitivity, psoriasis, rash

(maculopapular and vesiculobullous), pruritus, skin discoloration, urticaria

Endocrine & metabolic: **Metrorrhagia**, menorrhagia, dysmenorrhea, diabetes mellitus, diabetes insipidus, hypercalcemia, hyperglycemia, hypoglycemia, hypothyroidism, SIADH, hyperthyroidism, hyperuricemia, hypocalcemia, thyroid dysfunction, triglyceride increased

Gastrointestinal: **Nausea (27%), diarrhea (19%), abdominal pain (19%), constipation (20%), dyspepsia,** esophagitis, gastrointestinal hemorrhage, hematemesis, pancreatitis, vomiting

Genitourinary: **Urinary urgency,** impotence, pelvic pain, cystitis, urinary frequency, weight gain, prostatic disorder, vaginal hemorrhage, urosepsis, urinary tract infection

Hematologic: **Lymphopenia (88%), neutropenia, leukopenia,** lymphadenopathy, anemia, thrombocytopenia

Hepatic: **SGPT increased >5x baseline,** SGOT increased >5x baseline, cholecystitis, hepatitis, hepatomegaly, gamma GT increase

Local: **Injection site reaction (85%), inflammation (53%), pain,** injection site necrosis, edema, mass

Neuromuscular & skeletal: **Weakness (61%), myalgia (27%), hypertonia (50%), myasthenia (46%), arthralgia (31%), incoordination (21%),** leg cramps, tremor, paresthesia

Ocular: Blindness

Renal: Renal calculus

Respiratory: Dyspnea, apnea, asthma, pulmonary embolism, bronchospasm, pneumonia

Miscellaneous: **Flu-like symptoms (60%),** diaphoresis, hypersensitivity, anaphylactoid reaction, ethanol intolerance, sepsis

Signs and Symptoms of Overdose No human cases; probable response would be atrial tachycardia, confusion, cough, depression, disorientation, dry mouth, fever, hyperkalemia, hypocalcemia, hypotension, pemphigus, personality changes, nausea, vomiting

Pharmacodynamics/Kinetics

Limited data due to small doses used

Half-life elimination: 8 minutes to 4.3 hours

Time to peak, serum: 1-8 hours

Dosage

SubQ:

Children <18 years: Not recommended

Adults >18 years: 0.25 mg (8 million units) every other day

Monitoring Parameters Hemoglobin, liver function, and blood chemistries

Administration Withdraw 1 mL of reconstituted solution from the vial into a sterile syringe fitted with a 27-gauge needle and inject the solution subcutaneously; sites for self-injection include arms, abdomen, hips, and thighs

Contraindications Hypersensitivity to *E. coli*-derived products, natural or recombinant interferon beta, albumin human, or any other component of the formulation

Warnings Hepatotoxicity has been reported with all beta interferons, including rare reports of hepatitis (autoimmune) and hepatic failure requiring transplant. Interferons have been associated with severe psychiatric adverse events (psychosis, mania, depression, suicidal behavior/ideation) in patients with and without previous psychiatric symptoms, avoid use in severe psychiatric disorders and use caution in patients with a history of depression; patients exhibiting symptoms of depression should be closely monitored and discontinuation of therapy should be considered. Due to high incidence of flu-like adverse effects, use caution in patients with pre-existing cardiovascular disease, pulmonary disease, seizure disorders, myelosuppression, renal impairment or hepatic impairment. Severe injection site reactions (necrosis) may occur, which may or may not heal with continued therapy; patient and/or caregiver competency in injection technique should be confirmed and periodically re-evaluated. Safety and efficacy in patients <18 years of age have not been established.

Dosage Forms Injection, powder for reconstitution [preservative free]: 0.3 mg [9.6 million units] [contains albumin; packaged with prefilled syringe containing diluent]

Overdosage/Treatment

Decontamination: Not necessary

Supportive therapy: Fever/chills can be treated with acetaminophen or nonsteroidal anti-inflammatory agent (indomethacin); hypotension can be treated with crystalloid infusion

Enhancement of elimination: Hemodialysis is not useful

Drug Interactions

ACE inhibitors: Interferons may increase the adverse/toxic effects of ACE inhibitors, specifically the development of granulocytopenia. Risk: Monitor

Warfarin: Interferons may increase the anticoagulant effects of warfarin. Risk: Monitor

Zidovudine: Interferons may decrease the metabolism of zidovudine. Risk: Monitor

Pregnancy Risk Factor C

Pregnancy Implications A dose-related abortifacient activity was reported in Rhesus monkeys. There are no adequate and well-controlled studies in pregnant women. Treatment should be discontinued if a woman becomes pregnant, or plans to become pregnant during therapy.

Lactation Excretion in breast milk unknown/contraindicated

Nursing Implications Patient should be informed of possible side effects, especially depression, suicidal ideations, and the risk of abortion; flu-like symptoms such as chills, fever, malaise, sweating, and myalgia are common

Additional Information May be available only in small supplies

Interferon Gamma-1b

CAS Number 98059-61-1

U.S. Brand Names Actimmune®

Use Reduce frequency and severity of serious infections associated with chronic granulomatous disease; delay time to disease progression in patients with severe, malignant osteopetrosis

Unlabeled/Investigational Use Chronic lymphocytic leukemia, Hodgkin's disease, rheumatoid arthritis; may be useful in treatment for congenital osteopetrosis, toxoplasmosis, hyper-IgE states

Mechanism of Action Increases bone resorption in osteopetrosis

Adverse Reactions

Similar neurotoxic effects (neurobehavioral changes) as with interferon alfa

Cardiovascular: Tachycardia, cardiac arrhythmias, hypotension, edema, syncope, cardiac ectopy, chest pain, fibrillation (atrial), flutter (atrial), sinus tachycardia, tachycardia (supraventricular)

Central nervous system: **Fatigue/malaise, fever, headache, chills**, dizziness, CNS depression, confusion, sensory neuropathy, psychiatric effects, seizures, in patients with brain metastasis, EEG abnormalities, parkinsonian syndrome, memory disturbance, multiple sclerosis

Dermatologic: **Rash**, partial alopecia, pruritus, erythema nodosum leprosum, exacerbation of psoriasis

Endocrine & metabolic: Uric acid level (elevated)

Gastrointestinal: **Nausea, vomiting, diarrhea**, anorexia, xerostomia, abdominal cramps, stomatitis, sore throat, weight loss, flatulence, change in taste, flatulence

Hematologic: Leukopenia (mainly neutropenia), anemia, thrombocytopenia, decreased hemoglobin, hematocrit, platelets

Hepatic: Elevation of ALT and AST

Neuromuscular & skeletal: Myalgia, arthralgia, rigors, polymyositis (dermatomyositis)

Ocular: Blurred vision

Renal: Proteinuria, creatinine/BUN (elevated), oliguric or nonoliguric renal failure

Respiratory: Coughing, nasal congestion

Miscellaneous: Neutralizing antibodies, diaphoresis, systemic lupus erythematosus (SLE)

Signs and Symptoms of Overdose AV block, depression, hyperglycemia, hypertriglyceridemia, hypocalcemia, leukopenia or neutropenia (agranulocytosis, granulocytopenia), metallic taste, memory loss, wheezing

Pharmacodynamics/Kinetics

Absorption: I.M., SubQ: Slowly

Half-life elimination: I.V.: 38 minutes; I.M., SubQ: 3-6 hours

Time to peak, plasma: I.M.: 4 hours (1.5 ng/mL); SubQ: 7 hours (0.6 ng/mL)

Dosage

If severe reactions occur, modify dose (50% reduction) or therapy should be discontinued until adverse reactions abate.

Chronic granulomatous disease: Children >1 year and Adults: SubQ:

BSA ≤0.5 m^2: 1.5 mcg/kg/dose 3 times/week

BSA >0.5 m^2: 50 mcg/m^2 (1 million int. units/m^2) 3 times/week

Severe, malignant osteopetrosis: Children >1 year: SubQ:

BSA ≤0.5 m^2: 1.5 mcg/kg/dose 3 times/week

BSA >0.5 m^2: 50 mcg/m^2 (1 million int. units/m^2) 3 times/week

Note: Previously expressed as 1.5 million units/m^2; 50 mcg is equivalent to 1 million int. units/m^2.

Monitoring Parameters CBC with differential, platelets, LFTs, electrolytes, BUN, creatinine, and urinalysis prior to therapy and at 3-month intervals

Contraindications Hypersensitivity to interferon gamma, *E. coli* derived proteins, or any component of the formulation

Warnings Patients with pre-existing cardiac disease, seizure disorders, CNS disturbances, or myelosuppression should be carefully monitored; long-term effects on growth and development are unknown; safety and efficacy in children <1 year of age have not been established.

Dosage Forms Injection, solution [preservative free]: 100 mcg [2 million int. units] (0.5 mL)

Previously, 100 mcg was expressed as 3 million units. This is equivalent to 2 million int. units.

Reference Range Peak serum level after an I.V. dose of 3000 mcg/m^2: 7.4-9.6 ng/mL

Overdosage/Treatment

Supportive therapy: Indomethacin or acetaminophen can be given for fever; avoid glucocorticoids

---

Enhancement of elimination: Hemodialysis is not useful

Test Interactions

Hypertriglyceridemia; rarely causes hyponatremia, hyperglycemia, hypocalcemia

Drug Interactions Inhibits CYP1A2 (weak), 2E1 (weak)

Pregnancy Risk Factor C

Pregnancy Implications Safety and efficacy in pregnant women has not been established. Treatment should be discontinued if a woman becomes pregnant, or plans to become pregnant during therapy. A dose-related abortifacient activity was reported in Rhesus monkeys.

Lactation Excretion in breast milk unknown/contraindicated

Additional Information More heat- and acid-labile than alfa interferons

Iodine

Pronunciation (EYE oh dyne)

Related Information

● Toxins Which Should Be Lavaged with Solutions Other Than Water

CAS Number 7553-56-2

U.S. Brand Names Iodex [OTC]; Iodoflex™; Iodosorb®

Use Preoperatively to reduce vascularity of the thyroid gland prior to thyroidectomy; management of thyrotoxic crisis or recurrent hyperthyroidism; venous sclerosing agent; topical disinfectant; also found in marine life; as a water disinfectant

Mechanism of Action Free iodine oxidizes microbial protoplasm making it effective against bacteria, fungi, yeasts, protozoa, and viruses; complexes with amino groups in tissue compounds to form iodophors from which the iodine is slowly released causing a sustained action

Adverse Reactions

Cardiovascular: Sinus tachycardia

Central nervous system: Fever, headache, hyperthermia

Dermatologic: Skin rash, angioedema, acne, contact dermatitis, erythema, nonimmunologic contact urticaria

Endocrine & metabolic: Hypothyroidism, hypercalcemia, Hashimoto's disease, Graves' disease, autoimmune thyroid disease, thyroiditis, thyrotoxic periodic paralysis

Gastrointestinal: Diarrhea, metallic taste, fecal discoloration (black),

Hematologic: Eosinophilia, hemorrhage (mucosal)

Hepatic: Elevation of serum transaminases and bilirubin

Neuromuscular & skeletal: Arthralgia

Ocular: Edema of eyelids

Respiratory: Pulmonary edema

Miscellaneous: Lymph node enlargement, hypersalivation, lymphadenopathy

Signs and Symptoms of Overdose Acneiform rash, agranulocytosis, circulation collapse, cough, dysphagia, elevated serum osmolarity, fever, gastroenteritis, granulocytopenia, hypercalcemia, hypernatremia, hypotension, hypothyroidism, leukopenia, metabolic acidosis with increased lactic acid, nausea, neutropenia, periarteritis nodosa, renal failure (acute), sexual dysfunction, swelling of glottis or larynx, tachycardia, urine discoloration (blue-green), vomiting

Admission Criteria/Prognosis Any evidence of gastrointestinal or systemic toxicity, or any symptomatic patient should be admitted; asymptomatic patients after 6 hours of observation may be discharged if electrolyte status is normal

Pharmacodynamics/Kinetics

Absorption: Topical: Amount absorbed systemically depends upon concentration and characteristics of skin

Distribution: Primarily trapped by the thyroid

Bioavailability: Oral: >90%

Excretion: Urine (>90%)

Dosage Adults: RDA: 150 mg; apply topically as necessary to affected areas of skin

Monitoring Parameters Renal function, acid base status, electrolytes, CBC

Administration Topical: Iodosorb®: Apply $^1/_8$" to $^1/_4$" thickness to dry sterile gauze, then place prepared gauze onto clean wound. Change dressing when gel changes color from brown to yellow/gray (~3 times/week). Remove with sterile water, saline, or wound cleanser; gently blot fluid from surface leaving wound slightly moist before reapplying gel.

Contraindications Hypersensitivity to iodine or any component of the formulation

Iodosorb®, Iodoflex™: Hashimoto thyroiditis, history of Grave's disease, or nontoxic nodular goiter; pregnancy; breast-feeding

Warnings Not for application to large areas of the body or for use with tight or air-excluding bandages. Use caution with renal dysfunction. When used for self-medication (OTC), do not use on deep wounds, puncture wounds, animal bites, or serious burns without consulting with healthcare provider. Notify healthcare provider if condition does not improve within 7 days. Iodosorb® is for use as topical application to wet wounds only.

Dosage Forms

Dressing, topical [gel pad] (Iodoflex™): 0.9% (5 g, 10 g)

Gel, topical (Iodosorb®): 0.9% (40 g)

Ointment, topical (Iodex): 4.7% (30 g, 720 g)

Tincture, topical: 2% (30 mL, 480 mL); 7% (30 mL, 480 mL)

Reference Range

Iodide levels >200 mcg/L (1.6 µmol/L) can inhibit iodide uptake in the normal thyroid gland (Note: Iodide refers to the reduced form of iodine); postmortem blood iodine level of 146,000 mcg/L associated with fatality due to iodine overdose

Approximate normal range: Total blood iodine: 5-8 mcg/dL

Protein bound iodine: 3-6 mcg/dL

Postmortem protein bound iodine levels >1000 mcg/dL associated with suicidal fatalities due to iodine

Overdosage/Treatment

Decontamination: **Do not** use ipecac; activated charcoal is useful; gastric lavage (within 1 hour) with starch or 1% to 5% sodium thiosulfate will aid in removal (purple color of effluent)

Dermal: Wash skin with soap and water

Ocular: Irrigate copiously with saline

Supportive therapy: Endoscopy may be required to evaluate gastrointestinal hemorrhage or burns. Systemic corticosteroids may be useful in treating fungating ioderma, or gastrointestinal stricture formation.

Enhancement of elimination: Can be enhanced with sodium chloride induced diuresis

Antidote(s)

- Potassium Iodide [ANTIDOTE]
- Sodium Thiosulfate [ANTIDOTE]

Test Interactions Interferes with thyroid function tests; falsely elevates chloride concentrations; may cause false-positive urinary dipstick for hematuria

Pregnancy Risk Factor D

Pregnancy Implications May lead to cretinism

Lactation Enters breast milk/use caution (AAP rates "compatible")

Nursing Implications Avoid tight bandages because iodine may cause burns on occluded skin

Additional Information IDLH - 10 ppm; iodophors/iodoform have low toxicity; acrid odor with sharp taste; taste threshold: 1.5-2 mg/L; vapor is violet when heated; lithium blood levels increase during caffeine withdrawal; amount of iodine required for water disinfectant: 2-8 ppm

Specific References

Iyengar GV, Kawamura H, Dang HS, et al, "Dietary Intakes of Seven Elements of Importance in Radiological Protection by Asian Population: Comparison with ICRP Data," *Health Phys*, 2004, 86(6):557-64.

Jones CW, Kuntz DJ, and Feldman MS, "Urine Adulteration Testing for Iodine by HPLC," *J Anal Toxicol*, 2004, 28:297.

Kane MP and Busch RS, "Drug-Induced Thyrotoxic Periodic Paralysis," *Ann Pharmacother*, 2006, 40(4):778-81.

Paul BD and Jacobs A, "Spectrophotometric Detection of Iodide in Urine After Oxidation to Iodine," *J Anal Toxicol*, 2006, 30:153.

Iopanoic Acid

Pronunciation (eye oh pa NOE ik AS id)

CAS Number 96-83-3

U.S. Brand Names Biliopaco®; Cistobil®; Neocontrast®; Telepaque®

Synonyms Acidum Iopanoicum; Iodopanoic Acid

Use Radiocontrast agent for biliary tract

Mechanism of Toxic Action Contains ~66% iodine which is radiopaque

Adverse Reactions

Cardiovascular: Flushing

Central nervous system: Dizziness, headache

Dermatologic: Urticaria, pruritus

Endocrine & metabolic: Thyroid storm

Genitourinary: Dysuria

Hematologic: Thrombocytopenia

Renal: Renal failure, oliguria, proximal tubular necrosis

Miscellaneous: Anaphylactoid reactions, serum sickness

Signs and Symptoms of Overdose Diarrhea, hypotension, nausea, tachycardia, syncope, vomiting

Toxicodynamics/Kinetics

Absorption: 10 hours

Protein binding: 97%

Metabolism: Hepatic glucuronidation

Half-life: 12-20 hours

Elimination: Renal: 35%. Fecal: 22% to 65%

Peak opacification: 14-19 hours

Monitoring Parameters Kidney function, blood pressure, uric acid

Contraindications Known hypersensitivity to iopanoic acid

Use with caution in patients who have hyperthyroidism, hyperuricemia, cholangitis, renal impairment (maximum dose for renal impairment: 3 g), and coronary artery disease

Dosage Forms Tablet: 500 mg (6/package)

Reference Range Iodide levels >200 mcg/L (1.6 µmol/L) can inhibit iodide uptake in the normal thyroid gland. (Note that iodide refers to the reduced form of iodine.) Postmortem blood iodine level of 146,000 mcg/L associated with fatality due to iodine overdose.

Overdosage/Treatment

Decontamination: Lavage within 1 hour. Cholestyramine may aid in preventing absorption. **Do not** induce emesis. Activated charcoal may be useful in lieu of cholestyramine to prevent iodine absorption.

Supportive therapy: Corticosteroids can be utilized to treat thrombocytopenia; however, thrombocytopenia will usually resolve in 6-9 days.

Enhanced elimination: Urine output should be monitored to prevent renal blockage from uric acid. Alkalinization of the urine has been advocated to increase iopanoic acid solubility; however, this modality has not been proven in an overdose setting. Due to its glucuronide conjugate undergoing enterohepatic recirculation, multiple doses of activated charcoal or cholestyramine may be effective.

Test Interactions May produce falsely elevated TSH values (usually <10 units/L); causes a falsely increased free thyroxine level

Drug Interaction Aspirin can inhibit uricosuric effect of iopanoic acid as can pyrazinamide

Pregnancy Risk Factor D

Additional Information

Oral ingestions up to 75 g have been documented with complete recovery. Radiopaque; insoluble in water; contains 333 mg of iodine per tablet; has uricosuric and anticholinesterase effects agent.

How supplied: Tablets: 500 mg

Ipratropium

CAS Number 22254-24-6; 66985-17-9

U.S. Brand Names Atrovent®

Synonyms Ipratropium Bromide

Use Anticholinergic bronchodilator used in bronchospasm associated with COPD, bronchitis, and emphysema; symptomatic relief of rhinorrhea associated with the common cold and allergic and nonallergic rhinitis

Mechanism of Action Blocks the action of acetylcholine at parasympathetic sites in bronchial smooth muscle causing bronchodilation

Adverse Reactions

Cardiovascular: Palpitations, sinus tachycardia, tachycardia (supraventricular)

Central nervous system: **Nervousness**, anxiety, **dizziness, headache, fatigue**, insomnia, mania, paranoia

Dermatologic: Rash

Gastrointestinal: **Nausea, xerostomia, bitter taste**, buccal ulceration, paralytic ileus, **stomach upset**

Ocular: Blurred vision, exacerbation of closed-angle glaucoma, mydriasis

Respiratory: **Cough**, paradoxical wheezing

Pharmacodynamics/Kinetics

Onset of action: Bronchodilation: 1-3 minutes

Peak effect: 1.5-2 hours

Duration: ≤4 hours

Absorption: Negligible

Distribution: Inhalation: 15% of dose reaches lower airways

Dosage

Children >12 years and Adults: 2 inhalations 4 times/day up to 12 inhalations/24 hours

Rhinorrhea and sneezing due to the common cold: Ipratropium bromide nasal spray (0.06%) in buffered salt solution; two 42 mcg sprays/nostril

Administration Atrovent®: Shake inhaler before each use; rinsing mouth after each use decreases dry mouth side effect

Atrovent® HFA: Prime inhaler by releasing 2 test sprays into the air. If the inhaler has not been used for >3 days, reprime.

Contraindications Hypersensitivity to ipratropium, atropine, its derivatives, or any component of the formulation

In addition, Atrovent® inhalation aerosol is contraindicated in patients with hypersensitivity to soya lecithin or related food products (eg, soybean and peanut). **Note:** Other formulations may include these components; refer to product-specific labeling.

Warnings Not indicated for the initial treatment of acute episodes of bronchospasm; use with caution in patients with myasthenia gravis, narrow-angle glaucoma, benign prostatic hyperplasia (BPH), or bladder neck obstruction

Dosage Forms

[DSC] = Discontinued product

Aerosol for oral inhalation, as bromide (Atrovent®): 18 mcg/actuation (14 g) [contains soya lecithin and chlorofluorocarbons] [DSC]

Aerosol for oral inhalation, as bromide (Atrovent® HFA): 17 mcg/actuation (12.9 g)

Solution for nebulization, as bromide: 0.02% (2.5 mL)

Solution, intranasal, as bromide [spray] (Atrovent®): 0.03% (30 mL); 0.06% (15 mL)

Reference Range Inhalation of 555 mcg of ipratropium results in peak plasma concentration of 0.06 ng/mL (0.03% of inhaled dose)

Overdosage/Treatment Supportive therapy: Physostigmine should be administered for life-threatening anticholinergic poisoning, although formal studies are lacking; bethanechol (5-10 mg 3 times/day) can be given for peripheral anticholinergic side effects; esmolol can be used for tachyarrhythmia

Antidote(s)
- Physostigmine [ANTIDOTE]

Drug Interactions Anticholinergics: Concurrent use with ipratropium may increase risk of adverse events.

Pregnancy Risk Factor B

Pregnancy Implications Teratogenic effects were not observed in animal studies.

Lactation Excretion in breast milk unknown/use caution

Specific References
Peterson GM, Boyles PJ, Bleasel MD, et al, "Ipratropium Treatment of Acute Airways Disease," *Ann Pharmacother*, 2003, 37(3):339-44.

Irinotecan

U.S. Brand Names Camptosar®

Synonyms Camptothecin-11; CPT-11; NSC-616348

Use Treatment of metastatic carcinoma of the colon or rectum

Unlabeled/Investigational Use Lung cancer (small cell and nonsmall cell), cervical cancer, gastric cancer, pancreatic cancer, leukemia, lymphoma, breast cancer

Mechanism of Action A derivative of camptothecin from the Oriental tree *Camptotheca acuminata*; irinotecan inhibits the enzyme topoisomerase I which is involved in structural maintenance of DNA

Adverse Reactions
Cardiovascular: Flushing, sinus bradycardia, **vasodilation**
Central nervous system: **Insomnia, dizziness, fever**
Dermatologic: **Alopecia**, rash
Gastrointestinal: **Diarrhea** (may be severe), nausea, vomiting, **abdominal pain or cramps, anorexia, constipation, flatulence, stomatitis, dyspepsia**
Hematologic: **Myelosuppression**, anemia, thrombocytopenia, **neutropenia**
Neuromuscular & skeletal: **Weakness**
Ocular: Lacrimation
Respiratory: **Dyspnea, coughing, rhinitis**
Miscellaneous: **Diaphoresis**

Pharmacodynamics/Kinetics
Distribution: V_d: 33-150 L/m^2
Protein binding, plasma: Predominantly albumin; Parent drug: 30% to 68%, SN-38 (active drug): ~95%
Metabolism: Primarily hepatic to SN-38 (active metabolite) by carboxylesterase enzymes; SN-38 undergoes conjugation by UDP- glucuronosyl transferase 1A1 (UGT1A1) to form a glucuronide metabolite. SN-38 is increased by UGT1A1*28 polymorphism (10% of North Americans are homozygous for UGT1A1*28 allele). The lactones of both irinotecan and SN-38 undergo hydrolysis to inactive hydroxy acid forms.
Half-life elimination: SN-38: Mean terminal: 10-20 hours
Time to peak: SN-38: Following 90-minute infusion: ~1 hour
Excretion: Within 24 hours: Urine: Irinotecan (11% to 20%), metabolites (SN-38 <1%, SN-38 glucuronide, 3%)

Dosage Dosing regimens vary with usual dosage range of 40 mg/m^2/day to 250 mg/m^2/day up to a maximum of 750 mg/m^2/day; infusions are from 30-90 minutes and may vary from 3 times/week to weekly to every 3 weeks. See table.

Single-Agent Schedule: Recommended Dosage Modifications[1]

Toxicity NCI Grade[2] (Value)	During a Cycle of Therapy Weekly	At Start of Subsequent Cycles of Therapy (After Adequate Recovery), Compared to Starting Dose in Previous Cycle[1]	
		Weekly	Once Every 3 Weeks
No toxicity	Maintain dose level	↑ 25 mg/m^2 up to a maximum dose of 150 mg/m^2	Maintain dose level
Neutropenia			
1 (1500-1999/mm^3)	Maintain dose level	Maintain dose level	Maintain dose level
2 (1000-1499/mm^3)	↓ 25 mg/m^2	Maintain dose level	Maintain dose level

Table *(Continued)*

Toxicity NCI Grade[2] (Value)	During a Cycle of Therapy Weekly	At Start of Subsequent Cycles of Therapy (After Adequate Recovery), Compared to Starting Dose in Previous Cycle[1]	
		Weekly	Once Every 3 Weeks
3 (500-999/mm^3)	Omit dose until resolved to ≤ grade 2, then ↓ 25 mg/m^2	↓ 25 mg/m^2	↓ 50 mg/m^2
4 (<500/mm^3)	Omit dose until resolved to ≤ grade 2, then ↓ 50 mg/m^2	↓ 50 mg/m^2	↓ 50 mg/m^2
Neutropenic Fever (grade 4 neutropenia and ≥ grade 2 fever)	Omit dose until resolved, then ↓ 50 mg/m^2	↓ 50 mg/m^2	↓ 50 mg/m^2
Other Hematologic Toxicities	Dose modifications for leukopenia, thrombocytopenia, and anemia during a course of therapy and at the start of subsequent courses of therapy are also based on NCI toxicity criteria and are the same as recommended for neutropenia above.		
Diarrhea			
1 (2-3 stools/day > pretreatment)	Maintain dose level	Maintain dose level	Maintain dose level
2 (4-6 stools/day > pretreatment)	↓ 25 mg/m^2	Maintain dose level	Maintain dose level
3 (7-9 stools/day > pretreatment)	Omit dose until resolved to ≤ grade 2, then ↓ 25 mg/m^2	↓ 25 mg/m^2	↓ 50 mg/m^2
4 (≥10 stools/day > pretreatment)	Omit dose until resolved to ≤ grade 2, then ↓ 50 mg/m^2	↓ 50 mg/m^2	↓ 50 mg/m^2
Other Nonhematologic Toxicities[3]			
1	Maintain dose level	Maintain dose level	Maintain dose level
2	↓ 25 mg/m^2	↓ 25 mg/m^2	↓ 50 mg/m^2
3	Omit dose until resolved to ≤ grade 2, then ↓ 25 mg/m^2	↓ 25 mg/m^2	↓ 50 mg/m^2
4	Omit dose until resolved to ≤ grade 2, then ↓ 50 mg/m^2	↓ 50 mg/m^2	↓ 50 mg/m^2

[1]All dose modifications should be based on the worst preceding toxicity.
[2]National Cancer Institute Common Toxicity Criteria (version 1.0).
[3]Excludes alopecia, anorexia, asthenia.

Monitoring Parameters CBC with differential, platelet count, and hemoglobin with each dose

Administration Administer by I.V. infusion, usually over 90 minutes.

Contraindications Hypersensitivity to irinotecan or any component of the formulation; concurrent use of atazanavir, ketoconazole, St John's wort; pregnancy

Warnings
Hazardous agent – use appropriate precautions for handling and disposal. Severe hypersensitivity reactions have occurred.

[U.S. Boxed Warning]: May cause severe myelosuppression. Deaths due to sepsis following severe myelosuppression have been reported. Therapy should be temporarily discontinued if neutropenic fever occurs or if the absolute neutrophil count is <1000/mm^3. The dose of irinotecan should be reduced if there is a clinically significant decrease in the total WBC (<200/mm^3), neutrophil count (<1500/mm^3), hemoglobin (<8 g/dL), or platelet count (<100,000/mm^3). Routine administration of a colony-stimulating factor is generally not necessary, but may be considered for patients experiencing significant neutropenia.

Patients homozygous for the UGT1A1*28 allele are at increased risk of neutropenia; initial one-level dose reduction should be considered for both single-agent and combination regimens. Heterozygous carriers of the UGT1A1*28 allele may also be at increased risk; however, most patients have tolerated normal starting doses.

Patients with even modest elevations in total serum bilirubin levels (1.0-2.0 mg/dL) have a significantly greater likelihood of experiencing first-course grade 3 or 4 neutropenia than those with bilirubin levels that were <1.0 mg/dL. Patients with abnormal glucuronidation of bilirubin, such as those with Gilbert's syndrome, may also be at greater risk of myelosuppression when receiving therapy with irinotecan. Use caution when treating patients with known hepatic dysfunction or hyperbilirubinemia. Dosage adjustments should be considered.

Patients with diarrhea should be carefully monitored and treated promptly. **[U.S. Boxed Warning]: Severe diarrhea may be dose-limiting and potentially fatal; two severe (life-threatening) forms of diarrhea may occur.** Early diarrhea occurs during or within 24 hours of receiving irinotecan and is characterized by cholinergic symptoms (eg, increased salivation, diaphoresis, abdominal cramping); it is usually responsive to atropine. Late diarrhea occurs more than 24 hours after treatment which may lead to dehydration, electrolyte imbalance, or sepsis; it should be promptly treated with loperamide.

Patients should receive fluid and electrolyte replacement as indicated, or antibiotics if ileus, fever, or neutropenia develop. Hold diuretics during dosing due to potential risk of dehydration secondary to vomiting and/or diarrhea induced by irinotecan.

Use caution in patients who previously received pelvic/abdominal radiation, elderly patients with comorbid conditions, or baseline performance status of 2; close monitoring and dosage adjustments are recommended. **[U.S. Boxed Warning]: Should be administered under the supervision of an experienced cancer chemotherapy physician.**

Dosage Forms Injection, solution, as hydrochloride: 20 mg/mL (2 mL, 5 mL)
Camptosar®: 20 mg/mL (2 mL, 5 mL)

Overdosage/Treatment
Supportive therapy: Ondansetron (0.15 mg/kg I.V. or oral) with a corticosteroid is effective in preventing emesis; diphenhydramine can be used to decrease cholinergic reactions (lacrimation, sweating, flushing); loperamide (2 mg doses) is effective in treating diarrhea
Enhancement of elimination: Due to enterohepatic recirculation, multiple dosing of activated charcoal may be useful in enhancing clearance

Drug Interactions
Substrate (major) of CYP2B6, 3A4
Anticonvulsants (carbamazepine, phenobarbital, phenytoin): Decreases the therapeutic effect of irinotecan. Consider replacement of anticonvulsant with a nonenzyme-inducing agent ≥2 weeks prior to irinotecan therapy.
Atazanavir: May increase the levels/effects of irinotecan (SN-38) by CYP3A4 and UGT1A1 inhibition; avoid concurrent use.
Bevacizumab: May increase the adverse effects of irinotecan (eg, diarrhea, neutropenia).
CYP2B6 inducers: May decrease the levels/effects of irinotecan. Example inducers include carbamazepine, nevirapine, phenobarbital, phenytoin, and rifampin.
CYP2B6 inhibitors: May increase the levels/effects of irinotecan. Example inhibitors include desipramine, paroxetine, and sertraline.
CYP3A4 inducers: CYP3A4 inducers may decrease the levels/effects of irinotecan. Example inducers include aminoglutethimide, carbamazepine, nafcillin, nevirapine, phenobarbital, phenytoin, and rifamycins.
CYP3A4 inhibitors: May increase the levels/effects of irinotecan. Example inhibitors include azole antifungals, clarithromycin, diclofenac, doxycycline, erythromycin, imatinib, isoniazid, nefazodone, nicardipine, propofol, protease inhibitors, quinidine, telithromycin, and verapamil.
Ketoconazole: Increases the levels/effects of irinotecan and active metabolite. Discontinue ketoconazole 1 week prior to irinotecan therapy; **concurrent use is contraindicated.**
St John's wort: Decreases the therapeutic effect of irinotecan. Discontinue St John's wort ≥2 weeks prior to irinotecan therapy; **concurrent use is contraindicated.**

Pregnancy Risk Factor D
Pregnancy Implications Has shown to be teratogenic in animals. Teratogenic effects include a variety of external, visceral, and skeletal abnormalities. The patient should be warned of potential hazards to the fetus. Women of childbearing potential should avoid becoming pregnant while receiving treatment.
Lactation Excretion in breast milk unknown/not recommended
Additional Information Diarrhea is dose related; high doses of loperamide can increase tolerated dose of irinotecan; used in combination with fluorouracil and etoposide
Herb/Nutraceutical interaction: St John's wort may decrease the efficacy of irinotecan.

Specific References
Richards S, Umbreit JN, Fanucchi MP, et al, "Selective Serotonin Reuptake Inhibitor-Induced Rhabdomyolysis Associated with Irinotecan," *South Med J*, 2003, 96(10):1031-3.

Iron

CAS Number 1439-89-6
Synonyms Ferrous Fumarate; Ferrous Gluconate; Ferrous Sulfate; Iron Dextran Complex
Commonly Includes Ferrous sulfate, ferrous gluconate, ferrous fumarate, ferrous chloride, ferrous carbonate, ferrous chloride
Use Prevention and/or treatment of iron deficiency anemias; prenatal supplementation
Mechanism of Action Essential component of hemoglobin, myoglobin, and multiple enzymes; supplementation is given to replenish lost iron stores
Adverse Reactions
Anaphylactoid reactions: Respiratory difficulties and cardiovascular collapse have been reported and occur most frequently within the first several minutes of administration
Cardiovascular: Hypotension, myocardial depression, **flushing**, tachycardia, congestive heart failure, sinus tachycardia, vasodilation
Central nervous system: **Dizziness, fever, headache, chills**
Dermatologic: Urticaria, pustular drug eruption
Gastrointestinal: **Nausea, metallic taste, vomiting**, GI irritation, abdominal pain, diarrhea, dark stools, heartburn, esophagitis
Hematologic: Leukocytosis
Hepatic: Steatosis
Local: **Pain, staining of skin at the site of I.M. injection**, phlebitis
Neuromuscular & skeletal: Arthralgia
Renal: Hematuria
Respiratory: Aspiration
Miscellaneous: Lymphadenopathy, liquid preparations may temporarily stain the teeth, **diaphoresis**
Note: Diaphoresis, rash, arthralgia, fever, chills, dizziness, headache, and nausea may be delayed 24-48 hours after I.V. administration or 3-4 days after I.M. administration
Signs and Symptoms of Overdose Acidosis, acute GI irritation, bezoars, coagulopathy, coma, drowsiness, erosion of GI mucosa, esophageal ulceration, feces discoloration (black; green), fever, hematemesis, hematuria, hepatic and renal impairment, hyperthermia, hyperventilation, hypoglycemia, sedation, sweating, urine discoloration (black)
There are essentially five stages of iron poisoning:
Stage I (30 minutes to 6 hours): Predominately GI irritation, due primarily to the corrosive effect of iron; drowsiness, epigastric pain, GI bleeding, hypotension, nausea, and vomiting may occur. Hyperglycemia, leukocytosis, or metabolic acidosis may be present (due to vasodilatation).
Stage II (6-24 hours): A latent period of symptom quiescence during which symptomatic improvement may be noted; in severe poisonings, there may be no latent period
Stage III (6-48 hours): Metabolic and systemic derangement occur with cardiovascular collapse, coagulopathy (inhibition of thrombin and fibrinogen), coma, and seizures. Pulmonary edema may occur due to cardiac failure.
Stage IV (2-7 days): Hepatotoxicity (jaundice) and coagulopathy occur; metabolic acidosis is present, and renal insufficiency may occur
Stage V (1-8 weeks): Primarily delayed GI complications, including gastric/duodenal fibrosis resulting in obstructive pattern; achlorhydria may develop
Admission Criteria/Prognosis Admit patients with hypotension, abdominal pain, acidosis, nervous system abnormalities, serum iron levels >350 mcg/dL, positive abdominal radiographs, or ingestions >60 mg/kg of elemental iron
Pharmacodynamics/Kinetics
Total body stores are 3-4 g
Absorption: In ferrous state (Fe^{2+}) in duodenum and jejunum
Distribution: 70% as ferrous state in hemoglobin, 25% in ferric state as ferritin or hemosiderin, 0.1% in ferric state in plasma
Elimination: ≈1 mg/day of iron is lost via urinary excretion, skin desquamation; this may increase to 2 mg/day when iron accumulates
Dosage
Oral **(dose expressed in terms of elemental iron):**
Recommended daily allowance:
Male: 10 mg
Female: 18 mg
Pregnancy and lactation: 30-60 mg
Iron replacement:
Infants: 10-25 mg/day in 3-4 divided doses
Children:
6 months to 2 years: Up to 6 mg/kg/day in 3-4 divided doses
2-12 years: 3 mg/kg/day given 3-4 times/day
Adults: 2-3 mg/kg/day given 3 times/day

I.M. (Z-track method should be used for I.M. injection), **I.V.:**

A 0.5 mL test dose (0.25 mL in infants) should be given prior to starting iron dextran therapy; total dose should be divided into a daily schedule for I.M., total dose may be given as a single continuous infusion

Contraindications Hemosiderosis, hemochromatosis, hemolytic anemia, peptic ulcer disease, ulcerative colitis

Warnings Some products contain tartrazine which may cause allergic reactions

Dosage Forms

Amount of elemental iron is listed in brackets

Ferrous fumarate:

Capsule, controlled release (Span-FF®): 325 mg [106 mg]

Drops (Feostat®): 45 mg/0.6 mL [15 mg/0.6 mL] (60 mL)

Suspension, oral (Feostat®): 100 mg/5 mL [33 mg/5 mL] (240 mL)

Tablet: 325 mg [106 mg]

Chewable (chocolate flavor) (Feostat®): 100 mg [33 mg]

Femiron®: 63 mg [20 mg]

Fumerin®: 195 mg [64 mg]

Fumasorb®, Ircon®: 200 mg [66 mg]

Hemocyte®: 324 mg [106 mg]

Nephro-Fer™: 350 mg [115 mg]

Timed release (Ferro-Sequels®): Ferrous fumarate 150 mg [50 mg] and docusate sodium 100 mg

Ferrous gluconate:

Capsule, soft gelatin (Simron®): 86 mg [10 mg]

Elixir (Fergon®): 300 mg/5 mL [34 mg/5 mL] with alcohol 7% (480 mL)

Tablet: 300 mg [34 mg]; 325 mg [38 mg]

Fergon®, Ferralet®: 320 mg [37 mg]

Sustained release (Ferralet® Slow Release): 320 mg [37 mg]

Ferrous sulfate:

Capsule:

Exsiccated (Fer-In-Sol®): 190 mg [60 mg]

Exsiccated, timed release (Feosol®): 159 mg [50 mg]

Exsiccated, timed release (Ferralyn® Lanacaps®, Ferra-TD®): 250 mg [50 mg]

Ferospace®: 250 mg [50 mg]

Drops, oral:

Fer-In-Sol®: 75 mg/0.6 mL [15 mg/0.6 mL] (50 mL)

Fer-Iron®: 125 mg/mL [25 mg/mL] (50 mL)

Elixir (Feosol®): 220 mg/5 mL [44 mg/5 mL] with alcohol 5% (473 mL, 4000 mL)

Powder for injection: Deferoxamine: 500 mg vials

Syrup (Fer-In-Sol®): 90 mg/5 mL [18 mg/5 mL] with alcohol 5% (480 mL)

Tablet: 324 mg [65 mg]

Exsiccated (Feosol®) 200 mg [65 mg]

Exsiccated, timed release (Slow FE®): 160 mg [50 mg]

Feratab®: 300 mg [60 mg]

Mol-Iron®: 195 mg [39 mg]

Timed release (Fero-Gradumet®): 525 mg [105 mg]

Iron dextran complex: InFed™ injection: 50 mg/mL (2 mL, 10 mL)

Reference Range

Levels >500 mcg/dL associated with toxicity; consider treatment with symptomatic levels ≥350 mcg/dL; peak values are 2-4 hours after ingestion; standard measurement of total iron binding capacity (TIBC) are unreliable and should not be used to assess the patient

Therapeutic: Male: 75-175 mcg/dL (SI: 13.4-31.3 µmol/L). Female: 65-165 mcg/dL (SI: 11.6-29.5 µmol/L); iron levels >300 mcg/dL can be considered toxic and should be treated as an overdose

Overdosage/Treatment

Determine amount of drug ingested based on mg/kg of elemental iron; doses <20 mg/kg are minimal to no toxicity; 20-60 mg/kg are mild to moderate; >60 mg/kg are potentially serious. See table.

Iron	
Overdosage	**Elemental Iron**
Ferrous sulfate (hydrated)	20%
Ferrous fumarate	33%
Ferrous gluconate	12%
Ferrous chloride (hydrated)	28%
Ferric chloride (hydrated)	20%

Decontamination: Lavage within 1 hour with normal saline and/or whole bowel irrigation with polyethylene glycol electrolyte solution (GoLYTELY®); use WBI if radiopaque tablets present on KUB; charcoal is ineffective unless it is a multiple drug ingestion; oral deferoxamine is not effective

Supportive therapy: Shock can be treated with I.V. crystalloid fluids, blood products may be necessary; following treatment for fluid losses, metabolic acidosis, and shock, a severe iron overdose may be treated with deferoxamine. Deferoxamine may be administered I.V. (10-15 mg/kg/hour) or I.M. (40-90 mg/kg every 8 hours). Lethal dose of elemental iron is 180-300 mg/kg.

Antidote: Deferoxamine is a chelating agent for iron; it binds free iron and some iron bound to ferritin and hemosiderin; the complex of iron and deferoxamine (ferrioxamine) is then excreted renally with a "vin rosé" color; color change is dependent on pH and concentrations with basic pH and higher concentrations being positively associated with the change in color. Indications for deferoxamine therapy include asymptomatic serum iron concentrations >500 mcg/dL, radiopaque tablets on abdominal x-ray; symptomatic patients with iron levels >350 mcg/dL, persistent symptoms, acidosis, hypovolemia, mental status changes or abdominal pain.

Obtain baseline serum iron level and urine sample. Administration via I.V. route is preferred; give at 15 mg/kg/hour by continuous infusion. Doses up to 50 mg/kg/hour have been used for severe ingestion. Maximum recommended dose is 6 g/day; however, higher doses have been given. Continuous infusion of 15 mg/kg/hour should not be continued for longer than 24 hours without a "drug holiday." Monitor urine for "vin rosé" color change compared to baseline.

Endpoints of therapy include change in urine color back to baseline, serum concentrations of iron <100 mg/dL, and/or resolution of symptoms; chelation therapy typically requires <24-hour duration

Antidote(s)

- Deferoxamine [ANTIDOTE]
- Polyethylene Glycol - High Molecular Weight [ANTIDOTE]

Diagnostic Procedures

- Iron and Total Iron Binding Capacity/Transferrin

Test Interactions Measured serum iron concentrations will be lowered in face of deferoxamine therapy; high serum iron may falsely increase total iron binding capacity (TIBC) for most common assay. Hemoccult® and Gastroccult® tests may be unreliable in detecting GI bleeding in iron overdose treated with whole bowel irrigation (ferrous sulfate/ferrous gluconate: false-positive; ascorbic acid: false-negative)

Drug Interactions Antacids decrease iron absorption; vitamin C increases gastrointestinal absorption; iron can inhibit tetracycline and penicillamine absorption

Pregnancy Risk Factor A; Deferoxamine: C

Pregnancy Implications Although placental transport is poor and treatment of iron overdose in pregnancy should not be harmful, untreated patients may result in fetal and/or maternal morbidity and mortality

Nursing Implications Always obtain baseline urine before administration of deferoxamine; I.V. infusion may be prepared in saline or glucose

Additional Information Lethal dose: Elemental iron: 180-300 mg/kg.

Oral chelation with deferoxamine is not recommended; chelation with deferoxamine in parenteral overdoses of iron dextran solutions may not be as necessary as compared to oral ingestions at similar dosages since the elemental iron binds directly to dextran; liver transplantation has been used for iron-induced hepatic failure 5 days after ingestion; largest reported volume of polyethylene glycol electrolyte solution for use for whole bowel irrigation in a toxic ingestion was 44.3 L (2953 mL/kg) over a 5-day period in a 33-month old boy who ingested at least 160 mg/kg elemental iron (initial serum iron level: 367 mcg/dL); optimal bowel cleansing in pediatric patients (age 0.5-12 years): 6-10 hours of therapy at a rate of 25-35 mL/kg/hour of polyethylene glycol

Representative Iron Products		
Iron Product	**Dosage Form(s)**	**Approximate Elemental Iron per Dosage Unit**
Ferrous sulfate	250 mg tablets	50 mg/tablet
	325 mg tablets	65 mg/tablet
	Timed-release tablets	65-105 mg/tablet
	Elixir 220 mg/5 mL	44 mg/5 mL
	Drops 75 mg/0.6 mL	15 mg/0.6 mL
Ferrous gluconate	240 mg tablets	28 mg/tablet
	300 mg/tablets	36 mg/tablet
	325 mg tablets	40 mg/tablet
Ferrous fumarate	100 mg chewable tablets	33 mg/tablet
	Timed-release tablets	50-110 mg/tablet
	200 mg tablets	65 mg/tablet
	325 mg tablets	107 mg/tablet
	350 mg tablets	115 mg/tablet
	Suspension 350 mg/5 mL	33 mg/5 mL
Multivitamin hematinic products	Tablet or capsule	65-150 mg/tablet
Prenatal vitamins with iron	Tablet or capsule	9-106 mg/tablet

Table (*Continued*)

Iron Product	Dosage Form(s)	Approximate Elemental Iron per Dosage Unit
Adult multiple vitamin plus iron	Tablet or capsule	3-110 mg/tablet
Pediatric multiple vitamin plus iron	Chewable tablet	10-18 mg/tablet
	Drops	10 mg/mL
	Liquid	10 mg/5 mL
Carbonyl iron	Tablets and capsules	50-66 mg/tablet or capsule
	Liquid	15 mg/1.25 mL
Polysaccharide-iron complex	Tablets	50-150 mg/tablet
	Capsules	150 mg/capsule
	Elixir	100 mg/5 mL

Summary of Iron Deaths Reported to TESS 1985-2002

Age	Stated Iron Product Ingested	Stated Dose	Serum Iron Concentrations mcg/dL (mmol/L)	Time Serum Iron Drawn After Ingestion
3 y	Ferrous sulfate 325 mg tablets	Unknown	3805 (681)	3 h
18 mo	Ferrous sulfate	Unknown	23,000 (4119)	6 h
10 mo	Ferrous sulfate	22 g	>7000 (>1254)	Unknown
15 mo	Ferrous sulfate 325 mg tablets	Unknown	1200 (215)	1 h
17 mo	Prenatal iron tablets	Unknown	25,000 (4477)	6 h
17 mo	Ferrous sulfate 325 mg tablets	Unknown	1400 (251)	4 h
22 mo	Iron tablets	Unknown	4674 (837)	Unknown
10 mo	Ferrous sulfate tablets	Unknown	18,930 (3390)	Unknown
11 mo	Ferrous sulfate tablets	Unknown	>10,000 (>1790)	2 h?
14 mo	Ferrous sulfate tablets	Unknown	>10,000 (>1790)	2 h
15 mo	Iron tablets	Unknown	383 (68)	>10 h
16 mo	Ferrous sulfate 325 mg tablets	>30 tablets	8500 (1522)	Unknown
9 mo	Ferrous sulfate 325 mg tablets	>20 tablets	3730 (668)	>6 h
12 mo	Ferrous sulfate 325 mg tablets	35-40 tablets	4023 (720)	4 h
14 mo	Ferrous sulfte 325 mg tablets	Unknown	2088 (374)	3-4 h
18 mo	Ferrous sulfate 325 mg tablets	40 tablets	1651 (296)	9 h
2 y	Ferrous sulfate	90 tablets	14,000 (2507)	Unknown
2 y	Ferrous sulfate	35 tablets	6350 (1137)	4 h
3 y	Ferrous sulfate 325 mg tablets	30 tablets	>10,000 (>1790)	4 h
3 y	Ferrous sulfate	Unknown	377 (68)	3 h
15 mo	Iron tablets	Unknown	>400 (>72)	>24 h
17 mo	Prenatal vitamins with iron (65 mg Fe/tab)	"Whole bottle"	18,150 (3250)	Unknown
18 mo	Prenatal vitamins with iron (65 Fe/tab)	"4-5 tablets" (likely an underestimation)	>1000 (>179)	4.5 h
12 mo	Iron tablets	Unknown	1555 (278)	30 min
19 mo	Iron tablets (65 mg Fe)	35 tablets	6000 (1074)	1 h
15 mo	Prenatal vitamins with iron (325 mg ferrous sulfate/tab_	50 tablets	4500 (806)	6 h
16 mo	Prenatal vitamins with iron	Unknown	1200 (215)	Unknown

Table (*Continued*)

Age	Stated Iron Product Ingested	Stated Dose	Serum Iron Concentrations mcg/dL (mmol/L)	Time Serum Iron Drawn After Ingestion
16 mo	Prenatal vitamins with iron (325 mg ferrous sulfate/tab)	50 tablets	1440 (258)	Unknown
21 mo	Prenatal vitamins with iron (65 mg Fe/tab)	90 tablets	1858 (333)	10 h
20 mo	Ferrous sulfate 325 mg tablets	Unknown	1080 (193)	Unknown
11 mo	Iron tablets	50-70 tablets	8800 (1576)	2 h
23 mo	Prenatal vitamins with iron	Unknown	251 (45)	36 h
18 mo	Ferrous sulfate 325 mg tablets	Unknown	Not done	
22 mo	Ferrous sulfate 325 mg tablets	96 tablets	2583 (463)	6.5 h
1 y	Prenatal vitamins with iron	Unknown	5900 (1057)	12-14 h
16 mo	Prenatal vitamins with iron	Unknown	397 (71)	>3 days
17 mo	Prenatal vitamins with iron	>25 tablets	1055 (189)	6 h
16 mo	Ferrous sulfate	Unknown	12,000 (2149)	>4 h
14 mo	Iron tablets	Unknown	18,750 (3358)	3 h
36 y	Unknown iron preparation	Unknown	345 (62)	Unknown
14 y	Iron tablets	140 mg/kg	476 (85)	Unknown
34 y	Prenatal vitamins with iron	Unknown	92 (17)	Unknown

Specific References

Beuhler MC and Wallace KL, "Benign Outcome with Toxic Serum Iron Levels Following I.V. Iron Dextran Overdose in Three Patients," *J Toxicol Clin Toxicol*, 2003, 41(5):738.

Black J and Zenel JA, "Child Abuse by Intentional Iron Poisoning Presenting as Shock and Persistent Acidosis," *Pediatrics*, 2003, 111(1):197-9.

Finkelstein Y, Wahl MS, Bentur Y, et al, "Comparison of Iron Poisoning Patterns in 602 Preschool Children: A Population-Based Study from Illinois and Israel," *Clin Toxicol (Phila)*, 2005, 43:653.

Gades NM, Chyka PA, Butler AY, et al, "Activated Charcoal and the Absorption of Ferrous Sulfate in Rats," *Vet Hum Toxicol*, 2003, 45(4):183-7.

Goldstein LH and berkovitch M, "Ingestional of Slow-Release Iron Treated with Gastric Lavage - Never Say Late," *Clin Toxicol*, 2006, 44(3):343.

Habibe M, Matteucci MJ, Tanen DA, et al, "Effect of Oral Calcium Disodium EDTA on Iron Absorption in a Human Model of Mild Iron Overdose," *Acad Emerg Med*, 2003, 10:521b-22b.

Hayashi SA, Thundiyil J, Flori H, et al, "Acute Iron Toxicity from Accidental Intravenous Administration of an Oral Iron Preparation," *J Toxicol Clin Toxicol*, 2004, 42(5):821.

Manoguerra AS, Erdman AR, Booze LL, et al, "Iron Ingestion: An Evidence-Based Consensus Guideline for Out-of-Hospital Management," *Clin Toxicol*, 2005, 43(6):553-70.

Matteucci MJ, Habibe M, Robson K, et al, "Effect of Oral Calcium Disodium EDTA on Iron Absorption in a Human Model of Iron Overdose," *Clin Toxicol (Phila)*, 2006, 44(1):39-43.

Saadeh CE and Srkalovic G. "Acute Hypersensitivity Reaction to Ferric Gluconate in a Premedicated Patient," *Ann Pharmacother*, 2005, 39(12):2124-7.

Spiller HA, Wahlen HS, Stephens TL, et al, "Multi-Center Retrospective Evaluation of Carbonyl Iron Ingestions," *Vet Hum Toxicol*, 2002, 44(1):28-9.

Tenenbein M and Robertson A, "Hepatotoxicity in Acute Iron Poisoning," *J Toxicol Clin Toxicol*, 2004, 42(5):717.

Velez LI, Gracia R, Mills LD, et al, "Iron Bezoar Retained in Colon Despite 3 Days of Whole Bowel Irrigation," *J Toxicol Clin Toxicol*, 2004, 42(5):653-6.

Wheeler CJ and Kowdley KV, "Hereditary Hemochromatosis: A Review of the Genetics, Mechanism, Diagnosis, and Treatment of Iron Overload," *Comp Ther*, 2006, 32(1)10-6.

Wu ML, Tsai WJ, Ger J, et al, "Clinical Experience of Acute Ferric Chloride Poisoning," *Vet Hum Toxicol*, 2003, 45(5):243-6.

Isocarboxazid

Pronunciation (eye soe kar BOKS a zid)

CAS Number 59-63-2

U.S. Brand Names Marplan®

Use Symptomatic treatment of atypical, nonendogenous, or neurotic depression

Mechanism of Action Thought to act by increasing endogenous concentrations of epinephrine, norepinephrine, dopamine, and serotonin through inhibition of the enzyme (monoamine oxidase) responsible for the breakdown of these neurotransmitters

Adverse Reactions

Cardiovascular: **Hypotension**, hypertension, edema, ECG changes (peaked T waves), palpitations, vasoconstriction

Central nervous system: **Drowsiness**, excitement, mania, coma, hallucinations, seizures, delirium, hyperthermia

Dermatologic: Skin rash, hyperhidrosis

Endocrine & metabolic: Syndrome of inappropriate antidiuretic hormone

Gastrointestinal: Xerostomia, constipation, nausea

Genitourinary: Urinary retention, ejaculatory disturbances

Ocular: **Blurred vision**, photophobia, ptosis, diplopia, mydriasis, "ping-pong" gaze, nystagmus

Neuromuscular & skeletal: Muscle rigidity, hyperreflexia

Renal: Myoglobinuria leading to renal failure

Respiratory: Tachypnea

Miscellaneous: Diaphoresis

Dosage Adults: Oral: 10 mg 3 times/day; reduce to 10-20 mg/day in divided doses when condition improves

Monitoring Parameters Blood pressure

Contraindications Hypersensitivity to isocarboxazid or any component of the formulation; uncontrolled hypertension; pheochromocytoma; hepatic or renal disease; cerebrovascular defect; cardiovascular disease (CHF); CNS depressants, ethanol, meperidine, bupropion, buspirone, guanethidine, and serotonergic drugs (including SSRIs) - do not use within 5 weeks of fluoxetine discontinuation or 2 weeks of other antidepressant discontinuation; general anesthesia, local vasoconstrictors; spinal anesthesia (hypotension may be exaggerated); sympathomimetics (and related compounds); foods high in tyramine content; supplements containing tyrosine, phenylalanine, tryptophan, or caffeine

Warnings

[U.S. Boxed Warning]: Antidepressants increase the risk of suicidal thinking and behavior in children and adolescents with major depressive disorder (MDD) and other depressive disorders; consider risk prior to prescribing. Closely monitor for clinical worsening, suicidality, or unusual changes in behavior; the child's family or caregiver should be instructed to closely observe the patient and communicate condition with healthcare provider. Such observation would generally include at least weekly face-to-face contact with patients or their family members or caregivers during the first 4 weeks of treatment, then every other week visits for the next 4 weeks, then at 12 weeks, and as clinically indicated beyond 12 weeks. Additional contact by telephone may be appropriate between face-to-face visits. Adults treated with antidepressants should be observed similarly for clinical worsening and suicidality, especially during the initial few months of a course of drug therapy, or at times of dose changes, either increases or decreases. A medication guide should be dispensed with each prescription. **Isocarboxazid is FDA approved for the treatment of depression in children ≥16 years of age.**

The possibility of a suicide attempt is inherent in major depression and may persist until remission occurs. Monitor for worsening of depression or suicidality, especially during initiation of therapy or with dose increases or decreases. Worsening depression and severe abrupt suicidality that are not part of the presenting symptoms may require discontinuation or modification of drug therapy. Use caution in high-risk patients during initiation of therapy. Prescriptions should be written for the smallest quantity consistent with good patient care. The patient's family or caregiver should be alerted to monitor patients for the emergence of suicidality and associated behaviors such as anxiety, agitation, panic attacks, insomnia, irritability, hostility, impulsivity, akathisia, hypomania, and mania; patients should be instructed to notify their healthcare provider if any of these symptoms or worsening depression occur.

May worsen psychosis in some patients or precipitate a shift to mania or hypomania in patients with bipolar disorder. Monotherapy in patients with bipolar disorder should be avoided. Patients presenting with depressive symptoms should be screened for bipolar disorder. **Isocarboxazid is not FDA approved for the treatment of bipolar depression.**

Use with caution in patients who are hyperactive, hyperexcitable, or who have glaucoma, hyperthyroidism, or diabetes; avoid use of meperidine within 2 weeks of isocarboxazid use. Toxic reactions have occurred with dextromethorphan. Hypertensive crisis may occur with foods/supplements high in tyramine, tryptophan, phenylalanine, or tyrosine content.

Should not be used in combination with other antidepressants. Hypotensive effects of antihypertensives (beta-blockers, thiazides) may be exaggerated. May cause orthostatic hypotension (especially at dosages >30 mg/day) - use with caution in patients with hypotension or patients who would not tolerate transient hypotensive episodes - effects may be additive when used with other agents known to cause orthostasis (phenothiazines).

Discontinue at least 48 hours prior to myelography. May increase the risks associated with electroconvulsive therapy. Consider discontinuing, when possible, prior to elective surgery. Use with caution in patients receiving disulfiram. Use with caution in patients with renal impairment. The MAO inhibitors are effective and generally well tolerated by older patients. It is the potential interactions with tyramine-containing foods and other drugs, and their effects on blood pressure that have limited their use.

Dosage Forms Tablet: 10 mg

Overdosage/Treatment

Decontamination: Lavage (within 1 hour)/activated charcoal

Supportive therapy: Diazepam or lorazepam can be used for agitation/seizures; dantrolene (2.5 mg/kg every 6 hours) can be used for muscle rigidity and hyperthermia; norepinephrine is the preferred agent for treatment of hypotension. Avoid bretylium for ventricular dysrhythmia, lidocaine or procainamide are preferred. Hypertensive crisis can be treated with nitroprusside, phentolamine (2-10 mg slow I.V. injection in adults), diazoxide (50-100 mg I.V.). Dantrolene (2.5 mg/kg every 6 hours I.V.) can be used to treat hypermetabolic crisis; avoid use of succinoylcholine and bretylium.

Diagnostic Procedures

● Electrolytes, Blood

Test Interactions ↓ glucose

Drug Interactions

Amphetamines: MAO inhibitors in combination with amphetamines may result in severe hypertensive reaction; these combinations are best avoided.

Anorexiants: Concurrent use of anorexiants may result in serotonin syndrome; these combinations are best avoided; includes dexfenfluramine, fenfluramine, or sibutramine.

Barbiturates: MAO inhibitors may inhibit the metabolism of barbiturates and prolong their effect.

CNS stimulants: MAO inhibitors in combination with stimulants (methylphenidate) may result in severe hypertensive reaction; these combinations are best avoided

Dextromethorphan: Concurrent use of MAO inhibitors may result in serotonin syndrome; these combinations are best avoided.

Disulfiram: MAO inhibitors may produce delirium in patients receiving disulfiram; monitor.

Guanadrel and guanethidine: MAO inhibitors inhibit the antihypertensive response to guanadrel or guanethidine; use an alternative antihypertensive agent.

Hypoglycemic agents: MAO inhibitors may produce hypoglycemia in patients with diabetes; monitor.

Levodopa: MAO inhibitors in combination with levodopa may result in hypertensive reactions; monitor.

Lithium: MAO inhibitors in combination with lithium have resulted in malignant hyperpyrexia; this combination is best avoided.

Meperidine: May cause serotonin syndrome when combined with an MAO inhibitor; avoid this combination.

Nefazodone: Concurrent use of MAO inhibitors may result in serotonin syndrome; these combinations are best avoided.

Norepinephrine: MAO inhibitors may increase the pressor response of norepinephrine (effect is generally small); monitor.

Reserpine: MAO inhibitors in combination with reserpine may result in hypertensive reactions; monitor.

Serotonin agonists: Theoretically, may increase the risk of serotonin syndrome; includes sumatriptan, naratriptan, rizatriptan, and zolmitriptan.

SSRIs: May cause serotonin syndrome when combined with an MAO inhibitor; avoid this combination.

Succinylcholine: MAO inhibitors may prolong the muscle relaxation produced by succinylcholine via decreased plasma pseudocholinesterase.

Sympathomimetics (indirect-acting): MAO inhibitors in combination with sympathomimetics such as dopamine, metaraminol, phenylephrine, and decongestants (pseudoephedrine) may result in severe hypertensive reaction; these combinations are best avoided.

Tramadol: May increase the risk of seizures and serotonin syndrome in patients receiving an MAO inhibitor.

Trazodone: Concurrent use of MAO inhibitors may result in serotonin syndrome; these combinations are best avoided.

Tricyclic antidepressants: May cause serotonin syndrome when combined with an MAO inhibitor; avoid this combination.

Venlafaxine: Concurrent use of MAO inhibitors may result in serotonin syndrome; these combinations are best avoided.

Pregnancy Risk Factor C

Nursing Implications Watch for hypotension (orthostatic); monitor blood pressure carefully, especially at therapy onset or if other CNS drugs or cardiovascular drugs are added; check for dietary and drug restriction

Additional Information Avoid tyramine-containing foods: red wine, cheese (except cottage, ricotta, and cream), smoked or pickled fish, beef or chicken liver, dried sausage, fava or broad bean pods, yeast vitamin supplements

Isoniazid

Related Information
- Therapeutic Drugs Associated with Hallucinations

CAS Number 54-85-3

U.S. Brand Names Nydrazid®

Synonyms INH; Isonicotinic Acid Hydrazide

Use Treatment of susceptible tuberculosis infections and prophylactically to those individuals exposed to tuberculosis

Mechanism of Action Inhibits myocolic acid synthesis resulting in disruption of the bacterial cell wall; inhibits pyridoxine use as a cofactor in production of gamma-aminobutyric acid (GABA), an inhibitory neurotransmitter. Structurally related to nicotinic acid

Adverse Reactions

Cardiovascular: Myocarditis (hypersensitivity), pericardial effusion/pericarditis, sinus tachycardia, vasculitis

Central nervous system: Peripheral neuritis, vascular encephalopathy, seizures, stupor, dizziness, psychosis, fever, auditory and visual hallucinations, ataxia, memory disturbance, CNS depression, depression, mania, axonopathy

Dermatologic: Skin eruptions, angioedema, Stevens-Johnson syndrome, acute generalized exanthematous pustulosis, alopecia, toxic epidermal necrolysis, purpura, onycholysis, photosensitivity, pruritus, licheniform eruptions, exanthem

Endocrine & metabolic: Hyperglycemia

Gastrointestinal: Nausea, vomiting, stomach pain, loss of appetite, constipation, pancreatitis

Genitourinary: Urinary retention

Hematologic: Blood dyscrasias, hemolysis, eosinophilia, agranulocytosis, red blood cell aplasia, thrombocytopenia, aplastic anemia

Hepatic: Hepatitis, elevated liver transaminase levels, aminotransferase level elevation (asymptomatic)

Neuromuscular & skeletal: Weakness, peripheral neuritis, rhabdomyolysis

Ocular: Optic neuritis, photophobia, diplopia

Otic: Ototoxicity (deafness), tinnitus

Miscellaneous: Systemic lupus erythematosus

Signs and Symptoms of Overdose Arthralgia, blurred vision, coma, deafness, dizziness, encephalopathy, eosinophilia, exfoliative dermatitis, fever, hallucinations, hyperglycemia, hyperkalemia, hyperreflexia, hyperthermia, hypoglycemia, intractable seizures in acute overdose (>40 mg/kg), memory loss, meningitis, metabolic acidosis, myoclonus, myoglobinuria, nausea, neuropathy (peripheral), nystagmus, paresthesia, rhabdomyolysis, slurred speech, stupor, vomiting

Chronic overdosage has similar toxicities, though early signs of acute overdosage (nausea, vomiting) may not occur. Agranulocytosis, granulocytopenia, hypotension, leukocytosis, leukopenia, neutropenia, tachycardia

Admission Criteria/Prognosis Admit any patient who is symptomatic 6 hours postingestion or ingestions >20 mg/kg

Pharmacodynamics/Kinetics

Absorption: Rapid and complete; rate can be slowed with food

Distribution: All body tissues and fluids including CSF; crosses placenta; enters breast milk

Protein binding: 10% to 15%

Metabolism: Hepatic with decay rate determined genetically by acetylation phenotype

Half-life elimination: Fast acetylators: 30-100 minutes; Slow acetylators: 2-5 hours; may be prolonged with hepatic or severe renal impairment

Time to peak, serum: 1-2 hours

Excretion: Urine (75% to 95%); feces; saliva

Dosage

Oral, I.M. (recommendations often change due to resistant strains and newly developed information; consult *MMWR Morb Mortal Wkly Rep* for current CDC recommendations):

Children: 10-20 mg/kg/day in 1-2 divided doses (maximum: 300 mg total dose)

Prophylaxis: 10 mg/kg/day (up to 300 mg total dose) for 12 months

Adults: 5 mg/kg/day (usual dose is 300 mg)

Disseminated disease: 10 mg/kg/day in 1-2 divided doses

Treatment should be continued for 9 months with rifampin or for 6 months with rifampin and pyrazinamide

Prophylaxis: 300 mg/day for 12 months

American Thoracic Society and CDC currently recommend twice weekly therapy as part of a short-course regimen which follows 1-2 months of daily treatment for uncomplicated pulmonary tuberculosis in compliant patients

Children: 20-40 mg/kg/dose (up to 900 mg) twice weekly

Adults: 15 mg/kg/dose (up to 900 mg) twice weekly

Dosing adjustment in hepatic impairment: Dose should be reduced in severe hepatic disease

Stability Protect oral dosage forms from light

Monitoring Parameters Periodic liver function tests; monitoring for prodromal signs of hepatitis

Administration

Should be administered 1 hour before or 2 hours after meals on an empty stomach.

Contraindications Hypersensitivity to isoniazid or any component of the formulation; acute liver disease; previous history of hepatic damage during isoniazid therapy

Warnings Use with caution in patients with renal impairment and chronic liver disease. **[U.S. Boxed Warning]: Severe and sometimes fatal hepatitis may occur or develop even after many months of treatment.** Patients must report any prodromal symptoms of hepatitis, such as fatigue, weakness, malaise, anorexia, nausea, or vomiting. Malnourished patients should receive concomitant pyridoxine therapy. Periodic ophthalmic examinations are recommended even when usual symptoms do not occur; pyridoxine (10-50 mg/day) is recommended in individuals likely to develop peripheral neuropathies.

Dosage Forms

[DSC] = Discontinued product

Injection, solution (Nydrazid®): 100 mg/mL (10 mL) [DSC]

Syrup: 50 mg/5 mL (473 mL) [orange flavor]

Tablet: 100 mg, 300 mg

Reference Range

Therapeutic: 1-7 mcg/mL (SI: 7-51 µmol/L)

Toxic: >20 mcg/mL (SI: 146 µmol/L)

Overdosage/Treatment

Decontamination: **Do not** use ipecac; gastric lavage within 1 hour (protect airway if gag reflex is negative) with activated charcoal (lavage if obtuned)

Supportive therapy: Treat seizures with diazepam while awaiting pyridoxine; refractory seizures should be treated with thiopental or other short-acting barbiturates, phenytoin is **not** useful in treating isoniazid induced seizures; acidosis should be appropriately treated with sodium bicarbonate; early consideration of intubation is recommended. Pyridoxine has been shown to be effective in the treatment of intoxication, especially when seizures occur. Pyridoxine I.V. is administered on a milligram to milligram dose. If the amount of isoniazid ingested is unknown, 5 g of pyridoxine should be given over 3-5 minutes (70 mg/kg in children) and may be followed by an additional 5 g in 30 minutes; phenytoin is not useful; pyridoxine can also be useful for coma or optic neuropathy. Propofol use has not been studied. Because of the severe morbidity and high mortality rates with isoniazid overdose, patients who are asymptomatic after an overdose, should be monitored for 4-6 hours. Acute ingestions over 80 mg/kg should be given pyridoxine.

Enhancement of elimination: Dialysis may be useful (dialyzable 50% to 100%) as is hemoperfusion in refractory cases; exchange transfusion has been used successfully

Antidote(s)

- Pyridoxine [ANTIDOTE]

Test Interactions False-positive urinary glucose with Clinitest®

Drug Interactions

Substrate of CYP2E1 (major); Inhibits CYP1A2 (weak), 2A6 (moderate), 2C9 (weak), 2C19 (strong), 2D6 (moderate), 2E1 (moderate), 3A4 (strong); Induces CYP2E1 (after discontinuation) (weak)

Acetaminophen: Isoniazid may enhance the adverse/toxic effect of acetaminophen.

Antacids: Antacids may decrease the absorption of isoniazid.

Benzodiazepines (metabolized by oxidation): Isoniazid may decrease the metabolism, via CYP isoenzymes, of benzodiazepines (metabolized by oxidation).

Carbamazepine: Isoniazid may decrease the metabolism of carbamazepine.

Cycloserine: Cycloserine may enhance the CNS depressant effect of isoniazid.

CYP2A6 substrates: Isoniazid may increase the levels/effects of CYP2A6 substrates. Example substrates include dexmedetomidine and ifosfamide.

CYP2C19 substrates: Isoniazid may increase the levels/effects of CYP2C19 substrates. Example substrates include citalopram, diazepam, methsuximide, phenytoin, propranolol, and sertraline.

CYP2D6 substrates: Isoniazid may increase the levels/effects of CYP2D6 substrates. Example substrates include amphetamines, selected beta-blockers, dextromethorphan, fluoxetine, lidocaine, mirtazapine, nefazodone, paroxetine, risperidone, ritonavir, thioridazine, tricyclic antidepressants, and venlafaxine.

CYP2D6 prodrug substrates: Isoniazid may decrease the levels/effects of CYP2D6 prodrug substrates. Example prodrug substrates include codeine, hydrocodone, oxycodone, and tramadol.

CYP2E1 substrates: Isoniazid may increase the levels/effects of CYP2E1 substrates. Example substrates include inhalational anesthetics, theophylline, and trimethadione.

CYP3A4 substrates: Isoniazid may increase the levels/effects of CYP3A4 substrates. Example substrates include benzodiazepines, calcium channel blockers, mirtazapine, nateglinide, nefazodone, tacrolimus, and venlafaxine. Selected benzodiazepines (midazolam and triazolam), cisapride, ergot alkaloids, selected HMG-CoA reductase inhibitors (lovastatin and simvastatin), and pimozide are generally contraindicated with strong CYP3A4 inhibitors.

Disulfiram: Isoniazid may enhance the adverse/toxic effect of disulfiram.

Phenytoin: Isoniazid may decrease the metabolism, via CYP isoenzymes, of phenytoin.

Theophylline: Isoniazid may decrease the metabolism, via CYP isoenzymes, of theophylline derivatives.

Valproic Acid: Isoniazid may increase the serum concentration of valproic acid.

Pregnancy Risk Factor C

Pregnancy Implications Crosses the placenta

Lactation Enters breast milk/compatible

Additional Information Lethal dose: 80-150 mg/kg; Toxic dose: 1.5 g

Due to mild inhibition of monoamine oxidase by isoniazid, an interaction with tyramine containing foods may occur; children with low milk and low meat intake should receive concomitant pyridoxine therapy; most combination antituberculin products contain INH which generally should be regarded as the more significant toxin.

Specific References

Knapp JF, Johnson T, and Alander S, "Seizures in a 13-Year-Old Girl," *Pediatr Emerg Care*, 2003, 19(1):38-40.

Maw G and Aitken P, "Isoniazid Overdose: A Case Series, Literature Review and Survey of Antidote Availability," *Clin Drug Invest*, 2003, 23(7):479-85.

Noguera-Pons R, Borras-Blasco J, Romero-Crespo I, aet al, "Optic Neuritis with Concurrent Etanercept and Isoniazid Therapy," *Ann Pharmacother*, 2005, 39(12):2131-4.

Schier JG, Nelson LS, and Hoffman RS, "Inappropriate Laughter: An Isoniazid Adverse Drug Event," *J Toxicol Clin Toxicol*, 2003, 41(5):679.

Wills B and Erickson T, "Drug- and Toxin-Associated Seizures," *Med Clin North Am*, 2005, 89(6):1297-321 (review).

Isosorbide Dinitrate

Related Information

● Therapeutic Drugs Associated with Hallucinations

CAS Number 87-33-2

U.S. Brand Names Dilatrate®-SR; Isordil®

Synonyms ISD; ISDN

Use Prevention and treatment of angina pectoris; for congestive heart failure; to relieve pain, dysphagia, and spasm in esophageal spasm with GE reflux

Unlabeled/Investigational Use Esophageal spastic disorders

Mechanism of Action Reduces cardiac oxygen demand by decreasing left ventricular pressure and systemic vascular resistance by dilating coronary arteries and improving collateral flow to ischemic regions

Adverse Reactions

Cardiovascular: **Postural hypotension, cutaneous flushing of head, neck, and clavicular area**; tachycardia, sinus tachycardia, tachycardia (supraventricular)

Central nervous system: **Dizziness, headache, lightheadedness**, psychosis, visual hallucinations, seizures

Dermatologic: Rash, exfoliative dermatitis

Gastrointestinal: Nausea, GI upset, diarrhea, vomiting

Neuromuscular & skeletal: **Weakness**

Signs and Symptoms of Overdose Cough, cyanosis, dyspepsia, heart palpitations, hypotension, methemoglobin formation, ptosis, throbbing headache, urinary frequency, visual disturbances

Pharmacodynamics/Kinetics

Onset of action: Sublingual tablet: 2-10 minutes; Chewable tablet: 3 minutes; Oral tablet: 45-60 minutes

Duration: Sublingual tablet: 1-2 hours; Chewable tablet: 0.5-2 hours; Oral tablet: 4-6 hours

Metabolism: Extensively hepatic to conjugated metabolites, including isosorbide 5-mononitrate (active) and 2-mononitrate (active)

Half-life elimination: Parent drug: 1-4 hours; Metabolite (5-mononitrate): 4 hours

Excretion: Urine and feces

Dosage

Adults:

Oral: 5-40 mg every 6 hours or 40-80 mg every 8-12 hours in sustained release dosage form

Chewable: 5-10 mg every 2-3 hours

Sublingual: 2.5-10 mg every 4-6 hours

Monitoring Parameters Monitor for orthostasis

Administration Do not administer around-the-clock; the first dose of nitrates should be administered in a physician's office to observe for maximal cardiovascular dynamic effects and adverse effects (orthostatic blood pressure drop, headache); when immediate release products are prescribed twice daily (recommend 7 AM and noon); for 3 times/day dosing (recommend 7 AM, noon, and 5 PM); when sustained-release products are indicated, suggest once a day in morning or via twice daily dosing at 8 AM and 2 PM. Do not crush sublingual tablets.

Contraindications Hypersensitivity to isosorbide dinitrate or any component of the formulation; hypersensitivity to organic nitrates; concurrent use with phosphodiesterase-5 (PDE-5) inhibitors (sildenafil, tadalafil, or vardenafil); angle-closure glaucoma (intraocular pressure may be increased); head trauma or cerebral hemorrhage (increase intracranial pressure); severe anemia

Warnings Severe hypotension can occur. Use with caution in volume depletion, hypotension, and right ventricular infarctions. Paradoxical bradycardia and increased angina pectoris can accompany hypotension. Postural hypotension can also occur. Tolerance does develop to nitrates and appropriate dosing is needed to minimize this. Safety and efficacy have not been established in pediatric patients. Nitrate may aggravate angina caused by hypertrophic cardiomyopathy. Avoid concurrent use with sildenafil.

Dosage Forms

[DSC] = Discontinued product

Capsule, sustained release (Dilatrate®-SR): 40 mg

Tablet: 5 mg, 10 mg, 20 mg, 30 mg

Isordil®: 5 mg, 10 mg [DSC], 20 mg [DSC], 30 mg [DSC], 40 mg

Tablet, extended release (Isochron™): 40 mg

Tablet, sublingual: 2.5 mg, 5 mg

Isordil®: 2.5 mg, 5 mg, 10 mg [DSC]

Reference Range Peak isosorbide plasma levels after a 5 mg oral and sublingual dose: 3.1 mcg/L and 8.9 mcg/L, respectively

Overdosage/Treatment

Decontamination: Ipecac within 30 minutes or lavage (within 1 hour)/ activated charcoal

Supportive therapy: Formation of methemoglobinemia is dose related and unusual in normal doses; high levels can cause signs and symptoms of hypoxemia; treatment consists of placing patient in recumbent position and administering fluids; alpha-adrenergic vasopressors may be required; treat methemoglobinemia with oxygen and methylene blue at a dose of 1-2 mg/kg slow I.V.; treat hypotension with isotonic fluid and Trendelenburg positioning; pressors are rarely necessary unless ingestion is severe

Enhancement of elimination: Hemodialysis is not useful

Antidote(s)

● Methylene Blue [ANTIDOTE]

Diagnostic Procedures

● Methemoglobin, Blood

Test Interactions ↓ cholesterol (S)

Drug Interactions

Substrate of CYP3A4 (major)

CYP3A4 inducers: CYP3A4 inducers may decrease the levels/effects of isosorbide dinitrate. Example inducers include aminoglutethimide, carbamazepine, nafcillin, nevirapine, phenobarbital, phenytoin, and rifamycins.

CYP3A4 inhibitors: May increase the levels/effects of isosorbide dinitrate. Example inhibitors include azole antifungals, clarithromycin, diclofenac, doxycycline, erythromycin, imatinib, isoniazid, nefazodone, nicardipine, propofol, protease inhibitors, quinidine, telithromycin, and verapamil.

Sildenafil, tadalafil, vardenafil: Significant reduction of systolic and diastolic blood pressure with concurrent use (contraindicated). Do not administer sildenafil, tadalafil, or vardenafil within 24 hours of a nitrate preparation.

Pregnancy Risk Factor C

Lactation Excretion in breast milk unknown

Isosorbide Mononitrate

CAS Number 16051-77-7

U.S. Brand Names Imdur®; Ismo®; Monoket®

Synonyms ISMN

Use Long-acting metabolite of the vasodilator isosorbide dinitrate used for the prophylactic treatment of angina pectoris

Unlabeled/Investigational Use To prevent esophageal variceal bleeding

Mechanism of Action Prevailing mechanism of action for nitroglycerin (and other nitrates) is systemic venodilation, decreasing preload as measured by pulmonary capillary wedge pressure and left ventricular end diastolic volume and pressure; the average reduction in LVEDV is 25% at rest, with a corresponding increase in ejection fractions of 50% to 60%. This effect improves congestive symptoms in heart failure and improves the myocardial perfusion gradient in patients with coronary artery disease.

Adverse Reactions

Cardiovascular: Angina pectoris, arrhythmias, fibrillation (atrial), hypotension, palpitations, postural hypotension, premature ventricular contractions, supraventricular tachycardia, syncope, edema, sinus bradycardia, bundle branch block, flutter (atrial), chest pain, tachycardia (supraventricular)

Central nervous system: Headache (duration 2-3 hours), dizziness, malaise, agitation, anxiety, confusion, hypoesthesia, insomnia, nervousness, nightmares, vertigo

Dermatologic: Pruritus, rash

Gastrointestinal: Nausea, vomiting, abdominal pain, diarrhea, dyspepsia, tenesmus, increased appetite, tooth disorder, hemorrhoids

Genitourinary: Impotence, urinary frequency, dysuria

Hematologic: Methemoglobinemia (rarely), thrombocytopenia

Neuromuscular & skeletal: Neck stiffness, rigors, arthralgia, dyscoordination, weakness

Ocular: Blurred vision, diplopia

Respiratory: Bronchitis, pneumonia, upper respiratory tract infection, rhinitis

Miscellaneous: Cold sweat

Signs and Symptoms of Overdose Coma, diaphoresis, flushing, hypotension, metabolic acidosis, methemoglobinemia, palpitations, tachycardia, throbbing headache, visual disturbances. High levels or methemoglobinemia can cause signs and symptoms of hypoxemia.

Pharmacodynamics/Kinetics

Onset of action: 30-60 minutes

Absorption: Nearly complete and low intersubject variability in its pharmacokinetic parameters and plasma concentrations

Metabolism: Hepatic

Half-life elimination: Mononitrate: ~4 hours

Excretion: Urine and feces

Dosage

Adults: Oral:

Regular tablet: 20 mg twice daily separated by 7 hours

Extended release tablet (Imdur®): Initial: 30-60 mg once daily; after several days the dosage may be increased to 120 mg/day (given as two 60 mg tablets); daily dose should be taken in the morning upon arising; maximum: 240 mg/day

Asymmetrical dosing regimen of 7 AM and 3 PM or 9 AM and 5 PM to allow for a nitrate-free dosing interval to minimize nitrate tolerance

Esophageal variceal rebleeding: 80 mg once daily of nadolol (titrate until resting heart is reduced by 25% or at 55 beats/minute over a period of 5 days); following nadolol adjustment, isosorbide mononitrate can be added to a maximum oral dose of 40 mg twice daily

Dosing adjustment in renal impairment: Not necessary for elderly or patients with altered renal or hepatic function

Stability Tablets should be stored in a tight container at room temperature of 15°C to 30°C (59°F to 86°F)

Monitoring Parameters Monitor for orthostasis, increased hypotension

Administration Do not administer around-the-clock; Monoket® and Ismo® should be scheduled twice daily with doses 7 hours apart (8 AM and 3 PM); Imdur® may be administered once daily. Extended release tablets should not be chewed or crushed. Should be swallowed with a half-glassful of fluid.

Contraindications Hypersensitivity to isosorbide or any component of the formulation; hypersensitivity to organic nitrates; concurrent use with phosphodiesterase-5 (PDE-5) inhibitors (sildenafil, tadalafil, or vardenafil); angle-closure glaucoma (intraocular pressure may be increased); head trauma or cerebral hemorrhage (increase intracranial pressure); severe anemia

Warnings Severe hypotension can occur. Use with caution in volume depletion, hypotension, and right ventricular infarctions. Paradoxical bradycardia and increased angina pectoris can accompany hypotension. Orthostatic hypotension can also occur. Ethanol can accentuate this. Tolerance does develop to nitrates and appropriate dosing is needed to minimize this (drug-free interval). Safety and efficacy have not been established in pediatric patients. Nitrates may aggravate angina caused by hypertrophic cardiomyopathy. Avoid concurrent use with sildenafil.

Dosage Forms Tablet: 10 mg, 20 mg

Ismo®: 20 mg

Monoket®: 10 mg, 20 mg

Tablet, extended release (Imdur®): 30 mg, 60 mg, 120 mg

Reference Range Peak serum isosorbide mononitrate level after a 40 mg dose: ~706 ng/mL; serum levels of 100-500 ng/mL are considered therapeutic

Overdosage/Treatment

Decontamination: Ipecac within 30 minutes or lavage (within 1 hour)/ activated charcoal

Supportive therapy: Formation of methemoglobinemia is dose related and unusual in normal doses; high levels can cause signs and symptoms of hypoxemia; treatment consists of placing patient in recumbent position and administering fluids; alpha-adrenergic vasopressors may be required; treat methemoglobinemia with oxygen and methylene blue at a dose of 1-2 mg/kg I.V. slowly; treat hypotension with isotonic fluid and Trendelenburg position; pressors rarely necessary unless ingestion is severe

Enhancement of elimination: Hemodialysis is not useful; hemodialysis can decrease peak levels by 20% to 30% and result in plasma clearance of 81 mL/minute

Test Interactions May interfere with colorimetric cholesterol determinations resulting in falsely low cholesterol levels

Drug Interactions Substrate of CYP3A4 (major)

CYP3A4 inducers: CYP3A4 inducers may decrease the levels/effects of isosorbide mononitrate. Example inducers include aminoglutethimide, carbamazepine, nafcillin, nevirapine, phenobarbital, phenytoin, and rifamycins.

CYP3A4 inhibitors: May increase the levels/effects of isosorbide mononitrate. Example inhibitors include azole antifungals, clarithromycin, diclofenac, doxycycline, erythromycin, imatinib, isoniazid, nefazodone, nicardipine, propofol, protease inhibitors, quinidine, telithromycin, and verapamil.

Sildenafil, tadalafil, vardenafil: Significant reduction of systolic and diastolic blood pressure with concurrent use (contraindicated). Do not administer sildenafil, tadalafil, or vardenafil within 24 hours of a nitrate preparation.

Pregnancy Risk Factor C

Lactation Excretion in breast milk unknown

Additional Information Methemoglobin levels >10% may occur with ingestions >2 mg/kg; it appears that age and serum creatinine levels are inversely associated with development of vascular headache due to nitrates; risk for headache decreases by ~40% for at 10 year increase in age and is 5 times less likely in patients with serum creatinine levels >133 μmol/L as opposed to levels <97 μmol/L

Specific References

Jansen R, Cleophas TJ, Zwinderman AH, et al, "Chronic Nitrate Therapy in Patients with Angina with Comorbidity," *am J Ther*, 2006, 13: 188-91.

Isotretinoin

Related Information
● Vitamin A

CAS Number 4759-48-2

U.S. Brand Names Accutane®; Amnesteem™; Claravis™; Sotret®

Synonyms 13-*cis*-Retinoic Acid

Use Treatment of severe recalcitrant nodular acne unresponsive to conventional therapy

Unlabeled/Investigational Use Investigational: Treatment of children with metastatic neuroblastoma or leukemia that does not respond to conventional therapy

Mechanism of Action Reduces sebaceous gland size and reduces sebum production; regulates cell proliferation and differentiation

Adverse Reactions

Cardiovascular: Vasculitis

Central nervous system: CNS depression, headache, tiredness, mood changes, psychosis, pseudotumor cerebri

Dermatologic: **Dry skin**, skin rash, skin peeling on hands or soles of feet, **pruritus**, alopecia, **photosensitivity**, desquamation (scaling), pemphigus, Beau's lines, brittle fingernails, fingernail dystrophy, **cheilitis**, hypertrichosis, erythema multiforme, acne, toxic epidermal necrolysis, xerosis, erythema nodosum, exanthem, cutaneous vasculitis

Endocrine & metabolic: Growth suppression, hypertriglyceridemia, hypercalcemia, **increased serum concentration of triglycerides**, thyrotoxicosis, gynecomastia

Gastrointestinal: Stomach upset, abdominal pain, inflammatory bowel disease, anorexia, nausea, vomiting, ageusia, **xerostomia**, loss of sour taste, bleeding of gums, gastrointestinal vasculitis

Hematologic: Thrombocytopenia, agranulocytosis, hemolysis, decreased hemoglobin and hematocrit

Hepatic: Hepatitis

Local: **Burning**

Neuromuscular & skeletal: **Myalgia**, skeletal hyperostosis, acute myopathy, rhabdomyolysis (rare), **back pain** (29% in pediatric patients), decreased bone mineral density, acute arthritis, **bone pain, arthralgia**

Ocular: **Burning eyes**, conjunctivitis, **redness**, **itching of eye**, dry eyes, photophobia, optic neuropathy, cataract, blepharoconjunctivitis (dose related)

Renal: Hypercalciuria, renal vasculitis

Respiratory: **Epistaxis, dry nose**, pleural effusion, pulmonary vasculitis

Miscellaneous: Increased erythrocyte sedimentation rate, polyarteritis-nodosa-like vasculitis, fixed drug eruption, thyroglossal duct cyst, keloid formation, diaphoresis

Signs and Symptoms of Overdose All signs and symptoms have been transient. Abdominal pain, acrodynia, ataxia, cheilosis, depression, dermatitis, desquamation, dizziness, dry eyes, eczema, ejaculatory disturbances, flushing, headache, hematuria, hypercalcemia, hyperthyroidism, hyperuricemia, neutropenia, photophobia, tachypnea, vomiting

Pharmacodynamics/Kinetics

Distribution: Crosses placenta

Protein binding: 99% to 100%; primarily albumin

Metabolism: Hepatic via CYP2B6, 2C8, 2C9, 2D6, 3A4; forms metabolites; major metabolite: 4-oxo-isotretinoin (active)

Half-life elimination: Terminal: Parent drug: 21 hours; Metabolite: 21-24 hours

Time to peak, serum: 3-5 hours

Excretion: Urine and feces (equal amounts)

Dosage

Oral:

Children: Maintenance therapy for neuroblastoma (investigational): 100-250 mg/m^2/day in 2 divided doses

Children and Adults: Severe recalcitrant nodular acne: 0.5-2 mg/kg/day in 2 divided doses (dosages as low as 0.05 mg/kg/day have been reported to be beneficial) for 15-20 weeks or until the total cyst count decreases by 70%, whichever is sooner. A second course of therapy may be initiated after a period of ≥2 months off therapy.

Dosing adjustment in hepatic impairment: Dose reductions empirically are recommended in hepatitis disease

Stability Store at room temperature and protect from light

Monitoring Parameters CBC with differential and platelet count, baseline sedimentation rate, glucose, CPK

Pregnancy test (for all female patients of childbearing potential): Two negative tests with a sensitivity of at least 25 mIU/mL prior to beginning therapy (the second performed during the first five days of the menstrual period immediately preceding the start of therapy); monthly tests to rule out pregnancy prior to refilling prescription.

Lipids: Prior to treatment and at weekly or biweekly intervals until response to treatment is established. Test should not be performed <36 hours after consumption of ethanol.

Liver function tests: Prior to treatment and at weekly or biweekly intervals until response to treatment is established.

Administration Administer with food. Capsules can be swallowed, or chewed and swallowed. The capsule may be opened with a large needle and the contents placed on applesauce or ice cream for patients unable to swallow the capsule. Whole capsules should be swallowed with a full glass of liquid.

Contraindications Hypersensitivity to isotretinoin or any component of the formulation; sensitivity to parabens, vitamin A, or other retinoids; pregnancy

Warnings This medication should only be prescribed by prescribers competent in treating severe recalcitrant nodular acne, are experienced in the use of systemic retinoids, and are participating in the pregnancy prevention programs authorized by the FDA and product manufacturer. Use with caution in patients with diabetes mellitus, hypertriglyceridemia; acute pancreatitis and fatal hemorrhagic pancreatitis (rare) have been reported. Not to be used in women of childbearing potential unless woman is capable of complying with effective contraceptive measures. Patients must select and commit to two forms of contraception. Therapy is begun after two negative pregnancy tests; effective contraception must be used for at least 1 month before beginning therapy, during therapy, and for 1 month after discontinuation of therapy. Prescriptions should be written for no more than a 1-month supply, and pregnancy testing and counseling should be repeated monthly. **[U.S. Boxed Warning]: Because of the high likelihood of teratogenic effects (~20%), do not prescribe isotretinoin for women who are or who are likely to become pregnant while using the drug (see Additional Information for details).** Male and female patients must be enrolled in the manufacturer-sponsored and FDA-approved monitoring programs. Depression, psychosis, aggressive or violent behavior, and changes in mood. Rarely, suicidal thoughts and actions have been reported during isotretinoin usage. All patients should be observed closely for symptoms of depression or suicidal thoughts. Discontinuation of treatment alone may not be sufficient, further evaluation may be necessary. Cases of pseudotumor cerebri (benign intracranial hypertension) have been reported, some with concomitant use of tetracycline (avoid using together). Patients with papilledema, headache, nausea, vomiting, and visual disturbances should be referred to a neurologist and treatment with isotretinoin discontinued. Hearing impairment, which can continue after therapy is discontinued, may occur. Clinical hepatitis, elevated liver enzymes, inflammatory bowel disease, skeletal hyperostosis, premature epiphyseal closure, vision impairment, corneal opacities, and decreased night vision have also been reported with the use of isotretinoin. Bone mineral density may decrease; use caution in patients with a genetic predisposition to bone disorders (ie osteoporosis, osteomalacia) and with disease states or concomitant medications that can induce bone disorders. Patients may be at risk when participating in activities with repetitive impact (such as sports). Safety of long-term use is not established and is not recommended.

Dosage Forms

Capsule:

Accutane®: 10 mg, 20 mg, 40 mg [contains soybean oil and parabens]

Amnesteem™: 10 mg, 20 mg, 40 mg [contains soybean oil]

Claravis™: 10 mg, 20 mg, 40 mg

Sotret®: 10 mg, 20 mg, 30 mg, 40 mg [contains soybean oil]

Reference Range Therapeutic blood levels: 141-179 ng/mL

Overdosage/Treatment

Decontamination: Emesis within 30 minutes or lavage (within 1 hour)/ activated charcoal

Supportive therapy: Hyperventilation, furosemide or mannitol (0.25-2 g/kg every 3-4 hours) for increased intracranial pressure

Enhancement of elimination: Due to enterohepatic recirculation, multiple dosing of activated charcoal may be effective

Drug Interactions

Carbamazepine: Clearance of carbamazepine may be increased, leading to decreased levels.

Corticosteroids: Corticosteroids may cause osteoporosis. Interactive effect with isotretinoin unknown; use with caution.

Oral contraceptives: Retinoic acid derivatives may diminish the therapeutic effect of oral contraceptives. Two forms of contraception are recommended in females of childbearing potential during retinoic acid therapy.

Phenytoin: Phenytoin may cause osteomalacia. Interactive effect with isotretinoin unknown; use with caution.

Tetracycline: Cases of pseudotumor cerebri have been reported with concurrent use; avoid combination.

Pregnancy Risk Factor X

Pregnancy Implications Major fetal abnormalities (both internal and external), spontaneous abortion, premature births and low IQ scores in surviving infants have been reported. This medication is contraindicated in females of childbearing potential unless they are able to comply with the guidelines of pregnancy prevention programs put in place by the FDA and the manufacturer of isotretinoin.

Lactation Excretion in breast milk unknown/contraindicated

Nursing Implications Capsules can be swallowed, or chewed and swallowed. The capsule may be opened with a large needle and the contents placed on apple sauce or ice cream for patients unable to swallow the capsule; administer with meals

Additional Information

Females of childbearing potential must receive oral and written information reviewing the hazards of therapy and the effects that isotretinoin can have on a fetus. Therapy should not begin without two negative pregnancy tests, one to be performed in the physician's office when qualifying the patient for treatment, the second test performed on the second day of the next normal menstrual period or 11 days after the last unprotected intercourse, whichever is last. Two forms of contraception (a primary and secondary form as described in the pregnancy prevention program materials) must be used during treatment and limitations to their use must be explained. Prescriptions should be written for no more than a 1-month supply, and pregnancy testing and counseling should be repeated monthly. Urine pregnancy test kits (for monthly pregnancy testing) and a Pregnancy Prevention Program kit (to be given to the patient prior to therapy) are provided by the manufacturer. Any cases of accidental pregnancy should be reported to the manufacturer or the FDA MedWatch Program. All patients (male and female) must read and sign the informed consent material provided in the pregnancy prevention program. Prescriptions will not be honored unless they have the yellow qualification sticker affixed.

The manufacturers of isotretinoin have developed comprehensive educational programs for healthcare providers and patients. Prior to prescribing isotretinoin, healthcare providers must be registered in one of these programs. Additional information for Accutane® and the corresponding S.M.A.R.T. (System To Manage Accutane®-Related Teratogenicity) program may be obtained from Roche Laboratories. Additional information for Amnesteem™ and the S.P.I.R.I.T.™ program (System To Prevent Isotretinoin-Related Issues of Teratogenicity) program maybe obtained from Bertek Pharmaceuticals. Additional information for Sotret® and I.M.P.A.R.T.™ (Isotretinoin Medication Program: Alerting you to the Risks of Teratogenicity) may be obtained from Ranbaxy Pharmaceuticals.

Specific References

Looney M and Smith KM, "Isotretinoin in the Treatment of Granuloma Annulare," *Ann Pharmacother*, 2004, 38(3):494-7.

Moeller KE and Touma SC, "Prolonged Thrombocytopenia Associated with Isotretinoin," *Ann Pharmacother*, 2003, 37(11):1622-4.

O'Donnell J, "Overview of Existing Research and Information Linking Isotretinoin (Accutane®), Depression, Psychosis, and Suicide," *Am J Ther*, 2003, 10(2):148-59.

Itraconazole

CAS Number 84625-61-6

U.S. Brand Names Sporanox®

Use

Treatment of susceptible fungal infections in immunocompromised and immunocompetent patients including blastomycosis and histoplasmosis; indicated for aspergillosis, and onychomycosis of the toenail; treatment of onychomycosis of the fingernail without concomitant toenail infection via a pulse-type dosing regimen; has activity against *Aspergillus*, *Candida*, *Coccidioides*, *Cryptococcus*, *Sporothrix*, tinea unguium

Oral: Useful in superficial mycoses including dermatophytoses (eg, tinea capitis), pityriasis versicolor, sebopsoriasis, vaginal and chronic mucocutaneous candidiases; systemic mycoses including candidiasis, meningeal and disseminated cryptococcal infections, paracoccidioidomycosis, coccidioidomycoses; miscellaneous mycoses such as sporotrichosis, chromomycosis, leishmaniasis, fungal keratitis, alternariosis, zygomycosis

Oral solution: Treatment of oral and esophageal candidiasis

Intravenous solution: Indicated in the treatment of blastomycosis, histoplasmosis (nonmeningeal), and aspergillosis (in patients intolerant or refractory to amphotericin B therapy); empiric therapy of febrile neutropenic fever

Mechanism of Action Interferes with cytochrome P450 activity, decreasing ergosterol synthesis (principal sterol in fungal cell membrane) and inhibiting cell membrane formation

Adverse Reactions

Listed incidences are for higher doses appropriate for systemic fungal infections.

Cardiovascular: Edema, hypertension, arrhythmia, CHF

Central nervous system: Headache, fatigue, malaise, fever, dizziness, somnolence

Dermatologic: Rash, pruritus, angioedema, urticaria, alopecia, photosensitivity, Stevens-Johnson syndrome

Endocrine & metabolic: Decreased libido, hypertriglyceridemia, hypokalemia, adrenal suppression, gynecomastia, menstrual disorders

Gastrointestinal: **Nausea**, abdominal pain, anorexia, vomiting, diarrhea, constipation, gastritis

Genitourinary: Impotence

Hematologic: Neutropenia

Hepatic: Abnormal LFTs, hepatitis, hepatic failure

Neuromuscular & skeletal: Peripheral neuropathy

Otic: Tinnitus

Renal: Albuminuria

Respiratory: Pulmonary edema

Miscellaneous: Allergic reactions, anaphylactoid reactions, anaphylaxis

Pharmacodynamics/Kinetics

Absorption: Requires gastric acidity; capsule better absorbed with food, solution better absorbed on empty stomach

Distribution: V_d (average): 796 ± 185 L or 10 L/kg; highly lipophilic and tissue concentrations are higher than plasma concentrations. The highest concentrations: adipose, omentum, endometrium, cervical and vaginal mucus, and skin/nails. Aqueous fluids (eg, CSF and urine) contain negligible amounts.

Protein binding, plasma: 99.9%; metabolite hydroxy-itraconazole: 99.5%

Metabolism: Extensively hepatic via CYP3A4 into >30 metabolites including hydroxy-itraconazole (major metabolite); appears to have *in vitro* antifungal activity. Main metabolic pathway is oxidation; may undergo saturation metabolism with multiple dosing.

Bioavailability: Variable, ~55% (oral solution) in 1 small study; **Note:** Oral solution has a higher degree of bioavailability ($149\% \pm 68\%$) relative to oral capsules; should not be interchanged

Half-life elimination: Oral: After single 200 mg dose: 21 ± 5 hours; 64 hours at steady-state; I.V.: steady-state: 35 hours; steady-state concentrations are achieved in 13 days with multiple administration of itraconazole 100-400 mg/day.

Excretion: Feces (~3% to 18%); urine (~0.03% as parent drug, 40% as metabolites)

Dosage Note: Capsule: Absorption is best if taken with food, therefore, it is best to administer itraconazole after meals; Solution: Should be taken on an empty stomach.

Children: Efficacy and safety have not been established; a small number of patients 3-16 years of age have been treated with 100 mg/day for systemic fungal infections with no serious adverse effects reported. A dose of 5 mg/kg once daily was used in a pharmacokinetic study using the oral solution in patients 6 months-12 years; duration of study was 2 weeks.

Adults:

Oral:

Blastomycosis/histoplasmosis: 200 mg once daily, if no obvious improvement or there is evidence of progressive fungal disease, increase the dose in 100 mg increments to a maximum of 400 mg/day; doses >200 mg/day are given in 2 divided doses; length of therapy varies from 1 day to >6 months depending on the condition and mycological response

Aspergillosis: 200-400 mg/day

Onychomycosis: 200 mg once daily for 12 consecutive weeks

Life-threatening infections: Loading dose: 200 mg 3 times/day (600 mg/day) should be given for the first 3 days of therapy

Oropharyngeal candidiasis: Oral solution: 200 mg once daily for 1-2 weeks; in patients unresponsive or refractory to fluconazole: 100 mg twice daily (clinical response expected in 1-2 weeks)

Esophageal candidiasis: Oral solution: 100-200 mg once daily for a minimum of 3 weeks; continue dosing for 2 weeks after resolution of symptoms

I.V.: 200 mg twice daily for 4 doses, followed by 200 mg daily

Dosing adjustment in renal impairment: Not necessary; itraconazole injection is not recommended in patients with Cl_{cr} <30 mL/minute

Hemodialysis: Not dialyzable

Dosing adjustment in hepatic impairment: May be necessary, but specific guidelines are not available. Risk-to-benefit evaluation should be undertaken in patients who develop liver function abnormalities during treatment.

Monitoring Parameters Liver function in patients with pre-existing hepatic dysfunction, and in all patients being treated for longer than 1 month

Administration

Oral: Doses >200 mg/day are given in 2 divided doses; do not administer with antacids. Capsule absorption is best if taken with food, therefore, it is best to administer itraconazole after meals; solution should be taken on an empty stomach. When treating oropharyngeal and esophageal candidiasis, solution should be swished vigorously in mouth, then swallowed.

I.V.: Infuse 60 mL of the dilute solution (3.33 mg/mL = 200 mg itraconazole, pH ~4.8) over 60 minutes; flush with 15-20 mL of 0.9% sodium chloride over 30 seconds to 15 minutes

Contraindications Hypersensitivity to itraconazole, any component of the formulation, or to other azoles; concurrent administration with cisapride, dofetilide, ergot derivatives, levomethadyl, lovastatin, midazolam, pimozide, quinidine, simvastatin, or triazolam; treatment of onychomycosis in patients with evidence of left ventricular dysfunction, CHF, or a history of CHF

Warnings Discontinue if signs or symptoms of CHF or neuropathy occur during treatment. **[U.S. Boxed Warning]: Rare cases of serious cardiovascular adverse events (including death), ventricular tachycardia, and torsade de pointes have been observed due to increased cisapride, pimozide, quinidine, dofetilide or levomethadyl concentrations induced by itraconazole; concurrent use contraindicated. Use with caution in patients with left ventricular dysfunction or a history of CHF; not recommended for treatment of onychomycosis in these patients.** Not recommended for use in patients with active liver disease, elevated liver enzymes, or prior hepatotoxic reactions to other drugs. Itraconazole has been associated with rare cases of serious hepatotoxicity (including fatal cases and cases within the first week of treatment); treatment should be discontinued in patients who develop clinical symptoms of liver dysfunction or abnormal liver function tests during itraconazole therapy except in cases where expected benefit exceeds risk. Large differences in itraconazole pharmacokinetic parameters have been observed in cystic fibrosis patients receiving the solution; if a patient with cystic fibrosis does not respond to therapy, alternate therapies should be considered. Due to differences in bioavailability, oral capsules and oral solution **cannot be used interchangeably.** Intravenous formulation should be used with caution in renal impairment; consider conversion to oral therapy if renal dysfunction/toxicity is noted. Initiation of treatment with oral solution is not recommended in patients at immediate risk for systemic candidiasis (eg, patients with severe neutropenia).

Dosage Forms

Capsule: 100 mg

Injection, solution: 10 mg/mL (25 mL) [packaged in a kit containing sodium chloride 0.9% (50 mL); filtered infusion set (1)]

Solution, oral: 100 mg/10 mL (150 mL) [cherry flavor]

Reference Range Antifungal activity associated with serum itraconazole levels >500 mcg/L

Overdosage/Treatment

Decontamination: Ipecac within 30 minutes or lavage (within 1 hour)/activated charcoal

Enhancement of elimination: Multiple dosing of activated charcoal would not be expected to be helpful

Drug Interactions Substrate of CYP3A4 (major); **Inhibits** CYP3A4 (strong)

Antacids: May decrease serum concentration of itraconazole. Administer antacids 1 hour before or 2 hours after itraconazole capsules.

Alfentanil: Serum concentrations may be increased; monitor.

Anticonvulsants: Itraconazole may increase the serum concentration of carbamazepine; carbamazepine, phenobarbital, and phenytoin may decrease the serum concentration of itraconazole.

Benzodiazepines: Alprazolam, diazepam, temazepam, triazolam, and midazolam serum concentrations may be increased; consider a benzodiazepine not metabolized by CYP3A4 (such as lorazepam) or another antifungal that is metabolized by CYP3A4

Buspirone: Serum concentrations may be increased; monitor for sedation

Busulfan: Serum concentrations may be increased; avoid concurrent use

Calcium channel blockers: Serum concentrations may be increased (applies to those agents metabolized by CYP3A4, including felodipine, nifedipine, and verapamil); consider another agent instead of a calcium channel blocker, another antifungal, or reduce the dose of the calcium channel blocker; monitor blood pressure

Cisapride; Serum concentration is increased which may lead to malignant arrhythmias; concurrent use is contraindicated

Corticosteroids: Serum levels/effects of the corticosteroid may be increased; use caution.

CYP3A4 inducers: CYP3A4 inducers may decrease the levels/effects of itraconazole. Example inducers include aminoglutethimide, carbamazepine, nafcillin, nevirapine, phenobarbital, phenytoin, and rifamycins.

CYP3A4 substrates: Itraconazole may increase the levels/effects of CYP3A4 substrates. Example substrates include benzodiazepines, calcium channel blockers, mirtazapine, nateglinide, nefazodone, tacrolimus, and venlafaxine. Selected benzodiazepines (midazolam and triazolam), cisapride, ergot alkaloids, selected HMG-CoA reductase inhibitors (lovastatin and simvastatin), and pimozide are generally contraindicated with strong CYP3A4 inhibitors.

Didanosine: May decrease absorption of itraconazole (due to buffering capacity of oral solution); applies only to oral solution formulation of didanosine

Digoxin: Serum concentrations may be increased; monitor.

Disopyramide: Serum levels/effects (including QT_c prolongation) may be increased; use caution.

Docetaxel: Serum concentrations may be increased; avoid concurrent use

Dofetilide: Serum levels/toxicity may be increased; concurrent use is contraindicated.

Eletriptan: Serum level/toxicity of eletriptan may be increased; use caution.

Ergot alkaloids: Toxicity (vasospasm, ischemia) may be significantly increased by itraconazole; concurrent use is contraindicated.

Erythromycin (and clarithromycin): May increase serum concentrations of itraconazole.

H_2 blockers: May decrease itraconazole absorption. Itraconazole depends on gastric acidity for absorption. Avoid concurrent use.

Halofantrine: Serum levels/effects (including QT_c prolongation) may be increased; use caution.

HMG-CoA reductase inhibitors (except pravastatin and fluvastatin): Serum concentrations may be increased. The risk of myopathy/rhabdomyolysis may be increased. Switch to pravastatin/fluvastatin or suspend treatment during course of itraconazole therapy.

Hypoglycemic agents, oral: Serum concentrations may be increased; monitor.

Immunosuppressants: Cyclosporine, sirolimus, and tacrolimus: Serum concentrations may be increased; monitor serum concentrations and renal function.

Levomethadyl: Serum levels/effects may be increased by itraconazole, potentially resulting in malignant arrhythmia; concurrent use is contraindicated.

Nevirapine: May decrease serum concentrations of itraconazole; monitor

Oral contraceptives: Efficacy may be reduced by itraconazole (limited data); use barrier birth control method during concurrent use

Pimozide: Serum levels/toxicity may be increased; concurrent use is contraindicated.

Protease inhibitors: May increase serum concentrations of itraconazole. Includes amprenavir, indinavir, nelfinavir, ritonavir, and saquinavir; monitor. Serum concentrations of indinavir, ritonavir, or saquinavir may be increased by itraconazole.

Proton pump inhibitors: May decrease itraconazole absorption. Itraconazole depends on gastric acidity for absorption. Avoid concurrent use (includes omeprazole, lansoprazole).

Quinidine: Serum levels may be increased. Concurrent use is contraindicated.

Rifabutin: Serum concentrations may be increased; monitor.

Sildenafil: Serum concentrations may be increased by itraconazole; consider dosage reduction. A maximum sildenafil dose of 25 mg in 48 hours is recommended with other strong CYP3A4 inhibitors.

Tadalafil: Serum concentrations may be increased by itraconazole. A maximum tadalafil dose of 10 mg in 72 hours is recommended with strong CYP3A4 inhibitors.

Trimetrexate: Serum concentrations may be increased; monitor

Vardenafil: Serum concentrations may be increased by itraconazole. If itraconazole dose is 200 mg/day, limit vardenafil dose to a maximum of 5 mg/24 hours. If itraconazole dose is 400 mg/day, limit vardenafil dose to a maximum of 2.5 mg/24 hours.

Warfarin: Anticoagulant effects may be increased; monitor INR and adjust warfarin's dose as needed

Vinca alkaloids: Serum concentrations may be increased; avoid concurrent use

Zolpidem: Serum levels may be increased; monitor

Pregnancy Risk Factor C

Pregnancy Implications Should not be used to treat onychomycosis during pregnancy. Effective contraception should be used during treatment and for 2 months following treatment. Congenital abnormalities have been reported during postmarketing surveillance, but a causal relationship has not been established.

Lactation Enters breast milk/not recommended

Specific References

Koks CH, Huitema AD, Kroon ED, et al, "Population Pharmacokinetics of Itraconazole in Thai HIV-1-Infected Persons," *Ther Drug Monit*, 2003, 25(2):229-33.

Ivermectin

CAS Number 70161-11-4; 70209-81-3; 70288-86-7

U.S. Brand Names Stromectol®

Use Treatment of the following infections: Strongyloidiasis of the intestinal tract due to the nematode parasite *Strongyloides stercoralis*. Onchocerciasis due to the nematode parasite *Onchocerca volvulus*. Ivermectin is only active against the immature form of *Onchocerca volvulus*, and the intestinal forms of *Strongyloides stercoralis*.

Unlabeled/Investigational Use Has been used for other parasitic infections including *Ascaris lumbricoides*, Bancroftian filariasis, *Brugia malayi*, scabies, *Enterobius vermicularis*, *Mansonella ozzardi*, *Trichuris trichiura*.

Mechanism of Action Ivermectin is a semisynthetic antihelminthic agent; it binds selectively and with strong affinity to glutamate-gated chloride ion channels which occur in invertebrate nerve and muscle cells. This leads to increased permeability of cell membranes to chloride ions then hyperpolarization of the nerve or muscle cell, and death of the parasite.

Adverse Reactions

Frequency not defined.

Cardiovascular: Hypotension, mild ECG changes, orthostasis, peripheral and facial edema, transient tachycardia

Central nervous system: Dizziness, headache, hyperthermia, insomnia, somnolence, vertigo

Dermatologic: Pruritus, rash, urticaria, toxic epidermal necrolysis

Gastrointestinal: Abdominal pain, anorexia, constipation, diarrhea, nausea, vomiting

Hematologic: Anemia, eosinophilia, leukopenia

Hepatic: ALT/AST increased

Neuromuscular & skeletal: Myalgia, tremor, weakness

Ocular: Blurred vision, mild conjunctivitis, punctate opacity

Respiratory: Asthma exacerbation

Mazzotti reaction (with onchocerciasis): Arthralgia, edema, fever, lymphadenopathy, ocular damage, pruritus, rash, synovitis

Signs and Symptoms of Overdose Abdominal pain, hypotension, lethargy, pallor, pruritus, tachycardia, urticaria, vomiting

Pharmacodynamics/Kinetics

Onset of action: Peak effect: 3-6 months

Absorption: Well absorbed

Distribution: Does not cross blood-brain barrier

Half-life elimination: 16-35 hours

Metabolism: Hepatic (>97%)

Excretion: Urine (<1%); feces

Dosage

Oral: Children ≥15 kg and Adults:

Strongyloidiasis: 200 mcg/kg as a single dose; follow-up stool examinations

Onchocerciasis: 150 mcg/kg as a single dose; retreatment may be required every 3-12 months until the adult worms die

Monitoring Parameters Skin and eye microfilarial counts, periodic ophthalmologic exams

Administration Administer on an empty stomach with water.

Contraindications Hypersensitivity to ivermectin or any component of the formulation

Warnings Data have shown that antihelmintic drugs like ivermectin may cause cutaneous and/or systemic reactions (Mazzoti reaction) of varying severity including ophthalmological reactions in patients with onchocerciasis. These reactions are probably due to allergic and inflammatory responses to the death of microfilariae. Patients with hyper-reactive onchodermatitis may be more likely than others to experience severe adverse reactions, especially edema and aggravation of the onchodermatitis. Repeated treatment may be required in immunocompromised patients (eg, HIV); control of extraintestinal strongyloidiasis may necessitate suppressive (once monthly) therapy. Pretreatment assessment for *Loa loa* infection is recommended in any patient with significant exposure to endemic areas (West and Central Africa); serious and/or fatal encephalopathy has been reported during treatment in patients with loiasis. Safety and efficacy in children <15 kg have not been established.

Dosage Forms Tablet [scored]: 3 mg

Reference Range Doses of 50 mcg/kg can result in blood ivermectin levels of 9-13 ng/mL; adverse effects do not correlate with serum concentrations

Overdosage/Treatment

Decontamination: Ipecac within 30 minutes or lavage (within 1 hour)/activated charcoal

Supportive therapy: Hypotension can be treated with I.V. fluids (ie, saline) and placement in Trendelenburg position; dopamine or norepinephrine can be used for refractory hypotension; antihistamines can be used for urticaria or pruritus

Drug Interactions Substrate of CYP3A4 (minor)

Pregnancy Risk Factor C

Pregnancy Implications Safety and efficacy have not been established in pregnant women. The WHO considers use after the first trimester as "probably acceptable."

Lactation Enters breast milk/not recommended

Additional Information Often used for prophylaxis against heartworm (*Dirofilaria immitis*) in dogs

Specific References

Bagheri H, Simiani E, Montastruc JL, et al, "Adverse Drug Reactions to Anthelmintics," *Ann Pharmacother*, 2004, 38(3):383-8.

Fawcett RS, "Ivermectin Use in Scabies," *Am Fam Physician*, 2003, 68(6):1089-92.

Ketamine

Related Information

- Highlights of Recent Reports (2006) on Substance Abuse and Mental Health
- Phencyclidine
- Therapeutic Drugs Associated with Hallucinations

CAS Number 1867-66-9; 6740-88-1

U.S. Brand Names Ketalar®

Synonyms Ketamine Hydrochloride

Impairment Potential Yes

Use Induction of anesthesia; short surgical procedures; dressing changes

Mechanism of Action An N-methyl-D-aspartate (NMDA) neuroreceptor antagonist; some opiate agonist effect; while analgesic effect is rapid, laryngeal reflexes, muscle tone, and cardiopulmonary function is usually not affected; structurally related to phencyclidine

Adverse Reactions

Cardiovascular: **Tachycardia, increased cardiac output, paradoxical direct myocardial depression, hypertension**, edema, sinus tachycardia

Central nervous system: **Visual hallucinations, increased intracranial pressure, vivid dreams**, delirium, dysphoric states, dystonic reactions, psychosis, dizziness, insomnia, ataxia, malignant hyperthermia, electroencephalogram abnormalities, aggressive behavior

Gastrointestinal: Increased salivation, nausea, vomiting

Neuromuscular & skeletal: **Tonic-clonic movements, tremors**, clonus, myoclonus, muscle rigidity, hypertonus

Ocular: Diplopia, lacrimation, increased intraocular pressure, nystagmus

Respiratory: Bronchodilatation, laryngospasm

Miscellaneous: **Emergence reactions, vocalization**

Signs and Symptoms of Overdose Apnea, cardiac arrest, delirium, extrapyramidal reaction, fasciculations, hyperglycemia, insomnia, lacrimation, laryngospasm, polyneuropathy, seizures

Pharmacodynamics/Kinetics

Onset of action:

I.V.: General anesthesia: 1-2 minutes; Sedation: 1-2 minutes

I.M.: General anesthesia: 3-8 minutes

Duration: I.V.: 5-15 minutes; I.M.: 12-25 minutes

Metabolism: Hepatic via hydroxylation and N-demethylation; the metabolite norketamine is 25% as potent as parent compound

Half-life elimination: 11-17 minutes; Elimination: 2.5-3.1 hours

Excretion: Clearance: 18 mL/kg/minute

Dosage Illicit dose "snorted" by drug abusers: 50-100 mg

Anesthetic induction dose:

Oral: 4-5 mg/kg

I.M.: 5-10 mg/kg

I.V.: 1-2 mg/kg

Maintenance dose is $^1/_2$, up to total induction dose as needed to maintain anesthesia

Stability Do not mix with barbiturates or diazepam → precipitation may occur

Monitoring Parameters Cardiovascular effects, heart rate, blood pressure, respiratory rate, transcutaneous O_2 saturation

Administration Relative exclusion criteria to minimize the risk of sympathomimetic adverse events in adults:

- Avoid ketamine in patients with poorly controlled hypertension or ED blood pressures 140/90 or above.
- Avoid ketamine in patients with known coronary artery disease, or in older patients with risk factors for coronary artery disease

Relative exclusion criteria to minimize risk of emergence reactions in adults:

- Avoid ketamine in patients with known or suspected psychosis, even if currently stable or controlled with medications.

Drug administration in adults:

- The recommended ketamine dose is 1.5-2.0 mg/kg I.V., administered over at least 1 minute; 100 mg is a typical adult dose. There is no evidence of any greater safety or other advantage at lower doses.
- Consider prophylactic coadministration of midazolam (2-4 mg I.V.) to reduce the risk of emergence reactions and to enhance cardiovascular stability.
- I.V. access is desirable so that additional midazolam can be promptly administered in the rare event of a clinically important emergence reaction.
- Whenever possible, minimize lighting, noise, and physical contact during recovery until wakefulness is well established.

Contraindications Hypersensitivity to ketamine or any component of the formulation; elevated intracranial pressure; hypertension, aneurysms, thyrotoxicosis, congestive heart failure, angina, psychotic disorders; pregnancy

Warnings Use with caution in patients with coronary artery disease, catecholamine depletion, and tachycardia. **[U.S. Boxed Warning]: Postanesthetic emergence reactions which can manifest as vivid dreams, hallucinations, and/or frank delirium occur in 12% of patients; these reactions are less common in patients >65 years of age and when given I.M.** Emergence reactions, confusion, or irrational behavior may occur up to 24 hours postoperatively and may be reduced by pretreatment with a benzodiazepine. May cause dependence (withdrawal symptoms on discontinuation) and tolerance with prolonged use.

Dosage Forms

Injection, solution: 50 mg/mL (10 mL); 100 mg/mL (5 mL)

Ketalar®: 10 mg/mL (20 mL); 50 mg/mL (10 mL); 100 mg/mL (5 mL)

Reference Range

An I.V. dose of 2.5 mg/kg produces an average serum ketamine concentration of 1 mg/L at 12 minutes and 0.5 mg/L at 30 minutes, while doses of 4 mg/kg can produce a peak serum ketamine level of 6.3 mg/L

Postmortem blood and urine levels from a mixed-drug fatality were reported as 1.8 mg/L and 2 mg/L, respectively

Overdosage/Treatment

Decontamination: Lavage (within 1 hour)/activated charcoal

Supportive therapy: Benzodiazepines can be utilized for delirium, dysphoric reactions, or hallucinations; extrapyramidal reaction can be treated with diphenhydramine and/or benztropine. Benzodiazepines, alpha- and beta-adrenergic blockers, or verapamil can decrease cardiac stimulation; benzodiazepines are initial choice for seizure management and adverse cardiovascular events. Cardiovascular response to labetalol may not be predictable. Atropine can be used to prevent excess salivation; positive end expiratory pressure can be used to treat laryngospasm.

Test Interactions Except for ToxiLab™ system, commercial immunoassay urine screening tests do **not** detect ketamine as phencyclidine even though it is structurally related to PCP.

Drug Interactions

Substrate (major) of CYP2B6, 2C9, 3A4

CYP2B6 inhibitors: May increase the levels/effects of ketamine. Example inhibitors include desipramine, paroxetine, and sertraline.

CYP2C9 Inhibitors may increase the levels/effects of ketamine. Example inhibitors include delavirdine, fluconazole, gemfibrozil, ketoconazole, nicardipine, NSAIDs, sulfonamides and tolbutamide.

CYP3A4 inhibitors: May increase the levels/effects of ketamine. Example inhibitors include azole antifungals, clarithromycin, diclofenac, doxycycline, erythromycin, imatinib, isoniazid, nefazodone, nicardipine, propofol, protease inhibitors, quinidine, telithromycin, and verapamil.

Increased effect: Barbiturates, narcotics, hydroxyzine increase prolonged recovery; nondepolarizing may increase effects

Increased toxicity: Muscle relaxants, thyroid hormones may increase blood pressure and heart rate; halothane may decrease BP

Pregnancy Risk Factor D

Pregnancy Implications Crosses the placenta; fetal respiratory depression can occur

Additional Information Elevation of catecholamine levels occur. Illicit use is usually by intranasal insufflation.

Specific References

Adamowicz P and Kala M, "Urinary Excretion Rates of Ketamine and Norketamine Following Therapeutic Ketamine Administration: Method and Detection Window Considerations," *J Anal Toxicol*, 2005, 29(5):376-82.

Allen JY and Macias CG, "The Efficacy of Ketamine in Pediatric Emergency Department Patients Who Present with Acute Severe Asthma," *Ann Emerg Med*, 2005, 46(1):43-50.

Arican FO, Okan T, Badak O, et al, "An Unusual Presentation from Xylazine-Ketamine," *Vet Hum Toxicol*, 2004, 46(6):324-5.

Cheng PS, Fu CY, Lee CH, et al, "A GC-MS Method Development Study for the Determination of Ketamine or Its Metabolites and the Evaluation of the REMEDi Screening Method Using Real Urine Samples," *J Anal Toxicol*, 2006, 30:164.

Green SM and Krauss B, "Clinical Practice Guideline for Emergency Department Ketamine Dissociative Sedation in Children," *Ann Emerg Med*, 2004, 44(5):460-71.

Green SM and Sherwin TS, "Incidence and Severity of Recovery Agitation After Ketamine Sedation in Young Adults," *Am J Emerg Med*, 2005, 23(2):142-4.

Haroz R and Greenberg MI, "Emerging Drugs of Abuse," *Med Clin North Am*, 2005, 89(6):1259-76 (review).

Lalonde BR and Wallage HR, "Postmortem Blood Ketamine Distribution in Two Fatalities," *J Anal Toxicol*, 2004, 28(1):71-4.

Leong HS, Tan NL, Lui CP, et al, "Evaluation of Ketamine Abuse Using Hair Analysis: Concentration Trends in a Singapore Population," *J Anal Toxicol*, 2005, 29(5):314-8.

Lin HR and Lua AC, "Detection of Acid-Labile Conjugates of Ketamine and Its Metabolites in Urine Samples Collected from Pub Participants," *J Anal Toxicol*, 2004, 28:181-6.

Lua AC and Lin HR, "A Rapid and Sensitive ESI-MS Screening Procedure for Ketamine and Norketamine in Urine Samples," *J Anal Toxicol*, 2004, 28(8):680-4.

Miksa IR, Cummings MR, and Poppenga RH, "Determination of Acepromazine, Ketamine, Medetomidine, and Xylazine in Serum: Multi-Residue Screening by Liquid Chromatography-Mass Spectrometry," *J Anal Toxicol*, 2005, 29:544-51.

Negrusz A, Adamowicz P, Saini BK, et al, "Detection of Ketamine and Norketamine in Urine of Nonhuman Primates After a Single Dose of Ketamine Using Microplate Enzyme-linked Immunosorbent Assay (ELISA) and NCI-GC-MS," *J Anal Toxicol*, 2005, 29(3):163-8.

Sigillito RJ, Tuckler VE, Van Meter KW, et al, "Near Fatal Accidental Transdermal Overdose of Compounded Ketamine, Baclofen, Amitriptyline, Lidocaine, and Ketoprofen: A Case Report," *J Toxicol Clin Toxicol*, 2003, 41(5):672.

Ketobemidone

CAS Number 469-79-4

Use Pain relief in the postoperative period and during acute myocardial infarction; premedication for anesthesia

Mechanism of Action Opioid compound similar to meperidine structurally

Adverse Reactions

Central nervous system: Lethargy, headache, confusion, sedation, dizziness, euphoria

Gastrointestinal: Ileus, nausea, vomiting, xerostomia, obstipation, constipation

Genitourinary: Urinary retention

Neuromuscular & skeletal: Smooth muscle spasm

Ocular: Blurred vision

Respiratory: Cough, apnea

Signs and Symptoms of Overdose Apnea, coma

Toxicodynamics/Kinetics

Duration of effect: 4-5 hours

Distribution: V_d: 2-7.8 L/kg

Metabolism: Hepatic to norketobemidone and 4′-hydroxyketombemidone

Bioavailability: Oral (34%), rectal (44%)

Half-life: 2-2.4 hours

Elimination: Renal

Dosage

I.M.: 5-7.5 mg every 6 hours

I.V.:

Patient-controlled analgesia: 2-3 mg over one minute with each dose allowable per 15 minutes

Postoperative pain: 3 mg/hour decreasing to 0.75 mg/hour after shivering cessation

Oral: 5-15 mg every 3-6 hours

Rectal: 10 mg every 3-4 hours

Reference Range Following a 10 mg I.V. dose, peak serum levels are >500 ng/mL; following a 10 mg rectal dose, peak plasma levels range from 10-15 ng/mL; after a 10 mg oral dose, peak serum levels range from 10-30 ng/mL

Overdosage/Treatment Supportive therapy: Naloxone hydrochloride (0.4-2 mg I.V., SubQ, or through an endotracheal tube); a continuous infusion (at $^2/_3$ the response dose/hour) may be required

Antidote(s)

- Nalmefene [ANTIDOTE]
- Naloxone [ANTIDOTE]

Additional Information Often combined with a spasmolytic agent W-N-dimethyl-3,3-diphenyl 1-methylallylamine (A-29) due to its effects on smooth muscle spasm

Ketoconazole

CAS Number 65277-42-1

U.S. Brand Names Nizoral® A-D [OTC]; Nizoral®

Use Treatment of susceptible fungal infections, including candidiasis, oral thrush, blastomycosis, histoplasmosis, paracoccidioidomycosis, chronic mucocutaneous candidiasis, as well as certain recalcitrant cutaneous dermatophytoses; used topically for treatment of tinea corporis, tinea cruris, tinea versicolor and cutaneous candidiasis

Treatment of prostate cancer (androgen synthesis inhibitor)

Mechanism of Action Alters permeability of the cell wall; inhibits biosynthesis of triglycerides and phospholipids by fungi; inhibits several fungal enzymes that results in a build-up of toxic concentrations of hydrogen peroxide

Adverse Reactions

Cardiovascular: QT prolongation, vasculitis

Central nervous system: Psychosis, paranoid ideation

Dermatologic: Pruritus, rash, exfoliative dermatitis, alopecia, angioedema, xerosis, purpura, photosensitivity, exanthem, lichen planus

Endocrine & metabolic: Adrenal cortical insufficiency, gynecomastia

Gastrointestinal: Nausea, vomiting, abdominal pain, GI bleeding, anorexia, gingival hyperplasia

Hematologic: Thrombocytopenia

Hepatic: Hepatotoxicity, aminotransferase level elevation (asymptomatic)

Local: Irritation, stinging, phlebitis

Miscellaneous: Fixed drug eruption

Signs and Symptoms of Overdose Diarrhea, dizziness, headache, hypertriglyceridemia, hyperuricemia, hypothyroidism, myalgia, nausea, paresthesias, photophobia, sexual dysfunction, thrombocytopenia, vomiting

Pharmacodynamics/Kinetics

Absorption: Oral: Rapid (~75%); Shampoo: None; Gel: Minimal

Distribution: Well into inflamed joint fluid, saliva, bile, urine, breast milk, sebum, cerumen, feces, tendons, skin and soft tissues, and testes; crosses blood-brain barrier poorly; only negligible amounts reach CSF

Protein binding: 93% to 96%

Metabolism: Partially hepatic via CYP3A4 to inactive compounds

Bioavailability: Decreases as gastric pH increases

Half-life elimination: Biphasic: Initial: 2 hours; Terminal: 8 hours

Time to peak, serum: 1-2 hours

Excretion: Feces (57%); urine (13%)

Dosage

Oral:

Children ≥2 years: 3.3-6.6 mg/kg/day as a single dose for 1-2 weeks for candidiasis, for at least 4 weeks in recalcitrant dermatophyte infections, and for up to 6 months for other systemic mycoses

Adults: 200-400 mg/day as a single daily dose for durations as stated above

Shampoo: Apply twice weekly for 4 weeks with at least 3 days between each shampoo

Topical: Rub gently into the affected area once daily to twice daily

Dosing adjustment in hepatic impairment: Dose reductions should be considered in patients with severe liver disease

Hemodialysis: Not dialyzable (0% to 5%)

Monitoring Parameters Liver function tests

Administration

Administer oral tablets 2 hours prior to antacids to prevent decreased absorption due to the high pH of gastric contents. Cream, gel, and shampoo are for external use only.

Contraindications Hypersensitivity to ketoconazole or any component of the formulation; CNS fungal infections (due to poor CNS penetration); coadministration with ergot derivatives or cisapride is contraindicated due to risk of potentially fatal cardiac arrhythmias

Warnings

[U.S. Boxed Warning]: Ketoconazole has been associated with hepatotoxicity, including some fatalities; use with caution in patients with impaired hepatic function and perform periodic liver function tests.

[U.S. Boxed Warning]: Concomitant use with cisapride is contraindicated due to the occurrence of ventricular arrhythmias. High doses of ketoconazole may depress adrenocortical function.

Topical: Formulations may contain sulfites. Avoid exposure of gel to open flames during or immediately after application.

Dosage Forms

Cream, topical: 2% (15 g, 30 g, 60 g)

Kuric™: 2%: (25 g, 75 g)

Gel, topical:

Xolegel™: 2% (15 g)

Shampoo, topical: 1% (120 mL)

Nizoral® A-D: 1% (120 mL, 210 mL)

Tablet: 200 mg

Nizoral®: 200 mg

Reference Range Therapeutic: Peak: 1-4 mg/L; Trough: ≤1 mg/L

Overdosage/Treatment

Decontamination: Ipecac within 30 minutes or lavage (within 1 hour)/ activated charcoal

Enhancement of elimination: Multiple dosing of activated charcoal would not be expected to be helpful; not dialyzable (0% to 5%)

Drug Interactions Substrate of CYP3A4 (major); **Inhibits** CYP1A2 (strong), 2A6 (moderate), 2B6 (weak), 2C8 (weak), 2C9 (strong), 2C19 (moderate), 2D6 (moderate), 3A4 (strong)

Benzodiazepines: Alprazolam, diazepam, temazepam, triazolam, and midazolam serum concentrations may be increased; consider a benzodiazepine not metabolized by CYP3A4 (such as lorazepam) or another antifungal that is metabolized by CYP3A4. Concurrent use is contraindicated.

Buspirone: Serum concentrations may be increased; monitor for sedation

Busulfan: Serum concentrations may be increased; avoid concurrent use

Calcium channel blockers: Serum concentrations may be increased (applies to those agents metabolized by CYP3A4, including felodipine, nifedipine, and verapamil); consider another agent instead of a calcium channel blocker, another antifungal, or reduce the dose of the calcium channel blocker; monitor blood pressure

Cisapride: Serum concentration is increased which may lead to malignant arrhythmias; concurrent use is contraindicated

CYP1A2 substrates: Ketoconazole may increase the levels/effects of CYP1A2 substrates. Example substrates include aminophylline, fluvoxamine, mexiletine, mirtazapine, ropinirole, theophylline, and trifluoperazine.

CYP2A6 substrates: Ketoconazole may increase the levels/effects of CYP2A6 substrates. Example substrates include dexmedetomidine and ifosfamide.

CYP2C9 substrates: Ketoconazole may increase the levels/effects of CYP2C9 substrates. Example substrates include bosentan, dapsone, fluoxetine, glimepiride, glipizide, losartan, montelukast, nateglinide, paclitaxel, phenytoin, warfarin, and zafirlukast.

CYP2C19 substrates: Ketoconazole may increase the levels/effects of CYP2C19 substrates. Example substrates include citalopram, diazepam, methsuximide, phenytoin, propranolol, and sertraline.

CYP2D6 substrates: Ketoconazole may increase the levels/effects of CYP2D6 substrates. Example substrates include amphetamines, selected beta-blockers, dextromethorphan, fluoxetine, lidocaine, mirtazapine, nefazodone, paroxetine, risperidone, ritonavir, thioridazine, tricyclic antidepressants, and venlafaxine.

CYP2D6 prodrug substrates: Ketoconazole may decrease the levels/effects of CYP2D6 prodrug substrates. Example prodrug substrates include codeine, hydrocodone, oxycodone, and tramadol.

CYP3A4 inducers: CYP3A4 inducers may decrease the levels/effects of ketoconazole. Example inducers include aminoglutethimide, carbamazepine, nafcillin, nevirapine, phenobarbital, phenytoin, and rifamycins.

CYP3A4 substrates: Ketoconazole may increase the levels/effects of CYP3A4 substrates. Example substrates include benzodiazepines, calcium channel blockers, mirtazapine, nateglinide, nefazodone, tacrolimus, and venlafaxine. Selected benzodiazepines (midazolam and triazolam), cisapride, ergot alkaloids, selected HMG-CoA reductase inhibitors (lovastatin and simvastatin), and pimozide are generally contraindicated with strong CYP3A4 inhibitors.

Didanosine: May decrease absorption of ketoconazole (due to buffering capacity of oral solution); applies only to oral solution formulation of didanosine

Docetaxel: Serum concentrations may be increased; avoid concurrent use

Erythromycin (and clarithromycin): May increase serum concentrations of ketoconazole.

H_2 blockers: May decrease ketoconazole absorption. Ketoconazole depends on gastric acidity for absorption. Avoid concurrent use.

HMG-CoA reductase inhibitors (except pravastatin and fluvastatin): Serum concentrations may be increased. The risk of myopathy/rhabdomyolysis may be increased. Switch to pravastatin/fluvastatin or suspend treatment during course of ketoconazole therapy.

Immunosuppressants: Cyclosporine, sirolimus, and tacrolimus: Serum concentrations may be increased; monitor serum concentrations and renal function

Methylprednisolone: Serum concentrations may be increased; monitor

Nevirapine: May decrease serum concentrations of ketoconazole; monitor

Oral contraceptives: Efficacy may be reduced by ketoconazole (limited data); use barrier birth control method during concurrent use

Phenytoin: Serum concentrations may be increased; monitor phenytoin levels and adjust dose as needed

Protease inhibitors: May increase serum concentrations of ketoconazole. Includes amprenavir, indinavir, nelfinavir, ritonavir, and saquinavir; monitor

Proton pump inhibitors: May decrease ketoconazole absorption. Ketoconazole depends on gastric acidity for absorption. Avoid concurrent use (includes omeprazole, lansoprazole).

Quinidine: Serum levels may be increased; monitor

Rifampin: Rifampin decreases ketoconazole's serum concentration to levels which are no longer effective; avoid concurrent use.

Sildenafil: Serum concentrations may be increased by ketoconazole; consider dosage reduction. A maximum sildenafil dose of 25 mg in 48 hours is recommended with other strong CYP3A4 inhibitors.

Tadalafil: Serum concentrations may be increased by ketoconazole. A maximum tadalafil dose of 10 mg in 72 hours is recommended with strong CYP3A4 inhibitors.

Trimetrexate: Serum concentrations may be increased; monitor

Vardenafil: Serum concentrations may be increased by ketoconazole. If ketoconazole dose is 200 mg/day, limit vardenafil to a maximum of 5 mg/24 hours. If ketoconazole dose is 400 mg/day, limit vardenafil dose to a maximum of 2.5 mg/24 hours.

Warfarin: Anticoagulant effects may be increased; monitor INR and adjust warfarin's dose as needed

Vinca alkaloids: Serum concentrations may be increased; avoid concurrent use

Zolpidem: Serum levels may be increased; monitor

Pregnancy Risk Factor C

Pregnancy Implications Teratogenic effects were noted in animal studies. There are no adequate and well-controlled studies in pregnant women.

Lactation Enters breast milk/not recommended

Nursing Implications Administer 2 hours prior to antacids H_2-receptor antagonist to prevent decreased absorption due to the high pH of gastric contents

Specific References

Bulkowstein M, Mordish Y, Zimmerman DR, et al, "Ketoconazole-Induced Neurologic Sequelae," *Vet Hum Toxicol*, 2003, 45(5):239-40.

Liu PY, Lee CH, Lin LJ, et al, "Refractory Anaphylactic Shock Associated with Ketoconazole Treatment." *Ann Pharmacother*, 2005, 39(3):547-50.

Ketoprofen

Related Information

• Nonsteroidal Anti-inflammatory Drugs

CAS Number 22071-15-4 (Base); 57469-78-0 (Lysine); 57495-14-4 (Sodium)

U.S. Brand Names Orudis® KT [OTC]; Oruvail®

Use Acute or long-term treatment of rheumatoid arthritis and osteoarthritis; primary dysmenorrhea; mild to moderate pain

Mechanism of Action Inhibits prostaglandin synthesis by decreasing the activity of the enzyme, cyclooxygenase, which results in decreased formation of prostaglandin precursors

Adverse Reactions

Cardiovascular: Arrhythmias, congestive heart failure, hypertension, tachycardia

Central nervous system: Headache, nervousness, dizziness, somnolence, insomnia, malaise, depression, aseptic meningitis, confusion, drowsiness, hallucinations

Dermatologic: Rash, itching, angioedema, erythema multiforme, photosensitivity, Stevens-Johnson syndrome, toxic epidermal necrolysis, urticaria

Endocrine & metabolic: Fluid retention, hot flashes, polydipsia

Gastrointestinal: **Dyspepsia**, vomiting, diarrhea, nausea, constipation, abdominal distress/cramping/pain, flatulence, anorexia, stomatitis, gastritis, GI ulceration

Genitourinary: Urinary tract infection, cystitis

Hematologic: Agranulocytosis, anemia, bone marrow suppression, hemolytic anemia, leukopenia, thrombocytopenia

Hepatic: Hepatitis

Neuromuscular & skeletal: Peripheral neuropathy

Ocular: Visual disturbances, blurred vision, conjunctivitis, dry eyes, toxic amblyopia

Otic: Tinnitus, hearing decreased

Renal: Acute renal failure, renal function impairment, polyuria

Respiratory: Allergic rhinitis, dyspnea, epistaxis

Miscellaneous: Allergic reaction, anaphylaxis

Signs and Symptoms of Overdose Cognitive dysfunction, confusion, conjunctivitis, depression, drowsiness, dyspnea, eczema, exfoliative dermatitis, gastritis, GI bleeding, impotence, insomnia, myalgia, nausea, nephrotic syndrome, ototoxicity, photosensitivity, pseudotumor cerebri, purpura, tinnitus, vomiting, wheezing

Severe poisoning can manifest with apnea, coma, hypotension, leukocytosis, metabolic acidosis, nystagmus, renal and/or hepatic failure, respiratory depression, seizures

Pharmacodynamics/Kinetics

Absorption: Almost complete

Protein binding: >99%, primarily albumin

Metabolism: Hepatic via glucuronidation; metabolite can be converted back to parent compound; may have enterohepatic recirculation

Half-life elimination:
Capsule: 2-4 hours; moderate-severe renal impairment: 5-9 hours
Capsule, extended release: ~3-7.5 hours

Time to peak, serum:
Capsule: 0.5-2 hours

Capsule, extended release: 6-7 hours

Excretion: Urine (~80%, primarily as glucuronide conjugates)

Dosage

Oral:

Children ≥16 years and Adults:

Rheumatoid arthritis or osteoarthritis:

Capsule: 50-75 mg 3-4 times/day up to a maximum of 300 mg/day

Capsule, extended release: 200 mg once daily

Mild to moderate pain: Capsule: 25-50 mg every 6-8 hours up to a maximum of 300 mg/day

OTC labeling: 12.5 mg every 4-6 hours, up to a maximum of 6 tablets/24 hours

Elderly: Initial dose should be decreased in patients >75 years; use caution when dosage changes are made

Dosage adjustment in renal impairment:

Mild impairment: Maximum dose: 150 mg/day

Severe impairment: Maximum dose: 100 mg/day

Dosage adjustment in hepatic impairment and serum albumin <3.5 g/dL: Maximum dose: 100 mg/day

Administration

May take with food to reduce GI upset. Do not crush or break extended release capsules.

Contraindications Hypersensitivity to ketoprofen, aspirin, other NSAIDs, or any component of the formulation; perioperative pain in the setting of coronary artery bypass surgery (CABG); pregnancy (3rd trimester)

Warnings [U.S. Boxed Warning]: NSAIDs are associated with an increased risk of adverse cardiovascular events, including MI, stroke, and new onset or worsening of pre-existing hypertension. Risk may be increased with duration of use or pre-existing cardiovascular risk-factors or disease. Carefully evaluate individual cardiovascular risk profiles prior to prescribing. Use caution with fluid retention, CHF or hypertension.

Use of NSAIDs can compromise existing renal function. Renal toxicity can occur in patient with impaired renal function, dehydration, heart failure, liver dysfunction, those taking diuretics and ACEI and the elderly. Rehydrate patient before starting therapy. Monitor renal function closely. Ketoprofen is not recommended for patients with advanced renal disease.

[U.S. Boxed Warning]: NSAIDs may increase risk of gastrointestinal irritation, ulceration, bleeding, and perforation. These events may occur at any time during therapy and without warning. Use caution with a history of GI disease (bleeding or ulcers), concurrent therapy with aspirin, anticoagulants and/or corticosteroids, smoking, use of alcohol, the elderly or debilitated patients.

Use the lowest effective dose for the shortest duration of time, consistent with individual patient goals, to reduce risk of cardiovascular or GI adverse events. Alternate therapies should be considered for patients at high risk.

NSAIDs may cause serious skin adverse events including exfoliative dermatitis, Stevens-Johnson syndrome (SJS) and toxic epidermal necrolysis (TEN). Anaphylactoid reactions may occur, even without prior exposure; patients with "aspirin triad" (bronchial asthma, aspirin intolerance, rhinitis) may be at increased risk. Do not use in patients who experience bronchospasm, asthma, rhinitis, or urticaria with NSAID or aspirin therapy.

Use with caution in patients with decreased hepatic function. Closely monitor patients with any abnormal LFT. Severe hepatic reactions (eg, fulminant hepatitis, liver failure) have occurred with NSAID use, rarely; discontinue if signs or symptoms of liver disease develop, or if systemic manifestations occur.

Withhold for at least 4-6 half-lives prior to surgical or dental procedures. Safety and efficacy have not been established in pediatric patients.

Dosage Forms

[DSC] = Discontinued product

Capsule: 50 mg, 75 mg

Capsule, extended release: 200 mg

Tablet (Orudis® KT): 12.5 mg [contains tartrazine and sodium benzoate] [DSC]

Overdosage/Treatment

Decontamination: Ipecac within 30 minutes or lavage (within 1 hour)/ activated charcoal

Supportive therapy: Hypotension/dehydration can be managed with I.V. fluid therapy; acidosis should be treated with bicarbonates, seizures with benzodiazepines; antacids, blood products are indicated, as appropriate, for hemorrhage; famotidine (40 mg 2 times/day) can decrease incidence of gastric or duodenal ulcers in patients receiving long-term therapy of this drug

Enhancement of elimination: Dialysis or perfusion is indicated for secondary complications, acidosis, or renal failure and not toxin removal alone; multiple dosing of activated charcoal may be effective

Test Interactions ↑ chloride (S), sodium (S)

Drug Interactions

Inhibits CYP2C9 (weak)

ACE inhibitors: Antihypertensive effects may be decreased by concurrent therapy with NSAIDs; monitor blood pressure

Aminoglycosides: NSAIDs may decrease the excretion of aminoglycosides.

Angiotensin II antagonists: Antihypertensive effects may be decreased by concurrent therapy with NSAIDs; monitor blood pressure.

Anticoagulants (warfarin, heparin, LMWHs): In combination with NSAIDs can cause increased risk of bleeding.

Antiplatelet agents (ticlopidine, clopidogrel, aspirin, abciximab, dipyridamole, eptifibatide, tirofiban): In combination with NSAIDs can cause an increased risk of bleeding.

Beta-blockers: NSAIDs may decrease the antihypertensive effect of beta-blockers. Monitor.

Bisphosphonates: NSAIDs may increase the risk of gastrointestinal ulceration.

Cholestyramine (and other bile acid sequestrants): May decrease the absorption of NSAIDs. Separate by at least 2 hours.

Corticosteroids: May increase the risk of GI ulceration; avoid concurrent use.

Cyclosporine: NSAIDs may increase serum creatinine, potassium, blood pressure, and cyclosporine levels; monitor cyclosporine levels and renal function carefully.

Hydralazine: Antihypertensive effect is decreased; avoid concurrent use.

Lithium: Lithium levels can be increased; avoid concurrent use if possible or monitor lithium levels and adjust dose. Sulindac may have the least effect. When NSAID is stopped, lithium will need adjustment again.

Loop diuretics: Antihypertensive and diuretic effects may be diminished. Indomethacin reduces this efficacy, however, it may be anticipated with any NSAID.

Methotrexate: Severe bone marrow suppression, aplastic anemia, and GI toxicity have been reported with concomitant NSAID therapy. Avoid use during moderate or high-dose methotrexate (increased and prolonged methotrexate levels). NSAID use during low-dose treatment of rheumatoid arthritis has not been fully evaluated; extreme caution is warranted.

Pemetrexed: NSAIDs may decrease the excretion of pemetrexed. Patients with Cl_{cr} 45-79 mL/minute should avoid long acting NSAIDs for 5 days before and 2 days after pemetrexed treatment.

Probenecid: May increase the serum concentration of ketoprofen.

Thiazides: Antihypertensive effects may be decreased; avoid concurrent use.

Treprostinil: May enhance the risk of bleeding with concurrent use.

Vancomycin: NSAIDs may decrease the excretion of vancomycin.

Pregnancy Risk Factor B/D (3rd trimester)

Pregnancy Implications Teratogenic effects were not observed in animal studies. Embryotoxicity was observed in some, but not all, animal studies. Renal insufficiency and pulmonary hypertension have been noted in premature infants (case reports). Accumulation of the active enantiomer of ketoprofen has also been reported in premature neonates with renal insufficiency. Exposure to NSAIDs late in pregnancy may lead to premature closure of the ductus arteriosus and may inhibit uterine contractions.

Lactation Excretion in breast milk unknown/not recommended

Nursing Implications Do not crush capsule

Ketorolac

Related Information

- Nonsteroidal Anti-inflammatory Drugs

CAS Number 74103-06-3 (Base); 74103-07-4 (Tromethamine)

U.S. Brand Names Acular LS™; Acular® PF; Acular®; Toradol®

Synonyms Ketorolac Tromethamine

Use

Oral, injection: Short-term (≤5 days) management of moderately-severe acute pain requiring analgesia at the opioid level

Ophthalmic: Temporary relief of ocular itching due to seasonal allergic conjunctivitis; postoperative inflammation following cataract extraction; reduction of ocular pain and photophobia following incisional refractive surgery, reduction of ocular pain, burning and stinging following corneal refractive surgery

Mechanism of Action Inhibits prostaglandin synthesis by decreasing the activity of the enzyme, cyclooxygenase, which results in decreased formation of prostaglandin precursors

Adverse Reactions

Systemic:

Cardiovascular: Edema, hypertension, pallor, palpitation, syncope, flushing, hypotension

Central nervous system: **Headache**, dizziness, drowsiness, abnormal dreams, abnormal thinking, depression, euphoria, extrapyramidal symptoms, fever, hallucinations, inability to concentrate, insomnia, nervousness, stupor, aseptic meningitis, convulsions, psychosis

Dermatologic: Pruritus, purpura, rash, urticaria, exfoliative dermatitis, Lyell's syndrome, maculopapular rash, Stevens-Johnson syndrome, toxic epidermal necrolysis

Endocrine & metabolic: Hyperkalemia, hyponatremia

Gastrointestinal: **Gastrointestinal pain, dyspepsia, nausea**, diarrhea, constipation, flatulence, gastrointestinal fullness, vomiting, stomatitis, abnormal taste, anorexia, appetite increased, dry mouth, eructation, gastritis, rectal bleeding, weight gain, acute pancreatitis, esophagitis, GI hemorrhage, GI perforation, hematemesis, melena, peptic ulceration, tongue edema

Genitourinary: Urinary frequency increased, urinary retention

Hematologic: Anemia, eosinophilia, hemolytic uremic syndrome, leukopenia, thrombocytopenia, wound hemorrhage (postoperative)

Hepatic: Cholestatic jaundice, hepatitis, liver failure

Local: Injection site pain

Neuromuscular & skeletal: Hyperkinesis, paresthesia, tremors, weakness, flank pain, myalgia

Ocular: Abnormal vision, blurred vision

Otic: Hearing loss, tinnitus

Renal: Hematuria, oliguria, polyuria, proteinuria, acute renal failure, azotemia, nephritis

Respiratory: Cough, dyspnea, epistaxis, pulmonary edema, rhinitis, asthma, bronchospasm, laryngeal edema

Miscellaneous: Diaphoresis, excessive thirst, infections, anaphylactoid reaction, anaphylaxis, hypersensitivity reactions

Ophthalmic solution:

Central nervous system: Headache

Ocular: **Transient burning/stinging (Acular®: 40%; Acular® PF: 20%)**, conjunctival hyperemia, corneal infiltrates, iritis, ocular edema, ocular inflammation, ocular irritation, ocular pain, superficial keratitis, superficial ocular infection, dry eyes, corneal ulcer, blurred vision, corneal erosion, corneal perforation, corneal thinning, epithelial breakdown

Miscellaneous: Allergic reactions

Chills, coagulopathy, cognitive dysfunction, drowsiness, dry mouth, GI bleeding, nausea, nephrotic syndrome, ototoxicity, tinnitus, vomiting, wheezing

Severe poisoning can manifest with coma, hypotension, renal and/or hepatic failure, respiratory depression, seizures

Pharmacodynamics/Kinetics

Onset of action: Analgesic: I.M.: ~10 minutes

Peak effect: Analgesic: 2-3 hours

Duration: Analgesic: 6-8 hours

Absorption: Oral: Well absorbed

Distribution: Poor penetration into CSF; crosses placenta; enters breast milk

Protein binding: 99%

Metabolism: Hepatic

Half-life elimination: 2-8 hours; prolonged 30% to 50% in elderly

Time to peak, serum: I.M.: 30-60 minutes

Excretion: Urine (61% as unchanged drug)

Dosage

Children 2-16 years: **Do not exceed adult doses**

Single-dose treatment:

I.M.: 1 mg/kg (maximum: 30 mg)

I.V.: 0.5 mg/kg (maximum: 15 mg)

Oral (unlabeled): 1 mg/kg as a single dose reported in one study

Multiple-dose treatment (unlabeled): Limited pediatric studies. The maximum combined duration of treatment (for parenteral and oral) is 5 days.

I.V.: Initial dose: 0.5 mg/kg, followed by 0.25-1 mg/kg every 6 hours for up to 48 hours (maximum daily dose: 90 mg)

Oral: 0.25 mg/kg every 6 hours

Adults (pain relief usually begins within 10 minutes with parenteral forms):

Note: The maximum combined duration of treatment (for parenteral and oral) is 5 days; do not increase dose or frequency; supplement with low-dose opioids if needed for breakthrough pain. For patients <50 kg and/or ≥65 years, see Elderly dosing.

I.M.: 60 mg as a single dose or 30 mg every 6 hours (maximum daily dose: 120 mg)

I.V.: 30 mg as a single dose or 30 mg every 6 hours (maximum daily dose: 120 mg)

Oral: 20 mg, followed by 10 mg every 4-6 hours; do not exceed 40 mg/day; oral dosing is intended to be a continuation of I.M. or I.V. therapy only

Ophthalmic: Children ≥3 years and Adults:

Allergic conjunctivitis (relief of ocular itching) (Acular®): Instill 1 drop (0.25 mg) 4 times/day for seasonal allergic conjunctivitis

Inflammation following cataract extraction (Acular®): Instill 1 drop (0.25 mg) to affected eye(s) 4 times/day beginning 24 hours after surgery; continue for 2 weeks

Pain and photophobia following incisional refractive surgery (Acular® PF): Instill 1 drop (0.25 mg) 4 times/day to affected eye for up to 3 days

Pain following corneal refractive surgery (Acular LS™): Instill 1 drop 4 times/day as needed to affected eye for up to 4 days

Elderly >65 years: Renal insufficiency or weight <50 kg: **Note:** Ketorolac has decreased clearance and increased half-life in the elderly. In addition, the elderly have reported increased incidence of GI bleeding, ulceration, and perforation. The maximum combined duration of treatment (for parenteral and oral) is 5 days.

I.M.: 30 mg as a single dose or 15 mg every 6 hours (maximum daily dose: 60 mg)

I.V.: 15 mg as a single dose or 15 mg every 6 hours (maximum daily dose: 60 mg)

Oral: 10 mg every 4-6 hours; do not exceed 40 mg/day; oral dosing is intended to be a continuation of I.M. or I.V. therapy only

Dosage adjustment in renal impairment: Do not use in patients with advanced renal impairment. Patients with moderately-elevated serum creatinine should use half the recommended dose, not to exceed 60 mg/day I.M./I.V.

Dosage adjustment in hepatic impairment: Use with caution, may cause elevation of liver enzymes

Stability Do not mix with morphine sulfate, meperidine hydrochloride, promethazine hydrochloride, or hydroxyzine hydrochloride in that precipitation may occur

Monitoring Parameters Monitor response (pain, range of motion, grip strength, mobility, ADL function), inflammation; observe for weight gain, edema; monitor renal function (serum creatinine, BUN, urine output); observe for bleeding, bruising; evaluate gastrointestinal effects (abdominal pain, bleeding, dyspepsia); mental confusion, disorientation, CBC, liver function tests

Administration Oral: May take with food to reduce GI upset

I.M.: Administer slowly and deeply into the muscle. Analgesia begins in 30 minutes and maximum effect within 2 hours

I.V.: Administer I.V. bolus over a minimum of 15 seconds; onset within 30 minutes; peak analgesia within 2 hours

Ophthalmic solution: Contact lenses should be removed before instillation.

Contraindications Hypersensitivity to ketorolac, aspirin, other NSAIDs, or any component of the formulation; active or history of peptic ulcer disease; recent or history of GI bleeding or perforation; patients with advanced renal disease or risk of renal failure; labor and delivery; nursing mothers; prophylaxis before major surgery; suspected or confirmed cerebrovascular bleeding; hemorrhagic diathesis; concurrent ASA or other NSAIDs; epidural or intrathecal administration; concomitant probenecid; perioperative pain in the setting of coronary artery bypass surgery (CABG); pregnancy (3rd trimester)

Warnings

Systemic: Treatment should be started with I.V./I.M. administration then changed to oral only as a continuation of treatment. Total therapy is not to exceed 5 days. Should not be used for minor or chronic pain.

May prolong bleeding time; do not use when hemostasis is critical. Patients should be euvolemic prior to treatment. Low doses of narcotics may be needed for breakthrough pain.

[U.S. Boxed Warning]: NSAIDs are associated with an increased risk of adverse cardiovascular events, including MI, stroke, and new onset or worsening of pre-existing hypertension. Risk may be increased with duration of use or pre-existing cardiovascular risk-factors or disease. Carefully evaluate individual cardiovascular risk profiles prior to prescribing. Use caution with fluid retention, CHF or hypertension.

Use of NSAIDs can compromise existing renal function. Renal toxicity can occur in patient with impaired renal function, dehydration, heart failure, liver dysfunction, those taking diuretics and ACEI and the elderly. Rehydrate patient before starting therapy. Monitor renal function closely. Ketorolac is not recommended for patients with advanced renal disease.

[U.S. Boxed Warning]: NSAIDs may increase risk of gastrointestinal irritation, ulceration, bleeding, and perforation. These events may occur at any time during therapy and without warning. Use caution with a history of GI disease (bleeding or ulcers), concurrent therapy with aspirin, anticoagulants and/or corticosteroids, smoking, use of alcohol, the elderly or debilitated patients.

Use the lowest effective dose for the shortest duration of time, consistent with individual patient goals, to reduce risk of cardiovascular or GI adverse events. Alternate therapies should be considered for patients at high risk.

NSAIDs may cause serious skin adverse events including exfoliative dermatitis, Stevens-Johnson syndrome (SJS) and toxic epidermal necrolysis (TEN). Anaphylactoid reactions may occur, even without prior exposure; patients with "aspirin triad" (bronchial asthma, aspirin intolerance, rhinitis) may be at increased risk. Do not use in patients who experience bronchospasm, asthma, rhinitis, or urticaria with NSAID or aspirin therapy.

Use with caution in patients with decreased hepatic function. Closely monitor patients with any abnormal LFT. Severe hepatic reactions (eg, fulminant hepatitis, liver failure) have occurred with NSAID use, rarely;

discontinue if signs or symptoms of liver disease develop, or if systemic manifestations occur.

The elderly are at increased risk for adverse effects (especially peptic ulceration, CNS effects, renal toxicity) from NSAIDs even at low doses. Withhold for at least 4-6 half-lives prior to surgical or dental procedures.

Ophthalmic: May increase bleeding time associated with ocular surgery. Use with caution in patients with known bleeding tendencies or those receiving anticoagulants. Healing time may be slowed or delayed. Corneal thinning, erosion, or ulceration have been reported with topical NSAIDs; discontinue if corneal epithelial breakdown occurs. Use caution with complicated ocular surgery, corneal denervation, corneal epithelial defects, diabetes, rheumatoid arthritis, ocular surface disease, or ocular surgeries repeated within short periods of time; risk of corneal epithelial breakdown may be increased. Use for >24 hours prior to or for >14 days following surgery also increases risk of corneal adverse effects. Do not administer while wearing soft contact lenses. Safety and efficacy in pediatric patients <3 years of age have not been established.

Dosage Forms[DSC] = Discontinued product
Injection, solution, as tromethamine: 15 mg/mL (1 mL); 30 mg/mL (1 mL, 2 mL, 10 mL) [contains alcohol]
Solution, ophthalmic, as tromethamine:
Acular®: 0.5% (3 mL, 5 mL, 10 mL) [contains benzalkonium chloride]
Acular LS™: 0.4% (5 mL) [contains benzalkonium chloride]
Acular® P.F. [preservative free]: 0.5% (0.4 mL)
Tablet, as tromethamine: 10 mg
Toradol®: 10 mg [DSC]

Reference Range
Peak plasma level after a 60 mg dose (I.M.): 4-4.5 mcg/mL
Serum concentration:
Therapeutic: 0.3-5.0 mcg/mL
Toxic: >5.0 mcg/mL

Overdosage/Treatment
Decontamination: Ipecac within 30 minutes or lavage (within 1 hour)/ activated charcoal
Supportive therapy: Hypotension/dehydration can be managed with I.V. fluid therapy; dopamine is vasopressor of choice; acidosis should be treated with bicarbonates, seizures with benzodiazepines; antacids, blood products are indicated, as appropriate, for hemorrhage
Enhancement of elimination: Dialysis or perfusion is indicated for secondary complications, acidosis, or renal failure and not toxin removal alone

Test Interactions ↑ chloride (S), sodium (S), bleeding time

Drug Interactions ACE inhibitors: Antihypertensive effects may be decreased by concurrent therapy with NSAIDs; monitor blood pressure.
Angiotensin II antagonists: Antihypertensive effects may be decreased by concurrent therapy with NSAIDs; monitor blood pressure.
Anticoagulants: Increased risk of bleeding complications with concomitant use; monitor closely.
Antiepileptic drugs (carbamazepine, phenytoin): Sporadic cases of seizures have been reported with concomitant use.
Beta-blockers: NSAIDs may decrease the antihypertensive effect of beta-blockers. Monitor.
Cholestyramine (and other bile acid sequestrants): May decrease the absorption of NSAIDs. Separate by at least 2 hours.
Diuretics: May see decreased effect of diuretics.
Hydralazine's antihypertensive effect may be reduced; monitor.
Lithium: May increase lithium levels; monitor.
Methotrexate: Severe bone marrow suppression, aplastic anemia, and GI toxicity have been reported with concomitant NSAID therapy. Avoid use during moderate or high-dose methotrexate (increased and prolonged methotrexate levels). NSAID use during low-dose treatment of rheumatoid arthritis has not been fully evaluated; extreme caution is warranted.
Nondepolarizing muscle relaxants: Concomitant use has resulted in apnea.
NSAIDs, salicylates: Concomitant use increases NSAID-induced adverse effects; contraindicated.
Probenecid: Probenecid significantly decreases ketorolac clearance, increases ketorolac plasma levels, and doubles the half-life of ketorolac; concomitant use is contraindicated.
Psychoactive drugs (alprazolam, fluoxetine, thiothixene): Hallucinations have been reported with concomitant use.

Pregnancy Risk Factor C/D (3rd trimester)

Pregnancy Implications Ketorolac is contraindicated during labor and delivery (may inhibit uterine contractions and adversely affect fetal circulation). Avoid use of ketorolac ophthalmic solution during late pregnancy.

Lactation Enters breast milk/contraindicated (AAP rates "compatible")

Additional Information 30 mg provides the analgesia comparable to 12 mg of morphine or 100 mg of meperidine; postmarketing surveillance of ketorolac indicated that the risk of clinically serious GI bleeding was dose-dependent, particularly in elderly patients, who received doses >60 mg/day

Specific References

Meredith JT, Wait S, and Brewer KL, "A Prospective Double-Blind Study of Nasal Sumatriptan Versus I.V. Ketorolac in Migraine," *Am J Emerg Med*, 2003, 21(3):173-5.
Reinhart DJ, "Minimising the Adverse Effects of Ketorolac," *Drug Saf*, 2000, 22(6):487-97.
Singer AJ, Mynster CJ, and McMahon BJ, "The Effect of IM Ketorolac Tromethamine on Bleeding Time: A Prospective, Interventional, Controlled Study," *Am J Emerg Med*, 2003, 21(5):441-3.

Labetalol

CAS Number 32780-64-6; 36894-69-6
U.S. Brand Names Normodyne®; Trandate®
Synonyms Ibidomide Hydrochloride; Labetalol Hydrochloride
Use Treatment of mild to severe hypertension; I.V. for hypertensive emergencies

Mechanism of Action Blocks alpha-, beta$_1$-, and beta$_2$-adrenergic receptor sites; elevated renins are reduced; roughly 80% beta-blocker and 20% alpha-blocker; beta- to alpha-blocking ratio is 7:1 (I.V.) and 3:1 (oral)

Adverse Reactions
Cardiovascular: Hypotension (orthostatic) especially with I.V. administration, edema, congestive heart failure, AV conduction disturbances, bradycardia, sinus bradycardia, myocardial depression, arrhythmias (ventricular)
Central nervous system: Drowsiness, fatigue, dizziness, behavior disorders, headache
Dermatologic: Tingling in scalp or skin (transient with initiation of therapy), rash, alopecia, angioedema, urticaria, purpura, pruritus, psoriasis, licheniform eruptions, exanthem
Endocrine & metabolic: Sexual dysfunction
Gastrointestinal: Nausea, xerostomia, vomiting, diarrhea
Genitourinary: Urinary problems
Hematologic: Leukopenia
Hepatic: Hepatotoxicity (usually mild and reversible), cholestasis
Neuromuscular & skeletal: Paresthesia, reversible myopathy
Ocular: Diplopia (dose-related)
Respiratory: Wheezing, nasal congestion
Miscellaneous: Systemic lupus erythematosus

Signs and Symptoms of Overdose Agranulocytosis, bradycardia, cholestatic jaundice, claudication, depression, dyspepsia, ejaculatory disturbances, granulocytopenia, heart failure, hypoglycemia, hypotension, impotence, leukopenia, lightheadedness, neutropenia, night terrors, oliguric renal failure, priapism, wheezing

Admission Criteria/Prognosis Admit any hypotensive patient or adult ingestions >3.5 g

Pharmacodynamics/Kinetics
Onset of action: Oral: 20 minutes to 2 hours; I.V.: 2-5 minutes
Peak effect: Oral: 1-4 hours; I.V.: 5-15 minutes
Duration: Oral: 8-24 hours (dose dependent); I.V.: 2-4 hours
Distribution: V$_d$: Adults: 3-16 L/kg; mean: <9.4 L/kg; moderately lipid soluble, therefore, can enter CNS; crosses placenta; small amounts enter breast milk
Protein binding: 50%
Metabolism: Hepatic, primarily via glucuronide conjugation; extensive first-pass effect
Bioavailability: Oral: 25%; increased with liver disease, elderly, and concurrent cimetidine
Half-life elimination: Normal renal function: 2.5-8 hours
Excretion: Urine (<5% as unchanged drug)
Clearance: Possibly decreased in neonates/infants

Dosage
Due to limited documentation of its use, labetalol should be initiated cautiously in pediatric patients with careful dosage adjustment and blood pressure monitoring.
Children:
Oral: Limited information regarding labetalol use in pediatric patients is currently available in literature. Some centers recommend initial oral doses of 4 mg/kg/day in 2 divided doses. Reported oral doses have started at 3 mg/kg/day and 20 mg/kg/day and have increased up to 40 mg/kg/day.
I.V., intermittent bolus doses of 0.3-1 mg/kg/dose have been reported. For treatment of pediatric hypertensive emergencies, initial continuous infusions of 0.4-1 mg/kg/hour with a maximum of 3 mg/kg/hour have been used. Administration requires the use of an infusion pump.
Adults:
Oral: Initial: 100 mg twice daily, may increase as needed every 2-3 days by 100 mg until desired response is obtained; usual dose: 200-400 mg twice daily; may require up to 2.4 g/day.
Usual dose range (JNC 7): 200-800 mg/day in 2 divided doses
I.V.: 20 mg (0.25 mg/kg for an 80 kg patient) IVP over 2 minutes; may administer 40-80 mg at 10-minute intervals, up to 300 mg total dose.

I.V. infusion: Initial: 2 mg/minute; titrate to response up to 300 mg total dose, if needed. Administration requires the use of an infusion pump.

I.V. infusion (500 mg/250 mL D$_5$W) rates:
1 mg/minute: 30 mL/hour
2 mg/minute: 60 mL/hour
3 mg/minute: 90 mL/hour
4 mg/minute: 120 mL/hour
5 mg/minute: 150 mL/hour
6 mg/minute: 180 mL/hour

Dialysis: Not removed by hemo- or peritoneal dialysis; supplemental dose is not necessary.

Dosage adjustment in hepatic impairment: Dosage reduction may be necessary.

Stability Stable in D$_5$W, saline for 24 hours; **incompatible** with alkaline solutions, NaHCO$_3$; use only solutions that are clear or slightly yellow; may cause a precipitate if exposed to alkaline admixture; parenteral admixture at room temperature (25°C) or refrigeration (4°C): 24 hours

Monitoring Parameters Blood pressure, standing and sitting/supine, pulse, cardiac monitor and blood pressure monitor required for I.V. administration

Administration Bolus administered over 2 minutes. Loading infusions (2 mg/minute) require close monitoring of heart rate and blood pressure and are usually terminated after response or cumulative dose of 300 mg. There is limited documentation of prolonged continuous infusions. In clinical experience, prolonged continuous infusions have been used. In rare clinical situations, higher dosages (up to 6 mg/minute) have been used in the critical care setting (eg, aortic dissection). At the other extreme, continuous infusions at relatively low doses (2-6 mg/hour: note difference in units) have been used in some settings (following loading infusion in patients who are unable to be converted to oral regimens or in some cases as a continuation of outpatient oral regimens). These prolonged infusions should not be confused with loading infusions. Because of wide variation in the use of infusions, an awareness of institutional policies and practices is extremely important. Careful clarification of orders and specific infusion rates/units is required to avoid confusion. Due to the prolonged duration of action, careful monitoring should be extended for the duration of the infusion and for several hours after the infusion. Excessive administration may result in prolonged hypotension and/or bradycardia.

Contraindications Hypersensitivity to labetalol or any component of the formulation; sinus bradycardia; heart block greater than first degree (except in patients with a functioning artificial pacemaker); cardiogenic shock; bronchial asthma; uncompensated cardiac failure; pregnancy (2nd and 3rd trimesters)

Warnings Use only with extreme caution in compensated heart failure and monitor for a worsening of the condition. Avoid abrupt discontinuation in patients with a history of CAD; slowly wean while monitoring for signs and symptoms of ischemia. Use caution with concurrent use of beta-blockers and either verapamil or diltiazem; bradycardia or heart block can occur. Avoid concurrent I.V. use of both agents. Patients with bronchospastic disease should not receive beta-blockers. Labetalol may be used with caution in patients with nonallergic bronchospasm (chronic bronchitis, emphysema). Use cautiously in diabetics because it can mask prominent hypoglycemic symptoms. Can mask signs of thyrotoxicosis. Can cause fetal harm when administered in pregnancy. Use cautiously in the hepatically impaired. Use caution when using I.V. labetalol and inhalational anesthetics concurrently (significant myocardial depression).

Dosage Forms
Injection, solution, as hydrochloride: 5 mg/mL (4 mL, 20 mL, 40 mL)
Trandate®: 5 mg/mL (20 mL, 40 mL)
Tablet, as hydrochloride: 100 mg, 200 mg, 300 mg
Trandate®: 100 mg, 200 mg [contains sodium benzoate], 300 mg

Reference Range Toxic: Serum levels >500 ng/mL

Overdosage/Treatment
Decontamination: Gastric lavage (within 1 hour) with activated charcoal is recommended; **do not** use ipecac
Supportive therapy: Sympathomimetics (eg, epinephrine or dopamine), atropine, glucagon, or a pacemaker can be used to treat the toxic bradycardia, asystole, and/or hypotension; inamrinone may also be effective for labetalol-induced hypotension; initially fluids may be the best treatment for toxic hypotension with norepinephrine being used for second-line therapy
Enhancement of elimination: Multiple dosing of activated charcoal may be useful

Test Interactions False-positive urine catecholamines and VMA if measured by fluorometric or photometric methods; use HPLC or specific catecholamine radioenzymatic technique; can cause positive antinuclear antibody; a labetalol metabolite (3-amino-1-phenylbutane or APB) may cause a false-positive result with amphetamine/methamphetamine by thin-layer chromatography or immunoassay

Drug Interactions Substrate of CYP2D6 (major); **Inhibits** CYP2D6 (weak)

Alpha-blockers (prazosin, terazosin): Concurrent use of beta-blockers may increase risk of orthostasis.
Cimetidine increases the bioavailability of labetalol.
CYP2D6 inhibitors: May increase the levels/effects of labetalol. Example inhibitors include chlorpromazine, delavirdine, fluoxetine, miconazole, paroxetine, pergolide, quinidine, quinine, ritonavir, and ropinirole.
Halothane, isoflurane, enflurane (possibly other inhalational anesthetics): Excessive hypotension may occur.
NSAIDs may reduce antihypertensive efficacy of labetalol.
Salicylates may reduce the antihypertensive effects of beta-blockers.
Sulfonylureas: Effects may be decreased by beta-blockers.
Verapamil or diltiazem may have synergistic or additive pharmacological effects when taken concurrently with beta-blockers; avoid concurrent I.V. use.

Pregnancy Risk Factor C (manufacturer); D (2nd and 3rd trimesters - expert analysis)

Pregnancy Implications Labetolol crosses the placenta. Beta-blockers have been associated with persistent bradycardia, hypotension, and IUGR; IUGR is probably related to maternal hypertension. Available evidence suggests beta-blockers are generally safe during pregnancy (JNC-7). Cases of neonatal hypoglycemia have been reported following maternal use of beta-blockers at parturition or during breast-feeding.

Lactation Enters breast milk/use caution (AAP rates "compatible")

Additional Information Not shown to be effective for cocaine-cardiovascular toxicity

Specific References
Chobanian AV, Bakris GL, Black HR, et al, "The Seventh Report of the Joint National Committee on Prevention, Detection, Evaluation, and Treatment of High Blood Pressure: The JNC 7 Report," *JAMA*, 2003, 289(19):2560-71.
Schier JG, Howland MA, Hoffman RS, et al, "Fatality from Administration of Labetalol and Crushed Extended-Release Nifedipine," *Ann Pharmacother*, 2003, 37(10):1420-3.

Lamivudine

U.S. Brand Names Epivir-HBV®; Epivir®
Synonyms 3TC
Use
Epivir®: Treatment of HIV infection when antiretroviral therapy is warranted; should always be used as part of a multidrug regimen (at least three antiretroviral agents)
Epivir-HBV®: Treatment of chronic hepatitis B associated with evidence of hepatitis B viral replication and active liver inflammation

Unlabeled/Investigational Use Prevention of HIV following needlesticks (with or without protease inhibitor)

Mechanism of Action Lamivudine is a cytosine analog. After lamivudine is triphosphorylated, the principle mode of action is inhibition of HIV reverse transcription via viral DNA chain termination; inhibits RNA- and DNA-dependent DNA polymerase activities of reverse transcriptase. The monophosphate form of lamivudine is incorporated into the viral DNA by hepatitis B virus polymerase, resulting in DNA chain termination.

Adverse Reactions
(As reported in adults treated for HIV infection)
Central nervous system: **Headache, fatigue**; dizziness, depression, fever, chills, insomnia
Dermatologic: Rash, alopecia, pruritus, urticaria
Endocrine & metabolic: Hyperglycemia, lactic acidosis
Gastrointestinal: **Nausea, diarrhea, vomiting, pancreatitis (range: 0.5% to 18%; higher percentage in pediatric patients)**; anorexia, abdominal pain, heartburn, elevated amylase, splenomegaly, stomatitis
Hematologic: Neutropenia, anemia, thrombocytopenia, red cell aplasia
Hepatic: Elevated AST/ALT, hepatomegaly, hyperbilirubinemia, steatosis
Neuromuscular & skeletal: **Peripheral neuropathy, paresthesia, musculoskeletal pain**; myalgia, arthralgia, rhabdomyolysis, weakness, increased CPK
Respiratory: Nasal signs and symptoms, cough
Miscellaneous: Anaphylaxis, lymphadenopathy

Pharmacodynamics/Kinetics
Absorption: Rapid
Distribution: V$_d$: 1.3 L/kg
Protein binding, plasma: <36%
Metabolism: 5.2% to trans-sulfoxide metabolite
Bioavailability: Absolute; Cp$_{max}$ decreased with food although AUC not significantly affected
Children: 66%
Adults: 86% to 87%
Half-life elimination: Children: 2 hours; Adults: 5-7 hours
Time to peak, plasma: Fed: 3.2 hours; Fasted: 0.9 hours
Excretion: Primarily urine (as unchanged drug)

Dosage Note: The formulation and dosage of Epivir-HBV® are not appropriate for patients infected with both HBV and HIV. Use with at least two other antiretroviral agents when treating HIV

Oral:

Children 3 months to 16 years: HIV: 4 mg/kg twice daily (maximum: 150 mg twice daily)

Children 2-17 years: Treatment of hepatitis B (Epivir-HBV®): 3 mg/kg once daily (maximum: 100 mg/day)

Adolescents and Adults: Prevention of HIV following needlesticks (unlabeled use): 150 mg twice daily (with zidovudine with or without a protease inhibitor, depending on risk)

Adults:

HIV: 150 mg twice daily **or** 300 mg once daily

<50 kg: 4 mg/kg twice daily (maximum: 150 mg twice daily)

Treatment of hepatitis B (Epivir-HBV®): 100 mg/day

Dosing interval in renal impairment in pediatric patients: Insufficient data; however, dose reduction should be considered.

Dosing interval in renal impairment in patients >16 years for HIV:

Cl_{cr} 30-49 mL/minute: Administer 150 mg once daily

Cl_{cr} 15-29 mL/minute: Administer 150 mg first dose, then 100 mg once daily

Cl_{cr} 5-14 mL/minute: Administer 150 mg first dose, then 50 mg once daily

Cl_{cr} <5 mL/minute: Administer 50 mg first dose, then 25 mg once daily

Dosing interval in renal impairment in adult patients with hepatitis B:

Cl_{cr} 30-49: Administer 100 mg first dose then 50 mg once daily

Cl_{cr} 15-29: Administer 100 mg first dose then 25 mg once daily

Cl_{cr} 5-14: Administer 35 mg first dose then 15 mg once daily

Cl_{cr} <5: Administer 35 mg first dose then 10 mg once daily

Dialysis: Negligible amounts are removed by 4-hour hemodialysis or peritoneal dialysis. Supplemental dosing is not required.

Stability Store at 2°C to 25°C (68°F to 77°F) tightly closed.

Monitoring Parameters Amylase, bilirubin, liver enzymes, hematologic parameters, viral load, and CD4 count; signs and symptoms of pancreatitis

Administration May be taken with or without food. Adjust dosage in renal failure.

Contraindications Hypersensitivity to lamivudine or any component of the formulation

Warnings

Use caution with renal impairment; dosage reduction recommended. Use with extreme caution in children with history of pancreatitis or risk factors for development of pancreatitis. Do not use as monotherapy in treatment of HIV. Treatment of HBV in patients with unrecognized/untreated HIV may lead to rapid HIV resistance. In addition, treatment of HIV in patients with unrecognized/untreated HBV may lead to rapid HBV resistance. **[U.S. Boxed Warning]: Do not use Epivir-HBV® tablets or Epivir-HBV® oral solution for the treatment of HIV.**

[U.S. Boxed Warning]:Lactic acidosis and severe hepatomegaly with steatosis have been reported, including fatal cases. Use caution in hepatic impairment. Pregnancy, obesity, and/or prolonged therapy may increase the risk of lactic acidosis and liver damage.

Immune reconstitution syndrome may develop resulting in the occurrence of an inflammatory response to an indolent or residual opportunistic infection; further evaluation and treatment may be required. May be associated with fat redistribution (buffalo hump, increased abdominal girth, breast engorgement, facial atrophy, and dyslipidemia).

[U.S. Boxed Warning]: Monitor patients closely for several months following discontinuation of therapy for chronic hepatitis B; clinical exacerbations may occur.

Dosage Forms

Solution, oral:

Epivir®: 10 mg/mL (240 mL) [strawberry-banana flavor]

Epivir-HBV®: 5 mg/mL (240 mL) [strawberry-banana flavor]

Tablet:

Epivir®: 150 mg, 300 mg

Epivir-HBV®: 100 mg

Reference Range Peak serum concentrations after a 8 mg/kg I.V. and oral dose: 10,560 ng/mL and 5815 ng/mL, respectively

Overdosage/Treatment Decontamination: Emesis with ipecac within 30 minutes or lavage (within 1 hour)/activated charcoal; monitor hematologic parameters

Drug Interactions

Interferon alfa: Concomitant use of interferon alfa and nucleoside analogues may increase the risk of developing hepatic decompensation or other signs of mitochondrial toxicity, including pancreatitis or lactic acidosis.

Ganciclovir/valganciclovir: May increase the adverse effects/toxicity (eg, hematologic) of nucleoside reverse transcriptase inhibitors

Ribavirin: Concomitant use of ribavirin and nucleoside analogues may increase the risk of developing hepatic decompensation or other signs of mitochondrial toxicity, including pancreatitis or lactic acidosis.

Sulfamethoxazole/trimethoprim: Increased AUC and decreased clearance of lamivudine with concomitant use

Trimethoprim (and other drugs excreted by organic cation transport): May increase serum levels/effects of lamivudine.

Zalcitabine: Intracellular phosphorylation of lamivudine and zalcitabine may be inhibited if used together; concomitant use should be avoided.

Zidovudine: Plasma levels of zidovudine are increased by ~39% with concomitant use.

Pregnancy Risk Factor C

Pregnancy Implications Lamivudine crosses the placenta. It may be used in combination with zidovudine in HIV-infected women who are in labor, but have had no prior antiretroviral therapy, in order to reduce the maternal-fetal transmission of HIV. Cases of lactic acidosis/hepatic steatosis syndrome have been reported in pregnant women receiving nucleoside analogues. It is not known if pregnancy itself potentiates this known side effect; however, pregnant women may be at increased risk of lactic acidosis and liver damage. Hepatic enzymes and electrolytes should be monitored frequently during the 3rd trimester of pregnancy in women receiving nucleoside analogues. Health professionals are encouraged to contact the antiretroviral pregnancy registry to monitor outcomes of pregnant women exposed to antiretroviral medications (1-800-258-4263).

Lactation Enters breast milk/not recommended

Nursing Implications Monitor children for signs and symptoms of pancreatitis; evaluate frequently for opportunistic infection and other complications of HIV; administer on an empty stomach, if possible; adjust dosage in renal failure

Additional Information There are, as yet, no results from clinical trials evaluating the effect of lamivudine, in combination with zidovudine, on progression of HIV infection (eg, incidence of opportunistic infections or survival). Patients may continue to develop infections and other complications of HIV infection and should remain under close physician observation.

Specific References

De Santis M, Cavaliere AF, Caruso A, et al, "Hemangiomas and Other Congenital Malformations in Infants Exposed to Antiretroviral Therapy *in utero*," *JAMA*, 2004, 291(3):305.

Scotto G, Palumbom E, Fazio V, et al, "Prolonged Lamivudine Treatment in Patients with Chronic Active Anti-HBe-Positive Hepatitis," *Am J Ther*, 2006, 13(3):218-22.

Shiber JR, "Lactic Acidosis Caused by Nucleoside Analogues," *Am J Emerg Med*, 2005, 23(4):582-3.

Lamotrigine

CAS Number 84057-84-1

U.S. Brand Names Lamictal®

Synonyms BW-430C; LTG

Use Adjunctive therapy in the treatment of generalized seizures of Lennox-Gastaut syndrome and partial seizures in adults and children ≥2 years of age; conversion to monotherapy in adults with partial seizures who are receiving treatment with valproate or a single enzyme-inducing antiepileptic drug; maintenance treatment of bipolar disorder

Mechanism of Action Triazine derivative which inhibits release of glutamate (an excitatory amino acid)

Adverse Reactions

Reported in adults receiving adjunctive therapy:

Cardiovascular: Angina, atrial fibrillation, facial edema, hypertension, palpitations, postural hypotension, vasculitis, peripheral edema

Central nervous system: **Headache** (29%), **dizziness** (38%), **ataxia** (22%), **somnolence**, depression, anxiety, irritability, confusion, speech disorder, difficulty concentrating, malaise, seizure, incoordination, insomnia, pain, amnesia, hostility, memory decreased, nervousness, vertigo, chills, depersonalization, malaise, mania, migraine, movement disorder, stroke, suicidal ideation, Parkinson's disease exacerbation

Dermatologic: **Hypersensitivity rash** (10%; serious rash requiring hospitalization - adults 0.3%, children 0.8%), pruritus, acne, alopecia, angioedema, bruising, erythema multiforme, maculopapular rash, photosensitivity (rare), rash, Stevens-Johnson syndrome, urticaria, vesiculobullous rash, toxic epidermal necrolysis

Endocrine & metabolic: Hot flashes

Gastrointestinal: **Nausea**, abdominal pain, vomiting, diarrhea, dyspepsia, constipation, anorexia, tooth disorder, dysphagia, GI hemorrhage, gingival hyperplasia, halitosis, esophagitis, pancreatitis, xerostomia

Genitourinary: Vaginitis, dysmenorrhea, amenorrhea, impotence

Hematologic: Anemia, eosinophilia, hemorrhage, leukopenia, agranulocytosis, aplastic anemia, disseminated intravascular coagulation (DIC), hemolytic anemia, neutropenia, pancytopenia, red cell aplasia, thrombocytopenia

Hepatic: Hepatitis

Neuromuscular & skeletal: Tremor, arthralgia, neck pain, back pain, dysarthria, paralysis, tics

Ocular: **Diplopia** (28%), **blurred vision**, nystagmus, visual abnormality

Renal: Acute renal failure

Respiratory: **Rhinitis**, bronchospasm, dyspnea, apnea, epistaxis, bronchitis

Miscellaneous: Flu syndrome, fever, allergic reactions, hypersensitivity reactions (including rhabdomyolysis), immunosuppression (progressive), lupus-like reaction, multiorgan failure

Signs and Symptoms of Overdose QRS prolongation on ECG

Admission Criteria/Prognosis Admit any patient with nervous system or cardiac abnormalities (especially QRS prolongation over 100 msec on ECG), ingestions >1 g, or serum lamotrigine levels >10 mcg/mL

Pharmacodynamics/Kinetics

Distribution: V_d: 1.1 L/kg

Protein binding: 55%

Metabolism: Hepatic and renal; metabolized by glucuronic acid conjugation to inactive metabolites

Bioavailability: 98%

Half-life elimination: Adults: 25-33 hours; Concomitant valproic acid therapy: 59-70 hours; Concomitant phenytoin or carbamazepine therapy: 13-14 hours

Time to peak, plasma: 1-4 hours

Excretion: Urine (94%, ~90% as glucuronide conjugates and ~10% unchanged); feces (2%)

Dosage Note: Only whole tablets should be used for dosing, round calculated dose down to the nearest whole tablet: Oral:

Children 2-12 years: Lennox-Gastaut (adjunctive) or partial seizures (adjunctive): **Note:** Children 2-6 years will likely require maintenance doses at the higher end of recommended range:

Patients receiving AED regimens containing valproic acid:

Weeks 1 and 2: 0.15 mg/kg/day in 1-2 divided doses; round dose down to the nearest whole tablet. For patients >6.7 kg and <14 kg, dosing should be 2 mg every other day.

Weeks 3 and 4: 0.3 mg/kg/day in 1-2 divided doses; round dose down to the nearest whole tablet; may use combinations of 2 mg and 5 mg tablets. For patients >6.7 kg and <14 kg, dosing should be 2 mg/day.

Maintenance dose: Titrate dose to effect; after week 4, increase dose every 1-2 weeks by a calculated increment; calculate increment as 0.3 mg/kg/day rounded down to the nearest whole tablet; add this amount to the previously administered daily dose; usual maintenance: 1-5 mg/kg/day in 1-2 divided doses; maximum: 200 mg/day given in 1-2 divided doses

Patients receiving enzyme-inducing AED regimens without valproic acid:

Weeks 1 and 2: 0.6 mg/kg/day in 2 divided doses; round dose down to the nearest whole tablet

Weeks 3 and 4: 1.2 mg/kg/day in 2 divided doses; round dose down to the nearest whole tablet

Maintenance dose: Titrate dose to effect; after week 4, increase dose every 1-2 weeks by a calculated increment; calculate increment as 1.2 mg/kg/day rounded down to the nearest whole tablet; add this amount to the previously administered daily dose; usual maintenance: 5-15 mg/kg/day in 2 divided doses; maximum: 400 mg/day

Children >12 years: Lennox-Gastaut (adjunctive) or partial seizures (adjunctive): Refer to Adults dosing

Children ≥16 years: Conversion from single enzyme-inducing AED regimen to monotherapy: Refer to Adults dosing

Adults:

Lennox-Gastaut (adjunctive) or treatment of partial seizures (adjunctive):

Patients receiving AED regimens containing valproic acid: Initial dose: 25 mg every other day for 2 weeks, then 25 mg every day for 2 weeks. Dose may be increased by 25-50 mg every day for 1-2 weeks in order to achieve maintenance dose. Maintenance dose: 100-400 mg/day in 1-2 divided doses (usual range 100-200 mg/day).

Patients receiving enzyme-inducing AED regimens without valproic acid: Initial dose: 50 mg/day for 2 weeks, then 100 mg in 2 doses for 2 weeks; thereafter, daily dose can be increased by 100 mg every 1-2 weeks to be given in 2 divided doses. Usual maintenance dose: 300-500 mg/day in 2 divided doses; doses as high as 700 mg/day have been reported

Conversion to monotherapy (partial seizures in patients ≥16 years of age):

Adjunctive therapy with valproate: Initiate and titrate as per recommendations to a lamotrigine dose of 200 mg/day. Then taper valproate dose in decrements of not more than 500 mg/day at intervals of one week (or longer) to a valproate dosage of 500 mg/day; this dosage should be maintained for one week. The lamotrigine dosage should then be increased to 300 mg/day while valproate is decreased to 250 mg/day; this dosage should be maintained for one week. Valproate may then be discontinued, while the lamotrigine dose is increased by 100 mg/day at weekly intervals to achieve a lamotrigine maintenance dose of 500 mg/day.

Adjunctive therapy with enzyme-inducing AED: Initiate and titrate as per recommendations to a lamotrigine dose of 500 mg/day.

Concomitant enzyme-inducing AED should then be withdrawn by 20% decrements each week over a 4-week period. Patients should be monitored for rash.

Adjunctive therapy with non-enzyme inducing AED: No specific guidelines available

Bipolar disorder: 25 mg/day for 2 weeks, followed by 50 mg/day for 2 weeks, followed by 100 mg/day for 1 week; thereafter, daily dosage may be increased to 200 mg/day

Patients receiving valproic acid: Initial: 25 mg every other day for 2 weeks, followed by 25 mg/day for 2 weeks, followed by 50 mg/day for 1 week, followed by 100 mg/day (target dose) thereafter. **Note:** If valproate is discontinued, increase daily lamotrigine dose in 50 mg increments at weekly intervals until daily dosage of 200 mg is attained.

Patients receiving enzyme-inducing drugs (eg, carbamazepine): Initial: 50 mg/day for 2 weeks, followed by 100 mg/day (in divided doses) for 2 weeks, followed by 200 mg/day (in divided doses) for 1 week, followed by 300 mg/day (in divided doses) for 1 week. May increase to 400 mg/day (in divided doses) during week 7 and thereafter. **Note:** If carbamazepine (or other enzyme-inducing drug) is discontinued, decrease daily lamotrigine dose in 100 mg increments at weekly intervals until daily dosage of 200 mg is attained.

Discontinuing therapy: Children and Adults: Decrease dose by ~50% per week, over at least 2 weeks unless safety concerns require a more rapid withdrawal.

Restarting therapy after discontinuation: If lamotrigine has been withheld for >5 half-lives, consider restarting according to initial dosing recommendations.

Dosage adjustment in renal impairment: Decreased dosage may be effective in patients with significant renal impairment; use with caution

Dosage adjustment in hepatic impairment:

Child-Pugh Grade B: Reduce initial, escalation, and maintenance doses by 50%

Child-Pugh Grade C: Reduce initial, escalation, and maintenance doses by 75%

Monitoring Parameters Seizure, frequency and duration, serum levels of concurrent anticonvulsants, hypersensitivity reactions, especially rash

Administration Doses should be rounded down to the nearest whole tablet. Dispersible tablets may be chewed, dispersed in water, or swallowed whole. To disperse tablets, add to a small amount of liquid (just enough to cover tablet); let sit ~1 minute until dispersed; swirl solution and consume immediately. Do not administer partial amounts of liquid. If tablets are chewed, a small amount of water or diluted fruit juice should be used to aid in swallowing.

Contraindications Hypersensitivity to lamotrigine or any component of the formulation

Warnings [U.S. Boxed Warning]: Severe and potentially life-threatening skin rashes requiring hospitalization have been reported (children 0.8%, adults 0.3%); risk may be increased by coadministration with valproic acid, higher than recommended starting doses, and rapid dose titration. The majority of cases occur in the first 8 weeks; however, isolated cases may occur after prolonged treatment. Discontinue at first sign of rash unless rash is clearly not drug related. Use caution in patients with impaired renal, hepatic, or cardiac function. Avoid abrupt cessation, taper over at least 2 weeks if possible. May cause CNS depression, which may impair physical or mental abilities. Patients must be cautioned about performing tasks which require mental alertness (eg, operating machinery or driving). Effects with other sedative drugs or ethanol may be potentiated. Binds to melanin and may accumulate in the eye and other melanin-rich tissues; the clinical significance of this is not known. Safety and efficacy has not been established for use as initial monotherapy, conversion to monotherapy from nonenzyme-inducing antiepileptic drugs (AED) except valproate, or conversion to monotherapy from two or more AEDs. **Use caution in writing and/or interpreting prescriptions/orders; medication dispensing errors have occurred with similar-sounding medications (Lamisil®, ludiomil, lamivudine, labetalol, and Lomotil®).**

Dosage Forms

Tablet: 25 mg, 100 mg, 150 mg, 200 mg [contains lactose]

Tablet, combination package [each unit-dose starter kit contains]:

Lamictal® (blue kit; for patients taking valproate):

Tablet: Lamotrigine 25 mg (35s)

Lamictal® (green kit; for patients taking carbamazepine, phenytoin, phenobarbital, primidone, or rifampin and **not** taking valproate):

Tablet: Lamotrigine 25 mg (84s)

Tablet: Lamotrigine 100 mg (14s)

Lamictal® (orange kit; for patients **not** taking carbamazepine, phenytoin, phenobarbital, primidone, rifampin, or valproate; for use in bipolar patients only):

Tablet: Lamotrigine 25 mg (42s)

Tablet: Lamotrigine 100 mg (7s)

Tablet, dispersible/chewable: 2 mg, 5 mg, 25 mg [black currant flavor]

Reference Range

Not established

Postmortem levels in a related fatality were: Cardiac blood: 52 mg/L; liver: 220 mg/kg

Overdosage/Treatment

Decontamination: Lavage (within 1 hour)/activated charcoal

Supportive therapy: Cardiac monitoring should occur for 24 to 48 hours in the setting of acute overdose. Although no formal studies exist, I.V. sodium bicarbonate (1-2 mEq/kg) should be considered in treating wide complex tachycardia.

Enhancement of elimination: Multiple dosing of activated charcoal may be useful

Drug Interactions

Acetaminophen: May reduce serum concentrations of lamotrigine; mechanism not defined; of clinical concern only with chronic acetaminophen dosing (not single doses).

Carbamazepine: Lamotrigine may increase the epoxide metabolite of carbamazepine resulting in toxicity. Carbamazepine may decrease plasma levels of lamotrigine. Dosage adjustments may be needed when adding or withdrawing agents; monitor.

Oral contraceptives (estrogens): Oral contraceptives may decrease the serum concentration of lamotrigine; monitor. Dosage adjustment of lamotrigine may be required when starting/stopping oral contraceptives.

Phenytoin: May decrease plasma levels of lamotrigine. Dosage adjustments may be needed when adding or withdrawing agents; monitor.

Phenobarbital (barbiturates): May increase the metabolism of lamotrigine. Dosage adjustment may be needed when adding or withdrawing agent; monitor.

SSRIs (sertraline): Toxicity has been reported following the addition of sertraline; limited documentation; monitor.

Valproic acid: Inhibits the clearance of lamotrigine, dosage adjustment required when adding or withdrawing valproic acid. Inhibition appears maximal at valproic acid 250-500 mg/day. The incidence of serious rash may be increased by valproic acid.

Pregnancy Risk Factor C

Pregnancy Implications Lamotrigine has been found to decrease folate concentrations in animal studies. Teratogenic effects in animals were not observed. Safety and efficacy in pregnant women have not been established. Healthcare providers may enroll patients in the Lamotrigine Pregnancy Registry by calling (800) 336-2176. Patients may enroll themselves in the North American Antiepileptic Drug Pregnancy Registry by calling (888) 233-2334. Dose of lamotrigine may need adjusted during pregnancy to maintain clinical response; lamotrigine serum levels may decrease during pregnancy and return to prepartum levels following delivery.

Lactation Enters breast milk/not recommended (AAP rates "of concern")

Additional Information Low water solubility; not indicated for patients <16 years of age; when having the prescription refilled, patients should be advised to contact the prescriber if the medicine looks different or the label name has changed (see Warnings)

Specific References

Johannessen SI, Battino D, Berry DJ, et al, "Therapeutic Drug Monitoring of the Newer Antiepileptic Drugs," *Ther Drug Monit*, 2003, 25(3): 347-63.

Lancas FM, Sozza MA, and Queiroz ME, "Simultaneous Plasma Lamotrigine Analysis with Carbamazepine, Carbamazepine 10,11 Epoxide, Primidone, Phenytoin, Phenobarbital, and PEMA by Micellar Electrokinetic Capillary Chromatography (MECC)," *J Anal Toxicol*, 2003, 27(5):304-8.

Riley BD and Curry SC, "Lamotrigine Hypersensitivity Syndrome with Fatal Fulminant Hepatic Necrosis," *Clin Toxicol*, 2005, 43:635.

Thundiyil J, Stuart P, Anderson IB, et al, "Lamotrigine-Induced Seizures in a Pediatric Patient," *J Toxicol Clin Toxicol*, 2004, 42(5):716.

Lansoprazole

CAS Number 103577-45-3

U.S. Brand Names Prevacid® SoluTab™; Prevacid®

Use Short-term treatment of active duodenal ulcers; maintenance treatment of healed duodenal ulcers; as part of a multidrug regimen for *H. pylori* eradication to reduce the risk of duodenal ulcer recurrence; short-term treatment of active benign gastric ulcer; treatment of NSAID-associated gastric ulcer; to reduce the risk of NSAID-associated gastric ulcer in patients with a history of gastric ulcer who require an NSAID; short-term treatment of symptomatic GERD; short-term treatment for all grades of erosive esophagitis; to maintain healing of erosive esophagitis; long-term treatment of pathological hypersecretory conditions, including Zollinger-Ellison syndrome

Unlabeled/Investigational Use Active ulcer bleeding (parenteral formulation)

Mechanism of Action Similar to omeprazole; a proton pump inhibitor which decreases acid secretion in gastric parietal cells

Adverse Reactions

Cardiovascular: Angina, arrhythmia, bradycardia, cardiospasm, cerebrovascular accident, cerebral infarction, chest pain, edema, hypertension, hypotension, myocardial infarction, palpitations, peripheral edema, shock, syncope, tachycardia, vasodilation

Central nervous system: Abnormal dreams, agitation, amnesia, anxiety, apathy, chills, confusion, convulsion, depersonalization, depression, dizziness, emotional lability, fever, hallucinations, hostility aggravated, hypesthesia, insomnia, malaise, migraine, nervousness, neurosis, pain, sleep disorder, thinking abnormality, vertigo, dizziness, speech disorder

Dermatologic: Acne, alopecia, contact dermatitis, dry skin, maculopapular rash, photophobia, pruritus, skin carcinoma, urticaria, erythema multiforme, Stevens-Johnson syndrome, toxic epidermal necrolysis (some fatal)

Endocrine & metabolic: Breast enlargement, breast pain, breast tenderness, cholesterol increased, cholesterol decreased, dehydration, diabetes mellitus, electrolyte imbalance, glucocorticoids increased, goiter, gout, gynecomastia, hyperglycemia, hyperlipemia, hypoglycemia, hypothyroidism, menorrhagia, menstrual disorder

Gastrointestinal: Abdominal pain, diarrhea (4%, more likely at doses of 60 mg/day), constipation, nausea, enlarged abdomen, anorexia, appetite increased, bezoar, colitis, dry mouth, dyspepsia, dysphagia, enteritis, eructation, esophageal ulcer, esophagitis, fecal discoloration, flatulence, fundic gland polyps, gastric nodules, gastrin levels increased, gastritis, gastroenteritis, gastrointestinal anomaly, gastrointestinal disorder, gastrointestinal hemorrhage, glossitis, gum hemorrhage, halitosis, hematemesis, melena, mouth ulceration, pancreatitis, rectal disorder, rectal hemorrhage, salivation increased, stomatitis, taste loss, taste perversion, tenesmus, tongue disorder, ulcerative stomatitis, ulcerative colitis, vomiting, weight gain/loss, abnormal stools

Genitourinary: Abnormal menses, dysmenorrhea, dysuria, glycosuria, impotence, leukorrhea, libido decreased, pelvic pain, penis disorder, testis disorder, urethral pain, urinary frequency, urination impaired, vaginitis, urinary retention, increased libido

Hematologic: Anemia, eosinophilia, hemolysis, platelet abnormalities, RBC abnormal, WBC abnormal, agranulocytosis, aplastic anemia, leukopenia, neutropenia, pancytopenia, thrombocytopenia, thrombotic thrombocytopenic purpura

Hepatic: Increased alkaline phosphatase, increased ALT, AST increased, bilirubinemia, cholelithiasis, GGTP increased, GGTP decreased, globulins increased, abnormal liver function test, hepatotoxicity, LDH increased

Neuromuscular & skeletal: Asthenia, arthralgia, arthritis, back pain, bone disorder, hemiplegia, hyperkinesia, hypertonia, joint disorder, leg cramps, musculoskeletal pain, myalgia, myasthenia, neck pain, neck rigidity, paresthesia, synovitis, tremor

Ocular: Abnormal vision, blurred vision, conjunctivitis, diplopia, dry eyes, eye pain, retinal degeneration, visual field defect

Otic: Deafness, ear disorder, otitis media, parosmia, tinnitus

Renal: Creatinine increased, hematuria, kidney calculus, kidney pain, polyuria, albuminuria

Respiratory: Asthma, bronchitis, cough increased, dyspnea, epistaxis, hemoptysis, laryngeal neoplasia, pharyngitis, pleural disorder, pneumonia, respiratory disorder, rhinitis, sinusitis, stridor, upper respiratory inflammation, upper respiratory infection

Miscellaneous: Allergic reaction, candidiasis, carcinoma, fixed eruption, flu-like syndrome, hair disorder, hiccups, infection, moniliasis (oral), nail disorder, anaphylactoid reaction, lymphadenopathy, sweating, thirst

Pharmacodynamics/Kinetics

Duration: >1 day

Absorption: Rapid

Protein binding: 97%

Metabolism: Hepatic via CYP2C19 and 3A4, and in parietal cells to two inactive metabolites

Bioavailability: 80%; decreased 50% to 70% if given 30 minutes after food

Half-life elimination: 2 hours; Elderly: 2-3 hours; Hepatic impairment: ≤7 hours

Time to peak, plasma: 1.7 hours

Excretion: Feces (67%); urine (33%)

Dosage

Oral:

Children 1-11 years: GERD, erosive esophagitis:

≤30 kg: 15 mg once daily

>30 kg: 30 mg once daily

Adults:

Duodenal ulcer: Short-term treatment: 15 mg once daily for 4 weeks; maintenance therapy: 15 mg once daily

Gastric ulcer: Short-term treatment: 30 mg once daily for up to 8 weeks

NSAID-associated gastric ulcer (healing): 30 mg once daily for 8 weeks; controlled studies did not extend past 8 weeks of therapy

NSAID-associated gastric ulcer (to reduce risk): Oral: 15 mg once daily for up to 12 weeks; controlled studies did not extend past 12 weeks of therapy

Symptomatic GERD: Short-term treatment: 15 mg once daily for up to 8 weeks

Erosive esophagitis: Short-term treatment: 30 mg once daily for up to 8 weeks; continued treatment for an additional 8 weeks may be considered for recurrence or for patients that do not heal after the first 8 weeks of therapy; maintenance therapy: 15 mg once daily

Hypersecretory conditions: Initial: 60 mg once daily; adjust dose based upon patient response and to reduce acid secretion to <10 mEq/hour (5 mEq/hour in patients with prior gastric surgery); doses of 90 mg twice daily have been used; administer doses >120 mg/day in divided doses

Helicobacter pylori eradication: Currently accepted recommendations (may differ from product labeling): Dose varies with regimen: 30 mg once daily or 60 mg/day in 2 divided doses; requires combination therapy with antibiotics

Elderly: No dosage adjustment is needed in elderly patients with normal hepatic function

Dosage adjustment in renal impairment: No dosage adjustment is needed

Dosing adjustment in hepatic impairment: Dose reduction is necessary for severe hepatic impairment

Monitoring Parameters Patients with Zollinger-Ellison syndrome should be monitored for gastric acid output, which should be maintained at ≤10 mEq/hour during the last hour before the next lansoprazole dose; lab monitoring should include CBC, liver function, renal function, and serum gastrin levels

Administration

Oral: Administer before food; best if taken before breakfast. The intact granules should not be chewed or crushed; however, in addition to oral suspension, several options are available for those patients unable to swallow capsules:

Capsules may be opened and the intact granules sprinkled on 1 tablespoon of applesauce, Ensure® pudding, cottage cheese, yogurt, or strained pears. The granules should then be swallowed immediately.

Capsules may be opened and emptied into ~60 mL orange juice, apple juice, or tomato juice; mix and swallow immediately. Rinse the glass with additional juice and swallow to assure complete delivery of the dose.

Capsule granules may be mixed with apple, cranberry, grape, orange, pineapple, prune, tomato and V-8® juice and stored for up to 30 minutes.

Delayed release oral suspension granules should be mixed with 2 tablespoonfuls (30 mL) of water; no other liquid should be used; should not be administered through enteral administration tubes

Orally-disintegrating tablets: Should not be swallowed whole or chewed. Place tablet on tongue; allow to dissolve (with or without water) until particles can be swallowed.

Nasogastric tube administration: Capsules can be opened, the granules mixed (not crushed) with 40 mL of apple juice and then injected through the NG tube into the stomach, then flush tube with additional apple juice.

Contraindications Hypersensitivity to lansoprazole, substituted benzimidazoles (ie, esomeprazole, omeprazole, pantoprazole, rabeprazole), or any component of the formulation

Warnings Severe liver dysfunction may require dosage reductions. Symptomatic response does not exclude malignancy. Safety and efficacy have not been established in children <1 year of age.

Dosage Forms Capsule, delayed release (Prevacid®): 15 mg, 30 mg
Granules, for oral suspension, delayed release (Prevacid®): 15 mg/packet (30s), 30 mg/packet (30s) [strawberry flavor]
Injection, powder for reconstitution (Prevacid®): 30 mg
Tablet, orally disintegrating (Prevacid® SoluTab™): 15 mg [contains phenylalanine 2.5 mg; strawberry flavor]; 30 mg [contains phenylalanine 5.1 mg; strawberry flavor]

Reference Range Peak serum level after a 60 mg oral dose: 2.2 mcg/mL

Overdosage/Treatment

Decontamination: Emesis within 30 minutes or lavage (within 1 hour)/activated charcoal

Enhancement of elimination: Multiple dosing of activated charcoal may be effective

Not dialyzable

Test Interactions Possible increased plasma gastrin levels

Drug Interactions **Substrate** of CYP2C9 (minor), 2C19 (major), 3A4 (major); **Inhibits** CYP2C9 (weak), 2C19 (moderate), 2D6 (weak), 3A4 (weak); **Induces** CYP1A2 (weak)

CYP2C19 inducers: May decrease the levels/effects of lansoprazole. Example inducers include aminoglutethimide, carbamazepine, phenytoin, and rifampin.

CYP2C19 substrates: Lansoprazole may increase the levels/effects of CYP2C19 substrates. Example substrates include citalopram, diazepam, methsuximide, phenytoin, propranolol, and sertraline.

CYP3A4 inducers: CYP3A4 inducers may decrease the levels/effects of lansoprazole. Example inducers include aminoglutethimide, carbamazepine, nafcillin, nevirapine, phenobarbital, phenytoin, and rifamycins.

Itraconazole and ketoconazole: Proton pump inhibitors may decrease the absorption of itraconazole and ketoconazole.

Protease inhibitors: Proton pump inhibitors may decrease absorption of some protease inhibitors (atazanavir and indinavir).

Pregnancy Risk Factor B

Pregnancy Implications Animal studies have not shown teratogenic effects to the fetus. However, there are no adequate and well-controlled studies in pregnant women; use during pregnancy only if clearly needed.

Lactation Excretion in breast milk unknown/not recommended

Additional Information May have activity against *Helicobacter pylori*

Latanoprost

CAS Number 130209-82-4

U.S. Brand Names Xalatan®

Use Reduction of elevated intraocular pressure in patients with open-angle glaucoma and ocular hypertension

Mechanism of Action Latanoprost is a prostaglandin F_2-alpha analog of dinoprost believed to reduce intraocular pressure by increasing the outflow of the aqueous humor

Adverse Reactions

Cardiovascular: Chest pain, angina pectoris

Dermatologic: Rash, allergic skin reaction, toxic epidermal necrolysis

Neuromuscular & skeletal: Myalgia, arthralgia, back pain

Ocular: **Blurred vision, burning and stinging, conjunctival hyperemia, foreign body sensation, itching, increased pigmentation of the iris, punctate epithelial keratopathy**, dry eye, excessive tearing, eye pain, lid crusting, lid edema, lid erythema, lid discomfort/pain, photophobia, conjunctivitis, diplopia, eye discharge, retinal artery embolus, retinal detachment, vitreous hemorrhage from diabetic retinopathy, corneal edema, corneal erosion, eyelash change, eyelid skin darkening, herpes keratitis, iritis, keratitis, macular edema, uveitis

Respiratory: Upper respiratory tract infection, cold, flu, asthma, dyspnea

Pharmacodynamics/Kinetics

Onset of action: 3-4 hours

Peak effect: Maximum: 8-12 hours

Absorption: Through the cornea where the isopropyl ester prodrug is hydrolyzed by esterases to the biologically active acid. Peak concentration is reached in 2 hours after topical administration in the aqueous humor.

Distribution: V_d: 0.16 L/kg

Metabolism: Primarily hepatic via fatty acid beta-oxidation

Half-life elimination: 17 minutes

Excretion: Urine (as metabolites)

Dosage Adults: Ophthalmic: 1 drop (1.5 mcg) in the affected eye(s) once daily in the evening; do not exceed the once daily dosage because it has been shown that more frequent administration may decrease the IOP lowering effect

Stability Protect from light; store intact bottles under refrigeration (2°C to 8°C/36°F to 46°F). Once opened, the container may be stored at room temperature up to 25°C (77°F) for 6 weeks.

Administration If more than one topical ophthalmic drug is being used, administer the drugs at least 5 minutes apart

Contraindications Hypersensitivity to latanoprost or any component of the formulation

Warnings

Latanoprost may gradually change eye color, increasing the amount of brown pigment in the iris by increasing the number of melanosome in melanocytes. The long-term effects on the melanocytes and the consequences of potential injury to the melanocytes or deposition of pigment granules to other areas of the eye is currently unknown. Patients should be examined regularly, and depending on the clinical situation, treatment may be stopped if increased pigmentation ensues.

There have been reports of bacterial keratitis associated with the use of multiple-dose containers of topical ophthalmic products. Do not administer while wearing contact lenses.

Dosage Forms Solution, ophthalmic: 0.005% (2.5 mL) [contains benzalkonium chloride]

Overdosage/Treatment Decontamination: Ocular: Irrigate with saline

Drug Interactions May be used concomitantly with other topical ophthalmic drugs if administration is separated by at least 5 minutes.

Bimatoprost: Combination therapy may result in higher IOP than either agent alone.

Thimerosal-containing eye drops: Precipitation occurs when eye drops containing thimerosal are mixed with latanoprost. If such drugs are used, administer with an interval of at least 5 minutes between applications.

Pregnancy Risk Factor C

Additional Information Irreversible brown eye color change in individuals with blue-green eyes

Leflunomide

U.S. Brand Names Arava®

Use Treatment of active rheumatoid arthritis: indicated to reduce signs and symptoms, and to retard structural damage and improve physical function

Unlabeled/Investigational Use Treatment of cytomegalovirus (CMV) disease

Mechanism of Action An isoxazole derivative which inhibits pyrimidine synthesis, resulting in antiproliferative and anti-inflammatory effects; attenuates the immune response

Adverse Reactions

Cardiovascular: Hypertension, chest pain, palpitations, tachycardia, vasculitis, vasodilation, varicose veins, peripheral edema

Central nervous system: Headache, dizziness, pain, fever, malaise, migraine, anxiety, depression, insomnia, sleep disorder

Dermatologic: **Alopecia** (10%), rash, pruritus, dry skin, eczema, acne, dermatitis, hair discoloration, hematoma, nail disorder, skin disorder/discoloration, skin ulcer, bruising, urticaria, toxic epidermal necrolysis, urticaria, Stevens-Johnson syndrome, angioedema, erythema multiforme

Endocrine & metabolic: Hypokalemia, diabetes mellitus, hyperglycemia, hyperlipidemia, hyperthyroidism, menstrual disorder

Gastrointestinal: **Diarrhea**, nausea, abdominal pain, dyspepsia, weight loss, anorexia, gastroenteritis, stomatitis, vomiting, cholelithiasis, colitis, constipation, esophagitis, flatulence, gastritis, gingivitis, melena, enlarged salivary gland, tooth disorder, xerostomia, taste disturbance, pancreatitis

Genitourinary: Urinary tract infection, cystitis, dysuria, vaginal candidiasis, prostate disorder, urinary frequency, pelvic pain

Hematologic: Anemia, eosinophilia, thrombocytopenia, leukopenia, pancytopenia, agranulocytosis

Hepatic: Abnormal liver function test results, hepatotoxicity, hepatic failure, cholestasis, hepatic necrosis

Neuromuscular & skeletal: Back pain, joint disorder, weakness, tenosynovitis, synovitis, arthralgia, paresthesia, muscle cramps, neck pain, arthrosis, bursitis, myalgia, bone necrosis, bone pain, tendon rupture, neuralgia, neuritis, increased CPK, peripheral neuropathy

Ocular: Blurred vision, cataract, conjunctivitis, eye disorder

Renal: Albuminuria, hematuria

Respiratory: **Respiratory tract infection**, bronchitis, cough, pharyngitis, pneumonia, rhinitis, sinusitis, asthma, dyspnea, epistaxis, interstitial lung disease

Miscellaneous: Infection, accidental injury, allergic reactions, diaphoresis, anaphylaxis, herpes infection, subcutaneous nodule, oral candidiasis, sepsis, opportunistic infection

Pharmacodynamics/Kinetics

Distribution: V_d: 0.13 L/kg

Metabolism: Hepatic to A77 1726 (MI) which accounts for nearly all pharmacologic activity; further metabolism to multiple inactive metabolites; undergoes enterohepatic recirculation

Bioavailability: 80%

Half-life elimination: Mean: 14-15 days; enterohepatic recycling appears to contribute to the long half-life of this agent, since activated charcoal and cholestyramine substantially reduce plasma half-life

Time to peak: 6-12 hours

Excretion: Feces (48%); urine (43%)

Dosage

Oral:

Adults: Initial: 100 mg/day for 3 days, followed by 20 mg/day; dosage may be decreased to 10 mg/day in patients who have difficulty tolerating the 20 mg dose. Due to the long half-life of the active metabolite, plasma levels may require a prolonged period to decline after dosage reduction.

Elderly: Although hepatic function may decline with age, no specific dosage adjustment is recommended. Patients should be monitored closely for adverse effects which may require dosage adjustment.

Dosing adjustment in renal impairment: No specific dosage adjustment is recommended. There is no clinical experience in the use of leflunomide in patients with renal impairment. The free fraction of MI is doubled in dialysis patients. Patients should be monitored closely for adverse effects requiring dosage adjustment.

Dosing adjustment in hepatic impairment: No specific dosage adjustment is recommended. Since the liver is involved in metabolic activation and subsequent metabolism/elimination of leflunomide, patients with hepatic impairment should be monitored closely for adverse effects requiring dosage adjustment.

Dosing adjustment in hepatic toxicity: Guidelines for dosage adjustment or discontinuation based on the severity and persistence of ALT elevation secondary to leflunomide have been developed. If ALT elevations >2 times but ≤3 times ULN are noted, reduce dose to 10 mg/day, and monitor closely. If elevations persist or if elevations >3 times ULN are observed, discontinue leflunomide and initiate protocol to accelerate elimination. Cholestyramine (8 g 3 times/day for 1-3 days) or activated charcoal (50 g every 6 hours for 24 hours) may be administered

to decrease leflunomide concentrations rapidly. If elevations >3 times ULN persist additional cholestyramine and/or activated charcoal may be required.

Stability Protect from light; store at 25°C (77°F)

Monitoring Parameters A complete blood count (WBC, hemoglobin, hematocrit, and platelet count) as well as serum transaminase determinations should be monitored at baseline and monthly during the initial 6 months of treatment; if stable, monitoring frequency may be decreased to every 6-8 weeks thereafter (continue monthly when used in combination with other immunosuppressive agents). In addition, monitor for signs/symptoms of severe infection, abnormalities in hepatic function tests, or symptoms of hepatotoxicity.

Contraindications Hypersensitivity to leflunomide or any component of the formulation; pregnancy

Warnings Leflunomide has been associated with rare reports of hepatotoxicity, hepatic failure, and death. Multiple risk factors for hepatotoxicity including hepatic disease (including seropositive hepatitis B or C patients) and/or concurrent exposure to other hepatotoxins may increase the risk of hepatotoxicity. Most severe cases occur within 6 months of initiation. Monitoring of hepatic function is required.

Not recommended for patients with severe immune deficiency, bone marrow dysplasia, or uncontrolled infection. Has been associated with rare pancytopenia, agranulocytosis, and thrombocytopenia, particularly when given in combination with methotrexate or other immunosuppressive agents. Monitoring of hematologic function is required. Use with caution in patients with a prior history of significant hematologic abnormalities. Discontinue if evidence of bone marrow suppression or severe dermatologic reaction occurs, and begin procedure to accelerate elimination (cholestyramine or activated charcoal, see Overdosage/Toxicology). Interstitial lung disease has been associated (rarely) with leflunomide use. Discontinue in patients who develop new onset or worsening of pulmonary symptoms; accelerated elimination procedures should be considered if interstitial lung disease occurs; fatal outcomes have been reported. Consider interruption of therapy and accelerated elimination in patients who develop serious infections while receiving leflunomide. The use of live vaccines is not recommended.

[U.S. Boxed Warning]: Women of childbearing potential should not receive leflunomide until pregnancy has been excluded. Patients have been counseled concerning fetal risk and reliable contraceptive measures have been confirmed. Caution in renal impairment. Leflunomide will increase uric acid excretion. Immunosuppression may increase the risk of lymphoproliferative disorders or other malignancies.

Dosage Forms Tablet (Arava®): 10 mg, 20 mg

Overdosage/Treatment

Decontamination: Lavage within 1 hour. Activated charcoal without sorbitol or cholestyramine should then be given.

Enhanced elimination: Multiple dosing of activated charcoal without sorbitol (50 g every 6 hours for 24 hours) or cholestyramine (8 g every 8 hours for 1-3 days) may be useful. Cholestyramine and/or activated charcoal enhance elimination of leflunomide's active metabolite (MI). Cholestyramine reduces plasma levels by approximately 40% in 24 hours and 49% to 65% after 48 hours of dosing. Activated charcoal reduces plasma levels by 37% after 24 hours and 48% after 48 hours of continuous dosing.

Drug Interactions Inhibits CYP2C9 (weak)

Bile acid sequestrants (cholestyramine): May interfere with enterohepatic recycling of leflunomide. This is used emergently to remove drug from the circulation, but may decrease levels inadvertently if used concomitantly.

Hepatotoxic agents: Leflunomide may increase the risk of hepatotoxicity when combined with drugs which may cause hepatic injury; use caution.

Methotrexate: Concomitant treatment with leflunomide may increase the risk of hepatotoxicity or hematologic toxicity; monitor.

Rifampin: May increase the serum concentration of leflunomide's active metabolite; use caution.

Warfarin: Leflunomide may increase the effects of warfarin; monitor.

Pregnancy Risk Factor X

Pregnancy Implications Has been associated with teratogenic and embryolethal effects in animal models at low doses. Leflunomide is contraindicated in pregnant women or women of childbearing potential who are not using reliable contraception. Pregnancy must be excluded prior to initiating treatment. Following treatment, pregnancy should be avoided until undetectable plasma levels (< 0.02 mcg/mL) are verified. This may be accomplished by an extended drug elimination procedure: Administer cholestyramine 8 g 3 times/day for 11 days (the 11 days do not need to be consecutive). Plasma levels <0.02 mg/L should be verified by two separate tests performed at least 14 days apart. If plasma levels are >0.02 mg/L, additional cholestyramine treatment should be considered. Without this procedure, it may take up to 2 years to reach acceptable plasma concentrations.

Lactation Excretion in breast milk unknown/contraindicated

Additional Information Smoking increases plasma clearance by 38%.

Specific References

Chan J, Sanders DC, Du L, et al, "Leflunomide-Associated Pancytopenia with or without Methotrexate," *Ann Pharmacother*, 2004, 38(7):1206-11.

Levetiracetam

CAS Number 102767-28-2
U.S. Brand Names Keppra®
Use Indicated as adjunctive therapy in the treatment of partial onset seizures in adults with epilepsy
Unlabeled/Investigational Use Bipolar disorder; partial onset seizures in children with epilepsy
Mechanism of Action The precise mechanism by which levetiracetam exerts its antiepileptic effect is unknown and does not appear to derive from any interaction with known mechanisms involved in inhibitory and excitatory neurotransmission.
Adverse Reactions
Cardiovascular: Chest pain
Central nervous system: **Somnolence, headache**, pain, psychotic symptoms, amnesia, ataxia, depression, dizziness, emotional lability, nervousness, vertigo, agitation, anger, aggression, irritability, hostility, anxiety, apathy, depersonalization, confusion, convulsion, fever, insomnia, thinking abnormal
Dermatologic: Bruising, rash
Gastrointestinal: Anorexia, abdominal pain, constipation, diarrhea, dyspepsia, gastroenteritis, gingivitis, nausea, vomiting, weight gain
Hematologic: Decreased erythrocyte counts, decreased leukocytes, leukopenia, neutropenia, pancytopenia, thrombocytopenia
Neuromuscular & skeletal: **Weakness**, ataxia and other coordination difficulties, paresthesia, arthralgia, back pain, tremor
Ocular: Diplopia, amblyopia, otitis media
Respiratory: Pharyngitis, rhinitis, cough, sinusitis, bronchitis
Miscellaneous: **Infection**, flu-like symptoms
Signs and Symptoms of Overdose Coma, lethargy, respiratory depression, sedation
Admission Criteria/Prognosis Admit if somnolent, exhibiting respiratory depression, or if ingestion exceeds 10 g
Pharmacodynamics/Kinetics
Onset of action: Oral: Peak effect: 1 hour
Absorption: Oral: Rapid and complete
Distribution: V_d: Similar to total body water
Protein binding: <10%
Metabolism: Not extensive; primarily by enzymatic hydrolysis; forms metabolites (inactive)
Bioavailability: 100%
Half-life elimination: 6-8 hours
Excretion: Urine (66% as unchanged drug)
Dosage
Oral:
Children 4-16 years: Partial onset seizures (unlabeled use): 10-20 mg/kg/day in 2 divided doses; may increase weekly by 10-20 mg/kg, up to a maximum of 60 mg/kg
Children ≥16 years and Adults:
Partial onset seizure: Initial: 500 mg twice daily; additional dosing increments may be given (1000 mg/day additional every 2 weeks) to a maximum recommended daily dose of 3000 mg
Bipolar disorder (unlabeled use): Initial: 500 mg twice daily; if tolerated, increase to 500 mg twice daily; dose may be increased every 3 days until target dose of 3000 mg/day is reached; maximum: 4000 mg/day
Dosing adjustment in renal impairment:
Cl_{cr} >80 mL/minute: 500-1500 mg every 12 hours
Cl_{cr} 50-80 mL/minute: 500-1000 mg every 12 hours
Cl_{cr} 30-50 mL/minute: 250-750 mg every 12 hours
Cl_{cr} <30 mL/minute: 250-500 mg every 12 hours
End-stage renal disease patients using dialysis: 500-1000 mg every 24 hours; a supplemental dose of 250-500 mg following dialysis is recommended hours
Administration Tablets may be crushed and placed in food if unable to swallow whole (bitter taste may be expected).
Contraindications Hypersensitivity to levetiracetam or any component of the formulation
Warnings Psychotic symptoms (psychosis, hallucinations) and behavioral symptoms (including aggression, anger, anxiety, depersonalization, depression, personality disorder) may occur; incidence may be increased in children. Dose reduction may be required. Levetiracetam should be withdrawn gradually to minimize the potential of increased seizure frequency. Use caution with renal impairment; dosage adjustment may be necessary. Weakness, dizziness, and somnolence occur mostly during the first month of therapy. Safety and efficacy in children <4 years(oral formulation) or <16 years (I.V. formulation) have not been established.
Dosage Forms Injection, solution:
Keppra®: 100 mg/mL (5 mL)
Solution, oral:
Keppra®: 100 mg/mL (480 mL) [dye free; grape flavor]
Tablet:
Keppra®: 250 mg, 500 mg, 750 mg, 1000 mg

Reference Range Steady state serum levels following a 3000 mg daily dose: 10-37 mcg/mL. Peak serum levetiracetam after 5000 mg dose: 118 mcg/mL. Serum level after 30,000 mg overdose with resultant coma: 400 mcg/mL
Overdosage/Treatment
Decontamination: Lavage within 1 hour of ingestion with activated charcoal. Consider gastric decontamination if ingestion exceeds 10 g.
Supportive therapy: May require respiratory support for respiratory depression
Enhanced elimination: Multiple dosing of activated charcoal may be useful; hemodialysis can remove 50% of dose in 4 hours
Drug Interactions CNS depressants: May enhance the adverse/toxic effect of levetiracetam.
Pregnancy Risk Factor C
Pregnancy Implications Developmental toxicities were observed in animal studies. There are no adequate and well-controlled studies in pregnant women. Pregnant women exposed to levetiracetam may be enrolled in the Antiepileptic Drug Pregnancy Registry by calling 888-233-2334.
Lactation Enters breast milk/not recommended
Specific References
Stoner SC, Lea JW, Wolf AL, et al, "Levetiracetam for Mood Stabilization and Maintenance of Seizure Control Following Multiple Treatment Failures," *Ann Pharmacother*, 2005, 39(11):1928-31.

Levodopa

Related Information
• Therapeutic Drugs Associated with Hallucinations
CAS Number 59-92-7
U.S. Brand Names Dopar®; Larodopa®
Synonyms *L*-3-Hydroxytyrosine; *L*-Dopa
Use Treatment of Parkinson's disease
Diagnostic agent for growth hormone deficiency
Mechanism of Action Increases dopamine levels in the brain, then stimulates dopaminergic receptors in the basal ganglia to improve the balance between cholinergic and dopaminergic activity
Adverse Reactions
Cardiovascular: **Cardiac arrhythmias, hypotension (orthostatic)**, flutter (atrial), myocardial depression, tachycardia (supraventricular), palpitations
Central nervous system: **Anxiety, dizziness, confusion, nightmares**, memory loss, nervousness, insomnia, fatigue, psychosis, auditory and visual hallucinations, dystonic reactions, ataxia, electroencephalogram abnormalities, gustatory hallucinations, hyperthermia
Dermatologic: Urticaria, purpura, exanthem
Endocrine & metabolic: Hypoprolactinemia
Gastrointestinal: **Nausea, anorexia, constipation, vomiting**, GI bleeding, xerostomia, metallic taste
Genitourinary: **Dysuria**
Hematologic: Hemolytic anemia with positive direct and indirect Coombs' tests, leukopenia, neutropenia, agranulocytosis, granulocytopenia
Neuromuscular & skeletal: **Choreiform and involuntary movements**, clonus, myoclonus
Ocular: **Blepharospasm**, blurred vision
Miscellaneous: Bruxism, systemic lupus erythematosus
Signs and Symptoms of Overdose Agranulocytosis, alopecia, arrhythmias, chorea (extrapyramidal), congestive heart failure, confusion, delirium, dementia, depression, dysosmia, eosinophilia, euphoria, extrapyramidal reaction including choreoathetosis, feces discoloration (black), fibrillation (atrial), granulocytopenia, gout, hyperpigmented hair, hypertension, hyperuricemia, hypokalemia, hyponatremia, insomnia, leukocytosis, leukopenia, malignant hyperthermia (reported), mania, memory loss, myoclonus, nausea, neutropenia, night terrors, palpitations, Parkinson's-like symptoms, paroxysmal tachycardia (ventricular), pemphigus, respiratory dyskinesias, restlessness, pseudotumor cerebri, spasm, thrombocytopenia, urine discoloration (black; brown), vomiting
Pharmacodynamics/Kinetics
Duration: Variable, usually 6-12 hours
Absorption: May be decreased if given with a high protein meal
Metabolism: Peripheral decarboxylation to dopamine; small amounts reach brain and are decarboxylated to active dopamine
Half-life elimination: 1.2-2.3 hours
Time to peak, serum: 1-2 hours
Excretion: Primarily urine (80% as dopamine, norepinephrine, and homovanillic acid)
Dosage
Oral:
Children (given as a single dose to evaluate growth hormone deficiency): 0.5 g/m² **or**
<30 lbs: 125 mg
30-70 lbs: 250 mg
>70 lbs: 500 mg

Adults (administer with food): 500-1000 mg/day in divided doses every 6-12 hours; increase by 100-750 mg/day every 3-7 days until response or total dose of 8000 mg is reached

Significant therapeutic response may not be obtained for 6 months

Monitoring Parameters Serum growth hormone concentration

Administration

Administer with meals to decrease GI upset

Contraindications Hypersensitivity to levodopa or any component of the formulation; narrow-angle glaucoma; use of MAO inhibitors within prior 14 days (however, may be administered concomitantly with the manufacturer's recommended dose of an MAO inhibitor with selectivity for MAO type B); history of melanoma or any undiagnosed skin lesions

Warnings Use with caution in patients with history of cardiovascular disease (including myocardial infarction and arrhythmias); pulmonary diseases such as asthma, psychosis, wide-angle glaucoma, peptic ulcer disease; as well as in renal, hepatic, or endocrine disease. Sudden discontinuation of levodopa may cause a worsening of Parkinson's disease. Elderly may be more sensitive to CNS effects of levodopa. May cause or exacerbate dyskinesias. May cause orthostatic hypotension; Parkinson's disease patients appear to have an impaired capacity to respond to a postural challenge. Use with caution in patients at risk of hypotension (such as those receiving antihypertensive drugs) or where transient hypotensive episodes would be poorly tolerated (cardiovascular disease or cerebrovascular disease). Observe patients closely for development of depression with concomitant suicidal tendencies. Safety and effectiveness in pediatric patients have not been established. Some products may contain tartrazine. Dopaminergic agents have been associated with a syndrome resembling neuroleptic malignant syndrome on withdrawal or significant dosage reduction after long-term use. Pyridoxine may reverse effects of levodopa. Toxic reactions have occurred with dextromethorphan.

Dosage Forms Capsule: 100 mg, 250 mg, 500 mg
Tablet: 100 mg, 250 mg, 500 mg

Reference Range Peak serum level of 3.2 mg/L occurs after ingestion of 200 mg levodopa

Overdosage/Treatment

Decontamination: Emesis (within 30 minutes) may be of value in only very early ingestions; lavage (within 1 hour); activated charcoal of use

Supportive therapy: Deanol and pyridoxine of questionable use for dyskinesias, but have been tried; dantrolene and/or bromocriptine has been used in malignant hyperthermia; choreo-ballistic dyskinesia due to levodopa can improve with low dose propranolol (30-60 mg/day); levodopa-induced psychosis can be treated with remoxipride; amantadine at doses of 200-300 mg/day can help improve dyskinesia

Enhancement of elimination: Multiple dose activated charcoal has not been addressed

Test Interactions False-positive reaction for urinary glucose with Clinitest®; false-negative reaction using Clinistix®; false-positive urine ketones with Acetest®, Ketostix®, Labstix®; serum uric acid may be elevated; may cause false elevation of serum creatinine through interference with laboratory determination; may interfere with the TSH assay resulting in falsely low TSH levels

Drug Interactions

Antacids: Levodopa absorption may be increased; monitor

Anticholinergics: May reduce the efficacy of levodopa, possibly due to reduced gastrointestinal absorption (also see tricyclic antidepressants); limited evidence of clinical significance; monitor

Antipsychotics: May inhibit the antiparkinsonian effects of levodopa via dopamine receptor blockade; use antipsychotics with low dopamine blockade (clozapine, olanzapine, quetiapine)

Benzodiazepines: May inhibit the antiparkinsonian effects of levodopa; monitor for reduced effect

Clonidine: May reduce the efficacy of levodopa; monitor

Furazolidone: May increase the effect/toxicity of levodopa; hypertensive episodes have been reported; monitor

Iron salts: Binds levodopa and reduces its bioavailability; separate doses of iron and levodopa

Linezolid: Due to MAO inhibition (see note on MAO inhibitors), this agent is best avoided

MAO inhibitors: Concurrent use of levodopa with nonselective MAO inhibitors may result in hypertensive reactions via an increased storage and release of dopamine, norepinephrine, or both; use with carbidopa to minimize reactions if combination is necessary; otherwise avoid combination

L-methionine: May inhibit levodopa's antiparkinsonian effects; monitor for reduced effect

Metoclopramide: May increase the absorption/effect of levodopa; hypertensive episodes have been reported. Levodopa antagonizes metoclopramide's effects on lower esophageal sphincter pressure; avoid use of metoclopramide for reflux, monitor response to levodopa carefully if used.

Methyldopa: May potentiate the effects of levodopa; levodopa may increase the hypotensive response to methyldopa; monitor

Papaverine: May decrease the efficacy of levodopa; includes other similar agents (ethaverine); monitor

Penicillamine: May increase serum concentrations of levodopa; monitor for increased effect

Phenytoin: May inhibit levodopa's antiparkinsonian effects; monitor for reduced effect

Pyridoxine: May inhibit levodopa's antiparkinsonian effects; monitor for reduced effect (pyridoxine in doses >10-25 mg for levodopa alone, higher doses >200 mg/day may be a problem for levodopa/carbidopa)

Spiramycin: May inhibit levodopa's antiparkinsonian effects; monitor for reduced effect

Tacrine: May inhibit the effects of levodopa via enhanced cholinergic activity; monitor for reduced effect

Tricyclic antidepressants: May decrease the absorption (bioavailability) of levodopa; rare hypertensive episodes have also been attributed to this combination

Pregnancy Risk Factor C

Nursing Implications Sustained release product should not be crushed

Levofloxacin

Related Information
- Ciprofloxacin

CAS Number 100986-85-4; 138199-71-0

U.S. Brand Names Iquix®; Levaquin®; Quixin™

Use

Systemic: Treatment of mild, moderate, or severe infections caused by susceptible organisms. Includes the treatment of community-acquired pneumonia (including penicillin-resistant strains of *S. pneumoniae*); nosocomial pneumonia; chronic bronchitis (acute bacterial exacerbation); acute maxillary sinusitis; urinary tract infection (uncomplicated or complicated), including acute pyelonephritis caused by *E. coli*; prostatitis (chronic bacterial); skin or skin structure infections (uncomplicated or complicated)

Ophthalmic: Treatment of bacterial conjunctivitis caused by susceptible organisms (Quixin™ 0.5% ophthalmic solution); treatment of corneal ulcer caused by susceptible organisms (Iquix® 1.5% ophthalmic solution)

Unlabeled/Investigational Use Diverticulitis, enterocolitis, (*Shigella* sp), gonococcal infections, Legionnaires' disease, peritonitis, PID

Mechanism of Action As the S (-) enantiomer of the fluoroquinolone, ofloxacin, levofloxacin, inhibits DNA-gyrase in susceptible organisms thereby inhibiting relaxation of supercoiled DNA and promoting breakage of DNA strands. DNA gyrase (topoisomerase II), is an essential bacterial enzyme that maintains the superhelical structure of DNA and is required for DNA replication and transcription, DNA repair, recombination, and transposition.

Adverse Reactions

Systemic:

Cardiovascular: Cardiac failure, hypertension, bradycardia, tachycardia, arrhythmias (including ventricular tachycardia and torsade de pointes), QT_c prolongation

Central nervous system: Dizziness, fever, headache, insomnia, seizures, dysphonia

Dermatologic: Photosensitivity (<0.1%), erythema multiforme, rash, Stevens-Johnson syndrome

Genitourinary: Leukorrhea

Gastrointestinal: Nausea, vomiting, diarrhea, constipation, pseudomembranous colitis

Hematologic: Granulocytopenia, leukopenia, leukocytosis, thrombocytopenia, eosinophilia, hemolytic anemia, autoimmune hemolytic anemia (AIHA)

Hepatic: Elevated transaminases, hepatic failure, jaundice

Neuromuscular & skeletal: Tremor, arthralgia, tendon rupture

Renal: Acute renal failure

Respiratory: Pharyngitis, pulmonary embolism

Miscellaneous: Allergic reaction (including pneumonitis and anaphylaxis)

Ophthalmic solution:

Ocular: Decreased vision (transient), foreign body sensation, transient ocular burning, ocular pain or discomfort, photophobia, lid edema, ocular dryness, ocular itching

Miscellaneous: Allergic reaction

Signs and Symptoms of Overdose Acute renal failure, dizziness, diarrhea, seizures

Pharmacodynamics/Kinetics

Absorption: Rapid and complete

Distribution: V_d: 1.25 L/kg; CSF concentrations ~15% of serum levels; high concentrations are achieved in prostate, lung, and gynecological tissues, sinus, saliva

Protein binding: 50%

Metabolism: Minimally hepatic

Bioavailability: 99%

Half-life elimination: 6-8 hours
Time to peak, serum: 1-2 hours
Excretion: Primarily urine (as unchanged drug)

Dosage

Oral, I.V. (infuse I.V. solution over 60 minutes): Adults:
Chronic bronchitis (acute bacterial exacerbation): 500 mg every 24 hours for at least 7 days
Maxillary sinusitis (acute): 500 mg every 24 hours for 10-14 days
Pneumonia:
Community-acquired: 500 mg every 24 hours for 7-14 days or 750 mg every 24 hours for 5 days
Nosocomial: 750 mg every 24 hours for 7-14 days
Prostatitis (chronic bacterial): 500 mg every 24 hours for 28 days
Skin infections:
Uncomplicated: 500 mg every 24 hours for 7-10 days
Complicated: 750 mg every 24 hours for 7-14 days
Urinary tract infections:
Uncomplicated: 250 mg once daily for 3 days
Complicated, including acute pyelonephritis: 250 mg every 24 hours for 10 days

Ophthalmic:
Conjunctivitis (0.5% ophthalmic solution): Children ≥1 year and Adults:
Treatment day 1 and day 2: Instill 1-2 drops into affected eye(s) every 2 hours while awake, up to 8 times/day
Treatment day 3 through day 7: Instill 1-2 drops into affected eye(s) every 4 hours while awake, up to 4 times/day
Corneal ulceration (1.5% ophthalmic solution): Children ≥6 years and Adults:
Treatment day 1 through day 3: Instill 1-2 drops into affected eye(s) every 30 minutes to 2 hours while awake and ~4-6 hours after retiring.
Treatment day 4 to treatment completion: Instill 1-2 drops into affected eye(s) every 1-4 hours while awake.

Dosing adjustment in renal impairment:
Chronic bronchitis, acute maxillary sinusitis, uncomplicated skin infection, community-acquired pneumonia, chronic bacterial prostatitis, complicated UTI, or acute pyelonephritis: First dose as indicated in patients with normal renal function (250 mg or 500 mg), followed by:
Cl_{cr} 20-49 mL/minute: 250 mg every 24 hours
Cl_{cr} 10-19 mL/minute: 250 mg every 48 hours
Uncomplicated UTI: No dosage adjustment required
Complicated skin infection, community-acquired pneumonia, or nosocomial pneumonia:
Cl_{cr} 20-49 mL/minute: Administer 750 mg every 48 hours
Cl_{cr} 10-19 mL/minute: Administer 500 mg every 48 hours (initial: 750 mg)
Hemodialysis/CAPD: 250 mg every 48 hours (initial: 500 mg for most infections; initial: 750 mg for complicated skin/soft tissue infections followed by 500 mg every 48 hours)

Stability Injection: Stable for 72 hours when diluted to 5 mg/mL in a compatible I.V. fluid and stored at room temperature; stable for 14 days when stored under refrigeration; stable for 6 months when frozen, do not refreeze; do not thaw in microwave or by bath immersion; **incompatible** with mannitol and sodium bicarbonate
Ophthalmic solution: Store at 15°C to 25°C (59°F to 77°F)

Monitoring Parameters Evaluation of organ system functions (renal, hepatic, ophthalmologic, and hematopoietic) is recommended periodically during therapy; the possibility of crystalluria should be assessed; WBC and signs of infection

Administration
Oral: May be administered without regard to meals.
I.V.: Infuse I.V. solution over 60 minutes. Too rapid of infusion can lead to hypotension. Avoid administration through an intravenous line with a solution containing multivalent cations (ie, magnesium, calcium).

Contraindications Hypersensitivity to levofloxacin, any component of the formulation, or other quinolones

Warnings
Systemic: Not recommended in children <18 years of age; CNS stimulation may occur (tremor, restlessness, confusion, and very rarely hallucinations or seizures). Potential for seizures, although very rare, may be increased with concomitant NSAID therapy. Use with caution in individuals at risk of seizures, with known or suspected CNS disorders or renal dysfunction; use caution to avoid possible photosensitivity reactions during and for several days following fluoroquinolone therapy
Rare cases of torsade de pointes have been reported in patients receiving levofloxacin. Risk may be minimized by avoiding use in patients with known prolongation of QT interval, bradycardia, hypokalemia, hypomagnesemia, cardiomyopathy, or in those receiving concurrent therapy with Class Ia or Class III antiarrhythmics.
Severe hypersensitivity reactions, including anaphylaxis, have occurred with quinolone therapy. If an allergic reaction occurs (itching, urticaria, dyspnea or facial edema, loss of consciousness, tingling, cardiovascular collapse), discontinue drug immediately. Prolonged use may result in superinfection; pseudomembranous colitis may occur and should be considered in all patients who present with diarrhea. Tendon inflammation and/or rupture has been reported; risk may be increased with concurrent corticosteroids, particularly in the elderly. Discontinue at first sign of tendon inflammation or pain. Peripheral neuropathies have been linked to levofloxacin use; discontinue if numbness, tingling, or weakness develops. Quinolones may exacerbate myasthenia gravis; use with caution (rare, potentially life-threatening weakness of respiratory muscles may occur).
Ophthalmic solution: For topical use only. Do not inject subconjunctivally or introduce into anterior chamber of the eye. Contact lenses should not be worn during treatment for bacterial conjunctivitis. Safety and efficacy in children <1 year of age (Quixin™) or <6 years of age (Iquix®) have not been established. **Note:** Indications for ophthalmic solutions are product concentration-specific and should not be used interchangeably.

Dosage Forms Infusion [premixed in D_5W] (Levaquin®): 250 mg (50 mL); 500 mg (100 mL); 750 mg (150 mL)
Injection, solution [preservative free] (Levaquin®): 25 mg/mL (20 mL, 30 mL)
Solution, ophthalmic:
Iquix®: 1.5% (5 mL)
Quixin™: 0.5% (5 mL) [contains benzalkonium chloride]
Solution, oral (Levaquin®): 25 mg/mL (480 mL) [contains benzyl alcohol]
Tablet (Levaquin®): 250 mg, 500 mg, 750 mg
Levaquin® Leva-Pak: 750 mg (5s)

Overdosage/Treatment Treatment should include GI decontamination (for ingestions >5 g) and supportive care; not removed by peritoneal or hemodialysis

Test Interactions Can give a false-positive result for opiates by urine immunoassay screening

Drug Interactions Corticosteroids: Concurrent use may increase the risk of tendon rupture, particularly in elderly patients (overall incidence rare).
Glyburide: Quinolones may increase the effect of glyburide; monitor
Metal cations (aluminum, calcium, iron, magnesium, and zinc) bind quinolones in the gastrointestinal tract and inhibit absorption. Concurrent administration of most antacids, oral electrolyte supplements, quinapril, sucralfate, some didanosine formulations (chewable/buffered tablets and pediatric powder for oral suspension), and other highly-buffered oral drugs, should be avoided. Levofloxacin should be administered 2 hours before or 2 hours after these agents.
Probenecid: May decrease renal secretion of levofloxacin.
QT_c-prolonging agents: Effects may be additive with levofloxacin. Avoid concurrent use with Class Ia and Class III antiarrhythmics, erythromycin, cisapride, antipsychotics, and cyclic antidepressants.
Warfarin: The hypoprothrombinemic effect of warfarin may be enhanced by some quinolone antibiotics; monitor INR.

Pregnancy Risk Factor C

Pregnancy Implications Avoid use in pregnant women unless the benefit justifies the potential risk to the fetus

Lactation Excretion in breast milk unknown/not recommended

Nursing Implications Infuse I.V. solutions over 60 minutes

Additional Information Ophthalmic solution contains benzalkonium chloride 0.005% as a preservative.

Specific References

Coban S, Ceydilek B, Ekiz F, et al, "Levofloxacin-Induced Acute Fulminant Hepatic Failure in a Patient with Chronic Hepatitis B Infection," *Ann Pharmacother*, 2005, 39(10):1737-40.
Cunha BA, "Empiric Therapy of Community-Acquired Pneumonia: Guidelines for the Perplexed?" *Chest*, 2004, 125(5):1913-9 (review).
Hsiao SH, Chang CM, Tsao CJ, et al, "Acute Rhabdomyolysis Associated with Ofloxacin/levofloxacin Therapy," *Ann Pharmacother*, 2005, 39(1):146-9.
Mathis AS, Chan V, Gryszkiewicz M, et al, "Levofloxacin-Associated Achilles Tendon Rupture," *Ann Pharmacother*, 2003, 37(7-8):1014-7.
Nykamp DL, Blackmon CL, Schmidt PE, et al, "QTc Prolongation Associated with Combination Therapy of Levofloxacin, Imipramine, and Fluoxetine," *Ann Pharmacother*. 2005, 39(3):543-6.

Levonorgestrel

CAS Number 797-63-7
U.S. Brand Names Mirena®; Plan B®
Synonyms LNg 20
Use Prevention of pregnancy
Mechanism of Action Pregnancy may be prevented through several mechanisms: Thickening of cervical mucus, which inhibits sperm passage through the uterus and sperm survival; inhibition of ovulation, from a negative feedback mechanism on the hypothalamus, leading to reduced secretion of follicle stimulating hormone (FSH) and luteinizing hormone (LH); inhibition of implantation. Levonorgestrel is not effective once the implantation process has begun.

Adverse Reactions
Intrauterine system:
Cardiovascular: Hypertension
Central nervous system: Headache, depression, nervousness, migraine
Dermatologic: Acne, alopecia, eczema, induration
Endocrine & metabolic: Breast pain, dysmenorrhea, decreased libido, abnormal Pap smear, **amenorrhea, enlarged follicles**
Gastrointestinal: Abdominal pain, nausea, weight gain, vomiting
Genitourinary: Leukorrhea, vaginitis, cervicitis, dyspareunia
Hematologic: Anemia
Neuromuscular & skeletal: Back pain
Respiratory: Upper respiratory tract infection, sinusitis
Miscellaneous: Failed insertion, sepsis
Oral tablets:
Central nervous system: **Fatigue, headache, dizziness**
Endocrine & metabolic: **Heavier menstrual bleeding, lighter menstrual bleeding, breast tenderness**
Gastrointestinal: **Nausea, abdominal pain**, vomiting, diarrhea
Subdermal capsules:
Cardiovascular: Deep vein thrombosis, idiopathic intracranial hypertension, myocardial infarction, superficial venous thrombosis
Central nervous system: Anxiety, depression, dizziness, emotional lability, fatigue, headache, migraine, nervousness, stroke
Dermatologic: Acne, alopecia, blistering, bruising, cellulitis, dermatitis, hirsutism, hyperpigmentation, pruritus, rash, sloughing, ulcerations, urticaria
Endocrine & metabolic: **Increased/prolonged bleeding, spotting**, breast discharge, menstrual irregularities, dysmenorrhea, mastalgia
Gastrointestinal: Abdominal discomfort, appetite change, vomiting, weight gain
Genitourinary: Cervicitis, leukorrhea, vaginitis
Hematologic: Thrombotic thrombocytopenic purpura (TTP)
Local: Pain/itching at implant site (usually transient), infection at implant site, phlebitis
Neuromuscular & skeletal: Musculoskeletal pain, arm pain, nerve injury, numbness, tingling, weakness
Respiratory: Pulmonary embolism
Miscellaneous: Removal difficulties; these may include multiple incisions, remaining capsule fragments, pain, multiple visits, deep placement, lengthy procedure; abscess, adnexal enlargement, breast cancer, congenital anomalies, excessive scarring

Signs and Symptoms of Overdose Can result if >6 capsules are *in situ*; symptoms include uterine bleeding irregularities and fluid retention; benign intracranial hypertension

Pharmacodynamics/Kinetics
Duration: Intrauterine system: Up to 5 years
Absorption: Oral: Rapid and complete
Protein binding: Highly bound to albumin (~50%) and sex hormone-binding globulin (~47%)
Metabolism: To inactive metabolites
Half-life elimination: Oral: ~24 hours
Excretion: Primarily urine

Dosage Adults:
Long-term prevention of pregnancy: Intrauterine system: To be inserted into uterine cavity; should be inserted within 7 days of onset of menstruation or immediately after 1st trimester abortion; releases 20 mcg levonorgestrel/day over 5 years. May be removed and replaced with a new unit at anytime during menstrual cycle; do not leave any one system in place for >5 years
Emergency contraception: Oral tablet: One 0.75 mg tablet as soon as possible within 72 hours of unprotected sexual intercourse; a second 0.75 mg tablet should be taken 12 hours after the first dose; may be used at any time during menstrual cycle
Dosage adjustment in renal impairment: Safety and efficacy have not been established
Dosage adjustment in hepatic impairment: Safety and efficacy have not been established
Elderly: Not intended for use in postmenopausal women
Monitoring Parameters Monitor for prolonged menstrual bleeding, amenorrhea, irregularity of menses, Pap smear, blood pressure, serum glucose in patients with diabetes, LDL levels in patients with hyperlipidemias
Administration Intrauterine system: Inserted in the uterine cavity, to a depth of 6-9 cm, with the provided insertion device; should not be forced into the uterus
Contraindications Hypersensitivity to levonorgestrel or any component of the formulation; undiagnosed abnormal uterine bleeding, active hepatic disease or malignant tumors, known or suspected carcinoma of the breast; pregnancy

Additional product-specific contraindications: Intrauterine system: Congenital or acquired uterine anomaly, acute pelvic inflammatory disease, history of pelvic inflammatory disease (unless there has been a subsequent intrauterine pregnancy), postpartum endometritis, infected abortion within past 3 months, known or suspected uterine or cervical neoplasia, unresolved/abnormal Pap smear, untreated acute cervicitis or vaginitis, patient or partner with multiple sexual partners, conditions which increase susceptibility to infections (ie, leukemia, AIDS, I.V. drug abuse), unremoved IUD, history of ectopic pregnancy, conditions which predispose to ectopic pregnancy; genital actinomycosis
Note: A previously available levonorgestrel product also had the following contraindications: Active thrombophlebitis, or thromboembolic disorders (current or history of); history of intracranial hypertension

Warnings
Menstrual bleeding patterns may be altered, missed menstrual periods should not be used to identify early pregnancy. These products do not protect against HIV infection or other sexually-transmitted diseases. Patients presenting with lower abdominal pain should be evaluated for follicular atresia and ectopic pregnancy. Patients receiving enzyme-inducing medications should be evaluated for an alternative method of contraception. Levonorgestrel may affect glucose tolerance, monitor serum glucose in patients with diabetes. Safety and efficacy for use in renal or hepatic impairment have not been established. Use with caution in conditions that may be aggravated by fluid retention, depression, or history of migraine. Only for use in women of reproductive age.
Use of combination hormonal contraceptives increases the risk of cardiovascular side effects in women who smoke cigarettes, especially those who are >35 years of age; although this may be an estrogen-related effect, the risk with progestin-only contraceptives is not known and women should be strongly advised not to smoke. Combination hormonal contraceptives may lead to increased risk of myocardial infarction and should be used with caution in patients with risk factors for coronary artery disease; the actual risk with progestin-only contraceptives is not known, however, there have been postmarketing reports of myocardial infarction in women using levonorgestrel-only contraception. May increase the risk of thromboembolism; discontinue therapy if this occurs. Combination hormonal contraceptives may have a dose-related risk of vascular disease and hypertension; strokes have also been reported with postmarketing use of levonorgestrel-only contraception. Women with hypertension should be encouraged to use a nonhormonal form of contraception. The use of combination hormonal contraceptives has been associated with a slight increase in frequency of breast cancer (studies are not consistent); studies with progestin only contraceptives have been similar. Retinal thrombosis has been reported (rarely) with combination hormonal contraceptives and may be related to the estrogen component, however, progestin-only therapy should also be discontinued with unexplained partial or complete loss of vision.

Additional formulation-specific warnings:
Intrauterine system: Increased incidence of group A streptococcal sepsis and pelvic inflammatory disease (may be asymptomatic). May perforate uterus or cervix; risk of perforation is increased in lactating women. Partial penetration or embedment in the myometrium may decrease effectiveness and lead to difficult removal. Postpartum insertion should be delayed for 6 weeks or until uterine involution is complete. Use caution in patients with coagulopathy or receiving anticoagulants
Oral tablet: Not intended to be used for routine contraception and will not terminate an existing pregnancy
Dosage Forms Intrauterine device:
Mirena®: 52 mg levonorgestrel/unit [releases levonorgestrel 20 mcg/day]
Tablet:
Plan B®: 0.75 mg
Reference Range Contraceptive protection usually with plasma levonorgestrel concentrations of 0.29-0.35 ng/mL
Overdosage/Treatment Treatment includes removal of all implanted capsules. In single acute ingestion, acute toxic effects are unlikely. In pregnancy exposure, suggest decontamination by emesis within 30 minutes or lavage within 1 hour followed by activated charcoal.
Drug Interactions **Substrate** of CYP3A4 (major)
CYP3A4 inducers: CYP3A4 inducers may decrease the levels/effects of levonorgestrel. Example inducers include aminoglutethimide, carbamazepine, nafcillin, nevirapine, phenobarbital, phenytoin, and rifamycins.
Pregnancy Risk Factor X
Pregnancy Implications Epidemiologic studies have not shown an increased risk of birth defects when used prior to pregnancy or inadvertently during early pregnancy, although rare reports of congenital anomalies have been reported. Intrauterine system: Women who become pregnant with an IUD in place risk septic abortion (septic shock and death may occur), removal of IUD may result in pregnancy loss. In addition, miscarriage, premature labor, and premature delivery may occur if pregnancy is continued with IUD in place.
Lactation Enters breast milk/use caution (AAP rates "compatible")

Levorphanol

CAS Number 125-72-4; 5985-38-6; 77-07-6
U.S. Brand Names Levo-Dromoran®
Synonyms Levorphan Tartrate; Levorphanol Tartrate
Impairment Potential Yes
Use Relief of moderate to severe pain; also used parenterally for preoperative sedation and an adjunct to nitrous oxide/oxygen anesthesia; 2 mg levorphanol produces analgesia comparable to that produced by 10 mg of morphine
Mechanism of Action Levorphanol is a synthetic opioid agonist that is classified as a morphinan derivative. Opioids interact with stereospecific opioid receptors in various parts of the central nervous system and other tissues. Analgesic potency parallels the affinity for these binding sites. These drugs do not alter the threshold or responsiveness to pain, but the perception of pain.
Adverse Reactions
Cardiovascular: **Palpitations, hypotension, bradycardia, peripheral vasodilation**
Central nervous system: **CNS depression**, agitation, increased intracranial pressure, **fatigue, drowsiness, dizziness**
Dermatologic: **Pruritus**
Endocrine & metabolic: Syndrome of inappropriate antidiuretic hormone
Gastrointestinal: **Nausea, vomiting**, constipation, biliary tract spasm
Genitourinary: Urinary tract spasm
Neuromuscular & skeletal: **Weakness**
Ocular: Miosis
Respiratory: Apnea, respiratory depression
Miscellaneous: Physical and psychological dependence, histamine release
Pharmacodynamics/Kinetics
Onset of action: Oral: 10-60 minutes
Duration: 4-8 hours
Metabolism: Hepatic
Half-life elimination: 11-16 hours
Excretion: Urine (as inactive metabolite)
Dosage
Adults: **Note:** These are guidelines and do not represent the maximum doses that may be required in all patients. Doses should be titrated to pain relief/prevention.
Acute pain (moderate to severe):
Oral: Initial: Opiate-naive: 2 mg every 6-8 hours as needed; patients with prior opiate exposure may require higher initial doses; usual dosage range: 2-4 mg every 6-8 hours as needed
I.M., SubQ: Initial: Opiate-naive: 1 mg every 6-8 hours as needed; patients with prior opiate exposure may require higher initial doses; usual dosage range: 1-2 mg every 6-8 hours as needed
Slow I.V.: Initial: Opiate-naive: Up to 1 mg/dose every 3-6 hours as needed; patients with prior opiate exposure may require higher initial doses
Chronic pain: Patients taking opioids chronically may become tolerant and require doses higher than the usual dosage range to maintain the desired effect. Tolerance can be managed by appropriate dose titration. There is no optimal or maximal dose for levorphanol in chronic pain. The appropriate dose is one that relieves pain throughout its dosing interval without causing unmanageable side effects.
Premedication: I.M., SubQ: 1-2 mg/dose 60-90 minutes prior to surgery; older or debilitated patients usually require less drug
Dosing adjustment in hepatic disease: Reduction is necessary in patients with liver disease
Stability Store at room temperature, protect from freezing; I.V. is **incompatible** when mixed with aminophylline, barbiturates, heparin, methicillin, phenytoin, sodium bicarbonate
Monitoring Parameters Pain relief, respiratory and mental status, blood pressure
Administration I.V.: Inject 3 mg over 4-5 minutes
Contraindications Hypersensitivity to levorphanol or any component of the formulation; pregnancy (prolonged use or high doses at term)
Warnings
An opioid-containing analgesic regimen should be tailored to each patient's needs and based upon the type of pain being treated (acute versus chronic), the route of administration, degree of tolerance for opioids (naive versus chronic user), age, weight, and medical condition. The optimal analgesic dose varies widely among patients. Doses should be titrated to pain relief/prevention.
Use with caution in patients with hypersensitivity reactions to other phenanthrene derivative opioid agonists (morphine, hydrocodone, hydromorphone, levorphanol, oxycodone, oxymorphone); respiratory diseases including asthma, emphysema, COPD or severe liver or renal insufficiency; some preparations contain sulfites which may cause allergic reactions; tolerance or dependence may result from extended use; dextromethorphan has equivalent antitussive activity but has much lower toxicity in accidental overdose. Elderly may be particularly susceptible to the CNS depressant and constipating effects of narcotics.

Dosage Forms Injection, solution, as tartrate: 2 mg/mL (1 mL, 10 mL)
Tablet, as tartrate: 2 mg
Overdosage/Treatment Supportive therapy: Naloxone hydrochloride (0.4-2 mg I.V., SubQ, or through an endotracheal tube); a continuous infusion (at $^2/_3$ the response dose/hour) may be required
Antidote(s)
- Nalmefene [ANTIDOTE]
- Naloxone [ANTIDOTE]
Drug Interactions Increased toxicity: CNS depressants increase CNS depression
Pregnancy Risk Factor B/D (prolonged use or high doses at term)
Lactation Excretion in breast milk unknown/not recommended
Nursing Implications Observe patient for excessive sedation, respiratory depression, implement safety measures, assist with ambulation

Levothyroxine

Related Information
- Liothyronine
- Therapeutic Drugs Associated with Hallucinations
CAS Number 25416-65-3; 51-48-9; 55-03-8; 8065-29-0
U.S. Brand Names Levothroid®; Levoxyl®; Novothyrox; Synthroid®; Unithroid®
Synonyms L-Thyroxine Sodium; Levothyroxine Sodium; T_4
Use Replacement or supplemental therapy in hypothyroidism; pituitary TSH suppression
Mechanism of Action Exact mechanism of action is unknown; however, it is believed the thyroid hormone exerts its many metabolic effects through control of DNA transcription and protein synthesis; involved in normal metabolism, growth, and development; promotes gluconeogenesis, increases utilization and mobilization of glycogen stores, and stimulates protein synthesis, increases basal metabolic rate
Adverse Reactions
Cardiovascular: Angina, arrhythmias, blood pressure increased, cardiac arrest, flushing, heart failure, MI, palpitations, pulse increased, tachycardia
Central nervous system: Anxiety, emotional lability, fatigue, fever, headache, hyperactivity, insomnia, irritability, nervousness, pseudotumor cerebri (children), seizures (rare)
Dermatologic: Alopecia
Endocrine & metabolic: Fertility impaired, menstrual irregularities
Gastrointestinal: Abdominal cramps, appetite increased, diarrhea, vomiting, weight loss
Hepatic: Elevated liver function tests
Neuromuscular & skeletal: Bone mineral density decreased, muscle weakness, tremors, slipped capital femoral epiphysis (children)
Respiratory: Dyspnea
Miscellaneous: Diaphoresis, heat intolerance, hypersensitivity (to inactive ingredients - symptoms include urticaria, pruritus, rash, flushing, angioedema, GI symptoms, fever, arthralgia, serum sickness, wheezing)
Signs and Symptoms of Overdose Overdose may cause agitation, congestive heart failure, coma, fever, heat intolerance, hypertension, hyperthyroidism, hypoglycemia, insomnia, menstrual irregularities, nervousness, palpitations, psychosis, pseudotumor cerebri, seizures (may occur up to 1 week postingestion), sweating, tachycardia (may last 3 days), unrecognized adrenal insufficiency, and weight loss. Overtreatment of children may result in premature closure of epiphyses or craniosynostosis (infants). Acute massive overdose may be life-threatening.
Admission Criteria/Prognosis Admit any symptomatic patient, ingestion >4 mg, or serum total T_4 >75 mcg/dL
Pharmacodynamics/Kinetics
Onset of action: Therapeutic: Oral: 3-5 days; I.V. 6-8 hours
Peak effect: I.V.: ~24 hours
Absorption: Oral: Erratic (40% to 80%); decreases with age
Protein binding: >99%
Metabolism: Hepatic to triiodothyronine (active)
Time to peak, serum: 2-4 hours
Half-life elimination: Euthyroid: 6-7 days; Hypothyroid: 9-10 days; Hyperthyroid: 3-4 days
Excretion: Urine and feces; decreases with age
Dosage Doses should be adjusted based on clinical response and laboratory parameters.
Oral:
Children: Hypothyroidism:
Newborns: Initial: 10-15 mcg/kg/day. Lower doses of 25 mcg/day should be considered in newborns at risk for cardiac failure. Newborns with T_4 levels <5 mcg/dL should be started at 50 mcg/day. Adjust dose at 4- to 6-week intervals.
Infants and Children: Dose based on body weight and age as listed below. Children with severe or chronic hypothyroidism should be started at 25 mcg/day; adjust dose by 25 mcg every 2-4 weeks. In older children, hyperactivity may be decreased by starting with $^1/_4$ of the recommended dose and increasing by $^1/_4$ dose each week

until the full replacement dose is reached. Refer to adult dosing once growth and puberty are complete.

0-3 months: 10-15 mcg/kg/day
3-6 months: 8-10 mcg/kg/day
6-12 months: 6-8 mcg/kg/day
1-5 years: 5-6 mcg/kg/day
6-12 years: 4-5 mcg/kg/day
>12 years: 2-3 mcg/kg/day

Adults:

Hypothyroidism: 1.7 mcg/kg/day in otherwise healthy adults <50 years old, children in whom growth and puberty are complete, and older adults who have been recently treated for hyperthyroidism or who have been hypothyroid for only a few months. Titrate dose every 6 weeks. Average starting dose ~100 mcg; usual doses are ≤200 mcg/day; doses ≥300 mcg/day are rare (consider poor compliance, malabsorption, and/or drug interactions). **Note:** For patients >50 years or patients with cardiac disease, refer to Elderly dosing.

Severe hypothyroidism: Initial: 12.5-25 mcg/day; adjust dose by 25 mcg/day every 2-4 weeks as appropriate; **Note:** Oral agents are not recommended for myxedema (see I.V. dosing).

Subclinical hypothyroidism (if treated): 1 mcg/kg/day

TSH suppression:

Well-differentiated thyroid cancer: Highly individualized; Doses >2 mcg/kg/day may be needed to suppress TSH to <0.1 mU/L.

Benign nodules and nontoxic multinodular goiter: Goal TSH suppression: 0.1-0.3 mU/L

Elderly: Hypothyroidism:

>50 years without cardiac disease **or** <50 years with cardiac disease: Initial: 25-50 mcg/day; adjust dose at 6- to 8-week intervals as needed

>50 years with cardiac disease: Initial: 12.5-25 mcg/day; adjust dose by 12.5-25 mcg increments at 4- to 6-week intervals

Note: Elderly patients may require <1 mcg/kg/day

I.M., I.V.: Children, Adults, Elderly: Hypothyroidism: 50% of the oral dose

I.V.:

Adults: Myxedema coma or stupor: 200-500 mcg, then 100-300 mcg the next day if necessary; smaller doses should be considered in patients with cardiovascular disease

Elderly: Myxedema coma: Refer to Adults dosing; lower doses may be needed

Stability Protect tablets from light; do not mix I.V. solution with other I.V. infusion solutions; reconstituted solutions should be used immediately and any unused portions discarded

Monitoring Parameters Thyroid function test (serum thyroxine, thyrotropin concentrations), resin triiodothyronine uptake (rT_3U), free thyroxine index (FTI), T_4, TSH, heart rate, blood pressure, clinical signs of hypo- and hyperthyroidism; TSH is the most reliable guide for evaluating adequacy of thyroid replacement dosage. TSH may be elevated during the first few months of thyroid replacement despite patients being clinically euthyroid. In cases where T_4 remains low and TSH is within normal limits, an evaluation of "free" (unbound) T_4 is needed to evaluate further increase in dosage

Infants: Monitor closely for cardiac overload, arrhythmias, and aspiration from avid suckling

Infants/children: Monitor closely for under/overtreatment. Undertreatment may decrease intellectual development and linear growth, and lead to poor school performance due to impaired concentration and slowed mentation. Overtreatment may adversely affect brain maturation, accelerate bone age (leading to premature closure of the epiphyses and reduced adult height); craniosynostosis has been reported in infants. Treated children may experience a period of catch-up growth. Monitor TSH and total or free T_4 at 2 and 4 weeks after starting treatment; every 1-2 months for first year of life; every 2-3 months during years 1-3; every 3-12 months until growth completed.

Adults: Monitor TSH every 6-8 weeks until normalized; 8-12 weeks after dosage changes; every 6-12 months throughout therapy

Administration Dilute vial with 5 mL normal saline; use immediately after reconstitution; give by direct I.V. infusion over 2- to 3-minute period

Contraindications Hypersensitivity to levothyroxine sodium or any component of the formulation; recent MI or thyrotoxicosis; uncorrected adrenal insufficiency

Warnings [U.S. Boxed Warning]: Ineffective and potentially toxic for weight reduction. High doses may produce serious or even life-threatening toxic effects particularly when used with some anorectic drugs. Use with caution and reduce dosage in patients with angina pectoris or other cardiovascular disease; use cautiously in elderly since they may be more likely to have compromised cardiovascular functions. Patients with adrenal insufficiency, myxedema, diabetes mellitus and insipidus may have symptoms exaggerated or aggravated; thyroid replacement requires periodic assessment of thyroid status. Chronic hypothyroidism predisposes patients to coronary artery disease. Levoxyl® may rapidly swell and disintegrate causing choking or gagging

(should be administered with a full glass of water); use caution in patients with dysphagia or other swallowing disorders.

Dosage Forms Injection, powder for reconstitution, as sodium: 0.2 mg, 0.5 mg

Tablet, as sodium: 25 mcg, 50 mcg, 75 mcg, 88 mcg, 100 mcg, 112 mcg, 125 mcg, 150 mcg, 175 mcg, 200 mcg, 300 mcg

Levothroid®: 25 mcg, 50 mcg, 75 mcg, 88 mcg, 100 mcg, 112 mcg, 125 mcg, 150 mcg, 175 mcg, 200 mcg, 300 mcg

Levoxyl®, Synthroid®: 25 mcg, 50 mcg, 75 mcg, 88 mcg, 100 mcg, 112 mcg, 125 mcg, 137 mcg, 150 mcg, 175 mcg, 200 mcg, 300 mcg

Unithroid®: 25 mcg, 50 mcg, 75 mcg, 88 mcg, 100 mcg, 112 mcg, 125 mcg, 150 mcg, 175 mcg, 200 mcg, 300 mcg

Reference Range

Correlation is poor with symptomatology in acute overdose

Pediatrics: Cord T_4 and values in the first few weeks are much higher, falling over the first months and years

≥10 years: ~5.8-11.0 mcg/dL (SI: 75-142 nmol/L)

Borderline low: 4.5-5.7 mcg/dL (SI: 58-73 nmol/L) or less

Low: ≤4.4 mcg/dL (SI: ≤57 nmol/L); results <2.5 mcg/dL (SI: <32 nmol/L) are strong evidence for hypothyroidism

Adults:

Approximate normal range: 4.0-12.0 mcg/dL (SI: 51-154 nmol/L)

Borderline high: 11.1-13.0 mcg/dL (SI: 143-167 nmol/L)

High: ≥13.1 mcg/dL (SI: ≥169 nmol/L)

Normal range is increased in women on birth control pills (5.5-12.0 mcg/dL)

Normal range in pregnancy: ~5.5-16.0 mcg/dL (SI: ~71-206 nmol/L)

TSH: 0.4-10.0 (for those ≥80 years) mIU/L

T_4: 4.0-12.0 mcg/dL (51-154 nmol/L)

T_3 (RIA) (total T_3): 80-230 ng/dL (1.2-3.5 nmol/L)

T_4, free: 0.7-1.8 ng/dL (9-23 pmol/L)

Overdosage/Treatment

Decontamination: Gastric emptying indicated for ingestions >5 mg; lavage within 1 hour with activated charcoal; cholestyramine is an effective agent to decrease T_4 absorption; 50 mg of cholestyramine can bind at least 3 mg of thyroxine, therefore, 4 g of cholestyramine given 4 times/day should be administered in order to interrupt enterohepatic recirculation

Supportive therapy: Propranolol may be used for hyperadrenergic signs (1 mg I.V. in adults, 0.01-0.1 mg/kg in pediatrics); sodium ipodate (3 g/1.7 m²) has been used in acute ingestion to prevent T_4 to T_3 conversion

Enhancement of elimination: Plasmapheresis increases elimination 30-fold while charcoal hemoperfusion enhances T_4 elimination fivefold; plasmapheresis (36 minutes using 1 L of 5% human serum albumin and 1 L of fresh frozen plasma) has been utilized following thyroxine overdose with poor results (nearly complete rebound of thyroid hormone levels) and thus is not recommended

Test Interactions Many drugs may have effects on thyroid function tests (see Additional Information). Pregnancy, infectious hepatitis, and acute intermittent porphyria may increase thyroxine-binding globulin; nephrosis, severe hypoproteinemia, severe liver disease, and acromegaly may decrease thyroxine-binding globulin.

Drug Interactions Also refer to Additional Information.

Aluminum- and magnesium-containing antacids, calcium carbonate, simethicone, or sucralfate: May decrease T_4 absorption; separate dose from levothyroxine by at least 4 hours.

Antidiabetic agents (biguanides, meglitinides, sulfonylureas, thiazolidinediones, insulin): Changes in thyroid function may alter requirements of antidiabetic agent. Monitor closely at initiation of therapy, or when dose is changed or discontinued.

Cholestyramine and colestipol: Decrease T_4 absorption; separate dose from levothyroxine by at least 2 hours.

Digoxin: Digoxin levels may be reduced in hyperthyroidism; therapeutic effect may be reduced. Impact of thyroid replacement should be monitored.

Estrogens: May decrease serum free thyroxine concentrations.

Imatinib: May decrease the effects of thyroid replacement therapy; monitor.

Iron: Decreases T_4 absorption; separate dose from levothyroxine by at least 4 hours.

Kayexalate®: Decreases T_4 absorption; separate dose from levothyroxine by at least 4 hours.

Ketamine: May cause marked hypertension and tachycardia; monitor.

Theophylline, caffeine: Decreased theophylline clearance in hypothyroid patients; monitor during thyroid replacement.

Tricyclic and tetracyclic antidepressants: Therapeutic and toxic effects of levothyroxine and the antidepressant are increased.

Warfarin (and other oral anticoagulants): The hypoprothrombinemic response to warfarin may be altered by a change in thyroid function or replacement. Replacement may dramatically increase response to warfarin. However, initiation of warfarin in a patient stabilized on a dose of levothyroxine does not appear to require a significantly different approach.

Pregnancy Risk Factor A

Pregnancy Implications Untreated maternal hypothyroidism may have adverse effects on fetal growth and development and is associated with higher rate of complications (spontaneous abortion, pre-eclampsia, stillbirth, premature delivery). Treatment should not be discontinued during pregnancy. TSH levels should be monitored during each trimester and 6-8 weeks postpartum. Increased doses may be needed during pregnancy.

Lactation Enters breast milk/compatible

Nursing Implications I.V. form must be prepared immediately prior to administration; should not be admixed with other solutions

Additional Information Levothroid® tablets contain lactose; levothyroxine is soluble in water; horseradish can depress thyroid function

Equivalent doses: Thyroid USP 60 mg ~ levothyroxine 0.05-0.06 mg ~ liothyronine 0.015-0.0375 mg

50-60 mg thyroid ~ 50-60 mcg levothyroxine and 12.5-15 mcg liothyronine Liotrix®

Note: Several medications have effects on thyroid production or conversion. The impact in thyroid replacement has not been specifically evaluated, but patient response should be monitored:

Methimazole: Decreases thyroid hormone secretion, while propylthiouracil decreases thyroid hormone secretion and decreases conversion of T_4 to T_3.

Beta-adrenergic antagonists: Decrease conversion of T_4 to T_3 (dose related, propranolol ≥ 160 mg/day); patients may be clinically euthyroid.

Iodide, iodine-containing radiographic contrast agents may decrease thyroid hormone secretion; may also increase thyroid hormone secretion, especially in patients with Graves' disease.

Other agents reported to impact on thyroid production/conversion include aminoglutethimide, amiodarone, chloral hydrate, diazepam, ethionamide, interferon-alpha, interleukin-2, lithium, lovastatin (case report), glucocorticoids (dose-related), mercaptopurine, sulfonamides, thiazide diuretics, and tolbutamide.

In addition, a number of medications have been noted to cause transient depression in TSH secretion, which may complicate interpretation of monitoring tests for levothyroxine, including corticosteroids, octreotide, and dopamine. Metoclopramide may increase TSH secretion.

Specific References
Siraj ES, Gupta MK, and Reddy SS, "Raloxifene Causing Malabsorption of Levothyroxine," *Arch Intern Med*, 2003, 163(11):1367-70.

Lidocaine

CAS Number 6108-05-0; 73-78-9

U.S. Brand Names Anestacon®; Band-Aid® Hurt-Free™ Antiseptic Wash [OTC]; Burn Jel [OTC]; Burn-O-Jel [OTC]; Burnamycin [OTC]; L-M-X™ 4 [OTC]; L-M-X™ 5 [OTC]; LidaMantle®; Lidoderm®; Premjact® [OTC]; Solarcaine® Aloe Extra Burn Relief [OTC]; Topicaine® [OTC]; Xylocaine® MPF; Xylocaine® Viscous; Xylocaine®; Zilactin-L® [OTC]

Synonyms Lidocaine Hydrochloride; Lignocaine Hydrochloride

Use

Local anesthetic and acute treatment of ventricular arrhythmias from myocardial infarction, cardiac manipulation, digitalis intoxication; drug of choice for ventricular ectopy, ventricular tachycardia (VT), ventricular fibrillation (VF); for pulseless VT or VF preferably administer **after** defibrillation and epinephrine; control of premature ventricular contractions, wide-complex paroxysmal supraventricular tachycardia (PSVT); control of hemodynamically compromising PVCs; hemodynamically stable VT

Rectal: Temporary relief of pain and itching due to anorectal disorders

Topical: Local anesthetic for use in laser, cosmetic, and outpatient surgeries; minor burns, cuts, and abrasions of the skin

Orphan drug: Lidoderm® Patch: Relief of allodynia (painful hypersensitivity) and chronic pain in postherpetic neuralgia

Unlabeled/Investigational Use ACLS guidelines (not considered drug of choice): Stable monomorphic VT (preserved ventricular function), polymorphic VT (preserved ventricular function), drug-induced monomorphic VT

Mechanism of Action Class IB antiarrhythmic; suppresses automaticity of conduction tissue, by increasing electrical stimulation threshold of ventricle, His-Purkinje system, and spontaneous depolarization of the ventricles during diastole by a direct action on the tissues; blocks both the initiation and conduction of nerve impulses by decreasing the neuronal membrane's permeability to sodium ions, which results in inhibition of depolarization with resultant blockade of conduction

Adverse Reactions

Cardiovascular: Bradycardia, hypotension, heart block with sinus arrest, cardiac arrhythmias (tachycardia [ventricular]), cardiovascular collapse, torsade de pointes, sinus bradycardia, sinus tachycardia, arrhythmias (ventricular), vasoconstriction

Central nervous system: Lethargy, coma, agitation, slurred speech, seizures, psychosis, anxiety, euphoria, hallucinations, circumoral numbness, fever, hyperthermia, acute aphasia

Gastrointestinal: Nausea, vomiting

Hematologic: Porphyria, porphyrinogenic, methemoglobinemia, thrombocytopenia

Neuromuscular & skeletal: Paresthesia, clonus, myoclonus

Ocular: Blurred vision, diplopia, miosis

Otic: Ototoxicity, tinnitus

Respiratory: Depression or arrest

Miscellaneous: Fixed drug eruption, acute atraumatic compartment syndrome

Signs and Symptoms of Overdose Agitation, asystole, AV block, bradycardia, cardiovascular collapse, coma, convulsions, delirium, diplopia, disorientation, euphoria, heart block, hypokalemia, hypotension, methemoglobinemia, myasthenia gravis (exacerbation or precipitation), mydriasis, myoclonus, numbness, nystagmus, ototoxicity, ptosis, respiratory failure, slurred speech, tachycardia (ventricular), tinnitus, tremors

Admission Criteria/Prognosis Any patient with change in mental status, cardiopulmonary complaints, or methemoglobin levels >30% should be admitted; asymptomatic patients with methemoglobin levels <30% may be considered for discharge after 6 hours of observation and if methemoglobin levels fall to <15%

Pharmacodynamics/Kinetics

Onset of action: Single bolus dose: 45-90 seconds

Duration: 10-20 minutes

Distribution: V_d: 1.1-2.1 L/kg; alterable by many patient factors; decreased in CHF and liver disease; crosses blood-brain barrier

Protein binding: 60% to 80% to alpha$_1$ acid glycoprotein

Metabolism: 90% hepatic; active metabolites monoethylglycinexylidide (MEGX) and glycinexylidide (GX) can accumulate and may cause CNS toxicity

Half-life elimination: Biphasic: Prolonged with congestive heart failure, liver disease, shock, severe renal disease; Initial: 7-30 minutes; Terminal: Infants, premature: 3.2 hours, Adults: 1.5-2 hours

Dosage

Topical: Apply to affected area as needed; maximum: 3 mg/kg/dose; do not repeat within 2 hours.

L-M-X™ 4 cream: Apply $^1/_4$ inch thick layer to intact skin. Leave on until adequate anesthetic effect is obtained. Remove cream and cleanse area before beginning procedure.

Rectal: Relief of pain and itching (L-M-X™ 5): Children ≥ 12 years and Adults: Apply topically to clean, dry area **or** using applicator insert rectally, up to 6 times/day

Injectable local anesthetic: Varies with procedure, degree of anesthesia needed, vascularity of tissue, duration of anesthesia required, and physical condition of patient; maximum: 4.5 mg/kg/dose; do not repeat within 2 hours.

Patch: Postherpetic neuralgia: Apply patch to most painful area. Up to 3 patches may be applied in a single application. Patch may remain in place for up to 12 hours in any 24-hour period.

Antiarrhythmic:

I.V.: 1-1.5 mg/kg bolus over 2-3 minutes; may repeat doses of 0.5-0.75 mg/kg in 5-10 minutes up to a total of 3 mg/kg; continuous infusion: 1-4 mg/minute

I.V. (2 g/250 mL D$_5$W) infusion rates (infusion pump should be used for I.V. infusion administration):
1 mg/minute: 7.5 mL/hour
2 mg/minute: 15 mL/hour
3 mg/minute: 22.5 mL/hour
4 mg/minute: 30 mL/hour

Ventricular fibrillation (after defibrillation and epinephrine): Initial: 1-1.5 mg/kg. Repeat 0.5-0.75 mg/kg bolus may be given 3-5 minutes after initial dose. Total dose should not exceed 200-300 mg during a 1-hour period or 3 mg/kg total dose. Follow with continuous infusion after return of perfusion.

Endotracheal: 2-2.5 times the I.V. dose (2-4 mg/kg diluted with NS to a total volume of 10 mL)

Decrease dose in patients with CHF, shock, or hepatic disease.

Dosage adjustment in renal impairment: Not dialyzable (0% to 5%) by hemo- or peritoneal dialysis; supplemental dose is not necessary.

Dosage adjustment in hepatic impairment: Reduce dose in acute hepatitis and decompensated cirrhosis by 50%.

Monitoring Parameters Monitor ECG continuously, serum lidocaine concentration, obtain methemoglobin level

Administration Intratracheal: Dilute in NS or distilled water. Absorption is greater with distilled water, but causes more adverse effects on PaO$_2$. Pass catheter beyond tip of tracheal tube, stop compressions, spray drug quickly down tube. Follow immediately with several quick insufflations and continue chest compressions.

I.V.: Use microdrip (60 gtt/mL) or infusion pump to administer an accurate dose

Infusion rates: 2 g/250 mL D$_5$W (infusion pump should be used):
1 mg/minute: 7.5 mL/hour
2 mg/minute: 15 mL/hour
3 mg/minute: 22.5 mL/hour
4 mg/minute: 30 mL/hour

Buffered lidocaine for injectable local anesthetic: Add 2 mL of sodium bicarbonate 8.4% to 18 mL of lidocaine 1%

Topical:

Gel (Topicaine®): Avoid mucous membranes; remove prior to laser treatment.

Transdermal: Apply to painful area of skin immediately after removal from protective envelope. May be cut to appropriate size. After removal from skin, fold used transdermal systems so the adhesive side sticks to itself. Remove immediately if burning sensation occurs. Wash hands after application.

Contraindications Hypersensitivity to lidocaine or any component of the formulation; hypersensitivity to another local anesthetic of the amide type; Adam-Stokes syndrome; severe degrees of SA, AV, or intraventricular heart block (except in patients with a functioning artificial pacemaker); premixed injection may contain corn-derived dextrose and its use is contraindicated in patients with allergy to corn-related products

Warnings

Intravenous: Constant ECG monitoring is necessary during I.V. administration. Use cautiously in hepatic impairment, any degree of heart block, Wolff-Parkinson-White syndrome, CHF, marked hypoxia, severe respiratory depression, hypovolemia, history of malignant hyperthermia, or shock. Increased ventricular rate may be seen when administered to a patient with atrial fibrillation. Correct any underlying causes of ventricular arrhythmias. Monitor closely for signs and symptoms of CNS toxicity. The elderly may be prone to increased CNS and cardiovascular side effects. Reduce dose in hepatic dysfunction and CHF.

Injectable anesthetic: Follow appropriate administration techniques so as not to administer any intravascularly. Solutions containing antimicrobial preservatives should not be used for epidural or spinal anesthesia. Some solutions contain a bisulfite; avoid in patients who are allergic to bisulfite. Resuscitative equipment, medicine and oxygen should be available in case of emergency. Use products containing epinephrine cautiously in patients with significant vascular disease, compromised blood flow, or during or following general anesthesia (increased risk of arrhythmias). Adjust the dose for the elderly, pediatric, acutely ill, and debilitated patients.

Topical: L-M-X™ 4 cream: Do not leave on large body areas for >2 hours. Observe young children closely to prevent accidental ingestion. Not for use ophthalmic use or for use on mucous membranes.

Transdermal patch: May contain conducting metal (eg, aluminum); remove patch prior to MRI.

Dosage Forms [DSC] = Discontinued product

Cream, rectal (L-M-X™ 5): 5% (15 g) [contains benzyl alcohol; packaged with applicator]; (30 g) [contains benzyl alcohol]

Cream, topical (L-M-X™ 4): 4% (5 g) [contains benzyl alcohol; packaged with Tegaderm™ dressing]; (15 g, 30 g) [contains benzyl alcohol]

Cream, topical, as hydrochloride: 3% (30 g)

LidaMantle®: 3% (30 g, 85 g)

Gel, topical:

Burn-O-Jel: 0.5% (90 g)

Topicaine®: 4% (10 g, 30 g, 113 g) [contains alcohol 35%, benzyl alcohol, aloe vera, and jojoba]

Gel, topical, as hydrochloride:

Burn Jel: 2% (3.5 g, 120 g)

Solarcaine® Aloe Extra Burn Relief: 0.5% (113 g, 226 g) [contains aloe vera gel and tartrazine]

Infusion, as hydrochloride [premixed in D_5W]: 0.4% [4 mg/mL] (250 mL, 500 mL); 0.8% [8 mg/mL] (250 mL, 500 mL)

Injection, solution, as hydrochloride: 0.5% [5 mg/mL] (50 mL); 1% [10 mg/mL] (2 mL, 10 mL, 20 mL, 30 mL, 50 mL); 2% [20 mg/mL] (2 mL, 5 mL, 20 mL, 50 mL)

Xylocaine®: 0.5% [5 mg/mL] (50 mL); 1% [10 mg/mL] (10 mL, 20 mL, 50 mL); 2% [20 mg/mL] (1.8 mL, 10 mL, 20 mL, 50 mL)

Injection, solution, as hydrochloride [preservative free]: 0.5% [5 mg/mL] (50 mL); 1% [10 mg/mL] (2 mL, 5 mL, 30 mL); 1.5% [15 mg/mL] (20 mL); 2% [20 mg/mL] (2 mL, 5 mL, 10 mL); 4% [40 mg/mL] (5 mL)

Xylocaine®: 10% [100 mg/mL] (5 mL) [for ventricular arrhythmias]

Xylocaine® MPF: 0.5% [5 mg/mL] (50 mL); 1% [10 mg/mL] (2 mL, 5 mL, 10 mL, 30 mL); 1.5% [15 mg/mL] (10 mL, 20 mL); 2% [20 mg/mL] (2 mL, 5 mL, 10 mL); 4% [40 mg/mL] (5 mL)

Injection, solution, as hydrochloride [premixed in $D_{7.5}W$, preservative free]: 5% (2 mL)

Xylocaine® MPF: 1.5% (2 mL) [DSC]

Jelly, topical, as hydrochloride: 2% (5 mL, 30 mL)

Anestacon®: 2% (15 mL) [contains benzalkonium chloride]

Xylocaine®: 2% (5 mL, 30 mL)

Liquid, topical (Zilactin®-L): 2.5% (7.5 mL)

Lotion, topical, as hydrochloride (LidaMantle®): 3% (177 mL)

Ointment, topical: 5% (37 g, 50 g)

Solution, topical, as hydrochloride: 4% [40 mg/mL] (50 mL)

Band-Aid® Hurt-Free™ Antiseptic Wash: 2% (180 mL)

LTA® 360: 4% [40 mg/mL] (4 mL) [packaged with cannula for laryngotracheal administration]

Xylocaine®: 4% [40 mg/mL] (50 mL)

Solution, viscous, as hydrochloride: 2% [20 mg/mL] (20 mL, 100 mL)

Xylocaine® Viscous: 2% [20 mg/mL] (100 mL, 450 mL)

Spray, topical:

Burnamycin: 0.5% (60 mL) [contains aloe vera gel and menthol]

Premjact®: 9.6% (13 mL)

Solarcaine® Aloe Extra Burn Relief: 0.5% (127 g) [contains aloe vera]

Transdermal system, topical (Lidoderm®): 5% (30s)

Reference Range

Therapeutic: 1.5-4.0 mcg/mL (SI: 6.4-17.1 μmol/L), up to 6.0 mcg/mL (SI: 25.6 μmol/L) if necessary

Therapeutic level for tinnitus: 1.5-2.5 mcg/mL

Toxic: >6.0 mcg/mL (SI: >25.6 μmol/L)

Fatal: >15.0 mcg/mL

Overdosage/Treatment

Decontamination: Oral: **Do not** use ipecac due to possible development of seizures; lavage (within 1 hour)/activated charcoal

Supportive therapy: Termination of anesthesia by pneumatic tourniquet inflation should be attempted when the agent is administered by infiltration or regional injection. Seizures commonly respond to diazepam or lorazepam, while hypotension responds to I.V. fluids and Trendelenburg positioning. Refractory hypotension can be treated with norepinephrine, dopamine, dobutamine, or intra-aortic balloons. Bradyarrhythmias (when the heart rate is less than 60) can be treated with I.V. atropine 15 mcg/kg, isoproterenol, or a pacemaker. With the development of metabolic acidosis, I.V. sodium bicarbonate 0.5-2 mEq/kg and ventilatory assistance should be instituted. Methemoglobinemia should be treated with methylene blue 1-2 mg/kg in a 1% sterile aqueous solution I.V. push over 4-6 minutes repeated up to a total dose of 7 mg/kg. Cardiopulmonary bypass and cardiac pacing has been utilized. Phenobarbital can be also utilized for seizure treatment. Avoid use of phenytoin in that sinoatrial arrest may occur. Peripheral cardiopulmonary bypass support can be used to support hemodynamic compromise. Epidural phenylephrine 200 mcg reduces the incidence of hypotension induced by epidural lidocaine.

Enhancement of elimination: Arteriovenous hemofiltration is also not useful; not dialyzable (0% to 5%)

Diagnostic Procedures

• Lidocaine, Blood

Test Interactions Falsely lowered if blood makes contact with stopper of tube

Drug Interactions

Substrate of CYP1A2 (minor), 2A6 (minor), 2B6 (minor), 2C9 (minor), 2D6 (major), 3A4 (major); **Inhibits** CYP1A2 (strong), 2D6 (moderate), 3A4 (moderate)

Cimetidine increases lidocaine blood levels; monitor levels or use an alternative H_2 antagonist.

CYP1A2 substrates: Lidocaine may increase the levels/effects of CYP1A2 substrates. Example substrates include aminophylline, fluvoxamine, mexiletine, mirtazapine, ropinirole, theophylline, and trifluoperazine.

CYP2D6 inhibitors: May increase the levels/effects of lidocaine. Example inhibitors include chlorpromazine, delavirdine, fluoxetine, miconazole, paroxetine, pergolide, quinidine, quinine, ritonavir, and ropinirole.

CYP2D6 substrates: Lidocaine may increase the levels/effects of CYP2D6 substrates. Example substrates include amphetamines, selected beta-blockers, dextromethorphan, fluoxetine, mirtazapine, nefazodone, paroxetine, risperidone, ritonavir, thioridazine, tricyclic antidepressants, and venlafaxine.

CYP2D6 prodrug substrates: Lidocaine may decrease the levels/effects of CYP2D6 prodrug substrates. Example prodrug substrates include codeine, hydrocodone, oxycodone, and tramadol.

CYP3A4 inducers: CYP3A4 inducers may decrease the levels/effects of lidocaine. Example inducers include aminoglutethimide, carbamazepine, nafcillin, nevirapine, phenobarbital, phenytoin, and rifamycins.

CYP3A4 inhibitors: May increase the levels/effects of lidocaine. Example inhibitors include amiodarone (doses >400 mg/day), azole antifungals, clarithromycin, diclofenac, doxycycline, erythromycin, imatinib, isoniazid, nefazodone, nicardipine, propofol, protease inhibitors, quinidine, telithromycin, and verapamil.

CYP3A4 substrates: Lidocaine may increase the levels/effects of CYP3A4 substrates. Example substrates include benzodiazepines, calcium channel blockers, cyclosporine, mirtazapine, nateglinide, nefazodone, sildenafil (and other PDE-5 inhibitors), tacrolimus, and venlafaxine. Selected benzodiazepines (midazolam and triazolam), cisapride, ergot alkaloids, selected HMG-CoA reductase inhibitors (lovastatin and simvastatin), and pimozide are generally contraindicated with strong CYP3A4 inhibitors.

Propranolol: Increases lidocaine blood levels.

Protease inhibitors (eg, amprenavir, ritonavir): May increase lidocaine blood levels.

Pregnancy Risk Factor B (manufacturer); C (expert analysis)

Pregnancy Implications Animal studies with lidocaine have not shown teratogenic effects.

Lactation Enters breast milk (small amounts)/use caution (AAP rates "compatible")

Nursing Implications Local thrombophlebitis may occur in patients receiving prolonged I.V. infusions

Additional Information Odorless, bitter taste; intranasal use of 4% solution is 55% effective for migraine; child-resistant packaging ordered by the U.S. Consumer Product Safety Commission for products containing more than 5 mg of lidocaine

Specific References

Balit CR, Gilmore SP, and Isbister GK, "Paediatric Lidocaine (Lignocaine) Toxicity," *J Toxicol Clin Toxicol*, 2003, 41(5):686.

Chiu CY, Lin TY, Hsia SH, et al, "Systemic Anaphylaxis Following Local Lidocaine Administration During a Dental Procedure," *Pediatr Emerg Care*, 2004, 20(3):178-80.

Cullen L, Taylor D, Taylor S, et al, "Nebulized Lidocaine Decreases the Discomfort of Nasogastric Tube Insertion: A Randomized, Double-Blind Trial," *Ann Emerg Med*, 2004, 44(2):131-7.

Donald MJ and Derbyshire S, "Lignocaine Toxicity: A Complication of Local Anaesthesia Administered in the Community," *Emerg Med J*, 2004, 21(2):249-50.

Gimbel J, Linn R, Hale M, et al, "Lidocaine Patch Treatment in Patients with Low Back Pain: Results of an Open-Label, Nonrandomized Pilot Study," *Am J Ther*, 2005, 12(4):311-9.

Hahn IH, Hoffman RS, and Nelson LS, "EMLA-Induced Methemoglobinemia and Systemic Topical Anesthetic Toxicity," *J Emerg Med*, 2004, 26(1):85-8.

Kearns GL, Heacook J, Daly SJ, et al, "Percutaneous Lidocaine Administration via a New Iontophoresis System in Children: Tolerability and Absence of Systemic Bioavailability," *Pediatrics*, 2003, 112(3 Pt 1):578-82.

Perney P, Blanc F, Mourad G, et al, "Transitory Ataxia Related to Topically Administered Lidocaine," *Ann Pharmacother*, 2004, 38(5):828-30.

Lindane

CAS Number 58-89-9
UN Number 2761
Synonyms Benzene Hexachloride; Gamma Benzene Hexachloride; Hexachlorocyclohexane
Use Treatment of *Sarcoptes scabiei* (scabies), *Pediculus capitis* (head lice), and *Pthirus pubis* (crab lice); FDA recommends reserving lindane as a second-line agent or with inadequate response to other therapies
Mechanism of Action Directly absorbed by parasites and ova through the exoskeleton; stimulates the nervous system resulting in seizures and death of parasitic arthropods; interferes with the gamma-aminobutyric acid A receptor chloride channel complex in the synapse

Adverse Reactions
Frequency not defined (includes postmarketing and/or case reports).
Cardiovascular: Cardiac arrhythmia
Central nervous system: Ataxia, dizziness, headache, restlessness, seizures, pain
Dermatologic: Alopecia, contact dermatitis, skin and adipose tissue may act as repositories, eczematous eruptions, pruritus, urticaria
Gastrointestinal: Nausea, vomiting
Hematologic: Aplastic anemia
Hepatic: Hepatitis
Local: Burning and stinging
Neuromuscular & skeletal: Paresthesias
Renal: Hematuria
Respiratory: Pulmonary edema

Signs and Symptoms of Overdose Agitation, arrhythmia, ataxia, blindness, disseminated intravascular coagulation, hematuria, hepatitis, lactic acidosis, muscle necrosis, myoglobinuria, nausea, neutropenia, pulmonary edema, respiratory depression, restlessness, rhabdomyolysis, seizures, thrombocytopenia, vomiting

Pharmacodynamics/Kinetics
Absorption: ≤13% systemically
Distribution: Stored in body fat; accumulates in brain; skin and adipose tissue may act as repositories
Metabolism: Hepatic
Half-life elimination: Children: 17-22 hours
Time to peak, serum: Children: 6 hours
Excretion: Urine and feces

Dosage Children and Adults: Topical:
Scabies: Apply a thin layer of lotion and massage it on skin from the neck to the toes; after 8-12 hours, bathe and remove the drug
Head lice, crab lice: Apply shampoo to dry hair and massage into hair for 4 minutes; add small quantities of water to hair until lather forms, then rinse hair thoroughly and comb with a fine tooth comb to remove nits. Amount of shampoo needed is based on length and density of hair; most patients will require 30 mL (maximum: 60 mL).

Administration
For topical use only; never administer orally. Caregivers should apply with gloves (avoid natural latex, may be permeable to lindane). Rinse off with warm (not hot) water.
Lotion: Apply to dry, cool skin; do not apply to face or eyes. Wait at least 1 hour after bathing or showering (wet or warm skin increases absorption). Skin should be clean and free of any other lotions, creams, or oil prior to lindane application.
Shampoo: Apply to clean, dry hair. Wait at least 1 hour after washing hair before applying lindane shampoo. Hair should be washed with a shampoo not containing a conditioner; hair and skin of head and neck should be free of any lotions, oils, or creams prior to lindane application.

Contraindications Hypersensitivity to lindane or any component of the formulation; uncontrolled seizure disorders; crusted (Norwegian) scabies, acutely-inflamed skin or raw, weeping surfaces or other skin conditions which may increase systemic absorption

Warnings
[U.S. Boxed Warning]: Not considered a drug of first choice; use only in patients who have failed first-line treatments, or in patients who cannot tolerate these agents. Because of the potential for systemic absorption and CNS side effects, lindane should be used with caution; consider permethrin or crotamiton agent first. Oil-based hair dressing may increase toxic potential.

[U.S. Boxed Warning]: May be associated with severe neurologic toxicities (contraindicated in premature infants and uncontrolled seizure disorders). Seizures and death have been reported with use; use with caution in infants, small children, patients <50 kg, or patients with a history of seizures; use caution with conditions which may increase risk of seizures or medications which decrease seizure threshold; use caution with hepatic impairment; avoid contact with face, eyes, mucous membranes, and urethral meatus.

[U.S. Boxed Warning]: A lindane medication use guide must be given to all patients along with instructions for proper use. Patients should be informed that itching may occur following successful killing of lice and re-treatment may not be indicated. Should be used as a part of an overall lice management program

Dosage Forms Lotion, topical: 1% (60 mL)
Shampoo, topical: 1% (60 mL) [contains alcohol 0.5%]

Reference Range
In lindane-exposed workers, chronic symptoms can occur at blood levels >0.02 mcg/mL.
After acute ingestion: Blood levels >0.12 mcg/mL are correlated with sedation, seizures can occur at blood levels >0.2 mcg/mL (0.13 mcg/mL in patients with pre-existing seizure disorder), myonecrosis can occur at blood levels >0.6 mcg/mL and death can occur at blood levels exceeding 1.3 mcg/mL
Fatal oral dose: Adults: 28 g

Overdosage/Treatment
Decontamination:
Oral: Emesis should not be induced since seizures can occur within 15 minutes of ingestion; activated charcoal is effective; do not give with milk, oil, or fatty food since it may enhance absorption
Dermal: Use soap and water to decontaminate the skin; cholestyramine may be effective in hastening elimination; absorbed through skin and mucous membranes and gastrointestinal tract; has occasionally caused serious CNS, hepatic and renal toxicity when used excessively for prolonged periods, or when accidental ingestion has occurred
Supportive therapy: Diazepam and/or phenobarbital can be used to treat seizures
Enhancement of elimination: Hemoperfusion may be effective if performed early. Although it has not been formally studied, cholestyramine (4 g every 8 hours) may enhance the elimination of lindane.

Antidote(s)
• Cholestyramine Resin [ANTIDOTE]

Drug Interactions Increased toxicity: Drugs which lower seizure threshold

Pregnancy Risk Factor B
Pregnancy Implications There are no well-controlled studies in pregnant women
Lactation Enters breast milk/contraindicated
Nursing Implications Drug should not be administered orally
Additional Information Mean fatal oral dose: Adults: 28 g.
Consider alternative therapies (ie, crotamiton) for treatment of scabies in infants and children <10 years; drug has a bitter taste. TLV-TWA: 0.5 mg/m³; IDLH: 1000 ppm; OSHA PEL-TWA: 0.5 mg/m²

Specific References
Centers for Disease Control and Prevention (CDC), "Unintentional Topical Lindane Ingestions—United States, 1998-2003," *MMWR Morb Mortal Wkly Rep*, 2005, 3;54(21):533-5.

Forrester MB, Sievert JS, Stanley SK, et al, "Epidemiology of Lindane Exposures for Pediculosis Reported to Poison Centers in Texas, 1998-2002," *J Toxicol Clin Toxicol*, 2004, 42(1):55-60.

Singal A and Thami GP, "Lindane Neurotoxicity in Childhood," *Am J Ther*, 2006, 13(3):277-80.

Linezolid

CAS Number 165800-03-3

U.S. Brand Names Zyvox™

Use Treatment of vancomycin-resistant *Enterococcus faecium* (VRE) infections, nosocomial pneumonia caused by *Staphylococcus aureus* including MRSA or *Streptococcus pneumoniae* (penicillin-susceptible strains only), complicated and uncomplicated skin and skin structure infections (including diabetic foot infections without concomitant osteomyelitis), and community-acquired pneumonia caused by susceptible gram-positive organisms.

Mechanism of Action Inhibits bacterial protein synthesis by binding to bacterial 23S ribosomal RNA of the 50S subunit. This prevents the formation of a functional 70S initiation complex that is essential for the bacterial translation process. Linezolid is bacteriostatic against enterococci and staphylococci and bactericidal against most strains of streptococci.

Adverse Reactions

Cardiovascular: Hypertension

Central nervous system: **Headache** (27%), insomnia, dizziness, fever

Dermatologic: Rash, pruritus

Endocrine & metabolic: Lactic acidosis, serotonin symdrome

Gastrointestinal: **Nausea, diarrhea**, vomiting, constipation, taste alteration, **brownish tongue discoloration** (33%), oral moniliasis, pancreatitis, localized abdominal pain, dyspepsia

Genitourinary: **Vaginal yeast infection** (36% in a 5 day treatment course)

Hematologic: **Thrombocytopenia**, anemia, leukopenia, neutropenia; **Note:** Myelosuppression (including anemia, leukopenia, pancytopenia, and thrombocytopenia; may be more common in patients receiving linezolid for >2 weeks)

Hepatic: Abnormal LFTs

Neuromuscular & skeletal: Peripheral neuropathy

Ocular: Optic neuropathy

Renal: Increase in creatinine

Miscellaneous: *C. difficile*-related complications

Pharmacodynamics/Kinetics

Absorption: Rapid and extensive

Distribution: V_{dss}: Adults: 40-50 L

Protein binding: Adults: 31%

Metabolism: Hepatic via oxidation of the morpholine ring, resulting in two inactive metabolites (aminoethoxyacetic acid, hydroxyethyl glycine); does not involve CYP

Bioavailability: 100%

Half-life elimination: Children ≥1 week (full-term) to 11 years: 1.5-3 hours; Adults: 4-5 hours

Time to peak: Adults: Oral: 1-2 hours

Excretion: Urine (30% as parent drug, 50% as metabolites); feces (9% as metabolites)

Nonrenal clearance: 65%; increased in children ≥1 week to 11 years

Dosage VRE infections: Oral, I.V.:

Infants (excluding preterm neonates <1 week) and Children ≤11 years: 10 mg/kg every 8 hours for 14-28 days

Children ≥12 years and Adults: 600 mg every 12 hours for 14-28 days

Nosocomial pneumonia, complicated skin and skin structure infections, community acquired pneumonia including concurrent bacteremia: Oral, I.V.:

Infants (excluding preterm neonates <1 week) and Children ≤11 years: 10 mg/kg every 8 hours for 10-14 days

Children ≥12 years and Adults: 600 mg every 12 hours for 10-14 days

Uncomplicated skin and skin structure infections: Oral:

Infants (excluding preterm neonates <1 week) and Children <5 years: 10 mg/kg every 8 hours for 10-14 days

Children 5-11 years: 10 mg/kg every 12 hours for 10-14 days

Children ≥12-18 years: 600 mg every 12 hours for 10-14 days

Adults: 400 mg every 12 hours for 10-14 days

Elderly: No dosage adjustment required

Dosage adjustment in hepatic impairment: No dosage adjustment required for mild to moderate hepatic insufficiency (Child-Pugh Class A or B). Use in severe hepatic insufficiency has not been adequately evaluated.

Monitoring Parameters Weekly CBC and platelet counts, particularly in patients at increased risk of bleeding, with pre-existing myelosuppression, on concomitant medications that cause bone marrow suppression, in those who require >2 weeks of therapy, or in those with chronic infection who have received previous or concomitant antibiotic therapy.

Administration I.V.: Administer intravenous infusion over 30-120 minutes. Do not mix or infuse with other medications. When the same intravenous line is used for sequential infusion of other medications, flush line with D_5W, NS, or LR before and after infusing linezolid. The

yellow color of the injection may intensify over time without affecting potency.

Oral suspension: Invert gently to mix prior to administration, do not shake.

Contraindications Hypersensitivity to linezolid or any other component of the formulation

Warnings

Myelosuppression has been reported and may be dependent on duration of therapy (generally >2 weeks of treatment); use with caution in patients with pre-existing myelosuppression, in patients receiving other drugs which may cause bone marrow suppression, or in chronic infection (previous or concurrent antibiotic therapy). Weekly CBC monitoring is recommended. Discontinue linezolid in patients developing myelosuppression (or in whom myelosuppression worsens during treatment).

Lactic acidosis has been reported with use. Patients who develop recurrent nausea and vomiting, unexplained acidosis, or low bicarbonate levels need immediate evaluation.

Linezolid exhibits mild MAO inhibitor properties and has the potential to have the same interactions as other MAO inhibitors; use with caution in uncontrolled hypertension, pheochromocytoma, carcinoid syndrome, or untreated hyperthyroidism; avoid use with serotonergic agents such as TCAs, venlafaxine, trazodone, sibutramine, meperidine, dextromethorphan, and SSRIs; concomitant use has been associated with the development of serotonin syndrome. Unnecessary use may lead to the development of resistance to linezolid; consider alternatives before initiating outpatient treatment.

Peripheral and optic neuropathy (with vision loss) has been reported and may occur primarily with extended courses of therapy >28 days; any symptoms of visual change or impairment warrant immediate ophthalmic evaluation and possible discontinuation of therapy.

Due to inconsistent therapeutic concentrations in the CSF, empiric use in pediatric patients with CNS infections is not recommended.

Dosage Forms Infusion [premixed]: 200 mg (100 mL) [contains sodium 1.7 mEq]; 400 mg (200 mL) [contains sodium 3.3 mEq]; 600 mg (300 mL) [contains sodium 5 mEq]

Powder for oral suspension: 20 mg/mL (150 mL) [contains phenylalanine 20 mg/5 mL, sodium benzoate, and sodium 0.4 mEq/5 mL; orange flavor]

Tablet: 600 mg [contains sodium 0.1 mEq/tablet]

Reference Range Treatment serum range: 0.5-4 mcg/mL

Overdosage/Treatment

Decontamination: Oral: Activated charcoal

Supportive therapy: Metronidazole (250 mg 4 times/day for 10 days) can be used to treat pseudomembranous colitis

Enhanced elimination: Eliminated by dialysis (38% dialysis extraction ratio). Dialysis (along with sodium bicarbonate 1-2 meq/kg I.V.) should be used for severe lactic acidosis

Drug Interactions Adrenergic agents (eg, phenylpropanolamine, pseudoephedrine, sympathomimetic agents, vasopressor or dopaminergic agents) may cause hypertension.

Myelosuppressive medications: Concurrent use may increase risk of myelosuppression with linezolid.

Serotonergic agents (eg, TCAs, venlafaxine, trazodone, sibutramine, meperidine, dextromethorphan, and SSRIs) may cause a serotonin syndrome (eg, hyperpyrexia, cognitive dysfunction) when used concomitantly.

Tramadol: Concurrent use may increase risk of seizures.

Pregnancy Risk Factor C

Pregnancy Implications Teratogenic effects were not observed in animal studies. There are no adequate and well-controlled studies in pregnant women. Should be used in pregnancy only if the potential benefit justifies the risk to the fetus.

Lactation Excretion in breast milk unknown/use caution

Additional Information Avoid alcohol and foods (eg, cheese) containing tyramine (hypertensive crisis may result)

Specific References

Apodaca AA and Rakita RM, "Linezolid-Induced Lactic Acidosis," *N Engl J Med*, 2003, 348(1):86-7.

McKinnon PS, Sorensen SV, Liu LZ, et al, "Impact of Linezolid on Economic Outcomes and Determinants of Cost in a Clinical Trial Evaluating Patients with MRSA Complicated Skin and Soft-Tissue Infections," *Ann Pharmacother*, 2006, 40(6):1017-23.

Mogenet I, Raetz-Dillon S, Canonge JM, et al, "Successful Treatment of *Staphylococcus epidermidis* Hip Prosthesis Infection with Oral Linezolid," *Ann Pharmacother*, 2004, 38(6):986-8.

Ntziora F, Falagas ME, "Linezolid for the Treatment of Patients with Central Nervous System Infection," *Ann Pharmacotheraphy*, 2007, 41(2): 296-308.

Riley BD and Ruha AM, "Serotonin Syndrome in a Patient Treated with Linezolid," *Clin Toxicol*, 2005, 43:632.

Stein GE, Schooley S, Kak V, et al, "Oral Linezolid as Alternative Therapy in Patients with Cellulitis Who Have Been Referred to an Infusion Center," *P&T*, 2004, 29(8):510-2.

Sullivan J, Tobias J.D, "Preliminary Experience with the Use of Oral Linezolid in Infants for the Completion of Antibiotic Therapy in the Outpatient Setting After Admission to the Pediatric Intensive Care Unit," *Am J Therapeutics*, 2006, 13: 473-7.

Liothyronine

Related Information
- Levothyroxine

CAS Number 55-06-1; 6893-03-3

U.S. Brand Names Cytomel®; Triostat®

Synonyms Liothyronine Sodium; Sodium *L*-Triiodothyronine; T_3 Sodium (error-prone abbreviation)

Use

Oral: Replacement or supplemental therapy in hypothyroidism; management of nontoxic goiter; a diagnostic aid

I.V.: Treatment of myxedema coma/precoma

Mechanism of Action Primary active compound is T_3 (triiodothyronine), which may be converted from T_4 (thyroxine) and then circulates throughout the body to influence growth and maturation of various tissues; exact mechanism of action is unknown; however, it is believed the thyroid hormone exerts its many metabolic effects through control of DNA transcription and protein synthesis; involved in normal metabolism, growth, and development; promotes gluconeogenesis, increases utilization and mobilization of glycogen stores, and stimulates protein synthesis, increases basal metabolic rate

Adverse Reactions

Cardiovascular: Angina, arrhythmia, cardiopulmonary arrest, congestive heart failure, hypertension, hypotension, myocardial infarction, phlebitis, tachycardia

Central nervous system: Fever

Dermatologic: Allergic skin reactions

Neuromuscular & skeletal: Twitching

Signs and Symptoms of Overdose Hyperthyroidism, insomnia sweating, tachycardia

Admission Criteria/Prognosis Admit any symptomatic patient or serum total T_4 >75 mcg/dL

Pharmacodynamics/Kinetics

Onset of action: 2-4 hours

Peak response: 2-3 days

Absorption: Oral: Well absorbed (95% in 4 hours)

Half-life elimination: 2.5 days

Excretion: Urine

Dosage

Doses should be adjusted based on clinical response and laboratory parameters.

Children: Congenital hypothyroidism: Oral: 5 mcg/day increase by 5 mcg every 3-4 days until the desired response is achieved. Usual maintenance dose: 20 mcg/day for infants, 50 mcg/day for children 1-3 years of age, and adult dose for children >3 years.

Adults:

Hypothyroidism: Oral: 25 mcg/day increase by increments of 12.5-25 mcg/day every 1-2 weeks to a maximum of 100 mcg/day; usual maintenance dose: 25-75 mcg/day.

Patients with cardiovascular disease: Refer to Elderly dosing.

T_3 suppression test: Oral: 75-100 mcg/day for 7 days; use lowest dose for elderly

Myxedema: Oral: Initial: 5 mcg/day; increase in increments of 5-10 mcg/day every 1-2 weeks. When 25 mcg/day is reached, dosage may be increased at intervals of 5-25 mcg/day every 1-2 weeks. Usual maintenance dose: 50-100 mcg/day.

Myxedema coma: I.V.: 25-50 mcg

Patients with known or suspected cardiovascular disease: 10-20 mcg

Note: Normally, at least 4 hours should be allowed between doses to adequately assess therapeutic response and no more than 12 hours should elapse between doses to avoid fluctuations in hormone levels. Oral therapy should be resumed as soon as the clinical situation has been stabilized and the patient is able to take oral medication. If levothyroxine rather than liothyronine sodium is used in initiating oral therapy, the physician should bear in mind that there is a delay of several days in the onset of levothyroxine activity and that I.V. therapy should be discontinued gradually.

Simple (nontoxic) goiter: Oral: Initial: 5 mcg/day; increase by 5-10 mcg every 1-2 weeks; after 25 mcg/day is reached, may increase dose by 12.5-25 mcg. Usual maintenance dose: 75 mcg/day

Elderly: Oral: 5 mcg/day; increase by 5 mcg/day every 2 weeks

Stability Store between 2°C and 8°C (36°F to 46°F)

Monitoring Parameters T_3, TSH, heart rate, blood pressure, renal function, clinical signs of hypo- and hyperthyroidism; TSH is the most reliable guide for evaluating adequacy of thyroid replacement dosage. TSH may be elevated during the first few months of thyroid replacement despite patients being clinically euthyroid. In cases where T_4 remains low

and TSH is within normal limits, an evaluation of "free" (unbound) T_4 is needed to evaluate further increase in dosage.

Administration I.V. form must be prepared immediately prior to administration; dilute 200 mcg/mL vial with 2 mL of 0.9% sodium chloride injection and shake well until a clear solution is obtained; should not be admixed with other solutions

Contraindications Hypersensitivity to liothyronine sodium or any component of the formulation; undocumented or uncorrected adrenal insufficiency; recent myocardial infarction or thyrotoxicosis; artificial rewarming (injection)

Warnings [U.S. Boxed Warning]: Ineffective for weight reduction. High doses may produce serious or even life-threatening toxic effects particularly when used with some anorectic drugs. Use with extreme caution in patients with angina pectoris or other cardiovascular disease (including hypertension) or coronary artery disease; use with caution in elderly patients since they may be more likely to have compromised cardiovascular function. Patients with adrenal insufficiency, myxedema, diabetes mellitus and insipidus may have symptoms exaggerated or aggravated; thyroid replacement requires periodic assessment of thyroid status. Chronic hypothyroidism predisposes patients to coronary artery disease.

Dosage Forms Injection, solution, as sodium (Triostat®): 10 mcg/mL (1 mL) [contains alcohol 6.8%]

Tablet, as sodium (Cytomel®): 5 mcg, 25 mcg, 50 mcg

Reference Range Free T_3, serum: 250-390 pg/dL; TSH: 0.4 up to 10.0 (for those ≥80 years of age) mIU/L; remains normal in pregnancy

Overdosage/Treatment

Decontamination: Gastric emptying indicated for ingestions >2 mg; ipecac within 30 minutes or lavage within 1 hour with activated charcoal; 50 mg of cholestyramine can bind at least 3 mg of thyroxine, therefore, 4 g of cholestyramine given 4 times/day should be administered in order to interrupt enterohepatic recirculation

Supportive therapy: Propranolol may be used for hyperadrenergic signs (1 mg I.V. in adults, 0.01-0.1 mg/kg in pediatrics)

Enhancement of elimination: Plasmapheresis increases elimination 30-fold while charcoal hemoperfusion enhances T_4 elimination fivefold.

Test Interactions Many drugs may have effects on thyroid function tests; para-aminosalicylic acid, aminoglutethimide, amiodarone, barbiturates, carbamazepine, chloral hydrate, clofibrate, colestipol, corticosteroids, danazol, diazepam, estrogens, ethionamide, fluorouracil, I.V. heparin, insulin, lithium, methadone, methimazole, mitotane, nitroprusside, oxyphenbutazone, phenylbutazone, propylthiouracil, perphenazine, phenytoin, propranolol, salicylates, sulfonylureas, and thiazides

Drug Interactions Aluminum- and magnesium-containing antacids, calcium carbonate, simethicone, or sucralfate: May decrease T_4 absorption; separate dose from thyroid hormones by at least 4 hours.

Antidiabetic agents (biguanides, meglitinides, sulfonylureas, thiazolidinediones, insulin): Changes in thyroid function may alter requirements of antidiabetic agent. Monitor closely at initiation of therapy, or when dose is changed or discontinued.

Cholestyramine and colestipol: Decrease T_4 absorption; separate dose from thyroid hormones by at least 2 hours.

Digoxin: Digoxin levels may be reduced in hyperthyroidism; therapeutic effect may be reduced. Impact of thyroid replacement should be monitored.

Estrogens: May decrease serum free-thyroxine concentrations.

Iron: Decreases T_4 absorption; separate dose from thyroid hormones by at least 4 hours

Kayexalate®: Decreases T_4 absorption; separate dose from thyroid hormones by at least 4 hours

Ketamine: May cause marked hypertension and tachycardia; monitor

Theophylline, caffeine: Decreased theophylline clearance in hypothyroid patients; monitor during thyroid replacement.

Tricyclic and tetracyclic antidepressants: Therapeutic and toxic effects of thyroid hormones and the antidepressant are increased.

Warfarin (and other oral anticoagulants): The hypoprothrombinemic response to warfarin may be altered by a change in thyroid function or replacement. Replacement may dramatically increase response to warfarin. However, initiation of warfarin in a patient stabilized on a dose of thyroid hormones does not appear to require a significantly different approach.

Pregnancy Risk Factor A

Pregnancy Implications Untreated hypothyroidism may have adverse effects on fetal growth and development, and is associated with higher rate of complications; treatment should not be discontinued during pregnancy.

Lactation Enters breast milk (small amounts)/compatible

Additional Information Equivalent doses: Thyroid USP 60 mg ~ levothyroxine 0.05-0.06 mg ~ liothyronine 0.015-0.0375 mg

50-60 mg thyroid ~ 50-60 mcg levothyroxine and 12.5-15 mcg liothyronine

A synthetic form of *L*-Triiodothyronine (T_3) can be used in patients allergic to products derived from pork or beef.

Note: Several medications have effects on thyroid production or conversion. The impact in thyroid replacement has not been specifically evaluated, but patient response should be monitored:

Methimazole: Decreases thyroid hormone secretion, while propylthiouracil decreases thyroid hormone secretion and decreases conversion of T_4 to T_3.

Beta-adrenergic antagonists: Decrease conversion of T_4 to T_3 (dose related, propranolol ≥ 160 mg/day); patients may be clinically euthyroid.

Iodide, iodine-containing radiographic contrast agents may decrease thyroid hormone secretion; may also increase thyroid hormone secretion, especially in patients with Graves' disease.

Other agents reported to impact on thyroid production/conversion include aminoglutethimide, amiodarone, chloral hydrate, diazepam, ethionamide, interferon-alpha, interleukin-2, lithium, lovastatin (case report), glucocorticoids (dose-related), mercaptopurine, sulfonamides, thiazide diuretics, and tolbutamide.

In addition, a number of medications have been noted to cause transient depression in TSH secretion, which may complicate interpretation of monitoring tests for thyroid hormones, including corticosteroids, octreotide, and dopamine. Metoclopramide may increase TSH secretion.

Liotrix

CAS Number 8065-29-0
U.S. Brand Names Thyrolar®
Synonyms T_3/T_4 Liotrix
Use Replacement or supplemental therapy in hypothyroidism (uniform mixture of T_4:T_3 in 4:1 ratio by weight); little advantage to this product exists and cost is not justified

Mechanism of Action The primary active compound is T_3 (triiodothyronine), which may be converted from T_4 (thyroxine) and then circulates throughout the body to influence growth and maturation of various tissues. Liotrix is uniform mixture of synthetic T_4 and T_3 in 4:1 ratio; exact mechanism of action is unknown; however, it is believed the thyroid hormone exerts its many metabolic effects through control of DNA transcription and protein synthesis; involved in normal metabolism, growth, and development; promotes gluconeogenesis, increases utilization and mobilization of glycogen stores and stimulates protein synthesis, increases basal metabolic rate.

Adverse Reactions

Cardiovascular: Palpitations, tachycardia, cardiac arrhythmias, sinus tachycardia

Central nervous system: Nervousness, insomnia, fever, headache

Dermatologic: Hair loss

Gastrointestinal: Weight loss, increased appetite, diarrhea, abdominal cramps

Neuromuscular & skeletal: Tremors

Miscellaneous: Diaphoresis

Signs and Symptoms of Overdose Agitation, coma, hypertension, insomnia, seizures (may occur up to 1 week postingestion), tachycardia

Pharmacodynamics/Kinetics

Absorption: 50% to 95%

Metabolism: Partially hepatic, renal, and in intestines

Half-life elimination: 6-7 days

Time to peak, serum: 12-48 hours

Excretion: Partially feces (as conjugated metabolites)

Dosage

Oral:

Congenital hypothyroidism:

Children (dose/day):

0-6 months: 8-10 mcg/kg

6-12 months: 6-8 mcg/kg

1-5 years: 5-6 mcg/kg

6-12 years: 4-5 mcg/kg

>12 years: 2-3 mcg/kg

Hypothyroidism:

Adults: 30 mg/day, increasing by 15 mg/day at 2- to 3-week intervals to a maximum of 180 mg/day (usual maintenance dose: 60-120 mg/day)

Elderly: Initial: 15 mg, adjust dose at 2- to 4-week intervals by increments of 15 mg

Monitoring Parameters T_4, TSH, heart rate, blood pressure, clinical signs of hypo- and hyperthyroidism; TSH is the most reliable guide for evaluating adequacy of thyroid replacement dosage. TSH may be elevated during the first few months of thyroid replacement despite patients being clinically euthyroid. In cases where T_4 remains low and TSH is within normal limits, an evaluation of "free" (unbound) T_4 is needed to evaluate further increase in dosage.

Contraindications Hypersensitivity to liotrix or any component of the formulation; recent myocardial infarction or thyrotoxicosis, uncomplicated by hypothyroidism; uncorrected adrenal insufficiency, hypersensitivity to active or extraneous constituents

Warnings [U.S. Boxed Warning]: Ineffective for weight reduction; high doses may produce serious or even life-threatening toxic effects particularly when used with some anorectic drugs. Use cautiously in patients with pre-existing cardiovascular disease (angina, CHD), elderly since they may be more likely to have compromised cardiovascular function

Dosage Forms Tablet:

$1/4$ [levothyroxine sodium 12.5 mcg and liothyronine sodium 3.1 mcg]

$1/2$ [levothyroxine sodium 25 mcg and liothyronine sodium 6.25 mcg]

1 [levothyroxine sodium 50 mcg and liothyronine sodium 12.5 mcg]

2 [levothyroxine sodium 100 mcg and liothyronine sodium 25 mcg]

3 [levothyroxine sodium 150 mcg and liothyronine sodium 37.5 mcg]

Reference Range

TSH: 0.4-10.0 (for those ≥ 80 years) mIU/L

T_4: 4.0-12.0 mcg/dL (SI: 51-154 nmol/L)

T_3 (RIA) (total T_3): 80-230 ng/dL (SI: 1.2-3.5 nmol/L)

Free T_4: 0.7-1.8 ng/dL (SI: 9-23 pmol/L)

Overdosage/Treatment

Decontamination: Gastric emptying indicated for ingestions >2 mg; ipecac within 30 minutes or lavage within 1 hour with activated charcoal; 50 mg of cholestyramine can bind at least 3 mg of thyroxine, therefore, 4 g of cholestyramine given 4 times/day should be administered in order to interrupt enterohepatic recirculation

Supportive therapy: Propranolol may be used for hyperadrenergic signs (1 mg I.V. in adults, 0.01-0.1 mg/kg in pediatrics); sodium ipodate (3 g/ 1.7 m^2) has been used in acute ingestion to prevent T_4 to T_3 conversion.

Enhancement of elimination: Plasmapheresis increases elimination 30-fold while charcoal hemoperfusion enhances T_4 elimination fivefold

Test Interactions Many drugs may have effects on thyroid function tests; para-aminosalicylic acid, aminoglutethimide, amiodarone, barbiturates, carbamazepine, chloral hydrate, clofibrate, colestipol, corticosteroids, danazol, diazepam, estrogens, ethionamide, fluorouracil, I.V. heparin, insulin, lithium, methadone, methimazole, mitotane, nitroprusside, oxyphenbutazone, phenylbutazone, PTU, perphenazine, phenytoin, propranolol, salicylates, sulfonylureas, and thiazides

Drug Interactions Aluminum- and magnesium-containing antacids, calcium carbonate, simethicone, or sucralfate: May decrease T_4 absorption; separate dose from thyroid hormones by at least 4 hours.

Antidiabetic agents (biguanides, meglitinides, sulfonylureas, thiazolidinediones, insulin): Changes in thyroid function may alter requirements of antidiabetic agent. Monitor closely at initiation of therapy, or when dose is changed or discontinued.

Cholestyramine and colestipol: Decrease T_4 absorption; separate dose from thyroid hormones by at least 4 hours.

Digoxin: Digoxin levels may be reduced in hyperthyroidism; therapeutic effect may be reduced. Impact of thyroid replacement should be monitored.

Iron: Decreases T_4 absorption; separate dose from thyroid hormones by at least 4 hours

Kayexalate®: Decreases T_4 absorption; separate dose from thyroid hormones by at least 4 hours

Ketamine: May cause marked hypertension and tachycardia; monitor

Ritonavir: May alter response to thyroid hormones (limited documentation/case report); monitor

Somatrem, somatropin: Excessive thyroid hormone levels lead to accelerated epiphyseal closure; inadequate replacement interferes with growth response to growth hormone. Effect of thyroid replacement not specifically evaluated; use caution.

SSRI antidepressants: May need to increase dose of thyroid hormones when SSRI is added to a previously stabilized patient.

Sympathomimetics: Effects of sympathomimetic agent or thyroid hormones may be increased. Risk of coronary insufficiency is increased in patients with coronary artery disease when these agents are used together.

Theophylline, caffeine: Decreased theophylline clearance in hypothyroid patients; monitor during thyroid replacement.

Tricyclic and tetracyclic antidepressants: Therapeutic and toxic effects of thyroid hormones and the antidepressant are increased.

Warfarin (and other oral anticoagulants): The hypoprothrombinemic response to warfarin may be altered by a change in thyroid function or replacement. Replacement may dramatically increase response to warfarin. However, initiation of warfarin in a patient stabilized on a dose of thyroid hormones does not appear to require a significantly different approach.

Note: Several medications have effects on thyroid production or conversion. The impact in thyroid replacement has not been specifically evaluated, but patient response should be monitored:

Methimazole: Decreases thyroid hormone secretion, while propylthiouracil decrease thyroid hormone secretion and decreases conversion of T_4 to T_3.

Beta-adrenergic antagonists: Decrease conversion of T_4 to T_3 (dose related, propranolol ≥ 160 mg/day); patients may be clinically euthyroid.

Iodide, iodine-containing radiographic contrast agents may decrease thyroid hormone secretion; may also increase thyroid hormone secretion, especially in patients with Graves' disease.

Other agents reported to impact on thyroid production/conversion include aminoglutethimide, amiodarone, chloral hydrate, diazepam, ethionamide, interferon-alpha, interleukin-2, lithium, lovastatin (case report), glucocorticoids (dose-related), mercaptopurine, sulfonamides, thiazide diuretics, and tolbutamide.

In addition, a number of medications have been noted to cause transient depression in TSH secretion, which may complicate interpretation of monitoring tests for thyroid hormones, including corticosteroids, octreotide, and dopamine. Metoclopramide may increase TSH secretion.

Pregnancy Risk Factor A

Pregnancy Implications Untreated hypothyroidism may have adverse effects on fetal growth and development, and is associated with higher rate of complications; treatment should not be discontinued during pregnancy.

Nursing Implications Monitor T_4, TSH, heart rate, blood pressure, clinical signs of hypo- and hyperthyroidism; TSH is the most reliable guide for evaluating adequacy of thyroid replacement dosage. TSH may be elevated during the first few months of thyroid replacement despite patients being clinically euthyroid. In cases where T_4 remains low and TSH is within normal limits, an evaluation of "free" (unbound) T_4 is needed to evaluate further increase in dosage.

Additional Information No advantage over synthetic levothyroxine sodium; 1 grain (60 mg) liotrix is equivalent to 0.05-0.06 mg levothyroxine; 60 mg thyroid USP and thyroglobulin; and 45 mg of Thyroid Strong®

Lisinopril

Related Information
- Angiotensin Agents

CAS Number 76547-98-3; 83915-83-7

U.S. Brand Names Prinivil®; Zestril®

Use Treatment of hypertension, either alone or in combination with other antihypertensive agents; adjunctive therapy in treatment of CHF (afterload reduction); treatment of acute myocardial infarction within 24 hours in hemodynamically-stable patients to improve survival; treatment of left ventricular dysfunction after myocardial infarction

Mechanism of Action Competitive inhibition of angiotensin I being converted to angiotensin II, a potent vasoconstrictor, through the angiotensin I-converting enzyme (ACE) activity, with resultant lower levels of angiotensin II which causes an increase in plasma renin activity and a reduction in aldosterone secretion

Adverse Reactions

Cardiovascular: Hypotension (maximum hypotensive effect: 6 hours), syncope, chest pain, angina, palpitations, sinus tachycardia, vasodilation

Central nervous system: Fatigue, insomnia, dizziness, headache, mania

Dermatologic: Rash, angioedema, toxic epidermal necrolysis, bullous skin disease, purpura, photosensitivity, pruritus, licheniform eruptions, exanthem, cutaneous vasculitis

Endocrine & metabolic: Hypoglycemia, hyperkalemia, inappropriate antidiuretic hormone secretion

Gastrointestinal: Nausea, diarrhea, altered taste, pancreatitis

Genitourinary: Impotence

Hematologic: Leukopenia/neutropenia (agranulocytosis, granulocytopenia), anemia, aplastic anemia

Neuromuscular & skeletal: Muscle cramps, paresthesia

Renal: Deterioration in renal function, albuminuria, type IV renal tubular acidosis, renal vasculitis

Respiratory: Cough (dry), wheezing

Miscellaneous: Elevated antineutrophilic cytoplasmic antibodies (ANCA)

Signs and Symptoms of Overdose Hypotension is usually not severe in overdose and manifests itself within 1 hour with maximal effect at 4 hours. Azotemia, bradycardia, confusion, depression, diplopia, dry mouth, dyspnea, dyspepsia, eosinophilia, gout, hyperuricemia, hypoglycemia, insomnia, photophobia, thrombocytopenia

Pharmacodynamics/Kinetics

Onset of action: 1 hour

Peak effect: Hypotensive: Oral: ~6 hours

Duration: 24 hours

Absorption: Well absorbed; unaffected by food

Protein binding: 25%

Half-life elimination: 11-12 hours

Excretion: Primarily urine (as unchanged drug)

Dosage

Oral:

Hypertension:

Children ≥6 years: Initial: 0.07 mg/kg once daily (up to 5 mg); increase dose at 1- to 2-week intervals; doses >0.61 mg/kg or >40 mg have not been evaluated.

Adults: Initial: 10 mg/day; increase doses 5-10 mg/day at 1- to 2-week intervals; maximum daily dose: 40 mg

Elderly: Initial: 2.5-5 mg/day; increase doses 2.5-5 mg/day at 1- to 2-week intervals; maximum daily dose: 40 mg

Patients taking diuretics should have them discontinued 2-3 days prior to initiating lisinopril if possible. Restart diuretic after blood pressure is stable if needed. If diuretic cannot be discontinued prior to therapy, begin with 5 mg with close supervision until stable blood pressure. In patients with hyponatremia (<130 mEq/L), start dose at 2.5 mg/day,

Congestive heart failure: Adults: Initial: 5 mg; then increase by no more than 10 mg increments at intervals no less than 2 weeks to a maximum daily dose of 40 mg. Usual maintenance: 5-40 mg/day as a single dose. Patients should start/continue standard therapy, including diuretics, beta-blockers, and digoxin, as indicated.

Acute myocardial infarction (within 24 hours in hemodynamically stable patients): Oral: 5 mg immediately, then 5 mg at 24 hours, 10 mg at 48 hours, and 10 mg every day thereafter for 6 weeks. Patients should continue to receive standard treatments such as thrombolytics, aspirin, and beta-blockers.

Dosing adjustment in renal impairment:

Adults: Initial doses should be modified and upward titration should be cautious, based on response (maximum: 40 mg/day)

Cl_{cr} >30 mL/minute: Initial: 10 mg/day

Cl_{cr} 10-30 mL/minute: Initial: 5 mg/day

Hemodialysis: Initial: 2.5 mg/day; dialyzable (50%)

Children: Use in not recommended in pediatric patients with GFR <30 mL/1.73 m^2/minute

Monitoring Parameters BUN, serum creatinine, renal function, WBC, and potassium

Administration Watch for hypotensive effects within 1-3 hours of first dose or new higher dose.

Contraindications Hypersensitivity to lisinopril or any component of the formulation; angioedema related to previous treatment with an ACE inhibitor; bilateral renal artery stenosis; pregnancy (2nd and 3rd trimesters)

Warnings Anaphylactic reactions can occur. Angioedema can occur at any time during treatment (especially following first dose). It may involve head and neck (potentially affecting the airway) or the intestine (presenting with abdominal pain). Prolonged monitoring may be required especially if tongue, glottis, or larynx are involved as they are associated with airway obstruction. Those with a history of airway surgery in this situation have a higher risk. Careful blood pressure monitoring with first dose (hypotension can occur especially in volume-depleted patients). **[U.S. Boxed Warning]: Based on human data, ACEIs can cause injury and death to the developing fetus when used in the second and third trimesters. ACEIs should be discontinued as soon as possible once pregnancy is detected.** Dosage adjustment needed in renal impairment. Use with caution in hypovolemia; collagen vascular diseases; valvular stenosis (particularly aortic stenosis); hyperkalemia; or before, during, or immediately after anesthesia. Avoid rapid dosage escalation, which may lead to renal insufficiency. Rare toxicities associated with ACE inhibitors include cholestatic jaundice (which may progress to hepatic necrosis) and neutropenia/agranulocytosis with myeloid hyperplasia. If patient has renal impairment then a baseline WBC with differential and serum creatinine should be evaluated and monitored closely during the first 3 months of therapy. Hypersensitivity reactions may be seen during hemodialysis with high-flux dialysis membranes (eg, AN69). Deterioration in renal function can occur with initiation. Use with caution in unilateral renal artery stenosis and preexisting renal insufficiency. Safety and efficacy have not been established in children <6 years of age.

Dosage Forms [DSC] = Discontinued product

Tablet: 2.5 mg, 5 mg, 10 mg, 20 mg, 30 mg, 40 mg

Prinivil®: 5 mg, 10 mg, 20 mg, 30 mg; 40 mg [DSC]

Zestril®: 2.5 mg, 5 mg, 10 mg, 20 mg, 30 mg, 40 mg

Overdosage/Treatment

Decontamination: Ipecac within 30 minutes or lavage (within 1 hour)/ activated charcoal

Supportive therapy: Following initiation of essential overdose management, toxic symptom treatment and supportive treatment should be initiated. Hypotension usually responds to I.V. normal saline or Trendelenburg positioning. If unresponsive to these measures, the use of a parenteral inotrope may be required (eg, norepinephrine 0.1-0.2 mcg/kg/minute titrated to response). Seizures commonly respond to lorazepam or diazepam (I.V. 5-10 mg bolus in adults every 15 minutes if needed up to a total of 30 mg; I.V. 0.25-0.4 mg/kg/dose up to a total of 10 mg in children) or to phenytoin or phenobarbital. Naloxone may antagonize hypotensive effects. Inhaled sodium cromoglycate (total dose: 40 mg/day) can decrease ACE-inhibitor cough by 50%. For refractory hypotension, angiotensin amide infusion may be attempted.

Enhanced elimination: Multiple dosing of activated charcoal may be effective but not studied in an overdose setting; dialyzable (50%)

Antidote(s)

- Naloxone [ANTIDOTE]

Test Interactions ↑ BUN, creatinine, potassium; positive Coombs' [direct]; ↓ cholesterol (S); may cause false-positive urine acetone determinations using sodium nitroprusside reagent

Drug Interactions Allopurinol: Case reports (rare) indicate a possible increased risk of hypersensitivity reactions when combined with lisinopril.

Alpha$_1$ blockers: Hypotensive effect increased.

Aspirin: The effects of ACE inhibitors may be blunted by aspirin administration, particularly at higher dosages (see Cardiovascular Considerations) and/or increase adverse renal effects.

Diuretics: Hypovolemia due to diuretics may precipitate acute hypotensive events or acute renal failure.

Insulin: Risk of hypoglycemia may be increased.

Lithium: Risk of lithium toxicity may be increased; monitor lithium levels, especially the first 4 weeks of therapy.

Mercaptopurine: Risk of neutropenia may be increased.

NSAIDs: May attenuate hypertensive efficacy; effect has been seen with captopril and may occur with other ACE inhibitors; monitor blood pressure. May increase adverse renal effects.

Potassium-sparing diuretics (amiloride, spironolactone, triamterene): Increased risk of hyperkalemia.

Potassium supplements may increase the risk of hyperkalemia.

Trimethoprim (high dose) may increase the risk of hyperkalemia.

Pregnancy Risk Factor C (1st trimester)/D (2nd and 3rd trimesters)

Pregnancy Implications Decreased placental blood flow, low birth weight, fetal hypotension, preterm delivery, and fetal death have been noted with the use of some ACE inhibitors (ACEIs) in animal studies. Neonatal hypotension, skull hypoplasia, anuria, renal failure, oligohydramnios (associated with fetal limb contractures, craniofacial deformities, hypoplastic lung development), prematurity, intrauterine growth retardation, and patent ductus arteriosus have been reported with the use of ACEIs, primarily in the 2nd and 3rd trimesters. The risk of neonatal toxicity has been considered less when ACEIs have been used in the 1st trimester; however, major congenital malformations have been reported. The cardiovascular and/or central nervous systems are most commonly affected. Unless alternative agents are not appropriate, ACEIs should be discontinued as soon as possible once pregnancy is detected.

Lactation Excretion in breast milk unknown/not recommended

Nursing Implications May cause depression in some patients; discontinue if angioedema of the face, extremities, lips, tongue, or glottis occurs; watch for hypotensive effects within 1-3 hours of first dose or new higher dose

Additional Information Conversion factor from captopril to lisinopril is 5:1

Specific References

Cooper WO, Hernandez-Diaz S, Arbogast PG, et al, "Major Congenital Malformations After First-Trimester Exposure to ACE Inhibitors," *N Engl J Med*, 2006, 354(23):2443-51.

Dubey K, Balani DK, Tripathi CB, et al,. "Adverse Interactions of Rofecoxib with Lisinopril in Spontaneously Hypertensive Rats," *Clin Toxicol*, 2005, 43(5):361-73.

Graham MR, Allcock NM, and Lindsey CC, "Maintenance of Goal Blood Pressure Following Conversion from Lisinopril to Fosinopril," *J Pharm Technol*, 2003, 19:266-70.

Kao CD, Chang JB, Chen JT, et al, "Hypotension Due to Interaction Between Lisinopril and Tizanidine," *Ann Pharmacother*, 2004, 38(11):1840-3.

Mastrobattista J, "Angiontensin-Converting Enzyme Inhibitors in Pregnancy," *Semin Perinatol*, 1997, 21(2):124-34.

Nahata MC and Morosco RS, "Stability of Lisinopril in Two Liquid Dosage Forms," *Ann Pharmacother*, 2004, 38(3):396-9.

Quan A, "Fetopathy Associated with Exposure to Angiotensin-Converting Enzyme Inhibitors and Angiontensin Receptor Antagonists," *Early Hum Dev*, 2006, 82(1):23-8.

Lithium

Related Information

• Therapeutic Drugs Associated with Hallucinations

CAS Number 554-13-2

U.S. Brand Names Eskalith CR®; Eskalith®; Lithobid®

Synonyms Lithium Carbonate; Lithium Citrate

Impairment Potential Yes

Use Management of bipolar disorders; treatment of mania in individuals with bipolar disorder (maintenance treatment prevents or diminishes intensity of subsequent episodes)

Unlabeled/Investigational Use Potential augmenting agent for antidepressants; aggression, post-traumatic stress disorder, conduct disorder in children

Mechanism of Action Alters cation transport across cell membrane in nerve and muscle cells and influences reuptake of serotonin and/or norepinephrine

Adverse Reactions

Cardiovascular: Cardiac arrhythmias, hypotension, sinus node dysfunction, flattened or inverted T waves (reversible), edema, bradycardia, syncope

Central nervous system: Dizziness, vertigo, slurred speech, blackout spells, seizures, sedation, restlessness, confusion, psychomotor retardation, stupor, coma, dystonia, fatigue, lethargy, headache, pseudotumor cerebri, slowed intellectual functioning, tics

Dermatologic: Dry or thinning of hair, folliculitis, alopecia, exacerbation of psoriasis, rash

Endocrine & metabolic: Euthyroid goiter and/or hypothyroidism, hyperthyroidism, hyperglycemia, diabetes insipidus

Gastrointestinal: Polydipsia, anorexia, nausea, vomiting, diarrhea, xerostomia, metallic taste, weight gain, salivary gland swelling, excessive salivation

Genitourinary: Incontinence, polyuria, glycosuria, oliguria, albuminuria

Hematologic: Leukocytosis

Neuromuscular & skeletal: Tremor, muscle hyperirritability, ataxia, choreoathetoid movements, hyperactive deep tendon reflexes, myasthenia gravis (rare), peripheral neuropathy

cular: Nystagmus, blurred vision, transient scotoma, blepharospasm

Miscellaneous: Coldness and painful discoloration of fingers and toes

Signs and Symptoms of Overdose Alopecia, aphasia, arthralgia, ataxia, AV block, bradycardia, blurred vision, chorea (extrapyramidal), cognitive dysfunction, confusion, dementia, dysosmia, encephalopathy, fever, granulocytopenia, heart block, hepatic failure, hypercalcemia, hyperglycemia, hyperkalemia, hyperthyroidism, hypertonia, hypoglycemia, hypokalemia, hypotension, hypothyroidism, hypothermia, impotence, leukopenia, mania, myocardial infarction, myoglobinuria, neuroleptic malignant syndrome, neutropenia, nocturia, nystagmus, ototoxicity, Parkinson's-like symptoms, parotid pain, photophobia, polyuria, rhabdomyolysis, sedation, seizures, tinnitus, thrombocytosis, tremors, ventricular arrhythmia, visual changes. See table.

Lithium (Acute Ingestion)	
Serum Level	**Symptom**
1.5-2.0 mEq/L	Nausea, diarrhea
2.0-2.5 mEq/L	Polyuria, blurred vision, weakness, lethargy, dizziness, increased reflexes, fasiculations
2.5-3.0 mEq/L	Myoclonic twitching, incontinence, stupor, restlessness, coma
>3.0 mEq/L	Seizures, hypotension, cardiac arrhythmias

Admission Criteria/Prognosis For acute ingestions, admit any symptomatic patient or lithium level >2 mEq/L or acute ingestions >40 mg/kg

Pharmacodynamics/Kinetics

Absorption: Rapid and complete

Distribution: V$_d$: Initial: 0.3-0.4 L/kg; V$_{dss}$: 0.7-1 L/kg; crosses placenta; enters breast milk at 35% to 50% the concentrations in serum; distribution is complete in 6-10 hours

CSF, liver concentrations: $^1/_3$ to $^1/_2$ of serum concentration

Erythrocyte concentration: $\sim^1/_2$ of serum concentration

Heart, lung, kidney, muscle concentrations: Equivalent to serum concentration

Saliva concentration: 2-3 times serum concentration

Thyroid, bone, brain tissue concentrations: Increase 50% over serum concentrations

Protein binding: Not protein bound

Metabolism: Not metabolized

Bioavailability: Not affected by food; Capsule, immediate release tablet: 95% to 100%; Extended release tablet: 60% to 90%; Syrup: 100%

Half-life elimination: 18-24 hours; can increase to more than 36 hours in elderly or with renal impairment

Time to peak, serum: Nonsustained release: ~0.5-2 hours; slow release: 4-12 hours; syrup: 15-60 minutes

Excretion: Urine (90% to 98% as unchanged drug); sweat (4% to 5%); feces (1%)

Clearance: 80% of filtered lithium is reabsorbed in the proximal convoluted tubules; therefore, clearance approximates 20% of GFR or 20-40 mL/minute

Dosage

Oral: Monitor serum concentrations and clinical response (efficacy and toxicity) to determine proper dose

Children 6-12 years:

Bipolar disorder: 15-60 mg/kg/day in 3-4 divided doses; dose not to exceed usual adult dosage

Conduct disorder (unlabeled use): 15-30 mg/kg/day in 3-4 divided doses; dose not to exceed usual adult dosage

Adults: Bipolar disorder: 900-2400 mg/day in 3-4 divided doses or 900-1800 mg/day (sustained release) in 2 divided doses

Elderly: Bipolar disorder: Initial dose: 300 mg once or twice daily; increase weekly in increments of 300 mg/day, monitoring levels; rarely need >900-1200 mg/day

Dosing adjustment in renal impairment:
Cl$_{cr}$ 10-50 mL/minute: Administer 50% to 75% of normal dose
Cl$_{cr}$ <10 mL/minute: Administer 25% to 50% of normal dose
Hemodialysis: Dialyzable (50% to 100%)

Monitoring Parameters Serum lithium every 4-5 days during initial therapy; draw lithium serum concentrations 8-12 hours postdose; renal, thyroid, and cardiovascular function; fluid status; serum electrolytes; CBC with differential, urinalysis; monitor for signs of toxicity; b-HCG pregnancy test for all females not known to be sterile

Administration Administer with meals to decrease GI upset. Slow release tablets must be swallowed whole; do not crush or chew.

Contraindications Hypersensitivity to lithium or any component of the formulation; avoid use in patients with severe cardiovascular or renal disease, or with severe debilitation, dehydration, or sodium depletion; pregnancy

Warnings[U.S. Boxed Warning]: Lithium toxicity is closely related to serum levels and can occur at therapeutic doses; serum lithium determinations are required to monitor therapy. Use with caution in patients with thyroid disease, mild-moderate renal impairment, or mild-moderate cardiovascular disease. Use caution in patients receiving medications which alter sodium excretion (eg, diuretics, ACE inhibitors, NSAIDs), or in patients with significant fluid loss (protracted sweating, diarrhea, or prolonged fever); temporary reduction or cessation of therapy may be warranted. Some elderly patients may be extremely sensitive to the effects of lithium, see Dosage and Reference Range. Chronic therapy results in diminished renal concentrating ability (nephrogenic DI); this is usually reversible when lithium is discontinued. Changes in renal function should be monitored, and re-evaluation of treatment may be necessary. Use caution in patients at risk of suicide (suicidal thoughts or behavior).

Morphologic changes with glomerular and interstitial fibrosis and nephron atrophy have been reported in patients on chronic lithium therapy; morphologic changes have also been reported in manic-depressive patients never exposed to lithium. The relationship between morphologic changes and renal function, and the association with lithium therapy, have not been established.

Use with caution in patients receiving neuroleptic medications - a syndrome resembling NMS has been associated with concurrent therapy. Lithium may impair the patient's alertness, affecting the ability to operate machinery or driving a vehicle. Neuromuscular-blocking agents should be administered with caution; the response may be prolonged.

Higher serum concentrations may be required and tolerated during an acute manic phase; however, the tolerance decreases when symptoms subside. Normal fluid and salt intake must be maintained during therapy.

Safety and efficacy have not been established in children <12 years of age.

Dosage Forms [DSC] = Discontinued product
Capsule, as carbonate: 150 mg, 300 mg, 600 mg
Eskalith®: 300 mg [contains benzyl alcohol] [DSC]
Solution, as citrate: 300 mg/5 mL (5 mL, 500 mL) [equivalent to amount of lithium in lithium carbonate]
Syrup, as citrate: 300 mg/5 mL (480 mL) [equivalent to amount of lithium in lithium carbonate]
Tablet, as carbonate: 300 mg
Tablet, controlled release, as carbonate: 450 mg
Eskalith CR®: 450 mg [DSC]
Tablet, slow release, as carbonate: 300 mg
Lithobid®: 300 mg

Reference Range
Levels should be obtained twice weekly until both patient's clinical status and levels are stable then levels may be obtained every 1-3 months
Timing of serum samples: Draw trough just before next dose (8-12 hours after previous dose)
Therapeutic levels:
Acute mania: 0.6-1.2 mEq/L (SI: 0.6-1.2 mmol/L)
Protection against future episodes in most patients with bipolar disorder: 0.8-1 mEq/L (SI: 0.8-1.0 mmol/L); a higher rate of relapse is described in subjects who are maintained at <0.4 mEq/L (SI: 0.4 mmol/L)
Elderly patients can usually be maintained at lower end of therapeutic range (0.6-0.8 mEq/L)
Toxic concentration: >1.5 mEq/L (SI: >2 mmol/L)
Adverse effect levels:
GI complaints/tremor: 1.5-2 mEq/L
Confusion/somnolence: 2-2.5 mEq/L
Seizures/death: >2.5 mEq/L

Overdosage/Treatment
Decontamination: Lavage within 1 hour acute ingestions >40 mg/kg; 30-60 g of sodium polystyrene sulfonate may prevent absorption; whole bowel irrigation with polyethylene glycol (2 L/hour for 5 hours in adults),

may cause a 67% decrease in absorption; activated charcoal may not be effective in adsorbing lithium but is not harmful if used.

Supportive therapy: There is no specific antidote for lithium poisoning. In the acute ingestion, following initiation of essential overdose management, correction of fluid and electrolyte imbalances should be commenced. Lithium-induced tachycardia (ventricular) may respond to I.V. magnesium sulfate. Amiloride is an effective therapy in reducing lithium-induced polyuria by one-third. Lithium-induced nephrogenic diabetes insipidus can be treated with amiloride, hydrochlorothiazide, indomethacin, or I.V. ketorolac. Lithium-induced bradycardia may require transvenous pacemaker; may not respond to atropine or transcutaneous pacemaker.

Enhancement of elimination: Hemodialysis is the treatment of choice for severe intoxications; 50% to 100% dialyzable. Dialysis should be considered in a symptomatic patient with levels >4.0 mEq/L (acute ingestion), role of hemodialysis is controversial in chronic toxicity due to limited distribution out of CNS; other indications for dialysis include neurologic toxicity, renal failure, or ingestions of sustained release preparations. Four hours of hemodialysis should reduce lithium concentrations by ~1 mEq/L, but due to a rebound effect, a usual dialysis time of 10-12 hours is recommended. Dialysis using a bicarbonate bath (35 mM/L) may be more efficacious than an acetate bath in removing lithium.

Antidote(s)
- Ipecac Syrup [ANTIDOTE]
- Polyethylene Glycol - High Molecular Weight [ANTIDOTE]
- Sodium Polystyrene Sulfonate [ANTIDOTE]

Diagnostic Procedures
- Lithium RBC/Plasma Ratio
- Lithium, Blood

Test Interactions ↑ calcium (S), glucose, magnesium, potassium (S), serum bicarbonate, urea; ↓ thyroxine (S), serum bromide; causes leukopenia, thrombocytopenia

Drug Interactions ACE inhibitors: May increase the risk of lithium toxicity via sodium depletion; monitor
Angiotensin receptor antagonists (losartan): May reduce the renal clearance of lithium; monitor
Caffeine (xanthine derivatives): May lower lithium serum concentrations by increasing urinary lithium excretion; monitor.
Carbamazepine: Concurrent use of lithium with carbamazepine may increase the risk for neurotoxicity; monitor
Carbonic anhydrase inhibitors: May decrease lithium levels; includes acetazolamide; monitor
Calcium channel blockers (diltiazem and verapamil): May increase the risk for neurotoxicity (ataxia, tremors, nausea, vomiting, diarrhea, and/or tinnitus); monitor; does not appear to involve dihydropyridine class
Chlorpromazine: May lower serum concentrations of both drugs; monitor
COX-2 inhibitors (celecoxib): May increase lithium plasma concentrations (similar to NSAIDs); monitor.
Haloperidol: May increase the risk for neurotoxicity and encephalopathy; a rare encephalopathic syndrome resulting in irreversible brain damage has been reported in a few patients (causal relationship not established); monitor
Iodine salts: May enhance the hypothyroid effects of lithium; monitor
Loop diuretics: May decrease the renal excretion of lithium, leading to toxicity; monitor
MAO inhibitors: Should generally be avoided due to use reports of fatal malignant hyperpyrexia when combined with lithium
Methyldopa: May increase the risk for neurotoxicity; monitor
Metronidazole: May increase lithium toxicity (rare); monitor
Neuromuscular-blocking agents: Lithium may potentiate the response to neuromuscular blockade, resulting in prolonged blockade and possible delayed recovery
NSAIDs: Renal lithium excretion may be decreased leading to increased serum lithium concentrations; sulindac and aspirin may be the exceptions; monitor
Phenothiazines: May increase the risk for neurotoxicity; monitor
Phenytoin: May enhance lithium toxicity; monitor
Selegiline: Risk of severe reactions when combined with MAO inhibitors may be decreased when administered with selective MAO type B inhibitor, particularly at selegiline doses <10 mg/day; however, theoretical risk is still present
SSRIs: May increase the risk for neurotoxicity; monitor; effect noted with fluoxetine, fluvoxamine
Sibutramine: Combined use of lithium with sibutramine may increase the risk of serotonin syndrome; this combination is best avoided
Sodium-containing products: Bicarbonate and/or high sodium intake may reduce serum lithium concentrations via enhanced excretion; monitor.
Note: Reabsorption of lithium in the proximal convoluted tubule occurs against electrical and concentration gradients that do not distinguish between lithium and sodium. Therefore, lithium clearance may increase or decrease 30% to 50% with sodium load or depletion, respectively. Sodium depletion usually has the greater effect.

Sympathomimetics: Lithium may blunt the pressor response to sympathomimetics (epinephrine, phenylephrine, norepinephrine)

Tetracyclines: May increase lithium levels; monitor

Theophylline: May increase real clearance of lithium, resulting in a decrease in serum lithium concentrations; monitor

Thiazide diuretics: May increase serum lithium concentration via sodium depletion and decreased lithium clearance; a lithium dose reduction of 50% is commonly recommended

Tricyclic antidepressants: May increase the risk for neurotoxicity; monitor

Urea: May lower lithium serum concentrations by increasing urinary excretion; monitor.

Pregnancy Risk Factor D

Pregnancy Implications Cardiac malformations in the infant, including Ebstein's anomaly, are associated with use of lithium during the first trimester of pregnancy. Nontoxic effects to the newborn include shallow respiration, hypotonia, lethargy, cyanosis, diabetes insipidus, thyroid depression, and nontoxic goiter when lithium is used near term. Efforts should be made to avoid lithium use during the first trimester; if an alternative therapy is not appropriate, the lowest possible dose of lithium should be used throughout the pregnancy. Fetal echocardiography and ultrasound to screen for anomalies should be conducted between 16-20 weeks of gestation. Lithium levels should be monitored in the mother and may need adjusted following delivery. Enters breast milk/contraindicated

Lactation Enters breast milk/contraindicated

Nursing Implications Give with meals to decrease gastrointestinal upset

Specific References

Borovicka MC, Bond LC, and Gaughan KM, "Ziprasidone- and Lithium-induced Neuroleptic Malignant Syndrome," *Ann Pharmacother*, 2006, 40(1):139-42.

Bravo AE, Egger SS, Crespo S, et al, "Lithium Intoxication as a Result of an Interaction with Rofecoxib," *Ann Pharmacother*, 2004, 38(7):1189-91.

Hahn I, Pisupati D, Tarrer S, et al, "*In Vitro* Binding of Lithium Carbonate to Prussian Blue and Activated Charcoal," *Acad Emerg Med*, 2003, 10:519

Hung YM and Hung YM, "Acute Interstitial Nephritis on Chronic Lithium Nephropathy in a Lithium Overdose Patient," *Dial Transplant*, 2003, 32(9):568.

Kamijo Y, Soma K, Hamanaka S, et al, "Dural Sinus Thrombosis with Severe Hypernatremia Developing in a Patient on Long-Term Lithium Therapy," *J Toxicol Clin Toxicol*, 2003, 41(4):359-62.

Moretti ME, Koren G, Verjee Z, et al, "Monitoring Lithium in Breast Milk: An Individualized Approach for Breast-Feeding Mothers," *Ther Drug Monit*, 2003, 25(3):364-6.

Lodoxamide

CAS Number 53882-12-5; 53882-13-6; 63610-09-3

U.S. Brand Names Alomide®

Synonyms Lodoxamide Tromethamine

Use Treatment of allergic keratoconjunctivitis, allergic conjunctivitis, and allergic keratitis

Mechanism of Action Mast cell stabilizer (similar to sodium cromoglycate) that inhibits the *in vivo* type I immediate hypersensitivity reaction to increase cutaneous vascular permeability associated with IgE and antigen-mediated reactions

Adverse Reactions

Central nervous system: Headache, dizziness, somnolence

Dermatologic: Rash

Gastrointestinal: Nausea, stomach discomfort

Local: **Transient burning, stinging, discomfort**

Ocular: Blurred vision, corneal erosion/ulcer, eye pain, corneal abrasion, blepharitis, xerophthalmia

Respiratory: Sneezing, dry nose

Signs and Symptoms of Overdose Dizziness, fatigue, feeling of warmth, headache, nausea, sweating, and loose stools following oral administration.

Pharmacodynamics/Kinetics

Absorption: Topical: Negligible

Dosage Children >2 years and Adults: Instill 1-2 drops in eye(s) 4 times/day for up to 3 months

Contraindications Hypersensitivity to lodoxamide tromethamine or any component of the formulation

Warnings Safety and efficacy in children <2 years of age have not been established; not for injection; not for use in patients wearing soft contact lenses during treatment

Dosage Forms Solution, ophthalmic: 0.1% (10 mL) [contains benzalkonium chloride]

Overdosage/Treatment Decontamination: **Oral**: Lavage (within 1 hour)/activated charcoal. **Ocular**: Irrigate with normal saline through a Morgans lens

Drug Interactions No data reported

Pregnancy Risk Factor B

Loperamide

CAS Number 34552-83-5; 53179-11-6

U.S. Brand Names Imodium® A-D [OTC]

Synonyms Loperamide Hydrochloride

Use

Treatment of chronic diarrhea associated with inflammatory bowel disease; acute nonspecific diarrhea; increased volume of ileostomy discharge

OTC labeling: Control of symptoms of diarrhea, including Traveler's diarrhea

Unlabeled/Investigational Use Cancer treatment-induced diarrhea (eg, irinotecan induced); chronic diarrhea caused by bowel resection

Mechanism of Action Acts directly on intestinal muscles to inhibit peristalsis and prolong transit time

Adverse Reactions

Cardiovascular: Bradycardia

Central nervous system: Sedation, psychosis, restlessness, fatigue, dizziness, delirium

Dermatologic: Rash

Gastrointestinal: Nausea, vomiting, constipation, abdominal pain, abdominal cramping, xerostomia, appendicitis, pancreatitis

Genitourinary: Urinary retention, toxic megacolon

Signs and Symptoms of Overdose Bradycardia, CNS and respiratory depression, constipation, dry mouth, dystonic reactions, gastrointestinal cramping, headache, ileus, nausea, miosis, personality changes, vomiting

Admission Criteria/Prognosis Admit ingestions >1 mg/kg

Pharmacodynamics/Kinetics

Absorption: Poor

Distribution: Poor penetration into brain; low amounts enter breast milk

Metabolism: Hepatic via oxidative N-demethylation

Half-life elimination: 7-14 hours

Time to peak, plasma: Liquid: 2.5 hours; Capsule: 5 hours

Excretion: Urine and feces (1% as metabolites, 30% to 40% as unchanged drug)

Dosage

Oral:

Children:

Acute diarrhea: Initial doses (in first 24 hours):

2-5 years (13-20 kg): 1 mg 3 times/day

6-8 years (20-30 kg): 2 mg twice daily

8-12 years (>30 kg): 2 mg 3 times/day

Maintenance: After initial dosing, 0.1 mg/kg doses after each loose stool, but not exceeding initial dosage

Traveler's diarrhea:

6-8 years: 2 mg after first loose stool, followed by 1 mg after each subsequent stool (maximum dose: 4 mg/day)

9-11 years: 2 mg after first loose stool, followed by 1 mg after each subsequent stool (maximum dose: 6 mg/day)

≥12 years: See adult dosing.

Adults:

Acute diarrhea: Initial: 4 mg, followed by 2 mg after each loose stool, up to 16 mg/day

Chronic diarrhea: Initial: Follow acute diarrhea; maintenance dose should be slowly titrated downward to minimum required to control symptoms (typically, 4-8 mg/day in divided doses)

Traveler's diarrhea: Initial: 4 mg after first loose stool, followed by 2 mg after each subsequent stool (maximum dose: 8 mg/day)

Irinotecan-induced diarrhea (unlabeled use): 4 mg after first loose or frequent bowel movement, then 2 mg every 2 hours until 12 hours have passed without a bowel movement. If diarrhea recurs, then repeat administration

Dosage adjustment in hepatic impairment: No specific guidelines available.

Monitoring Parameters Stool frequency, fluid and electrolytes

Contraindications Hypersensitivity to loperamide or any component of the formulation; abdominal pain without diarrhea; children <2 years

Avoid use as primary therapy in acute dysentery, acute ulcerative colitis, bacterial enterocolitis, pseudomembranous colitis

Warnings

Should not be used if diarrhea is accompanied by high fever or blood in stool. Use caution in young children as response may be variable because of dehydration. Concurrent fluid and electrolyte replacement is often necessary in all age groups depending upon severity of diarrhea. Should not be used when inhibition of peristalsis is undesirable or dangerous. Discontinue if constipation, abdominal pain, or ileus develop. Use caution in patients with hepatic impairment because of reduced first pass metabolism. Use caution in treatment of AIDS patients; stop therapy at the sign of abdominal distention. Cases of toxic megacolon have occurred in this population. Loperamide is a symptom-directed treatment; if an underlying diagnosis is made, other disease-specific treatment may be indicated. Use caution in patients with hepatic impairment because of reduced first-pass metabolism; monitor for signs of CNS toxicity.

OTC labeling: If diarrhea lasts longer than 2 days, patient should stop taking loperamide and consult healthcare provider.

Dosage Forms Caplet, as hydrochloride: 2 mg
Diamode, Imodium® A-D, Kao-Paverin®: 2 mg
Capsule, as hydrochloride: 2 mg
Liquid, oral, as hydrochloride: 1 mg/5 mL (5 mL, 10 mL, 120 mL)
Imodium® A-D: 1 mg/5 mL (60 mL, 120 mL) [contains alcohol, sodium benzoate, benzoic acid; cherry mint flavor]
Imodium® A-D [new formulation]: 1 mg/7.5 mL (60 mL, 120 mL, 360 mL) [contains sodium 10 mg/30 mL, sodium benzoate; creamy mint flavor]
Tablet, as hydrochloride: 2 mg
K-Pek II: 2 mg

Reference Range Peak plasma loperamide level: ~0.75 ng/mL after a 4 mg oral dose

Overdosage/Treatment
Decontamination: Lavage (within 1 hour)/activated charcoal; **do not** use a cathartic if an ileus is present
Supportive therapy: Naloxone is useful to reverse CNS or apnea; dystonic reaction can be managed with benztropine (1-2 mg I.V.) or diphenhydramine (1 mg/kg up to 50 mg I.V.)

Antidote(s)
• Naloxone [ANTIDOTE]

Test Interactions ↑ glucose

Drug Interactions Substrate (minor) of CYP2B6
P-glycoprotein inhibitors: May increase CNS depressant effects of loperamide. Examples of inhibitors include cyclosporine, ketoconazole, quinidine, quinine, and ritonavir. Monitor.
Saquinavir: Loperamide may decrease levels/effects of saquinavir.

Pregnancy Risk Factor B

Pregnancy Implications Teratogenic effects were not observed in animal studies.

Lactation Enters breast milk/not recommended.

Additional Information Toxic dose: 2 mg/kg. If clinical improvement is not achieved after 16 mg/day for 10 days, control is unlikely with further use. Continue use if diet or other treatment does not control. Elderly are particularly sensitive to fluid and electrolyte loss. Drug therapy must be limited in order to avoid toxicity with this agent.

Specific References
Audi J, Layher J, and Morgan B, "Cardiac Conduction Disturbances Secondary to Chronic Abuse of Loperamide: An Initial Case Report," *J Toxicol Clin Toxicol*, 2004, 42(5):722.
Sklerov J, Levine B, Moore KA, et al, "Tissue Distribution of Loperamide and N-Desmethylloperamide Following a Fatal Overdose," *J Anal Toxicol*, 2006, 30:134.

Loracarbef

CAS Number 121961-22-6; 76470-66-1

U.S. Brand Names Lorabid®

Use Infections caused by susceptible organisms involving the respiratory tract, acute otitis media, sinusitis, skin and skin structure, bone and joint, and urinary tract and gynecologic

Mechanism of Action Inhibits bacterial cell wall synthesis by binding to one or more of the penicillin binding proteins (PBPs); inhibits the final transpeptidation step of peptidoglycan synthesis in bacterial cell walls, thus inhibiting cell wall biosynthesis. It is thought that beta-lactam antibiotics inactivate transpeptidase via acylation of the enzyme with cleavage of the CO-N bond of the beta-lactam ring. Upon exposure to beta-lactam antibiotics, bacteria eventually lyse due to ongoing activity of cell wall autolytic enzymes (autolysins and murein hydrolases) while cell wall assembly is arrested.

Adverse Reactions
Cardiovascular: Vasodilation
Central nervous system: Headache, somnolence, nervousness, dizziness
Dermatologic: Rashes, urticaria, pruritus
Endocrine & metabolic: Menorrhagia
Gastrointestinal: Diarrhea, nausea, vomiting, abdominal pain, anorexia
Genitourinary: **Vaginitis** (15%), vaginal moniliasis
Hematologic: Transient thrombocytopenia, leukopenia, and eosinophilia
Hepatic: Transient elevations of ALT, AST, alkaline phosphatase
Renal: Transient elevations of BUN/creatinine

Pharmacodynamics/Kinetics
Absorption: Rapid
Protein binding: ~25%
Bioavailability: ~90%; decreased by food
Half-life elimination: ~1 hour
Time to peak, serum: ~1 hour
Excretion: Clearance: Plasma: ~200-300 mL/minute

Dosage
Oral:
Children:
Impetigo: 15 mg/kg/day in divided doses for 10 days
Acute otitis media: 15 mg/kg twice daily for 10 days

Pharyngitis: 7.5-15 mg/kg twice daily for 10 days
Adults:
Pharyngitis: 200 mg every 12 hours for 10 days
Bronchitis: 200-400 mg every 12 hours for 7 days
Pneumonia: 400 mg every 12 hours for 14 days
Sinusitis: 200-400 mg every 12 hours for 10 days
Uncomplicated urinary tract infections: 200 mg once daily for 7 days
Skin and soft tissue: 200-400 mg every 12-24 hours
Adults, female:
Uncomplicated pyelonephritis: 400 mg every 12 hours for 14 days
Dosing comments in renal impairment:
$Cl_{cr} \geq 50$ mL/minute: Give usual dose
Cl_{cr} 10-49 mL/minute: 50% of usual dose at usual interval or usual dose given half as often
$Cl_{cr} < 10$ mL/minute: Give usual dose every 3-5 days
Hemodialysis: Doses should be administered after dialysis sessions

Stability Suspension may be kept at room temperature for 14 days

Administration Administer on an empty stomach at least 1 hour before or 2 hours after meals. Finish all medication. Shake suspension well before using.

Contraindications Hypersensitivity to loracarbef, any component of the formulation, or cephalosporins

Warnings Modify dosage in patients with severe renal impairment. Prolonged use may result in superinfection. Use with caution in patients with a previous history of hypersensitivity to other beta-lactam antibiotics (eg, penicillins, cephalosporins). Safety and efficacy in children <6 months of age have not been established.

Dosage Forms Capsule: 200 mg, 400 mg
Powder for oral suspension: 100 mg/5 mL (100 mL); 200 mg/5 mL (100 mL) [strawberry bubble gum flavor]

Reference Range Peak serum loracarbef levels range from 14-15.4 mcg/mL after a 400 mg oral dose

Overdosage/Treatment Decontamination: Emesis with ipecac within 30 minutes or lavage (within 1 hour)/activated charcoal

Drug Interactions Probenecid: May decrease cephalosporin elimination.

Pregnancy Risk Factor B

Pregnancy Implications Animal studies have not demonstrated teratogenicity. There are no adequate and well-controlled studies in pregnant women.

Lactation Excretion in breast milk unknown/use caution

Loratadine

CAS Number 79794-75-5

U.S. Brand Names Alavert™ [OTC]; Claritin® Hives Relief [OTC]; Claritin® [OTC]; Dimetapp® Children's ND [OTC]; Tavist® ND [OTC]

Impairment Potential Impairment may occur at double the therapeutic doses

Use Relief of nasal and non-nasal symptoms of seasonal allergic rhinitis with little sedative properties; urticaria (chronic); idiopathic chronic urticaria

Mechanism of Action Long-acting tricyclic antihistamine with selective peripheral histamine H_1 receptor antagonistic properties; derived from azatadine

Adverse Reactions
Cardiovascular: Hypotension, hypertension, palpitations, tachycardia, fibrillation (atrial), sinus tachycardia
Central nervous system: **Headache, somnolence, fatigue**, anxiety, CNS depression, ataxia
Dermatologic: Erythema multiforme, alopecia, angioedema, xerosis, urticaria, purpura, photosensitivity, pruritus, exanthem
Endocrine & metabolic: Breast pain, gynecomastia
Gastrointestinal: **Xerostomia**, stomatitis
Hepatic: Hepatotoxicity, liver necrosis
Neuromuscular & skeletal: Hyperkinesia, arthralgias, paresthesia
Respiratory: Dyspnea, pharyngitis, nasal dryness
Miscellaneous: Diaphoresis

Signs and Symptoms of Overdose Coma

Admission Criteria/Prognosis Admit any patient with cardiac abnormalities or ingestion >170 mg in children; admit any symptomatic patient or ingestion >35 mg.

Pharmacodynamics/Kinetics
Onset of action: 1-3 hours
Peak effect: 8-12 hours
Duration: >24 hours
Absorption: Rapid
Distribution: Significant amounts enter breast milk
Metabolism: Extensively hepatic via CYP2D6 and 3A4 to active metabolite
Half-life elimination: 12-15 hours
Excretion: Urine (40%) and feces (40%) as metabolites

Dosage
Oral: Seasonal allergic rhinitis, chronic idiopathic urticaria:
Children 2-5 years: 5 mg once daily

Children ≥6 years and Adults: 10 mg once daily

Elderly: Peak plasma levels are increased; elimination half-life is slightly increased; specific dosing adjustments are not available

Dosage adjustment in renal impairment: Cl$_{cr}$ ≤30 mL/minute:

Children 2-5 years: 5 mg every other day

Children ≥6 years and Adults: 10 mg every other day

Dosage adjustment in hepatic impairment: Elimination half-life increases with severity of disease

Children 2-5 years: 5 mg every other day

Children ≥6 years and Adults: 10 mg every other day

Administration Take on an empty stomach.

Contraindications Hypersensitivity to loratadine or any component of the formulation

Warnings Use with caution and modify dose in patients with liver or renal impairment; safety and efficacy in children <2 years of age have not been established

Dosage Forms Syrup: 1 mg/mL (120 mL)

Claritin®: 1 mg/mL (120 mL) [contains sodium benzoate; fruit flavor]; (60 mL, 120 mL) [alcohol free, dye free, sugar free; contains sodium 6 mg/5 mL and sodium benzoate; grape flavor]

Tablet: 10 mg

Alavert®, Claritin®, Claritin® Hives Relief, Claritin® 24 Hour Allergy, Tavist® ND: 10 mg

Tablet, rapidly disintegrating: 10 mg

Alavert®: 10 mg [contains phenylalanine 8.4 mg/tablet; mint and citrus burst flavors]

Claritin® RediTabs®: 10 mg [mint flavor]

Triaminic® Allerchews™: 10 mg

Reference Range Peak loratadine serum level of 18 ng/mL 1 hour after a single 40 mg dose

Overdosage/Treatment

Decontamination: Lavage (within 1 hour) ingestions >150 mg/activated charcoal

Enhancement of elimination: Hemodialysis is not useful; multiple dosing of activated charcoal may be useful

Drug Interactions Substrate (minor) of CYP2D6, 3A4; **Inhibits** CYP2C8 (weak), 2C19 (moderate), 2D6 (weak)

CYP2C19 substrates: Loratadine may increase the levels/effects of CYP2C19 substrates. Example substrates include citalopram, diazepam, methsuximide, phenytoin, propranolol, and sertraline.

Protease inhibitors (amprenavir, ritonavir, nelfinavir) may increase the serum levels of loratadine

Increased toxicity: Other antihistamines

Pregnancy Risk Factor B

Pregnancy Implications Loratadine was not found to be teratogenic in animal studies. There are no adequate and well-controlled studies in pregnant woman; use during pregnancy only if clearly needed.

Lactation Enters breast milk/not recommended (AAP rates "compatible")

Specific References

Manning B, Tai W, and Kearney T, "A Four Year Review of Pediatric Loratadine Ingestions; Implications for Poison Center Referral Guidelines," *J Toxicol Clin Toxicol*, 2003, 41(5):669.

Lorazepam

Related Information

- Seizures, Neonatal Guidelines
- Therapeutic Drugs Associated with Hallucinations

CAS Number 846-49-1

U.S. Brand Names Ativan®; Lorazepam Intensol®

Impairment Potential Yes. Cognitive and psychomotor impairment can occur in the elderly following acute single doses (0.5 and 1 mg) of oral lorazepam. (Pomara N, Tun H, DaSilva D, et al, "Benzodiazepine Use and Crash Risk in Older Patients," *JAMA*, 1998, 279(2):113-4.)

Use

Oral: Management of anxiety disorders or short-term relief of the symptoms of anxiety or anxiety associated with depressive symptoms

I.V.: Status epilepticus, preanesthesia for desired amnesia, antiemetic adjunct; pain/muscle spasm due to black widow spider bite

Unlabeled/Investigational Use Ethanol detoxification; insomnia; psychogenic catatonia; partial complex seizures; agitation (I.V.)

Mechanism of Action Depresses all levels of the CNS, including the limbic and reticular formation, probably through the increased action of gamma-aminobutyric acid (GABA), which is a major inhibitory neurotransmitter in the brain

Adverse Reactions

Cardiovascular: Hypotension

Central nervous system: Sedation (15.9%), headache, fatigue, depression, unsteadiness (3.4%), dizziness (6.9%), disorientation, sleep disturbances, agitation, aggressive behavior

Dermatologic: Hypertrichosis, erythema multiforme, alopecia, urticaria, purpura, Stevens-Johnson syndrome, pruritus, exanthem, lichen planus

Endocrine & metabolic: Menstrual irregularities

Gastrointestinal: Nausea, appetite changes, xerostomia, increased salivation

Hematologic: Blood dyscrasias

Neuromuscular & skeletal: Weakness (4.2%), reflex slowing

Miscellaneous: Fixed drug eruption, physical and psychological dependence with prolonged use, polyethylene glycol or propylene glycol poisoning (prolonged I.V. infusion)

Signs and Symptoms of Overdose Acute myoglobinuria, "alpha" coma (alpha frequency rhythm on EEG), ataxia, confusion, depression, disorientation, dyspnea, hypoactive reflexes, hyporeflexia, labored breathing, myalgia, nystagmus, rhabdomyolysis, visual and auditory hallucinations. Onset of effects may be delayed as long as 7 hours in acute overdosage.

Pharmacodynamics/Kinetics

Onset of action:

Hypnosis: I.M.: 20-30 minutes

Sedation: I.V.: 5-20 minutes

Anticonvulsant: I.V.: 5 minutes, oral: 30-60 minutes

Duration: 6-8 hours

Absorption: Oral, I.M.: Prompt

Distribution:

V$_d$: Neonates: 0.76 L/kg, Adults: 1.3 L/kg; crosses placenta; enters breast milk

Protein binding: 85%; free fraction may be significantly higher in elderly

Metabolism: Hepatic to inactive compounds

Half-life elimination: Neonates: 40.2 hours; Older children: 10.5 hours; Adults: 12.9 hours; Elderly: 15.9 hours; End-stage renal disease: 32-70 hours

Excretion: Urine; feces (minimal)

Dosage

Antiemetic:

Children 2-15 years: I.V.: 0.05 mg/kg (up to 2 mg/dose) prior to chemotherapy

Adults: Oral, I.V. (**Note:** May be administered sublingually; not a labeled route): 0.5-2 mg every 4-6 hours as needed

Anxiety and sedation:

Infants and Children: Oral, I.M., I.V.: Usual: 0.05 mg/kg/dose (range: 0.02-0.09 mg/kg) every 4-8 hours

I.V.: May use smaller doses (eg, 0.01-0.03 mg/kg) and repeat every 20 minutes, as needed to titrate to effect

Adults: Oral: 1-10 mg/day in 2-3 divided doses; usual dose: 2-6 mg/day in divided doses

Elderly: 0.5-4 mg/day; initial dose not to exceed 2 mg

Insomnia: Adults: Oral: 2-4 mg at bedtime

Preoperative: Adults:

I.M.: 0.05 mg/kg administered 2 hours before surgery (maximum: 4 mg/dose)

I.V.: 0.044 mg/kg 15-20 minutes before surgery (usual maximum: 2 mg/dose)

Operative amnesia: Adults: I.V.: Up to 0.05 mg/kg (maximum: 4 mg/dose)

Sedation (preprocedure): Infants and Children:

Oral, I.M., I.V.: Usual: 0.05 mg/kg (range: 0.02-0.09 mg/kg);

I.V.: May use smaller doses (eg, 0.01-0.03 mg/kg) and repeat every 20 minutes, as needed to titrate to effect

Status epilepticus: I.V.:

Infants and Children: 0.1 mg/kg slow I.V. over 2-5 minutes; do not exceed 4 mg/single dose; may repeat second dose of 0.05 mg/kg slow I.V. in 10-15 minutes if needed

Adolescents: 0.07 mg/kg slow I.V. over 2-5 minutes; maximum: 4 mg/dose; may repeat in 10-15 minutes

Adults: 4 mg/dose slow I.V. over 2-5 minutes; may repeat in 10-15 minutes; usual maximum dose: 8 mg

Rapid tranquilization of agitated patient (administer every 30-60 minutes):

Oral: 1-2 mg

I.M.: 0.5-1 mg

Average total dose for tranquilization: Oral, I.M.: 4-8 mg

Agitation in the ICU patient (unlabeled):

I.V.: 0.02-0.06 mg/kg every 2-6 hours

I.V. infusion: 0.01-0.1 mg/kg/hour

Monitoring Parameters Respiratory and cardiovascular status, blood pressure, heart rate, symptoms of anxiety

Administration May be administered by I.M., I.V., or orally

I.M.: Should be administered deep into the muscle mass

I.V.: Do not exceed 2 mg/minute or 0.05 mg/kg over 2-5 minutes; dilute I.V. dose with equal volume of compatible diluent (D$_5$W, NS, SWI).

Contraindications Hypersensitivity to lorazepam or any component of the formulation (cross-sensitivity with other benzodiazepines may exist); acute narrow-angle glaucoma; sleep apnea (parenteral); intra-arterial injection of parenteral formulation; severe respiratory insufficiency (except during mechanical ventilation); pregnancy

Warnings

Use with caution in elderly or debilitated patients, patients with hepatic disease (including alcoholics) or renal impairment. Use with caution in patients with respiratory disease or impaired gag reflex. Initial doses in elderly or debilitated patients should not exceed 2 mg. Prolonged lorazepam use may have a possible relationship to GI disease, including esophageal dilation.

The parenteral formulation of lorazepam contains polyethylene glycol and propylene glycol. Also contains benzyl alcohol - avoid in neonates. Concurrent administration with scopolamine results in an increased risk of hallucinations, sedation, and irrational behavior.

Causes CNS depression (dose-related) resulting in sedation, dizziness, confusion, or ataxia which may impair physical and mental capabilities. Patients must be cautioned about performing tasks which require mental alertness (eg, operating machinery or driving). Use with caution in patients receiving other CNS depressants or psychoactive agents. Effects with other sedative drugs or ethanol may be potentiated. Benzodiazepines have been associated with falls and traumatic injury and should be used with extreme caution in patients who are at risk of these events (especially the elderly).

Lorazepam may cause anterograde amnesia. Paradoxical reactions, including hyperactive or aggressive behavior have been reported with benzodiazepines, particularly in adolescent/pediatric or psychiatric patients. Does not have analgesic, antidepressant, or antipsychotic properties.

Use caution in patients with depression, particularly if suicidal risk may be present. Use with caution in patients with a history of drug dependence. Benzodiazepines have been associated with dependence and acute withdrawal symptoms on discontinuation or reduction in dose. Acute withdrawal, including seizures, may be precipitated after administration of flumazenil to patients receiving long-term benzodiazepine therapy.

As a hypnotic agent, should be used only after evaluation of potential causes of sleep disturbance. Failure of sleep disturbance to resolve after 7-10 days may indicate psychiatric or medical illness. A worsening of insomnia or the emergence of new abnormalities of thought or behavior may represent unrecognized psychiatric or medical illness and requires immediate and careful evaluation.

Dosage Forms Injection, solution (Ativan®): 2 mg/mL (1 mL, 10 mL); 4 mg/mL (1 mL, 10 mL) [contains benzyl alcohol]

Solution, oral concentrate (Lorazepam Intensol®): 2 mg/mL (30 mL) [alcohol free, dye free]

Tablet (Ativan®): 0.5 mg, 1 mg, 2 mg

Reference Range Therapeutic: Serum level: 50-240 ng/mL (SI: 156-746 nmol/L)

Overdosage/Treatment

Decontamination: Lavage (within 1 hour)/activated charcoal

Supportive therapy: Treatment for benzodiazepine overdose is supportive; rarely is mechanical ventilation required. Flumazenil (Romazicon™) has been shown to selectively block the binding of benzodiazepines to CNS receptors, resulting in a reversal of benzodiazepine-induced CNS depression. Do not use in concomitant tricyclic antidepressant ingestion; treat hypotension with isotonic crystalloids, place in Trendelenburg position or give dopamine or norepinephrine.

Enhancement of elimination: Multiple dose of activated charcoal may enhance elimination

Antidote(s)
- Flumazenil [ANTIDOTE]

Test Interactions May ↑ LFTs; Visine®, Drano®, and bleach can cause false-negative urine tests

Drug Interactions Clozapine: Benzodiazepines may enhance the adverse/toxic effect of Clozapine.

CNS depressants: Sedative effects and/or respiratory depression may be additive with CNS depressants; includes ethanol, barbiturates, narcotic analgesics, and other sedative agents; monitor for increased effect

Loxapine: There are rare reports of significant respiratory depression, stupor, and/or hypotension with concomitant use of loxapine and lorazepam; use caution if concomitant administration of loxapine and CNS drugs is required

Theophylline: May partially antagonize some of the effects of benzodiazepines; monitor for decreased response; may require higher doses for sedation

Pregnancy Risk Factor D

Pregnancy Implications Crosses the placenta; neonatal respiratory depression or hypotonia if administered near time of delivery

Lactation Enters breast milk/contraindicated (AAP rates "of concern")

Nursing Implications Keep injectable form in the refrigerator; inadvertent intra-arterial injection may produce arteriospasm resulting in gangrene which may require amputation; emergency resuscitative equipment should be available when administering by I.V.; prior to I.V. use, Ativan® injection must be diluted with an equal amount of compatible diluent; injection must be made slowly with repeated aspiration to make sure the injection is not intra-arterial and that perivascular extravasation has not occurred; provide safety measures (ie, side rails, night light, and call button); remove smoking materials from area; supervise ambulation

Additional Information Injectable form has a longer duration of action than diazepam; provides an amnestic effect, so is useful for preop and preadministration of chemotherapy; for psychotic agitation: 2 mg I.M.

With 5 mg of haloperidol I.M. may be particularly useful. **Note**: Prolonged infusions have been associated with toxicity from propylene glycol and/or polyethylene glycol.

Specific References

Clarkson JE, Gordon AM, and Logan BK, "Lorazepam and Driving Impairment," *J Anal Toxicol*, 2004, 28(6):475-80.

Dominguez KD, Crowley MR, Coleman DM, et al, "Withdrawal from Lorazepam in Critically Ill Children," *Ann Pharmacother*, 2006, 40(6):1035-9.

Honderick T, Williams D, Seaberg D, et al, "A Prospective, Randomized, Controlled Trial of Benzodiazepines and Nitroglycerine or Nitroglycerine Alone in the Treatment of Cocaine-Associated Acute Coronary Syndromes," *Am J Emerg Med*, 2003, 21(1):39-42.

Huffman JC and Stern TA, "The Use of Benzodiazepines in the Treatment of Chest Pain: A Review of the Literature," *J Emerg Med*, 2003, 25(4): 427-37.

Kent DA, Elko CJ, Gibson J, et al, "Use of Flumazenil for Lorazepam-Induced Paradoxical Reactions in Children," *J Toxicol Clin Toxicol*, 2003, 41(5):666.

Olshaker JS and Flanigan J, "Flumazenil Reversal of Lorazepam-Induced Acute Delirium," *J Emerg Med*, 2003, 24(2):181-3.

Thatcher JE, Gordon AM, and Logan BK, "Lorazepam and Driving Impairment," *J Anal Toxicol*, 2004, 28:281.

Verdel BM, Souverein PC, Egberts AG, et al, "Difference in Risks of Allergic Reaction to Sulfonamide Drugs Based on Chemical Structure," *Ann Pharmacother*, 2006, 40(6):1040-6.

Lorcainide

Related Information
- Flecainide

CAS Number 58934-46-6; 59729-31-6

Unlabeled/Investigational Use Management of ventricular/supraventricular arrhythmias

Mechanism of Action A class IC antiarrhythmic agent with similar actions as flecainide

Adverse Reactions

Cardiovascular: Bradycardia, heart block, P-R prolongation, QRS prolongation, QT$_c$ interval prolongation is minimal; worsening arrhythmias (ventricular), congestive heart failure, palpitations, chest pain, edema, cardiac arrest, hypotension, syncope, sinus bradycardia, angina, myocardial depression

Central nervous system: Dizziness, headache, sleep disturbance

Endocrine & metabolic: Hyponatremia

Miscellaneous: Diaphoresis

Signs and Symptoms of Overdose AV block, bradycardia, coma, hyponatremia, hypotension, insomnia, seizures, widened ventricular complexes

Toxicodynamics/Kinetics

Absorption: Oral: Well absorbed

Protein binding: 83%

Distribution: V$_d$: 5-10 L/kg

Metabolism: Hepatic to norlorcainide (active metabolite)

Bioavailability: 100%

Half-life: Lorcainide: 8 hours; norlorcainide: 27 hours

Elimination: Hepatic; clearance: 1500 mL/minute

Dosage

Oral: 100 mg twice daily; maximum daily oral dose: 400 mg

I.V.: Initial: 2 mg/kg with an infusion rate of 10 mg/minute under ECG control

Reference Range Serum therapeutic range: 150-400 ng/mL; serum lorcainide level of 1820 ng/mL and serum norlorcainide level of 450 ng/mL associated with fatality following an ingestion of 2.5 g

Overdosage/Treatment

Decontamination: Lavage (within 1 hour)/activated charcoal

Supportive therapy: Benzodiazepines can be used for seizure control; bradycardia or hypotension can be managed with catecholamines; cardiac pacing will probably not be effective; multiple dosing of activated charcoal may be effective

Losartan

U.S. Brand Names Cozaar®

Synonyms DuP 753; Losartan Potassium; MK594

Use Treatment of hypertension (HTN); treatment of diabetic nephropathy in patients with type 2 diabetes mellitus (noninsulin dependent, NIDDM) and a history of hypertension; stroke risk reduction in patients with HTN and left ventricular hypertrophy (LVH)

Mechanism of Action As a selective and competitive, nonpeptide angiotensin II receptor antagonist, losartan blocks the vasoconstrictor and aldosterone-secreting effects of angiotensin II; losartan interacts reversibly at the AT1 and AT2 receptors of many tissues and has slow dissociation kinetics; its affinity for the AT1 receptor is 1000 times greater than the AT2 receptor. Angiotensin II receptor antagonists may induce a more complete inhibition of the renin-angiotensin system than ACE inhibitors, they do not affect the response to bradykinin, and are less likely to be associated with nonrenin-angiotensin effects (eg, cough and angioedema). Losartan increases urinary flow rate and in addition to being natriuretic and kaliuretic, increases excretion of chloride, magnesium, uric acid, calcium, and phosphate.

Adverse Reactions

Cardiovascular: Angina, arrhythmias, AV block (second degree), bradycardia, CVA, **chest pain** (diabetic nephropathy), edema, facial edema, flushing, hypotension, orthostatic hypotension (hypertension/diabetic nephropathy), first-dose hypotension (dose-related: <1% with 50 mg, 2% with 100 mg), palpitations, syncope, tachycardia, ventricular arrhythmias, vasculitis

Central nervous system: Acute psychosis with paranoid delusions, anxiety, ataxia, confusion, depression, dizziness, **fatigue** (diabetic nephropathy), fever, headache, hypoesthesia (diabetic nephropathy), insomnia, memory impairment, MI, migraine, nervousness, sleep disorder, somnolence, vertigo

Dermatology: Alopecia, angioedema, cellulitis (diabetic nephropathy), dermatitis, dry skin, ecchymosis, erythema, Henoch-Schönlein purpura, maculopapular rash, photosensitivity, pruritus, rash, urticaria

Endocrine: Gout, hyperkalemia (hypertension/diabetic nephropathy), **hypoglycemia** (diabetic nephropathy), hyponatremia, impotence, libido decreased

Gastrointestinal: Abdominal pain, ageusia, anorexia, constipation, **diarrhea** (hypertension/diabetic nephropathy), dysgeusia, dyspepsia, flatulence, gastritis (diabetic nephropathy), nausea, pancreatitis, taste perversion, weight gain (diabetic nephropathy), vomiting, xerostomia

Genitourinary: Nocturia, **urinary tract infection** (diabetic nephropathy), urinary frequency

Hematologic: **Anemia** (diabetic nephropathy), hematocrit decreased, hemoglobin decreased, hyperkalemia

Hepatic: Bilirubin increased, hepatitis, transaminases increased

Neuromuscular & skeletal: Arm pain, arthralgia, arthritis, **back pain** (hypertension/diabetic nephropathy), hip pain, joint swelling, leg pain, muscle cramps, muscular weakness (diabetic nephropathy), knee pain (diabetic nephropathy), muscle weakness, myalgia, paresthesia, **weakness** (diabetic nephropathy), peripheral neuropathy, tremor

Ocular: Blurred vision, conjunctivitis, visual acuity decreased

Otic: Tinnitus

Renal: BUN increased, serum creatinine increased

Respiratory: Bronchitis, **cough** (diabetic nephropathy; hypertension, but similar to that associated with hydrochlorothiazide or placebo therapy), dyspnea, epistaxis, nasal congestion, pharyngitis, rhinitis, sinusitis (hypertension/diabetic nephropathy), upper respiratory infection

Miscellaneous: Allergic reaction, anaphylactic reactions, dental pain, diaphoresis, infection (diabetic nephropathy), flu-like syndrome (diabetic nephropathy)

Pharmacodynamics/Kinetics

Onset of action: 6 hours

Distribution: V_d: Losartan: 34 L; E-3174: 12 L; does not cross blood brain barrier

Protein binding, plasma: High

Metabolism: Hepatic (14%) via CYP2C9 and 3A4 to active metabolite, E-3174 (40 times more potent than losartan); extensive first-pass effect

Bioavailability: 25% to 33%; AUC of E-3174 is four times greater than that of losartan

Half-life elimination: Losartan: 1.5-2 hours; E-3174: 6-9 hours

Time to peak, serum: Losartan: 1 hour; E-3174: 3-4 hours

Excretion: Urine (4% as unchanged drug, 6% as active metabolite)
Clearance: Plasma: Losartan: 600 mL/minute; Active metabolite: 50 mL/minute

Dosage

Oral:

Hypertension:

Children 6-16 years: 0.7 mg/kg once daily (maximum: 50 mg/day); adjust dose based on response; doses >1.4 mg/kg (maximum: 100 mg) have not been studied

Adults: Usual starting dose: 50 mg once daily; can be administered once or twice daily with total daily doses ranging from 25-100 mg
Patients receiving diuretics or with intravascular volume depletion: Usual initial dose: 25 mg

Nephropathy in patients with type 2 diabetes and hypertension: Adults: Initial: 50 mg once daily; can be increased to 100 mg once daily based on blood pressure response

Stroke reduction (HTN with LVH): Adults: 50 mg once daily (maximum daily dose: 100 mg); may be used in combination with a thiazide diuretic

Dosing adjustment in renal impairment:
Children: Use is not recommended if Cl_{cr} <30 mL/minute.
Adults: No adjustment necessary.

Dosing adjustment in hepatic impairment: Reduce the initial dose to 25 mg/day; divide dosage intervals into two.

Monitoring Parameters Supine blood pressure, electrolytes, serum creatinine, BUN, urinalysis, symptomatic hypotension and tachycardia, CBC

Administration May be administered with or without food.

Contraindications Hypersensitivity to losartan or any component of the formulation; hypersensitivity to other A-II receptor antagonists; bilateral renal artery stenosis; pregnancy (2nd and 3rd trimesters)

Warnings

[U.S. Boxed Warning]: Based on human data, drugs that act on the angiotensin system can cause injury and death to the developing fetus when used in the second and third trimesters. Angiotensin receptor blockers should be discontinued as soon as possible once pregnancy is detected. Avoid use or use a smaller dose in patients who are volume depleted; correct depletion first. Deterioration in renal function can occur with initiation. May cause hyperkalemia; avoid potassium supplementation unless specifically required by healthcare provider. Use with caution in unilateral renal artery stenosis and pre-existing renal insufficiency; significant aortic/mitral stenosis. When used to reduce the risk of stroke in patients with HTN and LVH, may not be effective in the African-American population. Use caution with hepatic dysfunction, dose adjustment may be needed. Safety and efficacy in children <6 years of age have not been established.

Dosage Forms Tablet, as potassium: 25 mg, 50 mg, 100 mg

Overdosage/Treatment

Decontamination: Ipecac (within 30 minutes)/lavage (within 1 hour)/activated charcoal

Supportive therapy: Following initiation of essential overdose management, toxic symptom treatment and supportive treatment should be initiated. Hypotension usually responds to I.V. normal saline or Trendelenburg positioning. If unresponsive to these measures, the use of a parenteral inotrope may be required (eg, norepinephrine 0.1-0.2 mcg/kg/minute titrated to response). Seizures commonly respond to lorazepam or diazepam or to phenytoin or phenobarbital. Inhaled sodium cromoglycate (total dose: 40 mg/day) can decrease ACE-inhibitor cough by 50%.

Enhanced elimination: Multiple dosing of activated charcoal may be effective. Not removed via hemodialysis.

Drug Interactions **Substrate** (major) of CYP2C9, 3A4; **Inhibits** CYP1A2 (weak), 2C8 (moderate), 2C9 (moderate), 2C19 (weak), 3A4 (weak)

CYP2C9 inducers: May decrease the levels/effects of losartan. Example inducers include carbamazepine, phenobarbital, phenytoin, rifampin, rifapentine, and secobarbital.

CYP2C8 Substrates: Losartan may increase the levels/effects of CYP2C8 substrates. Example substrates include amiodarone, paclitaxel, pioglitazone, repaglinide, and rosiglitazone.

CYP2C9 Substrates: Losartan may increase the levels/effects of CYP2C9 substrates. Example substrates include bosentan, dapsone, fluoxetine, glimepiride, glipizide, montelukast, nateglinide, paclitaxel, phenytoin, warfarin, and zafirlukast.

CYP3A4 inducers: CYP3A4 inducers may decrease the levels/effects of losartan. Example inducers include aminoglutethimide, carbamazepine, nafcillin, nevirapine, phenobarbital, phenytoin, and rifamycins.

Fluconazole: Increases plasma levels of losartan via 2C8/9 inhibition (decreases the plasma levels of the active metabolite). Monitor for increased losartan efficacy.

Lithium: Risk of toxicity may be increased by losartan; monitor lithium levels.

NSAIDs: May decrease angiotensin II antagonist efficacy; effect has been seen with losartan, but may occur with other medications in this class; monitor blood pressure

Potassium-sparing diuretics (amiloride, potassium, spironolactone, triamterene): Increased risk of hyperkalemia.

Potassium supplements may increase the risk of hyperkalemia.

Rifampin may reduce antihypertensive efficacy of losartan.

Trimethoprim (high dose) may increase the risk of hyperkalemia.

Pregnancy Risk Factor C/D (2nd and 3rd trimesters)

Pregnancy Implications Discontinue as soon as possible when pregnancy is detected. Drugs which act directly on renin-angiotensin can cause fetal and neonatal morbidity and death.

Lactation Excretion in breast milk unknown/not recommended

Additional Information Maximal antihypertensive effect seen in 3-6 weeks; lowers serum uric acid levels

Specific References

Lindholm LH, Dahlöf B, Edelman JM, et al, "Effect of Losartan on Sudden Cardiac Death in People with Diabetes: Data from the LIFE Study," *Lancet*, 2003, 362(9384):619-20.

Lovastatin

CAS Number 75330-75-5
U.S. Brand Names Altocor™; Mevacor®
Synonyms Mevinolin; Monacolin K
Use

Adjunct to dietary therapy to decrease elevated serum total and LDL-cholesterol concentrations in primary hypercholesterolemia

Primary prevention of coronary artery disease (patients without symptomatic disease with average to moderately elevated total and LDL-cholesterol and below average HDL-cholesterol); slow progression of coronary atherosclerosis in patients with coronary heart disease

Adjunct to dietary therapy in adolescent patients (10-17 years of age, females >1 year post-menarche) with heterozygous familial hypercholesterolemia having LDL >189 mg/dL, **or** LDL >160 mg/dL with positive family history of premature cardiovascular disease (CVD), **or** LDL >160 mg/dL with the presence of at least two other CVD risk factors

Mechanism of Action Lovastatin acts by competitively inhibiting 3-hydroxyl-3-methylglutaryl-coenzyme A (HMG-CoA) reductase, the enzyme that catalyzes the rate-limiting step in cholesterol biosynthesis

Adverse Reactions

Cardiovascular: Chest pain

Central nervous system: Headache, dizziness, insomnia

Dermatologic: Alopecia, pruritus, dermatomyositis, rash

Gastrointestinal: Abdominal pain, acid regurgitation, constipation, diarrhea, dyspepsia, flatulence, nausea, xerostomia, vomiting

Neuromuscular & skeletal: **Increased CPK** (>2x normal), myalgia, weakness, muscle cramps, leg pain, arthralgia, paresthesia

Ocular: Blurred vision, eye irritation

Note: Additional class-related events or case reports (not necessarily reported with lovastatin therapy):

Cardiovascular: Angioedema, flushing, vasculitis

Central nervous system: Anxiety, chills, depression, fever, malaise, memory loss, psychic disturbance, vertigo

Dermatologic: Dryness of skin/mucous membranes, erythema multiforme, nail changes, nodules, photosensitivity, skin discoloration, Stevens-Johnson syndrome, toxic epidermal necrolysis, urticaria

Endocrine & metabolic: Decreased libido, erectile dysfunction, gynecomastia, impotence, thyroid dysfunction

Gastrointestinal: Alteration in taste, anorexia, pancreatitis

Hematologic: Eosinophilia, hemolytic anemia, leukopenia, thrombocytopenia, purpura

Hepatic: Alkaline phosphatase increased, cholestatic jaundice, cirrhosis, elevated transaminases, fatty liver, fulminant hepatic necrosis, hepatitis, hepatoma, hyperbilirubinemia, increased GGT

Neuromuscular & skeletal: Arthritis, facial paresis, increased CPK (>10x normal), myopathy, peripheral nerve palsy, peripheral neuropathy, polymyalgia rheumatica, rhabdomyolysis, tremor

Renal: Renal failure (secondary to rhabdomyolysis)

Ocular: Cataracts, impaired extraocular muscle movement, ophthalmoplegia

Respiratory: Dyspnea

Miscellaneous: Anaphylaxis, hypersensitivity reaction, increased ESR, positive ANA, systemic lupus erythematosus-like syndrome

Signs and Symptoms of Overdose Cholestatic jaundice, dyspepsia, gynecomastia, hyperthermia, myalgia, myoglobinuria, rhabdomyolysis

Admission Criteria/Prognosis Admit any ingestion >200 mg or admit any symptomatic patient

Pharmacodynamics/Kinetics

Onset of action: LDL-cholesterol reductions: 3 days

Absorption: 30%; increased with extended release tablets when taken in the fasting state

Protein binding: 95%

Metabolism: Hepatic; extensive first-pass effect; hydrolyzed to B-hydroxy acid (active)

Bioavailability: Increased with extended release tablets

Half-life elimination: 1.1-1.7 hours

Time to peak, serum: 2-4 hours

Excretion: Feces (~80% to 85%); urine (10%)

Dosage

Oral:

Adolescents 10-17 years: Immediate release tablet:

LDL reduction <20%: Initial: 10 mg/day with evening meal

LDL reduction ≥20%: Initial: 20 mg/day with evening meal

Usual range: 10-40 mg with evening meal, then adjust dose at 4-week intervals

Adults: Initial: 20 mg with evening meal, then adjust at 4-week intervals; maximum dose: 80 mg/day immediate release tablet **or** 60 mg/day extended release tablet; before initiation of therapy, patients should be placed on a standard cholesterol-lowering diet for 3-6 months and the diet should be continued during drug therapy. Patients receiving immunosuppressant drugs should start at 10 mg/day and not exceed 20 mg/day. Patients receiving concurrent therapy with fibrates should not exceed 20 mg lovastatin. Patients receiving amiodarone, niacin, or verapamil should not exceed 40 mg lovastatin daily.

Monitoring Parameters Obtain baseline LFTs and total cholesterol profile. LFTs should be performed before initiation of therapy, at 6- and 12 weeks after initiation or first dose, and periodically thereafter.

Administration Administer immediate release tablet with meals. Administer extended release tablet at bedtime; do not crush or chew.

Contraindications Hypersensitivity to lovastatin or any component of the formulation; active liver disease; unexplained persistent elevations of serum transaminases; pregnancy; breast-feeding

Warnings Liver function tests should be assessed before initiation of therapy in patients with a history of liver disease, prior to upwards dosage adjustment to ≥40 mg daily or when otherwise indicated; enzyme levels should be followed periodically thereafter as clinically warranted. Rhabdomyolysis with or without acute renal failure has occurred. Risk is dose-related and is increased with concurrent use of lipid-lowering agents which may cause rhabdomyolysis (gemfibrozil, fibric acid derivatives, or niacin at doses ≥1 g/day) or during concurrent use with potent CYP3A4 inhibitors. Avoid concurrent use of azole antifungals, macrolide antibiotics, and protease inhibitors. Use caution/limit dose with amiodarone, cyclosporine, danazol, gemfibrozil (or other fibrates), lipid-lowering doses of niacin, or verapamil. Patients should be instructed to report unexplained muscle pain or weakness; lovastatin should be discontinued if myopathy is suspected/confirmed. Temporarily discontinue in any patient experiencing an acute or serious condition predisposing to renal failure secondary to rhabdomyolysis. Use with caution in patients who consume large amounts of ethanol or have a history of liver disease. Safety and efficacy of the immediate release tablet have not been evaluated in prepubertal patients, patients <10 years of age, or doses >40 mg/day in appropriately-selected adolescents; extended release tablets have not been studied in patients <20 years of age.

Dosage Forms Tablet: 10 mg, 20 mg, 40 mg

Mevacor®: 20 mg, 40 mg

Tablet, extended release:

Altoprev®: 20 mg, 40 mg, 60 mg

Reference Range NCEP classification of pediatric patients with familial history of hypercholesterolemia or premature CVD: Acceptable total cholesterol: <170 mg/dL, LDL: <110 mg/dL

Overdosage/Treatment

Decontamination: Ipecac (within 30 minutes)/lavage (within 1 hour)/activated charcoal

Supportive therapy: If rhabdomyolysis occurs, alkaline diuresis (with sodium bicarbonate) and diuretics (mannitol preferably with furosemide as a second choice) in order to maintain urine flow may be needed

Test Interactions ↑ liver transaminases (S), HDL cholesterol, CPK; ↓ VLDL and LDL levels

Drug Interactions **Substrate** of CYP3A4 (major); **Inhibits** CYP2C9 (weak), 2D6 (weak), 3A4 (weak)

Amiodarone: Inhibits metabolism of lovastatin and may increase lovastatin-induced myopathy and rhabdomyolysis. Concurrent use is not recommended, but if unavoidable, dose of lovastatin should be limited.

Antacids: Plasma concentrations may be decreased when given with magnesium-aluminum hydroxide containing antacids (reported with atorvastatin and pravastatin). Clinical efficacy is not altered, no dosage adjustment is necessary

Azole antifungals: May decrease the metabolism, via CYP isoenzymes, of HMG-CoA reductase inhibitors and may increase risk of lovastatin-induced myopathy and rhabdomyolysis. Avoid concurrent use.

Cholestyramine reduces absorption of several HMG-CoA reductase inhibitors. Separate administration times by at least 4 hours.

Cholestyramine and colestipol (bile acid sequestrants): Cholesterol-lowering effects are additive.

Clofibrate and fenofibrate may increase the risk of myopathy and rhabdomyolysis; limit dose of lovastatin

Cyclosporine: Concurrent use may increase risk of myopathy; limit dose of lovastatin

CYP3A4 inhibitors: May increase the levels/effects of lovastatin. Example inhibitors include azole antifungals, clarithromycin, diclofenac, doxycycline, erythromycin, imatinib, isoniazid, nefazodone, nicardipine, propofol, protease inhibitors, quinidine, telithromycin, and verapamil. Avoid concurrent use.

Danazol: Concurrent use may increase risk of myopathy; limit dose of lovastatin.

Gemfibrozil: Increased risk of myopathy and rhabdomyolysis; limit dose of lovastatin

Grapefruit juice may inhibit metabolism of lovastatin via CYP3A4; avoid high dietary intakes of grapefruit juice.

Isradipine may decrease lovastatin blood levels.

Macrolide antibiotics: May decrease the metabolism, via CYP isoenzymes, of HMG-CoA reductase inhibitors and may increase risk of lovastatin-induced myopathy and rhabdomyolysis. Avoid concurrent use.

Nefazodone: May decrease the metabolism, via CYP isoenzymes, of HMG-CoA reductase inhibitors and may increase risk of lovastatin-induced myopathy and rhabdomyolysis. Avoid concurrent use.

Niacin (at higher dosages $\geq$ 1 g/day) may increase risk of myopathy and rhabdomyolysis; limit dose of lovastatin

Protease inhibitors: Concurrent use increases the risk of myopathy and rhabdomyolysis; concurrent use should be avoided.

Verapamil: Inhibits metabolism of lovastatin and may increase lovastatin-induced myopathy and rhabdomyolysis. Concurrent use is not recommended, but if unavoidable, dose of lovastatin should be limited.

Warfarin effect (hypoprothrombinemic response) may be increased; monitor INR closely when lovastatin is initiated or discontinued.

Pregnancy Risk Factor X

Pregnancy Implications Interferes with fetal steroid synthesis. Congenital abnormalities (VATER) have been associated with 1st trimester use. A case of bone deformity, tracheoesophageal fistula, and anal atresia has been noted in a fetus after first-trimester use of lovastatin and dextroamphetamine.

Lactation Excretion unknown/contraindicated

Nursing Implications Administer with meals, urge patient to adhere to cholesterol-lowering diet

Additional Information Before initiation of therapy, patients should be placed on a standard cholesterol-lowering diet for 6 weeks and the diet should be continued during drug therapy. Average length of time to development of rhabdomyolysis is one year; with an addition of a fibrate, the average time is about 32 days. Muscle pain (88%) or fatigue (74%) are the two most prominent symptoms in statin-induced rhabdomyolysis.

Specific References

Antons KA, Williams CD, Baker SK, et al, "Clinical Perspectives of Statin-Induced Rhabdomyolysis," *Am J Med*, 2006, 119):400-9.

Chan J, Hui RL, and Levin E, "Differential Association Between Statin Exposure and Elevated Levels of Creatine Kinase," *Ann Pharmacother*, 2005, 39(10):1611-6.

de Andrade Nishioka S and Guedes LQ, "Possible Lovastatin-Induced Fatal Necrotizing Pancreatitis," *J Pharm Technol*, 2003, 19:283-6.

Mukamal KJ, Smith CC, Karlamangla AS, et al, "Moderate Alcohol Consumption and Safety of Lovastatin and Warfarin Among Men: The Postcoronary Artery Bypass Graft Trial," *A, J Med*, 2006, 119:434-40.

Loxapine

Related Information
- Anticholinergic Effects of Common Psychotropics
- Antipsychotic Agents

CAS Number 27833-64-3

U.S. Brand Names Loxitane® C; Loxitane®

Synonyms Loxapine Succinate; Oxilapine Succinate

Impairment Potential Yes

Use Management of psychotic disorders

Mechanism of Action Unclear mechanism of action; a dibenzoxazepine thought to be similar to chlorpromazine

Adverse Reactions

Cardiovascular: **Hypotension (orthostatic)**, tachycardia, cardiac arrhythmias; abnormal T-waves with prolonged ventricular repolarization, severe hypotension, arrhythmias, flutter (atrial), fibrillation (atrial)

Central nervous system: **drowsiness, extrapyramidal reactions, pseudoparkinsonian signs and symptoms, tardive dyskinesia, confusion**, CNS depression, fever, sedation, restlessness, anxiety, psychosis, dystonic reactions, seizures, altered central temperature regulation, neuroleptic malignant syndrome, hyperthermia

Dermatologic: Hyperpigmentation, pruritus, rash, photosensitivity, alopecia, urticaria, purpura, exanthem

Endocrine & metabolic: Amenorrhea, galactorrhea, gynecomastia, syndrome of inappropriate antidiuretic hormone, sexual dysfunction

Gastrointestinal: **Xerostomia** (problem with denture users), adynamic ileus, constipation, GI upset, nausea, weight gain

Genitourinary: Urinary retention, overflow incontinence, priapism

Hematologic: Agranulocytosis (more often in women between fourth and tenth weeks of therapy), leukopenia (usually in patients with large doses for prolonged periods)

Hepatic: Cholestatic jaundice

Neuromuscular & skeletal: Paresthesia

Ocular: **Blurred vision**, retinal pigmentation

Miscellaneous: Systemic lupus erythematosus

Signs and Symptoms of Overdose Agitation, agranulocytosis, arrhythmias, CNS depression, deep sleep, dysphagia, dystonic reactions, extrapyramidal reaction, granulocytopenia, gynecomastia, hypertension followed by hypotension, hypothermia, leukocytosis, leukopenia, myoglobinuria, neuroleptic malignant syndrome, neutropenia, Parkinson's-like symptoms, ptosis, renal failure (acute), rhabdomyolysis, seizures, sinus tachycardia, syncope

Pharmacodynamics/Kinetics

Onset of action: Neuroleptic: Oral: 20-30 minutes

Peak effect: 1.5-3 hours

Duration: ~12 hours

Metabolism: Hepatic to glucuronide conjugates

Half-life elimination: Biphasic: Initial: 5 hours; Terminal: 12-19 hours

Excretion: Urine; feces (small amounts)

Dosage

Adults:

Oral: 10 mg twice daily, increase dose until psychotic symptoms are controlled; usual dose range: 60-100 mg/day in divided doses 2-4 times/day; dosages >250 mg/day are not recommended

I.M.: 12.5-50 mg every 4-6 hours or longer as needed and change to oral therapy as soon as possible

Monitoring Parameters Vital signs; lipid profile, fasting blood glucose/Hgb A_{1c}; BMI; mental status, abnormal involuntary movement scale (AIMS), extrapyramidal symptoms (EPS)

Contraindications Hypersensitivity to loxapine or any component of the formulation; severe CNS depression; coma

Warnings

May cause hypotension. Moderately sedating, use with caution in disorders where CNS depression is a feature. Use with caution in Parkinson's disease. Caution in patients with hemodynamic instability; bone marrow suppression; predisposition to seizures; subcortical brain damage; severe cardiac, hepatic, renal or respiratory disease. Esophageal dysmotility and aspiration have been associated with antipsychotic use - use with caution in patients at risk of pneumonia (ie, Alzheimer's disease). Caution in breast cancer or other prolactin-dependent tumors (may elevate prolactin levels). May alter temperature regulation or mask toxicity of other drugs due to antiemetic effects. May alter cardiac conduction; life-threatening arrhythmias have occurred with therapeutic doses of phenothiazines. May cause orthostatic hypotension - use with caution in patients at risk of this effect or those who would tolerate transient hypotensive episodes (cerebrovascular disease, cardiovascular disease, or other medications which may predispose). Safety and effectiveness of loxapine in pediatric patients have not been established.

Phenothiazines may cause anticholinergic effects (confusion, agitation, constipation, xerostomia, blurred vision, urinary retention); therefore, they should be used with caution in patients with decreased gastrointestinal motility, urinary retention, BPH, xerostomia, or visual problems. Conditions which also may be exacerbated by cholinergic blockade include narrow-angle glaucoma (screening is recommended) and worsening of myasthenia gravis. Relative to other antipsychotics, loxapine has a low potency of cholinergic blockade.

May cause extrapyramidal symptoms, including pseudoparkinsonism, acute dystonic reactions, akathisia, and tardive dyskinesia (risk of these reactions is moderate-high relative to other neuroleptics). May be associated with neuroleptic malignant syndrome (NMS) or pigmentary retinopathy.

Dosage Forms Capsule, as succinate: 5 mg, 10 mg, 25 mg, 50 mg

Reference Range Plasma loxapine level of 0.2 mg/L associated with stupor. Postmortem blood loxapine levels due to loxapine fatalities range from 1.2-9.5 mg/L.

Overdosage/Treatment

Decontamination: Lavage (within 1 hour)/activated charcoal

Supportive therapy: Hypotension usually responds to I.V. fluids or Trendelenburg positioning. If unresponsive to these measures, the use of a parenteral inotrope may be required (eg, norepinephrine 0.1-0.2 mcg/kg/minute titrated to response). Seizures commonly respond to lorazepam or diazepam (I.V. 5-10 mg bolus in adults every 15 minutes if needed up to a total of 30 mg; I.V. 0.25-0.4 mg/kg/dose up to a total of 10 mg in children) or to phenytoin or phenobarbital. Also critical cardiac arrhythmias often respond to I.V. phenytoin (15 mg/kg up to 1 gram), while other antiarrhythmics can be used. Neuroleptics often cause extrapyramidal reaction (eg, dystonic reactions) requiring management with diphenhydramine 1-2 mg/kg (adults) up to a maximum of 50 mg I.M. or I.V. slow push followed by a maintenance dose for 48-72 hours. When these reactions are unresponsive to diphenhydramine, benztropine mesylate I.V. 1-2 mg (adults) may be effective. These agents are generally effective within 2-5 minutes.

Enhancement of elimination: Multiple dosing of activated charcoal would not be expected to be useful

Test Interactions Increases glucose, increases plasma norepinephrine levels and epinephrine levels threefold to fivefold; false-positives for phenylketonuria, amylase, uroporphyrins, urobilinogen; EMIT assays may be false-positive in the presence of diphenhydramine, thioridazine, chlorpromazine, alimenazine, carbamazepine, cyclobenzaprine, or perphenazine

Drug Interactions

Acetylcholinesterase inhibitors (central): May increase the risk of antipsychotic-related extrapyramidal symptoms; monitor.

Aluminum salts: May decrease the absorption of antipsychotics; monitor

Amphetamines: Efficacy may be diminished by antipsychotics; in addition, amphetamines may increase psychotic symptoms; avoid concurrent use

Anticholinergics: May inhibit the therapeutic response to antipsychotics and excess anticholinergic effects may occur; includes benztropine, trihexyphenidyl, biperiden, and drugs with significant anticholinergic activity (TCAs, antihistamines, disopyramide)

Antihypertensives: Concurrent use of antipsychotics with an antihypertensive may produce additive hypotensive effects (particularly orthostasis)

Bromocriptine: Antipsychotics inhibit the ability of bromocriptine to lower serum prolactin concentrations

CNS depressants: Sedative effects may be additive with antipsychotics; monitor for increased effect; includes barbiturates, benzodiazepines, narcotic analgesics, ethanol, and other sedative agents

Epinephrine: Chlorpromazine (and possibly other low potency antipsychotics) may diminish the pressor effects of epinephrine

Guanethidine and guanadrel: Antihypertensive effects may be inhibited by antipsychotics

Levodopa: Antipsychotics may inhibit the antiparkinsonian effect of levodopa; avoid this combination

Lithium: Antipsychotics may produce neurotoxicity with lithium; this is a rare effect

Metoclopramide: May increase extrapyramidal symptoms (EPS) or risk.

Phenytoin: May reduce serum levels of antipsychotics; antipsychotics may increase phenytoin serum levels

Propranolol: Serum concentrations of antipsychotics may be increased; propranolol also increases antipsychotic concentrations

QT_c-prolonging agents: Effects on QT_c interval may be additive with antipsychotics, increasing the risk of malignant arrhythmias. Other QT_c-prolonging agents include type Ia antiarrhythmics, TCAs, and some quinolone antibiotics (sparfloxacin, moxifloxacin and gatifloxacin). Concomitant use with thioridazine is contraindicated.

Sulfadoxine-pyrimethamine: May increase antipsychotic concentrations

Tricyclic antidepressants: Concurrent use may produce increased toxicity or altered therapeutic response

Trazodone: Antipsychotics and trazodone may produce additive hypotensive effects

Valproic acid: Serum levels may be increased by antipsychotics

Pregnancy Risk Factor C

Pregnancy Implications Crosses placenta

Lactation Excretion in breast milk unknown/not recommended

Nursing Implications Injectable is for I.M. use only

Specific References

Moore KA, Levine B, Korell M, et al, "An Unusual Loxapine Intoxication," *J Anal Toxicol*, 2004, 28:300.

Malathion (Topical Lotion)

CAS Number 121-75-5

UN Number 2783

U.S. Brand Names Ovide®

Use Treatment of head lice and their ova (pediculosis)

Mechanism of Action A dimethoxy organophosphate insecticide with inherent toxicity

Adverse Reactions

Cardiovascular: Bradycardia, AV block, sinus bradycardia

Central nervous system: Anxiety, clumsiness, confusion, dizziness, drowsiness, seizures

Dermatologic: Contact dermatitis, irritation of scalp

Gastrointestinal: Abdominal cramps, diarrhea

Ocular: Nystagmus

Renal: Acute renal insufficiency

Signs and Symptoms of Overdose Paresthesia

Dosage Sprinkle Ovide™ lotion on dry hair and rub gently until the scalp is thoroughly moistened; pay special attention to the back of the head and neck. Allow to dry naturally - use no heat and leave uncovered. After 8-12 hours, the hair should be washed with a nonmedicated shampoo; rinse and use a fine-toothed comb to remove dead lice and eggs. If required, repeat with second application in 7-9 days. Further treatment is generally not necessary. Other family members should be evaluated to determine if infested and if so, receive treatment.

Overdosage/Treatment

Decontamination: Isolation, bagging, and disposal of all contaminated clothing and other articles; all emergency medical workers and hospital staff should follow appropriate precautions regarding exposure to hazardous material including the use of protective clothing, masks, goggles,and respiratory equipment

Dermal: Prompt thorough scrubbing of all affected areas with soap and water, including hair and nails

Gastric: Activated charcoal can be administered either orally or via a nasogastric tube; do not induce emesis because of danger of sudden respiratory compromise, alterations in mental status, seizures, coma, and possible aspiration of hydrocarbon vehicles; do not use any cathartic

Ocular: Irrigation with copious tepid sterile water or saline

Supportive therapy: Including airway management, ventilatory assistance, humidified oxygen administration, and close monitoring for sudden respiratory failure

Enhancement of elimination: Dialysis and hemoperfusion is not indicated due to effectiveness of the prescribed antidotal treatment and large volume of distribution of organophosphates

Antidote:

Atropine: Administration should be guided by respiratory status, starting at 2-5 mg I.V. every 5-10 minutes as needed and should be titrated to the resolution of excess pulmonary secretions; frequent administration of large doses (cumulative doses >100 mg) may be necessary in massive exposures

Glycopyrrolate: May be administered if atropine is unavailable at $\sim^1/_2$ the atropine dose

2-PAM: For more significant exposures (ie, exposures requiring large doses of atropine, or with recurring symptoms, or exposures to more lipid soluble agents), administration should follow: 1-2 g I.V. over 10-30 minutes, repeated in 1 hour if asthenia recurs, then every 4-12 hours for recurring symptoms

Antidote(s)

- Atropine [ANTIDOTE]
- Pralidoxime [ANTIDOTE]

Pregnancy Risk Factor B

Additional Information Contains 78% isopropyl alcohol

Maprotiline

Related Information

- Anticholinergic Effects of Common Psychotropics
- Therapeutic Drugs Associated with Hallucinations

CAS Number 10262-69-8; 10347-81-6

Synonyms Ludiomil; Maprotiline Hydrochloride

Impairment Potential Yes

Use Treatment of depression and anxiety associated with depression

Unlabeled/Investigational Use Bulimia; duodenal ulcers; enuresis; urinary symptoms of multiple sclerosis; pain; panic attacks; tension headache; cocaine withdrawal

Mechanism of Action Increases the synaptic concentration of serotonin and/or norepinephrine in the central nervous system by inhibition of their reuptake by the presynaptic neuronal membrane

Adverse Reactions

Cardiovascular: **Hypotension (orthostatic)**, heart block, tachycardia, torsade de pointes, sinus bradycardia, QRS prolongation

Central nervous system: **Drowsiness**, convulsions (dose-dependent), sedation, hand hypotonia, psychosis, dizziness, visual hallucinations, fever, hyperthermia

Dermatologic: **Rash**, cutaneous vasculitis

Endocrine & metabolic: Syndrome of inappropriate antidiuretic hormone

Gastrointestinal: **Extreme xerostomia**, constipation, increased appetite, weight gain

Genitourinary: **Urinary retention**

Hematologic: Leukocytosis, thrombocytopenia

Hepatic: Elevated liver function tests

Neuromuscular & skeletal: **Weakness**, tremor, clonus, myoclonus

Ocular: Blurred vision, increased intraocular pressure

Otic: Ototoxicity, tinnitus

Respiratory: Aspiration

Signs and Symptoms of Overdose Agitation, agranulocytosis, AV block, bradycardia, confusion, delirium, dental erosion, eosinophilia, granulocytopenia, hypnopompic hallucinations, hypotension, hypothermia, increased intraocular pressure, leukopenia, mania, neutropenia, photosensitivity, QT prolongation, respiratory depression, seizures, tachycardia, torsade de pointes, urinary retention, vasculitis

Pharmacodynamics/Kinetics

Absorption: Slow

Protein binding: 88%

Metabolism: Hepatic to active and inactive compounds

Half-life elimination, serum: 27-58 hours (mean: 43 hours)

Time to peak, serum: Within 12 hours

Excretion: Urine (70%); feces (30%)

Dosage

Oral:

Children 6-14 years: 10 mg/day, increase to a maximum daily dose of 75 mg

Adults: 75 mg/day to start, increase by 25 mg every 2 weeks up to 150-225 mg/day; given in 3 divided doses or in a single daily dose

Monitoring Parameters Monitor blood pressure and pulse rate prior to and during initial therapy; evaluate mood and somatic complaints; monitor appetite and weight; ECG in older adults

Contraindications Hypersensitivity to maprotiline or any component of the formulation; use of MAO inhibitors within 14 days; use in a patient during the acute recovery phase of MI

Warnings

[U.S. Boxed Warning]: Antidepressants increase the risk of suicidal thinking and behavior in children and adolescents with major depressive disorder (MDD) and other depressive disorders; consider risk prior to prescribing. Closely monitor for clinical worsening, suicidality, or unusual changes in behavior; the child's family or caregiver should be instructed to closely observe the patient and communicate condition with healthcare provider. Such observation would generally include at least weekly face-to-face contact with patients or their family members or caregivers during the first 4 weeks of treatment, then every other week visits for the next 4 weeks, then at 12 weeks, and as clinically indicated beyond 12 weeks. Additional contact by telephone may be appropriate between face-to-face visits. Adults treated with antidepressants should be observed similarly for clinical worsening and suicidality, especially during the initial few months of a course of drug therapy, or at times of dose changes, either increases or decreases. A medication guide should be dispensed with each prescription. **Maprotiline is not FDA approved for use in children.**

The possibility of a suicide attempt is inherent in major depression and may persist until remission occurs. Monitor for worsening of depression or suicidality, especially during initiation of therapy or with dose increases or decreases. Worsening depression and severe abrupt suicidality that are not part of the presenting symptoms may require discontinuation or modification of drug therapy. Use caution in high-risk patients during initiation of therapy. Prescriptions should be written for the smallest quantity consistent with good patient care. The patient's family or caregiver should be alerted to monitor patients for the emergence of suicidality and associated behaviors such as anxiety, agitation, panic attacks, insomnia, irritability, hostility, impulsivity, akathisia, hypomania, and mania; patients should be instructed to notify their healthcare provider if any of these symptoms or worsening depression occur.

May worsen psychosis in some patients or precipitate a shift to mania or hypomania in patients with bipolar disorder. Monotherapy in patients with bipolar disorder should be avoided. Patients presenting with depressive symptoms should be screened for bipolar disorder. **Maprotiline is not FDA approved for the treatment of bipolar depression.**

May cause sedation, resulting in impaired performance of tasks requiring alertness (eg, operating machinery or driving). Sedative effects may be additive with other CNS depressants and/or ethanol. The degree of sedation is high relative to other antidepressants. May increase the risks associated with electroconvulsive therapy. Consider discontinuing, when possible, prior to elective surgery. Therapy should not be abruptly discontinued in patients receiving high doses for prolonged periods.

May cause orthostatic hypotension (risk is moderate relative to other antidepressants) - use with caution in patients at risk of hypotension or in patients where transient hypotensive episodes would be poorly tolerated (cardiovascular disease or cerebrovascular disease). The degree of anticholinergic blockade produced by this agent is moderate relative to other cyclic antidepressants, however, caution should still be used in patients with urinary retention, benign prostatic hyperplasia, narrow-angle glaucoma, xerostomia, visual problems, constipation, or history of bowel obstruction.

Use with caution in patients with a history of cardiovascular disease (including previous MI, stroke, tachycardia, or conduction abnormalities). The risk conduction abnormalities with this agent is moderate relative to other antidepressants. Use caution in patients with a previous seizure disorder or condition predisposing to seizures such as brain damage, alcoholism, or concurrent therapy with other drugs which lower the seizure threshold. Use with caution in hyperthyroid patients or those receiving thyroid supplementation. Use with caution in patients with hepatic or renal dysfunction and in elderly patients.

Dosage Forms Tablet, as hydrochloride: 25 mg, 50 mg, 75 mg

Reference Range

Therapeutic: 100-150 ng/mL (SI: 361-540 nmol/L); levels >237 ng/mL can be associated with seizures

In the postmortem state, anatomical site concentration differences (ie, postmortem redistribution) may occur.

Overdosage/Treatment

Decontamination: Emesis is contraindicated, lavage (within 1 hour)/activated charcoal can be useful; multiple dosing of activated charcoal may be useful

Supportive therapy: Following initiation of essential overdose management, toxic symptoms should be treated. Ventricular arrhythmias may respond to systemic alkalinization (sodium bicarbonate 0.5-2 mEq/kg I.V.). Arrhythmias unresponsive to this therapy may respond to lidocaine 1 mg/kg I.V. followed by a titrated infusion. Seizures usually respond to benzodiazepines. If seizures are unresponsive or recur, phenytoin or phenobarbital may be required. For hypotension, isotonic saline is effective; norepinephrine (adults: 8-12 mcg/minute or children 0.1-0.2 mcg/kg/minute) is most effective pressor.

Antidote(s)

- Sodium Bicarbonate [ANTIDOTE]

Drug Interactions Substrate of CYP2D6 (major)

Altretamine: Concurrent use may cause orthostatic hypertension

Amphetamines: Cyclic antidepressants may enhance the effect of amphetamines; monitor for adverse CV effects

Anticholinergics: Combined use with cyclic antidepressants may produce additive anticholinergic effects

Antihypertensives: Cyclic antidepressants may inhibit the antihypertensive response to bethanidine, clonidine, debrisoquin, guanadrel, guanethidine, guanabenz, guanfacine; monitor BP; consider alternate antihypertensive agent

Beta-agonists: When combined with cyclic antidepressants may predispose patients to cardiac arrhythmias

Bupropion: May increase the levels of cyclic antidepressants; based on limited information; monitor response

Carbamazepine: Cyclic antidepressants may increase carbamazepine levels; monitor

Cholestyramine and colestipol: May bind cyclic antidepressants and reduce their absorption; monitor for altered response

Clonidine: Abrupt discontinuation of clonidine may cause hypertensive crisis, cyclic antidepressants may enhance the response

CNS depressants: Sedative effects may be additive with cyclic antidepressants; monitor for increased effect; includes benzodiazepines, barbiturates, antipsychotics, ethanol and other sedative medications

CYP2D6 inhibitors: May increase the levels/effects of maprotiline. Example inhibitors include chlorpromazine, delavirdine, fluoxetine, miconazole, paroxetine, pergolide, quinidine, quinine, ritonavir, and ropinirole.

Epinephrine (and other direct alpha-agonists): The pressor response to I.V. epinephrine, norepinephrine, and phenylephrine may be enhanced in patients receiving cyclic antidepressants; this combination is best avoided

Fenfluramine: May increase cyclic antidepressant levels/effects

Hypoglycemic agents (including insulin): Hypoglycemic effects may be enhanced, profound hypoglycemia has been reported; monitor for changes in blood glucose levels; reported with chlorpropamide, tolazamide, and insulin

Levodopa: Cyclic antidepressants may decrease the absorption (bioavailability) of levodopa; rare hypertensive episodes have also been attributed to this combination

Linezolid: Hyperpyrexia, hypertension, tachycardia, confusion, seizures, and **deaths have been reported** with agents which inhibit MAO (serotonin syndrome); this combination should be avoided

Lithium: Concurrent use with a cyclic antidepressant may increase the risk for neurotoxicity

MAO inhibitors: Hyperpyrexia, hypertension, tachycardia, confusion, seizures, and **deaths have been reported** (serotonin syndrome); this combination should be avoided

Methylphenidate: Metabolism of maprotiline may be decreased

Phenothiazines: Serum concentrations of some TCAs may be increased; in addition, TCAs may increase concentration of phenothiazines; monitor for altered clinical response

QT$_c$-prolonging agents: Concurrent use of cyclic agents with other drugs which may prolong QT$_c$ interval may increase the risk of potentially fatal arrhythmias; includes type Ia and type III antiarrhythmics agents, selected quinolones (sparfloxacin, gatifloxacin, moxifloxacin, grepafloxacin), cisapride, and other agents

Sucralfate: Absorption of cyclic antidepressants may be reduced with coadministration.

Sympathomimetics, indirect-acting: Cyclic antidepressants may result in a decreased sensitivity to indirect-acting sympathomimetics; includes dopamine and ephedrine; also see interaction with epinephrine (and direct-acting sympathomimetics)

Tramadol: Tramadol's risk of seizures may be increased with TCAs

Valproic acid: May increase serum concentrations/adverse effects of some cyclic antidepressants

Warfarin (and other oral anticoagulants): Cyclic antidepressants may increase the anticoagulant effect in patients stabilized on warfarin; monitor INR

Pregnancy Risk Factor B

Nursing Implications Monitor blood pressure and pulse rate prior to and during initial therapy; evaluate mental status; monitor weight, may increase appetite and possibly a craving for sweets

Additional Information Odorless, bitter tasting; seizures rarely seen 5-30 hours postdrug ingestion

Mecamylamine

Pronunciation (mek a MIL a meen)

CAS Number 60-40-2; 826-39-1

U.S. Brand Names Inversine®

Synonyms Mecamylamine Hydrochloride

Use Treatment of moderately severe to severe hypertension and in uncomplicated malignant hypertension

Unlabeled/Investigational Use Tourette's syndrome

Mechanism of Action Mecamylamine is a ganglionic blocker. This agent inhibits acetylcholine at the autonomic ganglia, causing a decrease in blood pressure. Mecamylamine also blocks central nicotinic cholinergic receptors, which inhibits the effects of nicotine and may suppress the desire to smoke.

Adverse Reactions

Cardiovascular: **Postural hypotension**, tachycardia, syncope, sinus tachycardia

Central nervous system: **Drowsiness**, dizziness, fatigue, hallucinations, confusion, sedation, psychosis

Endocrine & metabolic: **Decreased sexual ability**

Gastrointestinal: **Xerostomia**, loose stools, nausea, vomiting, anorexia, constipation,

Genitourinary: Impotence, urinary retention

Neuromuscular & skeletal: Tremors, choreiform movements, weakness

Ocular: **Blurred vision, mydriasis**

Signs and Symptoms of Overdose Constipation, diarrhea, hypotension, impotence, nausea, seizures, urinary retention, vomiting

Toxicodynamics/Kinetics

Absorption: Completely through gastrointestinal tract

Half-life, elimination: 6-8 hours

Time to peak plasma concentration: 1-2 hours

Elimination: 50% excreted renally within 1 day

Dosage Adults: Oral: 2.5 mg twice daily after meals for 2 days; increased by increments of 2.5 mg at intervals of ≥2 days until desired blood pressure response is achieved; average daily dose: 25 mg

Dosing adjustment/comments in renal impairment: Use with caution, if at all, although no specific guidelines are available

Monitoring Parameters Monitor for orthostatic hypotension; aid with ambulation

Contraindications Coronary insufficiency, pyloric stenosis, glaucoma, uremia, recent myocardial infarction, unreliable, uncooperative patients

Warnings Use with caution in patients receiving sulfonamides or antibiotics that cause neuromuscular blockade; use with caution in patients with impaired renal function, previous CNS abnormalities, prostatic hyperplasia, bladder obstruction, or urethral strictive; do not abruptly discontinue

Dosage Forms Tablet, as hydrochloride: 2.5 mg

Overdosage/Treatment

Decontamination: Lavage (within 1 hour)/activated charcoal

Supportive therapy: Signs and symptoms are a direct result of ganglionic blockade; pressor amines may be used to correct hypotension; use caution as patients will be unusually sensitive to these agents. Physostigmine (0.5-1 mg I.V.) may be utilized to reverse adverse effects

Enhancement of elimination: Multiple dosing of activated charcoal may be useful

Antidote(s)

● Physostigmine [ANTIDOTE]

Drug Interactions Increased effect with sulfonamides and antibiotics that cause neuromuscular blockade; action of mecamylamine may be increased by anesthesia, other antihypertensives, and ethanol

Pregnancy Risk Factor C

Nursing Implications Check frequently for hypotension (orthostatic); aid with ambulation

---

Mechlorethamine

CAS Number 51-75-2; 55-86-7

U.S. Brand Names Mustargen®

Synonyms Chlorethazine Mustard; Chlorethazine; HN₂; Mechlorethamine Hydrochloride; Mustine; Nitrogen Mustard; NSC-762

Use Combination therapy of Hodgkin's disease and malignant lymphomas; non-Hodgkin's lymphoma; may be used by intracavitary injection for treatment of metastatic tumors; pleural and other malignant effusions; topical treatment of mycosis fungoides

Mechanism of Action Bischloroethylamine which alkylates the N^7 position of guanine in DNA and RNA thus resulting in depurination of DNA-causing breakage

Adverse Reactions

Central nervous system: Headache, seizures

Dermatologic: Keratoacanthoma, hyperpigmentation

Endocrine & metabolic: Ovotoxic, **amenorrhea, delayed menses, oligomenorrhea, impaired spermatogenesis**

Gastrointestinal: **Nausea, vomiting**, dizziness, anorexia

Genitourinary: **Azoospermia**

Hematologic: **Leukopenia** (nadir: 6-8 days), **thrombocytopenia** (nadir: 10-16 days)

Hepatic: Jaundice

Local: Extravasation injury

Neuromuscular & skeletal: Tremors

Otic: Tinnitus, deafness, **ototoxicity**

Miscellaneous: **Precipitation of herpes zoster**

Signs and Symptoms of Overdose Deafness, diarrhea, nausea, suppression of all formed elements of the blood, uric acid crystals, vomiting

Pharmacodynamics/Kinetics

Duration: Unchanged drug is undetectable in blood within a few minutes

Absorption: Intracavitary administration: Incomplete secondary to rapid deactivation by body fluids

Metabolism: Rapid hydrolysis and demethylation, possibly in plasma

Half-life elimination: <1 minute

Excretion: Urine (50% as metabolites, <0.01% as unchanged drug)

Dosage

Refer to individual protocols.

Children and Adults: I.V.: 6 mg/m² on days 1 and 8 of a 28-day cycle (MOPP regimen)

Adults:

I.V.: 0.4 mg/kg **or** 12-16 mg/m² for one dose **or** divided into 0.1 mg/kg/day for 4 days, repeated at 4- to 6-week intervals

Intracavitary: 0.2-0.4 mg/kg (10-20 mg) as a single dose; may be repeated if fluid continues to accumulate.

Intrapericardially: 0.2-0.4 mg/kg as a single dose; may be repeated if fluid continues to accumulate.

Topical: 0.01% to 0.02% solution, lotion, or ointment

Hemodialysis: Not removed; supplemental dosing is not required.

Peritoneal dialysis: Not removed; supplemental dosing is not required.

Monitoring Parameters CBC with differential, hemoglobin, and platelet count

Administration

I.V. as a slow push through the side of a freely-flowing saline or dextrose solution. Due to the limited stability of the drug, and the increased risk of phlebitis and venous irritation and blistering with increased contact time, infusions of the drug are not recommended.

Mechlorethamine may cause extravasation. Use within 1 hour of preparation. Avoid extravasation since mechlorethamine is a potent vesicant. **Extravasation management:** Sodium thiosulfate ¹/₆ molar solution is the specific antidote for nitrogen mustard extravasations and should be used as follows: Mix 4 mL of 10% sodium thiosulfate with 6 mL of sterile water for injection. Inject 5-6 mL of this solution into the existing I.V. line. Remove the needle. Inject 2-3 mL of the solution SubQ clockwise into the infiltrated area using a 25-gauge needle. Change the needle with each new injection. Apply ice immediately for 6-12 hours.

Contraindications Hypersensitivity to mechlorethamine or any component of the formulation; pre-existing profound myelosuppression or infection; pregnancy

Warnings [U.S. Boxed Warnings]: Hazardous agent – use appropriate precautions for handling and disposal. Mechlorethamine is a potent vesicant; if extravasation occurs, severe tissue damage (leading to ulceration and necrosis) and pain may occur. Urate precipitation should be anticipated especially with lymphomas. **[U.S. Boxed Warning]: Should be administered under the supervision of an experienced cancer chemotherapy physician.**

Dosage Forms Injection, powder for reconstitution, as hydrochloride: 10 mg

Overdosage/Treatment

Decontamination: **Dermal**: Extravasation: Sodium thiosulfate ¹/₆ molar solution: Mix 4 mL of 10% sodium thiosulfate with 6 mL of sterile water injected with fine hypodermic needle into area of extravasation; apply ice packs for 6-12 hours; a 1% lidocaine solution may also be infiltrated. **Oral**: Dilute with milk or water

Supportive therapy: Colony stimulating factor may be utilized to treat granulocytopenia

Test Interactions ↑ potassium (S)

Drug Interactions Patients may experience impaired immune response to vaccines; possible infection after administration of live vaccines in patients receiving immunosuppressants

Pregnancy Risk Factor D

Lactation Excretion in breast milk unknown/not recommended

Nursing Implications Use within 1 hour of preparation

Additional Information Allopurinol may be given 2-3 days prior to treatment in lymphoma patients to prevent hyperuricemia; unused solutions can be neutralized by mixing with an equal volume of a solution containing 2.5% sodium bicarbonate and 2.5% sodium thiosulfate and letting stand for 45 minutes; equipment can be soaked (needles, gloves, etc) for 45 minutes in a 10% sodium thiosulfate bath before discarding; sodium thiosulfate has no effect on central nervous system effects

Specific References

Lemire SW, Ashley DL, and Calafat AM, "Quantitative Determination of the Hydrolysis Products of Nitrogen Mustards in Human Urine by Liquid Chromatography-Electrospray Ionization Tandem Mass Spectrometry," *J Anal Toxicol*, 2003, 27(1):1-6.

Meclizine

CAS Number 1104-22-9 (anhydrous); 31884-77-2 (monohydrate); 569-65-3

U.S. Brand Names Antivert®; Bonine® [OTC]; Dramamine® Less Drowsy Formula [OTC]

Synonyms Meclizine Hydrochloride; Meclozine Hydrochloride

Use Prevention and treatment of motion sickness; management of dizziness with diseases affecting the vestibular system

Mechanism of Action Has central anticholinergic action by blocking chemoreceptor trigger zone; decreases excitability of the middle ear labyrinth and blocks conduction in the middle ear vestibular-cerebellar pathways

Adverse Reactions

Cardiovascular: Sinus tachycardia

Central nervous system: **Drowsiness**, fatigue, sedation, dizziness, paranoia, extrapyramidal reaction, ataxia, memory disturbance

Gastrointestinal: Xerostomia, nausea, vomiting

Ocular: Blurred vision

Respiratory: **Thickening of bronchial secretions**

Signs and Symptoms of Overdose Confusion, disorientation, excitation alternating with drowsiness, flushing, hallucinations, memory loss, mydriasis, respiratory depression

Pharmacodynamics/Kinetics

Onset of action: ~1 hour

Duration: 8-24 hours

Metabolism: Hepatic

Half-life elimination: 6 hours

Excretion: Urine (as metabolites); feces (as unchanged drug)

Dosage

Children >12 years and Adults: Oral:

Motion sickness: 25-50 mg 1 hour before travel, repeat dose every 24 hours as needed

Vertigo: 25-100 mg/day in divided doses

Contraindications Hypersensitivity to meclizine or any component of the formulation

Warnings Use with caution in patients with angle-closure glaucoma, prostatic hyperplasia, pyloric or duodenal obstruction, or bladder neck obstruction; use with caution in hot weather, and during exercise; elderly may be at risk for anticholinergic side effects such as glaucoma, prostatic hyperplasia, constipation, gastrointestinal obstructive disease; if vertigo does not respond in 1-2 weeks, it is advised to discontinue use

Dosage Forms

Tablet, as hydrochloride: 12.5 mg, 25 mg

Antivert®: 12.5 mg, 25 mg, 50 mg

Dramamine® Less Drowsy Formula: 25 mg

Tablet, chewable, as hydrochloride (Bonine®): 25 mg

Reference Range Serum level of 10 ng/mL 12 hours after an oral dose of 75 mg

Overdosage/Treatment

Decontamination: Lavage (within 1 hour)/activated charcoal

Supportive therapy: There is no specific treatment for an antihistamine overdose, however, most of its clinical toxicity is due to anticholinergic effects. Anticholinesterase inhibitors may be useful by reducing acetylcholinesterase. Anticholinesterase inhibitors include physostigmine for central and peripheral effects, neostigmine, pyridostigmine and edrophonium. For anticholinergic overdose with severe life-threatening symptoms, physostigmine 1-2 mg (0.5 or 0.02 mg/kg for children) I.V., slowly may be given to reverse these effects.

Drug Interactions Increased toxicity: CNS depressants, neuroleptics, anticholinergics

Pregnancy Risk Factor B

Pregnancy Implications Crosses the placenta

Lactation Excretion in breast milk unknown/not recommended

Additional Information Moderately radiopaque

Meclofenamate

Related Information

• Nonsteroidal Anti-inflammatory Drugs

CAS Number 6385-02-0 (Sodium); 644-62-2 (Base)

Synonyms Meclofenamate Sodium

Use Treatment of inflammatory disorders

Mechanism of Action Inhibits prostaglandin synthesis by decreasing the activity of the enzyme, cyclooxygenase, which results in decreased formation of prostaglandin precursors

Adverse Reactions

Cardiovascular: Circulatory collapse, vasculitis

Central nervous system: **Dizziness**, headache, aseptic meningitis, psychosis, cognitive dysfunction, coma, seizures

Dermatologic: **Rash**, pruritus, exfoliative dermatitis, erythema multiforme, alopecia, angioedema, urticaria, purpura, photosensitivity, psoriasis, exanthem

Endocrine & metabolic: Hyperkalemia, anion gap metabolic acidosis, fluid retention

Gastrointestinal: **Abdominal cramps, heartburn, indigestion, nausea**, vomiting, GI bleeding, GI ulceration, constipation, diarrhea, dyspepsia, steatorrhea, xerostomia, stomatitis

Hematologic: Leukopenia, neutropenia, agranulocytosis, granulocytopenia; aplastic anemia (rare), platelet inhibition, hemolytic anemia

Hepatic: Elevated transaminases, hepatitis (fulminant), hepatic necrosis

Neuromuscular & skeletal: Paresthesia

Otic: Ototoxicity, tinnitus

Renal: Renal failure (acute), nephrotic syndrome, chronic renal failure, albuminuria

Respiratory: Wheezing, respiratory depression

Miscellaneous: Hypersensitivity, systemic lupus erythematosus (SLE), fixed drug eruption

Signs and Symptoms of Overdose Cognitive dysfunction, drowsiness, gastritis, GI bleeding, nausea, nephrotic syndrome, ototoxicity, tinnitus, vomiting, wheezing. Severe poisoning can manifest with coma, hypotension, renal and/or hepatic failure, respiratory depression, seizures

Pharmacodynamics/Kinetics

Duration: 2-4 hours

Distribution: Crosses placenta

Protein binding: 99%

Half-life elimination: 2-3.3 hours

Time to peak, serum: 0.5-1.5 hours

Excretion: Primarily urine and feces (as metabolites)

Dosage

Children >14 years and Adults: Oral:

Mild to moderate pain: 50 mg every 4-6 hours, not to exceed 400 mg/day

Rheumatoid arthritis/osteoarthritis: 200-400 mg/day in 3-4 equal doses

Contraindications Hypersensitivity to meclofenamate, aspirin, other NSAIDs, or any component of the formulation; perioperative pain in the setting of coronary artery bypass surgery (CABG); active GI bleeding, ulcer disease; pregnancy (3rd trimester)

Warnings

[U.S. Boxed Warning]: NSAIDs are associated with an increased risk of adverse cardiovascular events, including MI, stroke, and new onset or worsening of pre-existing hypertension. Risk may be increased with duration of use or pre-existing cardiovascular risk-factors or disease. Carefully evaluate individual cardiovascular risk profiles prior to prescribing. Use caution with fluid retention, CHF or hypertension.

Use of NSAIDs can compromise existing renal function. Renal toxicity can occur in patient with impaired renal function, dehydration, heart failure, liver dysfunction, those taking diuretics and ACEI and the elderly. Rehydrate patient before starting therapy. Monitor renal function closely. Use caution in patients with advanced renal disease.

[U.S. Boxed Warning]: NSAIDs may increase risk of gastrointestinal irritation, ulceration, bleeding, and perforation. These events may occur at any time during therapy and without warning. Use caution with a history of GI disease (bleeding or ulcers), concurrent therapy with aspirin, anticoagulants and/or corticosteroids, smoking, use of alcohol, the elderly or debilitated patients.

Use the lowest effective dose for the shortest duration of time, consistent with individual patient goals, to reduce risk of cardiovascular or GI adverse events. Alternate therapies should be considered for patients at high risk.

NSAIDs may cause serious skin adverse events including exfoliative dermatitis, Stevens-Johnson syndrome (SJS) and toxic epidermal necrolysis (TEN). Anaphylactoid reactions may occur, even without prior exposure; patients with "aspirin triad" (bronchial asthma, aspirin intolerance, rhinitis) may be at increased risk. Do not use in patients who experience bronchospasm, asthma, rhinitis, or urticaria with NSAID or aspirin therapy.

Use with caution in patients with decreased hepatic function. Closely monitor patients with any abnormal LFT. Severe hepatic reactions (eg, fulminant hepatitis, liver failure) have occurred with NSAID use, rarely; discontinue if signs or symptoms of liver disease develop, or if systemic manifestations occur.

The elderly are at increased risk for adverse effects (especially peptic ulceration, CNS effects, renal toxicity) from NSAIDs even at low doses.

Withhold for at least 4-6 half-lives prior to surgical or dental procedures. Safety and efficacy have not been established in children <14 years of age.

Dosage Forms Capsule, as sodium: 50 mg, 100 mg

Reference Range Steady-state meclofenamate plasma levels range from 10-20 mcg/mL at a dose of 100 mg 3 times/day; one 100 mg dose results in a peak plasma level of 8-9 mcg/mL

Overdosage/Treatment

Decontamination: Activated charcoal

Supportive therapy: Hypotension/dehydration can be managed with I.V. fluid therapy; acidosis should be treated with bicarbonates, seizures with benzodiazepines; antacids, blood products are indicated, as appropriate, for hemorrhage

Enhancement of elimination: Dialysis is indicated for secondary complications, acidosis, or renal failure and not toxin removal alone; multiple dosing of activated charcoal may be effective

Test Interactions ↑ chloride (S), sodium (S)

Drug Interactions ACE inhibitors: Antihypertensive effects may be decreased by concurrent therapy with NSAIDs; monitor blood pressure.

Angiotensin II antagonists: Antihypertensive effects may be decreased by concurrent therapy with NSAIDs; monitor blood pressure.

Anticoagulants (warfarin, heparin, LMWHs) in combination with NSAIDs can cause increased risk of bleeding.

Antiplatelet drugs (ticlopidine, clopidogrel, aspirin, abciximab, dipyridamole, eptifibatide, tirofiban) can cause an increased risk of bleeding.

Beta-blockers: NSAIDs may decrease the antihypertensive effect of beta-blockers. Monitor.

Cholestyramine (and other bile acid sequestrants): May decrease the absorption of NSAIDs. Separate by at least 2 hours.

Corticosteroids may increase the risk of GI ulceration; avoid concurrent use.

Cyclosporine: NSAIDs may increase serum creatinine, potassium, blood pressure, and cyclosporine levels; monitor cyclosporine levels and renal function carefully.

Gentamicin and amikacin serum concentrations are increased by indomethacin in premature infants. Results may apply to other aminoglycosides and NSAIDs.

Hydralazine's antihypertensive effect is decreased; avoid concurrent use.

Lithium levels can be increased; avoid concurrent use if possible or monitor lithium levels and adjust dose. Sulindac may have the least effect. When NSAID is stopped, lithium will need adjustment again.

Loop diuretics efficacy (diuretic and antihypertensive effect) is reduced. Indomethacin reduces this efficacy, however, it may be anticipated with any NSAID.

Methotrexate: Severe bone marrow suppression, aplastic anemia, and GI toxicity have been reported with concomitant NSAID therapy. Avoid use during moderate or high-dose methotrexate (increased and prolonged methotrexate levels). NSAID use during low-dose treatment of rheumatoid arthritis has not been fully evaluated; extreme caution is warranted.

Thiazides antihypertensive effects are decreased; avoid concurrent use.

Verapamil plasma concentration is decreased by diclofenac; avoid concurrent use.

Warfarin's INRs may be increased by piroxicam. Other NSAIDs may have the same effect depending on dose and duration. Monitor INR closely. Use the lowest dose of NSAIDs possible and for the briefest duration.

Pregnancy Risk Factor B/D (3rd trimester)

Pregnancy Implications Crosses the placenta

Lactation Enters breast milk/not recommended

Mefenamic Acid

Related Information
● Nonsteroidal Anti-inflammatory Drugs

CAS Number 61-68-7

U.S. Brand Names Ponstel®

Use Short-term relief of mild to moderate pain including primary dysmenorrhea

Mechanism of Action Inhibits prostaglandin synthesis by decreasing the activity of the enzyme, cyclooxygenase, which results in decreased formation of prostaglandin precursors

Adverse Reactions
Cardiovascular: Circulatory collapse, vasculitis

Central nervous system: Headache, aseptic meningitis, psychosis, cognitive dysfunction, insomnia, coma, seizures, **dizziness**, extrapyramidal reactions

Dermatologic: **Rash**, pruritus, exfoliative dermatitis, toxic epidermal necrolysis, urticaria, purpura, Stevens-Johnson syndrome, exanthem

Endocrine & metabolic: Hyperkalemia, anion gap metabolic acidosis, fluid retention

Gastrointestinal: **Abdominal cramps, nausea**, vomiting, GI bleeding, GI ulceration, constipation, diarrhea, dyspepsia, steatorrhea, feces discoloration (black), **heartburn, indigestion**

Hematologic: Leukopenia, neutropenia, agranulocytosis, granulocytopenia, aplastic anemia (rare), platelet inhibition, hemolytic anemia

Hepatic: Elevated transaminases, hepatitis (fulminant)

Otic: Ototoxicity, tinnitus

Renal: Renal failure (acute), nephrotic syndrome, chronic renal failure, albuminuria, glomerulonephritis

Respiratory: Wheezing, respiratory depression

Miscellaneous: Hypersensitivity

Signs and Symptoms of Overdose Bullous skin disease/pemphigoid, cognitive dysfunction, colitis, drowsiness, gastritis, GI bleeding, insomnia, nausea, nephrotic syndrome, ototoxicity, thrombocytopenia, tinnitus, vomiting, wheezing. Severe poisoning can manifest with coma, hypotension, renal and/or hepatic failure, respiratory depression, seizures (38%, 2-12 hours postingestion)

Admission Criteria/Prognosis Admit any patient with neurologic symptoms within 12 hours postingestion; pediatric ingestion >1 g or adult ingestion >3 g

Pharmacodynamics/Kinetics
Onset of action: Peak effect: 2-4 hours

Duration: ≤6 hours

Protein binding: High

Metabolism: Conjugated hepatically

Half-life elimination: 3.5 hours

Excretion: Urine (50%) and feces as unchanged drug and metabolites

Dosage
Oral:

Children >14 years and Adults: 500 mg to start then 250 mg every 4 hours as needed; maximum therapy: 1 week

Seizurgenic dose: Children: 2 g; Adults: 6 g

Dosing adjustment/comments in renal impairment: Not recommended for use

Administration
May be administered with food, milk, or antacids.

Contraindications Hypersensitivity to mefenamic acid, aspirin, other NSAIDs, or any component of the formulation; perioperative pain in the setting of coronary artery bypass surgery (CABG); active ulceration or chronic inflammation of the GI tract; renal disease; pregnancy (3rd trimester)

Warnings
[U.S. Boxed Warning]: NSAIDs are associated with an increased risk of adverse cardiovascular events, including MI, stroke, and new onset or worsening of pre-existing hypertension. Risk may be increased with duration of use or pre-existing cardiovascular risk-factors or disease. Carefully evaluate individual cardiovascular risk profiles prior to prescribing. Use caution with fluid retention, CHF or hypertension.

Use of NSAIDs can compromise existing renal function. Renal toxicity can occur in patient with impaired renal function, dehydration, heart failure, liver dysfunction, those taking diuretics and ACEI and the elderly. Rehydrate patient before starting therapy. Monitor renal function closely. Mefenamic acid is not recommended for patients with advanced renal disease.

[U.S. Boxed Warning]: NSAIDs may increase risk of gastrointestinal irritation, ulceration, bleeding, and perforation. These events may occur at any time during therapy and without warning. Use caution with a history of GI disease (bleeding or ulcers), concurrent therapy with aspirin, anticoagulants and/or corticosteroids, smoking, use of alcohol, the elderly or debilitated patients.

Use the lowest effective dose for the shortest duration of time, consistent with individual patient goals, to reduce risk of cardiovascular or GI adverse events. Alternate therapies should be considered for patients at high risk.

NSAIDs may cause serious skin adverse events including exfoliative dermatitis, Stevens-Johnson syndrome (SJS) and toxic epidermal necrolysis (TEN). Anaphylactoid reactions may occur, even without prior exposure; patients with "aspirin triad" (bronchial asthma, aspirin intolerance, rhinitis) may be at increased risk. Do not use in patients who experience bronchospasm, asthma, rhinitis, or urticaria with NSAID or aspirin therapy.

Use with caution in patients with decreased hepatic function. Closely monitor patients with any abnormal LFT. Severe hepatic reactions (eg, fulminant hepatitis, liver failure) have occurred with NSAID use, rarely; discontinue if signs or symptoms of liver disease develop, or if systemic manifestations occur.

The elderly are at increased risk for adverse effects (especially peptic ulceration, CNS effects, renal toxicity) from NSAIDs even at low doses.

Withhold for at least 4-6 half-lives prior to surgical or dental procedures. Safety and efficacy have not been established in children <14 years of age.

Dosage Forms Capsule: 250 mg

Reference Range Therapeutic mefenamic acid level: Up to 10 mcg/mL; levels >100 mcg/mL associated with severe neurological abnormalities

Overdosage/Treatment
Decontamination: Activated charcoal; **do not** induce emesis

Supportive therapy: Hypotension/dehydration can be managed with I.V. fluid therapy; acidosis should be treated with bicarbonates, seizures with benzodiazepines; antacids, blood products are indicated, as appropriate, for hemorrhage

Enhancement of elimination: Dialysis or perfusion is indicated for secondary complications, acidosis, or renal failure and not toxin removal alone; multiple dosing of activated charcoal may be effective

Test Interactions ↑ chloride (S), sodium (S); positive Coombs' [direct]

Drug Interactions
Substrate of CYP2C9 (minor); **Inhibits** CYP2C9 (strong)

ACE inhibitors: Antihypertensive effects may be decreased by concurrent therapy with NSAIDs; monitor blood pressure.

Angiotensin II antagonists: Antihypertensive effects may be decreased by concurrent therapy with NSAIDs; monitor blood pressure.

Anticoagulants (warfarin, heparin, LMWHs) in combination with NSAIDs can cause increased risk of bleeding.

Antiplatelet drugs (ticlopidine, clopidogrel, aspirin, abciximab, dipyridamole, eptifibatide, tirofiban) can cause an increased risk of bleeding.

Beta-blockers: NSAIDs may decrease the antihypertensive effect of beta-blockers. Monitor.

Cholestyramine (and other bile acid sequestrants): May decrease the absorption of NSAIDs. Separate by at least 2 hours.

Corticosteroids may increase the risk of GI ulceration; avoid concurrent use.

Cyclosporine: NSAIDs may increase serum creatinine, potassium, blood pressure, and cyclosporine levels; monitor cyclosporine levels and renal function carefully.

CYP2C9 Substrates: Mefenamic acid may increase the levels/effects of CYP2C9 substrates. Example substrates include bosentan, dapsone, fluoxetine, glimepiride, glipizide, losartan, montelukast, nateglinide, paclitaxel, phenytoin, warfarin, and zafirlukast.

Gentamicin and amikacin serum concentrations are increased by indomethacin in premature infants. Results may apply to other aminoglycosides and NSAIDs.

Hydralazine's antihypertensive effect is decreased; avoid concurrent use.

Lithium levels can be increased; avoid concurrent use if possible or monitor lithium levels and adjust dose. Sulindac may have the least effect. When NSAID is stopped, lithium will need adjustment again.

Loop diuretics efficacy (diuretic and antihypertensive effect) is reduced. Indomethacin reduces this efficacy, however, it may be anticipated with any NSAID.

Methotrexate: Severe bone marrow suppression, aplastic anemia, and GI toxicity have been reported with concomitant NSAID therapy. Avoid use during moderate or high-dose methotrexate (increased and prolonged methotrexate levels). NSAID use during low-dose treatment of rheumatoid arthritis has not been fully evaluated; extreme caution is warranted.

Thiazides antihypertensive effects are decreased; avoid concurrent use.

Verapamil plasma concentration is decreased by diclofenac; avoid concurrent use.

Warfarin's INRs may be increased by piroxicam. Other NSAIDs may have the same effect depending on dose and duration. Monitor INR closely. Use the lowest dose of NSAIDs possible and for the briefest duration.

Pregnancy Risk Factor C/D (3rd trimester)

Lactation Enters breast milk (trace amounts)/not recommended (AAP rates "compatible")

Specific References
Laredo P, Kupferschmidt H, Meier PJ, et al, "Acute Mefenamic Acid Poisoning in Switzerland," *Clin Toxicol (Phila)*, 2005, 43:744.

Mefloquine

CAS Number 51773-92-3; 53230-10-7

U.S. Brand Names Lariam®

Synonyms Mefloquine Hydrochloride

Use Treatment of acute malarial infections and prevention of malaria

Mechanism of Action Mefloquine is a quinoline-methanol compound structurally similar to quinine; mefloquine's effectiveness in the treatment and prophylaxis of malaria is due to the destruction of the asexual blood forms of the malarial pathogens that affect humans, *Plasmodium falciparum*, *P. vivax*, *P. malariae*, *P. ovale*

Adverse Reactions

Cardiovascular: Bradycardia, extrasystoles, syncope, AV block, chest pain, conduction abnormalities (transient), edema, hypotension, palpitations, tachycardia

Central nervous system: Headache, fever, chills, fatigue, neuropsychiatric events, dizziness, emotional lability, seizures, abnormal dreams, ataxia, aggressive behavior, agitation, anxiety, confusion, convulsions, depression, encephalopathy, hallucinations, insomnia, malaise, mood changes, panic attacks, paranoia, psychosis, somnolence, suicidal ideation and behavior (causal relationship not established), vertigo

Dermatologic: Rash, alopecia, pruritus, erythema multiforme, exanthema, Stevens-Johnson syndrome, urticaria

Gastrointestinal: Vomiting, diarrhea, stomach pain, nausea, appetite decreased, dyspepsia

Hematologic: Leukocytosis, thrombocytopenia

Neuromuscular & skeletal: Myalgia, arthralgia, muscle cramps/weakness, paresthesia, tremor

Ocular: Visual disturbances

Otic: Tinnitus, hearing impairment

Respiratory: Dyspnea

Miscellaneous: Anaphylaxis, diaphoresis (increased)

Pharmacodynamics/Kinetics

Absorption: Well absorbed

Distribution: V_d: 19 L/kg; blood, urine, CSF, tissues; enters breast milk

Protein binding: 98%

Metabolism: Extensively hepatic; main metabolite is inactive

Bioavailability: Increased by food

Half-life elimination: 21-22 days

Time to peak, plasma: 6-24 hours (median: ~17 hours)

Excretion: Primarily bile and feces; urine (9% as unchanged drug, 4% as primary metabolite)

Dosage

Oral (dose expressed as mg of mefloquine hydrochloride):

Children ≥6 months and >5 kg:

Malaria treatment: 20-25 mg/kg in 2 divided doses, taken 6-8 hours apart (maximum: 1250 mg) Take with food and an ample amount of water. If clinical improvement is not seen within 48-72 hours, an alternative therapy should be used for retreatment.

Malaria prophylaxis: 5 mg/kg/once weekly (maximum dose: 250 mg) starting 1 week before, arrival in endemic area, continuing weekly during travel and for 4 weeks after leaving endemic area. Take with food and an ample amount of water.

Adults:

Malaria treatment (mild to moderate infection): 5 tablets (1250 mg) as a single dose. Take with food and at least 8 oz of water. If clinical improvement is not seen within 48-72 hours, an alternative therapy should be used for retreatment.

Malaria prophylaxis: 1 tablet (250 mg) weekly starting 1 week before, arrival in endemic area, continuing weekly during travel and for 4 weeks after leaving endemic area. Take with food and at least 8 oz of water.

Dosage adjustment in renal impairment: No dosage adjustment needed in patients with renal impairment or on dialysis.

Dosage adjustment in hepatic impairment: Half-life may be prolonged and plasma levels may be higher.

Monitoring Parameters LFTS; ocular examination

Administration Administer with food and with at least 8 oz of water. When used for malaria prophylaxis, dose should be taken once weekly on the same day each week. If vomiting occurs within 30-60 minutes after dose, an additional half-dose should be given. Tablets may be crushed and suspended in a small amount of water, milk, or another beverage for persons unable to swallow tablets.

Contraindications Hypersensitivity mefloquine, related compounds (such as quinine and quinidine), or any component of the formulation; history of convulsions; cardiac conduction abnormalities; severe psychiatric disorder (including active or recent history of depression, generalized anxiety disorder, psychosis, or schizophrenia); use with halofantrine

Warnings Use with caution in patients with a previous history of depression (see Contraindications regarding severe psychiatric illness, including active/recent depression). May cause a range of psychiatric symptoms (anxiety, paranoia, depression, hallucinations and psychosis). Occasionally, symptoms have been reported to persist long after mefloquine has been discontinued. Rare cases of suicidal ideation and suicide have been reported (no causal relationship established). The appearance of psychiatric symptoms such as acute anxiety, depression, restlessness or confusion may be considered a prodrome to more serious events. When used as prophylaxis, substitute an alternative medication. Discontinue if unexplained neuropsychiatric disturbances occur. Use caution in patients with significant cardiac disease. If mefloquine is to be used for a prolonged period, periodic evaluations including liver function tests and ophthalmic examinations should be performed. (Retinal abnormalities have not been observed with mefloquine in humans; however, it has with long-term administration to rats.) In cases of life-threatening, serious, or overwhelming malaria infections due to *Plasmodium falciparum*, patients should be treated with intravenous antimalarial drug. Mefloquine may be given orally to complete the course. Dizziness, loss of balance, and other CNS disorders have been reported; due to long half-life, effects may persist after mefloquine is discontinued. Use caution in activities requiring alertness and fine motor coordination (driving, piloting planes, operating machinery, deep sea diving, etc).

Dosage Forms Tablet, as hydrochloride: 250 mg [equivalent to 228 mg base]

Reference Range Peak serum levels after a 250 mg oral dose in patients with malaria range from 0.7-1.4 mcg/mL (may be higher in healthy person, but lower in pregnancy)

Overdosage/Treatment Supportive therapy: Psychosis can be treated with diazepam and haloperidol

Drug Interactions **Substrate** of CYP3A4 (major); **Inhibits** CYP2D6 (weak), 3A4 (weak)

Anticonvulsants: Decreased effect of valproic acid, carbamazepine, phenobarbital, or phenytoin.

Antiarrhythmics: Chloroquine and quinidine may produce electrocardiographic changes and increase risk of convulsions. When used as initial treatment of severe malaria, delay mefloquine for 12 hours after the last dose. Use caution with other medications known to alter conduction.

CYP3A4 inducers: CYP3A4 inducers may decrease the levels/effects of mefloquine. Example inducers include aminoglutethimide, carbamazepine, nafcillin, nevirapine, phenobarbital, phenytoin, and rifamycins.

CYP3A4 inhibitors: May increase the levels/effects of mefloquine. Example inhibitors include azole antifungals, clarithromycin, diclofenac, doxycycline, erythromycin, imatinib, isoniazid, nefazodone, nicardipine, propofol, protease inhibitors, quinidine, telithromycin, and verapamil.

Halofantrine: Fatal prolongation of the QT_c interval reported; concomitant use is contraindicated.

Quinine: May produce electrocardiographic changes and increase risk of convulsions. When used as initial treatment of severe malaria, delay mefloquine for 12 hours after the last dose.

Vaccines: Vaccinations with attenuated live bacteria should be completed at least 3 days prior to first dose of mefloquine. Vaccination with oral live attenuated Ty21a vaccine should be delayed for at least 24 hours after the administration of mefloquine.

Pregnancy Risk Factor C

Pregnancy Implications Mefloquine crosses the placenta and is teratogenic in animals. There are no adequate and well-controlled studies in pregnant women, however, clinical experience has not shown teratogenic or embryotoxic effects; use with caution during pregnancy if travel to endemic areas cannot be postponed. Nonpregnant women of childbearing potential are advised to use contraception and avoid pregnancy during malaria prophylaxis and for 3 months thereafter. In case of an unplanned pregnancy, treatment with mefloquine is not considered a reason for pregnancy termination.

Lactation Enters breast milk/not recommended

Megestrol

CAS Number 595-33-5
U.S. Brand Names Megace®
Synonyms 5071-1DL(6); Megestrol Acetate; NSC-10363
Use
Palliative treatment of breast and endometrial carcinoma

Orphan drug: Treatment of anorexia, cachexia, or significant weight loss (≥10% baseline body weight) and confirmed diagnosis of AIDS

Mechanism of Action A synthetic progestin with antiestrogenic properties which disrupt the estrogen receptor cycle. Megestrol interferes with the normal estrogen cycle and results in a lower LH titer. May also have a direct effect on the endometrium. Megestrol is an antineoplastic progestin thought to act through an antileutenizing effect mediated via the pituitary.

Adverse Reactions
Cardiovascular: Cardiomyopathy, edema, hypertension, palpitations

Central nervous system: Confusion, convulsions, depression, fever, headache, insomnia, pain

Dermatologic: Allergic rash with or without pruritus, alopecia

Endocrine & metabolic: Adrenal insufficiency, amenorrhea, breakthrough bleeding, changes in menstrual flow, changes in cervical erosion and secretions, spotting, Cushing's syndrome, diabetes, fluid retention, HPA axis suppression, hyperglycemia, increased breast tenderness

Gastrointestinal: Constipation, diarrhea, flatulence, nausea, vomiting, weight gain (not attributed to edema or fluid retention)

Genitourinary: Decreased libido, impotence

Hepatic: Cholestatic jaundice, hepatotoxicity, hepatomegaly

Local: Thrombophlebitis

Neuromuscular & skeletal: Carpal tunnel syndrome, paresthesia, weakness

Respiratory: Cough, dyspnea, hyperpnea

Miscellaneous: Diaphoresis

Signs and Symptoms of Overdose Nausea, vomiting

Admission Criteria/Prognosis Admit any symptomatic ingestion or any ingestion >2 g orally

Pharmacodynamics/Kinetics
Absorption: Well absorbed orally

Metabolism: Completely hepatic to free steroids and glucuronide conjugates

Time to peak, serum: 1-3 hours

Half-life elimination: 15-100 hours

Excretion: Urine (57% to 78% as steroid metabolites and inactive compound); feces (8% to 30%)

Dosage
Adults: Oral (refer to individual protocols):
Female:
Breast carcinoma: 40 mg 4 times/day

Endometrial carcinoma: 40-320 mg/day in divided doses; use for 2 months to determine efficacy; maximum doses used have been up to 800 mg/day

Uterine bleeding (unlabeled use): 40 mg 2-4 times/day

Male/Female: HIV-related cachexia: Initial dose: 800 mg/day; daily doses of 400 and 800 mg/day were found to be clinically effective

Dosing adjustment in renal impairment: No data available; however, the urinary excretion of megestrol acetate administered in doses of 4-90 mg ranged from 56% to 78% within 10 days

Hemodialysis: Megestrol acetate has not been tested for dialyzability; however, due to its low solubility, it is postulated that dialysis would not be an effective means of treating an overdose

Monitoring Parameters Observe for signs of thromboembolic phenomena

Administration Megestrol acetate (Megace®) oral suspension is compatible with water, orange juice, apple juice, or Sustacal H.C. for immediate consumption.

Contraindications Hypersensitivity to megestrol or any component of the formulation; pregnancy

Warnings Use with caution in patients with a history of thrombophlebitis. Elderly females may have vaginal bleeding or discharge. May suppress hypothalamic-pituitary-adrenal (HPA) axis during chronic administration. Consider the possibility of adrenal suppression in any patient receiving or being withdrawn from chronic therapy when signs/symptoms suggestive of hypoadrenalism are noted (during stress or in unstressed state). Laboratory evaluation and replacement/stress doses of rapid-acting glucocorticoid should be considered.

Dosage Forms Suspension, oral, as acetate: 40 mg/mL (240 mL, 480 mL)
Megace®: 40 mg/mL (240 mL) [contains alcohol 0.06% and sodium benzoate; lemon-lime flavor]
Megace® ES: 125 mg/mL (150 mL) [contains alcohol 0.06% and sodium benzoate; lemon-lime flavor]
Tablet, as acetate: 20 mg, 40 mg

Reference Range Following a single 40 mg oral dose, peak plasma levels range from 10-56 ng/mL

Overdosage/Treatment
Decontamination: Emesis within 30 minutes or lavage (within 1 hour)/ activated charcoal

Test Interactions Altered thyroid and liver function tests; increased levels of prostate-specific antigen

Drug Interactions No data reported

Pregnancy Risk Factor X

Lactation Enters breast milk/contraindicated

Additional Information Herb/Nutraceutical: Avoid black cohosh, dong quai in estrogen-dependent tumors.

Melatonin

CAS Number 73-31-4
Synonyms N-Acetyl-5-methoxytryptamine
Use Sleep disorders (insomnia), circadian rhythm disturbances (ie, jet lag); only FDA approval (as an orphan drug) is for treatment of circadian rhythm sleep disorders in blind people with no light perception

Mechanism of Action A hormone produced and secreted in the pineal gland causes an increase in hypothalamus aminobutyric acid and serotonin. Increased secretion occurs during dark hours; decreases neopterin release; counteracts apoptosis; increases thymus activity

Adverse Reactions
Central nervous system: Drowsiness, dysphoria (especially in depressed patients), giddiness

Gastrointestinal: Nausea

Miscellaneous: Fixed drug eruption

Signs and Symptoms of Overdose Ataxia, drowsiness

Pharmacodynamics/Kinetics
Absorption: Rapid
Peak plasma level: 1 hour

Dosage
Oral:
Jet lag: 5 mg/day (at 1800 hours) for 1 week starting 3 days before the flight

Hypnotic effects: Oral: 0.1-0.3 mg (daytime); 1-10 mg (nighttime)

Insomnia: 5-75 mg at night have been used

Dosage Forms Tablet: 3 mg
Tablet, sublingual: 2.5 mg

Reference Range Mean baseline melatonin serum levels 80 pg/mL (range: 0-200) between 0200-0400 hours. Elevated endogenous levels seen after 0900 hours; after a 2.5 mg oral dose, plasma melatonin level may be as high as 8.50 pg/mL.

Overdosage/Treatment
Decontamination: Lavage (within 1 hour)/activated charcoal with sorbitol may be effective

Supportive: Need to monitor respiratory status; naloxone may be useful to reduce respiratory depression

Specific References
de Haan M, Macnab J, Kent DA, et al, "Melatonin Overdose Resulting in Respiratory Depression and Coma Responsive to Naloxone," *Clin Toxicol (Phila)*, 2005, 43:759.

Nelson LA, McGuire JM, and Hausafus SN, "Melatonin for the Treatment of Tardive Dyskinesia," *Ann Pharmacother*, 2003, 37(7-8):1128-31.

Todisco M, "Effectiveness of a Treatment Based on Melatonin in Five Patients with Systemic Sclerosis," *Am J Ther*, 2006, 13(1):84-7.

Todisco M, Casaccia P, and Rossi N, "Severe Bleeding Symptoms in Refractory Idiopathic Thrombocytopenic Purpura: A Case Successfully Treated with Melatonin," *Am J Ther*, 2003, 10(2):135-6.

Meloxicam

Related Information
- Nonsteroidal Anti-inflammatory Drugs

CAS Number 71125-38-7

U.S. Brand Names MOBIC®

Use Relief of signs and symptoms of osteoarthritis

Mechanism of Action Inhibits prostaglandin synthesis by decreasing the activity of the enzyme, cyclooxygenase, which results in decreased formation of prostaglandin precursors

Adverse Reactions

Cardiovascular: Angina, arrhythmia, cardiac failure, edema, hypertension, hypotension, myocardial infarction, palpitations, shock, tachycardia, vasculitis

Central nervous system: Abnormal dreams, anxiety, confusion, depression, headache and dizziness (occurred in 2% to 8% of patients, but occurred less frequently than placebo in controlled trials), malaise, nervousness, syncope, seizures, somnolence, vertigo

Dermatologic: Alopecia, angioedema, bullous eruption, erythema multiforme, photosensitivity reaction, pruritus, purpura, rash, Stevens-Johnson syndrome, toxic epidermal necrolysis, urticaria

Endocrine & metabolic: Hot flashes, dehydration

Gastrointestinal: Abdominal pain, colitis, diarrhea, duodenal ulcer, duodenal perforation, dyspepsia, flatulence, gastric ulcer, gastritis, gastric perforation, gastroesophageal reflux, gastrointestinal hemorrhage, hematemesis, intestinal perforation, melena, nausea, pancreatitis, taste perversion, weight changes, xerostomia, ulcerative stomatitis

Hematologic: Agranulocytosis, leukopenia, thrombocytopenia

Hepatic: Hepatitis, hepatic failure, hyperbilirubinemia, increased ALT, increased AST, increased GGT, jaundice

Neuromuscular & skeletal: Paresthesia, tremor

Ocular: Abnormal vision, conjunctivitis

Otic: Tinnitus

Renal: Albuminuria, increased BUN, increased creatinine, hematuria, interstitial nephritis, renal failure

Respiratory: Asthma, bronchospasm, cough, dyspnea, pharyngitis, upper respiratory infection

Miscellaneous: Allergic reaction, anaphylactic reaction, flu-like symptoms, falls

Signs and Symptoms of Overdose Drowsiness, epigastric pain, lethargy, nausea, vomiting

Pharmacodynamics/Kinetics

Distribution: 10 L

Protein binding: 99.4%

Metabolism: Hepatic via CYP2C9 and CYP3A4 (minor); forms 4 metabolites (inactive)

Bioavailability: 89%

Half-life elimination: Adults: 15-20 hours

Time to peak: Initial: 5-10 hours; Secondary: 12-14 hours

Excretion: Urine and feces (as inactive metabolites)

Dosage

Adult: Oral: Initial: 7.5 mg once daily; some patients may receive additional benefit from an increased dose of 15 mg once daily; maximum dose: 15 mg/day

Elderly: Increased concentrations may occur in elderly patients (particularly in females); however, no specific dosage adjustment is recommended

Dosage adjustment in renal impairment:

Mild to moderate impairment: No specific dosage recommendations

Significant impairment ($Cl_{cr} \leq 15$ mL/minute): Avoid use

Dosage adjustment in hepatic impairment:

Mild (Child-Pugh class A) to moderate (Child-Pugh class B) hepatic dysfunction: No dosage adjustment is necessary

Severe hepatic impairment: Patients with severe hepatic impairment have not been adequately studied

Stability Store at 25°C (77°F)

Monitoring Parameters CBC, periodic liver function, renal function (serum BUN, and creatinine)

Contraindications Hypersensitivity to meloxicam, aspirin, other NSAIDs, or any component of the formulation; perioperative pain in the setting of coronary artery bypass surgery (CABG); pregnancy (3rd trimester)

Warnings

[U.S. Boxed Warning]: NSAIDs are associated with an increased risk of adverse cardiovascular events, including MI, stroke, and new onset or worsening of pre-existing hypertension. Risk may be increased with duration of use or pre-existing cardiovascular risk-factors or disease. Carefully evaluate individual cardiovascular risk profiles prior to prescribing. Use caution with fluid retention, CHF or hypertension.

Use of NSAIDs can compromise existing renal function. Renal toxicity can occur in patient with impaired renal function, dehydration, heart failure, liver dysfunction, those taking diuretics and ACEI and the elderly. Rehydrate patient before starting therapy. Monitor renal function closely. Meloxicam is not recommended for patients with advanced renal disease

[U.S. Boxed Warning]: NSAIDs may increase risk of gastrointestinal irritation, ulceration, bleeding, and perforation. These events may occur at any time during therapy and without warning. Use caution with a history of GI disease (bleeding or ulcers), concurrent therapy with aspirin, anticoagulants and/or corticosteroids, smoking, use of alcohol, the elderly or debilitated patients.

Use the lowest effective dose for the shortest duration of time, consistent with individual patient goals, to reduce risk of cardiovascular or GI adverse events. Alternate therapies should be considered for patients at high risk.

NSAIDs may cause serious skin adverse events including exfoliative dermatitis, Stevens-Johnson syndrome (SJS) and toxic epidermal necrolysis (TEN). Anaphylactoid reactions may occur, even without prior exposure; patients with "aspirin triad" (bronchial asthma, aspirin intolerance, rhinitis) may be at increased risk. Do not use in patients who experience bronchospasm, asthma, rhinitis, or urticaria with NSAID or aspirin therapy.

Use with caution in patients with decreased hepatic function. Closely monitor patients with any abnormal LFT. Severe hepatic reactions (eg, fulminant hepatitis, liver failure) have occurred with NSAID use, rarely; discontinue if signs or symptoms of liver disease develop, or if systemic manifestations occur.

The elderly are at increased risk for adverse effects (especially peptic ulceration, CNS effects, renal toxicity) from NSAIDs even at low doses.

Withhold for at least 4-6 half-lives prior to surgical or dental procedures. Safety and efficacy have not been established in pediatric patients <2 years of age.

Dosage Forms Suspension:

Mobic®: 7.5 mg/5 mL (100 mL) [contains sodium benzoate; raspberry flavor]

Tablet: 7.5 mg, 15 mg

Mobic®: 7.5 mg, 15 mg

Overdosage/Treatment

Decontamination: Activated charcoal or cholestyramine may be used for decontamination of the GI tract.

Enhancement of elimination: Since meloxicam undergoes enterohepatic cycling, multiple doses of charcoal may be needed to reduce the potential for delayed toxicities. Cholestyramine has been shown to increase meloxicam clearance.

Drug Interactions Substrate (minor) of CYP2C9, 3A4; **Inhibits** CYP2C9 (weak)

ACE inhibitors: Antihypertensive effects may be decreased by concurrent therapy with NSAIDs; monitor blood pressure

Angiotensin II antagonists: Antihypertensive effects may be decreased by concurrent therapy with NSAIDs; monitor blood pressure

Anticoagulants (warfarin, heparin, LMWHs) in combination with NSAIDs can cause increased risk of bleeding.

Antiplatelet drugs (ticlopidine, clopidogrel, aspirin, abciximab, dipyridamole, eptifibatide, tirofiban) can cause an increased risk of bleeding.

Aspirin increases serum concentrations (AUC) of meloxicam (in addition to potential for additive adverse effects); concurrent use is not recommended.

Beta-blockers: NSAIDs may decrease the antihypertensive effect of beta-blockers. Monitor.

Cholestyramine (and other bile acid sequestrants): May decrease the absorption of NSAIDs. Separate by at least 2 hours.

Corticosteroids may increase the risk of GI ulceration; avoid concurrent use.

Cyclosporine: NSAIDs may increase serum creatinine, potassium, blood pressure, and cyclosporine levels; monitor cyclosporine levels and renal function carefully.

Hydralazine's antihypertensive effect is decreased; avoid concurrent use.

Lithium levels can be increased; avoid concurrent use if possible or monitor lithium levels and adjust dose. When NSAID is stopped, lithium will need adjustment again.

Loop diuretic's efficacy (diuretic and antihypertensive effect) may be reduced by NSAIDs.

Methotrexate: Severe bone marrow suppression, aplastic anemia, and GI toxicity have been reported with concomitant NSAID therapy. Avoid use during moderate or high-dose methotrexate (increased and prolonged methotrexate levels). NSAID use during low-dose treatment of rheumatoid arthritis has not been fully evaluated; extreme caution is warranted.

Thiazide diuretics: Antihypertensive effects of thiazide diuretics are decreased; avoid concurrent use.

Warfarin INRs may be increased by meloxicam. Monitor INR closely, particularly during initiation or change in dose. May increase risk of bleeding. Use lowest possible dose for shortest duration possible.

Pregnancy Risk Factor C/D (3rd trimester)

Pregnancy Implications May cause premature closure of the ductus arteriosus in the third trimester of pregnancy. It is not known whether meloxicam is excreted in human milk. Due to a potential for serious adverse reactions, the manufacturer recommends that a decision be made whether to discontinue nursing or discontinue the drug, taking into account the importance of the drug to the mother.

Lactation Excretion in breast milk unknown/not recommended

Melphalan

CAS Number 148-82-3

U.S. Brand Names Alkeran®

Synonyms L-PAM; L-Sarcolysin; NSC-8806; Phenylalanine Mustard

Use

Palliative treatment of multiple myeloma and nonresectable epithelial ovarian carcinoma; neuroblastoma, rhabdomyosarcoma, breast cancer, sarcoma; may be helpful in patients with primary amyloidosis

I.V. formulation: Use in patients in whom oral therapy is not appropriate

Unlabeled/Investigational Use Treatment of neuroblastoma, rhabdomyosarcoma, breast cancer; part of an induction regimen for marrow and stem cell transplantation

Mechanism of Action Alkylating agent which is a derivative of mechlorethamine that inhibits DNA and RNA synthesis via formation of carbonium ions; cross-links strands of DNA

Adverse Reactions

Cardiovascular: Vasculitis

Central nervous system: Fever

Dermatologic: **Alopecia, rash, pruritus**, vesiculation of skin, radiation recall dermatitis, scleroderma

Endocrine & metabolic: **Amenorrhea**, hyponatremia, ovarian failure

Gastrointestinal: Nausea, vomiting, diarrhea, stomatitis, oral ulceration, feces discoloration (black)

Genitourinary: Bladder irritation, hemorrhagic cystitis

Hematologic: **Thrombocytopenia, anemia, leukopenia**, neutropenia, **agranulocytosis**, granulocytopenia, **hemolytic anemia**

Hepatic: Increased transaminases (hepatitis, jaundice have been reported)

Local: Burning and discomfort at injection site

Respiratory: **Pulmonary fibrosis**, cough, dyspnea

Miscellaneous: Hypersensitivity

Pharmacodynamics/Kinetics

Absorption: Oral: Variable and incomplete

Distribution: V_d: 0.5-0.6 L/kg throughout total body water

Protein binding: 60% to 90%; primarily to albumin, 20% to α_1-acid glycoprotein

Metabolism: Hepatic; chemical hydrolysis to monohydroxymelphalan and dihydroxymelphalan

Bioavailability: Unpredictable; 61%±26%, decreasing with repeated doses

Half-life elimination: Terminal: I.V.: 1.5 hours; oral: 1-1.25 hours

Time to peak, serum: ~1-2 hours

Excretion: Oral: Feces (20% to 50%); urine (10% to 30% as unchanged drug)

Dosage Refer to individual protocols. Dose should always be adjusted to patient response and weekly blood counts.

Children:

Oral: 4-20 mg/m²/day for 1-21 days

Pediatric rhabdomyosarcoma: I.V.: 10-35 mg/m² bolus every 21-28 days

Bone marrow transplant for neuroblastoma: 70-140 mg/m² on days 7 and 6 before BMT or 140-220 mg/m² as a single dose before BMT

Adults:

Multiple myeloma:

Oral: 6 mg/day for 2-3 weeks or 10 mg/day for 7-10 days or 0.15 mg/kg/day for 7 days; labs should be carefully monitored during therapy and the drug may need to be discontinued after 2-3 weeks of treatment. Maintenance doses of 1-3 mg/day may be instituted after WBC recovery.

I.V.: 16 mg/m² over 15-20 minutes I.V. infusion and administered at 2-week intervals for 4 doses, then at 4-week intervals

Bone marrow transplant: I.V.: 50-60 mg/m² (up to 140 mg/m²)

Ovarian carcinoma: Oral: 0.2 mg/kg/day for 5 days, repeat every 4-5 weeks

Dosing adjustment in renal impairment:

Cl_{cr} 10-50 mL/minute: Administer at 75% of normal dose

Cl_{cr} <10 mL/minute: Administer at 50% of normal dose

Stability Dilute I.V. formulation with diluent (to 5 mg/mL), then immediately further dilute to ≤0.45 mg/mL with 0.9% sodium chloride injection in a glass bottle and administer within 60 minutes; store at room temperature; protect from light; do not refrigerate reconstituted product; use within 1 hour of reconstitution

Monitoring Parameters CBC with differential and platelet count, serum electrolytes, serum uric acid

Administration Reconstitute injection with special diluent 50 mg vial with special diluent to yield a 5 mg/mL solution; filter through a 0.45 μM Millex-HV filter; dilute the reconstituted solution with normal saline to a final concentration not to exceed 2 mg/mL; administer by I.V. infusion at a rate not to exceed 10 mg/minute, but total infusion should be given within 1 hour

Contraindications Hypersensitivity to melphalan or any component of the formulation; severe bone marrow suppression; patients whose disease was resistant to prior melphalan therapy; pregnancy

Warnings Hazardous agent – use appropriate precautions for handling and disposal. **[U.S. Boxed Warning]: Is potentially mutagenic, leukemogenic,** and carcinogenic. Suppresses ovarian function and produces amenorrhea; may also cause testicular suppression. **[U.S. Boxed Warning]: Bone marrow suppression is common.** Use with caution in patients with prior bone marrow suppression, impaired renal function (consider dose reduction), or who have received prior chemotherapy or irradiation. Toxicity to immunosuppressives is increased in elderly; start with lowest recommended adult doses. Signs of infection, such as fever and WBC rise, may not occur. Lethargy and confusion may be more prominent signs of infection. **[U.S. Boxed Warning]: Hypersensitivity has been reported with I.V. administration** and oral melphalan; may occur after multiple treatment cycles. **[U.S. Boxed Warning]: Should be administered under the supervision of an experienced cancer chemotherapy physician.** Safety and efficacy in children have not been established.

Dosage Forms Injection, powder for reconstitution: 50 mg [diluent contains ethanol and propylene glycol]

Tablet: 2 mg

Reference Range

At 0.6 mg/kg dose of melphalan, a peak plasma level of 280 ng/mL was obtained

Overdosage/Treatment

Decontamination: Lavage (within 1 hour)/activated charcoal

Supportive therapy: High-dose corticosteroids can be used for pulmonary fibrosis; ice pops if used during melphalan therapy can prevent oral stomatitis. Oral glutamine suspension as a swish and swallow, starting on day 7 every 4 hours around-the-clock for a total dose of 24 g daily, is effective in preventing oral mucositis. Filgrastim can be used to treat neutropenia.

Enhancement of elimination: Multiple dosing of activated charcoal may be effective

Test Interactions False-positive Coombs' test [direct]

Drug Interactions Cisplatin: May decrease I.V. melphalan clearance by altering renal function.

Cyclosporine: Risk of nephrotoxicity is increased by melphalan.

Digitalis glycosides: Melphalan may decrease plasma levels of digoxin.

Nalidixic acid: Concomitant use of I.V. melphalan with nalidixic acid may increase risk of necrotic enterocolitis (reported with pediatric patients).

Vaccine (live organism): Melphalan may increase the risk of vaccinal infection.

Pregnancy Risk Factor D

Pregnancy Implications Animal studies have demonstrated embryotoxicity and teratogenicity. Therapy may suppress ovarian function leading to amenorrhea. There are no adequate and well-controlled studies in pregnant women. Women of childbearing potential should be advised to avoid pregnancy while on melphalan therapy.

Lactation Excretion in breast milk unknown/not recommended

Nursing Implications Protect from light; avoid skin contact with I.V. formulation

Additional Information Myelosuppressive effects: **WBC**: Moderate. **Platelets**: Moderate. Onset (days): 7. Nadir (days): 10-18. Recovery (days): 42-50

Meperidine

CAS Number 50-13-5; 57-42-1

U.S. Brand Names Demerol®; Meperitab®

Synonyms Isonipecaine Hydrochloride; Meperidine Hydrochloride; Pethidine Hydrochloride

Impairment Potential Yes

Use Management of moderate to severe pain; adjunct to anesthesia and preoperative sedation

Unlabeled/Investigational Use Reduce postoperative shivering; reduce rigors from amphotericin

Mechanism of Action Binds to opiate receptors in the CNS, causing inhibition of ascending pain pathways, altering the perception of and response to pain; produces generalized CNS depression; a congenor of atropine

Adverse Reactions

Cardiovascular: **Hypotension**, palpitations, bradycardia, peripheral vasodilation, tachycardia (with I.V. injection), hypertension, sinus bradycardia, tachycardia (sinus);

Central nervous system: **Dizziness, fatigue, drowsiness**, sedation, seizures, psychosis, agitation, increased intracranial pressure, parkinsonism especially associated with synthetic analogues (MPPP, MPTP, PEPAP), electroencephalogram abnormalities, dysphoria, fever, CNS depression, hyperthermia

Dermatologic: Pruritus, angioedema, toxic epidermal necrolysis, urticaria

Endocrine & metabolic: Antidiuretic hormone release

Gastrointestinal: **Nausea, vomiting, constipation** (less likely than with morphine), licorice-like taste, biliary tract spasm, decreased esophageal sphincter tone, xerostomia

Genitourinary: Urinary tract spasm, urinary incontinence

Hematologic: Porphyria

Neuromuscular & skeletal: **Weakness**, myoclonus, tremors, hyperreflexia

Ocular: Miosis, mydriasis

Respiratory: Apnea, respiratory depression

Miscellaneous: **Histamine release**, physical and psychological dependence

Signs and Symptoms of Overdose Ejaculatory disturbances, myoglobinuria, rhabdomyolysis, seizures, syndrome of inappropriate antidiuretic hormone (SIADH)

Pharmacodynamics/Kinetics

Onset of action: Analgesic: Oral, SubQ: 10-15 minutes; I.V.: ~5 minutes

Peak effect: SubQ.: ~1 hour; Oral: 2 hours

Duration: Oral, SubQ.: 2-4 hours

Absorption: I.M.: Erratic and highly variable

Distribution: Crosses placenta; enters breast milk

Protein binding: 65% to 75%

Metabolism: Hepatic; hydrolyzed to meperidinic acid (inactive) or undergoes N-demethylation to normeperidine (active; has $^1/_2$ the analgesic effect and 2-3 times the CNS effects of meperidine)

Bioavailability: ~50% to 60%; increased with liver disease

Half-life elimination:

Parent drug: Terminal phase: Adults: 2.5-4 hours, Liver disease: 7-11 hours

Normeperidine (active metabolite): 15-30 hours; can accumulate with high doses or with decreased renal function

Excretion: Urine (as metabolites)

Dosage Note: Doses should be titrated to necessary analgesic effect. When changing route of administration, note that oral doses are about half as effective as parenteral dose. Oral route not recommended for chronic pain. These are guidelines and do not represent the maximum doses that may be required in all patients.

Children: Pain: Oral, I.M., I.V., SubQ: 1-1.5 mg/kg/dose every 3-4 hours as needed; 1-2 mg/kg as a single dose preoperative medication may be used; maximum 100 mg/dose

Adults: Pain:

Oral: Initial: Opiate-naive: 50 mg every 3-4 hours as needed; usual dosage range: 50-150 mg every 2-4 hours as needed

I.M., SubQ: Initial: Opiate-naive: 50-75 mg every 3-4 hours as needed; patients with prior opiate exposure may require higher initial doses; usual dosage range: 50-150 mg every 2-4 hours as needed

Preoperatively: 50-100 mg given 30-90 minutes before the beginning of anesthesia

Slow I.V.: Initial: 5-10 mg every 5 minutes as needed

Patient-controlled analgesia (PCA): Usual concentration: 10 mg/mL

Initial dose: 10 mg

Demand dose: 1-5 mg (manufacturer recommendations); range 5-25 mg (American Pain Society, 1999).

Lockout interval: 5-10 minutes

Elderly:

Oral: 50 mg every 4 hours

I.M.: 25 mg every 4 hours

Dosing adjustment in renal impairment: Avoid repeated administration of meperidine in renal dysfunction:

Cl_{cr} 10-50 mL/minute: Administer at 75% of normal dose

Cl_{cr} <10 mL/minute: Administer at 50% of normal dose

Dosing adjustment/comments in hepatic disease: Increased narcotic effect in cirrhosis; reduction in dose more important for oral than I.V. route

Stability Protect oral dosage forms from light; **incompatible** with aminophylline, heparin, phenobarbital, phenytoin, and sodium bicarbonate

Monitoring Parameters Pain relief, respiratory and mental status, blood pressure; observe patient for excessive sedation, CNS depression, seizures, respiratory depression

Administration Meperidine may be administered I.M. (preferably), SubQ, or I.V.; I.V. push should be administered slowly, use of a 10 mg/mL concentration has been recommended. For continuous I.V. infusions, a more dilute solution (eg, 1 mg/mL) should be used.

Contraindications Hypersensitivity to meperidine or any component of the formulation; use with or within 14 days of MAO inhibitors; pregnancy (prolonged use or high doses near term)

Warnings

Meperidine is not recommended for the management of chronic pain. When used for acute pain (in patients without renal or CNS disease), treatment should be limited to 48 hours and doses should not exceed 600 mg/24 hours. Oral meperidine is not recommended for acute pain management. Normeperidine (an active metabolite and CNS stimulant) may accumulate and precipitate anxiety, tremors, or seizures; risk increases with renal dysfunction and cumulative dose.

Use only with extreme caution (if at all) in patients with head injury or increased intracranial pressure (ICP); potential to elevate ICP may be greatly exaggerated in these patients. Use caution with pulmonary, hepatic, or renal disorders, supraventricular tachycardias, acute abdominal conditions, hypothyroidism, Addison's disease, BPH, or urethral stricture.

An opioid-containing analgesic regimen should be tailored to each patient's needs and based upon the type of pain being treated (acute versus chronic), the route of administration, degree of tolerance for opioids (naive versus chronic user), age, weight, and medical condition. The optimal analgesic dose varies widely among patients. Doses should be titrated to pain relief/prevention.

Some preparations contain sulfites which may cause allergic reaction. Tolerance or drug dependence may result from extended use.

Dosage Forms Injection, solution, as hydrochloride [ampul]: 25 mg/0.5 mL (0.5 mL); 25 mg/mL (1 mL); 50 mg/mL (1 mL, 1.5 mL, 2 mL); 75 mg/mL (1 mL); 100 mg/mL (1 mL)

Injection, solution, as hydrochloride [prefilled syringe]: 25 mg/mL (1 mL); 50 mg/mL (1 mL); 75 mg/mL (1 mL); 100 mg/mL (1 mL)

Injection, solution, as hydrochloride [for PCA pump]: 10 mg/mL (30 mL, 50 mL, 60 mL)

Injection, solution, as hydrochloride [vial]: 25 mg/mL (1 mL); 50 mg/mL (1 mL, 30 mL); 75 mg/mL (1 mL); 100 mg/mL (1 mL, 20 mL) [may contain sodium metabisulfite]

Syrup, as hydrochloride:

Demerol®: 50 mg/5 mL (480 mL) [contains benzoic acid; banana flavor]

Tablet, as hydrochloride: 50 mg, 100 mg

Demerol®, Meperitab®: 50 mg, 100 mg

Reference Range

Serum level:

Meperidine:

Therapeutic: 70-500 ng/mL (SI: 283-2020 nmol/L)

Toxic: >1000 ng/mL (SI: >4043 nmol/L)

Normeperidine: Toxic: >450 ng/mL

Urinary level: Meperidine: Therapeutic: 1-10 mg/L

In the postmortem state, anatomical site concentration differences (ie, postmortem redistribution) may occur.

Overdosage/Treatment Supportive therapy: Naloxone hydrochloride (0.4-2 mg I.V., SubQ, or through an endotracheal tube); a continuous infusion (at $^2/_3$ the response dose/hour) may be required; seizures are usually self-limited and can be managed with benzodiazepines. Naloxone is not useful in treating meperidine-induced seizures.

Antidote(s)

● Nalmefene [ANTIDOTE]

● Naloxone [ANTIDOTE]

Test Interactions ↑ amylase (S), BSP retention, CPK (I.M. injections)

Drug Interactions Substrate (minor) of CYP2B6, 2C19, 3A4

Acyclovir: May increase meperidine metabolite concentrations. Use caution.

Barbiturates: May decrease analgesic efficacy and increase sedative and/or respiratory depressive effects of meperidine.

Cimetidine: May increase meperidine metabolite concentrations; use caution.

CNS depressants (including benzodiazepines): May potentiate the sedative and/or respiratory depressive effects of meperidine.

MAO inhibitors: May enhance the serotonergic effect of meperidine, which may cause serotonin syndrome. Concurrent use with or within 14 days of an MAO inhibitor is contraindicated.

Phenothiazines: May potentiate the sedative and/or respiratory depressive effects of meperidine; may increase the incidence of hypotension.

Phenytoin: May decrease the analgesic effects of meperidine

Ritonavir: May increase meperidine metabolite concentrations; use caution.

Serotonin agonists: Serotonin agonists and meperidine may enhance serotonin levels in the brain. Serotonin syndrome may occur.

Serotonin reuptake inhibitors: May potentiate the effects of meperidine, increasing serotonin levels in the brain. Serotonin syndrome may occur.

Sibutramine: May enhance the serotonergic effect of meperidine. Serotonin syndrome may occur.

Tricyclic antidepressants: May potentiate the sedative and/or respiratory depressive effects of meperidine. In addition, potentially may increase the risk of serotonin syndrome.

Pregnancy Risk Factor B/D (prolonged use or high doses at term)

Pregnancy Implications Meperidine is known to cross the placenta, which may result in respiratory or CNS depression in the newborn.

Lactation Enters breast milk/contraindicated (AAP rates "compatible")

Additional Information Decrease the dose in patients with renal or hepatic impairment; equianalgesic doses: morphine 10 mg I.M. is equivalent to meperidine 75-100 mg I.M.

I.V. incompatible with barbiturates

Risk for meperidine-induced seizures includes renal insufficiency, alkaline urine, coadministration of phenothiazines and doses of meperidine >100 mg every 2 hours for longer than 24 hours.

Factors predisposing to normeperidine-induced seizures: Doses >100 mg every 2 hours for longer than 24 hours; renal failure; alkaline urine; coadministration of hepatic enzyme-inducing medications; coadministration of medications which can lower the seizure threshold (ie, phenothiazines); sickle cell anemia

Specific References
Bailey DN and Briggs JR, "Procainamide and Quinidine Inhibition of the Human Hepatic Degradation of Meperidine In Vitro," *J Anal Toxicol*, 2003, 27(3):142-4.
Felegi WB, Silverman ME, and Allegra JR, "Does the Distribution of Written Guidelines with Accompanying Educational Information for Appropriate Use of Meperidine Change Emergency Department Physicians' Prescribing Habits?" *Ann Emerg Med*, 2003, 42(4):S101.

Mephentermine

CAS Number 100-92-5; 1212-72-2; 6190-60-9
Synonyms Mephentermine Sulfate
Use Treatment of hypotension secondary to ganglionic blockade or spinal anesthesia; may be used as an emergency measure to maintain blood pressure until whole blood replacement becomes available
Mechanism of Action A sympathomimetic drug with similar properties as other paraphenylethylamines; an indirect-acting sympathomimetic that releases norepinephrine; the elevation in blood pressure is probably primarily related to an increased in cardiac output resulting from enhanced cardiac contraction and due to an increase in peripheral resistance from peripheral vasoconstriction to a lesser degree; may also stimulate beta-adrenergic receptors and the change in heart rate is variable, depending on vagal tone
Adverse Reactions
Cardiovascular: Arrhythmias
Central nervous system: Euphoria, weeping, nervousness, anxiety, convulsions, hallucinations (visual, auditory or olfactory), psychosis, paranoia, delirium
Gastrointestinal: Anorexia
Neuromuscular & skeletal: Tremor
Signs and Symptoms of Overdose Hallucinations, paranoia, seizures
Pharmacodynamics/Kinetics
Metabolism: Hepatic
Elimination: In urine
Dosage
Hypotension: I.M., I.V.:
Children: 0.4 mg/kg
Adults: 0.5 mg/kg
Hypotensive emergency: I.V. infusion: 20-60 mg
Administration May be given I.M.
Contraindications Known hypersensitivity to mephentermine, hypotension induced by drugs causing alpha blockade
Warnings Use with caution in patients with cardiovascular disease or hypertension
Dosage Forms Injection, as sulfate: 15 mg/mL (2 mL, 10 mL)
Overdosage/Treatment Supportive therapy: Agitation can be treated with diazepam (0.1 mg/kg); severe agitation can be treated with haloperidol (up to 0.1 mg/kg) or droperidol (up to 0.1 mg/kg I.V.); for treatment of distal extremity necrosis due to inadvertent intra-arterial administration, tolazoline (25 mg intra-arterial then 50 mg I.V.) may be useful; if this is not effective, stellate ganglion block may be necessary; seizures can be treated with benzodiazepines; hypertension can be treated with phentolamine or nitroprusside while ventricular arrhythmias can be treated with lidocaine
Antidote(s)
• Phentolamine [ANTIDOTE]
Drug Interactions Phenothiazines antagonize the pressor effects, MAO inhibitors potentiate the pressor effects
Pregnancy Risk Factor C
Pregnancy Implications Uterine stimulation may occur

Mephenytoin

CAS Number 50-12-4
Synonyms Methoin; Methylphenylethylhydantoin; Phenantoin
Impairment Potential Yes
Use Treatment of tonic-clonic and partial seizures in patients who are uncontrolled with less toxic anticonvulsants
Mechanism of Action Stabilizes neuronal membranes and decreases seizure activity by increasing efflux or decreasing influx of sodium ions across cell membranes in the motor cortex during generation of nerve impulses; prolongs effective refractory period and suppresses ventricular pacemaker automaticity, shortens action potential in the heart
Adverse Reactions
Cardiovascular: Hypotension, bradycardia, cardiac arrhythmias, cardiovascular collapse
Central nervous system: **Psychiatric changes, slurred speech, dizziness, drowsiness**, headache, insomnia, confusion, fever, ataxia,

psychotic episodes, complex partial epilepsy, simple partial epilepsy, tonic-clonic epilepsy
Dermatologic: Skin rash, Stevens-Johnson syndrome or SLE-like syndrome, alopecia, urticaria, purpura, toxic epidermal necrolysis, exfoliative dermatitis, acne, angioedema, bullous skin disease, pruritus, exanthem
Gastrointestinal: **Constipation, nausea, vomiting**, anorexia, weight loss, gingival hyperplasia (less common than with phenytoin)
Hematologic: Blood dyscrasias (neutropenia, thrombocytopenia, leukopenia, pancytopenia), aplastic anemia, Hodgkin's disease-like syndrome
Hepatic: Hepatitis, jaundice
Local: Venous irritation and pain, thrombophlebitis
Neuromuscular & skeletal: **Trembling**, paresthesia, neuropathy (peripheral)
Ocular: Diplopia, nystagmus, blurred vision, photophobia, conjunctivitis
Renal: Nephrotic syndrome, proteinuria, elevated serum creatinine, glomerulonephritis
Respiratory: Pulmonary fibrosis
Miscellaneous: Lymphadenopathy, serum sickness, periarteritis nodosa
Admission Criteria/Prognosis Admit any ingestion which results in a total mephenytoin serum level >50 mcg/mL
Pharmacodynamics/Kinetics
Onset of action: 30 minutes
Duration: 24-48 hours
Absorption: Oral: Rapid
Metabolism: In the liver
Half-life: 144 hours
Elimination: In urine
Dosage
Oral:
Children: 3-15 mg/kg/day in 3 divided doses; usual maintenance dose: 100-400 mg/day in 3 divided doses
Adults: Initial dose: 50-100 mg/day given daily; increase by 50-100 mg at weekly intervals; usual maintenance dose: 200-600 mg/day in 3 divided doses; maximum: 800 mg/day
Monitoring Parameters CBC and platelet count
Contraindications Hypersensitivity to mephenytoin, other hydantoins, or any component of the formulation
Warnings Fatal irreversible aplastic anemia has occurred; abrupt withdrawal may precipitate seizures; may increase frequency of petit mal seizures; use with caution in patients with liver disease or porphyria; usually listed in combination with other anticonvulsants
Dosage Forms Tablet: 100 mg
Reference Range Total mephenytoin (mephenytoin plus 5-ethyl-5-phenylhydantoin) of 25-40 mcg/mL produces optimal seizure control; serum levels >40 mcg/mL can produce central nervous system effects or exacerbate seizures
Overdosage/Treatment
Decontamination: Emesis within 30 minutes or lavage (within 1 hour)/ activated charcoal
Supportive therapy: Treatment is supportive for hypotension; treat with I.V. fluids and place patient in Trendelenburg position; seizures may be controlled with lorazepam or diazepam 5-10 mg (0.25-0.4 mg/kg in children); I.V. albumin (25 g every 6 hours has been used to increase bound fraction of drug); extravasation can be treated with compressive dressing, elevation and splinting of extremity
Enhancement of elimination: Multiple dosing of activated charcoal may be effective; peritoneal dialysis, diuresis, hemodialysis, hemoperfusion, and plasmapheresis is of little value
Test Interactions ↑ alkaline phosphatase (S); ↓ calcium (S)
Drug Interactions
CYP2C19 enzyme substrate
Acetaminophen: Hydantoins may enhance the hepatotoxic potential of acetaminophen overdoses
Acetazolamide: Concurrent use with hydantoins may result in an increased risk of osteomalacia
Acyclovir: May decrease hydantoin serum levels; limited documentation; monitor
Allopurinol: May increase hydantoin serum concentrations; monitor
Antacids: May decrease absorption of hydantoins; separate oral doses by several hours
Antiarrhythmics: Hydantoins may increase the metabolism of antiarrhythmics, decreasing their clinical effect; includes disopyramide, propafenone, and quinidine; amiodarone also may increase hydantoin concentrations (see CYP inhibitors)
Anticonvulsants: Hydantoins may increase the metabolism of anticonvulsants; includes barbiturates, carbamazepine, ethosuximide, felbamate, lamotrigine, tiagabine, topiramate, and zonisamide; does not appear to affect gabapentin or levetiracetam; felbamate and gabapentin may increase hydantoin levels; monitor
Antineoplastics: Several chemotherapeutic agents have been associated with a decrease in serum hydantoin levels; includes cisplatin, bleomycin, carmustine, methotrexate, and vinblastine; monitor hydantoin

serum levels. Limited evidence also suggest that enzyme-inducing anticonvulsant therapy may reduce the effectiveness of some chemotherapy regimens (specifically in ALL). Teniposide and methotrexate may be cleared more rapidly in these patients.

Antipsychotics: Hydantoins may enhance the metabolism (decrease the efficacy) of antipsychotics; monitor for altered response; dose adjustment may be needed; also see note on clozapine

Benzodiazepines: Hydantoins may decrease the serum concentrations of some benzodiazepines; monitor for decreased benzodiazepine effect

Beta-blockers: Metabolism of beta-blockers may be increased and clinical effect decreased; atenolol and nadolol are unlikely to interact given their renal elimination

Calcium channel blockers: Hydantoin may enhance the metabolism of calcium channel blockers, decreasing their clinical effect; nifedipine has been reported to increase hydantoin levels (case report); monitor

Capecitabine: May increase the serum concentrations of hydantoins; monitor

Chloramphenicol: Hydantoins may increase the metabolism of chloramphenicol and chloramphenicol may inhibit hydantoins metabolism; monitor for altered response

Ciprofloxacin: Case reports indicate ciprofloxacin may increase or decrease serum hydantoin concentrations; monitor

Clozapine: May decrease hydantoin serum concentrations; monitor

CNS depressants: Sedative effects may be additive with other CNS depressants; monitor for increased effect; includes ethanol, barbiturates, sedatives, antidepressants, narcotic analgesics, and benzodiazepines

Corticosteroids: Hydantoin may increase the metabolism of corticosteroids, decreasing their clinical effect; also see dexamethasone

Cyclosporine and tacrolimus: Levels may be decreased by hydantoin; monitor

CYP2C8/9 inhibitors: Serum levels and/or toxicity of hydantoin may be increased; inhibitors include amiodarone, cimetidine, fluvoxamine, some NSAIDs, metronidazole, ritonavir, sulfonamides, troglitazone, valproic acid, and zafirlukast; monitor for increased effect/toxicity

CYP2C19 inhibitors: Serum levels of hydantoin may be increased; inhibitors include cimetidine, felbamate, fluconazole, fluoxetine, fluvoxamine, omeprazole, teniposide, tolbutamide, and troglitazone

Dexamethasone: May decrease serum hydantoin due to increased metabolism; monitor

Digoxin: Effects and/or levels of digitalis glycosides may be decreased by hydantoin

Disulfiram: May increase serum hydantoin concentrations; monitor

Dopamine: I.V. hydantoins may increase the effect of dopamine (enhanced hypotension)

Doxycycline: Hydantoins may enhance the metabolism of doxycycline, decreasing its clinical effect; higher dosages may be required

Estrogens: Hydantoins may increase the metabolism of estrogens, decreasing their clinical effect; monitor

Enzyme inducers: The serum levels of hydantoins may be reduced by barbiturates, carbamazepine, chronic ethanol, dexamethasone, and rifampin

Folic acid: Replacement of folic acid has been reported to increase the metabolism of hydantoins, decreasing its serum concentrations and/or increasing seizures

Furosemide: Diuretic effect may be blunted by hydantoins (mechanism unclear); possibly due to decreased furosemide bioavailability

HMG-CoA reductase inhibitors: Hydantoins may increase the metabolism of these agents, reducing their clinical effect; monitor

Itraconazole: Hydantoins may decrease the effect of itraconazole

Levodopa: Hydantoins may inhibit the anti-Parkinson effect of levodopa

Lithium: Concurrent use of hydantoins and lithium has resulted in lithium intoxication

Methadone: Hydantoins may enhance the metabolism of methadone resulting in methadone withdrawal

Methylphenidate: May increase serum hydantoins concentrations; monitor

Neuromuscular blocking agents: Duration of effect may be decreased by hydantoins

Omeprazole: May increase serum hydantoins concentrations; monitor

Oral contraceptives: Hydantoins may enhance the metabolism of oral contraceptives, decreasing their clinical effect; an alternative method of contraception should be considered

Phenylbutazone: May increase hydantoin concentrations; monitor and adjust dosage

Primidone: Hydantoins enhance the conversion of primidone to phenobarbital resulting in elevated phenobarbital serum concentrations

Quetiapine: Serum concentrations may be substantially reduced by hydantoins, potentially resulting in a loss of efficacy; limited documentation; monitor

SSRIs: May increase hydantoin serum concentrations; fluoxetine and fluvoxamine are known to inhibit metabolism via CYP enzymes; sertraline and paroxetine have also been shown to increase concentrations in some patients; monitor

Sucralfate: May reduce the GI absorption of hydantoins; monitor

Theophylline: Hydantoins may increase metabolism of theophylline derivatives and decrease their clinical effect; theophylline may also increase hydantoin concentrations

Thyroid hormones (including levothyroxine): Hydantoins may alter the metabolism of thyroid hormones, reducing its effect; there is limited documentation of this interaction, but monitoring should be considered

Ticlopidine: May increase serum hydantoin concentrations and/or toxicity; monitor

Tricyclic antidepressants: Hydantoins may increase metabolism of tricyclic antidepressants and decrease their clinical effect; sedative effects may be additive; tricyclics may also increase hydantoin concentrations

Topiramate: Hydantoins may decrease serum levels of topiramate; topiramate may increase the effect of hydantoins

Trazodone: Serum levels of hydantoins may be increased; limited documentation; monitor

Trimethoprim: May increase serum hydantoin concentrations; monitor

Valproic acid (and sulfisoxazole): May displace hydantoins from binding sites; valproic acid may increase, decrease, or have no effect on hydantoin serum concentrations

Vigabatrin: May reduce hydantoin serum concentrations; monitor

Warfarin: Hydantoins transiently increased the hypothrombinemia response to warfarin initially; this is followed by an inhibition of the hypoprothrombinemic response

Pregnancy Risk Factor C

Nursing Implications Monitor CBC and platelet

Additional Information Usually used in combination with other anticonvulsants; **Note:** The company that makes Mesantoin® has **discontinued manufacturing** (July, 2000); the drug is currently available from Novartis under a transition program; small quantities may be obtained while transitioning patients to other antiepileptic agents.

Mephobarbital

CAS Number 115-38-8

U.S. Brand Names Mebaral®

Synonyms Methylphenobarbital

Impairment Potential Yes

Use Prophylactic management of tonic-clonic (grand mal) seizures and absence (petit mal) seizures

Mechanism of Action Increases seizure threshold in the motor cortex; depresses monosynaptic and polysynaptic transmission in the CNS

Adverse Reactions

Cardiovascular: Sinus tachycardia

Central nervous system: **Drowsiness, dizziness, lightheadedness, "hangover" effect**, paradoxical excitation (especially in children), sinus bradycardia

Dermatologic: Rash, including Stevens-Johnson syndrome or erythema multiforme

Gastrointestinal: Nausea, vomiting

Hematologic: Leukopenia/neutropenia (agranulocytosis, granulocytopenia), thrombocytopenic purpura

Miscellaneous: Psychological and physical dependence

Signs and Symptoms of Overdose CNS depression, cyclic coma, hypotension, hypothermia, nystagmus, ptosis, renal failure, respiratory depression, tachycardia, vision color changes (green tinge; yellow tinge)

Pharmacodynamics/Kinetics

Onset of action: 20-60 minutes

Duration: 6-8 hours

Absorption: ~50%

Half-life elimination, serum: 34 hours

Dosage

Oral:

Epilepsy:

Children: 6-12 mg/kg/day in 2-4 divided doses

Adults: 200-600 mg/day in 2-4 divided doses

Sedation:

Children:

<5 years: 16-32 mg 3-4 times/day

>5 years: 32-64 mg 3-4 times/day

Adults: 32-100 mg 3-4 times/day

Dosing adjustment in renal or hepatic impairment: Use with caution and reduce dosages

Monitoring Parameters Respiratory

Contraindications Hypersensitivity to mephobarbital, other barbiturates, or any component of the formulation; pre-existing CNS depression; respiratory depression; severe uncontrolled pain; history of porphyria; pregnancy

Dosage Forms Tablet: 32 mg, 50 mg, 100 mg

Reference Range Phenobarbital level should be in the range of 15-40 mcg/mL; levels >80 mcg/mL correlate with decreased mental status. Mephobarbital: therapeutic: 8-15 mg/L

Overdosage/Treatment

Decontamination: Ipecac within 30 minutes or lavage (within 1 hour)/ activated charcoal

Supportive therapy: Isotonic fluids for hypotension; dopamine or norepinephrine can be used

Enhancement of elimination: Repeated oral doses of activated charcoal significantly reduce the half-life of phenobarbital resulting from an enhancement of nonrenal elimination. Assure adequate hydration and renal function. Urinary alkalinization with I.V. sodium bicarbonate also helps to enhance elimination. Hemodialysis or hemoperfusion is of uncertain value. Patients in stage four coma due to high serum barbiturate levels may require charcoal hemoperfusion.

Test Interactions ↑ alkaline phosphatase (S), ammonia (B); ↓ bilirubin (S), calcium (S)

Drug Interactions **Substrate** of CYP2B6 (minor), 2C9 (minor), 2C19 (major); **Inhibits** CYP2C19 (weak); **Induces** CYP2A6 (weak)

Acetaminophen: Barbiturates may enhance the hepatotoxic potential of acetaminophen overdoses

CNS depressants: Sedative effects and/or respiratory depression with barbiturates may be additive with other CNS depressants; monitor for increased effect; includes ethanol, sedatives, antidepressants, narcotic analgesics, and benzodiazepines

Cyclosporine: Levels may be decreased by barbiturates; monitor

CYP2C19 inducers: May decrease the levels/effects of mephobarbital. Example inducers include aminoglutethimide, carbamazepine, phenytoin, and rifampin.

CYP2C19 inhibitors: May increase the levels/effects of mephobarbital. Example inhibitors include delavirdine, fluconazole, fluvoxamine, gemfibrozil, isoniazid, omeprazole, and ticlopidine.

Griseofulvin: Barbiturates may impair the absorption of griseofulvin, and griseofulvin metabolism may be increased by barbiturates, decreasing clinical effect

Guanfacine: Effect may be decreased by barbiturates

MAO inhibitors: Metabolism of barbiturates may be inhibited, increasing clinical effect or toxicity of the barbiturates

Methoxyflurane: Barbiturates may enhance the nephrotoxic effects of methoxyflurane

Valproic acid: Metabolism of barbiturates may be inhibited by valproic acid; monitor for excessive sedation; a dose reduction may be needed

Pregnancy Risk Factor D

Nursing Implications Observe patient for excessive sedation, apnea; raise bed rails, institute safety precautions, assist with ambulation

Additional Information Sometimes used in specific patients who have excessive sedation or hyperexcitability from phenobarbital; avoid abrupt discontinuation

Mepivacaine

CAS Number 1722-62-9; 96-88-8

U.S. Brand Names Carbocaine® [DSC]; Polocaine® MPF; Polocaine®

Synonyms Mepivacaine Hydrochloride

Use Local anesthesia by nerve block; infiltration in dental procedures

Mechanism of Action Mepivacaine is an amino amide local anesthetic similar to lidocaine; like all local anesthetics, mepivacaine acts by preventing the generation and conduction of nerve impulses

Adverse Reactions

Cardiovascular: Bradycardia, myocardial depression, hypotension, cardiovascular collapse, edema, sinus bradycardia, congestive heart failure

Central nervous system: Anxiety, restlessness, disorientation, confusion, seizures, drowsiness, unconsciousness, lightheadedness, headache, chills

Dermatologic: Urticaria

Gastrointestinal: Nausea, vomiting

Hematologic: Porphyria, porphyrinogenic

Local: Transient stinging or burning at injection site

Neuromuscular & skeletal: Tremors

Ocular: Blurred vision

Otic: Ototoxicity, tinnitus

Respiratory: Respiratory arrest

Miscellaneous: Neonatal CNS depression following paracervical blocks from delivery, shivering, anaphylactoid reactions

Signs and Symptoms of Overdose Apnea, bradycardia, bronchial spasm, cyanosis, depression, dizziness, muscle twitching, nystagmus, ototoxicity, seizures, tinnitus, tremors

Pharmacodynamics/Kinetics

Onset of action (route and dose dependent): Range: 3-20 minutes

Duration (route and dose dependent): 2-2.5 hours

Protein binding: ~75%

Metabolism: Primarily hepatic via N-demethylation, hydroxylation, and glucuronidation

Half-life elimination: Neonates: 8.7-9 hours; Adults: 1.9-3 hours

Excretion: Urine (95% as metabolites)

Dosage Children and Adults: Injectable local anesthetic: Varies with procedure, degree of anesthesia needed, vascularity of tissue, duration of anesthesia required, and physical condition of patient

Monitoring Parameters ECG, respiratory status

Administration Before injecting, withdraw syringe plunger to ensure injection is not into vein or artery

Contraindications Hypersensitivity to mepivacaine, other amide-type local anesthetics, or any component of the formulation

Warnings Use with caution in patients with cardiac disease, hepatic or renal disease, or hyperthyroidism. Local anesthetics have been associated with rare occurrences of sudden respiratory arrest; convulsions due to systemic toxicity leading to cardiac arrest have been reported presumably due to intravascular injection. A test dose is recommended prior to epidural administration and all reinforcing doses with continuous catheter technique. Do not use solutions containing preservatives for caudal or epidural block. Use caution in debilitated, elderly, or acutely ill patients; dose reduction may be required.

Dosage Forms Injection, solution, as hydrochloride [contains methylparabens]:

Carbocaine®: 1% (50 mL); 2% (50 mL)

Polocaine®: 1% (50 mL); 2% (50 mL)

Injection, solution, as hydrochloride [preservative free]:

Carbocaine®: 1% (30 mL); 1.5% (30 mL); 2% (20 mL); 3% (1.8 mL) [dental cartridge]

Polocaine® Dental: 3% (1.8 mL) [dental cartridge]

Polocaine® MPF: 1% (30 mL); 1.5% (30 mL); 2% (20 mL)

Reference Range

Therapeutic: Plasma levels are <5 mcg/mL

Fatal: Fatalities are associated with levels >10 mcg/mL

Overdosage/Treatment

Decontamination: Activated charcoal

Supportive therapy: Termination of anesthesia by pneumatic tourniquet inflation should be attempted when the agent is administered by infiltration or regional injection. Seizures commonly respond to diazepam, lorazepam or barbiturates, while hypotension responds to I.V. fluids and Trendelenburg positioning. Bradyarrhythmias (when the heart rate is less than 60) can be treated with I.V. atropine 15 mcg/kg. With the development of metabolic acidosis, I.V. sodium bicarbonate 0.5-2 mEq/kg and ventilatory assistance should be instituted.

Enhancement of elimination: Exchange transfusion is of minimal benefit

Pregnancy Risk Factor C

Pregnancy Implications May cause neonatal depression or seizures

Lactation Excretion in breast milk unknown/use caution

Nursing Implications Before injecting, withdraw syringe plunger to ensure injection is not into vein or artery; solution is acidic

Additional Information Numbing, bitter taste

Meprobamate

Related Information
- Carisoprodol

CAS Number 57-53-4

U.S. Brand Names Miltown®

Synonyms Equanil

Impairment Potential Yes. Serum meprobamate level >60 mg/L has been associated with impairment. (Baselt RC and Cravey RH, *Disposition of Toxic Drugs and Chemicals in Man*, 4th ed, Foster City, CA: Chemical Toxicology Institute, 1995, 460.) Driving impairment can occur if combined serum level of carisoprodol and meprobamate exceeds 10 mg/L.

Use Management of anxiety disorders

Unlabeled/Investigational Use Demonstrated value for muscle contraction, headache, premenstrual tension, external sphincter spasticity, muscle rigidity, opisthotonos-associated with tetanus

Mechanism of Action Precise mechanisms are not yet clear, but many effects have been ascribed to its central depressant actions

Adverse Reactions

Cardiovascular: Syncope, peripheral edema, cyanosis, sinus bradycardia, palpitations, sinus tachycardia, vasculitis

Central nervous system: **Drowsiness**, slurred speech, headache, euphoria, dizziness, paradoxical excitation, **ataxia**

Dermatologic: Exfoliative dermatitis, pityriasis rosea-like reaction, toxic epidermal necrolysis, urticaria, photosensitivity, pruritus, erythema nodosum

Endocrine & metabolic: Gynecomastia

Gastrointestinal: Xerostomia

Neuromuscular & skeletal: Paresthesia

Ocular: Nystagmus, miosis, mydriasis

Miscellaneous: Systemic lupus erythematosus, fixed drug eruption

Hypersensitivity reactions: **Mild**: Rash, leukopenia, purpura, angioedema, bullous dermatitis. **Severe**: Fever, chills, wheezing, renal failure, dermatitis, stomatitis, Stevens-Johnson syndrome, agranulocytosis

Signs and Symptoms of Overdose Agranulocytosis, areflexia, ataxia, bezoars, bradycardia, coma, drowsiness, granulocytopenia, hyporeflexia, hypotension, leukopenia, neutropenia, porphyria, respiratory depression, stupor, syncope, tachycardia, wheezing

Pharmacodynamics/Kinetics

Onset of action: Sedation: ~1 hour

Distribution: Crosses placenta; enters breast milk

Metabolism: Hepatic

Half-life elimination: 10 hours

Excretion: Urine (8% to 20% as unchanged drug); feces (10% as metabolites)

Dosage

Oral:

Children 6-12 years: Anxiety: 100-200 mg 2-3 times/day

Adults: Anxiety: 400 mg 3-4 times/day, up to 2400 mg/day

Dosing interval in renal impairment:

Cl_{cr} 10-50 mL/minute: Administer every 9-12 hours

Cl_{cr} <10 mL/minute: Administer every 12-18 hours

Hemodialysis: Moderately dialyzable (20% to 50%)

Dosing adjustment in hepatic impairment: Probably necessary in patients with liver disease

Monitoring Parameters Mental status

Contraindications Hypersensitivity to meprobamate, related compounds (including carisoprodol), or any component of the formulation; acute intermittent porphyria; pre-existing CNS depression; narrow-angle glaucoma; severe uncontrolled pain; pregnancy

Warnings Physical and psychological dependence and abuse may occur; abrupt cessation may precipitate withdrawal. Use with caution in patients with depression or suicidal tendencies, or in patients with a history of drug abuse. May cause CNS depression, which may impair physical or mental abilities. Patients must be cautioned about performing tasks which require mental alertness (eg, operating machinery or driving). Effects with other sedative drugs or ethanol may be potentiated. Not recommended in children <6 years of age; allergic reaction may occur in patients with history of dermatological condition (usually by fourth dose). Use with caution in patients with renal or hepatic impairment, or with a history of seizures. Use caution in the elderly as it may cause confusion, cognitive impairment, or excessive sedation.

Dosage Forms [DSC] = Discontinued product

Tablet: 200 mg, 400 mg

Miltown®: 200 mg, 400 mg [DSC]

Reference Range

Therapeutic: 6-12 mcg/mL (SI: 28-55 µmol/L); sedative dose 8-24 mcg/mL (SI: 37-110 µmol/L)

Toxic: >50 mcg/mL (SI: >229 µmol/L); coma is associated with levels >70 mcg/mL

Fatal: Fatalities can occur with levels >142 mcg/mL

Overdosage/Treatment

Decontamination: Lavage (within 1 hour)/activated charcoal

Supportive therapy: Following attempts to enhance drug elimination. Hypotension should be treated with I.V. fluids and/or Trendelenburg positioning.

Enhancement of elimination: Hemodialysis is recommended at plasma levels >20 mg/dL; charcoal hemoperfusion increases meprobamate clearance. Multiple dosing of activated charcoal may decrease half-life by 50%; forced diuresis with saline may be useful; moderately dialyzable (20% to 50%). Clearance through hemodialysis and hemoperfusion average 60 mL/minute and 153 mL/minute respectively. Continuous arteriovenous hemoperfusion clearance rates are 198 ± 16 mL/minute.

Drug Interactions CNS depressants: Sedative effects may be additive with other CNS depressants; monitor for increased effect; includes barbiturates, benzodiazepines, narcotic analgesics, ethanol, and other sedative agents

Pregnancy Risk Factor D

Pregnancy Implications Crosses the placenta

Lactation Enters breast milk/not recommended

Additional Information Can cause bezoars

Specific References

Daval S, Richard D, Souweine B, et al, "A One-Step and Sensitive GC-MS Assay for Meprobamate Determination in Emergency Situations," *J Anal Toxicol*, 2006, 30:302-5.

Meptazinol

CAS Number 34154-59-1; 54340-58-8; 59263-76-2

Unlabeled/Investigational Use In U.S.: Acute analgesic agent; also used to diminish Jarisch-Herxheimer reaction

Mechanism of Action A centrally acting opioid agonist-antagonist agent with cholinergic activity

Adverse Reactions

All adverse effects are seen frequently with parenteral administration as compared to oral administration

Central nervous system: Drowsiness, dizziness, euphoria, headache, amnesia, hallucinations, dysphoria

Gastrointestinal: **Nausea, vomiting**, xerostomia, dyspepsia

Ocular: Slight miosis, blurred vision

Miscellaneous: Diaphoresis

Signs and Symptoms of Overdose Respiratory depression

Toxicodynamics/Kinetics

Peak effect: Oral: 1-2 hours; Parenteral: 0.5-1 hour

Distribution: V_d: 2-3 L/kg

Protein binding: 23% to 27%

Metabolism: Hepatic

Bioavailability: Oral: 4% to 10%

Half-life: Neonates: 3.4 hours; Adults: 2 hours (adult men); 1.4-1.7 hours (adult women)

Elimination: Primarily renal (plasma clearance ~100 L/hour)

Effective analgesia: Oral: 4 hours

Dosage

Children: I.M. (in lateral thigh): 1 mg/kg

Analgesia:

Oral: 200 mg every 3-6 hours

Epidural: 30-90 mg (in 10 mL of normal saline)

I.M.: 75-100 mg every 2-4 hours

I.V.: 50-100 mg slowly every 2-4 hours; continuous I.V.: Loading dose of 50 mg I.V. followed by 0.5 mg/kg/hour for up to 1 day

Herxheimer reaction: I.V.: 300-500 mg

Reference Range Peak serum level after a 200 mg oral dose: 10-110 ng/mL; peak plasma level after a 50 mg I.V. dose: ~270 ng/mL

Overdosage/Treatment Supportive therapy: Naloxone hydrochloride (0.4-2 mg I.V., SubQ, or through an endotracheal tube); a continuous infusion (at $^2/_3$ the response dose/hour) may be required; opioid-induced myoclonus may respond to dantrolene (50-150 mg/day); higher than usual doses of naloxone may be necessary to treat respiratory depression

Antidote(s)

- Naloxone [ANTIDOTE]

Pregnancy Implications No teratogenic effects known; can cross the placenta

Additional Information $\sim^1/_{10}$ as potent as morphine with miosis and constipation occurring less frequently; structurally similar to pentazocine

---

Merbromin

Pronunciation (mer BROE min)

CAS Number 129-16-8

U.S. Brand Names Mercurochrome®

Use Dermal antiseptic

Mechanism of Action Bacteriostatic antimicrobial activity

Adverse Reactions

Central nervous system: Dizziness

Dermatologic: Contact dermatitis

Gastrointestinal: Abdominal pain, nausea, diarrhea in less than 4% of ingestions

Miscellaneous: Application to surgical wounds and decubitus ulcers has resulted in a fatality due to aplastic anemia; anaphylaxis

Dosage Apply freely, until injury has healed

Monitoring Parameters Renal function, liver function

Warnings Prolonged use or use on extensive areas should be under physician's directions

Dosage Forms Solution, topical: 2% (30 mL)

Reference Range Urinary and whole blood levels can be obtained; normally urinary values are <10 mcg/dL and whole blood <2 mcg/dL; whole blood levels <50 mcg/dL are usually associated with gastroenteritis and acute tubular necrosis; urinary levels for organic mercury are not useful since 90% is eliminated through bile in the feces; urinary mercury levels >56 mcg/L can result in neurotoxic effects (due to elemental mercury)

Overdosage/Treatment

Decontamination: **Oral:** Lavage ingestions >50 mg/kg within 1 hour/ activated charcoal is probably not useful. **Dermal:** Wash thoroughly with soap and water. **Ocular:** Irrigate with normal saline.

Supportive therapy: Succimer (10 mg/kg every 8 hours for 5 days, then every 12 hours for 14 days) may be useful in severe exposures; penicillamine or N-acetyl-penillamine can also be used; BAL may increase mercury levels in the central nervous system and is therefore contraindicated

Drug Interactions Incompatible with acids, most alkaloidal salts, many local anesthetics, metals, and sulfides

---

Mercaptopurine

Related Information

- Azathioprine

CAS Number 50-44-2; 6112-76-1

U.S. Brand Names Purinethol®

Synonyms 6-Mercaptopurine (error-prone abbreviation); 6-MP (error-prone abbreviation); NSC-755

Use Maintenance therapy in acute lymphoblastic leukemia (ALL); other (less common) uses include chronic granulocytic leukemia, induction therapy in ALL, and treatment of non-Hodgkin's lymphomas

Unlabeled/Investigational Use Steroid-sparing agent for corticosteroid-dependent Crohn's disease (CD) and ulcerative colitis (UC); maintenance of remission in CD; fistulizing Crohn's disease

Mechanism of Action Purine antagonist which inhibits DNA and RNA synthesis; acts as false metabolite and is incorporated into DNA and RNA, eventually inhibiting their synthesis; specific for the S phase of the cell cycle

Adverse Reactions

Central nervous system: Drug fever

Dermatologic: Hyperpigmentation, rash, alopecia, dry and scaling rash

Endocrine & metabolic: Hyperuricemia

Gastrointestinal: Nausea, vomiting, diarrhea, stomatitis, anorexia, stomach pain, mucositis, glossitis, tarry stools

Genitourinary: Oligospermia

Hematologic: **Myelosuppression**; **leukopenia**, **thrombocytopenia**, **anemia**, eosinophilia

Onset: 7-10 days

Nadir: 14-16 days

Recovery: 21-28 days

Hepatic: **Intrahepatic cholestasis and focal centralobular necrosis** (40%), characterized by hyperbilirubinemia, increased alkaline phosphatase and AST, jaundice, ascites, encephalopathy; more common at doses >2.5 mg/kg/day. Usually occurs within 2 months of therapy but may occur within 1 week, or be delayed up to 8 years.

Renal: Renal toxicity

Signs and Symptoms of Overdose Immediate symptoms are nausea and vomiting. Delayed symptoms include bone marrow suppression, hepatic necrosis, and gastroenteritis.

Pharmacodynamics/Kinetics

Absorption: Variable and incomplete (16% to 50%)

Distribution: V_d = total body water; CNS penetration is poor

Protein binding: 19%

Metabolism: Hepatic and in GI mucosa; hepatically via xanthine oxidase and methylation via TPMT to sulfate conjugates, 6-thiouric acid, and other inactive compounds; first-pass effect

Half-life elimination (age dependent): Children: 21 minutes; Adults: 47 minutes

Time to peak, serum: ~2 hours

Excretion: Urine (46% as mercaptopurine and metabolites)

Dosage

Oral (refer to individual protocols):

Children:

Induction: 2.5-5 mg/kg/day **or** 70-100 mg/m²/day given once daily

Maintenance: 1.5-2.5 mg/kg/day **or** 50-75 mg/m²/day given once daily

Adults:

Induction: 2.5-5 mg/kg/day (100-200 mg)

Maintenance: 1.5-2.5 mg/kg/day **or** 80-100 mg/m²/day given once daily

Elderly: Due to renal decline with age, start with lower recommended doses for adults

Note: In ALL, administration in the evening (vs morning administration) may lower the risk of relapse.

Dosing adjustment in renal or hepatic impairment: Dose should be reduced to avoid accumulation, but specific guidelines are not available.

Hemodialysis: Removed; supplemental dosing is usually required

Monitoring Parameters CBC with differential and platelet count, liver function tests, uric acid, urinalysis

Contraindications Hypersensitivity to mercaptopurine or any component of the formulation; patients whose disease showed prior resistance to mercaptopurine or thioguanine; severe liver disease, severe bone marrow suppression; pregnancy

Warnings Hazardous agent – use appropriate precautions for handling and disposal. Mercaptopurine is potentially carcinogenic, and may be teratogenic; use with caution in patients with prior bone marrow suppression. Common signs of infection, such as fever and leukocytosis may not occur; lethargy and confusion may be more prominent signs of infection. Use caution with other hepatotoxic drugs or in dosages >2.5 mg/kg/day; hepatotoxicity may occur. Patients with genetic deficiency of thiopurine methyltransferase (TPMT) or concurrent therapy with drugs which may inhibit TPMT (eg, olsalazine) or xanthine oxidase (eg, allopurinol) may be sensitive to myelosuppressive effects. Azathioprine is metabolized to mercaptopurine; concomitant use may result in profound myelosuppression and should be avoided.

To avoid potentially serious dosage errors, the terms "6-mercaptopurine" or "6-MP" should be avoided; use of these terms has been associated with sixfold overdosages.

Dosage Forms Tablet [scored]: 50 mg

Overdosage/Treatment Decontamination: Efforts to minimize absorption (charcoal, gastric lavage) may be ineffective unless instituted within 60 minutes of ingestion.

Drug Interactions Allopurinol: Can cause increased levels of mercaptopurine by inhibition of xanthine oxidase; decrease dose of mercaptopurine by 75% when both drugs are used concomitantly; may potentiate effect of bone marrow suppression (reduce mercaptopurine to 25% of dose).

Aminosalicylates (olsalazine, mesalamine, sulfasalazine): May inhibit TPMT, increasing toxicity/myelosuppression of mercaptopurine. Use caution.

Azathioprine: Metabolized to mercaptopurine, concomitant use may result in profound myelosuppression and should be avoided

Doxorubicin: Synergistic liver toxicity with mercaptopurine in >50% of patients, which resolved with discontinuation of the mercaptopurine.

Hepatotoxic drugs: Any agent which could potentially alter the metabolic function of the liver could produce higher drug levels and greater toxicities from either mercaptopurine or 6-TG.

Warfarin: mercaptopurine inhibits the anticoagulation effect of warfarin by an unknown mechanism.

Pregnancy Risk Factor D

Lactation Enters breast milk/contraindicated

Nursing Implications Adjust dosage in patients with renal insufficiency

Meropenem

Related Information

- Imipenem and Cilastatin

CAS Number 96036-03-2

U.S. Brand Names Merrem® I.V.

Use Carbapenem antibiotic useful against gram-positive and gram-negative (including *Pseudomonas aeruginosa*) organisms used in meningitis, skin, and soft tissue infections and in urinary tract infections

Unlabeled/Investigational Use Febrile neutropenia, urinary tract infections

Mechanism of Action Interacts with proteins in bacterial cytoplasmic membrane; similar to imipenem

Adverse Reactions

Central nervous system: Headache

Gastrointestinal: Abdominal pain, vomiting, diarrhea, nausea

Hepatic: Elevated liver function tests

Signs and Symptoms of Overdose Convulsions

Pharmacodynamics/Kinetics

Distribution: V_d: Adults: ~0.3 L/kg, Children: 0.4-0.5 L/kg; penetrates well into most body fluids and tissues; CSF concentrations approximate those of the plasma

Protein binding: 2%

Metabolism: Hepatic; metabolized to open beta-lactam form (inactive)

Half-life elimination:

Normal renal function: 1-1.5 hours

Cl_{cr} 30-80 mL/minute: 1.9-3.3 hours

Cl_{cr} 2-30 mL/minute: 3.82-5.7 hours

Time to peak, tissue: 1 hour following infusion

Excretion: Urine (~25% as inactive metabolites)

Dosage

I.V.:

Neonates:

Preterm: 20 mg/kg/dose every 12 hours (may be increased to 40 mg/kg/dose if treating a highly resistant organism such as *Pseudomonas aeruginosa*)

Full-term (<3 months of age): 20 mg/kg/dose every 8 hours (may be increased to 40 mg/kg/dose if treating a highly resistant organism such as *Pseudomonas aeruginosa*)

Children >3 months (<50 kg):

Complicated skin and skin structure infections: 10 mg/kg every 8 hours (maximum dose: 500 mg every 8 hours)

Intra-abdominal infections: 20 mg/kg every 8 hours (maximum dose: 1 g every 8 hours)

Meningitis: 40 mg/kg every 8 hours (maximum dose: 2 g every 8 hours)

Children >50 kg:

Complicated skin and skin structure infections: 500 mg every 8 hours

Intra-abdominal infections: 1 g every 8 hours

Meningitis: 2 g every 8 hours

Adults: 1 g every 8 hours

Elderly: No differences in safety or efficacy have been reported. However, increased sensitivity may occur in some elderly patients; adjust dose based on renal function; see Warnings/Precautions

Dosing adjustment in renal impairment: Adults:

Cl_{cr} 26-50 mL/minute: Administer recommended dose based on indication every 12 hours

Cl_{cr} 10-25 mL/minute: Administer one-half recommended dose every 12 hours

Cl_{cr} <10 mL/minute: Administer one-half recommended dose every 12 hours

Dialysis: Meropenem and its metabolites are readily dialyzable

Continuous arteriovenous or venovenous hemodiafiltration effects: Dose as Cl_{cr} 10-50 mL/minute

Monitoring Parameters Monitor for signs of anaphylaxis during first dose

Administration Administer I.V. infusion over 15-30 minutes; I.V. bolus injection over 3-5 minutes

Contraindications Hypersensitivity to meropenem, any component of the formulation, or other carbapenems (eg, imipenem); patients who have experienced anaphylactic reactions to other beta-lactams

Warnings Hypersensitivity reactions, including anaphylaxis, have occurred and often require immediate drug discontinuation. Seizures and other CNS adverse reactions have occurred, most commonly in patients with renal impairment and/or underlying neurologic disorders (less frequent than with Primaxin®). Use with caution in renal impairment; dose adjustment is necessary. Thrombocytopenia has been reported in patients with significant renal dysfunction. Pseudomembranous colitis has been associated with meropenem use. Superinfection is possible with long courses of therapy. Safety and efficacy have not been established for children <3 months of age

Dosage Forms Injection, powder for reconstitution: 500 mg [contains sodium 45.1 mg as sodium carbonate (1.96 mEq)]; 1 g [contains sodium 90.2 mg as sodium carbonate (3.92 mEq)]

Reference Range Peak serum meropenem levels after a 1 g dose: 55-62 mcg/mL 30 minutes postinfusion

Overdosage/Treatment
Supportive therapy: Benzodiazepines can be used for seizure control
Enhancement of elimination: Hemodialysis can effectively remove meropenem and its metabolite; dialysis clearance: 79-81 mL/minute

Drug Interactions Probenecid: May increase meropenem serum concentrations; use caution.
Valproic acid: Meropenem may decrease valproic acid serum concentrations to subtherapeutic levels; monitor.

Pregnancy Risk Factor B

Pregnancy Implications Teratogenic effects have not been found in animal studies; use during pregnancy only if clearly indicated.

Lactation Excretion in breast milk unknown/use caution

Mesalamine

CAS Number 89-57-6

U.S. Brand Names Asacol®; Canasa™; Pentasa®; Rowasa®

Synonyms 5-Aminosalicylic Acid; 5-ASA; Fisalamine; Mesalazine

Use
Oral: Remission and treatment of mildly to moderately active ulcerative colitis
Rectal: Treatment of active mild to moderate distal ulcerative colitis, proctosigmoiditis, or proctitis

Mechanism of Action Mesalamine (5-aminosalicylic acid) is the active component of sulfasalazine; the specific mechanism of action of mesalamine is unknown; however, it is thought that it modulates local chemical mediators of the inflammatory response, especially leukotrienes; action appears topical rather than systemic

Adverse Reactions
Adverse effects vary depending upon dosage form. Effects as reported with tablets, unless otherwise noted:
Cardiovascular: Chest pain, peripheral edema, edema, facial edema, myocarditis, pericarditis
Central nervous system: **Pain (14%)**, chills, dizziness (suppository: 3%), fever (enema: 3%; suppository: 1%), insomnia, malaise, confusion, depression, emotional lability, Guillain-Barré syndrome somnolence, transverse myelitis, T-wave abnormality, vertigo
Dermatologic: Rash (6%; suppository: 1%), pruritus (3%; enema: 1%), acne (2%; suppository: 1%), alopecia, dry skin, erythema nodosum, psoriasis, pyoderma gangrenosum, urticaria
Endocrine & metabolic: GGT elevated, gout, Kawasaki-like syndrome, menorrhagia
Gastrointestinal: **Eructation (16%)**, **abdominal pain (18%**; enema: 8%), dyspepsia, constipation (5%), vomiting (5%), colitis exacerbation (3%; suppository: 1%), nausea (capsule: 3%), flatulence (enema: 6%), hemorrhoids (enema: 1%), nausea and vomiting (capsule: 1%), rectal pain (enema: 1%; suppository: 2%), anorexia, appetite increased, bloody diarrhea, dry mouth, gastritis, oral ulcers, pancreatitis, perforated peptic ulcer, taste perversion
Genitourinary: Epididymitis, dysuria, urinary urgency
Hematologic: Agranulocytosis, aplastic anemia, eosinophilia, leukopenia, pancytopenia, anemia
Hepatic: Elevated alkaline phosphatase, elevated ALT, AST elevated, elevated bilirubin, cholestatic jaundice, cholecystitis, hepatitis, hepatocellular damage, hepatotoxicity, jaundice, LDH elevated, liver failure, minimal change nephrotic syndrome, hepatic necrosis
Hematologic: Thrombocytopenia
Local: Pain on insertion of enema tip (enema: 1%)
Neuromuscular & skeletal: Back pain (7%; enema: 1%), arthralgia, hypertonia, myalgia, arthritis, leg/joint pain (enema: 2%), hyperesthesia, neck pain, tremor, peripheral neuropathy
Ocular: Conjunctivitis, blurred vision, eye pain

Otic: Tinnitus
Respiratory: **Pharyngitis (11%)**, flu-like syndrome (3%; enema: 5%), cough increased, asthma exacerbation, eosinophilic pneumonia, fibrosing alveolitis, hypersensitivity pneumonitis, interstitial pneumonia, pleuritis
Renal: BUN elevated, hematuria, interstitial nephritis, serum creatinine elevated, urinary urgency
Miscellaneous: Lupus-like syndrome, lymphadenopathy, diaphoresis

Signs and Symptoms of Overdose Decreased motor activity, diarrhea, renal function impairment, tinnitus, vomiting

Pharmacodynamics/Kinetics
Absorption: Rectal: Variable and dependent upon retention time, underlying GI disease, and colonic pH; Oral: Tablet: ~28%, Capsule: ~20% to 30%
Metabolism: Hepatic and via GI tract to acetyl-5-aminosalicylic acid
Half-life elimination: 5-ASA: 0.5-1.5 hours; acetyl-5-ASA: 5-10 hours
Time to peak, serum: 4-7 hours
Excretion: Urine (as metabolites); feces (<2%)

Dosage
Adults (usual course of therapy is 3-6 weeks):
Oral:
Capsule: 1 g 4 times/day
Tablet: 800 mg 3 times/day
Retention enema: 60 mL (4 g) at bedtime, retained overnight, approximately 8 hours
Rectal suppository: Insert 1 suppository in rectum twice daily
Some patients may require rectal and oral therapy concurrently
Elderly: Postmarketing reports suggest an increased incidence of blood dyscrasias in patients >65 years of age; use with caution; monitor blood cell counts and renal function

Stability Unstable in presence of water or light; once foil has been removed, unopened bottles have an expiration of 1 year following the date of manufacture

Monitoring Parameters CBC and renal function, particularly in elderly patients

Administration Oral: Swallow capsules or tablets whole, do not chew or crush.
Rectal enema: Shake bottle well. Retain enemas for 8 hours or as long as practical.
Suppository: Remove foil wrapper; avoid excessive handling. Should be retained for at least 1-3 hours to achieve maximum benefit.

Contraindications Hypersensitivity to mesalamine, sulfasalazine, salicylates, or any component of the formulation; Canasa™ suppositories contain saturated vegetable fatty acid esters (contraindicated in patients with allergy to these components)

Warnings May cause an acute intolerance syndrome (cramping, acute abdominal pain, bloody diarrhea; sometimes fever, headache, rash); discontinue if this occurs. Patients with pyloric stenosis may have prolonged gastric retention of tablets, delaying the release of mesalamine in the colon. Pericarditis should be considered in patients with chest pain; pancreatitis should be considered in patients with new abdominal complaints. Symptomatic worsening of colitis/IBD may occur following initiation of therapy. Oligospermia (rare) has been reported in males. Use caution in patients with impaired renal or hepatic function. Renal impairment (including minimal change nephropathy and acute/chronic interstitial nephritis) has been reported; use caution with other medications converted to mesalamine. Postmarketing reports suggest an increased incidence of blood dyscrasias in patients >65 years of age. In addition, elderly may have difficulty administering and retaining rectal suppositories and decreased renal function; use with caution and monitor. Safety and efficacy in pediatric patients have not been established.
Rowasa® enema: Contains potassium metabisulfite; may cause severe hypersensitivity reactions (ie, anaphylaxis) in patients with sulfite allergies.

Dosage Forms Capsule, controlled release (Pentasa®): 250 mg, 500 mg
Suppository, rectal (Canasa™): 500 mg [DSC], 1000 mg [contains saturated vegetable fatty acid esters]
Suspension, rectal: 4 g/60 mL (7s, 28s) [contains potassium metabisulfite and sodium benzoate]
Rowasa®: 4 g/60 mL (7s, 28s) [contains potassium metabisulfite and sodium benzoate]
Tablet, delayed release [enteric coated] (Asacol®): 400 mg

Overdosage/Treatment
Decontamination: Oral: Activated charcoal is the preferred modality; consider decontamination for ingestions >3 g
Supportive therapy: Monitor fluid/electrolyte status along with renal function. Bradycardia may respond to I.V. fluids and atropine.

Drug Interactions Azathioprine, mercaptopurine, thioguanine: Risk of myelosuppression may be increased by aminosalicylates (due to inhibition of TPMT).
Digoxin: Mesalamine may decrease digoxin bioavailability.

Pregnancy Risk Factor B

Lactation Excretion in breast milk unknown/use caution

Nursing Implications Provide patient with copy of mesalamine administration instructions

Additional Information Mesalazine 400 mg is equivalent to sulfasalazine 1 g

Mesoridazine

Related Information
- Anticholinergic Effects of Common Psychotropics
- Antipsychotic Agents

CAS Number 32672-69-8; 5588-33-0

U.S. Brand Names Serentil® [DSC]

Synonyms Mesoridazine Besylate

Impairment Potential Yes

Use Symptomatic management of psychotic disorders, including schizophrenia, behavioral problems, alcoholism as well as reducing anxiety and tension occurring in neurosis

Unlabeled/Investigational Use Psychosis

Mechanism of Action Blockade of postsynaptic CNS dopamine receptors; a metabolite of thioridazine

Adverse Reactions

Cardiovascular: **Hypotension** (especially with I.V. use), **hypotension (orthostatic)**, tachycardia, cardiac arrhythmias, sinus tachycardia

Central nervous system: Sedation, drowsiness, restlessness, anxiety, extrapyramidal reactions, **pseudoparkinsonian signs and symptoms, tardive dyskinesia**, neuroleptic malignant syndrome, seizures, altered central temperature regulation, **akathisia, dystonias, dizziness**, hyperthermia

Dermatologic: Hyperpigmentation, pruritus, rash, photosensitivity

Endocrine & metabolic: Amenorrhea, galactorrhea, gynecomastia, syndrome of inappropriate antidiuretic hormone

Gastrointestinal: GI upset, xerostomia, **constipation**, weight gain

Genitourinary: Urinary retention, impotence

Hematologic: Agranulocytosis, leukopenia (usually in patients with large doses for prolonged periods), thrombocytopenia, hemolysis, eosinophilia

Hepatic: Cholestatic jaundice

Neuromuscular & skeletal: Trismus

Ocular: **Retinal pigmentation**, nystagmus, blurred vision

Respiratory: **Nasal congestion**

Miscellaneous: **Diaphoresis (decreased)**, systemic lupus erythematosus

Signs and Symptoms of Overdose Abnormal involuntary muscle movements, agranulocytosis, cardiac arrhythmias, coma, deep sleep, ejaculatory disturbances, enuresis, extrapyramidal reaction, galactorrhea, granulocytopenia, gynecomastia, hypotension, impotence, leukopenia, neuroleptic malignant syndrome, neutropenia, nystagmus, Parkinson's-like symptoms, photophobia, priapism, QRS prolongation, urine discoloration (pink; red; red-brown), vision color changes (brown tinge; yellow tinge)

Pharmacodynamics/Kinetics

Duration: 4-6 hours

Absorption: Tablet: Erratic; Liquid: More dependable

Protein binding: 91% to 99%

Half-life elimination: 24-48 hours

Time to peak, serum: 2-4 hours; Steady-state serum: 4-7 days

Excretion: Urine

Dosage

Concentrate may be diluted just prior to administration with distilled water, acidified tap water, orange or grape juice; do not prepare and store bulk dilutions

Adults:

Oral: 25-50 mg 3 times/day; maximum: 100-400 mg/day

I.M.: 25 mg initially, repeat in 30-60 minutes as needed; optimal dosage range: 25-200 mg/day

Monitoring Parameters Vital signs, orthostatic blood pressures; lipid profile, fasting blood glucose/Hgb A_{1c}, baseline (and periodic) serum potassium; BMI; mental status, abnormal involuntary movement scale (AIMS); tremors, gait changes, abnormal movement in trunk, neck, buccal area or extremities; monitor target behaviors for which the agent is given; monitor hepatic function (especially if fever with flu-like symptoms); baseline ECG, do not initiate if $QT_c > 450$ msec (discontinue in any patient with a $QT_c > 500$ msec)

Administration When administering I.M. or I.V., watch for hypotension. Dilute oral concentrate just prior to administration with distilled water, acidified tap water, orange or grape juice. Do not prepare and store bulk dilutions. Do not mix oral solutions of mesoridazine and lithium, these oral liquids are incompatible when mixed. **Note:** Avoid skin contact with oral medication; may cause contact dermatitis.

Contraindications Hypersensitivity to mesoridazine or any component of the formulation (cross-reactivity between phenothiazines may occur); severe CNS depression and coma; prolonged QT interval (>450 msec), including prolongation due to congenital causes; history of arrhythmias; concurrent use of medications which prolong QT_c (including type Ia and type III antiarrhythmics, cyclic antidepressants, some fluoroquinolones, cisapride)

Warnings

[U.S. Boxed Warning]: Has been shown to prolong QT_c interval in a dose-dependent manner (associated with an increased risk of torsade de pointes). Patients should have a baseline ECG prior to initiation, and should not receive mesoridazine if baseline $QT_c > 450$ msec. Mesoridazine should be discontinued in patients with a QT_c interval >500 msec. Potassium levels must be evaluated and normalized prior to and throughout treatment.

May cause hypotension, particularly with I.M. administration. Highly sedating, use with caution in disorders where CNS depression is a feature. Use with caution in Parkinson's disease. Caution in patients with hemodynamic instability; bone marrow suppression; predisposition to seizures; subcortical brain damage; severe cardiac, hepatic, renal, or respiratory disease. Esophageal dysmotility and aspiration have been associated with antipsychotic use; use with caution in patients at risk of pneumonia (ie, Alzheimer's disease). Caution in breast cancer or other prolactin-dependent tumors (may elevate prolactin levels). May alter temperature regulation or mask toxicity of other drugs due to antiemetic effects. May cause orthostatic hypotension - use with caution in patients at risk of this effect or those who would tolerate transient hypotensive episodes (cerebrovascular disease, cardiovascular disease, or other medications which may predispose).

Phenothiazines may cause anticholinergic effects (confusion, agitation, constipation, xerostomia, blurred vision, urinary retention). Therefore, they should be used with caution in patients with decreased gastrointestinal motility, urinary retention, BPH, xerostomia, or visual problems. Conditions which also may be exacerbated by cholinergic blockade include narrow-angle glaucoma (screening is recommended) and worsening of myasthenia gravis. Relative to other antipsychotics, mesoridazine has a high potency of cholinergic blockade.

May cause extrapyramidal symptoms, including pseudoparkinsonism, acute dystonic reactions, akathisia, and tardive dyskinesia (risk of these reactions is low relative to other neuroleptics). May be associated with neuroleptic malignant syndrome (NMS) or pigmentary retinopathy (particularly at doses >1 g/day).

Dosage Forms [DSC] = Discontinued product

Injection, solution, as besylate [DSC]: 25 mg/mL (1 mL)

Liquid, oral, as besylate [DSC]: 25 mg/mL (118 mL) [contains alcohol 0.61%]

Tablet, as besylate [DSC]: 10 mg, 25 mg, 50 mg, 100 mg

Overdosage/Treatment

Decontamination: Activated charcoal/lavage within 1 hour

Supportive therapy: Following initiation of essential overdose management, toxic symptom treatment and supportive treatment should be initiated. Hypotension usually responds to I.V. fluids or Trendelenburg positioning. If unresponsive to these measures, the use of a parenteral inotrope may be required. Seizures commonly respond to lorazepam or diazepam (I.V. 5-10 mg bolus in adults every 15 minutes if needed up to a total of 30 mg; I.V. 0.25-0.4 mg/kg/dose up to a total of 10 mg in children) or to phenytoin or phenobarbital. Also critical cardiac arrhythmias and prolonged QT interval on ECG often respond to I.V. phenytoin (15 mg/kg up to 1 g), while other antiarrhythmics can be used. Neuroleptics often cause extrapyramidal reaction (eg, dystonic reactions) requiring management with benztropine mesylate I.V. 1-2 mg (adults) may be effective. These agents are generally effective within 2-5 minutes. Avoid use of quinidine, procainamide, or disopyramide.

Enhancement of elimination: Multiple dosing of activated charcoal may be useful; not dialyzable (0% to 5%)

Test Interactions ↑ cholesterol (S), ↑ glucose; ↓ uric acid (S), calcium (S); may result in a false-positive when testing for tricyclic antidepressants through the EMIT system

Drug Interactions Acetylcholinesterase inhibitors (central): May increase the risk of antipsychotic-related extrapyramidal symptoms; monitor.

Aluminum salts: May decrease the absorption of phenothiazines; monitor

Amphetamines: Efficacy may be diminished by antipsychotics; in addition, amphetamines may increase psychotic symptoms; avoid concurrent use

Anticholinergics: May inhibit the therapeutic response to phenothiazines and excess anticholinergic effects may occur; includes benztropine, trihexyphenidyl, biperiden, and drugs with significant anticholinergic activity (TCAs, antihistamines, disopyramide)

Antihypertensives: Concurrent use of phenothiazines with an antihypertensive may produce additive hypotensive effects (particularly orthostasis)

Bromocriptine: Phenothiazines inhibit the ability of bromocriptine to lower serum prolactin concentrations

CNS depressants: Sedative effects may be additive with phenothiazines; monitor for increased effect; includes barbiturates, benzodiazepines, narcotic analgesics, ethanol, and other sedative agents

Epinephrine: Chlorpromazine (and possibly other low potency antipsychotics) may diminish the pressor effects of epinephrine

Guanethidine and guanadrel: Antihypertensive effects may be inhibited by chlorpromazine

Levodopa: Chlorpromazine may inhibit the antiparkinsonian effect of levodopa; avoid this combination

Lithium: Chlorpromazine may produce neurotoxicity with lithium; this is a rare effect

Metoclopramide: May increase extrapyramidal symptoms (EPS) or risk.

Polypeptide antibiotics: Rare cases of respiratory paralysis have been reported with concurrent use of phenothiazines

QT_c-prolonging agents: Effects on QT_c interval may be additive with phenothiazines, increasing the risk of malignant arrhythmias; includes type Ia antiarrhythmics, TCAs, and some quinolone antibiotics (sparfloxacin, moxifloxacin and gatifloxacin). **Concurrent use is contraindicated.**

Sulfadoxine-pyrimethamine: May increase phenothiazine concentrations

Tricyclic antidepressants: Concurrent use may produce increased toxicity or altered therapeutic response

Trazodone: Phenothiazines and trazodone may produce additive hypotensive effects

Valproic acid: Serum levels may be increased by phenothiazines

Pregnancy Risk Factor C

Lactation Enters breast milk/contraindicated (AAP rates "of concern")

Nursing Implications Watch for hypotension when administering I.M. or I.V.

Metaproterenol

Related Information
- Therapeutic Drugs Associated with Hallucinations

CAS Number 5874-97-5

U.S. Brand Names Alupent®

Synonyms Metaproterenol Sulfate; Orciprenaline Sulfate

Use Bronchodilator in reversible airway obstruction due to asthma or COPD; because of its delayed onset of action (one hour) and prolonged effect (4 or more hours), this may not be the drug of choice for assessing response to a bronchodilator

Mechanism of Action Relaxes bronchial smooth muscle by action on β_2-receptors with very little effect on heart rate

Adverse Reactions

Cardiovascular: **Tachycardia**, palpitations, hypertension, flushing, shortened P-R segment, lengthened QT segment, cardiac arrhythmias, chest pain, sinus tachycardia

Central nervous system: Dizziness, headache, **nervousness**, CNS stimulation, hyperactivity, insomnia, visual and gustatory hallucinations, mania

Dermatologic: Maculopapular rash, angioedema

Endocrine & metabolic: Hypokalemia, hyperglycemia

Gastrointestinal: GI upset

Neuromuscular & skeletal: **Tremors**

Signs and Symptoms of Overdose Angina, cardiac arrhythmias, dry mouth, insomnia, tremors, tachycardia, hypertension, seizures. Hypokalemia also may occur. Cardiac arrest and death may be associated with abuse of beta-agonist bronchodilators.

Pharmacodynamics/Kinetics

Onset of action: Bronchodilation: Oral: ~15 minutes; Inhalation: ~60 seconds

Peak effect: Oral: ~1 hour

Duration: ~1-5 hours

Dosage

Oral:

Children:

<2 years: 0.4 mg/kg/dose given 3-4 times/day; in infants, the dose can be given every 8-12 hours

2-6 years: 1-2.6 mg/kg/day divided every 6 hours

6-9 years: 10 mg/dose 3-4 times/day

Children >9 years and Adults: 20 mg 3-4 times/day

Elderly: Initial: 10 mg 3-4 times/day, increasing as necessary up to 20 mg 3-4 times/day

Inhalation: Children >12 years and Adults: 2-3 inhalations every 3-4 hours, up to 12 inhalations in 24 hours

Nebulizer:

Infants and Children: 0.01-0.02 mL/kg of 5% solution; minimum dose: 0.1 mL; maximum dose: 0.3 mL diluted in 2-3 mL normal saline every 4-6 hours (may be given more frequently according to need)

Adolescents and Adults: 5-20 breaths of full strength 5% metaproterenol **or** 0.2 to 0.3 mL 5% metaproterenol in 2.5-3 mL normal saline until nebulized every 4-6 hours (can be given more frequently according to need)

Stability Store in tight, light-resistant container

Monitoring Parameters Assess lung sounds, heart rate, and blood pressure before administration and during peak of medication; observe patient for wheezing after administration, if this occurs, call physician; monitor respiratory rate, arterial or capillary blood gases if applicable; FEV_1, peak flow, and/or other pulmonary function tests; CNS stimulation; serum glucose, serum potassium

Administration Inhalation: Do not use solutions for nebulization if they are brown or contain a precipitate. Shake inhaler well before using.

Oral: Administer around-the-clock to promote less variation in peak and trough serum levels

Contraindications Hypersensitivity to metaproterenol or any component of the formulation; pre-existing cardiac arrhythmias associated with tachycardia

Warnings

Optimize anti-inflammatory treatment before initiating maintenance treatment with metaproterenol. Do not use as a component of chronic therapy without an anti-inflammatory agent. Only the mildest form of asthma (Step 1 and/or exercise-induced) would not require concurrent use based upon asthma guidelines. Patient must be instructed to seek medical attention in cases where acute symptoms are not relieved or a previous level of response is diminished. The need to increase frequency of use may indicate deterioration of asthma, and treatment must not be delayed.

Use caution in patients with cardiovascular disease (arrhythmia or hypertension or CHF), convulsive disorders, diabetes, glaucoma, hyperthyroidism, or hypokalemia. Beta agonists may cause elevation in blood pressure, heart rate, and result in CNS stimulation/excitation. Beta$_2$ agonists may increase risk of arrhythmia, increase serum glucose, or decrease serum potassium.

Do not exceed recommended dose; serious adverse events including fatalities, have been associated with excessive use of inhaled sympathomimetics. Rarely, paradoxical bronchospasm may occur with use of inhaled bronchodilating agents; this should be distinguished from inadequate response. All patients should utilize a spacer device when using a metered-dose inhaler; additionally, a face mask should be used in children <4 years of age.

Metaproterenol has more beta$_1$ activity than beta$_2$-selective agents such as albuterol and, therefore, may no longer be the beta agonist of first choice. Oral use should be avoided due to the increased incidence of adverse effects.

Dosage Forms

Aerosol for oral inhalation, as sulfate (Alupent®): 0.65 mg/inhalation (14 g) [200 doses]

Solution for nebulization, as sulfate [preservative free]: 0.4% [4 mg/mL] (2.5 mL); 0.6% [6 mg/mL] (2.5 mL)

Syrup, as sulfate: 10 mg/5 mL (480 mL) [may contain sodium benzoate]

Tablet, as sulfate: 10 mg, 20 mg

Overdosage/Treatment Beta-adrenergic stimulation can cause increased heart rate, decreased blood pressure, and CNS stimulation; heart rate can be treated with beta-blockers; decreased blood pressure can be treated with pure beta-adrenergic agents; diazepam 0.07 mg/kg or lorazepam can be used for excitation, seizures

Test Interactions ↑ potassium (S)

Drug Interactions Beta-adrenergic blockers (eg, propranolol) antagonize metaproterenol's effects; avoid concurrent use.

Inhaled ipratropium may increase duration of bronchodilation.

MAO inhibitors may increase side effects; monitor heart rate and blood pressure.

TCAs may increase side effects; monitor heart rate and blood pressure.

Sympathomimetics may increase side effects; monitor heart rate and blood pressure.

Halothane may increase risk of malignant arrhythmias; avoid concurrent use.

Pregnancy Risk Factor C

Pregnancy Implications No data on crossing the placenta. Reported association with polydactyly in 1 study; may be secondary to severe maternal disease or chance.

Lactation Excretion in breast milk unknown

Additional Information Because of its delayed onset of action (1 hour) and prolonged effect (4 or more hours), this may not be the drug of choice for assessing response to a bronchodilator.

Metaxalone

Pronunciation (me TAKS a lone)

CAS Number 1665-48-1

U.S. Brand Names Skelaxin®

Impairment Potential Yes

Use Relief of discomfort associated with acute, painful musculoskeletal conditions

Mechanism of Action Does not have a direct effect on skeletal muscle; most of its therapeutic effect comes from actions on the central nervous system

Adverse Reactions

Frequency not defined.

Central nervous system: Paradoxical stimulation, headache, drowsiness, dizziness, irritability

Dermatologic: Allergic dermatitis

Gastrointestinal: Nausea, vomiting, stomach cramps

Hematologic: Leukopenia, hemolytic anemia

Hepatic: Hepatotoxicity

Miscellaneous: Anaphylaxis

Signs and Symptoms of Overdose Mydriasis, muscle rigidity, CNS depression

Pharmacodynamics/Kinetics
Onset of action: ~1 hour
Duration: ~4-6 hours
Metabolism: Hepatic
Bioavailability: Not established; food may increase
Half-life elimination: 9.2 hours
Time to peak: T_{max}: 3 hours
Excretion: Urine (as metabolites)

Dosage Children >12 years and Adults: Oral: 800 mg 3-4 times/day

Administration May be administered with or without food. However, serum concentrations may be increased when administered with food; clinical significance has not been established. Patients should be monitored.

Contraindications Hypersensitivity to metaxalone or any component of the formulation; impaired hepatic or renal function, history of drug-induced hemolytic anemias or other anemias

Warnings Use with caution in patients with impaired hepatic function

Dosage Forms [DSC] = Discontinued product
Tablet: 400 mg [DSC], 800 mg

Reference Range Mean peak serum metaxalone concentration (3.3 hours) after a 400 mg dose is about 856 mcg/L

Overdosage/Treatment
Decontamination: Lavage/activated charcoal with 3 hours of ingestion
Supportive care is mainstay of treatment

Test Interactions False-positive Benedict's test for urine glucose

Drug Interactions Increased effect of alcohol, CNS depressants

Pregnancy Risk Factor C

Pregnancy Implications Does not appear to be embryotoxic

Nursing Implications Raise bed rails, institute safety measures, assist with ambulation

Specific References
Nirog RS, Kandikere VN, Shukla M, et al, "Quantification of Metaxalone in Human Plasma by Liquid Chromatography Coupled to Tandem Mass Spectrometry," *J Anal Tox*, 2006, 30:245-51.

Metformin

CAS Number 657-24-9

U.S. Brand Names Glucophage® XR; Glucophage®; Riomet™

Synonyms Metformin Hydrochloride

Use Management of type 2 diabetes mellitus (noninsulin dependent, NIDDM) as monotherapy when hyperglycemia cannot be managed on diet alone. May be used concomitantly with a sulfonylurea or insulin to improve glycemic control.

Unlabeled/Investigational Use Treatment of HIV lipodystrophy syndrome

Mechanism of Action Unclear, requires some endogenous insulin to act as antidiabetic

Adverse Reactions
Cardiovascular: Vasculitis
Dermatologic: Cutaneous vasculitis
Endocrine & metabolic: Lactic acidosis, hyponatremia, hypoglycemia, acidosis, hyperinsulinemia, vitamin B_{12} deficiency
Gastrointestinal: **Diarrhea, anorexia, nausea, vomiting, constipation, heartburn, epigastric fullness**, metallic taste, pancreatitis
Hematologic: Megaloblastic anemia, porphyrinogenic, hemolytic anemia
Hepatic: Hepatitis, jaundice
Neuromuscular & skeletal: Fasciculations
Respiratory: Pulmonary vasculitis
Miscellaneous: Diaphoresis, hypersensitivity pneumonitis

Admission Criteria/Prognosis
Admit any ingestion >1700 mg.

Pharmacodynamics/Kinetics
Onset of action: Within days; maximum effects up to 2 weeks
Distribution: V_d: 654±358 L
Protein binding: Negligible
Bioavailability: Absolute: Fasting: 50% to 60%
Half-life elimination, plasma: 6.2 hours
Excretion: Urine (90% as unchanged drug)

Dosage Note: Allow 1-2 weeks between dose titrations: Generally, clinically significant responses are not seen at doses <1500 mg daily; however, a lower recommended starting dose and gradual increased dosage is recommended to minimize gastrointestinal symptoms

Children 10-16 years: Management of type 2 diabetes mellitus: Oral (500 mg tablet or oral solution): Initial: 500 mg twice daily (given with the morning and evening meals); increases in daily dosage should be made in increments of 500 mg at weekly intervals, given in divided doses, up to a maximum of 2000 mg/day

Adults ≥17 years: Management of type 2 diabetes mellitus: Oral:
Immediate release tablet or oral solution: Initial: 500 mg twice daily (give with the morning and evening meals) **or** 850 mg once daily; increase dosage incrementally.

Incremental dosing recommendations based on dosage form:
500 mg tablet: One tablet/day at weekly intervals
850 mg tablet: One tablet/day every other week
Oral solution: 500 mg twice daily every other week
Doses of up to 2000 mg/day may be given twice daily. If a dose > 2000 mg/day is required, it may be better tolerated in three divided doses. Maximum recommended dose 2550 mg/day.

Extended release tablet: Initial: 500 mg once daily (with the evening meal); dosage may be increased by 500 mg weekly; maximum dose: 2000 mg once daily. If glycemic control is not achieved at maximum dose, may divide dose to 1000 mg twice daily. If doses >2000 mg/day are needed, switch to regular release tablets and titrate to maximum dose of 2550 mg/day.

Elderly: The initial and maintenance dosing should be conservative, due to the potential for decreased renal function. Generally, elderly patients should not be titrated to the maximum dose of metformin. Do not use in patients ≥80 years of age unless normal renal function has been established.

Transfer from other antidiabetic agents: No transition period is generally necessary except when transferring from chlorpropamide. When transferring from chlorpropamide, care should be exercised during the first 2 weeks because of the prolonged retention of chlorpropamide in the body, leading to overlapping drug effects and possible hypoglycemia.

Concomitant metformin and oral sulfonylurea therapy: If patients have not responded to 4 weeks of the maximum dose of metformin monotherapy, consider a gradual addition of an oral sulfonylurea, even if prior primary or secondary failure to a sulfonylurea has occurred. Continue metformin at the maximum dose.

Failed sulfonylurea therapy: Patients with prior failure on glyburide may be treated by gradual addition of metformin. Initiate with glyburide 20 mg and metformin 500 mg daily. Metformin dosage may be increased by 500 mg/day at weekly intervals, up to a maximum of 2500 mg/day (dosage of glyburide maintained at 20 mg/day).

Concomitant metformin and insulin therapy: Initial: 500 mg metformin once daily, continue current insulin dose; increase by 500 mg metformin weekly until adequate glycemic control is achieved
Maximum dose: 2500 mg metformin; 2000 mg metformin extended release
Decrease insulin dose 10% to 25% when FPG <120 mg/dL; monitor and make further adjustments as needed

Dosing adjustment/comments in renal impairment: The plasma and blood half-life of metformin is prolonged and the renal clearance is decreased in proportion to the decrease in creatinine clearance. Per the manufacturer, metformin is contraindicated in the presence of renal dysfunction defined as a serum creatinine >1.5 mg/dL in males, or >1.4 mg/dL in females and in patients with abnormal clearance. Clinically, it has been recommended that metformin be avoided in patients with Cl_{cr} <60-70 mL/minute (DeFronzo, 1999).

Dosing adjustment in hepatic impairment: Avoid metformin; liver disease is a risk factor for the development of lactic acidosis during metformin therapy.

Monitoring Parameters Urine for glucose and ketones, fasting blood glucose, and hemoglobin A_{1c}. Initial and periodic monitoring of hematologic parameters (eg, hemoglobin/hematocrit and red blood cell indices) and renal function should be performed, at least annually. Check vitamin B_{12} and folate if anemia is present.

Administration Extended release dosage form should be swallowed whole; do not crush, break, or chew

Contraindications Hypersensitivity to metformin or any component of the formulation; renal disease or renal dysfunction (serum creatinine ≥1.5 mg/dL in males or ≥1.4 mg/dL in females or abnormal creatinine clearance from any cause, including shock, acute myocardial infarction, or septicemia); congestive heart failure requiring pharmacological management; acute or chronic metabolic acidosis with or without coma (including diabetic ketoacidosis)

Note: Temporarily discontinue in patients undergoing radiologic studies in which intravascular iodinated contrast materials are utilized.

Warnings [U.S. Boxed Warning]: Lactic acidosis is a rare, but potentially severe consequence of therapy with metformin. Lactic acidosis should be suspected in any diabetic patient receiving metformin who has evidence of acidosis when evidence of ketoacidosis is lacking. Discontinue metformin in clinical situations predisposing to hypoxemia, including conditions such as cardiovascular collapse, respiratory failure, acute myocardial infarction, acute congestive heart failure, and septicemia.

Metformin is substantially excreted by the kidney. The risk of accumulation and lactic acidosis increases with the degree of impairment of renal function. Patients with renal function below the limit of normal for their age should not receive metformin. In elderly patients, renal function should be monitored regularly; should not be used in any patient ≥80 years of age unless measurement of creatinine clearance verifies normal renal function. Use of concomitant medications that may affect renal function (ie, affect tubular secretion) may also affect metformin disposition. Metformin should be suspended in patients with dehydration and/or prerenal azotemia. Therapy should be suspended for any surgical procedures (resume only after normal intake resumed and normal renal function is verified). Metformin should also be temporarily discontinued for 48 hours in patients undergoing radiologic studies involving the intravascular administration of iodinated contrast materials (potential for acute alteration in renal function).

Avoid use in patients with impaired liver function. Patient must be instructed to avoid excessive acute or chronic ethanol use. Administration of oral antidiabetic drugs has been reported to be associated with increased cardiovascular mortality; metformin does not appear to share this risk. Safety and efficacy of metformin have been established for use in children ≥ 10 years of age; the extended release preparation is for use in patients ≥ 17 years of age.

Dosage Forms Solution, oral, as hydrochloride:
Riomet™: 100 mg/mL (118 mL, 473 mL) [contains saccharin; cherry flavor]
Tablet, as hydrochloride: 500 mg, 850 mg, 1000 mg
Glucophage®: 500 mg, 850 mg, 1000 mg
Tablet, extended release, as hydrochloride: 500 mg, 750 mg
Fortamet®: 500 mg, 1000 mg
Glucophage® XR: 500 mg, 750 mg
Glumetza™: 500 mg

Reference Range
Therapeutic serum level: 1-2 mg/L
Peak plasma metformin level after a 1.5 g dose: ~3.1 mg/L; levels >45 mg/L associated with toxicity

Overdosage/Treatment
Decontamination: Lavage (within 1 hour)/activated charcoal
Supportive therapy: Glucose for hypoglycemia; sodium bicarbonate for severe acidosis
Enhancement of elimination: Removed by hemodialysis; in presence of lactic acidosis, use nonlactate dialysate; hemodialysis with bicarbonate as the buffer can be used.

In one case report, continuous venovenous hemodialysis was performed with a blood flow of 180 mL/minute and dialysate flow of 2.5 L/hour. A Multiflow 60 kidney (Cobe) on a Prisma (Cobe) continuous renal replacement therapy machine was used. By continuous venovenous hemodialysis, an absolute clearance of 50.4 mL/minute was obtained in this case report.

Antidote(s)
- Dextrose [ANTIDOTE]
- Glucagon [ANTIDOTE]
- Sodium Bicarbonate [ANTIDOTE]

Drug Interactions Drugs which tend to produce hyperglycemia (eg, diuretics, corticosteroids, phenothiazines, thyroid products, estrogens, oral contraceptives, phenytoin, nicotinic acid, sympathomimetics, calcium channel blocking drugs, isoniazid) may lead to a loss of glycemic control
Cationic drugs (eg, amiloride, digoxin, morphine, procainamide, quinidine, quinine, ranitidine, triamterene, trimethoprim, and vancomycin) which are eliminated by renal tubular secretion could have the potential for interaction with metformin by competing for common renal tubular transport systems
Cimetidine increases (by 60%) peak metformin plasma and whole blood concentrations
Contrast agents: May increase the risk of metformin-induced lactic acidosis. Discontinue metformin prior to exposure and withhold for 48 hours.
Furosemide increased the metformin plasma and blood C_{max} without altering metformin renal clearance in a single dose study

Pregnancy Risk Factor B

Pregnancy Implications Abnormal blood glucose levels are associated with a higher incidence of congenital abnormalities. Insulin is the drug of choice for the control of diabetes mellitus during pregnancy.

Lactation Excretion in breast milk unknown/not recommended

Additional Information Related to withdrawn phenformin; average estimated incidence of lactic acidosis is 0.03 cases per 1000 patient-years; long-term therapy is associated with decreased intestinal absorption of vitamin B_{12} and folate

Specific References
Bouchard NC, Weisstuch JM, Hoffman RS, et al, "Metformin Clearance is Poor with Continuous Veno-Venous Hemodiafiltration (CVVHDF)," *J Toxicol Clin Toxicol*, 2004, 42(5):739.
Bryant SM, Cumpston K, Lipsky MS, et al, "Metformin-Associated Respiratory Alkalosis," *Am J Ther*, 2004, 11(3):236-7.
Criaco C, Bacis G, and Farina ML, "Severe Lactic Acidosis: Do Not Forget Phenformin," *J Toxicol Clin Toxicol*, 2003, 41(5):671.
Hoffman IS, Roa M, Torrico F, et al, "Ondansetron and Metformin-Induced Gastrointestinal Side Effects," *Am J Ther*, 2003, 10(6):447-51.
Khan JK, Pallaki M, Tolbert SR, et al, "Lactic Acidemia Associated with Metformin," *Ann Pharmacother*, 2003, 37(1):66-9.
LoVecchio F, Klemens J, Curry SC, et al, "Validation of a Metformin Poison Center Protocol: A 48-Month Experience in Toddlers," *J Toxicol Clin Toxicol*, 2003, 41(5):683.
Moore KA, Levine B, Titus JM, et al, "CASE REPORT: Analysis of Metformin in Antemortem Serum and Postmortem Specimens by a Novel HPLC Method and Application to an Intoxication Case," *J Anal Toxicol*, 2003, 27(8):592-4.
Nisse P, Mathieu-Nolf M, Deveaux M, et al, "A Fatal Case of Metformin Poisoning," *J Toxicol Clin Toxicol*, 2003, 41(7):1035-6.
Spiller HA and Quadrani DA, "Toxic Effects from Metformin Exposure," *Ann Pharmacother*, 2004, 38(5):776-80.

Methadone

Related Information
- Drugs Used in Addiction Treatment

CAS Number 1095-90-5; 125-56-4; 297-88-1; 76-99-3

U.S. Brand Names Dolophine®; Methadone Intensol™; Methadose®

Synonyms Methadone Hydrochloride

Impairment Potential Yes. No apparent impairment in complex tasks noted in patients on daily methadone maintenance (60-100 mg). (Moskowitz H and Robinson CD, "Methadone Maintenance and Tracking Performance," *Alcohol Drugs and Traffic Safety*, Kaye S and Meier GW, eds, Univ Puerto Rico, 1985, 995-1004.)

Use Management of severe pain; detoxification and maintenance treatment of narcotic addiction (must be part of an FDA-approved program)

Mechanism of Action Binds to opiate receptors in the CNS, causing inhibition of ascending pain pathways, altering the perception of and response to pain; produces generalized CNS depression

Adverse Reactions
Cardiovascular: **Hypotension, bradycardia, peripheral vasodilation, palpitations**, sinus bradycardia, torsade de pointes (methadone dose: >400 mg/day)
Central nervous system (toxicity may be delayed after 6 hours): CNS depression, increased intracranial pressure, agitation, psychosis, **drowsiness, dizziness**, sedation (marked sedation seen after repeated administration), **tiredness**, nervousness, headache, restlessness, malaise, confusion, hallucinations, paradoxical CNS stimulation, choreic movements
Dermatologic: Skin rash, hives, pruritus, angioedema, urticaria, purpura; bullous eruptions, exanthem
Endocrine & metabolic: Syndrome of inappropriate antidiuretic hormone, hypoadrenalism
Gastrointestinal: **Nausea, vomiting, constipation**, xerostomia, anorexia, stomach cramps, paralytic ileus, biliary tract spasm
Genitourinary: Decreased urination, ureteral spasm, urinary tract spasm
Local: Pain at injection site
Neuromuscular & skeletal: Rhabdomyolysis, **weakness**
Ocular: Miosis
Respiratory: Apnea, respiratory depression, dyspnea
Miscellaneous: **Histamine release**, physical and psychological dependence with prolonged use

Signs and Symptoms of Overdose Coma, ejaculatory disturbances, impotence, pulmonary edema, respiratory depression

Admission Criteria/Prognosis Admit all pediatric methadone overdoses.

Pharmacodynamics/Kinetics
Oral:
Onset of action: Within 30-60 minutes; Duration: 6-8 hours; with repeated doses, increases to 22-48 hours
Parenteral:
Onset of action: Within 10-20 minutes; Peak effect: Within 1-2 hours
Enhanced analgesia has been seen in elderly patients on therapeutic doses of narcotics; duration of action may be increased.
Absorption: Absorbed well from gastrointestinal tract
Distribution: V_d: 3.8 L/kg; distributes widely to tissues
Protein binding: 80% to 89%
Metabolism: Liver metabolism (N-demethylation)
Bioavailability, oral: 92%
Half-life: 15-25 hours, half-life may be prolonged with alkaline pH
Elimination: Urine (<10% as unchanged drug); increased renal excretion with urine pH <6; clearance: 0.08 L/hour/kg; oral clearance following one dose is 6.9 L/hour in nondrug users and 3.2 L/hour in drug addicts

Toxicodynamics/Kinetics
Oral:
Onset of action: Within 30-60 minutes; Duration: 6-8 hours; with repeated doses, increases to 22-48 hours
Parenteral:
Onset of action: Within 10-20 minutes; Peak effect: Within 1-2 hours
Enhanced analgesia has been seen in elderly patients on therapeutic doses of narcotics; duration of action may be increased.
Absorption: Absorbed well from gastrointestinal tract
Distribution: V_d: 3.8 L/kg; distributes widely to tissues
Protein binding: 80% to 89%

Metabolism: Liver metabolism (N-demethylation)

Bioavailability, oral: 92%

Half-life: 15-25 hours, half-life may be prolonged with alkaline pH

Elimination: Urine (<10% as unchanged drug); increased renal excretion with urine pH <6; clearance: 0.08 L/hour/kg; oral clearance following one dose is 6.9 L/hour in nondrug users and 3.2 L/hour in drug addicts

Dosage Note: These are guidelines and do not represent the maximum doses that may be required in all patients. Methadone accumulates with repeated doses and dosage may need reduction after 3-5 days to prevent CNS depressant effects. Some patients may benefit from every 8-12 hour dosing interval for chronic pain management. Doses should be titrated to appropriate effects.

Children:

Pain (analgesia):

Oral (unlabeled use): Initial: 0.1-0.2 mg/kg 4-8 hours initially for 2-3 doses, then every 6-12 hours as needed. Dosing interval may range from 4-12 hours during initial therapy; decrease in dose or frequency may be required (~ days 2-5) due to accumulation with repeated doses (maximum dose: 5-10 mg)

I.V. (unlabeled use): 0.1 mg/kg every 4-8 hours initially for 2-3 doses, then every 6-12 hours as needed. Dosing interval may range from 4-12 hours during initial therapy; decrease in dose or frequency may be required (~ days 2-5) due to accumulation with repeated doses (maximum dose: 5-8 mg)

Iatrogenic narcotic dependency (unlabeled): Oral: General guidelines: Initial: 0.05-0.1 mg/kg/dose every 6 hours; increase by 0.05 mg/kg/dose until withdrawal symptoms are controlled; after 24-48 hours, the dosing interval can be lengthened to every 12-24 hours; to taper dose, wean by 0.05 mg/kg/day; if withdrawal symptoms recur, taper at a slower rate

Adults:

Pain (analgesia):

Oral: Initial: 5-10 mg; dosing interval may range from 4-12 hours during initial therapy; decrease in dose or frequency may be required (~days 2-5) due to accumulation with repeated doses

Manufacturer's labeling: 2.5-10 mg every 3-4 hours as needed

I.V.: Manufacturers labeling: Initial: 2.5-10 mg every 8-12 hours in opioid-naive patients; titrate slowly to effect; may also be administered by SubQ or I.M. injection

Conversion from oral to parenteral dose: Initial dose: Oral: parenteral: 2:1 ratio

Detoxification: Oral: 15-40 mg/day

Maintenance treatment of opiate dependence: Oral: 20-120 mg/day

Dosage adjustment in renal impairment: Cl$_{cr}$ <10 mL/minute: Administer 50% to 75% of normal dose

Dosage adjustment in hepatic impairment: Avoid in severe liver disease

Stability Highly **incompatible** with all other I.V. agents when mixed together

Monitoring Parameters Pain relief, respiratory and mental status, blood pressure

Administration Oral dose for detoxification and maintenance may be administered in fruit juice or water.

Contraindications Hypersensitivity to methadone or any component of the formulation; respiratory depression (in the absence of resuscitative equipment or in an unmonitored setting); acute bronchial asthma or hypercarbia; pregnancy (prolonged use or high doses near term)

Warnings

An opioid-containing analgesic regimen should be tailored to each patient's needs and based upon the type of pain being treated (acute versus chronic), the route of administration, degree of tolerance for opioids (naive versus chronic user), age, weight, and medical condition. The optimal analgesic dose varies widely among patients. Doses should be titrated to pain relief/prevention. Patients maintained on stable doses of methadone may need higher and/or more frequent doses in case of acute pain (eg, postoperative pain, physical trauma). Methadone is ineffective for the relief of anxiety.

May prolong the QT interval; use caution in patients at risk for QT prolongation, with medications known to prolong the QT interval, or history of conduction abnormalities. QT interval prolongation and torsade de pointes may be associated with doses >200 mg/day, but have also been observed with lower doses. May cause severe hypotension; use caution with severe volume depletion or other conditions which may compromise maintenance of normal blood pressure. Use caution with cardiovascular disease or patients predisposed to dysrhythmias.

May cause respiratory depression. Use caution in patients with respiratory disease or pre-existing respiratory conditions (eg, severe obesity, asthma, COPD, sleep apnea, CNS depression). Because the respiratory effects last longer than the analgesic effects, slow titration is required. Abrupt cessation may precipitate withdrawal symptoms.

May cause CNS depression, which may impair physical or mental abilities. Patients must be cautioned about performing tasks which require mental alertness (eg, operating machinery or driving). Effects

with other sedative drugs or ethanol may be potentiated. Use with caution in patients with depression or suicidal tendencies, or in patients with a history of drug abuse. Tolerance or psychological and physical dependence may occur with prolonged use.

Use with caution in patients with head injury or increased intracranial pressure. May obscure diagnosis or clinical course of patients with acute abdominal conditions. Elderly may be more susceptible to adverse effects (eg, CNS, respiratory, gastrointestinal). Decrease initial dose and use caution in the elderly or debilitated; with hyper/hypothyroidism, prostatic hypertrophy, or urethral stricture; or with severe renal or hepatic failure. Safety and efficacy have not been established in patients <18 years of age. Tablets contain excipients to deter use by injection.

[U.S. Boxed Warning]: When used for treatment of narcotic addiction: May only be dispensed by opioid treatment programs certified by the Substance Abuse and Mental Health Services Administration (SAMHSA) and certified by the designated state authority. Exceptions include inpatient treatment of other conditions and emergency period (not >3 days) while definitive substance abuse treatment is being sought.

Dosage Forms Injection, solution, as hydrochloride: 10 mg/mL (20 mL)

Solution, oral, as hydrochloride: 5 mg/5 mL (500 mL); 10 mg/5 mL (500 mL) [contains alcohol 8%; citrus flavor]

Solution, oral concentrate, as hydrochloride: 10 mg/mL (946 mL)

Methadone Intensol™: 10 mg/mL (30 mL)

Methadose®: 10 mg/mL (1000 mL) [cherry flavor]

Methadose®: 10 mg/mL (1000 mL) [dye free, sugar free, unflavored]

Tablet, as hydrochloride (Dolophine®, Methadose®): 5 mg, 10 mg

Tablet, dispersible, as hydrochloride:

Methadose®: 40 mg

Methadone Diskets®: 40 mg [orange-pineapple flavor]

Reference Range

Therapeutic (pain control), serum: 0.1-0.4 mcg/mL (SI: 0.32-1.29 µmol/L); narcotic stabilization: 0.3-1.0 mcg/mL

Toxic: >2.0 mcg/mL (SI: >6.46 µmol/L)

Overdosage/Treatment

Decontamination: Lavage (within 1 hour)/activated charcoal

Supportive therapy: Naloxone hydrochloride (0.4-2 mg I.V., SubQ, or through an endotracheal tube); a continuous infusion (at $^2/_3$ the response dose/hour) may be required; opioid-induced myoclonus may respond to dantrolene (50-150 mg/day)

Antidote(s)

- Nalmefene [ANTIDOTE]
- Naloxone [ANTIDOTE]

Diagnostic Procedures

- Methadone, Urine

Test Interactions ↑ thyroxine (S), aminotransferases (ALT, AST) (S); brompheniramine, diphenhydramine, or doxylamine may cause a false-positive urinary immunoassay for methadone; disopyramide can cross react with methadone urinary immunoassays

Drug Interactions Substrate of CYP2C9 (minor), 2C19 (minor), 2D6 (minor), 3A4 (major); **Inhibits** CYP2D6 (moderate), 3A4 (weak)

Agonist/antagonist analgesics (buprenorphine, butorphanol, nalbuphine, pentazocine): May decrease analgesic effect of methadone and precipitate withdrawal symptoms; use is not recommended.

Antiretroviral agents, NNRTI: May decrease levels of methadone, opioid withdrawal syndrome has been reported. Effect reported with efavirenz and nevirapine.

Antiretroviral agents, NRTI: Methadone may increase bioavailability and toxic effects of zidovudine. Methadone may decrease bioavailability of didanosine and stavudine.

Antiretroviral agent, PI: Ritonavir (and combinations) may decrease levels of methadone; withdrawal symptoms have inconsistently been observed, monitor.

CNS depressants (including but not limited to opioid analgesics, general anesthetics, sedatives, hypnotics, ethanol): May cause respiratory depression, hypotension, profound sedation, or coma.

CYP2D6 substrates: Methadone may increase the levels/effects of CYP2D6 substrates. Example substrates include amphetamines, selected beta-blockers, dextromethorphan, fluoxetine, lidocaine, mirtazapine, nefazodone, paroxetine, risperidone, ritonavir, thioridazine, tricyclic antidepressants, and venlafaxine.

CYP2D6 prodrug substrates: Methadone may decrease the levels/effects of CYP2D6 prodrug substrates. Example prodrug substrates include codeine, hydrocodone, oxycodone, and tramadol.

CYP3A4 inducers: CYP3A4 inducers may decrease the levels/effects of methadone. Example inducers include aminoglutethimide, carbamazepine, nafcillin, nevirapine, phenobarbital, phenytoin, and rifamycins.

CYP3A4 inhibitors: May increase the levels/effects of methadone. Example inhibitors include azole antifungals, clarithromycin, diclofenac, doxycycline, erythromycin, imatinib, isoniazid, nefazodone, nicardipine, propofol, protease inhibitors, quinidine, telithromycin, and verapamil.

Desipramine: Levels of desipramine may be increased by methadone.

QT$_c$ interval-prolonging agents (including but may not be limited to amitriptyline, astemizole, bepridil, disopyramide, erythromycin, haloperidol, imipramine, quinidine, pimozide, procainamide, sotalol, and thioridazine): Effect/toxicity increased; use with caution.

Ritonavir: May increase levels/effects of methadone shortly after initiation. May decrease levels/effects of methadone with continued dosing.

Somatostatin: Therapeutic effect of methadone may be decreased; limited documentation; monitor

Zidovudine: serum concentrations may be increased by methadone; monitor

Pregnancy Risk Factor B/D (prolonged use or high doses at term)

Pregnancy Implications Crosses the placenta; neonatal respiratory depression

Lactation Amount of Methadone in breast milk is very low with mean relative infant dose as a percentage of maternal dose generally less than 3% (less than 0.1 mg daily). American Academy of pediatrics has deemed that methadone is compatable with breastfeeding

Nursing Implications Observe patient for excessive sedation, respiratory depression, implement safety measures, assist with ambulation

Additional Information Not detected as an opioid in most urine immunoassays; although narcotic-induced respiratory abnormalities with methadone are not as severe as with heroin, as little as 80 mg can cause pulmonary edema. In pediatric methadone exposures, 5 mg can cause coma, while 10 mg may be fatal. Pupillary signs (miosis) correlate well with plasma methadone levels in acute pediatric exposures. Ingestion of a single daily adult methadone maintenance dose has resulted in fatalities in children <6 years of age.

According to the Drug Abuse Warning Network, in 2004.

● An estimated 31,874 Emergency Department (ED) visits involved Methadone.

● An estimate 1,207 ED visits due to methadone involved a suicide attempt.

Specific References

Abdel-Latif, ME, Pinner J, Clews S, et al, "Effects of Breast Milk on the Severity and Outcome of Neonatal Abstinence Syndrome Among Infants of Drug-Dependent Mothers," *Pediatrics*, 2006, 117(6): e1163-e1168.

Biswas AK, Feldman BL, Davis DH, et al, "Myocardial Ischemia as a Result of Severe Benzodiazepine and Opioid Withdrawal," *Clin Toxicol (Phila)*, 2005, 43(3):207-9.

Centers for Disease Control and Prevention (CDC), "Increase in Poisoning Deaths Caused by Non-Illicit Drugs – Utah, 1991-2003," *MMWR Morb Mortal Wkly Rep*, 2005, 21;54(2):33-6.

Choo RE, Huestis MA, Schroeder JR, et al, "Neonatal Abstinence Syndrome in Methadone-Exposed Infants is Altered by Level of Prenatal Tobacco Exposure," *Drug Alcohol Depend*, 2004, 75(3):253-60.

Cooper G, Baldwin D, and Hand C, "Validation of the Cozart® Microplate ELISA for the Detection of Methadone in Hair," *J Anal Toxicol*, 2004, 28:294.

Cooper G, Wilson L, Reid C, et al, "Comparison of Cozart® Microplate ELISA and GC-MS Detection of Methadone and Metabolites in Human Hair," *J Anal Toxicol*, 2005, 29:678-81.

Ehret GB, Voide C, Gex-Fabry M, et al, "Drug-Induced Long QT Syndrome in Injection Drug Users Receiving Methadone," *Arch Intern Med*, 2006, 166:1280-7.

Friesen MS, Purssell RA, and Gair RD, "Aluminum Toxicity Following I.V. Use of Oral Methadone Solution," *Clin Toxicol*, 2006, 44(3):307-14.

Garcia-Repetto R, Soria-Sanchez ML, and Gimenez-Gracia MP, "A Retrospective Review of Methadone Deaths: A Toxicology Study," *J Anal Toxicol*, 2006, 30:132.

Hoch DK, Zhao J, Kreke K, et al, "An Online DAT II Immunoassay for the Detection of Methadone in Urine," *J Anal Toxicol*, 2003, 27(3):183.

Hon K, Cordery R, Haase W, et al, "A Multicenter Evaluation of Roche ONLINE® DAT II Methadone, Cocaine, and Cannabinoid Assays," *J Anal Toxicol*, 2004, 28:295-6.

Jansson LM, Velez M, Harrow C, "Methadone Maintenence and Lactation: A Review of the Literature and Current Management Guidelines," *J Hum Lact*, 2004: 20(1): 62-9.

Jennings JA, Jufer RA, Callery RT, et al, "Distribution of Methadone and EDDP in 100 Postmortem Cases," *J Anal Toxicol*, 2006, 30:150.

Johnson K, Gerada C, and Greenough A, "Treatment of Neonatal Abstinence Syndrome," *Arch Dis Child Fetal Neonatal Ed*, 2003, 88(1):F2-5 (review).

LoVecchio F, Sami A, Pizon AF, et al, "Isolated Methadone Overdose Typically Require Naloxone Within the First 9 Hours of Ingestion," *Clin Toxicol (Phila)*, 2005, 43:666.

Marraffa JM, Darko W, Stork CM, et al, "Methadone Causing Prolonged QTc Interval and Syncope After Paroxetine Initiation," *Clin Toxicol (Phila)*, 2005, 43:654.

Mycyk MB, Szyszko AL, and Aks SE, "Nebulized Naloxone Gently and Effectively Reverses Methadone Intoxication," *J Emerg Med*, 2003, 24(2):185-7.

Ondo WG, "Methadone for Refractory Restless Legs Syndrome," *Mov Disord*, 2005, 20(3):345-8.

Paterson S, Cordero R, McPhillips M, et al, "Interindividual Dose/Concentration Relationship for Methadone in Hair," *J Anal Toxicol*, 2003, 27(1):20-3.

Pfab R, Eyer F, Jetzinger E, et al, "Cause and Motivation in Cases of Non-Fatal Drug Overdoses in Opiate Addicts," *Clin Toxicol*, 2006, 44:255-9.

Philipp BL, Merewood A, and O'Brien S, "Methadone and Breastfeeding: New Horizons," *Pediatrics*, 2003, 111(6):1429-30.

Preston KL, Epstein DH, Davoudzadeh D, et al, "Methadone and Metabolite Urine Concentrations in Patients Maintained on Methadone," *J Anal Toxicol*, 2003, 27(6):332-41.

Rauber-Luthy C, Egli G, Bombeli T, et al, "A Case of Disseminated Intravascular Coagulation (DIC) After Intravenous Injection of Methadone Capsules," *J Toxicol Clin Toxicol*, 2004, 42(5):722.

Rock CM, Averin O, Day JE, et al, "Detection of Methadone and Two Major Metabolites in the Hair of Pregnant Women and Their Infants," *J Anal Toxicol*, 2006, 30:136.

Tennant F, "Tennant Blood Study - First Update," *Prac Pain Management*, 2006, 6(1):52-60.

Wong SH, Jin M, Shi R, et al, "Molecular Autopsy with Pharmacogenomics - A Multi-Center Study for Certifying Methadone Deaths: Preliminary Findings of Data Acquisition and Multiplex Genotyping CYP 450 2D6,2C9, 2C19, 3A4, and 3A5 by Pyrosequencing™," *J Anal Toxicol*, 2006, 30:160.

Wong SH, Wagner MA, Jentzen JM, et al, "Pharmacogenomics as an Aspect of Molecular Autopsy for Forensic Pathology/Toxicology: Does Genotyping CYP 2D6 Serve as an Adjunct for Certifying Methadone Toxicity?" *J Forensic Sci*, 2003, 48(6):1406-15.

Wunsch MJ, Behonick GS, and Massello W III, "Opioid Mortality in Southwestern Virginia," *J Anal Toxicol*, 2006, 30:159-60.

Methamphetamine

Related Information
● Highlights of Recent Reports (2006) on Substance Abuse and Mental Health

CAS Number 51-57-0; 537-46-2

U.S. Brand Names Desoxyn®

Synonyms Desoxyephedrine Hydrochloride; Methamphetamine Hydrochloride

Impairment Potential Yes. Blood methamphetamine levels >0.1 mg/L have been associated with driving impairment (typical driving behaviors noted include speeding, weaving, drifting out of lane of travel, and erratic driving). (Logan BK, "Methamphetamine and Driving Impairment," *J Forensic Sci*, 1996, 41(3):457-64.)

Use Treatment of attention-deficit/hyperactivity disorder (ADHD); exogenous obesity (short-term adjunct)

Unlabeled/Investigational Use Narcolepsy

Mechanism of Action A sympathomimetic amine related to ephedrine and amphetamine

Adverse Reactions

Cardiovascular: **Irregular heartbeat, cardiac arrhythmia,** hypertension, chest pain, dilated cardiomyopathy, vasculitis, sinus bradycardia, cardiomegaly, angina, sinus tachycardia, tachycardia (supraventricular), cerebral edema, myocardial infarction, Raynaud's phenomenon

Central nervous system: **False feeling of well being, nervousness, restlessness, insomnia,** mood or mental changes, dizziness, lightheadedness, headache, visual hallucinations, delusional perceptions, CNS stimulation (severe), hyperthermia, Tourette's syndrome, psychosis, irritability, seizures, paranoia, agitation, extrapyramidal reaction, bilateral putaminal involvement

Dermatologic: Skin rash, hives, licheniform eruptions, urticaria

Endocrine & metabolic: Changes in libido, growth suppression, hyponatremia, syndrome of inappropriate antidiuretic hormone

Gastrointestinal: Diarrhea, nausea, vomiting, stomach cramps, constipation, anorexia, weight loss, xerostomia, colonic ischemia, bitter dysgeusia

Hepatic: Hepatitis, jaundice, hepatomegaly, hepatic failure, centrilobular necrosis

Neuromuscular & skeletal: Tremor, choreoathetoid movements

Ocular: Blurred vision, mydriasis, cortical blindness

Miscellaneous: Tolerance and withdrawal with prolonged use, diaphoresis (increased), "washed-out" syndrome, fixed drug eruption, Pott puffy tumor (PPT)

Signs and Symptoms of Overdose Alopecia, confusion, delirium, feces discoloration (black), gynecomastia, hypertension, insomnia, mania, myoclonus, myoglobinuria, periarteritis nodosa, pulmonary edema, respiratory alkalosis, rhabdomyolysis, rigors, tachycardia or reflex bradycardia, tachypnea, tremors

Pharmacodynamics/Kinetics

Duration of action: 6-12 hours

Absorption: Rapid from GI tract

Metabolism: In liver to amphetamine (4% to 7%) and other metabolites

Half-life: 12-34 hours

Elimination: Renally

Dosage

Oral:

Children >6 years and Adults: ADHD: 2.5-5 mg 1-2 times/day; may increase by 5 mg increments at weekly intervals until optimum response is achieved, usually 20-25 mg/day

Children >12 years and Adults: Exogenous obesity: 5 mg 30 minutes before each meal; treatment duration should not exceed a few weeks

Monitoring Parameters Heart rate, respiratory rate, blood pressure, and CNS activity

Contraindications Hypersensitivity to methamphetamine, any component of the formulation, or idiosyncrasy to amphetamines or other sympathomimetic amines; patients with advanced arteriosclerosis, symptomatic cardiovascular disease, moderate to severe hypertension (stage II or III), hyperthyroidism, glaucoma, agitated states; patients with a history of drug abuse; use during or within 14 days following MAO inhibitor therapy; stimulant medications are contraindicated for use in children with attention-deficit/hyperactivity disorders and concomitant Tourette's syndrome or tics

Warnings

[U.S. Boxed Warning]: Dexamphetamine has been associated with serious cardiac cardiovascular events including sudden death in patients with pre-existing structural cardiac abnormalities or other serious heart problems. Using CNS stimulant treatment at usual doses in children and adolescents with serious heart problems and structural cardiac abnormalities has been associated with sudden death. In adults, stimulant use has been associated with sudden deaths, stroke, and myocardial infarction. Stimulant products should be avoided in the patients with known serious structural cardiac abnormalities, cardiomyopathy, serious heart rhythm abnormalities, or other serious heart problems that could increase the risk of sudden death that these conditions alone carry. Caution should be used in patients with hypertension and other cardiovascular conditions that might be exacerbated by increases in blood pressure or heart rate. Use of stimulants can cause an increase in blood pressure (average 2-4 mm Hg) and increases in heart rate (average 3-6 bpm), although some patients may have larger than average increases.

Use with caution in patients with bipolar disorder, cardiovascular disease, diabetes, seizure disorders, insomnia, porphyria, mild hypertension (stage I), or history of substance abuse. May exacerbate symptoms of behavior and thought disorder in psychotic patients. Stimulants may unmask tics in individuals with coexisting Tourette's syndrome. Potential for drug dependency exists - avoid abrupt discontinuation in patients who have received for prolonged periods. **[U.S. Boxed Warning]: Use in weight reduction programs only when alternative therapy has been ineffective; due to high potential for abuse and/or nontherapeutic use should be prescribed/dispensed sparingly.** Products may contain tartrazine - use with caution in potentially sensitive individuals. Stimulant use in children has been associated with growth suppression.

Dosage Forms Tablet, as hydrochloride: 5 mg

Reference Range

Therapeutic: Serum: 20-30 ng/mL

Psychosis can develop at serum levels of 150-500 ng/mL; serum levels >230 ng/mL can be fatal.

In the postmortem state, anatomical site concentration differences (ie, postmortem redistribution) may occur.

Overdosage/Treatment

Decontamination: Lavage (within 1 hour)/activated charcoal

Supportive therapy: Methamphetamine psychosis:

Haloperidol: I.V.: 5-10 mg

Diazepam: I.V.: 5-10 mg

Droperidol: I.M.: 2.5-5 mg can be used for psychosis if I.V. access is not available

Hypertension that is not responsive to sedation can be treated with phentolamine or nitroprusside

Enhancement of elimination: Multiple dosing of activated charcoal may be useful. While acid diuresis can increase excretion, it is not recommended due to renal effects.

Diagnostic Procedures

● Methamphetamines, Urine

Test Interactions A labetalol metabolite (3-amino-1-phenylbutane or APB) may cause a false-positive result with amphetamine/methamphetamine by thin-layer chromatography or immunoassay; false-positive by immunoassay may be seen with ranitidine, phenylpropanolamine, brompheniramine, chlorpromazine, fluspirilene or pipothiazine coingestion; alum (25 g/L) may elicit a false-negative urinary assay for methamphetamine; urine will be acidic in these cases. May interfere with the TSH assay resulting in falsely low TSH levels.

Drug Interactions **Substrate** of CYP2D6 (major)

Alkalinizers: Large doses of sodium bicarbonate or other alkalinizers may increase renal tubular reabsorption (decreased elimination) and enhance the effect of amphetamine; includes potassium or sodium citrate and acetate

CYP2D6 inhibitors: May increase the levels/effects of methamphetamine. Example inhibitors include chlorpromazine, delavirdine, fluoxetine, miconazole, paroxetine, pergolide, quinidine, quinine, ritonavir, and ropinirole.

False neurotransmitters (eg, guanethidine, methyldopa): Amphetamines may inhibit the antihypertensive response to these agents; monitor.

MAO inhibitors: Severe hypertensive episodes have occurred with amphetamine when used in patients receiving MAO inhibitors; concurrent use or use within 14 days is contraindicated

Sibutramine: Concurrent use of sibutramine and amphetamines may cause severe hypertension and tachycardia; use is contraindicated (benzphetamine)

SSRIs: Amphetamines may increase the potential for serotonin syndrome when used concurrently with selective serotonin reuptake inhibitors (including fluoxetine, fluvoxamine, paroxetine, and sertraline)

Tricyclic antidepressants: Concurrent use of amphetamines with TCAs may result in hypertension and CNS stimulation; avoid this combination

Pregnancy Risk Factor C

Pregnancy Implications Crosses the placenta; can cause low birth weight/premature birth; reportedly associated with increased obstetric complications and maternal death; preterm birth, intrauterine growth retardation, placental abruption

Lactation Enters breast milk/contraindicated

Additional Information Illicit methamphetamine may contain lead; alkalinizing urine can result in longer methamphetamine half-life and elevated blood level; ephedrine is a precursor in the illicit manufacture of methamphetamine

Mid-Year 2000 Emergency Department Drug Abuse Warning Network (DAWN) data: **Note:** Methamphetamine/speed is sometimes used in combination with other drugs; therefore, one Emergency Department (ED) episode can include mentions of one or more drugs.

● In the first half of 2000, methamphetamine/speed was mentioned in 2% of all drug-related episodes. This number was 48% greater than in the first half of 1999, which had 4730 mentions. It is important to remember that national estimates of methamphetamine/speed mentions tend to fluctuate substantially from year to year.

● The estimated number of amphetamine mentions rose 32% from 5668 mentions in the first half of 1999 to 7510 mentions in the first half of 2000.

● Methamphetamine/speed mentions increased 48% nationwide between the first halves of 1999 and 2000 (4730 to 6980). Among the 5 metropolitan areas with the greatest number of methamphetamine/speed mentions, there were significant increases for this period in Seattle (80%), San Diego (71%), and Phoenix (67%). Methamphetamine/speed mentions were statistically unchanged for the same period in Los Angeles-Long Beach and San Francisco.

Specific References

Baker G, Drez N, McFeeley P, et al, "Unusual Distribution of Methamphetamine in a Fatality," J Anal Toxicol, 2004, 28:293.

Barnes AJ, Kacinko SL, Schwilke EW, et al, "Methamphetamine and Amphetamine Disposition in Human Sweat Following Controlled Oral Methamphetamine Administration," J Anal Toxicol, 2006, 30:139.

Elliott SP, "MDMA and MDA Concentrations in Antemortem and Postmortem Specimens in Fatalities Following Hospital Admission," J Anal Toxicol, 2005, 29(5):296-300.

Haller C, Stone J, Chen K, et al, "Ephedrine Alkaloid Urine Concentrations and Cross Reactivities with Amphetamine/Methamphetamine Immunoassays," J Toxicol Clin Toxicol, 2004, 42(5):795.

Holler JM, Vorce SP, Bosy TZ, et al, "Quantitative and Isomeric Determination of Amphetamine and Methamphetamine from Urine Using a Nonprotic Elution Solvent and R(-)-α-Methoxy-α-Trifluoromethylphenylacetic Acid Chloride Derivatization," J Anal Toxicol, 2005, 29:652-63.

Kashani J and Ruha AM, "Methamphetamine Toxicity Secondary to Intravaginal Body Stuffing," J Toxicol Clin Toxicol, 2004, 42(7):987-9.

Kashani J and Ruha AM, "Severe Methamphetamine Toxicity Resulting from Intravaginal Body Stuffing," J Toxicol Clin Toxicol, 2004, 42(5):759-60.

Kim I, Oyler JM, Moolchan ET, et al, "Urinary Pharmacokinetics of Methamphetamine and Its Metabolite, Amphetamine Following Controlled Oral Administration to Humans," J Anal Toxicol, 2004, 28:288.

Kim JY, Suh SI, In MK, et al, "Gas Chromatography-High-Resolution Mass Spectrometric Method for Determination of Methamphetamine and Its Major Metabolite Amphetamine in Human Hair," J Anal Toxicol, 2005, 29(5):370-5.

Kimura H, Matsumoto K, and Mukaida M, "Rapid and Simple Quantitation of Methamphetamine by Using a Homogeneous Time-Resolved Fluoroimmunoassay Based on Fluorescence Resonance Energy Transfer from Europium to Cy5," J Anal Toxicol, 2005, 29(8):799-804.

Klette KL, Kettle AR, and Jamerson MH, "Prevalence of Use Study for Amphetamine (AMP), Methamphetamine (MAMP), 3,4-Methylenedioxy-Amphetamine (MDA), 3,4-Methylenedioxy-Methamphetamine (MDMA), and 3,4-Methylenedioxy-Ethylamphetamine (MDEA) in Military Entrance Processing Stations (MEPS) Specimens," J Anal Toxicol, 2006, 30:319-22.

Kronstrand R, Ahlner J, Dizdar N, et al, "Quantitative Analysis of Desmethylselegiline, Methamphetamine, and Amphetamine in Hair and Plasma from Parkinson Patients on Long-Term Selegiline Medication," *J Anal Toxicol*, 2003, 27(3):135-41.

Kronstrand R, Nystrom I, and Trygg T, "Amphetamine Enantiomer Distribution in Hair and Blood to Monitor Abstinence from Street Amphetamine in Adult Attention Deficit Hyperactivity Disorder (ADHD) Treatment," *J Anal Toxicol*, 2006, 30:158.

Kupiec T, DeCicco L, Spiehler V, et al, "Choice of an ELISA Assay for Screening Postmortem Blood for Amphetamine and/or Methamphetamine," *J Anal Toxicol*, 2003, 27:187.

Lavelle J, Brunelli B, A'Zary E, et al, "A Modified Method for the Liquid-Liquid Extraction and GC-MS Analysis of Amphetamine/Methamphetamine from Human Urine in a SAMHSA-Certified Drug Testing Laboratory," *J Anal Toxicol*, 2004, 28:303.

Levisky JA, Karch SB, Bowerman DL, et al, "False-Positive RIA for Methamphetamine Following Ingestion of an Ephedra-Derived Herbal Product," *J Anal Toxicol*, 2003, 27(2):123-4.

Lin DL, Yin RM, Liu HC, et al, "Deposition Characteristics of Methamphetamine and Amphetamine in Fingernail Clippings and Hair Sections," *J Anal Toxicol*, 2004, 28(6):411-21.

Lineberry TW and Bostwick JM, "Methamphetamine Abuse: A Perfect Storm of Complications," *Mayo Clin Proc*, 2006, 81(1):77-84.

Ling JM, Lopez GP, Cragin LS, et al, "Clinical Outcome of Unintentional Amphetamine Exposures," *Clin Toxicol (Phila)*. 2005, 43:648.

Marshall WP and Logan BK, "The Presence of N-Methyl-1-(1-(1,4 cyclohexadienyl))-2-Propanamine, a Birch Reduction Product, in Methamphetamine Positive Toxicology Samples," *J Anal Toxicol*, 2004, 28:299.

McGuinness T, "Methamphetanine Abuse," *AJN*, 2006, 106(12): 54-9.

Miki A, Katagi M, Shima N, et al, "Application of ORAL*screen™ Saliva Drug Test for the Screening of Methamphetamine, MDMA, and MDEA Incorporated in Hair," *J Anal Toxicol*, 2004, 28(2):132-4.

Miki A, Katagi M, and Tsuchihashi H, "Determination of Methamphetamine and Its Metabolites Incorporated in Hair by Column-Switching Liquid Chromatography-Mass Spectrometry," *J Anal Toxicol*, 2003, 27(2):95-102.

Moltz E, Crouch BI, and Caravati EM, "Hallucinogenic Amphetamines and Tryptamines: Analysis of TESS Data from 1997-2003," *J Toxicol Clin Toxicol*, 2004, 42(5):763-4.

Moore C, Feldman M, Giorgi N, et al, "Methamphetamine and Metabolites in Hair, Oral Fluid, and Urine," *J Anal Toxicol*, 2006, 30:148.

Moore C, Feldman M, Harrison E, et al, "Analysis of Amphetamines in Hair, Oral Fluid, and Urine," *Annale de Toxicologie Analytique*, 2005, 17(4):229-36.

O'Connor AD and Kao LW, "QRS Prolongation Following Massive Methamphetamine Ingestion," *Clin Toxicol (Phila)*, 2005, 43:662.

Peters FT, Samyn N, Wahl M, et al, "Concentrations and Ratios of Amphetamine, Methamphetamine, MDA, MDMA, and MDEA Enantiomers Determined in Plasma Samples from Clinical Toxicology and Driving Under the Influence of Drugs Cases by GC-NICI-MS," *J Anal Toxicol*, 2003, 27(8):552-9.

Robarge T, Lasater M, Edwards J, et al, "Use of GC and Tandem MS-MS for Confirmation and Quantitation of Amphetamines and Other Phenethylamines in Oral Fluid," *J Anal Toxicol*, 2006, 30:132.

Rhyee SH, Aks SE, DesLauriers C, et al, "Case Series of Methamphetamine Body Stuffers," *J Toxicol Clin Toxicol*, 2004, 42(5):763.

Sato M, Hida M, and Nagase H, "Analysis of Pyrolysis Products of Methamphetamine," *J Anal Toxicol*, 2004, 28(8):638-43.

Shakleya EM, Tarr SG, Kraner JC, et al, "Potential Marker for Smoked Methamphetamine Hydrochloride Based on a Gas Chromatography-Mass Spectrometry Quantification Method for Trans-Phenylpropene," *J Anal Toxicol*, 2005, 29:552-5.

Spivak LA, Hendrickson RG, Horowitz BZ, et al, "Parachuting: A Novel Delivery Method for Methamphetamine Use," *Clin Toxicol (Phila)*, 2005, 43:664.

Stout PR, Horn CK, Klette KL, et al, "Evaluation of Occupational Exposure to Methamphetamine in Workers Preparing Training Aids for Drug Detection Dogs," *J Anal Toxicol*, 2006, 30:153.

Stout PR, Wiegand R, and Klette K, "Comparison and Evaluation of DRI® Methamphetamine, DRI® Ecstasy, Abuscreen® Online, and a Modified Abuscreen® Online Screening Immunoassays for the Detection of AMP, MTH, MDA, and MDMA in Urine," *J Anal Toxicol*, 2003, 27:200.

Tirumalai PS, Shakleya DM, Gannett PM, et al, "Conversion of Methamphetamine to N-Methyl-Methamphetamine in Formalin Solutions," *J Anal Toxicol*, 2005, 29:48-53.

Uhl M and Scheufler F, "Effects of Hair Color on the Drug Incorporation Into Human Hair," *Annale de Toxicologie Analytique*, 2005, 17(4):279-84.

Villamor JL, Bermejo AM, Fernandez P, et al, "A New GC-MS Method for the Determination of Five Amphetamines in Human Hair," *J Anal Toxicol*, 2005, 29:135-44.

Wijetunga M, Seto T, Lindsay J, et al, "Crystal Methamphetamine-Associated Cardiomyopathy: Tip of the Iceberg?" *J Toxicol Clin Toxicol*, 2003, 41(7):981-6.

Wyman JF and Cody JT, "Determination of l-Methamphetamine: A Case History," *J Anal Toxicol* , 2005, 29:759-61.

Yang W, Barnes A, Moolchan ET, et al, "Simultaneous Quantification of Opiates, Methamphetamine, Cocaine, and Metabolites in Skin by Positive Chemical Ionization Gas Chromatography/Mass Spectrometry," *J Anal Toxicol*, 2004, 28:299.

Methaqualone

Pronunciation (meth A kwa lone)

Related Information

● Donor Victims of Poisoning in Whom Transplantation of Organs Occurred

CAS Number 340-56-7; 72-44-6

Synonyms Methaqualone Hydrochloride

Impairment Potential Yes. Plasma methaqualone levels >2 mg/L have been associated with erratic driving. (Baselt RC and Cravey RH, *Disposition of Toxic Drugs and Chemicals in Man*, 4th ed, Foster City, CA: Chemical Toxicology Institute, 1995, 484.)

Use Europeans use for insomnia; taken off the U.S. market in 1984

Mechanism of Action Nonbarbiturate hypnosedative

Adverse Reactions

Cardiovascular: Tachycardia, sinus tachycardia

Central nervous system: Euphoria, slurred speech, salivation, ataxia, electroencephalogram abnormalities

Dermatologic: Bullous lesions

Gastrointestinal: Vomiting, necrotizing cystitis

Neuromuscular & skeletal: Rhabdomyolysis

Ocular: Nystagmus

Renal: Hematuria

Respiratory: Aspiration

Signs and Symptoms of Overdose Apnea, AV block, coma, dyspnea, erythema multiforme, hematuria, hyperreflexia, hyperthermia, hypotension, myoclonus, respiratory depression, seizures, vision color changes (yellow tinge)

Pharmacodynamics/Kinetics

Absorption: Complete within 2 hours

Distribution: V_d: 2.4-6.4 L/kg

Protein binding: 70% to 90%

Metabolism: Hepatic

Half-life: 33-40 hours

Elimination: $\approx$8% of the drug is normally excreted in 4 hours in a normal patient

Toxicodynamics/Kinetics

Absorption: Complete within 2 hours

Distribution: V_d: 2.4-6.4 L/kg

Protein binding: 70% to 90%

Metabolism: Hepatic

Half-life: 33-40 hours

Elimination: ~8% of the drug is normally excreted in 4 hours in a healthy person

Dosage Insomnia: 150-300 mg at night

Reference Range A 600 mg dose will yield a peak plasma level of 7 mg/L; plasma level of methaqualone >10 mg/L is consistent with toxicity

Overdosage/Treatment

Decontamination: Lavage (within 1 hour)/activated charcoal

Supportive therapy: Treat seizures with diazepam, phenobarbital, or phenytoin

Enhancement of elimination: Hemodialysis or resin hemoperfusion can enhance elimination; do not use forced saline diuresis; multiple dosing of activated charcoal may be effective; level >40 mg/mL is an indication for consideration of extracorporeal removal of this drug; clearance by hemodialysis is estimated to be 23 mL/minute; by charcoal hemoperfusion it is 137 mL/minute

Drug Interactions Enhances codeine analgesia

Pregnancy Risk Factor D

Additional Information Lethal dose: 8 g. Mandrax® also contains diphenhydramine.

Metharbital

CAS Number 50-11-3

Impairment Potential Yes

Use Control of grand mal, petit mal, myoclonic and mixed types of seizures

Adverse Reactions

Cardiovascular: Hypotension, circulatory collapse

Central nervous system: Drowsiness, paradoxical excitement, hyperkinetic activity, cognitive impairment, defects in general comprehension, short-term memory deficits, decreased attention span, ataxia

Dermatologic: Skin eruptions, skin rash, exfoliative dermatitis

Hematologic: Megaloblastic anemia

Hepatic: Hepatitis

Ocular: Vision color changes (yellow tinge), ptosis

Respiratory: Apnea (especially with rapid I.V. use), respiratory depression
Miscellaneous: Psychological and physical dependence

Toxicodynamics/Kinetics
Metabolism: Demethylated to barbital (active)
Elimination: Renal, 1% excreted unchanged; 9% excreted as barbital

Dosage Oral:
Children: 5-15 mg/kg/day or 50 mg 1-3 times/day
Adults: 100 mg 1-3 times/day, adjust dosage to obtain optimal effect

Reference Range Therapeutic, serum: 5-10 mcg/mL

Overdosage/Treatment
Decontamination: Lavage (within 1 hour)/activated charcoal
Enhancement of elimination: Multiple dosing of activated charcoal may be helpful

Test Interactions ↑ alkaline phosphatase (S); ↓ calcium (S)
Pregnancy Risk Factor D
Nursing Implications Solution is slightly acidic
Additional Information Faint, aromatic odor

Methimazole

CAS Number 60-56-0
U.S. Brand Names Tapazole®
Synonyms Thiamazole
Use Palliative treatment of hyperthyroidism, to return the hyperthyroid patient to a normal metabolic state prior to thyroidectomy, and to control thyrotoxic crisis that may accompany thyroidectomy
Mechanism of Action A thiourea which inhibits the synthesis of thyroid hormones by blocking the oxidation of iodine in the thyroid gland, blocking iodine's ability to combine with tyrosine to form thyroxine and triiodothyronine (T_3), does not inactivate circulating T_4 and T_3

Adverse Reactions
Cardiovascular: Edema
Central nervous system: Headache, vertigo, drowsiness, CNS stimulation, depression
Dermatologic: Skin rash, urticaria, pruritus, erythema nodosum, skin pigmentation, exfoliative dermatitis, alopecia, cutaneous vasculitis
Endocrine & metabolic: Goiter
Gastrointestinal: Nausea, vomiting, stomach pain, abnormal taste, constipation, weight gain, salivary gland swelling
Hematologic: Leukopenia, agranulocytosis, granulocytopenia, thrombocytopenia, aplastic anemia, hypoprothrombinemia
Hepatic: Cholestatic jaundice, jaundice, hepatitis
Neuromuscular & skeletal: Arthralgia, paresthesia
Renal: Nephrotic syndrome, renal vasculitis
Respiratory: Pulmonary vasculitis
Miscellaneous: SLE-like syndrome, elevated antineutrophilic cytoplasmic antibodies (ANCA)

Pharmacodynamics/Kinetics
Onset of action: Antithyroid: Oral: 12-18 hours
Duration: 36-72 hours
Distribution: Concentrated in thyroid gland; crosses placenta; enters breast milk (1:1)
Protein binding, plasma: None
Metabolism: Hepatic
Bioavailability: 80% to 95%
Half-life elimination: 4-13 hours
Excretion: Urine (80%)

Dosage
Oral:
Children: Initial: 0.4 mg/kg/day in 3 divided doses; maintenance: 0.2 mg/kg/day in 3 divided doses up to 30 mg/24 hours maximum
Adults: Initial: 5 mg every 8 hours; maintenance dose: 5-15 mg/day up to 60 mg/day for severe hyperthyroidism
Adjust dosage as required to achieve and maintain serum T_3, T_4, and TSH levels in the normal range. An elevated T_3 may be the sole indicator of inadequate treatment. An elevated TSH indicates excessive antithyroid treatment.

Stability Protect from light
Monitoring Parameters Monitor for signs of hypothyroidism, hyperthyroidism, T_4, T_3; CBC with differential, liver function (baseline and as needed), serum thyroxine, free thyroxine index
Contraindications Hypersensitivity to methimazole or any component of the formulation; nursing mothers (per manufacturer; however, expert analysis and the AAP state this drug may be used with caution in nursing mothers); pregnancy
Warnings Use with extreme caution in patients receiving other drugs known to cause myelosuppression particularly agranulocytosis, patients >40 years of age; avoid doses >40 mg/day (increased myelosuppression); may cause acneiform eruptions or worsen the condition of the thyroid
Dosage Forms Tablet: 5 mg, 10 mg, 20 mg
Tapazole® 5 mg, 10 mg
Overdosage/Treatment
Decontamination: Lavage (within 1 hour)/activated charcoal

Supportive therapy: Recombinant human granulocyte-monocyte colony-stimulating factor (270 mcg SubQ/day combined with glucocorticosteroids and antibiotics) has been used successfully in order to treat methimazole agranulocytosis
Enhancement of elimination: Multiple dosing of activated charcoal may be effective

Drug Interactions Inhibits CYP1A2 (weak), 2A6 (weak), 2B6 (weak), 2C9 (weak), 2C19 (weak), 2D6 (moderate), 2E1 (weak), 3A4 (weak)
Beta-blockers: Methimazole may decrease beta-blocker clearance due to changes in thyroid function.
Digoxin: Methimazole may increase digoxin levels due to changes in thyroid function.
CYP2D6 substrates: Methimazole may increase the levels/effects of CYP2D6 substrates. Example substrates include amphetamines, selected beta-blockers, dextromethorphan, fluoxetine, lidocaine, mirtazapine, nefazodone, paroxetine, risperidone, ritonavir, thioridazine, tricyclic antidepressants, and venlafaxine.
CYP2D6 prodrug substrates: Methimazole may decrease the levels/effects of CYP2D6 prodrug substrates. Example substrates include codeine, hydrocodone, oxycodone, and tramadol.
Theophylline: Methimazole may decrease theophylline clearance due to changes in thyroid function.
Warfarin: Anticoagulant effect of warfarin may be decreased.
Pregnancy Risk Factor D
Pregnancy Implications Hypothyroidism and congenital defects (rare) may occur.
Lactation Enters breast milk/contraindicated (AAP rates "compatible")

Methocarbamol

CAS Number 532-03-6
U.S. Brand Names Robaxin®
Use Treatment of muscle spasm associated with acute painful musculoskeletal conditions, supportive therapy in tetanus
Mechanism of Action Causes skeletal muscle relaxation by reducing the transmission of impulses from the spinal cord to skeletal muscle
Adverse Reactions
Frequency not defined.
Cardiovascular: Flushing of face, bradycardia, hypotension, syncope
Central nervous system: Drowsiness, dizziness, lightheadedness, convulsion, vertigo, headache, fever, amnesia, confusion, insomnia, sedation, coordination impaired (mild)
Dermatologic: Allergic dermatitis, urticaria, pruritus, rash, angioneurotic edema
Gastrointestinal: Nausea, vomiting, metallic taste, dyspepsia
Hematologic: Leukopenia
Hepatic: Jaundice
Local: Pain at injection site, thrombophlebitis
Ocular: Nystagmus, blurred vision, diplopia, conjunctivitis
Renal: Renal impairment
Respiratory: Nasal congestion
Miscellaneous: Allergic manifestations, anaphylactic reaction
Signs and Symptoms of Overdose Apnea, cardiac arrhythmias, coma, drowsiness, hypotension, nausea, urine discoloration (black; blue; brown; green), vomiting
Pharmacodynamics/Kinetics
Onset of action: Muscle relaxation: Oral: ~30 minutes
Protein binding: 46% to 50%
Metabolism: Hepatic via dealkylation and hydroxylation
Half-life elimination: 1-2 hours
Time to peak, serum: ~2 hours
Excretion: Urine (as metabolites)
Dosage Tetanus: I.V.:
Children: Recommended **only** for use in tetanus: 15 mg/kg/dose or 500 mg/m²/dose, may repeat every 6 hours if needed; maximum dose: 1.8 g/m²/day for 3 days only
Adults: Initial dose: 1-3 g; may repeat dose every 6 hours until oral dosing is possible; injection should not be used for more than 3 consecutive days
Muscle spasm: Children ≥16 years and Adults:
Oral: 1.5 g 4 times/day for 2-3 days (up to 8 g/day may be given in severe conditions), then decrease to 4-4.5 g/day in 3-6 divided doses
I.M., I.V.: 1 g every 8 hours if oral not possible; injection should not be used for more than 3 consecutive days
Elderly: Muscle spasm: Oral: Initial: 500 mg 4 times/day; titrate to response
Dosing adjustment/comments in renal impairment: Do not administer parenteral formulation to patients with renal dysfunction.
Dosing adjustment in hepatic impairment: Specific dosing guidelines are not available; plasma protein binding and clearance are decreased; half-life is increased
Monitoring Parameters Cardiac/respiratory
Administration Injection: Maximum rate: 3 mL/minute; should not be used for more than 3 consecutive days; may be administered undiluted.

451

Monitor closely for extravasation. Administer I.V. while in recumbent position. Maintain position 15-30 minutes following infusion.

Tablet: May be crushed and mixed with food or liquid if needed. Avoid alcohol.

Contraindications Hypersensitivity to methocarbamol or any component of the formulation; renal impairment (injection formulation)

Warnings Oral: Use caution with renal or hepatic impairment.

Injection: Rate of injection should not exceed 3 mL/minute; solution is hypertonic; avoid extravasation. Use with caution in patients with a history of seizures. Use caution with hepatic impairment.

Dosage Forms Injection, solution: 100 mg/mL (10 mL) [in polyethylene glycol; vial stopper contains latex]

Tablet: 500 mg, 750 mg

Reference Range Peak serum level after 2 g: 25.8 mg/L; peak serum levels after 4 g: 41 mg/L; blood levels >320 mg/L have been associated with fatalities

Overdosage/Treatment

Decontamination: Activated charcoal

Supportive therapy: Following attempts to enhance drug elimination, hypotension should be treated with I.V. fluids and/or Trendelenburg positioning

Enhancement of elimination: Dialysis and hemoperfusion might be useful in reducing serum drug concentrations; patient should be observed for possible relapses due to incomplete gastric emptying

Test Interactions May cause color interference in certain screening tests for 5-HIAA using nitrosonaphthol reagent and in screening tests for urinary VMA using the Gitlow method.

Drug Interactions Increased effect/toxicity with CNS depressants; pyridostigmine (a single case of worsening myasthenia has been reported following methocarbamol administration)

Pregnancy Risk Factor C

Pregnancy Implications Animal reproduction studies have not been conducted. The manufacturer notes that fetal and congenital abnormalities have been rarely reported following *in utero* exposure. Use during pregnancy only if clearly needed.

Lactation Excretion in breast milk unknown/use caution

Nursing Implications Not recommended for SubQ administration; rate of injection should not exceed 3 mL/minute

Methohexital

CAS Number 309-36-4

U.S. Brand Names Brevital® Sodium

Synonyms Methohexital Sodium

Impairment Potential Yes

Use

Induction and maintenance of general anesthesia for short procedures

Can be used in pediatric patients ≥1 month of age as follows: For rectal or intramuscular induction of anesthesia prior to the use of other general anesthetic agents, as an adjunct to subpotent inhalational anesthetic agents for short surgical procedures, or for short surgical, diagnostic, or therapeutic procedures associated with minimal painful stimuli

Unlabeled/Investigational Use Wada test

Mechanism of Action Ultra short-acting I.V. barbiturate anesthetic

Adverse Reactions

Cardiovascular: Hypotension, peripheral vascular collapse, sinus bradycardia, sinus tachycardia

Central nervous system: Convulsions, CNS depression, headache, extrapyramidal reactions

Gastrointestinal: Nausea, vomiting

Local: **Pain on I.M. injection**, thrombophlebitis

Neuromuscular & skeletal: Involuntary muscle movement, myoclonus, rigidity, tremors

Respiratory: Apnea, respiratory depression, laryngospasm, coughing, rhinitis

Miscellaneous: Hiccups

Signs and Symptoms of Overdose Apnea, hypotension, ptosis, tachycardia, vision color changes (green tinge; yellow tinge), wheezing

Pharmacodynamics/Kinetics

Onset of action: I.V.: Immediately

Duration: Single dose: 10-20 minutes

Dosage Doses must be titrated to effect

Manufacturer's recommendations:

Infants <1 month: Safety and efficacy not established

Infants ≥1 month and Children:

I.M.: Induction: 6.6-10 mg/kg of a 5% solution

Rectal: Induction: Usual: 25 mg/kg of a 1% solution

Alternative pediatric dosing:

Children 3-12 years:

I.M.: Preoperative: 5-10 mg/kg/dose

I.V.: Induction: 1-2 mg/kg/dose

Rectal: Preoperative/induction: 20-35 mg/kg/dose; usual: 25 mg/kg/dose; maximum dose: 500 mg/dose; give as 10% aqueous solution

Adults: I.V.:

Induction: 50-120 mg to start; 20-40 mg every 4-7 minutes

Wada test (unlabeled): 3-4 mg over 3 second; following signs of recovery, administer a second dose of 2 mg over 2 seconds

Dosing adjustment/comments in hepatic impairment: Lower dosage and monitor closely

Stability Do not dilute with solutions containing bacteriostatic agents; solutions are alkaline (pH 9.5-11) and **incompatible** with acids (eg, atropine sulfate, succinylcholine), also **incompatible** with phenol-containing solutions and silicone

Administration Dilute to a maximum concentration of 1% for I.V. use; for Wada testing, a dilution of 1 mg/mL has been reported

Contraindications Hypersensitivity to methohexital or any component of the formulation; porphyria

Warnings Use with extreme caution in patients with liver impairment, asthma, cardiovascular instability. **[U.S. Boxed Warning]: Should only be administered in hospitals or ambulatory care settings.**

Dosage Forms Injection, powder for reconstitution, as sodium: 500 mg, 2.5 g, 5 g

Overdosage/Treatment

Decontamination: Activated charcoal

Supportive therapy: Treatment is primarily supportive with mechanical ventilation if needed

Enhancement of elimination: Charcoal hemoperfusion is unlikely to be of benefit due to rapid elimination; consider with fulminant hepatic failure

Drug Interactions Acetaminophen: Barbiturates may enhance the hepatotoxic potential of acetaminophen overdoses

Antiarrhythmics: Barbiturates may increase the metabolism of antiarrhythmics, decreasing their clinical effect; includes disopyramide, propafenone, and quinidine

Anticonvulsants: Barbiturates may increase the metabolism of anticonvulsants; includes ethosuximide, felbamate (possibly), lamotrigine, phenytoin, tiagabine, topiramate, and zonisamide; does not appear to affect gabapentin or levetiracetam

Antineoplastics: Limited evidence suggests that enzyme-inducing anticonvulsant therapy may reduce the effectiveness of some chemotherapy regimens (specifically in ALL); teniposide and methotrexate may be cleared more rapidly in these patients

Antipsychotics: Barbiturates may enhance the metabolism (decrease the efficacy) of antipsychotics; monitor for altered response; dose adjustment may be needed

Beta-blockers: Metabolism of beta-blockers may be increased and clinical effect decreased; atenolol and nadolol are unlikely to interact given their renal elimination

Calcium channel blockers: Barbiturates may enhance the metabolism of calcium channel blockers, decreasing their clinical effect

Chloramphenicol: Barbiturates may increase the metabolism of chloramphenicol and chloramphenicol may inhibit barbiturate metabolism; monitor for altered response

Cimetidine: Barbiturates may enhance the metabolism of cimetidine, decreasing its clinical effect

CNS depressants: Sedative effects and/or respiratory depression with barbiturates may be additive with other CNS depressants; monitor for increased effect; includes ethanol, sedatives, antidepressants, narcotic analgesics, and benzodiazepines

Corticosteroids: Barbiturates may enhance the metabolism of corticosteroids, decreasing their clinical effect

Cyclosporine: Levels may be decreased by barbiturates; monitor

Doxycycline: Barbiturates may enhance the metabolism of doxycycline, decreasing its clinical effect; higher dosages may be required

Estrogens: Barbiturates may increase the metabolism of estrogens and reduce their efficacy

Felbamate may inhibit the metabolism of barbiturates and barbiturates may increase the metabolism of felbamate

Griseofulvin: Barbiturates may impair the absorption of griseofulvin, and griseofulvin metabolism may be increased by barbiturates, decreasing clinical effect

Guanfacine: Effect may be decreased by barbiturates

Immunosuppressants: Barbiturates may enhance the metabolism of immunosuppressants, decreasing its clinical effect; includes both cyclosporine and tacrolimus

Loop diuretics: Metabolism may be increased and clinical effects decreased; established for furosemide, effect with other loop diuretics not established

MAO inhibitors: Metabolism of barbiturates may be inhibited, increasing clinical effect or toxicity of the barbiturates

Methadone: Barbiturates may enhance the metabolism of methadone resulting in methadone withdrawal

Methoxyflurane: Barbiturates may enhance the nephrotoxic effects of methoxyflurane

Oral contraceptives: Barbiturates may enhance the metabolism of oral contraceptives, decreasing their clinical effect; an alternative method of contraception should be considered

Theophylline: Barbiturates may increase metabolism of theophylline derivatives and decrease their clinical effect

Tricyclic antidepressants: Barbiturates may increase metabolism of tricyclic antidepressants and decrease their clinical effect; sedative effects may be additive

Valproic acid: Metabolism of barbiturates may be inhibited by valproic acid; monitor for excessive sedation; a dose reduction may be needed

Warfarin: Barbiturates inhibit the hypoprothrombinemic effects of oral anticoagulants via increased metabolism; this combination should generally be avoided

Pregnancy Risk Factor C

Nursing Implications Avoid extravasation or intra-arterial administration

Additional Information Lethal dose: 1-2 g

Methotrexate

Related Information
- Trimetrexate Glucuronate

CAS Number 59-05-2

U.S. Brand Names Rheumatrex®; Trexall™

Synonyms Amethopterin; Methotrexate Sodium; MTX (error-prone abbreviation) ; NSC-740

Use Treatment of trophoblastic neoplasms; leukemias; psoriasis; rheumatoid arthritis (RA), including polyarticular-course juvenile rheumatoid arthritis (JRA); breast, head and neck, and lung carcinomas; osteosarcoma; soft-tissue sarcomas; carcinoma of gastrointestinal tract, esophagus, testes; lymphomas

Unlabeled/Investigational Use Treatment and maintenance of remission in Crohn's disease

Mechanism of Action Methotrexate is a folate antimetabolite that inhibits DNA synthesis. Methotrexate irreversibly binds to dihydrofolate reductase, inhibiting the formation of reduced folates, and thymidylate synthetase, resulting in inhibition of purine and thymidylic acid synthesis. Methotrexate is cell cycle specific for the S phase of the cycle.

The MOA in the treatment of rheumatoid arthritis is unknown, but may affect immune function. In psoriasis, methotrexate is thought to target rapidly proliferating epithelial cells in the skin.

Adverse Reactions

Note: Adverse reactions vary by route and dosage. Hematologic and/or gastrointestinal toxicities may be common at dosages used in chemotherapy; these reactions are much less frequent when used at typical dosages for rheumatic diseases.

Cardiovascular: **Vasculitis**, pericarditis, pericardial effusion, serositis

Central nervous system: Malaise, fatigue, dizziness, **encephalopathy, seizures**, confusion, **fever**, chills, **headache**, hyperthermia, **arachnoiditis, coma, cranial nerve palsies**, leukoencephalopathy

Dermatologic: Alopecia, rash, depigmentation or hyperpigmentation of skin, photosensitivity, bullous acral erythema, toxic epidermal necrolysis, acne, bullous skin disease, urticaria, purpura, onycholysis, pruritus, yellow fingernail, exanthem, radiation recall dermatitis, cutaneous vasculitis

Endocrine & metabolic: Hypoglycemia, diabetes, gynecomastia, **hyperuricemia, defective oogenesis or spermatogenesis**

Gastrointestinal: **Ulcerative stomatitis, nausea**, abdominal distress, **vomiting, anorexia**, stomatitis, **diarrhea**, enteritis, fecal discoloration (black), metallic taste, **mucositis, glossitis, gingivitis, intestinal perforation**

Genitourinary: Cystitis

Hematologic: Myelosuppression, **leukopenia**, hemorrhage, pancytopenia (mean cumulative dose 675 mg), **thrombocytopenia**

Hepatic: Cirrhosis (especially noted in diabetics and obese patients), hepatic steatosis

Neuromuscular & skeletal: Rarely arthralgia, osteopathy, stress fractures, osteoporosis

Ocular: Blurred vision

Renal: **Renal failure, azotemia, nephropathy**, nephrotic syndrome

Respiratory: Interstitial pneumonitis, cough, dyspnea, crepitant rales, hyposmia, **pharyngitis**, eosinophilic pneumonia

Miscellaneous: Decreased resistance to infection, anaphylactic shock, accelerated nodulosis, Fournier's gangrene

Signs and Symptoms of Overdose Agranulocytosis, alopecia, ataxia, azotemia, bone marrow depression, cirrhosis, conjunctivitis, coma, cranial nerve palsies, dementia, diarrhea, elevated AST, encephalopathy, granulocytopenia, gynecomastia, hemiplegia, leukopenia, lymphoma, melena, myalgia, nausea, neutropenia, oligospermia, pleural effusion, sexual dysfunction, stomatitis, toxic epidermal necrolysis, tubular necrosis, vomiting

Pharmacodynamics/Kinetics

Onset of action: Antirheumatic: 3-6 weeks; additional improvement may continue longer than 12 weeks

Absorption: Oral: Rapid; well absorbed at low doses (<30 mg/m^2), incomplete after large doses; I.M.: Complete

Distribution: Penetrates slowly into 3rd space fluids (eg, pleural effusions, ascites), exits slowly from these compartments (slower than from plasma); crosses placenta; small amounts enter breast milk; sustained concentrations retained in kidney and liver

Protein binding: 50%

Metabolism: <10%; degraded by intestinal flora to DAMPA by carboxypeptidase; hepatic aldehyde oxidase converts methotrexate to 7-OH methotrexate; polyglutamates are produced intracellularly and are just as potent as methotrexate; their production is dose- and duration-dependent and they are slowly eliminated by the cell once formed

Half-life elimination: Low dose: 3-10 hours; High dose: 8-12 hours

Time to peak, serum: Oral: 1-2 hours; I.M.: 30-60 minutes

Excretion: Urine (44% to 100%); feces (small amounts)

Dosage Refer to individual protocols.

Note: Doses between 100-500 mg/m^2**may require** leucovorin rescue. Doses >500 mg/m^2**require** leucovorin rescue.

Children:

Dermatomyositis: Oral: 15-20 mg/m^2/week as a single dose once weekly **or** 0.3-1 mg/kg/dose once weekly

Juvenile rheumatoid arthritis: Oral, I.M.: 10 mg/m^2 once weekly, then 5-15 mg/m^2/week as a single dose **or** as 3 divided doses given 12 hours apart

Antineoplastic dosage range:

Oral, I.M.: 7.5-30 mg/m^2/week **or** every 2 weeks

I.V.: 10-18,000 mg/m^2 bolus dosing **or** continuous infusion over 6-42 hours

For dosing schedules, see table:

Methotrexate Dosing Schedules

Dose	Route	Frequency
Conventional		
15-20 mg/m^2	P.O.	Twice weekly
30-50 mg/m^2	P.O., I.V.	Weekly
15 mg/day for 5 days	P.O., I.M.	Every 2-3 weeks
Intermediate		
50-150 mg/m^2*	I.V. push	Every 2-3 weeks
240 mg/m^2*	I.V. infusion	Every 4-7 days
0.5-1 g/m^2**	I.V. infusion	Every 2-3 weeks
High		
1-25 g/m^2*	I.V. infusion	Every 1-3 weeks

*Doses between 100-500 mg/m^2 may require leucovorin rescue in some patients.

**Followed with leucovorin rescue - refer to Leucovorin monograph for details.

Pediatric solid tumors (high-dose): I.V.:

<12 years: 12-25 g/m^2

≥12 years: 8 g/m^2

Acute lymphocytic leukemia (intermediate-dose): I.V.: Loading: 100 mg/m^2 bolus dose, followed by 900 mg/m^2/day infusion over 23-41 hours.

Meningeal leukemia: I.T.: 10-15 mg/m^2 (maximum dose: 15 mg) **or** an age-based dosing regimen; one possible system is:

≤3 months: 3 mg/dose

4-11 months: 6 mg/dose

1 year: 8 mg/dose

2 years: 10 mg/dose

≥3 years: 12 mg/dose

Adults: I.V.: Range is wide from 30-40 mg/m^2/week to 100-12,000 mg/m^2 with leucovorin rescue

Trophoblastic neoplasms:

Oral, I.M.: 15-30 mg/day for 5 days; repeat in 7 days for 3-5 courses

I.V.: 11 mg/m^2 days 1 through 5 every 3 weeks

Head and neck cancer: Oral, I.M., I.V.: 25-50 mg/m^2 once weekly

Mycosis fungoides (cutaneous T-cell lymphoma): Oral, I.M.: Initial (early stages):

5-50 mg once weekly **or**

15-37.5 mg twice weekly

Bladder cancer: I.V.:

30 mg/m^2 day 1 and 8 every 3 weeks **or**

30 mg/m^2 day 1, 15, and 22 every 4 weeks

Breast cancer: I.V.: 30-60 mg/m^2 days 1 and 8 every 3-4 weeks

Gastric cancer: I.V.:1500 mg/m^2 every 4 weeks

Lymphoma, non-Hodgkin's: I.V.:

30 mg/m^2 days 3 and 10 every 3 weeks **or**

120 mg/m^2 day 8 and 15 every 3-4 weeks **or**

200 mg/m^2 day 8 and 15 every 3 weeks **or**
400 mg/m^2 every 4 weeks for 3 cycles **or**
1 g/m^2 every 3 weeks **or**
1.5 g/m^2 every 4 weeks
Sarcoma: I.V.: 8-12 g/m^2 weekly for 2-4 weeks
Rheumatoid arthritis: Oral: 7.5 mg once weekly **or** 2.5 mg every 12 hours for 3 doses/week, not to exceed 20 mg/week
Psoriasis:
  Oral: 2.5-5 mg/dose every 12 hours for 3 doses given weekly **or**
  Oral, I.M.: 10-25 mg/dose given once weekly
Ectopic pregnancy: I.M., I.V.: 50 mg/m^2 as a single dose
Elderly: Rheumatoid arthritis/psoriasis: Oral: Initial: 5-7.5 mg/week, not to exceed 20 mg/week

Dosing adjustment in renal impairment:
Cl$_{cr}$ 61-80 mL/minute: Reduce dose to 75% of usual dose
Cl$_{cr}$ 51-60 mL/minute: Reduce dose to 70% of usual dose
Cl$_{cr}$ 10-50 mL/minute: Reduce dose to 30% to 50% of usual dose
Cl$_{cr}$ <10 mL/minute: Avoid use
Hemodialysis: Not dialyzable (0% to 5%); supplemental dose is not necessary
Peritoneal dialysis: Supplemental dose is not necessary

Dosage adjustment in hepatic impairment:
Bilirubin 3.1-5 mg/dL **or** AST >180 units: Administer 75% of usual dose
Bilirubin >5 mg/dL: Do not use

Stability Store tablets and intact vials at room temperature (15°C to 25°C); protect from light. Dilute powder with D$_5$W or NS to a concentration of ≤25 mg/mL (20 mg and 50 mg vials) and 50 mg/mL (1 g vial). Intrathecal solutions may be reconstituted to 2.5-5 mg/mL with NS, D$_5$W, lactated Ringer's, or Elliott's B solution. Use preservative free preparations for intrathecal or high-dose administration. Further dilution in D$_5$W or NS is stable for 24 hours at room temperature (21°C to 25°C). Reconstituted solutions with a preservative may be stored under refrigeration for up to 3 months, and up to 4 weeks at room temperature. Intrathecal dilutions are stable at room temperature for 7 days, but it is generally recommended that they be used within 4-8 hours.

Monitoring Parameters For prolonged use (especially rheumatoid arthritis, psoriasis) a baseline liver biopsy, repeated at each 1-1.5 g cumulative dose interval, should be performed; WBC and platelet counts every 4 weeks; CBC and creatinine, LFTs every 3-4 months; chest x-ray

Administration Methotrexate may be administered I.M., I.V., or I.T.; I.V. administration may be as slow push, short bolus infusion, or 24- to 42-hour continuous infusion
Specific dosing schemes vary, but high dose should be followed by leucovorin calcium to prevent toxicity; refer to Leucovorin monograph

Contraindications Hypersensitivity to methotrexate or any component of the formulation; severe renal or hepatic impairment; pre-existing profound bone marrow suppression in patients with psoriasis or rheumatoid arthritis, alcoholic liver disease, AIDS, pre-existing blood dyscrasias; pregnancy (in patients with psoriasis or rheumatoid arthritis); breast-feeding

Warnings
Hazardous agent - use appropriate precautions for handling and disposal. May cause potentially life-threatening pneumonitis (may occur at any time during therapy and at any dosage); monitor closely for pulmonary symptoms, particularly dry, nonproductive cough. Methotrexate may cause photosensitivity and/or severe dermatologic reactions which are not dose-related. Methotrexate has been associated with acute and chronic hepatotoxicity, fibrosis, and cirrhosis. Risk is related to cumulative dose and prolonged exposure. Ethanol abuse, obesity, advanced age, and diabetes may increase the risk of hepatotoxic reactions.
Methotrexate may cause renal failure, gastrointestinal toxicity, or bone marrow depression. Use with caution in patients with renal impairment, peptic ulcer disease, ulcerative colitis, or pre-existing bone marrow suppression. Diarrhea and ulcerative stomatitis may require interruption of therapy; death from hemorrhagic enteritis or intestinal perforation has been reported. Methotrexate penetrates slowly into 3rd space fluids, such as pleural effusions or ascites, and exits slowly from these compartments (slower than from plasma). Dosage reduction may be necessary in patients with renal or hepatic impairment, ascites, and pleural effusion. Toxicity from methotrexate or any immunosuppressive is increased in the elderly.
Severe bone marrow suppression, aplastic anemia, and GI toxicity have occurred during concomitant administration with NSAIDs. Use caution when used with other hepatotoxic agents (azathioprine, retinoids, sulfasalazine). Methotrexate given concomitantly with radiotherapy may increase the risk of soft tissue necrosis and osteonecrosis. Immune suppression may lead to opportunistic infections.
For rheumatoid arthritis and psoriasis, immunosuppressive therapy should only be used when disease is active and less toxic; traditional therapy is ineffective. Discontinue therapy in RA or psoriasis if a significant decrease in hematologic components is noted. Methotrexate formulations and/or diluents containing preservatives should not be used for intrathecal or high-dose therapy. Methotrexate injection may contain benzyl alcohol and should not be used in neonates.

Dosage Forms Injection, powder for reconstitution [preservative free]: 20 mg, 1 g
Injection, solution: 25 mg/mL (2 mL, 10 mL) [contains benzyl alcohol]
Injection, solution [preservative free]: 25 mg/mL (2 mL, 4 mL, 8 mL, 10 mL)
Tablet: 2.5 mg
  Trexall™: 5 mg, 7.5 mg, 10 mg, 15 mg
Tablet, as sodium [dose pack] (Rheumatrex® Dose Pack): 2.5 mg (4 cards with 2, 3, 4, 5, or 6 tablets each)

Reference Range
Therapeutic levels: Variable; Toxic concentration: Variable; therapeutic range is dependent upon therapeutic approach.
High-dose regimens produce drug levels that are between 10^{-6} Molar and 10^{-7} Molar 24-72 hours after drug infusion
10^{-6} Molar unit = 1 micro Molar unit
  Toxic: Low-dose therapy: >9.1 ng/mL; high-dose therapy: >454 ng/mL

Overdosage/Treatment
Decontamination: (No cathartic) lavage (within 1 hour)/activated charcoal
Supportive therapy: Severe bone marrow toxicity can result from overdose; leucovorin rescue can reduce the toxicity; administer as quickly as possible 10 mg/m^2 every 6 hours for 72 hours, follow serum methotrexate levels; leucovorin treatment should be continued until methotrexate levels in serum fall below 50 mM/L. SubQ granulocyte colony stimulating factor may improve agranulocytosis (5 mcg/kg/day); aminophylline (2.5 mg/kg) has been used to treat methotrexate neurotoxicity in children; corticosteroids may be useful to treat methotrexate pulmonary hypersensitivity reaction; accelerated nodulosis has been successfully treated with penicillamine (250-500 mg/day); ondansetron (8 mg) improves methotrexate-induced nausea
  For intrathecal methotrexate overdose, cerebrospinal fluid washout procedure should be performed: Drain 30 mL of CSF as soon as possible; if >100 mg of methotrexate was administered, a neurosurgical consultation should be obtained; after a burrhole into the frontal horn of the right lateral ventricle with a Scott ventricular cannula is performed, 5 mL of warmed preservative-free normal saline is infused; simultaneously, 5 mL of CSF is drained from the lumbar puncture needle; over the next 4 hours, up to 550 mL of warmed normal saline is infused into the ventricles and subsequently removed through the lumbar puncture needle; the ventricular cannula is then attached to a intraventricular pressure transducer; leucovorin can be added to the final 100 mL of normal saline at a concentration of 0.02 mg/mL (however, its efficacy has not been determined); pentobarbital and phenytoin can be given to prevent seizures; 24 hours later, I.V. thymidylate rescue (8 g/m^2/day) can be given by continuous I.V. infusion (though this is investigational); alternatively, I.V. leucovorin (high-dose ~1 g) rescue can be given until the methotrexate levels in the blood and CSF are in nontoxic range; alkalinization of urine may help in enhancing elimination of methotrexate; monitor for cerebral edema; treat with mannitol if it is present. Dexamethasone can be given intravenously to limit meningeal irritation. Alternatively, a CSF exchange through the L.P. site can be performed (30 ml of Lactated Ringers in 30 ml of CSF with 3 exchanges. Maintain upright position).
Methotrexate can be precipitated in an acidic urine. The urine pH should be >6.5 by administering I.V. sodium bicarbonate (40-60 mEq/L in crystalloid fluids).
Carboxypeptidase G2 (CPG2) at a dose of 10-58 units/kg is an effective rescue treatment for patients with delayed elimination of methotrexate. It can be obtained through Dr. Matthew Boron at 301-496-5725 or page 1-888-720-0931.
Enhancement of elimination: Multiple dosing of activated charcoal is effective; renal excretion is optimized at a urinary pH over 7.0. Charcoal hemoperfusion, hydration, and urinary alkalinization may enhance elimination and prevent precipitation in renal tubules; not dialyzable (0% to 5%); clearance by hemoperfusion is estimated to be 54-137 mL/minute.

Antidote(s)
• Folic Acid [ANTIDOTE]
• Leucovorin [ANTIDOTE]
Test Interactions ↑ potassium (S)
Drug Interactions Acitretin: May enhance the hepatotoxic effect of methotrexate. Avoid concurrent use.
Cholestyramine: May decrease levels of methotrexate.
Corticosteroids: May decrease uptake of methotrexate into leukemia cells. Administration of these drugs should be separated by 12 hours. Dexamethasone has been reported to not affect methotrexate influx into cells.
Cyclosporine: Concomitant administration with methotrexate may increase levels and toxicity of each.

Cytarabine: Methotrexate, when administered prior to cytarabine, may enhance the efficacy and toxicity of cytarabine. Some combination treatment regimens (eg, hyper-CVAD) have been designed to take advantage of this interaction.

Hepatotoxic agents (azathioprine, retinoids, sulfasalazine) may increase the risk of hepatotoxic reactions

Mercaptopurine: Methotrexate may increase mercaptopurine levels. Dosage adjustment may be required.

NSAIDs: Severe bone marrow suppression, aplastic anemia, and GI toxicity have been reported with concomitant therapy. Should not be used during moderate or high-dose methotrexate due to increased and prolonged methotrexate levels (may increase toxicity); NSAID use during treatment of rheumatoid arthritis has not been fully explored, but continuation of prior regimen has been allowed in some circumstances, with cautious monitoring

Penicillins: May increase methotrexate concentrations (due to a reduction in renal tubular secretion). Primarily a concern with high doses of penicillins and higher dosages of methotrexate.

Probenecid: May increase methotrexate concentrations (due to a reduction in renal tubular secretion). Primarily a concern with higher dosages of methotrexate.

Salicylates: May increase the serum concentration of Methotrexate. Salicylate doses used for prophylaxis of cardiovascular events are not likely to be of concern.

Sulfonamides: May increase methotrexate concentrations (due to a reduction in renal tubular secretion). In addition, sulfonamides may reduce folate levels, increasing the risk/severity of bone marrow suppression. Particularly a concern with higher dosages of methotrexate.

Tetracyclines: May increase methotrexate toxicity; monitor

Theophylline: Methotrexate may increase theophylline levels.

Vaccines (live virus): Concurrent use with methotrexate may result in vaccinia infections.

Pregnancy Risk Factor D

Pregnancy Implications Fetal death or teratogenic effects may occur. Use is contraindicated in pregnant women with psoriasis or rheumatoid arthritis. Use for the treatment of neoplastic diseases only when the potential benefit to the mother outweighs the possible risk to the fetus. Pregnancy should be excluded prior to therapy in women of childbearing potential. Pregnancy should be avoided for ≥3 months following treatment in male patients and ≥1 ovulatory cycle in female patients.

Lactation Enters breast milk/contraindicated

Nursing Implications For intrathecal use, mix methotrexate without preservative with Elliott's B solution to concentration no greater than 2 mg/mL

Additional Information Toxic dose: I.V.: 1.5 mg/kg; Adults: I.T.: 12.5 mg Low-dose methotrexate (0.2 mg/kg/week) has been shown to be effective in treating idiopathic granulomatous hepatitis

Myelosuppressive effects: WBC: Mild; Platelets: Moderate; Onset (days): 7. Nadir (days): 10. Recovery (days): 21. Sodium content of 100 mg injection: 20 mg (0.86 mEq); Sodium content of 100 mg (low sodium) injection: 15 mg (0.65 mEq)

Risk factors for development of lung injury include older age, diabetes, rheumatoid pleuropulmonary involvement, previous use of disease modifying antirheumatic drugs, and hypoalbuminemia.

Specific References

Chang VC, Chen JD, Yen DT, et al, "Serious Pancytopenia from Methotrexate Treatment of Psoriatic Arthritis," *Am J Emerg Med*, 2006, 24:392-4.

Limelette N, Ferry M, Branger S, Thuillier A, et al, "In Vitro Stability Study of Methotrexate in Blood and Plasma Samples for Routine Monitoring," *Ther Drug Monit*, 2003, 25(1):81-7.

LoVecchio F, Watts D, and Katz K, "Four-Year Experience with Methotrexate Exposures," *J Toxicol Clin Toxicol*, 2003, 41(5):684.

Niven AS and Argyros G, "Alternate Treatments in Asthma," *Chest*, 2003, 123(4):1254-65.

Parshuram CS, Dupuis LL, To T, "Occurrence and Impact of Unanticipated Variation in Intravenous Methotrexate Dosing," *Ann Pharmacother*, 2006, 40(5):805-11.

Peyriere H, Cociglio M, Margueritte G, "Optimal Management of Methotrexate Intoxication in a Child with Osteosarcoma," *Ann Pharmacother*, 2004, 38(3):422-7.

Proudfoot AT, Krenzelok EP, Vale JA, et al, "AACT/EAPCCT Position Paper on Urine Alkalinization," *J Toxicol Clin Toxicol*, 2004, 42(1):1-26.

Schwartz S, Glover JF, Melton R, et al, "The Use of Recombinant Carboxypeptidase G2 in the Rescue of Patients with Methotrexate Induced Renal Insufficiency," *J Toxicol Clin Toxicol*, 2004, 42(5):713.

Methsuximide

CAS Number 77-41-8
U.S. Brand Names Celontin®
Impairment Potential Yes

Use Control of absence (petit mal) seizures that are refractory to other drugs

Unlabeled/Investigational Use Partial complex (psychomotor) seizures

Mechanism of Action Increases the seizure threshold and suppresses paroxysmal spike-and-wave pattern in absence seizures; depresses nerve transmission in the motor cortex

Adverse Reactions

Central nervous system: **Headache, dizziness, ataxia, drowsiness**, euphoria, nervousness, hallucinations, insomnia, agitation, behavioral changes, mental confusion, Parkinson-like symptoms, sedation

Dermatologic: **Stevens-Johnson syndrome**, rashes, hypertrichosis, alopecia, urticaria, purpura, pruritus, exanthem

Gastrointestinal: **Nausea, vomiting, anorexia, weight loss**, abdominal pain, flatulence, gingival hyperplasia

Hematologic: Leukopenia, aplastic anemia, thrombocytopenia, eosinophilia, pancytopenia, monocytosis

Ocular: Photophobia, periorbital edema

Miscellaneous: **Hiccups, SLE syndrome**

Signs and Symptoms of Overdose Agranulocytosis, ataxia, dizziness, dysarthria, granulocytopenia, hiccups, insomnia, neutropenia, leukopenia, relapsing coma, stupor

Pharmacodynamics/Kinetics

Metabolism: Hepatic; rapidly demethylated to N-desmethylmethsuximide (active metabolite)

Half-life elimination: 2-4 hours

Time to peak, serum: Within 1-3 hours

Excretion: Urine (<1% as unchanged drug)

Dosage

Oral:

Children: Anticonvulsant: Initial: 10-15 mg/kg/day in 3-4 divided doses; increase weekly up to maximum of 30 mg/kg/day

Adults: Anticonvulsant: 300 mg/day for the first week; may increase by 300 mg/day at weekly intervals up to 1.2 g/day in 2-4 divided doses/day

Stability Protect from high temperature

Monitoring Parameters CBC, hepatic function tests, urinalysis

Contraindications Hypersensitivity to succinimides or any component of the formulation

Warnings Use with caution in patients with hepatic or renal disease; abrupt withdrawal of the drug may precipitate absence status; methsuximide may increase tonic-clonic seizures in patients with mixed seizure disorders; methsuximide must be used in combination with other anticonvulsants in patients with both absence and tonic-clonic seizures. Succinimides have been associated with severe blood dyscrasias and cases of systemic lupus erythematosus.

Dosage Forms Capsule: 150 mg, 300 mg

Reference Range

Therapeutic (normethsuximide): 10-40 mcg/mL (SI: 53-212 μmol/L)

Toxic: >40 mcg/mL (SI: >212 μmol/L); N-desmethylmethsuximide levels >150 mcg/mL (SI: >738 μmol/L) associated with coma

Overdosage/Treatment

Decontamination: Activated charcoal

Enhancement of elimination: Charcoal hemoperfusion (useful in removal of toxic metabolite) and hemodialysis may be useful

Test Interactions ↑ alkaline phosphatase (S); ↓ calcium (S)

Drug Interactions **Substrate** of CYP2C19 (major); **Inhibits** CYP2C19 (weak)

CNS depressants: Sedative effects and/or respiratory depression may be additive with CNS depressants; includes ethanol, benzodiazepines, barbiturates, narcotic analgesics, and other sedative agents; monitor for increased effect

CYP2C19 inducers: May decrease the levels/effects of methsuximide. Example inducers include aminoglutethimide, carbamazepine, phenytoin, and rifampin.

CYP2C19 inhibitors: May increase the levels/effects of methsuximide. Example inhibitors include delavirdine, fluconazole, fluvoxamine, gemfibrozil, isoniazid, omeprazole, and ticlopidine.

Phenobarbital: Methsuximide may increase phenobarbital concentration.

Phenytoin: Methsuximide may increase phenytoin concentration.

Pregnancy Risk Factor C

Pregnancy Implications May be teratogenic

Nursing Implications Observe patient for excess sedation

Methyl Salicylate

CAS Number 119-36-8

Synonyms Betula Oil; Oil of Wintergreen; Sweet Birch Oil; Teaberry Oil

Use Flavoring agent in candy and rubefacient

Adverse Reactions

Cardiovascular: Circulatory collapse, pericardial effusion/pericarditis

Central nervous system: Headache, aseptic meningitis, psychosis, cognitive dysfunction, coma, seizures, electroencephalogram abnormalities

Dermatologic: Rash, pruritus, alopecia, pustular psoriasis, skin necrosis, nonimmunologic contact urticaria, Stevens-Johnson syndrome

Endocrine & metabolic: Hyperkalemia, anion gap metabolic acidosis, hypouricemia, fluid retention

Gastrointestinal: Abdominal pain, **nausea**, vomiting, GI bleeding, GI ulceration, constipation, diarrhea, **dyspepsia**, bezoars/concretions

Hematologic: Leukopenia, neutropenia, agranulocytosis, granulocytopenia, aplastic anemia (rare), platelet inhibition, hypoprothrombinemia

Hepatic: Elevated transaminases, hepatitis (fulminant)

Neuromuscular & skeletal: Rhabdomyolysis

Ocular: Diplopia

Otic: Ototoxicity, tinnitus

Renal: Renal failure (acute), albuminuria, nephrotic syndrome

Respiratory: Wheezing, adult respiratory distress syndrome, apnea, tachypnea, respiratory depression

Miscellaneous: Hypersensitivity

Signs and Symptoms of Overdose Bezoars, chest pain, coagulopathy, cognitive dysfunction, colitis, deafness, delirium, dementia, drowsiness, dry mouth, GI bleeding, gout, hematuria, hyperthermia, hypoglycemia, nausea, nephrotic syndrome, nystagmus, ototoxicity, stomatitis, tinnitus, vomiting, wheezing

Severe poisoning can manifest with agranulocytosis, confusion, coma, dizziness, feces discoloration (black; pink; red; tarry), fever, granulocytopenia, headache, hyperglycemia, hyponatremia, hypotension, leukopenia, neutropenia, metabolic acidosis, pylorospasm, respiratory depression, rhabdomyolysis, seizures, renal failure and/or hepatic failure, thirst, urine discoloration (pink)

Phases of aspirin poisoning:

Phase I (up to 12 hours after ingestion): Tachypnea and hyperventilation predominate (respiratory alkalosis) with increased renal secretion of sodium, potassium, and bicarbonate resulting in both an alkaline urine and serum pH

Phase II (12-24 hours after ingestion): Urine becomes more acidic as intracellular potassium decreases. While children <4 years of age may develop a pure metabolic acidosis, older patients will have significant respiratory compensation and thus serum pH can be alkalotic. Coagulation abnormalities may occur.

Phase III (over 24 hours after ingestion): Severe potassium and bicarbonate depletion occurs with hydrogen being excreted renally; serum pH becomes acidotic. Infants may reach this phase within 6 hours.

Admission Criteria/Prognosis Admit any child who has ingested over one "swallow" of oil of wintergreen

Pharmacodynamics/Kinetics

Absorption: Dermally can lead to systemic toxicity; absorption orally or dermally is incomplete

Distribution: V_d: ≈ 0.1-0.2 L/kg which increases in presence of acidosis

Protein binding: Significant

Metabolism: Hepatic, converts methyl salicylate to salicylic acid

Dosage See Additional Information.

Monitoring Parameters Salicylate concentrations, electrolytes, I & O, Aa gradient

Dosage Forms Solution, topical: 240 mL

Reference Range Not available for methyl salicylate; salicylate concentrations following acute ingestions as high as 1200 mg/L have been reported in survivors with deaths occurring in chronic exposures at concentrations as low as 100 mg/L; one swallow in an infant 21 months of age of oil of wintergreen resulted in a salicylate level of 81 mg/dL 6 hours postingestion

Overdosage/Treatment

Decontamination: Dermal: Wash with soap and water

Supportive therapy: Hypotension/dehydration can be managed with I.V. fluid therapy; acidosis should be treated with bicarbonates, seizures with benzodiazepines; blood products are indicated, as appropriate, for hemorrhage; antacids may promote gastric absorption

Enhancement of elimination: Forced alkaline diuresis with I.V. sodium bicarbonate to keep urine pH at 8 should be performed for salicylate levels >40 mg/dL; dialysis is indicated for secondary complications, acidosis, or renal failure and not toxin removal alone; consider hemodialysis for acute salicylate levels >100 mg/dL; multiple dosing of activated charcoal may not hasten elimination; dialyzable (50% to 100%); exchange transfusion has been used successfully in a child 2 years of age (elimination rate estimated to be 152 mg/hour) to treat a methyl salicylate intoxication

Drug Interactions Can potentiate bleeding when given with warfarin by platelet aggregation inhibition; elevation of international normalized ratio may result

Additional Information Lethal dose: Oral: Children: 7.5 mL; Adults: 30 mL

Always consider acetaminophen serum concentration in exposures to analgesics, mandatory in suicide attempts; 1 teaspoonful contains 7 g salicylate, most potent available salicylate product

Aspirin conversion factor (ACF) of methyl salicylate: 0.679

Specific gravity: 1.18

Specific References

Baxter AJ, Mrvos R, and Krenzelok EP, "Salicylism and Herbal Medicine," *Am J Emerg Med*, 2003, 21(5):448-9.

Parker D, Martinez C, Stanley C, et al, "The Analysis of Methyl Salicylate and Salicylic Acid from Chinese Herbal Medicine Ingestion," *J Anal Toxicol*, 2004, 28:214-7.

Wolowich WR, Hadley CM, Kelley MT, et al, "Plasma Salicylate from Methyl Salicylate Cream Compared to Oil of Wintergreen," *J Toxicol Clin Toxicol*, 2003, 41(4):355-8.

Methyldopa

Related Information

● Therapeutic Drugs Associated with Hallucinations

CAS Number 41372-08-1; 555-30-6

Synonyms Aldomet; Methyldopate Hydrochloride

Impairment Potential Yes

Use Management of moderate to severe hypertension

Mechanism of Action Stimulation of alpha-adrenergic receptors by a false transmitter that results in a decreased sympathetic outflow to the heart, kidneys and peripheral vasculature (similar to clonidine)

Adverse Reactions

Cardiovascular: **Peripheral edema**, hypotension (orthostatic), bradycardia, edema, myocarditis (hypersensitivity), sinus bradycardia, myocarditis, pericardial effusion/pericarditis, vasodilation

Central nervous system: Drowsiness, sedation, dizziness, headache, CNS depression, psychosis, seizures, fever, visual hallucinations, amnesia, paranoia, gustatory hallucinations, extrapyramidal reactions

Dermatologic: Rash, bullous lesions, erythema multiforme, toxic epidermal necrolysis, urticaria, purpura, seborrheic dermatitis, Stevens-Johnson syndrome, pruritus, erythema nodosum, exanthem, lichen planus

Endocrine & metabolic: Sodium retention, syndrome of inappropriate antidiuretic hormone, gynecomastia, parotitis, sexual dysfunction, nephrogenic diabetes insipidus

Gastrointestinal: Nausea, vomiting, diarrhea, xerostomia, "black" tongue, pancreatitis, metallic taste, lingua villosa nigra

Genitourinary: Retroperitoneal fibrosis, urinary incontinence

Hematologic: Hemolysis, positive Coombs' test, leukopenia, thrombocytopenia, red blood cell aplasia

Hepatic: Hepatitis, elevated liver enzymes, jaundice, cirrhosis, hepatic necrosis, hepatic vasculitis

Neuromuscular & skeletal: Weakness, paresthesia, Meige syndrome

Respiratory: Nasal congestion, asthma

Miscellaneous: Systemic lupus erythematosus, fixed drug eruption

Signs and Symptoms of Overdose Agranulocytosis, alopecia, AV block, bradycardia, cholestatic jaundice, circulatory collapse, CNS depression, cognitive dysfunction, colitis, constipation or diarrhea, delirium, dementia, depression, dermatitis, dizziness, eczema, ejaculatory disturbances, encephalopathy, flatus, galactorrhea, granulocytopenia, gynecomastia, hiccups, hyperprolactinemia, hypertension, hyperthermia, hypotension, hypothermia, impotence, leukopenia, lichenoid eruptions, memory loss, nausea, neutropenia, Parkinson's-like symptoms, parotid pain, photosensitivity, sedation, urine discoloration (black; brown; red; red-brown), vomiting

Pharmacodynamics/Kinetics

Onset of action: Peak effect: Hypotensive: Oral/parenteral: 3-6 hours

Duration: 12-24 hours

Distribution: Crosses placenta; enters breast milk

Protein binding: <15%

Metabolism: Intestinal and hepatic

Half-life elimination: 75-80 minutes; End-stage renal disease: 6-16 hours

Excretion: Urine (85% as metabolites) within 24 hours

Dosage

Children:

Oral: Initial: 10 mg/kg/day in 2-4 divided doses; increase every 2 days as needed to maximum dose of 65 mg/kg/day; do not exceed 3 g/day.

I.V.: 5-10 mg/kg/dose every 6-8 hours up to a total dose of 65 mg/kg/24 hours or 3 g/24 hours

Adults:

Oral: Initial: 250 mg 2-3 times/day; increase every 2 days as needed (maximum dose: 3 g/day): usual dose range (JNC 7): 250-1000 mg/day in 2 divided doses

I.V.: 250-500 mg every 6-8 hours; maximum dose: 1 g every 6 hours

Dosing interval in renal impairment:

Cl_{cr} >50 mL/minute: Administer every 8 hours.

Cl_{cr} 10-50 mL/minute: Administer every 8-12 hours.

Cl_{cr} <10 mL/minute: Administer every 12-24 hours.

Hemodialysis: Slightly dialyzable (5% to 20%)

Stability Injectable dosage form is most stable at acid to neutral pH; parenteral admixture at room temperature (25°C): 24 hours

Monitoring Parameters Blood pressure, standing and sitting/lying down, CBC, liver enzymes, Coombs' test (direct); blood pressure monitor required during I.V. administration

Administration When methyldopa is administered with antihypertensives other than thiazides, limit initial doses to 500 mg/day

Contraindications Hypersensitivity to methyldopa or any component of the formulation; active hepatic disease; liver disorders previously associated with use of methyldopa; on MAO inhibitors; bisulfite allergy if using oral suspension or injectable

Warnings May rarely produce hemolytic anemia and liver disorders; positive Coombs' test occurs in 10% to 20% of patients (perform periodic CBCs); sedation usually transient may occur during initial therapy or whenever the dose is increased. Use with caution in patients with previous liver disease or dysfunction, the active metabolites of methyldopa accumulate in uremia. Patients with impaired renal function may respond to smaller doses. Elderly patients may experience syncope (avoid by giving smaller doses). Tolerance may occur usually between the second and third month of therapy. Adding a diuretic or increasing the dosage of methyldopa frequently restores blood pressure control. Because of its CNS effects, methyldopa is not considered a drug of first choice in the elderly. Often considered the drug of choice for treatment of hypertension in pregnancy. Do not use injectable if bisulfite allergy.

Dosage Forms Injection, solution, as methyldopate hydrochloride: 50 mg/mL (5 mL) [contains sodium bisulfite]
Tablet: 250 mg, 500 mg

Reference Range
Therapeutic: 1-5 mcg/mL (SI: 4.7-23.7 µmol/L)
Toxic: >7 mcg/mL (SI: >33.0 µmol/L)

Overdosage/Treatment
Decontamination: Activated charcoal
Supportive therapy: Hypotension usually responds to I.V. fluids or Trendelenburg positioning. If unresponsive to these measures, the use of a parenteral vasoconstrictor may be required (eg, norepinephrine 0.1-0.2 mcg/kg/minute titrated to response). Treatment is primarily supportive and symptomatic. Use atropine to treat bradycardia. For treatment of lingua villosa nigra, discontinue causative agent. Clean the tongue with a toothbrush and rinse mouth with a half-strength solution of hydrogen peroxide or 10% carbamide peroxide. Symptoms should subside in a few days.
Enhancement of elimination: Dialysis/hemoperfusion may be of some use; slightly dialyzable (5% to 20%)

Test Interactions Methyldopa interferes with urinary uric acid, serum creatinine (alkaline picrate method), AST (colorimetric method), and urinary catecholamines (falsely high levels)

Drug Interactions Barbiturates and TCAs may reduce response to methyldopa.
Beta-blockers, MAO inhibitors, phenothiazines, and sympathomimetics: Hypertension, sometimes severe, may occur.
Iron supplements can interact and cause a significant **increase** in blood pressure.
Lithium: Methyldopa may increase lithium toxicity; monitor lithium levels.
Tolbutamide, haloperidol, anesthetics, and levodopa effects/toxicity are increased with methyldopa.

Pregnancy Risk Factor B
Pregnancy Implications Crosses the placenta
Lactation Enters breast milk/compatible
Nursing Implications Transient sedation or depression may be common for first 72 hours of therapy; usually disappears over time; infuse over 30-60 minutes

Specific References
Chobanian AV, Bakris GL, Black HR, et al, "The Seventh Report of the Joint National Committee on Prevention, Detection, Evaluation, and Treatment of High Blood Pressure: The JNC 7 Report," *JAMA*, 2003, 289(19):2560-71.

Methylergonovine

CAS Number 113-42-8; 57432-61-8
U.S. Brand Names Methergine®
Synonyms Methylergometrine Maleate; Methylergonovine Maleate
Use Prevention and control of uterine hemorrhage postpartum, usually administered in last stage of labor
Mechanism of Action A semisynthetic ergot alkaloid that directly stimulates alpha-adrenergic receptors. Less adrenergic effect than other ergot alkaloids. Directly contracts smooth muscle cells.

Adverse Reactions
Cardiovascular: Myocardial infarction, chest pain, hypertension, vasoconstriction
Central nervous system: Headache, vertigo
Gastrointestinal: Nausea, vomiting
Genitourinary: Uterine hypertonicity
Ocular: Blurred vision

Signs and Symptoms of Overdose Usually occurs within 4 hours; intranasal administration appears to exhibit fewer toxic effects
Paresthesia, nausea, vomiting, diarrhea, hypoperfusion of digits, tachycardia, hypertension, apnea, myocardial ischemia, coma

Admission Criteria/Prognosis Admit any symptomatic patient or asymptomatic ingestion >0.02 mg/kg

Pharmacodynamics/Kinetics
Onset of action: Oxytocic: Oral: 5-10 minutes; I.M.: 2-5 minutes; I.V.: Immediately
Duration: Oral: ~3 hours; I.M.: ~3 hours; I.V.: 45 minutes
Absorption: Rapid
Distribution: V_d: 39-73 L
Rapid; primarily to plasma and extracellular fluid following I.V. administration; tissues
Metabolism: Hepatic
Bioavailability: Oral: 60%; I.M.: 78%
Half-life elimination: Biphasic: Initial: 1-5 minutes; Terminal: 0.5-2 hours
Time to peak, serum: Oral: 0.3-2 hours; I.M.: 0.2-0.6 hours
Excretion: Urine and feces

Dosage I.M.: 0.2 mg postpartum, then 0.2 mg orally 3-4 times/day up to 7 days

Administration Administer over ≥60 seconds. Should not be routinely administered I.V. because of possibility of inducing sudden hypertension and cerebrovascular accident.

Contraindications Hypersensitivity to methylergonovine or any component of the formulation; ergot alkaloids are contraindicated with potent inhibitors of CYP3A4 (includes protease inhibitors, azole antifungals, and some macrolide antibiotics); hypertension; toxemia; pregnancy

Warnings Use caution in patients with sepsis, obliterative vascular disease, hepatic, or renal involvement, or second stage of labor; administer with extreme caution if using intravenously. Pleural and peritoneal fibrosis have been reported with prolonged daily use. Cardiac valvular fibrosis has also been associated with ergot alkaloids.

Dosage Forms Injection, solution, as maleate: 0.2 mg/mL (1 mL)
Tablet, as maleate: 0.2 mg

Reference Range Peak serum levels after a 0.2 mg dose: ~6 nmol/L

Overdosage/Treatment
Decontamination: Avoid ipecac; lavage within 1 hour/activated charcoal.
Supportive therapy: Terbutaline can be used to treat fetal bradycardia. Treat myocardial ischemia by traditional modalities.

Drug Interactions Substrate of CYP3A4 (major)
Antifungals, azole derivatives (itraconazole, ketoconazole) increase levels of ergot alkaloids by inhibiting CYP3A4 metabolism, resulting in toxicity; concomitant use is contraindicated.
Antipsychotics: May diminish the effects of methylergonovine (due to dopamine antagonism); these combinations should generally be avoided.
Beta blockers: Severe peripheral vasoconstriction has been reported with concomitant use of beta blockers and ergot derivatives. Monitor.
CYP3A4 inhibitors: May increase the levels/effects of methylergonovine. Example inhibitors include azole antifungals, clarithromycin, diclofenac, doxycycline, erythromycin, imatinib, isoniazid, nefazodone, nicardipine, propofol, protease inhibitors, quinidine, telithromycin, and verapamil.
Macrolide antibiotics: Erythromycin, clarithromycin, and troleandomycin may increase levels of ergot alkaloids by inhibiting CYP3A4 metabolism, resulting in toxicity (ischemia, vasospasm); concomitant use is contraindicated.
MAO inhibitors: The serotonergic effects of ergot derivatives may be increased by MAO inhibitors. Monitor for signs and symptoms of serotonin syndrome.
Metoclopramide: May diminish the effects of methylergonovine (due to dopamine antagonism); concurrent therapy should generally be avoided.
Protease inhibitors (ritonavir, amprenavir, atazanavir, indinavir, nelfinavir, and saquinavir) increase blood levels of ergot alkaloids by inhibiting CYP3A4 metabolism, acute ergot toxicity has been reported; concomitant use is contraindicated.
Serotonin agonists: Concurrent use with methylergonovine may increase the risk of serotonin syndrome (includes buspirone, SSRIs, TCAs, nefazodone, sumatriptan, and trazodone).
Sibutramine: May cause serotonin syndrome; concurrent use with ergot alkaloids is contraindicated.
Sumatriptan and other serotonin 5-HT$_1$ receptor agonists: Prolong vasospastic reactions; do not use sumatriptan or ergot-containing drugs within 24 hours of each other.
Vasoconstrictors: Concomitant use with peripheral vasoconstrictors may cause synergistic elevation of blood pressure; use is contraindicated.

Pregnancy Risk Factor C
Pregnancy Implications Fetal bradycardia and fetal acidosis can occur
Lactation Enters breast milk/use caution
Specific References
Aeby A, Johansson AB, De Schuiteneer B, et al, "Methylergometrine Poisoning in Children: Review of 34 Cases," *J Toxicol Clin Toxicol*, 2003, 41(3):249-53.

Methylphenidate

Related Information
- Therapeutic Drugs Associated with Hallucinations

CAS Number 113-45-1; 298-59-9

U.S. Brand Names Concerta®; Metadate® CD; Metadate™ ER; Methylin™ ER; Methylin™; Ritalin-SR®; Ritalin® LA; Ritalin®

Synonyms Methylphenidate Hydrochloride

Impairment Potential Yes. Urine methylphenidate levels >0.8 mg/L are consistent with driving impairment

Use Treatment of attention deficit disorder and symptomatic management of narcolepsy; multiple unlabeled uses

Unlabeled/Investigational Use Depression (especially elderly or medically ill)

Mechanism of Action Blocks the reuptake mechanism of dopaminergic neurons, appears to act at the cerebral cortex and subcortical structures

Adverse Reactions
Cardiovascular: **Tachycardia**, hypertension, hypotension, palpitations, cardiac arrhythmias, sinus tachycardia, vasculitis

Central nervous system: **Nervousness, insomnia**, dizziness, drowsiness, movement disorders, agitation, precipitation of Tourette's syndrome, toxic psychosis (rare), fever, headache, visual hallucinations, euphoria, psychosis, stuttering, neuroleptic malignant syndrome, cerebral vasculitis

Dermatologic: Rash, exfoliative dermatitis, erythema multiforme, alopecia, angioedema, urticaria, purpura, photosensitivity, exanthem

Endocrine & metabolic: Growth suppression

Gastrointestinal: **Anorexia**, nausea, abdominal pain, weight loss, xerostomia

Hematologic: Thrombocytopenia

Hepatic: Fulminant liver failure

Neuromuscular & skeletal: Choreoathetoid movements

Ocular: Talc retinopathy

Respiratory: Bilateral lung opacities

Miscellaneous: Hypersensitivity reactions, fixed drug eruption

Signs and Symptoms of Overdose Agitation, coma, insomnia, seizures, tachypnea

Admission Criteria/Prognosis Admit any patient with coingestants involved, acute cardiac or neurological effects, or dose >2 mg/kg of sustained release product in pediatric patients <6 years of age

Pharmacodynamics/Kinetics
Onset of action: Peak effect:

Immediate release tablet: Cerebral stimulation: ~2 hours

Extended release capsule (Metadate® CD): Biphasic; initial peak similar to immediate release product, followed by second rising portion (corresponding to extended release portion)

Sustained release tablet: 4-7 hours

Osmotic release tablet (Concerta®): Initial: 1-2 hours

Transdermal: ~2 hours

Duration: Immediate release tablet: 3-6 hours; Sustained release tablet: 8 hours; Extended release tablet: Methylin® ER, Metadate® ER: 8 hours, Concerta®: 12 hours

Absorption:

Oral: Readily absorbed

Transdermal: Absorption increased when applied to inflamed skin or exposed to heat. Absorption is continuous for 9 hours after application.

Metabolism: Hepatic via de-esterification to minimally active metabolite

Half-life elimination: d-methylphenidate: 3-4 hours; l-methylphenidate: 1-3 hours

Time to peak (Concerta®): C_{max}: 6-8 hours; Daytrana™: 7.5-10.5 hours

Excretion: Urine (90% as metabolites and unchanged drug)

Dosage
ADHD:

Oral (discontinue periodically to re-evaluate or if no improvement occurs within 1 month): Children ≥6 years and Adults: Initial: 0.3 mg/kg/dose or 2.5-5 mg/dose given before breakfast and lunch; increase by 0.1 mg/kg/dose or by 5-10 mg/day at weekly intervals; usual dose: 0.5-1 mg/kg/day; maximum dose: 2 mg/kg/day or 90 mg/day

Extended release products:

Metadate® ER, Methylin® ER, Ritalin® SR: Duration of action is 8 hours. May be given in place of regular tablets, once the daily dose is titrated using the regular tablets and the titrated 8-hour dosage corresponds to sustained release tablet size.

Metadate® CD, Ritalin® LA: Initial: 20 mg once daily; may be adjusted in 10-20 mg increments at weekly intervals; maximum: 60 mg/day

Concerta®: Duration of action is 12 hours:

Initial dose:

Children not currently taking methylphenidate: 18 mg once daily in the morning

Children currently taking methylphenidate: **Note:** Dosing based on current regimen and clinical judgment; suggested dosing listed below:

Patients taking methylphenidate 5 mg 2-3 times/day or 20 mg/day sustained release formulation: 18 mg once every morning

Patients taking methylphenidate 10 mg 2-3 times/day or 40 mg/day sustained release formulation: 36 mg once every morning

Patients taking methylphenidate 15 mg 2-3 times/day or 60 mg/day sustained release formulation: 54 mg once every morning

Dose adjustment: May increase dose in increments of 18 mg; dose may be adjusted at weekly intervals. A dosage strength of 27 mg is available for situations in which a dosage between 18-36 mg is desired. Maximum dose should not exceed 2 mg/kg/day **or** 54 mg/day in children 6-12 years or 72 mg/day in children 13-17 years.

Transdermal (Daytrana™): Children 6-12 years: Initial: 10 mg patch once daily; remove up to 9 hours after application. Titrate based on response and tolerability; may increase to next transdermal dose no more frequently than every week. **Note:** Application should occur 2 hours prior to desired effect. Drug absorption may continue for a period of time after patch removal.

Adults:

Narcolepsy: 10 mg 2-3 times/day, up to 60 mg/day

Depression (unlabeled use): Initial: 2.5 mg every morning before 9 AM; dosage may be increased by 2.5-5 mg every 2-3 days as tolerated to a maximum of 20 mg/day; may be divided (ie, 7 AM and 12 noon), but should not be given after noon; do not use sustained release product

Monitoring Parameters Blood pressure, heart rate, signs and symptoms of depression, CBC, differential and platelet counts, growth rate in children, signs of central nervous system stimulation

Administration
Do not crush or allow patient to chew sustained release dosage form. To effectively avoid insomnia, dosing should be completed by noon.

Concerta™: Administer dose once daily in the morning. May be taken with or without food, but must be taken with water, milk, or juice.

Metadate® CD, Ritalin® LA: Capsules may be opened and the contents sprinkled onto a small amount (equal to 1 tablespoon) of applesauce. Swallow applesauce without chewing. Do not crush or chew capsule contents.

Contraindications Hypersensitivity to methylphenidate, any component of the formulation, or idiosyncratic reactions to sympathomimetic amines; marked anxiety, tension, and agitation; glaucoma; use during or within 14 days following MAO inhibitor therapy; Tourette's syndrome or tics

Warnings [U.S. Boxed Warning]: Dexamphetamine has been associated with serious cardiac cardiovascular events including sudden death in patients with pre-existing structural cardiac abnormalities or other serious heart problems. Using CNS stimulant treatment at usual doses in children and adolescents with serious heart problems and structural cardiac abnormalities has been associated with sudden death. In adults, stimulant use has been associated with sudden deaths, stroke, and myocardial infarction. Stimulant products should be avoided in the patients with known serious structural cardiac abnormalities, cardiomyopathy, serious heart rhythm abnormalities, or other serious heart problems that could increase the risk of sudden death that these conditions alone carry. Caution should be used in patients with hypertension and other cardiovascular conditions that might be exacerbated by increases in blood pressure or heart rate. Use of stimulants can cause an increase in blood pressure (average 2-4 mm Hg) and increases in heart rate (average 3-6 bpm), although some patients may have larger than average increases.

Has demonstrated value as part of a comprehensive treatment program for ADHD. Use with caution in patients with bipolar disorder (may induce mixed/manic episode), diabetes mellitus, hyperthyroidism, seizure disorders (may reduce seizure threshold), insomnia, or porphyria. Use caution in patients with history of ethanol or drug abuse. May exacerbate symptoms of behavior and thought disorder in psychotic patients. **[U.S. Boxed Warning]: Potential for drug dependency exists - avoid abrupt discontinuation in patients who have received for prolonged periods.** Visual disturbances have been reported (rare). Stimulant use has been associated with growth suppression. Growth should be monitored during treatment. Stimulants may unmask tics in individuals with coexisting Tourette's syndrome. Concerta® should not be used in patients with esophageal motility disorders or pre-existing severe gastrointestinal narrowing (small bowel disease, short gut syndrome, history of peritonitis, cystic fibrosis, chronic intestinal pseudo-obstruction, Meckel's diverticulum). Safety and efficacy in children <6 years of age have not been established. Transdermal system may cause allergic contact sensitization, characterized by intense local reactions (edema, papules); sensitization may subsequently manifest systemically with other routes of methylphenidate administration; monitor closely. Avoid exposure of application site to any direct external heat sources (eg, heating pads, electric blankets). Efficacy of transdermal methylphenidate therapy for >7 weeks has not been established.

Dosage Forms Capsule, extended release, as hydrochloride:
Metadate® CD: 10 mg, 20 mg, 30 mg, 40 mg, 50 mg, 60 mg
Ritalin® LA: 10 mg, 20 mg, 30 mg, 40 mg

Solution, oral, as hydrochloride:
Methylin®: 5 mg/5 mL (500 mL) [grape flavor]; 10 mg/5 mL (500 mL) [grape flavor]

Tablet, as hydrochloride: 5 mg, 10 mg, 20 mg
Methylin®, Ritalin®: 5 mg, 10 mg, 20 mg

Tablet, chewable, as hydrochloride:
Methylin®: 2.5 mg [contains phenylalanine 0.42 mg; grape flavor]; 5 mg [contains phenylalanine 0.84 mg; grape flavor]; 10 mg [contains phenylalanine 1.68 mg; grape flavor]

Tablet, extended release, as hydrochloride: 20 mg
Concerta®: 18 mg, 27 mg, 36 mg, 54 mg [osmotic controlled release]
Metadate® ER, Methylin® ER: 10 mg, 20 mg

Tablet, sustained release, as hydrochloride:
Ritalin-SR®: 20 mg [dye free]

Transdermal system [once-daily patch]:
Daytrana™: 10 mg/9 hours (10s, 30s) [12.5 cm^2, total methylphenidate 27.5 mg]; 15 mg/9 hours (10s, 30s) [18.75 cm^2, total methylphenidate 41.3 mg]; 20 mg/9 hours (10s, 30s) [25 cm^2, total methylphenidate 55 mg]; 30 mg/9 hours (10s, 30s) [37.5 cm^2, total methylphenidate 82.5 mg]

Reference Range
Therapeutic: 5-40 ng/mL
After oral administration of 20 mg/day, concentration in plasma after 1 hour is 20 ng/mL
Toxic values (urine): 0.8-40 mcg/mL
Serum ritolinic acid level of 0.4 mg/L has been associated with a fatality following intranasal abuse of methylphenidate

Overdosage/Treatment
Decontamination: Lavage (within 1 hour)/activated charcoal
Supportive therapy: Nitroprusside may be used for hypertension while diazepam or lorazepam can be used for agitation. Haloperidol can be used for hallucinatory behavior.
Enhancement of elimination: Multiple dosing of activated charcoal may be useful; while acid diuresis can increase excretion, it is not recommended due to renal effects

Test Interactions False-positives by immunoassay can be seen with ranitidine, phenylpropanolamine, brompheniramine, chlorpromazine, fluspirilene, or pipothiazine coingestion

Drug Interactions **Substrate** of CYP2D6 (major); **Inhibits** CYP2D6 (weak)
Antihypertensive agents: Effectiveness of antihypertensive agent may be decreased; use with caution
Carbamazepine: Carbamazepine may decrease the serum concentration of methylphenidate.
Clonidine: Severe toxic reactions have been reported in combined use with methylphenidate.
CYP2D6 inhibitors: May increase the levels/effects of methylphenidate. Example inhibitors include chlorpromazine, delavirdine, fluoxetine, miconazole, paroxetine, pergolide, quinidine, quinine, ritonavir, and ropinirole.
Linezolid: Due to MAO inhibition (see note on MAO inhibitors), concurrent use with methylphenidate should generally be avoided.
MAO inhibitors: Severe hypertensive episodes have occurred with amphetamine when used in patients receiving nonselective MAO inhibitors; methylphenidate may be less likely to interact, or reactions may be less severe; use with caution only when warranted; wait 14 days following discontinuation of MAO inhibitor.
Phenytoin: Serum levels may be increased by methylphenidate (in some patients); monitor
Selegiline: When selegiline is used at low dosages (<10 mg/day), an interaction with methylphenidate is less likely than with nonselective MAO inhibitors (see MAO inhibitor information), but theoretically possible; monitor
Sibutramine: Potential for reactions noted with amphetamines (severe hypertension and tachycardia) appears to be low; use with caution
Tricyclic antidepressants: Methylphenidate may increase serum concentrations of some tricyclic agents; clinical reports of toxicity are limited; dosage reduction of tricyclic antidepressants may be required; monitor

Pregnancy Risk Factor C
Pregnancy Implications No increase in congenital malformations noted
Lactation Enters breast milk/use caution
Nursing Implications Do not crush or allow patient to chew sustained release dosage form
Additional Information Chewing tablets instead of swallowing can lead to decreased efficacy and increase in side effects

Specific References
Bailey B, Letarte A, and Abran MC, "Methylphenidate Ingestion in Preschool Children: A Case Series," *J Toxicol Clin Toxicol*, 2003, 41(5):657.
Lewis MG, Lewis JG, Elder PA, et al, "An Enzyme-Linked Immunosorbent Assay (ELISA) for Methylphenidate (Ritalin®) in Urine," *J Anal Toxicol*, 2003, 27(6):342-5.

Marquardt KA, Alsop JA, Lamb JP, et al, "Methylphenidate Ingestions: Comparison of Drug Formulations," *J Toxicol Clin Toxicol*, 2004, 42(5):728.
Padala PR, Petty F, and Bhatia SC, "Methylphenidate May Treat Apathy Independent of Depression," *Ann Pharmacother*, 2005, 39(11):1947-9.

MethylPREDNISolone

Related Information
- Corticosteroids

CAS Number 2375-03-5; 2921-57-5; 53-36-1; 83-43-2
U.S. Brand Names A-Methapred®; Depo-Medrol®; Medrol®; Solu-Medrol®
Synonyms 6-α-Methylprednisolone; A-Methapred; Methylprednisolone Acetate; Methylprednisolone Sodium Succinate

Use
Dental: Treatment of a variety of oral diseases of allergic, inflammatory or autoimmune origin
Medical: Primarily as an anti-inflammatory or immunosuppressant agent in the treatment of a variety of diseases including those of hematologic, allergic, inflammatory, neoplastic, and autoimmune origin. Prevention and treatment of graft-versus-host disease following allogeneic bone marrow transplantation.

Mechanism of Action In a tissue-specific manner, corticosteroids regulate gene expression subsequent to binding specific intracellular receptors and translocation into the nucleus. Corticosteroids exert a wide array of physiologic effects including modulation of carbohydrate, protein, and lipid metabolism and maintenance of fluid and electrolyte homeostasis. Moreover cardiovascular, immunologic, musculoskeletal, endocrine, and neurologic physiology are influenced by corticosteroids. Decreases inflammation by suppression of migration of polymorphonuclear leukocytes and reversal of increased capillary permeability.

Adverse Reactions
Cardiovascular: Edema, hypertension, arrhythmias
Central nervous system: Insomnia, nervousness, aseptic meningitis, vertigo, seizures, psychoses, pseudotumor cerebri, headache, mood swings, delirium, hallucinations, euphoria
Dermatologic: Hirsutism, acne, skin atrophy, hyperpigmentation
Endocrine & metabolic: Diabetes mellitus, adrenal suppression, hyperlipidemia, Cushing's syndrome, pituitary-adrenal axis suppression, growth suppression, glucose intolerance, hypokalemia, alkalosis, sodium and water retention, hyperglycemia, amenorrhea
Gastrointestinal: Increased appetite, indigestion, peptic ulcer, nausea, vomiting, abdominal distention, ulcerative esophagitis, pancreatitis
Hematologic: Transient leukocytosis
Neuromuscular & skeletal: Arthralgia, muscle weakness, osteoporosis, fractures, avascular necrosis
Ocular: Cataracts, glaucoma
Miscellaneous: Infections, hypersensitivity reactions, secondary malignancy, intractable hiccups

Signs and Symptoms of Overdose Arrhythmias (atrial fibrillation) and cardiovascular collapse are possible with rapid intravenous infusion of high-dose methylprednisolone. May mask signs and symptoms of infection. When consumed in high doses for prolonged periods, systemic hypercorticism and adrenal suppression may occur. In these cases, discontinuation should be done judiciously.

Pharmacodynamics/Kinetics
Onset of action: Peak effect (route dependent): Oral: 1-2 hours; I.M.: 4-8 days; Intra-articular: 1 week; methylprednisolone sodium succinate is highly soluble and has a rapid effect by I.M. and I.V. routes
Duration (route dependent): Oral: 30-36 hours; I.M.: 1-4 weeks; Intra-articular: 1-5 weeks; methylprednisolone acetate has a low solubility and has a sustained I.M. effect
Distribution: V_d: 0.7-1.5 L/kg
Half-life elimination: 3-3.5 hours; reduced in obese
Excretion: Clearance: Reduced in obese

Dosage Dosing should be based on the lesser of ideal body weight or actual body weight
Only sodium succinate may be given I.V.; methylprednisolone sodium succinate is highly soluble and has a rapid effect by I.M. and I.V. routes. Methylprednisolone acetate has a low solubility and has a sustained I.M. effect.
Children:
Anti-inflammatory or immunosuppressive: Oral, I.M., I.V. (sodium succinate): 0.5-1.7 mg/kg/day **or** 5-25 mg/m^2/day in divided doses every 6-12 hours; "Pulse" therapy: 15-30 mg/kg/dose over ≥30 minutes given once daily for 3 days
Status asthmaticus: I.V. (sodium succinate): Loading dose: 2 mg/kg/dose, then 0.5-1 mg/kg/dose every 6 hours for up to 5 days
Acute spinal cord injury: I.V. (sodium succinate): 30 mg/kg over 15 minutes, followed in 45 minutes by a continuous infusion of 5.4 mg/kg/hour for 23 hours
Lupus nephritis: I.V. (sodium succinate): 30 mg/kg over ≥30 minutes every other day for 6 doses

High-dose therapy for acute spinal cord injury: I.V. bolus: 30 mg/kg over 15 minutes, followed 45 minutes later by an infusion of 5.4 mg/kg/hour for 23 hours

Idiopathic thrombocytopenic purpura: Oral: 30 mg/kg daily for 3 days

Adults:

Anti-inflammatory or immunosuppressive: Oral: 2-60 mg/day in 1-4 divided doses to start, followed by gradual reduction in dosage to the lowest possible level consistent with maintaining an adequate clinical response

I.M. (sodium succinate): 10-80 mg/day once daily

I.M. (acetate): 10-80 mg every 1-2 weeks

I.V. (sodium succinate): 10-40 mg over a period of several minutes and repeated I.V. or I.M. at intervals depending on clinical response; when high dosages are needed, administer 30 mg/kg over a period of ≥30 minutes and may be repeated every 4-6 hours for 48 hours

Status asthmaticus: I.V. (sodium succinate): Loading dose: 2 mg/kg/dose, then 0.5-1 mg/kg/dose every 6 hours for up to 5 days

High-dose therapy for acute spinal cord injury: I.V. bolus: 30 mg/kg over 15 minutes, followed 45 minutes later by an infusion of 5.4 mg/kg/hour for 23 hours

Lupus nephritis: High-dose "pulse" therapy: I.V. (sodium succinate): 1 g/day for 3 days

Aplastic anemia: I.V. (sodium succinate): 1 mg/kg/day or 40 mg/day (whichever dose is higher) for 4 days. After 4 days, change to oral and continue until day 10 or until symptoms of serum sickness resolve, then rapidly reduce over approximately 2 weeks.

Hemodialysis: Slightly dialyzable (5% to 20%); administer dose post-hemodialysis

Intra-articular (acetate): Administer every 1-5 weeks

Large joints: 20-80 mg

Small joints: 4-10 mg

Intralesional (acetate): 20-60 mg every 1-5 weeks

Stability Intact vials of methylprednisolone sodium succinate should be stored at controlled room temperature

Reconstituted solutions of methylprednisolone sodium succinate should be stored at room temperature (15°C to 30°C) and used within 48 hours

Stability of parenteral admixture at room temperature (25°C) and at refrigeration temperature (4°C): 48 hours

Standard diluent (Solu-Medrol®): 40 mg/50 mL D₅W; 125 mg/50 mL D₅W

Minimum volume (Solu-Medrol®): 50 mL D₅W

Monitoring Parameters Blood pressure, blood glucose, electrolytes

Administration Oral: Administer after meals or with food or milk

Parenteral: Methylprednisolone sodium succinate may be administered I.M. or I.V.; I.V. administration may be IVP over one to several minutes or IVPB or continuous I.V. infusion

I.V.: Succinate:

Low dose: $\leq$1.8 mg/kg or $\leq$125 mg/dose: I.V. push over 3-15 minutes

Moderate dose: $\geq$2 mg/kg or 250 mg/dose: I.V. over 15-30 minutes

High dose: 15 mg/kg or $\geq$500 mg/dose: I.V. over $\geq$30 minutes

Doses >15 mg/kg or $\geq$1 g: Administer over 1 hour

Do **not** administer high-dose I.V. push; hypotension, cardiac arrhythmia, and sudden death have been reported in patients given high-dose methylprednisolone I.V. push over <20 minutes; intermittent infusion over 15-60 minutes; maximum concentration: I.V. push 125 mg/mL

Contraindications Hypersensitivity to methylprednisolone or any component of the formulation; viral, fungal, or tubercular skin lesions; administration of live virus vaccines; serious infections, except septic shock or tuberculous meningitis. Methylprednisolone formulations containing benzyl alcohol preservative are contraindicated in infants.

Warnings

Use with caution in patients with hyperthyroidism, cirrhosis, nonspecific ulcerative colitis, hypertension, osteoporosis, thromboembolic tendencies, CHF, convulsive disorders, myasthenia gravis, thrombophlebitis, peptic ulcer, diabetes, glaucoma, cataracts, or tuberculosis. Use caution in hepatic impairment. Because of the risk of adverse effects, systemic corticosteroids should be used cautiously in the elderly, in the smallest possible dose, and for the shortest possible time

Acute adrenal insufficiency may occur with abrupt withdrawal after long-term therapy or with stress; young pediatric patients may be more susceptible to adrenal axis suppression from topical therapy

Dosage Forms Injection, powder for reconstitution, as sodium succinate: 125 mg [strength expressed as base]

Solu-Medrol®: 40 mg, 125 mg, 500 mg, 1 g, 2 g [packaged with diluent; diluent contains benzyl alcohol; strength expressed as base]

Solu-Medrol®: 500 mg, 1 g

Injection, suspension, as acetate (Depo-Medrol®): 20 mg/mL (5 mL); 40 mg/mL (5 mL); 80 mg/mL (5 mL) [contains benzyl alcohol; strength expressed as base]

Injection, suspension, as acetate [single-dose vial] (Depo-Medrol®): 40 mg/mL (1 mL, 10 mL); 80 mg/mL (1 mL)

Tablet: 4 mg

Medrol®: 2 mg, 4 mg, 8 mg, 16 mg, 32 mg

Tablet, dose-pack: 4 mg (21s)

Medrol® Dosepack™: 4 mg (21s)

Overdosage/Treatment Supportive care is the primary treatment; toxic symptomatology rarely occurs with dosing of <3 weeks duration. Promethazine can be used to treat steroid-induced psychosis.

Test Interactions Interferes with skin tests

Drug Interactions **Substrate** of CYP3A4 (minor); **Inhibits** CYP2C8 (weak), 3A4 (weak)

Decreased effect:

Phenytoin, phenobarbital, rifampin increase clearance of methylprednisolone

Potassium depleting diuretics enhance potassium depletion

Increased toxicity:

Skin test antigens, immunizations decrease response and increase potential infections

Methylprednisolone may increase circulating glucose levels and may need adjustments of insulin or oral hypoglycemics

Pregnancy Risk Factor C

Lactation Excretion in breast milk unknown

Nursing Implications Acetate salt should not be given I.V.

Additional Information Sodium content of 1 g sodium succinate injection: 2.01 mEq; 53 mg of sodium succinate salt is equivalent to 40 mg of methylprednisolone base

Methylprednisolone acetate: Depo-Medrol®

Methylprednisolone sodium succinate: Solu-Medrol®

Specific References

Burry LD and Wax RS, "Role of Corticosteroids in Septic Shock," *Ann Pharmacother*, 2004, 38(3):464-72.

Giles FJ, Cortes JE, Halliburton TA, et al, "Intravenous Corticosteroids to Reduce Gemtuzumab Ozogamicin Infusion Reactions," *Ann Pharmacother*, 2003, 37(9):1182-5.

Ingram DG and Hagemann TM, "Promethazine Treatment of Steroid-Induced Psychosis in a Child," *Ann Pharmacother*, 2003, 37(7-8):1036-9.

MethylTESTOSTERone

CAS Number 58-18-4

U.S. Brand Names Android®; Methitest®; Testred®; Virilon®

Use

Male: Hypogonadism; delayed puberty; impotence and climacteric symptoms

Female: Palliative treatment of metastatic breast cancer; postpartum breast pain and/or engorgement

Mechanism of Action Stimulates receptors in organs and tissues to promote growth and development of male sex organs and maintains secondary sex characteristics in androgen-deficient males

Adverse Reactions

Cardiovascular: **Edema**

Central nervous system: Mania, paranoid psychosis

Dermatologic: **Acne (cystic), seborrheic dermatitis**; Female: Hirsutism (increase in pubic hair growth) atrophy, urticaria, purpura, pruritus, psoriasis, licheniform eruptions, exanthem

Endocrine & metabolic: Gynecomastia, amenorrhea, hypercalcemia

Male: **Virilism**

Female: **Virilism, menstrual problems (amenorrhea), breast soreness**

Gastrointestinal: GI irritation, nausea, vomiting, stomatitis

Genitourinary: Males: **Priapism**, prostatic hypertrophy, prostatic carcinoma, impotence

Hematologic: Leukopenia, polycythemia

Hepatic: Hepatic dysfunction, hepatic necrosis, cholestatic hepatitis, peliosis hepatitis, aminotransferase level elevation (asymptomatic)

Ocular: Night blindness

Miscellaneous: Hypersensitivity reactions, systemic lupus erythematosus

Pharmacodynamics/Kinetics

Metabolism: Hepatic

Excretion: Urine

Dosage Adults (buccal absorption produces twice the androgenic activity of oral tablets):

Male:

Oral: 10-40 mg/day

Buccal: 5-25 mg/day

Female:

Breast pain/engorgement:

Oral: 80 mg/day for 3-5 days

Buccal: 40 mg/day for 3-5 days

Breast cancer:

Oral: 50-200 mg/day

Buccal: 25-100 mg/day

Monitoring Parameters In prepubertal children, perform radiographic examination of the hand and wrist every 6 months to determine the rate of bone maturation and to assess the effect of treatment on the epiphyseal centers.

Contraindications Hypersensitivity to methyltestosterone or any component of the formulation; in males, known or suspected carcinoma of the breast or the prostate; pregnancy

Warnings Use with extreme caution in patients with liver or kidney disease or serious heart disease; may accelerate bone maturation without producing compensatory gain in linear growth

Dosage Forms Capsule (Android®, Testred®, Virilon®): 10 mg
Tablet (Methitest™): 10 mg

Reference Range Peak serum concentrations following a 10 mg ingestion: 24-39 ng/mL

Overdosage/Treatment Decontamination: Activated charcoal

Test Interactions Thyroxine-binding globulin levels may be decreased

Drug Interactions Anticoagulants, oral: May have increased effect; monitor INR

Cyclosporine: Toxicity may occur; avoid concurrent use

Hypoglycemics, oral: May have increased effect; monitor blood glucose

Pregnancy Risk Factor X

Lactation Excretion in breast milk unknown/contraindicated

Nursing Implications In prepubertal children, perform radiographic examination of the hand and wrist every 6 months to determine the rate of bone maturation and to assess the effect of treatment on the epiphyseal centers

Methyprylon

CAS Number 125-64-4

Impairment Potential Yes

Mechanism of Action Similar to glutethimide; it is a piperidineclione which has sedative/hypnotic properties; water and lipid soluble

Adverse Reactions

Cardiovascular: Tachycardia, hypotension, sinus tachycardia

Central nervous system: Headache, coma, dementia, seizures, hypothermia, hyperthermia

Gastrointestinal: Nausea, vomiting, diarrhea

Hematologic: Thrombocytopenia, neutropenia, porphyria, porphyrinogenic

Hepatic: Jaundice, mild elevation in liver function tests

Ocular: Miosis, nystagmus

Neuromuscular & skeletal: Hyperreflexia

Respiratory: Respiratory failure, apnea, pulmonary edema

Signs and Symptoms of Overdose Hypothermia, leukopenia or neutropenia (agranulocytosis, granulocytopenia)

Toxicodynamics/Kinetics

Distribution: V_d: 1 L/kg

Protein binding: 60%; parent compound: 38% metabolites

Metabolism: Hepatic

Half-life: 4-16 hours (in overdose: 50 hours)

Elimination: Urine 60%, feces 20%; ~50% of the drug is normally excreted in 4 hours in a healthy person

Dosage Usual daily dose: 200-400 mg at night

Reference Range Therapeutic serum level is ~8-10 mcg/mL; respiratory arrest can occur at plasma levels >60 mcg/mL

Overdosage/Treatment

Decontamination: Lavage (within 1 hour)/activated charcoal

Supportive therapy: Hypotension can be treated with isotonic saline/Trendelenburg; dopamine or norepinephrine can then be used

Enhancement of elimination: Multiple dosing of activated charcoal probably is not effective; forced diuresis does not play any role; hemodialysis can remove ~20% of the dose; charcoal hemoperfusion is not effective in enhancing elimination

Pregnancy Risk Factor B

Additional Information Minimum lethal dose: 6 g

Metoclopramide

CAS Number 364-62-5; 54143-57-6; 7232-21-5

U.S. Brand Names Reglan®

Use Prevention and/or treatment of nausea and vomiting associated with chemotherapy, radiation therapy, or postsurgery; symptomatic treatment of diabetic gastric stasis; gastroesophageal reflux; facilitation of intubation of the small intestine

Mechanism of Action Blocks dopamine receptors and (when given in higher doses) also blocks serotonin receptors in chemoreceptor trigger zone of the CNS; enhances the response to acetylcholine of tissue in upper GI tract causing enhanced motility and accelerated gastric emptying without stimulating gastric, biliary, or pancreatic secretions

Adverse Reactions

Cardiovascular: Bradycardia, hypotension/hypertension, hypertensive crisis, sinus bradycardia, palpitations, tachycardia (supraventricular)

Central nervous system: **Restlessness, drowsiness**, extrapyramidal reactions, fatigue, psychosis, anxiety, agitation, neuroleptic malignant syndrome, panic attacks, irritability, Chorea

Dermatologic: Rash

Endocrine & metabolic: Gynecomastia, hyperprolactinemia

Gastrointestinal: **Diarrhea**, constipation

Genitourinary: Priapism

Hematologic: Methemoglobinemia (particularly in neonates); leukopenia, neutropenia, agranulocytosis, granulocytopenia, sulfhemoglobinemia (especially in N-acetylcysteine therapy of acetaminophen overdose)

Neuromuscular & skeletal: **Weakness**, asterixis, trismus

Signs and Symptoms of Overdose Agitation, ataxia, AV block, chorea (extrapyramidal), cognitive dysfunction, delirium, depression, drowsiness, extrapyramidal reactions, fever, galactorrhea, gynecomastia, hyperprolactinemia, hypertension, hyperthermia, impotence, irritability, lactation, mania, metallic taste, methemoglobinemia (in infants), muscle hypertonia, neuroleptic malignant syndrome, nystagmus, Parkinson's-like symptoms, seizures, wheezing

Pharmacodynamics/Kinetics

Onset of action: Oral: 0.5-1 hour; I.V.: 1-3 minutes; I.M.: 10-15 minutes

Duration: Therapeutic: 1-2 hours, regardless of route

Distribution: V_d: 2-4 L/kg

Protein binding: 30%

Bioavailability: Oral: 65% to 95%

Half-life elimination: Normal renal function: 4-6 hours (may be dose dependent)

Time to peak, serum: Oral: 1-2 hours

Excretion: Urine (~85%)

Dosage

Children:

Gastroesophageal reflux: Oral: 0.1-0.2 mg/kg/dose up to 4 times/day; efficacy of continuing metoclopramide beyond 12 weeks in reflux has not been determined; total daily dose should not exceed 0.5 mg/kg/day

Gastrointestinal hypomotility (gastroparesis): Oral, I.M., I.V.: 0.1 mg/kg/dose up to 4 times/day, not to exceed 0.5 mg/kg/day

Antiemetic (chemotherapy-induced emesis): I.V.: 1-2 mg/kg 30 minutes before chemotherapy and every 2-4 hours, for a total of 5 doses (5-10 mg/kg) daily

Facilitate intubation: I.V.:
<6 years: 0.1 mg/kg
6-14 years: 2.5-5 mg

Adults:

Gastroesophageal reflux: Oral: 10-15 mg/dose up to 4 times/day 30 minutes before meals or food and at bedtime; single doses of 20 mg are occasionally needed for provoking situations; efficacy of continuing metoclopramide beyond 12 weeks in reflux has not been determined

Gastrointestinal hypomotility (gastroparesis):
Oral: 10 mg 30 minutes before each meal and at bedtime for 2-8 weeks
I.V. (for severe symptoms): 10 mg over 1-2 minutes; 10 days of I.V. therapy may be necessary for best response

Antiemetic (chemotherapy-induced emesis): I.V.: 1-2 mg/kg 30 minutes before chemotherapy and every 2-4 hours, for a total of 5 doses (5-10 mg/kg) daily

Postoperative nausea and vomiting: I.M.: 10 mg near end of surgery; 20 mg doses may be used

Facilitate intubation: I.V.: 10 mg

Elderly:

Gastroesophageal reflux: Oral: 5 mg 4 times/day (30 minutes before meals and at bedtime); increase dose to 10 mg 4 times/day if no response at lower dose

Gastrointestinal hypomotility:
Oral: Initial: 5 mg 30 minutes before meals and at bedtime for 2-8 weeks; increase if necessary to 10 mg doses
I.V.: Initiate at 5 mg over 1-2 minutes; increase to 10 mg if necessary

Postoperative nausea and vomiting: I.M.: 5 mg near end of surgery; may repeat dose if necessary

Dosing adjustment in renal impairment:

Cl_{cr} 10-40 mL/minute: Administer at 50% of normal dose

Cl_{cr} <10 mL/minute: Administer at 25% of normal dose

Hemodialysis: Not dialyzable (0% to 5%); supplemental dose is not necessary

Stability Injection: Store intact vial at controlled room temperature; injection is photosensitive and should be protected from light during storage; parenteral admixtures in D_5W or NS are stable for at least 24 hours, and do not require light protection if used within 24 hours.

Tablet: Store at controlled room temperature; protect from freezing

Monitoring Parameters Periodic renal function test; monitor for dystonic reactions; monitor for signs of hypoglycemia in patients using insulin and those being treated for gastroparesis; monitor for agitation and irritable confusion

Administration Injection solution may be given I.M., direct I.V. push, short infusion (15-30 minutes), or continuous infusion; lower doses (≤10 mg) of metoclopramide can be given I.V. push undiluted over 1-2 minutes; higher doses to be given IVPB over at least 15 minutes; continuous SubQ infusion and rectal administration have been reported

Contraindications Hypersensitivity to metoclopramide or any component of the formulation; GI obstruction, perforation or hemorrhage; pheochromocytoma; history of seizures

Warnings Use caution with a history of mental illness; has been associated with extrapyramidal symptoms (EPS) and depression. The frequency of EPS is higher in pediatric patients and adults <30 years of age; risk is increased at higher dosages. Extrapyramidal reactions typically occur within the initial 24-48 hours of treatment. Use caution with concurrent use of other drugs associated with EPS. Use caution in the elderly and with Parkinson's disease; may have increased risk of tardive dyskinesia. Use caution in patients with a history of seizures; risk of metoclopramide-associated seizures is increased. Neuroleptic malignant syndrome (NMS) has been reported (rarely) with metoclopramide. Use lowest recommended doses initially; may cause transient increase in serum aldosterone; use caution in patients who are at risk of fluid overload (CHF, cirrhosis). Use caution in patients with hypertension or following surgical anastomosis/closure. Patients with NADH-cytochrome b5 reductase deficiency are at increased risk of methemoglobinemia and/or sulfhemoglobinemia. Abrupt discontinuation may (rarely) result in withdrawal symptoms (dizziness, headache, nervousness). Use caution and adjust dose in renal impairment.

Dosage Forms Injection, solution (Reglan®): 5 mg/mL (2 mL, 10 mL, 30 mL)

Syrup: 5 mg/5 mL (10 mL, 480 mL)

Tablet (Reglan®): 5 mg, 10 mg

Reference Range Dose of 10 mg results in a mean plasma level of 65 ng/mL; following a 3 mg/kg overdose, a symptomatic infant exhibited blood metoclopramide level of 150 ng/mL

Overdosage/Treatment

Decontamination: Ipecac within 30 minutes or lavage (within 1 hour)/activated charcoal

Supportive therapy: Metoclopramide often causes extrapyramidal reaction (eg, dystonic reactions) requiring management with diphenhydramine 1-2 mg/kg (adults) up to a maximum of 50-100 mg I.M. or I.V. slow push followed by a maintenance dose (25-50 mg orally every 4-6 hours) for 48-72 hours. When these reactions are unresponsive to diphenhydramine, benztropine mesylate I.V. 1-2 mg (adults) may be effective. These agents are generally effective within 2-5 minutes. Treat methemoglobin with methylene blue.

Enhancement of elimination: Multiple dosing of activated charcoal may be useful; hemodialysis is not useful; not dialyzable (0% to 5%)

Antidote(s)

● Methylene Blue [ANTIDOTE]

Diagnostic Procedures

● Methemoglobin, Blood

Test Interactions ↑ aminotransferases (ALT, AST) (S), amylase (S); may produce falsely elevated TSH (usually <10 units/L).

Drug Interactions Substrate (minor) of CYP1A2, 2D6; **Inhibits** CYP2D6 (weak)

Anticholinergic agents antagonize metoclopramide's actions

Antipsychotic agents: Metoclopramide may increase extrapyramidal symptoms (EPS) or risk when used concurrently.

Cyclosporine: Metoclopramide may increase cyclosporine levels.

Opiate analgesics may increase CNS depression

Pregnancy Risk Factor B

Pregnancy Implications Crosses the placenta; available evidence suggests safe use during pregnancy

Lactation Enters breast milk/use caution

Additional Information Structurally similar to domperidone

Specific References

Dubow JS, Leikin J, Rezuk M, "Acute Chorea Associated with metoclopramide Use," *AM J Therapeutics*, 2006, 13:543-4.

Petroianu GA, Hasan MY, Kosanovic M, et al, "Metoclopramide Protection of Cholinesterase from Paraoxon Inhibition," *Vet Hum Toxicol*, 2003, 45(5):251-3.

Traub SJ, Su M, Hoffman RS, et al, "Use of Pharmaceutical Promotility Agents in the Treatment of Body Packers," *Am J Emerg Med*, 2003, 21(6):511-2.

Tzimenatos L and Bond GR, "198 Cases of Severe Injury or Death in Children Resulting from an Unintentional Therapeutic Error Outside of a Health Care Facilty," *Clin Toxicol*, 2005, 43:638.

Metoprolol

Related Information

● Selected Properties of Beta-Adrenergic Blocking Drugs

CAS Number 37350-58-6; 54163-88-1; 56392-17-7

U.S. Brand Names Lopressor®; Toprol-XL®

Synonyms Metoprolol Succinate; Metoprolol Tartrate

Use Treatment of hypertension and angina pectoris; prevention of myocardial infarction, atrial fibrillation, flutter, symptomatic treatment of hypertrophic subaortic stenosis; to reduce mortality/hospitalization in patients with congestive heart failure (NYHA class II or III) in patients already receiving ACE inhibitors, diuretics, and/or digoxin (sustained-release only)

Unlabeled/Investigational Use Treatment of ventricular arrhythmias, atrial ectopy, migraine prophylaxis, essential tremor, aggressive behavior

Mechanism of Action Selective inhibitor of beta$_1$-adrenergic receptors; competitively blocks beta$_1$-receptors, with little or no effect on beta$_2$-receptors at doses <100 mg

Adverse Reactions

Cardiovascular: Bradycardia, palpitations, edema, CHF, reduced peripheral circulation, arrhythmias, chest pain, heart block (second- and third-degree), orthostatic hypotension

Central nervous system: **Drowsiness, insomnia**, mental depression, confusion (especially in the elderly), hallucinations, headache, depression, nervousness

Dermatologic: Photosensitivity

Endocrine & metabolic: **Decreased sexual ability**

Gastrointestinal: Diarrhea or constipation, nausea, stomach discomfort, vomiting

Hematologic: Leukopenia, thrombocytopenia

Hepatic: Jaundice, hepatic dysfunction, hepatitis

Neuromuscular & skeletal: Arthralgia, paresthesia

Respiratory: Bronchospasm, dyspnea

Miscellaneous: Cold extremities

Signs and Symptoms of Overdose Apnea, asystole, ataxia, AV block, bradycardia, confusion, cyanosis, heart failure, hyperreflexia, hypotension, impotence, insomnia, metabolic acidosis, night terrors, respiratory arrest, seizures, wheezing

Pharmacodynamics/Kinetics

Onset of action: Peak effect: Antihypertensive: Oral: 1.5-4 hours

Duration: 10-20 hours

Absorption: 95%

Protein binding: 12%

Metabolism: Extensively hepatic via CYP2D6; significant first-pass effect

Bioavailability: Oral: 40% to 50%

Half-life elimination: 3-8 hours

Excretion: Urine (3% to 10% as unchanged drug)

Dosage

Children: Oral: 1-5 mg/kg/24 hours divided twice daily; allow 3 days between dose adjustments

Adults:

Hypertension: Oral: 100-450 mg/day in 2-3 divided doses, begin with 50 mg twice daily and increase doses at weekly intervals to desired effect; usual dosage range (JNC 7): 50-100 mg/day

Extended release: Same daily dose administered as a single dose

Angina, SVT, MI prophylaxis: Oral: 100-450 mg/day in 2-3 divided doses, begin with 50 mg twice daily and increase doses at weekly intervals to desired effect

Extended release: Same daily dose administered as a single dose

Hypertension/ventricular rate control: I.V. (in patients having nonfunctioning GI tract): Initial: 1.25-5 mg every 6-12 hours; titrate initial dose to response. Initially, low doses may be appropriate to establish response; however, up to 15 mg every 3-6 hours has been employed.

Congestive heart failure: Oral (extended release): Initial: 25 mg once daily (reduce to 12.5 mg once daily in NYHA class higher than class II); may double dosage every 2 weeks as tolerated, up to 200 mg/day

Myocardial infarction (acute): I.V.: 5 mg every 2 minutes for 3 doses in early treatment of myocardial infarction; thereafter give 50 mg orally every 6 hours 15 minutes after last I.V. dose and continue for 48 hours; then administer a maintenance dose of 100 mg twice daily.

Elderly: Oral: Initial: 25 mg/day; usual range: 25-300 mg/day

Extended release: 25-50 mg/day initially as a single dose; increase at 1- to 2-week intervals.

Hemodialysis: Administer dose posthemodialysis or administer 50 mg supplemental dose; supplemental dose is not necessary following peritoneal dialysis

Dosing adjustment/comments in hepatic disease: Reduced dose probably necessary

Monitoring Parameters Acute cardiac treatment: Monitor ECG and blood pressure with I.V. administration; heart rate and blood pressure with oral administration

Administration Oral: Do not crush or chew extended release tablets.

I.V.: When administered acutely for cardiac treatment, monitor ECG and blood pressure. May administer by rapid infusion (I.V. push) over 1 minute or by slow infusion (ie, 5-10 mg of metoprolol in 50 mL of fluid) over ~30 minutes. Necessary monitoring for surgical patients who are unable to take oral beta-blockers (prolonged ileus) has not been defined. Some institutions require monitoring of baseline and postinfusion heart rate and blood pressure when a patient's response to beta-blockade has not been characterized (ie, the patient's initial dose or following a change in dose). Consult individual institutional policies and procedures.

Contraindications Hypersensitivity to metoprolol or any component of the formulation; sick sinus syndrome; sinus bradycardia; heart block greater than first degree (except in patients with a functioning artificial pacemaker); cardiogenic shock; uncompensated cardiac failure; severe peripheral arterial disease; pheochromocytoma (without alpha blockade); pregnancy (2nd and 3rd trimesters)

Warnings

[U.S. Boxed Warning]: Beta-blocker therapy should not be withdrawn abruptly (particularly in patients with CAD), but gradually tapered to avoid acute tachycardia, hypertension, and/or ischemia. Beta-blockers may increase the risk of anaphylaxis (in predisposed patients) and blunt response to epinephrine. Use caution in patients with PVD (can aggravate arterial insufficiency). Use caution with concurrent use of beta-blockers and either verapamil or diltiazem; bradycardia or heart block can occur; avoid concurrent I.V. use of both agents. In general, beta-blockers should be avoided in patients with bronchospastic disease. Metoprolol, with B_1 selectivity, should be used cautiously in bronchospastic disease with close monitoring. Use cautiously in diabetics because it can mask prominent hypoglycemic symptoms. Can mask signs of thyrotoxicosis. In pheochromocytoma, initiate an alpha blocker prior to beta-blocker; beta-blocker alone may cause a paradoxical increase in blood pressure. Can cause fetal harm when administered in pregnancy. Use caution with hepatic dysfunction. Use care with anesthetic agents which decrease myocardial function. Use of beta-blockers may unmask cardiac failure in patients without a history of dysfunction

Extended release: Use care in compensated heart failure and monitor closely for a worsening of the condition. May need to increase diuretics and wait until clinically stable to advance dose to target.

Dosage Forms Injection, solution, as tartrate: 1 mg/mL (5 mL)
Lopressor®: 1 mg/mL (5 mL)
Tablet, as tartrate: 25 mg, 50 mg, 100 mg
Lopressor®: 50 mg, 100 mg
Tablet, extended release, as succinate: 25 mg, 50 mg, 100 mg, 200 mg [expressed as mg equivalent to tartrate]
Toprol-XL®: 25 mg, 50 mg, 100 mg, 200 mg [expressed as mg equivalent to tartrate]

Reference Range
Therapeutic: 20-340 ng/mL
Survival has occurred with levels as high as 7,140 ng/mL
In the postmortem state, anatomical site concentration differences (ie, postmortem redistribution) may occur.

Overdosage/Treatment
Decontamination: Ipecac within 30 minutes or lavage (within 1 hour)/activated charcoal
Supportive therapy: Sympathomimetics (eg, epinephrine or dopamine), atropine, glucagon, or a pacemaker can be used to treat the toxic bradycardia, asystole, and/or hypotension; initially fluids may be the best treatment for toxic hypotension; enoximone (0.5 mg/kg bolus then 15 mcg/kg/minute drip) can increase cardiac output and stroke volume in metoprolol overdose
Enhancement of elimination: Charcoal hemoperfusion can be used to lower serum levels

Test Interactions ↑ cholesterol (S), glucose

Drug Interactions **Substrate** of CYP2C19 (minor), 2D6 (major); **Inhibits** CYP2D6 (weak)
Acetylcholinesterase inhibitors (eg, donepezil, galantamine, neostigmine): May enhance the bradycardic effect of beta-blockers.
Alpha-/beta-agonists: Beta-blockers may enhance the vasopressor effect of alpha-/beta-agonists (direct-acting).
Alpha₁-blockers (prazosin, terazosin): Concurrent use of beta-blockers may increase risk of orthostasis.
Alpha₂-agonists: Beta-blockers may enhance the rebound hypertensive effect of alpha₂-agonists. This effect can occur when the alpha₂-agonist is abruptly withdrawn.
Aminoquinolines (antimalarial): May decrease the metabolism, via CYP isoenzymes, of beta-blockers.
Amiodarone: May enhance the bradycardic effect of beta-blockers.
Antipsychotic agents (phenothiazines): May enhance the hypotensive effect of beta-blockers. Beta-blockers may decrease the metabolism, via CYP isoenzymes, of antipsychotic agents (phenothiazines).
Barbiturates: May increase the metabolism, via CYP isoenzymes, of beta-blockers.
Beta₂-agonists: May diminish the bradycardic effect of beta-blockers (beta₁ selective).
Calcium channel blockers (nondihydropyridine): May enhance the hypotensive effect of beta-blockers. Bradycardia and signs of heart failure have also been reported.
Cardiac glycosides: Beta-blockers may enhance the bradycardic effect of cardiac glycosides.
CYP2D6 inhibitors: May increase the levels/effects of metoprolol. Example inhibitors include chlorpromazine, delavirdine, fluoxetine, miconazole, paroxetine, pergolide, quinidine, quinine, ritonavir, and ropinirole.
Dipyridamole: May enhance the bradycardic effect of beta-blockers.
Disopyramide: May enhance the bradycardic effect of beta-blockers.

Insulin: Beta-blockers may enhance the hypoglycemic effect of insulin. Tachycardia may be masked as a symptom of hypoglycemia.
Lidocaine: Beta-blockers may decrease the metabolism of lidocaine.
Nonsteroidal anti-inflammatory agents (NSAIDs): May diminish the antihypertensive effect of beta-blockers.
Propafenone: May decrease the metabolism, via CYP isoenzymes, of beta-blockers. Propafenone possesses some independent beta-blocking activity.
Propoxyphene: May decrease the metabolism, via CYP isoenzymes, of beta-blockers.
Quinidine: May decrease the metabolism, via CYP isoenzymes, of beta-blockers.
Rifamycin derivatives: May increase the metabolism, via CYP isoenzymes, of beta-blockers.
Selective serotonin reuptake inhibitors (SSRIs): May enhance the bradycardic effect of beta-blockers.
Sulfonylureas: Beta-blockers may enhance the hypoglycemic effect of sulfonylureas. Tachycardia may be masked as a symptom of hypoglycemia.
Theophylline: Beta-blockers (beta₁ selective) may diminish the bronchodilatory effect of theophylline derivatives.

Pregnancy Risk Factor C (manufacturer); D (2nd and 3rd trimesters - expert analysis)

Pregnancy Implications Metoprolol crosses the placenta. Beta-blockers have been associated with bradycardia, hypotension, and IUGR; IUGR is probably related to maternal hypertension. Available evidence suggests beta-blockers are generally safe during pregnancy (JNC-7). Cases of neonatal hypoglycemia have been reported following maternal use of beta-blockers at parturition or during breast-feeding.

Lactation Enters breast milk/use caution (AAP rates "compatible")

Nursing Implications Patient's therapeutic response may be evaluated by looking at blood pressure, apical and radial pulses, fluid I & O, daily weight, respirations, and circulation in extremities before and during therapy

Specific References
Allison S and Henderson SO, "Slow Supraventricular Tachycardia in a Patient on Beta-Blocker Therapy," *Am J Emerg Med*, 2005, 23(4):581-2.
Angier MK, Lewis RJ, Chaturvedi AK, et al, "Gas Chromatographic-Mass Spectrometric Confirmation of Beta-Blockers," *J Anal Toxicol*, 2004, 28:289.
Angier MK, Lewis RJ, Chaturvedi AK, et al, "Gas Chromatographic-Mass Spectrometric Differentiation of Atenolol, Metoprolol, Propranolol, and an Interfering Metabolite Product of Metoprolol," *J Anal Toxicol*, 2005, 29:517-21.
Dupuis C, Gaulier JM, Pelissier-Alicot AL, et al, "Determination of Three Beta-Blockers in Biofluids and Solid Tissues by Liquid Chromatography-electrospray-Mass Spectrometry," *J Anal Toxicol*, 2004, 28(8):674-9.
Fareed FN, Chan GM, and Hoffman RS, "Fatal Cocaine Metoprolol Interaction," *Clin Toxicol*, 2005, 43:641.
Wax PM, Erdman AR, Chyka PA, et al, "Beta-Blocker Ingestion: An Evidence-Based Consensus Guideline for Out-of-Hospital Management," *Clin Toxicol (Phila)*, 2005, 43(3):131-46.

Metronidazole

CAS Number 13182-89-3; 443-48-1; 69198-10-3
U.S. Brand Names Flagyl ER®; Flagyl®; MetroCream®; MetroGel-Vaginal®; MetroGel®; MetroLotion®; Noritate®; Rozex™
Synonyms Metronidazole Hydrochloride
Use
Treatment of susceptible anaerobic bacterial and protozoal infections in the following conditions: Amebiasis, symptomatic and asymptomatic trichomoniasis; skin and skin structure infections; CNS infections; intra-abdominal infections (as part of combination regimen); systemic anaerobic infections; treatment of antibiotic-associated pseudomembranous colitis (AAPC), bacterial vaginosis; as part of a multidrug regimen for *H. pylori* eradication to reduce the risk of duodenal ulcer recurrence
Topical: Treatment of inflammatory lesions and erythema of rosacea
Unlabeled/Investigational Use Crohn's disease
Mechanism of Action Reduced to a product by a nitroreductase enzyme which interacts with DNA to cause a loss of helical DNA structure and strand breakage resulting in inhibition of protein synthesis and cell death in susceptible organisms
Adverse Reactions
Systemic: Frequency not defined:
Cardiovascular: Flattening of the T-wave, flushing
Central nervous system: Ataxia, confusion, coordination impaired, dizziness, fever, headache, insomnia, irritability, seizures, vertigo
Dermatologic: Erythematous rash, urticaria
Endocrine & metabolic: Disulfiram-like reaction, dysmenorrhea, libido decreased

Gastrointestinal: **Nausea (~12%)**, anorexia, abdominal cramping, constipation, diarrhea, furry tongue, glossitis, proctitis, stomatitis, unusual/metallic taste, vomiting, xerostomia

Genitourinary: Cystitis, darkened urine (rare), dysuria, incontinence, polyuria, vaginitis

Hematologic: Neutropenia (reversible), thrombocytopenia (reversible, rare)

Neuromuscular & skeletal: Peripheral neuropathy, weakness

Respiratory: Nasal congestion, rhinitis, sinusitis, pharyngitis

Miscellaneous: Flu-like syndrome, moniliasis

Topical: Frequency not defined:

Central nervous system: Headache

Dermatologic: Burning, contact dermatitis, dryness, erythema, irritation, pruritus, rash

Gastrointestinal: Unusual/metallic taste, nausea, constipation

Local: Local allergic reaction

Neuromuscular & skeletal: Tingling/numbness of extremities

Ocular: Eye irritation

Vaginal:

Central nervous system: Headache, dizziness, depression, fatigue

Dermatologic: Itching, rash

Gastrointestinal: Gastrointestinal discomfort, nausea and/or vomiting, unusual/metallic taste, diarrhea, abdominal bloating, abdominal gas, xerostomia

Genitourinary: **Vaginitis, vaginal discharge**, vulva/vaginal irritation, pelvic discomfort, darkened urine

Hematologic: WBC increased

Miscellaneous: Thirst

Signs and Symptoms of Overdose Ataxia, cystitis, diplopia, dry skin, dysosmia, gynecomastia, hepatotoxicity (12.5 g ingestion), insomnia, nausea, neuropathy (peripheral), neutropenia, seizures, vomiting

Pharmacodynamics/Kinetics

Absorption: Oral: Well absorbed; Topical: Concentrations achieved systemically after application of 1 g topically are 10 times less than those obtained after a 250 mg oral dose

Distribution: To saliva, bile, seminal fluid, breast milk, bone, liver, and liver abscesses, lung and vaginal secretions; crosses placenta and blood-brain barrier

CSF: blood level ratio: Normal meninges: 16% to 43%; Inflamed meninges: 100%

Protein binding: <20%

Metabolism: Hepatic (30% to 60%)

Half-life elimination: Neonates: 25-75 hours; Others: 6-8 hours, prolonged with hepatic impairment; End-stage renal disease: 21 hours

Time to peak, serum: Oral: Immediate release: 1-2 hours

Excretion: Urine (20% to 40% as unchanged drug); feces (6% to 15%)

Dosage

Infants and Children:

Amebiasis: Oral: 35-50 mg/kg/day in divided doses every 8 hours for 10 days

Trichomoniasis: Oral: 15-30 mg/kg/day in divided doses every 8 hours for 7 days

Anaerobic infections:

Oral: 15-35 mg/kg/day in divided doses every 8 hours

I.V.: 30 mg/kg/day in divided doses every 6 hours

Clostridium difficile (antibiotic-associated colitis): Oral: 20 mg/kg/day divided every 6 hours

Maximum dose: 2 g/day

Adults:

Amebiasis: Oral: 500-750 mg every 8 hours for 5-10 days

Trichomoniasis: Oral: 250 mg every 8 hours for 7 days **or** 375 mg twice daily for 7 days **or** 2 g as a single dose

Anaerobic infections: Oral, I.V.: 500 mg every 6-8 hours, not to exceed 4 g/day

Antibiotic-associated pseudomembranous colitis: Oral: 250-500 mg 3-4 times/day for 10-14 days

Helicobacter pylori eradication: Oral: 250-500 mg with meals and at bedtime for 14 days; requires combination therapy with at least one other antibiotic and an acid-suppressing agent (proton pump inhibitor or H_2 blocker)

Bacterial vaginosis:

Oral: 750 mg (extended release tablet) once daily for 7 days

Vaginal: 1 applicatorful (~37.5 mg metronidazole) intravaginally once or twice daily for 5 days; apply once in morning and evening if using twice daily, if daily, use at bedtime

Acne rosacea: Topical:

0.75%: Apply and rub a thin film twice daily, morning and evening, to entire affected areas after washing. Significant therapeutic results should be noticed within 3 weeks. Clinical studies have demonstrated continuing improvement through 9 weeks of therapy.

1%: Apply thin film to affected area once daily

Elderly: Use lower end of dosing recommendations for adults, do not administer as a single dose

Dosing adjustment in renal impairment: Cl_{cr} <10 mL/minute: Administer 50% of dose or every 12 hours

Hemodialysis: Extensively removed by hemodialysis and peritoneal dialysis (50% to 100%); administer dose posthemodialysis

Peritoneal dialysis: Dose as for Cl_{cr} <10 mL/minute

Continuous arteriovenous or venovenous hemofiltration: Administer usual dose

Dosing adjustment/comments in hepatic disease: Unchanged in mild liver disease; reduce dosage in severe liver disease

Stability Reconstituted solution is stable for 96 hours when refrigerated; for I.V. infusion in normal saline or D_5W and neutralized (with sodium bicarbonate), solution is stable for 24 hours at room temperature; do not refrigerate neutralized solution because a precipitate will occur

Monitoring Parameters WBC count

Administration Oral: May be taken with food to minimize stomach upset. Extended release tablets should be taken on an empty stomach (1 hour before or 2 hours after meals).

I.V.: Avoid contact between the drug and aluminum in the infusion set.

Topical: No disulfiram-like reactions have been reported after **topical** application, although metronidazole can be detected in the blood. Apply to clean, dry skin. Cosmetics may be used after application (wait at least 5 minutes after using lotion).

Contraindications Hypersensitivity to metronidazole, nitroimidazole derivatives, or any component of the formulation; pregnancy (1st trimester - found to be carcinogenic in rats)

Warnings Use with caution in patients with liver impairment due to potential accumulation, blood dyscrasias; history of seizures, CHF, or other sodium retaining states; reduce dosage in patients with severe liver impairment, CNS disease, and severe renal failure (Cl_{cr} <10 mL/minute); if *H. pylori* is not eradicated in patients being treated with metronidazole in a regimen, it should be assumed that metronidazole-resistance has occurred and it should not again be used; seizures and neuropathies have been reported especially with increased doses and chronic treatment; if this occurs, discontinue therapy. **[U.S. Boxed Warning]: Possibly carcinogenic based on animal data.**

Dosage Forms [DSC] = Discontinued product

Capsule:

Flagyl®: 375 mg

Cream, topical: 0.75% (45 g)

MetroCream®: 0.75% (45 g) [contains benzyl alcohol]

Noritate®: 1% (60 g)

Gel, topical: 0.75% (45 g)

MetroGel®: 0.75% (45 g) [DSC], 1% (60 g)

Gel, vaginal:

MetroGel-Vaginal®, Vandazole™: 0.75% (70 g)

Infusion [premixed iso-osmotic sodium chloride solution]: 500 mg (100 mL)

Flagyl® I.V. RTU™: 500 mg (100 mL) [contains sodium 14 mEq]

Lotion, topical: 0.75% (60 mL)

MetroLotion®: 0.75% (60 mL) [contains benzyl alcohol]

Tablet: 250 mg, 500 mg

Flagyl®: 250 mg, 500 mg

Tablet, extended release:

Flagyl® ER: 750 mg

Reference Range 500 mg oral dose results in a peak plasma level of 12 mg/L (70 μmol/L)

Overdosage/Treatment

Decontamination: Activated charcoal; **do not** use a cathartic if an ileus is present

Supportive therapy: Benzodiazepines can be used for seizure control with phenobarbital in phenytoin used as second-line agent

Enhancement of elimination: Metronidazole and active metabolite are eliminated by hemodialysis; up to 45% of drug may be removed from 4 hours of hemodialysis; peritoneal dialysis can remove 10% of the dose (during a 7.5 hour period)

Test Interactions May cause falsely decreased AST and ALT

Drug Interactions Inhibits CYP2C9 (weak), 3A4 (moderate)

Cimetidine may increase metronidazole levels.

Cisapride: May inhibit metabolism of cisapride, causing potential arrhythmias; avoid concurrent use

CYP3A4 substrates: Metronidazole may increase the levels/effects of CYP3A4 substrates. Example substrates include benzodiazepines, calcium channel blockers, cyclosporine, mirtazapine, nateglinide, nefazodone, sildenafil (and other PDE-5 inhibitors), tacrolimus, and venlafaxine. Selected benzodiazepines (midazolam and triazolam), cisapride, ergot alkaloids, selected HMG-CoA reductase inhibitors (lovastatin and simvastatin), and pimozide are generally contraindicated with strong CYP3A4 inhibitors.

Ethanol: Ethanol results in disulfiram-like reactions.

Lithium: Metronidazole may increase lithium levels/toxicity; monitor lithium levels.

Phenytoin, phenobarbital may increase metabolism of metronidazole, potentially decreasing its effect.

Warfarin: Metronidazole increases P-T prolongation with warfarin.

Pregnancy Risk Factor B (may be contraindicated in 1st trimester)

Pregnancy Implications Crosses the placenta (carcinogenic in rats); contraindicated for the treatment of trichomoniasis during the first trimester of pregnancy, unless alternative treatment is inadequate. Until safety and efficacy for other indications have been established, use only during pregnancy when the benefit to the mother outweighs the potential risk to the fetus.

Lactation Enters breast milk/not recommended (AAP rates "of concern")

Nursing Implications No disulfiram-like reactions have been reported after **topical** application, although metronidazole can be detected in the blood; avoid contact between the drug and aluminum in the infusion set

Additional Information Sodium content of 500 mg (I.V.): 322 mg (14 mEq); D-lactic acidosis may develop in patients with short bowel syndrome due to overgrowth of D-lactate producing organisms (*Lactobacillus* species, *Streptococcus bovis*, *Bifidobacterium* species, or *Eubacterium* species); peripheral neuropathy usually does not occur in daily doses <800 mg but can occur at daily doses >2 g

Specific References

Burda A, Fischbein C, Howe T, et al, "Hemodialysis Clearance of Metronidazole Following Overdose," *J Toxicol Clin Toxicol*, 2004, 42(5):730.

Ofoefule SI, Ibezim EC, Esimone OC, et al, "Bioavailability of Metronidazole in Rabbits After Administration of a Rectal Suppository," *Am J Ther*, 2004, 11(3):190-3.

Mexiletine

CAS Number 31828-71-4; 5370-10-4

U.S. Brand Names Mexitil®

Use Management of serious ventricular arrhythmias; suppression of PVCs

Unlabeled/Investigational Use Diabetic neuropathy

Mechanism of Action Class IB antiarrhythmic, structurally related to lidocaine, which may cause increase in systemic vascular resistance and decrease in cardiac output; no significant negative inotropic effect

Adverse Reactions

Excessive doses: 1.8-2.4 g: CNS depression

Cardiovascular: Palpitations, bradycardia, chest pain, syncope, hypotension, arrhythmias (atrial or ventricular), fibrillation (atrial), flutter (atrial), AV block, sinus bradycardia, angina, myocardial depression, QT prolongation

Central nervous system: **Dizziness, lightheadedness, nervousness**, confusion, ataxia, memory disturbance

Dermatologic: Rash

Gastrointestinal: Nausea, vomiting, diarrhea, esophagitis associated with oral forms

Hematologic: Rarely thrombocytopenia

Hepatic: Hepatitis progressing to hepatic necrosis

Neuromuscular & skeletal: **Trembling, unsteady gait**, tremors, paresthesia

Ocular: Diplopia

Otic: Ototoxicity, tinnitus

Respiratory: Dyspnea

Miscellaneous: Positive antinuclear antibody, hiccup

Signs and Symptoms of Overdose Asystole, bradycardia, CNS depression, congestive heart failure, dry mouth, dysphagia, esophageal ulceration, hypotension, impotence, left bundle-branch block, lightheadedness, malaise, memory loss, nausea, neutropenia, paresthesia, QRS prolongation, seizures

Pharmacodynamics/Kinetics

Absorption: Elderly have a slightly slower rate, but extent of absorption is the same as young adults

Distribution: V_d: 5-7 L/kg

Protein binding: 50% to 70%

Metabolism: Hepatic; low first-pass effect

Half-life elimination: Adults: 10-14 hours (average: elderly: 14.4 hours, younger adults: 12 hours); prolonged with hepatic impairment or heart failure

Time to peak: 2-3 hours

Excretion: Urine (10% to 15% as unchanged drug); urinary acidification increases excretion, alkalinization decreases excretion

Dosage Adults: Oral: 400 mg to start, then 200 mg in 8 hours, then 200-400 mg every 8 hours; adjust dose in 50-100 mg increments with a minimum of 2-3 days between doses; do not exceed 1200 mg/day

Dosing adjustment in renal impairment: Cl_{cr} <10 mL/minute: Administer at 50% to 75% of normal dose

Dosing adjustment/comments in hepatic disease: Reduce maintenance dose to 25% to 30% of normal dose; patients with severe liver disease may require lower dosages and must be monitored closely

Administration Administer around-the-clock rather than 3 times/day to promote less variation in peak and trough serum levels; administer with food

Contraindications Hypersensitivity to mexiletine or any component of the formulation; cardiogenic shock; second- or third-degree AV block (except in patients with a functioning artificial pacemaker)

Warnings [U.S. Boxed Warning]: In the Cardiac Arrhythmia Suppression Trial (CAST), recent (>6 days but <2 years ago) myocardial infarction patients with asymptomatic, nonlife-threatening ventricular arrhythmias did not benefit and may have been harmed by attempts to suppress the arrhythmia with flecainide or encainide. An increased mortality or non-fatal cardiac arrest rate (7.7%) was seen in the active treatment group compared with patients in the placebo group (3%). The applicability of the CAST results to other populations is unknown. Antiarrhythmic agents should be reserved for patients with life-threatening ventricular arrhythmias. Can be proarrhythmic. Electrolyte disturbances alter response; should be corrected before initiating therapy. Use cautiously in patients with first-degree block, pre-existing sinus node dysfunction, intraventricular conduction delays, significant hepatic dysfunction, hypotension, or severe CHF. Alterations in urinary pH may change urinary excretion. Rare hepatic toxicity may occur; may cause acute hepatic injury.

Dosage Forms [DSC] = Discontinued product

Capsule, as hydrochloride: 150 mg, 200 mg, 250 mg

Mexitil®: 150 mg, 200 mg, 250 mg [DSC]

Reference Range

Therapeutic: 0.75-2.00 mcg/mL

Potentially toxic: >2.00 mcg/mL; level of 20 mcg/mL associated with seizures

In the postmortem state, anatomical site concentration differences (ie, postmortem redistribution) may occur.

Overdosage/Treatment

Decontamination: **Do not** use ipecac; lavage (within 1 hour)/activated charcoal is useful

Supportive therapy: Treatment includes supportive measures; atropine may be used for bradycardia; dopamine or norepinephrine can be used for hypotension. Seizures can be treated with benzodiazepines and phenytoin.

Enhancement of elimination: Forced diuresis with mannitol may be useful; do not alkalinize urine, this may delay excretion; hemodialysis may be useful, although there is no overdose experience of this modality

Diagnostic Procedures

- Mexiletine, Blood

Test Interactions Abnormal LFTs, positive ANA, thrombocytopenia; may cause false-positive amphetamine by urinary fluorescence polarization immunoassay

Drug Interactions **Substrate** (major) of CYP1A2, 2D6; **Inhibits** CYP1A2 (strong)

CYP1A2 inducers: May decrease the levels/effects of mexiletine. Example inducers include aminoglutethimide, carbamazepine, phenobarbital, and rifampin.

CYP1A2 inhibitors: May increase the levels/effects of mexiletine. Example inhibitors include ciprofloxacin, ketoconazole, norfloxacin, ofloxacin, and rofecoxib.

CYP1A2 substrates: Mexiletine may increase the levels/effects of CYP1A2 substrates. Example substrates include aminophylline, fluvoxamine, mirtazapine, ropinirole, theophylline, and trifluoperazine.

CYP2D6 inhibitors: May increase the levels/effects of mexiletine. Example inhibitors include chlorpromazine, delavirdine, fluoxetine, miconazole, paroxetine, pergolide, quinidine, quinine, ritonavir, and ropinirole.

Fluvoxamine: Clearance of mexiletine was reduced by 38% following coadministration with fluvoxamine. If used concurrently, mexiletine levels should be monitored.

Quinidine may increase mexiletine blood levels.

Theophylline blood levels are increased by mexiletine.

Urinary alkalinizers (antacids, sodium bicarbonate, acetazolamide) may increase mexiletine blood levels.

Pregnancy Risk Factor C

Lactation Enters breast milk/compatible

Additional Information I.V. form under investigation; bitter tasting

Mianserin

Related Information

- Antidepressant Agents

CAS Number 21535-47-7; 24219-97-4

Use Depression; has been used to treat fluvoxamine-induced akathisia

Mechanism of Action Tetracyclic piperazinoazepine antidepressant with few antimuscarinic effects; a central serotonin antagonist

Adverse Reactions

Cardiovascular: Bradycardia, hypotension (orthostatic), bundle branch block, sinus bradycardia, congestive heart failure, myocardial depression, sinus tachycardia, tachycardia (supraventricular)

Central nervous system: Drowsiness, seizures, restlessness

Dermatologic: Erythema multiforme, toxic epidermal necrolysis

Endocrine & metabolic: Hypokalemia, gynecomastia

Gastrointestinal: Glossitis

Hematologic: Leukopenia/neutropenia (agranulocytosis, granulocytopenia), aplastic anemia

Hepatic: Jaundice, elevated liver function tests

Neuromuscular & skeletal: Polyarthralgia

Miscellaneous: Diaphoresis, restless legs syndrome

Signs and Symptoms of Overdose Delirium, dizziness, gynecomastia, heart block, hypokalemia, hypotension, prolonged sedation, seizures, tachycardia/bradycardia with conduction disturbances leading to complete AV block, toxic epidermal necrolysis

Toxicodynamics/Kinetics

Distribution: V_d: 16 L/kg

Protein binding: 90%

Metabolism: Hepatic to two active metabolites

Bioavailability: 70%

Half-life: 6-40 hours

Time to peak plasma levels: 1-3 hours

Elimination: Clearance: 0.5 L/hour/kg

Dosage Initial dose: 30-40 mg/day; usual dose: 30-90 mg/day; maximum dose: 200 mg/day; for fluvoxamine-induced akathisia: 15 mg at night

Reference Range Peak serum level at a dose of 60 mg/day: 100-120 mcg/L; a peak plasma level of 439 mcg/L associated with heart block

Overdosage/Treatment

Decontamination: **Do not** induce emesis; activated charcoal

Supportive therapy: Treat seizures with diazepam or lorazepam; phenobarbital is second choice; atropine or isoproterenol can be used for bradycardia

Enhancement of elimination: Multiple dosing of activated charcoal or hemodialysis is not likely to be effective

Specific References

Martínez MA, Sánchez de la Torre C, and Almarza E, "A Comparative Solid-Phase Extraction Study for the Simultaneous Determination of Fluvoxamine, Mianserin, Doxepin, Citalopram, Paroxetine, and Etoperidone in Whole Blood by Capillary Gas-Liquid Chromatography with Nitrogen-Phosphorus Detection," *J Anal Toxicol*, 2004, 28(4):174-80.

Miconazole

CAS Number 22832-87-7; 22916-47-8

U.S. Brand Names Aloe Vesta® 2-n-1 Antifungal [OTC]; Baza® Antifungal [OTC]; Carrington Antifungal [OTC]; Femizol-M™ [OTC]; Fungoid® Tincture [OTC]; Lotrimin® AF Powder/Spray [OTC]; Micaderm® [OTC]; Micatin® [OTC]; Micro-Guard® [OTC]; Mitrazol™ [OTC]; Monistat-Derm®; Monistat® 1 Combination Pack [OTC]; Monistat® 3 [OTC]; Monistat® 7 [OTC]; Triple Care® Antifungal [OTC]; Zeasorb®-AF [OTC]

Synonyms Miconazole Nitrate

Use Treatment of vulvovaginal candidiasis and a variety of skin and mucous membrane fungal infections

Mechanism of Action Inhibits biosynthesis of ergosterol, damaging the fungal cell wall membrane, which increases permeability causing leaking of nutrients

Adverse Reactions

Topical: Allergic contact dermatitis, burning, maceration

Vaginal: Abdominal cramps, burning, irritation, itching

Pharmacodynamics/Kinetics

Absorption: Topical: Negligible

Distribution: Widely to body tissues; penetrates well into inflamed joints, vitreous humor of eye, and peritoneal cavity, but poorly into saliva and sputum; crosses blood-brain barrier but only to a small extent

Protein binding: 91% to 93%

Metabolism: Hepatic

Half-life elimination: Multiphasic: Initial: 40 minutes; Secondary: 126 minutes; Terminal: 24 hours

Excretion: Feces (~50%); urine (<1% as unchanged drug)

Dosage Topical: Children and Adults: **Note:** Not for OTC use in children <2 years:

Tinea pedis and tinea corporis: Apply twice daily for 4 weeks

Tinea cruris: Apply twice daily for 2 weeks

Vaginal: Adults: Vulvovaginal candidiasis:

Cream, 2%: Insert 1 applicatorful at bedtime for 7 days

Cream, 4%: Insert 1 applicatorful at bedtime for 3 days

Suppository, 100 mg: Insert 1 suppository at bedtime for 7 days

Suppository, 200 mg: Insert 1 suppository at bedtime for 3 days

Suppository, 1200 mg: Insert 1 suppository at bedtime (a one-time dose)

Note: Many products are available as a combination pack, with a suppository for vaginal instillation and cream to relieve external symptoms.

Contraindications Hypersensitivity to miconazole or any component of the formulation

Warnings For external use only; discontinue if sensitivity or irritation develop. Petrolatum-based vaginal products may damage rubber or latex condoms or diaphragms. Separate use by 3 days.

Dosage Forms [DSC] = Discontinued product

Combination products: Miconazole nitrate vaginal suppository 200 mg (3s) and miconazole nitrate external cream 2%

Monistat® 1 Combination Pack: Miconazole nitrate vaginal insert 1200 mg (1) and miconazole nitrate external cream 2% (5 g)

[Note: Do not confuse with 1-Day™ (formerly Monistat® 1) which contains tioconazole]

Monistat® 3 Combination Pack:

Miconazole nitrate vaginal suppository 200 mg (3s) and miconazole nitrate external cream 2%

Miconazole nitrate vaginal cream 4% and miconazole nitrate external cream 2%

Monistat® 7 Combination Pack:

Miconazole nitrate vaginal suppository 100 mg (7s) and miconazole nitrate external cream 2%

Miconazole nitrate vaginal cream 2% (7 prefilled applicators) and miconazole nitrate external cream 2%

Cream, topical, as nitrate: 2% (15 g, 30 g, 45 g)

Baza® Antifungal: 2% (4 g, 57 g, 142 g) [zinc oxide based formula]

Carrington Antifungal: 2% (150 g)

Micaderm®, Neosporin® AF, Podactin: 2% (30 g)

Micatin® Athlete's Foot, Micatin® Jock Itch: 2% (15 g)

Micro-Guard®, Mitrazol™: 2% (60 g)

Monistat-Derm®: 2% (15 g, 30 g, 85 g)

Secura® Antifungal: 2% (60 g, 98 g)

Cream, vaginal, as nitrate [prefilled or refillable applicator]: 2% (45 g)

Monistat® 3: 4% (15 g, 25 g)

Monistat® 7: 2% (45 g)

Liquid, spray, topical, as nitrate:

Micatin® Athlete's Foot: 2% (90 mL) [contains alcohol]

Neosporin AF®: 2% (105 mL)

Lotion, powder, as nitrate (Zeasorb®-AF): 2% (56 g) [contains alcohol 36%]

Ointment, topical, as nitrate:

Aloe Vesta® 2-n-1 Antifungal: 2% (60 g, 150 g)

DermaFungal: 2% (113 g)

Dermagran® AF: (113 g) [contains vitamin A and zinc]

Powder, topical, as nitrate:

Lotrimin® AF: 2% (160 g)

Micro-Guard®: 2% (90 g)

Mitrazol™: 2% (30 g)

Zeasorb®-AF: 2% (70 g)

Powder spray, topical, as nitrate:

Lotrimin® AF, Lotrimin® AF Jock Itch: 2% (140 g)

Micatin® Athlete's Foot, Micatin® Jock Itch: 2% (90 g) [contains alcohol]

Neosporin® AF: 2% (85 g)

Suppository, vaginal, as nitrate: 100 mg (7s); 200 mg (3s)

Monistat® 3: 200 mg (3s)

Monistat® 7: 100 mg (7s)

Tablet, effervescent, topical, as nitrate (DiabetAid™ Antifungal Foot Bath): 2% (10s)

Tincture, topical, as nitrate (Fungoid®): 2% (30 mL, 473 mL) [contains isopropyl alcohol 30%]; 30 mL size also available in a treatment kit which contains nail scrub and nail brush]

Overdosage/Treatment

Decontamination: Dermal: Wash with soap and water

Supportive therapy: Seizures and anaphylaxis can be treated with standard therapy

Enhancement of elimination: Not dialyzable (0% to 5%)

Drug Interactions Substrate of CYP3A4 (major); **Inhibits** CYP1A2 (moderate), 2A6 (strong), 2B6 (weak), 2C9 (strong), 2C19 (strong), 2D6 (strong), 2E1 (moderate), 3A4 (strong)

Note: The majority of reported drug interactions were observed following intravenous miconazole administration. Although systemic absorption following topical and/or vaginal administration is low, potential interactions due to CYP isoenzyme inhibition may occur (rarely). This may be particularly true in situations where topical absorption may be increased (eg, inflamed tissue).

Amphotericin B: Antifungal effects of both agents may be decreased

Cisapride: Risk of cardiotoxicity may be increased due to effect on metabolism; concurrent administration is contraindicated

CYP1A2 substrates: Miconazole may increase the levels/effects of CYP1A2 substrates. Example substrates include aminophylline, fluvoxamine, mexiletine, mirtazapine, ropinirole, theophylline, and trifluoperazine.

CYP2A6 substrates: Miconazole may increase the levels/effects of CYP2A6 substrates. Example substrates include dexmedetomidine and ifosfamide.

CYP2C9 Substrates: Miconazole may increase the levels/effects of CYP2C9 substrates. Example substrates include bosentan, dapsone, fluoxetine, glimepiride, glipizide, losartan, montelukast, nateglinide, paclitaxel, phenytoin, warfarin, and zafirlukast.

CYP2C19 substrates: Miconazole may increase the levels/effects of CYP2C19 substrates. Example substrates include citalopram, diazepam, methsuximide, phenytoin, propranolol, and sertraline.

CYP2D6 substrates: Miconazole may increase the levels/effects of CYP2D6 substrates. Example substrates include amphetamines, selected beta-blockers, dextromethorphan, fluoxetine, lidocaine, mirtazapine, nefazodone, paroxetine, risperidone, ritonavir, thioridazine, tricyclic antidepressants, and venlafaxine.

CYP2D6 prodrug substrates: Miconazole may decrease the levels/effects of CYP2D6 prodrug substrates. Example prodrug substrates include codeine, hydrocodone, oxycodone, and tramadol.

CYP2E1 substrates: Miconazole may increase the levels/effects of CYP2E1 substrates. Example substrates include inhalational anesthetics, theophylline, and trimethadione.

CYP3A4 inducers: CYP3A4 inducers may decrease the levels/effects of miconazole. Example inducers include aminoglutethimide, carbamazepine, nafcillin, nevirapine, phenobarbital, phenytoin, and rifamycins.

CYP3A4 substrates: Miconazole may increase the levels/effects of CYP3A4 substrates. Example substrates include benzodiazepines, calcium channel blockers, mirtazapine, nateglinide, nefazodone, tacrolimus, and venlafaxine. Selected benzodiazepines (midazolam and triazolam), cisapride, ergot alkaloids, selected HMG-CoA reductase inhibitors (lovastatin and simvastatin), and pimozide are generally contraindicated with strong CYP3A4 inhibitors.

Phenytoin: Serum concentration may be increased by miconazole

Sulfonylureas: Hypoglycemic effects may be increased

Warfarin: An increased anticoagulant effect may occur with coadministration, including reports associated with short-term (3-day) intravaginal miconazole therapy

Pregnancy Risk Factor C

Pregnancy Implications Benefits of use should outweigh possible risks

Lactation Excretion in breast milk unknown/use caution

Midazolam

CAS Number 59467-70-8; 59467-94-6; 59467-96-8

U.S. Brand Names Versed® [DSC]

Synonyms Midazolam Hydrochloride; Versed

Impairment Potential Yes

Use Preoperative sedation and provides conscious sedation prior to diagnostic or radiographic procedures; ICU sedation (continuous infusion); intravenous anesthesia (induction); intravenous anesthesia (maintenance)

Unlabeled/Investigational Use Anxiety, status epilepticus

Mechanism of Action A short-acting triazolobenzodiazepine which depresses all levels of the CNS, including the limbic and reticular formation, probably through the increased action of gamma-aminobutyric acid (GABA), which is a major inhibitory neurotransmitter in the brain

Adverse Reactions

Cardiovascular: Cardiac arrest, **hypotension**, bradycardia, ventricular dysrhythmia, sinus bradycardia, arrhythmias (ventricular)

Central nervous system: Drowsiness, amnesia, anxiety, dizziness, paradoxical excitation, psychosis, sedation, headache, delirium, ataxia, hypothermia, extrapyramidal reactions, aggressive behavior

Dermatologic: Angioedema, urticaria, pruritus, exanthem

Gastrointestinal: Nausea, vomiting

Local: **Pain and local reactions at injection site (severity less than diazepam)**

Neuromuscular & skeletal: Dysarthria, clonus, myoclonus, paresthesia

Ocular: Blurred vision, diplopia, mydriasis

Respiratory: **Apnea**, respiratory depression, laryngospasm, wheezing

Miscellaneous: Physical and psychological dependence with prolonged use, **hiccups**

Signs and Symptoms of Overdose Apnea, cardiovascular arrest, chills, coma, confusion, cough, dyspnea, encephalopathy, euphoria, hypotension, hypothermia, hyperactivity, respiratory depression, seizures, stupor

Pharmacodynamics/Kinetics

Onset of action: I.M.: Sedation: ~15 minutes; I.V.: 1-5 minutes
Peak effect: I.M.: 0.5-1 hour

Duration: I.M.: Up to 6 hours; Mean: 2 hours

Absorption: Oral: Rapid

Distribution: V_d: 0.8-2.5 L/kg; increased with congestive heart failure (CHF) and chronic renal failure

Protein binding: 95%

Metabolism: Extensively hepatic via CYP3A4

Bioavailability: Mean: 45%

Half-life elimination: 1-4 hours; prolonged with cirrhosis, congestive heart failure, obesity, and elderly

Excretion: Urine (as glucuronide conjugated metabolites); feces (~2% to 10%)

Dosage

The dose of midazolam needs to be individualized based on the patient's age, underlying diseases, and concurrent medications. Decrease dose (by ~30%) if narcotics or other CNS depressants are administered concomitantly. **Personnel and equipment needed for standard respiratory resuscitation should be immediately available during midazolam administration.**

Children <6 years may require higher doses and closer monitoring than older children; calculate dose on ideal body weight

Conscious sedation for procedures or preoperative sedation:

Oral: 0.25-0.5 mg/kg as a single dose preprocedure, up to a maximum of 20 mg; administer 30-45 minutes prior to procedure. Children <6 years or less cooperative patients may require as much as 1 mg/kg as a single dose; 0.25 mg/kg may suffice for children 6-16 years of age.

Intranasal (not an approved route): 0.2 mg/kg (up to 0.4 mg/kg in some studies), to a maximum of 15 mg; may be administered 30-45 minutes prior to procedure

I.M.: 0.1-0.15 mg/kg 30-60 minutes before surgery or procedure; range 0.05-0.15 mg/kg; doses up to 0.5 mg/kg have been used in more anxious patients; maximum total dose: 10 mg

I.V.:

Infants <6 months: Limited information is available in nonintubated infants; dosing recommendations not clear; infants <6 months are at higher risk for airway obstruction and hypoventilation; titrate dose in small increments to desired effect; monitor carefully

Infants 6 months to Children 5 years: Initial: 0.05-0.1 mg/kg; titrate dose carefully; total dose of 0.6 mg/kg may be required; usual maximum total dose: 6 mg

Children 6-12 years: Initial: 0.025-0.05 mg/kg; titrate dose carefully; total doses of 0.4 mg/kg may be required; usual maximum total dose: 10 mg

Children 12-16 years: Dose as adults; usual maximum total dose: 10 mg

Conscious sedation during mechanical ventilation: Children: Loading dose: 0.05-0.2 mg/kg, followed by initial continuous infusion: 0.06-0.12 mg/kg/hour (1-2 mcg/kg/minute); titrate to the desired effect; usual range: 0.4-6 mcg/kg/minute

Status epilepticus refractory to standard therapy (unlabeled use): Infants >2 months and Children: Loading dose: 0.15 mg/kg followed by a continuous infusion of 1 mcg/kg/minute; titrate dose upward every 5 minutes until clinical seizure activity is controlled; mean infusion rate required in 24 children was 2.3 mcg/kg/minute with a range of 1-18 mcg/kg/minute

Adults:

Preoperative sedation:

I.M.: 0.07-0.08 mg/kg 30-60 minutes prior to surgery/procedure; usual dose: 5 mg; **Note:** Reduce dose in patients with COPD, high-risk patients, patients ≥60 years of age, and patients receiving other narcotics or CNS depressants

I.V.: 0.02-0.04 mg/kg; repeat every 5 minutes as needed to desired effect or up to 0.1-0.2 mg/kg

Intranasal (not an approved route): 0.2 mg/kg (up to 0.4 mg/kg in some studies); administer 30-45 minutes prior to surgery/procedure

Conscious sedation: I.V.: Initial: 0.5-2 mg slow I.V. over at least 2 minutes; slowly titrate to effect by repeating doses every 2-3 minutes if needed; usual total dose: 2.5-5 mg; use decreased doses in elderly

Healthy Adults <60 years: Some patients respond to doses as low as 1 mg; no more than 2.5 mg should be administered over a period of 2 minutes. Additional doses of midazolam may be administered after a 2-minute waiting period and evaluation of sedation after each dose increment. A total dose >5 mg is generally not needed. If narcotics or other CNS depressants are administered concomitantly, the midazolam dose should be reduced by 30%.

Anesthesia: I.V.:

Induction:

Unpremedicated patients: 0.3-0.35 mg/kg (up to 0.6 mg/kg in resistant cases)

Premedicated patients: 0.15-0.35 mg/kg

Maintenance: 0.05-0.3 mg/kg as needed, or continuous infusion 0.25-1.5 mcg/kg/minute

Sedation in mechanically-ventilated patients: I.V. continuous infusion: 100 mg in 250 mL D_5W or NS (if patient is fluid-restricted, may concentrate up to a maximum of 0.5 mg/mL); initial dose: 0.02-0.08 mg/kg (~1 mg to 5 mg in 70 kg adult) initially and either repeated at 5-15 minute intervals until adequate sedation is achieved or continuous infusion rates of 0.04-0.2 mg/kg/hour and titrate to reach desired level of sedation

Elderly: I.V.: Conscious sedation: Initial: 0.5 mg slow I.V.; give no more than 1.5 mg in a 2-minute period; if additional titration is needed, give no more than 1 mg over 2 minutes, waiting another 2 or more minutes to evaluate sedative effect; a total dose of >3.5 mg is rarely necessary

Dosage adjustment in renal impairment:

Hemodialysis: Supplemental dose is not necessary

Peritoneal dialysis: Significant drug removal is unlikely based on physiochemical characteristics

Stability Admixtures do not require protection from light for short-term storage

Monitoring Parameters Respiratory and cardiovascular status, blood pressure, blood pressure monitor required during I.V. administration

Administration Intranasal: Administer using a 1 mL needleless syringe into the nostrils over 15 seconds; use the 5 mg/mL injection; $^1/_2$ of the dose may be administered to each nostril

Oral: Do not mix with any liquid (such as grapefruit juice) prior to administration

Parenteral:

I.M.: Administer deep I.M. into large muscle.

I.V.: Administer by slow I.V. injection over at least 2-5 minutes at a concentration of 1-5 mg/mL or by I.V. infusion. Continuous infusions should be administered via an infusion pump.

Contraindications Hypersensitivity to midazolam or any component of the formulation, including benzyl alcohol (cross-sensitivity with other benzodiazepines may exist); parenteral form is not for intrathecal or epidural injection; narrow-angle glaucoma; concurrent use of potent inhibitors of CYP3A4 (amprenavir, atazanavir, or ritonavir); pregnancy

Warnings [U.S. Boxed Warning]: May cause severe respiratory depression, respiratory arrest, or apnea. Use with extreme caution, particularly in noncritical care settings. Appropriate resuscitative equipment and qualified personnel must be available for administration and monitoring. Initial dosing must be cautiously titrated and individualized, particularly in elderly or debilitated patients, patients with hepatic impairment (including alcoholics), or in renal impairment, particularly if other CNS depressants (including opiates) are used concurrently. **[U.S. Boxed Warning]: Initial doses in elderly or debilitated patients should be conservative; as little as 1 mg, but not to exceed 2.5 mg.** Use with caution in patients with respiratory disease or impaired gag reflex. Use during upper airway procedures may increase risk of hypoventilation. Prolonged responses have been noted following extended administration by continuous infusion (possibly due to metabolite accumulation) or in the presence of drugs which inhibit midazolam metabolism.

Causes CNS depression (dose-related) resulting in sedation, dizziness, confusion, or ataxia which may impair physical and mental capabilities. Patients must be cautioned about performing tasks which require mental alertness (eg, operating machinery or driving). A minimum of 1 day should elapse after midazolam administration before attempting these tasks. Use with caution in patients receiving other CNS depressants or psychoactive agents. Effects with other sedative drugs or ethanol may be potentiated. Benzodiazepines have been associated with falls and traumatic injury and should be used with extreme caution in patients who are at risk of these events (especially the elderly).

May cause hypotension - hemodynamic events are more common in pediatric patients or patients with hemodynamic instability. Hypotension and/or respiratory depression may occur more frequently in patients who have received narcotic analgesics. Use with caution in obese patients, chronic renal failure, and CHF. Does not protect against increases in heart rate or blood pressure during intubation. Should not be used in shock, coma, or acute alcohol intoxication. **[U.S. Boxed Warning]: Parenteral form contains benzyl alcohol; avoid rapid injection in neonates or prolonged infusions.** Avoid intra-arterial administration or extravasation of parenteral formulation.

Midazolam causes anterograde amnesia. Paradoxical reactions, including hyperactive or aggressive behavior have been reported with benzodiazepines, particularly in adolescent/pediatric or psychiatric patients. Does not have analgesic, antidepressant, or antipsychotic properties.

Benzodiazepines have been associated with dependence and acute withdrawal symptoms on discontinuation or reduction in dose. Acute withdrawal, including seizures, may be precipitated after administration of flumazenil to patients receiving long-term benzodiazepine therapy.

Dosage Forms

Injection, solution: 1 mg/mL (2 mL, 5 mL, 10 mL); 5 mg/mL (1 mL, 2 mL, 5 mL, 10 mL) [contains benzyl alcohol 1%]

Injection, solution [preservative free]: 1 mg/mL (2 mL, 5 mL); 5 mg/mL (1 mL, 2 mL)

Syrup: 2 mg/mL (118 mL) [contains sodium benzoate; cherry flavor]

Reference Range Intranasal dose of 0.1-0.2 mg/kg result in serum midazolam levels of between 40-70 ng/mL within 3 minutes; plasma midazolam levels >100 ng/mL associated with sedation; plasma midazolam levels >200 ng/mL associated with sleep

Overdosage/Treatment

Supportive therapy: Rarely is mechanical ventilation required. Flumazenil (Romazicon™) has been shown to selectively block the binding of benzodiazepines to CNS receptors, resulting in a reversal of benzodiazepine-induced CNS depression. Resedation usually does not occur at midazolam adult doses <10 mg. Acetaminophen can be used to mask the metallic bitter taste.

Enhancement of elimination: Hemodialysis is not useful; multiple dosing of activated charcoal may be useful

Antidote(s)

• Flumazenil [ANTIDOTE]

Test Interactions Visine®, Drano®, bleach, and soap may result in a false-negative urine test

Drug InteractionsSubstrate of CYP2B6 (minor), 3A4 (major); **Inhibits** CYP2C8 (weak), 2C9 (weak), 3A4 (weak)

CNS depressants: Sedative effects and/or respiratory depression may be additive with CNS depressants; includes ethanol, barbiturates, narcotic analgesics, and other sedative agents; monitor for increased effect. **If narcotics or other CNS depressants are administered concomitantly, the midazolam dose should be reduced by 30% if <65 years of age, or by at least 50% if >65 years of age.**

CYP3A4 inducers: CYP3A4 inducers may decrease the levels/effects of midazolam. Example inducers include aminoglutethimide, carbamazepine, nafcillin, nevirapine, phenobarbital, phenytoin, and rifamycins.

CYP3A4 inhibitors: May increase the levels/effects of midazolam. Example inhibitors include azole antifungals, clarithromycin, diclofenac, doxycycline, erythromycin, imatinib, isoniazid, nefazodone, nicardipine, propofol, protease inhibitors, quinidine, telithromycin, and verapamil.

Levodopa: Therapeutic effects may be diminished in some patients following the addition of a benzodiazepine; limited/inconsistent data

Oral contraceptives: May decrease the clearance of some benzodiazepines (those which undergo oxidative metabolism); monitor for increased benzodiazepine effect

Saquinavir: A 56% reduction in clearance and a doubling of midazolam's half-life were seen with concurrent administration with saquinavir.

Theophylline: May partially antagonize some of the effects of benzodiazepines; monitor for decreased response; may require higher doses for sedation

Pregnancy Risk Factor D

Pregnancy Implications Crosses the placenta; not recommended for use during pregnancy

Lactation Enters breast milk/not recommended (AAP rates "of concern")

Additional Information Each mL contains 0.14 mEq of sodium. Flumazenil (0.4 mg I.V.) has been used successfully in reversing midazolam-induced laryngospasm.

Grapefruit juice may increase serum concentrations of midazolam; avoid concurrent use with oral form

Specific References

Everitt IJ and Barnett P, "Comparison of Two Benzodiazepines Used for Sedation of Children Undergoing Suturing of a Laceration in an Emergency Department," *Pediatr Emerg Care*, 2002, 18(2):72-4.

Jacoby J, Heller M, Nichoals J, et al, "Etomidate Versus Midazolam for Out-of-Hospital Intubation: A Prospective, Randomized Trial," *Ann Emerg Med*, 2006, 47:525-30.

Kanegaye JT, Favela JL, Acosta M, et al, "High-Dose Rectal Midazolam for Pediatric Procedures: A Randomized Trial of Sedative Efficacy and Agitation," *Pediatr Emerg Care*, 2003, 19(5):329-36.

Knott JC, Taylor DM, and Castle DJ, "Randomized Clinical Trial Comparing Intravenous Midazolam and Droperidol for Sedation of the Acutely Agitated Patient in the Emergency Department," *Ann Emerg Med*, 2006, 47(1):61-7.

McIntyre J, Robertson S, Norris E, et al, "Safety and Efficacy of Buccal Midazolam Versus Rectal Diazepam for Emergency Treatment of Seizures in Children: A Randomised Controlled Trial," *Lancet*, 2005, 366(9481):205-10.

Meinitzer A, Marz W, Mangge H, et al, "More Reliable Brain Death Diagnosis with Chromatographic Analysis of Midazolam, Diazepam, Thiopentone, and Active Metabolites," *J Anal Tox*, 2006, 30:196-201.

Sagarin MJ, Barton ED, Sakles JC, et al, "Underdosing of Midazolam in Emergency Endotracheal Intubation," *Acad Emerg Med*, 2003, 10(4):329-38.

Wolfe TR and Macfarlane TC, "Intranasal Midazolam Therapy for Pediatric Status Epilepticus," *Am J Emerg Med*, 2006, 24:343-6.

Midodrine

CAS Number 3092-17-9; 42794-76-3

U.S. Brand Names ProAmatine®

Synonyms Midodrine Hydrochloride

Use Orphan drug: Treatment of symptomatic orthostatic hypotension

Unlabeled/Investigational Use Investigational: Management of urinary incontinence

Mechanism of Action Oral sympathomimetic agent which is an alpha$_1$-adrenergic agonist resulting in vasoconstriction; essentially a prodrug

Adverse Reactions

Cardiovascular: Tachycardia, bradycardia, supine hypertension, flushing, sinus bradycardia, sinus tachycardia

Central nervous system: Headache, insomnia, sleep disturbance, irritability

Dermatologic: **Scalp pruritus**

Gastrointestinal: Nausea, xerostomia

Genitourinary: **Urinary urgency, retention**

Neuromuscular & skeletal: **Piloerection, paresthesia**

Renal: **Polyuria**

Miscellaneous: Diaphoresis

Pharmacodynamics/Kinetics

Onset of action: ~1 hour

Duration: 2-3 hours

Absorption: Rapid

Distribution: V_d (desglymidodrine): <1.6 L/kg; poorly across membrane (eg, blood brain barrier)

Protein binding: Minimal

Metabolism: Hepatic; midodrine is a prodrug which undergoes rapid deglycination to desglymidodrine (active metabolite); metabolism occurs in many tissues and plasma

Bioavailability: Desglymidodrine: 93%

Half-life elimination: Desglymidodrine: ~3-4 hours; Midodrine: 25 minutes

Time to peak, serum: Desglymidodrine: 1-2 hours; Midodrine: 30 minutes

Excretion: Urine (2% to 4%)

Clearance: Desglymidodrine: 385 mL/minute (predominantly by renal secretion)

Dosage

Adults: Oral: 10 mg 3 times/day during daytime hours (every 3-4 hours) when patient is upright (maximum: 40 mg/day)

Dosing adjustment in renal impairment: 2.5 mg 3 times/day, gradually increasing as tolerated

Monitoring Parameters Blood pressure, renal and hepatic parameters

Administration Doses may be given in approximately 3- to 4-hour intervals (eg, shortly before or upon rising in the morning, at midday, in the late afternoon not later than 6 PM). Avoid dosing after the evening meal or within 4 hours of bedtime. Continue therapy only in patients who appear to attain symptomatic improvement during initial treatment. Standing systolic blood pressure may be elevated 15-30 mm Hg at 1 hour after a 10 mg dose. Some effect may persist for 2-3 hours.

Contraindications Hypersensitivity to midodrine or any component of the formulation; severe organic heart disease; urinary retention; pheochromocytoma; thyrotoxicosis; persistent and significant supine hypertension

Warnings [U.S. Boxed Warning]: Indicated for patients for whom orthostatic hypotension significantly impairs their daily life despite standard clinical care. Use is not recommended with supine hypertension. Caution should be exercised in patients with diabetes, visual problems (especially if receiving fludrocortisone), urinary retention (reduce initial dose), or hepatic dysfunction; monitor renal and hepatic function prior to and periodically during therapy; safety and efficacy has not been established in children; discontinue and re-evaluate therapy if signs of bradycardia occur.

Dosage Forms Tablet, as hydrochloride: 2.5 mg, 5 mg, 10 mg

Reference Range After a 2.5 mg oral dose, peak serum level is ~11 mcg/L at 0.5 hour; serum deglymidodrine level is 5 mcg/L at 1-hour postingestion

Overdosage/Treatment

Decontamination: Activated charcoal

Supportive therapy: There is no specific antidote for midodrine intoxication and the bulk of the treatment is supportive. Hyperactivity and agitation usually respond to reduced sensory input, however with extreme agitation haloperidol (2-5 mg I.M. for adults) may be required. Hyperthermia is best treated with external cooling measures, or when severe or unresponsive, muscle paralysis with pancuronium may be needed. Hypertension is usually transient and generally does not require treatment unless severe. For diastolic blood pressures >110 mm Hg, a nitroprusside infusion should be initiated. Seizures usually respond to diazepam or lorazepam I.V. and/or phenytoin maintenance regimens.

Drug Interactions Increased effect: Concomitant fludrocortisone results in hypernatremia or an increase in intraocular pressure and glaucoma; bradycardia may be accentuated with concomitant administration of cardiac glycosides, psychotherapeutics, and beta-blockers; alpha-agonists may increase the pressure effects and alpha-antagonists may negate the effects of midodrine

Pregnancy Risk Factor C

Pregnancy Implications Increased rate of embryo resorption and decreased fetal weight were observed in animal studies. Use during pregnancy should be avoided unless the potential benefit outweighs the risk to the fetus.

Lactation Excretion in breast milk is unknown/use caution

Specific References

Young TM and Mathias CJ, "Taste and Smell Disturbance with the Alpha-Adrenoceptor Agonist Midodrine," *Ann Pharmacother*, 2004, 38(11):1868-70.

Mifepristone

CAS Number 84371-65-3

U.S. Brand Names Mifeprex®

Synonyms RU-38486; RU-486

Use Medical termination of intrauterine pregnancy, through day 49 of pregnancy. Patients may need treatment with misoprostol and possibly surgery to complete therapy

Unlabeled/Investigational Use Treatment of unresectable meningioma; has been studied in the treatment of breast cancer, ovarian cancer, and adrenal cortical carcinoma

Mechanism of Action An antiprogestin agent which interacts upon the decidua progesterone receptors resulting in increased release of endometrium prostaglandins and thus uterine bleeding, contraction and cervical dilation occurs thus promoting fetal evacuation

Adverse Reactions

Vaginal bleeding and uterine cramping are expected to occur when this medication is used to terminate a pregnancy; 90% of women using this medication for this purpose also report adverse reactions

Cardiovascular: Syncope, myocardial infarction

Central nervous system: **Headache, dizziness,** fatigue, fever, insomnia, anxiety, fainting

Gastrointestinal: **Abdominal pain (cramping), nausea, vomiting, diarrhea,** dyspepsia

Genitourinary: **Uterine cramping,** uterine hemorrhage, vaginitis, pelvic pain, ruptured ectopic pregnancy, leukorrhea

Hematologic: Decreased hemoglobin >2 g/dL, anemia

Hepatic: Significant SGOT, SGPT, alkaline phosphatase, and GT changes have been reported rarely

Neuromuscular & skeletal: Back pain, rigors, leg pain, weakness

Respiratory: Sinusitis

Miscellaneous: Viral infection, bacterial infection

In trials for unresectable meningioma, the most common adverse effects included fatigue, hot flashes, gynecomastia or breast tenderness, hair thinning, and rash. In premenopausal women, vaginal bleeding may be seen shortly after beginning therapy and cessation of menses is common. Thyroiditis and effects related to antiglucocorticoid activity have also been noted.

Pharmacodynamics/Kinetics

Absorption: Oral: rapid

Protein binding: 98% to albumin and α_1-acid glycoprotein

Metabolism: Hepatic via CYP3A4 to three metabolites (may possess some antiprogestin and antiglucocorticoid activity)

Bioavailability: Oral: 69%

Half-life elimination: Terminal: 18 hours following a slower phase where 50% eliminated between 12-72 hours

Time to peak: Oral: 90 minutes

Excretion: Feces (83%); urine (9%)

Dosage Oral:

Adults: Termination of pregnancy: Treatment consists of three office visits by the patient; the patient must read medication guide and sign patient agreement prior to treatment:

Day 1: 600 mg (three 200 mg tablets) taken as a single dose under physician supervision

Day 3: Patient must return to the healthcare provider 2 days following administration of mifepristone; if termination of pregnancy cannot be confirmed using ultrasound or clinical examination: 400 mcg (two 200 mcg tablets) of misoprostol; patient may need treatment for cramps or gastrointestinal symptoms at this time

Day 14: Patient must return to the healthcare provider ~14 days after administration of mifepristone; confirm complete termination of pregnancy by ultrasound or clinical exam. Surgical termination is recommended to manage treatment failures.

Elderly: Safety and efficacy have not been established

Dosage adjustment in renal impairment: Safety and efficacy have not been established

Dosage adjustment in hepatic impairment: Safety and efficacy have not been established; use with caution due to CYP3A4 metabolism

Unlabeled use: Refer to individual protocols. The dose used in meningioma is usually 200 mg/day, continued based on toxicity and response.

Monitoring Parameters Clinical exam and/or ultrasound to confirm complete termination of pregnancy; hemoglobin, hematocrit, and red blood cell count in cases of heavy bleeding

Contraindications Hypersensitivity to mifepristone, misoprostol, other prostaglandins, or any component of the formulation; chronic adrenal failure; porphyrias; hemorrhagic disorder or concurrent anticoagulant therapy; pregnancy termination >49 days; intrauterine device (IUD) in place; ectopic pregnancy or undiagnosed adnexal mass; concurrent long-term corticosteroid therapy; inadequate or lack of access to emergency medical services; inability to understand effects and/or comply with treatment

Warnings [U.S. Boxed Warning]: Patient must be instructed of the treatment procedure and expected effects. A signed agreement form must be kept in the patient's file. Physicians may obtain patient agreement forms, physician enrollment forms, and medical consultation directly from Danco Laboratories at 1-877-432-7596. Adverse effects (including blood transfusions, hospitalization, ongoing pregnancy, and other major complications) must be reported in writing to the medication distributor. To be administered only by physicians who can date pregnancy, diagnose ectopic pregnancies, provide access to surgical abortion (if needed), and can provide access to emergency care. Medication will be distributed directly to these physicians following signed agreement with the distributor. Must be administered under supervision by the qualified physician. Pregnancy is dated from day 1 of last menstrual period (presuming a 28-day cycle, ovulation occurring midcycle). Pregnancy duration can be determined using menstrual history and clinical examination. Ultrasound should be used if an ectopic pregnancy is suspected or if duration of pregnancy is uncertain. Ultrasonography may not identify all ectopic pregnancies, and healthcare providers should be alert for signs and symptoms which may be related to undiagnosed ectopic pregnancy in any patient who receives mifepristone

Bleeding occurs and should be expected (average 9-16 days, may be ≥30 days). In some cases, bleeding may be prolonged and heavy, potentially leading to hypovolemic shock. **[U.S. Boxed Warning]: Patients should be counseled to seek medical attention in cases of excessive bleeding;** the manufacturer cites soaking through two thick sanitary pads per hour for two consecutive hours as an example of excessive bleeding. Bleeding may require blood transfusion (rare), curettage, saline infusions, and/or vasoconstrictors. Use caution in patients with severe anemia. Confirmation of pregnancy termination by clinical exam or ultrasound must be made 14 days following treatment. Manufacturer recommends surgical termination of pregnancy when medical termination fails or is not complete. Prescriber should determine in advance whether they will provide such care themselves or through other providers. Preventative measures to prevent rhesus immunization must be taken prior to surgical abortion. Prescriber should also give the patient clear instructions on whom to call and what to do in the event of an emergency following administration of mifepristone

[U.S. Boxed Warning]: Bacterial infections have been reported following use of this product. In rare cases, these infections may be serious and/or fatal, with septic shock as a potential complication. A causal relationship has not been established. Sustained fever, abdominal pain, or pelvic tenderness should prompt evaluation; however, healthcare professionals are warned that atypical presentations of serious infection without these symptoms have also been noted. Patients presenting with nausea, vomiting, diarrhea, or weakness, with or without abdominal pain or fever, should be evaluated for serious bacterial infection when symptoms occur >24 hours after taking misoprostol. Treatment with antibiotics, including coverage for anaerobic bacteria (eg, *Clostridium sordellii*) should be initiated. **[U.S. Boxed Warning]: Patients undergoing treatment with mifepristone should be instructed to bring their Medication Guide with them when an obtaining treatment from an emergency room or healthcare provider that did not prescribe the medication initially in order to identify that they are undergoing a medical abortion.**

Safety and efficacy have not been established for use in women with chronic cardiovascular, hypertensive, hepatic, respiratory, or renal disease, insulin-dependent diabetes mellitus, severe anemia, or heavy smokers. Women >35 years of age and smokers (>10 cigarettes/day) were excluded from clinical trials. Safety and efficacy in pediatric patients have not been established.

Dosage Forms Tablet: 200 mg

Reference Range Peak serum mifepristone level 3 hours following a 25 mg/kg dose: ~7.5 μmol/L

Overdosage/Treatment
Decontamination: Activated charcoal
Supportive therapy: Transfusion and curettage may be required to treat uterine bleeding; acetaminophen can be used to treat headaches
Enhanced elimination: Multiple dosing of activated charcoal may be effective

Test Interactions May increase morning serum cortisol

Drug Interactions
 Substrate of CYP3A4 (minor); **Inhibits** CYP2D6 (weak), 3A4 (weak)
 There are no reported interactions. It might be anticipated that the concurrent administration of mifepristone and a progestin would result in an attenuation of the effects of one or both agents.

Pregnancy Risk Factor X

Pregnancy Implications This medication is used to terminate pregnancy; there are no approved treatment indications for its use during pregnancy. Prostaglandins (including mifepristone and misoprostol) may have teratogenic effects when used during pregnancy. It is unknown if mifepristone is excreted in human milk; breast-feeding contraindicated. Breast milk should be discarded for a few days following use of this medication.

Lactation Excretion in breast milk unknown/contraindicated

Additional Information An abortifacient approved in France in September 1988. Patients with prosthetic heart valves require chemoprophylaxis; avoid aspirin or other nonsteroidal anti-inflammatory drugs for 2 weeks

Specific Reference
Miech RP, "Pathophysiology of Mifepristone-Induced Septic Shock Due to *Clostridium sordellii*," *Ann Pharmacother*, 2005, 39(9):1483-8.

Milnacipran

Pronunciation (mil NAY ci pran)
CAS Number 101152-94-7; 17513-61-0; 92623-85-3
Impairment Potential Yes; particularly if daily dose is >100 mg
Use Treatment of major depression
Mechanism of Action A cyclopropanecarboxylic acid derivative which inhibits reuptake of both serotonin and noradrenaline neurotransmitters.
Adverse Reactions
Cardiovascular: Orthostatic hypotension (2% to 21%), tachycardia (2%), hypotension (1% to 2%)
Central nervous system: Headache (8%), dizziness (3% to 5%), tremor (3%), fatigue (2%), lethargy (2%), insomnia (5% to 6%), mania (rare)
Gastrointestinal: Nausea (11%), dry mouth (8%), abdominal pain (7%), constipation (7%)
Genitourinary: Dysuria (2%)
Hepatic: Transient elevation of transaminases
Ocular: Visual disturbances (2%)
Miscellaneous: Diaphoresis (3% to 4%)
Signs and Symptoms of Overdose CNS depression, coma, lethargy, tachycardia, tachypnea, vomiting
Admission Criteria/Prognosis Admit any symptomatic patient or adult ingestion >300 mg
Toxicodynamics/Kinetics
Volume of distribution: 5 L/kg
Protein binding: 13%
Metabolism: Hepatic glucuronidation to inactive metabolite
Half-life: 8 hours
Bioavailability: Oral: 85%
Time to peak concentration: 0.5-4 hours
Elimination: Renal clearance: 3.2 mL/kg/minute
 Renal: 90% (50% to 60% unchanged); 20% to 30% milnacipran glucuronide
 Fecal: <5%
Dosage Oral: 50 mg twice daily
 Dosing adjustment in renal insufficiency: 25 mg twice daily
Dosage Forms Capsule: 25 mg, 50 mg
Reference Range Therapeutic serum milnacipran level: 100-300 ng/mL; Lethal serum concentration: 3000 ng/mL
Overdosage/Treatment
Oral decontamination: Lavage within 1 hour with activated charcoal
Enhanced elimination: Hemodialysis is not likely to be helpful
Additional Information Brand names: Dalcipran, Ixel, Milneuron, Toledomin

Mineral Oil

CAS Number 8012-95-1
U.S. Brand Names Fleet® Mineral Oil Enema [OTC]; Kondremul® [OTC]; Liqui-Doss® [OTC]
Synonyms Heavy Mineral Oil; Liquid Paraffin; White Mineral Oil
Use Temporary relief of constipation, to relieve fecal impaction, preparation for bowel studies or surgery; baby oil can be used to remove tar/asphalt burns
Mechanism of Action An emollient laxative which eases passage of stool by decreasing water absorption and lubricating the intestine; low volatility; high viscosity
Adverse Reactions
Gastrointestinal: Nausea, vomiting, diarrhea, abdominal cramps, anal itching, intestinal obstruction from bezoar formation may result
Respiratory: Lipoid pneumonitis with aspiration
Signs and Symptoms of Overdose Aspiration of oils may cause chemical pneumonitis with fever, leukocytosis, x-ray changes
Pharmacodynamics/Kinetics
Onset of action: Oral: 6-8 hours; Rectal: 2-15 minutes
Distribution: Site of action is the colon
Excretion: Feces
Dosage
Children:
 Oral: 5-11 years: 5-20 mL once daily or in divided doses
 Rectal: 2-11 years: 30-60 mL as a single dose
Children >12 years and Adults:
 Oral: 15-45 mL/day once daily or in divided doses
 Rectal: Retention enema, contents of one enema (range 60-150 mL)/day as a single dose
Monitoring Parameters Monitor for response (stool frequency, consistency). Avoid use in patients who may aspirate.
Administration Oral: Mineral oil may be more palatable if refrigerated. Administer on an empty stomach in an upright position.
 Kondremul®: Shake well before use.
 Liqui-Doss®: Shake well before use. Prior to use, mix with 120 mL of any beverage; administer only at bedtime.
Rectal (Fleet® Mineral Oil): Gently insert enema rectally with patient lying on left side and left knee slightly bent, right knee drawn to chest.

Contraindications Patients with colostomy or an ileostomy, appendicitis, ulcerative colitis, diverticulitis

Warnings

Lipid pneumonitis results from aspiration of mineral oil. Aspiration risk increased in patients in prolonged supine position or conditions which interfere with swallowing or epiglottal function (eg, stroke, Parkinson's disease, Alzheimer's disease, esophageal dysmotility).

When used for self-medication (OTC): Healthcare provider should be contacted in case of sudden changes in bowel habits which last over 2 weeks; abdominal pain, nausea, vomiting; rectal bleeding following use; if needed for >1 week.

Dosage Forms

Liquid, oral:

Liqui-Doss®: 13.5 mL/15 mL (480 mL) [self-emulsifying oily liquid; alcohol free, sugar free]

Microemulsion, oral:

Kondremul®: 2.5 mL/5 mL (480 mL) [sugar free; mint flavor]

Oil, rectal [enema]:

Fleet® Mineral Oil: 100% (118 mL)

Oil, oral: 100% (480 mL, 3840 mL)

Overdosage/Treatment

Decontamination: **Do not** induce emesis; activated charcoal may be useful

Supportive therapy: Fluid/electrolyte replacement; pulmonary physiotherapy should be considered; corticosteroids are of unproven pulmonary benefit

Drug Interactions May impair absorption of fat-soluble vitamins (A, D, K, E), coumarin, sulfonamides; administration of surfactants (docusate) with mineral oil may increase mineral oil absorption and therefore enhance toxic potential of mineral oil resulting in a foreign body reaction in lymphoid tissue

Nursing Implications Administer on an empty stomach because of the risk of aspiration

Additional Information Associated with increased risk from bronchogenic carcinoma (from lipoid pneumonia), gastrointestinal tumors, and dermal tumors suppresses cough reflex; prolonged administration of mineral oil may decrease absorption of lipid-soluble vitamins A, D, E, and K. Light sterile mineral oils are not for injection. Gauze pads soaked with mineral oil compresses can be used to lyse eyelid adhesions due to cyanoacrylate adhesive; no ocular damage was reported over a $1^1/_2$-day period.

Minocycline

CAS Number 10118-90-8; 13614-98-7

U.S. Brand Names Dynacin®; Minocin®

Synonyms Minocycline Hydrochloride

Use Treatment of susceptible bacterial infections of both gram-negative and gram-positive organisms; treatment of anthrax (inhalational, cutaneous, and gastrointestinal); acne; meningococcal carrier state; Rickettsial diseases (including Rocky Mountain spotted fever, Q fever); nongonococcal urethritis, gonorrhea; acute intestinal amebiasis

Mechanism of Action Inhibits bacterial protein synthesis by binding with the 30S and possibly the 50S ribosomal subunit(s) of susceptible bacteria; cell wall synthesis is not affected

Adverse Reactions

Cardiovascular: Pericarditis, Raynaud's phenomenon, vasculitis

Central nervous system: Increased intracranial pressure, bulging fontanels in infants, vertigo, memory disturbance (1% to 14%), headache (1%), pseudotumor cerebri, fever, visual hallucination, lightheadedness

Dermatologic: Photosensitivity, dermatologic effects, pruritus, exfoliative dermatitis, rash, blue macular pigmentation (usually localized to legs, fingernails, and scars), pityriasis versicolor, pityriasis rosea-like reaction, onycholysis, neutrophilic dermatosis (Sweet's syndrome), erythema multiforme, angioedema, urticaria, purpura, Stevens-Johnson syndrome, yellow fingernails, erythema nodosum, licheniform eruptions, exanthem, cutaneous vasculitis

Endocrine & metabolic: Diabetes insipidus, black galactorrhea, black thyroid, thyroid dysfunction (extremely rare)

Gastrointestinal: Nausea, diarrhea, vomiting, esophagitis, anorexia, abdominal cramps, lingua villosa nigra

Genitourinary: Vaginal candidiasis

Hematologic: Leukemoid, eosinophilia, hemolytic anemia, neutropenia, thrombocytopenia

Hepatic: Hepatotoxicity, hepatitis (autoimmune), hepatic vasculitis, hepatic failure

Neuromuscular & skeletal: Paresthesia

Ocular: Scotoma

Otic: Ototoxicity, tinnitus

Renal: Acute renal failure, azotemia, interstitial nephritis, necrotizing vasculitis, renal vasculitis

Respiratory: Eosinophilic pneumonitis

Miscellaneous: **Discoloration of teeth in children**, superinfections, anaphylaxis, systemic lupus erythematosus (SLE), serum sickness-like reaction, fixed drug eruption, elevated antineutrophilic cytoplasmic antibodies (ANCA)

Pharmacodynamics/Kinetics

Absorption: Well absorbed

Distribution: Majority deposits for extended periods in fat; crosses placenta; enters breast milk

Protein binding: 70% to 75%

Half-life elimination: 16 hours (range: 11-23 hours)

Time to peak: Capsule, pellet filled: 1-4 hours; Extended release tablet: 3.5-4 hours

Excretion: Urine

Dosage

Children >8 years: Oral, I.V.: Initial: 4 mg/kg followed by 2 mg/kg/dose every 12 hours

Adults:

Infection: Oral, I.V.: 200 mg stat, 100 mg every 12 hours not to exceed 400 mg/24 hours

Acne: Oral: 50 mg 1-3 times/day

Dosage adjustment in renal impairment: Consider decreasing dose or increasing dosing interval with renal impairment.

Monitoring Parameters Culture and sensitivity testing prior to initiating therapy; LFTs, BUN, renal function with long-term treatment; if symptomatic for autoimmune disorder, include ANA, CBC

Administration Oral: May be taken with food or milk. Administer with adequate fluid to decrease the risk of esophageal irritation and ulceration. I.V.: Infuse slowly, usually over a 4- to 6-hour period.

Contraindications Hypersensitivity to minocycline, other tetracyclines, or any component of the formulation; pregnancy

Warnings May cause tissue hyperpigmentation or permanent tooth discoloration; avoid use during tooth development (children ≤8 years of age) unless other drugs are not likely to be effective or are contraindicated. May be associated with increases in BUN secondary to antianabolic effects; use caution in patients with renal impairment. Hepatotoxicity has been reported; use caution in patients with hepatic insufficiency. Autoimmune syndromes (eg, lupus-like, hepatitis, and vasculitis) have been reported; discontinue if symptoms. CNS effects (lightheadedness, vertigo) may occur; patients must be cautioned about performing tasks which require mental alertness (eg, operating machinery or driving). Has been associated (rarely) with pseudotumor cerebri. May cause photosensitivity; discontinue if skin erythema occurs. May cause overgrowth of nonsusceptible organisms, including fungi; discontinue if superinfection occurs. Avoid use in children ≤8 years of age.

Dosage Forms Capsule: 50 mg, 75 mg, 100 mg

Dynacin®: 75 mg, 100 mg

Capsule, pellet filled: 50 mg, 100 mg

Minocin®: 50 mg, 100 mg

Tablet: 50 mg, 75 mg, 100 mg

Dynacin®, myrac™: 50 mg, 75 mg, 100 mg

Tablet, extended release:

Solodyn™: 45 mg, 90 mg, 135 mg

Reference Range Maximum serum concentration after a single 200 mg oral dose: 2.7 mcg/mL; after a 200 mg I.V. dose; maximum serum concentration: 3.5 mcg/mL

Overdosage/Treatment

Decontamination: Activated charcoal

Supportive therapy: Antacids can be given for epigastric pain; acetazolamide (500 mg twice daily) can be used to treat pseudotumor cerebri. For treatment of lingua villosa nigra, discontinue causative agent. Clean the tongue with a toothbrush and rinse mouth with a half-strength solution of hydrogen peroxide or 10% carbamide peroxide. Symptoms should subside in a few days.

Enhancement of elimination: Multiple dosing of activated charcoal may be effective; not dialyzable (0% to 5%)

Test Interactions May cause false elevations on fluorescence test for urinary catecholamines

Drug Interactions Calcium-, magnesium-, or aluminum-containing antacids, bile acid sequestrants, bismuth, oral contraceptives, iron, zinc, sodium bicarbonate, penicillins, quinapril: May decrease absorption of tetracyclines.

Methoxyflurane anesthesia, when concurrent with tetracyclines, may cause fatal nephrotoxicity.

Penicillins: Tetracyclines may reduce bactericidal efficacy of penicillins and cephalosporins.

Retinoic acid derivatives: May increase risk of pseudotumor cerebri.

Typhoid vaccine: Antibacterial agents may decrease the therapeutic efficacy of the live, attenuated typhoid (Ty21a strain) vaccine

Warfarin: Hypoprothrombinemic response may be increased with tetracyclines; monitor INR closely during initiation or discontinuation.

Pregnancy Risk Factor D

Pregnancy Implications May cause permanent discoloration (brown-grey) of teeth. Animal studies indicate possible embryotoxicity.

Lactation Enters breast milk/not recommended (AAP rates "compatible")

Minoxidil

CAS Number 38304-91-5

U.S. Brand Names Loniten®; Rogaine® Extra Strength for Men [OTC]; Rogaine® for Men [OTC]; Rogaine® for Women [OTC]

Use Management of severe hypertension (usually in combination with a diuretic and beta-blocker); treatment (topical formulation) of alopecia androgenetica in males and females

Mechanism of Action Produces vasodilation by directly relaxing arteriolar smooth muscle, with little effect on veins, effects may be mediated by cyclic amp; stimulation of hair growth is secondary to vasodilation, increased cutaneous blood flow and stimulation of resting hair follicles

Adverse Reactions

Cardiovascular: **Edema**, chest pain, **congestive heart failure**, **tachycardia**, angina, pericardial effusion/pericarditis, **ECG changes**, myocardial depression, pulmonary hypertension, sinus tachycardia, vasodilation

Central nervous system: Dizziness, fatigue, headache

Dermatologic: **Hypertrichosis (commonly occurs within 1-2 months of therapy)**, coarsening facial features, dermatologic reactions, rash, Stevens-Johnson syndrome, sunburn, hirsutism, bullous lesions, acne, urticaria, exanthem

Endocrine & metabolic: Sodium and water retention, gynecomastia

Gastrointestinal: Vomiting, weight gain

Local: Topical burning, itching

Neuromuscular & skeletal: Paresthesia

Ocular: Optic neuritis

Respiratory: Pulmonary edema

Miscellaneous: Lupus erythematosus

Signs and Symptoms of Overdose Coma, erythema multiforme, hair discoloration (red), hyperglycemia, hypotension, hypertrichosis, ototoxicity, pericardial effusion, pericarditis, photosensitivity, tachycardia, thrombocytopenia, tinnitus

Admission Criteria/Prognosis Admit any ingestion >1 g

Pharmacodynamics/Kinetics

Onset of action: Hypotensive: Oral: ~30 minutes

Peak effect: 2-8 hours

Duration: 2-5 days

Protein binding: None

Metabolism: 88%, primarily via glucuronidation

Bioavailability: Oral: 90%

Half-life elimination: Adults: 3.5-4.2 hours

Excretion: Urine (12% as unchanged drug)

Dosage

Children <12 years: Hypertension: Oral: Initial: 0.1-0.2 mg/kg once daily; maximum: 5 mg/day; increase gradually every 3 days; usual dosage: 0.25-1 mg/kg/day in 1-2 divided doses; maximum: 50 mg/day

Children >12 years and Adults: Hypertension: Oral: Initial: 5 mg once daily, increase gradually every 3 days (maximum: 100 mg/day); usual dose range (JNC 7): 2.5-80 mg/day in 1-2 divided doses

Adults: Alopecia: Topical: Apply twice daily; 4 months of therapy may be necessary for hair growth.

Elderly: Initial: 2.5 mg once daily; increase gradually.

Note: Dosage adjustment is needed when added to concomitant therapy.

Dialysis: Supplemental dose is not necessary via hemo- or peritoneal dialysis.

Monitoring Parameters Blood pressure, standing and sitting/supine; fluid and electrolyte balance and body weight should be monitored

Contraindications Hypersensitivity to minoxidil or any component of the formulation; pheochromocytoma; acute MI; dissecting aortic aneurysm

Warnings Maximum therapeutic doses of a diuretic and two antihypertensives should be used before this drug is ever added. **[U.S. Boxed Warning]: It can cause pericardial effusion, tamponade, or exacerbate angina pectoris.** Monitor patients who are receiving guanethidine concurrently (orthostasis can be problematic). May need to add a diuretic to minimize fluid gain and a beta-blocker (if no contraindications) to treat tachycardia. Rapid control of blood pressure can lead to syncope, CVA, MI, ischemia. Hypersensitivity reactions occur rarely. Avoid use for a month after acute MI. Inform patients of hair growth patterns before initiating therapy. May take 1-6 months for hypertrichosis to reverse itself after discontinuation of the drug. Use with caution in patients with pulmonary hypertension, significant renal failure, CHF, or ischemic disease. Renal failure and dialysis patients may require a smaller dose.

Dosage Forms

[DSC] = Discontinued product

Solution, topical: 2% [20 mg/metered dose] (60 mL); 5% [50 mg/metered dose] (60 mL)

Rogaine® for Men, Rogaine® for Women: 2% [20 mg/metered dose] (60 mL)

Rogaine® Extra Strength for Men: 5% [50 mg/metered dose] (60 mL)

Tablet: 2.5 mg, 10 mg

Loniten®: 2.5 mg [DSC], 10 mg

Reference Range Mean serum level (oral) for 5 mg: 59.2 ng/mL

Overdosage/Treatment

Decontamination: Ipecac within 30 minutes or lavage (within 1 hour)/ activated charcoal

Supportive therapy: Hypotension usually responds to I.V. fluids or Trendelenburg positioning. If unresponsive to these measures, the use of a parenteral vasoconstrictor may be required (eg, phenylephrine or dopamine). Treatment is primarily supportive and symptomatic.

Enhancement of elimination: Multiple dosing of activated charcoal is useful; hemodialysis may be useful; dialyzable (50% to 100%)

Test Interactions ↑ alkaline phosphatase

Drug Interactions

Antihypertensives: Effects may be additive.

Guanethidine can cause severe orthostasis; avoid concurrent use - discontinue 1-3 weeks prior to initiating minoxidil.

Pregnancy Risk Factor C

Nursing Implications May cause hirsutism

Additional Information Usually given in combination with a diuretic and beta-blocker

Specific Reference

Chobanian AV, Bakris GL, Black HR, et al, "The Seventh Report of the Joint National Committee on Prevention, Detection, Evaluation, and Treatment of High Blood Pressure: The JNC 7 Report," *JAMA*, 2003, 289(19):2560-71.

Mirtazapine

Related Information

- Antidepressant Agents

CAS Number 61337-67-5

U.S. Brand Names Remeron SolTab®; Remeron®

Impairment Potential Yes

Use Treatment of depression

Mechanism of Action Strong alpha₂ antagonist with similar properties to mianserin; a tetracyclic piperazinoazepine that is a presynaptic alpha₂-adrenoreceptor antagonist as well as a 5-HT₂ and 5-HT₃ antagonist thus enhancing noradrenergic and serotonergic neurotransmission; does not inhibit serotonin reuptake

Adverse Reactions

Cardiovascular: Angina pectoris, atrial arrhythmia, bigeminy, bradycardia, cardiomegaly, cerebral ischemia, chest pain, edema, facial edema, hypertension, hypotension, left heart failure, myocardial infarction, peripheral edema, syncope, vasodilatation, ventricular extrasystoles, torsade de pointes, vascular headache

Central nervous system: Abnormal dreams, abnormal thoughts, confusion, malaise, agitation, akathisia, amnesia, anxiety, apathy, aphasia, ataxia, chills, coordination abnormal, delirium, delusions, dementia, depersonalization, depression, dizziness, dystonia, emotional lability, euphoria, extrapyramidal syndrome, fever, grand mal seizure, hallucinations, hostility, hypesthesia, hypotonia, manic reaction, migraine, neurosis, paranoid reaction, psychotic depression, **somnolence (54%)**, stupor, vertigo

Dermatologic: Acne, alopecia, cellulitis, dry skin, exfoliative dermatitis, petechia, photosensitivity reaction, pruritus, rash, seborrhea, skin hypertrophy, skin ulcer, urticaria

Endocrine & metabolic: Amenorrhea, breast engorgement, breast enlargement, breast pain, **cholesterol increased**, dehydration, diabetes mellitus, dysmenorrhea, goiter, gout, hypothyroidism, libido increased, menorrhagia, metrorrhagia, triglycerides increased

Gastrointestinal: Abdomen enlarged, abdominal pain, **appetite increased**, anorexia, aphthous stomatitis, colitis, constipation, eructation, gastroenteritis, gastritis, glossitis, gum hemorrhage, increased salivation, intestinal obstruction, nausea, oral moniliasis, pancreatitis, salivary gland enlargement, taste loss, tongue discoloration, tongue edema, ulcer, ulcerative stomatitis, vomiting, weight loss, **weight gain** (12%; weight gain of >7% reported in 8% of adults, ≤49% of pediatric patients) **xerostomia** (25%)

Genitourinary: Abnormal ejaculation, cystitis, dysuria, impotence, leukorrhea, urethritis, urinary frequency, urinary incontinence, urinary retention, urinary tract infection, urinary urgency, vaginitis

Hematologic: Agranulocytosis, anemia, leukopenia, pancytopenia, thrombocytopenia

Hepatic: Cholecystitis, cirrhosis, liver function tests abnormal

Local: Phlebitis

Neuromuscular & skeletal: Arthralgias, arthrosis, arthritis, back pain, bone pain, bursitis, dysarthria, dyskinesia, fracture, hypokinesia, hyperkinesias, myoclonus, myalgia, myositis, neck pain, neck rigidity, osteoporosis, paralysis, paresthesia, reflexes increased, tendon rupture, tenosynovitis, tremor, twitching, weakness

Ocular: Accomodation abnormality, blepharitis, conjunctivitis, diplopia, eye pain, glaucoma, keratoconjunctivitis, lacrimation disorder, nystagmus

Otic: Deafness, ear pain, hyperacusis, otitis media

Renal: Hematuria, kidney calculus, polyuria

Respiratory: Asphyxia, asthma, bronchitis, cough, dyspnea, epistaxis, laryngitis, pneumonia, pneumothorax, pulmonary embolus, sinusitis

Miscellaneous: Flu-like symptoms, thirst, drug dependence, hiccups, lymphadenopathy, lymphocytosis, herpes simplex, herpes zoster, parosmia, withdrawal syndrome

Signs and Symptoms of Overdose Coma, disorientation, drowsiness, sedation, lethargy, leukocytosis, somnolence, tachycardia (30%). Little or no cardiac complications.

Admission Criteria/Prognosis Admit any ingestion >100 mg or any symptomatic patient with change in mental status; for any polydrug overdose or ingestion >1 g, hospital admission should be considered.

Pharmacodynamics/Kinetics

Protein binding: 85%

Metabolism: Extensively hepatic via CYP1A2, 2C9, 2D6, 3A4 and via demethylation and hydroxylation

Bioavailability: 50%

Half-life elimination: 20-40 hours; hampered with renal or hepatic impairment

Time to peak, serum: 2 hours

Excretion: Urine (75%) and feces (15%) as metabolites

Dosage

Children: Safety and efficacy in children have not been established

Treatment of depression: Adults: Oral: Initial: 15 mg nightly, titrate up to 15-45 mg/day with dose increases made no more frequently than every 1-2 weeks; there is an inverse relationship between dose and sedation

Elderly: Decreased clearance seen (40% males, 10% females); no specific dosage adjustment recommended by manufacturer

Dosage adjustment in renal impairment:

Cl_{cr} 11-39 mL/minute: 30% decreased clearance

Cl_{cr} <10 mL/minute: 50% decreased clearance

Dosage adjustment in hepatic impairment: Clearance decreased by 30%

Monitoring Parameters Patients should be monitored for signs of agranulocytosis or severe neutropenia such as sore throat, stomatitis or other signs of infection or a low WBC; mental status for depression, suicidal ideation (especially at the beginning of therapy or when doses are increased or decreased), anxiety, social functioning, mania, panic attacks; lipid profile

Administration SolTab®: Open blister pack and place tablet on the tongue. Do not split tablet. Tablet is formulated to dissolve on the tongue without water.

Contraindications Hypersensitivity to mirtazapine or any component of the formulation; use of MAO inhibitors within 14 days

Warnings

[U.S. Boxed Warning]: Antidepressants increase the risk of suicidal thinking and behavior in children and adolescents with major depressive disorder (MDD) and other depressive disorders; consider risk prior to prescribing. Closely monitor for clinical worsening, suicidality, or unusual changes in behavior; the child's family or caregiver should be instructed to closely observe the patient and communicate condition with healthcare provider. Such observation would generally include at least weekly face-to-face contact with patients or their family members or caregivers during the first 4 weeks of treatment, then every other week visits for the next 4 weeks, then at 12 weeks, and as clinically indicated beyond 12 weeks. Additional contact by telephone may be appropriate between face-to-face visits. Adults treated with antidepressants should be observed similarly for clinical worsening and suicidality, especially during the initial few months of a course of drug therapy, or at times of dose changes, either increases or decreases. A medication guide should be dispensed with each prescription. **Mirtazapine is not FDA approved for use in children.**

The possibility of a suicide attempt is inherent in major depression and may persist until remission occurs. Monitor for worsening of depression or suicidality, especially during initiation of therapy or with dose increases or decreases. Worsening depression and severe abrupt suicidality that are not part of the presenting symptoms may require discontinuation or modification of drug therapy. Use caution in high-risk patients during initiation of therapy. Prescriptions should be written for the smallest quantity consistent with good patient care. The patient's family or caregiver should be alerted to monitor patients for the emergence of suicidality and associated behaviors such as anxiety, agitation, panic attacks, insomnia, irritability, hostility, impulsivity, akathisia, hypomania, and mania; patients should be instructed to notify their healthcare provider if any of these symptoms or worsening depression occur.

May worsen psychosis in some patients or precipitate a shift to mania or hypomania in patients with bipolar disorder. Monotherapy in patients with bipolar disorder should be avoided. Patients presenting with depressive symptoms should be screened for bipolar disorder. **Mirtazapine is not FDA approved for the treatment of bipolar depression.**

Discontinue immediately if signs and symptoms of neutropenia/agranulocytosis occur. May cause sedation, resulting in impaired performance of tasks requiring alertness (eg, operating machinery or driving). Sedative effects may be additive with other CNS depressants and/or ethanol. The degree of sedation is moderate-high relative to other antidepressants. The risks of orthostatic hypotension or anticholinergic effects are low relative to other antidepressants. The incidence of sexual dysfunction with mirtazapine is generally lower than with SSRIs.

May increase appetite and stimulate weight gain. Weight gain of >7% of body weight reported in 7.5% of patients treated with mirtazapine compared to 0% for placebo; 8% of patients receiving mirtazapine discontinued treatment due to the weight gain. In an 8-week pediatric clinical trial, 49% of mirtazapine-treated patients had a weight gain of at least 7% (mean increase 4 kg) as compared to 5.7% of placebo-treated patients (mean increase 1 kg).

May increase serum cholesterol and triglyceride levels. Use caution in patients with a previous seizure disorder or condition predisposing to seizures such as brain damage, alcoholism, or concurrent therapy with other drugs which lower the seizure threshold. Use with caution in patients with hepatic or renal dysfunction and in elderly patients. SolTab® formulation contains phenylalanine.

Dosage Forms Tablet (Remeron®): 15 mg, 30 mg, 45 mg

Tablet, orally disintegrating: 15 mg, 30 mg

Remeron SolTab®:

15 mg [contains phenylalanine 2.6 mg/tablet; orange flavor]

30 mg [contains phenylalanine 5.2 mg/tablet; orange flavor]

45 mg [contains phenylalanine 7.8 mg/tablet; orange flavor]

Reference Range Following a 20 mg oral dose, peak serum levels: ~100 ng/mL; serum level of 2300 ng/mL associated with a 900 mg ingestion and somnolence

Overdosage/Treatment

Decontamination: **Do not** induce emesis; lavage (within 1 hour)/activated charcoal

Supportive therapy: Treat seizures with diazepam or lorazepam; phenobarbital is second choice; atropine or isoproterenol can be used for bradycardia

Enhancement of elimination: Multiple dosing of activated charcoal or hemodialysis is not likely to be effective

Drug Interactions Substrate of CYP1A2 (major), 2C9 (minor), 2D6 (major), 3A4 (major); **Inhibits** CYP1A2 (weak), 3A4 (weak)

Clonidine: Antihypertensive effects of clonidine may be antagonized by mirtazapine (hypertensive urgency has been reported following addition of mirtazapine to clonidine); in addition, mirtazapine may potentially enhance the hypertensive response associated with abrupt clonidine withdrawal. Avoid this combination; consider an alternative agent.

CNS depressants: Sedative effects may be additive with other CNS depressants; monitor for increased effect; includes barbiturates, benzodiazepines, narcotic analgesics, ethanol and other sedative agents

CYP1A2 inducers: May decrease the levels/effects of mirtazapine. Example inducers include aminoglutethimide, carbamazepine, phenobarbital, and rifampin.

CYP1A2 inhibitors: May increase the levels/effects of mirtazapine. Example inhibitors include ciprofloxacin, fluvoxamine, ketoconazole, norfloxacin, ofloxacin, and rofecoxib.

CYP2D6 inhibitors: May increase the levels/effects of mirtazapine. Example inhibitors include chlorpromazine, delavirdine, fluoxetine, miconazole, paroxetine, pergolide, quinidine, quinine, ritonavir, and ropinirole.

CYP3A4 inducers: CYP3A4 inducers may decrease the levels/effects of mirtazapine. Example inducers include aminoglutethimide, carbamazepine, nafcillin, nevirapine, phenobarbital, phenytoin, and rifamycins.

CYP3A4 inhibitors: May increase the levels/effects of mirtazapine. Example inhibitors include azole antifungals, clarithromycin, diclofenac, doxycycline, erythromycin, imatinib, isoniazid, nefazodone, nicardipine, propofol, protease inhibitors, quinidine, telithromycin, and verapamil.

Linezolid: Due to MAO inhibition (see note on MAO inhibitors), this combination should be avoided

MAO inhibitors: Possibly serious or fatal reactions can occur when given with or when given within 14 days of an MAO inhibitor; use is contraindicated.

Selegiline: Interaction is less likely than with nonselective MAO inhibitors (see MAO inhibitor information), but theoretically possible; monitor

Sibutramine: Potential for serotonin syndrome when used in combination

Pregnancy Risk Factor C

Pregnancy Implications Animal studies did not show teratogenic effects, however, there was an increase in fetal loss and decrease in birth weight; use during pregnancy only if clearly needed.

Lactation Excretion in breast milk unknown/not recommended

Specific References

Garlipp P, Brüggemann BR, and Machleidt W, "A Non-Fatal Mirtazapine Overdose in a Suicide Attempt," *Australian and NZJ Psychiatry*, 2003, 37(4):244-5.

Kirkton C and McIntyre IM, "Therapeutic and Toxic Concentrations of Mirtazapine (Remeron®) in Postmortem Cases," *J Anal Toxicol*, 2006, 30:134.

Kirkton C and McIntyre IM, "Therapeutic and Toxic Concentrations of Mirtazapine," *J Anal Tox*, 2006, 30:687-91.

Langford NJ, Ferner RE, Patel H, et al, "Mirtazepine Overdose and Miosis," *J Toxicol Clin Toxicol*, 2003, 41(7):1037-8.

Meineke I, Kress I, Poser W, et al, "Therapeutic Drug Monitoring of Mirtazapine and Its Metabolite Desmethylmirtazapine by HPLC with Fluorescence Detection," *Ther Drug Monit*, 2004, 26(3):277-83.

Ranjan S, Chandra PS, and Chaturved SK, "Atypical Antipsychotic-Induced Akathisia with Depression: Therapeutic Role of Mirtazepine," *Ann Pharmacother*, 2006, 40(4):771-4.

Riley BD, LoVecchio F, Pizon AF, et al, "Isolated Mirtazapine Ingestions Typically Reult in Altered Mental Status," *Clin Toxicol (Phila)*, 2005, 43:743.

Shams M, Hiemke C, and HûÊrtter S, "Therapeutic Drug Monitoring of the Antidepressant Mirtazapine and Its N-Demethylated Metabolite in Human Serum," *Ther Drug Monit*, 2004, 26(1):78-84.

Waring WS, Good AM, and Bateman DN, "Lack of Significant Toxicity After Mirtazapine Overdose: Five-Year Review of Cases Admitted to a Regional Toxicology Unit," *Clin Toxicol (Phila)*, 2005, 43:728.

Waring WS, Good AM, and Bateman DN, "Lack of Significant Toxicity After Mirtazapine Overdose: A Five-Year Review of Cases Admitted to a Regional Toxicology Unit," *Clin Toxicol*, 2007, 45:45-50.

Misoprostol

CAS Number 59122-46-2

U.S. Brand Names Cytotec®

Use Prevention of NSAID-induced gastric ulcers; medical termination of pregnancy of ≤49 days (in conjunction with mifepristone)

Unlabeled/Investigational Use Cervical ripening and labor induction; NSAID-induced nephropathy; fat malabsorption in cystic fibrosis

Mechanism of Action Misoprostol is a synthetic prostaglandin E_1 analog that replaces the protective prostaglandins consumed with prostaglandin-inhibiting therapies (eg, nonsteroidal anti-inflammatory drugs); has been shown to induce uterine contractions

Adverse Reactions

Cardiovascular: Angina, chest pain, MI, arterial thrombosis

Central nervous system: Headache, CNS depression, depression, hyperthermia

Endocrine & metabolic: Abortifacient

Gastrointestinal: **Diarrhea (14% to 40%)**, **abdominal pain**, constipation, flatulence, nausea, vomiting, cramps

Genitourinary: Uterine stimulation, vaginal bleeding, uterine rupture

Respiratory: Pulmonary embolism

Miscellaneous: Thirst

Signs and Symptoms of Overdose Abdominal cramps, fever, hypertension, metabolic acidosis, rhabdomyolysis, tachycardia, tremor (3 g ingestion)

Admission Criteria/Prognosis Admit any adult ingestion >3 mg

Pharmacodynamics/Kinetics

Absorption: Rapid

Metabolism: Hepatic; rapidly de-esterified to misoprostol acid (active)

Half-life elimination: Metabolite: 20-40 minutes

Time to peak, serum: Active metabolite: Fasting: 15-30 minutes

Excretion: Urine (64% to 73%) and feces (15%) within 24 hours

Dosage Oral:

Children 8-16 years: Fat absorption in cystic fibrosis (unlabeled use): 100 mcg 4 times/day

Adults:

Prevention of NSAID-induced gastric ulcers: 200 mcg 4 times/day with food; if not tolerated, may decrease dose to 100 mcg 4 times/day with food or 200 mcg twice daily with food; last dose of the day should be taken at bedtime

Medical termination of pregnancy: Refer to Mifepristone.

Intravaginal: Adults: Labor induction or cervical ripening (unlabeled use): 25 mcg ($^1/_4$ of 100 mcg tablet); may repeat at intervals no more frequent than every 3-6 hours. Do not use in patients with previous cesarean delivery or prior major uterine surgery.

Administration Incidence of diarrhea may be lessened by having patient take dose right after meals. Therapy is usually begun on the second or third day of the next normal menstrual period.

Contraindications Hypersensitivity to misoprostol, prostaglandins, or any component of the formulation; pregnancy (when used to reduce NSAID-induced ulcers)

Warnings Safety and efficacy have not been established in children <18 years of age; use with caution in patients with renal impairment and the elderly. **[U.S. Boxed Warning]: Not to be used in women of child-bearing potential unless woman is capable of complying with effective contraceptive measures;** therapy is normally begun on the second or third day of next normal menstrual period. Uterine perforation and/or rupture have been reported in association with intravaginal use to induce labor or with combined oral/intravaginal use to induce abortion. The manufacturer states that Cytotec® should not be used as a cervical-ripening agent for induction of labor. However, The American College of Obstetricians and Gynecologists (ACOG) continues to support this off-label use.

Dosage Forms Tablet: 100 mcg, 200 mcg

Reference Range Peak blood misoprostol level after a 400 mcg oral dose is ~500 pg/mL

Overdosage/Treatment

Decontamination: Activated charcoal

Supportive therapy: Psyllium hydrophobic mucilliod (3.4 g twice daily) can be used to treat misoprostol-induced diarrhea

Drug Interactions Oxytocin: Misoprostol may increase the effect of oxytocin; wait 6-12 hours after misoprostol administration before initiating oxytocin.

Pregnancy Risk Factor X

Pregnancy Implications Misoprostol is an abortifacient. During pregnancy, use to prevent NSAID-induced ulcers is contraindicated. Reports of fetal death, congenital anomalies, uterine perforation, and abortion have been received after the use of misoprostol in pregnancy. Excretion in breast milk is unknown; breast-feeding is contraindicated. See Additional Information.

Lactation Excretion in breast milk unknown/contraindicated

Nursing Implications Incidence of diarrhea may be lessened by having patient take dose right after meals

Additional Information Has been utilized in self-abortion attempts; misoprostol (200 mcg) can prevent diclofenac-induced gastric ulcers (**not** duodenal ulcers)

When used to prevent NSAID-induced ulcers: Inform prescriber if you are pregnant. Do not get pregnant during or for 1 month following therapy. Male: Do not cause a female to become pregnant. Male/female: Consult prescriber for instruction on appropriate contraceptive measures. This drug may cause severe fetal defects, miscarriage, or abortion; do not share medication with others. Do not breast-feed.

Mitoxantrone

CAS Number 65271-80-9; 70476-82-3

U.S. Brand Names Novantrone®

Synonyms DAD; DHAD; DHAQ; Dihydroxyanthracenedione Dihydrochloride; Mitoxantrone Hydrochloride CL-232315; Mitozantrone; NSC-301739

Use Treatment of acute leukemias, lymphoma, breast cancer, pediatric sarcoma, progressive or relapsing-remitting multiple sclerosis, prostate cancer

Mechanism of Action Analogue of the anthracyclines, mitoxantrone intercalates DNA; binds to nucleic acids and inhibits DNA and RNA synthesis by template disordering and steric obstruction; replication is decreased by binding to DNA topoisomerase II and seems to inhibit the incorporation of uridine into RNA and thymidine into DNA; active throughout entire cell cycle

Adverse Reactions

Cardiovascular: **Arrhythmia (3% to 18%)**, **edema, nail bed changes**, CHF (2% to 3%; risk is much lower with anthracyclines, some reports suggest cumulative doses >160 mg/mL cause CHF in ~10% of patients), ECG changes, hypotension, ischemia, LVEF decreased (≤5%), tachycardia

Central nervous system: **Fatigue, fever, headache (6% to 13%)**, chills, anxiety, depression, seizures

Dermatologic: **Alopecia (20% to 61%)**, skin infection, irritant chemotherapy with blue skin discoloration, rash

Endocrine & metabolic: **Amenorrhea, menstrual disorder**, hypocalcemia, hypokalemia, hyponatremia, hyperglycemia

Gastrointestinal: **Abdominal pain, anorexia, nausea (29% to 76%), constipation, diarrhea (16% to 47%), GI bleeding, mucositis (10% to 29%), stomatitis, vomiting, weight gain/loss**, dyspepsia, aphthosis

Genitourinary: **Abnormal urine, urinary tract infection**, impotence, proteinuria, renal failure, sterility

Hematologic: **Hemoglobin decreased, leukopenia, lymphopenia, petechiae/bruising**, acute leukemia, anemia, granulocytopenia, hemorrhage; myelosuppressive effects of chemotherapy:

WBC: Mild

Platelets: Mild

Onset: 7-10 days

Nadir: 14 days

Recovery: 21 days

Hepatic: **Increased GGT**, jaundice, increased SGOT, increased SGPT

Local: Extravasation and phlebitis at the infusion site

Neuromuscular & skeletal: **Weakness (24%)**, back pain, myalgia, arthralgia

Ocular: Blurred vision, conjunctivitis

Renal: Hematuria

Respiratory: **Cough, dyspnea, upper respiratory tract infection**, pneumonia, rhinitis, sinusitis, interstitial pneumonitis (has occurred during combination chemotherapy)

Miscellaneous: **Fungal infections, infection, sepsis**, systemic infection, sweats, development of secondary leukemia (~1% to 2%), allergic reaction, anaphylactoid reactions, anaphylaxis

Signs and Symptoms of Overdose Leukopenia, marrow hypoplasia (pancytopenia), nausea, shaking chills, tachycardia, vomiting

Pharmacodynamics/Kinetics
Absorption: Oral: Poor
Distribution: V_d: 14 L/kg; distributes into pleural fluid, kidney, thyroid, liver, heart, and red blood cells
Protein binding: >95%, 76% to albumin
Metabolism: Hepatic; pathway not determined
Half-life elimination: Terminal: 23-215 hours; may be prolonged with hepatic impairment
Excretion: Urine (6% to 11%) and feces as unchanged drug and metabolites

Dosage Refer to individual protocols. I.V. (dilute in D_5W or NS):
Acute leukemias:
Children ≤2 years: 0.4 mg/kg/day once daily for 3-5 days
Children >2 years and Adults: 8-12 mg/m²/day once daily for 4-5 days
Solid tumors:
Children: 18-20 mg/m² every 3-4 weeks **or** 5-8 mg/m² every week
Adults: 12-14 mg/m² every 3-4 weeks **or** 2-4 mg/m²/day for 5 days every 4 weeks
Hormone-refractory prostate cancer: Adults: 12-14 mg/m²
Multiple sclerosis: Adults: 12 mg/m²
Dosing adjustment in renal impairment: Safety and efficacy have not been established
Hemodialysis: Supplemental dose is not necessary
Peritoneal dialysis: Supplemental dose is not necessary
Elderly: Clearance is decreased in elderly patients; use with caution
Dosing adjustment in hepatic impairment: Official dosage adjustment recommendations have not been established.
Moderate dysfunction (bilirubin 1.5-3 mg/dL): Some clinicians recommend a 50% dosage reduction
Severe dysfunction (bilirubin >3.0 mg/dL) may require a dosage adjustment to 8 mg/m²; some clinicians recommend a dosage reduction to 25% of dose

Stability Store intact vials at room temperature or refrigeration
Dilute in at least 50 mL of NS or D_5W; solution is stable for 7 days at room temperature or refrigeration
Incompatible with heparin and hydrocortisone
Standard I.V. dilution:
IVPB: Dose/100 mL D_5W or NS
Solution is stable for 7 days at room temperature and refrigeration

Monitoring Parameters CBC, serum uric acid (for treatment of leukemia), liver function tests, signs and symptoms of CHF; evaluate LVEF prior to start of therapy and regularly during treatment. In addition, for the treatment of multiple sclerosis, monitor LVEF prior to all doses following cumulative dose of ≥100 mg/m².

Administration Administered as a short (15-30 minutes) I.V. infusion; continuous 24-hour infusions are occasionally used. Although not generally recommended, mitoxantrone has been given as a rapid bolus over 1-3 minutes. High doses for bone marrow transplant are usually given as 1- to 4-hour infusions.

Contraindications Hypersensitivity to mitoxantrone or any component of the formulation; multiple sclerosis with left ventricular ejection fraction (LVEF) <50% or clinically significant decrease in LVEF; pregnancy

Warnings
Hazardous agent – use appropriate precautions for handling and disposal.
[U.S. Boxed Warning]: Do not use if baseline neutrophil count <1500 cells/mm³ (except for in the treatment of ANLL). Treatment may lead to severe myelosuppression; use with caution in patients with pre-existing myelosuppression.
[U.S. Boxed Warning]: May cause myocardial toxicity and potentially-fatal CHF; risk increases with cumulative dosing. Predisposing factors for mitoxantrone-induced cardiotoxicity include prior anthracycline therapy, prior cardiovascular disease, concomitant use of cardiotoxic drugs, and mediastinal/pericardial irradiation. Not recommended for use when left ventricular ejection fraction (LVEF) <50%. Use in multiple sclerosis should be limited to a cumulative dose of ≤140 mg/m², and discontinued if a significant decrease in LVEF is observed.
[U.S. Boxed Warnings]: For I.V. use only; may cause severe local tissue damage if extravasation occurs. Do not administer intrathecally; may cause serious and permanent neurologic damage. May cause urine, saliva, tears, and sweat to turn blue-green for 24 hours postinfusion. Whites of eyes may have blue-green tinge. **[U.S. Boxed Warning]: Has been associated with the development of secondary acute myelogenous leukemia and myelodysplasia.**
[U.S. Boxed Warning]: Should be administered under the supervision of an experienced cancer chemotherapy physician. Dosage should be reduced in patients with impaired hepatobiliary function; not for treatment of multiple sclerosis in patients with concurrent hepatic impairment. Not for treatment of primary progressive multiple sclerosis. Safety and efficacy in children have not been established.

Dosage Forms Injection, solution: 2 mg/mL (10 mL, 12.5 mL, 15 mL)
Novantrone®: 2 mg/mL (10 mL, 12.5 mL, 15 mL)

Overdosage/Treatment
No known antidote
Supportive therapy: Bradycardia may respond to atropine; consider reverse isolation; pancytopenia is usually reversible
Enhanced elimination: Hemoperfusion or hemodialysis is not useful

Test Interactions May cause a 50% reduction of prostate specific antigen, which does not correlate with response

Drug Interactions Inhibits CYP3A4 (weak)
Patients may experience impaired immune response to vaccines; possible infection after administration of live vaccines in patients receiving immunosuppressants

Pregnancy Risk Factor D

Pregnancy Implications May cause fetal harm if administered to a pregnant woman. Women with multiple sclerosis and who are biologically capable of becoming pregnant should have a pregnancy test prior to each dose.

Lactation Enters breast milk/contraindicated

Nursing Implications Vesicant; avoid extravasation
Mitoxantrone is excreted in human milk and significant concentrations (180 mg/mL) have been reported for 28 days after the last administration. Because of the potential for serious adverse reactions in infants from mitoxantrone, breast-feeding should be discontinued before starting treatment.

Additional Information Indications for stopping mitoxantrone due to cardiac toxicity include endomyocardial biopsy with evidence of characteristic changes of cardiomyopathy induced by an anthracycline (ie, distention of sarcoplasmic reticulum, vacuole formation and myofibrillar dropout), and/or a ≥20% decrease in cardiac ejection fraction

Moclobemide

CAS Number 71320-77-9
Use Symptomatic relief of depressive illness
Unlabeled/Investigational Use Depression; smoking cessation
Mechanism of Action Selective and reversible monoamine oxidase (type A) inhibitor

Adverse Reactions
Cardiovascular: Hypertension, tachycardia, sinus tachycardia, vasoconstriction
Central nervous system: Agitation, dizziness, headache, hypomania, insomnia, anxiety
Dermatologic: Rash, pruritus, alopecia
Gastrointestinal: **Xerostomia**, constipation, nausea, stomach pain
Hepatic: Cholestasis
Neuromuscular & skeletal: Tremor
Ocular: Blurred vision
Miscellaneous: **Diaphoresis**

Signs and Symptoms of Overdose Disorientation, tachycardia, tachypnea

Admission Criteria/Prognosis Any symptomatic patient or adult ingestion >1 g should be considered for admission to a cardiac-monitored bed or intensive care unit (ICU)

Pharmacodynamics/Kinetics
Absorption: 98% from GI tract
Distribution: 1.2 L/kg
Protein binding: ~50% to albumin
Metabolism: Oxidative reactions
Half-life elimination: Terminal: 1-2 hours
Excretion: Urine (95%, as metabolites)

Dosage
Oral:
Depression: Initial: 100 mg 3 times/day immediately following a meal; maximum dose/day: 600 mg; reduce dosage by 30% to 50% in patients with hepatic disease
Smoking cessation: 400 mg/day for 2 months, then, 200 mg/day for 1 month

Monitoring Parameters Blood pressure, warning signs of suicide
Administration Administer immediately after meals.
Contraindications Hypersensitivity to moclobemide or any component of the formulation; uncontrolled hypertension; hepatic disease; confusional states; concurrent use of sympathomimetics (and related compounds), MAO inhibitors, meperidine, tricyclic antidepressants, serotonergic drugs (including SSRIs) - do not use within 5 weeks of fluoxetine discontinuation or 2 weeks of other antidepressant discontinuation; general anesthesia, local vasoconstrictors; spinal anesthesia (hypotension may be exaggerated). Not approved for use in patients <18 years of age.

Warnings The possibility of a suicide attempt is inherent in major depression and may persist until remission occurs. Use caution in high-risk patients during initiation of therapy. Prescriptions should be written for the smallest quantity consistent with good patient care. Use caution in patients with thyrotoxicosis, pheochromocytoma, and renal dysfunction. Use caution in patients receiving concurrent CNS depressants, ethanol, or buspirone. Severe reactions may occur if MAO inhibitors and serotonergic agents, including SSRIs are used concurrently. Discontinue 2 days prior to local or general anesthesia. Use caution in hepatic impairment (dose adjustment required). Dietary restriction of tyramine does not appear to be necessary for patients receiving moclobemide (patients must be informed of signs/symptoms of reaction).

Dosage Forms Tablet: 150 mg, 300 mg

Reference Range Therapeutic serum range: 0.5-1.5 mg/L; plasma moclobemide levels as high as 62.5 mg/L associated with drowsiness

Overdosage/Treatment

Decontamination: Lavage within 2 hours of ingestion/activated charcoal

Supportive therapy: Competent supportive care is the most important treatment for an overdose with a monoamine oxidase (MAO) inhibitor. Both hypertension or hypotension can occur with intoxication. Hypotension may respond to I.V. fluids or vasopressors and hypertension usually responds to an alpha-adrenergic blocker. While treating the hypertension, care is warranted to avoid sudden drops in blood pressure, since this may worsen the MAO inhibitor toxicity. Muscle irritability and seizures often respond to diazepam or lorazepam, while hyperthermia is best treated antipyretics and cooling blankets. Cardiac arrhythmias are best treated with phenytoin or procainamide. Hypertensive crisis can be treated with nitroprusside, phentolamine (2-10 mg slow I.V. injection in adults), diazoxide (50-100 mg I.V.) or oral nifedipine (10 mg); dantrolene (2.5 mg/kg every 6 hours I.V.) can be used to treat hypermetabolic crisis.

Drug Interactions

Substrate (major) of CYP2C19, 2D6; **Inhibits** CYP1A2 (weak), 2C19 (weak), 2D6 (weak)

Anesthetics: Moclobemide should be stopped at least 2 days prior to using (local or general).

Antihypertensive agents: Moclobemide may decrease antihypertensive effect; use with caution. Monitor.

Antipsychotics: Moclobemide may exacerbate psychotic disorders.

Cimetidine: May increase moclobemide serum concentrations; consider 50% reduction in moclobemide dose.

CYP2C19 inducers: May decrease the levels/effects of moclobemide. Example inducers include aminoglutethimide, carbamazepine, phenytoin, and rifampin.

CYP2C19 inhibitors: May increase the levels/effects of moclobemide. Example inhibitors include delavirdine, fluconazole, fluvoxamine, gemfibrozil, isoniazid, omeprazole, and ticlopidine.

CYP2D6 inhibitors: May increase the levels/effects of moclobemide. Example inhibitors include chlorpromazine, delavirdine, fluoxetine, miconazole, paroxetine, pergolide, quinidine, quinine, ritonavir, and ropinirole.

Dextromethorphan: Concomitant use increases risk of serotonin syndrome; avoid concurrent use.

MAO inhibitors (conventional): Concomitant use increases risk of severe adverse reactions; concurrent use is contraindicated.

Meperidine: May increase the risk of severe adverse reactions; concurrent use is contraindicated.

Opiates: Moclobemide potentiates effects; avoid meperidine.

SSRIs: Concomitant use increases risk of serotonin syndrome. Do not use within 5 weeks of fluoxetine discontinuation or 2 weeks of other antidepressant discontinuation.

Sympathomimetic amines: Concomitant use may cause hypertension; concurrent use is contraindicated.

Tramadol: An increase risk of seizures and/or serotonin syndrome has been described with other MAO inhibitors; avoid concurrent use.

Tricyclic antidepressants: Concomitant use increases risk of severe adverse reactions; concurrent use is contraindicated.

Pregnancy Risk Factor Not available

Pregnancy Implications Safety has not been established, use only if benefits outweigh the risks.

Lactation Enters breast milk/use caution

Nursing Implications Monitor patients for signs of suicide risk; administer immediately after meals; monitor blood pressure

Specific Reference

Bleumink GS, van Vliet ACM, van der Tholen A, et al, "Fatal Combination of Moclobemide Overdose and Whisky," *Neth J Med*, 2003, 61(3): 88-90.

Molindone

Related Information

- Anticholinergic Effects of Common Psychotropics
- Antipsychotic Agents

CAS Number 15622-65-8; 7416-34-4

U.S. Brand Names Moban®

Synonyms Molindone Hydrochloride

Use Management of schizophrenia

Unlabeled/Investigational Use Management of psychotic disorders

Mechanism of Action Mechanism of action mimics that of chlorpromazine; however, it produces more extrapyramidal effects and less sedation than chlorpromazine

Adverse Reactions

Cardiovascular: **Hypotension (orthostatic)**, tachycardia, cardiac arrhythmias, sinus tachycardia

Central nervous system: **Extrapyramidal reactions, akathisia, persistent tardive dyskinesia**, pseudoparkinsonian signs and symptoms, seizures, altered central temperature regulation, neuroleptic malignant syndrome, restlessness, fever, sedation, drowsiness, restlessness, anxiety, hyperthermia

Dermatologic: Hyperpigmentation, pruritus, rash, photosensitivity

Endocrine & metabolic: Amenorrhea, galactorrhea, gynecomastia, syndrome of inappropriate antidiuretic hormone

Gastrointestinal: **Xerostomia, constipation**, GI upset, weight gain

Genitourinary: Urinary retention

Hematologic: Agranulocytosis (more often in women between fourth and tenth weeks of therapy); leukopenia (usually in patients with large doses for prolonged periods)

Hepatic: Elevated liver transaminases

Ocular: **Blurred vision**, retinal pigmentation

Miscellaneous: **Diaphoresis (decreased)**, systemic lupus erythematosus

Signs and Symptoms of Overdose Agranulocytosis, cardiac arrhythmias, deep sleep, extrapyramidal reaction, galactorrhea, granulocytopenia, gynecomastia, leukocytosis, leukopenia, myoglobinuria with oliguria, neuroleptic malignant syndrome, neutropenia, Parkinson's-like symptoms, priapism, renal failure, rhabdomyolysis

Pharmacodynamics/Kinetics

Metabolism: Hepatic

Half-life elimination: 1.5 hours

Time to peak, serum: ~1.5 hours

Excretion: Urine and feces (90%) within 24 hours

Dosage Oral:

Children: Schizophrenia/psychoses:

3-5 years: 1-2.5 mg/day in 4 divided doses

5-12 years: 0.5-1 mg/kg/day in 4 divided doses

Adults: Schizophrenia/psychoses: 50-75 mg/day increase at 3- to 4-day intervals up to 225 mg/day

Elderly: Behavioral symptoms associated with dementia: Initial: 5-10 mg 1-2 times/day; increase at 4- to 7-day intervals by 5-10 mg/day; increase dosing intervals (bid, tid, etc) as necessary to control response or side effects.

Monitoring Parameters Vital signs; lipid profile, fasting blood glucose/ Hgb A1$_c$; BMI; mental status, abnormal involuntary movement scale (AIMS), extrapyramidal symptoms (EPS)

Contraindications Hypersensitivity to molindone or any component of the formulation (cross-reactivity between phenothiazines may occur); severe CNS depression; coma

Warnings

May be sedating, use with caution in disorders where CNS depression is a feature. Use with caution in Parkinson's disease. Caution in patients with hemodynamic instability; bone marrow suppression; predisposition to seizures; subcortical brain damage; severe cardiac, hepatic, renal, or respiratory disease. Esophageal dysmotility and aspiration have been associated with antipsychotic use - use with caution in patients at risk of pneumonia (ie, Alzheimer's disease). Caution in breast cancer or other prolactin-dependent tumors (may elevate prolactin levels). May alter temperature regulation or mask toxicity of other drugs due to antiemetic effects. May alter cardiac conduction; life-threatening arrhythmias have occurred with therapeutic doses of neuroleptics. May cause orthostatic hypotension - use with caution in patients at risk of this effect or those who would tolerate transient hypotensive episodes (cerebrovascular disease, cardiovascular disease, or other medications which may predispose).

May cause anticholinergic effects (confusion, agitation, constipation, xerostomia, blurred vision, urinary retention); therefore, they should be used with caution in patients with decreased gastrointestinal motility, urinary retention, BPH, xerostomia, or visual problems. Conditions which also may be exacerbated by cholinergic blockade include narrow-angle glaucoma (screening is recommended) and worsening of myasthenia gravis. Relative to other neuroleptics, molindone has a low potency of cholinergic blockade.

May cause extrapyramidal symptoms, including pseudoparkinsonism, acute dystonic reactions, akathisia, and tardive dyskinesia (risk of these reactions is moderate-high relative to other neuroleptics). May be associated with neuroleptic malignant syndrome (NMS) or pigmentary retinopathy.

Dosage Forms Tablet, as hydrochloride: 5 mg, 10 mg, 25 mg, 50 mg

Reference Range Antipsychotic range: 27-69 ng/mL; level of 152 ng/mL seen with rhabdomyolysis

Overdosage/Treatment

Decontamination: **Oral**: Activated charcoal or gastric lavage for ingestions >500 mg in adults

Supportive therapy: Following initiation of essential overdose management, toxic symptom treatment and supportive treatment should be initiated. Hypotension usually responds to I.V. fluids or Trendelenburg positioning. If unresponsive to these measures, the use of a parenteral inotrope may be required (eg, norepinephrine 0.1-0.2 mcg/kg/minute titrated to response). Seizures commonly respond to lorazepam or diazepam (I.V. 5-10 mg bolus in adults every 15 minutes if needed up to a total of 30 mg; I.V. 0.25-0.4 mg/kg/dose up to a total of 10 mg in children) or to phenytoin or phenobarbital. Also critical cardiac arrhythmias often respond to I.V. phenytoin (15 mg/kg up to 1 gram), while other antiarrhythmics can be used. Neuroleptics often cause extrapyramidal reaction (eg, dystonic reactions) requiring management with diphenhydramine 1-2 mg/kg (adults) up to a maximum of 50 mg I.M. or I.V. slow push followed by a maintenance dose for 48-72 hours. When these reactions are unresponsive to diphenhydramine, benztropine mesylate I.V. 1-2 mg (adults) may be effective. These agents are generally effective within 2-5 minutes. Lidocaine is the first line agent for treatment of ventricular arrhythmias. Amiodarone may also be useful.

Test Interactions May result in false-positive tricyclics by the EMIT® system

Drug Interactions

Acetylcholinesterase inhibitors (central): May increase the risk of antipsychotic-related extrapyramidal symptoms; monitor.

Aluminum salts: May decrease the absorption of antipsychotics; monitor

Amphetamines: Efficacy may be diminished by antipsychotics; in addition, amphetamines may increase psychotic symptoms; avoid concurrent use

Anticholinergics: May inhibit the therapeutic response to antipsychotics and excess anticholinergic effects may occur; includes benztropine, trihexyphenidyl, biperiden, and drugs with significant anticholinergic activity (TCAs, antihistamines, disopyramide)

Antihypertensives: Concurrent use of antipsychotics with an antihypertensive may produce additive hypotensive effects (particularly orthostasis)

Bromocriptine: Antipsychotics inhibit the ability of bromocriptine to lower serum prolactin concentrations

CNS depressants: Sedative effects may be additive with antipsychotics; monitor for increased effect; includes barbiturates, benzodiazepines, narcotic analgesics, ethanol and other sedative agents

Epinephrine: Chlorpromazine (and possibly other low potency antipsychotics) may diminish the pressor effects of epinephrine

Guanethidine and guanadrel: Antihypertensive effects may be inhibited by antipsychotics Levodopa: Antipsychotics may inhibit the antiparkinsonian effect of levodopa; avoid this combination

Lithium: Antipsychotics may produce neurotoxicity with lithium; this is a rare effect

Metoclopramide: May increase extrapyramidal symptoms (EPS) or risk.

Propranolol: Serum concentrations of antipsychotics may be increased; propranolol also increases antipsychotic concentrations

QT$_c$-prolonging agents: Effects on QT$_c$ interval may be additive with antipsychotics, increasing the risk of malignant arrhythmias; includes type Ia antiarrhythmics, TCAs, and some quinolone antibiotics (sparfloxacin, moxifloxacin, and gatifloxacin)

Sulfadoxine-pyrimethamine: May increase antipsychotics concentrations

Tricyclic antidepressants: Concurrent use may produce increased toxicity or altered therapeutic response

Trazodone: Antipsychotics and trazodone may produce additive hypotensive effects

Valproic acid: Serum levels may be increased by antipsychotics

Pregnancy Risk Factor C

Pregnancy Implications Not known if crosses the placenta

Lactation Excretion in breast milk unknown

Nursing Implications May increase appetite and possibly a craving for sweets; recognize signs of neuroleptic malignant syndrome and tardive dyskinesia

Specific References

Flammia DD, Bateman HR, and Saady JJ, "Tissue Distribution of Molindone in a Multidrug Overdose," *J Anal Toxicol*, 2004, 28(6):533-6.

Flammia D, Christensen E, Bateman H, et al, "Fatal Overdose with Molindone and Lithium," *J Anal Toxicol*, 2003, 27:193.

Moricizine

CAS Number 29560-58-5; 31883-05-3

U.S. Brand Names Ethmozine®

Synonyms Moricizine Hydrochloride

Use Life-threatening ventricular arrhythmia

Unlabeled/Investigational Use PVCs, complete and nonsustained ventricular tachycardia, atrial arrhythmias

Mechanism of Action A phenothiazine compound with class I antiarrhythmic activity (myocardial membrane stabilizing effect); reduces fast inward sodium current of the action potential

Adverse Reactions

Cardiovascular: Heart failure, fibrillation (atrial), flutter (atrial), myocardial depression, arrhythmias (ventricular)

Central nervous system: Headache, fatigue, fever, hypothermia, **dizziness**

Dermatologic: Skin rash

Endocrine & metabolism: Impotence

Gastrointestinal: Nausea, abdominal pain, xerostomia, vomiting

Hematologic: Thrombocytopenia

Hepatic: Hepatic dysfunction

Ocular: Blurred vision

Respiratory: Dyspnea

Signs and Symptoms of Overdose Asystole, coma, exacerbation of heart failure, hypotension, junctional bradycardia, respiratory failure, sinus arrest, ventricular fibrillation, ventricular tachycardia

Admission Criteria/Prognosis Admit any patient exhibiting cardiotoxicity or adult ingestions >1 g

Pharmacodynamics/Kinetics

Protein binding, plasma: 95%

Metabolism: Significant first-pass effect; some enterohepatic recycling

Bioavailability: 38%

Half-life elimination: Healthy volunteers: 3-4 hours; Cardiac disease: 6-13 hours

Excretion: Feces (56%); urine (39%)

Dosage Oral: 600-900 mg/day in 2-3 divided doses

Dosing adjustment in renal/hepatic impairment: Reduce dosage in renal/hepatic insufficiency

Contraindications Hypersensitivity to moricizine or any component of the formulation; pre-existing second- or third-degree AV block (except in patients with a functioning artificial pacemaker); right bundle branch block when associated with left hemiblock or bifascicular block (unless functional pacemaker in place); cardiogenic shock

Warnings Can be proarrhythmic; watch for new rhythm disturbances or existing arrhythmias that worsen. Use cautiously in CAD, previous history of MI, CHF, and cardiomegaly. **[U.S. Boxed Warning]: The CAST II trial demonstrated a decreased trend in survival for patients receiving moricizine.** Dose-related increases in PR and QRS intervals occur. Use cautiously in patients with pre-existing conduction abnormalities, and significant hepatic impairment. Safety and efficacy have not been established in pediatric patients.

Dosage Forms Tablet, as hydrochloride: 200 mg, 250 mg, 300 mg

Overdosage/Treatment

Decontamination: **Do not** use ipecac; use lavage (within 1 hour)/activated charcoal

Supportive therapy: Avoid type IA antiarrhythmic agents (quinidine, procainamide, disopyramide); I.V. sodium bicarbonate (1-2 mEq/kg) can be used for hypotension or ventricular arrhythmia; phenytoin (15 mg/kg up to 1 g I.V. slow administration of 50 mg/minute) is antiarrhythmic of choice; magnesium sulfate, lidocaine, bretylium, or propranolol can also be used for ventricular arrhythmias

Enhancement of elimination: Hemodialysis is not useful

Drug Interactions Substrate of CYP3A4 (major); **Induces** CYP1A2 (weak), 3A4 (weak)

Cimetidine increases moricizine levels by 50%.

CYP3A4 inducers: CYP3A4 inducers may decrease the levels/effects of moricizine. Example inducers include aminoglutethimide, carbamazepine, nafcillin, nevirapine, phenobarbital, phenytoin, and rifamycins.

CYP3A4 inhibitors: May increase the levels/effects of moricizine. Example inhibitors include azole antifungals, clarithromycin, diclofenac, doxycycline, erythromycin, imatinib, isoniazid, nefazodone, nicardipine, propofol, protease inhibitors, quinidine, telithromycin, and verapamil.

Digoxin may result in additive prolongation of the PR interval when combined with moricizine (but not rate of second- and third-degree AV block).

Diltiazem increases moricizine levels resulting in an increased incidence of side effects. Moricizine decreases diltiazem plasma levels and decreases its half-life.

Drugs which may prolong QT interval (including cisapride, erythromycin, phenothiazines, cyclic antidepressants, and some quinolones) are contraindicated with Type Ia antiarrhythmics. Moricizine has some type Ia activity, and caution should be used.

Theophylline levels are decreased by 50% with moricizine due to increased clearance.

Pregnancy Risk Factor B

Lactation Enters breast milk/not recommended

Additional Information Based on adverse outcomes noted with moricizine in the CAST trial, the FDA recommends that use of moricizine be limited to patients with life-threatening ventricular arrhythmias

Morphine Sulfate

Related Information

- Heroin
- Highlights of Recent Reports (2006) on Substance Abuse and Mental Health

CAS Number 57-27-2; 6009-81-0; 6211-15-0; 64-31-3

U.S. Brand Names Astramorph/PF™; Avinza™; DepoDur™; Duramorph®; Infumorph®; Kadian®; MS Contin®; MSIR®; Oramorph SR®; RMS®; Roxanol 100®; Roxanol®-T; Roxanol®

Synonyms MSO$_4$ (error-prone abbreviation and should not be used)

Impairment Potential Yes

Use
Relief of moderate to severe acute and chronic pain; relief of pain of myocardial infarction; relief of dyspnea of acute left ventricular failure and pulmonary edema; preanesthetic medication

Orphan drug: Infumorph™: Used in microinfusion devices for intraspinal administration in treatment of intractable chronic pain

Mechanism of Action Binds to opiate receptors in the CNS, causing inhibition of ascending pain pathways, altering the perception of and response to pain; produces generalized CNS depression

Adverse Reactions
Cardiovascular: **Palpitations, hypotension, bradycardia,** peripheral vasodilation, sinus bradycardia, congestive heart failure

Central nervous system: CNS depression, psychosis, drowsiness, **dizziness,** sedation, agitation, increased intracranial pressure, Guillain-Barré syndrome, depression, dysphoria, paranoia, aggressive behavior

Dermatologic: Pruritus (more common with epidural or intrathecal administration)

Endocrine & metabolic: Syndrome of inappropriate antidiuretic hormone

Gastrointestinal: **Nausea, vomiting, constipation,** adynamic ileus, biliary tract spasm, Ogilvie's syndrome, decreased esophageal sphincter tone, intestinal obstruction

Genitourinary: Urinary retention, urinary tract spasm, urinary incontinence

Hematologic: Thrombocytopenia

Hepatic: Transaminases increased

Neuromuscular & skeletal: Clonus, myoclonus

Ocular: Miosis, nystagmus

Respiratory: Apnea, respiratory depression, aspiration, asthma, acute respiratory distress syndrome

Miscellaneous: Physical and psychological dependence, **histamine release,** anaphylaxis

Signs and Symptoms of Overdose Apnea, coma, constipation, dry mouth, dysuria, encephalopathy, hallucinations, hyponatremia, hypotension, hypothermia, impotence, miosis, myocardial depression, myoglobinuria, pulmonary edema, respiratory depression, rhabdomyolysis, seizures (in neonates), thirst

Pharmacodynamics/Kinetics
Onset of action: Oral (immediate release): ~30 minutes; I.V.: 5-10 minutes

Duration: Pain relief:
Immediate release formulations: 4 hours
Extended release epidural injection (DepoDur™): >48 hours

Toxicodynamics/Kinetics
Absorption: Oral: Variable
Distribution: V_d: 3-4 L/kg; lower in elderly patients
Protein binding: 35%
Metabolism: In the liver via glucuronide conjugation
Half-life: Neonates: Prolonged 6% to 10%; Adults: 1.5-2 hours
Elimination: Excreted unchanged in urine; renal clearance: 2 L/hour/kg
See table.

Morphine Sulfate		
Dosage Form/Route	**Analgesia**	
	Peak	**Duration**
Tablets	1 h	4-5 h
Oral solution	1 h	4-5 h
Extended release tablets	1 h	8-12 h
Suppository	20-60 min	3-7 h
Subcutaneous injection	50-90 min	4-5 h
I.M. injection	30-60 min	4-5 h
I.V. injection	20 min	4-5 h

Dosage **Note:** These are guidelines and do not represent the maximum doses that may be required in all patients. Doses should be titrated to pain relief/prevention.

Children >6 months and <50 kg: Acute pain (moderate-to-severe):
Oral (prompt release): 0.15-0.3 mg/kg every 3-4 hours as needed
I.M.: 0.1 mg/kg every 3-4 hours as needed
I.V.: 0.05-0.1 mg/kg every 3-4 hours as needed
I.V. infusion: Range: 10-30 mcg/kg/hour

Adolescents >12 years: Sedation/analgesia for procedures: I.V.: 3-4 mg and repeat in 5 minutes if necessary

Adults: Acute pain (moderate-to-severe):
Oral: Prompt release formulations: Opiate-naive: Initial: 10 mg every 3-4 hours as needed; patients with prior opiate exposure may require higher initial doses: usual dosage range: 10-30 mg every 3-4 hours as needed

Oral: Controlled-, extended-, or sustained-release formulations: **Note:** A patient's morphine requirement should be established using prompt-release formulations. Conversion to long-acting products may be considered when chronic, continuous treatment is required. Higher dosages should be reserved for use only in opioid-tolerant patients.

Capsules, extended release (Avinza™): Daily dose administered once daily (for best results, administer at same time each day)

Capsules, sustained release (Kadian®): Daily dose administered once daily or in 2 divided doses daily (every 12 hours)

Tablets, controlled release (MS Contin®), sustained release (Oramorph SR®), or extended release: Daily dose divided and administered every 8 or every 12 hours

I.V.: Initial: Opiate-naive: 2.5-5 mg every 3-4 hours; patients with prior opiate exposure may require higher initial doses. **Note:** Repeated doses (up to every 5 minutes if needed) in small increments (eg, 1-4 mg) may be preferred to larger and less frequent doses.

I.V., SubQ continuous infusion: 0.8-10 mg/hour; may increase depending on pain relief/adverse effects: usual range: up to 80 mg/hour although higher doses may be required

Mechanically-ventilated patients (based on 70 kg patient): 0.7-10 mg every 1-2 hours as needed; infusion: 5-35 mg/hour

Patient-controlled analgesia (PCA): (Opiate-naive: Consider lower end of dosing range):
Usual concentration: 1 mg/mL
Demand dose: Usual: 1 mg; range: 0.5-2.5 mg
Lockout interval: 5-10 minutes

Epidural: **Note:** Administer with extreme caution and in reduced dosage to geriatric or debilitated patients.
Infusion:
Bolus dose: 1-6 mg
Infusion rate: 0.1-1 mg/hour
Maximum dose: 10 mg/24 hours
Single-dose (extended release, Depo-Dur™):
Cesarean section: 10 mg
Lower abdominal/pelvic surgery: 10-15 mg
Note: Some patients may benefit from a 20 mg dose, however, the incidence of adverse effects may be increased.

Intrathecal (I.T.): One-tenth of epidural dose; **Note:** Administer with extreme caution and in reduced dosage to geriatric or debilitated patients.
Opiate-naive: 0.2-1 mg/dose (may provide adequate relief for 24 hours); repeat doses **not** recommended except to establish initial IT dose.

I.M., SubQ: **Note:** Repeated SubQ administration causes local tissue irritation, pain, and induration.
Initial: Opiate-naive: 5-10 mg every 3-4 hours as needed; patients with prior opiate exposure may require higher initial doses; usual dosage range: 5-20 mg every 3-4 hours as needed

Rectal: 10-20 mg every 3-4 hours

Chronic pain: Patients taking opioids chronically may become tolerant and require doses higher than the usual dosage range to maintain the desired effect. Tolerance can be managed by appropriate dose titration. There is no optimal or maximal dose for morphine in chronic pain. The appropriate dose is one that relieves pain throughout its dosing interval without causing unmanageable side effects.

Elderly or debilitated patients: Use with caution; may require dose reduction

Dosing adjustment in renal impairment:
Cl_{cr} 10-50 mL/minute: Administer at 75% of normal dose
Cl_{cr} <10 mL/minute: Administer at 50% of normal dose

Dosing adjustment/comments in hepatic disease: Unchanged in mild liver disease; substantial extrahepatic metabolism may occur; excessive sedation may occur in cirrhosis

Stability Refrigerate suppositories; do not freeze; degradation depends on pH and presence of oxygen; relatively stable in pH 4 and below; darkening of solutions indicate degradation; usual concentration for continuous I.V. infusion = 0.1-1 mg/mL in D_5W; **incompatible** with acyclovir, furosemide, heparin, pethidine, prochlorperazine, promethazine

Monitoring Parameters Pain relief, respiratory and mental status, blood pressure

Administration
Oral: Do not crush controlled release drug product, swallow whole. Kadian® can be opened and sprinkled on applesauce. Avinza™ can also be opened and sprinkled on applesauce; do not crush or chew the beads. Administration of oral morphine solution with food may increase bioavailability (not observed with Oramorph SR®).

I.V.: When giving morphine I.V. push, it is best to first dilute in 4-5 mL of sterile water, and then to administer slowly (eg, 15 mg over 3-5 minutes)

Epidural or intrathecal: Use preservative-free solutions

Contraindications Hypersensitivity to morphine sulfate or any component of the formulation; increased intracranial pressure; severe respiratory depression; acute or severe asthma; known or suspected paralytic ileus; sustained release products are not recommended with gastrointestinal obstruction or in acute/postoperative pain; pregnancy (prolonged use or high doses at term)

Warnings

An opioid-containing analgesic regimen should be tailored to each patient's needs and based upon the type of pain being treated (acute versus chronic), the route of administration, degree of tolerance for opioids (naive versus chronic user), age, weight, and medical condition. The optimal analgesic dose varies widely among patients. Doses should be titrated to pain relief/prevention. When used as an epidural injection, monitor for delayed sedation.

May cause respiratory depression; use with caution in patients (particularly elderly or debilitated) with impaired respiratory function or severe hepatic dysfunction and in patients with hypersensitivity reactions to other phenanthrene derivative opioid agonists (codeine, hydrocodone, hydromorphone, levorphanol, oxycodone, oxymorphone). Some preparations contain sulfites which may cause allergic reactions; infants <3 months of age are more susceptible to respiratory depression, use with caution and generally in reduced doses in this age group. Morphine shares the toxic potential of opiate agonists and usual precautions of opiate agonist therapy should be observed; may cause hypotension in patients with acute myocardial infarction, volume depletion, or concurrent drug therapy which may exaggerate vasodilation. Tolerance or drug dependence may result from extended use. Elderly may be particularly susceptible to the CNS depressant and constipating effects of narcotics.

Extended or sustained-release formulations:

[U.S. Boxed Warning]: Extended or sustained release dosage forms should not be crushed or chewed. Controlled-, extended-, or sustained-release products are not intended for "as needed (PRN)" use. MS Contin® 100 mg or 200 mg tablets are for use only in opioid-tolerant patients requiring >400 mg/day.

[U.S. Boxed Warning]: Avinza®: Do not administer with alcoholic beverages or ethanol-containing products, which may disrupt extended-release characteristic of product.

Injections: Note: Products are designed for administration by specific routes (I.V., intrathecal, epidural). Use caution when prescribing, dispensing, or administering to use formulations only by intended route(s).

[U.S. Boxed Warning]: Duramorph®: Due to the risk of severe and/or sustained cardiopulmonary depressant effects of Duramorph® must be administered in a fully equipped and staffed environment. Naloxone injection should be immediately available. Patient should remain in this environment for at least 24 hours following the initial dose.

Infumorph® solutions are **for use in microinfusion devices only**; not for I.V., I.M., or SubQ administration.

Depo-Dur™: Freezing may adversely affect modified-release mechanism of drug; check freeze indicator within carton prior to administration.

Dosage Forms

[DSC] = Discontinued product

Capsule, extended release (Avinza®): 30 mg, 60 mg, 90 mg, 120 mg

Capsule, sustained release (Kadian®): 20 mg, 30 mg, 50 mg, 60 mg, 100 mg

Infusion [premixed in D_5W]: 1 mg/mL (100 mL, 250 mL)

Injection, extended release liposomal suspension [lumbar epidural injection, preservative free] (DepoDur™): 10 mg/mL (1 mL, 1.5 mL, 2 mL)

Injection, solution: 2 mg/mL (1 mL); 4 mg/mL (1 mL); 5 mg/mL (1 mL); 8 mg/mL (1 mL); 10 mg/mL (1 mL, 10 mL); 15 mg/mL (1 mL, 20 mL); 25 mg/mL (4 mL, 10 mL, 20 mL, 40 mL, 50 mL, 100 mL, 250 mL); 50 mg/mL (20 mL, 40 mL) [some preparations contain sodium metabisulfite]

Injection, solution [epidural, intrathecal, or I.V. infusion; preservative free]: Astramorph/PF™: 0.5 mg/mL (2 mL, 10 mL); 1 mg/mL (2 mL, 10 mL)
  Duramorph®: 0.5 mg/mL (10 mL); 1 mg/mL (10 mL)

Injection, solution [epidural or intrathecal infusion via microinfusion device; preservative free] (Infumorph®): 10 mg/mL (20 mL); 25 mg/mL (20 mL)

Injection, solution [I.V. infusion via PCA pump]: 0.5 mg/mL (30 mL); 1 mg/mL (30 mL, 50 mL); 2 mg/mL (30 mL); 5 mg/mL (30 mL, 50 mL)

Injection, solution [preservative free]: 0.5 mg/mL (10 mL); 1 mg/mL (10 mL); 25 mg/mL (4 mL, 10 mL, 20 mL)

Solution, oral: 10 mg/5 mL (5 mL, 10 mL, 100 mL, 500 mL); 20 mg/5 mL (100 mL, 500 mL); 20 mg/mL (30 mL, 120 mL, 240 mL)
  Roxanol™: 20 mg/mL (30 mL, 120 mL)
  Roxanol 100™: 100 mg/5 mL (240 mL) [with calibrated spoon]
  Roxanol™-T: 20 mg/mL (30 mL, 120 mL) [tinted, flavored] [DSC]

Suppository, rectal (RMS®): 5 mg (12s), 10 mg (12s), 20 mg (12s), 30 mg (12s)

Tablet: 15 mg, 30 mg

Tablet, controlled release (MS Contin®): 15 mg, 30 mg, 60 mg, 100 mg, 200 mg

Tablet, extended release: 15 mg, 30 mg, 60 mg, 100 mg, 200 mg

Tablet, sustained release (Oramorph SR®): 15 mg, 30 mg, 60 mg, 100 mg

Reference Range

Therapeutic: Surgical anesthesia: 65-80 ng/mL (SI: 227-280 nmol/L)
Toxic: 200-5000 ng/mL (SI: 700-17,500 nmol/L)

Overdosage/Treatment

Supportive therapy: Naloxone hydrochloride (0.4-2 mg I.V., SubQ, or through an endotracheal tube); a continuous infusion (at $^2/_3$ the response dose/hour) may be required; opioid-induced myoclonus may respond to dantrolene (50-150 mg/day); ondansetron (4 mg I.V.) may be effective in treatment of morphine-induced pruritus. Severe chronic constipation may respond to oral naloxone 2-6 mg.

Antidote(s)

- Nalmefene [ANTIDOTE]
- Naloxone [ANTIDOTE]

Diagnostic Procedures

- Morphine, Urine
- Opiates, Qualitative, Urine

Test Interactions ↑ aminotransferases (ALT, AST) (S), amylase

Drug Interactions

Substrate of CYP2D6 (minor)

Antipsychotic agents: May increase hypotensive effects of morphine; monitor.

CNS depressants: May increase the effects/toxicity of morphine; monitor.

MAO inhibitors: May increase the effects/toxicity of morphine; some manufacturers recommend avoiding use within 14 days of MAO inhibitors

Pegvisomant: Therapeutic efficacy may be decreased by concomitant opiates, possibly requiring dosage adjustment of pegvisomant.

Rifamycin derivatives: May decrease levels/effects of morphine; monitor.

Selective serotonin reuptake inhibitors (SSRIs) and meperidine: Serotonergic effects may be additive, leading to serotonin syndrome.

Pregnancy Risk Factor B/D (prolonged use or high doses at term)

Pregnancy Implications Morphine crosses the placenta. The frequency of congenital malformations has not been reported to be greater than expected in children from mothers treated with morphine during pregnancy. Reduced growth and behavioral abnormalities in offspring have been observed in animal studies. Neonates born to mothers receiving chronic opioids during pregnancy should be monitored for neonatal withdrawal syndrome. DepoDur™ may be used in women undergoing cesarean section following clamping of the umbilical cord; not for use in vaginal labor and delivery.

Lactation Enters breast milk/use caution (AAP rates "compatible")

Nursing Implications Do not crush controlled release drug product, observe patient for excessive sedation, apnea; implement safety measures, assist with ambulation; use preservative-free solutions for intrathecal or epidural use

Additional Information

Stimulates prolactin release; addition of clonidine (75-150 mcg) increased duration of analgesia produced by epidural morphine (2 mg) for cesarean delivery; poppyseed use can be ruled out as a cause for a urinary morphine screen when codeine levels exceed 300 ng/mL; morphine to codeine ratio is <2 and high levels of morphine (>1000 ng/mL) are detected without codeine being present

International Olympic Committee urinary cutoff limit for morphine: 1 mcg/mL

Notable individuals in whom morphine was involved in their deaths: King George V (Britain) - 1936; Sigmund Freud (Psychiatrist) - 1939; Chris Farley (Comedian) - 1997

Mid-Year 2000 Preliminary Emergency Department Drug Abuse Warning Network (DAWN) data: **Note:** Heroin/morphine is sometimes used in combination with other drugs; therefore, one Emergency Department (ED) episode can include mentions of one or more drugs.

- Heroin/morphine mentions increased 22% from the first half of 1999 (38,565 mentions) to the first half of 2000 (47,008).

- From the first half of 1999 to the first half of 2000, heroin/morphine mentions increased:
  - 31% (from 9041 to 11,850) for adults age 26-34 and 22% (from 21,726 to 26,400) for adults age 35 and over.
  - 21% for males (from 26,048 to 31,472) and females (from 12,308 to 14,842); and
  - 27% for patients reported as white (from 15,364 to 19,455) and 17% for patients reported as black (from 13,292 to 15,487).

- During the same period, heroin/morphine mentions were unchanged for young adults age 18-25 and for patients reported as Hispanic.

- From the first half of 1999 to the first half of 2000, heroin/morphine mentions increased in 8 of the 21 metropolitan areas oversampled in DAWN and decreased in 1. The decrease came in Baltimore (18%). Increases were found in New Orleans (62%), Buffalo (58%), Miami-Hialeah (50%), San Francisco (34%), Detroit (33%), Boston (32%), Atlanta (25%), and San Diego (24%).

Specific References

Bhandari V, Bergqvist LL, Kronsberg SS, et al, "Morphine Administration and Short-Term Pulmonary Outcomes Among Ventilated Preterm Infants," *Pediatrics*, 2005, 116(2):352-9.

Bijur PE, Kenny MK, and Gallagher EJ, "Intravenous Morphine at 0.1 mg/kg Is Not Effective for Controlling Severe Acute Pain in the Majority of Patients," *Ann Emerg Med*, 2005, 46(4):362-7.

Brown SJ, Eichner SF, and Jones JR, "Nebulized Morphine for Relief of Dyspnea Due to Chronic Lung Disease," *Ann Pharmacother*, 2005, 39(6):1088-92.

Cone EJ, Heit HA, Caplan YH, et al, "Evidence of Morphine Metabolism to Hydromorphone in Pain Patients Chronically Treated with Morphine," *J Anal Toxicol*, 2006, 30:1-5.

Crandall CS, Kerrigan S, Aguerro RL, et al, "The Influerece of Collection Site and Methods on Postmortem Morphine Concentrations in a Porcine Model," *J Anal Tox*, 2006, 30:651-8.

Evans M, Terrell A, Foery R, et al, "New Report of a High-Dose Morphine Metabolite," *Prac Pain Management*, 2006, 6(1):84-5.

Gaudette KE and Weaver SJ, "Intraspinal Use of Morphine," *Ann Pharmacother*, 2003, 37(7-8):1132-5.

Greenwald PW, Provataris J, Coffey J, et al, "Low-Dose Naloxone Does Not Improve Morphine-Induced Nausea, Vomiting, or Pruritus," *Am J Emerg Med*, 2005, 23(1):35-9.

He Y, Lu J, Liu M, et al, "Determination of Morphine by Molecular Imprinting-Chemiluminescence Method," *J Anal Toxicol*, 2005, 29:528-38.

Hill V, Schaffer M, and Cairns T, "Absence of Hair Color Effects in Hair Analysis Results for Cocaine, Benzoylecgonine, Morphine, 6-monoacetylmorphine, Codeine, and 11-Nor-9-carboxy-△9-THC in Large Workplace Populations," *Annale de Toxicologie Analytique*, 2005, 17(4):285-98.

Kiely E, Bultman S, and Marinetti L, "The Analysis of Opiates in Hair in Postmortem Toxicology," *J Anal Toxicol*, 2006, 30:136.

McKinney PE, Crandall CS, Zumwalt R, et al, "Arterial and Venous Differences in Postmortem Morphine Concentrations in Heroin Overdose Deaths," *J Toxicol Clin Toxicol*, 2003, 41(5):734.

Miner JR, Fringer R, Siegel T, et al, "Serial Bispectral Index Scores in Patients Undergoing Observation for Sedative Overdose in the Emergency Department," *Am J Emerg Med*. 2006, 24(1):53-7.

Simons SH, van Dijk M, van Lingen RA, et al, "Routine Morphine Infusion in Preterm Newborns Who Received Ventilatory Support: A Randomized Controlled Trial," *JAMA*, 2003, 290(18):2419-27.

Taracha E, Habrat B, Chmielewska K, et al, "Excretion Profile of Opiates in Dependent Patients in Relation to Route of Administration and Type of Drug Measured in Urine with Immunoassay," *J Anal Toxicol*, 2005, 29:15-21.

Thevis M, Opfermann G, and Schanzer W, "Urinary Concentrations of Morphine and Codeine After Consumption of Poppy Seeds," *J Anal Toxicol*, 2003, 27(1):53-6.

Vinner E, Vignau J, Thibault D, et al, "Neonatal Hair Analysis Contribution to Establishing a Gestational Drug Exposure Profile and Predicting a Withdrawal Syndrome," *Ther Drug Monit*, 2003, 25(4):421-32.

Wang L, Irvan D, Kuntz DJ, et al, "Simultaneous Analysis of Morphine, Codeine, Oxymorphone, Hydromorphone, 6-Acetylmorphine, Oxycodone, Hydrocodone and Heroin in Hair and Oral Fluid," *J Anal Toxicol*, 2004, 28:285.

Warren RJ and Rajotte JW, "Significance of Blood Morphine Concentrations in Non-Heroin-Related Deaths," *J Anal Toxicol*, 2006, 30:156-7.

Wolfe JM, Smithline HA, Phipen S, et al, "Does Morphine Change the Physical Examination in Patients with Acute Appendicitis?" *Am J Emerg Med*, 2004, 22(4):280-5.

Moxonidine

CAS Number 75438-57-2

Synonyms Monoxidin

Unlabeled/Investigational Use Hypertension

Mechanism of Action Structurally similar to clonidine, moxonidine is a centrally active imidazoline and alpha$_2$-receptor antagonist; also promotes natriuresis

Adverse Reactions

Cardiovascular: **Hypotension (orthostatic)**, edema, facial flushing, hypertension

Central nervous system: Drowsiness (less sedation than clonidine), **dizziness**, headache, insomnia, vertigo

Gastrointestinal: **Xerostomia**

Hepatic: Cholestatic hepatitis

Renal: Diuresis

Miscellaneous: Thirst

Signs and Symptoms of Overdose Hypotension

Pharmacodynamics/Kinetics

Absorption: 80% to 90%

Distribution: V$_d$: 1.8-3 L/kg

Protein binding: 6% to 8% (not changed in renal failure)

Metabolism: To 4,5-dehydromoxonidine (10% to 20%)

Bioavailability: 89%

Half-life: 2.6 hours (increased in renal insufficiency)

Peak serum levels: 30-180 minutes

Elimination: Renal

Dosage Starting dose: 0.2-0.4 mg/day; may increase after 3 weeks to 0.2-0.4 mg twice daily; maximum single dose: 0.4 mg

Contraindications Bradycardia, sick sinus syndrome, atrioventricular block, arrhythmias, severe congestive heart failure, severe coronary ischemia, unstable angina pectoris, renal insufficiency (creatinine >1.8 mg/dL), angioedema, intermittent claudication, Raynaud's disease, Par-kinson's disease, epilepsy, glaucoma, depression, pregnancy, lactation, children <16 years of age

Warnings Use with caution in patients with mild to moderate renal impairment (serum creatinine: 1.2-1.8 mg/dL)

Dosage Forms Tablet: 0.2 mg, 0.3 mg, 0.4 mg

Reference Range Peak serum moxonidine levels after 0.2 mg oral and intravenous administration were 1495 pg/mL and 3965 pg/mL, respectively

Overdosage/Treatment

Decontamination: Activated charcoal

Supportive therapy: For hypotension, I.V. saline administration with placement of patient in Trendelenburg position; vasopressors may also be utilized

Enhancement of elimination: Multiple dosing of activated charcoal may be effective

Drug Interactions Concomitant use with beta-adrenergic blocking agents; abrupt withdrawal of moxonidine may lead to rebound hypertension

---

Nabilone

CAS Number 51022-71-0

U.S. Brand Names Cesamet®

Impairment Potential Yes

Use Treatment of nausea and vomiting associated with cancer chemotherapy

Mechanism of Action Nabilone is a synthetic cannabinoid utilized as an antiemetic drug in the control of nausea and vomiting in patients receiving cancer chemotherapy; like delta-9-tetrahydrocannabinol (the active principal of marijuana), nabilone is a dibenzo(b,d)pyrans and has central CNS antiemetic action thorough the dopaminergic pathway

Adverse Reactions

Cardiovascular: Hypotension, hypertension, tachycardia, sinus tachycardia

Central nervous system: Changes of mood, confusion, hallucinations, CNS depression, **dizziness, drowsiness**, headache, **euphoria, clumsiness**

Gastrointestinal: Loss of appetite or increased appetite, **xerostomia**

Ocular: Blurred vision

Respiratory: Difficulty breathing

Pharmacodynamics/Kinetics

Absorption: Rapid and complete

Distribution: ~12.5 L/kg

Metabolism: To several active metabolites by oxidation and stereospecific enzyme reduction; CYP450 enzymes may also be involved

Half-life elimination: Parent compound: 2 hours; Metabolites: 35 hours

Time to peak, serum: Within 2 hours

Excretion: Feces (~60%); renal (~24%)

Dosage Oral:

Children >4 years:

<18 kg: 0.5 mg twice daily

18-30 kg: 1 mg twice daily

>30 kg: 1 mg 3 times/day

Adults: 1-2 mg twice daily beginning 1-3 hours before chemotherapy is administered and continuing around-the-clock until 1 dose after chemotherapy is completed; maximum daily dose: 6 mg divided in 3 doses

Monitoring Parameters Blood pressure, heart rate; signs and symptoms of excessive use, abuse, or misuse

Administration Initial dose should be given 1-3 hours before chemotherapy; may be given 2-3 times a day during the entire chemotherapy course and for up to 48 hours after the last dose of chemotherapy; a dose of 1-2 mg the night before chemotherapy may be useful.

Contraindications Hypersensitivity to nabilone, cannabinoids, tetrahydrocannabinol, or any component of the formulation

Warnings May affect CNS function; use with caution in the elderly and those with pre-existing CNS depression. May cause additive CNS effects with sedatives, hypnotics, or other psychoactive agents; patients must be cautioned about performing tasks which require mental alertness (eg, operating machinery or driving). Use caution with current or previous history of mental illness; cannabinoid use may reveal symptoms of psychiatric disorders. Psychiatric adverse reactions may persist for up to 3 days after discontinuing treatment. Has potential for abuse and or dependence, use caution in patients with substance abuse history or potential. May cause tachycardia and orthostatic hypotension; use caution with cardiovascular disease. Safety and efficacy in children have not been established.

Dosage Forms Capsule:

Cesamet™: 1 mg

Reference Range Peak serum levels after a 2 mg dose: 10 ng/mL

Overdosage/Treatment

Decontamination: Oral: Lavage (within 1 hour)/activated charcoal

Supportive therapy: Benzodiazepines for agitation; hypotension can be treated with Trendelenburg/crystalloid infusion; tachycardia can be treated with beta-blockers

Drug Interactions

Anticholinergic agents (includes antihistamines, atropine, and scopolamine): Tachycardia and drowsiness may be additive.

CNS depressants (includes barbiturates, narcotic analgesics, and other sedative agents): Sedative effects may be additive with CNS depressants; monitor for increased effect.

Naltrexone: Oral cannabinoid effects may be enhanced via opioid receptor blockade.

Opioids: May have cross-tolerance and potentiation.

Sympathomimetic agents (includes amphetamines and cocaine): Hypertension, tachycardia, and cardiotoxicity may be additive.

Tricyclic antidepressants (includes amitriptyline, amoxapine, and desipramine): Tachycardia, hypertension, and drowsiness may be additive.

Pregnancy Risk Factor C

Pregnancy Implications Animal studies did not demonstrate teratogenic effects, however, dose-related decreased fetal weights and increased fetal resorptions were observed. There are no adequate and well-controlled studies in pregnant women. Use during pregnancy only if clearly needed.

Lactation Excretion in breast milk unknown/not recommended

Nursing Implications May cause drowsiness, euphoria; institute safety precautions

Nabumetone

Related Information

- Nonsteroidal Anti-inflammatory Drugs

CAS Number 42924-53-8

U.S. Brand Names Relafen®

Use Management of osteoarthritis and rheumatoid arthritis

Moderate pain

Mechanism of Action Nabumetone is a nonacidic, nonsteroidal anti-inflammatory drug that is rapidly metabolized after absorption to a major active metabolite, 6-methoxy-2-naphthylacetic acid. Nabumetone's active metabolite inhibits the cyclooxygenase enzyme which is indirectly responsible for the production of endoperoxides and prostaglandins E_2 and I_2 (prostacyclin). The active metabolite of nabumetone is felt to be the compound primarily responsible for therapeutic effect. Comparatively, the parent drug is a poor inhibitor of prostaglandin synthesis.

Adverse Reactions

Cardiovascular: Angina, arrhythmia, hypertension, myocardial infarction, syncope, vasculitis, congestive heart failure

Central nervous system: **Dizziness**, headache, nervousness, agitation, anxiety, confusion, depression, fever, malaise, nightmares, vertigo

Dermatologic: **Rash**, itching, acne, alopecia, angioneurotic edema, bullous eruptions, photosensitivity, urticaria, Stevens-Johnson syndrome, toxic epidermal necrolysis, erythema multiforme, pseudoporphyria cutanea tarda

Endocrine & metabolic: Fluid retention, hyperglycemia

Gastrointestinal: **Abdominal cramps, abdominal pain (12%), diarrhea (14%), dyspepsia (13%), heartburn, indigestion, nausea**, vomiting, anorexia, duodenal ulcer, dysphagia, gallstones, gastric ulcer, gastroenteritis, gingivitis, GI bleeding, melena, pancreatitis

Genitourinary: Hyperuricemia, hypokalemia, impotence

Hematologic: Anemia, granulocytopenia, leukopenia, thrombocytopenia, thrombophlebitis

Hepatic: Cholestatic jaundice, liver function abnormalities, hepatic failure, hepatitis

Neuromuscular & skeletal: Paresthesia, tremor, weakness

Ocular: Abnormal vision

Otic: Tinnitus

Renal: Albuminuria, azotemia, nephrolithiasis, interstitial nephritis, nephrotic syndrome, renal failure

Respiratory: Asthma, dyspnea, eosinophilic pneumonia, hypersensitivity pneumonitis, interstitial pneumonitis

Miscellaneous: Anaphylactoid reaction, anaphylaxis

Signs and Symptoms of Overdose Cognitive dysfunction, drowsiness, flatulence, gastritis, nausea, nephrotic syndrome, ototoxicity, photosensitivity, stomatitis, tinnitus, vomiting, wheezing. Severe poisoning can manifest with coma, hypotension, renal and/or hepatic failure, respiratory depression, and seizures.

Pharmacodynamics/Kinetics

Onset of action: Several days

Distribution: Diffusion occurs readily into synovial fluid

V_d: 6MNA: 29-82 L

Protein binding: 6MNA: >99%

Metabolism: Prodrug, rapidly metabolized in the liver to an active metabolite [6-methoxy-2-naphthylacetic acid (6MNA)] and inactive metabolites; extensive first-pass effect

Half-life elimination: 6MNA: ~24 hours

Time to peak, serum: 6MNA: Oral: 2.5-4 hours; Synovial fluid: 4-12 hours

Excretion: 6MNA: Urine (80%) and feces (9%)

Dosage

Adults: Oral: 1000 mg/day; an additional 500-1000 mg may be needed in some patients to obtain more symptomatic relief; may be administered once or twice daily

Dosing adjustment in renal impairment: None necessary; however, adverse effects due to accumulation of inactive metabolites of nabumetone that are renally excreted have not been studied and should be considered

Monitoring Parameters Patients with renal insufficiency: Baseline renal function followed by repeat test within weeks (to determine if renal function has deteriorated)

Contraindications Hypersensitivity to nabumetone, aspirin, other NSAIDs, or any component of the formulation; perioperative pain in the setting of coronary artery bypass surgery (CABG); pregnancy (3rd trimester)

Warnings

[U.S. Boxed Warning]: NSAIDs are associated with an increased risk of adverse cardiovascular events, including MI, stroke, and new onset or worsening of pre-existing hypertension. Risk may be increased with duration of use or pre-existing cardiovascular risk-factors or disease. Carefully evaluate individual cardiovascular risk profiles prior to prescribing. Use caution with fluid retention, CHF or hypertension.

Use of NSAIDs can compromise existing renal function. Renal toxicity can occur in patient with impaired renal function, dehydration, heart failure, liver dysfunction, those taking diuretics and ACEI and the elderly. Rehydrate patient before starting therapy. Monitor renal function closely. Not recommended for use in patients with advanced renal disease.

[U.S. Boxed Warning]: NSAIDs may increase risk of gastrointestinal irritation, ulceration, bleeding, and perforation. These events may occur at any time during therapy and without warning. Use caution with a history of GI disease (bleeding or ulcers), concurrent therapy with aspirin, anticoagulants and/or corticosteroids, smoking, use of alcohol, the elderly or debilitated patients.

Use the lowest effective dose for the shortest duration of time, consistent with individual patient goals, to reduce risk of cardiovascular or GI adverse events. Alternate therapies should be considered for patients at high risk.

NSAIDs may cause serious skin adverse events including exfoliative dermatitis, Stevens-Johnson syndrome (SJS) and toxic epidermal necrolysis (TEN). Anaphylactoid reactions may occur, even without prior exposure; patients with "aspirin triad" (bronchial asthma, aspirin intolerance, rhinitis) may be at increased risk. Do not use in patients who experience bronchospasm, asthma, rhinitis, or urticaria with NSAID or aspirin therapy.

Use with caution in patients with decreased hepatic function. Closely monitor patients with any abnormal LFT. Severe hepatic reactions (eg, fulminant hepatitis, liver failure) have occurred with NSAID use, rarely; discontinue if signs or symptoms of liver disease develop, or if systemic manifestations occur.

The elderly are at increased risk for adverse effects (especially peptic ulceration, CNS effects, renal toxicity) from NSAIDs even at low doses

Withhold for at least 4-6 half-lives prior to surgical or dental procedures. May cause photosensitivity reactions. Safety and efficacy have not been established in pediatric patients.

Dosage Forms

[DSC] = Discontinued product

Tablet: 500 mg, 750 mg

Relafen®: 500 mg, 750 mg [DSC]

Overdosage/Treatment

Decontamination: Activated charcoal

Supportive therapy: Hypotension/dehydration can be managed with I.V. fluid therapy; acidosis should be treated with bicarbonates, seizures with benzodiazepines; antacids, blood products are indicated, as appropriate, for hemorrhage

Enhancement of elimination: Dialysis or perfusion is indicated for secondary complications, acidosis, or renal failure and not toxin removal alone; multiple dosing of activated charcoal may be effective

Drug Interactions ACE inhibitors: Antihypertensive effects may be decreased by concurrent therapy with NSAIDs; monitor blood pressure.

Angiotensin II antagonists: Antihypertensive effects may be decreased by concurrent therapy with NSAIDs; monitor blood pressure.

Anticoagulants (warfarin, heparin, LMWHs) in combination with NSAIDs can cause increased risk of bleeding.

Antiplatelet drugs (ticlopidine, clopidogrel, aspirin, abciximab, dipyridamole, eptifibatide, tirofiban) can cause an increased risk of bleeding.

Beta-blockers: NSAIDs may decrease the antihypertensive effect of beta-blockers. Monitor.

Cholestyramine (and other bile acid sequestrants): May decrease the absorption of NSAIDs. Separate by at least 2 hours.

Corticosteroids may increase the risk of GI ulceration; avoid concurrent use.

Cyclosporine: NSAIDs may increase serum creatinine, potassium, blood pressure, and cyclosporine levels; monitor cyclosporine levels and renal function carefully.

Hydralazine's antihypertensive effect is decreased; avoid concurrent use.

Lithium levels can be increased; avoid concurrent use if possible or monitor lithium levels and adjust dose. Sulindac may have the least effect. When NSAID is stopped, lithium will need adjustment again.

Loop diuretics efficacy (diuretic and antihypertensive effect) is reduced.

Methotrexate: Severe bone marrow suppression, aplastic anemia, and GI toxicity have been reported with concomitant NSAID therapy. Avoid use during moderate or high-dose methotrexate (increased and prolonged methotrexate levels). NSAID use during low-dose treatment of rheumatoid arthritis has not been fully evaluated; extreme caution is warranted.

Thiazides antihypertensive effects are decreased; avoid concurrent use.

Warfarin's INRs may be increased by nabumetone. Monitor INR closely.

Use the lowest dose of NSAIDs possible and for the briefest duration.

Pregnancy Risk Factor C/D (3rd trimester)

Lactation Excretion in breast milk unknown/not recommended

Nadolol

Related Information
- Selected Properties of Beta-Adrenergic Blocking Drugs

CAS Number 42200-33-9

U.S. Brand Names Corgard®

Use Treatment of hypertension and angina pectoris; prophylaxis of migraine headaches

Mechanism of Action Competitively blocks response to beta-adrenergic stimulation; hydrophilic

Adverse Reactions

Cardiovascular: **Persistent bradycardia**, hypotension (orthostatic), Raynaud's syndrome, congestive heart failure, edema, sinus bradycardia, chest pain, angina, myocardial depression, QRS prolongation

Central nervous system: Fatigue, dizziness, malaise, ataxia

Dermatological: Rash, alopecia, toxic epidermal necrolysis, xerosis, urticaria, onycholysis, pruritus, psoriasis, licheniform eruptions

Gastrointestinal: Gastrointestinal discomfort, abdominal pain, flatulence, nausea, diarrhea, pancreatitis, xerostomia

Genitourinary: Impotence

Neuromuscular & skeletal: Paresthesia

Ocular: Optic atrophy

Respiratory: Wheezing, hypersensitivity, pneumonitis with elevated sedimentation rate, dyspnea, cough

Miscellaneous: Systemic lupus erythematosus

Signs and Symptoms of Overdose Ataxia, hyperglycemia, hyperkalemia, and impotence

Pharmacodynamics/Kinetics

Duration: 17-24 hours

Absorption: 30% to 40%

Distribution: Concentration in human breast milk is 4.6 times higher than serum

Protein binding: 28%

Half-life elimination: Adults: 10-24 hours; prolonged with renal impairment; End-stage renal disease: 45 hours

Time to peak, serum: 2-4 hours

Excretion: Urine (as unchanged drug)

Dosage Oral:

Adults: Initial: 40 mg/day, increase dosage gradually by 40-80 mg increments at 3- to 7-day intervals until optimum clinical response is obtained with profound slowing of heart rate; doses up to 160-240 mg/day in angina and 240-320 mg/day in hypertension may be necessary.

Hypertension: Usual dosage range (JNC 7): 40-120 mg once daily

Elderly: Initial: 20 mg/day; increase doses by 20 mg increments at 3- to 7-day intervals; usual dosage range: 20-240 mg/day.

Dosing adjustment in renal impairment:

Cl$_{cr}$ 31-40 mL/minute: Administer every 24-36 hours or administer 50% of normal dose.

Cl$_{cr}$ 10-30 mL/minute: Administer every 24-48 hours or administer 50% of normal dose.

Cl$_{cr}$ <10 mL/minute: Administer every 40-60 hours or administer 25% of normal dose.

Hemodialysis: Moderately dialyzable (20% to 50%); administer dose postdialysis or administer 40 mg supplemental dose.

Peritoneal dialysis: Supplemental dose is not necessary.

Dosing adjustment/comments in hepatic disease: Reduced dose probably necessary.

Monitoring Parameters Blood pressure, heart rate, fluid input and output, weight

Contraindications Hypersensitivity to nadolol or any component of the formulation; bronchial asthma; sinus bradycardia; sinus node dysfunction; heart block greater than first degree (except in patients with a functioning artificial pacemaker); cardiogenic shock; uncompensated cardiac failure

Warnings Administer only with extreme caution in patients with compensated heart failure, monitor for a worsening of the condition. Efficacy in heart failure has not been established for nadolol. **[U.S. Boxed Warning]:** **Beta-blocker therapy should not be withdrawn abruptly (particularly in patients with CAD), but gradually tapered to avoid acute tachycardia, hypertension, and/or ischemia.** Use caution with concurrent use of beta-blockers and either verapamil or diltiazem; bradycardia or heart block can occur. In general, patients with bronchospastic disease should not receive beta-blockers. Nadolol, if used at all, should be used cautiously in bronchospastic disease with close monitoring. Use cautiously in diabetics because it can mask prominent hypoglycemic symptoms. Can mask signs of thyrotoxicosis. Can cause fetal harm when administered in pregnancy. Use cautiously in the renally impaired (dosage adjustments are required). Use care with anesthetic agents which decrease myocardial function.

Dosage Forms [DSC] = Discontinued product

Tablet: 20 mg, 40 mg, 80 mg, 120 mg, 160 mg

Corgard®: 20 mg, 40 mg, 80 mg, 120 mg [DSC], 160 mg [DSC]

Reference Range Peak serum nadolol concentration of 5 ng/mL after a 2 mg dose; peak steady-state nadolol level after a 55 mg daily dose: 62 ng/mL

Overdosage/Treatment

Decontamination: Lavage (within 1 hour)/activated charcoal; **do not** use ipecac

Supportive therapy: Glucagon (50-150 mcg/kg followed by continuous drip of 1-5 mg/hour) for positive chronotropic effect; atropine/isoproterenol can be utilized to increase heart rate; calcium chloride may also be effective; do **not** use epinephrine

Enhancement of elimination: Multiple dosing of activated charcoal is effective; hemodialysis has been utilized with clinical improvement and increased clearance rate from 46-102 mL/minute (30% of drug can be fractionally removed during 4 hours of hemodialysis); in a nadolol overdose (6-20 mg of total drug removed); moderately dialyzable (20% to 50%)

Drug Interactions

Albuterol (and other beta$_2$ agonists): Effects may be blunted by nonspecific beta-blockers.

Alpha-blockers (prazosin, terazosin): Concurrent use of beta-blockers may increase risk of orthostasis.

Clonidine: Hypertensive crisis after or during withdrawal of either agent.

Drugs which slow AV conduction (digoxin): Effects may be additive with beta-blockers.

Epinephrine (including local anesthetics with epinephrine): Propranolol may cause hypertension.

Glucagon: Nadolol may blunt the hyperglycemic action of glucagon.

Insulin and oral hypoglycemics: Nadolol may mask symptoms of hypoglycemia.

Nadolol increases antipyrine's half-life.

NSAIDs (ibuprofen, indomethacin, naproxen, piroxicam) may reduce the antihypertensive effects of beta-blockers.

Salicylates may reduce the antihypertensive effects of beta-blockers.

Sulfonylureas: Beta-blockers may alter response to hypoglycemic agents.

Verapamil or diltiazem may have synergistic or additive pharmacological effects when taken concurrently with beta-blockers.

Pregnancy Risk Factor C

Pregnancy Implications No data available on crossing the placenta. Beta-blockers have been associated with bradycardia, hypotension, and IUGR; IUGR is probably related to maternal hypertension. Alternative beta-blockers are preferred for use during pregnancy due to limited data and prolonged half-life. Cases of neonatal hypoglycemia have been reported following maternal use of beta-blockers at parturition or during breast-feeding.

Lactation Enters breast milk/use caution (AAP rates "compatible")

Nursing Implications Patient's therapeutic response may be evaluated by looking at blood pressure, apical and radial pulses

Specific References

Chobanian AV, Bakris GL, Black HR, et al, "The Seventh Report of the Joint National Committee on Prevention, Detection, Evaluation, and Treatment of High Blood Pressure: The JNC 7 Report," *JAMA*, 2003, 289(19):2560-71.

Nalbuphine

CAS Number 20594-83-6; 23277-43-2

U.S. Brand Names Nubain®

Synonyms Nalbuphine Hydrochloride

Impairment Potential Yes

Use Relief of moderate to severe pain

Mechanism of Action Binds to opiate receptors in the CNS, causing inhibition of ascending pain pathways, altering the perception of and response to pain; produces generalized CNS depression. A 14-hydroxymorphine derivative. A kappa-receptor opioid agonist but a mcg-receptor antagonist.

Adverse Reactions

Cardiovascular: Hypotension, flushing, hypertension, tachycardia, sinus bradycardia, sinus tachycardia

Central nervous system: **CNS depression, narcotic withdrawal, drowsiness**, dizziness, headache, anxiety, agitation, hallucinations, confusion, nervousness, restlessness, night terrors, insomnia, paradoxical CNS stimulation

Dermatologic: Urticaria, skin rash

Gastrointestinal: Nausea, vomiting, anorexia, xerostomia, biliary tract spasm

Genitourinary: Ureteral spasm, decreased urination

Local: Pain at injection site

Neuromuscular & skeletal: Weakness

Ocular: Blurred vision

Respiratory: Apnea, respiratory depression, dyspnea, pulmonary edema

Miscellaneous: **Histamine release**, toxic megacolon, diaphoresis

Signs and Symptoms of Overdose Clammy skin, coma, depression, drowsiness, dyspepsia, dysphoria, hypotension, insomnia, miosis, night terrors

Pharmacodynamics/Kinetics

Onset of action: Peak effect: SubQ, I.M.: <15 minutes; I.V.: 2-3 minutes

Metabolism: Hepatic

Half-life elimination: 5 hours

Excretion: Feces; urine (~7% as metabolites)

Dosage I.M., I.V., SubQ:

Children 10 months to 14 years: Premedication: 0.2 mg/kg; maximum: 20 mg/dose

Adults: 10 mg/70 kg every 3-6 hours; maximum single dose: 20 mg; maximum daily dose: 160 mg

Dosing adjustment/comments in hepatic impairment: Use with caution and reduce dose

Stability Incompatible with nafcillin, diazepam, or pentobarbital

Monitoring Parameters Relief of pain, respiratory and mental status, blood pressure

Administration Administer I.M., SubQ, or I.V.

Contraindications Hypersensitivity to nalbuphine or any component of the formulation

Warnings Use caution in CNS depression. Sedation and psychomotor impairment are likely, and are additive with other CNS depressants or ethanol. May cause respiratory depression. Ambulatory patients must be cautioned about performing tasks which require mental alertness (eg, operating machinery or driving). Use with caution in patients with recent myocardial infarction, biliary tract surgery, head trauma, or increased intracranial pressure. Use caution in patients with decreased hepatic or renal function. May result in tolerance and/or drug dependence with chronic use; use with caution in patients with a history of drug dependence. Abrupt discontinuation following prolonged use may lead to withdrawal symptoms. May precipitate withdrawal symptoms in patients following prolonged therapy with mu opioid agonists. Use with caution in pregnancy (close neonatal monitoring required when used in labor and delivery). Safety and efficacy in pediatric patients (<18 years of age) have not been established.

Dosage Forms [DSC] = Discontinued product

Injection, solution, as hydrochloride: 10 mg/mL (10 mL); 20 mg/mL (10 mL)

Nubain®: 10 mg/mL (10 mL) [DSC]; 20 mg/mL (10 mL)

Injection, solution, as hydrochloride [preservative free]: 10 mg/mL (1 mL); 20 mg/mL (1 mL)

Nubain®: 10 mg/mL (1 mL); 20 mg/mL (1 mL)

Reference Range Peak blood nalbuphine level after a 30 mg oral dose in adults and elderly volunteers: 7 mcg/L and 49 mcg/L, respectively

Overdosage/Treatment Supportive therapy: Naloxone hydrochloride (0.4-2 mg I.V., SubQ, or through an endotracheal tube); a continuous infusion (at ²/₃ the response dose/hour) may be required. Risperidone (1 mg twice daily) can be used to treat nalbuphine-associated psychosis.

Antidote(s)
- Nalmefene [ANTIDOTE]
- Naloxone [ANTIDOTE]

Drug Interactions Increased toxicity: Barbiturate anesthetics may increase CNS depression

Pregnancy Risk Factor B/D (prolonged use or high doses at term)

Pregnancy Implications May cause neonatal bradycardia or respiratory depression when used during labor

Lactation Enters breast milk/use caution

Nursing Implications Observe patient for excessive sedation, apnea; implement safety measures, assist with ambulation; observe for narcotic withdrawal

Additional Information Little abuse potential

Specific Reference

Klinzing F, Vinner E, Brassart C, et al, "Hair Analysis by LC-MS as Evidence of Nalbuphine Abuse by a Nurse," *J Anal Tox*, 2007, 31: 62-5.

Nalidixic Acid

Related Information
- Therapeutic Drugs Associated with Hallucinations

CAS Number 389-08-2

U.S. Brand Names NegGram®

Synonyms Nalidixinic Acid

Use Urinary tract infections

Mechanism of Action Inhibits DNA polymerization in late stages of chromosomal replication; direct antagonist of gabanergic neurotransmission

Adverse Reactions

Central nervous system: Fever, chills, malaise, **drowsiness, dizziness**, confusion, toxic psychosis, seizures, **headache**, visual hallucinations, increased intracranial pressure, psychosis

Dermatologic: Rash, bullous eruptions, pruritus, photosensitivity reactions, exfoliative dermatitis, alopecia, angioedema, toxic epidermal necrolysis, urticaria, purpura, exanthem, photoallergic reaction

Endocrine & metabolic: Metabolic acidosis

Gastrointestinal: Nausea, vomiting, feces discoloration (greenish gray), feces discoloration (white/speckling)

Hematologic: Leukopenia, thrombocytopenia, hemolytic anemia, porphyrinogenic

Hepatic: Hepatotoxicity (cholestatic)

Neuromuscular & skeletal: Paresthesia

Ocular: Visual disturbances, nystagmus, color vision abnormalities

Miscellaneous: Systemic lupus erythematosus

Signs and Symptoms of Overdose Agranulocytosis, coma, dementia, dermatitis, diplopia, eosinophilia, erythema multiforme, granulocytopenia, hyperglycemia, hyperthermia, increased intracranial pressure, leukopenia, metabolic acidosis, nausea, neutropenia, photophobia, photosensitivity, pseudotumor cerebri, seizures, thrombocytopenia, toxic psychosis, vision color changes (blue tinge; violet tinge; yellow tinge), vomiting

Pharmacodynamics/Kinetics

Distribution: Achieves significant antibacterial concentrations only in the urinary tract; crosses placenta; enters breast milk

Protein binding: 90%

Metabolism: Partially hepatic; active metabolite, hydroxynalidixic acid

Half-life elimination: 6-7 hours; significantly prolonged with renal impairment

Time to peak, serum: 1-2 hours

Excretion: Urine (as unchanged drug, 80% as metabolites); feces (small amounts)

Dosage Oral:

Children 3 months to 12 years: 55 mg/kg/day divided every 6 hours; suppressive therapy is 33 mg/kg/day divided every 6 hours

Adults: 1 g 4 times/day for 2 weeks; then suppressive therapy of 500 mg 4 times/day

Dosing comments in renal impairment: Cl_cr <50 mL/minute: Avoid use

Monitoring Parameters Urinalysis, urine culture; CBC, renal, and hepatic function tests

Administration

May be administered with or without food; drink fluids liberally

Contraindications Hypersensitivity to nalidixic acid or any component of the formulation; infants <3 months of age; porphyria, seizures; concurrent melphalan or other alkylating agent; breast-feeding

Warnings

Use with caution in patients with impaired hepatic or renal function and prepubertal children; has been shown to cause cartilage degeneration in immature animals; may induce hemolysis in patients with G6PD deficiency; use caution in patients with seizure disorder. Potential for seizures, although very rare, may be increased with concomitant NSAID therapy. Tendon inflammation and/or rupture have been reported. Risk may be increased with concurrent corticosteroids, particularly in the elderly. Discontinue at first sign of tendon inflammation or pain. Peripheral neuropathy may rarely occur; prompt discontinuation is recommended in patients with signs and symptoms of neuropathy.

Severe hypersensitivity reactions, including anaphylaxis, have occurred with quinolone therapy. If an allergic reaction occurs (itching, urticaria, dyspnea, facial edema, loss of consciousness, tingling, cardiovascular collapse), discontinue drug immediately. Prolonged use may result in superinfection; pseudomembranous colitis may occur and should be considered in all patients who present with diarrhea. Quinolones may exacerbate myasthenia gravis, use with caution (rare, potentially life-threatening weakness of respiratory muscles may occur).

Dosage Forms

[DSC] = Discontinued product

Suspension, oral: 250 mg/5 mL (473 mL) [raspberry flavor] [DSC]

Tablet: 500 mg [DSC]

Reference Range Peak plasma level of 20-50 mcg/mL achieved 2 hours after oral dose of 1 g; urine concentration after 1 g oral dose can range from 25-250 mcg/mL

Overdosage/Treatment

Decontamination: Activated charcoal

Supportive therapy: Diazepam/lorazepam for seizures

Test Interactions False-positive urine glucose with Clinitest®, false increase in urinary VMA

Drug Interactions

Inhibits CYP1A2 (weak)

Corticosteroids: Concurrent use may increase the risk of tendon rupture, particularly in elderly patients (overall incidence rare).

Glyburide: Quinolones may increase the effect of glyburide; monitor.

Melphalan: Concomitant use of I.V. melphalan and nalidixic acid may increase the risk of developing necrotic enterocolitis (reported in pediatric patients).

Metal cations (aluminum, calcium, iron, magnesium, and zinc) bind quinolones in the gastrointestinal tract and inhibit absorption. Concurrent administration of most antacids, oral electrolyte supplements, quinapril, sucralfate, some didanosine formulations (chewable/buffered tablets and pediatric powder for oral suspension), and other highly-buffered oral drugs, should be avoided. Nalidixic acid should be administered 2 hours before or 2 hours after these agents.

Probenecid: May decrease renal secretion of nalidixic acid.

Warfarin: The hypoprothrombinemic effect of warfarin may be enhanced by some quinolone antibiotics; monitor INR.

Pregnancy Risk Factor B

Pregnancy Implications Teratogenic and embryocidal effects were observed in animal studies. One study suggests that use late in pregnancy may increase the risk of infantile pyloric stenosis in the newborn. However, this finding was based on a small number of cases and other causes such as chance could not be excluded. Other authors suggest that nalidixic acid is unlikely to be teratogenic at therapeutic doses, but that there is not enough data to state there is no risk.

Lactation Enters breast milk/contraindicated (AAP considers "compatible")

Naltrexone

Related Information
- Drugs Used in Addiction Treatment

CAS Number 16590-41-3; 16676-29-2

U.S. Brand Names Depade®; ReVia®; Vivitrol™

Synonyms Naltrexone Hydrochloride

Use Adjunct to the maintenance of an opioid-free state in detoxified individual; approved for use in the treatment of ethanol abuse; used in alternative medicine to treat HIV (T-cell count >500)

Mechanism of Action Naltrexone (a pure opioid antagonist) is a cyclopropyl derivative of oxymorphone similar in structure to naloxone and nalorphine (a morphine derivative); it acts as a competitive antagonist at opioid receptor sites, showing the highest affinity for mu receptors.

Adverse Reactions

Cardiovascular: Hypertension, tachycardia, sinus tachycardia

Central nervous system: **Insomnia, nervousness, headache**, irritability, anxiety, dysphoria, dizziness, panic attacks, delirium

Dermatologic: Rash, acne, pruritus, alopecia, oily skin

Gastrointestinal: **Nausea, abdominal cramping, vomiting**, anorexia

Hematologic: Thrombocytopenia, agranulocytosis, hemolysis

Hepatic: Hepatitis

Neuromuscular & skeletal: **Arthralgia**, myalgia

Ocular: Blurred vision

Otic: Tinnitus

Miscellaneous: Narcotic withdrawal

Signs and Symptoms of Overdose Agranulocytosis, dysphoria, granulocytopenia, hepatocellular damage, insomnia, leukopenia, neutropenia

Pharmacodynamics/Kinetics

Duration: Oral: 50 mg: 24 hours; 100 mg: 48 hours; 150 mg: 72 hours; I.M.: 4 weeks

Absorption: Oral: Almost complete

Distribution: V_d: 19 L/kg; widely throughout the body but considerable interindividual variation exists

Protein binding: 21%

Metabolism: Noncytochrome-mediated dehydrogenase conversion to 6-β-naltrexol and related minor metabolites; Oral: Extensive first-pass effect

Half-life elimination: Oral: 4 hours; 6-β-naltrexol: 13 hours; I.M.: naltrexone and 6-β-naltrexol: 5-10 days

Time to peak, serum: Oral: ~60 minutes; I.M.: Biphasic: 2 hours (first peak), 2-3 days (second peak)

Excretion: Primarily urine (as metabolites and unchanged drug)

Dosage

Adults: Do not give until patient is opioid-free for 7-10 days as determined by urinalysis

Oral: Alcohol dependence, opioid antidote: 25 mg; if no withdrawal signs within 1 hour give another 25 mg; maintenance regimen is flexible, variable and individualized (50 mg/day to 100-150 mg 3 times/week for 12 weeks); up to 800 mg/day has been tolerated in a small number of healthy adults without an adverse effect

I.M.: Alcohol dependence: 380 mg once every 4 weeks

Dosage adjustment in renal impairment: Use caution. No adjustment needed in mild impairment. Not adequately studied in moderate-to-severe renal impairment.

Dosage adjustment in hepatic impairment: Use caution. An increase in naltrexone AUC of approximately five- and 10-fold in patients with compensated or decompensated liver cirrhosis respectively, compared with normal liver function has been reported No adjustment required

with mild-to-moderate hepatic impairment. Not adequately studied in severe hepatic impairment.

Monitoring Parameters For narcotic withdrawal; liver function tests

Administration If there is any question of occult opioid dependence, perform a naloxone challenge test; do not attempt treatment until naloxone challenge is negative.

Oral: To minimize adverse gastrointestinal effects, administer with food or antacids or after meals; advise patient not to self-administer opiates while receiving naltrexone therapy.

I.M.: Vivitrol™: Administer I.M. into the upper outer quadrant of the gluteal area. Injection should alternate between the two buttocks. Do not substitute any components of the dose-pack; administer with needle provided.

Contraindications Hypersensitivity to naltrexone or any component of the formulation; narcotic dependence or current use of opioid analgesics; acute opioid withdrawal; failure to pass Narcan® challenge or positive urine screen for opioids; acute hepatitis; liver failure

Warnings[U.S. Boxed Warning]: Dose-related hepatocellular injury is possible; the margin of separation between the apparent safe and hepatotoxic doses appears to be only fivefold or less (contraindicated in acute hepatitis or hepatic failure).

May precipitate withdrawal symptoms in patients addicted to opiates, including pain, hypertension, sweating, agitation, irritability; in neonates: shrill cry, failure to feed. Patients should be opiate-free for a minimum of 7-10 days; use naloxone challenge test to confirm. Use with caution in patients with hepatic or renal impairment; not studied in severe hepatic or moderate-to-severe renal impairment.

Patients who had been treated with naltrexone may respond to lower opioid doses than previously used. This could result in potentially life-threatening opioid intoxication. Patients should be aware that they may be more sensitive to lower doses of opioids after naltrexone treatment is discontinued. Use of naltrexone does not eliminate or diminish withdrawal symptoms. Warn patients that attempts to overcome opioid blockade could lead to fatal overdose. Suicidal thoughts and depression have been reported; monitor closely.

Cases of eosinophilic pneumonia have been reported; monitor for hypoxia and dyspnea. Safety and efficacy in children have not been established.

Dosage Forms

Injection, powder for suspension [extended-release microspheres]:
Vivitrol™: 380 mg [diluent provided]

Tablet, as hydrochloride: 50 mg
Depade®: 25 mg, 50 mg, 100 mg
ReVia®: 50 mg

Reference Range Peak plasma naltrexone and 6-beta-naltrexol levels after a 100 mg oral dose: 27 ng/mL and 106 ng/mL, respectively

Overdosage/Treatment

Decontamination: Ipecac within 30 minutes or lavage (within 1 hour)/activated charcoal

Supportive therapy: Dysmorphic/irritability can be treated by titrating with morphine

Test Interactions ↑ gonadotropin, cortisol (S)

Drug Interactions Narcotic analgesics: Decreased effect of narcotic analgesics; may precipitate acute withdrawal reaction in physically dependent patients; concurrent use is contraindicated

Thioridazine: Lethargy and somnolence have been reported with the combination of naltrexone and thioridazine

Pregnancy Risk Factor C

Pregnancy Implications Evidence of early fetal loss has been observed in animal studies with oral naltrexone. There are no adequate and well-controlled studies in pregnant women.

Lactation Enters breast milk/not recommended

Nursing Implications Monitor for narcotic withdrawal

Additional Information Up to 800 mg/day has been tolerated in adults without an adverse effect

Specific References

Ameisen O, "Naltrexone Treatment for Alcohol Dependency," *JAMA*, 2005, 294(8):899-900.

ElChaar GM, Maisch NM, Augusto LM, et al, "Efficacy and Safety of Naltrexone Use in Pediatric Patients with Autistic Disorder," *Ann Pharmacother*, 2006, 40(6):1086-95.

O'Malley SS, Rounsaville BJ, Farren C, et al, "Initial and Maintenance Naltrexone Treatment for Alcohol Dependence Using Primary Care vs. Specialty Care: A Nested Sequence of 3 Randomized Trials," *Arch Intern Med*, 2003, 163(14):1695-704.

Naphazoline

CAS Number 550-99-2; 835-31-4

U.S. Brand Names AK-Con™; Albalon®; Allersol®; Clear Eyes® ACR [OTC]; Clear Eyes® [OTC]; Naphcon® [OTC]; Privine® [OTC]; VasoClear® [OTC]

Synonyms Naphazoline Hydrochloride

Use Topical ocular vasoconstrictor; will temporarily relieve congestion, itching, and minor irritation, and to control hyperemia in patients with superficial corneal vascularity; also has been used to treat myopathic ptosis

Mechanism of Action Stimulates alpha-adrenergic receptors in the arterioles of the conjunctiva and the nasal mucosa to produce vasoconstriction

Adverse Reactions

Cardiovascular: **Systemic cardiovascular stimulation, premature ventricular contractions (I.V.)**

Central nervous system: **Dizziness, headache, nervousness**, hypothermia

Gastrointestinal: **Nausea**

Local: **Transient stinging, nasal mucosa irritation, dryness, rebound congestion**

Ocular: **Mydriasis, increased intraocular pressure, blurring of vision**

Respiratory: **Sneezing**

Signs and Symptoms of Overdose Apnea, bradycardia, cardiovascular collapse, CNS depression, coma, hypothermia

Admission Criteria/Prognosis Patients may be discharged if asymptomatic 6 hours postingestion

Pharmacodynamics/Kinetics

Onset of action: Decongestant: Topical: ~10 minutes

Duration: 2-6 hours

Dosage Nasal:

Children:

<6 years: Intranasal: Not recommended (especially infants) due to CNS depression

6-12 years: 1 spray of 0.05% into each nostril every 6 hours if necessary; therapy should not exceed 3-5 days

Children >12 years and Adults: 0.05%, instill 1-2 drops or sprays every 6 hours if needed; therapy should not exceed 3-5 days

Ophthalmic:

Children <6 years: Not recommended for use due to CNS depression (especially in infants)

Children >6 years and Adults: Instill 1-2 drops into conjunctival sac of affected eye(s) every 3-4 hours; therapy generally should not exceed 3-4 days

Stability Store in tight, light-resistant containers

Administration Ophthalmic: Contact lenses should be removed prior to administering products containing benzalkonium chloride.

Contraindications Hypersensitivity to naphazoline or any component of the formulation; narrow-angle glaucoma

Warnings Rebound congestion may occur with extended use. Use with caution in the presence of hypertension, diabetes, hyperthyroidism, heart disease, coronary artery disease, cerebral arteriosclerosis, local infection or injury, benign prostatic hyperplasia, or long-standing bronchial asthma. Use in children, especially infants, may cause CNS depression, coma and marked reduction in body temperature. Products may contain benzalkonium chloride which may be absorbed by soft contact lenses.

When used for self-medication (OTC): Patients should notify healthcare provider if symptoms last >72 hours or if condition worsens. In addition with ophthalmic products, contact presciber in case of eye pain or if changes in vision occur.

Dosage Forms Solution, intranasal drops, as hydrochloride:

Privine®: 0.05% (25 mL)

Solution, intranasal spray, as hydrochloride:

Privine®: 0.05% (20 mL)

Solution, ophthalmic, as hydrochloride:

AK-Con™, Albalon®, Allersol®: 0.1% (15 mL) [contains benzalkonium chloride]

Clear Eyes® ACR: 0.012% (15 mL, 30 mL) [contains glycerin 0.2%, zinc sulfate 0.25%, and benzalkonium chloride]

Clear Eyes® Extra Relief: 0.012% (6 mL, 15 mL, 30 mL) [contains glycerin 0.2% and benzalkonium chloride]

Naphcon®: 0.012% (15 mL) [contains benzalkonium chloride]

Overdosage/Treatment

Decontamination: **Oral**: Do not induce emesis; lavage (with airway protection) may be useful if performed within 1 hour of ingestion; activated charcoal can be given. **Ocular**: Irrigation copiously with normal saline or water

Supportive therapy: Hypotension and/or bradycardia will usually respond to isotonic I.V. fluid administration (10-20 mL/kg); atropine can cause significant hypertension if given; nitroprusside or phentolamine can be given to treat hypertension while phentolamine can be used to treat localized vasoconstriction; seizures can be treated with lorazepam or diazepam; phenytoin or phenobarbital can be used in refractory cases; naloxone and flumazenil do not appear to be useful

Drug Interactions

Guanadrel: May enhance the therapeutic effect of alpha$_1$-agonists, in particular the mydriatic effects of ophthalmic products.

MAO inhibitors: MAO inhibitors may enhance the hypertensive effect of alpha$_1$-agonists; avoid use.

Methyldopa: May enhance the therapeutic effect of alpha$_1$-agonists, in particular the mydriatic effects of ophthalmic products.

Tricyclic antidepressants: Tricyclic antidepressants may enhance the vasopressor effect of alpha$_1$-agonists; avoid use.

Pregnancy Risk Factor C

Pregnancy Implications Animal reproduction studies have not been conducted.

Lactation Excretion in breast milk unknown/use caution

Nursing Implications Rebound congestion can result with continued use

Additional Information Recovery from overdose usually occurs within 36 hours

---

Naproxen

Related Information

• Nonsteroidal Anti-inflammatory Drugs

CAS Number 222-53-1; 26159-34-2

U.S. Brand Names Aleve® [OTC]; Anaprox® DS; Anaprox®; EC-Naprosyn®; Midol® Extended Relief; Naprelan®; Naprosyn®; Pamprin® Maximum Strength All Day Relief [OTC]

Synonyms Naproxen Sodium

Use Management of inflammatory disease and rheumatoid disorders (including juvenile rheumatoid arthritis); acute gout; mild to moderate pain; dysmenorrhea; fever, migraine headache

Mechanism of Action Inhibits prostaglandin synthesis by decreasing the activity of the enzyme, cyclooxygenase, which results in decreased formation of prostaglandin precursors

Adverse Reactions

Cardiovascular: Circulatory collapse, vasculitis

Central nervous system: Headache, aseptic meningitis, psychosis, cognitive dysfunction, **dizziness**, coma, seizures, exacerbation of Parkinson's disease

Dermatologic: **Rash, pruritus**, increased incidence of shallow facial scars (relative risk is 6) in children, exfoliative dermatitis, pityriasis rosea-like reaction, erythema multiforme, alopecia, angioedema, bullous skin disease, toxic epidermal necrolysis, Stevens-Johnson syndrome, erythema nodosum, exanthem, lichen planus, cutaneous vasculitis, phototoxicity

Endocrine & metabolic: Hyperkalemia, anion gap metabolic acidosis, parotiditis, parotitis, fluid retention

Gastrointestinal: **Abdominal discomfort, nausea**, vomiting, **GI bleeding, GI ulceration, constipation**, diarrhea, dyspepsia, pancreatitis, esophageal ulcerations, **heartburn, perforation, indigestion**, aphthous stomatitis, xerostomia, gastrointestinal vasculitis

Hematologic: Leukopenia, neutropenia, agranulocytosis, granulocytopenia, aplastic anemia (rare), platelet inhibition, eosinophilia, thrombocytopenia

Hepatic: Elevated transaminases, hepatitis (fulminant), aminotransferase level elevation (asymptomatic)

Ocular: Vortex keratopathy

Otic: Ototoxicity, tinnitus

Renal: Renal failure (acute), nephrotic syndrome, chronic renal failure, albuminuria, renal vasculitis

Respiratory: Wheezing, pulmonary infiltrate, respiratory depression, eosinophilic pneumonia

Miscellaneous: Hypersensitivity, systemic lupus erythematosus (SLE), fixed drug eruption, leukoclastic vasculitis

Signs and Symptoms of Overdose Coagulopathy, cognitive dysfunction, colitis, depression, drowsiness, ejaculatory disturbances, gastritis, GI bleeding, gout, impotence, increased intraocular pressure, lichenoid eruptions, lightheadedness, meningitis, nausea, nephrotic syndrome, night terrors, ototoxicity, photosensitivity, purpura, stomatitis, tinnitus, vomiting, wheezing. Severe poisoning can manifest with coma, hypotension, metabolic acidosis, renal and/or hepatic failure, respiratory depression, seizures

Pharmacodynamics/Kinetics

Onset of action: Analgesic: 1 hour; Anti-inflammatory: ~2 weeks

Peak effect: Anti-inflammatory: 2-4 weeks

Duration: Analgesic: ≤7 hours; Anti-inflammatory: ≤12 hours

Absorption: Almost 100%

Protein binding: >99%; increased free fraction in elderly

Half-life elimination: Normal renal function: 12-17 hours; End-stage renal disease: No change

Time to peak, serum: 1-4 hours

Excretion: Urine (95%)

Dosage Note: Dosage expressed as naproxen base; 200 mg naproxen base is equivalent to 220 mg naproxen sodium.

Oral:

Children >2 years: Juvenile arthritis: 10 mg/kg/day in 2 divided doses

Adults:

Gout, acute: Initial: 750 mg, followed by 250 mg every 8 hours until attack subsides. **Note:** EC-Naprosyn® is not recommended.

Migraine, acute (unlabeled use): Initial: 500-750 mg.; an additional 250-500 mg may be given if needed (maximum: 1250 mg in 24 hours). **Note:** EC-Naprosyn® is not recommended.

Pain (mild-to-moderate), dysmenorrhea, acute tendonitis, bursitis: Initial: 500 mg, then 250 mg every 6-8 hours; maximum: 1250 mg/day naproxen base

Rheumatoid arthritis, osteoarthritis, and ankylosing spondylitis: 500-1000 mg/day in 2 divided doses; may increase to 1.5 g/day of naproxen base for limited time period

OTC labeling: Pain/fever:

Children $\geq$ 12 years and Adults $\leq$ 65 years: 200 mg naproxen base every 8-12 hours; if needed, may take 400 mg naproxen base for the initial dose; maximum: 600 mg naproxen base/24 hours

Adults >65 years: 200 mg naproxen base every 12 hours

Dosing adjustment in renal impairment: Cl_{cr} <30 mL/minute: use is not recommended

Monitoring Parameters Occult blood loss, periodic liver function test, CBC, BUN, serum creatinine

Administration Administer with food, milk, or antacids to decrease GI adverse effects

Suspension: Shake suspension well before administration.

Tablet, extended release: Swallow tablet whole; do not break, crush, or chew.

Contraindications Hypersensitivity to naproxen, aspirin, other NSAIDs, or any component of the formulation; perioperative pain in the setting of coronary artery bypass surgery (CABG); pregnancy (3rd trimester)

Warnings

[U.S. Boxed Warning]: NSAIDs are associated with an increased risk of adverse cardiovascular events, including MI, stroke, and new onset or worsening of pre-existing hypertension. Risk may be increased with duration of use or pre-existing cardiovascular risk-factors or disease. Carefully evaluate individual cardiovascular risk profiles prior to prescribing. Use caution with fluid retention, CHF, or hypertension. Use the lowest effective dose for the shortest duration of time, consistent with individual patient goals, to reduce risk of cardiovascular or GI adverse events. Alternate therapies should be considered for patients at high risk.

[U.S. Boxed Warning]: NSAIDs may increase risk of gastrointestinal irritation, ulceration, bleeding, and perforation. These events may occur at any time during therapy and without warning. Use caution with a history of GI disease (bleeding or ulcers), concurrent therapy with aspirin, anticoagulants and/or corticosteroids, smoking, use of alcohol, the elderly or debilitated patients.

Use of NSAIDs can compromise existing renal function. Renal toxicity can occur in patient with impaired renal function, dehydration, heart failure, liver dysfunction, those taking diuretics and ACEI and the elderly. Rehydrate patient before starting therapy. Monitor renal function closely. Naproxen is not recommended for patients with advanced renal disease.

NSAIDs may cause serious skin adverse events including exfoliative dermatitis, Stevens-Johnson Syndrome (SJS) and toxic epidermal necrolysis (TEN). Anaphylactoid reactions may occur, even without prior exposure; patients with "aspirin triad" (bronchial asthma, aspirin intolerance, rhinitis) may be at increased risk. Do not use in patients who experience bronchospasm, asthma, rhinitis, or urticaria with NSAID or aspirin therapy.

Use with caution in patients with decreased hepatic function. Closely monitor patients with any abnormal LFT. Severe hepatic reactions (eg, fulminant hepatitis, liver failure) have occurred with NSAID use, rarely; discontinue if signs or symptoms of liver disease develop, or if systemic manifestations occur.

The elderly are at increased risk for adverse effects (especially peptic ulceration, CNS effects, renal toxicity) from NSAIDs even at low doses.

Withhold for at least 4-6 half-lives prior to surgical or dental procedures. Safety and efficacy have not been established in children <2 years of age.

OTC labeling: Prior to self-medication, patients should contact health care provider if they have had recurring stomach pain or upset, ulcers, bleeding problems, high blood pressure, heart or kidney disease, other serious medical problems, are currently taking a diuretic, or are $\geq$ 60 years of age. Recommended dosages should not be exceeded, due to an increased risk of GI bleeding. Consuming $\geq$ 3 alcoholic beverages/day or taking longer than recommended may increase the risk of GI bleeding. When used for self-medication, patients should be instructed to contact healthcare provider if used for fever lasting >3 days or for pain lasting >10 days in adults or >3 days in children. Not for self-medication (OTC use) in children <12 years of age.

Dosage Forms

Caplet, as sodium (Aleve®, Midol® Extended Relief, Pamprin® Maximum Strength All Day Relief): 220 mg [equivalent to naproxen 200 mg and sodium 20 mg]

Gelcap, as sodium (Aleve®): 220 mg [equivalent to naproxen 200 mg and sodium 20 mg]

Suspension, oral (Naprosyn®): 125 mg/5 mL (480 mL) [contains sodium 0.3 mEq/mL; orange-pineapple flavor]

Tablet (Naprosyn®): 250 mg, 375 mg, 500 mg

Tablet, as sodium: 220 mg [equivalent to naproxen 200 mg and sodium 20 mg]; 275 mg [equivalent to naproxen 250 mg and sodium 25 mg]; 550 mg [equivalent to naproxen 500 mg and sodium 50 mg]

Aleve®: 220 mg [equivalent to naproxen 200 mg and sodium 20 mg]

Anaprox®: 275 mg [equivalent to naproxen 250 mg and sodium 25 mg]

Anaprox® DS: 550 mg [equivalent to naproxen 500 mg and sodium 50 mg]

Tablet, controlled release, as sodium: 550 mg [equivalent to naproxen 500 mg and sodium 50 mg]

Naprelan®: 421.5 mg [equivalent to naproxen 375 mg and sodium 37.5 mg]; 550 mg [equivalent to naproxen 500 mg and sodium 50 mg]

Tablet, delayed release (EC-Naprosyn®): 375 mg, 500 mg

Reference Range

Trough concentrations of >50 mcg/L (217 μmol/L) are therapeutic in patients with rheumatoid arthritis; serum naproxen level of 414 mg/L associated with oral ingestion of 25 g and mild toxicity

Therapeutic range: 30-90 mcg/mL

Overdosage/Treatment

Decontamination: Activated charcoal

Supportive therapy: Hypotension/dehydration can be managed with I.V. fluid therapy; acidosis should be treated with bicarbonates, seizures with benzodiazepines; antacids, blood products are indicated, as appropriate, for hemorrhage; famotidine (40 mg 2 times/day) can decrease incidence of gastric or duodenal ulcers in patients receiving long-term therapy of this drug

Enhancement of elimination: Dialysis or perfusion is indicated for secondary complications, acidosis, or renal failure and not toxin removal alone; multiple dosing of activated charcoal may be effective

Test Interactions ↑ chloride (S), sodium (S); causes a falsely increased free thyroxine

Drug Interactions

Substrate (minor) of CYP1A2, 2C9

ACE inhibitors: Antihypertensive effects may be decreased by concurrent therapy with NSAIDs; monitor blood pressure.

Angiotensin II antagonists: Antihypertensive effects may be decreased by concurrent therapy with NSAIDs; monitor blood pressure.

Anticoagulants (warfarin, heparin, LMWHs) in combination with NSAIDs can cause increased risk of bleeding.

Antiplatelet drugs (ticlopidine, clopidogrel, aspirin, abciximab, dipyridamole, eptifibatide, tirofiban) can cause an increased risk of bleeding.

Beta-blockers: NSAIDs may decrease the antihypertensive effect of beta-blockers. Monitor.

Cholestyramine (and other bile acid sequestrants): May decrease the absorption of NSAIDs. Separate by at least 2 hours.

Corticosteroids may increase the risk of GI ulceration; avoid concurrent use.

Cyclosporine: NSAIDs may increase serum creatinine, potassium, blood pressure, and cyclosporine levels; monitor cyclosporine levels and renal function carefully.

Hydralazine's antihypertensive effect is decreased; avoid concurrent use.

Lithium levels can be increased; avoid concurrent use if possible or monitor lithium levels and adjust dose. Sulindac may have the least effect. When NSAID is stopped, lithium will need adjustment again.

Loop diuretics efficacy (diuretic and antihypertensive effect) is reduced. Indomethacin reduces this efficacy, however, it may be anticipated with any NSAID.

Methotrexate: Severe bone marrow suppression, aplastic anemia, and GI toxicity have been reported with concomitant NSAID therapy. Avoid use during moderate or high-dose methotrexate (increased and prolonged methotrexate levels). NSAID use during low-dose treatment of rheumatoid arthritis has not been fully evaluated; extreme caution is warranted.

Thiazides antihypertensive effects are decreased; avoid concurrent use.

Warfarin's INRs may be increased by naproxen. Other NSAIDs may have the same effect depending on dose and duration. Monitor INR closely. Use the lowest dose of NSAIDs possible and for the briefest duration.

Pregnancy Risk Factor B/D (3rd trimester)

Pregnancy Implications Crosses the placenta; maternal overdosage has lead to neonatal distress; drowsiness, hypotonia, edema

Lactation Enters breast milk/not recommended (AAP rates "compatible")

Nursing Implications Administer with food, milk, or antacids to decrease GI adverse effects

Additional Information Naproxen: Naprosyn® naproxen sodium: Anaprox®; 275 mg of Anaprox® equivalent to 250 mg of Naprosyn®

Specific References

Golden HE, Moskowitz RW, and Minic M, "Analgesic Efficacy and Safety of Nonprescription Doses of Naproxen Sodium Compared with Acetaminophen in the Treatment of Osteoarthritis of the Knee," *Am J Ther*, 2004, 11(2):85-94.

Mullen WM, Meier KM, Hagar SM, et al, "Severe Naproxen Overdose with Elevated Serum Levels," *J Toxicol Clin Toxicol*, 2003, 41(5):655.

N-Benzylpiperazine

Related Information
- Amphetamines, Qualitative, Urine

Use Hallucinogen; has been utilized as an antidepressant

Mechanism of Action Sympathomimetic: Similar autonomic effects of S(+)-amphetamine. Triggers release of dopamine and norepinephrine, and inhibits reuptake (in the CNS) of dopamine, norepinephrine, and serotonin

Adverse Reactions
Central nervous system: Seizures, insomnia, agitation, auditory/visual hallucinations
Ocular: Mydriasis

Toxicodynamics/Kinetics
Metabolism: Hepatic to benzylamine and N-benzylethylenediamine
Elimination: Renal

Dosage Hallucinogenic: Oral: 75-250 mg

Reference Range Whole blood (postmortem) N-benzylpiperazine level of 1.7 mcg/g blood associated with fatality

Overdosage/Treatment
Decontamination: Lavage (within 1 hour)/activated charcoal
Supportive therapy: Amphetamine psychosis:
Haloperidol: I.V.: 5-10 mg
Diazepam: I.V.: 5-10 mg
Droperidol: I.M.: 2.5-5 mg can be used for psychosis if I.V. access is not available
Oral: Risperidone 4 mgm and lorazepam 3 mg can aid in remission of neuropsychiatric effects
Hypertension that is not responsive to sedation can be treated with phentolamine or nitroprusside
Enhancement of elimination: Multiple dosing of activated charcoal may be useful. While acid diuresis can increase excretion, it is not recommended due to renal effects.

Additional Information Approximately 10% of the potency of S(+)-amphetamine; will test positive for amphetamines on urinary immunoassay

Specific Reference
Wikström M, Holmgren P, and Ahlner J, "A2 (N-Benzylpiperazine): A New Drug of Abuse in Sweden," *J Anal Tox*, 2004, 28(1):67-70.

Nebivolol

CAS Number 99200-09-6

Unlabeled/Investigational Use Hypertension

Mechanism of Action Selective beta$_1$-adrenoceptor antagonist which is mostly due to the D-isomer; L-isomer may improve left ventricular function

Adverse Reactions
Cardiovascular: Bradycardia, palpitations, sinus bradycardia
Central nervous system: Headache, dizziness, somnolence, insomnia
Endocrine & metabolic: Hypertriglyceridemia (doses >30 mg)
Gastrointestinal: Nausea
Genitourinary: Impotence
Neuromuscular & skeletal: Myalgia

Signs and Symptoms of Overdose Hypotension, impotence

Toxicodynamics/Kinetics
Distribution: V$_d$: 10.1-39.4 L/kg
Protein binding: 98%
Metabolism: Hepatic (aromatic hydroxylation) to nebivolol glucuronide
Bioavailability: 12% (fast metabolizers); 96% (slow metabolizers)
Half-life: 8 hours (27 hours in slow metabolizers)

Dosage Oral: 5 mg once daily

Reference Range Peak plasma level of 1 mcg/L in fast metabolizers and ~3 mcg/L in slow metabolizers following a 5 mg oral dose; no change in plasma catecholamine levels (either at rest or during exercise)

Overdosage/Treatment
Decontamination: Activated charcoal; **do not** use ipecac
Supportive therapy: Glucagon (50-150 mcg/kg followed by continuous drip of 1-5 mg/hour) for positive chronotropic effect; atropine/isoproterenol can be utilized to increase heart rate; calcium chloride may also be effective
Enhancement of elimination: Multiple dosing of activated charcoal is not likely to be of benefit; dialysis is not useful; not dialyzable (0% to 5%)

Antidote(s)
- Glucagon [ANTIDOTE]

Nedocromil Sodium

CAS Number 101626-68-0; 69049-73-6; 69049-74-7

Use
Aerosol: Maintenance therapy in patients with mild to moderate bronchial asthma
Ophthalmic: Treatment of itching associated with allergic conjunctivitis

Mechanism of Action Disodium salt of a pyranoquinolone dicarboxylic acid which inhibits mediator release from inflammatory cells; can decrease bronchial hyper-reactivity; greater effect in inhibiting histamine release than cromolyn

Adverse Reactions
Cardiovascular: Chest pain, angina, sinus tachycardia
Central nervous system: Dizziness, headache, fatigue
Gastrointestinal: **Bitter taste**, nausea, vomiting, xerostomia, diarrhea, unpleasant taste
Respiratory: Coughing, pharyngitis, rhinitis, bronchitis, dyspnea, bronchospasm

Signs and Symptoms of Overdose Bitter taste (13%), bronchospasm, dizziness, headache, nausea, vomiting

Pharmacodynamics/Kinetics
Duration of therapeutic effect: 2 hours
Protein binding, plasma: 89%
Bioavailability: Systemic: 7% to 9% absorption
Half-life: 1.5-2 hours
Elimination: Excreted unchanged in urine

Dosage Adults: Metered dose inhaler: 4 mg twice daily, up to 4 times/day

Monitoring Parameters Use of beta agonists (oral or inhaled), peak expiratory flow rates, frequency and severity of wheezing, coughing, chest tightness, shortness of breath or dyspnea

Contraindications Hypersensitivity to nedocromil or other ingredients in the preparation

Warnings Safety and efficacy in children <6 years of age have not been established; if systemic or inhaled steroid therapy is at all reduced, monitor patients carefully; nedocromil is **not** a bronchodilator and, therefore, should not be used for reversal of acute bronchospasm

Dosage Forms Aerosol, as sodium: 1.75 mg/activation (16.2 g)

Reference Range Peak plasma level after a 4 mg dose (inhalation): ~3.3 ng/mL in healthy person and 2.8 ng/mL in asthmatic patients; levels not relatable to effect

Overdosage/Treatment
Decontamination: Oral: Activated charcoal
Supportive therapy: Treat inhalation exposure with 100% humidified oxygen; treat anaphylaxis with epinephrine and corticosteroids; albuterol can be given for bronchospasm

Pregnancy Risk Factor B

Nursing Implications Nedocromil is **not** a bronchodilator and, therefore, should not be used for reversal of acute bronchospasm; has no known therapeutic systemic activity when delivered by inhalation

Additional Information Each canister provides ~112 inhalations; 1.75 g/actuation

Nefazodone

Related Information
- Antidepressant Agents

U.S. Brand Names Serzone®

Synonyms Nefazodone Hydrochloride; Serzone

Impairment Potential Yes

Use Treatment of depression

Unlabeled/Investigational Use Post-traumatic stress disorder

Mechanism of Action Chemically related to trazodone, 5-HT$_2$ receptor antagonist, also alpha$_1$-adrenergic antagonist; acts to inhibit neuronal uptake of serotonin and norepinephrine

Adverse Reactions
Cardiovascular: Postural hypotension, AV block
Central nervous system: **Headache, drowsiness, insomnia, agitation, dizziness**, lightheadedness, confusion, memory impairment, abnormal dreams, decreased concentration, ataxia, hallucinations, seizures, serotonin syndrome
Dermatologic: Pruritus, rash, angioedema, photosensitivity, Stevens-Johnson syndrome
Endocrine & metabolic: Galactorrhea, gynecomastia, increased prolactin, hyponatremia
Gastrointestinal: **Xerostomia, nausea, constipation**, vomiting, dyspepsia, diarrhea, increased appetite, thirst, taste perversion
Genitourinary: Impotence, priapism
Hematologic: Leukopenia, thrombocytopenia
Hepatic: Hepatic failure, hepatic necrosis
Neuromuscular & skeletal: **Weakness**, arthralgia, paresthesia, tremor, rhabdomyolysis (with lovastatin/simvastatin)
Ocular: Blurred vision, abnormal vision, visual field defect, eye pain
Otic: Tinnitus
Respiratory: Cough, bronchitis, dyspnea
Miscellaneous: Flu syndrome, allergic reaction

Signs and Symptoms of Overdose Bradycardia, diaphoresis, hypotension lethargy, nausea, vomiting

Admission Criteria/Prognosis Admit any adult ingestion >1 g.

Pharmacodynamics/Kinetics
Onset of action: Therapeutic: Up to 6 weeks

Metabolism: Hepatic to three active metabolites: Triazoledione, hydro-xynefazodone, and m-chlorophenylpiperazine (mCPP)

Bioavailability: 20% (variable)

Half-life elimination: Parent drug: 2-4 hours; active metabolites persist longer

Time to peak, serum: 1 hour, prolonged in presence of food

Excretion: Primarily urine (as metabolites); feces

Dosage Oral:

Children and Adolescents: Depression: Target dose: 300-400 mg/day (mean: 3.4 mg/kg)

Adults: Depression: 200 mg/day, administered in 2 divided doses initially, with a range of 300-600 mg/day in 2 divided doses thereafter

Monitoring Parameters If AST/ALT increase >3 times ULN, the drug should be discontinued and not reintroduced; mental status for depression, suicidal ideation (especially at the beginning of therapy or when doses are increased or decreased), anxiety, social functioning, mania, panic attacks

Administration Dosing after meals may decrease lightheadedness and postural hypotension, but may also decrease absorption and therefore effectiveness.

Contraindications Hypersensitivity to nefazodone, related compounds (phenylpiperazines), or any component of the formulation; liver injury due to previous nefazodone treatment, active liver disease, or elevated serum transaminases; concurrent use or use of MAO inhibitors within previous 14 days; use in a patient during the acute recovery phase of MI; concurrent use with carbamazepine, cisapride, or pimozide; concurrent therapy with triazolam or alprazolam is generally contraindicated (dosage must be reduced by 75% for triazolam and 50% for alprazolam; such reductions may not be possible with available dosage forms).

Warnings

[U.S. Boxed Warning]: Antidepressants increase the risk of suicidal thinking and behavior in children and adolescents with major depressive disorder (MDD) and other depressive disorders; consider risk prior to prescribing. Closely monitor for clinical worsening, suicidality, or unusual changes in behavior; the child's family or caregiver should be instructed to closely observe the patient and communicate condition with healthcare provider. Such observation would generally include at least weekly face-to-face contact with patients or their family members or caregivers during the first 4 weeks of treatment, then every other week visits for the next 4 weeks, then at 12 weeks, and as clinically indicated beyond 12 weeks. Additional contact by telephone may be appropriate between face-to-face visits. Adults treated with antidepressants should be observed similarly for clinical worsening and suicidality, especially during the initial few months of a course of drug therapy, or at times of dose changes, either increases or decreases. A medication guide should be dispensed with each prescription. **Nefazodone is not FDA approved for use in children.**

The possibility of a suicide attempt is inherent in major depression and may persist until remission occurs. Monitor for worsening of depression or suicidality, especially during initiation of therapy or with dose increases or decreases. Worsening depression and severe abrupt suicidality that are not part of the presenting symptoms may require discontinuation or modification of drug therapy. Use caution in high-risk patients during initiation of therapy. Prescriptions should be written for the smallest quantity consistent with good patient care. The patient's family or caregiver should be alerted to monitor patients for the emergence of suicidality and associated behaviors such as anxiety, agitation, panic attacks, insomnia, irritability, hostility, impulsivity, akathisia, hypomania, and mania; patients should be instructed to notify their healthcare provider if any of these symptoms or worsening depression occur.

May worsen psychosis in some patients or precipitate a shift to mania or hypomania in patients with bipolar disorder. Monotherapy in patients with bipolar disorder should be avoided. Patients presenting with depressive symptoms should be screened for bipolar disorder. **Nefazodone is not FDA approved for the treatment of bipolar depression.**

Cases of life-threatening hepatic failure have been reported (risk should be considered when choosing an agent for the treatment of depression); discontinue if clinical signs or symptoms suggest liver failure. May cause sedation, resulting in impaired performance of tasks requiring alertness (eg, operating machinery or driving). Sedative effects may be additive with other CNS depressants. Does not potentiate ethanol but use is not advised. The degree of sedation is low relative to other antidepressants.. May increase the risks associated with electroconvulsive therapy. Consider discontinuing, when possible, prior to elective surgery. Therapy should not be abruptly discontinued in patients receiving high doses for prolonged periods. Rare reports of priapism have occurred. The incidence of sexual dysfunction with nefazodone is generally lower than with SSRIs.

Use with caution in patients at risk of hypotension or in patients where transient hypotensive episodes would be poorly tolerated (cardiovascular disease or cerebrovascular disease). The risk of postural hypotension is low relative to other antidepressants. Use with caution in patients with urinary retention, benign prostatic hyperplasia, narrow-angle glaucoma, xerostomia, visual problems, constipation, or history of bowel obstruction (due to anticholinergic effects). The degree of anticholinergic blockade produced by this agent is very low relative to other cyclic antidepressants.

Use caution in patients with a previous seizure disorder or condition predisposing to seizures such as brain damage, alcoholism, or concurrent therapy with other drugs which lower the seizure threshold. Use with caution in patients with renal dysfunction and in elderly patients. Use with caution in patients with a history of cardiovascular disease (including previous MI, stroke, tachycardia, or conduction abnormalities). However, the risk of conduction abnormalities with this agent is very low relative to other antidepressants.

Dosage Forms Tablet, as hydrochloride: 50 mg, 100 mg, 150 mg, 200 mg, 250 mg

Reference Range

After a 150 mg oral dose, peak plasma nefazodone, HO-NEF, and meta-chlorophenylpiperazine levels were 1200 ng/mL, 400 ng/mL, and 25 ng/mL, respectively; serum level of 5.5 mcg/mL associated with drowsiness after a 3 g ingestion

TLC detection limit: 1 mcg/mL

HPLC detection limit: 1-10 ng/mL

Overdosage/Treatment

Decontamination: Oral: Adults with ingestions <3 g: Activated charcoal

Supportive therapy: Following initiation of essential overdose management, toxic symptoms should be treated. Ventricular arrhythmias often respond to phenytoin 15-20 mg/kg (adults) with concurrent systemic alkalinization (sodium bicarbonate 0.5-2 mEq/kg I.V.). Arrhythmias unresponsive to this therapy may respond to lidocaine 1 mg/kg I.V. followed by a titrated infusion. Treat bradycardia with atropine; benztropine may be useful to treat priapism. Seizures usually respond to lorazepam or diazepam I.V. boluses (5-10 mg for adults up to 30 mg or 0.25-0.4 mg/kg/dose for children up to 10 mg/dose). If seizures are unresponsive or recur, phenytoin or phenobarbital may be required. Priapism can be treated with alpha-adrenergic agonists.

Enhancement of elimination: Multiple dosing of activated charcoal may be effective; forced diuresis to remove active metabolite may not be beneficial

Drug Interactions

Substrate (major) of CYP2D6, 3A4; **Inhibits** CYP1A2 (weak), 2B6 (weak), 2C8 (weak), 2D6 (weak), 3A4 (strong)

Antiarrhythmics: Serum concentrations may be increased due to enzyme inhibition; monitor; includes amiodarone, lidocaine, propafenone, quinidine

Antipsychotics: Serum concentrations of some antipsychotics may be increased by nefazodone due to enzyme inhibition; includes clozapine, haloperidol, mesoridazine, pimozide, quetiapine, and risperidone

Benzodiazepines: Nefazodone inhibits the metabolism of triazolam (decrease dose by 75%) and alprazolam (decrease dose by 50%); triazolam is contraindicated per manufacturer

Buspirone: Concurrent use may result in serotonin syndrome; serum concentrations may be increased due to enzyme inhibition; these combinations are best avoided or limit buspirone to 2.5 mg/day

Calcium channel blockers: Serum concentrations may be increased due to enzyme inhibition; monitor for increased effect (hypotension)

Carbamazepine: Significantly reduces serum concentrations of nefazodone; coadministration is contraindicated

Cisapride: Nefazodone likely increases cisapride serum concentrations via CYP3A4 inhibition; this combination may lead to cardiac arrhythmias; concurrent use is contraindicated

Cyclosporine and tacrolimus: Serum levels and toxicity may be increased by nefazodone; monitor

CYP2D6 inhibitors: May increase the levels/effects of nefazodone. Example inhibitors include chlorpromazine, delavirdine, fluoxetine, miconazole, paroxetine, pergolide, quinidine, quinine, ritonavir, and ropinirole.

CYP3A4 inducers: CYP3A4 inducers may decrease the levels/effects of nefazodone. Example inducers include aminoglutethimide, carbamazepine (contraindicated), nafcillin, nevirapine, phenobarbital, phenytoin, and rifamycins.

CYP3A4 inhibitors: May increase the levels/effects of nefazodone. Example inhibitors include azole antifungals, clarithromycin, diclofenac, doxycycline, erythromycin, imatinib, isoniazid, nicardipine, propofol, protease inhibitors, quinidine, telithromycin, and verapamil.

CYP3A4 substrates: Nefazodone may increase the levels/effects of CYP3A4 substrates. Example substrates include benzodiazepines, calcium channel blockers, mirtazapine, nateglinide, nefazodone, tacrolimus, and venlafaxine. Selected benzodiazepines (midazolam and triazolam), cisapride, ergot alkaloids, selected HMG-CoA reductase inhibitors (lovastatin and simvastatin), and pimozide are generally contraindicated with strong CYP3A4 inhibitors.

Digoxin: Serum levels may be increased by nefazodone (modest increases); monitor for digoxin toxicity or increased serum levels

Donepezil: Serum concentrations may be increased due to enzyme inhibition; monitor

HMG-CoA reductase inhibitors (statins) have been associated with myositis and rhabdomyolysis when used in combination with nefazodone; this has been associated most strongly with lovastatin and simvastatin. Concomitant use of lovastatin with nefazodone should be avoided.

Linezolid: Due to MAO inhibition (see note on MAO inhibitors), this combination should be avoided

MAO inhibitors: Concurrent use may lead to serotonin syndrome; avoid concurrent use or use within 14 days

Meperidine: Combined use theoretically may increase the risk of serotonin syndrome

Methadone: Serum concentrations may be increased due to enzyme inhibition; monitor

Oral contraceptives: Serum concentrations may be increased due to enzyme inhibition; monitor

Pimozide: Serum concentrations may be increased due to enzyme inhibition; may result in life-threatening arrhythmias (also see note on antipsychotics); avoid use

Protease inhibitors: Indinavir, ritonavir saquinavir; serum concentrations may be increased due to enzyme inhibition; monitor

Quinidine: Metabolism is likely to be inhibited by nefazodone; avoid concurrent use

Selegiline: Concurrent use with nefazodone may be associated with a risk of serotonin syndrome, particularly at higher dosages (>10 mg/day)

Serotonin agonists: Theoretically may increase the risk of serotonin syndrome; includes sumatriptan, naratriptan, rizatriptan, and zolmitriptan

Sibutramine: Serum concentrations may be increased by nefazodone; monitor

Sildenafil, vardenafil: Serum concentrations may be increased by nefazodone via inhibition of CYP3A4; use caution. Specific dosage adjustment guidelines have not been established. Recommendations for other strong CYP3A4 inhibitors include single sildenafil dose not to exceed 25 mg in a 48-hour period, a single tadalafil dose not to exceed 10 mg in a 72-hour period, or a single vardenafil dose not to exceed 2.5 mg in a 24-hour period.

SSRIs: Combined use of nefazodone with an SSRI may produce serotonin syndrome; in addition, nefazodone may increase serum concentrations of some SSRIs due to enzyme inhibition (fluoxetine and citalopram)

Tricyclic antidepressants: Serum concentrations of some tricyclic antidepressants (amitriptyline, clomipramine) may be increased; monitor for increased effect or toxicity

Venlafaxine: Combined use with nefazodone may increase the risk of serotonin syndrome

Vinca alkaloids (vincristine and vinblastine): Serum concentrations may be increased due to enzyme inhibition; may result in increased toxicity

Zolpidem: Serum concentrations may be increased due to enzyme inhibition; monitor

Pregnancy Risk Factor C

Lactation Enters breast milk/not recommended

Additional Information May cause an increase in plasma prolactin levels; food delays absorption; inhibitor of cytochrome P450 III4A and IID6; women and elderly receiving single doses attain significant higher peak concentrations than male volunteers

Specific References

Goeringer K and Drummer O, "Postmortem Tissue Concentrations of Nefazodone," *J Anal Toxicol*, 2003, 27:192.

Isbister GK and Hackett LP, "Nefazodone Poisoning: Toxicokinetics and Toxicodynamics Using Continuous Data Collection," *J Toxicol Clin Toxicol*, 2003, 41(2):167-73.

Skrabal MZ, Stading JA, and Monaghan MS, "Rhabdomyolysis Associated With Simvastatin-Nefazodone Therapy," *South Med J*, 2003, 96(10):1034-5.

Staack RF and Maurer HH, "Piperazine-Derived Designer Drug 1-(3-Chlorophenyl)Piperazine (mCPP): GC-MS Studies on Its Metabolism and Its Toxicological Detection in Rat Urine Including Analytical Differentiation from Its Precursor Drugs Trazodone and Nefazodone," *J Anal Toxicol*, 2003, 27(8):560-8.

Nefopam Hydrochloride

CAS Number 13669-70-0; 23327-57-3

Use Moderate pain control - nonopiate analgesic

Mechanism of Action Nonopiate analgesic with anticholinergic effects; does not bind to opiate receptors, but appears to act at the spinal level

Adverse Reactions

Cardiovascular: Tachycardia

Central nervous system: Dizziness, drowsiness, euphoria, hallucinations, insomnia, seizures

Dermatologic: Diaphoresis, rash

Gastrointestinal: Dry mouth, nausea, vomiting

Genitourinary: Urinary retention

Respiratory: Respiratory depression

Signs and Symptoms of Overdose Deep coma with bundle branch block, fever, mydriasis, oliguria, renal failure, ventricular arrhythmia. Seizures can occur with ingestions >1.8 g.

Admission Criteria/Prognosis Admit any symptomatic patient or adult ingestions >300 mg.

Toxicodynamics/Kinetics

Absorption: Well absorbed

Distribution: V_d: 410-447 L

Protein binding: 71% to 76%

Metabolism: Hepatic to inactive metabolites

Half-life: 3-8 hours

Elimination: Renal: 92%; Fecal: 8%

Dosage Adults:

Oral: 30-60 mg three to four times/day; maximum daily dose: 300 mg

I.V.; I.M: 10-20 mg every 4-6 hours; slow I.V. With patient supine for at least 20 minutes following administration; maximum daily dose: 120 mg

Reference Range Oral 90 g doses result in plasma concentration range of 73-154 ng/mL. Postmortem blood level of 4380 ng/mL has been associated with self-injection of nefopam in a suicide attempt.

Overdosage/Treatment

Decontamination: Activated charcoal 50 g, can absorb up to 95% of a 10 g nefopam ingestion; lavage within 1 hour; avoid ipecac.

Supportive therapy: Naloxone is **not** expected to be useful. Seizures can be treated with benzodiazepines. Ventricular dysrhythmia can be treated with lidocaine or amiodarone. Sotalol can be used to treat monomorphic ventricular tachycardia. Atropine can be used to treat severe symptomatic bradycardia. Crystalloid fluids/vasopressors can be used to treat hypotension.

Pregnancy Risk Factor B; Animal studies have not demonstrated teratogenesis at doses up to 80 mg/kg/day

Pregnancy Implications Animal studies have not demonstrated teratogenesis at doses up to 80 mg/kg/day

Additional Information Brand names: Acupan®; AJAN; Nefadol; Nefam; Oxadol; Placadol; Silentan

Nesiritide

Pronunciation (ni SIR i tide)

Applies to Natrecor®

U.S. Brand Names Natrecor®

Synonyms B-type Natriuretic Peptide (Human); hBNP; Natriuretic Peptide

Use Treatment of acutely decompensated congestive heart failure (CHF) in patients with dyspnea at rest or with minimal activity

Mechanism of Action Binds to guanylate cyclase receptor on vascular smooth muscle and endothelial cells, increasing intracellular cyclic GMP, resulting in smooth muscle cell relaxation. Has been shown to produce dose-dependent reductions in pulmonary capillary wedge pressure (PCWP) and systemic arterial pressure.

Adverse Reactions

Note: Frequencies cited below were recorded in VMAC trial at dosages similar to approved labeling. Higher frequencies have been observed in trials using higher dosages of nesiritide.

>10%:

Cardiovascular: Hypotension (total: 11%; symptomatic: 4% at recommended dose, up to 30% at higher doses)

Renal: Increased serum creatinine (28% with >0.5 mg/dL increase over baseline)

1% to 10%:

Cardiovascular: Ventricular tachycardia (3%)*, ventricular extrasystoles (3%)*, angina (2%)*, bradycardia (1%), tachycardia, atrial fibrillation, AV node conduction abnormalities

Central nervous system: Headache (8%)*, dizziness (3%)*, insomnia (2%), anxiety (3%), fever, confusion, paresthesia, somnolence, tremor

Dermatologic: Pruritus, rash

Gastrointestinal: Nausea (4%)*, abdominal pain (1%)*, vomiting (1%)*

Hematologic: Anemia

Local: Injection site reaction

Neuromuscular & skeletal: Back pain (4%), leg cramps

Ocular: Amblyopia

Respiratory: Cough (increased), hemoptysis, apnea

Miscellaneous: Increased diaphoresis

*Frequency less than or equal to placebo or other standard therapy

Signs and Symptoms of Overdose Symptoms of overdose would be expected to include excessive and/or prolonged hypotension.

Treatment is symptomatic and supportive; dopamine is the vasopressor of choice

Drug discontinuation and/or dosage reduction may be required

Pharmacodynamics/Kinetics

Onset of action: 15 minutes (60% of 3-hour effect achieved)

Duration: >60 minutes (up to several hours) for systolic blood pressure; hemodynamic effects persist longer than serum half-life would predict

Distribution: V_{ss}: 0.19 L/kg

Metabolism: Proteolytic cleavage by vascular endopeptidases and proteolysis following receptor binding and cellular internalization

Half-life elimination: Initial (distribution) 2 minutes; Terminal: 18 minutes

Time to peak: 1 hour

Excretion: Urine

Dosage

Adults: I.V.: Initial: 2 mcg/kg (bolus); followed by continuous infusion at 0.01 mcg/kg/minute; **Note:** Should not be initiated at a dosage higher than initial recommended dose. At intervals of ≥3 hours, the dosage may be increased by 0.005 mcg/kg/minute (preceded by a bolus of 1 mcg/kg), up to a maximum of 0.03 mcg/kg/minute. Increases beyond the initial infusion rate should be limited to selected patients and accompanied by hemodynamic monitoring.

Patients experiencing hypotension during the infusion: Infusion should be interrupted. May attempt to restart at a lower dose (reduce initial infusion dose by 30% and omit bolus).

Dosage adjustment in renal impairment: No adjustment required

Stability

Vials may be stored at controlled room temperature of 20°C to 25°C (68°F to 77 °F) or under refrigeration at 2°C to 8°C (36°F to 46°F). Following reconstitution, vials are stable under these conditions for up to 24 hours.

Reconstitute 1.5 mg vial with 5 mL of diluent removed from a premixed plastic I.V. bag (compatible with 5% dextrose, 0.9% sodium chloride, 5% dextrose and 0.45% sodium chloride, or 5% dextrose and 0.2% sodium chloride). Do not shake vial to dissolve (roll gently). Withdraw entire contents of vial and add to 250 mL I.V. bag. Resultant concentration of solution approximately 6 mcg/mL.

Monitoring Parameters Blood pressure, hemodynamic responses (PCWP, RAP, CI)

Administration Do not administer through a heparin-coated catheter (concurrent administration of heparin via a separate catheter is acceptable, per manufacturer).

Prime I.V. tubing with 25 mL of infusion prior to connection with vascular access port and prior to administering bolus or starting the infusion. Withdraw bolus from the prepared infusion bag and administer over 60 seconds. Begin infusion immediately following administration of the bolus. Using a standard 6 mcg/mL concentration, bolus volume in mL = patient weight in kg × 0.33.

Physically incompatible with heparin, insulin, ethacrynate sodium, bumetanide, enalaprilat, hydralazine, and furosemide. Do not administer through the same catheter. Do not administer with any solution containing sodium metabisulfite. Catheter must be flushed between administration of nesiritide and physically incompatible drugs.

Contraindications Hypersensitivity to natriuretic peptide or any component of the formulation; cardiogenic shock (when used as primary therapy); hypotension (systolic blood pressure <90 mm Hg)

Warnings

May cause hypotension; administer in clinical situations when blood pressure may be closely monitored. Use caution in patients with systolic blood pressure <100 mm Hg (contraindicated if <90 mm Hg); more likely to experience hypotension. Effects may be additive with other agents capable of causing hypotension. Hypotensive effects may last for several hours.

Should not be used in patients with low filling pressures, or in patients with conditions which depend on venous return including significant valvular stenosis, restrictive or obstructive cardiomyopathy, constrictive pericarditis, and pericardial tamponade. May be associated with development of azotemia; use caution in patients with renal impairment or in patients where renal perfusion is dependent on renin-angiotensin-aldosterone system.

Atrial natriuretic peptide (ANP), a related peptide, has been associated with increased vascular permeability and decreased intravascular volume. This has not been observed in clinical trials with nesiritide, however, patients should be monitored for this effect.

Prepared through recombinant technology using E. coli; monitor for allergic or anaphylactic reactions. Use caution with prolonged infusions; limited experience for infusions >48 hours. Safety and efficacy in pediatric patients have not been established.

Dosage Forms Injection, powder for reconstitution: 1.5 mg

Reference Range Therapeutic drug concentration in heart failure patients is about 8-40 pmol/L

Drug Interactions

ACE inhibitors: An increased frequency of symptomatic hypotension was observed with concurrent administration.

Diuretics: Use caution in patients who may have decreased intravascular volume due to diuretic therapy (risk of hypotension and/or renal impairment may be increased). Nesiritide should be avoided in patients with low filling pressures.

Hypotensive agents: Effects on blood pressure are likely to be additive with nesiritide.

Pregnancy Risk Factor C

Pregnancy Implications Excretion in breast milk is unknown; use caution in breast-feeding women.

Lactation Excretion in breast milk unknown/use caution

Additional Information The duration of symptomatic improvement with nesiritide following discontinuation of the infusion has been limited (generally lasting several days). Atrial natriuretic peptide, which is related to nesiritide, has been associated with increased vascular permeability. This has not been observed in clinical trials with nesiritide, but patients should be monitored for this effect.

Nevirapine

CAS Number 129618-40-2

U.S. Brand Names Viramune®

Synonyms NVP

Use In combination therapy with other antiretroviral agents for the treatment of HIV-1

Mechanism of Action As a non-nucleoside reverse transcriptase inhibitor, nevirapine has activity against HIV-1 by binding to reverse transcriptase. It consequently blocks the RNA-dependent and DNA-dependent DNA polymerase activities including HIV-1 replication. It does not require intracellular phosphorylation for antiviral activity. Cross-resistance between nevirapine and HIV protease inhibitors is unlikely although emergence of HIV strains which are cross-resistant between non-nucleoside reverse transcriptase inhibitors have been observed in vitro. It is not immunosuppressive.

Adverse Reactions

Central nervous system: **Headache, fever**

Dermatologic: **Rash**, Stevens-Johnson syndrome, angioedema

Gastrointestinal: **Diarrhea**, ulcerative stomatitis, nausea, abdominal pain

Hematologic: **Neutropenia**, anemia, thrombocytopenia

Hepatic: Hepatitis, increased LFTs, hepatotoxicity, hepatic necrosis, cholestatic hepatitis

Neuromuscular & skeletal: Peripheral neuropathy, paresthesia, myalgia

Miscellaneous: Anaphylaxis

Hypersensitivity (frequency not defined): Symptoms of severe hypersensitivity/dermatologic reactions may include: Severe rash (or rash with fever), blisters, oral lesions, conjunctivitis, facial edema, muscle or joint aches, general malaise, hepatitis, eosinophilia, granulocytopenia, lymphadenopathy, or renal dysfunction. Nevirapine should be permanently discontinued.

Admission Criteria/Prognosis Admit any patient with liver function abnormalities following ingestion or an acute ingestion >1 g

Pharmacodynamics/Kinetics

Absorption: >90%

Distribution: Widely; V_d: 1.2-1.4 L/kg; CSF penetration approximates 40% to 50% of plasma

Protein binding, plasma: 60%

Metabolism: Extensively hepatic via CYP3A4 (hydroxylation to inactive compounds); may undergo enterohepatic recycling

Half-life elimination: Decreases over 2- to 4-week time with chronic dosing due to autoinduction (ie, half-life = 45 hours initially and decreases to 25-30 hours)

Time to peak, serum: 2-4 hours

Excretion: Urine (~81%, primarily as metabolites, <3% as unchanged drug); feces (~10%)

Dosage

Oral:

Children 2 months to <8 years: Initial: 4 mg/kg/dose once daily for 14 days; increase dose to 7 mg/kg/dose every 12 hours if no rash or other adverse effects occur; maximum dose: 200 mg/dose every 12 hours

Children ≥8 years: Initial: 4 mg/kg/dose once daily for 14 days; increase dose to 4 mg/kg/dose every 12 hours if no rash or other adverse effects occur; maximum dose: 200 mg/dose every 12 hours

Note: Alternative pediatric dosing (AIDSinfo guidelines): 120-200 mg/m² every 12 hours; this dosing has been proposed due to the fact that dosing based on mg/kg may result in an abrupt decrease in dose at the 8th birthday, which may be inappropriate.

Adults: Initial: 200 mg once daily for 14 days; maintenance: 200 mg twice daily (in combination with an additional antiretroviral agent)

Note: If patient experiences a rash during the 14-day lead-in period, dose should not be increased until the rash has resolved. Discontinue if severe rash, or rash with constitutional symptoms, is noted. If therapy is interrupted for >7 days, restart with initial dose for 14 days. Use of prednisone to prevent nevirapine-associated rash is not recommended. Permanently discontinue if symptomatic hepatic events occur.

Prevention of maternal-fetal HIV transmission in women with no prior antiretroviral therapy (AIDS information guidelines):

Mother: 200 mg as a single dose at onset of labor. May be used in combination with zidovudine.

Infant: 2 mg/kg as a single dose at age 48-72 hours. If a maternal dose was given <1 hour prior to delivery, administer a 2 mg/kg dose as soon as possible after birth and repeat at 48-72 hours. May be used in combination with zidovudine.

Dosage adjustment in renal impairment:
Cl$_{cr}$ ≥20 mL/minute: No adjustment required
Hemodialysis: An additional 200 mg dose is recommended following dialysis.

Dosage adjustment in hepatic impairment: Use not recommended with moderate-to-severe hepatic impairment. Permanently discontinue if symptomatic hepatic events occur.

Monitoring Parameters Liver function tests should be monitored at baseline, and intensively during the first 18 weeks of therapy (optimal frequency not established, some practitioners recommend more often than once a month, including prior to dose escalation, and at 2 weeks following dose escalation), then periodically throughout therapy; observe for CNS side effects. Assess/evaluate AST/ALT in any patients with a rash. Permanently discontinue if patient experiences severe rash, constitutional symptoms associated with rash, rash with elevated AST/ALT, or clinical hepatitis, Mild-to-moderate rash without AST/ALT elevation may continue treatment per discretion of prescriber. If mild-to-moderate urticarial rash, do not restart if treatment is interrupted.

Administration Oral: May be administered with or without food; may be administered with an antacid or didanosine; shake suspension gently prior to administration

Contraindications Hypersensitivity to nevirapine or any component of the formulation

Warnings

[U.S. Boxed Warning]: Severe hepatotoxic reactions may occur (fulminant and cholestatic hepatitis, hepatic necrosis) and, in some cases, have resulted in hepatic failure and death. The greatest risk of these reactions is within the initial 6 weeks of treatment. Patients with a history of chronic hepatitis (B or C) or increased baseline transaminase levels may be at increased risk of hepatotoxic reactions. Female gender and patients with increased CD4$^+$-cell counts may be at substantially greater risk of hepatic events (often associated with rash). Therapy should not be started with elevated CD4$^+$-cell counts unless the benefit of therapy outweighs the risk of serious hepatotoxicity (adult females: CD4$^+$-cell counts >250 cells/mm^3; adult males: CD4$^+$-cell counts >400 cells/mm^3).

[U.S. Boxed Warning]: Severe life-threatening skin reactions (eg, Stevens-Johnson syndrome, toxic epidermal necrolysis, hypersensitivity reactions with rash and organ dysfunction) have occurred; intensive monitoring is required during the initial 18 weeks of therapy to detect potentially life-threatening dermatologic, hypersensitivity, and hepatic reactions. Nevirapine must be initiated with a 14-day lead-in dosing period to decrease the incidence of adverse effects.

If a severe dermatologic or hypersensitivity reaction occurs, or if signs and symptoms of hepatitis occur, nevirapine should be permanently discontinued. These may include a severe rash, or a rash associated with fever, blisters, oral lesions, conjunctivitis, facial edema, muscle or joint aches, general malaise, hepatitis, eosinophilia, granulocytopenia, lymphadenopathy, or renal dysfunction.

Consider alteration of antiretroviral therapies if disease progression occurs while patients are receiving nevirapine. Safety and efficacy have not been established in neonates.

Dosage Forms Suspension, oral: 50 mg/5 mL (240 mL)
Tablet: 200 mg

Reference Range Peak serum nevirapine level after a 400 mg dose ranges from 2.9-3.4 mcg/mL

Overdosage/Treatment
Decontamination: Oral: Ipecac within 30 minutes or lavage within 1 hour/activated charcoal
Enhanced elimination: Due to enterohepatic circulation, multiple dosing of activated charcoal may be effective

Drug Interactions Substrate of CYP2B6 (minor), 2D6 (minor), 3A4 (major); Inhibits CYP1A2 (weak), 2D6 (weak), 3A4 (weak); Induces CYP2B6 (strong), 3A4 (strong)

Antiarrhythmics (includes amiodarone, disopyramide, lidocaine): Serum concentration/effects may be decreased by nevirapine.
Anticonvulsants (includes carbamazepine, clonazepam, ethosuximide): Serum concentration/effects may be decreased by nevirapine.
Calcium channel blockers: Serum concentration may be decreased by nevirapine.
Cimetidine may decrease the metabolism of nevirapine, potentially increasing levels/toxicity.
Clarithromycin: Serum concentration may be decreased by nevirapine; an alternative antimicrobial agent should be considered.
Cyclophosphamide: Serum concentration may be decreased by nevirapine.
CYP2B6 substrates: Nevirapine may decrease the levels/effects of CYP2B6 substrates. Example substrates include bupropion, efavirenz, promethazine, selegiline, and sertraline.
CYP3A4 inducers: CYP3A4 inducers may decrease the levels/effects of nevirapine. Example inducers include aminoglutethimide, carbamazepine, nafcillin, nevirapine, phenobarbital, phenytoin, and rifamycins.

CYP3A4 substrates: Nevirapine may decrease the levels/effects of CYP3A4 substrates. Example substrates include benzodiazepines, calcium channel blockers, clarithromycin, cyclosporine, erythromycin, estrogens, mirtazapine, nateglinide, nefazodone, protease inhibitors, tacrolimus, and venlafaxine
Efavirenz: Serum concentration may be decreased by nevirapine; specific adjustments not established
Immunosuppressants: Serum concentration may be decreased by nevirapine.
Ketoconazole: Nevirapine may inhibit ketoconazole absorption. Ketoconazole may inhibit metabolism of nevirapine. Avoid concurrent use.
Methadone: Plasma concentrations may be reduced by nevirapine. Acute withdrawal symptoms have been reported; monitor
Oral contraceptives: Nevirapine may decrease the clinical effect of oral contraceptives; recommend alternative form or additional method of contraception
Prednisone: Concurrent administration of prednisone for the initial 14 days of nevirapine therapy was associated with an increased incidence and severity of rash.
Protease inhibitors: Nevirapine may decrease serum concentrations of some protease inhibitors (AUC of indinavir, lopinavir, nelfinavir, and saquinavir may be decreased - no effect noted with ritonavir), specific dosage adjustments have not been recommended; no adjustment recommended for ritonavir, unless in combination with lopinavir (Kaletra™).
Rifampin, rifabutin: May decrease nevirapine concentrations; rifabutin concentrations may be increased by nevirapine; avoid concurrent use.
St John's wort: Concurrent use may reduce serum concentrations/efficacy of nevirapine. May lead to treatment failure and/or drug resistance. Avoid concurrent use.
Warfarin: Therapeutic effects may be increased; monitor.

Pregnancy Risk Factor C
Pregnancy Implications Nevirapine crosses the placenta. It may be used in combination with zidovudine in HIV-infected women who are in labor, but have had no prior antiretroviral therapy, in order to reduce the maternal-fetal transmission of HIV. Health professionals are encouraged to contact the antiretroviral pregnancy registry to monitor outcomes of pregnant women exposed to antiretroviral medications (1-800-258-4263).
Lactation Enters breast milk/contraindicated
Additional Information Potential compliance problems, frequency of administration, and adverse effects should be discussed with patients before initiating therapy to help prevent the emergence of resistance.

Niacin

CAS Number 59-67-6
U.S. Brand Names Niacor®; Niaspan®; Slo-Niacin® [OTC]
Synonyms Nicotinic Acid; Vitamin B$_3$
Use Adjunctive treatment of dyslipidemias (types IIa and IIb or primary hypercholesterolemia) to lower the risk of recurrent MI and/or slow progression of coronary artery disease, including combination therapy with other antidyslipidemic agents when additional triglyceride-lowering or HDL-increasing effects are desired; treatment of hypertriglyceridemia in patients at risk of pancreatitis; treatment of peripheral vascular disease and circulatory disorders; treatment of pellagra; dietary supplement
Mechanism of Action Component of two coenzymes which is necessary for tissue respiration, lipid metabolism, and glycogenolysis; inhibits the synthesis of very low density lipoproteins while increasing high density cholesterol; water soluble vitamin B complex
Adverse Reactions
Cardiovascular: Arrhythmias, atrial fibrillation, edema, flushing, hypotension, orthostasis, palpitations, syncope (rare), tachycardia
Central nervous system: Chills, dizziness, insomnia, migraine
Dermatologic: Acanthosis nigricans, dry skin, hyperpigmentation, maculopapular rash, pruritus, rash, urticaria
Endocrine & metabolic: Glucose tolerance decreased, gout, phosphorus levels decreased, uric acid level increased
Gastrointestinal: Abdominal pain, nausea, peptic ulcers, vomiting
Hepatic: Hepatic necrosis (rare), jaundice, liver enzymes elevated
Neuromuscular & skeletal: Myalgia, myopathy (with concurrent HMG-CoA reductase inhibitor), rhabdomyolysis (with concurrent HMG-CoA reductase inhibitor; rare), weakness
Ocular: Cystoid macular edema, toxic amblyopia
Respiratory: Dyspnea
Miscellaneous: Diaphoresis
Signs and Symptoms of Overdose Anorexia, arrhythmias, cholelithiasis, coagulopathy, delirium, diarrhea, hepatitis, nausea, hyperglycemia, hyperuricemia, thrombocytopenia
Pharmacodynamics/Kinetics
Absorption: Rapid and extensive (60% to 76%)
Distribution: Mainly to hepatic, renal, and adipose tissue
Metabolism: Extensive first-pass effects; converted to nicotinamide adenine dinucleotide, nicotinuric acid, and other metabolites
Half-life elimination: 45 minutes

Time to peak, serum: Immediate release formulation: ~45 minutes; extended release formulation: 4-5 hours

Excretion: Urine 60% to 88% (unchanged drug and metabolites)

Dosage Children: Oral:

Pellagra: 50-100 mg/dose 3 times/day

Recommended daily allowances:

0-0.5 years: 5 mg/day

0.5-1 year: 6 mg/day

1-3 years: 9 mg/day

4-6 years: 12 mg/day

7-10 years: 13 mg/day

Children and Adolescents: Recommended daily allowances:

Male:

11-14 years: 17 mg/day

15-18 years: 20 mg/day

19-24 years: 19 mg/day

Female: 11-24 years: 15 mg/day

Adults: Oral:

Recommended daily allowances:

Male: 25-50 years: 19 mg/day; >51 years: 15 mg/day

Female: 25-50 years: 15 mg/day; >51 years: 13 mg/day

Hyperlipidemia: Usual target dose: 1.5-6 g/day in 3 divided doses with or after meals using a dosage titration schedule; extended release: 375 mg to 2 g once daily at bedtime

Regular release formulation (Niacor®): Initial: 250 mg once daily (with evening meal); increase frequency and/or dose every 4-7 days to desired response or first-level therapeutic dose (1.5-2 g/day in 2-3 divided doses); after 2 months, may increase at 2- to 4-week intervals to 3 g/day in 3 divided doses

Extended release formulation (Niaspan®): 500 mg at bedtime for 4 weeks, then 1 g at bedtime for 4 weeks; adjust dose to response and tolerance; can increase to a maximum of 2 g/day, but only at 500 mg/day at 4-week intervals

With lovastatin: Maximum lovastatin dose: 40 mg/day

Pellagra: 50-100 mg 3-4 times/day, maximum: 500 mg/day

Niacin deficiency: 10-20 mg/day, maximum: 100 mg/day

Dosage adjustment in renal impairment: Use with caution

Dosage adjustment in hepatic impairment: Not recommended for use in patients with significant or unexplained hepatic dysfunction

Dosage adjustment for toxicity: Transaminases rise to 3 times ULN: Discontinue therapy.

Stability Injection has a pH 4-6

Monitoring Parameters Blood glucose; liver function tests (dyslipidemia, high dose, prolonged therapy) pretreatment and every 6-12 weeks for first year then periodically; lipid profile; elevated uric acid levels have been reported

Administration Administer with food. Niaspan® tablet strengths are not interchangeable. When switching from immediate release tablet, initiate Niaspan® at lower dose and titrate. Long-acting forms should not be crushed, broken, or chewed. Do not substitute long-acting forms for immediate release ones.

Contraindications Hypersensitivity to niacin, niacinamide, or any component of the formulation; active hepatic disease; active peptic ulcer; arterial hemorrhage

Warnings

Use caution in heavy ethanol users, unstable angina or MI, diabetes (interferes with glucose control), renal disease, active gallbladder disease (can exacerbate), gout, past history of hepatic disease, or with anticoagulants. Monitor glucose and liver function tests. Rare cases of rhabdomyolysis have occurred during concomitant use with HMG-CoA reductase inhibitors. With concurrent use or if symptoms suggestive of myopathy occur, monitor creatinine phosphokinase (CPK) and potassium. Immediate and extended or sustained release products should not be interchanged. Flushing is common and can be attenuated with a gradual increase in dose, and/or by taking aspirin 30-60 minutes before dosing. Compliance is enhanced with twice-daily dosing.

Note: Formulations of niacin (regular release versus extended release) are not interchangeable.

Niaspan®: 500 mg and 750 mg tablets are not interchangeable (eg, three 500 mg tablets are not equivalent to two 750 mg tablets).

Dosage Forms Capsule, extended release: 125 mg, 250 mg, 400 mg, 500 mg

Capsule, timed release: 250 mg

Tablet: 50 mg, 100 mg, 250 mg, 500 mg

Niacor®: 500 mg

Tablet, controlled release (Slo-Niacin®): 250 mg, 500 mg, 750 mg

Tablet, extended release (Niaspan®): 500 mg, 750 mg, 1000 mg

Note: 500 mg and 750 mg tablets are not interchangeable (eg, three 500 mg tablets are not equivalent to two 750 mg tablets)

Tablet, timed release: 250 mg, 500 mg, 750 mg, 1000 mg

Reference Range Serum niacin level after 11 g ingestion at 48 hours was 8.2 mcg/mL

Overdosage/Treatment

Decontamination: Activated charcoal

Supportive therapy: Aspirin (160 mg or 325 mg) can reduce flushing due to niacin when given in a prophylactic manner; ibuprofen (200 mg) is also effective

Enhancement of elimination: Multiple dosing of activated charcoal may be effective

Diagnostic Procedures

• Glucose, Random

Test Interactions False elevations in some fluorometric determinations of urinary catecholamines; false-positive urine glucose (Benedict's reagent); ↑ LFTs, glucose, and uric acid

Drug Interactions Bile acid sequestrants: May decrease the absorption of niacin; separate administration by 4-6 hours.

Pregnancy Risk Factor A/C (dose exceeding RDA recommendation)

Lactation Enters breast milk/consult prescriber

Nursing Implications Monitor closely for signs of hepatitis and myositis

Additional Information Pretreatment with 325 mg of aspirin prevents niacin-induced flushing; >61 mg/day may result in slower progression of HIV illness (RR=0.52)

Specific References

Mularski RA, Grazer RE, Santoni L, et al, "Treatment Advice on the Internet Leads to a Life-threatening Adverse Reaction: Hypotension Associated with Niacin Overdose," *Clin Toxicol (Phila)*, 2006, 44(1):81-4.

Santoni L, Strother JS, Grazer RE, et al, "Critically Ill Niacin Overdose," *J Toxicol Clin Toxicol*, 2003, 41(5):678.

Niacinamide

CAS Number 98-92-0

U.S. Brand Names Nicomide-T™

Synonyms Nicotinamide; Nicotinic Acid Amide; Vitamin B₃

Use Prophylaxis and treatment of pellagra; treatment of N-d-pyridimethyl-N-P-nitrophenyl urea (PNU/Vacor®) toxicity

Mechanism of Action Used by the body as a source of niacin; water soluble vitamin B complex; less vasodilatory action than niacin

Adverse Reactions

Cardiovascular: Flushing, hypotension, vasodilation

Central nervous system: Headache

Dermatologic: Pruritus, acanthosis nigricans

Gastrointestinal: Vomiting

Ocular: Blurred vision

Pharmacodynamics/Kinetics

Absorption: Oral: Rapid; Topical: Absorbed systemically

Metabolism: Hepatic

Half-life elimination: 45 minutes

Time to peak, serum: 20-70 minutes

Excretion: Urine (as metabolites)

Dosage

Oral:

Children: Pellagra: 100-300 mg/day in divided doses

Adults: 50 mg 3-10 times/day

Pellagra: 300-500 mg/day

Recommended daily allowance: 13-19 mg/day

Vacor® (PNU) toxicity: 500 mg I.M. or I.V. followed by 100-200 mg I.M. or I.V. every 4 hours up to 48 hours, then 100 mg orally 3-5 times/day for 2 weeks

Administration Topical: Prior to using cream or gel, wash face with mild cleanser. Apply thin layer to affected area. May apply under make-up or other medications. Re-evaluate after 8-12 weeks.

Contraindications Hypersensitivity to niacin, niacinamide, or any component of the formulation; liver disease; active peptic ulcer

Warnings Use caution in heavy ethanol users, unstable angina or CAD (risk of arrhythmias at high doses), diabetes (interfere with glucose control), renal disease, active gallbladder disease (can exacerbate), gout, or allergies. Avoid large pharmacological amounts in patients with a history of liver disease. Monitor liver function tests with high doses.

Dosage Forms Cream (Nicomide-T™): 4% (30 g) [contains benzyl alcohol]

Gel (Nicomide-T™): 4% (30 g) [contains alcohol]

Tablet: 100 mg, 250 mg, 500 mg

Overdosage/Treatment

Decontamination: Ipecac (within 30 minutes)/lavage (within 1 hour)/ activated charcoal

Enhancement of elimination: Multiple dosing of activated charcoal may be effective

Diagnostic Procedures

• Glucose, Random

Test Interactions False elevations of urinary catecholamines in some fluorometric determinations

Pregnancy Risk Factor A/C (dose exceeding RDA recommendation)

NiCARdipine

Related Information
- Calcium Channel Blockers

CAS Number 54527-84-3; 55985-32-5

U.S. Brand Names Cardene® I.V.; Cardene® SR; Cardene®

Synonyms Nicardipine Hydrochloride

Use Chronic stable angina (immediate-release product only); management of essential hypertension (immediate and sustained release; parenteral only for short time that oral treatment is not feasible)

Unlabeled/Investigational Use Congestive heart failure

Mechanism of Action Inhibits calcium ion from entering the "slow channels" or select voltage-sensitive areas of vascular smooth muscle and myocardium during depolarization, producing a relaxation of coronary vascular smooth muscle and coronary vasodilation; increases myocardial oxygen delivery in patients with vasospastic angina

Adverse Reactions
Cardiovascular: Flushing, palpitations, tachycardia, edema, syncope, abnormal ECG, chest pain, angina

Central nervous system: Headache, dizziness, somnolence, insomnia, malaise, abnormal dreams, CNS depression, depression

Dermatologic: Rash, urticaria, exanthem

Endocrine & metabolic: Parotitis

Gastrointestinal: Vomiting, constipation, dyspepsia, xerostomia, nausea

Genitourinary: Nocturia

Neuromuscular & skeletal: Tremor, erythromelalgia, weakness, paresthesia

Respiratory: Rhinitis

Miscellaneous: Pedal edema

Signs and Symptoms of Overdose Bradycardia, hypotension

Admission Criteria/Prognosis Admit any patient with cardiovascular symptoms; admit any ingestion in a child or ingestions >100 mg in an adult; asymptomatic patients (with normal ECG and blood pressure) can be discharged after 8 hours observation for nonsustained released preparation ingestions

Pharmacodynamics/Kinetics
Onset of action: Oral: 0.5-2 hours; I.V.: 10 minutes; Hypotension: ~20 minutes

Duration: ≤8 hours

Absorption: Oral: ~100%

Protein binding: >95%

Metabolism: Hepatic; CYP3A4 substrate (major); extensive first-pass effect (saturable)

Bioavailability: 35%

Half-life elimination: 2-4 hours

Time to peak, serum: 30-120 minutes

Excretion: Urine (60% as metabolites); feces (35%)

Dosage Adults:

Oral:

Immediate release: Initial: 20 mg 3 times/day; usual: 20-40 mg 3 times/day (allow 3 days between dose increases)

Sustained release: Initial: 30 mg twice daily, titrate up to 60 mg twice daily

Note: The total daily dose of immediate-release product may not automatically be equivalent to the daily sustained-release dose; use caution in converting.

I.V. (dilute to 0.1 mg/mL):

Acute hypertension: Initial: 5 mg/hour increased by 2.5 mg/hour every 15 minutes to a maximum of 15 mg/hour; consider reduction to 3 mg/hour after response is achieved. Monitor and titrate to lowest dose necessary to maintain stable blood pressure.

Substitution for oral therapy (approximate equivalents):

20 mg every 8 hours oral, equivalent to 0.5 mg/hour I.V. infusion

30 mg every 8 hours oral, equivalent to 1.2 mg/hour I.V. infusion

40 mg every 8 hours oral, equivalent to 2.2 mg/hour I.V. infusion

Dosing adjustment in renal impairment: Titrate dose beginning with 20 mg 3 times/day (immediate release) or 30 mg twice daily (sustained release). Specific guidelines for adjustment of I.V. nicardipine are not available, but careful monitoring/adjustment is warranted.

Dosing adjustment in hepatic impairment: Starting dose: 20 mg twice daily (immediate release) with titration. Specific guidelines for adjustment of I.V. nicardipine are not available, but careful monitoring/adjustment is warranted.

Stability Compatible with D$_5$W, D$_5$^{1}/$_2$NS, D$_5$NS, and D$_5$W with 40 mEq potassium chloride; 0.45% and 0.9% NS; **do not** mix with 5% sodium bicarbonate and lactated Ringer's solution; store at room temperature; protect from light; stable for 24 hours at room temperature

Monitoring Parameters ECG, blood pressure, electrolytes

Administration Oral: The total daily dose of immediate-release product may not automatically be equivalent to the daily sustained-release dose; use caution in converting. Do not chew or crush the sustained release formulation, swallow whole. Do not open or cut capsules.

I.V.: Ampuls must be diluted before use. Administer as a slow continuous infusion.

Contraindications Hypersensitivity to nicardipine or any component of the formulation; advanced aortic stenosis

Warnings
Blood pressure lowering should be done at a rate appropriate for the patient's condition. Rapid drops in blood pressure can lead to arterial insufficiency. Use with caution in CAD (can cause increase in angina), CHF (can worsen heart failure symptoms), and pheochromocytoma (limited clinical experience). Peripheral infusion sites (for I.V. therapy) should be changed ever 12 hours. Titrate I.V. dose cautiously in patients with CHF, renal, or hepatic dysfunction. Use the I.V. form cautiously in patients with portal hypertension (can cause increase in hepatic pressure gradient). Safety and efficacy have not been demonstrated in pediatric patients. Abrupt withdrawal may cause rebound angina in patients with CAD.

Dosage Forms Capsule (Cardene®): 20 mg, 30 mg

Capsule, sustained release (Cardene® SR): 30 mg, 45 mg, 60 mg

Injection, solution (Cardene® IV): 2.5 mg/mL (10 mL)

Reference Range Therapeutic blood nicardipine levels: 24-50 ng/mL

Overdosage/Treatment
Decontamination: Lavage (within 1 hour)/activated charcoal

Supportive therapy: The primary cardiac symptoms of calcium blocker overdose include hypotension and bradycardia. Hypotension is caused by peripheral vasodilation, myocardial depression, and bradycardia. Bradycardia results from sinus bradycardia, second- or third-degree atrioventricular block, or sinus arrest with junctional rhythm. Intraventricular conduction is usually not affected, so QRS duration is normal (verapamil does prolong the P-R interval and bepridil prolongs the QT interval and may cause ventricular arrhythmias, including torsade de pointes).

Noncardiac symptoms include confusion, stupor, nausea, vomiting, metabolic acidosis and hyperglycemia. Following initial gastric decontamination, if possible, repeated calcium administration may promptly reverse depressed cardiac contractility (but not sinus node depression or peripheral vasodilation); glucagon, epinephrine, and inamrinone may treat refractory hypotension; calcium chloride (1-3 g slow I.V. push) is considered a second-line agent for treatment of shock; glucagon and epinephrine also increase the heart rate (outside the U.S., 4-aminopyridine may be available as an antidote).

Enhanced elimination: Multiple dosing of activated charcoal may be useful for sustained release preparations; hemodialysis or hemoperfusion is not effective

Antidote(s)
- Glucagon [ANTIDOTE]

Drug Interactions
Substrate of CYP1A2 (minor), 2C9 (minor), 2D6 (minor), 2E1 (minor), 3A4 (major); **Inhibits** CYP2C9 (strong), 2C19 (moderate), 2D6 (moderate), 3A4 (strong)

Azole antifungals may inhibit the calcium channel blocker's metabolism; avoid this combination. Try an antifungal like terbinafine (if appropriate) or monitor closely for altered effect of the calcium channel blocker.

Calcium may reduce the calcium channel blocker's effects, particularly hypotension.

Cyclosporine's serum concentrations are increased by nicardipine; avoid this combination. Use another calcium channel blocker or monitor cyclosporine trough levels and renal function closely. Tacrolimus may be affected similarly.

CYP2C9 Substrates: Nicardipine may increase the levels/effects of CYP2C9 substrates. Example substrates include bosentan, dapsone, fluoxetine, glimepiride, glipizide, losartan, montelukast, nateglinide, paclitaxel, phenytoin, warfarin, and zafirlukast.

CYP2C19 substrates: Nicardipine may increase the levels/effects of CYP2C19 substrates. Example substrates include citalopram, diazepam, methsuximide, phenytoin, propranolol, and sertraline.

CYP2D6 substrates: Nicardipine may increase the levels/effects of CYP2D6 substrates. Example substrates include amphetamines, selected beta-blockers, dextromethorphan, fluoxetine, lidocaine, mirtazapine, nefazodone, paroxetine, risperidone, ritonavir, thioridazine, tricyclic antidepressants, and venlafaxine.

CYP2D6 prodrug substrates: Nicardipine may decrease the levels/effects of CYP2D6 prodrug substrates. Example prodrug substrates include codeine, hydrocodone, oxycodone, and tramadol.

CYP3A4 inducers: CYP3A4 inducers may decrease the levels/effects of nicardipine. Example inducers include aminoglutethimide, carbamazepine, nafcillin, nevirapine, phenobarbital, phenytoin, and rifamycins.

CYP3A4 inhibitors: May increase the levels/effects of nicardipine. Example inhibitors include azole antifungals, clarithromycin, diclofenac, doxycycline, erythromycin, imatinib, isoniazid, nefazodone, propofol, protease inhibitors, quinidine, telithromycin, and verapamil.

CYP3A4 substrates: Nicardipine may increase the levels/effects of CYP3A4 substrates. Example substrates include benzodiazepines, calcium channel blockers, mirtazapine, nateglinide, nefazodone, tacrolimus, and venlafaxine. Selected benzodiazepines (midazolam and triazolam), cisapride, ergot alkaloids, selected HMG-CoA reductase inhibitors (lovastatin and simvastatin), and pimozide are generally contraindicated with strong CYP3A4 inhibitors.

Metoprolol: Concentration of metoprolol is increased by 25% with concurrent use.

Nafcillin decreases plasma concentration of nicardipine; avoid this combination.

Propranolol: May decrease the metabolism of nicardipine.

Protease inhibitor like amprenavir and ritonavir may increase nicardipine's serum concentration.

Rifampin increases the metabolism of the calcium channel blocker; adjust the dose of the calcium channel blocker to maintain efficacy.

Sildenafil, tadalafil, vardenafil: Blood pressure-lowering effects may be additive; use caution.

Vecuronium: Clearance of vecuronium is decreased by 25% with use of I.V. nicardipine; reduce dose of muscle relaxant.

Pregnancy Risk Factor C

Pregnancy Implications Crosses the placenta; may exhibit tocolytic effect

Lactation Enters breast milk/not recommended

Nursing Implications Monitor closely for orthostasis; ampuls must be diluted before use; do not crush sustained release product

Nicergoline

CAS Number 27848-84-6

Use Transient ischemic attacks, cerebrovascular insufficiency, dementia

Mechanism of Action Ergot derivative with alpha-adrenergic blocking activity and vasodilatation

Adverse Reactions

Cardiovascular: Hypotension, syncope, bradycardia, flushing, sinus bradycardia

Central nervous system: Insomnia, agitation

Dermatologic: Urticaria

Gastrointestinal: Nausea, increased appetite, diarrhea

Hematologic: Inhibits platelet aggregation

Miscellaneous: Diaphoresis

Toxicodynamics/Kinetics

Onset of action: Oral: 1-1.5 hours

Protein binding: 82% to 87%

Half-life: Parent compound: 2.5 hours; MDL metabolite: 12-17 hours

Elimination: 80% renal, 20% fecal

Dosage

Oral: Initial: 10 mg 3 times/day; maintenance: 5-10 mg 3 times/day (before or during meals)

I.M.: 2-4 mg once or twice daily

I.V.: 4-8 mg diluted in 250 mL of normal saline and given over 30 minutes

Dosing adjustment in renal impairment: Reduce dose

Reference Range Oral dose of 70 mcg/kg results in plasma nicergoline level of 100-200 ng/mL

Overdosage/Treatment

Decontamination: Gastric lavage within 1 hour or induction of emesis within 30 minutes, activated charcoal; keep extremities warm

Supportive therapy: Treatment is symptomatic with captopril, nifedipine, prazosin, vasodilators (nitroprusside) or nitroglycerin for hypertension; phentolamine can also be used; diazepam can be utilized for seizures; heparin, dextran, or corticosteroids can be used for hypercoagulable state; hyperbaric oxygen can be used as an adjunct to treat localized tissue hypoxia

Enhancement of elimination: Multiple dosing of activated charcoal may be effective

Nicotine

Related Information

- Drugs Used in Addiction Treatment
- Substance-Related Disorders
- Toxins Which Should Be Lavaged with Solutions Other Than Water

CAS Number 54-11-5

UN Number 1654; 1655; 1656; 1657; 1658; 1659; 3144

U.S. Brand Names Commit™ [OTC]; NicoDerm® CQ® [OTC]; Nicorette® [OTC]; Nicotrol® Inhaler; Nicotrol® NS; Nicotrol® Patch [OTC]

Synonyms Habitrol

Commonly Includes Cigarettes (13-19 mg); nicotine gum (2-4 mg); cigars (15-40 mg); cigarette butt (5-7 mg); nicotine patch (8.3-114 mg); chewing tobacco (6-8 mg)

Use

Treatment to aid smoking cessation for the relief of nicotine withdrawal symptoms (including nicotine craving)

Insecticide (rarely), found in tobacco leaf (1% to 6% nicotine by weight) products.

Management of ulcerative colitis (transdermal)

Mechanism of Action Direct stimulant to nicotinic acetylcholine receptor causing either sympathetic or parasympathetic effects

Adverse Reactions

Chewing gum/lozenge:

Cardiovascular: Atrial fibrillation, **tachycardia**

Central nervous system: Dizziness, **headache (mild)**, insomnia, nervousness

Dermatologic: Erythema, itching

Endocrine & metabolic: Dysmenorrhea

Gastrointestinal: **Belching**, eructation, **excessive salivation**, GI distress, **increased appetite**, **indigestion**, **nausea**, **vomiting**

Neuromuscular & skeletal: Muscle pain

Respiratory: Hoarseness

Miscellaneous: Hiccups, hypersensitivity reactions, **jaw muscle ache**, **mouth or throat soreness**

Transdermal systems:

Cardiovascular: Atrial fibrillation, chest pain

Central nervous system: **Abnormal dreams**, anxiety, difficulty concentrating, dizziness, dysphoria, **insomnia**, nervousness, somnolence

Dermatologic: **Erythema**, itching, **pruritus**, rash

Gastrointestinal: Abdominal pain, anorexia, constipation, diarrhea, dyspepsia, nausea, taste perversion, xerostomia

Local: **Application site reaction**

Neuromuscular & skeletal: Arthralgia, myalgia, tremor

Respiratory: **Cough**, **pharyngitis**, **rhinitis**, **sinusitis**

Miscellaneous: Hypersensitivity reactions, thirst

Signs and Symptoms of Overdose Abdominal pain, apnea, AV block, blurred vision, cyanosis, dementia, diarrhea (may be delayed up to 24 hours in pediatric ingestion), dry mouth, dysosmia, dyspepsia, headache (early sign), hiccups, hyperglycemia, hypertension then bradycardia, hyperreflexia, hyperthermia, hyperventilation, hyponatremia, hypotension, hypotonia, increased bronchial secretions, insomnia, lacrimation, lightheadedness, mental confusion, muscle fasciculations/paralysis, myalgia, myasthenia gravis (exacerbation or precipitation), mydriasis, myoclonus, nausea, nystagmus, ototoxicity, paresthesia, respiratory depression, salivation, seizures, tachycardia, tinnitus, vomiting

Admission Criteria/Prognosis Admit pediatric ingestions >2 whole cigarettes, 6 cigarette butts or a total of >0.5 mg/kg of nicotine; symptomatic patients or patients with tachycardia or hypertension 4 hours postexposure should be admitted; survival after 4 hours is usually associated with complete recovery; any patient with change in mental status or cardiopulmonary complaints should be admitted

Pharmacodynamics/Kinetics

Onset of action: Intranasal: More closely approximate the time course of plasma nicotine levels observed after cigarette smoking than other dosage forms

Duration: Transdermal: 24 hours

Absorption: Transdermal: Slow

Metabolism: Hepatic, primarily to cotinine ($^1/_5$ as active)

Half-life elimination: 4 hours

Time to peak, serum: Transdermal: 8-9 hours

Excretion: Urine

Clearance: Renal: pH dependent

Dosage

Smoking deterrent: Patients should be advised to completely stop smoking upon initiation of therapy.

Oral:

Gum: Chew 1 piece of gum when urge to smoke, up to 24 pieces/day. Patients who smoke <25 cigarettes/day should start with 2-mg strength; patients smoking ≥25 cigarettes/day should start with the 4-mg strength. Use according to the following 12-week dosing schedule:

Weeks 1-6: Chew 1 piece of gum every 1-2 hours; to increase chances of quitting, chew at least 9 pieces/day during the first 6 weeks

Weeks 7-9: Chew 1 piece of gum every 2-4 hours

Weeks 10-12: Chew 1 piece of gum every 4-8 hours

Inhaler: Usually 6 to 16 cartridges per day; best effect was achieved by frequent continuous puffing (20 minutes); recommended duration of treatment is 3 months, after which patients may be weaned from the inhaler by gradual reduction of the daily dose over 6-12 weeks

Lozenge: Patients who smoke their first cigarette within 30 minutes of waking should use the 4 mg strength; otherwise the 2 mg strength is recommended. Use according to the following 12-week dosing schedule:

Weeks 1-6: One lozenge every 1-2 hours

Weeks 7-9: One lozenge every 2-4 hours

Weeks 10-12: One lozenge every 4-8 hours

Note: Use at least 9 lozenges/day during first 6 weeks to improve chances of quitting; do not use more than one lozenge at a time (maximum: 5 lozenges every 6 hours, 20 lozenges/day)

Topical:

Transdermal patch: Apply new patch every 24 hours to nonhairy, clean, dry skin on the upper body or upper outer arm; each patch should be applied to a different site. **Note:** Adjustment may be required during initial treatment (move to higher dose if experiencing withdrawal symptoms; lower dose if side effects are experienced).

NicoDerm CQ®:

Patients smoking ≥10 cigarettes/day: Begin with **step 1** (21 mg/day) for 4-6 weeks, followed by **step 2** (14 mg/day) for 2 weeks; finish with **step 3** (7 mg/day) for 2 weeks

Patients smoking <10 cigarettes/day: Begin with **step 2** (14 mg/day) for 6 weeks, followed by **step 3** (7 mg/day) for 2 weeks

Note: Initial starting dose for patients <100 pounds, history of cardiovascular disease: 14 mg/day for 4-6 weeks, followed by 7 mg/day for 2-4 weeks

Note: Patients receiving >600 mg/day of cimetidine: Decrease to the next lower patch size

Nicotrol®: One patch daily for 6 weeks

Note: Benefits of use of nicotine transdermal patches beyond 3 months have not been demonstrated.

Ulcerative colitis (unlabeled use): Transdermal: Titrated to 22-25 mg/day

Nasal: Spray: 1-2 sprays/hour; do not exceed more than 5 doses (10 sprays) per hour [maximum: 40 doses/day (80 sprays); each dose (2 sprays) contains 1 mg of nicotine

Monitoring Parameters Heart rate and blood pressure periodically during therapy; discontinue therapy if signs of nicotine toxicity occur (eg, severe headache, dizziness, mental confusion, disturbed hearing and vision, abdominal pain; rapid, weak and irregular pulse; salivation, nausea, vomiting, diarrhea, cold sweat, weakness); therapy should be discontinued if rash develops; discontinuation may be considered if other adverse effects of patch occur such as myalgia, arthralgia, abnormal dreams, insomnia, nervousness, dry mouth, sweating

Administration Gum: Should be chewed slowly to avoid jaw ache and to maximize benefit.

Lozenge: Allow to dissolve slowly in the mouth. Do not chew or swallow lozenge whole. Acidic foods/beverages decrease absorption of nicotine. Avoid coffee, orange juice, or soft drinks 15 minutes prior to, during, or after lozenge.

Contraindications Hypersensitivity to nicotine or any component of the formulation; patients who are smoking during the postmyocardial infarction period; patients with life-threatening arrhythmias, or severe or worsening angina pectoris; active temporomandibular joint disease (gum); pregnancy; not for use in nonsmokers

Warnings The risk versus the benefits must be weighed for each of these groups: patients with CAD, serious cardiac arrhythmias, vasospastic disease. Use caution in patients with hyperthyroidism, pheochromocytoma, or insulin-dependent diabetes. Use with caution in oropharyngeal inflammation and in patients with history of esophagitis, peptic ulcer, coronary artery disease, vasospastic disease, angina, hypertension, pheochromocytoma, severe renal dysfunction, and hepatic dysfunction. The inhaler should be used with caution in patients with bronchospastic disease (other forms of nicotine replacement may be preferred). Use of nasal product is not recommended with chronic nasal disorders (eg, allergy, rhinitis, nasal polyps, and sinusitis). Transdermal patch may contain conducting metal (eg, aluminum); remove patch prior to MRI. Cautious use of topical nicotine in patients with certain skin diseases. Hypersensitivity to the topical products can occur. Dental problems may be worsened by chewing the gum. Urge patients to stop smoking completely when initiating therapy. Safety and efficacy have not been established in pediatric patients.

Dosage Forms

Gum, chewing, as polacrilex: 2 mg (48s, 108s); 4 mg (48s, 108s)

Nicorette®:

2 mg (48s, 50s, 110s, 168s, 170s, 192s, 200s, 216s) [fruit chill flavor contains calcium 94 mg/gum and sodium 11 mg/gum; mint, fresh mint, fruit chill, orange, and original flavors]

4 mg (48s, 108s, 168s) [fruit chill flavor contains calcium 94 mg/gum and sodium 13 mg/gum; mint, fresh mint, fruit chill, orange, and original flavors]

Lozenge, as polacrilexL:

Commit®: 2 mg (48s, 72s) [contains phenylalanine 3.4 mg/lozenge, sodium 18 mg/lozenge; mint flavor]; 4 mg (48s, 72s) [contains phenylalanine 3.4 mg/lozenge, sodium 18 mg/lozenge; mint flavor]

Oral inhalation system:

Nicotrol® Inhaler: 10 mg cartridge [delivering 4 mg nicotine] (168s) [each unit consists of 5 mouthpieces, 28 storage trays each containing 6 cartridges, and 1 storage case]

Patch, transdermal: 7 mg/24 (30s); 14 mg/24 hours (30s); 21 mg/24 hours (30s)

NicoDerm® CQ®: 7 mg/24 hours (14s); 14 mg/24 hours (14s); 21 mg/24 hours (14s) [available in tan or clear patch]

Nicotrol®: 15 mg/16 hours (7s, 14s) [step 1]; 10 mg/16 hours (14s) [step 2]; 5 mg/16 hours (14s) [step 3]

Solution, intranasal spray (Nicotrol® NS): 10 mg/mL (10 mL) [delivers 0.5 mg/spray; 200 sprays]

Reference Range A serum nicotine level of 13,600 ng/mL has been associated with fatality. Mean plasma level after smoking one cigarette: 5-30 ng/mL. Mean plasma level after 6$\frac{1}{2}$ hours of smoking: 12-44 ng/mL. Pipe smoking can result in nicotine levels of 4-6 ng/mL. Plasma levels of cotinine averaged 0.001 mg/L in children from nonsmoking homes and 0.004 mg/L in children from homes with smoking cohabitants. Arterial levels are ∼6-8 times that of venous levels, thus leading to rapidly elevated brain levels. Cotinine serum levels as high as 800 ng/mL are associated with nausea, vomiting, and severe symptomatology. Steady state plasma nicotine level from transdermal patches: 12-17 ng/mL; steady state plasma nicotine level from chewing 4 mg nicotine gum: 23 ng/mL; urine cotinine levels in nonsmokers and smokers: <20 and >50 ng/mL, respectively. Therapeutic nicotine serum level for smoking cessation: 2-17 ng/mL. Accidental cigarette ingestion by children is a frequent occurrence in Japan where hundreds of cigarette brands (domestic and imported) are purchased. To evaluate the predictive value of the nicotine yield given on the label and determined by a smoking machine, measurement was done on the actual nicotine content of tobacco in 33 popular cigarette brands. See table.

Nicotine and Tobacco Content of 33 Cigarette Brands				
Japanese Domestic Cigarette Brands (n=16)				
Brand Names	Nicotine Content		Nicotine* Yield	Tobacco Content
	(mg)	(%)	(mg)	(g)
Peace**	23.97	2.35	2.4	1.02
Peace King Size	18.33	2.34	2.4	0.78
Hi-Light*	14.55	2.02	1.4	0.72
Echo	13.74	2.43	1.1	0.5
Hops	13.31	1.86	1.2	0.72
Caster Mild*	12.96	2.00	0.4	0.65
Marlboro	12.76	1.61	1.0	0.79
Cherry	12.62	1.96	1.2	0.68
Mild Seven*	12.57	1.87	0.9	0.67
SevenStar*	12.41	1.77	1.3	0.70
Cabin Mild*	11.99	1.86	0.7	0.65
Mild Seven Super Light*	11.77	1.76	0.5	0.67
MI-NE	11.51	1.70	1.0	0.68
Mild Seven Lights	10.88	1.63	0.8	0.67
Cabin Ultra Mild*	8.84	1.55	0.2	0.57
Frontier Lights	6.94	1.14	0.1	0.61
Salem Slim Lights	8.03	1.32	0.6	0.61
Average	13.07†	1.86	1.04††	0.70
(±SD)	(3.79)	(0.33)	(0.66)	(0.11)
Imported Cigarette Brands (n=17)				
Camel	15.38	2.04	0.8	0.75
Dunhill Ultimate Light	16.03	2.36	0.1	0.64
Next§	12.72	1.88	0.1	0.58
Parliament 100§	12.61	1.62	0.8	0.77
Lark Mild§	11.68	1.59	0.7	0.73
Lark	11.34	1.55	0.9	0.73
Kent1§	11.24	1.71	0.1	0.66
Vantage	11.07	1.78	0.7	0.62
Salem	10.94	1.63	1.0	0.67
Virginia Slims Lights§	10.65	1.63	0.5	0.67
Lucky Strike§	10.54	1.57	0.8	0.67
Island Super Lights	10.24	1.44	0.6	0.71
Kent	9.97	1.44	0.9	0.69
Lark Super Lights§	9.66	1.62	0.4	0.60
Philip Morris One§	9.53	1.95	0.1	0.49
Philip Morris Super Lights§	9.10	1.59	0.4	0.57
Average	11.16†	1.69	0.58††	0.66
(±SD)	(1.98)	(0.26)	(0.30)	(0.08)

*The advertised level determined by a smoking machine
**Nonfiltered cigarette
*The best ten brands sales in 1995
§The ten top-selling brands of imported cigarette in 1995
† p <0.05
†† p <0.01
From Fukumoto M, Kubo H, and Ogamo A, "Determination of Nicotine Content of Popular Cigarettes," *Vet Hum Toxicol*, 1997, 39(4):227, with permission.

Overdosage/Treatment

Decontamination: **Oral:** Emesis is not recommended due to seizure potential. For ingestions, lavage (within 1 hour) with 1:10,000 potassium permanganate (100 mg/L) is recommended after control of seizures. Use of activated charcoal for acute ingestions is not well established.

Dermal: Wash area well with cool water and dry; soap (especially alkaline soaps) may increase absorption; remove any remaining transdermal systems; nicotine will continue to be absorbed several hours after removal due to depot in skin. **Ocular:** Irrigate with saline.

Supportive therapy: Control seizures with benzodiazepines; if continuous, use phenobarbital; atropine can be utilized for cholinergic toxicity while phentolamine can be used for hypertension; avoid antacids due to increased nicotine absorption in alkali medium

Enhancement of elimination: Hemodialysis/hemoperfusion of unknown value. While acidifying the urine may enhance elimination, this modality is not recommended due to inherent dangers.

Antidote(s)
- Atropine [ANTIDOTE]

Diagnostic Procedures
- Nicotine Level

Drug InteractionsSubstrate (minor) of CYP1A2, 2A6, 2B6, 2C9, 2C19, 2D6, 2E1, 3A4; **Inhibits** CYP2A6 (weak), 2E1 (weak)

Adenosine: Nicotine increases the hemodynamic and AV blocking effects of adenosine; monitor

Bupropion: Monitor for treatment-emergent hypertension in patients treated with the combination of nicotine patch and bupropion

Cimetidine; May increases nicotine concentrations; therefore, may decrease amount of gum or patches needed

Pregnancy Risk Factor D (transdermal); X (chewing gum)

Pregnancy Implications Pregnant smokers are almost twice as likely to have a spontaneous abortion or a low birth weight neonate (<2500 g); prematurity, placenta previa, and abruption rates are also increased in the smoker; nicotine is present in breast milk

Lactation Excretion in breast milk unknown/use caution

Nursing Implications Patients should be instructed to chew slowly to avoid jaw ache and to maximize benefit

Additional Information
Lethal adult dose: 40 mg

Symptoms usually do not occur in pediatric ingestions <1 mg/kg; not useful as maintenance therapy for ulcerative colitis

Nicotine withdrawal is characterized by psychological distress, difficulty concentrating, tobacco craving, and hunger; average weight gain during smoking cessation is ~4 kg; 3% annual quit rate from smoking; contact the National Capital Poison Center (1-800-498-8666) with all cases of misuse, overdose or abuse of nicotine nasal spray; each actuation of Nicotrol® NS delivers a metered 50 µL spray containing 0.5 mg of nicotine

Tobacco harvesters absorbed ~0.8 mg nicotine per day.

Specific References
Bernert JT, Harmon TL, Sosnoff CS, et al, "Use of Continine Immunoassay Test Strips for Preclassifying Urine Samples from Smokers and Nonsmokers Prior to Analysis by LC-MS-MS," *J Anal Toxicol*, 2005, 29(8):814-8.

Centers for Disease Control and Prevention, "Nicotine Poisoning After Ingestion of Contaminated Ground Beef - Michigan, 2003," *MMWR Morb Mortal Wkly Rep*, 2003, 52(18):413-6.

Dahl B and Caravati EM, "Intracerebral Hemorrhage Associated with Ingestion of Tobacco Snuff," *J Toxicol Clin Toxicol*, 2003, 41(5):673.

Darwin WD and Huestis MA, "Simultaneous Assay for Nicotine, Nornicotine, Cotinine, Norcotinine, and 3-Hydroxycotinine in Oral Fluid by SPE and GC-MS-EI," *J Anal Toxicol*, 2004, 28:294.

Florescu A, Koren G, Klein J, et al, "Benchmarking Hair Cotinine as a Marker of Tobacco Smoke Exposure. Meta-Analysis of International Studies," *Annale de Toxicologie Analytique*, 2005, 17(4):253-62.

Garcia-Algar O, Vall O, Segura J, et al, "Nicotine Concentrations in Deciduous Teeth and Cumulative Exposure to Tobacco Smoke During Childhood," *JAMA*, 2003, 290(2):196-7.

"Nicotine Poisoning After Ingestion of Contaminated Ground Beef - Michigan, 2003," *MMWR Morb Mortal Wkly Rep*, 2003, 52(18):413.

Pietruszka M, Schaffer M, Chao O, et al, "Measurement of Nicotine and Cotinine in Hair of Children and Adults by GC-MS-MS," *J Anal Toxicol*, 2006, 30:162-3.

Warren RJ, "Fatal Nicotine Intoxication Resulting from the Ingestion of Ayahuasca," *J Anal Toxicol*, 2004, 28:287.

Wtsadik A, Kim I, Choo RE, et al, "Nicotine, Cotinine, Trans-3'-Hydroxycotinine, and Norcotinine as Biomarkers of Tobacco Smoke Exposure in Oral Fluid of Pregnant Smokers," *J Anal Toxicol*, 2006, 30:140-1.

Zevin S, Swed E, and Cahan C, "Clinical Effects of Locally Delivered Nicotine in Obstructive Sleep Apnea Syndrome," *Am J Ther*, 2003, 10(3):170-5.

NIFEdipine

Related Information
- Calcium Channel Blockers

CAS Number 21829-25-4

U.S. Brand Names Adalat® CC; Nifedical™ XL; Procardia XL®; Procardia®

Use Angina, hypertrophic cardiomyopathy, hypertension (sustained release only)

Mechanism of Action Inhibits calcium ion from entering the "slow channels" or select voltage-sensitive areas of vascular smooth muscle and myocardium during depolarization, producing a relaxation of coronary vascular smooth muscle and coronary vasodilation; increases myocardial oxygen delivery in patients with vasospastic angina

Adverse Reactions
Cardiovascular: **Flushing,** hypotension, tachycardia, palpitations, syncope, peripheral edema, chest pain, sinus bradycardia, angina, myocardial depression, QRS prolongation, sinus tachycardia, torsade de pointes, vasodilation, vasculitis

Central nervous system: **Dizziness, headache, lightheadedness, giddiness,** drowsiness, fever, chills, psychosis, memory disturbance

Dermatologic: Dermatitis, rash, photosensitivity reactions, flushing, purpura, bullous lesions, erythema multiforme, acute generalized exanthematous pustulosis, alopecia, angioedema, toxic epidermal necrolysis, urticaria, Stevens-Johnson syndrome, pruritus, erythema nodosum, licheniform eruptions, exanthem, pemphigoid nodularis

Endocrine & metabolic: Gynecomastia, parotitis

Gastrointestinal: **Nausea, heartburn,** diarrhea, constipation, gingival hyperplasia, vomiting, bezoars, intestinal infarction, concretions, metallic taste, loss of taste perception, decreased esophageal sphincter tone

Hematologic: Thrombocytopenia, leukopenia, anemia, hemolytic anemia

Neuromuscular & skeletal: **Weakness,** joint stiffness, arthritis with elevated ANA, clonus, myoclonus, erythromelalgia, rhabdomyolysis, paresthesia

Ocular: Blurred vision, transient blindness

Respiratory: Dyspnea, hyposmia

Miscellaneous: **Heat sensation,** diaphoresis, systemic lupus erythematosus, fixed drug eruption

Signs and Symptoms of Overdose Agranulocytosis, AV block, bradycardia, chest pain, congestive heart failure, constipation, depression, enuresis, exfoliative dermatitis, extrapyramidal reaction, gingival hyperplasia, granulocytopenia, gynecomastia, heart block, hyperglycemia, hyperthermia, hyperkalemia, hypokalemia, hypotension, leukopenia, lightheadedness, memory loss, neutropenia, nocturia, peripheral vasodilation, pulmonary edema, QT prolongation, Raynaud's (exacerbation), reflex tachycardia, wheezing

Pharmacodynamics/Kinetics
Onset of action: Immediate release: ~20 minutes

Protein binding (concentration dependent): 92% to 98%

Metabolism: Hepatic to inactive metabolites

Bioavailability: Capsule: 40% to 77%; Sustained release: 65% to 89% relative to immediate release capsules

Half-life elimination: Adults: Healthy: 2-5 hours, Cirrhosis: 7 hours; Elderly: 6.7 hours

Excretion: Urine (as metabolites)

Dosage Children: Oral:
Hypertensive emergencies: 0.25-0.5 mg/kg/dose
Hypertrophic cardiomyopathy: 0.6-0.9 mg/kg/24 hours in 3-4 divided doses

Adults: Oral: Initial: 10 mg 3 times/day as capsules or 30-60 mg once daily as sustained release tablet; maintenance: 10-30 mg 3-4 times/day (capsules); maximum: 180 mg/24 hours (capsules) or 120 mg/day (sustained release)

Dosing adjustment in hepatic impairment: Reduce oral dose by 50% to 60% in patients with cirrhosis

Monitoring Parameters Heart rate, blood pressure, signs and symptoms of CHF, peripheral edema

Administration Extended release tablets should be swallowed whole; do not crush or chew.

Contraindications Hypersensitivity to nifedipine or any component of the formulation; immediate release preparation for treatment of urgent or emergent hypertension; acute MI

Warnings
The use of sublingual short-acting nifedipine in hypertensive emergencies and pseudoemergencies is neither safe nor effective and SHOULD BE ABANDONED! Serious adverse events (cerebrovascular ischemia, syncope, heart block, stroke, sinus arrest, severe hypotension, acute myocardial infarction, ECG changes, and fetal distress) have been reported in relation to such use.

Blood pressure lowering should be done at a rate appropriate for the patient's condition. Rapid drops in blood pressure can lead to arterial insufficiency. Increased angina and/or MI has occurred with initiation or dosage titration of calcium channel blockers. Severe hypotension may occur in patients taking immediate release nifepine concurrently with beta blockers when undergoing CABG with high dose fentanyl anesthesia. When considering surgery with high dose fentanyl, may consider withdrawing nifedipine (>36 hours) before surgery if possible. Use caution in severe aortic stenosis. Use caution in patients with severe hepatic impairment (may need dosage adjustment). Abrupt withdrawal may cause rebound angina in patients with CAD. Use caution in CHF (may cause worsening of symptoms).

The extended release formulation consists of drug within a nondeformable matrix; following drug release/absorption, the matrix/shell is expelled in the stool. The use of nondeformable products in patients with known stricture/narrowing of the GI tract has been associated with symptoms of obstruction. Avoid grapefruit juice during treatment with nifedipine.

Dosage Forms Capsule, softgel: 10 mg, 20 mg
  Procardia®: 10 mg
  Tablet, extended release: 30 mg, 60 mg, 90 mg
    Adalat® CC, Procardia XL®: 30 mg, 60 mg, 90 mg
    Afeditab™ CR, Nifedical™ XL: 30 mg, 60 mg
    Nifediac™ CC: 30 mg, 60 mg, 90 mg [90 mg tablet contains tartrazine]

Reference Range Therapeutic: 25-100 ng/mL; although levels >28 ng/mL correlate with negative inotropic effect after I.V. use; serum nifedipine level of 1290 ng/mL associated with fatality (postmortem urine nifedipine level was 130 ng/mL)

Overdosage/Treatment
Decontamination: Avoid ipecac. Lavage (within 1 hour)/activated charcoal is useful. Whole bowel irrigation for sustained release preparations.

Supportive therapy: I.V. fluids and Trendelenburg positioning should be initiated as intoxication may cause hypotension. Calcium (calcium chloride I.V. 1-3 g in adults or 10-30 mg/kg in children over 5-10 minutes with repeats as needed) has been used as an "antidote" for acute intoxications, although its effectiveness is questionable in nifedipine overdose. Hyperinsulinemic therapy with 0.5-1.0 unit I.V. insulin bolus with an infusion of 0.2-1 unit/kg/hour plus a glucose bolus of 25 g I.V. and dextrose infusion to maintain a serum glucose >100 mg/dL may reverse cardiogenic shock due to calcium blockers. Heart block may respond to isoproterenol, glucagon, atropine and/or calcium, although a temporary pacemaker may be required. Inamrinone or dopamine may be required for hypotension and is considered to be first-line therapy in the treatment of shock. Glucagon may increase myocardial contractility.

Enhancement of elimination: Multiple dosing of activated charcoal is useful

Antidote(s)
- Glucagon [ANTIDOTE]

Drug Interactions Substrate of CYP2D6 (minor), 3A4 (major); **Inhibits** CYP1A2 (moderate), 2C9 (weak), 2D6 (weak), 3A4 (weak)
Alpha 1-blockers: May enhance the effects of calcium channel blockers; monitor blood pressure.
Azole antifungals: May inhibit the calcium channel blocker's metabolism; monitor for the toxic effects of calcium channel blocker and adjust accordingly.
Barbiturates: May increase metabolism of calcium channel blocker. Consider therapy modification.
Calcium may reduce the calcium channel blocker's effects.
Calcium channel blocker (nondihydropyridine): May enhance the hypotensive effects of calcium channel blocker (dihydropyridine).
Carbamazepine: May decrease nifedipine serum concentration.
Cimetidine: May increase nifedipine serum concentrations; monitor for toxic effects of calcium channel blocker or choose an alternative H$_2$ antagonist.
Cisapride: May increase nifedipine's effects; monitor blood pressure.
Cyclosporine: May decrease metabolism of calcium channel blocker (dihydropyridine); monitor for toxic effects of calcium channel blocker.
CYP1A2 substrates: Nifedipine may increase the levels/effects of CYP1A2 substrates. Example substrates include aminophylline, fluvoxamine, mexiletine, mirtazapine, ropinirole, theophylline, and trifluoperazine.
CYP3A4 inducers: CYP3A4 inducers may decrease the levels/effects of nifedipine. Example inducers include aminoglutethimide, carbamazepine, nafcillin, nevirapine, phenobarbital, phenytoin, and rifamycins.
CYP3A4 inhibitors: May increase the levels/effects of nifedipine. Example inhibitors include azole antifungals, clarithromycin, diclofenac, doxycycline, erythromycin, imatinib, isoniazid, nefazodone, nicardipine, propofol, protease inhibitors, quinidine, telithromycin, and verapamil.
Erythromycin: May increase nifedipine serum concentration; monitor blood pressure and adjust if necessary.
Grapefruit juice increases the bioavailability of nifedipine; avoid grapefruit juice.
Magnesium salts: Concurrent use may enhance the adverse/toxic effects of magnesium and enhance the hypotensive effects of the calcium channel blocker.
Nafcillin decreases plasma concentration of nifedipine; avoid this combination.
Neuromuscular-blocking agent (nondepolarizing): Calcium channel blockers may enhance the neuromuscular blocking effect; monitor.
Phenobarbital reduces the plasma concentration of nifedipine. May require much higher dose of nifedipine.
Phenytoin: May decrease nifedipine serum concentration; monitor and adjust if necessary.
Protease inhibitors like amprenavir and ritonavir may increase nifedipine's serum concentration.

Quinidine's serum concentration is reduced and nifedipine's is increased; adjust doses as needed.
Quinupristin/dalfopristin: May increase nifedipine serum concentration; monitor blood pressure and adjust if necessary.
Rifamycin derivatives: Increase the metabolism of the calcium channel blocker; adjust the dose of the calcium channel blocker to maintain efficacy.
Tacrolimus's serum concentrations are increased by nifedipine; monitor tacrolimus trough levels and renal function closely.
Vincristine's half-life is increased by nifedipine; monitor closely for vincristine dose adjustment.

Pregnancy Risk Factor C
Pregnancy Implications Late decelerations of fetal heart rate can occur
Lactation Enters breast milk/compatible
Nursing Implications May cause some patients to urinate frequently at night; may cause inflamed gums
Additional Information Tasteless; response to atropine may not be observed until after I.V. calcium administration
Specific References
Cantrell FL, Clark RF, and Manoguerra AS, "Determining Triage Guidelines for Unintentional Overdoses with Calcium Channel Antagonists, *Clin Toxicol (Phila)*, 2005, 43(7):849-53 (review).
Geronimo-Pardo M, Cuartero-Del-Pozo AB, Jimenez-Vizuete JM, et al, "Clarithromycin-Nifedipine Interaction as Possible Cause of Vasodilatory Shock," *Ann Pharmacother*, 2005, 39(3):538-42.
Olson KR, Erdman AR, Woolf AD, et al, "Calcium Channel Blocker Ingestion: An Evidence-based Consensus Guideline for Out-of-hospital Management," *Clin Toxicol (Phila)*, 2005, 43(7):797-822.
Schier JG, Howland MA, Hoffman RS, et al, "Fatality from Administration of Labetalol and Crushed Extended-Release Nifedipine," *Ann Pharmacother*, 2003, 37(10):1420-3.

Nilutamide

CAS Number 63612-50-0
U.S. Brand Names Nilandron®
Synonyms RU-23908
Use Treatment of metastatic prostate cancer
Mechanism of Action Nonsteroidal antiandrogen that inhibits androgen uptake or inhibits binding of androgen in target tissues. It specifically blocks the action of androgens by interacting with cytosolic androgen receptor F sites in target tissue
Adverse Reactions
Cardiovascular: Chest pain, edema, heart failure, hypertension, syncope
Central nervous system: Depression, dizziness, drowsiness, fever, **headache**, hypesthesia, **insomnia**, malaise
Dermatologic: Pruritus, alopecia, dry skin, rash
Endocrine & metabolic: Disulfiram-like reaction, **gynecomastia**, **hot flashes**
Gastrointestinal: **Abdominal pain**, **anorexia**, **constipation**, diarrhea, dyspepsia, GI hemorrhage, melena, **nausea**, vomiting, weight loss, xerostomia
Genitourinary: Hematuria, **libido decreased**, nocturia, **testicular atrophy**
Hematologic: Anemia, aplastic anemia
Hepatic: Hepatitis, **transient elevation in serum transaminases**
Neuromuscular & skeletal: Arthritis, paresthesia
Ocular: Abnormal vision, cataracts, chromatopsia, **impaired dark adaptation** (usually reversible with dose reduction, may require discontinuation in 1% to 2% of patients), photophobia
Respiratory: **Dyspnea**, interstitial pneumonitis (typically exertional dyspnea, cough, chest pain, and fever; most often occurring within the first 3 months of treatment); rhinitis
Miscellaneous: Diaphoresis, flu-like syndrome
Signs and Symptoms of Overdose Nausea, vomiting, malaise, headache, dizziness, elevated liver enzymes
Pharmacodynamics/Kinetics
Absorption: Rapid and complete
Protein binding: 72% to 85%
Metabolism: Hepatic, forms active metabolites
Half-life elimination: Terminal: 23-87 hours; Metabolites: 35-137 hours
Excretion: Urine (up to 78% at 120 hours; <1% as unchanged drug); feces (1% to 7%)
Dosage 300 mg/day (100 mg every 8 hours); consider reducing dose in hepatic insufficiency
Monitoring Parameters Obtain a chest x-ray if a patient reports dyspnea; if there are findings suggestive of interstitial pneumonitis, discontinue treatment with nilutamide. Measure serum hepatic enzyme levels at baseline and at regular intervals (3 months); if transaminases increase over 2-3 times the upper limit of normal, discontinue treatment. Perform appropriate laboratory testing at the first symptom/sign of liver injury (eg, jaundice, dark urine, fatigue, abdominal pain or unexplained GI symptoms).

Contraindications Hypersensitivity to nilutamide or any component of the formulation; severe hepatic impairment; severe respiratory insufficiency

Warnings

Hazardous agent - use appropriate precautions for handling and disposal.

[U.S. Boxed Warning]: Interstitial pneumonitis has been reported in 2% of patients exposed to nilutamide. Patients typically experienced progressive exertional dyspnea, and possibly cough, chest pain and fever. X-rays showed interstitial or alveolo-interstitial changes. The suggestive signs of pneumonitis most often occurred within the first 3 months of nilutamide treatment.

Hepatitis or marked increases in liver enzymes leading to drug discontinuation occurred in 1% of nilutamide patients. Rare cases of elevated hepatic enzymes followed by death have been reported.

Foreign postmarketing surveillance has revealed isolated cases of aplastic anemia in which a causal relationship with nilutamide could not be ascertained.

13% to 57% of patients receiving nilutamide reported a delay in adaptation to the dark, ranging from seconds to a few minutes. This effect sometimes does not abate as drug treatment is continued. Caution patients who experience this effect about driving at night or through tunnels. This effect can be alleviated by wearing tinted glasses.

Dosage Forms Tablet: 150 mg

Reference Range Peak plasma levels after a 100 mg and 300 mg oral dose: 0.8 mg/mL and 1.6 mg/mL, respectively

Overdosage/Treatment

Decontamination: Activated charcoal

Supportive therapy: Management is supportive

Enhancement of elimination: Dialysis is of no benefit

Drug Interactions **Substrate** of CYP2C19 (major); **Inhibits** CYP2C19 (weak)

CYP2C19 inducers: May decrease the levels/effects of nilutamide. Example inducers include aminoglutethimide, carbamazepine, phenytoin, and rifampin.

CYP2C19 inhibitors: May increase the levels/effects of nilutamide. Example inhibitors include delavirdine, fluconazole, fluvoxamine, gemfibrozil, isoniazid, omeprazole, and ticlopidine.

Pregnancy Risk Factor C; Not indicated for use in women

Pregnancy Implications Not indicated for use in women

Lactation Not indicated for use in women

Additional Information Other nonapproved uses: Treatment of acne, seborrhea, and transsexual hormonal feminization

Nilvadipine

Related Information
- Calcium Channel Blockers

CAS Number 75530-68-6

Synonyms Nivadipine

Unlabeled/Investigational Use Hypertension; also may be useful in patients with cerebrovascular disease or stable exertional or variant angina pectoris

Mechanism of Action Dihydropyridine calcium channel blocking agent with properties similar to nifedipine

Adverse Reactions

Cardiovascular: Flushing, tachycardia, edema, hypotension, ectopy (ventricular), shock, chest pain, angina, palpitations, sinus tachycardia, arrhythmias (ventricular)

Central nervous system: Headache, dizziness, sleep disturbances, insomnia

Gastrointestinal: Nausea

Ocular: Oscillopsia

Pharmacodynamics/Kinetics

Distribution: V_d: 24-40 L/kg

Protein binding: 98%

Bioavailability: Oral: 14% to 19%

Half-life elimination: 9.8-18.2 hours

Excretion: Urine

Clearance: 1.08 L/kg/hour

Dosage Hypertension: 4-16 mg/day; reduce dosage to a maximum dose of 8 mg in patients with cirrhosis or with concomitant use with cimetidine

Cerebrovascular disease: 2-4 mg twice daily

Angina pectoris: 8-16 mg/day

Contraindications Hypersensitivity to nilvadipine or any component of the formulation; acute apoplectic stroke; intracranial hemorrhage; raised intracranial pressure

Overdosage/Treatment

Decontamination: Avoid ipecac. Lavage (within 1 hour)/activated charcoal is useful. Whole bowel irrigation for sustained release preparations.

Supportive therapy: I.V. fluids and Trendelenburg positioning should be initiated as intoxication may cause hypotension. Calcium (calcium chloride I.V. 1-3 g in adults or 10-30 mg/kg in children over 5-10 minutes with repeats as needed) has been used as an "antidote" for acute intoxications, although its effectiveness is questionable in nifedipine overdose. Heart block may respond to isoproterenol, gluca-

gon, atropine and/or calcium, although a temporary pacemaker may be required. Inamrinone or dopamine may be required for hypotension and are considered first-line therapy in treatment of shock. Glucagon may increase myocardial contractility.

Enhancement of elimination: Multiple dosing of activated charcoal is useful

Drug Interactions Sildenafil, tadalafil, vardenafil: Blood pressure-lowering effects may be additive; use caution.

Additional Information Not available in U.S.

Nimodipine

Related Information
- Calcium Channel Blockers

CAS Number 66085-59-4

U.S. Brand Names Nimotop®

Use Improvement of neurological deficits due to spasm following subarachnoid hemorrhage from ruptured congenital intracranial aneurysms who are in good neurological condition postictus

Mechanism of Action Nimodipine is a calcium channel blocker; animal studies indicate that nimodipine has a greater effect on cerebral arterials than other arterials; this increased specificity may be due to the drug's increased lipophilicity and cerebral distribution as compared to nifedipine indicated for patients with subarachnoid hemorrhage

Adverse Reactions

Cardiovascular: Reductions in systemic blood pressure, flushing, tachycardia, palpitations, sinus bradycardia, QRS prolongation, sinus tachycardia, vasodilation

Central nervous system: Dizziness

Dermatologic: Acne, purpura, exanthem, pruritus

Gastrointestinal: Nausea, constipation

Hematologic: Bleeding

Neuromuscular & skeletal: Rhabdomyolysis

Respiratory: Wheezing

Signs and Symptoms of Overdose Depression, diarrhea, disorientation, gingival hyperplasia, hyponatremia, hypotension, lightheadedness, myalgia, peripheral vasodilation

Pharmacodynamics/Kinetics

Protein binding: >95%

Metabolism: Extensively hepatic

Bioavailability: 13%

Half-life elimination: 1-2 hours; prolonged with renal impairment

Time to peak, serum: ~1 hour

Excretion: Urine (50%) and feces (32%) within 4 days

Dosage **Note:** Capsules and contents are for oral administration **ONLY.**

Adults: Oral: 60 mg every 4 hours for 21 days, start therapy within 96 hours after subarachnoid hemorrhage.

Dialysis: Not removed by hemo- or peritoneal dialysis; supplemental dose is not necessary.

Dosing adjustment in hepatic impairment: Reduce dosage to 30 mg every 4 hours in patients with liver failure.

Monitoring Parameters Blood pressure

Administration For oral administration **ONLY.** If the capsules cannot be swallowed, the liquid may be removed by making a hole in each end of the capsule with an 18-gauge needle and extracting the contents into a syringe. If administered via NG tube, follow with a flush of 30 mL NS.

Contraindications Hypersensitivity to nimodipine or any component of the formulation

Warnings

May cause reductions in blood pressure. Use caution in hepatic impairment. Intestinal pseudo-obstruction and ileus have been reported during the use of nimodipine. Use caution in patients with decreased GI motility of a history of bowel obstruction. Use caution when treating patients with increased intracranial pressure.

[U.S. Boxed Warning]: Nimodipine has inadvertently been administered I.V. when withdrawn from capsules into a syringe for subsequent nasogastric administration. Severe cardiovascular adverse events, including fatalities, have resulted; precautions should be employed against such an event.

Dosage Forms Capsule, liquid filled: 30 mg

Overdosage/Treatment

Avoid ipecac.

Supportive therapy: Supportive and symptomatic treatment, including I.V. fluids and Trendelenburg positioning, should be initiated as intoxication may cause hypotension. Although calcium (calcium chloride I.V. 1-3 g in adults or 10-30 mg/kg in children over 5-10 minutes with repeats as needed) has been used as an "antidote" for acute intoxications, there is limited experience to support its routine use and should be reserved for those cases where definite signs of myocardial depression are evident. Heart block may respond to isoproterenol, glucagon, atropine and/or calcium, although a temporary pacemaker may be required; norepinephrine, dopamine, or inamrinone for treatment of refractory hypotension is considered first-line therapy in treatment of shock

Enhancement of elimination: Multiple dosing of activated charcoal may be useful

Antidote(s)
- Calcium Gluconate [ANTIDOTE]

Drug Interactions **Substrate** of CYP3A4 (major)

Antihypertensive agents: Effects may be potentiated by nimodipine.

Azole antifungals may inhibit the calcium channel blocker's metabolism; avoid this combination. Try an antifungal like terbinafine (if appropriate) or monitor closely for altered effect of the calcium channel blocker.

Calcium may reduce the calcium channel blocker's effects, particularly hypotension.

Calcium channel blockers: The effects of other calcium channel blockers may be potentiated by nimodipine.

CYP3A4 inducers: CYP3A4 inducers may decrease the levels/effects of nimodipine. Example inducers include aminoglutethimide, carbamazepine, nafcillin, nevirapine, phenobarbital, phenytoin, and rifamycins.

CYP3A4 inhibitors: May increase the levels/effects of nimodipine. Example inhibitors include azole antifungals, clarithromycin, diclofenac, doxycycline, erythromycin, imatinib, isoniazid, nefazodone, nicardipine, propofol, protease inhibitors, quinidine, telithromycin, and verapamil.

Grapefruit juice increases the bioavailability of nimodipine; monitor for altered nimodipine effects.

Protease inhibitor like amprenavir and ritonavir may increase nimodipine's serum concentration.

Rifampin increases the metabolism of the calcium channel blocker; adjust the dose of the calcium channel blocker to maintain efficacy.

Sildenafil, tadalafil, vardenafil: Blood pressure-lowering effects may be additive; use caution.

Valproic acid increased nimodipine's serum concentration; monitor altered effect of nimodipine.

Pregnancy Risk Factor C

Pregnancy Implications Use in pregnancy only when clearly needed and when the benefits outweigh the potential hazard to the fetus. Teratogenic and embryotoxic effects have been demonstrated in small animals. No well-controlled studies have been conducted in pregnant women.

Lactation Enters breast milk/not recommended

Nursing Implications If the capsules cannot be swallowed, the liquid may be removed by making a hole in each end of the capsule with an 18-gauge needle and extracting the contents into a syringe; if given via NG tube, follow with a flush of 30 mL NS

Nitrazepam

Related Information
- Clonazepam
- Flunitrazepam

CAS Number 146-22-5

Synonyms Nitrozepamum

Impairment Potential Yes. A brief or extended period (up to 1 year) of use is consistent with driving impairment in the elderly; impairment is greatest in the first 7 days of use.

Unlabeled/Investigational Use Short-term management of insomnia; treatment of infantile spasm and seizures

Mechanism of Action Facilitates gamma-aminobutyric acid neurotransmission; a 7-nitrobenzodiazepine derivative

Adverse Reactions

Central nervous system: Lethargy, disorientation, night terrors, opisthotonos, ataxia, headache, hypothermia

Dermatologic: Bullous eruptions

Endocrine & metabolic: Gout

Gastrointestinal: Salivation, dysphagia, anorexia

Hematologic: Porphyria

Neuromuscular & skeletal: Rhabdomyolysis

Ocular: Increased intraocular pressure

Signs and Symptoms of Overdose Apnea, aspiration

Pharmacodynamics/Kinetics

Peak serum levels: 1.4 hours

Duration of effect: 4-8 hours

Distribution: V_d: 2.4 L/kg (young patients); 4.8 L/kg (elderly)

Protein binding: 85% to 88%

Metabolism: Hepatic reduction

Bioavailability: 78%

Half-life: 24-29 hours

Elimination: Renal (80%), feces (20%)

Dosage

Oral:

Insomnia:

Children:

1-6 years: 2.5 mg

≥7 years: 5 mg

Adults: 5-10 mg at night

Epilepsy: Children and Adults: 1-6 mg/day; dosage should be decreased in elderly, hypothyroid patients, and cirrhosis

Children maximum dose: 60 mg

Adult maximum dose: 20 mg

Contraindications Hypersensitivity to nitrazepam, flunitrazepam, or clonazepam

Warnings Use with caution in patients with hypothyroidism, cirrhosis, elderly, pregnancy, and breast-feeding

Dosage Forms Capsule: 5 mg

Tablet: 5 mg

Reference Range Steady state plasma levels with a 5 mg/day oral dose: ~57(±17) ng/mL; fatalities associated with postmortem blood levels of 1.2-9 mg/L; therapeutic level: 0.035 + 0.084 mg/L

Overdosage/Treatment

Decontamination: Activated charcoal

Supportive therapy: Rarely is mechanical ventilation required; flumazenil has been shown to selectively block the binding of benzodiazepines to CNS receptors, resulting in a reversal of benzodiazepine-induced CNS depression and respiratory depression

Enhancement of elimination: Multiple dose of activated charcoal is effective

Antidote(s)
- Flumazenil [ANTIDOTE]

Test Interactions Nitrazepam can cause a false elevation (~15%) of clozapine serum levels

Drug Interactions Birth control pills, probenecid, and cimetidine can result in decreased nitrazepam clearance; rifampin can result in increased clearance of nitrazepam; hallucinations with concomitant erythromycin

Additional Information Hangover can occur at 20 mg oral doses; hallucinations from withdrawal can be treated with chlorpromazine

Nitrendipine

Related Information
- Calcium Channel Blockers

CAS Number 39562-70-6

Unlabeled/Investigational Use Hypertension

Mechanism of Action Dihydropyridine calcium channel blocking agent with actions similar to nifedipine

Adverse Reactions

Cardiovascular: Flushing, edema, tachycardia, palpitations, sinus tachycardia, vasodilation

Central nervous system: **Headache**, dizziness, fatigue

Gastrointestinal: Nausea, gingival hyperplasia

Otic: Tinnitus

Pharmacodynamics/Kinetics

Distribution: 6 L/kg

Protein binding: 98%

Metabolism: Hepatic to inactive metabolites

Bioavailability: 16% to 23%

Half-life elimination: 8.6 hours

Excretion: Urine (80%); feces (8%)

Dosage 20 mg/day (in patients with liver disease or in the elderly, an initial dose of 10 mg is recommended); maximum dose: 40 mg/day

Contraindications Hypersensitivity to any component of the formulation or other calcium channel blocking agents; hypotension; advanced aortic stenosis

Warnings Reduce dosage in elderly; use with caution in patients with liver insufficiency, digital ischemia, nonobstructive hypertrophic cardiomyopathy, Duchenne muscular dystrophy, or in combination with beta-blocking agents. Blood pressure lowering must be done at a rate appropriate for the patient's clinical condition.

Reference Range Peak plasma levels after a 20 mg oral dose: 5-40 mcg/L

Overdosage/Treatment

Decontamination: Avoid ipecac. Lavage (within 1 hour)/activated charcoal is useful. Whole bowel irrigation for sustained release preparations.

Supportive therapy: I.V. fluids and Trendelenburg positioning should be initiated as intoxication may cause hypotension. Calcium (calcium chloride I.V. 1-3 g in adults or 10-30 mg/kg in children over 5-10 minutes with repeats as needed) has been used as an "antidote" for acute intoxications and is considered a second-line agent (to traditional vasopressors) for treatment of shock. Heart block may respond to isoproterenol, glucagon, atropine and/or calcium, although a temporary pacemaker may be required. Inamrinone or dopamine may be required for hypotension. Glucagon may increase myocardial contractility.

Enhancement of elimination: Multiple dosing of activated charcoal is useful

Drug Interactions

Substrate of CYP3A4 (major); **Inhibits** CYP3A4 (weak)

Beta-blockers: Concomitant use may increase the hypotensive effects.

CYP3A4 inducers: CYP3A4 inducers may decrease the levels/effects of nitrendipine. Example inducers include aminoglutethimide, carbamazepine, nafcillin, nevirapine, phenobarbital, phenytoin, and rifamycins.

CYP3A4 inhibitors: May increase the levels/effects of nitrendipine. Example inhibitors include azole antifungals, clarithromycin, diclofenac, doxycycline, erythromycin, imatinib, isoniazid, nefazodone, nicardipine, propofol, protease inhibitors, quinidine, telithromycin, and verapamil.

Digoxin: At nitrendipine doses exceeding 20 mg/day, increased digoxin levels and toxicity can occur.

Sildenafil, tadalafil, vardenafil: Blood pressure-lowering effects may be additive; use caution.

Lactation Enters breast milk

Additional Information Not available in U.S.

Can cause an increase in plasma catecholamine, urinary aldosterone levels, and serum alkaline phosphatase levels. Natriuresis and diuresis may also occur on a short-term basis.

Nitric Oxide

CAS Number 10102-43-9

UN Number 1660

Use Orphan drug status for treatment of primary pulmonary hypertension in the newborn; may be useful for septic shock, ARDS, or treatment of pulmonary effects of paraquat; has been used to treat high altitude pulmonary edema (HAPE)

Mechanism of Action Produces selective pulmonary vasodilatation without systemic vasodilatation through direct effect on smooth muscle of pulmonary vasculature

Adverse Reactions

Cardiovascular: Vasodilation

Hematologic: Methemoglobinemia

Respiratory: Pulmonary fibrosis, rebound pulmonary hypertension from nitric oxide withdrawal

Admission Criteria/Prognosis Any patient with change in mental status, cardiopulmonary complaints, or methemoglobin levels >30% should be admitted; asymptomatic patients with methemoglobin levels <30% may be considered for discharge after 6 hours of observation and if methemoglobin levels fall to <15%

Pharmacodynamics/Kinetics

Onset of action: Inhalation: 2-5 minutes

Absorption: Rapidly absorbed via lungs; blood/gas partition coefficient is 0.47

Metabolism: Body: <0.004%

Excretion: Primarily exhaled gases; skin (minimal amounts)

Dosage High altitude pulmonary edema: 40 ppm of nitric oxide with room air

Contraindications Hypersensitivity to nitrous oxide or any component of the formulation; nitrous oxide should not be administered without oxygen; should not be given to patients after a full meal

Warnings Nausea and vomiting occurs postoperatively in ≈15% of patients. Prolonged use may produce bone marrow suppression and/or neurologic dysfunction. Oxygen should be briefly administered during emergence from prolonged anesthesia with nitrous oxide to prevent diffusion hypoxia. Patients with vitamin B_{12} deficiency (pernicious anemia) and those with other nutritional deficiencies (alcoholics) are at increased risk of developing neurologic disease and bone marrow suppression with exposure to nitrous oxide. May be addictive.

Dosage Forms Supplied in blue cylinders

Reference Range Normal plasma nitrate level: 24 μmol/L (range: 19-39 μmol/L); patients with congestive heart failure 56 μmol/L (range: 41-72 μmol/L)

Overdosage/Treatment Supportive therapy: Methylene blue for symptomatic methemoglobinemia

Antidote(s)

- Methylene Blue [ANTIDOTE]

Drug Interactions No data reported

Pregnancy Risk Factor No data reported

Additional Information Flammable, can inactivate surfactant; colorless gas; paralysis (motor neuropathy) may develop in alcoholics; TLV-TWA: 25 ppm; IDLH: 100 ppm

Nitrofurantoin

CAS Number 17140-81-7; 54-87-5; 67-20-9

U.S. Brand Names Furadantin®; Macrobid®; Macrodantin®

Use Prevention and treatment of urinary tract infections caused by susceptible gram-negative and some gram-positive organisms; *Pseudomonas*, *Serratia*, and most species of *Proteus* are generally resistant to nitrofurantoin

Mechanism of Action Inhibits several bacterial enzyme systems including acetyl coenzyme A interfering with metabolism and possibly cell wall synthesis

Adverse Reactions

Frequency not defined.

Cardiovascular: Chest pain, cyanosis, ECG changes (associated with pulmonary toxicity)

Central nervous system: Chills, depression, dizziness, drowsiness, fatigue, fever, headache, pseudotumor cerebri, psychotic reactions

Dermatologic: Alopecia, erythema multiforme, exfoliative dermatitis, pruritus, rash, Stevens-Johnson syndrome

Gastrointestinal: Abdominal pain, *C. difficile*-colitis, constipation, diarrhea, dyspepsia, loss of appetite, nausea (most common), pancreatitis, sore throat, vomiting

Hematologic: Agranulocytosis, aplastic anemia, eosinophilia, hemolytic anemia, methemoglobinemia, thrombocytopenia

Hepatic: Cholestasis, hepatitis, hepatic necrosis, serum transaminases increased, jaundice (cholestatic)

Neuromuscular & skeletal: Arthralgia, numbness, paresthesia, peripheral neuropathy, weakness

Ocular: Amblyopia, nystagmus, optic neuritis (rare)

Respiratory: Cough, dyspnea, pneumonitis, pulmonary fibrosis

Miscellaneous: Hypersensitivity (including acute pulmonary hypersensitivity), lupus-like syndrome

Signs and Symptoms of Overdose Apnea, cholestatic jaundice, crystalluria, erythema multiforme, hyperthermia, jaundice, leukopenia or neutropenia (agranulocytosis, granulocytopenia), methemoglobinemia, numbness, pseudotumor cerebri, sexual dysfunction, vision color changes (yellow tinge)

Admission Criteria/Prognosis Any patient with change in mental status, cardiopulmonary complaints, ingestion >10 mg/kg, or methemoglobin levels >30% should be admitted; asymptomatic patients with methemoglobin levels <30% may be considered for discharge after 6 hours of observation and if methemoglobin levels fall to <15%

Pharmacodynamics/Kinetics

Absorption: Well absorbed; macrocrystalline form absorbed more slowly due to slower dissolution (causes less GI distress)

Distribution: V_d: 0.8 L/kg; crosses placenta; enters breast milk

Protein binding: 60% to 90%

Metabolism: Body tissues (except plasma) metabolize 60% of drug to inactive metabolites

Bioavailability: Increased with food

Half-life elimination: 20-60 minutes; prolonged with renal impairment

Excretion:

Suspension: Urine (40%) and feces (small amounts) as metabolites and unchanged drug

Macrocrystals: Urine (20% to 25% as unchanged drug)

Dosage

Oral:

Children >1 month: 5-7 mg/kg/day in divided doses every 6 hours; maximum: 400 mg/day

UTI prophylaxis (chronic): 1-2 mg/kg/day in divided doses every 12-24 hours; maximum: 100 mg/day

Adults: 50-100 mg/dose every 6 hours

Macrocrystal/monohydrate: 100 mg twice daily

UTI prophylaxis (chronic): 50-100 mg/dose at bedtime

Dosing adjustment in renal impairment: Cl_{cr} <60 mL/minute: Contraindicated

Contraindicated in hemo- and peritoneal dialysis and continuous arteriovenous or venovenous hemofiltration

Monitoring Parameters Signs of pulmonary reaction, signs of numbness or tingling of the extremities, periodic liver function tests

Administration Administer with meals to slow the rate of absorption and decrease adverse effects; suspension may be mixed with water, milk, fruit juice, or infant formula

Contraindications Hypersensitivity to nitrofurantoin or any component of the formulation; renal impairment (anuria, oliguria, significantly elevated serum creatinine, or Cl_{cr}< 60 mL/minute); infants <1 month (due to the possibility of hemolytic anemia); pregnancy at term (38-42 weeks gestation), during labor and delivery, or when the onset of labor is imminent

Warnings Use with caution in patients with G6PD deficiency or in patients with anemia. Therapeutic concentrations of nitrofurantoin are not attained in urine of patients with Cl_{cr}<60 mL/minute. Use with caution if prolonged therapy is anticipated due to possible pulmonary toxicity. Acute, subacute, or chronic (usually after 6 months of therapy) pulmonary reactions have been observed in patients treated with nitrofurantoin; if these occur, discontinue therapy immediately; monitor closely for malaise, dyspnea, cough, fever, radiologic evidence of diffuse interstitial pneumonitis or fibrosis. Rare, but severe hepatic reactions have been associated with nitrofurantoin (onset may be insidious); discontinue immediately if hepatitis occurs. Has been associated with peripheral neuropathy (rare); risk may be increased by renal impairment, diabetes, vitamin B deficiency, or electrolyte imbalance; use caution.

Dosage Forms Capsule, macrocrystal: 50 mg, 100 mg

Macrodantin®: 25 mg, 50 mg, 100 mg

Capsule, macrocrystal/monohydrate (Macrobid®): 100 mg

Suspension, oral (Furadantin®): 25 mg/5 mL (470 mL)

Reference Range After an oral dose of 100 mg, urinary nitrofurantoin levels range from 50-100 mcg/mL and peak plasma level: ~0.72 mcg/mL

Overdosage/Treatment

Decontamination: Activated charcoal

Supportive therapy: Treat symptomatic methemoglobinemia with methylene blue

Enhancement of elimination: Multiple dosing of activated charcoal may be effective

Antidote(s)
- Methylene Blue [ANTIDOTE]

Diagnostic Procedures
- Methemoglobin, Blood

Test Interactions False-positive urine glucose (Benedict's and Fehling's methods); no false positives with enzymatic tests

Drug Interactions Decreased effect: Antacids, especially magnesium salts, decrease absorption of nitrofurantoin; nitrofurantoin may antagonize effects of norfloxacin

Increased toxicity: Probenecid (decreases renal excretion of nitrofurantoin); anticholinergic drugs increase absorption of nitrofurantoin

Pregnancy Risk Factor B

Pregnancy Implications Teratogenic effects have not been observed, however, may cause hemolytic anemia in infants. Use of nitrofurantoin is contraindicated at term (38-42 weeks gestation), during labor and delivery, or when the onset of labor is imminent.

Lactation Enters breast milk/not recommended (infants <1 month); AAP rates "compatible"

Nursing Implications Higher peak serum levels may cause increased gastritis; give with meals to slow the rate of absorption and thus decrease adverse effects

Nitroglycerin

CAS Number 55-63-0

U.S. Brand Names Minitran™; Nitrek®; Nitro-Bid®; Nitro-Dur®; Nitro-Tab®; Nitrogard®; Nitrolingual®; Nitrol® [DSC]; NitroQuick®; Nitrostat®; NitroTime®

Synonyms Glyceryl Trinitrate; Nitroglycerol; NTG

Use Angina pectoris; I.V. for congestive heart failure (especially when associated with acute myocardial infarction); hypertension due to ergotism; pulmonary hypertension; hypertensive emergencies occurring perioperatively (especially during cardiovascular surgery); industrial uses: dynamite, cordite; not FDA approved; topical use for relief of pain of anal fissures or ulcers

Unlabeled/Investigational Use Esophageal spastic disorders (sublingual)

Mechanism of Action Reduces cardiac oxygen demand by decreasing left ventricular pressure and systemic vascular resistance; dilates coronary arteries and improves collateral flow to ischemic regions

Adverse Reactions

Cardiovascular: **Flushing**, chest pain, **postural hypotension**, reflex tachycardia, severe hypotension, bradycardia, coronary vascular insufficiency, cardiac arrhythmias, palpitations, pallor, sinus bradycardia, angina, sinus tachycardia, vasodilation

Central nervous system: **Dizziness**, restlessness, **headache**, **lightheadedness**

Dermatologic: Allergic contact dermatitis, exfoliative dermatitis, urticaria, purpura, exanthem

Gastrointestinal: Nausea, vomiting, colic, diarrhea, loss of taste perception, xerostomia

Hematologic: Methemoglobinemia, thrombocytopenia

Neuromuscular & skeletal: **Weakness**

Miscellaneous: Alcohol intoxication, diaphoresis and collapse

Signs and Symptoms of Overdose Bloody diarrhea, bradycardia, circulatory collapse, clonic seizures, cyanosis, hypotension, methemoglobinemia, metabolic acidosis, palpitations, throbbing headache, tissue hypoxia

Admission Criteria/Prognosis Any patient with change in mental status, cardiopulmonary complaints, or methemoglobin levels >30% should be admitted; asymptomatic patients with methemoglobin levels <30% may be considered for discharge after 6 hours of observation and if methemoglobin levels fall to <15%

Pharmacodynamics/Kinetics Onset and duration of action is dependent upon dosage form administered. See table.

Nitroglycerin

Dosage Form	Onset of Effect	Peak Effect	Duration
Sublingual tablet	1-3 min	4-8 min	30-60 min
Lingual spray	2 min	4-10 min	30-60 min
Buccal tablet	2-5 min	4-10 min	2 h
Sustained release	20-45 min	45-120 min	4-8 h
Topical	15-60 min	30-120 min	2-12 h
Transdermal	40-60 min	60-180 min	8-24 h
I.V. drip	Immediate	Immediate	3-5 min

Absorption: Well from gastrointestinal tract

Distribution: V_d: 2.1-4.5 L/kg; distributed widely throughout the body

Protein binding: 60%

Metabolism: Extensive first-pass to inorganic nitrite

Half-life: S.L.: 1-4 minutes

Elimination: In urine; clearance: 140-320 mL/kg/minute

Dosage

Note: Hemodynamic and antianginal tolerance often develop within 24-48 hours of continuous nitrate administration

Children: Pulmonary hypertension: Continuous infusion: Start 0.25-0.5 mcg/kg/minute and titrate by 1 mcg/kg/minute at 20- to 60-minute intervals to desired effect; usual dose: 1-3 mcg/kg/minute; maximum: 5 mcg/kg/minute

Adults:

Buccal: Initial: 1 mg every 3-5 hours while awake (3 times/day); titrate dosage upward if angina occurs with tablet in place

Oral: 2.5-9 mg 2-4 times/day (up to 26 mg 4 times/day)

I.V.: 5 mcg/minute, increase by 5 mcg/minute every 3-5 minutes to 20 mcg/minute; if no response at 20 mcg/minute increase by 10 mcg/minute every 3-5 minutes, up to 200 mcg/minute

Ointment: 1" to 2" every 8 hours up to 4" to 5" every 4 hours

Patch, transdermal: Initial: 0.2-0.4 mg/hour, titrate to doses of 0.4-0.8 mg/hour; tolerance is minimized by using a patch-on period of 12-14 hours and patch-off period of 10-12 hours

Sublingual: 0.2-0.6 mg every 5 minutes for maximum of 3 doses in 15 minutes; may also use prophylactically 5-10 minutes prior to activities which may provoke an attack

Translingual: 1-2 sprays into mouth under tongue every 3-5 minutes for maximum of 3 doses in 15 minutes, may also be used 5-10 minutes prior to activities which may provoke an attack prophylactically

Anal fissure/ulcer pain: 200 mg applied topically to anal canal 4 times daily and after each bowel movement

May need to use nitrate-free interval (10-12 hours/day) to avoid tolerance development; tolerance may possibly be reversed with acetylcysteine; gradually decrease dose in patients receiving NTG for prolonged period to avoid withdrawal reaction

Stability I.V. infusion solution in NS or D_5W, is stable for 48 hours at room temperature, mixed and stored in glass containers; maximum concentration not to exceed 400 mcg/mL; do not mix with other drugs; store sublingual tablets and ointment in tightly closed container; store at 15°C to 30°C

Monitoring Parameters Blood pressure, heart rate

Administration I.V.: I.V. must be prepared in glass bottles; use special sets intended for nitroglycerin. glass I.V. bottles and administration sets provided by manufacturer.

Sublingual: Do not crush sublingual product (tablet). Place under tongue and allow to dissolve.

Translingual spray: Prime prior to first use (5 sprays into the air). If unused for 6 weeks, a single priming spray should be completed. Priming sprays should be directed away from patient and others. The end of the pump should be covered by the fluid in the bottle.

Contraindications

Hypersensitivity to organic nitrates; hypersensitivity to isosorbide, nitroglycerin, or any component of the formulation; concurrent use with phosphodiesterase-5 (PDE-5) inhibitors (sildenafil, tadalafil, or vardenafil); angle-closure glaucoma (intraocular pressure may be increased); head trauma or cerebral hemorrhage (increase intracranial pressure); severe anemia; allergy to adhesive (transdermal product)

Additional contraindications for I.V. product: Hypotension; uncorrected hypovolemia; inadequate cerebral circulation; constrictive pericarditis; pericardial tamponade

Warnings Severe hypotension can occur. Use with caution in volume depletion, hypotension, and right ventricular infarctions. Paradoxical bradycardia and increased angina pectoris can accompany hypotension. Orthostatic hypotension can also occur. Ethanol can accentuate this. Tolerance does develop to nitrates and appropriate dosing is needed to minimize this (drug-free interval). Safety and efficacy have not been established in pediatric patients. Avoid use of long-acting agents in acute MI or CHF; cannot easily reverse. Nitrate may aggravate angina caused by hypertrophic cardiomyopathy. Nitroglycerin transdermal patches should be removed prior to defibrillation or MRI study.

Dosage Forms Capsule, extended release: 2.5 mg, 6.5 mg, 9 mg

Nitro-Time®: 2.5 mg, 6.5 mg, 9 mg

Infusion [premixed in D_5W]: 25 mg (250 mL) [0.1 mg/mL]; 50 mg (250 mL) [0.2 mg/mL]; 50 mg (500 mL) [0.1 mg/mL]; 100 mg (250 mL) [0.4 mg/mL]; 200 mg (500 mL) [0.4 mg/mL]

Injection, solution: 5 mg/mL (5 mL, 10 mL) [contains alcohol and propylene glycol]

Ointment, topical:

Nitro-Bid®: 2% [20 mg/g] (1 g, 30 g, 60 g)

Solution, translingual spray:

Nitrolingual®: 0.4 mg/metered spray (4.9 g) [contains alcohol 20%; 60 metered sprays]; (12 g) [contains alcohol 20%; 200 metered sprays]

Tablet, sublingual:
NitroQuick®, Nitrostat®: 0.3 mg, 0.4 mg, 0.6 mg
Transdermal system [once daily patch]: 0.1 mg/hour (30s); 0.2 mg/hour (30s); 0.4 mg/hour (30s); 0.6 mg/hour (30s)
Minitran™: 0.1 mg/hour (30s); 0.2 mg/hour (30s); 0.4 mg/hour (30s); 0.6 mg/hour (30s)
Nitrek®: 0.2 mg/hour (30s); 0.4 mg/hour (30s); 0.6 mg/hour (30s)
Nitro-Dur®: 0.1 mg/hour (30s); 0.2 mg/hour (30s); 0.3 mg/hour (30s); 0.4 mg/hour (30s); 0.6 mg/hour (30s); 0.8 mg/hour (30s)

Reference Range Concentrations of 1.2-11.0 ng/mL produce 25% decrease in capillary wedge pressure

Overdosage/Treatment
Supportive therapy: Keep patient recumbent; elevate legs if needed; hypotension is treated with fluids and alpha-adrenergic pressors if needed; methylene blue treatment for symptomatic methemoglobin; if used topically, wipe off area of application
Enhancement of elimination: Forced diuresis may enhance elimination

Antidote(s)
- Methylene Blue [ANTIDOTE]

Diagnostic Procedures
- Methemoglobin, Blood

Test Interactions ↑ catecholamines (U)

Drug Interactions Alteplase (tissue plasminogen activator) has a lesser effect when used with I.V. nitroglycerin; avoid concurrent use.
Ergot alkaloids may cause an increase in blood pressure and decrease in antianginal effects; avoid concurrent use.
Ethanol can cause hypotension when nitrates are taken 1 hour or more after ethanol ingestion.
Heparin's effect may be reduced by I.V. nitroglycerin. May affect only a minority of patients.
Sildenafil, tadalafil, vardenafil: Significant reduction of systolic and diastolic blood pressure with concurrent use (contraindicated). Do not administer sildenafil, tadalafil, or vardenafil within 24 hours of a nitrate preparation.

Pregnancy Risk Factor C

Lactation Excretion in breast milk unknown/use caution

Nursing Implications I.V. must be prepared in glass bottles and use special sets intended for nitroglycerin; transdermal patches labeled as mg/hour

Additional Information I.V. preparations contain alcohol and/or propylene glycol; may need to use nitrate-free internal (10-12 hours/day) to avoid tolerance development; tolerance may possibly be reversed with acetylcysteine; gradually decrease dose in patients receiving NTG for prolonged period to avoid withdrawal reaction; monitor for ethanol toxicity due to diluent TLV-TWA 0.05 ppm; sweet, burning taste; tablets are not explosive.
Note: Nitroglycerin tabs is a slang for heroin with intravenous nitroglycerin.
It appears that age and serum creatinine levels are inversely associated with development of vascular headache due to nitrates. Risk for headache decreases by ~40% for a 10-year increase in age and is 5 times less likely in patients with serum creatinine levels >133 µmol/L as opposed to levels <97 µmol/L.
Lorazepam (2 mg I.V.) and nitroglycerin (I.V. infusion of 2 mg/kg/minute) have been used successfully to treat serotonin syndrome induced by sertraline.
Use of nitroglycerin patch (5 mg/day) near or distal to I.V. cannulation site may prevent intravenous infusion failure due to phlebitis or extravasation in patients requiring long-term (>50 hours) I.V. therapy.

Specific References
Brown TM, "Nitroglycerin in the Treatment of the Serotonin Syndrome," *Am J Emerg Med*, 2004, 22(6):510.
Diercks DB, Boghos E, Guzman H, et al, "Changes in the Numeric Descriptive Scale for Pain After Sublingual Nitroglycerin Do Not Predict Cardiac Etiology of Chest pain," *Ann Emerg Med*, 2005, 45(6):581-5.

Nitroprusside

CAS Number 13755-38-9; 14402-89-2
U.S. Brand Names Nitropress®
Synonyms Nitroprusside Sodium; Sodium Nitroferricyanide; Sodium Nitroprusside
Use Management of hypertensive crisis especially due to ergotism; congestive heart failure; used for controlled hypotension to reduce bleeding during surgery
Mechanism of Action Causes peripheral vasodilation by direct action on venous and arteriolar smooth muscle, thus reducing peripheral resistance; will increase cardiac output by decreasing afterload; reduces aortal and left ventricular impedance
Adverse Reactions
Cardiovascular: Excessive hypotensive response, palpitations, tachycardia followed by bradycardia, sinus bradycardia, sinus tachycardia, vasodilation

Central nervous system: Restlessness, disorientation, psychosis, intracranial hypertension (increased), headache, delirium
Endocrine & metabolic: Thyroid suppression, hypothyroidism
Gastrointestinal: Nausea, vomiting, adynamic ileus
Hematologic: Thrombocytopenia
Local: Transient phlebitis
Neuromuscular & skeletal: Muscle spasm, weakness
Otic: Ototoxicity, tinnitus
Respiratory: Substernal distress, hypoxia, tachypnea
Miscellaneous: Diaphoresis, thiocyanate toxicity
Signs and Symptoms of Overdose Azotemia, bradycardia, confusion, hyperventilation, hypotension, hypothyroidism, metabolic acidosis, methemoglobinemia, myoclonus, vomiting
Pharmacodynamics/Kinetics
Onset of action: BP reduction <2 minutes
Duration: 1-10 minutes
Metabolism: Nitroprusside is converted to cyanide ions in the bloodstream; decomposes to prussic acid which in the presence of sulfur donor is converted to thiocyanate (hepatic and renal rhodanase systems)
Half-life elimination: Parent drug: <10 minutes; Thiocyanate: 2.7-7 days
Excretion: Urine (as thiocyanate)
Dosage
I.V.:
Children: Continuous infusion:
Initial: 1 mcg/kg/minute by continuous I.V. infusion; increase in increments of 1 mcg/kg/minute at intervals of 20-60 minutes; titrating to the desired response
Usual dose: 3 mcg/kg/minute; rarely need >4 mcg/kg/minute
Maximum (short-term): 10 mcg/kg/minute. Dilute 15 mg × weight (kg) to 250 mL D₅W, then dose in mcg/kg/minute = infusion rate in mL/hour
Adults: Begin at 0.5 mcg/kg/minute; increase in increments of 2-4 mcg/kg/minute (up to 20 mcg/kg/minute), then in increments of 10-20 mcg/kg/minute; titrating to the desired hemodynamic effect or the appearance of headache or nausea. When >500 mcg/kg is administered by prolonged infusion of >2 mcg/kg/minute, cyanide is generated faster than an unaided patient can handle.
Cyanide risk for for nitroprusside administration:
Low risk:
Short-term (<8 hours) administration: 1.5 mg/kg total dose
Long-term (>8 hours) administration: 2-4 mcg/kg/minute (at a dose of 5-10 mcg/kg/minute, cyanide toxicity can result in 5-10 hours)
Thiocyanide toxicity usually does **not** occur at total nitroprusside doses <70 mg/kg
Stability Discard solution 24 hours after reconstitution and dilution in D₅W; promptly wrap in aluminum foil or other opaque material to protect from sunlight (incandescent light is safe); reconstituted solution should be very faint brown, discard if highly colored (blue, green or red); store powder in carton until use
Monitoring Parameters Blood pressure, heart rate; monitor for cyanide and thiocyanate toxicity; monitor acid-base status as acidosis can be the earliest sign of cyanide toxicity; monitor thiocyanate levels if requiring prolonged infusion (>3 days) or dose ≥4 mcg/kg/minute or patient has renal dysfunction; monitor cyanide blood levels in patients with decreased hepatic function; cardiac monitor and blood pressure monitor required
Administration I.V. infusion only, not for direct injection
Contraindications Hypersensitivity to nitroprusside or any component of the formulation; treatment of compensatory hypertension (aortic coarctation, arteriovenous shunting); high output failure; congenital optic atrophy or tobacco amblyopia
Warnings [U.S. Boxed Warning]: Continuous blood pressure monitoring is needed. Except when used briefly or at low (<2 mcg/kg/minute) infusion rates, nitroprusside gives rise to large cyanide quantities. Do not use the maximum dose for more than 10 minutes; if blood pressure not controlled then discontinue infusion. Monitor for cyanide toxicity via acid-base balance and venous oxygen concentration. Use with extreme caution in patients with elevated intracranial pressure. Use extreme caution in patients with hepatic or renal dysfunction. Use the lowest end of the dosage range with renal impairment. Thiocyanate toxicity occurs in patients with renal impairment or those on prolonged infusions. **[U.S. Boxed Warning]: Should not be administered by direct injection; must be further diluted with 5% dextrose in water.**
Dosage Forms Injection, solution, as sodium: 25 mg/mL (2 mL)
Reference Range
Cyanide levels
Whole blood levels: Smoker: ≤0.5 mg/L
Flushing and tachycardia seen at 0.5-1.0 mg/L; obtundation at 1.0-2.5 mg/L
Coma and death occur at >2.5 mg/L
Can also monitor thiocyanate levels if requiring prolonged infusion (>4 days) or ≥4 mcg/kg/minute; therapeutic: 6-29 mcg/mL (SI: 103-499 µmol/L)

Overdosage/Treatment

Supportive therapy: Thiocyanate toxicity includes psychosis, tremor, delirium, hypothyroidism, hyperreflexia, confusion, asthenia, tinnitus, and coma; no metabolic acidosis is noted with thiocyanate toxicity; cyanide toxicity includes acidosis (decreased HCO_3, decreased pH, increased lactate), increase in mixed venous blood oxygen tension, tachycardia, altered consciousness, seizures, and almond smell on breath. Nitroprusside has been shown to release cyanide *in vivo* with hemoglobin. Cyanide toxicity does not usually occur because of the rapid uptake of cyanide by erythrocytes and its eventual incorporation into cyanocobalamin. However, prolonged administration of nitroprusside or its reduced elimination can lead to cyanide intoxication. In these situations, airway support with oxygen therapy is germane, followed closely with antidotal therapy of amyl nitrate perles, sodium nitrate 300 mg I.V. (10 mg/kg for children) and sodium thiosulfate 12.5 g I.V. (1.5 mL/kg for children). Sodium bicarbonate (1 mEq/kg) for treatment of acidosis; hydroxocobalamin or cobalt EDTA (Kelocyanor®) may also be effective against cyanide toxicity. Cyanide toxicity can be prevented by coadministration with hydroxocobalamin (2.4 g or 80 vials of hydroxocobalamin for every 100 mg of nitroprusside) or more practically with coadministration with sodium thiosulfate (1 g of sodium thiosulfate for every 100 mg of nitroprusside). Propranolol can block the effect of rebound hypertension when nitroprusside is discontinued.

Enhancement of elimination: Hemodialysis may be effective when used in conjunction with above therapy

Antidote(s)
- Cyanide Antidote Kit [ANTIDOTE]
- Hydroxocobalamin [ANTIDOTE]

Diagnostic Procedures
- Cyanide, Blood

Drug Interactions None noted

Pregnancy Risk Factor C

Pregnancy Implications May decrease uterine blood flow by 25% to 35%

Lactation Excretion in breast milk unknown

Nursing Implications I.V. infusion only, not for direct injection; protect from light; brownish solution is usable, discard if bluish in color

Additional Information Nitroprusside is converted to cyanide ions by the endothelium in the bloodstream; decomposes to prussic acid which in the presence of sulfur donor is converted to thiocyanate (liver and kidney rhodanase systems); thiocyanate is then renally eliminated

Specific Reference
Devlin JW, Seta ML, Kanji S, et al, "Fenoldopam Versus Nitroprusside for the Treatment of Hypertensive Emergency," *Ann Pharmacother*, 2004, 38(5):755-9.

Nizatidine

CAS Number 76963-41-3

U.S. Brand Names Axid® AR [OTC]; Axid®

Use Treatment and maintenance of duodenal ulcer; meal-induced heartburn

Unlabeled/Investigational Use Part of a multidrug regimen for *H. pylori* eradication to reduce the risk of duodenal ulcer recurrence

Mechanism of Action Nizatidine is an H_2-receptor antagonist. In healthy volunteers, nizatidine has been effective in suppressing gastric acid secretion induced by pentagastrin infusion or food. Nizatidine reduces gastric acid secretion by 29.4% to 78.4%. This compares with a 60.3% reduction by cimetidine. Nizatidine 100 mg is reported to provide equivalent acid suppression as cimetidine 300 mg. There has been a significant correlation between plasma nizatidine concentrations and gastric acid suppression, although not always reliable. Following a single oral nighttime dose of nizatidine 300 mg, acid suppression has been shown to last at least 10 hours. Although there does appear to be a correlation between acid suppression and ulcer healing, the relationship dose not always hold. The amount of nighttime acid secretion is believed to be an important factor in the development of ulcer disease. Thus, the inhibition of nocturnal acid secretion may be an important consideration in the therapy of duodenal ulcers. In comparison with placebo, nizatidine doses of 150 mg or 300 mg at bedtime reduce nighttime hydrogen ion concentration by 70% and 79% respectively. Cimetidine 800 mg at bedtime and ranitidine 300 mg at bedtime reduce nocturnal acid secretion by 76% and 95% respectively. These differences are not significant.

Adverse Reactions

Cardiovascular: Chest pain, angina, leukocytoclastic vasculitis

Central nervous system: Somnolence, CNS depression, dizziness, headache, delirium

Dermatologic: Urticaria, pruritus, exanthem, cutaneous vasculitis

Endocrine & metabolic: Sexual dysfunction, gynecomastia

Hematologic: Leukocytosis, eosinophilia, thrombocytopenia

Hepatic: Hepatic failure

Neuromuscular & skeletal: Myalgia

Renal: Renal failure

Respiratory: Rhinitis

Miscellaneous: Diaphoresis, anaphylaxis

Signs and Symptoms of Overdose Dyspepsia, impotence, muscular tremors, rapid respiration, vomiting

Pharmacodynamics/Kinetics

Distribution: V_d: 0.8-1.5 L/kg

Protein binding: 35% to α_1-acid glycoprotein

Metabolism: Partially hepatic; forms metabolites

Bioavailability: >70%

Half-life elimination: 1-2 hours; prolonged with renal impairment

Time to peak, plasma: 0.5-3.0 hours

Excretion: Urine (90%; ~60% as unchanged drug); feces (<6%)

Dosage

Adults: Active duodenal ulcer: Oral:

Treatment: 300 mg at bedtime or 150 mg twice daily

Maintenance: 150 mg/day

Meal-induced heartburn: 75 mg before meals twice daily

Dosing adjustment in renal impairment:

Cl_{cr} 50-80 mL/minute: Administer 75% of normal dose

Cl_{cr} 10-50 mL/minute: Administer 50% of normal dose or 150 mg/day for active treatment and 150 mg every other day for maintenance treatment

Cl_{cr} <10 mL/minute: Administer 25% of normal dose or 150 mg every other day for treatment and 150 mg every 3 days for maintenance treatment

Contraindications Hypersensitivity to nizatidine or any component of the formulation; hypersensitivity to other H_2 antagonists (cross-sensitivity has been observed)

Warnings Use with caution in children <12 years of age; use with caution in patients with liver and renal impairment; dosage modification required in patients with renal impairment

Dosage Forms Capsule (Axid®): 150 mg, 300 mg

Solution, oral (Axid®): 15 mg/mL (120 mL, 480 mL) [bubble gum flavor]

Tablet (Axid® AR): 75 mg

Overdosage/Treatment

Decontamination: Activated charcoal

Supportive therapy: Treatment is primarily symptomatic and supportive

Enhancement of elimination: Multiple dosing of activated charcoal may be useful

Test Interactions

False-positive urine protein using Multistix®, gastric acid secretion test, skin test allergen extracts, serum creatinine, and serum transaminase concentrations

Drug Interactions Inhibits 3A4 (weak)

Antifungal agents (imidazole): Nizatidine may decrease the absorption of itraconazole or ketoconazole.

Pregnancy Risk Factor C

Pregnancy Implications No animal teratogenic effects at 1500 mg/kg/day

Lactation Enters breast milk/may be compatible

Nursing Implications Giving dose at 6 PM may better suppress nocturnal acid secretion than 10 PM

Additional Information LD_{50}: ~80 mg/kg

Specific Reference
Morisset M, Moneret-Vautrin DA, Loppinet V, et al, "Cross-Allergy to Ranitidine and Nizatidine," *Allergy*, 2000, 55(7):682-3.

Norfloxacin

CAS Number 70458-96-7

U.S. Brand Names Noroxin®

Use Uncomplicated urinary tract infections and cystitis caused by susceptible gram-negative and gram-positive bacteria; sexually-transmitted disease (eg, uncomplicated urethral and cervical gonorrhea) caused by *N. gonorrhoeae*; prostatitis due to *E. coli*

Mechanism of Action Norfloxacin is a DNA gyrase inhibitor. DNA gyrase is an essential bacterial enzyme that maintains the superhelical structure of DNA. DNA gyrase is required for DNA replication and transcription, DNA repair, recombination, and transposition; bactericidal

Adverse Reactions

Cardiovascular: Vasculitis

Central nervous system: Anxiety, ataxia, confusion, depression, dizziness, exacerbation of myasthenia gravis, fever, Guillain-Barré syndrome, headache, insomnia, psychotic reactions, seizures, somnolence,

Dermatologic: Angioedema, erythema, erythema multiforme, exfoliative dermatitis, photosensitivity, pruritus, rash, toxic epidermal necrolysis, Stevens-Johnson syndrome, urticaria

Endocrine & metabolic: Hyperhidrosis

Gastrointestinal: Abdominal pain, anorexia, bitter taste, constipation, diarrhea, dysgeusia, dyspepsia, flatulence, GI bleeding, heartburn, loose stools, nausea, pancreatitis, pseudomembranous colitis, vomiting, xerostomia

Hematologic: Hemolytic anemia (sometimes associated with G6PD deficiency), leukopenia, neutropenia, thrombocytopenia

Hepatic: Cholestatic jaundice, hepatitis, increased transaminases, jaundice

Neuromuscular & skeletal: Arthritis, arthralgia, back pain, myalgia, myoclonus, paresthesias, peripheral neuropathy, tremor, weakness; quinolones have been associated with tendonitis and tendon rupture

Ocular: Diplopia

Otic: Tinnitus, transient hearing loss

Renal: Acute renal failure, increased serum creatinine/BUN

Respiratory: Dyspnea

Miscellaneous: Anaphylactoid reactions

Pharmacodynamics/Kinetics

Absorption: Oral: Rapid, up to 40%

Distribution: Crosses placenta; small amounts enter breast milk

Protein binding: 15%

Metabolism: Hepatic

Half-life elimination: 3-4 hours; Renal impairment ($Cl_{cr} \leq 30$ mL/minute): 6.5 hours; Elderly: 4 hours

Time to peak, serum: 1-2 hours

Excretion: Urine (26% to 36%); feces (30%)

Dosage

Oral: Adults:

Urinary tract infections: 400 mg twice daily for 3-21 days depending on severity of infection or organism sensitivity; maximum: 800 mg/day

Uncomplicated gonorrhea: 800 mg as a single dose (CDC recommends as an alternative regimen to ciprofloxacin or ofloxacin)

Prostatitis: 400 mg every 12 hours for 4 weeks

Dosing interval in renal impairment: Cl_{cr} 10-30 mL/minute: Urinary tract infections: Administer 400 mg every 24 hours

Administration Hold antacids or sucralfate for 3-4 hours after giving norfloxacin; do not administer together. Best taken on an empty stomach with water (1 hour before or 2 hours after meals, milk, or other dairy products).

Contraindications Hypersensitivity to norfloxacin, quinolones, or any component of the formulation

Warnings Concurrent disease:

● Renal impairment: Use caution with renal impairment.

● Myasthenia gravis: Quinolones may exacerbate myasthenia gravis, use with caution (rare, potentially life-threatening weakness of respiratory muscles may occur).

● G6PD deficiency: Use caution in patients with glucose-6-phosphate dehydrogenase deficiency.

Key adverse reactions:

● Allergic reactions: Severe hypersensitivity reactions, including anaphylaxis, have occurred with quinolone therapy. If an allergic reaction occurs (itching, urticaria, dyspnea, facial edema, loss of consciousness, tingling, cardiovascular collapse), discontinue drug immediately.

● Tendon rupture: Tendon inflammation and/or rupture have been reported with norfloxacin and other quinolone antibiotics. Risk may be increased with concurrent corticosteroids, particularly in the elderly. Discontinue at first sign of tendon inflammation or pain.

● CNS effects: CNS stimulation may occur which may lead to tremor, restlessness, confusion, and very rarely to hallucinations or convulsive seizures. Potential for seizures, although very rare, may be increased with concomitant NSAID therapy. Use with caution in individuals at risk of seizures.

● QT_c prolongation: Use may be associated (rarely) with prolongation of QT_c interval; avoid concurrent use with class Ia and class III antiarrhythmics; use caution with other drugs which may cause QT_c prolongation.

● Photosensitization: Avoid excessive exposure to sunlight; other quinolones have been associated with phototoxicity.

● Neuropathy/paresthesia: May be associated with the development of peripheral neuropathy and/or paresthesias; discontinue in patients who develop symptoms consistent with neuropathy.

● Developmental effects: Not recommended in children <18 years of age; other quinolones have caused transient arthropathy in children; use with caution in patients with known or suspected CNS disorders.

● Superinfection: Prolonged use may result in superinfection; pseudomembranous colitis may occur and should be considered in all patients who present with diarrhea.

Dosage Forms Tablet: 400 mg

Reference Range Following a 400 mg oral dose, peak serum and urine levels: ~1.5 mcg/mL and >200 mcg/mL, respectively

Overdosage/Treatment

Decontamination: Activated charcoal

Supportive therapy: Do **not** use flumazenil; diazepam, phenobarbital, or phenytoin can be used for seizures

Enhancement of elimination: Multiple dosing of activated charcoal may be effective; only small amounts of ciprofloxacin are removed by dialysis (<10%)

Drug Interactions Inhibits CYP1A2 (strong), 3A4 (moderate)

Corticosteroids: Concurrent use may increase the risk of tendon rupture, particularly in elderly patients (overall incidence rare).

Cyclosporine: Norfloxacin may increase serum cyclosporine concentrations; monitor

CYP1A2 substrates: Norfloxacin may increase the levels/effects of CYP1A2 substrates. Example substrates include aminophylline, fluvoxamine, mexiletine, mirtazapine, ropinirole, and trifluoperazine.

CYP3A4 substrates: Norfloxacin may increase the levels/effects of CYP3A4 substrates. Example substrates include benzodiazepines, calcium channel blockers, mirtazapine, nateglinide, nefazodone, sildenafil (and other PDE-5 inhibitors), tacrolimus, and venlafaxine. Selected benzodiazepines (midazolam and triazolam), cisapride, ergot alkaloids, selected HMG-CoA reductase inhibitors (lovastatin and simvastatin), and pimozide are generally contraindicated with strong CYP3A4 inhibitors.

Glyburide: Quinolones may increase the effect of glyburide; monitor.

Metal cations (aluminum, calcium, iron, magnesium, and zinc) bind quinolones in the gastrointestinal tract and inhibit absorption. Concurrent administration of most antacids, oral electrolyte supplements, quinapril, sucralfate, some didanosine formulations (chewable/buffered tablets and pediatric powder for oral suspension), and other highly-buffered oral drugs, should be avoided. Norfloxacin should be administered 4 hours before or 8 hours after these agents.

Nitrofurantoin: May antagonize the activity of norfloxacin in treating UTIs.

Probenecid: May decrease renal secretion of norfloxacin.

QT_c-prolonging agents: Effects may be additive with norfloxacin. Avoid concurrent use with Class Ia and Class III antiarrhythmics; use caution with other drugs known to prolong QT_c, including erythromycin, cisapride, antipsychotics, and cyclic antidepressants.

Theophylline: Norfloxacin may increase serum levels/effects of theophylline; monitor.

Warfarin: The hypoprothrombinemic effect of warfarin may be enhanced by some quinolone antibiotics; monitor INR.

Pregnancy Risk Factor C

Pregnancy Implications Reports of arthropathy (observed in immature animals and reported rarely in humans) have limited the use of fluoroquinolones in pregnancy. Teratogenic effects have not been reported with norfloxacin in animal studies; however, embryonic loss has been reported with one species. Norfloxacin crosses the placenta. The Teratogen Information System concluded that therapeutic doses during pregnancy are unlikely to produce substantial teratogenic risk, but data are insufficient to say that there is no risk. There are no adequate and well-controlled studies in pregnant women. When considering treatment for life-threatening infection and/or prolonged duration of therapy, the potential risk to the fetus must be balanced against the severity of the potential illness.

Lactation Excretion in breast milk unknown/not recommended

Nursing Implications Hold antacids, sucralfate for 3-4 hours after giving

Specific Reference

Sahin MT, Ozturkcan S, Inanir I, et al, "Norfloxacin-Induced Toxic Epidermal Necrolysis," *Ann Pharmacother*, 2005, 39(4):768-70.

Nortriptyline

Related Information

● Anticholinergic Effects of Common Psychotropics

CAS Number 72-69-5; 894-71-3

U.S. Brand Names Aventyl® HCl; Pamelor®

Synonyms Nortriptyline Hydrochloride

Impairment Potential Yes

Use Treatment of symptoms of depression

Unlabeled/Investigational Use Chronic pain, anxiety disorders, enuresis, attention-deficit/hyperactivity disorder (ADHD); adjunctive therapy for smoking cessation

Mechanism of Action Increases the synaptic concentration of serotonin and/or norepinephrine in the central nervous system by inhibition of their reuptake by the presynaptic neuronal membrane

Adverse Reactions

Cardiovascular: Postural hypotension, cardiac arrhythmias, tachycardia, sudden death, bundle branch block, sinus tachycardia, tachycardia (supraventricular), torsade de pointes, exacerbation of Brugada syndrome

Central nervous system: **Dizziness, drowsiness, headache**, sedation, restlessness, fatigue, anxiety, psychosis, impaired cognitive function, and seizures have occurred occasionally, extrapyramidal reactions, neuroleptic malignant syndrome

Dermatologic: Alopecia, purpura, pruritus, exanthem

Endocrine & metabolic: Syndrome of inappropriate antidiuretic hormone, gynecomastia

Gastrointestinal: **Xerostomia, increased appetite, nausea, unpleasant taste, weight gain, constipation**, adynamic ileus, Ogilvie's syndrome, stomatitis, lingua villosa nigra

Genitourinary: Urinary retention

Hematologic: Rarely agranulocytosis, eosinophilia, porphyria

Hepatic: Jaundice, liver failure

Neuromuscular & skeletal: **Weakness**, tremors, clonus, myoclonus, paresthesia

Ocular: Blurred vision, photophobia, increased intraocular pressure, mydriasis, nystagmus, phototoxic

Renal: Renal vasculitis

Respiratory: Hyperventilation

Miscellaneous: Allergic reactions

Signs and Symptoms of Overdose Agitation, agranulocytosis, AV block, bone marrow depression, coma, confusion, delirium, dementia, dental erosion, depression, dysphagia, ejaculatory disturbances, granulocytopenia, heart block, hyperthermia, hypoglycemia, hyponatremia, hypotension, hypothermia, impotence, insomnia, increased intraocular pressure, leukopenia, mania, memory loss, neutropenia, night terrors, photosensitivity, P-R prolongation, pulmonary edema, QRS prolongation, QT prolongation, respiratory depression, seizures (within 3 hours of ingestion), tachycardia, thrombocytopenia, urinary retention, visual hallucinations. QRS interval >0.12 seconds may indicate significant toxicity.

Admission Criteria/Prognosis Admit any patient who is symptomatic 6 hours postingestion; admit any pediatric ingestion >5 mg/kg

Pharmacodynamics/Kinetics

Onset of action: Therapeutic: 1-3 weeks

Distribution: V_d: 21 L/kg

Protein binding: 93% to 95%

Metabolism: Primarily hepatic; extensive first-pass effect

Half-life elimination: 28-31 hours

Time to peak, serum: 7-8.5 hours

Excretion: Urine (as metabolites and small amounts of unchanged drug); feces (small amounts)

Dosage Oral:

Nocturnal enuresis:

Children:

6-7 years (20-25 kg): 10 mg/day

8-11 years (25-35 kg): 10-20 mg/day

>11 years (35-54 kg): 25-35 mg/day

Depression or ADHD (unlabeled use):

Children 6-12 years: 1-3 mg/kg/day or 10-20 mg/day in 3-4 divided doses

Adolescents: 30-100 mg/day in divided doses

Depression:

Adults: 25 mg 3-4 times/day up to 150 mg/day

Elderly (**Note:** Nortriptyline is one of the best tolerated TCAs in the elderly)

Initial: 10-25 mg at bedtime

Dosage can be increased by 25 mg every 3 days for inpatients and weekly for outpatients if tolerated

Usual maintenance dose: 75 mg as a single bedtime dose or 2 divided doses; however, lower or higher doses may be required to stay within the therapeutic window

Dosing adjustment in hepatic impairment: Lower doses and slower titration dependent on individualization of dosage is recommended

Stability Protect from light

Monitoring Parameters Blood pressure and pulse rate (ECG, cardiac monitoring) prior to and during initial therapy in older adults; weight; blood levels are useful for therapeutic monitoring

Contraindications Hypersensitivity to nortriptyline and similar chemical class, or any component of the formulation; use of MAO inhibitors within 14 days; use in a patient during the acute recovery phase of MI; pregnancy

Warnings

[U.S. Boxed Warning]: Antidepressants increase the risk of suicidal thinking and behavior in children and adolescents with major depressive disorder (MDD) and other depressive disorders; consider risk prior to prescribing. Closely monitor for clinical worsening, suicidality, or unusual changes in behavior; the child's family or caregiver should be instructed to closely observe the patient and communicate condition with healthcare provider. Such observation would generally include at least weekly face-to-face contact with patients or their family members or caregivers during the first 4 weeks of treatment, then every other week visits for the next 4 weeks, then at 12 weeks, and as clinically indicated beyond 12 weeks. Additional contact by telephone may be appropriate between face-to-face visits. Adults treated with antidepressants should be observed similarly for clinical worsening and suicidality, especially during the initial few months of a course of drug therapy, or at times of dose changes, either increases or decreases. A medication guide should be dispensed with each prescription. **Nortriptyline is not FDA approved for use in children.**

The possibility of a suicide attempt is inherent in major depression and may persist until remission occurs. Monitor for worsening of depression or suicidality, especially during initiation of therapy or with dose increases or decreases. Worsening depression and severe abrupt suicidality that are not part of the presenting symptoms may require discontinuation or modification of drug therapy. Use caution in high-risk patients during initiation of therapy. Prescriptions should be written for the smallest quantity consistent with good patient care. The patient's family or caregiver should be alerted to monitor patients for the emergence of suicidality and associated behaviors such as anxiety, agitation, panic attacks, insomnia, irritability, hostility, impulsivity, akathisia, hypomania, and mania; patients should be instructed to notify their healthcare provider if any of these symptoms or worsening depression occur.

May worsen psychosis in some patients or precipitate a shift to mania or hypomania in patients with bipolar disorder. Monotherapy in patients with bipolar disorder should be avoided. Patients presenting with depressive symptoms should be screened for bipolar disorder. **Nortriptyline is not FDA approved for the treatment of bipolar depression.**

May cause sedation, resulting in impaired performance of tasks requiring alertness (eg, operating machinery or driving). Sedative effects may be additive with other CNS depressants and/or ethanol. The degree of sedation is low-moderate relative to other antidepressants. May increase the risks associated with electroconvulsive therapy. Consider discontinuing, when possible, prior to elective surgery. Therapy should not be abruptly discontinued in patients receiving high doses for prolonged periods. May alter glucose regulation - use caution in patients with diabetes.

May cause orthostatic hypotension (risk is low relative to other antidepressants) - use with caution in patients at risk of hypotension or in patients where transient hypotensive episodes would be poorly tolerated (cardiovascular disease or cerebrovascular disease). The degree of anticholinergic blockade produced by this agent is moderate relative to other cyclic antidepressants, however, caution should still be used in patients with urinary retention, benign prostatic hyperplasia, narrow-angle glaucoma, xerostomia, visual problems, constipation, or history of bowel obstruction.

Use with caution in patients with a history of cardiovascular disease (including previous MI, stroke, tachycardia, or conduction abnormalities). The risk conduction abnormalities with this agent is moderate relative to other antidepressants. Use caution in patients with a previous seizure disorder or condition predisposing to seizures such as brain damage, alcoholism, or concurrent therapy with other drugs which lower the seizure threshold. Use with caution in hyperthyroid patients or those receiving thyroid supplementation. Use with caution in patients with hepatic or renal dysfunction and in elderly patients.

Dosage Forms Capsule, as hydrochloride: 10 mg, 25 mg, 50 mg, 75 mg

Pamelor®: 10 mg, 25 mg, 50 mg, 75 mg [may contain benzyl alcohol; 50 mg may also contain sodium bisulfite]

Solution, as hydrochloride (Pamelor®): 10 mg/5 mL (473 mL) [contains alcohol 4% and benzoic acid]

Reference Range

Therapeutic: 50-150 ng/mL (SI: 190-570 nmol/L)

Toxic: >500 ng/mL (SI: >1900 nmol/L)

In the postmortem state, anatomical site concentration differences (ie, postmortem redistribution) may occur.

Overdosage/Treatment

Decontamination: Lavage within 3 hours/activated charcoal; multiple dosing of activated charcoal would be expected to be useful to decontaminate gut adequately

Supportive therapy: Following initiation of essential overdose management, toxic symptoms should be treated. Ventricular arrhythmias and ventricular conduction defects often respond to concurrent systemic alkalinization (sodium bicarbonate 0.5-2 mEq/kg I.V.). Titrate to a serum pH of 7.45-7.55. Arrhythmias unresponsive to this therapy may respond to lidocaine 1 mg/kg I.V. followed by a titrated infusion. Phenytoin is also useful in treating ventricular dysrhythmias (15 mg/kg up to 1 g I.V.). Physostigmine (1-2 mg I.V. slowly for adults or 0.5 mg I.V. slowly for children) may be indicated for seizures or movement disorders but only as **a last resort**. Propranolol may also be utilized for supraventricular arrhythmias (rate: >160) at 1 mg/minute to a maximum of 5 mg in adults; pediatric dosage of 0.1 mg/kg/dose to 1 mg I.V.. Seizures usually respond to lorazepam or diazepam I.V. boluses (5-10 mg for adults up to 30 mg or 0.25-0.4 mg/kg/dose for children up to 10 mg/dose). If seizures are unresponsive or recur, phenytoin or phenobarbital may be required. Patients must be monitored for at least 24 hours if any signs or symptoms are exhibited. Dobutamine is preferred over dopamine for hypotension, although there is conflicting animal data. Norepinephrine appears effective in treating hypotension; glucagon (10 mg I.V.) can be given to treat hypotension. Flumazenil is contraindicated; magnesium has potentiated adverse cardiac effects (ie, asystole, decreased left ventricular pressure) in an animal model, although it was used successfully in treating refractory ventricular fibrillation at a dose of 20 nmol I.V. (a total of 2 doses). For treatment of lingua villosa nigra, discontinue causative agent. Clean the tongue with a toothbrush and rinse mouth with a half-strength solution of hydrogen peroxide or 10% carbamide peroxide. Oral symptoms should subside in a few days. Hypertonic saline (200 mL of 7.5% sodium chloride I.V. push) can improve antidepressant-induced cardiotoxicity that is **not** responding to other therapies.

TCA ovine antibody fragments (TCA Fab, Protherics Inc) have been developed and used investigationally at a dose of 1-2 g over 30 minutes I.V.; if QRS was >100 msec or terminal deflection of QRS in lead aVR was >3 mm, a second dose (2 g over 30 min or 4 g over 1 hour) was given. If no response, a third infusion (4 g over 60 minutes or 8 g over 2 hours) was given.

Enhanced elimination: Multiple dosing of activated charcoal may be effective

Antidote(s)
● Sodium Bicarbonate [ANTIDOTE]

Diagnostic Procedures
● Nortriptyline, Blood

Test Interactions Increases glucose; increases plasma norepinephrine levels and plasma epinephrine levels threefold to fivefold; EMIT assays may be false-positive in the presence of diphenhydramine, thioridazine, chlorpromazine, alimenazine, carbamazepine, cyclobenzaprine, or perphenazine

Drug Interactions Substrate of CYP1A2 (minor), 2C19 (minor), 2D6 (major), 3A4 (minor); **Inhibits** CYP2D6 (weak), 2E1 (weak)

Altretamine: Concurrent use may cause orthostatic hypertension

Amphetamines: TCAs may enhance the effect of amphetamines; monitor for adverse CV effects

Anticholinergics: Combined use with TCAs may produce additive anticholinergic effects

Antihypertensives: TCAs may inhibit the antihypertensive response to bethanidine, clonidine, debrisoquin, guanadrel, guanethidine, guanabenz, guanfacine; monitor BP; consider alternate antihypertensive agent

Beta-agonists: When combined with TCAs may predispose patients to cardiac arrhythmias

Bupropion: May increase the levels of tricyclic antidepressants; based on limited information; monitor response

Carbamazepine: Tricyclic antidepressants may increase carbamazepine levels; monitor

Cholestyramine and colestipol: May bind TCAs and reduce their absorption; monitor for altered response

Clonidine: Abrupt discontinuation of clonidine may cause hypertensive crisis, amitriptyline may enhance the response

CNS depressants: Sedative effects may be additive with TCAs; monitor for increased effect; includes benzodiazepines, barbiturates, antipsychotics, ethanol and other sedative medications

CYP2D6 inhibitors: May increase the levels/effects of nortriptyline. Example inhibitors include chlorpromazine, delavirdine, fluoxetine, miconazole, paroxetine, pergolide, quinidine, quinine, ritonavir, and ropinirole.

Epinephrine (and other direct alpha-agonists): Pressor response to I.V. epinephrine, norepinephrine, and phenylephrine may be enhanced in patients receiving TCAs (**Note:** Effect is unlikely with epinephrine or levonordefrin dosages typically administered as infiltration in combination with local anesthetics)

Fenfluramine: May increase tricyclic antidepressant levels/effects

Hypoglycemic agents (including insulin): TCAs may enhance the hypoglycemic effects of tolazamide, chlorpropamide, or insulin; monitor for changes in blood glucose levels; reported with chlorpropamide, tolazamide, and insulin

Levodopa: Tricyclic antidepressants may decrease the absorption (bioavailability) of levodopa; rare hypertensive episodes have also been attributed to this combination

Linezolid: Hyperpyrexia, hypertension, tachycardia, confusion, seizures, and **deaths have been reported** with agents which inhibit MAO (serotonin syndrome); this combination should be avoided

Lithium: Concurrent use with a TCA may increase the risk for neurotoxicity

MAO inhibitors: Hyperpyrexia, hypertension, tachycardia, confusion, seizures, and **deaths have been reported** (serotonin syndrome); this combination should be avoided

Methylphenidate: Metabolism of TCAs may be decreased

Phenothiazines: Serum concentrations of some TCAs may be increased; in addition, TCAs may increase concentration of phenothiazines; monitor for altered clinical response

QT$_c$-prolonging agents: Concurrent use of tricyclic agents with other drugs which may prolong QT$_c$ interval may increase the risk of potentially fatal arrhythmias; includes type Ia and type III antiarrhythmics agents, selected quinolones (sparfloxacin, gatifloxacin, moxifloxacin, grepafloxacin), cisapride, and other agents

Ritonavir: Combined use of high-dose tricyclic antidepressants with ritonavir may cause serotonin syndrome in HIV-positive patients; monitor

Sucralfate: Absorption of tricyclic antidepressants may be reduced with coadministration

Sympathomimetics, indirect-acting: Tricyclic antidepressants may result in a decreased sensitivity to indirect-acting sympathomimetics; includes dopamine and ephedrine; also see interaction with epinephrine (and direct-acting sympathomimetics)

Tramadol: Tramadol's risk of seizures may be increased with TCAs

Valproic acid: May increase serum concentrations/adverse effects of some tricyclic antidepressants

Warfarin (and other oral anticoagulants): TCAs may increase the anticoagulant effect in patients stabilized on warfarin; monitor INR

Pregnancy Risk Factor D

Lactation Enters breast milk/contraindicated (AAP rates "of concern")

Nursing Implications Offer patient sugarless hard candy for dry mouth

Additional Information Maximum antidepressant effect may not be seen for 2 or more weeks after initiation of therapy

Specific References

Barrueto F, Murr I, Meltzer A, et al, "Effects of Amiodarone in a Swine Model of Nortryptyline Toxicity," *J Med Tox*, 2006, 2(4):147-151.

Franssen EJ, Kunst PW, Bet PM, et al, "Toxicokinetics of Nortriptyline and Amitriptyline: Two Case Reports," *Ther Drug Monit*, 2003, 25(2):248-51.

Heard K, Dart RC, Bogdan G, et al, "A Preliminary Study of Tricyclic Antidepressant (TCA) Ovine FAB for TCA Toxicity," *J Toxicol Clin Toxicol*, 2006, 44:275-81.

McKinney PE and Rasmussen R, "Reversal of Severe Tricyclic Antidepressant-Induced Cardiotoxicity with Intravenous Hypertonic Saline Solution," *Ann Emerg Med*, 2003, 42(1):20-4.

Seger DL, Hantsch C, Zavoral T, et al, "Variability of Recommendations for Serum Alkalinization in Tricyclic Antidepressant Overdose: A Survey of U.S. Poison Center Medical Directors," *J Toxicol Clin Toxicol*, 2003, 41(4):331-8.

Spiller HA, Baker SD, Krenzelok EP, et al, "Use of Dosage as a Triage Guideline for Unintentional Cyclic Antidepressant (UCA) Ingestions in Children," *Am J Emerg Med*, 2003, 21(5):422-4.

Nystatin

CAS Number 1400-61-9

U.S. Brand Names Bio-Statin®; Mycostatin®; Nystat-Rx®; Nystop®; Pedi-Dri®

Use Treatment of susceptible cutaneous, mucocutaneous, and oral cavity fungal infections normally caused by the *Candida* species

Mechanism of Action Binds to sterols in fungal cell membrane, changing the cell wall permeability allowing for leakage of cellular contents

Adverse Reactions

Dose of 10,000,000/day can produce mild nausea

Dermatologic: Contact dermatitis, systemic contact dermatitis, Stevens-Johnson syndrome, acute generalized exanthematous pustulosis, urticaria, pruritus, exanthem

Gastrointestinal: Nausea, vomiting, diarrhea

Local: Irritation

Respiratory: Cough, wheezing

Miscellaneous: Fixed drug eruption

Signs and Symptoms of Overdose Diarrhea, nausea, vomiting, wheezing

Pharmacodynamics/Kinetics

Onset of action: Symptomatic relief from candidiasis: 24-72 hours

Absorption: Topical: None through mucous membranes or intact skin; Oral: Poorly absorbed

Excretion: Feces (as unchanged drug)

Dosage

Oral candidiasis: Suspension (swish and swallow orally):

Neonates: 100,000 units 4 times/day or 50,000 units to each side of mouth 4 times/day

Infants: 200,000 units 4 times/day or 100,000 units to each side of mouth 4 times/day

Children and Adults: 400,000-600,000 units 4 times/day; troche: 200,000-400,000 units 4-5 times/day

Mucocutaneous infections: Children and Adults: Topical: Apply 2-3 times/day to affected areas; very moist topical lesions are treated best with powder

Intestinal infections: Adults: Oral tablets: 500,000-1,000,000 units every 8 hours

Vaginal infections: Adults: Vaginal tablets: Insert 1 tablet/day at bedtime for 2 weeks

Stability Keep vaginal inserts in refrigerator; protect from temperature extremes, moisture and light

Administration

Suspension: Shake well before using. Should be swished about the mouth and retained in the mouth for as long as possible (several minutes) before swallowing.

Contraindications Hypersensitivity to nystatin or any component of the formulation

Dosage Forms

Capsule (Bio-Statin®): 500,000 units, 1 million units

Cream: 100,000 units/g (15 g, 30 g)

Mycostatin®: 100,000 units/g (30 g)

Ointment, topical: 100,000 units/g (15 g, 30 g)

Powder, for prescription compounding: 50 million units (10 g); 150 million units (30 g); 500 million units (100 g); 2 billion units (400 g)
Nystat-Rx®: 50 million units (10 g); 150 million units (30 g); 500 million units (100 g); 1 billion units (190 g); 2 billion units (350 g)
Powder, topical:
Mycostatin®: 100,000 units/g (15 g)
Nyamyc™: 100,000 units/g (15 g, 30 g)
Nystop®: 100,000 units/g (15 g, 30 g, 60 g)
Pedi-Dri®: 100,000 units/g (56.7 g)
Suspension, oral: 100,000 units/mL (5 mL, 60 mL, 480 mL)
Tablet: 500,000 units
Tablet, vaginal: 100,000 units (15s) [packaged with applicator]

Reference Range A dose of 2,700,000 units/kg produces a plasma level of 9.8 units/mL; mean salivary levels were 1000 units/mL 2 hours after dissolution of 2 nystatin pastilles (400,000 units)

Overdosage/Treatment Supportive therapy: General poison management

Drug Interactions No data reported

Pregnancy Risk Factor B/C (oral)

Lactation Does not enter breast milk/compatible (not absorbed orally)

Additional Information Very moist topical lesions are best treated with powder.

Ofloxacin

CAS Number 83380-47-6

U.S. Brand Names Floxin®; Ocuflox®

Synonyms Floxin Otic Singles

Use Quinolone antibiotic for skin and skin structure, lower respiratory, and urinary tract infections and sexually-transmitted diseases. Active against many gram-positive and gram-negative aerobic bacteria.
Ophthalmic: Treatment of superficial ocular infections involving the conjunctiva or cornea due to strains of susceptible organisms
Otic: Otitis externa, chronic suppurative otitis media, acute otitis media
Epididymitis (gonorrhea), leprosy, Traveler's diarrhea

Mechanism of Action Ofloxacin, a fluorinated quinolone, is a pyridone carboxylic acid derivative which exerts a broad spectrum antimicrobial effect. The primary target of the fluoroquinolones is DNA gyrase (topoisomerase II) an essential bacterial enzyme that maintains the superhelical structure of DNA. DNA gyrase is required for DNA replication and transcription, DNA repair, recombination, and transposition.

Adverse Reactions
Systemic:
Cardiovascular: Chest pain, syncope, vasculitis, edema, hypertension, palpitations, vasodilation, vasculitis
Central nervous system: Headache, insomnia, dizziness, fatigue, somnolence, sleep disorders, nervousness, pyrexia, pain, seizures, anxiety, cognitive changes, depression, dream abnormality, euphoria, hallucinations, vertigo, chills, malaise, Tourette's syndrome
Dermatologic: Rash/pruritus, Stevens-Johnson syndrome, photosensitivity
Gastrointestinal: Diarrhea, vomiting, GI distress, cramps, abdominal cramps, flatulence, abnormal taste, xerostomia, decreased appetite, nausea, weight loss
Genitourinary: Vaginitis, external genital pruritus in women
Hepatic: Hepatitis
Local: Pain at injection site
Neuromuscular & skeletal: Paresthesia, extremity pain, weakness; quinolones have been associated with tendonitis and tendon rupture
Ocular: Superinfection (ophthalmic), photophobia, lacrimation, dry eyes, stinging, visual disturbances
Otic: Decreased hearing acuity, tinnitus
Renal: Interstitial nephritis
Respiratory: Cough
Miscellaneous: Trunk pain, thirst
Ophthalmic: Frequency not defined:
Central nervous system: Dizziness
Gastrointestinal: Nausea
Ocular: Blurred vision, burning, chemical conjunctivitis/keratitis, discomfort, dryness, edema, eye pain, foreign body sensation, itching, photophobia, redness, stinging, tearing
Otic:
Central nervous system: Dizziness, transient neuropsychiatric disturbances, vertigo
Dermatologic: Pruritus, rash
Gastrointestinal: Taste perversion
Neuromuscular & skeletal: Paresthesia
Otic: Application site reaction, earache

Signs and Symptoms of Overdose Nausea, photosensitivity, pseudotumor cerebri, seizures, vomiting

Pharmacodynamics/Kinetics
Absorption: Well absorbed; food causes only minor alterations
Distribution: V_d: 2.4-3.5 L/kg
Protein binding: 20%
Bioavailability: Oral: 98%
Half-life elimination: Biphasic: 5-7.5 hours and 20-25 hours (accounts for <5%); prolonged with renal impairment
Excretion: Primarily urine (as unchanged drug)

Dosage
Oral, I.V.: Adults:
Lower respiratory tract infection: 400 mg every 12 hours for 10 days
Epididymitis (gonorrhea): 300 mg twice daily for 10 days
Cervicitis due to *C. trachomatis* and/or *N. gonorrhoeae*: 300 mg every 12 hours for 7 days
Skin/skin structure: 400 mg every 12 hours for 10 days
Urinary tract infection: 200-400 mg every 12 hours for 3-10 days
Prostatitis: 300 mg every 12 hours for 6 weeks
Ophthalmic: Children >1 year and Adults:
Conjunctivitis: Instill 1-2 drops in affected eye(s) every 2-4 hours for the first 2 days, then use 4 times/day for an additional 5 days
Corneal ulcer: Instill 1-2 drops every 30 minutes while awake and every 4-6 hours after retiring for the first 2 days; beginning on day 3, instill 1-2 drops every hour while awake for 4-6 additional days; thereafter, 1-2 drops 4 times/day until clinical cure.
Otic:
Acute otitis media with tympanostomy tubes: Children 1-12 years: Instill 5 drops into affected ear(s) twice daily for 10 days
Chronic suppurative otitis media with perforated tympanic membranes: Children >12 years and Adults: 10 drops into affected ear twice daily for 14 days
Otitis externa:
Children 6 months to 13 years: Instill 5 drops into affected ear(s) once daily for 7 days
Children ≥13 years and Adults: Instill 10 drops into affected ear(s) once daily for 7 days

Dosing adjustment/interval in renal impairment: Adults: I.V., Oral:
Cl_{cr} 10-50 mL/minute: Administer 200-400 mg every 24 hours
Cl_{cr} <10 mL/minute: Administer 100-200 mg every 24 hours
Continuous arteriovenous or venovenous hemodiafiltration effects: Administer 300 mg every 24 hours

Administration I.V.: Administer over at least 60 minutes. Infuse separately. Do not infuse through lines containing solutions with magnesium or calcium.
Ophthalmic: For ophthalmic use only; avoid touching tip of applicator to eye or other surfaces.
Oral: Do not take within 2 hours of food or any antacids which contain zinc, magnesium, or aluminum.
Otic: Prior to use, warm solution by holding bottle in hands for 1-2 minutes. Patient should lie down with affected ear upward and medication instilled. Pump tragus 4 times to ensure penetration of medication. Patient should remain in this position for 5 minutes.

Contraindications Hypersensitivity to ofloxacin or other members of the quinolone group such as nalidixic acid, oxolinic acid, cinoxacin, norfloxacin, and ciprofloxacin; hypersensitivity to any component of the formulation

Warnings
Use with caution in patients with epilepsy or other CNS diseases which could predispose seizures; potential for seizures, although very rare, may be increased with concomitant NSAID therapy. Use with caution in patients with renal or hepatic impairment. Tendon inflammation and/or rupture have been reported with quinolone antibiotics, including ofloxacin. Risk may be increased with concurrent corticosteroids, particularly in the elderly. Discontinue at first sign of tendon inflammation or pain. Peripheral neuropathies have been linked to ofloxacin use; discontinue if numbness, tingling, or weakness develops.
Rare cases of torsade de pointes have been reported in patients receiving ofloxacin and other quinolones. Risk may be minimized by avoiding use in patients with known prolongation of the QT interval, bradycardia, hypokalemia, hypomagnesemia, cardiomyopathy, or in those receiving concurrent therapy with Class Ia or Class III antiarrhythmics.
Severe hypersensitivity reactions, including anaphylaxis, have occurred with quinolone therapy. If an allergic reaction occurs (itching, urticaria, dyspnea, facial edema, loss of consciousness, tingling, cardiovascular collapse), discontinue drug immediately. Prolonged use may result in superinfection; pseudomembranous colitis may occur and should be considered in all patients who present with diarrhea. Quinolones may exacerbate myasthenia gravis, use with caution (rare, potentially life-threatening weakness of respiratory muscles may occur).

Dosage Forms
[DSC] = Discontinued product
Solution, ophthalmic (Ocuflox®): 0.3% (5 mL; 10 mL [DSC]) [contains benzalkonium chloride]
Solution, otic:
Floxin®: 0.3% (5 mL, 10 mL) [contains benzalkonium chloride]

Floxin® Otic Singles™: 0.3% (0.25 mL) [contains benzalkonium chloride; packaged as 2 single-dose containers per pouch, 10 pouches per carton, total net volume 5 mL]

Tablet (Floxin®): 200 mg, 300 mg, 400 mg

Reference Range Overdose of 3 g ofloxacin (I.V.) yielded a peak plasma level of 39.3 mcg/mL (patient had been administered 400 mg I.V. every 12 hours for 3 days previously)

Overdosage/Treatment

Decontamination: Activated charcoal

Supportive therapy: Phenytoin has been used successfully in treatment of ofloxacin-induced seizure

Enhancement of elimination: Multiple dosing of activated charcoal may be effective; not removed by dialysis

Test Interactions Can give a false-positive result for opiates by urine immunoassay screening

Drug Interactions

Inhibits CYP1A2 (strong)

Corticosteroids: Concurrent use may increase the risk of tendon rupture, particularly in elderly patients (overall incidence rare).

CYP1A2 substrates: Ofloxacin may increase the levels/effects of CYP1A2 substrates. Example substrates include aminophylline, fluvoxamine, mexiletine, mirtazapine, ropinirole, and trifluoperazine.

Glyburide: Quinolones may increase the effect of glyburide; monitor.

Metal cations (aluminum, calcium, iron, magnesium, and zinc) bind quinolones in the gastrointestinal tract and inhibit absorption. Concurrent administration of most antacids, oral electrolyte supplements, quinapril, sucralfate, some didanosine formulations (chewable/buffered tablets and pediatric powder for oral suspension), and other highly-buffered oral drugs, should be avoided. Ofloxacin should be administered 2 hours before or 2 hours after these agents.

Probenecid: May decrease renal secretion of ofloxacin.

QT$_c$-prolonging agents: Effects may be additive with ofloxacin. Avoid concurrent use with Class Ia and Class III antiarrhythmics; use caution with other drugs known to prolong QT$_c$, including erythromycin, cisapride, antipsychotics, and cyclic antidepressants.

Theophylline: Ofloxacin may increase plasma levels of theophylline. Monitor.

Warfarin: The hypoprothrombinemic effect of warfarin may be enhanced by some quinolone antibiotics; monitor INR.

Pregnancy Risk Factor C

Pregnancy Implications Reports of arthropathy (observed in immature animals and reported rarely in humans) have limited the use of fluoroquinolones in pregnancy. According to the FDA, the Teratogen Information System concluded that therapeutic doses during pregnancy are unlikely to produce substantial teratogenic risk, but data are insufficient to say that there is no risk. In general, reports of exposure have been limited to short durations of therapy in the first trimester. When considering treatment for life-threatening infection and/or prolonged duration of therapy, the potential risk to the fetus must be balanced against the severity of the potential illness.

Lactation Enters breast milk/not recommended (AAP rates "compatible")

Specific References

Wilkins DG, Mizuno A, Borges CR, et al, "Ofloxacin as a Reference Marker in Hair of Various Colors," *J Anal Toxicol*, 2003, 27(3):149-55.

Olanzapine

Related Information

• Antipsychotic Agents

CAS Number 132539-06-1

U.S. Brand Names Zyprexa® Zydis®; Zyprexa®

Synonyms LY170053; Zyprexa Zydis

Impairment Potential Yes

Use Treatment of the manifestations of schizophrenia; treatment of acute mania episodes associated with bipolar disorder (as monotherapy or in combination with lithium or valproate); maintenance treatment of bipolar disorder; acute agitation (patients with schizophrenia or bipolar mania)

Unlabeled/Investigational Use Treatment of psychotic symptoms; chronic pain

Mechanism of Action A thienobenzodiazepine with properties similar to clozapine; exact mechanism of action is unknown; olanzapine acts primarily as a dopamine (D$_1$, D$_2$, D$_4$ and D$_6$) and 5HT$_2$ antagonist; also inhibits serotonin type 3 and 6, muscarinic M$_{1-5}$, H$_1$, and adrenergic alpha$_1$-receptors

Adverse Reactions

Cardiovascular: Postural hypotension, tachycardia, hypotension, peripheral edema, chest pain, hypertension

Central nervous system: **Headache, somnolence, insomnia, agitation, nervousness, hostility, dizziness**, dystonic reactions, parkinsonian events, amnesia, euphoria, stuttering, akathisia, anxiety, personality changes, fever, abnormal dreams, speech disorder, neuroleptic malignant syndrome, seizures, tardive dyskinesia, diabetic coma

Dermatologic: Rash, bruising, photosensitivity reaction, angioedema, pruritus, urticaria

Endocrine & metabolic: Prolactin increased, amenorrhea, diabetes mellitus, hyperglycemia

Gastrointestinal: **Dyspepsia, constipation, weight gain** (clinically and long term), xerostomia, abdominal pain, appetite increased, vomiting, salivation increased, pancreatitis

Genitourinary: Premenstrual syndrome, incontinence, priapism

Hematologic: Leukopenia, agranulocytosis, neutropenia

Neuromuscular & skeletal: **Weakness**, arthralgia, neck rigidity, twitching, hypertonia, tremor, back pain, abnormal gait, akathisia, falling (particularly in older patients)

Ocular: Amblyopia

Respiratory: Rhinitis, cough, pharyngitis, dyspnea

Miscellaneous: Diaphoresis, allergic reactions, anaphylactoid reactions

Additional significant effects reported with I.M. administration: Articulation impairment, AV block, injection site pain, syncope

Signs and Symptoms of Overdose Coma, drowsiness, extrapyramidal movements, fasciculations, hypotension (possible, though not described), miosis, respiratory depression, rhinitis (10%), slurred speech, tachycardia, trismus

Pharmacodynamics/Kinetics

Absorption:

I.M.: Rapidly absorbed

Oral: Well absorbed; not affected by food; tablets and orally-disintegrating tablets are bioequivalent

Distribution: V$_d$: Extensive, 1000 L

Protein binding, plasma: 93% bound to albumin and alpha$_1$-glycoprotein

Metabolism: Highly metabolized via direct glucuronidation and cytochrome P450 mediated oxidation (CYP1A2, CYP2D6); 40% removed via first pass metabolism

Bioavailability: >57%

Half-life elimination: 21-54 hours; ~1.5 times greater in elderly

Time to peak, plasma: Maximum plasma concentrations after I.M. administration are 5 times higher than maximum plasma concentrations produced by an oral dose.

I.M.: 15-45 minutes

Oral: ~6 hours

Excretion: Urine (57%, 7% as unchanged drug); feces (30%)

Clearance: 40% increase in olanzapine clearance in smokers; 30% decrease in females

Dosage

Children: Schizophrenia/bipolar disorder: Oral: Initial: 2.5 mg/day; titrate as necessary to 20 mg/day (0.12-0.29 mg/kg/day)

Adults:

Schizophrenia: Oral:

Initial: 5-10 mg once daily (increase to 10 mg once daily within 5-7 days); thereafter, adjust by 5 mg/day at 1-week intervals, up to a recommended maximum of 20 mg/day. Maintenance: 10-20 mg once daily. **Note:** Doses of 30-50 mg/day have been used; however, doses >10 mg/day have not demonstrated better efficacy, and safety and efficacy of doses >20 mg/day have not been evaluated.

Bipolar I acute mixed or manic episodes: Oral:

Monotherapy: Initial: 10-15 mg once daily; increase by 5 mg/day at intervals of not less than 24 hours. Maintenance: 5-20 mg/day; recommended maximum dose: 20 mg/day

Combination therapy (with lithium or valproate): Initial: 10 mg once daily; dosing range: 5-20 mg/day

Agitation (acute, associated with bipolar I mania or schizophrenia): I.M.: Initial dose: 5-10 mg (a lower dose of 2.5 mg may be considered when clinical factors warrant); additional doses (2.5-10 mg) may be considered; however, 2-4 hours should be allowed between doses to evaluate response (maximum total daily dose: 30 mg, per manufacturer's recommendation)

Elderly: Oral, I.M.: Consider lower starting dose of 2.5-5 mg/day for elderly or debilitated patients; may increase as clinically indicated and tolerated with close monitoring of orthostatic blood pressure

Dosage adjustment in renal impairment: No adjustment required. Not removed by dialysis

Monitoring Parameters Vital signs; fasting lipid profile and fasting blood glucose/Hgb A$_{1c}$ (prior to treatment, at 3 months, then annually); periodic assessment of hepatic transaminases (in patients with hepatic disease); BMI, personal/family history of obesity, waist circumference; orthostatic blood pressure; mental status, abnormal involuntary movement scale (AIMS), extrapyramidal symptoms (EPS). Weight should be assessed prior to treatment, at 4 weeks, 8 weeks, 12 weeks, and then at quarterly intervals. Consider titrating to a different antipsychotic agent for a weight gain ≥5% of the initial weight.

Administration

Injection: For I.M. administration only; do not administer injection intravenously; inject slowly, deep into muscle. If dizziness and/or drowsiness are noted, patient should remain recumbent until examination indicates postural hypotension and/or bradycardia are not a problem.

Tablet: May be administered with or without food/meals.

Orally-disintegrating: Remove from foil blister by peeling back (do not push tablet through the foil); place tablet in mouth immediately upon removal; tablet dissolves rapidly in saliva and may be swallowed with or without liquid. May be administered with or without food/meals.

Contraindications Hypersensitivity to olanzapine or any component of the formulation

Warnings

[U.S. Boxed Warning]: Patients with dementia-related behavioral disorders treated with atypical antipsychotics are at an increased risk of death compared to placebo. An increased incidence of cerebrovascular adverse events (including fatalities) has been reported in elderly patients with dementia-related psychosis. Olanzapine is not approved for this indication.

Moderate to highly sedating, use with caution in disorders where CNS depression is a feature; patients must be cautioned about performing tasks which require mental alertness (eg, operating machinery or driving). Use with caution in Parkinson's disease; in patients with bone marrow suppression; predisposition to seizures; subcortical brain damage; severe hepatic, renal, or respiratory disease. Life-threatening arrhythmias have occurred with therapeutic doses of some neuroleptics. May induce orthostatic hypotension, especially during titration; use caution with history of MI, heart failure, conduction abnormalities, cerebrovascular disease, or conditions/medications which predispose to hypotension and/or bradycardia. Esophageal dysmotility and aspiration have been associated with antipsychotic use; use with caution in patients at risk of pneumonia (ie, Alzheimer's disease). Caution in breast cancer or other prolactin-dependent tumors (may elevate prolactin levels). Significant weight gain may occur. Impaired core body temperature regulation may occur; caution with strenuous exercise, heat exposure, dehydration, and concomitant medication possessing anticholinergic effects.

May cause anticholinergic effects (constipation, xerostomia, blurred vision, urinary retention); therefore, they should be used with caution in patients with decreased gastrointestinal motility, paralytic ileus, urinary retention, BPH, xerostomia, or visual problems. Conditions which also may be exacerbated by cholinergic blockade include narrow-angle glaucoma (screening is recommended) and worsening of myasthenia gravis. Relative to other neuroleptics, olanzapine has a moderate potency of cholinergic blockade.

May cause extrapyramidal symptoms, including pseudoparkinsonism, acute dystonic reactions, akathisia, and tardive dyskinesia (risk of these reactions is lower relative to other neuroleptics). May be associated with neuroleptic malignant syndrome (NMS). May cause hyperglycemia; in some cases may be extreme and associated with ketoacidosis, hyperosmolar coma, or death. Use with caution in patients with diabetes or other disorders of glucose regulation; monitor for worsening of glucose control. Olanzapine levels may be lower in patients who smoke, requiring dosage adjustment.

The possibility of a suicide attempt is inherent in psychotic illness or bipolar disorder; use caution in high-risk patients during initiation of therapy. Prescriptions should be written for the smallest quantity consistent with good patient care. Safety and efficacy in pediatric patients have not been established.

Dosage Forms Injection, powder for reconstitution (Zyprexa® IntraMuscular): 10 mg [contains lactose 50 mg]

Tablet (Zyprexa®): 2.5 mg, 5 mg, 7.5 mg, 10 mg, 15 mg, 20 mg

Tablet, orally disintegrating (Zyprexa® Zydis®): 5 mg [contains phenylalanine 0.34 mg/tablet], 10 mg [contains phenylalanine 0.45 mg/tablet], 15 mg [contains phenylalanine 0.67 mg/tablet], 20 mg [contains phenylalanine 0.9 mg/tablet]

Reference Range

Therapeutic serum range: 9-23 ng/mL; serum and urine olanzapine levels >600 ng/mL and 500 ng/mL, respectively, associated with coma following a 600 mg ingestion; toxicity may occur at blood olanzapine levels >100 ng/mL; death due to olanzapine toxicity can occur at postmortem blood olanzapine levels >160 ng/mL

Postmortem blood olanzapine level of 0.160 mg/L may indicate that this drug was the cause of death.

Olanzapine postmortem aorta blood concentrations of ≥0.8 mg/L or iliac blood values of ≥0.5 mg/L are sufficient to cause death. In instances of olanzapine overdose, liver concentrations can be expected to exceed 1.0 mg/kg.

Overdosage/Treatment

Decontamination: Oral: Activated charcoal

Supportive therapy: Hypotension should be treated with I.V. crystalloid fluids; avoid sympathomimetics with beta-agonist properties since this can theoretically worsen hypotension. Weight gain can be treated with nizatidine 150 mg twice daily. Ephedrine (25 mg/day) can be used to treat olanzapine- induced urinary incontinence. Physostigmine (2 mg I.V.) can reverse olanzapine-induced coma.

Enhanced elimination: Hemodialysis does not appear to be useful

Drug Interactions

Substrate of CYP1A2 (major), 2D6 (minor); **Inhibits** CYP1A2 (weak), 2C9 (weak), 2C19 (weak), 2D6 (weak), 3A4 (weak)

Acetylcholinesterase inhibitors (central): May increase the risk of antipsychotic-related extrapyramidal symptoms; monitor.

Anticholinergics: Adverse effects/toxicity may be additive with olanzapine.

Carbamazepine: May decrease olanzapine levels/effects; monitor.

Ciprofloxacin; May increase the levels/effects of olanzapine.

CNS depressants: Sedative effects and may be additive with CNS depressants; includes ethanol, barbiturates, narcotic analgesics, and other sedative agents; monitor for increased effect.

CYP1A2 inducers may decrease the levels/effects of olanzapine. Example inducers include aminoglutethimide, carbamazepine, phenobarbital, and rifampin.

CYP1A2 inhibitors: May increase the levels/effects of olanzapine. Example inhibitors include ciprofloxacin, fluvoxamine, ketoconazole, norfloxacin, ofloxacin, and rofecoxib.

Fluvoxamine: Increases olanzapine levels; consider using a lower dose of olanzapine in patients receiving concomitant treatment with fluvoxamine.

Lithium: Risk of extrapyramidal effects may be increased with concurrent therapy.

Pramlintide: Anticholinergic effects may be increased with concomitant therapy.

Pregnancy Risk Factor C

Pregnancy Implications No evidence of teratogenicity reported in animal studies. However, fetal toxicity and prolonged gestation have been observed. There are no adequate and well-controlled studies in pregnant women.

Lactation Enters breast milk/not recommended

Additional Information Antipsychotic efficacy was established in short-term (6 weeks) controlled trials of psychotic disorders; effectiveness in long-term use (>6 weeks) has not been systematically evaluated in controlled trial, therefore, the physician who uses olanzapine for extended periods should periodically re-evaluate the long-term usefulness of the drug for the individual patient; less extrapyramidal effects and adverse hematological effects as compared with clozapine. Postmortem blood olanzapine level of 0.160 mg/L may indicate that this drug was the cause of death.

Specific References

Avella J, Wetli CV, Wilson JC, et al, "Fatal Olanzapine-Induced Hyperglycemia Ketoacidosis," *Am J Forensic Med Pathol*, 2004, 25(2):172-5.

Battaglia J, Lindborg SR, Alaka K, et al, "Calming Versus Sedative Effects of Intramuscular Olanzapine in Agitated Patients," *Am J Emerg Med*, 2003, 21(3):192-8.

Boddy R, Ali R, and Dowsett R, "Use of Sublingual Olanzapine in Serotonin Syndrome," *J Toxicol Clin Toxicol*, 2004, 42(5):725.

Bonelli RM, "Olanzapine-Associated Seizure," *Ann Pharmacother*, 2003, 37(1):149-50.

Gex-Fabry M, Balant-Gorgia AE, and Balant LP, "Therapeutic Drug Monitoring of Olanzapine: The Combined Effect of Age, Gender, Smoking, and Comedication," *Ther Drug Monit*, 2003, 25(1):46-53.

Hester EK and Thrower MR, "Current Options in the Management of Olanzapine-Associated Weight Gain," *Ann Pharmacother*, 2005, 39(2):302-10.

Kinon BJ, Ahl J, Rotelli MD, et al, "Efficacy of Accelerated Dose Titration of Olanzapine with Adjunctive Lorazepam to Treat Acute Agitation in Schizophrenia," *Am J Emerg Med*, 2004, 22(3):181-6.

Lim CJ, Trevino C, and Tampi RR, "Can Olanzapine Cause Delirium in the Elderly?" 2006, *Ann Pharmacother*, 2006, 40(1):135-8.

O'Keeffe CW, Johnson WR, Ricksecker JK, et al, "Stability of Olanzapine in Stored Blood," *J Anal Toxicol*, 2003, 27(3):185.

Palenzona S, Meier PJ, Kupferschmidt H, et al, "The Clinical Picture of Olanzapine Poisoning with Special Reference to Fluctuating Mental Status," *J Toxicol Clin Toxicol*, 2004, 42(1):27-32.

Poklis JL, Winecker RE, and Poklis A, "Blood and Liver Olanzapine Findings in Fourteen Postmortem Cases," *J Anal Toxicol*, 2006, 30:135.

Reeves RR and Torres RA, "Orally Disintegrating Olanzapine for the Treatment of Psychotic and Behavioral Disturbances Associated with Dementia," *South Med J*, 2003, 96(7):699-701.

Rottinghaus D, Bryant S, and Harchelroad F, "The Serious Side of Olanzapine Overdose," *J Toxicol Clin Toxicol*, 2003, 41(5):673.

Schatz RA, "Olanzapine for Psychotic and Behavioral Disturbances in Alzheimer Disease," *Ann Pharmacother*, 2003, 37(9):1321-4.

Schneider LS, Dagerman KS, and Insel P, "Risk of Death with Atypical Antipsychotic Drug Treatment for Dementia: Meta-Analysis of Randomized Placebo-Controlled Trials," *JAMA*, 2005, 294(15):1934-43.

Suchard J and Erickson R, "Serotonin Syndrome from Acute Olanzapine Overdose," *J Toxicol Clin Toxicol*, 2004, 42(5):718.

Weizberg M, Mazzola JL, Bird SB,, et al, "Altered Mental Status from Olanzapine Overdose Treated with Physostigmine," *Clin Toxicol*, 2006, 44(3):319-25.

Wiener SE, Hoffman RS, and Nelson LS, "Smoking: A Novel Route of Olanzapine Abuse," *J Toxicol Clin Toxicol*, 2003, 41(5):741.

Olsalazine

CAS Number 15722-48-2
U.S. Brand Names Dipentum®
Synonyms Olsalazine Sodium
Use Maintenance of remission of ulcerative colitis in patients intolerant to sulfasalazine
Mechanism of Action The mechanism of action appears to be topical rather than systemic
Adverse Reactions
Cardiovascular: Palpitations, pericarditis
Central nervous system: Headache, fatigue, depression, fever
Dermatologic: Rash, itching, alopecia
Gastrointestinal: Nausea, dyspepsia, bloating, anorexia, **diarrhea** (secretory: dose dependent), **abdominal cramps**, **abdominal pain**, bloody diarrhea, pancreatitis
Hematologic: Blood dyscrasias
Hepatic: Hepatitis
Ocular: Dry eyes, blurred vision
Neuromuscular & skeletal: Arthralgia
Signs and Symptoms of Overdose Decreased motor activity, diarrhea
Pharmacodynamics/Kinetics
Absorption: <3%; very little intact olsalazine is systemically absorbed
Protein binding, plasma: >99%
Metabolism: Primarily via colonic bacteria to active drug, 5-aminosalicylic acid
Half-life elimination: 56 minutes
Time to peak: ~1 hour
Excretion: Primarily feces
Dosage Adults: Oral: 1 g/day in 2 divided doses; maximum dose: 3 g/day
Monitoring Parameters Stool frequency
Administration Take with food in evenly divided doses.
Contraindications Hypersensitivity to olsalazine, salicylates, or any component of the formulation
Warnings
Diarrhea is a common adverse effect of olsalazine; use with caution in patients with hypersensitivity to salicylates, sulfasalazine, or mesalamine
Dosage Forms Capsule, as sodium: 250 mg
Reference Range Olsalazine: 0-4.3 mM/L; olsalazine sodium: 3.3-12.4 mM/L. These are not therapeutic guideline levels. These are reported levels after administration that have been observed on study. No correlation to response is known at this time.
Overdosage/Treatment
Decontamination: For ingestions >3 g: Ipecac within 30 minutes or lavage within 1 hour; activated charcoal
Supportive therapy: Replace fluid losses with I.V. crystalloid solution
Drug Interactions Azathioprine, mercaptopurine, thioguanine: Aminosalicylates may increase the risk of myelosuppression (due to TPMT inhibition).
Warfarin: Olsalazine has been reported to increase the prothrombin time in patients taking warfarin.
Pregnancy Risk Factor C
Lactation Enters breast milk/use caution (monitor for diarrhea)
Additional Information Cross-reactivity with sulfasalazine allergy is probable

Omeprazole

CAS Number 73590-58-6
U.S. Brand Names Prilosec OTC™ [OTC]; Prilosec®
Use Short-term (4-8 weeks) treatment of active duodenal ulcer disease or active benign gastric ulcer; treatment of heartburn and other symptoms associated with gastroesophageal reflux disease (GERD); short-term (4-8 weeks) treatment of endoscopically-diagnosed erosive esophagitis; maintenance healing of erosive esophagitis; long-term treatment of pathological hypersecretory conditions; as part of a multidrug regimen for *H. pylori* eradication to reduce the risk of duodenal ulcer recurrence
OTC labeling: Short-term treatment of frequent, uncomplicated heartburn occurring ≥2 days/week
Unlabeled/Investigational Use Healing NSAID-induced ulcers; prevention of NSAID-induced ulcers
Mechanism of Action A benzimidazole compound prodrug which suppresses gastric acid secretion by inhibiting the parietal cell H^+/K^+ ATP pump
Adverse Reactions
Cardiovascular: Chest pain, tachycardia, bradycardia, hypertension, sinus bradycardia, angina, palpitations, sinus tachycardia
Central nervous system: Headache, dizziness, fever, fatigue, malaise, nervousness, lethargy
Dermatologic: Rash, dermatitis exfoliative, toxic epidermal necrolysis, alopecia, bullous skin disease, xerosis, purpura, pruritus, psoriasis, licheniform eruptions, exanthem
Endocrine & metabolic: Acute gout, hyponatremia, erythema nodosum
Gastrointestinal: Diarrhea, nausea, abdominal pain, vomiting, constipation, abdominal edema, anorexia, irritable colon, flatulence, xerostomia, gastric giardiasis, dysgeusia, weight gain
Genitourinary: Urinary tract infection, pyuria
Hematologic: Hypoglycemia, anemia, leukocytosis, pancytopenia, agranulocytosis, thrombocytopenia, neutropenia, megaloblastic anemia, hemolytic anemia
Hepatic: Hepatitis
Neuromuscular & skeletal: Back pain, myalgia, tremors, arthralgia, weakness, paresthesia
Ocular: Eye irritation
Renal: Proteinuria, interstitial nephritis (acute)
Respiratory: Cough
Miscellaneous: Lichen spinulosus, fixed drug eruption
Signs and Symptoms of Overdose Decreased respiratory rate has been demonstrated in animals only. Angioedema, blindness, confusion, depression, dermatitis, dry mouth, gout, gynecomastia, hematuria, hypoglycemia, hyperhidrosis, hyponatremia, hypothermia, nephritis, sedation, seizures, urinary frequency
Pharmacodynamics/Kinetics
Onset of action: Antisecretory: ~1 hour
  Peak effect: 2 hours
Duration: 72 hours
Protein binding: 95%
Metabolism: Extensively hepatic to inactive metabolites
Bioavailability: Oral: 30% to 40%; increased in Asian patients and patients with hepatic dysfunction
Half-life elimination: Delayed release capsule: 0.5-1 hour
Excretion: Urine (77% as metabolites, very small amount as unchanged drug); feces
Dosage
Oral:
Children ≥2 years: GERD or other acid-related disorders:
  <20 kg: 10 mg once daily
  ≥20 kg: 20 mg once daily
Adults:
  Active duodenal ulcer: 20 mg/day for 4-8 weeks
  Gastric ulcers: 40 mg/day for 4-8 weeks
  Symptomatic GERD: 20 mg/day for up to 4 weeks
  Erosive esophagitis: 20 mg/day for 4-8 weeks; maintenance of healing: 20 mg/day for up to 12 months total therapy (including treatment period of 4-8 weeks)
  Helicobacter pylori eradication: Dose varies with regimen: 20 mg once daily **or** 40 mg/day as single dose or in 2 divided doses; requires combination therapy with antibiotics
  Pathological hypersecretory conditions: Initial: 60 mg once daily; doses up to 120 mg 3 times/day have been administered; administer daily doses >80 mg in divided doses
  Frequent heartburn (OTC labeling): 20 mg/day for 14 days; treatment may be repeated after 4 months if needed
Dosage adjustment in hepatic impairment: Specific guidelines are not available; bioavailability is increased with chronic liver disease
Monitoring Parameters Improvement in gastrointestinal symptoms
Administration Capsule should be swallowed whole. Do not chew, crush, or open. Best if taken before breakfast. May be opened and contents added to applesauce. Administration via NG tube should be in an acidic juice.
Contraindications Hypersensitivity to omeprazole, substituted benzimidazoles (ie, esomeprazole, lansoprazole, pantoprazole, rabeprazole), or any component of the formulation
Warnings In long-term (2-year) studies in rats, omeprazole produced a dose-related increase in gastric carcinoid tumors. While available endoscopic evaluations and histologic examinations of biopsy specimens from human stomachs have not detected a risk from short-term exposure to omeprazole, further human data on the effect of sustained hypochlorhydria and hypergastrinemia are needed to rule out the possibility of an increased risk for the development of tumors in humans receiving long-term therapy. Bioavailability may be increased in the elderly, Asian population, and with hepatic dysfunction. Safety and efficacy have not been established in children <2 years of age. When used for self-medication (OTC), do not use for >14 days; treatment should not be repeated more often than every 4 months; OTC and oral suspension are not approved for use in children <18 years of age.
Dosage Forms Capsule, delayed release: 10 mg, 20 mg
  Prilosec®: 10 mg, 20 mg, 40 mg
Tablet, delayed release:
  Prilosec OTC™: 20 mg
Overdosage/Treatment
Decontamination: Activated charcoal
Enhancement of elimination: Multiple dosing of activated charcoal may be effective
Not dialyzable due to high protein binding although 1 case report in an anemic, anuric patient did describe removal by hemodialysis (Roggo)
Test Interactions May result in increased gastric levels

Drug Interactions Substrate of CYP2A6 (minor), 2C9 (minor), 2C19 (major), 2D6 (minor), 3A4 (minor); **Inhibits** CYP1A2 (weak), 2C9 (moderate), 2C19 (strong), 2D6 (weak), 3A4 (weak); **Induces** CYP1A2 (weak)

Benzodiazepines metabolized by oxidation (eg, diazepam, midazolam, triazolam): Esomeprazole and omeprazole may increase levels of benzodiazepines metabolized by oxidation.

Carbamazepine: Esomeprazole and omeprazole may increase carbamazepine levels.

Clozapine: Omeprazole may alter the concentrations/effects of clozapine; monitor.

CYP2C9 substrates: Omeprazole may increase the levels/effects of CYP2C9 substrates. Example substrates include amiodarone, fluoxetine, glimepiride, glipizide, nateglinide, phenytoin, pioglitazone, rosiglitazone, sertraline, and warfarin.

CYP2C19 inducers: May decrease the levels/effects of omeprazole. Example inducers include aminoglutethimide, carbamazepine, phenytoin, and rifampin.

CYP2C19 substrates: Omeprazole may increase the levels/effects of CYP2C19 substrates. Example substrates include citalopram, diazepam, methsuximide, phenytoin, propranolol, and sertraline.

Itraconazole and ketoconazole: Proton pump inhibitors may decrease the absorption of itraconazole and ketoconazole.

Methotrexate: Concurrent use with omeprazole may decrease the excretion of methotrexate. **Note:** Antirheumatic doses of methotrexate probably hold minimal risk.

Phenytoin: Elimination of phenytoin may be prolonged; monitor. Phenytoin may decrease omeprazole levels/effects.

Protease inhibitors: Proton pump inhibitors may decrease absorption of some protease inhibitors (atazanavir and indinavir). Avoid concurrent use.

Warfarin: Elimination of warfarin may be prolonged; monitor.

Pregnancy Risk Factor C

Pregnancy Implications Crosses the placenta; congenital abnormalities have been reported sporadically following omeprazole use during pregnancy. The manufacturer recommends use during pregnancy only if the potential benefit to the mother outweighs the possible risk to the fetus.

Lactation Enters breast milk/not recommended

Additional Information May be effective in preventing nonsteroidal anti-inflammatory drug-induced large gastric ulcers by inhibiting acid secretion; the incidence of side effects in elderly is not different than that of younger adults (≤ 65 years) despite slight decrease in elimination and increase in bioavailability. No dosage adjustments are necessary for elderly (≥ 65 years).

Specific References

El-Matary W and Dalzell M, "Omeprazole-Induced Hepatitis," *Pediatr Emerg Care*, 2005, 21(8):529-30.

Howaizi M and Delafosse C, "Omeprazole-Induced Intractable Cough," *Ann Pharmacother*, 2003, 37(11):1607-9.

Ondansetron

CAS Number 103639-04-9; 116002-70-1; 99614-02-5

U.S. Brand Names Zofran® ODT; Zofran®

Synonyms GR38032R; Ondansetron Hydrochloride

Use

Prevention of nausea and vomiting associated with moderately- to highly-emetogenic cancer chemotherapy; radiotherapy in patients receiving total body irradiation or fractions to the abdomen; prevention and treatment of postoperative nausea and vomiting

Generally **not** recommended for treatment of existing chemotherapy-induced emesis (CIE) or for prophylaxis of nausea from agents with a low emetogenic potential.

Unlabeled/Investigational Use Treatment of early-onset alcoholism; hyperemesis gravidarum

Mechanism of Action Selective 5-HT$_3$ receptor antagonist, blocking serotonin, both peripherally on vagal nerve terminals and centrally in the chemoreceptor trigger zone

Adverse Reactions

Cardiovascular: **Malaise/fatigue**, angina, cardiopulmonary arrest, ECG changes, flushing, hypotension, shock, tachycardia, vascular occlusive events

Central nervous system: **Headache**, drowsiness, fever, dizziness, anxiety, cold sensation, extrapyramidal reactions, grand mal seizures, oculogyric crisis

Dermatologic: Pruritus, rash, urticaria, angioedema

Endocrine & metabolic: Hypokalemia

Gastrointestinal: Constipation, diarrhea

Genitourinary: Gynecological disorder, urinary retention

Hepatic: Increased ALT/AST

Local: Injection site reaction

Neuromuscular & skeletal: Paresthesia, dystonic reactions

Respiratory: Hypoxia bronchospasm, laryngeal edema, laryngospasm, shortness of breath, stridor

Miscellaneous: Anaphylaxis, hypersensitivity reactions, hiccups

Signs and Symptoms of Overdose Sudden transient blindness, severe constipation, hypotension, flushing, and vasovagal episode with transient secondary heart block have been reported in some cases of overdose. I.V. doses of up to 252 mg/day have been inadvertently given without adverse effects.

Admission Criteria/Prognosis Admit any symptomatic patient or ingestion exceeding 1.5 mg/kg

Pharmacodynamics/Kinetics

Onset of action: ~30 minutes

Distribution: V$_d$: Children: 1.7-3.7 L/kg; Adults: 2.2-2.5 L/kg

Protein binding, plasma: 70% to 76%

Metabolism: Extensively hepatic via hydroxylation, followed by glucuronide or sulfate conjugation; CYP1A2, CYP2D6, and CYP3A4 substrate; some demethylation occurs

Bioavailability: Oral: 56% to 71%; Rectal: 58% to 74%

Half-life elimination: Children <15 years: 2-7 hours; Adults: 3-6 hours

Mild-to-moderate hepatic impairment: Adults: 12 hours

Severe hepatic impairment (Child-Pugh C): Adults: 20 hours

Time to peak: Oral: ~2 hours

Excretion: Urine (44% to 60% as metabolites, 5% to 10% as unchanged drug); feces (~25%)

Dosage Children:

I.V.:

Chemotherapy-induced emesis: 4-18 years: 0.15 mg/kg/dose administered 30 minutes prior to chemotherapy, 4 and 8 hours after the first dose **or** 0.45 mg/kg/day as a single dose

Postoperative nausea and vomiting: 2-12 years:

$\leq$40 kg: 0.1 mg/kg

>40 kg: 4 mg

Oral: Chemotherapy-induced emesis:

4-11 years: 4 mg 30 minutes before chemotherapy; repeat 4 and 8 hours after initial dose, then 4 mg every 8 hours for 1-2 days after chemotherapy completed

$\geq$12 years: Refer to adult dosing.

Oral: Gastroenteritis - ODT prep:

Weight 8-15 kg: 2 mg; 16-30 kg: 4 mg; >31 kg: 8 mg

Adults:

I.V.: Chemotherapy-induced emesis:

0.15 mg/kg 3 times/day beginning 30 minutes prior to chemotherapy **or**

0.45 mg/kg once daily **or**

8-10 mg 1-2 times/day **or**

24 mg or 32 mg once daily

I.M., I.V.: Postoperative nausea and vomiting: 4 mg as a single dose approximately 30 minutes before the end of anesthesia, or as treatment if vomiting occurs after surgery

Oral: Chemotherapy-induced emesis:

Highly-emetogenic agents/single-day therapy: 24 mg given 30 minutes prior to the start of therapy

Moderately-emetogenic agents: 8 mg every 12 hours beginning 30 minutes before chemotherapy, continuously for 1-2 days after chemotherapy completed

Total body irradiation: 8 mg 1-2 hours before daily each fraction of radiotherapy

Single high-dose fraction radiotherapy to abdomen: 8 mg 1-2 hours before irradiation, then 8 mg every 8 hours after first dose for 1-2 days after completion of radiotherapy

Daily fractionated radiotherapy to abdomen: 8 mg 1-2 hours before irradiation, then 8 mg 8 hours after first dose for each day of radiotherapy

Postoperative nausea and vomiting: 16 mg given 1 hour prior to induction of anesthesia

Elderly: No dosing adjustment required

Dosage adjustment in renal impairment: No dosing adjustment required

Dosage adjustment in hepatic impairment: Maximum daily dose: 8 mg in patients with severe liver disease (Child-Pugh score $\geq$10)

Monitoring Parameters Frequency of emesis

Administration Oral: Oral dosage forms should be administered 30 minutes prior to chemotherapy; 1-2 hours before radiotherapy; 1 hour prior to the induction of anesthesia

Orally-disintegrating tablets: Do not remove from blister until needed. Peel backing off the blister, do not push tablet through. Using dry hands, place tablet on tongue and allow to dissolve. Swallow with saliva.

I.M.: Should be administered undiluted

I.V.: Give first dose 30 minutes prior to beginning chemotherapy; the I.V. preparation has been successful when administered orally

IVPB: Infuse over 15-30 minutes; 24-hour continuous infusions have been reported, but are rarely used

Contraindications Hypersensitivity to ondansetron, other selective 5-HT$_3$ antagonists, or any component of the formulation

Warnings For chemotherapy, ondansetron should be used on a scheduled basis, not on an "as needed" (PRN) basis, since data support the use of this drug only in the prevention of nausea and vomiting (due to antineoplastic therapy) and not in the rescue of nausea and vomiting. Ondansetron should only be used in the first 24-48 hours of chemotherapy. Data do not support any increased efficacy of ondansetron in delayed nausea and vomiting. Does not stimulate gastric or intestinal peristalsis; may mask progressive ileus and/or gastric distension. Orally-disintegrating tablets contain phenylalanine. Safety and efficacy for children <1 month of age have not been established.

Dosage Forms [DSC] = Discontinued product
Infusion [premixed in D$_5$W, preservative free]:
Zofran®: 32 mg (50 mL)
Injection, solution:
Zofran®: 2 mg/mL (2 mL, 20 mL)
Solution, oral:
Zofran®: 4 mg/5 mL (50 mL) [contains sodium benzoate; strawberry flavor]
Tablet:
Zofran®: 4 mg; 8 mg; 24 mg [DSC]
Tablet, orally disintegrating:
Zofran® ODT: 4 mg, 8 mg [each strength contains phenylalanine <0.03 mg/tablet; strawberry flavor]

Overdosage/Treatment
Decontamination: Lavage (within 1 hour) oral ingestions >1.5 mg/kg; activated charcoal
Supportive therapy: Diphenhydramine can be used to manage pruritus, rashes, extrapyramidal signs (along with benztropine), and restlessness

Drug Interactions Substrate of CYP1A2 (minor), 2C9 (minor), 2D6 (minor), 2E1 (minor), 3A4 (major); **Inhibits** CYP1A2 (weak), 2C9 (weak), 2D6 (weak)
Apomorphine: Due to reports of profound hypotension during concomitant therapy, the manufacturer of apomorphine contraindicates its use with ondansetron.
CYP3A4 inducers: CYP3A4 inducers may decrease the levels/effects of ondansetron. Example inducers include aminoglutethimide, carbamazepine, nafcillin, nevirapine, phenobarbital, phenytoin, and rifamycins. The manufacturer does not recommend dosage adjustment in patients receiving CYP3A4 inducers.

Pregnancy Risk Factor B

Pregnancy Implications Clinical effects on the fetus: No data available on crossing the placenta; no effects on the fetus from two case reports.

Lactation Excretion in breast milk unknown/use caution

Nursing Implications First dose should be given 30 minutes prior to beginning chemotherapy

Additional Information I.V. product has been successful when used orally; elderly have a slightly decreased hepatic clearance rate; this does not, however, require a dose adjustment. Not effective in preventing motion sickness; more effective than metoclopramide in preventing emesis in cisplatin treatment; may be useful in treating acetaminophen-induced or theophylline-induced vomiting.

Specific References
Freedman SB, Adler M, Seshadri R, et al, "Oral Ondansetron for Gastroenteritis in a Pediatric Emergency Department," *N Engl J Med*, 2006, 354:1698-705.
Ng KH, "Chemotherapy-Induced Delayed Emesis: What Is the Role of 5-HT$_3$ Antagonists?" *J Pharm Technol*, 2003, 19:287-97.

Opium Alkaloids (Hydrochlorides)

Synonyms Opium Alkakoids

Impairment Potential Yes

Use Relief of severe pain

Adverse Reactions
Cardiovascular: **Hypotension**, bradycardia, peripheral vasodilation, sinus bradycardia, palpitations
Central nervous system: **Fatigue, drowsiness, dizziness**, CNS depression, agitation, increased intracranial pressure, cognitive dysfunction, paranoia
Dermatologic: Pruritus
Endocrine & metabolic: Syndrome of inappropriate antidiuretic hormone
Gastrointestinal: **Nausea, vomiting**, constipation (more constipating than morphine), biliary tract spasm
Genitourinary: Urinary tract spasm
Neuromuscular & skeletal: **Weakness**
Ocular: Miosis
Respiratory: Apnea, respiratory depression
Miscellaneous: Physical and psychological dependence, histamine release

Signs and Symptoms of Overdose Apnea, coma, delirium, dysphoria, hypotension, miosis, myoglobinuria, ptosis, pulmonary edema, respiratory depression, rhabdomyolysis, seizures (in neonates)

Pharmacodynamics/Kinetics
Absorption: Oral: Variable, more slowly absorbed than morphine
Distribution: V$_d$: 3-4 L/kg
Protein binding: 35%
Metabolism: In the liver via glucuronide conjugation
Half-life:
Neonates: Prolonged 6% to 10%
Adults: 2-4 hours
Elimination: Unchanged in urine

Dosage Adults: I.M., SubQ: 5-20 mg every 4-5 hours

Monitoring Parameters Pain relief, respiratory and mental status, blood pressure

Contraindications Hypersensitivity to opium alkaloids

Dosage Forms Injection: 20 mg/mL (1 mL)

Overdosage/Treatment Supportive therapy: Naloxone hydrochloride (0.4-2 mg I.V., SubQ, or through an endotracheal tube); a continuous infusion (at $^2/_3$ the response dose/hour) may be required

Antidote(s)
- Nalmefene [ANTIDOTE]
- Naloxone [ANTIDOTE]

Drug Interactions CNS depressants, MAO inhibitors may potentiate adverse effects

Pregnancy Risk Factor B/D (prolonged periods or high doses at term)

Nursing Implications Observe patient for excessive sedation, respiratory depression, implement safety measures, assist with ambulation

Specific References
Day J, Charles B, Slawson M, et al, "Determination of Five Opium-Related Compounds in Human Hair by LC-MS," *J Anal Toxicol*, 2004, 28:291.

Opium Tincture

Synonyms DTO (error-prone abbreviation); Opium Tincture, Deodorized

Impairment Potential Yes

Use Treatment of diarrhea or relief of pain

Mechanism of Action Contains many narcotic alkaloids including morphine; its mechanism for gastric motility inhibition is primarily due to this morphine content; it results in a decrease in digestive secretions, an increase in gastrointestinal muscle tone, and therefore a reduction in gastrointestinal propulsion

Adverse Reactions
Cardiovascular: **Palpitations**, **hypotension**, **bradycardia**, peripheral vasodilation
Central nervous system: CNS depression, agitation, increased intracranial pressure, dysphoria, paranoia, **drowsiness, dizziness**
Dermatologic: Pruritus
Endocrine & metabolic: Syndrome of inappropriate antidiuretic hormone
Gastrointestinal: Nausea, vomiting, constipation, biliary tract spasm
Genitourinary: Urinary tract spasm
Neuromuscular & skeletal: **Weakness**
Ocular: Miosis
Respiratory: Apnea, respiratory depression
Miscellaneous: Physical and psychological dependence, histamine release

Signs and Symptoms of Overdose Apnea, coma, hypotension, miosis, myasthenia gravis (exacerbation or precipitation), myoglobinuria, ptosis, pulmonary edema, respiratory depression, rhabdomyolysis, seizures (in neonates)

Pharmacodynamics/Kinetics
Duration: 4-5 hours
Absorption: Variable
Metabolism: Hepatic
Excretion: Urine

Dosage
Oral:
Children:
Diarrhea: 0.005-0.01 mL/kg/dose every 3-4 hours for a maximum of 6 doses/24 hours
Analgesia: 0.01-0.02 mL/kg/dose every 3-4 hours
Adults:
Diarrhea: 0.3-1 mL/dose every 2-6 hours to maximum of 6 mL/24 hours
Analgesia: 0.6-1.5 mL/dose every 3-4 hours

Monitoring Parameters Observe patient for excessive sedation, respiratory depression, implement safety measures, assist with ambulation

Contraindications Hypersensitivity to morphine sulfate or any component of the formulation; increased intracranial pressure; severe respiratory depression; severe hepatic or renal insufficiency; pregnancy (prolonged use or high dosages near term)

Warnings Opium shares the toxic potential of opiate agonists, and usual precautions of opiate agonist therapy should be observed; some preparations contain sulfites which may cause allergic reactions; infants <3 months of age are more susceptible to respiratory depression, use with caution and generally in reduced doses in this age group; this is **not** paregoric, dose accordingly

Dosage Forms Liquid: 10% (120 mL, 480 mL) [0.6 mL equivalent to morphine 6 mg; contains alcohol 19%]

Overdosage/Treatment Supportive therapy: Naloxone hydrochloride (0.4-2 mg I.V., SubQ, or through an endotracheal tube); a continuous infusion (at $^2/_3$ the response dose/hour) may be required

Antidote(s)
- Nalmefene [ANTIDOTE]
- Naloxone [ANTIDOTE]

Diagnostic Procedures
- Morphine, Urine
- Opiates, Qualitative, Urine

Test Interactions ↑ aminotransferases (ALT, AST) (S)

Drug Interactions Increased toxicity: CNS depressants, MAO inhibitors, tricyclic antidepressants may potentiate the effects of opiate agonists; dextroamphetamine may enhance the analgesic effect of opiate agonists

Pregnancy Risk Factor B/D (prolonged use or high doses at term)

Lactation Enters breast milk/use caution

Nursing Implications Observe patient for excessive sedation, respiratory depression, implement safety measures, assist with ambulation

Orlistat

U.S. Brand Names Xenical®

Use Management of obesity, including weight loss and weight management when used in conjunction with a reduced-calorie diet; reduce the risk of weight regain after prior weight loss; indicated for obese patients with an initial body mass index (BMI) $\geq$30 kg/m^2 or $\geq$27 kg/m^2 in the presence of other risk factors.

Mechanism of Action A reversible inhibitor of gastric and pancreatic lipases, thus inhibiting absorption of dietary fats by 30% (at doses of 120 mg 3 times/day).

Adverse Reactions

Central nervous system: **Headache (31%)**, fatigue, anxiety, sleep disorders

Dermatologic: Dry skin, angioedema, pruritus, rash, urticaria

Endocrine & metabolic: Menstrual irregularities

Gastrointestinal: **Oily spotting (27%), abdominal pain/discomfort (26%), flatus with discharge (24%), fatty/oily stool (20%), fecal urgency (22%), oily evacuation, increased defecation**, fecal incontinence, nausea, infectious diarrhea, rectal pain/discomfort, vomiting

Neuromuscular & skeletal: **Back pain**, arthritis, myalgia

Otic: Otitis

Respiratory: **Upper respiratory infection (38%)**

Miscellaneous: Allergic reactions, anaphylaxis

Pharmacodynamics/Kinetics

Absorption: Minimal

Metabolism: Metabolized within the gastrointestinal wall; forms inactive metabolites

Excretion: Feces (83% as unchanged drug)

Dosage Oral: Children $\geq$12 years and Adults: 120 mg 3 times/day with each main meal containing fat (during or up to 1 hour after the meal); omit dose if meal is occasionally missed or contains no fat.

Contraindications Hypersensitivity to orlistat or any component of the formulation; chronic malabsorption syndrome or cholestasis

Warnings Patients should be advised to adhere to dietary guidelines; gastrointestinal adverse events may increase if taken with a diet high in fat (>30% total daily calories from fat). The daily intake of fat should be distributed over three main meals. If taken with any one meal very high in fat, the possibility of gastrointestinal effects increases. Patients should be counseled to take a multivitamin supplement that contains fat-soluble vitamins to ensure adequate nutrition because orlistat has been shown to reduce the absorption of some fat-soluble vitamins and beta-carotene. Some patients may develop increased levels of urinary oxalate following treatment; caution should be exercised when prescribing it to patients with a history of hyperoxaluria or calcium oxalate nephrolithiasis. As with any weight-loss agent, the potential exists for misuse in appropriate patient populations (eg, patients with anorexia nervosa or bulimia). Safety and efficacy have not been established in children <12 years of age. Write/fill prescription carefully. Dispensing errors have been made between Xenical® (orlistat) and Xeloda® (capecitabine).

Dosage Forms Capsule: 120 mg

Overdosage/Treatment Essentially entirely supportive therapy, with most symptoms resolving spontaneously. For the patient who ingests >1 g, suggest observing for 24 hours or until GI symptoms abate.

Drug Interactions Amiodarone: Orlistat may decrease amiodarone absorption; monitor.

Cyclosporine: Cyclosporine serum levels may de decreased; administer cyclosporine 2 hours before or after orlistat; monitor.

Warfarin: Orlistat does not alter the pharmacokinetics of warfarin, however, vitamin K absorption may be decreased during orlistat therapy. Therefore, patients stabilized on warfarin should be monitored for changes in warfarin effects.

Pregnancy Risk Factor B

Pregnancy Implications There are no adequate and well-controlled studies of orlistat in pregnant women. Because animal reproductive studies are not always predictive of human response, orlistat is not recommended for use during pregnancy. Teratogenicity studies were conducted in rats and rabbits at doses up to 800 mg/kg/day. Neither study showed embryotoxicity or teratogenicity. This dose is 23 and 47 times the daily human dose calculated on a body surface area basis for rats and rabbits, respectively.

Lactation Excretion in breast milk unknown/not recommended

Additional Information Single doses of 800 mg and multiple doses of up to 400 mg 3 times/day for 15 days have been studied in normal weight and obese patients, without significant adverse findings; in case of significant overdose, it is recommended that the patient be observed for 24 hours.

Specific References

Chanoine JP, Hampl S, Jensen C, et al, "Effect of Orlistat on Weight and Body Composition in Obese Adolescents: A Randomized Controlled Trial," *JAMA*, 2005, 15;293(23):2873-83.

Graham MR, Landgraf CG, and Lindsey CC, "A Comparison of Orlistat Use in a Veteran Population: A Pharmacist-Managed Pharmacotherapy Weight-Loss Clinic Versus Standard Medical Care," *J Pharm Technol*, 2003, 19:343-8.

MacWalter RS, Fraser HW, and Armstrong KM, "Orlistat Enhances Warfarin Effect," *Ann Pharmacother*, 2003, 37(4):510-2.

Stafford RS and Radley DC, "National Trends in Antiobesity Medication Use," *Arch Intern Med*, 2003, 163(9):1046-50.

Orphenadrine

CAS Number 4682-36-4

U.S. Brand Names Norflex™

Synonyms Orphenadrine Citrate

Impairment Potential Yes

Use Treatment of muscle spasm associated with acute painful musculoskeletal conditions; supportive therapy in tetanus

Mechanism of Action Indirect skeletal muscle relaxant thought to work by central atropine-like effects; has some euphorigenic and analgesic properties

Adverse Reactions

Cardiovascular: Tachycardia, palpitations, sinus tachycardia

Central nervous system: **Dizziness**, fatigue, **drowsiness**

Gastrointestinal: Xerostomia, nausea, constipation

Neuromuscular & skeletal: Weakness

Ocular: **Blurred vision**

Signs and Symptoms of Overdose Anticholinergic symptoms, arrhythmias, blurred vision, confusion, dystonic reactions, hypertension, myoglobinuria, paralysis, psychosis, respiratory arrest, rhabdomyolysis, seizures, tachycardia, vasodilation

Pharmacodynamics/Kinetics

Onset of effect: Peak effect: Oral: 2-4 hours

Duration: 4-6 hours

Protein binding: 20%

Metabolism: Extensively hepatic

Half-life elimination: 14-16 hours

Excretion: Primarily urine (8% as unchanged drug)

Dosage

Adults:

Oral: 100 mg twice daily

I.M., I.V.: 60 mg every 12 hours

Administration

Do not crush sustained release drug product.

Contraindications Hypersensitivity to orphenadrine or any component of the formulation; glaucoma; GI obstruction; cardiospasm; myasthenia gravis

Warnings Use with caution in patients with CHF or cardiac arrhythmias; some products contain sulfites

Dosage Forms

Injection, solution, as citrate: 30 mg/mL (2 mL)

Norflex™: 30 mg/mL (2 mL) [contains sodium bisulfite]

Tablet, extended release, as citrate: 100 mg

Norflex™: 100 mg

Reference Range

Toxic: 2-3 mg/mL

Fatal: 4-8 mg/L

Overdosage/Treatment

Decontamination: Emesis not recommended due to potential for seizures; lavage (within 1 hour) in early ingestions after control of seizures; activated charcoal of benefit

Supportive therapy: Treatment is predominantly symptomatic and supportive; physostigmine has been used for life-threatening anticholinergic symptoms; bethanechol has been used to control peripheral symptoms; alkaline diuresis/mannitol has been used in rhabdomyolysis

Enhancement of elimination: Hemodialysis and peritoneal dialysis is ineffective; multiple-dose activated charcoal of unknown value, may be of benefit in ingestions of long-acting product

Drug Interactions

Substrate (minor) of CYP1A2, 2B6, 2D6, 3A4; **Inhibits** CYP1A2 (weak), 2A6 (weak), 2B6 (weak), 2C9 (weak), 2C19 (weak), 2D6 (weak), 2E1 (weak), 3A4 (weak)

Anticholinergic agents: May increase potential for anticholinergic adverse effects; includes drugs with high anticholinergic activity (diphenhydramine, TCAs, phenothiazines)

CNS depressants: Sedative effects may be additive. Monitor.

Levodopa: Effects may be decreased by orphenadrine. Monitor.

Pregnancy Risk Factor C

Lactation Excretion in breast milk unknown

Nursing Implications Do not crush sustained release drug product; raise bed rails, institute safety measures, assist with ambulation

Additional Information Aplastic anemia has occurred, rarely.

Oseltamivir

Pronunciation (oh sel TAM i vir)

U.S. Brand Names Tamiflu®

Use Treatment of uncomplicated acute illness due to influenza (A or B) infection in adults and children >1 year of age who have been symptomatic for no more than 2 days; prophylaxis against influenza (A or B) infection in adults and adolescents ≥13 years of age

Mechanism of Action Oseltamivir, a prodrug, is hydrolyzed to the active form, oseltamivir carboxylate. It is thought to inhibit influenza virus neuraminidase, with the possibility of alteration of virus particle aggregation and release. In clinical studies of the influenza virus, 1.3% of post-treatment isolates had decreased neuraminidase susceptibility to oseltamivir carboxylate.

Adverse Reactions

As seen with **treatment** doses: 1% to 10%:

Central nervous system: Insomnia (adults 1%), vertigo (adults 1%)

Gastrointestinal: Nausea (adults 10%), vomiting (adults 9%, children 15%), abdominal pain (children 5%)

Ocular: Conjunctivitis (children 1%)

Otic: Ear disorder (children 2%)

Respiratory: Epistaxis (children 3%)

Similar adverse effects were seen in **prophylactic** use, however, the incidence was generally less. The following reactions were seen more commonly with prophylactic use: Headache (20%), fatigue (8%), diarrhea (3%)

<1% and case reports (any indication): Aggravation of diabetes, anemia, arrhythmia, confusion, hepatitis, humerus fracture, peritonsillar abscess, pneumonia, pseudomembranous colitis, pyrexia, rash, seizure, transaminases increased, toxic epidermal necrolysis, unstable angina, swelling of face or tongue

Pharmacodynamics/Kinetics

Absorption: Well absorbed

Distribution: V_d: 23-26 L (oseltamivir carboxylate)

Protein binding, plasma: Oseltamivir carboxylate: 3%; Oseltamivir: 42%

Metabolism: Hepatic (90%) to oseltamivir carboxylate; neither the parent drug nor active metabolite has any effect on CYP

Bioavailability: 75% reaches systemic circulation in active form

Half-life elimination: Oseltamivir carboxylate: 6-10 hours; similar in geriatrics (68-78 years)

Time to peak: C_{max}: Oseltamivir: 65 ng/mL; Oseltamivir carboxylate: 348 ng/mL

Excretion: Urine (as carboxylate metabolite)

Dosage

Oral:

Treatment: Initiate treatment within 2 days of onset of symptoms; duration of treatment: 5 days:

Children: 1-12 years:

≤15 kg: 30 mg twice daily

>15 kg - ≤23 kg: 45 mg twice daily

>23 kg - ≤40 kg: 60 mg twice daily

>40 kg: 75 mg twice daily

Adolescents ≥13 years and Adults: 75 mg twice daily

Prophylaxis: Adolescents ≥13 years and Adults: 75 mg once daily for at least 7 days; treatment should begin within 2 days of contact with an infected individual. During community outbreaks, dosing is 75 mg once daily. May be used for up to 6 weeks; duration of protection lasts for length of dosing period

Dosage adjustment in renal impairment:

Cl_{cr} 10-30 mL/minute:

Treatment: Reduce dose to 75 mg once daily for 5 days

Prophylaxis: 75 mg every other day

Cl_{cr} <10 mL/minute: Has not been studied

Dosage adjustment in hepatic impairment: Has not been evaluated

Elderly: No adjustments required

Stability Capsules: Store at 25°C (77°F).

Oral suspension: Store powder for suspension at 25°C (77°F). Reconstitute with 23 mL of water (to make 25 mL total suspension). Once reconstituted, store suspension under refrigeration at 2°C to 8°C (36°F to 46°F); do not freeze. Use within 10 days of preparation.

Contraindications Hypersensitivity to oseltamivir or any component of the formulation

Warnings Oseltamivir is not a substitute for the influenza virus vaccine. Use caution with renal impairment; dosage adjustment is required for creatinine clearance between 10-30 mL/minute. Also consider primary or concomitant bacterial infections. Safety and efficacy for use in hepatic impairment or for treatment or prophylaxis in immunocompromised patients have not been established. Efficacy has not been established if treatment begins >40 hours after the onset of symptoms or in the treatment of patients with chronic cardiac and/or respiratory disease. Rare but severe hypersensitivity reactions (anaphylaxis, severe dermatologic reactions) have been associated with use. Safety and efficacy in children (<1 year of age) have not been established.

Dosage Forms Capsule, as phosphate:

Tamiflu®: 75 mg

Powder for oral suspension:

Tamiflu®: 12 mg/mL (25 mL) [contains sodium benzoate; tutti-frutti flavor]

Drug Interactions Influenza virus vaccine nasal spray (fluMist™): Safety and efficacy for use with influenza virus vaccine nasal spray have not been established. Do not administer nasal spray until 48 hours after stopping antiviral; do not administer antiviral for 2 weeks after receiving influenza virus vaccine nasal spray.

Pregnancy Risk Factor C

Pregnancy Implications There are insufficient human data to determine the risk to a pregnant woman or developing fetus. Studies evaluating the effects on embryo-fetal development in rats and rabbits showed a dose-dependent increase in the rates of minor skeleton abnormalities in exposed offspring. The rate of each abnormality remained within the background rate of occurrence in the species studied.

Lactation Excretion in breast milk unknown/not recommended

Nursing Implications Have patient take with food to decrease the nausea associated with this medicine; administer at breakfast and dinner when used for treatment (dosing is once daily when used for prophylaxis). Shake suspension well before using; may be stored under refrigeration or at room temperature.

Ouabain

CAS Number 11018-89-6; 630-60-4

Use Treatment of congestive heart failure; slows the ventricular rate in tachyarrhythmias such as fibrillation (atrial), flutter (atrial), tachycardia (ventricular), paroxysmal atrial tachycardia, cardiogenic shock; may not be as useful for tachyarrhythmias due to antegrade conduction

Mechanism of Action Derived from *Strophanthus gratus*; ouabain is a cardiac glycoside with actions similar to digitalis

Adverse Reactions

Cardiovascular: Sinus bradycardia, AV block, SA block, ectopic beats (atrial or nodal), tachycardia (ventricular), arrhythmias (ventricular), bigeminy, trigeminy, tachycardia (atrial) with AV block; congestive heart failure

Central nervous system: Drowsiness, fatigue, disorientation, dizziness, auditory and visual hallucinations, paranoia, headache

Neuromuscular & skeletal: Neuralgia, chorea (extrapyramidal)

Ocular: Vision color changes (blue tinge)

Toxicodynamics/Kinetics

Onset of action: 3-10 minutes

Peak effect: 0.5-2 hours

Half-life: 21 hours

Elimination: Renal (47%)

Dosage Average digitalizing dose: I.V.: 0.03-0.5 g

Stability Protect from light; not compatible with procaine

Overdosage/Treatment

Supportive therapy: Antidote: Life-threatening digoxin toxicity is treated with Digibind®; phenytoin, magnesium, and lidocaine are useful for cardiac arrhythmias; atropine is useful for bradycardia; avoid quinidine, bretylium, or cardioversion; ventricular pacing should be reserved for patients not responding to Digibind®; delirium can respond to Digibind®; torsade de pointes can be treated with magnesium sulfate and overdrive pacing (try to avoid isoproterenol)

Antidote(s)

● Atropine [ANTIDOTE]

● Digoxin Immune Fab [ANTIDOTE]

Oxazepam

CAS Number 604-75-1

U.S. Brand Names Serax®

Impairment Potential Yes. Serum oxazepam levels >0.2 mg/L are consistent with driving impairment. Brief or extended periods of exposure are less likely to cause driving impairment in the elderly compared with the longer half-life benzodiazepines. (Baselt RC and Cravey RH,

Disposition of Toxic Drugs and Chemicals in Man, 4th ed, Foster City, CA: Chemical Toxicology Institute, 1995, 569.)

Use Treatment of anxiety and management of alcohol withdrawal

Unlabeled/Investigational Use Anticonvulsant in management of simple partial seizures; hypnotic

Mechanism of Action Benzodiazepine anxiolytic sedative that produces CNS depression at the subcortical level, except at high doses, whereby it works at the cortical level

Adverse Reactions

Cardiovascular: Syncope

Central nervous system: **Drowsiness**, headache, dizziness, lethargy, slurred speech, ataxia

Dermatologic: Rash, erythema multiforme, urticaria, purpura, pruritus; bullous eruptions, exanthem

Endocrine & metabolic: Decreased libido

Gastrointestinal: Nausea, xerostomia

Hematologic: Leukopenia

Hepatic: Jaundice, hepatic dysfunction

Neuromuscular & skeletal: Tremor, paresthesia

Signs and Symptoms of Overdose Coma, confusion, dyspnea, hyperglycemia (spurious), hypoactive reflexes, hypochloremia, hyponatremia, hyporeflexia, nystagmus, slurred speech, unsteady gait

Pharmacodynamics/Kinetics

Absorption: Almost complete

Protein binding: 86% to 99%

Metabolism: Hepatic to inactive compounds (primarily as glucuronides)

Half-life elimination: 2.8-5.7 hours

Time to peak, serum: 2-4 hours

Excretion: Urine (as unchanged drug (50%) and metabolites)

Dosage Oral:

Children: 1 mg/kg/day has been administered

Adults:

Anxiety: 10-30 mg 3-4 times/day

Alcohol withdrawal: 15-30 mg 3-4 times/day

Hypnotic: 15-30 mg

Monitoring Parameters Respiratory and cardiovascular status

Administration Administer orally in divided doses

Contraindications Hypersensitivity to oxazepam or any component of the formulation (cross-sensitivity with other benzodiazepines may exist); narrow-angle glaucoma (not in product labeling, however, benzodiazepines are contraindicated); not indicated for use in the treatment of psychosis; pregnancy

Warnings

May cause hypotension (rare) - use with caution in patients with cardiovascular or cerebrovascular disease, or in patients who would not tolerate transient decreases in blood pressure. Serax® 15 mg tablet contains tartrazine; use is not recommended in pediatric patients <6 years of age; dose has not been established between 6-12 years of age.

Use with caution in elderly or debilitated patients, patients with hepatic disease (including alcoholics), or renal impairment. Use with caution in patients with respiratory disease or impaired gag reflex. Avoid use in patients with sleep apnea.

Causes CNS depression (dose-related) resulting in sedation, dizziness, confusion, or ataxia which may impair physical and mental capabilities. Patients must be cautioned about performing tasks which require mental alertness (eg, operating machinery or driving). Use with caution in patients receiving other CNS depressants or psychoactive agents. Effects with other sedative drugs or ethanol may be potentiated. Benzodiazepines have been associated with falls and traumatic injury and should be used with extreme caution in patients who are at risk of these events (especially the elderly).

Use caution in patients with depression, particularly if suicidal risk may be present. Use with caution in patients with a history of drug dependence. Benzodiazepines have been associated with dependence and acute withdrawal symptoms on discontinuation or reduction in dose. Acute withdrawal, including seizures, may be precipitated after administration of flumazenil to patients receiving long-term benzodiazepine therapy.

Benzodiazepines have been associated with anterograde amnesia. Paradoxical reactions, including hyperactive or aggressive behavior have been reported with benzodiazepines, particularly in adolescent/pediatric or psychiatric patients. Does not have analgesic, antidepressant, or antipsychotic properties.

Dosage Forms Capsule: 10 mg, 15 mg, 30 mg

Tablet: 15 mg [contains tartrazine]

Reference Range Therapeutic: 0.2-1.4 mcg/mL (SI: 0.7-4.9 μmol/L)

Overdosage/Treatment

Decontamination: Lavage pediatric ingestions >90 mg (within 1 hour)/activated charcoal

Supportive therapy: Treatment for benzodiazepine overdose is supportive. Rarely is mechanical ventilation required. Flumazenil has been shown to selectively block the binding of benzodiazepines to CNS receptors, resulting in a reversal of benzodiazepine-induced CNS depression.

Enhancement of elimination: Multiple dosing of activated charcoal may be useful; not dialyzable (0% to 5%)

Antidote(s)

● Flumazenil [ANTIDOTE]

Diagnostic Procedures

● Oxazepam, Serum

Test Interactions Visine®, Drano®, bleach may cause false-negative urine tests; oxazepam may interfere resulting in falsely elevated glucose

Drug Interactions Ethanol and other CNS depressants may increase the CNS effects of oxazepam

Levodopa: Therapeutic effects may be diminished in some patients following the addition of a benzodiazepine; limited/inconsistent data

Theophylline and other CNS stimulants may antagonize the sedative effects of oxazepam

Zidovudine: Increased incidence of headache with concurrent use.

Pregnancy Risk Factor D

Lactation Enters breast milk/not recommended

Nursing Implications Provide safety measures (ie, side rails, night light, and call button); remove smoking materials from area; supervise ambulation

Additional Information Excreted without need for liver metabolism

Oxcarbazepine

CAS Number 28721-07-5

U.S. Brand Names Trileptal®

Synonyms GP 47680; OCBZ

Use Monotherapy or adjunctive therapy in the treatment of partial seizures in adults and children (4-16 years of age) with epilepsy

Unlabeled/Investigational Use Bipolar disorder; treatment of neuropathic pain

Mechanism of Action Pharmacological activity results from both oxcarbazepine and its monohydroxy metabolite (MHD). Precise mechanism of anticonvulsant effect has not been defined. Oxcarbazepine and MHD block voltage sensitive sodium channels, stabilizing hyperexcited neuronal membranes, inhibiting repetitive firing, and decreasing the propagation of synaptic impulses. These actions are believed to prevent the spread of seizures. Oxcarbazepine and MHD also increase potassium conductance and modulate the activity of high-voltage activated calcium channels.

Adverse Reactions

As reported in adults with doses of up to 2400 mg/day (includes patients on monotherapy, adjunctive therapy, and those not previously on AEDs); incidence in children was similar.

Cardiovascular: Angioedema, bradycardia, cardiac failure, cerebral hemorrhage, chest pain, flushing, hypotension, hypertension, leg edema, palpitations, postural tachycardia

Central nervous system: Abnormal coordination, **abnormal gait**, abnormal thinking, abnormal feelings, agitation, aggressive reaction, amnesia, anguish, anxiety, apathy, aphasia, **ataxia**, aura, confusion, consciousness decreased, convulsions aggravated, delusion, delirium, **dizziness**, drunk feeling, dysmetria, dysphonia, dystonia, EEG abnormalities, emotional lability, euphoria, extrapyramidal disorder, **fatigue**, fever, **headache**, hypoesthesia, hysteria, insomnia, malaise, manic reaction, nervousness, oculogyric crisis, panic disorder, paralysis, paroniria, personality disorder, psychosis, **somnolence**, speech disorder, stupor, syncope, **vertigo**

Dermatologic: Acne, alopecia, bruising, contact dermatitis, eczema, erythema multiforme, erythematosus rash, facial rash, folliculitis, heat rash, maculopapular rash, photosensitivity reaction, psoriasis, purpura, rash, Stevens-Johnson syndrome, toxic epidermal necrolysis, ulcerative stomatitis, urticaria, vitiligo

Endocrine & metabolic: Hyponatremia, hot flushes, hyperglycemia, hypocalcemia, hypoglycemia, hypokalemia, intermenstrual bleeding, libido decreased/increased, menorrhagia

Gastrointestinal: **Abdominal pain**, appetite increased, biliary pain, blood in stool, cholelithiasis, colitis, constipation, diarrhea, dry mouth, duodenal ulcer, dysphagia, dyspepsia, enteritis, eructation, esophagitis, flatulence, gastritis, gastric ulcer, gingival bleeding, gum hyperplasia, hemorrhoids, **nausea**, rectal hemorrhage, retching, sialoadenitis, taste perversion, **vomiting**, weight gain, weight loss

Genitourinary: Dysuria, genital pruritus, micturition frequency, priapism

Hematologic: Eosinophilia, hematuria, hematemesis, leukopenia, leukorrhea, thrombocytopenia

Hepatic: GGT increased, liver enzymes elevated, serum transaminases increased

Neuromuscular & skeletal: Arthralgia, back pain, falling down, hemiplegia, hyperkinesia, hyperreflexia, hypertonia, hypokinesia, hyporeflexia, muscle contractions (involuntary), **muscle tremor**, neuralgia, rigors, sprains/strains, tetany, **tremor**, weakness

Ocular: Abnormal accommodation, **abnormal vision**, cataract, conjunctival hemorrhage, **diplopia**, eye edema, hemianopia, mydriasis, **nystagmus**, photophobia, ptosis, scotoma, xerophthalmia

Otic: Otitis externa, tinnitus

Renal: Renal calculus, renal pain, urinary tract pain

Respiratory: Asthma, dyspnea, epistaxis, laryngismus, pleurisy, rhinitis, sinusitis, upper respiratory tract infection

Miscellaneous: Chest infection, hiccups, hypersensitivity reaction, hypochondrium pain, lymphadenopathy, systemic lupus erythematosus

Signs and Symptoms of Overdose May include: Bradycardia, CNS depression (somnolence, ataxia), diplopia, hyponatremia, hypotension, nausea, tinnitus, vertigo, vomiting.

Pharmacodynamics/Kinetics

Absorption: Complete; food has no affect on rate or extent

Distribution: MHD: V_d: 49 L

Protein binding, serum: MHD: 40%

Metabolism: Hepatic to 10-monohydroxy metabolite (MHD; active); MHD is further conjugated to DHD (inactive)

Bioavailability: Decreased in children <8 years; increased in elderly >60 years

Half-life elimination: Parent drug: 2 hours; MHD: 9 hours; renal impairment (Cl_{cr} 30 mL/minute): MHD: 19 hours

Clearance of MHD is increased in younger children (~80% in children 2-4 years of age) and approaches that of adults by ~13 years of age

Time to peak, serum: 4.5 hours (3-13 hours)

Excretion: Urine (95%, <1% as unchanged oxcarbazepine, 27% as unchanged MHD, 49% as MHD glucuronides); feces (<4%)

Dosage Oral:

Children 4-16 years:

Adjunctive therapy: 8-10 mg/kg/day, not to exceed 600 mg/day, given in 2 divided daily doses. Maintenance dose should be achieved over 2 weeks, and is dependent upon patient weight, according to the following:

20-29 kg: 900 mg/day in 2 divided doses

29.1-39 kg: 1200 mg/day in 2 divided doses

>39 kg: 1800 mg/day in 2 divided doses

Conversion to monotherapy: Oxcarbazepine 8-10 mg/kg/day in twice daily divided doses, while simultaneously initiating the reduction of the dose of the concomitant antiepileptic drug; the concomitant drug should be withdrawn over 3-6 weeks. Oxcarbazepine dose may be increased by a maximum of 10 mg/kg/day at weekly intervals. See below for recommended total daily dose by weight.

Initiation of monotherapy: Oxcarbazepine should be initiated at 8-10 mg/kg/day in twice daily divided doses; doses may be titrated by 5 mg/kg/day every third day. See below for recommended total daily dose by weight.

Range of maintenance doses by weight during monotherapy:

20 kg: 600-900 mg/day

25-30 kg: 900-1200 mg/day

35-40 kg: 900-1500 mg/day

45 kg: 1200-1500 mg/day

50-55 kg: 1200-1800 mg/day

60-65 kg: 1200-2100 mg/day

70 kg: 1500-2100 mg/day

Adults:

Adjunctive therapy: Initial: 300 mg twice daily; dose may be increased by as much as 600 mg/day at weekly intervals; recommended daily dose: 1200 mg/day in 2 divided doses. Although daily doses >1200 mg/day demonstrated greater efficacy, most patients were unable to tolerate 2400 mg/day (due to CNS effects).

Conversion to monotherapy: Oxcarbazepine 600 mg/day in twice daily divided doses while simultaneously initiating the reduction of the dose of the concomitant antiepileptic drug. The concomitant dosage should be withdrawn over 3-6 weeks, while the maximum dose of oxcarbazepine should be reached in about 2-4 weeks. Recommended daily dose: 2400 mg/day.

Initiation of monotherapy: Oxcarbazepine should be initiated at a dose of 600 mg/day in twice daily divided doses; doses may be titrated upward by 300 mg/day every third day to a final dose of 1200 mg/day given in 2 daily divided doses

Dosing adjustment in renal impairment: Therapy should be initiated at one-half the usual starting dose (300 mg/day) and increased slowly to achieve the desired clinical response

Dosing adjustment in hepatic impairment: Adjustment not needed for mild-to-moderate impairment

Monitoring Parameters Seizure frequency, serum sodium (particularly during first 3 months of therapy), symptoms of CNS depression (dizziness, headache, somnolence). Additional serum sodium monitoring recommended during maintenance treatment in patients receiving other medications known to decrease sodium levels, in patients with signs/symptoms of hyponatremia, and in patients with an increase in seizure frequency or severity.

Administration Suspension: Prior to using for the first time, firmly insert the plastic adapter provided with the bottle. Cover adapter with child-resistant cap when not in use. Shake bottle for at least 10 seconds, remove child-resistant cap and insert the oral dosing syringe provided to withdraw appropriate dose. Dose may be taken directly from oral syringe or may be mixed in a small glass of water immediately prior to swallowing. Rinse syringe with warm water after use and allow to dry thoroughly. Discard any unused portion after 7 weeks of first opening bottle.

Contraindications Hypersensitivity to oxcarbazepine or any component of the formulation

Warnings Clinically significant hyponatremia (sodium <125 mmol/L) can develop during oxcarbazepine use; monitor serum sodium, particularly during the first 3 months of therapy or in patients at risk for hyponatremia. Potentially serious, sometimes fatal, dermatologic reactions (eg, Stevens-Johnson, toxic epidermal necrolysis) and multiorgan hypersensitivity reactions have been reported in adults and children; monitor for signs and symptoms of skin reactions and possible disparate manifestations associated with lymphatic, hepatic, renal and/or hematologic organ systems; gradual discontinuation and conversion to alternate therapy may be required. As with all antiepileptic drugs, oxcarbazepine should be withdrawn gradually to minimize the potential of increased seizure frequency. Use of oxcarbazepine has been associated with CNS related adverse events, most significant of these were cognitive symptoms including psychomotor slowing, difficulty with concentration, and speech or language problems, somnolence or fatigue, and coordination abnormalities, including ataxia and gait disturbances. Use caution in patients with previous hypersensitivity to carbamazepine (cross-sensitivity occurs in 25% to 30%). May reduce the efficacy of oral contraceptives (nonhormonal contraceptive measures are recommended).

Dosage Forms Suspension, oral: 300 mg/5 mL (250 mL) [contains ethanol; packaged with oral syringe]

Tablet: 150 mg, 300 mg, 600 mg

Reference Range Blood therapeutic range: 8-20 mg/L (20-200 µmol/L). Adverse effects occur with serum levels >35 mg/L. Serum oxcarbazepine (10-hydroxymetabolite) level of 45.6 mg/L is associated with bradycardia and hypotension.

Overdosage/Treatment

Treatment is symptomatic and supportive. Experience is limited; the largest reported overdose has been 24,000 mg.

Decontamination: Oral: Gastric lavage and/or activated charcoal for adult ingestions >2.5 g.

Supportive therapy: I.V. crystalloid infusion to treat hypotension; bradycardia responds to atropine

Enhanced elimination: Multiple dosing of activated charcoal is of uncertain benefit.

Drug Interactions **Inhibits** CYP2C19 (weak); **Induces** CYP3A4 (strong)

Carbamazepine: Oxcarbazepine serum concentrations may be reduced by a mean 40%

CYP3A4 substrates: Oxcarbazepine may decrease the levels/effects of CYP3A4 substrates. Example substrates include benzodiazepines, calcium channel blockers, clarithromycin, cyclosporine, erythromycin, estrogens, mirtazapine, nateglinide, nefazodone, nevirapine, protease inhibitors, tacrolimus, and venlafaxine.

Felodipine: Metabolism is increased due to enzyme induction; similar effects may be anticipated with other dihydropyridine calcium channel blockers

Hormonal contraceptives: Metabolism may be increased due to enzyme induction; use alternative contraceptive measures; oxcarbazepine with oral contraceptives has been shown to decrease plasma concentrations of the two hormonal components, ethinyl estradiol (48% and 52%) and levonorgestrel (32% and 52%).

Phenobarbital: Phenobarbital levels are increased (average of 14%); oxcarbazepine levels are decreased (average of 25%)

Phenytoin: Phenytoin levels may be increased (high dosages) by an average of 40%; oxcarbazepine levels may be decreased (by an average of 30%) during concurrent therapy; monitor phenytoin levels

Valproic acid decreases oxcarbazepine levels by an average of 18%

Verapamil's metabolism may be increased due to enzyme induction; verapamil may reduce blood levels of oxcarbazepine's active metabolite (MHD)

Pregnancy Risk Factor C

Pregnancy Implications Oxcarbazepine crosses the human placenta. Teratogenic effects have been observed in animal studies. Oxcarbazepine is structurally related to carbamazepine (teratogenic in humans), use during pregnancy only if the benefit to the mother outweighs the potential risk to the fetus. Nonhormonal forms of contraception should be used during therapy.

Lactation Enters breast milk/not recommended

Nursing Implications Inform those patients who have exhibited hypersensitivity reactions to carbamazepine that there is the possibility of cross-sensitivity reactions with oxcarbazepine. Inform patients of child-bearing age that hormonal contraceptives may be less effective when used with oxcarbazepine. Caution should be exercised if alcohol is taken with oxcarbazepine, due to the possible additive sedative effects. Advise patients that oxcarbazepine may cause dizziness and somnolence and that early in therapy they are advised not to drive or operate machinery.

Specific References

Barker MJ, Benitez JG, Ternullo S, et al, "Acute Oxcarbazepine and Atomoxetine Overdose with Quetiapine," *Vet Hum Toxicol*, 2004, 46(3):130-2.

Levine B, Green-Johnson D, Moore KA, et al, "Hydroxycarbazepine Distribution in Three Postmortem Cases," *J Anal Toxicol*, 2004, 28(6):509-11.

Malek-Ahmadi P and Hanretta AT, "Possible Reduction in Post-Traumatic Stress Disorder Symptoms with Oxcarbazepine in a Patient with Bipolar Disorder," *Ann Pharmacother*, 2004, 38(11):1852-4.

Miles MV, Tang PH, Ryan MA, et al, "Feasibility and Limitations of Oxcarbazepine Monitoring Using Salivary Monohydroxycarbamazepine (MHD)," *Ther Drug Monit*, 2004, 26(3):300-4.

Siniscalchi A, Mancuso F, Scornaienghi D, et al, "Acute Encephalopathy Induced by Oxcarbazepine and Furosemide," *Ann Pharmacother*, 2004, 38(3):509-10.

Oxitriptan

Related Information
- Tryptophan

CAS Number 4350-09-8; 56-69-9

Use Approved in U.S. as an orphan drug for use in postanoxic intention myoclonus

Unlabeled/Investigational Use Antidepressant, also used for sleep disorders, migraine headaches; epilepsy, Parkinsons, psychostimulant

Mechanism of Action A precursor of serotonin which is a neurotransmitter

Adverse Reactions

Cardiovascular: Transient hypotension

Central nervous system: Hypomania, agitation, anxiety, insomnia, akinesia

Dermatologic: Scleroderma

Gastrointestinal: Nausea, anorexia, diarrhea, vomiting

Respiratory: Dyspnea

Toxicodynamics/Kinetics

Absorption: 1-2 hours

Protein binding: 19%

Metabolism: Hepatic and peripheral decarboxylation to serotonin and 5-hydroxyindoleacetic acid

Bioavailability: 47% to 84%

Half-life: 4.3 hours

Elimination: Renal

Dosage Postanoxic myoclonus: Initial: 25 mg 4 times/day; can increase dose by 100 mg every 3-5 days

Depression: Initial: 10 mg/day; maximum daily dose: 600 mg

I.V.: 1-2 mg/kg

Monitoring Parameters CBC, ECG, electrolytes

Overdosage/Treatment

Decontamination: Lavage within 1 hour of ingestion (especially if coingestants involve drugs listed in "warning" section); activated charcoal

Supportive therapy: Nausea can be treated with prochlorperazine (5-10 mg); diarrhea can be treated with diphenoxylate

Additional Information An orphan drug for postanoxic intention myoclonus, available through Circa pharmaceuticals (516-842-8383), or in combination with carbidopa through Du Pont pharmaceuticals (1-800-474-2762). Has been used to treat LSD-induced psychosis

Oxycodone

CAS Number 124-90-3; 76-42-6

U.S. Brand Names OxyContin®; Oxydose™; OxyFast®; OxyIR®; Roxicodone™ Intensol™; Roxicodone™

Synonyms Dihydrohydroxycodeinone; Oxycodone Hydrochloride

Impairment Potential Yes

Use

Management of moderate to severe pain, normally used in combination with non-narcotic analgesics

OxyContin® is indicated for around-the-clock management of moderate to severe pain when an analgesic is needed for an extended period of time. **Note:** OxyContin® is not intended for use as an "as needed" analgesic or for immediately-postoperative pain management (should be used postoperatively only if the patient has received it prior to surgery or if severe, persistent pain is anticipated).

Mechanism of Action Binds to opiate receptors in the CNS, causing inhibition of ascending pain pathways, altering the perception of and response to pain; produces generalized CNS depression

Adverse Reactions

Cardiovascular: Postural hypotension, syncope, vasodilation

Central nervous system: **Fatigue, drowsiness, dizziness, somnolence**, nervousness, headache, restlessness, malaise, confusion, anxiety, abnormal dreams, euphoria, thought abnormalities, hallucinations,

intracranial pressure increased, mental depression, paradoxical CNS stimulation

Dermatologic: **Pruritus**, rash, exfoliative dermatitis, urticaria

Endocrine & metabolic: Hyponatremia, SIADH

Gastrointestinal: **Nausea, vomiting, constipation**, anorexia, stomach cramps, xerostomia, biliary spasm, abdominal pain, dyspepsia, gastritis, dysphagia, ileus, paralytic ileus

Genitourinary: Ureteral spasms, decreased urination, urinary retention

Local: Pain at injection site

Neuromuscular & skeletal: **Weakness**

Respiratory: Dyspnea, hiccoughs

Miscellaneous: Diaphoresis, anaphylaxis, anaphylactoid reactions, histamine release, physical and psychological dependence, withdrawal syndrome (may include seizures)

Note: Deaths due to overdose have been reported due to misuse/abuse after crushing the sustained release tablets.

Signs and Symptoms of Overdose CNS depression, coma, lightheadedness, miosis, noncardiogenic pulmonary edema, respiratory depression

Pharmacodynamics/Kinetics

Onset of action: Pain relief: 10-15 minutes

Peak effect: 0.5-1 hour

Duration: 3-6 hours; Controlled release: ≤12 hours

Metabolism: Hepatic

Half-life elimination: 2-3 hours

Excretion: Urine

Dosage

Oral:

Immediate release:

Children:

6-12 years: 1.25 mg every 6 hours as needed

>12 years: 2.5 mg every 6 hours as needed

Adults: 5 mg every 6 hours as needed

Controlled release: Adults:

Opioid naive (not currently on opioid): 10 mg every 12 hours

Currently on opioid/ASA or acetaminophen or NSAID combination:

1-5 tablets: 10-20 mg every 12 hours

6-9 tablets: 20-30 mg every 12 hours

10-12 tablets: 30-40 mg every 12 hours

May continue the nonopioid as a separate drug.

Currently on opioids: Use standard conversion chart to convert daily dose to oxycodone equivalent. Divide daily dose in 2 (for every 12-hour dosing) and round down to nearest dosage form.

Note: 80 mg or 160 mg tablets are for use **only** in opioid-tolerant patients. Special safety considerations must be addressed when converting to OxyContin® doses ≥160 mg every 12 hours. Dietary caution must be taken when patients are initially titrated to 160 mg tablets.

Dosing adjustment in hepatic impairment: Reduce dosage in patients with severe liver disease

Monitoring Parameters Pain relief, respiratory and mental status, blood pressure

Administration Do not crush controlled-release tablets; 80 mg and 160 mg tablets are for use **only** in opioid-tolerant patients. Do not administer OxyContin® 160 mg tablet with a high-fat meal.

Contraindications Hypersensitivity to oxycodone or any component of the formulation; significant respiratory depression; hypercarbia; acute or severe bronchial asthma; OxyContin® is also contraindicated in paralytic ileus (known or suspected); pregnancy (prolonged use or high doses at term)

Warnings

Use with caution in patients with hypersensitivity reactions to other phenanthrene derivative opioid agonists (morphine, hydrocodone, hydromorphone, levorphanol, oxycodone, oxymorphone), respiratory diseases including asthma, emphysema, and/or COPD. Use with caution in pancreatitis or biliary tract disease, acute alcoholism (including delirium tremens), adrenocortical insufficiency, CNS depression/coma, kyphoscoliosis (or other skeletal disorder which may alter respiratory function), hypothyroidism (including myxedema), prostatic hyperplasia, urethral stricture, and toxic psychosis.

Use with caution in the elderly, debilitated, severe hepatic or renal function. Hemodynamic effects (hypotension, orthostasis) may be exaggerated in patients with hypovolemia, concurrent vasodilating drugs, or in patients with head injury. Respiratory depressant effects and capacity to elevate CSF pressure may be exaggerated in presence of head injury, other intracranial lesion, or pre-existing intracranial pressure. Some preparations contain sulfites which may cause allergic reactions.

[U.S. Boxed Warning]: Healthcare provider should be alert to problems of abuse, misuse, and diversion. Tolerance or drug dependence may result from extended use.

Controlled-release formulations:

[U.S. Boxed Warnings]: Do NOT crush controlled-release tablets; 80 mg and 160 mg strengths are for use only in opioid-tolerant patients requiring high daily dosages >160 mg (80 mg formulation) or >320 mg (160 mg formulation). OxyContin® is not for use as an "as-needed" analgesic and is suitable only of continuous, around-the-clock management of moderate to severe pain.

Dosage Forms Capsule, immediate release, as hydrochloride: 5 mg
OxyIR®: 5 mg
Solution, oral, as hydrochloride: 5 mg/5 mL (500 mL)
Roxicodone®: 5 mg/5 mL (5 mL, 500 mL) [contains alcohol]
Solution, oral concentrate, as hydrochloride: 20 mg/mL (30 mL)
ETH-Oxydose™: 20 mg/mL (30 mL) [contains sodium benzoate; berry flavor]
OxyFast®: 20 mg/mL (30 mL) [contains sodium benzoate and dry natural rubber]
Roxicodone®: 20 mg/mL (30 mL) [contains sodium benzoate]
Tablet, as hydrochloride: 5 mg, 15 mg, 30 mg
Roxicodone®: 5 mg, 15 mg, 30 mg
Tablet, controlled release, as hydrochloride:
OxyContin®: 10 mg, 20 mg, 40 mg, 80 mg, 160 mg
Tablet, extended release, as hydrochloride: 10 mg, 20 mg, 40 mg, 80 mg

Reference Range Blood level of 5 mg/L associated with fatality

Overdosage/Treatment
Decontamination: Lavage (within 1 hour)/activated charcoal
Supportive therapy: Naloxone hydrochloride (0.4-2 mg I.V., SubQ, or through an endotracheal tube); a continuous infusion (at $^2/_3$ the response dose/hour) may be required

Antidote(s)
● Nalmefene [ANTIDOTE]
● Naloxone [ANTIDOTE]

Drug Interactions **Substrate** of CYP2D6 (major)
CNS depressants, MAO inhibitors, general anesthetics, and tricyclic antidepressants: May potentiate the effects of opiate agonists; dextroamphetamine may enhance the analgesic effect of opiate agonists
CYP2D6 inhibitors: May decrease the effects of oxycodone. Example inhibitors include chlorpromazine, delavirdine, fluoxetine, miconazole, paroxetine, pergolide, quinidine, quinine, ritonavir, and ropinirole.

Pregnancy Risk Factor B/D (prolonged use or high doses at term)
Pregnancy Implications Should be used in pregnancy only if clearly needed. Use of narcotics during pregnancy may produce physical dependence in the neonate; respiratory depression may occur in the newborn if narcotics are used prior to delivery (especially high doses).

Lactation Enters breast milk/use caution
Nursing Implications Observe patient for excessive sedation, respiratory depression, implement safety measures, assist with ambulation
Additional Information When taken with a high-fat meal, peak concentration is 25% greater following a single OxyContin® 160 mg tablet as compared to two 80 mg tablets. Prophylactic use of a laxative should be considered.

Specific References
Abadie JM, Allison KH, Black DA, et al, "Can an Immunoassay Become a Standard Technique in Detecting Oxycodone and Its Metabolites? *J Anal Toxicol*, 2005, 29(8):825-9.
Abadie JM and Bankson DD, "Can an Immunoassay Become a Standard Technique in Detecting Oxycodone and Its Metabolites?" *J Anal Toxicol*, 2006, 30:128.
Backer RC, Monforte JR, and Poklis A, "Evaluation of the DRI® Oxycodone Immunoassay for the Detection of Oxycodone in Urine," *J Anal Toxicol*, 2005, 29:675-7.
Burrows DL, Hagardorn AN, Harlan GC, et al, "A Fatal Drug Interaction Between Oxydocone and Clonazepam," *J Anal Toxicol*, 2003, 27(3):179.
Caplan YH, Cone EJ, Fant RV, et al, "Evidence for Toxic Multiple Drug-Drug Interactions in Oxycodone Deaths," *J Anal Toxicol*, 2004, 28:278-9.
Cone EJ, Fant RV, Rohay JM, et al, "Oxycodone Involvement in Drug Abuse Deaths: A DAWN-Based Classification Scheme Applied to an Oxycodone Postmortem Database Containing Over 1000 Cases," *J Anal Toxicol*, 2003, 27(2):57-67.
Cone EJ, Fant RV, Rohay JM, et al, "Oxycodone Involvement in Drug Abuse Deaths. II. Evidence for Toxic Multiple Drug-Drug Interactions," *J Anal Toxicol*, 2004, 28:616-24.
Haller CA, Stone J, Burke V, et al, "Comparison of an Automated and Point-of-Care Immunoassay to GC-MS for Urine Oxycodone Testing in the Clinical Laboratory," *J Anal Toxicol*, 2006, 30:106-11.
Hermos JA, Young MM, Gagnon DR, et al, "Characterizations of Long-term Oxycodone/Acetaminophen Prescriptions in Veteran Patients," *Arch Intern Med*, 2004, 164(21):2361-6.
Hughes AA, Bogdan GM, Dart RC, et al, "Comparative Rates of OxyContin® Abuse: Anecdotal Highs," *J Toxicol Clin Toxicol*, 2003, 41(5):746.
Hughes AA and Dart RC, "Seasons of Abuse? Temporal Trends of Prescription Opioids," *J Toxicol Clin Toxicol*, 2004, 42(5):762-3.
Jannetto PJ, Wong SH, Gock SB, et al, "Pharmacogenomics as Molecular Autopsy for Forensic Toxicology: Genotyping Oxycodone Cases for Cytochrome P450 2D6," *J Anal Toxicol*, 2003, 27:190.
Karunatilake H and Buckley NA, "Serotonin Syndrome Induced by Fluvoxamine and Oxycodone," *Ann Pharmacother*, 2006, 40(1):155-7.
Le NL, Reiter A, Tomlinson K, et al, "The Detection of Oxycodone in Meconium Specimens," *J Anal Toxicol*, 2005, 29:54-7.
Mildh LH, Piilonen A, and Kirvela OA, "Supplemental Oxygen Is Not Required in Trauma Patients Treated with IV Opiates," *Am J Emerg Med*, 2003, 21(1):35-8.
Miller NS and Greenfeld A, "Patient Characteristics and Risks Factors for Development of Dependence on Hydrocodone and Oxycodone," *Am J Ther*, 2004, 11(1):26-32.
Moore KA, Ramcharitar V, Levine B, et al, "Tentative Identification of Novel Oxycodone Metabolites in Human Urine," *J Anal Toxicol*, 2003, 27(6):346-52.
Wingert WR, Mundy L, and Chmara E, "Study of Oxycodone Occurrences at a Large City Medical Examiner's Office," *J Anal Toxicol*, 2006, 30:133.
Wolf BC, Lavezzi WA, Sullivan LM, et al, "One Hundred Seventy Two Deaths Involving the Use of Oxycodone in Palm Beach County," *J Forensic Sci*, 2005, 50(1):192-5.

Oxymetazoline

CAS Number 1491-59-4;2315-02-8
U.S. Brand Names 4-Way® Long Acting [OTC]; Afrin® Extra Moisturizing [OTC]; Afrin® Original [OTC]; Afrin® Severe Congestion [OTC]; Afrin® Sinus [OTC]; Afrin® [OTC]; Duramist® Plus [OTC]; Duration® [OTC]; Genasal [OTC]; Neo-Synephrine® 12 Hour Extra Moisturizing [OTC]; Neo-Synephrine® 12 Hour [OTC]; Néstrilla® [OTC]; OcuClear® [OTC] [DSC]; Twice-A-Day® [OTC]; Vicks Sinex® 12 Hour Ultrafine Mist [OTC]; Visine® L.R. [OTC]

Synonyms Oxymetazoline Hydrochloride
Use Symptomatic relief of nasal mucosal congestion and adjunctive therapy of middle ear infections, associated with acute or chronic rhinitis, the common cold, sinusitis, hay fever, or other allergies
Ophthalmic: Relief of redness of eye due to minor eye irritations, conjunctivitis

Mechanism of Action Sympathomimetic; stimulates alpha-adrenergic receptors in the arterioles of the nasal mucosa to produce vasoconstriction; imidazoline decongestant

Adverse Reactions
Primarily local **burning**, hypothermia, xerostomia; may be porphyrinogenic; intra-arterial injection can cause localized gangrene due to ischemia; peripheral vasoconstriction due to nasal application is very rare
Cardiovascular: Bradycardia, sinus bradycardia, sinus tachycardia
Central nervous system: Headache, psychosis, mania, seizures (in children), insomnia
Respiratory: **Dryness of the nasal mucosa, sneezing**

Signs and Symptoms of Overdose Apnea, bradycardia, cardiovascular collapse, CNS depression, coma, hypothermia

Pharmacodynamics/Kinetics
Onset of action: Intranasal: 5-10 minutes
Duration: 5-6 hours

Dosage Therapy should not exceed 3-5 days
Intranasal:
Children 2-5 years: 0.025% solution: Instill 2-3 drops in each nostril twice daily
Children ≥6 years and Adults: 0.05% solution: Instill 2-3 drops or 2-3 sprays into each nostril twice daily up to 3 days
Ophthalmic: Adults: 0.025% solution: Instill 1-2 drops into affected eye(s) every 6 hours up to 4 days

Stability Do not use if solution changes colors or becomes cloudy
Contraindications Hypersensitivity to oxymetazoline or any component of the formulation
Warnings
Nasal: Rebound congestion may occur with extended use (>3 days). Prior to self-medication (OTC use), contact healthcare provider in the presence of hypertension, diabetes, hyperthyroidism, heart disease, coronary artery disease, cerebral arteriosclerosis, or long-standing bronchial asthma.
Ophthalmic: Prior to OTC use, contact healthcare provider in the presence of glaucoma or if needed for >72 hours.

Dosage Forms Solution, intranasal, as hydrochloride [spray]: 0.05% (15 mL, 30 mL)
Afrin® Extra Moisturizing: 0.05% (15 mL) [contains benzyl alcohol and glycerin; regular or no drip formula]
Afrin® Original: 0.05% (15 mL, 30 mL) [contains benzalkonium chloride]
Afrin® Original: 0.05% (15 mL) [contains benzyl alcohol and benzalkonium chloride; no drip formula]
Afrin® Severe Congestion: 0.05% (15 mL) [contains benzyl alcohol and menthol; regular or no drip formula]
Afrin® Sinus: 0.05% (15 mL) [contains benzyl alcohol, benzalkonium chloride, camphor, phenol; regular or no drip formula]

Duramist® Plus, Neo-Synephrine® 12 Hour, Néstrilla®, Vicks Sinex® 12 Hour Ultrafine Mist, Vicks Sinex® 12 Hour, 4-Way® 12 Hour: 0.05% (15 mL) [contains benzalkonium chloride]

Duration®: 0.05% (30 mL) [contains benzalkonium chloride]

Genasal, NRS®: 0.05% (15 mL, 30 mL) [contains benzalkonium chloride]

Neo-Synephrine® 12 Hour Extra Moisturizing: 0.05% (15 mL) [contains glycerin]

Solution, ophthalmic, as hydrochloride (Visine® L.R.): 0.025% (15 mL, 30 mL) [contains benzalkonium chloride]

Overdosage/Treatment

Decontamination: Oral: Activated charcoal

Supportive therapy: Seizures can be treated with benzodiazepines or phenytoin; nitroprusside can be used to treat hypertension

Drug Interactions Increased toxicity with MAO inhibitors

Pregnancy Risk Factor C

Nursing Implications Spray/drops should not be used for >3 days without direct physician supervision

Additional Information Often best when used short-term in conjunction with long-term nasal corticosteroid

Oxymetholone

Pronunciation (oks i METH oh lone)

CAS Number 434-07-1

U.S. Brand Names Anadrol®

Use Anemias caused by the administration of myelotoxic drugs

Mechanism of Action Stimulates receptors in organs and tissues to promote growth and development of male sex organs and maintains secondary sex characteristics in androgen-deficient males

Adverse Reactions

Male:

Postpubertal:

Central nervous system: Insomnia, chills

Dermatologic: **Acne**

Endocrine & metabolic: **Gynecomastia**, decreased libido

Gastrointestinal: Nausea, diarrhea

Genitourinary: **Bladder irritability, priapism**, prostatic hypertrophy (elderly)

Hematologic: Iron deficiency anemia, suppression of clotting factors

Hepatic: Hepatic dysfunction, hepatic necrosis, hepatocellular carcinoma

Prepubertal:

Central nervous system: Chills, insomnia

Dermatologic: **Acne**, hyperpigmentation

Endocrine & metabolic: **Virilism**

Gastrointestinal: Diarrhea, nausea

Hematologic: Iron deficiency anemia, suppression of clotting factors

Hepatic: Hepatic necrosis, hepatocellular carcinoma, peliosis hepatitis

Female:

Central nervous system: Chills, insomnia

Endocrine & metabolic: **Virilism**, hypercalcemia

Gastrointestinal: Nausea, diarrhea

Hematologic: Iron deficiency anemia, suppression of clotting factors

Hepatic: Hepatic dysfunction, hepatic necrosis, hepatocellular carcinoma

Signs and Symptoms of Overdose Abnormal liver function test, confusion

Toxicodynamics/Kinetics

Half-life: 9 hours

Elimination: Primarily in urine

Dosage Adults: Erythropoietic effects: Oral: 1-5 mg/kg/day in 1 daily dose; maximum: 100 mg/day; give for a minimum trial of 3-6 months because response may be delayed

Monitoring Parameters Liver function, blood sugars, lipid profile, iron studies, hemoglobin/hematocrit, x-ray of bones every 6 months (prepubertal patients); signs of virilization (females)

Contraindications Hypersensitivity to oxymetholone or any component of the formulation; breast cancer in men; breast cancer in women with hypercalcemia; prostate cancer; severe liver dysfunction; nephrosis; pregnancy

Warnings [U.S. Boxed Warning]: Anabolic steroids may cause peliosis hepatis, liver cell tumors, and blood lipid changes with increased risk of arteriosclerosis; monitor diabetic patients carefully. Use with caution in elderly men; they may be at greater risk for prostate hyperplasia and cancer. Use caution with cardiac, renal, or hepatic disease; may develop edema. In breast cancer, may cause hypercalcemia by stimulating osteolysis. Use caution in children; may accelerate epiphyseal maturation thereby compromising adult height.

Dosage Forms Tablet: 50 mg

Overdosage/Treatment Decontamination: Oral: Ipecac within 30 minutes or lavage (within 1 hour)/activated charcoal

Test Interactions Altered glucose tolerance tests, thyroid function tests, and metyrapone tests

Drug Interactions Cyclosporine: Androgens may enhance the hepatotoxic effect of cyclosporine.

Warfarin: Androgens may enhance the anticoagulant effect of warfarin.

Pregnancy Risk Factor X

Pregnancy Implications Oligospermia or amenorrhea may occur resulting in an impairment of fertility

Lactation Excretion in breast milk unknown/not recommended

Additional Information May increase glucagon levels

Oxymorphone

CAS Number 357-07-3; 76-41-5

U.S. Brand Names Numorphan®

Synonyms Oxymorphone Hydrochloride

Impairment Potential Yes

Use Management of moderate to severe pain and preoperatively as a sedative and a supplement to anesthesia

Mechanism of Action Oxymorphone (Numorphan®) is a potent narcotic analgesic with uses similar to those of morphine. The drug is a semisynthetic derivative of morphine (phenanthrene derivative) and is closely related to hydromorphone chemically (Dilaudid®).

Adverse Reactions

Cardiovascular: **Hypotension**, palpitations, bradycardia, peripheral vasodilation, sinus bradycardia

Central nervous system: **Fatigue, drowsiness, dizziness**, CNS depression, agitation, increased intracranial pressure

Dermatologic: Pruritus

Endocrine & metabolic: Syndrome of inappropriate antidiuretic hormone

Gastrointestinal: **Nausea, vomiting, constipation**, biliary tract spasm

Genitourinary: Urinary tract spasm

Neuromuscular & skeletal: **Weakness**

Ocular: Miosis

Respiratory: Apnea, respiratory depression

Miscellaneous: **Histamine release**, physical and psychological dependence,

Pharmacodynamics/Kinetics

Onset of action: Analgesic: I.V., I.M., SubQ: 5-10 minutes

Duration: Analgesic: Parenteral: 3-4 hours

Protein binding: 10% to 12%

Metabolism: Hepatic via glucuronidation to active and inactive metabolites

Bioavailability: Oral: 10%

Half-life elimination: Oral: Immediate release: 7-9 hours; Extended release: 9-11 hours

Excretion: Urine

Dosage Adults: **Note:** More frequent dosing may be required.

I.M., SubQ: 0.5 mg initially, 1-1.5 mg every 4-6 hours as needed

I.V.: 0.5 mg initially

Rectal: 5 mg every 4-6 hours

Stability Refrigerate suppository

Monitoring Parameters Respiratory rate, heart rate, blood pressure, CNS activity

Administration Administer immediate release and extended release tablets 1 hour before or 2 hours after eating. Opana® ER tablet should be swallowed; do not break, crush. or chew.

Contraindications

Hypersensitivity to oxymorphone, other morphine analogs (phenanthrene derivatives) or any component of the formulation; paralytic ileus (known or suspected); increased intracranial pressure; severe respiratory depression (unless in monitored setting with resuscitative equipment); acute/severe bronchial asthma; hypercarbia; pregnancy (prolonged use or high doses at term.

Note: Oral formulations are also contraindicated in moderate-to-severe hepatic impairment

Warnings

An opioid-containing analgesic regimen should be tailored to each patient's needs and based upon the type of pain being treated (acute versus chronic), the route of administration, degree of tolerance for opioids (naive versus chronic user), age, weight, and medical condition. The optimal analgesic dose varies widely among patients. Doses should be titrated to pain relief/prevention.

May cause respiratory depression. Use extreme caution in patients with COPD or other chronic respiratory conditions characterized by hypoxia, hypercapnea, or diminished respiratory reserve (myexdema, cor pulmonale, kyphoscoliosis, obstructive sleep apnea, severe obesity). Use with caution in patients (particularly elderly or debilitated) with impaired respiratory function, adrenal disease, thyroid dysfunction, prostatic hypertrophy, renal impairment, or severe hepatic dysfunction. Use only with extreme caution (if at all) in patients with head injury or increased intracranial pressure (ICP); potential to elevate ICP and/or blunt papillary response may be greatly exaggerated in these patients. Use with caution in biliary tract disease or acute pancreatitis (may cause constriction of sphincter of Oddi).

Oxymorphone shares the toxic potential of opiate agonists and usual precautions of opiate agonist therapy should be observed; may cause hypotension in patients with acute myocardial infarction, volume depletion, or concurrent drug therapy which may exaggerate vasodilation. The elderly may be particularly susceptible to the CNS depressant and constipating effects of narcotics. Safety and efficacy have not been established in children <18 years of age.

[U.S. Boxed Warning]: Healthcare provider should be alert to problems of abuse, misuse, and diversion. Tolerance or drug dependence may result from extended use. Use caution in patients with a history of drug dependence or abuse. Abrupt discontinuation may precipitate withdrawal syndrome.

Extended release formulation:

[U.S. Boxed Warnings]: Opana® ER is an extended release oral formulation of oxymorphone and is not suitable for use as an "as needed" analgesic; tablets should not be broken, chewed, dissolved, or crushed; tablets should be swallowed whole. Opana® ER is intended for use in long-term, continuous management of moderate to severe chronic pain. It is not indicated for use in the immediate post-operative period (12-24 hours). [U.S. Boxed Warning]: The co-ingestion of ethanol or ethanol-containing medications with OPANA ER may result in accelerated release of drug from the dosage form, abruptly increasing plasma levels, which may have fatal consequences.

Dosage Forms Injection, solution, as hydrochloride:
  Numorphan®: 1 mg (1 mL)
Tablet, as hydrochloride:
  Oprana: 5 mg, 10 mg
Tablet, extended release, as hydrochloride:
  Oprana® ER: 5 mg, 10 mg, 20 mg, 40 mg

Overdosage/Treatment Supportive therapy: Naloxone hydrochloride (0.4-2 mg I.V., SubQ, or through an endotracheal tube); a continuous infusion (at $^2/_3$ the response dose/hour) may be required

Antidote(s)
● Nalmefene [ANTIDOTE]
● Naloxone [ANTIDOTE]

Drug Interactions CNS depressants (includes antipsychotics, benzodiazepines, barbiturates): May potentiate the CNS depressant effects of opiate agonists; reduce oxymorphone dosage in patients receiving other CNS depressants.

Dextroamphetamine: May enhance the analgesic effect of opiate agonists.

General anesthetics: May potentiate the CNS depressant effects of opiate agonists.

MAO inhibitors: May potentiate the CNS depressant effects of opiate agonists; monitor.

SSRIs: Analgesics (narcotic) may enhance the serotonergic effect of selective serotonin reuptake inhibitors. This may cause serotonin syndrome.

Tricyclic antidepressants: May potentiate the CNS depressant effects of opiate agonists; monitor.

Pregnancy Risk Factor B/D (prolonged use or high doses at term)

Pregnancy Implications Teratogenic effects were not observed in animal studies, however, decreased fetal weight, decreased litter size, increased stillbirths, and increased neonatal death were noted. Chronic opioid use during pregnancy may lead to a withdrawal syndrome in the neonate. Symptoms include irritability, hyperactivity, loss of sleep pattern, abnormal crying, tremor, vomiting, diarrhea, weight loss, or failure to gain weight. Opioid analgesics are considered pregnancy risk factor D if used for prolonged periods or in larger doses near term.

Lactation Excretion in breast milk unknown/use caution

Nursing Implications Observe patient for excessive sedation, respiratory depression, implement safety measures, assist with ambulation

Specific Reference
McIlwain H and Ahdieh H, "Safety, Tolerability, and Effectiveness of Oxymorphone Extended Release for Moderate to Severe Osteoarthritis Pain: A One-Year Study," *Am J Ther*, 2005, 12(2):106-12.

Oxyphencyclimine

Pronunciation (oks i fen SYE kli meen)
CAS Number 7081-38-1
Synonyms Oxyphencyclimine Hydrochloride
Use Management of inflammatory disorders, as an analgesic in the treatment of mild to moderate pain and as an antipyretic; I.V. form used as an alternate to surgery in management of patent ductus arteriosus in premature neonates; acute gouty arthritis; removed from U.S. market

Mechanism of Action Anti-inflammatory effect is a prominent feature of the drug's pharmacology. Several hypotheses have been presented for the mode of action. One of the main events in an inflammatory reaction is a leukocyte infiltration of the inflammatory site. An inhibition of leukocyte migration would restrict the entry of leukocytes and suppress, but not stop, the ensuing inflammation; has been observed to inhibit *in vitro* migration of total human leukocytes in a dose-dependent manner.

Adverse Reactions
Cardiovascular: Circulatory collapse
Central nervous system: Headache, aseptic meningitis, psychosis, cognitive dysfunction, coma, seizures
Dermatologic: **Rash, dry skin**, pruritus
Endocrine & metabolic: Hyperkalemia, anion gap metabolic acidosis, fluid retention
Gastrointestinal: **Abdominal pain, constipation, dry throat, xerostomia**, feces discoloration (black), nausea, vomiting, GI bleeding, GI ulceration, diarrhea, dyspepsia
Hematologic: Leukopenia, neutropenia, agranulocytosis, granulocytopenia, aplastic anemia (rare), platelet inhibition
Hepatic: Elevated transaminases, hepatitis (fulminant)
Otic: Ototoxicity, tinnitus
Renal: Renal failure (acute), nephrotic syndrome, chronic renal failure, albuminuria
Respiratory: **Dry nose**, wheezing, respiratory depression
Miscellaneous: **Diaphoresis (decreased)**, hypersensitivity

Signs and Symptoms of Overdose Arthralgia, cognitive dysfunction, drowsiness, gastritis, GI bleeding, hypothyroidism, nausea, nephrotic syndrome, ototoxicity, tinnitus, vomiting, wheezing. Severe poisoning can manifest with apnea, coma, feces discoloration (greenish gray; pink), hypotension, leukocytosis, metabolic acidosis, nystagmus, renal failure and/or hepatic failure, respiratory depression, seizures

Dosage
Adults: Oral:
Rheumatoid arthritis: 100-200 mg 3-4 times/day until desired effect, then reduce dose to not exceed 400 mg/day
Acute gouty arthritis: Initial: 400 mg then 100 mg every 4 hours until acute attack subsides, not longer than 1 week

Contraindications Hypersensitivity to oxyphencyclimine or any component of the formulation; angle-closure glaucoma; obstructive GI tract or uropathy; severe ulcerative colitis; myasthenia gravis; intestinal atony

Warnings Use with caution in patients with hepatic or renal disease, ulcerative colitis, hyperthyroidism, cardiovascular disease, hypertension, tachycardia, GI obstruction, obstruction of the urinary tract

Dosage Forms Tablet, as hydrochloride: 10 mg

Overdosage/Treatment
Decontamination: Ipecac within 30 minutes or lavage (within 1 hour)/ charcoal
Supportive therapy: Hypotension/dehydration can be managed with I.V. fluid therapy; acidosis should be treated with bicarbonates, seizures with benzodiazepines; antacids, blood products are indicated, as appropriate, for hemorrhage
Enhancement of elimination: Dialysis or perfusion is indicated for secondary complications, acidosis, or renal failure and not toxin removal alone

Test Interactions ↑ chloride (S), sodium (S), bleeding time

Drug Interactions Increased anticholinergic side effects by amantadine; decreased phenothiazines, antiparkinsonian drugs, Haldol® effects

Pregnancy Risk Factor C

Nursing Implications Do not crush tablet

Oxytocin

CAS Number 50-56-6
U.S. Brand Names Pitocin®
Synonyms Pit
Use Induction of labor at term; control of postpartum bleeding; adjunctive therapy in management of abortion

Mechanism of Action Produces the rhythmic uterine contractions characteristic to delivery and stimulates breast milk flow during nursing

Adverse Reactions
Frequency not defined.
Fetus or neonate:
  Cardiovascular: Arrhythmias (including premature ventricular contractions), bradycardia
  Central nervous system: Brain or CNS damage (permanent), neonatal seizures
  Hepatic: Neonatal jaundice
  Ocular: Neonatal retinal hemorrhage
  Miscellaneous: Fetal death, low Apgar score (5 minute)
Mother:
  Cardiovascular: Arrhythmias, hypertensive episodes, premature ventricular contractions
  Gastrointestinal: Nausea, vomiting
  Genitourinary: Pelvic hematoma, postpartum hemorrhage, uterine hypertonicity, tetanic contraction of the uterus, uterine rupture, uterine spasm
  Hematologic: Afibrinogenemia (fatal)
  Miscellaneous: Anaphylactic reaction, subarachnoid hemorrhage

Pharmacodynamics/Kinetics
Onset of action: Uterine contractions: I.M.: 3-5 minutes; I.V.: ~1 minute
Duration: I.M.: 2-3 hour; I.V.: 1 hour

Metabolism: Rapidly hepatic and via plasma (by oxytocinase) and to a smaller degree the mammary gland

Half-life elimination: 1-5 minutes

Excretion: Urine

Dosage

I.V. administration requires the use of an infusion pump. Adults:

Induction of labor: I.V.: 0.5-1 milliunits/minute; gradually increase dose in increments of 1-2 milliunits/minute until desired contraction pattern is established; dose may be decreased after desired frequency of contractions is reached and labor has progressed to 5-6 cm dilation. Infusion rates of 6 milliunits/minute provide oxytocin levels similar to those at spontaneous labor; rates of >9-10 milliunits/minute are rarely required.

Postpartum bleeding:

I.M.: Total dose of 10 units after delivery

I.V.: 10-40 units by I.V. infusion in 1000 mL of intravenous fluid at a rate sufficient to control uterine atony

Adjunctive treatment of abortion: I.V.: 10-20 milliunits/minute; maximum total dose: 30 units/12 hours

Monitoring Parameters Fluid intake and output during administration; fetal monitoring

Administration An infusion pump is required for administration

Contraindications Hypersensitivity to oxytocin or any component of the formulation; significant cephalopelvic disproportion; unfavorable fetal positions; fetal distress; hypertonic or hyperactive uterus; contraindicated vaginal delivery (invasive cervical cancer, active genital herpes, prolapse of the cord, cord presentation, total placenta previa, or vasa previa)

Warnings [U.S. Boxed Warning]: To be used for medical rather than elective induction of labor. May produce antidiuretic effect (ie, water intoxication and excess uterine contractions); high doses or hypersensitivity to oxytocin may cause uterine hypertonicity, spasm, tetanic contraction, or rupture of the uterus; severe water intoxication with convulsions, coma, and death is associated with a slow oxytocin infusion over 24 hours

Dosage Forms Injection, solution: 10 units/mL (1 mL, 10 mL)

Pitocin®: 10 units/mL (1 mL)

Reference Range Plasma oxytocin level following an infusion of 132 milliunits/minute ranges from 228-241 pg/mL

Overdosage/Treatment Supportive therapy: Ritodrine (6 mg I.V.) can be used to inhibit oxytocin-induced labor; while diazepam or lorazepam can be used to treat seizures, electrolytes (particularly sodium) need to be monitored and normalized for effective seizure control; arteriospasm has been treated successfully with intra-arterial injection of 1% lidocaine (3 mL), papaverine (2 mL) and heparin (10,000 units) following discontinuation of the drug

Drug Interactions Dinoprostone, misoprostol: May increase the effect of oxytocin; wait 6-12 hours after dinoprostone or misoprostol administration before initiating oxytocin.

Pregnancy Risk Factor X

Pregnancy Implications Reproduction studies have not been conducted. When used as indicated, teratogenic effects would not be expected. Nonteratogenic adverse reactions are reported in the neonate as well as the mother.

Lactation Excretion in breast milk unknown/use caution

Additional Information Sodium chloride 0.9% (NS) and dextrose 5% in water (D$_5$W) have been recommended as diluents; dilute 10-40 units to 1 L in NS, LR, or D$_5$W

Paclitaxel

Related Information

● Docetaxel

CAS Number 33069-62-4

U.S. Brand Names Onxol™; Taxol®

Synonyms NSC-125973; NSC-673089

Use Treatment of breast, lung (small cell and nonsmall cell), and ovarian cancers

Unlabeled/Investigational Use Treatment of bladder, cervical, prostate, and head and neck cancers

Mechanism of Action Derived from the rare Pacific yew tree (*Taxus brevifolia*), it induces microtubule formation while disrupting mitosis

Adverse Reactions

Allergic: Appear to be primarily nonimmunologically mediated release of histamine and other vasoactive substances; almost always seen within the first hour of an infusion (~75% occur within 10 minutes of starting the infusion); incidence is significantly reduced by premedication

Cardiovascular: **Bradycardia (transient, 25%),** myocardial infarction, atrial fibrillation

Central nervous system: Ataxia, neuroencephalopathy, seizures

Dermatologic: **Alopecia (87%), venous erythema, tenderness, discomfort,** phlebitis, pruritus, radiation recall, rash, Stevens-Johnson syndrome, toxic epidermal necrolysis

Gastrointestinal: **Severe, potentially dose-limiting mucositis, stomatitis (15%),** most common at doses >390 mg/m^2; mild nausea and

vomiting, diarrhea, enterocolitis, intestinal obstruction, pancreatitis, paralytic ileus

Hematologic: **Myelosuppression, leukopenia, neutropenia** (6% to 21%), **thrombocytopenia,** anemia

Onset: 8-11 days

Nadir: 15-21 days

Recovery: 21 days

Hepatic: **Mild increases in liver enzymes,** hepatic encephalopathy

Local: Necrotic changes and ulceration following extravasation

Neuromuscular & skeletal: **Arthralgia, myalgia**

Neurotoxicity: Peripheral neuropathy, **sensory and/or autonomic neuropathy (numbness, tingling, burning pain), myopathy or myopathic effects (25% to 55%), and central nervous system toxicity.** May be cumulative and dose-limiting. **Note:** Motor neuropathy is uncommon at doses <250 mg/m^2; sensory neuropathy is almost universal at doses >250 mg/m^2; myopathic effects are common with doses >250 mg/m^2, generally occurring within 2-3 days of treatment, resolving over 5-6 days; pre-existing neuropathy may increase the risk of neuropathy.

Ocular: Visual disturbances (scintillating scotomata)

Otic: Ototoxicity (tinnitus and hearing loss)

Respiratory: Interstitial pneumonia, pulmonary fibrosis, radiation pneumonitis

Signs and Symptoms of Overdose Agranulocytosis, chest pain, congestive heart failure, diplopia, dysphagia, dyspnea, erythema, granulocytopenia, leukopenia, myopathy, neuritis, neuropathy (peripheral), neutropenia, stomatitis, ventricular arrhythmias, wheezing

Pharmacodynamics/Kinetics

Distribution:

V$_d$: Widely distributed into body fluids and tissues; affected by dose and duration of infusion

V$_{dss}$:

1- to 6-hour infusion: 67.1 L/m^2

24-hour infusion: 227-688 L/m^2

Protein binding: 89% to 98%

Metabolism: Hepatic via CYP2C8 and 3A4; forms metabolites (primarily 6α-hydroxypaclitaxel)

Half-life elimination:

1- to 6-hour infusion: Mean (beta): 6.4 hours

3-hour infusion: Mean (terminal): 13.1-20.2 hours

24-hour infusion: Mean (terminal): 15.7-52.7 hours

Excretion: Feces (~70%, 5% as unchanged drug); urine (14%)

Clearance: Mean: Total body: After 1- and 6-hour infusions: 5.8-16.3 L/hour/m^2; After 24-hour infusions: 14.2-17.2 L/hour/m^2

Dosage

Premedication with dexamethasone (20 mg orally or I.V. at 12 and 6 hours **or** 14 and 7 hours before the dose), diphenhydramine (50 mg I.V. 30-60 minutes prior to the dose), and cimetidine, famotidine or ranitidine (I.V. 30-60 minutes prior to the dose) is recommended

Adults: I.V.: Refer to individual protocols

Ovarian carcinoma: 135-175 mg/m^2 over 3 hours every 3 weeks **or**

50-80 mg/m^2 over 1-3 hours weekly **or**

1.4-4 mg/m^2/day continuous infusion for 14 days every 4 weeks

Metastatic breast cancer: 175-250 mg/m^2 over 3 hours every 3 weeks **or**

50-80 mg/m^2 weekly **or**

1.4-4 mg/m^2/day continuous infusion for 14 days every 4 weeks

Nonsmall cell lung carcinoma: 135 mg/m^2 over 24 hours every 3 weeks

AIDS-related Kaposi's sarcoma: 135 mg/m^2 over 3 hours every 3 weeks **or**

100 mg/m^2 over 3 hours every 2 weeks

Dosage modification for toxicity (solid tumors, including ovary, breast, and lung carcinoma): Courses of paclitaxel should not be repeated until the neutrophil count is ≥1500 cells/mm^3 and the platelet count is ≥100,000 cells/mm^3; reduce dosage by 20% for patients experiencing severe peripheral neuropathy or severe neutropenia (neutrophil <500 cells/mm^3 for a week or longer)

Dosage modification for immunosuppression in advanced HIV disease: Paclitaxel should not be given to patients with HIV if the baseline or subsequent neutrophil count is <1000 cells/mm^3. Additional modifications include: Reduce dosage of dexamethasone in premedication to 10 mg orally; reduce dosage by 20% in patients experiencing severe peripheral neuropathy or severe neutropenia (neutrophil <500 cells/mm^3 for a week or longer); initiate concurrent hematopoietic growth factor (G-CSF) as clinically indicated

Dosage adjustment in hepatic impairment:Note: These recommendations are based upon the patient's first course of therapy where the usual dose would be 135 mg/m^2 dose over 24 hours or the 175 mg/m^2 dose over 3 hours in patients with normal hepatic function. Dosage in subsequent courses should be based upon individual tolerance. Adjustments for other regimens are not available.

24-hour infusion:

If transaminase levels <2 times upper limit of normal (ULN) and bilirubin level ≤1.5 mg/dL: 135 mg/m^2

If transaminase levels 2-<10 times ULN and bilirubin level ≤1.5 mg/dL: 100 mg/m^2
If transaminase levels <10 times ULN and bilirubin level 1.6-7.5 mg/dL: 50 mg/m^2
If transaminase levels ≥10 times ULN and bilirubin level >7.5 mg/dL: Avoid use
3-hour infusion:
If transaminase levels <10 times ULN and bilirubin level ≤1.25 times ULN: 175 mg/m^2
If transaminase levels <10 times ULN and bilirubin level 1.26-2 times ULN: 135 mg/m^2
If transaminase levels <10 times ULN and bilirubin level 2.01-5 times ULN: 90 mg/m^2
If transaminase levels ≥10 times ULN and bilirubin level >5 times ULN: Avoid use

Stability

Store intact vials at room temperature of 20°C to 25°C (68°F to 77°F). Dilute in NS or D$_5$W to a concentration of 0.3-1.2 mg/mL; reconstituted solution is stable for up to 27 hours at room temperature (25°C) and ambient light conditions. Solutions in D$_5$W, NS, D$_5$NS, and D$_5$LR are stable for up to 48 hours at room temperature (25°C).

Paclitaxel should be dispensed in either glass or Excel™/PAB™ containers. Should also use **nonpolyvinyl** (non-PVC) tubing (eg, polyethylene) to minimize leaching. Formulated in a vehicle known as Cremophor® EL (polyoxyethylated castor oil). Cremophor® EL has been found to leach the plasticizer DEHP from polyvinyl chloride infusion bags or administration sets. Contact of the undiluted concentrate with plasticized polyvinyl chloride (PVC) equipment or devices is not recommended. Administer through I.V. tubing containing an in-line (NOT >0.22 μ) filter; administration through IVEX-2® filters (which incorporate short inlet and outlet polyvinyl chloride-coated tubing) has not resulted in significant leaching of DEHP.

Monitoring Parameters Monitor for hypersensitivity reactions

Administration

Anaphylactoid-like reactions have been reported: Corticosteroids (dexamethasone), H$_1$-antagonists (diphenhydramine), and H$_2$-antagonists (famotidine), should be administered prior to paclitaxel administration to minimize potential for anaphylaxis

Administer I.V. infusion over 1-24 hours; use of a 0.22 micron in-line filter and nonsorbing administration set is recommended during the infusion

Nonpolyvinyl (non-PVC) tubing (eg, polyethylene) should be used to minimize leaching. Formulated in a vehicle known as Cremophor® EL (polyoxyethylated castor oil). Cremophor® EL has been found to leach the plasticizer DEHP from polyvinyl chloride infusion bags or administration sets. Contact of the undiluted concentrate with plasticized polyvinyl chloride (PVC) equipment or devices is not recommended. Administer through I.V. tubing containing an in-line (NOT >0.22 μ) filter; administration through IVEX-2® filters (which incorporate short inlet and outlet polyvinyl chloride-coated tubing) has not resulted in significant leaching of DEHP.

Contraindications Hypersensitivity to paclitaxel, Cremophor® EL (polyoxyethylated castor oil), or any component of the formulation; pregnancy

Warnings

Hazardous agent – use appropriate precautions for handling and disposal. **[U.S. Boxed Warning]: Severe hypersensitivity reactions have been reported;** prolongation of the infusion (to ≥6 hours) plus premedication may minimize this effect. Stop infusion and do not rechallenge for severe hypersensitivity reactions (hypotension requiring treatment, dyspnea requiring bronchodilators, angioedema, urticaria). Minor hypersensitivity reactions (flushing, skin reactions, dyspnea, hypotension, or tachycardia) do not require interruption of treatment. **[U.S. Boxed Warning]: Bone marrow suppression is the dose-limiting toxicity; do not administer if baseline absolute neutrophil count (ANC) is** <1500 cells/mm^3 (<1000 cells/mm^3 **for patients with AIDS-related KS);** reduce future doses by 20% for severe neutropenia (<500 cells/mm^3 for 7 days or more) and consider the use of supportive therapy, including growth factor treatment.

Use extreme caution with hepatic dysfunction (myelotoxicity may be worsened); dose reductions are recommended. Peripheral neuropathy may occur; patients with pre-existing neuropathies from chemotherapy or coexisting conditions (eg, diabetes mellitus) may be at a higher risk; reduce dose by 20% for severe neuropathy. Paclitaxel formulations contain dehydrated alcohol; may cause adverse CNS effects. Hypotension, bradycardia, and hypertension may occur; frequent monitoring of vital signs is recommended, especially during the first hour of the infusion. Rare but severe conduction abnormalities have been reported; conduct cardiac monitoring during subsequent infusions for these patients. When administered as sequential infusions, taxane derivatives (docetaxel, paclitaxel) should be administered before platinum derivatives (carboplatin, cisplatin) to limit myelosuppression. Elderly patients have an increased risk of toxicity (neutropenia, neuropathy). **[U.S. Boxed Warning]: Should be administered under the supervision of an experienced cancer chemotherapy physician.** Safety and efficacy in children have not been established.

Dosage Forms Injection, solution: 6 mg/mL (5 mL, 16.7 mL, 25 mL, 50 mL) [contains alcohol and purified Cremophor® EL (polyoxyethylated castor oil)]
Onxol™: 6 mg/mL (5 mL, 25 mL, 50 mL) [contains alcohol and purified Cremophor® EL (polyoxyethylated castor oil)]
Taxol®: 6 mg/mL (5 mL, 16.7 mL, 50 mL) [contains alcohol and purified Cremophor® EL (polyoxyethylated castor oil)]

Reference Range

Mean maximum serum concentrations: 435-802 ng/mL following 24-hour infusions of 200-275 mg/m^2 and were approximately 10% to 30% of those following 6-hour infusions of equivalent doses; not detected in cerebrospinal fluid

Overdosage/Treatment Supportive therapy: Amitriptyline may be helpful for neuropathy; epinephrine, crystalloid fluids, diphenhydramine (25-50 mg in adults) and methylprednisolone (125 mg in adults) should be given for anaphylaxis; high-dose corticosteroids can be given to treat pneumonitis; corticosteroids should be given for myositis; pulmonary infiltrates can be treated with steroids. Oral glutamine suspension as a swish and swallow, starting on day 7 every 4 hours around-the-clock for a total dose of 24 g daily, is effective in preventing oral mucositis; gabapentin can be used to treat myalgia. Atropine can be given for bradycardia.

Test Interactions ↑ serum triglyceride; minor increase of renal function or liver function tests

Drug Interactions Substrate (major) of CYP2C8, 2C9, 3A4; **Induces** CYP3A4 (weak)
Carboplatin, cisplatin (platinum derivatives): When administered as sequential infusions, taxane derivatives should be administered before platinum derivatives to limit myelosuppression and to enhance efficacy.
CYP2C8 inducers: May decrease the levels/effects of paclitaxel. Example inducers include carbamazepine, phenobarbital, phenytoin, rifampin, rifapentine, and secobarbital.
CYP2C9 inducers: May decrease the levels/effects of paclitaxel. Example inducers include carbamazepine, phenobarbital, phenytoin, rifampin, rifapentine, and secobarbital.
CYP2C8 Inhibitors may increase the levels/effects of paclitaxel. Example inhibitors include atazanavir, gemfibrozil, and ritonavir.
CYP2C9 Inhibitors may increase the levels/effects of paclitaxel. Example inhibitors include delavirdine, fluconazole, gemfibrozil, ketoconazole, nicardipine, NSAIDs, sulfonamides and tolbutamide.
CYP3A4 inducers: CYP3A4 inducers may decrease the levels/effects of paclitaxel. Example inducers include aminoglutethimide, carbamazepine, nafcillin, nevirapine, phenobarbital, phenytoin, and rifamycins.
CYP3A4 inhibitors: May increase the levels/effects of paclitaxel. Example inhibitors include azole antifungals, clarithromycin, diclofenac, doxycycline, erythromycin, imatinib, isoniazid, nefazodone, nicardipine, propofol, protease inhibitors, quinidine, telithromycin, and verapamil.
Doxorubicin: Paclitaxel may increase doxorubicin levels/toxicity.

Pregnancy Risk Factor D; Enters breast milk/contraindicated, antineoplastic agents are generally contraindicated.

Pregnancy Implications Teratogenic effects have been observed in animal studies; women of childbearing potential should be advised to avoid becoming pregnant

Lactation Excretion in breast milk unknown/contraindicated

Additional Information Skin necrosis can occur with subcutaneous extravasation. Products contain ethanol as a vehicle, which has caused intoxication in high-dose regimens.

Specific References

Beri R, Rosen FR, Pacini MJ, et al, "Severe Dermatologic Reactions at Multiple Sites After Paclitaxel Administration," *Ann Pharmacother*, 2004, 38(2):238-41.
The ICON and AGO Collaborators, "Paclitaxel Plus Platinum-Based Chemotherapy Versus Conventional Platinum-Based Chemotherapy in Women with Relapsed Ovarian Cancer: The ICON4/AGO-OVAR-2.2 Trial," *Lancet*, 2003, 361(9375):2099-106.

Pamidronate

CAS Number 109552-15-0; 40391-99-9

U.S. Brand Names Aredia®

Synonyms Pamidronate Disodium

Use Treatment of hypercalcemia associated with malignancy; treatment of osteolytic bone lesions associated with multiple myeloma or metastatic breast cancer; moderate to severe Paget's disease of bone

Unlabeled/Investigational Use Treatment of pediatric osteoporosis, treatment of osteogenesis imperfecta

Mechanism of Action Inhibits osteoclastic bone resorption of calcium

Adverse Reactions

As reported with hypercalcemia of malignancy; percentage of adverse effect varies upon dose and duration of infusion.
Cardiovascular: Atrial fibrillation, hypertension, syncope, tachycardia, atrial flutter, cardiac failure, hypotension
Central nervous system: **Fever, fatigue**, somnolence, psychosis, insomnia
Dermatologic: Angioedema

Endocrine & metabolic: **Hypophosphatemia** (9% to 18%), **hypokalemia** (4% to 18%), **hypomagnesemia** (4% to 12%), **hypocalcemia** (1% to 12%), hypothyroidism

Gastrointestinal: **Nausea, anorexia** (1% to 12%), constipation, stomatitis

Hematologic: Leukopenia, neutropenia, thrombocytopenia

Local: **Infusion site reaction**

Neuromuscular & skeletal: Myalgia, osteonecrosis (primarily jaws)

Ocular: Iritis, episcleritis, scleritis, uveitis

Renal: Uremia

Respiratory: Rales, rhinitis, upper respiratory tract infection, dyspnea

Miscellaneous: Allergic reactions, anaphylactic shock

Signs and Symptoms of Overdose Fever, hypocalcemia, hypokalemia, hypomagnesemia, hypophosphatemia, hypotension, taste perversion

Pharmacodynamics/Kinetics

Onset of action: 24-48 hours

  Peak effect: Maximum: 5-7 days

Absorption: Poor; pharmacokinetic studies lacking

Metabolism: Not metabolized

Half-life elimination: 21-35 hours

Excretion: Biphasic; urine ($\sim$50% as unchanged drug) within 120 hours

Dosage

Drug must be diluted properly before administration and infused intravenously slowly. Due to risk of nephrotoxicity, doses should not exceed 90 mg. I.V.: Adults:

Hypercalcemia of malignancy:

Moderate cancer-related hypercalcemia (corrected serum calcium: 12-13.5 mg/dL): 60-90 mg, as a single dose, given as a slow infusion over 2-24 hours; dose should be diluted in 1000 mL 0.45% NaCl, 0.9% NaCl, or D_5W

Severe cancer-related hypercalcemia (corrected serum calcium: >13.5 mg/dL): 90 mg, as a single dose, as a slow infusion over 2-24 hours; dose should be diluted in 1000 mL 0.45% NaCl, 0.9% NaCl, or D_5W

A period of 7 days should elapse before the use of second course; repeat infusions every 2-3 weeks have been suggested, however, could be administered every 2-3 months according to the degree and of severity of hypercalcemia and/or the type of malignancy.

Note: Some investigators have suggested a lack of a dose-response relationship. Courses of pamidronate for hypercalcemia may be repeated at varying intervals, depending on the duration of normocalcemia (median 2-3 weeks), but the manufacturer recommends a minimum interval between courses of 7 days. Oral etidronate at a dose of 20 mg/kg/day has been used to maintain the calcium lowering effect following I.V. bisphosphonates, although it is of limited effectiveness.

Osteolytic bone lesions with multiple myeloma: 90 mg in 500 mL D_5W, 0.45% NaCl or 0.9% NaCl administered over 4 hours on a monthly basis

Osteolytic bone lesions with metastatic breast cancer: 90 mg in 250 mL D_5W, 0.45% NaCl or 0.9% NaCl administered over 2 hours, repeated every 3-4 weeks

Paget's disease: 30 mg in 500 mL 0.45% NaCl, 0.9% NaCl or D_5W administered over 4 hours for 3 consecutive days

Dosing adjustment in renal impairment: Not recommended in severe renal impairment (patients with bone metastases)

Dosing adjustment in renal toxicity: In patients with bone metastases, treatment should be withheld in patients who experience deterioration in renal function (increase of serum creatinine $\geq$0.5 mg/dL in patients with normal baseline or $\geq$1.0 mg/dL in patients with abnormal baseline). Resumption of therapy may be considered when serum creatinine returns to within 10% of baseline.

Monitoring Parameters Serum electrolytes, monitor for hypocalcemia for at least 2 weeks after therapy; serum calcium, phosphate, magnesium, potassium, CBC with differential; monitor serum creatinine prior to each dose

Administration Administer in 0.5-1 L of normal saline or 5% dextrose; do not use Ringer's lactate. Drug must be properly diluted before administration and slowly infused intravenously (over at least 2 hours).

Contraindications Hypersensitivity to pamidronate, other bisphosphonates, or any component of the formulation; pregnancy

Warnings

Bisphosphonate therapy has been associated with osteonecrosis, primarily of the jaw; this has been observed mostly in cancer patients, but also in patients with postmenopausal osteoporosis and other diagnoses. Risk factors include a diagnosis of cancer, with concomitant chemotherapy, radiotherapy or corticosteroids; anemia, coagulopathy, infection or pre-existing dental disease. Symptoms included nonhealing extraction socket or an exposed jawbone. There are no data addressing whether discontinuation of therapy reduces the risk of developing osteonecrosis. However, as a precautionary measure, dental exams and preventative dentistry should be performed prior to placing patients with risk factors on chronic bisphosphonate therapy. Invasive dental procedures should be avoided during treatment.

Infrequently, severe (and occasionally debilitating) bone, joint, and/or muscle pain have been reported during bisphosphonate treatment. The onset of pain ranged from a single day to several months. Symptoms usually resolve upon discontinuation. Some patients experienced recurrence when rechallenged with same drug or another bisphosphonate; avoid use in patients with a history of these symptoms in association with bisphosphonate therapy.

May cause deterioration in renal function. Use caution in patients with renal impairment and avoid in severe renal impairment. Assess serum creatinine prior to each dose; withhold dose in patients with bone metastases who experience deterioration in renal function. Leukopenia has been observed with oral pamidronate and monitoring of white blood cell counts is suggested. Patients with pre-existing anemia, leukopenia, or thrombocytopenia should be closely monitored during the first 2 weeks of treatment.

Vein irritation and thrombophlebitis may occur with infusions. Monitor serum electrolytes, especially in the elderly.

Dosage Forms Injection, powder for reconstitution, as disodium: 30 mg, 90 mg

  Aredia®: 30 mg, 90 mg

Injection, solution: 3 mg/mL (10 mL); 6 mg/mL (10 mL); 9 mg/mL (10 mL)

Reference Range Calcium (total): Adults: 9.0-11.0 mg/dL (SI: 2.05-2.54 mM/L), may slightly decrease with aging; phosphorus: 2.5-4.5 mg/dL (SI: 0.81-1.45 mM/L)

Overdosage/Treatment Supportive therapy: Monitor for hypocalcemia; in one report (supplied by the drug company), fever and hypotension were corrected with use of steroids, but no formal studies could be found

Test Interactions $\downarrow$ calcium (S), phosphate

Drug Interactions Aminoglycosides: May lower serum calcium levels with prolonged administration. Concomitant use may have an additive hypocalcemic effect.

Antacids: May decrease the absorption of bisphosphonate derivatives; should be administered at a different time of the day. Antacids containing aluminum, calcium, or magnesium are of specific concern.

Calcium salts: May decrease the absorption of bisphosphonate derivatives. Separate oral dosing in order to minimize risk of interaction.

Iron salts: May decrease the absorption of bisphosphonate derivatives. Only oral iron salts and oral bisphosphonates are of concern.

Magnesium salts: May decrease the absorption of bisphosphonate derivatives. Only oral magnesium salts and oral bisphosphonates are of concern.

Nonsteroidal anti-inflammatory drugs (NSAIDs): May enhance the gastrointestinal adverse/toxic effects (increased incidence of GI ulcers) of bisphosphonate derivatives.

Phosphate supplements: Bisphosphonate derivatives may enhance the hypocalcemic effect of phosphate supplements.

Pregnancy Risk Factor C

Pregnancy Implications Pamidronate has been shown to cross the placenta and cause nonteratogenic embryo/fetal effects in animals. There are no adequate and well-controlled studies in pregnant women; manufacturer states pamidronate should not be used in pregnancy. Based on limited case reports, serum calcium levels in the newborn may be altered if pamidronate is administered during pregnancy. Bisphosphonates are incorporated into the bone matrix and gradually released over time. Theoretically, there may be a risk of fetal harm when pregnancy follows the completion of therapy.

Lactation Excretion in breast milk unknown/use caution

Additional Information Pamidronic acid causes severe bone pain in cystic fibrosis.

Specific References

Fraunfelder FW and Fraunfelder FT, "Bisphosphonates and Ocular Inflammation," *N Engl J Med*, 2003, 348(12):1187-8.

French AE, Kaplan N, Lishner M, et al, "Taking Bisphosphonates During Pregnancy," *Can Fam Physician*, 2003, 49:1281-2.

Whyte MP, Wenkert D, Clements KL, et al, "Bisphosphonate-Induced Osteopetrosis," *N Engl J Med*, 2003, 349(5):457-63.

Papaverine

CAS Number 32808-09-6; 39024-96-9; 58-74-2; 61-25-6

U.S. Brand Names Para-Time S.R.®

Synonyms Papaverine Hydrochloride; Pavabid [DSC]

Use Relief of peripheral and cerebral ischemia associated with arterial spasm

Unlabeled/Investigational Use Investigational: Parenteral: Various vascular spasms associated with muscle spasms as in myocardial infarction, angina, peripheral and pulmonary embolism, peripheral vascular disease, angiospastic states, and visceral spasm (ureteral, biliary, and GI colic); testing for impotence

Mechanism of Action Smooth muscle spasmolytic producing a generalized smooth muscle relaxation including vasodilatation, gastrointestinal sphincter relaxation, bronchiolar muscle relaxation and potentially a depressed myocardium; it is an inhibition of cellular respiration and phosphodiesterase along with being a calcium antagonist (inhibits uptake of adenosine)

Adverse Reactions

Cardiovascular: Flushing of the face, tachycardia, hypotension, cardiac arrhythmias with rapid I.V. use consisting of AV block, premature ventricular contraction, sinus tachycardia, arrhythmias (ventricular), vasodilation

Central nervous system: Depression, dizziness, drowsiness, sedation, headache

Dermatologic: Pruritus

Gastrointestinal: Xerostomia, nausea, constipation, vomiting, abdominal pain

Genitourinary: Priapism with intracavernous injection

Hematologic: Eosinophilia

Hepatic: Hepatic hypersensitivity, cirrhosis

Local: Thrombosis at the I.V. administration site

Respiratory: Apnea with rapid I.V. use

Miscellaneous: Diaphoresis

Signs and Symptoms of Overdose Asthenia, AV block, constipation, coma, diplopia, drowsiness, hyperglycemia, hypokalemia, lactic acidosis, liver damage, mydriasis, penile fibrosis, respiratory alkalosis

Pharmacodynamics/Kinetics

Onset of action: Oral: Rapid

Protein binding: 90%

Metabolism: Rapidly hepatic

Half-life elimination: 0.5-1.5 hours

Excretion: Primarily urine (as metabolites)

Dosage Children: I.M., I.V.: 1.5 mg/kg 4 times/day

Adults:

Oral: 100-300 mg 3-5 times/day

Oral, sustained release: 150-300 mg every 12 hours

I.M., I.V.: 30-120 mg every 3 hours as needed

Stability Protect from heat or freezing; not do refrigerate injection; solutions should be clear to pale yellow; precipitates with lactated Ringer's; **incompatible** with bromides and iodides

Administration Rapid I.V. administration may result in arrhythmias and fatal apnea; administer no faster than over 1-2 minutes.

Contraindications Hypersensitivity to papaverine or any component of the formulation

Warnings Use with caution in patients with glaucoma; administer I.V. cautiously since apnea and arrhythmias may result; may, in large doses, depress AV and intraventricular cardiac conduction leading to serious arrhythmias (eg, premature beats, paroxysmal tachycardia); chronic hepatitis noted with jaundice, eosinophilia, and abnormal LFTs

Dosage Forms Capsule, sustained release, as hydrochloride: 150 mg

Para-Time SR®: 150 mg

Injection, solution, as hydrochloride: 30 mg/mL (2 mL, 10 mL)

Reference Range Peak plasma papaverine level of 1 mg/L noted after 1 mg/kg intravenous dose

Overdosage/Treatment

Decontamination: Ipecac (within 30 minutes)/activated charcoal is useful

Supportive therapy: Lorazepam or diazepam 10-20 mg (0.25-0.4 mg/kg for children) is helpful for seizures; I.V. fluids and alpha-adrenergic pressors should be used for hypotension; sodium bicarbonate (1 mEq/kg) is useful to treat acidosis; calcium gluconate (10% I.V. solution; 0.2-0.5 mL/kg/dose up to 10 mL/dose over 5-10 minutes) can be used to treat hypotension or heart block; dopamine can also be used to treat hypotension while atropine, isoproterenol and/or glucagon can be used for heart block

Enhanced elimination: Multiple dosing of activated charcoal may be useful

Drug Interactions Decreased effect: Papaverine decreases the effects of levodopa

Increased toxicity: Additive effects with CNS depressants

Pregnancy Risk Factor C

Lactation Excretion in breast milk unknown/not recommended

Nursing Implications Rapid I.V. administration may result in arrhythmias and fatal apnea

Additional Information Therapeutic value is lacking

Specific References

Perk G, Hanna S, and Stalnikowicz R, "Lethal Oral Papaverine Overdose," *Am J Emerg Med*, 2003, 21(3):245.

Para-Aminosalicylate Sodium

CAS Number 133-10-8; 6018-19-5

Synonyms Aminosalicylate Sodium; PAS

Use Adjunctive treatment of tuberculosis

Adverse Reactions

Cardiovascular: Myocardial depression, congestive heart failure, sinus tachycardia

Central nervous system: Mania

Dermatologic: Alopecia, lichen planus

Endocrine & metabolic: Hypokalemia

Gastrointestinal: Nausea, vomiting, diarrhea

Hepatic: Hepatitis, jaundice

Miscellaneous: Allergy, mononucleosis-like syndrome

Pharmacodynamics/Kinetics

Absorption: Readily

Distribution: Widely distributed but appears in CSF only within inflamed meninges

Protein binding: 60% to 70%

Metabolism: Intestinal and liver

Half-life, elimination: ≈1 hour

Peak concentrations: Within 1-4 hours

Elimination: Primarily in urine within 12 hours

Dosage

Oral:

Children: 240-360 mg/kg/day in 3-4 divided doses

Adults: 12-15 g/day in 3-4 divided doses

Contraindications Known hypersensitivity to para-aminosalicylate

Warnings Avoid use in patients with hepatic or renal dysfunction, gastric bleeding disorders

Dosage Forms Tablet: 500 mg

Reference Range Inhibition of *Mycobacterium* tuberculosis at a level of 1 mcg/mL

Overdosage/Treatment

Decontamination: Lavage (within 1 hour)/activated charcoal

Enhancement of elimination: Multiple dosing of activated charcoal may be effective

Test Interactions Urine glucose

Drug Interactions Interferes with rifampin absorption; displaces phenytoin from albumin thus raising free phenytoin levels; probenecid can increase serum concentration

Pregnancy Risk Factor C

Additional Information Capsules contain bentonite which may decrease absorption of concomitantly ingested drugs.

Paraldehyde

Related Information

● Seizures, Neonatal Guidelines

CAS Number 123-63-7

UN Number 1264

U.S. Brand Names Paral®

Synonyms Paracetaldehyde

Impairment Potential Yes

Use Cyclic acetaldehyde trimer which is utilized as a treatment of status epilepticus and tetanus-induced seizures; has been used as a sedative/hypnotic, no longer used in the treatment of alcohol withdrawal symptoms

Mechanism of Action Unknown mechanism of action; causes depression of CNS, including the ascending reticular activating system to provide sedation/hypnosis and anticonvulsant activity

Adverse Reactions

Cardiovascular: Cardiovascular collapse, tachycardia, sinus bradycardia, sinus tachycardia

Central nervous system: **Drowsiness**, clumsiness, dizziness, "hangover effect"

Dermatologic: **Skin rash**

Endocrine & metabolic: Metabolic acidosis

Gastrointestinal: **Strong and unpleasant breath**, abdominal pain, **nausea, vomiting, stomach pain**, **irritation of mucous membrane**

Hematologic: Leukocytosis, porphyrinogenic

Hepatic: Hepatitis

Local: Thrombophlebitis

Renal: Acidosis (renal tubular), albuminuria, acute tubular necrosis

Respiratory: **Coughing**, respiratory depression, pulmonary edema, laryngeal spasm

Miscellaneous: Psychological and physical dependence with prolonged use

Signs and Symptoms of Overdose Acetone breath, coma (may last >30 hours), confusion, cough (seen early in the course of toxicity), dyspnea, feces discoloration (black), hemorrhagic gastritis, hyperventilation, mental confusion, metabolic acidosis, mild hypotension, myasthenia gravis (exacerbation or precipitation), pulmonary edema, pulmonary hemorrhage, renal failure, respiratory depression, stomatitis, tachypnea. Death has occurred with as little as 12-25 mL, usually due to pulmonary edema.

Pharmacodynamics/Kinetics

Onset of hypnosis:

Oral: Within 10-15 minutes

I.M.: Within 2-3 minutes

Duration: 6-8 hours

Distribution: Crosses the placenta

Metabolism: ≈70% to 80% of a dose metabolized in the liver

Half-life: Adults: 3.5-10 hours

Elimination: Up to 30% excreted as unchanged drug in expired air via the lungs; trace amounts excreted in urine unchanged

Dosage Oral: Sedation:
Children: 0.15-0.3 mL/kg
Adults: 4-8 mL

I.M., I.V.: I.V. use is rare and should be diluted (4% to 5% solution): 0.1-0.3 mL/kg

Rectal:
Children: 0.3 mL/kg to a maximum dose of 5 mL
Adults: 4-8 mL diluted with sodium chloride

Stability Decomposes with exposure to air and light to acetaldehyde which then oxidizes to acetic acid; store in tightly closed containers; protect from light

Administration Oral: Dilute in milk or iced fruit juice
Rectal: Mix paraldehyde 2:1 with oil (cottonseed or olive)
Do **not** use any plastic equipment for administration, use glass syringes and rubber tubing

Contraindications Hypersensitivity to paraldehyde or any component of the formulation; severe hepatic insufficiency; respiratory disease; GI inflammation or ulceration; concurrent disulfiram

Warnings Use with caution in patients with asthma or other bronchopulmonary disease; do not abruptly discontinue in patients receiving chronic therapy

Dosage Forms Liquid, oral or rectal: 1 g/mL (30 mL)

Reference Range Antiseizure therapeutic blood level: 100-200 mg/L; toxic level: >270 mg/L; blood level approaching 500 mg/L associated with fatality

Overdosage/Treatment
Decontamination: Lavage (within 30 minutes)/activated charcoal; **do not** induce emesis
Supportive therapy: Treat acidosis with sodium bicarbonate; for hypotension, fluid challenge with isotonic saline or placement of patient in Trendelenburg position; vasopressors (dopamine or norepinephrine) can be used for refractory cases

Test Interactions Ketonuria may be present

Drug Interactions CNS depressants: Sedative effects and/or respiratory depression may be additive with CNS depressants; includes ethanol, barbiturates, narcotic analgesics, and other sedative agents; monitor for increased effect
Disulfiram: Concurrent use of paraldehyde and disulfiram produces a "disulfiram reaction," this combination is contraindicated

Pregnancy Risk Factor C

Nursing Implications Discard unused contents of any container which has been opened for more than 24 hours; do **not** use discolored solution; do **not** use any plastic equipment for administration; parenteral solution may be given orally; should be given in milk or iced fruit juice or dilute to 200 mL with saline

Additional Information Minimal lethal dose: Oral: 25 mL; I.V.: 35 mL; Rectal: 12 mL
Do not abruptly discontinue in patients receiving chronic therapy; decomposes to acetic aid in air; 4-8 mL of paraldehyde is equivalent to 30 mg of phenobarbital; was used for the treatment of delirium, tremors, but its use has been supplanted by benzodiazepines; odor of acetic acid indicates that decomposition has occurred; may be irritating to mucosa

Paramethadione

CAS Number 115-67-3

Use Control absence (petit mal) seizures refractory to other drugs

Mechanism of Action Elevates the cortical and basal seizure thresholds, and reduces the synaptic response to low frequency impulses; similar properties to troxidone

Adverse Reactions
Central nervous system: **Drowsiness, dizziness, sedation, headache**
Dermatologic: Exfoliative dermatitis, rash, photosensitivity
Gastrointestinal: Feces discoloration (black)
Hematologic: Agranulocytosis, aplastic anemia, thrombocytopenia, exacerbation of porphyria
Hepatic: Hepatitis
Neuromuscular & skeletal: Myasthenia gravis (exacerbation)
Ocular: **Photophobia, diplopia**, blurred vision, nystagmus
Renal: Nephrosis, proteinuria
Miscellaneous: Systemic lupus erythematosus

Signs and Symptoms of Overdose Agranulocytosis, ataxia, granulocytopenia, leukopenia, nausea, neutropenia, visual disturbances, vision color changes (white tinge)

Toxicodynamics/Kinetics
Absorption: Rapid from gastrointestinal tract
Distribution: Widely throughout the body
Protein binding: Insignificant
Metabolism: Hepatic metabolism via microsomal enzymes
Half-life: 12-24 hours
Elimination: Slow renal excretion (primarily as active metabolites)

Dosage
Oral:
Children: 300-900 mg/day in 3-4 equally divided doses
Adults: Initial: 900 mg/day in 3-4 equally divided doses, increase by 300 mg at weekly intervals to maximum of 2.4 g/day

Dosing adjustment in renal/hepatic impairment: Avoid use in patients with Cl_{cr} <10 mL/minute or with severe liver disease

Reference Range Therapeutic: 5-50 mcg/mL

Overdosage/Treatment
Decontamination: Lavage (within 1 hour)/activated charcoal is useful. Consider gastric decontamination for ingestions >1 g.
Enhanced elimination: Alkalinization of the urine increases elimination of the active metabolite; multiple dosing of activated charcoal may be useful

Test Interactions ↑ alkaline phosphatase (S); ↓ calcium (S), thyroxine (S)

Pregnancy Implications Associated with high incidence of congenital malformations, 4 times more hazardous than ethosuximide

Nursing Implications Raise side rails, institute safety measures, assist with ambulation

Additional Information Lethal dose: 5 g. Only supplied graduated dropper should be used to measure oral solution; clean, colorless liquid with aromatic odor

Paregoric

CAS Number 8029-99-0

Synonyms Camphorated Tincture of Opium (error-prone synonym)

Impairment Potential Yes

Use Treatment of diarrhea or relief of pain; neonatal opiate withdrawal (heroin or methadone-induced withdrawal seizures)

Mechanism of Action Increases smooth muscle tone in gastrointestinal tract, decreases motility and peristalsis, diminishes digestive secretions

Adverse Reactions
Cardiovascular: **Hypotension**, bradycardia, vasodilation, sinus bradycardia
Central nervous system: **Drowsiness, dizziness**, CNS depression, increased intracranial pressure, agitation, sedation
Endocrine & metabolic: Syndrome of inappropriate antidiuretic hormone
Gastrointestinal: **Constipation**, nausea, vomiting, biliary tract spasm
Genitourinary: Urinary retention, ADH release, urinary tract spasm
Neuromuscular & skeletal: **Weakness**
Ocular: Miosis
Respiratory: Apnea, respiratory depression
Miscellaneous: Physical and psychological dependence, histamine release

Pharmacodynamics/Kinetics
In terms of opium:
Metabolism: Hepatic
Excretion: Urine (primarily as morphine glucuronide conjugates and unchanged drug - morphine, codeine, papaverine, etc)

Dosage
Oral:
Neonatal opiate withdrawal: 3-6 drops every 3-6 hours as needed, or initially 0.2 mL every 3 hours; increase dosage by approximately 0.05 mL every 3 hours until withdrawal symptoms are controlled; it is rare to exceed 0.7 mL/dose. Stabilize withdrawal symptoms for 3-5 days, then gradually decrease dosage over a 2- to 4-week period.
Children: 0.25-0.5 mL/kg 1-4 times/day
Adults: 5-10 mL 1-4 times/day

Stability Store in light-resistant, tightly closed container

Contraindications Hypersensitivity to opium or any component of the formulation; diarrhea caused by poisoning until the toxic material has been removed; pregnancy (prolonged use or high doses)

Warnings Use with caution in patients with respiratory, hepatic or renal dysfunction, severe prostatic hyperplasia, or history of narcotic abuse; opium shares the toxic potential of opiate agonists, and usual precautions of opiate agonist therapy should be observed; some preparations contain sulfites which may cause allergic reactions; infants <3 months of age are more susceptible to respiratory depression, use with caution and generally in reduced doses in this age group; tolerance or drug dependence may result from extended use

Dosage Forms Liquid, oral: Morphine equivalent 2 mg/5 mL (473 mL) [equivalent to opium 20 mg powder; contains alcohol 45% and benzoic acid]

Overdosage/Treatment Supportive therapy: Naloxone hydrochloride (0.4-2 mg I.V., SubQ, or through an endotracheal tube); a continuous infusion (at $^2/_3$ the response dose/hour) may be required

Antidote(s)
● Naloxone [ANTIDOTE]

Test Interactions ↑ aminotransferases (ALT, AST) (S)

Drug Interactions Increased effect/toxicity with CNS depressants (eg, alcohol, narcotics, benzodiazepines, TCAs, MAO inhibitors, phenothiazine)

Pregnancy Risk Factor B/D (prolonged use or high doses)

Lactation Enters breast milk/use caution

Nursing Implications Observe patient for excessive sedation, respiratory depression, implement safety measures, assist with ambulation

Additional Information Contains morphine 0.4 mg/mL and alcohol 45%

Paroxetine

Related Information
- Antidepressant Agents

CAS Number 61869-08-7; 78246-49-8

U.S. Brand Names Paxil CR™; Paxil®; Pexeva™

Synonyms Paroxetine Hydrochloride; Paroxetine Mesylate

Impairment Potential Yes

Use
Treatment of depression in adults; treatment of panic disorder with or without agoraphobia; obsessive-compulsive disorder (OCD) in adults; social anxiety disorder (social phobia); generalized anxiety disorder (GAD); post-traumatic stress disorder (PTSD)

Paxil CR™: Treatment of depression; panic disorder; premenstrual dysphoric disorder (PMDD), social anxiety disorder (social phobia)

Unlabeled/Investigational Use May be useful in eating disorders, impulse control disorders, self-injurious behavior; premenstrual disorders, vasomotor symptoms of menopause; treatment of depression and obsessive-compulsive disorder (OCD) in children

Mechanism of Action Paroxetine is a selective serotonin reuptake inhibitor (similar to fluvoxamine maleate), chemically unrelated to tricyclic, tetracyclic, or other antidepressants; presumably, the inhibition of serotonin reuptake from brain synapse stimulated serotonin activity in the brain; a phenylpiperidine derivative

Adverse Reactions
Cardiovascular: Bradycardia, hypotension, palpitations, vasodilation, hypotension (orthostatic), sinus bradycardia, sinus tachycardia, atrial fibrillation, bradycardia, bundle branch block, torsade de pointes, ventricular fibrillation, ventricular tachycardia

Central nervous system: **Headache, somnolence, dizziness, insomnia**, nervousness, anxiety, exacerbation of parkinsonism, extrapyramidal reaction, akathisia, electroencephalogram abnormalities, exacerbation of migraine headaches, fever, hyperthermia, somnambulism, mania, eclampsia, Guillain-Barré syndrome, neuroleptic malignant syndrome, seizures (including status epilepticus), dysphasia, agitation

Dermatologic: Alopecia, toxic epidermal necrolysis, acne, angioedema, xerosis, urticaria, purpura, photosensitivity, ecchymoses, erythema nodosum, exanthem, cutaneous vasculitis, erythema multiforme, exfoliative dermatitis

Endocrine & metabolic: Amenorrhea, syndrome of inappropriate antidiuretic hormone secretion leading to hyponatremia, serotonin syndrome, decreased libido, hyperglycemia, galactorrhea

Gastrointestinal: **Constipation, diarrhea, nausea, xerostomia**, anorexia, flatulence, vomiting, gastritis, aphthous stomatitis, stomatitis, colitis, dysphagia, pancreatitis

Genitourinary: **Ejaculatory disturbances**, priapism, scrotal pruritus

Hematologic: Granulocytopenia, anemia, leukopenia, neutropenia, agranulocytosis, aplastic anemia, bone marrow aplasia, hemolytic anemia, pancytopenia, porphyria, thrombocytopenia

Hepatic: Reversible elevation of liver enzymes, acute renal failure, hepatic necrosis

Neuromuscular & skeletal: **Weakness**, arthritis, tremors, paresthesia, clonus, myoclonus, chorea, akinesia, myasthenia

Ocular: Eye pain, acute angle-closure glaucoma, aggravation of glaucoma, optic neuritis, blurred vision

Otic: Ear pain

Respiratory: Asthma, rhinitis, allergic alveolitis, laryngospasm, pulmonary hypertension

Miscellaneous: **Diaphoresis**, bruxism, thirst, restless legs syndrome, withdrawal reactions (dizziness, sensory disturbances [eg, paresthesias such as electric shock sensations; agitation; anxiety; nausea; diaphoresis] particularly following abrupt withdrawal), anaphylactoid reaction

Signs and Symptoms of Overdose Anxiety, confusion, diarrhea, dyspepsia, ejaculatory disturbances, extrapyramidal reaction, fatigue, hyponatremia, hypotension, insomnia, priapism, tachycardia, urinary frequency

Admission Criteria/Prognosis Admit pediatric ingestions >120 mg

Pharmacodynamics/Kinetics
Absorption: Completely absorbed following oral administration

Distribution: V_d: 8.7 L/kg (3-28 L/kg)

Protein binding: 93% to 95%

Metabolism: Extensively hepatic via CYP enzymes via oxidation and methylation; nonlinear pharmacokinetics may be seen with higher doses and longer duration of therapy. Saturation of CYP2D6 appears to account for the nonlinearity. C_{min} concentrations 70% to 80% greater in the elderly compared to nonelderly patients; clearance is also decreased.

Half-life elimination: 21 hours (3-65 hours)

Time to peak, serum: Immediate release: 5.2 hours; controlled release: 6-10 hours

Excretion: Urine (64%, 2% as unchanged drug); feces (36% primarily via bile)

Dosage Oral:

Children:
Depression (unlabeled use; not recommended by FDA): Initial: 10 mg/day and adjusted upward on an individual basis to 20 mg/day

OCD (unlabeled use): Initial: 10 mg/day and titrate up as necessary to 60 mg/day

Self-injurious behavior (unlabeled use): 20 mg/day

Social phobia (unlabeled use): 2.5-15 mg/day

Adults:
Depression:
Paxil®, Pexeva™: Initial: 20 mg once daily, preferably in the morning; increase if needed by 10 mg/day increments at intervals of at least 1 week; maximum dose: 50 mg/day

Paxil CR™: Initial: 25 mg once daily; increase if needed by 12.5 mg/day increments at intervals of at least 1 week; maximum dose: 62.5 mg/day

GAD (Paxil®): Initial: 20 mg once daily, preferably in the morning; doses of 20-50 mg/day were used in clinical trials, however, no greater benefit was seen with doses >20 mg. If dose is increased, adjust in increments of 10 mg/day at 1-week intervals.

OCD (Paxil®, Pexeva™): Initial: 20 mg once daily, preferably in the morning; increase if needed by 10 mg/day increments at intervals of at least 1 week; recommended dose: 40 mg/day; range: 20-60 mg/day; maximum dose: 60 mg/day

Panic disorder:
Paxil®, Pexeva™: Initial: 10 mg once daily, preferably in the morning; increase if needed by 10 mg/day increments at intervals of at least 1 week; recommended dose: 40 mg/day; range: 10-60 mg/day; maximum dose: 60 mg/day

Paxil CR™: Initial: 12.5 mg once daily; increase if needed by 12.5 mg/day at intervals of at least 1 week; maximum dose: 75 mg/day

PMDD (Paxil CR™): Initial: 12.5 mg once daily in the morning; may be increased to 25 mg/day; dosing changes should occur at intervals of at least 1 week. May be given daily throughout the menstrual cycle or limited to the luteal phase.

PTSD (Paxil®): Initial: 20 mg once daily, preferably in the morning; increase if needed by 10 mg/day increments at intervals of at least 1 week; range: 20-50 mg

Social anxiety disorder:
Paxil®: Initial: 20 mg once daily, preferably in the morning; recommended dose: 20 mg/day; range: 20-60 mg/day; doses >20 mg may not have additional benefit

Paxil CR™: Initial: 12.5 mg once daily, preferably in the morning; may be increased by 12.5 mg/day at intervals of at least 1 week; maximum dose: 37.5 mg/day

Vasomotor symptoms of menopause (unlabeled use, Paxil CR™): 12.5-25 mg/day

Elderly: C_{min} concentrations 70% to 80% greater in the elderly compared to nonelderly patients; clearance is also decreased.
Paxil®, Pexeva™: Initial: 10 mg/day; increase if needed by 10 mg/day increments at intervals of at least 1 week; maximum dose: 40 mg/day

Paxil CR™: Initial: 12.5 mg/day; increase if needed by 12.5 mg/day increments at intervals of at least 1 week; maximum dose: 50 mg/day

Note: Upon discontinuation of paroxetine therapy, gradually taper dose:
Paxil®: Taper-phase regimen used in PTSD/GAD clinical trials involved an incremental decrease in the daily dose by 10 mg/day at weekly intervals; when 20 mg/day dose was reached, this dose was continued for 1 week before treatment was discontinued.

Paxil CR™: Patients receiving 37.5 mg/day in clinical trials had their dose decreased by 12.5 mg/day to a dose of 25 mg/day and remained at a dose of 25 mg/day for 1 week before treatment was discontinued.

Dosage adjustment in severe renal/hepatic impairment: Adults:
Cl_{cr} <30 mL/minute: Mean plasma concentration is ~4 times that seen in normal function.

Cl_{cr} 30-60 mL/minute and hepatic dysfunction: Plasma concentration is 2 times that seen in normal function.

Paxil®, Pexeva™: Initial: 10 mg/day; increase if needed by 10 mg/day increments at intervals of at least 1 week; maximum dose: 40 mg/day

Paxil CR™: Initial: 12.5 mg/day; increase if needed by 12.5 mg/day increments at intervals of at least 1 week; maximum dose: 50 mg/day

Monitoring Parameters Mental status for depression, suicidal ideation (especially at the beginning of therapy or when doses are increased or decreased), anxiety, social functioning, mania, panic attacks; akathisia

Administration May be administered with or without food. Do not crush, break, or chew controlled release tablets.

Contraindications Hypersensitivity to paroxetine or any component of the formulation; use of MAO inhibitors or within 14 days; concurrent use with thioridazine or pimozide

Warnings *Major psychiatric warnings:*

- **[U.S. Boxed Warning]: Antidepressants increase the risk of suicidal thinking and behavior in children and adolescents with major depressive disorder (MDD) and other depressive disorders;** consider risk prior to prescribing. Closely monitor for clinical worsening, suicidality, or unusual changes in behavior; the child's family or caregiver should be instructed to closely observe the patient and communicate condition with healthcare provider. A medication guide concerning the use of antidepressants in children and teenagers should be dispensed with each prescription. **Paroxetine is not FDA approved for use in children.**
- A higher incidence of suicidal behaviors has been observed in young adults receiving paroxetine for both depressive and nondepressive indications.
- The possibility of a suicide attempt is inherent in major depression and may persist until remission occurs. Patients treated with antidepressants (for any indication) should be observed for clinical worsening and suicidality, especially during the initial few months of a course of drug therapy, or at times of dose changes, either increases or decreases. Worsening depression and severe abrupt suicidality that are not part of the presenting symptoms may require discontinuation or modification of drug therapy. Use caution in high-risk patients during initiation of therapy.
- Prescriptions should be written for the smallest quantity consistent with good patient care. The patient's family or caregiver should be alerted to monitor patients for the emergence of suicidality and associated behaviors such as anxiety, agitation, panic attacks, insomnia, irritability, hostility, impulsivity, akathisia, hypomania, and mania; patients should be instructed to notify their healthcare provider if any of these symptoms or worsening depression or psychosis occur.
- May worsen psychosis in some patients or precipitate a shift to mania or hypomania in patients with bipolar disorder. Monotherapy in patients with bipolar disorder should be avoided. Patients presenting with depressive symptoms should be screened for bipolar disorder. **Paroxetine is not FDA approved for the treatment of bipolar depression.**

Key adverse effects:

- Serotonin syndrome: Symptoms of agitation, confusion, hallucinations, hyperreflexia, myoclonus, shivering, and tachycardia may occur with concomitant proserotonergic drugs or agents which reduce paroxetine's metabolism. Concurrent use of serotonin precursors (eg, tryptophan) is not recommended.
- Akathisia: Inability to remain still due to feelings of agitation or restlessness has been observed with paroxetine and other SSRIs. Usually occurs within the first few weeks of therapy.
- Anticholinergic effects: Has low potential for sedation and anticholinergic effects relative to cyclic antidepressants; however among the SSRI class these effects are relatively higher.
- CNS depression: Has a low potential to impair cognitive or motor performance; caution operating hazardous machinery or driving.
- SIADH and hyponatremia: Has been associated with the development of SIADH; hyponatremia has been reported rarely, predominately in the elderly

Concurrent disease:

- Cardiovascular disease: Use caution in patients with cardiovascular disease; paroxetine has not been systemically evaluated in patients with a recent history of MI or unstable heart disease.
- Hepatic impairment: Use caution; clearance is decreased and plasma concentrations are increased; a lower dosage may be needed.
- Narrow-angle glaucoma: Associated with an increased risk of mydriasis in patients with controlled narrow angle glaucoma.
- Platelet aggregation: May impair platelet aggregation, resulting in bleeding.
- Renal impairment: Use caution; clearance is decreased and plasma concentrations are increased; a lower dosage may be needed.
- Seizure disorders: Use caution with a previous seizure disorder or condition predisposing to seizures such as brain damage or alcoholism.
- Sexual dysfunction: May cause or exacerbate sexual dysfunction.

Concurrent drug therapy:

- Agents which lower seizure threshold: Concurrent therapy with other drugs which lower the seizure threshold.
- Anticoagulants/Antiplatelets: Use caution with concomitant use of NSAIDs, ASA, or other drugs that affect coagulation; the risk of bleeding is potentiated.
- CNS depressants: Use caution with concomitant therapy.
- MAO inhibitors: Potential for severe reaction when used with MAO inhibitors; autonomic instability, coma, death, delirium, diaphoresis, hyperthermia, mental status changes/agitation, muscular rigidity, myoclonus, neuroleptic malignant syndrome features, and seizures may occur. Concurrent use with paroxetine is contraindicated.

- Thioridazine and pimozide: Potential for QT_c prolongation and arrhythmia; concurrent use of paroxetine with either of these agents is contraindicated.

Special populations:

- Elderly: Use caution in elderly patients.
- Pregnancy: Avoid use in the first trimester.

Special notes:

- Electroconvulsive therapy: May increase the risks associated with electroconvulsive therapy; consider discontinuing, when possible, prior to ECT treatment.
- Withdrawal syndrome: May cause dysphoric mood, irritability, agitation, dizziness, sensory disturbances, anxiety, confusion, headache, lethargy, emotional lability, insomnia, hypomania, tinnitus, and seizures. Upon discontinuation of paroxetine therapy, gradually taper dose. If intolerable symptoms occur following a decrease in dosage or upon discontinuation of therapy, then resuming the previous dose with a more gradual taper should be considered.

Dosage Forms

Note: Available as paroxetine hydrochloride or mesylate; mg strength refers to paroxetine

Suspension, oral, as hydrochloride (Paxil®): 10 mg/5 mL (250 mL) [orange flavor]

Tablet, as hydrochloride (Paxil®): 10 mg, 20 mg, 30 mg, 40 mg

Tablet, as mesylate (Pexeva®): 10 mg, 20 mg, 30 mg, 40 mg

Tablet, controlled release, as hydrochloride (Paxil CR®): 12.5 mg, 25 mg, 37.5 mg

Reference Range
Oral doses of 40 mg produced a peak serum level of 26.6 ng/mL; postmortem blood levels following overdose range from 0.993-4.0 mg/L. Postmortem blood paroxetine level >0.4 mg/L may indicate that this drug was the cause of death.

Overdosage/Treatment

Decontamination: Activated charcoal

Supportive therapy: Crystalloid infusion for hypotension; amantadine (100-200 mg 2 times/day) has been used successfully in treating sexual dysfunction; bruxism can be treated with buspirone (5 mg at night)

Enhancement of elimination: Multiple dosing of activated charcoal may be effective

Test Interactions ↑ LFTs; ↓ sodium (especially in elderly)

Drug Interactions

Substrate of CYP2D6 (major); **Inhibits** CYP1A2 (weak), 2B6 (moderate), 2C9 (weak), 2C19 (weak), 2D6 (strong), 3A4 (weak)

Amphetamines: SSRIs may increase the sensitivity to amphetamines, and amphetamines may increase the risk of serotonin syndrome.

Aspirin (and other antiplatelet drugs): Concomitant use of paroxetine and NSAIDs, aspirin, or other drugs affecting coagulation has been associated with an increased risk of bleeding; monitor.

Atomoxetine: Paroxetine may increase the levels/effects; dose reduction of atomoxetine may be required.

Buspirone: Combined use with SSRIs may cause serotonin syndrome.

Carbamazepine: May increase levels/effects of paroxetine; monitor.

Carvedilol: Serum concentrations may be increased; monitor carefully for increased carvedilol effect (hypotension and bradycardia).

Cimetidine: Cimetidine may reduce the first-pass metabolism of paroxetine resulting in elevated paroxetine serum concentrations; consider an alternative H_2 antagonist.

Clozapine: May increase serum levels of clozapine; monitor for increased effect/toxicity.

CYP2B6 substrates: Paroxetine may increase the levels/effects of CYP2B6 substrates. Example substrates include bupropion, promethazine, propofol, selegiline, and sertraline.

CYP2D6 inhibitors: May increase the levels/effects of paroxetine. Example inhibitors include chlorpromazine, delavirdine, fluoxetine, miconazole, pergolide, quinidine, quinine, ritonavir, and ropinirole.

CYP2D6 substrates: Paroxetine may increase the levels/effects of CYP2D6 substrates. Example substrates include amphetamines, selected beta-blockers, dextromethorphan, fluoxetine, lidocaine, mirtazapine, nefazodone, risperidone, ritonavir, thioridazine, tricyclic antidepressants, and venlafaxine.

CYP2D6 prodrug substrates: Paroxetine may decrease the levels/effects of CYP2D6 prodrug substrates. Example prodrug substrates include codeine, hydrocodone, oxycodone, and tramadol.

Cyproheptadine: May inhibit the effects of serotonin reuptake inhibitors; monitor for altered antidepressant response; cyproheptadine acts as a serotonin agonist.

Dextromethorphan: Metabolism of dextromethorphan may be inhibited; visual hallucinations occurred; monitor.

Galantamine: Paroxetine may increase levels/effects; monitor.

Haloperidol: Metabolism may be inhibited and cause extrapyramidal symptoms (EPS); monitor patients for EPS if combination is utilized.

HMG-CoA reductase inhibitors: Metabolism may be inhibited by SSRIs; particularly lovastatin and simvastatin resulting in myositis and rhabdomyolysis; paroxetine appears to have weak interaction with CYP3A4, and therefore, appears to have a low risk of this interaction.

Lithium: Patients receiving SSRIs and lithium have developed neurotoxicity; if combination is used; monitor for neurotoxicity.

Loop diuretics: SSRIs may cause hyponatremia; additive hyponatremic effects may be seen with combined use of a loop diuretic (bumetanide, furosemide, torsemide); monitor for hyponatremia.

MAO inhibitors: SSRIs should not be used with nonselective MAO inhibitors (isocarboxazid, phenelzine); fatal reactions have been reported; this combination should be avoided.

Meperidine: Combined use may cause serotonin syndrome; monitor.

Nefazodone and trazodone: May increase the risk of serotonin syndrome with SSRIs; monitor.

NSAIDs: Concomitant use of paroxetine and NSAIDs, aspirin, or other drugs affecting coagulation has been associated with an increased risk of bleeding; monitor.

Phenytoin: Metabolism of phenytoin may be inhibited, resulting in phenytoin toxicity; monitor for toxicity (ataxia, confusion, dizziness, nystagmus, involuntary muscle movement).

Pimozide: Paroxetine may increase the levels/effects; concomitant use contraindicated.

Procyclidine: Paroxetine increases AUC of procyclidine by 35%; this may result in increased anticholinergic effects; procyclidine dose reduction may be necessary.

Risperidone: Paroxetine, a potent CYP2D6 inhibitor, inhibits the metabolism of risperidone (CYP2D6 substrate) resulting in elevated plasma risperidone levels. The clinical implications are unclear, but clinicians should monitor for potential extrapyramidal symptoms (EPS).

Ritonavir: Combined use of paroxetine with ritonavir may cause serotonin syndrome; monitor.

Selegiline: SSRIs have been reported to cause mania or hypertension when combined with selegiline; this combination is best avoided; concurrent use with SSRIs has also been reported to cause serotonin syndrome; as an MAO type B inhibitor, the risk of serotonin syndrome may be less than with nonselective MAO inhibitors.

Serotonergic uptake inhibitors: Combined use with other drugs which inhibit the reuptake may cause serotonin syndrome.

Sibutramine: May increase the risk of serotonin syndrome with SSRIs; avoid coadministration.

Sumatriptan (and other serotonin agonists): Concurrent use may result in toxicity; weakness, hyper-reflexia, and incoordination have been observed with sumatriptan and SSRIs. In addition, concurrent use may theoretically increase the risk of serotonin syndrome; includes sumatriptan, naratriptan, rizatriptan, and zolmitriptan.

Sympathomimetics: May increase the risk of serotonin syndrome with SSRIs.

Theophylline: Paroxetine may elevate serum levels of theophylline; monitor.

Thioridazine: Paroxetine may inhibit the metabolism of thioridazine, resulting in increased plasma levels and increasing the risk of QT_c interval prolongation. Concurrent use is contraindicated.

Tramadol: Combined use may cause serotonin syndrome; monitor.

Tricyclic antidepressants: The metabolism of tricyclic antidepressants (amitriptyline, desipramine, imipramine, nortriptyline) may be inhibited by SSRIs resulting is elevated serum levels; if combination is warranted, a low dose of TCA (10-25 mg/day) should be utilized.

Tryptophan: May increase serotonergic effects; concomitant use not recommended.

Venlafaxine: Combined use with paroxetine may increase the risk of serotonin syndrome.

Warfarin: May alter the hypoprothrombinemic response to warfarin; monitor INR.

Zolpidem: At least one case of acute delirium in association with combined therapy has been reported.

Pregnancy Risk Factor C

Pregnancy Implications Teratogenic effects were not observed in animal studies. Nonteratogenic effects including respiratory distress, cyanosis, apnea, seizures, temperature instability, feeding difficulty, and tremor have been reported in the neonate immediately following delivery. Adverse effects may be due to toxic effects of SSRI or drug discontinuation. There are no adequate and well-controlled studies in pregnant women. Use during pregnancy only if the potential benefit to the mother outweighs the possible risk to the fetus. If treatment during pregnancy is required, consider tapering therapy during the third trimester.

Lactation Enters breast milk/use caution (AAP rates "of concern")

Additional Information Paxil CR™ incorporates a degradable polymeric matrix (Geomatrix™) to control dissolution rate over a period of 4-5 hours. An enteric coating delays the start of drug release until tablets have left the stomach. Paroxetine has properties similar to fluvoxamine maleate. Buspirone (15-60 mg/day) may be useful in treatment of sexual dysfunction during treatment with a selective serotonin reuptake inhibitor.

Specific References

Arima Y, Kubo C, Tsujimoto M, et al, "Improvement of Dry Mouth by Replacing Paroxetine with Fluvoxamine," *Ann Pharmacother*, 2005, 39(3):567-71.

Baker SD, Vincent CB, and Morgan DL, "Paroxetine Exposures: Five-Year Analysis of Unintentional Ingestions in the Pediatric Population Reported to the Texas Poison Center Network," *J Toxicol Clin Toxicol*, 2003, 41(5):712.

Boyer EW and Shannon M, "The Serotonin Syndrome," *N Engl J Med*, 2005, 352(11):1112-20 (review).

Charlier C, Broly F, Lhermitte M, et al, "Polymorphisms in the CYP 2D6 Gene: Association with Plasma Concentrations of Fluoxetine and Paroxetine," *Ther Drug Monit*, 2003, 25(6):738-42.

Hemels ME, Einarson A, Koren G, et al, "Antidepressant Use During Pregnancy and the Rates of Spontaneous Abortions: A Meta-Analysis," *Ann Pharmacother*, 2005, 39(5):803-9.

Kumagai R, Ohnuma T, Nagata T, et al, "Visual and Auditory Hallucinations with Excessive Intake of Paroxetine," *Psychiatry Clin Neurosci*, 2003, 57(5):548-9.

Manos GH and Wechsler SM, "Transient Ischemic Attack Reported with Paroxetine Use," *Ann Pharmacother*, 2004, 38(4):617-20. Epub 2004 Feb 13.

Marcy TR and Britton ML, "Antidepressant-Induced Sweating," *Ann Pharmacother*, 2005, 39(4):748-52.

Marraffa JM, Darko W, Stork CM, et al, "Methadone Causing Prolonged QTc Interval and Syncope After Paroxetine Initiation," *Clin Toxicol (Phila)*, 2005, 43:654.

Martínez MA, Sánchez de la Torre C, and Almarza E, "A Comparative Solid-Phase Extraction Study for the Simultaneous Determination of Fluvoxamine, Mianserin, Doxepin, Citalopram, Paroxetine, and Etoperidone in Whole Blood by Capillary Gas-Liquid Chromatography with Nitrogen-Phosphorus Detection," *J Anal Toxicol*, 2004, 28(4):174-80.

Morag I, Batash D, Keidar R, et al, "Paroxetine Use Throughout Pregnancy: Does It Pose Any Risk to the Neonate?" *J Toxicol Clin Toxicol*, 2004, 42(1):97-100.

Paruchuri P, Godkar D, Anandacoomar swamy, D et al, "Rare Case of Serotonin Syndrome with Therapeuitic Doses of Paroxetine," *Am J Therapeutic*, 2006, 13:550-2.

Ramasubbu R, "SSRI Treatment-Associated Stroke: Causality Assessment in Two Cases," *Ann Pharmacother*, 2004, 38(7-8):1197-201.

Rodda KE and Drummer OH, "The Redistribution of Psychiatric Drugs in Postmortem Cases," *J Anal Toxicol*, 2004, 28:286.

Serebruany VL, "Selective Serotonin Reuptake Inhibitors and Increased Bleeding Risk: Are We Missing Something?" *Am J Med*, 2006, 119(2):113-6 (review).

Waksman JC, Heard K, Jolliff H, et al, "Serotonin Syndrome Associated with the Use of St John's Wort (*Hypericum perforatum*) and Paroxetine," *J Toxicol Clin Toxicol*, 2000, 38(5):521.

Zeskind PS and Stephens LE, "Maternal Selective Serotonin Reuptake Inhibitor Use During Pregnancy and Newborn Neurobehavior," *Pediatrics*, 2004, 113(2):368-75.

Pemoline

Related Information

● Therapeutic Drugs Associated with Hallucinations

CAS Number 18968-99-5; 2152-34-3; 68942-31-4

U.S. Brand Names Cylert®; PemADD® CT; PemADD®

Synonyms Phenylisohydantoin; PIO

Impairment Potential Yes

Use Controlling undirected hyperkinetic behavior; treat narcolepsy and antihistamine-induced drowsiness

Unlabeled/Investigational Use Narcolepsy

Mechanism of Action Sympathetic amine similar in action to amphetamines; central nervous system stimulant

Adverse Reactions

Central nervous system: **Insomnia**, stuttering

Endocrine & metabolic: Growth suppression

Gastrointestinal: **Anorexia, weight loss**

Hepatic: Fulminant liver failure (4-17 times general population rate)

Signs and Symptoms of Overdose Anorexia, choreoathetosis, dyskinesias, elevated liver function tests (1% to 2%), exacerbation of Tourette's syndrome, hallucinations (visual, tactile, and auditory), hyperthermia, insomnia, leukocytosis, mania, mydriasis, neutropenia, nystagmus, rhabdomyolysis, stuttering, vomiting

Pharmacodynamics/Kinetics

Onset of action: Peak effect: 4 hours

Duration: 8 hours

Protein binding: 50%

Metabolism: Partially hepatic

Half-life elimination: Children: 7-8.6 hours; Adults: 12 hours

Time to peak, serum: 2-4 hours

Excretion: Urine; feces (negligible amounts)

Dosage Oral: Initial: 37.5 mg increasing by 18.75 mg weekly; usual dose: 56.25-75 mg/day; maximum: 112.5 mg

Monitoring Parameters Liver enzymes (baseline and every 2 weeks)

Administration Administer medication in the morning.

Contraindications Hypersensitivity to pemoline or any component of the formulation; hepatic impairment (including abnormalities on baseline liver function tests); children <6 years of age; Tourette's syndrome; psychosis

Warnings

[U.S. Boxed Warning]: Not considered first-line therapy for ADHD due to association with hepatic failure. The manufacturer has recommended that signed informed consent following a discussion of risks and benefits must or should be obtained prior to the initiation of therapy. Therapy should be discontinued if a response is not evident after 3 weeks of therapy. Pemoline should not be started in patients with abnormalities in baseline liver function tests, and should be discontinued if clinically significant liver function test abnormalities are revealed at any time during therapy. Use with caution in patients with renal dysfunction or psychosis. In general, stimulant medications should be used with caution in patients with bipolar disorder, diabetes mellitus, cardiovascular disease, seizure disorders, insomnia, porphyria, or hypertension (although pemoline has been demonstrated to have a low potential to elevate blood pressure relative to other stimulants). May exacerbate symptoms of behavior and thought disorder in psychotic patients. Potential for drug dependency exists - avoid abrupt discontinuation in patients who have received for prolonged periods. Stimulant use has been associated with growth suppression, and careful monitoring is recommended. Stimulants may unmask tics in individuals with coexisting Tourette's syndrome.

Dosage Forms [DSC] = Discontinued product
Tablet (Cylert® [DSC], PemADD® [DSC]): 18.75 mg, 37.5 mg, 75 mg
Tablet, chewable (Cylert® [DSC], PemADD® CT [DSC]): 37.5 mg

Reference Range Therapeutic plasma range: 1-7 mcg/mL

Overdosage/Treatment
Decontamination: Lavage (within 1 hour)/activated charcoal
Supportive therapy: Diazepam can be used to treat choreoathetosis and may be more effective than benztropine; alkaline diuresis with a diuretic (mannitol or furosemide) should be used to prevent renal failure due to rhabdomyolysis

Test Interactions May produce false acid phosphatase elevations

Drug Interactions Anticonvulsants: Pemoline may decrease seizure threshold; efficacy of anticonvulsants may be decreased
CNS depressants: Effects may be additive; use caution when pemoline is used with other CNS acting medications

Pregnancy Risk Factor B

Lactation Excretion in breast milk unknown/not recommended

Additional Information Choreiform movements can occur in children at doses as low as 2 mg/kg; similar to dexamphetamine sulfate

---

Penbutolol

Related Information
● Selected Properties of Beta-Adrenergic Blocking Drugs

CAS Number 38363-32-5; 38363-40-5

U.S. Brand Names Levatol®

Synonyms Penbutolol Sulfate

Use Treatment of mild to moderate arterial hypertension

Mechanism of Action Blocks both beta$_1$- and beta$_2$-receptors and has mild intrinsic sympathomimetic activity; has negative inotropic and chronotropic effects and can significantly slow AV nodal conduction

Adverse Reactions
Cardiovascular: Exacerbation of Raynaud's phenomenon, hypotension, congestive heart failure, AV block, chest pain, edema, heart failure, sinus bradycardia, angina, myocardial depression, QRS prolongation
Central nervous system: Nightmares, fatigue, insomnia, ataxia, drowsiness, CNS depression, confusion, dizziness, headache
Dermatologic: Alopecia, purpura, pruritus, psoriasis, exanthem
Gastrointestinal: Constipation, abdominal pain, diarrhea, nausea, vomiting
Genitourinary: Impotence, nocturia, enuresis
Ocular: Diplopia
Miscellaneous: Cold extremities

Pharmacodynamics/Kinetics
Absorption: ~100%
Protein binding: 80% to 98%
Metabolism: Extensively hepatic (oxidation and conjugation)
Bioavailability: ~100%
Half-life elimination: 5 hours
Excretion: Urine

Dosage Adults: Oral: Initial: 20 mg once daily, full effect of a 20 or 40 mg dose is seen by the end of a 2-week period, doses of 40-80 mg have been tolerated but have shown little additional antihypertensive effects; usual dose range (JNC 7): 10-40 mg once daily

Contraindications Hypersensitivity to penbutolol or any component of the formulation; uncompensated congestive heart failure; cardiogenic shock; bradycardia or heart block (except in patients with a functioning artificial pacemaker); sinus node dysfunction; asthma; bronchospastic disease; COPD; pulmonary edema; pregnancy (2nd and 3rd trimester)

Warnings Avoid abrupt discontinuation in patients with a history of CAD; slowly wean while monitoring for signs and symptoms of ischemia. Use caution with concurrent use of beta-blockers and either verapamil or diltiazem; bradycardia or heart block can occur. Use caution in patients with PVD (can aggravate arterial insufficiency). Use cautiously in diabetics because it can mask prominent hypoglycemic symptoms. Can mask signs of thyrotoxicosis. Can cause fetal harm when administered in pregnancy. Beta-blockers with intrinsic sympathomimetic activity (including penbutolol) do not appear to be of benefit in CHF.

Dosage Forms Tablet, as sulfate: 20 mg

Reference Range 50 mg dose results in peak serum concentration of 770 ng/mL after 1 hour

Overdosage/Treatment
Decontamination: Lavage (within 1 hour)/activated charcoal
Supportive therapy: Sympathomimetics (eg, epinephrine or dopamine), atropine, glucagon, or a pacemaker can be used to treat the toxic bradycardia, asystole, and/or hypotension; initially fluids may be the best treatment for toxic hypotension
Enhancement of elimination: Charcoal hemoperfusion can be used to lower serum levels

Drug Interactions Alpha-blockers (prazosin, terazosin): Concurrent use of beta-blockers may increase risk of orthostasis.
Albuterol (and other beta$_2$ agonists): Effects may be blunted by nonspecific beta-blockers.
Clonidine: Hypertensive crisis after or during withdrawal of either agent.
Drugs which slow AV conduction (digoxin): Effects may be additive with beta-blockers.
Epinephrine (including local anesthetics with epinephrine): Penbutolol may cause hypertension.
Glucagon: Penbutolol may blunt the hyperglycemic action.
Insulin and oral hypoglycemics: May mask symptoms of hypoglycemia.
NSAIDs (ibuprofen, indomethacin, naproxen, piroxicam) may reduce the antihypertensive effects of beta-blockers.
Penbutolol masks the tachycardia that usually accompanies insulin-induced hypoglycemia.
Salicylates may reduce the antihypertensive effects of beta-blockers.
Sulfonylureas: beta-blockers may alter response to hypoglycemic agents.
Verapamil or diltiazem may have synergistic or additive pharmacological effects when taken concurrently with beta-blockers.

Pregnancy Risk Factor C (manufacturer); D (2nd and 3rd trimester - expert analysis)

Lactation Enters breast milk/use caution

Nursing Implications Advise against abrupt withdrawal
Monitor orthostatic blood pressures, apical and peripheral pulse and mental status changes (ie, confusion, depression)

Specific References
Chobanian AV, Bakris GL, Black HR, et al, "The Seventh Report of the Joint National Committee on Prevention, Detection, Evaluation, and Treatment of High Blood Pressure: The JNC 7 Report," *JAMA*, 2003, 289(19):2560-71.

Penicillin G (Parenteral/Aqueous)

CAS Number 113-98-4; 61-33-6; 69-57-8

U.S. Brand Names Pfizerpen®

Synonyms Benzylpenicillin Potassium; Benzylpenicillin Sodium; Crystalline Penicillin; Penicillin G Potassium; Penicillin G Sodium

Use Active against most gram-positive organisms except *Staphylococcus aureus*; some gram-negative such as *Neisseria gonorrhoeae* and some anaerobes and spirochetes; although ceftriaxone is now the drug of choice for Lyme disease and gonorrhea

Mechanism of Action Interferes with bacterial cell wall synthesis during active multiplication, causing cell wall death and resultant bactericidal activity against susceptible bacteria

Adverse Reactions
Cardiovascular: Myocarditis (hypersensitivity), myocarditis, vasculitis
Central nervous system: Convulsions, anxiety, confusion, drowsiness, fever, Jarisch-Herxheimer reaction, hyperthermia, aseptic meningitis
Dermatologic: Rash, angioedema, urticaria, dermatographism, cutis laxa, systemic contact dermatitis, immunologic contact urticaria, acute generalized exanthematous pustulosis, alopecia, toxic epidermal necrolysis, purpura, Stevens-Johnson syndrome, pruritus, exanthem
Endocrine & metabolic: Electrolyte imbalance, hypernatremia with sodium salt, hyperkalemia with potassium salt
Gastrointestinal: Nausea, diarrhea, pseudomembranous colitis, metallic taste, esophagitis
Hematologic: Hemolytic anemia, positive Coombs' reaction, neutropenia, thrombocytopenia
Hepatic: Granulomatous hepatitis, cholestasis, aminotransferase level elevation (asymptomatic)
Local: Thrombophlebitis
Neuromuscular & skeletal: Myoclonus
Renal: Acute interstitial nephritis (after large I.V. doses)
Respiratory: Asthma, bronchospasm

Miscellaneous: Hypersensitivity reactions, anaphylaxis (0.05% frequency with injection), total allergic reactions (1% to 10%), lymphadenopathy, mucocutaneous syndrome (febrile)

Signs and Symptoms of Overdose Colitis, dyspnea, eosinophilia, coagulopathy, leukopenia or neutropenia (agranulocytosis, granulocytopenia); pemphigus, periarteritis nodosa, pseudotumor cerebri, tongue discoloration

Pharmacodynamics/Kinetics

Distribution: Poor penetration across blood-brain barrier, despite inflamed meninges; crosses placenta; enters breast milk

Relative diffusion from blood into CSF: Good only with inflammation (exceeds usual MICs)

CSF:blood level ratio: Normal meninges: <1%; Inflamed meninges: 3% to 5%

Protein binding: 65%

Metabolism: Hepatic (30%) to penicilloic acid

Half-life elimination:

Neonates: <6 days old: 3.2-3.4 hours; 7-13 days old: 1.2-2.2 hours; >14 days old: 0.9-1.9 hours

Children and Adults: Normal renal function: 20-50 minutes

End-stage renal disease: 3.3-5.1 hours

Time to peak, serum: I.M.: ~30 minutes; I.V. ~1 hour

Excretion: Urine

Dosage

I.M., I.V. (do not give intrathecal):

Neonates:

Postnatal age <7 days:

<2000 g: 25,000 units/kg/dose every 12 hours; meningitis: 50,000 units/kg/dose every 12 hours

>2000 g: 20,000 units/kg/dose every 8 hours; meningitis: 50,000 units/kg/dose every 8 hours

Postnatal age >7 days:

<1200 g: 25,000 units/kg/dose every 12 hours; meningitis: 50,000 units/kg/dose every 12 hours

1200-2000 g: 25,000 units/kg/dose every 8 hours; meningitis: 75,000 units/kg/dose every 8 hours

>2000 g: 25,000 units/kg/dose every 6 hours; meningitis: 50,000 units/kg/dose every 6 hours

Infants and Children (sodium salt is preferred in children): 100,000-250,000 units/kg/day in divided doses every 4 hours; maximum: 4.8 million units/24 hours

Severe infections: Up to 400,000 units/kg/day in divided doses every 4 hours; maximum dose: 24 million units/day

Adults: 2-24 million units/day in divided doses every 4 hours

Dosing interval in renal impairment:

Cl$_{cr}$ 30-50 mL/minute: Administer every 6 hours

Cl$_{cr}$ 10-30 mL/minute: Administer every 8 hours

Cl$_{cr}$ <10 mL/minute: Administer every 12 hours

Stability Reconstituted parenteral solution is stable for 7 days when refrigerated; for I.V. infusion in NS or D$_5$W, solution is stable for 24 hours at room temperature; thawed solutions stable for 24 hours at room temperature or 14 days at refrigeration

Monitoring Parameters Observe for signs and symptoms of anaphylaxis during first dose

Administration Administer I.M. by deep injection in the upper outer quadrant of the buttock

Contraindications Hypersensitivity to penicillin or any component of the formulation

Warnings Avoid intra-arterial administration or injection into or near major peripheral nerves or blood vessels since such injections may cause severe and/or permanent neurovascular damage; use with caution in patients with renal impairment (dosage reduction required), pre-existing seizure disorders, or with a history of hypersensitivity to cephalosporins

Dosage Forms Infusion, as potassium [premixed iso-osmotic dextrose solution, frozen]: 1 million units (50 mL), 2 million units (50 mL), 3 million units (50 mL) [contains sodium 1.02 mEq and potassium 1.7 mEq per 1 million units]

Injection, powder for reconstitution, as potassium (Pfizerpen®): 5 million units, 20 million units [contains sodium 6.8 mg (0.3 mEq) and potassium 65.6 mg (1.68 mEq) per 1 million units]

Injection, powder for reconstitution, as sodium: 5 million units [contains sodium 1.68 mEq per 1 million units]

Reference Range After 500 mg oral dose, peak plasma level is 1.5-2.7 mg/L

Overdosage/Treatment

Decontamination: Emesis within 30 minutes or lavage within 1 hour (rarely necessary)/activated charcoal can be used

Supportive therapy: Allergic reactions can be treated with epinephrine, diphenhydramine, and corticosteroids

Enhancement of elimination: Hemodialysis or charcoal hemoperfusion can be useful in removing penicillin; moderately dialyzable (20% to 50%)

Antidote(s)

- Epinephrine [ANTIDOTE]

Diagnostic Procedures

- Electrolytes, Urine

Test Interactions False-positive or negative urinary glucose determination using Clinitest®; positive Coombs' [direct]; false-positive urinary and/or serum proteins; interferes with the Guthrie test for phenylketonuria

Drug Interactions Aminoglycosides: May be synergistic against selected organisms

Methotrexate: Penicillins may increase the exposure to methotrexate during concurrent therapy; monitor.

Oral contraceptives: Anecdotal reports suggesting decreased contraceptive efficacy with penicillins have been refuted by more rigorous scientific and clinical data.

Probenecid, disulfiram: May increase penicillin levels

Tetracyclines: May decrease penicillin effectiveness

Warfarin: Effects of warfarin may be increased

Pregnancy Risk Factor B

Pregnancy Implications Crosses the placenta

Lactation Enters breast milk/compatible

Nursing Implications Administer I.M. by deep injection in the upper outer quadrant of the buttock; dosage modification required in patients with renal insufficiency; give around-the-clock to promote less variation in peak and trough levels

Additional Information Toxic dose: 10,000,000 units (or 6 g)

1 million units is approximately equal to 625 mg.

Penicillin G potassium injection:

Potassium content per million units: 65.6 mg (1.7 mEq)

Sodium content per million units: 23.5 mg (1.02 mEq)

Specific References

Casey JR and Pichichero ME, "Meta-Analysis of Cephalosporin Versus Penicillin Treatment of Group A Streptococcal Tonsillopharyngitis in Children," *Pediatrics*, 2004, 113(4):866-82.

See S, Scott EK, and Levin MW, "Penicillin-Induced Jarisch-Herxheimer Reaction," *Ann Pharmacother*, 2005, 39(12):2128-30.

Pentamidine

CAS Number 140-64-7

U.S. Brand Names NebuPent®; Pentam-300®

Synonyms Pentamidine Isethionate

Use Treatment and prevention of pneumonia caused by *Pneumocystis carinii* (PCP)

Treatment of trypanosomiasis and visceral leishmaniasis

Mechanism of Action Interferes with RNA/DNA, phospholipids and protein synthesis, through inhibition of oxidative phosphorylation and/or interference with incorporation of nucleotides and nucleic acids into RNA and DNA, in protozoa

Adverse Reactions

Cardiovascular: **Chest pain**, hypotension, tachycardia, hypotension (orthostatic), torsade de pointes, sinus bradycardia, palpitations, sinus tachycardia, arrhythmias (ventricular), vasculitis

Central nervous system: Dizziness, fever, Jarisch-Herxheimer-like reaction, insomnia, gustatory hallucinations

Dermatologic: **Rash**, mucormycosis, Stevens-Johnson syndrome, bullous skin disease, xerosis, urticaria, purpura, pruritus, exanthem

Endocrine & metabolic: **Hyperkalemia**, hypoglycemia, hyperglycemia, hypocalcemia, hyperinsulinemia

Gastrointestinal: Vomiting, metallic taste in mouth, pancreatitis, gagging, hemorrhagic pancreatitis, xerostomia

Hematologic: Megaloblastic anemia, granulocytopenia, leukopenia, thrombocytopenia, eosinophilia

Local: **Pain at injection site**

Renal: Mild renal or hepatic injury, acidosis (renal tubular) type IV

Respiratory: **Cough, dyspnea, pharyngitis, wheezing**, irritation of the airway bronchospasm, rhinitis, eosinophilic pneumonia

Signs and Symptoms of Overdose No published cases of acute oral overdose. Agranulocytosis, anorexia, azotemia, cardiac arrhythmias, conjunctivitis, cough, granulocytopenia, hyperglycemia, hypocalcemia, hypoglycemia, hypomagnesemia, hypotension, leukopenia, myoglobinuria, neutropenia, QT prolongation, rhabdomyolysis, toxic epidermal necrolysis, wheezing

Pharmacodynamics/Kinetics

Absorption: I.M.: Well absorbed; Inhalation: Limited systemic absorption

Distribution: V$_d$: Steady state: 3-32 L/kg; systemic accumulation of pentamidine does not appear to occur following inhalation therapy

Protein binding: 69%

Half-life elimination: Terminal: 6.4-9.4 hours; may be prolonged with severe renal impairment

Excretion: Urine (33% to 66% as unchanged drug)

Dosage

Children:

Treatment of PCP pneumonia: I.M., I.V. (I.V. preferred): 4 mg/kg/day once daily for 10-14 days

Prevention of PCP pneumonia:

I.M., I.V.: 4 mg/kg monthly or every 2 weeks

Inhalation (aerosolized pentamidine in children ≥5 years): 300 mg/dose given every 3-4 weeks via Respirgard® II inhaler (8 mg/kg dose has also been used in children <5 years)

Treatment of trypanosomiasis (unlabeled use): I.V.: 4 mg/kg/day once daily for 10 days

Adults:

Treatment: I.M., I.V. (I.V. preferred): 4 mg/kg/day once daily for 14-21 days

Prevention: Inhalation: 300 mg every 4 weeks via Respirgard® II nebulizer

Dialysis: Not removed by hemo or peritoneal dialysis or continuous arteriovenous or venovenous hemofiltration; supplemental dosage is not necessary

Dosing adjustment in renal impairment: Adults: I.V.:

Cl$_{cr}$ 10-50 mL/minute: Administer 4 mg/kg every 24-36 hours

Cl$_{cr}$ <10 mL/minute: Administer 4 mg/kg every 48 hours

Monitoring Parameters Liver function tests, renal function tests, blood glucose, serum potassium and calcium, ECG, blood pressure

Administration

Inhalation: Deliver until nebulizer is gone (30-45 minutes)

I.V.: Infuse slowly over a period of at least 60 minutes or administer deep I.M.

Contraindications Hypersensitivity to pentamidine isethionate or any component of the formulation (inhalation and injection)

Warnings Use with caution in patients with diabetes mellitus, renal or hepatic dysfunction, hyper-/hypotension, leukopenia, thrombocytopenia, asthma, or hypo-/hyperglycemia.

Dosage Forms Injection, powder for reconstitution, as isethionate (Pentam-300®): 300 mg

Powder for nebulization, as isethionate (NebuPent®): 300 mg

Reference Range Peak plasma concentration after 2-hour I.V. infusion of 4 mg/kg pentamidine was 612 ng/mL; plasma concentration of 794 ng/mL obtained after an overdose of 160 mg/kg

Overdosage/Treatment

Supportive therapy: Bronchospasm can be treated with beta-adrenergic agonist agents; diphenhydramine (25 mg) or hydroxyzine hydrochloride (25 mg) can be used to treat pruritus or skin rash

Enhanced elimination: Charcoal hemoperfusion may be useful in enhancing elimination

Diagnostic Procedures

● Creatinine, Serum

Test Interactions ↑ insulin; ↓ glucose

Drug Interactions

Substrate of CYP2C19 (major); **Inhibits** CYP2C8/9 (weak), 2C19 (weak), 2D6 (weak), 3A4 (weak)

CYP2C19 inducers: May decrease the levels/effects of pentamidine. Example inducers include aminoglutethimide, carbamazepine, phenytoin, and rifampin.

CYP2C19 inhibitors: May increase the levels/effects of pentamidine. Example inhibitors include delavirdine, fluconazole, fluvoxamine, gemfibrozil, isoniazid, omeprazole, and ticlopidine.

QT$_c$-prolonging agents: Pentamidine may potentiate the effect of other drugs which prolong QT interval (cisapride, sparfloxacin, gatifloxacin, moxifloxacin, pimozide, and type Ia and type III antiarrhythmics).

Pregnancy Risk Factor C

Pregnancy Implications Based on animal data, the reference doses for embryolethality and for teratogenicity are estimated to be 0.08 mcg/kg/day and 4 mcg/kg/day, respectively. Aerosolized pentamidine can pass embryolethal doses to healthcare workers.

Lactation Excretion in breast milk unknown/contraindicated

Nursing Implications Infuse I.V. slowly over a period of at least 60 minutes or administer deep I.M.

Additional Information Do not use NS as a diluent; NS is incompatible with pentamidine; infuse over at least 1 hour; hypotension associated with I.V. administration

Pentazocine

Related Information

● Meptazinol

CAS Number 17146-95-1; 2276-52-0; 359-83-1; 64024-15-3

U.S. Brand Names Talwin® NX; Talwin®

Synonyms Naloxone Hydrochloride and Pentazocine Hydrochloride; Pentazocine Hydrochloride and Naloxone Hydrochloride; Pentazocine Hydrochloride; Pentazocine Lactate

Impairment Potential Yes

Use Relief of moderate to severe pain; has also been used as a sedative prior to surgery and as a supplement to surgical anesthesia

Mechanism of Action Binds to opiate receptors in the CNS, causing inhibition of ascending pain pathways, altering the perception of and response to pain; produces generalized CNS depression; partial agonist-antagonist

Adverse Reactions

Frequency not defined.

Cardiovascular: Hypotension, circulatory depression, shock, tachycardia, syncope, flushing

Central nervous system: Malaise, headache, nightmares, insomnia, CNS depression, sedation, hallucinations, confusion, disorientation, dizziness, euphoria, drowsiness, lightheadedness, irritability, chills, excitement

Dermatologic: Rash, pruritus, dermatitis, urticaria, Stevens-Johnson syndrome, toxic epidermal necrolysis, erythema multiforme

Gastrointestinal: Nausea, vomiting, xerostomia, constipation, anorexia, diarrhea, abdominal distress

Genitourinary: Urinary retention

Hematologic: WBCs decreased, eosinophilia

Local: Tissue damage and irritation with I.M./SubQ use

Neuromuscular & skeletal: Weakness, tremor, paresthesia

Ocular: Blurred vision, miosis

Otic: Tinnitus

Respiratory: Dyspnea, respiratory depression (rare)

Miscellaneous: Physical and psychological dependence, facial edema, diaphoresis, anaphylaxis

Signs and Symptoms of Overdose Asterixis, diarrhea, diplopia, dry mouth, erythema multiforme, hypertension, hyperthermia, miosis, myalgia, nephrotic syndrome, nystagmus, respiratory depression, seizures, tachycardia, toxic epidermal necrolysis

Pharmacodynamics/Kinetics

Onset of action: Oral, I.M., SubQ: 15-30 minutes; I.V.: 2-3 minutes

Duration: Oral: 4-5 hours; Parenteral: 2-3 hours

Protein binding: 60%

Metabolism: Hepatic via oxidative and glucuronide conjugation pathways; extensive first-pass effect

Bioavailability: Oral: ~20%; increased to 60% to 70% with cirrhosis

Half-life elimination: 2-3 hours; prolonged with hepatic impairment

Excretion: Urine (small amounts as unchanged drug)

Dosage Preoperative/pre-anesthestic: Children 1-16 years: I.M.: 0.5 mg/kg

Analgesia:

Children: I.M.:

5-8 years: 15 mg

8-14 years: 30 mg

Children >12 years and Adults: Oral: 50 mg every 3-4 hours; may increase to 100 mg/dose if needed, but should not exceed 600 mg/day

Adults:

I.M., SubQ: 30-60 mg every 3-4 hours, not to exceed total daily dose of 360 mg

I.V.: 30 mg every 3-4 hours (maximum: 360 mg/day)

Elderly: Elderly patients may be more sensitive to the analgesic and sedating effects. The elderly may also have impaired renal function. If needed, dosing should be started at the lower end of dosing range and adjust dose for renal function.

Dosing adjustment in renal impairment:

Cl$_{cr}$ 10-50 mL/minute: Administer 75% of normal dose

Cl$_{cr}$ <10 mL/minute: Administer 50% of normal dose

Dosing adjustment in hepatic impairment: Reduce dose or avoid use in patients with liver disease

Stability Store at room temperature, protect from heat and from freezing; I.V. form is **incompatible** with aminophylline, amobarbital (and all other I.V. barbiturates), glycopyrrolate (same syringe), heparin (same syringe), nafcillin (Y-site)

Monitoring Parameters Relief of pain, respiratory and mental status, blood pressure

Administration Rotate injection site for I.M., SubQ use; avoid intra-arterial injection; avoid SubQ use unless absolutely necessary (may cause tissue damage)

Contraindications Hypersensitivity to pentazocine, naloxone, or any component of the formulation; increased intracranial pressure (unless the patient is mechanically ventilated); pregnancy (prolonged use or high doses at term)

Warnings Use with caution in seizure-prone patients, acute myocardial infarction, patients undergoing biliary tract surgery, patients with renal and hepatic dysfunction, head trauma, increased intracranial pressure, and patients with a history of prior opioid dependence or abuse; pentazocine may precipitate opiate withdrawal symptoms in patients who have been receiving opiates regularly; injection contains sulfites which may cause allergic reaction; tolerance or drug dependence may result from extended use. **[U.S. Boxed Warning]: Talwin® NX is intended for oral administration only - severe vascular reactions have resulted from misuse by injection.**

Dosage Forms Injection, solution (Talwin®): 30 mg/mL (1 mL, 10 mL) [10 mL size contains sodium bisulfite]

Tablet (Talwin® NX): Pentazocine 50 mg and naloxone 0.5 mg

Reference Range

Therapeutic: 0.05-0.2 mg/L

Fatal: >1.0 mg/L

Overdosage/Treatment

Decontamination: Lavage (within 1 hour)/activated charcoal; **do not** induce emesis

Supportive therapy: Naloxone hydrochloride (large doses may be required); seizures can be treated with diazepam, lorazepam, phenytoin, or phenobarbital

Antidote(s)

- Nalmefene [ANTIDOTE]
- Naloxone [ANTIDOTE]

Drug Interactions May potentiate or reduce analgesic effect of opiate agonist (eg, morphine) depending on patients tolerance to opiates can precipitate withdrawal in narcotic addicts

Increased effect/toxicity with tripelennamine (can be lethal), CNS depressants (phenothiazines, tranquilizers, anxiolytics, sedatives, hypnotics, or alcohol)

Pregnancy Risk Factor B/D (prolonged use or high doses at term)

Pregnancy Implications Pentazocine was not found to be teratogenic in animal studies. Pentazocine and naloxone have been shown to cross the human placenta. Use should be avoided during labor and delivery of premature infants. Abstinence syndromes in the newborn have been reported after long-term use of pentazocine during pregnancy. Other adverse effects in the newborn have been reported following abuse of pentazocine during pregnancy; these effects may be due to pentazocine, other drugs abused, the mother's lifestyle, or a combination of all factors.

Lactation Excretion in breast milk unknown/use caution

Nursing Implications Rotate injection site for I.M., SubQ use; avoid intra-arterial injection; observe patient for excessive sedation, respiratory depression, implement safety measures, assist with ambulation; observe for narcotic withdrawal

Additional Information Lethal oral dose: 0.3 g. Pentazocine hydrochloride: Talwin® NX tablet (with naloxone); naloxone is used to prevent abuse by dissolving tablets in water and using as injection; may be combined with tripelennamine (Ts and blues)

Pentobarbital

CAS Number 57-33-0; 76-74-4
U.S. Brand Names Nembutal®
Synonyms Pentobarbital Sodium
Impairment Potential Yes
Use Sedative/hypnotic; preanesthetic; high-dose barbiturate coma for treatment of increased intracranial pressure or status epilepticus unresponsive to other therapy

Mechanism of Action Short-acting barbiturate with sedative, hypnotic, and anticonvulsant properties

Adverse Reactions

Cardiovascular: **Cardiac arrhythmias, hypotension**, sinus bradycardia, congestive heart failure, myocardial depression, **arterial spasm**, vasculitis

Central nervous system: **Drowsiness, CNS stimulation or CNS depression, impaired judgment**, decreased deep tendon reflexes, hypothermia, **lethargy, "hangover" effect**

Dermatologic: Rash, exfoliative dermatitis, erythema multiforme, angioedema, toxic epidermal necrolysis, urticaria, purpura, Stevens-Johnson syndrome, pruritus, erythema nodosum, exanthem, photoallergic reaction

Gastrointestinal: Nausea, vomiting

Local: **Pain at injection site, thrombophlebitis with I.V. use**

Renal: Oliguria

Respiratory: Laryngospasm, respiratory depression, apnea (especially with rapid I.V. use)

Miscellaneous: Physical and psychological dependency with chronic use; **gangrene with inadvertent intra-arterial injection**, systemic lupus erythematosus, fixed drug eruption

Signs and Symptoms of Overdose Bullous skin lesions, confusion, fever, hypoglycemia, hypotension, hypothermia, jaundice, myoglobinuria, ptosis, renal failure, rhabdomyolysis, slurred speech, unsteady gait, vision color changes (green tinge; yellow tinge)

Pharmacodynamics/Kinetics

Onset of action: I.M.: 10-15 minutes; I.V.: ~1 minute
Duration: I.V.: 15 minutes
Distribution: V_d: Children: 0.8 L/kg; Adults: 1 L/kg
Protein binding: 35% to 55%
Metabolism: Extensively hepatic via hydroxylation and oxidation pathways
Half-life elimination: Terminal: Children: 25 hours; Adults: Healthy: 22 hours (range: 15-50 hours)
Excretion: Urine (<1% as unchanged drug)

Dosage

Children:
Hypnotic: I.M.: 2-6 mg/kg; maximum: 100 mg/dose
Preoperative/preprocedure sedation: ≥6 months:
Note: Limited information is available for infants <6 months of age.
I.M.: 2-6 mg/kg; maximum: 100 mg/dose

I.V.: 1-3 mg/kg to a maximum of 100 mg until asleep
Conscious sedation prior to a procedure: Children 5-12 years: I.V.: 2 mg/kg 5-10 minutes before procedures, may repeat one time
Adolescents: Conscious sedation: I.V.: 100 mg prior to a procedure
Children and Adults: Barbiturate coma in head injury patients: I.V.: Loading dose: 5-10 mg/kg given slowly over 1-2 hours; monitor blood pressure and respiratory rate; Maintenance infusion: Initial: 1 mg/kg/hour; may increase to 2-3 mg/kg/hour; maintain burst suppression on EEG
Status epilepticus: I.V.: **Note:** Intubation required; monitor hemodynamics
Children: Loading dose: 5-15 mg/kg given slowly over 1-2 hours; maintenance infusion: 0.5-5 mg/kg/hour
Adults: Loading dose: 2-15 mg/kg given slowly over 1-2 hours; maintenance infusion: 0.5-3 mg/kg/hour
Adults:
Hypnotic:
I.M.: 150-200 mg
I.V.: Initial: 100 mg, may repeat every 1-3 minutes up to 200-500 mg total dose
Preoperative sedation: I.M.: 150-200 mg
Dosing adjustment in hepatic impairment: Reduce dosage in patients with severe liver dysfunction

Monitoring Parameters Respiratory status (for conscious sedation, includes pulse oximetry), cardiovascular status, CNS status; cardiac monitor and blood pressure monitor required

Administration Pentobarbital may be administered by deep I.M. or slow I.V. injection.
I.M.: No more than 5 mL (250 mg) should be injected at any one site because of possible tissue irritation.
I.V.: I.V. push doses can be given undiluted, but should be administered no faster than 50 mg/minute; parenteral solutions are highly alkaline; avoid extravasation; avoid rapid I.V. administration >50 mg/minute; avoid intra-arterial injection

Contraindications Hypersensitivity to barbiturates or any component of the formulation; marked hepatic impairment; dyspnea or airway obstruction; porphyria; pregnancy

Warnings

Tolerance to hypnotic effect can occur; do not use for >2 weeks to treat insomnia. Potential for drug dependency exists, abrupt cessation may precipitate withdrawal, including status epilepticus in epileptic patients. Do not administer to patients in acute pain. Use caution in elderly, debilitated, renally impaired, hepatic dysfunction, or pediatric patients. May cause paradoxical responses, including agitation and hyperactivity, particularly in acute pain and pediatric patients. Use with caution in patients with depression or suicidal tendencies, or in patients with a history of drug abuse. Tolerance, psychological and physical dependence may occur with prolonged use.

May cause CNS depression, which may impair physical or mental abilities. Patients must be cautioned about performing tasks which require mental alertness (eg, operating machinery or driving). Effects with other sedative drugs or ethanol may be potentiated. Use of this agent as a hypnotic in the elderly is not recommended due to its long half-life and potential for physical and psychological dependence.

May cause respiratory depression or hypotension, particularly when administered intravenously. Use with caution in hemodynamically unstable patients or patients with respiratory disease. High doses (loading doses of 15-35 mg/kg given over 1-2 hours) have been utilized to induce pentobarbital coma, but these higher doses often cause hypotension requiring vasopressor therapy.

Dosage Forms Injection, solution, as sodium: 50 mg/mL (20 mL, 50 mL) [contains alcohol 10% and propylene glycol 40%]

Reference Range

Hypnotic: 1-5 mcg/mL (SI: 4-22 µmol/L)
Drowsy: 6-10 mcg/mL (SI: 44 µmol/L)
Stuporous: 11-17 mcg/mL (SI: 46-76 µmol/L)
Coma: 20-50 mcg/mL (SI: 88-221 µmol/L)

Overdosage/Treatment

Decontamination: Lavage (within 1 hour)/activated charcoal
Supportive therapy: If hypotension occurs, administer I.V. fluids and place the patient in the Trendelenburg position. If unresponsive, an I.V. vasopressor (eg, dopamine, epinephrine) may be required.
Enhancement of elimination: Forced alkaline diuresis is of no value in the treatment of intoxications with short-acting barbiturates. Charcoal hemoperfusion or hemodialysis may be useful in the harder to treat intoxications, especially in the presence of very high serum barbiturate levels with coma; multiple dosing of activated charcoal may be effective. Hemodialysis clearance is ~22 mL/minute (18% fractional removal of drug during 4 hours); hemoperfusion clearance ranges from 50-300 mL/minute (27% fractional removal of drug in 4 hours)

Test Interactions ↑ ammonia (B); ↓ bilirubin (S)

Drug Interactions

Induces CYP2A6 (strong), 3A4 (strong)

Acetaminophen: Barbiturates may enhance the hepatotoxic potential of acetaminophen overdoses

Antiarrhythmics: Barbiturates may increase the metabolism of antiarrhythmics, decreasing their clinical effect; includes disopyramide, propafenone, and quinidine

Anticonvulsants: Barbiturates may increase the metabolism of anticonvulsants; includes ethosuximide, felbamate (possibly), lamotrigine, phenytoin, tiagabine, topiramate, and zonisamide; does not appear to affect gabapentin or levetiracetam

Antineoplastics: Limited evidence suggests that enzyme-inducing anticonvulsant therapy may reduce the effectiveness of some chemotherapy regimens (specifically in ALL); teniposide and methotrexate may be cleared more rapidly in these patients

Antipsychotics: Barbiturates may enhance the metabolism (decrease the efficacy) of antipsychotics; monitor for altered response; dose adjustment may be needed

Beta-blockers: Metabolism of beta-blockers may be increased and clinical effect decreased; atenolol and nadolol are unlikely to interact given their renal elimination

Calcium channel blockers: Barbiturates may enhance the metabolism of calcium channel blockers, decreasing their clinical effect

Chloramphenicol: Barbiturates may increase the metabolism of chloramphenicol and chloramphenicol may inhibit barbiturate metabolism; monitor for altered response

Cimetidine: Barbiturates may enhance the metabolism of cimetidine, decreasing its clinical effect

CNS depressants: Sedative effects and/or respiratory depression with barbiturates may be additive with other CNS depressants; monitor for increased effect; includes ethanol, sedatives, antidepressants, narcotic analgesics, and benzodiazepines

Corticosteroids: Barbiturates may enhance the metabolism of corticosteroids, decreasing their clinical effect

Cyclosporine: Levels may be decreased by barbiturates; monitor

CYP2A6 substrates: Pentobarbital may decrease the levels/effects of CYP2A6 substrates. Example substrates include ifosfamide and rifampin.

CYP3A4 substrates: Pentobarbital may decrease the levels/effects of CYP3A4 substrates. Example substrates include benzodiazepines, calcium channel blockers, clarithromycin, cyclosporine, erythromycin, estrogens, mirtazapine, nateglinide, nefazodone, nevirapine, protease inhibitors, tacrolimus, and venlafaxine.

Doxycycline: Barbiturates may enhance the metabolism of doxycycline, decreasing its clinical effect; higher dosages may be required

Estrogens: Barbiturates may increase the metabolism of estrogens and reduce their efficacy

Felbamate may inhibit the metabolism of barbiturates and barbiturates may increase the metabolism of felbamate

Griseofulvin: Barbiturates may impair the absorption of griseofulvin, and griseofulvin metabolism may be increased by barbiturates, decreasing clinical effect

Guanfacine: Effect may be decreased by barbiturates

Immunosuppressants: Barbiturates may enhance the metabolism of immunosuppressants, decreasing its clinical effect; includes both cyclosporine and tacrolimus

Loop diuretics: Metabolism may be increased and clinical effects decreased; established for furosemide, effect with other loop diuretics not established

MAO inhibitors: Metabolism of barbiturates may be inhibited, increasing clinical effect or toxicity of the barbiturates

Methadone: Barbiturates may enhance the metabolism of methadone resulting in methadone withdrawal

Methoxyflurane: Barbiturates may enhance the nephrotoxic effects of methoxyflurane

Oral contraceptives: Barbiturates may enhance the metabolism of oral contraceptives, decreasing their clinical effect; an alternative method of contraception should be considered

Theophylline: Barbiturates may increase metabolism of theophylline derivatives and decrease their clinical effect

Tricyclic antidepressants: Barbiturates may increase metabolism of tricyclic antidepressants and decrease their clinical effect; sedative effects may be additive

Valproic acid: Metabolism of barbiturates may be inhibited by valproic acid; monitor for excessive sedation; a dose reduction may be needed

Warfarin: Barbiturates inhibit the hypoprothrombinemic effects of oral anticoagulants via increased metabolism; this combination should generally be avoided

Pregnancy Risk Factor D

Lactation Enters breast milk/contraindicated

Pentostatin

CAS Number 53910-25-7
U.S. Brand Names Nipent®

Synonyms 2'-Deoxycoformycin; CL-825; Co-Vidarabine; dCF; Deoxycoformycin; NSC-218321

Use Treatment of hairy cell leukemia; non-Hodgkin's lymphoma, cutaneous T-cell lymphoma

Mechanism of Action An irreversible inhibitor of adenosine deaminase (ADA) in the erythrocyte and lymphatic tissue which causes a build-up of deoxyadenosine thus inhibiting purine metabolism; also inhibits ribonucleotide reductase which blocks DNA synthesis

Adverse Reactions

Cardiovascular: Chest pain, arrhythmia, peripheral edema

Central nervous system: **Fever, chills, headache**, opportunistic infections, anxiety, confusion, depression, dizziness, insomnia, nervousness, somnolence, myalgias, malaise, lethargy, seizures, coma (uncommon at doses <4 mg/m^2)

Dermatologic: **Skin rashes (25% to 30%), alopecia**, dry skin, eczema, pruritus

Gastrointestinal: **Mild to moderate nausea, vomiting (60%), stomatitis, diarrhea, anorexia**, constipation, flatulence, weight loss

Genitourinary: **Acute renal failure (35%)**, dysuria

Hematologic: **Thrombocytopenia (50%)**, dose-limiting in 25% of patients; **anemia (40% to 45%); neutropenia**, mild to moderate, not dose-limiting
    Nadir: 7 days
    Recovery: 10-14 days

Hepatic: **Mild to moderate increases in transaminase levels (30%)**, usually transient; **hepatitis (19%)**, usually reversible

Local: Thrombophlebitis

Neuromuscular & skeletal: Paresthesia, weakness

Ocular: Moderate to severe keratoconjunctivitis, abnormal vision, eye pain

Otic: Ear pain

Renal: Hematuria, BUN increased

Respiratory: **Pulmonary edema (15%)**, may be exacerbated by fludarabine; dyspnea, pneumonia, bronchitis, pharyngitis, rhinitis, epistaxis, sinusitis

Miscellaneous: **Infection (57%; 35% severe, life-threatening)**, hypersensitivity reactions

Pharmacodynamics/Kinetics

Distribution: I.V.: V_d: 36.1 L (20.1 L/m^2); rapidly to body tissues

Half-life elimination: Distribution half-life: 30-85 minutes; Terminal: 5-15 hours

Excretion: Urine ($\sim$50% to 96%) within 24 hours (30% to 90% as unchanged drug)

Dosage Refractory hairy cell leukemia: Adults (refer to individual protocols): 4 mg/m^2 every other week; I.V. bolus over $\geq$3-5 minutes in D$_5$W or normal saline at concentrations $\geq$2 mg/mL; patients should receive previous I.V. hydration with 500-1000 mL of 0.45% saline; patient should also receive 500 mL of 0.45% saline with 5% dextrose after infusion; reassess after usually 6 months of treatment

Monitoring Parameters CBC, renal function tests

Administration Administer I.V. as a 15- to 30-minute infusion; continuous infusion regimens have been reported, but are not commonly used I.V. bolus over $\geq$3-5 minutes in D$_5$W or NS at concentrations $\geq$2 mg/mL

Contraindications Hypersensitivity to pentostatin or any component; pregnancy

Warnings Hazardous agent - use appropriate precautions for handling and disposal. **[U.S. Boxed Warnings]: Severe renal, liver, pulmonary and CNS toxicities have occurred with doses higher than recommended; do not exceed the recommended dose. Do not administer concurrently with fludarabine; concomitant use has resulted in serious and fatal pulmonary toxicity.** Bone marrow suppression may occur, primarily early in treatment; if neutropenia persists beyond early cycles, evaluate for disease status. In patients who present with infections prior to treatment , infections should be resolved, if possible, prior to initiation of treatment. Use cautiously in patients with renal dysfunction; appropriate dosing guidelines in renal insufficiency have not been determined. May cause elevations (reversible) in liver function tests. Withhold treatment for CNS toxicity or severe rash. Pulmonary edema and hypotension have been reported in patients treated with pentostatin in combination with carmustine, etoposide or high dose cyclophosphamide as part of a myeloablative regimen for bone marrow transplant. **[U.S. Boxed Warning]: Should be administered under the supervision of an experienced cancer chemotherapy physician.** Safety and efficacy in children have not been established.

Dosage Forms Injection, powder for reconstitution: 10 mg

Reference Range Pentostatin plasma levels between 1-5 μM achieved after therapeutic dose

Overdosage/Treatment Supportive therapy: Keep patient hydrated; erythrocyte transfusions may be indicated when the erythrocyte deoxyadenosine triphosphate to ATP ratio exceeds 1.0

Drug Interactions Increased toxicity: Vidarabine, allopurinol; combined use with fludarabine may lead to severe, even fatal, pulmonary toxicity

Pregnancy Risk Factor D

Pregnancy Implications Pentostatin has been found to be teratogenic in animals. There are no adequate or well-controlled studies in humans.

Women of childbearing potential should be advised to avoid becoming pregnant. If used during pregnancy, the patient should be apprised of the potential risk to the fetus.

Lactation Excretion in breast milk unknown/contraindicated

Additional Information Treatment with pentostatin should either be avoided or administered with great caution in patients with a history of fludarabine-associated hemolytic anemia; may contain sodium hydroxide or hydrochloric acid for pH adjustment (pH of solution 7-8.5); infections (particularly disseminated herpes zoster) may occur; withhold dose if serum creatinine increases; polyethylene gloves should be utilized when administering this agent; extravasation injuries not reported

Pentoxifylline

CAS Number 6493-05-6
U.S. Brand Names Pentoxil®; Trental®
Synonyms Oxpentifylline

Use Treatment of intermittent claudication on the basis of chronic occlusive arterial disease of the limbs; may improve function and symptoms, but not intended to replace more definitive therapy

Unlabeled/Investigational Use AIDS patients with increased TNF, CVA, cerebrovascular diseases, diabetic atherosclerosis, diabetic neuropathy, gangrene, hemodialysis shunt thrombosis, vascular impotence, cerebral malaria, septic shock, sickle cell syndromes, and vasculitis

Mechanism of Action Mechanism of action remains unclear; is thought to reduce blood viscosity and improve blood flow by altering the rheology of red blood cells

Adverse Reactions
Cardiovascular: Chest pain, edema, hypotension
Central nervous system: Dizziness, headache, anxiety, arrhythmias, aseptic meningitis, confusion, depression, hallucinations, seizures
Dermatologic: Angioedema, rash
Gastrointestinal: Dyspepsia, nausea, vomiting
Hepatic: Cholecystitis, hepatitis, jaundice
Neuromuscular & skeletal: Tremor
Ocular: Blurred vision
Respiratory: Congestion, dyspnea
Miscellaneous: Anaphylactoid reactions

Signs and Symptoms of Overdose Agitation, atrioventricular block, dyspepsia, fever, flushing, hyperglycemia, hypokalemia (lasts for 12 hours), hypotension, laryngitis, mydriasis, myoclonus, seizures, syncope, tachycardia, thrombocytopenia

Admission Criteria/Prognosis Admit ingestions >50 mg/kg; monitor for seizures in ingestions >75 mg/kg; patients asymptomatic 12 hours postingestion can be discharged

Pharmacodynamics/Kinetics
Absorption: Well absorbed
Metabolism: Hepatic and via erythrocytes; extensive first-pass effect
Half-life elimination: Parent drug: 24-48 minutes; Metabolites: 60-96 minutes
Time to peak, serum: 2-4 hours
Excretion: Primarily urine (active metabolites); feces (4%)

Dosage
Adults: Oral: 400 mg 3 times/day with meals; may reduce to 400 mg twice daily if gastrointestinal or CNS side effects occur
Behçet disease: 600 mg 2 times/day for 2 weeks

Administration Tablets should be swallowed whole; do not chew, break, or crush.

Contraindications Hypersensitivity to pentoxifylline, xanthines (eg, caffeine, theophylline), or any component of the formulation; recent cerebral and/or retinal hemorrhage

Warnings Use with caution in patients with renal and hepatic impairment; start with lower doses in elderly patients and monitor renal function. Use caution in patients receiving anticoagulant therapy or at risk for bleeding complications; monitor PT/INR, hematocrit, and/or hemoglobin as necessary. May lower blood pressure; monitor with concomitant antihypertensive agent use. Safety and efficacy in pediatric patients have not been established.

Dosage Forms Tablet, extended release (Pentoxil®, Trental®): 400 mg

Reference Range
Therapeutic: 100-400 ng/mL; peak levels of 100 ng/mL obtained 2-3 hours after a 400 mg dose; serum level of 51,000 ng/mL associated with emesis, hypokalemia, and survival
Postmortem blood and urine levels of 0.63 mg/dL and 0.08 mg/dL found in a mixed pentoxifylline/diltiazem overdose.

Overdosage/Treatment
Decontamination: Lavage (within 1 hour) ingestions >50 mg/kg; activated charcoal; **do not** induce emesis
Supportive therapy: Seizures can be treated with diazepam, lorazepam, phenobarbital, or phenytoin. Hypotension can be treated with crystalloid infusion and Trendelenburg. Dopamine and norepinephrine can also be given for refractory hypotension. Atropine can be used to treat bradycardia.

Enhancement of elimination: Multiple dosing of activated charcoal may be effective; extracorporeal removal may also be effective although there is no experience with this modality

Test Interactions ↓ calcium (S), magnesium (S); false-positive theophylline levels are not likely

Drug Interactions Theophylline: Increased toxicity

Pregnancy Risk Factor C

Pregnancy Implications Teratogenic effects were not observed in animal studies. There are no adequate and well-controlled studies in pregnant women.

Lactation Enters breast milk/not recommended

Specific References
Chiao TB and Lee AJ, "Role of Pentoxifylline and Vitamin E in Attenuation of Radiation-Induced Fibrosis," *Ann Pharmacother*, 2005, 39(3):516-22.

Pergolide

CAS Number 66104-23-2; 66104-32-2
U.S. Brand Names Permax®
Synonyms Pergolide Mesylate

Use Adjunctive treatment to levodopa/carbidopa in the management of Parkinson's disease

Unlabeled/Investigational Use Tourette's disorder, chronic motor or vocal tic disorder

Mechanism of Action Pergolide is a semisynthetic ergot alkaloid similar to bromocriptine but stated to be more potent and longer-acting; it is a centrally-active dopamine agonist stimulating both D_1 and D_2 receptors

Adverse Reactions
Cardiovascular: Hypotension or postural hypotension, peripheral edema, chest pain, vasodilation, palpitation, syncope, arrhythmias, hypertension, MI, AV block, intracranial hypertension, pericarditis, pericardial effusion, vasculitis
Central nervous system: **Dizziness (19%), hallucinations, dystonia, somnolence, confusion**, insomnia, pain, anxiety, psychosis, EPS, incoordination, chills, facial paralysis, neuritis, neuroleptic malignant syndrome (NMS; associated with rapid discontinuation)
Dermatologic: Rash
Gastrointestinal: **Nausea (24%), constipation**, diarrhea, dyspepsia, abdominal pain, pancreatitis, anorexia, xerostomia, vomiting, dysphagia, nausea, intestinal obstruction
Genitourinary: Retroperitoneal fibrosis
Hematologic: Anemia
Neuromuscular & skeletal: **Dyskinesia (62%)**, myalgia, neuralgia
Ocular: Abnormal vision, diplopia
Respiratory: **Rhinitis**, dyspnea, epistaxis, laryngeal edema, pleural effusion, pleural fibrosis, pleuritis, pneumothorax
Miscellaneous: Flu syndrome, hiccups, valvular fibrosis

Pharmacodynamics/Kinetics
Absorption: Well absorbed
Protein binding, plasma: 90%
Metabolism: Extensively hepatic
Half-life elimination: 27 hours
Excretion: Urine (~50%); feces (50%)

Dosage When adding pergolide to levodopa/carbidopa, the dose of the latter can usually and should be decreased. Patients no longer responsive to bromocriptine may benefit by being switched to pergolide. Oral:
Children and Adolescents: Tourette's disorder, chronic motor or vocal disorder (unlabeled uses): Up to 300 mcg/day
Adults: Parkinson's disease: Start with 0.05 mg/day for 2 days, then increase dosage by 0.1 or 0.15 mg/day every 3 days over next 12 days, increase dose by 0.25 mg/day every 3 days until optimal therapeutic dose is achieved, up to 5 mg/day maximum; usual dosage range: 2-3 mg/day in 3 divided doses

Monitoring Parameters Blood pressure (both sitting/supine and standing), symptoms of parkinsonism, dyskinesias, mental status

Contraindications Hypersensitivity to pergolide mesylate, other ergot derivatives, or any component of the formulation; ergot alkaloids are contraindicated with potent inhibitors of CYP3A4 (includes protease inhibitors, azole antifungals, and some macrolide antibiotics)

Warnings
Symptomatic hypotension occurs in 10% of patients; use with caution in patients with a history of cardiac arrhythmias, hallucinations, or mental illness. Cardiac valvular, pleural, and peritoneal fibrosis have been reported with prolonged daily use. Avoid rapid dose reduction or abrupt discontinuation.
Pergolide has been associated with somnolence. Some patients have been reported to fall asleep during activities of daily living, including driving, while taking this medication. Not all patients exhibited somnolence prior to these events. Patients should be advised of this issue and factors which may increase risk (sleep disorders or other sedating medications) and instructed to report daytime somnolence or any episode of falling asleep during activities to the prescriber. Patients should use caution in performing activities which require alertness

(driving or operating machinery), and to avoid other medications which may cause CNS depression, including ethanol.

Dosage Forms Tablet: 0.05 mg, 0.25 mg, 1 mg

Overdosage/Treatment Decontamination: Lavage within 1 hour adult ingestions >5 mg/activated charcoal

Drug Interactions **Substrate** of CYP3A4 (major); **Inhibits** CYP2D6 (strong), 3A4 (weak)

Antifungals, azole derivatives (itraconazole, ketoconazole) increase levels of ergot alkaloids by inhibiting CYP3A4 metabolism, resulting in toxicity; concomitant use is contraindicated.

Antipsychotics: May diminish the effects of pergolide (due to dopamine antagonism); these combinations should generally be avoided.

CYP2D6 substrates: Pergolide may increase the levels/effects of CYP2D6 substrates. Example substrates include amphetamines, selected beta-blockers, dextromethorphan, fluoxetine, lidocaine, mirtazapine, nefazodone, paroxetine, risperidone, ritonavir, thioridazine, tricyclic antidepressants, and venlafaxine.

CYP2D6 prodrug substrates: Pergolide may decrease the levels/effects of CYP2D6 prodrug substrates. Example prodrug substrates include codeine, hydrocodone, oxycodone, and tramadol.

CYP3A4 inhibitors: May increase the levels/effects of pergolide. Example inhibitors include azole antifungals, clarithromycin, diclofenac, doxycycline, erythromycin, imatinib, isoniazid, nefazodone, nicardipine, propofol, protease inhibitors, quinidine, telithromycin, and verapamil.

Levodopa: Concurrent use may result in a higher frequency of hallucinations.

Macrolide antibiotics: Erythromycin, clarithromycin, and troleandomycin may increase levels of ergot alkaloids by inhibiting CYP3A4 metabolism, resulting in toxicity (ischemia, vasospasm); concomitant use is contraindicated.

MAO inhibitors: The serotonergic effects of ergot derivatives may be increased by MAO inhibitors. Monitor for signs and symptoms of serotonin syndrome.

Metoclopramide: May diminish the effects of pergolide (due to dopamine antagonism); concurrent therapy should generally be avoided.

Protease inhibitors (ritonavir, amprenavir, indinavir, nelfinavir, and saquinavir) increase blood levels of ergot alkaloids by inhibiting CYP3A4 metabolism, acute ergot toxicity has been reported; concomitant use is contraindicated.

Sibutramine: May cause serotonin syndrome; concurrent use with ergot alkaloids is contraindicated.

Serotonin agonists: Concurrent use with pergolide may increase the risk of serotonin syndrome (includes buspirone, SSRIs, TCAs, nefazodone, sumatriptan, and trazodone).

Pregnancy Risk Factor B

Lactation Excretion in breast milk unknown/not recommended

Nursing Implications Monitor closely for orthostasis and other adverse effects; raise bed rails and institute safety measures; aid patient with ambulation, may cause postural hypotension and drowsiness

Additional Information Lowers serum prolactin and growth hormone levels

---

Permethrin

CAS Number 52645-53-1

U.S. Brand Names A200® Lice [OTC]; Acticin®; Elimite®; Nix® [OTC]; Rid® Spray [OTC]

Use Single application treatment of infestation with *Pediculus humanus capitis* (head louse) and its nits, or *Sarcoptes scabiei* (scabies); also active against mosquitoes, blackflies, and tsetse flies

Mechanism of Action Inhibits sodium ion influx through nerve cell membrane channels in parasites resulting in delayed repolarization and thus paralysis of the pest (a pyrethroid)

Adverse Reactions

Cardiovascular: Edema, tachycardia, sinus tachycardia

Central nervous system: Convulsions, headache, dizziness, stuttering

Dermatologic: Pruritus, numbness or scalp discomfort, erythema, rash of the scalp

Gastrointestinal: Vomiting, sore throat

Local: Burning, stinging, tingling, cheek/perioral numbness

Neuromuscular & skeletal: Paresthesia

Ocular: Visual evoked potential abnormalities

Respiratory: Wheezing, dyspnea, sneezing

Signs and Symptoms of Overdose Oral ingestion: Anorexia, asthenia, coma, dizziness, fasciculations, headache, numbness, nausea, vomiting, and seizures can occur at doses >200 mL.

Pharmacodynamics/Kinetics

Absorption: <2%

Metabolism: Hepatic via ester hydrolysis to inactive metabolites

Excretion: Urine

Dosage

Topical:

Head lice: Children >2 months and Adults: After hair has been washed with shampoo, rinsed with water, and towel dried, apply a sufficient

volume of topical liquid to saturate the hair and scalp. Leave on hair for 10 minutes lice or nits still present.

Scabies: Apply cream from head to toe; leave on for 8-14 hours before washing off with water, a single application is usually adequate; may repeat in 1 week if lice or nits still present. For infants, also apply on the hairline, neck, scalp, temple, and forehead.

Administration Because scabies and lice are so contagious, use caution to avoid spreading or infecting oneself; wear gloves when applying

Cream: Apply from neck to toes. Bathe to remove drug after 8-14 hours. Repeat in 7 days if lice or nits are still present. Report if condition persists or infection occurs.

Cream rinse/lotion: Apply immediately after hair is shampooed, rinsed, and towel-dried. Apply enough to saturate hair and scalp (especially behind ears and on nape of neck). Leave on hair for 10 minutes before rinsing with water. Remove nits with fine-tooth comb. May repeat in 1 week if lice or nits are still present.

Contraindications Hypersensitivity to pyrethroid, pyrethrin, chrysanthemums, or any component of the formulation; lotion is contraindicated for use in infants <2 months of age

Warnings Treatment may temporarily exacerbate the symptoms of itching, redness, swelling; for external use only; use during pregnancy only if clearly needed

Dosage Forms Cream, topical (Acticin®, Elimite®): 5% (60 g) [contains coconut oil]

Lotion, topical: 1% (59 mL)

Liquid, topical [creme rinse formulation] (Nix®): 1% (60 mL) [contains isopropyl alcohol 20%]

Solution, spray [for bedding and furniture]:

A200® Lice: 0.5% (180 mL)

Nix®: 0.25% (148 mL)

Rid®: 0.5% (150 mL)

Overdosage/Treatment

Decontamination: Activated charcoal; wash exposed skin thoroughly with soap and water

Supportive therapy: Epinephrine or diphenhydramine for allergic reactions; nebulized bronchodilators for wheezing; treat seizures with diazepam, lorazepam, phenytoin, or phenobarbital

Drug Interactions No data reported

Pregnancy Risk Factor B

Lactation Effect on infant unknown

Nursing Implications Avoid contact with eyes during administration; shake well before using

Additional Information Available in 1% formulation; suitable for aircraft disinfection

Specific References

Centers for Disease Control and Prevention (CDC), "Human Exposure to Mosquito-Control Pesticides–Mississippi, North Carolina, and Virginia, 2002 and 2003," *MMWR Morb Mortal Wkly Rep*, 2005, 3;54(21): 529-32.

Perphenazine

Related Information

- Anticholinergic Effects of Common Psychotropics
- Antipsychotic Agents

CAS Number 58-39-9

U.S. Brand Names Trilafon® [DSC]

Impairment Potential Yes

Use Treatment of severe schizophrenia; nausea and vomiting

Unlabeled/Investigational Use Ethanol withdrawal; dementia in elderly; Tourette's syndrome; Huntington's chorea; spasmodic torticollis; Reye's syndrome; psychosis

Mechanism of Action Blocks postsynaptic mesolimbic dopaminergic receptors in the brain; exhibits a strong alpha-adrenergic blocking effect and depresses the release of hypothalamic and hypophyseal hormones

Adverse Reactions

Cardiovascular: **Hypotension**, tachycardia, cardiac arrhythmias, bradycardia, AV block, sinus bradycardia, sinus tachycardia, **orthostatic hypotension**

Central nervous system: Sedation, drowsiness, restlessness, anxiety, extrapyramidal reactions, **pseudoparkinsonian signs and symptoms**, seizures, altered central temperature regulation, **akathisia, dystonias, tardive dyskinesia, dizziness**, somnambulism

Dermatologic: Hyperpigmentation, pruritus, rash, photosensitivity reactions, Stevens-Johnson syndrome, exfoliative dermatitis, angioedema, urticaria, purpura, exanthem

Endocrine & metabolic: Amenorrhea, galactorrhea, gynecomastia, syndrome of inappropriate antidiuretic hormone, black galactorrhea

Gastrointestinal: Xerostomia, **constipation**, GI upset, weight gain

Genitourinary: Urinary retention

Hematologic: Agranulocytosis (more often in women between fourth and tenth weeks of therapy), leukopenia (usually in patients with large doses for prolonged periods)

Neuromuscular & skeletal: Torticollis, rhabdomyolysis

Ocular: Blurred vision, nystagmus, photophobia, **retinal pigmentation**

Respiratory: **Nasal congestion**

Miscellaneous: Systemic lupus erythematosus, **diaphoresis**, hiccups

Signs and Symptoms of Overdose Abnormal involuntary muscle movements, agitation, agranulocytosis, arrhythmias (QT_c prolongation), AV block, coma, deep sleep, dystonic reactions, extrapyramidal reaction, galactorrhea, granulocytopenia, gynecomastia, hypotension, impotence, jaundice, leukopenia, neuroleptic malignant syndrome, neutropenia, Parkinson's-like symptoms, seizures, thrombocytopenia, torsade de pointes, urine discoloration (pink; red; red-brown), ventricular tachycardia/fibrillation, vision color changes (brown tinge; yellow tinge). Children may have convulsive seizures.

Pharmacodynamics/Kinetics

Absorption: Oral: Well absorbed

Distribution: Crosses placenta

Metabolism: Extensively hepatic to metabolites via sulfoxidation, hydroxylation, dealkylation, and glucuronidation

Half-life elimination: Perphenazine: 9-12 hours; 7-hydroxyperphenazine: 11.3 hours

Time to peak, serum: Perphenazine: 1-3 hours; 7-hydroxyperphenazine: 2-4 hours

Excretion: Urine and feces

Dosage

Oral:

Children:

Schizophrenia/psychoses:

1-6 years: 4-6 mg/day in divided doses

6-12 years: 6 mg/day in divided doses

>12 years: 4-16 mg 2-4 times/day

Adults:

Schizophrenia/psychoses: 4-16 mg 2-4 times/day not to exceed 64 mg/day

Nausea/vomiting: 8-16 mg/day in divided doses up to 24 mg/day

Elderly: Behavioral symptoms associated with dementia: Initial: 2-4 mg 1-2 times/day; increase at 4- to 7-day intervals by 2-4 mg/day. Increase dose intervals (bid, tid, etc) as necessary to control behavior response or side effects. Maximum daily dose: 32 mg; gradual increase (titration) and bedtime administration may prevent some side effects or decrease their severity.

Hemodialysis: Not dialyzable (0% to 5%)

Dosing adjustment in hepatic impairment: Dosage reductions should be considered in patients with liver disease although no specific guidelines are available

Monitoring Parameters Vital signs; lipid profile, fasting blood glucose/Hgb A_{1c}; BMI; mental status, abnormal involuntary movement scale (AIMS), extrapyramidal symptoms (EPS)

Contraindications Hypersensitivity to perphenazine or any component of the formulation (cross-reactivity between phenothiazines may occur); severe CNS depression; subcortical brain damage; bone marrow suppression; blood dyscrasias; coma

Warnings

May cause hypotension. May be sedating, use with caution in disorders where CNS depression is a feature. Use with caution in Parkinson's disease. Caution in patients with hemodynamic instability; predisposition to seizures; severe cardiac, hepatic, renal, or respiratory disease. Esophageal dysmotility and aspiration have been associated with antipsychotic use - use with caution in patients at risk of pneumonia (ie, Alzheimer's disease). Caution in breast cancer or other prolactin-dependent tumors (may elevate prolactin levels). May alter temperature regulation or mask toxicity of other drugs due to antiemetic effects. May alter cardiac conduction - life-threatening arrhythmias have occurred with therapeutic doses of phenothiazines. May cause orthostatic hypotension - use with caution in patients at risk of this effect or those who would tolerate transient hypotensive episodes (cerebrovascular disease, cardiovascular disease, or other medications which may predispose).

Phenothiazines may cause anticholinergic effects (confusion, agitation, constipation, xerostomia, blurred vision, urinary retention); therefore, they should be used with caution in patients with decreased gastrointestinal motility, urinary retention, BPH, xerostomia, or visual problems. Conditions which also may be exacerbated by cholinergic blockade include narrow-angle glaucoma (screening is recommended) and worsening of myasthenia gravis. Relative to other neuroleptics, perphenazine has a low potency of cholinergic blockade.

May cause extrapyramidal symptoms, including pseudoparkinsonism, acute dystonic reactions, akathisia, and tardive dyskinesia (risk of these reactions is moderate-high relative to other neuroleptics). Older patients are at increased risk for developing tardive dyskinesia. May be associated with neuroleptic malignant syndrome (NMS) or pigmentary retinopathy.

Dosage Forms Tablet: 2 mg, 4 mg, 8 mg, 16 mg

Reference Range 0.004-0.064 mg/L (therapeutic serum level)

Overdosage/Treatment

Decontamination: Activated charcoal

Supportive therapy: Following initiation of essential overdose management, toxic symptom treatment and supportive treatment should be initiated. Hypotension usually responds to I.V. fluids or Trendelenburg positioning. If unresponsive to these measures, the use of a parenteral inotrope may be required (eg, norepinephrine 0.1-0.2 mcg/kg/minute titrated to response). Seizures commonly respond to lorazepam, diazepam, or phenobarbital. Also critical cardiac arrhythmics often respond to I.V. phenytoin (15 mg/kg up to 1 gram), while other antiarrhythmics can be used. Neuroleptics often cause extrapyramidal reaction (eg, dystonic reactions) requiring management with diphenhydramine 1-2 mg/kg (adults) up to a maximum of 50 mg I.M. or I.V. slow push followed by a maintenance dose for 48-72 hours. When these reactions are unresponsive to diphenhydramine, benztropine mesylate I.V. 1-2 mg (adults) may be effective. These agents are generally effective within 2-5 minutes.

Enhancement of elimination: Multiple dosing of activated charcoal may be useful; forced diuresis or hemodialysis is of no benefit; not dialyzable (0% to 5%)

Test Interactions ↑ cholesterol (S), glucose; ↓ uric acid (S)

Drug Interactions Substrate of CYP1A2 (minor), 2C9 (minor), 2C19 (minor), 2D6 (major), 3A4 (minor); **Inhibits** CYP1A2 (weak), 2D6 (weak)

Acetylcholinesterase inhibitors (central): May increase the risk of antipsychotic-related extrapyramidal symptoms; monitor.

Aluminum salts: May decrease the absorption of phenothiazines; monitor

Amphetamines: Efficacy may be diminished by antipsychotics; in addition, amphetamines may increase psychotic symptoms; avoid concurrent use

Anticholinergics: May inhibit the therapeutic response to phenothiazines and excess anticholinergic effects may occur; includes benztropine, trihexyphenidyl, biperiden, and drugs with significant anticholinergic activity (TCAs, antihistamines, disopyramide)

Antihypertensives: Concurrent use of phenothiazines with an antihypertensive may produce additive hypotensive effects (particularly orthostasis)

Bromocriptine: Phenothiazines inhibit the ability of bromocriptine to lower serum prolactin concentrations

CNS depressants: Sedative effects may be additive with phenothiazines; monitor for increased effect; includes barbiturates, benzodiazepines, narcotic analgesics, ethanol, and other sedative agents

CYP2D6 inhibitors: May increase the levels/effects of perphenazine. Example inhibitors include chlorpromazine, delavirdine, fluoxetine, miconazole, paroxetine, pergolide, quinidine, quinine, ritonavir, and ropinirole.

Epinephrine: Chlorpromazine (and possibly other low potency antipsychotics) may diminish the pressor effects of epinephrine

Guanethidine and guanadrel: Antihypertensive effects may be inhibited by phenothiazines

Levodopa: Phenothiazines may inhibit the antiparkinsonian effect of levodopa; avoid this combination

Lithium: Phenothiazines may produce neurotoxicity with lithium; this is a rare effect

Metoclopramide: May increase extrapyramidal symptoms (EPS) or risk.

Phenytoin: May reduce serum levels of phenothiazines; phenothiazines may increase phenytoin serum levels

Propranolol: Serum concentrations of phenothiazines may be increased; propranolol also increases phenothiazine concentrations

Polypeptide antibiotics: Rare cases of respiratory paralysis have been reported with concurrent use of phenothiazines

QT_c-prolonging agents: Effects on QT_c interval may be additive with phenothiazines, increasing the risk of malignant arrhythmias; includes type Ia antiarrhythmics, TCAs, and some quinolone antibiotics (sparfloxacin, moxifloxacin, and gatifloxacin)

Sulfadoxine-pyrimethamine: May increase phenothiazine concentrations

Tricyclic antidepressants: Concurrent use may produce increased toxicity or altered therapeutic response

Trazodone: Phenothiazines and trazodone may produce additive hypotensive effects

Valproic acid: Serum levels may be increased by phenothiazines

Pregnancy Risk Factor C

Pregnancy Implications Crosses the placenta

Lactation Enters breast milk/not recommended (AAP rates "of concern")

Phenazopyridine

CAS Number 136-40-3; 94-78-0

U.S. Brand Names Azo-Gesic® [OTC]; Azo-Standard® [OTC]; Prodium® [OTC]; Pyridium®; ReAzo [OTC]; Uristat® [OTC]; UTI Relief® [OTC]

Synonyms Phenazopyridine Hydrochloride; Phenylazo Diamino Pyridine Hydrochloride

Use Symptomatic relief of urinary burning, itching, frequency and urgency in association with urinary tract infection or following urologic procedures

Mechanism of Action An azo dye which exerts local anesthetic or analgesic action on urinary tract mucosa through an unknown mechanism

Adverse Reactions

Central nervous system: **Headache, dizziness**, aseptic meningitis

Gastrointestinal: **Stomach cramps, feces discoloration (orange-red)**

Genitourinary: Red-staining urine, urolithiasis

Dermatologic: Skin pigmentation (yellow-orange), rash, pruritus

Hematologic: Methemoglobinemia, hemolytic anemia, thrombocytopenia, neutropenia, methemoglobinemia followed by hemolysis

Hepatic: Hepatitis, hepatomegaly

Renal: Acute renal failure

Miscellaneous: Anaphylactoid reaction

Signs and Symptoms of Overdose Acute tubular necrosis, dyspnea, hepatic impairment, methemoglobinemia followed by hemolytic anemia, rhabdomyolysis (after a 6 g ingestion), yellow skin pigmentation

Admission Criteria/Prognosis Admit any ingestion >1 g; hematologic effects usually manifest itself within 4 hours; admit patients with symptomatic methemoglobinemia

Pharmacodynamics/Kinetics

Metabolism: Hepatic and via other tissues

Excretion: Urine (65% as unchanged drug)

Dosage Oral:

Children: 12 mg/kg/day in 3 divided doses administered after meals for 2 days

Adults: 100-200 mg 3 times/day after meals for 2 days when used concomitantly with an antibacterial agent

Dosing interval in renal impairment:

Cl_{cr} 50-80 mL/minute: Administer every 8-16 hours

Cl_{cr} <50 mL/minute: Avoid use

Monitoring Parameters Methemoglobin levels, CBC, renal/liver function, urine analysis

Contraindications Hypersensitivity to phenazopyridine or any component of the formulation; kidney or liver disease; patients with a Cl_{cr} <50 mL/minute

Warnings Does not treat infection, acts only as an analgesic; drug should be discontinued if skin or sclera develop a yellow color; use with caution in patients with renal impairment. Use of this agent in the elderly is limited since accumulation of phenazopyridine can occur in patients with renal insufficiency. Use is contraindicated in patients with a Cl_{cr} <50 mL/minute.

Dosage Forms Tablet, as hydrochloride: 100 mg, 200 mg

AZO-Gesic®, AZO-Standard®, Uristat®: 95 mg

Baridium®: 97.2 mg

ReAzo: 95 mg

Pyridium®: 100 mg, 200 mg

UTI Relief®: 97.2 mg

Overdosage/Treatment

Decontamination: Activated charcoal

Supportive therapy: Methylene blue (1-2 mg/kg) for symptomatic methemoglobin cases or methemoglobin levels >30%

Enhanced elimination: Exchange transfusion may be useful in infants

Antidote(s)

- Methylene Blue [ANTIDOTE]

Test Interactions Phenazopyridine may cause delayed reactions with glucose oxidase reagents (Clinistix®, Tes-Tape®); occasional false-positive tests occur with Tes-Tape®; cupric sulfate tests (Clinitest®) are not affected; interference may also occur with urine ketone tests (Acetest®, Ketostix®) and urinary protein tests; tests for urinary steroids and porphyrins may also occur. Can cause false elevation of serum total protein, and a false-negative leukocyte esterase on urine dipstick; may cause elevation of urinary vanillylmandelic acid assay

Drug Interactions No data reported

Pregnancy Risk Factor B

Lactation Excretion in breast milk unknown

Additional Information Stains on clothing due to phenazopyridine can be removed by soaking fabric in a 0.25% solution of sodium dithionite

Specific References

Gold NA and Bithoney WG, "Methemoglobinemia Due to Ingestion of At Most Three Pills of Pyridium in a 2-Year-Old: Case Report and Review," *J Emerg Med*, 2003, 25(2):143-8.

Gopalachar AS, Bowie VL, and Bharadwaj P, "Phenazopyridine-Induced Sulfhemoglobinemia," *Ann Pharmacother*, 2005, 39(6):1128-30.

Phenelzine

Related Information

- Selegiline
- Therapeutic Drugs Associated with Hallucinations

CAS Number 156-51-4; 51-71-8

U.S. Brand Names Nardil®

Synonyms Phenelzine Sulfate

Use Symptomatic treatment of atypical, nonendogenous or neurotic depression

Unlabeled/Investigational Use Selective mutism

Mechanism of Action Thought to act by increasing endogenous concentrations of epinephrine, norepinephrine, dopamine, and serotonin through inhibition of monoamine oxidase, which is responsible for the breakdown of these neurotransmitters

Adverse Reactions

Cardiovascular: **Orthostatic hypotension**, edema, vasoconstriction

Central nervous system: **Drowsiness**, psychosis, headache, auditory and visual hallucinations, vascular encephalopathy

Dermatologic: Skin rash

Endocrine & metabolic: **Decreased sexual ability**, syndrome of inappropriate antidiuretic hormone

Gastrointestinal: Xerostomia, constipation, nausea

Genitourinary: Urinary retention

Hematologic: Aplastic anemia

Hepatic: Jaundice, hepatic failure

Neuromuscular & skeletal: **Trembling, weakness**, clonus, myoclonus

Ocular: **Blurred vision**, photophobia, mydriasis, nystagmus, amblyopia, periodic gaze disturbance ("ping-pong gaze")

Miscellaneous: Lupus-like reaction, serotonin syndrome (flushing, diarrhea)

Signs and Symptoms of Overdose Coma, delirium, drowsiness, dry mouth, ejaculatory disturbances, exfoliative dermatitis, extrapyramidal reaction, fever, flushing, hallucinations, hyperthermia, hypotension, impotence, insomnia, mania, metabolic acidosis, methemoglobinemia, muscle myoclonus, muscle rigidity, mydriasis, myoglobinuria, neuroleptic malignant syndrome, nystagmus, palpitations, photosensitivity, ptosis, restlessness, rhabdomyolysis, seizures, sinus tachycardia, sweating, tachypnea, transient hypertension

Admission Criteria/Prognosis Any patient with change in mental status, cardiopulmonary complaints or hypotension should be admitted.

Pharmacodynamics/Kinetics

Onset of action: Therapeutic: 2-4 weeks; geriatric patients receiving an average of 55 mg/day developed a mean platelet MAO activity inhibition of about 85%.

Duration: May continue to have a therapeutic effect and interactions 2 weeks after discontinuing therapy

Absorption: Well absorbed

Metabolism: Oxidized via monoamine oxidase (primary pathway) and acetylation (minor pathway)

Half-life elimination: 11 hours

Excretion: Urine (primarily as metabolites and unchanged drug)

Dosage Oral:

Children: Selective mutism (unlabeled use): 30-60 mg/day

Adults: Depression: 15 mg 3 times/day; may increase to 60-90 mg/day during early phase of treatment, then reduce to dose for maintenance therapy slowly after maximum benefit is obtained; takes 2-4 weeks for a significant response to occur

Elderly: Depression: Initial: 7.5 mg/day; increase by 7.5-15 mg/day every 3-4 days as tolerated; usual therapeutic dose: 15-60 mg/day in 3-4 divided doses

Stability Protect from light

Monitoring Parameters Blood pressure, heart rate, diet, weight, mood (if depressive symptoms)

Contraindications Hypersensitivity to phenelzine or any component of the formulation; uncontrolled hypertension; pheochromocytoma; hepatic disease; congestive heart failure; CNS depressants, ethanol, meperidine, bupropion, buspirone, guanethidine, serotonergic drugs (including SSRIs) - do not use within 5 weeks of fluoxetine discontinuation or 2 weeks of other antidepressant discontinuation; general anesthesia, local vasoconstrictors; spinal anesthesia (hypotension may be exaggerated); sympathomimetics (and related compounds); foods high in tyramine content; supplements containing tyrosine, phenylalanine, tryptophan, or caffeine

Warnings

[U.S. Boxed Warning]: Antidepressants increase the risk of suicidal thinking and behavior in children and adolescents with major depressive disorder (MDD) and other depressive disorders; consider risk prior to prescribing. Closely monitor for clinical worsening, suicidality, or unusual changes in behavior; the child's family or caregiver should be instructed to closely observe the patient and communicate condition with healthcare provider. Such observation would generally include at least weekly face-to-face contact with patients or their family members or caregivers during the first 4 weeks of treatment, then every other week visits for the next 4 weeks, then at 12 weeks, and as clinically indicated beyond 12 weeks. Additional contact by telephone may be appropriate between face-to-face visits. Adults treated with antidepressants should be observed similarly for clinical worsening and suicidality, especially during the initial few months of a course of drug therapy, or at times of dose changes, either increases or decreases. A medication guide should be dispensed with each prescription. **Phenelzine is FDA approved for the treatment of depression in children ≥16 years of age.**

The possibility of a suicide attempt is inherent in major depression and may persist until remission occurs. Monitor for worsening of depression or suicidality, especially during initiation of therapy or with dose increases or decreases. Worsening depression and severe abrupt suicidality that are not part of the presenting symptoms may require discontinuation or modification of drug therapy. Use caution in high-risk patients during initiation of therapy. Prescriptions should be written for the smallest quantity consistent with good patient care. The patient's family or caregiver should be alerted to monitor patients for the emergence of suicidality and associated behaviors such as anxiety, agitation, panic attacks, insomnia, irritability, hostility, impulsivity, akathisia, hypomania, and mania; patients should be instructed to notify their healthcare provider if any of these symptoms or worsening depression occur.

May worsen psychosis in some patients or precipitate a shift to mania or hypomania in patients with bipolar disorder. Monotherapy in patients with bipolar disorder should be avoided. Patients presenting with depressive symptoms should be screened for bipolar disorder. Phenelzine is not FDA approved for the treatment of bipolar depression.

Use with caution in patients who are hyperactive, hyperexcitable, or who have glaucoma, hyperthyroidism, suicidal tendencies, or diabetes. Hypertensive crisis may occur with tyramine, tryptophan, or dopamine-containing foods. Should not be used in combination with other antidepressants. Hypotensive effects of antihypertensives (beta-blockers, thiazides) may be exaggerated. May cause orthostatic hypotension - use with caution in patients with hypotension or patients who would not tolerate transient hypotensive episodes (cardiovascular or cerebrovascular disease) - effects may be additive with other agents which cause orthostasis.. Use with caution in patients at risk of seizures, or in patients receiving other drugs which may lower seizure threshold. Toxic reactions have occurred with dextromethorphan. Discontinue at least 48 hours prior to myelography. May increase the risks associated with electroconvulsive therapy. Consider discontinuing, when possible, prior to elective surgery.

The MAO inhibitors are effective and generally well tolerated by older patients. It is the potential interactions with tyramine or tryptophan-containing foods and other drugs, and their effects on blood pressure that have limited their use.

Dosage Forms Tablet: 15 mg

Reference Range Suggested plasma therapeutic range for phenelzine is 8-55 ng/mL. Chronic daily dosing of 60 mg will usually produce plasma phenelzine levels <10 ng/mL.

Overdosage/Treatment

Decontamination: **Do not** induce emesis; activated charcoal is useful

Supportive therapy: Competent supportive care is the most important treatment for an overdose with a monoamine oxidase (MAO) inhibitor. Both hypertension or hypotension can occur with intoxication. Hypotension may respond to I.V. fluids or vasopressors; hypertension usually responds to an alpha-adrenergic blocker. While treating hypertension, care is warranted to avoid sudden drops in blood pressure, since this may worsen MAO inhibitor toxicity. Muscle irritability and seizures often respond to diazepam or lorazepam, while hyperthermia is best treated with antipyretics and cooling blankets. Dantrolene sodium (2.5 mg/kg I.V. every 6 hours) has been used successfully in treatment of hyperthermia/hypermetabolic state due to phenelzine overdose. Cardiac arrhythmias are best treated with phenytoin or procainamide. Hypertensive crisis can be treated with nitroprusside, phentolamine (2-10 mg slow I.V. injection in adults). Aortic counter-pulsation has been used to treat phenelzine-induced cardiogenic shock.

Enhancement of elimination: Charcoal hemoperfusion may be useful in decreasing phenelzine serum levels but there is no documentation of clinical improvement.

Test Interactions ↓ glucose; peaked T waves noted on ECG

Drug Interactions Amphetamines: MAO inhibitors in combination with amphetamines may result in severe hypertensive reaction; concurrent use is contraindicated.

Anorexiants: Concurrent use of anorexiants may result in serotonin syndrome; these combinations are best avoided; includes dexfenfluramine, fenfluramine, or sibutramine

Barbiturates: MAO inhibitors may inhibit the metabolism of barbiturates and prolong their effect

Bupropion: Concurrent use is contraindicated; allow at least 14 days between discontinuing MAO inhibitor and starting bupropion.

Buspirone: May cause hypertension; wait at least 10 days between discontinuing one agent and starting the other.

CNS stimulants: MAO inhibitors in combination with stimulants (methylphenidate) may result in severe hypertensive reaction; concurrent use is contraindicated.

Dextromethorphan: Concurrent use of MAO inhibitors may result in serotonin syndrome; concurrent use is contraindicated.

Disulfiram: MAO inhibitors may produce delirium in patients receiving disulfiram; monitor.

Guanadrel and guanethidine: MAO inhibitors inhibit the antihypertensive response to guanadrel or guanethidine; concurrent use is contraindicated; use an alternative antihypertensive agent.

Hypoglycemic agents: MAO inhibitors may produce hypoglycemia in patients with diabetes; monitor.

Levodopa: MAO inhibitors in combination with levodopa may result in hypertensive reactions; monitor.

Lithium: MAO inhibitors in combination with lithium have resulted in malignant hyperpyrexia; this combination is best avoided.

Meperidine: May cause serotonin syndrome when combined with an MAO inhibitor; concurrent use is contraindicated; avoid use of meperidine within 2 weeks of phenelzine use.

Nefazodone: Concurrent use of MAO inhibitors may result in serotonin syndrome; these combinations are best avoided

Norepinephrine: MAO inhibitors may increase the pressor response of norepinephrine (effect is generally small); monitor

Reserpine: MAO inhibitors in combination with reserpine may result in hypertensive reactions; monitor

Serotonin agonists: Theoretically may increase the risk of serotonin syndrome; includes sumatriptan, naratriptan, rizatriptan, and zolmitriptan

SSRIs: May cause serotonin syndrome when combined with an MAO inhibitor; avoid this combination. Allow 5 weeks between discontinuing fluoxetine and starting an MAO inhibitor; allow at least 10 days after discontinuing MAO inhibitor and starting fluoxetine.

Succinylcholine: MAO inhibitors may prolong the muscle relaxation produced by succinylcholine via decreased plasma pseudocholinesterase

Sympathomimetics (indirect-acting): MAO inhibitors in combination with sympathomimetics such as dopamine, metaraminol, phenylephrine, and decongestants (pseudoephedrine) may result in severe hypertensive reaction; concurrent use is contraindicated.

Tramadol: May increase the risk of seizures and serotonin syndrome in patients receiving an MAO inhibitor

Trazodone: Concurrent use of MAO inhibitors may result in serotonin syndrome; these combinations are best avoided

Tricyclic antidepressants: May cause serotonin syndrome when combined with an MAO inhibitor; avoid this combination

Venlafaxine: Concurrent use of MAO inhibitors may result in serotonin syndrome; these combinations are best avoided

Pregnancy Risk Factor C

Lactation Excretion in breast milk unknown/not recommended

Nursing Implications Watch for hypotension (orthostatic); monitor blood pressure carefully, especially at therapy onset or if other CNS drugs or cardiovascular drugs are added; check for dietary and drug restriction

Additional Information Tyramine-containing foods: red wine, cheese (except cottage, ricotta, and cream), smoked or pickled fish, beef or chicken liver, dried sausage, fava or broad bean pods, yeast vitamin supplements

Specific References

Gold DG and Fatemi SH, "Phenelzine-Opiate-Induced Delirium Complicated by Phenelzine Withdrawal," *J Pharm Technol*, 2003, 19:19-22.

Phenmetrazine

Related Information

- Dextroamphetamine

CAS Number 134-49-6; 13931-75-4; 1707-14-8

Synonyms Phenmetrazine Hydrochloride

Impairment Potential Yes. Blood and urine phenmetrazine levels >0.5 mg/L and 56 mg/L, respectively, may be associated with driving impairment.

Use Anorectic agent

Mechanism of Action A central nervous system stimulant similar to dexamphetamine; a methylchloroformate derivative

Adverse Reactions

Cardiovascular: Hypertension, tachycardia (ventricular), tachycardia, palpitations, cardiac arrhythmias, vasculitis, pulmonary hypertension

Central nervous system: **Insomnia**, headache, **nervousness**, dizziness, seizures, mania, may precipitate Tourette's syndrome, CNS depression, dysphonia, irritability, agitation, euphoria, hallucination, extrapyramidal reaction, movement disorders, paranoia

Endocrine & metabolic: Growth suppression, respiratory alkalosis, increased serum thyroxine (hyperthyroidism)

Gastrointestinal: Anorexia, nausea, vomiting, diarrhea, abdominal cramps, metallic taste, xerostomia

Genitourinary: Impotence

Hematologic: Porphyria

Neuromuscular & skeletal: Tremors, choreoathetoid movements, fasciculations

Ocular: Cataracts

Renal: Myoglobinuria

Respiratory: Tachypnea

Signs and Symptoms of Overdose Anxiety, coma, confusion, dizziness, dysrhythmias, hallucinations, headache, hypertension, noncardiogenic pulmonary edema, retinal vein occlusion, seizures, shock, tachycardia, tachypnea, tremor

Pharmacodynamics/Kinetics

Metabolism: Hepatic

Half-life: 8 hours

Elimination: Renal

Normal pH: 19%
Acidic pH: 46% within 16 hours
Dosage Oral: 12.5-75 mg/day
Dosage Forms Tablet: 25 mg, 75 mg
Reference Range
Therapeutic serum level: 60-130 ng/mL
Overdosage/Treatment
Decontamination: Lavage (within 1 hour)/activated charcoal
Supportive therapy: Seizures can be treated with diazepam or lorazepam; phenytoin or phenobarbital can be used for refractory seizures; sodium nitroprusside (initial dose: 3 mcg/kg/minute) can be used to treat hypertension; droperidol (up to 0.1 mg/kg) or haloperidol (up to 0.1 mg/kg) can be used to treat agitation
Enhanced elimination: **Do not** acidify urine
Additional Information Primarily found in Europe

Phenobarbital

Related Information
- Seizures, Neonatal Guidelines
- Therapeutic Drugs Associated with Hallucinations

CAS Number 50-06-6; 57-30-7
U.S. Brand Names Luminal® Sodium
Synonyms Phenobarbital Sodium; Phenobarbitone; Phenylethylmalonylurea
Impairment Potential Yes
Use Management of generalized tonic-clonic (grand mal) and partial seizures; sedative
Unlabeled/Investigational Use Febrile seizures in children; may also be used for prevention and treatment of neonatal hyperbilirubinemia and lowering of bilirubin in chronic cholestasis; neonatal seizures; management of sedative/hypnotic withdrawal
Mechanism of Action Interferes with transmission of impulses from the thalamus to the cortex of the brain resulting in an imbalance in central inhibitory and facilitatory mechanisms
Adverse Reactions
Cardiovascular: **Hypotension, cardiac arrhythmias, bradycardia, arterial spasm**, sinus bradycardia, vasodilation
Central nervous system: **Drowsiness, CNS stimulation or CNS depression, impaired judgment**, visual hallucinations, hypothermia, electroencephalogram abnormalities, depression, anticonvulsant hypersensitivity syndrome, **dizziness, lightheadedness, "hangover" effect, lethargy**
Dermatologic: Rash, bullous eruptions, systemic contact dermatitis, exfoliative dermatitis, erythema nodosum
Gastrointestinal: Nausea, vomiting, ileus
Hematologic: Thrombocytopenia
Hepatic: Hepatic dysfunction (idiosyncratic reaction), cholestasis
Local: **Thrombophlebitis** with I.V. use, **pain at injection site**
Ocular: Nystagmus
Renal: Oliguria, renal failure (secondary to hypotension), renal vasculitis
Respiratory: Laryngospasm, respiratory depression, apnea (especially with rapid I.V. use)
Miscellaneous: **Gangrene with inadvertent intra-arterial injection**, mucocutaneous syndrome (febrile), fixed drug eruption
Signs and Symptoms of Overdose Asterixis, ataxia, bullous lesions, cognitive dysfunction, confusion, dysarthria, extrapyramidal reaction, fever, focal neurological signs, gingival hyperplasia, hyperactivity, hyporeflexia, hypotension, hypothermia, hypothyroidism, jaundice, methemoglobinemia, miosis, myocardial depression, myoglobinuria, pemphigus, porphyria, ptosis, pulmonary edema, rhabdomyolysis, slurred speech, toxic epidermal necrolysis, unsteady gait, vision color changes (green tinge)
Admission Criteria/Prognosis Any patient with change in mental status, cardiopulmonary complaints, or phenobarbital levels >60 mcg/mL should be admitted
Pharmacodynamics/Kinetics
Onset of action: Oral: Hypnosis: 20-60 minutes; I.V.: ~5 minutes
Peak effect: I.V.: ~30 minutes
Duration: Oral: 6-10 hours; I.V.: 4-10 hours
Absorption: Oral: 70% to 90%
Protein binding: 20% to 45%; decreased in neonates
Metabolism: Hepatic via hydroxylation and glucuronide conjugation
Half-life elimination: Neonates: 45-500 hours; Infants: 20-133 hours; Children: 37-73 hours; Adults: 53-140 hours
Time to peak, serum: Oral: 1-6 hours
Excretion: Urine (20% to 50% as unchanged drug)
Dosage
Children:
Sedation: Oral: 2 mg/kg 3 times/day
Hypnotic: I.M., I.V., SubQ: 3-5 mg/kg at bedtime
Preoperative sedation: Oral, I.M., I.V.: 1-3 mg/kg 1-1.5 hours before procedure

Adults:
Sedation: Oral, I.M.: 30-120 mg/day in 2-3 divided doses
Hypnotic: Oral, I.M., I.V., SubQ: 100-320 mg at bedtime
Preoperative sedation: I.M.: 100-200 mg 1-1.5 hours before procedure
Anticonvulsant: Status epilepticus: **Loading dose:** I.V.:
Infants and Children: 10-20 mg/kg in a single or divided dose; in select patients may administer additional 5 mg/kg/dose every 15-30 minutes until seizure is controlled or a total dose of 40 mg/kg is reached
Adults: 300-800 mg initially followed by 120-240 mg/dose at 20-minute intervals until seizures are controlled or a total dose of 1-2 g
Anticonvulsant maintenance dose: Oral, I.V.:
Infants: 5-8 mg/kg/day in 1-2 divided doses
Children:
1-5 years: 6-8 mg/kg/day in 1-2 divided doses
5-12 years: 4-6 mg/kg/day in 1-2 divided doses
Children >12 years and Adults: 1-3 mg/kg/day in divided doses or 50-100 mg 2-3 times/day
Sedative/hypnotic withdrawal (unlabeled use): Initial daily requirement is determined by substituting phenobarbital 30 mg for every 100 mg pentobarbital used during tolerance testing; then daily requirement is decreased by 10% of initial dose
Dosing interval in renal impairment: Cl_{cr} <10 mL/minute: Administer every 12-16 hours
Hemodialysis: Moderately dialyzable (20% to 50%)
Dosing adjustment/comments in hepatic disease: Increased side effects may occur in severe liver disease; monitor plasma levels and adjust dose accordingly
Stability Protect elixir from light; not stable in aqueous solutions; use only clear solutions; do not add to acidic solutions, precipitation may occur
Monitoring Parameters Phenobarbital serum concentrations, mental status, CBC, LFTs, seizure activity
Administration Avoid rapid I.V. administration >50 mg/minute; avoid intra-arterial injection; parenteral solutions are highly alkaline; avoid extravasation
Contraindications Hypersensitivity to barbiturates or any component of the formulation; marked hepatic impairment; dyspnea or airway obstruction; porphyria; pregnancy
Warnings Potential for drug dependency exists, abrupt cessation may precipitate withdrawal, including status epilepticus in epileptic patients. Do not administer to patients in acute pain. Use caution in elderly, debilitated, renally or hepatic dysfunction, and pediatric patients. May cause paradoxical responses, including agitation and hyperactivity, particularly in acute pain and pediatric patients. Use with caution in patients with depression or suicidal tendencies, or in patients with a history of drug abuse. Tolerance, psychological and physical dependence may occur with prolonged use. May cause CNS depression, which may impair physical or mental abilities. Patients must cautioned about performing tasks which require mental alertness (eg, operating machinery or driving). Effects with other sedative drugs or ethanol may be potentiated. May cause respiratory depression or hypotension, particularly when administered intravenously. Use with caution in hemodynamically unstable patients (hypovolemic shock, CHF) or patients with respiratory disease. Due to its long half-life and risk of dependence, phenobarbital is not recommended as a sedative in the elderly. Use has been associated with cognitive deficits in children. Use with caution in patients with hypoadrenalism.
Dosage Forms Elixir: 20 mg/5 mL (473 mL) [contains alcohol]
Injection, solution, as sodium: 65 mg/mL (1 mL); 130 mg/mL (1 mL) [contains alcohol and propylene glycol]
Luminal® Sodium: 60 mg/mL (1 mL); 130 mg/mL (1 mL) [contains alcohol 10% and propylene glycol]
Tablet: 15 mg, 30 mg, 32 mg, 60 mg, 65 mg, 100 mg
Reference Range
Therapeutic:
Infants and children: 15-30 mcg/mL (SI: 65-129 μmol/L)
Adults: 20-40 mcg/mL (SI: 86-172 μmol/L)
Toxic: >40 mcg/mL (SI: >172 μmol/L); levels >80 mcg/mL (SI: 344 μmol/L) are associated with coma
Fatal: 50-130 mcg/mL (SI: 215-559 μmol/L)
Overdosage/Treatment
Decontamination: Gastric lavage for life-threatening overdoses within 1 hour; activated charcoal is effective
Supportive therapy: Hypotension: Isotonic I.V. fluid (10-20 mL/kg) is effective along with placement in Trendelenburg position; dopamine (2-5 mcg/kg progressing to 5-10 mcg/kg) or norepinephrine (0.1-0.2 mcg/kg/minute for children or 8-12 mcg/kg in adults to a maintenance dose of 2-4 mcg/minute) is effective. Exchange transfusion may be of benefit in treating a neonatal intoxication.
Enhancement of elimination: Repeated oral doses of activated charcoal significantly reduce the half-life of phenobarbital resulting from an enhancement of nonrenal elimination. The usual dose is 12.5-25 g every 1-2 hours until concentrations are <20 mg/L or unless the patient has no bowel movement, causing the charcoal to remain in the gastrointestinal tract. Assure adequate hydration and renal function.

Urinary alkalinization with I.V. sodium bicarbonate also helps to enhance elimination. Hemodialysis is of uncertain value. Patients in stage IV coma due to high serum barbiturate levels may require charcoal hemoperfusion; moderately dialyzable (20% to 50%). Hemodialysis clearance is ~80 mL/minute with 33% of drug removed in 4 hours. Hemoperfusion clearance ranges from 80-290 mL/minute with 39% of drug removed in 4 hours; continuous arteriovenous hemoperfusion clearance rates are 290 ± 25 mL/minute. Multiple dosing of activated charcoal is superior to urinary alkalinization in enhancing phenobarbital elimination.

Diagnostic Procedures
- Phenobarbital, Blood

Test Interactions ↑ alkaline phosphatase (S), ammonia (B); ↓ bilirubin (S), calcium (S)

Drug Interactions

Substrate of CYP2C9 (minor), 2C19 (major), 2E1 (minor); **Induces** CYP1A2 (strong), 2A6 (strong), 2B6 (strong), 2C8 (strong), 2C9 (strong), 3A4 (strong)

Acetaminophen: Barbiturates may enhance the hepatotoxic potential of acetaminophen overdoses

Antiarrhythmics: Barbiturates may increase the metabolism of antiarrhythmics, decreasing their clinical effect; includes disopyramide, propafenone, and quinidine

Anticonvulsants: Barbiturates may increase the metabolism of anticonvulsants; includes ethosuximide, felbamate (possibly), lamotrigine, phenytoin, tiagabine, topiramate, and zonisamide; does not appear to affect gabapentin or levetiracetam

Antineoplastics: Limited evidence suggests that enzyme-inducing anticonvulsant therapy may reduce the effectiveness of some chemotherapy regimens (specifically in ALL); teniposide and methotrexate may be cleared more rapidly in these patients

Antipsychotics: Barbiturates may enhance the metabolism (decrease the efficacy) of antipsychotics; monitor for altered response; dose adjustment may be needed

Beta-blockers: Metabolism of beta-blockers may be increased and clinical effect decreased; atenolol and nadolol are unlikely to interact given their renal elimination

Calcium channel blockers: Barbiturates may enhance the metabolism of calcium channel blockers, decreasing their clinical effect

Chloramphenicol: Barbiturates may increase the metabolism of chloramphenicol and chloramphenicol may inhibit barbiturate metabolism; monitor for altered response

Cimetidine: Barbiturates may enhance the metabolism of cimetidine, decreasing its clinical effect

CNS depressants: Sedative effects and/or respiratory depression with barbiturates may be additive with other CNS depressants; monitor for increased effect; includes ethanol, sedatives, antidepressants, narcotic analgesics, and benzodiazepines

Corticosteroids: Barbiturates may enhance the metabolism of corticosteroids, decreasing their clinical effect

Cyclosporine: Levels may be decreased by barbiturates; monitor

CYP1A2 substrates: Phenobarbital may decrease the levels/effects of CYP1A2 substrates. Example substrates include aminophylline, estrogens, fluvoxamine, mirtazapine, ropinirole, and theophylline.

CYP2A6 substrates: Phenobarbital may decrease the levels/effects of CYP2A6 substrates. Example substrates include ifosfamide and rifampin.

CYP2B6 substrates: Phenobarbital may decrease the levels/effects of CYP2B6 substrates. Example substrates include bupropion, efavirenz, promethazine, selegiline, and sertraline.

CYP2C8 Substrates: Phenobarbital may decrease the levels/effects of CYP2C8 substrates. Example substrates include amiodarone, paclitaxel, pioglitazone, repaglinide, and rosiglitazone.

CYP2C9 Substrates: Phenobarbital may decrease the levels/effects of CYP2C9 substrates. Example substrates include bosentan, celecoxib, dapsone, fluoxetine, glimepiride, glipizide, losartan, montelukast, nateglinide, paclitaxel, phenytoin, sulfonamides, trimethoprim, warfarin, and zafirlukast.

CYP2C19 inducers: May decrease the levels/effects of phenobarbital. Example inducers include aminoglutethimide, carbamazepine, phenytoin, and rifampin.

CYP2C19 inhibitors: May increase the levels/effects of phenobarbital. Example inhibitors include delavirdine, fluconazole, fluvoxamine, gemfibrozil, isoniazid, omeprazole, and ticlopidine.

CYP3A4 substrates: Phenobarbital may decrease the levels/effects of CYP3A4 substrates. Example substrates include benzodiazepines, calcium channel blockers, clarithromycin, cyclosporine, erythromycin, estrogens, mirtazapine, nateglinide, nefazodone, nevirapine, protease inhibitors, tacrolimus, and venlafaxine.

Doxycycline: Barbiturates may enhance the metabolism of doxycycline, decreasing its clinical effect; higher dosages may be required

Estrogens: Barbiturates may increase the metabolism of estrogens and reduce their efficacy

Felbamate may inhibit the metabolism of barbiturates and barbiturates may increase the metabolism of felbamate

Griseofulvin: Barbiturates may impair the absorption of griseofulvin, and griseofulvin metabolism may be increased by barbiturates, decreasing clinical effect

Guanfacine: Effect may be decreased by barbiturates

Immunosuppressants: Barbiturates may enhance the metabolism of immunosuppressants, decreasing its clinical effect; includes both cyclosporine and tacrolimus

Loop diuretics: Metabolism may be increased and clinical effects decreased; established for furosemide, effect with other loop diuretics not established

MAO inhibitors: Metabolism of barbiturates may be inhibited, increasing clinical effect or toxicity of the barbiturates

Methadone: Barbiturates may enhance the metabolism of methadone resulting in methadone withdrawal

Methoxyflurane: Barbiturates may enhance the nephrotoxic effects of methoxyflurane

Oral contraceptives: Barbiturates may enhance the metabolism of oral contraceptives, decreasing their clinical effect; an alternative method of contraception should be considered

Theophylline: Barbiturates may increase metabolism of theophylline derivatives and decrease their clinical effect

Tricyclic antidepressants: Barbiturates may increase metabolism of tricyclic antidepressants and decrease their clinical effect; sedative effects may be additive

Valproic acid: Metabolism of barbiturates may be inhibited by valproic acid; monitor for excessive sedation; a dose reduction may be needed

Warfarin: Barbiturates inhibit the hypoprothrombinemic effects of oral anticoagulants via increased metabolism; this combination should generally be avoided

Pregnancy Risk Factor D

Pregnancy Implications Crosses placenta; no direct causal relationship established with congenital malformations; folate deficiency and hypoprothrombinemia has been noted in infants of mothers receiving phenobarbital; exposure to phenobarbital in utero may result in significantly lower verbal intelligence scores in males (0.5 SD); exposure in the last trimester appears to cause the greatest detriment

Lactation Enters breast milk/not recommended (AAP recommends use "with caution")

Nursing Implications Parenteral solutions are highly alkaline; avoid extravasation; avoid rapid I.V. administration >50 mg/minute; avoid intra-arterial injection; institute safety measures to avoid injuries

Additional Information Sodium content of injection (65 mg, 1 mL): 6 mg (0.3 mEq); the elderly may be more sensitive to the sedative effects of phenobarbital

Specific References

Ali FE, Al-Bustan MA, Al-Busairi WA, et al, "Loss of Seizure Control Due to Anticonvulsant-Induced Hypocalcemia," Ann Pharmacother, 2004, 38(6):1002-5.

Cingolani M, Cippitelli M, Froldi R, et al, "Stability of Barbiturates in Fixed Tissues and Formalin Solutions," J Anal Toxicol, 2005, 29(3):205-8.

Kawasaki CI, Nishi R, Uekihara S, et al, "How Tightly Can a Drug Be Bound to a Protein and Still Be Removable by Charcoal Hemoperfusion in Overdose Cases?" Clin Toxicol (Phila), 2005, 43(2):95-9.

Proudfoot AT, Krenzelok EP, Vale JA, et al, "AACT/EAPCCT Position Paper on Urine Alkalinization," J Toxicol Clin Toxicol, 2004, 42(1):1-26.

Shalkham AS, Kirrane BM, Goldfarb D, et al, "The Availability and Use of Charcoal Hemoperfusion in the Treatment of Poisoned Patients," Clin Toxicol (Phila), 2005, 43:676.

van de Plas A, Stolk L, Verhoeven MA, et al, "Successful Treatment of Acute Phenobarbital Intoxication by Hemodiafiltration," Clin Toxicol (Phila), 2006, 44(1):93-4.

Phenol

Pronunciation (FEE nol)

CAS Number 108-95-2

UN Number 1671 (solid); 2312 (molten); 2821 (solution)

U.S. Brand Names Chloraseptic® Gargle [OTC]; Chloraseptic® Mouth Pain Spray [OTC]; Chloraseptic® Rinse [OTC]; Chloraseptic® Spray for Kids [OTC]; Chloraseptic® Spray [OTC]; Cá"pastat® Extra Strength [OTC]; Cá"pastat®[OTC]; Pain-A-Lay® [OTC]; Ulcerease® [OTC]

Synonyms Carbolic Acid

Commonly Includes Production of resin; industrial coatings, adhesives, dyes, perfumes, textiles, lubricating oils, antiseptic agents

Use Relief of sore throat pain, mouth, gum, and throat irritations, neurologic pain, rectal prolapse, hemorrhoids, hydrocele

Mechanism of Action Cardiac effects may be due to sodium channel blockage; at concentrations >5%, it can denature protein

Adverse Reactions

Cardiovascular: Hypotension, cardiovascular collapse, tachycardia, arrhythmias (atrial and ventricular), sinus tachycardia

Central nervous system: CNS depression, slurred speech, coma, agitation, confusion, seizures, panic attacks (with inhalation)

Dermatologic: Skin irritation, burns; white, red, or brown skin discoloration

Gastrointestinal: Nausea, vomiting, hemorrhage, GI ulceration, GI bleeding

Genitourinary: Urine discoloration (green)

Neuromuscular & skeletal: Rabbit syndrome

Renal: Nephritis

Respiratory: Pulmonary edema, wheezing, coughing, dyspnea, pneumonia

Miscellaneous: Oral burns

Signs and Symptoms of Overdose Cyanosis, dermal burns, hematuria, hypothermia, nephritis, seizures, urine discoloration (dark; brown; green), wheezing, Encephalopathy

Admission Criteria/Prognosis

Mild exposure: Asymptomatic patients may be discharged after 6 hours of observation

Serious exposure: Observe for 18-24 hours; death usually occurs within 24 hours of exposure

Can discharge patients who are asymptomatic 4 hours postexposure

Toxicodynamics/Kinetics

Absorption: Readily absorbed through the lungs (60% to 88%), orally (90%), through mucous membranes, and dermally ($\sim$0.35 m^3/hour)

Distribution: Not known

Metabolism: Hepatic hydroxylation and sulfate conjugation

Half-life: 13.86 hours (dermal exposure) Conjugated phenol: 1 hour; Elimination: 1-4.5 hours

Elimination: Renally with 52% unchanged

Dosage Allow to dissolve slowly in mouth; may be repeated every 2 hours as needed

Administration

Oral: Allow to lozenge dissolve slowly in mouth. Spray should be allowed to remain in mouth for $\sim$15 seconds, then expectorate.

Topical: Castellani Paint Modified: May stain skin and clothing; apply to clean area

Warnings

When used for self-medication (OTC) for sore throat: Not for use >7 days or if pain, redness, or irritation continues. If sore throat is severe, not for use >2 days or if followed by fever, headache, rash, nausea, or vomiting. Oral gargles and sprays should not be swallowed.

When used for self-medication (OTC) as a topical antiseptic: Do not use in eyes, or apply to large areas of the body, deep or puncture wounds, animal bites or burns. Do not use for >7 days; do not bandage affected area.

Dosage Forms

Lozenge, oral:

Cá"pastat®: 14.5 mg (18s) [sugar free; contains menthol; cherry flavor]

Cá"pastat® Extra Strength: 29 mg (18s) [sugar free; contains menthol; eucalyptus flavor]

Solution, oral: 1.4% (180 mL) [spray]

Cheracol® [spray]: Phenol 1.4% (180 mL) [alcohol and sugar free; contains tartrazine]

Chloraseptic® [gargle]: 1.4% (296 mL) [alcohol and sugar free; cool mint flavor]

Chloraseptic® Mouth Pain [rinse]: 1.4% (240 mL) [cinnamon flavor]

Chloraseptic® [spray]: 1.4% (20 mL, 30 mL) [alcohol and sugar free; cherry flavor]; (180 mL) [alcohol and sugar free; cherry, cool mint, and menthol flavors]

Chloraseptic® for Kids [spray]: 0.5% (177 mL) [grape flavor]

Pain-A-Lay® [gargle]: 1.4% (240 mL, 540 mL) [contains tartrazine]

Pain-A-Lay® [spray]: 1.4% (180 mL) [contains tartrazine]

Phenaseptic [spray]: 1.4% (180 mL) [cherry flavor]

Ulcerease® [gargle]: 0.6% (180 mL) [alcohol, dye, and sugar free; contains glycerin]

Solution, topical:

Castellani Paint Modified: Phenol 1.5% (30 mL) [contains alcohol 13%, acetone, basic fuchsin, resorcinol]

Castellani Paint Modified [colorless]: Phenol 1.5% (30 mL) [contains alcohol 13%, acetone, and resorcinol]

Swabs, topical (Phenol EZ®): 89% (30s) [$\sim$0.2 mL]

Reference Range

Lowest reported toxic serum phenol level: 27 mcg/mL

Toxic: >75 mg/L (urine)

Fatal: 3 g ingestion may be fatal

Dinitrophenol or hydroquinone may produce methemoglobin BEI (urine) is 250 mg/g creatinine; serum levels <20 mg/L not associated with acute toxicity

Urinary excretion of phenol (free plus conjugates) in humans with no known exposure: $\sim$8.7$\pm$2.0 mg/day

Mean phenol urine concentration of 214 mg/L (range 208-220 mg/L) associated with fatal phenol poisoning

Overdosage/Treatment

Decontamination:

Oral: Ipecac is contraindicated; lavage within 1 hour with water or polyethylene glycol/activated charcoal is useful for gastric decontamination

Dermal: Remove clothing, wash exposed skin with isopropyl alcohol, polyethylene glycol, or industrial methylated spirits

Inhalation: Remove from source and provide oxygen

Ocular: Flush eyes with copious amounts of water (if exposed); low or high (3500) molecular weight polyethylene glycol can be useful for dermal irrigation of affected areas

Supportive therapy: I.V. sodium bicarbonate (1-2 mEq/kg) can be used to treat acidosis

Enhanced elimination: Charcoal hemoperfusion has been used successfully and can be considered for blood phenol levels >175 mcg/mL (associated with a 0.44 mg/kg exposure)

Antidote(s)

- Methylene Blue [ANTIDOTE]

Diagnostic Procedures

- Electrolytes, Blood
- Methemoglobin, Blood

Pregnancy Risk Factor C

Additional Information Colorless or white crystals, acrid odor. Odor threshold of 0.05 ppm in air and 8 ppm in water; TLV-TWA: 5 ppm; IDLH: 100 ppm; PEL-TWA: 5 ppm. Atmospheric half-life: 0.6-1 day; soil half-life is <5 days. River water in the U.S. contains from 10-100 ppb of phenol; $\sim$64 square inches of body surface area exposure to phenol can be fatal.

Phenolphthalein

CAS Number 77-09-8

Synonyms Phenolphthalein, White; Phenolphthalein, Yellow

Use Stimulant laxative

Mechanism of Action A diphenylmethane compound which stimulates peristalsis by directly irritating the smooth muscle of the intestine, possibly the colonic intramural plexus

Adverse Reactions

Dermatologic: Rash, irritation and burning sensation of rectal mucosa, proctitis, toxic epidermal necrolysis, erythema multiforme, Stevens-Johnson syndrome, exfoliative dermatitis, angioedema, bullous skin disease, urticaria, pruritus, exanthem

Endocrine & metabolic: Electrolyte imbalance, hypoglycemia

Gastrointestinal: Abdominal cramps, nausea, vomiting

Miscellaneous: Systemic lupus erythematosus, fixed drug eruption

Signs and Symptoms of Overdose Abdominal pain, diarrhea, disseminated intravascular coagulation, feces discoloration (black; red), hypoglycemia, hypokalemia, hypotension, nephrotic syndrome, pancreatitis, pulmonary edema, seizures, tongue discoloration, toxic epidermal necrolysis

Pharmacodynamics/Kinetics

Onset of action: Within 6-8 hours

Elimination: In feces and skin, with up to 15% excreted in the urine as the conjugate; enterohepatically recycled

Dosage

Oral:

Children: 15-60 mg

Adults: 60-200 mg preferably at bedtime

Monitoring Parameters Monitor stools daily or weekly; fluid/electrolyte status

Contraindications Do not use in patients with abdominal pain, obstruction, nausea or vomiting; not to be used during pregnancy or lactation

Warnings Habit-forming and may result in laxative dependence and loss of normal bowel function with prolonged use, can cause skin hypersensitivity and fixed drug eruption

Dosage Forms Gum: 97.2 mg

Tablet: 60 mg, 90 mg, 97.2 mg, 130 mg

Tablet, chewable: 65 mg, 90 mg, 97.2 mg, 120 mg

Wafer: 64.8 mg

Wafer, chewable: 80 mg

Reference Range Serum phenolphthalein level of 0.4 mcg/L associated with fatality

Overdosage/Treatment

Decontamination: Activated charcoal is useful (**do not** use a cathartic)

Supportive therapy: I.V. fluid and electrolyte replacement

Enhancement of elimination: Multiple dosing of activated charcoal may be useful

Test Interactions ↓ calcium (S), potassium (S)

Pregnancy Risk Factor C

Additional Information Toxic dose: Children: 600 mg; Adults: 2 g

The chronic use of stimulant cathartics is inappropriate and should be avoided although constipation is a common complaint from elderly, such complaints require evaluation; short-term use of stimulants is best; if prophylaxis is desired, this can be accomplished with bulk agents (psyllium), stool softeners, and hyperosmotic agents (sorbitol 70%); stool softeners are unnecessary if stools are well hydrated, soft, or "mushy"

Phenolphthalein, white: Alophen Pills® [OTC], Medilax® [OTC], Modane® [OTC], Modane® Mild [OTC], Phenolax® [OTC], Prulet® [OTC]

Phenolphthalein, yellow: Evac-U-Gen® [OTC], Evac-U-Lax® [OTC], Ex-Lax® [OTC], Feen-A-Mint® [OTC], Lax-Pills® [OTC] Yellow is 2-3 times more potent than white. Urine or stool may be red or pink; produces an alkaline stool; does not decrease food absorption.

Phenoxybenzamine

CAS Number 59-96-1; 63-92-3
U.S. Brand Names Dibenzyline®
Synonyms Phenoxybenzamine Hydrochloride
Use Symptomatic management of pheochromocytoma; treatment of hypertensive crisis caused by sympathomimetic amines
Unlabeled/Investigational Use Micturition problems associated with neurogenic bladder, functional outlet obstruction, and partial prostate obstruction
Mechanism of Action Produces long-lasting noncompetitive alpha-adrenergic blockade of postganglionic synapses in exocrine glands and smooth muscle; relaxes urethra and increases opening of the bladder
Adverse Reactions
Cardiovascular: Postural hypotension, tachycardia (reflex), syncope, shock
Central nervous system: Lethargy, headache, confusion, fatigue, seizures (due to rapid administration of drug)
Gastrointestinal: Vomiting, nausea, diarrhea, xerostomia
Genitourinary: Inhibition of ejaculation
Neuromuscular & skeletal: Weakness
Ocular: Miosis
Respiratory: Nasal congestion
Signs and Symptoms of Overdose Dizziness, hypotension, lethargy, shock, tachycardia
Admission Criteria/Prognosis Admit any symptomatic patient or with ingestion >1.5 mg/kg
Pharmacodynamics/Kinetics
Onset of action: ~2 hours
Peak effect: 4-6 hours
Duration: ≥4 days
Half-life elimination: 24 hours
Excretion: Primarily urine and feces
Dosage
Oral:
Children: Initial: 0.2 mg/kg (maximum: 10 mg) once daily, increase by 0.2 mg/kg increments; usual maintenance dose: 0.4-1.2 mg/kg/day every 6-8 hours, higher doses may be necessary
Adults: Initial: 10 mg twice daily, increase by 10 mg every other day until optimum dose is achieved; usual range: 20-40 mg 2-3 times/day
Urinary retention: 10 mg twice daily
Monitoring Parameters Blood pressure, pulse, urine output, orthostasis
Administration GI irritation may be reduced by giving in divided doses
Contraindications Hypersensitivity to phenoxybenzamine or any component of the formulation; conditions in which a fall in blood pressure would be undesirable (eg, shock); concurrent use with phosphodiesterase-5 (PDE-5) inhibitors including sildenafil (>25 mg), tadalafil, or vardenafil
Warnings Use with caution in patients with renal impairment, cerebral, or coronary arteriosclerosis, can exacerbate symptoms of respiratory tract infections. Because of the risk of adverse effects, avoid the use of this medication in the elderly if possible.
Dosage Forms Capsule, as hydrochloride: 10 mg [contains benzyl alcohol]
Overdosage/Treatment
Decontamination: Oral: Activated charcoal should be administered. Lavage can be considered if ingestion occurred within 2 hours. Consider gastric decontamination at ingestions >1.5 mg/kg.
Supportive therapy: Hypotension and shock should be treated with fluids and by placing the patient in the Trendelenburg position; only alpha-adrenergic pressors such as norepinephrine (0.1-0.2 mcg/kg/minute; titrate to desired effect) should be used; mixed agents such as epinephrine, may cause more hypotension
Drug Interactions Alpha adrenergic agonists decrease the effect of phenoxybenzamine.
Beta-blockers may result in increased toxicity (hypotension, tachycardia).
Sildenafil, tadalafil, vardenafil: Blood pressure-lowering effects are additive. Use of vardenafil or tadalafil is contraindicated by the manufacturer. Use sildenafil with extreme caution (dose ≤25 mg).
Pregnancy Risk Factor C
Pregnancy Implications Placental transfer can occur resulting in fetal respiratory depression and transient hypotension
Nursing Implications Monitor for orthostasis; assist with ambulation

Phensuximide

CAS Number 86-34-0
Use Control of absence (petit mal) seizures; ethosuximide must be used in combination with other anticonvulsants in patients with both absence and tonic-clonic seizures
Mechanism of Action Increases the seizure threshold and suppresses paroxysmal spike-and-wave pattern in absence seizures; depresses nerve transmission in the motor cortex
Adverse Reactions
Central nervous system: **Dizziness, drowsiness, headache**, aggressiveness, CNS depression, night terrors, tiredness, paranoid psychosis, **ataxia**, psychosis
Dermatologic: **Stevens-Johnson syndrome**, rash, exfoliative dermatitis, hypertrichosis, alopecia, purpura, pruritus
Gastrointestinal: **Anorexia, nausea, vomiting, weight loss**, gingival hyperplasia
Genitourinary: Urine discoloration (pink/red to red/brown)
Hematologic: Agranulocytosis, leukopenia, aplastic anemia, thrombocytopenia, pancytopenia
Neuromuscular & skeletal: Weakness
Ocular: Photophobia
Miscellaneous: **Hiccups, systemic lupus erythematosus**
Signs and Symptoms of Overdose Acute: Ataxia, blood dyscrasias, CNS depression, coma, hypotension, night terrors, photophobia, stupor, urinary frequency
Chronic: Albuminuria, ataxia, confusion, hematuria, hepatic dysfunction, skin rash
Toxicodynamics/Kinetics
Absorption: Oral: Well absorbed
Protein binding: 0%
Metabolism: In the liver to norphensuximide (30%)
Half-life: 5-12 hours (8 hours for metabolite)
Time to peak serum concentration: Within 1-4 hours
Elimination: In urine as active and inactive metabolites
Dosage Children and Adults: Oral: 0.5-1 g 2-3 times/day
Reference Range Therapeutic: 10-20 mcg/mL (SI: 57-114 µmol/L)
Overdosage/Treatment
Decontamination: **Do not** induce emesis; lavage (within 1 hour)/activated charcoal
Enhancement of elimination: Forced diuresis is of no benefit; multiple dosing of activated charcoal may be useful; although data is lacking, hemodialysis or hemoperfusion may be effective
Test Interactions ↑ alkaline phosphatase (S); positive Coombs' [direct]; ↓ calcium (S)

Phentermine

CAS Number 1197-21-3; 122-09-8
U.S. Brand Names Adipex-P®; Ionamin®
Synonyms Phentermine Hydrochloride
Impairment Potential Yes
Use Short-term adjunct in a regimen of weight reduction based on exercise, behavioral modification, and caloric reduction in the management of exogenous obesity for patients with an initial body mass index ≥30 kg/m^2 or ≥27 kg/m^2 in the presence of other risk factors (diabetes, hypertension)
Mechanism of Action Phentermine is structurally similar to dextroamphetamine and is comparable to dextroamphetamine as an appetite suppressant, but is generally associated with a lower incidence and severity of CNS side effects. Phentermine, like other anorexiants, stimulates the hypothalamus to result in decreased appetite; anorexiant effects are most likely mediated via norepinephrine and dopamine metabolism. However, other CNS effects or metabolic effects may be involved.
Adverse Reactions
Cardiovascular: **Hypertension**, tachycardia, arrhythmias, palpitations, pulmonary hypertension, sinus tachycardia
Central nervous system: **Euphoria, nervousness, insomnia**, confusion, CNS depression, restlessness, headache, paranoid psychosis, psychosis, paranoia
Dermatologic: Alopecia
Endocrine & metabolic: Changes in libido
Gastrointestinal: Nausea, vomiting, diarrhea, abdominal cramps, constipation
Genitourinary: Dysuria
Hematologic: Blood dyscrasias
Neuromuscular & skeletal: Tremors, myalgia, rhabdomyolysis
Ocular: Blurred vision, mydriasis
Renal: Polyuria
Respiratory: Dyspnea
Miscellaneous: Diaphoresis (increased)
Signs and Symptoms of Overdose Agitation, hyperactivity, hypertension, hyperthermia, insomnia, seizures

Pharmacodynamics/Kinetics

Duration: Resin produces more prolonged clinical effects

Absorption: Well absorbed; resin absorbed slower

Half-life elimination: 20 hours

Excretion: Primarily urine (as unchanged drug)

Dosage

Oral:

Children 3-15 years: Obesity: 5-15 mg/day for 4 weeks

Adults: Obesity: 8 mg 3 times/day 30 minutes before meals or food or 15-37.5 mg/day before breakfast or 10-14 hours before retiring

Monitoring Parameters CNS

Contraindications Hypersensitivity or idiosyncrasy to sympathomimetic amines or any component of the formulation; patients with advanced arteriosclerosis, symptomatic cardiovascular disease, moderate to severe hypertension (stage II or III), hyperthyroidism, glaucoma, agitated states; patients with a history of drug abuse; use during or within 14 days following MAO inhibitor therapy; children <16 years of age (per manufacturer)

Warnings

Use with caution in patients with bipolar disorder, diabetes mellitus, cardiovascular disease, seizure disorders, insomnia, porphyria, or mild hypertension (stage I). May exacerbate symptoms of behavior and thought disorder in psychotic patients. Stimulants may unmask tics in individuals with coexisting Tourette's syndrome. Potential for drug dependency exists; avoid abrupt discontinuation in patients who have received for prolonged periods. Stimulant use has been associated with growth suppression, and careful monitoring is recommended.

Primary pulmonary hypertension (PPH), a rare and frequently fatal pulmonary disease, has been reported to occur in patients receiving a combination of phentermine and fenfluramine or dexfenfluramine. The possibility of an association between PPH and the use of phentermine alone cannot be ruled out.

Use in weight reduction programs only when alternative therapy has been ineffective. Serious, potentially life-threatening toxicities may occur when thyroid hormones (at dosages above usual daily hormonal requirements) are used in combination with sympathomimetic amines to induce weight loss. Treatment of obesity is not an approved use for thyroid hormone.

Dosage Forms Capsule, as hydrochloride: 15 mg, 30 mg

Adipex-P®: 37.5 mg

Capsule, resin complex:

Ionamin®: 15 mg; 30 mg [DSC]

Tablet, as hydrochloride: 37.5 mg

Adipex-P®: 37.5 mg

Reference Range Therapeutic plasma level: 30-90 ng/mL (does not correlate with weight loss)

Overdosage/Treatment

Decontamination: **Do not** induce emesis; lavage (within 1 hour)/activated charcoal

Supportive therapy: There is no specific antidote for phentermine intoxication and the bulk of the treatment is supportive. Hyperactivity and agitation usually respond to reduced sensory input, however with extreme agitation diazepam (10-20 mg orally in adults or 0.1 mg/kg in children) or I.V. droperidol (0.1 mg/kg) or haloperidol (0.1 mg/kg) may be required. Hyperthermia is best treated with external cooling measures, or when severe or unresponsive, muscle paralysis with pancuronium may be needed. Hypertension is usually transient and generally does not require treatment unless severe. For diastolic blood pressures >120 mm Hg, a nitroprusside infusion should be initiated. Seizures usually respond to diazepam IVP and/or phenytoin maintenance regimens. Alkaline diuresis with mannitol or furosemide may be required to treat rhabdomyolysis; do not acidify urine.

Enhancement of elimination: Multiple dosing of activated charcoal may be useful; extracorporeal removal has not been shown to be beneficial

Drug Interactions Antihypertensives: Phentermine may decrease the effect of antihypertensive medications

Antipsychotics: Efficacy of anorexiants may be decreased by antipsychotics; in addition, amphetamines or related compounds may induce an increase in psychotic symptoms in some patients

Furazolidone: Amphetamines (and related compounds) may induce hypertensive episodes in patients receiving furazolidone

Guanethidine: Amphetamines (and related compounds) inhibit the antihypertensive response to guanethidine; probably also may occur with guanadrel

Hypoglycemic agents: Dosage may need to be adjusted when phentermine is used in a diabetic receiving a special diet

Linezolid: Due to MAO inhibition (see note on MAO inhibitors), this combination should generally be avoided

MAO inhibitors: Concurrent use may be associated with hypertensive episodes

SSRIs: Concurrent use may be associated with a risk of serotonin syndrome

Pregnancy Risk Factor C

Nursing Implications Dose should not be given in evening or at bedtime

Phenylbutazone

CAS Number 50-33-9

Use As an analgesic in the treatment of mild to moderate pain and as an antipyretic; I.V. form used as an alternate to surgery in management of patent ductus arteriosus in premature neonates; acute gouty arthritis. Off the market since 1992.

Mechanism of Action Phenylbutazone is an anti-inflammatory, antipyretic, uricosuric, and analgesic; mechanism of action is thought to be due primarily to prostaglandin inhibition, leukocyte migration inhibition, and lysosomal enzyme stabilization

Adverse Reactions

Cardiovascular: Tachycardia, hypotension, myocarditis (hypersensitivity), fibrillation (atrial), flutter (atrial), angina, congestive heart failure, myocardial depression, pericardial effusion/pericarditis, sinus tachycardia

Central nervous system: Dizziness, drowsiness, headache, fatigue, seizures, gustatory hallucinations

Dermatologic: Rash, edema, erythema multiforme, toxic epidermal necrolysis, cutaneous vasculitis

Endocrine & metabolic: Parotitis

Gastrointestinal: Dyspepsia, heartburn, nausea, vomiting, abdominal pain, peptic ulcer, GI bleeding, GI perforation, loss of taste perception, esophagitis

Hematologic: Anemia, platelet inhibition, thrombocytopenia, coagulopathy, leukopenia, neutropenia, agranulocytosis, granulocytopenia, red blood cell aplasia

Hepatic: Hepatitis, granulomatous hepatitis, primary biliary cirrhosis

Ocular: Vision changes

Otic: Ototoxicity, tinnitus

Renal: Renal failure (acute), myoglobinuria, glomerulonephritis, renal vasculitis

Respiratory: Pulmonary edema, pulmonary vasculitis

Miscellaneous: Systemic lupus erythematosus, lymphadenopathy

Signs and Symptoms of Overdose Abdominal pain, agitation, ataxia, chest pain, cholestatic jaundice, coagulopathy, colitis, coma, dermatitis, diarrhea, drowsiness, dysosmia, erythema multiforme, exfoliative dermatitis, feces discoloration (black; greenish-gray; pink; red; red-brown), gastritis, hematuria, GI bleeding, hyperventilation, hypotension, hypothyroidism, jaundice, lichenoid eruptions, pemphigus, periarteritis nodosa, pericarditis, photosensitivity, respiratory arrest, rhabdomyolysis, seizures, stomatitis, toxic epidermal necrolysis, urine discoloration (red; red-brown)

Pharmacodynamics/Kinetics

Onset of action: 30-60 minutes

Duration: 3-5 days

Absorption: Oral: Well absorbed from gastrointestinal tract

Distribution: Most body tissues and synovial spaces

Protein binding: 98%

Metabolism: To oxyphenbutazone and hydroxyphenbutazone in the liver

Half-life: 50-100 hours (increases with hepatic impairment)

Time to peak serum concentration: Within 30-60 minutes

Elimination: Urinary excretion primarily as metabolites (99%)

Dosage

Adults: Oral: Initial:

Rheumatoid arthritis: 100-200 mg 3-4 times/day until desired effect, then reduce dose to not exceed 400 mg/day

Acute gouty arthritis: 400 mg, 100 mg every 4 hours until acute attack subsides, not to continue longer than 1 week

Dosing adjustment in hepatic impairment: Should not be administered to patients with liver dysfunction

Contraindications Active gastrointestinal bleeding, ulcer disease, hypersensitivity to phenylbutazone or any component

Warnings May cause agranulocytosis and aplastic anemia; is not just a simple analgesic; use only when other NSAIDs have failed; use with caution in patients with congestive heart failure, hypertension, decreased renal or hepatic function, history of gastrointestinal disease (bleeding or ulcers), or those receiving anticoagulants; safety and efficacy in children <6 months of age have not yet been established; because of severe hematologic adverse effects, discontinue use if no favorable response is seen

Dosage Forms Capsule: 100 mg

Tablet: 100 mg

Reference Range

Therapeutic: 50-100 mcg/mL (SI: 162-324 μmol/L)

Toxic: >100 mcg/mL (SI: >324 μmol/L)

Overdosage/Treatment

Supportive therapy: Management is primarily supportive and symptomatic. Fluid therapy is commonly effective in managing the hypotension except when this is due to an acute blood loss. Recurrent seizures should be treated with I.V. diazepam or lorazepam.

Enhancement of elimination: Multiple doses of charcoal may be needed to reduce the potential for delayed toxicities; charcoal hemoperfusion may remove 5% to 20% of drug

Test Interactions ↓ uric acid (S)

Drug Interactions May inhibit phenytoin or warfarin metabolism and methotrexate excretion

Pregnancy Risk Factor D

Pregnancy Implications Crosses the placenta

Specific References

Liang IE, Estes KE, Bird SB, et al, "Acute Phenylbutazone Toxicity: A Toxicokinetic Analysis," *J Toxicol Clin Toxicol*, 2004, 42(5):745-6.

Virji MA, Venkataraman ST, Lower DR, et al, "Role of Laboratory in the Management of Phenylbutazone Poisoning," *J Toxicol Clin Toxicol*, 2003, 41(7):1013-24.

Phenylephrine

CAS Number 59-42-7; 61-76-7

U.S. Brand Names AK-Dilate®; AK-Nefrin®; Formulation R™ [OTC]; Medicone® [OTC]; Mydfrin®; Neo-Synephrine® Extra Strength [OTC]; Neo-Synephrine® Mild [OTC]; Neo-Synephrine® Ophthalmic; Neo-Synephrine® Regular Strength [OTC]; Nostril® [OTC]; Phenoptic®; Prefrin™ [DSC]; Relief® [OTC]; Vicks® Sinex® Nasal Spray [OTC]; Vicks® Sinex® UltraFine Mist [OTC]

Synonyms Phenylephrine Hydrochloride; Phenylephrine Tannate

Use Treatment of hypotension, vascular failure in shock; as a vasoconstrictor in regional analgesia; symptomatic relief of nasal and nasopharyngeal mucosal congestion; as a mydriatic in ophthalmic procedures and treatment of wide-angle glaucoma; supraventricular tachycardia

Mechanism of Action Potent, direct-acting alpha-adrenergic stimulator with weak beta-adrenergic activity; causes vasoconstriction of the arterioles of the nasal mucosa and conjunctiva; activates the dilator muscle of the pupil to cause contraction; produces vasoconstriction of arterioles in the body

Adverse Reactions

Nasal:

Central nervous system: Psychosis, insomnia; visual, tactile, and auditory hallucinations; paranoid delusions, mania

Local: **Burning**

Respiratory: **Rebound congestion, sneezing**

Dermatologic: **Stinging, dryness**

Ophthalmic:

Central nervous system: Headache, browache

Dermatologic: Contact dermatitis, periorbital dermatitis

Ocular: **Transient stinging, mydriasis**, blurred vision, photophobia, lacrimation

Systemic:

Cardiovascular: Peripheral vasoconstriction, hypertension, angina, reflex bradycardia, arrhythmias

Central nervous system: Restlessness, excitability

Local: Extravasation injury

Neuromuscular & skeletal: **Tremor**

Pharmacodynamics/Kinetics

Onset of action: I.M., SubQ: 10-15 minutes; I.V.: Immediate; Ophthalmic: 10-15 minutes

Duration: I.M.: 0.5-2 hours; I.V.: 15-30 minutes; SubQ: 1 hour; Ophthalmic: Maximal mydriasis: 1 hour, recover time: 3-6 hours

Metabolism: Hepatic, via intestinal monoamine oxidase to phenolic conjugates

Excretion: Urine (90%)

Dosage

Ophthalmic procedures:

Infants <1 year: Instill 1 drop of 2.5% 15-30 minutes before procedures

Children and Adults: Instill 1 drop of 2.5% or 10% solution, may repeat in 10-60 minutes as needed

Nasal decongestant: (therapy should not exceed 5 continuous days)

Children:

2-6 years: Instill 1 drop every 2-4 hours of 0.125% solution as needed

6-12 years: Instill 1-2 sprays or instill 1-2 drops every 4 hours of 0.25% solution as needed

Children >12 years and Adults: Instill 1-2 sprays or instill 1-2 drops every 4 hours of 0.25% to 0.5% solution as needed; 1% solution may be used in adult in cases of extreme nasal congestion; do not use nasal solutions more than 3 days

Hypotension/shock:

Children:

I.M., SubQ: 0.1 mg/kg/dose every 1-2 hours as needed (maximum: 5 mg)

I.V. bolus: 5-20 mcg/kg/dose every 10-15 minutes as needed

I.V. infusion: 0.1-0.5 mcg/kg/minute

Adults:

I.M., SubQ: 2-5 mg/dose every 1-2 hours as needed (initial dose should not exceed 5 mg)

I.V. bolus: 0.1-0.5 mg/dose every 10-15 minutes as needed (initial dose should not exceed 0.5 mg)

I.V. infusion: 10 mg in 250 mL D$_5$W or normal saline (1:25,000 dilution) (40 mcg/mL); start at 100-180 mcg/minute (2-5 mL/

minute; 50-90 drops/minute) initially; when blood pressure is stabilized, maintenance rate: 40-60 mcg/minute (20-30 drops/minute)

Maternal hypotension: 0.1 mg/dose

Paroxysmal supraventricular tachycardia: I.V.:

Children: 5-10 mcg/kg/dose over 20-30 seconds

Adults: 0.25-0.5 mg/dose over 20-30 seconds

Stability Is stable for 48 hours in 5% dextrose in water at pH 3.5-7.5; do not use brown colored solutions

Monitoring Parameters Blood pressure, heart rate, arterial blood gases, central venous pressure

Administration Concentration and rate of infusion can be calculated using the following formulas: Dilute 0.6 mg × weight (kg) to 100 mL; then the dose in mcg/kg/minute = 0.1 × the infusion rate in mL/hour

Contraindications Hypersensitivity to phenylephrine or any component of the formulation; hypertension; ventricular tachycardia

Oral: Use with or within 14 days of MAO inhibitor therapy

Ophthalmic: Narrow-angle glaucoma

Warnings Some products contain sulfites which may cause allergic reactions in susceptible individuals.

Intravenous: Use with caution in the elderly, patients with hyperthyroidism, bradycardia, partial heart block, myocardial disease, or severe CAD. Not a substitute for volume replacement. Avoid hypertension; monitor blood pressure closely and adjust infusion rate. Infuse into a large vein if possible. Watch I.V. site closely. Avoid extravasation. **[U.S. Boxed Warning]: Should be administered by adequately trained individuals familiar with its use.**

Nasal, oral, rectal: Use caution with hyperthyroidism, diabetes mellitus, cardiovascular disease, ischemic heart disease, increased intraocular pressure, prostatic hyperplasia or in the elderly. Rebound congestion may occur when nasal products are discontinued after chronic use. When used for self-medication (OTC), notify healthcare provider if symptoms do not improve within 7 days (oral, rectal) or 3 days (nasal), are accompanied by fever (oral), or if bleeding occurs (rectal).

Ophthalmic: Use caution with or within 21 days of MAO inhibitor therapy. When used for self-medication (OTC), notify healthcare provider in case of vision changes, continued redness, or if symptoms worsen or do not improve within 3 days.

Dosage Forms [DSC] = Discontinued product

Cream, rectal, as hydrochloride (Formulation R™): 0.25% (54 g) [contains sodium benzoate]

Injection, solution, as hydrochloride: 1% [10 mg/mL] (1 mL, 5 mL) [may contain sodium metabisulfite]

Neo-Synephrine®: 1% (1 mL) [contains sodium metabisulfite]

Ointment, rectal, as hydrochloride:

Formulation R™: 0.25% (30 g, 60 g) [contains benzoic acid]

Rectacaine: 0.25% (30 g) [contains shark liver oil]

Solution, intranasal drops, as hydrochloride:

Neo-Synephrine® Extra Strength: 1% (15 mL) [contains benzalkonium chloride]

Neo-Synephrine® Regular Strength: 0.5% (15 mL) [contains benzalkonium chloride]

Rhinall: 0.25% (30 mL) [contains benzalkonium chloride and sodium bisulfite]

Solution, intranasal spray, as hydrochloride:

Neo-Synephrine® Extra Strength: 1% (15 mL) [contains benzalkonium chloride]

Neo-Synephrine® Mild: 0.25% (15 mL) [contains benzalkonium chloride]

Neo-Synephrine® Regular Strength: 0.5% (15 mL) [contains benzalkonium chloride]

Rhinall: 0.25% (40 mL) [contains benzalkonium chloride and sodium bisulfite]

Vicks® Sinex®, Vicks® Sinex® UltraFine Mist: 0.5% (15 mL) [contains benzalkonium chloride]

Solution, ophthalmic, as hydrochloride: 2.5% (1 mL, 2 mL, 3 mL, 5 mL, 15 mL) [may contain sodium bisulfite]

AK-Dilate®: 2.5% (2 mL, 15 mL); 10% (5 mL)

Altrafrin: 0.12% (15 mL) [OTC]; 2.5% (5 mL, 15 mL) [RX; contains benzalkonium chloride]; 10% (5 mL) [RX; contains benzalkonium chloride]

Mydfrin®: 2.5% (3 mL, 5 mL) [contains sodium bisulfite]

Neo-Synephrine®: 2.5% (15 mL); 10% (5 mL) [contains benzalkonium chloride] [DSC]

Neo-Synephrine® Viscous: 10% (5 mL) [contains benzalkonium chloride] [DSC]

Suppository, rectal, as hydrochloride: 0.25% (12s)

Anu-Med, Tronolane®: 0.25% (12s)

Medicone®: 0.25% (18s, 24s)

Rectacaine: 0.25% (12s) [contains shark liver oil]

Suspension, oral, as tannate (Ná Sop™): 7.5 mg/5 mL (120 mL) [orange flavor]

Tablet, as hydrochloride (Sudafed PE™): 10 mg

Tablet, chewable, as hydrochloride:

AH-chew® D: 10 mg [DSC]

Tablet, orally dissolving, as hydrochloride (Ná Sop™): 10 mg [contains phenylalanine 4 mg/tablet; bubble gum flavor]

Reference Range Peak plasma phenylephrine concentration after an oral dose of 9 mg: ~0.03 mg/L

Overdosage/Treatment Supportive therapy: Agitation can be treated with a benzodiazepine; propranolol (1 mg I.V. as needed to a total adult dose of 5 mg or 0.01-0.1 mg/kg in pediatrics to a total dose of 1 mg I.V.) or esmolol (50-100 mcg/kg/minute) can be given to treat tachycardia; atropine can be given for severe bradycardia with hypotension (not to be given for reflex bradycardia due to hypertension); nitroprusside, nifedipine, labetalol, hydralazine or esmolol can be used to treat hypertension

Drug Interactions Beta-blockers (nonselective) may increase hypertensive effect; avoid concurrent use.

MAO inhibitors: May potentiate hypertension and hypertensive crisis; avoid concurrent use.

Methyldopa can increase the pressor response; be aware of patient's drug regimen.

Tricyclic antidepressants: May enhance the vasopressor effect phenylephrine; avoid concurrent use.

Pregnancy Risk Factor C

Lactation Excretion in breast milk unknown/not recommended

Nursing Implications May cause necrosis or sloughing tissue if extravasation occurs during I.V. administration or SubQ administration

Extravasation: Use phentolamine as antidote; mix 5 mg with 9 mL of NS; inject a small amount of this dilution into extravasated area; blanching should reverse immediately. Monitor site; if blanching should recur, additional injections of phentolamine may be needed.

Additional Information Do not administer if the patient is exposed to chloroform, cyclopropane, halothane, trichloroethylene or other organic solvents in that ventricular arrhythmia may occur; pKa is ~8.8

Phenylpropanolamine *(Withdrawn from U.S. Market)*

CAS Number 154-41-6

Impairment Potential Yes

Use Anorexiant and nasal decongestant

Mechanism of Action Releases tissue stores of epinephrine and thereby produces an alpha- and beta-adrenergic stimulation; this causes vasoconstriction and nasal mucosa blanching; also appears to depress central appetite centers

Adverse Reactions

Cardiovascular: **Palpitations**, reflex bradycardia, cardiac arrhythmias, chest pain, **hypertension**, angina, vasculitis, AV block, sinus bradycardia, sinus tachycardia, arrhythmias (ventricular)

Central nervous system: Anxiety, psychosis, nervousness, restlessness, headache, insomnia, mania, paranoia, sympathetic storm, dystonia

Endocrine & metabolic: Hypokalemia

Genitourinary: Dysuria, urinary incontinence

Neuromuscular & skeletal: Rhabdomyolysis

Ocular: Mydriasis

Respiratory: Rhinitis

Miscellaneous: Fixed drug eruption

Signs and Symptoms of Overdose Anorexia, cognitive dysfunction, extrapyramidal reaction, hypertension, hyperthermia, palpitations, paresthesia, reflex bradycardia, renal failure, seizures, tachycardia, vomiting

Toxicodynamics/Kinetics

Onset of action: Nasal decongestion: 15-30 minutes

Duration: Tablet: 3 hours; Extended release: 12-16 hours

Absorption: Oral: Well absorbed

Distribution: V_d: 4.5 L/kg

Metabolism: In the liver to norephedrine

Bioavailability: ~100%

Half-life: 4.6-6.6 hours

Elimination: Primarily in urine as unchanged drug (80% to 90%)

Dosage

Oral:

Children: Decongestant:

2-6 years: 6.25 mg every 4 hours

6-12 years: 12.5 mg every 4 hours not to exceed 75 mg/day

Adults:

Decongestant: 25 mg every 4 hours or 50 mg every 8 hours, not to exceed 150 mg/day

Anorexic: 25 mg 3 times/day 30 minutes before meals or 75 mg (timed release) once daily in the morning

Precision release: 75 mg after breakfast

Reference Range Peak serum phenylpropanolamine: ~0.28 mg/L 6 hours after oral ingestion of 150 mg sustained release dose

Overdosage/Treatment

Decontamination: Lavage (within 1 hour)/activated charcoal

Supportive therapy: Lorazepam or diazepam 5-10 mg I.V. (0.25-0.4 mg/kg for children) or phenobarbital may be used for excitation and seizures; nitroprusside can be used for hypertension while labetalol or

esmolol can be used for tachycardia; ventricular ectopy can be treated with lidocaine

Enhancement of elimination: Multiple dosing of activated charcoal should be performed for sustained release preparation. Alkalinization can reduce the renal rate of elimination.

Nursing Implications Give dose early in day to prevent insomnia; observe for signs of nervousness, excitability

Phenytoin

Related Information

- Fosphenytoin
- Mephenytoin
- Seizures, Neonatal Guidelines
- Therapeutic Drugs Associated with Hallucinations

CAS Number 57-41-0

U.S. Brand Names Dilantin®; Phenytek™

Synonyms Diphenylhydantoin; DPH; Phenytoin Sodium, Extended; Phenytoin Sodium, Prompt; Phenytoin Sodium

Impairment Potential Yes; can be ergolytic (impair athletic performance)

Use Management of generalized tonic-clonic (grand mal), simple partial and complex partial seizures; prevention of seizures following head trauma/neurosurgery; ventricular arrhythmias, including those associated with digitalis intoxication; beneficial effects in the treatment of migraine or trigeminal neuralgia in some patients

Unlabeled/Investigational Use Ventricular arrhythmias, including those associated with digitalis intoxication, prolonged QT interval and surgical repair of congenital heart diseases in children; epidermolysis bullosa

Mechanism of Action Stabilizes neuronal membranes and decreases seizure activity by increasing efflux or decreasing influx of sodium ions across cell membranes in the motor cortex during generation of nerve impulses; prolongs effective refractory period and suppresses ventricular pacemaker automaticity, shortens action potential in the heart

Adverse Reactions

Effects not related to plasma phenytoin concentrations: Hypertrichosis, gingival hypertrophy, thickening of facial features, carbohydrate intolerance, folic acid deficiency, peripheral neuropathy, vitamin D deficiency, osteomalacia, systemic lupus erythematosus

Concentration-related effects: Nystagmus, blurred vision, diplopia, ataxia, slurred speech, dizziness, drowsiness, lethargy, coma, rash, fever, nausea, vomiting, gum tenderness, confusion, mood changes, folic acid depletion, osteomalacia, hyperglycemia

Rarely seen effects: SLE-like syndrome, lymphadenopathy, hepatitis, Stevens-Johnson syndrome, blood dyscrasias, dyskinesias, pseudolymphoma, venous irritation and pain, coarsening of the facial features, hypertrichosis

Dose related:

Cardiovascular: Myocarditis (hypersensitivity), AV block, facial edema

Central nervous system: **Slurred speech, psychiatric changes, dizziness, drowsiness**, psychosis, fever, visual hallucinations, ataxia, anticonvulsant hypersensitivity syndrome, insomnia

Dermatologic: Rash, exfoliative dermatitis, erythema multiforme, acne, acute generalized exanthematous pustulosis, linear IgA bullous dermatosis, hirsutism, hypertrichosis

Endocrine & metabolic: Folic acid depletion, osteomalacia, hyperglycemia, reduced plasma testosterone, gynecomastia, hypoglycemia

Gastrointestinal: **Nausea, constipation, vomiting, gingival hyperplasia**, burning tongue syndrome

Genitourinary: Priapism, possible urinary retention in children

Hematologic: Neutropenia, thrombocytopenia, anemia (megaloblastic), thrombocytopenia, megaloblastic anemia

Neuromuscular & skeletal: Sensory paresthesia (long-term treatment), choreoathetosis, chorea, osteoporosis

Ocular: Nystagmus, blurred vision, diplopia

Renal: Nephrotic syndrome

Miscellaneous: Mutism, pseudolymphoma, lymphadenopathy, mucocutaneous syndrome (febrile)

I.V.:

Cardiovascular: Hypotension, bradycardia, cardiac arrhythmias, cardiovascular collapse (especially with rapid I.V. use),

Local: Extravasation injury due to solvents and excipients

Signs and Symptoms of Overdose Acrodynia, agranulocytosis, chorea (extrapyramidal), cognitive dysfunction, coma, confusion, delirium, dementia, drowsiness, dysarthria, dysosmia, encephalopathy, enuresis, eosinophilia, extrapyramidal reaction, fever, granulocytopenia, gynecomastia, headache, hyperglycemia, hyperprolactinemia, hyperreflexia, hyperthermia, hypocalcemia, hypoglycemia, hypotension, hypothermia, hypothyroidism, leukemoid reaction, leukopenia, myasthenia gravis (exacerbation or precipitation), mydriasis, myocarditis, myoclonus, myoglobinuria, nausea, nephrotic syndrome, neutropenia, ophthalmoplegia, Parkinson's-like symptoms, periarteritis nodosa, pseudotumor cerebri, psychosis, respiratory depression, rhabdomyolysis, slurred speech, toxic epidermal necrolysis, tremors, unsteady gait, vision color changes (white tinge).

While toxicity from oral ingestion is relatively low, cardiac toxicity due to I.V. administration is primarily due to propylene glycol moiety. See table.

Manifestations of Phenytoin Toxicity

Levels	Manifestation
20 mcg/mL (79 µmol/L)	Nystagmus
30 mcg/mL (118.9 µmol/L)	Ataxia
40 mcg/mL (159 µmol/L)	Decreased mental status
50 mcg/mL (200 µmol/L)	Coma
95 mcg/mL (377 µmol/L)	Fatal

Admission Criteria/Prognosis Admit any patient with mental status changes or total phenytoin level >50 mcg/mL, or free phenytoin level >5 mcg/mL

Pharmacodynamics/Kinetics
Onset of action: I.V.: ~0.5-1 hour
Absorption: Oral: Slow
Distribution: V_d:
  Neonates: Premature: 1-1.2 L/kg; Full-term: 0.8-0.9 L/kg
  Infants: 0.7-0.8 L/kg
  Children: 0.7 L/kg
  Adults: 0.6-0.7 L/kg
Protein binding:
  Neonates: ≥80% (≤20% free)
  Infants: ≥85% (≤15% free)
  Adults: 90% to 95%
  Others: Decreased protein binding
    Disease states resulting in a decrease in serum albumin concentration: Burns, hepatic cirrhosis, nephrotic syndrome, pregnancy, cystic fibrosis
    Disease states resulting in an apparent decrease in affinity of phenytoin for serum albumin: Renal failure, jaundice (severe), other drugs (displacers), hyperbilirubinemia (total bilirubin >15 mg/dL), Cl_{cr} <25 mL/minute (unbound fraction is increased two- to threefold in uremia)
Metabolism: Follows dose-dependent capacity-limited (Michaelis-Menten) pharmacokinetics with increased V_{max} in infants >6 months of age and children versus adults; major metabolite (via oxidation), HPPA, undergoes enterohepatic recirculation
Bioavailability: Form dependent
Half-life elimination: Oral: 22 hours (range: 7-42 hours)
Time to peak, serum (form dependent): Oral: Extended-release capsule: 4-12 hours; Immediate release preparation: 2-3 hours
Excretion: Urine (<5% as unchanged drug); as glucuronides
  Clearance: Highly variable, dependent upon intrinsic hepatic function and dose administered; increased clearance and decreased serum concentrations with febrile illness

Dosage
Status epilepticus: I.V.:
  Neonates: Loading dose: 15-20 mg/kg in a single or divided dose; maintenance dose: Initial: 5 mg/kg/day in 2 divided doses; usual: 5-8 mg/kg/day in 2 divided doses; some patients may require dosing every 8 hours
  Infants and Children: Loading dose: 15-20 mg/kg in a single or divided dose; maintenance dose: Initial: 5 mg/kg/day in 2 divided doses, usual doses:
    6 months to 3 years: 8-10 mg/kg/day
    4-6 years: 7.5-9 mg/kg/day
    7-9 years: 7-8 mg/kg/day
    10-16 years: 6-7 mg/kg/day, some patients may require every 8 hours dosing
  Children with acute neurotrauma:
    0.5-9 years: 8-10 mg/kg/day
    10-16 years: 6-8 mg/kg/day
  Adults: Loading dose: 15-20 mg/kg in a single or divided dose, followed by 100-150 mg/dose at 30-minute intervals up to a maximum of 1500 mg/24 hours; maintenance dose: 300 mg/day or 5-6 mg/kg/day in 3 divided doses
Cocaine abuse treatment: 300 mg/day
Anticonvulsant: Children and Adults: Oral:
  Loading dose: 15-20 mg/kg; based on phenytoin serum concentrations and recent dosing history; administer oral loading dose in 3 divided doses given every 2-4 hours to decrease gastrointestinal adverse effects and to ensure complete oral absorption; maintenance dose: 300 mg/day or 5-6 mg/kg/day in 3 divided doses
Dosing adjustment/comments in renal impairment or hepatic disease: Safe in usual doses in mild liver disease; clearance may be substantially reduced in cirrhosis and plasma level monitoring with dose

adjustment advisable. Free phenytoin levels should be monitored closely.

Stability Capsule, tablet: Store below 30°C (86°F); protect from light and moisture
Oral suspension: Store at room temperature of 20°C to 25°C (68°F to 77°F); protect from freezing and light.
Solution for injection: Store at room temperature of 15°C to 30°C (59°F to 86°F); use only clear solutions free of precipitate and haziness, slightly yellow solutions may be used. Precipitation may occur if solution is refrigerated and may dissolve at room temperature.
  Further dilution of the solution for I.V. infusion is controversial and no consensus exists as to the optimal concentration and length of stability. Stability is concentration and pH dependent. Based on limited clinical consensus, NS or LR are recommended diluents; dilutions of 1-10 mg/mL have been used and should be administered as soon as possible after preparation (some recommend to discard if not used within 4 hours). Do not refrigerate.
  I.V. form is highly **incompatible** with many drugs and solutions. Mixing with other medications is not recommended.

Monitoring Parameters Blood pressure, vital signs (with I.V. use), plasma phenytoin level, CBC, liver function tests

Administration
Oral: Suspension: Shake well prior to use. Absorption is impaired when phenytoin suspension is given concurrently to patients who are receiving continuous nasogastric feedings. A method to resolve this interaction is to divide the daily dose of phenytoin and withhold the administration of nutritional supplements for 1-2 hours before and after each phenytoin dose.
I.M.: Although approved for I.M. use, I.M. administration is not recommended due to erratic absorption and pain on injection. Fosphenytoin may be considered.
I.V.: Vesicant. Fosphenytoin may be considered for loading in patients who are in status epilepticus, hemodynamically unstable, or develop hypotension/bradycardia with I.V. administration of phenytoin. Phenytoin may be administered by IVP or IVPB administration. The maximum rate of I.V. administration is 50 mg/minute. Highly sensitive patients (eg, elderly, patients with pre-existing cardiovascular conditions) should receive phenytoin more slowly (eg, 20 mg/minute). An in-line 0.22-5 micron filter is recommended for IVPB solutions due to the high potential for precipitation of the solution. Avoid extravasation. Following I.V. administration, NS should be injected through the same needle or I.V. catheter to prevent irritation.
pH: 10.0-12.3
SubQ: SubQ administration is not recommended because of the possibility of local tissue damage.

Contraindications Hypersensitivity to phenytoin, other hydantoins, or any component of the formulation; pregnancy

Warnings May increase frequency of petit mal seizures; I.V. form may cause hypotension, skin necrosis at I.V. site; avoid I.V. administration in small veins; use with caution in patients with porphyria; discontinue if rash or lymphadenopathy occurs; use with caution in patients with hepatic dysfunction, sinus bradycardia, SA block, or AV block; use with caution in elderly or debilitated patients, or in any condition associated with low serum albumin levels, which will increase the free fraction of phenytoin in the serum and, therefore, the pharmacologic response. Sedation, confusional states, or cerebellar dysfunction (loss of motor coordination) may occur at higher total serum concentrations, or at lower total serum concentrations when the free fraction of phenytoin is increased. Abrupt withdrawal may precipitate status epilepticus.

Dosage Forms Capsule, extended release, as sodium: 100 mg
  Dilantin®: 30 mg [contains sodium benzoate], 100 mg
  Phenytek™: 200 mg, 300 mg
Capsule, prompt release, as sodium: 100 mg
Injection, solution, as sodium: 50 mg/mL (2 mL, 5 mL) [contains alcohol and propylene glycol]
Suspension, oral: 125 mg/5 mL (240 mL)
  Dilantin®: 125 mg/5 mL (240 mL) [contains alcohol <0.6%, sodium benzoate; orange vanilla flavor]
Tablet, chewable:
  Dilantin®: 50 mg

Reference Range
Timing of serum samples: Because it is slowly absorbed, peak blood levels may occur 4-8 hours after ingestion of an oral dose. The serum half-life varies with the dosage and the drug follows Michaelis-Menten kinetics. The average adult half-life is about 24 hours. Steady-state concentrations are reached in 5-10 days.
Children and Adults: Toxicity is measured clinically, and some patients require levels outside the suggested therapeutic range
Therapeutic range:
  Total phenytoin: 10-20 mcg/mL (children and adults), 8-15 mcg/mL (neonates)
  Concentrations of 5-10 mcg/mL may be therapeutic for some patients but concentrations <5 mcg/mL are not likely to be effective

50% of patients show decreased frequency of seizures at concentrations >10 mcg/mL

86% of patients show decreased frequency of seizures at concentrations >15 mcg/mL

Add another anticonvulsant if satisfactory therapeutic response is not achieved with a phenytoin concentration of 20 mcg/mL

Free phenytoin: 1-2.5 mcg/mL

Toxic: <30-50 mcg/mL (SI: <120-200 µmol/L)

Lethal: >100 mcg/mL (SI: >400 µmol/L)

When to draw levels: This is dependent on the disease state being treated and the clinical condition of the patient

Key points:

Slow absorption of extended capsules and prolonged half-life minimize fluctuations between peak and trough concentrations, timing of sampling not crucial

Trough concentrations are generally recommended for routine monitoring. Daily levels are not necessary and may result in incorrect dosage adjustments. If it is determined essential to monitor free phenytoin concentrations, concomitant monitoring of total phenytoin concentrations is not necessary and expensive.

After a loading dose: Draw level within 48-96 hours

Rapid achievement: Draw within 2-3 days of therapy initiation to ensure that the patient's metabolism is not remarkably different from that which would be predicted by average literature-derived pharmacokinetic parameters; early levels should be used cautiously in design of new dosing regimens

Second concentration: Draw within 6-7 days with subsequent doses of phenytoin adjusted accordingly

If plasma concentrations have not changed over a 3- to 5-day period, monitoring interval may be increased to once weekly in the acute clinical setting

In stable patients requiring long-term therapy, generally monitor levels at 3- to 12-month intervals

Adjustment of serum concentration: See tables.

Adjustment of Serum Concentration in Patients with Low Serum Albumin

Measured Total Phenytoin Concentration (mcg/mL)	Patient's Serum Albumin (g/dL)			
	3.5	3	2.5	2
	Adjusted Total Phenytoin Concentration (mcg/mL)*			
5	6	7	8	10
10	13	14	17	20
15	19	21	25	30

*Adjusted concentration = measured total concentration divided by [(0.2 × albumin) + 0.1].

Adjustment of Serum Concentration in Patients with Renal Failure (Cl$_{cr}$ ≤10 mL/min)

Measured Total Phenytoin Concentration (mcg/mL)	Patient's Serum Albumin (g/dL)				
	4	3.5	3	2.5	2
	Adjusted Total Phenytoin Concentration (mcg/mL)*				
5	10	11	13	14	17
10	20	22	25	29	33
15	30	33	38	43	50

*Adjusted concentration = measured total concentration divided by [(0.1 × albumin) + 0.1].

Overdosage/Treatment

Decontamination: Activated charcoal

Supportive therapy: Treatment is supportive for hypotension; treat with I.V. fluids and place patient in Trendelenburg position; seizures may be controlled with lorazepam or diazepam 5-10 mg (0.25-0.4 mg/kg in children); extravasation can be treated with compressive dressing, elevation and splinting of extremity; systemic corticosteroids should be used for phenytoin hypersensitivity syndrome

Enhancement of elimination: Multiple dosing of activated charcoal may be effective; peritoneal dialysis, diuresis, hemodialysis, hemoperfusion, and plasmapheresis is of little value

Diagnostic Procedures

● Phenytoin, Blood

Test Interactions ↑ glucose, alkaline phosphatase (S); ↓ thyroxine (S), calcium (S); serum sodium increases in overdose setting; produces sustained reductions of both free thyroxine and free triodothyronine levels at therapeutic levels; oxaprozin falsely elevates plasma phenytoin concentrations

Drug Interactions

Substrate of CYP2C9 (major), 2C19 (major), 3A4 (minor); **Induces** CYP2B6 (strong), 2C8 (strong), 2C9 (strong), 2C19 (strong), 3A4 (strong)

Acetaminophen: Phenytoin may enhance the hepatotoxic potential of acetaminophen overdoses

Acetazolamide: Concurrent use with phenytoin may result in an increased risk of osteomalacia

Acyclovir: May decrease phenytoin serum levels; limited documentation; monitor

Allopurinol: May increase phenytoin serum concentrations; monitor

Antacids: May decrease absorption of phenytoin; separate oral doses by several hours

Antiarrhythmics: Phenytoin may increase the metabolism of antiarrhythmics, decreasing their clinical effect; includes disopyramide, propafenone, and quinidine; amiodarone also may increase phenytoin concentrations (see CYP inhibitors)

Anticonvulsants: Phenytoin may increase the metabolism of anticonvulsants; includes barbiturates, carbamazepine, ethosuximide, felbamate, lamotrigine, tiagabine, topiramate, and zonisamide; does not appear to affect gabapentin or levetiracetam; felbamate and gabapentin may increase phenytoin levels; monitor

Antineoplastics: Several chemotherapeutic agents have been associated with a decrease in serum phenytoin levels; includes cisplatin, bleomycin, carmustine, methotrexate, and vinblastine; monitor phenytoin serum levels. Limited evidence also suggest that enzyme-inducing anticonvulsant therapy may reduce the effectiveness of some chemotherapy regimens (specifically in ALL). Teniposide and methotrexate may be cleared more rapidly in these patients.

Antipsychotics: Phenytoin may enhance the metabolism (decrease the efficacy) of antipsychotics; monitor for altered response; dose adjustment may be needed; also see note on clozapine

Benzodiazepines: Phenytoin may decrease the serum concentrations of some benzodiazepines; monitor for decreased benzodiazepine effect

Beta-blockers: Metabolism of beta-blockers may be increased and clinical effect decreased; atenolol and nadolol are unlikely to interact given their renal elimination

Calcium channel blockers: Phenytoin may enhance the metabolism of calcium channel blockers, decreasing their clinical effect; calcium channel blockers (diltiazem, nifedipine) have been reported to increase phenytoin levels (case report); monitor.

Capecitabine: May increase the serum concentrations of phenytoin; monitor

Chloramphenicol: Phenytoin may increase the metabolism of chloramphenicol and chloramphenicol may inhibit phenytoin metabolism; monitor for altered response

Cimetidine: May increase the serum concentrations of phenytoin; monitor.

Ciprofloxacin: May decrease serum phenytoin concentrations; monitor.

Clozapine: Phenytoin may decrease levels/effects of clozapine; monitor.

CNS depressants: Sedative effects may be additive with other CNS depressants; monitor for increased effect; includes ethanol, barbiturates, sedatives, antidepressants, narcotic analgesics, and benzodiazepines

Corticosteroids: Phenytoin may increase the metabolism of corticosteroids, decreasing their clinical effect; also see dexamethasone

Cyclosporine and tacrolimus: Levels may be decreased by phenytoin; monitor

CYP2B6 substrates: Phenytoin may decrease the levels/effects of CYP2B6 substrates. Example substrates include bupropion, efavirenz, promethazine, selegiline, and sertraline.

CYP2C9 inducers: May decrease the levels/effects of phenytoin. Example inducers include carbamazepine, phenobarbital, rifampin, rifapentine, and secobarbital.

CYP2C9 Inhibitors may increase the levels/effects of phenytoin. Example inhibitors include delavirdine, fluconazole, gemfibrozil, ketoconazole, nicardipine, NSAIDs, sulfonamides and tolbutamide.

CYP2C8 Substrates: Phenytoin may decrease the levels/effects of CYP2C8 substrates. Example substrates include amiodarone, paclitaxel, pioglitazone, repaglinide, and rosiglitazone.

CYP2C9 Substrates: Phenytoin may decrease the levels/effects of CYP2C9 substrates. Example substrates include bosentan, celecoxib, dapsone, fluoxetine, glimepiride, glipizide, losartan, montelukast, nateglinide, paclitaxel, sulfonamides, trimethoprim, warfarin, and zafirlukast.

CYP2C19 inducers: May decrease the levels/effects of phenytoin. Example inducers include aminoglutethimide, carbamazepine, phenytoin, and rifampin.

CYP2C19 inhibitors: May increase the levels/effects of phenytoin. Example inhibitors include delavirdine, fluconazole, fluvoxamine, gemfibrozil, isoniazid, omeprazole, and ticlopidine.

CYP2C19 substrates: Phenytoin may decrease the levels/effects of CYP2C19 substrates. Example substrates include citalopram, diazepam, methsuximide, propranolol, proton pump inhibitors, sertraline, and voriconazole.

CYP3A4 substrates: Phenytoin may decrease the levels/effects of CYP3A4 substrates. Example substrates include benzodiazepines, calcium channel blockers, clarithromycin, cyclosporine, erythromycin, estrogens, mirtazapine, nateglinide, nefazodone, nevirapine, protease inhibitors, tacrolimus, and venlafaxine.

Digoxin: Effects and/or levels of digitalis glycosides may be decreased by phenytoin

Disulfiram: May increase serum phenytoin concentrations; monitor

Dopamine: Phenytoin (I.V.) may increase the effect of dopamine (enhanced hypotension)

Doxycycline: Phenytoin may enhance the metabolism of doxycycline, decreasing its clinical effect; higher dosages may be required

Estrogens: Phenytoin may increase the metabolism of estrogens, decreasing their clinical effect; monitor

Folic acid: Replacement of folic acid has been reported to increase the metabolism of phenytoin, decreasing its serum concentrations and/or increasing seizures

HMG-CoA reductase inhibitors: Phenytoin may increase the metabolism of these agents, reducing their clinical effect; monitor

Itraconazole: Phenytoin may decrease the effect of itraconazole

Levodopa: Phenytoin may inhibit the anti-Parkinson effect of levodopa

Lithium: Concurrent use of phenytoin and lithium has resulted in lithium intoxication

Methadone: Phenytoin may enhance the metabolism of methadone resulting in methadone withdrawal

Methylphenidate: May increase serum phenytoin concentrations; monitor

Metronidazole: May increase the serum concentrations of phenytoin; monitor.

Neuromuscular-blocking agents: Duration of effect may be decreased by phenytoin

Omeprazole: May increase serum phenytoin concentrations; monitor

Oral contraceptives: Phenytoin may enhance the metabolism of oral contraceptives, decreasing their clinical effect; an alternative method of contraception should be considered

Primidone: Phenytoin enhances the conversion of primidone to phenobarbital resulting in elevated phenobarbital serum concentrations

Quetiapine: Serum concentrations may be substantially reduced by phenytoin, potentially resulting in a loss of efficacy; limited documentation; monitor

SSRIs: May increase phenytoin serum concentrations; fluoxetine and fluvoxamine are known to inhibit metabolism via CYP enzymes; sertraline and paroxetine have also been shown to increase concentrations in some patients; monitor

Sucralfate: May reduce the GI absorption of phenytoin; monitor

Theophylline: Phenytoin may increase metabolism of theophylline derivatives and decrease their clinical effect; theophylline may also increase phenytoin concentrations

Thyroid hormones (including levothyroxine): Phenytoin may alter the metabolism of thyroid hormones, reducing its effect; there is limited documentation of this interaction, but monitoring should be considered

Ticlopidine: May increase serum phenytoin concentrations and/or toxicity; monitor

Tricyclic antidepressants: Phenytoin may increase metabolism of tricyclic antidepressants and decrease their clinical effect; sedative effects may be additive; tricyclics may also increase phenytoin concentrations

Topiramate: Phenytoin may decrease serum levels of topiramate; topiramate may increase the effect of phenytoin

Trazodone: Serum levels of phenytoin may be increased; limited documentation; monitor

Trimethoprim: May increase serum phenytoin concentrations; monitor

Valproic acid (and sulfisoxazole): May displace phenytoin from binding sites; valproic acid may increase, decrease, or have no effect on phenytoin serum concentrations

Vigabatrin: May reduce phenytoin serum concentrations; monitor

Warfarin: Phenytoin transiently increased the hypothrombinemia response to warfarin initially; this is followed by an inhibition of the hypoprothrombinemic response

Pregnancy Risk Factor D

Pregnancy Implications Crosses placenta with fetal serum concentrations equal to those of mother; eye, cardiac, cleft palate, and skeletal malformations have been noted; fetal hydantoin syndrome associated with maternal ingestion of 100-800 mg/kg during 1st trimester; lower IQ scores also documented in children born to mothers taking phenytoin during pregnancy

Lactation Enters breast milk/not recommended (AAP rates "compatible")

Nursing Implications I.V. injections should be followed by normal saline flushes through the same needle or I.V. catheter to avoid local irritation of the vein; must be diluted to concentrations <6 mg/mL, in normal saline, for I.V. infusion

Additional Information Less than 5% of total body phenytoin is removed by plasmapheresis and rapid re-equilibration after plasmapheresis can occur resulting in increased free phenytoin levels; intravenous phenytoin salt has poor water solubility (0.02 mg/mL at a pH of 7) with a high PTT (12) and requires 40% propylene glycol and 10% ethanol

Specific References

Adams BK, Mann MD, Aboo A, et al, "Prolonged Gastric Emptying Half-time and Gastric Hypomotility After Drug Overdose," *Am J Emerg Med*, 2004, 22(7):548-554.

Ali FE, Al-Bustan MA, Al-Busairi WA, et al, "Loss of Seizure Control Due to Anticonvulsant-Induced Hypocalcemia," *Ann Pharmacother*, 2004, 38(6):1002-5.

Altuntas Y, Ozturk B, Erdem L, et al, "Phenytoin-Induced Toxic Cholestatic Hepatitis in a Patient with Skin Lesions: Case Report," *South Med J*, 2003, 96(2):201-3.

Cave G and Sleigh JW, "ECG Features of Sodium Channel Blockade in Rodent Phenytoin Toxicity and Effect of Hypertonic Saline," *Vet Hum Toxicol*, 2003, 45(5):254-5.

Chan GM, Krief W, and Nelson LS, "A Five-Fold Phenytoin Pediatric Dosing Error," *Int J Med Toxicol*, 2004, 7(1):2.

Citerio G, Nobili A, Airoldi L, et al, "Severe Intoxication After Phenytoin Infusion: A Preventable Pharmacogenetic Adverse Reaction," *Neurology*, 2003, 60(4):1395-6.

Coffing MJ, Bertholf RL, Jones JB, et al, "Multicenter Evaluation of the Roche OnLine® TDM Phenytoin Assay on Roche/Hitachi Analyzer Systems," *J Anal Toxicol*, 2004, 28:289-90.

Fridell JA, Jain AK, Patel K, et al, "Phenytoin Decreases the Blood Concentrations of Sirolimus in a Liver Transplant Recipient: A Case Report," *Ther Drug Monit*, 2003, 25(1):117-9.

Gogtay NJ, Dalvi SS, Mhatre RB, et al, "A Randomized, Crossover, Assessor-Blind Study of the Bioequivalence of a Single Oral Dose of 200 mg of Four Formulations of Phenytoin Sodium in Healthy, Normal Indian Volunteers," *Ther Drug Monit*, 2003, 25(2):215-20.

Mostella J, Pieroni R, Jones R, et al, "Anticonvulsant Hypersensitivity Syndrome: Treatment with Corticosteroids and Intravenous Immunoglobulin," *South Med J*, 2004, 97(3):319-21.

Murphy A and Wilbur K, "Phenytoin-Diazepam Interaction," *Ann Pharmacother*, 2003, 37(5):659-63.

Rudis MI, Touchette DR, Swadron SP, et al, "Cost-Effectiveness of Oral Phenytoin, Intravenous Phenytoin, and Intravenous Fosphenytoin in the Emergency Department," *Ann Emerg Med*, 2004, 43(3):386-97.

Schwarz EB, Maselli J, Norton M, et al. "Prescription of Teratogenic Medications in United States Ambulatory Practices," *Am J Med*, 2005, 118(11):1240-9.

Pilocarpine

CAS Number 16509-56-1; 54-71-7; 92-13-7

U.S. Brand Names Isopto® Carpine; Pilocar®; Pilopine HS®; Salagen®

Synonyms Pilocarpine Hydrochloride

Use

Ophthalmic: Management of chronic simple glaucoma, chronic and acute angle-closure glaucoma

Oral: Symptomatic treatment of xerostomia caused by salivary gland hypofunction resulting from radiotherapy for cancer of the head and neck or Sjögren's syndrome

Unlabeled/Investigational Use Counter effects of cycloplegics

Mechanism of Action Stimulates parasympathetic receptors causing pupillary constriction and ciliary muscle contraction

Adverse Reactions

Ophthalmic:

Cardiovascular: Hypertension, tachycardia

Gastrointestinal: Diarrhea, nausea, salivation, vomiting

Ocular: Burning, ciliary spasm, conjunctival vascular congestion, **corneal granularity** (gel 10%), lacrimation, lens opacity, myopia, retinal detachment, visual acuity decreased, blepharospasm

Respiratory: Bronchial spasm, pulmonary edema

Miscellaneous: Diaphoresis

Oral (frequency varies by indication and dose):

Cardiovascular: Abnormal ECG, angina pectoris, arrhythmia, bradycardia, edema, **flushing**, facial edema, hypertension, hypotension, myocardial infarction, palpitations, peripheral edema, syncope, tachycardia, thrombosis

Central nervous system: Chills, **dizziness**, **headache**, pain, fever, somnolence, abnormal dreams, abnormal thinking, anxiety, aphasia, confusion, depression, emotional lability, hypothermia, insomnia, intracranial hemorrhage, migraine, nervousness, speech disorder, twitching, yawning, supraorbital or temporal headache

Dermatologic: Alopecia, contact dermatitis, dry skin, eczema, erythema nodosum, exfoliative dermatitis, photosensitivity reaction, pruritus, rash, seborrhea, skin ulcer, vesiculobullous rash

Endocrine & metabolic: Breast pain, hypoglycemia, lymphadenopathy, mastitis, menorrhagia, metrorrhagia, ovarian disorder

Gastrointestinal: Anorexia, appetite increased, colitis, constipation, diarrhea, dry mouth, dyspepsia, dysphagia, eructation, esophagitis, flatulence, gastritis, gastroenteritis, gastrointestinal disorder, gingivitis, glossitis, hiccup, melena, **nausea**, pancreatitis, parotid gland enlargement, salivary gland enlargement, salivation increased, stomatitis, taste loss, taste perversion, tongue disorder, vomiting

Genitourinary: Dysuria, hematuria, pyuria, urethral pain, urinary impairment, **urinary frequency**, urinary urgency, urinary incontinence, vaginal hemorrhage, vaginal moniliasis, vaginitis

Hematologic: Leukopenia, platelet abnormality, thrombocythemia, thrombocytopenia, WBC abnormality

Hepatic: Bilirubinemia, cholelithiasis, hepatitis, liver function test abnormal

Neuromuscular & skeletal: Arthralgia, arthritis, bone disorder, hyperkinesia, hypesthesia, leg cramps, myasthenia, neck pain, paresthesia, tremor, tendon disorder, tenosynovitis, **weakness**

Ocular: Amblyopia, abnormal vision, blurred vision, conjunctivitis, cataract, dry eyes, eye hemorrhage, eye pain, glaucoma, lacrimation

Otic: Deafness, ear pain, tinnitus

Respiratory: Bronchitis, cough increased, epistaxis, laryngismus, pneumonia, **rhinitis**, sputum increased, stridor, sinusitis

Miscellaneous: **Diaphoresis**, allergic reaction, body odor, herpes simplex, moniliasis, salpingitis, voice alteration

Signs and Symptoms of Overdose Abdominal cramps, bronchorrhea, dizziness, nausea, photophobia, third degree AV block (15%), vomiting

Admission Criteria/Prognosis Consider admission for ingestions of >20 mg or intraocular doses >30 drops

Pharmacodynamics/Kinetics

Onset of action:

Ophthalmic: Miosis: 10-30 minutes; Intraocular pressure reduction: 1 hour

Oral: 20 minutes

Duration:

Ophthalmic: Miosis: 4-8 hours; Intraocular pressure reduction: 4-12 hours

Oral: 3-5 hours

Half-life elimination: Oral: 0.76-1.35 hours; increased with hepatic impairment

Excretion: Urine

Dosage Adults:

Ophthalmic:

Glaucoma:

Solution: Instill 1-2 drops up to 6 times/day; adjust the concentration and frequency as required to control elevated intraocular pressure

Gel: Instill 0.5" ribbon into lower conjunctival sac once daily at bedtime

To counteract the mydriatic effects of sympathomimetic agents (unlabeled use): Solution: Instill 1 drop of a 1% solution in the affected eye

Oral: Xerostomia:

Following head and neck cancer: 5 mg 3 times/day, titration up to 10 mg 3 times/day may be considered for patients who have not responded adequately; do not exceed 2 tablets/dose

Sjögren's syndrome: 5 mg 4 times/day

Dosage adjustment in hepatic impairment: Oral: Patients with moderate impairment: 5 mg 2 times/day regardless of indication; adjust dose based on response and tolerability. Do not use with severe impairment (Child-Pugh score 10-15).

Monitoring Parameters Intraocular pressure, funduscopic exam, visual field testing

Administration Oral: Avoid administering with high-fat meal. Fat decreases the rate of absorption, maximum concentration, and increases the time it takes to reach maximum concentration.

Ophthalmic: If both solution and gel are used, the solution should be applied first, then the gel at least 5 minutes later. Following administration of the solution, finger pressure should be applied on the lacrimal sac for 1-2 minutes.

Contraindications Hypersensitivity to pilocarpine or any component of the formulation; acute inflammatory disease of the anterior chamber of the eye; in addition, tablets are also contraindicated in patients with uncontrolled asthma, angle-closure glaucoma, severe hepatic impairment

Warnings Use caution with cardiovascular disease; patients may have difficulty compensating for transient changes in hemodynamics or rhythm induced by pilocarpine.

Ophthalmic products: May cause decreased visual acuity, especially at night or with reduced lighting.

Oral tablets: Use caution with controlled asthma, chronic bronchitis or COPD; may increase airway resistance, bronchial smooth muscle tone, and bronchial secretions. Use caution with cholelithiasis, biliary tract disease, nephrolithiasis; adjust dose with moderate hepatic impairment.

Dosage Forms Gel, ophthalmic, as hydrochloride (Pilopine HS®): 4% (4 g) [contains benzalkonium chloride]

Solution, ophthalmic, as hydrochloride: 0.5% (15 mL); 1% (2 mL, 15 mL); 2% (2 mL, 15 mL); 3% (15 mL); 4% (2 mL, 15 mL); 6% (15 mL) [may contain benzalkonium chloride]

Isopto® Carpine: 1% (15 mL); 2% (15 mL); 4% (15 mL) [contains benzalkonium chloride]

Tablet, as hydrochloride: 5 mg

Salagen®: 5 mg, 7.5 mg

Reference Range After 2 days of oral dosage of 10 mg 3 times/day, maximum serum concentrations are ~41 ng/mL

Overdosage/Treatment

Decontamination: **Oral:** Due to spontaneous emesis, ipecac or lavage is usually not required; activated charcoal can be used. **Ocular:** Irrigate copiously with saline

Supportive therapy: Atropine will reverse most cardiac and muscarinic effects; chlorpromazine can be given for agitation, epinephrine (0.1-1 mg SubQ) or beta-adrenergic agonist agents can be used for bronchodilatation

Antidote(s)
- Atropine [ANTIDOTE]
- Epinephrine [ANTIDOTE]

Drug Interactions Inhibits CYP2A6 (weak), 2E1 (weak), 3A4 (weak)

Concurrent use with beta-blockers may cause conduction disturbances; pilocarpine may antagonize the effects of anticholinergic drugs

Pregnancy Risk Factor C

Lactation Excretion in breast milk unknown/not recommended

Additional Information Minimal lethal oral dose: 60 mg. Toxic ophthalmic dose: Systemic anticholinergic symptoms will occur after intraocular dose >30 drops (2% solution) or 60 drops (3% solution)

May exacerbate dementia of Alzheimer's disease; can reverse the mydriasis caused by sympathomimetic agents (phenylephrine, hydroxyamphetamine) but is not effective in reversing mydriasis due to antimuscarinic agents (ie, homatropine); no corneal effects due to pilocarpine use

Pimozide

CAS Number 2062-78-4

U.S. Brand Names Orap®

Use Suppression of severe motor and phonic tics in patients with Tourette's disorder who have failed to respond satisfactorily to standard treatment

Unlabeled/Investigational Use Psychosis; reported use in individuals with delusions focused on physical symptoms (ie, preoccupation with parasitic infestation); Huntington's chorea

Mechanism of Action A potent centrally-acting dopamine receptor antagonist resulting in its characteristic neuroleptic effects

Adverse Reactions

Reported with Tourette's disorder:

Cardiovascular: Abnormal ECG

Central nervous system: **Somnolence, sedation**, akathisia, drowsiness, hyperkinesias, insomnia, depression, headache, nervousness

Dermatologic: Rash

Gastrointestinal: **Xerostomia, constipation, increased salivation**, diarrhea, thirst, appetite increased, taste disturbance, dysphagia

Genitourinary: **Impotence**

Neuromuscular & skeletal: **Weakness, muscle tightness, rigidity**, myalgia, torticollis, tremor

Ocular: **Visual disturbance, accommodation decreased**

Miscellaneous: **Speech disorder**

Reported in disorders other than Tourette's disorder: Anorexia, blood dyscrasias, breast edema, chest pain, diaphoresis, dizziness, excitement; extrapyramidal symptoms (akathisia, akinesia, dystonia, pseudoparkinsonism, tardive dyskinesia); facial edema, gingival hyperplasia (case report); hypertension, hyponatremia, hypotension, jaundice, libido decreased, nausea, neuroleptic malignant syndrome, orthostatic hypotension, palpitations, periorbital edema, postural hypotension, QT_c prolongation, seizure, tachycardia, ventricular arrhythmias, vomiting, weight gain/loss

Signs and Symptoms of Overdose Drowsiness, ECG changes, enuresis, extrapyramidal reaction, galactorrhea, hypotension, impotence, numbness, Parkinson's-like symptoms, QT interval prolongation, respiratory depression, seizures, torsade de pointes

Admission Criteria/Prognosis Admit any ingestion >50 mg or exhibiting neurological sequelae

Pharmacodynamics/Kinetics

Absorption: 50%

Protein binding: 99%

Metabolism: Hepatic; significant first-pass effect

Half-life elimination: 50 hours

Time to peak, serum: 6-8 hours

Excretion: Urine

Dosage Oral: **Note:** An ECG should be performed baseline and periodically thereafter, especially during dosage adjustment:

Children ≤12 years: Tourette's disorder: Initial: 0.05 mg/kg preferably once at bedtime; may be increased every third day; usual range: 2-4 mg/day; do not exceed 10 mg/day (0.2 mg/kg/day)

Children >12 years and Adults: Tourette's disorder: Initial: 1-2 mg/day in divided doses, then increase dosage as needed every other day; range is usually 7-16 mg/day, maximum dose: 10 mg/day or 0.2 mg/kg/day are not generally recommended

Note: Sudden unexpected deaths have occurred in patients taking doses >10 mg. Therefore, dosages exceeding 10 mg/day are generally not recommended.

Dosing adjustment in hepatic impairment: Reduction of dose is necessary in patients with liver disease

Monitoring Parameters ECG should be performed baseline and periodically thereafter, especially during dosage adjustment; vital signs; lipid profile, fasting blood glucose/Hgb A_{1c}; BMI; mental status, abnormal involuntary movement scale (AIMS), extrapyramidal symptoms (EPS)

Contraindications Hypersensitivity to pimozide or any component of the formulation; severe CNS depression; coma; history of dysrhythmia; prolonged QT syndrome; concurrent use with QT_c-prolonging agents; hypokalemia or hypomagnesemia; concurrent use of drugs that are inhibitors of CYP3A4, including concurrent use of azole antifungals, fluvoxamine, macrolide antibiotics (such as clarithromycin or erythromycin [**Note:** The manufacturer lists azithromycin and dirithromycin in its list of contraindicated macrolides; however, these drugs do not inhibit CYP3A4 and are not expected to interact with pimozide]), mesoridazine, nefazodone, protease inhibitors (ie, atazanavir, indinavir, nelfinavir, ritonavir, saquinavir), sertraline, thioridazine, zileuton, and ziprasidone; simple tics other than Tourette's

Warnings May cause hypotension, use with caution in patients with autonomic instability. Moderately sedating, use with caution in disorders where CNS depression is a feature. Use with caution in Parkinson's disease. Caution in patients with hemodynamic instability; bone marrow suppression; predisposition to seizures; subcortical brain damage; severe cardiac, hepatic, renal, or respiratory disease. Esophageal dysmotility and aspiration have been associated with antipsychotic use - use with caution in patients at risk of pneumonia (ie, Alzheimer's disease). Caution in breast cancer or other prolactin-dependent tumors (may elevate prolactin levels). May alter temperature regulation or mask toxicity of other drugs due to antiemetic effects. May alter cardiac conduction - sudden unexplained deaths have occurred in patients taking high doses (>10 mg). This may be due to prolongation of the QT interval predisposing patients to ventricular arrhythmias. Monitor ECG at baseline and periodically during dosage titration. May cause orthostatic hypotension - use with caution in patients at risk of this effect or those who would tolerate transient hypotensive episodes (cerebrovascular disease, cardiovascular disease, or other medications which may predispose).

May cause anticholinergic effects (confusion, agitation, constipation, xerostomia, blurred vision, urinary retention); therefore, they should be used with caution in patients with decreased gastrointestinal motility, urinary retention, BPH, xerostomia, or visual problems. Conditions which also may be exacerbated by cholinergic blockade include narrow-angle glaucoma (screening is recommended) and worsening of myasthenia gravis. Relative to neuroleptics, pimozide has a moderate potency of cholinergic blockade.

May cause extrapyramidal symptoms, including pseudoparkinsonism, acute dystonic reactions, akathisia, and tardive dyskinesia (risk of these reactions is high relative to other neuroleptics). May be associated with neuroleptic malignant syndrome (NMS) or pigmentary retinopathy.

Avoid grapefruit juice due to potential inhibition of pimozide metabolism

Dosage Forms Tablet: 1 mg, 2 mg

Reference Range 3 mg dose produces a plasma level of 3.3 ng/mL

Overdosage/Treatment

Decontamination: Lavage (within 1 hour)/activated charcoal

Supportive therapy: Following initiation of essential overdose management, toxic symptom treatment and supportive treatment should be initiated. Hypotension usually responds to I.V. fluids or Trendelenburg positioning. If unresponsive to these measures, the use of a parenteral inotrope may be required (eg, norepinephrine 0.1-0.2 mcg/kg/minute titrated to response). Epinephrine should not be used. Seizures commonly respond to lorazepam, diazepam, or phenobarbital. Also critical cardiac arrhythmias often respond to I.V. phenytoin (15 mg/kg up to 1 gram), while other antiarrhythmics can be used. Neuroleptics often cause extrapyramidal reaction (eg, dystonic reactions) requiring management with diphenhydramine 1-2 mg/kg (adults) up to a maximum of 50 mg I.M. or I.V. slow push followed by a maintenance dose for 48-72 hours. When these reactions are unresponsive to diphenhydramine, benztropine mesylate I.V. 1-2 mg (adults) may be effective. These agents are generally effective within 2-5 minutes.

Enhancement of elimination: Multiple dosing of activated charcoal may be useful; forced diuresis or hemodialysis is of no benefit

Drug Interactions Substrate (major) of CYP1A2, 3A4; **Inhibits** CYP2C19 (weak), 2D6 (weak), 2E1 (weak), 3A4 (weak)

Acetylcholinesterase inhibitors (central): May increase the risk of antipsychotic-related extrapyramidal symptoms; monitor.

Aluminum salts: May decrease the absorption of antipsychotics; monitor

Amphetamines: Efficacy may be diminished by antipsychotics; in addition, amphetamines may increase psychotic symptoms; avoid concurrent use

Anticholinergics: May inhibit the therapeutic response to antipsychotics and excess anticholinergic effects may occur; includes benztropine, trihexyphenidyl, biperiden, and drugs with significant anticholinergic activity (TCAs, antihistamines, disopyramide)

Antihypertensives: Concurrent use of antipsychotics with an antihypertensive may produce additive hypotensive effects (particularly orthostasis)

Bromocriptine: Antipsychotics inhibit the ability of bromocriptine to lower serum prolactin concentrations

CNS depressants: Sedative effects may be additive with antipsychotics; monitor for increased effect; includes barbiturates, benzodiazepines, narcotic analgesics, ethanol, and other sedative agents

CYP1A2 inducers: May decrease the levels/effects of pimozide. Example inducers include aminoglutethimide, carbamazepine, phenobarbital, and rifampin.

CYP1A2 inhibitors: May increase the levels/effects of pimozide. Example inhibitors include ciprofloxacin, fluvoxamine, ketoconazole, norfloxacin, ofloxacin, and rofecoxib.

CYP3A4 inducers: CYP3A4 inducers may decrease the levels/effects of pimozide. Example inducers include aminoglutethimide, carbamazepine, nafcillin, nevirapine, phenobarbital, phenytoin, and rifamycins.

CYP3A4 inhibitors: May increase the levels/effects of pimozide. Example inhibitors include azole antifungals, clarithromycin, diclofenac, doxycycline, erythromycin, imatinib, isoniazid, nefazodone, nicardipine, propofol, protease inhibitors, quinidine, telithromycin, and verapamil. Concurrent use of strong CYP3A4 inhibitors with pimozide is contraindicated.

Epinephrine: Chlorpromazine (and possibly other low potency antipsychotics) may diminish the pressor effects of epinephrine

Guanethidine and guanadrel: Antihypertensive effects may be inhibited by antipsychotics

Levodopa: Antipsychotics may inhibit the antiparkinsonian effect of levodopa; avoid this combination

Lithium: Antipsychotics may produce neurotoxicity with lithium; this is a rare effect

Macrolide antibiotics: Concurrent use is contraindicated due to CYP inhibition and QT_c-prolonging effects. **Note:** The manufacturer lists azithromycin and dirithromycin in its list of contraindicated macrolides; however, these drugs do not inhibit CYP3A4 and are not expected to interact with pimozide.

Mesoridazine: Concurrent use with pimozide is contraindicated due to potential arrhythmias.

Metoclopramide: May increase extrapyramidal symptoms (EPS) or risk.

Phenytoin: May reduce serum levels of antipsychotics; antipsychotics may increase phenytoin serum levels

Propranolol: Serum concentrations of antipsychotics may be increased; propranolol also increases antipsychotics concentrations

QT_c-prolonging agents: Effects on QT_c interval may be additive with antipsychotics, increasing the risk of malignant arrhythmias; includes Class Ia and Class III antiarrhythmics, arsenic trioxide, chlorpromazine, dolasetron, droperidol, halofantrine, levomethadyl, mefloquine, pentamidine, probucol, tacrolimus, ziprasidone, tricyclic antidepressants, and some quinolone antibiotics (sparfloxacin, moxifloxacin, and gatifloxacin)

Sertraline: Concurrent use is contraindicated; may produce increased toxicity or attenuate therapeutic response.

Sulfadoxine-pyrimethamine: May increase antipsychotics concentrations

Thioridazine: Concurrent use with pimozide is contraindicated due to potential arrhythmias.

Tricyclic antidepressants: Concurrent use may produce increased toxicity or altered therapeutic response (also see note under QT_c prolonging agents)

Trazodone: Antipsychotics and trazodone may produce additive hypotensive effects

Valproic acid: Serum levels may be increased by antipsychotics

Ziprasidone: Concurrent use with pimozide is contraindicated due to potential arrhythmias.

Pregnancy Risk Factor C

Lactation Excretion in breast milk unknown

Nursing Implications Perform ECG at baseline and periodically thereafter, and with dose increases; refer to Contraindications for medicines which may predispose patients to potentially fatal cardiac arrhythmias

Additional Information Less sedation but more likely to cause extrapyramidal signs than chlorpromazine

Specific References

Gair RD, Friesen MS, Kent DA, et al, "Delayed Dystonia Following Pimozide Overdose in a Child," *J Toxicol Clin Toxicol*, 2004, 42(7): 977-81.

Pindolol

Related Information
- Selected Properties of Beta-Adrenergic Blocking Drugs
- Therapeutic Drugs Associated with Hallucinations

CAS Number 13523-86-9
U.S. Brand Names Visken®
Impairment Potential Yes
Use Management of hypertension

Unlabeled/Investigational Use Potential augmenting agent for antidepressants; ventricular arrhythmias/tachycardia, antipsychotic-induced akathisia, situational anxiety; aggressive behavior associated with dementia

Mechanism of Action Blocks both beta$_1$- and beta$_2$-receptors and has mild intrinsic sympathomimetic activity; pindolol has negative inotropic and chronotropic effects and can significantly slow AV nodal conduction

Adverse Reactions
Cardiovascular: Mesenteric arterial thrombosis, AV block, chest tightness, sinus bradycardia, palpitations, QRS prolongation, sinus tachycardia, Raynaud's phenomenon
Central nervous system: **Dizziness, anxiety, insomnia, fatigue**, auditory hallucinations
Dermatologic: Purpura, erythema multiforme, alopecia, toxic epidermal necrolysis, xerosis, urticaria, onycholysis, pruritus, psoriasis, licheniform eruptions, exanthem
Endocrine & metabolic: **Decreased sexual ability**
Gastrointestinal: Ischemic colitis, abdominal pain
Hematologic: Thrombocytopenia, leukopenia, neutropenia, agranulocytosis, granulocytopenia
Neuromuscular & skeletal: **Arthralgia, weakness, back pain**, fine tremors, paresthesia
Ocular: Diplopia
Respiratory: Wheezing
Miscellaneous: Systemic lupus erythematosus

Signs and Symptoms of Overdose Ataxia, AV block, bradycardia, cold extremities, colitis, coma, confusion, depression, dry mouth, edema (6%), heart block, heart failure and wheezing; hypertension and tachycardia also associated (due to beta agonist properties) followed by severe hypotension, hypoglycemia, impotence, insomnia, myasthenia gravis (exacerbation or precipitation)

Pharmacodynamics/Kinetics
Absorption: Rapid, 50% to 95%
Protein binding: 50%
Metabolism: Hepatic (60% to 65%) to conjugates
Half-life elimination: 2.5-4 hours; prolonged with renal impairment, age, and cirrhosis
Time to peak, serum: 1-2 hours
Excretion: Urine (35% to 50% as unchanged drug)

Dosage
Oral:
Adults:
Hypertension: Initial: 5 mg twice daily, increase as necessary by 10 mg/day every 3-4 weeks (maximum daily dose: 60 mg); usual dose range (JNC 7): 10-40 mg twice daily
Antidepressant augmentation: 2.5 mg 3 times/day
Elderly: Initial: 5 mg once daily, increase as necessary by 5 mg/day every 3-4 weeks
Dosing adjustment in renal and hepatic impairment: Reduction is necessary in severely impaired

Stability Protect from light
Monitoring Parameters Blood pressure, standing and sitting/supine, pulse, respiratory function

Contraindications Hypersensitivity to pindolol, beta-blockers, or any component of the formulation; uncompensated congestive heart failure; cardiogenic shock; bradycardia, sinus node dysfunction, or heart block (2nd or 3rd degree) except in patients with a functioning artificial pacemaker; pulmonary edema; severe hyperactive airway disease (asthma or COPD); Raynaud's disease

Warnings Administer very cautiously to patients with CHF, asthma, diabetes mellitus, hyperthyroidism. May mask signs and symptoms of thyrotoxicosis. Abrupt withdrawal of the drug should be avoided, drug should be discontinued over 1-2 weeks. Do not use in pregnant or nursing women. May potentiate hypoglycemia in a diabetic patient and mask signs and symptoms. Use with caution in patients with myasthenia gravis or peripheral vascular disease. May cause CNS depression; use caution in patients with a history of psychiatric illness. May potentiate anaphylactic reactions and/or blunt response to epinephrine treatment. Beta-blockers with intrinsic sympathomimetic activity (including pindolol) do not appear to be of benefit in CHF.

Dosage Forms Tablet: 5 mg, 10 mg
Reference Range Therapeutic: 0.02-0.04 mcg/mL; 250 mg ingestion was associated with a serum level of 0.66 mcg/mL; 500 mg ingestion produced a serum level of 1.5 mcg/mL

Overdosage/Treatment
Decontamination: **Do not** use ipecac; gastric lavage within 1 hour, activated charcoal should be utilized
Supportive therapy: Sympathomimetics (eg, epinephrine or dopamine), glucagon, atropine, or a pacemaker can be used to treat the toxic bradycardia, asystole, and/or hypotension; initially fluids may be the best treatment for toxic hypotension.
Enhancement of elimination: Multiple dosing of activated charcoal may be effective

Antidote(s)
- Glucagon [ANTIDOTE]

Test Interactions ↑ cholesterol (S), glucose; ↓ bilirubin (S)
Drug Interactions Substrate of CYP2D6 (major); **Inhibits** CYP2D6 (weak)
Albuterol (and other beta$_2$ agonists): Effects may be blunted by nonspecific beta-blockers
Alpha-blockers (prazosin, terazosin): Concurrent use of beta-blockers may increase risk of orthostasis
AV conduction-slowing agents (digoxin): Effects may be additive with beta-blockers
Calcium channel blockers (diltiazem, verapamil): May have synergistic or additive pharmacological effects when taken concurrently with beta-blockers
Clonidine: Hypertensive crisis after or during withdrawal of either agent
CYP2D6 inhibitors: May increase the levels/effects of pindolol. Example inhibitors include chlorpromazine, delavirdine, fluoxetine, miconazole, paroxetine, pergolide, quinidine, quinine, ritonavir, and ropinirole.
Epinephrine (including local anesthetics with epinephrine): Pindolol may cause hypertension
Glucagon: Pindolol may blunt the hyperglycemic action
Insulin and oral hypoglycemics: May mask symptoms of hypoglycemia
NSAIDs (ibuprofen, indomethacin, naproxen, piroxicam): May reduce the antihypertensive effects of beta-blockers
Salicylates: May reduce the antihypertensive effects of beta-blockers
Sulfonylureas: Beta-blockers may alter response to hypoglycemic agents

Pregnancy Risk Factor B
Pregnancy Implications Pindolol crosses the placenta. Beta-blockers have been associated with bradycardia, hypotension, and IUGR; IUGR is probably related to maternal hypertension. Available evidence suggests beta-blockers are generally safe during pregnancy (JNC-7). Cases of neonatal hypoglycemia have been reported following maternal use of beta-blockers at parturition or during breast-feeding.

Lactation Enters breast milk/use caution
Additional Information May cause hypoglycemia during hemodialysis
Specific References
Chobanian AV, Bakris GL, Black HR, et al, "The Seventh Report of the Joint National Committee on Prevention, Detection, Evaluation, and Treatment of High Blood Pressure: The JNC 7 Report," *JAMA*, 2003, 289(19):2560-71.

Piperacillin and Tazobactam Sodium

U.S. Brand Names Zosyn®
Synonyms Piperacillin Sodium and Tazobactam Sodium; Tazobactam and Piperacillin

Use Treatment of infections caused by susceptible organisms, including infections of the lower respiratory tract (community-acquired pneumonia, nosocomial pneumonia); urinary tract; skin and skin structures; gynecologic (endometritis, pelvic inflammatory disease); bone and joint infections; intra-abdominal infections (appendicitis with rupture/abscess, peritonitis); and septicemia. Tazobactam expands activity of piperacillin to include beta-lactamase producing strains of *S. aureus*, *H. influenzae*, *Bacteroides*, and other gram-negative bacteria.

Mechanism of Action Piperacillin interferes with bacterial cell wall synthesis during active multiplication, causing cell wall death and resultant bactericidal activity against susceptible bacteria; tazobactam prevents degradation of piperacillin by binding to the active side on beta-lactamase

Adverse Reactions
Cardiovascular: Hypertension, hypotension
Central nervous system: Insomnia, headache, agitation, fever, dizziness, confusion, seizures, paresthesia (painful)
Dermatologic: Erythema multiforme
Gastrointestinal: **Diarrhea**, *Clostridium difficile* colitis, pseudomembranous colitis
Dermatologic: Rash, pruritus, Stevens-Johnson syndrome
Gastrointestinal: Constipation, nausea, vomiting, dyspepsia
Hematologic: Hemolytic anemia, leukopenia, thrombocytopenia
Hepatic: Cholestatic jaundice, hepatitis, hepatotoxicity
Renal: Interstitial nephritis
Respiratory: Rhinitis, dyspnea, bronchospasm
Miscellaneous: Serum sickness-like reaction, fever
Several laboratory abnormalities have rarely been associated with piperacillin/tazobactam including reversible eosinophilia, and neutrope-

nia (associated most often with prolonged therapy), positive direct Coombs' test, prolonged PT and aPTT, transient elevations of LFTs, increased creatinine

Signs and Symptoms of Overdose Colitis, eosinophilia, hypokalemia, insomnia, leukopenia or neutropenia (agranulocytosis, granulocytopenia)

Pharmacodynamics/Kinetics
Both AUC and peak concentrations are dose proportional; hepatic impairment does not affect kinetics
Distribution: Well into lungs, intestinal mucosa, skin, muscle, uterus, ovary, prostate, gallbladder, and bile; penetration into CSF is low in subject with noninflamed meninges
Protein binding: Piperacillin and tazobactam: ~30%
Metabolism:
Piperacillin: 6% to 9% to desethyl metabolite (weak activity)
Tazobactam: ~26% to inactive metabolite
Half-life elimination: Piperacillin and tazobactam: 0.7-1.2 hours
Time to peak, plasma: Immediately following infusion of 30 minutes
Excretion: Clearance of both piperacillin and tazobactam are directly proportional to renal function
Piperacillin: Urine (68% as unchanged drug); feces (10% to 20%)
Tazobactam: Urine (80% as inactive metabolite)

Dosage Infants and Children ≥6 months: **Note:** Not FDA-approved for use in children <12 years of age:
I.V.: 240 mg of piperacillin component/kg/day in divided doses every 8 hours; higher doses have been used for serious pseudomonal infections: 300-400 mg of piperacillin component/kg/day in divided doses every 6 hours.
Children >12 years and Adults:
Nosocomial pneumonia: I.V.: Piperacillin/tazobactam 4/0.5 g every 6 hours for 7-14 days (when used empirically, combination with an aminoglycoside is recommended; consider discontinuation of aminoglycoside if *P. aeruginosa* is not isolated)
Severe infections: I.V.: Piperacillin/tazobactam 4/0.5 g every 8 hours or 3/0.375 g every 6 hours for 7-10 days
Moderate infections: I.M.: Piperacillin/tazobactam 2/0.25 g every 6-8 hours; treatment should be continued for ≥7-10 days depending on severity of disease (**Note:** I.M. route not FDA-approved)
Dosing interval in renal impairment:
Cl$_{cr}$ 20-40 mL/minute: Administer 2/0.25 g every 6 hours (3/0.375 g every 6 hours for nosocomial pneumonia)
Cl$_{cr}$ <20 mL/minute: Administer 2/0.25 g every 8 hours (2/0.25 g every 6 hours for nosocomial pneumonia)
Hemodialysis: Administer 2/0.25 g every 12 hours (every 8 hours for nosocomial pneumonia) with an additional dose of 0.75 g after each dialysis
Continuous arteriovenous or venovenous hemodiafiltration effects: Dose as for Cl$_{cr}$ 10-50 mL/minute

Stability Store at controlled room temperature; after reconstitution, stable for 24 hours at room temperature and 1 week when refrigerated; unused portions should be discarded after 24 hours at room temperature and 48 hours when refrigerated

Monitoring Parameters LFTs, creatinine, BUN, CBC with differential, serum electrolytes, urinalysis, PT, PTT; monitor for signs of anaphylaxis during first dose

Administration Administer by I.V. infusion over 30 minutes
Some penicillins (eg, carbenicillin, ticarcillin and piperacillin) have been shown to inactivate aminoglycosides *in vitro*. This has been observed to a greater extent with tobramycin and gentamicin, while amikacin has shown greater stability against inactivation. Concurrent use of these agents may pose a risk of reduced antibacterial efficacy *in vivo*, particularly in the setting of profound renal impairment. However, definitive clinical evidence is lacking. If combination penicillin/aminoglycoside therapy is desired in a patient with renal dysfunction, separation of doses (if feasible) and routine monitoring of aminoglycoside levels, CBC, and clinical response should be considered. **Note:** Reformulated Zosyn® containing EDTA has been shown to be compatible *in vitro* for Y-site infusion with amikacin and gentamicin, but not compatible with tobramycin.

Contraindications Hypersensitivity to penicillins, beta-lactamase inhibitors, or any component of the formulation

Warnings Bleeding disorders have been observed, particularly in patients with renal impairment; discontinue if thrombocytopenia or bleeding occurs. Due to sodium load and to the adverse effects of high serum concentrations of penicillins, dosage modification is required in patients with impaired or underdeveloped renal function; use with caution in patients with seizures or in patients with history of beta-lactam allergy; associated with an increased incidence of rash and fever in cystic fibrosis patients. Prolonged use may result in superinfection, including pseudomembranous colitis. Safety and efficacy have not been established in children <2 months of age.

Dosage Forms
Note: 8:1 ratio of piperacillin sodium/tazobactam sodium
Infusion [premixed iso-osmotic solution, frozen]:

2.25 g: Piperacillin 2 g and tazobactam 0.25 g (50 mL) [contains sodium 5.58 mEq (128 mg) and EDTA]
3.375 g: Piperacillin 3 g and tazobactam 0.375 g (50 mL) [contains sodium 8.38 mEq (192 mg) and EDTA]
4.5 g: Piperacillin 4 g and tazobactam 0.5 g (50 mL) [contains sodium 11.17 mEq (256 mg) and EDTA]
Injection, powder for reconstitution:
2.25 g: Piperacillin 2 g and tazobactam 0.25 g [contains sodium 5.58 mEq (128 mg) and EDTA]
3.375 g: Piperacillin 3 g and tazobactam 0.375 g [contains sodium 8.38 mEq (192 mg) and EDTA]
4.5 g: Piperacillin 4 g and tazobactam 0.5 g [contains sodium 11.17 mEq (256 mg) and EDTA]
40.5 g: Piperacillin 36 g and tazobactam 4.5 g [contains sodium 100.4 mEq (2304 mg) and EDTA; bulk pharmacy vial]

Reference Range After a dose of 4 g piperacillin/500 mg tazobactam, mean serum piperacillin and tazobactam levels were 223.7 mcg/mL and 27.2 mcg/mL, respectively

Overdosage/Treatment Enhancement of elimination: Combined charcoal hemoperfusion with hemodialysis may be useful, see Toxicodynamics

Test Interactions Increases ALT, AST; positive Coombs' [direct]

Drug Interactions Aminoglycosides: May be synergistic against selected organisms; physical inactivation of aminoglycosides in the presence of high concentrations of piperacillin and potential toxicity in patients with mild to moderate renal dysfunction
Heparin: Concomitant use with high-dose parenteral penicillins may result in increased risk of bleeding
Methotrexate: Penicillins may increase the exposure to methotrexate during concurrent therapy; monitor.
Neuromuscular blockers: May increase duration of blockade
Oral contraceptives: Anecdotal reports suggesting decreased contraceptive efficacy with penicillins have been refuted by more rigorous scientific and clinical data.
Probenecid: May increase levels of penicillins (piperacillin)
Tetracyclines: May decrease effectiveness of penicillins (piperacillin)
Warfarin: Effects of warfarin may be increased

Pregnancy Risk Factor B

Pregnancy Implications Piperacillin and tazobactam were not teratogenic in animal studies. Both piperacillin and tazobactam cross the human placenta.

Lactation Enters breast milk/use caution

Nursing Implications Administer 1 hour apart from aminoglycosides; give around-the-clock (ie, 6-12-6-12)

Additional Information Total sodium content: 108 mg/vial

Specific References
Lambourne J, Kitchen J, Hughes C, et al, "Piperacillin/Tazobactam-Induced Paresthesia," *Ann Pharmacother*, 2006, 40(5):977-9.
LeClaire AC, Martin CA, and Hoven AD, "Rash Associated with Piperacillin/Tazobactam Administration in Infectious Mononucleosis," *Ann Pharmacother*, 2004, 38(6):996-8.

Piperazine

CAS Number 110-85-0; 142-63-2; 142-88-1; 144-29-6; 14538-56-8; 18534-18-4; 41372-10-5

UN Number 2579

Synonyms Piperazine Citrate

Use Treatment of *Ascaris lumbricoides* (roundworm) and *Enterobius vermicularis*, (pinworm, threadworm); may be effective in treating tropical eosinophilia

Mechanism of Action Blocks acetylcholine response in smooth muscle causing flaccid paralysis; while the drug has its primary effect on the parasite in the gastrointestinal tract, there is no effect on larvae in tissues

Adverse Reactions
Central nervous system: Hypotonia, fever, dementia, CNS depression, depression, paranoia
Dermatologic: Urticaria, erythema multiforme, cutaneous vasculitis
Gastrointestinal: Vomiting, diarrhea
Hematologic: Hemolytic anemia, thrombocytopenia
Hepatic: Hepatitis
Neuromuscular & skeletal: Arthralgia
Ocular: Nystagmus, eye irritant on direct contact, cataract, lacrimation
Respiratory: Bronchospasm, cough, rhinorrhea, asthma

Signs and Symptoms of Overdose Ataxia, chorea, coma, confusion, headache, hyporeflexia, lethargy, myoclonus, nausea, seizures, tremors, vertigo

Pharmacodynamics/Kinetics
Absorption: Well absorbed
Time to peak, serum: 1 hour
Excretion: Urine (as unchanged drug and metabolites)

Dosage Oral (hexahydrate equivalent):
Ascaris lumbricoides:
Children: 75 mg/kg/day for 2 days (maximum daily dose: 3.5 g)

Adults: 3.5 g/day for 2 days
Enterobiasis:
Children: 65 mg/kg in one daily dose for 7 days (maximum daily dose: 2.5 g)
Adults: 65 mg/kg in one daily dose for 7 days (maximum daily dose: 2.5 g)
Tropical eosinophilia: Adults: 600 mg 3 times/day for 2 weeks
Monitoring Parameters Stool exam for worms and ova
Contraindications Hypersensitivity to piperazine or any component of the formulation; seizure disorders; liver or kidney impairment
Warnings Use with caution in patients with anemia or malnutrition; avoid prolonged use especially in children
Dosage Forms Piperazine citrate is available from Panorama Pharmacy (1-800-247-9767).
Overdosage/Treatment
Decontamination: Lavage (within 1 hour)/activated charcoal
Supportive therapy: Seizures can be treated with a benzodiazepine, phenytoin, or phenobarbital
Drug Interactions Pyrantel pamoate (antagonistic mode of action)
Pregnancy Risk Factor B

Piretanide

CAS Number 55837-27-9
Unlabeled/Investigational Use Congestive heart failure, hypertension
Mechanism of Action Inhibits reabsorption of sodium and chloride in the ascending loop of Henle and distal renal tubule, interfering with the chloride-binding cotransport system, thus causing increased excretion of water, sodium, chloride, magnesium, and calcium
Adverse Reactions
Cardiovascular: Hypotension (orthostatic)
Central nervous system: Dizziness, headache
Dermatologic: Eczema, psoriasis, pruritus, exanthema
Endocrine & metabolic: Hyperglycemia, hypokalemia (less than that with furosemide or hydrochlorothiazide), hypomagnesemia, hypercholesterolemia, hyperuricemia
Hepatic: Liver toxicity
Neuromuscular & skeletal: Arthralgia
Signs and Symptoms of Overdose Hyperglycemia, hyperuricemia, hypokalemia, hypomagnesemia, hypotension, muscle cramps
Toxicodynamics/Kinetics
Onset of diuresis: 30 minutes
Duration: Oral: 3-4 hours; I.V.: 90 minutes
Distribution: V_d: 0.17-0.53 L/kg (uremic patients)
Protein binding: 94%
Bioavailability: Oral: 80%
Half-life: 1 hour
Elimination: Renal (45%)
Dosage
Congestive heart failure:
Oral: 3-6 mg/day, up to 24 mg/day
I.V.: 6-12 mg every 12 hours
Hypertension: 6-12 mg/day
Renal failure: 6-96 mg/day
Reference Range Peak serum level after 12 mg oral dose: 775 ng/mL; peak serum level after 6 mg I.V. dose: 983 ng/mL
Overdosage/Treatment
Decontamination: Activated charcoal
Supportive therapy: I.V. hydration with 0.9% saline
Additional Information 6-12 mg of piretanide is equivalent to the antihypertensive effect of 100 mg of hydrochlorothiazide

Piroxicam

Related Information
- Nonsteroidal Anti-inflammatory Drugs
- Therapeutic Drugs Associated with Hallucinations
CAS Number 36322-90-4
U.S. Brand Names Feldene®
Use Symptomatic treatment of acute and chronic rheumatoid arthritis and osteoarthritis
Ankylosing spondylitis
Mechanism of Action Inhibits prostaglandin synthesis by decreasing the activity of the enzyme, cyclooxygenase, which results in decreased formation of prostaglandin precursors
Adverse Reactions
Cardiovascular: Circulatory collapse
Central nervous system: **Dizziness**, headache, aseptic meningitis, psychosis, cognitive dysfunction, coma, seizures
Dermatologic: **Rash**, pruritus, photosensitivity/phototoxicity, exfoliative dermatitis, alopecia, angioedema, urticaria, purpura, onycholysis, licheniform eruptions, exanthem
Endocrine & metabolic: Hyperkalemia, anion gap metabolic acidosis, fluid retention

Gastrointestinal: **Abdominal cramps, heartburn, indigestion, nausea**, vomiting, GI bleeding, GI ulceration, constipation, diarrhea, dyspepsia, esophagitis, aphthous stomatitis, xerostomia
Hematologic: Leukopenia, neutropenia, agranulocytosis, granulocytopenia, aplastic anemia (rare), platelet inhibition
Hepatic: Elevated transaminases, hepatitis (fulminant), hepatic necrosis
Neuromuscular & skeletal: Paresthesia
Otic: Ototoxicity, tinnitus
Renal: Renal failure (acute), nephrotic syndrome, chronic renal failure, albuminuria
Respiratory: Wheezing, respiratory depression
Miscellaneous: Hypersensitivity, systemic lupus erythematosus (SLE)
Signs and Symptoms of Overdose Coagulopathy, cognitive dysfunction, drowsiness, gastritis, GI bleeding, hyponatremia, nausea, nephrotic syndrome, ototoxicity, pemphigus, photosensitivity, stomatitis, syndrome of inappropriate antidiuretic hormone (SIADH), tinnitus, toxic epidermal necrolysis, vomiting, wheezing. Severe poisoning can manifest with blurred vision, coma, hypotension, renal and/or hepatic failure, respiratory depression, seizures, tremors.
Pharmacodynamics/Kinetics
Onset of action: Analgesic: ~1 hour
Peak effect: 3-5 hours
Protein binding: 99%
Metabolism: Hepatic
Half-life elimination: 45-50 hours
Excretion: Primarily urine and feces (small amounts) as unchanged drug (5%) and metabolites
Dosage
Oral:
Children: 0.2-0.3 mg/kg/day once daily; maximum dose: 15 mg/day
Adults: 10-20 mg/day once daily; although associated with increase in GI adverse effects, doses >20 mg/day have been used (ie, 30-40 mg/day)
Dosing adjustment in hepatic impairment: Reduction of dosage is necessary
Monitoring Parameters Occult blood loss, hemoglobin, hematocrit, and periodic renal and hepatic function tests; periodic ophthalmologic exams with chronic use
Contraindications Hypersensitivity to piroxicam, aspirin, other NSAIDs or any component of the formulation; perioperative pain in the setting of coronary artery bypass surgery (CABG); pregnancy (3rd trimester or near term)
Warnings
[U.S. Boxed Warning]: NSAIDs are associated with an increased risk of adverse cardiovascular events, including MI, stroke, and new onset or worsening of pre-existing hypertension. Risk may be increased with duration of use or pre-existing cardiovascular risk-factors or disease. Carefully evaluate individual cardiovascular risk profiles prior to prescribing. Use caution with fluid retention, CHF or hypertension.
Use of NSAIDs can compromise existing renal function. Renal toxicity can occur in patient with impaired renal function, dehydration, heart failure, liver dysfunction, those taking diuretics and ACEI and the elderly. Rehydrate patient before starting therapy. Monitor renal function closely. Not recommended for use in patients with advanced renal disease.
[U.S. Boxed Warning]: NSAIDs may increase risk of gastrointestinal irritation, ulceration, bleeding, and perforation. These events may occur at any time during therapy and without warning. Use caution with a history of GI disease (bleeding or ulcers), concurrent therapy with aspirin, anticoagulants and/or corticosteroids, smoking, use of alcohol, the elderly or debilitated patients.
Use the lowest effective dose for the shortest duration of time, consistent with individual patient goals, to reduce risk of cardiovascular or GI adverse events. Alternate therapies should be considered for patients at high risk.
NSAIDs may cause serious skin adverse events including exfoliative dermatitis, Stevens-Johnson syndrome (SJS) and toxic epidermal necrolysis (TEN). Anaphylactoid reactions may occur, even without prior exposure; patients with "aspirin triad" (bronchial asthma, aspirin intolerance, rhinitis) may be at increased risk. Do not use in patients who experience bronchospasm, asthma, rhinitis, or urticaria with NSAID or aspirin therapy. A serum sickness-like reaction can rarely occur; watch for arthralgias, pruritus, fever, fatigue, and rash.

Use with caution in patients with decreased hepatic function. Closely monitor patients with any abnormal LFT. Severe hepatic reactions (eg, fulminant hepatitis, liver failure) have occurred with NSAID use, rarely; discontinue if signs or symptoms of liver disease develop, or if systemic manifestations occur.
The elderly are at increased risk for adverse effects (especially peptic ulceration, CNS effects, renal toxicity) from NSAIDs even at low doses
Withhold for at least 4-6 half-lives prior to surgical or dental procedures.
Dosage Forms Capsule: 10 mg, 20 mg
Reference Range Therapeutic plasma piroxicam level: 5-10 mcg/mL; after a 1.8 g overdose, plasma piroxicam level was 241.6 mcg/mL

Overdosage/Treatment

Decontamination: Activated charcoal

Supportive therapy: Hypotension/dehydration can be managed with I.V. fluid therapy; acidosis should be treated with bicarbonates, seizures with benzodiazepines; antacids, blood products are indicated, as appropriate, for hemorrhage

Enhancement of elimination: Dialysis or perfusion is indicated for secondary complications, acidosis, or renal failure and not toxin removal alone; multiple dosing of activated charcoal may be effective; cholestyramine (4 g 3 times/day) may reduce the half-life of piroxicam

Test Interactions ↑ chloride (S), sodium (S), bleeding time

Drug Interactions Substrate of CYP2C9 (minor); **Inhibits** CYP2C9 (strong)

ACE inhibitors: Antihypertensive effects may be decreased by concurrent therapy with NSAIDs; monitor blood pressure.

Angiotensin II antagonists: Antihypertensive effects may be decreased by concurrent therapy with NSAIDs; monitor blood pressure.

Anticoagulants (warfarin, heparin, LMWHs) in combination with NSAIDs can cause increased risk of bleeding.

Antiplatelet drugs (ticlopidine, clopidogrel, aspirin, abciximab, dipyridamole, eptifibatide, tirofiban) can cause an increased risk of bleeding.

Beta-blockers: NSAIDs may decrease the antihypertensive effect of beta-blockers. Monitor.

Cholestyramine (and other bile acid sequestrants): May decrease the absorption of NSAIDs. Separate by at least 2 hours.

Corticosteroids may increase the risk of GI ulceration; avoid concurrent use.

Cyclosporine: NSAIDs may increase serum creatinine, potassium, blood pressure, and cyclosporine levels; monitor cyclosporine levels and renal function carefully.

CYP2C9 Substrates: Piroxicam may increase the levels/effects of CYP2C9 substrates. Example substrates include bosentan, dapsone, fluoxetine, glimepiride, glipizide, losartan, montelukast, nateglinide, paclitaxel, phenytoin, warfarin, and zafirlukast.

Hydralazine's antihypertensive effect is decreased; avoid concurrent use.

Lithium levels can be increased; avoid concurrent use if possible or monitor lithium levels and adjust dose.

Loop diuretics efficacy (diuretic and antihypertensive effect) is reduced. Indomethacin reduces this efficacy, however, it may be anticipated with any NSAID.

Methotrexate: Severe bone marrow suppression, aplastic anemia, and GI toxicity have been reported with concomitant NSAID therapy. Avoid use during moderate or high-dose methotrexate (increased and prolonged methotrexate levels). NSAID use during low-dose treatment of rheumatoid arthritis has not been fully evaluated; extreme caution is warranted.

Thiazides antihypertensive effects are decreased; avoid concurrent use.

Warfarin's INRs may be increased by piroxicam. Other NSAIDs may have the same effect depending on dose and duration. Monitor INR closely. Use the lowest dose of NSAIDs possible and for the briefest duration.

Pregnancy Risk Factor B/D (3rd trimester or near term)

Lactation Enters breast milk (small amounts)/not recommended (AAP rates "compatible")

Nursing Implications Administer with food to decrease GI adverse effect

Specific References

Wammack R, Remzi M, Seitz C, et al, "Efficacy of Oral Doxepin and Piroxicam Treatment for Interstitial Cystitis," *Eur Urol*, 41(6): 596-600.

Pizotifen

CAS Number 15574-96-6; 5189-11-7

Synonyms Pizotifen Malate

Impairment Potential Yes

Use Migraine prophylaxis

Unlabeled/Investigational Use Cyclical vomiting

Mechanism of Action A serotonin, histamine (H_1 receptor) and tryptamine antagonist; also has weak antimuscarinic actions

Adverse Reactions

Cardiovascular: Tachycardia, edema

Central nervous system: **Drowsiness** (up to 30%), dizziness, headache

Gastrointestinal: Weight gain (1-3 kg), nausea, xerostomia, appetite (increased)

Hepatic: Cholestatic jaundice

Ocular: Blurred vision

Neuromuscular & skeletal: Muscle cramps

Signs and Symptoms of Overdose Blurred vision, fever, mydriasis, tachycardia

Pharmacodynamics/Kinetics

Onset: May require several weeks of therapy

Half-life elimination: 26 hours

Time to peak: 5-7 hours

Dosage Migraine prophylaxis:

Children: Up to 1.5 mg/day in divided doses

Adult: Initial: 0.5 mg; usual adult daily dose: ~1.5 mg; maximum daily dose: 4.5 mg

Cyclical vomiting: Children: 1.5 mg nightly

Monitoring Parameters Hepatic function tests (prolonged use)

Contraindications Hypersensitivity to pizotifen or any component of the formulation; concurrent use of MAO inhibitors; gastric outlet obstruction (pyloroduodenal obstruction, stenosing pyloric ulcer)

Warnings Not for use in acute treatment of migraine attacks. May cause sedation; effects may be additive with other CNS depressants or ethanol. Patients must be cautioned to avoid operating machinery or driving until effects are known. Although anticholinergic effects are limited, use with caution in patients intolerant to anticholinergic agents, including tricyclic antidepressants, phenothiazines, or cyproheptadine. Use with caution in patients with narrow angle glaucoma, myasthenia gravis, bladder outlet obstruction (BPH), or other disorders in which anticholinergic effects may be poorly tolerated. Use caution in renal or hepatic disease/insufficiency, diabetes, cardiovascular disease, or in obese patients. Therapeutic response may require several weeks of therapy. Avoid abrupt discontinuation; taper dosage over 2 weeks prior to discontinuation. Tolerance may develop in some patients. Consider drug-free period after several months of treatment. Safety and efficacy have not been established in children <12 years of age.

Dosage Forms [CAN] = Canadian brand name

Tablet:

Sandomigran® [CAN]: 0.5 mg [pizotifen malate 0.73 mg]

Tablet, double strength:

Sandomigran® DS [CAN]: 1 mg [pizotifen malate 1.46 mg]

Overdosage/Treatment

Decontamination: Lavage within 1 hour ingestions >5 mg; activated charcoal

Supportive therapy: Fever can be controlled with cooling fan and tepid sponging

Drug Interactions CNS depressants: Sedative effects may be additive or synergistic with pizotifen. Includes sedative-hypnotics and drugs with significant sedative effects such as tricyclic antidepressants, antipsychotics, and ethanol.

MAO inhibitors: Concurrent use is contraindicated.

Pregnancy Risk Factor Not available

Pregnancy Implications Use only if potential benefit to the mother outweighs possible risk to the fetus.

Additional Information May prevent gastrointestinal adverse effects of calcitonin injections (at a dose of 0.5 mg 3 times/day)

Podophyllum Resin

Pronunciation (po DOF fil um REZ in)

CAS Number 518-28-5; 518-29-6; 568-53-6; 8050-60-0

U.S. Brand Names Podocon-25®

Synonyms Mandrake; May Apple; Podophyllin

Use Topical treatment of condyloma acuminata (venereal warts); therapeutically dispersed as 25% podophyllum resin in tincture of benzoin or alcohol

Mechanism of Action Arrests cells in the metaphase of mitosis

Adverse Reactions

Cardiovascular: Sinus tachycardia

Central nervous system: Memory disturbances

Neuromuscular & skeletal: Peripheral neuropathy

Signs and Symptoms of Overdose Develop 12-24 hours post-topical exposure but may develop 4-8 hours after ingestion. Anuria, ataxia, diarrhea, fever, hallucinations, hypotension, hypotonia, nausea, psychosis, tachycardia, and vomiting may occur. Within the first week, pancytopenia and hepatic dysfunction may occur and resolve in 2-3 weeks. Cardiotoxicity, coma, ileus, and memory loss may last 7-10 days. In the second week polyneuropathy may appear and last for 2-3 months. Hypotension (orthostatic) may last 6-9 months. Dermal burns (>0.5% concentration), contact dermatitis, blepharospasm, iritis, keratitis, hallucinations (visual or auditory) may occur.

Admission Criteria/Prognosis Admit any patient who develops symptoms within 8 hours of oral exposure; admit any pediatric oral ingestion >300 mg

Toxicodynamics/Kinetics Absorption: Absorbed well orally and cutaneously

Dosage Apply topically to lesion twice daily for no more than 3 days

Maximum topical exposure: 0.5 mL/day or 10 cm^2

Maximum tolerated dose: 2.8 g

Administration Shake well before using. Solution should be washed off within 1-4 hours for genital and perianal warts and within 1-2 hours for accessible meatal warts. Use protective occlusive dressing around warts to prevent contact with unaffected skin

Contraindications Not to be used on birthmarks, moles, or warts with hair growth; cervical, urethral, oral warts; not to be used by diabetic patient or patient with poor circulation; pregnancy

Warnings Use of large amounts of drug should be avoided; avoid contact with the eyes as it can cause severe corneal damage; do not apply to moles, birthmarks, or unusual warts; to be applied by a physician only; for external use only; 25% solution should not be applied to or near mucous membranes

Dosage Forms Liquid, topical: 25% (15 mL) [in benzoin tincture]

Overdosage/Treatment

Decontamination: **Oral:** Emesis within 30 minutes or lavage (within 1 hour)/activated charcoal **Dermal:** Wash with soap and water. **Ocular:** Copious irrigation with saline; mydriatic cycloplegic eye drops with topical corticosteroid application in severe cases

Supportive therapy: Thrombocytopenia and leukopenia should be treated as needed; hypotension should be treated with isotonic I.V. fluids, Trendelenburg positioning, and dopamine or norepinephrine drips

Enhancement of elimination: Resin/charcoal hemoperfusion may facilitate neurologic recovery but should be reserved for those patients who deteriorate despite supportive care; hemodialysis may be helpful for those who develop anuria

Drug Interactions No data reported

Pregnancy Risk Factor X

Pregnancy Implications May be teratogenic when used orally during first trimester of pregnancy; use is discouraged in pregnancy

Lactation Enters breast milk/contraindicated

Additional Information Minimum lethal exposure: Death has occurred with 350 mg (topical) or 10 g (oral)

Podophyllum is a mixture of 16 physiologic compounds: lignins (wood extracts) and flavonols; exists in rhizomes and roots of *Podophyllum peltatum* plant or "May apple" and contains at least 40% podophyllotoxin

---

Potassium Chloride

CAS Number 7447-40-7

U.S. Brand Names K+ Care®; K+10; K+8; K-Dur® 10; K-Dur® 20; K-Lor™; K-Tab®; Kaon-Cl-10®; Kaon-Cl® 20; Kay Ciel®; Klor-Con® 10; Klor-Con® 8; Klor-Con® M; Klor-Con®/25; Klor-Con®; Klotrix®; microK® 10; microK®; Rum-K®

Synonyms KCl

Use Replacement for potassium loss due to diuretics; treatment of hypokalemia and in metabolic acidosis; may be indicated in digitalis induced arrhythmias

Mechanism of Action As a principle intracellular ion, potassium serves as primary source for cellular electrical conduction

Adverse Reactions

Cardiovascular: Arrhythmias (ventricular)

Gastrointestinal: **Diarrhea, nausea, stomach pain, flatulence, vomiting,** esophagitis, bezoar

Signs and Symptoms of Overdose Apnea, bigeminy, confusion, diarrhea, esophageal ulceration, GI bleeding, hyporeflexia, hypotension, muscle cramps, nausea, paresthesia, peaked T waves, P-R prolongation, QRS prolongation, QT interval prolongation, ventricular arrhythmias, vomiting, weakness, widened QRS

Pharmacodynamics/Kinetics

Absorption: Well absorbed from upper GI tract

Distribution: Enters cells via active transport from extracellular fluid

Excretion: Primarily urine; skin and feces (small amounts); most intestinal potassium reabsorbed

Dosage Neonates: Oral, I.V.: 1-2 mEq/kg/day

Infants and older Children: 0.3 mEq/kg/hour; maximum hourly dose, I.V.: ~1 mEq/kg up to 40 mEq/hour; patient should be on a cardiac monitor for infusions over 0.5 mEq/kg/hour

Adults:

I.V.: 10-15 mEq/hour, not to exceed 300 mEq/day if serum potassium is >2.5 mEq/L; at serum potassium levels <2.0 mEq/L, I.V. dose may be at a rate of 40 mEq/hour not to exceed 400 mEq/day

Oral: Replacement therapy due to diuretics: Usual: 60 mEq/day is sufficient, although doses up to 100 mEq/day may be required

Dosing adjustment in renal impairment: Reduce dose and use with caution

Monitoring Parameters Serum potassium, glucose, chloride, pH, urine output (if indicated), cardiac monitor (if intermittent infusion or potassium infusion rates >0.25 mEq/kg/hour)

Administration Maximum concentration (peripheral line): 80 mEq/L

Contraindications Severe renal impairment, untreated Addison's disease, heat cramps, hyperkalemia, severe tissue trauma; solid oral dosage forms are contraindicated in patients in whom there is a structural, pathological, and/or pharmacologic cause for delay or arrest in passage through the GI tract; an oral liquid potassium preparation should be used in patients with esophageal compression or delayed gastric emptying time

Warnings Use with caution in patients with cardiac disease, severe renal impairment, hyperkalemia

Dosage Forms [DSC] = Discontinued product

Capsule, extended release: 10 mEq [750 mg]

microK® [microencapsulated]: 8 mEq [600 mg]

microK® 10 [microencapsulated]: 10 mEq [750 mg]

Infusion [premixed in D5W]: 20 mEq (1000 mL); 30 mEq (1000 mL); 40 mEq (1000 mL)

Infusion [premixed in D5W and LR]: 20 mEq (1000 mL); 30 mEq (1000 mL); 40 mEq (1000 mL)

Infusion [premixed in D5W and 1/4NS]: 10 mEq (500 mL, 1000 mL); 20 mEq (250 mL, 500 mL, 1000 mL); 30 mEq (1000 mL); 40 mEq (1000 mL)

Infusion [premixed in D5W and 1/2NS]: 10 mEq (500 mL, 1000 mL); 20 mEq (500 mL, 1000 mL); 30 mEq (1000 mL); 40 mEq (1000 mL)

Infusion [premixed in D5 and NS]: 20 mEq (1000 mL); 40 mEq (1000 mL)

Infusion [premixed in D5W and sodium chloride 0.3%]: 10 mEq (500 mL); 20 mEq (1000 mL); 30 mEq (1000 mL); 40 mEq (1000 mL)

Infusion [premixed in D10W and sodium chloride 0.2%]: 20 mEq (250 mL)

Infusion [premixed in NS]: 20 mEq (1000 mL); 40 mEq (1000 mL)

Infusion [premixed in SWFI; concentrate]: 10 mEq (50 mL, 100 mL); 20 mEq (50 mL, 100 mL); 30 mEq (100 mL); 40 mEq (100 mL)

Injection, solution [concentrate]: 2 mEq/mL (5 mL, 10 mL, 15 mL, 20 mL, 30 mL, 250 mL, 500 mL)

Powder, for oral solution: 20 mEq/packet (30s, 100s, 1000s)

K-Lor™: 20 mEq/packet (30s, 100s) [fruit flavor]

K+ Potassium: 20 mEq/packet (30s) [orange flavor]

Kay Ciel® 10%: 20 mEq/packet (30s, 100s) [sugar free]

Klor-Con®: 20 mEq/packet (30s, 100s) [sugar free; fruit flavor]

Klor-Con®/25: 25 mEq/packet (30s, 100s) [sugar free; fruit flavor]

Solution, oral: 20 mEq/15 mL (480 mL, 3840 mL); 40 mEq/15 mL (480 mL)

Kaon-Cl® 20: 40 mEq/15 mL (480 mL) [sugar free; contains alcohol; cherry flavor]

Kay Ciel®: 10%: 20 mEq/15 mL (480 mL) [sugar free; contains alcohol] [DSC]

Rum-K®: 20 mEq/10 mL (480 mL) [alcohol free, sugar free; butter/rum flavor]

Tablet, extended release: 8 mEq [600 mg]; 10 mEq [750 mg]; 20 mEq [1500 mg]

K-Dur® 10 [microencapsulated]: 10 mEq [750 mg]

K-Dur® 20 [microencapsulated]: 20 mEq [1500 mg; scored]

K-Tab®: 10 mEq [750 mg]

Kaon-Cl® 10: 10 mEq [750 mg]

Klor-Con® 8: 8 mEq [600 mg; wax matrix]

Klor-Con® 10: 10 mEq [750 mg; wax matrix]

Klor-Con® M10 [microencapsulated]: 10 mEq [750 mg]

Klor-Con® M15 [microencapsulated]: 15 mEq [1125 mg; scored]

Klor-Con® M20 [microencapsulated]: 20 mEq [1500 mg; scored]

Reference Range Normal serum potassium: 3.5-5 mEq/L; symptoms can occur with serum levels >6.5 mEq/L; levels >8 mEq/L can be fatal

Overdosage/Treatment

Decontamination: Ipecac within 30 minutes or lavage within 1 hour; activated charcoal does not appear to be useful

Supportive therapy: I.V. calcium (ie, 10 mL of 10% calcium chloride or gluconate given over 1-5 minutes, repeating as necessary) will antagonize adverse cardiac effects, but will not reduce serum potassium levels; while sodium bicarbonate (1-2 mEq/kg), insulin, and glucose will enhance intracellular shift of potassium; sodium polystyrene sulfonate (adult dose: 15 g orally or 30-50 g as an enema, pediatric dose: 1 g/kg) will exchange potassium for sodium; hyaluronidase can be used for extravasation; inhalation beta-adrenergic agonist agents (albuterol, salbutamol) can also result in rapid intravascular movement of potassium; calcium chloride is preferable since more ionized calcium is delivered as compared with the other calcium salts. Avoid the use of lidocaine in treating wide complex tachycardia due to hyperkalemia.

Enhancement of elimination: Dialysis (hemodialysis or peritoneal dialysis) is useful in enhancing elimination

Antidote(s)

● Sodium Bicarbonate [ANTIDOTE]

● Sodium Polystyrene Sulfonate [ANTIDOTE]

Test Interactions Hyperkalemia may cause depression of serum sodium; elevated serum ammonia levels may be falsely normalized during potassium repletion

Drug Interactions Increased effect/levels with potassium-sparing diuretics, salt substitutes, ACE inhibitors

Pregnancy Risk Factor A

Pregnancy Implications High levels are detrimental to fetal cardiac function

Additional Information Toxic oral dose with normal renal function: ~2 mEq/kg; lethal I.V. bolus dose: 0.75-0.9 mEq/kg

Alkalosis decreases serum potassium levels, acidosis elevates serum potassium levels; do not chew or crush tablets; salt substitutes contain from 50-70 mEq potassium per teaspoon; usually not irritating to the eye. Found in foods like cantaloupe, bananas, citrus fruits; foods with the highest potassium content (>1 g of potassium/100 g of food) include dried figs, molasses, and seaweed; other food products with potassium content >0.5 g of potassium/100 g of food include nuts, avocados, bran cereals, wheat germ, lima beans, dried dates or dried prunes. Potassium chloride is 13.3 mEq/g of salts (524 mg or 13.4 mM); average daily intake of potassium by adults is 2.8-3.9 g (70-100 mEq); radiopaque; liquid preparations should be used as opposed to solid forms in patients with esophageal compression due to left atrial enlargement or bowel hypomotility; total body potassium content is ~3500 mEq in an adult male with 50 mEq being in extracellular fluid compartment. Each 1 mEq/L decrease in serum potassium level can represent a total body potassium deficit of ~100-200 mEq. Whole blood specimen hemolysis can elevate serum potassium by ~0.5 mEq/L.

Specific References

Hoye A and Clark A, "Iatrogenic Hyperkalaemia," *Lancet*, 2003, 361(9375):2124.

Lu KC, Hsu YJ, Chiu JS, et al, "Effects of Potassium Supplementation on the Recovery of Thyrotoxic Periodic Paralysis," *Am J Emerg Med*, 2004, 22(7):544-547.

Owens H, Siparsky G, Bajaj L, et al, "Correction of Factitious Hyperkalemia in Hemolyzed Specimens," *Am J Emerg Med*, 2005, 23(7):872-5.

Wetherton AR, Corey TS, Buchino JJ, et al, "Fatal Intravenous Injection of Potassium in Hospitalized Patients," *Am J Forensic Med Pathol*, 2003, 24(2):128-31.

Povidone-Iodine

CAS Number 25655-41-8

U.S. Brand Names ACU-dyne® [OTC]; Betadine® Ophthalmic; Betadine® [OTC]; Minidyne® [OTC]; Operand® [OTC]; Summer's Eve® Medicated Douche [OTC]; Vagi-Gard® [OTC]

Synonyms Polyvinylpyrrolidone with Iodine; PVP-I

Use External antiseptic with broad microbicidal spectrum against bacteria, fungi, viruses, protozoa, and yeasts

Mechanism of Action Povidone-iodine is known to be a powerful broad spectrum germicidal agent effective against a wide range of bacteria, viruses, fungi, protozoa, and spores. It is an iodophor of which the polyvinylpyrrolidone is a solubilizing agent which liberates free iodine

Adverse Reactions

Central nervous system: Fever, headache

Dermatologic: Skin rash, angioedema, acne, contact dermatitis, erythema, chemical burn

Endocrine & metabolic: Hypothyroidism

Gastrointestinal: Diarrhea, metallic taste

Hematologic: Eosinophilia, hemorrhage (mucosal)

Hepatic: Elevation of serum transaminases and bilirubin

Neuromuscular & skeletal: Arthralgia

Ocular: Edema of eyelids

Otic: Ototoxicity

Respiratory: Pulmonary edema

Miscellaneous: Lymph node enlargement, anaphylactic shock

Signs and Symptoms of Overdose Agranulocytosis, circulation collapse, elevated serum osmolarity, gastroenteritis, granulocytopenia, hypernatremia, hypothyroidism, leukopenia, metabolic acidosis with increased lactic acid, neutropenia, renal failure (acute), swelling of glottis or larynx

Pharmacodynamics/Kinetics Absorption: Topical: Absorbed systemically as iodine; amount depends upon concentration, route of administration, characteristics of skin

Dosage

Shampoo: Apply 2 tsp to hair and scalp, lather and rinse; repeat application 2 times/week until improvement is noted, then shampoo weekly

Topical: Apply as needed for treatment and prevention of susceptible microbicidal infections

Monitoring Parameters Renal function, acid base status, electrolytes, CBC

Contraindications Hypersensitivity to iodine or any component of the formulation

Warnings Use caution in patients with thyroid disorders. Toxicity may occur following application of large or prolonged quantities; use caution with renal dysfunction, burns, pediatric patients. When used for self-medication (OTC use) do not apply to deep puncture wounds or serious burns; discontinue in case of redness, swelling, irritation or pain; do not use for longer than 1 week.

Dosage Forms [DSC] = Discontinued product

Gel, topical (Operand®): 10% (120 g)

Liquid, topical: 10% (30 mL)

Ointment, topical: 10% (1 g, 30 g)

Betadine®: 10% (0.9 g, 3.7 g, 30 g) [DSC]

Povidine™: 10% (30 g)

Pad [prep pads]: 10% (200s)

Betadine® SwabAids: 10% (100s)

Scrub brush [solution impregnated]: 7.5% (30s)

Solution, ophthalmic (Betadine®): 5% (50 mL)

Solution, perineal (Operand®): 10% (240 mL) [concentrate]

Solution, topical: 10% (240 mL, 480 mL, 3840 mL)

Betadine®: 10% (15 mL, 120 mL, 240 mL, 480 mL, 960 mL, 3840 mL)

Minidyne®: 10% (15 mL)

Operand®: 10% (60 mL, 120 mL, 240 mL, 480 mL, 960 mL, 3840 mL)

Solution, topical scrub:

Betadine® Surgical Scrub: 7.5% (120 mL, 480 mL, 960 mL, 3840 mL)

Betadine® Skin Cleanser: 7.5% (120 mL)

Operand®: 7.5% (60 mL, 120 mL, 240 mL, 480 mL, 960 mL, 3840 mL)

Solution, topical spray:

Betadine®: 5% (90 mL) [CFC free; contains dry natural rubber]

Operand®: 10% (59 mL)

Solution, vaginal douche:

Operand®: 10% (240 mL) [concentrate]

Summer's Eve® Medicated Douche: 0.3% (135 mL)

Vagi-Gard®: 10% (180 mL, 240 mL) [concentrate]

Solution, whirlpool (Operand®): 10% (3840 mL) [concentrate]

Swab [prep-swab ampul]: 10% (0.65 mL)

Swabsticks: 10% (25s, 50s)

Betadine®: 10% (50s, 150s, 200s)

Swabsticks [gel saturated]: 10% (50s)

Swabsticks, topical scrub: 7.5% (25s, 50s)

Reference Range RDA in adults is 150 mg

Overdosage/Treatment

Decontamination: **Do not** use ipecac; activated charcoal is useful; gastric lavage (within 1 hour) with starch will aid in removal (purple color of effluent)

Enhancement of elimination: Can be enhanced with osmotic diuresis or salt loading

Test Interactions Interferes with thyroid function tests; falsely elevates chloride concentrations

Drug Interactions No data reported

Pregnancy Risk Factor D

Pregnancy Implications Can cause fetal goiter and hypothyroidism

Lactation Enters breast milk/use caution (AAP rates "compatible")

Additional Information Antiseptic action is reduced by alkali solutions

Specific References

Azzam ZS, Farhat D, Braun E, et al, "Seizures: An Unusual Complication of Intrapleural Povidone-Iodine Irrigation," *J Pharm Technol*, 2003, 19:94-6.

Pramipexole

U.S. Brand Names Mirapex®

Use Treatment of the signs and symptoms of idiopathic Parkinson's disease

Unlabeled/Investigational Use Treatment of depression

Mechanism of Action Pramipexole is a nonergot dopamine agonist with specificity for the D_2 subfamily dopamine receptor, and has also been shown to bind to D_3 and D_4 receptors. By binding to these receptors, it is thought that pramipexole can stimulate dopamine activity on the nerves of the striatum and substantia nigra.

Adverse Reactions

Cardiovascular: **Postural hypotension**, edema, syncope, tachycardia, chest pain

Central nervous system: **Asthenia, dizziness, somnolence, insomnia, hallucinations, abnormal dreams**, malaise, confusion, amnesia, dystonias, akathisia, thinking abnormalities, myoclonus, hyperesthesia, paranoia; dose related: falling asleep during activities of daily living

Endocrine & metabolic: Decreased libido

Gastrointestinal: **Nausea, constipation**, anorexia, weight loss, xerostomia, dysphagia

Genitourinary: Urinary frequency (up to 6%), impotence, urinary incontinence

Hepatic: Elevated liver transaminase levels (<1%)

Neuromuscular & skeletal: **Weakness, dyskinesia, extrapyramidal symptoms (EPS)**, muscle twitching, leg cramps, arthritis, bursitis, myasthenia, hypertonia, gait abnormalities, rhabdomyolysis

Ocular: Vision abnormalities

Respiratory: Dyspnea, rhinitis

Signs and Symptoms of Overdose Lethargy, tachycardia, vomiting

Admission Criteria/Prognosis Admit any ingestion >10 mg in adults or >1 mg in infants, or any patient exhibiting postural hypotension in the setting of an overdose.

Pharmacodynamics/Kinetics

Protein binding: 15%

Bioavailability: 90%

Half-life elimination: ~8 hours; Elderly: 12-14 hours

Time to peak, serum: ~2 hours

Excretion: Urine (90% as unchanged drug)

Dosage Adults: Oral: Initial: 0.375 mg/day given in 3 divided doses, increase gradually by 0.125 mg/dose every 5-7 days; range: 1.5-4.5 mg/day

Dosage adjustment in renal impairment:

Cl_{cr} 35-59 mL/minute: Initial: 0.125 mg twice daily (maximum dose: 1.5 mg twice daily)

Cl$_{cr}$ 15-34 mL/minute: Initial: 0.125 mg once daily (maximum dose: 1.5 mg once daily)

Cl$_{cr}$ <15 mL/minute (or hemodialysis patients): Not adequately studied

Monitoring Parameters Monitor for improvement in symptoms of Parkinson's disease (eg, mentation, behavior, daily living activities, motor examinations), blood pressure, body weight changes, and heart rate

Administration Doses should be titrated gradually in all patients to avoid the onset of intolerable side effects. The dosage should be increased to achieve a maximum therapeutic effect, balanced against the side effects of dyskinesia, hallucinations, somnolence, and dry mouth.

Contraindications Hypersensitivity to pramipexole or any component of the formulation

Warnings Caution should be taken in patients with renal insufficiency and in patients with pre-existing dyskinesias. May cause orthostatic hypotension; Parkinson's disease patients appear to have an impaired capacity to respond to a postural challenge. Use with caution in patients at risk of hypotension (such as those receiving antihypertensive drugs) or where transient hypotensive episodes would be poorly tolerated (cardiovascular disease or cerebrovascular disease). Parkinson's patients being treated with dopaminergic agonists ordinarily require careful monitoring for signs and symptoms of postural hypotension, especially during dose escalation, and should be informed of this risk. May cause hallucinations, particularly in older patients. Pathologic degenerative changes were observed in the retinas of albino rats during studies with this agent, but were not observed in the retinas of pigmented rats or in other species. The significance of these data for humans remains uncertain.

Although not reported for pramipexole, other dopaminergic agents have been associated with a syndrome resembling neuroleptic malignant syndrome on withdrawal or significant dosage reduction after long-term use. Dopaminergic agents from the ergot class have also been associated with fibrotic complications, such as retroperitoneum, lungs, and pleura.

Pramipexole has been associated with somnolence, particularly at higher dosages (>1.5 mg/day). In addition, patients have been reported to fall asleep during activities of daily living, including driving, while taking this medication. Whether these patients exhibited somnolence prior to these events is not clear. Patients should be advised of this issue and factors which may increase risk (sleep disorders, other sedating medications, or concomitant medications which increase pramipexole concentrations) and instructed to report daytime somnolence or sleepiness to the prescriber. Patients should use caution in performing activities which require alertness (driving or operating machinery), and to avoid other medications which may cause CNS depression, including ethanol.

Dosage Forms Tablet, as dihydrochloride monohydrate: 0.125 mg, 0.25 mg, 0.5 mg, 1 mg, 1.5 mg

Overdosage/Treatment

Decontamination: Consider gastric decontamination for ingestions >6 mg; lavage within 1 hour for ingestions >10 mg

Supportive therapy: Dystonia can be treated with benztropine (1-4 mg I.V. or I.M. to a maximum daily dose of 6 mg) and/or diphenhydramine (children: 1.25 mg/kg; adults: 25-50 mg, up to 300 mg/day)

Enhancement of elimination: Hemodialysis is not likely to be useful

Drug Interactions Antipsychotics: May decrease the efficiency of pramipexole due to dopamine antagonism

Cationic drugs: Drugs secreted by the cationic transport system (diltiazem, triamterene, verapamil, quinidine, quinine, ranitidine) decrease the clearance of pramipexole by ~20%

Cimetidine: May increase serum concentrations; cimetidine in combination with pramipexole produced a 50% increase in AUC and a 40% increase in half-life

Metoclopramide: May decrease the efficiency of pramipexole due to dopamine antagonism

Pregnancy Risk Factor C

Pregnancy Implications Early embryonic loss and postnatal growth inhibition were observed in animal studies. There are no adequate and well-controlled studies in pregnant women.

Lactation Excretion in breast milk unknown/not recommended

Pramoxine

CAS Number 140-65-8; 637-58-1

U.S. Brand Names Anusol® Ointment [OTC]; Itch-X® [OTC]; Prax® [OTC]; ProctoFoam® NS [OTC]; Tronolane® [OTC]

Synonyms Pramoxine Hydrochloride

Use Temporary relief of pain and itching associated with anogenital pruritus or irritation; dermatosis, minor burns, or hemorrhoids

Mechanism of Action Pramoxine, like other anesthetics, decreases the neuronal membrane's permeability to sodium ions. Both initiation and conduction of nerve impulses are blocked, thus depolarization of the neuron is inhibited.

Adverse Reactions

Cardiovascular: Edema, sinus bradycardia

Dermatologic: Urticaria, rash, contact eczema

Local: Burning, stinging

Signs and Symptoms of Overdose Agitation, bradycardia, cardiovascular collapse, coma, convulsions, euphoria, hypotension, methemoglobinemia (may occur), myoclonus, ototoxicity, respiratory failure, slurred speech, tinnitus, tremors

Admission Criteria/Prognosis Any patient with change in mental status, cardiopulmonary complaints, or methemoglobin levels >30% should be admitted; asymptomatic patients with methemoglobin levels <30% may be considered for discharge after 6 hours of observation and if methemoglobin levels fall to <15%

Pharmacodynamics/Kinetics

Onset of action: Therapeutic: 2-5 minutes

Peak effect: 3-5 minutes

Duration: Several days

Dosage Adults: Topical: Apply as directed, usually every 3-4 hours to affected area (maximum adult dose: 200 mg)

Administration Apply sparingly, use the minimal effective dose.

Dosage Forms Cream, topical, as hydrochloride:

Tronolane®: 1% (30 g, 60 g) [contains zinc oxide 5%]

Foam, aerosol, topical, as hydrochloride: 1% (15 g)

ProctoFoam® NS: 1% (15 g)

Gel, topical, as hydrochloride:

Itch-X®: 1% (35.4 g) [contains benzyl alcohol]

Liquid, topical, as hydrochloride:

Curasore®: 1% (15 mL) [contains ethyl alcohol; packaged with cotton applicators]

Lotion, topical, as hydrochloride:

Caladryl® Clear: 1% (177 mL) [contains zinc acetate 0.1%]

Callergy Clear: 1% (180 mL) [contains zinc acetate 0.1%]

Prax®: 1% (15 mL, 120 mL, 240 mL)

Sarna® Sensitive: 1% (222 mL)

Ointment, rectal, as hydrochloride:

Anusol®, Tucks® Hemorrhoidal: 1% (30 g) [contains zinc oxide 12.5% and mineral oil; Anusol® Ointment renamed Tucks® Hemorrhoidal]

Solution, topical spray, as hydrochloride:

CalaMycin® Cool and Clear: 1% (60 mL) [contains zinc acetate 0.1%]

Itch-X®: 1% (60 mL) [contains zinc oxide 1% and benzyl alcohol]

Overdosage/Treatment

Decontamination: Lavage (within 1 hour)/activated charcoal

Supportive therapy: Seizures can be treated with diazepam, lorazepam, phenobarbital, or phenytoin; allergic reactions can be treated with epinephrine, diphenhydramine, and corticosteroids

Drug Interactions No data reported

Pregnancy Risk Factor C

Nursing Implications Apply sparingly, use the minimal effective dose

Additional Information Less sensitization than benzocaine

Pravastatin

CAS Number 81093-37-0; 81131-70-6

U.S. Brand Names Pravachol®

Synonyms Pravastatin Sodium

Use

Use with dietary therapy for the following:

Primary prevention of coronary events: In hypercholesterolemic patients without established coronary heart disease to reduce cardiovascular morbidity (myocardial infarction, coronary revascularization procedures) and mortality.

Secondary prevention of cardiovascular events in patients with established coronary heart disease: To slow the progression of coronary atherosclerosis; to reduce cardiovascular morbidity (myocardial infarction, coronary vascular procedures) and to reduce mortality; to reduce the risk of stroke and transient ischemic attacks

Hyperlipidemias: Reduce elevations in total cholesterol, LDL-C, apolipoprotein B, and triglycerides (elevations of 1 or more components are present in Fredrickson type IIa, IIb, III, and IV hyperlipidemias)

Heterozygous familial hypercholesterolemia (HeFH): In pediatric patients, 8-18 years of age, with HeFH having LDL-C ≥190 mg/dL or LDL ≥160 mg/dL with positive family history of premature cardiovascular disease (CVD) or 2 or more CVD risk factors in the pediatric patient

Mechanism of Action Pravastatin is a competitive inhibitor of 3-hydroxy-3-methylglutaryl coenzyme A (HMG-CoA) reductase, which is the rate-limiting enzyme involved in de novo cholesterol synthesis.

Adverse Reactions

As reported in short-term trials; safety and tolerability with long-term use were similar to placebo

Cardiovascular: Chest pain

Central nervous system: Cranial nerve dysfunction, headache, fatigue, fever, flushing, dizziness, insomnia, memory impairment, vertigo

Dermatologic: Alopecia, dermatitis, dermatomyositis, dry skin, edema, erythema multiforme, pruritus, purpura, Stevens-Johnson syndrome, urticaria

Endocrine & metabolic: Libido change, sexual dysfunction

Gastrointestinal: Appetite decreased, diarrhea, gynecomastia, heartburn, nausea, pancreatitis, taste disturbance, vomiting

Hematologic: Hemolytic anemia

Hepatic: Cholestatic jaundice, cirrhosis, elevated transaminases (>3x normal on two occasions - 1%), fulminant hepatic necrosis, hepatitis, hepatoma

Neuromuscular & skeletal: Muscle weakness, myalgia, myopathy, neuropathy, paresthesia, peripheral nerve palsy, polymyalgia rheumatica, rhabdomyolysis, tremor

Ocular: Lens opacity

Respiratory: Cough

Miscellaneous: Allergy, anaphylaxis, ESR increase, influenza, lupus erythematosus-like syndrome, positive ANA

Pharmacodynamics/Kinetics

Onset of action: Several days

Peak effect: 4 weeks

Absorption: Rapidly absorbed; average absorption 34%

Protein binding: 50%

Metabolism: Hepatic to at least two metabolites

Bioavailability: 17%

Half-life elimination: ~2-3 hours

Time to peak, serum: 1-1.5 hours

Excretion: Feces (70%); urine (≤20%, 8% as unchanged drug)

Dosage

Oral: **Note:** Doses should be individualized according to the baseline LDL-cholesterol levels, the recommended goal of therapy, and patient response; adjustments should be made at intervals of 4 weeks or more; doses may need adjusted based on concomitant medications

Children: HeFH:

8-13 years: 20 mg/day

14-18 years: 40 mg/day

Dosage adjustment for pravastatin based on concomitant immunosuppressants (ie, cyclosporine): Refer to Adults dosing section

Adults: Hyperlipidemias, primary prevention of coronary events, secondary prevention of cardiovascular events: Initial: 40 mg once daily; titrate dosage to response; usual range: 10-80 mg; (maximum dose: 80 mg once daily)

Dosage adjustment for pravastatin based on concomitant immunosuppressants (ie, cyclosporine): Initial: 10 mg/day, titrate with caution (maximum dose: 20 mg/day)

Elderly: No specific dosage recommendations. Clearance is reduced in the elderly, resulting in an increase in AUC between 25% to 50%. However, substantial accumulation is not expected.

Dosing adjustment in renal impairment: Initial: 10 mg/day

Dosing adjustment in hepatic impairment: Initial: 10 mg/day

Stability Store at 25°C (77°F); excursions permitted to 15°C to 30°C (59°F to 86°F). Protect from moisture and light.

Monitoring Parameters Obtain baseline LFTs and total cholesterol profile; creatine phosphokinase due to possibility of myopathy. Repeat LFTs prior to elevation of dose. May be measured when clinically indicated and/or periodically thereafter.

Administration May be taken without regard to meals.

Contraindications Hypersensitivity to pravastatin or any component of the formulation; active liver disease; unexplained persistent elevations of serum transaminases; pregnancy; breast-feeding

Warnings Secondary causes of hyperlipidemia should be ruled out prior to therapy. Liver function must be monitored by periodic laboratory assessment. Rhabdomyolysis with acute renal failure has occurred. Risk may be increased with concurrent use of other drugs which may cause rhabdomyolysis (including gemfibrozil, fibric acid derivatives, or niacin at doses ≥1 g/day). Temporarily discontinue in any patient experiencing an acute or serious condition predisposing to renal failure secondary to rhabdomyolysis. Use caution in patients with previous liver disease or heavy ethanol use. Treatment in patients <8 years of age is not recommended.

Dosage Forms Tablet, as sodium: 10 mg, 20 mg, 40 mg,

Pravachol®: 10 mg, 20 mg, 40 mg, 80 mg

Reference Range Peak plasma levels following a 19.2 mg oral dose: ~27 ng/mL

Overdosage/Treatment

Decontamination: Activated charcoal can be used

Supportive therapy: Treatment is symptomatic

Drug Interactions **Substrate** of CYP3A4 (minor); **Inhibits** CYP2C9 (weak), 2D6 (weak), 3A4 (weak)

Cholestyramine: Reduces pravastatin absorption; separate administration times by at least 4 hours.

Clofibrate and fenofibrate: May increase the risk of myopathy and rhabdomyolysis.

Colestipol: Reduces pravastatin absorption; separate administration by 1 hour.

Cyclosporine: Concurrent use may increase the risk of myopathy and rhabdomyolysis.

Gemfibrozil: Increased risk of myopathy and rhabdomyolysis.

Imidazole antifungals (itraconazole, ketoconazole): May modestly increase pravastatin concentrations (AUC).

Niacin: May increase the risk of myopathy and rhabdomyolysis.

P-glycoprotein inhibitors (eg, amiodarone, cyclosporine, ketoconazole): May increase pravastatin concentrations.

Pregnancy Risk Factor X

Pregnancy Implications Safety and efficacy have not been established for use during pregnancy (treatment should be discontinued if pregnancy is recognized). Administer to women of childbearing potential only if conception is unlikely; females should be counseled on appropriate contraceptive methods.

Lactation Enters breast milk/contraindicated

Nursing Implications Liver enzyme elevations may be observed during therapy with pravastatin; diet, weight reduction, and exercise should be attempted prior to therapy with pravastatin

Additional Information Before initiation of therapy, patients should be placed on a standard cholesterol-lowering diet for 6 weeks and the diet should be continued during drug therapy.

Prazepam

CAS Number 2955-38-6

Impairment Potential Yes

Use Treatment of anxiety

Unlabeled/Investigational Use Ethanol withdrawal; duodenal ulcer; narcotic addiction; spasticity; partial seizures

Mechanism of Action Benzodiazepine anxiolytic sedative that produces CNS depression at the subcortical level, except at high doses, whereby it works at the cortical level

Adverse Reactions

Cardiovascular: **Tachycardia, chest pain**, cardiac arrest, hypotension, bradycardia, cardiovascular collapse, sinus bradycardia

Central nervous system: **Drowsiness, fatigue, impaired coordination, lightheadedness, memory impairment, insomnia, depression, headache, anxiety, ataxia**, confusion, dizziness, amnesia, slurred speech, paradoxical excitation or rage, delirium, persecutory delusions

Dermatologic: **Rash**

Endocrine & metabolic: **Decreased libido**

Gastrointestinal: **Xerostomia, constipation, diarrhea, decreased salivation, nausea, vomiting, increased or decreased appetite**

Local: Phlebitis, pain with injection

Neuromuscular & skeletal: **Dysarthria**, orofacial dyskinesia

Ocular: **Blurred vision**, nystagmus, diplopia

Respiratory: Decreased respiratory rate, apnea, laryngospasm

Miscellaneous: **Diaphoresis**, physical and psychological dependence with prolonged use

Signs and Symptoms of Overdose Acute myoglobinuria, "alpha" coma (alpha frequency rhythm on EEG), ataxia, confusion, dry mouth, dyspnea, hypoactive reflexes, hyporeflexia, labored breathing, lightheadedness, rhabdomyolysis, visual and auditory hallucinations

Pharmacodynamics/Kinetics

Studies have shown that the elderly are more sensitive to the effects of benzodiazepines as compared to younger adults

Onset of action: Peak actions occur within 6 hours

Duration: 48 hours

Absorption: Readily from gastrointestinal tract

Distribution: V_d: 9.3-19.5 L/kg; distributed widely distributed throughout body

Protein binding: 85% to 97%

Metabolism: First-pass hepatic metabolism, primarily desmethyldiazepam (active)

Half-life: Parent: 78 minutes; Desmethyldiazepam: 30-100 hours; Half-life of desmethyldiazepam is significantly prolonged in elderly men (127.8 hours) as compared to young men (61.8 hours) and older women (75.4 hours); V_d is increased in the elderly

Time to peak serum concentration: Oral single dose: 2.5-6 hours

Elimination: Renal and feces (71%)

Dosage Adults: Oral: 30 mg/day in divided doses, may increase gradually to a maximum of 60 mg/day

Monitoring Parameters Respiratory and cardiovascular status

Contraindications Hypersensitivity to prazepam or any component of the formulation (cross-sensitivity with other benzodiazepines may exist); narrow-angle glaucoma; pregnancy

Warnings

Use with caution in elderly or debilitated patients, patients with hepatic disease (including alcoholics), or renal impairment. Use with caution in patients with respiratory disease, or impaired gag reflex. Avoid use in patients with sleep apnea.

Causes CNS depression (dose-related) resulting in sedation, dizziness, confusion, or ataxia which may impair physical and mental capabilities. Patients must be cautioned about performing tasks which require mental alertness (operating machinery or driving). Use with caution in patients receiving other CNS depressants or psychoactive agents. Effects with other sedative drugs or ethanol may be potentiated. Benzodiazepines have been associated with falls and traumatic injury and should be used with extreme caution in patients who are at risk of these events (especially the elderly).

Use caution in patients with depression, particularly if suicidal risk may be present. Use with caution in patients with a history of drug dependence. Benzodiazepines have been associated with dependence and acute withdrawal symptoms on discontinuation or reduction in dose. Acute withdrawal, including seizures, may be precipitated after administration of flumazenil to patients receiving long-term benzodiazepine therapy.

Benzodiazepines have been associated with anterograde amnesia. Paradoxical reactions, including hyperactive or aggressive behavior have been reported with benzodiazepines, particularly in adolescent/pediatric or psychiatric patients. Does not have analgesic, antidepressant, or antipsychotic properties.

Dosage Forms Capsule: 5 mg, 10 mg, 20 mg

Tablet: 5 mg, 10 mg

Reference Range Therapeutic: 50-240 ng/mL (SI: 156-746 nmol/L)

Overdosage/Treatment

Decontamination: Activated charcoal

Supportive therapy: Treatment for benzodiazepine overdose is supportive; rarely is mechanical ventilation required. Flumazenil (Romazicon™) has been shown to selectively block the binding of benzodiazepines to CNS receptors, resulting in a reversal of benzodiazepine-induced CNS depression. Do not use in concomitant tricyclic ingestion; treat hypotension with isotonic crystalloids, place in Trendelenburg position or give dopamine or norepinephrine.

Enhancement of elimination: Multiple dose of activated charcoal may enhance elimination

Antidote(s)

- Flumazenil [ANTIDOTE]

Test Interactions May ↑ LFTs. Visine®, Drano®, and bleach can cause false-negative urine tests.

Drug Interactions Substrate of CYP3A4 (minor)

CNS depressants: Sedative effects and/or respiratory depression may be additive with CNS depressants; includes ethanol, barbiturates, narcotic analgesics, and other sedative agents; monitor for increased effect

Oral contraceptives: May decrease the clearance of some benzodiazepines (those which undergo oxidative metabolism); monitor for increased benzodiazepine effect

Theophylline: May partially antagonize some of the effects of benzodiazepines; monitor for decreased response; may require higher doses for sedation

Pregnancy Risk Factor D

Pregnancy Implications Suggested to be teratogenic in animal and human data; can precipitate neonatal respiratory depression when given during delivery; crosses placenta

Nursing Implications Monitor for alertness

Additional Information Not available in U.S.

Prazepam offers no significant advantage over other benzodiazepines.

Prazosin

Related Information

- Bunazosin

CAS Number 19216-56-9; 19237-84-4

U.S. Brand Names Minipress®

Synonyms Furazosin; Prazosin Hydrochloride

Use Hypertension, severe congestive heart failure (in conjunction with diuretics and cardiac glycosides)

Unlabeled/Investigational Use Benign prostatic hyperplasia; Raynaud's syndrome

Mechanism of Action Competitively inhibits postsynaptic alpha-adrenergic receptors which results in vasodilation of veins and arterioles and a decrease in total peripheral resistance and blood pressure; effective for ergotism-induced hypertension

Adverse Reactions

Cardiovascular: **Hypotension (orthostatic)**, syncope, palpitations, tachycardia, edema, sinus bradycardia, chest pain, angina, sinus tachycardia, vasodilation

Central nervous system: **Dizziness, drowsiness, headache, malaise, lightheadedness**, night terrors, psychosis, hypothermia

Dermatologic: Rash, angioneurotic edema, alopecia, urticaria, pruritus, licheniform eruptions, exanthem

Endocrine & metabolic: Fluid retention, sexual dysfunction

Gastrointestinal: Nausea, xerostomia, fecal incontinence

Genitourinary: Urinary frequency, priapism, urinary incontinence

Neuromuscular & skeletal: Weakness, paresthesia

Respiratory: Nasal congestion

Miscellaneous: Positive ANA, systemic lupus erythematosus

Signs and Symptoms of Overdose Bone marrow depression, conjunctivitis, drowsiness, hypotension, hypothermia, impotence, enuresis, night terrors, ptosis, respiratory depression, syncope

Pharmacodynamics/Kinetics

Onset of action: BP reduction: ~2 hours

Maximum decrease: 2-4 hours

Duration: 10-24 hours

Distribution: Hypertensive adults: V_d: 0.5 L/kg

Protein binding: 92% to 97%

Metabolism: Extensively hepatic

Bioavailability: 43% to 82%

Half-life elimination: 2-4 hours; prolonged with congestive heart failure

Excretion: Urine (6% to 10% as unchanged drug)

Dosage Oral:

Children: Initial: 5 mcg/kg/dose (to assess hypotensive effects); usual dosing interval: every 6 hours; increase dosage gradually up to maximum of 25 mcg/kg/dose every 6 hours

Adults: Initial: 1 mg/dose 2-3 times/day; usual maintenance dose: 3-15 mg/day in divided doses 2-4 times/day; maximum daily dose: 20 mg

Stability Store in airtight container; protect from light

Monitoring Parameters Blood pressure, standing and sitting/supine

Contraindications Hypersensitivity to quinazolines (doxazosin, prazosin, terazosin) or any component of the formulation; concurrent use with phosphodiesterase-5 (PDE-5) inhibitors including sildenafil (>25 mg), tadalafil, or vardenafil

Warnings May cause significant orthostatic hypotension and syncope, especially with first dose. Risk is increased at doses >1 mg, hypovolemia, or in patients receiving concurrent beta-blocker therapy. Anticipate a similar effect if therapy is interrupted for a few days, if dosage is rapidly increased, or if another antihypertensive drug is introduced.

Dosage Forms Capsule, as hydrochloride: 1 mg, 2 mg, 5 mg

Reference Range Plasma level of 47.6 ng/mL was noted in an overdose setting 11 hours after a 120 mg ingestion

Overdosage/Treatment

Decontamination: Activated charcoal

Supportive therapy: Hypotension usually responds to I.V. fluids or Trendelenburg positioning. If unresponsive to these measures, the use of a parenteral vasoconstrictor may be required (eg, norepinephrine 0.1-0.2 mcg/kg/minute titrated to response). Treatment is primarily supportive and symptomatic.

Enhancement of elimination: Multiple dosing of activated charcoal may be effective

Antidote(s)

- Norepinephrine [ANTIDOTE]

Drug Interactions ACE inhibitors: Hypotensive effect may be increased.

Beta-blockers: Hypotensive effect may be increased.

Calcium channel blockers: Hypotensive effect may be increased.

NSAIDs may reduce antihypertensive efficacy.

Sildenafil, tadalafil, vardenafil: Blood pressure-lowering effects are additive. Use of tadalafil or vardenafil is contraindicated by the manufacturer. Use sildenafil with extreme caution (dose ≤25 mg).

Tricyclic antidepressants (TCAs) and low-potency antipsychotics: May increase risk of orthostasis.

Pregnancy Risk Factor C

Lactation Excretion in breast milk unknown/use caution

Nursing Implications Syncope may occur usually within 90 minutes of the initial dose

PrednisoLONE

CAS Number 1107-99-9; 125-02-0; 1715-33-9; 2920-86-7; 50-24-8; 5060-55-9; 52-21-1; 52438-85-4; 630-67-1; 7681-14-3

U.S. Brand Names AK-Pred®; Bubbli-Pred™ [DSC]; Econopred® Plus; Orapred ODT™; Orapred®; Pediapred®; Pred Forte®; Pred Mild®; Prelone®

Synonyms Deltahydrocortisone; Metacortandralone; Prednisolone Acetate, Ophthalmic; Prednisolone Acetate; Prednisolone Sodium Phosphate, Ophthalmic; Prednisolone Sodium Phosphate

Use Treatment of palpebral and bulbar conjunctivitis; corneal injury from chemical, radiation, thermal burns, or foreign body penetration; endocrine disorders, rheumatic disorders, collagen diseases, dermatologic diseases, allergic states, ophthalmic diseases, respiratory diseases, hematologic disorders, neoplastic diseases, edematous states, and gastrointestinal diseases; useful in patients with inability to activate prednisone (liver disease)

Mechanism of Action Decreases inflammation by suppression of migration of polymorphonuclear leukocytes and reversal of increased capillary permeability; suppresses the immune system by reducing activity and volume of the lymphatic system

Adverse Reactions

Cardiovascular: Edema, hypertension, QT prolongation, cardiomyopathy, cardiomegaly

Central nervous system: **Insomnia, nervousness**, vertigo, seizures, psychosis, pseudotumor cerebri, headache, mood swings, delirium, hallucinations, euphoria, cognitive dysfunction, depression, mania

Dermatologic: Hirsutism, acne, skin atrophy, bruising, hyperpigmentation, telangiectasia

Endocrine & metabolic: Diabetes mellitus, Cushing's syndrome, pituitary-adrenal axis suppression, growth suppression, glucose intolerance, hypokalemia, alkalosis, amenorrhea, sodium and water retention, hyperglycemia

Gastrointestinal: **Increased appetite, indigestion**, abdominal distention, ulcerative esophagitis, pancreatitis, peptic ulcer, nausea, vomiting

Neuromuscular & skeletal: Arthralgia, muscle weakness, osteoporosis, fractures, muscle wasting

Ocular: Cataracts, glaucoma

Respiratory: Epistaxis

Miscellaneous: Hypersensitivity reactions, Kaposi's sarcoma

Signs and Symptoms of Overdose When consumed in excessive quantities for prolonged periods, systemic hypercorticism and adrenal suppression may occur. In those cases discontinuation and withdrawal of the corticosteroid should be done judiciously.

Pharmacodynamics/Kinetics

Duration: 18-36 hours

Protein binding (concentration dependent): 65% to 91%; decreased in elderly

Metabolism: Primarily hepatic, but also metabolized in most tissues, to inactive compounds

Half-life elimination: 3.6 hours; End-stage renal disease: 3-5 hours

Excretion: Primarily urine (as glucuronides, sulfates, and unconjugated metabolites)

Dosage Dose depends upon condition being treated and response of patient; dosage for infants and children should be based on severity of the disease and response of the patient rather than on strict adherence to dosage indicated by age, weight, or body surface area. Consider alternate day therapy for long-term therapy. Discontinuation of long-term therapy requires gradual withdrawal by tapering the dose. Patients undergoing unusual stress while receiving corticosteroids, should receive increased doses prior to, during, and after the stressful situation.

Children:

Acute asthma:

Oral: 1-2 mg/kg/day in divided doses 1-2 times/day for 3-5 days

I.V. (sodium phosphate salt): 2-4 mg/kg/day divided 3-4 times/day

Anti-inflammatory or immunosuppressive dose: Oral, I.V., I.M. (sodium phosphate salt): 0.1-2 mg/kg/day in divided doses 1-4 times/day

Nephrotic syndrome: Oral:

Initial (first 3 episodes): 2 mg/kg/day **or** 60 mg/m^2/day (maximum: 80 mg/day) in divided doses 3-4 times/day until urine is protein free for 3 consecutive days (maximum: 28 days); followed by 1-1.5 mg/kg/dose **or** 40 mg/m^2/dose given every other day for 4 weeks

Maintenance (long-term maintenance dose for frequent relapses): 0.5-1 mg/kg/dose given every other day for 3-6 months

Adults:

Oral, I.V., I.M. (sodium phosphate salt): 5-60 mg/day

Multiple sclerosis (sodium phosphate): Oral: 200 mg/day for 1 week followed by 80 mg every other day for 1 month

Rheumatoid arthritis: Oral: Initial: 5-7.5 mg/day; adjust dose as necessary

Elderly: Use lowest effective dose

Dosing adjustment in hyperthyroidism: Prednisolone dose may need to be increased to achieve adequate therapeutic effects

Hemodialysis: Slightly dialyzable (5% to 20%); administer dose post-hemodialysis

Peritoneal dialysis: Supplemental dose is not necessary

Intra-articular, intralesional, soft-tissue administration:

Tebutate salt: 4-40 mg/dose

Sodium phosphate salt: 2-30 mg/dose

Ophthalmic suspension/solution: Children and Adults: Instill 1-2 drops into conjunctival sac every hour during day, every 2 hours at night until favorable response is obtained, then use 1 drop every 4 hours

Monitoring Parameters Blood pressure, blood glucose, electrolytes

Administration Sodium phosphate injection: For I.V., I.M., intra-articular, intralesional, or soft tissue administration

Tebutate injection: For intra-articular, intralesional, or soft tissue administration only

Contraindications Hypersensitivity to prednisolone or any component of the formulation; acute superficial herpes simplex keratitis; live or attenuated virus vaccines (with immunosuppressive doses of corticosteroids); systemic fungal infections; varicella

Warnings

Use with caution in patients with cirrhosis, nonspecific ulcerative colitis, hypertension, osteoporosis, thromboembolic tendencies, CHF, convulsive disorders, myasthenia gravis, thrombophlebitis, peptic ulcer, diabetes, or tuberculosis; acute adrenal insufficiency may occur with abrupt withdrawal after long-term therapy or with stress; young pediatric patients may be more susceptible to adrenal axis suppression from topical therapy. Changes in thyroid status may necessitate dosage adjustments; metabolic clearance of corticosteroids increases in hyperthyroid patients and decreases in hypothyroid ones.

Prolonged use of corticosteroids may result in glaucoma; damage to the optic nerve (not indicated for treatment of optic neuritis), defects in visual acuity and fields of vision, and posterior subcapsular cataract formation may occur. Prolonged use of corticosteroids may also increase the incidence of secondary infection, mask acute infection (including fungal infections) or prolong or exacerbate viral infections. Exposure to chickenpox should be avoided; corticosteroids should not be used to treat ocular herpes simplex. Use following cataract surgery may delay healing or increase the incidence of bleb formation.

Corticosteroids should not be used for cerebral malaria. Because of the risk of adverse effects, systemic corticosteroids should be used cautiously in the elderly, in the smallest possible dose, and for the shortest possible time.

Dosage Forms [DSC] = Discontinued product

Solution, ophthalmic, as sodium phosphate: 1% (5 mL, 10 mL, 15 mL) [contains benzalkonium chloride]

AK-Pred®: 1% (5 mL, 15 mL) [contains benzalkonium chloride]

Solution, oral, as sodium phosphate: Prednisolone base 5 mg/5 mL (120 mL)

Bubbli-Pred™: Prednisolone base 5 mg/5 mL (120 mL) [bubble gum flavor] [DSC]

Orapred®: 20 mg/5 mL (240 mL) [equivalent to prednisolone base 15 mg/5 mL; dye free; contains alcohol 2%, sodium benzoate; grape flavor]

Pediapred®: 6.7 mg/5 mL (120 mL) [equivalent to prednisolone base 5 mg/5 mL; dye free; raspberry flavor]

Suspension, ophthalmic, as acetate: 1% (5 mL, 10 mL, 15 mL) [contains benzalkonium chloride]

Econopred® Plus: 1% (5 mL, 10 mL) [contains benzalkonium chloride]

Pred Forte®: 1% (1 mL, 5 mL, 10 mL, 15 mL) [contains benzalkonium chloride and sodium bisulfite]

Pred Mild®: 0.12% (5 mL, 10 mL) [contains benzalkonium chloride and sodium bisulfite]

Syrup, as base: 5 mg/5 mL (120 mL); 15 mg/5 mL (240 mL, 480 mL)

Prelone®: 15 mg/5 mL (240 mL, 480 mL) [contains alcohol 5%, benzoic acid; cherry flavor]

Tablet, as base: 5 mg

Tablet, orally disintegrating, as base:

Orapred ODT™: 10 mg, 15 mg, 30 mg [grape flavor]

Overdosage/Treatment

Decontamination: Activated charcoal; acute overdose does not require tapering of dose

Supportive therapy: Psychosis can be treated with sertraline

Enhanced elimination: Its metabolite (prednisolone) is slightly dialyzable (5% to 20%)

Test Interactions Response to skin tests

Drug Interactions **Substrate** of CYP3A4 (minor); **Inhibits** CYP3A4 (weak)

Aminoglutethimide: May reduce the serum levels/effects of prednisolone; likely via induction of microsomal isoenzymes.

Antacids: May increase the absorption of corticosteroids; separate administration by ≥2 hours.

Aprepitant: May increase effects of systemic corticosteroids.

Azole antifungals: May increase the serum levels of corticosteroids; monitor.

Barbiturates: May decrease prednisolone levels; monitor.

Bile acid sequestrants: May decrease the absorption of corticosteroids (oral).

Calcium channel blockers (nondihydropyridine): May increase the serum levels of corticosteroids; monitor.

Cyclosporine: Corticosteroids may increase the serum levels of cyclosporine. In addition, cyclosporine may increase levels of corticosteroids; monitor.

Estrogens: May increase the serum levels of corticosteroids; monitor.

Fluoroquinolones: Concurrent use may increase the risk of tendon rupture, particularly in elderly patients (overall incidence rare).

Isoniazid: Serum concentrations may be decreased by corticosteroids.

Ketoconazole: May decrease metabolism of certain corticosteroids leading to increased levels (up to 60%) and increased risk of adverse effects; monitor.

Macrolide antibiotics: May decrease the metabolism of corticosteroids.

Neuromuscular-blocking agents: Concurrent use with corticosteroids may increase the risk of myopathy.

Nonsteroidal anti-inflammatory drugs (NSAIDs), ophthalmic: Concurrent use with ophthalmic corticosteroids may lead to delayed healing.

Potassium-depleting agents (eg, diuretics, amphotericin B): Concurrent use increases risk of hypokalemia (especially if digitalized); monitor.

Primidone: May increase the metabolism of corticosteroids.

Rifampin: May decrease serum levels/effects of prednisolone; monitor.

Salicylates: Salicylates may increase the gastrointestinal adverse effects of corticosteroids.

Skin tests: Corticosteroids may suppress reactions to skin tests.

Vaccines (dead organisms): Immunosuppressants may diminish the effect of these vaccines.

Vaccines (live organisms): Immunosuppressants may enhance the adverse/toxic effects of these vaccines.

Pregnancy Risk Factor C

Pregnancy Implications Animal studies have demonstrated teratogenic effects. There are no adequate and well-controlled studies in pregnant women.

Lactation Enters breast milk/use caution (AAP rates "compatible")

Nursing Implications Give oral formulation with food or milk to decrease GI effects; do not give acetate or tebutate salt I.V.

Additional Information Fluid and electrolyte effects are unlikely at daily prednisolone doses <30 mg.

Specific References
Mitchell JC and Counselman FL, "A Taste Comparison of Three Different Liquid Steroid Preparations: Prednisone, Prednisolone, and Dexamethasone," *Acad Emerg Med*, 2003, 10(4):400-3.

PredniSONE

Related Information
- Corticosteroids

CAS Number 53-03-1

U.S. Brand Names Deltasone®; Prednisone Intensol™; Sterapred® DS; Sterapred®

Synonyms Deltacortisone; Deltadehydrocortisone

Use Treatment of a variety of diseases including adrenocortical insufficiency, hypercalcemia, rheumatic and collagen disorders; dermatologic, ocular, respiratory, gastrointestinal, and neoplastic diseases; organ transplantation and a variety of diseases including those of hematologic, allergic, inflammatory, and autoimmune in origin; not available in injectable form, prednisolone must be used; acute urticaria

Unlabeled/Investigational Use Investigational: Prevention of postherpetic neuralgia and relief of acute pain in the early stages

Mechanism of Action Decreases inflammation by suppression of migration of polymorphonuclear leukocytes and reversal of increased capillary permeability; suppresses the immune system by reducing activity and volume of the lymphatic system; suppresses adrenal function at high doses

Adverse Reactions
Cardiovascular: Edema, hypertension, QT prolongation, cardiomegaly, cardiomyopathy
Central nervous system: Dizziness, seizures, psychosis, pseudotumor cerebri, headache, memory disturbance, mania, **insomnia, nervousness**
Dermatologic: Acne, purpura, skin atrophy, angioedema, acanthosis nigricans
Endocrine & metabolic: Cushing's syndrome, pituitary-adrenal axis suppression, amenorrhea, growth suppression, glucose intolerance, hypokalemia, alkalosis
Gastrointestinal: Peptic ulcer, nausea, vomiting, fecal discoloration (black), **increased appetite, indigestion**
Hematologic: Aplastic anemia (rate is 1 in every 3600 to 5000 patients), leukemoid reaction
Hepatic: Fatal hepatotoxicity (rate is 1 in every 24000 to 32000 patients)
Neuromuscular & skeletal: Osteoporosis, fractures, weakness
Ocular: Cataracts, glaucoma
Miscellaneous: Anaphylaxis

Signs and Symptoms of Overdose Primarily neuropsychiatric. Cognitive dysfunction, dementia, depression, eosinopenia, GI bleeding, hirsutism, hyperglycemia, hypertrichosis, hyperuricemia, hypokalemia, increased intraocular pressure, leukocytosis, lymphopenia, mania, memory loss, sexual dysfunction, thrombocytopenia

Pharmacodynamics/Kinetics
Protein binding (concentration dependent): 65% to 91%
Metabolism: Hepatically converted from prednisone (inactive) to prednisolone (active); may be impaired with hepatic dysfunction
Half-life elimination: Normal renal function: 2.5-3.5 hours
See Prednisolone monograph for complete information.

Dosage Dose depends upon condition being treated and response of patient; dosage for infants and children should be based on severity of the disease and response of the patient rather than on strict adherence to dosage indicated by age, weight, or body surface area. Consider alternate day therapy for long-term therapy. Discontinuation of long-term therapy requires gradual withdrawal by tapering the dose.
Children: Oral:
Anti-inflammatory or immunosuppressive dose: 0.05-2 mg/kg/day divided 1-4 times/day
Acute asthma: 1-2 mg/kg/day in divided doses 1-2 times/day for 3-5 days
Alternatively (for 3- to 5-day "burst"):
<1 year: 10 mg every 12 hours
1-4 years: 20 mg every 12 hours
5-13 years: 30 mg every 12 hours
>13 years: 40 mg every 12 hours
Asthma long-term therapy (alternative dosing by age):
<1 year: 10 mg every other day
1-4 years: 20 mg every other day
5-13 years: 30 mg every other day
>13 years: 40 mg every other day
Severe refractory asthma: 5-10 mg/dose every day or 10-30 mg every other day
Nephrotic syndrome: Initial: 2 mg/kg/day (maximum: 80 mg/day) in divided doses 3-4 times/day until urine is protein free for 5 days (maximum: 28 days); if albuminuria persists, use 4 mg/kg/dose every other day (maximum: 120 mg/day) for an additional 28 days; maintenance: 2 mg/kg/dose (maximum: 80 mg/dose) every other day for 28 days; then taper over 4-6 weeks
Children and Adults: Physiologic replacement: 4-5 mg/m²/day
Adults: 5-60 mg/day in divided doses 1-4 times/day
Urticaria: 20 mg every 12 hours for 4 days
Elderly: Use the lowest effective dose
Erythema multiforme major: I.V.: Cyclophosphamide 150 mg over 1 hour every 24 hours for 2-3 days with prednisone (15 mg every 6 hours)

Monitoring Parameters Blood pressure, blood glucose, electrolytes

Administration Administer with meals to decrease gastrointestinal upset

Contraindications Hypersensitivity to prednisone or any component of the formulation; serious infections, except tuberculous meningitis; systemic fungal infections; varicella

Warnings Withdraw therapy with gradual tapering of dose, may retard bone growth. Use with caution in patients with hypothyroidism, cirrhosis, CHF, ulcerative colitis, thromboembolic disorders, and patients at increased risk for peptic ulcer disease. Corticosteroids should be used with caution in patients with diabetes, hypertension, osteoporosis, glaucoma, cataracts, or tuberculosis. Use caution in hepatic impairment. Because of the risk of adverse effects, systemic corticosteroids should be used cautiously in the elderly, in the smallest possible dose, and for the shortest possible time.

Dosage Forms Solution, oral: 1 mg/mL (5 mL, 120 mL, 500 mL) [contains alcohol 5%, sodium benzoate; vanilla flavor]
Solution, oral concentrate (Prednisone Intensol™): 5 mg/mL (30 mL) [contains alcohol 30%]
Tablet: 1 mg, 2.5 mg, 5 mg, 10 mg, 20 mg, 50 mg
Sterapred®: 5 mg [supplied as 21 tablet 6-day unit-dose package or 48 tablet 12-day unit-dose package]
Sterapred® DS: 10 mg [supplied as 21 tablet 6-day unit-dose package or 48 tablet 12-day unit-dose package]

Overdosage/Treatment
Decontamination: Activated charcoal; acute overdose does not require tapering of dose
Enhanced elimination: Its metabolite (prednisolone) is slightly dialyzable (5% to 20%)

Test Interactions Skin tests

Drug Interactions **Substrate** of CYP3A4 (minor); **Induces** CYP2C19 (weak), 3A4 (weak)
Decreased effect:
Barbiturates, phenytoin, rifampin decrease corticosteroid effectiveness
Decreases salicylates
Decreases vaccines
Decreases toxoids effectiveness
Increased effect/toxicity: NSAIDs: Concurrent use of prednisone may increase the risk of GI ulceration

Pregnancy Risk Factor B

Pregnancy Implications Crosses the placenta. Immunosuppression reported in 1 infant exposed to high-dose prednisone plus azathioprine throughout gestation. One report of congenital cataracts. Available evidence suggests safe use during pregnancy.

Lactation Enters breast milk/compatible

Nursing Implications Give with meals to decrease gastritis; withdraw therapy with gradual tapering of dose

Specific References
Aaron SD, Vandemheen KL, Hebert P, et al, "Outpatient Oral Prednisone After Emergency Treatment of Chronic Obstructive Pulmonary Disease," *N Engl J Med*, 2003, 348(26):2618-25.
Mitchell JC and Counselman FL, "A Taste Comparison of Three Different Liquid Steroid Preparations: Prednisone, Prednisolone, and Dexamethasone," *Acad Emerg Med*, 2003, 10(4):400-3.
Watts DC, Slawson MH, Borges CR, et al, "The Analysis of Glucocorticoids by HPLC-MS (Quadrupole) and HPLC-MS (Time of Flight)," *J Anal Toxicol*, 2006, 30:146-7.

Primidone

Related Information
- Seizures, Neonatal Guidelines
- Therapeutic Drugs Associated with Hallucinations

CAS Number 125-33-7

U.S. Brand Names Mysoline®

Synonyms Desoxyphenobarbital; Primaclone

Impairment Potential Yes

Use Management of grand mal, psychomotor, and focal seizures

Unlabeled/Investigational Use Benign familial tremor (essential tremor)

Mechanism of Action Decreases neuron excitability, raises seizure threshold similar to phenobarbital

Adverse Reactions

Cardiovascular: **Hypertension**, edema, syncope, palpitations

Central nervous system: **Headache, ataxia, drowsiness, dizziness, lethargy, behavior changes, sedation**, psychosis, irritability, visual hallucinations

Dermatologic: Rash

Gastrointestinal: Nausea, vomiting

Genitourinary: Crystalluria

Hematologic: Leukopenia, malignant lymphoma-like syndrome, anemia (megaloblastic), thrombocytopenia

Neuromuscular & skeletal: Weakness

Ocular: Diplopia, nystagmus, strabismus

Miscellaneous: Systemic lupus-like syndrome

Signs and Symptoms of Overdose Agranulocytosis, ankle clonus, confusion, crystalluria (white, hexagonal crystals), dementia, fever, granulocytopenia, hypotension, hypothermia, hypothyroidism, jaundice, leukopenia, loss of deep tendon reflexes, neutropenia, nystagmus, ptosis, severe flapping tremors, slurred speech, unsteady gait, vision color changes (green tinge)

Admission Criteria/Prognosis Admit any patient with markedly depressed mental status changes, crystalluria or primidone level >40 mcg/mL

Pharmacodynamics/Kinetics

Distribution: Adults: V_d: 2-3 L/kg

Protein binding: 99%

Metabolism: Hepatic to phenobarbital (active) and phenylethylmalonamide (PEMA)

Bioavailability: 60% to 80%

Half-life elimination (age dependent): Primidone: 10-12 hours; PEMA: 16 hours; Phenobarbital: 52-118 hours

Time to peak, serum: ~4 hours

Excretion: Urine (15% to 25% as unchanged drug and active metabolites)

Dosage

Oral:

Neonates: Loading dose: 15-25 mg/kg/dose as a single dose; 12-20 mg/kg/day in divided doses 2-4 times/day; start with lower dosage and titrate upward

Children <8 years: Initial: 50-125 mg/day given at bedtime; increase by 50-125 mg/day increments every 3-7 days; usual dose: 10-25 mg/kg/day in divided doses 3-4 times/day

Children ≥8 years and Adults: Initial: 125-250 mg/day at bedtime; increase by 125-250 mg/day every 3-7 days; usual dose: 750-1500 mg/day in divided doses 3-4 times/day with maximum dosage of 2 g/day

Dosing interval in renal impairment:

Cl_{cr} 50-80 mL/minute: Administer every 8 hours

Cl_{cr} 10-50 mL/minute: Administer every 8-12 hours

Cl_{cr} <10 mL/minute: Administer every 12-24 hours

Hemodialysis: Moderately dialyzable (20% to 50%); administer dose postdialysis or administer supplemental 30% dose

Stability Protect from light

Monitoring Parameters Serum primidone and phenobarbital concentration, CBC, neurological status. Due to CNS effects, monitor closely when initiating drug in elderly. Monitor CBC at 6-month intervals to compare with baseline obtained at start of therapy. Since elderly metabolize phenobarbital at a slower rate than younger adults, it is suggested to measure both primidone and phenobarbital levels together.

Contraindications Hypersensitivity to primidone, phenobarbital, or any component of the formulation; porphyria; pregnancy

Warnings Use with caution in patients with renal or hepatic impairment, pulmonary insufficiency; abrupt withdrawal may precipitate status epilepticus. Potential for drug dependency exists. Do not administer to patients in acute pain. Use caution in elderly, debilitated, or pediatric patients - may cause paradoxical responses. May cause CNS depression, which may impair physical or mental abilities. Patients must cautioned about performing tasks which require mental alertness (eg, operating machinery or driving). Effects with other sedative drugs or ethanol may be potentiated. Use with caution in patients with depression or suicidal tendencies, or in patients with a history of drug abuse. Tolerance or psychological and physical dependence may occur with prolonged use. Primidone's metabolite, phenobarbital, has been associated with cognitive deficits in children. Use with caution in patients with hypoadrenalism.

Dosage Forms Tablet: 50 mg, 250 mg [generic tablet may contain sodium benzoate]

Dosage forms available in Canada: Tablet: 125 mg, 250 mg. **Note:** 50 mg tablet is **not** available in Canada.

Reference Range

Therapeutic:

Children <5 years: 7-10 mcg/mL (SI: 32-46 μmol/L)

Adults: 5-12 mcg/mL (SI: 23-55 μmol/L); toxic effects rarely present with levels <10 mcg/mL (SI: <46 μmol/L) if phenobarbital concentrations are low

Dosage of primidone is adjusted with reference mostly to the phenobarbital level

Toxic: >15 mcg/mL (SI: >69 μmol/L) associated with ataxia and/or drowsiness

Serum primidone level required for urinary crystal formation: ~80 mg/L

Overdosage/Treatment

Decontamination: Gastric lavage; activated charcoal is effective

Supportive therapy: Hypotension: Isotonic I.V. fluid (10-20 mL/kg) is effective along with placement in Trendelenburg position; dopamine (2-5 mg/kg progressing to 5-10 mcg/kg) or norepinephrine (0.1-0.2 mcg/kg/minute for children or 8-12 mcg/kg in adults to a maintenance dose of 2-4 mcg/minute) is effective

Enhancement of elimination: Repeated oral doses of activated charcoal significantly reduce the half-life of primidone resulting from an enhancement of nonrenal elimination. The usual dose is 12.5-25 g every 1-2 hours until concentrations are <20 mg/L or the patient has no bowel movement, causing the charcoal to remain in the gastrointestinal tract. Assure adequate hydration and renal function. Urinary alkalinization with I.V. sodium bicarbonate also helps to enhance elimination. Hemodialysis is of uncertain value. Patients in stage IV coma due to high serum drug levels may require charcoal hemoperfusion; moderately dialyzable (20% to 50%); clearance by hemodialysis and hemoperfusion is ~98 mL/minute (~55% of drug removed in 4 hours).

Diagnostic Procedures

• Primidone, Blood

Test Interactions ↑ alkaline phosphatase (S); ↓ calcium (S)

Drug Interactions Metabolized to phenobarbital; **Induces** CYP1A2 (strong), 2B6 (strong), 2C8 (strong), 2C9 (strong), 3A4 (strong)

Acetaminophen: Barbiturates may enhance the hepatotoxic potential of acetaminophen overdoses

Antiarrhythmics: Barbiturates may increase the metabolism of antiarrhythmics, decreasing their clinical effect; includes disopyramide, propafenone, and quinidine

Anticonvulsants: Barbiturates may increase the metabolism of anticonvulsants; includes ethosuximide, felbamate (possibly), lamotrigine, phenytoin, tiagabine, topiramate, and zonisamide; does not appear to affect gabapentin or levetiracetam

Antineoplastics: Limited evidence suggests that enzyme-inducing anticonvulsant therapy may reduce the effectiveness of some chemotherapy regimens (specifically in ALL); teniposide and methotrexate may be cleared more rapidly in these patients

Antipsychotics: Barbiturates may enhance the metabolism (decrease the efficacy) of antipsychotics; monitor for altered response; dose adjustment may be needed

Beta-blockers: Metabolism of beta-blockers may be increased and clinical effect decreased; atenolol and nadolol are unlikely to interact given their renal elimination

Calcium channel blockers: Barbiturates may enhance the metabolism of calcium channel blockers, decreasing their clinical effect

Chloramphenicol: Barbiturates may increase the metabolism of chloramphenicol and chloramphenicol may inhibit barbiturate metabolism; monitor for altered response

Cimetidine: Barbiturates may enhance the metabolism of cimetidine, decreasing its clinical effect

CNS depressants: Sedative effects and/or respiratory depression with barbiturates may be additive with other CNS depressants; monitor for increased effect. Includes ethanol, sedatives, antidepressants, narcotic analgesics, and benzodiazepines

Corticosteroids: Barbiturates may enhance the metabolism of corticosteroids, decreasing their clinical effect

Cyclosporine: Levels may be decreased by barbiturates; monitor

CYP1A2 substrates: Primidone may decrease the levels/effects of CYP1A2 substrates. Example substrates include aminophylline, estrogens, fluvoxamine, mirtazapine, ropinirole, and theophylline.

CYP2B6 substrates: Primidone may decrease the levels/effects of CYP2B6 substrates. Example substrates include bupropion, efavirenz, promethazine, selegiline, and sertraline.

CYP2C8 Substrates: Primidone may decrease the levels/effects of CYP2C8 substrates. Example substrates include amiodarone, paclitaxel, pioglitazone, repaglinide, and rosiglitazone.

CYP2C9 Substrates: Primidone may decrease the levels/effects of CYP2C9 substrates. Example substrates include bosentan, celecoxib, dapsone, fluoxetine, glimepiride, glipizide, losartan, montelukast, nateglinide, paclitaxel, phenytoin, sulfonamides, trimethoprim, warfarin, and zafirlukast.

CYP3A4 substrates: Primidone may decrease the levels/effects of CYP3A4 substrates. Example substrates include benzodiazepines, calcium channel blockers, clarithromycin, cyclosporine, erythromycin, estrogens, mirtazapine, nateglinide, nefazodone, nevirapine, protease inhibitors, tacrolimus, and venlafaxine.

Doxycycline: Barbiturates may enhance the metabolism of doxycycline, decreasing its clinical effect; higher dosages may be required

Estrogens: Barbiturates may increase the metabolism of estrogens and reduce their efficacy

Felbamate may inhibit the metabolism of barbiturates and barbiturates may increase the metabolism of felbamate

Griseofulvin: Barbiturates may impair the absorption of griseofulvin, and griseofulvin metabolism may be increased by barbiturates, decreasing clinical effect

Guanfacine: Effect may be decreased by barbiturates

Immunosuppressants: Barbiturates may enhance the metabolism of immunosuppressants, decreasing its clinical effect; includes both cyclosporine and tacrolimus

Loop diuretics: Metabolism may be increased and clinical effects decreased; established for furosemide, effect with other loop diuretics not established

MAO inhibitors: Metabolism of barbiturates may be inhibited, increasing clinical effect or toxicity of the barbiturates

Methadone: Barbiturates may enhance the metabolism of methadone resulting in methadone withdrawal

Methoxyflurane: Barbiturates may enhance the nephrotoxic effects of methoxyflurane

Oral contraceptives: Barbiturates may enhance the metabolism of oral contraceptives, decreasing their clinical effect; an alternative method of contraception should be considered

Theophylline: Barbiturates may increase metabolism of theophylline derivatives and decrease their clinical effect

Tricyclic antidepressants: Barbiturates may increase metabolism of tricyclic antidepressants and decrease their clinical effect; sedative effects may be additive

Valproic acid: Metabolism of barbiturates may be inhibited by valproic acid; monitor for excessive sedation; a dose reduction may be needed

Warfarin: Barbiturates inhibit the hypoprothrombinemic effects of oral anticoagulants via increased metabolism; this combination should generally be avoided

Pregnancy Risk Factor D

Pregnancy Implications Crosses the placenta. Dysmorphic facial features; hemorrhagic disease of newborn due to fetal vitamin K depletion, maternal folic acid deficiency may occur. Epilepsy itself, number of medications, genetic factors, or a combination of these probably influence the teratogenicity of anticonvulsant therapy. Benefit: risk ratio usually favors continued use during pregnancy.

Lactation Enters breast milk/not recommended (AAP recommends use "with caution")

Nursing Implications Observe patient for excessive sedation

Additional Information Hepatic metabolism to active products (phenylethylmalonamide and phenobarbital)

Probenecid

CAS Number 57-66-9

Synonyms Benemid [DSC]

Use Prevention of gouty arthritis; hyperuricemia; prolongation of beta-lactam effect (ie, serum levels)

Mechanism of Action Competitively inhibits the reabsorption of uric acid at the proximal convoluted tubule, thereby promoting its excretion and reducing serum uric acid levels; increases plasma levels of weak organic acids (penicillins, cephalosporins, or other beta-lactam antibiotics) by competitively inhibiting their renal tubular secretion

Adverse Reactions

Cardiovascular: Flushing of face

Central nervous system: **Headache**, dizziness, tonic-clonic epilepsy

Dermatologic: Rash, itching, lichen planus

Gastrointestinal: **Anorexia, nausea, vomiting**, sore gums

Genitourinary: Painful urination

Hematologic: Leukopenia, hemolytic anemia, aplastic anemia

Hepatic: Hepatic necrosis

Neuromuscular & skeletal: **Gouty arthritis (acute)**

Ocular: Retinal edema

Renal: Renal calculi, urate nephropathy, nephrotic syndrome

Miscellaneous: Anaphylaxis

Signs and Symptoms of Overdose Coma, nausea, tonic-clonic seizures, tremors, visual hallucinations, vomiting.

Pharmacodynamics/Kinetics

Onset of action: Effect on penicillin levels: 2 hours

Absorption: Rapid and complete

Metabolism: Hepatic

Half-life elimination (dose dependent): Normal renal function: 6-12 hours

Time to peak, serum: 2-4 hours

Excretion: Urine

Dosage

Oral:

Children:

<2 years: Not recommended

2-14 years: Prolong penicillin serum levels: 25 mg/kg starting dose, then 40 mg/kg/day given 4 times/day

Gonorrhea: <45 kg: 25 mg/kg × 1 (maximum: 1 g/dose) 30 minutes before penicillin, ampicillin or amoxicillin

Adults:

Hyperuricemia with gout: 250 mg twice daily for 1 week; increase to 250-500 mg/day; may increase by 500 mg/month, if needed, to maximum of 2-3 g/day (dosages may be increased by 500 mg every 6 months if serum urate concentrations are controlled)

Prolong penicillin serum levels: 500 mg 4 times/day

Gonorrhea: 1 g 30 minutes before penicillin, ampicillin or amoxicillin

Dosing adjustment in renal impairment: Cl_{cr} <50 mL/minute: Avoid use

Monitoring Parameters Uric acid, renal function, CBC

Administration Administer with food or antacids to minimize GI effects

Contraindications Hypersensitivity to probenecid or any component of the formulation; high-dose aspirin therapy; blood dyscrasias; uric acid kidney stones; children <2 years of age

Warnings Use with caution in patients with peptic ulcer. Salicylates may diminish the therapeutic effect of probenecid. This effect may be more pronounced with high, chronic doses, however, the manufacturer recommends the use of an alternative analgesic even in place of small doses of aspirin. Use of probenecid with penicillin in patients with renal insufficiency is not recommended. Probenecid monotherapy may not be effective in patients with a creatinine clearance <30 mL/minute. May cause exacerbation of acute gouty attack

Dosage Forms Tablet: 500 mg

Reference Range Peak plasma probenecid level following a 2 g dose: ~149 mcg/mL between 3 and 4 hours

Overdosage/Treatment

Decontamination: Do not induce emesis; activated charcoal is especially effective at binding probenecid for GI contamination

Supportive therapy: Seizures should be treated with benzodiazepines and barbiturates

Test Interactions False-positive glucose (U) with Clinitest®

Drug Interactions

Inhibits CYP2C19 (weak)

Carbapenems (ertapenem, imipenem, meropenem): Probenecid may decrease the excretion of carbapenem antibiotics.

Cephalosporins: Probenecid may decrease the excretion of cephalosporin antibiotics. This effect is used advantageously in selected cases to increase serum antibiotic concentrations.

Dapsone: Probenecid may decrease the excretion of dapsone.

Methotrexate: Probenecid may decrease the excretion of methotrexate; concomitant use should be avoided. If used concomitantly, the methotrexate dosage will likely need reduced. Monitor for evidence of methotrexate toxicity.

Nonsteroidal anti-inflammatory agents: Probenecid may increase the serum concentration of NSAIDs. The manufacturer of ketorolac contraindicates concomitant use.

Penicillins: Probenecid may decrease the excretion of penicillin antibiotics. This effect is used advantageously in selected cases to increase serum antibiotic concentrations.

Salicylates: Salicylates may diminish the therapeutic effect of probenecid.

Thiopental: Probenecid may enhance the therapeutic effect of thiopental.

Zidovudine: Probenecid may decrease the metabolism of zidovudine.

Pregnancy Risk Factor B

Lactation Excretion in breast milk unknown

Specific References

Spina SP and Dillon EC Jr, "Effect of Chronic Probenecid Therapy on Cefazolin Serum Concentrations," *Ann Pharmacother*, 2003, 37(5):621-4.

Procainamide

Related Information

● Therapeutic Drugs Associated with Hallucinations

CAS Number 51-06-9; 614-39-1

U.S. Brand Names Procanbid®; Pronestyl-SR® [DSC]; Pronestyl® [DSC]

Synonyms PCA (error-prone abbreviation); Procainamide Hydrochloride; Procaine Amide Hydrochloride

Use Treatment of ventricular tachycardia (VT), premature ventricular contractions, paroxysmal atrial tachycardia (PSVT), and atrial fibrillation (AF); prevent recurrence of ventricular tachycardia, paroxysmal supraventricular tachycardia, atrial fibrillation or flutter

Unlabeled/Investigational Use ACLS guidelines:

Stable monomorphic VT (EF >40%, no CHF)

Stable wide complex tachycardia, likely VT (EF >40%, no CHF, patient stable)

Atrial fibrillation or flutter, including pre-excitation syndrome (EF >40%, no CHF)

AV reentrant, narrow complex tachycardia (eg, reentrant SVT) [preserved ventricular function]

PALS guidelines: Tachycardia with pulses and poor perfusion (possible VT)

Mechanism of Action Decreases myocardial excitability and conduction velocity and depresses myocardial contractility, by increasing the electrical stimulation threshold of ventricle, His-Purkinje system and through direct cardiac effects; classified as a Class IA antiarrhythmic agent

Adverse Reactions

Cardiovascular: Pericardial effusion/pericarditis, hypotension, tachycardia, cardiac arrhythmias, AV block, QT prolongation, QRS prolongation, myocarditis, sinus tachycardia, exacerbation of Brugada syndrome

Central nervous system: Confusion, psychosis, disorientation, fever, visual hallucinations, ataxia, gustatory hallucinations

Dermatologic: Rash, angioedema, purpura, pruritus, licheniform eruptions, exanthem, cutaneous vasculitis

Endocrine & metabolic: Nephrogenic diabetes insipidus

Gastrointestinal: Nausea, vomiting, gastrointestinal complaints, diarrhea, xerostomia

Genitourinary: Urinary retention

Hematologic: Agranulocytosis, neutropenia, thrombocytopenia, hemolysis, positive Coombs' test, red blood cell aplasia

Hepatic: Granulomatous hepatitis

Neuromuscular & skeletal: Arthralgia, myalgia, myopathy, rhabdomyolysis

Ocular: Blurred vision

Respiratory: Pleural effusion

Miscellaneous: Drug-induced **systemic lupus erythematosus**

Signs and Symptoms of Overdose
Agranulocytosis, anticholinergic toxidrome, AV block, coagulopathy, confusion, drowsiness, granulocytopenia, hemoptysis, hyperthermia, hypotension, intraventricular conduction delay, junctional tachycardia, leukopenia, mania, myasthenia gravis (exacerbation or precipitation), neutropenia, oliguria, QRS prolongation, renal failure, respiratory failure, torsade de pointes

Pharmacodynamics/Kinetics

Onset of action: I.M. 10-30 minutes

Distribution: V_d: Children: 2.2 L/kg; Adults: 2 L/kg; Congestive heart failure or shock: Decreased V_d

Protein binding: 15% to 20%

Metabolism: Hepatic via acetylation to produce N-acetyl procainamide (NAPA) (active metabolite)

Bioavailability: Oral: 75% to 95%

Half-life elimination:
Procainamide (hepatic acetylator, phenotype, cardiac and renal function dependent):
Children: 1.7 hours; Adults: 2.5-4.7 hours; Anephric: 11 hours
NAPA (dependent upon renal function):
Children: 6 hours; Adults: 6-8 hours; Anephric: 42 hours

Time to peak, serum: Capsule: 45 minutes to 2.5 hours; I.M.: 15-60 minutes

Excretion: Urine (25% as NAPA)

Dosage
Must be titrated to patient's response

Children:
Oral: 15-50 mg/kg/24 hours divided every 3-6 hours
I.M.: 50 mg/kg/24 hours divided into doses of $1/8$ to $1/4$ every 3-6 hours in divided doses until oral therapy is possible
I.V. (infusion requires use of an infusion pump):
Load: 3-6 mg/kg/dose over 5 minutes not to exceed 100 mg/dose; may repeat every 5-10 minutes to maximum of 15 mg/kg/load
Maintenance as continuous I.V. infusion: 20-80 mcg/kg/minute; maximum: 2 g/24 hours
Possible VT (pulses and poor perfusion) [PALS 2005 Guidelines]: I.V.; I.O.: 15 mg/kg over 30-60 minutes

Adults:
Oral: Usual dose: 50 mg/kg/24 hours: maximum: 5 g/24 hours (**Note:** Twice-daily dosing approved for Procanbid®.)
Immediate release formulation: 250-500 mg/dose every 3-6 hours
Extended release formulation: 500 mg to 1 g every 6 hours; Procanbid®: 1000-2500 mg every 12 hours
I.M.: 0.5-1 g every 4-8 hours until oral therapy is possible
I.V. (infusion requires use of an infusion pump):
Loading dose: 15-18 mg/kg administered as slow infusion over 25-30 minutes **or** 100-200 mg/dose repeated every 5 minutes as needed to a total dose of 1 g. Reduce loading dose to 12 mg/kg in severe renal or cardiac impairment.
Maintenance dose: 1-4 mg/minute by continuous infusion. Maintenance infusions should be reduced by one-third in patients with moderate renal or cardiac impairment and by two-thirds in patients with severe renal or cardiac impairment.
ACLS guidelines: Infuse 20 mg/minute until arrhythmia is controlled, hypotension occurs, QRS complex widens by 50% of its original width, or total of 17 mg/kg is given.

Dosing interval in renal impairment:
Oral:
Cl_{cr} 10-50 mL/minute: Administer every 6-12 hours.
Cl_{cr} <10 mL/minute: Administer every 8-24 hours.
I.V.:
Loading dose: Reduce dose to 12 mg/kg in severe renal impairment.

Maintenance infusion: Reduce dose by one-third in patients with mild renal impairment. Reduce dose by two-thirds in patients with severe renal impairment.

Dialysis:
Procainamide: Moderately hemodialyzable (20% to 50%): 200 mg supplemental dose posthemodialysis is recommended.
N-acetylprocainamide: Not dialyzable (0% to 5%)
Procainamide/N-acetylprocainamide: Not peritoneal dialyzable (0% to 5%)
Procainamide/N-acetylprocainamide: Replace by blood level during continuous arteriovenous or venovenous hemofiltration

Dosing adjustment in hepatic impairment: Reduce dose by 50%.

Stability
Use only clear or slightly yellow solutions; store in airtight containers
Stability of parenteral admixture at room temperature (25°C): 24 hours
Stability of parenteral admixture at refrigeration temperature (4°C): 24 hours

Monitoring Parameters
ECG, blood pressure, CBC with differential, platelet count; cardiac monitor and blood pressure monitor required during I.V. administration; blood levels in patients with renal failure or receiving constant infusion >3 mg/minute for longer than 24 hours

Administration
Dilute I.V. With D_5W; maximum rate: 50 mg/minute; administer around-the-clock rather than 4 times/day to promote less variation in peak and trough serum levels. Do **not** crush or chew extended release drug product.

Contraindications
Hypersensitivity to procaine, other ester-type local anesthetics, or any component of the formulation; complete heart block (except in patients with a functioning artificial pacemaker); second-degree AV block (without a functional pacemaker); various types of hemiblock (without a functional pacemaker); SLE; torsade de pointes; concurrent cisapride use; QT prolongation

Warnings
Monitor and adjust dose to prevent QT_c prolongation. Watch for proarrhythmic effects. May precipitate or exacerbate CHF. Reduce dosage in renal impairment. May increase ventricular response rate in patients with atrial fibrillation or flutter; control AV conduction before initiating. Correct hypokalemia before initiating therapy. Hypokalemia may worsen toxicity. Use caution in digoxin-induced toxicity (can further depress AV conduction). Reduce dose if first-degree heart block occurs. Use caution with concurrent use of other antiarrhythmics. Avoid use in myasthenia gravis (may worsen condition). Hypersensitivity reactions can occur. Some tablets contain tartrazine; injection may contain bisulfite (allergens).

Potentially fatal blood dyscrasias have occurred with therapeutic doses; close monitoring is recommended during the first 3 months of therapy.

[U.S. Boxed Warning]: Long-term administration leads to the development of a positive antinuclear antibody (ANA) test in 50% of patients which may result in a drug-induced lupus erythematosus-like syndrome (in 20% to 30% of patients); discontinue procainamide with SLE symptoms and choose an alternative agent

Dosage Forms
Capsule, as hydrochloride: 250 mg, 500 mg
Injection, solution, as hydrochloride: 100 mg/mL (10 mL); 500 mg/mL (2 mL) [contains sodium metabisulfite]
Tablet, extended release, as hydrochloride: 500 mg, 750 mg, 1000 mg
Procanbid®: 500 mg, 1000 mg

Reference Range
Therapeutic: 4-10 mcg/mL for procainamide, <30 mcg/mL for sum of procainamide and N-acetyl procainamide; NAPA levels: 10-30 mcg/mL. Optimal ranges must be ascertained for individual patients, with ECG monitoring.
Toxic (procainamide): >14 mcg/mL (SI: >59.5 μmol/L)

Overdosage/Treatment
Decontamination: Ipecac within 30 minutes or lavage (within 1 hour)/ activated charcoal
Supportive therapy: Hypotension usually responds to I.V. fluids or Trendelenburg positioning. If unresponsive to these measures, the use of a parenteral inotrope may be required (eg, norepinephrine 0.1-0.2 mcg/kg/minute titrated to response). Concurrent sodium bicarbonate and sodium lactate infusions have been effective in reversing the drug-induced cardiac toxicity. Avoid quinidine, disopyramide, and beta-adrenergic blockers.
Enhancement of elimination: Multiple dosing of activated charcoal may be effective; hemodialysis or charcoal hemoperfusion are effective in decreasing half-life; NAPA is more effectively removed by hemoperfusion; forced diuresis or peritoneal dialysis is not effective; moderately dialyzable (20% to 50%); hemodialysis clearance of procainamide and NAPA: 65 mL/minute and 45 mL/minute respectively. ~78% of procainamide (and 49% of NAPA) concentration is fractionally removed during 4 hours of hemodialysis. Continuous arteriovenous hemodiafiltration using a high dialysate flow rate can enhance elimination of N-acetylprocainamide.

Drug Interactions
Substrate of CYP2D6 (major)

Amiodarone increases procainamide and NAPA blood levels; consider reducing procainamide dosage by 25% with concurrent use.

Cimetidine increases procainamide and NAPA blood concentrations; monitor blood levels closely or use an alternative H$_2$ antagonist.

Cisapride and procainamide may increase the risk of malignant arrhythmia; concurrent use is contraindicated.

CYP2D6 inhibitors: May increase the levels/effects of procainamide. Example inhibitors include chlorpromazine, delavirdine, fluoxetine, miconazole, paroxetine, pergolide, quinidine, quinine, ritonavir, and ropinirole.

Neuromuscular blocking agents: Procainamide may potentiate neuromuscular blockade.

Ofloxacin may increase procainamide levels due to an inhibition of renal secretion; monitor levels for procainamide closely.

QT$_c$-prolonging agents (eg, amiodarone, amitriptyline, bepridil, disopyramide, erythromycin, haloperidol, imipramine, pimozide, quinidine, sotalol, and thioridazine): Effects/toxicity may be increased; use with caution.

Sparfloxacin, gatifloxacin, and moxifloxacin may result in additional prolongation of the QT interval; concurrent use is contraindicated.

Trimethoprim increases procainamide and NAPA blood levels; closely monitor levels.

Pregnancy Risk Factor C

Lactation Enters breast milk/use caution (AAP rates "compatible")

Procaine

CAS Number 51-05-8; 59-46-1

U.S. Brand Names Novocain®

Synonyms Procaine Hydrochloride

Use Produce spinal anesthesia and epidural and peripheral nerve block by injection and infiltration methods

Mechanism of Action Blocks both the initiation and conduction of nerve impulses by decreasing the neuronal membrane's permeability to sodium ions, which results in inhibition of depolarization with resultant blockade of conduction

Adverse Reactions

Cardiovascular: Sinus bradycardia, sinus tachycardia

Central nervous system: Aseptic meningitis resulting in paralysis can occur, CNS stimulation followed by CNS depression, psychosis, paranoia, hallucinations, chills

Dermatologic: Skin discoloration; photoallergy

Gastrointestinal: Nausea, vomiting

Local: Burning sensation and pain at site of injection, tissue irritation

Ocular: Miosis, nystagmus, diplopia

Otic: Ototoxicity, tinnitus

Signs and Symptoms of Overdose Cardiac arrhythmias, coma, hypertension, mydriasis, seizures, tachycardia, tachypnea progressing to apnea

Pharmacodynamics/Kinetics

Onset of action: 2-5 minutes

Duration (patient, type of block, concentration, and method of anesthesia dependent); 0.5-1.5 hours

Metabolism: Rapidly hydrolyzed by plasma enzymes to para-aminobenzoic acid and diethylaminoethanol (80% conjugated before elimination)

Half-life elimination: 7.7 minutes

Excretion: Urine (as metabolites and some unchanged drug)

Dosage Dose varies with procedure, desired depth, and duration of anesthesia, desired muscle relaxation, vascularity of tissues, physical condition, and age of patient; maximum dose: 7 mg/kg; maximum dose with epinephrine: 9 mg/kg

Administration Prior to instillation of anesthetic agent, withdraw plunger to ensure needle is not in artery or vein; resuscitative equipment should be available when local anesthetics are administered

Contraindications Hypersensitivity to procaine, PABA, parabens, other ester local anesthetics, or any component of the formulation

Warnings Patients with cardiac diseases, hyperthyroidism, or other endocrine diseases may be more susceptible to toxic effects of local anesthetics; some preparations contain metabisulfite

Dosage Forms Injection, solution, as hydrochloride: 1% [10 mg/mL] (2 mL) [contains sodium bisulfite]; 10% (2 mL) [contains sodium bisulfite]

Reference Range

Therapeutic: 3-11 mcg/mL

Toxic: >20 mcg/mL are associated with toxicity

Overdosage/Treatment Supportive therapy: Termination of anesthesia by pneumatic tourniquet inflation should be attempted when the agent is administered by infiltration or regional injection. Seizures commonly respond to diazepam or lorazepam, while hypotension responds to I.V. fluids and Trendelenburg positioning. Bradyarrhythmias (when the heart rate is less than 60) can be treated with I.V., I.M., or SubQ atropine 15 mcg/kg. With the development of metabolic acidosis, I.V. sodium bicarbonate 0.5-2 mEq/kg and ventilatory assistance should be instituted. Chlorpromazine may be used to treat acute psychosis.

Drug Interactions Decreased effect of sulfonamides with the PABA metabolite of procaine, chloroprocaine, and tetracaine

Decreased/increased effect of vasopressors, ergot alkaloids, and MAO inhibitors on blood pressure when using anesthetic solutions with a vasoconstrictor

Pregnancy Risk Factor C

Lactation Excretion in breast milk unknown

Procarbazine

CAS Number 366-70-1; 671-16-9

U.S. Brand Names Matulane®

Synonyms Benzmethyzin; N-Methylhydrazine; NSC-77213; Procarbazine Hydrochloride

Use Treatment of Hodgkin's disease

Unlabeled/Investigational Use Treatment of non-Hodgkin's lymphoma, brain tumors, melanoma, lung cancer, multiple myeloma

Mechanism of Action Mechanism of action is not clear, methylating of nucleic acids; inhibits DNA, RNA, and protein synthesis; may damage DNA directly and suppress mitosis in the S phase of cell division; metabolic activation required by host

Adverse Reactions

Cardiovascular: Hypotension (orthostatic), hypertensive crisis

Central nervous system: **Manic reactions**, coma, **hallucinations**, psychosis, mania, **dizziness, headache, nervousness, insomnia, night terrors, disorientation**, foot drop, decreased reflexes, somnolence, **confusion, seizures**, hyperpyrexia, irritability, **ataxia**, CNS depression, **mental depression, CNS stimulation**, hyperthermia

Dermatologic: Alopecia, pruritus, dermatitis, alopecia, hypersensitivity rash, hyperpigmentation

Endocrine & metabolic: **Amenorrhea**

Gastrointestinal: Severe **nausea and vomiting** occur frequently and may be dose-limiting; **anorexia, abdominal pain, stomatitis, dysphagia, diarrhea**, and **constipation**; use a nonphenothiazine antiemetic, when possible

Genitourinary: Azoospermia, urinary frequency, nocturia

Hematologic: May be dose-limiting toxicity; procarbazine should be discontinued if leukocyte count is <4000 mL or platelet count <100,000 mL; leukopenia, **thrombocytopenia, hemolytic anemia**

Hepatic: Hepatotoxicity, jaundice

Neuromuscular & skeletal: Neuropathy (peripheral), arthralgia, myalgia, tremors, **paresthesia, weakness, tremors, decreased reflexes, foot drop**

Ocular: **Nystagmus**, diplopia, photophobia

Renal: Hematuria

Respiratory: **Pleural effusion, cough**, interstitial pneumonitis, hoarseness

Miscellaneous: Secondary malignancy, flu-like syndrome

Signs and Symptoms of Overdose Alopecia, arthralgia, bone marrow depression, coma, diarrhea, hallucinations, nausea, paresthesia, seizures, vomiting

Pharmacodynamics/Kinetics

Absorption: Rapid and complete

Distribution: Crosses blood-brain barrier; distributes into CSF

Metabolism: Hepatic and renal

Half-life elimination: 1 hour

Excretion: Urine and respiratory tract (<5% as unchanged drug, 70% as metabolites)

Dosage Refer to individual protocols. Dose based on patient's ideal weight if the patient is obese or has abnormal fluid retention. Oral (may be given as a single daily dose or in 2-3 divided doses):

Children:

BMT aplastic anemia conditioning regimen: 12.5 mg/kg/dose every other day for 4 doses

Hodgkin's disease: MOPP/IC-MOPP regimens: 100 mg/m^2/day for 14 days and repeated every 4 weeks

Neuroblastoma and medulloblastoma: Doses as high as 100-200 mg/m^2/day once daily have been used

Adults: Initial: 2-4 mg/kg/day in single or divided doses for 7 days then increase dose to 4-6 mg/kg/day until response is obtained or leukocyte count decreased <4000/mm^3 or the platelet count decreased <100,000/mm^3; maintenance: 1-2 mg/kg/day

Dosing in renal/hepatic impairment: Use with caution, may result in increased toxicity; decrease dose if serum creatinine >2 mg/dL or total bilirubin >3 mg/dL

Stability Protect from light

Monitoring Parameters CBC with differential, platelet and reticulocyte count, urinalysis, liver function test, renal function test.

Contraindications Hypersensitivity to procarbazine or any component of the formulation; pre-existing bone marrow aplasia; ethanol ingestion; pregnancy

Warnings Hazardous agent – use appropriate precautions for handling and disposal. Use with caution in patients with pre-existing renal or hepatic impairment; procarbazine possesses MAO inhibitor activity.

Procarbazine is a carcinogen which may cause acute leukemia; procarbazine may cause infertility. **[U.S. Boxed Warning]: Should be administered under the supervision of an experienced cancer chemotherapy physician.**

Dosage Forms Capsule, as hydrochloride: 50 mg

Overdosage/Treatment

Decontamination: Lavage (within 1 hour)/activated charcoal

Supportive therapy: Adverse effects, such as marrow toxicity may begin as late as 2-8 weeks after exposure. Hypotension can be treated with isotonic saline (10-20 mL/kg) and Trendelenburg positioning. Refractory hypotension can be treated with treated with dopamine or norepinephrine. Bone marrow depression can be treated with filgrastim (5 mcg/kg/day I.V. or SubQ) for 2 weeks or until absolute neutrophil count exceeds 10,000 cells/mm^3.

Test Interactions ↑ potassium (S)

Drug Interactions Increased toxicity:

Procarbazine exhibits weak monoamine oxidase (MAO) inhibitor activity; foods containing high amounts of tyramine should, therefore, be avoided (ie, beer, yogurt, yeast, wine, cheese, pickled herring, chicken liver, and bananas). When a MAO inhibitor is given with food high in tyramine, a hypertensive crisis, intracranial bleeding, and headache have been reported.

Sympathomimetic amines (epinephrine and amphetamines) and antidepressants (tricyclics) should be used cautiously with procarbazine.

Barbiturates, narcotics, phenothiazines, and other CNS depressants can cause somnolence, ataxia, and other symptoms of CNS depression

Ethanol has caused a disulfiram-like reaction with procarbazine; may result in headache, respiratory difficulties, nausea, vomiting, sweating, thirst, hypotension, and flushing

Pregnancy Risk Factor D

Pregnancy Implications Teratogenic with genitourinary malformations, oligodactyly, ventricular septal defects, cerebral hemorrhage, growth retardation, and hemangiomas present

Lactation Excretion in breast milk unknown/not recommended

Nursing Implications Protect from light

Additional Information Toxic dose: 1 g/m^2. Myelosuppressive effects: **WBC**: Moderate. **Platelets**: Moderate: Onset (days): 14. Nadir (days): 21. Recovery (days): 28

Prochlorperazine

CAS Number 58-38-8

U.S. Brand Names Compazine® [DSC]; Compro™

Synonyms Chlormeprazine; Compazine; Prochlorperazine Edisylate; Prochlorperazine Maleate

Impairment Potential Yes

Use Management of nausea and vomiting; psychosis; anxiety

Behavioral syndromes in dementia

Mechanism of Action Blocks postsynaptic mesolimbic dopaminergic receptors in the brain, including the medullary chemoreceptor trigger zone; exhibits a strong alpha-adrenergic blocking effect and depresses the release of hypothalamic and hypophyseal hormones

Adverse Reactions

Cardiovascular: **Hypotension** (especially with I.V. use), **hypotension (orthostatic), tachycardia, cardiac arrhythmias**, sinus tachycardia

Central nervous system: Sedation, drowsiness, restlessness, anxiety, extrapyramidal reactions, **pseudoparkinsonian signs and symptoms, tardive dyskinesia**, neuroleptic malignant syndrome, seizures, altered central temperature regulation, **dizziness, dystonias**

Dermatologic: **Hyperpigmentation**, pruritus, rash, photosensitivity, exfoliative dermatitis, toxic epidermal necrolysis, urticaria, purpura, exanthem

Endocrine & metabolic: Amenorrhea, galactorrhea, gynecomastia, syndrome of inappropriate antidiuretic hormone

Gastrointestinal: GI upset, **xerostomia, constipation**, weight gain

Genitourinary: **Urinary retention**, impotence

Hematologic: Leukopenia, neutropenia, agranulocytosis, granulocytopenia, (usually in patients with large doses for prolonged periods), thrombocytopenia, hemolysis, eosinophilia

Hepatic: Cholestatic jaundice

Ocular: **Retinal pigmentation**, photophobia, **blurred vision**, phototoxic

Miscellaneous: Anaphylactoid reactions, systemic lupus erythematosus, **diaphoresis (decreased)**, fixed drug eruption

Signs and Symptoms of Overdose Akathisia, coma, deep sleep, extrapyramidal reaction, photosensitivity, impotence, muscle spasm, neuroleptic malignant syndrome, nystagmus, Parkinson's-like symptoms, urine discoloration (pink; red; red-brown), vision color changes (brown tinge)

Pharmacodynamics/Kinetics

Onset of action: Oral: 30-40 minutes; I.M.: 10-20 minutes; Rectal: ~60 minutes

Peak antiemetic effect: I.V.: 30-60 minutes

Duration: Rectal: 12 hours; Oral: 3-4 hours; I.M., I.V.: Adults: 4-6 hours; I.M.: Children: 12 hours

Distribution: V$_d$: 1400-1548 L; crosses placenta; enters breast milk

Metabolism: Primarily hepatic; N-desmethyl prochlorperazine (major active metabolite)

Bioavailability: Oral: 12.5%

Half-life elimination: Oral: 3-5 hours; I.V.: ~7 hours

Dosage

Children >10 kg:

Oral, rectal: 0.4 mg/kg/24 hours in 3-4 divided doses; **or**

9-14 kg: 2.5 mg every 12-24 hours as needed; maximum: 7.5 mg/day

14-18 kg: 2.5 mg every 8-12 hours as needed; maximum: 10 mg/day

18-39 kg: 2.5 mg every 8 hours or 5 mg every 12 hours as needed; maximum: 15 mg/day

I.M.: 0.1-0.15 mg/kg/dose; usual: 0.13 mg/kg/dose; change to oral as soon as possible

I.V.: Not recommended in children <10 kg or <2 years

Adults:

Oral: 5-10 mg 3-4 times/day or sustained release twice daily; usual maximum: 40 mg/day; doses up to 150 mg/day may be required in some patients for treatment of severe psychotic disturbances

I.M.: 5-10 mg every 3-4 hours; usual maximum: 40 mg/day; doses up to 10-20 mg every 4-6 hours may be required in some patients for treatment of severe psychotic disturbances

I.V.: 2.5-10 mg; maximum 10 mg/dose or 40 mg/day; may repeat dose every 3-4 hours as needed

Rectal: 25 mg twice daily

Stability

Injection: Intact vials/ampuls for injection are stable at room temperature; protect from light; clear or slightly yellow solutions may be used.

I.V. infusion: Injection may be diluted in 50-100 mL NS or D$_5$W.

Suppository: May require refrigeration

Tablet: Stable at room temperature

Monitoring Parameters Vital signs; lipid profile, fasting blood glucose/Hgb A$_{1c}$; BMI; mental status, abnormal involuntary movement scale (AIMS); periodic ophthalmic exams (if chronically used); extrapyramidal symptoms (EPS)

Administration

May be administered orally, I.M., or I.V.: I.V. doses should be given as a short (~30 minute) infusion or by slow (5-10 minutes) IVP to avoid orthostatic hypotension.

Contraindications Hypersensitivity to prochlorperazine or any component of the formulation (cross-reactivity between phenothiazines may occur); severe CNS depression; coma; pediatric surgery; Reye's syndrome; should not be used in children <2 years of age or <9 kg

Warnings

May be sedating; use with caution in disorders where CNS depression is a feature. May obscure intestinal obstruction or brain tumor. May impair physical or mental abilities; patients must be cautioned about performing tasks which require mental alertness (eg, operating machinery or driving). Effects with other sedative drugs or ethanol may be potentiated. Use with caution in Parkinson's disease; hemodynamic instability; bone marrow suppression; predisposition to seizures; subcortical brain damage; and in severe cardiac, hepatic, renal or respiratory disease. Caution in breast cancer or other prolactin-dependent tumors (may elevate prolactin levels). May alter temperature regulation or mask toxicity of other drugs. Use caution with exposure to heat. May alter cardiac conduction; life-threatening arrhythmias have occurred with therapeutic doses of phenothiazines. May cause orthostatic hypotension; use with caution in patients at risk of hypotension or where transient hypotensive episodes would be poorly tolerated (cardiovascular disease or cerebrovascular disease). Hypotension may occur following administration, particularly when parenteral form is used or in high dosages.

Phenothiazines may cause anticholinergic effects (eg, constipation, xerostomia, blurred vision, urinary retention); therefore, they should be used with caution in patients with decreased gastrointestinal motility, urinary retention, BPH, xerostomia, or visual problems. Conditions which also may be exacerbated by cholinergic blockade include narrow-angle glaucoma (screening is recommended) and worsening of myasthenia gravis. May cause extrapyramidal symptoms, including pseudoparkinsonism, acute dystonic reactions, akathisia, and tardive dyskinesia (TD). Use caution in the the elderly; incidence of TD may be increased. Children with acute illness or dehydration are more susceptible to neuromuscular reactions (eg, dystonias); use cautiously. May be associated with neuroleptic malignant syndrome (NMS).

Dosage Forms

Injection, solution, as edisylate: 5 mg/mL (2 mL, 10 mL) [contains benzyl alcohol]

Suppository, rectal: 2.5 mg (12s), 5 mg (12s), 25 mg (12s) [may contain coconut and palm oil]

Compro™: 25 mg (12s) [contains coconut and palm oils]

Tablet, as maleate: 5 mg, 10 mg

Reference Range Blood level >1 mcg/mL associated with toxicity

Overdosage/Treatment

Decontamination: Activated charcoal; charcoal may need to be given in multiple doses for adequate decontamination

Supportive therapy: Initiate support with fluids, norepinephrine may be useful for hypotension; hypoperfusion states may respond to inotropic support with dobutamine. Bradyarrhythmia or ventricular dysrhythmia may respond to sodium bicarbonate or phenytoin; must avoid class IA and IC antiarrhythmics. Torsade de pointes may respond to magnesium; seizures should be managed with benzodiazepines or barbiturates; extrapyramidal reactions should be managed with diphenhydramine or benztropine.

Enhancement of elimination: Multiple dosing of charcoal may not be effective; not dialyzable

Test Interactions False-positives for phenylketonuria, urinary amylase, uroporphyrins, urobilinogen

Drug Interactions Acetylcholinesterase inhibitors (central): May increase the risk of antipsychotic-related extrapyramidal symptoms; monitor.

Alpha-/Beta- agonists: May enhance the arrhythmogenic effect of phenothiazines.

Analgesics (narcotic): Phenothiazines may enhance the hypotensive effect of narcotic analgesics.

Antacids: May decrease the absorption of phenothiazines; monitor.

Antidepressants (serotonin reuptake inhibitors/antagonist): Concurrent use may produce increased hypotension.

Anticholinergics: May inhibit the therapeutic response to phenothiazines and excess anticholinergic effects may occur; includes benztropine, trihexyphenidyl, biperiden, and drugs with significant anticholinergic activity (TCAs, antihistamines, disopyramide)

Antihistamines: May enhance the arrhythmogenic effect of phenothiazines.

Antimalarial agents: May increase phenothiazine concentrations.

Antiparkinson's Agents (dopamine agonists such as levodopa): Phenothiazines may inhibit the antiparkinsonian effect of levodopa; avoid this combination.

Attapulgite: May decrease absorption of phenothiazines.

Beta blockers: Serum concentrations of phenothiazines may be increased; phenothiazines may increase hypotensive effects of beta blockers.

CNS depressants: Sedative effects may be additive with phenothiazines; monitor for increased effect; includes barbiturates, benzodiazepines, narcotic analgesics, ethanol and other sedative agents.

Epinephrine: Chlorpromazine (and possibly other low potency antipsychotics) may diminish the pressor effects of epinephrine.

False Neurotransmitters (guanadrel, methyldopa): Antihypertensive effects may be inhibited by phenothiazines.

Lithium: Phenothiazines may produce neurotoxicity with lithium; this is a rare effect Phenytoin: Concurrent use may increase CNS depression.

Polypeptide antibiotics: Rare cases of respiratory paralysis have been reported with concurrent use of phenothiazines.

Pramlintide: May enhance the anticholinergic effects of phenothiazines.

QT_c-prolonging agents: Effects on QT_c interval may be additive with phenothiazines, increasing the risk of malignant arrhythmias; includes type Ia antiarrhythmics, TCAs, and some quinolone antibiotics (sparfloxacin, moxifloxacin, and gatifloxacin).

Pregnancy Risk Factor C

Pregnancy Implications Crosses the placenta

Lactation Excretion in breast milk unknown/use caution

Specific References

Walker M and Samii A, "Chronic Severe Dystonia After Single Exposure to Antiemetics," *Am J Emerg Med*, 2006, 24(1):125-7.

Proguanil

CAS Number 500-92-5; 637-32-1

Use Malarial prophylaxis (*Plasmodium falciparum* and *vivax*)

Mechanism of Action Proguanil's active metabolite (cycloguanil) inhibits nucleic acid synthesis by antagonizing *Plasmodium* dihydrofolate reductase; active against pre-erythrocytic forms with some sporontocidal activity

Adverse Reactions

Central nervous system: Dizziness

Dermatologic: Urticaria, alopecia (reversible), exanthema, photosensitivity

Gastrointestinal: Anorexia, vomiting, diarrhea, aphthous ulceration

Hematologic: Pancytopenia, megaloblastic anemia, thrombocytopenia, aplastic anemia (1:10,000 patient years), neutropenia

Miscellaneous: Thirst

Signs and Symptoms of Overdose Abdominal pain, hematuria (due to renal irritation), vomiting

Toxicodynamics/Kinetics

Absorption: 2-4 hours

Distribution: V_d: 30.7 L/kg

Protein binding: 75%

Metabolism: Hepatic metabolism to an active metabolite cycloguanil

Half-life: Proguanil: 18-40 hours; Cycloguanil: 11.7 hours

Elimination: Primary: Renal tubular secretion (renal clearance ~0.3 L/hour/kg); feces (10%)

Dosage Malaria prophylaxis may be used with chloroquine:

Adults: 200 mg/day beginning at least 1 day before entering a malarious region and for 6 weeks after leaving the area; lower dosage in renal failure

Children:

<1 year: 25 mg once daily

1-4 years: 50 mg once daily

5-8 years: 100 mg once daily

9-14 years: 150 mg once daily

>14 years: 200 mg once daily

Monitoring Parameters CBC

Reference Range Maximum proguanil and cycloguanil plasma levels after a 200 mg dose: ~170 ng/mL and 41 ng/mL, respectively

Overdosage/Treatment

Decontamination (for acute ingestions >5 mg/kg): Ipecac within 30 minutes or lavage (within 1 hour)/activated charcoal

Supportive therapy: Folate can be given to treat megaloblastic anemia

Enhanced elimination: Hemodialysis is not effective

Pregnancy Implications No adverse effects on fetus; documented folate supplements may need to be given

Promethazine

Related Information

• Therapeutic Drugs Associated with Hallucinations

CAS Number 58-33-3; 60-87-7

U.S. Brand Names Phenadoz™; Phenergan®

Synonyms Promethazine Hydrochloride

Impairment Potential Yes

Use Symptomatic treatment of various allergic conditions; antiemetic; motion sickness; sedative; postoperative pain (adjunctive therapy); anesthetic (adjunctive therapy); anaphylactic reactions (adjunctive therapy)

Mechanism of Action Blocks postsynaptic mesolimbic dopaminergic receptors in the brain; exhibits a strong alpha-adrenergic blocking effect and depresses the release of hypothalamic and hypophyseal hormones; competes with histamine for the H_1-receptor; reduces stimuli to the brainstem reticular system

Adverse Reactions

Cardiovascular: Bradycardia, hypertension, postural hypotension, tachycardia, nonspecific QT changes

Central nervous system: Catatonic states, confusion, disorientation, dizziness, drowsiness, dystonias, euphoria, excitation, extrapyramidal symptoms, fatigue, hallucinations, hysteria, insomnia, akathisia, pseudoparkinsonism, tardive dyskinesia, nervousness, neuroleptic malignant syndrome, sedation, seizures, somnolence

Dermatologic: Angioneurotic edema, photosensitivity, dermatitis, skin pigmentation (slate gray), urticaria

Endocrine & metabolic: Lactation, breast engorgement, amenorrhea, gynecomastia, hyper- or hypoglycemia

Gastrointestinal: Xerostomia, constipation, nausea, vomiting

Genitourinary: Urinary retention, ejaculatory disorder, impotence

Hematologic: Agranulocytosis, eosinophilia, leukopenia, hemolytic anemia, aplastic anemia, thrombocytopenia, thrombocytopenic purpura

Hepatic: Jaundice

Neuromuscular & skeletal: Incoordination, tremors

Ocular: Blurred vision, corneal and lenticular changes, diplopia, epithelial keratopathy, pigmentary retinopathy

Otic: Tinnitus

Respiratory: Apnea, respiratory depression

Signs and Symptoms of Overdose Agranulocytosis, anticholinergic hallucinations, anticholinergic toxidrome, CNS depression, coma, dry mouth, eclampsia, fever, flushing, granulocytopenia, hyperreflexia, hyperthermia, impotence, leukemoid reaction, leukopenia, mydriasis, myoclonus, neutropenia, seizures, tachycardia, urine discoloration (pink; red; red-brown), vision color changes (brown tinge)

Pharmacodynamics/Kinetics

Onset of action: I.M.: ~20 minutes; I.V.: 3-5 minutes

Peak effect: C_{max}: 9.04 ng/mL (suppository); 19.3 ng/mL (syrup)

Duration: 2-6 hours

Absorption:

I.M.: Bioavailability may be greater than with oral or rectal administration

Oral: Rapid and complete; large first pass effect limits systemic bioavailability

Distribution: V_d: 171 L

Protein binding: 93%

Metabolism: Hepatic; primarily oxidation; forms metabolites

Half-life elimination: 9-16 hours

Time to maximum serum concentration: 4.4 hours (syrup); 6.7-8.6 hours (suppositories)

Excretion: Primarily urine and feces (as inactive metabolites)

Dosage Children ≥2 years:

Allergic conditions: Oral, rectal: 0.1 mg/kg/dose (maximum: 12.5 mg) every 6 hours during the day and 0.5 mg/kg/dose (maximum: 25 mg) at bedtime as needed

Antiemetic: Oral, I.M., I.V., rectal: 0.25-1 mg/kg 4-6 times/day as needed (maximum: 25 mg/dose)

Motion sickness: Oral, rectal: 0.5 mg/kg/dose 30 minutes to 1 hour before departure, then every 12 hours as needed (maximum dose: 25 mg twice daily)

Sedation: Oral, I.M., I.V., rectal: 0.5-1 mg/kg/dose every 6 hours as needed (maximum: 50 mg/dose)

Adults:

Allergic conditions (including allergic reactions to blood or plasma): Oral, rectal: 12.5 mg 3 times/day and 25 mg at bedtime

I.M., I.V.: 25 mg, may repeat in 2 hours when necessary; switch to oral route as soon as feasible

Antiemetic: Oral, I.M., I.V., rectal: 12.5-25 mg every 4-6 hours as needed

Motion sickness: Oral, rectal: 25 mg 30-60 minutes before departure, then every 12 hours as needed

Sedation: Oral, I.M., I.V., rectal: 12.5-50 mg/dose

Monitoring Parameters Relief of symptoms, mental status

Administration Formulations available for oral, rectal, I.M./I.V. administration; not for SubQ or intra-arterial administration. Administer I.M. into deep muscle (preferred route of administration). Due to the possibility of orthostatic hypotension, I.V. administration is **not** the preferred route. Solution for injection may be diluted in 25-100 mL NS or D₅W (maximum concentration of 25 mg/mL) and infused over 15-30 minutes at a rate ≤25 mg/minute.

Contraindications Hypersensitivity to promethazine or any component of the formulation (cross-reactivity between phenothiazines may occur); coma; treatment of lower respiratory tract symptoms, including asthma; children <2 years of age

Warnings

[U.S. Boxed Warning]: Respiratory fatalities have been reported in children <2 years of age. In children ≥2 years, use the lowest possible dose; other drugs with respiratory depressant effects should be avoided. Not for SubQ or intra-arterial administration. Injection may contain sodium metabisulfite (may cause allergic reaction). I.M. is the preferred route of parenteral administration. I.V. use has been associated with severe tissue damage; discontinue immediately if burning or pain occurs with administration. May be sedating; use with caution in disorders where CNS depression is a feature. May impair physical or mental abilities; patients must be cautioned about performing tasks which require mental alertness (eg, operating machinery or driving). Use with caution in Parkinson's disease; hemodynamic instability; bone marrow suppression; subcortical brain damage; and in severe cardiac, hepatic, renal, or respiratory disease. Avoid use in Reye's syndrome. May lower seizure threshold; use caution in persons with seizure disorders or in persons using narcotics or local anesthetics which may also affect seizure threshold. May alter temperature regulation or mask toxicity of other drugs due to antiemetic effects. May alter cardiac conduction (life-threatening arrhythmias have occurred with therapeutic doses of phenothiazines). May cause orthostatic hypotension; use with caution in patients at risk of hypotension or where transient hypotensive episodes would be poorly tolerated (cardiovascular disease or cerebrovascular disease).

Phenothiazines may cause anticholinergic effects (constipation, xerostomia, blurred vision, urinary retention); therefore, they should be used with caution in patients with decreased gastrointestinal motility, urinary retention, BPH, xerostomia, or visual problems. Conditions which also may be exacerbated by cholinergic blockade include narrow-angle glaucoma (screening is recommended) and worsening of myasthenia gravis. May cause extrapyramidal symptoms, including pseudoparkinsonism, acute dystonic reactions, akathisia, and tardive dyskinesia. May be associated with neuroleptic malignant syndrome (NMS).

Dosage Forms [DSC] = Discontinued product

Injection, solution, as hydrochloride: 25 mg/mL (1 mL); 50 mg/mL (1 mL)

Phenergan®: 25 mg/mL (1 mL); 50 mg/mL (1 mL) [contains sodium metabisulfite]

Suppository, rectal, as hydrochloride: 12.5 mg, 25 mg, 50 mg

Phenadoz™: 12.5 mg, 25 mg

Phenergan®: 25 mg, 50 mg [DSC]

Promethegan™: 12.5 mg, 25 mg, 50 mg

Syrup, as hydrochloride: 6.25 mg/5 mL (120 mL, 480 mL) [contains alcohol]

Tablet, as hydrochloride: 12.5 mg, 25 mg, 50 mg

Phenergan®: 25 mg [DSC]

Reference Range

Therapeutic: 11-23 ng/mL

Toxic: >48 ng/mL

Fatal: 156 ng/mL (postmortem)

In the postmortem state, anatomical site concentration differences (ie, postmortem redistribution) may occur.

Overdosage/Treatment

Decontamination: Lavage (within 1 hour)/activated charcoal

Supportive therapy: Following initiation of essential overdose management, toxic symptom treatment and supportive treatment should be initiated. Hypotension usually responds to I.V. fluids or Trendelenburg positioning. If unresponsive to these measures, the use of a parenteral inotrope may be required (eg, norepinephrine 0.1-0.2 mcg/kg/minute titrated to response). Seizures commonly respond to lorazepam, diazepam, phenobarbital. Also critical cardiac arrhythmias often respond to I.V. phenytoin (15 mg/kg up to 1 gram), while other antiarrhythmics can be used. Neuroleptics often cause extrapyramidal reaction (eg, dystonic reactions) requiring management with diphenhydramine 1-2 mg/kg (adults) up to a maximum of 50 mg I.M. or I.V. slow push followed by a maintenance dose for 48-72 hours. When these reactions are unresponsive to diphenhydramine, benztropine mesylate I.V. 1-2 mg (adults) may be effective. These agents are generally effective within 2-5 minutes.

Enhancement of elimination: Multiple dosing of activated charcoal may be helpful; not dialyzable (0% to 5%)

Test Interactions Alters the flare response in intradermal allergen tests; HCG-based pregnancy tests may result in false-negatives or false-positives; increased serum glucose may be seen with glucose tolerance tests

Drug Interactions

Substrate (major) of CYP2B6, 2D6; **Inhibits** CYP2D6 (weak)

Aluminum salts: May decrease the absorption of phenothiazines; monitor

Amphetamines: Efficacy may be diminished by antipsychotics; in addition, amphetamines may increase psychotic symptoms; avoid concurrent use

Anticholinergics: May inhibit the therapeutic response to phenothiazines and excess anticholinergic effects may occur; includes benztropine, trihexyphenidyl, biperiden, and drugs with significant anticholinergic activity (TCAs, antihistamines, disopyramide)

Antihypertensives: Concurrent use of phenothiazines with an antihypertensive may produce additive hypotensive effects (particularly orthostasis)

Bromocriptine: Phenothiazines inhibit the ability of bromocriptine to lower serum prolactin concentrations

CNS depressants: Sedative effects may be additive with phenothiazines; monitor for increased effect; includes barbiturates, benzodiazepines, narcotic analgesics, ethanol, and other sedative agents

CYP2B6 inducers: May decrease the levels/effects of promethazine. Example inducers include carbamazepine, nevirapine, phenobarbital, phenytoin, and rifampin.

CYP2B6 inhibitors: May increase the levels/effects of promethazine. Example inhibitors include desipramine, paroxetine, and sertraline.

CYP2D6 inhibitors: May increase the levels/effects of promethazine. Example inhibitors include chlorpromazine, delavirdine, fluoxetine, miconazole, paroxetine, pergolide, quinidine, quinine, ritonavir, and ropinirole.

Epinephrine: Promethazine may diminish the pressor effects of epinephrine.

Guanethidine and guanadrel: Antihypertensive effects may be inhibited by phenothiazines

Levodopa: Phenothiazines may inhibit the antiparkinsonian effect of levodopa; avoid this combination

Lithium: Phenothiazines may produce neurotoxicity with lithium; this is a rare effect

Propranolol: Serum concentrations of phenothiazines may be increased; propranolol also increases phenothiazine concentrations

Polypeptide antibiotics: Rare cases of respiratory paralysis have been reported with concurrent use of phenothiazines

QTc-prolonging agents: Effects on QTc interval may be additive with phenothiazines, increasing the risk of malignant arrhythmias; includes type Ia antiarrhythmics, TCAs, and some quinolone antibiotics (sparfloxacin, moxifloxacin, and gatifloxacin)

Sulfadoxine-pyrimethamine: May increase phenothiazine concentrations

Tricyclic antidepressants: Concurrent use may produce increased toxicity or altered therapeutic response

Trazodone: Phenothiazines and trazodone may produce additive hypotensive effects

Valproic acid: Serum levels may be increased by phenothiazines

Pregnancy Risk Factor C

Pregnancy Implications Crosses the placenta; possible respiratory depression if drug is administered near time of delivery; behavioral changes, EEG alterations, impaired platelet aggregation reported with use during labor.

Lactation Excretion in breast milk unknown/not recommended

Specific References

Moreno R, Lowe RA, Brooks HS, et al, "Antiemetic Therapy in US Emergency Departments: Findings from the Year 2000 National

Hospital Ambulatory Medical Care Survey Database," *Ann Emerg Med*, 2003, 42(4):S98.

Sheth HS, Verrico MM, Skledar SJ, et al, "Promethazine Adverse Events After Implementation of a Medication Shortage Interchange," *Ann Pharmacother*, 2005, 39(2):255-61.

Propafenone

CAS Number 34183-22-7; 54063-53-5

U.S. Brand Names Rythmol® SR; Rythmol®

Synonyms Propafenone Hydrochloride

Use

Treatment of life-threatening ventricular arrhythmias

Rythmol® SR: Maintenance of normal sinus rhythm in patients with symptomatic atrial fibrillation

Unlabeled/Investigational Use Supraventricular tachycardias, including those patients with Wolff-Parkinson-White syndrome

Mechanism of Action Type 1C antiarrhythmic agent with sodium channel and weak beta-blocking activity

Adverse Reactions

Cardiovascular: Sinus arrest, bradycardia, heart block, hypotension, bundle branch block, fibrillation (atrial), flutter (atrial), sinus bradycardia, palpitations, sinus tachycardia, arrhythmias (ventricular)

Central nervous system: **Dizziness, drowsiness**, convulsions, psychosis, transient global amnesia, ataxia

Gastrointestinal: **Xerostomia**, bitter taste, constipation

Genitourinary: Impotence

Hepatic: Elevated liver function tests, cholestatic jaundice, cholestatic hepatitis

Neuromuscular & skeletal: Neuropathy (peripheral), clonus, myoclonus

Respiratory: Wheezing

Signs and Symptoms of Overdose AV block (third degree), blood dyscrasias, dizziness, granulocytopenia, hypotension, impotence, metallic taste, myoclonus, QRS prolongation, QT prolongation, seizures, tachycardia

Admission Criteria/Prognosis Admit any patient who is symptomatic or has ECG changes 6 hours postingestion

Pharmacodynamics/Kinetics

Absorption: Well absorbed

Metabolism: Hepatic; two genetically determined metabolism groups exist: fast or slow metabolizers; 10% of Caucasians are slow metabolizers; exhibits nonlinear pharmacokinetics; when dose is increased from 300-900 mg/day, serum concentrations increase tenfold; this nonlinearity is thought to be due to saturable first-pass effect

Bioavailability: 150 mg: 3.4%; 300 mg: 10.6%

Half-life elimination: Single dose (100-300 mg): 2-8 hours; Chronic dosing: 10-32 hours

Time to peak: 150 mg dose: 2 hours, 300 mg dose: 3 hours

Dosage Oral: Adults: **Note:** Patients who exhibit significant widening of QRS complex or second- or third-degree AV block may need dose reduction.

Immediate release tablet: Initial: 150 mg every 8 hours, increase at 3- to 4-day intervals up to 300 mg every 8 hours.

Extended release capsule: Initial: 225 mg every 12 hours; dosage increase may be made at a minimum of 5-day intervals; may increase to 325 mg every 12 hours; if further increase is necessary, may increase to 425 mg every 12 hours

Dosing adjustment in hepatic impairment: Reduction is necessary; however, specific guidelines are not available.

Monitoring Parameters ECG, blood pressure, pulse (particularly at initiation of therapy)

Administration Capsules should be swallowed whole; do not crush or chew.

Contraindications Hypersensitivity to propafenone or any component of the formulation; sinoatrial, AV, and intraventricular disorders of impulse generation and/or conduction (except in patients with a functioning artificial pacemaker); sinus bradycardia; cardiogenic shock; uncompensated cardiac failure; hypotension; bronchospastic disorders; uncorrected electrolyte abnormalities; concurrent use of ritonavir (see Drug Interactions)

Warnings

Monitor for proarrhythmic events. May prolong QT$_c$ interval; use caution with other QT$_c$-prolonging drugs. **[U.S. Boxed Warning]: In the Cardiac Arrhythmia Suppression Trial (CAST), recent (>6 days but <2 years ago) myocardial infarction patients with asymptomatic, nonlife-threatening ventricular arrhythmias did not benefit and may have been harmed by attempts to suppress the arrhythmia with flecainide or encainide. An increased mortality or nonfatal cardiac arrest rate (7.7%) was seen in the active treatment group compared with patients in the placebo group (3%). The applicability of the CAST results to other populations is unknown. Antiarrhythmic agents should be reserved for patients with life-threatening ventricular arrhythmias.** Can cause or unmask a variety of conduction disturbances. May alter pacing and sensing thresholds of artificial pacemakers. Patients with bronchospastic disease should generally not receive this drug. Monitor for worsening CHF if patient has underlying condition. Administer cautiously in significant hepatic dysfunction.

Dosage Forms Capsule, extended release, as hydrochloride (Rythmol® SR): 225 mg, 325 mg, 425 mg [contains soy lecithin]

Tablet, as hydrochloride (Rythmol®): 150 mg, 225 mg, 300 mg

Reference Range

Therapeutic: 500-2000 ng/mL

Serum propafenone level of 4839 ng/mL 5.5 hours postingestion is associated with severe toxicity; levels >7000 ng/mL are fatal

Overdosage/Treatment

Decontamination: Ipecac (within 30 minutes)/lavage (within 4 hours)/activated charcoal

Supportive therapy: Avoid flecainide, encainide; pacemaker may be useful; sodium bicarbonate may be useful for AV conduction disturbances or QRS prolongation along with reversing hypotension; atropine or isoproterenol for bradycardia; diazepam or lorazepam are useful to treat seizures

Enhanced elimination: Hemodialysis is not useful

Test Interactions May cause elevated antinuclear antibody titer

Drug Interactions

Substrate of CYP1A2 (minor), 2D6 (major), 3A4 (minor); **Inhibits** CYP1A2 (weak), 2D6 (weak)

Cimetidine: May increase propafenone levels.

CYP2D6 inhibitors: May increase the levels/effects of propafenone. Example inhibitors include chlorpromazine, delavirdine, fluoxetine, miconazole, paroxetine, pergolide, quinidine, quinine, ritonavir, and ropinirole.

Digoxin: Propafenone may increase digoxin levels; monitor for toxicity.

Metoprolol: Propafenone may increase metoprolol levels.

Phenobarbital: May decrease propafenone levels.

Propranolol: Propafenone may increase propranolol levels.

QT$_c$-prolonging agents: Effects may be additive with propafenone. Use caution with Class Ia and Class III antiarrhythmics, erythromycin, cisapride, antipsychotics, and cyclic antidepressants.

Quinidine: May increase propafenone levels.

Rifampin: May decrease propafenone levels.

Ritonavir: May increase propafenone levels; concurrent use is contraindicated.

Theophylline: Propafenone may increase theophylline levels.

Warfarin: Propafenone may increase warfarin levels/effects. Monitor INR closely.

Pregnancy Risk Factor C

Pregnancy Implications No adequate and well-controlled studies in pregnant women; use only if potential benefit to the mother justifies potential risk to the fetus.

Lactation Enters breast milk/use caution

Additional Information Sudden death noted in young postoperative heart patients either on propafenone or withdrawn from it

Specific References

Clarot F, Goulle JP, Horst M, et al, "Fatal Propafenone Overdoses: Case Reports and A Review of the Literature," *J Anal Toxicol*, 2003, 27(8):595-9.

Cocozzella D, Curciarello J, Corallini O, et al, "Propafenone Hepatotoxicity: Report of Two New Cases," *Dig Dis Sci*, 2003, 48(2):354-7.

Molia AC, Tholon J-P, Lamiable DL, et al, "Unintentional Pediatric Overdose of Propafenone," *Ann Pharmacother*, 2003, 37(7-8):1147-8.

Propofol

CAS Number 2078-24-8

U.S. Brand Names Diprivan®

Use Induction of anesthesia for inpatient or outpatient surgery in patients ≥3 years of age; maintenance of anesthesia for inpatient or outpatient surgery in patients >2 months of age; in adults, for the induction and maintenance of monitored anesthesia care sedation during diagnostic procedures; may be used (for patients >18 years of age who are intubated and mechanically ventilated) as an alternative to benzodiazepines for the treatment of agitation in the intensive care unit

Unlabeled/Investigational Use Postoperative antiemetic; refractory delirium tremens (case reports); conscious sedation

Mechanism of Action Propofol is a hindered phenolic (2,6-di-isopropyl-phenol) compound with intravenous general anesthetic properties. The drug is unrelated to any of the currently used barbiturate, opioid, benzodiazepine, arylcyclohexylamine, or imidazole intravenous anesthetic agents. It is a gamma-aminobutyric acid (GABA$_A$) neurotransmitter complex agonist, possibly a glycine (neurotransmitter) antagonist.

Adverse Reactions

Cardiovascular: **Hypotension**, hypertension, arrhythmia, bradycardia, decreased cardiac output, tachycardia, bigeminy, ECG abnormal, flushing, premature atrial contractions, premature ventricular contractions, somnolence, asystole, cardiac arrest, thrombosis, syncope

Central nervous system: **Movement**, agitation, anticholinergic syndrome, dizziness, delirium, fever, somnolence

Dermatologic: Pruritus, rash

Endocrine & metabolic: Hyperlipidemia, hypomagnesemia, increased serum triglycerides

Gastrointestinal: Hypersalivation, nausea, postoperative pancreatitis

Genitourinary: Cloudy urine, urine discoloration (green)

Hematologic: Leukocytosis, hemorrhage

Local: **Injection site burning, stinging, or pain**; swelling, blisters and/or tissue necrosis following accidental extravasation

Neuromuscular & skeletal: Dystonia, extremity pain, hypertonia, myalgia, paresthesia, perioperative myoclonia (rarely including convulsions and opisthotonos), rhabdomyolysis

Ocular: Amblyopia, vision abnormality

Respiratory: **Apnea, lasting 30-60 seconds; apnea, lasting >60 seconds**, respiratory acidosis during weaning, chills, cough, hypoxia, laryngospasm, lung function decreased, wheezing, pulmonary edema

Miscellaneous: Anaphylaxis, anaphylactoid reaction, perinatal disorder, phlebitis, postoperative unconsciousness with or without increase in muscle tone

Signs and Symptoms of Overdose Apnea, AV block, bradycardia, cardiovascular collapse, cough, hair discoloration (green), hiccups, hypotension, metabolic acidosis, myalgia, seizures

Pharmacodynamics/Kinetics

Onset of action: Anesthetic: Bolus infusion (dose dependent): 9-51 seconds (average 30 seconds)

Duration (dose and rate dependent): 3-10 minutes

Distribution: V_d: 2-10 L/kg; highly lipophilic

Protein binding: 97% to 99%

Metabolism: Hepatic to water-soluble sulfate and glucuronide conjugates

Half-life elimination: Biphasic: Initial: 40 minutes; Terminal: 4-7 hours (up to 1-3 days)

Excretion: Urine (~88% as metabolites, 40% as glucuronide metabolite); feces (<2%)

Clearance: 20-30 mL/kg/minute; total body clearance exceeds liver blood flow

Dosage Dosage must be individualized based on total body weight and titrated to the desired clinical effect; wait at least 3-5 minutes between dosage adjustments to clinically assess drug effects; smaller doses are required when used with narcotics; the following are general dosing guidelines:

General anesthesia:

Induction: I.V.:

Children 3-16 years, ASA I or II: 2.5-3.5 mg/kg over 20-30 seconds; use a lower dose for children ASA III or IV

Adults, ASA I or II, <55 years: 2-2.5 mg/kg (~40 mg every 10 seconds until onset of induction)

Elderly, debilitated, hypovolemic, or ASA III or IV: 1-1.5 mg/kg (~20 mg every 10 seconds until onset of induction)

Cardiac anesthesia: 0.5-1.5 mg/kg (~20 mg every 10 seconds until onset of induction)

Neurosurgical patients: 1-2 mg/kg (~20 mg every 10 seconds until onset of induction)

Maintenance: I.V. infusion:

Children 2 months to 16 years, ASA I or II: Initial: 200-300 mcg/kg/minute; decrease dose after 30 minutes if clinical signs of light anesthesia are absent; usual infusion rate: 125-150 mcg/kg/minute (range: 125-300 mcg/kg/minute; 7.5-18 mg/kg/hour); children ≤5 years may require larger infusion rates compared to older children

Adults, ASA I or II, <55 years: Initial: 150-200 mcg/kg/minute for 10-15 minutes; decrease by 30% to 50% during first 30 minutes of maintenance; usual infusion rate: 100-200 mcg/kg/minute (6-12 mg/kg/hour)

Elderly, debilitated, hypovolemic, ASA III or IV: 50-100 mcg/kg/minute (3-6 mg/kg/hour)

Cardiac anesthesia:

Low-dose propofol with primary opioid: 50-100 mcg/kg/minute (see manufacturer's labeling)

Primary propofol with secondary opioid: 100-150 mcg/kg/minute

Neurosurgical patients: 100-200 mcg/kg/minute (6-12 mg/kg/hour)

Maintenance: I.V. intermittent bolus: Adults, ASA I or II, <55 years: 20-50 mg increments as needed

Monitored anesthesia care sedation:

Initiation:

Adults, ASA I or II, <55 years: Slow I.V. infusion: 100-150 mcg/kg/minute for 3-5 minutes **or** slow injection: 0.5 mg/kg over 3-5 minutes

Elderly, debilitated, neurosurgical, or ASA III or IV patients: Use similar doses to healthy adults; avoid rapid I.V. boluses

Maintenance:

Adults, ASA I or II, <55 years: I.V. infusion using variable rates (preferred over intermittent boluses): 25-75 mcg/kg/minute **or** incremental bolus doses: 10 mg or 20 mg

Elderly, debilitated, neurosurgical, or ASA III or IV patients: Use 80% of healthy adult dose; **do not** use rapid bolus doses (single or repeated)

ICU sedation in intubated mechanically ventilated patients: Avoid rapid bolus injection; individualize dose and titrate to response

Adults: Continuous infusion: Initial: 0.3 mg/kg/hour; increase by 0.3-0.6 mg/kg/hour every 5-10 minutes until desired sedation level is achieved; usual maintenance: 0.3-3 mg/kg/hour or higher; reduce dose by 80% in elderly, debilitated, and ASA III or IV patients; reduce dose after adequate sedation established and adjust to response (ie, evaluate frequently to use minimum dose for sedation)

Stability Do not use if there is evidence of separation of phases of emulsion; discard any unused portions at end of the surgical procedure

Monitoring Parameters Cardiac monitor, blood pressure monitor, and ventilator required; serum triglyceride levels should be obtained prior to initiation of therapy (ICU setting) and every 3-7 days thereafter; daily sedation levels using standardized scale

Vital signs: Blood pressure, heart rate, cardiac output, pulmonary capillary wedge pressure should be monitored

Monitor zinc levels in patients predisposed to deficiency (burns, diarrhea, major sepsis). In patients at risk for renal impairment, urinalysis and urine sediment should be monitored prior to treatment and every other day of sedation.

Administration To reduce pain associated with injection, use larger veins of forearm or antecubital fossa; lidocaine I.V. (1 mL of a 1% solution) may also be used prior to administration. Do not use filter with <5 micron for administration. Soybean fat emulsion is used as a vehicle for propofol. Strict aseptic technique must be maintained in handling although a preservative has been added. Do not administer through the same I.V. catheter with blood or plasma. The American College of Critical Care Medicine recommends the use of a central vein for administration in an ICU setting.

Contraindications Hypersensitivity to propofol or any component of the formulation; propofol is also contraindicated when general anesthesia or sedation is contraindicated

Warnings

Use requires careful patient monitoring, should only be used by experienced personnel who are not actively engaged in the procedure or surgery. If used in a nonintubated and/or nonmechanically-ventilated patient, qualified personnel and appropriate equipment for rapid institution of respiratory and/or cardiovascular support must be immediately available.

Use a slower rate of induction and avoid rapid bolus administration in the elderly, debilitated, or ASA III/IV patients. Use with caution in patients who are hypotensive, hypovolemic, hemodynamically unstable, or have abnormally low vascular tone (eg, sepsis). Use caution in patients with severe cardiac disease (ejection fraction <50%) or respiratory disease; may have more profound adverse cardiovascular responses to propofol. Use caution in patients with a history of epilepsy or seizures; risk of seizure during recovery phase. Use caution in patients with increased intracranial pressure or impaired cerebral circulation - substantial decreases in mean arterial pressure and subsequent decreases in cerebral perfusion pressure may occur.

Use caution in patients with hyperlipidemia as evidenced by increased serum triglyceride levels or serum turbidity. Transient local pain may occur during I.V. injection; perioperative myoclonia has occurred. Not recommended for use in obstetrics, including cesarean section deliveries. Safety and efficacy in pediatric intensive care unit patients have not been established. Several deaths associated with severe metabolic acidosis have been reported in pediatric ICU patients on long-term propofol infusion. Concurrent use of fentanyl and propofol in pediatric patients may result in bradycardia.

Abrupt discontinuation prior to weaning or daily wake up assessments should be avoided. Abrupt discontinuation can result in rapid awakening, anxiety, agitation, and resistance to mechanical ventilation; titrate the infusion rate so the patient awakens slowly. Propofol does not have analgesic properties; pain should be treated with analgesic agents, propofol must be titrated separately from the analgesic agent. Propofol emulsion contains soybean oil, egg phosphatide, and glycerol; some formulations also contain sulfites. Some products may contain benzyl alcohol; benzyl alcohol has been associated with the "gasping syndrome" in neonates and low-birth-weight infants.

Dosage Forms Injection, emulsion: 10 mg/mL (20 mL, 50 mL, 100 mL) [products may contain egg lecithin, and soybean oil; may contain benzyl alcohol, sodium benzoate, or sodium metabisulfite]

Diprivan®: 10 mg/mL (20 mL, 50 mL, 100 mL) [contains egg lecithin, soybean oil, and disodium edetate]

Reference Range Propofol blood levels from 1.6-6.4 mcg/mL associated with anesthetic action; levels from 1.0-2.2 mcg/mL associated with regaining consciousness

Overdosage/Treatment Supportive therapy: Hypotension usually responds to I.V. fluids and/or Trendelenburg positioning; parenteral inotropes may be needed. Amiodarone can be used to treat propofol-induced ventricular tachycardia.

Test Interactions ↓ cholesterol (S)

Drug Interactions

Substrate of CYP1A2 (minor), 2A6 (minor), 2B6 (major), 2C9 (major), 2C19 (minor), 2D6 (minor), 2E1 (minor), 3A4 (minor); **Inhibits** CYP1A2

(moderate), 2C9 (weak), 2C19 (moderate), 2D6 (weak), 2E1 (weak), 3A4 (strong)

CNS depressants: Additive CNS depression and respiratory depression may necessitate dosage reduction when used with anesthetics, benzodiazepines, opiates, ethanol, phenothiazines.

CYP1A2 substrates: Propofol may increase the levels/effects of CYP1A2 substrates. Example substrates include aminophylline, fluvoxamine, mexiletine, mirtazapine, ropinirole, theophylline, and trifluoperazine.

CYP2B6 inhibitors: May increase the levels/effects of propofol. Example inhibitors include desipramine, paroxetine, and sertraline.

CYP2C9 Inhibitors may increase the levels/effects of propofol. Example inhibitors include delavirdine, fluconazole, gemfibrozil, ketoconazole, nicardipine, NSAIDs, sulfonamides and tolbutamide.

CYP2C19 substrates: Propofol may increase the levels/effects of CYP2C19 substrates. Example substrates include citalopram, diazepam, methsuximide, phenytoin, propranolol, and sertraline.

CYP3A4 substrates: Propofol may increase the levels/effects of CYP3A4 substrates. Example substrates include benzodiazepines, calcium channel blockers, mirtazapine, nateglinide, nefazodone, tacrolimus, and venlafaxine. Selected benzodiazepines (midazolam and triazolam), cisapride, ergot alkaloids, selected HMG-CoA reductase inhibitors (lovastatin and simvastatin), and pimozide are generally contraindicated with strong CYP3A4 inhibitors.

Narcotics: Concomitant use may lead to increased sedative or anesthetic effects of propofol, more pronounced decreases in systolic, diastolic, and mean arterial pressures and cardiac output. Lower doses of propofol may be needed. In addition, fentanyl may cause serious bradycardia when used with propofol in pediatric patients.

Vecuronium: Propofol may potentiate the neuromuscular blockade of vecuronium.

Pregnancy Risk Factor B

Pregnancy Implications Propofol is not recommended for obstetrics, including cesarean section deliveries. Propofol crosses the placenta and may be associated with neonatal depression.

Lactation Enters breast milk/not recommended

Nursing Implications Changes urine color to green with prolonged use

Additional Information On March 26, 2001, a specific warning was issued concerning the use of propofol in pediatric ICU patients. In the opinion of the FDA, a clinical trial evaluating the use of propofol as a sedative agent in this population was associated with a higher number of deaths as compared to standard sedative agents. The warning reminded healthcare professionals that propofol is not approved in the U.S. for sedation in pediatric ICU patients. A new clinical trial is planned to evaluate differences in safety within this population.

Specific References

Bassett KE, Anderson JL, Pribble CG, et al, "Propofol for Procedural Sedation in Children in the Emergency Department," *Ann Emerg Med*, 2003, 42(6): 773-82.

Frazee BW, Park RS, Lowery D, et al, "Propofol for Deep Procedural Sedation in the ED," *Am J Emerg Med*, 2005, 23(2):190-5.

Guenther E, Pribble CG, Junkins EP Jr, et al, "Propofol Sedation by Emergency Physicians for Elective Pediatric Outpatient Procedures," *Ann Emerg Med*, 2003, 42(6): 783-91.

Hofer KN, McCarthy MW, Buck ML, et al, "Possible Anaphylaxis After Propofol in a Child with Food Allergy," *Ann Pharmacother*, 2003, 37(3):398-401.

Miner JR, and Krauss B, "Procedural Sedation and Analgesia Research: State of the Art," *Academic Emergency Medicine*, 2007, 14:170-8.

Subramanian S, Kazzi Z, Schwartz M, et al, "Successful Treatment of Ventricular Tachycardia Associated with High-Dose Propofol Infusion," *J Toxicol Clin Toxicol*, 2004, 42(5):736.

Vesta KS, Martina S, and Kozlowski EA, "Propofol-Induced Priapism, A Case Confirmed with Rechallenge," *Ann Pharmacother*, 2006, 40(5):980-2.

Walker BH Jr, "Is Capnography Necessary for Propofol Sedation?" *Ann Emerg Med*, 2004, 44(5):549-50.

Wiegand TJ, Zvosec DL, and Smith SW, "Use of Propofol for Severe GHB Withdrawal: Two Cases," *Clin Toxicol (Phila)*, 2005, 43:665.

Propoxyphene

Related Information

- Therapeutic Drugs Associated with Hallucinations

CAS Number 1639-60-7; 469-62-5

U.S. Brand Names Darvon-N®; Darvon®

Synonyms Dextropropoxyphene; Propoxyphene Hydrochloride; Propoxyphene Napsylate

Impairment Potential Yes

Use Management of mild to moderate pain

Mechanism of Action Binds to opiate receptors in the CNS, causing inhibition of ascending pain pathways, altering the perception of and response to pain; produces generalized CNS depression

Adverse Reactions

Cardiovascular: **Hypotension**, sinus tachycardia

Central nervous system: **Dizziness, lightheadedness, sedation, paradoxical excitation and insomnia**, headache, **fatigue**, psychosis, **drowsiness**, agitation, nervousness, restlessness, malaise, confusion, CNS depression, auditory hallucinations, increased intracranial pressure

Dermatologic: Skin rash, hives, pruritus, exanthem

Gastrointestinal: GI upset, **nausea, vomiting, constipation**, anorexia, stomach cramps, xerostomia, paralytic ileus, biliary tract spasm

Genitourinary: Ureteral spasm, decreased urination

Hepatic: Elevated liver enzymes

Neuromuscular & skeletal: Hyperreflexia, **weakness**

Respiratory: Dyspnea, apnea

Miscellaneous: Psychologic and physical dependence, **histamine release**

Signs and Symptoms of Overdose Cardiac arrhythmia (ventricular), coma, cyanosis, deafness, dementia, diabetes insipidus, disorientation, dizziness, hypernatremia, hyperreflexia, hyperthermia, hypothermia, impotence, insomnia, jaundice, miosis, myoglobinuria, neutropenia, nodal tachycardia, nystagmus, primary atrioventricular block, ptosis, pulmonary edema, rhabdomyolysis, seizures, thrombocytopenia, tremors, vomiting. Death can occur within 1 hour.

Admission Criteria/Prognosis Admit any adult ingestion > 1 g or > 500 mg if taken in conjunction with another CNS depressive agent

Pharmacodynamics/Kinetics

Onset of effect: Oral: Within 30-60 minutes

Duration: 4-6 hours

Distribution: V_d: 12-26 L/kg

Protein binding: 78%

Metabolism: First-pass effect; metabolized in the liver to an active metabolite (norpropoxyphene) and inactive metabolites

Bioavailability: Oral: 30% to 70%

Half-life:

Adults: Parent drug: 8-24 hours (mean: ~15 hours); Norpropoxyphene: 34 hours;

Elderly: Parent drug: 37 hours; Norpropoxyphene: 42 hours

Elimination: 20% to 25% excreted in urine

Dosage Oral:

Children: Doses for children are not well established; doses of the hydrochloride of 2-3 mg/kg/d divided every 6 hours have been used

Adults:

Hydrochloride: 65 mg every 3-4 hours as needed for pain; maximum: 390 mg/day

Napsylate: 100 mg every 4 hours as needed for pain; maximum: 600 mg/day

Elderly: Refer to Adults dosing; consider increasing dosing interval

Dosing adjustment in renal impairment: Serum concentrations of propoxyphene may be increased or elimination may be delayed. Avoid use in Cl_{cr} <10 mL/minute. Specific dosing recommendations not available for less severe impairment.

Not dialyzable (0% to 5%)

Dosing adjustment in hepatic impairment: Serum concentrations of propoxyphene may be increased or elimination may be delayed; specific dosing recommendations not available.

Monitoring Parameters Pain relief, respiratory and mental status, blood pressure

Administration Should be administered with glass of water on an empty stomach. Food may decrease rate of absorption, but may slightly increase bioavailability.

Contraindications Hypersensitivity to propoxyphene or any component of the formulation

Warnings

[U.S. Boxed Warning]: When given in excessive doses, either alone or in combination with other CNS depressants (including alcohol), propoxyphene is a major cause of drug-related deaths; recommended dosage must not be exceeded and alcohol intake should be limited. Avoid use in severely depressed or suicidal patients. Should not be prescribed in patients who are addiction prone or suicidal. Use caution in patients taking CNS depressant medications or antidepressants, and in patients who use alcohol in excess.

Use caution in patients dependent on opiates, substitution may result in acute opiate withdrawal symptoms. Tolerance or drug dependence may result from extended use. Propoxyphene should be used with caution in patients with renal or hepatic dysfunction or in the elderly; consider dosing adjustment.

Dosage Forms Capsule, as hydrochloride (Darvon®): 65 mg

Tablet, as napsylate (Darvon-N®): 100 mg

Reference Range

Therapeutic: 0.1-0.4 mcg/mL, ranges published vary and may not correlate with clinical effect

Toxic: >0.5 mcg/mL (SI: >1.5 μmol/L)

Fatal: >1 mcg/mL (SI: 2.9 μmol/L)

In the postmortem state, anatomical site concentration differences (ie, postmortem redistribution) may occur

Hair Dextropropoxyphene and norpropoxyphene concentrations at concentrations of 26.4 ng/mg and 71 ng/mg of hair respectively are associated with overdose.

Overdosage/Treatment
Decontamination: Lavage/activated charcoal within 2 hours of ingestion
Supportive therapy: Naloxone hydrochloride for CNS depression, may also stop seizures and alleviate hypotension. Lidocaine or sodium bicarbonate can reverse QRS prolongation and ventricular arrhythmias.
Enhancement of elimination: Multiple dosing of activated charcoal is useful; not dialyzable (0% to 5%)

Antidote(s)
- Nalmefene [ANTIDOTE]
- Naloxone [ANTIDOTE]

Test Interactions False-positive methadone test; ↑ LFTs, ↓ glucose (S), 17-OHCS (U); diphenhydramine may cause a false-positive urinary assay for propoxyphene on the EMIT II immunoassay

Drug Interactions Inhibits CYP2C9 (weak), 2D6 (weak), 3A4 (weak)
Decreased effect with charcoal, cigarette smoking
Increased toxicity: CNS depressants may potentiate pharmacologic effects; propoxyphene may inhibit the metabolism and increase the serum concentrations of carbamazepine, phenobarbital, MAO inhibitors, tricyclic antidepressants, and warfarin

Pregnancy Risk Factor C/D (prolonged use)
Pregnancy Implications Withdrawal symptoms have been reported in the neonate following propoxyphene use during pregnancy. Teratogenic effects have also been noted in case reports. Opioid analgesics are considered pregnancy risk factor D if used for prolonged periods or in large doses near term.
Lactation Enters breast milk/use caution (AAP rates "compatible")

Specific References
Afshari R, Maxwell S, Dawson A, et al, "ECG Abnormalities in Co-proxamol (Paracetamol/Dextropropoxyphene) Poisoning," Clin Toxicol (Phila), 2005, 43(4):255-9.
Barkin RL, Barkin SJ, and Barkin DS, "Propoxyphene (Dextropropoxyphene): A Critical Review of a Weak Opioid Analgesic That Should Remain in Antiquity," Am J Therapeutics, 2006, 13:534-42.
Poklis A, Poklis JL, Tarnai L, et al, "Evaluation of the Triage PPY On-Site Testing Device for Detection of Dextropropoxyphene in Urine," J Anal Toxicol, 2004, 28(6):485-8.

Propranolol

Related Information
- Selected Properties of Beta-Adrenergic Blocking Drugs
- Therapeutic Drugs Associated with Hallucinations

CAS Number 13013-17-7; 13071-11-9; 318-98-9; 3506-09-0; 4199-10-4; 5051-22-9; 525-66-6
U.S. Brand Names Inderal® LA; Inderal®InnoPran XL™; Propranolol Intensol™
Synonyms Propranolol Hydrochloride
Impairment Potential Yes
Use Management of hypertension; angina pectoris; pheochromocytoma; essential tremor; tetralogy of Fallot cyanotic spells; arrhythmias (such as atrial fibrillation and flutter, AV nodal re-entrant tachycardias, and catecholamine-induced arrhythmias); prevention of myocardial infarction; migraine headache; symptomatic treatment of hypertrophic subaortic stenosis
Unlabeled/Investigational Use Tremor due to Parkinson's disease; ethanol withdrawal; aggressive behavior; antipsychotic-induced akathisia; prevention of bleeding esophageal varices; anxiety; schizophrenia; acute panic; gastric bleeding in portal hypertension; thyrotoxicosis
Mechanism of Action Nonselective beta-adrenergic blocker (class II antiarrhythmic); competitively blocks response to $beta_1$- and $beta_2$-adrenergic stimulation which results in decreases in heart rate, myocardial contractility, blood pressure, and myocardial oxygen demand

Adverse Reactions
Cardiovascular: **Bradycardia**, hypotension, impaired myocardial contractility, congestive heart failure, worsening of AV conduction disturbances, abnormal T-wave inversion, claudication, syncope, myocardial depression, QRS prolongation, Raynaud's phenomenon
Central nervous system: **Mental depression**, lightheadedness, psychosis, insomnia, vivid dreams, drowsiness, auditory and visual hallucinations, agitation, paranoia
Dermatologic: Exfoliative dermatitis, erythema multiforme, acne, angioedema, toxic epidermal necrolysis, Stevens-Johnson syndrome, onycholysis, photosensitivity, pruritus, licheniform eruptions, exanthem, cutaneous vasculitis
Endocrine & metabolic: **Decreased sexual ability**, hypoglycemia, hyperglycemia
Gastrointestinal: Nausea, vomiting, diarrhea, abdominal pain, gastrointestinal distress, loss of taste perception, xerostomia
Genitourinary: Impotence, penile fibrosis, retroperitoneal fibrosis
Hematologic: Agranulocytosis, thrombocytopenic purpura

Neuromuscular & skeletal: Myotonia, myasthenia gravis (exacerbation), arthralgia, weakness, paresthesia
Ocular: Diplopia, phototoxic
Respiratory: Wheezing, rhinitis
Miscellaneous: Cold extremities, systemic lupus erythematosus

Signs and Symptoms of Overdose Agranulocytosis, alopecia, ataxia, AV block, cardiovascular collapse, cognitive dysfunction, dementia, depression, dyspnea, granulocytopenia, Graves' disease, heart/respiratory failure and wheezing, hyperglycemia, hyperreflexia, hyperthyroidism, hypoglycemia, hypothyroidism, impotence, leukopenia, mesenteric ischemia, myasthenia gravis (exacerbation or precipitation), neutropenia, paranoia, pemphigus, pulmonary edema, purpura, retroperitoneal fibrosis, rhinorrhea, seizures (>1.5 g ingestion in adults), severe hypotension, sexual dysfunction, shock, sinus bradycardia, urticaria

Admission Criteria/Prognosis Admit an adult ingestion >1 g, or QRS duration on ECG >100 ms; patients asymptomatic 6 hours postingestion may be discharged

Pharmacodynamics/Kinetics
Onset of action: Beta-blockade: Oral: 1-2 hours
Duration: ~6 hours
Distribution: V_d: 3.9 L/kg in adults; crosses placenta; small amounts enter breast milk
Protein binding: Newborns: 68%; Adults: 93%
Metabolism: Hepatic to active and inactive compounds; extensive first-pass effect
Bioavailability: 30% to 40%; may be increased in Down syndrome
Half-life elimination: Neonates and Infants: Possible increased half-life; Children: 3.9-6.4 hours; Adults: 4-6 hours
Excretion: Urine (96% to 99%)

Dosage Akathisia: Oral: Adults: 30-120 mg/day in 2-3 divided doses
Angina: Oral: Adults: 80-320 mg/day in doses divided 2-4 times/day
Long-acting formulation: Initial: 80 mg once daily; maximum dose: 320 mg once daily
Essential tremor: Oral: Adults: 20-40 mg twice daily initially; maintenance doses: usually 120-320 mg/day
Hypertension:
Oral:
Children: Initial: 0.5-1 mg/kg/day in divided doses every 6-12 hours; increase gradually every 5-7 days; maximum: 16 mg/kg/24 hours
Adults: Initial: 40 mg twice daily; increase dosage every 3-7 days; usual dose: ≤320 mg divided in 2-3 doses/day; maximum daily dose: 640 mg; usual dosage range (JNC 7): 40-160 mg/day in 2 divided doses
Long-acting formulation: Initial: 80 mg once daily; usual maintenance: 120-160 mg once daily; maximum daily dose: 640 mg; usual dosage range (JNC 7): 60-180 mg/day once daily
I.V.: Children: 0.01-0.05 mg/kg over 1 hour; maximum dose: 10 mg
Hypertrophic subaortic stenosis: Oral: Adults: 20-40 mg 3-4 times/day
Long-acting formulation: 80-160 mg once daily
Migraine headache prophylaxis: Oral:
Children: Initial: 2-4 mg/kg/day **or**
≤35 kg: 10-20 mg 3 times/day
>35 kg: 20-40 mg 3 times/day
Adults: Initial: 80 mg/day divided every 6-8 hours; increase by 20-40 mg/dose every 3-4 weeks to a maximum of 160-240 mg/day given in divided doses every 6-8 hours; if satisfactory response not achieved within 6 weeks of starting therapy, drug should be withdrawn gradually over several weeks
Long-acting formulation: Initial: 80 mg once daily; effective dose range: 160-240 mg once daily
Myocardial infarction prophylaxis: Oral: Adults: 180-240 mg/day in 3-4 divided doses
Pheochromocytoma: Oral: Adults: 30-60 mg/day in divided doses
Tachyarrhythmias:
Oral:
Children: Initial: 0.5-1 mg/kg/day in divided doses every 6-8 hours; titrate dosage upward every 3-7 days; usual dose: 2-6 mg/kg/day; higher doses may be needed; do not exceed 16 mg/kg/day or 60 mg/day
Adults: 10-30 mg/dose every 6-8 hours
Elderly: Initial: 10 mg twice daily; increase dosage every 3-7 days; usual dosage range: 10-320 mg given in 2 divided doses
I.V.:
Children: 0.01-0.1 mg/kg/dose slow IVP over 10 minutes; maximum dose: 1 mg for infants; 3 mg for children
Adults (in patients having nonfunctional GI tract): 1 mg/dose slow IVP; repeat every 5 minutes up to a total of 5 mg; titrate initial dose to desired response
Tetralogy spells: Children:
Oral: Palliation: Initial: 1 mg/kg/day every 6 hours; if ineffective, may increase dose after 1 week by 1 mg/kg/day to a maximum of 5 mg/kg/day; if patient becomes refractory, may increase slowly to a maximum of 10-15 mg/kg/day. Allow 24 hours between dosing changes.

I.V.: 0.01-0.2 mg/kg/dose infused over 10 minutes; maximum initial dose: 1 mg

Thyrotoxicosis:

Oral:

Children: 2 mg/kg/day, divided every 6-8 hours, titrate to effective dose

Adolescents and Adults: Oral: 10-40 mg/dose every 6 hours

I.V.: Adults: 1-3 mg/dose slow IVP as a single dose

Dosing adjustment/comments in renal impairment:

Not dialyzable (0% to 5%); supplemental dose is not necessary.

Peritoneal dialysis effects: Supplemental dose is not necessary.

Dosing adjustment/comments in hepatic disease: Marked slowing of heart rate may occur in cirrhosis with conventional doses; low initial dose and regular heart rate monitoring

Stability Compatible in saline, **incompatible** with HCO_3^-; protect injection from light

Monitoring Parameters Acute cardiac treatment: Monitor ECG and blood pressure with I.V. administration; heart rate and blood pressure with oral administration

Administration I.V. dose is much smaller than oral dose. When administered acutely for cardiac treatment, monitor ECG and blood pressure. May administer by rapid infusion (I.V. push) at a rate of 1 mg/minute or by slow infusion over ~30 minutes. Necessary monitoring for surgical patients who are unable to take oral beta-blockers (prolonged ileus) has not been defined. Some institutions require monitoring of baseline and postinfusion heart rate and blood pressure when a patient's response to beta-blockade has not been characterized (ie, the patient's initial dose or following a change in dose). Consult individual institutional policies and procedures. Do not crush long-acting oral forms.

Contraindications Hypersensitivity to propranolol, beta-blockers, or any component of the formulation; uncompensated congestive heart failure (unless the failure is due to tachyarrhythmias being treated with propranolol), cardiogenic shock, bradycardia or heart block (2nd or 3rd degree), pulmonary edema, severe hyperactive airway disease (asthma or COPD), Raynaud's disease; pregnancy (2nd and 3rd trimesters)

Warnings Administer cautiously in compensated heart failure and monitor for a worsening of the condition (efficacy of propranolol in CHF has not been demonstrated). **[U.S. Boxed Warning]: Beta-blocker therapy should not be withdrawn abruptly (particularly in patients with CAD), but gradually tapered (over 2 weeks) to avoid acute tachycardia, hypertension, and/or ischemia.** Use caution in patient with PVD. Use caution with concurrent use of beta-blockers and either verapamil or diltiazem; bradycardia or heart block can occur. Avoid concurrent I.V. use of both agents. Use cautiously in diabetics because it can mask prominent hypoglycemic symptoms. Can mask signs of thyrotoxicosis. Can cause fetal harm when administered in pregnancy. Use cautiously in hepatic dysfunction (dosage adjustment required). Use care with anesthetic agents which decrease myocardial function. Not indicated for hypertensive emergencies.

Dosage Forms Capsule, extended release, as hydrochloride (InnoPran XL™): 80 mg, 120 mg

Capsule, sustained release, as hydrochloride (Inderal® LA): 60 mg, 80 mg, 120 mg, 160 mg

Injection, solution, as hydrochloride (Inderal®): 1 mg/mL (1 mL)

Solution, oral, as hydrochloride: 4 mg/mL (5 mL, 500 mL); 8 mg/mL (500 mL) [strawberry-mint flavor; contains alcohol 0.6%]

Tablet, as hydrochloride (Inderal®): 10 mg, 20 mg, 40 mg, 60 mg, 80 mg

Reference Range

Therapeutic: 50-100 ng/mL (SI: 190-390 nmol/L) at end of dose interval

Fatal: Levels >2000 ng/mL (SI: >7702 nmol/L)

In the postmortem state, anatomical site concentration differences (ie, postmortem redistribution) may occur

Overdosage/Treatment

Decontamination: Lavage (within 1 hour)/activated charcoal; **do not** use ipecac

Supportive therapy: Glucagon (50-150 mcg/kg followed by continuous drip of 1-5 mg/hour) for positive chronotropic effect, inamrinone may need to be added; atropine/isoproterenol can be utilized to increase heart rate; calcium chloride may also be effective but this approach has not been thoroughly been investigated; do **not** use epinephrine in that unopposed alpha effects may occur; pacemaker or intra-aortic balloon counter pulsation may be required; calcium chloride may improve the hemodynamic depression or electromechanical disassociation caused by propranolol toxicity but will not affect the heart rate

Enhancement of elimination: Multiple dosing of activated charcoal may be effective; not dialyzable (0% to 5%)

Antidote(s)

● Glucagon [ANTIDOTE]

Test Interactions ↑ thyroxine (S), cholesterol (S), glucose

Drug Interactions **Substrate** of CYP1A2 (major), 2C19 (minor), 2D6 (major), 3A4 (minor); **Inhibits** CYP1A2 (weak), 2D6 (weak)

Albuterol (and other beta₂ agonists): Effects may be blunted by nonspecific beta-blockers.

Alpha-blockers (prazosin, terazosin): Concurrent use of beta-blockers may increase risk of orthostasis.

Aluminum hydroxide: Absorption of propranolol may be decreased.

Cholestyramine, colestipol: Plasma levels of propranolol may be decreased.

Cimetidine increases the plasma concentration of propranolol and its pharmacodynamic effects may be increased.

Clonidine: Hypertensive crisis after or during withdrawal of either agent

CYP1A2 inducers: May decrease the levels/effects of propranolol. Example inducers include aminoglutethimide, carbamazepine, phenobarbital, and rifampin.

CYP1A2 inhibitors: May increase the levels/effects of propranolol. Example inhibitors include ciprofloxacin, fluvoxamine, ketoconazole, norfloxacin, ofloxacin, and rofecoxib.

CYP2D6 inhibitors: May increase the levels/effects of propranolol. Example inhibitors include chlorpromazine, delavirdine, fluoxetine, miconazole, paroxetine, pergolide, quinidine, quinine, ritonavir, and ropinirole.

Diazepam: Metabolism of diazepam may be inhibited; concentrations of diazepam and metabolites may be increased.

Drugs which slow AV conduction (digoxin): Effects may be additive with beta-blockers.

Epinephrine (including local anesthetics with epinephrine): Propranolol may cause hypertension.

Flecainide: Pharmacological activity of both agents may be increased when used concurrently.

Fluoxetine may inhibit the metabolism of propranolol, resulting in cardiac toxicity.

Glucagon: Propranolol may blunt hyperglycemic action.

Haloperidol: Hypotensive effects may be potentiated.

Hydralazine: The bioavailability propranolol (rapid release) and hydralazine may be enhanced with concurrent dosing.

Insulin: Propranolol inhibits recovery and may cause hypertension and bradycardia following insulin-induced hypoglycemia; also masks the tachycardia that usually accompanies insulin-induced hypoglycemia.

Lidocaine: Metabolism of lidocaine may be decreased.

NSAIDs (ibuprofen, indomethacin, naproxen, piroxicam) may reduce the antihypertensive effects of beta-blockers.

Phenothiazines (chlorpromazine, phenothiazine): Plasma levels of propranolol and phenothiazine may both be increased.

Propafenone: May increase the concentrations/effects of propranolol.

Quinidine: May increase plasma levels of propranolol by decreasing metabolism.

Rifampin: May decrease plasma levels of propranolol by increasing metabolism.

Salicylates may reduce the antihypertensive effects of beta-blockers

Serotonin 5-HT₁D receptor agonists (such as rizatriptan, zolmitriptan): Propranolol may increase bioavailability of serotonin 5-HT₁D receptor agonists.

Sulfonylureas: Beta-blockers may alter response to hypoglycemic agents.

Theophylline: Theophylline clearance may be decreased by propranolol.

Verapamil or diltiazem may have synergistic or additive pharmacological effects when taken concurrently with beta-blockers; avoid concurrent I.V. use of both.

Warfarin: Propranolol may increase bioavailability of warfarin and PT may be increased.

Pregnancy Risk Factor C (manufacturer); D (2nd and 3rd trimesters - expert analysis)

Pregnancy Implications Propranolol crosses the placenta. Beta-blockers have been associated with bradycardia, hypotension, and IUGR. IUGR is probably related to maternal hypertension. Available evidence suggests beta-blockers are generally safe during pregnancy (JNC-7). Cases of neonatal hypoglycemia have been reported following maternal use of beta-blockers at parturition or during breast-feeding.

Lactation Enters breast milk/use caution (AAP rates "compatible")

Nursing Implications I.V. dose much smaller than oral dose; I.V. administration should not exceed 1 mg/minute

Additional Information Healthy African-American individuals are more sensitive to beta-blockade effects of propranolol than healthy white individuals

Specific References

Bania TC, Chu J, and Wosolowski M, "The Hemodynamic Effect of Intralipid on Propranolol Toxicity," *Acad Emerg Med*, 2006, 13(5):S109.

Cave G, Harvey MG, and Castle CD, "The Role of Fat Emulsion Therapy in a Rodent Model of Propranolol Toxicity: A Preliminary Study," *J Med Toxicol*, 2006, 2(1):4-7.

Chobanian AV, Bakris GL, Black HR, et al, "The Seventh Report of the Joint National Committee on Prevention, Detection, Evaluation, and Treatment of High Blood Pressure: The JNC 7 Report," *JAMA*, 2003, 289(19):2560-71.

De Rosa G, Delogu AB, Piastra M, et al, "Catecholaminergic Polymorphic Ventricular Tachycardia: Successful Emergency Treatment with Intravenous Propranolol," *Pediatr Emerg Care*, 2004, 20(3):175-7.

DeWitt CR and Waksman JC, "Pharmacology, Pathophysiology and Management of Calcium Channel Blocker and Beta-Blocker Toxicity," *Toxicol Rev*, 2004, 23(4):223-38.

Koksal AS, Uskudar O, Koklu S, et al, "Propranolol-Exacerbated Mesenteric Ischemia in a Patient with Hyperthyroidism," *Ann Pharmacother*, 2005, 39(3):559-62.

Megarbane B, Karyo S, and Baud FJ, "The Role of Insulin and Glucose (Hyperinsulinaemia/Euglycaemia) Therapy in Acute Calcium Channel Antagonist and Beta-Blocker Poisoning," *Toxicol Rev*, 2004, 23(4): 215-22.

Satar S, Acikalin A, and Akpinar O, "Unusual Electrocardiographic Changes with Propranolol and Diltiazem Overdosage: A Case Report," *Am J Ther*, 2003, 10(4):299-302.

Sheth PP, Morgan DL, Vincent CB, et al, "Beta-Blocker Ingestion by Young Children: One Pill May Make You Mildly Ill," *Clin Toxicol (Phila)*. 2005, 43:645.

Spitz DJ, "An Unusual Death in an Asthmatic Patient," *Am J Forensic Med Pathol*, 2003, 24(3):271-2.

Wax PM, Erdman AR, Chyka PA, et al, "Beta-Blocker Ingestion: An Evidence-Based Consensus Guideline for Out-of-Hospital Management," *Clin Toxicol (Phila)*, 2005, 43(3):131-46.

Propylhexedrine

Pronunciation (proe pil HEKS e dreen)
CAS Number 1007-33-6; 101-40-6; 3595-11-7; 6192-95-6
U.S. Brand Names Benzedrex® [OTC]
Impairment Potential Yes
Use Topical nasal decongestant
Mechanism of Action Related to amphetamine, propylhexedrine causes vasoconstriction of dilated arterioles (potent alpha-adrenergic agonist)
Adverse Reactions
Local: Nasal: Burning, stinging
Respiratory: Sneezing, nasal discharge increased
Signs and Symptoms of Overdose Chronic abuse has caused cardiomyopathy, dyspnea, foreign body granulation, pulmonary hypertension, and sudden death.
Admission Criteria/Prognosis Consider admission for ingestions over 250 mg, or symptomatic patients 4 hours postexposure
Toxicodynamics/Kinetics
Onset of action: Intranasal: 10 minutes
Duration: Intranasal: 1-2 hours
Elimination: Renal
Dosage Nasal: Children 6-12 years and Adults: Two inhalations in each nostril, not more frequently than every 2 hours
Administration For nasal inhalation only.
Contraindications Hypersensitivity to propylhexedrine or any component of the formulation
Warnings Do not exceed recommended dosage; do not use for more than 3 days; for nasal use only
Dosage Forms Inhaler, nasal: 0.4-0.5 mg/inhalation (1s) [total content 250 mg]
Reference Range Blood propylhexedrine levels with normal therapeutic use range around 0.01 mg/L; serum and urine level of 30 mg/L and 60 mg/L, respectively, associated with fatality
Overdosage/Treatment
Decontamination: **Oral**: Activated charcoal. **Ocular**: Irrigate copiously with saline
Supportive therapy: Propranolol or esmolol can be utilized for tachyarrhythmias
Nursing Implications Drug has been extracted from inhaler and injected I.V. as an amphetamine substitute
Additional Information Drug has been extracted from inhaler and injected I.V. as an amphetamine substitute; often utilized as a drug of abuse (similar to amphetamines) in which sudden death can occur due to heart failure or cardiac arrhythmia; PKA of solution: ~10.4; has been ingested by soaking fibrous interior of inhaler in hot water; exhibits ~10% of effect of CNS stimulation as amphetamine

Propylthiouracil

CAS Number 51-52-5
Synonyms PTU (error-prone abbreviation)
Use Palliative treatment of hyperthyroidism as an adjunct to ameliorate hyperthyroidism in preparation for surgical treatment or radioactive iodine therapy and in the management of thyrotoxic crisis
Mechanism of Action Inhibits the synthesis of thyroid hormones by blocking the oxidation of iodine in the thyroid gland; blocks synthesis of thyroxine and triiodothyronine
Adverse Reactions
Cardiovascular: Edema, leukocytoclastic vasculitis, ANCA-positive vasculitis
Central nervous system: Fever, drowsiness, vertigo, headache, drug fever, dizziness, neuritis

Dermatologic: Skin rash, urticaria, pruritus, exfoliative dermatitis, alopecia, erythema nodosum, cutaneous vasculitis
Endocrine & metabolic: Goiter, weight gain, swollen salivary glands
Gastrointestinal: Nausea, vomiting, loss of taste perception, stomach pain, constipation
Hematologic: Leukopenia, agranulocytosis, thrombocytopenia, bleeding, aplastic anemia
Hepatic: Cholestatic jaundice, hepatitis
Renal: Nephritis, glomerulonephritis, acute renal failure, renal vasculitis
Respiratory: Interstitial pneumonitis, alveolar hemorrhage, pulmonary vasculitis
Neuromuscular & skeletal: Arthralgia, paresthesia
Miscellaneous: SLE-like syndrome, elevated antineutrophilic cytoplasmic antibodies (ANCA)
Signs and Symptoms of Overdose Deafness, dysosmia, enuresis, galactorrhea, hyperthermia, leukopenia or neutropenia (agranulocytosis, granulocytopenia), myopathy
Pharmacodynamics/Kinetics
Onset of action: Therapeutic: 24-36 hours
Peak effect: Remission: 4 months of continued therapy
Duration: 2-3 hours
Distribution: Concentrated in the thyroid gland
Protein binding: 75% to 80%
Metabolism: Hepatic
Bioavailability: 80% to 95%
Half-life elimination: 1.5-5 hours; End-stage renal disease: 8.5 hours
Time to peak, serum: ~1 hour
Excretion: Urine (35%)
Dosage Oral: Administer in 3 equally divided doses at approximately 8-hour intervals; adjust dosage to maintain T_3, T_4, and TSH levels in normal range; elevated T_3 may be sole indicator of adequate treatment, elevated TSH indicates excessive antithyroid treatment
Neonates: 5-10 mg/kg/day in divided doses every 8 hours
Children: Initial: 5-7 mg/kg/day in divided doses every 8 hours **or**
6-10 years: 50-150 mg/day
>10 years: 150-300 mg/day
Maintenance: $^1/_3$ to $^2/_3$ of the initial dose in divided doses every 8-12 hours; this usually begins after 2 months on an effective initial dosage
Adults: Initial: 300-450 mg/day in divided doses every 8 hours (severe hyperthyroidism may require 600-1200 mg/day); maintenance: 100-150 mg/day in divided doses every 8-12 hours
Elderly: Use lower dose recommendations; initial dose: 150-300 mg/day
Dosing adjustment in renal impairment:
Cl_{cr} 10-50 mL/minute: Administer at 75% of normal dose
Cl_{cr} <10 mL/minute: Administer at 50% of normal dose
Monitoring Parameters CBC with differential, prothrombin time, liver function tests, thyroid function tests (TSH, T_3, T_4); periodic blood counts are recommended chronic therapy
Contraindications Hypersensitivity to propylthiouracil or any component of the formulation; pregnancy
Warnings Use with caution in patients >40 years of age because PTU may cause hypoprothrombinemia and bleeding; use with extreme caution in patients receiving other drugs known to cause agranulocytosis; may cause agranulocytosis, thyroid hyperplasia, thyroid carcinoma (usage >1 year). Discontinue in the presence of agranulocytosis, aplastic anemia, ANCA-positive vasculitis, hepatitis, unexplained fever, or exfoliative dermatitis. Safety and efficacy have not been established in children <6 years of age.
Dosage Forms Tablet: 50 mg
Reference Range Peak serum level of 10 mcg/mL following 400 mg ingestion
Overdosage/Treatment Decontamination: Ipecac within 30 minutes or lavage (within 1 hour)/activated charcoal; consider gastrointestinal decontamination for ingestions >5 g
Diagnostic Procedures
● Thyroxine, Blood
Test Interactions ↑ alkaline phosphatase; reverse T_3; ↓ T_3
Drug Interactions Anticoagulants: Anticoagulants may be potentiated by antivitamin-K effect of propylthiouracil. Oral anticoagulant activity is increased only until metabolic effect stabilizes.
Correction of hyperthyroidism may alter disposition of beta-blockers, digoxin, and theophylline, necessitating a dose reduction of these agents.
Pregnancy Risk Factor D
Pregnancy Implications Crosses the placenta and may induce goiter and hypothyroidism in the developing fetus (cretinism). May need to monitor infant's thyroid function periodically.
Lactation Enters breast milk/use caution (AAP rates "compatible")
Additional Information The use of antithyroid thioamides is as effective in elderly as in younger adults; however, the expense, potential adverse effects, and inconvenience (compliance, monitoring) make them undesirable. The use of radioiodine, due to ease of administration and less concern for long-term side effects and reproduction problems, makes it a more appropriate therapy.

Specific References

Ruiz JK, Rossi GV, Vallejos HA, et al, "Fulminant Hepatic Failure Associated with Propylthiouracil," *Ann Pharmacother*, 2003, 37(2): 224-8.

Protriptyline

Related Information
- Antidepressant Agents

CAS Number 1225-55-4; 438-60-8

U.S. Brand Names Vivactil®

Synonyms Protriptyline Hydrochloride

Impairment Potential Yes

Use Treatment of various forms of depression, often in conjunction with psychotherapy

Mechanism of Action Increases the synaptic concentration of serotonin and/or norepinephrine in the central nervous system by inhibition of their reuptake by the presynaptic neuronal membrane

Adverse Reactions

Cardiovascular: Arrhythmias, hypotension, hypotension (orthostatic), palpitations, exacerbation of Brugada syndrome

Central nervous system: **Dizziness, drowsiness, headache**, confusion, delirium, hallucinations, nervousness, restlessness, parkinsonian syndrome, anxiety, seizures, insomnia, nightmares, psychosis, fever, hyperthermia, extrapyramidal reactions

Dermatologic: Alopecia, photosensitivity, petechiae, angioedema, urticaria, purpura, pruritus

Endocrine & metabolic: Breast enlargement, galactorrhea, gynecomastia, syndrome of inappropriate antidiuretic hormone secretion, sexual function impairment

Gastrointestinal: **Xerostomia, constipation, unpleasant taste, weight gain, increased appetite, nausea**, diarrhea, heartburn, trouble with gums, decreased lower esophageal sphincter, tone may cause GE reflux, stomatitis, lingua villosa nigra

Genitourinary: Dysuria, testicular edema

Hematologic: Agranulocytosis, leukopenia, eosinophilia, thrombocytopenia

Hepatic: Cholestatic jaundice, elevated liver enzymes

Neuromuscular & skeletal: **Weakness**, fine muscle tremors, rhabdomyolysis, paresthesia

Ocular: Blurred vision, eye pain, increased intraocular pressure, mydriasis, phototoxic

Otic: Tinnitus

Miscellaneous: Diaphoresis (excessive), allergic reactions

Admission Criteria/Prognosis Admit any patient with neurologic or cardiovascular symptoms occurring 6 hours postingestion

Pharmacodynamics/Kinetics

Distribution: Crosses placenta

Protein binding: 92%

Metabolism: Extensively hepatic via N-oxidation, hydroxylation, and glucuronidation; first-pass effect (10% to 25%)

Half-life elimination: 54-92 hours (average: 74 hours)

Time to peak, serum: 24-30 hours

Excretion: Urine

Dosage

Oral:

Adolescents: 15-20 mg/day in 3 divided doses

Adults: 15-60 mg in 3-4 divided doses

Elderly: 15-20 mg/day

Maximum dose: 60 mg/day

Monitoring Parameters Monitor for cardiac abnormalities in elderly patients receiving doses >20 mg

Administration Make any dosage increase in the morning dose

Contraindications Hypersensitivity to protriptyline (cross-reactivity to other cyclic antidepressants may occur) or any component of the formulation; use of MAO inhibitors within 14 days; use of cisapride; use in a patient during the acute recovery phase of MI

Warnings

[U.S. Boxed Warning]: **Antidepressants increase the risk of suicidal thinking and behavior in children and adolescents with major depressive disorder (MDD) and other depressive disorders;** consider risk prior to prescribing. Closely monitor for clinical worsening, suicidality, or unusual changes in behavior; the child's family or caregiver should be instructed to closely observe the patient and communicate condition with healthcare provider. Such observation would generally include at least weekly face-to-face contact with patients or their family members or caregivers during the first 4 weeks of treatment, then every other week visits for the next 4 weeks, then at 12 weeks, and as clinically indicated beyond 12 weeks. Additional contact by telephone may be appropriate between face-to-face visits. Adults treated with antidepressants should be observed similarly for clinical worsening and suicidality, especially during the initial few months of a course of drug therapy, or at times of dose changes, either increases or decreases. A medication guide should be dispensed with each prescription. **Protriptyline is FDA approved for the treatment of depression in adolescents.**

The possibility of a suicide attempt is inherent in major depression and may persist until remission occurs. Monitor for worsening of depression or suicidality, especially during initiation of therapy or with dose increases or decreases. Worsening depression and severe abrupt suicidality that are not part of the presenting symptoms may require discontinuation or modification of drug therapy. Use caution in high-risk patients during initiation of therapy. Prescriptions should be written for the smallest quantity consistent with good patient care. The patient's family or caregiver should be alerted to monitor patients for the emergence of suicidality and associated behaviors such as anxiety, agitation, panic attacks, insomnia, irritability, hostility, impulsivity, akathisia, hypomania, and mania; patients should be instructed to notify their healthcare provider if any of these symptoms or worsening depression occur.

May worsen psychosis in some patients or precipitate a shift to mania or hypomania in patients with bipolar disorder. Monotherapy in patients with bipolar disorder should be avoided. Patients presenting with depressive symptoms should be screened for bipolar disorder. **Protriptyline is not FDA approved for the treatment of bipolar depression.**

May cause sedation, resulting in impaired performance of tasks requiring alertness (eg, operating machinery or driving). Sedative effects may be additive with other CNS depressants and/or ethanol. The degree of sedation is low relative to other antidepressants. May aggravate aggressive behavior. May increase the risks associated with electroconvulsive therapy. Consider discontinuing, when possible, prior to elective surgery. Therapy should not be abruptly discontinued in patients receiving high doses for prolonged periods. May alter glucose regulation - use with caution in patients with diabetes.

May cause orthostatic hypotension (risk is moderate relative to other antidepressants) - use with caution in patients at risk of hypotension or in patients where transient hypotensive episodes would be poorly tolerated (cardiovascular disease or cerebrovascular disease). The degree of anticholinergic blockade produced by this agent is moderate relative to other cyclic antidepressants, however, caution should still be used in patients with urinary retention, benign prostatic hyperplasia, narrow-angle glaucoma, xerostomia, visual problems, constipation, or history of bowel obstruction.

Use with caution in patients with a history of cardiovascular disease (including previous MI, stroke, tachycardia, or conduction abnormalities). The risk of conduction abnormalities with this agent is moderate-high relative to other antidepressants. Use caution in patients with a previous seizure disorder or condition predisposing to seizures such as brain damage, alcoholism, or concurrent therapy with other drugs which lower the seizure threshold. Use with caution in hyperthyroid patients or those receiving thyroid supplementation. Use with caution in patients with hepatic or renal dysfunction and in elderly patients.

Dosage Forms Tablet, as hydrochloride: 5 mg, 10 mg

Reference Range Therapeutic: 70-250 ng/mL (SI: 266-950 nmol/L); Toxic: >500 ng/mL (SI: >1900 nmol/L); levels >1000 ng/mL (SI: >3800 nmol/L) associated with cardiotoxic effects

Overdosage/Treatment

Decontamination: **Do not** induce emesis; lavage is effective if performed within 90 minutes and may be effective if performed within 6 hours/ activated charcoal

Supportive therapy: Following initiation of essential overdose management, toxic symptoms should be treated. Ventricular arrhythmias and ventricular conduction defects often respond to concurrent systemic alkalinization (sodium bicarbonate 0.5-2 mEq/kg I.V.). Titrate to a serum pH of 7.45-7.55. Arrhythmias unresponsive to this therapy may respond to lidocaine 1 mg/kg I.V. followed by a titrated infusion. Phenytoin is also useful in treating ventricular dysrhythmias (15 mg/kg up to 1 g I.V.). Physostigmine (1-2 mg I.V. slowly for adults or 0.5 mg I.V. slowly for children) may be indicated for seizures or movement disorders but only as **a last resort**. Propranolol may also be utilized for supraventricular arrhythmias (rate: >160) at 1 mg/minute to a maximum of 5 mg in adults; pediatric dosage of 0.1 mg/kg/dose to 1 mg I.V.. Seizures usually respond to lorazepam or diazepam I.V. boluses (5-10 mg for adults up to 30 mg or 0.25-0.4 mg/kg/dose for children up to 10 mg/ dose). If seizures are unresponsive or recur, phenytoin or phenobarbital may be required. Patients must be monitored for at least 24 hours if any signs or symptoms are exhibited. Dobutamine is preferred over dopamine for hypotension, although there is conflicting animal data. Norepinephrine appears effective in treating hypotension; glucagon (10 mg I.V.) can be given to treat hypotension. Flumazenil is contraindicated; magnesium has potentiated adverse cardiac effects (ie, asystole, decreased left ventricular pressure) in an animal model, although it was used successfully in treating refractory ventricular fibrillation at a dose of 20 nmol I.V. (a total of 2 doses). For treatment of lingua villosa nigra, discontinue causative agent. Clean the tongue with a toothbrush and rinse mouth with a half-strength solution of hydrogen peroxide or 10% carbamide peroxide. Oral symptoms should subside in a few days.

Test Interactions ↑ glucose

Drug Interactions

Substrate of CYP2D6 (major)

Altretamine: Concurrent use may cause orthostatic hypertension

Amphetamines: TCAs may enhance the effect of amphetamines; monitor for adverse CV effects

Anticholinergics: Combined use with TCAs may produce additive anticholinergic effects

Antihypertensives: Cyclic antidepressants may inhibit the antihypertensive response to bethanidine, clonidine, debrisoquin, guanadrel, guanethidine, guanabenz, guanfacine; monitor BP; consider alternate antihypertensive agent

Beta-agonists: When combined with TCAs may predispose patients to cardiac arrhythmias

Bupropion: May increase the levels of tricyclic antidepressants; based on limited information; monitor response

Carbamazepine: Tricyclic antidepressants may increase carbamazepine levels; monitor

Cholestyramine and colestipol: May bind TCAs and reduce their absorption; monitor for altered response

Clonidine: Abrupt discontinuation of clonidine may cause hypertensive crisis, cyclic antidepressants may enhance the response

CNS depressants: Sedative effects may be additive with TCAs; monitor for increased effect; includes benzodiazepines, barbiturates, antipsychotics, ethanol, and other sedative medications

CYP2D6 inhibitors: May increase the levels/effects of protriptyline. Example inhibitors include chlorpromazine, delavirdine, fluoxetine, miconazole, paroxetine, pergolide, quinidine, quinine, ritonavir, and ropinirole.

Epinephrine (and other direct alpha-agonists): Pressor response to I.V. epinephrine, norepinephrine, and phenylephrine may be enhanced in patients receiving TCAs (**Note:** Effect is unlikely with epinephrine or levonordefrin dosages typically administered as infiltration in combination with local anesthetics)

Fenfluramine: May increase tricyclic antidepressant levels/effects

Hypoglycemic agents (including insulin): TCAs may enhance the hypoglycemic effects of tolazamide, chlorpropamide, or insulin; monitor for changes in blood glucose levels; reported with chlorpropamide, tolazamide, and insulin

Levodopa: tricyclic antidepressants may decrease the absorption (bioavailability) of levodopa; rare hypertensive episodes have also been attributed to this combination

Linezolid: Hyperpyrexia, hypertension, tachycardia, confusion, seizures, and **deaths have been reported** with agents which inhibit MAO (serotonin syndrome); this combination should be avoided

Lithium: Concurrent use with a TCA may increase the risk for neurotoxicity

MAO inhibitors: Hyperpyrexia, hypertension, tachycardia, confusion, seizures, and **deaths have been reported** (serotonin syndrome); this combination should be avoided

Methylphenidate: Metabolism of tricyclic antidepressants may be decreased

Phenothiazines: Serum concentrations of some TCAs may be increased; in addition, TCAs may increase concentration of phenothiazines; monitor for altered clinical response

QT$_c$-prolonging agents: Concurrent use of tricyclic agents with other drugs which may prolong QT$_c$ interval may increase the risk of potentially fatal arrhythmias; includes type Ia and type III antiarrhythmics agents, selected quinolones (sparfloxacin, gatifloxacin, moxifloxacin, grepafloxacin), cisapride, and other agents

Ritonavir: Combined use of high-dose tricyclic antidepressants with ritonavir may cause serotonin syndrome in HIV-positive patients; monitor

Sucralfate: Absorption of tricyclic antidepressants may be reduced with coadministration

Sympathomimetics, indirect-acting: Tricyclic antidepressants may result in a decreased sensitivity to indirect-acting sympathomimetics; includes dopamine and ephedrine; also see interaction with epinephrine (and direct-acting sympathomimetics)

Tramadol: Tramadol's risk of seizures may be increased with TCAs

Valproic acid: May increase serum concentrations/adverse effects of some tricyclic antidepressants

Warfarin (and other oral anticoagulants): Tricyclic antidepressants may increase the anticoagulant effect in patients stabilized on warfarin; monitor INR

Pregnancy Risk Factor C

Lactation Excretion in breast milk unknown/not recommended

Nursing Implications Offer patient sugarless hard candy or gum for dry mouth. Clean the tongue with a toothbrush and rinse mouth with a half-strength solution of hydrogen peroxide or 10% carbamide peroxide. Symptoms should subside in a few days.

Pseudoephedrine

CAS Number 345-78-8

U.S. Brand Names Biofed [OTC]; Decofed® [OTC]; Dimetapp® 12-Hour Non-Drowsy Extentabs® [OTC]; Dimetapp® Decongestant [OTC]; Genaphed® [OTC]; Kidkare Decongestant [OTC]; Kodet SE [OTC]; Oranyl [OTC]; PediaCare® Decongestant Infants [OTC]; Silfedrine Children's [OTC]; Sudafed® 12 Hour [OTC]; Sudafed® 24 Hour [OTC]; Sudafed® Children's [OTC]; Sudafed® [OTC]; Sudodrin [OTC]; Triaminic® Allergy Congestion [OTC]

Synonyms d-Isoephedrine Hydrochloride; Pseudoephedrine Hydrochloride; Pseudoephedrine Sulfate

Impairment Potential Yes

Use Temporary symptomatic relief of nasal congestion due to common cold, upper respiratory allergies, and sinusitis; also promotes nasal or sinus drainage; prevention of barotrauma during air travel

Mechanism of Action Directly stimulates alpha-adrenergic receptors of respiratory mucosa causing vasoconstriction; directly stimulates beta-adrenergic receptors causing bronchial relaxation, increased heart rate and contractility

Adverse Reactions

Cardiovascular: **Tachycardia, palpitations, cardiac arrhythmias**, chest pain, myocardial ischemia, angina, sinus tachycardia

Central nervous system: **Nervousness, excitation, dizziness, insomnia, headache, drowsiness, transient stimulation**, psychosis, mania, paranoia, CNS depression, seizures

Dermatologic: Systemic contact dermatitis, exfoliative dermatitis, angioedema, urticaria, exanthem, toxic epidermal necrolysis

Endocrine & metabolic: Hypokalemia

Gastrointestinal: Nausea, vomiting, ischemic colitis

Genitourinary: Dysuria

Neuromuscular & skeletal: **Tremors**

Miscellaneous: Fixed drug eruption

Signs and Symptoms of Overdose Arrhythmias, convulsions, depression, insomnia, mydriasis, nausea, vomiting

Pharmacodynamics/Kinetics

Onset of action: Decongestant: Oral: 15-30 minutes

Duration: Immediate release tablet: 4-6 hours; Extended release: ≤12 hours

Absorption: Rapid

Metabolism: Partially hepatic

Half-life elimination: 9-16 hours

Excretion: Urine (70% to 90% as unchanged drug, 1% to 6% as active norpseudoephedrine); dependent on urine pH and flow rate; alkaline urine decreases renal elimination of pseudoephedrine

Dosage

Oral:

Children (do not give sustained release tablets):

<2 years: 4 mg/kg/day in divided doses every 6 hours

2-5 years: 15 mg every 6 hours; maximum: 60 mg/24 hours

6-12 years: 30 mg every 6 hours; maximum: 120 mg/24 hours

Adults: 30-60 mg every 4-6 hours, sustained release: 120 mg every 12 hours; maximum: 480 mg/24 hours

Prevention of barotrauma during air travel: 120 mg at least 30 minutes before air travel

Dosing adjustment in renal impairment: Reduce dose

Administration

Do not crush extended release drug product, swallow whole.

Contraindications Hypersensitivity to pseudoephedrine or any component of the formulation; with or within 14 days of MAO inhibitor therapy

Warnings Use with caution in patients >60 years of age; administer with caution to patients with hypertension, hyperthyroidism, diabetes mellitus, cardiovascular disease, ischemic heart disease, increased intraocular pressure, or prostatic hyperplasia. Elderly patients are more likely to experience adverse reactions to sympathomimetics. Overdosage may cause hallucinations, seizures, CNS depression, and death. When used for self-medication (OTC), notify healthcare provider if symptoms do not improve within 7 days or are accompanied by fever.

Dosage Forms

Caplet, extended release, as hydrochloride (Contact® Cold, Sudafed® 12 Hour): 120 mg

Liquid, as hydrochloride: 30 mg/5 mL (120 mL, 480 mL)

Silfedrine Children's: 15 mg/5 mL (120 mL, 480 mL) [alcohol and sugar free; grape flavor]

Simply Stuffy™: 15 mg/5 mL (120 mL) [alcohol free; contains sodium benzoate; cherry berry flavor]

Sudafed® Children's: 15 mg/5 mL (120 mL) [alcohol and sugar free; contains sodium benzoate; grape flavor]

Liquid, oral drops, as hydrochloride:

Dimetapp® Decongestant Infant Drops: 7.5 mg/0.8 mL (15 mL) [alcohol free; contains sodium benzoate; grape flavor]

Kidkare Decongestant: 7.5 mg/0.8 mL (30 mL) [alcohol free; contains benzoic acid and sodium benzoate; cherry flavor]

PediaCare® Decongestant: 7.5 mg/0.8 mL (15 mL) [alcohol free, dye free; contains benzoic acid, sodium benzoate; fruit flavor]

Syrup, as hydrochloride:

Biofed: 30 mg/5 mL (120 mL, 240 mL, 480 mL, 3840 mL) [alcohol free; contains sodium benzoate]

ElixSure™ Congestion: 15 mg/5 mL (120 mL) [grape bubble gum flavor]

Tablet, as hydrochloride: 30 mg, 60 mg

Genaphed®, Kodet SE, Oranyl, Sudafed®, Sudodrin, Sudo-Tab®: 30 mg

SudoGest: 30 mg, 60 mg

Tablet, chewable, as hydrochloride (Sudafed® Children's): 15 mg [sugar free; contains phenylalanine 0.78 mg/tablet; orange flavor]

Tablet, extended release, as hydrochloride:

Dimetapp® 12-Hour Non-Drowsy Extentabs®: 120 mg

Sudafed® 24 Hour: 240 mg

Reference Range Following an oral dose of 180 mg, peak plasma pseudoephedrine levels range from 0.5-0.9 mcg/mL

Overdosage/Treatment

Decontamination: Activated Charcoal.

There is no specific antidote. Treatment is supportive. Hyperactivity and agitation usually respond to reduced sensory input; however, with extreme agitation, haloperidol (2-5 mg I.M. for adults) may be required. Hyperthermia is best treated with external cooling measures, or when severe or unresponsive, muscle paralysis with pancuronium may be needed. Hypertension is usually transient and generally does not require treatment unless severe. For diastolic blood pressures >110 mm Hg, a nitroprusside infusion should be initiated. Seizures usually respond to lorazepam or diazepam I.V. and/or phenytoin maintenance regimens.

Drug Interactions

Decreased effect of methyldopa, reserpine

Increased toxicity: MAO inhibitors may increase blood pressure effects of pseudoephedrine; propranolol, sympathomimetic agents may increase toxicity

Pregnancy Risk Factor C

Lactation Enters breast milk/use caution (AAP rates "compatible")

Nursing Implications Do not crush extended release drug product

Additional Information Pseudoephedrine hydrochloride: Cenafed® syrup [OTC], Decofed® syrup [OTC], Neofed® [OTC], Novafed®, Sudafed® [OTC], Sudafed® 12 Hour [OTC], Sudafed® tablet [OTC], Sufedrin® [OTC]

Pseudoephedrine sulfate: Afrinol® [OTC]

Specific References

Boland DM, Rein J, Lew EO, et al, "Fatal Cold Medication Intoxication in an Infant," *J Anal Toxicol*, 2003, 27:523-6.

Pyrazinamide

CAS Number 98-96-4

Synonyms Pyrazinoic Acid Amide

Use Adjunctive treatment of tuberculosis in combination with other antituberculosis agents

Mechanism of Action Converted to pyrazinoic acid in susceptible strains of *Mycobacterium* which lowers the pH of the environment structurally related to nicitinamide

Adverse Reactions

Cardiovascular: Hypertension

Central nervous system: Malaise, seizures, fever, headache

Dermatologic: Urticaria, rash, photosensitivity, lichenoid photodermatitis

Endocrine & metabolic: Gout, hyperuricemia

Gastrointestinal: Nausea, vomiting, anorexia

Hematologic: Thrombocytopenia

Hepatic: Hepatotoxicity, jaundice (40 mg/kg)

Neuromuscular & skeletal: Arthralgia, rhabdomyolysis

Renal: Interstitial nephritis, urate retention

Signs and Symptoms of Overdose Gout, GI upset, hepatitis (>3 g/day dosage), hyperuricemia, photophobia

Pharmacodynamics/Kinetics

Bacteriostatic or bactericidal depending on drug's concentration at infection site

Absorption: Well absorbed

Distribution: Widely into body tissues and fluids including liver, lung, and CSF

Relative diffusion from blood into CSF: Adequate with or without inflammation (exceeds usual MICs)

CSF:blood level ratio: Inflamed meninges: 100%

Protein binding: 50%

Metabolism: Hepatic

Half-life elimination: 9-10 hours

Time to peak, serum: Within 2 hours

Excretion: Urine (4% as unchanged drug)

Dosage

Oral (calculate dose on ideal body weight rather than total body weight):

Note: A four-drug regimen (isoniazid, rifampin, pyrazinamide, and either streptomycin or ethambutol) is preferred for the initial, empiric treatment of TB. When the drug susceptibility results are available, the regimen should be altered as appropriate. For the treatment of latent TB infection (LTBI), combination pyrazinamide/rifampin therapy should not generally be offered (*MMWR* Aug 8, 2003).

Children and Adults:

Daily therapy: 15-30 mg/kg/day (maximum: 2 g/day)

Directly observed therapy (DOT):

Twice weekly: 50-70 mg/kg (maximum: 4 g)

Three times/week: 50-70 mg/kg (maximum: 3 g)

Elderly: Start with a lower daily dose (15 mg/kg) and increase as tolerated

Dosing adjustment in renal impairment: Cl_{cr} <50 mL/minute: Avoid use or reduce dose to 12-20 mg/kg/day

Dosing adjustment in hepatic impairment: Reduce dose

Monitoring Parameters Periodic liver function tests, serum uric acid, sputum culture, chest x-ray 2-3 months into treatment and at completion

Contraindications Hypersensitivity to pyrazinamide or any component of the formulation; acute gout; severe hepatic damage

Warnings Use with caution in patients with renal failure, chronic gout, diabetes mellitus, or porphyria. Use with caution in patients receiving concurrent medications associated with hepatotoxicity (particularly with rifampin), or in patients with a history of alcoholism (even if ethanol consumption is discontinued during therapy).

Dosage Forms Tablet: 500 mg

Overdosage/Treatment

Decontamination: Activated charcoal

Enhancement of elimination: Multiple dosing of activated charcoal may be effective

Drug Interactions Combination therapy with rifampin and pyrazinamide has been associated with severe and fatal hepatotoxic reactions.

Pregnancy Risk Factor C

Lactation Enters breast milk/use caution

Pyrimethamine

CAS Number 58-14-0

U.S. Brand Names Daraprim®

Use Prophylaxis of malaria due to susceptible strains of plasmodia; used in conjunction with quinine and sulfadiazine for the treatment of uncomplicated attacks of chloroquine-resistant *P. falciparum* malaria; used in conjunction with fast-acting schizonticide to initiate transmission control and suppression cure; synergistic combination with sulfonamide in treatment of toxoplasmosis

Mechanism of Action Inhibits parasitic dihydrofolate reductase, resulting in inhibition of tetrahydrofolic acid synthesis

Adverse Reactions

Frequency not defined.

Cardiovascular: Arrhythmias (large doses)

Central nervous system: Depression, fever, insomnia, lightheadedness, malaise, seizures

Dermatologic: Abnormal skin pigmentation, dermatitis, erythema multiforme, rash, Stevens-Johnson syndrome, toxic epidermal necrolysis

Gastrointestinal: Anorexia, abdominal cramps, vomiting, diarrhea, xerostomia, atrophic glossitis

Hematologic: Megaloblastic anemia, leukopenia, pancytopenia, thrombocytopenia, pulmonary eosinophilia

Genitourinary: Hematuria

Miscellaneous: Anaphylaxis

Signs and Symptoms of Overdose Apnea, fever, megaloblastic anemia, seizures, tachycardia, vomiting

Pharmacodynamics/Kinetics

Onset of action: ~1 hour

Absorption: Well absorbed

Distribution: Widely, mainly in blood cells, kidneys, lungs, liver, and spleen; crosses into CSF; crosses placenta; enters breast milk

Protein binding: 80% to 87%

Metabolism: Hepatic

Half-life elimination: 80-95 hours
Time to peak, serum: 1.5-8 hours
Excretion: Urine (20% to 30% as unchanged drug)

Dosage
Malaria chemoprophylaxis (for areas where chloroquine-resistant *P. falciparum* exists): Begin prophylaxis 2 weeks before entering endemic area:
Children: 0.5 mg/kg once weekly; not to exceed 25 mg/dose
or
Children:
<4 years: 6.25 mg once weekly
4-10 years: 12.5 mg once weekly
Children >10 years and Adults: 25 mg once weekly
Dosage should be continued for all age groups for at least 6-10 weeks after leaving endemic areas
Chloroquine-resistant *P. falciparum* malaria (when used in conjunction with quinine and sulfadiazine):
Children:
<10 kg: 6.25 mg/day once daily for 3 days
10-20 kg: 12.5 mg/day once daily for 3 days
20-40 kg: 25 mg/day once daily for 3 days
Adults: 25 mg twice daily for 3 days
Toxoplasmosis:
Infants (congenital toxoplasmosis): Oral: 1 mg/kg once daily for 6 months with sulfadiazine then every other month with sulfa, alternating with spiramycin.
Children: Loading dose: 2 mg/kg/day divided into 2 equal daily doses for 1-3 days (maximum: 100 mg/day) followed by 1 mg/kg/day divided into 2 doses for 4 weeks; maximum: 25 mg/day
With sulfadiazine or trisulfapyrimidines: 2 mg/kg/day divided every 12 hours for 3 days, followed by 1 mg/kg/day once daily or divided twice daily for 4 weeks given with trisulfapyrimidines or sulfadiazine
Adults: 50-75 mg/day together with 1-4 g of a sulfonamide for 1-3 weeks depending on patient's tolerance and response, then reduce dose by 50% and continue for 4-5 weeks **or** 25-50 mg/day for 3-4 weeks
Prophylaxis for first episode of *Toxoplasma gondii*:
Children ≥1 month of age: 1 mg/kg/day once daily with dapsone, plus oral folinic acid 5 mg every 3 days
Adolescents and Adults: 50 mg once weekly with dapsone, plus oral folinic acid 25 mg once weekly
Prophylaxis to prevent recurrence of *Toxoplasma gondii*:
Children ≥1 month of age: 1 mg/kg/day once daily given with sulfadiazine or clindamycin, plus oral folinic acid 5 mg every 3 days
Adolescents and Adults: 25-50 mg once daily in combination with sulfadiazine or clindamycin, plus oral folinic acid 10-25 mg daily; atovaquone plus oral folinic acid has also been used in combination with pyrimethamine.

Monitoring Parameters CBC, including platelet counts
Administration
Administer with meals to minimize GI distress.
Contraindications Hypersensitivity to pyrimethamine or any component of the formulation; chloroguanide; resistant malaria; megaloblastic anemia secondary to folate deficiency
Warnings When used for more than 3-4 days, it may be advisable to administer leucovorin to prevent hematologic complications; monitor CBC and platelet counts every 2 weeks; use with caution in patients with impaired renal or hepatic function or with possible G6PD. Use caution in patients with seizure disorders or possible folate deficiency (eg, malabsorption syndrome, pregnancy, alcoholism).
Dosage Forms Tablet: 25 mg
Overdosage/Treatment
Decontamination: Lavage within 1 hour, activated charcoal
Supportive therapy: Initiate with I.V. fluids; assure respiratory patency; treat seizures aggressively with benzodiazepines, follow with barbiturates, if necessary; other complications of seizures (acid base, etc), treat conventionally as necessary
Antidote: Leucovorin 10 mg/m² every 6 hours daily for 3 days followed by folic acid 10 mg/day if hematologic toxicity is present
Antidote(s)
• Leucovorin [ANTIDOTE]
Drug Interactions Inhibits CYP2C9 (moderate), 2D6 (moderate)
Antipsychotic agents: Serum levels may be increased by pyrimethamine.
Bone marrow suppressive agents: Sulfonamides (synergy), methotrexate, TMP/SMZ, zidovudine may increase the risk of bone marrow suppression.
CYP2C9 Substrates: Pyrimethamine may increase the levels/effects of CYP2C9 substrates. Example substrates include bosentan, dapsone, fluoxetine, glimepiride, glipizide, losartan, montelukast, nateglinide, paclitaxel, phenytoin, warfarin, and zafirlukast.
CYP2D6 substrates: Pyrimethamine may increase the levels/effects of CYP2D6 substrates. Example substrates include amphetamines, selected beta-blockers, dextromethorphan, fluoxetine, lidocaine, mirtazapine, nefazodone, paroxetine, risperidone, ritonavir, thioridazine, tricyclic antidepressants, and venlafaxine.

CYP2D6 prodrug substrates: Pyrimethamine may decrease the levels/effects of CYP2D6 prodrug substrates. Example prodrug substrates include codeine, hydrocodone, oxycodone, and tramadol.
Pregnancy Risk Factor C
Pregnancy Implications There are no adequate or well-controlled studies in pregnant women. Teratogenicity has been reported in animal studies. If administered during pregnancy (ie, for toxoplasmosis), supplementation of folate is strongly recommended. Pregnancy should be avoided during therapy.
Lactation Enters breast milk/not recommended (AAP rates "compatible")
Nursing Implications Monitor complete blood counts and platelet counts twice weekly
Additional Information Leucovorin may be given to prevent hematologic problems due to folic acid deficiency.

Quazepam

CAS Number 36735-22-5
U.S. Brand Names Doral®
Impairment Potential Yes
Use Short-term treatment of insomnia
Mechanism of Action Depresses all levels of the CNS, including the limbic and reticular formation, probably through the increased action of gamma-aminobutyric acid (GABA), which is a major inhibitory neurotransmitter in the brain
Adverse Reactions
Central nervous system: **Drowsiness** (12%), headache (4.5%), fatigue (1.9%), dizziness (1.5%), slurred speech, irritability, dystonia
Dermatologic: Hypertrichosis, alopecia, urticaria, purpura, pruritus
Endocrine & metabolic: Changes in libido
Gastrointestinal: Xerostomia (1.5%), dyspepsia (1.1%)
Genitourinary: Urinary retention, incontinence
Hematologic: Leukocytosis, thrombocytosis
Hepatic: Jaundice, elevated total bilirubin, elevated SGPT (ALT), elevated alkaline phosphatase
Neuromuscular & skeletal: Dysarthria, paresthesia
Renal: Elevated creatinine, elevated BUN
Signs and Symptoms of Overdose Ataxia, confusion, coma, dyspnea, hypoactive reflexes, hyporeflexia, hypotension, slurred speech, somnolence
Pharmacodynamics/Kinetics
Studies have shown that the elderly are more sensitive to the effects of benzodiazepines as compared to younger adults
Absorption: Rapid through gastrointestinal tract
Distribution: V_d: 5-8.6 L/kg; distributed widely throughout body
Protein binding: 95%
Metabolism: In the liver to two active compounds (2-oxoquazepam and N-desalkyl-2-oxoquazepam)
Half-life: Parent: 25-41 hours; Active metabolite: 40-114 hours
In the elderly: Parent: 53 hours; Active metabolite: 39-73 hours
Time to peak serum concentration: 2 hours
Elimination: Excreted in urine (31%) and feces (23%)
Dosage Adults: Oral: Initial: 15 mg at bedtime, in some patients the dose may be reduced to 7.5 mg after a few nights
Elderly: Dosing should be cautious; begin at lower end of dosing range (ie, 7.5 mg)
Dosing adjustment in hepatic impairment: Dose reduction may be necessary
Monitoring Parameters Respiratory and cardiovascular status
Contraindications Hypersensitivity to quazepam or any component of the formulation (cross-sensitivity with other benzodiazepines may exist); narrow-angle glaucoma (not in product labeling, however, benzodiazepines are contraindicated); pregnancy
Warnings
Should be used only after evaluation of potential causes of sleep disturbance. Failure of sleep disturbance to resolve after 7-10 days may indicate psychiatric or medical illness. A worsening of insomnia or the emergence of new abnormalities of thought or behavior may represent unrecognized psychiatric or medical illness and requires immediate and careful evaluation. Use with caution in elderly or debilitated patients, patients with hepatic disease (including alcoholics), or renal impairment. Use with caution in patients with respiratory disease or impaired gag reflex. Avoid use in patients with sleep apnea.
Causes CNS depression (dose-related) resulting in sedation, dizziness, confusion, or ataxia which may impair physical and mental capabilities. Patients must be cautioned about performing tasks which require mental alertness (operating machinery or driving). Use with caution in patients receiving other CNS depressants or psychoactive agents. Effects with other sedative drugs or ethanol may be potentiated. Benzodiazepines have been associated with falls and traumatic injury and should be used with extreme caution in patients who are at risk of these events (especially the elderly).
Use caution in patients with depression, particularly if suicidal risk may be present. Use with caution in patients with a history of drug dependence.

Benzodiazepines have been associated with dependence and acute withdrawal symptoms on discontinuation or reduction in dose. Acute withdrawal, including seizures, may be precipitated after administration of flumazenil to patients receiving long-term benzodiazepine therapy.

Benzodiazepines have been associated with anterograde amnesia. Paradoxical reactions, including hyperactive or aggressive behavior have been reported with benzodiazepines, particularly in adolescent/ pediatric or psychiatric patients. Does not have analgesic, antidepressant, or antipsychotic properties.

Dosage Forms Tablet: 7.5 mg, 15 mg

Reference Range Mean plasma level of 148 ng/mL 1.5 hours after ingestion of 25 mg

Overdosage/Treatment

Decontamination: Activated charcoal

Supportive therapy: Treatment is supportive. Rarely is mechanical ventilation required. Flumazenil has been shown to reverse benzodiazepine induced CNS depression.

Enhancement of elimination: Multiple dosing of activated charcoal may be useful

Antidote(s)

● Flumazenil [ANTIDOTE]

Drug Interactions Substrate of CYP3A4 (minor)

CNS depressants: Sedative effects and/or respiratory depression may be additive with CNS depressants; includes ethanol, barbiturates, narcotic analgesics, and other sedative agents; monitor for increased effect

Levodopa: Therapeutic effects may be diminished in some patients following the addition of a benzodiazepine; limited/inconsistent data

Oral contraceptives: May decrease the clearance of some benzodiazepines (those which undergo oxidative metabolism); monitor for increased benzodiazepine effect

Theophylline: May partially antagonize some of the effects of benzodiazepines; monitor for decreased response; may require higher doses for sedation

Pregnancy Risk Factor X

Lactation Enters breast milk/not recommended (AAP rates "of concern")

Nursing Implications Provide safety measures (ie, side rails, night light, call button); remove smoking materials from area; supervise ambulation

Additional Information More likely than triazolam to cause daytime sedation and fatigue; classified as a long-acting benzodiazepine hypnotic, therefore, may prevent withdrawal symptoms with discontinuation of therapy

Specific References

Kato K, Yasui-Furukori N, Fukasawa T, et al, "Effects of Itraconazole on the Plasma Kinetics of Quazepam and Its Two Active Metabolites After a Single Oral Dose of the Drug," *Ther Drug Monit*, 2003, 25(4):473-7.

Quetiapine

Related Information

● Antipsychotic Agents

U.S. Brand Names Seroquel®

Synonyms Quetiapine Fumarate

Use Treatment of schizophrenia; treatment of acute manic episodes associated with bipolar disorder (as monotherapy or in combination with lithium or valproate)

Unlabeled/Investigational Use Autism, psychosis (children)

Mechanism of Action

Mechanism of action of quetiapine, as with other antipsychotic drugs, is unknown. However, it has been proposed that this drug's antipsychotic activity is mediated through a combination of dopamine type 2 (D_2) and serotonin type 2 ($5-HT_2$) antagonism. It is an antagonist at multiple neurotransmitter receptors in the brain: serotonin $5-HT_{1A}$ (IC_{50}=717nM) and $5-HT_2$ (IC_{50}=148nM), dopamine D_1 (IC_{50}=1268nM) and D_2 (IC_{50}=329nM), histamine H_1 (IC_{50}=30nM), and adrenergic alpha$_1$- (IC_{50}=94nM) and alpha$_2$- (IC_{50}=271nM) receptors; but appears to have no appreciable affinity at cholinergic muscarinic and benzodiazepine receptors.

Antagonism at receptors other than dopamine and $5-HT_2$ with similar receptor affinities may explain some of the other effects of quetiapine. The drug's antagonism of histamine H_1-receptors may explain the somnolence observed with it. The drug's antagonism of adrenergic alpha$_1$-receptors may explain the orthostatic hypotension observed with it.

Adverse Reactions

Cardiovascular: Postural hypotension, tachycardia, palpitations, peripheral edema, bradycardia, QT prolongation

Central nervous system: **Agitation, dizziness, headache, somnolence**, anxiety, fever, pain, abnormal dreams, tardive dyskinesia

Dermatologic: Rash, photosensitivity, Stevens-Johnson syndrome

Endocrine & metabolic: **Cholesterol increased, triglycerides increased**, diabetes mellitus, hyperglycemia, hyperlipidemia, hypothyroidism, hyponatremia, SIADH

Gastrointestinal: **Weight gain (≥7% body weight, dose related), xerostomia**, abdominal pain (dose related), constipation, dyspepsia (dose related), anorexia, vomiting, gastroenteritis, appetite increased, salivation increased

Hematologic: Leukopenia, anemia, leukocytosis, agranulocytosis

Hepatic: AST increased, ALT increased, GGT increased, alkaline phosphatase increased

Neuromuscular & skeletal: Dysarthria, back pain, weakness, tremor, hypertonia, dysarthria, involuntary movements, rhabdomyolysis

Ocular: Amblyopia

Respiratory: Rhinitis, pharyngitis, cough, dyspnea, epistaxis

Miscellaneous: Diaphoresis, flu-like syndrome, anaphylaxis

Signs and Symptoms of Overdose Agitation, coma, hypotension, tachycardia

Admission Criteria/Prognosis Admit any symptomatic patient or asymptomatic ingestion >25 mg/kg.

Pharmacodynamics/Kinetics

Absorption: Rapidly absorbed following oral administration

Distribution: V_d: 10 ± 4 L/kg; V_{dss}: ~2 days

Protein binding, plasma: 83%

Metabolism: Primarily hepatic; via CYP3A4; forms two inactive metabolites

Bioavailability: 9% ± 4%; tablet is 100% bioavailable relative to solution

Half-life elimination: Mean: Terminal: ~6 hours

Time to peak, plasma: 1.5 hours

Excretion: Urine (73% as metabolites, <1% as unchanged drug); feces (20%)

Dosage

Oral:

Children and Adolescents:

Autism (unlabeled use): 100-350 mg/day (1.6-5.2 mg/kg/day)

Psychosis and mania (unlabeled use): Initial: 25 mg twice daily; titrate as necessary to 450 mg/day

Adults:

Schizophrenia/psychoses: Initial: 25 mg twice daily; increase in increments of 25-50 mg 2-3 times/day on the second and third day, if tolerated, to a target dose of 300-400 mg in 2-3 divided doses by day 4. Make further adjustments as needed at intervals of at least 2 days in adjustments of 25-50 mg twice daily. Usual maintenance range: 300-800 mg/day

Mania: Initial: 50 mg twice daily on day 1, increase dose in increments of 100 mg/day to 200 mg twice daily on day 4; may increase to a target dose of 800 mg/day by day 6 at increments of ≤200 mg/day. Usual dosage range: 400-800 mg/day

Elderly: 40% lower mean oral clearance of quetiapine in adults >65 years of age; higher plasma levels expected and, therefore, dosage adjustment may be needed; elderly patients usually require 50-200 mg/day

Dosing comments in renal insufficiency: 25% lower mean oral clearance of quetiapine than normal subjects; however, plasma concentrations similar to normal subjects receiving the same dose; no dosage adjustment required

Dosing comments in hepatic insufficiency: 30% lower mean oral clearance of quetiapine than normal subjects; higher plasma levels expected in hepatically impaired subjects; dosage adjustment may be needed

Initial: 25 mg/day, increase dose by 25-50 mg/day to effective dose, based on clinical response and tolerability to patient

Monitoring Parameters Vital signs; fasting lipid profile and fasting blood glucose/Hgb A_{1c} (prior to treatment, at 3 months, then annually); BMI, personal/family history of obesity, waist circumference; blood pressure; mental status, abnormal involuntary movement scale (AIMS); Weight should be assessed prior to treatment, at 4 weeks, 8 weeks, 12 weeks, and then at quarterly intervals. Consider titrating to a different antipsychotic agent for a weight gain ≥5% of the initial weight. Patients should have eyes checked for cataracts every 6 months while on this medication.

Contraindications Hypersensitivity to quetiapine or any component of the formulation; severe CNS depression; bone marrow suppression; blood dyscrasias; severe hepatic disease, coma

Warnings

[U.S. Boxed Warning]: Patients with dementia-related behavioral disorders treated with atypical antipsychotics are at an increased risk of death compared to placebo. Quetiapine is not approved for this indication.

Has been noted to cause cataracts in animals, lens examination on initiation of therapy and every 6 months is recommended. May be sedating, use with caution in disorders where CNS depression is a feature. Use with caution in Parkinson's disease. Caution in patients with hemodynamic instability; prior myocardial infarction or ischemic heart disease; hypercholesterolemia; thyroid disease; predisposition to seizures; subcortical brain damage; hepatic impairment; severe cardiac, renal, or respiratory disease. May alter temperature regulation or mask toxicity of other drugs due to antiemetic effects. May alter cardiac conduction - life-threatening arrhythmias have occurred with therapeutic doses of antipsychotics. May cause orthostatic hypotension - use with caution in patients at risk of this effect or those who would tolerate transient hypotensive episodes (cerebrovascular disease, cardiovascular disease, or other medications which may predispose). Esophageal dysmotility and aspiration have been associated with antipsychotic use - use with caution in patients at risk of pneumonia (ie, Alzheimer's disease).

May cause anticholinergic effects (confusion, agitation, constipation, xerostomia, blurred vision, urinary retention); therefore, they should be used with caution in patients with decreased gastrointestinal motility, urinary retention, BPH, xerostomia, or visual problems. Conditions which also may be exacerbated by cholinergic blockade include narrow-angle glaucoma (screening is recommended) and worsening of myasthenia gravis. Relative to other antipsychotics, quetiapine has a moderate potency of cholinergic blockade. The risk of extrapyramidal symptoms, tardive dyskinesia, and neuroleptic malignant syndrome (NMS) in association with quetiapine is very low relative to other antipsychotics. May cause hyperglycemia; in some cases may be extreme and associated with ketoacidosis, hyperosmolar coma, or death. Use with caution in patients with diabetes or other disorders of glucose regulation; monitor for worsening of glucose control.

The possibility of a suicide attempt is inherent in psychotic illness or bipolar disorder; use caution in high-risk patients during initiation of therapy. Prescriptions should be written for the smallest quantity consistent with good patient care.

Dosage Forms Tablet, as fumarate:
Seroquel®: 25 mg, 50 mg, 100 mg, 200 mg, 300 mg, 400 mg

Reference Range Serum range for quetiapine doses from 300-600 mg: ~44-91 ng/mL. Serum quetiapine level following a 20 g overdose (and associated with deep coma) was 12,700 ng/mL. Postmortem cavity blood and liver quetiapine levels of 170,000 ng/mL and 190 mg/kg, respectively, were found in a quetiapine fatality. Quetiapine may undergo postmortem redistribution.

Overdosage/Treatment

Decontamination: Lavage/activated charcoal can be given for ingestions >25 mg/kg. Care is primarily supportive.

Supportive therapy: Hypotension can be treated initially with isotonic saline and Trendelenburg positioning. Refractory hypotension can be treated with alpha adrenergic agonists such as norepinephrine or phenylephrine. Avoid bretylium due to its alpha adrenergic blocking activity.

Supportive therapy for phenelzine: Quetiapine (50 mg) can be given for phenelzine-induced insomnia.

Test Interactions Quetiapine recipients may exhibit false-positive results on tricyclic antidepressants assays. There is interference by quetiapine with antibodies used in some TCA immunoassays (Syva®, Microgenics®, and Triage®).

Drug Interactions

Substrate of CYP2D6 (minor), 3A4 (major)

Acetylcholinesterase inhibitors (central): May increase the risk of anti-psychotic-related extrapyramidal symptoms; monitor.

Antihypertensives: Concurrent use with an antihypertensive may produce additive hypotensive effects (particularly orthostasis)

Azole antifungals (fluconazole, itraconazole, ketoconazole): Administration with ketoconazole increases serum concentration of quetiapine by 335%; use with caution.

Cimetidine: May decrease quetiapine's clearance by 20%; increasing serum concentrations.

CNS depressants: Quetiapine may enhance the sedative effects of other CNS depressants; includes antidepressants, benzodiazepines, barbiturates, ethanol, narcotic analgesics, and other sedative agents; monitor for increased effect.

CYP3A4 inducers: CYP3A4 inducers may decrease the levels/effects of quetiapine. Example inducers include aminoglutethimide, carbamazepine, nafcillin, nevirapine, phenobarbital, phenytoin, and rifamycins. Higher maintenance doses of quetiapine may be required.

CYP3A4 inhibitors: May increase the levels/effects of quetiapine. Example inhibitors include azole antifungals, clarithromycin, diclofenac, doxycycline, erythromycin, imatinib, isoniazid, nefazodone, nicardipine, propofol, protease inhibitors, quinidine, telithromycin, and verapamil.

Divalproex: Concomitant use of quetiapine and divalproex increased the mean maximum plasma concentration of quetiapine at by 17% at steady state. The mean oral clearance of valproic acid was increased by 11%.

Levodopa: Quetiapine may inhibit the antiparkinsonian effect of levodopa; monitor.

Lorazepam: Metabolism of lorazepam may be reduced by quetiapine; clearance is reduced 20% in the presence of quetiapine; monitor for increased sedative effect.

Metoclopramide: May increase extrapyramidal symptoms (EPS) or risk.

Phenytoin: Metabolism/clearance of quetiapine may be increased; five-fold changes have been noted. Higher maintenance doses of quetiapine may be required.

Thioridazine: May increase clearance of quetiapine, decreasing serum concentrations; clearance may be increased by 65%.

Pregnancy Risk Factor C

Lactation Excretion in breast milk unknown/not recommended

Specific References

Balit CR, Isbister GK, Hackett LP, et al, "Quetiapine Poisoning: A Case Series," *Ann Emerg Med*, 2003, 42(6):751-8.

Barker MJ, Benitez JG, Ternullo S, et al, "Acute Oxcarbazepine and Atomoxetine Overdose with Quetiapine," *Vet Hum Toxicol*, 2004, 46(3):130-2.

Caravati EM, Juenke JM, and Crouch BI, "*In Vitro* Effects of Quetiapine on Tricyclic Antidepressant Immunoassays," *J Toxicol Clin Toxicol*, 2003, 41(5):735.

Dogu O, Sevim S, and Kaleagasi HS, "Seizures Associated with Quetiapine Treatment," *Ann Pharmacother*, 2003, 37(9):1224-7.

Flammia DD, Valouch T, and Venuti S, "Tissue Distribution of Quetiapine in 20 Cases in Virginia," *J Anal Tox*, 2006, 30:287-92.

Hendrickson RG and Morocco AP, "Quetiapine Cross-Reactivity Among Three Tricyclic Antidepressant Immunoassays," *J Toxicol Clin Toxicol*, 2003, 41(2):105-8.

Hopenwasser J, Mozayani A, Danielson TJ, et al, "Postmortem Distribution of the Novel Antipsychotic Drug Quetiapine," *J Anal Toxicol*, 2004, 28:264-8.

Jabeen S, Polli SI, and Gerber DR, "Acute Respiratory Failure with a Single Dose of Quetiapine Fumarate," *Ann Pharmacother*, 2006, 40(3):559-62.

Langman LJ, Kaliciak HA, and Carlyle S, "Fatal Overdoses Associated with Quetiapine," *J Anal Toxicol*, 2004, 28(6):520-5.

Lin SN, Chang Y, Moody DE, et al, "A Liquid Chromatographic-Electrospray-Tandem Mass Spectrometric Method for Quantitation of Quetiapine in Human Plasma and Liver Microsomes: Application to a Study of *in vitro* Metabolism," *J Anal Toxicol*, 2004, 28(6):443-8.

Parker DR and McIntyre IM, "Case Studies of Postmortem Quetiapine: Therapeutic or Toxic Concentrations?" *J Anal Toxicol*, 2005, 29(5):407-12.

Precourt A, Dunewicz M, Gregoire G, et al, "Multiple Complications and Withdrawal Syndrome Associated with Quetiapine/Venlafaxine Intoxication," *Ann Pharmacother*, 2005, 39(1):153-6.

Slattery A, King WD, and Dorough L, "Quetiapine Overdose in an 8-Year-Old," *Clin Toxicol (Phila)*, 2005, 43:656.

Sokolski KN and Brown BJ, "Quetiapine for Insomnia Associated with Refractory Depression Exacerbated by Phenelzine," *Ann Pharmacother*, 2006, 40(3):567-70.

Watts D and Wax P, "Physostigmine Administration for Quetiapine Toxicity," *J Toxicol Clin Toxicol*, 2003, 41(5):646.

Quinagolide

CAS Number 87056-78-8; 94424-50-7

Use Treat hyperprolactinemia

Mechanism of Action Potent nonergot dopamine-D_2 receptor agonist; octahydrobenzoyl (g) quinolone compound

Adverse Reactions

Cardiovascular: Hypotension (orthostatic), palpitations, pre-eclampsia, sinus bradycardia

Central nervous system: Headache, dizziness, lethargy, psychosis, delusions, CNS depression, depression

Endocrine & metabolic: Hot flashes

Gastrointestinal: Weight loss, **nausea**, **vomiting**, constipation, anorexia, xerostomia

Neuromuscular & skeletal: Muscle cramps

Respiratory: Nasal congestion

Toxicodynamics/Kinetics

Onset of action: 2 hours

Peak onset: 4 hours

Dosage Hyperprolactinemia: 0.03-0.5 mg/day; usual dosage range: 0.05-0.1 mg/day at bedtime with food; maximum dose: 1.65 mg/day

Overdosage/Treatment

Decontamination: Lavage (within 1 hour)/activated charcoal with sorbitol
Enhancement of elimination: Multiple dosing of activated charcoal may be effective

Test Interactions May ↑ serum estradiol levels; ↓ prolactin level (S); may reduce thyroxine level (S)

Additional Information Especially useful in patients resistant to bromocriptine; may be useful in the treatment of acromegaly, Parkinson's disease, or for use in lactation inhibition; promotes reduction in pituitary microadenoma size; decreases galactorrhea

Quinapril

Related Information

● Angiotensin Agents

CAS Number 82586-55-8; 85441-61-8

U.S. Brand Names Accupril®

Synonyms Quinapril Hydrochloride

Use Management of hypertension; treatment of congestive heart failure

Unlabeled/Investigational Use Treatment of left ventricular dysfunction after myocardial infarction

Mechanism of Action Competitive inhibition of angiotensin I being converted to angiotensin II, a potent vasoconstrictor, through the angiotensin I-converting enzyme (ACE) activity, with resultant lower levels of angiotensin II which causes an increase in plasma renin activity and a reduction in aldosterone secretion

Adverse Reactions

Cardiovascular: Hypotension, myocardial infarction, angina pectoris, hypotension (orthostatic), rhythm disturbances, tachycardia, vasculitis, palpitations, syncope, flushing, peripheral edema, chest discomfort, sinus tachycardia, vasodilation

Central nervous system: Dizziness, headache, fatigue, malaise, CNS depression, somnolence, insomnia, fever, depression

Dermatologic: Urticaria, pruritus, angioneurotic edema, exfoliative dermatitis, photosensitivity, exanthem, pemphigus vulgaris

Endocrine & metabolic: Hypoglycemia

Gastrointestinal: Diarrhea, abdominal pain, anorexia, constipation, flatulence, xerostomia, pancreatitis

Hematologic: Neutropenia, bone marrow suppression

Hepatic: Hepatitis

Neuromuscular & skeletal: Gout, arthralgia, shoulder pain, paresthesia

Ocular: Blurred vision, visual hallucinations

Renal: Elevated BUN/serum creatinine

Respiratory: Upper respiratory symptoms, cough, bronchospasm, bronchitis, sinusitis, pharyngeal pain

Miscellaneous: Diaphoresis

Pharmacodynamics/Kinetics

Onset of action: 1 hour

Duration: 24 hours

Absorption: Quinapril: $\geq 60\%$

Protein binding: Quinapril: 97%; Quinaprilat: 97%

Metabolism: Rapidly hydrolyzed to quinaprilat, the active metabolite

Half-life elimination: Quinapril: 0.8 hours; Quinaprilat: 3 hours; increases as Cl_{cr} decreases

Time to peak, serum: Quinapril: 1 hour; Quinaprilat: ~2 hours

Excretion: Urine (50% to 60% primarily as quinaprilat)

Dosage

Adults: Oral:

Hypertension: Initial: 10-20 mg once daily, adjust according to blood pressure response at peak and trough blood levels; initial dose may be reduced to 5 mg in patients receiving diuretic therapy if the diuretic is continued; usual dose range (JNC 7): 10-40 mg once daily

Congestive heart failure or post-MI: Initial: 5 mg once daily, titrated at weekly intervals to 20-40 mg daily in 2 divided doses

Elderly: Initial: 2.5-5 mg/day; increase dosage at increments of 2.5-5 mg at 1- to 2-week intervals.

Dosing adjustment in renal impairment: Lower initial doses should be used; after initial dose (if tolerated), administer initial dose twice daily; may be increased at weekly intervals to optimal response:

Hypertension: Initial:

$Cl_{cr} > 60$ mL/minute: Administer 10 mg/day

Cl_{cr} 30-60 mL/minute: Administer 5 mg/day

Cl_{cr} 10-30 mL/minute: Administer 2.5 mg/day

Congestive heart failure: Initial:

$Cl_{cr} > 30$ mL/minute: Administer 5 mg/day

Cl_{cr} 10-30 mL/minute: Administer 2.5 mg/day

Dosing comments in hepatic impairment: In patients with alcoholic cirrhosis, hydrolysis of quinapril to quinaprilat is impaired; however, the subsequent elimination of quinaprilat is unaltered.

Stability Store at room temperature

Monitoring Parameters BUN, serum creatinine, renal function; nausea, headache, diarrhea, change in taste, cough

Contraindications Hypersensitivity to quinapril or any component of the formulation; angioedema related to previous treatment with an ACE inhibitor; bilateral renal artery stenosis; patients with idiopathic or hereditary angioedema; pregnancy (2nd and 3rd trimesters)

Warnings

Anaphylactic reactions can occur. Angioedema can occur at any time during treatment (especially following first dose). It may involve head and neck (potentially affecting the airway) or the intestine (presenting with abdominal pain). Prolonged monitoring may be required especially if tongue, glottis, or larynx are involved as they are associated with airway obstruction. Those with a history of airway surgery in this situation have a higher risk. Careful blood pressure monitoring with first dose (hypotension can occur especially in volume-depleted patients).

[U.S. Boxed Warning]: Based on human data, ACEIs can cause injury and death to the developing fetus when used in the second and third trimesters. ACEIs should be discontinued as soon as possible once pregnancy is detected. Dosage adjustment needed in renal impairment. Use with caution in hypovolemia; collagen vascular diseases; valvular stenosis (particularly aortic stenosis); hyperkalemia; or before, during, or immediately after anesthesia. Avoid rapid dosage escalation, which may lead to renal insufficiency. Rare toxicities associated with ACE inhibitors include cholestatic jaundice (which may progress to hepatic necrosis) and neutropenia/agranulocytosis with myeloid hyperplasia. If patient has renal impairment, a baseline

WBC with differential and serum creatinine should be evaluated and monitored closely during the first 3 months of therapy.

Hypersensitivity reactions may be seen during hemodialysis with high-flux dialysis membranes (eg, AN69). Patients receiving ACE inhibitors have experienced rare life-threatening anaphylactoid reactions during desensitization. Rare hepatic reactions, progressing from cholestatic jaundice to hepatic necrosis, have been reported with ACE inhibitors. Discontinue if marked elevation of hepatic transaminases or jaundice occurs. Use with caution in unilateral renal artery stenosis and pre-existing renal insufficiency. Deterioration in renal function can occur with initiation.

Dosage Forms Tablet: 5 mg, 10 mg, 20 mg, 40 mg

Accupril®: 5 mg, 10 mg, 20 mg, 40 mg

Reference Range Following a 10 mg dose, peak serum levels of quinapril and quinaprilat are 65 mg/mL and 223 ng/mL, respectively

Overdosage/Treatment

Decontamination: Activated charcoal

Supportive therapy: Following initiation of essential overdose management, toxic symptom treatment and supportive treatment should be initiated. Hypotension usually responds to I.V. fluids or Trendelenburg positioning. If unresponsive to these measures, the use of a parenteral inotrope may be required (eg, norepinephrine 0.1-0.2 mcg/kg/minute titrated to response). Naloxone has been shown to antagonize hypotensive effects of captopril, but routine use in an overdose situation due to this agent is uncertain. For refractory hypotension, angiotensin amide infusion may be attempted.

Enhancement of elimination: Multiple dosing of activated charcoal may be effective; hemodialysis is not effective

Test Interactions ↑ potassium (S)

Drug Interactions Alpha$_1$ blockers: Hypotensive effect increased.

Aspirin: The effects of ACE inhibitors may be blunted by aspirin administration, particularly at higher dosages (see Cardiovascular Considerations) and/or increase adverse renal effects.

Diuretics: Hypovolemia due to diuretics may precipitate acute hypotensive events or acute renal failure.

Insulin: Risk of hypoglycemia may be increased.

Lithium: Risk of lithium toxicity may be increased; monitor lithium levels, especially the first 4 weeks of therapy.

Mercaptopurine: Risk of neutropenia may be increased.

NSAIDs: May attenuate hypertensive efficacy; effect has been seen with captopril and may occur with other ACE inhibitors; monitor blood pressure. May increase risk of adverse renal effects.

Potassium-sparing diuretics (amiloride, spironolactone, triamterene): Increased risk of hyperkalemia.

Potassium supplements may increase the risk of hyperkalemia.

Quinolones: Absorption may be decreased by quinapril; separate administration by at least 2-4 hours.

Tetracyclines: Absorption may be reduced by quinapril; separate administration by at least 2-4 hours.

Trimethoprim (high dose) may increase the risk of hyperkalemia.

Pregnancy Risk Factor C (1st trimester)/D (2nd and 3rd trimesters)

Pregnancy Implications Decreased placental blood flow, low birth weight, fetal hypotension, preterm delivery, and fetal death have been noted with the use of some ACE inhibitors (ACEIs) in animal studies. Neonatal hypotension, skull hypoplasia, anuria, renal failure, oligohydramnios (associated with fetal limb contractures, craniofacial deformities, hypoplastic lung development), prematurity, intrauterine growth retardation, and patent ductus arteriosus have been reported with the use of ACEIs, primarily in the 2nd and 3rd trimesters. The risk of neonatal toxicity has been considered less when ACEIs have been used in the 1st trimester; however, major congenital malformations have been reported. The cardiovascular and/or central nervous systems are most commonly affected. Unless alternative agents are not appropriate, ACEIs should be discontinued as soon as possible once pregnancy is detected.

Lactation Enters breast milk/use caution

Nursing Implications May cause depression in some patients; discontinue if angioedema of the face, extremities, lips, tongue, or glottis occurs; watch for hypotensive effects within 1-3 hours of first dose or new higher dose

Additional Information Patients taking diuretics are at risk for developing hypotension on initial dosing; to prevent this, discontinue diuretics 2-3 days prior to initiating quinapril; may restart diuretics if blood pressure is not controlled by quinapril alone

Due to frequent decreases in glomerular filtration (also creatinine clearance) with aging, elderly patients may have exaggerated responses to ACE inhibitors; differences in clinical response due to hepatic changes are not observed. ACE inhibitors may be preferred agents in elderly patients with CHF and diabetes mellitus. Diabetic proteinuria is reduced and insulin sensitivity is enhanced. In general, the side effect profile is favorable in elderly and causes little or no CNS confusion; use lowest dose recommendations initially.

Specific References

Chobanian AV, Bakris GL, Black HR, et al, "The Seventh Report of the Joint National Committee on Prevention, Detection, Evaluation, and

Treatment of High Blood Pressure: The JNC 7 Report," *JAMA*, 2003, 289(19):2560-71.

Cooper W, Hernandez-Diaz S, Arbogast P, et al, "Major Congenital Malformations After First Trimester Exposure to ACE Inhibitors," *N Engl J Med*, 2006, 354:2443-51.

Mastrobattista J, "Angiontensin-Converting Enzyme Inhibitors in Pregnancy," *Semin Perinatol*, 1997, 21(2):124-34.

Quan A, "Fetopathy Associated with Exposure to Angiontensin-Converting Enzyme Inhibitors and Angiontensin Receptor Antagonists," *Early Hum Dev*, 2006, 82(1):23-8.

Quinidine

Related Information
- Therapeutic Drugs Associated with Hallucinations

CAS Number 27555-34-6; 50-54-4; 56-52-2; 6151-39-9; 63717-04-4; 65484-56-2; 6591-63-5; 7054-25-3; 72402-50-7; 747-45-4

U.S. Brand Names Quinaglute® Dura-Tabs® [DSC]

Synonyms Quinidine Gluconate; Quinidine Polygalacturonate; Quinidine Sulfate

Use Prophylaxis after cardioversion of atrial fibrillation and/or flutter to maintain normal sinus rhythm; prevent recurrence of paroxysmal supraventricular tachycardia, paroxysmal AV junctional rhythm, paroxysmal ventricular tachycardia, paroxysmal atrial fibrillation, and atrial or ventricular premature contractions; has activity against *Plasmodium falciparum* malaria

Mechanism of Action Depresses phase O of the action potential; decreases myocardial excitability and conduction velocity, and myocardial contractility by decreasing sodium influx during depolarization and potassium efflux in repolarization; also reduces calcium transport across cell membrane; class I antiarrhythmic

Adverse Reactions
Cardiovascular: Syncope, hypotension, tachycardia, heart block, fibrillation (ventricular), vascular collapse, severe hypotension with rapid I.V. administration, torsade de pointes, sinus bradycardia, sinus tachycardia, vasculitis

Central nervous system: Dizziness, confusion, delirium, hallucinations, agitation, psychosis, headache, memory disturbance, insomnia, paranoia

Dermatologic: Angioedema, pruritus, rash, may exacerbate psoriasis, eczematous dermatitis, skin discoloration (blue-gray), exfoliative dermatitis, erythema multiforme, acne, acute generalized exanthematous pustulosis, alopecia, bullous skin disease, toxic epidermal necrolysis, photoallergy, exanthem, cutaneous vasculitis

Endocrine & metabolic: Hyperinsulinemia

Gastrointestinal: **Nausea, vomiting, stomach cramps, bitter taste, anorexia, diarrhea**, esophagitis, abdominal pain

Hematologic: Blood dyscrasias, thrombocytopenic purpura, hemolysis, agranulocytosis, aplastic anemia

Hepatic: Cholestatic jaundice, granulomatous hepatitis

Ocular: Impaired vision, photophobia, diplopia

Otic: Ototoxicity, tinnitus

Renal: Renal vasculitis

Respiratory: Apnea, respiratory depression, eosinophilic pneumonia

Miscellaneous: Fever with leukocytosis; can cause drug-induced systemic lupus erythematosus or SICCA syndrome or drug fever; cinchonism, lymphadenopathy, fixed drug eruption

Signs and Symptoms of Overdose Absence of P waves, agranulocytosis, anuria, apnea, ataxia, AV block, bradycardia, coma, dementia, depression, drowsiness, granulocytopenia, hallucinations, heart block, hyperthermia, hypoglycemia, leukopenia, lichenoid eruptions, memory loss, myasthenia gravis (exacerbation or precipitation), mydriasis, myoglobinuria, neutropenia, photosensitivity, P-R prolongation, respiratory distress with shallow respirations, QRS prolongation, QT prolongation, rhabdomyolysis, seizures, severe hypotension, syncope, thrombocytopenia, ventricular arrhythmias

Pharmacodynamics/Kinetics
Onset of action: I.M.: 15 minutes

Duration: Oral: Regular tablets or capsules: 6-8 hours; Extended-release tablets: ~12 hours

Absorption: Well from gastrointestinal tract; peak oral absorption: 60-90 minutes

Distribution: V_d: Adults: 2-3.5 L/kg, decreased V_d with congestive heart failure, malaria, increased V_d with cirrhosis; cirrhosis, or acute myocardial infarction; all tissues except brain; concentrates in heart, liver, kidneys, and skeletal muscle

Protein binding: Newborns: 60% to 70%; Adults: 80% to 90%
Decreased protein-binding with cyanotic congenital heart disease

Metabolism: Extensive in the liver

Bioavailability: Sulfate: 80%; Gluconate: 70%

Half-life: Children: 2.5-6.7 hours; Adults: 6-8 hours
Increased half-life with elderly, cirrhosis and congestive heart failure

Time to peak plasma concentration: 1-3 hours

Elimination: Urine (15% to 25% as unchanged drug); clearance: 4.7 mL/kg/minute; ~37% of the drug is normally excreted in 4 hours in a healthy person

Dosage Dosage expressed in terms of the salt: 267 mg of quinidine gluconate = 200 mg of quinidine sulfate.

Children: Test dose for idiosyncratic reaction (sulfate, oral or gluconate, I.M.): 2 mg/kg or 60 mg/m^2
Oral (quinidine sulfate): 15-60 mg/kg/day in 4-5 divided doses or 6 mg/kg every 4-6 hours; usual 30 mg/kg/day or 900 mg/m^2/day given in 5 daily doses
I.V. **not** recommended (quinidine gluconate): 2-10 mg/kg/dose given at a rate ≤10 mg/minute every 3-6 hours as needed

Adults: Test dose: Oral, I.M.: 200 mg administered several hours before full dosage (to determine possibility of idiosyncratic reaction)
Oral (for malaria):
Sulfate: 100-600 mg/dose every 4-6 hours; begin at 200 mg/dose and titrate to desired effect (maximum daily dose: 3-4 g)
Gluconate: 324-972 mg every 8-12 hours
I.M.: 400 mg/dose every 2-6 hours; initial dose: 600 mg (gluconate)
I.V.: 200-400 mg/dose diluted and given at a rate ≤10 mg/minute; may require as much as 500-750 mg

Dosing adjustment in renal impairment: Cl_{cr} <10 mL/minute: Administer 75% of normal dose.

Hemodialysis: Slightly hemodialyzable (5% to 20%); 200 mg supplemental dose posthemodialysis is recommended.

Peritoneal dialysis: Not dialyzable (0% to 5%)

Dosing adjustment/comments in hepatic impairment: Larger loading dose may be indicated, reduce maintenance doses by 50% and monitor serum levels closely.

Stability Do not use discolored parenteral solution

Monitoring Parameters Cardiac monitor required during I.V. administration; CBC, liver and renal function tests, should be routinely performed during long-term administration

Administration Administer around-the-clock to promote less variation in peak and trough serum levels
Oral: Do not crush, chew, or break sustained release dosage forms.
Parenteral: When injecting I.M., aspirate carefully to avoid injection into a vessel; maximum I.V. infusion rate: 10 mg/minute

Contraindications Hypersensitivity to quinidine or any component of the formulation; thrombocytopenia; thrombocytopenic purpura; myasthenia gravis; heart block greater than first degree; idioventricular conduction delays (except in patients with a functioning artificial pacemaker); those adversely affected by anticholinergic activity; concurrent use of quinolone antibiotics which prolong QT interval, cisapride, amprenavir, or ritonavir

Warnings Monitor and adjust dose to prevent QT_c prolongation. Watch for proarrhythmic effects. Correct hypokalemia before initiating therapy. Hypokalemia may worsen toxicity. **[U.S. Boxed Warning]: Antiarrhythmic drugs have not been shown to enhance survival in nonlife-threatening ventricular arrhythmias and may increase mortality; the risk is greatest with structural heart disease. Quinidine may increase mortality in treatment of atrial fibrillation/flutter.** May precipitate or exacerbate CHF. Reduce dosage in hepatic impairment. Use may cause digoxin-induced toxicity (adjust digoxin's dose). Use caution with concurrent use of other antiarrhythmics. Hypersensitivity reactions can occur. Can unmask sick sinus syndrome (causes bradycardia). Has been associated with severe hepatotoxic reactions, including granulomatous hepatitis. Hemolysis may occur in patients with G6PD (glucose-6-phosphate dehydrogenase) deficiency. Different salt products are not interchangeable.

Dosage Forms Injection, solution, as gluconate: 80 mg/mL (10 mL) [equivalent to quinidine base 50 mg/mL]
Tablet, as sulfate: 200 mg, 300 mg
Tablet, extended release, as gluconate: 324 mg [equivalent to quinidine base 202 mg]
Tablet, extended release, as sulfate: 300 mg [equivalent to quinidine base 249 mg]

Reference Range Therapeutic: 2-5 mcg/mL (SI: 6.2-15.4 μmol/L). Patient dependent therapeutic response occurs at levels of 3-6 mcg/mL (SI: 9.2-18.5 μmol/L). Optimal therapeutic level is method dependent; >8 mcg/mL (SI: >24 μmol/L) are associated with cinchonism while levels >14 ng/L are associated with cardiac toxicity

Overdosage/Treatment
Decontamination: Emesis within 30 minutes or lavage (within 1 hour)/ activated charcoal

Supportive therapy: Electrolyte balance should be monitored and treated, especially when refractory arrhythmias develop. Sodium bicarbonate 1-2 mEq/kg I.V. (or 0.5-1 mEq/kg in children) may decrease conduction defects. Phenytoin or lidocaine are often effective at controlling drug-induced arrhythmias, while phenytoin is preferred due to its beneficial effects on AV conduction velocity. Torsade de pointes can be treated with magnesium sulfate or overdrive pacemaker. Cholestyramine (4-8 g/day) is effective for treating quinidine-induced diarrhea. Dopamine and/or norepinephrine can be used to treat refractory hypotension.

Extracorporeal membrane oxygenation has been used successfully to establish and maintain cardiovascular stability.

Enhancement of elimination: Multiple dosing of activated charcoal is effective; hemodialysis or charcoal hemoperfusion have little effect, although hemoperfusion can be considered in patients with hepatic failure; slightly dialyzable (5% to 20%)

Antidote(s)

- Sodium Bicarbonate [ANTIDOTE]

Test Interactions ↑ prothrombin time; ↓ glucose; may interfere with urinary analysis of catecholamines; triamterene can interfere with the fluorescent measurement of quinidine, leading to falsely elevated quinidine assays

Drug Interactions Substrate of CYP2C9 (minor), 2E1 (minor), 3A4 (major); **Inhibits** CYP2C9 (weak), 2D6 (strong), 3A4 (strong)

Amiloride may cause prolonged ventricular conduction leading to arrhythmias.

Amiodarone may increase quinidine blood levels; monitor quinidine levels.

Cimetidine: Increase quinidine blood levels; closely monitor levels or use an alternative H_2 antagonist.

Cisapride and quinidine may increase risk of malignant arrhythmias; concurrent use is contraindicated.

Codeine: Analgesic efficacy may be reduced.

CYP2D6 substrates: Quinidine may increase the levels/effects of CYP2D6 substrates. Example substrates include amphetamines, selected beta-blockers, dextromethorphan, fluoxetine, lidocaine, mirtazapine, nefazodone, paroxetine, risperidone, ritonavir, thioridazine, tricyclic antidepressants, and venlafaxine.

CYP2D6 prodrug substrates: Quinidine may decrease the levels/effects of CYP2D6 prodrug substrates. Example prodrug substrates include codeine, hydrocodone, oxycodone, and tramadol.

CYP3A4 inducers: CYP3A4 inducers may decrease the levels/effects of quinidine. Example inducers include aminoglutethimide, carbamazepine, nafcillin, nevirapine, phenobarbital, phenytoin, and rifamycins.

CYP3A4 inhibitors: May increase the levels/effects of quinidine. Example inhibitors include azole antifungals, clarithromycin, diclofenac, doxycycline, erythromycin, imatinib, isoniazid, nefazodone, nicardipine, propofol, protease inhibitors, telithromycin, and verapamil.

CYP3A4 substrates: Quinidine may increase the levels/effects of CYP3A4 substrates. Example substrates include benzodiazepines, calcium channel blockers, mirtazapine, nateglinide, nefazodone, tacrolimus, and venlafaxine. Selected benzodiazepines (midazolam and triazolam), cisapride, ergot alkaloids, selected HMG-CoA reductase inhibitors (lovastatin and simvastatin), and pimozide are generally contraindicated with strong CYP3A4 inhibitors.

Digoxin blood levels may be increased. Monitor digoxin blood levels.

Metoprolol: Increased metoprolol blood levels.

Mexiletine blood levels may be increased.

Nifedipine blood levels may be increased by quinidine; nifedipine may decrease quinidine blood levels.

Propafenone blood levels may be increased.

Propranolol blood levels may be increased.

QT_c-prolonging agents (eg, amiodarone, amitriptyline, bepridil, disopyramide, erythromycin, haloperidol, imipramine, pimozide, procainamide, sotalol, thioridazine): Effects may be additive; use with caution.

Ritonavir, nelfinavir and amprenavir may increase quinidine levels and toxicity; concurrent use is contraindicated.

Sparfloxacin, gatifloxacin, and moxifloxacin may result in additional prolongation of the QT interval; concurrent use is contraindicated.

Timolol blood levels may be increased.

Urinary alkalinizers (antacids, sodium bicarbonate, acetazolamide) increase quinidine blood levels.

Verapamil and diltiazem increase quinidine blood levels.

Warfarin effects may be increased by quinidine; monitor INR closely during addition or withdrawal of quinidine.

Pregnancy Risk Factor C

Lactation Enters breast milk/compatible

Nursing Implications When injecting I.M., aspirate carefully to avoid injection into a vessel; do not crush sustained release drug product

Additional Information Doses >250 mg/day of quinidine result in **increased serum digoxin concentrations about 2.5 times the digoxin concentration before quinidine was added.** The new steady-state of digoxin concentration occurs in 7-14 days, with signs of toxicity beginning to appear in 3-7 days after initiation of quinidine therapy. Therefore, **serum digoxin concentrations should be measured before initiation of quinidine therapy and again in 4-6 days.** Measure trough because of variability of peak interval. **Renal failure** prolongs apparent half-life, perhaps through accumulation of fluorescent metabolites. Severe heart failure also prolongs half-life, as does liver disease. Concomitant administration of **phenytoin** increases hepatic metabolism, and therefore decreases half-life and serum quinidine concentrations. Clearance may be diminished in the elderly.

Specific References

Cubeddu LX, "QT Prolongation and Fatal Arrhythmias: A Review of Clinical Implications and Effects of Drugs," *Am J Ther*, 2003, 10(6):452-7.

Kao LW and Furbee RB, "Drug-Induced Q-T Prolongation," *Med Clin N Am*, 2005, 89(6):1125-44 (review).

Quinine

Related Information

- Toxins Which Should Be Lavaged with Solutions Other Than Water

CAS Number 130-95-0

Synonyms Quinine Sulfate

Use Suppression or treatment of chloroquine-resistant *P. falciparum* malaria; treatment of *Babesia microti* infection

Prevention and treatment of nocturnal recumbency leg muscle cramps

Mechanism of Action Not completely understood; depresses oxygen uptake and carbohydrate metabolism; intercalates into DNA, disrupting the parasite's replication and transcription; affects calcium distribution within muscle fibers and decreases the excitability of the motor end-plate region; interferes with function of plasmodial DNA; also, recent evidence suggests it may also do this through increased pH of plasmodial organelles; local anesthetic action and analgesic properties

Adverse Reactions

Cardiovascular: Flushing of the skin, angina, syncope, cardiac arrhythmias, hypotension, sinus bradycardia, chest pain, QRS prolongation

Central nervous system: **Severe headache**, CNS depression, seizures, fever, fear, restlessness, psychosis, dizziness, ataxia, insomnia, hyperthermia

Dermatologic: Rash, pruritus, acne, exfoliative dermatitis, angioedema, bullous skin disease, urticaria, purpura, photoallergy, licheniform eruptions, exanthem, cutaneous vasculitis

Endocrine & metabolic: Hypoglycemia, hyperinsulinemia, abortifacient

Gastrointestinal: **Nausea, diarrhea, vomiting**, abdominal pain, altered taste, bitter taste

Hematologic: Thrombocytopenia, leukopenia, neutropenia, agranulocytosis, granulocytopenia, blackwater fever, hemolytic/uremic syndrome, disseminated intravascular coagulation

Hepatic: Hepatitis, elevated liver function test results, granulomatous hepatitis

Neuromuscular & skeletal: Myasthenia gravis (exacerbation or precipitation of)

Ocular: **Blurred vision**, night blindness, diplopia, optic atrophy, photophobia

Otic: **Tinnitus**, ototoxicity

Respiratory: Apnea, respiratory depression

Miscellaneous: Symptoms of cinchonism, hypersensitivity reactions, diaphoresis, fixed drug eruption

Signs and Symptoms of Overdose Abdominal pain, AV block, blindness (with a dose >5 g), blood dyscrasias, bradycardia, cardiac arrhythmias, cinchonism-ototoxicity, coma, confusion, deafness, erythema multiforme, headache, hemolysis, hypoglycemia, hypokalemia, hypoprothrombinemia, hypotension, methemoglobinemia, mydriasis, myoglobinuria, nausea, nephritis, nystagmus, photosensitivity, renal injury, rhabdomyolysis, tinnitus (38%), toxic epidermal necrolysis, urine discoloration (black; brown; dark; red-brown), vision color changes (green tinge; red tinge), visual disturbance

Admission Criteria/Prognosis Any patient with change in mental status, cardiopulmonary complaints, or methemoglobin levels >30% should be admitted; asymptomatic patients with methemoglobin levels <30% may be considered for discharge after 6 hours of observation and if methemoglobin levels fall to <15%

Pharmacodynamics/Kinetics

Onset of action: 1-3 hours

Duration: Regular: 6-8 hours; Extended: ~12 hours

Absorption: Oral: Readily absorbed, mainly from the upper small intestine even in diarrhea

Distribution: V_d: 1.2-1.7 L/kg; higher in convalescent malaria; distributed in all tissues except brain; concentrates in heart, liver, kidneys, and skeletal muscle

Protein binding: 70% to 95%

Metabolism: Primarily in the liver

Half-life: 6-12 hours; lower in active or convalescent malaria; Adults: 8-14 hours; Patients with liver failure: 66-99 hours

Time to peak serum concentration: Oral: 1-1.5 hours; I.M.: 1 hour

Elimination: Not effectively removed by peritoneal dialysis, removed by hemodialysis; excreted in bile and saliva with <5% excreted unchanged in urine; excretion in urine is twice as rapid if urine is acidic

Dosage

Oral:

Children: Chloroquine-resistant malaria and babesiosis: 25 mg/kg/day in divided doses every 8 hours for 7 days; maximum: 650 mg/dose

Adults:

Chloroquine-resistant malaria: 650 mg every 8 hours for 7 days in conjunction with another agent

Babesiosis: 650 mg every 6-8 hours for 7 days

Leg cramps: 200-300 mg at bedtime

Dosing interval/adjustment in renal impairment:

Cl_{cr} 10-50 mL/minute: Administer every 8-12 hours or 75% of normal dose

Cl_{cr} <10 mL/minute: Administer every 24 hours or 30% to 50% of normal dose

Monitoring Parameters Monitor CBC with platelet count, liver function tests, blood glucose, ophthalmologic examination

Administration

Avoid use of aluminum-containing antacids because of drug absorption problems. Swallow dose whole to avoid bitter taste. May be administered with food.

Contraindications Hypersensitivity to quinine or any component of the formulation; tinnitus, optic neuritis, G6PD deficiency; history of black water fever; thrombocytopenia with quinine or quinidine; pregnancy

Warnings Use with caution in patients with cardiac arrhythmias (quinine has quinidine-like activity) and in patients with myasthenia gravis

Dosage Forms Capsule, as sulfate: 200 mg, 325 mg

Tablet, as sulfate: 260 mg

Reference Range Therapeutic: 2.5-9.6 mcg/mL; Toxic: >10.0 mcg/mL; Fatal: >15.0 mcg/mL

Overdosage/Treatment

Decontamination: Emesis not recommended; lavage (within 1 hour) with 1:10,000 potassium permanganate 100 mg in 1 L water, indicated if early in ingestion

Supportive therapy: Stellate ganglion block procedure has not been shown to be of clear benefit as blindness is usually reversible; effect of nitrates uncertain; treat acidosis, hypoglycemia accordingly; treat cardiac conduction defects with sodium bicarbonate (I.V. 1-3 mEq/kg), titrate to serum pH 7.45-7.50; control seizures with benzodiazepine prior to lavage. Quinine-induced hypoglycemia can be treated with octreotide (50 mcg I.V. every 12 hours)

Arrhythmias: Avoid disopyramide/procainamide (class IA and IC)

Ventricular tachycardia: Pacing, conversion, isoproterenol 2-10 mcg/minute (0.1-1 mcg/kg/minute (children))

Torsade de pointes: $MgSO_4$ 2 g, then drip at 3-20 mg/minute

Bradycardia: Pacing, standard therapy

Hypotension: Norepinephrine, isoproterenol effective

Enhancement of elimination: Studies have demonstrated enhanced elimination with multiple dose charcoal; hemodialysis minimally effective (not recommended)

Antidote(s)

- Norepinephrine [ANTIDOTE]

Test Interactions ↑ prothrombin time; positive Coombs' [direct]

Drug Interactions Substrate (minor) of CYP1A2, 2C19, 3A4; **Inhibits** CYP2C8 (moderate), 2C9 (moderate), 2D6 (strong), 3A4 (weak)

CYP2C8 Substrates: Quinine may increase the levels/effects of CYP2C8 substrates. Example substrates include amiodarone, paclitaxel, pioglitazone, repaglinide, and rosiglitazone.

CYP2C9 Substrates: Quinine may increase the levels/effects of CYP2C9 substrates. Example substrates include bosentan, dapsone, fluoxetine, glimepiride, glipizide, losartan, montelukast, nateglinide, paclitaxel, phenytoin, warfarin, and zafirlukast.

CYP2D6 substrates: Quinine may increase the levels/effects of CYP2D6 substrates. Example substrates include amphetamines, selected beta-blockers, dextromethorphan, fluoxetine, lidocaine, mirtazapine, nefazodone, paroxetine, risperidone, ritonavir, thioridazine, tricyclic antidepressants, and venlafaxine.

CYP2D6 prodrug substrates: Quinine may decrease the levels/effects of CYP2D6 prodrug substrates. Example prodrug substrates include codeine, hydrocodone, oxycodone, and tramadol.

Decreased effect: Phenobarbital, phenytoin, aluminum salt antacids, and rifampin may decrease quinine serum concentrations

Increased toxicity:

To avoid risk of seizures and cardiac arrest, delay mefloquine dosing at least 12 hours after last dose of quinine

Beta-blockers + quinine may increase bradycardia

Quinine may enhance coumarin anticoagulants and potentiate non-depolarizing and depolarizing muscle relaxants

Quinine may increase plasma concentration of digoxin by as much as twofold; closely monitor digoxin concentrations and decrease digoxin dose with initiation of quinine by $^1/_2$

Verapamil, amiodarone, urinary alkalinizing agents, and cimetidine may increase quinine serum concentrations

Pregnancy Risk Factor X Oxytoxic action

Lactation Enters breast milk/compatible

Nursing Implications Administer by slow I.V. infusion

Additional Information

Adults: Minimum lethal dose: 5 g. Toxic dose: 2 g

Parenteral dosage form may be obtained from the Centers for Disease Control if needed; a common adulterant in street drugs. The FDA does not allow more than 2.45 mg/ounce of quinine in any carbonated beverage (CRF 21 part 172.575).

Specific References

Morrison LD, Velez LI, Shepherd G, et al, "Death by Quinine," *Vet Hum Toxicol*, 2003, 45(6):303-6.

Radiological/Contrast Media (Nonionic)

Pronunciation (ray deo LOG ik al/KON trast MEE dia non eye ON ik)

Related Information

- Contrast Media Reactions, Premedication for Prophylaxis

U.S. Brand Names Amipaque® [DSC]; Isovue®; Omnipaque®; Optiray®; ProHance®

Synonyms Iohexol; Iopamidol; Ioversol; Metrizamide

Impairment Potential None

Use Enhance visualization of structures during radiologic procedures

Mechanism of Action Iodine content is radiopaque and thus allows for radiographic visualization.

Adverse Reactions

Cardiovascular: Hypotension, bradycardia, flushing

Central nervous system: Headache, seizures, aphasia

Dermatologic: Pruritus, pallor, urticaria

Endocrine & metabolic: Dehydration

Gastrointestinal: Nausea, vomiting, diarrhea, metallic taste

Hematologic: Hemolysis

Ocular: Cortical blindness

Renal: Renal insufficiency, proteinuria

Respiratory: Cough

Neuromuscular & skeletal: Weakness

Miscellaneous: Hypersensitivity reaction, anaphylaxis

Contraindications Known hypersensitivity

Warnings Anaphylactic-like reactions and hypotension; acute severe back, leg or groin pain; decision to use contrast enhancement should include consideration of risk of the drug, risk of the procedure, expected benefit of the image and patient's underlying disorder

Dosage Forms

[DSC] = Discontinued product

Injection, solution:

Gadoteridol (ProHance®): 279.3 mg/mL (15 mL, 30 mL, 50 mL) [single use vial]; 279.3 mg/mL (20 mL) [prefilled syringe]

Iohexol (Omnipaque®): 140 mg/mL, 180 mg/mL, 210 mg/mL, 240 mg/mL, 300 mg/mL, 350 mg/mL

Iopamidol:

Isovue-128®

Isovue-200®

Isovue-300®

Isovue-370®

Isovue-M 200®

Isovue-M 300®

Ioversol:

Optiray® 160

Optiray® 240

Optiray® 320

Metrizamide: Amipaque® [DSC]

Overdosage/Treatment

Supportive therapy: Ensure adequate hydration; monitor for electrolyte disturbances. Hypotension can be treated with 10-20 mL/kg of crystalloid infusion and placement in Trendelenburg position. Dopamine or norepinephrine can be used for blood pressure support. Bradycardia can be treated with atropine. Hypersensitivity reactions and anaphylaxis can be treated with standard therapy. N-acetylcysteine may be renoprotective.

Enhanced elimination: Hemodialysis can remove most contrast media.

Antidote(s)

- Acetylcysteine [ANTIDOTE]

Test Interactions May interfere with thyroid function tests (especially protein-bound iodine assays).

Drug Interactions Interleukins: Risk of hypersensitivity reactions may be increased.

Metformin: Risk of metformin-induced acidosis may be increased by iodinated contrast agents. Discontinue metformin prior to contrast exposure and withhold for 48 hours.

Pregnancy Implications Diatrizonate D can cross the placenta; no specific fetal abnormalities noted

Specific References

Fedutes BA and Ansani NT, "Seizure Potential of Concomitant Medications and Radiographic Contrast Media Agents," *Ann Pharmacother*, 2003, 37(10):1506-10.

Raloxifene

CAS Number 82640-04-8; 84449-90-1
U.S. Brand Names Evista®
Synonyms Keoxifene Hydrochloride; NSC-706725; Raloxifene Hydrochloride
Use Prevention and treatment of osteoporosis in postmenopausal women
Unlabeled/Investigational Use Risk reduction for invasive breast cancer in postmenopausal women at increased risk for breast cancer
Mechanism of Action A selective estrogen receptor modulator, meaning that it affects some of the same receptors that estrogen does, but not all, and in some instances, it antagonizes or blocks estrogen; it acts like estrogen to prevent bone loss and improve lipid profiles (decreases total and LDL cholesterol but does not raise triglycerides), but it has the potential to block some estrogen effects such as those that lead to breast cancer and uterine cancer

Adverse Reactions
Note: Has been associated with increased risk of thromboembolism (DVT, PE) and superficial thrombophlebitis; risk is similar to reported risk of HRT
Cardiovascular: Chest pain
Central nervous system: Migraine, depression, insomnia, fever
Dermatologic: Rash
Endocrine & metabolic: Hot flashes, hypertriglyceridemia (in women with a history of increased triglycerides in response to oral estrogens)
Gastrointestinal: Nausea, dyspepsia, vomiting, flatulence, gastroenteritis, weight gain
Genitourinary: Vaginitis, urinary tract infection, cystitis, leukorrhea
Neuromuscular & skeletal: Leg cramps, arthralgia, myalgia, arthritis
Ocular: Retinal vein occlusion
Respiratory: Sinusitis, pharyngitis, cough, pneumonia, laryngitis
Miscellaneous: Infection, flu syndrome, diaphoresis

Signs and Symptoms of Overdose Incidence of overdose in humans has not been reported. In an 8-week study of postmenopausal women, a dose of raloxifene 600 mg/day was safely tolerated. No mortality was seen after a single oral dose in rats or mice at 810 times the human dose for rats and 405 times the human dose for mice.

Pharmacodynamics/Kinetics
Onset of action: 8 weeks
Absorption: ~60%
Distribution: 2348 L/kg
Protein binding: >95% to albumin and α-glycoprotein
Metabolism: Hepatic, extensive first-pass effect; metabolized to glucuronide conjugates
Bioavailability: ~2%
Half-life elimination: 27.7-32.5 hours
Excretion: Primarily feces; urine (0.2%)

Dosage Adults: Female: Oral: 60 mg/day which may be administered any time of the day without regard to meals
Monitoring Parameters Radiologic evaluation of bone mineral density (BMD) is the best measure of the treatment of osteoporosis; to monitor for the potential toxicities of raloxifene, complete blood counts should be evaluated periodically.
Administration May be administered any time of the day without regard to meals
Contraindications Hypersensitivity to raloxifene or any component of the formulation; active or history of venous thromboembolic events; pregnancy; breast-feeding
Warnings Use caution in patients at high risk for venous thromboembolism (deep vein thrombosis, pulmonary embolism); patients with cardiovascular disease; history of cervical/uterine carcinoma; renal/hepatic insufficiency (however, pharmacokinetic data are lacking); concurrent use of estrogens; women with a history of elevated triglycerides in response to treatment with oral estrogens (or estrogen/progestin). Discontinue at least 72 hours prior to and during prolonged immobilization (postoperative recovery or prolonged bedrest). Safety and efficacy in premenopausal women or men have not been established.
Dosage Forms Tablet, as hydrochloride:
Evista®: 60 mg
Overdosage/Treatment
Decontamination: Oral: Lavage, activated charcoal are preferred modalities; cholestyramine can also decrease oral absorption; consider gastric decontamination for ingestions >1 g
Drug Interactions Cholestyramine: May decrease the absorption of raloxifene.
Levothyroxine: Raloxifene may decrease levothyroxine absorption; separate doses by several hours.
Pregnancy Risk Factor X
Pregnancy Implications Raloxifene should not be used by pregnant women or by women planning to become pregnant in the immediate future
Lactation Excretion in breast milk unknown/contraindicated
Additional Information The decrease in estrogen-related adverse effects with the selective estrogen-receptor modulators in general and raloxifene in particular should improve compliance and decrease the incidence of cardiovascular events and fractures while not increasing breast cancer

Ramipril

Related Information
• Angiotensin Agents
CAS Number 87333-19-5
U.S. Brand Names Altace®
Use Treatment of hypertension, alone or in combination with thiazide diuretics; congestive heart failure treatment postmyocardial infarction
Unlabeled/Investigational Use Treatment of heart failure
Mechanism of Action Ramipril is a prodrug that is converted to ramiprilat in the serum (HOE 498); ramiprilat is an angiotensin-converting enzyme (ACE) inhibitor which prevents the formation of angiotensin II from angiotensin I and exhibits pharmacologic effects that are similar to captopril

Adverse Reactions
Higher rates of adverse reactions have generally been noted in patients with CHF. However, the frequency of adverse effects associated with placebo is also increased in this population.
Cardiovascular: Angina, edema, hypotension, postural hypotension, myocardial infarction, palpitations, symptomatic hypotension, syncope
Central nervous system: Agitation, amnesia, anxiety, cerebrovascular events, convulsions, depression, dizziness, fatigue, headache, insomnia, malaise, nervousness, somnolence, vertigo
Dermatologic: Angioedema, erythema multiforme, onycholysis, pemphigoid, pemphigus, photosensitivity, purpura, Stevens-Johnson syndrome, toxic epidermal necrolysis
Endocrine & metabolic: Hyperkalemia, hyponatremia, impotence
Hematologic: Agranulocytosis, bone marrow depression, decreased hematocrit, decreased hemoglobin, eosinophilia, hemolytic anemia, pancytopenia, thrombocytopenia
Hepatic: Elevated transaminase levels
Gastrointestinal: Abdominal pain, anorexia, constipation, diarrhea, dyspepsia, dysphagia, gastroenteritis, increased salivation, nausea, pancreatitis, taste disturbance, vomiting, weight gain, xerostomia
Neuromuscular & skeletal: Arthralgia, arthritis, chest pain (noncardiac), myalgia, neuralgia, neuropathy, paresthesia, tremor
Ocular: Vision disturbances
Otic: Hearing loss, tinnitus
Renal: Elevated serum creatinine, elevated BUN, renal dysfunction, proteinuria; transient elevations of creatinine and/or BUN may occur more frequently
Respiratory: **Cough (increased)**, dyspnea, epistaxis
Miscellaneous: Anaphylactoid reaction, hypersensitivity reactions (fever, rash, urticaria), increased diaphoresis
Worsening of renal function may occur in patients with bilateral renal artery stenosis or in hypovolemia. In addition, a syndrome which may include fever, myalgia, arthralgia, interstitial nephritis, vasculitis, rash, eosinophilia with positive ANA, and elevated ESR has been reported with ACE inhibitors. Risk of pancreatitis and agranulocytosis may be increased in patients with collagen vascular disease or renal impairment.

Signs and Symptoms of Overdose Hyperuricemia, hyponatremia, insomnia, severe hypotension
Pharmacodynamics/Kinetics
Onset of action: 1-2 hours
Duration: 24 hours
Absorption: Well absorbed (50% to 60%)
Distribution: Plasma levels decline in a triphasic fashion; rapid decline is a distribution phase to peripheral compartment, plasma protein and tissue ACE (half-life 2-4 hours); 2nd phase is an apparent elimination phase representing the clearance of free ramiprilat (half-life: 9-18 hours); and final phase is the terminal elimination phase representing the equilibrium phase between tissue binding and dissociation
Metabolism: Hepatic to the active form, ramiprilat
Half-life elimination: Ramiprilat: Effective: 13-17 hours; Terminal: >50 hours
Time to peak, serum: ~1 hour
Excretion: Urine (60%) and feces (40%) as parent drug and metabolites
Dosage
Adults: Oral: 2.5-5 mg once daily, maximum: 20 mg/day
Dosing adjustment in renal impairment:
Cl$_{cr}$ 10-50 mL/minute: Administer 50% to 75% of normal dose
Cl$_{cr}$ <40 mL/minute: Patients should be started on 1.25 mg/day and titrated up to 5 mg/day maximum
Cl$_{cr}$ <10 mL/minute: Administer 25% to 50% of normal dose
Monitoring Parameters BUN, serum creatinine, renal function; nausea, headache, diarrhea, change in taste, cough
Administration Capsule is usually swallowed whole, but may be may be mixed in water, apple juice, or applesauce.

Contraindications Hypersensitivity to ramipril or any component of the formulation; prior hypersensitivity (including angioedema) to ACE inhibitors; bilateral renal artery stenosis; pregnancy (2nd and 3rd trimesters)

Warnings Anaphylactic or anaphylactoid reactions can occur. Angioedema can occur at any time during treatment (especially following first dose). It may involve head and neck (potentially affecting the airway) or the intestine (presenting with abdominal pain). Prolonged monitoring may be required especially if tongue, glottis, or larynx are involved as they are associated with airway obstruction. Those with a history of airway surgery in this situation have a higher risk. Careful blood pressure monitoring with first dose (hypotension can occur especially in volume-depleted patients). **[U.S. Boxed Warning]: Based on human data, ACEIs can cause injury and death to the developing fetus when used in the second and third trimesters. ACEIs should be discontinued as soon as possible once pregnancy is detected.** Dosage adjustment needed in renal impairment. Use with caution in hypovolemia; collagen vascular diseases; valvular stenosis (particularly aortic stenosis); hyperkalemia; or before, during, or immediately after anesthesia. Avoid rapid dosage escalation, which may lead to renal insufficiency. Rare toxicities associated with ACE inhibitors include cholestatic jaundice (which may progress to hepatic necrosis) and neutropenia/agranulocytosis with myeloid hyperplasia. If patient has renal impairment then a baseline WBC with differential and serum creatinine should be evaluated and monitored closely during the first 3 months of therapy. Hypersensitivity reactions may be seen during hemodialysis with high-flux dialysis membranes (eg, AN69). Use with caution in unilateral renal artery stenosis and pre-existing renal insufficiency.

Dosage Forms Capsule: 1.25 mg, 2.5 mg, 5 mg, 10 mg

Reference Range Serum ramipril blood level range: 4.7-8.8 ng/mL associated with a hypotensive effect (~20 mm Hg drop) in patients with severe hypertension; levels up to 357 ng/mL have been reported without adverse effects during long-term therapy

Overdosage/Treatment
Decontamination: Activated charcoal

Supportive therapy: Following initiation of essential overdose management, toxic symptom treatment and supportive treatment should be initiated. Hypotension usually responds to I.V. fluids or Trendelenburg positioning. If unresponsive to these measures, the use of a parenteral inotrope may be required (eg, norepinephrine 0.1-0.2 mcg/kg/minute titrated to response). For refractory hypotension, angiotensin amide infusion may be attempted.

Enhancement of elimination: Multiple dosing of activated charcoal may be useful

Test Interactions ↑ BUN, creatinine, potassium, ESR; positive Coombs' [direct]; ↓ cholesterol (S), reduces plasma aldosterone level by 50%; may cause false-positive urine acetone determinations using sodium nitroprusside reagent

Drug Interactions Alpha$_1$ blockers: Hypotensive effect increased.
Aspirin: The effects of ACE inhibitors may be blunted by aspirin administration, particularly at higher dosages (see Cardiovascular Considerations) and/or increase adverse renal effects.
Diuretics: Hypovolemia due to diuretics may precipitate acute hypotensive events or acute renal failure.
Insulin: Risk of hypoglycemia may be increased.
Lithium: Risk of lithium toxicity may be increased; monitor lithium levels, especially the first 4 weeks of therapy.
Mercaptopurine: Risk of neutropenia may be increased.
NSAIDs: May attenuate hypertensive efficacy; effect has been seen with captopril and may occur with other ACE inhibitors; monitor blood pressure. May increase risk of adverse renal effects or hyperkalemia.
Potassium-sparing diuretics (amiloride, spironolactone, triamterene): Increased risk of hyperkalemia.
Potassium supplements may increase the risk of hyperkalemia.
Trimethoprim (high dose) may increase the risk of hyperkalemia.

Pregnancy Risk Factor C (1st trimester)/D (2nd and 3rd trimesters)

Pregnancy Implications Decreased placental blood flow, low birth weight, fetal hypotension, preterm delivery, and fetal death have been noted with the use of some ACE inhibitors (ACEIs) in animal studies. Neonatal hypotension, skull hypoplasia, anuria, renal failure, oligohydramnios (associated with fetal limb contractures, craniofacial deformities, hypoplastic lung development), prematurity, intrauterine growth retardation, and patent ductus arteriosus have been reported with the use of ACEIs, primarily in the 2nd and 3rd trimesters. The risk of neonatal toxicity has been considered less when ACEIs have been used in the 1st trimester; however, major congenital malformations have been reported. The cardiovascular and/or central nervous systems are most commonly affected. Unless alternative agents are not appropriate, ACEIs should be discontinued as soon as possible once pregnancy is detected.

Lactation Excretion in breast milk unknown/not recommended

Nursing Implications May cause depression in some patients; discontinue if angioedema of the face, extremities, lips, tongue, or glottis occurs; watch for hypotensive effects within 1-3 hours of first dose or new higher dose

Additional Information Some patients may have a decreased hypotensive effect between 12 and 16 hours; consider dividing total daily dose into 2 doses 12 hours apart; if the patient is receiving a diuretic, a potential for first-dose hypotension is increased; to decrease this potential, stop diuretic for 2-3 days prior to initiating ramipril; continue diuretic if needed to control blood pressure. Due to frequent decreases in glomerular filtration (also creatinine clearance) with aging, elderly patients may have exaggerated responses to ACE inhibitors. In general, the side effect profile is favorable in elderly and causes little or no CNS confusion; use lowest dose recommendations initially. Ramipril is effective and safe in reducing arterial pressure and reducing microalbuminuria in single-kidney patients without renovascular hypertension. Reduces mortality by 27% when given 3-10 days postmyocardial infarction.

Ranitidine

Related Information
- Therapeutic Drugs Associated with Hallucinations

CAS Number 66357-35-5

U.S. Brand Names Zantac® 75 [OTC]; Zantac®

Synonyms Ranitidine Hydrochloride

Use
Zantac®: Short-term and maintenance therapy of duodenal ulcer, gastric ulcer, gastroesophageal reflux, active benign ulcer, erosive esophagitis, and pathological hypersecretory conditions; as part of a multidrug regimen for *H. pylori* eradication to reduce the risk of duodenal ulcer recurrence

Zantac® 75 [OTC]: Relief of heartburn, acid indigestion, and sour stomach

Unlabeled/Investigational Use Recurrent postoperative ulcer, upper GI bleeding, prevention of acid-aspiration pneumonitis during surgery, and prevention of stress-induced ulcers

Mechanism of Action Competitive inhibition of histamine at H$_2$-receptors of the gastric parietal cells, which inhibits gastric acid secretion

Adverse Reactions
Cardiovascular: Bradycardia, sinus bradycardia, angina, vasoconstriction, vasculitis
Central nervous system: Dizziness, sedation, malaise, mental confusion, auditory and visual hallucinations, psychosis, delirium, dystonic reactions, headache, restlessness, aseptic meningitis, memory disturbance, drug fever, paranoia, AV block
Dermatologic: Contact dermatitis, rash, toxic epidermal necrolysis, photosensitivity, toxic pustuloderma, acute generalized exanthematous pustulosis, erythema multiforme, angioedema, xerosis, urticaria, purpura, pruritus, psoriasis, exanthem, cutaneous vasculitis
Endocrine & metabolic: Gynecomastia (may be unilateral), parotitis
Gastrointestinal: Constipation, nausea, vomiting, hypergastrinemia, pancreatitis
Genitourinary: Impotence
Hematologic: Thrombocytopenia, bone marrow hypoplasia (especially in renal failure)
Hepatic: Hepatitis (may be hypersensitivity reaction)
Neuromuscular & skeletal: Arthralgias, choreiform movements
Renal: Allergic interstitial nephritis
Respiratory: Wheezing, eosinophilic pneumonia
Miscellaneous: Fixed drug eruption

Signs and Symptoms of Overdose Agranulocytosis, bradycardia, chest pain, cholestatic jaundice, chorea (extrapyramidal), cognitive dysfunction, depression, diarrhea, disorientation, extrapyramidal reaction, granulocytopenia, gynecomastia, hyperprolactinemia, impotence, insomnia, increased intraocular pressure, leukemoid reaction, leukopenia, mania, memory loss, migraine headache (exacerbation), muscular tremors, neutropenia, parotid pain, rapid respiration, vomiting

Pharmacodynamics/Kinetics
Absorption: Oral: 50%
Distribution: Normal renal function: V$_d$: 1.7 L/kg; Cl$_{cr}$ 25-35 mL/minute: 1.76 L/kg minimally penetrates the blood-brain barrier; enters breast milk
Protein binding: 15%
Metabolism: Hepatic to N-oxide, S-oxide, and N-desmethyl metabolites
Bioavailability: Oral: 48%
Half-life elimination:
Oral: Normal renal function: 2.5-3 hours; Cl$_{cr}$ 25-35 mL/minute: 4.8 hours
I.V.: Normal renal function: 2-2.5 hours
Time to peak, serum: Oral: 2-3 hours; I.M.: ≤15 minutes
Excretion: Urine: Oral: 30%, I.V.: 70% (as unchanged drug); feces (as metabolites)

Dosage Children 1 month to 16 years:
Duodenal and gastric ulcer:
Oral:
Treatment: 2-4 mg/kg/day divided twice daily; maximum treatment dose: 300 mg/day
Maintenance: 2-4 mg/kg once daily; maximum maintenance dose: 150 mg/day
I.V.: 2-4 mg/kg/day divided every 6-8 hours; maximum: 150 mg/day

GERD and erosive esophagitis:
Oral: 5-10 mg/kg/day divided twice daily; maximum: GERD: 300 mg/day, erosive esophagitis: 600 mg/day
I.V.: 2-4 mg/kg/day divided every 6-8 hours; maximum: 150 mg/day
or as an alternative
Continuous infusion: Initial: 1 mg/kg/dose for one dose followed by infusion of 0.08-0.17 mg/kg/hour or 2-4 mg/kg/day
Children $\geq$ 12 years: Prevention of heartburn: Oral: Zantac® 75 [OTC]: 75 mg 30-60 minutes before eating food or drinking beverages which cause heartburn; maximum: 150 mg/24 hours; do not use for more than 14 days
Adults:
Duodenal ulcer: Oral: Treatment: 150 mg twice daily, or 300 mg once daily after the evening meal or at bedtime; maintenance: 150 mg once daily at bedtime
Helicobacter pylori eradication: 150 mg twice daily; requires combination therapy
Pathological hypersecretory conditions:
Oral: 150 mg twice daily; adjust dose or frequency as clinically indicated; doses of up to 6 g/day have been used
I.V.: Continuous infusion for Zollinger-Ellison: 1 mg/kg/hour; measure gastric acid output at 4 hours, if >10 mEq or if patient is symptomatic, increase dose in increments of 0.5 mg/kg/hour; doses of up to 2.5 mg/kg/hour have been used
Gastric ulcer, benign: Oral: 150 mg twice daily; maintenance: 150 mg once daily at bedtime
Erosive esophagitis: Oral: Treatment: 150 mg 4 times/day; maintenance: 150 mg twice daily
Prevention of heartburn: Oral: Zantac® 75 [OTC]: 75 mg 30-60 minutes before eating food or drinking beverages which cause heartburn; maximum: 150 mg in 24 hours; do not use for more than 14 days
Patients not able to take oral medication:
I.M.: 50 mg every 6-8 hours
I.V.: Intermittent bolus or infusion: 50 mg every 6-8 hours
Continuous I.V. infusion: 6.25 mg/hour
Elderly: Ulcer healing rates and incidence of adverse effects are similar in the elderly, when compared to younger patients; dosing adjustments not necessary based on age alone
Dosing adjustment in renal impairment: Adults: Cl_{cr} <50 mL/minute:
Oral: 150 mg every 24 hours; adjust dose cautiously if needed
I.V.: 50 mg every 18-24 hours; adjust dose cautiously if needed
Hemodialysis: Adjust dosing schedule so that dose coincides with the end of hemodialysis
Dosing adjustment/comments in hepatic disease: Patients with hepatic impairment may have minor changes in ranitidine half-life, distribution, clearance, and bioavailability; dosing adjustments not necessary, monitor
Stability Solution for I.V. infusion in NS or D_5W is stable for 48 hours at room temperature or 30 days when frozen; is stable for 24 hours in TPN solutions; is stable only for 12 hours in total nutrient admixtures (TPN) when lipids are added
Monitoring Parameters AST, ALT, serum creatinine; when used to prevent stress-related GI bleeding, measure the intragastric pH and try to maintain pH >4; signs and symptoms of peptic ulcer disease, occult blood with GI bleeding, monitor renal function to correct dose; monitor for side effects
Administration Ranitidine injection may be administered I.M. or I.V.:
I.M.: Injection is administered undiluted
I.V.: Must be diluted; may be administered IVP or IVPB or continuous I.V. infusion
IVP: Ranitidine (usually 50 mg) should be diluted to a total of 20 mL with NS or D_5W and administered over at least 5 minutes
IVPB: Administer over 15-20 minutes
Continuous I.V. infusion: Administer at 6.25 mg/hour and titrate dosage based on gastric pH by continuous infusion over 24 hours
EFFERdose®:
25 mg tablet: Dissolve in at least 5 mL (1 teaspoonful) of water; wait until completely dissolved before administering
150 mg tablet: Dissolve each dose in 6-8 ounces of water before drinking
Contraindications Hypersensitivity to ranitidine or any component of the formulation
Warnings Use with caution in patients with hepatic impairment; use with caution in renal impairment, dosage modification required; avoid use in patients with history of acute porphyria (may precipitate attacks); long-term therapy may be associated with vitamin B_{12} deficiency; EFFERdose® formulations contain phenylalanine; safety and efficacy have not been established for pediatric patients <1 month of age
Dosage Forms Capsule 150 mg, 300 mg
Infusion [premixed in NaCl 0.45%; preservative free]:
Zantac®: 50 mg (50 mL)
Injection, solution: 25 mg/mL (2 mL, 6 mL)
Zantac®: 25 mg/mL (2 mL, 6 mL, 40 mL) [contains phenol 0.5% as preservative]

Syrup: 15 mg/mL (10 mL) [contains alcohol 7.5%; peppermint flavor]
Zantac®: 15 mg/mL (473 mL) [contains alcohol 7.5%; peppermint flavor]
Tablet: 75 mg [OTC], 150 mg, 300 mg
Zantac®: 150 mg, 300 mg
Zantac 75®: 75 mg
Zantac 150™: 150 mg
Tablet, effervescent:
Zantac® EFFERdose®: 25 mg [contains sodium 1.33 mEq/tablet, phenylalanine 2.81 mg/tablet, and sodium benzoate]; 150 mg [contains sodium 7.96 mEq/tablet, phenylalanine 16.84 mg/tablet, and sodium benzoate]
Reference Range Plasma level of 100 ng/mL will cause 50% inhibition of gastric acid secretion
Overdosage/Treatment
Decontamination: Activated charcoal
Supportive therapy: Treatment is primarily symptomatic and supportive
Test Interactions False-positive urine protein using Multistix®, gastric acid secretion test, skin test allergen extracts, serum creatinine and serum transaminase concentrations
Drug Interactions Substrate (minor) of CYP1A2, 2C19, 2D6; **Inhibits** CYP1A2 (weak), 2D6 (weak)
Propantheline: Slight delay and increase in peak ranitidine levels
Triazolam: Ranitidine increases bioavailability of triazolam (10% to 30%), possibly by reducing gastric acidity
Warfarin: May increase or decrease prothrombin time when used concomitantly; monitor
Pregnancy Risk Factor B
Pregnancy Implications Ranitidine crosses the placenta, teratogenic effects to the fetus have not been reported. Use with caution during pregnancy.
Lactation Enters breast milk/use caution
Nursing Implications I.M. solution does not need to be diluted before use; monitor creatinine clearance for renal impairment; observe caution in patients with renal function impairment and hepatic function impairment
Additional Information Giving dose at 6 PM be may better than 10 PM bedtime, the highest acid production usually starts at approximately 7 PM, thus giving at 6 PM controls acid secretion better; give I.V. administration over a 30-minute period to avoid bradycardia; causes fewer adverse reactions and interactions than cimetidine; most patient's ulcers have healed within 4 weeks; long-term therapy may cause vitamin B_{12} deficiency; Cimetidine (400 mg orally twice daily) has been used to treat ranitidine-induced hypergastrinemia
Specific References

Burda A, Razo M, and Wahl M, "Therapeutic Errors with Ranitidine in Pediatric Patients," *Clin Toxicol*, 2005, 43:639.
Salinger LS, Webster CW, Sangali B, et al, "Zantac® (Ranitidine) Therapeutic Errors in Infants," *J Toxicol Clin Toxicol*, 2004, 42(5):749-50.

Rauwolfia serpentina

CAS Number 8063-17-0
Impairment Potential Yes
Use Mild essential hypertension; relief of agitated psychotic states
Adverse Reactions
Cardiovascular: Hypotension, tachycardia, flushing, sinus bradycardia, sinus tachycardia
Central nervous system: Drowsiness, fatigue, CNS depression, coma, parkinsonism, hypothermia
Endocrine & metabolic: Sodium and water retention, gynecomastia, galactorrhea
Gastrointestinal: Abdominal cramps, nausea, vomiting, increased gastric acid secretion, xerostomia, diarrhea
Ocular: Miosis, conjunctival flushing
Respiratory: Nasal congestion
Signs and Symptoms of Overdose Bradycardia, CNS depression, coma, extensor plantar response, facial flushing, galactorrhea, gynecomastia, hypotension, hypothermia, miosis, Parkinson's-like symptoms, tremors, and vomiting
Dosage Adults: Oral: 200-400 mg/day in 2 divided doses
Stability Protect from light
Monitoring Parameters Blood pressure, standing and sitting/supine, ECG for 72 hours after ingestion
Overdosage/Treatment
Decontamination: Activated charcoal
Supportive therapy: Hypotension usually responds to I.V. fluids or Trendelenburg positioning. If unresponsive to these measures, the use of a parenteral inotrope may be required (eg, norepinephrine 0.1-0.2 mcg/kg/minute titrated to response). Anticholinergic agents may be useful in reducing the parkinsonian effects. Avoid the use of digoxin in these patients.
Enhancement of elimination: Multiple dosing of activated charcoal may be effective

Pregnancy Risk Factor C

Pregnancy Implications Effects on neurobehavioral development in rodents

Remifentanil

CAS Number 132539-07-2

U.S. Brand Names Ultiva®

Synonyms GI87084B

Use Analgesic for use during the induction and maintenance of general anesthesia; for continued analgesia into the immediate postoperative period; analgesic component of monitored anesthesia

Unlabeled/Investigational Use Management of pain in mechanically - ventilated patients

Mechanism of Action Binds with stereospecific mu-opioid receptors at many sites within the CNS, increases pain threshold, alters pain reception, inhibits ascending pain pathways

Adverse Reactions

Cardiovascular: Hypotension and bradycardia (dose dependent), tachycardia, hypertension, arrhythmias, heart block, syncope, CPK-MB increased, asystole

Central nervous system: Dizziness, headache, agitation, fever, anxiety, confusion, hallucinations, prolonged emergence from anesthesia

Dermatologic: Pruritus

Endocrine & metabolic: Electrolyte disorders

Gastrointestinal: **Nausea, vomiting**, constipation, diarrhea, dysphagia, gastrointestinal

Hematologic: Anemia, thrombocytopenia

Neuromuscular & skeletal: Muscle rigidity (dose dependent)

Ocular: Visual disturbances

Respiratory: Respiratory depression, apnea, hypoxia, bronchospasm, pleural effusion, pulmonary edema

Miscellaneous: Shivering, postoperative pain, anaphylactic/anaphylactoid reactions

Pharmacodynamics/Kinetics

Onset of action: I.V.: 1-3 minutes

Distribution: V_d: 100 mL/kg; increased in children

Protein binding: ~70% (primarily alpha$_1$ acid glycoprotein)

Metabolism: Rapid via blood and tissue esterases

Half-life elimination (dose dependent): Terminal: 10-20 minutes; effective: 3-10 minutes

Excretion: Urine

Dosage I.V. continuous infusion: Dose should be based on ideal body weight (IBW) in obese patients (>30% over IBW).

Children birth to 2 months: Maintenance of anesthesia with nitrous oxide (70%): 0.4 mcg/kg/minute (range: 0.4-1 mcg/kg/minute); supplemental bolus dose of 1 mcg/kg may be administered, smaller bolus dose may be required with potent inhalation agents, potent neuraxial anesthesia, significant comorbidities, significant fluid shifts, or without atropine pretreatment. Clearance in neonates is highly variable; dose should be carefully titrated.

Children 1-12 years: Maintenance of anesthesia with halothane, sevoflurane or isoflurane: 0.25 mcg/kg/minute (range 0.05-1.3 mcg/kg/minute); supplemental bolus dose of 1 mcg/kg may be administered every 2-5 minutes. Consider increasing concomitant anesthetics with infusion rate >1 mcg/kg/minute. Infusion rate can be titrated upward in increments up to 50% or titrated downward in decrements of 25% to 50%. May titrate every 2-5 minutes.

Adults:

Induction of anesthesia: 0.5-1 mcg/kg/minute; if endotracheal intubation is to occur in <8 minutes, an initial dose of 1 mcg/kg may be given over 30-60 seconds

Coronary bypass surgery: 1 mcg/kg/minute

Maintenance of anesthesia: **Note:** Supplemental bolus dose of 1 mcg/kg may be administered every 2-5 minutes. Consider increasing concomitant anesthetics with infusion rate >1 mcg/kg/minute. Infusion rate can be titrated upward in increments of 25% to 100% or downward in decrements of 25% to 50%. May titrate every 2-5 minutes.

With nitrous oxide (66%): 0.4 mcg/kg/minute (range: 0.1-2 mcg/kg/minute)

With isoflurane: 0.25 mcg/kg/minute (range: 0.05-2 mcg/kg/minute)

With propofol: 0.25 mcg/kg/minute (range: 0.05-2 mcg/kg/minute)

Coronary bypass surgery: 1 mcg/kg/minute (range: 0.125-4 mcg/kg/minute); supplemental dose: 0.5-1 mcg/kg

Continuation as an analgesic in immediate postoperative period: 0.1 mcg/kg/minute (range: 0.025-0.2 mcg/kg/minute). Infusion rate may be adjusted every 5 minutes in increments of 0.025 mcg/kg/minute. Bolus doses are not recommended. Infusion rates >0.2 mcg/kg/minute are associated with respiratory depression.

Coronary bypass surgery, continuation as an analgesic into the ICU: 1 mcg/kg/minute (range: 0.05-1 mcg/kg/minute)

Analgesic component of monitored anesthesia care: **Note:** Supplemental oxygen is recommended:

Single I.V. dose given 90 seconds prior to local anesthetic:

Remifentanil alone: 1 mcg/kg over 30-60 seconds

With midazolam: 0.5 mcg/kg over 30-60 seconds

Continuous infusion beginning 5 minutes prior to local anesthetic:

Remifentanil alone: 0.1 mcg/kg minute

With midazolam: 0.05 mcg/kg/minute

Continuous infusion given after local anesthetic:

Remifentanil alone: 0.05 mcg/kg/minute (range: 0.025-0.2 mcg/kg/minute)

With midazolam: 0.025 mcg/kg/minute (range: 0.025-0.2 mcg/kg/minute)

Note: Following local or anesthetic block, infusion rate should be decreased to 0.05 mcg/kg/minute; rate adjustments of 0.025 mcg/kg/minute may be done at 5-minute intervals

Mechanically-ventilated patients: Acute pain (moderate-to-severe) (unlabeled use): 0.6-15 mcg/kg/hour

Elderly: Elderly patients have an increased sensitivity to effect of remifentanil, doses should be decreased by $^1/_2$ and titrated

Monitoring Parameters Respiratory and cardiovascular status, blood pressure, heart rate

Administration An infusion device should be used to administer continuous infusions. During the maintenance of general anesthesia, I.V. boluses may be administered over 30-60 seconds. Injections should be given into I.V. tubing close to the venous cannula; tubing should be cleared after treatment to prevent residual effects when other fluids are administered through the same I.V. line.

Contraindications Not for intrathecal or epidural administration, due to the presence of glycine in the formulation; hypersensitivity to remifentanil, fentanyl, or fentanyl analogs, or any component of the formulation

Warnings Remifentanil is not recommended as the sole agent in general anesthesia, because the loss of consciousness cannot be assured and due to the high incidence of apnea, hypotension, tachycardia and muscle rigidity; it should be administered by individuals specifically trained in the use of anesthetic agents and should not be used in diagnostic or therapeutic procedures outside the monitored anesthesia setting; resuscitative and intubation equipment should be readily available.

Interruption of an infusion will result in offset of effects within 5-10 minutes; the discontinuation of remifentanil infusion should be preceded by the establishment of adequate postoperative analgesia orders, especially for patients in whom postoperative pain is anticipated. Use caution in the morbidly obese.

Dosage Forms Injection, powder for reconstitution: 1 mg, 2 mg, 5 mg [contains glycine 15 mg]

Reference Range Plasma remifentanil level in 50% of patients unresponsive to surgical stimuli ranges from 1.5-2 ng/mL

Overdosage/Treatment

Decontamination: Activated charcoal for oral ingestion

Supportive therapy: Naloxone in large doses and/or a continuous infusion may be necessary

Antidote(s)

- Nalmefene [ANTIDOTE]
- Naloxone [ANTIDOTE]

Drug Interactions Anesthetics: Synergistic with other anesthetics, may need to decrease thiopental, propofol, isoflurane and midazolam by up to 75%

CNS depressants: Increased effect of CNS depressants

Pregnancy Risk Factor C

Pregnancy Implications Remifentanil has been shown to cross the placenta. Neonatal respiratory depression and sedation may occur.

Lactation Excretion in breast milk unknown/use caution

Repaglinide

CAS Number 135062-02-1

U.S. Brand Names Prandin®

Use Management of type 2 diabetes mellitus (noninsulin dependent, NIDDM); may be used in combination with metformin or thiazolidinediones

Mechanism of Action Nonsulfonylurea hypoglycemic agent of the meglitinide class (the nonsulfonylurea moiety of glyburide) used in the management of type 2 diabetes mellitus; stimulates insulin release from pancreatic beta cells

Adverse Reactions

Cardiovascular: Chest pain

Central nervous system: **Headache**

Dermatologic: Alopecia, Stevens-Johnson syndrome

Gastrointestinal: Nausea, heartburn, vomiting, constipation, diarrhea, tooth disorder, pancreatitis

Endocrine & metabolic: **Hypoglycemia**

Genitourinary: Urinary tract infection

Hematologic: Leukopenia, thrombocytopenia, hemolytic anemia

Hepatic: Elevated liver function test results, hepatic dysfunction (severe)

Neuromuscular & skeletal: Arthralgia, back pain, paresthesia

Respiratory: **Upper respiratory tract infection**, sinusitis, rhinitis, bronchitis

Miscellaneous: Allergy, anaphylactoid reaction

Signs and Symptoms of Overdose Agitation, cerebral damage, coma, confusion, convulsions, nausea, severe hypoglycemia, seizures, stupor, sweating, tachycardia, tingling of lips and tongue, yawning

Admission Criteria/Prognosis Admit any symptomatic patient or asymptomatic normoglycemic patient after 8 hours of observation. Admit any ingestion >100 mg.

Pharmacodynamics/Kinetics

Onset of action: Single dose: Increased insulin levels: ~15-60 minutes

Duration: 4-6 hours

Absorption: Rapid and complete

Distribution: V_d: 31 L

Protein binding, plasma: >98%

Metabolism: Hepatic via CYP3A4 isoenzyme and glucuronidation to inactive metabolites

Bioavailability: Mean absolute: ~56%

Half-life elimination: 1 hour

Time to peak, plasma: ~1 hour

Excretion: Within 96 hours: Feces (~90%, <2% as parent drug); Urine (~8%)

Dosage Adults: Oral: Should be taken within 15 minutes of the meal, but time may vary from immediately preceding the meal to as long as 30 minutes before the meal

Initial: For patients not previously treated or whose Hb A_{1c} is <8%, the starting dose is 0.5 mg. For patients previously treated with blood glucose-lowering agents whose Hb A_{1c} is ≥8%, the initial dose is 1 or 2 mg before each meal.

Dose adjustment: Determine dosing adjustments by blood glucose response, usually fasting blood glucose. Double the preprandial dose up to 4 mg until satisfactory blood glucose response is achieved. At least 1 week should elapse to assess response after each dose adjustment.

Dose range: 0.5-4 mg taken with meals. Repaglinide may be dosed preprandial 2, 3 or 4 times/day in response to changes in the patient's meal pattern. Maximum recommended daily dose: 16 mg.

Patients receiving other oral hypoglycemic agents: When repaglinide is used to replace therapy with other oral hypoglycemic agents, it may be started the day after the final dose is given. Observe patients carefully for hypoglycemia because of potential overlapping of drug effects. When transferred from longer half-life sulfonylureas (eg, chlorpropamide), close monitoring may be indicated for up to ≥1 week.

Combination therapy: If repaglinide monotherapy does not result in adequate glycemic control, metformin or a thiazolidinedione may be added. Or, if metformin or thiazolidinedione therapy does not provide adequate control, repaglinide may be added. The starting dose and dose adjustments for combination therapy are the same as repaglinide monotherapy. Carefully adjust the dose of each drug to determine the minimal dose required to achieve the desired pharmacologic effect. Failure to do so could result in an increase in the incidence of hypoglycemic episodes. Use appropriate monitoring of FPG and Hb A_{1c} measurements to ensure that the patient is not subjected to excessive drug exposure or increased probability of secondary drug failure. If glucose is not achieved after a suitable trial of combination therapy, consider discontinuing these drugs and using insulin.

Dosing adjustment in renal impairment:

Cl_{cr} 40-80 mL/minute (mild to moderate renal dysfunction): Initial dosage adjustment does not appear to be necessary.

Cl_{cr} 20-40 mL/minute: Initiate 0.5 mg with meals; titrate carefully.

Dosing adjustment in hepatic impairment: Use conservative initial and maintenance doses. Use longer intervals between dosage adjustments.

Monitoring Parameters Periodically monitor fasting blood glucose and glycosylated hemoglobin (Hb A_{1c}) levels with a goal of decreasing these levels towards the normal range. During dose adjustment, fasting glucose can be used to determine response.

Administration Administer repaglinide 15-30 minutes before meals. Patients who are anorexic or NPO, may need to have their dose held to avoid hypoglycemia.

Contraindications Hypersensitivity to repaglinide or any component of the formulation; diabetic ketoacidosis, with or without coma (treat with insulin); type 1 diabetes (insulin dependent, IDDM)

Warnings Use with caution in patients with hepatic or renal impairment. May cause hypoglycemia; appropriate patient selection, dosage, and patient education are important to avoid hypoglycemic episodes. It may be necessary to discontinue repaglinide and administer insulin if the patient is exposed to stress (fever, trauma, infection, surgery). Safety and efficacy have not been established in pediatric patients. Not indicated for use in combination with NPH insulin due to potential cardiovascular events.

Dosage Forms Tablet:

Prandin®: 0.5 mg, 1 mg, 2 mg

Reference Range Target range: Adults: Fasting blood glucose: <120 mg/dL. Glycosylated hemoglobin: <7%

Overdosage/Treatment

Decontamination: Oral: Lavage within 1 hour/activated charcoal can be used.

Supportive therapy: 25 g dextrose should be given for hypoglycemia; octreotide (30 ng/kg I.V.) can also be given. (Hypoglycemia usually will be of shorter duration as compared with sulfonylureas.)

Drug Interactions Substrate of CYP2C8 (major), 3A4 (major)

CYP2C8 inducers: May decrease the levels/effects of repaglinide. Example inducers include carbamazepine, phenobarbital, phenytoin, rifampin, rifapentine, and secobarbital.

CYP2C8 Inhibitors may increase the levels/effects of repaglinide. Example inhibitors include atazanavir, gemfibrozil, and ritonavir.

CYP3A4 inducers: CYP3A4 inducers may decrease the levels/effects of repaglinide. Example inducers include aminoglutethimide, carbamazepine, nafcillin, nevirapine, phenobarbital, phenytoin, and rifamycins.

CYP3A4 inhibitors: May increase the levels/effects of repaglinide. Example inhibitors include azole antifungals, clarithromycin, diclofenac, doxycycline, erythromycin, imatinib, isoniazid, nefazodone, nicardipine, propofol, protease inhibitors, quinidine, telithromycin, and verapamil.

Gemfibrozil: Gemfibrozil may increase the serum concentration of repaglinide (prolonged, severe hypoglycemia has been reported). The addition of itraconazole may augment the effects of gemfibrozil on repaglinide. Consider alternative therapy.

HMG-CoA reductase inhibitors (eg, atorvastatin, fluvastatin, lovastatin, pravastatin, simvastatin): May increase repaglinide concentrations by decreasing metabolism.

Macrolide antibiotics (eg, clarithromycin, erythromycin, troleandomycin): May increase repaglinide concentrations by decreasing metabolism.

Oral contraceptives (estrogens, such as estradiol, ethinyl estradiol, mestranol): May increase repaglinide concentrations. Repaglinide may increase oral contraceptive (estrogens) serum concentration.

Oral contraceptives (progestins): May increase repaglinide concentrations. Repaglinide may increase oral contraceptive (progestins) serum concentration.

Rifampin: May decrease levels/effects of repaglinide; monitor serum glucose.

Trimethoprim: May increase repaglinide concentrations; monitor serum glucose carefully.

Pregnancy Risk Factor C

Pregnancy Implications Clinical effects on the fetus: Safety in pregnant women has not been established. Use during pregnancy only if clearly needed. Abnormal blood glucose levels are associated with a higher incidence of congenital abnormalities. Insulin is the drug of choice for the control of diabetes mellitus during pregnancy.

Lactation Excretion in breast milk unknown/not recommended

Nursing Implications Patients who are anorexic or NPO, may need to have their dose held to avoid hypoglycemia

Additional Information Avoid ethanol, gymnema, and garlic (may cause hypoglycemia). When given with food, the AUC of repaglinide is decreased. St John's wort may decrease repaglinide levels.

Reserpine

Related Information

● *Rauwolfia serpentina*

CAS Number 50-55-5

Impairment Potential Yes

Use Management of mild-to-moderate hypertension; treatment of agitated psychotic states (schizophrenia)

Unlabeled/Investigational Use Management of tardive dyskinesia

Mechanism of Action Reduces blood pressure via depletion of sympathetic biogenic amines (norepinephrine and dopamine); this also commonly results in sedative effects

Adverse Reactions

Cardiovascular: Hypotension, tachycardia, hypotension (orthostatic), fibrillation (atrial), flutter (atrial), sinus bradycardia, cardiomyopathy, cardiomegaly, pericardial effusion/pericarditis, sinus tachycardia, vasodilation

Central nervous system: **Dizziness**, drowsiness, fatigue, coma, psychosis, hallucinations, parkinsonism, hypothermia, CNS depression, insomnia, fever, hyperthermia, neuroleptic malignant syndrome, extrapyramidal reactions

Dermatologic: Pruritus

Endocrine & metabolic: Sodium and water retention, gynecomastia, galactorrhea, hyperprolactinemia

Gastrointestinal: **Nausea, xerostomia, diarrhea, anorexia, vomiting**, increased gastric acid secretion, fecal discoloration (black), abdominal cramps

Ocular: Miosis, conjunctival flushing

Respiratory: **Nasal congestion**, rhinitis

Miscellaneous: Systemic lupus erythematosus, breast cancer

Signs and Symptoms of Overdose Bradycardia, CNS depression, coma, depression, extensor plantar response, flushing, galactorrhea, gynecomastia, hyperglycemia, hypertension, hypothermia, hypotension, impotence, miosis, Parkinson's-like symptoms, ptosis, sexual dysfunction, syncope, tremors, vomiting, wheezing

Pharmacodynamics/Kinetics
Onset of action: Antihypertensive: 3-6 days
Duration: 2-6 weeks
Absorption: ~40%
Distribution: Crosses placenta; enters breast milk
Protein binding: 96%
Metabolism: Extensively hepatic (>90%)
Half-life elimination: 50-100 hours
Excretion: Feces (30% to 60%); urine (10%)

Dosage Note: When used for management of hypertension, full antihypertensive effects may take as long as 3 weeks.
Oral:
Children: Hypertension: 0.01-0.02 mg/kg/24 hours divided every 12 hours; maximum dose: 0.25 mg/day (not recommended in children)
Adults:
Hypertension: Initial: 0.5 mg/day for 1-2 weeks; usual dose range (JNC 7): 0.05-0.25 mg once daily; 0.1 mg every other day may be given to achieve 0.05 mg once daily
Tardive dyskinesia/schizophrenia: Initial: 0.5 mg/day; usual range: 0.1-1 mg
Elderly: Initial: 0.05 mg once daily, increasing by 0.05 mg every week as necessary

Dosing adjustment in renal impairment: Cl_{cr} <10 mL/minute: Avoid use
Dialysis: Not removed by hemo or peritoneal dialysis; supplemental dose is not necessary

Stability Protect oral dosage forms from light; **incompatible** with ethacrynic acid

Monitoring Parameters Blood pressure, standing and sitting/supine

Contraindications Hypersensitivity to reserpine or any component of the formulation; active peptic ulcer disease, ulcerative colitis; history of mental depression (especially with suicidal tendencies); patients receiving electroconvulsive therapy (ECT)

Warnings Use with caution in patients with impaired renal function, inflammatory bowel disease, asthma, Parkinson's disease, gallstones, or history of peptic ulcer disease, and the elderly. At high doses, significant mental depression, anxiety, or psychosis may occur (uncommon at dosages <0.25 mg/day). May cause orthostatic hypotension; use with caution in patients at risk of hypotension or in patients where transient hypotensive episodes would be poorly tolerated (cardiovascular disease or cerebrovascular disease). Avoid concurrent use of MAO inhibitors and/or drugs with MAO-inhibiting properties. Some products may contain tartrazine.

Dosage Forms Tablet: 0.1 mg, 0.25 mg

Overdosage/Treatment
Decontamination: Lavage within 1 hour, activated charcoal
Supportive therapy: Hypotension usually responds to I.V. fluids or Trendelenburg positioning. If unresponsive to these measures, the use of a parenteral inotrope may be required (eg, norepinephrine 0.1-0.2 mcg/kg/minute titrated to response). Anticholinergic agents may be useful in reducing the parkinsonian effects. Avoid the use of digoxin in these patients. Alprazolam can reverse reserpine-induced depression.
Enhancement of elimination: Multiple dosing of activated charcoal may be effective

Test Interactions ↑ catecholamines (U) 1 or 2 days postingestion; ↑ prolactin

Drug Interactions Antihypertensives: Hypotensive effects may be increased.
CNS depressants, ethanol: Additive CNS effects may occur.
Digitalis glycosides: Concomitant administration may predispose some patients to cardiac arrhythmias.
MAO inhibitors: Reserpine may cause hypertensive reactions; concurrent use is not recommended. Theoretically, risk is decreased if reserpine is initiated several days prior to MAO inhibitors.
Quinidine, procainamide: Reserpine may increase the risk of cardiac arrhythmias effects.
Sympathomimetics: The effects of direct-acting sympathomimetics (eg, epinephrine, norepinephrine) may be modestly increased/prolonged. However, the effects of indirect-acting sympathomimetics (amphetamines, dopamine) may be blocked by reserpine.

Pregnancy Risk Factor C
Pregnancy Implications Crosses the placenta; appears in breast milk
Lactation Enters breast milk/use caution
Nursing Implications Observe for mental depression and alert family members to report any symptoms
Additional Information Full antihypertensive effects may take as long as 3 weeks; at high doses, mental depression is possible and might lead to suicide

Specific References
Chobanian AV, Bakris GL, Black HR, et al, "The Seventh Report of the Joint National Committee on Prevention, Detection, Evaluation, and Treatment of High Blood Pressure: The JNC 7 Report," *JAMA*, 2003, 289(19):2560-71.

Reteplase

U.S. Brand Names Retavase®
Synonyms r-PA; Recombinant Plasminogen Activator
Use Acute myocardial infarction (thrombolytic agent)
Mechanism of Action Catalyzes cleavage of endogenous plasminogen to generate plasmin; can decrease fibrinogen levels to <100 mg/dL within 2 hours of injection

Adverse Reactions
Cardiovascular: Pericardial hemorrhage, **hypotension, arrhythmias, trauma arrhythmias**
Central nervous system: Intracranial hemorrhage (0.8%), fever
Gastrointestinal: **GI bleeding** (5% to 49%), nausea, vomiting
Genitourinary: Bleeding (2% to 10%)
Hematologic: Anemia (1% to 3%), **bleeding**

Pharmacodynamics/Kinetics
Onset of action: Thrombolysis: 30-90 minutes
Half-life elimination: 13-16 minutes
Excretion: Feces and urine
Clearance: Plasma: 250-450 mL/minute

Dosage I.V.: 10 units over 2 minutes followed by a second 10 unit bolus dose in 30 minutes

Monitoring Parameters Monitor for signs of bleeding (hematuria, GI bleeding, gingival bleeding)

Administration Reteplase should be reconstituted using the diluent, syringe, needle and dispensing pin provided with each kit and the each reconstituted dose should be administered I.V. over 2 minutes; no other medication should be added to the injection solution

Contraindications Hypersensitivity to reteplase or any component of the formulation; active internal bleeding; history of cerebrovascular accident; recent intracranial or intraspinal surgery or trauma; intracranial neoplasm, arteriovenous malformations, or aneurysm; known bleeding diathesis; severe uncontrolled hypertension

Warnings
Concurrent heparin anticoagulation can contribute to bleeding; careful attention to all potential bleeding sites. I.M. injections and nonessential handling of the patient should be avoided. Venipunctures should be performed carefully and only when necessary. If arterial puncture is necessary, use an upper extremity vessel that can be manually compressed. If serious bleeding occurs then the infusion of anistreplase and heparin should be stopped.
For the following conditions the risk of bleeding is higher with use of reteplase and should be weighed against the benefits of therapy: recent major surgery (eg, CABG, obstetrical delivery, organ biopsy, previous puncture of noncompressible vessels), cerebrovascular disease, recent gastrointestinal or genitourinary bleeding, recent trauma including CPR, hypertension (systolic BP >180 mm Hg and/or diastolic BP >110 mm Hg), high likelihood of left heart thrombus (eg, mitral stenosis with atrial fibrillation), acute pericarditis, subacute bacterial endocarditis, hemostatic defects including ones caused by severe renal or hepatic dysfunction, significant hepatic dysfunction, pregnancy, diabetic hemorrhagic retinopathy or other hemorrhagic ophthalmic conditions, septic thrombophlebitis or occluded AV cannula at seriously infected site, advanced age (eg, >75 years), patients receiving oral anticoagulants, any other condition in which bleeding constitutes a significant hazard or would be particularly difficult to manage because of location.
Coronary thrombolysis may result in reperfusion arrhythmias. Follow standard MI management. Rare anaphylactic reactions can occur. Safety and efficacy in pediatric patients have not been established.

Dosage Forms Injection, powder for reconstitution [preservative free]: 10.4 units [equivalent to reteplase 18.1 mg; contains sucrose and polysorbate 80; packaged with sterile water for injection]

Reference Range Maximal serum Retavase™ levels after a 15 unit bolus: 1536 int. unit/mL

Overdosage/Treatment Supportive therapy: Treat bleeding complications with transfusions of red blood cells, fresh frozen plasma, and cryoprecipitate; do not administer dextran; although human overdose data is lacking, administration of aminocaproic acid (Amicar®) at a dose of 3-5 g I.V. followed by an infusion rate of 1-1.25 g/hour may be useful

Drug Interactions Aminocaproic acid (antifibrinolytic agent) may decrease effectiveness.
Drugs which affect platelet function (eg, NSAIDs, dipyridamole, ticlopidine, clopidogrel, IIb/IIIa antagonists) may potentiate the risk of hemorrhage; use with caution.
Heparin and aspirin: Use with aspirin and heparin may increase bleeding. However, aspirin and heparin were used concomitantly with reteplase in the majority of patients in clinical studies.
Warfarin or oral anticoagulants: Risk of bleeding may be increased during concurrent therapy.

Pregnancy Risk Factor C
Pregnancy Implications Abortifacient in rabbits

Lactation Excretion in breast milk unknown/use caution

Additional Information Not antigenic; a nonglycosylated deletion mutant of wild type t-PA lacking the kringle-1, finger and growth factor domains of t-PA not compatible with heparin in solution

Specific Reference

Simpson D, Siddiqui AA, Scott CJ, and Hilleman DE, "Reteplase: A Review of Its use in the Management of Thrombotic Occlusive Disorders," *Am J Cardiovasc Drugs*, 2006, 6(4):265-85.

Ribavirin

CAS Number 36791-04-5

U.S. Brand Names Copegus®; Rebetol®; Ribasphere™; Virazole®

Synonyms RTCA; Tribavirin

Use

Inhalation: Treatment of patients with respiratory syncytial virus (RSV) infections; specially indicated for treatment of severe lower respiratory tract RSV infections in patients with an underlying compromising condition (prematurity, bronchopulmonary dysplasia and other chronic lung conditions, congenital heart disease, immunodeficiency, immunosuppression), and recent transplant recipients

Oral capsule:

In combination with interferon alfa-2b (Intron® A) injection for the treatment of chronic hepatitis C in patients with compensated liver disease who have relapsed after alpha interferon therapy or were previously untreated with alpha interferons

In combination with peginterferon alfa-2b (PEG-Intron®) injection for the treatment of chronic hepatitis C in patients with compensated liver disease who were previously untreated with alpha interferons

Oral solution: In combination with interferon alfa 2b (Intron® A) injection for the treatment of chronic hepatitis C in patients ≥3 years of age with compensated liver disease who were previously untreated with alpha interferons or patients ≥18 years of age who have relapsed after alpha interferon therapy

Oral tablet: In combination with peginterferon alfa-2a (Pegasys®) injection for the treatment of chronic hepatitis C in patients with compensated liver disease who were previously untreated with alpha interferons (includes patients with histological evidence of cirrhosis [Child-Pugh class A] and patients with clinically-stable HIV disease)

Unlabeled/Investigational Use Used in other viral infections including influenza A and B and adenovirus

Mechanism of Action Inhibits replication of RNA and DNA viruses; inhibits influenza virus RNA polymerase activity and inhibits the initiation and elongation of RNA fragments resulting in inhibition of viral protein synthesis

Adverse Reactions

Inhalation:

Cardiovascular: Hypotension, cardiac arrest

Central nervous system: Fatigue, headache, insomnia

Gastrointestinal: Nausea, anorexia

Hematologic: Anemia

Ocular: Conjunctivitis

Respiratory: Mild bronchospasm, worsening of respiratory function, apnea

Miscellaneous: Digitalis toxicity

Note: Incidence of adverse effects (approximate) in healthcare workers: Headache 51%; conjunctivitis 32%; rhinitis, nausea, rash, dizziness, pharyngitis, and lacrimation 10% to 20%

Oral (all adverse reactions are documented while receiving combination therapy with interferon alpha-2b):

Cardiovascular: Chest pain*

Central nervous system: **Dizziness, headache*, fatigue*, fever*, insomnia, irritability, depression*, emotional lability*, impaired concentration***, nervousness*; suicidal ideation, vertigo

Dermatologic: **Alopecia, rash, pruritus**

Endocrine & metabolic: Diabetes mellitus, gout, thyroid function test abnormalities

Gastrointestinal: **Nausea, anorexia, dyspepsia, vomiting***, taste perversion, pancreatitis

Hematologic: **Decreased hemoglobin, decreased WBC, absolute neutrophil count** <0.5 × 10⁹/L, **thrombocytopenia, hemolysis**, hemolytic anemia

Hepatic: Hyperbilirubinemia

Neuromuscular & skeletal: **Myalgia*, arthralgia*, musculoskeletal pain, rigors**, weakness

Otic: Hearing disorder

Respiratory: **Dyspnea, sinusitis***, **nasal congestion**, pulmonary dysfunction

Miscellaneous: **Flu-like syndrome***, sarcoidosis

*Similar to interferon alone

Incidence of anorexia, headache, fever, suicidal ideation, and vomiting are higher in children.

Pharmacodynamics/Kinetics

Absorption: Inhalation: Systemic; dependent upon respiratory factors and method of drug delivery; maximal absorption occurs with the use of aerosol generator via endotracheal tube; highest concentrations in respiratory tract and erythrocytes

Distribution: Oral capsule: Single dose: V_d 2825 L; distribution significantly prolonged in the erythrocyte (16-40 days), which can be used as a marker for intracellular metabolism

Protein binding: Oral: None

Metabolism: Hepatically and intracellularly (forms active metabolites); may be necessary for drug action

Bioavailability: Oral: 64%

Half-life elimination, plasma:

Children: Inhalation: 6.5-11 hours

Adults: Oral:

Capsule, single dose (Rebetol®, Ribasphere™): 24 hours in healthy adults, 44 hours with chronic hepatitis C infection (increases to ~298 hours at steady state)

Tablet, single dose (Copegus®): 120-170 hours

Time to peak, serum: Inhalation: At end of inhalation period; Oral capsule: Multiple doses: 3 hours; Tablet: 2 hours

Excretion: Inhalation: Urine (40% as unchanged drug and metabolites); Oral capsule: Urine (61%), feces (12%)

Dosage Aerosol inhalation: Infants and children: Use with Viratek® small particle aerosol generator (SPAG-2) at a concentration of 20 mg/mL (6 g reconstituted with 300 mL of sterile water without preservatives). Continuous aerosol administration: 12-18 hours/day for 3 days, up to 7 days in length

Oral capsule or solution:

Children ≥3 years: Chronic hepatitis C (in combination with interferon alfa-2b):

25-36 kg: 400 mg/day (200 mg twice daily)

37-49 kg: 600 mg/day (200 mg in morning and 400 mg in evening)

50-61 kg: 800 mg/day (400 mg twice daily)

>61 kg: Refer to adult dosing

Note: Duration of therapy is 48 weeks in pediatric patients with genotype 1 and 24 weeks in patients with genotype 2,3. Discontinue treatment in any patient if HCV-RNA is not below the limit of detection of the assay after 24 weeks of therapy.

Oral capsule:

Adults:

Chronic hepatitis C (in combination with interferon alfa-2b):

≤75 kg: 400 mg in the morning, then 600 mg in the evening

>75 kg: 600 mg in the morning, then 600 mg in the evening

Note: If HCV-RNA is undetectable at 24 weeks, duration of therapy is 48 weeks. In patients who relapse following interferon therapy, duration of dual therapy is 24 weeks.

Chronic hepatitis C (in combination with peginterferon alfa-2b): 400 mg twice daily; duration of therapy is 1 year; after 24 weeks of treatment, if serum HCV-RNA is not below the limit of detection of the assay, consider discontinuation.

Oral tablet: Adults:

Chronic hepatitis C, genotype 1,4 (in combination with peginterferon alfa-2a):

<75kg: 1000 mg/day in 2 divided doses for 48 weeks

≥75kg: 1200 mg/day in 2 divided doses for 48 weeks

Chronic hepatitis C, genotype 2,3 (in combination with peginterferon alfa-2a): 800 mg/day in 2 divided doses for 24 weeks

Dosage adjustment in renal impairment: Cl_{cr} <50 mL/minute: Oral route is contraindicated

Dosage adjustment for toxicity: Oral: Capsule, solution, tablet:

Patient **without** cardiac history:

Hemoglobin <10 g/dL:

Children: 7.5 mg/kg/day

Adults: Decrease dose to 600 mg/day

Hemoglobin <8.5 g/dL: Children and Adults: Permanently discontinue treatment

Patient **with** cardiac history:

Hemoglobin has ≥2 g/dL decrease during any 4-week period of treatment:

Children: 7.5 mg/kg/day

Adults: Decrease dose to 600 mg/day

Hemoglobin <12 g/dL after 4 weeks of reduced dose: Children and Adults: Permanently discontinue treatment

Monitoring Parameters Inhalation: Respiratory function, hemoglobin, reticulocyte count, CBC, I & O

Oral: CBC with differential (pretreatment, 2- and 4 weeks after initiation); pretreatment and monthly pregnancy test for women of childbearing age; LFTs, TSH, HCV-RNA after 24 weeks of therapy; ECG in patients with pre-existing cardiac disease

Administration Inhalation: Ribavirin should be administered in well-ventilated rooms (at least 6 air changes/hour). In mechanically-ventilated patients, ribavirin can potentially be deposited in the ventilator delivery system depending on temperature, humidity, and electrostatic forces; this deposition can lead to malfunction or obstruction of the expiratory valve, resulting in inadvertently high positive end-expiratory pressures. The use of one-way valves in the inspiratory lines, a breathing circuit filter in the expiratory line, and frequent monitoring and filter replacement have been effective in preventing these problems. Solutions in SPAG-2 unit should be discarded at least every 24 hours and when the liquid level is low before adding newly reconstituted solution. Should not be mixed with other aerosolized medication.

Oral: Administer concurrently with interferon alfa injection.
- Capsule, in combination with interferon alfa-2b: May be administered with or without food, but always in a consistent manner in regard to food intake.
- Capsule, in combination with peginterferon alfa 2b: Administer with food.
- Solution, in combination with interferon alfa-2b: May be administered with or without food, but always in a consistent manner in regard to food intake.
- Tablet: Should be administered with food.

Contraindications Hypersensitivity to ribavirin or any component of the formulation; women of childbearing age who will not use contraception reliably; pregnancy

Additional contraindications for oral formulation: Male partners of pregnant women; $Cl_{cr}<$ 50 mL/minute; hemoglobinopathies (eg, thalassemia major, sickle cell anemia); as monotherapy for treatment of chronic hepatitis C; patients with autoimmune hepatitis, anemia, severe heart disease

Refer to individual monographs for Interferon Alfa-2b (Intron® A) and Peginterferon Alfa-2a (Pegasys®) for additional contraindication information.

Warnings

[U.S. Boxed Warning]: Negative pregnancy test is required before initiation and monthly thereafter. Avoid pregnancy in female patients and female partners of male patients, during therapy, and for at least 6 months after treatment; two forms of contraception should be used. Elderly patients are more susceptible to adverse effects; use caution. Safety and efficacy have not been established in patients who have failed other alpha interferon therapy, received organ transplants, or been coinfected with hepatitis B or HIV (Copegus® may be used in HIV coinfected patients unless CD4+ cell count is <100 cells/microL). **[U.S. Boxed Warning]: Monotherapy not effective for chronic hepatitis C infection.** Safety and efficacy have not been established in patients <3 years of age.

Inhalation: **[U.S. Boxed Warning]: Use with caution in patients requiring assisted ventilation because precipitation of the drug in the respiratory equipment may interfere with safe and effective patient ventilation; sudden deterioration of respiratory function has been observed;** monitor carefully in patients with COPD and asthma for deterioration of respiratory function. Ribavirin is potentially mutagenic, tumor-promoting, and gonadotoxic. Although anemia has not been reported with inhalation therapy, consider monitoring for anemia 1-2 weeks post-treatment. Pregnant healthcare workers may consider unnecessary occupational exposure; ribavirin has been detected in healthcare workers' urine. Healthcare professionals or family members who are pregnant (or may become pregnant) should be counseled about potential risks of exposure and counseled about risk reduction strategies.

Oral: Severe psychiatric events have occurred including depression and suicidal behavior during combination therapy. Avoid use in patients with a psychiatric history; discontinue if severe psychiatric symptoms occur. **[U.S. Boxed Warning]: Hemolytic anemia is a significant toxicity; usually occurring within 1-2 weeks.** Assess cardiac disease before initiation. Anemia may worsen underlying cardiac disease; use caution. If any deterioration in cardiovascular status occurs, discontinue therapy. Use caution in pulmonary disease; pulmonary symptoms have been associated with administration. Discontinue therapy in suspected/confirmed pancreatitis or if hepatic decompensation occurs. Use caution in patients with sarcoidosis (exacerbation reported).

Hemolytic anemia (hemoglobin <10 g/dL) was observed in up to 10% of treated patients in clinical trials when alfa interferons were combined with ribavirin; anemia occurred within 1-2 weeks of initiation of therapy.

Dosage Forms Capsule: 200 mg
Rebetol®, Ribasphere™: 200 mg
Powder for solution, inhalation [for aerosol administration]:
Virazole®: 6 g [reconstituted product provides 20 mg/mL]
Solution, oral:
Rebetol®: 40 mg/mL (100 mL) [contains sodium benzoate; bubble-gum flavor]
Tablet: 200 mg
Copegus®: 200 mg
Tablet [dose pack]:
RibaPak™: 400 mg (14s), 600 mg (14s)

Reference Range Cytotoxic at plasma levels >200 mcg/mL; a 3 mg/kg dose produced a peak plasma level of 1-2 mcg/mL

Overdosage/Treatment
Decontamination: Activated charcoal for oral ingestion
Enhancement of elimination: Hemodialysis is not useful
Test Interactions May cause transient elevation of serum iron level
Drug Interactions Antiretroviral (nucleoside): Concomitant use of ribavirin and nucleoside analogues may increase the risk of developing lactic acidosis (includes adefovir, didanosine, lamivudine, stavudine, zalcitabine, zidovudine). Concurrent use with didanosine has been noted to increase the risk of pancreatitis, peripheral neuropathy in addition to lactic acidosis. Suspend therapy if signs/symptoms of toxicity are present.
Interferons (alfa): Concurrent therapy may increase the risk of hemolytic anemia.
Lamivudine, stavudine: Antagonistic in vitro; use with caution (per manufacturer)
Zidovudine: Antagonistic in vitro; use with caution (per manufacturer). Concurrent therapy with ribavirin/interferon alfa-2a may cause increased risk of severe anemia and/or severe neutropenia.
Pregnancy Risk Factor X
Pregnancy Implications Produced significant embryocidal and/or teratogenic effects in all animal studies at ~0.01 times the maximum recommended daily human dose. Use is contraindicated in pregnancy. Negative pregnancy test is required before initiation and monthly thereafter. Avoid pregnancy in female patients and female partners of male patients during therapy by using two effective forms of contraception; continue contraceptive measures for at least 6 months after completion of therapy. If patient or female partner becomes pregnant during treatment, she should be counseled about potential risks of exposure. If pregnancy occurs during use or within 6 months after treatment, report to company (Copegus™: 800-526-6367; Rebetol®: 800-727-7064).
Lactation Excretion in breast milk unknown/not recommended
Nursing Implications Inhalation: Keep accurate I & O record; discard solutions placed in the SPAG-2 unit at least every 24 hours and before adding additional fluid; healthcare workers who are pregnant or who may become pregnant should be advised of the potential risks of exposure and counseled about risk reduction strategies including alternate job responsibilities; ribavirin may adsorb to contact lenses
Oral: Educate female patients about prevention of pregnancy and need for monthly pregnancy testing. Educate male patients about protection of female sexual partners from pregnancy.
Additional Information RSV season is usually December to April; viral shedding period for RSV is usually 3-8 days; surgical masks do not prevent inhalation
Food: Oral: High-fat meal increases the AUC and C_{max}

Rifabutin

CAS Number 72559-06-9
U.S. Brand Names Mycobutin®
Synonyms Ansamycin
Use Prevention of disseminated *Mycobacterium avium* complex (MAC) in patients with advanced HIV infection
Unlabeled/Investigational Use Utilized in multidrug regimens for treatment of MAC
Mechanism of Action Inhibits DNA-dependent RNA polymerase at the beta subunit which prevents chain initiation
Adverse Reactions
Cardiovascular: Chest pain, angina
Central nervous system: Fever, headache, seizures, confusion, insomnia
Dermatologic: **Rash**, skin erythema
Gastrointestinal: Abdominal pain, diarrhea, dyspepsia, nausea, vomiting, epigastric pain, anorexia, flatulence, eructation, loss of taste perception
Genitourinary: **Urine discoloration**
Hematologic: Thrombocytopenia, anemia, **leukopenia, neutropenia**
Hepatic: Elevated liver enzymes, jaundice
Neuromuscular & skeletal: Arthralgia, myalgia
Ocular: Anterior uveitis
Signs and Symptoms of Overdose Agranulocytosis, granulocytopenia, leukopenia, neutropenia, polyarthralgia (at doses >1 g/day)
Pharmacodynamics/Kinetics
Absorption: Readily, 53%
Distribution: V_d: 9.32 L/kg; distributes to body tissues including the lungs, liver, spleen, eyes, and kidneys
Protein binding: 85%
Metabolism: To active and inactive metabolites
Bioavailability: Absolute: HIV: 20%
Half-life elimination: Terminal: 45 hours (range: 16-69 hours)
Time to peak, serum: 2-4 hours
Excretion: Urine (10% as unchanged drug, 53% as metabolites); feces (10% as unchanged drug, 30% as metabolites)
Dosage
Oral:
Children >1 year:

Prophylaxis: 5 mg/kg daily; higher dosages have been used in limited trials

Treatment (unlabeled use): Patients not receiving NNRTIs or protease inhibitors:

Initial phase (2 weeks to 2 months): 10-20 mg/kg daily (maximum: 300 mg).

Second phase: 10-20 mg/kg daily (maximum: 300 mg) or twice weekly

Adults:

Prophylaxis: 300 mg once daily (alone or in combination with azithromycin)

Treatment (unlabeled use):

Patients not receiving NNRTIs or protease inhibitors:

Initial phase: 5 mg/kg daily (maximum: 300 mg)

Second phase: 5 mg/kg daily or twice weekly

Patients receiving nelfinavir, amprenavir, indinavir: Reduce dose to 150 mg/day; no change in dose if administered twice weekly

Dosage adjustment in renal impairment: $Cl_{cr} < 30$ mL/minute: Reduce dose by 50%

Monitoring Parameters Periodic liver function tests, CBC with differential, platelet count

Administration Should be administered on an empty stomach, but may be taken with meals to minimize nausea or vomiting.

Contraindications Hypersensitivity to rifabutin, any other rifamycins, or any component of the formulation; rifabutin is contraindicated in patients with a WBC $< 1000/mm^3$ or a platelet count $< 50,000/mm^3$

Warnings Rifabutin as a single agent must not be administered to patients with active tuberculosis since its use may lead to the development of tuberculosis that is resistant to both rifabutin and rifampin; rifabutin should be discontinued in patients with AST > 500 units/L or if total bilirubin is > 3 mg/dL. Use with caution in patients with liver impairment; modification of dosage should be considered in patients with renal impairment.

Dosage Forms Capsule: 150 mg

Reference Range Peak and trough plasma levels of a 600 mg dose twice daily is 900 ng/mL and 200 ng/mL, respectively

Overdosage/Treatment

Decontamination: Lavage within 1 hour, activated charcoal

Enhancement of elimination: Multiple dosing of activated charcoal may be effective; hemodialysis or charcoal hemoperfusion may be effective

Drug Interactions Substrate of CYP3A4 (major); Induces CYP3A4 (strong)

Alfentanil: Rifamycin derivatives may increase the metabolism, via CYP isoenzymes, of alfentanil.

Amiodarone: Rifamycin derivatives may increase the metabolism, via CYP isoenzymes, of amiodarone.

Angiotensin II receptor blockers (irbesartan, losartan): Rifamycin derivatives may increase the metabolism, via CYP isoenzymes, of angiotensin II receptor blockers.

Antiemetics (5-HT$_3$ antagonists): Rifamycin derivatives may increase the metabolism, via CYP isoenzymes, of antiemetics (5-HT$_3$ antagonists).

Antifungal agents (imidazole): Rifamycin derivatives may increase the metabolism, via CYP isoenzymes, of antifungal agents (imidazole). Antifungal agents (imidazole) may decrease the metabolism, via CYP isoenzymes, of rifabutin.

Aprepitant: Rifamycin derivatives may increase the metabolism, via CYP isoenzymes, of aprepitant.

Barbiturates: Rifamycin derivatives may increase the metabolism, via CYP isoenzymes, of barbiturates.

Benzodiazepines (metabolized by oxidation): Rifamycin derivatives may increase the metabolism, via CYP isoenzymes, of benzodiazepines (metabolized by oxidation).

Beta-blockers: Rifamycin derivatives may increase the metabolism, via CYP isoenzymes, of beta-blockers.

Buspirone: Rifamycin derivatives may increase the metabolism, via CYP isoenzymes, of buspirone.

Calcium channel blockers: Rifamycin derivatives may increase the metabolism, via CYP isoenzymes, of calcium channel blockers.

Clopidogrel: Rifamycin derivatives may enhance the therapeutic effect of clopidogrel.

Corticosteroids (systemic): Rifamycin derivatives may increase the metabolism, via CYP isoenzymes, of corticosteroids (systemic).

Cyclosporine: Rifamycin derivatives may increase the metabolism, via CYP isoenzymes, of cyclosporine.

CYP3A4 inducers: CYP3A4 inducers may decrease the levels/effects of rifabutin. Example inducers include aminoglutethimide, carbamazepine, nafcillin, nevirapine, phenobarbital, and phenytoin.

CYP3A4 substrates: Rifabutin may decrease the levels/effects of CYP3A4 substrates. Example substrates include benzodiazepines, calcium channel blockers, clarithromycin, cyclosporine, erythromycin, estrogens, mirtazapine, nateglinide, nefazodone, nevirapine, protease inhibitors, tacrolimus, and venlafaxine.

Dapsone: Rifamycin derivatives may increase the metabolism, via CYP isoenzymes, of dapsone.

Disopyramide: Rifamycin derivatives may increase the metabolism, via CYP isoenzymes, of disopyramide.

Estrogens (oral contraceptives): Rifamycin derivatives may decrease the serum concentration of oral contraceptive (estrogens); contraceptive failure is possible.

Fluconazole: Rifamycin derivatives may increase the metabolism, via CYP isoenzymes, of fluconazole. Fluconazole may decrease the metabolism, via CYP isoenzymes, of rifabutin.

Gefitinib: Rifamycin derivatives may increase the metabolism, via CYP isoenzymes, of gefitinib.

HMG-CoA reductase inhibitors: Rifamycin derivatives may increase the metabolism, via CYP isoenzymes, of HMG-CoA reductase inhibitors.

Isoniazid: Rifamycin derivatives may enhance the hepatotoxic effect of isoniazid; however, this is a frequently employed combination regimen.

Macrolide antibiotics: Macrolide antibiotics may decrease the metabolism, via CYP isoenzymes, of rifamycin derivatives.

Morphine: Rifamycin derivatives may decrease the serum concentration of morphine sulfate.

Phenytoin: Rifamycin derivatives may increase the metabolism, via CYP isoenzymes, of phenytoin.

Progestins (contraceptives): Rifamycin derivatives may decrease the serum concentration of contraceptives (progestins); contraceptive failure is possible.

Propafenone: Rifamycin derivatives may increase the metabolism, via CYP isoenzymes, of propafenone.

Protease inhibitors: Rifamycin derivatives may increase the metabolism, via CYP isoenzymes, of protease inhibitors. Protease inhibitors may decrease the metabolism, via CYP isoenzymes, of rifabutin. Dosage adjustments of both rifabutin and the protease inhibitors are necessary if used together.

Quinidine: Rifamycin derivatives may increase the metabolism, via CYP isoenzymes, of quinidine.

Repaglinide: Rifamycin derivatives may increase the metabolism, via CYP isoenzymes, of repaglinide.

Reverse transcriptase inhibitors (non-nucleoside): Rifamycin derivatives may increase the metabolism, via CYP isoenzymes, of reverse transcriptase inhibitors (non-nucleoside).

Tacrolimus: Rifamycin derivatives may increase the metabolism, via CYP isoenzymes, of tacrolimus.

Tamoxifen: Rifamycin derivatives may increase the metabolism, via CYP isoenzymes, of tamoxifen.

Terbinafine: Rifamycin derivatives may increase the metabolism of terbinafine.

Tocainide: Rifamycin derivatives may increase the metabolism, via CYP isoenzymes, of tocainide.

Tricyclic antidepressants: Rifamycin derivatives may increase the metabolism, via CYP isoenzymes, of tricyclic antidepressants.

Warfarin: Rifamycin derivatives may increase the metabolism, via CYP isoenzymes, of warfarin.

Zaleplon: Rifamycin derivatives may increase the metabolism, via CYP isoenzymes, of zaleplon.

Zolpidem: Rifamycin derivatives may increase the metabolism, via CYP isoenzymes, of zolpidem.

Pregnancy Risk Factor B

Lactation Excretion in breast milk unknown

Nursing Implications Administer with meals

Additional Information May discolor urine, saliva, and tears a brown-orange color; synergistic effects against *Mycobacterium avium* intracellular complex (MAC) reported when combined with clarithromycin or clofazimine; rifabutin-associated (over 1.2 g/day) uveitis usually resolves within 2 months

---

Rifampin

CAS Number 13292-46-1

U.S. Brand Names Rifadin®; Rimactane®

Synonyms Rifampicin

Use Management of active tuberculosis in combination with other agents; eliminate meningococci from asymptomatic carriers

Prophylaxis of *Haemophilus influenzae* type b infection; *Legionella* pneumonia; used in combination with other anti-infectives in the treatment of staphylococcal infections; treatment of *M. leprae* infections

Mechanism of Action Inhibits bacterial RNA synthesis by binding to the beta subunit of DNA-dependent RNA polymerase, blocking RNA transcription

Adverse Reactions

Cardiovascular: Chest pain, angina

Central nervous system: Drowsiness, fatigue, confusion, fever, headache, ataxia, electroencephalogram abnormalities, psychosis

Dermatologic: Rash, pruritus, Stevens-Johnson syndrome, cutaneous vasculitis, red discoloration

Gastrointestinal: Nausea, abdominal pain, vomiting, diarrhea, stomatitis, pseudomembranous colitis

Hematologic: Eosinophilia, blood dyscrasias (leukopenia, thrombocytopenia), agranulocytosis, granulocytopenia, red blood cell aplasia
Hepatic: Hepatitis, hepatic vasculitis
Local: Irritation at the I.V. site
Renal: Renal failure, glomerulosclerosis, renal vasculitis
Miscellaneous: Flu-like syndrome

Signs and Symptoms of Overdose Abdominal pain, cholelithiasis, colitis, coma, dyspnea, erythema multiforme, facial edema, feces discoloration (orange-red; red-brown), hepatitis, hyperglycemia, hypersensitivity, leukopenia, myopathy, nausea, nephritis, pemphigus, pruritus, pulmonary edema, red man syndrome, renal failure (acute), scleral discoloration (after 6-10 hours), skin discoloration, stomatitis, thrombocytopenia, toxic epidermal necrolysis, urine discoloration (brown; orange; orange-red; orange-yellow; red), vomiting, wheezing

Pharmacodynamics/Kinetics
Duration: ≤24 hours
Absorption: Oral: Well absorbed; food may delay or slightly reduce peak
Distribution: Highly lipophilic; crosses blood-brain barrier well
Relative diffusion from blood into CSF: Adequate with or without inflammation (exceeds usual MICs)
CSF: blood level ratio: Inflamed meninges: 25%
Protein binding: 80%
Metabolism: Hepatic; undergoes enterohepatic recirculation
Half-life elimination: 3-4 hours; prolonged with hepatic impairment; End-stage renal disease: 1.8-11 hours
Time to peak, serum: Oral: 2-4 hours
Excretion: Feces (60% to 65%) and urine (~30%) as unchanged drug

Dosage
Oral (I.V. infusion dose is the same as for the oral route):
Tuberculosis therapy: Note: A four-drug regimen (isoniazid, rifampin, pyrazinamide, and either streptomycin or ethambutol) is preferred for the initial, empiric treatment of TB. When the drug susceptibility results are available, the regimen should be altered as appropriate.
Infants and Children <12 years:
Daily therapy: 10-20 mg/kg/day usually as a single dose (maximum: 600 mg/day)
Directly observed therapy (DOT): Twice weekly: 10-20 mg/kg (maximum: 600 mg); 3 times/week: 10-20 mg/kg (maximum: 600 mg)
Adults:
Daily therapy: 10 mg/kg/day (maximum: 600 mg/day)
Directly observed therapy (DOT): Twice weekly: 10 mg/kg (maximum: 600 mg); 3 times/week: 10 mg/kg (maximum: 600 mg)
Latent tuberculosis infection (LTBI): As an alternative to isoniazid:
Children: 10-20 mg/kg/day (maximum: 600 mg/day)
Adults: 10 mg/kg/day (maximum: 600 mg/day) for 2 months. **Note:** Combination with pyrazinamide should not generally be offered (*MMWR*, Aug 8, 2003).
H. influenzae **prophylaxis** (unlabeled use):
Infants and Children: 20 mg/kg/day every 24 hours for 4 days, not to exceed 600 mg/dose
Adults: 600 mg every 24 hours for 4 days
Leprosy: Adults:
Multibacillary: 600 mg once monthly for 24 months in combination with ofloxacin and minocycline
Paucibacillary: 600 mg once monthly for 6 months in combination with dapsone
Single lesion: 600 mg as a single dose in combination with ofloxacin 400 mg and minocycline 100 mg
Meningococcal meningitis prophylaxis:
Infants <1 month: 10 mg/kg/day in divided doses every 12 hours for 2 days
Infants ≥1 month and Children: 20 mg/kg/day in divided doses every 12 hours for 2 days
Adults: 600 mg every 12 hours for 2 days
Nasal carriers of *Staphylococcus aureus* (unlabeled use):
Children: 15 mg/kg/day divided every 12 hours for 5-10 days in combination with other antibiotics
Adults: 600 mg/day for 5-10 days in combination with other antibiotics
Synergy for *Staphylococcus aureus* **infections** (unlabeled use): Adults: 300-600 mg twice daily with other antibiotics
Dosing adjustment in hepatic impairment: Dose reductions may be necessary to reduce hepatotoxicity
Hemodialysis or peritoneal dialysis: Plasma rifampin concentrations are not significantly affected by hemodialysis or peritoneal dialysis.

Stability Reconstituted I.V. solution is stable for 24 hours at room temperature; rifampin oral suspension can be compounded with simple syrup or wild cherry syrup at a concentration of 10 mg/mL; the suspension is stable for 4 weeks at room temperature or in a refrigerator when stored in a glass amber prescription bottle

Monitoring Parameters Periodic (baseline and every 2-4 weeks during therapy) monitoring of liver function (AST, ALT, bilirubin), CBC; hepatic status and mental status, sputum culture, chest x-ray 2-3 months into treatment

Administration I.V.: Administer I.V. preparation once daily by slow I.V. infusion over 30 minutes to 3 hours at a final concentration not to exceed 6 mg/mL.
Oral: Administer on an empty stomach (ie, 1 hour prior to, or 2 hours after meals or antacids) to increase total absorption. The compounded oral suspension must be shaken well before using. May mix contents of capsule with applesauce or jelly.

Contraindications Hypersensitivity to rifampin, any rifamycins, or any component of the formulation; concurrent use of amprenavir, saquinavir/ritonavir (possibly other protease inhibitors)

Warnings
Use with caution and modify dosage in patients with liver impairment; observe for hyperbilirubinemia; discontinue therapy if this in conjunction with clinical symptoms or any signs of significant hepatocellular damage develop; since rifampin has enzyme-inducing properties, porphyria exacerbation is possible; use with caution in patients with porphyria; do not use for meningococcal disease, only for short-term treatment of asymptomatic carrier states. Use with caution in patients receiving concurrent medications associated with hepatotoxicity (particularly with pyrazinamide), or in patients with a history of alcoholism (even if ethanol consumption is discontinued during therapy).
Monitor for compliance and effects including hypersensitivity, thrombocytopenia in patients on intermittent therapy; urine, feces, saliva, sweat, tears, and CSF may be discolored to red/orange; do not administer I.V. form via I.M. or SubQ routes; restart infusion at another site if extravasation occurs; remove soft contact lenses during therapy since permanent staining may occur; regimens of 600 mg once or twice weekly have been associated with a high incidence of adverse reactions including a flu-like syndrome.

Dosage Forms
Capsule: 150 mg, 300 mg
Injection, powder for reconstitution: 600 mg

Overdosage/Treatment
Decontamination: Immediate administration of activated charcoal inhibits absorption by 90%; lavage (within 1 hour) useful in early ingestions; activated charcoal may be of value
Supportive therapy: Mainly supportive and symptomatic treatment; overdose is rare and experience is limited; monitor hepatic and renal function
Enhancement of elimination: Multiple dosing of activated charcoal may be effective due to enterohepatic circulation

Test Interactions ↑ bilirubin (S); positive Coombs' [direct]; rifampicin can cause false-positive urine assay of opiates by kinetic interaction of microparticles in solution (KIMS) method up to a concentration of 0.9 mcg/mL

Drug Interactions Induces CYP1A2 (strong), 2A6 (strong), 2B6 (strong), 2C8 (strong), 2C9 (strong), 2C19 (strong), 3A4 (strong)
Acetaminophen: Rifampin may increase the metabolism of acetaminophen.
Alfentanil: Rifamycin derivatives may increase the metabolism, via CYP isoenzymes, of alfentanil.
Amiodarone: Rifamycin derivatives may increase the metabolism, via CYP isoenzymes, of amiodarone
Angiotensin II receptor blockers (irbesartan, losartan): Rifamycin derivatives may increase the metabolism, via CYP isoenzymes, of angiotensin II receptor blockers.
Antiemetics (5-HT$_3$ antagonists): Rifamycin derivatives may increase the metabolism, via CYP isoenzymes, of antiemetics (5-HT$_3$ antagonists).
Antifungal Agents (imidazole): Rifamycin derivatives may increase the metabolism, via CYP isoenzymes, of antifungal agents (imidazole).
Aprepitant: Rifamycin derivatives may increase the metabolism, via CYP isoenzymes, of aprepitant.
Barbiturates: Rifamycin derivatives may increase the metabolism, via CYP isoenzymes, of barbiturates.
Benzodiazepines (metabolized by oxidation): Rifamycin derivatives may increase the metabolism, via CYP isoenzymes, of benzodiazepines (metabolized by oxidation).
Beta-blockers: Rifamycin derivatives may increase the metabolism, via CYP isoenzymes, of beta-blockers.
Buspirone: Rifamycin derivatives may increase the metabolism, via CYP isoenzymes, of buspirone.
Calcium channel blockers: Rifamycin derivatives may increase the metabolism, via CYP isoenzymes, of calcium channel blockers.
Chloramphenicol: Rifampin may increase the metabolism, via CYP isoenzymes, of chloramphenicol.
Clopidogrel: Rifamycin derivatives may enhance the therapeutic effect of Clopidogrel.
Corticosteroids (systemic): Rifamycin derivatives may increase the metabolism, via CYP isoenzymes, of corticosteroids (systemic).
Cyclosporine: Rifamycin derivatives may increase the metabolism, via CYP isoenzymes, of cyclosporine.
CYP1A2 substrates: Rifampin may decrease the levels/effects of CYP1A2 substrates. Example substrates include aminophylline, estrogens, fluvoxamine, mirtazapine, ropinirole, and theophylline.

CYP2A6 substrates: Rifampin may decrease the levels/effects of CYP2A6 substrates (eg, ifosfamide).

CYP2B6 substrates: Rifampin may decrease the levels/effects of CYP2B6 substrates. Example substrates include bupropion, efavirenz, promethazine, selegiline, and sertraline.

CYP2C8 substrates: Rifampin may decrease the levels/effects of CYP2C8 substrates. Example substrates include amiodarone, paclitaxel, pioglitazone, repaglinide, and rosiglitazone.

CYP2C9 substrates: Rifampin may decrease the levels/effects of CYP2C9 substrates. Example substrates include bosentan, celecoxib, dapsone, fluoxetine, glimepiride, glipizide, losartan, montelukast, nateglinide, paclitaxel, phenytoin, sulfonamides, trimethoprim, warfarin, and zafirlukast.

CYP2C19 substrates: Rifampin may decrease the levels/effects of CYP2C19 substrates. Example substrates include citalopram, diazepam, methsuximide, phenytoin, propranolol, proton pump inhibitors, sertraline, and voriconazole.

CYP3A4 substrates: Rifampin may decrease the levels/effects of CYP3A4 substrates. Example substrates include benzodiazepines, calcium channel blockers, clarithromycin, cyclosporine, erythromycin, estrogens, mirtazapine, nateglinide, nefazodone, nevirapine, protease inhibitors, tacrolimus, and venlafaxine.

Dapsone: Rifamycin derivatives may increase the metabolism, via CYP isoenzymes, of dapsone.

Disopyramide: Rifamycin derivatives may increase the metabolism, via CYP isoenzymes, of disopyramide.

Estrogens (oral contraceptives): Rifamycin derivatives may decrease the serum concentration of oral contraceptive (estrogens); contraceptive failure is possible.

Fexofenadine: Rifampin may decrease the serum concentration of fexofenadine.

Fluconazole: Rifamycin derivatives may increase the metabolism, via CYP isoenzymes, of fluconazole.

Fusidic Acid: Rifampin may decrease the excretion of fusidic acid.

Gefitinib: Rifamycin derivatives may increase the metabolism, via CYP isoenzymes, of gefitinib.

HMG-CoA reductase inhibitors: Rifamycin derivatives may increase the metabolism, via CYP isoenzymes, of HMG-CoA reductase inhibitors.

Isoniazid: Rifamycin derivatives may enhance the hepatotoxic effect of isoniazid; however, this is a frequently employed combination regimen.

Macrolide antibiotics: Macrolide antibiotics may decrease the metabolism, via CYP isoenzymes, of rifamycin derivatives.

Methadone: Rifamycin derivatives may increase the metabolism, via CYP isoenzymes, of methadone.

Morphine: Rifamycin derivatives may decrease the serum concentration of morphine sulfate.

Phenytoin: Rifamycin derivatives may increase the metabolism, via CYP isoenzymes, of phenytoin.

Progestins (contraceptives): Rifamycin derivatives may decrease the serum concentration of contraceptive (progestins); contraceptive failure is possible.

Propafenone: Rifamycin derivatives may increase the metabolism, via CYP isoenzymes, of propafenone.

Protease inhibitors: Rifamycin derivatives may increase the metabolism, via CYP isoenzymes, of protease inhibitors. Concurrent use with saquinavir/ritonavir increases risk of hepatotoxicity. Rifampin administration should be avoided.

Pyrazinamide: Pyrazinamide may enhance the hepatotoxic effect of rifampin.

Quinidine: Rifamycin derivatives may increase the metabolism, via CYP isoenzymes, of quinidine.

Repaglinide: Rifamycin derivatives may increase the metabolism, via CYP isoenzymes, of repaglinide.

Reverse transcriptase inhibitors (non-nucleoside): Rifamycin derivatives may increase the metabolism, via CYP isoenzymes, of reverse transcriptase inhibitors (non-nucleoside).

Sulfonylureas: Rifampin may increase the metabolism, via CYP isoenzymes, of sulfonylureas.

Tacrolimus: Rifamycin derivatives may increase the metabolism, via CYP isoenzymes, of tacrolimus.

Tamoxifen: Rifamycin derivatives may increase the metabolism, via CYP isoenzymes, of tamoxifen.

Terbinafine: Rifamycin derivatives may increase the metabolism of terbinafine.

Tocainide: Rifamycin derivatives may increase the metabolism, via CYP isoenzymes, of tocainide.

Tricyclic antidepressants: Rifamycin derivatives may increase the metabolism, via CYP isoenzymes, of tricyclic antidepressants.

Warfarin: Rifamycin derivatives may increase the metabolism, via CYP isoenzymes, of warfarin.

Zaleplon: Rifamycin derivatives may increase the metabolism, via CYP isoenzymes, of zaleplon.

Zidovudine: Rifamycin derivatives may increase the metabolism, via CYP isoenzymes, of zidovudine.

Zolpidem: Rifamycin derivatives may increase the metabolism, via CYP isoenzymes, of zolpidem.

Pregnancy Risk Factor C

Pregnancy Implications Teratogenic rate is 4.4% (hydro-cephalus, congenital limb changes)

Lactation Enters breast milk/not recommended (AAP rates "compatible")

Nursing Implications Evaluate hepatic status and mental status; give on an empty stomach (ie, 1 hour prior to, or 2 hours after meals) to increase total absorption

Additional Information Lethal dose: 14 g. Normally used with other anti-TB drugs since resistant strains occur rapidly

Specific References

Orisakwe OE, Afonne OJ, Agbasi PU, et al, "Urinary Excretion of Rifampicin in the Presence of Ciprofloxacin," *Am J Ther*, 2004, 11(3):171-4.

Orisakwe OE, Agbasi PU, Ofoefule SI, et al, "Effect of Pefloxacin on the Urinary Excretion of Rifampicin," *Am J Ther*, 2004, 11(1):13-6.

Rilmenidine

CAS Number 54187-04-1

Unlabeled/Investigational Use Hypertension

Mechanism of Action Oxazoline derivative which has alpha$_2$-adrenergic receptor antagonist and an imidazoline receptor agonist with less sedation than clonidine

Adverse Reactions

Cardiovascular: Hypotension, shock

Respiratory: Bronchospasm

Toxicodynamics/Kinetics

Distribution: V_d: 5 L/kg

Protein binding: <10%

Half-life: 8.31 hours

Time to peak plasma concentration: 2 hours

Elimination: Renal

Dosage Oral: 1-2 mg/day in divided doses

Overdosage/Treatment

Decontamination: Lavage (within 1 hour)/activated charcoal

Supportive therapy: For hypotension, give I.V. saline; vasopressors may be necessary. Bronchospasm can be treated with beta-adrenergic agonist agents

Enhancement of elimination: Multiple dosing of activated charcoal may be effective

Test Interactions May decrease plasma norepinephrine and epinephrine

Riluzole

CAS Number 1744-22-5

U.S. Brand Names Rilutek®

Synonyms 2-Amino-6-Trifluoromethoxy-benzothiazole; RP-54274

Use Treatment of amyotrophic lateral sclerosis (ALS); riluzole can extend survival or time to tracheostomy

Mechanism of Action Glutamate neuroreceptor antagonist which promotes GABA activity

Adverse Reactions

Central nervous system: CNS depression, depression, vertigo

Gastrointestinal: **Nausea, abdominal pain, constipation**, pancreatitis

Hematologic: Neutropenia (within first 2 months of therapy), methemoglobinemia

Hepatic: **ALT (SGPT) elevations**, elevated liver function tests, hepatitis

Neuromuscular & skeletal: Myalgia, worsening of weakness spasticity or stiffness

Pharmacodynamics/Kinetics

Absorption: 90%; high-fat meal decreases AUC by 20% and peak blood levels by 45%

Protein binding, plasma: 96%, primarily to albumin and lipoproteins

Metabolism: Extensively hepatic to six major and a number of minor metabolites via CYP1A2 dependent hydroxylation and glucuronidation

Bioavailability: Oral: Absolute: 60%

Half-life elimination: 12 hours

Excretion: Urine (90%; 85% as metabolites, 2% as unchanged drug) and feces (5%) within 7 days

Dosage

Adults: Oral: 50 mg every 12 hours; no increased benefit can be expected from higher daily doses, but adverse events are increased

Dosage adjustment in smoking: Cigarette smoking is known to induce CYP1A2; patients who smoke cigarettes would be expected to eliminate riluzole faster. There is no information, however, on the effect of, or need for, dosage adjustment in these patients.

Dosage adjustment in special populations: Females and Japanese patients may possess a lower metabolic capacity to eliminate riluzole compared with male and Caucasian subjects, respectively

Dosage adjustment in renal impairment: Use with caution in patients with concomitant renal insufficiency

Dosage adjustment in hepatic impairment: Use with caution in patients with current evidence or history of abnormal liver function indicated by significant abnormalities in serum transaminase, bilirubin or GGT levels. Baseline elevations of several LFTs (especially elevated bilirubin) should preclude use of riluzole.

Monitoring Parameters Monitor serum aminotransferases including ALT levels before and during therapy. Evaluate serum ALT levels every month during the first 3 months of therapy, every 3 months during the remainder of the first year and periodically thereafter. Evaluate ALT levels more frequently in patients who develop elevations. Maximum increases in serum ALT usually occurred within 3 months after the start of therapy and were usually transient when <5 times ULN (upper limits of normal).

In trials, if ALT levels were <5 times ULN, treatment continued and ALT levels usually returned to below 2 times ULN within 2-6 months. Treatment in studies was discontinued, however, if ALT levels exceed 5 times ULN, so that there is no experience with continued treatment of ALS patients once ALT values exceed 5 times ULN.

If a decision is made to continue treatment in patients when the ALT exceeds 5 times ULN, frequent monitoring (at least weekly) of complete liver function is recommended. Discontinue treatment if ALT exceeds 10 times ULN or if clinical jaundice develops.

Administration Administer at the same time each day, 1 hour before or 2 hours after a meal.

Contraindications Severe hypersensitivity reactions to riluzole or any component of the formulation

Warnings Among 4000 patients given riluzole for ALS, there were 3 cases of marked neutropenia (ANC <500/mm^3), all seen within the first 2 months of treatment. Use with caution in patients with concomitant renal insufficiency. Use with caution in patients with current evidence or history of abnormal liver function; do not administer if baseline liver function tests are elevated. The elderly, female, or Japanese patients may have decreased clearance of riluzole; use with caution. May cause dizziness or somnolence; caution should be used performing tasks which require alertness (operating machinery or driving).

Dosage Forms Tablet: 50 mg

Overdosage/Treatment

Decontamination: Lavage (within 1 hour)/activated charcoal

Supportive therapy: Methemoglobin which is symptomatic or a methemoglobin level >30% should be treated with methylene blue (50 mg I.V. in adults).

Antidote(s)
- Methylene Blue [ANTIDOTE]

Drug Interactions **Substrate** of CYP1A2 (major)

CYP1A2 inducers: May decrease the levels/effects of riluzole. Example inducers include aminoglutethimide, carbamazepine, phenobarbital, and rifampin.

CYP1A2 inhibitors: May increase the levels/effects of riluzole. Example inhibitors include amiodarone, ciprofloxacin, fluvoxamine, ketoconazole, norfloxacin, ofloxacin, and rofecoxib.

Pregnancy Risk Factor C

Pregnancy Implications Impaired fertility, decreased implantation, increased intrauterine death, and adverse effects on offspring growth and viability were observed in animal studies. There are no adequate or well-controlled studies in pregnant women.

Lactation Excretion in breast milk unknown/not recommended

Additional Information May be obtained through Rhone-Poulenc Rorer Inc (Collegeville, PA) for compassionate use (through treatment IND process) by calling 800-727-6737 for treatment of amyotrophic lateral sclerosis; may be more effective for amyotrophic lateral sclerosis of bulbar onset; in animal models, riluzole was a potent inhibitor of seizures induced by ouabain

Specific References

Woolf A, Carstairs SD, Tanen DA, "Riluzole-Induced Methemoglobinemia," *Ann Emerg Med*, 2004, 43(2):294-5.

Rimantadine

CAS Number 13392-28-4; 1501-84-4

U.S. Brand Names Flumadine®

Synonyms Rimantadine Hydrochloride

Use Prophylaxis (adults and children) and treatment (adults) of influenza A viral infection (not influenza B)

Mechanism of Action Similar to amantadine; inhibits viral RNA and protein synthesis

Adverse Reactions

Cardiovascular: Hypotension (orthostatic), edema

Central nervous system: Dizziness, confusion, headache, insomnia, difficulty in concentrating, anxiety, restlessness, irritability, hallucinations

Gastrointestinal: Nausea, vomiting, xerostomia

Genitourinary: Urinary retention

Signs and Symptoms of Overdose Convulsions (especially in the elderly), sedation

Pharmacodynamics/Kinetics

Onset of action: Antiviral activity: No data exist establishing a correlation between plasma concentration and antiviral effect

Absorption: Tablet and syrup formulations are equally absorbed

Metabolism: Extensively hepatic

Half-life elimination: 25.4 hours; prolonged in elderly

Time to peak: 6 hours

Excretion: Urine (<25% as unchanged drug)

Clearance: Hemodialysis does not contribute to clearance

Dosage Oral:

Prophylaxis:

Children <10 years: 5 mg/kg give once daily

Children >10 years and Adults: 100 mg twice/day

Treatment: Adults: 100 mg twice/day

In patients with severe hepatic dysfunction or renal function, and in elderly nursing home patients, the dosage should be reduced to 100 mg/day

Monitoring Parameters Monitor for CNS or GI effects in elderly or patients with renal or hepatic impairment

Administration Initiation of rimantadine within 48 hours of the onset of influenza A illness halves the duration of illness and significantly reduces the duration of viral shedding and increased peripheral airways resistance; continue therapy for 5-7 days after symptoms begin

Contraindications Hypersensitivity to drugs of the adamantine class, including rimantadine and amantadine, or any component of the formulation

Warnings Use with caution in patients with renal and hepatic dysfunction; avoid use, if possible, in patients with recurrent and eczematoid dermatitis, uncontrolled psychosis, or severe psychoneurosis. An increase in seizure incidence may occur in patients with seizure disorders; discontinue drug if seizures occur; resistance may develop during treatment; viruses exhibit cross-resistance between amantadine and rimantadine. Due to increased resistance, in June 2006, the CDC recommended that rimantadine no longer be used for the treatment or prophylaxis of influenza A in the United States until susceptibility has been re-established.

Dosage Forms Syrup, as hydrochloride:

Flumadine®: 50 mg/5 mL (240 mL) [raspberry flavor]

Tablet, as hydrochloride: 100 mg

Flumadine®: 100 mg

Reference Range Peak serum levels: 240-320 ng/mL after a 200 mg dose

Overdosage/Treatment

Decontamination: Lavage (within 1 hour)/activated charcoal

Enhancement of elimination: Multiple dosing of activated charcoal may not be useful

Drug Interactions Acetaminophen: Small reduction in AUC and peak concentration of rimantadine.

Aspirin: Peak plasma and AUC concentrations of rimantadine are slightly reduced.

Cimetidine: Rimantadine clearance is decreased (~18%).

Pregnancy Risk Factor C

Pregnancy Implications Embryotoxic in high dose rat studies.

Lactation Excretion in breast milk unknown/ not recommended

Specific References

Singer C, Papapetropoulos S, Gonzalez MA, et al, "Rimantadine in Parkinson's Disease Patients Experiencing Peripheral Adverse Effects from Amantadine: Report of a Case Series," *Mov Disord*, 2005, 20(7):873-7.

Risedronate

CAS Number 105462-24-6; 115436-72-1

U.S. Brand Names Actonel®

Synonyms Risedronate Sodium

Use Paget's disease of the bone; treatment and prevention of glucocorticoid-induced osteoporosis; treatment and prevention of osteoporosis in postmenopausal women

Mechanism of Action A potent bisphosphonate which inhibits bone resorption via actions on osteoclasts or on osteoclast precursors; decreases the rate of bone resorption direction, leading to an indirect decrease in bone formation

Adverse Reactions

Cardiovascular: Chest pain

Central nervous system: Headache, dizziness

Dermatological: Rash

Gastrointestinal: Abdominal pain, diarrhea, belching, colitis, constipation, nausea

Neuromuscular & skeletal: Arthralgia, bone pain, leg cramps, myasthenia

Respiratory: Bronchitis, rales/rhinitis

Pharmacodynamics/Kinetics

Onset of action: May require weeks

Absorption: Rapid

Distribution: V$_d$: 6.3 L/kg

Protein binding: ~24%

Metabolism: None
Bioavailability: Poor, ~0.54% to 0.75%
Half-life elimination: Initial: 1.5 hours; Terminal: 480 hours
Excretion: Urine (up to 85%); feces (as unabsorbed drug)

Dosage
Oral:
Adults (patients should receive supplemental calcium and vitamin D if dietary intake is inadequate):
Paget's disease of bone: 30 mg once daily for 2 months
Treatment and prevention of postmenopausal osteoporosis or gluco-corticoid-induced osteoporosis: 5 mg once daily (efficacy for use longer than 1 year has not been established)
Elderly: No dosage adjustment is necessary
Dosage adjustment in renal impairment: Cl_{cr} <30 mL/minute: **Not** recommended

Monitoring Parameters Alkaline phosphatase should be periodically measured; serum calcium, phosphorus, and possibly potassium due to its drug class; use of absorptiometry may assist in noting benefit in osteoporosis; monitor pain and fracture rate

Administration It is imperative to administer risedronate 30-60 minutes before the patient takes any food, drink, or other medications orally to avoid interference with absorption. The patient should take alendronate on an empty stomach with a full glass (8 oz) of **plain water** (not mineral water) and avoid lying down for 30 minutes after swallowing the tablet to help delivery to stomach.

Contraindications Hypersensitivity to risedronate, bisphosphonates, or any component of the formulation; hypocalcemia; abnormalities of the esophagus which delay esophageal emptying such as stricture or achalasia; inability to stand or sit upright for at least 30 minutes; severe renal impairment (Cl_{cr} <30 mL/minute)

Warnings
Bisphosphonates may cause upper gastrointestinal disorders such as dysphagia, esophagitis, esophageal ulcer, and gastric ulcer. Use caution in patients with renal impairment. Hypocalcemia must be corrected before therapy initiation with risedronate. Ensure adequate calcium and vitamin D intake, especially for patients with Paget's disease in whom the pretreatment rate of bone turnover may be greatly elevated.

Bisphosphonate therapy has been associated with osteonecrosis, primarily of the jaw; this has been observed mostly in cancer patients, but also in patients with postmenopausal osteoporosis and other diagnoses. There are no data addressing whether discontinuation of therapy reduces the risk of developing osteonecrosis. However, as a precautionary measure, dental exams and preventative dentistry should be performed prior to placing patients with risk factors (eg, chemotherapy, corticosteroids, poor oral hygiene) on chronic bisphosphonate therapy. Invasive dental procedures should be avoided during treatment.

Infrequently, severe (and occasionally debilitating) bone, joint, and/or muscle pain have been reported during bisphosphonate treatment. The onset of pain ranged from a single day to several months. Symptoms usually resolve upon discontinuation. Some patients experienced recurrence when rechallenged with same drug or another bisphosphonate; avoid use in patients with a history of these symptoms in association with bisphosphonate therapy.

Safety and efficacy in pediatric patients have not been established.

Dosage Forms Tablet, as sodium:
Actonel®: 5 mg, 30 mg, 35 mg

Reference Range Calcium (total): Adults: 9.0-11.0 mg/dL (2.05-2.54 mM/L), may slightly decrease with aging; phosphorus: 2.5-4.5 mg/dL (0.81-1.45 mM/L)

Overdosage/Treatment
Decontamination: Activated charcoal
Supportive therapy: Monitor serum calcium and phosphorous; give I.V. hydration

Drug Interactions Aminoglycosides: May lower serum calcium levels with prolonged administration. Concomitant use may have an additive hypocalcemic effect.
Antacids: May decrease the absorption of bisphosphonate derivatives; should be administered at a different time of the day. Antacids containing aluminum, calcium, or magnesium are of specific concern.
Calcium salts: May decrease the absorption of bisphosphonate derivatives. Separate oral dosing in order to minimize risk of interaction.
Iron salts: May decrease the absorption of bisphosphonate derivatives. Only oral iron salts and oral bisphosphonates are of concern.
Magnesium salts: May decrease the absorption of bisphosphonate derivatives. Only oral magnesium salts and oral bisphosphonates are of concern.
Nonsteroidal anti-inflammatory drugs (NSAIDs): May enhance the gastrointestinal adverse/toxic effects (increased incidence of GI ulcers) of bisphosphonate derivatives.
Phosphate supplements: Bisphosphonate derivatives may enhance the hypocalcemic effect of phosphate supplements.

Pregnancy Risk Factor C
Pregnancy Implications Teratogenic and nonteratogenic embryo/fetal effects have been reported in animal studies. There are no adequate and well-controlled studies in pregnant women. Bisphosphonates are incorporated into the bone matrix and gradually released over time. Theoretically, there may be a risk of fetal harm when pregnancy follows the completion of therapy. Based on limited case reports with pamidronate, serum calcium levels in the newborn may be altered if administered during pregnancy.
Lactation Excretion in breast milk unknown/not recommended
Specific References
French AE, Kaplan N, Lishner M, et al, "Taking Bisphosphonates During Pregnancy," *Can Fam Physician*, 2003, 49:1281-2.

Risperidone

Related Information
● Antipsychotic Agents
CAS Number 106266-06-2
U.S. Brand Names Risperdal® Consta™; Risperdal® M-Tab®; Risperdal®
Synonyms Risperdal M-Tab®
Impairment Potential Yes
Use Treatment of schizophrenia; treatment of acute mania or mixed episodes associated with bipolar I disorder (as monotherapy or in combination with lithium or valproate)
Unlabeled/Investigational Use Behavioral symptoms associated with dementia in elderly; treatment of Tourette's disorder; treatment of pervasive developmental disorder and autism in children and adolescents
Mechanism of Action Risperidone is a benzisoxazole derivative, mixed serotonin-dopamine antagonist; binds to $5-HT_2$-receptors in the CNS and in the periphery with a very high affinity; binds to dopamine-D_2 receptors with less affinity. The binding affinity to the dopamine-D_2 receptor is 20 times lower than the $5-HT_2$ affinity. The addition of serotonin antagonism to dopamine antagonism (classic neuroleptic mechanism) is thought to improve negative symptoms of psychoses and reduce the incidence of extrapyramidal side effects. Alpha$_1$, alpha$_2$ adrenergic, and histaminergic receptors are also antagonized with high affinity. Risperidone has low to moderate affinity for $5-HT_{1C}$, $5-HT_{1D}$, and $5-HT_{1A}$ receptors, weak affinity for D_1 and no affinity for muscarinics or beta$_1$ and beta$_2$ receptors

Adverse Reactions
Frequency not defined: Gastrointestinal: Dysphagia, esophageal dysmotility
Cardiovascular: Hypotension (especially orthostatic), tachycardia
Central nervous system: **Insomnia, agitation, anxiety, headache, extrapyramidal symptoms (dose dependent), dizziness (I.M. injection)**, sedation, dizziness (oral formulation), restlessness, dystonic reactions, pseudoparkinsonism, tardive dyskinesia, neuroleptic malignant syndrome, altered central temperature regulation, nervousness, fatigue, somnolence, hallucination, tremor, hypoesthesia, akathisia, stroke
Dermatologic: Photosensitivity (rare), rash, dry skin, seborrhea, acne
Endocrine & metabolic: Amenorrhea, galactorrhea, gynecomastia, sexual dysfunction, diabetes mellitus, hyperglycemia
Gastrointestinal: **Weight gain**, constipation, GI upset, xerostomia, dyspepsia, vomiting, abdominal pain, nausea, anorexia, diarrhea, weight changes
Genitourinary: Polyuria
Neuromuscular & skeletal: Myalgia
Ocular: Abnormal vision
Respiratory: **Rhinitis (I.M. injection)**
Neuromuscular & skeletal: Myalgia
Ocular: Abnormal vision
Respiratory: Rhinitis (oral formulation), coughing, sinusitis, pharyngitis, dyspnea
Miscellaneous: Anaphylactic reaction
Signs and Symptoms of Overdose Dystonia, ejaculatory disturbances, enuresis, hallucinations, hypotension, mania, muscle spasms, neuroleptic malignant syndrome, palpitations, prolonged QT interval, tachycardia, hyponatremia
Pharmacodynamics/Kinetics
Absorption:
Oral: Rapid and well absorbed; food does not affect rate or extent
Injection: <1% absorbed initially; main release occurs at ~3 weeks and is maintained from 4-6 weeks
Distribution: V_d: 1-2 L/kg
Protein binding, plasma: Risperidone 90%; 9-hydroxyrisperidone: 77%
Metabolism: Extensively hepatic via CYP2D6 to 9-hydroxyrisperidone (similar pharmacological activity as risperidone); *N*-dealkylation is a second minor pathway
Bioavailability: Solution: 70%; Tablet: 66%; orally-disintegrating tablets and oral solution are bioequivalent to tablets
Half-life elimination: Active moiety (risperidone and its active metabolite 9-hydroxyrisperidone)

Oral: 20 hours (mean)

Extensive metabolizers: Risperidone: 3 hours; 9-hydroxyrisperidone: 21 hours

Poor metabolizers: Risperidone: 20 hours; 9-hydroxyrisperidone: 30 hours

Injection: 3-6 days; related to microsphere erosion and subsequent absorption of risperidone

Time to peak, plasma: Oral: Risperidone: Within 1 hour; 9-hydroxyrisperidone: Extensive metabolizers: 3 hours; Poor metabolizers: 17 hours

Excretion: Urine (70%); feces (15%)

Dosage

Oral:

Children and Adolescents:

Pervasive developmental disorder (unlabeled use): Initial: 0.25 mg twice daily; titrate up 0.25 mg/day every 5-7 days; optimal dose range: 0.75-3 mg/day

Autism (unlabeled use): Initial: 0.25 mg at bedtime; titrate to 1 mg/day (0.1 mg/kg/day)

Schizophrenia (unlabeled use): Initial: 0.5 mg once or twice daily; titrate as necessary up to 2-6 mg/day

Bipolar disorder (unlabeled use): Initial: 0.5 mg; titrate to 0.5-3 mg/day

Tourette's disorder (unlabeled use): Initial: 0.5 mg; titrate to 2-4 mg/day

Adults:

Schizophrenia:

Initial: 1 mg twice daily; may be increased by 2 mg/day to a target dose of 6 mg/day; usual range: 4-8 mg/day; may be given as a single daily dose once maintenance dose is achieved; daily dosages >6 mg do not appear to confer any additional benefit, and the incidence of extrapyramidal symptoms is higher than with lower doses. Further dose adjustments should be made in increments/decrements of 1-2 mg/day on a weekly basis. Dose range studied in clinical trials: 4-16 mg/day.

Maintenance: Target dose: 4 mg once daily (range 2-8 mg/day)

Bipolar mania:

Initial: 2-3 mg once daily; if needed, adjust dose by 1 mg/day in intervals $\geq$24 hours; dosing range: 1-6 mg/day

Maintenance: No dosing recommendation available for treatment >3 weeks duration.

Elderly: A starting dose of 0.5 mg twice daily, and titration should progress slowly in increments of no more than 0.5 mg twice daily; increases to dosages >1.5 mg twice daily should occur at intervals of $\geq$1 week.

Additional monitoring of renal function and orthostatic blood pressure may be warranted. If once-a-day dosing in the elderly or debilitated patient is considered, a twice daily regimen should be used to titrate to the target dose, and this dose should be maintained for 2-3 days prior to attempts to switch to a once-daily regimen.

I.M.: Adults: Schizophrenia (Risperdal® Consta™): 25 mg every 2 weeks; some patients may benefit from larger doses; maximum dose not to exceed 50 mg every 2 weeks. Dosage adjustments should not be made more frequently than every 4 weeks.

Note: Oral risperidone (or other antipsychotic) should be administered with the initial injection of Risperdal® Consta™ and continued for 3 weeks (then discontinued) to maintain adequate therapeutic plasma concentrations prior to main release phase of risperidone from injection site. When switching from depot administration to a short-acting formulation, administer short-acting agent in place of the next regularly-scheduled depot injection.

Dosing adjustment in renal impairment: Oral: Starting dose of 0.5 mg twice daily; clearance of the active moiety is decreased by 60% in patients with moderate to severe renal disease compared to healthy subjects.

Dosing adjustment in hepatic impairment: Oral: Starting dose of 0.5 mg twice daily; the mean free fraction of risperidone in plasma was increased by 35% compared to healthy subjects.

Monitoring Parameters Vital signs; lipid profile, fasting blood glucose/Hgb A_{1c}; BMI; mental status, abnormal involuntary movement scale (AIMS), extrapyramidal symptoms; orthostatic blood pressure changes for 3-5 days after starting or increasing dose

Administration Oral: Oral solution can be mixed with water, coffee, orange juice, or low-fat milk, but is **not compatible** with cola or tea. May be administered with or without food.

Risperdal® M-Tabs™ should not be removed from blister pack until administered. Using dry hands, place immediately on tongue. Tablet will dissolve within seconds, and may be swallowed with or without liquid. Do not split or chew.

I.M.: Risperdal® Consta™ should be administered into the upper outer quadrant of the gluteal area. Injection should alternate between the two buttocks. Do not combine two different dosage strengths into one single administration. Do not substitute any components of the dose-pack; administer with needle provided.

Contraindications Hypersensitivity to risperidone or any component of the formulation

Warnings

[U.S. Boxed Warning]: Elderly patients with dementia-related behavioral disorders treated with atypical antipsychotics are at an increased risk of cerebrovascular adverse events and death compared to placebo; risk may be increased with dehydration (increased risk of death observed with concurrent furosemide). Risperidone is not approved for the treatment of dementia-related psychosis.

Low to moderately sedating, use with caution in disorders where CNS depression is a feature. Use with caution in Parkinson's disease. Caution in patients with hemodynamic instability; bone marrow suppression; predisposition to seizures; subcortical brain damage; severe cardiac, hepatic, or respiratory disease. Use with caution in renal or hepatic dysfunction; dose reduction recommended. Esophageal dysmotility and aspiration have been associated with antipsychotic use; use with caution in patients at risk of aspiration pneumonia (ie, Alzheimer's disease). Caution in breast cancer or other prolactin-dependent tumors (elevates prolactin levels). May alter temperature regulation or mask toxicity of other drugs due to antiemetic effects.

May cause orthostasis. Use with caution in patients with cardiovascular diseases (eg, heart failure, history of myocardial infarction or ischemia, cerebrovascular disease, conduction abnormalities). Use caution in patients receiving medications for hypertension (orthostatic effects may be exacerbated) or in patients with hypovolemia or dehydration. May alter cardiac conduction (low risk relative to other neuroleptics); life-threatening arrhythmias have occurred with therapeutic doses of neuroleptics.

May cause anticholinergic effects (confusion, agitation, constipation, xerostomia, blurred vision, urinary retention); therefore, they should be used with caution in patients with decreased gastrointestinal motility, urinary retention, BPH, xerostomia, or visual problems. Conditions which also may be exacerbated by cholinergic blockade include narrow-angle glaucoma (screening is recommended) and worsening of myasthenia gravis. Relative to other neuroleptics, risperidone has a low potency of cholinergic blockade.

May cause extrapyramidal symptoms, including pseudoparkinsonism, acute dystonic reactions, akathisia, and tardive dyskinesia (risk of these reactions is low relative to other neuroleptics, and is dose dependent). Risk of neuroleptic malignant syndrome (NMS) may be increased in patients with Parkinson's disease or Lewy Body Dementia; monitor for symptoms of confusion, obtundation, postural instability and extrapyramidal symptoms. May cause hyperglycemia; in some cases may be extreme and associated with ketoacidosis, hyperosmolar coma, or death. Use with caution in patients with diabetes or other disorders of glucose regulation; monitor for worsening of glucose control.

The possibility of a suicide attempt is inherent in psychotic illness or bipolar disorder; use caution in high-risk patients during initiation of therapy. Prescriptions should be written for the smallest quantity consistent with good patient care. Safety and efficacy in children have not been established.

Dosage Forms Injection, microspheres for reconstitution, extended release (Risperdal® Consta™): 25 mg, 37.5 mg, 50 mg [supplied in a dose-pack containing vial with active ingredient in microsphere formulation, prefilled syringe with diluent, needle-free vial access device, and safety needle]

Solution, oral: 1 mg/mL (30 mL) [contains benzoic acid]

Tablet: 0.25 mg, 0.5 mg, 1 mg, 2 mg, 3 mg, 4 mg

Tablet, orally disintegrating (Risperdal® M-Tabs™): 0.5 mg [contains phenylalanine 0.42 mg]; 3 mg [contains phenylalanine 0.63 mg]; 4 mg [contains phenylalanine 0.84 mg]

Reference Range

Within 2 hours of a 1 mg oral dose, peak plasma level: 3-8 mcg/L; postmortem blood and urinary risperidone levels following a suicidal ingestion: 1.8 mg/L and 14.4 mg/L, respectively

Overdosage/Treatment

Decontamination: Lavage/activated charcoal within 1 hour

Supportive therapy: Lidocaine or phenytoin for ventricular arrhythmia; magnesium sulfate (I.V.: 2 g) may cause resolution of prolonged QT_c dispersion; sertraline can be used to treat risperidone-induced obsessive compulsive symptoms

Enhancement of elimination: Multiple dosing of activated charcoal may be effective

Asymptomatic patients with normal EKG may be discharged after a 6-hour period of observation. Symptomatic patients should be admitted to a setting where careful monitoring of their cardiac rhythm and mental status can occur.

Test Interactions ↑ prolactin

Drug Interactions

Substrate of CYP2D6 (major), 3A4 (minor); **Inhibits** CYP2D6 (weak), 3A4 (weak)

Acetylcholinesterase inhibitors (central): May increase the risk of antipsychotic-related extrapyramidal symptoms; monitor.

Carbamazepine: Plasma concentrations of risperidone and 9-hydroxyrisperidone were decreased by ~50% with concomitant use. The dose of risperidone may need to be titrated accordingly when carbamazepine is added or discontinued.

Clozapine: Decreases clearance of risperidone, increasing its serum concentrations

CNS depressants: May increase adverse effects/toxicity of other CNS depressants.

CYP2D6 inhibitors: May increase the levels/effects of risperidone. Example inhibitors include chlorpromazine, delavirdine, fluoxetine, miconazole, paroxetine, pergolide, quinidine, quinine, ritonavir, and ropinirole.

Lithium: May increase the neurotoxic effects (eg, EPS) of risperidone; monitor.

Pramlintide: May enhance the anticholinergic effect of risperidone. These effects are specific to the GI tract.

SSRIs: May increase the levels/effects of risperidone; monitor.

Verapamil: May increase the levels and effects of risperidone.

Pregnancy Risk Factor C; Enters breast milk/contraindicated

Pregnancy Implications Risperidone and its metabolite are excreted in breast milk; it is recommended that women not breast feed during therapy or for 12 weeks after the last injection if using Risperdal® Consta™.

Lactation Enters breast milk/not recommended

Additional Information Temazepam (30 mg) can be used to treat insomnia due to risperidone. Avoid ethanol, kava kava, gotu kola, valerian, and St John's wort (may increase CNS depression). Risperdal® M-Tabs™ contain phenylalanine.

Risperdal Consta™ is an injectable formulation of risperidone using the extended release Medisorb® drug-delivery system; small polymeric microspheres degrade slowly, releasing the medication at a controlled rate.

Specific References

Kane JM, Eerdekens M, Lindenmayer JP, et al, "Long-Acting Injectable Risperidone: Efficacy and Safety of the First Long-Acting Atypical Antipsychotic," *Am J Psychiatry*, 2003, 160(6):1125-32.

Karki SD and Masood GR, "Combination Risperidone and SSRI-Induced Serotonin Syndrome," *Ann Pharmacother*, 2003, 37(3):388-91.

Kunwar AR and Megna JL, "Resolution of Risperidone-Induced Hyperprolactinemia with Substitution of Quetiapine," *Ann Pharmacother*, 2003, 37(2):206-8.

Moody DE, Laycock JD, Huang W, et al, "A High-Performance Liquid Chromatographic-Atmospheric Pressure Chemical Ionization-Tandem Mass Spectrometric Method for Determination of Risperidone and 9-Hydroxyrisperidone in Human Plasma," *J Anal Toxicol*, 2004, 28(6):494-7.

Norris B, Angeles V, Eisenstein R, Seale JP, "Neuroleptic Malignant Syndrome with Delayed Onset of Fever Following Risperidone Administration," *Ann Pharmacother*, 2006, 40(12):2260-4.

Razaq M and Samma M, "A Case of Risperidone-induced Hypothermia," *Am J Ther*, 2004, 11(3):229-30.

Ritodrine

CAS Number 23239-51-2; 26652-09-5

Synonyms Ritodrine Hydrochloride

Use Inhibits uterine contraction in preterm labor

Mechanism of Action Tocolysis due to its uterine beta$_2$-adrenergic receptor stimulating effects; this agent's beta$_2$ effects can also cause bronchial relaxation and vascular smooth muscle stimulation

Adverse Reactions

Cardiovascular: Tachycardia, **hypertension** (increases in maternal and fetal heart rates and maternal hypertension), **palpitations**, angina, chest pain, sinus tachycardia, tachycardia (supraventricular)

Central nervous system: Headache, migraine headache (exacerbation of), mania

Endocrine & metabolic: **Hyperglycemia** (temporary) and insulin concentrations, galactorrhea, decreases serum potassium concentrations, parotitis, hypokalemia

Gastrointestinal: **Vomiting, nausea**

Hematologic: Leukocytosis, leukemoid reaction, neutropenia

Neuromuscular & skeletal: **Tremors**

Respiratory: Pulmonary edema

Signs and Symptoms of Overdose Parotid pain

Pharmacodynamics/Kinetics

Distribution: Crosses placenta

Protein binding: 32%

Metabolism: Hepatic

Half-life elimination: 15 hours

Time to peak, serum: 0.5-1 hour

Excretion: Urine (as unchanged drug and inactive conjugates)

Dosage

Adults:

I.V.: 50-100 mcg/minute; increase by 50 mcg/minute every 10 minutes; continue for 12 hours after contractions have stopped

Oral: Start 30 minutes before stopping I.V. infusion; 10 mg every 2 hours for 24 hours, then 10-20 mg every 4-6 hours up to 120 mg/day

Stability Stable for 48 hours at room temperature after dilution in 500 mL of NS, D$_5$W, or LR I.V. solutions

Monitoring Parameters Hematocrit, serum potassium, glucose, colloidal osmotic pressure, heart rate, and uterine contractions

Administration Monitor amount of I.V. fluid administered to prevent fluid overload; place patient in left lateral recumbent position to reduce risk of hypotension; use microdrip chamber or I.V. pump to control infusion rate

Contraindications Cardiac arrhythmias; pheochromocytoma; pregnancy (before 20th week)

Warnings Monitor hydration status and blood glucose concentrations; fatal maternal pulmonary edema has been reported, sometimes after delivery; fluid overload must be avoided, hydration levels should be monitored closely; if pulmonary edema occurs, the drug should be discontinued; use with caution in patients with moderate pre-eclampsia, diabetes, or migraine; some products may contain sulfites; maternal deaths have been reported in patients treated with ritodrine and concurrent corticosteroids (pulmonary edema)

Dosage Forms Ritodrine hydrochloride:

Injection: 10 mg/mL (5 mL); 15 mg/mL (10 mL)

Tablet: 10 mg

Reference Range After an oral 120 mg dose, maximum blood ritodrine level is 32 ng/mL

Overdosage/Treatment

Decontamination: Lavage (within 1 hour)/activated charcoal

Supportive therapy: Diazepam or lorazepam can be given for agitation; esmolol (50-100 mcg/kg I.V.) can be used for tachyarrhythmia

Enhancement of elimination: Multiple dosing of activated charcoal may be effective; hemodialysis may be effective

Drug Interactions Decreased effect with beta-blockers

Increased effect/toxicity with meperidine, sympathomimetics, diazoxide, magnesium, betamethasone (pulmonary edema), potassium-depleting diuretics, general anesthetics

Pregnancy Risk Factor B (contraindicated before 20th week)

Pregnancy Implications Increased fetal heart rate; transient fetal hypoglycemia, hyperbilirubinemia in neonates have been noted; crosses the placenta

Nursing Implications Monitor amount of I.V. fluid administered to prevent fluid overload; place patient in left lateral recumbent position to reduce risk of hypotension; use microdrip chamber or I.V. pump to control infusion rate

Ritonavir

U.S. Brand Names Norvir®

Use Treatment of HIV infection; should always be used as part of a multidrug regimen (at least 3 antiretroviral agents)

Mechanism of Action Peptidomimetic inhibitor of HIV-1 and HIV-2 proteases

Adverse Reactions

Protease inhibitors cause dyslipidemia which includes elevated cholesterol and triglycerides and a redistribution of body fat centrally to cause increased abdominal girth, buffalo hump, facial atrophy, and breast enlargement. These agents also cause hyperglycemia.

Cardiovascular: Vasodilation

Central nervous system: Fever, headache, malaise, dizziness, insomnia, somnolence, thinking abnormally

Dermatologic: Rash

Endocrine & metabolic: **Increased triglycerides**, hyperlipidemia, increased uric acid, increased glucose

Gastrointestinal: **Diarrhea, nausea, vomiting, taste perversion**, abdominal pain, anorexia, constipation, dyspepsia, flatulence, local throat irritation

Hematologic: **Anemia, decreased WBCs**, neutropenia, eosinophilia, neutrophilia, prolonged PT, leukocytosis

Hepatic: **Increased GGT**, increased liver function test results

Neuromuscular & skeletal: **Weakness**, increased CPK, myalgia, paresthesia

Respiratory: Pharyngitis

Miscellaneous: Diaphoresis, increased potassium, increased calcium

Pharmacodynamics/Kinetics

Absorption: Variable; increased with food

Distribution: High concentrations in serum and lymph nodes

Protein binding: 98% to 99%

Metabolism: Hepatic via CYP3A4 and 2D6; five metabolites, low concentration of an active metabolite achieved in plasma (oxidative)

Half-life elimination: 3-5 hours

Time to peak, plasma: 2 hours (fasted); 4 hours (nonfasted)

Excretion: Urine (~11%); feces (~86%)

Dosage Treatment of HIV infection: Oral:

Children >1 month: 350-400 mg/m^2 twice daily (maximum dose: 600 mg twice daily). Initiate dose at 250 mg/m^2 twice daily; titrate dose upward every 2-3 days by 50 mg/m^2 twice daily.

Adults: 600 mg twice daily; dose escalation tends to avoid nausea that many patients experience upon initiation of full dosing. Escalate the dose as follows: 300 mg twice daily for 1 day, 400 mg twice daily for 2 days, 500 mg twice daily for 1 day, then 600 mg twice daily. Ritonavir may be better tolerated when used in combination with other antiretrovirals by initiating the drug alone and subsequently adding the second agent within 2 weeks.

Pharmacokinetic "booster" in combination with other protease inhibitors: 100-400 mg/day

Refer to individual monographs; specific dosage recommendations often require adjustment of both agents.

Note: Dosage adjustments for ritonavir when administered in combination therapy:

Amprenavir: Adjustments necessary for each agent:
Amprenavir 1200 mg with ritonavir 200 mg once daily **or**
Amprenavir 600 mg with ritonavir 100 mg twice daily
Amprenavir plus efavirenz (3-drug regimen): Amprenavir 1200 mg twice daily plus ritonavir 200 mg twice daily plus efavirenz at standard dose
Indinavir: Adjustments necessary for both agents:
Indinavir 800 mg twice daily plus ritonavir 100-200 mg twice daily **or**
Indinavir 400 mg twice daily plus ritonavir 400 mg twice daily
Nelfinavir: Ritonavir 400 mg twice daily
Rifabutin: Decrease rifabutin dose to 150 mg every other day
Saquinavir: Ritonavir 400 mg twice daily

Dosing adjustment in renal impairment: None necessary
Dosing adjustment in hepatic impairment: No adjustment required in mild or moderate impairment; however, careful monitoring is required in moderate hepatic impairment (levels may be decreased); caution advised with severe impairment (no data available)

Monitoring Parameters Triglycerides, cholesterol, CBC, LFTs, CPK, uric acid, basic HIV monitoring, viral load, and CD4 count, glucose

Administration Administer with food. Liquid formulations usually have an unpleasant taste. Consider mixing it with chocolate milk or a liquid nutritional supplement. Whenever possible, administer oral solution with calibrated dosing syringe.

Contraindications Hypersensitivity to ritonavir or any component of the formulation; concurrent alfuzosin, amiodarone, cisapride, dihydroergotamine, ergonovine, ergotamine, flecainide, methylergonovine, midazolam, pimozide, propafenone, quinidine, triazolam, and voriconazole (when ritonavir ≥800 mg/day)

Warnings
[U.S. Boxed Warning]: Ritonavir may interact with many medications, resulting in potentially serious and/or life-threatening adverse events; careful review is required. A listing of medications that should not be used is available with each bottle and patients should be provided with this information. Avoid concurrent use with lovastatin, simvastatin, and St John's wort; atorvastatin should be used at the lowest possible dose, while fluvastatin or pravastatin may be safer alternatives. Cushing's syndrome and adrenal suppression have been reported in patients receiving concomitant ritonavir and fluticasone; avoid concurrent use unless benefit outweighs risk. Dosage adjustment is required for combination therapy with amprenavir and ritonavir; in addition, the risk of hyperlipidemia may be increased during concurrent therapy. Cardiac and neurological events have been reported with concurrent use of disopyramide, mexiletine, nefazodone, fluoxetine or beta blockers. Pancreatitis has been observed; use with caution in patients with increased triglycerides; monitor serum lipase and amylase.

Use with caution in patients with hemophilia A or B; increased bleeding during protease inhibitor therapy has been reported. Changes in glucose tolerance, hyperglycemia, exacerbation of diabetes, DKA, and new-onset diabetes mellitus have been reported in patients receiving protease inhibitors. May be associated with fat redistribution (buffalo hump, increased abdominal girth, breast engorgement, facial atrophy, and dyslipidemia). Immune reconstitution syndrome may develop resulting in the occurrence of an inflammatory response to an indolent or residual opportunistic infection; further evaluation and treatment may be required. May cause hepatitis or exacerbate pre-existing hepatic dysfunction; use with caution in patients with hepatitis B or C and in hepatic disease. Safety and efficacy have not been established in children <1 month of age.

Dosage Forms Capsule: 100 mg [contains ethanol and polyoxyl 35 castor oil]
Solution: 80 mg/mL (240 mL) [contains ethanol and polyoxyl 35 castor oil; peppermint and caramel flavor]

Reference Range After a 400 mg oral dose, peak serum ritonavir level: ~5.3 mcg/mL

Overdosage/Treatment
Decontamination: Activated charcoal
Supportive therapy: Treatment is supportive.

Drug Interactions
Substrate of CYP1A2 (minor), 2B6 (minor), 2D6 (major), 3A4 (major);
Inhibits CYP2C8 (strong), 2C9 (weak), 2C19 (weak), 2D6 (strong), 2E1 (weak), 3A4 (strong); **Induces** CYP1A2 (weak), 2C8 (weak), 2C9 (weak), 3A4 (weak)

Alfuzosin: Serum concentrations may be increased by ritonavir; concurrent use is contraindicated.

Amprenavir: The serum concentrations of ritonavir may be increased by amprenavir. In addition, the risk of cholesterol/triglyceride elevations may be increased. Specific dosing has been recommended for both agents.

Analgesics (eg, tramadol, meperidine, propoxyphene): Serum levels of parent drug or metabolite may be increased by ritonavir.

Antiarrhythmics (eg, disopyramide, mexiletine, lidocaine): Toxicity may be greatly increased; concurrent use of ritonavir is contraindicated with amiodarone, flecainide, propafenone, and quinidine.

Anticonvulsants: Ritonavir may increase levels (carbamazepine, ethosuximide) or decrease levels (lamotrigine, divalproex, phenytoin); monitor.

Antidepressants (eg, bupropion, trazodone, nefazodone, fluoxetine, and possibly other SSRIs): Ritonavir may increase the levels/effects of these agents.

Antipsychotics (clozapine, perphenazine, risperidone, thioridazine): Serum concentrations may be increased by ritonavir. Avoid use with thioridazine.

Benzodiazepines (clorazepate, diazepam, estazolam, flurazepam midazolam, triazolam) toxicity may be increased; concurrent use of midazolam and triazolam is specifically contraindicated.

Beta-blockers: Serum concentrations/effects may be increased by ritonavir.

Calcium channel blockers: Serum concentrations/effects may be increased by ritonavir.

Cimetidine: May increase the levels/effects of ritonavir; monitor.

Cisapride toxicity (arrhythmia) may be increased by ritonavir; concurrent use is contraindicated.

Clarithromycin serum concentrations are increased by ritonavir; dosage adjustment required (based on Cl$_{cr}$).

CYP2C8 substrates: Ritonavir may increase the levels/effects of CYP2C89 substrates. Example substrates include amiodarone, paclitaxel, pioglitazone, repaglinide, and rosiglitazone.

CYP2D6 substrates: Ritonavir may increase the levels/effects of CYP2D6 substrates. Example substrates include amphetamines, selected beta-blockers, dextromethorphan, fluoxetine, lidocaine, mirtazapine, nefazodone, paroxetine, risperidone, thioridazine, tricyclic antidepressants, and venlafaxine.

CYP2D6 prodrug substrates: Ritonavir may decrease the levels/effects of CYP2D6 prodrug substrates. Example prodrug substrates include codeine, hydrocodone, oxycodone, and tramadol.

CYP3A4 inducers: CYP3A4 inducers may decrease the levels/effects of ritonavir. Example inducers include aminoglutethimide, carbamazepine, nafcillin, nevirapine, phenobarbital, phenytoin, and rifamycins.

CYP3A4 substrates: Ritonavir may increase the levels/effects of CYP3A4 substrates. Example substrates include benzodiazepines, calcium channel blockers, mirtazapine, nateglinide, nefazodone, tacrolimus, and venlafaxine. Selected benzodiazepines (midazolam and triazolam), cisapride, ergot alkaloids, and pimozide are generally contraindicated with strong CYP3A4 inhibitors.

Delavirdine: Ritonavir may increase the levels/toxicity of delavirdine.

Desipramine (and possibly other TCAs at high doses) serum levels may be increased by ritonavir in HIV-positive patients, requiring dosage adjustment; monitor.

Didanosine: Administration should be separated by 2.5 hours to avoid formulation incompatibility.

Digoxin: Serum concentrations may be increased by ritonavir; monitor.

Disulfiram: May cause disulfiram reaction (oral solution contains 43% ethanol)

Eplerenone: Ritonavir may increase the levels/effects of eplerenone; monitor.

Ergot alkaloids (dihydroergotamine, ergotamine, ergonovine, methylergonovine) toxicity (peripheral ischemia, vasospasm) is increased by ritonavir; concurrent use is contraindicated.

Estrogen (oral or transdermal contraceptives): Effects may be decreased (not well characterized). Use alternative contraceptive measures.

Fentanyl: Ritonavir may increase the levels/effects; monitor.

HMG-CoA reductase inhibitors (atorvastatin, cerivastatin, lovastatin, simvastatin) serum concentrations may be increased by ritonavir, increasing the risk of myopathy/rhabdomyolysis. Lovastatin or simvastatin should not be used with ritonavir. Use lowest possible dose of atorvastatin. Fluvastatin and pravastatin may be safer alternatives.

Immunosuppressants (cyclosporine, sirolimus, tacrolimus): Serum levels/effects may be increased by ritonavir; monitor.

Indinavir serum concentrations are increased by ritonavir.

Inhaled corticosteroids (eg, budesonide, fluticasone): Serum concentrations may be increased by ritonavir, resulting in decreased serum cortisol, HPA axis suppression; concurrent use is not recommended.

Itraconazole, ketoconazole serum concentrations are increased by ritonavir. Limit ketoconazole dose to ≤200 mg/day.

Meperidine: Serum concentrations of metabolite (normeperidine) are increased by ritonavir, which may increase the risk of CNS toxicity.

Methadone: Serum concentrations may be decreased by ritonavir; dose adjustment of methadone may be necessary.

Metronidazole: May cause disulfiram reaction (oral solution contains 43% ethanol).

Pimozide toxicity is significantly increased by ritonavir; concurrent use is contraindicated.

Rifabutin and rifabutin metabolite serum concentrations may be increased by ritonavir; reduce rifabutin dose to 150 mg every other day.

Rifampin: May decrease levels/effects of ritonavir; alternative antimycobacterial agent recommended.

Saquinavir: Serum concentrations are increased by ritonavir; dosage of both agents should be adjusted.

Sildenafil: Serum concentrations may be increased by ritonavir; when used concurrently, do not exceed a maximum sildenafil dose of 25 mg in a 48-hour period.

Tadalafil: Serum concentrations may be increased by ritonavir. A maximum tadalafil dose of 10 mg in 72 hours is recommended with strong CYP3A4 inhibitors.

Theophylline: Serum concentrations may be decreased by ritonavir.

Trazodone: Serum concentrations/effects may be increased by ritonavir; use caution and reduce trazodone dose.

Vardenafil: Serum concentrations may be increased by ritonavir; do not exceed vardenafil dose of 2.5 mg in 72 hours.

Voriconazole: Serum levels are reduced by ritonavir. Concurrent use is contraindicated with ritonavir dose $\geq$ 800 mg/day. Concomitant use not recommended with lower doses of ritonavir unless benefit outweighs risk.

Zolpidem: Serum levels/effects may be increased by ritonavir; monitor.

Pregnancy Risk Factor B

Pregnancy Implications According to preliminary data, placental passage of ritonavir is minimal. Pregnancy and protease inhibitors are both associated with an increased risk of hyperglycemia. Glucose levels should be closely monitored. Healthcare professionals are encouraged to contact the antiretroviral pregnancy registry to monitor outcomes of pregnant women exposed to antiretroviral medications (1-800-258-4263).

Lactation Excretion in breast milk unknown/not recommended

Additional Information Oral solution contains 43% ethanol by volume.

Specific References

Bergshoeff AS, Wolfs TF, Geelen SP, et al, "Ritonavir-Enhanced Pharmacokinetics of Nelfinavir/M8 During Rifampin Use," *Ann Pharmacother*, 2003, 37(4):521-5.

Rivastigmine

CAS Number 123441-03-2

U.S. Brand Names Exelon®

Synonyms ENA 713; Rivastigmine Tartrate; SDZ ENA 713

Use Mild to moderate dementia from Alzheimer's disease

Mechanism of Action A deficiency of cortical acetylcholine is thought to account for some of the symptoms of Alzheimer's disease; rivastigmine increases acetylcholine in the central nervous system through reversible inhibition of its hydrolysis by cholinesterase

Adverse Reactions

Cardiovascular: Syncope, hypertension, chest pain, peripheral edema, edema, periorbital or facial edema, hypotension, postural hypotension, cardiac failure, atrial fibrillation, bradycardia, AV block, bundle branch block, sick sinus syndrome, cardiac arrest, supraventricular tachycardia, tachycardia, angina pectoris, myocardial infarction, peripheral ischemia, thrombosis, intracranial hemorrhage

Central nervous system: **Dizziness, headache**, fatigue, insomnia, confusion, depression, anxiety, malaise, somnolence, hallucinations, aggressiveness, vertigo, pain, agitation, nervousness, delusion, paranoid reaction, ataxia, convulsions, apraxia, aphasia, dysphonia, fever, hypothermia, migraine, neuralgia, delirium, emotional lability, psychosis

Dermatologic: Rash, rashes (maculopapular, eczema, bullous, exfoliative, psoriaform, erythematous), urticaria, Stevens-Johnson syndrome

Endocrine & metabolic: Hypothyroidism, dehydration

Gastrointestinal: **Nausea, vomiting, diarrhea, anorexia, abdominal pain**; dyspepsia, constipation, flatulence, weight loss, eructation, peptic ulcer, gastroesophageal reflux, GI hemorrhage, intestinal obstruction, pancreatitis, colitis, severe vomiting with esophageal rupture (following inappropriate reinitiation of dose)

Genitourinary: Urinary tract infection

Hematologic: Hematoma, thrombocytopenia, purpura, anemia, leukocytosis

Hepatic: Abnormal hepatic function, cholecystitis

Local: Thrombophlebitis

Neuromuscular & skeletal: Weakness, tremor, back pain, arthralgia, bone fracture, hypokinesia, hyperkinesia, hypertonia, arthritis, peripheral neuropathy

Ocular: Conjunctival hemorrhage, diplopia, glaucoma

Renal: Urinary incontinence, acute renal failure

Respiratory: Rhinitis, upper respiratory tract infections, cough, pharyngitis, bronchitis, epistaxis, bronchospasm, apnea, pulmonary embolism

Miscellaneous: Increased diaphoresis, flu-like syndrome, infection, allergy, lymphadenopathy

Pharmacodynamics/Kinetics

Duration: Anticholinesterase activity (CSF): ~10 hours (6 mg dose)

Absorption: Fasting: Rapid and complete within 1 hour

Distribution: V_d: 1.8-2.7 L/kg

Protein binding: 40%

Metabolism: Extensively via cholinesterase-mediated hydrolysis in the brain; metabolite undergoes N-demethylation and/or sulfate conjugation hepatically; CYP minimally involved; linear kinetics at 3 mg twice daily, but nonlinear at higher doses

Bioavailability: 36% to 40%

Half-life elimination: 1.5 hours

Time to peak: 1 hour

Excretion: Urine (97% as metabolites); feces (0.4%)

Dosage Adults: Mild to moderate Alzheimer's dementia: Oral: Initial: 1.5 mg twice daily to start; if dose is tolerated for at least 2 weeks then it may be increased to 3 mg twice daily; increases to 4.5 mg twice daily and 6 mg twice daily should only be attempted after at least 2 weeks at the previous dose; maximum dose: 6 mg twice daily. If adverse events such as nausea, vomiting, abdominal pain, or loss of appetite occur, the patient should be instructed to discontinue treatment for several doses then restart at the same or next lower dosage level; antiemetics have been used to control GI symptoms. If treatment is interrupted for longer than several days, restart the treatment at the lowest dose and titrate as previously described.

Elderly: Clearance is significantly lower in patients older than 60 years of age, but dosage adjustments are not recommended. Titrate dose to individual's tolerance.

Dosage adjustment in renal impairment: Dosage adjustments are not recommended, however, titrate the dose to the individual's tolerance.

Dosage adjustment in hepatic impairment: Clearance is significantly reduced in mild to moderately impaired patients. Although dosage adjustments are not recommended, use lowest possible dose and titrate according to individual's tolerance. May consider waiting >2 weeks between dosage adjustments.

Stability Store below 25°C (77°F); store solution in an upright position and protect from freezing

Monitoring Parameters Cognitive function at periodic intervals

Administration Should be administered with meals (breakfast or dinner). Capsule should be swallowed whole. Liquid form is available for patients who cannot swallow capsules (can be swallowed directly from syringe or mixed with water, soda, or cold fruit juice). Stir well and drink within 4 hours of mixing.

Contraindications Hypersensitivity to rivastigmine, other carbamate derivatives (eg, neostigmine, pyridostigmine, physostigmine), or any component of the formulation

Warnings Significant nausea, vomiting, anorexia, and weight loss are associated with use; occurs more frequently in women and during the titration phase. If treatment is interrupted for more than several days, reinstate at the lowest daily dose. Use caution in patients with a history of peptic ulcer disease or concurrent NSAID use. Use caution in patients undergoing anesthesia who will receive succinylcholine-type muscle relaxation, patients with sick sinus syndrome, bradycardia or supraventricular conduction conditions, urinary obstruction, seizure disorders, or pulmonary conditions such as asthma or COPD. Safety and efficacy in children have not been established.

Dosage Forms Capsule:

Exelon®: 1.5 mg, 3 mg, 4.5 mg, 6 mg

Solution, oral:

Exelon®: 2 mg/mL (120 mL) [contains sodium benzoate]

Overdosage/Treatment

Decontamination: Oral: Activated charcoal

Supportive therapy: In cases of asymptomatic overdoses, rivastigmine should be held for 24 hours. Cholinergic crisis, caused by significant acetylcholinesterase inhibition, is characterized by severe nausea, vomiting, salivation, sweating, bradycardia, hypotension, respiratory depression, collapse, and convulsions. Treatment is supportive and symptomatic. Atropine (initial dose: 0.03 mg/kg I.M.) can be used for symptomatic treatment. Dialysis would not be helpful. Overdoses as high as 46 mg have resulted in full recovery within 24 hours with supportive care.

Drug Interactions Anticholinergics: Effects may be reduced with rivastigmine

Antipsychotic agents: Acetylcholinesterase inhibitors (central) may increase the risk of antipsychotic-related extrapyramidal symptoms; monitor.

Beta-blockers without ISA activity: May increase risk of bradycardia

Calcium channel blockers (diltiazem or verapamil): May increase risk of bradycardia

Cholinergic agonists: Effects may be increased with rivastigmine

Digoxin: Increased risk of bradycardia with concurrent use

Neuromuscular blockers: Depolarizing neuromuscular blocking agents effects may be increased with rivastigmine

NSAIDs: Although not seen in clinical studies, patients may be at increased risk for peptic ulcers or gastrointestinal bleeding with concomitant use; monitor

Pregnancy Risk Factor B

Pregnancy Implications There are no adequate studies in pregnant women. Should be used only if the benefit outweighs the potential risk to the fetus. It is unknown if rivastigmine is excreted in human breast milk. There is no indication for use in nursing mothers.

Lactation Excretion in breast milk unknown/use caution

Nursing Implications Educate patient or caregiver about medicine.

Specific References

Brvar M, Mozina M, and Bunc M, "Poisoning with Rivastigmine," *Clin Toxicol (Phila)*. 2005, 43(7):891-2

Lai MW and Burns EM, "Pediatric "Pesticide" Poisoning in a Pill: Predominant Nicotinic Cholinergic Effects After Exposure to a Therapeutic Carbamate," *Clin Toxicol (Phila)*. 2005, 43:643.

Rizatriptan

U.S. Brand Names Maxalt-MLT®; Maxalt®

Synonyms MK462

Use Acute treatment of migraine with or without aura

Mechanism of Action Selective agonist for serotonin (5-HT$_{1D}$ receptor) in cranial arteries to cause vasoconstriction and reduce sterile inflammation associated with antidromic neuronal transmission correlating with relief of migraine

Adverse Reactions

Cardiovascular: Systolic/diastolic blood pressure increases (5-10 mm Hg), chest pain, palpitations, angina, arrhythmia, facial edema, bradycardia, tachycardia, myocardial ischemia, myocardial infarction, syncope

Central nervous system: Dizziness, drowsiness, fatigue (13% to 30% - dose related), akinesia, decreased mental activity, chills, hangover effect, neurological/psychiatric abnormalities, stroke

Dermatologic: Skin flushing, pruritus, toxic epidermal necrolysis

Endocrine & metabolic: Mild increase in growth hormone, hot flashes

Gastrointestinal: Nausea, abdominal pain, dry mouth, diarrhea, dysgeusia

Neuromuscular & skeletal: Arthralgia, muscle weakness, myalgia, neck pain, neck stiffness, bradykinesia

Ocular: Blurred vision, dry eyes, eye pain

Otic: Tinnitus

Renal: Polyuria

Respiratory: Dyspnea, nasopharyngeal irritation, pharyngitis

Miscellaneous: Diaphoresis, heat sensitivity

Pharmacodynamics/Kinetics

Onset of action: ~30 minutes

Duration: 14-16 hours

Protein binding: 14%

Metabolism: Via monoamine oxidase-A; first-pass effect

Bioavailability: 40% to 50%

Half-life elimination: 2-3 hours

Time to peak: 1-1.5 hours

Excretion: Urine (82%, 8% to 16% as unchanged drug); feces (12%)

Dosage

Note: In patients with risk factors for coronary artery disease, following adequate evaluation to establish the absence of coronary artery disease, the initial dose should be administered in a setting where response may be evaluated (physician's office or similarly staffed setting). ECG monitoring may be considered.

Oral: 5-10 mg, repeat after 2 hours if significant relief is not attained; maximum: 30 mg in a 24-hour period (use 5 mg dose in patients receiving propranolol with a maximum of 15 mg in 24 hours)

Note: For orally-disintegrating tablets (Maxalt-MLT™): Patient should be instructed to place tablet on tongue and allow to dissolve. Dissolved tablet will be swallowed with saliva.

Stability Store in blister pack until administration

Monitoring Parameters Headache severity, signs/symptoms suggestive of angina; consider monitoring blood pressure, heart rate, and/or ECG with first dose in patients with likelihood of unrecognized coronary disease, such as patients with significant hypertension, hypercholesterolemia, obese patients, diabetics, smokers with other risk factors or strong family history of coronary artery disease

Contraindications Hypersensitivity to rizatriptan or any component of the formulation; documented ischemic heart disease or Prinzmetal's angina; uncontrolled hypertension; basilar or hemiplegic migraine; during or within 2 weeks of MAO inhibitors; during or within 24 hours of treatment with another 5-HT$_1$ agonist, or an ergot-containing or ergot-type medication (eg, methysergide, dihydroergotamine)

Warnings

Use only in patients with a clear diagnosis of migraine. May cause vasospastic reactions resulting in colonic, peripheral, or coronary ischemia. Use with caution in elderly or patients with hepatic or renal impairment (including dialysis patients), history of hypersensitivity to sumatriptan or adverse effects from sumatriptan, and in patients at risk of coronary artery disease (as predicted by presence of risk factors) unless cardiovascular evaluation provides evidence that the patient is free of cardiovascular disease. In patients with risk factors for coronary artery disease, following adequate evaluation to establish the absence of coronary artery disease, the initial dose should be administered in a setting where response may be evaluated (physician's office or similarly staffed setting). ECG monitoring may be considered. Do not use with ergotamines. May increase blood pressure transiently; may cause coronary vasospasm (less than sumatriptan); avoid in patients with signs/symptoms suggestive of reduced arterial flow (ischemic bowel, Raynaud's) which could be exacerbated by vasospasm.

Patients who experience sensations of chest pain/pressure/tightness or symptoms suggestive of angina following dosing should be evaluated for coronary artery disease or Prinzmetal's angina before receiving additional doses.

Reconsider diagnosis of migraine if no response to initial dose. Long-term effects on vision have not been evaluated.

Dosage Forms Tablet, as benzoate (Maxalt®): 5 mg, 10 mg

Tablet, orally disintegrating, as benzoate (Maxalt-MLT®): 5 mg [contains phenylalanine 1.05 mg/tablet; peppermint flavor]; 10 mg [contains phenylalanine 2.1 mg/tablet; peppermint flavor]

Overdosage/Treatment

Decontamination for oral ingestion: Lavage within 1 hour/activated charcoal

Supportive therapy: Nitroprusside, nifedipine, or hydralazine for hypertensive crisis; lidocaine or procainamide for ventricular ectopy; nitroglycerin can reverse sumatriptan-induced coronary artery vasoconstriction

Drug Interactions Use within 24 hours of another selective 5-HT$_1$ agonist or ergot-containing drug should be avoided due to possible additive vasoconstriction

MAO inhibitors and nonselective MAO inhibitors increase concentration of rizatriptan

Propranolol: Plasma concentration of rizatriptan increased 70%

SSRIs: Rarely, concurrent use results in weakness and incoordination; monitor closely

Pregnancy Risk Factor C

Pregnancy Implications There are no adequate and well-controlled studies using rizatriptan in pregnant women. Use only if potential benefit to the mother outweighs the potential risk to the fetus. A pregnancy registry has been established to monitor outcomes of women exposed to rizatriptan during pregnancy (800-986-8999). In some animal studies, administration was associated with decreased weight gain, developmental toxicity and increased mortality in the offspring. Teratogenic effects were not observed.

Lactation Excretion in breast milk unknown/use caution

Rosuvastatin

Pronunciation (roe SOO va sta tin)

U.S. Brand Names Crestor®

Synonyms Rosuvastatin Calcium

Use Used with dietary therapy for hyperlipidemias to reduce elevations in total cholesterol (TC), LDL-C, apolipoprotein B, and triglycerides (TG) in patients with primary hypercholesterolemia (elevations of 1 or more components are present in Fredrickson type IIa, IIb, and IV hyperlipidemias); treatment of homozygous familial hypercholesterolemia (FH)

Mechanism of Action Inhibitor of 3-hydroxy-3-methylglutaryl coenzyme A (HMG-CoA) reductase, the rate-limiting enzyme in cholesterol synthesis (reduces the production of mevalonic acid from HMG-CoA); this then results in a compensatory increase in the expression of LDL receptors on hepatocyte membranes and a stimulation of LDL catabolism

Adverse Reactions

2% to 10%:

Cardiovascular: Chest pain, hypertension, peripheral edema, angina, palpitation, arrhythmia, syncope

Central nervous system: Headache, depression, dizziness, insomnia, pain, anxiety, vertigo

Dermatologic: Rash, bruising, pruritus, photosensitivity

Gastrointestinal: Pharyngitis (9%), abdominal pain, constipation, gastroenteritis, vomiting, pancreatitis

Hematologic: Anemia

Hepatic: Hepatitis

Neuromuscular & skeletal: Myalgia, arthritis, arthralgia, hypertonia, paresthesia, neuralgia, myasthenia, myositis, myopathy, rhabdomyolysis

Renal: Kidney failure

Respiratory: Bronchitis, cough

Miscellaneous: Hypersensitivity reactions

Pharmacodynamics/Kinetics

Onset: Within 1 week; maximal at 4 weeks

Distribution: V$_d$: 134 L

Protein binding: 90%

Metabolism: Hepatic (10%), via CYP2C9 (1 active metabolite identified)

Bioavailability: 20% (high first-pass extraction by liver)

Asian patients have been noted to have increased bioavailability.

Half-life elimination: 19 hours

Time to peak, plasma: 3-5 hours

Excretion: Feces (90%), primarily as unchanged drug

Dosage

Adults: Oral:

Heterozygous familial and nonfamilial hypercholesterolemia; mixed dyslipidemia: Initial: 10 mg once daily (20 mg in patients with severe hypercholesterolemia); after 2 weeks, may be increased to 20 mg once daily; dosing range: 5-40 mg/day (maximum dose: 40 mg once daily)

Homozygous FH: Initial: 20 mg once daily (maximum dose: 40 mg/day)

Dosage adjustment with concomitant medications:

Cyclosporine: Rosuvastatin dose should not exceed 5 mg/day

Gemfibrozil: Rosuvastatin dose should not exceed 10 mg/day

Dosage adjustment in renal impairment:

Mild to moderate impairment: No dosage adjustment required.

Cl_{cr} <30 mL/minute/1.73 m^2: Initial: 5 mg/day; do not exceed 10 mg once daily

Monitoring Parameters Total cholesterol, LDL, and HDL cholesterol; liver function tests should be determined at baseline (prior to initiation), 3 months following initiation, and 3 months after any increase in dose; baseline CPK (recheck CPK in any patient with symptoms suggestive of myopathy)

Administration May be administered with or without food.

Contraindications Hypersensitivity to rosuvastatin or any component of the formulation; active liver disease; unexplained persistent elevations of serum transaminases (>3 times ULN); pregnancy; breast-feeding

Warnings Secondary causes of hyperlipidemia should be ruled out prior to therapy. Liver function must be monitored by periodic laboratory assessment. Use with caution in patients who consume large amounts of ethanol or have a history of liver disease. Rhabdomyolysis with acute renal failure has occurred. Discontinue in any patient in which CPK levels are markedly elevated (>10 times ULN) or if myopathy is suspected/diagnosed. An increased incidence of rosuvastatin-associated myopathy has been reported during concomitant therapy with fibric acid derivatives, niacin, cyclosporine, and in certain subgroups of the Asian population. Risk is also elevated at higher dosages of rosuvastatin. Patients should be instructed to report unexplained muscle pain, tenderness, or weakness, particularly if associated with fever and/or malaise. Use caution in patients predisposed to myopathy (eg, renal failure, advanced age, inadequately treated hypothyroidism). Temporarily withhold in patients experiencing an acute or serious condition predisposing to renal failure secondary to rhabdomyolysis (sepsis, hypotension, major surgery, trauma, severe metabolic or endocrine or electrolyte disorders, uncontrolled seizures). Safety and efficacy have not been established in children (limited experience with homozygous FH in patients >8 years of age).

Dosage Forms Tablet, as calcium: 5 mg, 10 mg, 20 mg, 40 mg

Drug Interactions Substrate (minor) of CYP2C9, 3A4

Antacids: Plasma concentrations may be decreased when given with magnesium/aluminum hydroxide-containing antacids. Antacids should be administered at least 2 hours after rosuvastatin.

Cholestyramine and colestipol (bile acid sequestrants): Reduce absorption of several HMG-CoA reductase inhibitors; separate administration times by at least 4 hours. Cholesterol-lowering effects are additive.

Clofibrate and fenofibrate may increase the risk of myopathy and rhabdomyolysis with HMG-CoA reductase inhibitors. Effects on lipid levels may be additive.

Cyclosporine: May increase serum concentrations of rosuvastatin (up to 10 times usual concentrations). Limit dose to 5 mg/day.

Gemfibrozil: Serum concentrations of rosuvastatin may be increased (doubled) during concurrent administration; combination should be avoided. Limit dose to 10 mg/day.

Hormonal contraceptives: Rosuvastatin increases serum concentrations of ethinyl estradiol and norgestrel.

Niacin: May increase the risk of myopathy and rhabdomyolysis with HMG-CoA reductase inhibitors.

Warfarin: Effects may be increased by rosuvastatin. Monitor.

Pregnancy Risk Factor X

Pregnancy Implications Use in women of childbearing potential only if they are highly unlikely to conceive; discontinue if pregnancy occurs.

Lactation Excretion in breast milk unknown/contraindicated

Salicylate

Related Information
- Methyl Salicylate

CAS Number 50-78-2

Use Treatment of mild to moderate pain, inflammation and fever; may be used as a prophylaxis of myocardial infarction and transient ischemic attacks (TIA)

Mechanism of Action Inhibits prostaglandin synthesis, acts on the hypothalamus heat-regulating center to reduce fever, blocks prostaglandin synthetase action which prevents formation of the platelet-aggregating substance thromboxane A$_2$; inhibits both vitamin K-dependent and independent clotting factors

Adverse Reactions

Cardiovascular: Circulatory collapse, pericardial effusion/pericarditis, fibrillation (atrial), flutter (atrial), angina, sinus tachycardia, vasculitis

Central nervous system: Headache, aseptic meningitis, psychosis, cognitive dysfunction, coma, seizures, electroencephalogram abnormalities, mania, aseptic meningitis

Dermatologic: Rash, pruritus, alopecia, systemic contact dermatitis, immunologic contact urticaria, Stevens-Johnson syndrome, exfoliative dermatitis, pityriasis rosea-like reaction, erythema multiforme, acute generalized exanthematous pustulosis, angioedema, bullous skin disease, toxic epidermal necrolysis, urticaria, purpura, psoriasis, erythema nodosum, licheniform eruptions

Endocrine & metabolic: Hyperkalemia, anion gap metabolic acidosis, hypouricemia, fluid retention

Gastrointestinal: Abdominal pain, **nausea**, vomiting, GI bleeding, GI ulceration, constipation, diarrhea, **dyspepsia**, esophagitis, aphthous stomatitis

Hematologic: Leukopenia, neutropenia, agranulocytosis, granulocytopenia, aplastic anemia (rare), platelet inhibition, hypoprothrombinemia, thrombocytopenia

Hepatic: Elevated transaminases, hepatitis (fulminant), impaired gluconeogenesis

Neuromuscular & skeletal: Rhabdomyolysis

Ocular: Diplopia, color vision abnormalities

Otic: Ototoxicity, tinnitus (serum levels > 30 mg/dl)

Renal: Renal failure (acute), albuminuria, nephrotic syndrome, acute tubular necrosis

Respiratory: Wheezing, adult respiratory distress syndrome, apnea, tachypnea, respiratory depression, rhinitis, hyposmia, eosinophilic pneumonia

Miscellaneous: Hypersensitivity, bezoars/concretions, Henoch-Schönlein purpura, fixed drug eruption

Bezoars, chest pain, coagulopathy, cognitive dysfunction, colitis, deafness, delirium, dementia, drowsiness, dry mouth, GI bleeding, gout, hematuria, hyperthermia, hypoglycemia, nausea, nephrotic syndrome, nystagmus, ototoxicity, stomatitis, tinnitus, vomiting, wheezing.

Severe poisoning can manifest with agranulocytosis, coma, confusion, dizziness, feces discoloration (black; pink; red; tarry), fever, granulocytopenia, headache, hyperglycemia, hyponatremia, hypotension, leukopenia, metabolic acidosis, neutropenia, pylorospasm, thirst, renal failure and/or hepatic failure, respiratory depression, rhabdomyolysis, seizures, urine discoloration (pink).

Phases of salicylate poisoning:

Phase I (up to 12 hours after ingestion): Tachypnea and hyperventilation predominate (respiratory alkalosis) with increased renal secretion of sodium, potassium, and bicarbonate resulting in both an alkaline urine and serum pH

Phase II (12-24 hours after ingestion): Urine becomes more acidic as intracellular potassium decreases. While children <4 years of age may develop a pure metabolic acidosis, older patients will have significant respiratory compensation and thus serum pH can be alkalotic. Coagulation abnormalities may occur.

Phase III (over 24 hours after ingestion): Severe potassium and bicarbonate depletion occurs with hydrogen being excreted renally; serum pH becomes acidotic; infants may reach this phase within 6 hours

Admission Criteria/Prognosis Admit any patient with acidosis, mental status changes, thermoregulatory abnormality, glucose abnormality, serum salicylate >50 mg/dL following an acute ingestion

Pharmacodynamics/Kinetics

Absorption: From the stomach and small intestine

Distribution: V_d: 0.2 L/kg (increases in overdose); distributes readily into most body fluids and tissues

Protein binding: 75% to 90%; salicylic acid: 80% at low serum concentrations; 50% at 70 mg/dL and 30% at 120 mg/dL

Metabolism: Hydrolyzed to salicylate (active) by esterases in the gastrointestinal mucosa, red blood cells, synovial fluid and blood; occurs primarily by hepatic microsomal enzymes; metabolic pathways are saturable

Half-life: 15-20 minutes; half-life is dose-dependent ranging from 3 hours at lower doses (300-600 mg), 5-6 hours (after 1 g) and 10 hours with higher doses

Time to peak serum concentration: About 1-2 hours

Elimination: Renal; primarily as free salicylic acid and conjugated metabolites; ≈52% of the drug is normally excreted in 4 hours in a normal patient

Dosage

Children:

Analgesic and antipyretic: Oral, rectal: 10-15 mg/kg/dose every 4-6 hours, up to a total of 60-80 mg/kg/24 hours

Anti-inflammatory: Oral: Initial: 60-90 mg/kg/day in divided doses; usual maintenance: 80-100 mg/kg/day divided every 6-8 hours, maximum dose: 3.6 g/day; monitor serum concentrations

Antirheumatic: Oral: 60-100 mg/kg/day in divided doses every 4 hours

Kawasaki disease: Oral: 80-100 mg/kg/day divided every 6 hours; after fever resolves: 8-10 mg/kg/day once daily; monitor serum concentrations

Adults:

Analgesic and antipyretic: Oral, rectal: 325-650 mg every 4-6 hours up to 4 g/day

Anti-inflammatory: Oral: Initial: 2.4-3.6 g/day in divided doses; usual maintenance: 3.6-5.4 g/day; monitor serum concentrations

TIA: Oral: 1.3 g/day in 2-4 divided doses

Myocardial infarction and stroke prophylaxis: 160 mg/day

Dosing adjustment in renal impairment: Cl_{cr} <10 mL/minute: Avoid use

Dosing adjustment in hepatic disease: Avoid use in severe liver disease

Stability Keep suppositories in refrigerator, do not freeze; hydrolysis of aspirin occurs upon exposure to water or moist air, resulting in salicylate and acetate, which possess a vinegar-like odor; do not use if a strong odor is present

Monitoring Parameters Serum concentrations, renal function; hearing changes or tinnitus; monitor for response (ie, pain, inflammation, range of motion, grip strength); observe for abnormal bleeding, bruising, weight gain

Contraindications Bleeding disorders, hypersensitivity to salicylates or other nonsteroidal anti-inflammatory drugs (NSAIDs)

Warnings Do not use aspirin in children <16 years of age for chickenpox or flu symptoms due to the association with Reye's syndrome; use with caution in patients with platelet and bleeding disorders, renal dysfunction

Dosage Forms

Suppository, rectal: 60 mg, 120 mg, 125 mg, 130 mg, 195 mg, 200 mg, 300 mg, 325 mg, 600 mg, 650 mg, 1200 mg

Tablet: 325 mg, 500 mg, 650 mg

Tablet:

Buffered:

325 mg with aluminum hydroxide 75 mg and magnesium hydroxide 75 mg

325 mg with aluminum hydroxide 150 mg and magnesium hydroxide 150 mg

500 mg with aluminum hydroxide 33 mg and magnesium hydroxide 150 mg

Chewable: 81 mg

Chewing gum: 227 mg

Controlled release: 800 mg

Enteric coated (delayed release): 80 mg, 165 mg, 325 mg, 500 mg, 650 mg, 975 mg

Timed release: 650 mg

Tablet, with caffeine 400 mg and caffeine 32 mg; 500 mg and caffeine 32 mg

Reference Range

Sample size: 1.5-2 mL blood (lavender top (EDTA) tube)

Timing of serum samples: Peak levels usually occur 2 hours after ingestion; half-life increases with dosage (eg, the half-life after 300 mg is 3 hours, and after 1 g is 5-6 hours, and after 8-10 g is 10 hours) Salicylate serum concentrations correlate with the pharmacological actions and adverse effects observed. See table.

Serum Salicylate: Clinical Correlations

Serum Salicylate Concentration (mg/dL)	Desired Effects	Adverse Effects / Intoxication
~10	Antiplatelet	GI intolerance and bleeding, hypersensitivity, hemostatic defects
	Antipyresis	
	Analgesia	
15-20	Anti-inflammatory	Mild salicylism
25-40	Treatment of rheumatic fever	Nausea/vomiting, hyperventilation, salicylism, flushing, sweating, thirst, headache, diarrhea and tachycardia
>40		Respiratory alkalosis, hemorrhage, excitement, confusion, asterixis, pulmonary edema, convulsions, tetany, metabolic acidosis, fever, coma, cardiovascular collapse, renal and respiratory failure

Overdosage/Treatment

Decontamination: Activated charcoal with cathartic is quite effective; each gram of activated charcoal can bind up to 550 mg of salicylic acid; whole bowel irrigation can also be used; gastric decontamination should occur with ingestions over 150 mg/kg

Supportive therapy: Hypotension/dehydration can be managed with I.V. fluid therapy; acidosis should be treated with I.V. sodium bicarbonate, hypokalemia will need to be corrected, seizures with benzodiazepines; blood products are indicated, as appropriate, for hemorrhage; antacids may promote gastric absorption

Enhancement of elimination: Forced alkaline diuresis with I.V. sodium bicarbonate to keep urine pH at 8 should be performed for salicylate levels >40 mg/dL; dialysis is indicated for secondary complications, seizures acidosis, or renal failure and not toxin removal alone; consider hemodialysis for acute salicylate levels >100 mg/dL or chronic salicylate levels >60 mg/dL; multiple dosing of activated charcoal may not hasten elimination; dialyzable (50% to 100%); exchange transfusion has been used in a 2-year-old child (elimination rate estimated to be 152 mg/hour) to treat a methyl salicylate intoxication

Test Interactions False-negative results for glucose oxidase urinary glucose tests (Clinistix®); false-positives using the cupric sulfate method (Clinitest®); also, interferes with Gerhardt test (VMA determination), 5-HIAA, xylose tolerance test, T_3, and T_4; can cause false elevations of serum carbon dioxide assays (using the Technicon® RA-1000 system); high salicylate levels can falsely cause hyperchloremia by direct potentiometry; >2 g/day causes a falsely increased free thyroxine level

Drug Interactions Aspirin decreases serum concentrations probably by protein-binding displacement; there is an increased bleeding potential with concomitant warfarin therapy; may increase lithium and methotrexate concentrations by decreasing renal clearance; may decrease diuretic and hypotensive effects of thiazides, loop diuretics, ACE inhibitors, and beta-blockers; may increase nephrotoxicity of cyclosporine; salicylate absorption can be delayed with aluminum hydroxide, antihistamines, tricyclic antidepressants, isoniazid, opiates, neuroleptics, or sedative-hypnotics

By inhibiting gastric alcohol dehydrogenase, aspirin can increase the bioavailability and peak concentrations of ethyl alcohol. Aspirin (1 g) has been shown to increase bioavailability of ethanol (0.3 g/kg) in the fed state but not in the fasting state.

Toluene abuse with aspirin can increase the risk for toluene-induced ototoxicity

Concomitant administration of glyburide and aspirin can cause an increase of insulin levels resulting in transient hypoglycemia; concurrent intake of ethanol and aspirin can reduce the peak aspirin concentration by 25%

Pregnancy Risk Factor C (D if full-dose aspirin in 3rd trimester)

Pregnancy Implications Late term fetus is more sensitive to adverse (acidotic) effects of aspirin; but with low-dose aspirin, no evidence for increased frequency of abruptio placentae or perinatal mortality noted

Nursing Implications Administer with food or a full glass of water to minimize GI distress; do not crush sustained release tablet; previous nonreaction does not guarantee future safe taking of medication

Additional Information

Lethal dose: 300 mg/kg; Toxic dose (acute): 200 mg/kg

To help evaluate the toxicity of nonaspirin salicylate agents, conversion to an aspirin equivalent dose (AED) may be necessary; by multiplying the dose ingested by the aspirin conversion factor (ACF) described in the table, the AED can be calculated. This calculation assumes that the nonaspirin salicylate is 100% absorbed, and there is 100% conversion to salicylate and that the potency of the nonaspirin salicylate is equipotent with aspirin on a mole for mole basis. Zileuton (600 mg 4 times/day orally) can protect asthmatics from idiosyncratic reactions (ie, bronchoconstriction) due to aspirin. Aspirin is not very water soluble, pharmacobezoars/concretions have been reported with overdosage. Ketonuria is seen in ~41% of salicylate-poisoned patients.

Specific References

Balit CR, Isbister GK, and Buckley NA, "Randomized Controlled Trial of Topical Aspirin in the Treatment of Bee and Wasp Stings," *J Toxicol Clin Toxicol*, 2003, 41(6):801-8.

Bhutta AT, Van Savell H, and Schexnayder SM, "Reye's Syndrome: Down but Not Out," *South Med J*, 2003, 96(1):43-5.

Boullata JI, McDonnell PJ, and Oliva CD, "Anaphylactic Reaction to a Dietary Supplement Containing Willow Bark," *Ann Pharmacother*, 2003, 37(6):832-5.

Cantrell FL, Nordt SP, and Farson-Collier M, "Low-Dose Aspirin Poisoning in a Child - How Accurate Are Existing Triage Guidelines?" *Clin Toxicol (Phila)*, 2005, 43:647.

Cull M and Vicas IM-O, "Salicylate Toxicity with Topical Exposure on Intact Skin," *Clin Toxicol*, 2005, 43:640.

Dalen JE, "Aspirin to Prevent Heart Attack and Stroke: What's the Right Dose?" *Am J Emerg Med*, 2006, 119:198-202.

Gorelick PB, Richardson D, Kelly M, et al, "Aspirin and Ticlopidine for Prevention of Recurrent Stroke in Black Patients: A Randomized Trial," *JAMA*, 2003 289(22):2947-57.

Judge BS, "Metabolic Acidosis: Differentiating the Causes in the Poisoned Patient," *Med Clin N Am*, 2005, 89(6):1107-24 (review).

Lewis TV, Schaeffer SE, Hagemann TM, et al, "Misleading Product Packaging Contributing to Salicyalte Toxicity in an Infant," *Clin Toxicol (Phila)*, 2005, 43:651.

Pena-Alonso YR, Montoya-Cabrera MA, Bustos-Cordoba E, et al, "Aspirin Intoxication in a Child Associated with Myocardial Necrosis: Is This a Drug-Related Lesion?" *Pediatr Dev Pathol*, 2003, 6(4):342-7.

Proudfoot AT, Krenzelok EP, Brent J, et al, "Does Urine Alkalinization Increase Salicylate Elimination? If So, Why?" *Toxicol Rev*, 2003, 22(3):129-36.

Proudfoot AT, Krenzelok EP, Vale JA, et al, "AACT/EAPCCT Position Paper on Urine Alkalinization," *J Toxicol Clin Toxicol*, 2004, 42(1):1-26.

Schaper A, Renneberg B, and Desel H, "Dangerous Drugs - An Analysis of 142 Fatalities Due to Poisoning in Northern Germany," *J Toxicol Clin Toxicol*, 2003, 41(5):713.

Smolinske S, Temple K, Lada P, et al, "Take Too (Many) ASA and Call Me from the Morgue," *J Toxicol Clin Toxicol*, 2004, 42(5):724.

Song W and Dou C, "One-Step Immunoassay for Acetaminophen and Salicylate in Serum, Plasma, and Whole Blood," *J Anal Toxicol*, 2003, 27(6):366-71.

Wood DM, Dargan PI, and Jones AL, "Should All Patients with Drug Overdose Have a Salicylate Level?" *J Toxicol Clin Toxicol*, 2003, 41(5):651.

Salmeterol

CAS Number 89365-50-4; 94749-08-3
U.S. Brand Names Serevent® Diskus®; Serevent® [DSC]
Synonyms Salmeterol Xinafoate
Use Maintenance treatment of asthma and in prevention of bronchospasm (inhalation aerosol in patients >12 years of age; inhalation powder in patients ≥4 years of age) with reversible obstructive airway disease, including patients with symptoms of nocturnal asthma, who require regular treatment with inhaled, short-acting beta$_2$ agonists; prevention of exercise-induced bronchospasm; maintenance treatment of bronchospasm associated with COPD
Mechanism of Action Relaxes bronchial smooth muscle by action on beta$_2$-receptors with little effect on heart rate; longer-acting than albuterol
Adverse Reactions
Cardiovascular: Tachycardia (slight), palpitations, hypertension, flushing, shortened P-R segment, lengthened QT segment, cardiac arrhythmias, sinus tachycardia, torsade de pointes
Central nervous system: **Headache**, dizziness, nervousness, CNS stimulation, hyperactivity, insomnia, mania
Dermatologic: Maculopapular rash, urticaria, pruritus
Endocrine & metabolic: Hypokalemia, hyperglycemia
Gastrointestinal: GI upset
Neuromuscular & skeletal: Tremor
Respiratory: **Pharyngitis**, bronchospasm
Pharmacodynamics/Kinetics
Onset of action: Asthma: 30-48 minutes, COPD: 2 hours
Peak effect: 2-4 hours, COPD: 3.27-4.75 hours
Duration: 12 hours
Protein binding: 96%
Metabolism: Hepatically hydroxylated
Half-life elimination: 5.5 hours
Excretion: Feces (60%), urine (25%)
Dosage
Note: Do **not** use spacer with inhalation powder
Asthma, maintenance and prevention:
Inhalation, aerosol: Children ≥12 years and Adults: 42 mcg (2 puffs) twice daily (12 hours apart)
Inhalation, powder (Serevent® Diskus®): Children ≥4 years and Adults: One inhalation (50 mcg) twice daily
Exercise-induced asthma, prevention:
Inhalation, aerosol: Children ≥12 years and Adults: 42 mcg (2 puffs) 30-60 minutes prior to exercise; additional doses should not be used for 12 hours
Inhalation, powder (Serevent® Diskus®): Children ≥4 years and Adults: One inhalation (50 mcg) at least 30 minutes prior to exercise; additional doses should not be used for 12 hours
COPD (maintenance treatment of associated bronchospasm):
Inhalation, aerosol: Adults: 42 micrograms (2 puffs) twice daily (morning and evening, 12 hours apart)
Inhalation, powder (Serevent® Diskus®): Adults: One inhalation (50 mcg) twice daily, ~12 hours apart
Stability Aerosol: Store at 15°C to 30°C (59°F to 86°F); store canister with nozzle down; shake well before each use. Protect from freezing temperature. The therapeutic effect may decrease when the canister is cold therefore the canister should remain at room temperature. Do not store at temperatures >120°F.

Inhalation powder: Store at controlled room temperature 20°C to 25°C (68°F to 77°F) in a dry place away from direct heat or sunlight. Stable for 6 weeks after removal from foil pouch.
Monitoring Parameters FEV$_1$, peak flow, and/or other pulmonary function tests; blood pressure, heart rate; CNS stimulation; serum glucose, serum potassium. Monitor for increased use of short-acting beta$_2$-agonist inhalers; may be marker of a deteriorating asthma condition.
Administration Inhalation: Shake well before use. **Not** to be used for the relief of acute attacks.
Contraindications Hypersensitivity to salmeterol, adrenergic amines, or any component of the formulation; need for acute bronchodilation
Warnings
Asthma treatment:[U.S. Boxed Warning]: Long-acting beta$_2$ agonists may increase the risk of asthma-related deaths. In a large, randomized clinical trial (SMART, 2006), salmeterol was associated with a small, but statistically significant increase in asthma-related deaths (when added to usual asthma therapy); risk may be greater in African-American patients versus Caucasians. Should only be used as adjuvant therapy in patients not adequately controlled on inhaled corticosteroids or whose disease requires two maintenance therapies. Salmeterol is not meant to relieve acute asthmatic symptoms, should not be initiated in patients with significantly worsening or acutely deteriorating asthma, and is not a substitute for inhaled or oral corticosteroids. Short-acting beta$_2$ agonist should be used for acute symptoms and symptoms occurring between treatments. Corticosteroids should not be stopped or reduced when salmeterol is initiated. During the initiation of salmeterol watch for signs of worsening asthma.
Concurrent diseases: Use caution in patients with cardiovascular disease (eg, arrhythmia, hypertension, or CHF), seizure disorders, diabetes, glaucoma, hyperthyroidism, hepatic impairment, or hypokalemia. Beta agonists may cause elevation in blood pressure, heart rate, and result in CNS stimulation/excitation. Beta$_2$ agonists may increase risk of arrhythmia, increase serum glucose, or decrease serum potassium.
Adverse events: Salmeterol should not be used more than twice daily; do not exceed recommended dose; do not use with other long-acting beta$_2$ agonists; serious adverse events including fatalities, have been associated with excessive use of inhaled sympathomimetics. Rarely, paradoxical bronchospasm may occur with use of inhaled bronchodilating agents; this should be distinguished from inadequate response. Powder for oral inhalation contains lactose; very rare anaphylactic reactions have been reported in patients with severe milk protein allergy.
Safety and efficacy have not been established in children <4 years of age.
Dosage Forms Powder for oral inhalation: 50 mcg (28s, 60s) [delivers 50 mcg/inhalation; contains lactose]
Overdosage/Treatment
Decontamination: Activated charcoal for oral ingestion
Supportive therapy: Beta-blockers can be used for hyperadrenergic signs (use with caution in patients with wheezing); mexiletine can be used to treat ventricular arrhythmia
Drug Interactions Substrate of CYP3A4 (major)
Atomoxetine: May enhance the tachycardia effect of beta$_2$-agonists.
Beta$_2$-agonists: May diminish the bradycardia effect of beta-blockers (beta$_1$ selective).
Beta-blockers (nonselective): May diminish the bronchodilator effect of beta$_2$-agonists.
CYP3A4 inhibitors: May increase the levels/effects of salmeterol. Example inhibitors include amprenavir, atazanavir, clarithromycin, delavirdine, diclofenac, fosamprenavir, imatinib, indinavir, isoniazid, itraconazole, ketoconazole, miconazole, nefazodone, nelfinavir, nicardipine, propofol, quinidine, ritonavir, and telithromycin.
Sympathomimetics: May enhance the adverse/toxic effect of salmeterol.
Pregnancy Risk Factor C
Pregnancy Implications Benefits of use should outweigh risks
Lactation Enters breast milk/use caution
Additional Information Tachyphylaxis usually does not occur

Salsalate

CAS Number 552-94-3
U.S. Brand Names Amigesic®; Disalcid® [DSC]; Mono-Gesic®; Salflex®
Synonyms Disalicylic Acid; Salicylsalicylic Acid
Use Treatment of minor pain or fever; rheumatoid arthritis, osteoarthritis, and related inflammatory conditions
Mechanism of Action Inhibits prostaglandin synthesis, acts on the hypothalamus heat-regulating center to reduce fever, blocks prostaglandin synthetase action which prevents formation of the platelet-aggregating substance thromboxane A$_2$
Adverse Reactions
Cardiovascular: Circulatory collapse, sinus tachycardia

Central nervous system: Headache, aseptic meningitis, psychosis, cognitive dysfunction, dizziness, coma, seizures, mania

Dermatologic: Rash, pruritus

Endocrine & metabolic: Hyperkalemia, anion gap metabolic acidosis, fluid retention

Gastrointestinal: **Stomach pain, dyspepsia, heartburn, nausea**, vomiting, GI bleeding, GI ulceration, constipation, diarrhea

Hematologic: Leukopenia, neutropenia, agranulocytosis, granulocytopenia, aplastic anemia (rare), platelet inhibition

Hepatic: Elevated transaminases, hepatitis (fulminant), hepatic necrosis

Otic: Ototoxicity, tinnitus

Renal: Renal failure (acute), nephrotic syndrome, chronic renal failure, albuminuria

Respiratory: Wheezing, respiratory depression

Miscellaneous: Hypersensitivity

Signs and Symptoms of Overdose Bezoars, cognitive dysfunction, drowsiness, gastritis, GI bleeding, hyperthermia, hypoglycemia, hyponatremia, nausea, nephrotic syndrome, nystagmus, ototoxicity, respiratory alkalosis, tachypnea, tinnitus, vomiting, wheezing, Severe poisoning can manifest with coma, feces discoloration (black; pink; red; tarry), hyperglycemia, hypotension, renal failure and/or hepatic failure, respiratory depression, seizures, urine discoloration (pink)

Pharmacodynamics/Kinetics

Onset of action: Therapeutic: 3-4 days of continuous dosing

Absorption: Complete from small intestine

Metabolism: Hepatically hydrolyzed to two moles of salicylic acid (active)

Half-life elimination: 7-8 hours

Excretion: Primarily urine

Dosage

Adults: Oral: 3 g/day in 2-3 divided doses

Dosing comments in renal impairment: In patients with end stage renal disease undergoing hemodialysis: 750 mg twice daily with an additional 500 mg after dialysis

Contraindications Hypersensitivity to salsalate or any component of the formulation; GI ulcer or bleeding; pregnancy (3rd trimester)

Warnings Use with caution in patients with platelet and bleeding disorders, renal dysfunction, erosive gastritis, or peptic ulcer disease, dehydration, previous nonreaction does not guarantee future safe taking of medication; do not use aspirin in children <16 years of age for chickenpox or flu symptoms due to the association with Reye's syndrome

Dosage Forms Tablet: 500 mg, 750 mg

Amigesic®: 500 mg, 750 mg

Overdosage/Treatment

Decontamination: Ipecac within 30 minutes or lavage (within 1 hour)/activated charcoal

Supportive therapy: Hypotension/dehydration can be managed with I.V. fluid therapy; acidosis should be treated with bicarbonates, seizures with benzodiazepines; antacids, blood products are indicated, as appropriate, for hemorrhage

Enhancement of elimination: Dialysis or perfusion is indicated for secondary complications, acidosis, or renal failure and not toxin removal alone; multiple dosing of activated charcoal may be effective; forced alkaline diuresis with I.V. bicarbonate to keep a urine pH >8 can hasten elimination

Test Interactions False-negative results for glucose oxidase urinary glucose tests (Clinistix®); false-positives using the cupric sulfate method (Clinitest®); also, interferes with Gerhardt test (VMA determination), 5-HIAA, xylose tolerance test, T₃, and T₄; a serum level of salicylate (by immunoassay) may underestimate salsalate levels; degradation of salsalate to salicylate can occur if specimens are allow to sit at room temperature; >1.5 g/day causes a falsely increased free thyroxine level

Drug Interactions Decreased effect with urinary alkalinizers, antacids, corticosteroids; decreased effect of uricosurics, spironolactone; ACE inhibitor effects may be decreased by concurrent therapy with NSAIDs Increased effect/toxicity of oral anticoagulants, hypoglycemics, methotrexate

Pregnancy Risk Factor C/D (3rd trimester)

Lactation Enters breast milk/contraindicated

Additional Information Does not appear to inhibit platelet aggregation; total dose (mg) multiplied by 1.4 gives aspirin equivalent dose

Saquinavir

CAS Number 127779-20-8; 149845-06-7

U.S. Brand Names Fortovase®; Invirase®

Synonyms Saquinavir Mesylate

Use Treatment of HIV infection; used in combination with at least two other antiretroviral agents

Mechanism of Action As an inhibitor of HIV protease, saquinavir prevents the cleavage of viral polyprotein precursors which are needed to generate functional proteins in and maturation of HIV-infected cells

Adverse Reactions

Protease inhibitors cause dyslipidemia which includes elevated cholesterol and triglycerides and a redistribution of body fat centrally to cause increased abdominal girth, buffalo hump, facial atrophy, and breast enlargement. These agents also cause hyperglycemia.

Cardiovascular: Chest pain, portal hypertension, syncope

Central nervous system: Anxiety, depression, fatigue, headache, insomnia, pain, ataxia, confusion, seizures

Dermatologic: Rash, verruca, bullous skin eruption, Stevens-Johnson syndrome

Endocrine & metabolic: Hyperglycemia, hypoglycemia, hyperkalemia, libido disorder, serum amylase increased, calcium increased, hypokalemia, triglycerides increased, serum phosphate decreased

Gastrointestinal: **Diarrhea, nausea**, abdominal discomfort, abdominal pain, appetite decreased, buccal mucosa ulceration, constipation, dyspepsia, flatulence, taste alteration, vomiting, pancreatitis, upper quadrant abdominal pain

Hematologic: Acute myeloblastic leukemia, hemoglobin decreased, hemolytic anemia, thrombocytopenia

Hepatic: AST increased, ALT increased, bilirubin increased, alkaline phosphatase increased, ascites, chronic liver disease exacerbation, hepatitis, cholangitis, jaundice, LFTs increased

Local: Thrombophlebitis

Neuromuscular & skeletal: Paresthesia, weakness, CPK increased, neuropathy, polyarthritis

Renal: Creatinine kinase increased

Miscellaneous: Allergic reactions

Pharmacodynamics/Kinetics

Absorption: Poor; increased with high fat meal; Fortovase® has improved absorption over Invirase®

Distribution: V_d: 700 L; does not distribute into CSF

Protein binding, plasma: ~98%

Metabolism: Extensively hepatic via CYP3A4; extensive first-pass effect

Bioavailability: Invirase®: ~4%; Fortovase®: 12% to 15%

Excretion: Feces (81% to 88%), urine (1% to 3%) within 5 days

Dosage Oral: Children ≥16 years and Adults: **Note:** Fortovase® and Invirase® are not bioequivalent and should not be used interchangeably; only Fortovase® should be used to initiate therapy:

Unboosted regimen: Fortovase®: 1200 mg (six 200 mg capsules) 3 times/day or 1600 mg twice daily within 2 hours after a meal in combination with a nucleoside analog

Note: Saquinavir hard-gel capsules (Invirase®) should not be used in "unboosted regimens."

Ritonavir-boosted regimens:

Fortovase®: 1000 mg (five 200 mg capsules) twice daily in combination with ritonavir 100 mg twice daily

Invirase®: 1000 mg (five 200 mg capsules or two 500 mg tablets) twice daily given in combination with ritonavir 100 mg twice daily. This combination should be given together and within 2 hours after a full meal in combination with a nucleoside analog.

Dosage adjustments of Fortovase® when administered in combination therapy:

Delavirdine: Fortovase® 800 mg 3 times/day

Lopinavir and ritonavir (Kaletra™): Fortovase® or Invirase® 1000 mg twice daily

Nelfinavir: Fortovase®: 1200 mg twice daily

Elderly: Clinical studies did not include sufficient numbers of patients ≥65 years of age; use caution due to increased frequency of organ dysfunction

Monitoring Parameters Monitor viral load, CD4 count, triglycerides, cholesterol, glucose

Administration Take saquinavir within 2 hours after a full meal. Avoid direct sunlight when taking saquinavir. When used with ritonavir, saquinavir and ritonavir should be administered at the same time.

Contraindications Hypersensitivity to saquinavir or any component of the formulation; exposure to direct sunlight without sunscreen or protective clothing; severe hepatic impairment; coadministration with amiodarone, bepridil, cisapride, flecainide, midazolam, pimozide, propafenone, quinidine, rifampin, triazolam, or ergot derivatives

Warnings Use caution in patients with hepatic insufficiency. May exacerbate pre-existing hepatic dysfunction; use with caution in patients with hepatitis B or C and in cirrhosis. May be associated with fat redistribution (buffalo hump, increased abdominal girth, breast engorgement, facial atrophy). Use caution in hemophilia. May increase cholesterol and/or triglycerides; hypertriglyceridemia may increase risk of pancreatitis.

Saquinavir interacts with multiple medications (including herbal products) when given concurrently; refer to Drug Interactions. **[U.S. Boxed Warning]: Fortovase® and Invirase® are not bioequivalent and should not be used interchangeably; only Fortovase® should be used to initiate therapy.** Fortovase® is recommended when saquinavir will be given as the sole protease inhibitor; Invirase® may be used only if combined with ritonavir. Safety and efficacy have not been established in children <16 years of age.

Dosage Forms Note: Strength expressed as base; [DSC] = Discontinued product

Capsule, as mesylate:

Invirase®: 200 mg [contains lactose 63.3 mg/capsule]
Capsule, soft gelatin, as base:
Fortovase®: 200 mg [DSC]
Tablet, as mesylate:
Invirase®: 500 mg

Reference Range Peak serum saquinavir levels after a 600 mg oral dose and 12 mg I.V. dose: ~66 ng/mL and 87 ng/mL, respectively

Overdosage/Treatment
Decontamination: Activated charcoal
Enhanced elimination: Multiple dosing of activated charcoal may be beneficial

Drug Interactions Substrate of CYP2D6 (minor), 3A4 (major); **Inhibits** CYP2C9 (weak), 2C19 (weak), 2D6 (weak), 3A4 (moderate)

Antiarrhythmics: Serum levels/toxicity may be increased by saquinavir; serious and/or life-threatening reactions may occur. Concurrent use with amiodarone, bepridil, flecainide, propafenone, or quinidine is contraindicated. Use caution with systemic lidocaine.

Anticonvulsants: Saquinavir serum concentrations may be decreased by carbamazepine, phenobarbital, or phenytoin; use with caution.

Azole antifungals (itraconazole, ketoconazole): Serum concentrations of saquinavir may be increased. Dose adjustment was not needed at the study dose when used for a limited time (ketoconazole 400 mg once daily and Fortovase® 1200 mg 3 times daily).

Benzodiazepines: An increase in midazolam and triazolam serum levels may occur resulting in significant over sedation when administered with saquinavir. Concurrent use is contraindicated. A decreased dose may be considered when used with alprazolam, clorazepate, diazepam, or flurazepam.

Calcium channel blockers: Use with caution; serum concentrations of calcium channel blockers may be increased.

Cisapride: Saquinavir inhibits the metabolism of cisapride and should not be administered concurrently due to risk of life-threatening cardiac arrhythmias.

Clarithromycin: Serum concentrations of saquinavir and clarithromycin may both be increased. Dose adjustment not was not needed at the study dose when used for 7 days (clarithromycin 500 mg twice daily and Fortovase® 1200 mg 3 times/day); dosage adjustment of clarithromycin is recommended in patients with renal impairment.

Corticosteroids: Dexamethasone may decrease serum concentrations of saquinavir; use with caution.

CYP3A4 inducers: CYP3A4 inducers may decrease the levels/effects of saquinavir. Example inducers include aminoglutethimide, carbamazepine, nafcillin, nevirapine, phenobarbital, phenytoin, and rifamycins.

CYP3A4 substrates: Saquinavir may increase the levels/effects of CYP3A4 substrates. Example substrates include benzodiazepines, calcium channel blockers, cyclosporine, mirtazapine, nateglinide, nefazodone, sildenafil (and other PDE-5 inhibitors), tacrolimus, and venlafaxine. Selected benzodiazepines (midazolam and triazolam), cisapride, ergot alkaloids, selected HMG-CoA reductase inhibitors (lovastatin and simvastatin), and pimozide are generally contraindicated with strong CYP3A4 inhibitors.

Ergot alkaloids (dihydroergotamine, ergonovine, ergotamine and methylergonovine): Serum levels/toxicity may be increased by saquinavir; serious and/or life-threatening reactions may occur; concurrent use is contraindicated.

HMG-CoA reductase inhibitors: Saquinavir increased serum concentrations of simvastatin, lovastatin, and atorvastatin; risk of myopathy/rhabdomyolysis may be increased. Avoid use with simvastatin and lovastatin. Use caution with atorvastatin and cerivastatin (fluvastatin, pravastatin, and rosuvastatin are not appreciably metabolized by CYP3A4).

Immunosuppressants: Saquinavir may increase the serum levels of cyclosporine, sirolimus, or tacrolimus.

Methadone: Serum concentrations of methadone may be decreased; an increased dose may be needed when administered with saquinavir

Non-nucleoside reverse transcriptase inhibitors: Saquinavir serum concentrations may be increased by delavirdine. Serum levels of saquinavir and efavirenz may be decreased with concurrent use; saquinavir should not be used as the sole protease inhibitor with efavirenz or nevirapine.

Oral contraceptives: Serum levels of the hormones in oral contraceptives may decrease significantly with administration of saquinavir. Patients should use alternative methods of contraceptives during saquinavir therapy.

PDE-5 inhibitors: Serum concentrations may be increased by saquinavir; dosing adjustment is required. Limit sildenafil dose to 25 mg/48 hours. The maximum dose of tadalafil is 10 mg/72 hours. Vardenafil dosing should not exceed 2.5 mg/24 hours.

Pimozide: Serum levels/toxicity may be increased by saquinavir; serious and/or life-threatening reactions may occur; concurrent use is contraindicated.

Protease inhibitors: Atazanavir, indinavir, and ritonavir may increase serum levels of saquinavir. Serum levels of saquinavir and nelfinavir may be increased with concurrent use. Lopinavir/ritonavir (combination product) may increase serum levels of saquinavir. Refer to Dosage section. Dosage adjustment recommendations with atazanavir have not been established.

Rifabutin: Serum concentrations of saquinavir are decreased and levels of rifabutin are increased. Saquinavir should not be used as the sole protease inhibitor when given with rifabutin.

Rifampin: Serum concentrations of saquinavir are markedly decreased. Risk of hepatotoxicity is increased with concurrent use of ritonavir-boosted saquinavir therapy. Concurrent use is contraindicated.

Tricyclic antidepressants: Serum concentrations of amitriptyline and imipramine may be increased; monitor.

Warfarin: Serum concentrations of warfarin may be affected; monitor.

Pregnancy Risk Factor B

Pregnancy Implications Preliminary data show that saquinavir pharmacokinetics may be affected by pregnancy; studies are not yet complete. Pregnancy and protease inhibitors are both associated with an increased risk of hyperglycemia. Glucose levels should be closely monitored. Health professionals are encouraged to contact the antiretroviral pregnancy registry to monitor outcomes of pregnant women exposed to antiretroviral medications (1-800-258-4263).

Lactation Excretion in breast milk unknown/contraindicated

Nursing Implications Observe for signs of opportunistic infections and other illnesses associated with HIV; administer on a full stomach, if possible

Additional Information A high-fat meal maximizes bioavailability. Saquinavir levels may increase if taken with grapefruit juice. Saquinavir serum concentrations may be decreased by St John's wort; avoid concurrent use. Garlic capsules may decrease saquinavir serum concentrations; avoid use if saquinavir is the only protease inhibitor.

Scopolamine

Related Information
● Therapeutic Drugs Associated with Hallucinations

CAS Number 114-49-8; 51-34-3; 6533-68-2

U.S. Brand Names Isopto® Hyoscine; Scopace™; Transderm Scōp®

Synonyms Hyoscine Butylbromide; Hyoscine Hydrobromide; Scopolamine Butylbromide; Scopolamine Hydrobromide

Impairment Potential Yes

Use Preoperative medication to produce amnesia and decrease salivation and respiratory secretions to produce cycloplegia and mydriasis; treatment of iridocyclitis, prevention of nausea and vomiting by motion; produces more CNS depression, mydriasis, and cycloplegia but less effective in preventing reflex bradycardia and effecting the intestines than atropine

Mechanism of Action Blocks the action of acetylcholine at parasympathetic sites in smooth muscle, secretory glands and the CNS; increases cardiac output, dries secretions, antagonizes histamine and serotonin; a tropane alkaloid

Adverse Reactions
Cardiovascular: Tachycardia, palpitations, sinus tachycardia, tachycardia (supraventricular), sinus bradycardia
Central nervous system: Disorientation, drowsiness, hallucinations, confusion, anxiety, psychosis, delirium, electroencephalogram abnormalities, amnesia, lilliputian hallucinations, mania, paranoia
Dermatologic: **Dry skin**
Gastrointestinal: **Xerostomia, dry throat, constipation**
Genitourinary: Urinary retention
Local: **Irritation at injection site**
Ocular: **Blurred vision, photophobia**, cycloplegia, mydriasis, increased intraocular pressure, esotropia
Respiratory: **Dry nose**
Miscellaneous: **Diaphoresis (decreased)**, anaphylactoid reactions, allergic reactions
Note: Systemic adverse effects have been reported with both the topical and ophthalmic preparations

Signs and Symptoms of Overdose Bradycardia, bronchospasm, coma, confusion, delirium, dementia, dysuria, hypertension, hyperthermia, increased intraocular pressure, memory loss, mydriasis, photophobia, seizures, tachycardia, visual hallucinations

Pharmacodynamics/Kinetics
Onset of action: Oral, I.M.: 0.5-1 hour; I.V.: 10 minutes
Peak effect: 20-60 minutes; may take 3-7 days for full recovery; transdermal: 24 hours
Duration: Oral, I.M.: 4-6 hours; I.V.: 2 hours
Absorption: Tertiary salts (hydrobromide) are well absorbed; quaternary salts (butylbromide) are poorly absorbed (local concentrations in the GI tract following oral dosing may be high)
Metabolism: Hepatic
Half-life elimination: 4.8 hours
Excretion: Urine (as metabolites)

Dosage
Preoperatively:
Children: I.M., SubQ: 6 mcg/kg/dose (maximum: 0.3 mg/dose) or 0.2 mg/m² may be repeated every 6-8 hours **or** alternatively:

4-7 months: 0.1 mg
7 months to 3 years: 0.15 mg
3-8 years: 0.2 mg
8-12 years: 0.3 mg
Adults:
I.M., I.V., SubQ: 0.3-0.65 mg; may be repeated every 4-6 hours
Transdermal patch: Apply 2.5 cm² patch to hairless area behind ear the night before surgery or 1 hour prior to cesarean section (the patch should be applied no sooner than 1 hour before surgery for best results and removed 24 hours after surgery)
Motion sickness: Transdermal: Children >12 years and Adults: Apply 1 disc behind the ear at least 4 hours prior to exposure and every 3 days as needed; effective if applied as soon as 2-3 hours before anticipated need, best if 12 hours before
Ophthalmic:
Refraction:
Children: Instill 1 drop of 0.25% to eye(s) twice daily for 2 days before procedure
Adults: Instill 1-2 drops of 0.25% to eye(s) 1 hour before procedure
Iridocyclitis:
Children: Instill 1 drop of 0.25% to eye(s) up to 3 times/day
Adults: Instill 1-2 drops of 0.25% to eye(s) up to 4 times/day
Parkinsonism, spasticity, motion sickness: Oral: 0.4-0.8 mg as a range; the dosage may be cautiously increased in parkinsonism and spastic states.
Gastrointestinal/genitourinary spasm (Buscopan® [available in Canada; not available in the U.S.]): Adults:
Oral: 10-20 mg daily (1-2 tablets); maximum: 6 tablets/day
I.M., I.V., SubQ: 10-20 mg; maximum: 100 mg/day

Stability Avoid acid solutions, because hydrolysis occurs at pH <3

Administration When giving I.V., must first be diluted with sterile water for injection

Contraindications Hypersensitivity to scopolamine or any component of the formulation; narrow-angle glaucoma; acute hemorrhage; paralytic ileus, GI or GU obstruction; thyrotoxicosis; tachycardia secondary to cardiac insufficiency; myasthenia gravis

Warnings Use with caution with hepatic or renal impairment since adverse CNS effects occur more often in these patients; use with caution in infants and children since they may be more susceptible to adverse effects of scopolamine; use with caution in patients with GI obstruction, prostatic hyperplasia (nonobstructive), or urinary retention. Discontinue if patient reports unusual visual disturbances or pain within the eye. Use caution in hiatal hernia, reflux esophagitis, and ulcerative colitis. Scopolamine (hyoscine) hydrobromide should not be interchanged with scopolamine butylbromide formulations; dosages are not equivalent. Transdermal patch may contain conducting metal (eg, aluminum); remove patch prior to MRI.

Dosage Forms [CAN] = Canadian brand name
Injection, solution, as hydrobromide: 0.4 mg/mL (1 mL)
Injection, solution, as hyoscine-N-butylbromide:
Buscopan® [CAN]: 20 mg/mL [not available in U.S.]
Solution, ophthalmic, as hydrobromide:
Isopto® Hyoscine: 0.25% (5 mL, 15 mL) [contains benzalkonium chloride]
Tablet, as hyoscine-N-butylbromide:
Buscopan® [CAN]: 10 mg [not available in U.S.]
Tablet, soluble, as hydrobromide:
Maldemar™, Scopace™: 0.4 mg
Transdermal system:
Transderm Scōp®: 1.5 mg (4s, 10s, 24s) [releases ~1 mg over 72 hours]

Reference Range Serum level of 890 pg/mL (SI: 7.93 nmol/L) correlated with psychosis

Overdosage/Treatment
Decontamination: Activated charcoal
Supportive therapy: Physostigmine can be utilized in life-threatening anticholinergic symptoms and has been used to treat paranoia and agitated states; seizures can be treated with diazepam, lorazepam, phenobarbital, or phenytoin
Enhancement of elimination: Multiple dosing of activated charcoal may be useful

Antidote(s)
● Physostigmine [ANTIDOTE]

Drug Interactions Anticholinergic agents: Adverse anticholinergic effects may be additive with other anticholinergic agents (includes tricyclic antidepressants, antihistamines, and phenothiazines).
CNS depressants: Sedative effects may be additive with scopolamine; use caution.

Pregnancy Risk Factor C

Pregnancy Implications Can cause neonatal drowsiness and tachycardia

Lactation Enters breast milk/use caution (AAP rates "compatible")

Nursing Implications Topical disc is programmed to deliver in vivo 0.5 mg over 3 days; wash hands before and after applying the disc to avoid drug contact with eyes

Additional Information Used as a chemical submissive agent in South America

Secobarbital

CAS Number 76-73-3
U.S. Brand Names Seconal®
Synonyms Quinalbarbitone Sodium; Secobarbital Sodium
Impairment Potential Yes. A 200 mg dose results in driving impairment. (O'Hanlon JF, "Driving Performance Under the Influence of Drugs: Rationale for, and Application of, a New Test," *Br J Clin Pharmacol*, 1984, 18(Suppl 1): 121S-9S.)
Use Short-term treatment of insomnia and as preanesthetic agent
Mechanism of Action Interferes with transmission of impulses from the thalamus to the cortex of the brain resulting in an imbalance in central inhibitory and facilitatory mechanisms
Adverse Reactions
Cardiovascular: Hypotension, cardiac arrhythmias, bradycardia, sinus bradycardia
Central nervous system: **Drowsiness, dizziness, lightheadedness, hangover effect**, impaired judgment, CNS stimulation or CNS depression, hypothermia, electroencephalogram abnormalities
Dermatologic: Rash, mucosal ulcerations, bullous eruptions, exfoliative dermatitis, erythema nodosum
Gastrointestinal: Nausea, vomiting
Local: **Pain at injection site**, arterial spasm and gangrene with inadvertent intra-arterial injection; thrombophlebitis with I.V. use
Renal: Oliguria
Respiratory: Laryngospasm, respiratory depression, apnea (especially with rapid I.V. use)
Miscellaneous: Acute atraumatic compartment syndrome
Signs and Symptoms of Overdose CNS depression, confusion, fever, jaundice, hypotension, hypothermia, myasthenia gravis (exacerbation or precipitation), nystagmus, possible bezoars, ptosis, unsteady gait, slurred speech, vision color changes (green tinge)
Pharmacodynamics/Kinetics
Onset of hypnosis: 15-30 minutes
Duration: 3-4 hours with 100 mg dose
Distribution: 1.5 L/kg; crosses the placenta; appears in breast milk
Protein binding: 45% to 60%
Metabolism: Hepatic, by microsomal enzyme system
Half-life elimination: 15-40 hours, mean: 28 hours
Time to peak, serum: Within 2-4 hours
Excretion: Urine (as inactive metabolites, small amounts as unchanged drug)
Dosage
Children:
Hypnotic: I.M.: 3-5 mg/kg/dose; maximum: 100 mg/dose
Preoperative sedation:
Oral: 50-100 mg 1-2 hours before procedure
Rectal: 5 mg/kg **or** <6 months: 30-60 mg; 6 months to 3 years: 60 mg; >3 years: 60-120 mg
Sedation: Oral: 6 mg/kg/day divided every 8 hours
Adults:
Hypnotic:
Oral, I.M.: 100-200 mg/dose
I.V.: 50-250 mg/dose
Preoperative sedation: Oral: 100-300 mg 1-2 hours before procedure
Sedation: Oral: 20-40 mg/dose 2-3 times/day
Fatal dose: 2-3 g
Stability Do not shake vial during reconstitution, rotate ampul; aqueous solutions are not stable reconstitute with aqueous polyethylene glycol; aqueous (sterile water) solutions should be used within 30 minutes; do not use bacteriostatic water for injection or lactated Ringer's; precipitates when used in solution with cimetidine
Monitoring Parameters Blood pressure, heart rate, respiratory rate, CNS status
Contraindications Hypersensitivity to barbiturates or any component of the formulation; marked hepatic impairment; dyspnea or airway obstruction; porphyria; pregnancy
Warnings Should be used only after evaluation of potential causes of sleep disturbance. Failure of sleep disturbance to resolve after 7-10 days may indicate psychiatric or medical illness. Potential for drug dependency exists, abrupt cessation may precipitate withdrawal, including status epilepticus in epileptic patients. Do not administer to patients in acute pain. Use caution in elderly, debilitated, renally impaired, or pediatric patients. May cause paradoxical responses, including agitation and hyperactivity, particularly in acute pain and pediatric patients. Use with caution in patients with depression or suicidal tendencies, or in patients with a history of drug abuse. Tolerance, psychological and physical dependence may occur with prolonged use. Use with caution in patients with hepatic function impairment. May cause CNS depression, which may impair physical or mental abilities. Patients must cautioned about performing tasks which require mental alertness (eg, operating machinery

or driving). Effects with other sedative drugs or ethanol may be potentiated. May cause respiratory depression or hypotension, Use with caution in hemodynamically unstable patients or patients with respiratory disease.

Dosage Forms Capsule, as sodium: 100 mg

Reference Range

Therapeutic (serum): 3-5 mcg/mL (SI: 12.6-21.0 μmol/L)

Toxic (serum): >5 mcg/mL (SI: >21.0 μmol/L)

Lethal (serum): ≥20 mcg/mL (SI: >84 μmol/L)

In the postmortem state, anatomical site concentration differences (ie, postmortem redistribution) may occur.

Overdosage/Treatment

Decontamination: Lavage (within 1 hour)/activated charcoal

Supportive therapy: If hypotension occurs, administer I.V. fluids and place the patient in the Trendelenburg position. If unresponsive, an I.V. vasopressor (eg, dopamine, epinephrine) may be required.

Enhancement of elimination: Forced alkaline diuresis is of no value in the treatment of intoxications with short-acting barbiturates. Charcoal hemoperfusion may be useful in the harder to treat intoxications, especially in the presence of very high serum barbiturate levels. Hemodialysis is less useful; slightly dialyzable (5% to 20%); hemoperfusion clearance ranges from 20-119 mL/minute; fractional removal of secobarbital by hemoperfusion is ~16% in 4 hours (as compared to 1% in 4 hours with hemodialysis)

Drug Interactions

Induces CYP2A6 (strong), 2C8 (strong), 2C9 (strong)

Acetaminophen: Barbiturates may enhance the hepatotoxic potential of acetaminophen overdoses

Antiarrhythmics: Barbiturates may increase the metabolism of antiarrhythmics, decreasing their clinical effect; includes disopyramide, propafenone, and quinidine

Anticonvulsants: Barbiturates may increase the metabolism of anticonvulsants; includes ethosuximide, felbamate (possibly), lamotrigine, phenytoin, tiagabine, topiramate, and zonisamide; does not appear to affect gabapentin or levetiracetam

Antineoplastics: Limited evidence suggests that enzyme-inducing anticonvulsant therapy may reduce the effectiveness of some chemotherapy regimens (specifically in ALL); teniposide and methotrexate may be cleared more rapidly in these patients

Antipsychotics: Barbiturates may enhance the metabolism (decrease the efficacy) of antipsychotics; monitor for altered response; dose adjustment may be needed

Beta-blockers: Metabolism of beta-blockers may be increased and clinical effect decreased; atenolol and nadolol are unlikely to interact given their renal elimination

Calcium channel blockers: Barbiturates may enhance the metabolism of calcium channel blockers, decreasing their clinical effect

Chloramphenicol: Barbiturates may increase the metabolism of chloramphenicol and chloramphenicol may inhibit barbiturate metabolism; monitor for altered response

Cimetidine: Barbiturates may enhance the metabolism of cimetidine, decreasing its clinical effect

CNS depressants: Sedative effects and/or respiratory depression with barbiturates may be additive with other CNS depressants; monitor for increased effect; includes ethanol, sedatives, antidepressants, narcotic analgesics, and benzodiazepines

Corticosteroids: Barbiturates may enhance the metabolism of corticosteroids, decreasing their clinical effect

Cyclosporine: Levels may be decreased by barbiturates; monitor

CYP2A6 substrates: Secobarbital may decrease the levels/effects of CYP2A6 substrates. Example substrates include ifosfamide and rifampin.

CYP2C8 Substrates: Secobarbital may decrease the levels/effects of CYP2C8 substrates. Example substrates include amiodarone, paclitaxel, pioglitazone, repaglinide, and rosiglitazone.

CYP2C9 Substrates: Secobarbital may decrease the levels/effects of CYP2C9 substrates. Example substrates include bosentan, celecoxib, dapsone, fluoxetine, glimepiride, glipizide, losartan, montelukast, nateglinide, paclitaxel, phenytoin, sulfonamides, trimethoprim, warfarin, and zafirlukast.

Doxycycline: Barbiturates may enhance the metabolism of doxycycline, decreasing its clinical effect; higher dosages may be required

Estrogens: Barbiturates may increase the metabolism of estrogens and reduce their efficacy

Felbamate may inhibit the metabolism of barbiturates and barbiturates may increase the metabolism of felbamate

Griseofulvin: Barbiturates may impair the absorption of griseofulvin, and griseofulvin metabolism may be increased by barbiturates, decreasing clinical effect

Guanfacine: Effect may be decreased by barbiturates

Immunosuppressants: Barbiturates may enhance the metabolism of immunosuppressants, decreasing its clinical effect; includes both cyclosporine and tacrolimus

Loop diuretics: Metabolism may be increased and clinical effects decreased; established for furosemide, effect with other loop diuretics not established

MAO inhibitors: Metabolism of barbiturates may be inhibited, increasing clinical effect or toxicity of the barbiturates

Methadone: Barbiturates may enhance the metabolism of methadone resulting in methadone withdrawal

Methoxyflurane: Barbiturates may enhance the nephrotoxic effects of methoxyflurane

Oral contraceptives: Barbiturates may enhance the metabolism of oral contraceptives, decreasing their clinical effect; an alternative method of contraception should be considered

Theophylline: Barbiturates may increase metabolism of theophylline derivatives and decrease their clinical effect

Tricyclic antidepressants: Barbiturates may increase metabolism of tricyclic antidepressants and decrease their clinical effect; sedative effects may be additive

Valproic acid: Metabolism of barbiturates may be inhibited by valproic acid; monitor for excessive sedation; a dose reduction may be needed

Warfarin: Barbiturates inhibit the hypoprothrombinemic effects of oral anticoagulants via increased metabolism; this combination should generally be avoided

Pregnancy Risk Factor D

Pregnancy Implications Crosses the placenta

Lactation Enters breast milk/use caution (AAP rates "compatible")

Nursing Implications I.V.: Give undiluted or diluted with sterile water for injection, normal saline, or Ringer's injection; maximum infusion rate: 50 mg/15 seconds

Selegiline

CAS Number 14611-51-9; 2079-54-1

U.S. Brand Names Eldepryl®

Synonyms Deprenyl; L-Deprenyl; Selegiline Hydrochloride

Use Adjunct in the management of parkinsonian patients in which levodopa/carbidopa therapy is deteriorating

Unlabeled/Investigational Use Early Parkinson's disease; attention-deficit/hyperactivity disorder (ADHD); negative symptoms of schizophrenia; extrapyramidal symptoms; Alzheimer's disease (studies have shown some improvement in behavioral and cognitive performance)

Mechanism of Action Potent monoamine oxidase (MAO) type-B inhibitor; MAO-B plays a major role in the metabolism of dopamine; selegiline may also increase dopaminergic activity by interfering with dopamine reuptake at the synapse

Adverse Reactions

Cardiovascular: Hypotension (orthostatic), arrhythmias, hypertension, tachycardia, angina, syncope, hypotension, chest pain, palpitations, vasoconstriction

Central nervous system: **Mood changes, dizziness, dyskinesias** (13%), confusion, CNS depression, insomnia, agitation, loss of balance, psychosis, visual hallucinations

Dermatologic: Hypertrichosis, photosensitivity

Endocrine & metabolic: Hyperprolactinemia

Gastrointestinal: **Nausea, vomiting, xerostomia, abdominal pain,** anorexia

Genitourinary: Urinary retention, nocturia

Neuromuscular & skeletal: **Dyskinesias,** involuntary movements (increased), bradykinesia, muscle twitches, paresthesia

Ocular: Blurred vision

Miscellaneous: Bruxism

Admission Criteria/Prognosis Admit any symptomatic patient or ingestion >20 mg

Pharmacodynamics/Kinetics

Onset of action: Therapeutic: Oral: Within 1 hour

Duration: Oral: 24-72 hours

Absorption:

Orally disintegrating tablet: Rapid; greater bioavailability than capsule/tablet

Transdermal: 25% to 30% (of total selegiline content) over 24 hours

Protein binding: ~90%

Metabolism: Hepatic, primarily via CYP2B6 to active (N-desmethylselegiline, amphetamine, methamphetamine) and inactive metabolites

Half-life elimination: Oral: 10 hours; Transdermal: 18-25 hours

Excretion: Urine (primarily metabolites); feces

Dosage

Oral:

Children and Adolescents: ADHD (unlabeled use): 5-15 mg/day

Adults: Parkinson's disease: 5 mg twice daily with breakfast and lunch or 10 mg in the morning

Elderly: Parkinson's disease: Initial: 5 mg in the morning, may increase to a total of 10 mg/day

Monitoring Parameters Blood pressure, symptoms of parkinsonism

Administration Oral: Orally disintegrating tablet (Zelapar™): Take in morning before breakfast; place on top of tongue and allow to dissolve. Avoid food or liquid 5 minutes before and after administration.

Topical: Transdermal (Emsam®): Apply to clean, dry, intact skin to the upper torso (below the neck and above the waist), upper thigh, or outer surface of the upper arm. Avoid exposure of application site to external heat source, which may increase the amount of drug absorbed. Apply at the same time each day and rotate application sites. Wash hands with soap and water after handling. Avoid touching the sticky side of the patch.

Contraindications Hypersensitivity to selegiline or any component of the formulation; concomitant use of meperidine

Orally disintegrating tablet: Additional contraindications: Concomitant use of dextromethorphan, methadone, propoxyphene, tramadol, oral selegiline, other MAO inhibitors

Transdermal: Additional contraindications: Pheochromocytoma; concomitant use of bupropion, selective or dual serotonin reuptake inhibitors (including SSRIs and SNRIs), tricyclic antidepressants, buspirone, tramadol, propoxyphene, methadone, dextromethorphan, St. John's wort, mirtazapine, cyclobenzaprine, oral selegiline and other MAO inhibitors; carbamazepine, and oxcarbazepine; elective surgery requiring general anesthesia, local anesthesia containing sympathomimetic vasoconstrictors; sympathomimetics (and related compounds); foods high in tyramine content; supplements containing tyrosine, phenylalanine, tryptophan, or caffeine

Warnings

Oral: MAO-B selective inhibition should not pose a problem with tyramine-containing products as long as the typical oral doses are employed, however, rare reactions have been reported. Increased risk of nonselective MAO inhibition occurs with oral capsule/tablet doses >10 mg/day or orally disintegrating tablet doses >2.5 mg/day. Use of oral selegiline with tricyclic antidepressants and SSRIs has also been associated with rare reactions and should generally be avoided. Addition to levodopa therapy may result in exacerbation of levodopa adverse effects, requiring a reduction in levodopa dosage.

Transdermal: Nonselective MAO inhibition occurs with transdermal delivery and is necessary for antidepressant efficacy. Hypertensive crisis as a result of ingesting tyramine-rich foods is always a concern with nonselective MAO inhibition. Although transdermal delivery minimizes inhibition of MAO-A in the gut, there is limited data with higher transdermal doses; dietary restrictions are recommended with doses >6 mg/24hours. Monitor for worsening of depression, suicidality and/or associated behaviors such as anxiety, agitation, panic attacks, insomnia, irritability, hostility, impulsivity, hypomania, and mania; worsening depression and severe abrupt suicidality that are not part of the presenting symptoms may require discontinuation or modification of drug therapy. Use caution in high-risk patients during initiation of therapy; prescriptions should be written for the smallest quantity. The patient's family or caregiver should be alerted to monitor patients for the emergence of suicidality and associated behaviors such as anxiety, agitation, panic attacks, insomnia, irritability, hostility, impulsivity, akathisia, hypomania, and mania; patients should be instructed to notify their healthcare provider if any of these symptoms or worsening depression occur.

Transdermal selegiline may worsen psychosis in some patients or precipitate a shift to mania or hypomania in patients with bipolar disorder. Monotherapy in patients with bipolar disorder should be avoided. Patients presenting with depressive symptoms should be screened for bipolar disorder. Selegiline is not FDA approved for the treatment of bipolar depression. **[U.S. Boxed Warning]: Antidepressants increase the risk of suicidal thinking and behavior in children and adolescents with major depressive disorder (MDD) and other depressive disorders. Selegiline is not FDA approved for use in children.**

Should not be used in combination with other antidepressants. Do not use within 5 weeks of fluoxetine discontinuation or 1 week of other antidepressant discontinuation. Wait 2 weeks after discontinuing transdermal selegiline before initiating therapy with buspirone or any other contraindicated drug. May cause orthostatic hypotension - use with caution in patients with hypotension or patients who would not tolerate transient hypotensive episodes (cardiovascular or cerebrovascular disease) - effects may be additive with other agents which cause orthostasis. Discontinue at least 10 days prior to elective surgery. Use with caution in renal and hepatic impairment.

Medication should not be stopped abruptly; taper off as rapidly as possible. Safety and efficacy in children <16 years of age have not been established.

Dosage Forms Capsule, as hydrochloride: 5 mg

Eldepryl®: 5 mg

Tablet, as hydrochloride: 5 mg

Tablet, orally-disintegrating:

Zelapar™: 1.25 mg [contains phenylalanine 1.25 mg/tablet]

Transdermal system [once-daily patch]:

Emsam®: 6 mg/24 hours (30s); 9 mg/24 hours (30s); 12 mg/24 hours (30s)

Reference Range Postmortem blood methamphetamine level following a 60 mg ingestion ranged from 0.17-0.28 mcg/mL

Overdosage/Treatment

Decontamination: **Do not** induce emesis; lavage (within 1 hour)/activated charcoal is useful

Supportive therapy: Competent supportive care is the most important treatment for an overdose with a monoamine oxidase (MAO) inhibitor. Both hypertension or hypotension can occur with intoxication. Hypotension may respond to I.V. fluids or vasopressors and hypertension usually responds to an alpha-adrenergic blocker. While treating the hypertension, care is warranted to avoid sudden drops in blood pressure, since this may worsen the MAO inhibitor toxicity. Muscle irritability and seizures often respond to diazepam or lorazepam, while hyperthermia is best treated antipyretics and cooling blankets. Cardiac arrhythmias are best treated with phenytoin or procainamide. Hypertensive crisis can be treated with nitroprusside, phentolamine (2-10 mg slow I.V. injection in adults), diazoxide (50-100 mg I.V.) or oral nifedipine (10 mg). Dantrolene (2.5 mg/kg every 6 hours I.V.) can be used to treat hypermetabolic crisis. Hypertensive crisis can be treated with nitroprusside, phentolamine (2-10 mg slow I.V. injection in adults), diazoxide (50-100 mg I.V.) or oral nifedipine (10 mg); dantrolene (2.5 mg/kg every 6 hours I.V.) can be used to treat hypermetabolic crisis. Avoid phenothiazines.

Drug Interactions Substrate of CYP1A2 (minor), 2A6 (minor), 2B6 (major), 2C8 (minor), 2C19 (minor), 2D6 (minor), 3A4 (minor); **Inhibits** CYP1A2 (weak), 2A6 (weak), 2C9 (weak), 2C19 (weak), 2D6 (weak), 2E1 (weak), 3A4 (weak)

Note: Many drug interactions involving selegiline are theoretical, primarily based on interactions with nonspecific MAO inhibitors; at oral (capsule/tablet) doses <10 mg/day and orally disintegrating tablet doses <2.5 mg, the risk of these interactions with selegiline may be very low. Transdermal selegiline results in higher plasma levels and nonselective MAO inhibition.

Amphetamines: MAO inhibitors in combination with amphetamines may result in severe hypertensive reaction or serotonin syndrome; these combinations are best avoided (contraindicated with transdermal selegiline).

Anorexiants: Concurrent use of selegiline (high dose) in combination with CNS stimulants or anorexiants may result in serotonin syndrome; these combinations are best avoided; includes dexfenfluramine, fenfluramine, or sibutramine

Atomoxetine: MAO inhibitors may increase the toxicity of atomoxetine; avoid concomitant use.

Barbiturates: MAO inhibitors may inhibit the metabolism of barbiturates and prolong their effect

Bupropion: MAO inhibitors may increase the toxicity of bupropion; avoid concomitant use.

Buspirone: Concomitant use with selegiline may cause increased blood pressure; avoid combination.

Carbamazepine: May increase levels/effects of selegiline; concomitant use of transdermal selegiline is contraindicated.

CNS stimulants: MAO inhibitors in combination with stimulants (methylphenidate, dexmethylphenidate) may result in serotonin syndrome; these combinations are best avoided (contraindicated with transdermal selegiline).

COMT inhibitors (eg, entacapone, tolcapone): May increase to toxicity of MAO inhibitors; avoid concomitant use.

CYP2B6 inducers: May decrease the levels/effects of selegiline. Example inducers include carbamazepine, nevirapine, phenobarbital, phenytoin, and rifampin.

CYP2B6 inhibitors: May increase the levels/effects of selegiline. Example inhibitors include desipramine, paroxetine, and sertraline.

Dextromethorphan: Concurrent use of selegiline (high dose) may result in serotonin syndrome; these combinations are best avoided (contraindicated with transdermal and orally disintegrating tablet selegiline).

Disulfiram: MAO inhibitors may produce delirium in patients receiving disulfiram; monitor.

False neurotransmitters (eg, guanadrel and guanethidine): MAO inhibitors inhibit the antihypertensive response to guanadrel or guanethidine; use an alternative antihypertensive agent.

Hypoglycemic agents: MAO inhibitors may produce hypoglycemia in patients with diabetes; monitor.

Levodopa: MAO inhibitors in combination with levodopa may result in hypertensive reactions; monitor.

Lithium: MAO inhibitors in combination with lithium have resulted in malignant hyperpyrexia; this combination is best avoided.

Meperidine: Use with selegiline (high dose) may result in serotonin syndrome; concurrent use contraindicated.

Methadone: Concomitant use with an MAO inhibitor may increase the risk of serotonin syndrome (contraindicated with transdermal and orally disintegrating tablet selegiline).

Mirtazapine, nefazodone: Concurrent use of selegiline (high dose) may result in serotonin syndrome; these combinations are best avoided (contraindicated with transdermal selegiline).

Norepinephrine: MAO inhibitors may increase the pressor response of norepinephrine (effect is generally small); monitor (contraindicated with transdermal selegiline).

Oral contraceptives: Increased selegiline levels have been noted with concurrent administration; monitor

Propoxyphene: Concomitant use with an MAO inhibitor may increase the risk of serotonin syndrome (contraindicated with transdermal and orally disintegrating tablet selegiline).

Reserpine: MAO inhibitors in combination with reserpine may result in hypertensive reactions; monitor.

Sibutramine: May cause serotonin syndrome when combined with an MAO inhibitor; avoid this combination.

SSRIs/SNRIs: Concurrent use of selegiline with a selective serotonin or serotonin/norepinephrine reuptake inhibitor may result in mania or hypertension. It is generally best to avoid these combinations (contraindicated with transdermal selegiline).

St John's wort: May cause serotonin syndrome when combined with an MAO inhibitor; avoid this combination.

Sympathomimetics (indirect-acting): MAO inhibitors in combination with sympathomimetics such as dopamine, metaraminol, phenylephrine, and decongestants (pseudoephedrine) may result in severe hypertensive reaction; these combinations are best avoided (contraindicated with transdermal selegiline).

Tramadol: May increase the risk of seizures and serotonin syndrome in patients receiving an MAO inhibitor (contraindicated with transdermal and orally disintegrating tablet selegiline).

Trazodone: Concurrent use of selegiline (high dose) may result in serotonin syndrome; these combinations are best avoided.

Tricyclic antidepressants: May cause serotonin syndrome when combined with an MAO inhibitor; avoid this combination (contraindicated with transdermal selegiline).

Venlafaxine: Concurrent use of selegiline (high dose) may result in serotonin syndrome; these combinations are best avoided (contraindicated with transdermal selegiline).

Pregnancy Risk Factor C

Pregnancy Implications Teratogenic and adverse behavioral events were noted in animal studies. There are no adequate and well-controlled studies in pregnant women.

Lactation Excretion in breast milk unknown/use caution

Nursing Implications Monoamine oxidase inhibitor type "B"; there should **not** be a problem with tyramine-containing products as long as the typical doses are employed

Specific References

Goetz CG, Poewe W, Rascol O, et al, "Evidence-Based Medical Review Update: Pharmacological and Surgical Treatments of Parkinson's Disease: 2001 to 2004," *Mov Disord*, 2005, 20(5):523-39.

Sertindole

Related Information
● Antipsychotic Agents

Unlabeled/Investigational Use Antipsychotic agent

Mechanism of Action Antagonist of dopamine (d$_2$), serotonin, and norepinephrine (alpha$_1$-receptors); has limbic selectivity, somewhat similar to clozapine

Adverse Reactions

Cardiovascular: Hypotension (orthostatic), syncope

Central nervous system: Lethargy, drowsiness, dizziness, **headache**, dystonia

Genitourinary: Dry ejaculation

Neuromuscular & skeletal: Tremor, cogwheel rigidity

Respiratory: Nasal congestion

Toxicodynamics/Kinetics

Peak plasma level: 8-10 hours

Half-life: 60 hours (may exceed 100 hours in >10% of patients)

Protein binding: 99%

Metabolism: Hepatic to norsertindole and Lu28-092

Elimination: Fecal

Dosage 4-32 mg/day; usual therapeutic dosage range: 16-20 mg/day

Overdosage/Treatment

Decontamination: Activated charcoal

Enhancement of elimination: Multiple dosing of activated charcoal may be effective

Additional Information Potent anxiolytic activity, low extrapyramidal reaction; no anticholinergic effects

Sertraline

Related Information
● Antidepressant Agents

CAS Number 79559-97-0; 79617-96-2

U.S. Brand Names Zoloft®

Synonyms Sertraline Hydrochloride

Impairment Potential Yes, at doses >500 mg. Serum sertraline level of 1285 mcg/L associated with driving impairment. Although no cases of fatal overdose with only sertraline have been reported, symptoms of nonfatal sertraline-only overdoses include somnolence, nausea, vomiting, tachycardia, ECG changes, anxiety, and dilated pupils with the amounts ingested ranging from 500-6000 mg.

Use Treatment of major depression; obsessive-compulsive disorder (OCD); panic disorder; post-traumatic stress disorder (PTSD); premenstrual dysphoric disorder (PMDD); social anxiety disorder

Unlabeled/Investigational Use Eating disorders; generalized anxiety disorder (GAD); impulse control disorders

Mechanism of Action Antidepressant with selective inhibitory effects on presynaptic serotonin (5-HT) reuptake; it is a naphthylamine derivative

Adverse Reactions

Cardiovascular: Palpitations, atrial arrhythmias, AV block, bradycardia, QT$_c$ prolongation, vasculitis, ventricular tachycardia (including torsade de pointes)

Central nervous system: **Insomnia**, **somnolence**, **dizziness**, **headache**, **fatigue**, agitation, anxiety, nervousness, dystonia, extrapyramidal symptoms, hallucinations, neuroleptic malignant syndrome, oculogyric crisis, psychosis

Dermatologic: Rash, angioedema, Stevens-Johnson syndrome (and other severe dermatologic reactions), photosensitivity

Endocrine & metabolic: Libido decreased, galactorrhea, gynecomastia, hyperglycemia, hyperprolactinemia, hypothyroidism, serotonin syndrome, SIADH

Gastrointestinal: **Xerostomia**, **diarrhea**, **nausea**, constipation, anorexia, dyspepsia, flatulence, vomiting, weight gain, abdominal pain, gum hyperplasia, pancreatitis (rare)

Genitourinary: **Ejaculatory disturbances**, micturition disorders, priapism

Hematologic: Agranulocytosis, aplastic anemia, leukopenia, thrombocytopenia, PT/INR increased

Hepatic: Bilirubin increased, hepatic failure, hepatitis, hepatomegaly, jaundice, transaminases increased

Neuromuscular & skeletal: Tremors, paresthesia

Ocular: Visual difficulty, abnormal vision, blindness, cataract, optic neuritis

Otic: Tinnitus

Renal: Acute renal failure

Respiratory: Pulmonary hypertension

Miscellaneous: Diaphoresis (increased), allergic reaction, anaphylactoid reaction, lupus-like syndrome, serum sickness

Additional adverse reactions reported in pediatric patients (frequency >2%): Aggressiveness, epistaxis, hyperkinesia, purpura, sinusitis, urinary incontinence

Signs and Symptoms of Overdose Agitation, amenorrhea, bone marrow depression, chest pain, conjunctivitis, dermatitis, drowsiness, dysphagia, dysuria, ejaculatory disturbances, fatigue, gynecomastia, hallucinations, hirsutism, hypertension, hypertonia, hypertrichosis, hypertriglyceridemia, hypoglycemia, hypotension, insomnia, lacrimation, mania, muscle twitching, myalgia, myoclonus, purpura, sinus tachycardia (which usually resolves in 12 hours), stomatitis, tachycardia

Pharmacodynamics/Kinetics

Absorption: Slow

Protein binding: 98%

Metabolism: Hepatic; extensive first-pass metabolism

Bioavailability: 88%

Half-life elimination: Parent drug: 26 hours; Metabolite N-desmethylsertraline: 66 hours (range: 62-104 hours)

Time to peak, plasma: 4.5-8.4 hours

Excretion: Urine and feces

Dosage

Oral:

Children and Adolescents: OCD:

6-12 years: Initial: 25 mg once daily

13-17 years: Initial: 50 mg once daily

Note: May increase daily dose, at intervals of not less than 1 week, to a maximum of 200 mg/day. If somnolence is noted, give at bedtime.

Adults:

Depression/OCD: Oral: Initial: 50 mg/day (see "Note" above)

Panic disorder, PTSD, social anxiety disorder: Initial: 25 mg once daily; increase to 50 mg once daily after 1 week (see "Note" above)

PMDD: 50 mg/day either daily throughout menstrual cycle **or** limited to the luteal phase of menstrual cycle, depending on physician assessment. Patients not responding to 50 mg/day may benefit from dose increases (50 mg increments per menstrual cycle) up to 150 mg/day when dosing throughout menstrual cycle **or** up to 100 mg day when dosing during luteal phase only. If a 100 mg/day dose has been established with luteal phase dosing, a 50 mg/day titration step for 3 days should be utilized at the beginning of each luteal phase dosing period.

Elderly: Depression/OCD: Start treatment with 25 mg/day in the morning and increase by 25 mg/day increments every 2-3 days if tolerated to 50-100 mg/day; additional increases may be necessary; maximum dose: 200 mg/day

Dosage adjustment/comment in renal impairment: Multiple-dose pharmacokinetics are unaffected by renal impairment.
Hemodialysis: Not removed by hemodialysis

Dosage adjustment/comment in hepatic impairment: Sertraline is extensively metabolized by the liver; caution should be used in patients with hepatic impairment; a lower dose or less frequent dosing should be used.

Monitoring Parameters Monitor nutritional intake and weight; mental status for depression, suicidal ideation, anxiety, social functioning, mania, panic attacks; akathisia; growth in pediatric patients

Administration Oral concentrate: Must be diluted before use. Immediately before administration, use the dropper provided to measure the required amount of concentrate; mix with 4 ounces ($^1/_2$ cup) of water, ginger ale, lemon/lime soda, lemonade, or orange juice **only**. Do not mix with any other liquids than these. The dose should be taken immediately after mixing; do not mix in advance. A slight haze may appear after mixing; this is normal. **Note:** Use with caution in patients with latex sensitivity; dropper dispenser contains dry natural rubber.

Contraindications Hypersensitivity to sertraline or any component of the formulation; use of MAO inhibitors within 14 days; concurrent use of pimozide; concurrent use of sertraline oral concentrate with disulfiram

Warnings *Major psychiatric warnings:*
- **[U.S. Boxed Warning]: Antidepressants increase the risk of suicidal thinking and behavior in children and adolescents with major depressive disorder (MDD) and other depressive disorders;** consider risk prior to prescribing. Closely monitor for clinical worsening, suicidality, or unusual changes in behavior; the child's family or caregiver should be instructed to closely observe the patient and communicate condition with healthcare provider. A medication guide concerning the use of antidepressants in children and teenagers should be dispensed with each prescription. **Sertraline is not FDA approved for use in children with major depressive disorder (MDD). However, it is approved for the treatment of obsessive-compulsive disorder (OCD) in children ≥6 years of age.**
- The possibility of a suicide attempt is inherent in major depression and may persist until remission occurs. Patients treated with antidepressants should be observed for clinical worsening and suicidality, especially during the initial few months of a course of drug therapy, or at times of dose changes, either increases or decreases. Worsening depression and severe abrupt suicidality that are not part of the presenting symptoms may require discontinuation or modification of drug therapy. Use caution in high-risk patients during initiation of therapy.
- Prescriptions should be written for the smallest quantity consistent with good patient care. The patient's family or caregiver should be alerted to monitor patients for the emergence of suicidality and associated behaviors such as anxiety, agitation, panic attacks, insomnia, irritability, hostility, impulsivity, akathisia, hypomania, and mania; patients should be instructed to notify their healthcare provider if any of these symptoms or worsening depression or psychosis occur.
- May worsen psychosis in some patients or precipitate a shift to mania or hypomania in patients with bipolar disorder. Monotherapy in patients with bipolar disorder should be avoided. Patients presenting with depressive symptoms should be screened for bipolar disorder. **Sertraline is not FDA approved for the treatment of bipolar depression.**

Key adverse effects:
- Anticholinergic effects: Relatively devoid of these side effects
- CNS depression: Has a low potential to impair cognitive or motor performance; caution operating hazardous machinery or driving.
- SIADH and hyponatremia: Has been associated with the development of SIADH; hyponatremia has been reported rarely, predominately in the elderly

Concurrent disease:
- Hepatic impairment: Use caution; clearance is decreased and plasma concentrations are increased; a lower dosage may be needed.
- Other concurrent illness: Use caution in patients with certain concomitant systemic illness; due to limited experience.
- Platelet aggregation: May impair platelet aggregation, resulting in bleeding.
- Renal impairment: Use caution; clearance is decreased and plasma concentrations are increased; a lower dosage may be needed.
- Seizure disorders: Use caution with a previous seizure disorder or condition predisposing to seizures such as brain damage or alcoholism.
- Sexual dysfunction: May cause or exacerbate sexual dysfunction.
- Uric acid nephropathy: Use caution in patients at risk of uric acid nephropathy; sertraline acts as a mild uricosuric.
- Weight loss: May cause weight loss. Use caution in patients where weight loss is undesirable.

Concurrent drug therapy:
- Agents which lower seizure threshold: Concurrent therapy with other drugs which lower the seizure threshold.
- Anticoagulants/Antiplatelets: Use caution with concomitant use of NSAIDs, ASA, or other drugs that affect coagulation; the risk of bleeding is potentiated.
- CNS depressants: Use caution with concomitant therapy.
- MAO inhibitors: Potential for severe reaction when used with MAO inhibitors; autonomic instability, coma, death, delirium, diaphoresis, hyperthermia, mental status changes/agitation, muscular rigidity, myoclonus, neuroleptic malignant syndrome features, and seizures may occur.

Special populations:
- Elderly: Use caution in elderly patients.
- Latex sensitivity: Use oral concentrate formulation with caution in patients with latex sensitivity; dropper dispenser contains dry, natural rubber.
- Pediatrics: Monitor growth in pediatric patients.

Special notes:
- Electroconvulsive therapy: May increase the risks associated with electroconvulsive therapy; consider discontinuing, when possible, prior to ECT treatment.
- Withdrawal syndrome: May cause dysphoric mood, irritability, agitation, dizziness, sensory disturbances, anxiety, confusion, headache, lethargy, emotional lability, insomnia, hypomania, tinnitus, and seizures. Upon discontinuation of sertraline therapy, gradually taper dose. If intolerable symptoms occur following a decrease in dosage or upon discontinuation of therapy, then resuming the previous dose with a more gradual taper should be considered.

Dosage Forms Note: Available as sertraline hydrochloride; mg strength refers to sertraline
Solution, oral concentrate:
Zoloft®: 20 mg/mL (60 mL) [contains alcohol 12%]
Tablet: 25 mg, 50 mg, 100 mg
Zoloft®: 25 mg, 50 mg, 100 mg

Reference Range Six hours after doses of 400 mg and 200 mg, peak plasma levels were 253.2 ng/mL and 105.4 ng/mL, respectively; plasma levels correlate poorly to clinical presentation; therapeutic clinical trials: 0.03-0.19 mg/L; postmortem peripheral blood sertraline levels range from 0.23-1 mg/L. Serum sertraline level of 2930 mcg/L and desmethylsertraline level of 1678 mcg/L were recorded after a maximum ingestion of 8 g of sertraline; the patient survived with supportive care. Postmortem blood sertraline level >1.5 mg/L may indicate that this drug was the cause of death.

Overdosage/Treatment
Overdose of <100 mg in children <5 years of age are tolerated well with decontamination and minimal supportive care
Decontamination: Lavage ingestions >1 g in adults (within 1 hour)/ activated charcoal
Supportive therapy: Amantadine (100-200 mg 2 times/day) has been used successfully in treating sexual dysfunction; lorazepam (2 mg I.V.) and nitroglycerin (I.V. infusion of 2 mg/kg/minute) have been used successfully to treat serotonin syndrome induced by sertraline; bruxism can be treated with buspirone (5 mg at night); sildenafil (50-100 mg) can be used to treat sexual dysfunction; nefazodone (100 mg at bedtime) has been used successfully in treating sertraline-induced anorgasmia
Enhancement of elimination: Multiple dosing of activated charcoal may be effective

Diagnostic Procedures
- Sertraline, Blood

Test Interactions ↑ LFTs, cholesterol, triglycerides; ↓ uric acid, glucose; sertraline may cause a false-positive urinary benzodiazepine assay using the original cloned enzyme donor immunoassay system

Drug Interactions Substrate of CYP2B6 (minor), 2C9 (minor), 2C19 (major), 2D6 (major), 3A4 (minor); **Inhibits** CYP1A2 (weak), 2B6 (moderate), 2C8 (weak), 2C9 (weak), 2C19 (moderate), 2D6 (moderate), 3A4 (moderate)
Amphetamines: SSRIs may increase the sensitivity to amphetamines, and amphetamines may increase the risk of serotonin syndrome
Benzodiazepines: Sertraline may inhibit the metabolism of alprazolam and diazepam resulting in elevated serum levels; monitor for increased sedation and psychomotor impairment
Buspirone: Sertraline inhibits the reuptake of serotonin; combined use with a serotonin agonist (buspirone) may cause serotonin syndrome
Carbamazepine: Sertraline may inhibit the metabolism of carbamazepine resulting in increased carbamazepine levels and toxicity; monitor for altered carbamazepine response
Cimetidine: Concurrent use resulted in an increase in sertraline's AUC, C_{max}, and half-life; monitor.
Clozapine: Sertraline may increase serum levels of clozapine; monitor for increased effect/toxicity
Cyclosporine: Sertraline may increase serum levels of cyclosporine (and possibly tacrolimus); monitor

CYP2B6 substrates: Sertraline may increase the levels/effects of CYP2B6 substrates. Example substrates include bupropion, promethazine, propofol, and selegiline.

CYP2C19 inducers: May decrease the levels/effects of sertraline. Example inducers include aminoglutethimide, carbamazepine, phenytoin, and rifampin.

CYP2C19 inhibitors: May increase the levels/effects of sertraline. Example inhibitors include delavirdine, fluconazole, fluvoxamine, gemfibrozil, isoniazid, omeprazole, and ticlopidine.

CYP2C19 substrates: Sertraline may increase the levels/effects of CYP2C19 substrates. Example substrates include citalopram, diazepam, methsuximide, phenytoin, and propranolol.

CYP2D6 inhibitors: May increase the levels/effects of sertraline. Example inhibitors include chlorpromazine, delavirdine, fluoxetine, miconazole, paroxetine, pergolide, quinidine, quinine, ritonavir, and ropinirole.

CYP2D6 substrates: Sertraline may increase the levels/effects of CYP2D6 substrates. Example substrates include amphetamines, selected beta-blockers, dextromethorphan, fluoxetine, lidocaine, mirtazapine, nefazodone, paroxetine, risperidone, ritonavir, thioridazine, tricyclic antidepressants, and venlafaxine.

CYP2D6 prodrug substrates: Sertraline may decrease the levels/effects of CYP2D6 prodrug substrates. Example prodrug substrates include codeine, hydrocodone, oxycodone, and tramadol.

CYP3A4 substrates: Sertraline may increase the levels/effects of CYP3A4 substrates. Example substrates include benzodiazepines, calcium channel blockers, cyclosporine, mirtazapine, nateglinide, nefazodone, sildenafil (and other PDE-5 inhibitors), tacrolimus, and venlafaxine. Selected benzodiazepines (midazolam and triazolam), cisapride, ergot alkaloids, selected HMG-CoA reductase inhibitors (lovastatin and simvastatin), and pimozide are generally contraindicated with strong CYP3A4 inhibitors.

Cyproheptadine: May inhibit the effects of serotonin reuptake inhibitors (fluoxetine); monitor for altered antidepressant response; cyproheptadine acts as a serotonin agonist

Dextromethorphan: Some SSRIs inhibit the metabolism of dextromethorphan; visual hallucinations occurred; monitor for serotonin syndrome

Erythromycin: Serotonin syndrome has been reported when added to sertraline; limited documentation

Haloperidol: Serum concentrations may be increased by sertraline (small increase); monitor

HMG-CoA reductase inhibitors: Sertraline may inhibit the metabolism of lovastatin and simvastatin (metabolized by CYP3A4) resulting in myositis and rhabdomyolysis; although its inhibition is weak, these combinations are best avoided

Lamotrigine: Toxicity has been reported following the addition of sertraline; monitor

Lithium: Patients receiving SSRIs and lithium have developed neurotoxicity; if combination is used, monitor for neurotoxicity

Loop diuretics: Sertraline may cause hyponatremia; additive hyponatremic effects may be seen with combined use of a loop diuretic (bumetanide, furosemide, torsemide); monitor for hyponatremia

MAO inhibitors: Sertraline should not be used with nonselective MAO inhibitors (isocarboxazid, phenelzine); fatal reactions have been reported; this combination is contraindicated.

Meperidine: Concurrent use may result in serotonin syndrome; these combinations are best avoided

Nefazodone: May increase the risk of serotonin syndrome

NSAIDs: Concomitant use of sertraline and NSAIDs, aspirin, or other drugs affecting coagulation has been associated with an increased risk of bleeding; monitor.

Phenothiazines: Sertraline may inhibit metabolism of thioridazine or mesoridazine, potentially leading to malignant ventricular arrhythmias. Avoid concurrent use. Wait at least 5 weeks after discontinuing sertraline prior to starting thioridazine.

Phenytoin: Sertraline may inhibit the metabolism of phenytoin and may result in phenytoin toxicity. Studies have demonstrated minimal impact with concurrent dosing, however, monitoring of levels/effects is recommended.

Pimozide: Sertraline may increase serum levels of pimozide. Concurrent use is contraindicated.

Ritonavir: Combined use of sertraline with ritonavir may cause serotonin syndrome in HIV-positive patients; monitor

Selegiline: SSRIs have been reported to cause mania or hypertension when combined with selegiline; this combination is best avoided. Concurrent use with SSRIs has been reported to cause serotonin syndrome. As an MAO type B inhibitor, the risk of serotonin syndrome may be less than with nonselective MAO inhibitors.

Sibutramine: May increase the risk of serotonin syndrome with SSRIs; monitor.

SSRIs: Combined use with other drugs which inhibit the reuptake may cause serotonin syndrome

Sumatriptan (and other serotonin agonists): Concurrent use may result in toxicity; weakness, hyper-reflexia, and incoordination have been observed with sumatriptan and SSRIs. In addition, concurrent use may theoretically increase the risk of serotonin syndrome; includes sumatriptan, naratriptan, rizatriptan, and zolmitriptan.

Sympathomimetics: May increase the risk of serotonin syndrome with SSRIs

Tolbutamide: Sertraline may decrease the metabolism of tolbutamide; monitor for changes in glucose control.

Tramadol: Sertraline combined with tramadol (serotonergic effects) may cause serotonin syndrome; monitor

Trazodone: Sertraline may inhibit the metabolism of trazodone resulting in increased toxicity; monitor

Tricyclic antidepressants: Sertraline may inhibit the metabolism of tricyclic antidepressants (amitriptyline, desipramine, imipramine, nortriptyline) resulting is elevated serum levels; if combination is warranted, a low dose of TCA (10-25 mg/day) should be utilized

Tryptophan: Sertraline may inhibit the reuptake of serotonin; combination with tryptophan, a serotonin precursor, may cause agitation and restlessness; this combination is best avoided

Venlafaxine: Sertraline may increase the risk of serotonin syndrome

Warfarin: Sertraline may alter the hypoprothrombinemic response to warfarin; monitor

Zolpidem: Onset of hypnosis may be shortened in patients receiving sertraline; monitor

Pregnancy Risk Factor C

Pregnancy Implications There are no adequate and well-controlled studies in pregnant women; use only if potential benefit to the mother justifies potential risk to the fetus.

Lactation Enters breast milk/not recommended (AAP rates "of concern")

Additional Information Buspirone (15-60 mg/day) may be useful in treatment of sexual dysfunction during treatment with a selective serotonin reuptake inhibitor; may exacerbate tics in Tourette's syndrome

Specific References

Boyer EW and Shannon M, "The Serotonin Syndrome," *N Engl J Med*, 2005, 352(11):1112-20 (review).

Hartnell NR, Wilson JP, Patel NC, et al, "Adverse Event Reporting with Selective Serotonin-Reuptake Inhibitors," *Ann Pharmacother*, 2003, 37(10):1387-91.

Rohrig TP and Goodson LJ, "A Sertraline-Intoxicated Driver," *J Anal Toxicol*, 2004, 28(8):689-91.

Serebruany VL, "Selective Serotonin Reuptake Inhibitors and Increased Bleeding Risk: Are We Missing Something?" *Am J Med*, 2006, 119(2):113-6 (review).

Zeskind PS and Stephens LE, "Maternal Selective Serotonin Reuptake Inhibitor Use During Pregnancy and Newborn Neurobehavior," *Pediatrics*, 2004, 113(2):368-75.

Sildenafil

CAS Number 0139755-83-2

U.S. Brand Names Viagra®

Synonyms UK92480

Impairment Potential Unknown

Use Treatment of erectile dysfunction; may be useful to reverse psychotropic-induced erectile dysfunction in men or reduced arousal/delayed orgasm in women

Unlabeled/Investigational Use Psychotropic-induced sexual dysfunction; pulmonary arterial hypertension in children

Mechanism of Action Does not directly cause penile erections, but affects the response to sexual stimulation. The physiologic mechanism of erection of the penis involves release of nitric oxide (NO) in the corpus cavernosum during sexual stimulation. NO then activates the enzyme guanylate cyclase, which results in increased levels of cyclic guanosine monophosphate (cGMP), producing smooth muscle relaxation and inflow of blood to the corpus cavernosum. Sildenafil enhances the effect of NO by inhibiting phosphodiesterase type 5 (PDE5), which is responsible for degradation of cGMP in the corpus cavernosum. When sexual stimulation causes local release of NO, inhibition of PDE5 by sildenafil causes increased levels of cGMP in the corpus cavernosum, resulting in smooth muscle relaxation and inflow of blood to the corpus cavernosum. At recommended doses, it has no effect in the absence of sexual stimulation.

Adverse Reactions

Cardiovascular: Atrial fibrillation, flushing

Central nervous system: Dizziness, **headache**, aggressive behavior, insomnia, pyrexia

Dermatologic: Rash, erythema

Gastrointestinal: Diarrhea, **dyspepsia** , gastritis

Genitourinary: Urinary tract infection

Hematologic: Anemia, leukopenia

Hepatic: LFTs increased

Neuromuscular & skeletal: Myalgia, paresthesia

Ocular: Abnormal vision (color changes, blurred or increased sensitivity to light 3%; up to 11% with doses >100 mg)

Respiratory: Dyspnea exacerbated, epistaxis, nasal congestion, rhinitis, sinusitis

Admission Criteria/Prognosis

Admit any symptomatic patient or ingestion >1 g.

Pharmacodynamics/Kinetics

Onset of action: ~60 minutes

Duration: 2-4 hours

Absorption: Rapid; slower with a high-fat meal

Distribution: V_{dss}: 105 L

Protein binding, plasma: ~96%

Metabolism: Hepatic via CYP3A4 (major) and CYP2C9 (minor route)

Bioavailability: 40%

Half-life elimination: 4 hours

Time to peak: 30-120 minutes; delayed by 60 minutes with a high-fat meal

Excretion: Feces (80%); urine (13%)

Dosage

Adults: Oral:

Erectile dysfunction (Viagra®): For most patients, the recommended dose is 50 mg taken as needed, approximately 1 hour before sexual activity. However, sildenafil may be taken anywhere from 30 minutes to 4 hours before sexual activity. Based on effectiveness and tolerance, the dose may be increased to a maximum recommended dose of 100 mg or decreased to 25 mg. The maximum recommended dosing frequency is once daily.

Pulmonary arterial hypertension (Revatio™): 20 mg 3 times/day, taken 4-6 hours apart

Dosage adjustment for patients >65 years of age: Hepatic impairment (cirrhosis), severe renal impairment (creatinine clearance <30 mL/minute): Higher plasma levels have been associated which may result in increase in efficacy and adverse effects; Viagra®: Starting dose of 25 mg should be considered

Dosage considerations for patients taking alpha blockers: Viagra®: Doses of 50 or 100 mg, should not be taken within 4 hours of an alpha blocker; doses of 25 mg may be given at any time

Dosage adjustment for concomitant use of potent CYP34A inhibitors:

Revatio™:

Erythromycin, saquinavir: No dosage adjustment

Itraconazole, ketoconazole, ritonavir: Not recommended

Viagra®:

Erythromycin, itraconazole, ketoconazole, saquinavir: Starting dose of 25 mg should be considered

Ritonavir: Maximum: 25 mg every 48 hours

Stability Store tablets at controlled room temperature 15°C to 30°C (59°F to 86°F)

Administration Administer 30 minutes to 4 hours before sexual activity (optimally 1 hour before).

Contraindications Hypersensitivity to sildenafil or any component of the formulation; concurrent use of organic nitrates (nitroglycerin) in any form (potentiates the hypotensive effects)

Warnings

Decreases in blood pressure may occur due to vasodilator effects; use caution in patients with resting hypotension (BP <90/50), hypertension (BP >170/110), fluid depletion, severe left ventricular outflow obstruction, or autonomic dysfunction, and patients receiving alpha-blockers or other antihypertensive medication. Not recommended for use with pulmonary veno-occlusive disease.

Use caution in patients with cardiovascular disease, including cardiac failure, unstable angina, or a recent history (within the last 6 months) of myocardial infarction, stroke, or life-threatening arrhythmia. Use caution in patients receiving concurrent bosentan. Use caution in patients with bleeding disorders or with active peptic ulcer disease; safety and efficacy have not been established.

There is a degree of cardiac risk associated with sexual activity; therefore, physicians may wish to consider the cardiovascular status of their patients prior to initiating any treatment for erectile dysfunction. Sildenafil should be used with caution in patients with anatomical deformation of the penis (angulation, cavernosal fibrosis, or Peyronie's disease), or in patients who have conditions which may predispose them to priapism (sickle cell anemia, multiple myeloma, leukemia).

Rare cases of nonarteritic ischemic optic neuropathy (NAION) have been reported; risk may be increased with history of vision loss. Other risk factors for NAION include low cup-to-disc ratio ("crowded disc"), coronary artery disease, diabetes, hypertension, hyperlipidemia, smoking, and age >50 years.

The safety and efficacy of sildenafil with other treatments for erectile dysfunction have not been established; use is not recommended. May cause dose-related impairment of color discrimination. Use caution in patients with retinitis pigmentosa; a minority have generic disorders of retinal phosphodiesterases (no safety information available). Safety and efficacy in pediatric patients have not been established.

Dosage Forms

Tablet:

Revatio™: 20 mg

Viagra®: 25 mg, 50 mg, 100 mg

Overdosage/Treatment

Decontamination: Activated charcoal

Supportive therapy: Avoid organic nitrate products

Enhancement of elimination: Dialysis is not expected to be useful

Drug Interactions

Substrate of CYP2C9 (minor), 3A4 (major); **Inhibits** CYP1A2 (weak), 2C9 (weak), 2C19 (weak), 2D6 (weak), 2E1 (weak), 3A4 (weak)

Azole antifungals: May increase the serum concentrations of sildenafil; reduce starting dose to 25 mg.

Alpha-blockers (doxazosin): Concomitant use may lead to symptomatic hypotension in some patients. Patient should be stable on an alpha-blocker prior to initiation of PDE-5 inhibitor. Sildenafil should be started at 25 mg. If patient is taking an optimal dose of PDE-5 inhibitor, alpha-blocker should be initiated at lowest dose.

Bosentan: May decrease serum concentration and effect of sildenafil.

CYP3A4 inhibitors: May increase the levels/effects of sildenafil. Example inhibitors include azole antifungals, clarithromycin, diclofenac, doxycycline, erythromycin, imatinib, isoniazid, nefazodone, nicardipine, propofol, protease inhibitors, quinidine, telithromycin, and verapamil.

Macrolide antibiotics: May increase serum concentrations of sildenafil; reduce starting dose of Viagra® to 25 mg if used with clarithromycin, erythromycin, telithromycin, or troleandomycin. No adjustments with Revatio™ are required.

Nitroglycerin (other nitrates): Concurrent use with sildenafil is contraindicated due to the potential for severe, potentially fatal, hypotensive responses.

Protease inhibitors: May increase the serum concentrations of sildenafil; reduce dose of Viagra® to 25 mg/24 hours; use of Revatio™ is not recommended.

Pregnancy Risk Factor B

Pregnancy Implications There are no adequate and well-controlled studies in pregnant women.

Lactation Excretion in breast milk unknown/use caution

Specific References

Bratt G and Stahle L, "Sildenafil Does Not Alter Nelfinavir Pharmacokinetics," *Ther Drug Monit*, 2003, 25(2):240-2.

Cantrell FL, "Sildenafil Citrate Ingestion in a Pediatric Patient," *Pediatr Emerg Care*, 2004, 20(5):314-5.

Kekilli M, Beyazit Y, Purnak T, et al, "Acute Myocardial Infarction After Sildenafil Citrate Ingestion," *Ann Pharmacother*, 2005, 39(7):1362-4.

Lewis RJ, Johnson RD, and Blank CL, "Quantitative Determination of Sildenafil (Viagra®) and Its Metabolite (UK-103,320) in Fluid and Tissue Specimens Obtained from Six Aviation Fatalities," *J Anal Toxicol*, 2006, 30:14-20.

Marquardt KA, Alsop JA, and Albertson TE, "Sildenafil in Children - Send into the ED or Watch at Home?" *Clin Toxicol (Phila)*, 2005, 43:644.

Nahata M, Morosco R, and Brady M, "Extemporaneous Sildenafil Citrate Oral Suspensions for the Treatment of Pulmonary Hypertension in Children," *Am J Health Syst Pharm*, 2006, 63:254-7.

Nurnberg HG and Duttagupta S, "Economic Analysis of Sildenafil Citrate (Viagra®) Add-on to Treat Erectile Dysfunction Associated with Selective Serotonin Reuptake Inhibitor Use," *Am J Ther*, 2004, 11(1):9-12.

Pagani S, Mirtella D, Mencarelli R, et al, "Postmortem Distribution of Sildenafil in Histological Material," *J Anal Toxicol*, 2005, 29(4):254-7.

Romanelli F and Smith KM, "Recreational Use of Sildenafil by HIV-Positive and -Negative Homosexual/Bisexual Males," *Ann Pharmacother*, 2004, 38(6):1024-30.

Tracqui A and Ludes B, "HPLC-MS for the Determination of Sildenafil Citrate (Viagra) in Biological Fluids: Application to the Salivary Excretion of Sildenafil After Oral Intake," *J Anal Toxicol*, 2003, 27(2):88-94.

Wills BK, Albinson C, Clifton J, et al, "Sildenafil Citrate Ingestion and Prolonged Priapism and Tachycardia in a Pediatric Patient," *Clin Toxicol*, 2005, 43:633.

Silver Nitrate

CAS Number 7761-88-8

UN Number 1493

Synonyms $AgNO_3$

Use Cauterization of wounds and sluggish ulcers, removal of granulation tissue and warts; aseptic prophylaxis of burns. Industrial uses include cosmetics (at a concentration of up to 4%), photography, manufacture of silver salts, hair dyeing, ivory etching, and as a laboratory reagent.

Mechanism of Action Free silver ions precipitate bacterial proteins by combining with chloride in tissue forming silver chloride; coagulates cellular protein to form an eschar; silver ions or salts or colloidal silver preparations can inhibit the growth of both gram-positive and gram-negative bacteria. This germicidal action is attributed to the precipitation of bacterial proteins by liberated silver ions. Silver nitrate coagulates cellular protein to form an eschar, and this mode of action is the postulated mechanism for control of benign hematuria, rhinitis, and recurrent pneumothorax.

Adverse Reactions
Dermatologic: Burning and skin irritation, staining of the skin
Endocrine & metabolic: Hyponatremia
Hematologic: Methemoglobinemia

Signs and Symptoms of Overdose Blackening of skin and mucous membranes, coma, convulsions, death, diarrhea, pain and burning of mouth, salivation, shock, vomiting. Absorbed nitrate can cause methemoglobinemia. Prolonged silver nitrate administration (topically) can result in hyperchloremia, hyponatremia, and late hyperchloremia. If taken orally, gastrointestinal burns with esophageal strictures can occur.

Pharmacodynamics/Kinetics
Absorption: Because silver ions readily combine with protein, there is minimal GI and cutaneous absorption of the 0.5% and 1% preparations
Excretion: Highest amounts of silver noted on autopsy have been in kidneys, excretion in urine is minimal

DosageChildren and Adults:
Sticks: Apply to mucous membranes and other moist skin surfaces only on area to be treated 2-3 times/week for 2-3 weeks
Topical solution: Apply a cotton applicator dipped in solution on the affected area 2-3 times/week for 2-3 weeks

Stability Must be stored in a dry place; exposure to light causes silver to oxidize and turn brown, dipping in water causes oxidized film to readily dissolve

Monitoring Parameters With prolonged use, monitor methemoglobin levels

Administration Applicators are **not** for ophthalmic use.

Contraindications Hypersensitivity to silver nitrate or any component of the formulation; not for use on broken skin, cuts, or wounds

Warnings Do not use applicator sticks on the eyes. Prolonged use may result in skin discoloration.

Dosage Forms Applicator sticks, topical: Silver nitrate 75% and potassium nitrate 25% (6", 12", 18")
Solution, topical: 10% (30 mL); 25% (30 mL); 50% (30 mL)

Overdosage/Treatment
Decontamination:
Ocular: Irrigation of eyes for at least 15 minutes with normal saline. Sodium chloride can precipitate the silver as insoluble silver chloride.
Dermal: Irrigate for at least 15 minutes with saline. Remove all clothes and jewelry. Clothing can be washed but shoes should be discarded. Pay particular attention to scalp and nail decontamination.
Oral: Rinse out mouth with water. Give milk or water to dilute. Avoid ipecac or lavage since silver is corrosive. Note that patient's vomitus may be caustic and stain on contact.
Supportive therapy: Diazepam or lorazepam can be given to treat seizures. Methylene blue should be considered if cyanosis develops or if methemoglobin levels exceed 30%. Silver antidotes are probably of little to no clinical use.

Pregnancy Risk Factor C

Nursing Implications Silver nitrate solutions stain skin and utensils

Additional Information Fatal dose: As low as 2 g. Applicators are **not** for ophthalmic use.

Simvastatin

CAS Number 79902-63-9
U.S. Brand Names Zocor®
Use
Used with dietary therapy for the following:
Secondary prevention of cardiovascular events in hypercholesterolemic patients with established coronary heart disease (CHD) or at high risk for CHD: To reduce cardiovascular morbidity (myocardial infarction, coronary revascularization procedures) and mortality; to reduce the risk of stroke and transient ischemic attacks
Hyperlipidemias: To reduce elevations in total cholesterol, LDL-C, apolipoprotein B, and triglycerides in patients with primary hypercholesterolemia (elevations of 1 or more components are present in Fredrickson type IIa, IIb, III, and IV hyperlipidemias); treatment of homozygous familial hypercholesterolemia
Heterozygous familial hypercholesterolemia (HeFH): In adolescent patients (10-17 years of age, females >1 year postmenarche) with HeFH having LDL-C ≥190 mg/dL **or** LDL ≥160 mg/dL with positive family history of premature cardiovascular disease (CVD), or 2 or more CVD risk factors in the adolescent patient

Mechanism of Action Simvastatin acts by competitively inhibiting 3-hydroxyl-3-methylglutaryl-coenzyme A (HMG-CoA) reductase, the enzyme that catalyzes the rate-limiting step in cholesterol biosynthesis

Adverse Reactions
Cardiovascular: Symptomatic hypotension, shock, chest pain, angina, vasculitis
Central nervous system: Headache, psychosis, CNS depression, depression

Dermatologic: Photosensitivity, erythema multiforme, alopecia, angioedema, toxic epidermal necrolysis, urticaria, purpura, Stevens-Johnson syndrome, pruritus, licheniform eruptions, exanthem
Endocrine & metabolic: Gynecomastia
Gastrointestinal: Constipation, dyspepsia, flatulence
Genitourinary: Impotence (onset: 2 days to 27 months)
Hepatic: Persistent elevations in liver enzymes, aminotransferase level elevation (asymptomatic)
Neuromuscular & skeletal: Polymyositis (dermatomyositis), CPK elevations (rarely) in the absence of clinical myopathy, rhabdomyolysis at doses >160 mg, paresthesia
Ocular: Esotropia
Respiratory: Interstitial lung disease with pleural effusion
Miscellaneous: Systemic lupus erythematosus

Pharmacodynamics/Kinetics
Onset of action: >3 days
Peak effect: 2 weeks
Absorption: 85%
Protein binding: ~95%
Metabolism: Hepatic via CYP3A4; extensive first-pass effect
Bioavailability: <5%
Half-life elimination: Unknown
Time to peak: 1.3-2.4 hours
Excretion: Feces (60%); urine (13%)

Dosage Oral: **Note:** Doses should be individualized according to the baseline LDL-cholesterol levels, the recommended goal of therapy, and the patient's response; adjustments should be made at intervals of 4 weeks or more; doses may need adjusted based on concomitant medications
Children 10-17 years (females >1 year postmenarche): HeFH: 10 mg once daily in the evening; range: 10-40 mg/day (maximum: 40 mg/day)
Dosage adjustment for simvastatin with concomitant cyclosporine, fibrates, niacin, amiodarone, or verapamil: Refer to drug-specific dosing in Adults dosing section
Adults:
Homozygous familial hypercholesterolemia: 40 mg once daily in the evening **or** 80 mg/day (given as 20 mg, 20 mg, and 40 mg evening dose)
Prevention of cardiovascular events, hyperlipidemias: 20-40 mg once daily in the evening; range: 5-80 mg/day
Patients requiring only moderate reduction of LDL-cholesterol may be started at 10 mg once daily
Patients requiring reduction of >45% in low-density lipoprotein (LDL) cholesterol may be started at 40 mg once daily in the evening
Patients with CHD or at high risk for CHD: Dosing should be started at 40 mg once daily in the evening; simvastatin may be started simultaneously with diet
Dosage adjustment with concomitant medications:
Cyclosporine: Initial: 5 mg simvastatin, should **not** exceed 10 mg/day
Fibrates or niacin: Simvastatin dose should **not** exceed 10 mg/day
Amiodarone or verapamil: Simvastatin dose should **not** exceed 20 mg/day

Dosing adjustment/comments in renal impairment: Because simvastatin does not undergo significant renal excretion, modification of dose should not be necessary in patients with mild to moderate renal insufficiency.
Severe renal impairment: Cl_{cr} <10 mL/minute: Initial: 5 mg/day with close monitoring.

Stability Tablets should be stored in well-closed containers at temperatures between 5°C to 30°C (41°F to 86°F)

Monitoring Parameters Creatine phosphokinase levels due to possibility of myopathy; serum cholesterol (total and fractionated)
Obtain liver function tests prior to initiation, dose, and thereafter when clinically indicated. Patients titrated to the 80 mg dose should be tested prior to initiation and 3 months after initiating the 80 mg dose. Thereafter, periodic monitoring (ie, semiannually) is recommended for the first year of treatment. Patients with elevated transaminase levels should have a second (confirmatory) test and frequent monitoring until values normalize. Discontinue if increase in ALT/AST is persistently >3 times ULN.

Administration May be taken without regard to meals.

Contraindications Hypersensitivity to simvastatin or any component of the formulation; acute liver disease; unexplained persistent elevations of serum transaminases; pregnancy; breast-feeding

Warnings Secondary causes of hyperlipidemia should be ruled out prior to therapy. Liver function must be monitored by laboratory assessment. Rhabdomyolysis with acute renal failure has occurred. Risk is dose-related and is increased with concurrent use of lipid-lowering agents which may cause rhabdomyolysis (gemfibrozil, fibric acid derivatives, or niacin at doses ≥1 g/day), during concurrent use with danazol or strong CYP3A4 inhibitors (including amiodarone, clarithromycin, cyclosporine, erythromycin, telithromycin, itraconazole, ketoconazole, nefazodone, grapefruit juice in large quantities, verapamil, or protease inhibitors such as indinavir, nelfinavir, or ritonavir. Weigh the risk versus benefit when combining any of these drugs with simvastatin. Do not initiate simvastatin-containing treatment in a patient with pre-existing therapy of cyclosporine or danazol, unless the patient has previously demonstrated tolerance to ≥5 mg/day simvastatin. Temporarily discontinue in any patient experiencing an acute or serious major medical or surgical condition which may increase the risk of rhabdomyolysis. Discontinue temporarily for elective surgical procedures. Use caution in patients with renal insufficiency. Use with caution in patients who consume large amounts of ethanol or have a history of liver disease. Safety and efficacy have not been established in patients <10 years or in premenarcheal girls.

Dosage Forms Tablet: 5 mg, 10 mg, 20 mg, 40 mg
  Zocor®: 5 mg, 10 mg, 20 mg, 40 mg, 80 mg

Overdosage/Treatment
  Decontamination: Activated charcoal
  Enhanced elimination: Multiple dosing of activated charcoal may be effective

Drug Interactions
  Substrate of CYP3A4 (major); **Inhibits** CYP2C8 (weak), 2C9 (weak), 2D6 (weak)
  Amiodarone may increase the risk of myopathy and rhabdomyolysis; dose of simvastatin should not exceed 20 mg/day.
  Antacids: Plasma concentrations may be decreased when given with magnesium-aluminum hydroxide containing antacids (reported with atorvastatin and pravastatin). Clinical efficacy is not altered, no dosage adjustment is necessary
  Cholestyramine reduces absorption of several HMG-CoA reductase inhibitors. Separate administration times by at least 4 hours.
  Cholestyramine and colestipol (bile acid sequestrants): Cholesterol-lowering effects are additive.
  Clofibrate and fenofibrate may increase the risk of myopathy and rhabdomyolysis; dose of simvastatin should not exceed 10 mg/day
  Cyclosporine: Concurrent use may increase the risk of myopathy and rhabdomyolysis; dose of simvastatin should not exceed 10 mg/day
  CYP3A4 inhibitors: May increase the levels/effects of simvastatin. Example inhibitors include azole antifungals, clarithromycin, diclofenac, doxycycline, erythromycin, imatinib, isoniazid, nefazodone, nicardipine, propofol, protease inhibitors, quinidine, telithromycin, and verapamil.
  Danazol: May increase risk of myopathy and rhabdomyolysis; dose of simvastatin should not exceed 10 mg/day.
  Gemfibrozil: Increased risk of myopathy and rhabdomyolysis; dose of simvastatin should not exceed 10 mg/day.
  Grapefruit juice may inhibit metabolism of simvastatin via CYP3A4; avoid high dietary intakes of grapefruit juice.
  Niacin (≥1 g/day): Concurrent use may increase the risk of myopathy and rhabdomyolysis; dose of simvastatin should not exceed 10 mg/day.
  Verapamil may increase the risk of myopathy and rhabdomyolysis; dose of simvastatin should not exceed 20 mg/day.
  Warfarin effects (hypoprothrombinemic response) may be increased; monitor INR closely when simvastatin is initiated or discontinued.

Pregnancy Risk Factor X
Pregnancy Implications Cholesterol biosynthesis may be important in fetal development. Contraindicated in pregnancy. Administer to women of childbearing potential only when conception is highly unlikely and patients have been informed of potential hazards.

Lactation Excretion in breast milk unknown/contraindicated
Nursing Implications Liver enzyme elevations may be observed during simvastatin therapy; combination therapy with other hypolipidemic agents may be required to achieve optimal reductions of LDL cholesterol; diet, weight reduction, and exercise should be attempted to control hypercholesterolemia before the institution of simvastatin therapy
Additional Information Average length of time to development of rhabdomyolysis is one year; with an addition of a fibrate, the average time is about 32 days. Muscle pain (88%) or fatigue (74%) are the two most prominent symptoms in statin-induced rhabdomyolysis.

Specific References
Antons KA, Williams CD, Baker SK, et al, "Clinical Perspectives of Statin-Induced Rhabdomyolysis," *Am J Med*, 2006, 119):400-9..
Ho MR, Baker JE, and Miller AL, "Simvastatin-Induced Rhabdomyolysis," *Am J Emerg Med*, 2004, 22(3):234-5.
Rosenson RS, "Current Overview of Statin-Induced Myopathy," *Am J Med*, 2004, 116(6):408-16.
Roten L, Schoenenberger RA, Krahenbuhl S, et al, "Rhabdomyolysis in Association with Simvastatin and Amiodarone," *Ann Pharmacother*, 2004, 38(6):978-81.
Shaukat A, Benekli M, Vladutiu GD, et al, "Simvastatin-Fluconazole Causing Rhabdomyolysis," *Ann Pharmacother*, 2003, 37(7-8):1032-5.
Skrabal MZ, Stading JA, and Monaghan MS, "Rhabdomyolysis Associated with Simvastatin-Nefazodone Therapy," *South Med J*, 2003, 96(10):1034-5.

Sodium Benzoate

CAS Number 532-32-1
Use Adjunctive therapy for the prevention and treatment of hyperammonemia due to suspected or proven urea cycle defects; used to treat urea cycle enzyme deficiency in combination with arginine
Mechanism of Action Assists in lowering serum ammonia levels by activation of a nonurea cycle pathway (the benzoate-hippurate pathway); ammonia in the presence of benzoate will conjugate with glycine to form hippurate which is excreted by the kidney
Adverse Reactions
  Cardiovascular: Chest pain, angina
  Dermatologic: Urticaria, rash
  Gastrointestinal: Nausea, vomiting
  Miscellaneous: Anaphylaxis
Pharmacodynamics/Kinetics
  Half-life: 0.75-7.4 hours
  Elimination: Clearance is largely attributable to metabolism with urinary excretion of hippurate, the major metabolite
Dosage Investigational use (not FDA approved): Children: Oral, I.V.: 0.25 g/kg bolus followed by 0.25-0.5 g/kg/day as continuous infusion or divided every 6-8 hours
Monitoring Parameters Serum ammonia level
Warnings Use with caution in patients with Reye's syndrome, propionic or methylmalonic acidemia; use with caution in neonates with hyperbilirubinemia due to potential displacement of bilirubin from albumin binding sites
Dosage Forms Powder: 454 g
Overdosage/Treatment
  Supportive therapy: Treat urticarial rash with epinephrine, diphenhydramine and corticosteroids
Additional Information Not available commercially; oral solutions must be compounded using powder form. I.V. solutions must also be compounded and tested for sterility and pyrogenicity prior to use.

Sodium Chloride

CAS Number 7647-14-5
U.S. Brand Names Altamist [OTC]; Ayr® Baby Saline [OTC]; Ayr® Saline Mist [OTC]; Ayr® Saline [OTC]; Breathe Right® Saline [OTC]; Broncho Saline® [OTC]; Entsol® [OTC]; Muro 128® [OTC]; Na-Zone® [OTC]; Nasal Moist® [OTC]; NaSal™ [OTC]; Ocean® [OTC]; Pediamist® [OTC]; Pretz® Irrigation [OTC]; SalineX® [OTC]; SeaMist® [OTC]; Simply Saline™ [OTC]; Wound Wash Saline™ [OTC]
Synonyms NaCl; Normal Saline; Salt
Use
  Parenteral: Restores sodium ion in patients with restricted oral intake (especially hyponatremia states or low salt syndrome). In general, parenteral saline uses:
    Bacteriostatic sodium chloride: Dilution or dissolving drugs for I.M., I.V., or SubQ injections
    Essential in lithium or bromide toxicity (I.V. sodium chloride)
    Concentrated sodium chloride: Additive for parenteral fluid therapy
    Hypertonic sodium chloride: For severe hyponatremia and hypochloremia
    Hypotonic sodium chloride: Hydrating solution
    Normal saline: Restores water/sodium losses
    Pharmaceutical aid/diluent for infusion of compatible drug additives
  Ophthalmic: Reduces corneal edema
  Oral: Restores sodium losses
  Inhalation: Restores moisture to pulmonary system; loosens and thins congestion caused by colds or allergies; diluent for bronchodilator solutions that require dilution before inhalation
  Intranasal: Restores moisture to nasal membranes
  Irrigation: Wound cleansing, irrigation, and flushing
  Traumatic brain injury (hypertonic sodium chloride)
Mechanism of Action There is a fluid shift from intracellular to extracellular space centrally with acute salt poisoning resulting in dehydration of brain cells; principal extracellular cation; functions in fluid and electrolyte balance, osmotic pressure control, and water distribution
Adverse Reactions
  Cardiovascular: Thrombosis, hypervolemia, sinus tachycardia
  Endocrine & metabolic: Hypernatremia, dilution of serum electrolytes, overhydration, hypokalemia
  Gastrointestinal: Salty taste
  Local: Phlebitis, extravasation
  Renal: Tubular necrosis (acute)
  Respiratory: Congestive conditions, pulmonary edema
Signs and Symptoms of Overdose Coma, congestive heart failure, cramps, diarrhea, dizziness, flat anterior fontanelle (infants), fluid retention, hypokalemia, irritability, nausea, obtundation, pulmonary edema, restlessness, seizures, tachycardia, thirst, vomiting

Admission Criteria/Prognosis Ingestions >0.5 g/kg, symptomatic patients or asymptomatic patients with serum sodium levels >160 mEq/L should be considered for admission

Pharmacodynamics/Kinetics

Absorption: Oral, I.V.: Rapid

Distribution: Widely distributed

Excretion: Primarily urine; also sweat, tears, saliva

Dosage

Children: I.V.: Hypertonic solutions (>0.9%) should only be used for the initial treatment of acute serious symptomatic hyponatremia; maintenance: 3-4 mEq/kg/day; maximum: 100-150 mEq/day; dosage varies widely depending on clinical condition

Replacement: Determined by laboratory determinations mEq

Sodium deficiency (mEq/kg) = [% dehydration (L/kg)/100 × 70 (mEq/L)] + [0.6 (L/kg) × (140 - serum sodium) (mEq/L)]

Children ≥2 years and Adults:

Intranasal: 2-3 sprays in each nostril as needed

Irrigation: Spray affected area

Children and Adults: Inhalation: Bronchodilator diluent: 1-3 sprays (1-3 mL) to dilute bronchodilator solution in nebulizer prior to administration

Adults:

GU irrigant: 1-3 L/day by intermittent irrigation

Heat cramps: Oral: 0.5-1 g with full glass of water, up to 4.8 g/day

Replacement I.V.: Determined by laboratory determinations mEq

Sodium deficiency (mEq/kg) = [% dehydration (L/kg)/100 × 70 (mEq/L) + [0.6 (L/kg) × (140 - serum sodium) (mEq/L)]

To correct acute, serious hyponatremia: mEq sodium = [desired sodium (mEq/L) - actual sodium (mEq/L)] × [0.6 × wt (kg)]; for acute correction use 125 mEq/L as the desired serum sodium; acutely correct serum sodium in 5 mEq/L/dose increments; more gradual correction in increments of 10 mEq/L/day is indicated in the asymptomatic patient

Chloride maintenance electrolyte requirement in parenteral nutrition: 2-4 mEq/kg/24 hours or 25-40 mEq/1000 kcals/24 hours; maximum: 100-150 mEq/24 hours

Sodium maintenance electrolyte requirement in parenteral nutrition: 3-4 mEq/kg/24 hours or 25-40 mEq/1000 kcals/24 hours; maximum: 100-150 mEq/24 hours.

Ophthalmic:

Ointment: Apply once daily or more often

Solution: Instill 1-2 drops into affected eye(s) every 3-4 hours

Stability Store injection at room temperature; protect from heat and from freezing; use only clear solutions

Monitoring Parameters Serum sodium, potassium, chloride, and bicarbonate levels; I & O, weight

Contraindications Hypersensitivity to sodium chloride or any component of the formulation; hypertonic uterus, hypernatremia, fluid retention

Warnings Use with caution in patients with CHF, renal insufficiency, liver cirrhosis, hypertension, edema; sodium toxicity is almost exclusively related to how fast a sodium deficit is corrected; both rate and magnitude are extremely important; do not use bacteriostatic sodium chloride in newborns since benzyl alcohol preservatives have been associated with toxicity. Wound Wash Saline™ is for single-patient use only.

Dosage Forms

Gel, intranasal:

Ayr® Saline No-Drip: 0.5% (22 mL) [spray gel; contains benzalkonium chloride, benzyl alcohol and soybean oil]

Ayr® Saline: 0.5% (14 g) [contains soybean oil]

Entsol®: 3% (20 g) [contains aloe, benzalkonium chloride, and vitamin E]

Simply Saline® Nasal Moist®: 0.65% (30 g)

Injection, solution [preservative free]: 0.9% (2 mL, 5 mL, 10 mL, 20 mL, 100 mL)

Injection, solution [preservative free, prefilled I.V. flush syringe]: 0.9% (2 mL, 2.5 mL, 3 mL, 5 mL, 10 mL)

Injection, solution: 0.45% (25 mL, 50 mL, 100 mL, 250 mL, 500 mL, 1000 mL); 0.9% (3 mL, 5 mL, 10 mL, 20 mL, 25 mL, 30 mL, 50 mL, 100 mL, 150 mL, 250 mL, 500 mL, 1000 mL); 3% (500 mL); 5% (500 mL)

Syrex: 0.9% (2.5 mL, 5 mL, 10 mL) [prefilled syringe]

Injection, solution [bacteriostatic]: 0.9% (10 mL, 20 mL, 30 mL) [contains benzyl alcohol]

Injection, solution [concentrate]: 14.6% (2.5 mEq/mL) (20 mL, 40 mL); 23.4% (4 mEq/mL) (30 mL, 100 mL, 200 mL, 250 mL)

Ointment, ophthalmic: 5% (3.5 g)

Altachlore, Muro 128®: 5% (3.5 g)

Powder for nasal solution (Entsol®): 3% (10.5 g)

Solution for inhalation: 0.45% (3 mL, 5 mL); 0.9% (3 mL, 5 mL, 15 mL); 3% (15 mL); 10% (15 mL)

Broncho® Saline: 0.9% (90 mL, 240 mL) [for dilution of bronchodilator solutions]

Solution, intranasal: 0.65% (45 mL)

Altamist: 0.65% (60 mL) [spray; contains benzalkonium chloride]

Ayr® Baby Saline: 0.65% (30 mL) [spray/drops; contains benzalkonium chloride]

Ayr® Saline: 0.65% (50 mL) [drops; contains benzalkonium chloride]

Ayr® Saline: 0.65% (50 mL) [mist, contains benzalkonium chloride]

Breathe Right® Saline: 0.65% (44 mL) [spray; contains benzalkonium chloride]

Deep Sea: 0.65% (45 mL) [spray; contains benzalkonium chloride]

Entsol® Mist: 3% (30 mL) [spray; contains benzalkonium chloride]

Entsol® [preservative free]: 3% (100 mL) [spray]

Entsol® [preservative free]: 3% (240 mL) [nasal wash]

Mycinaire™: 0.65% (30 mL) [mist; contains benzalkonium chloride]

Na-Zone®: 0.65% (60 mL) [spray; contains benzalkonium chloride]

NaSal™: 0.65% (15 mL) [drops; contains benzalkonium chloride], (30 mL) [spray; contains benzalkonium chloride]

Nasal Moist®: 0.65% (45 mL) [spray]

Ocean®: 0.65% (45 mL) [mist/spray/drops; contains benzalkonium chloride]; (473 mL) [refill bottle; contains benzalkonium chloride]

Ocean® for Kids: 0.65% (37.5 mL) [drops/spray/stream; contains benzalkonium chloride]

Pretz®: 0.75% (50 mL) [spray; contains benzalkonium chloride and yerba santa]; (240 mL) [irrigation; contains benzalkonium chloride and yerba santa]; (960 mL) [refill bottle; contains benzalkonium chloride and yerba santa]

SalineX®: 0.4% (15 mL) [drops]; (50 mL) [spray]

Simply Saline®: 0.9% (44 mL, 90 mL) [mist]

Simply Saline® Baby: 0.9% (45 mL) [mist]

4-Way® Saline Moisturizing Mist: 0.74% (30 mL) [alcohol free; contains benzalkonium chloride, eucalyptol, and menthol]

Solution for irrigation: 0.45% (1500 mL, 2000 mL); 0.9% (250 mL, 500 mL, 1000 mL, 1500 mL, 2000 mL, 3000 mL, 4000 mL, 5000 mL)

Wound Wash Saline™: 0.9% (90 mL, 210 mL)

Solution, ophthalmic: 5% (15 mL)

Altachlore: 5% (15 mL, 30 mL)

Muro 128®: 2% (15 mL); 5% (15 mL, 30 mL)

Reference Range

Serum/plasma levels:

Neonates: Full-term: 133-142 mEq/L; Premature: 132-140 mEq/L

Children 2 months to Adults: 135-145 mEq/L

Neurologic symptoms occur when serum sodium reaches 150-160 mEq/L; serum sodium levels from 160-185 mEq/L will commonly cause seizures, especially if an attempt is made to rapidly lower serum sodium; >185 mEq/L, death will likely result

Overdosage/Treatment

Decontamination: **Oral**: Emesis within 30 minutes or lavage within 1 hour; activated charcoal probably is not useful. **Ocular**: Irrigate copiously with water.

Supportive therapy: For hypernatremia, give 30-50 mEq/L of sodium (half chloride, half bicarbonate) by slow I.V. infusion; prepare solution by adding 15-25 mEq/L sodium chloride (2.5 mEq/mL) and 15-25 mEq sodium bicarbonate (1 mEq/mL) to 1 liter D_5W; administer at a rate of $^2/_3$ maintenance with a goal of achieving normal serum sodium at 24-36 hours after initiating treatment; seizures may occur if serum sodium is lowered too quickly; I.V. mannitol (0.5-1 g/kg) should be used to treat cerebral edema; seizures can be treated with lorazepam or diazepam 0.1-0.25 mg/kg

Enhancement of elimination: Hypernatremia is resolved through the use of diuretics and free water replacement. Peritoneal dialysis should be considered in infants who are salt poisoned; hemodialysis should be considered in patients who are refractory to other therapies or in patients with renal impairment.

Drug Interactions Decreased levels of lithium

Pregnancy Risk Factor C

Pregnancy Implications Most of dose is concentrated in the decidua and fetal part of the placenta; some diffuses into maternal blood. When hypertonic sodium chloride is injected into the amniotic fluid, the following may result: Disseminated intravascular coagulation, renal necrosis, uterine and cervical lesions, pulmonary embolism, pneumonia, hemorrhage, death.

Nursing Implications Bacteriostatic NS should not be used for diluting or reconstituting drugs for administration in neonates; I.V. infusion of 3% or 5% sodium chloride should not exceed 100 mL/hour and should be administered in a central line only; presence or worsening of rales and degree of peripheral edema with infusions

Additional Information

Lethal dose: 3 g/kg

Deaths have been reported in patients who have consumed salt water as an emetic; ingestion of 0.5-1 g/kg sodium chloride is likely to be toxic; tablets can be radiopaque; 1 tablespoon of tablet salt contains ~305 mEq of sodium and can cause an elevation of serum sodium by 30.5 mEq/L in a child 3 years of age; sodium content of human milk: 7 mEq/L; cow's milk: 21 mEq/L

Specific References

Barr J, Khan S, McCullough S, et al, "Homemade Play Dough Toxicoses in Dogs: 14 Cases (1998-2001)," *J Toxicol Clin Toxicol*, 2003, 41(5):666.

Casavant MJ and Fitch JA, "Fatal Hypernatremia from Saltwater Used as an Emetic," *J Toxicol Clin Toxicol*, 2003, 41(6):861-3.

Kupiec TC, Goldenring JM, and Raj V, "A Non-Fatal Case of Sodium Toxicity," *J Anal Toxicol*, 2004, 28(6):525-8.

Sodium Dichloroacetate

CAS Number 2156-56-1; 79-43-6

Impairment Potential Yes, at doses >50 mg/kg

Use Treatment of chronic or congenital forms of lactic acidosis; also has been used to treat homozygous familial hypercholesterolemia

Mechanism of Action An organohalide which activates the enzyme pyruvate dehydrogenase which results in pyruvate and lactate catabolism and inhibits glycolysis

Signs and Symptoms of Overdose Drowsiness, elevation of liver enzymes, elevation of serum urate and ketone levels, sedation (at doses >50 mg/kg), peripheral neuropathy (with chronic daily dosing of 50-100 mg/kg)

Toxicodynamics/Kinetics
Distribution: V_d: 0.3 L/kg
Metabolism: Hepatic to glycine, oxalate, and CO_2
Bioavailability: High
Half-life: ~1 hour (single dose); 8 hours (chronic doses)
Time to peak plasma levels: Oral: 15-30 minutes

Dosage Oral: Daily doses of 25-100 mg/kg
I.V.: 50 mg/kg over 30 minutes followed by a second dose in 2 hours
Highest reported dose:
Children: 1.5 g
Adults: 34 g
Should not be given chronically

Reference Range Following a 50 mg/kg intravenous dose, peak plasma DCA concentration is ~116 mcg/mL

Overdosage/Treatment
Decontamination: Oral: Activated charcoal/lavage at doses >100 mg/kg within 1 hour
Supportive therapy: Peripheral neuropathy usually resolves upon discontinuation of drug

Test Interactions Elevates acetoacetate and beta hydroxybutyrate levels

Additional Information DCA is a production of water chlorination; usual daily dose ingested through drinking water is 2-4 mcg/kg

Sodium Salicylate

CAS Number 54-21-7

Use Treatment of minor pain or fever; arthritis

Mechanism of Action Inhibits prostaglandin synthesis, acts on the hypothalamus heat-regulating center to reduce fever; decreases pain receptor sensitivity. Other proposed mechanisms of action for salicylate anti-inflammatory action are lysosomal stabilization, kinin and leukotriene production, alteration of chemotactic factors, and inhibition of neutrophil activation. This latter mechanism may be the most significant pharmacologic action to reduce inflammation.

Adverse Reactions
Dermatologic: Rash
Gastrointestinal: Nausea, vomiting, GI distress, GI bleeding, ulcers
Hematologic: Platelet inhibition
Hepatic: Hepatotoxicity
Respiratory: Wheezing

Signs and Symptoms of Overdose Bezoars, drowsiness, gastritis, GI bleeding, hyperthermia, hypoglycemia, nausea, nystagmus, ototoxicity, tinnitus, vomiting, wheezing. Severe poisoning can manifest with agranulocytosis, coma, confusion, dizziness, feces discoloration (black; pink; red; tarry), fever, granulocytopenia, headache, hyperglycemia, hyponatremia, hypotension, leukopenia, metabolic acidosis, neutropenia, pylorospasm, rhabdomyolysis, renal failure and/or hepatic failure, respiratory depression, seizures, urine discoloration (pink)

Admission Criteria/Prognosis Admit any patient with acidosis, mental status changes, thermoregulatory abnormality, glucose abnormality, serum salicylate >40 mg/dL following an acute ingestion

Pharmacodynamics/Kinetics
Absorption: From stomach and small intestine
Half-life elimination, serum: Aspirin: 15-20 minutes; metabolic pathways are saturable such that salicylates half-life is dose-dependent ranging from 3 hours at lower doses (300-600 mg), 5-6 hours (after 1 g) and 15-30 hours with higher doses; in therapeutic anti-inflammatory doses, half-lives generally range from 6-12 hours

Dosage Adults: Oral: 325-650 mg every 4 hours

Monitoring Parameters Serum concentrations, renal function; hearing changes or tinnitus; monitor for response (ie, pain, inflammation, range of motion, grip strength); observe for abnormal bleeding, bruising, weight gain

Contraindications Bleeding disorders (factor VII or IX deficiencies), hypersensitivity to salicylates or other nonsteroidal anti-inflammatory drugs (NSAIDs); tartrazine dye and asthma

Warnings Tinnitus or impaired hearing may indicate toxicity; discontinue use 1 week prior to surgical procedures

Dosage Forms Tablet, enteric coated: 325 mg, 650 mg

Reference Range
Sample size: 1.5-2 mL blood (purple top tube)
Timing of serum samples: Peak levels usually occur 2 hours after ingestion; half-life increases with dosage (eg, the half-life after 300 mg is 3 hours, and after 1 g is 5-6 hours, and after 8-10 g is 10 hours) Salicylate serum concentrations correlate with the pharmacological actions and adverse effects observed. See table.

Serum Salicylate: Clinical Correlations		
Serum Salicylate Concentration (mg/dL)	**Desired Effects**	**Adverse Effects / Intoxication**
~10	Antiplatelet	GI intolerance and bleeding, hypersensitivity, hemostatic defects
	Antipyresis	
	Analgesia	
15-20	Anti-inflammatory	Mild salicylism
25-40	Treatment of rheumatic fever	Nausea/vomiting, hyperventilation, salicylism, flushing, sweating, thirst, headache, diarrhea and tachycardia
>40		Respiratory alkalosis, hemorrhage, excitement, confusion, asterixis, pulmonary edema, convulsions, tetany, metabolic acidosis, fever, coma, cardiovascular collapse, renal and respiratory failure

Overdosage/Treatment
Decontamination: Activated charcoal is quite effective; each gram of activated charcoal can bind up to 550 mg of salicylic acid; whole bowel irrigation can also be used
Supportive therapy: Hypotension/dehydration can be managed with I.V. fluid therapy; acidosis should be treated with I.V. sodium bicarbonate (hypokalemia will need to be corrected), seizures with benzodiazepines; blood products are indicated, as appropriate, for hemorrhage; antacids may promote gastric absorption
Enhancement of elimination: Forced alkaline diuresis with I.V. sodium bicarbonate to keep urine pH at 8 should be performed for salicylate levels >40 mg/dL; dialysis is indicated for secondary complications, acidosis, or renal failure and not toxin removal alone; consider hemodialysis for acute salicylate levels >100 mg/dL; multiple dosing of activated charcoal may not hasten elimination; dialyzable (50% to 100%)

Drug Interactions Ammonium chloride, vitamin C (high dose), methionine, antacids, urinary alkalinizers, carbonic anhydrase inhibitors, corticosteroids, nizatidine, alcohol, ACE inhibitors, beta-blockers, loop diuretics, methotrexate, probenecid, sulfinpyrazone, spironolactone, sulfonylureas

Pregnancy Risk Factor C

Nursing Implications Sodium content of 1 g: 6.25 mEq; less effective than an equal dose of aspirin in reducing pain or fever; patients hypersensitive to aspirin may be able to tolerate

Additional Information Sodium content of 1 g: 6.25 mEq; less effective than an equal dose of aspirin in reducing pain or fever; patients hypersensitive to aspirin may be able to tolerate; total dose (mg) multiplied by 1.1 provides aspirin equivalent dose

Sorbinil

CAS Number 68367-52-2

Unlabeled/Investigational Use Decrease the adverse effects of diabetes mellitus, specifically diabetic, nephropathy, retinopathy, neuropathy, and cataract formation

Mechanism of Action Aldose reductase inhibitor structurally related to hydantoin, decreased amounts of sorbitol and fructose are formed from glucose; thus, less water is drawn into the lens (through osmosis) and neurons, thus possibly leading to less diabetic complications

Adverse Reactions
Dermatologic: Toxic epidermal necrolysis
Hematologic: Leukopenia, thrombocytopenia
Hepatic: Elevated liver function tests
Neuromuscular & skeletal: Myalgia
Respiratory: Adult respiratory distress syndrome
Miscellaneous: Hypersensitivity syndrome (maculopapular rash)

Toxicodynamics/Kinetics

Distribution: V_d: 0.7-1 L/kg

Half-life: 38-52 hours

Elimination: Renal (33%); renal clearance: 5.99 mL/1.73 m²/minute

Dosage 200-250 mg once daily

Reference Range After a single 250 mg dose, peak plasma levels were 3.3 mcg/mL in healthy young males, 5.4 mcg/mL in elderly males, and 6.3 mcg/mL in elderly females; after 5 days on above dose, plasma sorbinil levels can reach 10.6 mcg/mL

Overdosage/Treatment

Decontamination: Activated charcoal

Enhancement of elimination: Multiple dosing of activated charcoal may be effective

Sotalol

Related Information

● Selected Properties of Beta-Adrenergic Blocking Drugs

CAS Number 959-24-0

U.S. Brand Names Betapace AF®; Betapace®; Sorine®

Synonyms Sotalol Hydrochloride

Use Treatment of documented life-threatening ventricular arrhythmias (ie, sustained ventricular tachycardia), maintenance of normal sinus rhythm in patients with symptomatic atrial fibrillation and atrial flutter currently in sinus rhythm. Manufacturer states substitutions should not be made for Betapace AF™ since Betapace AF™ is distributed with a patient package insert specific for atrial fibrillation/flutter.

Mechanism of Action Has both B- and B_2-receptor blocking activity; also passes some type III antiarrhythmic activity

Adverse Reactions

Cardiovascular: **Bradycardia, chest pain, palpitations**, congestive heart failure, peripheral vascular disorders, edema, abnormal ECG, hypotension, proarrhythmia, Raynaud's phenomenon, syncope, leukocytoclastic vasculitis

Central nervous system: **Fatigue, dizziness, lightheadedness**, mental confusion, anxiety, headache, sleep problems, depression, emotional lability, clouded sensorium, incoordination, vertigo, paralysis, fever

Dermatologic: Itching/rash, cutaneous vasculitis, red crusted skin, photosensitivity reaction, pruritus, alopecia

Endocrine & metabolic: Decreased sexual ability, hyperlipidemia

Gastrointestinal: Diarrhea, nausea/vomiting, stomach discomfort, flatulence, xerostomia

Genitourinary: Impotence, retroperitoneal fibrosis

Hematologic: Bleeding, thrombocytopenia, eosinophilia, leukopenia

Hepatic: Increased serum transaminases

Local: Phlebitis, skin necrosis after extravasation

Neuromuscular & skeletal: **Weakness**, paresthesia, extremity pain, back pain, myalgia

Ocular: Visual problems

Respiratory: **Dyspnea**, upper respiratory problems, asthma, pulmonary edema, bronchiolitis obliterans with organized pneumonia

Miscellaneous: Diaphoresis, cold extremities

Signs and Symptoms of Overdose Bleeding, depression, eosinophilia, heart block, hypoglycemia, impotence, insomnia, leukopenia or neutropenia (agranulocytosis, granulocytopenia), lightheadedness, myasthenia gravis (exacerbation or precipitation), QT prolongation, thrombocytopenia

Admission Criteria/Prognosis Admit any patient with QT prolongation, cardiac arrhythmia; admit any pediatric ingestion >8 mg/kg or adult ingestion >1 g

Pharmacodynamics/Kinetics

Onset of action: Rapid, 1-2 hours

Peak effect: 2.5-4 hours

Duration: 8-16 hours

Absorption: Decreased 20% to 30% by meals compared to fasting

Distribution: Low lipid solubility; enters milk of laboratory animals and is reported to be present in human milk

Protein binding: None

Metabolism: None

Bioavailability: 90% to 100%

Half-life elimination: 12 hours; Children: 9.5 hours; terminal half-life decreases with age <2 years (may by ≥1 week in neonates)

Excretion: Urine (as unchanged drug)

Dosage Sotalol should be initiated and doses increased in a hospital with facilities for cardiac rhythm monitoring and assessment. Proarrhythmic events can occur after initiation of therapy and with each upward dosage adjustment.

Children: Oral: The safety and efficacy of sotalol in children have not been established

Note: Dosing per manufacturer, based on pediatric pharmacokinetic data; wait at least 36 hours between dosage adjustments to allow monitoring of QT intervals

≤2 years: Dosage should be adjusted (decreased) by plotting of the child's age on a logarithmic scale; see graph or refer to manufacturer's package labeling.

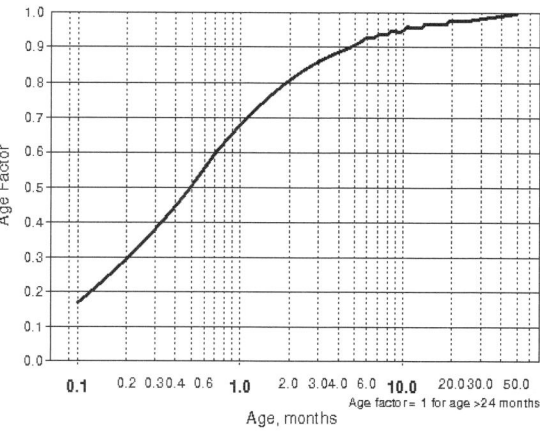

Age Factor Nomogram

Adapted from U.S. Food and Drug Administration.
http://www.fda.gov/cder/foi/label/2001/2115s3lbl.PDF

>2 years: Initial: 90 mg/m²/day in 3 divided doses; may be incrementally increased to a maximum of 180 mg/m²/day

Adults: Oral:

Ventricular arrhythmias (Betapace®, Sorine™):

Initial: 80 mg twice daily

Dose may be increased gradually to 240-320 mg/day; allow 3 days between dosing increments in order to attain steady-state plasma concentrations and to allow monitoring of QT intervals

Most patients respond to a total daily dose of 160-320 mg/day in 2-3 divided doses.

Some patients, with life-threatening refractory ventricular arrhythmias, may require doses as high as 480-640 mg/day; however, these doses should only be prescribed when the potential benefit outweighs the increased of adverse events.

Atrial fibrillation or atrial flutter (Betapace AF™): Initial: 80 mg twice daily

If the initial dose does not reduce the frequency of relapses of atrial fibrillation/flutter and is tolerated without excessive QT prolongation (not >520 msec) after 3 days, the dose may be increased to 120 mg twice daily. This may be further increased to 160 mg twice daily if response is inadequate and QT prolongation is not excessive.

Elderly: Age does not significantly alter the pharmacokinetics of sotalol, but impaired renal function in elderly patients can increase the terminal half-life, resulting in increased drug accumulation

Dosage adjustment in renal impairment:

Children: Safety and efficacy in children with renal impairment have not been established.

Adults: Impaired renal function can increase the terminal half-life, resulting in increased drug accumulation. Sotalol (Betapace AF™) is contraindicated per the manufacturer for treatment of atrial fibrillation/flutter in patients with a Cl_{cr} <40 mL/minute.

Ventricular arrhythmias (Betapace®, Sorine™):

Cl_{cr} >60 mL/minute: Administer every 12 hours

Cl_{cr} 30-60 mL/minute: Administer every 24 hours

Cl_{cr} 10-30 mL/minute: Administer every 36-48 hours

Cl_{cr} <10 mL/minute: Individualize dose

Atrial fibrillation/flutter (Betapace AF™):

Cl_{cr} >60 mL/minute: Administer every 12 hours

Cl_{cr} 40-60 mL/minute: Administer every 24 hours

Cl_{cr} <40 mL/minute: Use is contraindicated

Dialysis: Hemodialysis would be expected to reduce sotalol plasma concentrations because sotalol is not bound to plasma proteins and does not undergo extensive metabolism; administer dose postdialysis or administer supplemental 80 mg dose; peritoneal dialysis does not remove sotalol; supplemental dose is not necessary

Monitoring Parameters Serum magnesium, potassium, ECG

Administration Food may decrease adsorption

Contraindications Hypersensitivity to sotalol or any component of the formulation; bronchial asthma; sinus bradycardia; second- and third-degree AV block (unless a functioning pacemaker is present); congenital or acquired long QT syndromes; cardiogenic shock; uncontrolled congestive heart failure. Betapace AF® is contraindicated in patients with significantly reduced renal filtration (Cl_{cr} <40 mL/minute).

Warnings

Manufacturer recommends initiation (or reinitiation) and doses increased in a hospital setting with continuous monitoring and staff familiar with the recognition and treatment of life-threatening arrhythmias. Dosage of sotalol should be adjusted gradually with 3 days between dosing increments to achieve steady-state concentrations, and to allow time to monitor QT intervals. Some experts will initiate therapy on an outpatient basis in a patient without heart disease or bradycardia, who has a baseline uncorrected QT interval <450 msec, and normal serum potassium and magnesium levels; close EKG monitoring during this time is necessary. ACC/AHA guidelines for management of atrial fibrillation also recommend that for outpatient initiation the patient not have risk factors predisposing to drug-induced ventricular proarrhythmia (Fuster, 2001). Creatinine clearance must be calculated prior to dosing. Use cautiously in the renally-impaired (dosage adjustment required).

Monitor and adjust dose to prevent QT_c prolongation. Concurrent use with other QT_c-prolonging drugs (including Class I and Class III antiarrhythmics) is generally not recommended; withhold for 3 half-lives. Watch for proarrhythmic effects. Correct electrolyte imbalances before initiating (especially hypokalemia and hyperkalemia). Consider pre-existing conditions such as sick sinus syndrome before initiating. Conduction abnormalities can occur particularly sinus bradycardia. Use cautiously within the first 2 weeks post-MI (experience limited). Administer cautiously in compensated heart failure and monitor for a worsening of the condition. Use caution in patients with PVD (can aggravate arterial insufficiency). Beta-blocker therapy should not be withdrawn abruptly (particularly in patients with CAD), but gradually tapered to avoid acute tachycardia, hypertension, and/or ischemia. Use caution with concurrent use of beta-blockers and either verapamil or diltiazem; bradycardia or heart block can occur. Use cautiously in diabetics because it can mask prominent hypoglycemic symptoms. Can mask signs of thyrotoxicosis. Use care with anesthetic agents which decrease myocardial function.

[U.S. Boxed Warning]: Betapace® should not be substituted for Betapace® AF; Betapace® AF is distributed with an educational insert specifically for patients with atrial fibrillation/flutter.

Dosage Forms Tablet, as hydrochloride: 80 mg, 80 mg [AF], 120 mg, 120 mg [AF], 160 mg, 160 mg [AF], 240 mg

Betapace® [light blue]: 80 mg, 120 mg, 160 mg, 240 mg

Betapace AF® [white]: 80 mg, 120 mg, 160 mg

Sorine® [white]: 80 mg, 120 mg, 160 mg, 240 mg

Reference Range Peak serum level: ∼1.7 mg/L after 160 mg oral dose; peak serum sotalol level following a 11.2 g overdose: 20.6 mg/L

Overdosage/Treatment

Decontamination: Lavage (within 1 hour)/activated charcoal; do not use ipecac

Supportive therapy: Glucagon (50-150 mcg/kg followed by continuous drip of 1-5 mg/hour) for positive chronotropic effect; glucagon can correct bradycardia and sinus arrest; atropine/isoproterenol can be utilized to increase heart rate; calcium chloride may also be effective; doses >320 mg are at risk for torsade de pointes; lidocaine has also been used successfully in treating torsade de pointes due to a 3-4 g ingestion of sotalol

Enhancement of elimination: Multiple dosing of activated charcoal is likely to be of benefit; hemodialysis or hemoperfusion may be effective

Antidote(s)

- Glucagon [ANTIDOTE]

Drug Interactions Amiodarone: May cause additive effects on QT_c prolongation as well as decreased heart rate, and has been associated with cardiac arrest in patients receiving beta-blockers.

Antacids (aluminum/magnesium) decrease sotalol blood levels; separate administration by 2 hours.

Antiarrhythmics: Concurrent use of Class Ia or Class III antiarrhythmics may result in additive QT_c prolongation; concurrent use is not recommended.

Beta$_2$ agonists: Effects may be diminished by concurrent sotalol; use caution.

Beta-blockers: Due to shared pharmacological effects, heart rate reductions may be additive; concurrent use is not recommended.

Calcium channel blockers: Concurrent use may lead to additive effects on AV conduction, ventricular contractility, and/or hypotension; use caution.

Cisapride: Concurrent use with sotalol increases malignant arrhythmias; contraindicated.

Clonidine: Sotalol may cause rebound hypertension after discontinuation of clonidine.

QT_c-prolonging drugs: Concurrent use may result in additive QT_c prolongation, potentially increasing the risk of malignant arrhythmias. Use of cisapride, mesoridazine, thioridazine, and pimozide with other QT_c-prolonging agents is contraindicated. Concurrent use of sotalol with Class I and Class III antiarrhythmics is not recommended; withhold for 3 half-lives. Use caution with other QT_c-prolonging agents (including bepridil, erythromycin, clarithromycin), fluoroquinolones (including sparfloxacin, gatifloxacin, and moxifloxacin), haloperidol, and TCAs.

Phenothiazines (mesoridazine and thioridazine): Concurrent use may result in additive QT_c prolongation, potentially increasing the risk of malignant arrhythmias; contraindicated.

Pimozide: Concurrent use may result in additive QT_c prolongation, potentially increasing the risk of malignant arrhythmias; contraindicated.

Pregnancy Risk Factor B

Pregnancy Implications There are no adequate and well-controlled studies in pregnant women. Beta-blockers have been associated with bradycardia, hypotension, and IUGR; IUGR is probably related to maternal hypertension. Sotalol has been shown to cross the placenta, and is found in amniotic fluid, therefore, sotalol should be used during pregnancy only if the potential benefit outweighs the potential risk. Cases of neonatal hypoglycemia have been reported following maternal use of beta-blockers at parturition or during breast-feeding.

Lactation Enters breast milk/use caution (AAP rates "compatible")

Nursing Implications Initiation of therapy and dose escalation should be done in a hospital with cardiac monitoring; lidocaine and other resuscitative measures should be available

Additional Information Risk factors for development of sotalol-induced torsade de pointes include female gender, sustained ventricular tachycardia or fibrillation on presentation, medical history of congestive heart failure, and a daily dose >320 mg

Specific References

Cubeddu LX, "QT Prolongation and Fatal Arrhythmias: A Review of Clinical Implications and Effects of Drugs," *Am J Ther*, 2003, 10(6): 452-7.

Nahata MC and Morosco RS, "Stability of Sotalol in Two Liquid Formulations at Two Temperatures," *Ann Pharmacother*, 2003, 37(4):506-9.

Singh BN, Singh SN, Reda DJ, et al, Sotalol Amiodarone Atrial Fibrillation Efficacy Trial (SAFE-T) Investigators, "Amiodarone Versus Sotalol for Atrial Fibrillation," *N Engl J Med*, 2005, 352(18):1861-72.

Sparfloxacin

CAS Number 110871-86-8

U.S. Brand Names Zagam®

Use Treatment of adults with community-acquired pneumonia caused by *C. pneumoniae*, *H. influenzae*, *H. parainfluenzae*, *M. catarrhalis*, *M. pneumoniae* or *S. pneumoniae*; treatment of acute bacterial exacerbations of chronic bronchitis caused by *C. pneumoniae*, *E. cloacae*, *H. influenzae*, *H. parainfluenzae*, *K. pneumoniae*, *M. catarrhalis*, *S. aureus* or *S. pneumoniae*

Mechanism of Action Inhibits DNA-gyrase in susceptible organisms; inhibits relaxation of supercoiled DNA and promotes breakage of double-stranded DNA

Adverse Reactions

Cardiovascular: QT_c interval prolongation, vasodilation, angina pectoris, arrhythmias, atrial fibrillation, atrial flutter, complete AV block, postural hypotension, torsade de pointes

Central nervous system: Insomnia, dizziness, headache, anxiety, confusion, hallucinations, migraine, sleep disorder, vertigo

Dermatologic: Photosensitivity reaction, pruritus, angioedema, ecchymosis, exfoliative dermatitis, rash, Stevens-Johnson syndrome, toxic epidermal necrolysis

Gastrointestinal: Diarrhea, dyspepsia, nausea, abdominal pain, vomiting, flatulence, taste perversion, dry mouth

Hematologic: Anemia, eosinophilia, leukopenia, pancytopenia

Hepatic: Increased LFTs, hepatic failure

Neuromuscular & skeletal: Tendon rupture, tendonitis

Respiratory: Asthma, dyspnea

Miscellaneous: Allergic reaction, anaphylactoid reaction, anaphylactic shock

Signs and Symptoms of Overdose Symptoms of overdose include acute renal failure, seizures

Pharmacodynamics/Kinetics

Absorption: Unaffected by food or milk; reduced ∼50% by concurrent administration of aluminum- and magnesium-containing antacids

Distribution: Widely throughout the body; V_d: 3.9 L/kg

Protein binding: 45%

Metabolism: Hepatic, primarily by phase II glucuronidation

Half-life elimination: Mean terminal: 20 hours (range: 16-30 hours)

Time to peak, serum: 3-5 hours

Excretion: Urine (50%; ∼10% as unchanged drug); feces (50%)

Dosage

Adults: Oral:

Loading dose: 2 tablets (400 mg) on day 1

Maintenance: 1 tablet (200 mg) daily for 10 additional days (total 11 tablets)

Leprosy: Loading dose: 400 mg followed by 200 mg/day for 12 weeks

Dosing adjustment in renal impairment: Cl_{cr} <50 mL/minute: Administer 400 mg on day 1, then 200 mg every 48 hours for a total of 9 days of therapy (total 6 tablets)

Monitoring Parameters Evaluation of organ system functions (renal, hepatic, ophthalmologic, and hematopoietic) is recommended periodically during therapy; the possibility of crystalluria should be assessed; WBC and signs and symptoms of infection

Administration May be taken without regard to meals, however, should be administered at the same time each day. Antacids containing aluminum or magnesium; products containing iron, zinc, or calcium; and sucralfate and didanosine should all be given >4 hours after sparfloxacin.

Contraindications Hypersensitivity to sparfloxacin, any component of the formulation, or other quinolones; a concurrent administration with drugs which increase the QT interval including amiodarone, bepridil, bretylium, cisapride, disopyramide, furosemide, procainamide, quinidine, sotalol, albuterol, chloroquine, halofantrine, phenothiazines, prednisone, and tricyclic antidepressants

Warnings Not recommended in children <18 years of age, other quinolones have caused transient arthropathy in children; CNS stimulation may occur (tremor, restlessness, confusion, and very rarely hallucinations or seizures); potential for seizures, although very rare, may be increased with concomitant NSAID therapy. Use with caution in individuals at risk of seizures. Use with caution in patients with known or suspected CNS disorder or renal dysfunction; prolonged use may result in superinfection. Moderate to severe photosensitivity reactions may occur in patients exposed to direct or indirect sunlight, or to artificial ultraviolet light. Patients should avoid unnecessary sunlight exposure during treatment and for 5 days following therapy. Pseudomembranous colitis may occur and should be considered in patients who present with diarrhea. Tendon inflammation and/or rupture have been reported with other quinolone antibiotics. Risk may be increased with concurrent corticosteroids, particularly in the elderly. Discontinue at first sign of tendon inflammation or pain.

Severe hypersensitivity reactions, including anaphylaxis, have occurred with quinolone therapy. If an allergic reaction occurs (itching, urticaria, dyspnea, facial edema, loss of consciousness, tingling, cardiovascular collapse), discontinue drug immediately. Although quinolones may exacerbate myasthenia gravis, sparfloxacin appears to be an exception; caution is still warranted.

Dosage Forms [DSC] = Discontinued product
Tablet: 200 mg [DSC]

Reference Range Following a 400 mg oral dose, peak sparfloxacin plasma level: 1.3 mcg/mL

Overdosage/Treatment GI decontamination and supportive care; not removed by peritoneal or hemodialysis

Drug Interactions Corticosteroids: Concurrent use may increase the risk of tendon rupture, particularly in elderly patients (overall incidence rare).

Glyburide: Quinolones may increase the effect of glyburide; monitor

Metal cations (aluminum, calcium, iron, magnesium and zinc) bind quinolones in the gastrointestinal tract and inhibit absorption. Concurrent administration of most antacids, oral electrolyte supplements, quinapril, sucralfate, some didanosine formulations (chewable/buffered tablets and pediatric powder for oral suspension), and other highly-buffered oral drugs, should be avoided. Sparfloxacin should be administered 2 hours before or 4 hours after these agents.

Probenecid: May decrease renal secretion of sparfloxacin.

QT$_c$-prolonging agents: Effects may be additive with sparfloxacin. Avoid concurrent use with Class Ia and Class III antiarrhythmics, erythromycin, cisapride, antipsychotics, and cyclic antidepressants.

Warfarin: The hypoprothrombinemic effect of warfarin may be enhanced by some quinolone antibiotics; monitor INR.

Pregnancy Risk Factor C

Pregnancy Implications Quinolones are known to distribute well into breast milk; consequently use during lactation should be avoided if possible; avoid use in pregnant women unless the benefit justifies the potential risk to the fetus

Lactation Enters breast milk/not recommended

Spirapril

CAS Number 83647-97-6; 94841-17-5

Use Treatment of hypertension, congestive heart failure

Mechanism of Action Angiotensin-converting enzyme inhibitor; inhibits renin-angiotensin system

Adverse Reactions
Cardiovascular: Hypotension (orthostatic), QT prolongation, vasodilation
Central nervous system: Headache, dizziness, migraine headache (exacerbation of), hypoesthesia
Dermatologic: Skin rash
Gastrointestinal: Nausea, diarrhea, vomiting
Neuromuscular & skeletal: Back pain
Ocular: Conjunctivitis
Respiratory: Cough

Pharmacodynamics/Kinetics
Absorption: Oral: 53% to 60% (delayed by high fat meals)
Distribution: V$_d$: Oral: 270 L; I.V.: 28 L

Protein binding: 86% to 91%
Metabolism: Hepatic to active metabolite spiraprilat
Half-life: 1-2 hours
Elimination: Renal

Dosage Congestive heart failure: Oral: 1.5-6.25 mg
Hypertension: Starting dose: Oral: 12 mg/day in 1-2 divided doses; may increase dose in 2- to 4-week intervals

Contraindications Hypersensitivity to spirapril or any component of the formulation; angioedema or other sensitivity to any ACE inhibitor; bilateral renal artery stenosis; pregnancy (2nd and 3rd trimesters)

Warnings Anaphylactic reactions can occur. Angioedema can occur at any time during treatment (especially following first dose). It may involve head and neck (potentially affecting the airway) or the intestine (presenting with abdominal pain). Prolonged monitoring may be required especially if tongue, glottis, or larynx are involved as they are associated with airway obstruction. Those with a history of airway surgery in this situation have a higher risk. Careful blood pressure monitoring with first dose (hypotension can occur especially in volume-depleted patients). Dosage adjustment needed in renal impairment. Use with caution in hypovolemia; collagen vascular diseases; valvular stenosis (particularly aortic stenosis); hyperkalemia; or before, during, or immediately prior to anesthesia. Avoid rapid dosage escalation which may lead to renal insufficiency. Rare toxicities associated with ACE inhibitors include cholestatic jaundice (which may progress to hepatic necrosis) and neutropenia/agranulocytosis with myeloid hyperplasia. If patient has renal impairment then a baseline WBC with differential and serum creatinine should be evaluated and monitored closely during the first 3 months of therapy. Hypersensitivity reactions may be seen during hemodialysis with high-flux dialysis membranes (eg, AN69). Deterioration in renal function can occur with initiation. Use with caution in unilateral renal artery stenosis and pre-existing renal insufficiency.

Dosage Forms Tablet: 3 mg, 6 mg, 12 mg, 24 mg

Reference Range After a 6 mg oral dose, peak plasma spirapril and spiraprilat level is ~20 ng/mL and 23 ng/mL, respectively; after a 6 mg I.V. dose, peak serum spiraprilat level is ~45 ng/mL

Overdosage/Treatment
Decontamination: Activated charcoal
Supportive therapy: Following initiation of essential overdose management, toxic symptom treatment and supportive treatment should be initiated. Hypotension usually responds to I.V. normal saline or Trendelenburg positioning. If unresponsive to these measures, the use of a parenteral inotrope may be required (eg, norepinephrine 0.1-0.2 mcg/kg/minute titrated to response). Naloxone may antagonize hypotensive effects. Inhaled sodium cromoglycate (total dose: 40 mg/day) can decrease ACE-inhibitor cough by 50%.
Enhanced elimination: Multiple dosing of activated charcoal may be effective

Drug Interactions Alpha$_1$ blockers: Hypotensive effect increased.
Aspirin: May decrease ACE inhibitor efficacy and/or increase risk of renal effects.
Diuretics: Hypovolemia due to diuretics may precipitate acute hypotensive events or acute renal failure.
Insulin: Risk of hypoglycemia may be increased.
Lithium: Risk of lithium toxicity may be increased; monitor lithium levels, especially the first 4 weeks of therapy.
Mercaptopurine: Risk of neutropenia may be increased.
NSAIDs: May attenuate hypertensive efficacy; effect has been seen with captopril and may occur with other ACE inhibitors; monitor blood pressure. May increase risk of renal effects.
Potassium-sparing diuretics (amiloride, potassium, spironolactone, triamterene): Increased risk of hyperkalemia.
Potassium supplements may increase the risk of hyperkalemia.
Trimethoprim (high dose) may increase the risk of hyperkalemia.

Pregnancy Risk Factor C (1st trimester); D (2nd and 3rd trimesters)

Pregnancy Implications Cranial defects, hypocalvaria/acalvaria, oligohydramnios, persistent anuria following delivery, hypotension, renal defects, renal dysgenesis/dysplasia, renal failure, pulmonary hypoplasia, limb contractures secondary to oligohydramnios, and stillbirth reported. ACE inhibitors should be avoided during pregnancy, particularly in the 2nd and 3rd trimesters.

Additional Information Not available in U.S.

Spironolactone

CAS Number 52-01-7

U.S. Brand Names Aldactone®

Use Management of edema associated with excessive aldosterone excretion; hypertension; congestive heart failure; primary hyperaldosteronism; hypokalemia; treatment of hirsutism; cirrhosis of liver accompanied by edema or ascites

Unlabeled/Investigational Use Female acne (adjunctive therapy); hirsutism; hypertension (pediatric); diuretic (pediatric)

Mechanism of Action Competes with aldosterone for receptor sites in the distal renal tubules, increasing sodium chloride and water excretion while conserving potassium and hydrogen ions; may block the effect of aldosterone on arteriolar smooth muscle as well

Adverse Reactions

Cardiovascular: Myocarditis (hypersensitivity), myocarditis, vasculitis, Raynaud's phenomenon

Central nervous system: Lethargy, headache, mental confusion, fever, ataxia, CNS depression, depression

Dermatologic: Rash, alopecia, hypertrichosis, erythema multiforme, xerosis, urticaria, purpura, photosensitivity, pruritus, bullous pemphigoid, licheniform eruptions, exanthem

Endocrine & metabolic: Hyperkalemia (especially in patients with azotemia or receiving potassium supplements), dehydration, hyponatremia, hypokalemia, hyperchloremic metabolic acidosis, postmenopausal bleeding, amenorrhea, gynecomastia

Gastrointestinal: Anorexia, nausea, vomiting, diarrhea, gastritis, loss of taste perception, xerostomia

Hematologic: Eosinophilia

Hepatic: Hepatotoxicity

Neuromuscular & skeletal: Paresthesia

Ocular: Myopia

Renal: Elevated BUN

Miscellaneous: Development of systemic lupus erythematosus

Pharmacodynamics/Kinetics

Duration of action: 2-3 days

Protein binding: 91% to 98%

Metabolism: Hepatic to multiple metabolites, including canrenone (active)

Half-life elimination: 78-84 minutes

Time to peak, serum: 1-3 hours (primarily as the active metabolite)

Excretion: Urine and feces

Dosage To reduce delay in onset of effect, a loading dose of 2 or 3 times the daily dose may be administered on the first day of therapy. Oral:

Neonates: Diuretic: 1-3 mg/kg/day divided every 12-24 hours

Children:

Diuretic, hypertension: 1.5-3.5 mg/kg/day **or** 60 mg/m^2/day in divided doses every 6-24 hours

Diagnosis of primary aldosteronism: 125-375 mg/m^2/day in divided doses

Vaso-occlusive disease: 7.5 mg/kg/day in divided doses twice daily (not FDA approved)

Adults:

Edema, hypokalemia: 25-200 mg/day in 1-2 divided doses

Hypertension (JNC 7): 25-50 mg/day in 1-2 divided doses

Diagnosis of primary aldosteronism: 100-400 mg/day in 1-2 divided doses

Hirsutism in women: 50-200 mg/day in 1-2 divided doses

CHF, severe (with ACE inhibitor and a loop diuretic $\pm$ digoxin): 12.5-25 mg/day; maximum daily dose: 50 mg (higher doses may occasionallly be used). In the RALES trial, 25 mg every other day was the lowest maintenance dose possible.

Note: If potassium >5.4 mEq/L, consider dosage reduction.

Elderly: Initial: 25-50 mg/day in 1-2 divided doses, increasing by 25-50 mg every 5 days as needed.

Dosing interval in renal impairment:

Cl$_{cr}$ 10-50 mL/minute: Administer every 12-24 hours.

Cl$_{cr}$ <10 mL/minute: Avoid use.

Monitoring Parameters Blood pressure, serum electrolytes (potassium, sodium), renal function, I & O ratios and daily weight throughout therapy

Contraindications Hypersensitivity to spironolactone or any component of the formulation; anuria; acute renal insufficiency; significant impairment of renal excretory function; hyperkalemia; pregnancy (pregnancy-induced hypertension - per expert analysis)

Warnings Avoid potassium supplements, potassium-containing salt substitutes, a diet rich in potassium, or other drugs that can cause hyperkalemia. Monitor for fluid and electrolyte imbalances. Gynecomastia is related to dose and duration of therapy. Diuretic therapy should be carefully used in severe hepatic dysfunction; electrolyte and fluid shifts can cause or exacerbate encephalopathy. Discontinue use prior to adrenal vein catheterization. When evaluating a heart failure patient for spironolactone treatment, creatinine should be ≤2.5 mg/dL in men or ≤2 mg/dL in women and potassium <5 mEq/L. **[U.S. Boxed Warning]: Shown to be a tumorigen in chronic toxicity animal studies. Avoid unnecessary use.**

Dosage Forms Tablet: 25 mg, 50 mg, 100 mg

Reference Range Steady-state of canrenone levels (of spironolactone dosing 50 mg twice daily) are 50-70 ng/mL (trough) and 146-250 ng/mL (peak)

Overdosage/Treatment

Decontamination: Activated charcoal

Supportive therapy: Hyperkalemia can be treated with glucose/insulin and sodium bicarbonate (1 mEq/kg); sodium polystyrene sulfonate can also be given; I.V. fluids administration of 0.45% sodium chloride with furosemide (1 mg/kg, up to 40 mg) can be used to promote urine flow

Test Interactions May cause false elevation in serum digoxin concentrations measured by RIA

Drug Interactions ACE inhibitors can cause hyperkalemia, especially in patients with renal impairment, potassium-rich diets, or on other drugs causing hyperkalemia; avoid concurrent use or monitor closely.

Cholestyramine can cause hyperchloremic acidosis in cirrhotic patients; avoid concurrent use.

Digoxin's positive inotropic effect may be reduced; serum levels of digoxin may increase.

Mitotane loses its effect; avoid concurrent use.

Potassium supplements may increase potassium retention and cause hyperkalemia; avoid concurrent use.

Salicylates and NSAIDs may interfere with the natriuretic action of spironolactone.

Pregnancy Risk Factor D

Pregnancy Implications Teratogenic effects were not observed in animal studies; however, doses used were less than or equal to equivalent doses in humans. The antiandrogen effects of spironolactone have been shown to cause feminization of the male fetus in animal studies. Two case reports did not demonstrate this effect in humans however, the authors caution that adequate data is lacking. Diuretics are generally avoided in pregnancy due to the theoretical risk that decreased plasma volume may cause placental insufficiency. Diuretics should not be used during pregnancy in the presence of reduced placental perfusion (eg, pre-eclampsia, intrauterine growth restriction).

Lactation Enters breast milk/not recommended (AAP rates "compatible")

Additional Information May be used in patients with hyperuricemia or gout

Specific References

Bozkurt B, Agoston I, and Knowlton AA, "Complications of Inappropriate Use of Spironolactone in Heart Failure: When an Old Medicine Spirals Out of New Guidelines," *J Am Coll Cardiol*, 2003, 41(2):211-4.

Buck ML, "Clinical Experience with Spironolactone in Pediatrics," *Ann Pharmacother*, 2005, 39(5):823-8.

Chobanian AV, Bakris GL, Black HR, et al, "The Seventh Report of the Joint National Committee on Prevention, Detection, Evaluation, and Treatment of High Blood Pressure: The JNC 7 Report," *JAMA*, 2003, 289(19):2560-71.

Christy NA, Franks AS, and Cross LB, "Spironolactone for Hirsutism in Polycystic Ovary Syndrome," *Ann Pharmacother*, 2005, 39(9):1517-21.

Raebel MA, McClure DL, Chan KA, et al, "Laboratory Evalution of Potassium and Creatinine Among Ambulatory Patients Prescribed Spirono-Lactone: Are We Monitoring for Hyperkalemia," *Annals of Pharmacotherapy*, 2007, 41(2):193-200.

Stanozolol

CAS Number 10418-03-8

U.S. Brand Names Winstrol®

Use Prophylactic use against hereditary angioedema

Mechanism of Action Synthetic testosterone derivative with similar androgenic and anabolic actions

Adverse Reactions

Male:

Postpubertal:

Central nervous system: Insomnia, chills

Dermatologic: **Acne (cystic)**, seborrheic dermatitis, hypertrichosis

Endocrine & metabolic: **Gynecomastia**, decreased libido

Gastrointestinal: Nausea, diarrhea

Genitourinary: **Priapism, bladder irritability**, prostatic hypertrophy (elderly)

Hematologic: Iron deficiency anemia, suppression of clotting factors

Hepatic: Hepatic necrosis, hepatocellular carcinoma, hepatic dysfunction

Miscellaneous: Antiphospholipid syndrome

Prepubertal:

Central nervous system: Chills, insomnia, factors

Dermatologic: **Acne**, hyperpigmentation

Endocrine & metabolic: **Virilism**

Gastrointestinal: Diarrhea, nausea

Hematologic: Iron deficiency anemia, suppression of clotting

Hepatic: Hepatic necrosis, hepatocellular carcinoma

Female:

Cardiovascular: Edema

Central nervous system: Chills, insomnia, paranoid psychosis, mania, CNS depression, depression

Dermatologic: Hypertrichosis

Endocrine & metabolic: **Virilism**, hypercalcemia

Gastrointestinal: Nausea, diarrhea

Hematologic: Iron deficiency anemia, suppression of clotting factors

Hepatic: Hepatic dysfunction, hepatic necrosis, hepatocellular carcinoma, peliosis hepatitis

Pharmacodynamics/Kinetics

Metabolism: Hepatic

Excretion: Urine (90%); feces (6%)

Dosage Children: Acute attacks:
<6 years: 1 mg/day
6-12 years: 2 mg/day
Adults: Oral: Initial: 2 mg 3 times/day, may then reduce to a maintenance dose of 2 mg/day or 2 mg every other day after 1-3 months
Dosing adjustment in hepatic impairment: Avoid use in patients with severe liver dysfunction

Contraindications Hypersensitivity to stanozolol or any component of the formulation; nephrosis; carcinoma of breast or prostate; pregnancy

Warnings May stunt bone growth in children; anabolic steroids may cause peliosis hepatis, liver cell tumors, and blood lipid changes with increased risk of arteriosclerosis; monitor diabetic patients carefully; use with caution in elderly patients, they may be at greater risk for prostatic hyperplasia; use with caution in patients with cardiac, renal, or hepatic disease or epilepsy

Dosage Forms Tablet: 2 mg

Overdosage/Treatment Decontamination: Activated charcoal

Drug Interactions Increased toxicity: ACTH, adrenal steroids may increase risk of edema and acne; stanozolol enhances the hypoprothrombinemic effects of oral anticoagulants; enhances the hypoglycemic effects of insulin and sulfonylureas (oral hypoglycemics)

Pregnancy Risk Factor X

Lactation Enters breast milk/contraindicated

Stavudine

CAS Number 3056-17-5
U.S. Brand Names Zerit®
Synonyms d4T

Use Treatment of adults with advanced HIV infection who are intolerant to approved therapies with proven clinical benefit or who have experienced significant clinical or immunologic deterioration while receiving these therapies, or for whom such therapies are contraindicated

Mechanism of Action Inhibits reverse transcriptase of the human immunodeficiency virus (HIV)

Adverse Reactions
All adverse reactions reported below were similar to comparative agent, zidovudine, except for peripheral neuropathy, which was greater for stavudine.
Central nervous system: **Headache, chills/fever, malaise, insomnia, anxiety, depression, pain,** insomnia
Dermatologic: **Rash**
Endocrine & metabolic: Lactic acidosis, redistribution/accumulation of body fat
Gastrointestinal: **Nausea, vomiting, diarrhea, pancreatitis, abdominal pain,** anorexia, pancreatitis
Hematologic: Neutropenia, thrombocytopenia, anemia, leukopenia
Hepatic: Increased hepatic transaminases, increased bilirubin, hepatomegaly, hepatic failure, hepatic steatosis
Neuromuscular & skeletal: **Peripheral neuropathy,** myalgia, back pain, weakness, motor weakness (severe)
Miscellaneous: Allergic reaction

Admission Criteria/Prognosis Admit any patient symptomatic after 6 hours postingestion, liver function test abnormalities or ingested dose >2 mg/kg

Pharmacodynamics/Kinetics
Distribution: V_d: 0.5 L/kg
Bioavailability: 86.4%
Metabolism: Undergoes intracellular phosphorylation to an active metabolite
Half-life elimination: 1-1.6 hours
Time to peak, serum: 1 hour
Excretion: Urine (40% as unchanged drug)

Dosage Oral:
Newborns (Birth to 13 days): 0.5 mg/kg every 12 hours
Children:
>14 days and <30 kg: 1 mg/kg every 12 hours
≥30 kg: Refer to Adults dosing
Adults:
≥60 kg: 40 mg every 12 hours
<60 kg: 30 mg every 12 hours
Dosing adjustment for toxicity: If symptoms of peripheral neuropathy occur, discontinue until symptoms resolve. Treatment may then be resumed at 50% the recommended dose. If symptoms recur at lower dose, permanent discontinuation should be considered.
Dosing adjustment in renal impairment:
Children: Specific recommendations not available. Reduction in dose or increase in dosing interval should be considered.
Adults:
Cl_{cr} >50 mL/minute:
≥60 kg: 40 mg every 12 hours
<60 kg: 30 mg every 12 hours
Cl_{cr} 26-50 mL/minute:
≥60 kg: 20 mg every 12 hours

<60 kg: 15 mg every 12 hours
Cl_{cr} 10-25 mL/minute, hemodialysis (administer dose after hemodialysis on day of dialysis):
≥60 kg: 20 mg every 24 hours
<60 kg: 15 mg every 24 hours
Elderly: Older patients should be closely monitored for signs and symptoms of peripheral neuropathy; dosage should be carefully adjusted to renal function

Monitoring Parameters Monitor liver function tests and signs and symptoms of peripheral neuropathy; monitor viral load and CD4 count

Administration May be administered without regard to meals. Oral solution should be shaken vigorously prior to use.

Contraindications Hypersensitivity to stavudine or any component of the formulation

Warnings Use with caution in patients who demonstrate previous hypersensitivity to zidovudine, didanosine, zalcitabine, pre-existing bone marrow suppression, renal insufficiency, or peripheral neuropathy. Peripheral neuropathy may be the dose-limiting side effect. Zidovudine should not be used in combination with stavudine. **[U.S. Boxed Warning]: Lactic acidosis and severe hepatomegaly with steatosis have been reported with stavudine use, including fatal cases.** Risk may be increased in obesity, prolonged nucleoside exposure, or in female patients. Suspend therapy in patients with suspected lactic acidosis; consider discontinuation of stavudine if lactic acidosis is confirmed. Pregnant women may be at increased risk of lactic acidosis and liver damage. Severe motor weakness (resembling Guillain-Barré syndrome) has also been reported (including fatal cases, usually in association with lactic acidosis); manufacturer recommends discontinuation if motor weakness develops (with or without lactic acidosis). **[U.S. Boxed Warning]: Pancreatitis (including some fatal cases) has occurred during combination therapy (didanosine with or without hydroxyurea).** Risk increased when used in combination regimen with didanosine and hydroxyurea. Suspend therapy with agents toxic to the pancreas (including stavudine, didanosine, or hydroxyurea) in patients with suspected pancreatitis.

Dosage Forms Capsule: 15 mg, 20 mg, 30 mg, 40 mg
Powder, for oral solution: 1 mg/mL (200 mL) [dye free; fruit flavor]

Reference Range Peak serum level after an oral dose of 4 mg/kg is 4.2 mcg/mL

Overdosage/Treatment
Decontamination: Ipecac within 30 minutes or lavage (within 1 hour)/ activated charcoal
Enhancement of elimination: Multiple dosing of activated charcoal may be effective

Drug Interactions Didanosine: Risk of pancreatitis may be increased with concurrent use. Cases of fatal lactic acidosis have been reported with this combination when used during pregnancy; use only if clearly needed.
Doxorubicin: May inhibit intracellular phosphorylation of stavudine; use with caution.
Hydroxyurea: Risk of hepatotoxicity or pancreatitis may be increased with concurrent use.
Ribavirin: Concomitant use of ribavirin and nucleoside analogues may increase the risk of developing hepatic decompensation or other signs of mitochondrial toxicity, including pancreatitis or lactic acidosis. May inhibit intracellular phosphorylation of stavudine; use with caution.
Zalcitabine: May increase risk of peripheral neuropathy; concurrent use not recommended.
Zidovudine: Inhibits intracellular phosphorylation of stavudine; concurrent use not recommended.

Pregnancy Risk Factor C

Pregnancy Implications Cases of fatal and nonfatal lactic acidosis, with or without pancreatitis, have been reported in pregnant women. It is not known if pregnancy itself potentiates this known side effect; however, pregnant women may be at increased risk of lactic acidosis and liver damage. Hepatic enzymes and electrolytes should be monitored frequently during the 3rd trimester of pregnancy. Pharmacokinetics of stavudine are not significantly altered during pregnancy; dose adjustments are not needed. The Perinatal HIV Guidelines Working Group considers stavudine to be an alternative NRTI in dual nucleoside combination regimens; use with didanosine only if no alternatives are available, do not use with zidovudine. Health professionals are encouraged to contact the antiretroviral pregnancy registry to monitor outcomes of pregnant women exposed to antiretroviral medications (1-800-258-4263 or www.APRegistry.com).

Lactation Excretion in breast milk unknown/contraindicated

Streptokinase

Related Information
● Therapeutic Drugs Associated with Hallucinations
CAS Number 9002-01-1
U.S. Brand Names Streptase®
Synonyms SK

Use Thrombolytic agent used in treatment of recent severe or massive deep vein thrombosis (within 7 days), pulmonary emboli, peripheral arterial thrombosis, myocardial infarction, and occluded arteriovenous cannulas; can prevent venous valvular damage and development of venous hypertension; not effective for strokes

Mechanism of Action Activates the conversion of plasminogen to plasmin by forming a complex, exposing plasminogen-activating site, and clearing a peptide bond that converts plasminogen to plasmin; plasmin degrades fibrin, fibrinogen and other procoagulant proteins into soluble fragments; effective both outside and within the formed thrombus/embolus

Adverse Reactions

Cardiovascular: **Hypotension, trauma arrhythmias, arrhythmias**, chest pain, pericardial effusion/pericarditis, angina

Central nervous system: Headache, chills, hallucinations, Guillain-Barré syndrome, fever, hyperthermia

Dermatologic: **Angioneurotic edema**, rash, cutaneous vasculitis

Gastrointestinal: Nausea, vomiting

Hematologic: **Bleeding (surface), internal bleeding, cerebral hemorrhage**, hemolytic anemia, anemia

Hepatic: Liver hemorrhage

Local: Extravasation injury

Ocular: **Periorbital edema**, ocular hemorrhage,

Renal: Renal failure due to acute tubular necrosis, glomerulonephritis

Respiratory: **Bronchospasm**, epistaxis, alveolar hemorrhage, pulmonary hemorrhage

Miscellaneous: **Anaphylaxis, bleeding at sites of percutaneous trauma**, diaphoresis, acute atraumatic compartment syndrome

Signs and Symptoms of Overdose Bleeding gums, coagulopathy, confusion, depression, eczema, epistaxis, hematoma, hematuria, hemoptysis, intracranial hemorrhage, jaundice, leukocytosis, ocular hemorrhage, oozing at catheter site, spontaneous ecchymosis, tubular necrosis, wheezing

Pharmacodynamics/Kinetics

Onset of action: Activation of plasminogen occurs almost immediately

Duration: Fibrinolytic effect: Several hours; Anticoagulant effect: 12-24 hours

Half-life elimination: 83 minutes

Excretion: By circulating antibodies and the reticuloendothelial system

Dosage I.V.:

Children: Safety and efficacy not established; limited studies have used 3500-4000 units/kg over 30 minutes followed by 1000-1500 units/kg/hour

Clotted catheter: 25,000 units, clamp for 2 hours then aspirate contents and flush with normal saline

Adults: Antibodies to streptokinase remain for at least 3-6 months after initial dose: Administration requires the use of an infusion pump

An intradermal skin test of 100 int. units has been suggested to predict allergic response to streptokinase. If a positive reaction is not seen after 15-20 minutes, a therapeutic dose may be administered.

Guidelines for acute myocardial infarction (AMI): 1.5 million units over 60 minutes

Administration:

Dilute two 750,000 unit vials of streptokinase with 5 mL dextrose 5% in water (D$_5$W) each, gently swirl to dissolve

Add this dose of the 1.5 million units to 150 mL D$_5$W

This should be infused over 60 minutes; an in-line filter $\geq$ 0.45 micron should be used

Monitor for the first few hours for signs of anaphylaxis or allergic reaction. **Infusion should be slowed if lowering of 25 mm Hg in blood pressure or terminated if asthmatic symptoms appear.**

Begin heparin 5000-10,000 unit bolus followed by 1000 units/hour approximately 3-4 hours after completion of streptokinase infusion or when PTT is <100 seconds

Guidelines for acute pulmonary embolism (APE): 3 million unit dose over 24 hours

Administration:

Dilute four 750,000 unit vials of streptokinase with 5 mL dextrose 5% in water (D$_5$W) each, gently swirl to dissolve

Add this dose of 3 million units to 250 mL D$_5$W, an in-line filter $\geq$ 0.45 micron should be used

Administer 250,000 units (23 mL) over 30 minutes followed by 100,000 units/hour (9 mL/hour) for 24 hours

Monitor for the first few hours for signs of anaphylaxis or allergic reaction. **Infusion should be slowed if blood pressure is lowered by 25 mm Hg or if asthmatic symptoms appear.**

Begin heparin 1000 units/hour ~3-4 hours after completion of streptokinase infusion or when PTT is <100 seconds

Monitor PT, PTT, and fibrinogen levels during therapy

Thromboses: 250,000 units to start, then 100,000 units/hour for 24-72 hours depending on location

Cannula occlusion: 250,000 units into cannula, clamp for 2 hours, then aspirate contents and flush with normal saline; **Not recommended; see Warnings**

Stability Keep in refrigerator, use reconstituted solutions within 24 hours; store unopened vials at room temperature

Monitoring Parameters Blood pressure, PT, aPTT, platelet count, hematocrit, fibrinogen concentration, signs of bleeding

Administration I.V. infusion requires an infusion pump; streptokinase is administered by I.V., intra-arterial, or intracoronary infusion; may also be used to clear an occluded arteriovenous cannula

Contraindications Hypersensitivity to anistreplase, streptokinase, or any component of the formulation; active internal bleeding; history of CVA; recent (within 2 months) intracranial or intraspinal surgery or trauma; intracranial neoplasm, arteriovenous malformation, or aneurysm; known bleeding diathesis; severe uncontrolled hypertension

Warnings

Concurrent heparin anticoagulation can contribute to bleeding; careful attention to all potential bleeding sites. I.M. injections and nonessential handling of the patient should be avoided. Venipunctures should be performed carefully and only when necessary. If arterial puncture is necessary, use an upper extremity vessel that can be manually compressed. If serious bleeding occurs then the infusion of streptokinase and heparin should be stopped.

For the following conditions the risk of bleeding is higher with use of thrombolytics and should be weighed against the benefits of therapy: recent (within 10 days) major surgery (eg, CABG, obstetrical delivery, organ biopsy, previous puncture of noncompressible vessels), cerebrovascular disease, recent (within 10 days) gastrointestinal or genitourinary bleeding, recent trauma (within 10 days) including CPR, hypertension (systolic BP >180 mm Hg and/or diastolic BP >110 mm Hg), high likelihood of left heart thrombus (eg, mitral stenosis with atrial fibrillation), acute pericarditis, subacute bacterial endocarditis, hemostatic defects including ones caused by severe renal or hepatic dysfunction, significant hepatic dysfunction, pregnancy, diabetic hemorrhagic retinopathy or other hemorrhagic ophthalmic conditions, septic thrombophlebitis or occluded AV cannula at seriously infected site, advanced age (eg, >75 years), patients receiving oral anticoagulants, any other condition in which bleeding constitutes a significant hazard or would be particularly difficult to manage because of location.

Coronary thrombolysis may result in reperfusion arrhythmias. Hypotension, occasionally severe, can occur (not from bleeding or anaphylaxis). Follow standard MI management. Rare anaphylactic reactions can occur. Cautious repeat administration in patients who have received anistreplase or streptokinase within 1 year (streptokinase antibody may decrease effectiveness or risk of allergic reactions). Safety and efficacy in pediatric patients has not been established.

Streptokinase is not indicated for restoration of patency of intravenous catheters. Serious adverse events relating to the use of streptokinase in the restoration of patency of occluded intravenous catheters have involved the use of high doses of streptokinase in small volumes (250,000 international units in 2 mL). Uses of lower doses of streptokinase in infusions over several hours, generally into partially occluded catheters, or local instillation into the catheter lumen and subsequent aspiration, have been described in the medical literature. Healthcare providers should consider the risk for potentially life-threatening reactions (hypersensitivity, apnea, bleeding) associated with the use of streptokinase in the management of occluded intravenous catheters.

Dosage Forms [DSC] = Discontinued product

Injection, powder for reconstitution: 250,000 int. units; 750,000 int. units; 1,500,000 int. units [DSC]

Reference Range

Partial thromboplastin time (PTT) activated: 20.4-33.2 seconds

Prothrombin time (PT): 10.9-13.7 seconds (same as control)

Fibrinogen: 200-400 mg/dL

Overdosage/Treatment Supportive therapy: Treat bleeding complications with transfusions of red blood cells, fresh frozen plasma, and cryoprecipitate; do not administer dextran; although human overdose data is lacking, administration of aminocaproic acid (Amicar®) at a dose of 3-5 g I.V. followed by an infusion rate of 1-1.25 g/hour may be useful

Drug Interactions Aminocaproic acid (antifibrinolytic agent) may decrease effectiveness of thrombolytic agents.

Drugs which affect platelet function (eg, NSAIDs, dipyridamole, ticlopidine, clopidogrel, IIb/IIIa antagonists) may potentiate the risk of hemorrhage; use with caution.

Heparin and aspirin: Use with aspirin and heparin may increase bleeding over aspirin and heparin alone. However, aspirin and heparin were used concurrently in the majority of patients in some major clinical studies of streptokinase.

Warfarin or oral anticoagulants: Risk of bleeding may be increased during concurrent therapy.

Pregnancy Risk Factor C

Pregnancy Implications If streptokinase is used near term, delivery by Cesarean section should be considered

Lactation Excretion in breast milk unknown

Nursing Implications For I.V. or intracoronary use only; avoid I.M. injections; do not mix with other drugs

Additional Information Best results are realized if used within 5-6 hours of myocardial infarction; antibodies to streptokinase remain for 3-6 months after initial dose, use another thrombolytic enzyme (ie, urokinase) if repeat thrombolytic therapy is indicated; 6-month mortality rate in use for ischemic strokes is 44% higher in streptokinase group. Investigators applied analysis to data for patients ≥75 years of age from two large trials studying the impact of streptokinase on patient outcome after acute myocardial infarction; their conclusion was that age alone is not a contraindication to the use of streptokinase and that thrombolytic therapy is cost-effective and is beneficial toward the survival of elderly patients. Additional studies are needed to determine if a weight-adjusted dose will maintain efficacy but decrease adverse events such as stroke. Incidence of streptokinase-induced Guillain-Barré syndrome is ~5 cases/30,000-40,000 doses.

Streptomycin

CAS Number 3810-74-0; 57-92-1

Synonyms Streptomycin Sulfate

Use Combination therapy of active tuberculosis; used in combination with other agents for treatment of streptococcal or enterococcal endocarditis, mycobacterial infections, plague, tularemia, and brucellosis. Streptomycin is indicated for persons from endemic areas of drug-resistant *Mycobacterium tuberculosis* or who are HIV infected.

Mechanism of Action Inhibits bacterial protein synthesis by binding directly to the 30S ribosomal subunits causing faulty peptide sequence to form in the protein chain

Adverse Reactions

Cardiovascular: Hypotension, myocarditis (hypersensitivity), angina, chest pain, myocarditis, sinus tachycardia

Central nervous system: Drug fever, headache, drowsiness, Jarisch-Herxheimer reaction

Dermatologic: Rash, systemic contact dermatitis, immunologic contact urticaria, lichen planus

Gastrointestinal: Nausea, vomiting

Hematologic: Eosinophilia, anemia, hemolytic anemia

Neuromuscular & skeletal: Neuromuscular blockade, paresthesia, tremor, arthralgia, weakness

Ocular: Oscillating vision

Otic: Ototoxicity (auditory), ototoxicity (vestibular), tinnitus

Renal: Nephrotoxicity

Respiratory: Difficulty breathing, hyposmia

Miscellaneous: Anaphylactoid reactions

Pharmacodynamics/Kinetics

Absorption:

Oral: Poorly absorbed

I.M.: Well absorbed

Distribution: To extracellular fluid including serum, abscesses, ascitic, pericardial, pleural, synovial, lymphatic, and peritoneal fluids; poorly distributed into CSF; crosses placenta; small amounts enter breast milk

Protein binding: 34%

Half-life elimination: Newborns: 4-10 hours; Adults: 2-4.7 hours, prolonged with renal impairment

Time to peak: I.M.: Within 1 hour

Excretion: Urine (90% as unchanged drug); feces, saliva, sweat, and tears (<1%)

Dosage Intramuscular (may also be given intravenous piggyback):

Tuberculosis therapy: **Note:** A four-drug regimen (isoniazid, rifampin, pyrazinamide and either streptomycin or ethambutol) is preferred for the initial, empiric treatment of TB. When the drug susceptibility results are available, the regimen should be altered as appropriate.

Patients with TB and without HIV infection:

OPTION 1:

Isoniazid resistance rate <4%: Administer daily isoniazid, rifampin, and pyrazinamide for 8 weeks followed by isoniazid and rifampin daily or directly observed therapy (DOT) 2-3 times/week for 16 weeks

If isoniazid resistance rate is not documented, ethambutol or streptomycin should also be administered until susceptibility to isoniazid or rifampin is demonstrated. Continue treatment for at least 6 months or 3 months beyond culture conversion.

OPTION 2: Administer daily isoniazid, rifampin, pyrazinamide, and either streptomycin or ethambutol for 2 weeks followed by DOT 2 times/week administration of the same drugs for 6 weeks, and subsequently, with isoniazid and rifampin DOT 2 times/week administration for 16 weeks

OPTION 3: Administer isoniazid, rifampin, pyrazinamide, and either ethambutol or streptomycin by DOT 3 times/week for 6 months

Patients with TB and with HIV infection: Administer any of the above OPTIONS 1, 2, or 3; however, treatment should be continued for a total of 9 months and at least 6 months beyond culture conversion

Note: Some experts recommend that the duration of therapy should be extended to 9 months for patients with disseminated disease, miliary disease, disease involving the bones or joints, or tuberculosis lymphadenitis

Children:

Daily therapy: 20-30 mg/kg/day (maximum: 1 g/day)

Directly observed therapy (DOT): Twice weekly: 25-30 mg/kg (maximum: 1.5 g)

DOT: 3 times/week: 25-30 mg/kg (maximum: 1 g)

Adults:

Daily therapy: 15 mg/kg/day (maximum: 1 g)

Directly observed therapy (DOT): Twice weekly: 25-30 mg/kg (maximum: 1.5 g)

DOT: 3 times/week: 25-30 mg/kg (maximum: 1 g)

Enterococcal endocarditis: 1 g every 12 hours for 2 weeks, 500 mg every 12 hours for 4 weeks in combination with penicillin

Streptococcal endocarditis: 1 g every 12 hours for 1 week, 500 mg every 12 hours for 1 week

Tularemia: 1-2 g/day in divided doses for 7-10 days or until patient is afebrile for 5-7 days

Plague: 2-4 g/day in divided doses until the patient is afebrile for at least 3 days

Elderly: 10 mg/kg/day, not to exceed 750 mg/day; dosing interval should be adjusted for renal function; some authors suggest not to give more than 5 days/week or give as 20-25 mg/kg/dose twice weekly

Dosing interval in renal impairment:

Cl_{cr} 10-50 mL/minute: Administer every 24-72 hours

Cl_{cr} <10 mL/minute: Administer every 72-96 hours

Removed by hemo and peritoneal dialysis: Administer dose postdialysis

Stability Depending upon manufacturer, reconstituted solution remains stable for 2-4 weeks when refrigerated and 24 hours at room temperature; exposure to light causes darkening of solution without apparent loss of potency

Monitoring Parameters Hearing (audiogram), BUN, creatinine; serum concentration of the drug should be monitored in all patients; eighth cranial nerve damage is usually preceded by high-pitched tinnitus, roaring noises, sense of fullness in ears, or impaired hearing and may persist for weeks after drug is discontinued

Administration Inject deep I.M. into large muscle mass; I.V. administration is not recommended

Contraindications Hypersensitivity to streptomycin or any component of the formulation; pregnancy

Warnings [U.S. Boxed Warning]: May cause neurotoxicity, nephrotoxicity, and/or neuromuscular blockade and respiratory paralysis; usual risk factors include pre-existing renal impairment, concomitant neuro-/nephrotoxic medications, advanced age and dehydration. The drug's neurotoxicity can result in respiratory paralysis from neuromuscular blockade, especially when the drug is given soon after anesthesia or muscle relaxants. Use with caution in patients with pre-existing vertigo, tinnitus, hearing loss, neuromuscular disorders, or renal impairment; modify dosage in patients with renal impairment; ototoxicity is directly proportional to the amount of drug given and the duration of treatment; tinnitus or vertigo are indications of vestibular injury and impending bilateral irreversible damage; renal damage is usually reversible. **[U.S. Boxed Warning]: Parenteral form should be used only where appropriate audiometric and laboratory testing facilities are available.**

Dosage Forms Injection, powder for reconstitution: 1 g

Reference Range Peak serum streptomycin level after a 15 mg/kg I.M. dose: ~40 mcg/mL

Therapeutic: Peak: 15-40 mcg/mL; Trough: <5 mcg/mL

Toxic: Peak: >50 mcg/mL; Trough: >10 mcg/mL

Overdosage/Treatment

Supportive therapy: Neuromuscular blockade can be reversed by calcium

Enhanced elimination: Can be removed by hemodialysis

Test Interactions False-positive urine glucose with Benedict's solution

Drug Interactions Increased/prolonged effect: Depolarizing and nondepolarizing neuromuscular blocking agents

Increased toxicity: Concurrent use of amphotericin may increase nephrotoxicity

Pregnancy Risk Factor D

Pregnancy Implications Neonatal hearing deficits have been noted

Lactation Enters breast milk/compatible

Additional Information Incidence of cochleotoxicity is ~10% to 63% with loop diuretics and noise exposure being ototoxic synergistic. Inhaled tobramycin appears to exhibit minimal ototoxic effects. There may be a genetic basis (in the mitochondrial 12 S ribosomal RNA gene) for ototoxicity in 17% to 33% of cases. Suggested evaluation for ototoxicity with aminoglycoside treatment includes:

● baseline audiometric evaluation (tonal air conduction thresholds from 250-20,000 Hz)

● monitoring during aminoglycoside treatment (to a tonal-air conduction threshold at frequency >8000 Hz)

● follow-up audiometric assessment (tonal air conduction thresholds at frequencies >8000 Hz) until the threshold stabilizes

Strontium-89

Pronunciation (STRON shee um atey nine)

Related Information
● Toxins Which Should Be Lavaged with Solutions Other Than Water

CAS Number 14158-27-1

U.S. Brand Names Metastron®

Synonyms Strontium-89 Chloride

Use Relief of bone pain in patients with skeletal metastases

Mechanism of Action Similar to calcium; deposits in bone and teeth; stimulates bone formation while inhibiting bone resorption

Adverse Reactions
Most severe reactions of marrow toxicity can be managed by conventional means;

Dermatologic: Flushing sensation following rapid administration (usually over <30 seconds)

Hematologic: Thrombocytopenia (nadir: 4-8 weeks) with a mean reduction of platelets (~20% to 50% reduction)

Signs and Symptoms of Overdose Bone marrow suppression, chills, diarrhea, nausea, vomiting

Toxicodynamics/Kinetics
Half-life: 50.6 days

Elimination (once released from bone): Renal: 70% to 80%; Fecal: 20% to 30%

Dosage Adults: I.V.: 148 megabecquerel (4 millicurie) administered by slow I.V. injection over 1-2 minutes or 1.5-2.2 megabecquerel (40-60 microcurie)/kg; repeated doses are generally not recommended at intervals <90 days; measure the patient dose by a suitable radioactivity calibration system immediately prior to administration

Stability Store vial and its contents inside its transportation container at room temperature

Monitoring Parameters Routine blood tests

Contraindications Hypersensitivity to any strontium-containing compounds or any other component of the formulation; pregnancy; breast-feeding

Warnings Use caution in patients with bone marrow compromise; incontinent patients may require urinary catheterization. Body fluids may remain radioactive up to one week after injection. Not indicated for use in patients with cancer not involving bone and should be used with caution in patients whose platelet counts fall <60,000 or whose white blood cell counts fall <2400. A small number of patients have experienced a transient increase in bone pain at 36-72 hours postdose; this reaction is generally mild and self-limiting. It should be handled cautiously, in a similar manner to other radioactive drugs. Appropriate safety measures to minimize radiation to personnel should be instituted.

Dosage Forms Injection, solution, as chloride [preservative free]: 10.9-22.6 mg/mL [148 megabecquerel, 4 millicurie] (10 mL)

Overdosage/Treatment Decontamination: Oral ingestion: Since absorption is rapid and water should not theoretically be used for gastric lavage, removal is probably not efficacious; give 1.5-10 g of sodium alginate (then 2-4 tablets every 2-4 hours for 24 hours) or 50-100 mL of aluminum phosphate gel (followed by 40 mL every 2 hours) or 65 mL of aluminum hydroxide orally (followed by 40 mL every 1-2 hours)

Pregnancy Risk Factor D

Nursing Implications During the first week after injection, strontium-89 will be present in the blood and urine, therefore, the following common sense precautions should be instituted:
● Where a normal toilet is available, use in preference to a urinal, flush the toilet twice
● Wipe away any spilled urine with a tissue and flush it away
● Have patient wash hands after using the toilet
● Immediately wash any linen or clothes that become stained with blood or urine
● Wash away any spilled blood if a cut occurs

Additional Information Reacts with water (thermic reaction); does not emit gamma radiation

Specific References
Kirrane BM, Hoffman RS, and Nelson LS, "Massive Strontium Ferrate Ingestion Does Not Produce Acute Toxicity," *Clin Toxicol (Phila)*, 2005, 43:749.

Sucralfate

CAS Number 54182-58-0

U.S. Brand Names Carafate®

Synonyms Aluminum Sucrose Sulfate, Basic

Use Short-term management of duodenal ulcers; maintenance for duodenal ulcers; suspension may be used topically for treatment of stomatitis due to cancer chemotherapy and other causes of esophageal and gastric erosions

Unlabeled/Investigational Use Gastric ulcers; suspension may be used topically for treatment of stomatitis due to cancer chemotherapy and other causes of esophageal and gastric erosions; GERD, esopha-gitis; treatment of NSAID mucosal damage; prevention of stress ulcers; postsclerotherapy for esophageal variceal bleeding

Mechanism of Action Forms a complex, a paste-like, cytoprotective substance, when combined with gastric acid that adheres to the damaged mucosal area. This selectively forms a protective coating that protects the lining against peptic acid, pepsin, and bile salts.

Adverse Reactions
Central nervous system: Dizziness, sleepiness

Dermatologic: Rash, pruritus

Gastrointestinal: Constipation, diarrhea, nausea, gastric discomfort, indigestion, xerostomia, intestinal obstruction may occur secondary to bezoars

Neuromuscular & skeletal: Back pain, dysarthria

Signs and Symptoms of Overdose Toxicity is minimal; may cause bezoars, constipation, encephalopathy

Pharmacodynamics/Kinetics
Onset of action: Paste formation and ulcer adhesion: 1-2 hours

Duration: Up to 6 hours

Absorption: Oral: <5%

Distribution: Acts locally at ulcer sites; unbound in GI tract to aluminum and sucrose octasulfate

Metabolism: None

Excretion: Urine (small amounts as unchanged compounds)

Dosage Oral:
Children: Dose not established; doses of 40-80 mg/kg/day divided every 6 hours have been used
Stomatitis: 2.5-5 mL (1 g/10 mL suspension), swish and spit or swish and swallow 4 times/day

Adults:
Duodenal ulcer treatment: 1 g 4 times/day, 1 hour before meals or food and at bedtime for 4-8 weeks, or alternatively 2 g twice daily
Duodenal ulcer maintenance therapy: 1 g twice daily
Stomatitis: 1 g/10 mL suspension, swish and spit or swish and swallow 4 times/day

Stability Shake well and refrigerate suspension

Monitoring Parameters Aluminum

Administration Tablet may be broken or dissolved in water before ingestion. Administer with water on an empty stomach.

Contraindications Hypersensitivity to sucralfate or any component of the formulation

Warnings Successful therapy with sucralfate should not be expected to alter the posthealing frequency of recurrence or the severity of duodenal ulceration; use with caution in patients with chronic renal failure who have an impaired excretion of absorbed aluminum. Because of the potential for sucralfate to alter the absorption of some drugs, separate administration (take other medication 2 hours before sucralfate) should be considered when alterations in bioavailability are believed to be critical

Dosage Forms Suspension, oral: 1 g/10 mL (10 mL)
Carafate®: 1 g/10 mL (420 mL)
Tablet: 1 g
Carafate®: 1 g

Reference Range Normal serum aluminum levels are <15 mcg/L (SI: <555 nmol/L); toxicity can occur at levels >100 mcg/L (SI: >3706 nmol/L)

Overdosage/Treatment Enhancement of elimination: Deferoxamine, traditionally used as an iron chelator, has been shown to increase urinary aluminum output. Deferoxamine chelation of aluminum has resulted in improvements of clinical symptoms and bone histology. Hemofiltration or hemodialysis can lower serum aluminum concentrations.

Drug Interactions Decreased effect: Digoxin, phenytoin (hydantoins), warfarin, ketoconazole, quinidine, ciprofloxacin, norfloxacin (quinolones), tetracycline, theophylline; because of the potential for sucralfate to alter the absorption of some drugs, separate administration (take other medications 2 hours before sucralfate) should be considered when alterations in bioavailability are believed to be critical

Note: When given with aluminum-containing antacids, may increase serum/body aluminum concentrations (see Warnings/Precautions)

Pregnancy Risk Factor B

Pregnancy Implications No data available; available evidence suggests safe use during pregnancy.

Lactation Enters breast milk/compatible

Nursing Implications Monitor for constipation; give 2 hours before or after administration of other oral drugs

Additional Information May decrease gastric emptying; little overdose experience; increased serum aluminum levels can occur after inadvertent I.V. administration

Sufentanil

CAS Number 56030-54-7; 60561-17-3

U.S. Brand Names Sufenta®

Synonyms Sufentanil Citrate

Impairment Potential Yes

Use Analgesic supplement in maintenance of balanced general anesthesia

Mechanism of Action Binds with stereospecific receptors at many sites within the CNS, increases pain threshold, alters pain reception, inhibits ascending pain pathways; ultra short-acting narcotic; not a partial opiate antagonist

Adverse Reactions

Cardiovascular: **Hypotension, bradycardia,** hypertension, tachycardia, arrhythmia, shock, sinus tachycardia

Central nervous system: **Drowsiness,** electroencephalogram abnormalities, agitation, CNS depression

Dermatologic: Pruritus

Endocrine & metabolic: Sexual dysfunction

Gastrointestinal: **Nausea, vomiting**

Neuromuscular & skeletal: Skeletal muscle rigidity, clonus, myoclonus, hyporeflexia

Respiratory: **Respiratory depression,** wheezing, apnea

Miscellaneous: Physical and psychological dependence with prolonged use

Signs and Symptoms of Overdose Biliary tract spasm, coma, convulsions, myoclonus

Pharmacodynamics/Kinetics

Onset of action: 1-3 minutes

Duration: Dose dependent; usually 30-60 minutes, may be up to 3.5 hours

Distribution: V_d: 2.9 L/kg

Protein binding: 92.5%

Metabolism: Primarily by the liver

Half-life: 158 minutes Patients with cardiac surgery: 595 minutes; Patients with abdominal aortic surgery: 12 hours; Patients hyperventilating: 232 minutes; Obese patients: Increased half-life

Dosage Children <12 years: 10-25 mcg/kg with 100% O_2, maintenance: 25-50 mcg as needed

Adults: Dose should be based on body weight; **Note:** In obese patients (ie, >20% above ideal body weight), use lean body weight to determine dosage

1-2 mcg/kg with N_2O/O_2 for endotracheal intubation; maintenance: 10-25 mcg as needed

2-8 mcg/kg with N_2O/O_2 more complicated major surgical procedures; maintenance: 10-50 mcg as needed

8-30 mcg/kg with 100% O_2 and muscle relaxant produces sleep; at doses of ≥8 mcg/kg maintains a deep level of anesthesia; maintenance: 10-50 mcg as needed

Administration Parenteral: I.V.: Slow I.V. injection or by infusion

Contraindications Hypersensitivity to sufentanil or any component of the formulation

Warnings Sufentanil can cause severely compromised respiratory depression; use with caution in patients with head injuries, hepatic or renal impairment or with pulmonary disease; sufentanil shares the toxic potential of opiate agonists, precaution of opiate agonist therapy should be observed; rapid I.V. infusion may result in skeletal muscle and chest wall rigidity, impaired ventilation, respiratory distress/arrest; nondepolarizing skeletal muscle relaxant may be required

Dosage Forms Injection, solution [preservative free]: 50 mcg/mL (1 mL, 2 mL, 5 mL)

Reference Range Peak serum sufentanil levels are ~11 mcg/L 10 minutes after I.V. administration of 1.5 mcg/kg of the drug

Overdosage/Treatment Supportive therapy: Naloxone hydrochloride (0.4-2 mg I.V., SubQ, or through an endotracheal tube); a continuous infusion (at $^2/_3$ the response dose/hour) may be required

Antidote(s)

- Nalmefene [ANTIDOTE]
- Naloxone [ANTIDOTE]

Drug Interactions **Substrate** of CYP3A4 (major)

CYP3A4 inhibitors: May increase the levels/effects of sufentanil. Example inhibitors include azole antifungals, clarithromycin, diclofenac, doxycycline, erythromycin, imatinib, isoniazid, nefazodone, nicardipine, propofol, protease inhibitors, quinidine, telithromycin, and verapamil.

Increased effect/toxicity with CNS depressants, beta-blockers

Pregnancy Risk Factor C

Nursing Implications Patient may develop rebound respiratory depression postoperatively

Specific References

Boitquin LP, Hecq JD, Vanbeckbergen DF, et al, "Stability of Sufentanil Citrate with Levobupivacaine HCl in NaCl 0.9% Infusion After Microwave Freeze-Thaw Treatment," *Ann Pharmacother,* 2004, 38(11): 1836-9.

Sulfamethoxazole and Trimethoprim

CAS Number 8064-90-2

U.S. Brand Names Bactrim™ DS; Bactrim™; Septra® DS; Septra®

Synonyms Co-Trimoxazole; SMZ-TMP; Sulfatrim; TMP-SMZ; Trimethoprim and Sulfamethoxazole

Use

Oral treatment of urinary tract infections due to *E. coli, Klebsiella* and *Enterobacter* sp, *M. morganii, P. mirabilis* and *P. vulgaris;* acute otitis media in children and acute exacerbations of chronic bronchitis in adults due to susceptible strains of *H. influenzae* or *S. pneumoniae;* prophylaxis of *Pneumocystis carinii* pneumonitis (PCP), traveler's diarrhea due to enterotoxigenic *E. coli* or *Cyclospora*

I.V. treatment or severe or complicated infections when oral therapy is not feasible, for documented PCP, empiric treatment of PCP in immune compromised patients; treatment of documented or suspected shigellosis, typhoid fever, *Nocardia asteroides* infection, or other infections caused by susceptible bacteria

Unlabeled/Investigational Use Cholera and *Salmonella*-type infections and nocardiosis; chronic prostatitis; as prophylaxis in neutropenic patients with *P. carinii* infections, in leukemics, and in patients following renal transplantation, to decrease incidence of PCP; treatment of *Cyclospora* infection, typhoid fever, *Nocardia asteroides* infection

Mechanism of Action Sulfamethoxazole interferes with bacterial folic acid synthesis and growth via inhibition of dihydrofolic acid formation from para-aminobenzoic acid; trimethoprim inhibits dihydrofolic acid reduction to tetrahydrofolate resulting in sequential inhibition of enzymes of the folic acid pathway

Adverse Reactions

Cardiovascular: QT prolongation, torsade de pointes

Central nervous system: Confusion, dizziness, CNS depression, hallucinations, seizures, fever, ataxia, aseptic meningitis, kernicterus in neonates, psychosis, Jarisch-Herxheimer reaction

Dermatologic: **Allergic skin reactions, rash, urticaria, photosensitivity** (more common in patients taking large dosages or in patients with AIDS), erythema multiforme, epidermal necrolysis, Stevens-Johnson syndrome, neutrophilic dermatosis (Sweet's syndrome), nail discoloration (brown); overall risk for skin disorders is ~2.8/100,000, exfoliative dermatitis, acute generalized exanthematous pustulosis, angioedema, bullous skin disease, purpura, pruritus, psoriasis, erythema nodosum, licheniform eruptions, exanthem, cutaneous vasculitis

Endocrine & metabolic: Hypoglycemia (lasting ~12 hours), hyponatremia, hyperkalemia

Gastrointestinal: **Nausea, anorexia, vomiting,** glossitis, stomatitis, diarrhea, pseudomembranous colitis, pancreatitis, splenomegaly, fecal discoloration (black), esophagitis, vanishing bile duct syndrome, aphthous stomatitis, lingua villosa nigra, gastrointestinal vasculitis

Genitourinary: Urine discoloration (black, brown, rust, yellow-brown), crystalluria

Hematologic: Thrombocytopenia, anemia (megaloblastic), granulocytopenia, aplastic anemia, porphyria, red blood cell aplasia; overall risk for blood disorders is ~5.6/100,000

Hepatic: Hepatitis, cholestasis, granulomatous hepatitis, hepatic vasculitis

Local: Irritation, pain, phlebitis

Neuromuscular & skeletal: Tremor (at doses >15 mg/kg/day), rhabdomyolysis

Ocular: Iritis

Otic: Ototoxicity, tinnitus

Renal: Interstitial nephritis, renal vasculitis

Respiratory: Cough, pulmonary vasculitis

Miscellaneous: Serum sickness, periarteritis nodosa, systemic lupus erythematosus, fixed drug eruption

Signs and Symptoms of Overdose Blood dyscrasias, cholestatic jaundice, coagulopathy, colitis, depression, erythema multiforme, jaundice, hyperkalemia, hypoglycemia, leukopenia or neutropenia (agranulocytosis, granulocytopenia), meningitis, methemoglobinemia, pseudotumor cerebri, toxic epidermal necrolysis

Admission Criteria/Prognosis Any patient with change in mental status, cardiopulmonary complaints, or methemoglobin levels >30% should be admitted; asymptomatic patients with methemoglobin levels <30% may be considered for discharge after 6 hours of observation and if methemoglobin levels fall to <15%; admit adult ingestions >10 tablets

Pharmacodynamics/Kinetics

Absorption: Oral: Almost completely, 90% to 100%

Protein binding: SMX: 68%, TMP: 45%

Metabolism: SMX: N-acetylated and glucuronidated; TMP: Metabolized to oxide and hydroxylated metabolites

Half-life elimination: SMX: 9 hours, TMP: 6-17 hours; both are prolonged in renal failure

Time to peak, serum: Within 1-4 hours

Excretion: Both are excreted in urine as metabolites and unchanged drug

Effects of aging on the pharmacokinetics of both agents has been variable; increase in half-life and decreases in clearance have been associated with reduced creatinine clearance

Dosage Dosage recommendations are based on the trimethoprim component

Children >2 months:

Mild to moderate infections: Oral, I.V.: 8 mg TMP/kg/day in divided doses every 12 hours

Serious infection/*Pneumocystis*: I.V.: 20 mg TMP/kg/day in divided doses every 6 hours

Urinary tract infection prophylaxis: Oral: 2 mg TMP/kg/dose daily

Prophylaxis of *Pneumocystis*: Oral, I.V.: 10 mg TMP/kg/day or 150 mg TMP/m^2/day in divided doses every 12 hours for 3 days/week; dose should not exceed 320 mg trimethoprim and 1600 mg sulfamethoxazole 3 days/week

Cholera: Oral, I.V.: 5 mg TMP/kg twice daily for 3 days

Cyclospora: Oral, I.V.: 5 mg TMP/kg twice daily for 7 days

Adults:

Urinary tract infection/chronic bronchitis: Oral: 1 double strength tablet every 12 hours for 10-14 days

Sepsis: I.V.: 20 TMP/kg/day divided every 6 hours

Pneumocystis carinii:

Prophylaxis: Oral: 1 double strength tablet daily or 3 times/week

Treatment: Oral, I.V.: 15-20 mg TMP/kg/day in 3-4 divided doses

Cholera: Oral, I.V.: 160 mg TMP twice daily for 3 days

Cyclospora: Oral, I.V.: 160 mg TMP twice daily for 7 days

Nocardia: Oral, I.V.: 640 mg TMP/day in divided doses for several months (duration is controversial; an average of 7 months has been reported)

Dosing adjustment in renal impairment: Adults:

I.V.:

Cl$_{cr}$ 15-30 mL/minute: Administer 2.5-5 mg/kg every 12 hours

Cl$_{cr}$ <15 mL/minute: Administer 2.5-5 mg/kg every 24 hours

Oral:

Cl$_{cr}$ 15-30 mL/minute: Administer 1 double strength tablet every 24 hours or 1 single strength tablet every 12 hours

Cl$_{cr}$ <15 mL/minute: Not recommended

Stability Do not refrigerate injection; is less soluble in more alkaline pH; protect from light; do not use NS as a diluent; injection vehicle contains benzyl alcohol and sodium metabisulfite

Stability of parenteral admixture at room temperature (25°C):

5 mL/125 mL D$_5$W = 6 hours

5 mL/100 mL D$_5$W = 4 hours

5 mL/75 mL D$_5$W = 2 hours

Administration Infuse I.V. co-trimoxazole over 60-90 minutes; must be further diluted 1:25 (5 mL drug to 125 mL diluent, ie, D$_5$W); in patients who require fluid restriction, a 1:15 dilution (5 mL drug to 75 mL diluent, ie, D$_5$W) or a 1:10 dilution (5 mL drug to 50 mL diluent, ie, D$_5$W) can be administered

Contraindications Hypersensitivity to any sulfa drug, trimethoprim, or any component of the formulation; porphyria; megaloblastic anemia due to folate deficiency; infants <2 months of age; marked hepatic damage; severe renal disease; pregnancy (at term)

Warnings

Use with caution in patients with G6PD deficiency, impaired renal or hepatic function or potential folate deficiency (malnourished, chronic anticonvulsant therapy, or elderly); maintain adequate hydration to prevent crystalluria; adjust dosage in patients with renal impairment. Injection vehicle contains benzyl alcohol and sodium metabisulfite.

Chemical similarities are present among sulfonamides, sulfonylureas, carbonic anhydrase inhibitors, thiazides, and loop diuretics (except ethacrynic acid). Use in patients with sulfonamide allergy is specifically contraindicated in product labeling, however, a risk of cross-reaction exists in patients with allergy to any of these compounds; avoid use when previous reaction has been severe.

Fatalities associated with severe reactions including Stevens-Johnson syndrome, toxic epidermal necrolysis, hepatic necrosis, agranulocytosis, aplastic anemia and other blood dyscrasias; discontinue use at first sign of rash. Elderly patients appear at greater risk for more severe adverse reactions. May cause hypoglycemia, particularly in malnourished, or patients with renal or hepatic impairment. Use with caution in patients with porphyria or thyroid dysfunction. Slow acetylators may be more prone to adverse reactions. Caution in patients with allergies or asthma. May cause hyperkalemia (associated with high doses of trimethoprim). Incidence of adverse effects appears to be increased in patients with AIDS.

Dosage Forms

Note: The 5:1 ratio (SMX:TMP) remains constant in all dosage forms.

Injection, solution: Sulfamethoxazole 80 mg and trimethoprim 16 mg per mL (5 mL, 10 mL, 30 mL) [contains propylene glycol ~400 mg/mL, alcohol, benzyl alcohol, and sodium metabisulfite]

Suspension, oral: Sulfamethoxazole 200 mg and trimethoprim 40 mg per 5 mL (480 mL) [contains alcohol]

Septra®: Sulfamethoxazole 200 mg and trimethoprim 40 mg per 5 mL (480 mL) [contains alcohol 0.26% and sodium benzoate; cherry and grape flavors] [DSC]

Tablet: Sulfamethoxazole 400 mg and trimethoprim 80 mg

Bactrim™: Sulfamethoxazole 400 mg and trimethoprim 80 mg [contains sodium benzoate]

Septra®: Sulfamethoxazole 400 mg and trimethoprim 80 mg

Tablet, double strength: Sulfamethoxazole 800 mg and trimethoprim 160 mg

Bactrim™ DS: Sulfamethoxazole 800 mg and trimethoprim 160 mg [contains sodium benzoate]

Septra® DS: Sulfamethoxazole 800 mg and trimethoprim 160 mg

Reference Range Peak plasma concentrations of 20-50 mg/L (79-198 µmol/L) of SMZ and 0.9-1.9 mg/L (3.1-6.5 µmol/L) of TMP occur after oral ingestion of 800 mg of SMZ and 160 mg of TMP; plasma trimethoprim levels >5 mg/L (17 µmol/L) may be needed to treat *P. carinii* pneumonia

Overdosage/Treatment

Decontamination: Lavage (within 1 hour)/activated charcoal

Supportive therapy: Leucovorin (10 mg/m^2 every 6 hours for 72 hours) for trimethoprim bone marrow toxicity. For treatment of lingua villosa nigra, discontinue causative agent. Clean the tongue with a toothbrush and rinse mouth with a half-strength solution of hydrogen peroxide or 10% carbamide peroxide. Symptoms should subside in a few days.

Enhancement of elimination: Multiple dosing of activated charcoal may be effective

Test Interactions Falsely increases creatinine (Jaffé alkaline picrate reaction); increased serum methotrexate by dihydrofolate reductase method; does not interfere with RIA method; may cause elevation of serum creatinine due to interference with tubular secretion of creatinine

Drug Interactions Sulfamethoxazole: **Substrate** of CYP2C9 (major), 3A4 (minor); **Inhibits** CYP2C9 (moderate)

Trimethoprim: **Substrate** (major) of CYP2C9, 3A4; **Inhibits** CYP2C8 (moderate) 2C9 (moderate)

ACE Inhibitors and angiotensin receptor antagonists: May increase the risk of hyperkalemia with sulfamethoxazole/trimethoprim.

Amantadine: Concurrent use with sulfamethoxazole/trimethoprim has been associated with toxic delirium (rare).

Cyclosporine: May result in an increased risk of nephrotoxicity when used with sulfamethoxazole/trimethoprim. Sulfonamides may decrease the serum concentrations of cyclosporine.

CYP2C9 inducers: May decrease the levels/effects of sulfamethoxazole and trimethoprim. Example inducers include carbamazepine, phenobarbital, phenytoin, rifampin, rifapentine, and secobarbital.

CYP2C8 Substrates: Trimethoprim may increase the levels/effects of CYP2C8 substrates. Example substrates include amiodarone, paclitaxel, pioglitazone, repaglinide, and rosiglitazone.

CYP2C9 Substrates: Sulfmethoxazole and trimethoprim may increase the levels/effects of CYP2C9 substrates. Example substrates include bosentan, dapsone, fluoxetine, glimepiride, glipizide, losartan, montelukast, nateglinide, paclitaxel, phenytoin, warfarin, and zafirlukast.

Dapsone: Trimethoprim may increase the serum concentration of dapsone.

Diuretics, potassium-sparing: May increase the risk of hyperkalemia with sulfamethoxazole/trimethoprim.

Leucovorin: Although occasionally recommended to limit or reverse hematologic toxicity of high-dose sulfamethoxazole/trimethoprim, concurrent use has been associated with a decreased effectiveness in treating *Pneumocystis carinii*.

Methotrexate: Sulfamethoxazole/trimethoprim may increase toxicity of methotrexate (due to displacement from binding sites and/or decreased renal secretion).

Phenytoin: Sulfamethoxazole/trimethoprim may increase phenytoin levels/toxicity. Phenytoin may decrease sulfamethoxazole/trimethoprim levels.

Procainamide: Trimethoprim may decrease the excretion of procainamide.

Pyrimethamine: Concurrent therapy with pyrimethamine (in doses >25 mg/week) may be at increased risk of megaloblastic anemia.

Sulfonylureas: Sulfamethoxazole/trimethoprim may increase the hypoglycemic effect of sulfonylureas; monitor.

Warfarin: Sulfamethoxazole/trimethoprim may increase the hypoprothrombinemic effect of warfarin; monitor INR closely.

Pregnancy Risk Factor C/D (at term - expert analysis)

Pregnancy Implications Do not use at term to avoid kernicterus in the newborn; use during pregnancy only if risks outweigh the benefits since folic acid metabolism may be affected

Lactation Enters breast milk/contraindicated (AAP rates "compatible with restrictions")

Additional Information Injection vehicle contains benzyl alcohol and sodium metabisulfite; folinic acid should be given if bone marrow depression occurs; one double-strength tablet of trimethoprim-sulfamethoxazole 5 times/week has been demonstrated to aid in preventing spontaneous bacterial peritonitis in cirrhotic patients. Alkalinization of urine pH to >7.5 with sodium bicarbonate or acetazolamide may help prevent trimethoprim-induced hyperkalemia.

Specific References

Dib EG, Bernstein S, and Benesch C, "Multifocal Myoclonus Induced by Trimethoprim-Sulfamethoxazole Therapy in a Patient with *Nocardia* Infection," *N Eng J Med*, 2004, 350(1):88-9.

Therrien R, "Possible Trimethoprim/Sulfamethoxazole-Induced Aseptic Meningitis," *Ann Pharmacother*, 2004, 38(11):1863-7.

Sulfasalazine

Related Information
- Therapeutic Drugs Associated with Hallucinations

CAS Number 599-79-1

U.S. Brand Names Azulfidine® EN-tabs®; Azulfidine®

Synonyms Salicylazosulfapyridine

Use Management of ulcerative colitis, Crohn's disease; also may be effective in ankylosing spondylitis, scleroderma, rheumatoid arthritis, Behūlet's disease and psoriasis; also may be useful in radiation, enteritis, and dermatitis herpetiformis

Unlabeled/Investigational Use Ankylosing spondylitis, collagenous colitis, Crohn's disease, psoriasis, psoriatic arthritis, juvenile chronic arthritis

Mechanism of Action Acts locally in the colon to decrease the inflammatory response and systemically interferes with secretion by inhibiting prostaglandin synthesis

Adverse Reactions

Cardiovascular: Sinus tachycardia

Central nervous system: **Fever, dizziness**, encephalopathy, CNS depression, **headache**, malaise, myopathy, visual hallucinations, confusion, Jarisch-Herxheimer reaction, depression, gustatory hallucinations, extrapyramidal reactions

Dermatologic: **Itching**, toxic epidermal necrolysis, **skin rash**, **photosensitivity**, Lyell's syndrome, Stevens-Johnson syndrome, alopecia, exfoliative dermatitis, acute generalized exanthematous pustulosis, bullous skin disease, xerosis, urticaria, purpura, psoriasis, erythema nodosum, licheniform eruptions, exanthem, cutaneous vasculitis

Endocrine & metabolic: Thyroid function disturbance

Gastrointestinal: **Anorexia, nausea**, abdominal pain, **vomiting, diarrhea**, colitis, xerostomia

Genitourinary: Crystalluria, urine discoloration (orange, orange-yellow), **reversible oligospermia**

Hematologic: Granulocytopenia, leukopenia, thrombocytopenia, aplastic anemia, hemolytic anemia (Coombs' positive), lymphocytosis, porphyrinogenic

Hepatic: Hepatitis, jaundice

Neuromuscular & skeletal: Chorea

Ocular: Vision color changes (red tinge)

Renal: Interstitial nephritis, acute nephrotoxicity, hematuria, proteinuria

Respiratory: Bronchiolitis obliterans organizing pneumonia, pneumonitis, bilateral lung opacities

Miscellaneous: Systemic lupus erythematosus, serum sickness-like reactions, lymphadenopathy, fixed drug eruption

Signs and Symptoms of Overdose Doses of as little as 2-5 g/day may produce toxicity. The aniline radical is responsible for hematologic toxicity. Abdominal pain, acidosis, agranulocytosis, anorexia, confusion, diarrhea, dizziness, drowsiness, fever, headache, hemolytic anemia, jaundice, nausea, vomiting

Pharmacodynamics/Kinetics

Absorption: 10% to 15% as unchanged drug from small intestine

Distribution: Small amounts enter feces and breast milk

Metabolism: Via colonic intestinal flora to sulfapyridine and 5-aminosalicylic acid (5-ASA); following absorption, sulfapyridine undergoes N-acetylation and ring hydroxylation while 5-ASA undergoes N-acetylation

Half-life elimination: 5.7-10 hours

Excretion: Primarily urine (as unchanged drug, components, and acetylated metabolites)

Dosage

Oral:

Children ≥2 years: Ulcerative colitis: Initial: 40-60 mg/kg/day in 3-6 divided doses; maintenance dose: 20-30 mg/kg/day in 4 divided doses

Children ≥6 years: Juvenile rheumatoid arthritis: Enteric coated tablet: 30-50 mg/kg/day in 2 divided doses; Initial: Begin with $^1/_4$ to $^1/_3$ of expected maintenance dose; increase weekly; maximum: 2 g/day typically

Adults:

Ulcerative colitis: Initial: 1 g 3-4 times/day, 2 g/day maintenance in divided doses; may initiate therapy with 0.5-1 g/day

Rheumatoid arthritis: Enteric coated tablet: Initial: 0.5-1 g/day; increase weekly to maintenance dose of 2 g/day in 2 divided doses; maximum: 3 g/day (if response to 2 g/day is inadequate after 12 weeks of treatment)

Dosing interval in renal impairment:

Cl_{cr} 10-30 mL/minute: Administer twice daily

Cl_{cr} <10 mL/minute: Administer once daily

Dosing adjustment in hepatic impairment: Avoid use

Stability Protect from light; shake suspension well

Monitoring Parameters Stool frequency, hematocrit, reticulocyte count, CBC, urinalysis, renal function tests, liver function tests

Administration GI intolerance is common during the first few days of therapy (administer with meals).

Contraindications Hypersensitivity to sulfasalazine, sulfa drugs, salicylates, or any component of the formulation; porphyria; GI or GU obstruction; pregnancy (at term)

Warnings Use with caution in patients with renal impairment; impaired hepatic function or urinary obstruction, blood dyscrasias, severe allergies or asthma, or G6PD deficiency; may cause folate deficiency (consider providing 1 mg/day folate supplement). Chemical similarities are present among sulfonamides, sulfonylureas, carbonic anhydrase inhibitors, thiazides, and loop diuretics (except ethacrynic acid). Use in patients with sulfonamide allergy is specifically contraindicated in product labeling, however, a risk of cross-reaction exists in patients with allergy to any of these compounds; avoid use when previous reaction has been severe. Safety and efficacy have not been established in children <2 years of age.

Dosage Forms Tablet (Azulfidine®, Sulfazine): 500 mg

Tablet, delayed release, enteric coated (Azulfidine® EN-tabs®, Sulfazine EC): 500 mg

Reference Range Toxic level of sulfapyridine: >50 mg/L (200 µmol/L)

Overdosage/Treatment

Decontamination: Emesis within 30 minutes or lavage (within 1 hour)/ activated charcoal or cholestyramine can reduce sulfasalazine absorption

Supportive therapy: Anaphylaxis can be treated with standard therapy; acetylcysteine (24 g I.V. over 36 hours) has been used to treat sulfasalazine-induced hepatitis; sulfasalazine-induced agranulocytosis can be treated with filgrastim (300 mcg/day)

Enhancement of elimination: Multiple dosing of activated charcoal may be effective

Drug Interactions Azathioprine, mercaptopurine, sulfasalazine: May increase the risk of myelosuppression (due to TPMT inhibition).

Cyclosporine concentrations may be decreased; monitor levels and renal function

Digoxin's absorption may be decreased

Folic acid's absorption may be decreased

Hydantoin levels may be increased; monitor levels and adjust as necessary

Hypoglycemics: Increased effect of oral hypoglycemics (rare, but severe); monitor blood sugar

Methenamine: Combination may result in crystalluria; avoid use

Methotrexate-induced bone marrow suppression may be increased

NSAIDs and salicylates: May increase sulfonamide concentrations

PABA (para-aminobenzoic acid - may be found in some vitamin supplements): Interferes with the antibacterial activity of sulfonamides; avoid concurrent use

Sulfinpyrazone: May increase sulfonamide concentrations

Thiazide diuretics: May increase the incidence of thrombocytopenia purpura

Thiopental's effect may be enhanced; monitor for possible dosage reduction

Uricosuric agents: Actions of these agents are potentiated

Warfarin and other oral anticoagulants: Anticoagulant effect may be increased; decrease dose and monitor INR closely

Pregnancy Risk Factor B/D (at term)

Lactation Enters breast milk/use caution (AAP recommends use "with caution")

Nursing Implications Gastrointestinal intolerance is common during the first few days of therapy; drug commonly imparts an orange-yellow discoloration to urine and skin. This drug should be administered after food to reduce gastrointestinal irritation; may cause orange-yellow discoloration of urine and skin.

Additional Information Since sulfasalazine impairs folate absorption, consider providing 1 mg/day folate supplement

Specific References

Borras-Blasco J, Navarro-Ruiz A, Matarredona J, et al, "Photo-Induced Stevens-Johnson Syndrome Due to Sulfasalazine Therapy," *Ann Pharmacother*, 2003, 37(9):1241-3.

SulfiSOXAZOLE

CAS Number 80-74-0

U.S. Brand Names Gantrisin®

Synonyms Sulfisoxazole Acetyl; Sulphafurazole

Use Treatment of lower, uncomplicated urinary tract infections, otitis media, *Chlamydia*; nocardiosis; treatment of acute pelvic inflammatory disease in prepubertal children

Mechanism of Action Interferes with bacterial growth by inhibiting bacterial folic acid synthesis through competitive antagonism of PABA

Adverse Reactions

Cardiovascular: Myocarditis (hypersensitivity), myocarditis

Central nervous system: **Fever, dizziness, headache**, psychosis, Jarisch-Herxheimer reaction, gustatory hallucinations

Dermatologic: **Itching, skin rash, photosensitivity**, Lyell's syndrome, Stevens-Johnson syndrome, nail discoloration (brown), toxic epidermal necrolysis

Endocrine & metabolic: Parotitis, thyroid function disturbance

Gastrointestinal: **Anorexia, nausea,** abdominal pain, **vomiting, diarrhea**

Genitourinary: Crystalluria

Hematologic: Granulocytopenia, leukopenia, thrombocytopenia, aplastic anemia, hemolytic anemia, methemoglobinemia

Hepatic: Hepatitis, jaundice, cholestasis, granulomatous hepatitis

Renal: Interstitial nephritis, acute nephropathy, hematuria

Respiratory: Cough

Miscellaneous: Serum sickness-like reactions, periarteritis nodosa

Signs and Symptoms of Overdose Doses of as little as 2-5 g/day may produce toxicity. The aniline radical is responsible for hematologic toxicity. Abdominal pain, acidosis, agranulocytosis, anorexia, dizziness, drowsiness, fever, hematuria, hemolytic anemia, jaundice, nausea, nephrotoxicity, vomiting.

Pharmacodynamics/Kinetics

Absorption: Sulfisoxazole acetyl is hydrolyzed in GI tract to sulfisoxazole which is readily absorbed

Distribution: Crosses placenta; enters breast milk

CSF:blood level ratio: Normal meninges: 50% to 80%; Inflamed meninges: 80+%

Protein binding: 85% to 88%

Metabolism: Hepatic via acetylation and glucuronide conjugation to inactive compounds

Half-life elimination: 4-7 hours; prolonged with renal impairment

Time to peak, serum: 2-3 hours

Excretion: Urine (95%, 40% to 60% as unchanged drug) within 24 hours

Dosage

Not for use in patients <2 months of age

Children >2 months: Oral: 75 mg/kg stat, 120-150 mg/kg/day in divided doses every 4-6 hours; not to exceed 6 g/day

Adults: Oral: 2-4 g stat, 4-8 g/day in divided doses every 4-6 hours

Dosing interval in renal impairment:

Cl_{cr} 10-50 mL/minute: Administer every 8-12 hours

Cl_{cr} <10 mL/minute: Administer every 12-24 hours

>50% removed by hemodialysis

Children and Adults: Ophthalmic:

Ointment: Apply small amount to affected eye 1-3 times/day and at bedtime

Solution: Instill 1-2 drops to affected eye every 2-3 hours

Stability Protect from light

Monitoring Parameters CBC, urinalysis, renal function tests, temperature

Administration Administer around-the-clock to promote less variation in peak and trough serum levels.

Contraindications Hypersensitivity to sulfisoxazole, any sulfa drug, or any component of the formulation; porphyria; infants <2 months of age (sulfas compete with bilirubin for protein binding sites); patients with urinary obstruction; sunscreens containing PABA; pregnancy (at term)

Warnings Use with caution in patients with G6PD deficiency (hemolysis may occur), hepatic or renal impairment; dosage modification required in patients with renal impairment; risk of crystalluria should be considered in patients with impaired renal function. Chemical similarities are present among sulfonamides, sulfonylureas, carbonic anhydrase inhibitors, thiazides, and loop diuretics (except ethacrynic acid). Use in patients with sulfonamide allergy is specifically contraindicated in product labeling, however, a risk of cross-reaction exists in patients with allergy to any of these compounds; avoid use when previous reaction has been severe.

Dosage Forms Suspension, oral, pediatric, as acetyl (Gantrisin®): 500 mg/5 mL (480 mL) [contains alcohol 0.3%; raspberry flavor]

Tablet: 500 mg

Reference Range 2 g oral dose results in peak plasma level of 10-15 mg/L (37-56 µmol/L)

Overdosage/Treatment

Decontamination: Activated charcoal

Enhancement of elimination: Multiple dosing of activated charcoal may be effective; alkalinizing the urine decreases serum half-life by almost 30%; hemodialysis can enhance sulfisoxazole elimination

Test Interactions False-positive protein in urine; false-positive urine glucose with Clinitest®; can interfere in serum calcium assays, thus giving the appearance of hypocalcemia

Drug Interactions

Substrate of CYP2C9 (major); **Inhibits** CYP2C9 (strong)

Cyclosporine concentrations may be decreased; monitor levels and renal function

CYP2C9 Inducers may decrease the levels/effects of Sulfisoxazole. Example inducers include carbamazepine, phenobarbital, phenytoin, rifampin, rifapentine, and secobarbital.

CYP2C9 Substrates: Sulfisoxazole may increase the levels/effects of CYP2C9 substrates. Example substrates include bosentan, dapsone, fluoxetine, glimepiride, glipizide, losartan, montelukast, nateglinide, paclitaxel, phenytoin, warfarin, and zafirlukast.

Hydantoin levels may be increased; monitor levels and adjust as necessary

Hypoglycemics: Increased effect of oral hypoglycemics (rare, but severe); monitor blood sugar

Methenamine: Combination may result in crystalluria; avoid use

Methotrexate-induced bone marrow suppression may be increased

NSAIDs and salicylates: May increase sulfonamide concentrations

PABA (para-aminobenzoic acid - may be found in some vitamin supplements): Interferes with the antibacterial activity of sulfonamides; avoid concurrent use

Sulfinpyrazone: May increase sulfonamide concentrations

Thiazide diuretics: May increase the incidence of thrombocytopenia purpura

Thiopental's effect may be enhanced; monitor for possible dosage reduction

Uricosuric agents: Actions of these agents are potentiated

Warfarin and other oral anticoagulants: Anticoagulant effect may be increased; decrease dose and monitor INR closely

Pregnancy Risk Factor B/D (near term)

Pregnancy Implications Can cause kernicterus in neonates

Lactation Enters breast milk/compatible

Nursing Implications Give around-the-clock to promote less variation in peak and trough serum levels; maintain adequate fluid intake

---

Sulindac

Related Information

● Nonsteroidal Anti-inflammatory Drugs

CAS Number 38194-50-2

U.S. Brand Names Clinoril®

Use Management of inflammatory disease, rheumatoid disorders; acute gouty arthritis; structurally similar to indomethacin but acts like aspirin; safest NSAID for use in mild renal impairment

Mechanism of Action Inhibits prostaglandin synthesis by decreasing the activity of the enzyme, cyclooxygenase, which results in decreased formation of prostaglandin precursors

Adverse Reactions

Cardiovascular: Circulatory collapse, hypotension, vasculitis, Raynaud's phenomenon

Central nervous system: **Dizziness,** headache, aseptic meningitis, psychosis, cognitive dysfunction, coma, seizures, paranoia, gustatory hallucinations

Dermatologic: **Rash,** pruritus, Stevens-Johnson syndrome, exfoliative dermatitis, angioedema, urticaria, licheniform eruption, exanthem, phototoxicity

Endocrine & metabolic: Hyperkalemia, anion gap metabolic acidosis, fluid retention, gynecomastia

Gastrointestinal: **Abdominal cramps, heartburn, indigestion, nausea,** vomiting, GI bleeding, GI ulceration, constipation, diarrhea, dyspepsia, metallic taste, loss of taste perception, aphthous stomatitis, xerostomia, stomatitis

Hematologic: Leukopenia, neutropenia, agranulocytosis, granulocytopenia, aplastic anemia (rare), platelet inhibition, erythroblastopenia

Hepatic: Elevated transaminases, hepatitis (fulminant), hepatic necrosis, cholestasis, cholelithiasis

Neuromuscular & skeletal: Paresthesia

Otic: Ototoxicity, tinnitus

Renal: Renal failure (acute), nephrotic syndrome, chronic renal failure, albuminuria

Respiratory: Wheezing, respiratory depression

Miscellaneous: Hypersensitivity, anaphylactoid reactions, fixed drug eruption

Signs and Symptoms of Overdose Azotemia, chills, coagulopathy, cognitive dysfunction, drowsiness, gastritis, GI bleeding, hyperthermia, insomnia, leukemoid reaction, leukocytosis, nausea, nephritis, nephrotic syndrome, ototoxicity, photosensitivity, purpura, thrombocytopenia, tinnitus, toxic epidermal necrolysis, vomiting, wheezing. Severe poisoning can manifest with alopecia coma, hypotension, renal and/or hepatic failure, respiratory depression, and seizures.

Pharmacodynamics/Kinetics

Onset of action: Analgesic: ~1 hour

Duration: 12-24 hours

Absorption: 90%

Metabolism: Hepatic; prodrug metabolized to sulfide metabolite (active) for therapeutic effects and to sulfone metabolites (inactive)

Half-life elimination: Parent drug: ~8 hours; Active metabolite: ~16 hours

Excretion: Urine (50%, primarily as inactive metabolites); feces (25%, primarily as metabolites)

Dosage

Maximum therapeutic response may not be realized for up to 3 weeks. Oral:

Children: Dose not established

Adults: 150-200 mg twice daily or 300-400 mg once daily; not to exceed 400 mg/day

Dosing adjustment in hepatic impairment: Dose reduction is necessary

Monitoring Parameters Liver enzymes, BUN, serum creatinine, CBC, blood pressure; signs and symptoms of GI bleeding

Administration
Should be administered with food or milk.

Contraindications Hypersensitivity to sulindac, aspirin, other NSAIDs, or any component of the formulation; perioperative pain in the setting of coronary artery bypass surgery (CABG); pregnancy (3rd trimester)

Warnings

[U.S. Boxed Warning]: NSAIDs are associated with an increased risk of adverse cardiovascular events, including MI, stroke, and new onset or worsening of pre-existing hypertension. Risk may be increased with duration of use or pre-existing cardiovascular risk-factors or disease. Carefully evaluate individual cardiovascular risk profiles prior to prescribing. Use caution with fluid retention, CHF or hypertension.

Use of NSAIDs can compromise existing renal function. Renal toxicity can occur in patient with impaired renal function, dehydration, heart failure, liver dysfunction, those taking diuretics and ACEI and the elderly. Rehydrate patient before starting therapy. Monitor renal function closely. Sulindac is not recommended for patients with advanced renal disease. Use caution in patients with renal lithiasis; sulindac metabolites have been reported as components of renal stones. Use hydration in patients with a history of renal stones.

[U.S. Boxed Warning]: NSAIDs may increase risk of gastrointestinal irritation, ulceration, bleeding, and perforation. These events may occur at any time during therapy and without warning. Use caution with a history of GI disease (bleeding or ulcers), concurrent therapy with aspirin, anticoagulants and/or corticosteroids, smoking, use of alcohol, the elderly or debilitated patients.

Use the lowest effective dose for the shortest duration of time, consistent with individual patient goals, to reduce risk of cardiovascular or GI adverse events. Alternate therapies should be considered for patients at high risk.

NSAIDs may cause serious skin adverse events including exfoliative dermatitis, Stevens-Johnson syndrome (SJS) and toxic epidermal necrolysis (TEN). Anaphylactoid reactions may occur, even without prior exposure; patients with "aspirin triad" (bronchial asthma, aspirin intolerance, rhinitis) may be at increased risk. Do not use in patients who experience bronchospasm, asthma, rhinitis, or urticaria with NSAID or aspirin therapy.

Use with caution in patients with decreased hepatic function. Closely monitor patients with any abnormal LFT. Severe hepatic reactions (eg, fulminant hepatitis, liver failure) have occurred with NSAID use, rarely; discontinue if signs or symptoms of liver disease develop, or if systemic manifestations occur. May require dosage adjustment in hepatic dysfunction; sulfide and sulfone metabolites may accumulate.

Withhold for at least 4-6 half-lives prior to surgical or dental procedures. Safety and efficacy in pediatric patients have not been established.

Dosage Forms Tablet: 150 mg, 200 mg
Clinoril®: 200 mg

Reference Range Peak plasma levels after a 200 mg oral dose: ~4 mg/L (parent compound); 3 mg/L (sulfide metabolite); and 2 mg/L (sulfone metabolite)

Overdosage/Treatment
Decontamination: Activated charcoal

Supportive therapy: Hypotension/dehydration can be managed with I.V. fluid therapy; acidosis should be treated with bicarbonates, seizures with benzodiazepines; antacids, blood products are indicated, as appropriate, for hemorrhage

Enhancement of elimination: Dialysis or perfusion is indicated for secondary complications, acidosis, or renal failure and not toxin removal alone; multiple dosing of activated charcoal may be effective

Test Interactions ↑ chloride (S), sodium (S), bleeding time

Drug Interactions ACE inhibitors: Antihypertensive effects may be decreased by concurrent therapy with NSAIDs; monitor blood pressure.

Aminoglycosides: NSAIDs may decrease the excretion of aminoglycosides.

Angiotensin II antagonists: Antihypertensive effects may be decreased by concurrent therapy with NSAIDs; monitor blood pressure.

Anticoagulants (warfarin, heparin, LMWHs): When used with NSAIDs can cause increased risk of bleeding.

Antiplatelet drugs (ticlopidine, clopidogrel, aspirin, abciximab, dipyridamole, eptifibatide, tirofiban): Concurrent use may cause an increased risk of bleeding.

Beta-blockers: NSAIDs may decrease the antihypertensive effect of beta-blockers. Monitor.

Bisphosphonates: NSAIDs may increase the risk of gastrointestinal ulceration.

Cholestyramine (and other bile acid sequestrants): May decrease the absorption of NSAIDs. Separate by at least 2 hours.

Corticosteroids: May increase the risk of GI ulceration; avoid concurrent use.

Cyclosporine: NSAIDs may increase serum creatinine, potassium, blood pressure, and cyclosporine levels; monitor cyclosporine levels and renal function carefully.

Dimethyl sulfoxide: May reduce plasma levels of sulindac's active metabolite. Combination may cause peripheral neuropathy; avoid concurrent use.

Hydralazine's antihypertensive effect is decreased; avoid concurrent use.

Lithium: NSAIDs may increase lithium levels; avoid concurrent use if possible or monitor lithium levels and adjust dose. Sulindac may have the least effect. When NSAID is stopped, lithium will need adjustment again.

Loop diuretic: NSAIDs may decrease the efficacy (diuretic and antihypertensive effect) of loop diuretics.

Methotrexate: Severe bone marrow suppression, aplastic anemia, and GI toxicity have been reported with concomitant NSAID therapy. Avoid use during moderate or high-dose methotrexate (increased and prolonged methotrexate levels). NSAID use during low-dose treatment of rheumatoid arthritis has not been fully evaluated; extreme caution is warranted.

Pemetrexed: NSAIDs may decrease the excretion of pemetrexed. Patients with Cl$_{cr}$ 45-79 mL/minute should avoid long-acting NSAIDs for 5 days before and 2 days after pemetrexed treatment.

Thiazides antihypertensive effects are decreased; avoid concurrent use.

Treprostinil: May enhance the risk of bleeding with concurrent use.

Vancomycin: NSAIDs may decrease the excretion of vancomycin.

Pregnancy Risk Factor B/D (3rd trimester)

Pregnancy Implications Animal studies have not documented teratogenic effects. However, known effects of NSAIDs suggest the potential for premature ductus arteriosus closeure, particularly in late pregnancy.

Lactation Excretion in breast milk unknown/not recommended

Additional Information Structurally similar to indomethacin but acts like aspirin; associated with the highest incidence of upper GI bleeds among NSAIDs

Sulpiride

Related Information
- Antipsychotic Agents
- Tiapride

CAS Number 15676-16-1; 23672-07-3

Impairment Potential Blood sulpiride level of 2.1 mg/L consistent with driving impairment

Unlabeled/Investigational Use Antidepressive agent and antipsychotic agent

Mechanism of Action Substituted benzamide with selective dopamine receptor antagonism

Adverse Reactions

Cardiovascular: Palpitations, hypertension

Central nervous system: Dizziness, headache, neuroleptic malignant syndrome, sedation, Parkinson symptoms, **extrapyramidal effects**, tardive dyskinesia, agitation

Endocrine & metabolic: Galactorrhea, sexual dysfunction, hyperprolactinemia

Gastrointestinal: Nausea, vomiting, xerostomia, constipation

Genitourinary: Impotence

Hematologic: Porphyrinogenic

Hepatic: Cholestatic jaundice, primary biliary cirrhosis

Ocular: Blurred vision

Miscellaneous: Anticholinergic effects, diaphoresis

Toxicodynamics/Kinetics

Distribution: V$_d$: 1-2.7 L//kg

Protein binding: <40%

Bioavailability: Oral: 35% (food lowers absorption)

Half-life: 6-8 hours; 20-26 hours in renal failure

Elimination: Renal (clearance: 310 mL/minute)

Dosage Oral: 200-400 mg twice daily; may increase gradually to a maximum dose of 1.2 g/day
I.M.: 600-800 mg/day

Reference Range

Therapeutic steady-state serum range for sulpiride: 0.071-1.121 mcg/mL

Postmortem blood sulpiride level of 38 mcg/mL associated with suicidal ingestion of ~12 g

Overdosage/Treatment

Decontamination: Emesis within 30 minutes or lavage (within 1 hour)/activated charcoal

Enhancement of elimination: Multiple dosing of activated charcoal may be effective

Additional Information Stimulates prolactin secretion; can exacerbate hypertension caused by pheochromocytoma, cross-hypersensitivity may exist with metoclopramide, tiapride, sultopride

Sulthiamine

CAS Number 61-56-3
Synonyms RP10248; Sultiame; Tetrahydro-2-para-sulfamoylphenyl-1,2-thiazine 1,1 dioxide
Impairment Potential Yes
Use Anticonvulsant agent used for generalized seizures temporal lobe seizures, myoclonic or focal seizures; not useful for absence seizures
Mechanism of Action Antiepileptic agent and a weak carbonic anhydrase inhibitor; a synthetic sulfonamide
Adverse Reactions
Central nervous system: Headache, lethargy, ataxia, vertigo
Genitourinary: Crystalluria
Neuromuscular & skeletal: Paresthesia
Ocular: Ptosis
Respiratory: Hyperpnea, dyspnea
Signs and Symptoms of Overdose Catatonia, crystalluria (in acidic urine), drowsiness, hyperreflexia, hypotension, prolonged extensor plantar reflexes, vomiting
Admission Criteria/Prognosis Admit symptomatic patient or any ingestion >4 g
Pharmacodynamics/Kinetics
Protein binding: 29%
Half-life: 30 hours
Elimination: Renal
Dosage Oral:
Children: Initial: 3-5 mg/kg/day; can increase daily dose: 10-15 mg/kg; maximum daily dose: 1.2 g
Adults: Initial: 100 mg 2 times/day; can be increased to 200 mg 3 times/day
Monitoring Parameters Urine pH, urine output
Warnings Use with caution in patients with renal impairment
Dosage Forms Suspension: 50 mg/5 mL
Tablets: 50 mg, 200 mg
Reference Range
Therapeutic plasma level is up to 12 mcg/mL; severe toxicity is associated with plasma levels >30 mcg/mL
Overdosage/Treatment
Decontamination: Lavage (within 1 hour)/activated charcoal
Supportive therapy: Urine pH should be kept alkaline (by use of I.V. sodium bicarbonate: 1-2 mEq/kg) in order to avoid crystalluria and renal impairment
Drug Interactions By inhibiting its metabolism, sulthiamine can raise phenytoin serum levels

Sumatriptan Succinate

CAS Number 103628-46-2; 103628-47-3; 103628-48-4
U.S. Brand Names Imitrex®
Synonyms Sumatriptan Succinate
Impairment Potential Yes
Use
Acute treatment of migraine with or without aura
Sumatriptan injection: Acute treatment of cluster headache episodes
Mechanism of Action Selective agonist for serotonin (5HT, ID subtype receptor) in cranial arteries to cause vasoconstriction and reduces sterile inflammation associated with antidromic neuronal transmission correlating with relief of migraine
Adverse Reactions
Cardiovascular: Chest pain, tightness, heaviness, pressure, flushing (injection); abdominal aortic aneurysm, arrhythmia, atrial fibrillation, cerebral ischemia, cerebrovascular accident, ECG changes, flushing, heart block, Prinzmetal's angina, Raynaud syndrome, shock, thrombosis, transient myocardial ischemia, syncope
Central nervous system: **Dizziness, warm/hot sensation**, drowsiness, malaise, fatigue, headache, anxiety (injection); dizziness, drowsiness, malaise, fatigue, nonspecified pain, vertigo, migraine, sleepiness (tablet); dizziness, vertigo (nasal spray); agitation, convulsions, dystonic reaction, hallucinations, increased intracranial pressure, sensation changes, subarachnoid hemorrhage
Dermatologic: Angioneurotic edema, photosensitivity, pruritus, rash
Endocrine & metabolic: Abnormal menstrual cycle, fluid disturbances (including retention), increased TSH
Gastrointestinal: Nausea, vomiting, hyposalivation, abdominal discomfort, dysphagia; mouth, tongue discomfort (injection); **bad taste, nausea, vomiting** (nasal spray); abdominal discomfort, decreased appetite, diarrhea, dyspeptic symptoms, dysphagia, gastrointestinal pain, intestinal obstruction, ischemic colitis, numbness of tongue, swallowing disorders, xerostomia
Hematologic: Anemia, hemolytic anemia, pancytopenia, thrombocytopenia
Hepatic: Abnormal liver function tests
Local: **Pain at the injection site**, thrombophlebitis
Neuromuscular & skeletal: **Tingling**, numbness; neck, throat, and jaw: pain, tightness, pressure; muscle cramps, weakness, myalgia (injection); neck, throat, and jaw: pain, tightness, pressure (tablet); paresthesia (tablet); joint ache, muscle stiffness, paresthesia
Ocular: Vision alterations (injection); accommodation disorders
Renal: Acute renal failure, hematuria
Respiratory: Nasal disorder, nasal discomfort (nasal spray, injection); throat discomfort (injection, nasal spray); bronchospasm, nose/throat hemorrhage, pulmonary embolism
Miscellaneous: Burning, feeling of heaviness, pressure sensation, feeling of tightness, strange feeling, cold sensation, diaphoresis (injection); nonspecified pressure, tightness, heaviness (tablet); warm sensation, cold sensation, death, dental pain, hiccups, hypersensitivity reactions, phlebitis, psychomotor disorders, severe anaphylaxis/anaphylactoid reactions
Signs and Symptoms of Overdose Angina, chest pain, hypertension, numbness. Fatalities due to myocardial infarction usually occur 3 or more hours after treatment.
Pharmacodynamics/Kinetics
Onset of action: ~30 minutes
Distribution: V_d: 2.4 L/kg
Protein binding: 14% to 21%
Metabolism: Hepatic, primarily via MAO-A isoenzyme
Bioavailability: SubQ: 97% ± 16% of that following I.V. injection; Oral: 15%
Half-life elimination: Injection, tablet: 2.5 hours; Nasal spray: 2 hours
Time to peak, serum: 5-20 minutes
Excretion:
Injection: Urine (38% as indole acetic acid metabolite, 22% as unchanged drug)
Nasal spray: Urine (42% as indole acetic acid metabolite, 3% as unchanged drug)
Tablet: Urine (60% as indole acetic acid metabolite, 3% as unchanged drug); feces (40%)
Dosage
Adults:
Oral: A single dose of 25 mg, 50 mg, or 100 mg (taken with fluids). If a satisfactory response has not been obtained at 2 hours, a second dose may be administered. Results from clinical trials show that initial doses of 50 mg and 100 mg are more effective than doses of 25 mg, and that 100 mg doses do not provide a greater effect than 50 mg and may have increased incidence of side effects. Although doses of up to 300 mg/day have been studied, the total daily dose should not exceed 200 mg. The safety of treating an average of >4 headaches in a 30-day period have not been established.
Intranasal: A single dose of 5 mg, 10 mg, or 20 mg administered in one nostril. A 10 mg dose may be achieved by administering a single 5 mg dose in each nostril. If headache returns, the dose may be repeated once after 2 hours, not to exceed a total daily dose of 40 mg. The safety of treating an average of >4 headaches in a 30-day period has not been established.
SubQ: 6 mg; a second injection may be administered at least 1 hour after the initial dose, but not more than 2 injections in a 24-hour period. If side effects are dose-limiting, lower doses may be used.
Dosage adjustment in renal impairment: Dosage adjustment not necessary
Dosage adjustment in hepatic impairment: Bioavailability of oral sumatriptan is increased with liver disease. If treatment is needed, do not exceed single doses of 50 mg. The nasal spray has not been studied in patients with hepatic impairment, however, because the spray does not undergo first-pass metabolism, levels would not be expected to alter. Use of all dosage forms is contraindicated with severe hepatic impairment.
Elderly: Due to increased risk of CAD, decreased hepatic function, and more pronounced blood pressure increases, use of the tablet dosage form in elderly patients is not recommended. Use of the nasal spray has not been studied in the elderly. Pharmacokinetics of injectable sumatriptan in the elderly are similar to healthy patients.
Stability Store at 2°C to 20°C (36°F to 86°F); protect from light
Administration Oral: Should be taken with fluids as soon as symptoms to appear
Injection solution: For SubQ administration; do not administer I.V.; may cause coronary vasospasm
Contraindications Hypersensitivity to sumatriptan or any component of the formulation; patients with ischemic heart disease or signs or symptoms of ischemic heart disease (including Prinzmetal's angina, angina pectoris, myocardial infarction, silent myocardial ischemia); cerebrovascular syndromes (including strokes, transient ischemic attacks); peripheral vascular syndromes (including ischemic bowel disease); uncontrolled hypertension; use within 24 hours of ergotamine derivatives; use within 24 hours of another 5-HT_1 agonist; concurrent administration or within 2 weeks of discontinuing an MAO inhibitor, specifically MAO type A inhibitors; management of hemiplegic or basilar

migraine; prophylactic treatment of migraine; severe hepatic impairment; not for I.V. administration

Warnings

Sumatriptan is indicated only in patients ≥18 years of age with a clear diagnosis of migraine or cluster headache.

Cardiac events (coronary artery vasospasm, transient ischemia, myocardial infarction, ventricular tachycardia/fibrillation, cardiac arrest and death), cerebral/subarachnoid hemorrhage and stroke have been reported with 5-HT$_1$ agonist administration.

Do not give to patients with risk factors for CAD until a cardiovascular evaluation has been performed; if evaluation is satisfactory, the healthcare provider should administer the first dose and cardiovascular status should be periodically evaluated.

Significant elevation in blood pressure, including hypertensive crisis, has also been reported on rare occasions in patients with and without a history of hypertension. Vasospasm-related reactions have been reported other than coronary artery vasospasm. Peripheral vascular ischemia and colonic ischemia with abdominal pain and bloody diarrhea have occurred.

Use with caution in patients with history of seizure disorder or in patients with a lowered seizure threshold. Safety and efficacy in pediatric patients have not been established.

Dosage Forms

Note: Strength expressed as sumatriptan base

Injection, solution, as succinate: 8 mg/mL (0.5 mL) [disposable cartridge for use with STATdose System®]; 12 mg/mL (0.5 mL) [disposable cartridge for use with STATdose System® or vial]

Solution, intranasal spray: 5 mg (100 μL unit dose spray device); 20 mg (100 μL unit dose spray device)

Tablet, as succinate: 25 mg, 50 mg, 100 mg

Reference Range Therapeutic range: 18-60 ng/mL

Overdosage/Treatment

Decontamination for oral ingestion: Ipecac within 30 minutes or lavage within 30 minutes/activated charcoal

Supportive therapy: Nitroprusside, nifedipine, or hydralazine for hypertensive crisis; lidocaine or procainamide for ventricular ectopy; nitroglycerin can reverse sumatriptan-induced coronary artery vasoconstriction

Drug Interactions Note: Use cautiously in patients receiving concomitant medications that can lower the seizure threshold.

Ergot-containing drugs: Prolong vasospastic reactions; do not use sumatriptan or ergot-containing drugs within 24 hours of each other.

MAO inhibitors (MAO type A inhibitors, nonspecific MAO inhibitors): Reduce sumatriptan clearance; concurrent use is contraindicated; wait at least 2 weeks after discontinuing MAO type A inhibitor to start sumatriptan.

Selegiline: Selegiline is a selective MAO type B inhibitor; while not specifically contraindicated, combination may best be avoided until further study.

SSRIs: Can lead to symptoms of hyper-reflexia, weakness, and incoordination; monitor.

Pregnancy Risk Factor C

Pregnancy Implications There are no adequate and well-controlled studies using sumatriptan in pregnant women. Use only if potential benefit to the mother outweighs the potential risk to the fetus.

Lactation Enters breast milk/use caution (AAP rates "compatible")

Nursing Implications Do not administer I.V., may cause coronary vasospasm; pain at injection site lasts <1 hour

Additional Information May increase growth hormone level; oral dose of 100 mg is investigational; oral sumatriptan (100 mg) may prevent headache recurrence; may exacerbate depression. Hypertension is a risk factor for sumatriptan-associated chest pain for men in particular, as is a family history of acute myocardial infarction. Raynaud's phenomenon is a risk factor for sumatriptan-associated chest pain in women, but not in men. Chest pain due to sumatriptan usually lasts for <2 hours duration.

Specific References

Hoffman RJ, Ginsburg BY, Nelson LS, et al, "Acute Coronary Syndrome Following Subcutaneous Sumatriptam Administration in a Child," *Clin Toxicol*, 2005, 43:634.

Meredith JT, Wait S, and Brewer KL, "A Prospective Double-Blind Study of Nasal Sumatriptan Versus I.V. Ketorolac in Migraine," *Am J Emerg Med*, 2003, 21(3):173-5.

Tacrine

CAS Number 1684-40-8; 321-64-2

U.S. Brand Names Cognex®

Synonyms Tacrine Hydrochloride; Tetrahydroaminoacrine; THA

Use Treatment of mild to moderate dementia of the Alzheimer's type

Mechanism of Action Inhibits cholinesterase activity similar to neostigmine

Adverse Reactions

Cardiovascular: Chest pain, shock, angina, sinus bradycardia

Central nervous system: Agitation, dizziness, seizures, insomnia

Dermatologic: Purpura, acne, alopecia, bullous skin disease, xerosis, urticaria, pruritus, psoriasis, exanthem

Gastrointestinal: Nausea, abdominal pain, vomiting, diarrhea, belching

Hepatic: Dose-related hepatitis

Ocular: Lacrimation

Respiratory: Asthma, bronchospasm

Signs and Symptoms of Overdose Bradycardia, confusion, depression, hallucination, hypotension, purpura, tachypnea

Pharmacodynamics/Kinetics

Absorption: Oral: Rapid

Distribution: V$_d$: Mean: 349 L; reduced by food

Protein binding, plasma: 55%

Metabolism: Extensively by CYP450 to multiple metabolites; first pass effect

Bioavailability: Absolute: 17%

Half-life elimination, serum: 2-4 hours; Steady-state: 24-36 hours

Time to peak, plasma: 1-2 hours

Dosage

Adults: Initial: 10 mg 4 times/day; may increase by 40 mg/day adjusted every 6 weeks; maximum: 160 mg/day; best administered separate from meal times.

Dose adjustment based upon transaminase elevations:

ALT ≤3 times ULN*: Continue titration

ALT >3 to ≤5 times ULN*: Decrease dose by 40 mg/day, resume when ALT returns to normal

ALT >5 times ULN*: Stop treatment, may rechallenge upon return of ALT to normal

*ULN = upper limit of normal

Patients with clinical jaundice confirmed by elevated total bilirubin (>3 mg/dL) should not be rechallenged with tacrine

Monitoring Parameters ALT (SGPT) levels and other liver enzymes weekly for at least the first 18 weeks, then monitor once every 3 months

Contraindications Hypersensitivity to tacrine, acridine derivatives, or any component of the formulation; patients previously treated with tacrine who developed jaundice

Warnings The use of tacrine has been associated with elevations in serum transaminases; serum transaminases (specifically ALT) must be monitored throughout therapy; use extreme caution in patients with current evidence of a history of abnormal liver function tests; use caution in patients with urinary tract obstruction (bladder outlet obstruction or prostatic hyperplasia), asthma, and sick-sinus syndrome, bradycardia, or conduction abnormalities (tacrine may cause bradycardia and/or heart block). Also, patients with cardiovascular disease, asthma, or peptic ulcer should use cautiously. Adverse cardiovascular events may also occur in patients without known cardiac disease. Use with caution in patients with a history of seizures. May cause nausea, vomiting, or loose stools. Abrupt discontinuation or dosage decrease may worsen cognitive function. May be associated with neutropenia.

Dosage Forms Capsule, as hydrochloride: 10 mg, 20 mg, 30 mg, 40 mg

Reference Range

In clinical trials, serum concentrations >20 ng/mL were associated with a much higher risk of development of symptomatic adverse effects

Peak level: 6.5 ng/mL in 90 minutes after 50 mg dose

Overdosage/Treatment Antidote is atropine for muscarinic symptoms; pralidoxime (2-PAM) may also be needed to reverse severe muscle asthenia or paralysis

Antidote(s)

• Atropine [ANTIDOTE]

• Pralidoxime [ANTIDOTE]

Drug Interactions Substrate of CYP1A2 (major); **Inhibits** CYP1A2 (weak)

Anticholinergic agents: Tacrine may antagonize the therapeutic effect of anticholinergic agents (benztropine, trihexyphenidyl); a peripherally-acting agent (glycopyrrolate) has been reported to reduce tacrine-associated gastrointestinal complaints

Antipsychotic agents: Acetylcholinesterase inhibitors (central) may increase the risk of antipsychotic-related extrapyramidal symptoms; monitor.

Beta-blockers: Tacrine in combination with beta-blockers may produce additive bradycardia

Calcium channel blockers: Tacrine in combination with heart rate lowering calcium channel blockers (diltiazem and verapamil) may produce additive bradycardia

Cholinergic agents: Tacrine in combination with other cholinergic agents (eg, ambenonium, edrophonium, neostigmine, pyridostigmine, bethanechol), will likely produce additive cholinergic effects

CYP1A2 inducers: May decrease the levels/effects of tacrine. Example inducers include aminoglutethimide, carbamazepine, phenobarbital, and rifampin.

CYP1A2 inhibitors: May increase the levels/effects of tacrine. Example inhibitors include ciprofloxacin, fluvoxamine, ketoconazole, norfloxacin, ofloxacin, and rofecoxib.

Digoxin: Tacrine, in combination with digoxin, may produce additive bradycardia

Haloperidol: Tacrine may worsen Parkinson's disease and inhibit the effects of haloperidol.

Levodopa: Tacrine may worsen Parkinson's disease and inhibit the effects of levodopa

Neuromuscular blocking agents (nondepolarizing): Theoretically, tacrine may antagonize the effect of nondepolarizing neuromuscular blocking agents

Succinylcholine: Tacrine may prolong the effect of succinylcholine

Theophylline: Tacrine may inhibit the metabolism of theophylline resulting in elevated plasma levels; dose adjustment will likely be needed

Pregnancy Risk Factor C

Lactation Excretion in breast milk unknown/not recommended

Additional Information Discontinue tacrine if ALT exceeds 3 times the upper limit of normal

Tacrolimus

CAS Number 104987-11-3

U.S. Brand Names Prograf®; Protopic®

Synonyms FK506

Use

Oral/injection: Potent immunosuppressive drug used in heart, kidney, or liver transplant recipients

Topical: Moderate-to-severe atopic dermatitis in patients not responsive to conventional therapy or when conventional therapy is not appropriate

Unlabeled/Investigational Use Potent immunosuppressive drug used in lung, small bowel transplant recipients; immunosuppressive drug for peripheral stem cell/bone marrow transplantation

Mechanism of Action Suppresses cellular immunity (inhibits T-lymphocyte activation), possibly by binding to an intracellular protein, FKBP-12

Adverse Reactions

Oral, I.V.:

≥15%:

Cardiovascular: Chest pain, hypertension

Central nervous system: Dizziness, headache, insomnia, tremor (headache and tremor are associated with high whole blood concentrations and may respond to decreased dosage)

Dermatologic: Pruritus, rash

Endocrine & metabolic: Diabetes mellitus, hyperglycemia, hyper-/hypokalemia, hyperlipemia, hypomagnesemia, hypophosphatemia

Gastrointestinal: Abdominal pain, constipation, diarrhea, dyspepsia, nausea, vomiting

Genitourinary: Urinary tract infection

Hematologic: Anemia, leukocytosis, thrombocytopenia

Hepatic: Ascites

Neuromuscular & skeletal: Arthralgia, back pain, weakness, paresthesia

Renal: Abnormal kidney function, increased creatinine, oliguria, urinary tract infection, increased BUN

Respiratory: Atelectasis, dyspnea, increased cough, pleural effusion

<15%:

Cardiovascular: Abnormal ECG (QRS or ST segment abnormal), angina pectoris, cardiopulmonary failure, deep thrombophlebitis, heart rate decreased, hemorrhage, hemorrhagic stroke, hypervolemia, hypotension, generalized edema, peripheral vascular disorder, phlebitis, postural hypotension, tachycardia, thrombosis, vasodilation

Central nervous system: Abnormal dreams, abnormal thinking, agitation, amnesia, anxiety, chills, confusion, depression, dizziness, elevated mood, emotional lability, encephalopathy, hallucinations, nervousness, paralysis, psychosis, quadriparesis, seizure, somnolence

Dermatologic: Acne, alopecia, cellulitis, exfoliative dermatitis, fungal dermatitis, hirsutism, increased diaphoresis, photosensitivity reaction, skin discoloration, skin disorder, skin ulcer

Endocrine & metabolic: Acidosis, alkalosis, Cushing's syndrome, decreased bicarbonate, decreased serum iron, diabetes mellitus, hypercalcemia, hypercholesterolemia, hyperphosphatemia, hypoproteinemia, increased alkaline phosphatase

Gastrointestinal: Anorexia, appetite increased, cramps, duodenitis, dysphagia, enlarged abdomen, esophagitis (including ulcerative), flatulence, gastritis, gastroesophagitis, GI perforation/hemorrhage, ileus, oral moniliasis, pancreatic pseudocyst, rectal disorder, stomatitis, weight gain

Genitourinary: Bladder spasm, cystitis, dysuria, nocturia, oliguria, urge incontinence, urinary frequency, urinary incontinence, urinary retention, vaginitis

Hematologic: Bruising, coagulation disorder, decreased prothrombin, hypochromic anemia, leukopenia, polycythemia

Hepatic: Abnormal liver function tests, ALT/AST increased, bilirubinemia, cholangitis, cholestatic jaundice, GGT increased, hepatitis (including granulomatous), jaundice, liver damage, increase LDH

Neuromuscular & skeletal: Hypertonia, incoordination, joint disorder, leg cramps, myalgia, myasthenia, myoclonus, nerve compression, neuropathy, osteoporosis

Ocular: Abnormal vision, amblyopia

Otic: Ear pain, otitis media, tinnitus

Renal: Albuminuria, renal tubular necrosis, toxic nephropathy

Respiratory: Asthma, bronchitis, lung disorder, pharyngitis, pneumonia, pneumothorax, pulmonary edema, respiratory disorder, rhinitis, sinusitis, voice alteration

Miscellaneous: Abscess, abnormal healing, allergic reaction, crying, flu-like syndrome, generalized spasm, hernia, herpes simplex, peritonitis, sepsis, writing impaired

Postmarketing and/or case reports (limited to important or life-threatening): Acute renal failure, anaphylaxis, ARDS, arrhythmia, atrial fibrillation, atrial flutter, blindness, cardiac arrest, cerebral infarction, coma, deafness, delirium, DIC, hearing loss, hemiparesis, hemolytic-uremic syndrome, hemorrhagic cystitis, hepatic necrosis, hepatotoxicity, leukoencephalopathy, lymphoproliferative disorder (related to EBV), myocardial hypertrophy (associated with ventricular dysfunction; reversible upon discontinuation), MI, neutropenia, pancreatitis (hemorrhagic and necrotizing), pancytopenia, quadriplegia, QT_c prolongation, respiratory failure, seizure, Stevens-Johnson syndrome, syncope, toxic epidermal necrolysis, thrombocytopenic purpura, torsade de pointes, TTP, veno-occlusive hepatic disease, venous thrombosis, ventricular fibrillation. Calcineurin inhibitor-induced hemolytic uremic syndrome/thrombotic thrombocytopenic purpura/thrombotic microangiopathy (HUS/TTP/TMA) have been reported (with concurrent sirolimus).

Topical (as reported in children and adults, unless otherwise noted):

>10%:

Central nervous system: Headache (5% to 20%), fever (1% to 21%)

Dermatologic: Skin burning (43% to 58%; tends to improve as lesions resolve), pruritus (41% to 46%), erythema (12% to 28%)

Respiratory: Increased cough (18% children)

Miscellaneous: Flu-like syndrome (23% to 28%), allergic reaction (4% to 12%)

1% to 10%:

Cardiovascular: Peripheral edema (3% to 4% adults)

Central nervous system: Hyperesthesia (3% to 7% adults), pain (1% to 2%)

Dermatologic: Skin tingling (2% to 8%), acne (4% to 7% adults), localized flushing (following ethanol consumption 3% to 7% adults), folliculitis (2% to 6%), urticaria (1% to 6%), rash (2% to 5%), pustular rash (2% to 4%), vesiculobullous rash (4% children), contact dermatitis (3% to 4%), cyst (1% to 3% adults), eczema herpeticum (1% to 2%), fungal dermatitis (1% to 2% adults), sunburn (1% to 2% adults), dry skin (1% children)

Endocrine & metabolic: Dysmenorrhea (4% women)

Gastrointestinal: Diarrhea (3% to 5%), dyspepsia (1% to 4% adults), abdominal pain (3% children), vomiting (1% adults), gastroenteritis (adults 2%), nausea (1% children)

Neuromuscular & skeletal: Myalgia (2% to 3% adults), weakness (2% to 3% adults), back pain (2% adults)

Ocular: Conjunctivitis (2% adults)

Otic: Otitis media (12% children)

Respiratory: Rhinitis (6% children), sinusitis (2% to 4% adults), bronchitis (2% adults), pneumonia (1% adults)

Miscellaneous: Varicella/herpes zoster (1% to 5%), lymphadenopathy (3% children)

≥1%: Alopecia, increased ALT, increased AST, anaphylactoid reaction, angina pectoris, angioedema, anorexia, anxiety, arrhythmia, arthralgia, arthritis, bilirubinemia, breast pain, cellulitis, cerebrovascular accident, cheilitis, chills, constipation, increased creatinine, dehydration, depression, dizziness, dyspnea, ear pain, ecchymosis, edema, epistaxis, exacerbation of untreated area, eye pain, furunculosis, gastritis, hernia, hyperglycemia, hypertension, hypoglycemia, hypoxia, laryngitis, leukocytosis, leukopenia, abnormal liver function tests, lymphadenopathy (0.8%), malaise, migraine, neck pain, neuritis, palpitation, paresthesia, peripheral vascular disorder, photosensitivity reaction, skin discoloration, diaphoresis, taste perversion, unintended pregnancy, vaginal moniliasis, vasodilation, vertigo. Calcineurin inhibitor-induced hemolytic uremic syndrome/thrombotic thrombocytopenic purpura/thrombotic microangiopathy (HUS/TTP/TMA) have been reported (with concurrent sirolimus).

Signs and Symptoms of Overdose Circumoral numbness, coma, delirium, diarrhea, dyspnea, encephalopathy, hirsutism, hyperglycemia, hyperuricemia, hypokalemia, hypomagnesemia, insomnia, leukocytosis, night terrors, pleural effusion, thrombocytopenia

Admission Criteria/Prognosis Admit ingestions >1.5 mg/kg

Pharmacodynamics/Kinetics

Absorption: Better in resected patients with a closed stoma; unlike cyclosporine, clamping of the T-tube in liver transplant patients does not alter trough concentrations or AUC

Oral: Incomplete and variable; food within 15 minutes of administration decreases absorption (27%)

Topical: Serum concentrations range from undetectable to 20 ng/mL (<5 ng/mL in majority of adult patients studied)

Protein binding: 99%

Metabolism: Extensively hepatic via CYP3A4 to eight possible metabolites (major metabolite, 31-demethyl tacrolimus, shows same activity as tacrolimus *in vitro*)

Bioavailability: Oral: Adults: 7% to 28%, Children: 10% to 52%; Topical: <0.5%; Absolute: Unknown

Half-life elimination: Variable, 21-61 hours in healthy volunteers

Time to peak: 0.5-4 hours

Excretion: Feces (~92%); feces/urine (<1% as unchanged drug)

Dosage

Oral:

Children: **Note:** Patients without pre-existing renal or hepatic dysfunction have required (and tolerated) higher doses than adults to achieve similar blood concentrations. It is recommended that therapy be initiated at high end of the recommended adult I.V. and oral dosing ranges; dosage adjustments may be required. If switching from I.V. to oral, the oral dose should be started 8-12 hours after stopping the infusion. Adjunctive therapy with corticosteroids is recommended early post-transplant.

Liver transplant: Initial dose: 0.15-0.20 mg/kg/day in 2 divided doses, given every 12 hours; begin oral dose no sooner than 6 hours post-transplant

Adults: **Note:** If switching from I.V. to oral, the oral dose should be started 8-12 hours after stopping the infusion. Adjunctive therapy with corticosteroids is recommended early post-transplant.

Heart transplant: Initial dose: 0.075 mg/kg/day in 2 divided doses, given every 12 hours; begin oral dose no sooner than 6 hours post-transplant

Kidney transplant: Initial dose: 0.2 mg/kg/day in 2 divided doses, given every 12 hours; initial dose may be given within 24 hours of transplant, but should be delayed until renal function has recovered; African-American patients may require larger doses to maintain trough concentration

Liver transplant: Initial dose: 0.1-0.15 mg/kg/day in 2 divided doses, given every 12 hours; begin oral dose no sooner than 6 hours post-transplant

I.V.: Children and Adults: **Note:** I.V. route should only be used in patients not able to take oral medications and continued only until oral medication can be tolerated; anaphylaxis has been reported. Begin no sooner than 6 hours post-transplant; adjunctive therapy with corticosteroids is recommended.

Heart transplant: Initial dose: 0.01 mg/kg/day as a continuous infusion

Kidney, liver transplant: Initial dose: 0.03-0.05 mg/kg/day as a continuous infusion

Prevention of graft-vs-host disease: 0.03 mg/kg/day as continuous infusion

Topical: Children ≥2 years and Adults: Atopic dermatitis (moderate to severe): Apply minimum amount of 0.03% or 0.1% ointment to affected area twice daily; rub in gently and completely. Discontinue use when symptoms have cleared. If no improvement within 6 weeks, patients should be re-examined to confirm diagnosis.

Dosing adjustment in renal impairment: Evidence suggests that lower doses should be used; patients should receive doses at the lowest value of the recommended I.V. and oral dosing ranges; further reductions in dose below these ranges may be required.

Tacrolimus therapy should usually be delayed up to 48 hours or longer in patients with postoperative oliguria.

Hemodialysis: Not removed by hemodialysis; supplemental dose is not necessary.

Peritoneal dialysis: Significant drug removal is unlikely based on physiochemical characteristics.

Dosing adjustment in hepatic impairment: Use of tacrolimus in liver transplant recipients experiencing post-transplant hepatic impairment may be associated with increased risk of developing renal insufficiency related to high whole blood levels of tacrolimus. The presence of moderate-to-severe hepatic dysfunction (serum bilirubin >2 mg/dL; Child-Pugh score ≥10) appears to affect the metabolism of tacrolimus. The half-life of the drug was prolonged and the clearance reduced after I.V. administration. The bioavailability of tacrolimus was also increased after oral administration. The higher plasma concentrations as determined by ELISA, in patients with severe hepatic dysfunction are probably due to the accumulation of metabolites of lower activity. These patients should be monitored closely and dosage adjustments should be considered. Some evidence indicates that lower doses could be used in these patients.

Stability Twenty-four hours in dextrose 5% solutions or normal saline; tacrolimus is completely available from plastic syringes, glass or polyolefin containers; polyvinyl-containing sets (eg, Venoset®, Accuset®) adsorb significant amounts of the drug, and their use may lead to a lower dose being delivered to the patient

Monitoring Parameters Renal function, hepatic function, serum electrolytes, glucose and blood pressure, measure 3 times/week for first few weeks, then gradually decrease frequency as patient stabilizes. Whole blood concentrations should be used for monitoring (trough for oral

therapy). Signs/symptoms of anaphylactic reactions during infusion should also be monitored.

Administration

I.V.: Administer by I.V. continuous infusion only. Do not use PVC tubing when administering dilute solutions. Usually intended to be administered as a continuous infusion over 24 hours.

Oral: If dosed once daily (not common), administer in the morning. If dosed twice daily, doses should be 12 hours apart. If the morning and evening doses differ, the larger dose (differences are never >0.5-1 mg) should be given in the morning. If dosed 3 times/day, separate doses by 8 hours.

Topical: Do not use with occlusive dressings. Burning at the application site is most common in first few days; improves as atopic dermatitis improves. Limit application to involved areas. Continue as long as signs and symptoms persist; discontinue if resolution occurs; re-evaluate if symptoms persist >6 weeks.

Contraindications Hypersensitivity to tacrolimus or any component of the formulation

Warnings

Oral/injection: Insulin-dependent post-transplant diabetes mellitus (PTDM) has been reported (1% to 20%); risk increases in African-American and Hispanic kidney transplant patients. **[U.S. Boxed Warning]: Increased susceptibility to infection and the possible development of lymphoma may occur after administration of tacrolimus.** Nephrotoxicity and neurotoxicity have been reported, especially with higher doses; to avoid excess nephrotoxicity do not administer simultaneously with cyclosporine; monitoring of serum concentrations (trough for oral therapy) is essential to prevent organ rejection and reduce drug-related toxicity; tonic clonic seizures may have been triggered by tacrolimus. A period of 24 hours should elapse between discontinuation of cyclosporine and the initiation of tacrolimus. Use caution in renal or hepatic dysfunction, dosing adjustments may be required. Delay initiation if postoperative oliguria occurs. Use may be associated with the development of hypertension (common). Myocardial hypertrophy has been reported (rare). Each mL of injection contains polyoxyl 60 hydrogenated castor oil (HCO-60) (200 mg) and dehydrated alcohol USP 80% v/v. Anaphylaxis has been reported with the injection, use should be reserved for those patients not able to take oral medications.

Topical: [U.S. Boxed Warning]: Topical calcineurin inhibitors have been associated with rare cases of malignancy. Avoid use on malignant or skin conditions (eg cutaneous T-cell lymphoma). Topical calcineurin agents are considered second-line therapies in the treatment of atopic dermatitis/eczema, and should be limited to use in patients who have failed treatment with other therapies. **[U.S. Boxed Warning]: They should be used for short-term and intermittent treatment using the minimum amount necessary for the control of symptoms should be used.** Application should be limited to involved areas. Safety of intermittent use for >1 year has not been established.

Should not be used in immunocompromised patients. Do not apply to areas of active viral infection; infections at the treatment site should be cleared prior to therapy. Patients with atopic dermatitis are predisposed to skin infections, and tacrolimus therapy has been associated with risk of developing eczema herpeticum, varicella zoster, and herpes simplex. May be associated with development of lymphadenopathy; possible infectious causes should be investigated. Discontinue use in patients with unknown cause of lymphadenopathy or acute infectious mononucleosis. Not recommended for use in patients with skin disease which may increase systemic absorption (eg, Netherton's syndrome). Avoid artificial or natural sunlight exposure, even when Protopic® is not on the skin. Safety not established in patients with generalized erythroderma. **[U.S. Boxed Warning]: The use of Protopic® in children <2 years of age is not recommended,** particularly since the effect on immune system development is unknown.

Dosage Forms Capsule (Prograf®): 0.5 mg, 1 mg, 5 mg

Injection, solution (Prograf®): 5 mg/mL (1 mL) [contains dehydrated alcohol 80% and polyoxyl 60 hydrogenated castor oil]

Ointment, topical (Protopic®): 0.03% (30 g, 60 g, 100 g); 0.1% (30 g, 60 g, 100 g)

Reference Range Whole blood trough therapeutic level: 9.8-19.4 ng/mL. Tacrolimus whole blood trough concentrations should be kept below 20 ng/mL to avoid adverse events in renal transplant recipients. The incidence of adverse events is 76% with tacrolimus whole blood trough concentrations >30 ng/mL, compared with only 5.3% with concentrations <10 ng/mL

Overdosage/Treatment

Decontamination: Lavage (within 1 hour)/activated charcoal

Enhancement of elimination: Multiple dosing of activated charcoal may be effective; dialysis/plasmapheresis not effective

Drug Interactions

Substrate of CYP3A4 (major); **Inhibits** CYP3A4 (weak)

Antacids: Separate administration by at least 2 hours

Anticonvulsants: Carbamazepine, phenobarbital, phenytoin: May decrease tacrolimus blood levels.

Calcium channel blockers: May increase tacrolimus serum concentrations; monitor.

Caspofungin: May decrease tacrolimus serum concentrations.

Cisapride (and metoclopramide): May increase serum concentration of tacrolimus

Cyclosporine: Concomitant use is associated with synergistic immunosuppression and increased nephrotoxicity; give first dose of tacrolimus no sooner than 24 hours after last cyclosporine dose. In the presence of elevated tacrolimus or cyclosporine concentration, dosing of the other usually should be delayed longer.

CYP3A4 inducers: CYP3A4 inducers may decrease the levels/effects of tacrolimus. Example inducers include aminoglutethimide, carbamazepine, nafcillin, nevirapine, phenobarbital, phenytoin, and rifamycins.

CYP3A4 inhibitors: May increase the levels/effects of tacrolimus. Example inhibitors include azole antifungals, clarithromycin, diclofenac, doxycycline, erythromycin, imatinib, isoniazid, nefazodone, nicardipine, propofol, protease inhibitors, quinidine, telithromycin, and verapamil.

Ganciclovir: Nephrotoxicity may be additive with tacrolimus; use caution.

Macrolides: May increase tacrolimus serum concentrations (limited documentation); monitor.

Potassium-sparing diuretics: Tacrolimus use may lead to hyperkalemia; avoid concomitant use

Rifabutin, rifampin: May decrease serum levels of tacrolimus.

Sirolimus: May decrease tacrolimus serum concentrations. Concurrent therapy may increase the risk of HUS/TTP/TMA.

St John's wort: May decrease tacrolimus serum concentrations; avoid concurrent use.

Sucralfate: Separate administration by at least 2 hours

Vaccines (live): Vaccine may be less effective; avoid vaccination during treatment if possible

Voriconazole: Tacrolimus serum concentrations may be increased; monitor serum concentrations and renal function. Decrease tacrolimus dosage by 66% when initiating voriconazole.

Pregnancy Risk Factor C

Pregnancy Implications Crosses the placenta

Lactation Enters breast milk/contraindicated

Additional Information Overdoses up to 7 mg/kg have produced little acute symptomatology. A whole blood tacrolimus level of 42.6 ng/mL was obtained after an ingestion of 0.8 mg/kg, with minimal side effects.

Specific References

French AE, Soldin SJ, Soldin OP, et al, "Milk Transfer and Neonatal Safety of Tacrolimus," *Ann Pharmacother*, 2003, 37(6):815-8.

O'Connor AD and Rusyniak D, "Tacrolimus Overdose Resulting in Metabolic Acidosis and Renal Failure," *Clin Toxicol*, 2005, 43:635.

Page RL 2nd, Klem PM, and Rogers C, "Potential Elevation of Tacrolimus Trough Concentrations with Concomitant Metronidazole Therapy," *Ann Pharmacother*, 2005, 39(6):1109-13.

Takahashi K, Motohashi H, Yonezawa A, et al, "Lansoprazole-Tacrolimus Interaction in Japanese Transplant Recipient with CYP2C19 Polymorphism," *Ann Pharmacother*, 2004, 38(5):791-4.

Tamoxifen

CAS Number 10540-29-1; 54965-24-1

U.S. Brand Names Nolvadex®; Soltamox™

Synonyms ICI-46474; NSC-180973; TAM; Tamoxifen Citrate

Use Palliative or adjunctive treatment of advanced breast cancer; reduce the incidence of breast cancer in women at high risk; reduce risk of invasive breast cancer in women with ductal carcinoma in situ (DCIS); metastatic female and male breast cancer

Unlabeled/Investigational Use Treatment of mastalgia, gynecomastia, pancreatic carcinoma, melanoma and desmoid tumors; induction of ovulation; treatment of precocious puberty in females, secondary to McCune-Albright syndrome

Mechanism of Action Competitively binds to estrogen receptors on tumors and other tissue targets, producing a nuclear complex that decreases DNA synthesis and inhibits estrogen effects; nonsteroidal agent with potent antiestrogenic properties which compete with estrogen for binding sites in breast and other tissues; cells accumulate in the G_0 and G_1 phases; therefore, tamoxifen is cytostatic rather than cytocidal

Adverse Reactions

Cardiovascular: **Flushing**, arterial thrombosis, superior mesenteric artery thrombosis, vasculitis

Central nervous system: Dizziness, psychosis, headache

Dermatologic: **Rash**, pruritus, leiomyoma growth, radiation recall dermatitis, alopecia, hypertrichosis, xerosis, urticaria, purpura, exanthem, cutaneous vasculitis

Endocrine & metabolic: Vaginal bleeding or discharge, menstrual irregularities, hypercalcemia in patients with bony metastasis, galactorrhea, hot flashes, ovarian cysts, hypoprolactinemia, hypertriglyceridemia

Gastrointestinal: **Nausea, weight gain, vomiting** is rare, cholestasis, steatohepatitis, xerostomia

Genitourinary: Priapism, endometriosis, recurrent vulvovaginal candidiasis, uterine leiomyosarcoma

Hematologic: **Occasional leukopenia, thrombocytopenia**, porphyria, agranulocytosis, thromboembolism (3.8% to 6.8%), porphyrinogenic, **anemia, hepatotoxicity**

Hepatic: Steatosis hepatitis, cirrhosis

Neuromuscular & skeletal: **Increased bone and tumor pain**

Ocular: Corneal opacification, reduced visual acuity, retinopathy at high doses (120 mg/day for 1 year)

Renal: Nephrotic syndrome

Respiratory: Eosinophilic pneumonia

Miscellaneous: Antiphospholipid syndrome

Signs and Symptoms of Overdose Azoospermia, cataract, depression, galactorrhea, hirsutism, hypercalcemia, lactation, leukopenia or neutropenia (agranulocytosis, granulocytopenia), mental confusion, oligospermia, priapism, sexual dysfunction

Pharmacodynamics/Kinetics

Absorption: Well absorbed; tablet and oral solution are bioequivalent

Distribution: High concentrations found in uterus, endometrial and breast tissue

Protein binding: 99%

Metabolism: Hepatic (via CYP3A4) to major metabolites, N-desmethyl tamoxifen (major) and 4-hydroxytamoxifen (minor), and a tamoxifen derivative (minor); undergoes enterohepatic recirculation

Half-life elimination: Distribution: 7-14 hours; Elimination: 5-7 days; Metabolites: 14 days

Time to peak, serum: 5 hours

Excretion: Feces (26% to 51%); urine (9% to 13%)

Dosage

Oral (refer to individual protocols):

Children: Female: Precocious puberty and McCune-Albright syndrome (unlabeled use): A dose of 20 mg/day has been reported in patients 2-10 years of age; safety and efficacy have not been established for treatment of longer than 1 year duration

Adults:

Breast cancer:

Metastatic (males and females) or adjuvant therapy (females): 20-40 mg/day; daily doses >20 mg should be given in 2 divided doses (morning and evening)

Prevention (high-risk females): 20 mg/day for 5 years

DCIS (females): 20 mg once daily for 5 years

Note: Higher dosages (up to 700 mg/day) have been investigated for use in modulation of multidrug resistance (MDR), but are not routinely used in clinical practice

Induction of ovulation (unlabeled use): 5-40 mg twice daily for 4 days

Monitoring Parameters Monitor WBC and platelet counts, serum calcium, LFTs; abnormal vaginal bleeding

Contraindications Hypersensitivity to tamoxifen or any component of the formulation; concurrent warfarin therapy or history of deep vein thrombosis or pulmonary embolism (when tamoxifen is used for cancer risk reduction); pregnancy

Warnings

Hazardous agent - use appropriate precautions for handling and disposal.

[U.S. Boxed Warning]: Serious and life-threatening events (including stroke, pulmonary emboli, and uterine malignancy) have occurred at an incidence greater than placebo during use for cancer risk reduction; these events are rare, but require consideration in risk:benefit evaluation. An increased incidence of thromboembolic events has been associated with use for breast cancer; risk may increase with chemotherapy addition; use caution in individuals with a history of thromboembolic events. Use with caution in patients with leukopenia, thrombocytopenia, or hyperlipidemias. Decreased visual acuity, retinopathy, corneal changes, and increased incidence of cataracts have been reported. Hypercalcemia has occurred in patients with bone metastasis. Significant bone loss of the lumbar spine and hip was associated with use in premenopausal women. Liver abnormalities such as cholestasis, fatty liver, hepatitis, and hepatic necrosis have occurred. Hepatocellular carcinomas have been reported in some studies; relationship to treatment is unclear. Endometrial hyperplasia, polyps, endometriosis, uterine fibroids, and ovarian cysts have occurred. Increased risk of uterine or endometrial cancer; monitor. Safety and efficacy in children <2 years of age, or for treatment durations >1 year in children 2-10 years, have not been established.

Dosage Forms Solution, oral: 10 mg/5 mL (150 mL) [licorice flavor]

Tablet: 10 mg, 20 mg

Reference Range

Oral dose of 0.3 mg/kg yields a peak blood level of 0.06-0.14 mcg/mL

Peak level of tamoxifen after a 20 mg dose: 42 mcg/L

Peak level of N-desmethyltamoxifen after a 20 mg dose: 12 mcg/L

Overdosage/Treatment

Decontamination: Lavage (within 1 hour)/activated charcoal

Supportive therapy: Oral clonidine, 0.1 mg/d is effective against tamoxifen-induced hot flashes in postmenopausal women with breast cancer.

Enhancement of elimination: Multiple dosing of activated charcoal may be effective.

Test Interactions False T_4 elevation (no clinical evidence of hyperthyroidism)

Drug Interactions
Substrate of CYP2A6 (minor), 2B6 (minor), 2C9 (major), 2D6 (major), 2E1 (minor), 3A4 (major); **Inhibits** CYP2B6 (weak), 2C8 (moderate), 2C9 (weak), 3A4 (weak)

Anastrozole: Tamoxifen may reduce the levels/effects of anastrozole. Concurrent therapy is not recommended (per manufacturer).

CYP2C8 substrates: Tamoxifen may increase the levels/effects of CYP2C8 substrates. Example substrates include amiodarone, paclitaxel, pioglitazone, repaglinide, and rosiglitazone.

CYP2C9 inducers: May decrease the levels/effects of tamoxifen. Example inducers include carbamazepine, phenobarbital, phenytoin, rifampin, rifapentine, and secobarbital.

CYP2C9 inhibitors: May increase the levels/effects of tamoxifen. Example inhibitors include delavirdine, fluconazole, gemfibrozil, ketoconazole, nicardipine, NSAIDs, sulfonamides, and tolbutamide.

CYP2D6 inhibitors: May increase the levels/effects of tamoxifen. Example inhibitors include chlorpromazine, delavirdine, fluoxetine, miconazole, paroxetine, pergolide, quinidine, quinine, ritonavir, and ropinirole.

CYP3A4 inducers: CYP3A4 inducers may decrease the levels/effects of tamoxifen. Example inducers include aminoglutethimide, carbamazepine, nafcillin, nevirapine, phenobarbital, phenytoin, and rifamycins.

CYP3A4 inhibitors: May increase the levels/effects of tamoxifen. Example inhibitors include azole antifungals, clarithromycin, diclofenac, doxycycline, erythromycin, imatinib, isoniazid, nefazodone, nicardipine, propofol, protease inhibitors, quinidine, telithromycin, and verapamil.

Rifamycins: Rifamycin derivatives may increase the metabolism (via CYP isoenzymes) of tamoxifen.

Warfarin: Concomitant use is contraindicated when used for risk reduction; results in significant enhancement of the anticoagulant effects of warfarin

Pregnancy Risk Factor D

Pregnancy Implications No adequate or well-controlled studies in pregnant women. For sexually-active women of childbearing age, initiate during menstruation (negative β-hCG immediately prior to initiation in women with irregular cycles). Pregnancy should be avoided for 2 months after treatment has been discontinued.

Lactation Excretion in breast milk unknown/contraindicated

Nursing Implications Increase of bone pain usually indicates a good therapeutic response

Specific References
Bergh J, "Breast-Cancer Prevention: Is the Risk-Benefit Ratio in Favour of Tamoxifen?" *Lancet*, 2003, 362(9379):183-4.
Cersosimo RJ, "Tamoxifen for Prevention of Breast Cancer," *Ann Pharmacother*, 2003, 37(2):268-73.
Kreher NC, Eugster EA, and Shankar RR, "The Use of Tamoxifen to Improve Height Potential in Short Pubertal Boys," *Pediatrics*, 2005, 116(6):1513-5.
Paik S, Shak S, Tang G, et al, "A Multigene Assay to Predict Recurrence of Tamoxifen-Treated, Node-Negative Breast Cancer," *N Engl J Med*, 2004, 351(27):2817-26.

Tamsulosin

Pronunciation (tam SOO loe sin)
CAS Number 106463-17-6
U.S. Brand Names Flomax®
Synonyms Tamsulosin Hydrochloride
Use Treatment of signs and symptoms of benign prostatic hyperplasia (BPH)

Mechanism of Action Tamsulosin is an antagonist of alpha$_{1A}$ adrenoreceptors in the prostate. Smooth muscle tone in the prostate is mediated by alpha$_{1A}$ adrenoreceptors; blocking them leads to relaxation of smooth muscle in the bladder neck and prostate causing an improvement of urine flow and decreased symptoms of BPH. Approximately 75% of the alpha$_1$ receptors in the prostate are of the alpha$_{1A}$ subtype.

Adverse Reactions
>10%:
Cardiovascular: Studies specific for orthostatic hypotension: Overall, at least one positive test was observed in 16% of patients receiving 0.4 mg and 19% of patients receiving the 0.8 mg dose. "First-dose" orthostatic hypotension following a 0.4 mg dose was reported as 7% at 4 hours postdose and 6% at 8 hours postdose.
Central nervous system: Headache (19% to 21%), dizziness (15% to 17%)
Genitourinary: Abnormal ejaculation (8% to 18%)
Respiratory: Rhinitis (13% to 18%)
1% to 10%:
Cardiovascular: Chest pain (~4%)
Central nervous system: Somnolence (3% to 4%), insomnia (1% to 2%), vertigo (0.6% to 1%)

Endocrine & metabolic: Libido decreased (1% to 2%)
Gastrointestinal: Diarrhea (4% to 6%), nausea (3% to 4%), stomach discomfort (2% to 3%), bitter taste (2% to 3%)
Neuromuscular & skeletal: Weakness (8% to 9%), back pain (7% to 8%)
Ocular: Amblyopia (0.2% to 2%)
Respiratory: Pharyngitis (5% to 6%), cough (3% to 5%), sinusitis (2% to 4%)
Miscellaneous: Infection (9% to 11%), tooth disorder (1% to 2%)
<1% (Limited to important or life-threatening): Orthostasis (symptomatic) (0.2% to 0.4%), syncope (0.2% to 0.4%)
Postmarketing and/or case reports: Allergic reactions (rash, angioedema, pruritus, urticaria) priapism; constipation, palpitation, transaminases increased, vomiting

Signs and Symptoms of Overdose Headache, dizziness, syncope, bradycardia, orthostasis, hypotonia

Pharmacodynamics/Kinetics
Absorption: >90%
Protein binding: 94% to 99%, primarily to alpha$_1$ acid glycoprotein (AAG)
Metabolism: Hepatic via CYP; metabolites undergo extensive conjugation to glucuronide or sulfate
Bioavailability: Fasting: 30% increase
Distribution: V_d: 16 L
Steady-state: By the fifth day of once-daily dosing
Half-life elimination: Healthy volunteers: 9-13 hours; Target population: 14-15 hours
Time to peak: Fasting: 4-5 hours; with food: 6-7 hours
Excretion: Urine (76%, <10% as unchanged drug); feces (21%)

Dosage
Oral: Adults: 0.4 mg once daily ~30 minutes after the same meal each day; dose may be increased after 2-4 weeks to 0.8 mg once daily in patients who fail to respond. If therapy is interrupted for several days, restart with 0.4 mg once daily.
Dosage adjustment in renal impairment:
Cl$_{cr}$ ≥10 mL/minute: No adjustment needed
Cl$_{cr}$ <10 mL/minute: Not studied

Administration Capsules should be swallowed whole; do not crush, chew, or open.

Contraindications Hypersensitivity to tamsulosin or any component of the formulation; concurrent use with phosphodiesterase-5 (PDE-5) inhibitors including sildenafil (>25 mg), tadalafil (if tamsulosin dose >0.4 mg/day), or vardenafil

Warnings Not intended for use as an antihypertensive drug. May cause orthostasis, syncope or dizziness. Patients should avoid situations where injury may occur as a result of syncope. Rule out prostatic carcinoma before beginning therapy with tamsulosin. Intraoperative Floppy Iris Syndrome occurred most often in patients taking their alpha-1 blocker at the time of cataract surgery, but some cases occurred when the alpha-1 blocker blocker was stopped 2-14 days prior to surgery and as long as 5 weeks to 9 months prior to surgery. The benefit of stopping an alpha-1 blocker prior to cataract surgery has not been established. Rarely, patients with a sulfa allergy have also developed an allergic reaction to tamsulosin; avoid use when previous reaction has been severe.

Dosage Forms Capsule, as hydrochloride: 0.4 mg

Overdosage/Treatment
Decontamination: Oral: Administer activated charcoal
Supportive therapy: To treat hypotension, first administer 10-20 mL/kg of isotonic crystalloid solution and then place in Trendelenberg position. If vasopressor is needed, norepinephrine (0.5-1 mcg/minute initial dose in adults; 0.1 mcg/kg/minute initial dose in children - titrate to desired effect) is preferred agent. Seizures can be treated with benzodiazepine or phenobarbital.

Drug Interactions
Substrate (major) of CYP2D6, 3A4
Alpha-adrenergic blockers: Risk of hypotension may increase in combination with other alpha-adrenergic blocking agents.
Beta-blockers: Beta-blockers may increase risk of first-dose orthostatic hypotension of tamsulosin
Calcium channel blockers: Risk of hypotension may increase
Cimetidine: Cimetidine may decrease tamsulosin clearance.
CYP2D6 inhibitors: May increase the levels/effects of tamsulosin. Example inhibitors include chlorpromazine, delavirdine, fluoxetine, miconazole, paroxetine, pergolide, quinidine, quinine, ritonavir, and ropinirole.
CYP3A4 inducers: CYP3A4 inducers may decrease the levels/effects of tamsulosin. Example inducers include aminoglutethimide, carbamazepine, nafcillin, nevirapine, phenobarbital, phenytoin, and rifamycins.
CYP3A4 inhibitors: May increase the levels/effects of tamsulosin. Example inhibitors include azole antifungals, clarithromycin, diclofenac, doxycycline, erythromycin, imatinib, isoniazid, nefazodone, nicardipine, propofol, protease inhibitors, quinidine, telithromycin, and verapamil.
Sildenafil, tadalafil, vardenafil: Blood pressure-lowering effects are additive. Use of vardenafil is contraindicated by the manufacturer.

Use sildenafil with extreme caution (dose ≤25 mg). Tadalafil may be used when tamsulosin dose is ≤0.4 mg/day.

Pregnancy Risk Factor B

Pregnancy Implications Teratogenic effects were not observed in animal studies, however, tamsulosin is not indicated for use in women.

Lactation Not indicated for use in women

Specific References

Anand JS, Chodorowski Z, Wisniewski M, et al, "Acute Intoxication with Tamsulosin Hydrochloride," *J Tox Clin Tox*, 2005, 43:311.

Temazepam

CAS Number 846-50-4

U.S. Brand Names Restoril®

Impairment Potential Yes. A single oral 20 mg dose at bedtime may cause driving impairment for as long as 12-24 hours. Brief or extended periods of exposure are less likely to cause driving impairment in the elderly compared with the longer half-life benzodiazepines. (Betts TA and Birtle J, "Effect of Two Hypnotic Drugs on Actual Driving Performances Next Morning," *Br Med J*, 1982, 285(6345):852.)

Use Treatment of anxiety and as an adjunct in the treatment of depression; also may be used in the management of panic attacks; transient insomnia and sleep latency

Unlabeled/Investigational Use Treatment of anxiety; adjunct in the treatment of depression; management of panic attacks

Mechanism of Action Benzodiazepine anxiolytic sedative that produces CNS depression at the subcortical level, except at high doses, whereby it works at the cortical level

Adverse Reactions

Cardiovascular: Palpitations

Central nervous system: Drowsiness (9.1%), anxiety (2%), ataxia, fatigue (4.8%), depression (1.7%), headache (8.5%), confusion (1.7%), dizziness (4.5%), amnesia, night terrors (1.2%), nervousness (4.6%), lethargy (4.5%), "hangover" effect (2.5%), euphoria (1.5%), vertigo (1.2%), hallucinations, aggressive behavior

Dermatologic: Urticaria, purpura, bullous eruptions, licheniform eruptions, exanthem

Gastrointestinal: Xerostomia (1.7%), diarrhea (1.7%), abdominal discomfort (1.5%), nausea (3.1%), vomiting, anorexia

Neuromuscular & skeletal: Weakness (1.4%), tremor, backache, paresthesia

Ocular: Blurred vision (1.3%), burning eyes

Respiratory: Dyspnea

Miscellaneous: Diaphoresis, fixed drug eruption, acute atraumatic compartment syndrome

Signs and Symptoms of Overdose Ataxia, cognitive dysfunction, coma, dyspnea, confusion, diarrhea, hypoactive reflexes, hyporeflexia, hypotension, hypothermia, night terrors, slurred speech, somnolence

Pharmacodynamics/Kinetics

Distribution: V$_d$: 1.4 L/kg

Protein binding: 96%

Metabolism: Hepatic

Half-life elimination: 9.5-12.4 hours

Time to peak, serum: 2-3 hours

Excretion: Urine (80% to 90% as inactive metabolites)

Dosage Adults: Oral: 15-30 mg at bedtime; 15 mg in elderly or debilitated patients

Monitoring Parameters Respiratory and cardiovascular status

Contraindications Hypersensitivity to temazepam or any component of the formulation (cross-sensitivity with other benzodiazepines may exist); narrow-angle glaucoma (not in product labeling, however, benzodiazepines are contraindicated); pregnancy

Warnings

Should be used only after evaluation of potential causes of sleep disturbance. Failure of sleep disturbance to resolve after 7-10 days may indicate psychiatric or medical illness. A worsening of insomnia or the emergence of new abnormalities of thought or behavior may represent unrecognized psychiatric or medical illness and requires immediate and careful evaluation.

Use with caution in elderly or debilitated patients, patients with hepatic disease (including alcoholics), or renal impairment. Use with caution in patients with respiratory disease, or impaired gag reflex. Avoid use inpatients with sleep apnea.

Causes CNS depression (dose-related) resulting in sedation, dizziness, confusion, or ataxia which may impair physical and mental capabilities. Patients must be cautioned about performing tasks which require mental alertness (eg, operating machinery or driving). Use with caution in patients receiving other CNS depressants or psychoactive agents. Effects with other sedative drugs or ethanol may be potentiated. Benzodiazepines have been associated with falls and traumatic injury and should be used with extreme caution in patients who are at risk of these events (especially the elderly).

Use caution in patients with depression, particularly if suicidal risk may be present. Use with caution in patients with a history of drug dependence.

Benzodiazepines have been associated with dependence and acute withdrawal symptoms on discontinuation or reduction in dose (may occur after as little as 10 days). Acute withdrawal, including seizures, may be precipitated after administration of flumazenil to patients receiving long-term benzodiazepine therapy.

Benzodiazepines have been associated with anterograde amnesia. Paradoxical reactions, including hyperactive or aggressive behavior, have been reported with benzodiazepines, particularly in adolescent/pediatric or psychiatric patients. Does not have analgesic, antidepressant, or antipsychotic properties.

Dosage Forms Capsule: 15 mg, 30 mg

Restoril®: 7.5 mg, 15 mg, 30 mg

Reference Range Therapeutic: 26 ng/mL after 24 hours; can be quantified by high performance liquid chromatography; postmortem levels >88.5 ng/mL have been correlated with fatalities

Overdosage/Treatment

Decontamination: Activated charcoal

Supportive therapy: Treatment for benzodiazepine overdose is supportive. Rarely is mechanical ventilation required. Flumazenil has been shown to reverse benzodiazepine-induced CNS depression.

Enhancement of elimination: Multiple dosing of activated charcoal is effective; hemodialysis/forced diuresis is of no utility

Antidote(s)

● Flumazenil [ANTIDOTE]

Test Interactions Visine®, Drano®, bleach may cause false-negative urine tests; oxazepam may interfere giving falsely elevated glucose results

Drug Interactions Substrate (minor) of CYP2B6, 2C9, 2C19, 3A4

CNS depressants: Sedative effects and/or respiratory depression may be additive with CNS depressants; includes ethanol, barbiturates, narcotic analgesics, and other sedative agents; monitor for increased effect

Theophylline: May partially antagonize some of the effects of benzodiazepines; monitor for decreased response; may require higher doses for sedation

Pregnancy Risk Factor X

Lactation Enters breast milk/not recommended (AAP rates "of concern")

Nursing Implications Provide safety measures (ie, side rails, night light, and call button); remove smoking materials from area; supervise ambulation

Additional Information Causes minimal change in REM sleep patterns

---

Tenecteplase

CAS Number 191588-94-0

U.S. Brand Names TNKase™

Use Thrombolytic agent used in the management of acute myocardial infarction for the lysis of thrombi in the coronary vasculature to restore perfusion and reduce mortality

Unlabeled/Investigational Use Acute MI – combination regimen of tenecteplase (unlabeled dose), abciximab, and heparin (unlabeled dose)

Mechanism of Action Initiates fibrinolysis by binding to fibrin and converting plasminogen to plasmin; more fibrin-specific than alteplase or reteplase. Produced by recombinant DNA technology through Chinese hamster ovary cells.

Adverse Reactions

As with all drugs which may affect hemostasis, bleeding is the major adverse effect associated with tenecteplase. Hemorrhage may occur at virtually any site. Risk is dependent on multiple variables, including the dosage administered, concurrent use of multiple agents which alter hemostasis, and patient predisposition. Rapid lysis of coronary artery thrombi by thrombolytic agents may be associated with reperfusion-related arterial and/or ventricular arrhythmias. The incidence of stroke and bleeding increase in patients >65 years.

Central nervous system: Stroke, intracranial hemorrhage (0.9%)

Dermatologic: Angioedema, rash, urticaria

Gastrointestinal: GI hemorrhage, retroperitoneal bleeding

Genitourinary: GU bleeding

Hematologic: **Bleeding** (22% minor: ASSENT-2 trial; 5% major: ASSENT-2 trial)

Local: Bleeding at catheter puncture site, **hematoma**

Respiratory: Pharyngeal bleeding, respiratory tract bleeding, laryngeal edema, epistaxis

Miscellaneous: Anaphylaxis, cholesterol embolism (clinical features may include livedo reticularis, "purple toe" syndrome, acute renal failure, gangrenous digits, hypertension, pancreatitis, myocardial infarction, cerebral infarction, spinal cord infarction, retinal artery occlusion, bowel infarction, rhabdomyolysis)

Additional effects associated with use in myocardial infarction:

Cardiovascular: Cardiogenic shock, arrhythmias, AV block, heart failure, cardiac arrest, recurrent myocardial ischemia, myocardial reinfarction, myocardial rupture, cardiac tamponade, pericarditis, pericardial effusion, mitral regurgitation, thrombosis, embolism, electromechanical dissociation, hypotension

Central nervous system: Fever

Gastrointestinal: Nausea, vomiting
Respiratory: Pulmonary edema

Pharmacodynamics/Kinetics
Distribution: V_d is weight related and approximates plasma volume
Metabolism: Primarily hepatic
Half-life elimination: 90-130 minutes
Excretion: Clearance: Plasma: 99-119 mL/minute

Dosage
I.V.:
Adult: Recommended total dose should not exceed 50 mg and is based on patient's weight; administer as a bolus over 5 seconds
If patient's weight is:
    <60 kg, dose: 30 mg (6 mL in volume)
    ≥60 to <70 kg, dose: 35 mg (7 mL in volume)
    ≥70 to <80 kg, dose: 40 mg (8 mL in volume)
    ≥80 to <90 kg, dose: 45 mg (9 mL in volume)
    ≥90 kg, dose: 50 mg (10 mL in volume)
All patients should receive 150-325 mg of aspirin as soon as possible and then daily. Intravenous heparin should be initiated as soon as possible and aPTT maintained between 50-70 seconds.

Dosage adjustment in renal impairment: No formal recommendations for renal impairment

Dosage adjustment in hepatic impairment: Severe hepatic failure is a relative contraindication. Recommendations were not made for mild to moderate hepatic impairment.

Elderly: Although dosage adjustments are not recommended, the elderly have a higher incidence of morbidity and mortality with the use of tenecteplase. The 30-day mortality in the ASSENT-2 trial was 2.5% for patients <65 years, 8.5% for patients 65-74 years, and 16.2% for patients ≥75 years. The intracranial hemorrhage rate was 0.4% for patients <65, 1.6 % for patients 65-74 years, and 1.7 % for patients ≥75. The risks and benefits of use should be weighed carefully in the elderly.

Stability Store at room temperature not to exceed 30°C (86°F) or under refrigeration 2°C to 8°C (36°F to 46°F). If reconstituted and not used immediately, store in refrigerator and use within 8 hours.

Monitoring Parameters CBC, aPTT, signs and symptoms of bleeding, ECG monitoring

Administration Tenecteplase should be reconstituted using the supplied 10 cc syringe with TwinPak™ dual cannula device and 10 mL sterile water for injection. Do not shake when reconstituting. Slight foaming is normal and will dissipate if left standing for several minutes. The reconstituted solution is 5 mg/mL. Any unused solution should be discarded. Tenecteplase is **incompatible** with dextrose solutions. Dextrose-containing lines must be flushed with a saline solution before and after administration. Administer as a single I.V. bolus over 5 seconds.

Contraindications Hypersensitivity to tenecteplase or any component of the formulation; active internal bleeding; history of stroke; intracranial/intraspinal surgery or trauma within 2 months; intracranial neoplasm; arteriovenous malformation or aneurysm; bleeding diathesis; severe uncontrolled hypertension

Warnings Stop antiplatelet agents and heparin if serious bleeding occurs. Avoid I.M. injections and nonessential handling of the patient for a few hours after administration. Monitor for bleeding complications. Venipunctures should be performed carefully and only when necessary. If arterial puncture is necessary, then use an upper extremity that can be easily compressed manually. For the following conditions, the risk of bleeding is higher with use of tenecteplase and should be weighed against the benefits: Recent major surgery, cerebrovascular disease, recent GI or GU bleed, recent trauma, uncontrolled hypertension (systolic BP ≥180 mm Hg and/or diastolic BP ≥110 mm Hg), suspected left heart thrombus, acute pericarditis, subacute bacterial endocarditis, hemostatic defects, severe hepatic dysfunction, pregnancy, hemorrhagic diabetic retinopathy or other hemorrhagic ophthalmic conditions, septic thrombophlebitis or occluded arteriovenous cannula at seriously infected site, advanced age (see Usual Dosing, Elderly), anticoagulants, recent administration of GP IIb/IIIa inhibitors. Coronary thrombolysis may result in reperfusion arrhythmias. Caution with readministration of tenecteplase. Safety and efficacy have not been established in pediatric patients. Cholesterol embolism has rarely been reported.

Dosage Forms Injection, powder for reconstitution, recombinant: 50 mg [packaged with diluent and syringe]

Reference Range Peak plasma tenecteplase usually exceeds 1000 ng/mL

Overdosage/Treatment Supportive therapy: Treat bleeding complications with transfusions of red blood cells, fresh frozen plasma, and cryoprecipitate; do not administer dextran; although human overdose data is lacking, administration of aminocaproic acid (Amicar®) at a dose of 3-5 g I.V. followed by an infusion rate of 1-1.25 g/hour may be useful

Drug Interactions Aminocaproic acid (antifibrinolytic agent) may decrease effectiveness.
Drugs which affect platelet function (eg, NSAIDs, dipyridamole, ticlopidine, clopidogrel, IIb/IIIa antagonists) may potentiate the risk of hemorrhage; use with caution.

Heparin and aspirin: Use with aspirin and heparin may increase bleeding. However, aspirin and heparin were used concomitantly with tenecteplase in the majority of patients in clinical studies.
Warfarin or oral anticoagulants: Risk of bleeding may be increased during concurrent therapy.

Pregnancy Risk Factor C

Pregnancy Implications Administer to pregnant women only if the potential benefits justify the risk to the fetus. Exercise caution when administering to a nursing woman. No embryo toxicity noted in rodent studies.

Lactation Use caution

Nursing Implications Dextrose-containing lines must be flushed with a saline solution before and after administration. Check frequently for signs of bleeding. Avoid I.M. injections and nonessential handling of patient.

Additional Information Intracranial hemorrhage associated with higher doses of heparin (which is coadministered) and with bolus administration of thrombolytics. Information can be obtained as needed through Genentec, Inc: (800) 551-2231 or (650) 225-1100.

Tenidap

Unlabeled/Investigational Use Rheumatoid arthritis, osteoarthritis

Mechanism of Action Inhibits cyclooxygenase and 5-lipoxygenase impairing prostaglandin and leukotriene production

Adverse Reactions
Central nervous system: Dizziness, headache
Gastrointestinal (noted in ~25% of patients): Nausea, constipation
Otic: Tinnitus
Renal: Reversible proteinuria

Toxicodynamics/Kinetics
Onset of action: Within 24 hours
Protein binding: 99%

Dosage 120 mg/day (usually given in the morning)

Overdosage/Treatment
Decontamination: Activated charcoal
Supportive therapy: Hypotension/dehydration can be managed with I.V. fluid therapy; acidosis should be treated with bicarbonates, seizures with benzodiazepines; antacids, blood products are indicated, as appropriate, for hemorrhage
Enhancement of elimination: Multiple doses of activated charcoal; dialysis or perfusion is indicated for secondary complications, acidosis, or renal failure and not toxin removal alone

Additional Information Oxindole-type nonsteroidal agent similar to indomethacin; may slow progressive joint erosion

Terazosin

CAS Number 63074-08-8; 63590-64-7; 70024-40-7

U.S. Brand Names Hytrin®

Impairment Potential Yes

Use Management of mild to moderate hypertension; alone or in combination with other agents such as diuretics or beta-blockers; benign prostate hyperplasia (BPH)

Mechanism of Action An alpha₁-specific blocking agent with minimal alpha₂ effects; this allows peripheral postsynaptic blockade, with the resultant decrease in arterial tone, while preserving the negative feedback loop which is mediated by the peripheral presynaptic alpha₂-receptors (similar in action to prazosin but longer duration of action)

Adverse Reactions
Cardiovascular: **Hypotension (orthostatic)**, syncope, palpitations, tachycardia, edema, sinus tachycardia, atrial fibrillation
Central nervous system: **Dizziness, lightheadedness**, night terrors, **drowsiness, malaise, headache**, hypothermia
Dermatologic: Rash, licheniform eruptions
Endocrine & metabolic: Fluid retention, sexual dysfunction
Gastrointestinal: Nausea, xerostomia
Genitourinary: Urinary frequency, priapism
Hematologic: Thrombocytopenia
Neuromuscular & skeletal: Weakness, paresthesia
Ocular: Blurred vision, phototoxic
Respiratory: Nasal congestion
Miscellaneous: Allergic reactions, anaphylaxis

Signs and Symptoms of Overdose Drowsiness, dyspnea, hypotension, hypothermia, impotence, night terrors, shock, syncope

Pharmacodynamics/Kinetics
Onset of action: 1-2 hours
Absorption: Rapid
Protein binding: 90% to 95%
Metabolism: Extensively hepatic
Half-life elimination: 9.2-12 hours
Time to peak, serum: ~1 hour
Excretion: Feces (60%); urine (40%)

Dosage

Oral: Adults:

Hypertension: Initial: 1 mg at bedtime; slowly increase dose to achieve desired blood pressure, up to 20 mg/day; usual dose range (JNC 7): 1-20 mg once daily

Dosage reduction may be needed when adding a diuretic or other antihypertensive agent; if drug is discontinued for greater than several days, consider beginning with initial dose and retitrate as needed; dosage may be given on a twice daily regimen if response is diminished at 24 hours and hypotensive is observed at 2-4 hours following a dose

Benign prostatic hyperplasia: Initial: 1 mg at bedtime, increasing as needed; most patients require 10 mg day; if no response after 4-6 weeks of 10 mg/day, may increase to 20 mg/day

Monitoring Parameters Standing and sitting/supine blood pressure, especially following the initial dose at 2-4 hours following the dose and thereafter at the trough point to ensure adequate control throughout the dosing interval; urinary symptoms

Contraindications Hypersensitivity to quinazolines (doxazosin, prazosin, terazosin) or any component of the formulation; concurrent use with phosphodiesterase-5 (PDE-5) inhibitors including sildenafil (>25 mg), tadalafil, or vardenafil

Warnings Can cause significant orthostatic hypotension and syncope, especially with first dose; anticipate a similar effect if therapy is interrupted for a few days, if dosage is rapidly increased, or if another antihypertensive drug (particularly vasodilators) or a PDE5 inhibitor is introduced. Patients should be cautioned about performing hazardous tasks when starting new therapy or adjusting dosage upward. Prostate cancer should be ruled out before starting for BPH. Use with caution in hepatic impairment. Intraoperative floppy iris syndrome has been observed in cataract surgery patients who were on or were previously treated with alpha₁ blockers. Causality has not been established and there appears to be no benefit in discontinuing alpha blocker therapy prior to surgery. Safety and efficacy in children have not been established.

Dosage Forms Capsule: 1 mg, 2 mg, 5 mg, 10 mg

Reference Range Single dose of 5 mg produces a peak concentration of 45 mcg/L at 2 hours

Overdosage/Treatment

Decontamination: Activated charcoal

Supportive therapy: Hypotension usually responds to I.V. fluids or Trendelenburg positioning. If unresponsive to these measures, the use of a parenteral vasoconstrictor may be required (eg, norepinephrine 0.1-0.2 mcg/kg/minute titrated to response). Treatment is primarily supportive and symptomatic.

Enhancement of elimination: Multiple dosing of activated charcoal would not be expected to be effective

Test Interactions No effect on lipid profile

Drug Interactions

ACE inhibitors: Hypotensive effect may be increased.

Beta-blockers: Hypotensive effect may be increased.

Calcium channel blockers: Hypotensive effect may be increased.

NSAIDs may reduce antihypertensive efficacy.

Sildenafil, tadalafil, vardenafil: Blood pressure-lowering effects are additive. Use of tadalafil or vardenafil is contraindicated by the manufacturer. Use sildenafil with extreme caution (dose ≤25 mg).

Pregnancy Risk Factor C

Lactation Excretion in breast milk unknown

Additional Information Considered a step 2 drug in stepped approach to hypertension

Specific References

Chobanian AV, Bakris GL, Black HR, et al, "The Seventh Report of the Joint National Committee on Prevention, Detection, Evaluation, and Treatment of High Blood Pressure: The JNC 7 Report," *JAMA*, 2003, 289(19):2560-71.

Terbinafine

CAS Number 78628-80-5; 91161-71-6

U.S. Brand Names Lamisil® AT™ [OTC]; Lamisil®

Synonyms Terbinafine Hydrochloride

Use

Active against most strains of *Trichophyton mentagrophytes*, *Trichophyton rubrum*; may be effective for infections of *Microsporum gypseum* and *M. nanum*, *Trichophyton verrucosum*, *Epidermophyton floccosum*, *Candida albicans*, and *Scopulariopsis brevicaulis*

Oral: Onychomycosis of the toenail or fingernail due to susceptible dermatophytes

Topical: Antifungal for the treatment of tinea pedis (athlete's foot), tinea cruris (jock itch), and tinea corporis (ringworm) [OTC/prescription formulations]; tinea versicolor [prescription formulations]

Mechanism of Action Synthetic alkylamine derivative which inhibits squalene epoxidases which is a key enzyme in sterol biosynthesis in fungi to result in a deficiency in ergosterol within fungal cell wall and result in fungal cell death

Adverse Reactions

Oral:

Central nervous system: Headache, dizziness, vertigo, fatigue, malaise

Dermatologic: Rash, pruritus, urticaria, angioedema, alopecia, precipitation/exacerbation of cutaneous lupus erythematosus, Stevens-Johnson syndrome, toxic epidermal necrolysis

Gastrointestinal: Diarrhea, dyspepsia, abdominal pain, appetite decreased, taste disturbance, vomiting

Hematologic: Lymphocytopenia, agranulocytosis, neutropenia, thrombocytopenia

Hepatic: Liver enzymes increased, hepatic failure

Neuromuscular & skeletal: Arthralgia, myalgia

Ocular: Visual disturbances, changes in ocular lens and retina

Miscellaneous: Allergic reactions, anaphylaxis, precipitation/exacerbation of systemic lupus erythematosus

Topical:

Dermatologic: Pruritus, contact dermatitis, irritation, burning, dryness

Local: Irritation, stinging

Pharmacodynamics/Kinetics

Absorption: Topical: Limited (<5%); Oral: >70%

Distribution: V_d: 2000 L; distributed to sebum and skin predominantly

Protein binding, plasma: >99%

Metabolism: Hepatic; no active metabolites; first-pass effect; little effect on CYP

Bioavailability: Oral: 40%

Half-life elimination:

Topical: 22-26 hours

Oral: Terminal half-life: 200-400 hours; very slow release of drug from skin and adipose tissues occurs; effective half-life: ~36 hours

Time to peak, plasma: 1-2 hours

Excretion: Urine (70% to 75%)

Dosage

Children ≥12 years and Adults:

Topical cream, solution:

Athlete's foot (tinea pedis): Apply to affected area twice daily for at least 1 week, not to exceed 4 weeks [OTC/prescription formulations]

Ringworm (tinea corporis) and jock itch (tinea cruris): Apply cream to affected area once or twice daily for at least 1 week, not to exceed 4 weeks; apply solution once daily for 7 days [OTC formulations]

Adults:

Oral:

Superficial mycoses: Fingernail: 250 mg/day for up to 6 weeks; toenail: 250 mg/day for 12 weeks; doses may be given in two divided doses

Systemic mycosis: 250-500 mg/day for up to 16 months

Topical solution: Tinea versicolor: Apply to affected area twice daily for 1 week [prescription formulation]

Dosing adjustment in renal impairment: GFR <50 mL/minute: Oral administration is not recommended.

Dosing adjustment in hepatic impairment: Clearance is decreased by ~50% with hepatic cirrhosis; use is not recommended.

Stability Cream: Store at 5°C to 30°C (41°F to 86°F).

Solution: Store at 5°C to 25°C (41°F to 77°F); do not refrigerate

Tablet: Store below 25°C (77°F); protect from light

Monitoring Parameters CBC and LFTs at baseline and repeated if use is for >6 weeks

Contraindications Hypersensitivity to terbinafine, naftifine, or any component of the formulation

Warnings While rare, the following complications have been reported and may require discontinuation of therapy: Changes in the ocular lens and retina, pancytopenia, neutropenia, Stevens-Johnson syndrome, toxic epidermal necrolysis. Rare cases of hepatic failure (including fatal cases) have been reported following oral treatment of onychomycosis. Not recommended for use in patients with active or chronic liver disease. Discontinue if symptoms or signs of hepatobiliary dysfunction or cholestatic hepatitis develop. If irritation/sensitivity develop with topical use, discontinue therapy. Oral products are not recommended for use with pre-existing liver or renal disease (≤50 mL/minute GFR). **Use caution in writing and/or filling prescription/orders. Confusion between Lamictal® (lamotrigine) and Lamisil® (terbinafine) has occurred.**

Dosage Forms Cream, as hydrochloride:

Lamisil® AT™: 1% (12 g) [contains benzyl alcohol]

Solution, as hydrochloride [topical spray]:

Lamisil® [DSC], Lamisil® AT™: 1% (30 mL)

Tablet:

Lamisil®: 250 mg

Reference Range Peak terbinafine level after a 250 mg oral dose is ~1 mcg/mL

Overdosage/Treatment Decontamination: Activated charcoal

Drug Interactions

Substrate (minor) of 1A2, 2C9, 2C19, 3A4; **Inhibits** CYP2D6 (strong); **Induces** CYP3A4 (weak)

Effects of drugs metabolized by CYP2D6 (including beta-blockers, SSRIs, MAO inhibitors, tricyclic antidepressants) may be increased; warfarin effects may be increased

CYP2D6 substrates: Terbinafine may increase the levels/effects of CYP2D6 substrates. Example substrates include amphetamines, selected beta-blockers, dextromethorphan, fluoxetine, lidocaine, mirtazapine, nefazodone, paroxetine, risperidone, ritonavir, thioridazine, tricyclic antidepressants, and venlafaxine.

CYP2D6 prodrug substrates: Terbinafine may decrease the levels/effects of CYP2D6 prodrug substrates. Example prodrug substrates include codeine, hydrocodone, oxycodone, and tramadol.

Rifampin: Rifampin increases terbinafine clearance (100%).

Pregnancy Risk Factor B

Pregnancy Implications Avoid use in pregnancy since treatment of onychomycosis is postponable

Lactation Enters breast milk/not recommended

Additional Information Fungistatic against *Candida albicans*

Specific References

Aksakal BA, Ozsoy E, Arnavut O, et al, "Oral Terbinafine-Induced Bullous Pemphigoid," *Ann Pharmacother*, 2003, 37(11):1625-7.

't Jong GW, Stricker BH, and Sturkenboom MC, "Marketing in the Lay Media and Prescriptions of Terbinafine in Primary Care: Dutch Cohort Study," *BMJ*, 2004, 328(7445):931.

Walter RB, Lukaschek J, Renner EL, et al, "Fatal Hepatic Veno-Occlusive Disease Associated with Terbinafine in a Liver Transplant Recipient," *J Hepatol*, 2003, 38(3):373-4.

Terbutaline

CAS Number 23031-32-5

U.S. Brand Names Brethine®

Synonyms Brethaire [DSC]; Bricanyl [DSC]

Use Bronchodilator in reversible airway obstruction and bronchial asthma Tocolytic agent (management of preterm labor)

Mechanism of Action Relaxes bronchial smooth muscle by action on β_2-receptors with less effect on heart rate

Adverse Reactions

Cardiovascular: Tachycardia (slight), palpitations, hypertension, flushing, shortened P-R segment, angina, lengthened QT segment, cardiac arrhythmias, fibrillation (atrial), chest pain, flutter (atrial), sinus tachycardia

Central nervous system: **Restlessness, nervousness**, dizziness, headache, CNS stimulation, hyperactivity, insomnia, mania

Dermatologic: Maculopapular rash

Endocrine & metabolic: Hypokalemia, hyperglycemia

Gastrointestinal: GI upset

Neuromuscular & skeletal: **Trembling**, tremors

Signs and Symptoms of Overdose Arrhythmias, chest pain convulsions, hepatitis, hyperglycemia, hypocalcemia, hypokalemia, insomnia, myoglobinuria, nausea, rhabdomyolysis, vomiting

Pharmacodynamics/Kinetics

Onset of action: Oral: 30-45 minutes; SubQ: 6-15 minutes

Protein binding: 25%

Metabolism: Hepatic to inactive sulfate conjugates

Bioavailability: SubQ doses are more bioavailable than oral

Half-life elimination: 11-16 hours

Excretion: Urine

Dosage

Children <12 years: Bronchoconstriction:

Oral: Initial: 0.05 mg/kg/dose 3 times/day, increased gradually as required; maximum: 0.15 mg/kg/dose 3-4 times/day or a total of 5 mg/24 hours

SubQ: 0.005-0.01 mg/kg/dose to a maximum of 0.3 mg/dose every 15-20 minutes for 3 doses

Children >12 years and Adults: Bronchoconstriction:

Oral:

12-15 years: 2.5 mg every 6 hours 3 times/day; not to exceed 7.5 mg in 24 hours

>15 years: 5 mg/dose every 6 hours 3 times/day; if side effects occur, reduce dose to 2.5 mg every 6 hours; not to exceed 15 mg in 24 hours

SubQ: 0.25 mg/dose repeated in 15-30 minutes for one time only; a total dose of 0.5 mg should not be exceeded within a 4-hour period inhalations

Adults: Premature labor (tocolysis; unlabeled use):

Acute: I.V. 2.5-10 mcg/minute; increased gradually every 10-20 minutes; effective maximum dosages from 17.5-30 mcg/minute have been used with caution. Duration of infusion is at least 12 hours.

Maintenance: Oral: 2.5-10 mg every 4-6 hours for as long as necessary to prolong pregnancy depending on patient tolerance

Dosing adjustment/comments in renal impairment:

Cl_{cr} 10-50 mL/minute: Administer at 50% of normal dose

Cl_{cr} <10 mL/minute: Avoid use

Stability Store injection at room temperature; protect from heat, light, and from freezing; use only clear solutions

Monitoring Parameters Serum potassium, glucose; heart rate, blood pressure, respiratory rate; monitor for signs and symptoms of pulmonary edema (when used as a tocolytic); monitor FEV_1, peak flow, and/or other pulmonary function tests (when used as bronchodilator)

Administration I.V.: Use infusion pump.

Oral: Administer around-the-clock to promote less variation in peak and trough serum levels

Contraindications Hypersensitivity to terbutaline or any component of the formulation; cardiac arrhythmias associated with tachycardia; tachycardia caused by digitalis intoxication

Warnings

When used for tocolysis, there is some risk of maternal pulmonary edema, which has been associated with the following risk factors, excessive hydration, multiple gestation, occult sepsis and underlying cardiac disease. To reduce risk, limit fluid intake to 2.5-3 L/day, limit sodium intake, maintain maternal pulse to <130 beats/minute.

Use caution in patients with cardiovascular disease (arrhythmia or hypertension or CHF), convulsive disorders, diabetes, glaucoma, hyperthyroidism, or hypokalemia. Beta agonists may cause elevation in blood pressure, heart rate, and result in CNS stimulation/excitation. $Beta_2$ agonists may increase risk of arrhythmia, increase serum glucose, or decrease serum potassium.

When used as a bronchodilator, optimize anti-inflammatory treatment before initiating maintenance treatment with terbutaline. Do not use as a component of chronic therapy without an anti-inflammatory agent. Only the mildest form of asthma (Step 1 and/or exercise-induced) would not require concurrent use based upon asthma guidelines. Patient must be instructed to seek medical attention in cases where acute symptoms are not relieved or a previous level of response is diminished. The need to increase frequency of use may indicate deterioration of asthma, and treatment must not be delayed.

Do not exceed recommended dose; serious adverse events including fatalities, have been associated with excessive use of inhaled sympathomimetics. Rarely, paradoxical bronchospasm may occur with use of inhaled bronchodilating agents; this should be distinguished from inadequate response.

Dosage Forms Injection, solution, as sulfate: 1 mg/mL (1 mL)

Tablet, as sulfate: 2.5 mg, 5 mg

Additional dosage forms available in Canada: Powder for oral inhalation (Bricanyl® Turbuhaler): 500 mcg/actuation [50 or 200 metered doses]

Reference Range Peak plasma level after a 0.75 mg SubQ dose: ~10 mcg/L 30 minutes after injection

Overdosage/Treatment

Decontamination: Activated charcoal

Supportive therapy: Prudent use of a cardioselective beta-adrenergic blocker can be considered, keeping in mind the potential for induction of bronchoconstriction in an asthmatic individual; esmolol (150-300 mg/hour) can be safely used to treat tachycardia with hypotension even during pregnancy

Enhancement of elimination: Dialysis has not been shown to be of value

Drug Interactions

Decreased effect with beta-blockers

Increased toxicity with MAO inhibitors, TCAs

Pregnancy Risk Factor B

Lactation Enters breast milk/compatible

Nursing Implications Injection with SubQ use

Additional Information Used unofficially to delay delivery in preterm labor; has short-lived clinical effectiveness with development of tolerance with chronic use

Testosterone

Related Information

● Androstenedione

CAS Number 1045-69-8; 1255-49-8; 14191-92-5; 15262-86-9; 2697-92-9; 315-37-7; 57-85-2; 5721-91-5; 58-20-8; 58-22-0; 5949-44-0

U.S. Brand Names Androderm®; AndroGel®; Delatestryl®; Depo®-Testosterone; Striant™; Testim™; Testoderm® with Adhesive [DSC]; Testoderm® [DSC]; Testopel®

Synonyms Testosterone Cypionate; Testosterone Enanthate

Use

Injection: Androgen replacement therapy in the treatment of delayed male puberty; male hypogonadism (primary or hypogonadotropic); inoperable female breast cancer (enanthate only)

Pellet: Androgen replacement therapy in the treatment of delayed male puberty; male hypogonadism (primary or hypogonadotropic)

Buccal, topical: Male hypogonadism (primary or hypogonadotropic)

Mechanism of Action Principal endogenous androgen responsible for promoting the growth and development of the male sex organs and maintaining secondary sex characteristics in androgen-deficient males

Adverse Reactions

Frequency not defined.

Cardiovascular: Flushing, edema

Central nervous system: Excitation, aggressive behavior, sleeplessness, anxiety, mental depression, headache

Dermatologic: Hirsutism (increase in pubic hair growth), acne

Endocrine & metabolic: Menstrual problems (amenorrhea), virilism, breast soreness, gynecomastia, hypercalcemia, hypoglycemia

Gastrointestinal: Nausea, vomiting, GI irritation

Following buccal administration: Bitter taste, gum edema, gum or mouth irritation, gum tenderness, taste perversion

Genitourinary: Prostatic hyperplasia, prostatic carcinoma, impotence, testicular atrophy, epididymitis, priapism, bladder irritability

Hepatic: Hepatic dysfunction, cholestatic hepatitis, hepatic necrosis

Hematologic: Leukopenia, polycythemia, suppression of clotting factors

Miscellaneous: Hypersensitivity reactions

Signs and Symptoms of Overdose Cholestatic jaundice, depression, gynecomastia, hirsutism, hypercalcemia, hypertension, hypertrichosis, impotence, jaundice, leukopenia or neutropenia (agranulocytosis, granulocytopenia), oligospermia

Pharmacodynamics/Kinetics

Duration (route and ester dependent): I.M.: Cypionate and enanthate esters have longest duration, ≤2-4 weeks

Absorption: Transdermal gel: ~10% of applied dose

Distribution: Crosses placenta; enters breast milk

Protein binding: 98%; bound to sex hormone-binding globulin (40%) and albumin

Metabolism: Hepatic; forms metabolites, including dihydrotestosterone (DHT) and estradiol (both active)

Half-life elimination: 10-100 minutes

Excretion: Urine (90%); feces (6%)

Dosage

Adolescents: I.M.:

Male hypogonadism:

Initiation of pubertal growth: 40-50 mg/m^2/dose (cypionate or enanthate ester) monthly until the growth rate falls to prepubertal levels

Terminal growth phase: 100 mg/m^2/dose (cypionate or enanthate ester) monthly until growth ceases

Maintenance virilizing dose: 100 mg/m^2/dose (cypionate or enanthate ester) twice monthly

Delayed male puberty: 40-50 mg/m^2/dose monthly (cypionate or enanthate ester) for 6 months

Adolescents and Adults: Pellet (for subcutaneous implantation): Delayed male puberty, male hypogonadism: 150-450 mg every 3-6 months

Adults:

I.M.:

Female: Inoperable breast cancer: Testosterone enanthate: 200-400 mg every 2-4 weeks

Male: Long-acting formulations: Testosterone enanthate (in oil)/testosterone cypionate (in oil):

Hypogonadism: 50-400 mg every 2-4 weeks

Delayed puberty: 50-200 mg every 2-4 weeks for a limited duration

Transdermal: Primary male hypogonadism **or** hypogonadotropic hypogonadism:

Testoderm®: Apply 6 mg patch daily to scrotum (if scrotum is inadequate, use a 4 mg daily system)

Androderm®: Apply two systems nightly to clean, dry area on the back, abdomen, upper arms, or thighs for 24 hours for a total of 5 mg day

AndroGel®, Testim™: 5 g (to deliver 50 mg of testosterone with 5 mg systemically absorbed) applied once daily (preferably in the morning) to clean, dry, intact skin of the shoulder and upper arms. AndroGel® may also be applied to the abdomen. Dosage may be increased to a maximum of 10 g (100 mg). **Do not apply testosterone gel to the genitals**.

Oral (buccal): Hypogonadism or hypogonadotropic hypogonadism: 30 mg twice daily (every 12 hours) applied to the gum region above the incisor tooth

Dosing adjustment/comments in hepatic disease: Reduce dose

Monitoring Parameters Periodic liver function tests, PSA, cholesterol, hemoglobin and hematocrit; radiologic examination of wrist and hand every 6 months (when using in prepubertal children)

Gel: Morning serum testosterone levels 14 days after start of therapy

Administration

I.M.: Warm to room temperature; shaking vial will help redissolve crystals that have formed after storage. Administer by deep I.M. injection into the upper outer quadrant of the gluteus maximus.

Oral: Striant™: One mucoadhesive for buccal application (buccal system) should be applied to a comfortable area above the incisor tooth. Apply flat side of system to gum. Rotate to alternate sides of mouth with each application. Hold buccal system firmly in place for 30 seconds to ensure adhesion. The buccal system should adhere to gum for 12 hours. If the buccal system falls out, replace with a new system. If the system falls out within 4 hours of next dose, the new buccal system should remain in place until the time of the following scheduled dose. System will soften and mold to shape of gum as it absorbs moisture from mouth. Do not

chew or swallow the buccal system. The buccal system will not dissolve; gently remove by sliding downwards from gum; avoid scratching gum.

Transdermal:

Androderm®: Apply to clean, dry area of skin on the arm, back, or upper buttocks.

Testoderm®: Apply to clean, dry scrotal skin. Dry shave scrotal hair for optimal skin contact. Do not use chemical depilatories.

AndroGel®, Testim™: Apply (preferably in the morning) to clean, dry, intact skin of the shoulder and upper arms (AndroGel® may also be applied to the abdomen). Upon opening the packet(s), the entire contents should be squeezed into the palm of the hand and immediately applied to the application site(s). Alternatively, a portion may be squeezed onto palm of hand and applied, repeating the process until entire packet has been applied. Application sites should be allowed to dry for a few minutes prior to dressing. Hands should be washed with soap and water after application. **Do not apply testosterone gel to the genitals**.

Contraindications Hypersensitivity to testosterone, soy, or any component of the formulation; males with carcinoma of the breast or prostate; pregnancy or women who may become pregnant

Systemic use is contraindicated in hepatic, renal, or cardiac disease; benign prostatic hyperplasia with obstruction; undiagnosed genital bleeding; hypercalcemia

Warnings When used to treat delayed male puberty, perform radiographic examination of the hand and wrist every 6 months to determine the rate of bone maturation. May cause hypercalcemia in patients with prolonged immobilization. May accelerate bone maturation without producing compensating gain in linear growth. Has both androgenic and anabolic activity, the anabolic action may enhance hypoglycemia. Use caution in elderly patients or patients with other demographic factors which may increase the risk of prostatic carcinoma; careful monitoring is required. May cause fluid retention; use caution in patients with cardiovascular disease or other edematous conditions. Prolonged use of orally-active androgens has been associated with serious hepatic effects (hepatitis, hepatic neoplasms, cholestatic hepatitis, jaundice). May potentiate sleep apnea in some male patients (obesity or chronic lung disease). Transdermal patch may contain conducting metal (eg, aluminum); remove patch prior to MRI. Gels and buccal system have not been evaluated in males <18 years of age; safety and efficacy of injection have not been established in males <12 years of age.

Dosage Forms [CAN] = Canadian brand name

Capsule, gelatin, as deconate (Andriol™ [CAN]): 40 mg (10s) [not available in U.S.]

Gel, topical:

AndroGel®:

1.25 g/actuation (75 g) [1% metered-dose pump; delivers 5 g/4 actuations; provides 60 1.25 g actuations; contains ethanol]

2.5 g (30s) [1% unit dose packets; contains ethanol]

5 g (30s) [1% unit dose packets; contains ethanol]

Testim®: 5 g (30s) [1% unit-dose tube; contains ethanol]

Injection, in oil, as cypionate: 200 mg/mL (10 mL)

Depo®-Testosterone: 100 mg/mL (10 mL); 200 mg/mL (1 mL, 10 mL) [contains benzyl alcohol, benzyl benzoate, and cottonseed oil]

Injection, in oil, as enanthate: 200 mg/mL (5 mL)

Delatestryl®: 200 mg/mL (1 mL) [prefilled syringe; contains sesame oil]; (5 mL) [multidose vial; contains sesame oil]

Kit [for prescription compounding testosterone 2%; kits also contain mixing jar and stirrer]:

First® Testosterone:

Injection, in oil: Testosterone propionate 100 mg/mL (12 mL) [contains sesame oil and benzyl alcohol]

Ointment: White petroleum (48 g)

First® Testosterone MC:

Injection, in oil: Testosterone propionate 100 mg/mL (12 mL) [contains sesame oil and benzyl alcohol]

Cream: Moisturizing cream (48 g)

Mucoadhesive, for buccal application [buccal system] (Striant®): 30 mg (10s)

Pellet, for subcutaneous implantation (Testopel®): 75 mg (1 pellet/vial)

Transdermal system (Androderm®): 2.5 mg/day (60s); 5 mg/day (30s) [contains ethanol]

Reference Range

Testosterone, urine:

Male: 100-1500 ng/24 hours

Female: 100-500 ng/24 hours

Normal serum ranges (male): 12.1-35.7 nmol/L

Normal ratio of testosterone to epitestosterone: <6

Injected agents can be detectable in urine for 2 months while oral agents can be detectable for 2 weeks

Overdosage/Treatment

Decontamination: Oral: Activated charcoal

Supportive therapy: Clomiphene (100 mg/day) may restore pituitary hormone levels (and free testosterone levels) following recreational steroid-induced pituitary-gonadal failure. Pruritic rash due to transdermal testosterone can be treated with topical corticosteroids.

Test Interactions May cause a decrease in creatinine and creatine excretion and an increase in the excretion of 17-ketosteroids; decreases total T_4 serum level due to a decrease in thyroxine-binding globulin (free T_4 is unchanged)

Drug Interactions

Substrate (minor) of CYP2B6, 2C9, 2C19, 3A4; **Inhibits** CYP3A4 (weak)
Warfarin: Testosterone may increase the effects warfarin.

Pregnancy Risk Factor X

Pregnancy Implications Testosterone may cause adverse effects, including masculinization of the female fetus, if used during pregnancy. Females who are or may become pregnant should also avoid skin-to-skin contact to areas where testosterone has been applied topically on another person.

Lactation Enters breast milk/contraindicated

Nursing Implications Warm injection to room temperature and shaking vial will help redissolve crystals that have formed after storage; administer by deep I.M. injection into the upper outer quadrant of the gluteus maximus. Transdermal system (Testoderm®) should be applied on clean, dry, scrotal skin. Dry-shave scrotal hair for optimal skin contact. Do not use chemical depilatories. Androderm® and Testoderm® TTS should be applied to clean dry area of skin on the arm, back, or upper buttocks.

Additional Information Relative potency values: Methyltestosterone*: 1.15; mesterolone: 1.15; methandrostenolone: 1.7; metanozolol*: 5; oxandrolone*: 11.3; nandrolone decanoate: 11.3
*Associated with severe hepatic toxicity

Specific References

Maitre A, Saudan C, Mangin P, et al, "Urinary Analysis of Four Testosterone Metabolites and Pregnanediol by Gas Chromatography-Combustion-Isotope Ratio Mass Spectrometry After Oral Administrations of Testosterone," *J Anal Toxicol*, 2004, 28(6):426-31.

Tetracaine

CAS Number 136-47-0; 94-24-6

U.S. Brand Names AK-T-Caine™; Cepacol Viractin® [OTC]; Opticaine®; Pontocaine®

Synonyms Amethocaine Hydrochloride; Tetracaine Hydrochloride

Use Spinal anesthesia; local anesthesia in the eye for various diagnostic and examination purposes; topically applied to nose and throat for various diagnostic procedures; topical gel [OTC] for treatment of pain associated with cold sores and fever blisters; **approximately 10 times more potent than procaine**

Mechanism of Action Blocks both the initiation and conduction of nerve impulses by decreasing the neuronal membrane's permeability to sodium ions, which results in inhibition of depolarization with resultant blockade of conduction

Adverse Reactions

Injection:

Cardiovascular: Cardiac arrest, hypotension

Central nervous system: Chills, convulsions, dizziness, drowsiness, nervousness, unconsciousness

Gastrointestinal: Nausea, vomiting

Neuromuscular & skeletal: Tremors

Ocular: Blurred vision, pupil constriction

Otic: Tinnitus

Respiratory: Respiratory arrest

Miscellaneous: Allergic reaction

Ophthalmic: Ocular: Chemosis, lacrimation, photophobia, transient stinging

With chronic use: Corneal erosions, corneal healing retardation, corneal opacification (permanent), corneal scarring, keratitis (severe)

Signs and Symptoms of Overdose Apnea, bradycardia, cataract, hypotension, lacrimation, ototoxicity, respiratory depression, seizures, tinnitus

Pharmacodynamics/Kinetics

Onset of action: Anesthetic: Rhinolaryngology: 5-10 minutes

Duration: Rhinolaryngology: ~30 minutes

Metabolism: Hepatic; detoxified by plasma esterases to aminobenzoic acid

Excretion: Urine

Dosage Children ≥2 years and Adults: Topical gel [OTC]: Cold sores and fever blisters: Apply to affected area up to 3-4 times/day for up to 7 days

Adults:

Ophthalmic solution (not for prolonged use): Instill 1-2 drops

Spinal anesthesia:

High, medium, low, and saddle blocks: 0.2% to 0.3% solution

Prolonged (2-3 hours): 1% solution

Subarachnoid injection: 5-20 mg

Saddle block: 2-5 mg; a 1% solution should be diluted with equal volume of CSF before administration

Topical mucous membranes (2% solution): Apply as needed; dose should not exceed 20 mg

Stability Store the solutions in the refrigerator; **incompatible** with alkalis

Administration Before injection, withdraw syringe plunger to make sure injection is not into vein or artery

Contraindications Hypersensitivity to tetracaine, ester-type anesthetics, aminobenzoic acid, or any component of the formulation; injection should not be used when spinal anesthesia is contraindicated

Warnings Use with caution in patients with cardiac disease, hyperthyroidism, abnormal or decreased levels of plasma esterases. Use of the lowest effective dose is recommended. Acutely ill, elderly, debilitated, obstetric patients, or patients with increased intra-abdominal pressure may require decreased doses. Products may contain sodium bisulfite which may cause allergic reactions in some individuals.
Ophthalmic: May delay wound healing. Prolonged use is not recommended. The anesthetized eye should be protected from irritation, foreign bodies, and rubbing to prevent inadvertent damage.

Dosage Forms [DSC] = Discontinued product

Injection, solution, as hydrochloride [preservative free] (Pontocaine®): 1% [10 mg/mL] (2 mL) [contains sodium bisulfite]

Injection, solution, as hydrochloride [premixed in dextrose 6%] (Pontocaine®): 0.3% [3 mg/mL] (5 mL) [DSC]

Injection, powder for reconstitution, as hydrochloride [preservative free] (Pontocaine® Niphanoid®): 20 mg

Solution, ophthalmic, as hydrochloride: 0.5% [5 mg/mL] (15 mL)

Solution, topical, as hydrochloride (Pontocaine®): 2% [20 mg/mL] (30 mL, 118 mL) [for rhinolaryngology]

Overdosage/Treatment

Decontamination: Lavage (within 1 hour)/irrigate/activated charcoal

Supportive therapy: Treatment is primarily symptomatic and supportive. Termination of anesthesia by pneumatic tourniquet inflation should be attempted when the agent is administered by infiltration or regional injection. Seizures commonly respond to diazepam or lorazepam, while hypotension responds to I.V. fluids and Trendelenburg positioning. With the development of metabolic acidosis, I.V. sodium bicarbonate 0.5-2 mEq/kg and ventilatory assistance should be instituted.

Enhancement of elimination: Multiple dosing of activated charcoal may be effective

Pregnancy Risk Factor C

Pregnancy Implications Animal reproduction studies have not been conducted.

Lactation Excretion in breast milk unknown/use caution

Additional Information Approximately 10 times more potent than procaine

Tetracycline

Related Information

- Minocycline
- Therapeutic Drugs Associated with Hallucinations

CAS Number 1336-20-5; 60-54-8; 64-75-5; 6416-04-2

U.S. Brand Names Sumycin®; Wesmycin®

Synonyms Achromycin; TCN; Tetracycline Hydrochloride

Use Treatment of susceptible bacterial infections of both gram-positive and gram-negative organisms; also some unusual organisms including *Mycoplasma*, *Chlamydia*, and *Rickettsia*; may also be used for acne, exacerbations of chronic bronchitis, treatment of "seal finger", *Helicobacter pylori*, and treatment of gonorrhea and syphilis in patients that are allergic to penicillin

Mechanism of Action Inhibits bacterial protein synthesis by binding with the 30S and possibly the 50S ribosomal subunit(s) of susceptible bacteria; may also cause alterations in the cytoplasmic membrane

Adverse Reactions

Cardiovascular: Intracranial hypertension, myocarditis (hypersensitivity), congestive heart failure, myocardial depression, myocarditis, vasculitis

Central nervous system: Pseudotumor cerebri, visual hallucinations, drug fever, Jarisch-Herxheimer reaction, hyperthermia

Dermatologic: Rash, exfoliative dermatitis, photosensitivity, toxic epidermal necrolysis, angioedema, Stevens-Johnson syndrome, bullous skin disease, urticaria, purpura, psoriasis, yellow fingernail, exanthem, solar urticaria, lichen planus, cutaneous vasculitis

Gastrointestinal: Discoloration of teeth and enamel hypoplasia (infants), nausea, vomiting, diarrhea, stomatitis, glossitis, antibiotic-associated pseudomembranous colitis, esophagitis, xerostomia, pancreatitis, esophageal ulceration, fecal discoloration (black, greenish gray, red, white/speckling), peritoneal adhesions, lingua villosa nigra, photo-onycholysis

Hematologic: Neutropenia, hemolysis, hypoprothrombinemia, aplastic anemia

Hepatic: Hepatic steatosis (at doses >1 g/day I.V.); fatty degeneration of liver

Local: Extravasation injury

Neuromuscular & skeletal: Myasthenia gravis (exacerbation), paresthesia

Ocular: Myopia, phototoxic

Renal: Renal damage, Fanconi-like syndrome, renal tubular acidosis type II, uremia

Respiratory: Pulmonary infiltrates with eosinophilia, asthma, bronchospasm

Miscellaneous: Hypersensitivity reactions, incidence of *Candida* superinfection (increased), exacerbation of systemic lupus erythematosus, injury to growing bones and teeth, fixed drug eruption

Signs and Symptoms of Overdose Azotemia, coagulopathy, colitis, diplopia, dysphagia, Fanconi syndrome, hypoglycemia, hypothermia, lichenoid eruptions, metallic taste, myasthenia gravis (exacerbation or precipitation), nausea, thrombocytopenia, tongue discoloration, toxic epidermal necrolysis, vomiting

Pharmacodynamics/Kinetics

Absorption: Oral: 75%

Distribution: Small amount appears in bile

Relative diffusion from blood into CSF: Good only with inflammation (exceeds usual MICs)

CSF:blood level ratio: Inflamed meninges: 25%

Protein binding: ~65%

Half-life elimination: Normal renal function: 8-11 hours; End-stage renal disease: 57-108 hours

Time to peak, serum: Oral: 2-4 hours

Excretion: Urine (60% as unchanged drug); feces (as active form)

Dosage

Oral:

Children >8 years: 25-50 mg/kg/day in divided doses every 6 hours

Adults: 250-500 mg/dose every 6 hours

Helicobacter pylori eradication: 500 mg 2-4 times/day depending on regimen; requires combination therapy with at least one other antibiotic and an acid-suppressing agent (proton pump inhibitor or H$_2$ blocker)

Dosing interval in renal impairment:

Cl$_{cr}$ 50-80 mL/minute: Administer every 8-12 hours

Cl$_{cr}$ 10-50 mL/minute: Administer every 12-24 hours

Cl$_{cr}$ <10 mL/minute: Administer every 24 hours

Dialysis: Slightly dialyzable (5% to 20%) via hemo- and peritoneal dialysis or via continuous arteriovenous or venovenous hemofiltration; no supplemental dosage necessary

Dosing adjustment in hepatic impairment: Avoid use or maximum dose is 1 g/day

Stability Outdated tetracyclines have caused a Fanconi-like syndrome

Monitoring Parameters Renal, hepatic, and hematologic function test, temperature, WBC, cultures and sensitivity, appetite, mental status

Administration Should be administered on an empty stomach (ie, 1 hour prior to, or 2 hours after meals) to increase total absorption. Administer at least 1-2 hours prior to, or 4 hours after antacid because aluminum and magnesium cations may chelate with tetracycline and reduce its total absorption.

Contraindications Hypersensitivity to tetracycline or any component of the formulation; do not administer to children ≤8 years of age; pregnancy

Warnings Use of tetracyclines during tooth development may cause permanent discoloration of the teeth and enamel, hypoplasia and retardation of skeletal development and bone growth with risk being the greatest for children <4 years and those receiving high doses; use with caution in patients with renal or hepatic impairment (eg, elderly); dosage modification required in patients with renal impairment since it may increase BUN as an antianabolic agent; pseudotumor cerebri has been reported with tetracycline use (usually resolves with discontinuation); outdated drug can cause nephropathy; superinfection possible; use protective measure to avoid photosensitivity

Dosage Forms Capsule, as hydrochloride: 250 mg, 500 mg

Suspension, oral, as hydrochloride (Sumycin®): 125 mg/5 mL (480 mL) [contains sodium benzoate and sodium metabisulfite; fruit flavor]

Tablet, as hydrochloride (Sumycin®): 250 mg, 500 mg

Reference Range

Therapeutic: Not established

Toxic: >16 mcg/mL

Overdosage/Treatment

Decontamination: Activated charcoal

Supportive therapy: Antacids can be given for epigastric pain; acetazolamide (500 mg twice daily) can be used to treat pseudotumor cerebri. For treatment of lingua villosa nigra, discontinue causative agent. Clean the tongue with a toothbrush and rinse mouth with a half-strength solution of hydrogen peroxide or 10% carbamide peroxide. Symptoms should subside in a few days.

Enhancement of elimination: Multiple dosing of activated charcoal may be effective; slightly dialyzable (5% to 20%)

Test Interactions False-negative urine glucose with Clinistix®; may cause an elevation of BUN through a catabolic effect and **not** through renal impairment

Drug Interactions **Substrate** of CYP3A4 (major); **Inhibits** CYP3A4 (moderate)

Antacids: May decrease tetracycline absorption; separate doses.

Calcium supplements (oral): May decrease tetracycline absorption; separate doses.

CYP3A4 inducers: CYP3A4 inducers may decrease the levels/effects of tetracycline. Example inducers include aminoglutethimide, carbamazepine, nafcillin, nevirapine, phenobarbital, phenytoin, and rifamycins.

CYP3A4 substrates: Tetracycline may increase the levels/effects of CYP3A4 substrates. Example substrates include benzodiazepines, calcium channel blockers, cyclosporine, mirtazapine, nateglinide, nefazodone, sildenafil (and other PDE-5 inhibitors), tacrolimus, and venlafaxine. Selected benzodiazepines (midazolam and triazolam), cisapride, ergot alkaloids, selected HMG-CoA reductase inhibitors (lovastatin and simvastatin), and pimozide are generally contraindicated with strong CYP3A4 inhibitors.

Didanosine: May decrease tetracycline absorption; separate doses.

Digoxin: Tetracyclines may rarely increase digoxin serum levels.

Iron: May decrease tetracycline absorption; separate doses.

Methoxyflurane anesthesia when concurrent with tetracycline may cause fatal nephrotoxicity.

Oral contraceptives: Anecdotal reports suggesting decreased contraceptive efficacy with tetracyclines have been refuted by more rigorous scientific and clinical data.

Quinapril: May decrease tetracycline absorption; separate doses.

Warfarin with tetracyclines may result in increased anticoagulation.

Pregnancy Risk Factor D (systemic)/B (topical)

Pregnancy Implications Crosses the placenta and enters fetal circulation; may cause permanent discoloration of teeth if used during the last half of pregnancy. Fatty liver may occur during pregnancy with daily ingestions over 4 grams.

Lactation Enters breast milk/not recommended (AAP rates "compatible")

Nursing Implications Give around-the-clock (ie, 6-12-6-12)

Additional Information May reduce serum vitamin B concentrations; D-lactic acidosis may develop in patients with short bowel syndrome due to overgrowth of D-lactate producing organisms (*Lactobacillus* species, *Streptococcus bovis*, *Bifidobacterium* species, or *Eubacterium* species).

Specific References

Cham G, Pan J, Lim F, et al, "Topical Heparin with Tetracycline Versus Heparin or Tetracycline Alone, in Preventing Ocular Scarring Due to the Venom of the Black Spitting Cobra (Naja Sumatrana)," *Clin Toxicol (Phila)*, 2005, 43:775.

Morison WL, "Clinical Practice: Photosensitivity," *N Engl J Med*, 2004, 350(11):1111-7.

Tetrahydrozoline

CAS Number 522-48-5; 84-22-0

U.S. Brand Names Eye-Sine™ [OTC]; Geneye® [OTC]; Murine® Tears Plus [OTC]; Optigene® 3 [OTC]; Tyzine® Pediatric; Tyzine®; Visine® Advanced Relief [OTC]; Visine® Original [OTC]

Synonyms Tetrahydrozoline Hydrochloride; Tetryzoline

Use Symptomatic relief of nasal congestion and conjunctival congestion

Mechanism of Action Stimulates alpha-adrenergic receptors in the arterioles of the conjunctiva and the nasal mucosa to produce vasoconstriction

Adverse Reactions

Cardiovascular: Tachycardia, palpitations, increased blood pressure, increased heart rate

Central nervous system: Headache

Local: **Transient stinging**

Neuromuscular & skeletal: Tremor

Ocular: Blurred vision

Respiratory: **Sneezing**

Signs and Symptoms of Overdose Bradycardia, cardiovascular collapse, coma, CNS depression, hypothermia

Admission Criteria/Prognosis Patients may be discharged if asymptomatic 6 hours postingestion

Pharmacodynamics/Kinetics

Onset of action: Decongestant: Intranasal: 4-8 hours

Duration: Ophthalmic vasoconstriction: 2-3 hours

Dosage Nasal congestion: Intranasal:

Children 2-6 years: Instill 2-3 drops of 0.05% solution every 4-6 hours as needed, no more frequent than every 3 hours

Children >6 years and Adults: Instill 2-4 drops or 3-4 sprays of 0.1% solution every 3-4 hours as needed, no more frequent than every 3 hours

Conjunctival congestion: Ophthalmic: Adults: Instill 1-2 drops in each eye 2-4 times/day

Monitoring Parameters Blood pressure, heart rate, symptom response

Dosage Forms Solution, intranasal, as hydrochloride:

Tyzine®: 0.1% (15 mL) [spray bottle; contains benzalkonium chloride]; (30 mL) [dropper bottle; contains benzalkonium chloride]

Tyzine® Pediatric: 0.05% (15 mL) [spray bottle; contains benzalkonium chloride]

Solution, ophthalmic, as hydrochloride: 0.05% (15 mL)

Eye-Sine™, Geneye®, Optigene® 3: 0.05% (15 mL) [may contain benzalkonium chloride]

Murine® Tears Plus: 0.05% (15 mL, 30 mL) [contains benzalkonium chloride]

Visine® Advanced Relief: 0.05% (30 mL) [contains benzalkonium chloride and polyethylene glycol]

Visine® Original: 0.05% (15 mL, 30 mL) [contains benzalkonium chloride; 15 mL size also available with dropper]

Overdosage/Treatment

Decontamination:

Oral: Do not induce emesis; lavage (with airway protection) may be useful if performed within 1 hour of ingestion; activated charcoal can be given

Ocular: Irrigation copiously with normal saline or water

Supportive therapy: Hypotension and/or bradycardia will usually respond to isotonic I.V. fluid administration (10-20 mL/kg); atropine can cause significant hypertension if given; nitroprusside or phentolamine can be given to treat hypertension while phentolamine can be used to treat localized vasoconstriction; seizures can be treated with lorazepam or diazepam; phenytoin or phenobarbital can be used in refractory cases; naloxone and flumazenil do not appear to be useful

Drug Interactions Increased toxicity: MAO inhibitors can cause an exaggerated adrenergic response if taken concurrently or within 21 days of discontinuing MAO inhibitor; beta-blockers can cause hypertensive episodes and increased risk of intracranial hemorrhage; anesthetics

Pregnancy Risk Factor C

Nursing Implications Do not use for >3-4 days without direct physician supervision

Specific References

Daggy A, Kaplan R, Roberge R, et al, "Pediatric Visine® (Tetrahydrozoline) Ingestion: Case Report and Review of Imidazoline Toxicity," *Vet Hum Toxicol*, 2003, 45(4):210-2.

Thalidomide

CAS Number 50-35-1

U.S. Brand Names Thalomid®

Synonyms NSC-66847

Use Treatment and maintenance of cutaneous manifestations of erythema nodosum leprosum

Unlabeled/Investigational Use Treatment of Crohn's disease; graft-versus-host reactions after bone marrow transplantation; AIDS-related aphthous stomatitis; Behûlet's syndrome; Waldenström's macroglobulinemia; Langerhans cell histiocytosis; may be effective in rheumatoid arthritis, discoid lupus erythematosus, and erythema multiforme

Mechanism of Action A derivative of glutethimide; mode of action for immunosuppression is unclear; inhibition of neutrophil chemotaxis and decreased monocyte phagocytosis may occur; may cause 50% to 80% reduction of tumor necrosis factor - alpha

Adverse Reactions

Controlled clinical trials: ENL:

Cardiovascular: Peripheral edema

Central nervous system: **Somnolence, headache**, dizziness, vertigo, chills, malaise

Dermatologic: **Rash**, dermatitis (fungal), nail disorder, pruritus, maculopapular rash

Gastrointestinal: Constipation, diarrhea, nausea, moniliasis, tooth pain, abdominal pain

Genitourinary: Impotence

Neuromuscular & skeletal: Asthenia, pain, back pain, neck pain, neck rigidity, tremor

Respiratory: Pharyngitis, rhinitis, sinusitis

HIV-seropositive:

General: An increased viral load has been noted in patients treated with thalidomide. This is of uncertain clinical significance.

Cardiovascular: Peripheral edema

Central nervous system: **Somnolence, dizziness, fever, headache**, nervousness, insomnia, agitation, chills, neuropathy (up to 8% in HIV-seropositive patients)

Dermatologic: **Rash, maculopapular rash, acne** (3.1% to 11.1%), dermatitis (fungal), nail disorder, pruritus

Gastrointestinal: **AST increase** (2.8% to 12.5%), **diarrhea, nausea** (≤12.5%), **oral moniliasis** (6.3% to 11.1%), anorexia, constipation, dry mouth, flatulence, LFT multiple abnormalities, abdominal pain

Hematologic: **Leukopenia, anemia** (5.6% to 12.5%)

Neuromuscular & skeletal: **Paresthesia** (5.6% to 15.6%), **weakness** (5.6% to 21.9%), back pain, pain

Respiratory: Pharyngitis, sinusitis

Miscellaneous: **Diaphoresis** (≤12.5%), **lymphadenopathy** (5.6% to 12.5%), accidental injury, infection

Postmarketing and/or case reports (limited to important or life-threatening): Acute renal failure, arrhythmias, bradycardia, CML, dyspnea, electrolyte imbalances, erythema multiforme, erythema nodosum, Hodgkin's disease, hypersensitivity, hyperthyroidism, intestinal perforation, lethargy, lymphopenia, mental status changes, myxedema, neutropenia, orthostatic hypotension, pancytopenia, paresthesia, peripheral neuritis, photosensitivity, pleural effusion, psychosis, Raynaud's syndrome, seizures, Stevens-Johnson syndrome, suicide attempt, syncope, thrombosis, toxic epidermal necrolysis, tumor lysis syndrome

Pharmacodynamics/Kinetics

Distribution: V_d: 120 L

Protein binding: 55% to 66%

Metabolism: Nonenzymatic hydrolysis in plasma; forms multiple metabolites

Half-life elimination: 5-7 hours

Time to peak, plasma: 3-6 hours

Excretion: Urine (<1% as unchanged drug)

Dosage

Oral:

Multiple myeloma: 200 mg once daily (with dexamethasone 40 mg daily on days 1-4, 9-12, and 17-20 of a 28-day treatment cycle)

Cutaneous ENL:

Initial: 100-300 mg/day taken once daily at bedtime with water (at least 1 hour after evening meal)

Patients weighing <50 kg: Initiate at lower end of the dosing range

Severe cutaneous reaction or patients previously requiring high dose may be initiated at 400 mg/day; doses may be divided, but taken 1 hour after meals

Maintenance: Dosing should continue until active reaction subsides (usually at least 2 weeks), then tapered in 50 mg decrements every 2-4 weeks

Patients who flare during tapering or with a history or requiring prolonged maintenance should be maintained on the minimum dosage necessary to control the reaction. Efforts to taper should be repeated every 3-6 months, in increments of 50 mg every 2-4 weeks.

Behûlet's syndrome (unlabeled use): 100-400 mg/day

Graft-vs-host reactions (unlabeled use): 100-1600 mg/day; usual initial dose: 200 mg 4 times/day for use up to 700 days

AIDS-related aphthous stomatitis (unlabeled use): 200 mg twice daily for 5 days, then 200 mg/day for up to 8 weeks

Discoid lupus erythematosus (unlabeled use): 100-400 mg/day; maintenance dose: 25-50 mg

Stability Store at 15°C to 30°C (50°F to 86°F). Protect from light. Keep in original package.

Monitoring Parameters CBC with differential, platelets; signs of neuropathy monthly for the first 3 months, then periodically during treatment; consider monitoring of sensory nerve application potential amplitudes (at baseline and every 6 months) to detect asymptomatic neuropathy. In HIV-seropositive patients: viral load after 1 and 3 months, then every 3 months. Pregnancy testing (sensitivity of at least 50 mIU/mL) is required within 24 hours prior to initiation of therapy, weekly during the first 4 weeks, then every 4 weeks in women with regular menstrual cycles or every 2 weeks in women with irregular menstrual cycles.

Administration Avoid extensive handling of capsules; capsules should remain in blister pack until ingestion. If exposed to the powder content from broken capsules or body fluids from patients receiving thalidomide, the exposed area should be washed with soap and water.

Contraindications Hypersensitivity to thalidomide or any component of the formulation; neuropathy (peripheral); patient unable to comply with STEPS® program (including males); women of childbearing potential unless alternative therapies are inappropriate and adequate precautions are taken to avoid pregnancy; pregnancy

Warnings

Hazardous agent – use appropriate precautions for handling and disposal. **[U.S. Boxed Warning]: Thalidomide is a known teratogen; effective contraception must be used for at least 4 weeks before initiating therapy, during therapy, and for 4 weeks following discontinuation of thalidomide for women of childbearing potential.** Use caution with drugs which may decrease the efficacy of hormonal contraceptives.

[U.S. Boxed Warning]: Thrombotic events have been reported, generally in patients with other risk factors for thrombosis (neoplastic disease, inflammatory disease, or concurrent therapy with combination chemotherapy). Use in combination with dexamethasone is associated with increased risk for deep vein thrombosis (DVT) and pulmonary embolism (PE). Monitor for signs and symptoms of thromboembolism; patients at risk may benefit from prophylactic anticoagulation or aspirin.

May cause sedation; patients must be warned to use caution when performing tasks which require alertness. Use caution in patients with renal or hepatic impairment, neurological disorders, or constipation. Thalidomide has been associated with the development of peripheral neuropathy, which may be irreversible; use caution with other medications which may cause peripheral neuropathy. Consider immediate discontinuation (if clinically appropriate) in patients who develop neuropathy. May cause seizures; use caution in patients with a history of seizures, concurrent therapy with drugs which alter seizure threshold, or conditions which predispose to seizures. May cause neutropenia;

discontinue therapy if absolute neutrophil count decreases to <750/mm³. Use caution in patients with HIV infection; has been associated with increased viral loads. May cause orthostasis and/or bradycardia; use with caution in patients with cardiovascular disease or in patients who would not tolerate transient hypotensive episodes. Hypersensitivity, Stevens-Johnson syndrome (SJS) and toxic epidermal necrolysis (TEN) have been reported; withhold therapy and evaluate with skin rashes; permanently discontinue if rash is exfoliative, purpuric, bullous or if SJS or TEN is suspected. Safety and efficacy have not been established in children <12 years of age.

Dosage Forms Capsule:
Thalomid®: 50 mg, 100 mg, 200 mg

Reference Range Therapeutic plasma thalidomide levels in graft-vs-host reactions are 5-8 mcg/mL, although it has been suggested that lower plasma levels (0.5-1.5 mcg/mL) may be therapeutic; peak serum thalidomide level after a 200 mg dose: 1.2 mcg/mL

Overdosage/Treatment
Decontamination: Activated charcoal with sorbitol
Supportive therapy: Bisacodyl suppositories can be used for constipation

Drug Interactions Abatacept: Thalidomide may be associated with increased risk of serious infection when used in combination with abatacept.
Anakinra: Thalidomide may be associated with increased risk of serious infection when used in combination with anakinra.
CNS depressants: Thalidomide may enhance the sedative activity of other drugs such as ethanol, barbiturates, reserpine, and chlorpromazine
Vaccine (killed): Thalidomide may decrease the effect of vaccines (killed).
Vaccine (live attenuated): Thalidomide may increase the risk of vaccinal infection.

Pregnancy Risk Factor X

Pregnancy Implications Embryotoxic with limb defects noted from the 27th to 40th gestational day of exposure; all cases of phocomelia occur from the 27th to 42nd gestational day; fetal cardiac, gastrointestinal, and genitourinary tract abnormalities have also been described. Effective contraception must be used for at least 4 weeks before initiating therapy, during therapy, and for 4 weeks following discontinuation of thalidomide. Males (even those vasectomized) must use a latex condom during any sexual contact with women of childbearing age. Risk to the fetus from semen of male patients is unknown.

Lactation Excretion in breast milk unknown/not recommended

Additional Information Thalidomide is approved for marketing only under a special distribution program. This program, called the "System for Thalidomide Education and Prescribing Safety" (STEPS™), has been approved by the FDA. Prescribing and dispensing of thalidomide is restricted to prescribers and pharmacists registered with the program. Prior to dispensing, an authorization number must be obtained (1-888-423-5436) from Celgene (write authorization number on prescription). No more than a 4-week supply should be dispensed. Blister packs should be dispensed intact (do not repackage capsules). Prescriptions must be filled within 7 days.

Specific References
Barlogie B, Tricot G, Anaissie E, et al, "Thalidomide and Hematopoietic-cell Transplantation for Multiple Myeloma," *N Engl J Med*, 2006, 354(15):1021-30.
Behrens RJ, Gulley JL, and Dahut WL, "Pulmonary Toxicity During Prostate Cancer Treatment with Docetaxel and Thalidomide," *Am J Ther*, 2003, 10(3):228-32.
Duyvendak M, Naunton M, Kingma BJ, et al, "Thalidomide-Associated Thrombocytopenia," *Ann Pharmacother*, 2005, 39(11):1936-9.
Gordinier ME and Dizon DS, "Dyspnea During Thalidomide Treatment for Advanced Ovarian Cancer," *Ann Pharmacother*, 2005, 39(5):962-5.
Hussein MA, Baz R, Srkalovic G, et al, "Phase 2 Study of Pegylated Liposomal Doxorubicin, Vincristine, Decreased-Frequency Dexamethasone, and Thalidomide in Newly Diagnosed and Relapsed-Refractory Multiple Myeloma," *Mayo Clin Proc*, 2006, 81(7):889-95.
Kaur A, Yu SS, Lee AJ, et al, "Thalidomide-Induced Sinus Bradycardia," *Ann Pharmacother*, 2003, 37(7-8):1040-3.
Nasca MR, Micali G, Cheigh NH, et al, "Dermatologic and Nondermatologic Uses of Thalidomide," *Ann Pharmacother*, 2003, 37(9):1307-20.
Sayarlioglu M, Kotan MC, Topcu N, et al, "Treatment of Recurrent Perforating Intestinal Ulcers with Thalidomide in Behcet's Disease," *Ann Pharmacother*, 2004, 38(5):808-11.
Thompson JL and Hansen LA, "Thalidomide Dosing in Patients with Relapsed or Refractory Multiple Myeloma," *Ann Pharmacother*, 2003, 37(4):571-6.

Theophylline

Related Information
- Aminophylline
- Therapeutic Drugs Associated with Hallucinations

CAS Number 58-55-9

U.S. Brand Names Elixophyllin®; Quibron®-T/SR; Quibron®-T; T-Phyl®; Theo-24®; Theochron®; Theolair-SR® [DSC]; Theolair™; Uniphyl®

Synonyms Theophylline Anhydrous

Use Bronchodilator in reversible airway obstruction due to asthma or COPD as maintenance therapy only; for neonatal apnea/bradycardia
Use for clinically-significant atrioventricular nodal blockade following acute inferior myocardial infarction

Mechanism of Action Exact mechanism is unknown; probable mechanism involves increasing tissue concentrations of cAMP and/or occupying adenosine receptors as an antagonist and/or inhibition of phosphodiesterases, PDE III, PDE IV

Adverse Reactions
Uncommon at serum theophylline concentrations ≤20 mcg/mL
Central nervous system: Stuttering
Cardiovascular: Palpitations, sinus tachycardia, tachycardia (ventricular), tachycardia (supraventricular), flutter (atrial), chest pain, angina, arrhythmias (ventricular), vasodilation, sinus bradycardia
Central nervous system: Insomnia, irritability, agitation, seizures, nervousness, psychosis, restlessness, visual hallucinations, sympathetic storm, hyperthermia
Dermatologic: Skin rash
Endocrine & metabolic: SIADH
Gastrointestinal: Nausea, vomiting, abdominal pain, bezoars/concretions, Ogilvie's syndrome, decreased esophageal sphincter tone
Neuromuscular & skeletal: Tremors, rhabdomyolysis
Miscellaneous: Allergic reactions, acute atraumatic compartment syndrome

Signs and Symptoms of Overdose Anorexia, bezoars, delirium, diuresis, esophageal ulceration, exfoliative dermatitis, feces discoloration (black), fibrillation (atrial), hypercalcemia, hyperglycemia, hypertension, hypokalemia, hypophosphatemia, hypomagnesemia, hyponatremia, hypotension, insomnia, intestinal pseudo-obstruction (Ogilvie's syndrome), irritability, lactic acidosis, leg cramps, nausea, paroxysmal tachycardia (ventricular), tachycardia, seizures, vomiting. Repetitive vomiting is an indication to hold theophylline therapy and rule out toxicity by serum concentrations.

Pharmacodynamics/Kinetics
Absorption: Oral: Dosage form dependent
Distribution: 0.45 L/kg based on ideal body weight
Metabolism: Children >1 year and Adults: Hepatic; involves CYP1A2, 2E1 and 3A4; forms active metabolites (caffeine and 3-methylxanthine)
Half-life elimination: Highly variable and dependent upon age, liver function, cardiac function, lung disease, and smoking history
Time to peak, serum:
Oral: Liquid: 1 hour; Tablet, enteric-coated: 5 hours; Tablet, uncoated: 2 hours
I.V.: Within 30 minutes
Excretion: Urine
Neonates: 50% unchanged
Children >3 months and Adults: 10% unchanged

Dosage
Use ideal body weight for obese patients
Neonates:
Apnea of prematurity: Oral, I.V.: Loading dose: 4 mg/kg (theophylline); 5 mg/kg (aminophylline)
There appears to be a delay in theophylline elimination in infants <1 year of age, especially neonates; both the initial dose and maintenance dosage should be conservative
I.V.: Initial: Maintenance infusion rates:
Neonates:
≤24 days: 0.08 mg/kg/hour theophylline
>24 days: 0.12 mg/kg/hour theophylline
Children >1 year and Adults:
Treatment of acute wheezing: I.V.: Loading dose (in patients not currently receiving aminophylline or theophylline): 6 mg/kg (based on aminophylline) given I.V. over 20-30 minutes; administration rate should not exceed 25 mg/minute (aminophylline).
Approximate I.V. maintenance dosages are based upon **continuous infusions**; bolus dosing (often used in children <6 months of age) may be determined by multiplying the hourly infusion rate by 24 hours and dividing by the desired number of doses/day.
Dosage should be adjusted according to serum level measurements during the first 12- to 24-hour period.
Oral theophylline: Treatment of acute wheezing: Initial dosage recommendation: Loading dose (to achieve a serum level of ~10 mcg/mL; loading doses should be given using a rapidly absorbed oral product **not** a sustained release product):
If no theophylline has been administered in the previous 24 hours: 4-6 mg/kg theophylline
If theophylline has been administered in the previous 24 hours, administer ¹/₂ the loading dose or 2-3 mg/kg theophylline can be given in emergencies when serum levels are not available.
On the average, for every 1 mg/kg theophylline given, blood levels will rise 2 mcg/mL. Ideally, defer the loading dose if a serum theophylline concentration can be obtained rapidly. However, if

this is not possible, exercise clinical judgment. If the patient is not experiencing theophylline toxicity, this is unlikely to result in dangerous adverse effects.

These recommendations, based on mean clearance rates for age or risk factors, were calculated to achieve a serum level of 10 mcg/mL (5 mcg/mL for newborns with apnea/bradycardia). In newborns and infants, a fast-release oral product can be used. The total daily dose can be divided every 12 hours in newborns and every 6-8 hours in infants. In children and healthy adults, a slow-release product can be used. The total daily dose can be divided every 8-12 hours.

Bronchial asthma: Oral theophylline: See table.

Oral Theophylline Dosage for Bronchial Asthma*

Age	Initial 3 Days	Second 3 Days	Steady-State Maintenance
<1 y	0.2 × (age in weeks) + 5		0.3 × (age in weeks) + 8
1-9 y	16 up to a maximum of 400 mg/24 h	20	22
9-12 y	16 up to a maximum of 400 mg/24 h	16 up to a maximum of 600 mg/24 h	20 up to a maximum of 800 mg/24 h
12-16 y	16 up to a maximum of 400 mg/24 h	16 up to a maximum of 600 mg/24 h	18 up to a maximum of 900 mg/24 h
Adults	400 mg/24 h	600 mg/24 h	900 mg/24 h

*Dose in mg/kg/24 hours of theophylline.

Increasing dose: The dosage may be increased in approximately 25% increments at 2- to 3-day intervals so long as the drug is tolerated or until the maximum dose is reached.

Maintenance dose: See table.

Maintenance Dose for Acute Symptoms

Population Group	Oral Theophylline (mg/kg/day)	I.V. Aminophylline
Premature infant or newborn - 6 wk (for apnea/bradycardia)	4	5 mg/kg/day
6 wk - 6 mo	10	12 mg/kg/day or continuous I.V. infusion*
Infants 6 mo-1 y	12-18	15 mg/kg/day or continuous I.V. infusion*
Children 1-9 y	20-24	1 mg/kg/hour
Children 9-12 y, and adolescent daily smokers of cigarettes or marijuana, and otherwise healthy adult smokers under 50 y	16	0.9 mg/kg/hour
Adolescents 12-16 y (nonsmokers)	13	0.7 mg/kg/hour
Otherwise healthy nonsmoking adults (including elderly patients)	10 (not to exceed 900 mg/day)	0.5 mg/kg/hour
Cardiac decompensation, cor pulmonale and/or liver dysfunction	5 (not to exceed 400 mg/day)	0.25 mg/kg/hour

*For continuous I.V. infusion divide total daily dose by 24 = mg/kg/hour.

These recommendations, based on mean clearance rates for age or risk factors, were calculated to achieve a serum level of 10 mcg/mL (5 mcg/mL for newborns with apnea/bradycardia). In newborns and infants, a fast-release oral product can be used. The total daily dose can be divided every 12 hours in newborns and every 6-8 hours in infants. In children and healthy adults, a slow-release product can be used. The total daily dose can be divided every 8-12 hours.

Dose should be further adjusted based on serum levels; see table.

Dosage Adjustment After Serum Theophylline Measurement

Serum Theophylline		Guidelines
Within normal limits	10-20 mcg/mL	Maintain dosage if tolerated. Recheck serum theophylline concentration at 6-12 mo intervals.*
Too high	20-25 mcg/mL	Decrease doses by about 10%. Recheck serum theophylline concentration after 3 d and then at 6-12 mo intervals.*
	25-30 mcg/mL	Skip next dose and decrease subsequent doses by about 25%. Recheck serum theophylline.
	>30 mcg/mL	Skip next 2 doses and decrease subsequent doses by 50%. Recheck serum theophylline.
Too low	7.5-10 mcg/mL	Increase dose by about 25%.† Recheck serum theophylline concentration after 3 d and then at 6-12 mo intervals.*
	5-7.5 mcg/mL	Increase dose by about 25% to the nearest dose increment† and recheck serum theophylline for guidance in further dosage adjustment (another increase will probably be needed, but this provides a safety check).

From Weinberger M and Hendeles L, "Practical Guide to Using Theophylline," *J Resp Dis*, 1981, 2:12-27.
*Finer adjustments in dosage may be needed for some patients.
†Dividing the daily dose into 3 doses administered at 8-hour intervals may be indicated if symptoms occur repeatedly at the end of a dosing interval.

Dosing adjustment/comments in hepatic disease: Higher incidence of toxic effects including seizures in cirrhosis; plasma levels should be monitored closely during long-term administration in cirrhosis and during acute hepatitis, with dose adjustment as necessary.

Rectal: Adults: 500 mg 3 times/day; avoid using suppositories due to erratic, unreliable absorption

Clinically significant atrioventricular nodal blockade following acute inferior myocardial infarction: 100 mg/minute; I.V. to a maximum: 250 mg

Stability Store injection at room temperature, do not refrigerate; protect from heat and from freezing; use only clear solutions; stability of parenteral admixture at room temperature (25°C): 30 days

Administration
Oral: Long-acting preparations should be taken with a full glass of water, swallowed whole, or cut in half if scored. Do **not** crush. Extended release capsule forms may be opened and the contents sprinkled on soft foods; do **not** chew beads.

Contraindications Hypersensitivity to theophylline or any component of the formulation; premixed injection may contain corn-derived dextrose and its use is contraindicated in patients with allergy to corn-related products

Warnings If a patient develops signs and symptoms of theophylline toxicity (eg, persistent, repetitive vomiting), a serum theophylline level should be measured and subsequent doses held. Due to potential saturation of theophylline clearance at serum levels in or (in some patients) less than the therapeutic range, dosage adjustment should be made in small increments (maximum: 25%). Due to wider interpatient variability, theophylline serum level measurements must be used to optimize therapy and prevent serious toxicity. Use with caution in patients with peptic ulcer, hyperthyroidism, seizure disorders, hypertension, and patients with cardiac arrhythmias (excluding bradyarrhythmias).

Dosage Forms

Capsule, extended release: 100 mg, 125 mg, 200 mg, 300 mg
  TheoCap™: 125 mg, 200 mg, 300 mg [12 hour]
  Theo-24®: 100 mg, 200 mg, 300 mg, 400 mg [24 hours]
Elixir:
  Elixophyllin®: 80 mg/15 mL (480 mL) [contains alcohol 20%; fruit flavor]
Infusion [premixed in D$_5$W]: 200 mg (50 mL, 100 mL); 400 mg (100 mL, 250 mL, 500 mL); 800 mg (250 mL, 500 mL, 1000 mL)
Tablet, controlled release:
  Uniphyl®: 400 mg, 600 mg [24 hours; contains cetostearyl alcohol]
Tablet, extended release: 100 mg, 200 mg, 300 mg, 450 mg
  Theochron®: 100 mg, 200 mg, 300 mg, 450 mg [12-24 hours]
Tablet, immediate release:
  Quibron®-T: 300 mg [DSC]
Tablet, sustained release:
  Quibron®-T/SR: 300 mg [8-12 hours] [DSC]

Reference Range

Timing of serum samples: If toxicity is suspected, draw a level at any time; if lack of therapeutic is effected, draw a trough immediately before the next oral dose
Therapeutic (theophylline): Neonatal apnea: 6-13 mcg/mL; Therapeutic: 10-20 mcg/mL; Toxic: 10-15 mcg/mL

Overdosage/Treatment

Decontamination: **Do not** use ipecac; lavage should be performed if <1 hour after ingestion and >50 mg/kg was ingested; activated charcoal; whole bowel irrigation should be considered for significant sustained release preparation ingestion
Supportive therapy: Metoclopramide or ondansetron can be used for vomiting; 50% of severe theophylline toxic patients respond to 10 mg of metoclopramide to control vomiting; hypotension should be treated with I.V. normal saline hydration. Phenylephrine or levarterenol are preferred vasopressors that can be utilized for hypotension although an I.V. beta-adrenergic blocker (propranolol or esmolol) can be utilized in the patient without a history of bronchospastic disease. Seizures may require diazepam/lorazepam along with phenobarbital; phenytoin is contra-indicated. Lidocaine can be used for ventricular arrhythmias; must monitor for hypoglycemia. Nitrazepam can be given if infantile spasm occur due to theophylline toxicity.
Enhancement of elimination: Multiple doses of activated charcoal can reduce the half-life of aminophylline/theophylline to 2-3 hours; do not use if an ileus is present. Charcoal hemoperfusion can increase the clearance of aminophylline/theophylline by approximately twofold to threefold over that of hemodialysis and is thus the extracorporeal modality of choice. Guidelines for charcoal hemoperfusion include a theophylline level >100 mcg/mL in an acute overdose setting (or 50 mcg/mL in a chronic setting), or the following signs if the level is >35 mcg/mL: ventricular arrhythmias, metabolic acidosis, hypotension, refractory to vasopressors or fluid therapy, seizures, ileus. If a sustained release preparation is ingested or patient with chronic ingestion is >60 years of age, the threshold for using charcoal hemoperfusion should be lower. If the patient is experiencing fluid overload due to congestive heart failure, hemodialysis can be performed to remove both theophylline/aminophylline and fluid; continuous arteriovenous hemoperfusion rates are 193±2 mL/minute; drug clearance rate of hemodialysis and hemoperfusion is 185 and 295 mL/kg/hour respectively.

Diagnostic Procedures

• Theophylline, Blood

Test Interactions Caffeine in high concentrations on selected procedures cross reacts as theophylline

Drug Interactions

Substrate of CYP1A2 (major), 2C9 (minor), 2D6 (minor), 2E1 (major), 3A4 (major); **Inhibits** CYP1A2 (weak)
CYP1A2 inducers: May decrease the levels/effects of theophylline. Example inducers include aminoglutethimide, carbamazepine, phenobarbital, and rifampin.
CYP1A2 inhibitors: May increase the levels/effects of theophylline. Example inhibitors include ciprofloxacin, fluvoxamine, ketoconazole, norfloxacin, ofloxacin, and rofecoxib.
CYP2E1 inhibitors: May increase the levels/effects of theophylline. Example inhibitors include disulfiram, isoniazid, and miconazole.
CYP3A4 inducers: CYP3A4 inducers may decrease the levels/effects of theophylline. Example inducers include aminoglutethimide, carbamazepine, nafcillin, nevirapine, phenobarbital, phenytoin, and rifamycins.
CYP3A4 inhibitors: May increase the levels/effects of theophylline. Example inhibitors include azole antifungals, clarithromycin, diclofenac, doxycycline, erythromycin, imatinib, isoniazid, nefazodone, nicardipine, propofol, protease inhibitors, quinidine, telithromycin, and verapamil.

Pregnancy Risk Factor C

Pregnancy Implications Theophylline crosses the placenta; adverse effects may be seen in the newborn. Theophylline metabolism may change during pregnancy; monitor serum levels.

Lactation Enters breast milk/compatible (AAP rates "compatible")

Nursing Implications Do not crush sustained release or enteric coated drug products

Additional Information Elderly, acutely ill, and patients with severe respiratory problems, pulmonary edema, or liver dysfunction are at greater risk of toxicity because of reduced drug clearance. Saliva levels are approximately equal to 60% of plasma levels; infantile spasm can occur; charcoal-broiled foods may increase elimination, reducing half-life by 50%; cigarette smoking may require an increase of dosage by 50% to 100%; aminophylline 100 mg is equivalent to theophylline 79 mg

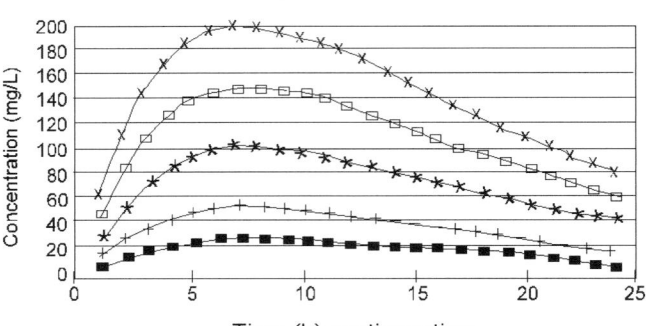

SERUM THEOPHYLLINE OVERDOSE
Nonsmokers

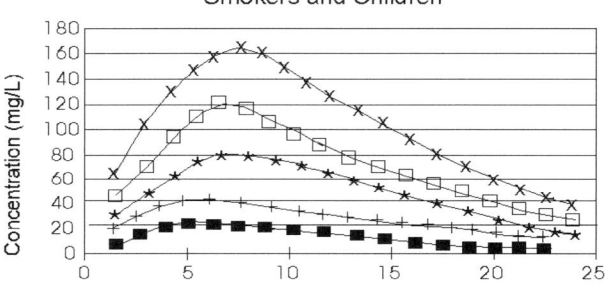

SERUM THEOPHYLLINE OVERDOSE
Smokers and Children

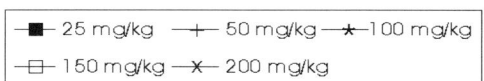

Nomogram for overdose of sustained-release theophylline in 1) nonsmoking adults, and 2) smokers and children. (Courtesy of Frank Paloucek, PharmD, College of Pharmacy, University of Illinois, Chicago.)

Specific References

Davis E, Perez A, and McKay CA, "A Novel Self-Contained Hemoperfusion Device for the Treatment of Theophylline Overdose in a Swine Model," *J Toxicol Clin Toxicol*, 2003, 41(5):695.

Juárez-Olguin H, Flores-Pérez J, Pérez-Guillé G, et al, "Therapeutic Monitoring of Theophylline in Newborns with Apnea," *P&T*, 2004, 29(5): 322-3.

Nenov VD, Marinov P, Sabeva J, et al, "Current Applications of Plasmapheresis in Clinical Toxicology," *Nephrol Dial Transplant*, 2003, 18(Suppl 5):v56-8.

Wills B and Erickson T, "Drug- and Toxin-Associated Seizures," *Med Clin North Am*, 2005, 89(6):1297-321 (review).

Thiamine

CAS Number 59-43-8; 67-03-8
U.S. Brand Names Thiamilate® [OTC]
Synonyms Aneurine Hydrochloride; Thiamine Hydrochloride; Thiaminium Chloride Hydrochloride; Vitamin B$_1$
Use Treatment of thiamine deficiency including beriberi, Wernicke's encephalopathy syndrome, and peripheral neuritis associated with pellagra, alcoholic patients with altered sensorium; various genetic

metabolic disorders; dietary sources include legumes, pork, beef, whole grains, yeast, fresh vegetables; a deficiency state can occur in as little 3 weeks following total dietary absence

Mechanism of Action An essential coenzyme in carbohydrate metabolism by combining with adenosine triphosphate to form thiamine pyrophosphate

Adverse Reactions
Hypersensitivity is rare
Cardiovascular: Cardiovascular collapse and death (primarily following repeated I.V. administration), shock
Dermatologic: Rash, pigmented purpura, angioedema, purpura, dermatitis
Neuromuscular & skeletal: Tingling
Respiratory: Sneezing
Miscellaneous: Warmth, radiopaque

Pharmacodynamics/Kinetics
Absorption: Oral: Adequate; I.M.: Rapid and complete
Excretion: Urine (as unchanged drug and as pyrimidine after body storage sites become saturated)

Dosage Overall caloric requirement of thiamine: 0.5 mg/1000 calories; dietary supplement (depends on caloric or carbohydrate content of the diet):
Infants: 0.3-0.5 mg/day
Children: 0.5-1 mg/day
Adults: 1-2 mg/day
Note: The above doses can be found as a combination in multivitamin preparations
Children:
Noncritically ill thiamine deficiency: Oral: 10-50 mg/day in divided doses every day for 2 weeks followed by 5-10 mg/day for one month
Beriberi: I.M.: 10-25 mg/day for 2 weeks, then 5-10 mg orally every day for one month (oral as therapeutic multivitamin)
Adults:
Wernicke's encephalopathy: I.M., I.V.: 50 mg as a single dose, then 50 mg I.M. every day until normal diet resumed; alternatively: I.V.: 100 mg/day for 5 days can be given
Noncritically ill thiamine deficiency: Oral: 10-50 mg/day in divided doses
Beriberi: I.M., I.V.: 10-30 mg 3 times/day for 2 weeks, then switch to 5-10 mg orally every day for one month (oral as therapeutic multivitamin)

Stability Protect oral dosage forms from light; **incompatible** with alkaline or neutral solutions and with oxidizing or reducing agents; exposure to heat may inactivate vitamin; **incompatible** with neutral or alkaline solutions; **incompatible** with barbiturates

Administration Administer by slow I.V. injection

Contraindications Hypersensitivity to thiamine or any component of the formulation

Warnings Use with caution with parenteral route (especially I.V.) of administration

Dosage Forms Injection, solution, as hydrochloride: 100 mg/mL (2 mL)
Tablet, as hydrochloride: 50 mg, 100 mg, 250 mg, 500 mg

Reference Range Therapeutic: 1.6-4 mg/dL

Test Interactions False-positive for uric acid using the phosphotungstate method and for urobilinogen using the Ehrlich's reagent; large doses may interfere with the spectrophotometric determination of serum theophylline concentration

Drug Interactions Neuromuscular blocking agents; high carbohydrate diets or I.V. dextrose solutions increase thiamine requirement

Pregnancy Risk Factor A/C (dose exceeding RDA recommendation)

Lactation Enters breast milk/compatible

Nursing Implications Parenteral form may be administered by I.M. or slow I.V. injection

Additional Information Found in green vegetables, pork, liver, fish, eggs; requires adequate magnesium for use as a coenzyme; >4.9 mg/day may result in slower progression of HIV illness (RR=0.6)

Specific References
Chung SP, Kim SW, Yoo IS, et al, "Magnetic Resonance Imaging as a Diagnostic Adjunct to Wernicke Encephalopathy in the ED," *Am J Emerg Med*, 2003, 21(6):497-502.
Kumar PD, "Thiamine Shortage - Plight of Low-Cost, Lifesaving Orphan Drugs," *N Engl J Med*. 2006, 354(5):532-3.

Thiamphenicol

CAS Number 15318-45-3; 2393-92-2; 2611-61-2; 847-25-6

Unlabeled/Investigational Use Gonorrhea, chancroid, *Gardnerella vaginalis*, vaginitis

Mechanism of Action Reversibly binds to 50S ribosomal subunits of susceptible organisms preventing amino acids from being transferred to growing peptide chains thus inhibiting protein synthesis

Adverse Reactions
Dose-dependent reversible myelosuppression is more frequent than with chloramphenicol; not seen after single-dose use

Central nervous system: Headache, drowsiness, dizziness, polyneuropathy
Dermatologic: Pruritus
Gastrointestinal: Epigastric pain, abdominal pain, nausea, vomiting
Neuromuscular & skeletal: Neuropathy (peripheral) with long-term use
Ocular: Optic neuritis

Toxicodynamics/Kinetics
Absorption: Oral: 75% to 91%; I.M.: 100%
Distribution: V_d: ~0.5 L/kg
Protein binding: 10% to 20%
Half-life: 2.6-7 hours
Elimination: Renal

Dosage Oral: Single dose of 2.5 g (for uncomplicated gonorrhea) or 500 mg 3 times/day for 6 days
I.M.:
Children: 25-30 mg/kg/day
Adults: 1-3 g/day
I.V.: 750 mg to 1 g 3 times/day

Reference Range Serum levels after an I.V. dose of 10 mg/kg: ~13-14 mcg/mL; after an oral dose of 2.5 g, peak serum thiamphenicol levels range from 16-18 mcg/mL

Overdosage/Treatment
Decontamination: Oral: Activated charcoal
Enhancement of elimination: Multiple dosing of activated charcoal may be effective; although there is no human overdose experience, hemodialysis or hemoperfusion may be effective

Pregnancy Implications Crosses the placenta

Additional Information Less likely than chloramphenicol to cause "gray syndrome" in neonates

Thiethylperazine

CAS Number 1179-69-7

U.S. Brand Names Torecan® [DSC]

Use Relief of nausea and vomiting
Treatment of vertigo

Mechanism of Action Blocks postsynaptic mesolimbic dopaminergic receptors in the brain; exhibits a strong alpha-adrenergic blocking effect and depresses the release of hypothalamic and hypophyseal hormones; acts directly on chemoreceptor trigger zone and vomiting center; may also inhibit impulses from peripheral autonomic afferents to the vomiting center

Adverse Reactions
Cardiovascular: Tachycardia, orthostatic hypotension, peripheral edema
Central nervous system: **Drowsiness, dizziness**, confusion, convulsions, extrapyramidal symptoms, tardive dyskinesia, fever, headache
Gastrointestinal: **Xerostomia**, anorexia
Hematologic: Agranulocytosis
Hepatic: Cholestatic jaundice
Ocular: Blurred vision
Otic: Tinnitus
Respiratory: **Dry nose**

Signs and Symptoms of Overdose Abnormal involuntary muscle movements, coma, deep sleep, extrapyramidal reaction, hypotension or hypertension, urine discoloration (pink; red; red-brown)

Toxicodynamics/Kinetics
Following administration antiemetic effects occur within 30 minutes and continue for approximately 4 hours
Absorption: Oral: Well absorbed
Metabolism: Hepatic
Elimination: Renal

Dosage
Children >12 years and Adults:
Oral, I.M., I.V.: 10 mg 1-6 times/day as needed
Hemodialysis: Not dialyzable (0% to 5%)
Dosing comments in hepatic impairment: Use with caution

Administration
Inject I.M. deeply into large muscle mass, patient should be lying down and remain so for at least 1 hour after administration; although not generally recommended, thiethylperazine can be given as an I.V. infusion over 15-30 minutes; should **not** be given I.V. push; SubQ administration not recommended

Overdosage/Treatment
Decontamination: Activated charcoal; charcoal may need to be given in multiple doses for adequate decontamination
Supportive therapy: Initiate support with fluids, norepinephrine may be useful for hypotension; hypoperfusion states may respond to inotropic support with dobutamine. Bradyarrhythmia or ventricular dysrhythmia may respond to sodium bicarbonate or phenytoin; must avoid class 1A and 1C antiarrhythmics. Torsade de pointes may respond to magnesium; seizures should be managed with benzodiazepines or barbiturates; extrapyramidal reactions should be managed with diphenhydramine or benztropine.

Enhancement of elimination: Multiple dosing of charcoal may not be effective

Pregnancy Risk Factor X

Nursing Implications Inject I.M. deeply into large muscle mass, patient should be lying down and remain so for at least 1 hour after administration; help with ambulation

Thimerosal

Pronunciation (thye MER oh sal)

CAS Number 54-64-8

U.S. Brand Names Mersol® [OTC]; Merthiolate® [OTC]

Use Organomercurial antiseptic with sustained bacteriostatic and fungistatic activity; 49.6% mercury by weight; currently not used as a preservative in any U.S. based vaccines

Mechanism of Action Weakly bacteriostatic

Adverse Reactions

Central nervous system: Agitation (from chronic use)

Endocrine & metabolic: Hypokalemia (from chronic use)

Gastrointestinal: Nausea, vomiting, hemorrhagic gastritis

Neuromuscular & skeletal: Dysarthria

Ocular: Ocular irritation

Renal: Neuropathy (peripheral), renal failure

Respiratory: Laryngeal obstruction

Elemental mercury is poorly absorbed orally with minimal adverse effects. Inhalation acutely can cause chemical pneumonitis, gingivostomatitis, and noncardiogenic pulmonary edema. Chronic exposure to mercury vapor causes acrodynia, fatigue, insomnia, memory loss, and tremor.

Inorganic mercury: Abdominal pain, GI irritation, GI bleeding, shock, renal failure, and acute tubular necrosis will develop after oral administration, with possible CNS toxicity.

Organic mercury: Causes CNS toxicity including ataxia, dysarthria, gastrointestinal distress, hearing and visual loss, and paresthesias.

Dosage Apply 1-3 times/day

Contraindications Hypersensitivity to thimerosal

Warnings Prolonged administration can result in mercury toxicity; contains 49% mercury

Dosage Forms Solution, topical (Merthiolate®): 0.1% [1 mg/mL = 1:1000] (30 mL)

Solution, topical spray (Merthiolate®): 0.1% [1 mg/mL = 1:1000] (60 g)

Tincture, topical (Mersol®): 0.1% [1 mg/mL = 1:1000] (120 mL, 480 mL, 4000 mL)

Reference Range Urinary and whole blood levels can be obtained; normally urinary values are <10 mcg/dL and whole blood <2 mcg/dL; whole blood levels <50 mcg/dL are usually associated with gastroenteritis and acute tubular necrosis; urinary levels for organic mercury are not useful since 90% is eliminated through bile in the feces; urinary mercury levels >56 mcg/L can result in neurotoxic effects (due to elemental mercury)

Overdosage/Treatment

Decontamination:

Gastrointestinal: Lavage if ingested within 1 hour; **do not** induce emesis; charcoal has been shown to decrease inorganic mercury absorption in rats and should be used; milk or egg white may also be useful to bind mercury; whole bowel irrigation with GoLYTELY® may be beneficial if abdominal x-ray shows evidence of mercury

Inhalation: Patients with inhalation exposures should be monitored for pulmonary edema and pneumonitis; give oxygen if necessary

Dermal: Skin decontamination with soap and water

Ocular: Irrigate ocular exposures with saline

Supportive therapy:

Organic mercury: Oral DMSA (succimer) 10 mg/kg every 8 hours for 5 days then 10 mg/kg every 12 hours for 2 or more weeks will enhance urinary mercury excretion

BAL is not recommended for elemental and organic mercury poisoning since BAL may cause redistribution of mercury to the brain which is the primary target organ in these poisonings

Enhancement of elimination: Generally ineffective

Drug Interactions Increased ocular hypersensitivity may occur with tetracycline exposure

Additional Information Some brands of HBIG, IVIG, and some vaccines have thimerosal as a preservative. High-dose therapy with HBIG and IVIG have caused suspected nephrotoxicity.

Thioridazine

Related Information

- Anticholinergic Effects of Common Psychotropics
- Antipsychotic Agents

CAS Number 13-61-0; 50-52-2

U.S. Brand Names Mellaril® [DSC]; Thioridazine Intensol™

Synonyms Thioridazine Hydrochloride

Use Management of schizophrenic patients who fail to respond adequately to treatment with other antipsychotic drugs, either because of insufficient effectiveness or the inability to achieve an effective dose due to intolerable adverse effects from those medications

Unlabeled/Investigational Use Psychosis

Mechanism of Action Blocks postsynaptic mesolimbic dopaminergic receptors in the brain; exhibits a strong alpha-adrenergic blocking effect and depresses the release of hypothalamic and hypophyseal hormones

Adverse Reactions

Anticholinergic toxidrome

Cardiovascular: **Hypotension** (especially with I.V. use), **hypotension (orthostatic)**, AV block edema, tachycardia, cardiac arrhythmias, QRS prolongation, T-wave abnormality, ectopy, torsade de pointes, prolonged QT interval, sinus tachycardia, arrhythmias (ventricular), sinus bradycardia

Central nervous system: **Pseudoparkinsonian signs and symptoms, tardive dyskinesia, akathisia, dystonias, dizziness**, sedation, drowsiness, restlessness, Parkinson's, anxiety, extrapyramidal reactions, neuroleptic malignant syndrome, seizures, altered central temperature regulation

Dermatologic: Hyperpigmentation, pruritus, rash, photosensitivity, Stevens-Johnson syndrome, hypertrichosis, alopecia, angioedema, urticaria, purpura, acanthosis nigricans, exanthem

Endocrine & metabolic: Amenorrhea, galactorrhea, gynecomastia, syndrome of inappropriate antidiuretic hormone, parotitis, hyperprolactinemia

Gastrointestinal: **Constipation**, GI upset, xerostomia, abdominal distention, weight gain, Ogilvie's syndrome

Genitourinary: Urinary retention, impotence, priapism

Hematologic: Agranulocytosis, leukopenia (usually in patients with large doses for prolonged periods), thrombocytopenia, hemolysis, eosinophilia, neutropenia, granulocytopenia

Hepatic: Cholestatic jaundice

Neuromuscular & skeletal: Myoclonus, rhabdomyolysis, paresthesia, Meige syndrome

Ocular: **Retinal pigmentation**, blurred vision, mydriasis, retinopathy

Respiratory: **Nasal congestion**, epistaxis

Miscellaneous: **Diaphoresis**, anaphylactoid reaction, pseudolymphoma, systemic lupus erythematosus

Signs and Symptoms of Overdose Abnormal involuntary muscle movements, AV block (first degree), coma, deep sleep, dysphagia, ejaculatory disturbances, extrapyramidal reaction, galactorrhea, gynecomastia, hepatic failure, hirsutism, hyperprolactinemia, hyperreflexia, hypertonia, hypotension or hypertension, hypothermia or hyperthermia, hyponatremia, impotence, myoclonus, neuroleptic malignant syndrome, nystagmus, priapism, QRS prolongation, QT prolongation, renal disorders (oliguria) at overdoses >2.5 g, tachycardia (ventricular), urine discoloration (pink; red; red-brown), vision color changes (brown tinge)

Admission Criteria/Prognosis Admit any symptomatic ingestion >5 mg/kg in children or a total of 500 mg in adults

Pharmacodynamics/Kinetics

Onset of action: 30-60 minutes

Duration: 4-6 hours

Absorption: Absorbed well from gastrointestinal tract

Distribution: V_d: 18 L/kg

Protein binding: ≥90%

Metabolism: Hepatic

Half-life: 26-36 hours

Time to peak serum concentration: Within 1 hour

Elimination: Kidneys (up to 17%)

Dosage

Oral:

Children >2-12 years: Range: 0.5-3 mg/kg/day in 2-3 divided doses; usual: 1 mg/kg/day; maximum: 3 mg/kg/day

Behavior problems: Initial: 10 mg 2-3 times/day, increase gradually

Severe psychoses: Initial: 25 mg 2-3 times/day, increase gradually

Children >12 years and Adults:

Schizophrenia/psychoses: Initial: 50-100 mg 3 times/day with gradual increments as needed and tolerated; maximum: 800 mg/day in 2-4 divided doses; if >65 years, initial dose: 10 mg 3 times/day

Depressive disorders/dementia: Initial: 25 mg 3 times/day; maintenance dose: 20-200 mg/day

Elderly: Behavioral symptoms associated with dementia: Oral: Initial: 10-25 mg 1-2 times/day; increase at 4- to 7-day intervals by 10-25 mg/day; increase dose intervals (qd, bid, etc) as necessary to control response or side effects. Maximum daily dose: 400 mg; gradual increases (titration) may prevent some side effects or decrease their severity.

Hemodialysis: Not dialyzable (0% to 5%)

Stability Protect all dosage forms from light

Monitoring Parameters Baseline and periodic ECG; vital signs; serum potassium, lipid profile, fasting blood glucose/Hgb A$_{1c}$; BMI; mental status, abnormal involuntary movement scale (AIMS); periodic eye exam; do not initiate if QT$_c$ >450 msec

Administration Oral concentrate must be diluted in 2-4 oz of liquid (eg, water, fruit juice, carbonated drinks, milk, or pudding) before administration. Do not take antacid within 2 hours of taking drug. **Note:** Avoid skin contact with oral suspension or solution; may cause contact dermatitis.

Contraindications Hypersensitivity to thioridazine or any component of the formulation (cross-reactivity between phenothiazines may occur); severe CNS depression; circulatory collapse; severe hypotension; bone marrow suppression; blood dyscrasias; coma; in combination with other drugs that are known to prolong the QT$_c$ interval; in patients with congenital long QT syndrome or a history of cardiac arrhythmias; concurrent use with medications that inhibit the metabolism of thioridazine (fluoxetine, paroxetine, fluvoxamine, propranolol, pindolol); patients known to have genetic defect leading to reduced levels of activity of CYP2D6

Warnings

[U.S. Boxed Warning]: Thioridazine has dose-related effects on ventricular repolarization leading to QT$_c$ prolongation, a potentially life-threatening effect. Therefore, it should be reserved for patients with schizophrenia who have failed to respond to adequate levels of other antipsychotic drugs. May cause orthostatic hypotension - use with caution in patients at risk of this effect or those who would tolerate transient hypotensive episodes (cerebrovascular disease, cardiovascular disease, or other medications which may predispose).

Highly sedating, use with caution in disorders where CNS depression is a feature. Use with caution in Parkinson's disease. Caution in patients with hemodynamic instability; bone marrow suppression; predisposition to seizures; subcortical brain damage; severe cardiac, hepatic, renal, or respiratory disease. Esophageal dysmotility and aspiration have been associated with antipsychotic use - use with caution in patients at risk of pneumonia (ie, Alzheimer's disease). Caution in breast cancer or other prolactin-dependent tumors (may elevate prolactin levels). May alter temperature regulation or mask toxicity of other drugs due to antiemetic effects.

Phenothiazines may cause anticholinergic effects (confusion, agitation, constipation, xerostomia, blurred vision, urinary retention); therefore, they should be used with caution in patients with decreased gastrointestinal motility, urinary retention, BPH, xerostomia, or visual problems. Conditions which also may be exacerbated by cholinergic blockade include narrow-angle glaucoma (screening is recommended) and worsening of myasthenia gravis. Relative to other neuroleptics, thioridazine has a high potency of cholinergic blockade.

May cause extrapyramidal symptoms, including pseudoparkinsonism, acute dystonic reactions, akathisia, and tardive dyskinesia (risk of these reactions is low relative to other neuroleptics). May be associated with neuroleptic malignant syndrome (NMS). Doses exceeding recommended doses may cause pigmentary retinopathy.

Dosage Forms Tablet, as hydrochloride: 10 mg, 15 mg, 25 mg, 50 mg, 100 mg, 150 mg, 200 mg

Reference Range

Therapeutic: 1.0-1.5 mcg/mL (SI: 2.7-4.1 μmol/L)

Toxic: >10.0 mcg/mL (SI: >27.0 μmol/L); no relationship between serum levels and cardiac toxicity

In the postmortem state, anatomical site concentration differences (ie, postmortem redistribution) may occur.

Overdosage/Treatment

Decontamination: Lavage (within 1 hour)/activated charcoal. Consider gastrointestinal decontamination for pediatric ingestions >4 mg/kg or adult ingestions >400mg.

Supportive therapy: Following initiation of essential overdose management, toxic symptom treatment and supportive treatment should be initiated. Hypotension usually responds to I.V. fluids or Trendelenburg positioning. If unresponsive to these measures, the use of a parenteral inotrope may be required. Seizures commonly respond to lorazepam, diazepam, or phenobarbital. Also critical cardiac arrhythmias often respond to I.V. phenytoin (15 mg/kg up to 1 g), while other antiarrhythmics can be used. Lidocaine is usually **not** effective. Cardiac pacing may need to be performed to treat ventricular arrhythmias. Neuroleptics often cause extrapyramidal reaction (eg, dystonic reactions) requiring management with diphenhydramine 1-2 mg/kg (adults) up to a maximum of 50 mg I.M. or I.V. slow push followed by a maintenance dose for 48-72 hours. When these reactions are unresponsive to diphenhydramine, benztropine mesylate I.V. 1-2 mg (adults) may be effective. These agents are generally effective within 2-5 minutes. Sodium bicarbonate (1-3 mEq/kg I.V.) can be used for cardiac conduction abnormalities. Priapism can be treated with 0.2-0.4 mL of phenylephrine (1 mg/mL) intracorporeal every 15 minutes until resolution.

Enhancement of elimination: Multiple dosing of activated charcoal may not be effective; forced diuresis is not effective; not dialyzable (0% to 5%)

Antidote(s)

• Physostigmine [ANTIDOTE]

Diagnostic Procedures

• Thioridazine, Quantitative

Test Interactions False-positives for phenylketonuria, urinary amylase, uroporphyrins, urobilinogen; lowers testosterone levels and serum luteinizing hormone concentrations; may interfere with serum tricyclic levels; high doses of thioridazine can cause a false-positive EMIT urinary immunoassay

Drug Interactions

Substrate of CYP2C19 (minor), 2D6 (major); **Inhibits** CYP1A2 (weak), 2C9 (weak), 2D6 (moderate), 2E1 (weak)

Acetylcholinesterase inhibitors (central): May increase the risk of antipsychotic-related extrapyramidal symptoms; monitor.

Aluminum salts: May decrease the absorption of phenothiazines; monitor

Amphetamines: Efficacy may be diminished by antipsychotics; in addition, amphetamines may increase psychotic symptoms; avoid concurrent use

Anticholinergics: May inhibit the therapeutic response to phenothiazines and excess anticholinergic effects may occur; includes benztropine, trihexyphenidyl, biperiden, and drugs with significant anticholinergic activity (TCAs, antihistamines, disopyramide)

Antihypertensives: Concurrent use of phenothiazines with an antihypertensive may produce additive hypotensive effects (particularly orthostasis)

Beta-blockers: May increase the risk of arrhythmia; propranolol and pindolol are **contraindicated**

Bromocriptine: Phenothiazines inhibit the ability of bromocriptine to lower serum prolactin concentrations

Carvedilol: Serum concentrations may be increased, leading to hypotension and bradycardia; avoid concurrent use

CNS depressants: Sedative effects may be additive with phenothiazines; monitor for increased effect; includes barbiturates, benzodiazepines, narcotic analgesics, ethanol, and other sedative agents

CYP2D6 inhibitors: May increase the levels/effects of thioridazine. Example inhibitors include chlorpromazine, delavirdine, fluoxetine, miconazole, paroxetine, pergolide, quinidine, quinine, ritonavir, and ropinirole. **Thioridazine is contraindicated with inhibitors of this enzyme.**

CYP2D6 substrates: Thioridazine may increase the levels/effects of CYP2D6 substrates. Example substrates include amphetamines, selected beta-blockers, dextromethorphan, fluoxetine, lidocaine, mirtazapine, nefazodone, paroxetine, risperidone, ritonavir, tricyclic antidepressants, and venlafaxine.

CYP2D6 prodrug substrates: Thioridazine may decrease the levels/effects of CYP2D6 prodrug substrates. Example prodrug substrates include codeine, hydrocodone, oxycodone, and tramadol.

Epinephrine: Chlorpromazine (and possibly other low potency antipsychotics) may diminish the pressor effects of epinephrine

Guanethidine and guanadrel: Antihypertensive effects may be inhibited by phenothiazines

Levodopa: Phenothiazines may inhibit the antiparkinsonian effect of levodopa; avoid this combination

Lithium: Phenothiazines may produce neurotoxicity with lithium; this is a rare effect

Metoclopramide: May increase extrapyramidal symptoms (EPS) or risk.

Phenytoin: May reduce serum levels of phenothiazines; phenothiazines may increase phenytoin serum levels

Polypeptide antibiotics: Rare cases of respiratory paralysis have been reported with concurrent use of phenothiazines

Potassium-depleting agents: May increase the risk of serious arrhythmias with thioridazine; includes many diuretics, aminoglycosides, and amphotericin; monitor serum potassium closely

Propranolol: Serum concentrations of phenothiazines may be increased; propranolol also increases phenothiazine concentrations; may also occur with pindolol. **These agents are contraindicated with thioridazine.**

QT$_c$-prolonging agents: Effects on QT$_c$ interval may be additive with phenothiazines, increasing the risk of malignant arrhythmias; includes type Ia antiarrhythmics, TCAs, and some quinolone antibiotics (sparfloxacin, moxifloxacin and gatifloxacin). **These agents are contraindicated with thioridazine.**

Sulfadoxine-pyrimethamine: May increase phenothiazine concentrations

Trazodone: Phenothiazines and trazodone may produce additive hypotensive effects

Tricyclic antidepressants: Concurrent use may produce increased toxicity or altered therapeutic response

Valproic acid: Serum levels may be increased by phenothiazines

Pregnancy Risk Factor C

Pregnancy Implications Crosses the placenta

Lactation Excretion in breast milk unknown/not recommended

Nursing Implications Dilute the oral concentrate with water or juice before administration; avoid skin contact with oral suspension or solution; may cause contact dermatitis

Additional Information Lethal dose: ~1 g

Thioridazine may exhibit an increased risk for cardiac arrest and ventricular arrhythmia at doses >600 mg.

Oral formulations may cause stomach upset; may cause thermoregulatory changes; extrapyramidal reactions are lower with thioridazine than with other phenothiazines due to high antimuscarinic potency
- Thioridazine: Mellaril-S® oral suspension
- Thioridazine hydrochloride: Mellaril® oral solution and tablet

Specific References

Greene T and Dougherty T, "Thioridazine Induced Torsades de Pointes Treated with Sodium Bicarbonate and Transvenous Pacing," *J Toxicol Clin Toxicol*, 2003, 41(5):663.

Thiothixene

Related Information
- Anticholinergic Effects of Common Psychotropics
- Antipsychotic Agents

CAS Number 22189-31-7; 49746-04-5; 49746-09-0; 5591-45-7; 58513-59-0

U.S. Brand Names Navane®

Synonyms Tiotixene

Impairment Potential Yes

Use Management of schizophrenia

Unlabeled/Investigational Use Psychotic disorders

Mechanism of Action Elicits antipsychotic activity by postsynaptic blockade of CNS dopamine receptors resulting in inhibition of dopamine-mediated effects; also has alpha-adrenergic blocking activity

Adverse Reactions

Cardiovascular: **Hypotension** (especially with I.V. use), **hypotension (orthostatic)**, tachycardia, cardiac arrhythmias, sinus tachycardia

Central nervous system: **Pseudoparkinsonian signs and symptoms, tardive dyskinesia, akathisia, dystonias, dizziness**, sedation, drowsiness, restlessness, anxiety, extrapyramidal reactions, neuroleptic malignant syndrome, seizures, altered central temperature regulation, electroencephalogram abnormalities, hyperthermia

Dermatologic: Hyperpigmentation, pruritus, rash, photosensitivity

Endocrine & metabolic: Amenorrhea, galactorrhea, gynecomastia, syndrome of inappropriate antidiuretic hormone (may cause hyponatremia due to inappropriate secretion of antidiuretic hormone)

Gastrointestinal: **Constipation**, GI upset, xerostomia, weight gain

Genitourinary: Urinary retention, impotence

Hematologic: Agranulocytosis, leukopenia (usually in patients with large doses for prolonged periods), thrombocytopenia, hemolysis, eosinophilia

Hepatic: Cholestatic jaundice

Neuromuscular & skeletal: Rhabdomyolysis

Ocular: Retinal pigmentation, blurred vision

Respiratory: **Nasal congestion**

Miscellaneous: **Diaphoresis**, anaphylactoid reactions, systemic lupus erythematosus

Signs and Symptoms of Overdose Agranulocytosis, blood dyscrasias, dizziness, drowsiness, ejaculatory disturbances, eosinophilia, extrapyramidal reaction, galactorrhea, granulocytopenia, gynecomastia, hyponatremia, hypotension, impotence, leukocytosis, leukopenia, myoclonus, neuroleptic malignant syndrome, neutropenia, Parkinson's-like symptoms, priapism, rigidity, tremors, urine discoloration (pink; red; red-brown)

Pharmacodynamics/Kinetics

Onset of action: I.M.: 10-30 minutes

Duration: Up to 12 hours

Absorption: Rapid

Distribution: Widely distributed into body

Protein binding: 91% to 99%

Metabolism: Extensive liver metabolism

Half-life: 34 hours

Time to peak serum concentration: 1-3 hours

Elimination: Bile and feces

Dosage Oral:

Children <12 years (unlabeled): Schizophrenia/psychoses: 0.25 mg/kg/24 hours in divided doses (dose not well established; use not recommended)

Children >12 years and Adults:

Mild to moderate psychosis: 2 mg 3 times/day, up to 20-30 mg/day; more severe psychosis: Initial: 5 mg 2 times/day, may increase gradually, if necessary; maximum: 60 mg/day

Rapid tranquilization of the agitated patient (administered every 30-60 minutes): 5-10 mg; average total dose for tranquilization: 15-30 mg

Hemodialysis: Not dialyzable (0% to 5%)

Stability Refrigerate

Monitoring Parameters Vital signs; lipid profile, fasting blood glucose/Hgb A$_{1c}$; BMI; mental status, abnormal involuntary movement scale (AIMS), extrapyramidal symptoms (EPS)

Contraindications Hypersensitivity to thiothixene or any component of the formulation; severe CNS depression; circulatory collapse; blood dyscrasias; coma

Warnings

May be sedating, use with caution in disorders where CNS depression is a feature. Use with caution in Parkinson's disease. Caution in patients with hemodynamic instability; predisposition to seizures; subcortical brain damage; bone marrow suppression; severe cardiac, hepatic, renal, or respiratory disease. Esophageal dysmotility and aspiration have been associated with antipsychotic use - use with caution in patients at risk of pneumonia (ie, Alzheimer's disease). Caution in breast cancer or other prolactin-dependent tumors (may elevate prolactin levels). May alter temperature regulation or mask toxicity of other drugs due to antiemetic effects. May alter cardiac conduction - life-threatening arrhythmias have occurred with therapeutic doses of neuroleptics. May cause orthostatic hypotension - use with caution in patients at risk of this effect or those who would tolerate transient hypotensive episodes (cerebrovascular disease, cardiovascular disease, or other medications which may predispose). Safety and efficacy in children <12 years of age have not been established.

May cause anticholinergic effects (confusion, agitation, constipation, xerostomia, blurred vision, urinary retention); therefore, they should be used with caution in patients with decreased gastrointestinal motility, urinary retention, BPH, xerostomia, or visual problems. Conditions which also may be exacerbated by cholinergic blockade include narrow-angle glaucoma (screening is recommended) and worsening of myasthenia gravis. Relative to other neuroleptics, thiothixene has a low potency of cholinergic blockade.

May cause extrapyramidal symptoms, including pseudoparkinsonism, acute dystonic reactions, akathisia, and tardive dyskinesia (risk of these reactions is high relative to other neuroleptics). May be associated with neuroleptic malignant syndrome (NMS) or pigmentary retinopathy.

Dosage Forms [DSC] = Discontinued product

Capsule: 1 mg, 2 mg, 5 mg, 10 mg

Navane®: 1 mg [DSC], 2 mg, 5 mg, 10 mg, 20 mg

Reference Range At 2.5 hours after dosing of 15-60 mg/day, serum levels ranged from 10.0-22.5 ng/mL; therapeutic: 10-40 ng/mL

Overdosage/Treatment

Decontamination: Lavage (within 1 hour)/activated charcoal

Supportive therapy: Following initiation of essential overdose management, toxic symptom treatment and supportive treatment should be initiated. Hypotension usually responds to I.V. fluids or Trendelenburg positioning. If unresponsive to these measures, the use of a parenteral inotrope may be required (eg, norepinephrine 0.1-0.2 mcg/kg/minute titrated to response). Seizures commonly respond to lorazepam, diazepam, or phenobarbital. Also critical cardiac arrhythmias often respond to I.V. phenytoin (15 mg/kg up to 1 g), while other antiarrhythmics can be used. Neuroleptics often cause extrapyramidal reaction (eg, dystonic reactions) requiring management with diphenhydramine 1-2 mg/kg (adults) up to a maximum of 50 mg I.M. or I.V. slow push followed by a maintenance dose for 48-72 hours. When these reactions are unresponsive to diphenhydramine, benztropine mesylate I.V. 1-2 mg (adults) may be effective. These agents are generally effective within 2-5 minutes. Sodium bicarbonate (1-3 mEq/kg) can be used for cardiac conduction for abnormalities.

Enhancement of elimination: Multiple dosing of activated charcoal may not be effective; forced diuresis is not effective; not dialyzable (0% to 5%)

Diagnostic Procedures
- Thiothixene, Blood

Test Interactions ↑ cholesterol (S), glucose; ↓ uric acid (S)

Drug Interactions

Substrate of CYP1A2 (major); **Inhibits** CYP2D6 (weak)

Acetylcholinesterase inhibitors (central): May increase the risk of antipsychotic-related extrapyramidal symptoms; monitor.

Aluminum salts: May decrease the absorption of antipsychotics; monitor.

Amphetamines: Efficacy may be diminished by antipsychotics; in addition, amphetamines may increase psychotic symptoms; avoid concurrent use.

Anticholinergics: May inhibit the therapeutic response to antipsychotics and excess anticholinergic effects may occur; includes benztropine, trihexyphenidyl, biperiden, and drugs with significant anticholinergic activity (TCAs, antihistamines, disopyramide).

Antihypertensives: Concurrent use of antipsychotics with an antihypertensive may produce additive hypotensive effects (particularly orthostasis).

Bromocriptine: Antipsychotics inhibit the ability of bromocriptine to lower serum prolactin concentrations.

CNS depressants: Sedative effects may be additive with antipsychotics; monitor for increased effect; includes barbiturates, benzodiazepines, narcotic analgesics, ethanol, and other sedative agents.

CYP1A2 inducers: May decrease the levels/effects of thiothixene. Example inducers include aminoglutethimide, carbamazepine, phenobarbital, and rifampin.

CYP1A2 inhibitors: May increase the levels/effects of thiothixene. Example inhibitors include ciprofloxacin, fluvoxamine, ketoconazole, norfloxacin, ofloxacin, and rofecoxib.

Epinephrine: Chlorpromazine (and possibly other low potency antipsychotics) may diminish the pressor effects of epinephrine.

Guanethidine and guanadrel: Antihypertensive effects may be inhibited by antipsychotics.

Levodopa: Antipsychotics may inhibit the antiparkinsonian effect of levodopa; avoid this combination.

Lithium: Antipsychotics may produce neurotoxicity with lithium; this is a rare effect.

Metoclopramide: May increase extrapyramidal symptoms (EPS) or risk.

Propranolol: Serum concentrations of antipsychotics may be increased; propranolol also increases antipsychotics concentrations.

QT_c-prolonging agents: Effects on QT_c interval may be additive with antipsychotics, increasing the risk of malignant arrhythmias; includes type Ia antiarrhythmics, TCAs, and some quinolone antibiotics (sparfloxacin, moxifloxacin, and gatifloxacin).

Sulfadoxine-pyrimethamine: May increase antipsychotics concentrations.

Trazodone: Antipsychotics and trazodone may produce additive hypotensive effects.

Tricyclic antidepressants: Concurrent use may produce increased toxicity or altered therapeutic response.

Valproic acid: Serum levels may be increased by antipsychotics.

Pregnancy Risk Factor C
Pregnancy Implications Crosses placenta
Lactation Excretion in breast milk unknown/not recommended

Thyroid

U.S. Brand Names Armour® Thyroid; Nature-Throid® NT; Westhroid®
Synonyms Desiccated Thyroid; Thyroid Extract; Thyroid USP
Use Replacement or supplemental therapy in hypothyroidism; pituitary TSH suppressants (thyroid nodules, thyroiditis, multinodular goiter, thyroid cancer), thyrotoxicosis, diagnostic suppression tests

Mechanism of Action The primary active compound is T_3 (triiodothyronine), which may be converted from T_4 (thyroxine) and then circulates throughout the body to influence growth and maturation of various tissues; exact mechanism of action is unknown; however, it is believed the thyroid hormone exerts its many metabolic effects through control of DNA transcription and protein synthesis; involved in normal metabolism, growth, and development; promotes gluconeogenesis, increases utilization and mobilization of glycogen stores and stimulates protein synthesis, increases basal metabolic rate

Adverse Reactions
Cardiovascular: Palpitations, tachycardia, cardiac arrhythmias, chest pain, sinus tachycardia, tachycardia (supraventricular)
Central nervous system: Nervousness, insomnia, fever, headache, psychosis
Dermatologic: Hair loss
Gastrointestinal: Weight loss, increased appetite, diarrhea, abdominal cramps
Neuromuscular & skeletal: Tremors
Miscellaneous: Diaphoresis

Signs and Symptoms of Overdose Angina, CHF, delayed tachycardia, fever (within 12-24 hours), flushing, heat intolerance, hyperthermia, insomnia, menstrual irregularities, mild hypertension, mydriasis, nausea, nervousness, sweating, vomiting, weight loss

Admission Criteria/Prognosis Admit any symptomatic patient or if total serum T_4 exceeds 75 mcg/dL

Pharmacodynamics/Kinetics
Absorption: T_4 is 48% to 79% absorbed; T_3 is 95% absorbed; desiccated thyroid contains thyroxine, liothyronine, and iodine (primarily bound); following absorption thyroxine is largely converted to liothyronine
Protein binding: 99% (bound to albumin, thyroxine-binding globulin, and thyroxin-binding prealbumin); desiccated thyroid contains thyroxine, liothyronine, and iodine (primarily bound)
Metabolism: Largely converted to liothyronine; liothyronine is metabolized in the liver to inactive compounds
Half-life: Liothyronine: 1-2 days; Thyroxine: 6-7 days
Elimination: Excreted in urine as conjugated forms

Dosage Oral:
Children: See table.

Recommended Pediatric Dosage for Congenital Hypothyroidism

Age	Daily Dose (mg)	Daily Dose/kg (mg)
0-6 mo	15-30	4.8-6
6-12 mo	30-45	3.6-4.8
1-5 y	45-60	3-3.6
6-12 y	60-90	2.4-3
>12 y	>90	1.2-1.8

Adults: Start at 15 mg/day and titrate by 15 mg/day in increments of 2- to 4-week intervals; usual maintenance dose: 60-120 mg/day

Monitoring Parameters T_3, T_4, TSH, heart rate, blood pressure, clinical signs of hypo- and hyperthyroidism; in cases where T_4 remains low and TSH is within normal limits, an evaluation of "free" (unbound) T_4 is needed to evaluate further increase in dosage. Check levels of T_3 and T_4 after ingestion, and then every 3 days. Thyroid replacement requires periodic assessment of thyroid status; TSH is the most reliable guide for evaluating adequacy of thyroid replacement dosage. TSH may be elevated during the first few months of thyroid replacement despite patients being clinically euthyroid.

Contraindications Hypersensitivity to beef or pork or any component of the formulation; recent myocardial infarction; thyrotoxicosis uncomplicated by hypothyroidism; uncorrected adrenal insufficiency

Warnings [U.S. Boxed Warning]: Ineffective for weight reduction. High doses may produce serious or even life-threatening toxic effects particularly when used with some anorectic drugs. Use cautiously in patients with pre-existing cardiovascular disease (angina, CHD), elderly since they may be more likely to have compromised cardiovascular function. Chronic hypothyroidism predisposes patients to coronary artery disease. Desiccated thyroid contains variable amounts of T_3, T_4, and other triiodothyronine compounds which are more likely to cause cardiac signs or symptoms due to fluctuating levels. Should avoid use in the elderly for this reason. Drug of choice is levothyroxine in the minds of many clinicians.

Dosage Forms
Tablet: 30 mg, 32.5 mg, 60 mg, 65 mg, 90 mg, 120 mg, 130 mg, 180 mg, 240 mg, 300 mg
Armour® Thyroid: 15 mg, 30 mg, 60 mg, 90 mg, 120 mg, 180 mg, 240 mg, 300 mg
Nature-Throid® NT, Westhroid®: 32.5 mg, 65 mg, 130 mg, 195 mg
Reference Range
See table.

Laboratory Ranges

	Normal Values
T_4, Total	5.8-11.0 mcg/dL
T_3	85-185 ng/dL
T_3 resin uptake (RT$_3$ U)	25%-35%
Free thyroxine index (FT$_4$ I)	1.3-4.2
TSH	0.4-4.8 µIU/mL

Overdosage/Treatment
Decontamination: Gastric emptying indicated for ingestions >5 mg; ipecac within 30 minutes or (lavage within 1 hour) activated charcoal; cholestyramine is an effective agent to decrease T_4 absorption; 50 mg cholestyramine can bind at least 3 mg of thyroxine, therefore, 4 g of cholestyramine given 4 times/day should be administered in order to interrupt enterohepatic recirculation
Supportive therapy: Propranolol may be used for hyperadrenergic signs (1 mg I.V. in adults, 0.01-0.1 mg/kg in pediatrics); sodium ipodate (3 g/1.7 m^2) has been used in acute ingestion to prevent T_4 to T_3 conversion
Enhancement of elimination: Plasmapheresis increases elimination 30-fold while charcoal hemoperfusion enhances T_4 elimination fivefold

Diagnostic Procedures
• Thyroxine, Blood

Test Interactions Many drugs may affect thyroid function tests; para-aminosalicylic acid, aminoglutethimide, amiodarone, barbiturates, carbamazepine, chloral hydrate, clofibrate, colestipol, corticosteroids, danazol, diazepam, estrogens, ethionamide, fluorouracil, I.V. heparin, insulin, lithium, methadone, methimazole, mitotane, nitroprusside, oxyphenbutazone, phenylbutazone, PTU, perphenazine, phenytoin, propranolol, salicylates, sulfonylureas, and thiazides

Drug Interactions Decreased effect:
Beta-blocker effect is decreased when patients become euthyroid
Thyroid hormones increase the therapeutic need for oral hypoglycemics or insulin
Estrogens increase TBG, thereby decreasing effect of thyroid replacement
Cholestyramine and colestipol decrease the effect of orally administered thyroid replacement
Serum digitalis concentrations are reduced in hyperthyroidism or when hypothyroid patients are converted to a euthyroid state
Theophylline levels decrease when hypothyroid patients converted to a euthyroid state
Increased toxicity: Thyroid may potentiate the hypoprothrombinemic effect of oral anticoagulants

Pregnancy Risk Factor A
Lactation Enters breast milk/compatible
Nursing Implications Monitor pulse rate and blood pressure

Tiagabine

CAS Number 115103-54-3
U.S. Brand Names Gabitril®
Synonyms Tiagabine Hydrochloride
Use Adjunctive therapy in adults and children ≥12 years of age in the treatment of partial seizures
Mechanism of Action Prolongs action of GABA by inhibiting its reuptake into presynaptic neurons
Adverse Reactions

All adverse effects are dose related

Central nervous system: Dizziness, headache, somnolence, CNS depression, ataxia, amnesia, coma, dizziness (27% to 31%), seizures (5%)

Gastrointestinal: Gingivitis, stomatitis, nausea (11%), vomiting (7%), diarrhea (2% to 10%), abdominal pain (5% to 7%)

Hematologic: Thrombocytopenia

Neuromuscular & skeletal: Tremor (9% to 21%), weakness, myoclonus, myalgia (2% to 5%)

Ocular: Amblyopia (4% to 9%)

Signs and Symptoms of Overdose Seizures can occur with ingestions over one gram in adults or more than 100 mgm in children.

Clinical Effects Reported After Overdose with Tiagabine

Symptom	No. of Patients with Reported Effect	Percent of Total
Lethargy	32	56%
Seizures		
Multiple discrete	16	28%
Status epilepticus	3	5%
Single	2	4%
Agitation	18	32%
Confusion	17	30%
Coma	16	28%
Tachycardia	15	26%
Respiratory depression	12	21%
Tremors	11	19%
Dizziness	6	11%
Dystonias/abnormal posturing	6	11%
Hallucinations	3	5%
Hypertension	3	5%
Hypotension	2	4%

Admission Criteria/Prognosis Admit any ingestion >300 mg.
Pharmacodynamics/Kinetics

Absorption: Rapid (45 minutes); prolonged with food

Protein binding: 96%, primarily to albumin and α_1-acid glycoprotein

Metabolism: Hepatic via CYP (primarily 3A4)

Bioavailability: Oral: Absolute: 90%

Half-life elimination: 2-5 hours when administered with enzyme inducers; 7-9 hours when administered without enzyme inducers

Time to peak, plasma: 45 minutes

Excretion: Feces (63%); urine (25%); 2% as unchanged drug; primarily as metabolites

Dosage Oral (administer with food):

Patients receiving enzyme-inducing AED regimens:

Children 12-18 years: 4 mg once daily for 1 week; may increase to 8 mg daily in 2 divided doses for 1 week; then may increase by 4-8 mg weekly to response or up to 32 mg daily in 2-4 divided doses

Adults: 4 mg once daily for 1 week; may increase by 4-8 mg weekly to response or up to 56 mg daily in 2-4 divided doses; usual maintenance: 32-56 mg/day

Patients **not** receiving enzyme-inducing AED regimens: The estimated plasma concentrations of tiagabine in patients not taking enzyme-inducing medications is twice that of patients receiving enzyme-inducing AEDs. Lower doses are required; slower titration may be necessary.

Monitoring Parameters A reduction in seizure frequency is indicative of therapeutic response to tiagabine in patients with partial seizures; complete blood counts, renal function tests, liver function tests, and routine blood chemistry should be monitored periodically during therapy

Contraindications Hypersensitivity to tiagabine or any component of the formulation

Warnings

New-onset seizures and status epilepticus have been associated with tiagabine use when taken for unlabeled indications. Often these seizures have occurred shortly after the initiation of treatment or shortly after a dosage increase. Seizures have also occurred with very low doses or after several months of therapy. In most cases, patients were using concomitant medications (eg, antidepressants, antipsychotics, stimulants, narcotics). In these instances, the discontinuation of tiagabine, followed by an evaluation for an underlying seizure disorder, is suggested. Use for unapproved indications, however, has not been proven to be safe or effective and is not recommended. When tiagabine is used as an adjunct in partial seizures (an FDA-approved indication), it should not be abruptly discontinued because of the possibility of increasing seizure frequency, unless safety concerns require a more rapid withdrawal. Rarely, nonconvulsive status epilepticus has been reported following abrupt discontinuation or dosage reduction.

Use with caution in patients with hepatic impairment. Experience in patients not receiving enzyme-inducing drugs has been limited; caution should be used in treating any patient who is not receiving one of these medications (decreased dose and slower titration may be required). Weakness, sedation, and confusion may occur with tiagabine use. Patients must be cautioned about performing tasks which require mental alertness (eg, operating machinery or driving). Effects with other sedative drugs or ethanol may be potentiated. Animal studies suggest that tiagabine may bind to retina and uvea; however, no treatment-related ophthalmoscopic changes were seen long-term; periodic monitoring may be considered. May cause serious rash, including Stevens-Johnson syndrome. Safety and efficacy have not been established in children <12 years of age.

Dosage Forms Tablet, as hydrochloride: 2 mg, 4 mg, 6 mg, 8 mg, 10 mg, 12 mg, 16 mg

Reference Range

Maximal plasma level after a 24 mg/dose: 552 ng/mL

Serum level of 710 ng/mL has been associated with status epilepticus following an overdose.

Overdosage/Treatment

Decontamination: Lavage (within 1 hour)/activated charcoal

Supportive therapy: Myoclonus and seizures responds to I.V. benzodiazepines.

Enhancement of elimination: Due to this drug undergoing enterohepatic recirculation, multiple dosing of activated charcoal may be effective

Drug Interactions Substrate of 3A4 (major)

CNS depressants: Sedative effects may be additive with other CNS depressants; monitor for increased effect; includes ethanol, sedatives, antidepressants, narcotic analgesics, other anticonvulsants, and benzodiazepines

CYP3A4 inducers: CYP3A4 inducers may decrease the levels/effects of tiagabine. Example inducers include aminoglutethimide, carbamazepine, nafcillin, nevirapine, phenobarbital, phenytoin, and rifamycins.

CYP3A4 inhibitors: May increase the levels/effects of tiagabine. Example inhibitors include azole antifungals, clarithromycin, diclofenac, doxycycline, erythromycin, imatinib, isoniazid, nefazodone, nicardipine, propofol, protease inhibitors, quinidine, telithromycin, and verapamil.

Valproate: Increased free tiagabine concentrations (*in vitro*) by 40%

Pregnancy Risk Factor C
Lactation Enters breast milk/not recommended
Specific References

Fulton JA, Hoffman RS, and Nelson LS, "Tiagabine Overdose: A Case of Status Epilepticus in a Non-Epileptic Patient," *Clin Toxicol (Phila)*. 2005, 43(7):869-71

Kazzi SN, Jones CM, Cragin LS, et al, "Retrospective Review of Exposures to Tiagabine as Reported to a Regional Poison Center," *Clin Toxicol (Phila)*, 2005, 43:728.

Kazzi ZN, Jones CC, and Morgan BW, "Seizures in a Pediatric Patient with a Tiagabine Overdose," *J Med Toxicol*, 2006, 2(4):160-2.

Kazzi Z, Jones C, Hamilton E, et al, "Tiagabine Overdose in a Toddler Resulting in Seizure Activity," *J Toxicol Clin Toxicol*, 2004, 42(5):721.

Spiller HA, Winter ML, Ryan M, et al, "Retrospective Evaluation of Tiagabine Overdose," *Clin Toxicol (Phila)*, 2005, 43(7):855-9 (review).

Tsutaoka BT and Wiegand TJ, "Seizures Associated with Tiagabine Overdose: A Case Series," *Clin Toxicol (Phila)*, 2005, 43:734.

Tiapride

CAS Number 51012-32-9; 51012-33-0
Impairment Potential Yes
Unlabeled/Investigational Use Management of behavioral disorders and dyskinesias; also used for alcohol withdrawal
Mechanism of Action A dopamine (D_2 receptor) antagonist (a substituted benzamide)
Adverse Reactions

Cardiovascular: Orthostatic hypotension, torsade de pointes

Central nervous system: Drowsiness, tardive dyskinesia (in the elderly), malignant neuroleptic syndrome, dystonia

Dermatologic: Erythema

Endocrine & metabolic: Hyperprolactinemia

Admission Criteria/Prognosis Admit ingestion >3 g

Toxicodynamics/Kinetics
Absorption: 1.4 hours
Distribution: V_d: 1.43 L/kg
Protein binding: Low
Metabolism: Hepatic to N-monodesethyl tiapride
Bioavailability: 75%
Half-life: 3-4 hours
Elimination: Urine (50% to 75%)

Dosage Alcohol detoxification: 100 mg 3 times/day
Extrapyramidal symptomatology: 100-300 mg/day (reduce dosage in renal insufficiency)

Reference Range Following 100 mg oral dose, peak plasma tiapride level is ~1.47 mcg/mL

Overdosage/Treatment
Decontamination: Oral: Activated charcoal
Supportive therapy: Dystonia can be treated with tetrabenzamide and clozapine; biperidine and sulpiride has been also used to treat dystonia with less effect

Ticlopidine

CAS Number 53885-35-1; 55142-85-3
U.S. Brand Names Ticlid®
Synonyms Ticlopidine Hydrochloride
Use Prophylaxis of thromboembolic complications; intermittent claudication; prevention of platelet loss during extracorporeal circulatory procedures; may improve graft patency in coronary artery bypass grafts, improves exercise performance in patients with coronary artery disease. May prevent vaso-occlusive crisis in sickle cell disease; may improve mortality in postmyocardial infarction patients; may offer postoperative protective against deep vein thrombosis; may have some antirheumatic activity. Reduces risk for stroke or transient ischemic attacks. Can reduce proteinuria and hematuria while elevating creatinine clearance in patients with glomerulonephritis.
Unlabeled/Investigational Use Protection of aortocoronary bypass grafts, diabetic microangiopathy, ischemic heart disease, prevention of postoperative DVT, reduction of graft loss following renal transplant
Mechanism of Action Ticlopidine is an inhibitor of platelet function with a mechanism which is different from other antiplatelet drugs. The drug significantly increases bleeding time. This effect may not be solely related to ticlopidine's effect on platelets. The prolongation of the bleeding time caused by ticlopidine is further increased by the addition of aspirin; no inhibition on prostaglandin metabolism is noted.

Adverse Reactions
Central nervous system: Dizziness
Dermatologic: **Skin rash**, ecchymosis, dermatitis, urticaria, pruritus, acute generalized exanthematous pustulosis, toxic erythroderma, angioneurotic edema
Gastrointestinal: Diarrhea, nausea, vomiting, GI pain, GI bleed, anorexia, flatulence
Hematologic: Neutropenia, thrombocytopenia (usually within 3 months of starting therapy), agranulocytosis, anemia, prolonged bleeding time, aplastic anemia, hemolytic/uremic syndrome; thrombotic thrombocytopenic purpura (develops within 1 month of therapy)
Hepatic: Elevated liver function tests, cholestatic jaundice, cholestasis, cholestatic hepatitis
Ocular: Retinal vasculitis
Otic: Tinnitus
Renal: Hematuria, interstitial nephritis, renal insufficiency
Respiratory: Epistaxis, bronchiolitis obliterans

Signs and Symptoms of Overdose Abdominal pain, ataxia, confusion, hematologic abnormalities, hypotension, metabolic acidosis, retinal vasculitis, seizures, tachycardia, vomiting

Pharmacodynamics/Kinetics
Onset of action: Within 6 hours
Peak: Achieved after 3-5 days of oral therapy; serum levels do not correlate with clinical antiplatelet activity
Duration of action: 4-10 days
Protein binding: 98%
Metabolism: Extensively in the liver and has at least one active metabolite, a 2-keto derivative (PCR 3787)
Bioavailability: Oral: 80% to 90%
Half-life, elimination: 24 hours (acute); 30-50 hours (chronic)
Elimination: Fecal: 60%; Urine: 25%

Dosage Adults: Oral: 1 tablet twice daily with food; maximum daily dose: 750 mg
Monitoring Parameters Signs of bleeding; CBC with differential every 2 weeks starting the second week through the third month of treatment; more frequent monitoring is recommended for patients whose absolute neutrophil counts have been consistently declining or are 30% less than baseline values. The peak incidence of TTP occurs between 3-4 weeks, the peak incidence of neutropenia occurs at approximately 4-6 weeks, and the incidence of aplastic anemia peaks after 4-8 weeks of therapy.

Few cases have been reported after 3 months of treatment. Liver function tests (alkaline phosphatase and transaminases) should be performed in the first 4 months of therapy if liver dysfunction is suspected.
Administration Oral: Administer with food.
Contraindications Hypersensitivity to ticlopidine or any component of the formulation; active pathological bleeding such as PUD or intracranial hemorrhage; severe liver dysfunction; hematopoietic disorders (neutropenia, thrombocytopenia, a past history of TTP)
Warnings Use with caution in patients who may have an increased risk of bleeding (such as, ulcers). Consider discontinuing 10-14 days before elective surgery. Use caution in mixing with other antiplatelet drugs. Use with caution in patients with severe liver disease or severe renal impairment (experience is limited). **[U.S. Boxed Warning]: May cause life-threatening hematologic reactions, including neutropenia, agranulocytosis, thrombotic thrombocytopenia purpura (TTP), and aplastic anemia.** Routine monitoring is required (see Monitoring Parameters). Monitor for signs and symptoms of neutropenia including WBC count. Discontinue if the absolute neutrophil count falls to <1200/mm^3 or if the platelet count falls to <80,000/mm^3.
Dosage Forms Tablet, as hydrochloride: 250 mg
Reference Range An oral dose of 1 g produces a peak blood ticlopidine concentration of 1.2 mg/L

Overdosage/Treatment
Decontamination: Activated charcoal
Supportive therapy: Seizures should initially be treated with diazepam or lorazepam; if recurrent, phenobarbital or phenytoin can be given; monitor fluid and electrolyte status; granulocyte-stimulating factor can be used to treat neutropenia; high-dose corticosteroid therapy can be useful against aplastic anemia or prolongation of bleeding time; plasmapheresis should be considered for patients exhibiting thrombocytopenic purpura

Test Interactions ↑ cholesterol (S) (8% to 10%), alkaline phosphatase, transaminases (S)
Drug Interactions Substrate of CYP3A4 (major); **Inhibits** CYP1A2 (weak), 2C9 (weak), 2C19 (strong), 2D6 (moderate), 2E1 (weak), 3A4 (weak)
Antacids reduce absorption of ticlopidine (~18%).
Anticoagulants or other antiplatelet agents may increase the risk of bleeding; use with caution.
Carbamazepine blood levels may be increased by ticlopidine.
Cimetidine increases ticlopidine levels.
Cyclosporine blood levels may be reduced by ticlopidine.
CYP2C19 substrates: Ticlopidine may increase the levels/effects of CYP2C19 substrates. Example substrates include citalopram, diazepam, methsuximide, phenytoin, propranolol, and sertraline.
CYP2D6 substrates: Ticlopidine may increase the levels/effects of CYP2D6 substrates. Example substrates include amphetamines, selected beta-blockers, dextromethorphan, fluoxetine, lidocaine, mirtazapine, nefazodone, paroxetine, risperidone, ritonavir, thioridazine, tricyclic antidepressants, and venlafaxine.
CYP2D6 prodrug substrates: Ticlopidine may decrease the levels/effects of CYP2D6 prodrug substrates. Example prodrug substrates include codeine, hydrocodone, oxycodone, and tramadol.
CYP3A4 inducers: CYP3A4 inducers may decrease the levels/effects of ticlopidine. Example inducers include aminoglutethimide, carbamazepine, nafcillin, nevirapine, phenobarbital, phenytoin, and rifamycins.
Digoxin blood levels may be decreased by ticlopidine.
Phenytoin blood levels may be increased by ticlopidine (case reports).
Theophylline blood levels may be increased by ticlopidine.
Pregnancy Risk Factor B
Pregnancy Implications No evidence for teratogenesis in mice/rabbit studies
Lactation Excretion in breast milk unknown
Additional Information Discontinue use 10-14 days prior to surgery; ingestion of 10 g in an adult can cause metabolic acidosis; ingestion of 6 g in an adult resulted in liver function test abnormalities

Specific References
Gorelick PB, Richardson D, Kelly M, et al, "Aspirin and Ticlopidine for Prevention of Recurrent Stroke in Black Patients: A Randomized Trial," *JAMA*, 2003 289(22):2947-57.
Makkar K, Wilensky RL, Julien MB, et al, "Rash with Both Clopidogrel and Ticlopidine in Two Patients Following Percutaneous Coronary Intervention with Drug-Eluting Stents," *Ann Pharmacother*, 2006, 40(6):1204-7.
Skurnik YD, Tcherniak A, Edlan K, et al, "Ticlopidine-Induced Cholestatic Hepatitis," *Ann Pharmacother*, 2003, 37(3):371-5.

Tilidine

CAS Number 20380-58-9; 2107-79-5; 24357-97-9
Impairment Potential Yes
Unlabeled/Investigational Use Treat moderate to severe pain
Mechanism of Action Binds to opiate receptors in the CNS, causing inhibition of ascending pain pathways, altering the perception of and

response to pain; produces generalized CNS depression; a cogenor of atropine

Adverse Reactions

Central nervous system: Hallucinations, dizziness, confusion

Dermatologic: Pruritus

Gastrointestinal: Nausea, vomiting, salivation

Hematologic: Porphyrinogenic

Neuromuscular & skeletal: Tremors, hyperreflexia, hyperactive deep tendon reflexes, clonus, myoclonus

Ocular: Miosis

Respiratory: Apnea, respiratory depression

Toxicodynamics/Kinetics

Onset of action: Oral: 15-30 minutes

Duration of action: 4-6 hours

Distribution: V_d: 3.71 L/kg

Metabolism: Hepatic to nortilidine (active metabolite) and bis-nortilidine

Half-life: 5 hours

Dosage Oral:

Children >2 years: 5 mg plus 2.5 mg per year of age, not to exceed 1 mg/kg

Adults: 50-100 mg up to 4 times/day; maximum daily dose: 400 mg

Parenteral: Up to 400 mg

Rectal: 75 mg 4 times/day

Dosing adjustment in renal impairment: Reduce dose

Reference Range Maximum tilidine plasma concentration of 907 ng/mL achieved after 50 mg dose (I.V.); nortilidine peak plasma level after a 50 mg dose: 69 ng/mL

Overdosage/Treatment

Decontamination: Activated charcoal

Supportive therapy: Naloxone hydrochloride (0.4-2 mg I.V., SubQ, or through an endotracheal tube); a continuous infusion (at $^2/_3$ the response dose/hour) may be required

Antidote(s)

- Nalmefene [ANTIDOTE]
- Naloxone [ANTIDOTE]

Additional Information Often combined orally with naloxone (ie, Valoron N®)

Timolol

Related Information

- Selected Properties of Beta-Adrenergic Blocking Drugs
- Therapeutic Drugs Associated with Hallucinations

CAS Number 26839-75-8; 26921-17-5

U.S. Brand Names Betimol®; Blocadren®; Timoptic-XE®; Timoptic® OcuDose®; Timoptic®

Synonyms Timolol Hemihydrate; Timolol Maleate

Use Ophthalmic dosage form used to treat elevated intraocular pressure such as glaucoma or ocular hypertension; orally for treatment of hypertension and angina and reduce mortality following myocardial infarction and prophylaxis of migraine; may exacerbate myasthenia gravis

Mechanism of Action Blocks both beta$_1$-adrenergic and beta$_2$-adrenergic receptors, reduces intraocular pressure by reducing aqueous humor production or possibly outflow; reduces blood pressure by blocking adrenergic receptors and decreasing sympathetic outflow, produces a negative chronotropic and inotropic activity through an unknown mechanism

Adverse Reactions

Ophthalmic:

Ocular: **Conjunctival hyperemia**, anisocoria, corneal punctate keratitis, keratitis, corneal staining, decreased corneal sensitivity, eye pain, vision disturbances

Miscellaneous: Systemic allergic reaction (anaphylaxis, angioedema, rash, urticaria)

Systemic:

Cardiovascular: Arrhythmias, chest pain, bradycardia, palpitations, edema, congestive heart failure, reduced peripheral circulation, orthostatic hypotension, Raynaud's phenomenon

Central nervous system: **Drowsiness, insomnia**, mental depression, confusion (especially in the elderly), hallucinations, headache, nervousness, memory loss, nightmares

Dermatologic: Angioedema, psoriasis, rash, urticaria

Endocrine & metabolic: **Decreased sexual ability**

Gastrointestinal: Diarrhea or constipation, nausea, vomiting, stomach discomfort

Genitourinary: Retroperitoneal fibrosis

Hematologic: Leukopenia, thrombocytopenia

Respiratory: Bronchospasm, dyspnea

Miscellaneous: Cold extremities, anaphylaxis

Signs and Symptoms of Overdose Ataxia, bradycardia, confusion, depression, dyspnea, heart failure, hypertension, hypoglycemia, impotence, myasthenia gravis (exacerbation or precipitation), severe hypotension, wheezing

Pharmacodynamics/Kinetics

Onset of action:

Hypotensive: Oral: 15-45 minutes

Peak effect: 0.5-2.5 hours

Intraocular pressure reduction: Ophthalmic: 30 minutes

Peak effect: 1-2 hours

Duration: ~4 hours; Ophthalmic: Intraocular: 24 hours

Protein binding: 60%

Metabolism: Extensively hepatic; extensive first-pass effect

Half-life elimination: 2-2.7 hours; prolonged with renal impairment

Excretion: Urine (15% to 20% as unchanged drug)

Dosage Children and Adults: Ophthalmic:

Solution: Initial: 0.25% solution, instill 1 drop twice daily; increase to 0.5% solution if response not adequate; decrease to 1 drop/day if controlled; do not exceed 1 drop twice daily of 0.5% solution

Gel-forming solution (Timoptic-XE®): Instill 1 drop (either 0.25% or 0.5%) once daily

Adults: Oral:

Hypertension: Initial: 10 mg twice daily, increase gradually every 7 days, usual dosage: 20-40 mg/day in 2 divided doses; maximum: 60 mg/day

Prevention of myocardial infarction: 10 mg twice daily initiated within 1-4 weeks after infarction

Migraine headache: Initial: 10 mg twice daily, increase to maximum of 30 mg/day

Monitoring Parameters Blood pressure, apical and radial pulses, fluid I & O, daily weight, respirations, mental status, and circulation in extremities before and during therapy

Administration Ophthalmic: Administer other topically-applied ophthalmic medications at least 10 minutes before Timoptic-XE®; wash hands before use; invert closed bottle and shake once before use; remove cap carefully so that tip does not touch anything; hold bottle between thumb and index finger; use index finger of other hand to pull down the lower eyelid to form a pocket for the eye drop and tilt head back; place the dispenser tip close to the eye and gently squeeze the bottle to administer 1 drop; remove pressure after a single drop has been released; **do not allow the dispenser tip to touch the eye**; replace cap and store bottle in an upright position in a clean area; do **not** enlarge hole of dispenser; do **not** wash tip with water, soap, or any other cleaner. Some ophthalmic solutions contain benzalkonium chloride; wait at least 10 minutes after instilling solution before inserting soft contact lenses.

Contraindications Hypersensitivity to timolol or any component of the formulation; sinus bradycardia; sinus node dysfunction; heart block greater than first degree (except in patients with a functioning artificial pacemaker); cardiogenic shock; uncompensated cardiac failure; bronchospastic disease; pregnancy (2nd and 3rd trimesters)

Warnings

Administer cautiously in compensated heart failure and monitor for a worsening of the condition. **[U.S. Boxed Warning]: Beta-blocker therapy should not be withdrawn abruptly (particularly in patients with CAD), but gradually tapered to avoid acute tachycardia, hypertension, and/or ischemia.** Use caution with concurrent use of beta-blockers and either verapamil or diltiazem; bradycardia or heart block can occur. Beta-blockers can aggravate symptoms in patients with PVD. Patients with bronchospastic disease should generally not receive beta-blockers; monitor closely if used in patients with potential risk of bronchospasm. Use cautiously in diabetics because it can mask prominent hypoglycemic symptoms. Can mask signs of thyrotoxicosis. Can cause fetal harm when administered in pregnancy. Use cautiously in severe renal impairment: marked hypotension can occur in patients maintained on hemodialysis. Use care with anesthetic agents which decrease myocardial function. Can worsen myasthenia gravis.

Ophthalmic: Systemic absorption and adverse effects may occur, including bradycardia and/or hypotension. Should not be used alone in angle-closure glaucoma (has no effect on pupillary constriction). Multidose vials have been associated with development of bacterial keratitis; avoid contamination.

Dosage Forms

Note: Unless otherwise specified, strength expressed as base.

Gel-forming solution, ophthalmic, as maleate: 0.25% (5 mL); 0.5% (2.5 mL, 5 mL)

Timoptic-XE®: 0.25% (5 mL); 0.5% (5 mL)

Solution, ophthalmic, as hemihydrate:

Betimol®: 0.25% (5 mL, 10 mL, 15 mL); 0.5% (5 mL, 10 mL, 15 mL) [contains benzalkonium chloride]

Solution, ophthalmic, as maleate: 0.25% (5 mL, 10 mL, 15 mL); 0.5% (5 mL, 10 mL, 15 mL) [contains benzalkonium chloride]

Istalol™: 0.5% (10 mL) [contains benzalkonium chloride and potassium sorbate]

Timoptic®: 0.25% (5 mL); 0.5% (5 mL, 10 mL) [contains benzalkonium chloride]

Solution, ophthalmic, as maleate [preservative free]:

Timoptic® in OcuDose®: 0.25% (0.2 mL); 0.5% (0.2 mL) [single use]

Tablet, as maleate: 5 mg, 10 mg, 20 mg [strength expressed as salt]

Blocadren®: 20 mg [strength expressed as salt]

Reference Range Following single 20 mg dose, levels may range from 60-114 ng/mL

Overdosage/Treatment

Decontamination: Lavage (within 1 hour)/activated charcoal; **do not** use ipecac

Supportive therapy: Sympathomimetics (eg, epinephrine or dopamine), glucagon, atropine or a pacemaker can be used to treat the toxic bradycardia, asystole, and/or hypotension; initially, fluids may be the best treatment for toxic hypotension

Enhancement of elimination: Multiple dosing of activated charcoal may be effective

Test Interactions ↑ cholesterol (S), glucose

Drug Interactions Substrate of CYP2D6 (major); Inhibits CYP2D6 (weak)

Albuterol (and other beta$_2$ agonists): Effects may be blunted by nonspecific beta-blockers.

Alpha-blockers (prazosin, terazosin): Concurrent use of beta-blockers may increase risk of orthostasis.

AV conduction-slowing agents (digoxin): Effects may be additive with beta-blockers.

Clonidine: Hypertensive crisis after or during withdrawal of either agent (not reported with timolol ophthalmic solution)

CYP2D6 inhibitors: May increase the levels/effects of timolol. Example inhibitors include chlorpromazine, delavirdine, fluoxetine, miconazole, paroxetine, pergolide, quinidine, quinine, ritonavir, and ropinirole.

Epinephrine (including local anesthetics with epinephrine): Timolol may cause hypertension.

Glucagon: Timolol may blunt hyperglycemic action.

Insulin and oral hypoglycemics: May mask symptoms of hypoglycemia.

NSAIDs (ibuprofen, indomethacin, naproxen, piroxicam) may reduce the antihypertensive effects of beta-blockers.

Salicylates may reduce the antihypertensive effects of beta-blockers.

Sulfonylureas: Beta-blockers may alter response to hypoglycemic agents.

Verapamil or diltiazem may have synergistic or additive pharmacological effects when taken concurrently with beta-blockers.

Pregnancy Risk Factor C (manufacturer); D (2nd and 3rd trimesters - expert analysis)

Pregnancy Implications No data available on whether timolol crosses the placenta. Beta-blockers have been associated with bradycardia, hypotension, hypoglycemia, and intrauterine growth rate (IUGR); IUGR is probably related to maternal hypertension. Available evidence suggests beta-blockers are generally safe during pregnancy (JNC-7). Cases of neonatal hypoglycemia have been reported following maternal use of beta-blockers at parturition or during breast-feeding.

Lactation Enters breast milk/use caution (AAP rates "compatible")

Nursing Implications Apply gentle pressure to lacrimal sac during and immediately following instillation (1 minute) to avoid systemic absorption; stop drug if breathing difficulty occurs

Additional Information First beta-blocker approved for treatment of the postmyocardial infarction patient; does not cause night blindness.

Tirilazad

Unlabeled/Investigational Use Subarachnoid hemorrhage, spinal cord injury, stroke, head traumas

Mechanism of Action A 21-aminosteroid with antioxidant effects similar to methylprednisolone; inhibits lipid peroxidation

Adverse Reactions

Cardiovascular: Tachycardia (supraventricular), tachycardia (ventricular), palpitations, tachycardia, sinus tachycardia, arrhythmias (ventricular)

Central nervous system: Lightheadedness, drowsiness, headache

Gastrointestinal: Nausea, abdominal pain

Hepatic: Elevated liver function tests

Neuromuscular & skeletal: Muscle cramps, leg cramps

Toxicodynamics/Kinetics

Distribution: V$_d$:3 L/kg (single dose); 16-30 L/kg (multiple doses)

Protein binding: 99%

Metabolism: Hepatic

Half-life: 16 hours

Elimination: Feces

Dosage Subarachnoid hemorrhage: I.V.: 2-6 mg/kg/day up to 10 days

Spinal cord injury: 10 mg/kg/day for 2 days is being investigated

Reference Range Peak serum levels after a 3 mg/kg dose: 11.2 mcg/L in men and 7.4 mcg/mL in women

Overdosage/Treatment

Supportive therapy: Supportive and symptomatic treatment, including I.V. fluids and Trendelenburg positioning, should be initiated as intoxication may cause hypotension. Although calcium (calcium chloride I.V. 1-2 g in adults or 10-30 mg/kg in children over 5-10 minutes with repeats as needed) has been used as an "antidote" for acute intoxications, there is limited experience to support its routine use and should be reserved for those cases where definite signs of myocardial depression are evident. Heart block may respond to isoproterenol, glucagon, atropine and/or calcium, although a temporary pacemaker may be required; norepinephrine, dopamine, or inamrinone for refractory hypotension.

Additional Information As of December 28, 1994, clinical trials of this agent were suspended in treatment of head trauma due to increase in mortality compared to placebo; no glucocorticoid activity; probably most effective when used within 4 hours postinjury

Tirofiban

CAS Number 142373-60-2; 144494-65-5; 150915-40-5

U.S. Brand Names Aggrastat®

Synonyms MK383; Tirofiban Hydrochloride

Use In combination with heparin, indicated for the treatment of acute coronary syndrome, including patients who are to be managed medically and those undergoing PTCA or atherectomy. In this setting, it has been shown to decrease the rate of a combined endpoint of death, new myocardial infarction or refractory ischemia/repeat cardiac procedure.

Mechanism of Action Blocks platelet glycoprotein IIb/IIIa receptors; an antiplatelet agent. A reversible antagonist of fibrinogen binding to the GP IIb/IIIa receptor, the major platelet surface receptor involved in platelet aggregation. When administered intravenously, it inhibits *ex vivo* platelet aggregation in a dose- and concentration-dependent manner. When given according to the recommended regimen, >90% inhibition is attained by the end of the 30-minute infusion. Platelet aggregation inhibition is reversible following cessation of the infusion.

Adverse Reactions

Bleeding is the major drug-related adverse effect. Major bleeding was reported in 1.4% to 2.2%, minor bleeding in 10.5% to 12%, transfusion was required in 4.0% to 4.3%.

>1% (nonbleeding adverse events):

Cardiovascular: Bradycardia, coronary artery dissection, edema (2%)

Central nervous system: Dizziness, fever (>1%), headache (>1%), vasovagal reaction

Gastrointestinal: Nausea (>1%)

Genitourinary: Pelvic pain

Hematologic: Thrombocytopenia: <90,000/mm^3 (1.5%)

Neuromuscular & skeletal: Leg pain

Miscellaneous: Diaphoresis

<1%: Intracranial bleeding (0.0% to 0.1%), GI bleeding (0.1% to 0.2%), retroperitoneal bleeding (0.0% to 0.6%), GU bleeding (0.0% to 0.1%), thrombocytopenia: <50,000/mm^3 (0.3%)

Signs and Symptoms of Overdose Bleeding is the most frequent manifestation of overdose

Pharmacodynamics/Kinetics

Distribution: 35% unbound

Metabolism: Minimally hepatic

Half-life elimination: 2 hours

Excretion: Urine (65%) and feces (25%) primarily as unchanged drug

Clearance: Elderly: Reduced by 19% to 26%

Dosage

Adults: I.V.: Initial rate of 0.4 mcg/kg/minute for 30 minutes and then continued at 0.1 mcg/kg/minute; dosing should be continued through angiography and for 12-24 hours after angioplasty or atherectomy. See table.

Tirofiban Dosing (Using 50 mcg/mL Concentration)				
Patient Weight (kg)	Patients with Normal Renal Function		Patients with Renal Dysfunction	
	30-Min Loading Infusion Rate (mL/h)	Maintenance Infusion Rate (mL/h)	30-Min Loading Infusion Rate (mL/h)	Maintenance Infusion Rate (mL/h)
30-37	16	4	8	2
38-45	20	5	10	3
46-54	24	6	12	3
55-62	28	7	14	4
63-70	32	8	16	4
71-79	36	9	18	5
80-87	40	10	20	5
88-95	44	11	22	6
96-104	48	12	24	6
105-112	52	13	26	7
113-120	56	14	28	7
121-128	60	15	30	8
128-137	64	16	32	8
138-145	68	17	34	9
146-153	72	18	36	9

Dosing adjustment in severe renal impairment: $Cl_{cr} < 30$ mL/minute: Reduce dose to 50% of normal rate

Stability Store at 25°C (77°F); do not freeze. Protect from light during storage.

Monitoring Parameters Platelet count. Hemoglobin and hematocrit should be monitored prior to treatment, within 6 hours following loading infusion, and at least daily thereafter during therapy. Platelet count may need to be monitored earlier in patients who received prior glycoprotein IIb/IIIa antagonists. Persistent reductions of platelet counts $< 90,000/mm^3$ may require interruption or discontinuation of infusion. Because tirofiban requires concurrent heparin therapy, aPTT levels should also be followed. Monitor vital signs and laboratory results prior to, during, and after therapy. Assess infusion insertion site during and after therapy (every 15 minutes or as institutional policy). Observe and teach patient bleeding precautions (avoid invasive procedures and activities that could result in injury). Monitor closely for signs of unusual or excessive bleeding (eg, CNS changes, blood in urine, stool, or vomitus, unusual bruising or bleeding). Breast-feeding is contraindicated.

Administration Intended for intravenous delivery using sterile equipment and technique. Do not add other drugs or remove solution directly from the bag with a syringe. Do not use plastic containers in series connections; such use can result in air embolism by drawing air from the first container if it is empty of solution. Discard unused solution 24 hours following the start of infusion. May be administered through the same catheter as heparin. Tirofiban injection must be diluted to a concentration of 50 mcg/mL (premixed solution does not require dilution).

Contraindications Hypersensitivity to tirofiban or any component of the formulation; active internal bleeding or a history of bleeding diathesis within the previous 30 days; history of intracranial hemorrhage, intracranial neoplasm, arteriovenous malformation, or aneurysm; history of thrombocytopenia following prior exposure; history of CVA within 30 days or any history of hemorrhagic stroke; major surgical procedure or severe physical trauma within the previous month; history, symptoms, or findings suggestive of aortic dissection; severe hypertension (systolic BP >180 mm Hg and/or diastolic BP >110 mm Hg); concomitant use of another parenteral GP IIb/IIIa inhibitor; acute pericarditis

Warnings Bleeding is the most common complication. Watch closely for bleeding, especially the arterial access site for the cardiac catheterization. Prior to pulling the sheath, heparin should be discontinued for 3-4 hours and ACT <180 seconds or aPTT <45 seconds. Use standard compression techniques after sheath removal. Watch the site closely afterwards for further bleeding. Use with extreme caution in patients with platelet counts <150,000/mm³, patients with hemorrhagic retinopathy, and chronic dialysis patients. Use caution with administration of other drugs affecting hemostasis. Adjust the dose with severe renal dysfunction (Cl_{cr} <30 mL/minute). The use of tirofiban, aspirin and heparin together causes more bleeding than aspirin and heparin alone. Do not administer in the same I.V. line as diazepam.

Dosage Forms
Infusion [premixed in sodium chloride]: 50 mcg/mL (100 mL, 250 mL)
Injection, solution: 250 mcg/mL (50 mL)

Overdosage/Treatment
Decontamination: Oral: Lavage (within 1 hour)/activated charcoal
Supportive therapy: Cessation of therapy and assessment for transfusion. Tirofiban has a relatively short half-life and its platelet effects dissipate rather quickly. However, when immediate reversal is required, platelet transfusions can be useful. Tirofiban is dialyzable. Seizures should initially be treated with diazepam or lorazepam; if recurrent, phenobarbital or phenytoin can be given; monitor fluid and electrolyte status; granulocyte-stimulating factor can be used to treat neutropenia; high-dose corticosteroid therapy can be useful against aplastic anemia or prolongation of bleeding time

Drug Interactions
Cephalosporins which contain the MTT side chain may theoretically increase the risk of hemorrhage.
Drugs which affect platelet function (eg, aspirin, NSAIDs, dipyridamole, ticlopidine, clopidogrel) may potentiate the risk of hemorrhage.
Heparin and aspirin: Use with aspirin and heparin is associated with an increase in bleeding over aspirin and heparin alone. However, the concurrent use of aspirin and heparin has also improved the efficacy of tirofiban.
Levothyroxine and omeprazole increase tirofiban clearance; however, the clinical significance of this interaction remains to be demonstrated.
Thrombolytic agents theoretically may increase the risk of hemorrhage.
Warfarin and oral anticoagulants: Risk of bleeding may be increased during concurrent therapy.
Other IIb/IIIa antagonists: Concomitant use of other injectable glycoprotein IIb/IIIa antagonists is contraindicated (see Contraindications).

Pregnancy Risk Factor B
Lactation Excretion in breast milk unknown/contraindicated

Tizanidine

CAS Number 51322-75-9
U.S. Brand Names Zanaflex®
Synonyms Sirdalud®
Impairment Potential Yes
Use Skeletal muscle relaxant used for treatment of muscle spasticity, tension headaches
Unlabeled/Investigational Use Tension headaches, low back pain, and trigeminal neuralgia
Mechanism of Action An alpha$_2$-adrenergic agonist agent which decreases excitatory input to alpha motor neurons; an imidazole derivative which acts as a centrally acting muscle relaxant with alpha$_2$-adrenergic agonist properties; acts on the level of the spinal cord
Adverse Reactions
Cardiovascular: **Hypotension**, bradycardia, palpitations, sinus bradycardia
Central nervous system: Insomnia, fatigue, headache, dizziness, **drowsiness, sedation, somnolence**
Dermatologic: Pruritus
Gastrointestinal: Nausea, vomiting, **xerostomia**
Neuromuscular & skeletal: Tremor, **muscle weakness**
Signs and Symptoms of Overdose Bradycardia, dry mouth, hypotension
Pharmacodynamics/Kinetics
Duration: 3-6 hours
Bioavailability: 40%
Metabolism: Extensively hepatic
Half-life elimination: 2 hours
Time to peak, serum:
Fasting state: Capsule, tablet: 1 hour
Fed state: Capsule: 3-4 hours, Tablet: 1.5 hours
Excretion: Urine (60%); feces (20%)
Dosage Muscle spasm: Initial: Oral: 2-4 mg 3 times/day; maximum daily dose:
36 mg
Tension headache: Initial: 2 mg 3 times/day; can titrate after 2 week intervals to a maximum daily dose: 18 mg
Reduce dosage in renal or hepatic impairment
Monitoring Parameters Monitor liver function (aminotransferases) at baseline, 1, 3, 6 months and then periodically thereafter; monitor ophthalmic function
Administration Capsules may be opened and contents sprinkled on food; however, extent of absorption is increased up to 20% relative to administration of the capsule under fasted conditions.
Contraindications Hypersensitivity to tizanidine or any component of the formulation; concomitant therapy with ciprofloxacin or fluvoxamine or other potent inhibitors of CYP1A2
Warnings Reduce dose in patients with liver or renal disease. May cause significant orthostatic hypotension or bradycardia; use with caution in patients with hypotension or cardiac disease. Tizanidine clearance is reduced by more than 50% in elderly patients with renal insufficiency (Cl_{cr} <25 mL/minute) compared to healthy elderly subjects; this may lead to a longer duration of effects and, therefore, should be used with caution in renally impaired patients. Due to extensive hepatic metabolism, avoid use or use extreme caution in patents with hepatic impairment.
Dosage Forms Capsule:
Zanaflex®: 2 mg, 4 mg, 6 mg
Tablet: 2 mg, 4 mg
Zanaflex®: 2 mg [DSC], 4 mg
Reference Range
Peak serum level after a 12 mg oral dose: ~12 ng/mL
Postortem heart blood tizanidine level was 2.3 mg/L in a fatality.
Overdosage/Treatment
Decontamination: Activated charcoal
Supportive therapy: Benzodiazepines for seizure control; atropine can be given for treatment of bradycardia; flumazenil has been used to reverse coma successfully; hypotension may respond to I.V. crystalloid infusion
Enhancement of elimination: Forced diuresis is not helpful; multiple dosing of activated charcoal may be helpful. Following attempts to enhance drug elimination, hypotension should be treated with I.V. fluids and/or Trendelenburg positioning
Antidote(s)
● Flumazenil [ANTIDOTE]
Drug Interactions
Substrate of CYP1A2 (major)
Baclofen, other CNS depressants: Additive CNS depression may occur.
CYP1A2 inhibitors (potent): May increase the levels/effects of tizanidine. Significant effects (hypotension) may occur. Example inhibitors include ketoconazole, norfloxacin, ofloxacin, and rofecoxib. Concurrent use is contraindicated.
Ciprofloxacin: May increase the levels/effects (eg, hypotension) of tizanidine. Concurrent use is contraindicated.

Diuretics, other alpha adrenergic agonists, antihypertensives: Additive hypotensive effects may occur.

Fluvoxamine: May increase levels/effects (eg, hypotension) of tizanidine. Contraindicated.

Mirtazapine: May antagonize the alpha-agonist effects of tizanidine.

Oral contraceptives: May decrease the clearance of tizanidine.

Pregnancy Risk Factor C

Lactation Excretion in breast milk unknown/not recommended

Additional Information Food increases maximum concentration of tizanidine by 33% and reduces the time to peak by 40 minutes; extent of absorption is unchanged

Tizanidine, 20 mg/day, is similar in efficacy to baclofen, 50 mg/day, in treating spasticity due to cerebrovascular lesions

Specific References

Adamson LA, Spiller HA, and Bosse GM, "Tizanidine (Zanaflex®) Exposure," *J Toxicol Clin Toxicol*, 2003, 41(5):664.

Cox D, Sklerov JH, Moore KA, et al, "Tizanidine Distribution in a Postmortem Case," *J Anal Toxicol*, 2006, 30:153.

Sklerov JH, Cox DE, Moore KA, et al, "Tizanidine Distribution in a Postmortem Case," *J Anal Toxicol*, 2006, 30:331.

Spiller HA, Bosse GM, and Adamson LA, "Retrospective Review of Tizanidine (Zanaflex®) Overdose," *J Toxicol Clin Toxicol*, 2004, 42(5):593-6.

Tocainide

Related Information

● Therapeutic Drugs Associated with Hallucinations

CAS Number 35891-93-1; 41708-72-9

U.S. Brand Names Tonocard® [DSC]

Synonyms Tocainide Hydrochloride

Use Suppresses and prevents symptomatic ventricular arrhythmias; limited effectiveness in tachycardia (ventricular)

Unlabeled/Investigational Use Trigeminal neuralgia

Mechanism of Action Suppresses automaticity of conduction tissue, by increasing electrical stimulation threshold of ventricle, His-Purkinje system, and spontaneous depolarization of the ventricles during diastole by a direct action on the tissues; blocks both the initiation and conduction of nerve impulses by decreasing the neuronal membrane's permeability to sodium ions, which results in inhibition of depolarization with resultant blockade of conduction

Adverse Reactions

Similar to lidocaine and mexiletine

Cardiovascular: Hypotension, bradycardia, tachycardia, tachycardia (ventricular), palpitations, heart block, pericardial effusion, sinus tachycardia, arrhythmias (ventricular), sinus bradycardia

Central nervous system: **Dizziness, nervousness, confusion, ataxia**, lightheadedness, visual hallucinations, seizures, paranoid psychosis, memory disturbance, paranoia, psychosis

Dermatologic: Rash, skin lesions, Stevens-Johnson syndrome, erythema multiforme

Gastrointestinal: **Nausea, anorexia**, vomiting, diarrhea

Hematologic: Agranulocytosis, anemia, leukopenia, neutropenia, aplastic anemia, thrombocytopenia

Hepatic: Granulomatous hepatitis

Neuromuscular & skeletal: **Tremors**, paresthesia

Ocular: Nystagmus, diplopia

Otic: Tinnitus

Renal: Glomerulonephritis

Respiratory: **Pulmonary fibrosis**, respiratory arrest,

Miscellaneous: Exacerbation of lupus erythematosus, diaphoresis, systemic lupus erythematosus

Signs and Symptoms of Overdose Anorexia, AV block, delirium, diuresis, exfoliative dermatitis, heart block, hematuria, leukopenia or neutropenia (agranulocytosis, granulocytopenia), metallic taste, pericarditis, tachycardia (ventricular), tinnitus

Pharmacodynamics/Kinetics

Absorption: Oral: 99% to 100%

Distribution: V_d: 1.62-3.2 L/kg

Protein binding: 10% to 20%

Metabolism: Hepatic to inactive metabolites; negligible first-pass effect

Half-life elimination: 11-14 hours; Renal and hepatic impairment: 23-27 hours

Time to peak, serum: 30-160 minutes

Excretion: Urine (40% to 50% as unchanged drug)

Dosage Adults: Oral: 1200-1800 mg/day in 3 divided doses, up to 2400 mg/day

Dosing adjustment in renal impairment: Cl_{cr} <30 mL/minute: Administer 50% of normal dose or 600 mg once daily

Dosing adjustment in hepatic impairment: Maximum daily dose: 1200 mg

Monitoring Parameters Monitor for tremor; titration of dosing and initiation of therapy require cardiac monitoring

Contraindications Hypersensitivity to tocainide, any component of the formulation, or any local anesthetics of the amide type; second- or third-degree heart block (except in patients with a functioning artificial pacemaker)

Warnings Watch for proarrhythmic effects. Correct electrolyte imbalances before initiating (especially hypokalemia and hyperkalemia). Use cautiously in heart failure. Adjust dose in patients with significant renal or hepatic impairment. Bone marrow depression can rarely occur during the first 3 months of therapy.

Dosage Forms [DSC] = Discontinued product

Tablet, as hydrochloride [DSC]: 400 mg, 600 mg

Reference Range Therapeutic: 4-10 mcg/mL (SI: 18-43 μmol/L); toxic: >12 mcg/mL (SI: 52 μmol/L)

Overdosage/Treatment

Decontamination: Lavage (within 1 hour)/activated charcoal

Supportive therapy: Seizures can be treated with lorazepam or diazepam, phenytoin, or phenobarbital; do not use isoproterenol for arrhythmia treatment. Hypotension can be managed with isotonic saline, with placement in Trendelenburg position; dopamine or norepinephrine can also be used for refractory hypotension; pacemaker placement may need to be performed for heart block.

Enhancement of elimination: Hemodialysis (for 4 hours) or hemoperfusion are effective; moderately dialyzable (20% to 50%)

Drug Interactions

Inhibits CYP1A2 (weak)

Rifampin may reduce tocainide blood levels.

Urinary alkalinizers (antacids, sodium bicarbonate, acetazolamide) may increase tocainide blood levels.

Pregnancy Risk Factor C

Pregnancy Implications Does not appear to be teratogenic

Lactation Enters breast milk/contraindicated

Nursing Implications Monitor for tremor; titration of dosing and initiation of therapy require cardiac monitoring

Additional Information Minimum lethal dose: 16 g; response correlates with response to lidocaine

---

TOLAZamide

CAS Number 1156-19-0

U.S. Brand Names Tolinase®

Use Adjunct to diet for the management of mild to moderately severe, stable, noninsulin-dependent (type II) diabetes mellitus

Mechanism of Action Stimulates insulin release from the pancreatic beta cells; reduces glucose output from the liver; insulin sensitivity is increased at peripheral target sites

Adverse Reactions

Cardiovascular: Sinus tachycardia, tachycardia (supraventricular)

Central nervous system: **Headache**, ataxia, **dizziness**

Dermatologic: Rash, hives, photosensitivity, purpura, pruritus, exanthem

Endocrine & metabolic: Disulfiram reactions, hypoglycemia, hyperinsulinemia

Gastrointestinal: **Anorexia, vomiting, nausea**, abdominal pain, **diarrhea, constipation, heartburn, epigastric fullness**

Genitourinary: Porphyrinogenic

Hematologic: Leukopenia, thrombocytopenia, aplastic anemia, hemolysis, bone marrow suppression, agranulocytosis, porphyria

Hepatic: Jaundice, cholestasis

Neuromuscular & skeletal: Weakness, fasciculations, paresthesia

Miscellaneous: Systemic lupus erythematosus

Signs and Symptoms of Overdose Diuresis, hypoglycemia, hyponatremia, leukopenia or neutropenia (agranulocytosis, granulocytopenia), lichenoid eruptions, photophobia

Pharmacodynamics/Kinetics

Onset of action: 4-6 hours

Duration: 10-24 hours

Protein binding: >98%

Metabolism: Extensively hepatic to one active and three inactive metabolites

Half-life elimination: 7 hours

Excretion: Urine

Dosage Oral (doses >1000 mg/day normally do not improve diabetic control):

Adults: Initial: 100 mg/day, increase at 2- to 4-week intervals; maximum dose: 1000 mg; give as a single or twice daily dose

Conversion from insulin → tolazamide

10 units day = 100 mg/day

20-40 units/day = 250 mg/day

>40 units/day = 250 mg/day and 50% of insulin dose

Doses >500 mg/day should be given in 2 divided doses

Dosing comments in hepatic impairment: Initial and maintenance doses should be conservative

Monitoring Parameters Signs and symptoms of hypoglycemia (fatigue, sweating, numbness of extremities); urine for glucose and ketones; fasting blood glucose; hemoglobin A_{1c} or fructosamine

Contraindications Hypersensitivity to tolazamide, sulfonylureas, or any component of the formulation; type 1 diabetes mellitus (insulin dependent, IDDM) therapy; diabetes complicated by ketoacidosis; pregnancy

Warnings

False-positive response has been reported in patients with liver disease, idiopathic hypoglycemia of infancy, severe malnutrition, acute pancreatitis, renal dysfunction. Transferring a patient from one sulfonylurea to another does not require a priming dose; doses >1000 mg/day normally do not improve diabetic control. Has not been studied in older patients; however, except for drug interactions, it appears to have a safe profile and decline in renal function does not affect its pharmacokinetics. How "tightly" an elderly patient's blood glucose should be controlled is controversial; however, a fasting blood sugar <150 mg/dL is now an acceptable end point. Such a decision should be based on the patient's functional and cognitive status, how well they recognize hypoglycemic or hyperglycemic symptoms, and how to respond to them and their other disease states.

Chemical similarities are present among sulfonamides, sulfonylureas, carbonic anhydrase inhibitors, thiazides, and loop diuretics (except ethacrynic acid). Use in patients with sulfonylurea allergy is specifically contraindicated in product labeling, however, a risk of cross-reaction exists in patients with allergy to any of these compounds; avoid use when previous reaction has been severe.

Product labeling states oral hypoglycemic drugs may be associated with an increased cardiovascular mortality as compared to treatment with diet alone or diet plus insulin. Data to support this association are limited, and several studies, including a large prospective trial (UKPDS) have not supported an association.

Dosage Forms [DSC] = Discontinued product

Tablet: 100 mg, 250 mg, 500 mg

Tolinase® [DSC]: 100 mg, 250 mg

Reference Range Fasting blood glucose: Adults: 80-140 mg/dL; Elderly: 100-180 mg/dL

Overdosage/Treatment

Decontamination: Lavage (within 1 hour)/activated charcoal

Supportive therapy: Glucose (25 g I.V.) is mainstay of therapy. Glucagon (1-5 mg I.V., I.M., or SubQ) (0.03-0.1 mg/kg in pediatrics) will have limited benefit; diazoxide is a third-line agent (3-8 mg/kg/24 hours); octreotide (50 mcg SubQ every 12 hours) may be helpful in sulfonylurea overdose.

Enhancement of elimination: Multiple dosing of activated charcoal may be effective; not dialyzable (0% to 5%)

Antidote(s)

- Dextrose [ANTIDOTE]
- Glucagon [ANTIDOTE]
- Octreotide [ANTIDOTE]

Diagnostic Procedures

- Electrolytes, Blood
- Glucose, Random

Drug Interactions Increased toxicity: Monitor patient closely; large number of drugs interact with sulfonylureas including salicylates, anticoagulants, H_2 antagonists, TCAs, MAO inhibitors, beta-blockers, thiazides

Pregnancy Risk Factor D

Pregnancy Implications Can cause neonatal hypoglycemia

Lactation Excretion in breast milk unknown

Nursing Implications Patients who are anorexic or NPO may need to have their dose held to avoid hypoglycemia

Specific References

Johnson KK, Green DL, Rife JP, et al, "Sulfonamide Cross-Reactivity: Fact or Fiction?" *Ann Pharmacother*, 2005, 39(2):290-301.

Tolazoline

CAS Number 59-97-2; 59-98-3

U.S. Brand Names Priscoline® [DSC]

Synonyms Benzazoline Hydrochloride; Tolazoline Hydrochloride

Use Treatment of persistent pulmonary vasoconstriction and hypertension of the newborn (persistent fetal circulation), peripheral vasospastic disorders

Mechanism of Action Competitively blocks alpha-adrenergic receptors to produce brief antagonism of circulating epinephrine and norepinephrine; reduces hypertension caused by catecholamines and causes vascular smooth muscle relaxation (direct action); results in peripheral vasodilation and decreased peripheral resistance

Adverse Reactions

Cardiovascular: **Hypotension**, peripheral vasodilation, tachycardia, palpitations (5%), hypertension, arrhythmias, edema, flushing, pulmonary hypertension, vasodilation

Central nervous system: Vertigo (5%)

Endocrine & metabolic: **Hypochloremic alkalosis**

Gastrointestinal: **GI bleeding, abdominal pain**, vomiting, nausea, diarrhea

Hematologic: **Thrombocytopenia**, agranulocytosis (increased), pancytopenia, leukopenia

Local: **Burning at injection site**

Neuromuscular & skeletal: Increased pilomotor activity, piloerection

Ocular: Mydriasis (in premature infants), ptosis

Renal: **Acute renal failure, oliguria**

Respiratory: Alveolar hemorrhage, pulmonary hemorrhage, dyspnea

Miscellaneous: Secretions (increased)

Pharmacodynamics/Kinetics

Half-life elimination: Neonates: 3-10 hours; prolonged with renal impairment

Time to peak, serum: Within 30 minutes

Excretion: Urine (primarily as unchanged drug)

Dosage

Neonates: Initial: I.V.: 1-2 mg/kg over 10-15 minutes via scalp vein or upper extremity; maintenance: 1-2 mg/kg/hour; use lower maintenance doses in patients with decreased renal function. Also used in neonates for acute vasospasm "cath toes" at 0.25 mg/kg/hour (no load); maximum dose: 6-8 mg/kg/hour

Dosing interval in renal impairment in newborns: Urine output <0.9 mL/kg/hour: Decrease dose to 0.08 mg/kg/hour for every 1 mg/kg of loading dose

Adults: Peripheral vasospastic disorder:

Oral: 25-50 mg 4 times/day

I.M., I.V., SubQ: 10-50 mg 4 times/day

Stability Compatible in D_5W, $D_{10}W$, and saline solutions

Monitoring Parameters Vital signs, blood gases, cardiac monitor

Administration I.V.: Usual maximum concentration: 0.1 mg/mL

Contraindications Hypersensitivity to tolazoline or any component of the formulation; known or suspected coronary artery disease

Warnings Stimulates gastric secretion and may activate stress ulcers; therefore, use with caution in patients with gastritis, peptic ulcer; use with caution in patients with mitral stenosis

Dosage Forms [DSC] = Discontinued product

Injection, solution, as hydrochloride [DSC]: 25 mg/mL (4 mL)

Overdosage/Treatment

Supportive therapy: For treatment of hypotension, I.V. crystalloid infusion while lowering the head can be performed; for refractory cases, intravenous ephedrine (10-25 mg slow I.V. push in adults or 0.2-0.3 mg/kg every 4-6 hours in children) can be used.

Drug Interactions

Decreased effect (vasopressor) of epinephrine followed by a rebound increase in blood pressure

Increased toxicity: Disulfiram reaction may possibly be seen with concomitant ethanol use

Pregnancy Risk Factor C

Nursing Implications Dilute in D_5W; monitor blood pressure for hypotension; observe limbs for change in color; do not mix with any other drug in syringe or bag

---

TOLBUTamide

CAS Number 473-41-6; 64-77-7

U.S. Brand Names Orinase Diagnostic® [DSC]; Tol-Tab®

Synonyms Tolbutamide Sodium

Use Adjunct to diet for the management of mild to moderately severe, stable, noninsulin-dependent (type II) diabetes mellitus

Mechanism of Action A sulfonylurea hypoglycemic agent; its ability to lower elevated blood glucose levels in patients with functional pancreatic beta cells is similar to the other sulfonylurea agents; stimulates synthesis and release of endogenous insulin from pancreatic islet tissue. The hypoglycemic effect is attributed to an increased sensitivity of insulin receptors and improved peripheral utilization of insulin. Suppression of glucagon secretion may also contribute to the hypoglycemic effects of tolbutamide.

Adverse Reactions

Cardiovascular: Venospasm, tachycardia, tachycardia (atrial), sinus tachycardia, tachycardia (supraventricular)

Central nervous system: **Headache, dizziness**, ataxia, seizures

Dermatologic: Pruritus, systemic contact dermatitis, Stevens-Johnson syndrome, toxic epidermal necrolysis, urticaria, purpura, licheniform eruptions, exanthem, photoallergic reaction

Endocrine & metabolic: Hypoglycemia, disulfiram-type reactions, syndrome of inappropriate antidiuretic hormone, hyperinsulinemia, hyponatremia

Gastrointestinal: **Anorexia, constipation, heartburn, epigastric fullness, diarrhea**, nausea, vomiting

Hematologic: Leukopenia, thrombocytopenia, porphyria

Hepatic: Jaundice, cholestasis, granulomatous liver disease (noncaseating), elevated transaminases, primary biliary cirrhosis

Local: Thrombophlebitis, phlebitis

Neuromuscular & skeletal: Weakness, fasciculations, paresthesia

Ocular: Retrobulbar neuritis

Otic: Ototoxicity, tinnitus, otic neuropathy

Respiratory: Eosinophilic pneumonia
Miscellaneous: Hypersensitivity reaction, scotoma, fixed drug eruption

Signs and Symptoms of Overdose Eczema, hypoglycemia, hypothyroidism, leukopenia or neutropenia (agranulocytosis, granulocytopenia), photophobia, photosensitivity

Pharmacodynamics/Kinetics
Onset of action: Peak effect: Hypoglycemic action: Oral: 1-3 hours
Duration: Oral: 6-24 hours
Absorption: Oral: Rapid
Distribution: V_d: 6-10 L; increased with decreased albumin concentrations
Protein binding: 95% to 97%, primarily to albumin
Metabolism: Hepatic to hydroxymethyltolbutamide (mildly active) and carboxytolbutamide (inactive); metabolism does not appear to be affected by age
Half-life elimination: Plasma: 4-25 hours; Elimination: 4-9 hours
Time to peak, serum: 3-5 hours
Excretion: Urine (<2% as unchanged drug, primarily as metabolites)

Dosage Divided doses may improve gastrointestinal tolerance
Adults:
Oral: Initial: 1-2 g/day as a single dose in the morning or in divided doses throughout the day. Total doses may be taken in the morning; however, divided doses may allow increased gastrointestinal tolerance. Maintenance dose: 0.25-3 g/day; however, a maintenance dose >2 g/day is seldom required.
I.V. bolus: 1 g over 2-3 minutes
Elderly: Oral: Initial: 250 mg 1-3 times/day; usual: 500-2000 mg; maximum: 3 g/day

Dosing adjustment in renal impairment: Adjustment is not necessary
Hemodialysis: Not dialyzable (0% to 5%)

Dosing adjustment in hepatic impairment: Reduction of dose may be necessary in patients with impaired liver function

Stability Use parenteral formulation within 1 hour following reconstitution

Monitoring Parameters Fasting blood glucose, hemoglobin A_{1c} or fructosamine

Administration Oral: Entire dose can be administered in AM, divided doses may improve GI tolerance

Contraindications Hypersensitivity to tolbutamide, sulfonylureas, or any component of the formulation; diabetes complicated by ketoacidosis; treatment of type 1 diabetes; pregnancy

Warnings
False-positive response has been reported in patients with liver disease, idiopathic hypoglycemia of infancy, severe malnutrition, acute pancreatitis. Because of its low potency and short duration, it is a useful agent in the elderly if drug interactions can be avoided. How "tightly" an elderly patient's blood glucose should be controlled is controversial; however, a fasting blood sugar <150 mg/dL is now an acceptable end point. Such a decision should be based on the patient's functional and cognitive status, how well they recognize hypoglycemic or hyperglycemic symptoms, and how to respond to them and their other disease states.
Chemical similarities are present among sulfonamides, sulfonylureas, carbonic anhydrase inhibitors, thiazides, and loop diuretics (except ethacrynic acid). Use in patients with sulfonylurea allergy is specifically contraindicated in product labeling, however, a risk of cross-reaction exists in patients with allergy to any of these compounds; avoid use when previous reaction has been severe.
Product labeling states oral hypoglycemic drugs may be associated with an increased cardiovascular mortality as compared to treatment with diet alone or diet plus insulin. Data to support this association are limited, and several studies, including a large prospective trial (UKPDS) have not supported an association.

Dosage Forms Tablet: 500 mg

Reference Range Fasting blood glucose: Adults: 80-140 mg/dL; Elderly: 100-180 mg/dL

Overdosage/Treatment
Decontamination: Lavage (within 1 hour)/activated charcoal
Supportive therapy: Glucose (25 g I.V.) is mainstay of therapy. Glucagon (1-5 mg I.V., I.M., or SubQ) (0.03-0.1 mg/kg in pediatrics) will have limited benefit; diazoxide is a third-line agent (3-8 mg/kg/24 hours); octreotide (50 mcg SubQ every 12 hours) may be helpful in sulfonylurea overdose.
Enhancement of elimination: Multiple dosing of activated charcoal may be effective; not dialyzable (0% to 5%)

Antidote(s)
• Dextrose [ANTIDOTE]
• Glucagon [ANTIDOTE]
• Octreotide [ANTIDOTE]

Diagnostic Procedures
• Electrolytes, Blood
• Glucose, Random

Drug InteractionsSubstrate of CYP2C9 (major), 2C19 (minor); **Inhibits** CYP2C8 (weak), 2C9 (strong)
CYP2C9 inducers: May decrease the levels/effects of tolbutamide. Example inducers include carbamazepine, phenobarbital, phenytoin, rifampin, rifapentine, and secobarbital.

CYP2C9 Inhibitors may increase the levels/effects of tolbutamide. Example inhibitors include delavirdine, fluconazole, gemfibrozil, ketoconazole, nicardipine, NSAIDs, and sulfonamides.
CYP2C9 Substrates: Tolbutamide may increase the levels/effects of CYP2C9 substrates. Example substrates include bosentan, dapsone, fluoxetine, glimepiride, glipizide, losartan, montelukast, nateglinide, paclitaxel, phenytoin, warfarin, and zafirlukast.
Increased effects with salicylates, probenecid, MAO inhibitors, chloramphenicol, insulin, phenylbutazone, antidepressants, metformin, H_2 antagonists, and others
Decreased effects:
Hypoglycemic effects may be decreased by beta-blockers, cholestyramine, hydantoins, thiazides, rifampin, and others
Ethanol may decrease the half-life of tolbutamide

Pregnancy Risk Factor D

Pregnancy Implications Abnormal blood glucose levels are associated with a higher incidence of congenital abnormalities. Insulin is the drug of choice for the control of diabetes mellitus during pregnancy.

Lactation Enters breast milk/compatible

Nursing Implications Patients who are anorexic or NPO may need to have their dose held to avoid hypoglycemia

Additional Information Sodium content of 1 g vial: 3.5 mEq

Specific References
Johnson KK, Green DL, Rife JP, et al, "Sulfonamide Cross-Reactivity: Fact or Fiction?" *Ann Pharmacother*, 2005, 39(2):290-301.

Tolmetin

Related Information
• Nonsteroidal Anti-inflammatory Drugs

CAS Number 26171-23-3 (Base); 35711-34-3 (Anhydrous Sodium); 64490-92-2 (Dihydrate Sodium)

U.S. Brand Names Tolectin® DS; Tolectin®

Synonyms Tolmetin Sodium

Use Treatment of rheumatoid arthritis and osteoarthritis, juvenile rheumatoid arthritis

Mechanism of Action Inhibits prostaglandin synthesis by decreasing the activity of the enzyme, cyclooxygenase, which results in decreased formation of prostaglandin precursors

Adverse Reactions
Cardiovascular: Circulatory collapse
Central nervous system: **Dizziness**, headache, aseptic meningitis, psychosis, cognitive dysfunction, coma, seizures
Dermatologic: **Rash**, pruritus, angioedema, toxic epidermal necrolysis, purpura, exanthem
Endocrine & metabolic: Hyperkalemia, anion gap metabolic acidosis, fluid retention, gynecomastia
Gastrointestinal: **Abdominal cramps, heartburn, indigestion, nausea**, vomiting, GI bleeding, GI ulceration, constipation, diarrhea, dyspepsia, esophageal ulceration, aphthous stomatitis, xerostomia, stomatitis
Hematologic: Leukopenia, neutropenia, agranulocytosis, granulocytopenia, aplastic anemia (rare), platelet inhibition
Hepatic: Elevated transaminases, hepatitis (fulminant), hepatic necrosis
Otic: Ototoxicity, tinnitus
Renal: Renal failure (acute), nephrotic syndrome, proteinuria, chronic renal failure, albuminuria
Respiratory: Wheezing, respiratory depression
Miscellaneous: Hypersensitivity, systemic lupus erythematosus

Signs and Symptoms of Overdose Cognitive dysfunction, drowsiness, gastritis, GI bleeding, nausea, nephrotic syndrome, ototoxicity, thrombocytopenia, tinnitus, vomiting, wheezing. Severe poisoning can manifest with coma, hypotension, renal and/or hepatic failure, respiratory depression, seizures

Pharmacodynamics/Kinetics
Onset of action: Analgesic: 1-2 hours; Anti-inflammatory: Days to weeks
Absorption: Well absorbed
Bioavailability: Reduced 16% with food or milk
Half-life elimination: Biphasic: Rapid: 1-2 hours; Slow: 5 hours
Time to peak, serum: 30-60 minutes
Excretion: Urine (as inactive metabolites or conjugates) within 24 hours

Dosage
Oral:
Children ≥2 years:
Anti-inflammatory: Initial: 20 mg/kg/day in 3 divided doses, then 15-30 mg/kg/day in 3 divided doses
Analgesic: 5-7 mg/kg/dose every 6-8 hours
Adults: 400 mg 3 times/day; usual dose: 600-1.8 g/day; maximum: 2 g/day

Monitoring Parameters Occult blood loss, CBC, liver enzymes, BUN, serum creatinine, periodic liver function test

Contraindications Hypersensitivity to tolmetin, aspirin, other NSAIDs, or any component of the formulation; perioperative pain in the setting of coronary artery bypass surgery (CABG); pregnancy (3rd trimester or near term)

Warnings

[U.S. Boxed Warning]: NSAIDs are associated with an increased risk of adverse cardiovascular events, including MI, stroke, and new onset or worsening of pre-existing hypertension. Risk may be increased with duration of use or pre-existing cardiovascular risk-factors or disease. Carefully evaluate individual cardiovascular risk profiles prior to prescribing. Use caution with fluid retention, CHF or hypertension.

Use of NSAIDs can compromise existing renal function. Renal toxicity can occur in patient with impaired renal function, dehydration, heart failure, liver dysfunction, those taking diuretics and ACEI and the elderly. Rehydrate patient before starting therapy. Monitor renal function closely. Use caution in patients with advanced renal disease.

[U.S. Boxed Warning]: NSAIDs may increase risk of gastrointestinal irritation, ulceration, bleeding, and perforation. These events may occur at any time during therapy and without warning. Use caution in patients with a history of GI disease (bleeding or ulcers), concurrent therapy with aspirin, anticoagulants and/or corticosteroids, smoking, use of alcohol, the elderly or debilitated patients.

Use the lowest effective dose for the shortest duration of time, consistent with individual patient goals, to reduce risk of cardiovascular or GI adverse events. Alternate therapies should be considered for patients at high risk.

NSAIDs may cause serious skin adverse events including exfoliative dermatitis, Stevens-Johnson syndrome (SJS) and toxic epidermal necrolysis (TEN). Anaphylactoid reactions may occur, even without prior exposure; patients with "aspirin triad" (bronchial asthma, aspirin intolerance, rhinitis) may be at increased risk. Do not use in patients who experience bronchospasm, asthma, rhinitis, or urticaria with NSAID or aspirin therapy.

Use with caution in patients with decreased hepatic function. Closely monitor patients with any abnormal LFT. Severe hepatic reactions (eg, fulminant hepatitis, liver failure) have occurred with NSAID use, rarely; discontinue if signs or symptoms of liver disease develop, or if systemic manifestations occur.

The elderly are at increased risk for adverse effects (especially peptic ulceration, CNS effects, renal toxicity) from NSAIDs even at low doses.

Withhold for at least 4-6 half-lives prior to surgical or dental procedures. Safety and efficacy have not been established in children <2 years of age.

Dosage Forms

Capsule: 400 mg

Tablet: 200 mg, 600 mg

Tolectin®: 600 mg [contains sodium 54 mg (2.35 mEq)]

Overdosage/Treatment

Decontamination: Activated charcoal

Supportive therapy: Hypotension/dehydration can be managed with I.V. fluid therapy; acidosis should be treated with bicarbonates, seizures with benzodiazepines; antacids, blood products are indicated, as appropriate, for hemorrhage

Enhancement of elimination: Dialysis or perfusion is indicated for secondary complications, acidosis, or renal failure and not toxin removal alone; multiple dosing of activated charcoal may be effective

Test Interactions ↑ protein

Drug Interactions

ACE inhibitors: Antihypertensive effects may be decreased by concurrent therapy with NSAIDs; monitor blood pressure.

Angiotensin II antagonists: Antihypertensive effects may be decreased by concurrent therapy with NSAIDs; monitor blood pressure.

Anticoagulants (warfarin, heparin, LMWHs) in combination with NSAIDs can cause increased risk of bleeding.

Antiplatelet drugs (ticlopidine, clopidogrel, aspirin, abciximab, dipyridamole, eptifibatide, tirofiban) can cause an increased risk of bleeding.

Beta-blockers: NSAIDs may decrease the antihypertensive effect of beta-blockers. Monitor.

Cholestyramine (and other bile acid sequestrants): May decrease the absorption of NSAIDs. Separate by at least 2 hours.

Corticosteroids may increase the risk of GI ulceration; avoid concurrent use.

Cyclosporine: NSAIDs may increase serum creatinine, potassium, blood pressure, and cyclosporine levels; monitor cyclosporine levels and renal function carefully.

Hydralazine's antihypertensive effect is decreased; avoid concurrent use.

Lithium levels can be increased; avoid concurrent use if possible or monitor lithium levels and adjust dose. Sulindac may have the least effect. When NSAID is stopped, lithium will need adjustment again.

Loop diuretics efficacy (diuretic and antihypertensive effect) may be reduced.

Methotrexate: Severe bone marrow suppression, aplastic anemia, and GI toxicity have been reported with concomitant NSAID therapy. Avoid use during moderate or high-dose methotrexate (increased and prolonged methotrexate levels). NSAID use during low-dose treatment of rheumatoid arthritis has not been fully evaluated; extreme caution is warranted.

Thiazides antihypertensive effects are decreased; avoid concurrent use.

Warfarin's INRs may be increased by piroxicam. Other NSAIDs may have the same effect depending on dose and duration. Monitor INR closely. Use the lowest dose of NSAIDs possible and for the briefest duration.

Pregnancy Risk Factor C/D (3rd trimester or at term)

Lactation Enters breast milk/not recommended (AAP rates "compatible")

Nursing Implications Assess audiometric and ophthalmic exam before, during, and after treatment

Additional Information Sodium content of 200 mg: 0.8 mEq. The only NSAID affected by food/milk, which decreases total bioavailability by 16%. If GI upset occurs with tolmetin, take with antacids other than sodium bicarbonate.

Tolrestat

CAS Number 82964-04-3

Unlabeled/Investigational Use Decrease the adverse effects of diabetes mellitus, specifically diabetic, nephropathy, retinopathy, neuropathy, and cataract formation

Mechanism of Action Carboxylic acid; decreased amounts of sorbitol and fructose are formed from glucose; thus, less water is drawn into the lens (through osmosis) and neurons, thus possibly leading to less diabetic complications

Adverse Reactions

Overdose experience has not been reported

Central nervous system: **Dizziness**

Dermatologic: Rash

Endocrine & metabolic: Hyperchloremic acidosis may occur

Hepatic: Elevated liver enzymes

Toxicodynamics/Kinetics

Absorption: Within 2 hours

Protein binding: 99%

Half-life: 10-13 hours

Elimination: Renal (63% to 68%) and fecal (25% to 27%)

Dosage 200 mg before breakfast or 100 mg twice daily

Reference Range Peak plasma level after a 100 mg oral dose: 5.3-8.8 mcg/mL

Overdosage/Treatment

Decontamination: Lavage (within 1 hour) if >1.2 g ingested; activated charcoal can be given

Enhancement of elimination: Multiple dosing of activated charcoal may be effective

Tolterodine

U.S. Brand Names Detrol® LA; Detrol®

Synonyms Tolterodine Tartrate

Use Treatment of patients with an overactive bladder with symptoms of urinary frequency, urgency, or urge incontinence

Mechanism of Action Tolterodine is a competitive antagonist of muscarinic receptors. In animal models, tolterodine demonstrates selectivity for urinary bladder receptors over salivary receptors. Urinary bladder contraction is mediated by muscarinic receptors. Tolterodine increases residual urine volume and decreases detrusor muscle pressure.

Adverse Reactions

As reported with immediate release tablet, unless otherwise specified

Cardiovascular: Chest pain, tachycardia, peripheral edema, palpitations

Central nervous system: Headache (extended release capsules), somnolence (extended release capsules), fatigue (extended release capsules), dizziness (extended release capsules), anxiety (extended release capsules), hallucinations

Dermatologic: Dry skin, angioedema

Gastrointestinal: **Dry mouth** (extended release capsules), abdominal pain (extended release capsules), constipation (extended release capsules), dyspepsia (extended release capsules), diarrhea, weight gain

Genitourinary: Dysuria (extended release capsules)

Neuromuscular & skeletal: Arthralgia

Ocular: Abnormal vision (extended release capsules), dry eyes (extended release capsules)

Respiratory: Bronchitis, sinusitis (extended release capsules)

Miscellaneous: Anaphylactoid reactions

Admission Criteria/Prognosis Admit any symptomatic patient or with ingestion >5 mg.

Pharmacodynamics/Kinetics

Absorption: Immediate release tablet: Rapid; ≥77%

Distribution: I.V.: V_d: 113±27 L

Protein binding: >96% (primarily to alpha$_1$-acid glycoprotein)

Metabolism: Extensively hepatic, primarily via CYP2D6 (some metabolites share activity) and 3A4 usually (minor pathway). In patients with a genetic deficiency of CYP2D6, metabolism via 3A4 predominates. Forms three active metabolites.

Bioavailability: Immediate release tablet: Increased 53% with food

Half-life elimination:

Immediate release tablet: Extensive metabolizers: ~2 hours; Poor metabolizers: ~10 hours

Extended release capsule: Extensive metabolizers: ~7 hours; Poor metabolizers: ~18 hours

Time to peak: Immediate release tablet: 1-2 hours; Extended release tablet: 2-6 hours

Excretion: Urine (77%); feces (17%); excreted primarily as metabolites (<1% unchanged drug) of which the active 5-hydroxymethyl metabolite accounts for 5% to 14% (<1% in poor metabolizers)

Dosage

Adults: Oral: Initial: 2 mg twice daily; the dose may be lowered to 1 mg twice daily based on individual response and tolerability

Dosing adjustment in patients concurrently taking cytochrome P450 3A4 inhibitors: 1 mg twice daily

Dosing adjustment in renal impairment: Use with caution

Dosing adjustment in hepatic impairment: Administer 1 mg twice daily

Administration Extended release capsule: Swallow whole; do not crush, chew, or open

Contraindications Hypersensitivity to tolterodine or any component of the formulation; urinary retention; gastric retention; uncontrolled narrow-angle glaucoma; myasthenia gravis

Warnings Use with caution in patients with bladder flow obstruction, may increase the risk of urinary retention. Use with caution in patients with gastrointestinal obstructive disorders (ie, pyloric stenosis), may increase the risk of gastric retention. Use with caution in patients with controlled (treated) narrow-angle glaucoma; metabolized in the liver and excreted in the urine and feces, dosage adjustment is required for patients with renal or hepatic impairment. Tolterodine has been associated with QT_c prolongation at high (supratherapeutic) doses. The manufacturer recommends caution in patients with congenital prolonged QT or in patients receiving concurrent therapy with QT_c-prolonging drugs (class Ia or III antiarrhythmics). However, the extent of QT_c prolongation even at supratherapeutic dosages was less than 15 msec. Individuals who are poor metabolizers via CYP2D6 or in the presence of inhibitors of CYP2D6 and CYP3A4 may be more likely to exhibit prolongation. Dosage adjustment is recommended in patients receiving CYP3A4 inhibitors (a lower dose of tolterodine is recommended). Safety and efficacy in pediatric patients have not been established.

Dosage Forms Capsule, extended release, as tartrate (Detrol® LA): 2 mg, 4 mg

Tablet, as tartrate (Detrol®): 1 mg, 2 mg

Reference Range 50% inhibitory blood tolterodine level for salivary stimulation is 6-8 mcg/L

Overdosage/Treatment Decontamination: Lavage within 1 hour/activated charcoal

Drug Interactions

Substrate of CYP2C9 (minor), 2C19 (minor), 2D6 (major), 3A4 (major)

Acetylcholinesterase inhibitors (central): May reduce the therapeutic efficacy of tolterodine.

Anticholinergic agents: Concomitant use with tolterodine may increase the risk of anticholinergic side effects.

Antifungal agents (eg, ketoconazole, fluconazole): May increase the levels/effects of tolterodine; monitor.

CYP2D6 inhibitors: May increase the levels/effects of tolterodine, which may include QT_c prolongation. Example inhibitors include chlorpromazine, delavirdine, fluoxetine, miconazole, paroxetine, pergolide, quinidine, quinine, ritonavir, and ropinirole.

CYP3A4 inducers: CYP3A4 inducers may decrease the levels/effects of tolterodine. Example inducers include aminoglutethimide, carbamazepine, nafcillin, nevirapine, phenobarbital, phenytoin, and rifamycins.

CYP3A4 inhibitors: May increase the levels/effects of tolterodine, which may include QT_c prolongation. Example inhibitors include azole antifungals, clarithromycin, diclofenac, doxycycline, erythromycin, imatinib, isoniazid, nefazodone, nicardipine, propofol, protease inhibitors, quinidine, telithromycin, and verapamil.

Pramlintide: Concomitant use with tolterodine may increase the risk of anticholinergic gastrointestinal adverse effects (eg, reduced gut motility).

Warfarin: Tolterodine may increase the effects of warfarin.

Pregnancy Risk Factor C

Pregnancy Implications Teratogenic effects were observed in some animal studies. There are no adequate and well-controlled studies in pregnant women. Use during pregnancy only if the potential benefit to the mother outweighs the possible risk to the fetus.

Lactation Excretion in breast milk unknown/not recommended

Topiramate

CAS Number 97240-79-4

U.S. Brand Names Topamax®

Use In adults and pediatric patients, adjunctive therapy for partial onset seizures and adjunctive therapy of primary generalized tonic-clonic seizures; treatment of seizures associated with Lennox-Gastaut syndrome

Unlabeled/Investigational Use Infantile spasms, neuropathic pain, cluster headache

Mechanism of Action Blocks voltage-activated sodium neuronal channels thus enhancing the inhibiting neurotransmitter gamma aminobutyric acid (GABA) activity at $GABA_a$ receptors; also attenuates activation of glutamate neuronal receptors

Adverse Reactions

Cardiovascular: Chest pain, edema, AV block

Central nervous system: **Dizziness, ataxia, somnolence, psychomotor slowing, nervousness, memory difficulties, speech problems, fatigue**, language problems, abnormal coordination, confusion, depression, difficulty concentrating, hypoesthesia, hallucinations, psychosis, suicide attempts, delirium, encephalopathy, manic reaction, paranoid reaction, psychosis, suicidal behavior, hyperthermia (severe)

Dermatologic: Photosensitivity, erythema multiforme, pemphigus, Stevens-Johnson syndrome, toxic epidermal necrolysis, alopecia, rash

Endocrine & metabolic: **Serum bicarbonate decreased** (up to 67%; marked reductions to <17 mEq/L have been reported in up to 11% of patients); hot flashes; metabolic acidosis (hyperchloremia, nonanion gap); dehydration

Gastrointestinal: **Nausea**, dyspepsia, abdominal pain, anorexia, constipation, xerostomia, gingivitis, weight loss, diarrhea, vomiting, pancreatitis

Genitourinary: Impotence, dysuria

Hematologic: Bone marrow depression, eosinophilia, granulocytopenia, pancytopenia

Hepatic: Hepatic failure, hepatitis

Neuromuscular & skeletal: **Paresthesia, tremor**, myalgia, weakness, back pain, leg pain, rigors, hypertonia, arthralgia, apraxia, dyskinesia, neuropathy, vertigo, tremor, migraine (aggravated)

Ocular: **Nystagmus, diplopia, abnormal vision**, conjunctivitis, syndrome of acute myopia/secondary angle-closure glaucoma, eye pain

Otic: Hearing decreased, tinnitus

Renal: Nephrolithiasis, renal calculus, renal tubular acidosis

Respiratory: **Upper respiratory infection**, pharyngitis, sinusitis, epistaxis

Miscellaneous: Flu-like symptoms, oligohydrosis

Admission Criteria/Prognosis Overdosage experience is limited; suggest admission if acute neurological symptoms are present or if ingestions exceed 2 g

Pharmacodynamics/Kinetics

Absorption: Good, rapid; unaffected by food

Protein binding: 15% to 41% (inversely related to plasma concentrations)

Metabolism: Hepatic via P450 enzymes

Bioavailability: 80%

Half-life elimination: Mean: Adults: Normal renal function: 21 hours; shorter in pediatric patients; clearance is 50% higher in pediatric patients

Time to peak, serum: ~2-4 hours

Excretion: Urine (~70% to 80% as unchanged drug)

Dialyzable: ~30%

Dosage Oral:

Children 2-16 years: Partial seizures (adjunctive therapy), primary generalized tonic-clonic seizures (adjunctive therapy), or seizure associated with Lennox-Gastaut syndrome: Initial dose titration should begin at 25 mg (or less, based on a range of 1-3 mg/kg/day) nightly for the first week; dosage may be increased in increments of 1-3 mg/kg/day (administered in 2 divided doses) at 1- or 2-week intervals to a total daily dose of 5-9 mg/kg/day.

Adults:

Partial onset seizures (adjunctive therapy), primary generalized tonic-clonic seizures (adjunctive therapy): Initial: 25-50 mg/day; titrate in increments of 25-50 mg per week until an effective daily dose is reached; the daily dose may be increased by 25 mg at weekly intervals for the first 4 weeks; thereafter, the daily dose may be increased by 25-50 mg weekly to an effective daily dose (usually at least 400 mg); usual maximum dose: 1600 mg/day

Note: A more rapid titration schedule has been previously recommended (ie, 50 mg/week), and may be attempted in some clinical situations; however, this may reduce the patient's ability to tolerate topiramate.

Migraine, cluster headache (unlabeled uses): Initial: 25 mg/day, titrated at weekly intervals in 25 mg increments, up to 200 mg/day

Dosing adjustment in renal impairment: Cl_{cr} <70 mL/minute: Administer 50% dose and titrate more slowly

Hemodialysis: Supplemental dose may be needed during hemodialysis

Dosing adjustment in hepatic impairment: Clearance may be reduced

Monitoring Parameters Seizure frequency, hydration status; electrolytes (recommended monitoring includes serum bicarbonate at baseline and periodically during treatment); monitor for symptoms of acute acidosis and complications of long-term acidosis (nephrolithiasis, osteomalacia, and reduced growth rates in children); ammonia level in patients with unexplained lethargy, vomiting, or mental status changes; symptoms of secondary angle closure glaucoma

Administration Oral: May be administered without regard to meals

Capsule sprinkles: May be swallowed whole or opened to sprinkle the contents on soft food (drug/food mixture should not be chewed).

Tablet: Because of bitter taste, tablets should not be broken.

Contraindications Hypersensitivity to topiramate or any component of the formulation

Warnings Key Adverse Reactions:

- Metabolic acidosis (hyperchloremic, nonanion gap): Topiramate may decrease serum bicarbonate concentrations, due to inhibition of carbonic anhydrase and increased renal bicarbonate loss. Decreases in serum bicarbonate are relatively common (7% to 67%) but usually mild to moderate (average decrease of 4 mEq/L at dose of 400 mg/day in adults and 6 mg/kg/day in children). Treatment-emergent metabolic acidosis is less common; however, risk may be increased in patients with a predisposing condition (renal, respiratory and/or hepatic impairment), ketogenic diet, or concurrent treatment with other drugs which may cause acidosis. Metabolic acidosis may occur at dosages as low as 50 mg/day. Serum bicarbonate should be monitored, as well as potential complications of chronic acidosis (nephrolithiasis, osteomalacia, and reduced growth rates in children). Dose reduction or discontinuation (by tapering dose) should be considered in patients with persistent or severe metabolic acidosis. If treatment is continued, alkali supplementation should be considered.
- Kidney stones: The risk of kidney stones is about 2-4 times that of the untreated population, the risk of this event may be reduced by increasing fluid intake.
- Hyperthermia: May be associated (rarely) with severe oligohydrosis and hyperthermia, most frequently in children; use caution and monitor closely during strenuous exercise, during exposure to high environmental temperature, or in patients receiving drugs with anticholinergic activity.
- CNS Effects: Cognitive dysfunction, psychiatric disturbances (mood disorders), and sedation (somnolence or fatigue) may occur with topiramate use; incidence may be related to rapid titration and higher doses. Topiramate may also cause paresthesia and ataxia.
- Withdrawal: Avoid abrupt withdrawal of topiramate therapy, it should be withdrawn/tapered slowly to minimize the potential of increased seizure frequency.

Concurrent Disease:

- Organ dysfunction: Use cautiously in patients with hepatic or renal impairment; dosage adjustment may be required
- Glaucoma: Has been associated with secondary angle-closure glaucoma in adults and children, typically within 1 month of initiation. Discontinue in patients with acute onset of decreased visual acuity or ocular pain.

Concurrent Drug Therapy:

- Valproate: Hyperammonemia with or without encephalopathy may occur and has been documented in patients who have tolerated each drug alone. Risk may be increased in patients with inborn errors of metabolism or decreased hepatic mitochondrial activity. Monitor for lethargy, vomiting, or unexplained changes in mental status.

Special populations:

- Safety and efficacy have not been established in children <2 years of age for adjunctive treatment and <10 years of age for monotherapy.
- Pregnancy: No adequate and well-controlled studies have been conducted; use only if benefit clearly outweighs risk

Dosage Forms Capsule, sprinkle: 15 mg, 25 mg
Tablet: 25 mg, 50 mg, 100 mg, 200 mg

Reference Range

Peak plasma topiramate level after a 1.2 g dose: ~29 mcg/mL
Postmortem blood (central) and vitreous fluid levels following a topiramate overdose was 170 mg/L (490 μmole/L) and 65 mg/L (190 μmole/L), respectively

Overdosage/Treatment

Decontamination: Lavage ingestions >1 g/activated charcoal
Enhanced elimination: Multiple dosing of activated charcoal may be beneficial; topiramate is cleared by hemodialysis at a rate that is almost 6 times that of normal individuals

Drug Interactions

Inhibits CYP2C19 (weak); **Induces** CYP3A4 (weak)
Acetazolamide: Coadministration may increase the chance of nephrolithiasis and/or hyperthermia.
Anticholinergic drugs: Concurrent administration may increase the risk of oligohydrosis and/or hyperthermia; includes drugs with high anticholinergic activity such as antihistamines, cyclic antidepressants, and antipsychotics; use caution
Carbamazepine: May reduce topiramate levels 40%
CNS depressants: Sedative effects may be additive with topiramate; monitor for increased effect; includes barbiturates, benzodiazepines, narcotic analgesics, ethanol, and other sedative agents.
Digoxin: Blood levels of digoxin are decreased when coadministered with topiramate.
Estrogens: Blood levels of estrogens are decreased when coadministered with topiramate, this may lead to a loss of efficacy.
Oral contraceptives: See interaction with Estrogens; use of alternative nonhormonal contraception is recommended.

Phenytoin: May decrease topiramate levels by as much as 48%; topiramate may increase phenytoin concentration by 25%
Valproic acid: Hyperammonemia with or without encephalopathy has been reported in patients who tolerated either drug alone. These drugs may modestly decrease the serum concentrations of the other drug.

Pregnancy Risk Factor C

Pregnancy Implications Topiramate was found to be teratogenic in animal studies; however, there is limited information in pregnant women; use only if benefit to the mother outweighs the risk to the fetus. Based on limited data, topiramate was found to cross the placenta. Postmarketing experience includes reports of hypospadias following *in vitro* exposure to topiramate.

Lactation Enters breast milk/not recommended

Specific References

Adin J, Gomez MC, Blanco Y, et al, "Topiramate Serum Concentration-to-Dose Ratio: Influence of Age and Concomitant Antiepileptic Drugs and Monitoring Implications," *Ther Drug Monit*, 2004, 26(3):251-7.

Bray GA, Hollander P, Klein S, et al, "A 6-Month Randomized, Placebo-Controlled, Dose-Ranging Trial of Topiramate for Weight Loss in Obesity," *Obes Res*, 2003, 11(6):722-33.

Britzi M, Soback S, Isoherranen N, et al, "Analysis of Topiramate and Its Metabolites in Plasma and Urine of Healthy Subjects and Patients with Epilepsy by Use of a Novel Liquid Chromatography-Mass Spectrometry Assay," *Ther Drug Monit*, 2003, 25(3):314-22.

Chung AM and Reed MD, "Intentional Topiramate Ingestion in an Adolescent Female," *Ann Pharmacother*, 2004, 38(9):1439-42.

Cumpston KL and Jones-Lovato H, "Fatal Topiramate Overdose with Antemortem Cardiac Conduction Abnormality and Seizures," *Clin Toxicol (Phila)*, 2005, 43:734.

de Carolis P, Magnifico F, Pierangeli G, et al, "Transient Hypohidrosis Induced by Topiramate," *Epilepsia*, 2003, 44(7):974-6.

Dodson WE, Kamin M, Kraut L, et al, "Topiramate Titration to Response: Analysis of Individualized Therapy Study (TRAITS)," *Ann Pharmacother*, 2003, 37(5):615-20.

Doose DR, Wang SS, Padmanabhan M, et al, "Effect of Topiramate or Carbamazepine on the Pharmacokinetics of an Oral Contraceptive Containing Norethindrone and Ethinyl Estradiol in Healthy Obese and Nonobese Female Subjects," *Epilepsia*, 2003, 44(4):540-9.

Garris SS and Oles KS, "Impact of Topiramate on Serum Bicarbonate Concentrations in Adults," *Ann Pharmacother*, 2005, 39(3):424-6.

Langman LJ, Kaliciak HA, and Boone SA, "Fatal Acute Topiramate Toxicity," *J Anal Toxicol*, 2003, 27(3):323-4.

Lin G and Lawrence R, "Pediatric Case Report of Topiramate Toxicity," *Clin Toxicol (Phila).* , 2006, 44(1):67-9.

Lin G and Lawrence R, "Topamax Toxicity in the Pediatric Population," *J Toxicol Clin Toxicol*, 2004, 42(5):718.

Lindsay S, Mrvos R, and Krenzelok EP, "Toxicity Associated With Pediatric Topiramate Ingestions," *Clin Toxicol (Phila)*. 2005, 43:643.

Marquardt KA, Alsop JA, and Albertson TE, "Unreported Symptoms Seen in a Series of Topiramate Overdoses," *J Toxicol Clin Toxicol*, 2004, 42(5):726.

Perez Bravo A, "Topiramate Use as Treatment in Restless Legs Syndrome," *Actas Esp Psiquiatr*, 2004, 32(3):132-7.

Tebb Z and Tobias JD, "Newer Anticonvulsants - New Adverse Effects," *So Med J*, 2006, 99:375-7.

Traub SJ, Howland MA, Hoffman RS, et al, "Acute Topiramate Toxicity," *J Toxicol Clin Toxicol*, 2003, 41(7):987-90.

Torsemide

CAS Number 56211-40-6; 72810-59-4

U.S. Brand Names Demadex®

Use Management of edema associated with congestive heart failure and hepatic or renal disease; used alone or in combination with antihypertensives in treatment of hypertension; I.V. form is indicated when rapid onset is desired

Mechanism of Action Inhibits reabsorption of sodium and chloride in the ascending loop of Henle and distal renal tubule, interfering with the chloride-binding cotransport system, thus causing increased excretion of water, sodium, chloride, magnesium, and calcium; less potassium loss than furosemide

Adverse Reactions

Cardiovascular: **Orthostatic hypotension**, vasculitis
Central nervous system: Dizziness, headache
Dermatologic: Urticaria, photosensitivity, angioedema, cutaneous vasculitis
Endocrine & metabolic: Hypokalemia, hyponatremia, hypochloremia, alkalosis, dehydration, hyperuricemia
Gastrointestinal: Pancreatitis, nausea, oral solutions may cause diarrhea due to sorbitol content
Hematologic: Agranulocytosis, anemia, thrombocytopenia
Otic: Potential ototoxicity, tinnitus

Renal: Nephrocalcinosis, interstitial nephritis, hypercalciuria, prerenal azotemia, renal vasculitis
Respiratory: Rhinitis, pulmonary vasculitis

Signs and Symptoms of Overdose Agranulocytosis, disorientation, diuresis, granulocytopenia, hyperuricemia, hypokalemia, hyponatremia, hypotension, leukopenia, neutropenia, nocturia

Pharmacodynamics/Kinetics
Onset of action: Diuresis: 30-60 minutes
    Peak effect: 1-4 hours
Duration: ~6 hours
Absorption: Oral: Rapid
Protein binding, plasma: ~97% to 99%
Metabolism: Hepatic (80%) via CYP
Bioavailability: 80% to 90%
Half-life elimination: 2-4; Cirrhosis: 7-8 hours
Excretion: Urine (20% as unchanged drug)

Dosage Adults: Oral, I.V.:
Congestive heart failure: 10-20 mg once daily; may increase gradually for chronic treatment by doubling dose until the diuretic response is apparent (for acute treatment, I.V. dose may be repeated every 2 hours with double the dose as needed)
Chronic renal failure: 20 mg once daily; increase as described above
Hepatic cirrhosis: 5-10 mg once daily with an aldosterone antagonist or a potassium-sparing diuretic; increase as described above
Hypertension: 2.5-5 mg once daily; increase to 10 mg after 4-6 weeks if an adequate hypotensive response is not apparent; if still not effective, an additional antihypertensive agent may be added

Monitoring Parameters Renal function, electrolytes, and fluid status (weight and I & O), blood pressure

Administration I.V. injections should be administered over ≥2 minutes; the oral form may be administered regardless of meal times; patients may be switched from the I.V. form to the oral and vice versa with no change in dose; no dosage adjustment is needed in the elderly or patients with hepatic impairment

To administer as a continuous infusion: 50 mg or 200 mg torsemide should be diluted in 250 mL or 500 mL of compatible solution in plastic containers

Contraindications Hypersensitivity to torsemide, any component of the formulation, or any sulfonylureas; anuria

Warnings
Adjust dose to avoid dehydration. In cirrhosis, avoid electrolyte and acid/base imbalances that might lead to hepatic encephalopathy. Ototoxicity is associated with rapid I.V. administration of other loop diuretics and has been seen with oral torsemide. Do not administer intravenously in less than 2 minutes; single doses should not exceed 200 mg. Hypersensitivity reactions can rarely occur. Monitor fluid status and renal function in an attempt to prevent oliguria, azotemia, and reversible increases in BUN and creatinine. Close medical supervision of aggressive diuresis is required. Monitor closely for electrolyte imbalances particularly hypokalemia and correct when necessary. Coadministration with antihypertensives may increase the risk of hypotension.
Chemical similarities are present among sulfonamides, sulfonylureas, carbonic anhydrase inhibitors, thiazides, and loop diuretics (except ethacrynic acid). Use in patients with sulfonylurea allergy is specifically contraindicated in product labeling, however, a risk of cross-reaction exists in patients with allergy to any of these compounds; avoid use when previous reaction has been severe.

Dosage Forms Injection, solution: 10 mg/mL (2 mL, 5 mL)
Tablet: 5 mg, 10 mg, 20 mg, 100 mg

Reference Range
Peak serum level:
Healthy person: 4 mcg/mL 1 hour after 20 mg dose
Edematous patient: 3.7 mcg/mL 1 hour after 20 mg dose

Overdosage/Treatment
Decontamination: Lavage (within 1 hour)/activated charcoal
Supportive therapy: Crystalloid (normal saline) with Trendelenburg position for hypotension; dopamine or norepinephrine for refractory hypotension
Enhancement of elimination: Multiple dosing of activated charcoal may be effective; not dialyzable

Antidote(s)
- DOPamine [ANTIDOTE]
- Norepinephrine [ANTIDOTE]

Test Interactions ↑ uric acid, creatinine

Drug Interactions **Substrate** of CYP2C8 (minor), 2C9 (major); **Inhibits** CYP2C19 (weak)
ACE inhibitors: Hypotensive effects and/or renal effects are potentiated by hypovolemia.
Aminoglycosides: Ototoxicity may be increased.
Anticoagulant activity is enhanced.
Antidiabetic agents: Glucose tolerance may be decreased.
Antihypertensive agents: Effects may be enhanced.

Beta-blockers: Plasma concentrations of beta-blockers may be increased with torsemide.
Chloral hydrate: Transient diaphoresis, hot flashes, hypertension may occur.
Cisplatin: Ototoxicity may be increased.
CYP2C9 inducers: May decrease the levels/effects of torsemide. Example inducers include carbamazepine, phenobarbital, phenytoin, rifampin, rifapentine, and secobarbital.
Digitalis: Arrhythmias may occur with diuretic-induced electrolyte disturbances.
Lithium: Plasma concentrations of lithium may be increased; monitor lithium levels.
NSAIDs: Torsemide efficacy may be decreased.
Probenecid: Torsemide action may be reduced.
Salicylates: Diuretic action may be impaired in patients with cirrhosis and ascites.
Thiazides: Synergistic effects may result.

Pregnancy Risk Factor B
Pregnancy Implications A decrease in fetal weight, an increase in fetal resorption, and delayed fetal ossification has occurred in animal studies.
Lactation Excretion in breast milk unknown/use caution
Nursing Implications Monitor renal function, electrolytes, and fluid states closely including weight and I & O
Additional Information 10-20 mg torsemide is approximately equivalent to: Furosemide: 40 mg; bumetanide: 1 mg; piretanide: 12 mg

Tramadol

CAS Number 22204-88-2; 27203-92-5; 36282-47-0
U.S. Brand Names Ultram® ER; Ultram®
Synonyms Tramadol Hydrochloride
Impairment Potential Yes
Use Relief of moderate to moderately severe pain
Treatment of restless legs syndrome
Mechanism of Action Centrally acting analgesic with selective (mu) opioid receptor agonist and norepinephrine and serotonin reuptake inhibition; ~1.5-3 times less potent than morphine but more antitussive effect than codeine

Adverse Reactions
Cardiovascular: Hypotension (orthostatic), shock, tachycardia, sinus tachycardia, sinus bradycardia
Central nervous system: Headache, dizziness, lethargy, stimulation, euphoria, seizures, depression and suicidal ideation, hyperthermia, panic attacks, mania
Dermatologic: Pruritus, erythema, urticaria, exanthem
Gastrointestinal: Constipation, nausea, vomiting, xerostomia
Neuromuscular & skeletal: Hyperreflexia, hyporeflexia, tremor, rhabdomyolysis
Otic: Tinnitus
Respiratory: Respiratory depression, laryngospasm
Miscellaneous: Diaphoresis, anaphylactoid reactions, trismus

Signs and Symptoms of Overdose Coma, miosis, respiratory depression, seizures (at oral doses >700 mg or I.V. doses >300 mg), sleepiness
Admission Criteria/Prognosis Admit any patient with CNS depression, seizures, or ingestions >600 mg.

Pharmacodynamics/Kinetics
Onset of action: ~1 hour
Duration of action: 9 hours
Absorption: Rapid and complete
Distribution: V_d: 2.5-3 L/kg
Protein binding, plasma: 20%
Metabolism: Extensively hepatic via demethylation, glucuronidation, and sulfation; has pharmacologically active metabolite formed by CYP2D6 (M1; O-desmethyl tramadol)
Bioavailability: Immediate release: 75%; Extended release: 85% to 90% as compared to immediate release.
Half-life elimination: Tramadol: ~6-8 hours; Active metabolite: 7-9 hours; prolonged in elderly, hepatic or renal impairment
Time to peak: Immediate release: 2 hours; Extended release: 12 hours
Excretion: Urine (30% as unchanged drug; 60% as metabolites)

Dosage
Moderate-to-severe chronic pain: Oral:
Adults:
Immediate release formulation: 50-100 mg every 4-6 hours (not to exceed 400 mg/day)
    For patients not requiring rapid onset of effect, tolerability may be improved by starting dose at 25 mg/day and titrating dose by 25 mg every 3 days, until reaching 25 mg 4 times/day. Dose may then be increased by 50 mg every 3 days as tolerated, to reach dose of 50 mg 4 times/day.
Extended release formulation: 100 mg once daily; titrate every 5 days (maximum: 300 mg/day)
Elderly: >75 years:

Immediate release: 50 mg every 6 hours (not to exceed 300 mg/day); see dosing adjustments for renal and hepatic impairment.

Extended release formulation: See adult dosing.

Restless legs syndrome: Oral: 50 mg 1 hour before bedtime and as needed for daytime symptoms; maximum daily dose 150 mg

Dosing adjustment in renal impairment:

Immediate release: Cl_{cr} <30 mL/minute: Administer 50-100 mg dose every 12 hours (maximum: 200 mg/day)

Extended release: Should not be used in patients with Cl_{cr} < 30 mL/minute

Dosing adjustment in hepatic impairment:

Immediate release: Cirrhosis: Recommended dose: 50 mg every 12 hours

Extended release: Should not be used in patients with severe (Child-Pugh Class C) hepatic dysfunction

Monitoring Parameters Pain relief, respiratory rate, blood pressure, and pulse; signs of tolerance or abuse

Administration

Do not crush or chew extended release tablet.

Contraindications

Hypersensitivity to tramadol, opioids, or any component of the formulation; opioid-dependent patients; acute intoxication with alcohol, hypnotics, centrally-acting analgesics, opioids, or psychotropic drugs

Ultram® ER (extended release formulation): Additional contraindications: Severe (Cl_{cr} <30 mL/minute) renal dysfunction, severe (Child-Pugh Class C) hepatic dysfunction

Warnings Should be used only with extreme caution in patients receiving MAO inhibitors. May cause CNS depression and/or respiratory depression, particularly when combined with other CNS depressants. Use with caution and reduce dosage when administered to patients receiving other CNS depressants. An increased risk of seizures may occur in patients receiving serotonin reuptake inhibitors (SSRIs or anorectics), tricyclic antidepressants, other cyclic compounds (including cyclobenzaprine, promethazine), neuroleptics, MAO inhibitors, or drugs which may lower seizure threshold. Patients with a history of seizures, or with a risk of seizures (head trauma, metabolic disorders, CNS infection, or malignancy, or during ethanol/drug withdrawal) are also at increased risk.

Elderly patients and patients with chronic respiratory disorders may be at greater risk of adverse events. Use with caution in patients with increased intracranial pressure or head injury. Avoid use in patients who are suicidal or addiction prone. Use caution in heavy alcohol users. Use caution in treatment of acute abdominal conditions; may mask pain. Use tramadol with caution and reduce dosage in patients with liver disease or renal dysfunction. Not recommended during pregnancy or in nursing mothers. Tolerance or drug dependence may result from extended use (withdrawal symptoms have been reported); abrupt discontinuation should be avoided. Tapering of dose at the time of discontinuation limits the risk of withdrawal symptoms. Safety and efficacy in pediatric patients <18 years of age have not been established; use in this population is not recommended.

Dosage Forms

Tablet, as hydrochloride: 50 mg

Ultram®: 50 mg

Tablet, extended release, as hydrochloride:

Ultram® ER: 100 mg, 200 mg, 300 mg

Reference Range Serum tramadol levels ranging from 100-300 ng/mL can be considered therapeutic; blood (postmortem) tramadol levels >13 mg/L associated with fatality by suicide attempt

Overdosage/Treatment

Decontamination: Activated charcoal/sorbitol

Supportive therapy: Treat seizures with benzodiazepines or barbiturates; naloxone is probably not effective in treating seizures but may be of some use in treating CNS depression (naloxone may increase the risk for seizures); naloxone is effective in $\sim^1/_2$ the cases

Elimination: Multiple doses of activated charcoal; hemodialysis or hemoperfusion not likely to be beneficial after absorption and distribution are completed (hemodialysis removes only ~7% of the dose)

Antidote(s)

• Nalmefene [ANTIDOTE]

• Naloxone [ANTIDOTE]

Test Interactions Generally does not interfere with urine opiate screens; false-positive tramadol urinary assay can occur with venlafaxine by tandem mass spectrometry

Drug Interactions

Substrate of CYP2B6 (minor), 2D6 (major), 3A4 (minor)

Carbamazepine: Tramadol metabolism is increased by carbamazepine. Avoid concurrent use; increases risk of seizures.

Cyclobenzaprine: May enhance the neuroexcitatory and/or seizure-potentiating effect of tramadol.

CYP2D6 inhibitors: May decrease the effects of tramadol. Example inhibitors include chlorpromazine, delavirdine, fluoxetine, miconazole, paroxetine, pergolide, quinidine, quinine, ritonavir, and ropinirole.

Ethanol: Tramadol may enhance the CNS depressant effect of ethanol.

MAO inhibitors: May increase the neuroexcitatory effects or risk of seizures. Examples of inhibitors include isocarboxazid, linezolid, phenelzine, selegiline, and tranylcypromine.

Naloxone: May increase the risk of seizures (if administered in tramadol overdose).

Quinidine: May increase the tramadol serum concentrations and decrease serum concentrations of M1

SSRIs: May increase the neuroexcitatory effects or risk of seizures with tramadol. Examples of SSRIs include citalopram, escitalopram, fluoxetine, fluvoxamine, paroxetine, sertraline.

Serotonin modulators: May enhance the adverse/toxic effects of tramadol. The development of serotonin syndrome may occur.

Sibutramine: May enhance the serotonergic effects of tramadol. Avoid concurrent use.

Tricyclic antidepressants: May increase the risk of seizures.

Pregnancy Risk Factor C

Pregnancy Implications Crosses placenta with umbilical/maternal venous concentration ratio of 80%

Lactation Enters breast milk/contraindicated

Additional Information Fatal dose: ~3 g. Metoclopramide can be used to treat tramadol-induced nausea and vomiting. Ultracet®, a short-term (≤5 days) combination product for management of acute pain, contains 37.5 mg of tramadol hydrochloride and 325 mg acetaminophen

Specific References

Allen KR, "Interference by Venlafaxine Ingestion in the Detection of Tramadol by Liquid Chromatography Linked to Tandem Mass Spectrometry for the Screening of Illicit Drugs in Human Urine," *Clin Toxicol*, 2006, 44:147-53.

Barsotti CE, Mycyk MB, and Reyes J, "Withdrawal Syndrome from Tramadol Hydrochloride," *Am J Emerg Med*, 2003 21(1):87-8.

Bynum ND, Poklis JL, Gaffney-Kraft M, et al, "Postmortem Distribution of Tramadol, Amitriptyline, and Their Metabolites in a Suicidal Overdose," *J Anal Toxicol*, 2005, 29(5):401-6.

Houlihan DJ, "Serotonin Syndrome Resulting from Coadministration of Tramadol, Venlafaxine, and Mirtazapine," *Ann Pharmacother*, 2004, 38(3):411-3.

Jovanovic-Cupic V, Martinovic Z, and Nesic N, "Seizures Associated with Intoxication and Abuse of Tramadol," *Clin Toxicol*, 2006, 44:143-6.

Marquardt KA, Alsop JA, and Albertson TE, "Tramadol Exposures Reported to Statewide Poison Control System," *Ann Pharmacother*, 2005, 39(6):1039-44.

Rowden AK, Calise AG, and Holstege CP, "Influence of Marketing on Tramadol Prescribing Practices in an Urban Teaching Hospital," *Clin Toxicol (Phila)*, 2005, 43:667.

Tranylcypromine

CAS Number 13492-01-8; 155-09-9

U.S. Brand Names Parnate®

Synonyms Transamine Sulphate; Tranylcypromine Sulfate

Impairment Potential Yes

Use Symptomatic treatment of atypical, nonendogenous or neurotic depression

Unlabeled/Investigational Use Post-traumatic stress disorder

Mechanism of Action Thought to act by increasing endogenous concentrations of epinephrine, norepinephrine, dopamine and serotonin through inhibition of the enzyme (monoamine oxidase) responsible for the breakdown of these neurotransmitters

Adverse Reactions

Cardiovascular: Orthostatic hypotension, edema

Central nervous system: Dizziness, headache, drowsiness, sleep disturbances, fatigue, hyperreflexia, twitching, ataxia, mania, akinesia, confusion, disorientation, memory loss

Dermatologic: Rash, pruritus, urticaria, localized scleroderma, cystic acne (flare), alopecia

Endocrine & metabolic: Sexual dysfunction (anorgasmia, ejaculatory disturbances, impotence), hypernatremia, hypermetabolic syndrome, SIADH

Gastrointestinal: Xerostomia, constipation, weight gain

Genitourinary: Urinary retention, incontinence

Hematologic: Leukopenia, agranulocytosis

Hepatic: Hepatitis

Neuromuscular & skeletal: Weakness, tremor, myoclonus

Ocular: Blurred vision, glaucoma

Miscellaneous: Diaphoresis

Signs and Symptoms of Overdose Agranulocytosis, delirium, extrapyramidal reaction, fever, granulocytopenia, hypertension, impotence, insomnia, leukopenia, neutropenia, numbness, ptosis, thrombocytopenia

Pharmacodynamics/Kinetics

Onset of action: Therapeutic: 2 days to 3 weeks continued dosing

Half-life elimination: 90-190 minutes

Time to peak, serum: ~2 hours

Excretion: Urine

Dosage Adults: Oral: 10 mg twice daily, increase by 10 mg increments at 1- to 3-week intervals; maximum: 60 mg/day

Monitoring Parameters Blood pressure, mental status

Contraindications Hypersensitivity to tranylcypromine, other MAO inhibitors, dibenzazepine derivatives, or any component of the formulation; cardiovascular disease; cerebrovascular defect; headache history; hepatic disease; hypertension; pheochromocytoma; renal disease; concurrent use of antihistamines, antiparkinson drugs, antihypertensives, bupropion, buspirone, CNS depressants, dexfenfluramine, dextromethorphan, diuretics, ethanol, meperidine, and SSRIs; general anesthesia (discontinue 10 days prior to elective surgery); local vasoconstrictors; spinal anesthesia (hypotension may be exaggerated); sympathomimetics (and related compounds); foods high in tyramine content; supplements containing tyrosine, phenylalanine, tryptophan, or caffeine

Warnings

Risk of suicide: [U.S. Boxed Warning]: Antidepressants increase the risk of suicidal thinking and behavior in children and adolescents with major depressive disorder (MDD) and other depressive disorders; consider risk prior to prescribing. Closely monitor for clinical worsening, suicidality, or unusual changes in behavior such as anxiety, agitation, panic attacks, insomnia, irritability, hostility, impulsivity, akathisia, hypomania, and mania. The child's family or caregiver should be instructed to closely observe the patient and communicate condition with healthcare provider. Such observation would generally include at least weekly face-to-face contact with patients or their family members or caregivers during the first 4 weeks of treatment, then every other week visits for the next 4 weeks, then at 12 weeks, and as clinically indicated beyond 12 weeks. Additional contact by telephone may be appropriate between face-to-face visits. A medication guide should be dispensed with each prescription. **Tranylcypromine is not FDA approved for treatment of children and adolescents.**

Adults treated with antidepressants should be observed similarly for clinical worsening and suicidality, especially during the initial few months of a course of drug therapy, or at times of dose changes, either increases or decreases. The possibility of a suicide attempt is inherent in major depression and may persist until remission occurs. Worsening depression and severe abrupt suicidality that are not part of the presenting symptoms may require discontinuation or modification of drug therapy. Use caution in high-risk patients during initiation of therapy. Prescriptions should be written for the smallest quantity consistent with good patient care.

Disease state precautions: Use with caution in patients who are hyperactive, hyperexcitable, or who have glaucoma, hyperthyroidism, diabetes or hypotension. May cause orthostatic hypotension (especially at dosages >30 mg/day); use with caution in patients who would not tolerate transient hypotensive episodes. Use with caution in patients at risk of seizures, or in patients receiving other drugs which may lower seizure threshold. Discontinue at least 48 hours prior to myelography. May increase the risks associated with electroconvulsive therapy. Consider discontinuing, when possible, prior to elective surgery. Use with caution in patients with renal impairment. May worsen psychosis in some patients or precipitate a shift to mania or hypomania in patients with bipolar disorder. Monotherapy in patients with bipolar disorder should be avoided. Patients presenting with depressive symptoms should be screened for bipolar disorder. **Tranylcypromine is not FDA approved for the treatment of bipolar depression.**

Elderly patients: The MAO inhibitors are effective and generally well tolerated by older patients. It is the potential interactions with tyramine or tryptophan-containing foods and other drugs, and their effects on blood pressure that have limited their use.

Dosage Forms Tablet: 10 mg

Reference Range Therapeutic blood level: 0.1 mg/L; serum level of 1 mg/L has been associated with coma

Overdosage/Treatment

Decontamination: Lavage (within 1 hour)/activated charcoal

Supportive therapy: Diazepam or lorazepam can be used for agitation/seizures. Dantrolene (2.5 mg/kg every 6 hours) can be used for muscle rigidity and hyperthermia. Labetalol may be useful for hypertension, while norepinephrine is the preferred agent for treatment of hypotension. Avoid bretylium for ventricular dysrhythmia, lidocaine or procainamide are preferred. Hypertensive crisis can be treated with nitroprusside, phentolamine (2-10 mg slow I.V. injection in adults), diazoxide (50-100 mg I.V.). Dantrolene (2.5 mg/kg every 6 hours I.V.) can be used to treat hypermetabolic crisis.

Enhancement of elimination: Hemodialysis may be useful.

Diagnostic Procedures

• Electrolytes, Blood

Drug Interactions Inhibits CYP1A2 (moderate), 2A6 (strong), 2C8 (weak), 2C9 (weak), 2C19 (moderate), 2D6 (moderate), 2E1 (weak), 3A4 (weak)

Acetylcholinesterase inhibitors: May diminish the anticholinergic side effects of tranylcypromine.

Alpha-/beta-agonists: MAO inhibitors may enhance the vasopressor effect. Alpha-/beta-agonists (indirect-acting): MAO inhibitors may enhance the vasopressor effect.

Alpha$_1$-agonist: MAO inhibitors may enhance the hypertensive effects.

Altretamine: May enhance the orthostatic effect of MAO inhibitors.

Amphetamines: MAO inhibitors in combination with amphetamines may result in severe hypertensive reaction; these combinations are best avoided.

Anesthetics, general: Discontinue tranylcypromine 10 days prior to elective surgery.

Anorexiants: Concurrent use of anorexiants may result in serotonin syndrome; contraindicated with dexfenfluramine; avoid use with fenfluramine or sibutramine.

Anticholinergics: May enhance the adverse/toxic anticholinergic effects of tranylcypromine.

Atomoxetine: MAO Inhibitors may enhance the neurotoxic (central) effect of atomoxetine. Avoid combination. Atomoxetine should not be used within 14 days of an MAO inhibitor.

Bupropion: May cause hypertensive crisis; at least 14 days should elapse before initiating bupropion; concurrent use with an MAO inhibitor is contraindicated.

Buspirone: May cause increased blood pressure; concurrent use with an MAO inhibitor should be avoided.

COMT Inhibitors: May enhance the adverse/toxic effect of MAO inhibitors. Avoid concurrent use.

Cyclobenzaprine: May enhance the serotonergic effect of MAO Inhibitors. This could result in serotonin syndrome. Avoid combination.

CYP1A2 substrates: Tranylcypromine may increase the levels/effects of CYP1A2 substrates. Example substrates include aminophylline, fluvoxamine, mexiletine, mirtazapine, ropinirole, theophylline, and trifluoperazine.

CYP2A6 substrates: Tranylcypromine may increase the levels/effects of CYP2A6 substrates. Example substrates include dexmedetomidine and ifosfamide.

CYP2C19 substrates: Tranylcypromine may increase the levels/effects of CYP2C19 substrates. Example substrates include citalopram, diazepam, methsuximide, phenytoin, and trimipramine.

CYP2D6 substrates: Tranylcypromine may increase the levels/effects of CYP2D6 substrates. Example substrates include amphetamines, selected beta-blockers, dextromethorphan, fluoxetine, lidocaine, mirtazapine, nefazodone, paroxetine, risperidone, thioridazine, tricyclic antidepressants, and venlafaxine.

CYP2D6 prodrug substrates: Tranylcypromine may decrease the levels/effects of CYP2D6 prodrug substrates. Example prodrug substrates include codeine, hydrocodone, oxycodone, and tramadol.

Dexmethylphenidate: MAO inhibitors may enhance the hypertensive effect of dexmethylphenidate; avoid concurrent use.

Dextromethorphan: Concurrent use of MAO inhibitors may result in serotonin syndrome; concurrent use is contraindicated.

Disulfiram: MAO inhibitors may produce delirium in patients receiving disulfiram; monitor.

Ethanol: Tranylcypromine may enhance CNS depressant effect of ethanol.

False neurotransmitters: MAO inhibitors inhibit the antihypertensive response to guanadrel or methyldopa; monitor therapy.

Levodopa: MAO inhibitors in combination with levodopa may result in hypertensive reactions; monitor.

Lithium: MAO inhibitors in combination with lithium have resulted in CNS toxicity (malignant hyperpyrexia, tardive dyskinesias); monitor therapy.

Meperidine: May cause serotonin syndrome when combined with an MAO inhibitor; concurrent use is contraindicated; should not be used within 14 days of an MAO inhibitor.

Methylphenidate: MAO inhibitors may enhance the hypertensive effect of methylphenidate. Avoid combination.

Mirtazapine: MAO inhibitors may enhance the neurotoxic (central) effect of mirtazapine. Avoid combination.

Pramlintide: Pramlintide may enhance the anticholinergic effect of tranylcypromine. Additive effects on reduced GI motility may occur.

Rauwolfia alkaloids: MAO inhibitors may enhance the adverse/toxic effect of rauwolfia alkaloids. If a rauwolfia alkaloid is added to existing MAOI therapy, a burst of catecholamine stimulation (eg, excitation, hypertension) may occur.

Serotonin/norepinephrine reuptake inhibitors (SNRIs): MAO inhibitors may enhance the serotonergic effect of SNRI antidepressants. This may cause serotonin syndrome.

Selective serotonin reuptake inhibitors (SSRIs): MAO Inhibitors may enhance the serotonergic effect of SSRIs. This may cause serotonin syndrome. Avoid concurrent use. Do not use within 5 weeks of fluoxetine discontinuation or 2 weeks of other antidepressant discontinuation.

Serotonin 5-HT$_{1D}$ receptor agonists: May increase the risk of serotonin syndrome. The manufacturers of rizatriptan, sumatriptan, and zolmitriptan state that concurrent use (or use within 2 weeks of MAO therapy) is contraindicated.

Serotonin modulators: May enhance the adverse/toxic effect of other serotonin modulators, such as tranylcypromine. The development of serotonin syndrome may occur.

Sibutramine: May enhance the serotonergic effect of tranylcypromine. This may cause serotonin syndrome. Avoid concurrent use.

Thioridazine: Tranylcypromine may decrease the metabolism of thioridazine. Avoid concurrent use.

Tramadol: May enhance the neuroexcitatory and/or seizure-potentiating effect of MAO Inhibitors.

Tricyclic antidepressants: MAO inhibitors may enhance the serotonergic effect of tricyclic antidepressants. This may cause serotonin syndrome. Avoid concurrent use.

Pregnancy Risk Factor C
Lactation Enters breast milk/not recommended
Additional Information Minimum lethal dose: 170 mg
Chronic overdosage (a reported 550 mg/day) has resulted in only reversible thrombocytopenia and delirium.

Trazodone

Related Information
- Anticholinergic Effects of Common Psychotropics
- Antidepressant Agents

CAS Number 19794-93-5; 25332-39-2
U.S. Brand Names Desyrel®
Synonyms Trazodone Hydrochloride
Impairment Potential Yes
Use Treatment of depression
Unlabeled/Investigational Use Potential augmenting agent for antidepressants, hypnotic
Mechanism of Action Inhibits reuptake of serotonin and norepinephrine; hypotension may be due to alpha-receptor blockade

Adverse Reactions

Cardiovascular: Postural hypotension, cardiac arrhythmias, edema, prolongation of QT interval, decreases amplitude of T wave, sinus bradycardia, vasculitis

Central nervous system: **Dizziness, confusion, headache**, drowsiness, sedation, insomnia, agitation, seizures, extrapyramidal reactions, mania, psychosis, gustatory hallucinations, fever, hyperthermia

Dermatologic: Leukocytoclastic dermatitis, erythema multiforme, exacerbation of plaque, psoriasis, bullous lesions, exfoliative dermatitis, alopecia, urticaria, purpura, pruritus, exanthem, cutaneous vasculitis

Endocrine & metabolic: Syndrome of inappropriate antidiuretic hormone, serotonin syndrome, spontaneous orgasm (when yawning) may occur, hypoprolactinemia, gynecomastia

Gastrointestinal: **Xerostomia, bad taste in mouth, nausea**, constipation, vomiting

Genitourinary: Urinary retention, prolonged priapism

Hepatic: Hepatitis

Neuromuscular & skeletal: **Muscle tremors**, clonus, myoclonus, weakness, paresthesia

Ocular: Blurred vision

Respiratory: Eosinophilic pneumonia

Signs and Symptoms of Overdose Ataxia, AV block (first degree), bradycardia, clitoral hypertrophy, coma, delirium, drowsiness, dry mouth, ejaculation disturbances, erythema multiforme, extrapyramidal reaction, heart block, hepatic failure, hypotension, incontinence, insomnia, muscle asthenia, myoclonus, ototoxicity, photosensitivity, priapism, prolonged QT interval, respiratory depression, seizures (rarely), tinnitus, torsade de pointes, vomiting

Pharmacodynamics/Kinetics

Onset of action: Therapeutic (antidepressant): 1-3 weeks; sleep aid: 1-3 hours

Protein binding: 85% to 95%

Metabolism: Hepatic via CYP3A4 to an active metabolite (mCPP)

Half-life elimination: 7-8 hours, two compartment kinetics

Time to peak, serum: 30-100 minutes; delayed with food (up to 2.5 hours)

Excretion: Primarily urine; secondarily feces

Dosage

Therapeutic effects may take up to 4 weeks to occur; therapy is normally maintained for several months after optimum response is reached to prevent recurrence of depression

Oral:

Adolescents: Initial: 25-50 mg/day; increase to 100-150 mg/day in divided doses

Adults: Initial: 150 mg/day in 3 divided doses (may increase by 50 mg/day every 3-7 days); maximum: 600 mg/day

Maximum tolerated dose:

Children: 200 mg

Adults: 9 g

Monitoring Parameters ECG for at least 4 hours
Administration Dosing after meals may decrease lightheadedness and postural hypotension
Contraindications Hypersensitivity to trazodone or any component of the formulation

Warnings

[U.S. Boxed Warning]: Antidepressants increase the risk of suicidal thinking and behavior in children and adolescents with major depressive disorder (MDD) and other depressive disorders; consider risk prior to prescribing. Closely monitor for clinical worsening, suicidality, or unusual changes in behavior; the child's family or caregiver should be instructed to closely observe the patient and communicate condition with healthcare provider. Such observation would generally include at least weekly face-to-face contact with patients or their family members or caregivers during the first 4 weeks of treatment, then every other week visits for the next 4 weeks, then at 12 weeks, and as clinically indicated beyond 12 weeks. Additional contact by telephone may be appropriate between face-to-face visits. Adults treated with antidepressants should be observed similarly for clinical worsening and suicidality, especially during the initial few months of a course of drug therapy, or at times of dose changes, either increases or decreases. A medication guide should be dispensed with each prescription. **Trazodone is not FDA approved for use in children.**

The possibility of a suicide attempt is inherent in major depression and may persist until remission occurs. Monitor for worsening of depression or suicidality, especially during initiation of therapy or with dose increases or decreases. Worsening depression and severe abrupt suicidality that are not part of the presenting symptoms may require discontinuation or modification of drug therapy. Use caution in high-risk patients during initiation of therapy. Prescriptions should be written for the smallest quantity consistent with good patient care. The patient's family or caregiver should be alerted to monitor patients for the emergence of suicidality and associated behaviors such as anxiety, agitation, panic attacks, insomnia, irritability, hostility, impulsivity, akathisia, hypomania, and mania; patients should be instructed to notify their healthcare provider if any of these symptoms or worsening depression occur.

May worsen psychosis in some patients or precipitate a shift to mania or hypomania in patients with bipolar disorder. Monotherapy in patients with bipolar disorder should be avoided. Patients presenting with depressive symptoms should be screened for bipolar disorder. **Trazodone is not FDA approved for the treatment of bipolar depression.**

Priapism, including cases resulting in permanent dysfunction, has occurred with the use of trazodone. Not recommended for use in a patient during the acute recovery phase of MI. Trazodone should be initiated with caution in patients who are receiving concurrent or recent therapy with a MAO inhibitor. May cause sedation, resulting in impaired performance of tasks requiring alertness (eg, operating machinery or driving). Sedative effects may be additive with other CNS depressants and ethanol. The degree of sedation is very high relative to other antidepressants. May increase the risks associated with electroconvulsive therapy. Consider discontinuing, when possible, prior to elective surgery. Therapy should not be abruptly discontinued in patients receiving high doses for prolonged periods.

Use with caution in patients at risk of hypotension or in patients where transient hypotensive episodes would be poorly tolerated (cardiovascular disease or cerebrovascular disease). The risk of postural hypotension is high relative to other antidepressants.

Use caution in patients with a previous seizure disorder or condition predisposing to seizures such as brain damage, alcoholism, or concurrent therapy with other drugs which lower the seizure threshold. Use with caution in patients with hepatic or renal dysfunction and in elderly patients. Use with caution in patients with a history of cardiovascular disease (including previous MI, stroke, tachycardia, or conduction abnormalities). However, the risk of conduction abnormalities with this agent is low relative to other antidepressants.

Dosage Forms Tablet, as hydrochloride: 50 mg, 100 mg, 150 mg, 300 mg

Reference Range

Therapeutic: 0.5-2.5 mcg/mL (SI: 1-6 μmol/L)

Overdoses of 4-5 g are associated with levels of 15-19 mcg/mL

In the postmortem state, anatomical site concentration differences (ie, postmortem redistribution) may occur.

Overdosage/Treatment

Decontamination: Lavage (within 1 hour)/activated charcoal

Supportive therapy: Following initiation of essential overdose management, toxic symptoms should be treated supportively. Treat bradycardia with atropine; benztropine may be useful to treat priapism. Seizures usually respond to lorazepam or diazepam I.V. boluses (5-10 mg for adults up to 30 mg or 0.25-0.4 mg/kg/dose for children up to 10 mg/dose). If seizures are unresponsive or recur, phenobarbital may be required. Priapism can be treated with alpha-adrenergic agonists, aspiration and irrigation of corpora cavernosa with epinephrine solutions and a Winters' shunt.

Diagnostic Procedures
- Trazodone, Blood

Test Interactions Spurious positive amphetamine urinary immunoassay screen can result from trazodone therapy.

Drug Interactions

Substrate of CYP2D6 (minor), 3A4 (major); **Inhibits** CYP2D6 (moderate), 3A4 (weak)

Antipsychotics: Trazodone, in combination with other psychotropics (low potency antipsychotics), may result in additional hypotension (isolated case reports); monitor.

Azole antifungals: Serum concentrations of trazodone may be increased by azole antifungals, via inhibition of CYP3A4. Ketoconazole has been specifically studied. Consider a lower dose of trazodone.

Buspirone: Serotonergic effects may be additive (limited documentation); monitor.

Carbamazepine: Serum concentrations of trazodone may be decreased by carbamazepine, due to induction of CYP3A4. Other CYP inducers are likely to share this effect.

CNS depressants: Sedative effects may be additive with CNS depressants. Includes ethanol, barbiturates, benzodiazepines, narcotic analgesics, and other sedative agents; monitor for increased effect

CYP2D6 substrates: Trazodone may increase the levels/effects of CYP2D6 substrates. Example substrates include amphetamines, selected beta-blockers, dextromethorphan, fluoxetine, lidocaine, mirtazapine, nefazodone, paroxetine, risperidone, ritonavir, thioridazine, tricyclic antidepressants, and venlafaxine.

CYP2D6 prodrug substrates: Trazodone may decrease the levels/effects of CYP2D6 prodrug substrates. Example prodrug substrates include codeine, hydrocodone, oxycodone, and tramadol.

CYP3A4 inducers: CYP3A4 inducers may decrease the levels/effects of trazodone. Example inducers include aminoglutethimide, carbamazepine, nafcillin, nevirapine, phenobarbital, phenytoin, and rifamycins.

CYP3A4 inhibitors: May increase the levels/effects of trazodone. Example inhibitors include azole antifungals, clarithromycin, diclofenac, doxycycline, erythromycin, imatinib, isoniazid, nefazodone, nicardipine, propofol, protease inhibitors, quinidine, telithromycin, and verapamil.

Linezolid: Due to MAO inhibition (see note on MAO inhibitors), this combination should be avoided

MAO inhibitors: Concurrent use may lead to serotonin syndrome; avoid concurrent use or use within 14 days

Meperidine: Combined use, theoretically, may increase the risk of serotonin syndrome

Protease inhibitors: Serum concentrations of trazodone may be increased by protease inhibitors, via inhibition of CYP3A4. Consider a lower dose of trazodone.

Serotonin agonists: Theoretically, may increase the risk of serotonin syndrome; includes sumatriptan, naratriptan, rizatriptan, and zolmitriptan

SSRIs: Combined use of trazodone with an SSRI may, theoretically, increase the risk of serotonin syndrome; in addition, some SSRIs may inhibit the metabolism of trazodone resulting in elevated plasma levels and increased sedation; includes fluoxetine and fluvoxamine (see CYP inhibition); low doses of trazodone appear to represent little risk

Venlafaxine: Combined use with trazodone may increase the risk of serotonin syndrome

Pregnancy Risk Factor C

Lactation Enters breast milk/use caution (AAP rates "of concern")

Nursing Implications Use side rails on bed if administered to the elderly; observe patient's activity and compare with admission level

Additional Information Therapeutic effects may take up to 4 weeks to occur; therapy is normally maintained for several months after optimum response is reached to prevent recurrence of depression

Adult ingestions over two grams usually are symptomatic

Specific References

Margolese HC and Chouinard G, "Serotonin Syndrome from Addition of Low-Dose Trazodone to Nefazodone," *Am J Psychiatry*, 2000, 157(6):1022.

Martinez MA, Ballesteros S, Sanchez de la Torre C, et al, "Investigation of a Fatality Due to Trazodone Poisoning: Case Report and Literature Review," *J Anal Toxicol*, 2005, 29(4):262-8.

Staack RF and Maurer HH, "Piperazine-Derived Designer Drug 1-(3-Chlorophenyl)Piperazine (mCPP): GC-MS Studies on Its Metabolism and Its Toxicological Detection in Rat Urine Including Analytical Differentiation from Its Precursor Drugs Trazodone and Nefazodone," *J Anal Toxicol*, 2003, 27(8):560-68.

Tretinoin (Topical)

CAS Number 302-79-4

U.S. Brand Names Altinac™; Avita®; Renova®; Retin-A® Micro; Retin-A®

Synonyms *trans*-Retinoic Acid; Retinoic Acid; Vitamin A Acid

Use Treatment of acne vulgaris, photodamaged skin, and some skin cancers

Unlabeled/Investigational Use Some skin cancers

Mechanism of Action Keratinocytes in the sebaceous follicle become less adherent which allows for easy removal; decreases microcomedone formation

Adverse Reactions

Cardiovascular: Edema, leukocytoclastic vasculitis, cardiomyopathy, cardiomegaly, pericardial effusion/pericarditis, pulmonary hypertension

Central nervous system: Pseudotumor cerebri, insomnia, confusion, anxiety, agitation, truncal ataxia, psychosis, cerebellar hemorrhage, hypothermia

Dermatologic: Excessive dryness, erythema, scaling of the skin, hyperpigmentation or hypopigmentation, photosensitivity, initial acne flare-up, **alopecia** (14%), neutrophilic dermatosis (Sweet's syndrome)

Endocrine & metabolic: Hypercalcemia

Gastrointestinal: Gastric ulcer (3%)

Hematologic: Basophilia, thrombocytosis, intravascular hemolysis

Local: Stinging, blistering

Ocular: Papilledema

Otic: Hearing loss (6%)

Renal: Acute renal failure

Respiratory: Epistaxis

Signs and Symptoms of Overdose Dyspnea, fever, hypotension, leukocytosis, tachycardia

Pharmacodynamics/Kinetics

Absorption: Minimal

Metabolism: Hepatic for the small amount absorbed

Excretion: Urine and feces

Dosage Topical:

Children >12 years and Adults: Acne vulgaris: Begin therapy with a weaker formulation of tretinoin (0.025% cream, 0.04% microsphere gel, or 0.01% gel) and increase the concentration as tolerated; apply once daily to acne lesions before retiring or on alternate days; if stinging or irritation develop, decrease frequency of application

Adults ≥18: Palliation of fine wrinkles, mottled hyperpigmentation, and tactile roughness of facial skin: Pea-sized amount of the 0.02% or 0.05% cream applied to entire face once daily in the evening

Elderly: Use of the 0.02% cream in patients 65-71 years of age showed similar improvement in fine wrinkles as seen in patients <65 years. Safety and efficacy of the 0.02% cream have not been established in patients >71 years of age. Safety and efficacy of the 0.05% cream have not been established in patients >50 years of age.

Monitoring Parameters Calcium (serum)

Administration Palliation of fine wrinkles, mottled hyperpigmentation, and tactile roughness of facial skin: Cream: Prior to application, gently wash face with a mild soap. Pat dry. Wait 20-30 minutes to apply cream. Avoid eyes, ears, nostrils, and mouth.

Contraindications Hypersensitivity to tretinoin or any component of the formulation; sunburn

Warnings Use with caution in patients with eczema; avoid excessive exposure to sunlight and sunlamps; avoid contact with abraded skin, mucous membranes, eyes, mouth, angles of the nose. Palliation of fine wrinkles, mottled hyperpigmentation, and tactile roughness of facial skin: Do not use the 0.05% cream for longer than 48 weeks or the 0.02% cream for longer than 52 weeks. Not for use on moderate- to heavily-pigmented skin. Gel is flammable; do not expose to high temperatures or flame.

Dosage Forms [DSC] = Discontinued product

Cream, topical: 0.025% (20 g, 45 g); 0.05% (20 g, 45 g); 0.1% (20 g, 45 g)

Avita®: 0.025% (20 g, 45 g)

Renova®: 0.02% (40 g); 0.05% (40 g, 60 g)

Retin-A®: 0.025% (20 g, 45 g); 0.05% (20 g, 45 g); 0.1% (20 g, 45 g)

Gel, topical: 0.025% (15 g, 45 g)

Avita®: 0.025% (20 g, 45 g) [contains ethanol 83%]

Retin-A®: 0.01% (15 g, 45 g); 0.025% (15 g, 45 g) [contains alcohol 90%]

Retin-A® Micro [microsphere gel]: 0.04% (20 g, 45 g); 0.1% (20 g, 45 g) [contains benzyl alcohol]

Liquid, topical (Retin-A®): 0.05% (28 mL) [contains alcohol 55%] [DSC]

Overdosage/Treatment

Decontamination: Emesis within 30 minutes or lavage (within 1 hour)/activated charcoal

Supportive therapy: Sweet's syndrome can be treated with methylprednisolone (1 g/day for 3 days); retinoic acid syndrome can be treated with dexamethasone (10 mg I.V. every 12 hours for 3 or more days); tachycardia can be treated with beta-adrenergic blockers while hypotension can be treated with crystalloid fluid bolus (10-20 mL/kg) and Trendelenburg placement; dopamine or norepinephrine can be used for refractory hypotension

Drug Interactions Substrate of CYP2A6 (minor), 2B6 (minor), 2C8 (major), 2C9 (minor); **Inhibits** CYP2C9 (weak); **Induces** CYP2E1 (weak)

Increased toxicity: Sulfur, benzoyl peroxide, salicylic acid, resorcinol, any product with strong drying effects (potentiates adverse reactions seen with tretinoin)

Photosensitizing medications (thiazides, tetracyclines, fluoroquinolones, phenothiazines, sulfonamides): Augment phototoxicity; should not be used when treating palliation of fine wrinkles, mottled hyperpigmentation, and tactile roughness of facial skin

Pregnancy Risk Factor C

Pregnancy Implications Oral tretinoin is teratogenic and fetotoxic in rats at doses 1000 and 500 times the topical human dose, respectively; however, tretinoin does not appear to be teratogenic when used topically since it is rapidly metabolized by the skin; ear malformations have been noted

Lactation Enters breast milk/compatible

Nursing Implications Observe for signs of hypersensitivity, blistering, excessive dryness; do not apply to mucous membranes

Additional Information "Retinoic acid syndrome" is seen in patients with acute promyelocytic leukemia taking tretinoin (>45 mg/m^2/day); it consists of dyspnea (60%), pleural effusion (20%), bone pain, cardiac failure (6%), fever, tachycardia, nausea and vomiting (57%), renal insufficiency (11%), leukocytosis, and disseminated intravascular coagulation

---

Triamcinolone

Related Information
- Corticosteroids

CAS Number 124-94-7; 1997-15-5; 5611-51-8; 67-78-7; 76-25-5; 989-96-8

U.S. Brand Names Aristocort® A; Aristocort® Forte; Aristocort®; Aristospan®; Azmacort®; Kenalog-10®; Kenalog-40®; Kenalog® in Orabase®; Kenalog®; Nasacort® AQ; Nasacort® [DSC]; Tri-Nasal®; Triderm®

Synonyms Triamcinolone Acetonide, Aerosol; Triamcinolone Acetonide, Parenteral; Triamcinolone Diacetate, Oral; Triamcinolone Diacetate, Parenteral; Triamcinolone Hexacetonide; Triamcinolone, Oral

Use

Nasal inhalation: Management of seasonal and perennial allergic rhinitis in patients $\geq$6 years of age

Oral inhalation: Control of bronchial asthma and related bronchospastic conditions

Oral topical: Adjunctive treatment and temporary relief of symptoms associated with oral inflammatory lesions and ulcerative lesions resulting from trauma

Systemic: Adrenocortical insufficiency, rheumatic disorders, allergic states, respiratory diseases, systemic lupus erythematosus (SLE), and other diseases requiring anti-inflammatory or immunosuppressive effects

Topical: Inflammatory dermatoses responsive to steroids

Mechanism of Action Decreases inflammation by suppression of migration of polymorphonuclear leukocytes and reversal of increased capillary permeability; suppresses the immune system by reducing activity and volume of the lymphatic system; suppresses adrenal function at high doses

Adverse Reactions
Systemic:

Cardiovascular: CHF, hypertension

Central nervous system: Convulsions, fever, headache, intracranial pressure increased, vertigo

Dermatologic: Bruising, facial erythema, petechiae, photosensitivity, rash, thin/fragile skin, wound healing impaired

Endocrine & metabolic: Adrenocortical/pituitary unresponsiveness (particularly during stress), carbohydrate tolerance decreased, cushingoid state, diabetes mellitus (manifestations of latent disease), fluid retention, growth suppression (children), hypokalemic alkalosis, menstrual irregularities, negative nitrogen balance, potassium loss, sodium retention

Gastrointestinal: Abdominal distention, diarrhea, dyspepsia, nausea, oral *Monilia* (oral inhaler), pancreatitis, peptic ulcer, ulcerative esophagitis, weight gain

Local: Skin atrophy (at the injection site)

Neuromuscular & skeletal: Femoral/humeral head aseptic necrosis, muscle mass decreased, muscle weakness, osteoporosis, pathologic fracture of long bones, steroid myopathy, vertebral compression fractures

Ocular: Cataracts, intraocular pressure increased, exophthalmus, glaucoma

Respiratory: Cough increased (nasal spray), epistaxis (nasal inhaler/spray), pharyngitis (nasal spray/oral inhaler), sinusitis (oral inhaler), voice alteration (oral inhaler)

Miscellaneous: Anaphylaxis, diaphoresis increased, suppression of skin test reactions

Topical:

Dermatologic: Itching, allergic contact dermatitis, dryness, folliculitis, skin infection (secondary), hypertrichosis, acneiform eruptions, hypopigmentation, skin maceration, skin atrophy, striae, miliaria, perioral dermatitis, atrophy of oral mucosa

Local: Burning, irritation

Signs and Symptoms of Overdose When consumed in excessive quantities, systemic hypercorticism and adrenal suppression may occur.

In those cases discontinuation and withdrawal of the corticosteroid should be done judiciously.

Pharmacodynamics/Kinetics
Duration: Oral: 8-12 hours
Absorption: Topical: Systemic
Time to peak: I.M.: 8-10 hours
Half-life elimination: Biologic: 18-36 hours

Dosage
The lowest possible dose should be used to control the condition; when dose reduction is possible, the dose should be reduced gradually. Parenteral dose is usually $^1/_3$ to $^1/_2$ the oral dose given every 12 hours. In life-threatening situations, parenteral doses larger than the oral dose may be needed.

Injection:

Acetonide:

Intra-articular, intrabursal, tendon sheaths: Adults: Initial: Smaller joints: 2.5-5 mg, larger joints: 5-15 mg

Intradermal: Adults: Initial: 1 mg

I.M.: Range: 2.5-60 mg/day

Children 6-12 years: Initial: 40 mg

Children >12 years and Adults: Initial: 60 mg

Diacetate: Adults:

Intra-articular, intrasynovial: Range: 5-40 mg; duration of effect varies from 1 week to 2 months, although more frequent dosing may be needed in acutely-inflamed joints

Average dose: Knee: 25 mg, finger: 2-5 mg

Intralesional, sublesional: Range: 5-48 mg, dependent upon size of lesion

Maximum: 12.5 mg/injection site, 25 mg/lesion, 75 mg/week

Usual treatment course: 2-3 injections at 1- to 2-week intervals

I.M.: Initial range: 3-48 mg/day; average dose: 40 mg/week

Hexacetonide: Adults:

Intralesional, sublesional: Up to 0.5 mg/square inch of affected skin

Intra-articular: Range: 2-20 mg

Triamcinolone Dosing		
	Acetonide	**Hexacetonide**
Intrasynovial	5-40 mg	
Intralesional	1-30 mg (usually 1 mg per injection site); 10 mg/mL suspension usually used	Up to 0.5 mg/sq inch affected area
Sublesional	1-30 mg	
Systemic I.M.	2.5-60 mg/dose (usual adult dose: 60 mg; may repeat with 20-100 mg dose when symptoms recur)	
Intra-articular	2.5-40 mg	2-20 mg average
large joints	5-15 mg	10-20 mg
small joints	2.5-5 mg	2-6 mg
Tendon sheaths	2.5-10 mg	
Intradermal	1 mg/site	

Intranasal: Perennial allergic rhinitis, seasonal allergic rhinitis:

Nasal spray:

Children 6-11 years: 110 mcg/day as 1 spray in each nostril once daily.

Children $\geq$12 years and Adults: 220 mcg/day as 2 sprays in each nostril once daily

Nasal inhaler:

Children 6-11 years: Initial: 220 mcg/day as 2 sprays in each nostril once daily

Children $\geq$12 years and Adults: Initial: 220 mcg/day as 2 sprays in each nostril once daily; may increase dose to 440 mcg/day (given once daily or divided and given 2 or 4 times/day)

Oral: Adults:

Acute rheumatic carditis: Initial: 20-60 mg/day; reduce dose during maintenance therapy

Acute seasonal or perennial allergic rhinitis: 8-12 mg/day

Adrenocortical insufficiency: Range 4-12 mg/day

Bronchial asthma: 8-16 mg/day

Dermatological disorders, contact/atopic dermatitis: Initial: 8-16 mg/day

Ophthalmic disorders: 12-40 mg/day

Rheumatic disorders: Range: 8-16 mg/day

SLE: Initial: 20-32 mg/day, some patients may need initial doses $\geq$48 mg; reduce dose during maintenance therapy

Oral inhalation: Asthma:

Children 6-12 years: 100-200 mcg 3-4 times/day **or** 200-400 mcg twice daily; maximum dose: 1200 mg/day

Children >12 years and Adults: 200 mcg 3-4 times/day **or** 400 mcg twice daily; maximum dose: 1600 mcg/day

Oral topical: Oral inflammatory lesions/ulcers: Press a small dab (about $^1/_4$ inch) to the lesion until a thin film develops. A larger quantity may be required for coverage of some lesions. For optimal results use only enough to coat the lesion with a thin film; do not rub in.

Topical:
Cream, Ointment: Apply thin film to affected areas 2-4 times/day
Spray: Apply to affected area 3-4 times/day

Monitoring Parameters Blood pressure, blood glucose, electrolytes

Administration Injection: Avoid injecting into a previously infected joint; do not inject into unstable joints
I.M.: Inject deep in large muscle mass, avoid deltoid.
Nasal spray, inhalation: Shake well prior to use. Gently blow nose to clear nostrils.
Oral inhalation: Shake well prior to use. Rinse mouth and throat after using inhaler to prevent candidiasis. Use spacer device provided with Azmacort®.
Oral topical: Apply small dab to lesion until a thin film develops; do not rub in. Apply at bedtime or after meals if applications are needed throughout the day.
Tablet: Once-daily doses should be given in the morning.
Topical: Apply a thin film sparingly and avoid topical application on the face. Do not use on open skin or wounds. Do not occlude area unless directed.

Contraindications Hypersensitivity to triamcinolone or any component of the formulation; systemic fungal infections; serious infections (except septic shock or tuberculous meningitis); primary treatment of status asthmaticus; fungal, viral, or bacterial infections of the mouth or throat (oral topical formulation)

Warnings
May cause suppression of hypothalamic-pituitary-adrenal (HPA) axis, particularly in younger children or in patients receiving high doses for prolonged periods. Particular care is required when patients are transferred from systemic corticosteroids to inhaled products due to possible adrenal insufficiency or withdrawal from steroids, including an increase in allergic symptoms. Patients receiving 20 mg per day of prednisone (or equivalent) may be most susceptible. Fatalities have occurred due to adrenal insufficiency in asthmatic patients during and after transfer from systemic corticosteroids to aerosol steroids; aerosol steroids do **not** provide the systemic steroid needed to treat patients having trauma, surgery, or infections. Withdrawal and discontinuation of the corticosteroid should be done slowly and carefully

Use with caution in patients with hypothyroidism, cirrhosis, nonspecific ulcerative colitis and patients at increased risk for peptic ulcer disease. Corticosteroids should be used with caution in patients with diabetes, hypertension, osteoporosis, glaucoma, cataracts, or tuberculosis. Use caution in hepatic impairment. Do not use occlusive dressings on weeping or exudative lesions and general caution with occlusive dressings should be observed; discontinue if skin irritation or contact dermatitis should occur; do not use in patients with decreased skin circulation; avoid the use of high potency steroids on the face.

Because of the risk of adverse effects, systemic corticosteroids should be used cautiously in the elderly, in the smallest possible dose, and for the shortest possible time. Azmacort® (metered dose inhaler) comes with its own spacer device attached and may be easier to use in older patients.

Controlled clinical studies have shown that orally-inhaled and intranasal corticosteroids may cause a reduction in growth velocity in pediatric patients. (In studies of orally-inhaled corticosteroids, the mean reduction in growth velocity was approximately 1 centimeter per year [range 0.3-1.8 cm per year] and appears to be related to dose and duration of exposure.) The growth of pediatric patients receiving inhaled corticosteroids, should be monitored routinely (eg, via stadiometry). To minimize the systemic effects of orally-inhaled and intranasal corticosteroids, each patient should be titrated to the lowest effective dose.

May suppress the immune system, patients may be more susceptible to infection. Use with caution in patients with systemic infections or ocular herpes simplex. Avoid exposure to chickenpox and measles. Injection suspension contains benzyl alcohol; benzyl alcohol has been associated with the "gasping syndrome" in neonates and low-birth-weight infants.

Oral topical: Discontinue if local irritation or sensitization should develop. If significant regeneration or repair of oral tissues has not occurred in seven days, re-evaluation of the etiology of the oral lesion is advised.

Dosage Forms
Aerosol for oral inhalation, as acetonide (Azmacort®): 100 mcg per actuation (20 g) [240 actuations]
Aerosol, topical, as acetonide (Kenalog®): 0.2 mg/2-second spray (63 g)
Cream, as acetonide: 0.025% (15 g, 80 g, 454 g); 0.1% (15 g, 80 g, 454 g, 2270 g); 0.5% (15 g)
Aristocort® A: 0.025% (15 g, 60 g); 0.1% (15 g, 60 g); 0.5% (15 g) [contains benzyl alcohol]
Triderm®: 0.1% (30 g, 85 g)
Injection, suspension, as acetonide:

Kenalog-10®: 10 mg/mL (5 mL) [contains benzyl alcohol; not for I.V. or I.M. use]
Kenalog-40®: 40 mg/mL (1 mL, 5 mL, 10 mL) [contains benzyl alcohol; not for I.V. or intradermal use]
Injection, suspension, as hexacetonide (Aristospan®): 5 mg/mL (5 mL); 20 mg/mL (1 mL, 5 mL) [contains benzyl alcohol; not for I.V. use]
Lotion, as acetonide: 0.025% (60 mL); 0.1% (60 mL)
Ointment, topical, as acetonide: 0.025% (15 g, 80 g, 454 g); 0.1% (15 g, 80 g, 454 g); 0.5% (15 g)
Aristocort® A: 0.1% (15 g, 60 g)
Paste, oral, topical, as acetonide: 0.1% (5 g)
Solution, intranasal, as acetonide [spray] (Tri-Nasal®): 50 mcg/inhalation (15 mL) [120 doses]
Suspension, intranasal, as acetonide [spray] (Nasacort® AQ): 55 mcg/inhalation (16.5 g) [120 doses]
Tablet (Aristocort®): 4 mg [contains lactose and sodium benzoate]

Overdosage/Treatment
Decontamination: Activated charcoal; acute overdose does not require tapering of dose
Enhanced elimination: Its metabolite (prednisolone) is slightly dialyzable (5% to 20%)

Drug Interactions
Decreased effect: Barbiturates, phenytoin, rifampin increase metabolism of triamcinolone; vaccine and toxoid effects may be reduced
Increased effect: Salmeterol: The addition of salmeterol has been demonstrated to improve response to inhaled corticosteroids (as compared to increasing steroid dosage)
Increased toxicity: Salicylates may increase risk of GI ulceration

Pregnancy Risk Factor C
Pregnancy Implications There are no adequate studies in pregnant women, however, triamcinolone is teratogenic in animals; use during pregnancy with caution. Increased incidence of cleft palate, neonatal adrenal suppression, low birth weight, and cataracts in the infant has been reported following corticosteroid use during pregnancy. In general, the use of large amounts, or prolonged use, of topical corticosteroids during pregnancy should be avoided. In the mother, corticosteroids may increase calcium and potassium excretion, elevate blood pressure, and cause salt and water retention.

Lactation Excretion in breast milk unknown/use caution

Nursing Implications Once daily doses should be given in the morning; evaluate clinical response and mental status; may mask signs and symptoms of infection; inject I.M. dose deep in large muscle mass, avoid deltoid; avoid SubQ dose; a thin film is effective topically and avoid topical application on the face; do not occlude area unless directed

Additional Information 16 mg triamcinolone is equivalent to 100 mg cortisone (no mineralocorticoid activity); adrenal insufficiency can occur with intramuscular injections >400 mg

Specific References
Kumar S, Singh RJ, Reed AM, et al, "Cushing's Syndrome After Intra-articular and Intradermal Administration of Triamcinolone Acetonide in Three Pediatric Patients," *Pediatrics*, 2004, 113(6):1820-4.
Mistlin A and Gibson T, "Osteonecrosis of the Femoral Head Resulting from Excessive Corticosteroid Nasal Spray Use," *J Clin Rheumatol*, 2004, 10(1):45-7.

Triamterene

CAS Number 396-01-0
U.S. Brand Names Dyrenium®
Use Alone or in combination with other diuretics in treatment of edema and hypertension; decreases potassium excretion caused by kaliuretic diuretics
Mechanism of Action Competes with aldosterone for receptor sites in the distal renal tubules, increasing sodium, chloride, and water excretion while conserving potassium and hydrogen ions; may block the effect of aldosterone on arteriolar smooth muscle as well

Adverse Reactions
Cardiovascular: Bradycardia, sinus bradycardia
Central nervous system: Headache, hyperthermia
Dermatologic: Photosensitivity, purpura
Endocrine & metabolic: Hyperkalemia, hyperuricemia
Gastrointestinal: Nausea, vomiting, diarrhea
Hematologic: Pancytopenia, anemia (megaloblastic)
Renal: Reversible renal failure, renal stone formation, interstitial nephritis, acute tubular necrosis
Genitourinary: Urine discoloration (blue), urine discoloration (fluorescent)

Pharmacodynamics/Kinetics
Onset of action: Diuresis occurs within 2-4 hours
Duration: 7-9 hours
Absorption: Oral: Unreliable
Distribution: V_d: 2.5 L/kg
Protein binding: 55% (parent compound); 90% (active metabolite)

Metabolism: Hepatic to an active metabolite (hydroxytriamterene sulfate)

Bioavailability: 52%

Half-life: 1.5-2.5 hours

Dosage Adults: Oral: 100-300 mg/day in 1-2 divided doses; maximum dose: 300 mg/day; usual dosage range (JNC 7): 50-100 mg/day

Dosing comments in renal impairment: Cl_{cr} <10 mL/minute: Avoid use.

Dosing adjustment in hepatic impairment: Dose reduction is recommended in patients with cirrhosis.

Monitoring Parameters Blood pressure, serum electrolytes (especially potassium), renal function, weight, I & O

Contraindications Hypersensitivity to triamterene or any component of the formulation; patients receiving other potassium-sparing diuretics; anuria; severe hepatic disease; hyperkalemia or history of hyperkalemia; severe or progressive renal disease; pregnancy (expert analysis)

Warnings

[U.S. Boxed Warning]: Hyperkalemia can occur; patients at risk include those with renal impairment, diabetes, the elderly, and the severely ill. Serum potassium levels must be monitored at frequent intervals especially when dosages are changed or with any illness that may cause renal dysfunction. Avoid potassium supplements, potassium-containing salt substitutes, a diet rich in potassium, or other drugs that can cause hyperkalemia. Monitor for fluid and electrolyte imbalances. Diuretic therapy should be carefully used in severe hepatic dysfunction; electrolyte and fluid shifts can cause or exacerbate encephalopathy. Use cautiously in patients with history of kidney stones and diabetes. Can cause photosensitivity.

Dosage Forms Capsule: 50 mg, 100 mg [contains benzyl alcohol]

Reference Range Peak plasma levels after a 50 mg oral dose: 25 ng/mL (of hydroxytriamterene sulfate - 770 ng/mL)

Overdosage/Treatment

Decontamination: Activated charcoal

Supportive therapy: Hyperkalemia can be treated with glucose/insulin and sodium bicarbonate (1 mEq/kg); sodium polystyrene sulfonate can also be given; I.V. fluids administration of 0.45% sodium chloride with furosemide (1 mg/kg, up to 40 mg) can be used to promote urine flow

Test Interactions Triamterene can interfere with the fluorescent measurement of quinidine, leading to falsely elevated quinidine assays

Drug Interactions

ACE inhibitors can cause hyperkalemia, especially in patients with renal impairment, potassium-rich diets, or on other drugs causing hyperkalemia; avoid concurrent use or monitor closely.

Potassium supplements may further increase potassium retention and cause hyperkalemia; avoid concurrent use.

Pregnancy Risk Factor B (manufacturer); D (expert analysis)

Pregnancy Implications No data available. Generally, use of diuretics during pregnancy is avoided due to risk of decreased placental perfusion.

Lactation Excretion in breast milk unknown

Nursing Implications Observe for hyperkalemia; assess weight and I & O daily to determine weight loss; if ordered once daily, dose should be given in the morning

Additional Information Abrupt discontinuation of therapy may result in rebound kaliuresis; taper off gradually; can discolor urine to bluish color; has antifolate activity

Specific References

Chobanian AV, Bakris GL, Black HR, et al, "The Seventh Report of the Joint National Committee on Prevention, Detection, Evaluation, and Treatment of High Blood Pressure: The JNC 7 Report," *JAMA*, 2003, (19)289:2560-71.

Triazolam

Related Information

• Therapeutic Drugs Associated with Hallucinations

CAS Number 28911-01-5

U.S. Brand Names Halcion®

Impairment Potential Yes. Blood triazolam levels >4 mcg/L are consistent with driving impairment. Brief or extended periods of exposure are less likely to cause driving impairment in the elderly compared with the longer half-life benzodiazepines. (Joynt BP, "Triazolam Blood Concentrations in Forensic Cases in Canada," *J Anal Toxicol*, 1993, 17(3):171-7.)

Use Short-term treatment of insomnia

Mechanism of Action Depresses all levels of the CNS, including the limbic and reticular formation, probably through the increased action of gamma-aminobutyric acid (GABA), which is a major inhibitory neurotransmitter in the brain

Adverse Reactions

Cardiovascular: Tachycardia, chest pain

Central nervous system: **Drowsiness** (14%), ataxia, confusional states/ memory impairment, tiredness, lightheadedness, insomnia, depression, headache (9.7%), transient global amnesia (TGA), dizziness, nervousness, euphoria, night terrors, coordination disorders, amnesia

Dermatologic: Dermatitis, hypertrichosis, alopecia, purpura, photosensitivity, pruritus, exanthem

Gastrointestinal: Xerostomia, constipation, diarrhea, nausea/vomiting, taste alteration

Neuromuscular & skeletal: Paresthesia

Ocular: Visual disturbances

Otic: Tinnitus

Signs and Symptoms of Overdose Ataxia, cholestatic jaundice, cognitive dysfunction, coma, confusion, diminished reflexes, hypotension, hypothermia, mania, myoglobinuria, night terrors, respiratory depression, rhabdomyolysis, slurred speech, somnolence, visual or auditory hallucinations

Admission Criteria/Prognosis Admit any patient with mental status changes or ingestion >3 mg

Pharmacodynamics/Kinetics

Onset of action: Hypnotic: 15-30 minutes

Duration: 6-7 hours

Distribution: V_d: 0.8-1.8 L/kg

Protein binding: 89%

Metabolism: Extensively hepatic

Half-life elimination: 1.7-5 hours

Excretion: Urine as unchanged drug and metabolites

Dosage

Oral (onset of action is rapid, patient should be in bed when taking medication):

Children <18 years: Dosage not established

Adults:

Hypnotic: 0.125-0.25 mg at bedtime (maximum dose: 0.5 mg/day)

Preprocedure sedation (dental): 0.25 mg taken the evening before oral surgery; or 0.25 mg 1 hour before procedure

Elderly: Insomnia (short-term use): 0.0625-0.125 mg at bedtime; maximum dose: 0.25 mg/day. Due to the higher incidence of CNS adverse reactions and its short half-life, this benzodiazepine is not a drug of first choice. For short-term only.

Dosing adjustment/comments in hepatic impairment: Reduce dose or avoid use in cirrhosis

Monitoring Parameters Respiratory and cardiovascular status

Administration May take with food. Tablet may be crushed or swallowed whole. Onset of action is rapid, patient should be in bed when taking medication.

Contraindications Hypersensitivity to triazolam or any component of the formulation (cross-sensitivity with other benzodiazepines may exist); concurrent therapy with atazanavir, ketoconazole, itraconazole, nefazodone, and ritonavir; pregnancy

Warnings

Should be used only after evaluation of potential causes of sleep disturbance. Failure of sleep disturbance to resolve after 7-10 days may indicate psychiatric or medical illness. A worsening of insomnia or the emergence of new abnormalities of thought or behavior may represent unrecognized psychiatric or medical illness and requires immediate and careful evaluation. Prescription should be written for a maximum of 7-10 days and should not be prescribed in quantities exceeding a 1-month supply. Abrupt discontinuation after sustained use (generally >10 days) may cause withdrawal symptoms.

An increase in daytime anxiety may occur after as few as 10 days of continuous use, which may be related to withdrawal reaction in some patients. Anterograde amnesia may occur at a higher rate with triazolam than with other benzodiazepines. Use with caution in elderly or debilitated patients, patients with hepatic disease (including alcoholics), or renal impairment. Use with caution in patients with respiratory disease or impaired gag reflex. Avoid use in patients with sleep apnea.

Causes CNS depression (dose-related) resulting in sedation, dizziness, confusion, or ataxia which may impair physical and mental capabilities. Patients must be cautioned about performing tasks which require mental alertness (eg, operating machinery or driving). Use with caution in patients receiving other CNS depressants or psychoactive agents. Effects with other sedative drugs or ethanol may be potentiated. Benzodiazepines have been associated with falls and traumatic injury and should be used with extreme caution in patients who are at risk of these events (especially the elderly).

Use caution with potent CYP3A4 inhibitors, as they may significantly decreased the clearance of triazolam. Use caution in patients with depression, particularly if suicidal risk may be present. Use with caution in patients with a history of drug dependence. Benzodiazepines have been associated with dependence and acute withdrawal symptoms on discontinuation or reduction in dose. Acute withdrawal, including seizures, may be precipitated after administration of flumazenil to patients receiving long-term benzodiazepine therapy.

Paradoxical reactions, including hyperactive or aggressive behavior have been reported with benzodiazepines, particularly in adolescent/pediatric or psychiatric patients. Does not have analgesic, antidepressant, or antipsychotic properties.

Dosage Forms Tablet: 0.125 mg, 0.25 mg [contains sodium benzoate]

Reference Range Therapeutic serum triazolam level: 5-20 ng/mL (14.5-58.3 nmol/L); fatalities have been associated with postmortem blood level >47 nmol/L

Overdosage/Treatment

Decontamination: Lavage ingestions >2 mg (within 1 hour)/activated charcoal

Supportive therapy: Treatment for benzodiazepine overdose is supportive. Rarely is mechanical ventilation required. Flumazenil (Romazicon™) may be used to reverse benzodiazepine-induced CNS depression.

Enhancement of elimination: Multiple dose of activated charcoal may be effective

Antidote(s)
- Flumazenil [ANTIDOTE]

Test Interactions Visine®, Drano®, bleach may cause false-negative urine tests; oxazepam may interfere giving falsely elevated glucose results

Drug Interactions Substrate of CYP3A4 (major); **Inhibits** CYP2C8 (weak), 2C9 (weak)

Clozapine: Benzodiazepines may enhance the adverse/toxic effect of clozapine.

CNS depressants: Sedative effects and/or respiratory depression may be additive with CNS depressants; includes ethanol, barbiturates, narcotic analgesics, and other sedative agents; monitor for increased effect

CYP3A4 inducers: CYP3A4 inducers may decrease the levels/effects of triazolam. Example inducers include aminoglutethimide, carbamazepine, nafcillin, nevirapine, phenobarbital, phenytoin, and rifamycins.

CYP3A4 inhibitors: May increase the levels/effects of triazolam. Example inhibitors include azole antifungals, clarithromycin, diclofenac, doxycycline, erythromycin, imatinib, isoniazid, nefazodone, nicardipine, propofol, protease inhibitors, quinidine, telithromycin, and verapamil.

Disulfiram: May decrease the metabolism, via CYP isoenzymes, of triazolam.

Isoniazid: Isoniazid may increase triazolam levels.

Oral contraceptives: May decrease the clearance and increase the half-life of triazolam; monitor for increased triazolam effect

Proton Pump Inhibitors: May increase the serum concentration of triazolam.

Theophylline: May partially antagonize some of the effects of benzodiazepines; monitor for decreased response; may require higher doses for sedation

Pregnancy Risk Factor X

Pregnancy Implications Other benzodiazepines are known to cross the placenta and accumulate in the fetus. Teratogenic effects have been reported. Use of triazolam is contraindicated in pregnancy.

Lactation Excretion in breast milk unknown/not recommended

Nursing Implications Provide safety measures (ie, side rails, night light, call button); remove smoking materials from area; supervise ambulation

Additional Information Triazolam serum concentration may be increased by grapefruit juice; avoid concurrent use.

Specific References

Lin D-L, Huang T-Y, Liu H-C, et al, "Urinary Excretion of α-Hydroxytriazolam Following a Single Dose of Halcion®," *J Anal Toxicol*, 2005, 29:118-23.

Tsujikawa K, Kuwayama K, Miyaguchi H, et al, "Urinary Excretion Profiles of Two Major Triazolam Metabolites, alpha-Hydroxytriazolam and 4-Hydroxytriazolam," *J Anal Toxicol*, 2005, 29(4):240-4.

Trifluoperazine

Related Information
- Anticholinergic Effects of Common Psychotropics
- Antipsychotic Agents

CAS Number 117-89-5; 440-17-5

U.S. Brand Names Stelazine® [DSC]

Synonyms Trifluoperazine Hydrochloride

Impairment Potential Yes

Use Treatment of psychoses and management of anxiety

Unlabeled/Investigational Use Management of psychotic disorders

Mechanism of Action Blocks postsynaptic mesolimbic dopaminergic receptors in the brain; exhibits a strong alpha-adrenergic blocking effect and depresses the release of hypothalamic and hypophyseal hormones

Adverse Reactions

Cardiovascular: **Hypotension** (especially with I.V. use), **hypotension (orthostatic)**, tachycardia, cardiac arrhythmias, sinus tachycardia

Central nervous system: **Pseudoparkinsonian signs and symptoms, dizziness, akathisia, dystonia, tardive dyskinesia**, sedation, drowsiness, restlessness, anxiety, extrapyramidal reactions, neuroleptic malignant syndrome, seizures, altered central temperature regulation, gustatory hallucinations, tardive dystonia

Dermatologic: Hyperpigmentation, pruritus, rash, photosensitivity

Endocrine & metabolic: Amenorrhea, galactorrhea, gynecomastia, syndrome of inappropriate antidiuretic hormone, hyperprolactinemia

Gastrointestinal: **Constipation**, GI upset, xerostomia, Ogilvie's syndrome, weight gain

Genitourinary: Urinary retention, impotence

Hematologic: Agranulocytosis, leukopenia, aplastic anemia

Hepatic: Cholestatic jaundice

Ocular: **Retinal pigmentation**, nystagmus, blurred vision, lenticular opacities, blepharospasm

Respiratory: **Nasal congestion**

Miscellaneous: **Diaphoresis (decreased)**, anaphylactoid reactions, systemic lupus erythematosus

Signs and Symptoms of Overdose Abnormal involuntary muscle movements, agranulocytosis, coma, deep sleep, dysphagia, extrapyramidal reaction, facial grimacing, galactorrhea, generalized rigidity, granulocytopenia, gynecomastia, hepatic failure, hyperthermia, hypotension or hypertension, impotence, leukopenia, neuroleptic malignant syndrome, neutropenia, nystagmus, Parkinson's-like symptoms, slurred speech, stridor, torticollis, trismus, urine discoloration (pink; red; red-brown), vision color changes (brown tinge)

Pharmacodynamics/Kinetics

Onset of action: Rapid

Duration: ≥12 hours

Distribution: Widely distributed into body

Protein binding: ≥90%

Metabolism: Extensive liver metabolism

Half-life: >24 hours with chronic use; 7-18 hours with one dose

Time to peak plasma concentration: 2-4 hours

Elimination: Primarily excreted renally; biliary

Dosage

Children 6-12 years: Psychoses:

Oral: Hospitalized or well supervised patients: Initial: 1 mg 1-2 times/day, gradually increase until symptoms are controlled or adverse effects become troublesome; maximum: 15 mg/day

I.M.: 1 mg twice daily

Adults:

Psychoses:

Outpatients: Oral: 1-2 mg twice daily

Hospitalized or well supervised patients: Initial: 2-5 mg twice daily with optimum response in the 15-20 mg/day range; do not exceed 40 mg/day

I.M.: 1-2 mg every 4-6 hours as needed up to 10 mg/24 hours maximum

Nonpsychotic anxiety: Oral: 1-2 mg twice daily; maximum: 6 mg/day; therapy for anxiety should not exceed 12 weeks; do not exceed 6 mg/day for longer than 12 weeks when treating anxiety; agitation, jitteriness, or insomnia may be confused with original neurotic or psychotic symptoms

Stability Store injection at room temperature; protect from heat and from freezing; use only clear or slightly yellow solutions

Monitoring Parameters Vital signs; lipid profile, fasting blood glucose/Hgb A$_{1c}$; BMI; mental status, abnormal involuntary movement scale (AIMS)

Contraindications Hypersensitivity to trifluoperazine or any component of the formulation (cross-reactivity between phenothiazines may occur); severe CNS depression; bone marrow suppression; blood dyscrasias; severe hepatic disease; coma

Warnings

May be sedating, use with caution in disorders where CNS depression is a feature. Use with caution in Parkinson's disease. Caution in patients with hemodynamic instability; predisposition to seizures; subcortical brain damage; hepatic impairment; severe cardiac, renal, or respiratory disease. Esophageal dysmotility and aspiration have been associated with antipsychotic use - use with caution in patients at risk of pneumonia (ie, Alzheimer's disease). Caution in breast cancer or other prolactin-dependent tumors (may elevate prolactin levels). May alter temperature regulation or mask toxicity of other drugs due to antiemetic effects. May alter cardiac conduction - life-threatening arrhythmias have occurred with therapeutic doses of phenothiazines. May cause orthostatic hypotension - use with caution in patients at risk of this effect or those who would tolerate transient hypotensive episodes (cerebrovascular disease, cardiovascular disease or other medications which may predispose). Safety in children <6 months of age has not been established.

Phenothiazines may cause anticholinergic effects (confusion, agitation, constipation, xerostomia, blurred vision, urinary retention); therefore, they should be used with caution in patients with decreased gastrointestinal motility, urinary retention, BPH, xerostomia, or visual problems. Conditions which also may be exacerbated by cholinergic blockade include narrow-angle glaucoma (screening is recommended) and worsening of myasthenia gravis. Relative to other antipsychotics, trifluoperazine has a low potency of cholinergic blockade.

May cause extrapyramidal symptoms, including pseudoparkinsonism, acute dystonic reactions, akathisia, and tardive dyskinesia (risk of these reactions is high relative to other neuroleptics). May be associated with neuroleptic malignant syndrome (NMS) or pigmentary retinopathy.

Dosage Forms Tablet: 1 mg, 2 mg, 5 mg, 10 mg

Reference Range Therapeutic level: 0.002-0.060 mg/L

Overdosage/Treatment

Decontamination: Lavage (within 1 hour)/activated charcoal

Supportive therapy: Following initiation of essential overdose management, toxic symptom treatment and supportive treatment should be initiated. Hypotension usually responds to I.V. fluids or Trendelenburg positioning. If unresponsive to these measures, the use of a parenteral inotrope may be required (eg, norepinephrine 0.1-0.2 mcg/kg/minute titrated to response). Seizures commonly respond to lorazepam, diazepam, or phenobarbital. Also critical cardiac arrhythmias often respond to I.V. phenytoin (15 mg/kg up to 1 g), while other antiarrhythmics can be used. Neuroleptics often cause extrapyramidal reaction (eg, dystonic reactions) requiring management with diphenhydramine 1-2 mg/kg (adults) up to a maximum of 50 mg I.M. or I.V. slow push followed by a maintenance dose for 48-72 hours. When these reactions are unresponsive to diphenhydramine, benztropine mesylate I.V. 1-2 mg (adults) may be effective. These agents are generally effective within 2-5 minutes.

Enhancement of elimination: Multiple dosing of activated charcoal may be effective; not dialyzable (0% to 5%)

Test Interactions ↑ cholesterol (S), glucose; ↓ uric acid (S); may cross react with serum tricyclic assay

Drug Interactions Substrate of CYP1A2 (major)

Acetylcholinesterase inhibitors (central): May increase the risk of antipsychotic-related extrapyramidal symptoms; monitor

Aluminum salts: May decrease the absorption of phenothiazines; monitor

Amphetamines: Efficacy may be diminished by antipsychotics; in addition, amphetamines may increase psychotic symptoms; avoid concurrent use

Anticholinergics: May inhibit the therapeutic response to phenothiazines and excess anticholinergic effects may occur; includes benztropine, trihexyphenidyl, biperiden, and drugs with significant anticholinergic activity (TCAs, antihistamines, disopyramide)

Antihypertensives: Concurrent use of phenothiazines with an antihypertensive may produce additive hypotensive effects (particularly ortho-stasis)

Bromocriptine: Phenothiazines inhibit the ability of bromocriptine to lower serum prolactin concentrations

CNS depressants: Sedative effects may be additive with phenothiazines; monitor for increased effect; includes barbiturates, benzodiazepines, narcotic analgesics, ethanol, and other sedative agents

CYP1A2 inducers: May decrease the levels/effects of trifluoperazine. Example inducers include aminoglutethimide, carbamazepine, phenobarbital, and rifampin.

CYP1A2 inhibitors: May increase the levels/effects of trifluoperazine. Example inhibitors include ciprofloxacin, fluvoxamine, ketoconazole, norfloxacin, ofloxacin, and rofecoxib.

Epinephrine: Chlorpromazine (and possibly other low potency antipsychotics) may diminish the pressor effects of epinephrine

Guanethidine and guanadrel: Antihypertensive effects may be inhibited by phenothiazines

Levodopa: Phenothiazines may inhibit the antiparkinsonian effect of levodopa; avoid this combination

Lithium: Phenothiazines may produce neurotoxicity with lithium; this is a rare effect.

Metoclopramide: May increase extrapyramidal symptoms (EPS) or risk.

Polypeptide antibiotics: Rare cases of respiratory paralysis have been reported with concurrent use of phenothiazines

Propranolol: Serum concentrations of phenothiazines may be increased; propranolol also increases phenothiazine concentrations

QT$_c$-prolonging agents: Effects on QT$_c$ interval may be additive with phenothiazines, increasing the risk of malignant arrhythmias; includes type Ia antiarrhythmics, TCAs, and some quinolone antibiotics (sparfloxacin, moxifloxacin, and gatifloxacin)

Sulfadoxine-pyrimethamine: May increase phenothiazine concentrations

Trazodone: Phenothiazines and trazodone may produce additive hypotensive effects

Tricyclic antidepressants: Concurrent use may produce increased toxicity or altered therapeutic response

Valproic acid: Serum levels may be increased by phenothiazines

Pregnancy Risk Factor C

Lactation Enters breast milk/not recommended (AAP rates "of concern")

Nursing Implications Give I.M. injection deep in upper outer quadrant of buttock; watch for hypotension when administering I.M. or I.V.

Additional Information Do not exceed 6 mg/day for longer than 12 weeks when treating anxiety; agitation, jitteriness or insomnia may be confused with original neurotic or psychotic symptoms; radiopaque

Trimeprazine

CAS Number 4330-99-8; 84-96-8

Impairment Potential Yes

Use Cough suppressant; relief of pruritus; anesthesia induction; useful for plant-induced dermatitis; allergic rhinitis; sleep disorders

Mechanism of Action A phenothiazine derivation with antimuscarinic and antihistaminic (H$_1$- receptor) effects

Adverse Reactions

Cardiovascular: Hypotension (orthostatic), bradycardia, sinus tachycardia

Central nervous system: **Drowsiness**, nightmares, headache, CNS depression, sedation, malignant hyperthermia, dystonia, ataxia

Dermatologic: Angioedema, urticaria, purpura, photosensitivity, pruritus, exanthem

Endocrine & metabolic: Gynecomastia

Gastrointestinal: Xerostomia, constipation, stomatitis

Hematologic: Leukopenia, pancytopenia

Neuromuscular & skeletal: Tremors, paresthesia

Ocular: Mydriasis, diplopia

Otic: Tinnitus

Respiratory: **Thickening of bronchial secretions**, respiratory depression

Miscellaneous: Systemic lupus erythematosus

Signs and Symptoms of Overdose Akathisia, CNS depression, coma, hypotension, parkinsonism

Pharmacodynamics/Kinetics

Absorption: Well absorbed

Metabolism: Extensively hepatically metabolized largely to n-desalkyl metabolites

Bioavailability: Tablet: 70%; the sustained release capsules give closely comparable serum and urinary levels

Half-life, elimination: 4.78 hours

Time to peak serum concentration:

Syrup: 3.5 hours

Tablet: 4.5 hours

Dosage Oral, (maximum daily dose): 100 mg

Children:

>3 years: 2.5 mg up to 3 times/day

>6 years: Sustained release (Spansule®) capsule: 5 mg/day

Night walking: 6 mg/kg up to 60 mg

Preoperative anesthesia (children >2 years): 2-5 mg/kg

Adults:

Pruritus: 2.5 mg 4 times/day

Sustained release (Spansule®) capsule: 5 mg every 12 hours; decrease dose in elderly

Monitoring Parameters ECG, CBC, blood pressure, arterial blood gases

Contraindications Hypersensitivity to trimeprazine or any component

Warnings Phenothiazines elevate prolactin levels and may be associated with breast tumorigenesis. Because phenothiazines lower the seizure threshold, trimeprazine should not be administered for 48 hours before and after myelography. Use with caution in patients with history of narrow-angle glaucoma, bladder neck obstruction, symptomatic prostate hypertrophy, asthma, sleep apnea, and stenosing peptic ulcer

Dosage Forms Tablet, as tartrate: 2.5 mg, 5 mg

Reference Range Therapeutic plasma level: 0.05-4.0 mcg/mL; postmortem blood level of 6.52 mcg/mL associated with fatality due to overdose of trimeprazine (postmortem urine was 6.22 mcg/mL)

Overdosage/Treatment

Decontamination: Lavage (within 1 hour)/activated charcoal

Supportive therapy: Following initiation of essential overdose management, toxic symptom treatment and supportive treatment should be initiated. Hypotension usually responds to I.V. fluids or Trendelenburg positioning. If unresponsive to these measures, the use of a parenteral inotrope may be required (eg, norepinephrine 0.1-0.2 mcg/kg/minute titrated to response). Seizures commonly respond to lorazepam, diazepam, or phenobarbital. Also critical cardiac arrhythmias often respond to I.V. phenytoin (15 mg/kg up to 1 gram), while other antiarrhythmics can be used. Neuroleptics often cause extrapyramidal reaction (eg, dystonic reactions) requiring management with diphenhydramine 1-2 mg/kg (adults) up to a maximum of 50 mg I.M. or I.V. slow push followed by a maintenance dose for 48-72 hours. When these reactions are unresponsive to diphenhydramine, benztropine mesylate I.V. 1-2 mg (adults) may be effective. These agents are generally effective within 2-5 minutes.

Enhancement of elimination: Multiple dosing of activated charcoal may be helpful; not dialyzable (0% to 5%)

Drug Interactions Increased effect/toxicity with CNS depressants, alcohol, MAO inhibitors (avoid concomitant use), oral contraceptives, progesterone, reserpine, nylidrin; reduce narcotic or barbiturate concurrent dosage by 25% to 50%

Pregnancy Risk Factor C

Additional Information Chronic use can cause an increase in prolactin levels

Trimethaphan Camsylate

CAS Number 68-91-7; 7187-66-8

Synonyms Trimetaphan Camsilate; Trimethaphan Camphorsulfonate

Use Immediate and temporary reduction of blood pressure in patients with hypertensive emergencies; controlled hypotension during surgery

Mechanism of Action Blocks transmission in both adrenergic and cholinergic ganglia by blocking stimulation from presynaptic receptors to postsynaptic receptors mediated by acetylcholine; possesses direct peripheral vasodilatory activity and is a weak histamine releaser

Adverse Reactions

Cardiovascular: Hypotension (especially orthostatic), tachycardia, left bundle-branch block, first degree AV block, reduced cardiac output, chest pain, angina, sinus tachycardia, tachycardia (supraventricular), vasodilation

Central nervous system: Restlessness, anxiety, mania, paranoia

Dermatologic: Itching, rash

Endocrine & metabolic: Sodium and water retention

Gastrointestinal: Anorexia, nausea, vomiting, xerostomia, adynamic ileus, constipation

Genitourinary: Urinary retention, impotence

Neuromuscular & skeletal: Weakness

Ocular: Mydriasis, cycloplegia

Respiratory: Apnea, respiratory arrest

Miscellaneous: Anhidrosis

Signs and Symptoms of Overdose AV block, hypotension, impotence, respiratory arrest, tachycardia

Pharmacodynamics/Kinetics

Onset of action: Immediate

Peak effect: 5 minutes

Duration: 10-30 minutes

Metabolism: Primarily by postganglionic pseudocholinesterase

Elimination: Urine

Dosage Administration requires the use of an infusion pump

Severe hypertension and hypertensive emergencies: I.V.:

Children: 50-150 mcg/kg/minute; dilute 150 mg × weight (kg) to 250 mL in D_5W then dose in mcg/kg/minute = 10 × infusion rate in mL/hour

Adults: Initial rate: 0.5-1 mg/minute; titrate dose to the desired effect

Hypertension due to acute dissecting aneurysms: Initial rate: 1-2 mg/minute, adjusting as needed to keep systolic blood pressure of 100-120 mm Hg

Controlled hypotension during surgery: Initial rate: 3-4 mg/minute adjusted to maintain blood pressure at a desirable level; usual dosage needed 0.3-6 mg/minute

Stability Refrigerate; however, is stable for up to 14 days at room temperature

Monitoring Parameters Blood pressure and heart rate

Administration Must be diluted; usually mixed as 1 mg/mL concentration in 5% dextrose

Contraindications Hypersensitivity to trimethaphan camsylate or any component; hypovolemia or shock; anemia; respiratory insufficiency

Warnings Use with caution in patients with arteriosclerosis, cardiac, hepatic and renal dysfunction, diabetes mellitus, or Addison's disease. Pupillary dilation does not necessarily indicate anoxia or the depth of anesthesia since the drug appears to have a specific effect on the pupil.

Dosage Forms Injection: 50 mg/mL (10 mL)

Overdosage/Treatment Supportive therapy: Following initiation of essential overdose management, toxic symptoms should be treated. Seizures usually respond to lorazepam or diazepam I.V. boluses (5-10 mg for adults up to 30 mg or 0.25-0.4 mg/kg/dose for children up to 10 mg/dose). If seizures are unresponsive or recur, phenytoin or phenobarbital may be required. Hypotension usually responds to I.V. fluids or Trendelenburg positioning. If unresponsive to these measures, the use of a parenteral inotrope may be required (eg, dopamine 10 mcg/kg/minute starting dose or norepinephrine 0.1-0.2 mcg/kg/minute titrated to response). Physostigmine or neostigmine 0.5-1 mg I.V. slow push reverses many of the drug's acute toxic effects, while bethanechol has proven useful in treating the drug-induced urinary retention.

Test Interactions ↓ potassium (S)

Drug Interactions Increased effect with anesthetics; increased effect of nondepolarizing neuromuscular blocking agents

Pregnancy Risk Factor C

Pregnancy Implications Can cause meconium ileus in neonates; crosses placenta

Nursing Implications Must be diluted; usually mixed as 1 mg/mL concentration in 5% dextrose; solution should be freshly prepared and any unused portion discarded

Additional Information Pupillary dilation does not necessarily indicate depth of anesthesia; discontinue drug before wound closure

Trimethobenzamide

CAS Number 554-92-7

U.S. Brand Names Tigan®

Synonyms Trimethobenzamide Hydrochloride

Impairment Potential Yes

Use Treatment of nausea and vomiting

Mechanism of Action Acts centrally to inhibit the medullary chemoreceptor trigger zone

Adverse Reactions

Cardiovascular: Hypotension

Central nervous system: Coma, depression, disorientation, dizziness, drowsiness, extrapyramidal symptoms, headache, opisthotonos, Parkinson-like syndrome, seizures

Hematologic: Blood dyscrasias

Hepatic: Jaundice

Neuromuscular & skeletal: Muscle cramps

Ocular: Blurred vision

Miscellaneous: Hypersensitivity reactions

Signs and Symptoms of Overdose CNS depression, hypotension, seizures

Pharmacodynamics/Kinetics

Onset of action: Antiemetic: Oral: 10-40 minutes; I.M.: 15-35 minutes

Duration: 3-4 hours

Absorption: Rectal: ~60%

Bioavailability: Oral: 60% to 100%

Half-life elimination: 7-9 hours

Time to peak: Oral: 45 minutes; I.M.: 30 minutes

Excretion: Urine (30% to 50%)

Dosage

Rectal use is contraindicated in neonates and premature infants

Children:

<14 kg: Oral, rectal: 100 mg 3-4 times/day

14-40 kg: Oral, rectal: 100-200 mg 3-4 times/day

Adults:

Oral: 250-300 mg 3-4 times/day

I.M., rectal: 200 mg 3-4 times/day

Stability Store capsules, injection solution, and suppositories at room temperature.

Administration

Administer I.M. only; not for I.V. administration. Inject deep into upper outer quadrant of gluteal muscle.

Contraindications Hypersensitivity to trimethobenzamide, benzocaine (or similar local anesthetics), or any component of the formulation; injection contraindicated in children; suppositories contraindicated in premature infants or neonates

Warnings May mask emesis due to Reye's syndrome or mimic CNS effects of Reye's syndrome in patients with emesis of other etiologies; use in patients with acute vomiting should be avoided. May cause drowsiness; patient should avoid tasks requiring alertness (eg, driving, operating machinery). May cause extrapyramidal symptoms (EPS) which may be confused with CNS symptoms of primary disease responsible for emesis. Risk of adverse effects (eg, EPS, seizure) may be increased in patients with acute febrile illness, dehydration, or electrolyte imbalance; use caution.

Dosage Forms

Capsule, as hydrochloride (Tigan®): 300 mg

Injection, solution, as hydrochloride: 100 mg/mL (2 mL)

Tigan®: 100 mg/mL (2 mL [preservative free], 20 mL)

Suppository, rectal, as hydrochloride: 100 mg, 200 mg

Tebamide™: 100 mg, 200 mg [contains benzocaine]

Tigan®, Trimazide [DSC]: 200 mg [contains benzocaine]

Overdosage/Treatment

Decontamination: Lavage (within 1 hour)/activated charcoal; charcoal may need to be given in multiple doses for adequate decontamination

Supportive therapy: Initiate support with fluids, norepinephrine may be useful for hypotension; hypoperfusion states may respond to inotropic support with dobutamine. Seizures should be managed with benzodiazepines or barbiturates.

Enhancement of elimination: Multiple dosing of charcoal may not be effective

Pregnancy Risk Factor C

Pregnancy Implications Teratogenic effects were not observed in animal studies. Safety and efficacy have not been established in pregnant patients. Trimethobenzamide has been used to treat nausea and vomiting of pregnancy.

Lactation Excretion in breast milk unknown

Nursing Implications Use only clear solution

Additional Information Note: Less effective than phenothiazines but may be associated with fewer side effects; rectal is ~60% absorbed. Concomitant ethanol use should be avoided.

Trimetrexate Glucuronate

Related Information
- Methotrexate

CAS Number 52128-38-5; 82952-64-5

U.S. Brand Names Neutrexin®

Synonyms NSC-352122; Trimetrexate Glucuronate

Use Alternative therapy for the treatment of moderate-to-severe *Pneumocystis carinii* pneumonia (PCP) in immunocompromised patients, including patients with acquired immunodeficiency syndrome (AIDS), who are intolerant of, or are refractory to, co-trimoxazole therapy or for whom co-trimoxazole and pentamidine are contraindicated. **Concurrent folinic acid (leucovorin) must always be administered.**

Unlabeled/Investigational Use Treatment of nonsmall cell lung cancer, metastatic colorectal cancer, metastatic head and neck cancer, pancreatic adenocarcinoma, cutaneous T-cell lymphoma

Mechanism of Action Trimetrexate is a folate antimetabolite that inhibits DNA synthesis by inhibition of dihydrofolate reductase (DHFR); DHFR inhibition reduces the formation of reduced folates and thymidylate synthetase, resulting in inhibition of purine and thymidylic acid synthesis.

Adverse Reactions
Central nervous system: Convulsions, fever

Dermatologic: Rash, hyperpigmentation, radiation recall dermatitis

Gastrointestinal: Stomatitis, nausea, vomiting

Hematologic: Neutropenia, thrombocytopenia, anemia

Hepatic: Elevated liver function tests

Neuromuscular & skeletal: Paresthesia

Renal: Elevated serum creatinine

Miscellaneous: Flu-like illness, hypersensitivity reactions

Signs and Symptoms of Overdose Leukopenia or neutropenia (agranulocytosis, granulocytopenia)

Pharmacodynamics/Kinetics
Distribution: V_d: 0.62 L/kg

Protein binding: 80% to 90% (concentration dependent)

Metabolism: Extensively hepatic: O-demethylation followed by conjugation to glucuronide or sulfate (major); N-demethylation and oxidation (minor)

Half-life elimination: 9-18 hours (11 hours with leucovorin)

Excretion: Urine (10% to 40% as unchanged drug); feces (<1% to 8%)

Dosage
Note: Concurrent leucovorin 20 mg/m² every 6 hours must be administered daily (oral or I.V.) during treatment and for 72 hours past the last dose of trimetrexate glucuronate.

Adults: I.V.:

Pneumocystis carinii: 45 mg/m² once daily for 21 days; **alternative dosing based on weight:**

<50 kg:Trimetrexate glucuronate 1.5 mg/kg/day; leucovorin 0.6 mg/kg 4 times/day

50-80 kg:Trimetrexate glucuronate 1.2 mg/kg/day; leucovorin 0.5 mg/kg/4 times/day

>80 kg: Trimetrexate glucuronate 1 mg/kg/day; leucovorin 0.5 mg/kg/4 times/day

Note: Oral doses of leucovorin should be rounded up to the next higher 25 mg increment.

Antineoplastic: 6-16 mg/m² once daily for 5 days every 21-28 days **or** 150-200 mg/m² every 2 weeks

Dosage adjustment in hepatic impairment: Although it may be necessary to reduce the dose in patients with liver dysfunction, no specific recommendations exist.

Stability Reconstituted I.V. solution is stable for 24 hours at room temperature or 7 days when refrigerated; intact vials should be refrigerated at 2°C to 8°C

Monitoring Parameters Check and record patient's temperature daily; absolute neutrophil counts (ANC), platelet count, renal function tests (serum creatinine, BUN), hepatic function tests (ALT, AST, alkaline phosphatase)

Administration Reconstituted solution should be filtered (0.22 µM) prior to further dilution; final solution should be clear, hue will range from colorless to pale yellow; trimetrexate forms a precipitate instantly upon contact with chloride ion or leucovorin, therefore it should not be added to solutions containing sodium chloride or other anions; trimetrexate and leucovorin solutions **must** be administered separately; intravenous lines should be flushed with at least 10 mL of D₅W between trimetrexate and leucovorin

Contraindications Hypersensitivity to trimetrexate, methotrexate, leucovorin, or any component of the formulation; severe existing myelosuppression; pregnancy

Warnings Hazardous agent - use appropriate precautions for handling and disposal. **[U.S. Boxed Warning]: Must be administered with concurrent leucovorin to avoid potentially serious or life-threatening toxicities.** Leucovorin therapy must extend for 72 hours past the last dose of trimetrexate. Hypersensitivity/allergic-type reactions have been reported, primarily when given as a bolus infusion, at higher than recommended doses for PCP, or in combination with fluorouracil or leucovorin. May cause anaphylactoid reactions (rarely) including acute hypotension and loss of consciousness. Epinephrine should be available for treatment of acute allergic symptoms. Use with caution in patients with mild myelosuppression, severe hepatic or renal dysfunction, hypoproteinemia, hypoalbuminemia, or previous extensive myelosuppressive therapies. Withhold zidovudine during trimetrexate treatment.

Dosage Forms Injection, powder for reconstitution [preservative free]: 25 mg, 200 mg

Reference Range Peak plasma level: Oral: 3 mcg/L after 60 mg/m² dose; I.V.: 12 nmol/L after 30 mg/m² dose

Overdosage/Treatment
Decontamination: Ipecac within 30 minutes or lavage (within 1 hour)/ activated charcoal

Supportive therapy: Severe bone marrow toxicity can result from overdose; leucovorin rescue can reduce the toxicity; administer as quickly as possible 10 mg/m² (5-15 mg) every 6 hours for 72 hours

Enhancement of elimination: Multiple dosing of activated charcoal is effective; renal excretion is optimized at a urinary pH of 7.0. Charcoal hemoperfusion, hydration, and urinary alkalinization may enhance elimination and prevent precipitation in renal tubules; not dialyzable (0% to 5%)

Antidote(s)
- Folic Acid [ANTIDOTE]
- Leucovorin [ANTIDOTE]

Test Interactions Mild creatinine elevation, mild liver function test elevation

Drug Interactions Live virus vaccines (ie, yellow fever, BCG, MMP): Trimetrexate, due to immunosuppressive effects, may increase vaccine toxicity (eg, infection).

Zidovudine: May increase the myelotoxicity of trimetrexate. Discontinue zidovudine during trimetrexate treatment.

Pregnancy Risk Factor D

Pregnancy Implications Teratogenic effects and fetal loss were observed in animal studies. May cause fetal harm when administered to pregnant women. Women of childbearing potential should avoid becoming pregnant while receiving treatment. If used in pregnancy, or if patient becomes pregnant during treatment, the patient should be apprised of potential hazard to the fetus.

Lactation Excretion in breast milk unknown/not recommended

Nursing Implications Notify primary physician of fever ≥103°F, generalized rash, seizures, bleeding from any site, uncontrolled nausea/ vomiting, laboratory abnormalities which warrant dose modification; or any other clinical adverse event or laboratory abnormality occurring in therapy which is judged as serious for that patient, or which causes unexplained effects or concern.

Initiate "Bleeding Precautions" for platelet counts ≤50,000/mm³

Initiate "Infection Control Measures" for absolute neutrophil counts (ANC) ≤1000/mm³

Additional Information Not a vesicant; methotrexate derivative; incompatible with foscarnet

---

Trimipramine

Pronunciation (trye MI pra meen)

CAS Number 521-78-8; 739-71-9

U.S. Brand Names Surmontil®

Synonyms Trimipramine Maleate

Impairment Potential Yes

Use Treatment of various forms of depression, often in conjunction with psychotherapy

Mechanism of Action Increases the synaptic concentration of serotonin and/or norepinephrine in the central nervous system by inhibition of their reuptake by the presynaptic neuronal membrane

Adverse Reactions
Cardiovascular: Postural hypotension, cardiac arrhythmias, tachycardia, sudden death, sinus tachycardia, tachycardia (supraventricular), exacerbation of Brugada syndrome

Central nervous system: **Dizziness, drowsiness, headache,** sedation, fatigue, anxiety, impaired cognitive function, seizures have occurred occasionally, psychosis, gustatory hallucinations, hyperthermia

Dermatologic: Alopecia, urticaria, purpura, photosensitivity, pruritus, exanthem

Endocrine & metabolic: Syndrome of inappropriate antidiuretic hormone, parotitis, gynecomastia

Gastrointestinal: **Xerostomia, increased appetite, nausea, unpleasant taste, weight gain, constipation,** stomatitis

Genitourinary: Urinary retention

Hematologic: Agranulocytosis, eosinophilia, may cause alterations in bleeding time, thrombocytopenia

Hepatic: Jaundice

Neuromuscular & skeletal: **Weakness,** tremors, paresthesia

Ocular: Blurred vision, increased intraocular pressure, mydriasis, nystagmus

Miscellaneous: Allergic reactions

Signs and Symptoms of Overdose Agitation, agranulocytosis, coma, confusion, dementia, granulocytopenia, hallucinations, hypotension, hypothermia, increased intraocular pressure, leukopenia, neuroleptic malignant syndrome, neutropenia, seizures, tachycardia, urinary retention

Admission Criteria/Prognosis Admit any patient who is symptomatic 6 hours postingestion

Pharmacodynamics/Kinetics

Distribution: V_d: 17-48 L/kg

Protein binding: 95%; free drug: 3% to 7%

Metabolism: Hepatic; significant first-pass effect

Bioavailability: 18% to 63%

Half-life elimination: 16-40 hours

Excretion: Urine

Toxicodynamics/Kinetics

Absorption: Rapid from the gastrointestinal tract

Distribution: V_d: 17-48 L/kg; distributed widely in the body

Protein binding: 95%

Metabolism: Undergoes significant first-pass metabolism metabolized in the liver to desmethyl trimipramine

Half-life: 6-20 hours

Time to peak serum concentration: Within 6 hours

Elimination: Urine

Dosage Adults: Oral: 50-150 mg/day as a single bedtime dose up to a maximum of 200 mg/day outpatient and 300 mg/day inpatient

Monitoring Parameters Blood pressure and pulse rate prior to and during initial therapy; evaluate mental status; monitor weight; ECG in older adults

Contraindications Hypersensitivity to trimipramine, any component of the formulation, or other dibenzodiazepines; use of MAO inhibitors within 14 days; use in a patient during the acute recovery phase of MI

Warnings

[U.S. Boxed Warning]: Antidepressants increase the risk of suicidal thinking and behavior in children and adolescents with major depressive disorder (MDD) and other depressive disorders; consider risk prior to prescribing. Closely monitor for clinical worsening, suicidality, or unusual changes in behavior; the child's family or caregiver should be instructed to closely observe the patient and communicate condition with healthcare provider. Such observation would generally include at least weekly face-to-face contact with patients or their family members or caregivers during the first 4 weeks of treatment, then every other week visits for the next 4 weeks, then at 12 weeks, and as clinically indicated beyond 12 weeks. Additional contact by telephone may be appropriate between face-to-face visits. Adults treated with antidepressants should be observed similarly for clinical worsening and suicidality, especially during the initial few months of a course of drug therapy, or at times of dose changes, either increases or decreases. A medication guide should be dispensed with each prescription. **Trimipramine is not FDA approved for use in children.**

The possibility of a suicide attempt is inherent in major depression and may persist until remission occurs. Monitor for worsening of depression or suicidality, especially during initiation of therapy or with dose increases or decreases. Worsening depression and severe abrupt suicidality that are not part of the presenting symptoms may require discontinuation or modification of drug therapy. Use caution in high-risk patients during initiation of therapy. Prescriptions should be written for the smallest quantity consistent with good patient care. The patient's family or caregiver should be alerted to monitor patients for the emergence of suicidality and associated behaviors such as anxiety, agitation, panic attacks, insomnia, irritability, hostility, impulsivity, akathisia, hypomania, and mania; patients should be instructed to notify their healthcare provider if any of these symptoms or worsening depression occur.

May worsen psychosis in some patients or precipitate a shift to mania or hypomania in patients with bipolar disorder. Monotherapy in patients with bipolar disorder should be avoided. Patients presenting with depressive symptoms should be screened for bipolar disorder. **Trimipramine is not FDA approved for the treatment of bipolar depression.**

Often causes sedation, resulting in impaired performance of tasks requiring alertness (eg, operating machinery or driving). Sedative effects may be additive with other CNS depressants and/or ethanol. The degree of sedation is very high relative to other antidepressants. May increase the risks associated with electroconvulsive therapy. Consider discontinuing, when possible, prior to elective surgery. Therapy should not be abruptly discontinued in patients receiving high doses for prolonged periods. Use with caution in patients with hepatic or renal dysfunction and in elderly patients.

May cause orthostatic hypotension (risk is high relative to other antidepressants) - use with caution in patients at risk of hypotension or in patients where transient hypotensive episodes would be poorly tolerated (cardiovascular disease or cerebrovascular disease). The degree of anticholinergic blockade produced by this agent is very high relative to other cyclic antidepressants - use caution in patients with urinary retention, benign prostatic hyperplasia, narrow-angle glaucoma,

xerostomia, visual problems, constipation, or history of bowel obstruction. May cause alteration in glucose regulation - use with caution in patients with diabetes.

Use with caution in patients with a history of cardiovascular disease (including previous MI, stroke, tachycardia, or conduction abnormalities). The risk of conduction abnormalities with this agent is high relative to other antidepressants. Use caution in patients with a previous seizure disorder or condition predisposing to seizures such as brain damage, alcoholism, or concurrent therapy with other drugs which lower the seizure threshold. Use with caution in hyperthyroid patients or those receiving thyroid supplementation.

Dosage Forms Capsule: 25 mg, 50 mg, 100 mg

Reference Range An oral dose of 50 mg yields a peak serum level of 260 nmol/L; in the postmortem state, anatomical site concentration differences (ie, postmortem redistribution) may occur.

Overdosage/Treatment

Decontamination: Do **not** induce emesis; gastric lavage (within 2-3 hours)/activated charcoal is useful

Supportive therapy: Following initiation of essential overdose management, toxic symptoms should be treated. Ventricular arrhythmias often respond to systemic alkalinization (sodium bicarbonate 0.5-2 mEq/kg I.V.). Arrhythmias unresponsive to this therapy may respond to lidocaine 1 mg/kg I.V. followed by a titrated infusion. Seizures usually respond to lorazepam or diazepam I.V. boluses (5-10 mg for adults up to 30 mg or 0.25-0.4 mg/kg/dose for children up to 10 mg/dose). If seizures are unresponsive or recur, phenytoin or phenobarbital may be required.

Enhanced elimination: Multiple dosing of activated charcoal may be useful

Antidote(s)

- Sodium Bicarbonate [ANTIDOTE]

Test Interactions ↑ glucose; may cross react with phenothiazine assay

Drug Interactions

Substrate (major) of CYP2C19, 2D6, 3A4

Altretamine: Concurrent use may cause orthostatic hypertension

Amphetamines: TCAs may enhance the effect of amphetamines; monitor for adverse CV effects

Anticholinergics: Combined use with TCAs may produce additive anticholinergic effects

Antihypertensives: TCAs may inhibit the antihypertensive response to bethanidine, clonidine, debrisoquin, guanadrel, guanethidine, guanabenz, guanfacine; monitor BP; consider alternate antihypertensive agent

Beta-agonists: When combined with TCAs may predispose patients to cardiac arrhythmias

Bupropion: May increase the levels of tricyclic antidepressants; based on limited information; monitor response

Carbamazepine: Tricyclic antidepressants may increase carbamazepine levels; monitor

Cholestyramine and colestipol: May bind TCAs and reduce their absorption; monitor for altered response

Clonidine: Abrupt discontinuation of clonidine may cause hypertensive crisis, amitriptyline may enhance the response (also see note on antihypertensives)

CNS depressants: Sedative effects may be additive with TCAs; monitor for increased effect; includes benzodiazepines, barbiturates, antipsychotics, ethanol, and other sedative medications

CYP2D6 inhibitors: May increase the levels/effects of trimipramine. Example inhibitors include chlorpromazine, delavirdine, fluoxetine, miconazole, paroxetine, pergolide, quinidine, quinine, ritonavir, and ropinirole.

CYP2C19 inducers: May decrease the levels/effects of trimipramine. Example inducers include aminoglutethimide, carbamazepine, phenytoin, and rifampin.

CYP2C19 inhibitors: May increase the levels/effects of trimipramine. Example inhibitors include delavirdine, fluconazole, fluvoxamine, gemfibrozil, isoniazid, omeprazole, and ticlopidine.

CYP3A4 inducers: CYP3A4 inducers may decrease the levels/effects of trimipramine. Example inducers include aminoglutethimide, carbamazepine, nafcillin, nevirapine, phenobarbital, phenytoin, and rifamycins.

CYP3A4 inhibitors: May increase the levels/effects of trimipramine. Example inhibitors include azole antifungals, clarithromycin, diclofenac, doxycycline, erythromycin, imatinib, isoniazid, nefazodone, nicardipine, propofol, protease inhibitors, quinidine, telithromycin, and verapamil.

Epinephrine (and other direct alpha-agonists): Pressor response to I.V. epinephrine, norepinephrine, and phenylephrine may be enhanced in patients receiving TCAs (**Note:** Effect is unlikely with epinephrine or levonordefrin dosages typically administered as infiltration in combination with local anesthetics).

Fenfluramine: May increase tricyclic antidepressant levels/effects

Hypoglycemic agents (including insulin): TCAs may enhance the hypoglycemic effects of tolazamide, chlorpropamide, or insulin; monitor for changes in blood glucose levels; reported with chlorpropamide, tolazamide, and insulin

677

Levodopa: Tricyclic antidepressants may decrease the absorption (bioavailability) of levodopa; rare hypertensive episodes have also been attributed to this combination

Linezolid: Hyperpyrexia, hypertension, tachycardia, confusion, seizures, and **deaths have been reported** with agents which inhibit MAO (serotonin syndrome); this combination should be avoided

Lithium: Concurrent use with a TCA may increase the risk for neurotoxicity

MAO inhibitors: Hyperpyrexia, hypertension, tachycardia, confusion, seizures, and **deaths have been reported** (serotonin syndrome); this combination should be avoided

Methylphenidate: Metabolism of TCAs may be decreased

Phenothiazines: Serum concentrations of some TCAs may be increased; in addition, TCAs may increase concentration of phenothiazines; monitor for altered clinical response

QT_c-prolonging agents: Concurrent use of tricyclic agents with other drugs which may prolong QT_c interval may increase the risk of potentially fatal arrhythmias; includes type Ia and type III antiarrhythmics agents, selected quinolones (sparfloxacin, gatifloxacin, moxifloxacin, grepafloxacin), cisapride, and other agents

Ritonavir: Combined use of high-dose tricyclic antidepressants with ritonavir may cause serotonin syndrome in HIV-positive patients; monitor

Sucralfate: Absorption of tricyclic antidepressants may be reduced with coadministration

Sympathomimetics, indirect-acting: Tricyclic antidepressants may result in a decreased sensitivity to indirect-acting sympathomimetics; includes dopamine and ephedrine; also see interaction with epinephrine (and direct-acting sympathomimetics)

Valproic acid: May increase serum concentrations/adverse effects of some tricyclic antidepressants

Warfarin (and other oral anticoagulants): TCAs may increase the anticoagulant effect in patients stabilized on warfarin; monitor INR

Pregnancy Risk Factor C

Lactation Enters breast milk/contraindicated

Additional Information May cause alterations in bleeding time

Tryptophan

Related Information
- Oxitriptan

CAS Number 73-22-3

Synonyms L-Tryptophan

Use Antidepressant, insomnia, dietary supplement, postanoxic myoclonus

Mechanism of Action An essential amino acid which is a precursor to serotonin

Adverse Reactions

Eosinophilia-myalgia syndrome has been associated with L-tryptophan use manufactured by a single Japanese company (Showa-Denko). Thought to be related by presence of impurities (3-phenylaminoalanine) this syndrome is characterized by an early phase (0-2 months) which consists of **myalgia, skin rash, edema, fever, arthralgia, and dyspnea**. Tachycardia may also be present. Later manifestations may include **weight loss, muscle weakness**, progressing ascending axonal polyneuropathy, **paresthesias, alopecia, scleroderma-like cutaneous induration**, liver function abnormalities. Leukocytosis with eosinophilia (eosinophil counts ranging from 1000-36,000/mm^3) usually occur. Eosinophilic fascitis may also occur. Doses associated with development of this syndrome involve 1.2-2.4 g/day for 2 weeks to 8 years.

Cardiovascular: Vasculitis

Central nervous system: Headache, drowsiness, fever, euphoria

Endocrine & metabolic: Sexual dysfunction

Gastrointestinal: Nausea, pancreatitis

Neuromuscular & skeletal: Dyskinesias

Ocular: Nystagmus

Respiratory: Pneumonitis, pleural effusion, eosinophilic pneumonia, pulmonary vasculitis

Signs and Symptoms of Overdose Dizziness, headache, hypoglycemia, nausea (>5 g intake)

Pharmacodynamics/Kinetics

Distribution: V_d: 0.3-3 L/kg

Protein binding: 65% to 78%

Metabolism: In the brain (to serotonin) and in the liver (via kynurenine pathway to quinolinic acid, tryptamine, niacin among other metabolites)

Half-life: 1-3 hours

Dosage Insomnia: 1-2 g at bedtime; doses up to 6 g/day in divided doses have been used to treat depression

Dosage Forms Tablet: 500 mg

Overdosage/Treatment

Decontamination: **Do not** induce emesis; lavage within 1 hour if coingestion (ie, MAO inhibitors, selective serotonin reuptake inhibitors) have occurred; activated charcoal may be useful

Supportive therapy: Although its long-term benefits have not been proven, prednisone (15-60 mg/day) may provide some relief of myalgias and other acute manifestations of eosinophilia-myalgia syndrome. While total eosinophil counts may decrease following high-dose steroid therapy, no effect on neurologic or skin induration complications appear to occur. Cyproheptadine (4 mg twice daily) can be used to treat muscle spasms or cramps. (Do **not** use cyproheptadine if serotonin syndrome is present.)

Drug Interactions Fluoxetine → restlessness, agitation, nausea, diarrhea

Additional Information Usual daily dietary intake: 0.5-2 g; minimum daily requirement: ~3 mg/kg; may exacerbate Huntington's disease; 60 mg of L-tryptophan provide the equivalent of 1 mg of niacin; 1 glass of cow's milk contains ~100 mg tryptophan

Ubidecarenone

CAS Number 303-98-0

Synonyms Mitoquinone; Ubidecarenone

Unlabeled/Investigational Use In U.S.: Congestive heart failure, angina, periodontal disease, also used in treatment of warfarin-induced alopecia, breast cancer, chronic lung disease; prevention of doxorubicin-induced cardiac toxicity

Mechanism of Action A fat soluble quinone which acts as a coenzyme in mitochondrial electron transport and adenosine triphosphate (ATP) synthesis; may affect prostaglandin synthesis

Adverse Reactions

Central nervous system: Headache, agitation, dizziness

Dermatologic: Pruritus

Gastrointestinal: Nausea, diarrhea, anorexia

Pharmacodynamics/Kinetics

Half-life: 34 hours

Peak plasma level: 5-10 hours

Elimination: Biliary (fecal)

Dosage Chronic lung disease: 90 mg/day for 8 weeks

Breast cancer: 90-390 mg/day

Heart failure:
Oral: 50-150 mg/day in 2-3 divided doses
I.V.: 50-100 mg/day

Angina:
Oral: 150-600 mg/day in divided doses
I.V.: 1.5 mg/day for 1 week

Periodontal disease: Oral: 25 mg twice daily

Warfarin-induced alopecia: 30 mg/day

Prevention of doxorubicin cardiac toxicity: 50 mg/day

Contraindications Previous hypersensitivity to ubidecarenone

Warnings Use with caution in patients with diabetes mellitus, liver/biliary disease, renal insufficiency

Dosage Forms Capsule: 10 mg, 30 mg, 50 mg, 75 mg, 100 mg, 150 mg

Liquid: 30 mg/5 mL (480 mL)

Tablet: 25 mg, 60 mg, 200 mg

Tablet, chewable: 100 mg, 200 mg

Reference Range

Normal endogenous blood level of ubidecarenone: 0.3-1.6 mcg/mL

Therapeutic blood levels for congestive heart failure: 2-2.5 mcg/mL

Overdosage/Treatment

Decontamination: **Oral**: Emesis within 30 minutes or lavage (within 1 hour)/activated charcoal. **Ocular**: Irrigate eyes copiously with saline.

Additional Information Total body ubidecarenone content is 1-1.5 g; available as a food supplement in the U.S.; not water soluble

Urapidil

CAS Number 34661-75-1; 64887-14-5

Synonyms Urapidil Hydrochloride

Use Hypertension

Mechanism of Action Alpha$_1$-adrenoceptor antagonist (peripheral vasodilator); a phenylpiperazine derivative of 4-aminouracil

Adverse Reactions

Cardiovascular: Palpitations, bradycardia, hypotension (orthostatic), sinus bradycardia

Central nervous system: Headache, dizziness, fatigue

Dermatologic: Allergic skin reactions, pruritus

Gastrointestinal: Nausea

Renal: Enuresis

Respiratory: Nasal congestion

Signs and Symptoms of Overdose Coagulopathy, diarrhea, drowsiness, enuresis, eosinophilia, hypotension

Pharmacodynamics/Kinetics

Protein binding: 80%

Metabolism: Hepatic to p-hydroxylated urapidil; first-pass effect (20%)

Bioavailability: 70%

Half-life elimination: Oral: 4.7 hours; I.V.: 2.7 hours

Excretion: Urine (15% to 30%) as unchanged drug

Dosage Oral: 30-90 mg twice daily
I.V.: 25 mg over 20 seconds

Reference Range Dose of 120 mg can cause a urapidil blood level of 750 ng/mL 3-5 hours postingestion

Overdosage/Treatment

Decontamination: Ipecac within 30 minutes or lavage (within 1 hour)/charcoal

Supportive therapy: Treat hypotension with fluids or Trendelenburg positioning; vasopressors may be required to support blood pressure (eg, phenylephrine or dopamine)

Drug Interactions Cimetidine modifies pharmacokinetics such that dosage reduction is necessary

Additional Information 20% as potent as prazosin; may increase plasma renin and catecholamine level

Urokinase

CAS Number 9039-53-6

U.S. Brand Names Abbokinase®

Synonyms UK

Use Thrombolytic agent for the lysis of acute massive pulmonary emboli or pulmonary emboli with unstable hemodynamics

Unlabeled/Investigational Use Thrombolytic agent used in treatment of recent severe or massive deep vein thrombosis, myocardial infarction, and occluded I.V. or dialysis cannulas

Mechanism of Action Promotes thrombolysis by directly activating plasminogen to plasmin, which degrades fibrin, fibrinogen, and other procoagulant plasma proteins

Adverse Reactions

Cardiovascular: **Arrhythmias, hypotension**

Central nervous system: Headache, chills, hyperthermia

Dermatologic: Rash, **angioneurotic edema**

Gastrointestinal: Nausea, vomiting

Hematologic: Anemia, eye hemorrhage

Local: **Bleeding at sites of percutaneous trauma**, extravasation injury

Ocular: **Periorbital edema**

Respiratory: **Bronchospasm**, epistaxis

Miscellaneous: **Anaphylaxis**, diaphoresis

Signs and Symptoms of Overdose Bleeding gums, coagulopathy, epistaxis, GI bleeding, hematoma, hematuria, hemoptysis, intracranial hemorrhage, ocular hemorrhage, oozing at catheter site, spontaneous ecchymosis

Pharmacodynamics/Kinetics

Onset of action: I.V.: Fibrinolysis occurs rapidly

Duration: ≥4 hours

Distribution: 11.5 L

Half-life elimination: 6.4-18.8 minutes

Excretion: Urine and feces (small amounts)

Dosage

Children and Adults: Deep vein thrombosis (unlabeled use): I.V.: Loading: 4400 units/kg over 10 minutes, then 4400 units/kg/hour for 12 hours

Adults:

Myocardial infarction (unlabeled use): Intracoronary: 750,000 units over 2 hours (6000 units/minute over up to 2 hours)

Occluded I.V. catheters (unlabeled use):

5000 units in each lumen over 1-2 minutes, leave in lumen for 1-4 hours, then aspirate; may repeat with 10,000 units in each lumen if 5000 units fails to clear the catheter; **do not infuse into the patient**; volume to instill into catheter is equal to the volume of the catheter

I.V. infusion: 200 units/kg/hour in each lumen for 12-48 hours at a rate of at least 20 mL/hour

Dialysis patients: 5000 units is administered in each lumen over 1-2 minutes; leave urokinase in lumen for 1-2 days, then aspirate

Acute pulmonary embolism: I.V.: Loading: 4400 int. units/kg over 10 minutes; maintenance: 4400 int. units/kg/hour for 12 hours. Following infusion, anticoagulation treatment is recommended to prevent recurrent thrombosis. Do not start anticoagulation until aPTT has decreased to less than twice the normal control value. If heparin is used, do not administer loading dose. Treatment should be followed with oral anticoagulants.

Stability Store in refrigerator; reconstitute by gently rolling and tilting; do not shake; contains no preservatives, should not be reconstituted until immediately before using, discard unused portion; stable at room temperature for 24 hours after reconstitution

Monitoring Parameters Blood pressure, pulse; CBC, platelet count, aPTT, urinalysis

Administration I.V. infusion: Usual concentration: 1250-1500 units/mL; maximum concentration not yet defined

Contraindications Hypersensitivity to urokinase or any component of the formulation; active internal bleeding; history of CVA; recent (within 2 months) intracranial or intraspinal surgery or trauma; intracranial neoplasm, arteriovenous malformation, or aneurysm; known bleeding diathesis; severe uncontrolled hypertension

Warnings

Concurrent heparin anticoagulation can contribute to bleeding; careful attention to all potential bleeding sites. I.M. injections and nonessential handling of the patient should be avoided. Venipunctures should be performed carefully and only when necessary. If arterial puncture is necessary, use an upper extremity vessel that can be manually compressed. If serious bleeding occurs, then the infusion of urokinase and heparin should be stopped.

For the following conditions the risk of bleeding is higher with use of thrombolytics and should be weighed against the benefits of therapy: recent (within 10 days) major surgery (eg, CABG, obstetrical delivery, organ biopsy, previous puncture of noncompressible vessels), cerebrovascular disease, recent (within 10 days) gastrointestinal or genitourinary bleeding, recent trauma (within 10 days) including CPR, hypertension (systolic BP >180 mm Hg and/or diastolic BP >110 mm Hg), high likelihood of left heart thrombus (eg, mitral stenosis with atrial fibrillation), acute pericarditis, subacute bacterial endocarditis, hemostatic defects including ones caused by severe renal or hepatic dysfunction, significant hepatic dysfunction, pregnancy, diabetic hemorrhagic retinopathy or other hemorrhagic ophthalmic conditions, septic thrombophlebitis or occluded AV cannula at seriously infected site, advanced age (eg, >75 years), patients receiving oral anticoagulants, any other condition in which bleeding constitutes a significant hazard or would be particularly difficult to manage because of location.

Coronary thrombolysis may result in reperfusion arrhythmias. Follow standard MI management. Rare anaphylactoid reactions can occur. Formulated in human albumin; products made from human sources have a theoretical risk of transmitting infectious agents. Safety and efficacy in pediatric patients have not been established.

Dosage Forms [DSC] = Discontinued product

Injection, powder for reconstitution: 250,000 int. units [contains human albumin 250 mg and mannitol 25 mg] [DSC]

Overdosage/Treatment Supportive therapy: Treat bleeding complications with transfusions of red blood cells, fresh frozen plasma, and cryoprecipitate; do not administer dextran; although human overdose data is lacking, administration of aminocaproic acid (Amicar®) at a dose of 3-5 g I.V. followed by an infusion rate of 1-1.25 g/hour may be useful

Test Interactions Earlier peaks of creatine phosphokinase isoenzyme can occur

Drug Interactions Aminocaproic acid (antifibrinolytic agent) may decrease effectiveness.

Drugs which affect platelet function (eg, aspirin, NSAIDs, dipyridamole, ticlopidine, clopidogrel, IIb/IIIa antagonists) may potentiate the risk of hemorrhage; use with caution.

Heparin: Concurrent use may increase risk of bleeding; use caution.

Warfarin or oral anticoagulants: Risk of bleeding may be increased during concurrent therapy.

Pregnancy Risk Factor B

Pregnancy Implications Urokinase was not found to be teratogenic in animal studies; it is not known if it crosses the human placenta. Placental separation and hemorrhage have been reported in one patient treated at 3 months gestation. Use during pregnancy only if clearly needed.

Lactation Excretion in breast milk unknown/use caution

Nursing Implications Use 0.22 or 0.45 micron filter during I.V. therapy

Additional InformationNote: Not currently being manufactured; contact Abbott Labs (800-615-0187) for further information.

Abbokinase® Open Cath 5000 unit product is **not** for systemic administration; it must be aspirated out of the catheter

Valacyclovir

Related Information

● Acyclovir

U.S. Brand Names Valtrex®

Synonyms Valacyclovir Hydrochloride

Use Treatment of herpes zoster (shingles) in immunocompetent patients; treatment of first-episode genital herpes; episodic treatment of recurrent genital herpes; suppression of recurrent genital herpes and reduction of heterosexual transmission of genital herpes in immunocompetent patients; suppression of genital herpes in HIV-infected individuals; treatment of herpes labialis (cold sores)

Mechanism of Action Inhibits DNA synthesis and viral replication by competing with deoxyguanosine triphosphate for viral DNA polymerase (thymidine kinase) and being incorporated into viral DNA

Adverse Reactions

Cardiovascular: Facial edema, hypertension, tachycardia

Central nervous system: **Headache** (14% to 35%), dizziness, depression, agitation, coma, confusion, consciousness decreased, encephalopathy, auditory hallucinations, visual hallucinations, mania, psychosis

Dermatologic: Alopecia, erythema multiforme, photosensitivity reaction, rash

Endocrine: Dysmenorrhea

Gastrointestinal: Abdominal pain, nausea, vomiting, diarrhea

Hematologic: Leukopenia, thrombocytopenia, anemia, aplastic anemia, hemolytic uremic syndrome (HUS), thrombotic thrombocytopenic purpura/hemolytic uremic syndrome

Hepatic: AST increased, hepatitis

Neuromuscular & skeletal: Arthralgia, tremor

Ocular: Visual disturbances

Renal: Creatinine increased, renal failure

Miscellaneous: Acute hypersensitivity reactions, anaphylaxis

Pharmacodynamics/Kinetics

Absorption: Rapid

Distribution: Acyclovir is widely distributed throughout the body including brain, kidney, lungs, liver, spleen, muscle, uterus, vagina, and CSF

Protein binding: 13.5% to 17.9%

Metabolism: Hepatic; valacyclovir is rapidly and nearly completely converted to acyclovir and L-valine by first-pass effect; acyclovir is hepatically metabolized to a very small extent by aldehyde oxidase and by alcohol and aldehyde dehydrogenase (inactive metabolites)

Bioavailability: ~55% once converted to acyclovir

Half-life elimination: Normal renal function: Adults: Acyclovir: 2.5-3.3 hours, Valacyclovir: ~30 minutes; End-stage renal disease: Acyclovir: 14-20 hours

Excretion: Urine, primarily as acyclovir (88%); **Note:** Following oral administration of radiolabeled valacyclovir, 46% of the label is eliminated in the feces (corresponding to nonabsorbed drug), while 47% of the radiolabel is eliminated in the urine.

Dosage Oral:

Adolescents and Adults: Herpes labialis (cold sores): 2 g twice daily for 1 day (separate doses by ~12 hours)

Adults:

Herpes zoster (shingles): 1 g 3 times/day for 7 days

Genital herpes:

Initial episode: 1 g twice daily for 10 days

Recurrent episode: 500 mg twice daily for 3 days

Reduction of transmission: 500 mg once daily (source partner)

Suppressive therapy:

Immunocompetent patients: 1000 mg once daily (500 mg once daily in patients with <9 recurrences per year)

HIV-infected patients (CD4 ≥100 cells/mm^3): 500 mg twice daily

Dosing interval in renal impairment:

Herpes zoster: Adults:

Cl$_{cr}$ 30-49 mL/minute: 1 g every 12 hours

Cl$_{cr}$ 10-29 mL/minute: 1 g every 24 hours

Cl$_{cr}$ <10 mL/minute: 500 mg every 24 hours

Genital herpes: Adults:

Initial episode:

Cl$_{cr}$ 10-29 mL/minute: 1 g every 24 hours

Cl$_{cr}$ <10 mL/minute: 500 mg every 24 hours

Recurrent episode: Cl$_{cr}$ <10-29 mL/minute: 500 mg every 24 hours

Suppressive therapy: Cl$_{cr}$ <10-29 mL/minute:

For usual dose of 1 g every 24 hours, decrease dose to 500 mg every 24 hours

For usual dose of 500 mg every 24 hours, decrease dose to 500 mg every 48 hours

HIV-infected patients: 500 mg every 24 hours

Herpes labialis: Adolescents and Adults:

Cl$_{cr}$ 30-49 mL/minute: 1 g every 12 hours for 2 doses

Cl$_{cr}$ 10-29 mL/minute: 500 mg every 12 hours for 2 doses

Cl$_{cr}$ <10 mL/minute: 500 mg as a single dose

Hemodialysis: Dialyzable (~33% removed during 4-hour session); administer dose postdialysis

Chronic ambulatory peritoneal dialysis/continuous arteriovenous hemofiltration dialysis: Pharmacokinetic parameters are similar to those in patients with ESRD; supplemental dose not needed following dialysis

Stability Store at 15°C to 25°C (59°F to 77°F).

Monitoring Parameters Urinalysis, BUN, serum creatinine, liver enzymes, and CBC

Administration If GI upset occurs, administer with meals.

Contraindications Hypersensitivity to valacyclovir, acyclovir, or any component of the formulation

Warnings Hazardous agent - use appropriate precautions for handling and disposal. Thrombotic thrombocytopenic purpura/hemolytic uremic syndrome has occurred in immunocompromised patients (at doses of 8 g/day); use caution and adjust the dose in elderly patients or those with renal insufficiency and in patients receiving concurrent nephrotoxic agents. For genital herpes, treatment should begin as soon as possible after the first signs and symptoms (within 72 hours of onset of first diagnosis or within 24 hours of onset of recurrent episodes). For herpes zoster, treatment should begin within 72 hours of onset of rash. For cold sores, treatment should begin at with earliest symptom (tingling, itching, burning). Safety and efficacy in prepubertal patients have not been established.

Dosage Forms Caplet: 500 mg, 1000 mg

Reference Range After a 1 g oral dose, peak serum acyclovir levels were ~5.65 mcg/mL

Overdosage/Treatment

Decontamination: Activated charcoal

Supportive therapy: Renal toxicity and crystalluria can be managed with I.V. fluid hydration

Enhancement of elimination: Multiple dosing of activated charcoal may be effective; hemodialysis can remove ~60% of total body burden; exchange transfusion is not useful

Drug Interactions Cimetidine: Decreased renal clearance of acyclovir; no dosage adjustment needed in patients with normal renal function

Probenecid: Decreased renal clearance of acyclovir; no dosage adjustment needed in patients with normal renal function

Pregnancy Risk Factor B

Pregnancy Implications Teratogenicity registry has shown no increased rate of birth defects than that of the general population; however, the registry is small and use during pregnancy is only warranted if the potential benefit to the mother justifies the risk of the fetus.

Lactation Enters breast milk/use caution

Additional Information Due to higher bioavailability than acyclovir, plasma acyclovir levels are 3-5 times higher with valacyclovir administration as compared with acyclovir administration

Specific References

Katiyar A, Daubert GP, and Aaron C, "Acute Renal Failure Following Acute Oral Valacyclovir Overdose," *Clin Toxicol (Phila)*, 2005, 43:732.

Valproic Acid and Derivatives

CAS Number 1069-66-5; 2430-27-5; 76584-70-8; 77372-61-3; 99-66-1

U.S. Brand Names Depacon®; Depakene®; Depakote® Delayed Release; Depakote® ER; Depakote® Sprinkle®

Synonyms 2-Propylpentanoic Acid; 2-Propylvaleric Acid; Dipropylacetic Acid; Divalproex Sodium; DPA; Valproate Semisodium; Valproate Sodium; Valproic Acid

Use

Monotherapy and adjunctive therapy in the treatment of patients with complex partial seizures; monotherapy and adjunctive therapy of simple and complex absence seizures; adjunctive therapy patients with multiple seizure types that include absence seizures

Mania associated with bipolar disorder (Depakote®)

Migraine prophylaxis (Depakote®, Depakote® ER)

Unlabeled/Investigational Use Behavior disorders (eg, agitation, aggression) in patients with dementia (based on the results of several randomized, controlled trials, there is little evidence to support this use); status epilepticus

Mechanism of Action Causes increased availability of gamma-aminobutyric acid (GABA), an inhibitory neurotransmitter, to brain neurons or may enhance the action of GABA or mimic its action at postsynaptic receptor sites

Adverse Reactions

Central nervous system: Drowsiness, irritability, confusion, restlessness, hyperactivity, psychosis, malaise, visual hallucinations, extrapyramidal syndrome, headache, ataxia

Dermatologic: Alopecia, erythema multiforme

Endocrine & metabolic: Hyperammonemia, hypernatremia with sodium valproate, metabolic acidosis

Gastrointestinal: Nausea, vomiting, diarrhea, pancreatitis, abdominal cramps, anorexia, hemorrhage, weight gain, gingival hyperplasia

Hematologic: Thrombocytopenia, prolongation of bleeding time, leukopenia, pancytopenia, eosinophilia, red blood cell aplasia, factor X deficiency, transient myeloid dysplasia

Hepatic: Transient elevated liver enzymes, liver failure (especially noted in children <2 years of age), fatty degeneration of liver, cholestatic hepatitis, impaired gluconeogenesis, cholecystitis, hyperammonemic encephalopathy (in patients with UCD)

Neuromuscular & skeletal: Tremors, chorea, clonus, myoclonus, osteoporosis (long-term therapy)

Ocular: Nystagmus

Renal: Enuresis, anuria

Respiratory: Pleural effusion

Miscellaneous: Systemic lupus erythematosus

Signs and Symptoms of Overdose Agranulocytosis, cerebral edema, cholestatic jaundice, coagulopathy, coma, confusion, dementia, encephalopathy, enuresis, extrapyramidal reaction, Fanconi syndrome, granulocytopenia, hyperactivity, hyperglycemia, hyperthermia, hyporeflexia, hypothermia, hypothyroidism, ileus, irritability, jaundice, leukopenia (3%), mania, metabolic acidosis (at serum levels >50 mcg/mL), migraine headache (exacerbation), miosis, myoclonus, nephritis, neutropenia, night terrors, nystagmus, optic nerve atrophy, photophobia, pseudotumor cerebri, tachycardia (17%), thrombocytopenia (8%), tremors

Admission Criteria/Prognosis Admit any patient with central nervous system abnormality associated with the ingestion, hepatic toxicity, or ingestions >100 mg/kg

Pharmacodynamics/Kinetics

Absorption: Nearly 100%

Distribution: Total valproate: 11 L/1.73 m^2; free valproate 92 L/1.73 m^2

Protein binding (dose dependent): 80% to 90%

Metabolism: Extensively hepatic via glucuronide conjugation and mitochondrial beta-oxidation. The relationship between dose and total valproate concentration is nonlinear; concentration does not increase proportionally with the dose, but increases to a lesser extent due to saturable plasma protein binding. The kinetics of unbound drug are linear.

Bioavailability: Extended release: 90% of I.V. dose and 81% to 90% of delayed release dose

Half-life elimination: (increased in neonates and with liver disease): Children: 4-14 hours; Adults: 9-16 hours

Time to peak, serum: 1-4 hours; Divalproex (enteric coated): 3-5 hours

Excretion: Urine (30% to 50% as glucuronide conjugate, 3% as unchanged drug)

Dosage Seizures:

Children >10 years and Adults:

Oral: Initial: 10-15 mg/kg/day in 1-3 divided doses; increase by 5-10 mg/kg/day at weekly intervals until therapeutic levels are achieved; maintenance: 30-60 mg/kg/day. Adult usual dose: 1000-2500 mg/day. **Note:** Regular release and delayed release formulations are usually given in 2-4 divided doses/day, extended release formulation (Depakote® ER) is usually given once daily. Conversion to Depakote® ER from a stable dose of Depakote® may require an increase in the total daily dose between 8% and 20% to maintain similar serum concentrations.

Children receiving more than one anticonvulsant (ie, polytherapy) may require doses up to 100 mg/kg/day in 3-4 divided doses

I.V.: Administer as a 60-minute infusion (≤20 mg/minute) with the same frequency as oral products; switch patient to oral products as soon as possible. Alternatively, rapid infusions have been given: ≤15 mg/kg over 5-10 minutes (1.5-3 mg/kg/minute).

Rectal (unlabeled): Dilute syrup 1:1 with water for use as a retention enema; loading dose: 17-20 mg/kg one time; maintenance: 10-15 mg/kg/dose every 8 hours

Status epilepticus (unlabeled use): Adults:

Loading dose: I.V.: 15-25 mg/kg administered at 3 mg/kg/minute.

Maintenance dose: I.V. infusion: 1-4 mg/kg/hour; titrate dose as needed based upon patient response and evaluation of drug-drug interactions

Mania: Adults: Oral: 750-1500 mg/day in divided doses; dose should be adjusted as rapidly as possible to desired clinical effect; a loading dose of 20 mg/kg may be used; maximum recommended dosage: 60 mg/kg/day

Migraine prophylaxis: Adults: Oral:

Extended release tablets: 500 mg once daily for 7 days, then increase to 1000 mg once daily; adjust dose based on patient response; usual dosage range 500-1000 mg/day

Delayed release tablets: 250 mg twice daily; adjust dose based on patient response, up to 1000 mg/day

Elderly: Elimination is decreased in the elderly. Studies of elderly patients with dementia show a high incidence of somnolence. In some patients, this was associated with weight loss. Starting doses should be lower and increases should be slow, with careful monitoring of nutritional intake and dehydration. Safety and efficacy for use in patients >65 years have not been studied for migraine prophylaxis.

Dosing adjustment in renal impairment: A 27% reduction in clearance of unbound valproate is seen in patients with Cl$_{cr}$ <10 mL/minute. Hemodialysis reduces valproate concentrations by 20%, therefore no dose adjustment is needed in patients with renal failure. Protein binding is reduced, monitoring only total valproate concentrations may be misleading.

Dosing adjustment/comments in hepatic impairment: Reduce dose. Clearance is decreased with liver impairment. Hepatic disease is also associated with decreased albumin concentrations and 2- to 2.6-fold increase in the unbound fraction. Free concentrations of valproate may be elevated while total concentrations appear normal.

Monitoring Parameters Liver enzymes, CBC with platelets

Administration Depakote® ER: Swallow whole, do not crush or chew. Patients who need dose adjustments smaller than 500 mg/day for migraine prophylaxis should be changed to Depakote® delayed release tablets. Sprinkle capsules may be swallowed whole or open cap and sprinkle on small amount (1 teaspoonful) of soft food and use immediately (do not store or chew).

Depacon®: Following dilution to final concentration, administer over 60 minutes at a rate of ≤20 mg/minute. Alternatively, single doses up to 15 mg/kg have been administered as a rapid infusion over 5-10 minutes (1.5-3 mg/kg/minute).

Contraindications Hypersensitivity to valproic acid, derivatives, or any component of the formulation; hepatic dysfunction; urea cycle disorders

Warnings

[US Boxed Warning]: Hepatic failure resulting in fatalities has occurred in patients; children <2 years of age are at considerable risk. Other risk factors include organic brain disease, mental retardation with severe seizure disorders, congenital metabolic disorders, and patients on multiple anticonvulsants. Hepatotoxicity has been reported after 3 days to 6 months of therapy. Monitor patients closely for appearance of malaise, weakness, facial edema, anorexia, jaundice, and vomiting.

[US Boxed Warning]: May cause teratogenic effects such as neural tube defects (eg, spina bifida). Use in women of childbearing potential requires that benefits of use in mother be weighed against the potential risk to fetus, especially when used for conditions not associated with permanent injury or risk of death (eg, migraine).

May cause severe thrombocytopenia, inhibition of platelet aggregation and bleeding; tremors may indicate overdosage; use with caution in patients receiving other anticonvulsants. Cases of life-threatening pancreatitis, occurring at the start of therapy or following years of use, have been reported in adults and children. Some cases have been hemorrhagic with rapid progression of initial symptoms to death. Hypersensitivity reactions affecting multiple organs have been reported in association with valproic acid use; may include dermatologic and/or hematologic changes (eosinophilia, neutropenia, thrombocytopenia) or symptoms of organ dysfunction.

Hyperammonemia and/or encephalopathy, sometimes fatal, have been reported following the initiation of valproate therapy and may be present with normal transaminase levels. Ammonia levels should be measured in patients who develop unexplained lethargy and vomiting, or changes in mental status. Discontinue therapy if ammonia levels are increased and evaluate for possible urea cycle disorder (UCD). Although rare genetic disorders, UCD evaluation should be considered for the following patients, prior to the start of therapy: History of unexplained encephalopathy or coma; encephalopathy associated with protein load; pregnancy or postpartum encephalopathy; unexplained mental retardation; history of elevated plasma ammonia or glutamine; history of cyclical vomiting and lethargy; episodic extreme irritability, ataxia; low BUN or protein avoidance; family history of UCD or unexplained infant deaths (particularly male); signs or symptoms of UCD (hyperammonemia, encephalopathy, respiratory alkalosis).

In vitro studies have suggested valproate stimulates the replication of HIV and CMV viruses under experimental conditions. The clinical consequence of this is unknown, but should be considered when monitoring affected patients.

Anticonvulsants should not be discontinued abruptly because of the possibility of increasing seizure frequency; valproate should be withdrawn gradually to minimize the potential of increased seizure frequency, unless safety concerns require a more rapid withdrawal. Concomitant use with clonazepam may induce absence status.

CNS depression may occur with valproate use. Patients must be cautioned about performing tasks which require mental alertness (operating machinery or driving). Effects with other sedative drugs or ethanol may be potentiated.

Dosage Forms

Note: Strength expressed as valproic acid

Capsule, as valproic acid (Depakene®): 250 mg

Capsule, sprinkles, as divalproex sodium (Depakote® Sprinkle®): 125 mg

Injection, solution, as valproate sodium (Depacon®): 100 mg/mL (5 mL) [contains edetate disodium]

Syrup, as valproic acid: 250 mg/5 mL (480 mL)

Depakene®: 250 mg/5 mL (480 mL)

Tablet, delayed release, as divalproex sodium (Depakote®): 125 mg, 250 mg, 500 mg

Tablet, extended release, as divalproex sodium (Depakote® ER): 250 mg, 500 mg

Reference Range

Therapeutic: 50-100 mcg/mL (SI: 350-690 μmol/L); seizure control may improve at levels >100 mcg/mL (SI: >690 μmol/L)

Toxic: Toxicity may occur at levels of 100-150 mcg/mL (SI: 690-1040 μmol/L)

Postmortem blood valproic acid levels from valproic acid overdoses range from 520 mg/L to 1970 mg/L.

Overdosage/Treatment

Decontamination: Lavage (within 1 hour)/activated charcoal within 14 hours of ingestion

Supportive therapy: Supportive treatment is necessary; intubation will probably be required at serum VPA levels >850 mcg/mL; naloxone has been used to reverse CNS depressant effects, but may block action of other anticonvulsants; carnitine (1 g 3 times/day) is useful in reducing ammonia level; L-carnitine (100 mg/kg loading dose then 250 mg every 8 hours for 4 days) has been used to treat hepatic dysfunction in children due to valproic acid overdose. Additionally, its use has been advocated in the treatment of Reye's or Reye's-like syndrome due to valproic acid

Enhancement of elimination: Multiple dosing of activated charcoal is effective; hemoperfusion and/or hemodialysis may be effective in treating persistent hypotension or acidosis; hemodialyzer clearance is ~23 mL/minute; not hemodialyzed in a normal dose situation due to high protein-binding of valproic acid, but in an overdose situation, whereupon protein binding is decreased, hemodialysis may be effective. Simultaneous "in series" hemodialysis/hemoperfusion has been demonstrated to decrease valproate half-life to <2 hours; hemodialysis has been used successfully in decreasing valproic acid serum level from 949-113 mcg/mL postdialysis. Charcoal hemoperfusion has been used successfully (plasma clearance: 54.5 mL/minute); forced diuresis (4 mL/kg/hour of I.V. fluid with a urine flow of 3.5-4 mL/kg/hour) has been advocated to increase urinary valproic acid clearance 5.5 fold in massive valproic acid overdose (serum level >1000 mcg/mL); it should be noted that this modality has not been extensively studied

Antidote(s)
- Levocarnitine [ANTIDOTE]
- Naloxone [ANTIDOTE]

Diagnostic Procedures
- Valproic Acid, Blood

Test Interactions False-positive urine ketones; ↑ sodium, glucose; ↓ calcium

Drug Interactions For valproic acid: **Substrate** (minor) of CYP2A6, 2B6, 2C9, 2C19, 2E1; **Inhibits** CYP2C9 (weak), 2C19 (weak), 2D6 (weak), 3A4 (weak); **Induces** CYP2A6 (weak)

Carbamazepine: Valproic acid may increase, decrease, or have no effect on carbamazepine levels; valproic acid may increase serum concentrations of carbamazepine - epoxide (active metabolite); valproic acid may induce the metabolism of carbamazepine; monitor.

Carbapenem antibiotics (ertapenem, imipenem, meropenem): May decrease valproic acid concentrations to subtherapeutic levels; monitor.

Felbamate: May increase the levels/effects of valproic acid; monitor.

Isoniazid: May decrease valproic acid metabolism (limited documentation).

Lamotrigine: Valproic acid inhibits the metabolism of lamotrigine; combination therapy has been proposed to increase the risk of toxic epidermal necrolysis; monitor.

Macrolide antibiotics: May decrease valproic acid metabolism (limited documentation); includes clarithromycin, erythromycin, troleandomycin; monitor.

Primidone, phenobarbital: Valproic acid appears to inhibit the metabolism of phenobarbital; monitor for increased effect.

Salicylates: May displace valproic acid from plasma proteins, leading to acute toxicity.

Topiramate: Hyperammonemia with or without encephalopathy has been reported in patients who tolerated either drug alone. These drugs may modestly decrease the serum concentrations of the other drug.

Tricyclic antidepressants: Valproate may increase serum concentrations and/or toxicity of tricyclic antidepressants.

Zidovudine: Valproic acid may increase the levels/effects of zidovudine; monitor.

Pregnancy Risk Factor D

Pregnancy Implications Crosses the placenta; 1 to 2% incidence of spina bifida

Lactation Enters breast milk/use caution (AAP considers "compatible")

Nursing Implications Do not crush enteric-coated drug product or capsules

Additional Information Tremors may indicate overdosage; monitor serum ammonium; may cause increase in alkaline phosphatase in pediatric patients; long-term or high-dose valproic acid treatment can induce hypocarnitinemia

Sodium content of valproate sodium syrup (5 mL): 23 mg (1 mEq): Divalproex sodium: Depakote®; valproate sodium: Depakene® syrup; valproic acid: Depakene® capsule

Specific References
Coves-Orts FJ, Borras-Blasco J, Navarro-Ruiz A, et al, "Acute Seizures Due to a Probable Interaction Between Valproic Acid and Meropenem," *Ann Pharmacother*. 2005, 39(3):533-7.

Cuturic M and Abramson RK, "Acute Hyperammonemic Coma with Chronic Valproic Acid Therapy," *Ann Pharmacother*, 2005, 39(12): 2119-22.

Panomvana Na Ayudhya D, Suwanmanee J, and Visudtibhan A, "Pharmacokinetic Parameters of Total and Unbound Valproic Acid and Their Relationships to Seizure Control in Epileptic Children," *Am J Ther*, 2006, 13(3):211-7

Kielstein JT, Woywodt A, Schumann G, et al, "Efficiency of High-Flux Hemodialysis in the Treatment of Valproic Acid Intoxication," *J Toxicol Clin Toxicol*, 2003, 41(6):873-6.

Lum E, Gorman SK, and Slavik RS, "Valproic Acid Management of Acute Alcohol Withdrawal," *Ann Pharmacother*, 2006, 40(3):441-8.

Mallet L, Babin S, and Morais JA, "Valproic Acid-Induced Hyperammonemia and Thrombocytopenia in an Elderly Woman," *Ann Pharmacother*, 2004, 38(10):1643-7.

Muñiz AE, "Electrocardiographic Changes with Valproic Acid Overdose," Virginia Commonwealth University Health System, Richmond, Virginia, *South Med*, 2003, 96(10 Suppl 1):11-2.

O'Bryan EC, Veser FH, Veser B, et al, "Depacon in the Acute Treatment of Mania," *Ann Emerg Med*, 2004, 44:S23.

Perez A and McKay CA, "Role of Carnitine in Valproic Acid Toxicity," *J Toxicol Clin Toxicol*, 2003, 41(6):899.

Sheehan NL, Brouillette MJ, Delisle MS, et al, "Possible Interaction Between Lopinavir/Ritonavir and Valproic Acid Exacerbates Bipolar Disorder," *Ann Pharmacother*, 2006, 40(1):147-50.

Weng T, Shih FF, and Chen WJ, "Unusual Causes of Hyperammonemia in the ED," *Am J Emerg Med*, 2004, 22:105-7.

Valsartan

CAS Number 137862-53-4

U.S. Brand Names Diovan®

Use Alone or in combination with other antihypertensive agents in treating essential hypertension; treatment of heart failure (NYHA Class II-IV) in patients intolerant to angiotensin converting enzyme (ACE) inhibitors

Mechanism of Action As a prodrug, valsartan produces direct antagonism of the angiotensin II (AT2) receptors, unlike the angiotensin-converting enzyme inhibitors. It displaces angiotensin II from the AT1 receptor and produces its blood pressure lowering effects by antagonizing AT1-induced vasoconstriction, aldosterone release, catecholamine release, arginine vasopressin release, water intake, and hypertrophic responses. This action results in more efficient blockade of the cardiovascular effects of angiotensin II and fewer side effects than the ACE inhibitors.

Adverse Reactions
Hypertension:
    Cardiovascular: Edema
    Central nervous system: Dizziness, fatigue, headache
    Endocrine & metabolic: Serum potassium increased
    Gastrointestinal: Abdominal pain, diarrhea, nausea
    Hematologic: Neutropenia
    Neuromuscular & skeletal: Arthralgia
    Respiratory: Cough, pharyngitis, rhinitis, sinusitis, upper respiratory infection
    Miscellaneous: Viral infection
Heart failure:
    Central nervous system: **Dizziness**
    Cardiovascular: Hypotension, postural hypotension
    Central nervous system: Fatigue
    Endocrine & metabolic: Hyperkalemia
    Gastrointestinal: Diarrhea
    Neuromuscular & skeletal: Arthralgia, back pain
    Renal: Creatinine elevated >50%
All indications:
    Cardiovascular: Chest pain, orthostatic effects, palpitations
    Central nervous system: Anxiety, insomnia, somnolence, syncope, vertigo
    Dermatologic: Angioedema, alopecia, pruritus, rash
    Endocrine & metabolic: Hyperkalemia (hypertensive patients)
    Gastrointestinal: Anorexia, constipation, dyspepsia, flatulence, vomiting, xerostomia
    Genitourinary: Impotence
    Hematologic: Anemia, hematocrit decreased, hemoglobin decreased
    Hepatic: Serum transaminases increased, hepatitis
    Neuromuscular & skeletal: Asthenia, back pain, muscle cramps, myalgia, paresthesia
    Renal: Creatinine increased, impaired renal function; may be associated with worsening of renal function in patients dependent on renin-angiotensin-aldosterone system
    Respiratory: Dyspnea
    Miscellaneous: Allergic reactions

Pharmacodynamics/Kinetics
Onset of antihypertensive effect: 2 weeks (maximal: 4 weeks)
Distribution: V_d: 17 L (adults)
Protein binding: 95%, primarily albumin
Metabolism: To inactive metabolite
Bioavailability: 25% (range 10% to 35%)
Half-life elimination: 6 hours
Time to peak, serum: 2-4 hours
Excretion: Feces (83%) and urine (13%) as unchanged drug

Dosage
Adults: Oral:
Hypertension: Initial: 80 mg or 160 mg once daily (in patients who are not volume depleted); majority of effect within 2 weeks, maximal effects in 4-6 weeks; dose may be increased to achieve desired effect; maximum recommended dose: 320 mg/day
Heart failure: Initial: 40 mg twice daily; titrate dose to 80-160 mg twice daily, as tolerated; maximum daily dose: 320 mg. **Note:** Do not use with ACE inhibitors and beta blockers.

Dosing adjustment in renal impairment: No dosage adjustment necessary if Cl_{cr} >10 mL/minute.

Dosing adjustment in hepatic impairment (mild - moderate): ≤80 mg/day

Dialysis: Not significantly removed

Monitoring Parameters Baseline and periodic electrolyte panels, renal and liver function tests, urinalysis; symptoms of hypotension or hypersensitivity

Administration Administer with or without food.

Contraindications Hypersensitivity to valsartan or any component of the formulation; hypersensitivity to other A-II receptor antagonists; bilateral renal artery stenosis; pregnancy (2nd and 3rd trimesters)

Warnings

[U.S. Boxed Warning]: Based on human data, drugs that act on the angiotensin system can cause injury and death to the developing fetus when used in the second and third trimesters. Angiotensin receptor blockers should be discontinued as soon as possible once pregnancy is detected. During the initiation of therapy, hypotension may occur, particularly in patients with heart failure or post-MI patients. Avoid use or use a smaller dose in patients who are volume depleted; correct depletion first.

Deterioration in renal function can occur with initiation. Use with caution in unilateral renal artery stenosis and pre-existing renal insufficiency; significant aortic/mitral stenosis. Use caution in patients with severe renal impairment or significant hepatic dysfunction. Monitor renal function closely in patients with severe heart failure; changes in renal function should be anticipated and dosage adjustments of valsartan or concomitant medications may be needed.

Dosage Forms Tablet: 40 mg, 80 mg, 160 mg, 320 mg

Overdosage/Treatment

Decontamination: Ipecac (within 30 minutes)/lavage (within 1 hour)/activated charcoal

Supportive therapy: Following initiation of essential overdose management, toxic symptom treatment and supportive treatment should be initiated. Hypotension usually responds to I.V. normal saline or Trendelenburg positioning. If unresponsive to these measures, the use of a parenteral inotrope may be required (eg, norepinephrine 0.1-0.2 mcg/kg/minute titrated to response). Seizures commonly respond to lorazepam or diazepam or to phenytoin or phenobarbital. Inhaled sodium cromoglycate (total dose: 40 mg/day) can decrease ACE-inhibitor cough by 50%.

Enhanced elimination: Multiple dosing of activated charcoal may be effective

Test Interactions Increased serum potassium with potassium-sparing diuretics

Drug Interactions

Inhibits CYP2C9 (weak)

Lithium: Risk of toxicity may be increased by valsartan; monitor lithium levels.

NSAIDs: May decrease angiotensin II antagonist efficacy; effect has been seen with losartan, but may occur with other medications in this class; monitor blood pressure

Potassium-sparing diuretics (amiloride, potassium, spironolactone, triamterene): Increased risk of hyperkalemia.

Potassium supplements may increase the risk of hyperkalemia.

Trimethoprim (high dose) may increase the risk of hyperkalemia.

Pregnancy Risk Factor C/D (2nd and 3rd trimesters)

Pregnancy Implications Medications which act on the renin-angiotensin system are reported to have the following fetal/neonatal effects: Hypotension, neonatal skull hypoplasia, anuria, renal failure, and death; oligohydramnios is also reported. These effects are reported to occur with exposure during the 2nd and 3rd trimesters. Valsartan should be discontinued as soon as possible after pregnancy is detected.

Lactation Excretion in breast milk unknown/contraindicated

Additional Information Valsartan may have an advantage over losartan due to minimal metabolism requirements and consequent use in mild to moderate hepatic impairment.

Specific References

Irons BK and Kumar A, "Valsartan-Induced Angioedema," *Ann Pharmacother*, 2003, 37(7-8):1024-7.

Ripley TL, "Valsartan in Chronic Heart Failure," *Ann Pharmacother*, 2005, 39(3):460-9.

Vancomycin

CAS Number 1404-93-9

U.S. Brand Names Vancocin®

Synonyms Vancomycin Hydrochloride

Use

Treatment of patients with the following infections or conditions:
- Infections due to documented or suspected methicillin-resistant *S. aureus* or beta-lactam resistant coagulase-negative *Staphylococcus*
- Serious or life-threatening infections (ie, endocarditis, meningitis) due to documented or suspected staphylococcal or streptococcal infections in patients who are allergic to penicillins and/or cephalosporins
- Empiric therapy of infections associated with gram-positive organisms; used orally for staphylococcal enterocolitis or for antibiotic-associated pseudomembranous colitis produced by *C. difficile*

The Centers for Disease Control and Prevention (CDC) recently published a document on the spread of vancomycin resistance with a special focus on resistant enterococci.

When vancomycin is appropriate:
- Treatment of serious infections due to β-lactam-resistant gram-positive microorganisms
- Treatment of gram-positive infections in patients with allergies to β-lactam antimicrobials
- When antibiotic-associated colitis (AAC) fails to respond to metronidazole or if it is severe and life threatening
- Prophylaxis, as recommended by the American Heart Association, for endocarditis after certain procedures in patients at high risk for endocarditis
- Prophylaxis for surgical procedures involving implantation of prosthetic materials or devices at institutions with a high rate of infections due to methicillin-resistant *Staphylococcus aureus* (MRSA) or methicillin-resistant *Staphylococcus epidermidis* (MRSE)

When use of vancomycin should be discouraged:
- Routine surgical prophylaxis
- Empiric antimicrobial therapy for a febrile neutropenic patient, unless there is strong evidence that the patient has an infection due to gram-positive microorganisms, and the prevalence of β-lactam-resistant organisms in the hospital is substantial
- Treatment in response to a single blood culture positive for coagulase-negative staphylococci, if other blood cultures drawn in the same time frame are negative
- Continued empiric use for presumed infections in patients whose cultures are negative for β-lactam-resistant gram-positive microorganisms
- Systemic or local prophylaxis for infection or colonization of indwelling central or peripheral intravascular catheters or vascular grafts
- Selective decontamination of the digestive tract
- Eradication of MRSA colonization
- Primary treatment of AAC
- Routine prophylaxis for very low-birth-weight infants
- Routine prophylaxis for patients on continuous ambulatory peritoneal dialysis

Mechanism of Action Inhibits bacterial cell wall synthesis by blocking glycopeptide polymerization through binding tightly to D-alanyl-D-alanine portion of cell wall precursor

Adverse Reactions

Rapid infusion associated with red neck or red man syndrome: Erythema multiforme-like reaction with intense pruritus, tachycardia, hypotension, rash involving face, neck, upper trunk, back and upper arms

Cardiovascular: Cardiac arrest, **hypotension, flushing**, sinus tachycardia, vasculitis, leukocytoclastic vasculitis

Central nervous system: Fever, chills, hyperthermia

Dermatologic: **Redneck or redman syndrome, rash**, macular skin rash, linear IgA bullous dermatosis, Stevens-Johnson syndrome, acute generalized exanthematous pustulosis, angioedema, bullous skin disease, toxic epidermal necrolysis, urticaria, exanthem, Henoch-Schönlein purpura, cutaneous vasculitis

Gastrointestinal: **Nausea, bitter taste, vomiting**

Genitourinary: Priapism

Hematologic: Neutropenia, eosinophilia, thrombocytopenia

Local: Phlebitis

Neuromuscular & skeletal: Lower back pain, paresthesia

Otic: Ototoxicity, tinnitus associated with prolonged serum concentration >40 mcg/mL - may be permanent

Renal: Nephrotoxicity (higher incidence with trough concentrations >10 mcg/mL), renal vasculitis

Miscellaneous: Hypersensitivity reactions, systemic lupus erythematosus,

Signs and Symptoms of Overdose Colitis, deafness, dermatitis, exfoliative dermatitis, lacrimation, leukopenia or neutropenia (agranulocytosis, granulocytopenia), thrombocytopenia, tubular necrosis

Pharmacodynamics/Kinetics

Absorption: Oral: Poor; I.M.: Erratic; Intraperitoneal: ~38%

Distribution: Widely in body tissues and fluids. except for CSF

Relative diffusion from blood into CSF: Good only with inflammation (exceeds usual MICs)

CSF:blood level ratio: Normal meninges: Nil; Inflamed meninges: 20% to 30%

Protein binding: 10% to 50%

Half-life elimination: Biphasic: Terminal:

Newborns: 6-10 hours

Infants and Children 3 months to 4 years: 4 hours

Children >3 years: 2.2-3 hours

Adults: 5-11 hours; significantly prolonged with renal impairment

End-stage renal disease: 200-250 hours

Time to peak, serum: I.V.: 45-65 minutes

Excretion: I.V.: Urine (80% to 90% as unchanged drug); Oral: Primarily feces

Dosage Initial dosage recommendation: I.V.:

Neonates:

Postnatal age <7 days:
  <1200 g: 7.5 mg/kg/dose given every 24 hours
  1200-2000 g: 10 mg/kg/dose given every 12 hours
  >2000 g: 15 mg/kg/dose given every 12 hours

Postnatal age >7 days:
  <1200 g: 7.5 mg/kg/dose given every 24 hours
  ≥1200 g: 10 mg/kg/dose given every 8 hours

Infants >1 month and Children: 40 mg/kg/day in divided doses every 6 hours

Infants >1 month and Children with staphylococcal central nervous system infection: 60 mg/kg/day in divided doses every 6 hours

Note: Some patients may require larger or more frequent doses if serum levels document the need (ie, febrile granulocytopenic patients)

Adults:
  <60 kg: 750 mg every 12 hours
  60-100 kg: 1 g every 12 hours
  100-120 kg: 1.25 g every 12 hours
  >120 kg: 1.5 g every 12 hours

Intrathecal:
  Neonates: 5-10 mg/day
  Children: 5-20 mg/day
  Adults: 20 mg/day

Oral: Pseudomembranous colitis produced by *C. difficile*:
  Neonates: 10 mg/kg/day in divided doses
  Children: 40 mg/kg/day in divided doses, added to fluids
  Adults: 250-500 mg 3 times/day in divided doses

Dosing interval in renal impairment: Following a usual loading dose, dosages and frequency of administration are best determined by measurement of serum levels and assessment of renal insufficiency

Dosing adjustments/comments in hepatic impairment: Reduce dose by 60%

Monitoring Parameters Periodic renal function tests, urinalysis, serum vancomycin concentrations, WBC, audiogram

Administration Administer vancomycin by I.V. intermittent infusion over at least 60 minutes at a final concentration not to exceed 5 mg/mL. If a maculopapular rash appears on the face, neck, trunk, and/or upper extremities (Red man syndrome), slow the infusion rate to over $1^1/_2$ to 2 hours and increase the dilution volume. Hypotension, shock, and cardiac arrest (rare) have also been reported with too rapid of infusion. Reactions are often treated with antihistamines and steroids.

Extravasation treatment: Monitor I.V. site closely; extravasation will cause serious injury with possible necrosis and tissue sloughing. Rotate infusion site frequently.

Contraindications Hypersensitivity to vancomycin or any component of the formulation; avoid in patients with previous severe hearing loss

Warnings Use with caution in patients with renal impairment or those receiving other nephrotoxic or ototoxic drugs; dosage modification required in patients with impaired renal function (especially elderly)

Dosage Forms Capsule (Vancocin®): 125 mg, 250 mg

Infusion [premixed in iso-osmotic dextrose] (Vancocin®): 500 mg (100 mL); 1 g (200 mL)

Injection, powder for reconstitution: 500 mg, 1 g, 5 g, 10 g

Overdosage/Treatment

Decontamination: Ipecac within 30 minutes or lavage (within 1 hour)/ activated charcoal

Supportive therapy: Hypotension can respond to fluids; has responded to diphenhydramine (12.5 mg I.V.) in one case

Enhancement of elimination: Peritoneal dialysis can remove 40% of drug in 15 hours; continuous arteriovenous or intermittent hemofiltration may also be useful; multiple dosing of activated charcoal may be useful; hemodialysis (using polysulfone dialyzers) may increase elimination of vancomycin (mean clearance: 85 mL/minute with 49.5% extent of vancomycin removal); multiple dosing of activated charcoal may reduce vancomycin half-life by $^2/_3$ (under 10 hours); charcoal hemoperfusion is **not** useful. Plasma exchange transfusions may result in clinically significant removal of vancomycin from the plasma.

Diagnostic Procedures

• Vancomycin Level

Test Interactions Fluorescence polarization immunoassay (FPIA) may result in overestimation of vancomycin in patients with renal failure. This overestimation is caused by interference of the degradation product, CDP-1, in this assay.

Drug Interactions Increased toxicity: Anesthetic agents; other ototoxic or nephrotoxic agents

Pregnancy Risk Factor C

Pregnancy Implications Can cause fetal bradycardia

Lactation Enters breast milk/use caution

Additional Information Symptoms of red man symdrom include Facial flushing, Urticaria (usually of upper body), chest pain, and dyspnea. It is usually related to rate of vancomycin infusion (14% incidence if one gram is given over ten minutes) and is treated by slowing the rate of infusion, vancomycin dilution and antihistamines.

Specific References

Cadle RM, Mansouri MD, and Darouiche RO, "Vancomycin-Induced Elevation of Liver Enzyme Levels," *Ann Pharmacother*, 2006, 40(6):1186-9.

Dager WE and King JH, "Aminoglycosides in Intermittent Hemodialysis: Pharmacokinetics with Individual Dosing," *Ann Pharmacother*, 2006, 40(1):9-14.

Klibanov OM, Filicko JE, DeSimone JA Jr, et al, "Sensorineural Hearing Loss Associated with Intrathecal Vancomycin," *Ann Pharmacother*, 2003, 37(1):61-5.

Nornoo AO, and Elwel RJ, "Stability of Vancomycin in Icodextrin Peritoneal Dialysis Solution," *Ann Pharmacol*, 40(11):1950-4.

Pai MP, Mercier RC, and Allen SE, "Using Vancomycin Concentrations for Dosing Daptomycin in a Morbidly Obese Patient with Renal Insufficiency," *Ann Pharmacother*, 2006, 40(3):553-8.

Patrick BN, Rivey MP, and Allington DR, "Acute Renal Failure Associated with Vancomycin- and Tobramycin-Laden Cement in Total Hip Arthroplasty," *Ann Pharmacol*, 2006, 40(11):2037-42.

Segarra-Newnham M and Tagoff SS, "Probable Vancomycin-Induced Neutropenia," *Ann Pharmacother*, 2004, 38(11):1855-9.

Taber DJ, Fann AL, Malat G, et al, "Evaluation of Estimated and Measured Creatinine Clearances for Predicting the Pharmacokinetics of Vancomycin in Adult Liver Transplant Recipients," *Ther Drug Monit*, 2003, 25(1):67-72.

Vinken AG, Li JZ, Balan DA, et al, "Comparison of Linezolid with Oxacillin or Vancomycin in the Empiric Treatment of Cellulitis in U.S. Hospitals," *Am J Ther*, 2003, 10(4):264-74.

Vasopressin

CAS Number 11000-17-2; 113-79-1; 50-57-7

U.S. Brand Names Pitressin®

Synonyms 8-Arginine Vasopressin; ADH; Antidiuretic Hormone

Use

Treatment of diabetes insipidus; prevention and treatment of postoperative abdominal distention; differential diagnosis of diabetes insipidus

Useful to increase blood pressure in calcium channel blocker and caffeine overdose

Unlabeled/Investigational Use Adjunct in the treatment of GI hemorrhage and esophageal varices; pulseless arrest (ventricular tachycardia [VT]/ventricular fibrillation [VF], asystole/pulseless electrical activity [PEA]); vasodilatory shock (septic shock)

Mechanism of Action Increases cyclic adenosine monophosphate (cAMP) which increases water permeability at the renal tubule resulting in decreased urine volume and increased osmolality; causes peristalsis by directly stimulating the smooth muscle in the GI tract

Adverse Reactions

Cardiovascular: Elevated blood pressure, bradycardia, arrhythmias, venous thrombosis, vasoconstriction with higher doses, angina, myocardial infarction, tachycardia (ventricular), torsade de pointes, chest pain, peripheral gangrene, superior mesenteric artery thrombosis, arrhythmias (ventricular), sinus bradycardia

Central nervous system: Pounding in the head, fever, headache, vertigo

Dermatologic: Urticaria, cutaneous gangrene, circumoral pallor, bullous lesions, skin necrosis

Endocrine & metabolic: Hyponatremia, water intoxication, hyperprolactinemia

Gastrointestinal: Flatulence, abdominal cramps, nausea, vomiting, mesenteric occlusion, ischemic colitis, diarrhea, colonic ischemia

Hepatic: Hepatic steatosis

Neuromuscular & skeletal: Tremor, rhabdomyolysis

Miscellaneous: Diaphoresis, anaphylaxis, allergic reaction, anaphylactic shock

Pharmacodynamics/Kinetics

Onset of action: Nasal: 1 hour

Duration: Nasal: 3-8 hours; I.M., SubQ: 2-8 hours

Metabolism: Nasal/Parenteral: Hepatic, renal

Half-life elimination: Nasal: 15 minutes; Parenteral: 10-20 minutes

Excretion: Nasal: Urine; SubQ: Urine (5% as unchanged drug) after 4 hours

Dosage

Diabetes insipidus (highly variable dosage; titrated based on serum and urine sodium and osmolality in addition to fluid balance and urine output): I.M., SubQ:

Children: 2.5-10 units 2-4 times/day as needed

Adults: 5-10 units 2-4 times/day as needed (dosage range 5-60 units/day)

Continuous I.V. infusion: Children and Adults: 0.5 milliunit/kg/hour (0.0005 unit/kg/hour); double dosage as needed every 30 minutes to a maximum of 0.01 unit/kg/hour

Intranasal: Administer on cotton pledget, as nasal spray, or by dropper

Abdominal distention: Adults: I.M.: 5 units stat, 10 units every 3-4 hours

GI hemorrhage (unlabeled use): I.V. infusion: Dilute in NS or D$_5$W to 0.1-1 unit/mL
- Children: Initial: 0.002-0.005 units/kg/minute; titrate dose as needed; maximum: 0.01 unit/kg/minute; continue at same dosage (if bleeding stops) for 12 hours, then taper off over 24-48 hours
- Adults: Initial: 0.2-0.4 unit/minute, then titrate dose as needed, if bleeding stops; continue at same dose for 12 hours, taper off over 24-48 hours

Pulseless arrest (unlabeled use) [ACLS protocol]: Adults: I.V; I.O.: 40 units; may give one dose to replace first or second dose of epinephrine. I.V./I.O. drug administration is preferred, but if no access, may give endotracheally at 2 to 2 $^1/_2$ times the I.V. dose. Mix with 5-10 mL of water or normal saline, and administer down the endotracheal tube.

Vasodilatory shock/septic shock (unlabeled use): Adults: I.V.: 0.01-0.04 units/minute for the treatment of septic shock. Doses >0.04 units/minute may have more cardiovascular side effects. Most case reports have used 0.04 units/minute continuous infusion as a fixed dose.

Dosing adjustment in hepatic impairment: Some patients respond to much lower doses with cirrhosis for calcium channel blocker

Stability Store injection at room temperature; protect from heat and from freezing; use only clear solutions

Monitoring Parameters Serum and urine sodium, urine specific gravity, urine and serum osmolality; urine output, fluid input and output, blood pressure, heart rate

Administration I.V.: Use extreme caution to avoid extravasation because of risk of necrosis and gangrene. In treatment of varices, infusions are often supplemented with nitroglycerin infusions to minimize cardiac effects.
- GI hemorrhage: Administration requires the use of an infusion pump and should be administered in a peripheral line.
- Vasodilatory shock: Administration through a central catheter is recommended.
  - **Infusion rates:** 100 units in 500 mL D$_5$W rate
    - 0.1 unit/minute: 30 mL/hour
    - 0.2 unit/minute: 60 mL/hour
    - 0.3 unit/minute: 90 mL/hour
    - 0.4 unit/minute: 120 mL/hour
    - 0.5 unit/minute: 150 mL/hour
    - 0.6 unit/minute: 180 mL/hour

Intranasal (topical administration on nasal mucosa): Administer injectable vasopressin on cotton plugs, as nasal spray, or by dropper. Should not be inhaled.

Contraindications Hypersensitivity to vasopressin or any component of the formulation

Warnings Use with caution in patients with seizure disorders, migraine, asthma, vascular disease, renal disease, cardiac disease; chronic nephritis with nitrogen retention. Goiter with cardiac complications, arteriosclerosis; I.V. infiltration may lead to severe vasoconstriction and localized tissue necrosis; also, gangrene of extremities, tongue, and ischemic colitis. Elderly patients should be cautioned not to increase their fluid intake beyond that sufficient to satisfy their thirst in order to avoid water intoxication and hyponatremia; under experimental conditions, the elderly have shown to have a decreased responsiveness to vasopressin with respect to its effects on water homeostasis

Dosage Forms Injection, solution: 20 units/mL (0.5 mL, 1 mL, 10 mL)
Pitressin®: 20 units/mL (1 mL)

Reference Range Plasma: 0-2 pg/mL (SI: 0-2 ng/L) if osmolality <285 mOsm/L; 2-12 pg/mL (SI: 2-12 ng/L) if osmolality >290 mOsm/L

Overdosage/Treatment 20 IU bolus IV and titrate to blood pressure (about 4 to 5 IU per hour IV)

Drug Interactions Decreased effect: Lithium, epinephrine, demeclocycline, heparin, and ethanol block antidiuretic activity to varying degrees
Increased effect: Chlorpropamide, phenformin, urea and fludrocortisone potentiate antidiuretic response

Pregnancy Risk Factor B

Pregnancy Implications Animal reproduction studies have not been conducted. Vasopressin and desmopressin have been used safely during pregnancy and nursing based on case reports.

Lactation Enters breast milk/use caution

Nursing Implications Watch for signs of I.V. infiltration and gangrene; elderly patients should be cautioned not to increase their fluid intake beyond that sufficient to satisfy their thirst in order to avoid water intoxication and hyponatremia; under experimental conditions, the elderly have shown to have a decreased responsiveness to vasopressin with respect to its effects on water homeostasis

Additional Information Due to prolongation of QT$_c$ interval on ECG, avoid vasopressin in arsenic poisoning; not useful in treating lithium-induced diabetes insipidus

Specific References
Koshman SL, Zed PJ, and Abu-Laban RB, "Vasopressin in Cardiac Arrest," *Circulation*, 2005, 39(10):1687-92.

Obritsch MD, Jung R, Fish DN, et al, "Effects of Continuous Vasopressin Infusion in Patients with Septic Shock," *Ann Pharmacother*, 2004, 38(7):1117-22.

Wenzel V, Krismer AC, Arntz HR, et al, "A Comparison of Vasopressin and Epinephrine for Out-of-Hospital Cardiopulmonary Resuscitation," *N Engl J Med*, 2004, 350(2):105-13.

Wyer PC, Perera P, Jin Z, et al, "Vasopressin or Epinephrine for Out-of-Hospital Cardiac Arrest," *Ann Emerg Med*, 2006, 48:86-97.

Venlafaxine

CAS Number 99300-78-4
U.S. Brand Names Effexor® XR; Effexor®
Impairment Potential Yes
Use Treatment of major depressive disorder; generalized anxiety disorder (GAD), social anxiety disorder (social phobia), panic disorder
Unlabeled/Investigational Use Obsessive-compulsive disorder (OCD); hot flashes; neuropathic pain; attention-deficit/hyperactivity disorder (ADHD)
Mechanism of Action Venlafaxine and its active metabolite o-desmethylvenlafaxine (ODV) are potent inhibitors of neuronal serotonin and norepinephrine reuptake and weak inhibitors of dopamine reuptake. Venlafaxine and ODV have no significant activity for muscarinic cholinergic, H$_1$-histaminergic, or alpha$_2$-adrenergic receptors. Venlafaxine and ODV do not possess MAO-inhibitory activity.

Adverse Reactions
Cardiovascular: Vasodilation, hypertension (dose-related; 3% in patients receiving <100 mg/day, up to 13% in patients receiving >300 mg/day), tachycardia, chest pain, postural hypotension, ventricular tachycardia
Central nervous system: **Headache (25%), somnolence (23%), dizziness, insomnia, nervousness**, anxiety, abnormal dreams, yawning, agitation, confusion, abnormal thinking, depersonalization, depression, akathisia, catatonia, delirium, emotional lability, extrapyramidal symptoms, hallucinations, manic reaction, psychosis, seizure, tardive dyskinesia, vertigo, hostility (up to 1% in children/adolescents), suicidal ideation (reported at a frequency of 2% in children/adolescents with major depressive disorder)
Dermatologic: Rash, pruritus, epidermal necrolysis, erythema multiforme, erythema nodosum, exfoliative dermatitis, hirsutism, rash (maculopapular, pustular, or vesiculobullous), Stevens-Johnson syndrome, ecchymosis
Endocrine & metabolic: Decreased libido, increased transaminases/GGT, metrorrhagia, serotonin syndrome, SIADH, hyponatremia
Gastrointestinal: **Nausea (37%), xerostomia (22%), constipation, anorexia**, diarrhea, vomiting, dyspepsia, flatulence, taste perversion, weight loss, hemorrhage, pancreatitis
Genitourinary: **Abnormal ejaculation/orgasm**, impotence, urinary frequency, impaired urination, orgasm disturbance, urinary retention, prostatitis, vaginitis
Hematologic: Agranulocytosis, aplastic anemia, abnormal bleeding
Hepatic: Hepatic failure, hepatic necrosis
Neuromuscular & skeletal: **Weakness**, tremor, hypertonia, paresthesia, twitching, torticollis, dyskinesias, rhabdomyolysis
Ocular: Blurred vision, mydriasis, abnormal vision, ophthalmic hemorrhage
Otic: Tinnitus
Respiratory: Asthma, bronchitis, dyspnea
Miscellaneous: **Diaphoresis**, infection, chills, trauma, anaphylaxis

Signs and Symptoms of Overdose Profound CNS depression can occur with concomitant ingestions of other CNS depressants. Sedation, seizures (7%), tachycardia (sinus)

Admission Criteria/Prognosis Monitor asymptomatic immediate release and sustained release overdoses for 6 and 18 hours, respectively, before discharge.

Pharmacodynamics/Kinetics
Absorption: Oral: 92% to 100%; food has no significant effect on the absorption of venlafaxine or formation of the active metabolite O-desmethylvenlafaxine (ODV)
Distribution: At steady state: Venlafaxine 7.5 ± 3.7 L/kg, ODV 5.7 ± 1.8 L/Kg
Protein binding: Bound to human plasma protein: Venlafaxine 27%, ODV 30%
Metabolism: Hepatic via CYP2D6 to active metabolite, O-desmethylvenlafaxine (ODV); other metabolites include N-desmethylvenlafaxine and N,O-didesmethylvenlafaxine
Bioavailability: Absolute: ~45%
Half-life elimination: Venlafaxine: 3-7 hours; ODV: 9-13 hours; Steady-state, plasma: Venlafaxine/ODV: Within 3 days of multiple-dose therapy; prolonged with cirrhosis (Adults: Venlafaxine: ~30%, ODV: ~60%) and with dialysis (Adults: Venlafaxine: ~180%, ODV: ~142%)
Time to peak:
Immediate release: Venlafaxine: 2 hours, ODV: 3 hours
Extended release: Venlafaxine: 5.5 hours, ODV: 9 hours
Excretion: Urine (~87%, 5% as unchanged drug, 29% as unconjugated ODV, 26% as conjugated ODV, 27% as minor inactive metabolites) within 48 hours

Clearance at steady state: Venlafaxine: 1.3 $\pm$ 0.6 L/hour/kg, ODV: 0.4 $\pm$ 0.2 L/hour/kg

Clearance decreased with:

Cirrhosis: Adults: Venlafaxine: ~50%, ODV: ~30%

Severe cirrhosis: Adults: Venlafaxine: ~90%

Renal impairment (Cl$_{cr}$ 10-70 mL/minute): Adults: Venlafaxine: ~24%

Dialysis: Adults: Venlafaxine: ~57%, ODV: ~56%; due to large volume of distribution, a significant amount of drug is not likely to be removed.

Dosage Oral:

Children and Adolescents:

ADHD (unlabeled use): Initial: 12.5 mg/day

Children <40 kg: Increase by 12.5 mg/week to maximum of 50 mg/day in 2 divided doses

Children ≥40 kg: Increase by 25 mg/week to maximum of 75 mg/day in 3 divided doses.

Mean dose: 60 mg or 1.4 mg/kg administered in 2-3 divided doses

Adults:

Depression:

Immediate-release tablets: 75 mg/day, administered in 2 or 3 divided doses, taken with food; dose may be increased in 75 mg/day increments at intervals of at least 4 days, up to 225-375 mg/day

Extended-release capsules: 75 mg once daily taken with food; for some new patients, it may be desirable to start at 37.5 mg/day for 4-7 days before increasing to 75 mg once daily; dose may be increased by up to 75 mg/day increments every 4 days as tolerated, up to a maximum of 225 mg/day

GAD, social anxiety disorder: Extended-release capsules: 75 mg once daily taken with food; for some new patients, it may be desirable to start at 37.5 mg/day for 4-7 days before increasing to 75 mg once daily; dose may be increased by up to 75 mg/day increments every 4 days as tolerated, up to a maximum of 225 mg/day

Panic disorder: Extended-release capsules: 37.5 mg once daily for 1 week; may increase to 75 mg daily, with subsequent weekly increases of 75 mg/day up to a maximum of 225 mg/day.

Obsessive-compulsive disorder (unlabeled use): Titrate to usual dosage range of 150-300 mg/day; however, doses up to 375 mg daily have been used; response may be seen in 4 weeks

Neuropathic pain (unlabeled use): Dosages evaluated varied considerably based on etiology of chronic pain, but efficacy has been shown for many conditions in the range of 75-225 mg/day; onset of relief may occur in 1-2 weeks, or take up to 6 weeks for full benefit.

Hot flashes (unlabeled use): Doses of 37.5-75 mg/day have demonstrated significant improvement of vasomotor symptoms after 4-8 weeks of treatment; in one study, doses >75 mg/day offered no additional benefit; however, higher doses (225 mg/day) may be beneficial in patients with perimenopausal depression.

Attention-deficit disorder (unlabeled use): Initial: Doses vary between 18.75 to 75 mg/day; may increase after 4 weeks to 150 mg/day; if tolerated, doses up to 225 mg/day have been used

Note: When discontinuing this medication after more than 1 week of treatment, it is generally recommended that the dose be tapered. If venlafaxine is used for 6 weeks or longer, the dose should be tapered over 2 weeks when discontinuing its use.

Dosing adjustment in renal impairment: Cl$_{cr}$ 10-70 mL/minute: Decrease dose by 25%; decrease total daily dose by 50% if dialysis patients; dialysis patients should receive dosing after completion of dialysis

Dosing adjustment in moderate hepatic impairment: Reduce total daily dosage by 50%

Monitoring Parameters Blood pressure should be regularly monitored, especially in patients with a high baseline blood pressure; may cause mean increase in heart rate of 4-9 beats/minute; cholesterol; mental status for depression, suicidal ideation (especially at the beginning of therapy or when doses are increased or decreased), anxiety, social functioning, mania, panic attacks; height and weight should be monitored in children

Administration Administer with food.

Extended release capsule: Swallow capsule whole; do not crush or chew. Alternatively, contents may be sprinkled on a spoonful of applesauce and swallowed immediately without chewing; followed with a glass of water to ensure complete swallowing of the pellets.

Contraindications Hypersensitivity to venlafaxine or any component of the formulation; use of MAO inhibitors within 14 days; should not initiate MAO inhibitor within 7 days of discontinuing venlafaxine

Warnings *Major psychiatric warnings:*

* **[U.S. Boxed Warning]: Antidepressants increase the risk of suicidal thinking and behavior in children and adolescents with major depressive disorder (MDD) and other depressive disorders;** consider risk prior to prescribing. Closely monitor for clinical worsening, suicidality, or unusual changes in behavior; the child's family or caregiver should be instructed to closely observe the patient and communicate condition with healthcare provider. A medication guide concerning the use of antidepressants in children and teenagers should be dispensed with each prescription. **Venlafaxine is not FDA approved for use in children.**

- The possibility of a suicide attempt is inherent in major depression and may persist until remission occurs. Patients treated with antidepressants should be observed for clinical worsening and suicidality, especially during the initial few months of a course of drug therapy, or at times of dose changes, either increases or decreases. Worsening depression and severe abrupt suicidality that are not part of the presenting symptoms may require discontinuation or modification of drug therapy. Use caution in high-risk patients during initiation of therapy.

- Prescriptions should be written for the smallest quantity consistent with good patient care. The patient's family or caregiver should be alerted to monitor patients for the emergence of suicidality and associated behaviors such as anxiety, agitation, panic attacks, insomnia, irritability, hostility, impulsivity, akathisia, hypomania, and mania; patients should be instructed to notify their healthcare provider if any of these symptoms or worsening depression or psychosis occur.

- May worsen psychosis in some patients or precipitate a shift to mania or hypomania in patients with bipolar disorder. Monotherapy in patients with bipolar disorder should be avoided. Patients presenting with depressive symptoms should be screened for bipolar disorder. **Venlafaxine is not FDA approved for the treatment of bipolar depression.**

Key adverse effects:

- CNS depression: Has a low potential to impair cognitive or motor performance; caution operating hazardous machinery or driving.

- SIADH and hyponatremia: Has been associated with the development of SIADH; hyponatremia has been reported rarely, predominately in the elderly

- Weight loss and anorectic effects: Have been observed in both pediatric and adult patients; weight loss was not limited to those experiencing reduced appetite

- Reduced growth rate (pediatric): Small differences in height have been observed in pediatric patients receiving venlafaxine, particularly those <12 years of age, compared to placebo

Concurrent disease:

- Anxiety/Insomnia: May cause increase in anxiety, nervousness, and insomnia.

- Hepatic impairment: Use caution; clearance is decreased and plasma concentrations are increased; a lower dosage may be needed.

- Hypercholesterolemia: May cause increases to serum cholesterol.

- Hypertension/Tachycardia: May cause sustained increase in blood pressure or tachycardia. Control pre-existing hypertension prior to initiation of venlafaxine. Use caution in patients with recent history of MI, unstable heart disease, or hyperthyroidism. Effect is dose related and increases are generally modest (12-15 mm Hg diastolic).

- Narrow-angle glaucoma: May cause mydriasis; use caution in patients with increased intraocular pressure or at risk of acute narrow-angle glaucoma.

- Platelet aggregation: May impair platelet aggregation, resulting in bleeding.

- Renal impairment: Use caution; clearance is decreased and plasma concentrations are increased; a lower dosage may be needed.

- Seizure disorders: Use caution with a previous seizure disorder or condition predisposing to seizures such as brain damage or alcoholism.

- Sexual dysfunction: May cause or exacerbate sexual dysfunction.

- Weight loss: May cause weight loss; use caution in patients where weight loss is undesirable.

Concurrent drug therapy:

- Agents which lower seizure threshold: Concurrent therapy with other drugs which lower the seizure threshold.

- Anticoagulants/Antiplatelets: Use caution with concomitant use of NSAIDs, ASA, or other drugs that affect coagulation; the risk of bleeding is potentiated.

- CNS depressants: Use caution with concomitant therapy.

- MAO inhibitors: Potential for severe reaction when used with MAO inhibitors; autonomic instability, coma, death, delirium, diaphoresis, hyperthermia, mental status changes/agitation, muscular rigidity, myoclonus, neuroleptic malignant syndrome features, and seizures may occur.

- Agents causing weight loss or anorectic effects should be avoided.

Special notes:

- Electroconvulsive therapy: May increase the risks associated with electroconvulsive therapy; consider discontinuing, when possible, prior to ECT treatment.

- Withdrawal syndrome: May cause dysphoric mood, irritability, agitation, dizziness, sensory disturbances, anxiety, confusion, headache, lethargy, emotional lability, insomnia, hypomania, tinnitus, and seizures. Upon discontinuation of venlafaxine therapy, gradually taper dose. If intolerable symptoms occur following a decrease in dosage or upon discontinuation of therapy, then resuming the previous dose with a more gradual taper should be considered.

Dosage Forms Capsule, extended release:
Effexor® XR: 37.5 mg, 75 mg, 150 mg
Tablet: 25 mg, 37.5 mg, 50 mg, 75 mg, 100 mg
Effexor®: 25 mg, 37.5 mg, 50 mg, 75 mg, 100 mg

Reference Range Peak serum level of 163 ng/mL (325 ng/mL of ODV metabolite) obtained after a 150 mg oral dose; 4-hour postingestion serum level of 6100 ng/mL (1800 ng/mL of ODV metabolite) associated with coma; a venlafaxine plasma level of 7040 ng/mL (ODV of 1000 ng/mL) was associated with seizures

Overdosage/Treatment
Decontamination: Lavage (within 1 hour)/activated charcoal
Supportive therapy: Sodium bicarbonate (1-2 mEq/kg) can be given for cardiac conduction disturbances; lidocaine can be used for ventricular arrhythmias; lorazepam can be helpful for seizure control while benztropine (0.5 mg twice daily) can be useful to treat hot flashes and excessive sweating caused by venlafaxine; night sweats can be treated with 0.5 mg benzatropine at bedtime
Enhancement of elimination: Multiple dosing of activated charcoal may be of some benefit; forced diuresis/extracorporeal removal is not expected to be of any benefit

Test Interactions ↑ serum cholesterol

Drug Interactions
Substrate of CYP2C9 (minor), 2C19 (minor), 2D6 (major), 3A4 (major); **Inhibits** CYP2B6 (weak), 2D6 (weak), 3A4 (weak)
Buspirone: Concurrent use may result in serotonin syndrome; these combinations are best avoided
Clozapine: Addition of venlafaxine has been associated with case reports of increased clozapine serum concentrations and seizures.
CYP2D6 inhibitors: May increase the levels/effects of venlafaxine. Example inhibitors include chlorpromazine, delavirdine, fluoxetine, miconazole, paroxetine, pergolide, quinidine, quinine, ritonavir, and ropinirole.
CYP3A4 inducers: CYP3A4 inducers may decrease the levels/effects of venlafaxine. Example inducers include aminoglutethimide, carbamazepine, nafcillin, nevirapine, phenobarbital, phenytoin, and rifamycins.
CYP3A4 inhibitors: May increase the levels/effects of venlafaxine. Example inhibitors include azole antifungals, clarithromycin, diclofenac, doxycycline, erythromycin, imatinib, isoniazid, nefazodone, nicardipine, propofol, protease inhibitors, quinidine, telithromycin, and verapamil.
Haloperidol: Serum levels may be increased during concurrent administration; AUC may be increased by as much as 70%
Indinavir: Serum levels may be reduced by venlafaxine (AUC reduced by 28%); clinical significance unknown
Lithium: Concurrent use may increase risk of serotonin syndrome.
MAO inhibitors: Serotonin syndrome may result when venlafaxine is used in combination or within 2 weeks of an MAO inhibitor; these combinations should be avoided
Meperidine: Concurrent use may increase risk of serotonin syndrome
Mirtazapine: Concurrent use may increase risk of serotonin syndrome
Nefazodone: Concurrent use may increase risk of serotonin syndrome; in addition, nefazodone may inhibit the metabolism of venlafaxine
Selegiline: Concurrent use may predispose to serotonin syndrome; avoid concurrent use.
Serotonin agonists: Theoretically, may increase the risk of serotonin syndrome; includes sumatriptan, naratriptan, rizatriptan, and zolmitriptan
Sibutramine: Concurrent use may increase risk of serotonin syndrome; avoid concomitant use.
SSRIs: Concurrent use may increase risk of serotonin syndrome.
Tramadol: Concurrent use may increase risk of serotonin syndrome.
Trazodone: Concurrent use may increase risk of serotonin syndrome.
Tricyclic antidepressants: Concurrent use may increase risk of serotonin syndrome
Warfarin: Case reports of increased INR when venlafaxine was added to therapy.

Pregnancy Risk Factor C

Pregnancy Implications There are no adequate or well-controlled studies in pregnant women. Use only in pregnancy if clearly needed. If used during pregnancy (until or shortly before birth), monitor newborn for discontinuation effects.

Lactation Enters breast milk/not recommended

Additional Information Avoid ethanol (may increase CNS effects). Avoid valerian, St John's wort, SAMe, kava kava, tryptophan (may increase risk of serotonin syndrome and/or excessive sedation).

Specific References
Bond GR, Steele PE, and Uges DR, "Massive Venlafaxine Overdose Resulted in a False Positive Abbott AxSYM® Urine Immunoassay for Phencyclidine," *J Toxicol Clin Toxicol*, 2003, 41(7):999-1002.

Bradley RH, Barkin RL, Jerome J, et al, "Efficacy of Venlafaxine for the Long Term Treatment of Chronic Pain with Associated Major Depressive Disorder," *Am J Ther*, 2003, 10(5):318-23.
Cumpston K, Chao M, and Pallasch E, "Massive Venlafaxine Overdose Resulting in Arrhythmogenic Death," *J Toxicol Clin Toxicol*, 2003, 41(5):659.
Marraffa JM, Stork CM, Hodgman MJ, et al, "Venlafaxine Overdose Resulting in Seizures and QRS Widening 16 H After Exposure," *J Toxicol Clin Toxicol*, 2004, 42(5):739.
Mazur JE, Doty JD, and Krygiel AS, "Fatality Related to a 30-g Venlafaxine Overdose," *Pharmacotherapy*, 2003, 23(12):1668-72.
Pan JJ and Shen WW, "Serotonin Syndrome Induced by Low-Dose Venlafaxine," *Ann Pharmacother.*, 2003, 37(2):209-11.
Phelps NJ and Cates ME, "The Role of Venlafaxine in the Treatment of Obsessive-compulsive Disorder," *Ann Pharmacother*, 2005, 39(1):136-40.
Phillips BB, Digmann RR, and Beck MG, "Hepatitis Associated with Low-dose Venlafaxine for Postmenopausal Vasomotor Symptoms," *Ann Pharmacother*, 2006, 40(2):323-7.
Precourt A, Dunewicz M, Gregoire G, et al, "Multiple Complications and Withdrawal Syndrome Associated with Quetiapine/Venlafaxine Intoxication," *Ann Pharmacother*, 2005, 39(1):153-6.
Sarandol A and Taneli B, "Seizure Activity After Venlafaxine Overdose," *J Pharm Technol*, 2003, 19:358-60.
Sayar K, Aksu G, Ak I, et al, "Venlafaxine Treatment of Fibromyalgia," *Ann Pharmacother*, 2003, 37(11):1561-5.
Vis PM, van Baardewijk M, and Einarson TR, "Duloxetine and Venlafaxine-XR in the Treatment of Major Depressive Disorder: A Meta-Analysis of Randomized Clinical Trials," *Ann Pharmacother*, 2005, 39(11):1798-807.

Verapamil

Related Information
- Calcium Channel Blockers

CAS Number 152-11-4; 52-53-9

U.S. Brand Names Calan® SR; Calan®; Covera-HS®; Isoptin® SR; Verelan® PM; Verelan®

Synonyms Iproveratril Hydrochloride; Verapamil Hydrochloride

Use Orally for treatment of angina pectoris (vasospastic, chronic stable, unstable) and hypertension; I.V. for supraventricular tachyarrhythmias (PSVT, atrial fibrillation, atrial flutter)

Unlabeled/Investigational Use Migraine; hypertrophic cardiomyopathy; bipolar disorder (manic manifestations)

Mechanism of Action Inhibits calcium ion from entering the "slow channels" or select voltage-sensitive areas of vascular smooth muscle and myocardium during depolarization; produces a relaxation of coronary vascular smooth muscle and coronary vasodilation; increases myocardial oxygen delivery in patients with vasospastic angina

Adverse Reactions
Cardiovascular: Hypotension, bradycardia; first, second, or third degree AV block; worsening heart failure, fibrillation (atrial), flutter (atrial), myocardial depression, tachycardia (supraventricular), sinus bradycardia, vasculitis
Central nervous system: Dizziness, psychosis, fatigue, seizures, (occasionally with I.V. use), headache, parkinsonism
Dermatologic: Hypertrichosis, exfoliative dermatitis, erythema multiforme, alopecia, angioedema, urticaria, purpura, Stevens-Johnson syndrome, photosensitivity, pruritus, licheniform eruptions, exanthem
Endocrine & metabolic: Polydipsia, hyperkalemia, hyperprolactinemia, hypokalemia, nephrogenic diabetes insipidus
Gastrointestinal: Constipation, nausea, abdominal pain, abdominal discomfort, vomiting, GI bleeding (relative risk: 2.39), decreased esophageal sphincter tone, xerostomia
Hepatic: Elevated hepatic enzymes, cholestasis
Neuromuscular & skeletal: Erythromelalgia, paresthesia
Respiratory: May precipitate insufficiency of respiratory muscle function in Duchenne muscular dystrophy

Signs and Symptoms of Overdose Acidosis, asthenia, asystole, AV block, bundle-branch block, cardiac arrhythmias, cholestatic jaundice, coagulopathy, colonic ischemia, colon perforation, coma, confusion, constipation, drowsiness, dyspnea, eosinophilia, esophageal ulceration, extrapyramidal reaction, flatulence, gingival hyperplasia, gynecomastia, hyperkalemia, hypoglycemia, heart block, hyperglycemia, hypotension, impotence, junctional bradycardia, myoglobinuria, nausea, possible bezoars with resultant bowel infarction, rhabdomyolysis, seizures, skin flushing, syncope

Pharmacodynamics/Kinetics
Onset of action: Peak effect: Oral: Immediate release: 1-2 hours; I.V.: 1-5 minutes
Duration: Oral: Immediate release tablets: 6-8 hours; I.V.: 10-20 minutes
Protein binding: 90%
Metabolism: Hepatic via multiple CYP isoenzymes; extensive first-pass effect

Bioavailability: Oral: 20% to 35%

Half-life elimination: Infants: 4.4-6.9 hours; Adults: Single dose: 2-8 hours, Multiple doses: 4.5-12 hours; prolonged with hepatic cirrhosis

Excretion: Urine (70%, 3% to 4% as unchanged drug); feces (16%)

Dosage Children: SVT:

I.V.:

<1 year: 0.1-0.2 mg/kg over 2 minutes; repeat every 30 minutes as needed

1-15 years: 0.1-0.3 mg/kg over 2 minutes; maximum: 5 mg/dose, may repeat dose in 15 minutes if adequate response not achieved; maximum for second dose: 10 mg/dose

Oral (dose not well established):

1-5 years: 4-8 mg/kg/day in 3 divided doses **or** 40-80 mg every 8 hours

>5 years: 80 mg every 6-8 hours

Adults:

SVT: I.V.: 2.5-5 mg (over 2 minutes); second dose of 5-10 mg (~0.15 mg/kg) may be given 15-30 minutes after the initial dose if patient tolerates, but does not respond to initial dose; maximum total dose: 20 mg

Angina: Oral: Initial dose: 80-120 mg 3 times/day (elderly or small stature: 40 mg 3 times/day); range: 240-480 mg/day in 3-4 divided doses

Hypertension: Oral:

Immediate release: 80 mg 3 times/day; usual dose range (JNC 7): 80-320 mg/day in 2 divided doses

Sustained release: 240 mg/day; usual dose range (JNC 7): 120-360 mg/day in 1-2 divided doses; 120 mg/day in the elderly or small patients (no evidence of additional benefit in doses >360 mg/day).

Extended release:

Covera-HS®: Usual dose range (JNC 7): 120-360 mg once daily (once-daily dosing is recommended at bedtime)

Verelan® PM: Usual dose range: 200-400 mg once daily at bedtime

Dosing adjustment in renal impairment: Cl_{cr} <10 mL/minute: Administer at 50% to 75% of normal dose.

Dialysis: Not dialyzable (0% to 5%) via hemo- or peritoneal dialysis; supplemental dose is not necessary.

Dosing adjustment/comments in hepatic disease: Reduce dose in cirrhosis, reduce dose to 20% to 50% of normal and monitor ECG.

Stability Store injection at room temperature; protect from heat and from freezing; use only clear solutions; **compatible** in solutions of pH of 3-6, but may precipitate in solutions having a pH of ≥6

Monitoring Parameters Monitor blood pressure closely

Administration Oral: Do not crush or chew sustained or extended release products.

Calan® SR, Isoptin® SR: Administer with food.

Verelan®, Verelan® PM: Capsules may be opened and the contents sprinkled on 1 tablespoonful of applesauce, then swallowed without chewing.

I.V.: Rate of infusion: Over 2 minutes.

Contraindications Hypersensitivity to verapamil or any component of the formulation; severe left ventricular dysfunction; hypotension (systolic pressure <90 mm Hg) or cardiogenic shock; sick sinus syndrome (except in patients with a functioning artificial pacemaker); second- or third-degree AV block (except in patients with a functioning artificial pacemaker); atrial flutter or fibrillation and an accessory bypass tract (WPW, Lown-Ganong-Levine syndrome)

Warnings Avoid use in heart failure; can exacerbate condition. Can cause hypotension. Rare increases in liver function tests can be observed. Can cause first-degree AV block or sinus bradycardia. Other conduction abnormalities are rare. Use caution when using verapamil together with a beta-blocker. Avoid use of I.V. verapamil with an I.V. beta-blocker; can result in asystole. Use caution in patients with hypertrophic cardiomyopathy (IHSS). Use with caution in patients with attenuated neuromuscular transmission (Duchenne's muscular dystrophy, myasthenia gravis). Adjust the dose in severe renal dysfunction and hepatic dysfunction. Verapamil significantly increases digoxin serum concentrations (adjust digoxin's dose). May prolong recovery from nondepolarizing neuromuscular-blocking agents.

Dosage Forms Caplet, sustained release: 120 mg, 180 mg, 240 mg

Calan® SR: 120 mg, 180 mg, 240 mg

Capsule, extended release, controlled onset, as hydrochloride:

Verelan® PM: 100 mg, 200 mg, 300 mg

Capsule, sustained release, as hydrochloride: 120 mg, 180 mg, 240 mg, 360 mg

Verelan®: 120 mg, 180 mg, 240 mg, 360 mg

Injection, solution, as hydrochloride: 2.5 mg/mL (2 mL, 4 mL)

Tablet, as hydrochloride: 80 mg, 120 mg

Calan®: 40 mg, 80 mg, 120 mg

Tablet, extended release: 120 mg, 180 mg, 240 mg

Tablet, extended release, controlled onset, as hydrochloride:

Covera-HS®: 180 mg, 240 mg

Tablet, sustained release, as hydrochloride: 120 mg, 180 mg, 240 mg

Isoptin® SR: 120 mg, 180 mg, 240 mg

Reference Range

A ratio of verapamil/norverapamil >2.3 may be a predictor for fatal outcome

Therapeutic: 50-200 ng/mL (SI: 100-410 nmol/L) for parent; under normal conditions norverapamil concentration is the same as parent drug

Toxic: >845 ng/mL

Fatal: >2000 ng/mL

Levels of 2200 ng/mL and 2700 ng/mL associated with ingestions of 3.2 and 4 g, respectively

In the postmortem state, anatomical site concentration differences (ie, postmortem redistribution) may occur.

Overdosage/Treatment

Decontamination: Ipecac-induced emesis can hypothetically worsen calcium antagonist toxicity, since it can produce vagal stimulation. The potential for seizures precipitously following acute ingestion of large doses of a calcium antagonist may also contraindicate the use of ipecac. Lavage (within 1 hour)/activated charcoal; whole bowel irrigation may be effective for sustained release preparations

Supportive therapy: Supportive and symptomatic treatment, including I.V. fluids and Trendelenburg positioning, should be initiated as intoxication may cause hypotension. Although calcium (calcium chloride I.V. 1-3 g in adults or 10-30 mg/kg in children over 5-10 minutes with repeats as needed) has been used as an "antidote" for acute intoxications, inamrinone or dopamine may be needed for hypotension and traditional use of vasopressors is the first-line therapy for shock, with calcium chloride being the second-line agent. Hyperinsulinemic therapy with 0.5-1.0 unit I.V. insulin bolus with an infusion of 0.2-1 unit/kg/hour plus a glucose bolus of 25 g I.V. and dextrose infusion to maintain a serum glucose >100 mg/dL may reverse cardiogenic shock due to calcium blockers. Heart block may respond to isoproterenol, glucagon, atropine and/or calcium, although a temporary pacemaker may be required; sodium bicarbonate should be given for acidosis. Glucagon may increase myocardial contractility. In an animal model, the therapy of hyperinsulinemia with euglycemia allowed for larger increases in myocardial contractility than calcium chloride, epinephrine, and glucagon. In a swine model, hypertonic sodium bicarbonate (4 mEq/kg over 4 minutes) reversed myocardial depression and increased mean arterial pressure.

Enhancement of elimination: Multiple dosing of activated charcoal may be effective; not dialyzable (0% to 5%); charcoal hemoperfusion (mean plasma clearance: 73 mL/minute) is ~10 times more efficient than hemodialysis (mean plasma clearance: 8.3 mL/minute) in removal of verapamil; even so, hemoperfusion clearance is only ~1% that of normal hepatic clearance. Thus, the only indication for prolonged charcoal hemoperfusion in verapamil overdose is in the setting of concomitant hepatic dysfunction.

Antidote(s)

● Glucagon [ANTIDOTE]

Test Interactions ↑ glucose (S)

Drug Interactions Substrate of CYP1A2 (minor), 2B6 (minor), 2C9 (minor), 2C18 (minor), 2E1 (minor), 3A4 (major); **Inhibits** CYP1A2 (weak), 2C9 (weak), 2D6 (weak), 3A4 (moderate)

Alfentanil's plasma concentration is increased. Fentanyl and sufentanil may be affected similarly.

Amiodarone use may lead to bradycardia and decreased cardiac output. Monitor closely if using together.

Aspirin and concurrent verapamil use may increase bleeding times; monitor closely, especially if on other antiplatelet agents or anticoagulants.

Azole antifungals may inhibit the calcium channel blocker's metabolism; avoid this combination. Try an antifungal like terbinafine (if appropriate) or monitor closely for altered effect of the calcium channel blocker.

Barbiturates reduce the plasma concentration of verapamil. May require much higher dose of verapamil.

Beta-blockers may have increased pharmacodynamic interactions with verapamil (see Warnings/Precautions).

Buspirone's serum concentration may increase. May require dosage adjustment.

Calcium may reduce the calcium channel blocker's effects, particularly hypotension.

Carbamazepine's serum concentration is increased and toxicity may result; avoid this combination.

Cimetidine reduced verapamil's metabolism; consider an alternative H_2 antagonist.

Colchicine: Verapamil may increase colchicine toxicity (especially nephrotoxicity).

Cyclosporine's serum concentrations are increased by verapamil; avoid this combination. Use another calcium channel blocker or monitor cyclosporine trough levels and renal function closely.

CYP3A4 inducers: CYP3A4 inducers may decrease the levels/effects of verapamil. Example inducers include aminoglutethimide, carbamazepine, nafcillin, nevirapine, phenobarbital, phenytoin, and rifamycins.

688

CYP3A4 inhibitors: May increase the levels/effects of verapamil. Example inhibitors include azole antifungals, clarithromycin, diclofenac, doxycycline, erythromycin, imatinib, isoniazid, nefazodone, nicardipine, propofol, protease inhibitors, telithromycin, and quinidine.

CYP3A4 substrates: Verapamil may increase the levels/effects of CYP3A4 substrates. Example substrates include benzodiazepines, calcium channel blockers, cyclosporine, mirtazapine, nateglinide, nefazodone, sildenafil (and other PDE-5 inhibitors), tacrolimus, and venlafaxine. Selected benzodiazepines (midazolam and triazolam), cisapride, ergot alkaloids, selected HMG-CoA reductase inhibitors (lovastatin and simvastatin), and pimozide are generally contraindicated with strong CYP3A4 inhibitors.

Digoxin's serum concentration is increased; reduce digoxin's dose when adding verapamil.

Doxorubicin's clearance was reduced; monitor for altered doxorubicin's effect.

Erythromycin may increase verapamil's effects; monitor altered verapamil effect.

Ethanol's effects may be increased by verapamil; reduce ethanol consumption.

Flecainide may have additive negative effects on conduction and inotropy.

Grapefruit juice: Verapamil serum concentrations may be increased by grapefruit juice. Avoid concurrent use.

HMG-CoA reductase inhibitors (atorvastatin, cerivastatin, lovastatin, simvastatin): Serum concentration will likely be increased; consider pravastatin/fluvastatin or a dihydropyridine calcium channel blocker. If concurrent use with lovastatin is unavoidable, dose of lovastatin should not exceed 40 mg/day.

Lithium neurotoxicity may result when verapamil is added; monitor lithium levels.

Midazolam's plasma concentration is increased by verapamil; monitor for prolonged CNS depression.

Nafcillin decreases plasma concentration of verapamil; avoid this combination.

Nondepolarizing muscle relaxant: Neuromuscular blockade may be prolonged. Monitor closely.

Prazosin's serum concentration increases; monitor blood pressure.

Quinidine's serum concentration is increased; adjust quinidine's dose as necessary.

Rifampin increases the metabolism of calcium channel blockers; adjust the dose of the calcium channel blocker to maintain efficacy.

Risperidone: Verapamil may increase the levels and effects of risperidone.

Sildenafil, tadalafil, vardenafil: Blood pressure-lowering effects may be additive; use caution.

Tacrolimus's serum concentrations are increased by verapamil; avoid the combination. Use another calcium channel blocker or monitor tacrolimus trough levels and renal function closely.

Theophylline's serum concentration may be increased by verapamil. Those at increased risk include children and cigarette smokers.

Pregnancy Risk Factor C

Pregnancy Implications Use in pregnancy only when clearly needed and when the benefits outweigh the potential risk to the fetus. Crosses the placenta. One report of suspected heart block when used to control fetal supraventricular tachycardia. May exhibit tocolytic effects.

Lactation Enters breast milk (small amounts)/not recommended

Nursing Implications Help patient with ambulation; monitor blood pressure closely; I.V. rate of infusion is over 2 minutes; do not crush sustained release drug product

Additional Information Incidence of adverse reactions is most common with I.V. administration; discontinue disopyramide 48 hours before starting therapy, do not restart therapy until 24 hours after verapamil has been discontinued; response to atropine may not be observed until after I.V. calcium administration; largest survivable ingestion: 24 g (slow-release capsules)

Specific References

Bania TC, Chu J, Perez E, et al, "Hemodynamic Effects of Intravenous Fat Emulsion in an Animal Model of Severe Verapamil Toxicity Resuscitated with Atropine, Calcium and Saline," *Academic Emergency Medicine*, 2007, 14:105-111.

Barry JD, Durkovitch DW, Richardson WH, et al, "Vasopressin Treatment of Verapamil Toxicity in the Porcine Model," *J Toxicol Clin Toxicol*, 2003, 41(5):694.

Cantrell FL, Clark RF, and Manoguerra AS, "Determining Triage Guidelines for Accidental Overdose with Calcium Channel Antagonists," *J Toxicol Clin Toxicol*, 2004, 42(5):734-5.

Cantrell FL, Clark RF, and Manoguerra AS, "Determining Triage Guidelines for Unintentional Overdoses with Calcium Channel Antagonists," *Clin Toxicol (Phila)*, 2005, 43(7):849-53 (review).

Chobanian AV, Bakris GL, Black HR, et al, "The Seventh Report of the Joint National Committee on Prevention, Detection, Evaluation, and Treatment of High Blood Pressure: The JNC 7 Report," *JAMA*, 2003, 289(19):2560-71.

Chu J, Bania TC, Perez E, et al, "Glibenclamide as a Treatment for Severe Verapamil Toxicity," *Acad Emerg Med*, 2003, 10:511a.

Chu J, Bania TC, Perez E, et al, "Glibenclamide (GLB) Does Not Produce a Dose-Dependent Improvement of Hemodynamics in Verapamil (VER) Toxicity," *J Toxicol Clin Toxicol*, 2004, 42(5):799.

DeWitt CR and Waksman JC. "Pharmacology, Pathophysiology and Management of Calcium Channel Blocker and Beta-Blocker Toxicity," *Toxicol Rev*, 2004, 23(4):223-38.

Eisenberg MJ, Brox A, and Bestawros AN, "Calcium Channel Blockers: An Update," *Am J Med*, 2004, 116(1):35-43.

Kinoshita H, Taniguchi T, Nishiguchi M, et al, "An Autopsy Case of Combined Drug Intoxication Involving Verapamil, Metoprolol and Digoxin," *Forensic Sci Int*, 2003, 133(1-2):107-12.

Manoguerra AS and Cantrell FL, "Therapeutic Errors with Calcium Channel Blockers: Who? What? Where? And Why?" *J Toxicol Clin Toxicol*, 2003, 41(5):703.

Megarbane B, Karyo S, and Baud FJ, "The Role of Insulin and Glucose (Hyperinsulinaemia/Euglycaemia) Therapy in Acute Calcium Channel Antagonist and Beta-Blocker Poisoning," *Toxicol Rev*, 2004, 23(4):215-22.

Michael JB and Sztajnkrycer MD, "Deadly Pediatric Poisons: Nine Common Agents That Kill at Low Doses," *Emerg Med Clin N Am*, 2004, 22:1019-50.

Olson KR, Erdman AR, Woolf AD, et al, "Calcium Channel Blocker Ingestion: An Evidence-Based Consensus Guideline for Out-of-Hospital Management," *Clin Toxicol (Phila)*. 2005, 43(7):797-822.

Pizon AF, LoVecchio F, and Matesick LD, "Calcium Channel Blocker Overdose: One Center's Experience," *Clin Toxicol (Phila)*, 2005, 43:679.

Reed M, Wall GC, Shah NP, et al, "Verapamil Toxicity Resulting from a Probable Interaction with Telithromycin," *Ann Pharmacother*, 2005, 39(2):357-60.

Rogers JJ and Waksman JC, "Normal LV Function and BNP Levels in a Case of Severe Verapamil Poisoning: Time to Look at the Role of Vasodilatation as the Cause of Toxicity," *Clin Toxicol (Phila)*, 2005, 43:745.

Schaeffer TH, Waksman JC, and Schaffer MS, "Accidental OD of Verapamil in an Infant from Medical Error," *Clin Toxicol (Phila)*, 2005, 43:656.

Schwartz MD and Morgan BW, "Massive Verapamil Pharmacobezoar Resulting in Esophageal Perforation," *Int J Med Toxicol*, 2004, 7(1):4.

Shepherd G and Klein-Schwartz W, "High-Dose Insulin Therapy for Calcium-Channel Blocker Overdose," *Ann Pharmacother*, 2005, 39(5):923-30.

Summers MA, Moore JL, and McAuley JW, "Use of Verapamil as a Potential P-Glycoprotein Inhibitor in a Patient with Refractory Epilepsy," *Ann Pharmacother*, 2004, 38(10):1631-4.

Sztajnkrycer MD, Bond GR, Johnson SB, et al, "Use of Vasopressin in a Canine Model of Severe Verapamil Poisoning: A Pilot Study," *Acad Emerg Med*, 2004, 11(5):469-70.

Tan CKD, Chan BSH, Nanavati Z, et al, "Extracorporeal Albumin Dialysis Does Not Reduce Serum Drug Concentrations After Overdose with Sustained-Release Verapamil," *J Toxicol Clin Toxicol*, 2004, 42(5):718.

Varoni MV, Palomba D, Satta M, et al, "Low Urinary Kallikrein Rats: Different Sensitivity of Verapamil on Hypertensive Response to Central Acute Cadmium Administration," *Vet Hum Toxicol*, 2003, 45(4):202-6.

Wilimowska J, Piekoszewski W, Krzyanowska-Kierepka E, et al, "Monitoring of Verapamil Enantiomers Concentration in Overdose," *Clin toxicol*, 2006, 44:169-71.

Vigabatrin

CAS Number 60643-86-9

Impairment Potential Yes

Use Active management of partial or secondary generalized seizures not controlled by usual treatments; treatment of infantile spasms

Unlabeled/Investigational Use Spasticity, tardive dyskinesias

Mechanism of Action Irreversible inhibitor of GABA transaminase - a structural analog of GABA

Adverse Reactions

Cardiovascular: Facial flushing

Central nervous system: Lethargy, mania, confusion, CNS depression, insomnia, fatigue, dizziness, sedation (at onset of therapy), psychosis (especially in patients with behavioral abnormalities, acute and reversible), headache, mania, paranoia, aggressive behavior

Dermatologic: Alopecia

Gastrointestinal: Xerostomia, gingival hyperplasia

Hepatic: Liver failure, hepatic necrosis

Neuromuscular & skeletal: Myoclonus

Ocular: Diplopia

Signs and Symptoms of Overdose Delirium

Pharmacodynamics/Kinetics

Duration (rate of GABA-T resynthesis dependent): Variable (not strictly correlated to serum concentrations)

Absorption: Rapid
Metabolism: Minimal
Half-life elimination: 5-8 hours; Elderly: Up to 13 hours
Time to peak: 2 hours
Excretion: Urine (70%, as unchanged drug)

Dosage
Initial dose: 1-2 g/day then titrate to maintenance dose of 2-4 g/day in 1-2 divided doses (lower initial doses in the elderly, patients with renal insufficiency, or patients with psychiatric illnesses)
Infantile spasm: 50-200 mg/kg/day
Spasticity: 2-3 g/day
Tardive dyskinesia: 2-8 g/day

Monitoring Parameters Ophthalmologic examination at baseline and periodically during therapy (every 3 months); including mydriatic peripheral fundus examination and visual field perimetry. Observe patient for excessive sedation, especially when instituting or increasing therapy.

Administration May be administered with or without food.
Sachet: Dissolve powder in 10 mL of water, juice, infant formula, or milk immediately before administration. The appropriate aliquot may be administered using an oral syringe.

Contraindications Hypersensitivity to vigabatrin of any component of the formulation; pregnancy or breast-feeding

Warnings May be associated with ophthalmologic toxicities, which may be permanent; baseline and periodic monitoring is required. Patients must be instructed to report changes in vision. Patients must be closely monitored for potential neurotoxicity (observed in animal models but not established in humans). Use caution in patients with a history of psychosis (psychotic/agitated reactions may occur more frequently), depression, or behavioral problems. Use caution in elderly patients and in patients with renal impairment (Cl_{cr} <60 mL/minute). May cause an increase in seizure frequency in some patients, use particular caution in patients with myoclonic seizures, which may be more prone to this effect. Do not discontinue abruptly; gradually reduce dose over a 2- to 4-week period.

Dosage Forms Powder for oral suspension [sachets]: 0.5 g [contains povidone]
Tablet: 500 mg

Reference Range
Peak S+ enantiomer: 93 nmol/mL after 1.5 g dose
Peak R- enantiomer: 169 nmol/mL after 1.5 g dose

Overdosage/Treatment
Decontamination: Lavage (within 1 hour)/activated charcoal
Enhancement of elimination: Multiple dosing of activated charcoal may be useful; hemodialysis may be useful

Drug Interactions
Phenobarbital: Serum concentrations of phenobarbital may be decreased by vigabatrin (9% to 21%).
Phenytoin: Serum concentrations of phenytoin may be decreased by vigabatrin (16% to 33%).

Pregnancy Risk Factor Not assigned; contraindicated per manufacturer
Pregnancy Implications Cleft palate observed in rabbit studies
Lactation Excretion in breast milk unknown/contraindicated
Additional Information Water soluble; may worsen myoclonic seizures; rodent studies showed intramyelinic edema (reversible on cessation of treatment)

VinBLAStine

CAS Number 143-67-9; 865-21-4
U.S. Brand Names Velban® [DSC]
Synonyms NSC-49842; Vinblastine Sulfate; VLB
Use Treatment of Hodgkin's and non-Hodgkin's lymphoma, testicular, lung, head and neck, breast, and renal carcinomas, Mycosis fungoides, Kaposi's sarcoma, histiocytosis, choriocarcinoma, and idiopathic thrombocytopenic purpura
Mechanism of Action Vinblastine binds to tubulin and inhibits microtubule formation, therefore, arresting the cell at metaphase by disrupting the formation of the mitotic spindle; it is specific for the M and S phases. Vinblastine may also interfere with nucleic acid and protein synthesis by blocking glutamic acid utilization; extracted from *Vinca rosea* (periwinkle)

Adverse Reactions
Cardiovascular: Hypertension, Raynaud's phenomenon
Central nervous system: Depression, malaise, headache, seizures
Dermatologic: **Alopecia**, rash, photosensitivity, dermatitis
Endocrine & metabolic: **SIADH**, hyperuricemia
Gastrointestinal: **Diarrhea** (less common), **stomatitis, anorexia, metallic taste**, constipation, abdominal pain, nausea (mild), vomiting (mild), paralytic ileus, stomatitis
Genitourinary: Urinary retention
Hematologic: May cause severe **bone marrow suppression** and is the dose-limiting toxicity of VLB (unlike vincristine); severe **granulocytopenia** and **thrombocytopenia** may occur following the administration of VLB and nadir 5-10 days after treatment
Myelosuppression (primarily **leukopenia**, may be dose limiting)

Onset: 4-7 days
Nadir: 5-10 days
Recovery: 4-21 days
Neuromuscular & skeletal: Jaw pain, myalgia, paresthesia
Respiratory: Bronchospasm
VLB rarely produces neurotoxicity at clinical doses; however, neurotoxicity may be seen, especially at high doses; if it occurs, symptoms are similar to VCR toxicity (ie, peripheral neuropathy, loss of deep tendon reflexes, headache, weakness, urinary retention, and GI symptoms, tachycardia, orthostatic hypotension, convulsions); hemorrhagic colitis

Signs and Symptoms of Overdose Agranulocytosis, ataxia, bleeding, colitis, deafness, diarrhea, fever, granulocytopenia, hypertension, hyperuricemia, hyponatremia, leukopenia, neutropenia, paresthesia, Parkinson's-like symptoms, ptosis, tachycardia, thrombocytopenia

Pharmacodynamics/Kinetics
Distribution: V_d: 27.3 L/kg; binds extensively to tissues; does not penetrate CNS or other fatty tissues; distributes to liver
Protein binding: 99%
Metabolism: Hepatic to active metabolite
Half-life elimination: Biphasic: Initial: 0.164 hours; Terminal: 25 hours
Excretion: Feces (95%); urine (<1% as unchanged drug)

Dosage Refer to individual protocols.
Children and Adults: I.V.: 4-20 mg/m² (0.1-0.5 mg/kg) every 7-10 days **or** 5-day continuous infusion of 1.5-2 mg/m²/day **or** 0.1-0.5 mg/kg/week
Dosing adjustment in hepatic impairment:
Serum bilirubin 1.5-3.0 mg/dL or AST 60-180 units: Administer 50% of normal dose
Serum bilirubin 3.0-5.0 mg/dL: Administer 25% of dose
Serum bilirubin >5.0 mg/dL or AST >180 units: Omit dose

Monitoring Parameters CBC with differential and platelet count, serum uric acid, hepatic function tests

Administration FATAL IF GIVEN INTRATHECALLY. Administer vinblastine I.V., usually as a slow (2-3 minutes) push, or a bolus (5- to 15-minute) infusion. It is occasionally given as a 24-hour continuous infusion. Avoid extravasation; may cause sloughing. Solution should be administered only by qualified personnel. Do not allow to come in contact with skin; if contact occurs, wash well with soap and water.
Extravasation management: Mix 250 units hyaluronidase with 6 mL of NS. Inject the hyaluronidase solution subcutaneously through 6 clockwise injections into the infiltrated area using a 25-gauge needle; change the needle with each new injection. Apply heat immediately for 1 hour. Repeat 4 times/day for 3-5 days. Elevate extremity. Application of cold or hydrocortisone is contraindicated. Aspirate infusate from IV site.

Contraindications For I.V. use only; **I.T. use may result in death**; hypersensitivity to vinblastine or any component of the formulation; pregnancy

Warnings
Hazardous agent - use appropriate precautions for handling and disposal.
[U.S. Boxed Warning]: Vinblastine is a moderate vesicant; avoid extravasation. Dosage modification required in patients with impaired liver function and neurotoxicity. Using small amounts of drug daily for long periods may cause neurotoxicity and is therefore not advised. **[U.S. Boxed Warning]: For I.V. use only. Intrathecal administration may result in death.** Monitor closely for shortness of breath or bronchospasm in patients receiving mitomycin C. **[U.S. Boxed Warning]: Should be administered under the supervision of an experienced cancer chemotherapy physician.**

Dosage Forms Injection, powder for reconstitution, as sulfate: 10 mg
Injection, solution, as sulfate: 1 mg/mL (10 mL) [contains benzyl alcohol]

Overdosage/Treatment
Supportive therapy: Seizures can be treated with diazepam, lorazepam, or barbiturates; extravasation can be treated with warm compresses with infiltration of hyaluronidase (150 units in saline in a concentration of 15 units/mL); surgical debridement may be necessary. Ocular exposure should be treated with oral prednisone and dexamethasone eye drops.
Intrathecal overdose: Maintain upright posture for gravitational protection. Maintain lumbar puncture site for CSF exchange/drainage, Give 30 ml of Lactated Ringers per 30 ml of CSF for three exchanges.
Enhancement of elimination: Exchange transfusion (2 volume) has been performed in a child 3 years of age who received ten times the therapeutic dose; not removed by hemodialysis

Drug Interactions
Substrate of CYP2D6 (minor), 3A4 (major); **Inhibits** CYP2D6 (weak), 3A4 (weak)
CYP3A4 inducers: CYP3A4 inducers may decrease the levels/effects of vinblastine. Example inducers include aminoglutethimide, carbamazepine, nafcillin, nevirapine, phenobarbital, phenytoin, and rifamycins.
CYP3A4 inhibitors: May increase the levels/effects of vinblastine. Example inhibitors include azole antifungals, clarithromycin, diclofenac, doxycycline, erythromycin, imatinib, isoniazid, nefazodone, nicardipine, propofol, protease inhibitors, quinidine, telithromycin, and verapamil.
Mitomycin-C: Previous or simultaneous use with mitomycin-C has resulted in acute shortness of breath and severe bronchospasm within minutes or several hours after vinca alkaloid injection and may occur up to 2 weeks

after the dose of mitomycin. Mitomycin-C, in combination with administration of VLB, may cause acute shortness of breath and severe bronchospasm, onset may be within minutes or several hours after VLB injection Phenytoin may reduce vinblastine serum concentrations.

Pregnancy Risk Factor D

Lactation Enters breast milk/not recommended

Additional Information Urine (for 4 days) and feces (for 7 days) should be handled with care

Myelosuppressive effects: Onset (days): 4-7. Nadir (days): 10. Recovery (days): 17

VinCRIStine

Related Information

● Therapeutic Drugs Associated with Hallucinations

CAS Number 2068-78-2; 57-22-7

U.S. Brand Names Oncovin® [DSC]; Vincasar PFS®

Synonyms LCR; Leurocristine Sulfate; NSC-67574; VCR; Vincristine Sulfate

Use Treatment of leukemias, Hodgkin's disease, non-Hodgkin's lymphomas, Wilms' tumor, neuroblastoma, rhabdomyosarcoma

Mechanism of Action Binds to microtubular protein of the mitotic spindle causing metaphase arrest; cell-cycle phase specific in the M and S phases; extracted from *Vinca rosea* (periwinkle)

Adverse Reactions

Cardiovascular: Hypotension (orthostatic), myocardial infarction,

Central nervous system: Neurotoxicity, seizures, CNS depression, psychosis, hallucinations, cranial nerve paralysis, visual hallucinations, fever, ataxia, dysphoria, axonopathy (ascending)

Dermatologic: **Alopecia** (occurs in 20% to 70% of patients and is reversible), rash, radiation recall dermatitis

Endocrine & metabolic: Hyperuricemia, syndrome of inappropriate antidiuretic hormone, parotitis

Gastrointestinal: Constipation (at doses of 12.5-75 mcg/kg), paralytic ileus secondary to neurologic toxicity (particularly in the elderly), nausea, vomiting, diarrhea, stomatitis

Local: Pain, cellulitis and tissue necrosis if infiltrated; phlebitis

Neuromuscular & skeletal: Jaw pain, leg pain, myalgias, cramping, motor difficulties, numbness, Charcot-Marie-Tooth disease, weakness

Neurologic: Effects of VCR may be additive with those of other neurotoxic agents and spinal cord irradiation. Dose related: Begins at 5-6 g and is significant at 15-20 g

Ocular: Optic atrophy with cortical blindness has been reported, **ptosis/ diplopia**

Respiratory: Dyspnea

Signs and Symptoms of Overdose Ascending paralysis, coma with intrathecal injection, confusion, deafness, fever, hypertension, hyperuricemia, leukopenia, Mees' lines, migraine headache (exacerbation), muscle atrophy, myopathy, numbness, occipital headache, paresthesia, thrombocytosis, thrombocytopenia

Pharmacodynamics/Kinetics

Absorption: Oral: Poor

Distribution: V_d: 163-165 L/m^2; Poor penetration into CSF; rapidly removed from bloodstream and tightly bound to tissues; penetrates blood-brain barrier poorly

Protein binding: 75%

Metabolism: Extensively hepatic

Half-life elimination: Terminal: 24 hours

Excretion: Feces (~80%); urine (<1% as unchanged drug)

Dosage

I.V.: Refer to individual protocols; orders for single doses >2.5 mg or >5 mg/treatment cycle should be verified with the specific treatment regimen and/or an experienced oncologist prior to dispensing. Doses are often capped at 2 mg; however, this may reduce the efficacy of the therapy, and may not be advisable.

Children ≤10 kg or BSA <1 m^2: Initial therapy: 0.05 mg/kg once weekly then titrate dose; maximum single dose: 2 mg

Children >10 kg or BSA ≥1 m^2: 1-2 mg/m^2, may repeat once weekly for 3-6 weeks; maximum single dose: 2 mg

Neuroblastoma: I.V. continuous infusion with doxorubicin: 1 mg/m^2/day for 72 hours

Adults: 0.4-1.4 mg/m^2, may repeat every week **or**
0.4-0.5 mg/day continuous infusion for 4 days every 4 weeks **or**
0.25-0.5 mg/m^2/day for 5 days every 4 weeks

Dosing adjustment in hepatic impairment:

Serum bilirubin 1.5-3.0 mg/dL or AST 60-180 units: Administer 50% of normal dose

Serum bilirubin 3.0-5.0 mg/dL: Administer 25% of dose

Serum bilirubin >5.0 mg/dL or AST >180 units: Omit dose

Monitoring Parameters Serum electrolytes (sodium), hepatic function tests, neurologic examination, CBC, serum uric acid

Administration FATAL IF GIVEN INTRATHECALLY.

I.V.: Usually administered as slow (1-2 minutes) push or as short (10-15 minutes) infusion; 24-hour continuous infusions are occasionally used Intralesional injection has been reported for Kaposi's sarcoma

Extravasation management: Mix 250 units hyaluronidase with 6 mL of NS. Inject the hyaluronidase solution subcutaneously through 6 clockwise injections into the infiltrated area using a 25-gauge needle. Change the needle with each new injection. Elevate extremity. Apply heat immediately for 1 hour. Repeat 4 times/day for 3-5 days. Application of cold or hydrocortisone is contraindicated.

Contraindications Hypersensitivity to vincristine or any component of the formulation; **for I.V. use only, fatal if given intrathecally;** patients with demyelinating form of Charcot-Marie-Tooth syndrome; pregnancy

Warnings

Hazardous agent – use appropriate precautions for handling and disposal. **[U.S. Boxed Warning]: Vincristine is a vesicant; avoid extravasation. (Individuals administering should be experienced in vincristine administration.)**

Dosage modification required in patients with impaired hepatic function or who have pre-existing neuromuscular disease. Use with caution in the elderly; avoid eye contamination; observe closely for shortness of breath, bronchospasm, especially in patients treated with mitomycin C. Alterations in mental status such as depression, confusion, or insomnia; constipation, paralytic ileus, and urinary tract disturbances may occur. All patients should be on a prophylactic bowel management regimen.

[U.S. Boxed Warning]: Intrathecal administration of vincristine has uniformly caused death; vincristine should never be administered by this route. For I.V. use only. Neurologic effects of vincristine may be additive with those of other neurotoxic agents and spinal cord irradiation.

Dosage Forms Injection, solution, as sulfate: 1 mg/mL (1 mL, 2 mL)

Reference Range 5-day continuous infusion (total dose: 4 mg/m^2) produced plasma level of 1.8-10.9 ng/mL at 1 hour and <0.25 ng/mL at 24 hours after discontinuation of therapy

Overdosage/Treatment

Supportive therapy: Constipation resolves after 2 weeks; neurotoxicity can be decreased with pretreatment during induction period with glutamic acid (1.5 g/day); folinic acid has been utilized but efficacy is not known (100 mg every 3 hours for 1 day, then 100 mg every 6 hours for 2 days); seizures can be treated with benzodiazepines or barbituates.

Intrathecal overdose: Maintain upright posture for gravitational protection. Maintain lumbar puncture site for CSF exchange/drainage, Give 30 ml of Lactated Ringers per 30 ml of CSF for three exchanges.

Enhancement of elimination: For intrathecal route, remove contaminated CNS fluid and flush with lactated Ringer's solution with fresh frozen plasma to maintain a protein level of 150 mg/dL; glutamic acid 10 g I.V. over 1 day followed by 500 mg/day orally until neurotoxicity is stabilized

Extravasation treatment: Inject 3-5 mL of hyaluronidase (10 units/mL) SubQ clockwise into the infiltrated area using a 25-gauge needle; change the needle with each injection; apply heat immediately for 1 hour, repeat 4 times/day for 3-5 days (application of cold and injection of hydrocortisone is contraindicated). Use warm, drug compresses. Aspirate infusate from i.v. site. Elevate extremity.

Drug Interactions

Substrate of CYP3A4 (major); **Inhibits** CYP3A4 (weak)

CYP3A4 inducers: CYP3A4 inducers may decrease the levels/effects of vincristine. Example inducers include aminoglutethimide, carbamazepine, nafcillin, nevirapine, phenobarbital, phenytoin, and rifamycins.

CYP3A4 inhibitors: May increase the levels/effects of vincristine. Example inhibitors include azole antifungals, clarithromycin, diclofenac, doxycycline, erythromycin, imatinib, isoniazid, nefazodone, nicardipine, propofol, protease inhibitors, quinidine, telithromycin, and verapamil.

Digoxin plasma levels and renal excretion may decrease with combination chemotherapy including vincristine

Mitomycin-C: Acute pulmonary reactions may occur with mitomycin-C. Previous or simultaneous use with mitomycin-C has resulted in acute shortness of breath and severe bronchospasm within minutes or several hours after vinca alkaloid injection and may occur up to 2 weeks after the dose of mitomycin.

Nifedipine: May increase the levels/effects of vincristine; monitor.

Phenytoin levels may decrease with combination chemotherapy.

Vincristine should be given 12-24 hours before asparaginase to minimize toxicity (may decrease the hepatic clearance of vincristine)

Pregnancy Risk Factor D

Lactation Enters breast milk/not recommended

Nursing Implications Maintain adequate hydration; allopurinol may be given to prevent uric acid nephropathy; observe for life-threatening wheezing after administration; use of rectal thermometer or rectal tubing should be avoided to prevent injury to rectal mucosa

Additional Information Urine (for 4 days) and feces (for 1 week) must be handled with care

Vinorelbine

CAS Number 71486-22-1

U.S. Brand Names Navelbine®

Synonyms Dihydroxydeoxynorvinkaleukoblastine; NVB; Vinorelbine Tartrate

Use Treatment of nonsmall cell lung cancer

Unlabeled/Investigational Use Treatment of breast cancer, ovarian carcinoma, Hodgkin's disease, non-Hodgkin's lymphoma

Mechanism of Action Semisynthetic vinca alkaloid which binds to tubulin and inhibits microtubule formation, therefore, arresting the cell at metaphase by disrupting the formation of the mitotic spindle; it is specific for the M and S phases. Vinorelbine may also interfere with nucleic acid and protein synthesis by blocking glutamic acid utilization.

Adverse Reactions

Cardiovascular: Chest pain, deep vein thrombosis, flushing, hypertension, hypotension, vasodilation, tachycardia

Central nervous system: **Fatigue (27%)**, headache

Dermatologic: **Alopecia (12%)**, angioedema, radiation recall (dermatitis, esophagitis)

Endocrine & metabolic: Syndrome of inappropriate ADH secretion, hyponatremia

Gastrointestinal: **Nausea (44%, severe <2%) and vomiting (20%) are most common and are easily controlled with standard antiemetics; constipation (35%), diarrhea (17%)**, paralytic ileus, abdominal pain, dysphagia, esophagitis, mucositis, pancreatitis

Emetic potential: Moderate (30% to 60%)

Genitourinary: Hemorrhagic cystitis

Hematologic: **May cause severe bone marrow suppression and is the dose-limiting toxicity of vinorelbine; severe granulocytopenia (90%) may occur following the administration of vinorelbine; leukopenia (92%), anemia (83%)**, thrombocytopenia

Myelosuppressive:

WBC: Moderate - severe

Onset (days): 4-7

Nadir (days): 7-10

Recovery (days): 14-21

Hepatic: **Elevated AST (SGOT) (67%), elevated total bilirubin (13%)**

Local: **Injection site reaction (28%), injection site pain (16%)**, vesicant and can cause tissue irritation and necrosis if infiltrated (if extravasation occurs, follow institutional policy, which may include hyaluronidase and hot compresses), phlebitis

Neuromuscular & skeletal: **Weakness (36%), peripheral neuropathy (20% to 25%)**; mild to moderate peripheral neuropathy manifested by paresthesia and hyperesthesia, loss of deep tendon reflexes (<5%); severe peripheral neuropathy (generally reversible); myalgia (<5%), arthralgia (<5%), jaw pain (<5%), back pain, gait instability, muscle weakness

Respiratory: Dyspnea, pneumonia, pulmonary edema, pulmonary embolus

Miscellaneous: Anaphylaxis, tumor pain

Pharmacodynamics/Kinetics

Absorption: Unreliable; must be given I.V.

Distribution: V_d: 25.4-40.1 L/kg; binds extensively to human platelets and lymphocytes (79.6% to 91.2%)

Protein binding: 80% to 90%

Metabolism: Extensively hepatic to two metabolites, deacetylvinorelbine (active) and vinorelbine N-oxide

Bioavailability: Oral: 26% to 45%

Half-life elimination: Triphasic: Terminal: 27.7-43.6 hours

Excretion: Feces (46%); urine (18%, 10% to 12% as unchanged drug)

Clearance: Plasma: Mean: 0.97-1.26 L/hour/kg

Dosage Refer to individual protocols.

Adults: I.V.:

Single-agent therapy: 30 mg/m² every 7 days

Combination therapy with cisplatin: 25 mg/m² every 7 days (with cisplatin 100 mg/m² every 4 weeks); **Alternatively:** 30 mg/m² in combination with cisplatin 120 mg/m² on days 1 and 29, then every 6 weeks

Dosage adjustment in hematological toxicity: Granulocyte counts should be ≥1000 cells/mm³ prior to the administration of vinorelbine. Adjustments in the dosage of vinorelbine should be based on granulocyte counts obtained on the day of treatment as follows:

Granulocytes ≥1500 cells/mm³ on day of treatment: Administer 100% of starting dose

Granulocytes 1000-1499 cells/mm³ on day of treatment: Administer 50% of starting dose

Granulocytes <1000 cells/mm³ on day of treatment: Do not administer. Repeat granulocyte count in one week; if 3 consecutive doses are held because granulocyte count is <1000 cells/mm³, discontinue vinorelbine

For patients who, during treatment, have experienced fever and/or sepsis while granulocytopenic or had 2 consecutive weekly doses held due to granulocytopenia, subsequent doses of vinorelbine should be:

75% of starting dose for granulocytes ≥1500 cells/mm³

37.5% of starting dose for granulocytes 1000-1499 cells/mm³

Dosage adjustment in renal impairment: No dose adjustments are required for renal insufficiency.

Dosing adjustment in hepatic impairment: Vinorelbine should be administered with caution in patients with hepatic insufficiency. In patients who develop hyperbilirubinemia during treatment with vinorelbine, the dose should be adjusted for total bilirubin as follows:

Serum bilirubin ≤2 mg/dL: Administer 100% of starting dose

Serum bilirubin 2.1-3 mg/dL: Administer 50% of starting dose

Serum bilirubin >3 mg/dL: Administer 25% of starting dose

Dosing adjustment in patients with concurrent hematologic toxicity and hepatic impairment: Administer the lower doses determined from the above recommendations

Monitoring Parameters CBC with differential and platelet count, hepatic function tests

Administration FATAL IF GIVEN INTRATHECALLY. Administer as a direct intravenous push or rapid bolus, over 6-10 minutes (up to 30 minutes). Longer infusions may increase the risk of pain and phlebitis. Intravenous doses should be followed by 150-250 mL of saline or dextrose to reduce the incidence of phlebitis and inflammation. **CENTRAL LINE ONLY** for IVPB administration. Avoid extravasation; may cause sloughing.

Extravasation management: Mix 250 units hyaluronidase with 6 mL of NS. Inject the hyaluronidase solution subcutaneously through 6 clockwise injections into the infiltrated area using a 25-gauge needle. Change the needle with each new injection. Elevate extremities. Apply heat immediately for 1 hour. Repeat 4 times/day for 3-5 days. Application of cold or hydrocortisone is contraindicated.

Contraindications For I.V. use only; **I.T. use may result in death**; hypersensitivity to vinorelbine or any component of the formulation; pregnancy

Warnings

Hazardous agent - use appropriate precautions for handling and disposal. **[U.S. Boxed Warning]: Avoid extravasation**; dosage modification required in patients with impaired liver function and neurotoxicity. Frequently monitor patients for myelosuppression both during and after therapy. **[U.S. Boxed Warnings]: Granulocytopenia is dose-limiting. Intrathecal administration may result in death.** Use with caution in patients with cachexia or ulcerated skin.

Acute shortness of breath and severe bronchospasm have been reported, most commonly when administered with mitomycin. Fatal cases of interstitial pulmonary changes and ARDS have also been reported. May cause severe constipation (grade 3-4), paralytic ileus, intestinal obstruction, necrosis, and/or perforation. **[U.S. Boxed Warning]: Should be administered under the supervision of an experienced cancer chemotherapy physician.**

Dosage Forms Injection, solution [preservative free]: 10 mg/mL (1 mL, 5 mL)

Reference Range Peak serum level of 1130 ng/mL achieved 15 minutes after a 30 mg/m² I.V. dose

Overdosage/Treatment

Supportive therapy: Seizures can be treated with diazepam, lorazepam, phenytoin, or barbiturates; extravasation can be treated with warm compresses with infiltration of hyaluronidase (150 units in saline in a concentration of 15 units/mL); surgical debridement may be necessary

Enhancement of elimination: Not dialyzable

Drug Interactions

Substrate of CYP2D6 (minor), 3A4 (major); **Inhibits** CYP2D6 (weak), 3A4 (weak)

Cisplatin: Incidence of granulocytopenia is significantly higher than with single-agent vinorelbine.

CYP3A4 inducers: CYP3A4 inducers may decrease the levels/effects of vinorelbine. Example inducers include aminoglutethimide, carbamazepine, nafcillin, nevirapine, phenobarbital, phenytoin, and rifamycins.

CYP3A4 inhibitors: May increase the levels/effects of vinorelbine. Example inhibitors include azole antifungals, clarithromycin, diclofenac, doxycycline, erythromycin, imatinib, isoniazid, nefazodone, nicardipine, propofol, protease inhibitors, quinidine, telithromycin, and verapamil.

Mitomycin-C: Previous or simultaneous use with mitomycin-C has resulted in acute shortness of breath and severe bronchospasm within minutes or several hours after vinca alkaloid injection and may occur up to 2 weeks after the dose of mitomycin.

Pregnancy Risk Factor D

Lactation Excretion in breast milk unknown/contraindicated

Additional Information Not useful in renal cell carcinoma; metoclopramide (20-40 mg) can be given prophylactically as an antiemetic agent; I.V. route usually utilized, although oral weekly doses of 50-160 mg have been used in patients with advanced breast cancer; less neurotoxic than vincristine or vinblastine

Vitamin A

Related Information
- Isotretinoin

CAS Number 68-26-8

U.S. Brand Names Aquasol A®; Palmitate-A® [OTC]

Synonyms Oleovitamin A

Use Treatment and prevention of vitamin A deficiency

Mechanism of Action Needed for bone development, growth, visual adaptation to darkness, testicular and ovarian function, and as a cofactor in many biochemical processes

Adverse Reactions

Reactions are only seen with doses exceeding physiologic replacement

Central nervous system: Irritability, sedation, drowsiness, dizziness, delirium, headache due to increased intracranial pressure, coma, psychosis, ataxia (truncal), insomnia

Dermatologic: Erythema, peeling skin, alopecia, yellow pigmentation (increased)

Gastrointestinal: Vomiting, diarrhea

Hematologic: Normochromic macrocytic anemia

Hepatic: Hepatomegaly

Ocular: Visual disturbances, papilledema

Otic: Ototoxicity, tinnitus

Miscellaneous: Perioral fissures

Signs and Symptoms of Overdose Anorexia, ascites, coagulopathy, diplopia, dizziness, erythema, fatigue, hypercalcemia, hypoprothrombinemia, increased intracranial pressure, low grade fever, myoglobinuria, nausea, nystagmus, portal hypertension, pruritus, pseudotumor cerebri, rhabdomyolysis, skin desquamation over hands and feet, vomiting

Pharmacodynamics/Kinetics

Absorption: Vitamin A in dosages **not** exceeding physiologic replacement is well absorbed after oral administration; water miscible preparations are absorbed more rapidly than oil preparations; large oral doses, conditions of fat malabsorption, low protein intake, or hepatic or pancreatic disease reduces oral absorption

Distribution: Large amounts concentrate for storage in the liver; enters breast milk

Metabolism: Conjugated with glucuronide; undergoes enterohepatic recirculation

Excretion: Feces

Dosage RDA:

<1 year: 375 mcg

1-3 years: 400 mcg

4-6 years: 500 mcg*

7-10 years: 700 mcg*

>10 years: 800-1000 mcg*

Supplementation in measles: Children: Oral:

<1 year: 100,000 units/day for 2 days

>1 year: 200,000 units/day for 2 days

Severe deficiency with xerophthalmia:

Children 1-8 years:

Oral: 5000-10,000 units/kg/day for 5 days or until recovery occurs

I.M.: 5000-15,000 units/day for 10 days

Children >8 years and Adults:

Oral: 500,000 units/day for 3 days, then 50,000 units/day for 14 days, then 10,000-20,000 units/day for 2 months

I.M.: 50,000-100,000 units/day for 3 days, 50,000 units/day for 14 days

Deficiency (without corneal changes): Oral:

Infants <1 year: 10,000 units/kg/day for 5 days, then 7500-15,000 units/day for 10 days

Children 1-8 years: 5000-10,000 units/kg/day for 5 days, then 17,000-35,000 units/day for 10 days

Children >8 years and Adults: 100,000 units/day for 3 days then 50,000 units/day for 14 days

Malabsorption syndrome (prophylaxis): Children >8 years and Adults: Oral: 10,000-50,000 units/day of water miscible product

Dietary supplement: Oral:

Infants up to 6 months: 1500 units/day

Children:

6 months to 3 years: 1500-2000 units/day

4-6 years: 2500 units/day

7-10 years: 3300-3500 units/day

Children >10 years and Adults: 4000-5000 units/day

Hepatotoxic dose: 600,000 units (acute); 25,000-50,000 units/day (chronic)

Stability Protect from light

Monitoring Parameters Monitor calcium; serum alkaline phosphatase, bilirubin, and prothrombin time may be elevated

Administration Do not give by I.V. push.

Contraindications Hypersensitivity to vitamin A or any component of the formulation; hypervitaminosis A; pregnancy (dose exceeding RDA)

Warnings Evaluate other sources of vitamin A while receiving this product; patients receiving >25,000 units/day should be closely mon-

itored for toxicity. Parenteral vitamin A: In low birth weight infants, polysorbates have been associated with thrombocytopenia, renal dysfunction, hepatomegaly, cholestasis, ascites, hypotension, and metabolic acidosis (E-Ferol syndrome).

Dosage Forms Capsule [softgel]: 10,000 units; 25,000 units

Injection, solution (Aquasol A®): 50,000 units/mL (2 mL) [contains polysorbate 80]

Tablet (Palmitate-A®): 5000 units, 15,000 units

Reference Range

RDA: Male: 1000 mcg retinol equivalent (RE); Female: 800 mcg RE; 1 RE = 1 retinol equivalent; 1 RE = 1 mcg retinol or 6 mg beta-carotene

Normal levels: >0.67 units/mL or 20-60 mcg/dL; levels >100 mcg/dL are associated with the toxic state

Overdosage/Treatment

Decontamination: Emesis within 30 minutes or lavage (within 1 hour) if ingestion is acute and >12,000 units/kg in children or >840,000 units in adults/cholestyramine or activated charcoal

Supportive therapy: Hypercalcemia can be treated with furosemide (20-40 mg I.V.), saline hydration and prednisone (10-40 mg orally)

Drug Interactions Decreased effect: Cholestyramine decreases absorption of vitamin A; neomycin and mineral oil may also interfere with vitamin A absorption

Increased toxicity: Retinoids may have additive adverse effects

Pregnancy Risk Factor A/X (dose exceeding RDA recommendation)

Pregnancy Implications Excessive use of vitamin A shortly before and during pregnancy could be harmful to babies. Facial/ear deformities can occur.

Lactation Enters breast milk/compatible at normal daily doses

Nursing Implications Do not give by I.V. push; patients receiving >25,000 units/day should be closely monitored for toxicity

Additional Information 1 mg equals 3333 units

Specific References

Benn CS, Martins C, Rodrigues A, et al, "Randomised Study of Effect of Different Doses of Vitamin A on Childhood Morbidity and Mortality," *BMJ*, 2006, 331(7530):1428-32.

Jackson HA and Sheehan AH. "Effect of Vitamin A on Fracture Risk," *Ann Pharmacother*, 2005, 39(12):2086-90.

Michaelsson K, Lithell H, Vessby B, et al, "Serum Retinol Levels and the Risk of Fracture," *N Engl J Med*, 2003, 348(4):287-94.

O'Donnell J, "Polar Hysteria: An Expression of Hypervitaminosis A," *Am J Ther*, 2004, 11(6):507-16.

Vitamin D

CAS Number 19356-17-3; 32222-06-3; 41294-56-8; 50-14-6; 63283-36-3; 67-96-9; 67-97-0

Synonyms Activated Ergosterol; Alfacalcidol; Calcifediol; Calcitriol; Cholecalciferol; Dihydrotachysterol; Ergocalciferol; Viosterol

Use Treatment of refractory rickets, hypophosphatemia, hypoparathyroidism; vitamin D-deficient states

Mechanism of Action Fat soluble vitamin; stimulates calcium and phosphate absorption from the small intestine, promotes secretion of calcium from bone to blood

Adverse Reactions

Cardiovascular: Hypertension, arrhythmias, cardiomyopathy, cardiomegaly

Central nervous system: Drowsiness, irritability, headache

Dermatologic: Pruritus

Endocrine & metabolic: Acidosis

Gastrointestinal: Nausea, diarrhea, vomiting, anorexia, xerostomia, metallic taste

Neuromuscular & skeletal: Weakness, muscle and bone pain

Renal: Polyuria, nephrocalcinosis, renal tubular acidosis type I

Signs and Symptoms of Overdose Albuminuria, anemia, anorexia, azotemia, confusion, drowsiness, dysosmia, ectopic calcification, headache, hypercalcemia, hyperphosphatemia, hypertension, hypomagnesemia, muscle asthenia, nausea, nystagmus, pancreatitis, renal failure, vomiting

Pharmacodynamics/Kinetics

Peak effect: In ≈1 month following daily doses

Absorption: Readily absorbed from gastrointestinal tract; absorption requires intestinal presence of bile

Metabolism: Inactive until hydroxylated in the liver and the kidney to calcifediol and then to calcitriol (most active form)

Dosage Dietary supplementation: Oral:

Infants, premature: 10-20 mcg/day (400-800 units), up to 750 mcg/day (30,000 units)

Infants and healthy Children: 10 mcg/day (400 units)

Adults:

<25 years: 400 units

>25 years: 200 units

Renal failure: Oral:

Children: 0.1-1 mg/day (4000-40,000 units)

Adults: 0.5 mg/day (20,000 units)

Hypoparathyroidism: Oral:

Children: 1.25-5 mg/day (50,000-200,000 units) and calcium supplements (500 mg elemental calcium 6 times/day)

Adults: 625 mcg to 5 mg/day (25,000-200,000 units) and calcium supplements (500 mg elemental calcium 6 times/day)

Vitamin D-dependent rickets: Oral:

Children: 75-125 mcg/day (3000-5000 units)

Adults: 250 mcg to 1.5 mg/day (10,000-60,000 units)

Nutritional rickets and osteomalacia:

Children and Adults (with normal absorption): Oral: 25 mcg/day (1000 units)

Children with malabsorption: Oral: 250-625 mcg/day (10,000-25,000 units)

Adults: I.M.: 250 mcg/day

Monitoring Parameters Serum calcium and phosphorous levels, BUN, renal status

Dosage Forms Capsule (Drisdol®): 50,000 units [1.25 mg]

Injection (Calciferol™): 500,000 units/mL [12.5 mg/mL] (1 mL)

Liquid (Calciferol™, Drisdol®): 8000 units/mL [200 mcg/mL] (60 mL)

Tablet (Calciferol™): 50,000 units [1.25 mg]

Reference Range

Normal serum range of vitamin D and 25-hydroxy D_3: 10-50 pg/mL

Normal serum range of 1.25-hydroxy D_3: 10-20 pg/mL; free 1,25 dihydroxy vitamin D levels that are elevated (mean level 852 fmol/L with a reference range of 305-523 fmol/L) may contribute to pathogenesis of hypercalcemia

Toxicity is associated with serum 25-hydroxy D_3 >850 nmol/L and free 1,25 dihydroxy D_3 >280 fmol/L; overdosage is associated with normal serum total 1,25 dihydroxy D_3 and elevated serum 25-hydroxy D_3 and free 1,25 dihydroxy D_3 due to protein binding interaction

Overdosage/Treatment Supportive therapy: Hypercalcemia can be treated with saline, diuresis, furosemide (20-40 mg I.V.) and hydrocortisone (100 mg I.V. every 6 hours); calcitonin (4-8 int. units/kg I.M. every 6-12 hours) can be used for persistent or severe hypercalcemia; hemodialysis can also be used for severe hypercalcemia; pamidronate disodium (90 mg I.V.) can be given to treat hypercalcemia due to vitamin D intoxication

Test Interactions Serum cholesterol may be falsely elevated by vitamin D

Drug Interactions Hepatic metabolism is increased with glutethimide/phenytoin; effects of vitamin D are decreased with concomitant administration of phenobarbital

Pregnancy Risk Factor A (D if dose exceeds RDA recommendation)

Pregnancy Implications Large doses (10,000 int. units/kg) can produce arterial stenosis, abnormal bone mineralization, elfin facies, and nephrocalcinosis in the neonate

Additional Information Cholecalciferol (vitamin D_3) is a potent rodenticide containing 13,000 int. units of vitamin D per g; marketed as Rampage or Quintox; present in fish, cod liver oils, butter, eggs, liver; 1.25 mg ergocalciferol provides 50,000 units of vitamin D activity; elimination of vitamin D metabolites delayed in hypothyroid individuals; insoluble in water; increased milk consumption is associated with increased serum levels of 25-hydroxy-vitamin D and increased urinary calcium

Specific References

Barrueto F Jr, Howland MH, Hoffman RS, et al, "Unintentional Pediatric Vitamin D Intoxication," *J Toxicol Clin Toxicol*, 2003, 41(5):662.

Vitamin E

CAS Number 10191-41-0; 17407-37-3; 4345-03-3; 58-95-7; 59-02-9; 7695-91-2

U.S. Brand Names Aqua Gem E® [OTC]; Aquasol E® [OTC]; E-Gems® [OTC]; Key-E® Kaps [OTC]; Key-E® [OTC]

Synonyms d-Alpha Tocopherol; dl-Alpha Tocopherol

Use Prevention and treatment of hemolytic anemia secondary to vitamin E deficiency, dietary supplement

Unlabeled/Investigational Use To reduce the risk of bronchopulmonary dysplasia or retrolental fibroplasia in infants exposed to high concentrations of oxygen; prevention and treatment of tardive dyskinesia and Alzheimer's disease; prevention and treatment of hemolytic anemia secondary to vitamin E deficiency

Mechanism of Action Prevents oxidation of vitamin A and C; protects polyunsaturated fatty acids in membranes from attack by free radicals and protects red blood cells against hemolysis

Adverse Reactions

Central nervous system: Headache

Dermatologic: Rash, contact dermatitis and erythema multiforme with topical preparation

Endocrine & metabolic: Creatinuria, gonadal dysfunction, decreased serum thyroxine and triiodothyronine

Gastrointestinal: Nausea, diarrhea, abdominal pain, intestinal cramps

Genitourinary: Increased urinary estrogens and androgens

Hepatic: Increased cholesterol and hypertriglyceridemia

Neuromuscular & skeletal: Weakness

Ocular: Blurred vision

Signs and Symptoms of Overdose Abdominal pain, asthenia, azotemia, cholestatic jaundice, diarrhea, nausea

Pharmacodynamics/Kinetics

Absorption: Oral: Depends on presence of bile; reduced in conditions of malabsorption, in low birth weight premature infants, and as dosage increases; water miscible preparations are better absorbed than oil preparations

Distribution: To all body tissues, especially adipose tissue, where it is stored

Metabolism: Hepatic to glucuronides

Excretion: Feces

Dosage RDA: Oral:

Infants:

Premature, ≤3 months: 25 units/day

≤6 months: 4.5 units/day

6-12 months: 6 units/day

Children:

1-3 years: 9 units/day

4-10 years: 10.5 units/day

Children >11 years and Adults:

Male: 15 units/day

Female: 12 units/day

Prevention of vitamin E deficiency: Neonates, premature, low birthweight (results in normal levels within 1 week): Oral: 25-50 units/24 hours until 6-10 weeks of age or 125-150 units/kg total in 4 doses on days 1, 2, 7, and 8 of life

Vitamin E deficiency treatment: Adults: Oral: 50-200 units/24 hours for 2 weeks

Topical: Apply a thin layer over affected areas as needed

Stability Protect from light

Monitoring Parameters Monitor plasma tocopherol concentrations (normal range: 6-14 mcg/mL)

Administration Swallow capsules whole, do not crush or chew.

Contraindications Hypersensitivity to vitamin E or any component of the formulation

Warnings May induce vitamin K deficiency; necrotizing enterocolitis has been associated with oral administration of large dosages (eg, >200 units/day) of a hyperosmolar vitamin E preparation in low birth weight infants

Dosage Forms Capsule: 400 int. units, 1000 int. units

Key-E® Kaps: 200 int. units, 400 int. units

Capsule, softgel: 200 int. units, 400 int. units, 600 int. units, 1000 int. units

Alph-E: 200 int. units, 400 int. units

Alph-E-Mixed: 200 int. units [contains mixed tocopherols]; 400 int. units [contains mixed tocopherols], 1000 int. units [sugar free; contains mixed tocopherols]

Aqua Gem E®: 200 units, 400 units

d-Alpha-Gems™: 400 int. units [derived from soybean oil]

E-Gems®: 30 int. units, 100 int. units, 200 int. units, 400 int. units, 600 int. units, 800 int. units, 1000 int. units, 1200 int. units [derived from soybean oil]

E-Gems Plus®: 200 int. units, 400 int. units, 800 int. units [contains mixed tocopherols]

E-Gems Elite®: 400 int. units [contains mixed tocopherols]

Ester-E™: 400 int. units

Gamma E-Gems®: 90 int. units [also contains mixed tocopherols]

Gamma-E Plus: 200 int. units [contains soybean oil]

High Gamma Vitamin E Complete™: 200 int. units [contains soybean oil, mixed tocopherols]

Cream: 50 int. units/g (60 g), 100 int. units/g (60 g), 1000 int. units/120 g (120 g), 30,000 int. units/57 g (57 g)

Key-E®: 30 int. units/g (60 g, 120 g, 600 g)

Lip balm (E-Gem® Lip Care): 1000 int. units/tube [contains vitamin A and aloe]

Oil, oral/topical: 100 int. units/0.25 mL (60 mL, 75 mL); 1150 units/0.25 mL (30 mL, 60 mL, 120 mL); 28,000 int. units/30 mL (30 mL)

Alph-E: 28,000 int. units/30 mL (30 mL) [topical]

E-Gems®: 100 units/10 drops (15 mL, 60 mL)

Ointment, topical (Key-E®): 30 units/g (60 g, 120 g, 480 g)

Powder (Key-E®): 700 int. units per 1/4 teaspoon (15 g, 75 g, 1000 g) [derived from soybean oil]

Solution, oral drops: 15 int. units/0.3 mL (30 mL)

Aquasol E®: 15 int. units/0.3 mL (12 mL, 30 mL) [latex free]

Aquavit-E: 15 int. units/0.3 mL (30 mL) [butterscotch flavor]

Suppository, rectal/vaginal (Key-E®): 30 int. units (12s, 24s) [contains coconut oil]

Tablet: 100 int. units, 200 int. units, 400 int. units, 500 int. units

Key-E®: 200 int. units, 400 int. units

Reference Range

Therapeutic: 0.8-2.5 mg/dL (SI: 19-35 μmol/L), some method variation

Toxic: >3.5 mg/dL; levels >4.5 mg/dL associated with necrotizing enterocolitis

Overdosage/Treatment Decontamination: Oral: Activated charcoal

Drug Interactions Cholestyramine (and colestipol): May reduce absorption of vitamin E

Iron: Vitamin E may impair the hematologic response to iron in children with iron-deficiency anemia; monitor

Orlistat: May reduce absorption of vitamin E

Warfarin: Vitamin E may alter the effect of vitamin K actions on clotting factors resulting in an increase hypoprothrombinemic response to warfarin; monitor

Pregnancy Risk Factor A/C (dose exceeding RDA recommendation)

Lactation Enters breast milk/compatible

Additional Information Cluster of deaths in low-birth-weight infants in 1984 (~38) secondary to injectable vitamin E (E-Ferol); ascribed to large amount of polysorbates injected; found in sunflower oil, vegetable oils, eggs, wheat germ oil

Specific References

Miller ER 3rd, Pastor-Barriuso R, Dalal D, et al, "Meta-Analysis: High-Dosage Vitamin E Supplementation May Increase All-Cause Mortality," *Ann Intern Med*, 2005, 142(1):37-46.

Pham DQ and Plakogiannis R, "Vitamin E Supplementation in Cardiovascular Disease and Cancer Prevention: Part 1," *Ann Pharmacother*, 2005, 39(11):1870-8.

Pham DQ and Plakogiannis R, "Vitamin E Supplementation in Alzheimer's Disease, Parkinson's Disease, Tardive Dyskinesia, and Cataract: Part 2," *Ann Pharmacother*, 2005, 39(12):2065-71.

Warfarin

Related Information

● Dicumarol

CAS Number 129-06-6; 2610-86-8; 81-81-2

U.S. Brand Names Coumadin®; Jantoven™

Synonyms Warfarin Sodium

Use Prophylaxis and treatment of venous thrombosis, pulmonary embolism and thromboembolic disorders; atrial fibrillation with risk of embolism and as an adjunct in the prophylaxis of systemic embolism after myocardial infarction

Unlabeled/Investigational Use Prevention of recurrent transient ischemic attacks and to reduce risk of recurrent myocardial infarction

Mechanism of Action Interferes with hepatic synthesis of vitamin K-dependent coagulation factors (II, VII, IX, X)

Adverse Reactions

As with all anticoagulants, bleeding is the major adverse effect of warfarin. Hemorrhage may occur at virtually any site. Risk is dependent on multiple variables, including the intensity of anticoagulation and patient susceptibility.

Additional adverse effects are often related to idiosyncratic reactions, and the frequency cannot be accurately estimated.

Cardiovascular: Vasculitis, edema, hemorrhagic shock

Central nervous system: Fever, lethargy, malaise, asthenia, pain, headache, dizziness, stroke

Dermatologic: Rash, dermatitis, bullous eruptions, urticaria, pruritus, alopecia

Gastrointestinal: Anorexia, nausea, vomiting, stomach cramps, abdominal pain, diarrhea, flatulence, gastrointestinal bleeding, taste disturbance, mouth ulcers

Genitourinary: Priapism, hematuria

Hematologic: Hemorrhage, leukopenia, unrecognized bleeding sites (eg, colon cancer) may be uncovered by anticoagulation, retroperitoneal hematoma, agranulocytosis

Hepatic: Increased transaminases, hepatic injury, jaundice

Neuromuscular & skeletal: Paresthesia, osteoporosis

Respiratory: Hemoptysis, epistaxis, pulmonary hemorrhage, tracheobronchial calcification

Miscellaneous: Hypersensitivity/allergic reactions

Skin necrosis/gangrene, due to paradoxical local thrombosis, is a known but rare risk of warfarin therapy. Its onset is usually within the first few days of therapy and is frequently localized to the limbs, breast or penis. The risk of this effect is increased in patients with protein C or S deficiency.

"Purple toes syndrome," caused by cholesterol microembolization, also occurs rarely. Typically, this occurs after several weeks of therapy, and may present as a dark, purplish, mottled discoloration of the plantar and lateral surfaces. Other manifestations of cholesterol microembolization may include rash; livedo reticularis; gangrene; abrupt and intense pain in lower extremities; abdominal, flank, or back pain; hematuria; renal insufficiency; hypertension; cerebral ischemia; spinal cord infarction; or other symptom of vascular compromise.

Signs and Symptoms of Overdose Alopecia, bleeding gums, cholelithiasis, circulatory collapse, coagulopathy, esophageal ulceration, eosinophilia, feces discoloration (black; light brown; pink; red; tarry), hematuria, hepatitis, intracranial hemorrhage, numbness, ocular hemorrhage, pericardial effusion/pericarditis, urine discoloration (orange)

Admission Criteria/Prognosis Patients with bleeding, prolonged prothrombin time, or history of a large ingestion (>0.5 mg/kg) should be considered for admission.

Pharmacodynamics/Kinetics

Onset of action: Anticoagulation: Oral: 36-72 hours

Peak effect: Full therapeutic effect: 5-7 days; INR may increase in 36-72 hours

Peak effect after one dose - 3 hours

Duration: 2-5 days

Absorption: Oral: Rapid

Metabolism: Hepatic

Half-life elimination: 20-60 hours; Mean: 40 hours; highly variable among individuals

Protein Binding - 98%

Dosage Oral:

Infants and Children: 0.05-0.34 mg/kg/day; infants <12 months of age may require doses at or near the high end of this range; consistent anticoagulation may be difficult to maintain in children <5 years of age

Adults: Initial dosing must be individualized. Consider the patient (hepatic function, cardiac function, age, nutritional status, concurrent therapy, risk of bleeding) in addition to prior dose response (if available) and the clinical situation. Start 5-10 mg daily for 2 days. Adjust dose according to INR results; usual maintenance dose ranges from 2-10 mg daily (individual patients may require loading and maintenance doses outside these general guidelines).

Note: Lower starting doses may be required for patients with hepatic impairment, poor nutrition, CHF, elderly, or a high risk of bleeding. Higher initial doses may be reasonable in selected patients (ie, receiving enzyme-inducing agents and with low risk of bleeding).

I.V. (administer as a slow bolus injection): 2-5 mg/day

Dosing adjustment/comments in hepatic disease: Monitor effect at usual doses; the response to oral anticoagulants may be markedly enhanced in obstructive jaundice (due to reduced vitamin K absorption) and also in hepatitis and cirrhosis (due to decreased production of vitamin K-dependent clotting factors); prothrombin index should be closely monitored

Monitoring Parameters Prothrombin time, hematocrit, INR

Administration Oral: Do not take with food. Take at the same time each day.

I.V.: Administer as a slow bolus injection over 1-2 minutes; avoid all I.M. injections

Contraindications Hypersensitivity to warfarin or any component of the formulation; hemorrhagic tendencies; hemophilia; thrombocytopenia purpura; leukemia; recent or potential surgery of the eye or CNS; major regional lumbar block anesthesia or surgery resulting in large, open surfaces; patients bleeding from the GI, respiratory, or GU tract; threatened abortion; aneurysm; ascorbic acid deficiency; history of bleeding diathesis; prostatectomy; continuous tube drainage of the small intestine; polyarthritis; diverticulitis; emaciation; malnutrition; cerebrovascular hemorrhage; eclampsia/pre-eclampsia; blood dyscrasias; severe uncontrolled or malignant hypertension; severe hepatic disease; pericarditis or pericardial effusion; subacute bacterial endocarditis; visceral carcinoma; following spinal puncture and other diagnostic or therapeutic procedures with potential for significant bleeding; history of warfarin-induced necrosis; an unreliable, noncompliant patient; alcoholism; patient who has a history of falls or is a significant fall risk; pregnancy

Warnings

Use care in the selection of patients appropriate for this treatment. Ensure patient cooperation especially from the alcoholic, illicit drug user, demented, or psychotic patient. Use with caution in trauma, acute infection (antibiotics and fever may alter affects), renal insufficiency, prolonged dietary insufficiencies (vitamin K deficiency), moderate-severe hypertension, polycythemia vera, vasculitis, open wound, active TB, history of PUD, anaphylactic disorders, indwelling catheters, severe diabetes, thyroid disease, severe renal disease, and menstruating and postpartum women. Use with caution in protein C deficiency.

Hemorrhage is the most serious risk of therapy. Patient must be instructed to report bleeding, accidents, or falls. Patient must also report any new or discontinued medications, herbal or alternative products used, significant changes in smoking or dietary habits. Necrosis or gangrene of the skin and other tissues can occur (rarely) due to early hypercoagulability. "Purple toes syndrome," due to cholesterol microembolization, may rarely occur (often after several weeks of therapy). Women may be at risk of developing ovarian hemorrhage at the time of ovulation. The elderly may be more sensitive to anticoagulant therapy.

Dosage Forms Injection, powder for reconstitution, as sodium (Coumadin®): 5 mg

Tablet, as sodium (Coumadin®, Jantoven™): 1 mg, 2 mg, 2.5 mg, 3 mg, 4 mg, 5 mg, 6 mg, 7.5 mg, 10 mg

Reference Range

Therapeutic serum warfarin levels: 2-5 mcg/mL (SI: 6.5-16.2 μmol/L)
Prothrombin time should be $1\frac{1}{2}$ to 2 times the control or INR should be ↑ 2 to 3 times based upon indication
Normal prothrombin time: 10-13 seconds
INR ranges based upon indication: See table.

INR Ranges Based Upon Indication

Indication	Targeted INR Range	Targeted INR
Acute myocardial infarction with risk factor[1]	2.0-3.0	2.5
Atrial fibrillation (moderate- to high-risk patients)	2.0-3.0	2.5
Bileaflet or tilting disk mechanical aortic valve (NSR, NL LA)	2.0-3.0	2.5
Bileaflet mechanical aortic valve with atrial fibrillation	2.5-3.5	3
Bileaflet mechanical aortic valve with atrial fibrillation with ASA 80-100 mg/day	2.0-3.0	2.5
Bileaflet or tilting disk mechanical mitral valve	2.5-3.5	3
Bileaflet or tilting disk mechanical mitral valve with ASA 80-100 mg/day	2.0-3.0	2.5
Bioprosthetic mitral or aortic valve[2]	2.0-3.0	2.5
Bioprosthetic mitral or aortic valve with atrial fibrillation	2.0-3.0	2.5
Cardioembolic cerebral ischemic events	2.0-3.0	2.5
Mechanical heart valve (caged ball, caged disk) with ASA 80-100 mg/day	2.5-3.5	3
Mechanical prosthetic valve with systemic embolism despite adequate anticoagulation[3]	2.5-3.5	3
Rheumatic mitral valve disease and NSR (left atrial diameter >5.5 cm)	2.0-3.0	2.5
Venous thromboembolism	2.0-3.0	2.5

[1]Up to 3 months of therapy following heparin or LMWH in patients with anterior Q-wave infarction, severe left-ventricular dysfunction, mural thrombus on 2D echo, atrial fibrillation, history of systemic or pulmonary embolism, congestive heart failure.
[2]Maintained for 3 months; chronic low-dose aspirin (80 mg/day) after warfarin therapy.
[3]Add ASA 80-100 mg/day.
For complete discussion, *See Chest,* 2001, 119(Suppl):1S-370S

Warfarin levels are not used for monitoring degree of anticoagulation. They may be useful if a patient with unexplained coagulopathy is using the drug surreptitiously or if it is unclear whether clinical resistance is due to true drug resistance or lack of drug intake.

Normal prothrombin time (PT): 10.9-12.9 seconds. Healthy premature newborns have prolonged coagulation test screening results (eg, PT, aPTT, TT) which return to normal adult values at approximately 6 months of age. Healthy prematures, however, do not develop spontaneous hemorrhage or thrombotic complications because of a balance between procoagulants and inhibitors

The World Health Organization (WHO), in cooperation with other regulatory-advisory bodies, has developed system of standardizing the reporting of PT values through the determination of the International

Normalized Ratio (INR). The INR involves the standardization of the PT by the generation of two pieces of information: the PT ratio and the International Sensitivity Index (ISI)

Therapeutic ranges are now available or being developed to assist practicing physicians in their treatment of patients with a wide variety of thrombotic disorders

Overdosage/Treatment

Decontamination: Activated charcoal should be given for ingestions >4 mg/kg

Supportive therapy: Critically prolonged INR and bleeding complications can be treated successfully with recombinant factor (dose range: 15-90 mcg/kg body weight). Indications for use of rFVIIa have included an INR >10 in high-risk persons or clinical hemorrhage. Check urine and stool for blood; fresh frozen plasma (15 mL/kg) should be administered; vitamin K$_1$ should be given in doses as outlined: See table.

For active bleeding: Prothrombin complex concentrate (which contains Factors II, VII, IX and X) at 50 units per kg IV can be given. Alternatively recombinant coagulation activated factor VII at doses of 70 to 90 mcg/kg or 1.2 to 4.8 mg total can also be given. Either complex should be given in conjunction with Vitamin K.

Management of Elevated INR

INR	Patient Situation	Action
>3 and <5	No bleeding or need for rapid reversal (ie, no need for surgery)	Omit next few warfarin doses and/or restart at lower dose when INR approaches desired range. If only minimally above range, then no dosage reduction may be required.
>5 and <9.0	No bleeding or need for rapid reversal	Omit next 1-2 doses, monitor INR more frequently, and restart at lower dose when INR approaches target range **or** omit dose and give 1-2.5 mg vitamin K orally (use this if patient has risk factors for bleeding).
	No bleeding but reversal needed for surgery or dental extraction within 24 hours	Vitamin K 2-4 mg orally (expected reversal within 24 hours); give additional 1-2 mg if INR remains high at 24 hours.
>9.0 and <20.0	No bleeding	Stop warfarin, give vitamin K 3-5 mg orally; follow INR closely; repeat vitamin K if needed. Reassess need and dose of warfarin when INR approaches desirable range.
Rapid reversal required (ie, INR >20)	Serious bleeding or major warfarin overdose	Stop warfarin, give vitamin K 10 mg by slow I.V. infusion. May repeat vitamin K every 12 hours and give fresh plasma transfusion or prothrombin complex concentrate as needed. When appropriate, heparin can be given until the patient becomes responsive to warfarin.

Enhancement of elimination: Cholestyramine or multiple dosing of activated charcoal may be useful

Antidote(s)

- Cholestyramine Resin [ANTIDOTE]
- Phytonadione [ANTIDOTE]

Diagnostic Procedures

- Warfarin, Blood

Test Interactions ↑ aPTT

Drug Interactions Substrate of CYP1A2 (minor), 2C9 (major), 2C19 (minor), 3A4 (minor); **Inhibits** CYP2C9 (moderate), 2C19 (weak)

Acetaminophen: May enhance the anticoagulant effect of warfarin. Most likely to occur with daily acetaminophen doses >1.3 g for >1 week.

Allopurinol: May enhance the anticoagulant effect of warfarin. Reductions in warfarin will likely be required.

Aminoglutethimide: May increase the metabolism, via CYP isoenzymes, of warfarin. Monitor therapy for decreased warfarin effect.

Amiodarone: May enhance the anticoagulant effect of warfarin. An empiric warfarin dosage reduction of 30% to 50% at the initiation of warfarin may be considered.

Androgens: May enhance the anticoagulant effect of warfarin. Significant reductions in warfarin dosage may be needed during concomitant therapy.

Antifungal agents (imidazole): May decrease the metabolism, via CYP isoenzymes, of warfarin. Monitor for increased therapeutic/toxic effects of warfarin.

Antithyroid agents: May diminish the anticoagulant effects of warfarin. Monitor for decreased therapeutic effects.

Aprepitant: May decrease the serum concentration of warfarin. Monitor closely for 2 weeks following each course of aprepitant.

Azathioprine: May decrease the anticoagulant effect of warfarin. An adjustment in warfarin dose may be needed.

Barbiturates: May increase the metabolism, via CYP isoenzymes, of warfarin. Monitor for decreased therapeutic effect of warfarin. Anticoagulation dosage increase of 30% to 60% may be needed based upon monitored PT.

Bile acid sequestrants: May decrease absorption of warfarin. Separating the administration of doses by >2 hours may reduce the risk of interaction.

Bosentan: May increase metabolism, via CYP isoenzymes, of warfarin. Monitor for decreased effects.

Capecitabine: May decrease metabolism of warfarin. Monitor for evidence of excess anticoagulation.

Carbamazepine: May increase the metabolism, via CYP isoenzymes, of warfarin. Monitor for decreased therapeutic effect of warfarin.

Cephalosporins: May enhance the anticoagulant effect of warfarin. Monitor for increased evidence of bleeding especially in cephalosporins that have NMTT side chain.

Cimetidine: May enhance the anticoagulant effect of warfarin. Monitor for increased therapeutic effects of warfarin.

Contraceptives, hormonal (estrogens and progestins): May diminish the anticoagulant effect of warfarin. Monitor for changes in coagulation status.

COX-2 inhibitor: May enhance the anticoagulant effect of warfarin. Monitor for increased signs and symptoms of bleeding.

CYP2C9 inducers (strong): May increase the metabolism of warfarin. Examples of inducers include: Carbamazepine, fosphenytoin, phenobarbital, phenytoin, primidone, rifampin, rifapentine, secobarbital. Monitor for decreased effect of warfarin.

CYP2C9 Inhibitors may increase the levels/effects of warfarin. Example inhibitors include delavirdine, fluconazole, gemfibrozil, ketoconazole, nicardipine, NSAIDs, sulfonamides and tolbutamide.

Dicloxacillin: May increase the metabolism, via CYP isoenzymes, of warfarin. Monitor for decreased therapeutic effect of warfarin.

Disulfiram: May increase the serum concentration of warfarin. Monitor for increased therapeutic effects of warfarin.

Drotrecogin Alfa: Warfarin may enhance the adverse/toxic effect of drotrecogin alfa. Monitor for increased risk of bleeding during concomitant therapy. If possible, avoid use of drotrecogin within 7 days of warfarin therapy, or if INR ≥3.

Etoposide: May enhance the anticoagulant effect of warfarin. Monitor for increased effects of warfarin.

Fibric acid derivatives: May enhance the anticoagulant effect of warfarin. Monitor for toxic effects of warfarin; may warrant a 25% to 33% reduction in the warfarin dosage.

Fluconazole: May decrease the metabolism, via CYP isoenzymes, of warfarin. Monitor for increased therapeutic/toxic effects warfarin.

Fluorouracil: May enhance the anticoagulant effect of warfarin. Monitor for increased effects of warfarin.

Glucagon: May enhance the anticoagulant effect of warfarin. Monitor for toxic effects of warfarin, especially if glucagon is administered in high doses.

Glutethimide: May increase the metabolism, via CYP isoenzymes, of warfarin. Consider alternative sedative-hypnotic. Monitor for decreased therapeutic effects of warfarin.

Griseofulvin: May increase the metabolism, via CYP isoenzymes, of warfarin. Monitor for decreased therapeutic effects of warfarin.

HMG-CoA reductase inhibitors: May enhance the anticoagulant effect of warfarin. Monitor for increased effects of warfarin.

Ifosfamide: May enhance the anticoagulant effect of warfarin. Monitor for increased effects of warfarin.

Leflunomide: May enhance the anticoagulant effect of warfarin. Monitor for increased effects of warfarin.

Macrolide antibiotics: May decrease the metabolism, via CYP isoenzymes, of warfarin. Monitor for increased therapeutic effects of warfarin. CYP inhibitors (eg, clarithromycin, erythromycin, and troleandomycin) appear to pose the greatest risk. Azithromycin and telithromycin have also been implicated in a few cases.

Mercaptopurine: May diminish the anticoagulant effect of warfarin. Monitor for decreased therapeutic effects of warfarin.

Metronidazole: May decrease the metabolism, via CYP isoenzymes, of warfarin. If concomitant therapy is necessary, consider an empiric reduction in warfarin dosage of approximately one-third. Monitor for increased therapeutic/toxic effects of warfarin.

Nafcillin: May increase the metabolism of warfarin. Consider choosing an alternative antibiotic if available. Monitor for decreased therapeutic effect of warfarin if nafcillin is initiated. The effects on warfarin dosing may persist long after the nafcillin is discontinued. Close monitoring is required even after nafcillin is discontinued.

NSAID (nonselective): May enhance the anticoagulant effect of warfarin. Monitor for increased signs and symptoms of bleeding.

Orlistat: May enhance the anticoagulant effect of warfarin. Monitor for changes in effects of warfarin.

Phenytoin: May enhance the anticoagulant effect of warfarin. Warfarin may increase the serum concentration of phenytoin. Monitor for increased effects of warfarin and for increased serum concentrations/toxic effects of phenytoin.

Phytonadione: May antagonize the effects of warfarin. Monitor for decreased therapeutic effect of warfarin.

Propafenone: May increase the serum concentration of warfarin. Monitor for increased prothrombin times (PT)/therapeutic effects of warfarin.

Propoxyphene: May decrease the metabolism, via CYP isoenzymes, of warfarin. Monitor for increased prothrombin time/toxic effects of warfarin.

Proton pump inhibitors (omeprazole): May increase the serum concentration of warfarin. Monitor for increased effects of warfarin.

Quinidine: May enhance the anticoagulant effect of warfarin. Monitor for increased prothrombin times (PT)/therapeutic effects of warfarin.

Quinolone antibiotics: May enhance the anticoagulant effect of warfarin. Monitor for increased prothrombin time/toxic effects of warfarin.

Rifamycin derivatives: May increase the metabolism, via CYP isoenzymes, of warfarin. Monitor for decreased prothrombin times (PT)/therapeutic effects of warfarin.

Ropinirole: May enhance the anticoagulant effect of warfarin. Monitor for increased INR/effects of warfarin.

Salicylates: May enhance the anticoagulant effect of warfarin. Monitor for increased signs and symptoms of bleeding if used concomitantly.

Selective serotonin reuptake inhibitors (SSRIs): May enhance the anticoagulant effect of warfarin. Monitor for increased therapeutic/toxic effects of warfarin.

Sulfasalazine: May diminish the anticoagulant effect of warfarin. Monitor for decreased INR/effects of warfarin

Sulfinpyrazone: May decrease the metabolism, via CYP isoenzymes, of warfarin and may decrease the protein binding of warfarin. Monitor for increased prothrombin time (PT)/toxic effects of warfarin.

Sulfonamide derivatives: May enhance the anticoagulant effect of warfarin. Monitor for increased prothrombin time (PT)/toxic effects of warfarin.

Tetracycline derivatives: May enhance the anticoagulant effect of warfarin. Monitor for toxic effects of warfarin.

Thyroid products: May enhance the anticoagulant effect of warfarin. Monitor for increased hypoprothrombinemic effects of warfarin.

Tigecycline: May increase the serum concentration of warfarin. Monitor for increased effects of warfarin.

Tolterodine: May increase the effects of warfarin.

Treprostinil: May enhance the adverse/toxic effect of warfarin. Monitor for increased risk of bleeding when used concomitantly.

Tricyclic antidepressants: May enhance the anticoagulant effect of warfarin. Monitor for increased prothrombin times (PT)/toxic effects of warfarin.

Vitamin A: May enhance the anticoagulant effect of warfarin. Monitor for increased prothrombin time (PT)/effects of warfarin.

Vitamin E: May enhance the anticoagulant effect of warfarin. Monitor for increased prothrombin time (PT)/effects of warfarin. Likely only of significant concern with higher doses of vitamin E (eg, 1200 int. units/day).

Voriconazole: May increase the serum concentration of warfarin. Monitor for increased effects (eg, INR, bleeding) of warfarin.

Zafirlukast: May decrease the metabolism, via CYP isoenzymes, of warfarin. Monitor for increased prothrombin time (PT)/effects of warfarin.

Zileuton: May increase the serum concentration of warfarin. Monitor for increased effects of warfarin.

Pregnancy Risk Factor D

Pregnancy Implications Oral anticoagulants cross the placenta and produce fetal abnormalities. Warfarin should not be used during pregnancy because of significant risks. Adjusted-dose heparin can be given safely throughout pregnancy in patients with venous thromboembolism.

Lactation Does not enter breast milk, only metabolites are excreted (AAP rates "compatible")

Additional Information High intensity warfarin therapy (titrated to an internal normalized ratio ≥3) can prevent thrombosis in patients with antiphospholipid antibody syndrome; for I.V. injection, reconstitute with 2.7 mL of sterile water to yield 2 mg/mL.

The chart provides information about the amount of reconstituted solution of Coumadin® for injection that corresponds to a specific dose

Warfarin Dosage	
Desired Dose of Coumadin® (mg)	Coumadin® for Injection Administration Volume (mL)
0.5	0.25
1	0.50
1.5	0.75
2	1
2.5	1.25
3	1.50
3.5	1.75
4	2
4.5	2.25
5	2.50
5.5	2.75*
6	3*
6.5	3.25*
7	3.50*
7.5	3.75*
8	4*
8.5	4.25*
9	4.50*
9.5	4.75*
10	5*

*More than 1 vial required for this dose.

Further information can be obtained by calling Bristol-Myers Squibb: 800-321-1335

TLV-TWA: 0.1 mg/m^3; IDLH: 200 mg/m^3 (industrial exposure)

The first month of therapy appears to be the period of highest risk of bleeding (1.6% incidence).

Herbal Products with Coumarin Constituents

Alfalfa
Angelica
Aniseed
Arnica
Asafoetida
Bogbean
Boldo
Bromelain
Buchu
Capsicum
Cassia
Celery
Chamomile (German)
Chamomile (Roman)
Cinchona
Fenugreek
Fucus
Horse - chestnut
Horseradish
Mango
Meadowsweet
Nettle
Parsley
Passion flower
Prickly ash (northern and southern)
Quassia
Quilinggao (essence of tortoise shell)
Wild carrot
Wild lettuce

Onset of coagulopathy after an acute ingestion (over 4 mg/kg) is 18 to 48 hours. Skin Necrosis due to Protein C deficiency occurs within ten days of use with a female predominance. Starts as painful red patches (hemorrhage) in high fat areas (Breasts, Buttocks). Purple toe syndrome is due to cholesterol crystal emboli from bleeding into atherosclerotic plaques. It occurs 3 to ten weeks after start of therapy and usually appears as a purple discoloration of the plantan surface of the toes.

Specific References

Alpert JS, "How Can We Improve Our Use of Oral Anticoagulant?" *Am J Med*, 2006, 119:101-2.

Atreja A, El-Sameed YA, Jneid H, et al, "Elevated International Normalized Ratio in the ED: Clinical Course and Physician Adherence to the Published Recommendations," *Am J Emerg Med*, 2005, 23(1):40-4.

Beatty SJ, Mehta BH, and Rodis JL, "Decreased Warfarin Effect After Initiation of High-Protein, Low-Carbohydrate Diets," *Ann Pharmacother*, 2005, 39(4):744-7.

Boulanger L, Hauch O, Friedman M, et al, "Warfarin Exposure and the Risk of Thromboembolic and Major Bleeding Events Among Medicaid Patients with Atrial Fibrillation," *Ann Pharmacother*, 2006, 40(6):1024-9.

Brazier NC and Levine MA, "Drug-Herb Interaction Among Commonly Used Conventional Medicines: A Compendium for Health Care Professionals," *Am J Ther*, 2003, 10(3):163-9.

Brody DL, Alyagari V, Shachleford AM, Diringer MN, "Use of Recombinant Factor VIIa in Patients with Warfarin-Associated Intracranial Hemorrhage," *Neurocrit Care*, 2005, 2(3):263-7.

Busenbark LA and Cushnie SA, "Effect of Graves' Disease and Methimazole on Warfarin Anticoagulation," *Ann Pharmacother*, 2006, 40(6):1200-3.

Choudhry NK, Anderson GM, Laupacis A, et al, "Impact of Adverse Events on Prescribing Warfarin in Patients with Atrial Fibrillation: Matched Pair Analysis," *BMJ*, 2006, 332(7534):141-5.

Choudhry NK, Soumerai SB, Normand ST, et al, "Warfarin Prescribing in Atrial Fibrillation: The Impact of Physician, Patient, and Hospital Characteristics," *Am J Med*, 2006, 119(7):607-15.

Davydov L, Yermolnik M, and Cuni LJ, "Warfarin and Amoxicillin/Clavulanate Drug Interaction," *Ann Pharmacother*, 2003, 37(3):367-70.

Eikelboom J and Hankey G, "Ximelagatran or Warfarin in Atrial Fibrillation?" *Lancet*, 2004, 363(9410):734.

Elbe DH and Chang SW, "Moxifloxacin-Warfarin Interaction: A Series of Five Case Reports," *Ann Pharmacother*, 2005, 39(2):361-4.

Feldstein C, Smith DH, Perrin N, et al, "Reducing Warfarin Medication Interactions," *Arch Intern Med*, 2006, 166:1009-15.

Gras-Champel V, Voyer A, Guillaume N, et al, "Quality Evaluation of the Management of Oral Anticoagulation Therapy (OAT): The Awareness of Treating Physicians and the Education of Patients Needs to Be Improved," *Am J Ther*, 2006, 13(3):223-8.

Holbrook AM, Pereira JA, Labiris R, et al, "Systematic Overview of Warfarin and Its Drug and Food Interactions," *Arch Intern Med*, 2005, 23;165(10):1095-106 (review).

Isbister GK, Hackett LP, and Whyte IM, "Intentional Warfarin Overdose," *Ther Drug Monit*, 2003, 25(6):715-22.

Janney LM and Waterbury NV, "Capecitabine-Warfarin Interaction," *Ann Pharmacother*, 2005, 39(9):1546-51.

Johnston JA, Cluxton RJ Jr, Heaton PC, et al, "Predictors of Warfarin Use Among Ohio Medicaid Patients with New-Onset Nonvalvular Atrial Fibrillation," *Arch Intern Med*, 2003, 163(14):1705-10.

Kassebaum PJ, Shaw DL, and Tomich DJ, "Possible Warfarin Interaction with Menthol Cough Drops," *Ann Pharmacother*, 2005, 39(2):365-7.

Kim KY and Mancano MA, "Fenofibrate Potentiates Warfarin Effects," *Ann Pharmacother*, 2003, 37(2):212-5.

Knijff-Dutmer EA, Schut GA, and van de Laar MA, "Concomitant Coumarin-NSAID Therapy and Risk for Bleeding," *Ann Pharmacother*, 2003, 37(1):12-6.

Kolilekas L, Anagnostopoulos GK, Lampaditis I, et al, "Potential Interaction Between Telithromycin and Warfarin," *Ann Pharmacother*, 2004, 38(9):1424-7.

Kovacs MJ, Kearon C, Julian JA, et al, "Influence of Warfarin on Symptoms of Fatigue: Findings of a Randomized Trial," *Ann Pharmacother*, 2005, 39(5):840-2.

Kovacs MJ, Rodger M, Anderson DR, et al, "Comparison of 10-mg and 5-mg Warfarin Initiation Nomograms Together with Low-Molecular-Weight Heparin for Outpatient Treatment of Acute Venous Thromboembolism: A Randomized, Double-Blind, Controlled Trial," *Ann Intern Med*, 2003, 138(9):714-9.

Kuykendall JR, Houle MD, and Rhodes RS, "Possible Warfarin Failure Due to Interaction with Smokeless Tobacco," *Ann Pharmacother*, 2004, 38(4):595-7. Epub 2004 Feb 06.

Lee DC, Johnson AB, and Rudolph GS, "Outcome of Emergency Department (ED) Patients with Elevated International Normalization Ratio (INR)," *Clin Toxicol*, 2005, 43:637.

MacWalter RS, Fraser HW, and Armstrong KM, "Orlistat Enhances Warfarin Effect," *Ann Pharmacother*, 2003, 37(4):510-2.

Margolin L, "Increased Warfarin Sensitivity Complicated by Retroperitoneal Haemorrhage in a Patient with Merkel Cell Carcinoma," *Clinical Drug Investigation*, 2003, 23:217-8.

Martin LA and Mehta SD, "Diminished Anticoagulant Effects of Warfarin with Concomitant Mercaptopurine Therapy," *Pharmacotherapy*, 2003, 23(2):260-4.

Matsumoto K, Ueno K, Nakabayashi T, et al, "Amiodarone Interaction Time Differences with Warfarin and Digoxin," *J Pharm Technol*, 2003, 19:83-90.

Menzin J, Boulanger L, Hauch O, et al, "Quality of Anticoagulation Control and Costs of Monitoring Warfarin Therapy Among Patients with Atrial Fibrillation in Clinic Settings: A Multi-Site Managed-Care Study," *Ann Pharmacother*, 2005, 39(3):446-51.

Mukamal KJ, Smith CC, Karlamangla AS, et al, "Moderate Alcohol Consumption and Safety of Lovastatin and Warfarin Among Men: The Postcoronary Artery Bypass Graft Trial," *A, J Med*, 2006, 119:434-40.

Murphey LM and Hood EH, "Bosentan and Warfarin Interaction," *Ann Pharmacother*, 2003, 37(7-8):1028-31.

Polat C, Dervisoglu A, Guven H, et al, "Anticoagulant-Induced Intramural Intestinal Hematoma," *Am J Emerg Med*, 2003, 21(3):208-11.

Rao KB, Pallaki M, Tolbert SR, et al, "Enhanced Hypoprothrombinemia with Warfarin Due to Azithromycin," *Ann Pharmacother*, 2004, 38(6):982-5.

Rindone JP and Murphy TW, "Warfarin-Cranberry Juice Interaction Resulting in Profound Hypoprothrombinemia and Bleeding," *Am J Ther*, 2006, 13(3):203-4

Rudnicka AR, Ashby D, Brennan P, et al, "Thrombosis Prevention Trial: Compliance with Warfarin Treatment and Investigation of a Retained Effect," *Arch Intern Med*, 2003, 163(12):1454-60.

Schulman S and Bijsterveld NR, "Anticoagulants and The Reversal," *Transfus Med Rev*, 2007, 21(1):37-48.

Suvarna R, Pirmohamed M, and Henderson L, "Possible Interaction Between Warfarin and Cranberry Juice," *BMJ*, 2003, 327(7429):1454.

Tai CM, Liu KL, Chen CC, et al, "Lateral Abdominal Wall Hematoma Due to Tear of Internal Abdominal Oblique Muscle in a Patient Under Warfarin Therapy," *Am J Emerg Med*, 2005, 23(7):911-2.

Xylazine

CAS Number 7361-61-7

Use Animal tranquilizing agent

Mechanism of Action Structurally similar to clonidine and phenothiazines, this agent acts by stimulation of alpha$_2$ receptors in the central and peripheral nervous systems

Signs and Symptoms of Overdose Apnea, bradycardia, coma (at doses >1 g), drowsiness, hyperglycemia (mild), hyporeflexia, hypotension (although transient paradoxical hypertension has been described), hypotonia, incontinence, miosis

Admission Criteria/Prognosis Admit any symptomatic patient or exposure to concentrations >0.5 mg/kg

Toxicodynamics/Kinetics

Onset of action: Within 30 minutes

Absorption: Well-absorbed orally

Metabolism: Hepatic; primary metabolite is 2,6-dimethylaniline

Half-life: 4.9 hours (after I.M. overdose)

Elimination: Primarily renal

Dosage Animals: I.V./I.M.: 0.5-5 mg/kg

Reference Range Following injection (I.M.) of 1.5 g xylazine and resultant coma, serum and urinary concentrations were 4.6 mg/L and 194 mg/L, respectively

Overdosage/Treatment

Decontamination: Oral: Activated charcoal

Supportive therapy: Hypotension can initially be treated with I.V. isotonic saline (10-20 mL/kg) and Trendelenburg positioning. Dopamine or norepinephrine can be used for refractory hypotension. Tolazoline (10 mg I.V. repeated every 5-10 minutes to a maximum of 40 mg I.V.) may also be useful. Atropine is useful in treatment of bradycardia. For treatment of nontransient hypertension, phentolamine is the drug of choice. Naloxone is **not** useful in reversing coma.

Specific References

Moore K, Ripple M, Sakinedzad S, et al, "Tissue Distribution of Xylazine in a Suicide by Hanging," *J Anal Toxicol*, 2003, 27:193.

Wolowich WR, McPeak J, Good TG, et al, "Xylazine Injection in Man," *J Toxicol Clin Toxicol*, 2003, 41(5):646.

Yohimbine

CAS Number 146-48-5; 65-19-0

U.S. Brand Names Aphrodyne®; Yocon®

Synonyms Yohimbine Hydrochloride

Impairment Potential Yes. Doses of 10-30 mg can produce central nervous system stimulation including mydriasis; dissociative state similar to phencyclidine can occur with excessive dosages (~250 mg). (Linden CH, Vellman WP, and Rumack B, "Yohimbine: A New Street Drug," *Ann Emerg Med*, 1985, 14(10):1002-4.)

Unlabeled/Investigational Use Treatment of SSRI-induced sexual dysfunction; weight loss; impotence; sympatholytic and mydriatic; may have activity as an aphrodisiac; used in veterinary medicine as a reversal agent for xylazine

Mechanism of Action Derived from the bark of the yohimbe tree (*Pausinystalia yohimbe*), this indole alkaloid produces an alpha$_2$-adrenergic blockade; also is a weak MAO inhibitor; parasympathetic tone is also decreased

Adverse Reactions

Cardiovascular: Tachycardia, bradycardia, hypertension, hypotension (orthostatic), flushing, shock, sinus tachycardia, vasodilation, sinus bradycardia

Central nervous system: Anxiety, mania, hallucinations, irritability, dizziness, psychosis, insomnia, headache, panic attacks

Gastrointestinal: Nausea, vomiting, anorexia

Hematologic: Neutropenia, agranulocytosis

Neuromuscular & skeletal: Tremors, paresthesia

Ocular: Lacrimation, mydriasis

Respiratory: Bronchospasm, sinusitis

Miscellaneous: Antidiuretic action, salivation, diaphoresis, systemic lupus erythematosus

Pharmacodynamics/Kinetics

Duration of action: Usually 3-4 hours, but may last 36 hours

Absorption: 33%

Distribution: V_d: 0.3-3 L/kg

Half-life elimination: 0.6 hour

Dosage Adults: Oral: Impotence: 5.4 mg 3 times/day

Contraindications Hypersensitivity to yohimbine or any component of the formulation; renal disease

Warnings Do not use in pregnancy; do not use in children; not for use in geriatric, psychiatric, or cardio-renal patients with a history of gastric or duodenal ulcer; generally not for use in females. Should not be used in kidney disease or psychiatric disorders; can cause high blood pressure and anxiety, tachycardia, nausea, or vomiting.

Dosage Forms Tablet, as hydrochloride: 5.4 mg

Reference Range After a 10 mg oral dose, peak plasma yohimbine level achieved was ~75 mcg/L after 45 minutes

Overdosage/Treatment

Decontamination: Activated charcoal

Supportive therapy: For hypertension, nifedipine or labetalol may be useful; for hypertensive emergencies, phentolamine with nitroprusside is useful; benzodiazepines can be used for agitation; clonidine (5 mcg/kg) may be particularly useful in treating hypertension or anxiety; phenothiazines and tricyclic antidepressants can potentiate psychic effects and thus should be avoided

Test Interactions Possible ↑ catecholamine levels

Drug Interactions

Substrate of CYP2D6 (minor); **Inhibits** CYP2D6 (weak)

Antihypertensives: Effect of antihypertensives may be reduced by yohimbine

CNS active agents: Caution with other CNS acting drugs

Linezolid: Due to MAO inhibition (see note on MAO inhibitors), combinations with this agent should generally be avoided

MAO inhibitors: Theoretically may increase toxicity or adverse effects

Additional Information Also a street drug of abuse that can be smoked; has a bitter taste; dissociative state may resemble phencyclidine intoxication

Specific References

Dargan PI, Shiew CM, Greene SL, et al, "Yohimbine Poisoning from Slimming Pills Bought over the Internet," *Clin Toxicol (Phila)*, 2005, 43:661.

Zafirlukast

U.S. Brand Names Accolate®

Synonyms ICI-204,219

Use Prophylaxis and chronic treatment of asthma in adults and children ≥5 years of age

Mechanism of Action An inhibitor of the sulfidopeptide leukotrienes which can cause bronchoconstriction

Adverse Reactions

Central nervous system: **Headache**

Dermatologic: Alopecia, cutaneous vasculitis

Gastrointestinal: Xerostomia

Hepatic: Elevation of hepatic enzymes

Neuromuscular & skeletal: Weakness

Respiratory: **Pharyngitis**, rhinitis, pulmonary vasculitis

Miscellaneous: Churg-Strauss syndrome (rare), lupus

Pharmacodynamics/Kinetics

Protein binding: >99%, primarily to albumin

Metabolism: Extensively hepatic via CYP2C9

Bioavailability: Reduced 40% with food

Half-life elimination: 10 hours

Time to peak, serum: 3 hours

Excretion: Urine (10%); feces

Dosage

Oral:

Children <5 years: Safety and effectiveness have not been established

Children 5-11 years: 10 mg twice daily

Children ≥12 years and Adults: 20 mg twice daily

Elderly: The mean dose (mg/kg) normalized AUC and C_{max} increase and plasma clearance decreases with increasing age. In patients >65 years of age, there is a two- to threefold greater C_{max} and AUC compared to younger adults.

Dosing adjustment in renal impairment: There are no apparent differences in the pharmacokinetics between renally impaired patients and normal subjects.

Dosing adjustment in hepatic impairment: In patients with hepatic impairment (ie, biopsy-proven cirrhosis), there is a 50% to 60% greater C_{max} and AUC compared to normal subjects.

Monitoring Parameters Monitor for improvements in air flow; monitor closely for sign/symptoms of hepatic injury; periodic monitoring of LFTs may be considered (not proved to prevent serious injury, but early detection may enhance recovery)

Administration Administer at least 1 hour before or 2 hours after a meal

Contraindications Hypersensitivity to zafirlukast or any component of the formulation

Warnings

Zafirlukast is not indicated for use in the reversal of bronchospasm in acute asthma attacks, including status asthmaticus. Therapy with zafirlukast can be continued during acute exacerbations of asthma.

Hepatic adverse events (including hepatitis, hyperbilirubinemia, and hepatic failure) have been reported; female patients may be at greater risk. Discontinue immediately if liver dysfunction is suspected. Periodic testing of liver function may be considered (early detection is generally believed to improve the likelihood of recovery). If hepatic dysfunction is suspected (due to clinical signs/symptoms), liver function tests should be measured immediately. Do not resume or restart if hepatic function studies are consistent with dysfunction. Use caution in patients with alcoholic cirrhosis; clearance is reduced.

Rare cases of eosinophilic vasculitis (Churg-Strauss) have been reported in patients receiving zafirlukast (usually, but not always, associated with reduction in concurrent steroid dosage). No causal relationship established. Monitor for eosinophilic vasculitis, rash, pulmonary symptoms, cardiac symptoms, or neuropathy.

An increased proportion of zafirlukast patients >55 years of age reported infections as compared to placebo-treated patients. These infections were mostly mild or moderate in intensity and predominantly affected the respiratory tract. Infections occurred equally in both sexes, were dose-proportional to total milligrams of zafirlukast exposure, and were associated with coadministration of inhaled corticosteroids.

Dosage Forms Tablet: 10 mg, 20 mg

Reference Range Peak serum levels after a 20 mg and 40 mg oral dose: ~150 ng/mL and 250 ng/mL, respectively; plasma zafirlukast levels >5 ng/mL are associated with inhibition of leukotriene D_4-induced bronchoconstriction

Overdosage/Treatment

Decontamination: Activated charcoal

Enhanced elimination: Multiple dosing of activated charcoal may be effective

Test Interactions May interfere with plasma bilirubin assay

Drug Interactions **Substrate** of CYP2C9 (major); **Inhibits** CYP1A2 (weak), 2C8 (weak), 2C9 (moderate), 2C19 (weak), 2D6 (weak), 3A4 (weak)

Aspirin: Coadministration of zafirlukast with aspirin results in mean increased plasma levels of zafirlukast by 45%

CYP2C9 inducers: May decrease the levels/effects of zafirlukast. Example inducers include carbamazepine, phenobarbital, phenytoin, rifampin, rifapentine, and secobarbital.

CYP2C9 substrates: Zafirlukast may increase the levels/effects of CYP2C9 substrates. Example substrates include bosentan, dapsone, fluoxetine, glimepiride, glipizide, losartan, montelukast, nateglinide, paclitaxel, phenytoin, warfarin, and zafirlukast.

Erythromycin: Coadministration of a single dose of zafirlukast with erythromycin to steady state results in decreased mean plasma levels of zafirlukast by 40% due to a decrease in zafirlukast bioavailability.

Theophylline: Coadministration of zafirlukast at steady state with a single dose of liquid theophylline preparations results in decreased mean plasma levels of zafirlukast by 30%, but no effects on plasma theophylline levels were observed. Cases of increased theophylline serum concentrations have been reported.

Warfarin: Coadministration of zafirlukast with warfarin results in a clinically significant increase in prothrombin time (PT). Closely monitor prothrombin times of patients on oral warfarin anticoagulant therapy and zafirlukast, and adjust anticoagulant dose accordingly.

Pregnancy Risk Factor B

Pregnancy Implications There are no adequate and well-controlled trials in pregnant women. Teratogenic effects not observed in animal studies; fetal defects were observed when administered in maternally toxic doses.

Lactation Enters breast milk/contraindicated

Additional Information Food decreases bioavailability of zafirlukast by 40%. Questions regarding use can be directed to AstraZeneca Pharmaceuticals, Wilmington, Delaware; (800) 456-3669

Zalcitabine

CAS Number 7481-89-2

U.S. Brand Names Hivid®

Synonyms ddC; Dideoxycytidine

Use Orphan drug use in the treatment of AIDS

Mechanism of Action Purine nucleoside (cytosine) analog, zalcitabine or 2′,3′-dideoxycytidine (ddC) is converted to active metabolite ddCTP; lack the presence of the 3′-hydroxyl group necessary for phosphodiester linkages during DNA replication. As a result viral replication is prematurely terminated. ddCTP acts as a competitor for binding sites on the HIV-RNA dependent DNA polymerase (reverse transcriptase) to further contribute to inhibition of viral replication.

Adverse Reactions

Cardiovascular: Fibrillation (atrial), flutter (atrial), cardiomegaly, cardiomyopathy, palpitations, sinus tachycardia, arrhythmias (ventricular)

Central nervous system: Fever, malaise, amnesia

Dermatologic: Pruritus, urticaria, angioedema

Endocrine & metabolic: Hypoglycemia, hyperglycemia, hypophosphatemia, hypernatremia, hyponatremia, hypocalcemia, hypomagnesemia

Gastrointestinal: **Oral ulcers**, anorexia, pancreatitis, diarrhea, nausea, vomiting, aphthous stomatitis

Hematologic: **Neutropenia**, eosinophilia, anemia, thrombocytopenia

Hepatic: Hepatotoxicity

Neuromuscular & skeletal: Distal neuropathy (peripheral), arthralgias

Otic: Tinnitus

Miscellaneous: Night sweats

Pharmacodynamics/Kinetics

Absorption: Well, but variable; decreased 39% with food

Distribution: Minimal data available; variable CSF penetration

Protein binding: <4%

Metabolism: Intracellularly to active triphosphorylated agent

Bioavailability: >80%

Half-life elimination: 2.9 hours; Renal impairment: ≤8.5 hours

Excretion: Urine (>70% as unchanged drug)

Dosage

Oral:

Neonates: Dose unknown

Infants and Children <13 years: Safety and efficacy have not been established; investigational dose: 0.01 mg/kg every 8 hours

Adolescents and Adults: 0.75 mg 3 times/day

Dosing adjustment in renal impairment: Adults:

Cl_{cr} 10-40 mL/minute: 0.75 mg every 12 hours

Cl_{cr} <10 mL/minute: 0.75 mg every 24 hours

Moderately dialyzable (20% to 50%)

Monitoring Parameters Renal function, viral load, liver function tests, CD4 counts, CBC, serum amylase, triglycerides, calcium

Administration Food decreases absorption; take on an empty stomach. Administer around-the-clock. Do not take at the same time with dapsone.

Contraindications Hypersensitivity to zalcitabine or any component of the formulation

Warnings Careful monitoring of pancreatic enzymes and liver function tests in patients with a history of pancreatitis, increased amylase, those on parenteral nutrition or with a history of ethanol abuse. **[U.S. Boxed Warning]: Discontinue use immediately if pancreatitis is suspected. [U.S. Boxed Warning]: Lactic acidosis and severe hepatomegaly and failure have rarely occurred with zalcitabine resulting in fatality (stop treatment if lactic acidosis or hepatotoxicity occur); some cases may possibly be related to underlying hepatitis B;** use with caution in patients on digitalis, or with CHF, renal failure, or hyperphosphatemia. **[U.S. Boxed Warning]: Zalcitabine can cause severe peripheral neuropathy;** avoid use, if possible, in patients with preexisting neuropathy or at risk of developing neuropathy. Risk factors include CD4 counts <50 cells/mm³, diabetes mellitus, weight loss, other drugs known to cause peripheral neuropathy.

Dosage Forms [DSC] = Discontinued product

Tablet:

Hivid®: 0.375 mg [DSC], 0.75 mg

Reference Range Therapeutic blood level: ~0.5 μmol/L

Overdosage/Treatment

Decontamination: Lavage (within 1 hour)/activated charcoal

Enhancement of elimination: Multiple dosing of activated charcoal may be effective; dialysis may be effective, although there is no data in an overdosage setting

Drug Interactions Antacids: Magnesium/aluminum-containing antacids may reduce zalcitabine absorption.

Doxorubicin: Decreases zalcitabine phosphorylation *in vitro*; clinical relevance unknown.

Metoclopramide: May reduce zalcitabine absorption.

Nephrotoxic drugs: Amphotericin, foscarnet, cimetidine, probenecid, and aminoglycosides may potentiate the risk of developing peripheral neuropathy or other toxicities associated with zalcitabine by interfering with the renal elimination of zalcitabine.

Neurotoxic drugs: Drugs associated with peripheral neuropathy which should be avoided, if possible; includes chloramphenicol, cisplatin, dapsone, disulfiram, ethionamide, glutethimide, didanosine, gold, hydralazine, iodoquinol, isoniazid, metronidazole, nitrofurantoin, phenytoin, ribavirin, and vincristine.

Reverse transcriptase inhibitors: It is not recommended that zalcitabine be given in combination with didanosine, stavudine, or lamivudine due to overlapping toxicities, virologic interactions, or lack of clinical data. Lamivudine has also been shown to decrease zalcitabine phosphorylation *in vitro*.

Ribavirin: Concomitant use of ribavirin and nucleoside analogues may increase the risk of developing hepatic decompensation or other signs of mitochondrial toxicity, including pancreatitis or lactic acidosis.

Pregnancy Risk Factor C

Pregnancy Implications It is not known if zalcitabine crosses the human placenta. Animal studies have shown zalcitabine to be teratogenic, developmental toxicities were also observed. Cases of lactic acidosis/hepatic steatosis syndrome have been reported in pregnant women receiving nucleoside analogue drugs. It is not known if pregnancy itself potentiates this known side effect; however, pregnant women may be at increased risk of lactic acidosis and liver damage. Hepatic enzymes and electrolytes should be monitored frequently during the 3rd trimester of pregnancy in women receiving nucleoside analogues. Health professionals are encouraged to contact the antiretroviral pregnancy registry to monitor outcomes of pregnant women exposed to antiretroviral medications (1-800-258-4263 or www.APRegistry.com).

Lactation Excretion in breast milk unknown/contraindicated

Additional Information Can be combined with zidovudine (at a zidovudine dose of 200 mg every 8 hours); limiting dosage for distal, symmetrical neuropathy (peripheral) is 0.01 mg/kg every 8 hours; less bone marrow suppression than with zidovudine

Zaleplon

CAS Number 151319-34-5
U.S. Brand Names Sonata®
Impairment Potential Yes: Doses exceeding 10 mg
Use Short-term (7-10 days) treatment of insomnia (has been demonstrated to be effective for up to 5 weeks in controlled trial)
Mechanism of Action Zaleplon is unrelated to benzodiazepines, barbiturates, or other hypnotics. However, it interacts with the benzodiazepine GABA receptor complex. Nonclinical studies have shown that it binds selectively to the brain omega-1 receptor situated on the alpha subunit of the GABA-A receptor complex.

Adverse Reactions

Cardiovascular: Peripheral edema, chest pain, angina, bundle branch block, pericardial effusion, syncope, ventricular tachycardia

Central nervous system: Amnesia, anxiety, depersonalization, dizziness, hallucinations, hypesthesia, somnolence, vertigo, malaise, depression, lightheadedness, impaired coordination, fever, migraine, ataxia, dystonia

Dermatologic: Photosensitivity reaction, rash, pruritus, alopecia

Gastrointestinal: Abdominal pain, anorexia, colitis, dyspepsia, nausea, constipation, xerostomia, intestinal obstruction

Genitourinary: Dysmenorrhea, urinary retention

Hematologic: Eosinophilia

Neuromuscular & skeletal: Paresthesia, tremor, myalgia, weakness, back pain, arthralgia, dysarthria, facial paralysis, circumoral paresthesia

Ocular: Abnormal vision (at doses over 40 mg), eye pain, glaucoma, ptosis

Otic: Hyperacusis

Respiratory: Epistaxis, pulmonary embolus

Miscellaneous: Parosmia

Signs and Symptoms of Overdose CNS depression, ranging from drowsiness to coma. Mild overdose is associated with drowsiness, confusion, and lethargy. Serious case may result in ataxia, respiratory depression, hypotension, hypotonia, coma, and rarely death.

Pharmacodynamics/Kinetics

Onset of action: Rapid

Peak effect: ~1 hour

Duration: 6-8 hours

Absorption: Rapid and almost complete

Distribution: V_d: 1.4 L/kg

Protein binding: 60% ±15%

Metabolism: Extensive, primarily via aldehyde oxidase to form 5-oxozaleplon and to a lesser extent by CYP3A4 to desethylzaleplon; all metabolites are pharmacologically inactive

Bioavailability: 30%

Half-life elimination: 1 hour

Time to peak, serum: 1 hour

Excretion: Urine (primarily metabolites, <1% as unchanged drug)

Clearance: Plasma: Oral: 3 L/hour/kg

Dosage Oral:

Adults: 10 mg at bedtime (range: 5-20 mg); has been used for up to 5 weeks of treatment in controlled trial setting

Elderly: 5 mg at bedtime

Dosage adjustment in renal impairment: No adjustment for mild to moderate renal impairment; use in severe renal impairment has not been adequately studied

Dosage adjustment in hepatic impairment: Mild to moderate impairment: 5 mg; not recommended for use in patients with severe hepatic impairment

Administration Immediately before bedtime or when the patient is in bed and cannot fall asleep

Contraindications Hypersensitivity to zaleplon or any component of the formulation

Warnings

Symptomatic treatment of insomnia should be initiated only after careful evaluation of potential causes of sleep disturbance. Failure of sleep disturbance to resolve after 7-10 days may indicate psychiatric and/or medical illness.

Use with caution in patients with depression, particularly if suicidal risk may be present. Use with caution in patients with a history of drug dependence. Abrupt discontinuance may lead to withdrawal symptoms. May impair physical and mental capabilities. Patients must be cautioned about performing tasks which require mental alertness (operating machinery or driving). Use with caution in patients receiving other CNS depressants or psychoactive medications. Effects with other sedative drugs or ethanol may be potentiated.

Use with caution in the elderly, those with compromised respiratory function, or renal and hepatic impairment. Because of the rapid onset of action, zaleplon should be administered immediately prior to bedtime or after the patient has gone to bed and is having difficulty falling asleep. Capsules contain tartrazine (FDC yellow #5); avoid in patients with sensitivity (caution in patients with asthma).

Dosage Forms Capsule: 5 mg, 10 mg [contains tartrazine]

Reference Range Single oral zaleplon doses of 10 mg or 20 mg give an average zaleplon peak serum level of 26 mcg/L and 49 mcg/L, respectively, at 1.1 hours

Overdosage/Treatment

Decontamination: Activated charcoal or lavage within one hour at doses exceeding 1 mg/kg

Supportive therapy: Treatment is supportive. Flumazenil use is of uncertain benefit.

Drug Interactions

Substrate of CYP3A4 (minor)

Cimetidine: May increase zaleplon levels/effects; use 5 mg zaleplon as starting dose in patients receiving cimetidine

CNS depressants: Sedative effects may be additive with psychotropics; monitor for increased effect; includes anticonvulsants, antipsychotics, barbiturates, benzodiazepines, narcotic analgesics, and other sedative agents

Flumazenil: May diminish the sedative effect of zaleplon.

Rifamycin Derivatives: May decrease the levels/effects of zaleplon.

Pregnancy Risk Factor C

Pregnancy Implications Not recommended for use during pregnancy

Lactation Enters breast milk/not recommended

Additional Information Prescription quantities should not exceed a 1-month supply.

Zanamivir

Pronunciation (za NA mi veer)
CAS Number 139110-80-8
U.S. Brand Names Relenza®
Use Treatment of uncomplicated acute illness due to influenza virus A and B; treatment should only be initiated in patients who have been symptomatic for no more than 2 days. Prophylaxis against influenza virus A and B
Mechanism of Action Zanamivir inhibits influenza virus neuraminidase enzymes (sialidase), potentially altering virus particle aggregation and release. It is effective against influenza A and B replication.

Adverse Reactions

Most adverse reactions occurred at a frequency which was less than or equal to the control (lactose vehicle).

>10%:

Central nervous system: Headache (prophylaxis 13% to 24%; treatment 2%)

Gastrointestinal: Throat/tonsil discomfort/pain (prophylaxis 8% to 19%)

Respiratory: Cough (prophylaxis 7% to 17%; treatment ≤2%), nasal signs and symptoms (prophylaxis 12%; treatment 2%)

Miscellaneous: Viral infection (prophylaxis 3% to 13%)

1% to 10%:

Central nervous system: Fever/chills (prophylaxis 5% to 9%; treatment <1.5%), fatigue (prophylaxis 5% to 8%; treatment

<1.5%), malaise (prophylaxis 5% to 8%; treatment <1.5%), dizziness (treatment 1% to 2%)

Dermatologic: Urticaria (treatment <1.5%)

Gastrointestinal: Anorexia/appetite decreased (prophylaxis 2% to 4%), nausea (prophylaxis 1% to 2%; treatment ≤3%), diarrhea (prophylaxis 2%; treatment 2% to 3%), vomiting (prophylaxis 1% to 2%; treatment 1% to 2%) abdominal pain (treatment <1.5%)

Hepatic:Liver function test, enzyme elevation

Neuromuscular & skeletal: Muscle pain (prophylaxis 3% to 8%), musculoskeletal pain (prophylaxis 6%), arthralgia/articular rheumatism (prophylaxis 2%), arthralgia (treatment <1.5%), myalgia (treatment <1.5%)

Respiratory: Infection (ear/nose/throat; prophylaxis 2%; treatment 2% to 5%), sinusitis (treatment 3%), bronchitis (treatment 2.3%), nasal inflammation (prophylaxis 1%)

<1%: Asthma (worsening bronchospasm), transient lymphopenia, hemorrhage (ear/nose/throat)

Postmarketing and/or case reports: Allergic or allergic-like reaction (including oropharyngeal edema), arrhythmia, syncope, seizure, bronchospasm, dyspnea, facial edema, rash (including serious cutaneous reactions)

Pharmacodynamics/Kinetics

Absorption: Inhalation: 4% to 17%; oral: 2%

Protein binding, plasma: <10%

Metabolism: None

Half-life elimination, serum: 1.6-5.1 hours
Intravenous: 1.6 hours
Inhalation: 2.9 hours
Intranasal: 3.4 hours

Excretion: Urine (as unchanged drug); feces (unabsorbed drug)

Dosage

Oral inhalation:

Children ≥5 years and Adults: Prophylaxis (household setting): Two inhalations (10 mg) once daily for 10 days. Begin within 1$^{1}/_{2}$ days following onset of signs or symptoms of index case.

Children ≥7 years and Adults: Treatment: Two inhalations (10 mg total) twice daily for 5 days. Doses on first day should be separated by at least 2 hours; on subsequent days, doses should be spaced by ~12 hours. Begin within 2 days of signs or symptoms.

Adolescents and Adults: Prophylaxis (community outbreak): Two inhalations (10 mg) once daily for 28 days. Begin within 5 days of outbreak.

Stability Store at room temperature (25°C) 77°F; do not puncture blister until taking a dose using the Diskhaler®

Administration Inhalation: Must be used with Diskhaler® delivery device. Patients who are scheduled to use an inhaled bronchodilator should use their bronchodilator prior to zanamivir. With the exception of the initial dose when used for treatment, administer at the same time each day.

Contraindications Hypersensitivity to zanamivir or any component of the formulation

Warnings Patients must be instructed in the use of the delivery system. No data are available to support the use of this drug in patients who begin use for treatment after 48 hours of symptoms. Effectiveness has not been established in patients with significant underlying medical conditions or for prophylaxis of influenza in nursing home patients. Not recommended for use in patients with underlying respiratory disease, such as asthma or COPD, due to lack of efficacy and risk of serious adverse effects. Bronchospasm, decreased lung function, and other serious adverse reactions, including those with fatal outcomes, have been reported in patients with and without airway disease; discontinue with bronchospasm or signs of decreased lung function. For a patient with an underlying airway disease where a medical decision has been made to use zanamivir, a fast-acting bronchodilator should be made available, and used prior to each dose. Not a substitute for the flu vaccine. Consider primary or concomitant bacterial infections. Powder for oral inhalation contains lactose. Safety and efficacy of repeated courses or use with severe renal impairment have not been established; efficacy in children <5 years of age have not been established.

Dosage Forms Powder for oral inhalation: 5 mg/blister (20s) [4 blisters per Rotadisk® foil pack, 5 Rotadisk® per package; packaged with Diskhaler® inhalation device; contains lactose]

Reference Range Median serum zanamivir concentration from 3.6 mg twice daily to 16 mg 6 times/day (intranasal) range from 46-67 ng/mL

Overdosage/Treatment

Supportive therapy: Treatment is limited, and symptoms appear similar to reported adverse events from clinical studies.

Treatment: Symptom-directed and supportive. I.V. doses of 600 mg have been well tolerated in adults. Bronchospasm can be treated with beta$_2$ inhaled adrenergic agonists.

Drug Interactions Influenza virus vaccine: Zanamivir may diminish the therapeutic effect of live, attenuated influenza virus vaccine (FluMist™). The manufacturer of FluMist™ recommends that the administration of anti-influenza virus medications be avoided during the period beginning

48 hours prior to vaccine administration and ending 2 weeks after vaccine.

Pregnancy Risk Factor C

Pregnancy Implications Zanamivir has been shown to cross the placenta in animal models, however, no evidence of fetal malformations has been demonstrated. There are no adequate and well-controlled studies in pregnant women; not mutagenic

Lactation Excretion in breast milk unknown/use caution

Additional Information Majority of patients included in clinical trials were infected with influenza A, however, a number of patients with influenza B infections were also enrolled. Patients with lower temperature or less severe symptoms appeared to derive less benefit from therapy. No consistent treatment benefit was demonstrated in patients with chronic underlying medical conditions.

Ziconotide

CAS Number 107452-89-1

U.S. Brand Names Ziconal

Use Management of severe chronic pain in patients requiring intrathecal (I.T.) therapy and are intolerant or refractory to other therapies

Unlabeled/Investigational Use Pain management (especially neuropathic or cancer)

Mechanism of Action A peptide derived from sea snails that is a neuronal calcium antagonist

Adverse Reactions

Cardiovascular: Orthostatic hypotension, syncope (within 6 hours of dose), bradycardia, tachycardia, nonspecific T-wave changes

Central nervous system: Vestibular toxicity, ataxia, auditory hallucinations, sedation, dizziness at doses of 10 mcg/kg/hour; agitation seen at lower doses

Dermatologic: Rash

Gastrointestinal: Nausea, diarrhea

Ocular: Nystagmus

Respiratory: Cough, nasal congestion

Pharmacodynamics/Kinetics

Distribution: I.T.: V_d: ~140 mL

Protein binding: 50%

Metabolism: Metabolized via endopeptidases and exopeptidases present on multiple organs including kidney, liver, lung; degraded to peptide fragments and free amino acids

Half-life elimination: I.V.: 1-1.6 hours (plasma); I.T.: 2.9-6.5 hours (CSF)

Excretion: I.V.: Urine (<1%)

Dosage Administered intrathecally (careful dose titration needed):

Neuropathic/malignant pain: 0.3-300 ng/kg/hr

Head trauma: 60 mg over 3 hours

Monitoring Parameters Monitor for psychiatric or neurological impairment; signs and symptoms of meningitis or other infection; serum CPK (every other week for first month then monthly); pain relief

Administration Not for I.V. administration.For I.T. administration only using Medtronic SynchroMed® EL, SynchroMed® II Infusion System, or CADD-Micro® ambulatory infusion pump.

Medtronic SynchroMed® EL or SynchroMed® II Infusion Systems:

Naive pump priming (first time use with ziconotide): Use 2 mL of undiluted ziconotide 25 mcg/mL solution to rinse the internal surfaces of the pump; repeat twice for a total of 3 rinses

Initial pump fill: Use only undiluted 25 mcg/mL solution and fill pump after priming. Following the initial fill only, adsorption on internal device surfaces will occur, requiring the use of the undiluted solution and refill within 14 days.

Pump refills: Contents should be emptied prior to refill. Subsequent pump refills should occur at least every 40 days if using diluted solution or every 60 days if using undiluted solution

CADD-Micro® ambulatory infusion pump: Refer to manufacturers' manual for initial fill and refill instructions

Contraindications Hypersensitivity to ziconotide or any component of the formulation; history of psychosis; I.V. administration

I.T. administration is contraindicated in patients with infection at the injection site, uncontrolled bleeding, or spinal canal obstruction that impairs CSF circulation

Warnings [U.S Boxed Warning]: Severe psychiatric symptoms and neurological impairment have been reported; interrupt or discontinue therapy if cognitive impairment, hallucinations, mood changes, or changes in consciousness occur. Cognitive impairment may appear gradually during treatment and is generally reversible after discontinuation. Use caution in the elderly; may experience confusion. Patients should be instructed to use caution in performing tasks which require alertness (eg, operating machinery or driving). May have additive effects with opiates or other CNS-depressant medications. Does not potentiate opiate-induced respiratory depression. Will not prevent or relieve symptoms associated with opiate withdrawal and opiates should not be abruptly discontinued. Unlike opioids, ziconotide therapy can be interrupted abruptly or discontinued without evidence of withdrawal. Meningitis may occur with use of I.T. pumps and treatment may require removal of system and discontinuation of therapy. Safety and efficacy have not been established with renal or hepatic dysfunction, or in pediatric patients.

Dosage Forms Injection, solution, as acetate [preservative free]: 25 mcg/mL (20 mL); 100 mcg/mL (1 mL, 2 mL, 5 mL)

Overdosage/Treatment Supportive therapy: Symptomatic treatment upon drug discontinuation

Drug Interactions CNS depressants: Ziconotide may enhance the adverse/toxic effects of other CNS depressants.

Pregnancy Risk Factor C

Pregnancy Implications Teratogenic effects were not observed in animal studies, but increased postimplantation pup loss was reported. Maternal toxicity was also noted. There are no adequate and well-controlled studies in pregnant women.

Lactation Excretion in breast milk unknown/not recommended

Additional Information Ziconotide is a synthetic form of sea snail venom found in the piscivorous marine snail *Congus magus*, which lives in shallow, tropical salt water

Zidovudine

CAS Number 30516-87-1
U.S. Brand Names Retrovir®
Synonyms Azidothymidine; AZT (error-prone abbreviation); Compound S; ZDV
Use Management of patients with HIV infections in combination with at least two other antiretroviral agents; for prevention of maternal/fetal HIV transmission as monotherapy
Unlabeled/Investigational Use Postexposure prophylaxis for HIV exposure as part of a multidrug regimen
Mechanism of Action Zidovudine is a thymidine analog which interferes with the HIV viral RNA dependent DNA polymerase by competing with thymidine triphosphate resulting in inhibition of viral replication
Adverse Reactions
Cardiovascular: Cardiomyopathy, chest pain, syncope, vasculitis
Central nervous system: **Severe headache** (42%), **fever**, malaise, dizziness, insomnia, somnolence, anxiety, confusion, depression, dizziness, loss of mental acuity, mania, seizures, somnolence, vertigo
Dermatologic: **Rash**, hyperpigmentation of nails (bluish-brown), pruritus, angioedema, skin and nail pigmentation changes, Stevens-Johnson syndrome, toxic epidermal necrolysis, urticaria
Endocrine & metabolic: Gynecomastia, lactic acidosis
Gastrointestinal: **Nausea** (46% to 61%), **anorexia, diarrhea, pain, vomiting**, dyspepsia, constipation, dysphagia, flatulence, mouth ulcer, oral mucosal pigmentation, pancreatitis, taste perversion
Genitourinary: Urinary frequency, urinary hesitancy
Hematologic: **Anemia** (23% in children), **leukopenia, granulocytopenia** (39% in children), changes in platelet count, aplastic anemia, hemolytic anemia, leukopenia, pancytopenia with marrow hypoplasia, pure red cell aplasia
Hepatic: Hepatitis, hepatomegaly with steatosis, jaundice, LDH increased
Neuromuscular & skeletal: **Weakness**, paresthesia, back pain, CPK increased, muscle spasm, myopathy and myositis with pathological changes (similar to that produced by HIV disease), paresthesia, rhabdomyolysis, tremor
Ocular: Amblyopia, macular edema, photophobia
Otic: Hearing loss
Respiratory: Cough, dyspnea, rhinitis, sinusitis
Miscellaneous: Diaphoresis, flu-like syndrome, generalized pain, lymphadenopathy, sensitization reactions, anaphylaxis

Signs and Symptoms of Overdose Agranulocytosis, ataxia, cardiomyopathy, cholestatic jaundice, drowsiness (after 20 g ingestion), generalized seizures, granulocytopenia, gynecomastia, headache, insomnia, leukopenia, lymphoma, mania, nausea, neutropenia, nystagmus

Pharmacodynamics/Kinetics
Distribution: Significant penetration into the CSF; crosses placenta
V_d: 1-2.2 L/kg
Relative diffusion from blood into CSF: Adequate with or without inflammation (exceeds usual MICs)
CSF:blood level ratio: Normal meninges: ~60%
Protein binding: 25% to 38%
Metabolism: Hepatic via glucuronidation to inactive metabolites; extensive first-pass effect
Bioavailability: 54% to 74%
Half-life elimination: Terminal: 0.5-3 hours
Time to peak, serum: 30-90 minutes
Excretion:
Oral: Urine (72% to 74% as metabolites, 14% to 18% as unchanged drug)
I.V.: Urine (45% to 60% as metabolites, 18% to 29% as unchanged drug)

Dosage
Prevention of maternal-fetal HIV transmission:

Neonatal: **Note:** Dosing should begin 8-12 hours after birth and continue for the first 6 weeks of life.
Oral:
Full-term infants: 2 mg/kg/dose every 6 hours
Infants ≥30 weeks and <35 weeks gestation at birth: 2 mg/kg/dose every 12 hours; at 2 weeks of age, advance to 2 mg/kg/dose every 8 hours
Infants <30 weeks gestation at birth: 2 mg/kg/dose every 12 hours; at 4 weeks of age, advance to 2 mg/kg/dose every 8 hours
I.V.: Infants unable to receive oral dosing:
Full term: 1.5 mg/kg/dose every 6 hours
Infants ≥30 weeks and <35 weeks gestation at birth: 1.5 mg/kg/dose every 12 hours; at 2 weeks of age, advance to 1.5 mg/kg/dose every 8 hours
Infants <30 weeks gestation at birth: 1.5 mg/kg/dose every 12 hours; at 4 weeks of age, advance to 1.5 mg/kg/dose every 8 hours
Maternal: Oral (per AIDSinfo guidelines): 100 mg 5 times/day **or** 200 mg 3 times/day **or** 300 mg twice daily. Begin at 14-34 weeks gestation and continue until start of labor.
During labor and delivery, administer zidovudine I.V. at 2 mg/kg over 1 hour followed by a continuous I.V. infusion of 1 mg/kg/hour until the umbilical cord is clamped
Treatment of HIV infection:
Children 3 months to 12 years:
Oral: 160 mg/m²/dose every 8 hours; dosage range: 90 mg/m²/dose to 180 mg/m²/dose every 6-8 hours; some Working Group members use a dose of 180 mg/m² to 240 mg/m² every 12 hours when using in drug combinations with other antiretroviral compounds, but data on this dosing in children is limited
I.V. continuous infusion: 20 mg/m²/hour
I.V. intermittent infusion: 120 mg/m²/dose every 6 hours
Adults:
Oral: 300 mg twice daily or 200 mg 3 times/day
I.V.: 1-2 mg/kg/dose (infused over 1 hour) administered every 4 hours around-the-clock (6 doses/day)
Prevention of HIV following needlesticks (unlabeled use): Oral: Adults: 200 mg 3 times/day plus lamivudine 150 mg twice daily; a protease inhibitor (eg, indinavir) may be added for high risk exposures; begin therapy within 2 hours of exposure if possible
Patients should receive I.V. therapy only until oral therapy can be administered
Dosing interval in renal impairment: Cl_{cr} <10 mL/minute: May require minor dose adjustment
Hemodialysis: At least partially removed by hemo- and peritoneal dialysis; administer dose after hemodialysis or administer 100 mg supplemental dose; during CAPD, dose as for Cl_{cr} <10 mL/minute
Continuous arteriovenous or venovenous hemodiafiltration effects: Administer 100 mg every 8 hours
Dosing adjustment in hepatic impairment: Reduce dose by 50% or double dosing interval in patients with cirrhosis
Monitoring Parameters Monitor CBC and platelet count at least every 2 weeks, MCV, serum creatinine kinase, viral load, and CD4 count; observe for appearance of opportunistic infections
Administration Oral: Administer around-the-clock to promote less variation in peak and trough serum levels; may be administered without regard to food
I.M.: Do not administer I.M.
I.V.: Avoid rapid infusion or bolus injection
Neonates: Infuse over 30 minutes
Adults: Infuse over 1 hour
Contraindications Life-threatening hypersensitivity to zidovudine or any component of the formulation
Warnings [U.S. Boxed Warning]: Often associated with hematologic toxicity including granulocytopenia, severe anemia requiring transfusions, or (rarely) pancytopenia. Use with caution in patients with bone marrow compromise (granulocytes <1000 cells/mm³ or hemoglobin <9.5 mg/dL); dosage adjustment may be required in patients who develop anemia or neutropenia. **[U.S. Boxed Warning]: Lactic acidosis and severe hepatomegaly with steatosis have been reported, including fatal cases;** use with caution in patients with risk factors for liver disease (risk may be increased in obese patients or prolonged exposure) and suspend treatment with zidovudine in any patient who develops clinical or laboratory findings suggestive of lactic acidosis (transaminase elevation may/may not accompany hepatomegaly and steatosis). Use caution in combination with interferon alfa with or without ribavirin in HIV/HBV coinfected patients; monitor closely for hepatic decompensation, anemia, or neutropenia; dose reduction or discontinuation of interferon and/or ribavirin may be required if toxicity evident. **[U.S. Boxed Warning]: Prolonged use has been associated with symptomatic myopathy and myositis.** Immune reconstitution syndrome may develop resulting in the occurrence of an inflammatory response to an indolent or residual opportunistic infection; further evaluation and treatment may be required. Reduce dose in patients with severe renal impairment.

Dosage Forms Capsule:
Retrovir®: 100 mg
Injection, solution [preservative free]:
Retrovir®: 10 mg/mL (20 mL)
Syrup:
Retrovir®: 50 mg/5 mL (240 mL) [contains sodium benzoate; strawberry flavor]
Tablet: 300 mg
Retrovir®: 300 mg

Reference Range Peak serum level after 200 mg dose: ~0.9 mcg/mL; serum level taken 12 hours after a 20 g overdose: 49.4 mcg/mL

Overdosage/Treatment
Decontamination: Lavage (within 1 hour)/activated charcoal
Supportive therapy: Transfusions with blood component; vitamin B_{12} administration may assist in preventing anemia; seizures can be treated with diazepam or lorazepam
Enhancement of elimination: Multiple dosing of activated charcoal may be effective; while hemodialysis may remove its metabolites, it has no effect on the parent compound and cannot be routinely recommended

Antidote(s)
• Filgrastim [ANTIDOTE]

Diagnostic Procedures
• Zidovudine, Blood

Drug Interactions Substrate (minor) of CYP2A6, 2C9, 2C19, 3A4
Acyclovir, valacyclovir: May increase CNS depression of zidovudine; monitor.
Bone marrow suppressants/cytotoxic agents: Concomitant use may increase risk of hematologic toxicity. (May be seen with adriamycin, dapsone, flucytosine, vincristine, vinblastine.)
Fluconazole: Fluconazole may increase levels/effects of zidovudine.
Ganciclovir, valganciclovir: Concomitant use may increase risk of hematologic toxicities; monitor hemoglobin, hematocrit, and white blood cell count with differential frequently; dose reduction or interruption of either agent may be needed
Interferon-alfa: Concomitant use may increase risk of hepatic decompensation or hematologic toxicities; monitor hemoglobin, hematocrit, and white blood cell count with differential frequently; dose reduction or interruption of either agent may be needed.
Methadone: May increase serum levels/effects of zidovudine; monitor.
Probenecid: Probenecid may increase zidovudine levels/effects. Myalgia, malaise, and/or fever and maculopapular rash have been reported with concomitant use.
Ribavirin: Concomitant use of ribavirin and nucleoside analogues may increase the risk of developing hepatic decompensation or other signs of mitochondrial toxicity, including pancreatitis or lactic acidosis. May decrease the antiviral activity of zidovudine (based on *in vitro* data); monitor closely.
Rifampin: May decrease levels of zidovudine; monitor.
Stavudine: Zidovudine may decrease the antiviral activity of stavudine (based on *in vitro* data). Avoid concurrent use.
Trimetrexate: Zidovudine may increase the myelosuppressive effects of trimetrexate; avoid concomitant use.
Valproic acid: Valproic acid may increase plasma levels of zidovudine; monitor for possible increase in side effects (AUC increased by 80%)

Pregnancy Risk Factor C

Pregnancy Implications Zidovudine crosses the placenta. The use of zidovudine reduces the maternal-fetal transmission of HIV by ~70% and should be considered for antenatal and intrapartum therapy whenever possible. In HIV infected mothers not previously on antiretroviral therapy, treatment may be delayed until after 10-12 weeks gestation. Cases of lactic acidosis/hepatic steatosis syndrome have been reported in pregnant women receiving nucleoside analogues. It is not known if pregnancy itself potentiates this known side effect; however, pregnant women may be at increased risk of lactic acidosis and liver damage. Hepatic enzymes and electrolytes should be monitored frequently during the 3rd trimester of pregnancy in women receiving nucleoside analogues. Health professionals are encouraged to contact the antiretroviral pregnancy registry to monitor outcomes of pregnant women exposed to antiretroviral medications (1-800-258-4263).

Lactation Enters breast milk/not recommended

Nursing Implications Monitor complete blood count and platelet count at least every 2 weeks; observe for appearance of opportunistic infections; give around-the-clock to promote less variation in peak and trough serum levels

Specific References
De Santis M, Cavaliere AF, Caruso A, et al, "Hemangiomas and Other Congenital Malformations in Infants Exposed to Antiretroviral Therapy In Utero," *JAMA*, 2004, 291(3):305.

Zileuton

CAS Number 11406-87-2
U.S. Brand Names Zyflo™ [DSC]

Use Prophylaxis and chronic treatment of asthma in children ≥12 years of age and adults

Mechanism of Action Specific inhibitor of 5-lipoxygenase and thus inhibits leukotriene (LTB4, LTC4, LTD4 and LTE4) formation. Leukotrienes are substances that induce numerous biological effects including augmentation of neutrophil and eosinophil migration, neutrophil and monocyte aggregation, leukocyte adhesion, increased capillary permeability and smooth muscle contraction.

Adverse Reactions
Central nervous system: Insomnia, dizziness, **headache**
Dermatologic: Urticaria
Gastrointestinal: diarrhea, dyspepsia, abdominal pain
Ocular: Increased intraocular pressure
Hepatic: Reversible transaminase increases, **ALT elevation**

Pharmacodynamics/Kinetics
Absorption: Rapid
Distribution: 1.2 L/kg
Protein binding: 93%
Metabolism: Several metabolites in plasma and urine; metabolized by CYP1A2, 2C9, and 3A4
Bioavailability: Unknown
Half-life elimination: 2.5 hours
Time to peak, serum: 1.7 hours
Excretion: Urine (~95% primarily as metabolites); feces (~2%)

Dosage Oral:
Children <12 years: Safety and effectiveness have not been established
Children ≥12 years and Adults: 600 mg 4 times/day

Monitoring Parameters Evaluate hepatic transaminases at initiation of and during therapy with zileuton. Monitor serum ALT before treatment begins, once-a-month for the first 3 months, every 2-3 months for the remainder of the first year, and periodically thereafter for patients receiving long-term zileuton therapy. If symptoms of liver dysfunction (right upper quadrant pain, nausea, fatigue, lethargy, pruritus, jaundice or "flu-like" symptoms) develop or transaminase elevations >5 times ULN occur, discontinue therapy and follow transaminase levels until normal.

Administration May be administered without regard to meals (eg, with or without food)

Contraindications Hypersensitivity to zileuton or any component of the formulation; active liver disease or transaminase elevations greater than or equal to three times the upper limit of normal (≥3 times ULN)

Warnings Not indicated for the reversal of bronchospasm in acute asthma attacks; therapy may be continued during acute asthma exacerbations. Hepatic adverse effects have been reported (elevated transaminase levels); females >65 years and patients with pre-existing elevated transaminases may be at greater risk. Serum ALT should be monitored. Discontinue zileuton and follow transaminases until normal if patients develop clinical signs/symptoms of liver dysfunction or with transaminase levels >5 times ULN (use caution with history of liver disease and/or in those patients who consume substantial quantities of ethanol.)

Dosage Forms Tablet: 600 mg

Reference Range Peak plasma level after an 800 mg dose: 3.4-4.5 mcg/mL

Overdosage/Treatment
Decontamination: Activated charcoal
Supportive therapy: Urticaria can be treated with epinephrine and antihistamines

Antidote(s)
• Epinephrine [ANTIDOTE]

Drug Interactions Substrate (minor) of CYP1A2, 2C9, 3A4; **Inhibits** CYP1A2 (moderate)
CYP1A2 Substrates: Zileuton may increase the levels/effects of CYP1A2 substrates. Example substrates include aminopylline, fluvoxamine, mexiletine, mirtazapine, ropinirole, theophylline, and trifluoperazine.
Propranolol: Concomitant use results in a doubling of propranolol AUC and increased beta-blocker activity. Monitor patient closely; reduce propranolol dose if necessary.
Theophylline: Concomitant use results in an approximate doubling of serum theophylline concentrations. Monitor concentrations closely; reduce theophylline dose.
Warfarin: Concomitant use results in a significant increase in prothrombin time. PT/INR should be closely monitored; adjust warfarin dose.

Pregnancy Risk Factor C

Pregnancy Implications Clinical effects on the fetus: Developmental studies indicated adverse effects (reduced body weight and increased skeletal variations) in rats at an oral dose of 300 mg/kg/day. There are no adequate and well-controlled studies in pregnant women.

Lactation Excretion in breast milk unknown/not recommended

Additional Information No effect on release of prostaglandin D_2 or histamine; in April, 1995, the Advisory Committee of the FDA Division of Pulmonary and Allergy Drugs unanimously voted to recommend that zileuton be approved for marketing; zileuton (600 mg 4 times/day orally) can protect asthmatics from idiosyncratic reactions (ie, bronchoconstriction) due to aspirin

Zinc Chloride

Pronunciation (zink KLOR ide)
Related Information
• Toxins Which Should Be Lavaged with Solutions Other Than Water
CAS Number 7440-66-6
UN Number 1436
Adverse Reactions Respiratory, gastrointestinal, ocular, pancreatic
Signs and Symptoms of Overdose Hypertension, metal fume fever, nephritis (hematuria), pancreatic insufficiency, pancreatitis. Inhalation of zinc chloride fumes from soldering has also caused asthma. Ingestion of zinc salts has produced gastritis, diarrhea, hyperthermia, shock, vomiting, and death. Eye exposure may result in corneal damage, cough, and lens opacification. Zinc chloride is highly corrosive.
Toxicodynamics/Kinetics
Absorption: In small intestine (20% to 30%); iron and dairy products decrease absorption
Protein binding: Highly protein bound
Elimination: Primarily fecal; urinary excretion is 0.3-0.4 mg/day
Injection, solution: 1 mg/mL (10 mL, 50 mL)
Dosage Forms Injection, solution: 1 mg/mL (10 mL, 50 mL)
Reference Range Normal blood levels of zinc: 68-136 mcg/dL; plasma zinc concentration following ingestion of ~193 g zinc chloride was 3915 mcg/dL (599 µmol/L), resulting in gastric necrotic lesions
Overdosage/Treatment
Decontamination: **Do not** evacuate gastric contents with zinc chloride or phosphide because they are corrosive. Dilute with milk.
    Ocular: Copious irrigation, especially if zinc concentration exceeds 10%.
Enhancement elimination: Calcium disodium, ethylene diaminetetraacetate, or dimercaprol has been used with success. N-acetylcysteine has been used to increase urinary excretion of zinc sulfate.
Pregnancy Risk Factor C
Nursing Implications Patients on TPN therapy should have periodic serum copper and serum zinc levels
Additional Information Toxic dose of zinc chloride in a child: 1 g/kg or zinc concentrations >20%
Radiopaque. Taste threshold: 15 ppm. Opacification of water: 30 ppm. Zinc chloride is the most toxic form.
Average ambient air zinc concentration: <1 mcg/m^3. Average concentration of surface water: <50 mcg/L.
Average daily intake in diet: 0.14-0.21 mg/kg
Zinc chloride fume: TLV-TWA: 1 mg/m^3; TLV-STEL: 2 mg/m^3. Zinc oxide fume: TLV-TWA: 5 mg/m^3; TLV-STEL: 10 mg/m^3. Zinc oxide dust: TLV-TWA: 10 mg/m^3
Specific References
Kazzi Z, Price G, Eaton S, et al, "Pneumonitis and Respiratory Failure Secondary to Civiian Exposure to a Smoke Bomb in a Partially Enclosed Space," *J Toxicol Clin Toxicol*, 2004, 42(5):716.

Zinc Oxide

Related Information
• Metal Fume Fever
CAS Number 1314-13-2; 8051-03-4
U.S. Brand Names Ammens® Medicated Deodorant [OTC]; Balmex® [OTC]; Boudreaux's® Butt Paste [OTC]; Critic-Aid Skin Care® [OTC]; Desitin® Creamy [OTC]; Desitin® [OTC]
Synonyms Base Ointment; Lassar's Zinc Paste
Use Protective coating for mild skin irritations and abrasions, soothing and protective ointment to promote healing of chapped skin, diaper rash, and superficial (but not deep) skin ulcers; used with coal tar in treatment of eczema; also used in sunscreens; used in dental cements as a temporary filling
Mechanism of Action Mild astringent with weak antiseptic properties; blocks ultraviolet A and B along with long-wave light; when heated over 900°F, can be a cause of metal fume fever (at an exposure of 5 mg/m^3 for 2 hours)
Adverse Reactions
Central nervous system: Chills
Dermatologic: Skin sensitivity, dermal irritation
Miscellaneous: Solitary aspergillosis of maxillary sinus associated with zinc oxide from overfilled teeth
Toxicodynamics/Kinetics Absorption: May be absorbed dermally in burns
Dosage Infants, Children, and Adults: Topical: Apply as required to affected areas several times/day
Stability Avoid prolonged storage at temperatures >30°C
Contraindications Hypersensitivity to zinc oxide or any component of the formulation
Dosage Forms Cream:
    Balmex®: 11.3% (60 g, 120 g, 480 g) [contains aloe and vitamin E]
    Ointment, topical: 20% (30 g, 60 g, 480 g); 40% (120 g)

Desitin®: 40% (30 g, 60 g, 90 g, 120 g, 270 g, 480 g) [contains cod liver oil and lanolin]
Desitin® Creamy: 10% (60 g, 120 g)
Paste, topical:
    Boudreaux's® Butt Paste: 16% (30 g, 60 g, 120 g, 480 g) [contains castor oil, boric acid, mineral oil, and Peruvian balsam]
    Critic-Aid Skin Care®: 20% (71 g, 170 g)
    Powder, topical (Ammens® Medicated Deodorant): 9.1% (187.5 g, 330 g) [original and shower fresh scent]
Overdosage/Treatment Decontamination: Dermal: Irrigate with soap and water. For treatment of metal fume fever see Metal Fume Fever. **Do not** evacuate gastric contents with zinc oxide or phosphide because they are corrosive. Dilute with milk.
Additional Information Black discoloration when exposed to light can accelerate growth of *Aspergillus fumigatus*, calamine is a combination of zinc oxide with ferric oxide; may result in a radiopacity on a KUB
Specific References
Liu CH, Lee CT, Tsai FC, et al, "Gastroduodenal Corrosive Injury After Oral Zinc Oxide," *Ann Emerg Med*, 2006, 47(3):296.

Zinc Sulfate

Pronunciation (zink SUL fate)
CAS Number 4468-02-4 (zinc gluconate); 7440-66-6; 7446-20-0 (zinc sulfate); 7733-02-0 (zinc sulfate)
U.S. Brand Names Orazinc® [OTC]; Zincate®
Synonyms ZnSO$_4$ (error-prone abbreviation)
Use Supplement for correction of zinc deficiency; used in treatment of acrodermatitis enteropathica
Mechanism of Action Needed for DNA and RNA synthesis and other enzyme symptoms
Adverse Reactions
Central nervous system: Lethargy, chills
Gastrointestinal: Vomiting, pancreatitis, metallic taste
Hematologic: Sideroblastic anemia (due to zinc-induced copper deficiency), thrombocytopenia, leukopenia
Signs and Symptoms of Overdose Blurred vision, decreased consciousness, diarrhea, hyperamylasemia, hypotension, hypothermia, jaundice, profuse sweating, pulmonary edema, oliguria, tachycardia, vomiting
Toxicodynamics/Kinetics
Absorption: Zinc sulfate: 20% to 30%
Protein binding: 99%
Half-life: 3 hours
Elimination: Through small bowel excretion
Dosage Maximum daily dose:
    Zinc gluconate: 230 mg
    Zinc sulfate: 660 mg
Stability Store oral liquid (injectable used orally) in refrigerator
Monitoring Parameters Patients on TPN therapy should have periodic serum copper and serum zinc levels
Dosage Forms Capsule (Orazinc®, Zincate®): 220 mg [elemental zinc 50 mg]
Injection, solution [preservative free]: 1 mg elemental zinc/mL (10 mL); 5 mg elemental zinc/mL (5 mL)
Tablet (Orazinc®): 110 mg [elemental zinc 25 mg]
Reference Range Normal serum zinc: 9.2-23.0 µmol/L; levels >30.0 µmol/L associated with bone marrow suppression; normal urinary zinc levels: 0.3-0.4 mg/day (increased to 2.1 mg/day in patients with proteinuria)
Overdosage/Treatment
Decontamination:
    Dermal: Wash with soap and water
    Ocular: Irrigate copiously with saline following exposure to zinc salt concentrations >0.5%; for zinc chloride exposure following water irrigating, irrigation with 0.5 molar (1.7%) edetate disodium solution for 15 minutes within 2 minutes of exposure may be helpful
    Oral: Lavage within 1 hour may be useful; dilute with milk; whole bowel irrigation has been utilized
Supportive therapy: Removal of excess zinc will eventually lead to normal hematopoiesis, although copper levels should be monitored and copper replaced as needed
Enhancement of elimination: Calcium disodium, ethylene diamine tetraacetate, dimercaprol or BAL has been used with some success; acetylcysteine has been used to increase the urinary excretion of zinc sulfate
Antidote(s)
• Succimer [ANTIDOTE]
• Unithiol [ANTIDOTE]
Pregnancy Risk Factor C
Pregnancy Implications Zinc deficiency during pregnancy can lead to intrauterine growth retardation during last trimester of pregnancy; has been associated with increased incidence of premature deliveries and stillborns at zinc ingestion of 0.6 mg/kg/day

Nursing Implications Do not give undiluted by direct injection into a peripheral vein because of potential for phlebitis, tissue irritation, and potential to increase renal loss of minerals from a bolus injection

Additional Information Lethal dose: Zinc sulfate: I.V.: 7.4 g

Daily consumption of 100-150 mg of zinc results in a negative copper balance; can cause a decrease in HDL cholesterol

RDA requirement of zinc: Infants: 5 mg; Children: 10 mg; Adults: Male: 15 mg; Female: 12 mg; During pregnancy: 15 mg; Lactating females: 16-19 mg

Historically, zinc sulfate was used as an emetic agent and is radiopaque; may result in radiopacity on KUB with oral ingestion; elevated zinc levels can occur from chronic ingestion of coins (especially pennies); zinc gluconate (20 mg of elemental zinc) may decrease duration and severity of infant diarrhea; >20 mg/day can be twice as likely in resulting in faster progression of HIV illness

Specific References

Bobat R, Coovadia H, Stephen C, et al, "Safety and Efficacy of Zinc Supplementation for Children with HIV-1 Infection in South Africa: A Randomised Double-Blind Placebo-Controlled Trial," *Lancet*, 2005, 366(9500):1862-7

Volmer PA, Roberts J, and Meerdink GL, "Canine Zinc Toxicosis from Ingestion of a Decorative Bathroom Fixture," *J Toxicol Clin Toxicol*, 2003, 41(5):741.

Zipeprol

Related Information
- Therapeutic Drugs Associated with Hallucinations

CAS Number 34758-83-3; 34758-84-4

Impairment Potential Yes

Unlabeled/Investigational Use Cough suppressant; often used as a drug of abuse (not FDA approved in U.S.)

Mechanism of Action A substituted, nonopiate piperazine with centrally acting antitussive action and peripheral actions on bronchospasm; also has antihistaminic and antiserotonin properties

Adverse Reactions

Central nervous system: Drowsiness, dizziness, auditory and visual hallucinations, ataxia, retrograde amnesia (with doses >300 mg), CNS depression, pseudotumor cerebri, extrapyramidal reactions, amnesia, opisthotonos, cognitive dysfunction

Gastrointestinal: Nausea, constipation

Neuromuscular & skeletal: Chorea

Respiratory: Apnea

Miscellaneous: Abuse potential

Signs and Symptoms of Overdose Ataxia, coma, headache, lethargy, opisthotonic crisis, respiratory depression, restlessness, seizures, tremor

Admission Criteria/Prognosis Admit any ingestion >600 mg; admit any ingestion >1g in an adult

Toxicodynamics/Kinetics

Absorption: 15 minutes

Metabolism: Hepatic

Half-life: 6 hours

Elimination: Renal (1% to 5% excreted unchanged)

Dosage Children:

Oral: 3-5 mg/kg/day in divided doses

Rectal: 100-150 mg/day

Adults:

Oral: 150-300 mg/day in divided doses

Rectal: 150 mg 1-2 times/day

Monitoring Parameters Respiratory states, arterial blood gases

Reference Range Postmortem blood zipeprol level after ~1.5 g ingestion ranges from 2 mcg/mL to 20.5 mcg/mL; liver to blood postmortem distribution ranges from 2.5-6.3; after a 175 mg oral dose, peak serum level approximates 0.75 mcg/mL

Overdosage/Treatment

Decontamination: **Do not** induce emesis; lavage (within 1 hour)/activated charcoal

Supportive therapy: Benzodiazepines or barbiturates can be used for seizure although human data is lacking, pyridoxine may be useful in treating seizures; high doses of naloxone (>6 mg) may antagonize CNS depressant effects

Antidote(s)
- Naloxone [ANTIDOTE]
- Pyridoxine [ANTIDOTE]

Additional Information Minimum lethal dose: 2 g

Abusers use 750 mg to 1 g for euphoric effect. Seizurgenic dose is 1.5 g in adults or 25 mg/kg in children; mechanism for seizures may be GABA Inhibition; cerebral edema can occur

Ziprasidone

CAS Number 138982-67-9; 146939-27-7

U.S. Brand Names Geodon®

Synonyms Zeldox; Ziprasidone Hydrochloride; Ziprasidone Mesylate

Use Treatment of schizophrenia

Unlabeled/Investigational Use Tourette's syndrome

Mechanism of Action The exact mechanism of action is unknown. However, *in vitro* radioligand studies show that ziprasidone has high affinity for D_2, $5-HT_{2a}$, $5-HT_{1A}$, $5-HT_{2c}$ and $5-HT_{1d}$, moderate affinity for alpha$_1$ adrenergic and histamine H_1 receptors, and low affinity for alpha$_2$ adrenergic, beta adrenergic, $5-HT_3$, $5-HT_4$, cholinergic, mu, sigma, or benzodiazepine receptors. Ziprasidone moderately inhibits the reuptake of serotonin and norepinephrine.

Adverse Reactions

Note: Although minor QT_c prolongation (mean 10 msec at 160 mg/day) may occur more frequently (incidence not specified), clinically relevant prolongation (>500 msec) was rare (0.06%).

Cardiovascular: Angina, atrial fibrillation, AV block (first degree), bradycardia, bundle branch block, cardiomegaly, facial edema, hypertension, myocarditis, peripheral edema, postural hypotension, QT prolongation, syncope, tachycardia, vasodilation

Central nervous system: Abnormal gait, accidental fall, agitation, akinesia, akathisia, amnesia, anxiety, ataxia, buccoglossal syndrome, cerebral infarction, chills, circumoral paresthesia, confusion, delirium, dizziness, dystonia, extrapyramidal symptoms, fever, hostility, hypertonia, hypesthesia, incoordination, insomnia, opisthotonos, psychosis, seizures, speech disorder, **somnolence (13% at 2 mg doses and 20% at 20 mg doses)**, stroke, vertigo

Dermatologic: Alopecia, contact dermatitis, eczema, exfoliative dermatitis, ecchymosis, fungal dermatitis, furunculosis, maculopapular rash, photosensitivity reaction, rash, urticaria, vesiculobullous rash

Endocrine & metabolic: Amenorrhea, anorgasmia, dehydration, dysmenorrhea, gout, gynecomastia, hypercholesterolemia, hyperglycemia, hyperkalemia, hyperlipemia, hyperthyroidism, hyperuricemia, hypocalcemia, hypoglycemia, hypokalemia, hypomagnesemia, hyponatremia, hypoproteinemia, hypothyroidism, ketosis, lactation (female), menorrhagia, metrorrhagia, sexual dysfunction (male and female), thirst, thyroiditis

Gastrointestinal: Anorexia, abdominal pain, constipation, dyspepsia, diarrhea, flank pain, dysphagia, fecal impaction, gingival bleeding, hematemesis, leukoplakia (mouth), nausea, melena, rectal hemorrhage, tongue edema, vomiting, weight gain, xerostomia

Genitourinary: Abnormal ejaculation, impotence, nocturia, polyuria, priapism, uterine hemorrhage, vaginal hemorrhage

Hematologic: Anemia, basophilia, eosinophilia, leukocytosis, lymphocytosis, monocytosis, polycythemia, thrombocytopenia, thrombocythemia

Hepatic: Cholestatic jaundice, fatty liver, hepatitis, hepatomegaly, increased alkaline phosphatase, increased GGT, increased LDH, increased transaminases, jaundice

Local: Phlebitis, thrombophlebitis, pain at injection site

Neuromuscular & skeletal: Cogwheel rigidity, choreoathetosis, dyskinesia, hypokinesia, hypotonia, increased CPK myalgia, myoclonus, myopathy, neuropathy, paresthesia, tenosynovitis, torticollis, tremor, trismus, weakness

Ocular: Abnormal vision, blepharitis, cataract, conjunctivitis, diplopia, dry eyes, keratitis, keratoconjunctivitis, nystagmus, ocular hemorrhage, oculogyric crisis, photophobia, visual field defect

Otic: Tinnitus

Renal: Albuminuria, hematuria, increased BUN, increased creatinine (serum), oliguria, urinary retention

Respiratory: Dyspnea, epistaxis, hemoptysis, increased cough, laryngismus, pneumonia, pulmonary embolism, respiratory alkalosis, respiratory disorder (primarily cold symptoms, upper respiratory infection), rhinitis

Miscellaneous: Accidental injury, diaphoresis, flu syndrome, lactate dehydrogenase elevated, lymphadenopathy, lymphedema, motor vehicle accident, withdrawal syndrome

Pharmacodynamics/Kinetics

Absorption: Well absorbed

Distribution: V_d: 1.5 L/kg

Protein binding: 99%, primarily to albumin and alpha$_1$-acid glycoprotein

Metabolism: Extensively hepatic, primarily via aldehyde oxidase; less than $1/3$ of total metabolism via CYP3A4 and CYP1A2 (minor)

Bioavailability: Oral (with food): 60% (up to twofold increase with food); I.M.: 100%

Half-life elimination: Oral: 7 hours; I.M.: 2-5 hours

Time to peak: Oral: 6-8 hours; I.M.: ≤60 minutes

Excretion: Feces (66%) and urine (20%) as metabolites; little as unchanged drug (1% urine, 4% feces)

Clearance: 7.5 mL/minute/kg

Dosage Oral:

Children and Adolescents: Tourette's syndrome (unlabeled use): 5-40 mg/day

Adults: Psychosis: Initial: 20 mg twice daily (with food)

Adjustment: Increases (if indicated) should be made no more frequently than every 2 days; ordinarily patients should be observed for improvement over several weeks before adjusting the dose

Maintenance: Range 20-100 mg twice daily; however, dosages >80 mg twice daily are generally not recommended

I.M.: Adults: Psychosis: 10 mg every 2 hours **or** 20 mg every 4 hours; maximum: 40 mg/day; oral therapy should replace I.M. administration as soon as possible

Elderly: No dosage adjustment is recommended; consider initiating at a low end of the dosage range, with slower titration

Dosage adjustment in renal impairment:
Oral: No dosage adjustment is recommended
I.M.: Cyclodextrin, an excipient in the I.M. formulation, is cleared by renal filtration; use with caution.

Dosage adjustment in hepatic impairment: No dosage adjustment is recommended

Stability Store at controlled room temperature of 15°C to 30°C (59°F to 86°F)

Monitoring Parameters Vital signs; serum potassium and magnesium; fasting lipid profile and fasting blood glucose/Hgb A_{1c} (prior to treatment, at 3 months, then annually); BMI, personal/family history of obesity, waist circumference; blood pressure; mental status, abnormal involuntary movement scale (AIMS), extrapyramidal symptoms. Weight should be assessed prior to treatment, at 4 weeks, 8 weeks, 12 weeks, and then at quarterly intervals. Consider titrating to a different antipsychotic agent for a weight gain ≥5% of the initial weight. The value of routine ECG screening or monitoring has not been established.

Administration Administer with food

Contraindications Hypersensitivity to ziprasidone or any component of the formulation; history (or current) prolonged QT; congenital long QT syndrome; recent myocardial infarction; history of arrhythmias; uncompensated heart failure; concurrent use of other QT_c-prolonging agents including amiodarone, arsenic trioxide, bretylium, chlorpromazine, cisapride, class Ia antiarrhythmics (quinidine, procainamide), dofetilide, dolasetron, droperidol, halofantrine, ibutilide, levomethadyl, mefloquine, mesoridazine, pentamidine, pimozide, probucol, some quinolone antibiotics (moxifloxacin, sparfloxacin, gatifloxacin), sotalol, tacrolimus, and thioridazine

Warnings

[U.S. Boxed Warning]: Patients with dementia-related behavioral disorders treated with atypical antipsychotics are at an increased risk of death compared to placebo. Ziprasidone is not approved for this indication.

May result in QT_c prolongation (dose-related), which has been associated with the development of malignant ventricular arrhythmias (torsade de pointes) and sudden death. Observed prolongation was greater than with other atypical antipsychotic agents (risperidone, olanzapine, quetiapine), but less than with thioridazine. Avoid hypokalemia, hypomagnesemia. Use caution in patients with bradycardia. Discontinue in patients found to have persistent QT_c intervals >500 msec. Patients with symptoms of dizziness, palpitations, or syncope should receive further cardiac evaluation.

May cause extrapyramidal symptoms, including pseudoparkinsonism, acute dystonic reactions, akathisia, and tardive dyskinesia. Disturbances of temperature regulation have been reported with antipsychotics (not reported in premarketing trials of ziprasidone). Antipsychotic use may also be associated with neuroleptic malignant syndrome (NMS). Use with caution in patients at risk of seizures, including those with a history of seizures, head trauma, brain damage, alcoholism, or concurrent therapy with medications which may lower seizure threshold. Elderly patients may be at increased risk of seizures due to an increased prevalence of predisposing factors.

May cause orthostatic hypotension; use with caution in patients at risk of this effect or in those who would tolerate transient hypotensive episodes (cerebrovascular disease, cardiovascular disease, hypovolemia, or other medications which may predispose).

Atypical antipsychotics have been associated with development of hyperglycemia; in some cases, may be extreme and associated with ketoacidosis, hyperosmolar coma, or death. There is limited documentation with ziprasidone and specific risk associated with this agent is not known. Use caution in patients with diabetes or other disorders of glucose regulation; monitor for worsening of glucose control.

Cognitive and/or motor impairment (sedation) is common with ziprasidone, resulting in impaired performance of tasks requiring alertness (eg, operating machinery or driving). Use with caution in disorders where CNS depression is a feature. Use with caution in Parkinson's disease. Esophageal dysmotility and aspiration have been associated with antipsychotic use; use with caution in patients at risk of aspiration pneumonia (ie, Alzheimer's disease). Caution in breast cancer or other prolactin-dependent tumors (may elevate prolactin levels). Use caution in patients with renal or hepatic impairment. Ziprasidone has been associated with a fairly high incidence of rash (5%); discontinue if alternative etiology is not identified. Safety and efficacy have not been established in pediatric patients.

The possibility of a suicide attempt is inherent in psychotic illness or bipolar disorder; use caution in high-risk patients during initiation of therapy. Prescriptions should be written for the smallest quantity consistent with good patient care.

Dosage Forms Capsule, as hydrochloride: 20 mg, 40 mg, 60 mg, 80 mg
Injection, powder for reconstitution, as mesylate: 20 mg

Overdosage/Treatment
Decontamination: Activated charcoal
Supportive therapy: Reported symptoms include somnolence, slurring of speech, and hypertension. Acute extrapyramidal reactions may also occur, and should be treated with benztropine or diphenhydramine. Akathisia should be treated with beta adrenergic blocking agents. Not removed by dialysis.

Test Interactions ↓ cholesterol, triglycerides; may cause transient elevation of prolactin levels

Drug Interactions Substrate (minor) of CYP1A2, 3A4; **Inhibits** CYP2D6 (weak), 3A4 (weak)

Acetylcholinesterase inhibitors (central): May increase the risk of antipsychotic-related extrapyramidal symptoms; monitor.

Amphetamines: Efficacy may be diminished by antipsychotics; in addition, amphetamines may increase psychotic symptoms; avoid concurrent use

Antihypertensives: Concurrent use of ziprasidone with an antihypertensive may produce additive hypotensive effects (particularly orthostasis)

Carbamazepine: May decrease serum concentrations of ziprasidone (AUC is decreased by 35%); other enzyme-inducing agents may share this potential

CNS depressants: Sedative effects may be additive with ziprasidone; monitor for increased effect; includes barbiturates, benzodiazepines, narcotic analgesics, ethanol, and other sedative agents

Ketoconazole: May increase serum concentrations of ziprasidone (AUC is increased by 35% to 40%); other CYP3A4 inhibitors may share this potential. QT_c prolongation was not demonstrated.

Levodopa: Ziprasidone may inhibit the antiparkinsonian effect of levodopa; avoid this combination

Metoclopramide: May increase extrapyramidal symptoms (EPS) or risk.

Potassium- or magnesium-depleting agents: May increase the risk of serious arrhythmias with ziprasidone; includes many diuretics, aminoglycosides, cyclosporine, and amphotericin; monitor serum potassium and magnesium levels closely

QT_c-prolonging agents: May result in additive effects on cardiac conduction, potentially resulting in malignant or lethal arrhythmias; concurrent use is contraindicated. Includes amiodarone, arsenic trioxide, bretylium, chlorpromazine, cisapride; class Ia antiarrhythmics (quinidine, procainamide); dofetilide, dolasetron, droperidol, halofantrine, ibutilide, levomethadyl, mefloquine, mesoridazine, pentamidine, pimozide, probucol; some quinolone antibiotics (moxifloxacin, sparfloxacin, gatifloxacin); sotalol, tacrolimus, and thioridazine.

Pregnancy Risk Factor C

Pregnancy Implications Developmental toxicity demonstrated in animals. There are no adequate and well-controlled studies in pregnant women. Use only if potential benefit justifies risk to the fetus.

Lactation Excretion in breast milk unknown/not recommended

Additional Information The increased potential to prolong QT_c, as compared to other available antipsychotic agents, should be considered in the evaluation of available alternatives.

Specific References

Biswas AK, Zabrocki LA, Mayes KL, et al, "Cardiotoxicity Associated with Intentional Ziprasidone and Bupropion Overdose," *J Toxicol Clin Toxicol*, 2003, 41(2):101-4.

Borovicka MC, Bond LC, and Gaughan KM, "Ziprasidone- and Lithium-Induced Neuroleptic Malignant Syndrome," *Ann Pharmacother*, 2006, 40(1):139-42.

Citrome L, Brook S, Warrington L, et al, "Ziprasidone Versus Haloperidol for the Treatment of Agitation," *Ann Emerg Med*, 2004, 44:S22.

Daniel DG, Brook S, Warrington L, et al, "Intramuscular Ziprasidone in Agitated Patients with Bipolar Diagnoses," *Ann Emerg Med*, 2004, 44:S22.

Francis A, Preval H, Klotz SG, et al, "Intramuscular Ziprasidone in the Psychiatric Emergency Department Expanded Sample," *Ann Emerg Med*, 2004, 44:S22.

Klotz SG, Preval H, Southard R, et al, "Use of Intramuscular Ziprasidone in the Psychiatric Emergency Service," *Ann Emerg Med*, 2003, 42(4):S101.

Krier S, Heard K, DeWitt C, et al, "Effect of Subacute Ziprasidone Administration and Withdrawal on Acute Cocaine Intoxication," *Clin Toxicol (Phila)*, 2005, 43:730.

Lofton AL, Klein-Schwartz W, Spiller HA, et al, "Prospective Multi-Poison Center Study of Ziprasidone Exposures," *J Toxicol Clin Toxicol*, 2004, 42(5):726.

Lovecchio F, Watts D, and Eckholdt P, "Three-Year Experience with Ziprasidone Exposures," *Am J Emerg Med*, 2005, 23(4):586-7.

Martel ML, "Ziprasidone for Sedation of the Agitated ED Patient," *Am J Emerg Med*, 2004, 22(3):238.

Potkin SG, Keck P, Giller E, et al, "Ziprasidone in Bipolar Mania: Efficacy Across Patient Subgroups," *Ann Emerg Med*, 2004, 44:S23.

Watts D and Lovecchio F, "Three-Year Experience with Ziprasidone Exposures," *J Toxicol Clin Toxicol*, 2004, 42(5):813.

Zolpidem

CAS Number 82626-48-0; 99294-93-6
U.S. Brand Names Ambien®
Synonyms Zolpidem Tartrate
Impairment Potential Yes. Serum zolpidem levels >100 mcg/L are associated with driving impairment. (Baselt RC and Cravey RH, *Disposition of Toxic Drugs and Chemicals in Man*, 4th ed, Foster City, CA: Chemical Toxicology Institute, 1995, 788.)
Use Hypnotic for short-term management of insomnia
Mechanism of Action Selective agonist of the omega-1 receptor at the CNS gamma amino butyric acid (GABA)/chloride channel complex; not a benzodiazepine, but an imidazopyridin
Adverse Reactions
Cardiovascular: Bradycardia, sinus bradycardia
Central nervous system: Headache, drowsiness, dizziness, slurred speech, hallucinations, anterograde amnesia, headache, night terrors, confusion, drowsiness, coma, ataxia, visual hallucinations, auditory hallucinations, paranoia, psychosis, somnolence, delirium
Dermatologic: Pruritus, bullous skin disease, urticaria, purpura, photosensitivity
Gastrointestinal: Nausea, vomiting, diarrhea, xerostomia
Hepatic: Hepatitis
Neuromuscular & skeletal: Myalgia, hyporeflexia
Ocular: Miosis
Respiratory: Apnea, respiratory depression
Signs and Symptoms of Overdose Coma, diplopia, esophageal ulceration, hypotension, miosis, night terrors, respiratory depression
Pharmacodynamics/Kinetics
Onset of action: 30 minutes
Duration: 6-8 hours
Absorption: Rapid
Distribution: Very low amounts enter breast milk
Protein binding: 92%
Metabolism: Hepatic, primarily via CYP3A4 (~60%), to inactive metabolites
Half-life elimination: 2.5-2.8 hours (range 1.4-4.5 hours); Cirrhosis: Up to 9.9 hours
Time to peak, plasma: 2 hours; 4 hours with food
Excretion: As metabolites in urine, bile, feces
Dosage Adults: Oral: 10 mg immediately before bedtime; 5 mg in elderly patients or patients with renal/liver disease; maximum dose: 20 mg
Monitoring Parameters Daytime alertness; respiratory and cardiac status
Administration Ingest immediately before bedtime due to rapid onset of action. Ambien CR™ tablets should not be divided, crushed, or chewed.
Contraindications Hypersensitivity to zolpidem or any component of the formulation
Warnings Should be used only after evaluation of potential causes of sleep disturbance. Failure of sleep disturbance to resolve after 7-10 days may indicate psychiatric or medical illness. Use with caution in patients with depression. Abnormal thinking and behavioral changes have been associated with sedative-hypnotics. Sedative/hypnotics may produce withdrawal symptoms following abrupt discontinuation. Causes CNS depression, which may impair physical and mental capabilities. Effects with other sedative drugs or ethanol may be potentiated. Use caution in the elderly; dose adjustment recommended. Closely monitor elderly or debilitated patients for impaired cognitive or motor performance. Avoid use in patients with sleep apnea or a history of sedative-hypnotic abuse. Use caution with hepatic impairment; dose adjustment required. Prescriptions should be written for the smallest effective dose (especially in the elderly) and for the smallest quantity consistent with good patient care (especially with depression). Safety and efficacy have not been established in pediatric patients.
Dosage Forms [DSC] = Discontinued product
Tablet, as tartrate:
Ambien®: 5 mg, 10 mg
Ambien® PAK™ [dose pack]: 5 mg (30s); 10 mg (30s) [DSC]
Tablet, extended release, as tartrate (Ambien CR™): 6.25 mg, 12.5 mg
Reference Range
Therapeutic: 80-150 ng/mL; serum levels of 500 ng/mL associated with coma
Autopsy blood zolpidem level of 4.1 mcg/mL associated with fatality
Postmortem blood and urine levels: 7.9 mcg/mL and 4.41 mcg/mL, respectively, following zolpidem overdose
Overdosage/Treatment
Decontamination: Activated charcoal for adult ingestions >100 mg
Supportive therapy: Flumazenil effectively antagonizes CNS depressant effects
Enhancement of elimination: Not dialyzable; multiple dosing of activated charcoal may be effective
Antidote(s)
- Flumazenil [ANTIDOTE]

Drug Interactions
Substrate of CYP1A2 (minor), 2C9 (minor), 2C19 (minor), 2D6 (minor), 3A4 (major)
Antipsychotics: Sedative effects may be additive with antipsychotics, including phenothiazines; monitor for increased effect
CNS depressants: Sedative effects may be additive with other CNS depressants; monitor for increased effect; includes barbiturates, benzodiazepines, narcotic analgesics, ethanol, and other sedative agents
CYP3A4 inducers: CYP3A4 inducers may decrease the levels/effects of zolpidem. Example inducers include aminoglutethimide, carbamazepine, nafcillin, nevirapine, phenobarbital, phenytoin, and rifamycins.
CYP3A4 inhibitors: May increase the levels/effects of zolpidem. Example inhibitors include azole antifungals, clarithromycin, diclofenac, doxycycline, erythromycin, imatinib, isoniazid, nefazodone, nicardipine, propofol, protease inhibitors, quinidine, telithromycin, troleandomycin, and verapamil.
Rifamycin derivatives: May decrease levels/effects of zolpidem.
Pregnancy Risk Factor B
Pregnancy Implications Incomplete calcification of fetal skull bones in rats at levels of 20-100 mg/kg
Lactation Enters breast milk/not recommended (AAP rates "compatible")
Nursing Implications Patients may require assistance with ambulation; lower doses in the elderly are usually effective; institute safety measures
Specific References
Chang MY and Lin JL, "Irreversible Ischemic Hand Following Intraarterial Injection of Zolpidem Powder," *J Toxicol Clin Toxicol*, 2003, 41(7): 1025-8.
Cheze M, Deveaux M, Lenoan A, et al, "Clonazepam, Bromazepam, and Zolpidem in Hair of Victims of Drug-Facilitated Crimes: Quantitative Analysis by LC-MS/MS and Correlation with Self-Report," *Annale de Toxicologie Analytique*, 2005, 17(4):269-74.
Huang CL, Chang CJ, Hung CF, et al, "Zolpidem-Induced Distortion in Visual Perception," *Ann Pharmacother*, 2003, 37(5):683-6.
Johnson W, Harding P, Cochems A, et al, "Zolpidem-Impaired Drivers in Wisconsin - A Six-Year Retrospective," *J Anal Toxicol*, 2006, 30:161.
Kintz P, Villain M, Dumestre-Toulet V, et al, "Usefulness of LC-MS/MS in Drug-Facilitated Sexual Assault Evidence: A Case Study Involving Zolpidem," *Annale de Toxicologie Analytique*, 2005, 17(4):263-8.
Laloup M, Fernandez M, De Boeck G, et al, "Validation of a Liquid Chromatography-Tandem Mass Spectrometry Method for the Simultaneous Determination of 26 Benzodiazepines and Metabolites, Zolpidem and Zopiclone, in Blood, Urine, and Hair," *J Anal Toxicol*, 2005, 29: 616-26.
Morley SR, Galloway JG, Forrest AR, et al, "Zolpidem as a Primary Cause of Death: A Case Report," *J Anal Toxicol*, 2006, 30:133.
Rappa LR, Larose-Pierre M, Payne DR, et al, "Detoxification from High-Dose Zolpidem Using Diazepam," *Ann Pharmacother*, 2004, 38(4):590-4. Epub 2004 Feb 13.
Tsai MJ, Huang YB, and Wu PC, "A Novel Clinical Pattern of Visual Hallucination After Zolpidem Use," *J Toxicol Clin Toxicol*, 2003, 41(6):869-72.

Zopiclone

CAS Number 43200-80-2
Impairment Potential Yes
Use Symptomatic relief of transient and short-term insomnia
Unlabeled/Investigational Use In U.S.: Insomnia (<1-month duration)
Mechanism of Action A nonbenzodiazepine sedative hypnotic agent which facilitates gamma aminobutyric acid function
Adverse Reactions
Cardiovascular: Palpitations
Central nervous system: Dizziness, headache, confusion, slurred speech, ataxia, nightmares, memory disturbance, psychosis, drowsiness, lethargy, insomnia, aggressive behavior
Gastrointestinal: **Bitter taste**, xerostomia, nausea, vomiting, loss of taste perception, bitter taste
Genitourinary: Urinary retention
Neuromuscular & skeletal: Dysarthria, tremor
Ocular: Blurred vision
Miscellaneous: Dependence
Signs and Symptoms of Overdose CNS depression, coma, hyperglycemia, hyperkalemia, respiratory depression
Admission Criteria/Prognosis Asymptomatic patients may be discharged 8 hours postingestion; admit any ingestion >30 mg
Pharmacodynamics/Kinetics
Absorption: Elderly: 75% to 94%
Distribution: Rapidly from vascular compartment
Protein binding: ~45%
Metabolism: Extensively hepatic
Half-life elimination: 5 hours; Elderly: 7 hours; Hepatic impairment: 11.9 hours
Time to peak, serum: <2 hours; Hepatic impairment: 3.5 hours
Excretion: Urine (75%); feces (16%)

Dosage Oral: 7.5 mg 30-60 minutes before bedtime

Monitoring Parameters Monitor for confusion, excessive drowsiness especially in elderly, and monitor patients with hepatic insufficiency closely

Administration Administer just before bedtime.

Contraindications Hypersensitivity to zopiclone or any component of the formulation; patients with severe respiratory impairment (eg, sleep apnea); pregnancy (similar agents)

Warnings Causes CNS depression; use with caution in patients who previously manifested paradoxical reactions to ethanol or other sedatives. Should not be administered for more than 7-10 days consecutively; failure of insomnia to remit after 7-10 days may indicate presence of a primary psychiatric or mental illness. Use with caution in elderly patients and in patients with myasthenia gravis, hepatic dysfunction, renal dysfunction, severe pulmonary insufficiency, and depression. Anterograde amnesia can occur, do not take unless a full night's sleep and clearance of the drug from the body are possible. Abnormal thinking and psychotic behaviors may occur with use; confusion may occur, especially in the elderly. Elderly are more susceptible to adverse reactions. Increased daytime anxiety and/or restlessness have been observed with use. May cause dependence; withdrawal symptoms can occur with abrupt discontinuation; the risk of dependence is increased in patients with a history of alcoholism and drug abuse. Not recommended for use in patients <18 years of age.

Dosage Forms Tablet: 5 mg, 7.5 mg

Reference Range After a 7.5 mg oral dose, peak serum levels are ~60-70 mcg/L at 1-1.5 hours and decline to 3 mcg/L at 24 hours; postmortem levels associated with fatal overdoses of zopiclone: 1.4-3.9 mg/L

Overdosage/Treatment

Decontamination: Activated charcoal

Supportive therapy: Monitor respiratory status; rarely is mechanical ventilation required; flumazenil has been used successfully in one case; flumazenil has been shown to selectively block the binding of benzodiazepines to CNS receptors, resulting in a reversal of benzodiazepine-induced CNS depression and respiratory depression

Enhancement of elimination: Hemodialysis/hemoperfusion are not expected to be useful; multiple dosing of activated charcoal may be effective

Antidote(s)

- Flumazenil [ANTIDOTE]

Drug Interactions

Substrate (major) of CYP2C9, 3A4

CNS depressants: Zopiclone may produce additive CNS depressant effects when coadministered with ethanol; sedatives, antihistamines, anticonvulsants, or psychotropic medications.

CYP2C9 inducers: May decrease the levels/effects of zopiclone. Example inducers include carbamazepine, phenobarbital, phenytoin, rifampin, rifapentine, and secobarbital.

CYP2C9 Inhibitors may increase the levels/effects of zopiclone. Example inhibitors include delavirdine, fluconazole, gemfibrozil, ketoconazole, nicardipine, NSAIDs, sulfonamides and tolbutamide.

CYP3A4 inducers: CYP3A4 inducers may decrease the levels/effects of zopiclone. Example inducers include aminoglutethimide, carbamazepine, nafcillin, nevirapine, phenobarbital, phenytoin, and rifamycins.

CYP3A4 inhibitors: May increase the levels/effects of zopiclone. Example inhibitors include azole antifungals, clarithromycin, diclofenac, doxycycline, erythromycin, imatinib, isoniazid, nefazodone, nicardipine, propofol, protease inhibitors, quinidine, telithromycin, and verapamil.

Pregnancy Risk Factor Not assigned; similar agents rated D

Pregnancy Implications There is insufficient data on safety in pregnancy, however, benzodiazepines may cause congenital malformations during the 1st trimester and neonatal CNS depression during the last few weeks of pregnancy; it is expected zopiclone may do the same.

Lactation Enters breast milk/not recommended

Nursing Implications Monitor for effectiveness and excessive drowsiness or confusion the next day; administer just prior to sleep

Specific References

Cienki JJ, Burkhart KK, and Donovan JW, "Zopiclone Overdose Responsive to Flumazenil," *Clin Toxicol* , 2005, 43(5):385-6.

Laloup M, Fernandez M, De Boeck G, et al, "Validation of a Liquid Chromatography-Tandem Mass Spectrometry Method for the Simultaneous Determination of 26 Benzodiazepines and Metabolites, Zolpidem and Zopiclone, in Blood, Urine, and Hair," *J Anal Toxicol*, 2005, 29:616-26.

Maguire R, Moran C, Talbot D, et al, "Determination of Zopiclone Misuse in the Republic of Ireland Using GC-MS," *J Anal Toxicol*, 2003, 27(3):184.

Nordgren HK, Holmgren P, Liljeberg P, et al, "Application of Direct Urine LC-MS-MS Analysis for Screening of Novel Substances in Drug Abusers," *J Anal Toxicol*, 2005, 29(4):234-9.

Reith DM, Fountain J, McDowell R, et al, "Comparison of the Fatal Toxicity Index of Zopiclone with Benzodiazepines," *J Toxicol Clin Toxicol*, 2003, 41(7):975-80.

Zuclopenthixol

CAS Number 633-59-0; 64053-00-5; 85721-05-7

Synonyms Z-Chlopenthixol; Zuclopenthixol Acetate; Zuclopenthixol Decanoate; Zuclopenthixol Dihydrochloride

Use Management of schizophrenia; acetate injection is intended for short-term acute treatment; decanoate injection is for long-term management; dihydrochloride tablets may be used in either phase

Unlabeled/Investigational Use Bipolar disorder, psychoses; agitated states

Mechanism of Action A thioxanthene with a piperazine sidechain; related to fluphenazine; the cis(z)-clopenthixol is the active isomer of this neuroleptic; blocks postsynaptic dopaminergic brain receptors

Adverse Reactions

Cardiovascular: Palpitations

Central nervous system: Dystonia, akinesia, sedation, extrapyramidal effects

Endocrine & metabolic: Elevated serum triglyceride levels

Gastrointestinal: Reduced salivation, weight gain, constipation, xerostomia

Genitourinary: Uricosuric, priapism

Hematologic: Eosinophilia

Hepatic: Liver enzyme elevation

Neuromuscular & skeletal: Rigidity, tremors

Ocular: Blurred vision

Signs and Symptoms of Overdose Dry mouth, extrapyramidal effects, hypotension, respiratory depression, sedation, seizures, tachycardia

Admission Criteria/Prognosis Admit any ingestion >1 g or any patient exhibiting neurologic symptoms

Pharmacodynamics/Kinetics

Onset: Acetate injection: Sedation within 2 hours

Duration of action: Acetate injection: 2-3 days; Decanoate injection: 2 weeks

Distribution: V_d: 15-20 L/kg

Metabolism: Hepatic via N-dealkylation

Half-life elimination: Terminal: Oral: 20 hours; Depot: 19 days

Time to peak: Acetate injection: 24-36 hours; Dihydrochloride tablet: 3 hours; Depot: 3-7 days

Dosage Oral: Zuclopenthixol hydrochloride: Initial: 20-30 mg/day in divided doses; usual maintenance dose: 20-75 mg/day; maximum daily dose: 150 mg

I.M.:

Zuclopenthixol acetate: 50-150 mg; may be repeated in 2-3 days; no more than 4 injections should be given in the course of treatment; maximum dose during course of treatment: 400 mg

Zuclopenthixol decanoate: 100 mg by deep I.M. injection; additional doses of 100-200 mg (I.M.) may be given over the following 1-4 weeks; maximum weekly dose: 600 mg

Monitoring Parameters Vital signs; lipid profile, fasting blood glucose/Hgb A$_{1c}$; BMI; mental status, abnormal involuntary movement scale (AIMS), extrapyramidal symptoms (EPS)

Contraindications Hypersensitivity to zuclopenthixol, thioxanthenes, or any component of the formulation; acute intoxication (ethanol, barbiturate, or opioid); severe CNS depression; coma; suspected or established subcortical brain damage; circulatory collapse; blood dyscrasias; pheochromocytoma

Warnings

May be sedating, use with caution in disorders where CNS depression is a feature. Use with caution in Parkinson's disease. Caution in patients with hemodynamic instability; predisposition to seizures; bone marrow suppression; severe cardiac, hepatic, renal, or respiratory disease. Esophageal dysmotility and aspiration have been associated with antipsychotic use - use with caution in patients at risk of pneumonia (ie, Alzheimer's disease). Caution in breast cancer or other prolactin-dependent tumors (may elevate prolactin levels). May alter temperature regulation or mask toxicity of other drugs due to antiemetic effects. May alter cardiac conduction - life-threatening arrhythmias have occurred with therapeutic doses of neuroleptics. May cause orthostatic hypotension - use with caution in patients at risk of this effect or those who would tolerate transient hypotensive episodes (cerebrovascular disease, cardiovascular disease, or other medications which may predispose). Safety and efficacy in children <18 years of age have not been established.

May cause anticholinergic effects (confusion, agitation, constipation, dry mouth, blurred vision, urinary retention); therefore, they should be used with caution in patients with decreased gastrointestinal motility, urinary retention, BPH, xerostomia, or visual problems. Conditions which also may be exacerbated by cholinergic blockade include narrow-angle glaucoma (screening is recommended) and worsening of myasthenia gravis. Relative to other neuroleptics, zuclopenthixol has a low potency of cholinergic blockade.

May cause extrapyramidal reactions, including pseudoparkinsonism, acute dystonic reactions, akathisia, and tardive dyskinesia (risk of these reactions is high relative to other neuroleptics). May be associated with neuroleptic malignant syndrome (NMS) or pigmentary retinopathy.

Dosage Forms [CAN] = Canadian brand name
Injection, as acetate:
Clopixol Acuphase® [CAN]: 50 mg/mL [zuclopenthixol 42.5 mg/mL] (1 mL, 2 mL) [not available in the U.S.]
Injection, as decanoate:
Clopixol® Depot [CAN]: 200 mg/mL [zuclopenthixol 144.4 mg/mL] (10 mL) [not available in the U.S.]
Tablet, as dihydrochloride:
Clopixol® [CAN]: 10 mg, 25 mg, 40 mg [not available in the U.S.]

Reference Range Therapeutic z-chlopenthixol serum levels are 2-12 ng/mL; ingestion of 2.5 g resulted in a peak blood level of 900 ng/mL

Overdosage/Treatment
Decontamination: **Do not** induce emesis; lavage (within 6 hours) with activated charcoal may be useful
Supportive therapy: Benzodiazepines can be useful to control agitation or seizures

Drug Interactions Substrate of CYP2D6 (major)
Acetylcholinesterase inhibitors (central): May increase the risk of antipsychotic-related extrapyramidal symptoms; monitor.
Aluminum salts: May decrease the absorption of antipsychotics; monitor.
Amphetamines: Efficacy may be diminished by antipsychotics; in addition, amphetamines may increase psychotic symptoms. Avoid concurrent use.
Anticholinergics: May inhibit the therapeutic response to antipsychotics and excess anticholinergic effects may occur; includes benztropine, trihexyphenidyl, biperiden, and drugs with significant anticholinergic activity (TCAs, antihistamines, disopyramide).
Antihypertensives: Concurrent use of antipsychotics with an antihypertensive may produce additive hypotensive effects (particularly orthostasis).
Bromocriptine: Antipsychotics inhibit the ability of bromocriptine to lower serum prolactin concentrations.

CNS depressants: Sedative effects may be additive with antipsychotics; monitor for increased effect; includes barbiturates, benzodiazepines, narcotic analgesics, ethanol, and other sedative agents.
CYP2D6 inhibitors: May increase the levels/effects of zuclopenthixol. Example inhibitors include chlorpromazine, delavirdine, fluoxetine, miconazole, paroxetine, pergolide, quinidine, quinine, ritonavir, and ropinirole.
Epinephrine: Chlorpromazine (and possibly other low potency antipsychotics) may diminish the pressor effects of epinephrine.
Guanethidine and guanadrel: Antihypertensive effects may be inhibited by antipsychotics.
Levodopa: Antipsychotics may inhibit the antiparkinsonian effect of levodopa; avoid this combination.
Lithium: Antipsychotics may produce neurotoxicity with lithium; this is a rare effect.
Metoclopramide: May increase extrapyramidal symptoms (EPS) or risk.
Phenytoin: May reduce serum levels of antipsychotics; phenothiazines may increase phenytoin serum levels.
Polypeptide antibiotics (polymyxin): Rare cases of respiratory paralysis have been reported with concurrent use of antipsychotics.
Propranolol: Serum concentrations of antipsychotics may be increased; propranolol also increases some antipsychotic concentrations.
Sulfadoxine/pyrimethamine: May increase antipsychotic concentrations.
Tricyclic antidepressants: Concurrent use may produce increased toxicity or altered therapeutic response.
Trazodone: Antipsychotics and trazodone may produce additive hypotensive effects.
Valproic acid: Serum levels may be increased by antipsychotics.

Pregnancy Risk Factor C
Lactation Enters breast milk/not recommended

SECTION II

NONMEDICINAL AGENTS

ACIDS AND ALKALIS

Jack C. Clifton II, MD and Steven E. Aks, DO, FACMT

Description

Acids and alkalis are ubiquitous in the household and the workplace. Acids commonly stored and shipped in bulk include the inorganic acids: hydrochloric, sulfuric, phosphoric, and nitric acid. Commonly encountered inorganic alkalis are sodium hydroxide and ammonium hydroxide. Common organic acids and bases include such agents as acetic acid and diethylamine (Table 1).

Table 1. Acid and Base Classifications With Selected Common Examples		
Class	**Common Examples**	**Chemical Formula**
Inorganic Acids and Bases		
Strong acids	Sulfuric	H_2SO_4
	Hydrochloric	HCl
Weak acids	Phosphoric	H_3PO_4
	Carbonic	H_2CO_3
Weak bases	Ammonia	NH_3
	Magnesium hydroxide	$Mg(OH)_2$
Strong bases	Potassium hydroxide	KOH
	Sodium hypochlorite	NaClO
Organic Acids and Bases		
Saturated acids	Acetic (ethanoic) acid	$C_2H_4O_2$
	Butyric (butanoic) acid	$C_4H_8O_2$
Unsaturated acids	Valeric (pentanoic) acid	$C_5H_{10}O_2$
	Acrylic acid	$C_3H_4O_2$
Alkylamine bases	Diethylamine	$C_4H_{11}N$
Alkanolamine bases	Ethanolamine	C_2H_7NO

Since these agents can be so familiar, great care must be taken to identify these agents using identification numbers (CAS; UN/D.O.T.) or by precisely spelling the commonly used identifiers; in particular, it is important to avoid confusing hydrochloric and hydrofluoric acids — as the latter has a specific antidote. The toxicity of standard acids and bases is through contact (dermal and ocular), and respiratory irritation, typically through mists.

The concentration, form, and quantity of acids and bases are critical when assessing the significance of a spill or exposure. Acids and bases may exist in pure form, as salts (partial replacement of H^+ or ^-OH ions with another ion), or as an anhydride (metal or metalloid oxide), though properties are generally similar across forms.

Strong acids and bases, particularly anhydrides, can be strongly exothermic when neutralized, especially when water is added to a larger quantity of product. Heated acids can also release potent fumes. While this is a concern in fire suppression, this should not deter use of water decontamination of patients exposed to corrosives, once clothes are removed and most of the product has been gently brushed or blotted away. Copious tepid fluids will keep exothermic reactions manageable, and most quickly restore tissue pH toward normal.

Acids in particular are also a threat because of their propensity to cause generation of toxic gases when mixed with salts and other compounds (Table 2). A number of the organic bases are notable for their flammability and may release toxic nitrous oxides when heated. Incidents involving poorly managed chemical warehouses can be a hazardous material nightmare because of the proximity of so many incompatible substances.

Table 2. Selected Important Chemical Reactions Involving Acids and Bases

Agent Exposed	Toxic Product Generated
Cyanide salts with acids	Hydrocyanic gas
Metals with acids	Hydrogen gas
Arsenic with acids	Arsine gas
Metal phosphides	Phosphine gas
Bleach (NaClO) with acid	Chlorine gas
Bleach (NaClO) with ammonia	Chloramine gas

With the preceding as background, this section will focus on a few of the very common acids and bases.

Sources of Exposure

Hydrochloric acid (CAS #7647-01-0) is used for metal etching, as a bleach, and for various industrial uses in chemical synthesis. Hydrochloric acid is a nonflammable, colorless gas or fuming liquid with a characteristic suffocating odor. After reacting with metals, it can form hydrogen gas, which is highly flammable. A concentration of 100 ppm is considered immediately life-threatening due to its ability to cause asphyxiation and chemical injury. Its vapor pressure is 3240 mm Hg at 18°C (64°F), nearly 70 times the vapor pressure of water at these conditions.

Hydrofluoric acid (CAS #7664-39-3) in a concentration of 1% to 100% is commonly utilized in industrial settings for etching (ceramics, microchips, and glass), electroplating, and rust removal. Commercial products (1% to 12%) for home use include rust removers and chrome cleaners. Anhydrous HF (100%) is a colorless liquid with a boiling point of 19.4°C (67°F) and a vapor pressure of 400 mm Hg at 2.5°C (36.5°F) that fumes at concentrations >48%; therefore, vapor formation at a spill site may be hazardous to workers. A concentration of 20 ppm may be immediately dangerous to life and health.

Sulfuric acid (CAS #7664-93-9) is utilized in chemical and fertilizer manufacturing. It represents the most commonly used chemical in the United States. Two examples of sulfuric acid's use in common products are battery acid (30% solution) and toilet bowl cleaners (10% solution). Sulfuric acid is a clear, colorless, nonflammable liquid when pure. Although nonflammable by itself, this acid can ignite other combustible materials, such as wood or paper. A concentration of 10-20 ppm is nearly unbearable because of its extreme irritant effect. Sulfuric acid has a vapor pressure of 1 mm Hg at 146°C (295°F).

Nitric acid (CAS #7697-37-2; fuming, CAS #52583-42-3) is used in the engraving process, metal refining, and electroplating. Nitric acid is a transparent, colorless, or yellowish fuming liquid. It is nonflammable, but when combined with other materials, can accelerate their burning. Its vapor pressure is 760 mm Hg at 25°C (77°F). Mists of nitric acid cannot be tolerated – even at low concentrations. A concentration of 100 ppm is considered immediately life-threatening because of its potential to cause asphyxiation.

Phosphoric acid (CAS #7664-38-2) is utilized for metal cleaning and rustproofing. In low concentrations, it can be used as a disinfectant. In very low concentrations it can have a pleasant taste, and is in fact found in Coca Cola™. Phosphoric acid is a colorless liquid or rhombic crystal as a solid. It becomes anhydrous when heated to 150°C (3020°F). Phosphoric acid has a low vapor pressure [0.0285 mm Hg at 20°C (68°F)]. When used as an agent for metal cleaning, phosphoric acid may react with impurities in the metal and release phosphine gas, which is highly flammable. Phosphine gas may explode in the presence of high temperatures; rescue workers must therefore use extreme caution if fires are burning at an accident site. In addition to its flammability, phosphine is a noncompetitive inhibitor of cytochrome oxidase resulting in the subsequent blockade of electron transfer and oxidative phosphorylation, particularly in the myocardium where cardiac arrhythmias and cardiovascular collapse may result.

Sodium hydroxide (CAS #1310-73-2) is used as a drain cleaner and as lye (96% to 100% solution). It is available commercially in Drano® (56% solution) and in Clinitest® tablets (54.2% sodium hydroxide). Sodium hydroxide is usually in the form of a whitish, lumpy solid that is easily liquefied. It is a prototype of alkaline caustics. This base can react violently with other chemical products (eg, acetic acid). By itself it is corrosive. It has a vapor pressure of 1 mm Hg at 739°C (1362°F).

Ammonium hydroxide (CAS #1336-21-6) can be found in common household cleaning products in concentrations ranging from 3% to 10%. It is also used in industry in the production of fertilizers, fibers, and other chemicals. Ammonium hydroxide is a colorless, alkaline liquid with a very pungent odor. In its anhydrous form (NH_3) it is a colorless alkaline gas.

Given the wide range of uses for these agents, it is hardly surprising that over 57,000 exposures to acidic and alkaline compounds are reported annually to reporting poison control centers.[58] Large quantities of these agents are produced yearly in the U.S. According to 1999 data reported in *Chemical and Engineering News*,[94] the following amounts of chemicals were produced in the U.S. that year (Table 3).

Table 3. Production Quantities of Selected Acids and Bases in U.S. in 2004	
Chemical	Amount (thousand tons)
Sulfuric acid	37,515
Hydrochloric acid	5,012
Nitric acid	6,703
Phosphoric acid	11,463
Sodium hydroxide	9,508
Anhydrous ammonia	10,762

Target Organs and Mechanisms of Action

Exposure is possible via ocular, dermal, inhalational, and oral routes; the eye, skin, and mucous membranes of the gastrointestinal and respiratory tracts constitute the major sites for caustic damage. The clinical syndrome observed will reflect the route, concentration, amount, and duration of exposure. Low concentrations of acids or alkalis act as irritants to the skin, eyes, and mucous membranes when exposure is brief. At higher concentrations or with prolonged exposure, these substances are corrosive. Systemic effects of caustic exposure may be manifested following severe burns, inhalation of fumes, or ingestion.

By definition, an acid is a proton donor while a base is a proton acceptor.[11,60] There are important differences between the burns induced by acidic and alkaline compounds. Alkali burns cause more significant and persistent changes in corneal, mucous membrane (GI and respiratory tract), and skin pH than do acid burns. Through the process of liquefactive necrosis, alkalis penetrate and destroy tissue to deeper levels via protein hydrolysis and lipid saponification. In contrast, acid burns tend to be dryer and more superficial since the affected tissue proteins upon desiccation and denaturation coagulate into an eschar which prevents deeper tissue damage.[6,8,14,15,24,81,83]

Deserving special attention, HF, a relatively weak inorganic acid ($pK_a = 3.8$) that is desiccating and corrosive like other acids, will produce coagulation necrosis of tissues; however, unique to HF is its ability to deeply penetrate tissues in a manner similar to alkalis where it exerts additional toxicity resulting in hypocalcemia, hypomagnesemia, and hyperkalemia.

Clinical Presentation

Common symptoms after exposure to caustic mists include tearing and burning of mucous membranes. Inhalation of acid mists can cause cough, dyspnea, choking, bronchoconstriction, and even pulmonary edema, sometimes delayed for 6-12 hours after the exposure. A chemical pneumonitis may also develop with many similarities to that caused by the nitrogen oxides.

Ocular and dermal exposure are painful, with erythema and vesicle formation initially, followed by obvious burns. Dermal burns progress rapidly within minutes necessitating rapid intervention, particularly for the more deeply penetrating alkali injuries. Tearing is noted initially after ocular injuries, and is followed by development of corneal erosions.

Acid or alkali ingestion may produce a variety of signs and/or symptoms including stridor, dyspnea, drooling, vomiting, dysphagia, odynophagia, perioral or oral burns, and pain in the chest, epigastrium, or abdomen. However, in a patient with a caustic ingestion history, the absence of these signs and/or symptoms, including oropharyngeal pain or burns, does not preclude serious injury to GI tract.[16,24,26,32,76,84,101,114-116] In adults, the most severe injuries are reported after suicidal ingestions. Acids are thought not to result in esophageal injury as often as with alkaline ingestions.[31,109] However, many studies have demonstrated acid-induced esophageal damage to be as frequent and severe as alkaline-induced esophageal damage.[27,43,63,115] Gastric and duodenal burns secondary to caustic ingestion are also quite common.[7,9,14,19,21,29,42,46,54,66,75,77,93,96,100,111,115] In either case, extensive tissue involvement may lead to perforation anywhere along the upper GI tract with life-threatening complications.[4,9,27,40,43,53,77,83,115] Respiratory distress in the patient following a caustic ingestion may be due to aspiration of the caustic, perforation of the GI tract resulting in mediastinitis, air, and/or fluid in the chest, or edema of the larynx and/or epiglottis.[21,23,52,71,73,83,92,99] There is generally little systemic absorption of these chemicals except infrequently in the case of severe nitric acid exposure associated with methemoglobinemia presenting clinically with cyanosis and respiratory distress.[36] Sulfuric acid and hydrochloric acid through their gastric absorption may also lead to a more severe metabolic acidosis accompanied by an increased anion gap or normal anion gap, respectively. More serious presentations subsequent to caustic ingestion may include signs and/or symptoms related to GI bleeding, DIC, or shock.[16,20,21,35,40,44,47,48,93,116]

Management Guidelines

Field Stabilization and Triage

In incidents with multiple casualties and/or limited transport or treatment facilities, some triage will be required.[95] At the site of a spill, rescue workers must be careful to wear protective clothing so they do not become secondarily contaminated by the caustic; polyvinylchloride or natural rubber gloves will protect the hands from serious HF dermal exposure. Respiratory protection should also be worn if mists are present.

The patient should be removed from the source of exposure. Assuming no traumatic or other injuries, serious extensive chemical burns will be evident if each victim's clothes are removed. All clothing must be removed to uncover any traumatic injuries or chemical burns.

Inhalational injury is an important consideration. Acid mists are heavier than air, but tend to disperse rapidly. If the patient's exposure is by inhalation, he or she should be moved into fresh air and given 100% oxygen. Attention to basic resuscitation principles is essential. Airway control (bag-valve-mask or intubation) is necessary if the patient has inadequate ventilatory effort or poor air exchange. Immediate transport is mandated if the patient is exhibiting signs of respiratory distress or is hypotensive.

For ocular or dermal exposure, the affected area should be copiously irrigated with water for at least 15 minutes; alkali burns require longer periods of irrigation.[15,97,102] Burns may become more severe if flushing is delayed for more than 1-2 minutes;[112] the final outcome of any chemically induced ocular injury is directly related to the duration of contact between the eye and the caustic substance.[97,102] Using a base to neutralize an acid (or vice versa) is not advised, because the heat of reaction may exacerbate the burn.[91] Contact lenses, rings, and other jewelry should be removed. Timely transport of the patient to an emergency department after decontamination and irrigation of external burns is essential. If only minor eye irritation is present without other symptoms, once adequate ocular irrigation is complete, evacuation may be delayed in deference to more seriously injured patients.

The history of exposure, vital signs, and predisposing medical conditions must be considered; if doubt remains, prompt emergency department observation is optimal. Patients with no evidence of respiratory distress, dermal, or ocular irritation are unlikely to have received a serious exposure at the spill site.

Emergency Department Management

The adequacy of field decontamination will usually be apparent – keys are removal of clothes, removal of gross contamination, and then copious irrigation with tepid water to stop the burning. The potential for secondary contamination is limited, but appropriate gloves (rubber or nitrile) and goggles are useful during gross decontamination.

In the emergency department, the physician should assume any dermal or ocular irrigation administered at the time of the injury to be inadequate. Immediate copious irrigation should be initiated for any acid or alkali burn. Ideally, this should be done in a decontamination room to minimize exposure to healthcare workers and other patients. Testing of dermal or ocular pH may be helpful after irrigation, which should continue until the pH is normalized.[15,17,97,102] Ocular findings may range from mere erythema of the conjunctivae in mild avid exposure to complete corneal opacification with permanent visual impairment and increased intraocular pressure in severe acid and alkali exposures. Ophthalmologic consultation is necessary for significant ocular burns.

Alkali burns of the skin and mucous membranes may range from white or gray areas with erythematous borders to complete tissue loss. Acid-induced dermal injuries appear as thermal burns with erythema, blistering, or full-thickness loss of skin.[108] Dermal injuries require standard burn management, except some would favor draining the acid-containing fluid from the acid-induced blisters. Patients with extensive dermal involvement require meticulous attention to the judiciously aggressive replacement of fluids.[78]

For patients with documented inhalational injuries or those presenting with stridor, rales, rhonchi, or dyspnea, chest x-rays and arterial blood gas level determinations are useful; however, changes may not be evident for several hours after exposure. One-hundred percent oxygen should be administered and airway intervention should be performed as necessary. Bronchodilators may be of some benefit in patients with bronchospasm. For HF inhalation, nebulized calcium gluconate (2.5%) may also be considered.

The clinician must view all caustic ingestions as life-threatening. A methodical strategy in the evaluation and treatment of the patient with a caustic ingestion must be followed (see Figure). The history must include the caustic's name and concentration along with the amount ingested and the time of ingestion. The signs and symptoms listed in the figure below should be sought. However, the clinician must remember that the absence of the signs and/or symptoms in a patient with a caustic ingestion does not necessarily indicate the absence of severe or life-threatening GI injury.

Emergency Management of Ingested Caustics

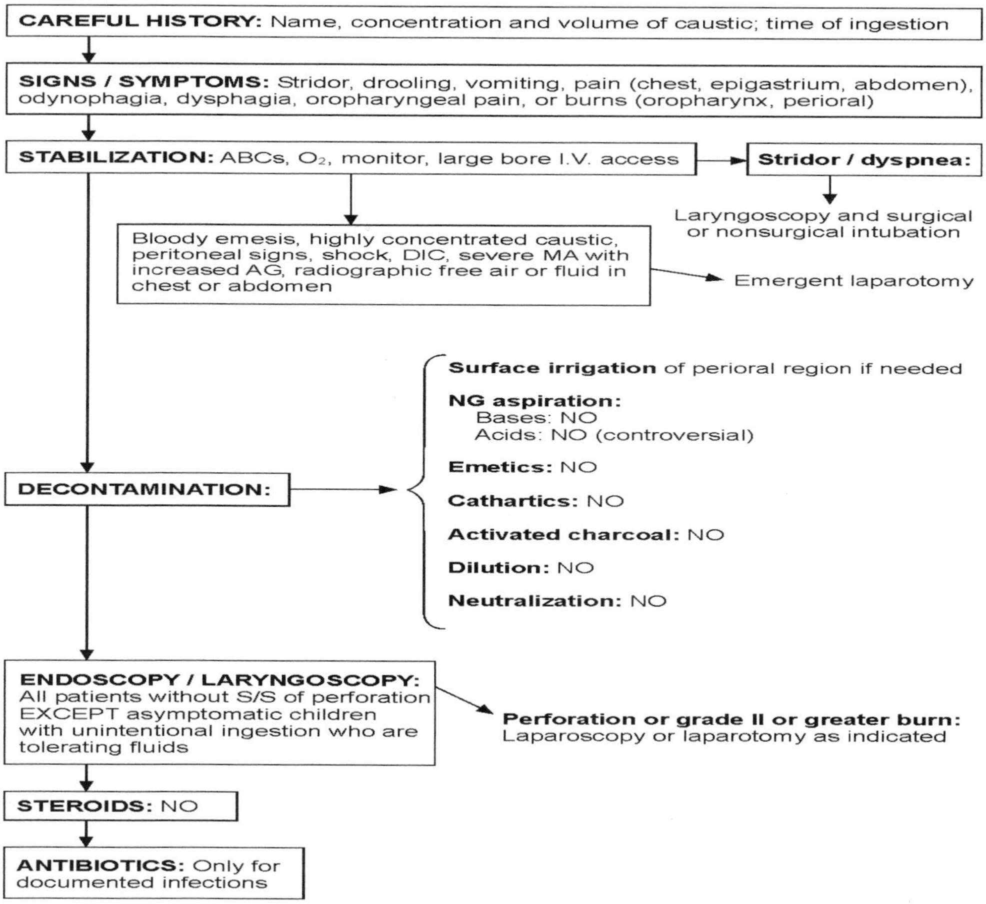

CAREFUL HISTORY: Name, concentration and volume of caustic; time of ingestion

SIGNS / SYMPTOMS: Stridor, drooling, vomiting, pain (chest, epigastrium, abdomen), odynophagia, dysphagia, oropharyngeal pain, or burns (oropharynx, perioral)

STABILIZATION: ABCs, O$_2$, monitor, large bore I.V. access → **Stridor / dyspnea:**

Laryngoscopy and surgical or nonsurgical intubation

Bloody emesis, highly concentrated caustic, peritoneal signs, shock, DIC, severe MA with increased AG, radiographic free air or fluid in chest or abdomen → Emergent laparotomy

DECONTAMINATION:
- **Surface irrigation** of perioral region if needed
- **NG aspiration:**
  - Bases: NO
  - Acids: NO (controversial)
- **Emetics:** NO
- **Cathartics:** NO
- **Activated charcoal:** NO
- **Dilution:** NO
- **Neutralization:** NO

ENDOSCOPY / LARYNGOSCOPY: All patients without S/S of perforation EXCEPT asymptomatic children with unintentional ingestion who are tolerating fluids → **Perforation or grade II or greater burn:** Laparoscopy or laparotomy as indicated

STEROIDS: NO

ANTIBIOTICS: Only for documented infections

Stabilization: An aggressive approach to airway stabilization in the symptomatic patient must be executed. Laryngoscopy with surgical or nonsurgical airway placement may be required. Continual monitoring of the respiratory and cardiovascular status of all caustic ingestion patients is essential. Immediate I.V. access should be established for fluid administration. Emergent surgical consultation is necessary in any ingestion patient with bloody emesis, peritoneal signs, metabolic acidosis (pH < 7.2) with an increased anion gap or air, and/or fluid in the chest or abdomen.[18,29,48,61,64,69,110,113]

Decontamination: Dermal irrigation of the perioral region may be necessary in the caustic ingestion patient with facial burns. Decontamination procedures should not include emetics which may result in esophageal re-exposure to the caustic, cathartics which may actually extend the area of injury along the GI tract, or activated charcoal which does not adsorb caustics and will interfere with subsequent endoscopy. Even though nasogastric suction of alkali from the stomach is contraindicated, some authors advocate gentle suction of acid which has pooled in the stomach.[20,30,31,50,74] This practice remains controversial due to the risk of perforation within the GI tract.

Dilution: Dilutional techniques in the caustic ingestion patient are unproven since they have never been adequately studied in humans.[21,30,39,51,104] In that dilutional therapy increases the risk of vomiting in the poisoned patient resulting in esophageal re-exposure to the caustic and possible aspiration and perforation, diluents should be utilized very cautiously, if at all.

Neutralization: Neutralization therapy is controversial and should not be utilized in the routine ED management of patients with caustic ingestions.[24,80,84,91,98,104]

Endoscopy/Laryngoscopy: Unless signs of GI tract perforation are present which mandate emergent surgical intervention, immediate laryngoscopy/endoscopy is necessary in all patients who have ingested acidic or alkaline compounds, except for the child with an unintentional ingestion who is asymptomatic and tolerating liquids.[3,4,9,16,18,32,39,40,48,49,55,56,59,66,76,79,82,83,93,100,106,113,115,116] The majority of studies involving caustic ingestions have demonstrated that the presence or absence of a patient's signs and/or symptoms at presentation does not reliably predict the presence or absence of serious injury to the GI tract.[21,22,26,29,33,43,70,80,84,87,101,111,114,116] A qualified endoscopist should evaluate the laryngeal region as well as the esophagus, stomach, and duodenum utilizing Zargar's classification of any observed burns (Table 4).[116] Any necrotic areas or perforations of the GI tract noted during endoscopy should result in an immediate surgical consultation.

Corticosteroid administration: The use of corticosteroids may prevent the recognition of gastrointestinal tract perforation.[20,31] Patient studies of caustic ingestions have also revealed that first degree burns (grade 1) do not progress to stricture formation in the esophagus, while all third degree burns (grade 3) progress to stricture formation in patients receiving or not receiving corticosteroids. No study has appropriately evaluated the effect of steroids in patients with grade 2 (a or b) burns. Therefore, corticosteroid administration to the patient with a caustic ingestion can not be recommended.[1,2,10,12-14,29,41,43,65,67,85,105,116]

Antibiotics: Antibiotic therapy should be reserved only for documented infections.

Routine labs should include a complete blood cell count, electrolytes, blood urea nitrogen, creatinine, coagulation studies, liver function tests, arterial blood gas, chest and abdominal radiographs (rule out aspiration pneumonitis, free air, or effusion), and stool for Hemoccult®. Methemoglobin levels should be obtained in patients with known nitric acid exposure and in those patients presenting with cyanosis.

The assessment of HF exposure deserves special mention. The patient's presentation depends on the amount and concentration of HF as well as the route and duration of exposure. Patients exposed to <20% HF may not be symptomatic for up to 24 hours postexposure; 20% to 50% HF usually produces symptoms within 8 hours, while >50% HF results in immediate symptoms. Dermal exposure constitutes the most common route with the majority of HF injuries involving the hands. Progressive itching, burning, and pain with signs ranging from early erythema to blisters and necrotic (eschar) areas occur. Topical application of a 2.5% calcium gluconate gel (3.5 g calcium gluconate powder in 150 mL of K-Y® jelly) should be initiated with pain elimination as the goal. Should the calcium gluconate gel fail, then subcutaneous injection of 10% calcium gluconate should follow. The area of injured tissue may be infiltrated subcutaneously with a small gauge needle utilizing 0.5 mL/cm^2. Use of subcutaneous injection in digits is limited because of the potential to compromise local circulation. In the case of more severe burns to the hands or feet, intra-arterial (radial, brachial, posterior tibial, femoral) calcium gluconate infusion may be required. 10 mL of 10% calcium gluconate solution added to 40 mL of NS or $_5$W may be infused into the artery over 4 hours with pain resolution as the goal. Tissues of the eye are very sensitive to HF. Symptoms include tearing, injection of the conjunctivae, and pain. Corneal denudation and scarring may result. HF is a mucosal irritant of both the upper and lower respiratory tract. Mild, non-life-threatening irritation of the upper airway to florid pulmonary edema ending in death may be observed. In HF ingestions, abdominal pain associated with nausea and vomiting are commonly observed. Erosions of the upper GI tract to severe colitis with perforation may occur. Theoretically, HF's systemic effects can be seen following any route of exposure, but are rare after ocular exposure. Most commonly, hypocalcemia, hypomagnesemia, and hyperkalemia may lead to respiratory failure, hypotension, and cardiac arrhythmias.

Sequelae

The short term complications of serious chemical burns to be cognizant of are similar to those of thermal burns, including pneumonia, cellulitis, sepsis, gastrointestinal bleeding, renal failure, and thromboembolism. Possible systemic effects of ingestion to be anticipated include metabolic acidosis, hypotension, disseminated intravascular coagulation, shock, and potentially death.

The long-term effects of caustic exposure that may be observed are numerous. Severe caustic burns to the eye may result in corneal scarring, cataracts, glaucoma, or blindness. Dermal burns may persist as indolent ulcers or permanent scars. Inhalational caustic injuries may produce long-term morbidity ranging from pulmonary fibrosis and bronchiectasis to chronic obstructive airway disease. Ingestion of caustics resulting in severe gastrointestinal burns may lead to strictures of the esophagus, stomach, and duodenum.[19,25,46,96,111] Esophageal shortening and motility dysfunction as well as a gastric dumping syndrome or achlorhydria with a resultant pernicious anemia may also result from caustic ingestions.[8,37,38,47,62,68,89,90] Caustic-induced injury to the laryngeal region may result in dysphonia, aphonia, and aspiration-related problems in the patient.[23,34,52,71,86,88,92,99,103,107] There are no reported teratogenic properties associated with either acids or bases; however, squamous cell carcinoma and adenocarcinoma of the esophagus and stomach have been reported up to 40 years after the ingestion of corrosives.[5,28,45,57,72]

Disposition

Patients should be admitted to the hospital for evidence of functionally significant burns to the hand, foot, or perineum, any circumferential burn where vascular compromise may occur, or for a burn with >25% involvement of body surface area. The patient should be admitted at a center where there are qualified burn specialists, or plastic and hand surgeons. Parenteral antibiotics should not be initiated until positive cultures document the presence of an infection. Also, a patient with significant inhalation injury with evidence of an elevated arterial-alveolar gradient should be kept for observation. Appropriate disposition of the caustic ingestion patient may be based on the burn grade discovered during endoscopic evaluation (Table 4).[116] Grade 0 (normal exam) or grade 1 burns: admit to the regular floor, allow P.O. intake as tolerated, prescribe antacids, and administer analgesics as needed. Most of these patients will return home within 48 hours on antacids. Grade 2a burns: hospital management is identical to the grade 0 and grade 1 burns, but the patient's discharge home on antacids occurs somewhat later (5-11 days). Grade 2b and grade 3 (a or b) burns: these patients require a much more prolonged hospitalization in the ICU, NPO status with I.V. hydration, and appropriate nutritional support. Close monitoring for possible complications such as perforation, airway obstruction, and shock is essential.

Table 4. Endoscopic Caustic Burn Classification	
Grade 0	Normal exam
Grade 1	Edema and hyperemia of the mucosa
Grade 2a	Mucosal friability, blisters, hemorrhages, erosions, whitish membranes, exudates, superficial ulcerations
Grade 2b	Grade 2a plus deep discrete or circumferential ulceration
Grade 3a	Small scattered areas of multiple ulcerations and necrosis
Grade 3b	Extensive necrosis

From Zargar SA, Kochhar R, Mehta S, et al, "The Role of Fiberoptic Endoscopy in the Management of Corrosive Ingestion and Modified Endoscopic Classification of Burns," *Gastrointest Endosc*, 1991, 37(2):165-9.

References

1. Alford BR and Harris HH, "Chemical Burns of the Mouth, Pharynx and Esophagus," *Ann Otol*, 1959, 66:122-8.
2. Anderson KD, Rouse TM, and Randolph JG, "A Controlled Trial of Corticosteroids in Children with Corrosive Injury of the Esophagus," *N Eng J Med*, 1990, 323(10):637-40.
3. Andreoni B, Farina ML, Biffi R, et al, "Esophageal Perforation and Caustic Injury: Emergency Management of Caustic Ingestion," *Dis Esophagus*, 1997, 10(2):95-100.
4. Andreoni B, Marini A, Gavinelli M, et al, "Emergency Management of Caustic Ingestion in Adults," *Surg Today*, 1995, 25(2):119-24.

5. Appelqvist P and Salmo M, "Lye Corrosion Carcinoma of the Esophagus: A Review of 63 Cases," *Cancer*, 1980, 45(10):2655-8.

6. Ashcraft KW and Padula RT, "The Effect of Dilute Corrosives on the Esophagus," *Pediatrics*, 1974, 53(2):226-32.

7. Aviram G, Kessler A, Reif S, et al, "Corrosive Gastritis: Sonographic Findings in the Acute Phase and Follow-up," *Pediatr Radiol*, 1997, 27(10):805-6.

8. Bautista A, Varela R, Villanueva A, et al, "Motor Function of the Esophagus After Caustic Burn," *Eur J Pediatr Surg*, 1996, 6(4):204-7.

9. Berthet B, Castellani P, Brioche MI, et al, "Early Operation for Severe Corrosive Injury of the Upper Gastrointestinal Tract," *Eur J Surg*, 1996, 162(12):951-5.

10. Bikhazi HB, Thompson ER, and Shumrick DA, "Caustic Ingestion: Current Status: A Report of 105 Cases," *Arch Otolaryngol*, 1969, 89(5):770-3.

11. Bronsted JN, "Some Remarks on the Concept of Acids and Bases," *Recueil des Travaux Chimiques des Pays-Bas*, 1923, 42:718-28.

12. Byrne WJ, "Foreign Bodies, Bezoars, and Caustic Ingestion," *Gastrointest Endosc Clin N Am*, 1994, 4(1):99-119.

13. Cannon S and Chandler JR, "Corrosive Burns of the Esophagus: Analysis of 100 Patients," *Eye Ear Nose Throat Mon*, 1963, 42:35-44.

14. Cardona JC and Daly JF, "Current Management of Corrosive Esophagitis," *Ann Otol Rhinol Laryngol*, 1971, 80:521-7.

15. Cartotto RC, Peters WJ, Neligan PC, et al, "Chemical Burns," *Can J Surg*, 1996, 39(3):205-11.

16. Casasnovas AB, Martinez EE, Cives RV, et al, "A Retrospective Analysis of Ingestion of Caustic Substances by Children: Ten-Year Statistics in Galicia," *Eur J Pediatr*, 1997, 156(5):410-4.

17. Catalano RA, *Ocular Emergencies*, Philadelphia, PA: WB Saunders Company, 1992, 179-90.

18. Celerier M, "Management of Caustic Esophagitis in Adults," *Ann Chir* 1996, 50(6):449-55.

19. Chaudhary A, Puri AS, Dhar P, et al, "Elective Surgery for Corrosive-Induced Gastric Injury," *World J Surg*, 1996 20(6):703-6.

20. Chodak GW and Passaro E Jr, "Acid Ingestion: Need for Gastic Resection," *JAMA*, 1978, 239(3):225-6.

21. Christesen HB, "Prediction of Complications Following Caustic Ingestion in Adults," *Clin Otolaryngol*, 1995, 20(3):272-8.

22. Christesen HB, "Prediction of Complications Following Unintentional Caustic Ingestion in Children: Is Endoscopy Always Necessary?" *Acta Paediatr*, 1995, 84(10):1177-82.

23. Clausen JO, Nielsen TL, and Fogh A, "Admission to Danish Hospitals After Suspected Ingestion of Corrosives: A Nationwide Survey (1984-1988) Comprising Children Aged 0-14 Years," *Dan Med Bull*, 1994, 41(2):234-7.

24. Clifton JC II, "Acid Ingestion," Ford M, Delaney K, Ling L, et al, eds, *Clinical Toxicology*, Philadelphia, PA: W.B. Saunders Company, 2001, 1009-18.

25. Cochran ST, Fonkalsrud EW, and Gyepes MT, "Complete Obstruction of the Gastric Antrum in Children Following Acid Ingestion," *Arch Surg*, 1978, 113(3):308-10.

26. Crain EF, Gershel JC, and Mezey AP, "Caustic Ingestions: Symptoms as Predictors of Esophageal Injury," *Am J Dis Child*, 1984, 138(9):863-5.

27. Dilawari JB, Singh S, Rao PN, et al, "Corrosive Acid Ingestion in Man – A Clinical and Endoscopic Study," *Gut*, 1984, 25(2):183-7.

28. Eaton H and Tennekoon GE, "Squamous Carcinoma of the Stomach Following Corrosive Acid Burns," *Br J Surg*, 1972, 59(5):382-7.

29. Estrera A, Taylor W, Mills LJ, et al, "Corrosive Burns of the Esophagus and Stomach: A Recommendation for an Aggressive Surgical Approach," *Ann Thorac Surg*, 1986, 41(3):276-83.

30. Fisher RA, Eckhauser ML, and Radivoyevitch M, "Acid Ingestion in an Experimental Model," *Surg Gynecol Obstet*, 1985, 161(1):91-9.

31. Ford M, "Alkali and Acid Injuries of the Upper Gastrointestinal Tract," Hoffman RS and Goldfrank LR, eds, *Critical Care Toxicology*, New York, NY: Churchill Livingston, 1991, 225-49.

32. Gaudreault P, Parent M, McGuigan MA, et al, "Predictability of Esophageal Injury from Signs and Symptoms: A Study of Caustic Ingestion in 378 Children," *Pediatrics*, 1983, 71(5):767-70.

33. Gorman RL, Khin-Maung-Gyi MT, Klein-Schwartz W, et al, "Initial Symptoms as Predictors of Esophageal Injury in Alkaline Corrosive Ingestions," *Am J Emerg Med*, 1992, 10(3):189-94.

34. Gregor RT, "The Use of Carbon Dioxide Laser in Dealing with Fibrous Strictures of the Larynx and Trachea," *J Otolaryngol*, 1988, 17(1):16-8.

35. Greif F and Kaplan O, "Acid Ingestion: Another Cause of Disseminated Intravascular Coagulopathy," *Crit Care Med*, 1986, 14(11):990-1.

36. Griffin JP, "Methaemoglobinaemia," *Adverse Drug React Toxicol Rev*, 1997, 16(1):45-63.

37. Guelrud M, "Esophageal Motor Abnormalities After Lye Ingestion," *Am J Gastroenterol*, 1996, 91(11):2450.

38. Guelrud M and Arocha M, "Motor Function Abnormalities in Acute Caustic Esophagitis," *J Clin Gastroenterol*, 1980, 2(3):247-50.

39. Gumaste VV and Dave PB, "Ingestion of Corrosive Substances by Adults," *Am J Gastroenterol*, 1992, 87(1):1-5.

40. Guth AA, Pachter HL, Albanese C, et al, "Combined Duodenal and Colonic Necrosis: An Unusual Sequela of Caustic Ingestion," *J Clin Gastroenterol*, 1994, 19(4):303-5.

41. Haller JA Jr, Andrews HG, White JJ, et al, "Pathophysiology and Management of Acute Corrosive Burns of the Esophagus: Results of Treatment of 285 Children," *J Pediatr Surg*, 1971, 6(5):578-84.

42. Harness J, "Surgery Grand Rounds: Diagnosis and Treatment of Acid Gastric Burns, *New Physician*, 1976 25:70-4.

43. Hawkins DB, Demeter MJ, and Barnett TE, "Caustic Ingestion: Controversies in Management: A Review of 214 Cases," *Laryngoscope*, 1980, 90(1):98-109.

44. Holinger PH, "Corrosive Esophagitis Due to Nitric Acid," *Laryngoscope*, 1953, 63:789-807.

45. Hopkins RA and Postlethwait RW, "Caustic Burns and Carcinoma of the Esophagus," *Ann Surg* 1981, 194(2):146-8.

46. Hsu CP, Chen CY, Hsu NY, et al, "Surgical Treatment and Its Long-Term Result for Caustic-Induced Prepyloric Obstruction," *Eur J Surg*, 1997, 163:(4)275-9.

47. Jelenko C 3rd, Story J, and Ellison RG Jr, "Ingestion of Mineral Acid," *South Med J*, 1972, 65(7):868-71.

48. Jeng LB, Chen HY, Chen SC, et al, "Upper Gastrointestinal Tract Ablation for Patients with Extensive Injury After Ingestion of Strong Acid," *Arch Surg*, 1994, 129(10):1086-90.

49. Karjoo M, "Caustic Ingestion and Foreign Bodies in the Gastrointestinal System," *Curr Opin Pediatr*, 1998, 10(5):516-22.

50. Kikendall JW, "Caustic Ingestion Injuries," *Gastroenterol Clin North Am*, 1991, 20(4):847-57.

51. Knopp R, "Caustic Ingestions," *JACEP*, 1979, 8(8):329-36.

52. Kornak JM, Freije JE, and Campbell BH, "Caustic and Thermal Epiglottitis in the Adult," *Otolaryngol Head Neck Surg*, 1996, 114(2):310-2.

53. Kushimo T and Ekanem MM, "Acid Ingestion in a 2-Day Old Baby," *West Afr J Med*, 1997, 16(2):121-3.

54. Lai KH, Huang BS, Huang MH, et al, "Emergency Surgical Intervention for Severe Corrosive Injuries of the Upper Digestive Tract," *Chung Hua I Hsueh Tsa Chih* (Taipei), 1995, 56(l):40-6.

55. Lambert H, Renaud D, Weber M, et al, "Current Treatment of Poisoning by Ingestion of Caustic Substances," *J Toxicol Clin Exp*, 1992, 12(1):11-26.

56. Lamireau T, Llanas B, Deprez C, et al, "Severity of Ingestion of Caustic Substance in Children," *Arch Pediatr*, 1997, 4(6):529-34.

57. Linden CH, "Inorganic Acids and Bases," *Hazardous Materials Toxicology: Clinical Principles of Environmental Disease*, 1st ed, Sullivan J and Krieger G, eds, Baltimore, MD: Williams and Wilkins, 1992.

58. Litovitz TL, Klein-Schwartz W, White S, et al, "1999 Annual Report of the American Association of Poison Control Centers Toxic Exposure Surveillance System," *Am J Emerg Med*, 2000, 18(5):517-74.

59. Lovejoy FH Jr and Woolf AD, "Corrosive Ingestions," *Pediatr Rev*, 1995, 16(12):473-4.

60. Lowry TM, "The Uniqueness of Hydrogen," *Chemistry and Industry*, 1923, 42:43-7.

61. Martel W, "Radiologic Features of Esophagogastritis Secondary to Extremely Caustic Agents," *Radiology*, 1972, 103(1):31-6.

62. Maull KI, Scher LA, and Greenfield LJ, "Surgical Implications of Acid Ingestion," *Surg Gynecol Obstet*, 1979, 148(6):895-8.

63. Muhletaler CA, Gerlock AJ Jr, DeSoto L, et al, "Acid Corrosive Esophagitis: Radiographic Findings," *AJR Am J Roentgenol*, 1980, 134(6):1137-40.

64. Meredith JW, Kon ND, and Thompson JN, "Management of Injuries from Liquid Lye Ingestion," *J Trauma*, 1988, 28(8):1173-80.

65. Middelkamp JN, Ferguson TB, Roper CL, et al, "The Management and Problems of Caustic Burns in Children," *J Thorac Cardiovasc Surg*, 1969, 57(4):341-7.

66. Mitani M, Hirata K, Fukuda M, et al, "Endoscopic Ultrasonography in Corrosive Injury of the Upper Gastrointestinal Tract by Hydrochloric Acid," *J Clin Ultrasound*, 1996, 24(1):40-2.

67. Moazam F, Talbert JL, Miller D, et al, "Caustic Ingestion and Its Sequelae in Children," *South Med J*, 1987, 80(2):187-90.

68. Mutaf O, Genc A, Herek O, et al, "Gastroesophageal Reflux: A Determinant in the Outcome of Caustic Esophageal Burns," *J Pediatr Surg*, 1996, 31(11):1494-5.

69. Noirclerc M, DiCostanzo J, Sastre B, et al, "Surgical Management of Caustic Injuries to the Upper Gastrointestinal Tract," DeMeester TR and Matthews HR, eds, *International Trends in General Thoracic Surgery*, St Louis, MO: CV Mosby, 1987, 261-5.

70. Nuutinen M, Uhari M, Karvali T, et al, "Consequences of Caustic Ingestions in Children," *Acta Paediatr*, 1994, 83(11):1200-5.

71. Ochi K, Ohashi T, Sato S, et al, "Surgical Treatment for Caustic Ingestion Injury of the Pharynx, Larynx, and Esophagus," *Acta Otolaryngol Suppl*, (Stockh), 1996, 522:116-9.

72. O'Donnell CH, Abbott WE, and Hirshfield JW, "Surgical Treatment of Corrosive Gastritis," *Am J Surg*, 1949, 78:251-5.

73. Parsons DS, Smith RB, Mair EA, et al, "Unique Case Presentations of Acute Epiglottic Swelling and a Protocol for Acute Airway Compromise," *Laryngoscope*, 1996, 106(10):1287-91.

74. Penner GE, "Acid Ingestion: Toxicology and Treatment," *Ann Emerg Med*, 1980, 9(7):374-9.

75. Phelps G, Srinivasa A, and Sengupta SK, "Gastric Stenosis Following the Ingestion of Car Battery Acid," *PNG Med J*, 1991, 34(l):61-4.

76. Previtera C, Giusti F, and Guglielmi M, "Predictive Value of Visible Lesions (Cheeks, Lips, Oropharynx) in Suspected Caustic Ingestion: May Endoscopy Reasonably Be Omitted in Completely Negative Pediatric Patients?" *Pediatr Emerg Care*, 1990, 6(3):176-8.

77. Ribet ME, "Esophagogastrectomy for Acid Injury," *Ann Thorac Surg*, 1992, 53(4):739.

78. Richard R and Staley M, eds, *Burn Care and Rehabilitation: Principles and Practice*, Philadelphia, PA: FA Davis, 1994.

79. Romanczuk W and Korczowski R, "The Significance of Early Panendoscopy in Caustic Ingestion in Children," *Turk J Pediatr*, 1992, 34(2):93-8.

80. Rothstein FC, "Caustic Injuries to the Esophagus in Children," *Pediatr Clin North Am*, 1986, 33(3): 665-74.

81. Rubin MM, Jui V, and Cozzi GM, "Treatment of Caustic Ingestion," *J Oral Maxillofac Surg*, 1989, 47(3):286-90.

82. Sarfati E, Gossot D, Assens P, et al, "Management of Caustic Ingestion in Adults," *Br J Surg*, 1987, 74(2):146-8.

83. Sarfati E, Jacob L, Servant JM, et al, "Tracheobronchial Necrosis After Caustic Ingestion," *J Thorac Cardiovasc Surg*, 1992, 103(3):412-3.

84. Scher LA and Maull KI, "Emergency Management and Sequelae of Acid Ingestions," *JACEP*, 1978, 7(5):206-8.

85. Schild JA, "Caustic Ingestion in Adult Patients," *Laryngoscope*, 1985, 95(10):1199-201.

86. Scott JC, Jones B, Eisele DW, et al, "Caustic Ingestion Injuries of the Upper Aerodigestive Tract," *Laryngoscope*, 1992, 102(1):1-8.

87. Sellars SL and Spence RA, "Chemical Burns of the Oesophagus," *J Laryngol Otol*, 1987, 101(11): 1211-3.

88. Shikowitz MJ, Levy J, Villano D, et al, "Speech and Swallowing Rehabilitation Following Devastating Caustic Ingestion: Techniques and Indicators for Success," *Laryngoscope*, 1996, 106(2 Pt 2 Su 78): 1-12.

89. Shirazi S, Schulze-Delrieu K, Custer-Hagen T, et al, "Motility Changes in Opossum Esophagus From Experimental Esophagitis," *Dig Dis Sci*, 1989, 34(11):1668-76.

90. Sinar DR, Fletcher JR, Cordova CC, et al, "Acute Acid-Induced Esophagitis Impairs Esophageal Peristalsis in Baboons," *Gastroenterol*, 1981, 80:1286.

91. Smilkstein MJ, "Should We Add an Acid to an Alkali Injury? For Now, Let's Remain Neutral!" *Acad Emerg Med*, 1995, 2(11):945-6.

92. Soo G and van Hasselt CA, "Caustic Injury of the Larynx," *Otolaryngol Head Neck Surg*, 1998, 119(4):425-6.

93. Stiff G, Alwafi A, Rees BI, et al, "Corrosive Injuries of the Oesophagus and Stomach: Experience in Management at a Regional Paediatric Centre," *Ann R Coll Surg Engl* , 1996, 78(2):119-23.

94. McCoy M, Reisch M, and Tullo AH, "Facts and Figures for the Chemical Industry: Production," *C&EN*, 2005, 83(28):67-76.

95. Stutz DR and Ulin S, *Hazardous Materials Injuries: A Handbook for Prehospital Care*, 4th ed, Beltsville, MD: Bradford Communications Corp, 1997.

96. Tamisani AM, Di Noto C, and Di Rovasenda E, "A Rare Complication Due to Sulfuric Acid Ingestion," *Eur J Pediatr Surg*, 1992, 2(3):162-4.

97. Terzidou C and Georgiadis N, "A Simple Ocular Irrigation System for Alkaline Burns of the Eye," *Ophthalmic Surg Lasers*, 1997, 28(3):255-7.

98. Tucker JA and Yarrington CT Jr, "The Treatment of Caustic Ingestion," *Otolaryngol Clin North Am*, 1979, 12(2):343-50.

99. Vergauwen P, Moulin D, Buts JP, et al, "Caustic Burns of the Upper Digestive and Respiratory Tracts," *Eur J Pediatr*, 1991, 150(10):700-3.

100. Vila Carbo JJ, Gutierrez San Roman C, Garcia-Sala Viguer C, et al, "Caustic Burns of the Stomach Secondary to Ingestion of Acid in Infants: Importance of Fibro-Endoscopy," *An Esp Pediatr*, 1990, 32(5):451-4.

101. Viscomi GJ, Jan Beekhius G, and Whitten CF, "An Evaluation of Early Esophagoscopy and Corticosteroid Therapy in the Management of Corrosive Injury of the Esophagus," *J Pediatrics*, 1961, 59:356-60.

102. Wagoner MD, "Chemical Injuries of the Eye: Current Concepts in Pathophysiology and Therapy," *Surv Ophthalmol*, 1997, 41(4):275-313.

103. Wang Z, "Dilation of Simultaneous Laryngeal and Esophageal Stricture With Two T-Tubes," *J Laryngol Otol*, 1994, 108(1):42-3.

104. Wasserman RL and Ginsburg CM, "Caustic Substance Injuries," *J Pediatrics*, 1985, 107(2):169-74.

105. Webb WR, Koutras P, Ecker RR, et al, "An Evaluation of Steroids and Antibiotics in Caustic Burns of the Esophagus," *Ann Thorac Surg*, 1970, 9(2):95-102.

106. Wijburg FA, Heymans HS, and Urbanus NA, "Caustic Esophageal Lesions in Childhood: Prevention of Stricture Formation," *J Pediatr Surg*, 1989, 24(2):171-3.

107. Williams DC, "Acute Respiratory Obstruction Caused by Ingestion of a Caustic Substance," *Br Med J (Clin Res Ed)*, 1985, 291(6491):313-4.

108. Winder C, "Medical Treatment of Caustic Burns," *Med J Aust*, 1997, 167(9):511-2.

109. Wormald PJ and Wilson DA, "Battery Acid Burns of the Upper Gastrointestinal Tract," *Clin Otolaryngol*, 1993, 18(2):112-4.

110. Wu MH and Lai WW, "Surgical Management of Extensive Corrosive Injuries of the Alimentary Tract," *Surg Gynecol Obstet*, 1993, 177(1):12-6.

111. Yamataka A, Pringle KC, and Wyeth J, "A Case of Zinc Chloride Ingestion," *J Pediatr Surg*, 1998, 33(4):660-2.

112. Yano K, Hata Y, Matsuka K, et al, "Experimental Study on Alkaline Skin Injuries: Periodic Changes in Subcutaneous Tissue pH and the Effects Exerted by Washing," *Burns*, 1993, 19(4):320-3.

113. Yararbai O, Osmanodlu H, Kaplan H, et al, "Esophagocoloplasty in the Management of Postcorrosive Strictures of the Esophagus," *Hepatogastroenterology*, 1998, 45(19):59-64.

114. Yarington CT Jr, "Ingestion of Caustic: A Pediatric Problem," *J Pediatr*, 1965, 67(4):674-7.

115. Zargar SA, Kochhar R, Nagi B, et al, "Ingestion of Corrosive Acids. Spectrum of Injury to Upper Gastrointestinal Tract and Natural History," *Gastroenterology*, 1989, 97(3):702-7.

116. Zargar SA, Kochhar R, Mehta S, et al, "The Role of Fiberoptic Endoscopy in the Management of Corrosive Ingestion and Modified Endoscopic Classification of Burns," *Gastrointest Endosc*, 1991, 37(2):165-9.

117. Jovic-Stosic J, Babic G, Todorvic V, et al, "Treatment of Esophageal Stricture Due to Corrosive Substance Ingestion," *J Toxicol Clin Toxicol*, 2001, 39(3):296.

EXAMPLES OF MASS EXPOSURES INVOLVING THE PEDIATRIC POPULATION

Carl R. Baum, MD, FAAP, FACMT

The Case of the Hapless Hyperventilating Hockey Players

In Massachusetts, 12 school-age children and some of their family members went to an away peewee league hockey tournament in the western part of the state, where they stayed in a local hotel, swam in the hotel pool, and had meals within the town. Over the course of the next 2-5 weeks, 16 of the children, 12 boys and 4 girls, some hockey players, and some siblings of the players, presented to a regional toxicology clinic on referral from their pediatricians with a similar constellation of symptoms, most noting fatigue as well as skin and respiratory problems, and most of the symptoms had persisted since the hockey weekend. The children, whose ages ranged from 7 to 14 years, had some or all of the following: fatigue with significantly decreased tolerance for exercise; a subtle white or ashy-appearing rash; a dry, nonproductive hacking cough; chest tightness; wheezing; irritated mucous membranes, mostly involving the eyes with some nasal irritation; diffuse abdominal pain; nausea; and some emesis. The patients were afebrile, with vital signs within the normal ranges, and their physical exams were otherwise unremarkable, other than the aforementioned rash and irritated mucous membranes. With the exception of one child who had asthma, none of the others had significant medical histories, and all were healthy and active prior to the hockey weekend. Some of the children experienced onset of symptoms during the hockey weekend, and some within 1-2 days after the weekend. None of the adults who attended the hockey tournament were known to have any of these symptoms.[1]

Consider the following:

1. How would you plan and organize the assessment and evaluation of multiple patients with multiple symptoms?
2. What further information and what laboratory evaluations, if any, would you need to obtain?
3. What would you tell the patients, their parents, and their pediatricians?

This article describes a series of incidents in this century during which large numbers of people have become ill or even died because of the exposures to a variety of toxins. This "world tour" will bring us to a number of sites, beginning in the United States (1937); Minamata Bay, Japan (1956); Seveso, Italy (1976); Port Pirie, S. Australia (1979-82); New Orleans, LA (1981); Bhopal, India (1984); Chernobyl, Ukraine (1986); Tokyo, Japan (1995); and Haiti (1996).

What can be learned from mass exposures? While these events may not reflect the day-to-day experiences of physicians in the clinic or emergency room, much can be learned from the way the incidents are reported and studied, which helps us describe and understand the effect of these toxins over the very long term, the importance of regulatory agencies, and the elements of an environmental history. Finally, mass exposures remind us that there are no accidents; rather, series of errors occur, sometimes over many years, that go unnoticed and culminate in catastrophic events.

United States (1937)

This was an important year in infectious diseases because the antibiotic sulfanilamide was introduced. Pharmaceutical companies rushed to produce this miracle drug. Among them was the Massengill Company, which anticipated a need, especially among children, for a liquid preparation. The company knew that the drug could not simply be dissolved without the use of a solvent. In this case, they chose diethylene glycol (DEG) to help develop the elixir of sulfanilamide. DEG, like ethylene glycol, is an antifreeze and solvent and was an inexpensive and effective solvent for the elixir. The elixir was subjected to and passed Massengill's tests for appearance, flavor, and fragrance. The company did not test the safety of the new product.

DEG, discovered in 1869, is a condensation product of ethylene glycol manufacture. It did not become commercially available until 1928. By 1937, the entire world literature on DEG consisted of a few rodent studies that suggested probable toxicity. These data were ignored, and production of 228 gallons of the DEG-based elixir proceeded. Over the subsequent 4 weeks, 353 patients received the elixir for a variety of indications, such as gonorrhea, tonsillitis, otitis, and soft-tissue infections. The instructions read as follows:

... begin with 2-3 teaspoonfuls in water every 4 hours. Decrease in 24-48 hours to 1-2 teaspoonfuls and continue at this dose until recovery.

Many did not recover. In fact, a number of patients taking the elixir developed new symptoms, including nausea and emesis, followed by flank pain, anuria, coma, and seizures. Gastrointestinal disturbances may have limited absorption of the elixir. Some died. It was estimated that a fatal cumulative dose was 10 teaspoonfuls for children or 20 teaspoonfuls for adults. Mean survival after the first dose was 9 days (range 2-22 days). There were clusters of cases around the country, in East St Louis, Tulsa, and Charleston. Only 6 gallons of elixir were eventually distributed, but the death toll was 34 children and 71 adults. Postmortem examination revealed "hydropic tubular nephrosis," or vacuolar nephropathy. Unlike ethylene glycol poisoning, no calcium oxalate deposition was observed in the renal tubules. A centrilobular hepatic degeneration was seen.

The disaster did have some beneficial effects. Until this time, federal regulation of pharmaceuticals was limited to the 1906 Pure Food and Drug Act, which prohibited misbranding and adulteration of food, beverages, and drugs. There were no safety requirements. Planned revision of the Act was stalled in Congress, but the emotion aroused by this disaster led to the 1938 Food, Drug, and Cosmetic Act, which led to the modern Food and Drug Administration.[2]

Minamata Bay, Japan (1956)

Like the events described above, this story actually begins many years before and represents a typical pattern of errors which culminate in disaster. In 1932, the Chisso Corporation began using mercury as a catalyst in the synthesis of acetaldehyde. This reaction produced a toxic organic form of mercury, methyl mercury chloride, which was discharged into Minamata Bay. Fish living in the contaminated waters of the Bay were consumed by larger fish. Over the years, through a process known as bioaccumulation, methyl mercury was incorporated progressively into animal tissues and the food chain. By the 1950s, small animals, such as cats, were dying mysteriously, and in 1956, humans began presenting to hospitals with a variety of neurologic symptoms. Within 5 months, methyl mercury was implicated as the cause for what became known as "Minamata Disease." In the 1960s, methyl mercury levels in fish peaked at 60 times normal background levels. Cases of intrauterine intoxication became known as "fetal Minamata disease."[3] Masumoto[4] described this toxic encephalopathy which was acquired prenatally and resulted in cerebral palsy. Harada[5] examined EEGs in 32 children; in 19 with congenital disease, 10 had abnormal findings; among 13 with acquired disease, 8 had abnormal studies. No focal abnormalities were seen on the EEGs. Methyl mercury is postulated to interfere with migration of neural cells from the neural tubule during embryogenesis. A syndrome of microcephaly, cerebral palsy, and contractures resulted, portrayed in the famous *Life* magazine photograph depicting a Japanese mother cradling an affected child.

An expert panel convened to assess the net impact of fish consumption on cognitive development concluded that prenatal exposure to methyl mercury might account for a loss of up to 1.5 intelligence-quotient (IQ) points.[6]

Seveso, Italy (1976)

In this story, a disinfectant, trichlorophenol, was produced from a variety of starting materials at a Roche plant. On July 9, a Friday, the night shift arrived at the plant and went to work around 10:00 in the evening. On Saturday at 4:45 AM, a foreman shut down the heat in a reaction vessel in an attempt to interrupt the distillation. His shift ended at 6:00 AM, but the reaction did not. The last recorded temperature in the vessel was 158°C, and pressure continued to build until just after noon that day. With only the cleaning staff on hand, the excessive pressure burst a safety valve, and an aerosol cloud escaped toward the southeast. Inhabitants of the surrounding area were warned not to touch fruits and vegetables, although the warning efforts were delayed because it was now the weekend. Within 5 days, obvious skin inflammation was noted among some inhabitants, particularly in children. Ultimately, dioxin was found in the plant and from the surrounding areas. Children began presenting with a late-occurring acne, known as chloracne.[7] Later studies revealed indirect markers of hepatic microsomal enzyme activity, as well as modest elevations of liver function tests (GGT and ALT), which persisted for up to 6 years after the accident.[8]

Dioxin is actually a family of chemicals. The particular species was identified as tetrachlorodibenzo-p-dioxin, a contaminant of herbicide and germicide production. Most of the childhood exposures around Seveso resulted from consumption of contaminated foods or contact with soil. The U.S. Environmental Protection Agency estimates that a lifetime exposure of 1 ng/kg/day could result in 1560 additional cases of cancer per 10,000 population. Children, therefore, may bear out this legacy in years to come.[9] A study conducted in Seveso, approximately 20 years after the accident, revealed that dioxin toxicity was confined to acute dermatological effects, and that chloracne occurrence was related to younger age and light hair color.[10]

Port Pirie, S. Australia (1979-82)

This exposure occurred over many years. This industrial town, with a population of 16,000, was situated immediately downwind of a large lead-smelting factory. There was extensive lead contamination in the town's topsoil and yard and house dust. McMichael et al[11] undertook a large, prospective study of inhabitants. They followed over 500 children who were born in the period 1979-82, and measured blood lead levels in both the birth mothers, antenatally and at delivery, and in the children at birth, at 6, 15, and 24 months, and then annually. The investigators used one of the well-known instruments for assessing childhood development, the McCarthy Scales of Children's Abilities. They found that mean lead levels in midpregnancy among the mothers was 9 g/dL; the peak at age 2 years among the children was 21 g/dL. At that time, the CDC's "cut-off" level for lead in the United States was 30 g/dL. McMichael and coworkers found that the blood lead was inversely related to development at age 4 years. This study was one of a series that suggested even low levels of lead had adverse effects on development and helped provide impetus to further lower "acceptable" lead levels subsequently, to 25 g/dL in 1985 and to 10 g/dL in 1991.

New Orleans, Louisiana (1981)

In the spring of 1981, a neonatologist named Juan Gershanik joined the staff of a small Louisiana hospital, where he cared for a 750 g infant who suddenly died. This was a child who otherwise had been doing quite well and had every reason to survive. Gershanik thought that a poison might have been responsible. His colleagues did not agree with this theory, but Gershanik persisted and noticed a pattern with other deaths: the victims were small and ill, but many had been improving before a rapid demise. He described a syndrome of multi-system disease, characterized by severe metabolic acidosis and gasps that signaled impending death. This became known as the gasping syndrome, or "gasping baby syndrome."[12] A postmortem urinalysis for organic acids on a GC-MS revealed large amounts of benzoic acid and hippuric acid. That same evening Gershanik returned to the nursery and discovered, to his horror, a vial of bacteriostatic water atop one of the isolettes contained 0.9% benzyl alcohol, a preservative. He realized that benzyl alcohol was converted via alcohol dehydrogenase to benzoic acid and hippuric acid. He immediately removed these vials (and others) containing benzyl alcohol from the nursery and, abruptly, there were no new cases of the syndrome. Gershanik corresponded with the manufacturer of the bacteriostatic water and with the FDA. Both largely ignored his concerns about its safety. In January of 1982, he reported his findings, and other institutions began to corroborate the pattern of unexpected deaths. Similar urinary organic acid profiles were found among these victims. Nearly 1 year after Gershanik removed the offending vials from his nursery, the FDA issued a "Dear Doctor" letter warning of the association between benzyl alcohol and the syndrome, and in September 1983, the AAP issued a position statement warning of the dangers of benzyl alcohol as a preservative in very sick children. After knowledge of the association became widespread, there were dramatic falls in mortality and intraventricular hemorrhage; overall, benzyl alcohol was blamed for about 3000 deaths and countless permanent disabilities. During the period in which its use was limited, there were dramatic falls in the incidence of cerebral palsy, kernicterus, especially significant among small ($<$1000 g) and premature ($<$27 weeks gestation) infants.

Why did these events occur in 1981? This was a period of aggressive respiratory therapy. With limited transcutaneous monitoring available, therapists performed frequent blood gas testing, which required frequent flushing of arterial lines. Ironically, as an infant became more ill, more blood gases were obtained, leading to greater benzyl alcohol exposure and risk for the syndrome.

Bhopal, India (1984)

Once again, a large corporation was involved in this story. Years before, in 1969, Union Carbide built a plant in Bhopal to package U.S.-produced pesticides. In 1980, expansion allowed for production of carbamate insecticides, requiring a chemical known as methyl isocyanate, or MIC. By 1984, squatters' rights had been granted to inhabitants of the area, and 100,000 of the city's population of 900,000 lived within 1 km of the plant. Shortly after midnight on December 3, water inadvertently entered a tank containing 41,000 kg of liquid MIC. This led to an exothermic reaction, and a cloud of MIC gas, an irritant that causes an obstructive pattern in the lung, was explosively released. A total of 1000 were dead by morning. A number of studies were done on victims in the area. In one, the death rate among 1337 affected children was 8.9% (119 dead);[13] another study of 211 victims found that respiratory symptoms at 100 days were persistent among over 50% of those within 2 km of the plant compared to 8.5% of those beyond 8 km of the plant. Apprehension and depression was noted among older children, some of whom awoke after the accident to find themselves on a pile of dead bodies.[14] A follow-up study 3 years later revealed persistent eye complaints among those exposed to MIC.[15]

Chernobyl, Ukraine (1986)

In the former Soviet Union, one of the nuclear power reactors in use was known as an RBMK type. This particular design, which was used to produce both electrical power and weapon-grade plutonium, required a tall structure that precluded the usual containment shell. This resulted in a somewhat unforgiving design, because production of steam increased plant reactivity, unlike other reactors, in which steam inhibited the nuclear reaction. Xenon, another reactor product, tended to shut down the reactor if control rods were in place. In a test designed to prevent plant shutdown, the control rods were removed. But the control rods were also required as a safety feature to prevent a runaway nuclear reaction. Needless to say, steam accumulated, causing an enormous increase in the nuclear reaction. This caused a steam explosion that blew the top off the reactor. The story might have ended at this point, because the reaction stopped, but another design feature, a graphite moderator, caught fire and burned for 9 days. This helped spread radionuclides, resulting in the largest known release of radioactive material. The reactor was subsequently encased in a concrete tomb, but not before over 21,000 km^2 of soil were contaminated. In the first few months, the radioisotope iodine-131 (half-life 8 days) was most responsible for exposures and is blamed for causing thyroid cancers. Cesium-137 was responsible for longer-term exposures. Much of the radiation was spread to the northwest, as far as Scandinavia. Overall, an estimated 17 million people were exposed; 2.5 million were younger than 5 years of age. Delayed acknowledgment of the disaster complicated the aftermath and resulted in needless exposures. Most at risk were the so-called liquidators, who went to the scene to clean up the site and encase the reactor. Also at risk were inhabitants of the area living within 30 km, and children, whose rapidly growing bodies and long lives leave them especially susceptible to both immediate and latent effects of radiation.[16]

Most of the research done in the first decade following the accident looked at short- and medium-term effects. Language barriers and the fact that few studies appeared in western journals hampered interpretation of these studies. Furthermore, the breakup of the Soviet Union led to many small republics that guarded their data, which did not facilitate progress. An overdiagnosis bias resulted from poor monitoring, especially among liquidators. Baseline levels of radiation and rates of cancers were not well known for the region. Weinberg et al[16] examined the plight of numerous groups who have emigrated from the Soviet Union, including 250,000 Soviet Jews. These investigators note that many èmigrès are seeking, to this day, healthcare for perceived long-term illness. How do we assess these problems? The Japanese model of radiation released at Hiroshima and Nagasaki cannot be applied because different radionuclides were released at Chernobyl. Furthermore, the above-noted fire in the graphite moderator sustained the release of radionuclides over a 9-day period, leading to more significant exposures via inhalation and ingestion. A U.S. National Chernobyl Registry has been established to sort out the details of the exposure and has recommended regular physical examinations in exposed children, with attention to the thyroid gland and overall body growth. If clinically indicated, complete blood counts, thyroid function tests, and neuropsychiatric evaluations are recommended. Another study by Dubrova[17] found a higher-than-normal mutation rate in the genome of children born in the region near the reactor after the accident compared to a control group in the United Kingdom. This difference could not be attributed to either parent or to genetic differences. A follow-up study of thyroid cancer incidence revealed significant radiation risk only for those exposed at an age of 0-9 years, with higher risk associated with younger age.[18]

Tokyo, Japan (1995)

In the mid-1990s, this populous city of 12 million had 3 million commuters per day. During the rush hour on the morning of March 20, 1995, the group Aum Shinrikyo planted a toxic substance on five subway cars on 3 different lines that converged beneath the government offices. Okamura[19] reported the events: 11 people died in this exposure, and 5000 required emergency evaluation. At St Luke's Hospital, 640 patients were seen in the Emergency Department within a few hours. Five patients were pregnant, and 3 presented in cardiac arrest. The gaseous chemical agent was quickly identified as sarin, developed in the 1930s as a potent organophosphate insecticide, which blocks the effect of the enzyme acetylcholinesterase at the myoneural junction, leading to a cholinergic crisis. Lethal effects result from respiratory insufficiency, with a lethal dose estimated at 1 mg. Treatment strategy revolves around blocking cholinergic activity with atropine, as well as regeneration of acetylcholinesterase with 2-pyridine aldoxime methiodide (2-PAM). Decontamination and supportive care are essential, along with prevention of secondary contamination among healthcare providers. In the post-9/11 era, terrorism preparedness has included a focus on sarin and other "nerve" agents.

Haiti (1996)

During an epidemic of renal failure, Haiti's Ministry of Health called upon the U.S. Centers for Disease Control to investigate the situation. Many children were found to have had emesis, abdominal pain, lethargy, and malaise. Some children were flown to the centers in the U.S. for renal dialysis. Parents of two of the deceased children provided samples of antipyretic elixirs, sold under the brand names "Afebril" and "Valodon." These elixirs were found to contain acetaminophen as an active ingredient, with DEG as an excipient. One 7-year-old transferred to the U.S. had a renal ultrasound which revealed enlarged, swollen kidneys consistent with classic DEG changes. In this case, investigators learned DEG had been inappropriately substituted for propylene glycol as a diluent. Ultimately, 30 children died.[20]

In another occurrence, 33 children died following treatment with a DEG-containing cough expectorant in Gurgaon, India.[21]

There have been other fatal DEG contaminations of pharmaceutical products since the 1937 elixir of sulfanilamide disaster; sedative mixtures in South Africa (1969), glycerine in India (1986), and acetaminophen in Nigeria (1990) and Bangladesh (1990-2). In each case, deliberate or accidental substitution of a diluent with the less expensive DEG was responsible.[2]

The Case of the Hapless Hyperventilating Hockey Players, Revisited (1996)

The children presented in the first case had played in a hotel swimming pool that, in fact, had been excessively brominated. Bromine is used as a pool disinfectant and is generally less irritating than chlorine to mucous membranes. Adults exposed to excessive bromine have developed a constellation of findings known as reactive airways dysfunction syndrome (RADS), which includes asthma-like symptoms and rash. In order to sort out these hockey players, data obtained on each patient included a complete history, a standardized patient inventory of symptoms consistent with RADS, a physical examination, and a laboratory evaluation. The latter included a complete blood count, tests of renal function, quantitative immunoglobulins, and pulmonary function testing

On physical examination, a few had dry, excoriated skin; examinations were otherwise unremarkable. One boy had an IgE that was marginally elevated, and in 3 (19%) children, PFTs were abnormal, with bronchial hyperactivity to cold-air challenge. This hyperactivity was consistent with RADS. All of the children had follow-up visits at least 3 months later. The one boy with past medical history significant for asthma remained asymptomatic, while the patient with elevated IgE at the first visit demonstrated persistent RADS, despite use of inhaled β_2 agonists and steroids.[1]

The Environmental History

What are the elements of an environmental history? Questions about home, occupation, tobacco smoke, food, and lead should be included when interviewing parents, other caregivers, and older children themselves. The timing of questions varies; in the prenatal months, ask about renovations, smoking, and feeding. When the child is 6 months of age, ask about possible poison exposures; in preschool, arts and crafts. In the teenage years, ask about hobbies and occupational exposures. Other timing issues concern the season of the year; lawn, garden, and other chemical applications in the spring and summer; wood and gas stoves and fireplaces in the fall and winter.[22]

Conclusion

In summary, much can be learned from mass exposures. We learn how to report these events and conduct research in the aftermath. Regulatory agencies may play a role in investigating these disasters and preventing their recurrence. A properly obtained environmental history may help sort out the details of an exposure. Finally, we learn something about the nature of "accidents"; most of these events occur not because of an isolated catastrophic failure but because of a series of less significant failures that may go unnoticed.

Footnotes

1. Perry HE, Shannon MW, Baum CR, et al, "Persistent Symptoms in Sixteen Children Following Bromine Exposure from A Pool," Presented at the Ambulatory Pediatric Association Annual Meeting, Washington, DC, May, 1997.

2. Wax PM, "It's Happening Again – Another Diethylene Glycol Mass Poisoning," *Clin Toxicol*, 1996, 34(5):517-20.

3. Powell PP, "Minamata Disease: A Story of Mercury's Malevolence," *South Med J*, 1991, 84(11):1352-8.

4. Matsumoto H, Koya G, and Takeuchi T, "Fetal Minamata Disease. A Neuropathological Study of Two Cases of Intrauterine Intoxication by a Methyl Mercury Compound," *J Neuropathol Exp Neurol*, 1965, 24(4):563-74.

5. Harada Y, Miyamoto Y, Nonaka I, et al, "Electroencephalographic Studies on Minamata Disease in Children," *Dev Med Child Neurol*, 1968, 10(2):257-8.

6. Cohen JT, Bellinger DC, and Shaywitz BA, "A Quantitative Analysis of Prenatal Methyl Mercury Exposure and Cognitive Development," *Am J Prev Med*, 2005, 29(4):353-65.

7. Caputo R, Monti M, Ermacora E, et al, "Cutaneous Manifestations of Tetrachlorodibenzo-p-Dioxin in Children and Adolescents: Follow-Up 10 Years After the Seveso, Italy Accident," *J Am Acad Dermatol*, 1988, 19 (5 Pt 1):812-9.

8. Ideo G, Bellati G, Bellobuono A, et al, "Increased Urinary D-Glucaric Acid Excretion by Children Living in an Area Polluted with Tetrachlorodibenzoparadioxin (TCDD)," *Clin Chim Acta*, 1982, 120(3):273-83.

9. "TCDD," Agency for Toxic Substances and Disease Registry, Atlanta, GA, June, 1989.

10. Baccarelli A, Pesatori AC, Consonni D, et al, "Health Status and Plasma Dioxin Levels in Chloracne Cases 20 Years After the Seveso, Italy Accident," *Br J Derm*, 2005, 152:459-65.

11. McMichael AJ, Baghurst PA, Wigg NR, et al, "Port Pirie Cohort Study: Environmental Exposure to Lead and Children's Abilities at the Age of Four Years," *N Engl J Med*, 1988, 319:468-75.

12. Gershanik J, Boecler B, Ensley H, et al, "The Gasping Syndrome and Benzyl Alcohol Poisoning," *N Engl J Med*, 1982, 307(22):1384-8.

13. Sutcliffe M, "An Eyewitness in Bhopal," *BMJ*, 1985, 290:1883-4.

14. Irani SF and Mahashur AA, "A Survey of Bhopal Children Affected by Methyl Isocyanate Gas," *J Postgrad Med*, 1986, 32(4):195-8.

15. Andersoon N, Ajwani MK, Mahashabde S, et al, "Delayed Eye and Other Consequences From Exposure to Methyl Isocyanate: 93% Follow Up of Exposed and Unexposed Cohorts in Bhopal," *Br J Ind Med*, 1990, 47(8):553-8.

16. Weinberg AD, Kripalani S, McCarthy PL, et al, "Caring for Survivors of the Chernobyl Disaster: What the Clinician Should Know," *JAMA*, 1995, 274(5):408-12.

17. Dubrova YE, Nesterov VN, Krouchinsky NG, et al, "Human Minisatellite Mutation Rate After the Chernobyl Accident," *Nature*, 1996, 380:686-6.

18. Ivanov VK, Gorski AI, Tsyb AF, et al, "Radiation-Epidemiological Studies of Thyroid Cancer Incidence Among Children and Adolescents in the Bryansk Oblast of Russia After the Chernobyl Accident (1991-2001 Follow-up Period)," *Radiat Environ Biophys*, 2006, 45(1):9-16.

19. Okumura T, Takasu N, Ishimatsu S, et al, "Report on 640 Victims of the Tokyo Subway Sarin Attack," *Ann Emerg Med*, 1996, 28(2):129-35.

20. Scalzo AJ, "Diethylene Glycol Toxicity Revisited: The 1996 Haitian Epidemic," *Clin Toxicol*, 1996, 34(5):513-6.

21. Singh J Dutta AK, and Khare S, "Diethylene Glycol Poisoning in Gurgaon, India, 1998" *Bull World Health Organ*, 2001, 79(2):88-95.

22. Balk SJ, "The Environmental History: Asking the Right Questions," *Contemp Ped*, 1996, 13(2):19-36.

TOXICOLOGY BASICS OF NONMEDICINAL AGENT EXPOSURES

Edward P. Krenzelok, PharmD, FAACT, DABAT

Introduction

New chemical compounds, mixtures, and products are produced throughout the world at an astounding rate. Production of a substance often precedes adequate toxicological testing to fully assess its hazards to man and the environment. Even for chemicals used in commerce for decades, there may be surprisingly little data to help clinicians plan immediate treatment and answer exposed patients' questions about long-term effects. Following a chemical exposure incident, this lack of information may produce confusion, anxiety, and anger in patients, caregivers, and the public. Rarely are there absolute answers to all the health-related questions that arise from such incidents. Health care providers, however, can obtain valuable assistance from poison information centers, toxicologists, and occupational medicine experts, and through the use of toxicology references and databases. Physicians charged with acute treatment and subsequent management need to understand certain toxicological principles as well as the strengths and limitations of the toxicology literature. This chapter is intended to aid clinicians in applying this knowledge to patient care.

What is Toxicity?

Stedman's Medical Dictionary defines toxicity as "the state of being poisonous" and toxin as a "noxious or poisonous substance..."[1] These definitions are nonspecific and reflect the ambiguity and art that exists within the field of toxicology. It is important to remember that everything is potentially toxic. Dose is the factor that principally determines whether a chemical exposure produces obvious harm to health, no demonstrable effect, or even beneficial effects. Exposure level, duration of exposure, and rate of absorption determine dose; tissue and plasma binding, excretion, and metabolism of an agent all modify its toxicity. Other potential modifying factors are listed in Table 1. Toxins also come in a variety of physical forms (Table 2).

Table 1. Factors That Modify Toxic Effect of a Given Dose
Host factors (age, sex, genomics, body fat, nutritional status)
Health behaviors (EtOH, smoking)
Other medical conditions, medications
Reproductive status
Repair
Biotransformation and excretion
Incident factors
Route of entry
Environmental factors

Table 2. Physical Forms of Toxins	
Solid	Gas
Liquid	Mist
Aerosol	Vapor
Dust	Fumes
Smoke	Fog

Every individual has a unique threshold that must be attained after exposure to most agents for an adverse effect to become manifest. Adverse effects can be overly clinical, damaging but not apparent clinically, or cumulative. This dose-response relationship for a chemical can be altered by many factors (Table 1); subclinical, latent, and idiosyncratic nondose-related effects must also be considered. Published acceptable exposure limits are not absolute; even when they have safety margins added, they are often designed for average groups of healthy workers. Furthermore, data may be based upon *in vitro* or animal testing models.

These models are frequently controversial and their validity must be considered when the data are extrapolated to human exposures.

In addition, these exposure limits are designed for workplace exposures by adults. Brief, acute, high-dose exposures, exposures to children, women, or the elderly, and continuous low-level residential exposures are less well understood. Limits for these variables are less common and less applicable.

Dose-response relationships are based upon bell-shaped curves with intense and minimal responses at the tails of the curves. While the majority of individuals in a population respond within two standard deviations of the mean dose of an agent, it is imperative that clinicians use reported toxic doses and air concentrations merely as guidelines. They are but one more factor to be added to the history, physical examination, and other laboratory data in planning patient evaluation and treatment.

The word hazard in the context of a chemical exposure incident is used commonly, but often inappropriately. Whereas toxicity reflects the ability of a substance to cause injury in an exposed individual, hazard to responders and the public depends on many factors beyond its simple toxicity (Table 3). If one can be confident that there will be no exposure to a highly toxic substance, then there is little hazard. Conversely, an agent of low toxicity can be very harmful, given sufficient exposure—consider prolonged painting in the confined space of an unventilated room. Conveying these concepts is especially important when communicating with the "worried well" and the media.

Table 3: Contributors to the Hazard Factor

Agent and Release Factors

- Amount, concentration, physical state, and density
- Volatility and reactivity under accident conditions
- Potential for explosion, thermal and corrosive injury
- Presence of ignition sources or fire
- Weather, terrain, and ventilation conditions

Exposure Factors

- Number, age, and health of potentially exposed populations
- Robustness of storage and containment structures
- Adequacy of identification, monitoring, and warning
- Adequacy of shelter and evacuation
- Threat to water supplies and environment

Human and Planning Factors

- Maintenance of equipment and facilities for the agent and response
- Adequacy of pre-planning and coordination
- Adequacy of emergency response and medical services
- Training, number, and quality of operational and response personnel
- Adequacy of actions for containment, mitigation, and medical care

Finally, it is useful for health care providers to have some knowledge of the physicochemical properties of a chemical involved in an incident. Vapor density indicates the weight of a gas or vapor relative to dry air and provides clues as to the degree of patient exposure in inhalation injuries. For example, chlorine is heavier than air and anhydrous ammonia is lighter. This has obvious, though imperfect, exposure implications for a victim who remained flat on the ground until rescued. A liquid with a high vapor pressure will volatilize easily into the air from a contaminated patient; inadequate decontamination of the patient may pose a threat to health care providers in a poorly ventilated ambulance or decontamination room. Lipid and water solubility bear on absorption and decontamination methods. Other physicochemical properties such as boiling point, ignition point, and upper and lower explosive limits help define hazard, particularly to workers, first responders, and the public near an incident scene. Fire services, and especially their hazardous materials units, are usually very knowledgeable in this area.

Acute vs Chronic Toxicity

There are three types of exposures that can lead to toxicity: acute, subchronic, and chronic. Acute exposure is a single exposure to a chemical that may occur momentarily, briefly over several minutes, or for up to approximately 8 hours. Inhalations or dermal exposures occurring over the course of a workday or a single exposure episode can be classified in this manner. Toxic manifestations that develop secondary to short, nonrepeated exposures are classified as acute toxicity. Subchronic exposures are intermittent acute exposures that do not exceed 90 days. The terms subchronic or subacute are applied rarely to toxicity in the clinical setting, and such exposures are usually labeled inappropriately as chronic exposures. It is important to properly characterize the temporal nature of a toxic exposure, since the literature differentiates carefully between the toxic manifestations that may ensue from acute, subchronic, and chronic exposures to poisons and toxins. Misinterpretation of these classifications and the information regarding them can lead to inaccurate diagnosis and prognosis. For example, an acute exposure to toluene may produce narcosis but not the renal and hepatic pathology that is associated with chronic toluene exposure. There are significant medical, psychological, and financial consequences to such errors. Chronic exposures are repeated acute or continuous exposures that occur over an extended temporal period, which may be days, weeks, or years. Lead poisoning in bridge painters, silicosis in miners, and neuropathies secondary to prolonged solvent exposure are examples of chronic toxicity.

Toxin Identification and Toxicity Rating Systems

The toxicology and industrial hygiene literature is replete with abbreviations, numeric, and alpha-numeric codes that serve as identifiers and indicators of safety as well as toxicity. What is a TLV? How are CAS numbers used? Can an LD_{50} be used prognostically in humans? Awareness of the most clinically relevant terms will help the clinician identify toxins, assess toxicity, and perform hazard risk assessments.

Toxin Descriptors

Community and worker right to know legislation as well as SARA Title III regulations have spawned the wide distribution of Material Safety Data Sheets (MSDS). These documents contain limited information about an individual product's composition, adverse health effects and their treatment, physicochemical properties, and provide guidance on spill containment and clean-up. MSDS may be inaccurate and are usually inadequate for comprehensive medical care. However, they are useful in product identification and frequently accompany exposed patients to the emergency department. Chemical ingredients are listed usually by name and by the Chemical Abstracts Service (CAS) Registry number, the most common numeric code used to identify toxins in the United States. The CAS number is a unique identifier that enables immediate identification of the substance, and helps avoid the confusion inherent in the many synonyms, closely related compounds, and "sound-alikes" present in chemical nomenclature. For instance, the CAS number of nitric acid is 7697-37-2. A call to a regional poison information center with this number allows their personnel to identify immediately the toxin and to provide toxicity and hazard information. Another commonly used identifier is the Registry of Toxic Effects of Chemical Substances (RTECS) number, which also uniquely identifies chemicals. It is found rarely on Material Safety Data Sheets; its primary use is to search databases for the toxicity literature. Field information such as data from truck placards and shipping labels may provide general hazard classifications (eg, poisonous versus corrosive chemicals) and tentative identification of a substance. However, these numbers are often not specific and must be used with caution. Again, using the example of nitric acid, its placard (for some forms and concentrations) is United Nations number 1760. This number is shared by some 30 other product groups, including aluminum sulfate solution, some weed killers, and some cosmetics!

When possible, it is judicious to use one of the specific numbers (especially the CAS number) to identify what chemicals may have been implicated in an exposure. Synonyms should be avoided since they may be regional or colloquial terms that are inadequate and possibly dangerous in decision-making and treatment. For example, an exposure to "alcohol" could involve ethanol, methanol, or isopropanol, all of which have unique chemical and toxicological properties.

Toxicity Rating

A variety of descriptive terms are used to describe dose-response relationships in the literature. These terms usually reflect animal mortality data and may be based upon acute, subchronic, or chronic exposures. The term used most commonly is the Lethal Dose 50 (LD_{50}). This is the amount of chemical required to kill 50% of an experimental animal population and is commonly referred to simply as the "lethal dose." The limitation of this value lies in the uncertainty of extrapolating it to a human exposure. However, if the value is either very low or very high, an assumption is generally made that a given chemical is either relatively safe or toxic to humans. This assumption must be tempered by existing human data, usually in the form of case reports, and even then, caution must be exercised. For example, the LD_{50}'s of the organophosphate insecticides, parathion and malathion, in rats are 5 mg/kg and 1000 mg/kg, respectively. This means that considerably smaller amounts of parathion caused 50% of the rats to die. However, exposure to either of these can produce significant human cholinergic toxicity, though it may require a larger amount of malathion to do so. Similarly, the Lethal Dose Low (LD$_{LO}$) is the lowest amount known to be fatal when dose-response testing is conducted. Human toxicity data is reported as the Toxic Dose Low (TD$_{LO}$). This is the lowest amount that has actually been reported to produce toxicity in a human. Unfortunately, there is a conspicuous absence of this information in the literature. Inhalation toxicity is described by similar terminology – Lethal Concentration-$_{50}$, Lethal Concentration-$_{Low}$, Toxic Concentration-$_{Low}$, etc.

Modifications of the Hodge-Sterner Toxicity Table are published in many toxicology references and rate the degree of toxicity from "Dangerously Toxic" (LD$_{50}$ <1 mg/kg) in six gradations to "Practically Nontoxic" (LD$_{50}$ >15 g/kg). These data are supposed to be applicable to a 70 kg male. This type of rating system provides limited insight into the potential toxicity of an agent, but it does not consider the acute or chronic nature of the exposure, has rather broad ranges, and is supported by neither scientific nor clinical data. Reliance solely upon this system may result in either complacency or inappropriate therapy.

Exposure Standards

What is a permissible exposure level? Ideally, there should be no exposures to potentially noxious chemicals. However, given the ubiquity of noxious chemicals in industrialized society, reality dictates that a risk to benefit ratio exists for most products. Levels of acceptable exposure have been established by both the Occupational Safety and Health Administration (OSHA) and the American Conference of Governmental Industrial Hygienists (ACGIH). It is of paramount importance to understand that these values are arbitrary, and are designed to protect nearly all workers. Some individuals are more sensitive than others, that is, dose-response relationships vary within similar populations. The values, unless otherwise specified, reflect the air concentrations to which an individual can be exposed over a specific period of time and are customarily reported in parts per million (ppm). Caution must be exercised when interpreting OSHA and ACGIH exposure limits, since these values do not take into consideration factors such as underlying health problems or performance of demanding work (which may increase respiration and accordingly increase the amount of inhaled toxin). The most commonly used exposure standard is referred to as the Threshold Limit Value (TLV), which reflects the maximum allowable exposure over a specific period of time. The TLV-Time-Weighted Average (TWA) (also referred to as the Permissible Exposure Limit (PEL)) is the average concentration to which an individual can be exposed in the workplace over a standard 8-hour day or 40-hour work week without developing any adverse effects. For example, the TLV-TWA for formaldehyde is 3 ppm. However, sensitive individuals may develop mucosal irritation at air concentrations of <0.5 ppm. The TLV-Short-Term Exposure Limit (STEL) is the maximum concentration to which a worker can be exposed for 15 continuous minutes without developing intolerable irritation, chronic or irreversible tissue damage, or narcosis that may impair work efficiency or endanger the worker. This standard allows an individual to have four such exposures separated by at least 60 minutes per day. The TLV-Ceiling (TLV-C) is the concentration that should never be exceeded, even instantaneously. Special attention should be paid to the Immediately Dangerous to Life or Health (IDLH) Level. The IDLH is the maximum concentration from which one could escape without impairment of judgment or the development of irreversible health effects. These values are rarely available when patients with toxic effects are being treated in an emergency department or when first responders are at a hazardous materials incident. However, if the values are known, they can assist the health care provider in making both diagnostic and prognostic decisions regarding the patient.

Toxicokinetics

The absorption, distribution, metabolism, and elimination of drugs is called pharmacokinetics. The application of those principles to toxicology is referred to as toxicokinetics. An appreciation of the basic principles of toxicokinetics can facilitate patient assessment and management. Only factors that affect the route of absorption are addressed here.

Routes of Exposure

- Oral
- Ocular
- Dermal
- Inhalation
- Injection

Due to the nature of hazardous materials incidents, many of the exposures to noxious agents are inhalational and can result in both local and systemic toxicity. A variety of factors dictate how well a chemical is absorbed via the inhalational route; of considerable importance is particle size. Particulate matter with particle diameters >10 microns tend to lodge in the pharynx or nasal cavity; they generally do not produce effects in the lower respiratory tract. Particles smaller than 10 microns are respirable and, depending upon their size and shape, tend to gain access to the lower respiratory tract. If the diameter of a particle is in the range of 1-5 microns, it may be deposited in the bronchioles; those particles <1 micron may reach the alveoli.

Solubility also plays an important role in the inhalational absorption of chemicals. Respirable particles that are water-soluble may be scrubbed out partially by the mucous membranes of the upper respiratory tract. This tends to limit an injury to the upper respiratory tract. In contrast, respirable substances that have lower water solubility, such as nitrogen dioxide (Silo Filler's Disease), can be inspired into the alveoli. There they may be converted to nitrous acid and lead to the development of pulmonary edema.

The skin is not impervious to the absorption of toxins. Lipid-soluble chemicals such as solvents can penetrate the dermis and cause systemic toxicity. It is important to know the solubility and corrosive characteristics of a chemical, as well as the duration of contact, to determine its potential for toxicity. Skin damaged by abrasions, burns, or wounds permits greater absorption and requires special attention during decontamination.

Summary

As stated previously, toxicology is more of an art than a science. However, some of the mystery of toxicology can be eliminated by understanding terminology and a few basic concepts. A considerable amount of knowledge exists about the toxicology of drug overdoses but there is a paucity of human data regarding hazardous materials. Common sense, basic life support considerations, and the incorporation of toxicological principles allows health care providers to make informed decisions in patient management and to contribute to important community decisions such as evacuation.

Footnote

1. *Stedman's Medical Dictionary*, Philadelphia, PA: Lippincott Williams and Wilkins, 2006.

1-Propanol

Applies to Antiseptic Agents; Cleaners; Cosmetics; Lacquer; Polishes

CAS Number 71-23-8

UN Number 1274

Synonyms n-Propyl Alcohol; Optal; Propanol; Propyl Alcohol; Propylic Alcohol

Use In lacquers, cosmetics, cleaners, polishes, and antiseptic agents

Mechanism of Toxic Action Central nervous system depression

Adverse Reactions

Central nervous system: Delirium, coma, personality changes

Dermatologic: Dermal irritation

Gastrointestinal: Nausea, vomiting, mucous membrane irritation

Ocular: Eye irritation

Signs and Symptoms of Overdose Cutaneous erythema, diarrhea, feces discoloration (black), GI irritation, hypotension, nausea, porphyria, vomiting; seizures and coma may develop

Toxicodynamics/Kinetics Absorption: Quick from GI tract; can be absorbed dermally

Overdosage/Treatment

Decontamination: Lavage (within 1 hour)/activated charcoal

Enhancement of elimination: Hemodialysis for patients in deep and persistent coma

Diagnostic Procedures

- Glucose, Random
- Osmolality, Serum

Additional Information More toxic than isopropyl alcohol; 20 mL of 1-propanol with water can cause hypotension

1,1-Dichloroethene

Applies to Coating (Steel Pipes); Packaging Materials/Food Wraps; Retardant Coating (Carpet Backing)

CAS Number 75-35-4

UN Number 1303

Synonyms 1,1 DCE; VCD; Vinylidene Chloride

Use Chemical intermediate in polyvinylidene chloride production; found in food wraps and other packaging materials; also as a coating for steel pipes, retardant coating in carpet backing, and adhesives

Mechanism of Toxic Action Mucosal irritant and CNS depressant

Adverse Reactions

Central nervous system: Narcosis, cranial nerve palsies

Dermatologic: Leukoderma

Endocrine & metabolic: Hypoglycemia

Hepatic: Elevated liver enzymes

Ocular: Eye irritant

Signs and Symptoms of Overdose Lethargy

Toxicodynamics/Kinetics

Metabolism: By way of oxidation .

Elimination: Renal

Overdosage/Treatment

Decontamination: **Do not** induce emesis; lavage (within 1 hour)/activated charcoal; dilute with water or milk

Enhancement of elimination: Forced diuresis may be beneficial (although there is no human data).

Additional Information Levels of 4000 ppm associated with narcosis; possible increased toxicity with acetaminophen, ethanol, or phenobarbital. TLV-TWA: 5 ppm

1,2-Dibromoethane

Applies to Fire Extinguishers; Flue Gases; Gasoline (Antiknocking Additive); Mechanical Gauge Fluid; Soil Fumigant (Europe)

CAS Number 106-93-4

UN Number 1605

Synonyms Bromofume; DBE; EDB; Ethylene Dibromide; Glycol Dibromide

Use Acts as a lead scavenger in gasoline (at a level of ~179 mg/dL); therefore, its use is as an antiknocking additive. It has also been used as a soil fumigant (for nematode removal) in Europe, but this use was banned in the U.S. in 1994; also used as a chemical intermediate for bromide synthesis and is an ingredient in fire extinguishers and mechanical gauge fluid; found as a contaminant in flue gases.

Mechanism of Toxic Action Cytotoxic metabolites (bromoacetaldehyde and free bromide ions) can cause lipid peroxidation and result in tissue lesions. Bromide toxicity can also occur resulting in cell membrane damage and displacement of body chloride ions. Glutathione depletion can result. Binds directly to DNA.

Adverse Reactions

Central nervous system: CNS depression

Dermatologic: Vesiculation, rash

Endocrine & metabolic: Metabolic acidosis

Gastrointestinal: GI ulceration

Hepatic: Hepatic failure within 2 days

Local: Inflammation

Neuromuscular & skeletal: Muscle necrosis

Renal: Renal failure within 2 days

Respiratory: Pulmonary edema, respiratory depression

Signs and Symptoms of Overdose Agitation, anorexia, bradycardia, CNS depression, cough, dermal blisters, dermal blisters, diarrhea, dizziness, drowsiness, GI upset, hepatic necrosis (centrilobular hepatic necrosis), hepatomegaly, hypotension, jaundice, mydriasis, ocular irritation, skin erythema and pruritus, tachycardia, tachypnea, thirst, vomiting

Toxicodynamics/Kinetics

Absorption: By inhalation, ingestion of dermal routes. Inhalation absorption is 58% in rodents.

Metabolism: Oxidized in hepatic cytochrome P450 enzymes to 2-bromo-acetaldehyde and free bromide ions.

Elimination: Renal, as glutothione conjugates, bromide or bromoacetic acids. Slight amounts are excreted as carbon dioxide (by inhalation) interactions.

Reference Range

Normal bromide levels are <40 mg/L. Moderate toxicity is encountered at bromide levels of 200 mg/L, while fatalities can occur at levels >330 mg/L.

Serum bromide levels of 830 mg/L and 380 mg/L have been correlated with fatalities.

Overdosage/Treatment

Decontamination:

Oral: Lavage/administer activated charcoal within 2 hours of exposure.

Dermal: **Note:** 1,2-dibromoethane can penetrate polyvinyl chloride, surgical rubber or leather gloves. Nylon appears somewhat protective. Remove all contaminated clothing. Wash the skin with soap and water for 15-20 minutes.

Inhalation: Administer high flow humidified 100% oxygen.

Ocular: Irrigate with saline or water for at least 15-20 minutes.

Supportive therapy: Corticosteroids can be used to treat symptomatic bradycardia; intravenous bicarbonate for metabolic acidosis.

Enhancement of elimination: Multiple dosing of activated charcoal may be useful in enhancing elimination.

Diagnostic Procedures

- Bromide, Serum
- Glucose, Random

Drug Interaction Ethanol can potentiate the cytotoxic effect of 1,2-dibromoethane. Disulfiram, cyanamide, and chloral hydrate, which are aldehyde dehydrogenase inhibitors, can also potentiate the toxicity of DBE.

Additional Information A probable carcinogen (lymphoma). A brownish liquid with a sweet chloroform-like odor. Cooking of food with DBE causes decomposition to ethylene glycol and bromide. Air DBE concentrations >75 ppm are associated with gastrointestinal and respiratory irritation. IDLH: 400 ppm. PEL-TWA: 20 ppm have been implicated as causing male sterility with reduction in sperm count

1,2-Dibromo-3-Chloropropane

Applies to Fumigant (Soil); Nematocide (Soil)

CAS Number 96-12-8

UN Number 2872

U.S. Brand Names Fumagon®; Fumazone®; Nemafume®; Nemagon®; Nemapax®; Nemazon®

Synonyms BBC12; DBCP

Use Soil fumigant and nematocide to protect field crops; also used as an intermediate in organic chemical synthesis; was the preferred fumigant for pineapples in Hawaii, although this practice was stopped by the EPA in 1985

Mechanism of Toxic Action Possibly inhibits carbohydrate metabolism of sperm at the level of nicotinamide adenine dinucleotide dehydrogenase

Adverse Reactions

Endocrine & metabolic: Spermatogenesis preponderate of female off-spring to male workers; sterilization may occur due to necrosis of seminiferous tubule cells

Gastrointestinal: Abdominal pain

Ocular: Eye irritant

Respiratory: Pulmonary edema

Signs and Symptoms of Overdose Azoospermia, epigastric pain, eye irritation, headache, lightheadedness, nausea

Toxicodynamics/Kinetics

Absorption: Can be absorbed by dermal, GI, or inhalation

Elimination: Inhalation: Feces (14%)

Overdosage/Treatment Decontamination: **Oral:** Dilute with milk or water; **do not** induce emesis. Activated charcoal may be useful. **Dermal:** Wash with soap and water. **Ocular:** Irrigate with saline.

Additional Information FSH and LH elevations may occur. Azoospermia correlates with elevated FSH levels and usually is reversible. Pungent odor. Taste threshold: 0.01 mg/L. TLV: 0.01 ppm.

1,2,3-Trichloropropane

CAS Number 96-18-4
Synonyms Allyl Trichloride; Glycerol Trichlorohydrin; Trichlorohydrin
Use Primarily as a paint or varnish remover, cleaning or degreasing agent
Mechanism of Toxic Action Metabolites may lead to DNA/protein adducts or lipid peroxidation; a respiratory irritant
Adverse Reactions Throat and ocular irritation at levels ~100 ppm; has caused squamous cell carcinomas in rodent models
Toxicodynamics/Kinetics
Absorption: Probably by inhalation, oral (up to 80%), and dermal routes
Metabolism: To carbon dioxide (which is expired) and glutathione conjugated (mercapturic acid)
Elimination: Urine and fecal
Overdosage/Treatment Decontamination: **Oral:** Dilute with milk or water; activated charcoal may be used with a cathartic. **Dermal:** Wash with soap and water. **Ocular:** Irrigate with saline.
Additional Information Found in soil in California and Hawaii at levels ranging from 0.2-2 ppb. Combustion products include chloride fumes. Drinking water concentrations: <0.2 mcg/L. Atmospheric half-life: 15.3 days. Water half-life: 44 days (hydrolysis). TLV-TWA (skin): 10 ppm

1,3-Butadiene

Applies to Carpet Backing; Foams; Fungicides (Production); Paper Coating
CAS Number 106-99-0
UN Number 1010
Synonyms Biethylene; Bivinyl; Butadiene Divinyl
Use In the manufacture of foams, carpet backing, paper coating, production of fungicides
Mechanism of Toxic Action Asphyxiant - anesthesia at high concentrations; no cumulative toxicity
Adverse Reactions
Cardiovascular: Bradycardia, hypotension, sinus bradycardia
Central nervous system: CNS depression
Endocrine & metabolic: Ovotoxic
Hematologic: Possibly leukemogenic
Signs and Symptoms of Overdose Blurred vision, cough, drowsiness, hallucinations, headache, skin irritation, upper airway irritation
Toxicodynamics/Kinetics
Metabolism: Though not studied in humans, major metabolites appear to be diepoxybutane and 3,4-epoxy-1,2-butanediol; glutathione-S-tranferase appears to be one detoxifying pathway
Half-life (animal model): 2-10 hours
Monitoring Parameters Blood glucose
Overdosage/Treatment
Although there is no experimental data, there is a theoretical basis to utilize acetylcysteine to help detoxify this substance
Decontamination: **Oral:** Basic poison management. **Inhalation:** Move patient to fresh air; treat with 100% humidified oxygen.
Diagnostic Procedures
• Glucose, Random
Additional Information
Colorless; mild aromatic odor at >1.3 ppm; carcinogenic and genotoxic; metabolites are active alkylating agents
TLV-TWA: 10 ppm; IDLH: 20,000 ppm; PEL-TWA: 1000 ppm
Organic vapor cartridges can adsorb up to 1000 ppm of butadiene.
Atmospheric half-life: 6 hours
Median 1,3-butadiene concentration in ambient air: 0.3 ppb in urban areas and 0.1 ppb in rural areas; indoor air concentrations may be higher (1-9 ppb) due to cigarette smoke, thus leading to an estimated daily intake of ~13 mcg per person
Specific References
McDonald JD, Bechtold WE, Krone JR, et al, "Analysis of Butadiene Urinary Metabolites by Liquid Chromatography-Triple Quadrupole Mass Spectrometry," *J Anal Toxicol*, 2004, 28:168-73.

1,3-Dichloropropene

Applies to DD-92; Fumigant (Soil)
CAS Number 10061-01-5; 10061-02-6; 542-75-6
U.S. Brand Names Telone®; Terr-o-cide® 15-D; Terr-O-Gas® 57/43T
Synonyms 1,3-Dichloropropylene
Use Soil fumigant for nematodes used primarily on soil of vegetable or tobacco crops (preplanting); also used as a solvent
Mechanism of Toxic Action Mucous membrane irritant; chemical structure is similar to vinyl chloride
Adverse Reactions
Dermatologic: Skin vesicant
Respiratory: Respiratory irritant, bronchospasm
Miscellaneous: Hypersensitivity (delayed)
Signs and Symptoms of Overdose Cough, dizziness, diarrhea, dyspnea, headache, hypotension, malaise, metabolic acidosis, nausea, neck pain, pancreatitis, pleuritic chest pain, pruritus (dermal contact), vomiting

Toxicodynamics/Kinetics
Absorbed by inhalation and/or dermal exposure
Metabolism: Hepatic to an N-acetyl cysteine conjugate through glutathione pathway
Reference Range Excretion of N-acetyl glucosaminidase (NAG) >1.5 mg/day is considered elevated
Overdosage/Treatment Decontamination: **Oral: Do not** induce emesis; dilute with milk or water; lavage (within 1 hour)/activated charcoal. **Dermal:** Wash with soap and water. **Inhalation:** Administer 100% oxygen. **Ocular:** Irrigate with normal saline.
Additional Information Possible association with development of histiocytic lymphoma and acute myelomonocytic leukemia; lung tumors noted in rodents; penetrates rubber protective gear. Odor threshold: 1-3 ppm (garlic-like). PEL-TWA (skin): 1 ppm; TWA-TLV: 1 ppm

1,3-Dinitrobenzene

CAS Number 99-65-0
UN Number 1597
Synonyms 1,3 DNB; Dinitrobenzene; Meta-Dinitrobenzene
Use Primarily used as an explosive, as a camphor substitute in nitrocellulose; medicinally, has been used as an indicator for 17-ketosteroid detection
Mechanism of Toxic Action Causes methemoglobinemia through oxidation of ferrous hemoglobin to ferric derivative
Adverse Reactions
Dermal: Skin/hair yellowing
No apparent long-term effects
Cardiovascular: Hypotension, tachycardia, cyanosis, sinus tachycardia
Central nervous system: Dizziness, headache, fatigue, ataxia, fever, hyperthermia
Gastrointestinal: Nausea, vomiting, bitter almond smell
Hematologic: Anemia, methemoglobinemia, Aplastic anemia
Ocular: Nystagmus, optic neuropathy
Respiratory: Dyspnea
Hepatic: Subacute hepatic necrosis
Admission Criteria/Prognosis Any patient with change in mental status, cardiopulmonary complaints, or methemoglobin levels >30% should be admitted; asymptomatic patients with methemoglobin levels <30% may be considered for discharge after 6 hours of observation and if methemoglobin levels fall to <15%
Toxicodynamics/Kinetics Absorption: Oral, inhalation, and dermal (well absorbed)
Monitoring Parameters Methemoglobinemia
Overdosage/Treatment
Decontamination: **Dermal:** Wash with soap and water. **Ocular:** Irrigate copiously with saline.
Supportive therapy: Treat symptomatic methemoglobinemia with methylene blue. Ascorbic acid (3 g/day during periods of cyanosis) has been used to improve oxygen delivery, although its efficacy is not proven. Administer 100% humidified oxygen.
Antidote(s)
• Methylene Blue [ANTIDOTE]
Additional Information Penetrates latex gloves; odor of bitter almonds in vomitus or urine may be noted: IDLH-50 mg/m³

1,4-Dioxane

CAS Number 123-91-1
UN Number 1165
Synonyms 1,4-Diethylene Dioxide
Use A solvent for chemical processing (adhesives, cosmetics, deodorants, lacquers, pulping of wood, waxes); laboratory reagent; chemical intermediate used in pharmaceuticals/pesticides. Formerly used as a stabilizer of 1,1;1-trichlorabethane, 1-4-dioxane is manufactured by acid catalyzed conversion of diethylene glycol; it is formed by ethylene glycol breakdown
Adverse Reactions Ocular irritation (50 ppm for 6 hours); nose/throat irritation (300 ppm for 15 minutes); vomiting, abdominal pain, elevated liver function tests, cerebral edema
Reference Range Following inhalation exposure of 1.6 ppm for 7.5 hours, urinary 1,4-dioxane and HEAA levels were 3.5 umol/L and 414 umol/L, respectively
Overdosage/Treatment
Inhalation: Give 100% humidified oxygen
Ocular: Irrigate with copious amounts of water or saline
Additional Information
A colorless, volatile liquid which is miscible in water; considered possibly carcinogenic in humans
Odor threshold: 24 ppm (ethereal odor)
Ambient atmospheric levels: 0.1-0.4 mcg/m³
Ambient water level: 1 mcg/L
Atmospheric half-life: 1-3 days
TLV (8-hour TWA): 20 ppm (skin)
IDLH: 500 ppm; minimal lethal exposure: 470 ppm for 3 days
PEL: 100 ppm

Maximum permitted concentration in food/spermicidal/medicinal products: 10 ppm

Half-life in soils: 4 weeks to 6 months; does not bioconcentrate in aquatic organisms

Specific References

CDC/ATSDR: Toxicological Profile for 1,4-Dioxane, U.S. Department of Health and Human Services, Sept 2004.

2-Butoxyethanol

Applies to Butyl Cellulosolve
CAS Number 111-76-2
UN Number 2369
Synonyms 2-Butoxy-1-Ethanol; BUCS; Ethylene Glycol Monobutyl Ether
Use Solvent/cleaning agent; dry cleaning, textile (dyeing), in inks, paint thinners, and protective coatings; often found in window/glass cleaners (usually 9% to 12% concentrations)
Mechanism of Toxic Action Both 2-butoxyethanol and its metabolite 2-butoxyacetic acid cause elevated osmotic fragility of red blood cells resulting in hemolysis; butoxyacetic acid is responsible for the metabolic acidosis.
Adverse Reactions

Cardiovascular: Tachycardia, hypotension

Central nervous system: Headache, coma

Dermatologic: Photo-onycholysis, cherry angiomas

Endocrine & metabolic: Metabolic acidosis, hypokalemia

Gastrointestinal: Eructation

Hematologic: Hemolytic anemia

Ocular: Eye irritation, mydriasis (reacts to light)

Renal: Hematuria, albuminuria, oxaluria

Respiratory: Nasal/pharyngeal irritation

Admission Criteria/Prognosis For oral ingestions of liquids containing >10% ethyl glycol butyl ether, admit any child who ingests >10 mL
Toxicodynamics/Kinetics

Absorption: Inhalation (57%), oral and dermal (within two hours)

Distribution: V_d: 54 L

Metabolism: Hepatic oxidation via alcohol dehydrogenase to butoxyacetaldehyde with further oxidation to 2-butoxyacetic acid

Half-life: Oral: 210 minutes. Dermal: 34 minutes. Elimination: Renal

Overdosage/Treatment

Decontamination: Oral: Lavage within 1 hour. Activated charcoal has not been demonstrated to be useful.

Supportive therapy: Use of ethanol or 4-methylpyrazole as an inhibitor of alcohol dehydrogenase has been useful in animal models, but human data are lacking. Acidosis can be treated with 1-2 mEq/kg of sodium bicarbonate. Dopamine can be used to treat hypotension. Fomepizole (15 mg/kg I.V., then 10 mg/kg I.V. in twelve hours) may assist in resolving metabolic acidosis, if administered within six hours.

Enhanced elimination: Hemodialysis is of unknown effectiveness, it should be considered in patients with acidosis or renal failure.

Additional Information

A colorless liquid with a faint odor; does not produce osmolar gap.

Irritant symptoms occur at air concentrations of 200 ppm, while levels >300 ppm can cause narcosis, renal or hepatic injury

Density: 0.9 g/mL; does not affect serum osmolarity. Average indoor air concentration: 0.2 ppb. Odor threshold: 0.1-0.4 ppm. Atmospheric half-life: <1 day. Water half-life: ~5 days. Soil half-life: 1 week to 1 month. TWA-TLV: 25 ppm; PEL-TWA: 50 ppm (skin)

Specific References

Gualtieri JF, DeBoer L, Harris CR, et al, "Repeated Ingestion of 2-Butoxyethanol: Case Report and Literature Review," *J Toxicol Clin Toxicol*, 2003, 41(1):57-62.

Hippolyte T, Andollo W, and Ohr J, "Acute Poisoning with Brake Fluid," *J Anal Toxicol*, 2006, 30:131.

2-Hexanone

CAS Number 591-78-6
Synonyms 2-Oxohexane; Butyl Methyl Ketone; MBK; Methyl-n-Butyl Ketone; Propylacetone
Commonly Found In Coated fabrics, paints, solvents
Mechanism of Toxic Action Metabolite 2,5-hexanedione can cause distal neuronal swelling and axonal degeneration
Adverse Reactions

Cardiovascular: Tachycardia, sinus tachycardia

Central nervous system: Polyneuropathy (distal sensory), CNS depression, axonopathy

Respiratory: Respiratory depression

Signs and Symptoms of Overdose Asthenia, dyspnea, lacrimation, nausea, ocular irritation, paresthesia, upper airway irritation, vomiting
Admission Criteria/Prognosis Symptomatic patients or patients with abnormal chest x-rays should be admitted

Toxicodynamics/Kinetics

Absorption: Through lungs (75% to 92%), oral (66%), and dermal (rate of 4.8-8.0 mcg/cm^2/minute)

Metabolism: To 2,5-hexanedione (neurotoxic agent)

Elimination: Through lungs, in urine

Reference Range 2,5-hexanedione: urine: <5.0 mg/L; blood: <10.0 mcg/L
Overdosage/Treatment Decontamination: Lavage within 1 hour; dilute with 4-8 oz milk or water. Irrigate skin with soap and water.
Additional Information Very soluble in water; has been found in milk and cream at levels of 7-18 ppb. Odor threshold: 0.076 ppm (acetone). TLV-TWA: 5 ppm; PEL-TWA: 5 ppm; IDLH: 1000 ppm. Atmospheric half-life: 36 hours. River water half-life: 10-15 days

2-Methyl-4-Chlorophenoxyacetic Acid

CAS Number 94-74-6
U.S. Brand Names Agritox®; Agroxone®; Chiptox®; Cornex®; Dedweed®; Empal®; Hedonal® M; Homotuho®; Kilsen®; Mephanac®; Phenoxylene®; Ruonox®; Shamrok®; Weed Control; Weedar®; Weedone®
Synonyms MCP; MCPA; Methylchlorophenoxy Acetic Acid
Use Controls annual/perennial weeds in cereals, grasslands and turf
Mechanism of Toxic Action A chlorophenoxy herbicide used to control broadleaf weeds; an auxin which causes abnormal plant growth
Signs and Symptoms of Overdose Vomiting is usually the first symptom, followed by oropharyngeal burning and hypotension. Agitation, coma, lethargy, leukocytosis, mild rhabdomyolysis, miosis, muscle spasms, proteinuria, seizures, tachycardia, and twitching can occur.
Toxicodynamics/Kinetics

Half-life: 133 hours (12.6 hours with forced alkaline diuresis)

Elimination: Renal

Reference Range Fatal MCPA serum level (after a 0.25 g/kg ingestion): ~180 mg/L; recovery has occurred following ingestion of 0.8-1.67 g/kg (and associated serum MCPA level of 546 mg/L)
Overdosage/Treatment

Decontamination: Oral: Do not administer syrup of ipecac. Gastric lavage should be performed and activated charcoal should be administered.

Supportive therapy: Hypotension can be treated with isotonic saline (10-20 mL/kg) and placement in Trendelenburg position. Dopamine or norepinephrine can be given for refractory cases. Seizures can be treated with diazepam.

Enhanced elimination: Forced alkaline diuresis can decrease the half-life of MCPA. Sodium bicarbonate (1-2 mEq/kg) with potassium chloride (20-40 mEq/L) can be used to maintain alkaline urine. Furosemide or mannitol can be used to maintain diuresis. Hemodialysis is not expected to be useful.

Additional Information Colorless crystals

2-Octyl Cyanoacrylate

Pronunciation (too ok til sye AN oh ah kril ate)
Use Topical skin adhesive
Mechanism of Action Polymerizes on skin in an exothermic reaction to form a strong flexible bond
Adverse Reactions Local: Burning sensation
Dosage Topical: Apply to affected area on skin in three layers; wound should be clean and dry before application; wound should be held in a horizontal position
Contraindications Use is contraindicated in any infected wound, decubiti, on mucous membranes or mucocutaneous junction, skin which is exposed to body fluids or dense hair, or patients allergic to cyanoacrylate or formaldehyde; do not apply to wet or actively bleeding wounds, or below the skin surface; should also not be utilized in wounds of high tension area
Dosage Forms Liquid: 0.5 ml in a sterile, prefilled, single-use applicator (with colorant: D and C violet #2)
Overdosage/Treatment Decontamination: **Dermal**: Bond is active within 15-20 seconds; petroleum jelly or acetone may help loosen the bond; water, soap, Betadine®, or saline would not be expected to have any effect. **Ocular**: Immediately flush eye with copious amounts of water or normal saline
Additional Information Should be stored under 30°C; more information can be obtained at 1-877-337-6226; as effective as 5-0 monofilament sutures; adhesive sloughs off in 1-2 weeks; avoid washing or soaking the affected area; wound should be held for 30-40 seconds for full polymerization to occur; full tensile strength occurs in 2 minutes

2,3-Benzofuran

Applies to Adhesives (Food Container); Asphalt Floor Tiles; Cigarette Smoke; Coating on Citrus Fruits; Paint Production
CAS Number 271-89-6
Synonyms Benzofuran; Benzofurfuran; Coumarone; Cumaron

Use Found in cigarette smoke, as a coating on citrus fruits, asphalt floor tiles, food container adhesives; used in paint production

Mechanism of Toxic Action Produced by destructive distillation of coal (naphtha fraction) and fossil fuels

Adverse Reactions Little human adverse effect experience

Overdosage/Treatment

Decontamination: Flush skin or eyes with copious amounts of water.
Supportive therapy: Give oxygen if the patient is exposed to heated decomposition products; monitor pulmonary status.

Additional Information Aromatic odor, colorless liquid, insoluble in water. FDA regulation for protective coating on citrus fruits: maximum: 200 ppm. When heated, can emit acrid fumes

2,4-D

Related Information

- 2-Methyl-4-Chlorophenoxyacetic Acid

CAS Number 94-75-7

UN Number 2765

Synonyms 2,4-Dichlorophenoxyacetic Acid

Commonly Found In Choroxone®; Esteron®; Salvo®; Weedar®; Weedone®

Mechanism of Toxic Action A chlorophenoxy herbicide used to control broadleaf weeds; an auxin which causes abnormal plant growth; a weak uncoupler of oxidative phosphorylation

Adverse Reactions

Cardiovascular: Cardiac arrhythmias, bradycardia, sinus bradycardia, sinus tachycardia
Dermatologic: Concentrated solutions ($>$12%) can cause dermal burns
Endocrine: Hypokalemia
Gastrointestinal: Acute nausea, diarrhea, vomiting
Hematologic: Thrombocytopenia
Neuromuscular & skeletal: Myoclonus, peripheral (sensory) neuropathy, myotonia, hyperthermia
Respiratory: Pulmonary edema

Signs and Symptoms of Overdose Elevated liver function tests, hypophosphatemia, miosis, myoglobinuria, myotonia (rare), rhabdomyolysis, tachycardia

Admission Criteria/Prognosis Any ingestion $>$50 mg/kg should be admitted

Toxicodynamics/Kinetics

Absorption: Absorbed through skin/oral/inhalation routes
Distribution: V_d: 0.1 L/kg; 10 L/kg in overdose
Protein binding: Extensive
Half-life: 4-140 hours - prolonged in acidic urine
Peak effect: 4-24 hours
Elimination: Urine; does not bioaccumulate

Reference Range

At an oral ingested dose of 5 mg/kg, peak plasma level was 35 mg/L at 24 hours; plasma levels $>$100 mg/L associated with coma
Urine 2,4-D concentration of 314 mg/L (range 111-670 mg/L) associated with fatal poisoning

Overdosage/Treatment

Decontamination: **Oral:** Lavage/activated charcoal for ingestions within 4 hours exceeding 40 mg/kg. **Dermal:** Irrigate with saline. **Ocular:** Flush eyes with water or saline for 10-15 minutes.
Supportive therapy: Hypotension can be treated with 10-20 mL/kg of isotonic saline and Trendelenburg positioning; dopamine or norepinephrine can be used. Quinidine may be helpful for cardiac arrhythmias.
Enhancement of elimination: Alkaline diuresis for patients with metabolic acidosis, mental status changes, or a serum level $>$500 mg/L. Keep urine pH $>$7.6 by use of sodium bicarbonate (I.V.: 44-88 mEq/L). Alkaline diuresis can enhance elimination by decreasing 2,4-D half-life by 90%. Clearance by hemodialysis is 64 mL/minute. Renal clearance with a pH of 8.3 (urinary) is 63 mL/minute. Furosemide can be given to maintain diuresis.

Additional Information Minimum lethal dose: 80 mg/kg. Slight phenol odor when heated; does not contain tetrachlorodibenzoparadioxin (TCDD); does not accumulate in food chain

Specific References

Bradberry SM, Proudfoot AT, and Vale JA, "Poisoning Due to Chlorophenoxy Herbicides," *Toxicol Rev*, 2004, 23(2):65-73 (review).
Brahmi N, Mokhtar HB, Thabet H, et al, "2,4-D (Chlorophenoxy) Herbicide Poisoning," *Vet Hum Toxicol*, 2003, 45(6):321-2.
Gardner M, Spruill-McCombs M, Beach J, et al, "Quantification of 2,4-D on Solid-phase Exposure Sampling Media by LC-MS-MS," *J Anal Toxicol*, 2005, 29(3):188-92.
Greve KW, Bianchini KJ, Doane BM, et al, "Psychological Evaluation of the Emotional Effects of a Community Toxic Exposure," *J Occup Environ Med*, 2005, 47(1):51-9.
Horswell J and Dickson S, "Use of Biosensors to Screen Urine Samples for Potentially Toxic Chemicals," *J Anal Toxicol*, 2003, 27(6):372-6.
Letcher RJ, Li HX, and Chu SG, "Determination of Hydroxylated Polychlorinated Biphenyls (HO-PCBs) in Blood Plasma by High-Performance Liquid Chromatography-Electrospray Ionization-Tandem Quadrupole Mass Spectrometry," *J Anal ToxicolM*, 2005, 29(4):209-16.
Pont AR, Charron AR, and Brand RM, "Transdermal Penetration of the Herbicide 2,4-D Is Enhanced by UV Absorbers Found in Commercial Sunscreens," *J Toxicol Clin Toxicol*, 2003, 41(5): 722-3.

2,4-Dichlorophenol

Applies to Antiseptics (Production); Bactericides (Production); Disinfectant (Production); Fungicides (Production); Mothproofing

CAS Number 120-83-2

UN Number 2020 (solid)

Synonyms 2,4-DCP; 4,6-Dichlorophenol

Use Intermediate in production of 2,4-dichlorophenoxy acetic acid (2,4-D), bifenox, and dichloroprop herbicides; also used in production of pentachlorophenol and other disinfectants, fungicides, bactericides, and antiseptics; a waterborne contaminant of the kraft pulping process; also used as a mitocide and for mothproofing

Mechanism of Toxic Action Interferes with cell division by disrupting spindle formation and interfering with oxidative phosphorylation; can cause CNS depression

Adverse Reactions

Dermatologic: Chloracne, hyperpigmentation, hirsutism
Hematologic: Porphyria cutanea tarda
Miscellaneous: Sarcoma

Signs and Symptoms of Overdose CNS depression, lethargy, seizures, tremors

Admission Criteria/Prognosis Admit any patient exhibiting neurologic changes

Toxicodynamics/Kinetics

Absorption: Dermally, orally, and by inhalation
Half-life: ~10 minutes
Metabolism: Hepatic sulfation and glucuronidation

Reference Range Death due to dermal exposure (~10% total body surface area); postmortem blood, urine, bile, and stomach levels were 24.3 mg/L, 5.3 mg/L; 18.7 mg/L, and 1.2 mg/L, respectively

Overdosage/Treatment

Decontamination: **Oral:** **Do not** induce emesis; lavage (within 1 hour)/ activated charcoal. **Dermal:** Wash with soap and water. **Inhalation:** Give 100% humidified oxygen. **Ocular:** Irrigate with saline or water; anesthetic use may follow copious irrigation
Supportive therapy: Seizures can be treated with benzodiazepines, phenobarbital, or phenytoin.

Additional Information

Human exposure may occur from drinking contaminated water.
Human water quality criteria (EPA): 0.3 mcg/L
Half-life in water: 62 hours at a pH of 8 with a mean concentration of 0.2 mcg/L
Average daily intake of 2,3-dichlorophenol: ~0.4 mcg
Taste threshold (medicinal): ~2-8 mcg/L. Odor threshold in water: 0.0003 to 0.04 mg/L
Solid at room temperature; photolytic degradation is 0.11% per hour; decomposition rate in neutral clay-loam soil at 20°C is 81% in 40 days.
Average atmospheric concentration (during rain) in Portland, Oregon, is ~0.23 ppt.
Combustion products can contain hydrochloric acid.

2,4-Dinitrotoluene

CAS Number 121-14-2

UN Number 1600 (molten); 2038 (solid or liquid)

Synonyms 2,4-DNT

Use In the production of polyurethane polymers, explosives, and automobile air bags; an isomer of DNT

Mechanism of Toxic Action Producer of methemoglobin in rodent studies; not reported in humans; cytotoxic to hepatocytes

Adverse Reactions

Cardiovascular: Cyanosis
Central nervous system: Headache, vertigo, dizziness
Dermatologic: Dermatitis, turns skin yellow
Gastrointestinal: Nausea, vomiting
Hematologic: Anemia, hemolysis, although not described in humans, methemoglobinemia may occur (onset may be delayed for 4 hours)
Hepatic: Hepatitis
Neuromuscular & skeletal: Arthralgia (especially in the knees)
Miscellaneous: Cutaneous T-cell lymphoma

Toxicodynamics/Kinetics

Absorption: By oral (rapid and complete) and inhalation routes
Elimination: Renal

Monitoring Parameters CBC, methemoglobin

Reference Range Urinary 2,4 DNT levels in ammunition plant workers range from 2-9 mcg/L

Overdosage/Treatment

Decontamination: **Oral:** Do not induce emesis. Lavage within 4 hours. Activated charcoal may be useful. **Dermal:** Wash with soap and water. **Ocular:** Irrigate with water and saline.

Supportive therapy: Symptomatic methemoglobinemia (or methemoglobin levels >30%) can be treated with methylene blue.

Antidote(s)

- Methylene Blue [ANTIDOTE]

Drug Interaction Reduced tolerance to ethanol; ethanol many intensify symptoms of 2,4-dinitrotoluene: IDLH-50 mg/m^3

Additional Information

Water soluble; mean concentration in U.S. waters is <10 mcg/L. TWA (skin): 1.5 mg/m^3; IDLH: 200 ng/m^3

Boiling point: 300°C; An oily liquid

2,4,5-T

CAS Number 93-76-5

Synonyms 2,4,5-Trichlorophenoxyacetic Acid

Mechanism of Toxic Action Has been banned by the EPA in 1979

Adverse Reactions

Dermatologic: More irritating to the skin and mucous membranes than 2,4-D

Neuromuscular & skeletal: Paresthesia

Signs and Symptoms of Overdose Paresthesia

Toxicodynamics/Kinetics Half-life: 23-33 hours, 90 hours in acidic urine

Overdosage/Treatment

Decontamination: Irrigate with saline; lavage (within 1 hour)/activated charcoal for ingestions >400 mg/kg

Supportive therapy: Hypotension can be treated with 10-20 mL/kg of isotonic saline and Trendelenburg positioning; dopamine or norepinephrine can be used; quinidine may be helpful for cardiac arrhythmias

Enhancement of elimination: Alkaline diuresis for patients with metabolic acidosis, mental status changes, or a serum level >500 mg/L; keep urine pH between 7.6-8.8; furosemide can be given to maintain diuresis

Additional Information 2,3,7,8-tetrachlorodibenzoparadioxin (TCDD) is a contaminant of 2,4,5-T. 2,3,5-T and 2,3-D was used as a 50:50 mixture in agent orange. 2,4,5-T alone usually contains <0.1 ppm of TCDD; does not affect cholinesterase level

2,4,6-Trichlorophenol

CAS Number 25167-82-2; 88-06-2

UN Number 2020

U.S. Brand Names Caswell No 880C®; Dowicide 2S®; Omal®; Phenachlor®

Use Antiseptic and pesticide; used as a wood and glue preservative; antimildew agent in textile manufacture

Mechanism of Toxic Action Chemical which is actually a metabolite of lindane, 2,4,6-trichlorophenol is a respiratory irritant

Adverse Reactions

Respiratory: Bronchospasm and cough on inhalation

Miscellaneous: Chronic oral exposure has produced liver cancer and leukemia in rodent models

Toxicodynamics/Kinetics

Absorption: Probably by oral or dermal (9.9×10^{-4} cm/minute) routes

Metabolism: Hepatic

Elimination: Urine

Overdosage/Treatment Decontamination: **Ocular:** Irrigate with saline. **Dermal:** Wash with soap and water. **Inhalation:** Administer 100% humidified oxygen.

Additional Information

Fish and shellfish may concentrate 2,4,6-trichlorophenol and it has been estimated that a daily ingestion of 21 g of fish can result in an intake of 95 mcg of this agent.

Daily intake from drinking water: 0.4-100 mcg. Taste threshold: 2 ppb. Odor threshold: 2.6 ppb. Atmospheric half-life: 1 day to 3 weeks. Water half-life: 1-19 days

2,4,6-Trinitrotoluene

CAS Number 118-96-7

UN Number 0209 (<30% water); 1356 (>30% water)

Synonyms Alpha TNT; TNT; Tolit; Trilit; Tritol; Triton

Use High explosive agent used in military or civilian blasting procedures; chemical intermediate in production of dyes and photographic chemicals

Mechanism of Toxic Action Cause of methemoglobin; dermal irritant

Adverse Reactions Hematologic: Glucose-6-phosphate dehydrogenase deficiency-induced hemolytic anemia

Signs and Symptoms of Overdose Altered taste, anemia (aplastic), cataract, constipation, dermal burns, elevated liver enzymes, hemolytic anemia (especially in individuals deficient in G6PD enzyme), methemoglobinemia, paresthesia, red color to urine, toxic hepatitis

Admission Criteria/Prognosis Any patient with change in mental status, cardiopulmonary complaints, or methemoglobin levels >30% should be admitted. Asymptomatic patients with methemoglobin levels <30% may be considered for discharge after 6 hours of observation and if methemoglobin levels fall to <15%.

Toxicodynamics/Kinetics

Absorption: Inhalation, oral, and dermal exposure

Metabolism: Hepatic to nitro reduction to 2,6-dinitro-4-aminotoluene (DNAT)

Elimination: Renal

Overdosage/Treatment

Decontamination: **Dermal:** Wash with soap and water. **Ocular:** Irrigate with saline.

Supportive therapy: Methylene blue for symptomatic methemoglobinemia

Antidote(s)

- Methylene Blue [ANTIDOTE]

Additional Information Combustible, pale yellow solid. Atmospheric half-life: 18-184 days. Water half-life: 14-84 hours. PEL-TWA (skin designation): 0.5 mg/m^3. TLV-TWA (skin designation): 0.5 mg/m^3

Specific References

Vorisek V, Pour M, Ubik K, et al, "Analytical Monitoring of Trinitrotoluene Metabolites in Urine by GC-MS. Part I: Semiquantitative Determination of 4-Amino-2,6-Dinitrotoluene in Human Urine," *J Anal Toxicol*, 2005, 29:62-5.

3-3'-Dichlorobenzidine

CAS Number 91-94-1

U.S. Brand Names Curithane®

Synonyms Dichlorobenzidine

Use Production of pigments (primarily yellow and red) for ink, paper, paint, textiles, and plastics

Mechanism of Toxic Action Can cause DNA and protein adduction resulting in genotoxicity

Signs and Symptoms of Overdose Bladder cancer, dermatitis, dizziness, headache, pharyngitis

Toxicodynamics/Kinetics

Absorption: By inhalation and oral routes

Metabolism: Hepatic N-acetylation

Elimination: Renal

Overdosage/Treatment Decontamination: **Dermal:** Remove clothing, wash skin with soap and water. **Ocular:** Irrigate with copious amounts of water. **Inhalation:** Administer 100% humidified oxygen.

Additional Information Slightly soluble in water; not volatile

Atmospheric half-life: 2 hours to 60 days

Average air concentration in Canada: $\sim 7.6 \times 10^{-16}$ mcg/m^3

Estimated water level in Canada: 3.4×10^{-7} ng/L

Estimated soil concentration in Canada: $\sim 1.1 \times 10^{-16}$ mcg/g

Average daily intake of Canadian infants and adults: 3.6×10^{-8} ng/kg and 7.4×10^{-9} ng/kg respectively

EPA ambient water quality criteria for human health: 0.01 mcg/L for water and fish and 0.02 mcg/L for fish only

3,4-Methylenedioxymethamphetamine

Related Information

- Highlights of Recent Reports (2006) on Substance Abuse and Mental Health

CAS Number 4764-17-4; 51497-09-7

Synonyms Ecstasy; MDMA

Use Originally used as an appetite suppressant in 1913; also has been utilized in psychotherapy

Mechanism of Toxic Action A sympathomimetic that is structurally related to amphetamine and mescaline; this drug blocks serotonin reuptake while causing serotonin release, which is calcium mediated; exhibits $\sim 10\%$ of the CNS stimulant effect as amphetamine

Adverse Reactions

Cardiovascular: Tachycardia; hypertension, chest pain, ventricular fibrillation, ventricular tachycardia

Central nervous system: Euphoria, headache, hyperthermia, seizures, coma, fatigue, serotonin syndrome, paranoia, cognitive impairment, depression, insomnia, dystonia, hallucinations, leukoencephalopathy

Endocrine & metabolic: Hyponatremia due to SIADH, hypoglycemia

Gastrointestinal: Dry mouth, anorexia, diarrhea, nausea, vomiting

Hematologic: Disseminated intravascular coagulation, thrombocytopenia,

Hepatic: Hepatitis, aminotransferase level elevation (asymptomatic)

Neuromuscular & skeletal: Trismus, muscle rigidity, rhabdomyolysis, piloerection, clonus

Ocular: Mydriasis

Renal: Acute renal failure

Miscellaneous: Sweating, bruxism, thirst

Signs and Symptoms of Overdose Agitation, hyperthermia

Toxicodynamics/Kinetics

Onset of effect: 30-45 minutes (oral)

Duration of effect: 4-6 hours

Metabolism: Hepatic, through cytochrome P450 isoenzyme CYP2D6 into 3,4-methylenedioxyamphetamine (MDA)

Half-life: MDMA: 7.6-9 hours; MDA: 16-38 hours

Elimination: Renal

Reference Range MDMA serum concentrations >1 mg/L are associated with fatality; peak serum MDMA and MDA concentrations following an oral dose of 1.5 mg/kg: ~0.33 mg/L and 0.015 mg/L, respectively

Overdosage/Treatment

Supportive therapy: Severe hyponatremia (serum sodium <120 mM/L) can be treated with either continuous infusion of 0.9% normal saline or 3% normal saline at 50 mL/hour, with furosemide 40 mg twice daily. Seizures should be treated with a benzodiazepine or barbiturate. Hyperthermia should be aggressively treated with cooling blankets, ice packs, and cooling fans. The role of chlorpromazine, cyprohepta-dine, dantrolene, or beta-adrenergic blockers is uncertain in treating hyperthermia. Ventricular arrhythmias may respond to lidocaine. Benzodiazepines can be given for agitation. Nitroprusside or phentola-mine can be given for hypertensive emergency. Hypotension should be treated with crystaloid fluids.

Test Interactions Positive amphetamine result on urinary immunoassay

Drug Interaction Hypertension, diaphoresis, and hypertonicity lasting for 6 hours has occurred with concomitant use of phenelzine.

Additional Information Psychotherapy dose: 2 mg/kg initially with a booster dose of 0.5 mg/kg to 1 mg/kg in 3-4 hours. Recreational dose: 75-160 mg with a booster dose of 50-75 mg after 3-4 hours

Specific References

Baltarowich L, Smolinske S, and Thomas R, "Fatal Complications of Ecstasy and Amphetamine Abuse," *J Toxicol Clin Toxicol*, 2003, 41(5):744.

Bordo DJ and Dorfman MA, "Ecstasy Overdose: Rapid Cooling Leads to Successful Outcome," *Am J Emerg Med*, 2004, 22(4):326-7.

Dams R, De Letter EA, Mortier KA, et al, "Fatality Due to Combined Use of the Designer Drugs MDMA and PMA: A Distribution Study," *J Anal Toxicol*, 2003, 27(5):318-22.

de la Torre R, Farre M, Roset PN, et al, "Human Pharmacology of MDMA: Pharmacokinetics, Metabolism, and Disposition," *Ther Drug Monit*, 2004, 26(2):137-44.

Goldstein LH, Mordish Y, Abu-Kishak I, et al, "Acute Paralysis Following Recreational MDMA (Ecstasy) Use," *Clin Toxicol*, 2006, 44(3):39-41.

Hendrickson RG, Horowitz BZ, and Norton RL, "Parachuting Meth: A Novel Delivery Method for Methamphetamine and Delayed-Onset Toxicity from Body Stuffing," *Clin Toxicol*, 2006, 44:379-82.

Hsu J, Liu C, Hsu CP, et al, "Performance Characteristics of Selected Immunoassays for Preliminary Test of 3,4-Methylenedioxymethamphe-tamine, Methamphetamine, and Related Drugs in Urine Specimens," *J Anal Toxicol*, 2003, 27:471-8.

Jenkins KM, Young MS, Mallet CR, et al, "Mixed-Mode Solid-Phase Extraction Procedures for the Determination of MDMA and Metabolites in Urine Using LC-MS, LC-UV, or GC-NPD," *J Anal Toxicol*, 2004, 28(1):50-8.

Klette KL, Jamerson MH, Morris-Kukoski CL, et al, "Rapid Simultaneous Determination of Amphetamine, Methamphetamine, 3,4-Methylene-dioxyamphetamine, 3,4-Methylenedioxymethamphetamine, and 3,4-Methylenedioxyethylamphetamine in Urine by Fast Gas Chromatogra-phy-Mass Spectrometry," *J Anal Toxicol*, 2006, 30:151.

Klette KL, Kettle AR, and Jamerson MH, "Prevalence of Use Study for Amphetamine (AMP), Methamphetamine (MAMP), 3,4-Methylene-dioxy-amphetamine (MDA), 3,4-Methylenedioxy-methamphetamine (MDMA), and 3,4-Methylenedioxy-ethylamphetamine (MDEA) in Mili-tary Entrance Processing Stations (MEPS) Specimens," *J Anal Toxicol*, 2006, 30:319-22.

Lai TI, Hwang JJ, Fang CC, et al, "Methylene 3,4 Dioxymethampheta-mine-Induced Acute Myocardial Infarction," *Ann Emerg Med*, 2003, 42(6):759-62.

Lin DL and Liu RH, "Abuse of Methylenedioxymethamphetamine in Taiwan - Analytical Approaches and Analytes Distribution in Antemor-tem and Postmortem Specimens," *J Anal Toxicol*, 2004, 28:296.

Lin DL, Liu HC, Yin RM, et al, "Effectiveness of Multiple Internal Standards: Deuterated Analogues of Methylenedioxymethampheta-mine, Methylenedioxyamphetamine, Methamphetamine, and Amphetamine," *J Anal Toxicol*, 2004, 28(8):650-4.

Logan BK, Luthi R, and Gordon AM, "A Short Series of Deaths Involving MDMA," *J Anal Toxicol*, 2004, 28:279.

Lu H, Kirkland PD, Heninger MM, et al, "Myocardial Hypertrophy in Users of Methylenedioxymethamphetamine MDMA," *J Toxicol Clin Toxicol*, 2003, 41(5):693.

Madhok A, Boxer R, and Chowdhury D, "Atrial Fibrillation in an Adolescent: The Agony of Ecstasy," *Pediatr Emerg Care*, 2003, 19(5):348-9.

Maresova V, Hampl J, Chundela Z, et al, "The Identification of a Chlorinated MDMA," *J Anal Toxicol*, 2005, 29(5):353-8.

McGowan KF, Quang LS, Sadasivan S, et al, "A Murine Model for *In Vivo* Neurotoxicity of Gamma-Hydroxybutyrate (GHB) and 3,4-Methylene-
dioxymethamphetamine (MDMA; Ectasy)," *J Toxicol Clin Toxicol*, 2003, 41(5):724.

Monks TJ, Jones DC, Bai F, et al, "The Role of Metabolism in 3,4-(+)-Methylenedioxyamphetamine and 3,4-(+)-Methylenedioxymethamphe-tamine (Ecstasy) Toxicity," *Ther Drug Monit*, 2004, 26(2):132-6.

Muntain CD and Tuckler V, "Cerebrovascular Accident Following MDMA Ingestion," *J Med Toxicol*, 2006, 2(1):16-8.

Nordgren HK and Beck O, "Direct Screening of Urine for MDMA and MDA by Liquid Chromatography - Tandem Mass Spectrometry," *J Anal Toxicol*, 2003, 27(1):15-9.

Pichini S, Navarro M, Pacifici R, et al, "Usefulness of Sweat Testing for the Detection of MDMA After a Single-Dose Administration," *J Anal Toxicol*, 2003, 27(5):294-303.

Rella JG and Murano T, "Ecstasy and Acute Myocardial Infarction," *Ann Emerg Med*, 2004, 44(5):550-1.

Rusyniak DE, Scruggs SL, Kamendulis LM, et al, "Ecstasy's (MDMA's) Effect on Oxidative Phosphorylation in Isolated Rat Liver Mitochondria," *Acad Emerg Med*, 2003, 10:510.

Rusyniak DE, Scruggs SL, and Sprague JE, "Ecstasy's Effect on *In-Vitro* and *Ex-Vivo* Oxidative Phosphorylation in Rodent Skeletal," *Acad Emerg Med*, 2004, 11(5):469.

Rusyniak DE and Sprague JE, "Toxin-Induced Hyperthermic Syn-dromes," *Med Clin North Am*, 2005, 89(6):1277-96 (review).

Shakleya DM, Kraner JC, Kaplan JA, et al, "Methylation of 3,4-Methylenedioxymethamphetamine in Formalin-Fixed Human Liver Tis-sue," *J Anal Toxicol*, 2006, 30:141.

Smolinske S, Baltarowich L, and Thomas R, "Ecstasy and Methamphe-tamine Related Hyperthermia," *J Toxicol Clin Toxicol*, 2003, 41(5):655.

Villamor JL, Bermejo AM, Fernandez P, et al, "A New GC-MS Method for the Determination of Five Amphetamines in Human Hair," *J Anal Toxicol*, 2005, 29:135-44.

3,4-Methylenedioxy-N-Methyl-Butanamine

Synonyms MBDB

Use Similar to hallucinogenic amphetamines, less hallucinogenic: an "entactogen"

Mechanism of Toxic Action Central nervous system stimulant

Adverse Reactions

(+)-isomer is probably more potent

Cardiovascular: Tachycardia, hypertension

Central nervous system: Seizures

Miscellaneous: Diaphoresis

Toxicodynamics/Kinetics

Metabolism: Hepatic demethylation to 3,4-methylene-dioxybutanamine (BDB)

Elimination: Urinary, as parent compound and as 3,4-methylene-dioxy-butanamine (BDB) within 36 hours; also eliminated via saliva and sweat

Dosage 100 mg

Overdosage/Treatment

Decontamination: Oral: Gastric lavage within 1 hour with activated charcoal

Supportive therapy: Treat agitation with diazepam (0.1 mg/kg I.V. or 0.3 mg/kg orally in children; 5 mg I.V. or 10 mg orally in adults). Seizures can be treated with benzodiazepines or barbiturate. Nitroprusside can be used to treat hypertension. Monitor for rhabdomyolysis.

Additional Information A controlled substance in U.S. and France.

4-Aminopyridine

CAS Number 504-24-5

UN Number 2671

Use In Europe: Bird repellent and as a pesticide. Has possible utility as a antagonist of nondepolarizing neuromuscular blocking agents, verapamil overdose, botulism, and aminoglycoside neuromuscular blockade

Unlabeled/Investigational Use In the United States: Multiple sclerosis, Eaton-Lambert syndrome, Alzheimer's disease, myasthenia gravis, and spinal cord trauma

Mechanism of Action Enhances transmembrane calcium in flux which thus facilitates synaptic transmission; also blocks neuronal potassium channels which results in acetylcholine release

Adverse Reactions

Neurological effects are dose related occurring at daily doses >0.5 mg/kg

Cardiovascular: Tachycardia

Central nervous system: **Dizziness**, insomnia, generalized seizures (within 15 minutes of exposure), psychosis, headache, confusion, extrapyramidal symptoms

Gastrointestinal: **Nausea**, thirst, xerostomia, vomiting

Hepatic: Elevated liver enzymes

Neuromuscular & skeletal: Weakness, tremors, **paresthesias**, **gait instability**

Respiratory: Dyspnea

Miscellaneous: Diaphoresis

Signs and Symptoms of Overdose Choreoathetoid movements, confusion, diaphoresis, dizziness, dyspnea, dystonia, extrapyramidal effects, metabolic acidosis, seizures, tremor, weakness

Admission Criteria/Prognosis Admit any symptomatic patient or ingestion >0.5 mg/kg

Toxicodynamics/Kinetics

Distribution: V_d: 2.6 L/kg

Protein binding: Negligible; <5%

Bioavailability: Oral: 95%; poorly absorbed dermally

Half-life: 3.6 hours

Total serum clearance: 0.6 L/hour/kg

Elimination: Renal (87% to 91% of the drug is eliminated unchanged)

Dosage

Botulism: I.V.: 0.5 mg/kg; continuous infusion of 0.25 mg/kg/hour (monitor for seizures; will not improve respiratory parameters; may improve peripheral paralysis)

Eaton-Lambert syndrome:
Oral: 40-200 mg/day in divided doses
I.V.: 0.3-0.6 mg/kg

Multiple sclerosis:
Oral: 10-50 mg in 2-4 divided doses
I.V.: 1-5 mg every 10-60 minutes, over 1.5-3.5 hours to a maximum dose of 35 mg

Myasthenia gravis:
Oral: 40-200 mg/day in 2 to 4 divided doses
I.V.: 10-20 mg

Reversal of neuromuscular blockade: Oral: 0.3-0.6 mg/kg

Verapamil overdose: I.V. (separated by a 10-minute interval): 2 doses of 10 mg I.V. slowly dose: 18-33.5 mg

Spinal cord injury: Acute: Continuous I.V. infusion: 9-15 mg/hour; total

Spinal cord injury: Chronic: Investigational: Oral: 10 mg

Reference Range Peak serum 4-aminopyridine level after a 20 mg I.V. and oral dose: ~300 ng/mL and 62 ng/mL, respectively. Therapeutic serum 4-AP: 30-59 ng/mL. A 266 ng/mL serum level has been associated with severe toxicity in an infant.

Overdosage/Treatment

Decontamination: Do not induce emesis; lavage (within 1 hour)/activated charcoal

Supportive therapy: Seizures can be initially managed with diazepam; phenobarbital or phenytoin can be used as second-line therapy. Nondepolarizing neuromuscular blocking agents can be used if seizures persist (after the patient is intubated with assisted ventilation). d-Tubocurarine (10-15 mg slowly I.V. followed by additional doses up to 5 mg every 25 minutes in adults or 0.4 mg/kg bolus in children with additional doses of 15% to 20% of the initial dose used as needed to maintain muscle relaxation) or metocurine (1.5-8 mg slow I.V. push in adults with 0.5-1 mg as needed or 0.2 mg/kg in children with additional doses of 15% to 20% of the initial dose) can be used to counteract skeletal muscle effects of prolonged seizures. Due to its cardiac effects, avoid pancuronium. Sodium bicarbonate (1-3 mEq/kg) can be used to treat metabolic acidosis. Propranolol can be used for cardiac toxicity while atropine (0.01 mg/kg/dose slow I.V. up to 0.4 mg/dose) can be used to treat abdominal cramps and diarrhea.

Enhanced elimination: Although human data are lacking, charcoal hemoperfusion may be useful for ingestion of >500 mg. Since enterohepatic recirculation may take place, multiple dosing of activated charcoal may be useful.

Additional Information

Toxic dose: 0.6 mg/kg

Transiently beneficial for peripheral paralysis (but **not** respiratory paralysis) in botulism; may be a competitive antagonist for verapamil hypotension

4-Bromo-2,5-Dimethoxyphenylethylamine

Related Information
● Mescaline

Synonyms 2C-B

Impairment Potential Yes

Use Psychoactive drug often combined with ecstasy and ketamine

Mechanism of Toxic Action Structurally related to mescaline; binds to central nervous system serotonin receptors

Adverse Reactions Central nervous system: Visual, auditory, olfactory, tactile hallucinations (dose related), euphoria

Toxicodynamics/Kinetics

Duration of action: 4-8 hours

Metabolism, hepatic: 2-(4-bromo-2,5-dimethoxyphenyl)-ethanol, 4-bromo-2,5-dimethoxyphenylacetic acid, 2-(2-hydroxy-4-bromo-5-methoxyphenyl)-ethylamine, 2-(2-methoxy-4-bromo-5-hydroxyphenyl)-ethylamine, 1-acetoamino-2-(2-hydroxy-4-bromo-5-methoxyphenyl)-ethane, and 1-acetoamino-2-(2-methoxy-4-bromo-5-hydroxyphenyl)-ethane

Overdosage/Treatment

Decontamination: Lavage (within 1 hour)/activated charcoal with cathartic

---

Supportive therapy: Benzodiazepines are useful for agitation. Haloperidol or chlorpromazine can be used if psychiatric symptoms are not responsive to benzodiazepines. Do not use phenothiazines for treatment of flashback.

Additional Information Supplied as white tablets (3-8 mg). Hallucinogenic doses range from 4-30 mg.

4-Methylthioamphetamine

Use Drug of abuse in Europe

Mechanism of Action A dose-dependent releasing agent of serotonin; a reversible inhibitor of rodent monoamine-oxidase A (MAO-A)

Adverse Reactions

Central nervous system: Tremors, ataxia, seizures

Gastrointestinal: Abdominal cramps, nausea

Miscellaneous: Diaphoresis

Admission Criteria/Prognosis Admit any patient who ingests >300 mg.

Dosage Tablets are 100 mg

Reference Range Blood levels of 4-MTA >4 mg/L are consistent with an overdose. No postmortem redistribution is noted.

Overdosage/Treatment

Decontamination: Oral: Lavage any ingestion in children or ingestion >300 mg in adults. Activated charcoal may be utilized.

Supportive therapy: Benzodiazepines can be given to treat seizures.

4,4′-Methylenebis (2-Chloroaniline)

Applies to DAC; MOCA

CAS Number 191-14-4

U.S. Brand Names Activator-M®; Bis-Amine A®; CA-800®; Cuamine-M®; Curene® 442

Synonyms DACPM; MCOVA

Use Primarily as a curing agent in polymers containing isocyanate; also used in manufacture of epoxy resins; involved in manufacture of belt drives in computers, elevator or escalator wheels, gun mounts, radar systems, and shoe soles

Mechanism of Toxic Action Forms adducts with hemoglobin, serum albumin, and tissue DNA; may be tumor promoter similar to benzidine

Adverse Reactions Cutaneous T-cell lymphoma and proteinuria in humans; carcinogenic in animals with lungs, liver, breast, and bladder being the target organs in a dose-dependent manner

Toxicodynamics/Kinetics

Absorption: Inhalation, oral (40% in animal models), and dermal

Metabolism: Hepatic N-hydroxylation and N-acetylation to toxic metabolites

Half-life: 23 hours

Elimination: Renal and fecal

Overdosage/Treatment Decontamination: **Dermal:** Remove contaminated clothing; wash with soap and water. Penetration of gloves is concentration-dependent and can occur from 2-35 hours, with natural latex gloves appearing to be most effective. **Ocular:** Irrigate copiously with saline.

Drug Interaction Phenobarbital can accelerate metabolism (hydroxylation)

Additional Information Atmospheric half-life: 0.3-2.9 hours (photoxidation). Water half-life: 1-72 days (surface); 8 weeks to 1 year (groundwater). PEL-TWA (skin designation): 0.2 ppm. TLV-TWA (skin designation): 0.2 ppm

5-Methoxy-N,N-Diisopropyltryptamine

Synonyms 5-OMe-DIPT; Foxy

Use A designer hallucinogen and aphrodisiac

Mechanism of Toxic Action An indolealkylamine which stimulates dopaminergic and tryptaminergic receptors

Signs and Symptoms of Overdose Visual hallucinations, mydriasis, muscle spasms, agitation

Toxicodynamics/Kinetics

Absorption: Well absorbed orally

Metabolism: Degraded by monoamine oxidase (oxidative deamination)

Peak effect: 1-1.5 hours

Elimination: Renal

Reference Range Following oral dose of 4 mg, urine level (obtained 4 hours postingestion in a symptomatic male) of 5-methoxy-N,N-diisopropyltryptamine and its metabolite (5-methoxy-indole acetic acid) was 1.7 mcg/mL and 1.3 mcg/mL, respectively

Overdosage/Treatment

Decontamination: Oral: Activated charcoal within 1 hour

Supportive therapy: Anxiety/agitation can be treated with benzodiazepines (such as lorazepam 0.05 mg I.M. or I.V.; up to 4 mg total in adults)

Drug Interaction Synergistic with cannabinoid

Additional Information Threshold hallucinogenic dose: 4 mg; usual dosage range: 6-10 mg. Recovery usually seen within 6 hours.

Specific References

Meatherall R and Sharma P, "Foxy, A Designer Tryptamine Halluci-nogen," *J Anal Toxicol*, 2003, 27(5):313-7.

Sklerov J, Levine B, Moore KA, et al, "A Fatal Intoxication Following the Ingestion of 5-Methoxy-N,N-Dimethyltryptamine in an Ayahuasca Preparation," *J Anal Toxicol*, 2005, 29(8):838-41.

Smolinske S, Rastogi R, and Schenkel S, "Foxy Methoxy: A New Drug of Abuse," *J Toxicol Clin Toxicol*, 2003, 41(5):641.

Abciximab

U.S. Brand Names ReoPro®

Synonyms 7E3; C7E3

Use Prevention of acute cardiac ischemic complications in patients at high risk for abrupt closure of the treated coronary vessel and patients at risk of restenosis; an adjunct with heparin to prevent cardiac ischemic complications in patients with unstable angina not responding to conventional therapy when a percutaneous coronary intervention is scheduled within 24 hours

Unlabeled/Investigational Use Acute MI – combination regimen of abciximab (full dose), tenecteplase (half dose), and heparin (unlabeled dose)

Mechanism of Action Fab antibody fragment of the chimeric human-murine monoclonal antibody 7E3; this agent binds to platelets resulting in steric hindrance, thus inhibiting platelet aggregation

Adverse Reactions

Cardiovascular: **Hypotension**, fibrillation (atrial) or flutter (atrial), tachy-cardia (ventricular), complete AV block

Central nervous system: Dizziness, coma, insomnia, hyperesthesia, dysphonia

Dermatologic: Pruritus

Gastrointestinal: Diarrhea, ileus

Genitourinary: Urinary retention, urinary tract infection

Hematologic: **Bleeding**, thrombocytopenia (0.5%)

Neuromuscular & skeletal: Myopathy

Miscellaneous: Anaphylaxis

Signs and Symptoms of Overdose Thrombocytopenia

Pharmacodynamics/Kinetics Half-life elimination: ~30 minutes

Dosage

I.V.: 0.25 mg/kg bolus administered 10-60 minutes before the start of intervention followed by an infusion of 0.125 mcg/kg/minute (to a maximum of 10 mcg/minute) for 12 hours

Patients with unstable angina not responding to conventional medical therapy and who are planning to undergo percutaneous coronary intervention within 24 hours may be treated with abciximab 0.25 mg/kg intravenous bolus followed by an 18- to 24-hour intravenous infusion of 10 mcg/minute, concluding 1 hour after the percutaneous coronary intervention.

Monitoring Parameters Prothrombin time, activated partial thrombo-plastin time, hemoglobin, hematocrit, platelet count, fibrinogen, fibrin split products, transfusion requirements, signs of hypersensitivity reactions, guaiac stools, and Hemastix® urine

Administration

Abciximab is intended for coadministration with aspirin postangioplasty and heparin infused and weight adjusted to maintain a therapeutic bleeding time (eg, ACT 300-500 seconds). Solution must be filtered prior to administration. Do not shake the vial.

Bolus dose: Aseptically withdraw the necessary amount of abciximab for the bolus dose into a syringe using a 0.2 or 5 micron low protein-binding syringe filter (or equivalent); the bolus should be administered 10-60 minutes before the procedure.

Continuous infusion: Aseptically withdraw 4.5 mL (9 mg) of abciximab for the infusion through a 0.2 or 5 micron low protein-binding syringe filter into a syringe; inject this into 250 mL of NS or D_5W to make a solution with a final concentration of 35 mcg/mL. Infuse at the rate of 17 mL/hour (10 mcg/minute) for 12 hours via pump. If a syringe filter was not used when preparing the infusion, administer using an in-line 0.02 or 0.22 low protein-binding filter.

Contraindications Hypersensitivity to abciximab, to murine proteins, or any component of the formulation; active internal hemorrhage or recent (within 6 weeks) clinically-significant GI or GU bleeding; history of cerebrovascular accident within 2 years or cerebrovascular accident with significant neurological deficit; clotting abnormalities or administra-tion of oral anticoagulants within 7 days unless prothrombin time (PT) is ≤1.2 times control PT value; thrombocytopenia (<100,000 cells/µL); recent (within 6 weeks) major surgery or trauma; intracranial tumor, arteriovenous malformation, or aneurysm; severe uncontrolled hyperten-sion; history of vasculitis; use of dextran before PTCA or intent to use dextran during PTCA; concomitant use of another parenteral GP IIb/IIIa inhibitor

Warnings

Administration of abciximab is associated with increased frequency of major bleeding complications, including retroperitoneal bleeding, pul-monary bleeding, spontaneous GI or GU bleeding, and bleeding at the arterial access. Risk may be increased with patients weighing <75 kilograms, elderly patients (>65 years of age), history of previous GI disease, and recent thrombolytic therapy. Avoid the creation of venous access at noncompressible sites.

The risk of major bleeds may increase with concurrent use of thrombo-lytics. Anticoagulation, such as with heparin, may contribute to the risk of bleeding. In serious, uncontrolled bleeding, abciximab and heparin should be stopped. Increased risk of hemorrhage during or following angioplasty is associated with unsuccessful PTCA, PTCA procedure >70 minutes duration, or PTCA performed within 12 hours of symptom onset for acute myocardial infarction.

Administration of abciximab may result in human antichimeric antibody formation that can cause hypersensitivity reactions (including anaphy-laxis), thrombocytopenia, or diminished efficacy. Readministration of abciximab within 30 days or in patients with human antichimeric antibodies (HACA) increases the incidence and severity of thrombocytopenia.

Dosage Forms Injection, solution: 2 mg/mL (5 mL)

Overdosage/Treatment Supportive therapy: Essentially no overdose experience; anaphylaxis may be treated with standard treatment; discontinue heparin; use pressure techniques if bleeding develops; consider platelet transfusion for patients with serious, uncontrolled bleeding and if bleeding time is >10 minutes

Drug Interactions

Heparin and aspirin: Use with aspirin and heparin may increase bleeding over aspirin and heparin alone. However, aspirin and heparin were used concurrently in the majority of patients in the major clinical studies of abciximab.

Monoclonal antibodies: Allergic reactions may be increased in patients who have received diagnostic or therapeutic monoclonal antibodies due to the presence of HACA antibodies.

Thrombolytic agents theoretically may increase the risk of bleeding; use with caution.

Warfarin and oral anticoagulants: Risk of bleeding may be increased during concurrent therapy.

Other IIb/IIIa antagonists: Avoid concomitant use of other glycoprotein IIb/IIIa antagonists (see Contraindications).

Pregnancy Risk Factor C

Pregnancy Implications Animal reproduction studies have not been conducted. *In vitro* studies have shown only small amounts of abciximab to cross the placenta. It is not known whether abciximab can cause fetal harm when administered to a pregnant woman or can affect reproduction capacity.

Lactation Excretion in breast milk unknown/use caution

Additional Information Platelet aggregation returns to ≥50% of base-line within 24 hours in 62% of patients and within 48 hours in 88% of patients; bleeding time falls to <12 minutes within 12 hours in 75% of patients and within 24 hours in 90% of patients; may reduce restenosis rate. Risk factors for major bleeding episodes: Female gender, increasing age, low body weight

Acetaldehyde

CAS Number 75-07-0

UN Number 1089

Synonyms Acetic Aldehyde; Ethanal; Ethyl Aldehyde

Use Production of plastics, mirrors, aniline, disinfectants, explosives, varnishes, synthetics, acetic acid, acetic anhydride, food flavorings; also a combustion product of wood and fuels; found in tobacco smoke and car exhaust; found as a fermentation product in beer or wine; a metabolite of ethanol

Mechanism of Toxic Action Pulmonary/mucosal irritant (~$^1/_{10}$ of an irritant as formaldehyde); can cause CNS depression; also may affect mitochondrial phosphorylation and inhibit myocardial protein synthesis

Adverse Reactions Gastrointestinal: Metallic taste

Signs and Symptoms of Overdose Hypertension/tachycardia at low concentrations; hypotension/bradycardia at high concentrations; ocular irritation (at 50 ppm) with photophobia and lacrimation; bronchitis, cough, dermal burns, dyspnea, vomiting (when ingested as a liquid), erythema, pulmonary edema

Toxicodynamics/Kinetics

Absorption: Oral/dermal/inhalation routes

Metabolism: Hepatic oxidation by aldehyde dehydrogenase to acetate

Overdosage/Treatment Decontamination: **Oral:** Lavage (within 1 hour)/activated charcoal. **Dermal:** Wash with soap and water. **Inhalation:** Administer 100% humidified oxygen

Additional Information A colorless liquid with a fruity taste. Specific gravity: 0.78 as a liquid and 1.52 as a gas. In cigarette smoke, acetaldehyde content may approach 1 mg. TLA-TWA: 100 ppm; IDLH: 10,000 ppm. Odor threshold: 0.21 ppm

Acetic Acid

Pronunciation (a SEE tik AS id)
CAS Number 64-19-7
U.S. Brand Names VoSol®
Synonyms Ethanoic Acid
Use Continuous or intermittent irrigation of the bladder; treatment of superficial bacterial infections of the external auditory canal; may be useful in jellyfish sting

Adverse Reactions
Dermatologic: Erythema/edema may occur, nonimmunologic contact urticaria
Endocrine & metabolic: Systemic acidosis
Gastrointestinal (ingestion): Epigastric pain, abdominal pain, pyloric stenosis, gastric perforation, achlorhydria
Ocular: Corneal irritation
Renal: Urologic pain; hematuria has occurred in patients receiving irrigation
Respiratory: Reactive airways disease syndrome

Signs and Symptoms of Overdose Hemolysis, disseminated intravascular coagulopathy
Inhalation: Coagulopathy, cough, hematuria, tachypnea, wheezing
Ingestion: Headache, nausea, vomiting

Dosage
Irrigation: For continuous irrigation of the urinary bladder with 0.25% acetic acid irrigation, the rate of administration will approximate the rate of urine flow; usually 500-1500 mL/24 hours; for periodic irrigation of an indwelling urinary catheter to maintain patency, approximately 50 mL of 0.25% acetic acid irrigation is required. (Note: Dosage of an irrigating solution depends on the capacity or surface area of the structure being irrigated.)
Otic: Insert saturated wick, keep moist 24 hours; remove wick and instill 5 drops 3-4 times/day

Administration Not for internal intake or I.V. infusion; topical use or irrigation use only.

Contraindications Hypersensitivity to acetic acid or any component of the formulation; during transurethral procedures

Warnings Not for internal intake or I.V. infusion; topical use or irrigation use only. Use of irrigation in patients with mucosal lesions of urinary bladder may cause irritation. Systemic acidosis may result from absorption.

Dosage Forms
[DSC] = Discontinued product
Solution for irrigation: 0.25% (250 mL, 500 mL, 1000 mL)
Solution, otic (VéSol® [DSC]): 2% (15 mL)

Overdosage/Treatment
Decontamination: Dilution of affected area; **do not** use ipecac or induce emesis
Supportive therapy: Inhalation 100% oxygen

Pregnancy Risk Factor C

Nursing Implications For continuous or intermittent irrigation of the urinary bladder, urine pH should be checked at least 4 times/day and the irrigation rate adjusted to maintain a pH of 4.5-5; topical use or irrigation use only

Additional Information Clear liquid with pungent odor; similar effects as hydrochloric acid but less corrosive
The frequency of pneumonia cases is about 8%. Lethality in the case of pneumonia development was 50%.

Specific References
Sarmanaev SK, "Risk Factors of Pneumonia Development in Cases of Poisonings by Acetic Acid (AAP)," *J Toxicol Clin Toxicol*, 2003, 41(5):664.
Sarmanaev SK and Akhmetov IR, "The Use of Tables for Prognosis of Life-Threatening States Requiring ICU Hospitalization in Cases of Acetic Acid Poisonings (AAP)," *J Toxicol Clin Toxicol*, 2003, 41(5):661.

Acetone

Pronunciation (A se tone)
Applies to Defatting Agent; Solvent
CAS Number 67-64-1
UN Number 1090
Synonyms 2-Propanone; Dimethyl Formaldehyde; Dimethyl Ketone
Use Volatile solvent (ie, fingernail polish remover, glues, rubber cement); defatting agent in semiconductor industry
Mechanism of Toxic Action Release of norepinephrine on heart; narcotic properties

Adverse Reactions
Cardiovascular: Tachycardia, sinus tachycardia
Central nervous system: Depression
Ocular: Eye irritation, lacrimation
Respiratory: Respiratory depression

Signs and Symptoms of Overdose Ataxia, bronchial irritation, cough, coma, headache, hyperglycemia, hypoglycemia, hypotension, narcosis, sedation, seizures (in children), vomiting

Admission Criteria/Prognosis Patients with mental status or respiratory abnormalities or blood acetone levels >330 mg/L should be admitted; any patient with change in mental status or cardiopulmonary complaints should be admitted

Toxicodynamics/Kinetics
Absorption: Readily through the lungs (75% to 80%) and skin (more slowly) and the GI tract (74% to 83%)
Distribution: V_d: 0.8 L/kg
Metabolism: Hepatic oxidation to acetate and formate at a rate of 1-3 mg/kg/hour
Half-life, elimination: 17-24 hours
Elimination: Excreted through the lungs and urine

Monitoring Parameters Blood glucose, serum/urine acetone, arterial pH
Dosage Forms Liquid: 120 mL, 480 mL
Reference Range Toxic: Blood levels >330 mg/L; urinary acetone levels correlating to air acetone levels of 200 ppm and 750 ppm are 21.6 mg/L and 76.6 mg/L, respectively; blood acetone levels associated with air acetone levels of 200 ppm and 750 ppm are 41.4 mg/L and 118 mg/L respectively; average amount of acetone in expired air of a healthy subject is ~1 mcg/L

Overdosage/Treatment
Decontamination: Oral: **Do not** induce vomiting. Activated charcoal can adsorb 42% to 44% of acetone.
Supportive therapy: Inhalation: Airway support and 100% humidified oxygen

Diagnostic Procedures
- Glucose, Random

Test Interactions May cause a false elevation of serum creatinine through interference with laboratory determination

Additional Information
Ingestion: Toxic dose: 2-3 mL/kg
Fruity odor, sweet taste. Acetone is a metabolite of isopropyl alcohol. Cigarette smoke contains <0.5 mg acetone per cigarette; no increased cancer risk; very water soluble; potentiates CNS toxicity of ethanol
Odor threshold: 13-20 ppm. Atmospheric half-life: ~22 days. Inhalation: TLV-TWA: 750 ppm; IDLH: 20,000 ppm; PEL-TWA: 1000 ppm
Estimated inhalational dose of acetone in an adult: ~0.37 mg/day
Average acetone levels in urban areas: ~7 ppb in the troposphere.
Average amount in drinking water: ~1 ppb

Specific References
Gunia P, Gray J, Gottsch S, et al, "Treatment of Dermal Exposure to Common Household Items," *J Toxicol Clin Toxicol*, 2003, 41(5):650.
Laakso O, Haapla M, Kuitunen T, et al, "Screening of Exhaled Breath by Low-Resolution Multicomponent FT-IR Spectrometry in Patients Attending Emergency Departments," *J Anal Toxicol*, 2004, 28(2):111-7.

Acetonitrile

Applies to Solvent
CAS Number 75-05-8
UN Number 1648
U.S. Brand Names Ardell Instant Glue Remover®; Artificial Nail Tip and Glue Remover®; Super Nail Glue Off®; Super Nail Off®
Synonyms Cyanomethane; Methyl Cyanide
Use Highly polar solvent used in cosmetic nail remover
Mechanism of Toxic Action Converts to cyanide by hepatic metabolism
Signs and Symptoms of Overdose CNS stimulation followed by CNS depression, congestive heart failure, myocardial depression, respiratory depression, seizures

Toxicodynamics/Kinetics
Absorption: Dermal, oral, and inhalation
Distribution: V_d: 0.7 L/kg
Protein binding: 0%
Metabolism: Hepatic hydrolysis to hydrogen cyanide
Half-life: Acetonitrile: 32 hours. Cyanide: 15 hours

Reference Range Whole blood cyanide level of 6 mcg/mL (2310 μmol/L) reported 12 hours after exposure in a 16-month of age boy

Overdosage/Treatment
Decontamination:
Oral: Basic poison management. Emesis is contraindicated due to the rapid course of neurologic symptoms. Activated charcoal may be useful.
Inhalation: Give 100% oxygen.
Supportive therapy: Give sodium bicarbonate for acidosis, otherwise treat as cyanide exposures.
Enhancement of elimination: Hemodialysis and charcoal hemoperfusion have been utilized; hyperbaric oxygen may also be utilized. Hydroxocobalamin and dicobalt-EDTA are used for chelation in Europe.

Antidote(s)
- Amyl Nitrite [ANTIDOTE]
- Sodium Nitrite [ANTIDOTE]
- Sodium Thiosulfate [ANTIDOTE]

Diagnostic Procedures
- Anion Gap, Blood
- Electrolytes, Blood
- Methemoglobin, Blood

Additional Information Decomposes to hydrogen cyanide gas at 120°C

Specific References

Mateus FH, Lepera JS, and Lanchote VL, "Determination of Acetonitrile and Cyanide in Rat Blood: Application to an Experimental Study," *J Anal Toxicol*, 2005, 29:105-10.

Tsutaoka BT, Anderson IB, and Olson KR, "A Case Series of Dermal Acetonitrile Exposures," *J Toxicol Clin Toxicol*, 2003, 41(5):643.

Acetylene

CAS Number 74-86-2
Synonyms Ethyne; Welding Gas
Use Primarily used for welding when mixed with oxygen
Mechanism of Toxic Action Central nervous system depressant combined with asphyxiation
Signs and Symptoms of Overdose Coma, dizziness, garlic-like odor, headache, incoordination, lethargy
Overdosage/Treatment Decontamination: Remove from site of exposure; administer 100% humidified oxygen; monitor carboxyhemoglobin level and if significantly elevated, treat as per carbon monoxide exposure
Additional Information May cause elevation of urine and serum acetone; may present as diabetic coma; contaminants may include phosphine ($<$95 ppm), arsine ($<$3 ppm), and hydrogen sulfide. See table.

Air Concentration Levels and Symptoms
10%: Intoxication
20%: Staggering gait
30%: Incoordination
33% (at 7 minutes): Coma

Acetylene Dichloride

Applies to Dye (Production); Perfume (Production); Thermoplastics (Production)
CAS Number 156-59-2; 156-60-5; 540-59-0
UN Number 1150
U.S. Brand Names Dioform®
Synonyms 1,2 DCE; 1,2-Dichloroethene
Use Chemical intermediate in the production of chlorinated solvents; used in production of dyes, perfumes, and thermoplastics
Mechanism of Toxic Action Mucosal irritant and CNS depressant
Adverse Reactions
Central nervous system: CNS depression
Dermatologic: Dermal irritation
Ocular: Eye irritation at concentrations of 1000 ppm
Signs and Symptoms of Overdose Dizziness, lethargy, nausea (at concentrations of ~2000 ppm), muscle cramps, tremor
Toxicodynamics/Kinetics
Absorption: Through inhalation (75%)
Metabolism: Hepatic (cytochrome P450) epoxidation to dichloroethanol and dichloroacetic acid
Overdosage/Treatment
Decontamination: **Oral:** Lavage within 1 hour of ingestion. **Dermal:** Wash with soap and water. **Inhalation:** Remove from source and administer 100% humidified oxygen.
Supportive therapy: Calcium gluconate may relieve muscle cramping.
Additional Information Very flammable. Odor threshold: 17 ppm (acrid). TLV-TWA: 200 ppm. Usual general population exposure: 0.013 to 0.076 ppb (1-6 mcg/day). EPA water maximum containment level: 0.07 mg/L (cis-isomer); 0.1 mg/L (trans-isomer). Half-life: Atmospheric: 8.3 days (cis-isomer); 3.6 days (trans-isomer). Water: 3-6 hours

Acrolein

Related Information
- Allyl Alcohol

Applies to Biocide (Paper Industry); Herbicides (Manufacture); Pharmaceuticals (Manufacture); Slimicide (Paper Industry); Tear Gas; Textiles (Manufacture); Tissue Fixative (Paper Industry)
CAS Number 100-73-2; 107-02-8; 869-29-4
UN Number 1092; 2607
U.S. Brand Names Aqualin®; Magnacide H®
Synonyms Propylene Aldehyde; Pyran Aldehyde: 2-Propenal
Use Manufacture of pharmaceuticals, herbicides, textiles, and as a tear gas; found as an irritant gas generated by fire; production of acrylic acid; as a tissue fixative, biocide, and slimicide in paper industry
Mechanism of Toxic Action Irritation of mucous membranes; suppresses glycolysis and reacts with sulfhydryl groups of proteins; release of catecholamines is noted; high water stability can lead to primary upper airway damage

Adverse Reactions
Eye: Irritation
Cardiovascular: Sinus tachycardia
Respiratory: Pulmonary edema
Signs and Symptoms of Overdose Bronchial constriction, coma, cough, dyspnea, erythema, hypertension, lacrimation, tachycardia, tachypnea at air levels of 0.6 ppm
Admission Criteria/Prognosis Patients with persistent respiratory symptoms or elevation of liver alkaline phosphatase (which may be a biomarker of exposure) should be considered for hospital admission
Toxicodynamics/Kinetics
Absorption: Through ingestion and inhalation
Metabolism: Hepatic to S-carboxy ethyl mercapturic acid methyl ester
Overdosage/Treatment
Decontamination: Oral: Lavage (within 1 hour)/activated charcoal
Supportive therapy: Inhalation: Humidified oxygen, inhaled beta-adrenergic agonist agents for wheezing; treat for pulmonary edema
Additional Information
Toxic dose for irritation: 10 ppm
One of the major irritants in smog; yellow liquid with pungent odor (acrid)
Acrolein is present in cigarette smoke: 3-220 mcg/cigarette and marijuana: 92-145 mcg/joint
Odor threshold: Water: 0.11 ppm. Air: 0.16 ppm. TLV-TWA: 0.1 ppm; IDLH: 2 ppm; PEL-TWA: 0.1 ppm. Atmospheric half-life: 15-20 hours. Ambient air level: ~0.3 ppb
Newer concepts: N-acetylcysteine protected against hepatitis in laboratory animals

Acrylamide

CAS Number 79-06-1
UN Number 2074
U.S. Brand Names Nyloprint®
Synonyms 2-Propenamide; Acrylic Amide; Ethylene Carboxamide; Propenamide
Use Vinyl monomer synthesized from acetonitrile; it is polymerized to produce flocculators used in waste water treatment, paper strengtheners, grouting agents, gels, and adhesive agents
Mechanism of Toxic Action Causes progressive degeneration by sensory neurons ("dying back"), starting distally and progressing proximally; thought to be due to activation of activity of sulfhydryl-dependent glycolytic enzymes inhibiting axonal energy production
Adverse Reactions
Central nervous system: Ataxia, axonopathy
Dermatologic: Dermal irritation, desquamation of palms and soles
Gastrointestinal: Anorexia
Neuromuscular & skeletal: Hyporeflexia, neuritis, paresthesia
Respiratory: Cough
Miscellaneous: Palm diaphoresis
Signs and Symptoms of Overdose
Dependent on time and duration, total dose, and rate of exposure
High-dose:
Acute: Ataxia, cardiovascular collapse, confusion, disorientation, hallucinations, hypothermia, possible seizures, somnolence, tremor
Subacute (days/weeks): Decreased concentration, drowsiness, dysarthria, nystagmus, paresthesia (may follow in 2-3 weeks), somnolence, truncal ataxia, urinary retention
Chronic: Sensorimotor and proprioceptive neuropathy
Complete recovery over weeks to months in mild exposure but in severe exposure, recovery may be incomplete. Elevated liver transaminases and decreased urinary output have been reported. Severe thrombocytopenia has been reported. Exfoliated erythematous rash (especially on hands) occurs with chronic exposure.
Toxicodynamics/Kinetics
Absorption: Rapid through oral, dermal, and inhalation
Distribution: Rapid to blood and then tissue
Metabolism: Hepatic
Half-life: 2 hours
Time to peak blood levels: 1 hour
Elimination: Renal
Warnings/Precautions When vapors are present, must use impervious body protector as significant toxicity may occur through dermal absorption
Overdosage/Treatment
Decontamination: Lavage (within 1 hour)/activated charcoal
Supportive therapy: Pyridoxine (vitamin B_6) 3-10 g of 10% solution in D_5W over 30-60 minutes; may delay neurotoxic effect. N-acetylcysteine has been utilized, but it is of unproven benefit.
Antidote(s)
- Pyridoxine [ANTIDOTE]

Additional Information Acrylamide may be measured in tissue and blood by HPLC; considered a suspected human skin carcinogen. Odorless, colorless, white flake-like powder

Specific References
Mucci LA, Sandin S, Balter K, et al, "Acrylamide Intake and Breast Cancer Risk in Swedish Women," *JAMA*, 2005, 293(11):1326-7.

Acrylonitrile

Applies to Acrylic/Modacrylic Fibers; Acrylics; Adhesives; Fumigant; Pesticide; Plastics; Rubber

CAS Number 107-13-1

UN Number 1093

Synonyms 2-Propenenitrile; Cyanoethylene; Vinyl Cyanide

Use Raw material in acrylic/modacrylic fibers; also used in the manufacture of plastics, rubber, acrylics, and adhesives; used as a fumigant and pesticide

Mechanism of Toxic Action Produced through the process of propylene amoxidation; hepatic conversion to cyanide can produce signs and symptoms of cyanide

Adverse Reactions
Cardiovascular: Tachycardia
Central nervous system: Dizziness, headache, seizures
Dermatologic: Dermal irritation, desquamation, toxic epidermal necrosis may develop in 3 weeks
Endocrine & metabolic: Lactic acidosis
Gastrointestinal: Nausea, diarrhea, vomiting
Hematologic: Anemia
Hepatic: Jaundice, hepatic injury
Neuromuscular & skeletal: Limb weakness
Ocular: Conjunctivitis
Respiratory: Irregular breathing, dyspnea

Admission Criteria/Prognosis All symptomatic patients should probably be admitted to an intensive care unit for 1-2 days; asymptomatic patients should be observed for at least 2 hours and then can be discharged; survival after 4 hours (in an acute exposure) is usually associated with recovery

Toxicodynamics/Kinetics
Absorption: Inhalation: 52%. Dermal: 0.6 mg/cm^2/hour
Metabolism: To 2-cyanoethylene oxide then converted to cyanide
Half-life: 7-8 hours
Elimination: Renal (68%)

Reference Range Plasma thiocyanate level >20 mg/L in nonsmokers or 30 mg/L in smokers is consistent with exposure to acrylonitrile; exposure to an average air level of 4.2 ppm of acrylonitrile over an 8-hour day produces a urine acrylonitrile level of 360 mcg/L and a urinary thiocyanate level of 11.4 mg/L

Overdosage/Treatment
Decontamination: Basic poison management (lavage within 1 hour/ activated charcoal). Emesis is contraindicated due to the rapid course of neurologic symptoms. Give 100% oxygen.
Supportive therapy: Give sodium bicarbonate for acidosis; cyanide antidote kit (amyl nitrate, sodium nitrate followed by sodium thiosulfate); N-acetylcysteine has been effective in rodent models
Enhancement of elimination: Hemodialysis and charcoal hemoperfusion have been utilized; hyperbaric oxygen may also be utilized. Hydroxocobalamin, dicobalt-EDTA, and 4-dimethylaminophenol used for chelation in Europe

Antidote(s)
- Amyl Nitrite [ANTIDOTE]
- Cyanide Antidote Kit [ANTIDOTE]
- Hydroxocobalamin [ANTIDOTE]
- Oxygen (Hyperbaric) [ANTIDOTE]
- Sodium Nitrite [ANTIDOTE]
- Sodium Thiosulfate [ANTIDOTE]

Diagnostic Procedures
- Anion Gap, Blood
- Cyanide, Blood
- Electrolytes, Blood
- Methemoglobin, Blood
- Thiocyanate, Blood or Urine

Additional Information
Levels of 16-100 ppm for 20-45 minutes can produce symptoms.
Children are more susceptible than adults.
Associated with increase in prostate, colon, lung, and stomach cancer.
Full recovery will usually occur if the patient survives for 4 hours.
Pungent odor (onion/garlic-like).
Odor threshold in water: 19 ppm. Atmospheric half-life: 12 hours.
TLV-TWA: 2 ppm; IDLH: 4000 ppm
Typical acrylonitrile level in margarine: 25 mcg/kg; in cigarettes: 1-2 mg/cigarette.
Acrylonitrile can be absorbed through leather products.

Specific References
Hung D, Hsu C, and Chen Y, "Cyanide Intoxication in an Acrylonitrile Chemical Accident," *Clin Toxicol (Phila)*, 2005, 43:751.
Swaen GM, Bloemen LJ, Twisk J, et al, "Mortality Update of Workers Exposed to Acrylonitrile in the Netherlands," *J Occup Environ Med*, 2004, 46(7):691-8.

Acyclovir

Pronunciation (ay SYE kloe veer)

Related Information
- Famciclovir
- Therapeutic Drugs Associated with Hallucinations
- Valacyclovir

CAS Number 59277-89-3; 69657-51-8

U.S. Brand Names Zovirax®

Synonyms Aciclovir; ACV; Acycloguanosine

Use Treatment of genital herpes simplex virus (HSV), herpes labialis (cold sores), herpes zoster (shingles), HSV encephalitis, neonatal HSV, mucocutaneous HSV, varicella-zoster (chickenpox)

Unlabeled/Investigational Use Prevention of HSV reactivation in HIV-positive patients; prevention of HSV reactivation in hematopoietic stem-cell transplant (HSCT); prevention of HSV reactivation during periods of neutropenia in patients with acute leukemia

Mechanism of Action Inhibits DNA synthesis and viral replication by competing with deoxyguanosine triphosphate for viral DNA polymerase (thymidine kinase) and by being incorporated into viral DNA

Adverse Reactions
Systemic: Oral:
Central nervous system: Lightheadedness, headache
Gastrointestinal: Diarrhea, nausea, vomiting, abdominal pain
Systemic: Parenteral:
Central nervous system: **Lightheadedness**
Dermatologic: Hives, itching, rash
Gastrointestinal: **Anorexia**, nausea, vomiting
Hepatic: Liver function tests increased
Local: Inflammation at injection site or phlebitis
Renal: Acute renal failure, BUN increased, creatinine increased
Topical:
Dermatologic: **Mild pain, burning, stinging**, itching
All forms: Postmarketing and/or case reports (<1%): Aggression, agitation, alopecia, anaphylaxis, anemia, angioedema, anorexia, ataxia, coma, confusion, consciousness decreased, delirium, diarrhea, dizziness, encephalopathy, erythema multiforme, fever, gastrointestinal distress, hallucinations, hematuria, hepatitis, hyperbilirubinemia, insomnia, jaundice, leukocytoclastic vasculitis, leukopenia, local tissue necrosis (following extravasation), mental depression, myalgia, paresthesia, peripheral edema, photosensitization, pruritus, psychosis, renal failure, seizures, somnolence, sore throat, Stevens-Johnson syndrome, thrombocytopenia, thrombocytopenic purpura/hemolytic uremic syndrome (TTP/HUS), toxic epidermal necrolysis, tremor, urticaria, visual disturbances

Pharmacodynamics/Kinetics
Absorption: Oral: 15% to 30%
Distribution: V$_d$: 0.8 L/kg (63.6 L): Widely (eg, brain, kidney, lungs, liver, spleen, muscle, uterus, vagina, CSF)
Protein binding: 9% to 33%
Metabolism: Converted by viral enzymes to acyclovir monophosphate, and further converted to diphosphate then triphosphate (active form) by cellular enzymes
Bioavailability: Oral: 10% to 20% with normal renal function (bioavailability decreases with increased dose)
Half-life elimination: Terminal: Neonates: 4 hours; Children 1-12 years: 2-3 hours; Adults: 3 hours
Time to peak, serum: Oral: Within 1.5-2 hours
Excretion: Urine (62% to 90% as unchanged drug and metabolite)

Dosage
Note: Obese patients should be dosed using ideal body weight
Genital HSV:
I.V.: Children ≥12 years and Adults (immunocompetent): Initial episode, severe: 5 mg/kg every 8 hours for 5-7 days
Oral:
Children:
Initial episode (unlabeled use): 40-80 mg/kg/day divided into 3-4 doses for 5-10 days (maximum: 1 g/day)
Chronic suppression (unlabeled use; limited data): 80 mg/kg/day in 3 divided doses (maximum: 1 g/day), re-evaluate after 12 months of treatment
Adults:
Initial episode: 200 mg every 4 hours while awake (5 times/day) for 10 days (per manufacturer's labeling); 400 mg 3 times/day for 5-10 days has also been reported
Recurrence: 200 mg every 4 hours while awake (5 times/day) for 5 days (per manufacturer's labeling; begin at earliest signs of disease); 400 mg 3 times/day for 5 days has also been reported
Chronic suppression: 400 mg twice daily or 200 mg 3-5 times/day, for up to 12 months followed by re-evaluation (per manufacturer's labeling); 400-1200 mg/day in 2-3 divided doses has also been reported

Topical: Adults (immunocompromised): Ointment: Initial episode: $^1/_2$" ribbon of ointment for a 4" square surface area every 3 hours (6 times/day) for 7 days

Herpes labialis (cold sores): Topical: Children ≥12 years and Adults: Cream: Apply 5 times/day for 4 days

Herpes zoster (shingles):

Oral: Adults (immunocompetent): 800 mg every 4 hours (5 times/day) for 7-10 days

I.V.:

Children <12 years (immunocompromised): 20 mg/kg/dose every 8 hours for 7 days

Children ≥12 years and Adults (immunocompromised): 10 mg/kg/dose or 500 mg/m^2/dose every 8 hours for 7 days

HSV encephalitis: I.V.:

Children 3 months to 12 years: 20 mg/kg/dose every 8 hours for 10 days (per manufacturer's labeling); dosing for 14-21 days also reported

Children ≥12 years and Adults: 10 mg/kg/dose every 8 hours for 10 days (per manufacturer's labeling); 10-15 mg/kg/dose every 8 hours for 14-21 days also reported

Mucocutaneous HSV:

I.V.:

Children <12 years (immunocompromised): 10 mg/kg/dose every 8 hours for 7 days

Children ≥12 years and Adults (immunocompromised): 5 mg/kg/dose every 8 hours for 7 days (per manufacturer's labeling); dosing for up to 14 days also reported

Oral: Adults (immunocompromised, unlabeled use): 400 mg 5 times a day for 7-14 days

Topical: Ointment: Adults (nonlife-threatening, immunocompromised): $^1/_2$" ribbon of ointment for a 4" square surface area every 3 hours (6 times/day) for 7 days

Neonatal HSV: I.V.: Neonate: Birth to 3 months: 10 mg/kg/dose every 8 hours for 10 days (manufacturer's labeling); 15 mg/kg/dose or 20 mg/kg/dose every 8 hours for 14-21 days has also been reported

Varicella-zoster (chickenpox): Begin treatment within the first 24 hours of rash onset:

Oral:

Children ≥2 years and ≤40 kg (immunocompetent): 20 mg/kg/dose (up to 800 mg/dose) 4 times/day for 5 days

Children >40 kg and Adults (immunocompetent): 800 mg/dose 4 times a day for 5 days

I.V.:

Children <1 year (immunocompromised, unlabeled use): 10 mg/kg/dose every 8 hours for 7-10 days

Children ≥1 year and Adults (immunocompromised, unlabeled use): 1500 mg/m^2/day divided every 8 hours or 10 mg/kg/dose every 8 hours for 7-10 days

Prevention of HSV reactivation in HIV-positive patients, for use only when recurrences are frequent or severe (unlabeled use): Oral:

Children: 80 mg/kg/day in 3-4 divided doses

Adults: 200 mg 3 times/day or 400 mg 2 times/day

Prevention of HSV reactivation in HSCT (unlabeled use): Note: Start at the beginning of conditioning therapy and continue until engraftment or until mucositis resolves (~30 days)

Oral: Adults: 200 mg 3 times/day

I.V.:

Children: 250 mg/m^2/dose every 8 hours or 125 mg/m^2/dose every 6 hours

Adults: 250 mg/m^2/dose every 12 hours

Bone marrow transplant recipients (unlabeled use): I.V.: Children and Adults: Allogeneic patients who are HSV and CMV seropositive: 500 mg/m^2/dose (10 mg/kg) every 8 hours; for clinically-symptomatic CMV infection, consider replacing acyclovir with ganciclovir

Dosing adjustment in renal impairment:

Oral:

Cl_{cr} 10-25 mL/minute: Normal dosing regimen 800 mg every 4 hours: Administer 800 mg every 8 hours

Cl_{cr} <10 mL/minute:

Normal dosing regimen 200 mg every 4 hours, 200 mg every 8 hours, or 400 mg every 12 hours: Administer 200 mg every 12 hours

Normal dosing regimen 800 mg every 4 hours: Administer 800 mg every 12 hours

I.V.:

Cl_{cr} 25-50 mL/minute: Administer recommended dose every 12 hours

Cl_{cr} 10-25 mL/minute: Administer recommended dose every 24 hours

Cl_{cr} <10 mL/minute: Administer 50% of recommended dose every 24 hours

Hemodialysis: Administer dose after dialysis

Peritoneal dialysis: No supplemental dose needed

CAVH: 3.5 mg/kg/day

CVVHD/CVVH: Adjust dose based upon Cl_{cr} 30 mL/minute

Monitoring Parameters Urinalysis, BUN, serum creatinine, liver enzymes, CBC

Administration

Oral: May be administered with or without food.

I.V.: Avoid rapid infusion; infuse over 1 hour to prevent renal damage; maintain adequate hydration of patient; check for phlebitis and rotate infusion sites

Topical: Not for use in the eye. Apply using a finger cot or rubber glove to avoid transmission to other parts of the body or to other persons.

Contraindications Hypersensitivity to acyclovir, valacyclovir, or any component of the formulation

Warnings

Use with caution in immunocompromised patients; thrombocytopenic purpura/hemolytic uremic syndrome (TTP/HUS) has been reported. Use caution in the elderly, pre-existing renal disease, or in those receiving other nephrotoxic drugs. Maintain adequate hydration during oral or intravenous therapy. Use I.V. preparation with caution in patients with underlying neurologic abnormalities, serious hepatic or electrolyte abnormalities, or substantial hypoxia.

Safety and efficacy of oral formulations have not been established in pediatric patients <2 years of age.

Chickenpox: Treatment should begin within 24 hours of appearance of rash; oral route not recommended for routine use in otherwise healthy children with varicella, but may be effective in patients at increased risk of moderate to severe infection (>12 years of age, chronic cutaneous or pulmonary disorders, long-term salicylate therapy, corticosteroid therapy).

Genital herpes: Physical contact should be avoided when lesions are present; transmission may also occur in the absence of symptoms. Treatment should begin with the first signs or symptoms.

Herpes labialis: For external use only to the lips and face; do not apply to eye or inside the mouth or nose. Treatment should begin with the first signs or symptoms.

Herpes zoster: Acyclovir should be started within 72 hours of appearance of rash to be effective.

Dosage Forms

[DSC] = Discontinued product

Capsule: 200 mg

Zovirax®: 200 mg

Cream, topical:

Zovirax®: 5% (2 g, 5 g)

Injection, powder for reconstitution, as sodium: 500 mg, 1000 mg

Zovirax®: 500 mg [DSC]

Injection, solution, as sodium [preservative free]: 25 mg/mL (20 mL, 40 mL); 50 mg/mL (10 mL, 20 mL)

Ointment, topical:

Zovirax®: 5% (15 g)

Suspension, oral: 200 mg/5 mL (480 mL)

Zovirax®: 200 mg/5 mL (480 mL) [banana flavor]

Tablet: 400 mg, 800 mg

Zovirax®: 400 mg, 800 mg

Reference Range Neurotoxicity is associated with plasma levels of 470 μmol/mL

Overdosage/Treatment

Decontamination: Ipecac within 30 minutes or lavage (within 1 hour)/activated charcoal

Supportive therapy: Renal toxicity and crystalluria can be managed with I.V. fluid hydration

Enhancement of elimination: Multiple dosing of activated charcoal may be effective; hemodialysis can remove ~60% of total body burden; exchange transfusion is not useful

Pregnancy Risk Factor B B

Pregnancy Implications Teratogenic effects were not observed in animal studies. Acyclovir has been shown to cross the human placenta. Results from a pregnancy registry, established in 1984 and closed in 1999, did not find an increase in the number of birth defects with exposure to acyclovir when compared to those expected in the general population. However, due to the small size of the registry and lack of long-term data, the manufacturer recommends using during pregnancy with caution and only when clearly needed. Data from the pregnancy registry may be obtained from GlaxoSmithKline.

Lactation Enters breast milk/use with caution (AAP rates "compatible")

Nursing Implications Infuse over 1 hour; maintain adequate hydration of patient; check infusion site for phlebitis, rotate site to prevent phlebitis; wear gloves when applying ointment for self-protection

Additional Information Not effective against cytomegalovirus. Injection formulations: Sodium content of 1 g: 96.6 mg (4.2 mEq)

Specific References

Benson PC and Swadron SP, "Empiric Acyclovir is Infrequently Initiated in the Emergency Department to Patients Ultimately Diagnosed with Encephalitis," *Ann Emerg Med*, 2006, 47(1):100-5.

Hsu CC, Lai TI, Lien WC, et al, "Emergent Hemodialysis for Acyclovir Toxicity," *Am J Emerg Med*, 2005, 23(7):899-900.

Aldicarb

CAS Number 116-06-3
U.S. Brand Names Temik®
Use Marketed in solutions of up to 100% aldicarb; insecticide
Mechanism of Toxic Action Potent, reversible inhibition of acetylcholinesterase and plasma cholinesterase, resulting in excess accumulation of acetylcholine at muscarinic and nicotinic receptors, and in the central nervous system

Adverse Reactions

Cardiovascular: **Hyperdynamic** (~18% to 21%) or hypodynamic (~7% to 10%) states, edema, QT prolongation, sinus bradycardia, sinus tachycardia

Central nervous system: Toxicity is limited because carbamates do not significantly cross the blood-brain barrier; CNS changes occur with most severe intoxications, hyperactivity, hypothermia

Genitourinary: Incontinence

Neuromuscular & skeletal: Weakness, paralysis

Respiratory: Respiratory depression

Miscellaneous: Flu-like symptoms (especially with chronic exposure)

Signs and Symptoms of Overdose Abdominal pain, agitation, generalized asthenia, AV block, asystole, bradycardia, bronchorrhea, coma, confusion, cranial nerve palsy, decreased hemoglobin, decreased red blood cell count, decreased platelet count, diaphragmatic paralysis, dysarthria, fecal incontinence, flaccid paralysis, excessive sweating, headache, heart block, hyperglycemia (severe intoxication), hypertension, hypotension, lacrimation, metabolic acidosis (severe intoxication), miosis (unreactive to light), mydriasis (rarely), skeletal muscle fasciculation, nausea, pallor, pulmonary edema, QT prolongation, respiratory depression, salivation, seizures, tachycardia, tachypnea, urinary incontinence, vomiting

Toxicodynamics/Kinetics

Absorption: Readily through oral, dermal, or respiratory exposure

Metabolism: Rapidly metabolized to weakly active compounds through hepatic hydrolysis and other pathways, and may undergo enterohepatic recirculation

Half-life: 5.75 hours

Elimination: Metabolites are excreted in urine

Warnings/Precautions Aldicarb translocates from soil into food sources in significant quantity; readily absorbed through intact skin; risk of aspiration pneumonitis exists with agents having a hydrocarbon vehicle

Reference Range

Highest survivable aldicarb concentrations: Serum: 3.22 mcg/mL; Urine: 1 mcg/mL

Following a 10 g ingestion, peak serum aldicarb level was 3.22 mcg/L (at 3 hours) and associated with severe toxicity; serum aldicarb >0.1 mcg/mL is associated with symptoms

Overdosage/Treatment

Decontamination: Isolation, bagging, and disposal of all contaminated clothing and other articles. All emergency medical workers and hospital staff should follow appropriate precautions regarding exposure to hazardous material including the use of protective clothing, masks, goggles, and respiratory equipment.

Oral: Activated charcoal can be administered either orally or via a nasogastric tube. **Do not** induce emesis because of danger of sudden respiratory compromise, alterations in mental status, seizures, coma, and possible aspiration of hydrocarbon vehicles. Do not utilize cathartics.

Dermal: Prompt thorough scrubbing of all affected areas with soap and water, including hair and nails; 5% bleach may also be used

Ocular: Irrigation with copious tepid sterile water or saline

Supportive therapy: Airway management, ventilatory assistance, humidified oxygen administration, and close monitoring for sudden respiratory failure

Antidote:

Atropine: Administration should be guided by respiratory status, starting at 2-5 mg I.V. every 5-10 minutes as needed, and should be titrated to the resolution of excess pulmonary secretions. Frequent administration of large doses (cumulative doses >100 mg) may be necessary in massive exposures.

Glycopyrrolate: May be administered if atropine is unavailable (200-400 mcg I.V. or I.M. initially, or ~$\frac{1}{2}$ the dose of atropine).

2-PAM: Although not specifically indicated, 2-PAM may be considered in the following situations:

Life-threatening symptoms such as respiratory paralysis

Continued excessive atropine requirements

Concomitant organophosphate and carbamate exposure

Enhancement of elimination: Dialysis and hemoperfusion are not indicated due to effectiveness of the prescribed treatment and large volumes of distribution of organophosphates.

Antidote(s)
- Atropine [ANTIDOTE]

Diagnostic Procedures
- Creatinine, Serum
- Pseudocholinesterase, Serum

Drug Interaction Paralysis is potentiated by neuromuscular blockade (ie, pancuronium, vecuronium, succinylcholine, atracurium, doxacurium, mivacurium); inhibition of serum esterase prolongs the half-life of succinylcholine, cocaine, and other ester anesthetics; cholinergic toxicity is potentiated by cholinesterase inhibitors such as physostigmine

Additional Information

Red blood cell cholinesterase and serum pseudocholinesterase may be depressed following acute or chronic organophosphate exposure and are theoretically useful for differentiating between carbamate and organophosphate exposures; RBC cholinesterase is typically not analyzed by in-house laboratories and is usually not available for consideration during acute management. Pseudocholinesterase levels may be rapidly available from some in-house laboratories, but are not as reliable a marker of organophosphate exposure because of variability secondary to variant genotypes, hepatic disease, oral estrogen use, or malnutrition, thus they may not be useful in ruling out carbamate exposure.

The intermediate syndrome is not related to delayed neuropathy.

QT_c prolongation on ECG in the setting of organophosphate poisoning is associated with a high incidence of respiratory failure and mortality.

Spray solutions are balanced to pH = 7.0 and also contain dichloromethane and methyl isocyanate;

Other information concerning pesticide exposures is available through the EPA-funded National Pesticide Telecommunications Network: 1-800-858-7378 (weekdays, 8 AM to 6 PM, Central Standard time)

Specific References

Mendes CA, Mendes GE, Cipullo JP, et al, "Acute Intoxication Due to Ingestion of Vegetables Contaminated with Aldicarb," *Clin Toxicol (Phila)*, 2005, 43(2):117-8.

Aldrin

Related Information
- Dieldrin

CAS Number 309-00-2
U.S. Brand Names Aldrec®; Aldrex®; Aldrite®; Compound 118®; Drinox®; Octalene®; Seedrin®
Synonyms HHDN
Use Insecticide - general crop protection, used against termites, EPA discontinued use in 1970s
Mechanism of Toxic Action Cyclodiene organochlorine agent which may be a competitive inhibitor of the inhibitory neurotransmitter GABA at the GABA A receptor

Adverse Reactions

Central nervous system: Convulsions, headache, dizziness, seizures

Gastrointestinal: Nausea, vomiting, anorexia

Hematologic: Hemolysis

Neuromuscular & skeletal: Muscle twitching

Renal: Hematuria, albuminuria, elevated blood urea nitrogen

Toxicodynamics/Kinetics

Absorption: Absorbed by oral or dermal routes; also by inhalation

Metabolism: Epoxidized to dieldrin (by mono-oxygenase) then to pentachloroketone and aldrin dicarboxylic acid (among other metabolites)

Elimination: Feces

Reference Range Blood aldrin levels taken from general population in El Paso, TX (1982-3) demonstrated presence of aldrin in 34% of subjects at a mean level of 4.6 ppb

Overdosage/Treatment

Decontamination: Oral: Activated charcoal. **Dermal:** Soap and water wash. **Ocular:** Irrigate with saline.

Supportive therapy: Beta-adrenergic blocking agents may be used for tachycardia or hypertension. Benzodiazepines, phenobarbital, or phenytoin can be used for seizures.

Enhancement of elimination: Multiple dosing of activated charcoal may be effective.

Additional Information Lethal dose: Oral: 71 mg/kg. Odor threshold: 0.02 mg/kg

Allyl Alcohol

Related Information
- Acrolein

CAS Number 107-18-6
UN Number 1098
Synonyms Propenol; Vinylcarbinol
Use

Industrial: Synthetic chemical intermediate

Agriculture: Weed killer

Mechanism of Toxic Action A mucosal and skin irritant; the metabolite acrolein can produce cardiotoxicity and rapid onset of coma

Adverse Reactions

Central nervous system: Headache, rapid onset of coma

Dermatologic: Dermal irritation, bullous eruption

Gastrointestinal: Nausea, vomiting

Ocular: Lacrimation, irritation, photophobia, corneal ulceration

Renal: Hematuria

Respiratory: Cough, dyspnea, hemoptysis

Toxicodynamics/Kinetics Hepatic metabolism to acrolein through alcohol dehydrogenase enzyme (ADH)

Reference Range Postmortem blood allyl alcohol level of 309 mg/L and acrolein level of 7.2 mg/L were noted in a suicide fatality after an ~200 g allyl alcohol ingestion

Overdosage/Treatment

Decontamination: **Oral**: Dilute with 4-8 ounces of milk or water; activated charcoal may be helpful. Consider gastric lavage if patient presents within 2 hours. **Dermal**: Irrigate and wash with soap and water. **Inhalation**: Administer 100% humidified oxygen. **Ocular**: Administer copious amounts of saline in water through irrigation.

Supportive therapy: Although no human studies exist, fomepizole or ethanol therapy to inhibit ADH enzyme and acrolein formation may be useful. N-acetylcysteine administration may also be helpful (no human data).

Enhancement of elimination: Hemodialysis may enhance elimination (no human data).

Additional Information

Oral lethal dose: 50-500 mg/kg

Odor threshold: 0.8 ppm. Eye irritation can occur at 5 ppm. IDLH: 20 ppm. Atmospheric half-life: 6 hours.

A colorless liquid with a mustard-like odor; soluble with water

Aluminum

CAS Number 7429-90-5

UN Number 1309; 1383; 1396

Commonly Found In Packaging, building, transportation, and electrical applications

Use Primarily used in metallurgical purposes (ie, production of alloy castings)

Mechanism of Toxic Action Can cause neurotoxicity through an unknown mechanism. Proposed mechanisms include inhibition of neuronal microtubule formation and competition with cations (especially magnesium).

Signs and Symptoms of Overdose Asterixis, asthma, dialysis dementia (dysarthria, stammering, seizures, and motor disturbances), encephalopathy, microcytic anemia, myoclonus, osteomalacia, pulmonary fibrosis, seizures, slurred speech

Toxicodynamics/Kinetics

Absorption: Oral: 0.1% to 0.3%

Elimination: Renal (up to 0.5 mg/24 hours)

Reference Range Normal serum level: 0.35-0.85 mcg/dL (0.13-0.32 μmol/L). Aluminum bone disease occurs with aluminum levels >3 mcg/dL.

Overdosage/Treatment

Decontamination: Oral: Ranitidine (300 mg/day) may decrease aluminum absorption

Supportive therapy: Benzodiazepines should be utilized for seizure control. Deferoxamine is the chelator of choice. Aluminum neurotoxicity in dialysis patients can be treated with deferoxamine 1 g I.M. on the evening prior to dialysis and a high-flux dialyzer or charcoal cartridge to remove DFO-aluminum complex during dialysis. Anemia can be treated with a 3-month course of deferoxamine (30 mg/kg I.V. over the last 2 hours of dialysis 3 times per week).

Additional Information

Insoluble in water and alcohol; iron deficiency may increase aluminum absorption, possible association with dialysis, dementia, and renal osteodystrophy

Aluminum is the most abundant metallic component (~8%) of the Earth's crust. Bauxite is the main source of environmental aluminum.

Aluminum content of tobacco and cannabis is about 0.4% by weight

Aluminum only has one oxidation state (+3); background atmospheric aluminum levels range from 0.005-0.2 mg/m³; baseline drinking water aluminum levels range from 0.003-1.6 mg/L; soil aluminum levels range from 700 mg/kg to over 100,000 mg/kg

Foods containing highest aluminum levels are ground coffee beans (52 mg/kg), salt (31-37 mg/kg), natural peanut butter (26-94 mg/kg), pumpernickel bread (13.2 mg/kg), chocolate cookie, Oreo® (12.7 mg/kg), spinach (8.7 mg/kg), and lettuce (7.2 mg/kg). Calcium gluconate contains 38.8 mcg aluminum per 8 mL volume; potassium acid phosphate contains 2.8 mcg aluminum per 1.3 mL total volume.

Aluminum is not bioconcentrated in plants or terrestrial food chain; antacids/buffered aspirin can contain from 4-562 mg/kg of aluminum. Daily intake of aluminum is ~2-14 mg by food ingestion, 0.2 mg through drinking water, and 0.2 mg by inhalation. Normal dietary

aluminum is 5 mg/day with ~15 mcg absorbed, thus the total body burden of aluminum is ~30-50 mg (50% in bone, 25% in lungs). Atmospheric aluminum levels range from 0.005-0.18 ng/mg (higher in the summer). Typical aluminum soil concentration is 71,000 mg/kg. See table.

Estimated Number of Workers Potentially Exposed to Aluminum and Compounds in the Workplace

Aluminum Compound	Number of Potentially Exposed Workers
Aluminum — pure	31,369
Aluminum dust	1833
Aluminum — unknown	1,033,235
Aluminum oxide	1,345,659
Aluminum oxide, powder	172,756
Aluminum hydroxide	325,788
Aluminum hydroxide, gel	37,772
Dried aluminum hydroxide gel	7006
Aluminum chloride	49,913
Aluminum chloride hydroxide	1579
Aluminum sulfate	212,239
Aluminum sulfate, liquid	23,354
Aluminum sulfate, powder	1496
Aluminum nitrate	34,929
Aluminum phosphide	622
Aluminum phosphate	19,526
Aluminum phosphate, gel	4228
Aluminum fluoride	175
Aluminum, calcined	27,670

Source: National Occupational Exposure Study (NOES); NIOSH 1991
Reference: U.S. Department of Health and Human Services, "Toxicological Profile for Aluminum," Agency for Toxic Substances and Disease Registry, September 1997.

Specific References

Bouchard NC, Malostvoker I, Harbord N, et al, "Acute Aluminum Encephalopathy from Alum Bladder Irrigation: Aluminum Extraction with High Flux Henodialysis Is Superior to Charcoal Hemoperfusion," Clin Toxicol (Phila), 2005, 43:677.

Esley C, Begum A, Woolley MP, et al, "Aluminum in Tobacco and Cannabis and Smoking-Related Disease," Am J Med, 2006, 119(3):276.

Friesen MS, Purssell RA, and Gair RD, "Aluminum Toxicity Following I.V. Use of Oral Methadone Solution," Clin Toxicol, 2006, 44(3):307-14.

Liao YH, Yu HS, Ho CK, et al, "Biological Monitoring of Exposures to Aluminum, Gallium, Indium, Arsenic, and Antimony in Optoelectronic Industry Workers," J Occup Environ Med, 2004, 46(9):931-6.

Aluminum Phosphide

Related Information

- Phosphine
- Toxins Which Should Be Lavaged with Solutions Other Than Water

CAS Number 20859-73-8; 7803-51-2

UN Number 1397; 3048

U.S. Brand Names Al-Phos®; Celphos®; Delicia®; Detia®; Phostoxin®; Quickphos®

Synonyms Aluminum Monophosphide

Use Fumigation of grain, rodenticide

Mechanism of Toxic Action Liberates phosphine gas in the GI tract which blocks cytochrome C thus uncoupling oxidative phosphorylation and electron transport in the mitochondria

Adverse Reactions

Cardiovascular: Hypotension (within 6 hours), myocardial injury with widening of QRS complex on ECG, fibrillation (atrial), tachycardia (ventricular), cyanosis, pericarditis, edema, tachycardia, arrhythmias (ventricular)

Central nervous system: Headache, ataxia, dizziness

Endocrine & metabolic: Hyperkalemia, metabolic acidosis, adrenal dysfunction may occur, hypomagnesemia and hypermagnesemia have been reported

Gastrointestinal: Stomach pain, vomiting, watery diarrhea

Hematologic: Bleeding, intravascular hemolysis, methemoglobinemia

Hepatic: Hepatic failure

Ocular: Diplopia

Neuromuscular & skeletal: Tremors, paresthesia

Renal: Renal failure, oliguria

Respiratory: Tachypnea, pulmonary edema

Miscellaneous: Diathesis

Toxicodynamics/Kinetics Protein binding: 60% to 70%

Overdosage/Treatment

Decontamination: Gastric lavage within 1 hour with 1:5000 potassium permanganate to oxidize unabsorbed toxin. Sodium bicarbonate (2% solution) can also be utilized to neutralize gastric hydrochloric acid, thus inhibiting release of phosphine.

Supportive therapy: Sodium bicarbonate should be used to treat acidosis. Dopamine can be used to treat hypotension. If hypotension does not respond to vasopressors, hydrocortisone (400 mg every 4-6 hours) or dexamethasone (4 mg I.V. every 4 hours) can be used to treat adrenal dysfunction. Magnesium should be administered in order to prevent cardiac arrhythmia; suggested dose: 3 g (I.V. continuous infusion) over 3 hours followed by 6 g I.V. over 24 hours for the next 3 to 5 days. Ventricular arrhythmias can be treated successfully with trimetazidine (20 mg orally twice daily). Treat symptomatic methemoglobinemia with 1-2 mL/kg of 1% methylene blue. Endoscopic dilation may be required to treat esophageal structures (which can develop two weeks post ingestion).

Additional Information Decomposes in water; dark gray or dark yellow crystals; oral estimate of daily human exposure that is likely to be without risk of deleterious effects during a lifetime: 0.0004 mg/kg/day.

Specific References

"Cytochrome-C Oxidase Inhibition in 26 Aluminum Phosphide Posioned Patients," *Clin Toxicol (Phila)*, 2006, 44:155-8.

Kapoor S, Naik S, Kumar et al, "Benign Esophageal Structure Following Aluminium Phosphide Poisoning," *Indian J Gastroenterol*, 2005, 24(6):261-262.

Talukdar R, Singal DK, and Tandon RK, "Aluminium Phosphide Induced Esophageal Structure," *Indian J Gastroenterol*, 2006, 25(2):98-99.

Americum

CAS Number 7440-35-9

Use In ionization smoke detectors (0.9 microcuries of ^{241}Am in household detectors). No stable isotopes. Also used in diagnosis of thyroid disorders.

Mechanism of Toxic Action Emission of alpha particles during radio-active decay. Since there is very limited alpha particle penetration, cellular damage is located over the immediate vicinity of exposure.

Adverse Reactions Hematologic: Lymphopenia/thrombocytopenia from inhalation of 100 g of ^{124}Am exposure

Toxicodynamics/Kinetics

Absorption: By inhalation; <0.1% absorbed orally; <20% absorbed dermally

Elimination: Fecal (>50%)

Overdosage/Treatment

Decontamination: Inhalation: Administer 100% humidified oxygen.

Supportive therapy: Enhanced urinary excretion may be accomplished with DTPA (diethylenetriamine pentacetic acid) (1 g I.V. in 250 mL isotonic saline or D_5W).

Additional Information Ambient air concentration: <1 aCi/m^3. Surface seawater concentration: 270 pCi/m^3. Primarily taken up in skeleton and liver. Total skeletal burden is 0.27 pCi; found in shellfish, grain, fruits, and vegetables. Call Radiation Emergency Assistance Center/Training Site in Oak Ridge, Tennessee (800) 576-1004 for exposure information.

Amikacin

CAS Number 39831-55-5

U.S. Brand Names Amikin®

Synonyms Amikacin Sulfate

Use Treatment of documented gram-negative enteric infection resistant to gentamicin and tobramycin; documented infection of mycobacterial organisms susceptible to amikacin

Mechanism of Action Inhibits protein synthesis in susceptible bacteria by binding to ribosomal subunits

Adverse Reactions

Cardiovascular: Chest pain

Central nervous system: Anxiety

Dermatologic: Rash

Neuromuscular & skeletal: Neuromuscular blockade, myasthenia gravis (exacerbation or precipitation of)

Otic: Ototoxicity, deafness, tinnitus

Renal: Nephrotoxicity, Fanconi-like syndrome

Signs and Symptoms of Overdose Hypomagnesemia

Pharmacodynamics/Kinetics

Absorption:

I.M.: Rapid

Oral: Poorly absorbed

Distribution: Primarily into extracellular fluid (highly hydrophilic); penetrates blood-brain barrier when meninges inflamed; crosses placenta

Relative diffusion of antimicrobial agents from blood into CSF: Good only with inflammation (exceeds usual MICs)

CSF: blood level ratio: Normal meninges: 10% to 20%; Inflamed meninges: 15% to 24%

Protein-binding: 0% to 11%

Half-life elimination (renal function and age dependent):

Infants: Low birth weight (1-3 days): 7-9 hours; Full-term >7 days: 4-5 hours

Children: 1.6-2.5 hours

Adults: Normal renal function: 1.4-2.3 hours; Anuria/end-stage renal disease: 28-86 hours

Time to peak, serum: I.M.: 45-120 minutes

Excretion: Urine (94% to 98%)

Dosage

Individualization is critical because of the low therapeutic index. Use of ideal body weight (IBW) for determining the mg/kg/dose appears to be more accurate than dosing on the basis of total body weight (TBW). In morbid obesity, dosage requirement may best be estimated using a dosing weight of IBW + 0.4 (TBW - IBW). Initial and periodic peak and trough plasma drug levels should be determined, particularly in critically ill patients with serious infections or in disease states known to significantly alter aminoglycoside pharmacokinetics (eg, cystic fibrosis, burns, or major surgery).

Neonates: I.V.:

<1200 g, 0-4 weeks: 7.5 mg/kg/dose every 12 hours

Postnatal age <7 days:

1200-2000 g: 7.5 mg/kg/dose every 12 hours

>2000 g: 10 mg/kg/dose every 12 hours

Postnatal age >7 days:

1200-2000 g: 7 mg/kg/dose every 8 hours

>2000 g: 7.5-10 mg/kg/dose every 8 hours

Infants, Children, and Adults: I.M., I.V.: 7.5 mg/kg/dose every 8 hours

Dosing interval in renal impairment: Loading dose: 5-7.5 mg/kg; subsequent dosages and frequency of administration are best determined by measurement of serum levels and assessment of renal insufficiency

Some patients may require larger or more frequent doses if serum levels document the need (ie, cystic fibrosis or febrile granulocytopenic patients)

Stability Stable for 24 hours at room temperature when mixed in D_5W, $D_5\frac{1}{4}$NS, $D_5\frac{1}{2}$NS, NS, LR

Monitoring Parameters Urinalysis, BUN, serum creatinine, appropriately timed peak and trough concentrations, vital signs, temperature, weight, I & O, hearing parameters

Administration Administer by intermittent I.V. infusion over 30 minutes at a final concentration not to exceed 5 mg amikacin/mL

Contraindications Hypersensitivity to amikacin sulfate or any component of the formulation; cross-sensitivity may exist with other aminoglycosides

Warnings [U.S. Boxed Warning]: Amikacin may cause neurotoxicity, nephrotoxicity, and/or neuromuscular blockade and respiratory paralysis; usual risk factors include pre-existing renal impairment, concomitant neuro-/nephrotoxic medications, advanced age and dehydration. Dose and/or frequency of administration must be monitored and modified in patients with renal impairment. Drug should be discontinued if signs of ototoxicity, nephrotoxicity, or hypersensitivity occur. Ototoxicity is proportional to the amount of drug given and the duration of treatment. Tinnitus or vertigo may be indications of vestibular injury and impending bilateral irreversible damage. Renal damage is usually reversible.

Dosage Forms

[DSC] = Discontinued product

Injection, solution, as sulfate: 50 mg/mL (2 mL, 4 mL); 62.5 mg/mL (8 mL) [DSC]; 250 mg/mL (2 mL, 4 mL)

Amikin®: 50 mg/mL (2 mL); 250 mg/mL (2 mL, 4 mL) [contains metabisulfite]

Reference Range

Therapeutic: Peak: 25-30 mcg/mL, trough: 4-8 mcg/mL

Toxic: Peak: >35 mcg/mL; trough: >10 mcg/mL

Overdosage/Treatment Enhancement of elimination: Ticarcillin complexation or exchange transfusion does not appear to be of added benefit; saline diuresis may be of benefit; dialyzable (50% to 100%)

Drug Interactions

Decreased effect of aminoglycoside: High concentrations of penicillins and/or cephalosporins (*in vitro* data)

Increased toxicity of aminoglycoside: Indomethacin I.V., amphotericin, loop diuretics, vancomycin, enflurane, methoxyflurane; increased effect of neuromuscular-blocking agents and polypeptide antibiotics with administration of aminoglycosides

Pregnancy Risk Factor C

Lactation Enters breast milk/compatible

Nursing Implications Aminoglycoside levels measured from blood taken from Silastic® central catheters can sometimes give falsely high readings; administer I.M. injection in large muscle mass; obtain culture for culture and sensitivity before first dose; weigh patient and obtain baseline renal function before therapy begins; monitor vital signs, serum levels are reportedly lower in patients with fever. Give around-the-clock rather than 3 times/day, to promote less variation in peak and trough serum levels; give other antibiotics at least 1 hour before or after amikacin.

Additional Information

Sodium content of 1 g: 29.9 mg (1.3 mEq)

Incidence of cochleotoxicity is ~10% to 63% with loop diuretics; noise exposure is ototoxic synergistic. Inhaled tobramycin appears to exhibit minimal ototoxic effects. There may be a genetic basis (in the mitochondrial 12 S ribosomal RNA gene) for ototoxicity in 17% to 33% of cases. Suggested evaluation for ototoxicity with aminoglycoside treatment includes:

- baseline audiometric evaluation (tonal air conduction thresholds from 250-20,000 Hz)
- monitoring during aminoglycoside treatment (to a tonal-air conduction threshold at frequency >8000 Hz)
- follow-up audiometric assessment (tonal air conduction thresholds at frequencies >8000 Hz) until the threshold stabilizes

Specific References

Corpus KA, Weber KB, and Zimmerman CR, "Intrathecal Amikacin for the Treatment of Pseudomonal Meningitis," *Ann Pharmacother*, 2004, 38(6):992-5.

Amitraz

Related Information
- Xylene

CAS Number 33089-61-1
U.S. Brand Names BAAM®; Ectodex®; Mitac®; Taktic®; Triatox®
Synonyms U-36059
Use A topical ectoparasiticide in veterinary practice; effective against lice, mites, and ticks; used on fruit, trees, cattle, sheep, pigs, and honey bee hives; an acaricide and insect repellent
Mechanism of Toxic Action An α_2 adrenoceptor agonist (similar to clonidine). Reduces insulin secretion and heat production. Often combined with various solvents which contribute to CNS toxicity (particularly xylene).
Adverse Reactions Ocular: Visual evoked potential abnormalities
Signs and Symptoms of Overdose Onset of symptoms is usually within 4 hours. Coma (55% to 100%), bradycardia (10% to 62%), seizures (7% to 14%), CNS depression, drowsiness, vomiting (50% to 62%), flushing, headache, hyperglycemia (48% to 72%), hypokalemia, hypotonia, hypotension (42% to 67%), miosis, hypothermia (9% to 33%), respiratory depression (17% to 43%), glycosuria (21% to 42%), minor elevations in liver transaminases, polyuria, ataxia
Admission Criteria/Prognosis Admit any symptomatic patient or ingestion over 0.2 mg/kg to a cardiac monitored bed
Toxicodynamics/Kinetics
Absorption: Oral: 2 hours; dermal absorption may occur
Metabolism: Hepatic to an aromatic amine (2,4-dimethyl aniline)
Half-life: 4 hours
Elimination: Renal
Monitoring Parameters Glucose, potassium, ECG
Reference Range Blood amitraz concentration of 3.7 mg/L associated with deep coma following an ingestion of up to 12.5 g of amitraz; CNS symptoms may occur at plasma amitraz concentrations over 500 mcg/L; plasma amitraz level under 100 mcg/L not associated with symptoms
Overdosage/Treatment
Decontamination: **Oral:** Lavage/activated charcoal within 2 hours. **Dermal:** Remove contaminated clothing and wash thoroughly with soap and water. **Ocular:** Irrigate copiously with saline.
Supportive therapy: Diazepam or lorazepam for seizure control. Atropine for bradycardia (multiple doses may be needed). Isotonic crystalloid fluid 10-20 mL/kg I.V. and Trendelenburg positioning for hypotension. Dopamine or norepinephrine are vasopressors of choice. Hyperglycemia is usually transient and does not require specific treatment.
Antidote(s)
- Atropine [ANTIDOTE]
Additional Information
First marketed in 1974; concentrations (emulsifiable) solutions contain 20-200 g/L. Usually associated with a xylene vehicle; found in concentrations of 1 g of amitraz/5 mL of solution. When heated can decompose to nitrogen oxide fumes. LD50 in dogs: 100 mg/kg. Ingestion of 2.5 mg/kg can produce severe symptoms.
How supplied: Emulsifiable concentrate: 50-200 g/L; Powder: Wettable: 500 g/L; Dog shampoo (dispersal powder): 250 or 500 g/L
Specific References
Avsarogullari L, Ikizceli I, Sungur M, et al, "Acute Amitraz Poisoning in Adults: Clinical Features, Laboratory Findings, and Management," *Clin Toxicol (Phila)*, 2006, 44(1):19-23.
Gursoy S, Kunt N, Kaygusuz K, et al, "Intravenous Amitraz Poisoning," *Clin Toxicol (Phila)*, 2005, 43(2):113-6.
Proudfoot AT, "Poisoning with Amitraz," *Toxicol Rev*, 2003, 22(2):71-4.
Yilmaz HL and Yildizdas DR, "Amitraz Poisoning, An Emerging Problem: Epidemiology, Clinical Features, Management, and Preventive Strategies," *Arch Dis Child*, 2003, 88(2):130-4.

Ammonia

CAS Number 7664-41-7
UN Number 1005; 2073; 2672

Synonyms Spirit of Hartshorn
Commonly Found In Household cleaners (5% to 10%) and bleach
Use Primarily in fertilizers; manufacture of nitrous oxide; petroleum refining
Mechanism of Toxic Action Tissue injury of moist mucosal membranes caused by reaction with water to form ammonia hydroxide; can cause burns by liquefaction necrosis
Adverse Reactions
Cardiovascular: Chest pain
Dermatologic: Immunologic contact urticaria
Gastrointestinal: Salivation
Respiratory: Reactive airways disease syndrome, hyposmia
Miscellaneous: Mucosal irritation
Signs and Symptoms of Overdose Burns, chest pain, coma, conjunctivitis, corneal defects, cough, dyspnea, GI irritation, headache, lacrimation, nausea, pulmonary edema, salivation, swelling, upper airway irritation, urticaria, wheezing, vomiting. Long-term sequelae include bronchiolitis obliterans and peribronchial fibrosis.
Admission Criteria/Prognosis Patient may be discharged if asymptomatic 6-8 hours postexposure
Toxicodynamics/Kinetics
Absorption: Not well absorbed
Metabolism: Hepatic to urea and glutamine
Overdosage/Treatment
Decontamination:
Oral: **Do not** induce emesis or perform gastric lavage; dilute with water or milk (4 oz in children, 8 oz in adults).
Ocular: Irrigate eyes copiously with normal saline.
Inhalation: Administer 100% humidified oxygen.
Supportive therapy: Flush injured surfaces with water. Treat for pulmonary edema. Use steroids for third degree esophageal burns. Inverse-ratio ventilation using lower tidal volume mechanical ventilation (6 mL/kg) and plateau pressures of 30 cm water may decrease mortality. While positive end expiratory pressures should be considered, oxygen toxicity should be monitored. Use of perfluorocarbon partial liquid ventilation and exogenous surfactant in chemical-induced ARDS is investigational.
Additional Information Irritation can occur at 400 ppm. Stomatitis can occur at ammonia concentrations of 50 ppm. The mixture of ammonia with hypochlorite bleach can result in chloramine which can produce pulmonary edema.
Colorless liquid; penetrating pungent odor; stable, colorless gas; highly water soluble; alkali (pH 11.6). Odor threshold: 25-48 ppm (air); 1.5 ppm (water). Atmospheric half-life: 2-3 days. TLV-TWA: 25 ppm; IDLH: 500 ppm
Specific References
Cavender FL, Millner GC, and Goad PT, "Use of Toxicity Data in Determining In-House Concentrations Following a Catastrophic Release of Ammonia in a Derailment of Tankcars," *Clin Toxicol (Phila)*, 2005, 43:750.
Haroz R and Greenberg MI, "Bowel Necrosis Following the Intentional Administration of an Ammonia-Containing Enema," *Clin Toxicol (Phila)*, 2005, 43:745.
Lee JH, Farley CL, Brodrick CD, et al, "Anhydrous Ammonia Eye Injuries Associated with Illicit Methamphetamine Production," *Ann Emerg Med*, 2003, 41(1):157.
Weisskopf MG, Drew JM, Hanrahan LP, et al, "Hazardous Ammonia Releases: Public Health Consequences and Risk Factors for Evacuation and Injury, United States, 1993-1998," *J Occup Environ Med*, 2003, 45(2):197-204.

Ammonium Bifluoride

CAS Number 1341-49-7
UN Number 1727 (solid); 2817 (solution)
Use Magnesium manufacture, wheel cleaner, herbicide enhancer
Mechanism of Toxic Action Since approximately two-thirds of this agent is fluoride, most of its toxicity is relatable to fluoride at a cellular level; fluoride binds serum calcium (thus causing hypocalcemia) and decreases oxygen consumption; also causes direct mucosal damage
Adverse Reactions Cardiovascular: Fibrillation (ventricular), arrhythmias (ventricular)
Signs and Symptoms of Overdose Abdominal pain, choking, CNS depression, diarrhea, disconjugate eye movements, dyspnea, gastric ulcer, hyperkalemia, hyperreflexia, hypocalcemia, hypomagnesemia, metabolic acidosis, muscle spasms, muscle weakness, nausea, ocular irritation, prolonged QT interval on ECG, pustular skin rash, vomiting (hematemesis), salivation, seizures, tachycardia, ventricular fibrillation
Admission Criteria/Prognosis Admit any ingestion of this agent
Toxicodynamics/Kinetics
Distribution: V_d (fluoride): 0.5-0.7 L/kg
Half-life: 2-9 hours
Elimination: Primarily renal (fecal elimination is up to 10%)
Monitoring Parameters ECG, electrolytes, calcium, magnesium

Reference Range Normal plasma fluoride range: 0.01-0.2 mg/L; urine fluoride following an ingestion resulting in cardiac arrest was 110 mg/L (toxic >10 mg/L)

Overdosage/Treatment

Decontamination:

Oral: Dilute with milk. Calcium carbonate tablets or milk of magnesia may inhibit absorption by binding fluoride. Lavage (within 1 hour) with a soft nasogastric tube (with 10% calcium gluconate) may be useful. Do not induce emesis.

Dermal/ocular: As first aid, the affected extremity can be irrigated with water and bathed in an iced solution of 25% magnesium sulfate. Calcium gluconate gel 2.5% can also be utilized.

Supportive therapy: Monitor electrolytes, calcium and magnesium. Benzodiazepines should be used to control seizures.

Additional Information Density: 1.5 g/mL

Ammonium Chloride

Pronunciation (a MOE nee um KLOR ide)

CAS Number 12125-02-9

Use Treatment of hypochloremic states or metabolic alkalosis; industrial use: galvanizing procedures, fertilizer, electroplating, soldering, manufacture of dry batteries, deodorizer cleaners (Lysol®, Swish Toilet Bowl Cleaner®); may be useful in bromide toxicity

Mechanism of Action Increases acidity by increasing free hydrogen ion concentration; as an expectorant by irritating, the mucosa, causing reflex stimulation of the bronchial mucosal glands

Adverse Reactions

Frequency not defined.

Central nervous system: Headache, coma, drowsiness, EEG abnormalities, mental confusion, seizures

Dermatologic: Rash

Endocrine & metabolic: Calcium-deficient tetany, hyperchloremia, hypokalemia, metabolic acidosis, potassium and sodium may be decreased

Gastrointestinal: Abdominal pain, gastric irritation, nausea, vomiting

Hepatic: Ammonia may be increased

Local: Pain at site of injection

Neuromuscular & skeletal: Twitching

Respiratory: Hyperventilation

Signs and Symptoms of Overdose Apnea, bradycardia, diuresis, headache, hyperchloremic hypokalemic metabolic acidosis, hyperventilation, hypomagnesemia, nausea, pulmonary edema, vomiting

Pharmacodynamics/Kinetics

Metabolism: Hepatic; forms urea and hydrochloric acid

Excretion: Urine

Toxicodynamics/Kinetics

Absorption: Rapid from the GI tract with absorption being complete in 3-6 hours

Distribution: Unknown

Elimination: In urine (1% to 3% in feces)

Dosage

Metabolic alkalosis: The following equations represent different methods of correction utilizing either the serum HCO_3^-, the serum chloride, or the base excess

Dosing of mEq NH₄Cl via the chloride-deficit method (hypochloremia):

Dose of mEq NH₄Cl = [0.2 L/kg × body weight (kg)] × [103 - observed serum chloride]; administer 50% of dose over 12 hours, then re-evaluate

Note: 0.2 L/kg is the estimated chloride volume of distribution and 103 is the average normal serum chloride concentration (mEq/L)

Dosing of mEq NH₄Cl via the bicarbonate-excess method (refractory hypochloremic metabolic alkalosis):

Dose of NH₄Cl = [0.5 L/kg × body weight (kg)] × (observed serum HCO_3^- - 24); administer 50% of dose over 12 hours, then re-evaluate

Note: 0.5 L/kg is the estimated bicarbonate volume of distribution and 24 is the average normal serum bicarbonate concentration (mEq/L)

These equations will yield different requirements of ammonium chloride

Monitoring Parameters Serum bicarbonate; signs and symptoms of ammonia toxicity

Administration Administer by slow intravenous infusion to avoid local irritation and adverse effects. Rate of infusion should not exceed 5 mL/minute in an adult.

Contraindications Severe hepatic or renal dysfunction

Warnings Use caution in patients with primary respiratory acidosis or pulmonary insufficiency. Safety and efficacy have not been established in children.

Dosage Forms Injection, solution: Ammonium 5 mEq/mL and chloride 5 mEq/mL (20 mL) [equivalent to ammonium chloride 267.5 mg/mL]

Overdosage/Treatment

Decontamination: Activated charcoal

Supportive therapy: I.V. sodium bicarb for acidosis; replenish potassium

Test Interactions ↑ ammonia (B), glucose (S); ↓ potassium (S), sodium (S), urine pH

Pregnancy Risk Factor C

Pregnancy Implications Reproduction studies have not been conducted.

Nursing Implications Rapid I.V. injection may increase the likelihood of ammonia toxicity; rate should not exceed 1 mEq/kg/hour; 26.75% solution must be diluted prior to administration

Additional Information Odorless, may produce an explosive reaction (with potassium chlorate, nitrates, hydrogen cyanide); TLV-TWA: 10 mg/m³; PEL-TWA: 10 mg/m³

Aniline

Related Information

- Methemoglobin, Blood

CAS Number 62-53-3

UN Number 1547

Synonyms Aminobenzene; Aminophen; Analine; Aniline Oil; Benzeneamine; Blue Oil; Krystalline; Kyanor; Phenylamine

Use Prepared from indigo and potash; used in manufacture of dyes, resins, varnishes, perfumes, shoe blacks, vulcanizing rubber, paint removers, herbicides, fungicides, explosives, photographic chemicals, isocyanates, rigid polyurethane, and as a solvent

Adverse Reactions

Hematologic: Methemoglobinemia followed by hemolysis

Miscellaneous: Cutaneous T-cell lymphoma

Signs and Symptoms of Overdose Mild skin and eye irritant. Inducement of methemoglobinemia causing headache, tinnitus, confusion, seizures, dizziness, drowsiness, loss of consciousness, and coma in the absence of respiratory compromise. Methemoglobinemia may be followed by hemolysis. Central cyanosis is evident which does not improve with 100% oxygen. Blood is noted to be "chocolate brown" and will not become red while bubbling in 100% oxygen. Hemolysis may also occur causing heart, kidney, and liver damage; renal failure may ensue.

Admission Criteria/Prognosis Any patient with change in mental status, cardiopulmonary complaints, or methemoglobin levels >30% should be admitted; asymptomatic patients with methemoglobin levels <30% may be considered for discharge after 6 hours of observation and if methemoglobin levels fall to <15%

Toxicodynamics/Kinetics

Absorption: Readily through all routes; delay rate up to 4 hours, the development of methemoglobinemia; methemoglobin is caused by oxidation of iron in hemoglobin Fe^{+2} to Fe^{+3} which is incapable of transporting oxygen; hemolysis then occurs 2-7 days after exposure

Metabolism: By ring hydroxylation and then conjugated to glucuronides and sulfates

Half-life: 2-7 hours

Elimination: Metabolites are renally cleared

Monitoring Parameters Methemoglobin levels; aniline levels have not been measured in blood or serum; urinary p-aminophenol can be measured by colorimetry; CBC, WBC smear, renal function, myoglobin, urinalysis and other indices of hemolysis may be required

Warnings/Precautions Persons with hemoglobin M, G6PD deficiency or NADH-cytochrome B_5 reductase deficiency may be more sensitive; patients exposed to other methemoglobin inducers are at increased risks; patients with cardiovascular disease are at greater risk from consequences; when vapors are present, must use impervious body protector as significant toxicity may occur through dermal absorption

Reference Range Urinary p-aminophenol >10 mg/L may indicate potential toxic dose with 20 mg/L indicating the need for medical intervention; as little as 1 g can be fatal in human; aniline vapor concentrations >100-160 ppm cause serious disturbances

Overdosage/Treatment

Decontamination: Emesis within 30 minutes, lavage (within 1 hour)/ activated charcoal; remove patient from inhalation and administer 100% humidified air; exposed skin and eyes should be irrigated with water

Supportive therapy: Methemoglobinemia: Treat symptomatic patients or if level is >20%, administer 100% oxygen. If required, methylene blue: 1-2 mg/kg/dose I.V. over a few minutes; may repeat in 4 hours if needed; doses >15 mg/kg may cause hemolysis. High doses of methylene blue may precipitate Heinz body formation and hemolysis. Transfusion of PRBCs may be needed. Treatment for myoglobinuria may require urine alkalinization and maintenance of adequate urinary output to prevent renal damage.

Enhanced elimination: One reported case of hemodialysis was used in an aniline exposure which was refractory to supportive care. Hemodialysis should be instituted for those who develop renal failure. Exchange transfusion has been used after unsuccessful treatment with methylene blue.

Antidote(s)

- Methylene Blue [ANTIDOTE]

Diagnostic Procedures
- Methemoglobin, Blood
- N,N-Dimethyl-P-Toluidine

Additional Information
Estimated lethal dose: 15-30 g

Inadequate information concerning human carcinogenicity (bladder cancer); limited evidence that has been carcinogenic in animals (splenic sarcomas, bladder carcinoma)

How supplied: Colorless to brown, oil, combustible liquid with a characteristic amine-like odor; turns brown when exposed to air and light; when heated, forms toxic fumes of nitrogen oxide

Specific References
Bomhard EM and Herbold BA., "Genotoxic Activities of Aniline and Its Metabolites and Their Relationship to the Carcinogenicity of Aniline in the Spleen of Rats," *Crit Rev Toxicol*. 2005, 35(10):783-835 (review).

Katz K, Ruha AM, Curry S, et al, "Aniline and Methanol Toxicity After Shoe Dye Ingestion," *J Toxicol Clin Toxicol*, 2003, 41(5):644.

Anisole

Synonyms Methoxybenzene; Methyl Phenyl Ether; Phenyl Methyl Ether
Use As a food additive, solvent; in perfumes, detergents
Mechanism of Toxic Action Mucosal irritation
Signs and Symptoms of Overdose Erythema, conjunctivitis
Overdosage/Treatment Decontamination: **Oral:** Lavage within 1 hour with activated charcoal; **Dermal:** Irrigate with water; **Ocular:** Irrigate with water
Additional Information Pleasant aromatic odor

Anticoagulant Rodenticide

CAS Number 117-52-2; 56073-07-5; 56073-10-1; 82-66-6; 83-26-1
U.S. Brand Names Bromone®; Caid®; d-Con®; Dipazin®; Diphacin®; Drat®; Endox®; Endrocide®; Foumarin®; Havoc®; Krumkil®; Lurat®; Maki®; Microzul®; Pivacin®; Pival®; Racumin®; Ramucide®; Ratafin®; Ratak®; Ratimus®; Ratindan®; Raviac®; Rodentin®; SuperCaid®; Talon-G®; Talon®; Topitox®; Tri-Ban®
Synonyms Brodifacoum; Bromadiolone; Chlorphacinone; Coumafuryl; Coumatetralyl; Difenacoum; Diphacinone; Hydroxycoumarin; Indanedione; Phytonadione; Pindone; Pivaldione
Mechanism of Toxic Action Inhibition of synthesis of vitamin K_1-dependent clotting factors II, VII, IX, and X through potent inhibition of vitamin K_1-2,3-epoxide reductase; resulting hypoprothrombinemia and decreased coagulation predisposes toward hemorrhage; benzylacetone metabolite of hydroxycoumarins also induces direct capillary injury, further predisposing toward hemorrhage

Adverse Reactions
Cardiovascular: Hypovolemic/hemorrhagic hypotension and shock, pericardial effusion/pericarditis

Central nervous system: Dizziness, subarachnoid, intracerebral and intraventricular hemorrhage

Dermatologic: Easy bruising, petechial rash, ecchymosis, skin necrosis, "purple toe" syndrome

Gastrointestinal: Bleeding gums, punctate or frank hemorrhage of mucosal surfaces, abdominal pain, hematemesis, hematochezia, melena

Genitourinary: Uterine bleed, cystitis

Hepatic: Cholestasis

Renal: Hematuria

Respiratory: Hemoptysis, epistaxis

Signs and Symptoms of Overdose Easy bruising, ecchymosis, bleeding gums, epistaxis, and mucosal hemorrhage progressing to symptoms of upper and lower GI bleeding; hypotension and hypovolemic shock may follow hemorrhage. Intracranial hemorrhage may occur, especially following trauma. Indanediones may also cause neurologic and cardiopulmonary symptoms independent of anticoagulant activity.

Admission Criteria/Prognosis Patients with bleeding, prolonged prothrombin time, or a history of a large ingestion (warfarin >0.5 mg/kg ingested, hydroxycoumarin >0.05 mg ingested, or indandione >5 mg ingested) should be considered for admission; usually a few mouthfuls of this product does not require hospitalization

Toxicodynamics/Kinetics
Onset of anticoagulation: Typically within 24-48 hours

Maximum effect: 36-72 hours

Duration: Following repeated doses, may persist up to 45-300 days

Absorption: Complete and rapid following oral exposure

Distribution: V_d of 0.12-0.9 L/kg; rapid tissue distribution

Protein binding: Extensive plasma protein binding (97% to 99%)

Metabolism: Hepatic microsomal hydroxylation and conjugation of the inactive metabolites

Half-life: Brodifacoum: 25 days. Difenacoum: 12 days; Bromadiolone: 140 hours

Elimination: Extensive renal elimination of metabolites, with some biliary excretion

Monitoring Parameters Hemoglobin, hematocrit, INR, partial thromboplastin time (PTT), prothrombin time (PT), stool guaiac

Reference Range Serum brodifacoum level of 254 ng/mL associated with prothrombin and partial thromboplastin times of 189 seconds, along with bleeding; plasma difenacoum levels of 0.97 mg/L associated with severe bleeding; low factor II, VII, IX and X levels are diagnostic. Serum bromadiolone level of 440 mcg/L associated with INr value >10.

Overdosage/Treatment
Decontamination is usually not required for one-time acute ingestions in pediatric patients. In suicide attempts, decontamination should be performed.

Decontamination:

Emesis is contraindicated in patients who may experience alterations in consciousness, or who have prolonged PT values. In anticoagulated patients, intracranial hemorrhage may follow vomiting-induced elevations in intracranial pressures.

Activated charcoal administration should follow large ingestions of long-acting anticoagulants, unless otherwise contraindicated.

Supportive therapy:

Consider treatment if INR>4.

Obtain PT values immediately postingestion, then 24 and 48 hours postingestion. If significant prolongation occurs, obtain PT values every 6-12 hours thereafter; repeat PT may be obtained 4-5 days postevent. The patient should be closely monitored for signs and symptoms of bleeding for several weeks postingestion.

Vitamin K_1: Oral, SubQ, I.M., I.V.: Children: 1-5 mg; Adults: 15 mg Up to 600 mg per day divided every 6 to 12 hours may be required in adults. If INR >5, begin with an oral dose of 50 mg and then titrate 9-12 hours dosing.

I.V. doses of up to 0.6 mg/kg diluted in saline or dextrose may be administered to refractory cases. I.V. infusion rates should not exceed 1 mg/minute or 5% of total dose/minute. I.M. administration of phytonadione may lead to significant hematoma formation. I.V. administration may elicit a hypotensive anaphylactoid reaction, and steps should be taken to anticipate hemodynamic and ventilatory support, as well as decreasing or discontinuation of the infusion.

Prophylactic oral vitamin K_1 is not indicated for accidental non-suicidal ingestions because it may further delay the onset of PT prolongation thereby masking the need for long-term vitamin K_1 therapy

Packed red blood cells (PRBCs) and intravenous crystalloids and colloids will provide immediate hemodynamic support in hypovolemia and hemorrhage. Fresh frozen plasma (FFP) (15 ml per kg), and in extreme cases pooled clotting factors, may be used for cases of refractory hemorrhage.

If active bleeding occurs: Recombinant coagulation activated factor VII at doses of 70 to 90 mcg/kg or 1.2 to 4.8 mg total with vitamin K (10 mg or 100 mcg/kg IV) can also be considered. Alternatively, Prothrombin complex concentrate (which contains factors II, VII, IX and X) at 50 units per kg IV can be given.

Enhancement of elimination: Plasmapheresis has been used to increase brodifacoum clearance

Antidote(s)
- Charcoal [ANTIDOTE]
- Ipecac Syrup [ANTIDOTE]
- Phytonadione [ANTIDOTE]

Diagnostic Procedures
- Urinalysis

Additional Information Single small ingestions of long-acting agents rarely lead to clinically significant anticoagulation and bleeding. Prolonged PT values will identify chronic ingestions, massive ingestions, or patients who were previously anticoagulated. Anticoagulant ingestion may exacerbate underlying diseases such as peptic ulceration. These agents may be absorbed through intact skin, or by inhalation of powders, sprays, or concentrates. Rodent baits and pellets are usually colored with water-soluble blue or green dye to facilitate recognition of oral exposure. No deaths reported in the American Association of Poison Control Centers annual data reports from 1987 to 1993 among children <6 years of age (encompassing ~72,060 warfarin-related exposures in rodenticides).

How supplied: Rodent bait (corn or grain pellets), cake, powder, or liquid concentrate

For comparison: See table.

For Brodifacoum, the toxic dose is about 1 mg (or 0.01 mg/kg) and duration of INR increase of at least 6 weeks.

Anticoagulant Rodenticides

Class	Drug	Notes
Hydroxycoumarins		
Short-acting	Coumafuryl (Foumarin,® Lurat,® Krumkil,® Ratafin®)	
Long-acting	Brodifacoum (d-Con,® Talon,® Talon-G,® Havoc®)	$t_{1/2}$ = 120 d (dogs) $t_{1/2}$ = 156 h (rats) 0.005% grain-based pellets
	Bromadiolone (Bromone,® Super-Caid,® Ratimus,® Maki®)	Grain-based pellets
	Coumatetralyl (Endox,® Endrocide,® Racumin,® Rodentin®)	Little human experience
	Difenacoum (Ratak®)	0.005% grain-based pellets
Indanediones (may be considered long-acting)	Chlorphacinone (Caid,® Drat,® Microzul,® Ramucide,® Raviac,® Topitox®)	$t_{1/2}$ = 5.9-11 d (human) 0.005%, 0.25%, or 2.5% bait, solution, or concentrate
	Diphacinone (Dipazin,® Diphacin,® Ratindan®)	0.005%, 0.05%, 0.1%, 0.2%, or 2% cake, bait, or concentrate
	Pindone/pivaldione (Pival,® Pivacin,® Tri-Ban®)	0.025%, 0.1%, 0.2%, 0.5%, 1.5%, or 2% powder or concentrate

Specific References
Alsop JA, Tegzes JM, and Ferguson TJ, "Unexplained Prolonged INRs in a College Student," *J Toxicol Clin Toxicol*, 2003, 41(5):649.

Caravati EM, Erdman AR, Scharman EJ, et al, "Practice Guideline: Long-acting Anticoagulant Rodenticide Poisoning: An Evidence-Based Consensus Guideline for Out-of-Hospital Management," *Clin Toxicol*, 2007, 45(1):1-23.

Grobosch T, Angelow B, Schonberg C, et al, "Acute Bromadiolone Intoxication," *J Anal Toxicol*, 2006, 30:281-6.

Meiser H, "Detection of Anticoagulant Residues by a New HPLC Method in Specimens of Poisoned Animals and a Poison Control Case Study," *J Anal Toxicol*, 2005, 29:556-63.

Osterhoudt KC and Henretig FM, "Bias in Pediatric Brodifacoum Exposure Data," *Pediatr Emerg Care*, 2003, 19(1):62.

Watt BE, Proudfoot AT, Bradberry SM, Vale JA, "Anticoagulant Rodenticides," *Toxicol Rev*, 2005, 24(4):259-69.

Zupancic-Salek S, Kovacevic-Metelko J, Radman I, "Successful Reversal of Anticoagulant Effect of Superwarfarin Poisoning with Recombinant Activated Factor VII," *Blood Coagul Fibrinolysis*, 2005 June, 16(4):239-44.

Antimony

CAS Number 10025-91-9; 1309-64-4; 1314-60-9; 1315-04-4; 1345-04-6; 28300-74-5; 7440-36-0; 7803-52-3

UN Number 1549; 1551; 1733; 2676; 2871

Synonyms Sb(+3); Sb(+5); Sb(-3); Sb(0)

Use Naturally brittle metal usually alloyed with lead or other metals; used in grid metal for lead storage batteries, solder, sheet/pipe metal, castings, ammunition, cable sheathing, pewter; antimony trioxide is used as a fire retardant; trivalent organic antimony was used in therapy for schistosomiasis

Mechanism of Toxic Action Primarily an irritant, inhibits the enzyme phosphofructokinase

Adverse Reactions
Cardiovascular: High blood pressure, AV block, cardiomegaly, cardiomyopathy, angina, chest pain, QT prolongation, torsade de pointes, arrhythmias (ventricular)
Central nervous system: Dementia
Dermatological: Dermal irritation
Endocrine & metabolic: Menstruation disturbances
Gastrointestinal: Abdominal pain, vomiting, diarrhea, peptic ulceration
Genitourinary: Crystalluria
Hematologic: Hemolytic anemia, leukopenia, thrombocytopenia, anemia
Neuromuscular & skeletal: Myalgia
Ocular: Eye irritation

Renal: Proteinuria, renal failure
Respiratory: Inhalation can cause pneumoconiosis, cough
Miscellaneous: Thirst

Signs and Symptoms of Overdose ECG abnormalities (elevation of S-T segment, flat T waves). Vomiting can occur with oral ingestion of 0.5 mg/kg antimony tartrate.

Toxicodynamics/Kinetics
Absorption: Oral: 2% to 7% (antimony tartrate/antimony trichloride)
Half-life: 38 days
Elimination: Renal (faster with pentavalent than trivalent compounds)

Reference Range Baseline antimony levels: 0.4 mcg/L (blood); 0.096-0.12 mcg/g (hair); 0.6 mcg/L (urine)

Overdosage/Treatment
Decontamination: Oral: Dilute with milk or water.
Enhancement of elimination: Chelation therapy with BAL may mitigate the toxicity of trivalent antimony compounds. Hemodialysis may be useful in increasing clearance of pentavalent (but not trivalent) antimony, although human experience in this modality is lacking.

Antidote(s)
- Dimercaprol [ANTIDOTE]

Additional Information Silvery white powder. OSHA-PEL-TWA: 0.5 mg/m³ (air). Water standard: 145 mcg/L. Average daily intake: Ingestion: ~5 mcg; inhalation: ~0.04 mcg

Specific References
Schwaner RA, Beuhler MC, and Wax PM, "Comparison of "Normal" Reference Ranges for Selected Heavy Metals with Biomonitoring Exposure Data of US Population," *J Toxicol Clin Toxicol*, 2003, 41(5):741.

Tarabar AF, Khan Y, Nelson LS, et al, "Antimony Toxicity from the Use of Tartar Emetic for the Treatment of Alcohol Abuse," *Vet Hum Toxicol*, 2004, 46(6):331-3.

Arsenic

Related Information
- Copper
- Lewisite

CAS Number 7440-38-2

UN Number 1554; 1558; 1573

Synonyms Arsenate; Arsenite

Commonly Found In Pesticides, rodenticides, ant poisons, wood preservative, microchips, well water, seafood

Mechanism of Toxic Action Multisystem disease secondary to inhibition of oxidative phosphorylation
Enzymes inhibited by As^{+3} include pyruvated dehydrogenase complex, alpha-ketoglutarate dehydrogenase complex, thiolase, Glucose 6-phosphate dehydrogenase and glutathione synthetase and reductase

Adverse Reactions
Cardiovascular: Cardiotoxicity, tachycardia, acrocyanosis, Raynaud's phenomenon, congestive heart failure, myocardial depression, myocarditis, pericardial effusion/pericarditis, sinus tachycardia, tachycardia (supraventricular), vasodilation
Central nervous system: Neurotoxicity, axonopathy (peripheral), fever, hyperthermia, memory disturbance, Jarisch-Herxheimer reaction, delirium, psychosis, leukoencephalopathy
Dermatologic: Desquamation (scaling), hyperpigmentation, alopecia (patchy); airborne contact dermatitis, exanthem; dermal effects are usually not seen with inhalation exposure, lichen planus
Gastrointestinal: Gastrointestinal pathology, nausea, vomiting, metallic taste, salivation, feces discoloration (black), bloody diarrhea, abdominal pain, garlic odor
Hematologic: Bone marrow suppression, neutropenia, pancytopenia (leukopenia, thrombocytopenia, aplastic anemia)
Renal: Tubular necrosis (acute), hematuria
Miscellaneous: Basal cell carcinoma, cutaneous T-cell lymphoma

Signs and Symptoms of Overdose Agranulocytosis, alopecia, blindness, cough, encephalopathy, fasciculations, fever, garlic-like breath, hematuria, hemolytic anemia, hypotension, lacrimation, leukopenia, Mees' lines (on nail beds; forms at 4-6 weeks postexposure), myoglobinuria, neuritis, nystagmus, pancytopenia, paresthesia, radiopacity, seizures, stocking-glove sensory neuropathy, sweating, tachycardia, torsade de pointes, tremor

Admission Criteria/Prognosis All suspected patients should be admitted; survival >1 week after an acute exposure is usually associated with recovery, although peripheral neuropathy may be long term

Toxicodynamics/Kinetics
Absorption: Oral, inhalation (60% to 90%), and dermal (most arsenic compounds absorption is low except for arsenic trichloride and arsenic acid)
Distribution: V_d: 0.2 L/kg
Metabolism: Reduction/oxidation reactions that interconvert arsenate and arsenite and methylation reactions to monomethyl arsonic acid and cacodylic acid
Half-life: 4-5 days
Elimination: Renal, degree of metabolism is ingestant dependent

Absorption: Oral, inhalation (60 to 90%) and dermal (most arsenic compounds, absorption is low except for arsenic trichloride and arsenic acid)

Reference Range

Urine concentrations in nonexposed individuals ≤50 mcg/L; hair concentrations detectable 30 hours postingestion; urine ≥100 mcg/L is suggestive for chronic exposure; blood not usually helpful, although blood arsenic levels >1000 mcg/L are usually associated with fatality; background whole blood arsenic level is usually <1 mcg/dl

Mean urine concentration of arsenic 0.2 mg/L associated with fatal poisoning

Seafood (methylated arsenic) can elevate, urinary arsenic levels for 2 to 3 days

Hair/nail arsenic levels in unexposed individuals <1 ppm

Overdosage/Treatment

Decontamination:

Oral: Lavage (within 1 hour)/activated charcoal. Aluminum hydroxide may prevent absorption of pentavalent arsenic compounds (due to its phosphate-binding abilities), although this has not been investigated in humans. Whole bowel irrigation is effective.

Dermal: Remove contaminated clothing; wash with soap and water.

Ocular: Copious irrigation with saline

Supportive therapy: Succimer (at standard doses to treat lead poisoning) is probably the treatment of choice. 2,3-Dimercaptopropane sulphonate (DMPS or unithiol) is also useful to enhance this metal's elimination at a dose of 100 mg 3 times/day orally for 5 days. 2,3-Dimercaptopropane-sulphonate (DMPS), a water soluble derivative of dimercaprol, has been recently demonstrated to prevent polyneuropathy when started within 48 hours of exposure at a dose of 5 mg/kg I.V. every 4 hours for 24 hours, and then 400 mg orally every 4 hours for 5-7 days. BAL should be utilized for severe acute exposures except for arsine gas. Penicillamine provides long-term therapy or alternatives to BAL. Oral spirulina extract (250 mg) plus zinc (2 mg) twice daily for 16 weeks may be useful in treating chronic arsenic poisoning (with melanosis and keratosis).

Enhanced elimination: Hemodialysis clearance of arsenic ranges from 76-87 mL/minute; the clinical utility of this modality is unknown. No studies have been performed regarding hemodialysis with metal-chelate compound. Clearance of arsenic through hemodialysis is estimated to range from 76-87 mL/minute. Due to tissue binding of arsenic, this is not felt to be a useful modality for removal of arsenic. No current studies exist on the use of chelation with extracorporeal removal methods.

Antidote(s)

- Dimercaprol [ANTIDOTE]
- Penicillamine [ANTIDOTE]
- Succimer [ANTIDOTE]
- Unithiol [ANTIDOTE]

Diagnostic Procedures

- Arsenic, Blood
- Arsenic, Hair, Nails
- Arsenic, Urine
- Electrolytes, Blood
- Heavy Metal Screen, Blood

Additional Information

Toxic oral dose: 120-200 mg

Causes garlic odor; seafood contains arsenobetaine and arsenocholine; dietary history is important.

A radiopaque compound, but rapid absorption makes observation unlikely. Arsine gas is the most toxic, then trivalent arsenite, then pentavalent arsenate. Acute exposure can cause chronic symptoms. Bone marrow, skin, and peripheral nervous system are usual targets of chronic exposure.

Found in some homeopathic medications; Chinese herbal balls may contain from 7.8-621.3 mg of mercury and from 0.1-36.6 mg of arsenic.

TLV-TWA: 0.2 mg/m^3

Urban arsenic levels of ambient air: 20-30 ng/m^3. Arsenic levels in groundwater: 1-2 ppb; found in the earth's crust at an arsenic level of 2 ppm.

Arsenic levels in selected media: Grains: 0.22 ppm; Meat: 0.14 ppm; Seafood: 4-5 ppm; Cigarette: 1.5 ppm

Estimated daily intake of arsenic (adult): Nonsmoker: 51.5 mcg; smoker (2 packs/day): 63.5 mcg; Drinking water: 10 mcg; Food: 45 mcg

Cancers associated with inorganic arsenic exposure: Lung (oat cell, adenocarcinoma), Skin (Basal cell, Bower's disease), Bladder and hepatic angiosarcoma

Specific References

Belson M, Holmes A, Funk A, et al, "Cross-Sectional Exposure Assessment of Environmental Contaminants in Churchill County, Nevada," *J Toxicol Clin Toxicol*, 2003, 41(5):722.

Burgess JL, Josyula AB, Montenegro M, et al, "Low Dose Arsenic Exposure and Urinary 8-OHdG in Arizona and Sonora," *Clin Toxicol (Phila)*, 2005, 43:748.

Burgess JL, Rowland H, Josyula A, et al, "Reduction in Total Inorganic Urinary Arsenic and Toenail Arsenic with Provision of Bottled Water," *J Toxicol Clin Toxicol*, 2004, 42(5):807.

Cantrell FL, "Look What I Found! - Poison Hunting on eBay®," *Clin Toxicol*, 2005, 43(5):375-9.

Chakraborti D, Mukherjee SC, Saha KC, et al, "Arsenic Toxicity from Homeopathic Treatment," *J Toxicol Clin Toxicol*, 2003, 41(7):963-7.

Cohen SM, Arnold LL, Eldan M, et al, "Methylated Arsenicals: The Implications of Metabolism and Carcinogenicity Studies in Rodents to Human Risk Assessment," *Crit Rev Toxicol*, 2006, 36:99-133.

Goulle JP, Mahieu L, and Kintz P, "The Murder Weapon Was Found in the Hair!" *Annale de Toxicologie Analytique*, 2005, 17(4):243-6.

Hantson P, Haufroid V, Buchet JP, et al, "Acute Arsenic Poisoning Treated by Intravenous Dimercaptosuccinic Acid (DMSA) and Combined Extrarenal Epuration Techniques," *J Toxicol Clin Toxicol*, 2003, 41(1):1-6.

Hopehayn C, Bush HM, Bingcang A, et al, "Association Between Arsenic Exposure from Drinking Water and Anemia During Pregnancy," *J Occup Environ Med*, 2006, 48(6):635-43.

Josyula AB, Rowland H, Kurzius-Spencer M, et al, "Environmental Arsenic Exposure and Sputum Metalloproteinase Concentrations," *Clin Toxicol (Phila)*, 2005, 43:753.

Kales SN, Huyck KL, and Goldman RH, "Elevated Urine Arsenic: Unspeciated Results Lead to Unnecessary Concern and Further Evaluations," *J Anal Toxicol*, 2006, 30:80-5.

Kinoshita H, Hirose Y, Tanaka T, et al, "Oral Arsenic Trioxide Poisoning and Secondary Hazard from Gastric Content," *Ann Emerg Med*, 2004, 44(6):625-7.

Krause E, Nussle P, Santana D, et al, "Arsenic and Lead Soil Contamination near a Heavy Metal Refinery in the Andes Mountains," *J Toxicol Clin Toxicol*, 2003, 41(5):739.

Kumagai Y, Sumi D, "Arsenic: Signal Transduction, Transcription Factor, and Biotransformation Involved in Cellular Response and Toxicity," *Ann Rev of Pharmacol Toxicol*, 2007, 47:243-62.

Lamm SH, Engel A, Kruse MB, et al, "Arsenic in Drinking Water and Bladder Cancer Mortality in the United States: An Analysis Based on 133 U.S. Counties and 30 Years of Observation," *J Occup Environ Med*, 2004, 46:298-306.

Misbahuddin M, Islan AM, Khardker S, et al, "Efficacy of Spirulina Extract Plus Zinc in Patients of Chronic Arsenic Poisoning: A Randomized Placebo-Controlled Study," *Clin Toxicol*, 2006, 44:135-41.

Morton J and Mason H, "Speciation of Arsenic Compounds in Urine from Occupationally Unexposed and Exposed Persons in the U.K. Using a Routine LC-ICP-MS Method," *J Anal Toxicol*, 2006, 30:293-301.

Mukherjee SC, Saha KC, Pati S, "Murshidabad – One of the Nine Groundwater Arsenic-Affected Districts of West Bengal, India. Part II: Dermatological, Neurological, and Obstetric Findings," *Clin Toxicol (Phila)*. 2005, 43(7):835-48.

Mycyk MB, Crulcich M, Mucha A, et al, "Exposure Assessment of Children Exposed to Arsenic in an Urban Playlot," *J Toxicol Clin Toxicol*, 2003, 41(5):737.

Poklis A, "A Case of Homicide by Chronic Arsenic Poisoning with Apparent Radiographic Evidence of Arsenic Administration," *J Anal Toxicol*, 2003, 27:192.

Rahman MM, Sengupta MK, Ahamed S, et al, "Murshidabad – One of the Nine Groundwater Arsenic-Affected Districts of West Bengal, India. Part I: Magnitude of Contamination and Population at Risk," *Clin Toxicol (Phila)*. 2005, 43(7):823-34

Rahman M, Vahter M, Sohel N, et al, "Arsenic Exposure and Age- and Sex-Specific Risk for Skin Lesions: A Population-Based Case-Reference Study in Bangladesh," *Environ Health Perspect*, 2006, 114:1847-52.

Sawyer TS, Moran D, and Lowry JA, "Accidental Ingestion of Sodium Sulfur Arsenate Proves Rapidly Fatal," *Clin Toxicol (Phila)*, 2005, 43:747.

Sethi NK, Sethi PF, and Anand I, "Acute Arsenic Poisoning Mimicking Guillain Barré Syndrome," *Int J Med Toxicol*, 2003, 6(2):11.

Steinmaus C, Bates M, Yuan Y, et al, "Arsenic Methylation and Bladder Cancer Risk in Case-Control Studies in Argentina and the United States," *J Occup Environ Med*, 2006, 48(5):478-88.

Vantroyen B, Heilier JF, Meulemans A, et al, "Survival After a Lethal Dose of Arsenic Trioxide," *J Toxicol Clin Toxicol*, 2004, 42(6)889-95.

Verret WJ, Chen Y, Ahmed A, et al, "A Randomized, Double-Blind Placebo-Controlled Trial Evaluating the Effects of Vitamin E and Selenium on Arsenic-Induced Skin Lesions in Bangladesh," *J Occup Environ Med*, 2005, 47:1026-35.

Wang RY, Paschal DC, Osterloh J, et al, "Urinary-Speciated Arsenic Levels from Selected U.S. Regions," *J Toxicol Clin Toxicol*, 2004, 42(5):770-1.

Arsine

Applies to Etchers; Jewelry; Lead Burners; Silicone Chips

CAS Number 7784-42-1

UN Number 2188

Synonyms Arsenic Trihydride; Arsenous Hydride; Hydrogen Arsenide; AsH$_3$

Use Produced when water comes into contact with molten arsenic; used in the semiconductor industry; also found in jewelry, lead burners, etchers, silicone chips, fertilizer makers, aniline workers

Mechanism of Toxic Action Decline of erythrocyte glutathione concentrations after arsine binds to hemoglobin

Signs and Symptoms of Overdose Abdominal cramping, abdominal tenderness, asthenia, dizziness, headache, hemolysis (potent), hypotension, jaundice (2-24 hrs. postexposure), pulmonary edema, nausea, oliguria may occur later, painless hemoglobinuria, seizures, shivering, vomiting, bone marrow depression has been reported. Renal failure within 72 hours.

Admission Criteria/Prognosis Any symptomatic patient or evidence of hemolysis should be admitted; patients may be discharged after 24 hours if the patient is asymptomatic without signs of hemolysis

Toxicodynamics/Kinetics

Absorption: Inhalation: Well absorbed

Metabolism: To arsenic and trimethylarsine

Elimination: Excreted as arsenic in urine, feces, hair, fingernails, and by the lungs

Reference Range Toxic: Blood: >200 mcg/dL; urine: >1000 mcg/L. A plasma free hemoglobin level >1.5 g/dL indicates the need for definitive treatment (possibly exchange transfusion).

Overdosage/Treatment

Decontamination: **Dermal:** Wash with soap and water. **Inhalation:** Administer 100% humidified oxygen.

Supportive therapy: Immediate removal from victim; alkalinization of urine to prevent renal failure; exchange transfusions helpful in severe hemolysis with a free plasma hemoglobin over 1.5 g/dL; heavy metal chelators are ineffective. Maintain good urine output.

Elimination: Hemodialysis may be required for renal failure but will not remove the arsine-hemoglobin complex.

Additional Information One of the most potent hemolytic toxins known; odorless, colorless, nonirritating at low concentrations (<2 ppm); garlic-like odor at higher concentrations. Immediate lethal air concentration: 250 ppm. Case fatality rate: 25%. Potential human carcinogen. Hemolysis is blocked by carbon monoxide and partially blocked by methemoglobin. One hour exposure: 5 ppm TLV-TWA: 0.05 ppm; IDLH: 6 ppm; PEL-TWA: 0.05 ppm

Specific References

Goetz R, Sweeney R, Snook CP, et al, "Case Series: A New Source of Arsine," *Clin Toxicol (Phila)*, 2005, 43:746.

O'Connor AD, Kao LW, and Furbee RB, "Arsine Gas Poisoning After Occupational Exposure," *Clin Toxicol (Phila)*, 2005, 43:746.

Skinner CG, Kneewicz AA, Coon TP, et al, "Arsine Gas Exposure Presenting as Back Pain and Hematuria: A Case Series," *Clin Toxicol (Phila)*, 2005, 43:747.

Asbestos

Related Information

- Gastrointestinal Cancer Risks from Asbestos

Applies to Auto Repair; Brake/Clutch Linings; Building Demolition; Cement Pipe; Chemical Filters; Electrical Insulation; Fireproof Clothing; Gaskets; Locomotive Repair; Power Plants

CAS Number 1332-21-4

UN Number 2212; 2590

U.S. Brand Names Avibest® (Chrysotile type)

Synonyms Magnesium Silicate

Use Found in manufacture of cement pipe or panels, electrical insulation, fireproof clothing, locomotive repair, power plants, building demolition, car repair, chemical filters, gaskets, brake/clutch linings, transmission component

Mechanism of Toxic Action

Not well delineated; asbestos is fibrogenic with accumulation of macrophage and fiber phagocytosis occurring; it is unclear whether asbestos fibers induce carcinogenesis or are tumor promoting agents; lipid peroxidation can occur with chrysotile agents

Half-life (fibers >10 um): 7.9 years (chrysotile); 150 years (tremolite)

Adverse Reactions

Cardiovascular: Chest pain, angina

Renal: Renal cell cancer

Respiratory: Cough, Bronchogenic Carcinoma (Risk is over tenfold for smokers), Mesothelioma

Signs and Symptoms of Overdose Asbestosis: Bilateral interstitial fibrosis affecting lower $^2/_3$ of lung; symptoms include dyspnea, rales (usually occur 10-40 years after exposure), renal failure, acute myelocytic leukemia, and skin warts

Toxicodynamics/Kinetics

Fibers >3 μm in diameter or longer than 100 μm are not rapidly cleared from pulmonary tract

Absorption: No dermal or GI absorption

Elimination: Mucociliary transport through lung

Clearance: Upper airways: 2-3 hours. Lower airways: 10-160 days

Overdosage/Treatment Supportive therapy: There is no specific treatment for asbestosis. Traditional antineoplastic therapy for tumors is the mainstay of treatment. Certainly, patients with asbestos exposure should avoid cigarette smoking.

Additional Information

Levels of airborne asbestos (fibers measured by phase contrast microscopy/L of air): School: 0.00024; Rural: 0.000002; Urban: 0.003-0.000003; Industrial operations: 0.15-0.0015

Chrysotile exposures do not appear to increase the risk of mesothelioma; risk of mesiothelioma to amphiboles exposure is about 1.23%.

Serpentine asbestos (extended sheet polysilicate structure): Chrysotile (white asbestos)* - TLV: 2 fibers/mL of air

Amphibole group (linear double chain polysilicate structure): Actinolite TLV: 2 fibers/mL of air; Amosite (brown asbestos)* - TLV: 0.5 fibers/mL of air; Anthophyllite (gray asbestos)* - TLV: 2 fibers/mL of air; Crocidolite (blue asbestos)* - TLV: 0.2 fibers/mL of air; Mullite - TLV: 2 fibers/mL of air; Tremolite (silicic acid: calcium magnesium salt) - TLV: 2 fibers/mL of air

*Associated with high fibrogenic potential

OSHA-PEL: 0.2 fibers/nL of air

Carcinomas associated with asbestos include lung (especially in smokers), pleural mesothelioma (not increased in smokers), peritoneum mesothelioma, laryngeal carcinoma; carcinomas of questionable association with asbestos include colon, renal, pancreas, ovary, esophagus, and lymphomas

While all types of fibers can cause lung cancer, amphibole group fibers are more potent for inducing mesotheliomas than serpentine fibers; EPA estimates that lifetime exposure of asbestos dust (0.001 fiber >3 μm in length per mL of air) could result in 2-4 excess lung cancer or mesothelioma deaths per 100,000 individuals.

Pulmonary function tests may show restrictive pattern; open lung biopsy may be required; gallium scanning or bronchoalveolar lavage may be helpful

In older homes (built from 1920s to 1970s), asbestos may be located around boilers, steam pipes, ductwork, floor coverings (especially 9" vinyl tiles), "popcorn" ceiling finishes, exterior siding, roofing shingles, and acoustical ceiling tiles

Specific References

Alfonso HS, Fritschi L, de Klerk NH, et al, "Plasma Concentrations of Retinol, Carotene, and Vitamin E and Mortality in Subjects with Asbestosis in a Cohort Exposed to Crocidolite in Wittenoom, Western Australia," *J Occup Environ Med*, 2005, 47(6):573-79.

Hemminki K and Li X, "Time Trends and Occupational Risk Factors for Peritoneal Mesothelioma in Sweden," *J Occup Environ Med*, 2003, 45(4):451-5.

Hemminki K and Li X, "Time Trends and Occupational Risk Factors for Pleural Mesothelioma in Sweden," *J Occup Environ Med*, 2003, 45(4):456-61.

Muller JG, Rudolph WG, Liekse JM, et al, "Changes in B-Readings over Time in the United States Navy Asbestos Medical Surveillance Program," *J Occup Environ Med*, 2007, 49:194-203.

Osinubi OY, Moline J, Rovner E, et al, "A Pilot Study of Telephone-Based Smoking Cessation Intervention in Asbestos Workers," *J Occup Environ Med*, 2003, 45(5):569-74.

Wang LI, Neuberg D, and Christiani DC, "Asbestos Exposure, Manganese Superoxide Dismutase (MnSOD) Genotype, and Lung Cancer Risk," *J Occup Environ Med*, 2004, 46(6):556-64.

Yarborough CM, "Chrysotile as a Cuase of Mesothelioma: An Assessment Based on Epidemiology," *Crit Rev Toxicol*, 2006, 36:165-87.

Asphalt

CAS Number 8052-42-4

UN Number 1999

Synonyms Road Tar

Use Road surfacing or roof sealant agent; also used in paints, electrical adhesive, radioactive waste disposal

Mechanism of Toxic Action Can cause thermal injury; generally exhibits high viscosity, low volatility and high surface tension

Adverse Reactions

Central nervous system: Headache, hyperthermia

Dermatologic: Thermal burns, oil acne, hyperpigmentation, fingernail discoloration (black)

Gastrointestinal: Upon ingestion, concretions and bezoars can develop

Ocular: Eye irritation

Respiratory: Cough

Monitoring Parameters Carboxyhemoglobin (inhalation)

Overdosage/Treatment

Decontamination:

Dermal: Initially immerse affected area in cool water; emulsifying agents can assist in debridement. Bacitracin can be used as a topical antibiotic. Liquid Tween® 80 (polysorbate 80), can be applied to affected area; cover with wet dressings for 6 hours and then irrigate with saline. This procedure may be repeated until tar is removed. Alternatively a neosporin-based cream (Neosporin®-G-Cream) can be used in the above manner, while covering the affected area with sterile wet dressing for 24 hours, then irrigate with saline (complete removal may take 3 days). Other, less effective agents include Neosporin® ointment, mineral oil, petro-latum, or lanolin. Additionally, butter or mayonnaise has been used as an emulsifier with some success. Medi-Sol (De-Solv-it; Orange-Sol) or Unibase® with triple-antibiotic ointments can also be used. Thermal burns should be treated in the traditional manner after removal. Do **not** debride tar mechanically without using an emulsifying agent. **Do not** use gasoline, kerosene, or acetone to irrigate.

Inhalation: Administer 100% humidified oxygen.

Ocular: Initially copiously irrigate with saline. Irrigation can also include sterile surface active solvents (ie, Shur-Clens®) with saline to facilitate tar removal. Additionally, a polysorbate with neomycin sulfate can be used to remove tar from conjunctivae.

Additional Information TLV-TWA (Fume): 5 mg/m³; fumes from asphalt may contain carbon monoxide, hydrocarbons or hydrogen sulfide; specific gravity: 0.95-1.1

Specific References

Schultz OE and Stephens TL, "Don't Hold the Mayo," *Clin Toxicol (Phila)*, 2005, 43:678.

Barium

Pronunciation (BA ree um)

Related Information

- Barium Nitrate
- Toxins Which Should Be Lavaged with Solutions Other Than Water

CAS Number 7440-39-3

UN Number 1339; 1400; 1854

U.S. Brand Names Anatrast; Baricon™; Baro-Cat®; Barobag®; Barosperse®; Bear-E-Yum® CT; Bear-E-Yum® GI; CheeTah®; Digital HD; Enhancer; Entrobar®; EntroEase®; Flo-Coat; HD 200® Plus; HD 85®; Intropaste; Liqui-Coat HD®; Liquid Barosperse®; Medebar® Plus; Medescan; Prepcat; Tomocat® 1000; Tomocat®; Tonopaque

Synonyms Ba, Barium Sulfate

Mechanism of Toxic Action Barium can sequester potassium (thus producing potassium redistribution) within muscle cells resulting in decreased ionic potential (under 60 mV) and paralysis. Potassium efflux is blocked by barium.

Adverse Reactions

Cardiovascular: Hypertension, tachycardia (ventricular), sinus bradycardia, sinus tachycardia, arrhythmias (ventricular), vasoconstriction

Central nervous system: Hypothermia, bilateral putaminal involvement

Dermatologic: Angioedema

Endocrine and metabolic: Hypokalemia, hypophosphatemia

Gastrointestinal: Abdominal pain, diarrhea, nausea, vomiting, feces discoloration (black), feces discoloration (clay/putty), feces discoloration (red), feces discoloration (white/speckling), xerostomia, appendicitis

Neuromuscular & skeletal: Muscle paralysis, myopathy, paresthesia, rhabdomyolysis areflexic flaccid quadriplegia

Ocular: Mydriasis,

Respiratory: Wheezing, apnea, allergic rhinitis (benign pneumoconiosis)

Signs and Symptoms of Overdose Abdominal pain, allergic rhinitis, angioedema, apnea, areflexia, AV block, dermal burns, diaphoresis, diarrhea, fasciculations, feces discoloration (black; clay/putty; red; white/speckling), flaccid muscle paralysis, hypertension, hypokalemia, hypophosphatemia, hyporeflexia, hypothermia, mydriasis, nausea, paresthesia, rhabdomyolysis, tachycardia (ventricular), vomiting, wheezing

Admission Criteria/Prognosis Patients who are symptomatic or develop hypokalemia should be admitted; asymptomatic patients can be discharged after 8 hours postexposure

Toxicodynamics/Kinetics

Absorption: Oral absorption from food sources: 1% to 15% (average 6%)

Distribution: Primarily to skeleton and teeth

Half-life: 3.6 days (2 hours on dialysis)

Elimination: Primarily fecal

Contraindications

Hypersensitivity to barium or any component of the formulation; known or suspected obstruction of the colon, known or suspected GI tract perforation, suspected tracheoesophageal fistula, obstructing lesions of small intestine, pyloric stenosis

Specific agents may also be contraindicated with inflammation or neoplastic lesions of the rectum, recent rectal biopsy; use in infants with swallowing disorders; newborns with complete duodenal or jejunal obstruction with suspected distal small bowel or colon obstruction; very small preterm infants and young babies requiring small volumes of contrast media; infants and young children with possible leakage from GI tract (eg, necrotizing enterocolitis, unexplained pneumoperitoneum, gasless abdomen, bowel or esophageal perforation, postoperative anastomosea)

Dosage Forms

Suspension, oral, as sulfate:

Bear-E-Yum® CT: 1.5% (200 mL) [bubble gum flavor]

Bear-E-Yum® GI: 60% (200 mL, 1900 mL) [bubble gum flavor]

EntroEase®: 13% (600 mL) [marshmallow flavor]

Intropaste: 44% (454 g) [suspension paste; raspberry flavor]

Liqui-Coat HD®: 210% (150 mL) [vanilla-raspberry flavor]

Suspension, oral/rectal, as sulfate:

Baro-Cat®: 1.5% (300 mL, 900 mL, 1900 mL) [banana-pineapple flavor]

CheeTah®: 2.2% (250 mL, 450 mL, 900 mL, 1900 mL) [butterscotch vanilla flavor]

Liquid Barosperse®: 60% (355 mL, 1900 mL) [vanilla flavor]

Medescan: 2.2% (250 mL, 450 mL, 1900 mL) [raspberry flavor]

Prepcat: 1.5% (450 mL) [strawberry flavor]

Tomocat®: 5% (145 mL) [concentrate to make a 1.5% solution; strawberry flavor]

Tomocat® 1000: 5% (225 mL) [concentrate; strawberry flavor]

Suspension, rectal, as sulfate:

Anatrast: 100% (500 g) [suspension paste; packaged with enema tips]

Entrobar®: 50% (500 mL) [packaged in administration kit]

Flo-Coat: 100% (1850 mL)

Medebar® Plus: 100% (1900 mL)

Powder for suspension, oral, as sulfate:

Baricon™: 98% (340 g) [lemon-vanilla flavor]

Digital HD: 96% (245 g) [citrus flavor]

Enhancer: 98% (312 g) [lemon-vanilla flavor]

HD 200® Plus: 98% (312 g) [strawberry flavor]

Tonopaque: 95% (180 g) [cherry flavor]

Powder for suspension, oral/rectal, as sulfate:

Barosperse®: 95% (225 g, 900 g) [vanilla flavor]

HD 85®: 85% (1900 mL) [raspberry flavor]

Powder for suspension, rectal, as sulfate (Barobag®): 97% (340 g, 454 g) [packaged as an enema kit]

Reference Range Ingestion of barium carbonate resulting in muscle paralysis was associated with a peak barium level of 150 mEq/L; normal serum barium levels: 3-29 mcg/dL; normal urinary excretion of barium in unexposed patients: 26 mcg of barium daily; serum and urine barium levels following a symptomatic inhalation injury were 370 mcg/dL and 1600 mcg/dL, respectively. Serum barium level of 133 mcg/dL is associated with severe symptoms.

Overdosage/Treatment

Decontamination: Lavage (within 1 hour)/activated charcoal will not bind barium. Magnesium sulfate or sodium sulfate is the preferred cathartic in order to convert barium to inabsorbable barium sulfate.

Supportive therapy: Monitor potassium. Paralysis and ventricular arrhythmia will respond to large doses of potassium (may require 120 mEq IV over 30 minutes or 400 mEq per day). Rebound hyperkamua (upto 9 MEq/L) may occur without cardiac effects. Avoid the use of I.V. sulfate or magnesium salts since this may cause precipitation of barium in the kidneys. Hypertension can be treated with nitroglycerin.

Enhancement of elimination: Forced diuresis with I.V. saline solution with furosemide (1 mg/kg I.V.) to keep a urine flow of 3-6 mL/kg/hour will hasten elimination. Hemodialysis with a high flux filter and a sodium bicarbonate/potassium dialysate may also be useful.

Pregnancy Implications Safety and efficacy for use during pregnancy have not been established. In general, elective radiography of the abdomen is avoided during pregnancy unless essential for diagnosis.

Additional Information

Found in most soils ranging from 15-3000 ppm; average atmospheric barium concentration in North America is 0.012 mcg/m³; in seawater it is ~13 mcg/L. Brazil nuts have high concentrations of barium (3000-4000 ppm).

TLV-TWA: Barium: 0.5 mg/m³; Barium sulfate: 10 mg/m³

Total daily barium intake: 650-1770 mg

Average amount of barium ingested through drinking water: 1-2 mg/kg/day

Average amount of barium intake through inhalation: 1-30 mg/day (75% absorbed)

Specific References

Centers for Disease Control and Prevention (CDC), "Barium Toxicity After Exposure to Contaminated Contrast Solution - Goias State, Brazil, 2003," *MMWR Morb Mortal Wkly Rep*, 2003, 52(43):1047-8.

Koch M, Appoloni O, Haufroid V, et al, "Acute Barium Intoxication and Hemodiafiltration," *J Toxicol Clin Toxicol*, 2003, 41(4):363-7.

Rivera W, Hail S, Hall W, et al, "Accidental Intravenous Barium Sulfate Infusion," *J Toxicol Clin Toxicol*, 2003, 41(5):673.

Szajewski J and Praski S, "High-Potassium Haemodialysis in Barium Poisoning," *J Toxicol Clin Toxicol*, 2004, 42(1):117.

Barium Nitrate

CAS Number 10022-31-8

UN Number 1446

Synonyms Barium Dinitrate; Nitrobarite

Use Sparklers, fireworks; incendiaries, ceramic glazes

Mechanism of Toxic Action A soluble barium salt; a direct muscle stimulant which produces nitrogen oxides upon combustion

Adverse Reactions
Cardiovascular: Hypertension, tachyarrhythmias (ventricular)
Central nervous system: Headache
Endocrine & metabolism: May cause hypokalemia
Gastrointestinal: Nausea, vomiting, diarrhea, abdominal cramping
Hematologic: Leukocytosis
Neuromuscular & skeletal: Motor weakness
Respiratory: Hypoventilation

Admission Criteria/Prognosis Admit any symptomatic patient or any ingestion >10 g.

Monitoring Parameters Serum electrolytes

Reference Range Normal serum barium levels: 0.08-0.4 mg/L; normal urinary excretion of barium in unexposed patients: 26 mcg of barium daily

Overdosage/Treatment
Decontamination: **Oral:** Emesis within 30 minutes or lavage within 1 hour; activated charcoal. **Dermal:** Wash the exposed area with soap and water. **Inhalation:** Administer 100% humidified oxygen. **Ocular:** Irrigate copiously with saline or water.
Supportive therapy: Lidocaine or procainamide can be used to treat ventricular arrhythmias.

Additional Information TLV-TWA: 0.5 mg/m^3; IDLH: 250 mg/m^3. Specific gravity: 3.24

Benomyl

Applies to 50 DF; Fungicide
CAS Number 17804-35-2
U.S. Brand Names Benex®; Benlate®; Tersan® 1991
Synonyms BBC; MBC
Use A fungicide used on ornamental plants, vegetables, fruits
Mechanism of Toxic Action A benzimidazole carbamate which has no effect on cholinesterase; a dermal irritant

Adverse Reactions
Cardiovascular: Edema
Dermatologic: Contact dermatitis, eczema, photosensitization, hyperpigmentation, dermal erythema
Ocular: Conjunctivitis
Respiratory: Cough
Miscellaneous: Aneuploidy induction

Signs and Symptoms of Overdose Lethargy, somnolence

Toxicodynamics/Kinetics
Absorption: Poor
Metabolism: Carbendazim and methyl 5-hydroxy-2-benzimidazole (or 5-HBC)
Elimination: Primarily renal (within 72 hours)

Reference Range Exposed, asymptomatic nursery workers had 5-HBC urine levels ranging from 3-87 µmol/mol creatinine

Overdosage/Treatment
Decontamination: **Oral:** Lavage (within 1 hour)/activated charcoal. **Dermal:** Wash copiously with soap and water; remove all clothing (especially leather clothing). **Ocular:** Irrigate with saline copiously.
Supportive therapy: Topical steroid preparations can be used for contact dermatitis.

Additional Information TLV-TWA: 0.84 ppm; a white powder with an acrid odor; no evidence for human carcinogenicity; does not accumulate in soil

Bentazon

Applies to Herbicide
CAS Number 25057-89-0
Synonyms Basagran; Bentazone
Use Selective contact postemergent herbicide used on growing grains such as rice, corn, peanuts, beans, peas, and peppers
Mechanism of Toxic Action Irritant
Signs and Symptoms of Overdose Vomiting, diarrhea, tachycardia, dyspnea, weakness, tremors, muscle rigidity, rhabdomyolysis, coma, diaphoresis have all been noted on ingestion
Reference Range Following a 240 g ingestion in a fatal suicide attempt, plasma and urine levels of bentazon was 1500 mg/L and 1000 mg/L respectively

Overdosage/Treatment
Decontamination: **Oral:** Activated charcoal; consider gastric lavage for ingestions over 50 g. **Respiratory:** Administer 100% oxygen
Supportive therapy: Bromocriptine (2.5 mg 3 times/day for 3 days) has been used to treat muscle rigidity and signs of neuroleptic malignant syndrome; otherwise, therapy is supportive

Additional Information An odorless, white/colorless crystalline powder usually diluted in water. Water half-life <1 day; soil half-life <1 month

Specific References
Turcant A, Harry P, Cailleux A, et al, "Fatal Acute Poisoning by Bentazon," *J Anal Toxicol*, 2003, 27(2):113-7.

Benzene

Applies to Dyes; Lacquer; Oil Cloths; Varnishes
CAS Number 71-43-2
UN Number 1114
U.S. Brand Names Polystream®
Synonyms (6)-Annulene; Carbon Oil; Mineral Naphtha; Phene; Phenyl Hydride
Commonly Found In Industrial solvent, gasoline (0.81% to 1.35%, higher percentage in Europe)
Use In lacquers, manufacture of dyes, oil cloths, varnishes, gasoline additive, natural rubber
Mechanism of Toxic Action Hematotoxicity, CNS depression, leukemogenic

Adverse Reactions
Cardiovascular: Cardiac toxicity
Central nervous system: CNS depression, euphoria
Gastrointestinal: Feces discoloration (black), burning sensation of mucous membranes
Hematologic: Acute Myelogenous Leukemia, usually after chronic exposure, aplastic anemia, neutropenia, megaloblastic anemia, agranulocytosis, malignant lymphoma
Hepatic: Hepatotoxicity
Respiratory: Bronchial irritation, pulmonary edema
Miscellaneous: Aneuploidy induction, cutaneous T-cell lymphoma

Signs and Symptoms of Overdose Aspiration, ataxia, blistering, coma (3000 ppm), cough, dementia, dizziness, lethargy, headache, hematuria, hoarseness, leukopenia, mydriasis, ototoxicity, paresthesia, seizures, tinnitus, tremors, tachycardia, erythema, vomiting (ingestion of 9 g)

Admission Criteria/Prognosis Symptomatic patients 12 hours postinhalation exposure should be admitted; patients who have ingested a significant amount of benzene should be admitted

Toxicodynamics/Kinetics
Absorption: Inhalation: Rapid (70% to 80% within first 5 minutes). Oral: 90% to 97% of dose in rodent models. Dermal: <1%; absorption rate: 0.4 mg/cm^2/hour
Metabolism: Hepatic via cytochrome P450-dependent mixed function oxidase through two detoxification pathways: 1) via glutathione to mercapturic acid, and 2) through sulfate/glucuronide conjugation. Hematotoxic metabolites include hydroquinone, phenol, muconic dialdehyde, and catechol.
Half-life: 8 hours
Elimination: Renal (<1%) and by inhalation (16% to 42%). Through dermal absorption as much as 30% can be excreted through the kidneys as phenol. Oral ingestion (rabbit model): 43% was eliminated through the lungs (1.5% as carbon dioxide), with urinary excretion accounting for 33%.

Monitoring Parameters Obtain baseline complete blood count; if abnormal, perioxidase, leukocyte alkaline phosphatase, an iron level, and a reticulocyte count should be performed. Urinary levels of muconic and S-phenylmercapturic acid samples at the end of work shift are better exposure indicators for benzene than phenol. The BEI for S-phenylmercapturic acid muconic acid are 25 mcg/g creatinine and 500 mcg/g creatinine at the end of shift respectively.

Reference Range Normal urine phenol level <10 mg/L, blood benzene level of 0.2 mg/L is consistent with exposure of 25 ppm as is a urinary phenol level of 200 mg/L

Overdosage/Treatment
Decontamination:
Oral: Basic poison management. Lavage within 2 hours of ingestion with respiratory protection. Activated charcoal may be useful. Diazepam and/or phenytoin may be helpful in controlling seizures. Indomethacin has been demonstrated to decrease myelotoxicity in rodent models, but human data are lacking. Due to the possibility of arrhythmias, avoid epinephrine.
Inhalation: Move patient to fresh air; give 100% humidified oxygen
Ocular: Irrigate with copious amounts of water or saline
Dermal: Remove contaminated clothing and wash area thoroughly with soap and water
Enhancement of elimination: Although there is no experience in its use, acetylcysteine has a theoretical role in increasing glutathione stores and enhancing elimination.

Drug Interaction
Ethyl alcohol can potentiate the severity of benzene-induced hematological abnormalities
Weak genotoxicity; can cross the placenta

Additional Information
Estimated oral lethal dose: 1 mL/kg and lethal (rapidly) air concentration over 20,000 ppm. Serious health effects can occur with one hour exposure at air concentrations >150 ppm
Daily benzene intake of a smoker (32 cigarettes daily) is ~10 times (1.8 mg/day) that of a nonsmoker. Median benzene levels in homes with smokers is ~50% greater than that of nonsmokers (3.3 ppb vs 2.2 ppb).

Atmospheric half-life of benzene is ~5.6 days. In water, it is ~17 days, although the half-life of its hydroxyl radicals in water may be 8-9 months.

Benzene was substantially reduced in automotive gasoline after 1995 (see Gasoline monograph). It has been estimated that benzene exposure to pumping gasoline at service stations is ~1 ppm. Ambient median benzene levels in urban areas is ~12.6 ppb, while California's median benzene levels are much lower (3.3 ppb) due to stricter gasoline requirements.

Biomarkers indicative for significant benzene (below 4000/mm^3), low erythrocyte counts (below 4,000,000/m^3), or elevated leukocyte alkaline phosphatase levels.

TLV-TWA: 0.5 ppm; IDLH: 500 ppm; STEL: 1 ppm

Gas density: 2.8

Specific gravity: 0.88

Slightly water soluble

Odor threshold: 1.5-5 ppm

Median level of benzene found in snow samples (near Denver, Colorado): 0.02 mcg/L

Blood testing: Use lavender top (EDTA) tube and refrigerate (minimum volume 7 mL)

In November 2005, FDA received private laboratory results reporting low levels of benzene in a small number of soft drinks that contained benzoate salts (an antimicrobial) and ascorbic acid (vitamin C). FDA has no regulatory limits for benzene in beverages other than bottles water, for which FDA uses the US Environmental Protection Agency (EPA) maximum contaminant level (MCL) of 5 ppb for drinking water, as a quality standard.

Benzene is found in the air from emissions from burning coal and oil, gasoline service stations, and motor vehicle exhaust. Benzene is a carcinogen and has caused cancer in workers exposed to high levels from workplace air. Benzene can form at the parts per billion (ppb) level in some beverages that contain both benzoate salts and ascorbic acid (vitamin C) or erythorbic acid (a closely related substance (isomer) also known as d-ascorbic acid). Elevated temperatures and light can stimulate benzene formation in the presence of benzoate salts and vitamin C, while sugar and EDTA salts inhibit benzene formation.

As follow-up to the November 2005 benzene findings, FDA's Center for Food Safety and Applied Nutrition (CFSAN) initiated a limited survey of beverages with a focus on soft drinks that contain both benzoate and ascorbic or erythorbic acid. The vast majority of beverages sampled to date (including those containing both benzoate preservative and ascorbic acid) contain either no detectable benzene or levels below the 5 ppb limit for drinking water.

The follow table lists benzene levels in particular beverages that are >1 ppb only. For method 1, the estimated limit of detection (LOD) is 0.2 ppb when benzene is determined with cryogenic focusing using the m/z 78 ion in the scan mode. For method 2, the estimated LOD is 0.02 ppb when benzene is determined without cryogenic focusing using the m/z 78 ion in the SIm mode. Multiple results reported for the same lot of a soft drink wee usually obtained from a resampling of the same bottle at a later time. Results indicate benzene levels measured on individual purchased beverages.

Benzene Levels >1 ppb in Beverage Product Samples

PRODUCT		FOUND, ppb	
		Method 1	Method 2
Products Containing Benzoate Only	Safeway Select Diet Cola, lot 1	1.3	
	Food Lion Caffeine Free Diet Cola with Splena	1.1	
	Giant Diet Sun Pop Orange, lot 1	3.5	

Table   (*Continued*)

PRODUCT		FOUND, ppb	
		Method 1	Method 2
Products Containing Benzoate + Ascorbic Acid (Vitamin C) or Erythorbic Acid	Safeway Select Diet Orange, lot 1	79.2	
	Safeway Select Diet Orange, lot 2	15.2	10.7
	Safeway Select Diet Orange, lot 3	13.2	11.4
	Safeway Select Diet Orange, lot 4		1.2
	Shasta Caffeine Free Orange Soda	1.2	
	Crush Pineapple		9.2
	Sunny D Citrus Punch, lot 1	1.1	
	Sunny D Citrus Punch, lot 2	3.5	
	AquaCal Strawberry Flavored Water Beverage, lot 1	23.4	
	AquaCal Strawberry Flavored Water Beverage, lot 2	10.4	9.2
	AquaCal Peach Mango Flavored Water Beverage, lot 1	2.6	
	AquaCal Peach Mango Flavored Water Beverage, lot 2	4.0	3.4
	AquaCal Concord Grape Flavored Water Beverage	4.6	4.0
	Belly Washers Black Cherry Blast Vitamin C Juice Drink, lot 1	2.3	2.0
	Belly Washers Black Cherry Blast Vitamin C Juice Drink, lot 2		1.6
	Belly Washers Battle Berry Vitamin C Juice Drink, lot 1	2.0	1.6
	Belly Washers Battle Berry Vitamin C Juice Drink, lot 2		1.3
	Belly Washers Web Berry Vitamin C Juice Drink		1.8
	Belly Washers Eerie Berry Vitamin C Juice Drink		2.8
	Faygo Moon Mist*	2.8	1.4
	Crystal Light Sunrise Class Orange, lot 1**	76.6	87.9
	Crystal Light Sunrise Class Orange, lot 2**	1.4	1.1
	Crystal Light Sunrise Class Orange, lot 3**		73.9
	Rush! Energy Lite Drink**	1.4	
	Kool-Aid Jammers 10 Juice Drink Tropical Punch**	2.9	2.3
	Kool-Aid Jammers Juice Drink Kiwi-Strawberry, lot 1**	2.0	1.5

Table (*Continued*)

PRODUCT		FOUND, ppb	
		Method 1	Method 2
Other	Ocean Spray Light Cranberry Juice Cocktail, lot 1 (ascorbate only)***	3.0	2.5
	Ocean Spray Light Cranberry Juice Cocktail, lot 2 (ascorbate only)***		4.8
	Giant Light Cranberry Juice Cocktail, lot 1 (ascorbate only)***	10.7	9
	Giant Light Cranberry Juice Cocktail, lot 2 (ascorbate only)***		5.4
	New Crystal Light Sunrise Classic Orange, (ascorbate, EDTA)		1.6

*Contains erythorbic acid (d-ascorbic acid, an isomer of vitamin C)
**Contains EDTA (a food ingredient used to promote flavor retention)
***May contain natural benzoic acid (benzoate)

Specific References

Buffler PA, Kelsh M, Chapman P, et al, "Primary Brain Tumor Mortality at a Petroleum Exploration and Extraction Research Facility," *J Occup Environ Med*, 2004, 46:257-70.

Lin Y-S, Vermeulen R, Tsai CH, et al, "Albumin Adducts of Electrophilic Benzene Metabolites in Benzene-Exposed and Control Workers," *Environ Health Perspectives*, 2007, 115(1):28-34.

Marrs TC, "Diazepam in the Treatment of Organophosphorus Ester Pesticide Poisoning," *Toxicol Rev*, 2003, 22(2):75-81.

Olmos V, Lenzken SC, Lopez CM, et al, "High Performance Liquid Chromatography Method for Urinary Trans, Trans-Muconic Acid: Application to Environmental Exposure to Benzene," *J Anal Toxicol*, 2006, 30:258-61.

Wennborg H, Magnusson LL, Bonde JP, et al, "Congenital Malformations Related to Maternal Exposure to Specific Agents in Biomedical Research Laboratories," *J Occup Environ Med*, 2005, 47(1):11-9.

Wong O, "Is There a Causal Relationship Between Exposure to Diesel Exhaust and Multiple Myeloma?" *Toxicol Rev*, 2003, 22(2):91-102.

Benzidine

Related Information
• 4,4'-Methylenebis (2-Chloroaniline)

Applies to Fast Corinth Base B
CAS Number 92-87-5
UN Number 1885
Synonyms 4,4'-Diphenylediamine; Benzidin
Use In the production of azo dyes for leathers, textiles, and paper; not produced in the U.S. for dye manufacture
Mechanism of Toxic Action Intermediate metabolites through hepatic degradation; may be carcinogenic
Adverse Reactions
Dermatologic: Allergic eczematous dermatitis
Miscellaneous: Cutaneous T-cell lymphoma
Toxicodynamics/Kinetics
Absorption: Through intact skin, lungs, intestine
Metabolism: Hepatic to N-acetylbenzidine; undergoes enterohepatic recirculation
Half-life: 5 hours
Elimination: Renal and bile
Reference Range
Urine levels in workers exposed to benzidine based dyes ranged from:
Benzidine: 0-363 lmcg/L
Monoacetylbenzidine: 6-1117 mcg/L
Diacetylbenzidine: 4-160 mcg/L
Overdosage/Treatment
Decontamination: **Oral:** Lavage (within 1 hour)/activated charcoal. **Do not** use mineral oil as a cathartic in that oils may enhance intestinal absorption. **Dermal:** Irrigate with soap and water; remove contaminated clothing. **Ocular:** Irrigate with saline.
Supportive therapy: While no human treatment data exists, interruption of benzidine metabolism by such agents as aspirin or indomethacin (through inhibition of cyclooxygenase) may reduce peroxide formation. Similarly, a reducing agent such as ascorbic acid may decrease levels of toxic oxidized reactive metabolites which can be carcinogenic.
Enhancement of elimination: Due to enterohepatic recirculation, multiple dosing of activated charcoal may be effective.

Additional Information Occupationally exposed workers may have a higher incidence of bladder (transitional cell) carcinoma; may alter natural killer cell activity. Atmospheric half-life: 12 hours. Water half-life: 100 days

Beryllium

CAS Number 1304-56-9; 13327-32-7; 13510-48-0; 13510-49-1; 13597-99-4; 14215-00-0; 35089-00-0; 66104-24-3; 7440-41-7; 7787-47-5; 7787-49-7; 7787-56-6
UN Number 1566; 1567; 2464
Synonyms Beryl; Glucinium
Commonly Found In Ore processing, aircraft disc brakes, space vehicles, optics, microwave oven components, automotive electronics, fuel containers
Mechanism of Toxic Action Acute (rare) and chronic toxicities most commonly seen with inhalation exposure of soluble compounds in occupational setting; inhibits phosphatases, hexokinase, lactate dehydrogenase
Adverse Reactions
Cardiovascular: Chest pain, angina, cor pulmonale
Dermatologic: Skin ulceration
Gastrointestinal: Salty taste
Hematologic: Granulomas
Hepatic: Granulomatous hepatitis
Renal: Kidney stones, nephritis
Respiratory: Chronic "sarcoid-like" pulmonary disease; acute bronchitis after exposure to soluble to be at levels of 25 to 600 mg/m^3; lung cancer
Signs and Symptoms of Overdose Conjunctivitis (acute), dermatotoxicity (dermal irritation, granuloma, skin ulcers), nausea, pneumonitis, pulmonary fibronodular disease, right-sided heart failure, seizures, vomiting
Admission Criteria/Prognosis Significant, acute exposure should be admitted for 3 days due to delayed onset of pneumonitis
Toxicodynamics/Kinetics
Absorption: Inhalation (primarily); oral and dermal (poorly absorbed)
Protein binding: 70%
Metabolism: Not biotransformed
Half-life: 2-8 weeks
Reference Range Urine concentrations: 0.4-1.0 mcg/L in controls
Overdosage/Treatment
Decontamination: Remove from exposure source; oxygen indicated for symptomatic inhalation exposure
Dermal: Beryllium foreign body residues need to be removed for skin ulceration to heal.
Supportive therapy: Chronic pulmonary symptoms may respond to corticosteroids. Oral exposure should be treated by diluting with milk or water. Chelation is not effective. A high calcium diet might displace beryllium from bones. Bronchodilators such as albuterol may be useful. Persons with chronic beryllium disease have had a variable response to corticosteroid treatment.
Additional Information
Beryllium is odorless; chronic beryllium poisoning requires at least four of these findings:
1. Exposure
2. Beryllium in lung/granulomas
3. Respiratory disease
4. Radiograph of fibronodular disease
5. Restrictive pulmonary function
6. Consistent lung/lymph pathology
Up to 16% of individuals are sensitized following exposure
Average concentration of beryllium: Atmospheric air: <0.1 ng/m^3; fresh water: 10-1000 ng/L; soil: 2.8-5 mg/kg; cigarette smoke: 2% to 10%
Idiosyncratically affects 5% of heavily exposed workers after 1- to 20-year latency
TLV: 0.002 mg/m^3
Beryllium measurable in lung and granulomas of chronic beryllium disease patients; also useful in lymphoblast transformation test from bronchoalveolar lavage fluid
Insoluble in water
Air beryllium levels >100 mcg/m^3 can result in acute beryllium disease. Appropriate rescuer personnel protective equipment incude a dust mist respirator.
Specific References

Bekris LM, Viernes HM, Farin FM, et al, "Chronic Beryllium Disease and Glutathione Biosynthesis Genes," *J Occup Environ Med*, 2006, 48(6):599-606.

Newman LS, Mroz MM, Balkissoon R, et al, "Beryllium Sensitization Progresses to Chronic Beryllium Disease," *Am J Respir Crit Care Med*, 2005, 171(1):54-60.

Sackett HM, Maier LA, Silveira LJ, et al, "Beryllium Medical Surveillance at a Former Nuclear Weapons Facility During Cleanup Operations," *J Occup Environ Med*, 2004, 46(9):953-61.

Sawyer RT, Abraham JL, Daniloff E, et al, "Secondary Ion Mass Spectroscopy Demonstrates Retention of Beryllium in Chronic Beryllium Disease Granulomas," *J Occup Environ Med*, 2005, 47:1218-26.

Silver K and Sharp RR, "Ethical Considerations in Testing Workers for the Glu60 Marker of Genetic Susceptibility to Chronic Beryllium Disease," *J Occup Environ Med*, 2006, 48:434-43.

Biphenyl

CAS Number 92-52-4

Synonyms Difenilo; Diphenyl; E230; Phenylbenzene

Use Fungistatic agent for fruits; used in petroleum refineries as a heat transfer agent and used as an insulating oil

Mechanism of Toxic Action An irritant; also may be an inhibitor of the enzyme adenosine transaminase which accounts for fungistatic properties

Signs and Symptoms of Overdose Cirrhosis, cough, epistaxis, fatigue, headache, hepatic necrosis, insomnia, nausea, numbness, ocular/oral irritation, Parkinsonium symptoms, throat irritation, tremor, vomiting

Admission Criteria/Prognosis Admit any patient with symptomatic gastrointestinal signs or exposures >20 ppm; TLV-TWA is 0.2 ppm

Toxicodynamics/Kinetics
Absorption: Dermal absorption may occur
Metabolism: Hepatic
Elimination: Renal, biliary

Monitoring Parameters Renal function, liver function tests

Overdosage/Treatment Decontamination: **Dermal:** Wash area with soap and water. **Inhalation:** Administer 100% humidified oxygen. **Ocular:** Irrigate with water or saline.

Pregnancy Implications No adverse effects documented

Additional Information GI symptoms can occur at concentrations >20 ppm; TLV-TWA: 0.2 ppm; IDLH: ~60 ppm
Colorless and solid at room termperature

Specific References
Wastensson G, Hagberg S, Andersson E, et al, "Parkinson's Disease in Diphenyl-Exposed Workers: A Causal Association?" *Parkinsonism and Related Disorders*, 2006, 12:29-34.

Borates

CAS Number 10043-35-3; 10294-33-4; 1303-86-2; 1303-96-4; 7440-42-8; 7637-07-2

UN Number 1008; 1458; 2692

U.S. Brand Names Borax®; Dobill's Solution®

Synonyms Boric Anhydride; Boron Oxide; Boron Sesquioxide; Boron Trioxide; Magnesium Perborate; Sodium Biborate; Sodium Borate; Sodium Metaborate; Sodium Perborate; Sodium Pyroborate; Sodium Tetraborate

Use Various; used in herbicides; common ingredient of medicated powders, skin lotions, mouthwashes, toothpastes, powders, water softeners, topical astringents and antiseptics; also used in making glass fibers, enamels, glazes, fire-resistant materials, pigments, paints, catalysts, photographic agents, and insecticides; found in rodent and ant poisons

Adverse Reactions
Central nervous system: Fever, hyperthermia
Miscellaneous: Toxic shock-like syndrome

Signs and Symptoms of Overdose Toxicity may be delayed for hours. Gastrointestinal upset, vomiting (has been described as blue-green), retching, CNS depression, restlessness, irritability, and seizures occur from chronic exposure. Death results from dehydration, shock, circulatory collapse and renal failure. Renal failure, oliguria, and anuria occur several days after exposure. Metabolic acidosis may occur. Erythematous rash (usually on buttocks and scrotum) with desquamation occurring where rash is persistent and on mucous membranes, perianal and anal surfaces. Alopecia totalis can occur with acute or chronic poisoning.

Admission Criteria/Prognosis Patients with acidosis, renal impairment, or ingestions >200 mg/kg in children or >6 g in adults, should be admitted.

Toxicodynamics/Kinetics
Absorption: Through gastrointestinal tract, mucous membranes, and abraded and denuded skin
Distribution: V_d: 0.17-0.5 L/kg; distributes to all tissues except brain in 30 minutes
Half-life: 5-27 hours
Peak CNS concentration: In 3 hours
Elimination: 50% excreted in urine within 12 hours and 80% to 100% over 5-7 days

Warnings/Precautions High affinity for brain, liver, and kidney; damage to tissues, especially renal tubular epithelium may be irreversible

Reference Range Normal: 0.0-0.72 mg/dL in children; 0.0-0.2 mg/dL in adults; levels do not seem to correlate well with severity of symptoms; levels >40 mg/dL associated with fatality in infants

Overdosage/Treatment
Decontamination: **Oral:** Ipecac within 30 minutes or lavage within 1 hour; activated charcoal will probably not be useful. Gastric decontamination should occur with ingestions >200 mg/kg in a child or >6 g in an adult. **Dermal:** Wash skin with soap and water. **Ocular:** Irrigate with saline.
Supportive therapy: Monitor for hypotension, shock, seizures
Enhancement of elimination: Hemodialysis or exchange transfusion may enhance elimination. Saline diuresis may be of some benefit. Early institution of peritoneal dialysis, in asymptomatic patients ingesting a large dose, has been advocated.

Additional Information
Average daily boron intake in humans: 10-25 mg
Average amount of boron in surface water: ~0.1 mg/L
Mean boron level in soil in U.S.: 26 mg/kg
FDA tolerance limit for boron in citrus fruit: 8 ppm
Concentration of boron in sea water: ~4.5 mg/L
How supplied: Boric acid: White powder or crystalline solid. Sodium tetraborate anhydrous: Light gray and odorless. Sodium tetraborate decahydrate and pentahydrate: White, odorless, crystalline solids.

Boric Acid

CAS Number 10043-35-3

Use
Food preservatives, emulsifiers, neutralizers, antifungal water softeners, contact lens cleaner, antiseptics, pesticides (for cockroaches)
Ophthalmic: Mild antiseptic used for inflamed eyelids
Topical ointment: Temporary relief of chapped, chafed, or dry skin, diaper rash, abrasions, minor burns, sunburn, insect bites, and other skin irritations

Mechanism of Action Disinfectant, astringent

Adverse Reactions
Central nervous system: CNS stimulation followed by CNS depression, fever
Dermatologic: Erythematous skin eruptions, pruritus, alopecia, erythrodermic desquamation (2-3 days after exposure) (boiled lobster appearance)
Gastrointestinal: Gastrointestinal disturbance, vomiting, nausea, diarrhea, feces discoloration (black), feces discoloration (blue), feces discoloration (blue-green)
Hepatic: Elevated liver function test results
Renal: Acute tubular necrosis

Signs and Symptoms of Overdose Cardiovascular collapse, confusion, dermatitis, desquamation, elevated liver function test results, circulatory collapse, diarrhea, dry skin, hyperthermia, toxic epidermal necrolysis, seizures, urine discoloration (blue-green)

Pharmacodynamics/Kinetics
Absorption: Not well absorbed through intact skin; absorbed well through inflamed skin
Half-life: 12 hours
Elimination: Renal, within 96 hours of ingestion

Dosage Apply to lower eyelid 1-2 times/day

Contraindications Hypersensitivity to boric acid or any component

Warnings If irritation persists or increases, discontinue use

Dosage Forms Ointment, topical: 10% (30 g)

Reference Range Normal boric acid levels: Children: 0.0-0.7 mg/dL; Adults: 0.0-0.2 mg/dL; levels of 2.0-15.0 mg/dL are associated with survival; levels >40.0 mg/dL are associated with lethality

Overdosage/Treatment
Decontamination: Emesis within 30 minutes or lavage within 1 hour for ingestions >200 mg/kg or 12 g total ingestion/activated charcoal will not adsorb boric acid well; irrigate skin with soap and water for dermal exposure
Supportive therapy: Treat hypotension with isotonic saline, dopamine, or norepinephrine
Enhancement of elimination: Exchange transfusion or hemodialysis should be considered for serious toxic manifestations or if renal failure develops. Boric acid serum levels >200 µmol/mL should be considered as indication for hemodialysis.

Drug Interactions Increases riboflavin excretion

Nursing Implications Application to abraded skin or open wounds has caused fatal poisonings in infants

Additional Information Not a corrosive substance

Specific References
Sabuncuoglu BT, Kocaturk PA,, Yaman O, et al, "Effects of Subacute Boris Acid Administration on Rat Kidney Tissue," *Clin Toxicol*, 2006, 44:249-53.

Bromates

Related Information
• Toxins Which Should Be Lavaged with Solutions Other Than Water

CAS Number 7758-01-2; 7789-38-0

UN Number 1450; 3213

Use Found in permanent wave hair neutralizers as potassium bromate (2%) or sodium bromate (10%), and bread preservatives

Mechanism of Toxic Action Mucosal irritant; oxidizing effect on renal tubule can cause renal failure; potassium bromate may be more toxic than sodium bromate

Signs and Symptoms of Overdose Albuminuria, deafness, diarrhea, dizziness, hemolysis, hiccups, hypotension, nausea, ototoxicity, renal failure, seizures, tachypnea, tinnitus (more common in adults than children), vomiting

Admission Criteria/Prognosis Admit any pediatric or adult ingestion >30 mg/kg body weight.

Toxicodynamics/Kinetics Distribution: V_d: 0.24 L/kg

Overdosage/Treatment

Decontamination: Lavage within 1 hour with sodium bicarbonate (2% to 5%) to prevent formation of hydrobromic acid.

Supportive therapy: Give sodium thiosulfate (10-50 mL of a 10% solution over 30-60 minutes) to convert bromate to less toxic bromide; monitor with audiograms.

Enhancement of elimination: Hemodialysis can be used if renal failure ensues, but is not effective in reducing bromide levels.

Bromethalin

Applies to Assault (0.01%); Vengeance (0.01%)

CAS Number 63333-35-7

Synonyms EL-614

Use Rodenticide in concentrations of ~0.01%

Mechanism of Toxic Action A neurotoxin which acts by uncoupling oxidative phosphorylation particularly in the central nervous system

Adverse Reactions

Cardiovascular: Cerebral edema has occurred in animal studies

Central nervous system: Coma, seizures

Neuromuscular & skeletal: Myoclonus, tremors

Admission Criteria/Prognosis Admit any symptomatic patient; asymptomatic patients need to be observed for up to 24 hours; ingestions >0.5 mg/kg may require observation

Toxicodynamics/Kinetics

Absorption: Oral: Absorbed well; not well absorbed dermally

Metabolism: Metabolized to desmethyl bromethalin which is as active as the parent compound in uncoupling oxidative phosphorylation

Half-life: 135 hours (animals)

Overdosage/Treatment

Decontamination: **Oral:** Do **not** induce emesis. Lavage within 1 hour ingestions >1 bait package (0.5 mg/kg). Activated charcoal with sorbitol may be useful. **Ocular:** Irrigate with saline.

Supportive therapy: Monitor for cerebral edema. Supportive care includes phenytoin (or a benzodiazepine), mannitol, and dexamethasone with hyperventilation to decrease increased intracranial pressure.

Additional Information Bait pellets are green in color

Bromides

Related Information

• Bromisovalerylurea

Impairment Potential Yes

Commonly Includes Sodium, potassium, and ammonium bromide; also in multiple medications as salt form of drug; dextromethorphan hydrobromide, homatropine hydrobromide, neostigmine, potassium, propantheline, pyridostigmine, quinine hydrobromide, scopolamine hydrobromide; although this source of bromism has been rare in the U.S. since 1974.

Mechanism of Action Central nervous system depressant

Adverse Reactions

Central nervous system: Headache, slurred speech, hallucinations, retrograde amnesia, memory disturbance, hyperesthesia, CNS depression, depression

Dermatologic: Papules (erythematous, pustular) usually on legs, acneiform eruptions

Endocrine & metabolic: Hypochloremia, hypothyroidism

Gastrointestinal: Nausea, vomiting, anorexia, feces discoloration (black)

Neuromuscular & skeletal: Hypo- or areflexia, tremors, clonus

Signs and Symptoms of Overdose Chronic toxicity often causes acne-like rash; amnesia, ataxia, decreased anion gap, dementia, erythema multiforme, gastric bezoar, hallucinations, hypothyroidism, mydriasis, nausea, nystagmus, papilledema, photophobia, pseudotumor cerebri, sedation, slurred speech, tremors, vomiting

Admission Criteria/Prognosis Symptomatic patients, patients with impairment of renal function, serum bromide levels >150 mcg/mL (in chronic ingestions) or acute oral ingestions >10 g should be admitted

Toxicodynamics/Kinetics

Absorption: ≥90%, can form bezoar

Distribution: V_d: 0.35-0.48 L/kg

Protein binding: 0%

Half-life: 9-15 days

Elimination: Via tubular secretion, renal clearance: 26 mL/kg/day

Reference Range Therapeutic serum bromide levels: 750-1500 mcg/mL; symptoms of toxicity from bromides usually occur at serum bromine levels >1500 mcg/mL; coma >2000 mcg/mL; fatal levels >3000 mcg/mL; background blood bromide level averages ~5.3 mcg/mL (range: 2.5-11.7 mcg/mL); urine bromide levels >0.25 mg/dL are associated with exposure

Overdosage/Treatment

Decontamination: Emesis within 30 minutes or lavage (within 1 hour)/ activated charcoal may be useful for organic bromide compounds (carbromal). Consider whole bowel irrigation

Supportive therapy: I.V. administration of sodium chloride or oral sodium chloride (2-3 g) 3-4 times daily with 4-10 liters of fluid

Enhancement of elimination: Forced saline diuresis to maintain a urine flow of 3-5 mL/kg/hour; hemodialysis can reduce half-life to 1-2 hours; indications for hemodialysis include depressed mental status, cardiac failure, renal failure, or bromide serum levels >2000 mcg/mL; furosemide (1 mg/kg up to 40 mg) can be added to ensure adequate urine output of 3-6 mL\kg\hour; mannitol and ethacrynic acid can also be used

Diagnostic Procedures

• Anion Gap, Blood

Test Interactions Causes negative anion gap: Bromide can interfere with chloride determinations on virtually all standard laboratory tests (including sequential multiple analyzers). It can also interfere with bicarbonate determinations in some analyzers.

Pregnancy Implications Can cause fetal CNS depression; microcephaly, heart malformations, intrauterine growth retardation, club foot, hypotonia, polydactyly have been documented

Additional Information Transient rise in concentrations are often seen in initial days of treatment; radiopaque; daily dietary intake: 0.1-0.3 mg/kg body weight

Bromisovalerylurea

Related Information

• Bromides

CAS Number 496-67-3

Use A sedative-hypnotic agent primarily used in Japan for sleep disorders

Mechanism of Action CNS depressant similar to bromides

Signs and Symptoms of Overdose Amnesia, ataxia, confusion, delirium, dysarthria, gastric atony, hepatitis, pancreatitis, rhabdomyolysis, toxic epidermal necrolysis, vasculitis, vomiting

Toxicodynamics/Kinetics Elimination: Renal: 3-5 hours

Dosage Oral: 600-900 mg

Reference Range Total BVU serum levels >10 mcg/mL associated with toxicity; if (+)-BVU/total BVU ratio is >35%, a considerable amount of the drug remains in the GI tract, not yet absorbed

Overdosage/Treatment

Decontamination: Oral: Avoid gastric lavage due to the fact that dissolution and absorption of the remaining BVU can be accelerated by lavage. Suggested mode for gastric decontamination is oral use of activated charcoal.

Supportive therapy: Intravenous administration of sodium chloride

Enhanced elimination: Although no formal studies exist, charcoal hemoperfusion may remove a significant amount of drug.

Pregnancy Implications Bromism can occur in the fetus

Bromoform

Related Information

• Adipose Tissue Ranges of Toxins

• Dibromochloromethane

CAS Number 75-25-2

UN Number 2515

Synonyms Methenyl Tribromide; Tribromomethane

Use Not produced in the U.S.; used as a fluid for mineral ore separation, a laboratory reagent and used in quality control in the electronics industry; formerly used medicinally as a sedative or antitussive agent

Mechanism of Toxic Action Central nervous depressant; can be generated during water chlorination when water reacts with organic acids; thus, exposure can occur through drinking water (levels usually ~5 mcg/L)

Adverse Reactions

Central nervous system: Depression

Miscellaneous: On inhalation, can be a mucosal irritant and lacrimator

Signs and Symptoms of Overdose May be hepatotoxic and nephrotoxic; coma, miosis, respiratory depression, stupor, tremor

Toxicodynamics/Kinetics

Absorption: Absorbed by inhalation and oral routes (60% to 90%)

Metabolism: Oxidation in liver

Elimination: Pulmonary hepatotoxic in animal models

Reference Range Background blood levels in individuals exposed to bromoform only through drinking water is ~0.6 ppb

Overdosage/Treatment

Decontamination (oral overdose): Lavage (within 1 hour)/activated charcoal

Supportive therapy: Although human overdose experience has been virtually nonexistent over the past 90 years, respiratory support appears to be a crucial modality. Naloxone may be of some benefit; otherwise, treat as for bromides.

Drug Interaction Rate of metabolism may be increased with phenobarbital

Additional Information

Fatal oral dose: 250-500 mg/kg

Colorless liquid with a sweet odor; not flammable. Prepared by mixing acetone with sodium hypobromite or by treating chloroform with aluminum bromide. Anesthetic properties similar to chloroform. Upon heating, it decomposes to bromide ion fumes.

Odor threshold: Air: 13.45 mg/m^3; Water: 0.5 mg/L. OSHA: PEL-TWA: 0.5 ppm; TLV-TWA: 0.5 ppm. Mean urban ambient air concentration of bromoform: 3.6 ppt

FDA: Bottled water regulation for total trihalomethanes: 0.1 mg/L

Atmospheric half-life: Possibly 1-2 months; estimated daily dose to an average adult: <1 mcg

---

Bromophos

CAS Number 2104-96-3

U.S. Brand Names Brofene®; Nexion®

Synonyms O,O-Dimethyl-O-(2,5-Dichloro-4-Bromophenyl) Phosphorothioate

Use Marketed as insecticide granules, dusting agent, or spray liquid with or without petroleum derivative as a solvent

Mechanism of Toxic Action Irreversible inhibition of acetylcholinesterase and plasma cholinesterase, resulting in excess accumulation of acetylcholine at muscarinic and nicotinic receptors, and in the central nervous system

Adverse Reactions

Cardiovascular: **Hyperdynamic** (~18% to 21%) or hypodynamic (~7% to 10%) states, QT prolongation, sinus bradycardia, sinus tachycardia

Central nervous system: Depression, seizures, hyperactivity, cognitive dysfunction, hypothermia

Genitourinary: Incontinence

Neuromuscular & skeletal: Weakness (delayed), paralysis, delayed paresthesia

Respiratory: Pulmonary edema, respiratory depression

Miscellaneous: Flu-like symptoms (especially with chronic exposure), intermediate syndrome

Signs and Symptoms of Overdose

Abdominal pain, agitation, asystole, AV block, bradycardia, bronchorrhea, coma, confusion, cranial nerve palsies, diaphragmatic paralysis, dysarthria, excessive sweating, generalized asthenia, headache, heart block, decreased hemoglobin, decreased red blood cell count, decreased platelet count, fecal incontinence, hypertension, hypotension, lacrimation, metabolic acidosis and hyperglycemia (severe intoxication), miosis (unreactive to light), mydriasis (rarely), nausea, pallor, pulmonary edema, QT prolongation, respiratory depression, salivation, seizures, skeletal muscle fasciculation and flaccid paralysis, tachycardia, tachypnea, urinary incontinence, vomiting

An "intermediate syndrome" of limb asthenia and respiratory paralysis has been reported to occur between 24 and 96 hours postorganophosphate exposure, and is independent of the acute cholinergic crisis. Late paresthesia characterized by stocking and glove paresthesia, anesthesia, and asthenia are infrequently observed weeks to months following acute exposure to certain organophosphates.

Toxicodynamics/Kinetics

Absorption: Readily through oral, dermal, or respiratory exposure

Metabolism: Rapid to weakly active compounds through hepatic hydrolysis and other pathways

Elimination: Metabolites are excreted in urine

Warnings/Precautions Risk of aspiration pneumonitis exists following oral exposure to agents having a hydrocarbon vehicle; severe laryngeal irritation and violent coughing may result from exposure to dusting powders; exposure to dusting powders and insecticide granules may cause contact dermatitis

Overdosage/Treatment

Decontamination: Isolation, bagging, and disposal of all contaminated clothing and other articles. All emergency medical workers and hospital staff should follow appropriate precautions regarding exposure to hazardous material including the use of protective clothing, masks, goggles, and respiratory equipment.

Oral: Activated charcoal can be administered either orally or via a nasogastric tube. **Do not** induce emesis because of danger of sudden respiratory compromise, alterations in mental status, seizures, coma, and possible aspiration of hydrocarbon vehicles. **Do not** give a cathartic.

Dermal: Prompt thorough scrubbing of all affected areas with soap and water, including hair and nails; 5% bleach also may be used

Ocular: Irrigation with copious tepid sterile water or saline

Supportive therapy: Airway management, ventilatory assistance, humidified oxygen administration, and close monitoring for sudden respiratory failure

Antidote:

Atropine: Administration should be guided by respiratory status, starting at 2-5 mg I.V. every 5-10 minutes as needed, and should be titrated to the resolution of excess pulmonary secretions. Frequent administration of large doses (cumulative doses >100 mg) may be necessary in massive exposures.

Glycopyrrolate: May be administered if atropine is unavailable (200-400 mcg I.M. or I.V. initially, or ~$^1/_2$ the dose of atropine).

2-PAM: For more significant exposures (ie, exposures requiring large doses of atropine, or with recurring symptoms, or exposures to more lipid soluble agents), administration should follow: 1-2 g I.V. over 10-30 minutes, repeated in 1 hour if asthenia recurs, then every 4-12 hours for recurring symptoms.

Enhancement of elimination: Dialysis and hemoperfusion are not indicated due to effectiveness of the prescribed antidotal treatment and large volumes of distribution of organophosphates.

Antidote(s)

- Atropine [ANTIDOTE]
- Glycopyrrolate [ANTIDOTE]
- Pralidoxime [ANTIDOTE]

Diagnostic Procedures

- Creatinine, Serum
- Pseudocholinesterase, Serum

Drug Interaction Paralysis is potentiated by neuromuscular blockade (ie, pancuronium, vecuronium, succinylcholine, atracurium, doxacurium, mivacurium); inhibition of serum esterase prolongs the half-life of succinylcholine, cocaine, and other ester anesthetics; cholinergic toxicity is potentiated by cholinesterase inhibitors such as physostigmine

Additional Information

Red blood cell cholinesterase and serum pseudocholinesterase may be depressed following acute or chronic organophosphate exposure; RBC cholinesterase is typically not analyzed by in-house laboratories and is usually not available for consideration during acute management. Pseudocholinesterase levels may be rapidly available from some in-house laboratories, but are not as reliable a marker of organophosphate exposure because of variability secondary to variant genotypes, hepatic disease, oral estrogen use, or malnutrition. Because of this variability, true indication of suppression of either of these enzymes can only be estimated through comparison to pre-exposure values; these enzymes may be useful in measuring a patient's recovery postexposure, especially if the recovery is not progressing as expected.

The intermediate syndrome is not related to delayed neuropathy.

QT$_c$ prolongation on ECG in the setting of organophosphate poisoning is associated with a high incidence of respiratory failure and mortality.

Other information concerning pesticide exposures is available through the EPA-funded National Pesticide Telecommunications Network: 1-800-858-7378 (weekdays, 8 AM to 6 PM, Central Standard time)

Button Batteries (Discontinued)

Synonyms Disc Battery; Watch Battery

Mechanism of Toxic Action Leakage of mercury, potassium, lithium thionyl chloride, or sodium hydroxide at the site of the battery seal can cause gastrointestinal burns; electrical burns or pressure necrosis can occur in the gastrointestinal tract

Adverse Reactions

Gastrointestinal: Esophageal impaction for larger cells (>20 mm in diameter); can also occur in infants <1 year of age for cells >16 mm in diameter: dysphagia, odynophagia, intestinal obstruction

Respiratory: Tachypnea, tracheoesophageal fistula, nasal septal perforation

Signs and Symptoms of Overdose Abdominal pain, dysphagia, esophageal ulceration, fever, tachypnea

Admission Criteria/Prognosis Asymptomatic patients with batteries that have passed beyond the esophagus may be discharged on a regular diet

Monitoring Parameters Mercury levels (for mercury-based batteries) and radiographs

Overdosage/Treatment

Supportive therapy: Avoid emetics. Withhold nasal or otic drops for exposure to nose or ear. Remove promptly if located in airway or in esophagus. Obtain plain radiographs to localize and estimate size of battery. Mercury level for mercury-containing cells may be required. Endoscopic removal for esophageal impaction. If the battery is beyond the esophagus, it is likely (85%) to pass within 96 hours, with 99% of all ingested batteries passing within 7 days. Batteries >15 mm in diameter are less likely to pass through the gastrointestinal tract spontaneously, in children younger than 6 years of age. Cimetidine can be used to reduce corrosion.

Enhancement of elimination: Metoclopramide may be utilized when there are no signs for obstruction or peritonitis. Similarly, one dose of a saline cathartic or sorbitol can be utilized, although these modalities have not been proven to be of value. Polyethylene glycol use has not been well defined and can be considered for batteries located (in asymptomatic patients) distal to the esophagus. Symptomatic patients require surgery or endoscopy. Repeat radiograph in 4-7 days.

Additional Information Strain all stools. Button battery hotline: 202-625-3333

Specific References

Kirk MA, Baer AB, Holstege CP, et al, "Nasal Button Battery Impaction as Cause of Periorbital Cellulitis and Corrosive Tissue Injury," *J Toxicol Clin Toxicol*, 2003, 41(5):679.

Butyl Alcohol

Applies to Lacquer; Paint; Pharmaceuticals (Extractant in Manufacture); Resin

CAS Number 71-36-3

UN Number 1120

Synonyms Butan-l-ol; Butanol; Butyl Hydroxide; Propylcarbinol; Propylmethanol

Use In solvents in paints, lacquers, and resins; also used as extractants in the manufacture of pharmaceuticals; has been used as a sedative

Mechanism of Toxic Action Central nervous system depression

Adverse Reactions

Central nervous system: Depression

Gastrointestinal: Irritant to mucous membranes

Signs and Symptoms of Overdose Ataxia, coma, corneal abnormalities, cough, confusion, dermal erythema, diarrhea, dizziness, drowsiness, fatigue, eye irritation (at 50 ppm), feces discoloration (black), headache (slight), keratitis, porphyria, respiratory depression, vomiting

Toxicodynamics/Kinetics

Absorption: Rapid from the GI tract and dermally

Elimination: By the kidneys faster than ethanol

Overdosage/Treatment

Decontamination: Ipecac/activated charcoal may be useful

Enhancement of elimination: Use hemodialysis for persistent coma.

Diagnostic Procedures

- Electrolytes, Blood
- Glucose, Random
- Osmolality, Serum

Additional Information Minimum toxic dose: 3-7 oz. Fuel oil odor is irritating. In pregnancy, tert-butyl alcohol may be fetotoxic. Odor threshold: 50 ppm. TLV-TWA: 100 ppm

Cadmium

CAS Number 7440-43-9

UN Number 2570

Commonly Found In Solder, metal ores, amalgams, alkaline storage batteries (nickel cadmium batteries), polyvinyl chloride pigments, electroplating processes, cigarette smoke; production of phosphate fertilizers

Mechanism of Toxic Action Local irritation with system toxic effects, primarily proximal renal tubular dysfunction causing impaired regulation of calcium, uric acid and phosphorus, along with proteinuria and glucosuria.

Adverse Reactions

Cardiovascular: Hypertension, shock, cardiomegaly, cardiomyopathy, cor pulmonale

Central nervous system: Fever, seizures, chills

Dermatologic: Photosensitivity

Endocrine & metabolic: Sexual dysfunction, hypokalemia

Gastrointestinal: Diarrhea, vomiting, metallic taste, bad taste, salivation

Genitourinary: Urine discoloration (dark)

Hematologic: Anemia

Hepatic: Hepatic necrosis

Neuromuscular & skeletal: Osteomalacia, myoclonus

Ocular: Visual evoked potential abnormalities

Renal: Nephrotoxicity, renal tubular necrosis, renal failure, proteinuria, acidosis (renal tubular), Fanconi syndrome, glomerulonephritis, renal cell cancer - Nephrolithiasis

Respiratory: Emphysema, bronchitis, cough, bronchiolitis obliterans, hyposmia

Miscellaneous: Tooth discoloration, cutaneous T-cell lymphoma

Signs and Symptoms of Overdose Acute inhalational exposure resembles metal fume fever. Acute oral exposure causes albuminuria, diarrhea, glycosuria, hepatic necrosis, hypochromic anemia, hypokalemia, hypotension, metallic taste, myoclonus, nephritis, photosensitivity, respiratory arrest, seizures, and vomiting. Chemical pneumonitis can be progressive.

Admission Criteria/Prognosis Acutely symptomatic individuals or chronically exposed patients with blood cadmium levels >15 mcg/L or urinary cadmium excretion >100 mcg/day should be admitted; survival after 4 days postexposure is usually associated with recovery

Toxicodynamics/Kinetics

Potential carcinogen

Absorption: 10% either pulmonary or gastrointestinal (increased G.I. absorption in iron-deficient patients)

Distribution: Concentrates in liver and kidney; does not cross placenta; low concentrations in breast milk

Protein binding: Bound primarily to metallothionein and albumin in the +2 valence

Half-life, elimination: 7 to 30 years

Reference Range

Suggested significant exposure with urinary levels >20 mcg/L (concentrations fourfold higher in smokers than nonsmokers) or blood levels >10 mcg/L.

Normal range of whole blood Cd levels:

Smokers: 1.4-4.5 mcg/L

Nonsmokers: 0.4-1 mcg/L

Normal Hair Cd levels:

Smokers:1 mg/kg

Nonsmokers: 0.5 mg/kg

Normal Cd urinary level is <1 mcg/L

Overdosage/Treatment

Decontamination: Ipecac within 30 minutes or lavage within 1 hour; whole bowel irrigation may be helpful; can dilute with milk or water. Activated charcoal does not appear to be effective.

Supportive therapy: No treatment for chronic intoxication. BAL and calcium disodium EDTA are contraindicated due to increased incidence of cadmium-induced renal disease. Dimercaptosuccinic acid (150 mg 3 times/day for 5 days, then twice daily for 14 days) has been shown to increase cadmium excretion by ~30%.

Enhancement of elimination: Hemoperfusion would not be expected to be effective.

Antidote(s)

- Succimer [ANTIDOTE]

Diagnostic Procedures

- Cadmium, Blood
- Cadmium, Hair
- Cadmium, Urine

Additional Information

Environmental exposure in Japan resulted in Itai-Itai disease. Increased beta$_2$-microglobulin excretion is a nonspecific marker for cadmium renal toxicity. Diabetic patients appear to be particularly prone to the adverse renal effects of cadmium.

Foods which contain the highest levels of cadmium include potatoes (0.04 ppm), leafy vegetables (0.03 ppm), grain and cereal products (0.02 ppm); total daily intake from food is ~30 mcg of cadmium.

Content of cadmium in cigarettes averages from 1-2 mcg per cigarette. Mean body burden of cadmium: 1.65 mg in nonsmokers; 11.34 mg in smokers (0.03-0.04 mg of cadmium/pack-year).

Zinc deficiency may exacerbate cadmium-induced nephrotoxicity. High doses of deferoxamine may reduce cadmium induced liver and renal toxicity (in a rodent model).

Lethal oral amount of Cd salts - 5 grams

Specific References

Schmidt B, Roberts RS, Davis P, et al, "Caffeine Therapy for Apnea of Prematurity," *N Engl J Med*, 2006, 254:2112-21.

Sethi PK, Khandelwal D, and Sethi N, "Cadmium Exposure: Health Hazards of Silver Cottage Industry in Developing Countries," *J Med Toxicol*, 2006, 2(1):14-5.

Tarabar AF and Su M, "Mercury and Cadmium Toxicity in a Haitian Voodoo Minister That Resulted in Acute Renal Failure," *J Toxicol Clin Toxicol*, 2003, 41(5):741.

Calcium Hypochlorite

Related Information

- Sodium Hypochlorite

CAS Number 7778-54-3

UN Number 1748; 2208; 2880

Synonyms B-K Powder; Bleaching Powder; Calcium Hypochloride; Chlorinated Lime; Lo-Bax; Losantin Lime Chloride

Use Bleaching agent, algicide, oxidizing agent, fungicide, deodorant, disinfectant; used in sugar refining and preparation of surgical chlorinated soda solution (Dakin's solution)

Mechanism of Toxic Action Corrosive - oxidizing agent directly related to concentration of chlorine

Adverse Reactions

Cardiovascular: Chest pain, angina

Dermatologic: Dermatitis

Ocular: Eye irritation

Signs and Symptoms of Overdose Chest pain, erythema, dyspnea, local edema, pain, sore throat, vomiting

Overdosage/Treatment

Decontamination: **Oral**: **Do not** induce vomiting. **Do not** use gastric lavage. Dilute with milk or water. Endoscopy may be useful for oral ingestions. (Endoscopy is usually not required with a 3% to 6% solution ingestion.) **Do not** neutralize. **Dermal**: Irrigate skin with saline. **Ocular**: Irrigate copiously with water or saline.

Supportive therapy: Ocular: Topical mydriatic agents (ie, 1% atropine twice daily) and topical antibiotics with topical steroids (1% prednisolone tapered over 10 days) can be used.

Additional Information Whitish granular powder with strong odor of chlorine; usually found in concentrations >50%. Specific gravity 2.35. Decomposed by water and alcohol and may ignite when in contact with acids or organic materials

Calcium Oxide

CAS Number 1305-78-8
UN Number 1910
U.S. Brand Names Stomylex™
Synonyms Calcium Monoxide; Calx; Quick Lime
Commonly Found In Manufacture of steel, aluminum, glass; used in sewage treatments; found in dry cement (60% to 67%)
Mechanism of Toxic Action Strong alkaline irritant; can be formed when calcium reacts with water; calcium oxide reacts with water to form calcium hydroxide
Adverse Reactions

Cardiovascular: Tachycardia

Dermatologic: Dermal burns, erythema, skin edema

Gastrointestinal: Esophageal ulceration, dysphagia, vomiting, abdominal pain

Ocular: Ocular burns, glaucoma, conjunctivitis, corneal ulceration (may be delayed for 1 week), corneal opacification, lacrimation, blinking

Renal: Oliguria

Respiratory: Dyspnea, tachypnea, nasal ulceration, stridor, bronchospasm
Monitoring Parameters CBC, electrolytes, chest x-ray, ocular pH
Overdosage/Treatment

Decontamination:

Oral: Dilute with small amounts of milk or water (not >8 ounces in adults or 4 ounces in children). Do not give syrup of ipecac. **Do not** lavage. **Do not** give activated charcoal.

Dermal: Brush off particles of calcium oxide. Irrigate with saline or water under low pressure. Monitor pH of runoff.

Inhalation: Administer 100% oxygen.

Ocular: Irrigate with copious amounts of saline or water. Particles may need to be removed mechanically. Follow saline or water irrigation with irrigation of 0.01-0.05 M EDTA solution for 15 minutes. Cycloplegics (1% atropine twice daily) can be used to prevent ciliary spasm and topical antibiotics should be used.

Supportive therapy: For oral ingestion, perform endoscopy within 24 hours if a significant ingestion occurs, or when stridor, dysphagia, or drooling are present. Corticosteroids (0.1 mg/kg of dexamethasone daily or 1-2 mg/kg of prednisone daily for 3 weeks and then taper) may be useful for second or third degree gastrointestinal burns, although their usefulness has not been investigated in controlled human trials. Use of sucralfate or H$_2$-blockers is also unproven. Albuterol or other beta-adrenergic agonist agents can be used to treat bronchospasm.

Antidote(s)
- Edetate Disodium [ANTIDOTE]

Additional Information Exposure to 9 mg/m^3 can cause lacrimation; found in various dermatological preparations in Europe. pH in a water solution of calcium oxide: ~12.5. Specific gravity: 3.3. IDLH: 25 mg/m^3; TWA: 2 mg/m^3

Calcium Polysulfide

Synonyms Lime Sulfur
Use Control tree fungus
Mechanism of Toxic Action Mucosal caustic agent; can cause metabolic acidosis
Adverse Reactions

Cardiovascular: Sinus tachycardia

Central nervous system: Coma

Dermatologic: Dermal irritation

Endocrine & metabolism: Metabolic acidosis

Gastrointestinal: Esophageal stricture, perioral cyanosis

Hepatic: Liver failure

Neuromuscular & skeletal: Rhabdomyolysis

Renal: Renal failure

Miscellaneous: Sulfur or rotten egg odor
Admission Criteria/Prognosis Admit any symptomatic patient or ingestion >100 mL
Toxicodynamics/Kinetics Elimination: Renal

Reference Range Normal serum sulfate level: 0.5-1.5 mEq/L; levels >2.3 mEq/L may be associated with acidosis
Overdosage/Treatment

Decontamination: **Oral:Do not** induce emesis; lavage (within 1 hour)/ activated charcoal. **Dermal**: Wash with soap and water. **Inhalation:** Administer 100% humidified oxygen. **Ocular**: Irrigate with copious amounts of water.

Supportive therapy: Treatment similar to hydrogen sulfide: Treat acidosis with sodium bicarbonate (1-2 mEq/kg); sodium nitrite (300 mg in adults) may be useful.

Additional Information Releases hydrogen sulfide upon contact with water or acids; 400 mL can be fatal if taken orally

Camphor

CAS Number 21368-68-3; 464-48-2; 464-49-3; 76-22-2
UN Number 2717
Synonyms 2-Camphanone; Anemone Camphor; Formosa Camphor; Gum Camphor; Huile de Camphre; Kampfer; Laurel Camphor; Matricaria Camphor
Use Plasticizer, moth repellent, preservative in pharmaceuticals and cosmetics, in lacquers and varnishes, explosives, and pyrotechnics; used as an antipruritic, topical rubefacient, aphrodisiac, abortifacient, contraceptive, cold remedy, suppressor of lactation, and antiseptic; camphorated liniment or oil usually contains 20% camphor; camphor spirits usually 10%
Mechanism of Action Stimulant of cerebral cortex
Adverse Reactions

Cardiovascular: Tachycardia, Reye's syndrome, sinus tachycardia

Central nervous system: Headache, dizziness, delirium, seizures, coma

Dermatologic: Nonimmunologic contact urticaria, eczema

Gastrointestinal: Nausea, vomiting

Hepatic: Elevated liver function tests

Neuromuscular & skeletal: Myoclonus, fasciculations

Ocular: Mydriasis, strabismus

Renal: Albuminuria

Respiratory: Tachypnea
Signs and Symptoms of Overdose A distinctive oral odor may be apparent; tachycardia, CNS depression, renal failure. Convulsions may occur suddenly without warning or may be preceded by dementia, fasciculations, hyperventilation, irritability, mental confusion, neuromuscular hyperactivity, tremors, and jerky extremity movement. Seizures may be followed by coma and apnea. Vomiting may occur shortly after ingestion (a gastrointestinal irritant). Hepatic transaminases may be mildly and briefly elevated. Most symptoms occur within 30 minutes. Chronic ingestion may cause granulomatous hepatitis.
Admission Criteria/Prognosis Ingestions of >1 g in adults (or 30 mg/kg in a child), or symptomatic patients, should be admitted, probably into an intensive care unit; if asymptomatic for 4 hours after a small ingestion, the patient can probably be safely discharged
Pharmacodynamics/Kinetics

Absorption: Readily through skin and mucous membranes

Distribution: V$_d$: 2-4 L/kg

Protein binding: 61%

Metabolism: Rapidly oxidized and conjugated in liver; metabolites may accumulate in fat stores

Half-life: 93-167 minutes

Peak effect: 90 minutes

Elimination: Odor of camphor may appear in urine; excreted primarily in urine; can also be excreted through the lungs
Dosage See Additional Information.
Monitoring Parameters Liver/renal function; monitor neurologic status
Contraindications Do not use in infants
Dosage Forms Translucent crystalline mass, blocks, or powder
Reference Range Levels >14.5 ng/L associated with seizures
Overdosage/Treatment

Decontamination: Lavage (within 1 hour for ingestions >30 mg/kg)

Eye: Irrigate with room temperature tap water for 15 minutes

Dermal: Wash affected area thoroughly with soap and water; systemic toxicity from dermal exposure is unlikely

Supportive therapy: Treat seizures with benzodiazepines; if seizures are refractory, phenobarbital or pentobarbital should be initiated; ventilatory support may be required; do not give alcohols, oils, or fats because this will increase absorption

Enhancement of elimination: Lipid hemoperfusion and resin hemoperfusion has been reported to decrease levels in patients with refractory seizures; hemodialysis is ineffective; charcoal hemoperfusion may be helpful, although not as clear a benefit as resin hemoperfusion; all of these techniques are somewhat controversial
Pregnancy Risk Factor C
Pregnancy Implications Crosses placenta and has been associated with one fetal death; three other cases report healthy outcomes

Additional Information Minimum lethal dose: 1 g (50 mg/kg). Odor is aromatic and pungent; aromatic taste produces sensation of cold; may mimic Reye's syndrome; TLV-TWA: 5 ppm; IDLH: 200 mg/m^3

Specific References
Manoguerra AS, Erdman AR, Wax PM, et al, "Camphor Poisoning: An Evidence-Based Practice Guideline for Out-of-Hospital Management," *Clin Tox*, 2006, 44:357-70.

Capecitabine

U.S. Brand Names Xeloda®
Synonyms NSC-712807
Use Treatment of metastatic colorectal cancer, metastatic breast cancer
Mechanism of Action Capecitabine is a prodrug of fluorouracil. It undergoes hydrolysis in the liver and tissues to form fluorouracil which is the active moiety. Fluorouracil is a fluorinated pyrimidine antimetabolite that inhibits thymidylate synthetase, blocking the methylation of deoxyuridylic acid to thymidylic acid, interfering with DNA, and to a lesser degree, RNA synthesis. Fluorouracil appears to be phase specific for the G$_1$ and S phases of the cell cycle.

Adverse Reactions
Cardiovascular: Angina, atrial fibrillation, bradycardia, cardiac arrest, cardiac failure, cardiomyopathy, cerebrovascular accident, chest pain, deep vein thrombosis, dysrhythmia, **edema**, electrocardiogram changes, hypertension, hypotension, myocardial infarction, myocardial ischemia, myocarditis, pericardial effusion, tachycardia, venous thrombosis, ventricular extrasystoles

Central nervous system: Ataxia, confusion, depression, dizziness, encephalopathy, **fatigue**, **fever**, headache, insomnia, irritability, loss of consciousness, mood alteration, **pain**, sedation, vertigo

Dermatologic: Alopecia, **dermatitis**, ecchymoses, nail disorders, **palmarplantar erythrodysesthesia** (hand-and-foot syndrome) (may be dose limiting), photosensitivity reaction, pruritus, radiation recall syndrome, skin discoloration, skin ulceration

Endocrine & metabolic: Dehydration, hot flush, hypokalemia, hypomagnesemia, hypertriglyceridemia

Gastrointestinal: Abdominal distension, **anorexia**, **abdominal pain**, colitis, **constipation**, **decreased appetite**, **diarrhea (may be dose limiting)**, duodenitis, dyspepsia, dysphagia, esophagitis, gastric ulcer, gastritis, gastroenteritis, GI hemorrhage, hematemesis, hemorrhage, ileus, increased appetite, intestinal obstruction, **mild to moderate nausea**, motility disorder, necrotizing enterocolitis, oral candidiasis, oral discomfort, proctalgia, **stomatitis**, taste disturbance upper GI inflammatory disorders, toxic dilation of intestine, **vomiting**, weight gain

Genitourinary: Nocturia

Hematologic: **Anemia**, idiopathic thrombocytopenic purpura, **lymphopenia**, leukopenia, **neutropenia**, pancytopenia, **thrombocytopenia**

Hepatic: Ascites, **increased bilirubin**, cholestasis, hepatitis, hepatic failure, hepatic fibrosis

Local: Thrombophlebitis

Neuromuscular & skeletal: Arthralgia, arthritis, back pain, bone pain, dysarthria, joint stiffness, limb pain, myalgia, neuropathy, **paresthesia**, tremor

Ocular: Abnormal vision, conjunctivitis, **eye irritation**, keratoconjunctivitis

Renal: Renal impairment

Respiratory: Asthma, bronchitis, bronchopneumonia, bronchospasm, cough, **dyspnea**, epistaxis, hemoptysis, hoarseness, laryngitis, pneumonia, pulmonary embolism, respiratory distress, sore throat

Miscellaneous: Cachexia, diaphoresis increased, fibrosis, fungal infection, influenza-like illness, hypersensitivity, lymphedema, viral infection, sepsis, thirst

Signs and Symptoms of Overdose Alopecia, diarrhea, myelosuppression, nausea, vomiting

Pharmacodynamics/Kinetics
Absorption: Rapid and extensive
Protein binding: <60%; ~35% to albumin
Metabolism:
  Hepatic: Inactive metabolites: 5'-deoxy-5-fluorocytidine, 5'-deoxy-5-fluorouridine
  Tissue: Active metabolite: Fluorouracil
Half-life elimination: 0.5-1 hour
Time to peak: 1.5 hours; Fluorouracil: 2 hours
Excretion: Urine (96%, 57% as α-fluoro-β-alanine); feces (<3%)

Dosage Oral:
Adults: 2500 mg/m^2/day in 2 divided doses (~12 hours apart) at the end of a meal for 2 weeks followed by a 1- or 2-week rest period
Elderly: The elderly may be pharmacodynamically more sensitive to the toxic effects of fluorouracil. Insufficient data are available to provide dosage modifications.

Dosing adjustment in renal impairment:
Cl$_{cr}$ 50-80 mL/minute: No adjustment of initial dose
Cl$_{cr}$ 30-50 mL/minute: Reduce dose by 25%
Cl$_{cr}$ <30 mL/minute: Do not use

Dosing adjustment in hepatic impairment:
Mild to moderate impairment: No starting dose adjustment is necessary; however, carefully monitor patients
Severe hepatic impairment: Patients have not been studied

Dosage modification guidelines:

Recommended Dose Modifications

Toxicity NCI Grades	During a Course of Therapy (Monotherapy)	Dose Adjustment for Next Cycle (% of starting dose)
Grade 1	Maintain dose level	Maintain dose level
Grade 2		
1st appearance	Interrupt until resolved to grade 0-1	100%
2nd appearance	Interrupt until resolved to grade 0-1	75%
3rd appearance	Interrupt until resolved to grade 0-1	50%
4th appearance	Discontinue treatment permanently	
Grade 3		
1st appearance	Interrupt until resolved to grade 0-1	75%
2nd appearance	Interrupt until resolved to grade 0-1	50%
3rd appearance	Discontinue treatment permanently	
Grade 4		
1st appearance	Discontinue permanently	50%
	or	
	If physician deems it to be in the patient's best interest to continue, interrupt until resolved to grade 0-1	

Stability Store tablets at room temperature of 25°C (77°F).
Monitoring Parameters Renal function should be estimated at baseline to determine initial dose; during therapy, CBC with differential, hepatic function, and renal function should be monitored
Administration Capecitabine is administered orally, usually in two divided doses taken 12 hours apart. Doses should be taken after meals with water.
Contraindications Hypersensitivity to capecitabine, fluorouracil, or any component of the formulation; known deficiency of dihydropyrimidine dehydrogenase (DPD); severe renal impairment (Cl$_{cr}$ <30 mL/minute); pregnancy

Warnings
Hazardous agent - use appropriate precautions for handling and disposal. Use with caution in patients with bone marrow suppression, poor nutritional status, ≥80 years of age, or renal or hepatic dysfunction. Patients with baseline moderate renal impairment require dose reduction. Patients with mild-to-moderate renal impairment require careful monitoring and subsequent dose reduction with any grade 2 or higher adverse event. Use with caution in patients who have received extensive pelvic radiation or alkylating therapy. Use cautiously with warfarin; altered coagulation parameters and bleeding have been reported. Rare and unexpected severe toxicity (stomatitis, diarrhea, neutropenia, neurotoxicity) may be attributed to dihydropyrimidine dehydrogenase (DPD) deficiency.

Capecitabine can cause severe diarrhea; median time to first occurrence is 34 days. Subsequent doses should be reduced after grade 3 or 4 diarrhea or recurrence of grade 2 diarrhea. Necrotizing enterocolitis (typhlitis) has been reported.

Hand-and-foot syndrome (palmar-plantar erythrodysesthesia or chemotherapy-induced acral erythema) is characterized by numbness, dysesthesia/paresthesia, tingling, painless or painful swelling, erythema, desquamation, blistering, and severe pain. If grade 2 or 3 hand-and-foot syndrome occurs, interrupt administration of capecitabine until the event resolves or decreases in intensity to grade 1. Following grade 3 hand-and-foot syndrome, decrease subsequent doses of capecitabine.

There has been cardiotoxicity associated with fluorinated pyrimidine therapy, including myocardial infarction, angina, dysrhythmias, cardiogenic shock, sudden death, ECG changes, and cardiomyopathy. These adverse events may be more common in patients with a history of coronary artery disease. **[U.S. Boxed Warning]: Capecitabine may increase the anticoagulant effects of warfarin; monitor closely.**

Safety and efficacy in children <18 years of age have not been established.

Dosage Forms Tablet: 150 mg, 500 mg

Overdosage/Treatment

Decontamination: Emesis within 30 minutes or lavage (within 1 hour)/ activated charcoal for oral ingestion

Supportive therapy: Monitor hematologically for at least 4 weeks. Allopurinol (300 mg 3 times/day) may be useful in decreasing toxicity; for treatment of acute encephalopathy, dexamethasone (10 mg every 6 hours I.V.) and thiamine may expedite neurologic recovery.

Enhancement of elimination: Forced diuresis or hemodialysis may enhance elimination

Drug Interactions Phenytoin: Concomitant use may increase the levels/ effects of phenytoin; monitor.

Warfarin: Capecitabine may decrease the metabolism of warfarin; monitor closely.

Pregnancy Risk Factor D

Pregnancy Implications There are no adequate and well-controlled studies using capecitabine in pregnant women; however, fetal harm may occur. Women of childbearing potential should avoid pregnancy.

Lactation Excretion in breast milk unknown/not recommended

Additional Information Food reduced the rate and extent of absorption of capecitabine.

Captan

Applies to Foliage Protection

CAS Number 133-06-2

U.S. Brand Names Orthocide® 406; Orthocide®; Vancide® 89

Synonyms Captane; Captano

Use Foliage protection

Mechanism of Toxic Action A phthalimide (chloroalkyl thio) fungicide which is not phytotoxic is a dermal sensitizer which causes allergic dermatitis through a cell-mediated (type IV) immunologic reaction.

Signs and Symptoms of Overdose Conjunctivitis, dermatitis, desquamation, persistent erythema, photosensitivity

Toxicodynamics/Kinetics

Absorption: Poor through the GI tract (60%)

Metabolism: Hepatic

Elimination: Urine (52%), feces (16%), air (23%)

Overdosage/Treatment Decontamination: **Oral:** Emesis within 30 minutes or lavage (within 1 hour)/activated charcoal. **Dermal:** Irrigate skin with soap and water. **Inhalation:** Administer 100% humidified oxygen

Specific References

Chodorowski Z and Anand JS, "Acute Oral Suicidal Intoxication with Captan: A Case Report," *J Toxicol Clin Toxicol*, 2003, 41(5):603.

Carbaryl

CAS Number 63-25-2

UN Number 2757

U.S. Brand Names Arilate®; Carbatox®; Crunch®; Hexavin®; Sevin®; Vioxan®

Synonyms 1-Naphthyl N-Methylcarbamate

Use Marketed as an insecticide dusting agent or spray liquid

Mechanism of Toxic Action Reversible inhibition of acetylcholinesterase and plasma cholinesterase, resulting in excess accumulation of acetylcholine at muscarinic and nicotinic receptors, and in the central nervous system

Adverse Reactions

Cardiovascular: **Hyperdynamic** (~18% to 21%) or hypodynamic (~7% to 10%) states, edema, sinus bradycardia, sinus tachycardia

Central nervous system: Toxicity is limited because carbamates do not significantly cross the blood-brain barrier; CNS changes occur with most severe intoxications, hyperactivity

Endocrine & metabolism: Hypoglycemia

Genitourinary: Urinary incontinence

Neuromuscular & skeletal: Weakness, paralysis

Ocular: Diplopia

Respiratory: Cough, respiratory depression

Miscellaneous: Flu-like symptoms (especially with chronic exposure)

Signs and Symptoms of Overdose Delayed neurotoxicity manifesting as limb asthenia has been reported following a massive ingestion of carbaryl (~500 mg/kg). Abdominal pain, agitation, asystole, AV block, bradycardia, bronchorrhea, coma, cranial nerve palsies, confusion, decreased hemoglobin, decreased platelet count, decreased red blood cell count, diaphragmatic paralysis, dysarthria, excessive sweating, fecal and urinary incontinence, flaccid paralysis, generalized asthenia, headache, heart block, hypertension, hypotension, lacrimation, metabolic acidosis and hyperglycemia (severe intoxication), miosis (unreactive to light), mydriasis (rarely), nausea, pallor, pulmonary edema, QT prolongation, respiratory depression, salivation, seizures, tachycardia, tachypnea, skeletal muscle fasciculation, vomiting

Overdosage/Treatment

Decontamination: Isolation, bagging, and disposal of all contaminated clothing and other articles. All emergency medical workers and hospital staff should follow appropriate precautions regarding exposure to hazardous material including the use of protective clothing, masks, goggles, and respiratory equipment.

Oral: Activated charcoal can be administered either orally or via a nasogastric tube. **Do not** induce emesis because of danger of sudden respiratory compromise, alterations in mental status, seizures, coma, and possible aspiration of hydrocarbon vehicles. **Do not** use a cathartic.

Dermal: Prompt thorough scrubbing of all affected areas with soap and water, including hair and nails; 5% bleach may also be used

Ocular: Irrigation with copious tepid sterile water or saline

Supportive therapy: Airway management, ventilatory assistance, humidified oxygen administration, and close monitoring for sudden respiratory failure. Diazepam is the agent of choice for seizure control and should be given as pretreatment in seriously ill patients.

Antidote:

Atropine: Administration should be guided by respiratory status, starting at 2-5 mg I.V. every 5-10 minutes as needed, and should be titrated to the resolution of excess pulmonary secretions. Frequent administration of large doses (cumulative doses > 100 mg) may be necessary in massive exposures.

Glycopyrrolate: May be administered if atropine is unavailable (200-400 mcg I.V. or I.M. initially, or ~1/2 the dose of atropine).

2-PAM: Experimental data has indicated that carbaryl toxicity may be potentiated by oxime therapy. Do not use 2-PAM for a known or strongly suspected single ingestion of carbaryl.

Enhancement of elimination: Dialysis and hemoperfusion are not indicated due to effectiveness of the prescribed antidotal treatment and large volumes of distribution of organophosphates.

Antidote(s)

- Atropine [ANTIDOTE]

Diagnostic Procedures

- Creatinine, Serum
- Pseudocholinesterase, Serum

Drug Interaction Paralysis is potentiated by neuromuscular blockade (ie, pancuronium, vecuronium, succinylcholine, atracurium, doxacurium, mivacurium); inhibition of serum esterase prolongs the half-life of succinylcholine, cocaine, and other ester anesthetics; cholinergic toxicity is potentiated by cholinesterase inhibitors such as physostigmine; administration of oxime antidotes (2-PAM and obidoxime) has been shown to increase carbaryl toxicity in animal models

Additional Information

Odorless and colorless, white, or gray solid

Red blood cell cholinesterase, and serum pseudocholinesterase may be depressed following acute or chronic organophosphate exposure and are theoretically useful for differentiating between carbamate and organophosphate exposures.

RBC cholinesterase is typically not analyzed by in-house laboratories and is usually not available for consideration during acute management. Pseudocholinesterase levels may be rapidly available from some in-house laboratories, but are not as reliable a marker of organophosphate exposure because of variability secondary to variant genotypes, hepatic disease, oral estrogen use, or malnutrition, thus they may not be useful in ruling out carbamate exposure.

Decreased sperm counts and sperm motility have been noted in a rodent model.

Vapor pressure: 0.005 mm Hg at 20°C

ACGIH TLV: 5 mg/m³; PEL-TWA: 5 mg/m³; IDLH: 625 mg/m³

Other information concerning pesticide exposures is available through the EPA-funded National Pesticide Telecommunications Network: 1-800-858-7378 (weekdays, 8 AM to 6 PM, Central Standard time)

Specific References

Long H, Kirrane B, Nelson LS, et al, "Carbaryl Inhibition of Plasma Cholinesterase Activity," *J Toxicol Clin Toxicol*, 2003, 41(5):737.

Santinelli R, Tolone C, D'Avanzo A, et al, "Pontine Myelinolysis in a Child with Carbamate Poisoning," *Clin Toxicol*, 2006, 44(3):327-8.

Carbinoxamine

CAS Number 3505-38-2; 486-16-8

U.S. Brand Names CarbihistCarbinoxamine PD; Carboxine; Histex™ CT; Histex™ I/E; Histex™ PD; Palgic; Pediatiex™

Synonyms Carbinoxamine Maleate; Carbinoxamine Tannate

Use Allergic rhinitis

Mechanism of Action An ethanolamine antihistamine which blocks acetylcholine at muscarinic receptors; also has serotonin antagonist effects

Adverse Reactions

Central nervous system: **Drowsiness**, dizziness

Dermatologic: Contact dermatitis

Gastrointestinal: Anorexia, diarrhea, nausea, xerostomia, vomiting

Genitourinary: Dysuria

Renal: Polyuria

Respiratory: **Thickening of bronchial secretions**

Signs and Symptoms of Overdose Usually occur within 2 hours of ingestion; ataxia, coma, diplopia, dry mouth, fever, mydriasis, seizures, tachycardia, tremor, visual hallucinations

Pharmacodynamics/Kinetics Half-life elimination: 10-20 hours

Dosage Children: 0.2-0.4 mg/kg/day
Adults: 4-8 mg given 3 or 4 times/day

Administration Shake suspension well before use.

Contraindications Hypersensitivity to carbinoxamine or any component of the formulation; use with or within 14 days of MAO inhibitor therapy

Warnings Use caution with asthma, increased intraocular pressure, hypothyroidism, cardiovascular disease, hypertension, pyloroduodenal obstruction, symptomatic prostatic hyperplasia, or bladder neck obstruction. Causes sedation; caution must be used in performing tasks which require mental alertness (eg, operating machinery or driving). May cause paradoxical excitation in pediatric patients. Safety and efficacy have not been established in children <9 months of age.

Dosage Forms
[DSC] = Discontinued product
Capsule, variable release:
Histex™ I/E: Carbinoxamine maleate 2 mg [immediate release] and carbinoxamine maleate 8 mg [extended release] [DSC]
Liquid, as maleate:
Carbihist: 4 mg/5 mL (120 mL) [cotton candy flavor] [DSC]
Carbinoxamine PD: 4 mg/5 mL (480 mL) [bubble gum flavor] [DSC]
Carboxine: 1.75 mg/5 mL (480 mL) [bubble gum flavor] [DSC]
Histex™ PD: 4 mg/5 mL (480 mL) [alcohol free, dye free, sugar free; bubble gum flavor]
Pediatex™: 1.75 mg/5 mL (480 mL) [alcohol free, dye free, sugar free; cotton candy flavor] [DSC]
Solution, as maleate:
Palgic: 4 mg/5 mL (480 mL) [bubble gum flavor]
Suspension, as tannate:
Pediatex™ 12: Carbinoxamine 3.6 mg per 5 mL (480 mL) [contains sodium benzoate; candy apple flavor] [DSC]
Suspension, variable release:
Histex™ PD-12: Carbinoxamine maleate 2 mg [immediate release] and carbinoxamine tannate 6 mg [extended release] per 5 mL (120 mL, 480 mL) [alcohol free, dye free, sugar free; contains sodium benzoate; bubble gum flavor]
Tablet, as maleate [scored]:
Palgic: 4 mg

Overdosage/Treatment
Decontamination: Oral: Do **not** induce emesis; lavage (within 2 hours)/activated charcoal
Supportive therapy: Physostigmine has been useful to successfully reverse visual hallucination; this agent should be reserved for life-threatening anticholinergic symptoms; benzodiazepines can be used for seizure control or for treatment of agitation
Enhanced elimination: Multiple dosing of activated charcoal may be effective

Drug Interactions
Barbiturates (and other CNS depressants): CNS depressant effects may be increased.
MAO inhibitors: Anticholinergic effects of the antihistamine may be increased and prolonged.
Tricyclic antidepressants: CNS depressant effects may be increased.

Pregnancy Risk Factor C

Pregnancy Implications Animal reproduction studies have not been conducted.

Lactation Excretion in breast milk unknown/use caution

Carbon Dioxide

CAS Number 124-38-9

UN Number 1013; 1845 (dry ice)

Synonyms Carbonic Acid Gas; Carbonic Anhydride; CO_2; Dry Ice

Use In urea synthesis; manufacture of soft drinks; used in fire extinguishers; dry ice; exposure can also occur from brewing, mining, and foundry work; dry ice has been used for cryotherapy (to treat warts/nevi)

Mechanism of Toxic Action
Inhalation: Simple asphyxiant (a colorless, odorless gas)
Solid form (as dry ice): Can cause freeze injury

Adverse Reactions
Cardiovascular: Tachycardia, hypotension, cyanosis, edema, chest pain, angina
Central nervous system: Insomnia, headache, dizziness, confusion, lightheadedness, memory loss, ataxia, coma, seizures, delirium, panic attacks, psychosis
Endocrine & metabolic: Metabolic acidosis (dry ice)
Gastrointestinal: Nausea, throat irritation
Ocular: Decreased vision, photophobia, eye irritation, color vision abnormalities, diplopia, ptosis, visual evoked potential abnormalities
Respiratory: Cough, respiratory acidosis, apnea, tachypnea, hyposmia

Monitoring Parameters Arterial blood gases

Overdosage/Treatment
Inhalation: Administer 100% humidified oxygen
Supportive: Seizures can be treated with benzodiazepine or phenobarbital. A freeze injury due to dermal exposure to dry ice should be managed with rapid rewarming (water bath 40°C to 42°C for $\frac{1}{2}$ hour), with digit or extremity elevation. Management is otherwise similar to that of a thermal burn.

Additional Information
Signs of asphyxia can occur at oxygen concentrations <16%; oxygen levels <10% may be lethal; ambient carbon dioxide concentrations >35% can cause circulatory and respiratory depression; symptoms can occur at 1% concentration; TLV: 5000 ppm; IDLH: 50,000 ppm lethal carbon dioxide concentration in one minute inhalation: 100,000 ppm; specific gravity: 1.101
Carbon dioxide build-up due to inadequate ventilation is one of the major causes of "sick building syndrome" (~52% of cases of sick building syndrome). Recommended indoor ventilation rate for general office environment is 20 cfm (0.56 m³/min), which allows for indoor carbon dioxide to rise ~0.05 volume % above outdoor carbon dioxide levels
For seven occupants per 1000 square feet (93 m²) with 10 feet (3 m) of office ceiling, there should be 0.84 air changes per hour (8400 cubic foot/hour of outdoor air).
Dry ice is solid carbon dioxide maintained at -80°F (-26°C); can cause freeze injury if directly applied to skin and can cause asphyxiation if gas sublimes in an enclosed room; can combine with moisture to condense in thick, low lying fog
60% of carbon dioxide production remains in atmosphere (where upon it is used for plant photosynthesis). The green house effect occurs from increases in carbon dioxide (~1 ppm yearly) due to increased formation (combustion) and reduced decomposition (deforestation). Carbon dioxide does not support combustion soluble in water (1:1 ratio); with no caustic effect.
Inhalation of carbon dioxide (10% concentration) can raise intraocular pressure

Specific References
Centers for Disease Control and Prevention (CDC), "Acute Illness from Dry Ice Exposure During Hurricane Ivan—Alabama, 2004," *MMWR Morb Mortal Wkly Rep*, 2004, 53(50):1182-3.
Centers for Disease Control and Prevention (CDC), "Investigation of a Home with Extremely Elevated Carbon Dioxide Levels—West Virginia, December 2003," *MMWR Morb Mortal Wkly Rep*, 2004, 53(50):1181-2.
Halpern P, Raskin Y, Sorkine P, et al, "Exposure to Extremely High Concentrations of Carbon Dioxide: A Clinical Description of a Mass Casualty Incident," *Ann Emerg Med*, 2004, 43(2):196-9.
Hsieh CC, Shih CL, Fang CC, et al, "Carbon Dioxide Asphyxiation Caused by Special-Effect Dry Ice in an Election Campaign," *Am J Emerg Med*, 2005, 23(4):567-8.

Carbon Disulfide

Applies to Corrosion Inhibitors; Gold Plating; Matches (Manufacture); Nickel Plating; Photography (Instant Color); Rayon; Solvent (Gums, Resins)

CAS Number 75-15-0

UN Number 1131

U.S. Brand Names Caswell No 162; Weeviltox®

Synonyms Carbon Bisulfide; Carbon Sulfide; Dithiocarbonic Anhydride

Use Organic solvent used in gums and resins; used in manufacture of matches, instant color photography, corrosion inhibitors, gold and nickel plating, and rayon

Mechanism of Toxic Action Reacts with amino and thiols to inhibit cellular functions; damages the hepatic enzyme systems

Adverse Reactions
Cardiovascular: May be atherosclerogenic, angina, chest pain
Central nervous system: CNS depression, polyneuropathy, parkinsonism, hypothermia, seizures, memory disturbance, depression, mania, extrapyramidal reactions, axonopathy
Dermatologic: Burns on dermal contact
Hepatic: Fatty degeneration of liver
Neuromuscular & skeletal: Paresthesia, tremors
Ocular: Color vision abnormalities, visual evoked potential abnormalities
Respiratory: Dyspnea, hyposmia

Signs and Symptoms of Overdose Possibly diabetogenic; death can occur from respiratory paralysis. Burning of upper airway, cranial nerve palsies, diplopia, dizziness, dyspnea, headache, hypertension, nausea, neuritis, nystagmus, psychosis, rotten egg breath, seizures, tremor, vomiting, Decreased Spermatogenesis

Toxicodynamics/Kinetics
Absorption: Dermal absorption does occur; lipid soluble
Metabolism: Hepatic cytochrome P450 to carbonyl sulfide; also detoxified by glutathione pathway
Half-life: <1 hour
Elimination: Excreted by the lungs

Reference Range Monitor urine level of 2-thiothiazolidine-4-carboxylic acid; blood carbon disulfide levels ranging from 0.1-0.78 mg/L associated with air levels of ~80 ppm

Overdosage/Treatment

Decontamination: Emesis within 30 minutes or lavage (within 1 hour)/activated charcoal

Supportive therapy: Avoid catecholamines due to probable monoamine oxidase inhibition; diazepam/lorazepam can be used for seizures. Pyridoxine use for neurologic toxicity is unproven. Although its use is unproven, there is a theoretical basis in which to use acetylcysteine to help detoxify carbon disulfide.

Additional Information

Fatal oral dose: 15 mL

Colorless liquid; may have aromatic, sweet odor; similar effect of disulfiram; parkinsonism has been described; may cause a reduction of urine homovanillic acid and vanillylmandelic acid concentrations

TLV-TWA: 10 ppm; IDLH: 5000 ppm; PEL-TWA: 4 ppm

Odor threshold: 0.1 ppm. Atmospheric half-life: 12 days. Water half-life: ~1 year

Ambient carbon disulfide levels average 65 ppt in urban areas and 41 ppt in rural areas

Specific References

Chang SJ, Shih TS, Chou TC, et al, "Electrocardiographic Abnormality for Workers Exposed to Carbon Disulfide at a Viscose Rayon Plant," *J Occup Environ Med*, 2006, 48(1):394-99.

Luo JC, Chang HY, Chang SJ, et al, "Elevated Triglyceride and Decreased High Density Lipoprotein Level in Carbon Disulfide Workers in Taiwan," *J Occup Environ Med*, 2003, 45(1):73-8.

Carbon Monoxide

Related Information

● Asphalt

CAS Number 630-08-0

UN Number 1016

Synonyms Carbon Oxide; Carbonic Oxide; CO; Exhaust Gas; Flue Gas

Commonly Found In Auto exhaust, byproduct of methylene chloride; produced in a closed space fire due to incomplete combustion of materials

Mechanism of Toxic Action Causes tissue hypoxia and inhibition of cellular respiration; binds to myoglobin, cytochrome a, a_3 and also increases xanthine oxidase and nitric oxide production resulting in oxidative stress; may cause cerebral glutamate elevation along with lipid peroxidation and cerebral edema

Adverse Reactions

Cardiovascular: Cardiac abnormalities most pronounced, syncope, sinus bradycardia, cardiomyopathy, cardiomegaly, chest pain, palpitations, sinus tachycardia

Central nervous system: CNS effects, acute neurological abnormalities including dementia, drowsiness, coma, seizures, headache, confabulation, Parkinson-like syndrome, memory disturbance, depression, psychosis, bilateral putaminal involvement, leukoencephalopathy

Delayed neurological sequelae observed within 40 days of significant carbon monoxide poisoning (12% to 43% incidence) including disorientation, bradykinesia, chorea (extrapyramidal), equilibrium disturbances, apathy, cogwheel rigidity, aphasia, incontinence, personality changes, short-term memory deficit, seizure disorders, and chronic headaches

Dermatologic: Bullous eruptions

Neuromuscular & skeletal: Chorea, apraxia, neuropathy (peripheral), rhabdomyolysis

Ocular: Cortical blindness, visual evoked potential abnormalities

Otic: Deafness

Signs and Symptoms of Overdose

Acute effects of carbon monoxide poisoning (adapted from Ernst A and Zibrak JD, "Carbon Monoxide Poisoning," *N Engl J Med*, 1998, 339(22):1603-8): Abdominal pain and muscle cramping (5%); chest pain (9%); concentration difficulties, confusion, or disorientation (43%); loss of consciousness (6%); nausea and vomiting (47%); shortness of breath (usually associated with hyperventilation) (40%); throbbing, bitemporal headache (91%); dizziness or vertigo (77%); visual changes (25%); weakness primarily in the legs (53%)

Other (<5%): Arrhythmias, AV block, bradycardia, cortical blindness in children, fever, hallucinations, hearing loss (sensorineural), hot flashes, hypotension, hypothermia, muscle necrosis, myoglobinuria, tinnitus, tachycardia

Other effects commonly seen are lethargy, mydriasis, nystagmus, tachycardia

Carbon monoxide presentation in 140 children (from Mathieu D and Mathieu-Nolf M, *J Toxicol Clin Toxicol*, 2001, 39:266): Abnormal extensor plantar response (8%); cerebellar impairment (8%); flaccidity (17%); headache (37%); hyperreflexia (42%); lethargy/coma (19%); loss of consciousness (37%); seizures (5%); vomiting (22%)

Admission Criteria/Prognosis Acute neurologic symptoms, abnormal ECG, metabolic acidosis, chest pain, rhabdomyolysis, carboxyhemoglo-

bin levels >25%, or if patient remains symptomatic after 4 hours on 100% oxygen, should be considered for admission; ~$^2/_3$ of comatose patients will recover

Toxicodynamics/Kinetics

Absorption: Readily through the lungs; does not accumulate over time

Half-life: 5-6 hours in room air; 30-90 minutes in 100% oxygen; 30 minutes in hyperbaric oxygen; 100% oxygen in children: 44 minutes

Elimination: Through the lungs

Effect of anemia and carboxyhemoglobin on oxyhemoglobin dissociation curve. Note that 60% carboxyhemoglobin has a greater affinity for oxygen than an equivalent physiological anemia which indicates that carbon monoxide shifts the oxygen dissociation curve leftward.

Monitoring Parameters Arterial blood gases, carboxyhemoglobin

Reference Range Carboxyhemoglobin level by CO-Oximeter™: Endogenous level: ≤0.65; smokers may have from 3% to 8%. Severe symptoms may start at 10%; >35% is associated with fatalities from acute exposure; BEI is <8%; venous and arterial samples are equivalent

Overdosage/Treatment

Decontamination: 100% humidified oxygen by nonrebreather face mask until asymptomatic if patient is not pregnant. If pregnant, the patient should be on 100% nonrebreather face mask for 5 times the length of time needed for the carboxyhemoglobin level to be <5%. Continue therapy until carboxyhemoglobin level is <5%. Hyperbaric oxygen for patients with acute neurotoxicity, patients with angina, maternal carboxyhemoglobin of 15% in pregnant patients, or asymptomatic carboxyhemoglobin of 25%. **Do not** consider hypothermia or exchange transfusion. Hyperbaric oxygen should be administered at 2.8 ATA within 6 hours of exposure to carbon monoxide for maximum benefit.

Supportive therapy: Dopamine (17 mcg/kg/minute) has been shown in a case report to reverse carbon monoxide-induced blindness.

Antidote(s)

● Oxygen (Hyperbaric) [ANTIDOTE]

Diagnostic Procedures

● Carboxyhemoglobin, Blood
● Computed Transaxial Tomography, Head Studies
● Electrolytes, Blood
● Glucose, Random
● Urea Nitrogen, Blood

Additional Information

Colorless, odorless gas. Delayed neurotoxicity consisting of short-term memory deficit, ataxia, cognitive impairment may occur 2-3 weeks after an acute exposure. Parkinson syndrome may occur.

Carbon monoxide detectors are usually set to alarm at 85 decibels at indoor carbon monoxide air concentrations of 70 ppm (within 189 minutes), 150 ppm (within 50 minutes) or 400 ppm (within 15 minutes). Essentially, these concentrations, with corresponding time exposure, will result in a carboxyhemoglobin level of 10% during periods of heavy exertion. A carbon monoxide detector shall operate at or below the plotted limits for the 10% COHb curve as shown in the figure. If the detector employs a variable sensitivity setting, test measurements are to be made at maximum and minimum settings. For this test, three carbon monoxide concentrations (100, 200, 400 ppm) are to be used as specified in the figure.

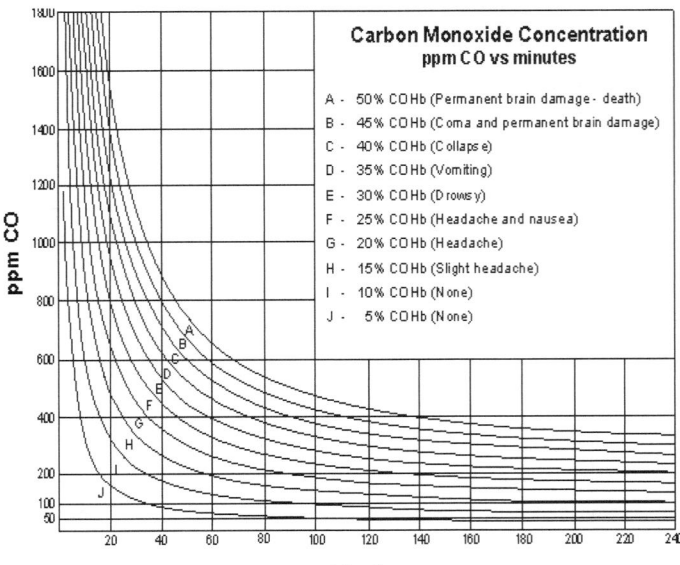

Carbon Monoxide Concentration
ppm CO vs minutes

A - 50% COHb (Permanent brain damage - death)
B - 45% COHb (Coma and permanent brain damage)
C - 40% COHb (Collapse)
D - 35% COHb (Vomiting)
E - 30% COHb (Drowsy)
F - 25% COHb (Headache and nausea)
G - 20% COHb (Headache)
H - 15% COHb (Slight headache)
I - 10% COHb (None)
J - 5% COHb (None)

Minutes

According to estimates from the Bureau of Labor statistics, carbon monoxide accounted for 867 nonfatal work-related carbon monoxide exposures in private industry and 32 work-related deaths in 1992.

TLV-TWA: 50 ppm; IDLH: 1200 ppm; PEL-TWA: 35 ppm

Carbon monoxide intoxication may also result from methylene chloride exposure.

Half-life for carboxyhemoglobin elimination is ~27.5 minutes with use of an inflatable portable hyperbaric chamber (modified Ganow bag) at 1.58 ATA

Automobile exhaust may contain as high as 7% carbon monoxide.

Occupations particularly at risk from exposure to carbon monoxide: Blast furnace operators; bus drivers; carbide manufacturers; cooks/bakers; fire fighters; formaldehyde manufacturers; garage mechanics; iron/steel foundry (cupola); kraft paper pulp mills (Kraft recovery furnaces); lead molders; liners; operators of snow melting machines; petroleum-refining plants (catalytic cracking units); pulmonary function test practitioners; skating rinks (from Zamboni ice cleaners); tollway booth collectors; traffic policeman; warehouse storage and loading facilities (forklift operators); welders

Xenobiotics in which carbon monoxide is a metabolic byproduct:
- Methylene chloride (peak of 50% COHb described in humans)
- Dibromomethane (peak of 27% COHb in rodents)*
- Diiodomethane (peak of 14.2% COHb described postingestion in a girl, 20 months of age)
- Bromochloromethane (peak of 11% COHb in rodents)*
- 1,3-Benzodioxoles*
- Tetrahalomethane (?)*
- Dibromochlormethane*
  (?) = Possible
  *Noted in rodents only

Suggested indications for hyperbaric oxygen include: Coma or any period of loss of consciousness; COHb >25% or >15% if pregnant; signs of cardiac abnormality; history of ischemic heart disease and COHb >20%; recurrent symptoms for up to 3 weeks; nonresolution of symptoms on oxygen after 6 hours; neurologic symptoms other than a transient headache; metabolic acidosis; abnormal and persistent psychometric testing; muscle necrosis, pulmonary edema, dysrhythmias, EKG changes, brain changes on neuroimaging

Risk of CO poisoning due to outdoor generators can be minimized by:

Placement of outdoor generator over 8 feet from building

Locate generators on the opposite side of building away from window air conditioners

Avoid connecting generator to a central electric panel

Celebrities in whom carbon monoxide was involved in their deaths: Ron Luciano (baseball umpire) 1995; Kevin Carter (photojournalist) 1994; Vitas Gerulaitis (tennis player) 1994; Jug McSpadden (golfer); Thelma Todd (actress) 1935; Dan White (murderer) 1985; Don Wilson (baseball pitcher) 1975; Emile Zola (novelist) 1902; Flora Disney (1938); Jimmy Campbell (bluegrass fiddle player) 2003; Rosey Nix Adams (daughter of June Carter Cash) 2003; Steve Neal (political writer, Chicago) 2004; Nick and Mary Yankovic (parents of "Weird Al" Yankovic) 2004; Zurab Zhvania (Prime Minister of Georgia) 2005; William Inge (playwright), 1973; Brad Delp (lead singer for the group Boston), 2007.

Specific References

Aslan S, Karcioglu O, Bilge F, et al, "Post-interval Syndrome After Carbon Monoxide Poisoning," *Vet Hum Toxicol*, 2004, 46(4):183-5.

Bayer M, Hanoian A, and Caperino CL, "A Documented Association of Poison Control Center Media Interactions and Carbon Monoxide Calls," *J Toxicol Clin Toxicol*, 2003, 41(5):708.

Below E and Lignitz E, "Cases of Fatal Poisoning in Post-mortem Examinations at the Institute of Forensic Medicine in Greifswald – Analysis of Five Decades of Post-Mortems," *Forensic Sci Int*, 2003, 23(133(1-2):125-31.

Bianchini KJ, Houston RJ, Greve KW, et al, "Malingered Neurocognitive Dysfunction in Neurotoxic Exposure: An Application of the Slick Criteria," *J Occup Environ Med*, 2003, 45(10):1087-99.

Brent RL, "Environmental Causes of Human Congenital Malformations: The Pediatrician's Role in Dealing with These Complex Clinical Problems Caused by a Multiplicity of Environmental and Genetic Factors," *Pediatrics*, 2004, 113(4 Suppl):957-68.

Centers for Disease Control and Prevention (CDC), "Carbon Monoxide Poisoning After Hurricane Katrina - Alabama, Louisiana, and Missisipi, August-September 2005," *MMWR Morb Mortal Wkly Rep*, 2005, 54(39):996-8.

Centers for Disease Control and Prevention (CDC), "Carbon Monoxide Poisonings After Two Major Hurricanes - Alabama and Texas - August-October 2005," *MMWR Morb Mortal Wkly Rep*, 2006, 55(9):236-9.

Centers for Disease Control and Prevention (CDC), "Carbon Monoxide Poisonings Resulting from Open Air Exposures to Operating Motorboats - Lake Havasu City, Arizona, 2003," *MMWR Morb Mortal Wkly Rep*, 2004, 53(15):314-18.

Centers for Disease Control and Prevention (CDC), "Carbon Monoxide Release and Poisonings Attributed to Underground Utiity Cable Fires - New York, January 2000-June 2004," *MMWR Morb Mortal Wkly Rep*, 2004, 53(39):920-2.

Centers for Disease Control and Prevention (CDC), "Use of Carbon Monoxide Alarms to Prevent Poisonings During a Power Outage - North Carolina, December 2002," *MMWR Morb Mortal Wkly Rep*, 2004, 53(9):189-92.

Centers for Disease Control and Prevention (CDC), "Unintentional Non-Fire-Related Carbon Monoxide Exposures – United States, 2001-2003," *MMWR Morb Mortal Wkly Rep*, 2005, 21;54(2):36-9.

Chang SJ, Shih TS, Chou TC, et al, "Electrocardiographic Abnormality for Workers Exposed to Carbon Disulfide at a Viscose Rayon Plant," *J Occup Environ Med*, 2006, 48:394-9.

Czogala J and Goniewicz ML, "The Complex Analytical Method for Assessment of Passive Smokers' Exposure to Carbon Monoxide," *J Anal Toxicol*, 2005, 29(8):830-4.

Dales R, "Ambient Carbon Monoxide May Influence Heart Rate Variability in Subjects with Coronary Artery Disease," *J Occup Environ Med*, 2004, 46(12):1217-21.

Delgado J, McKay C. Frankel J, et al, "Potential Carbon Monoxide Exposures: The Relationship Between Call Origin and Carboxyhemoglobin Levels," *Clin Toxicol (Phila)*, 2005, 43:718.

Domachevsky L, Adir Y, Grupper M, et al, "Hyperbaric Oxygen in the Treatment of Carbon Monoxide Poisoning," *Clin Toxicol (Phila)*, 2005, 43(3):181-8 (review).

Dueñas-Laita A, Pèrez-Castrillòn JL, Martin-Escudero JC, et al, "Study of Some Controversies in Carbon Monoxide Poisoning," *Clin Toxicol (Phila)*, 2005, 43:755.

Erdogan MS, Islam SS, Chaudhari A, et al, "Occupational Carbon Monoxide Poisoning Among West Virginia Workers' Compensation Claims: Diagnosis, Treatment Duration, and Utilization," *J Occup Environ Med*, 2004, 46(6):577-83.

Frankel J, Delgado J, Adamcewicz M, et al, "Carbon Monoxide Poisoning in Connecticut: An Analysis of Three Databases," *Clin Toxicol (Phila)*, 2005, 43:718.

Gupta A, Pasquale-Styles MA, Hepler BR, et al, "Apparent Suicidal Carbon Monoxide Poisonings with Concomitant Prescription Drug Overdoses," *J Anal Toxicol*, 2005, 29:744-9.

Hampson NB, "Trends in the Incidence of Carbon Monoxide Poisoning in the United States," *Am J Emerg Med*, 2005, 23(7):838-41

Hampson NB and Zmaeff JL, "Carbon Monoxide Poisoning from Portable Electric Generators," *J Am Coll Cardiol*, 2005, 28:123-5.

Henry CR, Satran D, Adkinson CD, et al, "Myocardial Injury Associated with Carbon Monoxide Poisoning Predicts Long-Term Mortality," *Acad Emerg Med*, 2004, 11(5):469.

Hoffman RJ and Hoffman RS, "Effect of Mandated Residential Carbon Monoxide Detector Use on the Morbidity of Reported Cases," *Clin Toxicol (Phila)*, 2005, 43:703.

Hoffman RJ and Hoffman RS, "Mandatory Reporting of Carbon Monoxide Poisoning by Health Care Providers: Effect on Poison Center Calls," *Clin Toxicol (Phila)*, 2005, 43:719.

Holstege CP, Baer AB, Eldridge DL, et al, "Case Series of Elevated Troponin I Following Carbon Monoxide Poisoning," *J Toxicol Clin Toxicol*, 2004, 42(5):742.

Horton DK, Berkowitz Z, and Kaye WE, "Secondary Contamination of ED Personnel from Hazardous Materials Events, 1995-2001," *Am J Emerg Med*, 2003, 21(3):199-204.

Jenkins AJ, Homer CD, Engelhart DA, et al, "Carbon Monoxide-Related Deaths in Cuyahoga County, Ohio, 1988 to 1998," *J Anal Toxicol*, 2003, 27(3):178-9.

Johnson-Arbor KK and McKay CA, "Prolonged Increases in Troponin T After Carbon Monoxide Poisoning," *Clin Toxicol (Phila)*, 2005, 43:757.

Kales SN and Christiani DC, "Acute Chemical Emergencies," *N Engl J Med*, 2004, 350(8):800-8.

Kao LW and Nanagas KA, "Carbon Monoxide Poisoning," *Emerg Med Clin N Am*, 2004, 22:985-1018.

Kao LW and Nanagas KA, "Carbon Monoxide Poisoning," *Med Clin N Am*, 2005, 89(6):1161-94 (review).

Klein KR, White SR, Herzog P, et al, "Demand for PCC Services 'Surged' During the 2003 Blackout," *J Toxicol Clin Toxicol*, 2004, 42(5):814-5.

Laakso O, Haapla M, Kuitunen T, et al, "Screening of Exhaled Breath by Low-Resolution Multicomponent FT-IR Spectrometry in Patients Attending Emergency Departments," *J Anal Toxicol*, 2004, 28(2):111-7.

Lavonas E, Tomaszewski C, Kerns W, et al, "Epidemic Carbon Monoxide Poisoning Despite a CO Alarm Law," *J Toxicol Clin Toxicol*, 2003, 41(5):711-2.

Lewis RJ, Johnson RD, and Canfield DV, "An Accurate Method for the Determination of Carboxyhemoglobin in Postmortem Blood Using GC-TCD," *J Anal Toxicol*, 2003, 27(3):182.

Maready E Jr, Holstege C, Brady W, et al, "Electrocardiographic Abnormality in Carbon Monoxide–Poisoned Patients," *Ann Emerg Med*, 2004, 44:S92.

Ong JR, Hou SW, Shu HT, et al, "Diagnostic Pitfall: Carbon Monoxide Poisoning Mimicking Hyperventilation Syndrome," *Am J Emerg Med*, 2005, 23(7):903-4.

Petersen HW and Windberg CN, "Comparison of Measurements of Carboxymyoglobin in Muscles in Relation to Carbon Monoxide in Blood," *J Anal Toxicol*, 2006, 30:143.

Powell A, Eberhradt M, Bonfante G, et al, "Noninvasive Measurement of Carbon Monoxide Levels in Patients with Headaches," *Ann Emerg Med*, 2004, 44:S90.

Pulsipher DT, Hopkins RO, and Weaver LK, "Basal Ganglia Volumes Following CO Poisoning: A Prospective Longitudinal Study," *Undersea Hyperb Med*, 2006, 33:245-256.

Sam-Lai NF, Saviuc P, and Danel V, "Carbon Monoxide Poisoning Monitoring Network: A Five-Year Experience of Household Poisonings in Two French Regions," *J Toxicol Clin Toxicol*, 2003, 41(4):349-53.

Sarmanaev SKh, Samolova RG, and Aidarova LF, "Epidemiology of Carbon Monoxide (CM) Poisonings in UFA," *J Toxicol Clin Toxicol*, 2003, 41(5):713.

Satran D, Henry CR, Adkinson C, et al, "Cardiovascular Manifestations of Moderate to Severe Carbon Monoxide Poisoning," *J Am Coll Cardiol*, 2005 45(9):1513-6.

Schwartz L, Martinez L, Louie J, et al, "An Evaluation of a Carbon Monoxide Poisoning Education Program," *Clin Toxicol (Phila)*, 2005, 43:703.

Stefanidou M and Athanaselis S, "Toxicological Aspects of Fire," *Vet Hum Toxicol*, 2004, 46(4):196-8.

Thomassen O, Brattebo G, and Rostrup M, "Carbon Monoxide Poisoning While Using a Small Cooking Stove in a Tent," *Am J Emerg Med*, 2004, 22(3):204-6.

Tomaszewski C, Lavonas E, Kerns R, et al, "Effect of a Carbon Monoxide Alarm Regulation on CO Poisoning," *J Toxicol Clin Toxicol*, 2003, 41(5):710.

Wills B and Erickson T, "Drug- and Toxin-Associated Seizures," *Med Clin North Am*, 2005, 89(6):1297-321 (review).

Wolowich WR, Hadley CM, Kelley MT, et al, "Plasma Salicylate from Methyl Salicylate Cream Compared to Oil of Wintergreen," *J Toxicol Clin Toxicol*, 2003, 41(4):355-8.

Wood DM, Dargan PI, and Jones AL, "Poisoned Patients as Potential Organ Donors: A Postal Survey of Transplant Centres and Intensive Care Units," *J Toxicol Clin Toxicol*, 2003, 41(5):651.

Yeoh MJ and Braitberg G, "Carbon Monoxide and Cyanide Poisoning in Fire Related Deaths in Victoria, Australia," *J Toxicol Clin Toxicol*, 2004, 42(6):855-63.

Carbon Tetrachloride

Applies to Fluorocarbons; Fumigation of Grain; Insecticide

CAS Number 56-23-5

UN Number 1846

U.S. Brand Names Benzinoform®; Fasciolin®; Flukoids®; Freon 10®; Halon 104®; Tetraform®

Synonyms Carbon Chloride; Perchlormethane; Tetrachloromethane; Tetrasol

Use In the production of fluorocarbons, fumigation of grain, and as an insecticide

Mechanism of Toxic Action Antihelmintic; cirrhosis of liver, renal insufficiency; free radicals bind to hepatocytes which lead to lipid peroxidation and cell death

Adverse Reactions
Cardiovascular: Tachycardia, sinus tachycardia
Central nervous system: Memory disturbance, leukoencephalopathy
Gastrointestinal: Feces discoloration (clay/putty)
Hepatic: Hepatotoxicity, centrilobular hepatic necrosis
Ocular: Eye irritation
Miscellaneous: Suspected human carcinogen (liver cancer and leukemia), cutaneous T-cell lymphoma

Signs and Symptoms of Overdose Aplastic anemia, anuria, ataxia, coma, confusion, delirium, dementia, hematuria, jaundice, nausea, seizures, skin erythema, tremor (intention), vomiting

Admission Criteria/Prognosis Any symptomatic patient, or any patient with radiopaque solvent on abdominal radiograph should be admitted

Toxicodynamics/Kinetics
Absorption: Readily from the skin, lungs, and the GI tract (85%; rapid, within 10 minutes); can produce renal or hepatic toxicity from any of these sites
Metabolism: In the liver, metabolites include hexachloroethane, carbon dioxide, and phosgene
Half-life: Oral: 40-85 hours. Inhalation: 1-40 hours
Elimination: Excreted through the lungs (50% to 80%) as carbon dioxide

Reference Range Toxic: 2.0-5.0 mg/dL

Overdosage/Treatment
Decontamination: **Inhalation:** Administer 100% humidified oxygen. **Dermal:** Remove contaminated clothing (especially leather), shoes, belts, hats, etc and place in a sealed plastic bag. Wash skin thoroughly with soap and water. **Oral:** Basic poison management; avoid ipecac. **Do not** use catecholamines due to enhancement of ventricular arrhythmia. Avoid enzyme-inducing agents such as phenobarbital.

Supportive therapy: Hyperbaric oxygen may be of benefit to prevent hepatitis. N-acetylcysteine (at 140 mg/kg oral loading dose, followed by 70 mg/kg every 4 hours for 17 doses) may be of benefit to prevent hepatitis if given within 16 hours postexposure. Due to the fact that these agents induce cytochrome P450, avoid the use of ethanol or phenobarbital.

Antidote(s)
- Acetylcysteine [ANTIDOTE]
- Oxygen (Hyperbaric) [ANTIDOTE]

Diagnostic Procedures
- Electrolytes, Blood
- Electrolytes, Urine

Additional Information
Lethal dose: 43 mg/kg
Colorless liquid with odor of chloroform; N-acetylcysteine may be of benefit (research studies); radiopaque
TLV-TWA: 5 ppm; IDLH: 300 ppm; PEL-TWA: 2 ppm
Atmospheric half-life: Over 30 years. Water half-life: ~6-12 months. Soil half-life: 6-12 months
Average urban ambient carbon tetrachloride levels: 0.1-0.3 ppb; average indoor carbon tetrachloride level: 0.2-0.4 ppb; median drinking water carbon tetrachloride level: 0.3-0.7 mcg/L; average daily exposure of carbon tetrachloride: ~0.11 mcg/kg

Specific References
Weber LW, Boll M, and Stampfl A, "Hepatotoxicity and Mechanism of Action of Haloalkanes: Carbon Tetrachloride as a Toxicological Model," *Crit Rev Toxicol*, 2003, 33(2):105-36.

Cesium

CAS Number 7440-46-2

UN Number 1407

Synonyms Cs

Use In manufacture of photoelectric cells; as a gamma ray source (^{137}Cs) for wheat, potato, and flour sterilization

Mechanism of Toxic Action Radioactive cesium emits gamma radiation which can result in tissue damage; may enhance brain levels of norepinephrine and dopamine

Adverse Reactions
Cardiovascular: Torsade de pointes
Central nervous system: Euphoria
Dermatologic: Skin erythema
Endocrine: Reduced male fertility
Gastrointestinal: Vomiting, diarrhea, nausea
Ocular: Lacrimation, conjunctivitis

Toxicodynamics/Kinetics
Absorption: Oral: 78%; Dermal: 3% (^{137}Cs)
Half-life: ^{134}Cs: 2 years; ^{137}Cs: 30 years
Elimination: Urinary

Overdosage/Treatment Decontamination: Oral: Prussian blue (10 g or 125 mg/kg orally twice daily) may be efficacious

Additional Information Cesium acts similar to potassium. It is naturally occurring as a stable isotope (^{133}Cs) at an average of 1 ppm in granite rock and 4 ppm in sedimentary rock. Seawater concentration: 0.5 mcg/L. Concentration of ^{134}Cs in Poland, 1975: 1.1 pCi/m^3. Concentration of ^{134}Cs above Chernobyl, May 8, 1986: 1,756 pCi/m^3

Decay Properties of the Radioactive Isotopes of Cesium

Isotope	Half-life (years)	Decay mode	Intensity percent	Beta particle energy (MeV)
^{134}Cs	2.062	β_1^-	27	0.02309
		β_2^-	2.5	0.1234
		β_3^-	70	0.2101
^{137}Cs	30	β_1^-	94.6	0.1734
		β_2^-	5.4	0.4246

Specific References
Dainiak N, Waselenko JK, Armitage JO, et al, "The Hematologist and Radiation Casualties," *Hematology (Am Soc Hematol Educ Program)*, 2003, 473-96 (review).

Lydon TJ, DeRoos FJ, and Perrone J, "Pulseless Ventricular Tachycardia Secondary to Alternative Cancer Therapy with Cesium Chloride," *J Toxicol Clin Toxicol*, 2004, 42(5):731.

Lyon AW and Mayhew WJ, "Cesium Toxicity: A Case of Self-Treatment by Alternate Therapy Gone Awry," *Ther Drug Monit*, 2003, 25(1):114-6.

Ring JP, "Radiation Risks and Dirty Bombs," *Health Phys*, 2004, 86(2 Suppl):S42-7.

Chenopodium Oils

CAS Number 8006-99-3
Synonyms Oil of American Wormseed; Volatile Oil
Adverse Reactions Cardiovascular: Sinus bradycardia
Signs and Symptoms of Overdose Abdominal pain, dizziness, flushing, headache, nausea, salivation (start several hours after ingestion); tinnitus, vomiting; followed by ataxia, coma, deafness, drowsiness, and in some cases progresses to tachycardia, seizures, and death
Respiratory depression is seen with large ingestions and pulmonary edema is a common finding in fatal cases. Renal damage (hematuria and albuminuria) and hepatitis. Mucous membrane irritant, CNS depressant or CNS stimulant. CNS depression may be rapid (30 minutes) or delayed (up to 4 hours) and may continue for up to 3 days; chemical pneumonitis and pulmonary edema are possible
Camphor causes mydriasis while eucalyptus oil may cause miosis; seizures may occur with eucalyptus oil; tachycardia and bradycardia have been reported. Camphor causes sudden seizures, abdominal pain, diarrhea, sudden seizures, and vomiting; mild elevation of liver enzymes
Toxicodynamics/Kinetics
Absorption: Well absorbed through mucous membranes
Metabolism: By the liver
Elimination: Excreted primarily through kidney
Reference Range No toxic levels established
Overdosage/Treatment
Decontamination: Emesis is not recommended because as an essential oil, *Chenopodium* oil may be aspirated and there is potential for CNS depression and seizures. Gastric lavage within 1 hour is preferred. Activated charcoal is recommended. For products with a thick hydrocarbon base, gastric lavage may decrease systemic effects.
Supportive therapy: Liver function and renal function should be monitored. Cardiac and respiratory systems should be supported. CNS depression and electrolytes should be followed closely.
Enhancement of elimination: Eucalyptus oil has been successfully treated with mannitol and peritoneal and hemodialysis. Camphor has been reported to be extracted with amberlite resin hemoperfusion. Use of enhanced elimination techniques for these overdoses should be based on the amount ingested, the clinical picture, and/or symptoms that are failing to respond to supportive care.
Drug Interaction Enhances the penetration of fluorouracil on excised skin
Additional Information Volatile oils: Camphor, cedar leaf, cinnamon oil, eucalyptus, lavender, menthol, myristica, peppermint oil, sandalwood oil, sassafras oil, thymol, turpentine oil; may explode when heated

Chloralose

CAS Number 15879-93-3
Use Rodent, mole, crow poison
Mechanism of Toxic Action A central nervous system depressant which acts as a stimulant on spinal reflexes (similar to strychnine).
Adverse Reactions
Cardiovascular: Tachycardia, facial flushing
Central nervous system: Ataxia, coma, hypothermia, hyperthermia, headache
Hematologic: Leukocytosis
Neuromuscular & skeletal: Rhabdomyolysis, myoclonus
Ocular: Miosis
Respiratory: Apnea, respiratory depression
Toxicodynamics/Kinetics
Metabolism: Hepatic to urochloralic acid
Elimination: Renal (urochloralic acid)
Reference Range Plasma chloralose >3.5 mg/L is associated with coma. Postmortem blood level of 151 mg/L has been associated with chloralose-induced fatality. Urine chloralose concentration of 15.2 mg/L is associated with seizures. May undergo postmortem redistribution.
Overdosage/Treatment
Decontamination: **Oral**: Do not induce emesis. Gastric lavage (within 1 hour)/activated charcoal should be considered. **Inhalation**: Administer 100% humidified oxygen.
Supportive therapy: Seizures should be managed with benzodiazepines. Barbiturates or phenytoin are second-line agents. Propofol has been used to treat myoclonus.
Additional Information Oral toxic dose: Infants: 20 mg/kg. Adults: 1 g.

Chlorate Salts

CAS Number 7775-09-0
UN Number 1461; 3210
Synonyms Asex; B-Herbtox; Chlorate of Soda; Chlorate Salt of Sodium; Chlorax; Chloric Acid-Sodium Salt; De-fol-ate; Desolat; Drexel Acetol; Evalu-Super; Grain Sorghum Harvest Aid; Granex O; Harvest-Aid; Klorex; Kusa-Tohru; Ortho C-1 Defoliant and Weed Killer; Rasikal; Shed-a-Leaf; Sodium Chlorate; Travex; Tumbleaf; Val-Drop

Use Historically used as antiseptics, it is primarily found in weed killers (sodium chlorate), and in the manufacture of matches and explosives.
Adverse Reactions Cardiovascular: Sinus tachycardia
Signs and Symptoms of Overdose Cyanosis resistant to oxygen therapy; nausea, vomiting, and abdominal cramping; diarrhea or colic usually precede pallor; methemoglobinemia and hemolysis may occur; drowsiness, coma, and seizures have been reported. Moderate elevations of LFTs with hepatomegaly and jaundice have been reported. Chlorates are nephrotoxic; acute renal insufficiency with oliguria or anuria is common. Severe exposure may cause subacute intravascular coagulation and leukocytosis lasting 40 days. Chronic exposure to chlorates of 5-10 days will also follow a similar pattern.
Admission Criteria/Prognosis Any patient with change in mental status, cardiopulmonary complaints, or methemoglobin levels >30% should be admitted; asymptomatic patients with methemoglobin levels <30% may be considered for discharge after 6 hours of observation and if methemoglobin levels fall to <15% or patients with hyperkalemia. These symptoms usually occur within 4 hours of exposure.
Toxicodynamics/Kinetics
Absorption: Good through respiratory and gastrointestinal tract; poor through skin
Elimination: Slow through the kidneys
Monitoring Parameters When 1 mL of a 1% (w/v) solution of diphenylamine in concentrated sulfuric acid is added to material containing chlorates, a blue color is produced; urine is probably the fluid of choice, but blood can also be measured through spectrophotometry for chlorate
Overdosage/Treatment
Decontamination: Lavage (within 1 hour)/activated charcoal with sorbitol
Supportive therapy: Obtain baseline hemoglobin, hematocrit, and methemoglobin; monitor urinalysis, BUN, creatinine, CBC, and methemoglobin; transfuse if needed. Alkaline diuresis may be required if significant hemoglobinuria; methylene blue 1-2 mg/kg/dose of 1% slow I.V. for those patients who are symptomatic or with methemoglobin >30%; additional doses may be required. A DIC profile may be needed. Sodium thiosulfate should be considered (2-5 g oral or in 100 mL of 5% sodium hydrochloride) for symptomatic patients to attempt to inactivate the chlorate ion, although this modality is not proven to be effective. Methemoglobinemia produced by chlorates may be refractory to methylene blue.
Enhancement of elimination: Exchange transfusion combined with hemodialysis or peritoneal dialysis should be considered in severely intoxicated patients.
Antidote(s)
- Methylene Blue [ANTIDOTE]
- Sodium Thiosulfate [ANTIDOTE]
Additional Information How supplied: Potassium chlorate: Colorless or white crystals or powder. Sodium chlorate: Colorless to pale yellow crystals or powder

Chlordane

CAS Number 12789-03-6; 5103-71-9; 5103-74-2; 57-74-9
U.S. Brand Names Chlordan®; Niran®; Octachlor®; Ortho-Klor®; Velsicol® 1068
Use Organochlorine subterranean termiticide by which all commercial use was discontinued by the EPA in April, 1988
Mechanism of Toxic Action Neurotoxic mechanism unknown; may involve competitive inhibition of GABA or reduced levels of norepinephrine involved in neuronal transmission
Adverse Reactions
Cardiovascular: Tachycardia, Raynaud's phenomenon, sinus tachycardia, Reye's-like syndrome
Central nervous system: Headache, dizziness, irritability, seizures (usually within 3 hours of exposure), paresthesia
Dermatologic: Scleroderma
Gastrointestinal: Nausea, diarrhea, anorexia
Genitourinary: Oliguria
Hematologic: Aplastic anemia
Hepatic: Jaundice, elevated liver function test results
Neuromuscular & skeletal: Paresthesia
Ocular: Blurred vision, diplopia
Respiratory: Dyspnea
Toxicodynamics/Kinetics
Absorption: By inhalation (76%), oral, and dermal routes
Metabolism: Hepatic; active metabolites include heptachlor and oxychlordane
Half-life: 88 days
Elimination: Primarily fecal
Reference Range Ingestion of 215 g (3 g/kg) of chlordane resulted in a chlordane blood level of 5 mg/L (patient recovered); seizures can occur at chlorane serum levels of 2-4 mcg/L
Overdosage/Treatment
Decontamination: **Oral:** Lavage (within 1 hour)/activated charcoal or cholestyramine; **do not** use oil-based cathartics. **Dermal:** Repeated and copious scrubbing with soap and water

Supportive therapy: Since barbiturates hasten the elimination of oxychlordane, this may be the antiseizure drug of choice. Benzodiazepines can also be used.

Enhancement of elimination: Multiple doses of activated charcoal or cholestyramine may be useful.

Additional Information Lethal oral dose: 25 mg/kg. Can cause sclerodermatous changes of the hands. World Health Organization guideline limit for drinking water: 0.3 mcg/L TWA-TLV: 0.5 mg/m^3

Specific References

Hardell L, Andersson SO, Carlberg M, et al, "Adipose Tissue Concentrations of Persistent Organic Pollutants and the Risk of Prostate Cancer," *J Occup Environ Med*, 2006, 48:700-7.

Chlordecone

CAS Number 143-50-0

U.S. Brand Names Compound 1189®; Kepone®; Merex®

Synonyms Decachloroketone

Use Insecticide (fire ant, slugs, grass mole cricket, tobacco fireworm) on tobacco, shrubs, and banana plants

Mechanism of Toxic Action Increases permeability of neuronal membrane; has estrogenic properties

Adverse Reactions

Cardiovascular: Pleuritic chest pain, edema, angina

Central nervous system: Auditory and visual hallucinations, headache, slurred speech, ataxia, increased intracranial pressure, axonopathy

Dermatologic: Rash, maculopapular rash

Gastrointestinal: Nausea

Genitourinary: Oligospermia

Hepatic: Elevated alkaline phosphatase

Neuromuscular & skeletal: Tremors, arthralgia, neuropathy (peripheral)

Ocular: Cataracts, nystagmus, papilledema

Toxicodynamics/Kinetics

Absorption: Inhalation, oral (90%), and dermal

Metabolism: Hepatic reduction to chlordecone alcohol

Half-life: 63-148 days

Elimination: Primarily fecal (biliary)

Monitoring Parameters Alkaline phosphatase

Reference Range Blood chlordecone levels >1 ppm associated with neurotoxicity; blood levels >2000 ng/mL associated with tremor

Overdosage/Treatment

Decontamination: **Oral:** Lavage (within 1 hour)/activated charcoal or cholestyramine. **Dermal:** Wash with soap and water. **Ocular:** Copious irrigation with saline

Supportive therapy: **Do not** use phenytoin for tremor since it may exacerbate tremor. Propranolol may be effective in alleviating tremor. Prednisolone has been used to alleviate headache due to increased intracerebral pressure.

Enhancement of elimination: Due to enterohepatic recirculation, multiple dosing with cholestyramine (4 g every 8 hours) has been shown to be effective.

Additional Information FDA action level for oysters, clams, mussels, and fin fish: 0.03 ppm; crabs: 0.4 ppm; high bioaccumulation potential in fish

Chlorfenvinphos

CAS Number 18708-86-6; 18708-87-7; 470-90-6

UN Number 2783

U.S. Brand Names Apachlor®; Birlane®; Dermaton®; Supone®; Unitox®

Synonyms O,O-Diethyl O-(2-Chloro-1(2',4'-Dichlorophenyl)Vinyl) Phosphate

Use Marketed as insecticide granules, dusting agent, or spray liquid with or without petroleum derivative as a solvent

Mechanism of Toxic Action Potent, irreversible inhibition of acetylcholinesterase and plasma cholinesterase, resulting in excess accumulation of acetylcholine at muscarinic and nicotinic receptors, and in the central nervous system

Adverse Reactions

Cardiovascular: **Hyperdynamic** (~18% to 21%) or hypodynamic (~7% to 10%) states, QT prolongation, sinus bradycardia, sinus tachycardia

Central nervous system: Depression, seizures, hyperactivity, cognitive dysfunction, hypothermia

Genitourinary: Urinary incontinence

Neuromuscular & skeletal: Weakness (delayed), paralysis, delayed paresthesia

Respiratory: Pulmonary edema, respiratory depression

Miscellaneous: Flu-like symptoms (especially with chronic exposure)

Signs and Symptoms of Overdose

Abdominal pain, agitation, asystole, AV block, bradycardia, bronchorrhea, coma, confusion, cranial nerve palsies, decreased hemoglobin, decreased platelet count, decreased red blood cell count, diaphragmatic paralysis, dysarthria, excessive sweating, fecal and urinary incontinence, generalized asthenia, headache, heart block, hypertension,

hypotension, lacrimation, miosis (unreactive to light), mydriasis (rarely), metabolic acidosis and hyperglycemia (severe intoxication), pallor, nausea, pulmonary edema, QT prolongation, respiratory depression, salivation, seizures skeletal muscle fasciculation and flaccid paralysis, tachycardia, tachypnea, vomiting

An "intermediate syndrome" of limb asthenia and respiratory paralysis has been reported to occur between 24 and 96 hours postorganophosphate exposure, and is independent of the acute cholinergic crisis. Late paresthesia characterized by stocking and glove paresthesia, anesthesia, and asthenia is infrequently observed weeks to months following acute exposure to certain organophosphates.

Toxicodynamics/Kinetics

Absorption: Readily through oral, dermal, or respiratory exposure. Dermal rate: 0.06-1.43 cm^2/hour

Metabolism: Rapidly metabolized to weakly active compounds through hepatic hydrolysis and other pathways

Half-life: 12-15 hours

Elimination: Metabolites are excreted in urine

Warnings/Precautions Environmentally persistent; chlorfenvinphos is a soil applied insecticide used for arable crops, and may translocate into plants, fruits, and vegetables grown in treated soil; risk of aspiration pneumonitis exists with agents having a hydrocarbon vehicle; severe laryngeal irritation and violent coughing may result from exposure to dusting powders; exposure to dusting powders and insecticide granules may cause contact dermatitis

Reference Range Serum concentration: Chlorfenvinphos level of 300 ng/mL associated with severe respiratory distress and bronchial hypersecretion; blood chlorfenvinphos level 3 hours after oral ingestion of 50 mL of 50% chlorfenvinphos is ~300 ng/mL

Overdosage/Treatment

Decontamination: Isolation, bagging, and disposal of all contaminated clothing and other articles. All emergency medical workers and hospital staff should follow appropriate precautions regarding exposure to hazardous material including the use of protective clothing, masks, goggles, and respiratory equipment.

Oral: Lavage within 1 hour with a 5% sodium bicarbonate or 2% potassium permanganate. Activated charcoal can be administered either orally or via a nasogastric tube. **Do not** induce emesis because of danger of sudden respiratory compromise, alterations in mental status, seizures, coma, and possible aspiration of hydrocarbon vehicles. When using activated charcoal, **do not** use a cathartic.

Dermal: Prompt thorough scrubbing of all affected areas with soap and water, including hair and nails; 5% bleach can also be used

Ocular: Irrigation with copious tepid sterile water or saline

Supportive therapy: Airway management, ventilatory assistance, humidified oxygen administration, and close monitoring for sudden respiratory failure

Antidote:

Atropine: Administration should be guided by respiratory status, starting at 2-5 mg I.V. every 5-10 minutes as needed, and should be titrated to the resolution of excess pulmonary secretions. Frequent administration of large doses (cumulative doses >100 mg) may be necessary in massive exposures.

Glycopyrrolate: May be administered if atropine is unavailable (200-400 mcg I.V. or I.M. initially, or ~$^1\!/_2$ the dose of atropine).

2-PAM: For more significant exposures (ie, exposures requiring large doses of atropine, or with recurring symptoms, or exposures to more lipid soluble agents), administration should follow: 1-2 g I.V. over 10-30 minutes, repeated in 1 hour if asthenia recurs, then every 4-12 hours for recurring symptoms.

Enhancement of elimination: Dialysis and hemoperfusion are not indicated due to effectiveness of the prescribed treatment and large volumes of distribution of organophosphates. Hemoperfusion clearance was used successfully in one case report (68 mL/minute), with the highest value of clearance observed during the fourth hour of hemoperfusion.

Antidote(s)

- Atropine [ANTIDOTE]
- Pralidoxime [ANTIDOTE]

Diagnostic Procedures

- Creatinine, Serum
- Pseudocholinesterase, Serum

Drug Interaction Paralysis is potentiated by neuromuscular blockade (ie, pancuronium, vecuronium, succinylcholine, atracurium, doxacurium, mivacurium); inhibition of serum esterase prolongs the half-life of succinylcholine, cocaine, and other ester anesthetics; cholinergic toxicity is potentiated by cholinesterase inhibitors such as physostigmine

Additional Information

Toxic dose (dermal): 10 mg/kg

Red blood cell cholinesterase, and serum pseudocholinesterase may be depressed following acute or chronic organophosphate exposure; RBC cholinesterase is typically not analyzed by in-house laboratories, and is usually not available for consideration during acute management.

Pseudocholinesterase levels may be rapidly available from some in-house laboratories, but are not as reliable a marker of organophosphate exposure because of variability secondary to variant genotypes, hepatic disease, oral estrogen use, or malnutrition. Because of this variability, true indication of suppression of either of these enzymes can only be estimated through comparison to pre-exposure values; these enzymes may be useful in measuring a patient's recovery postexposure, especially if the recovery is not progressing as expected.

The intermediate syndrome is not related to delayed neuropathy.

QT_c prolongation on ECG in the setting of organophosphate poisoning is associated with a high incidence of respiratory failure and mortality.

An amber liquid with a mild odor

Specific gravity: 1.36

Half-life in soil: 9-210 days; Atmospheric half-life: 7-92 hours; Water half-life: 170 days (pH 6); 80 days (pH 8)

Cooking will partially reduce chlorfenvinphos residues

Other information concerning pesticide exposures is available through the EPA-funded National Pesticide Telecommunications Network: 1-800-858-7378 (weekdays, 8 AM to 6 PM, Central Standard time)

Chlorine

Related Information
- Chlorine Dioxide
- Sodium Hypochlorite

Applies to Bleach; Disinfectant (Water); Pulp Mills; Swimming Pools

CAS Number 7782-50-5

UN Number 1017

U.S. Brand Names Clorox®

Synonyms Bertholite

Commonly Found In War gas used in World War I; can be produced by mixing bleach with acid

Use In pulp mills and for swimming pools; also used in bleaching; used as a water disinfectant

Mechanism of Toxic Action Converted to hydrogen chloride in lung parenchyma, strong irritant and corrosive agent; free radical generation may be present

Adverse Reactions

Cardiovascular: Cardiovascular collapse, chest pain, angina

Ocular: Lacrimation

Respiratory: Pulmonary edema, bronchoconstriction, reactive airways dysfunction syndrome, bronchiectasis

Miscellaneous: Increased risk for lymphoma

Signs and Symptoms of Overdose Airway irritation, chest pain, cough, dermal burns, dyspnea, eye irritation, headache, hyperchloremic metabolic acidosis, hypertension, hypotension, stomatitis, vomiting, wheezing

Admission Criteria/Prognosis Ongoing pulmonary symptoms 6 hours postexposure requires hospital admission

Toxicodynamics/Kinetics Absorption: Not well absorbed, low solubility

Reference Range Not measurable

Overdosage/Treatment

Supportive therapy: Administer 100% humidified oxygen. A 3.5% to 5% sodium bicarbonate solution by nebulization may be helpful for acute respiratory symptoms. Wheezing can be treated with beta-adrenergic agonists. Steroids are of no proven benefit. Avoid use of intravenous sodium bicarbonate.

Endoscope is not necessary when the subject accidentally swallows a small quantity (<40 mL) of diluted bleach, the clinical examination is normal, the bleach contains <3% of available chlorine, and bleach pH is <12. Otherwise, endoscopy should be performed within 6-12 hours after ingestion. Inverse-ratio ventilation using lower tidal volume mechanical ventilation (6 mL/kg) and plateau pressures of 30 cm water may decrease mortality. While positive end expiratory pressures should be considered, oxygen toxicity should be monitored. Use of perfluorocarbon partial liquid ventilation and exogenous surfactant in chemical-induced ARDS is investigational.

Diagnostic Procedures
- Lung Scan, Ventilation

Additional Information

Green-yellow gas. Taste threshold: 5 ppm. Odor threshold: 3.5 ppm. TLV-TWA: 0.5 ppm; IDLH: 30 ppm; PEL-TWA: 0.5 ppm

Mixing hypochlorite (bleach) with an acid can release chlorine gas; mixing hypochlorite (bleach) with ammonia can release chloramine gas.

As a water disinfectant, chlorine is bactericidal at levels of 0.2 mg/L and cysticidal at 1.5-2 residual free chlorine (pH 7).

Environmental persistence: Low

Specific References

Bania TC and Chu J, "Effect of Intravenous NaHCO₃ on Toxicity from Inhaled Chlorine Gas in an Animal Model," *Acad Emerg Med*, 2006, 13(5):S178.

Bania TC and Chu J, "Sucrose as a Potential Therapy for Chlorine-Induced Pulmonary Edema," *Acad Emerg Med*, 2006, 13(5):S177-8.

Eldridge DL, Richardson W, Michels JE, et al, "The Role of Poison Centers in a Mass Chlorine Exposure," *Clin Toxicol (Phila)*, 2005, 43:766.

Horton DK, Berkowitz Z, and Kaye WE, "Secondary Contamination of ED Personnel from Hazardous Materials Events, 1995-2001," *Am J Emerg Med*, 2003, 21(3):199-204.

Kales SN and Christiani DC, "Acute Chemical Emergencies," *N Engl J Med*, 2004, 350(8):800-8.

Rosenman KD, Reilly MJ, Schill DP, et al, "Cleaning Products and Work-Related Asthma," *J Occup Environ Med*, 2003, 45(5):556-63.

Chlorine Dioxide

CAS Number 10049-04-4

UN Number 9191

Synonyms Alcide; Anthium Dioxide

Use An intermediate, from water treatment and disinfecting applications (eg, pulp bleaching) when generated from sodium chlorite utilization (usually with sulfuric acid)

Mechanism of Toxic Action Mucosal irritation; a strong oxidizer

Signs and Symptoms of Overdose Bronchospasm, conjunctivitis, cough, dyspnea, headache, leukocytosis, rhinitis, tachycardia

Toxicodynamics/Kinetics Elimination: Urinary

Overdosage/Treatment

Decontamination: **Inhalation**: Administer 100% humidified oxygen; **Ocular**: Irrigate with copious amounts of saline or water

Supportive therapy: Treat bronchospasm with beta-adrenergic agonist agents; corticosteroids may be useful

Additional Information A yellow gas with pungent odor; decomposes rapidly in sunlight and carbon monoxide. Maximum residual disinfectant level for chlorine dioxide in water is 0.8 mg/L. Daily exposure to chlorine dioxide via drinking water: 1.6-2 mg/day. Minimal IDLH: 5 ppm. Lethal concentration in air: 19 ppm. TLV: 0.1 ppm. Air levels of 2-5 ppm are irritating.

Chloroacetophenone

Related Information
- Chlorobenzylidene Malononitrile

Applies to Tear Gas

CAS Number 532-27-4

UN Number 1697

Synonyms CAF; CN; MACE; Phenacyl Chloride

Use Active ingredient in tear gas; riot control

Mechanism of Toxic Action Lacrimator - irritation due to the active halogen group reacting transiently with sulfhydryl groups

Adverse Reactions

Dermal: Allergic contact dermatitis, burning sensation of the skin, dermal erythema, bullous dermatitis

Gastrointestinal: Metallic taste, vomiting

Ocular: Ocular burning, blepharospasms, lacrimation (eye symptoms may last for 30 minutes)

Respiratory: Bronchospasm (may be delayed for 36 hours), pulmonary edema (may be delayed for 24 hours), cough, sneezing

Signs and Symptoms of Overdose Agitation, bronchospasm, cough, erythema, eye pain, lacrimation, laryngospasm (may be delayed for 2 days), nausea, pharyngitis, rhinorrhea, skin irritation, sneezing, tearing, vomiting

Toxicodynamics/Kinetics

Onset of effect: Rapid

Duration: Usually resolves in 30 minutes, skin effects may last for 2-3 hours

Absorption: Not absorbed

Overdosage/Treatment

Decontamination: Move patient rapidly to fresh air and monitor for wheezing. Administer 100% humidified oxygen. Personnel should avoid contaminating themselves. Wash skin with soap and at least two liters of water.

Ocular: Avoid rubbing eyes as it may prolong effect. Copious irrigation with water or saline is needed.

Supportive therapy: Solution of antacid (magnesium hydroxide - aluminum hydroxide - simethicone) gently blotted topically over exposed facial areas (avoiding eyes) may help resolve symptoms. Bronchospasm can be treated with inhaled beta₂ agonists. Inverse-ratio ventilation using lower tidal volume mechanical ventilation (6 mL/kg) and plateau pressures of 30 cm water may decrease mortality. While positive end expiratory pressures should be considered, oxygen toxicity should be monitored. Use of perfluorocarbon partial liquid ventilation and exogenous surfactant in chemical-induced ARDS is investigational.

Additional Information

Colorless to white vapor with a fragrant odor of apple blossoms; insoluble in water. Can be detected using gas chromatography/mass spectrophotometry (GC/MS). TLV-TWA: 0.05 ppm; IDLH: 100 mg/m³; PEL-TWA: 0.05 ppm. Vapor density: 5.3 (with air). Atmospheric half-life: 9.2 days

Threshold for eye irritation: 0.3 mg/m³ (permanent eye injury may occur)

Incapacitating dose: 5-20 mg/m³

Median incapacitating dose: 80 mg/m³/minute

Median lethal dose: 7000 mg/m³/minute (dispersed from solvent); 14,000 mg/m³/minute (from thermal grenade)

Decomposes to chlorine when heated; no bioconcentration
Environmental persistence: Short
Action on metal: Tarnishes steel, mild corrosion

Specific References

Blain PG, "Tear Gases and Irritant Incapacitants, 1-Chloroacetophenone, 2-Chlorobenzylidene Malononitrile and Dibenz[b,f]-1,4-Oxazepine," *Toxicol Rev*, 2003, 22(2):103-10 (review).

Chlorobenzene

Applies to Caswell No 183A; DDT (Production); Degreaser (Car Parts); Solvent
CAS Number 108-90-7
UN Number 1134
Synonyms Benzene Chloride; MCB; Monochlorobenzene
Use Solvent used in production of DDT, phenol compounds (replaced primarily by cumene), diisocyanate, nitrochlorobenzene, and degreasing car parts

Adverse Reactions

Cardiovascular: Cyanosis
Central nervous system: CNS depression, seizures, coma, hyperesthesia
Hematologic: Methemoglobinemia
Neuromuscular & skeletal: Muscle spasms, neuritis, myoclonus
Miscellaneous: Mucosal irritant (at levels >200 ppm)

Toxicodynamics/Kinetics

Absorption: Inhalation: 38% to 45%. Gastrointestinal: 31%
Metabolism: Hepatic transition to 4-chlorophenol and through glutathione conjugation to parachlorophenyl mercapturic acid

Reference Range Levels of residents living near a former toxic chemical dump ranged from 25-120 mcg/L of chlorobenzene in the urine and 0.05-17 ng/L of chlorobenzene in blood

Overdosage/Treatment

Decontamination: **Dermal:** Wash with soap and water. **Ocular:** Irrigate with normal saline.
Supportive therapy: Respiratory support with administration of 100% humidified oxygen

Additional Information This compound can decompose through heating to chlorine gas. Odor threshold: 0.21 ppm; IDLH: 2400 ppm; PEL-TWA: 75 ppm

Chlorobenzylidene Malononitrile

Applies to Deep Freeze; Paralyzer
CAS Number 2698-41-1
Synonyms CS; Ortho-Chlorobenzylidene Malonitrile
Use Active ingredient in tear gas
Mechanism of Toxic Action Lacrimator: May be metabolized to thiocyanate in peripheral tissues

Adverse Reactions

Dermatologic: Dermal burns
Ocular: Ocular burning, blepharospasms, cataract
Respiratory: Bronchospasm (may be delayed for 36 hours), pulmonary edema (may be delayed for 24 hours)

Signs and Symptoms of Overdose Agitation, bronchospasm, cough, erythema, eye pain, lacrimation, laryngospasm, nausea, pharyngitis, reactive airway disease, rhinorrhea, skin irritation, sneezing, tearing, vomiting

Toxicodynamics/Kinetics

Onset of action: Immediate
Metabolism: Hepatic hydrolysis to O-chlorobenzaldehyde and malononitrile; peripheral metabolism may produce thiocyanate

Overdosage/Treatment

Decontamination: Move patient to fresh air and monitor for wheezing. Personnel should avoid contaminating themselves. Wash skin with soap and water. Avoid rubbing of eyes as it may prolong effect. Copious irrigation is needed. Recovery usually will occur within 10-20 minutes.
Dermal: Skin can be washed with a mild alkaline solution (6% sodium bicarbonate, 3% sodium carbonate and 1% benzalkonium chloride) to hasten elimination.
Supportive therapy: Monitor for cyanide in cases of ingestion or extremely high exposure. Inverse-ratio ventilation using lower tidal volume mechanical ventilation (6 mL/kg) and plateau pressures of 30 cm water may decrease mortality. While positive end expiratory pressures should be considered, oxygen toxicity should be monitored. Use of perfluorocarbon partial liquid ventilation and exogenous surfactant in chemical-induced ARDS is investigational.

Additional Information LD-50 (respiratory concentration) is estimated to be 25,000-150,000 mg/m³/minute. Soft contact lenses may minimize exposure. A white crystalline solid (density: 1.3) with a pepper odor. IDLH: 2 mg/m³; PEL-TWA: 0.05 ppm

Specific References

Blain PG, "Tear Gases and Irritant Incapacitants, 1-Chloroacetophenone, 2-Chlorobenzylidene Malononitrile and Dibenz[b,f]-1,4-Oxazepine," *Toxicol Rev*, 2003, 22(2):103-10 (review).

Horton DK, Berkowitz Z, and Kaye WE, "Secondary Contamination of ED Personnel from Hazardous Materials Events, 1995-2001," *Am J Emerg Med*, 2003, 21(3):199-204.
Horton DK, Burgess P, Rossiter S, et al, "Secondary Contamination of Emergency Department Personnel from O-Chlorobenzylidene Malononitrile Exposure," 2002, *Ann Emerg Med*, 2005, 45(6):655-8.

Chloroform

Pronunciation (KLOR oh form)
Related Information
• Adipose Tissue Ranges of Toxins
CAS Number 67-66-3
UN Number 1888
Synonyms Formyl Trichloride; Freon 20; Methane Trichloride; TCM; Trichloroform; Trichloromethane
Synonyms Thrichloromethane
Use Solvent, grain fumigant, found in emulsions, spirits, tinctures; has been used as an anesthetic agent, refrigerant, and aerosol propellant
Mechanism of Toxic Action A direct depressant on the respiratory center in the brain stem; interferes with gangliosides in neuronal membranes and phospholipids on surfactant layer in lungs; can cause lipid peroxidation

Adverse Reactions

Cardiovascular: Sinus bradycardia, sinus tachycardia, arrhythmias (ventricular), vasodilation
Central nervous system: Psychosis
Dermatologic: Nonimmunologic contact urticaria
Gastrointestinal: Nausea and vomiting can occur at doses of 22-237 ppm
Hepatic: Centrilobular hepatic necrosis, aminotransferase level elevation (asymptomatic)
Ocular: Blepharospasm
Miscellaneous: Aneuploidy induction, cutaneous T-cell lymphoma

Signs and Symptoms of Overdose

Bradycardia, CNS depression, dizziness, drowsiness, dry mouth, fibrillation, nausea, headache, hemolysis, hepatitis, hepatomegaly, hypotension, tachycardia (ventricular), vomiting
Burning, corneal injury, conjunctivitis, and urticaria may occur with eye exposure. Acetone breath, cardiac arrest, cardiac arrhythmias, mydriasis, and nystagmus have been reported. Chemical pneumonitis, pulmonary edema, and respiratory depression may occur. Chronic use may produce degenerative brain changes and psychotic behavior.

Admission Criteria/Prognosis Significant, acute exposures should be admitted; see Additional Information

Toxicodynamics/Kinetics

Absorption: Well through inhalation, oral, and dermal exposure
Distribution: V_d: 2.6 L/kg; throughout and soluble in adipose tissue
Metabolism: To chlormethanol, hydrochloric acid, phosgene, chloride, and CO_2
Half-life: Inhalation: 8 hours
Elimination: Primarily from lungs in the form of chloroform and carbon dioxide; <1% excreted in urine

Monitoring Parameters Gas chromatograph and flame ionization detector as well as HPLC have been used to determine levels in blood; blood levels in fatalities range from 1-12 mg/dL

Dosage Forms Liquid: 480 mL

Reference Range Blood chloroform levels with anesthesia: 0.07-0.165 mg/mL. Postmortem blood and urine chloroform level of 18.1 mg and 1.5 mg/L has been associated with fatality. Ranges of blood chloroform (postmortem) levels in fatalities are 10-194 mg/L.

Overdosage/Treatment

Decontamination: Emesis within 30 minutes, lavage (within 1 hour)/ activated charcoal. Remove from area of exposure and remove clothing; wash thoroughly.
Supportive therapy: Treatment of cardiac and respiratory status. Lidocaine, propranolol, bretylium, phenytoin, disopyramide, or overdrive pacing has been used in treatment of PVCs. Atropine may be used if severe bradycardia is present. If oral ingestion, radiograph may show radiopacity. Monitor blood glucose, urinalysis, LFTs and renal function. Administration of N-acetylcysteine for treatment of hepatitis is still theoretical.

Antidote(s)
• Atropine [ANTIDOTE]

Drug Interaction Thiopentone can increase incidence of hypotension

Additional Information

Lethal dose: Oral: 0.5 g/kg (as little as 10 mL may cause death). Fatal dose: 40,000 ppm. Anesthetic dose: 8000-10,000 ppm.
Listed as a suspected carcinogen; radiopaque
Odor threshold: Air: 85 ppm; Water: 2.4 ppm; TLV-TWA: 10 ppm
Atmospheric half-life: 80 days. Water (pH 9) half-life: 25-37 years
Average atmospheric chloroform levels in urban areas: 0.00002-0.002 ppm. Average indoor chloroform levels: 0.0002-0.004 ppm. Average chloroform levels near indoor, heated swimming pools: 0.035-0.2 ppm. Average daily intake of chloroform through drinking water: 4-88 mcg; from urban ambient atmosphere: 6-200 mcg

Foods containing chloroform include: Butter: 1100 mcg/kg; mixed cereal: 220 mcg/kg; infant food: 230 mcg/kg; cheddar cheese: 83 mcg/kg; grains: 1.4-3000 mcg/kg; dried legumes: 6.1-57 mcg/kg; dairy products: 7-1100 mcg/kg

Specific References

Bania TC and Chu J, "Sucrose as a Potential Therapy for Chlorine-Induced Pulmonary Edema," *Acad Emerg Med*, 2006, 13(5):S177-8.

Lykissa ED, Gonzales C, Kearney J, et al, "Chloroform and Hydrochloric Acid Identified in Human Remains," *J Anal Toxicol*, 2006, 30:163.

Singer PP and Jones GR, "An Unusual Autoerotic Fatality Associated with Chloroform Inhalation," *J Anal Tox*, 2006, 30:216-8.

Chloromethane

Applies to Butyl Rubber (Production); Freon 40; Herbicide; Methyl Cellulose (Production); Oil Extractant; Polystyrene Foam (Molding); Polyurethane Foam (Molding); Propellant; R40; Refrigerant; Silicone (Production)

CAS Number 74-87-3

UN Number 1063

U.S. Brand Names Artic®

Synonyms Methyl Chloride; Monochloromethane

Use Chlorinated hydrocarbon used in the production of silicones, butyl rubber, methyl cellulose; was also used as a refrigerant (although this use has declined over the past 30 years), as a propellant, and as a herbicide; also used in molding polystyrene and polyurethane foams and as an oil extractant

Mechanism of Toxic Action Hepatically and renally toxic through probably glutathione depletion and lipid peroxidation; also a neurotoxic agent

Adverse Reactions

Cardiovascular: Sinus tachycardia

Central nervous system: Fever

Respiratory: Primarily from inhalation with a latent period of up to 2 days postinhalation; respiratory depression, nephritis

Signs and Symptoms of Overdose Neurological effects will usually occur at air concentrations >30,000 ppm. Asthenia, albuminuria, anemia, ataxia, blurred vision, cirrhosis (long-term exposure), coma, confusion, depression, dermal erythema, diarrhea, diplopia, dizziness, drowsiness, elevated BUN, elevated creatinine, fatigue, headache, hematuria, hypotension, jaundice, mydriasis, nausea, oliguria, proteinuria, seizures, sleep disturbances, slurred speech, tachycardia, tremor, vertigo, vomiting, wheezing

Toxicodynamics/Kinetics

Absorption: Not absorbed through intact skin; can be absorbed through the lungs by a rate of between 1.4-3.7 mcg/kg/minute

Protein binding: 0%

Metabolism: Hepatic and erythrocyte conjugation with glutathione to S-methylcysteine

Half-life: 50-90 minutes (beta phase)

Elimination: Primarily pulmonary; less than 0.01% per minute is renally excreted

Monitoring Parameters CBC, liver enzymes, renal tests, urine analysis

Reference Range After exposure to 50 ppm, chloromethane breath levels range from 50-80 mcg/L; while chloromethane blood levels range from 35-100 mcg/L

Overdosage/Treatment

Decontamination: Inhalation: Move patient out of environment; administer 100% humidified oxygen

Supportive therapy: Benzodiazepines for seizure control; symptoms usually abate after 6 hours

Drug Interaction Lethargy may be more pronounced in patients also taking a benzodiazepine

Additional Information Lethal concentration: 20,000 ppm. Toxic symptoms: 200 ppm.

Colorless gas with a sweet odor. Odor threshold: 10 ppm. IDLH: 10,000 ppm; TLV-TWA: 50 ppm. Atmospheric half-life: ~1 year. Ground water half-life: ~2 years. Natural background air concentration: ~1 ppb. U.S. chloromethane production in 1994 was ~451.3 million kg.

Chloropicrin

Applies to Fumigant (Stored Grain); Fungicide; Insecticide; Tear Gas (World War I)

CAS Number 76-06-2

UN Number 1580

Synonyms C.P.; Nitrochloroform; Pepper Gas; Trichloronitromethane; Vomiting Gas

Use Used as a tear gas in World War I; now used as a stored grain fumigant, insecticide, and fungicide; often used as a warning agent for fumigants

Mechanism of Toxic Action Lacrimator, mucous membrane irritant

Signs and Symptoms of Overdose Abdominal pain (10%), agitation, anxiety, cough, dizziness, dyspnea, dysuria (3%), headache (48%), eye irritation, nausea (19%), pulmonary edema, pleuritic chest pain (19%), rhabdomyolysis, sore throat, vomiting

Admission Criteria/Prognosis Admit any patient with prolonged dyspnea or rhabdomyolysis

Overdosage/Treatment

Decontamination: Remove from exposure; administer 100% humidified oxygen. **Dermal**: Remove all clothing and wash skin with at least 2 L of cold water. **Ocular**: Irrigate with water or saline for at least 15 minutes.

Supportive therapy: Nonsteroidal anti-inflammatory agents can be used to treat pleuritic chest pain.

Additional Information Can penetrate any standard gas mask. Lacrimation can occur at levels of 3-37 ppm within 30 seconds. Lethal concentration is 119 ppm at 30 minutes. Thermal decompensation products include phosgene, nitrosyl chloride, chlorine, carbon monoxide, and nitrogen oxides. Odor threshold: 1.1 ppm. Irritant effect threshold: 0.3 ppm. IDLH: 4 ppm; TLV-TWA: 0.1 ppm

Number* and Percentage of Persons with Acute Chloropicrin-Related Illness, by Selected Characteristics Kern County, CA, October 2003		
Characteristic	**No.**	**(%)**
Age group (yrs)		
0-5	22	(13)
6-9	17	(10)
10-14	23	(14)
15-19	15	(9)
20-29	18	(11)
30-39	21	(13)
40-64	26	(16)
Unknown	23	(14)
Sex		
Female	77	(47)
Male	88	(53)
Severity†		
Low	163	(99)
Moderate	2	(1)
Date of exposure		
October 3	9	(6)
October 4	135	(82)
Both dates	22	(14)
Occupation		
Firefighter	9	(6)
Applicator / Grower	4	(2)
Day care worker	2	(1)
Nonoccupational (community resident)	150	(91)
Symptoms		
Eye	164	(99)
Lacrimation	125	(82)
Pain / burning	89	(54)
Skin (pruritus or rash)	3	(2)
Gastrointestinal	77	(47)
Vomiting	37	(22)
Nausea	35	(21)
Abdominal pain	10	(6)
Diarrhea	5	(3)
Hematochezia	1	(1)
Respiratory	85	(51)
Cough	53	(32)
Dyspnea	27	(16)
Upper respiratory irritation	22	(13)
Chest pain	8	(5)
Asthma exacerbation	6	(4)
Neurologic	40	(24)
Headache	39	(25)
Dizziness	1	(1)
Fatigue	1	(1)

*N = 165.

†Using CDC's severity index for use in state-based surveillance of acute pesticide-related illness and injury. Available at http://www.cdc.gov/niosh/topics/pesticides/pdfs/pest-sevindexv6.pdf.

Specific References

Centers for Disease Control and Prevention (CDC), "Exposure to Tear Gas from A Theft-Deterrent Device on a Safe," *MMWR Morb Mortal Wkly Rep*, 2004, 53(8):176-7.

Chloroxylenol

CAS Number 88-04-0
Synonyms PCMX
Commonly Includes Disinfectant agents (4.8% concentration in Dettol®)
Use Effective against gram-positive bacteria; a chlorinated phenol compound
Mechanism of Action Central nervous system and cardiac depression
Signs and Symptoms of Overdose Aspiration pneumonia, bronchospasm, coma, laryngeal edema, nodal tachycardia, pulmonary edema, respiratory failure
Pharmacodynamics/Kinetics Elimination: Renal
Monitoring Parameters Electrolytes, renal function, chest x-ray
Dosage Forms Solution: 4.8%
Reference Range Postmortem blood chloroxylenol level of 2.3 mg/100 mL associated with fatality
Overdosage/Treatment
Decontamination: **Oral:** Do not induce emesis; lavage may be considered if airway is protected; activated charcoal is of uncertain efficacy. **Ocular:** Irrigate with saline.
Supportive therapy: Hypotension can be treated with I.V. crystalloid solutions and Trendelenburg placement; dopamine can be used for refractory cases; verapamil can be used for nodal tachycardia
Additional Information Not a caustic agent

Chlorpyrifos

CAS Number 2921-88-2
UN Number 2783
U.S. Brand Names Dursban TC®; Dursban®; Lorsban®; Pyrinex®
Synonyms O,O-Diethyl-O-(3,5,6-Trichloro-2-Pyridyl) Phosphorothioate; Phosphorothioic Acid; Trichlorpyriphos (Discontinued)
Use Broad spectrum insecticide for control of mosquitoes, flies, cockroaches, fleas, and termites (TC formulation); has been used as an ascaricide and a veterinary ectoparasiticide
Adverse Reactions
Cardiovascular: QT prolongation, sinus bradycardia, sinus tachycardia
Central nervous system: Anxiety, restlessness, dizziness, dystonic reactions, cognitive dysfunction, hypothermia
Dermatologic: Mild skin irritant
Neuromuscular & skeletal: Choreoathetosis
Ocular: **Miosis** (82%), mydriasis can be present in severely affected individuals; conjunctivitis, photophobia, opsoclonus
Respiratory: Rhinorrhea
Miscellaneous: Diaphoresis, intermediate syndrome
Signs and Symptoms of Overdose
Abdominal pain, agitation, asystole, AV block, bradycardia, bronchorrhea, coma, confusion, decreased hemoglobin, decreased platelet count, decreased red blood cell count, diaphragmatic paralysis, dysarthria, excessive sweating, fecal and urinary incontinence, generalized asthenia, headache, heart block, hypertension, hypotension, lacrimation, metabolic acidosis and hyperglycemia (severe intoxication), miosis (unreactive to light), mydriasis (rarely), nausea, pallor, pulmonary edema, QT prolongation, respiratory depression, salivation, seizures, skeletal muscle fasciculation and flaccid paralysis, tachycardia, tachypnea, vomiting
An "intermediate syndrome" of limb asthenia and respiratory paralysis has been reported to occur between 24 and 96 hours postorganophosphate exposure, and is independent of the acute cholinergic crisis. Late paresthesia characterized by stocking and glove paresthesia, anesthesia, and asthenia is infrequently observed weeks to months following acute exposure to certain organophosphates. Cases of delayed neurotoxicity have been described.
Toxicodynamics/Kinetics
Absorption: Oral: 70%. Dermal: <3%
Metabolism: Hepatic to diethylphosphate, diethylthiophosphate, and 3,5,6-trichloro-2-pyridinol (TCP)
Half-life: 27 hours
Reference Range Oral dose of 5 mg/kg followed by dermal exposures between 0.5-5 mg/kg 2 weeks later produced blood chlorpyrifos levels <30 mcg/L (blood TCP levels were 0.9 mg/L 6 hours after oral ingestion and 0.06 mg/L 24 hours after dermal administration); a single oral dose of 0.5 mg/kg can depress plasma cholinesterase levels by 85%; urine 3,5,6-trichloro 2-pyridinol (TCP) level of 25 mcg/mg creatinine is associated with a 30% decrease of cholinesterase level
Overdosage/Treatment
Decontamination: Isolation, bagging, and disposal of all contaminated clothing and other articles. All emergency medical workers and hospital staff should follow appropriate precautions regarding exposure to hazardous material including the use of protective clothing, masks, goggles, and respiratory equipment.
Oral: Activated charcoal can be administered either orally or via a nasogastric tube. **Do not** induce emesis because of danger of sudden respiratory compromise, alterations in mental status, seizures, coma, and possible aspiration of hydrocarbon vehicles. **Do not** give a cathartic.
Dermal: Prompt thorough scrubbing of all affected areas with soap and water, including hair and nails; 5% bleach can also be used
Ocular: Irrigation with copious tepid sterile water or saline
Supportive therapy: Airway management, ventilatory assistance, humidified oxygen administration, and close monitoring for sudden respiratory failure
Antidote:
Atropine: Administration should be guided by respiratory status, starting at 2-5 mg I.V. every 5-10 minutes as needed, and should be titrated to the resolution of excess pulmonary secretions. Frequent administration of large doses (cumulative doses >100 mg) may be necessary in massive exposures.
Glycopyrrolate: May be administered if atropine is unavailable (200-400 mcg I.V. or I.M. initially, or ~$^1/_2$ the dose of atropine).
2-PAM: For more significant exposures (ie, exposures requiring large doses of atropine, or with recurring symptoms, or exposures to more lipid soluble agents), administration should follow: 1-2 g I.V. over 10-30 minutes, repeated in 1 hour if asthenia recurs, then every 4-12 hours for recurring symptoms.
Enhancement of elimination: Dialysis and hemoperfusion are not indicated due to effectiveness of the prescribed treatment and large volumes of distribution of organophosphates.
Antidote(s)
• Atropine [ANTIDOTE]
• Pralidoxime [ANTIDOTE]
Diagnostic Procedures
• Creatinine, Serum
• Pseudocholinesterase, Serum
Additional Information Toxic dose: 300 mg/kg
Red blood cell cholinesterase, and serum pseudocholinesterase may be depressed following acute or chronic organophosphate exposure; RBC cholinesterase is typically not analyzed by in-house laboratories, and is usually not available for consideration during acute management. Pseudocholinesterase levels may be rapidly available from some in-house laboratories, but are not as reliable a marker of organophosphate exposure because of variability secondary to variant genotypes, hepatic disease, oral estrogen use, or malnutrition. Because of this variability, true indication of suppression of either of these enzymes can only be estimated through comparison to pre-exposure values; these enzymes may be useful in measuring a patient's recovery postexposure, especially if the recovery is not progressing as expected.
The intermediate syndrome is not related to delayed neuropathy.
QT_c prolongation on ECG in the setting of organophosphate poisoning is associated with a high incidence of respiratory failure and mortality.
Less likely than other organophosphates to induce organophosphate-induced delayed neuropathy
Emits a sulfur (garlic) odor at airborne concentrations >1 ppb
Atmospheric half-life: 6.34 hours
EPA tolerance range for agriculture products: 0.05-15 ppm
Estimated daily dietary intake for a 14-16 year old male in the U.S.: ~3.4 ng/kg body weight
Tolerance in food: Citrus oil: 25 ppm; Corn oil: 3 ppm; Mint oil: 10 ppm; Peanut oil: 1.5 ppm; Animal feeds: 0.5-15 ppm
TLV-TWA: 0.2 mg/m^3
Other information concerning pesticide exposures is available through the EPA-funded National Pesticide Telecommunications Network: 1-800-858-7378 (weekdays, 8 AM to 6 PM, Central Standard time)

Specific References

Albers JW, Berent S, Garabrant DH, et al, "The Effects of Occupational Exposure to Chlorpyrifos on the Neurologic Examination of Central Nervous System Function: A Prospective Cohort Study," *J Occup Environ Med*, 2004, 46(4):367-78.
Baker BA, Alexander BH, Mandel JS, et al, "Pesticide Exposure in Spouses from the Farm Family Exposure Study," *J Toxicol Clin Toxicol*, 2004, 42(5):802.
Dalvi RR, Dalvi PS, and Lane C, "Cytochrome P450-mediated Activation and Toxicity of Chlorpyrifos in Male and Female Rats," *Vet Hum Toxicol*, 2004, 46(6):297-9.
Eddleston M, Eyer P, Worek F, et al, "Differences Between Organophosphorus Insecticides in Human Self-Poisoning: A Prospective Cohort Study," *Lancet*, 2005, 366(9495):1452-9.
Kventsel I, Berkovitch M, Reiss A, et al, "Scopolamine Treatment for Severe Extra-pyramidal Signs Following Organophosphate (Chlorpyrifos) Ingestion," *Clin Toxicol (Phila)*. 2005, 43(7):877-9.
Li AA, Mink PJ, McIntosh LJ, et al, "Evaluation of Epidemiologic and Animal Data Associating Pesticides with Parkinson's Disease," *J Occup Environ Med*, 2005, 47(10):1059-87.

Martinez MA, Ballesteros S, de la Torre CS, et al, "Attempted Suicide by Ingestion of Chlorpyrifos: Identificatin in Serum and Gastric Content by GC-FID/GC-MS," *J Anal Toxicol*, 2004, 28:609-15.

Mattingly JE, Sullivan JE, Spiller HA, et al, "Intermediate Syndrome After Exposure to Chlorpyrifos in a 16-Month-Old Girl," *J Emerg Med*, 2003, 25(4): 379-81.

Meggs WJ, Means L, Brewer KL, et al, "Preliminary Report: Toxicity of Chronic Low-Level Exposures to Organophosphorus Insecticides," *Clin Toxicol (Phila)*, 2005, 43:693.

Morrissey BF, Harter LC, Cropley JM, et al, "Residential Phaseout of Chlorpyrifos and Diazinon: Reductions in Reported Human Exposure Cases in Washington State," *J Toxicol Clin Toxicol*, 2004, 42(5):806-7.

van Wijngaarden E, "Mortality of Mental Disorders in Relation to Potential Pesticide Exposure," *J Occup Environ Med*, 2003, 45(5):564-8.

Weiss B, Amler S, and Amler RW, "Pesticides," *Pediatrics*, 2004, 113(4 Suppl):1030-6.

Chromium

Related Information
- Toxins Which Should Be Lavaged with Solutions Other Than Water

CAS Number 10025-73-7; 10060-12-5; 10101-53-8; 12018-01-8; 12314-42-0; 13530-65-9; 25013-82-5; 7440-47-3; 7775-11-3; 7778-50-9; 7789-02-8; 7789-09-5; 7789-12-0

UN Number 1439; 1463; 1758; 2720

U.S. Brand Names Chrometrace®

Synonyms Cr; Hexaquachromium Chloride

Commonly Found In Chromium exposure may be found in battery manufacturers, painters, printers, welders, jewelers, steel workers, oil drillers, match manufacturers, leather workers, lithographers, tanners, cement workers

Mechanism of Action Chromium picolinate is the only active form of chromium. It appears that chromium, in its trivalent form, increases insulin sensitivity and improves glucose transport into cells. The mechanism by which this happens could include one or more of the following:
Increase the number of insulin receptors
Enhance insulin binding to target tissues
Promote activation of insulin-receptor tyrosine kinase activity
Enhance beta cell sensitivity in the pancreas

Mechanism of Toxic Action Dermatologic and pulmonary sensitizers; possibly carcinogenic with compounds of valence +6 (hexavalent)

Adverse Reactions
Dermatologic: Dermal sensitization, systemic contact dermatitis
Gastrointestinal: Gastroenteritis
Hematologic: Hemolysis, methemoglobinemia
Hepatic: Hepatic necrosis
Renal: Acute tubular necrosis
Respiratory: Asthma, bronchospasm, hyposmia
Miscellaneous: Anaphylactoid reactions, cutaneous T-cell lymphoma

Signs and Symptoms of Overdose Acute nausea, coma, dark red urine and stool, hypotension, skin burns, thrombocytopenia, vomiting

Toxicodynamics/Kinetics
Absorption, chromium III: Oral: 3%; also absorbed dermally and through inhalation; gut absorption: <2%
Half-life: Inhalation: 4-10 hours
  Hexavalent: Urinary: 15-41 hours
Elimination: Inhalation and dermal: Renal. Oral: Primarily fecal

Reference Range
Serum: Normal population urine range: 0.24-1.80 mcg/L; Whole blood chromium concentrations >2mg/L are lethal

Some laboratories report much higher "normals" because the methods they use or the collection technique is not adequate to prevent substantial contamination. If a laboratory reports "<1 ng/mL" or some similar figure without a lower level for normal, the value can be relied upon to discover toxic states, perhaps, but not deficiency states. Serum levels of 10 ng/mL correspond to short-term atmospheric exposure limit of 0.1 mg/m³ of chromium trioxide. Serum levels even higher would be expected in acute systemic toxicity. Almost a twofold diurnal variation is noted in serum chromium levels, with the level highest in the morning and falling after each meal as insulin levels rise. Serum chromium levels are ~60% of normal in diabetic patients, which overlaps the normal range.

Normal urinary concentration is <10 mcg/L in healthy adults receiving 30-100 mcg chromium daily. Levels vary with the laboratory and have declined with improved methods of avoiding contamination. Levels two- to threefold above this may reflect supplementation or excess losses. Levels elevated tenfold and higher have been seen in exposed asymptomatic tannery workers. Spot levels of chromium in urine of 30 ng/g creatinine correspond to the short-term atmospheric exposure limit of 0.1 mg/m³ of chromium trioxide in industrial exposure situations.

Median hair chromium content: 0.234 mg/kg; median nail chromium content: 0.52 mg/kg.

Mean Breast Milk Concentration: 0.3 mg/Liter

Overdosage/Treatment
Decontamination:
  Oral: Lavage within 1 hour with 1% ascorbic acid solution (10 g ascorbic acid orally for every L of lavage fluid). **Do not** use antacids since antacids may increase absorption.
  Dermal: Copious irrigation. Use 10% ascorbic acid topically to convert hexavalent chromium to a less toxic trivalent form.
Supportive therapy: Nephrotoxicity can be managed with ascorbic acid (1 g I.V. every 10-20 minutes up to 3 g), although this therapy has not been supported in clinical trials. Monitor serum/urine pH during treatment with ascorbic acid. Topical ascorbic acid may be effective in treating chromium dermatitis. 2,3-Dimercaptopropane sulphonate (DMPS or unithiol) is also useful to enhance this metal's elimination at a dose of 100 mg 3 times/day orally for 5 days, or 250 mg I.V. every 4 hours for 24 hours, then 250 mg every 6 hours.
Enhancement of elimination: Acetylcysteine may be an effective therapy in enhancing chromium elimination. Hemodialysis should also be employed, especially if renal insufficiency is present. Double volume exchange transfusion can lower plasma chromium concentration by 75% in infants. Due to accumulation of chromium in the liver, orthotopic cadaveric liver transplantation has been performed successfully in a comatose patient with hepatic necrosis, 5 days after ingesting potassium dichromate. Peritoneal dialysis is *not* effective.

Antidote(s)
- Unithiol [ANTIDOTE]

Diagnostic Procedures
- Chromium, Serum
- Chromium, Urine

Drug Interaction Chromium can cause a decrease in insulin requirements.

Drug Interactions Any medications that may also affect blood sugars; (eg, beta-blockers, thiazides, any medications prescribed to treat diabetes); discuss chromium use prior to initiating

Additional Information
Minimum lethal dose: Potassium dichromate: 0.1 g; Lethal dose: Hexavalent chromium: Oral: ~1 g.

Increased lung cancer mortality identiied among workers with cumulative urinalysis measure >200 mcg/L - years chromium.

Determination of the amount of chromium in the serum or urine of normal persons is extremely difficult, due to the very low levels present. Levels observed are in the 0.1 ng/mL range, equivalent to one part in 10 billion. Extreme caution must be taken to avoid contamination by dust (from skin, leather, cloth) and contact with steel (which contains chromium). See figure.

Linear Relationship Between Water Soluble Chromium Concentrations in Workroom Air and the Chromium Concentrations in Blood and Urine at the End of a 5-Day Shift in Workers of a Dichromate Plant

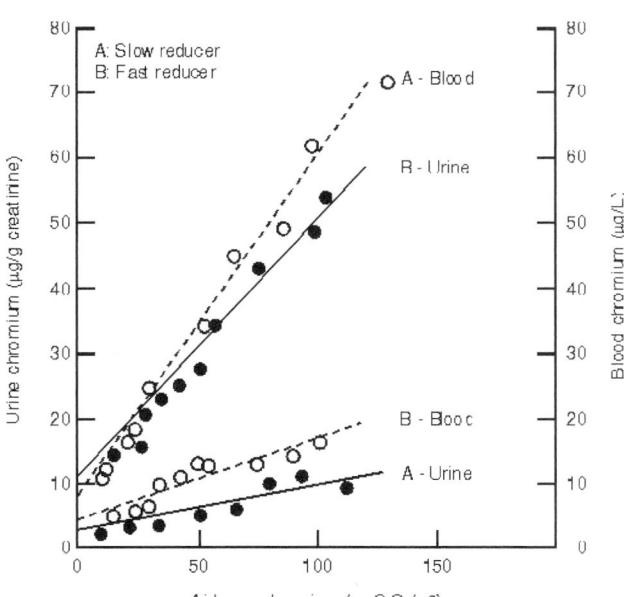

From "Toxicological Profile for Chromium," U.S. Department of Health and Human Services, Agency for Toxic Substances and Disease Registry, August 1998.

Chromium is felt to be an essential element in the human, with chromium III purported to be an integral part of "glucose tolerance factor," a partially characterized complex that has been suggested to contain two molecules of nicotinic acid and a small oligopeptide complexed to chromium III. This organic moiety is thought necessary for insulin action on the cell surface. Deficiency of chromium can cause an acquired insulin resistance or diabetes mellitus with associated hyperlipidemia in otherwise well-nourished patients. The classic cases, however, were reported prior to the availability of accurate serum levels of chromium, and reported levels then in "deficiency" were tenfold or more higher than we now know to be "normal". Chromium deficiency with associated glucose intolerance and fasting hypoglycemia has been most often observed during refeeding of malnourished individuals after famine starvation in relief programs. In infants, one or more oral doses of chromium, 250 mcg, have been curative. Chromium deficiency with associated glucose intolerance has also been observed in long-term parenteral nutrition when inadequate chromium was included. Neuropathy, encephalopathy, and abnormalities of amino acid profile (serum low in branched-chain amino acids and high in aromatic amino acids) have been noted in conjunction with this condition.

With regard to toxicity, pure metallic chromium is nontoxic. Chromium III is poorly absorbed and much less toxic than chromium VI. Industrial monitoring for toxicity in the past has relied on air samples largely for total and hexavalent chromium, the major species of concern. Workers are potentially exposed in tanneries, mines, and industries for metal plating, welding, photography, paint, dye, and explosives. Skin exposure may lead to dermatitis, and respiratory exposure to bronchitis, asthma, and lung cancer. Hair contains 1000-fold more chromium than serum or urine, and hair chromium content does correlate with industrial exposure; but more data are needed before hair chromium monitoring can replace industrial air monitoring and samples of blood and urine in cases of suspected toxicity or deficiency. Acute systemic chromate toxicity may cause acute tubular necrosis, acute hepatitis, seizures, and coma. Acute respiratory or gastrointestinal symptoms relate to the locus of absorption. Intermediate levels of long-term exposure may cause tubular albuminuria in industrial workers.

Chromium supplementation has been shown by some workers to improve glucose tolerance and improve insulin efficiency in glucose intolerant (but not in normal or overtly diabetic) patients on diets equivalent to the lower quartile of ordinary chromium intake in the United States. The implication is that many individuals in the U.S. population have a marginal chromium intake. We may, therefore, anticipate increased self-medication and supplementation in the future, and greater medical interest in this trace metal. The literature regarding chromium was for many years confused due to difficulties with analysis and contamination. Much old work needs to be repeated, and this field is still very much in flux.

The main excretory pathway for chromium III is renal. Estimated safe and adequate, oral intake recommended by the U.S. National Academy of Sciences range from 50-200 mcg/day, but in the U.S. 90% of people eat less, the mean intake being 25-33 mcg/day. Such intake recommendations likely derive from the 1980s when average estimated intake was determined to be 50-100 mcg/day. With increasingly accurate assays, new recommended ranges may be set lower. Absorption of chromium III is on the order of 0.5%, by radioisotope studies. One hospital pharmacy supplies 12 mcg of chromium from MTE5® trace mineral parenteral nutrition supplement per day. We are unaware of a large survey.

Cigarette tobacco contains 0.24-6.3 mg/kg of chromium. Atmospheric total chromium levels in the U.S. are 0.01-0.03 mcg/m^3 in urban areas and <0.01 mcg/m^3 in rural areas. River and lake chromium content is <30 mcg/L and 5 mcg/L, respectively.

Expected residence in air is <10 days; concentration in U.S. drinking water of chromium is 0.4-8 mcg/L; concentration in tobacco is 0.24-14.6 mg/kg.

See tables.

Industries That May Be Sources of Chromium Exposure*

Abrasives manufacturers	Laboratory workers
Acetylene purifiers	Leather finishers
Adhesives workers	Linoleum workers
Aircraft sprayers	Lithographers
Alizarin manufacturers	Magnesium treaters
Alloy manufacturers	Match manufacturers
Aluminum anodizers	Metal cleaners
Anodizers	Metal workers
Battery manufacturers	Milk preservers
Biologists	Oil drillers
Blueprint manufacturers	Oil purifiers
Boiler scalers	Painters
Candle manufacturers	Palm-oil bleachers
Cement workers	Paper waterproofers
Ceramic workers	Pencil manufacturers
Chemical workers	Perfume manufacturers
Chromate workers	Photoengravers
Chromium-alloy workers	Photographers
Chromium-alum workers	Platinum polishers
Chromium platers	Porcelain decorators
Copper etchers	Pottery frosters
Copper-plate strippers	Pottery glazers
Corrosion-inhibitor workers	Printers
Crayon manufacturers	Railroad engineers
Diesel locomotive repairmen	Refractory-brick manufacturers
Drug manufacturers	Rubber manufacturers
Dye manufacturers	Shingle manufacturers
Dyers	Silk-screen manufacturers
Electroplaters	Smokeless-powder manufacturers
Enamel workers	Soap manufacturers
Explosive manufacturers	Sponge bleachers
Fat purifiers	Steel workers
Fireworks manufacturers	Tanners
Flypaper manufacturers	Textile workers
Furniture polishers	Wallpaper printers
Fur processors	Wax workers
Glass-fibre manufacturers	Welders
Glue manufacturers	Wood-preservative workers
Histology technicians	Wood stainers
Jewelers	

*IARC 1990
Reference: U.S. Department of Health and Human Services, "Toxicological Profile for Chromium," Agency for Toxic Substances and Disease Registry, August 1998.

Chromium Content in Various U.S. Foods

Sample	Mean Concentration (mcg/kg)
Fresh vegetables	30-140
Frozen vegetables	230
Canned vegetables	230
Fresh fruits	90-190
Fruits	20
Canned fruits	510
Dairy products	100
Chicken eggs	160-520
Chicken eggs	60
Whole fish	50-80
Edible portion of fresh finfish	<100-160
Meat and fish	110-230
Seafoods	120-470
Grains and cereals	40-220
Sugar, refined*	<20

*Value in Finnish sugar
Reference: U.S. Department of Health and Human Services, "Toxicological Profile for Chromium," Agency for Toxic Substances and Disease Registry, August 1998.

Specific References

Bania TC and Chu J, "Sucrose as a Potential Therapy for Chlorine Induced Pulmonary Edema," *Acad Emerg Med*, 2006, 13(5):S177-8.

Birk T, Mundt KA, Dell L, et al, "Lung Cancer Mortality in the German Chromate Industry, 1958-1998," *J Occup Environ Med*, 2006, 48:426-33.

Costa M and Klein CB, "Toxicity and Carcinogenicity of Chromium Compounds in Humans," *Crit Rev Toxicol*, 2006, 36:155-63.

Hantson P, Van Caenegem O, Decordier I, et al, "Hexavalent Chromium Ingestion: Biological Markers of Nephrotoxicity and Genotoxicity," *Clin Toxicol (Phila)*, 2005, 43(2):111-2.

Schwenk TL and Costley CD, "When Food Becomes a Drug: Nonanabolic Nutritional Supplement Use in Athletes," *Am J Sports Med*, 2002, 30(6):907-16.

Wani S, Weskamp C, Marple J, et al, "Acute Tubular Necrosis Associated with Chromium Picolinate-Containing Dietary Supplement," *Ann Pharmacother*, 2006, 40(3):563-6.

Cobalt

Related Information
- Adipose Tissue Ranges of Toxins

CAS Number 10026-22-9; 10724-43-4; 1307-96-6; 1308-04-9; 1308-06-1; 513-79-1; 7440-48-4; 7646-79-9

UN Number 1318; 2001

Synonyms Cobalt Chloride; Cobalt Oxide; Cobalt Sulfate

Commonly Found In Superalloys as a paint drier, magnets, in pigment manufacture, glass decolorizer; industries with significant exposure to cobalt include tool sharpeners, miners, grinders; component in hard metal

Mechanism of Toxic Action Essential element in vitamin B_{12} which acts as a coenzyme in hemopoiesis

Adverse Reactions
Cardiovascular: Cardiomyopathy

Dermatologic: Contact dermatitis, allergic dermatitis, eczema, nonimmunologic contact urticaria, systemic contact dermatitis, airborne contact dermatitis

Endocrine & metabolic: Metabolic acidosis, hypothyroidism, hyperlipidemia, goiter

Gastrointestinal: Nausea, vomiting, diarrhea

Hematologic: Anemia or polycythemia (not noted after inhalation exposure), methemoglobinemia, neutropenia

Ocular: Optic atrophy, conjunctivitis

Respiratory: Wheezing, interstitial fibrosis, and giant cell pneumonitis, pulmonary fibrosis, bronchospasm, asthma

Renal: Goodpasture's syndrome

Signs and Symptoms of Overdose Cardiomegaly, cyanosis, hypothyroid goiter, hypertension, polycythemia, pruritus

Toxicodynamics/Kinetics
Absorption: Variable gastrointestinal absorption (18% to 97%); absorbed through skin and also by inhalation

Half-life: 5-10 years

Elimination: Through lungs and renal feces

Reference Range Normal levels of urine: Up to 2.2 mcg/L; Plasma: Up to 1.2 mcg/L; Hair: 0.047 mg/kg; Nails: 0.06 mg/kg

Overdosage/Treatment
Decontamination: Lavage (within 1 hour)/activated charcoal. In oral ingestion, iron can decrease cobalt absorption.

Supportive therapy: Sodium bicarbonate for metabolic acidosis. Restrictive pulmonary symptoms (hard metal disease) can be treated with prednisone (40-60 mg/day) and cyclophosphamide (25 mg twice daily).

Enhancement of elimination: Calcium disodium EDTA (50 mg/kg/day for 5 days) can increase cobalt excretion fourfold. BAL, acetylcysteine, or succimer has been shown experimentally to increase fecal excretion of cobalt. Hemodialysis may be of some value.

Antidote(s)
- Acetylcysteine [ANTIDOTE]
- Dimercaprol [ANTIDOTE]
- Edetate Calcium Disodium [ANTIDOTE]
- Succimer [ANTIDOTE]

Diagnostic Procedures
- Cobalt, Serum
- Cobalt, Urine

Drug Interaction Iron deficiency leads to increased oral absorption; oral iron can reduce amounts of cobalt absorbed

Additional Information
Cobalt, a metallic element, is a component of vitamin B_{12} and is found in most foods. The daily requirement is unknown, as is deficiency in humans. Cobalt has the capacity to cause polycythemia, and for that reason, cobaltous chloride is used to successfully treat certain types of anemia. Accidental overdose of cobaltous chloride, especially in children, may lead to cyanosis, coma, and death. Cobalt dust inhaled in industrial settings may produce asthma and pulmonary symptoms. Long-term exposure may result in accumulation and cause polycythemia, goiter, cardiomyopathy, and nerve damage. Epidemic of lethal cardiomyopathy due to ingestion of 0.04-0.14 mg/kg/day of cobalt which was added as a foam stabilizer, occurred in the U.S. and Canada in the 1960s.

Total body content of cobalt: 1-1.5 mg

Normal amounts of cobalt ingested from food: 50-40 mcg/day

Daily intake >6 mg can cause cardiomyopathy; air concentrations >100 mcg/m^3 can cause pulmonary fibrosis.

Mean urban air concentrations range from 1-2 ng/m^3; concentration of in drinking water is <5 mcg/L; average concentration in the earth's crust is 25 mg/kg.

Tobacco contains <2.3 mg cobalt/kg dry weight.

IDLH: 20 mg/m^3; PEL-TWA: 0.05 mg/m^3; TLV-TWA: 0.05 mg/m^3

Copper

Related Information
- Copper Content of Human Tissues and Body Fluids
- Copper Content of Selected Foods

CAS Number 10290-12-7; 12002-03-8; 12069-69-1; 12258-96-7; 1317-39-1; 1332-40-7; 142-71-2; 20427-59-2; 26506-47-8; 3251-23-8; 544-92-3; 7288-92-0; 7440-50-8; 7758-89-6; 7758-99-8; 866-82-0

UN Number 1479; 1578; 1585; 1586; 2630; 2721; 2775; 2776; 3009; 3010

Commonly Found In Elemental copper, and as the following hydrated or anhydrous salts: acetate, arsenate, chlorate, chloride, citrate, cyanide, dinitrate, fluoroborate, hydrate, hydroxide, malonate, oxide, oxychloride, selenate, silicate, sulfate, and copper in association with organochlorine (DDT), or carbamate insecticide; used in electrical industry, plumbing, industrial valves and fittings, pigments, furniture polish

Mechanism of Toxic Action Copper is a cofactor for ascorbic acid oxidase, catalase, peroxidase, lactase, and tyrosinase; copper may induce hemolysis through oxidation of hemoglobin sulfhydryl groups, thereby increasing permeability of the red blood cell. Copper also inhibits the sulfhydryl moieties of G6PD and glutathione, thereby reducing their free radical scavenging activities.

Adverse Reactions
Cardiovascular: Shock and cardiovascular collapse

Central nervous system: Lethargy, confusion, coma, drowsiness, hyperthermia, fever, extrapyramidal reactions, bilateral putaminal involvement

Dermatologic: Delayed allergic contact dermatitis, immunologic contact urticaria - Green hair shafts

Gastrointestinal: Oral thermal injury, GI ulceration, gastroenteritis (at ingestions >15 mg of copper sulfate)

Hematologic: Hemolysis

Hepatic: Hepatitis, aminotransferase level elevation (asymptomatic), granulomatous liver disease (noncaseating)

Neuromuscular & skeletal: Rhabdomyolysis

Ocular: Corneal discoloration (chalcosis), eye irritation, conjunctivitis, corneal ulceration

Renal: Renal tubular necrosis, renal failure

Respiratory: Irritation, nasal ulceration, wheezing, rales

Miscellaneous: Metal fume fever

Signs and Symptoms of Overdose Acute tubular necrosis and renal failure, allergic contact dermatitis, blue-green vomitus, cardiovascular collapse, corneal discoloration and ulceration, diarrhea, feces discoloration (black), fibrosis, gastroenteritis, hair discoloration (green), hemolysis, hepatomegaly and hepatitis with centrilobular necrosis and biliary stasis, hypotension, jaundice, metallic taste, mucous membrane irritation, nasal ulceration, nausea, oral ulceration, pulmonary edema, shock, ulceration and burns, urticaria, vomiting. Methemoglobinemia is a rare finding, occurring only in severe cases (hemolysis and shock).

Admission Criteria/Prognosis Admit any adult ingestion >1 g or pediatric ingestion >25 mg or if hemolysis is present.

Toxicodynamics/Kinetics
Onset of reaction: Hemorrhagic gastritis, diarrhea, hemolytic anemia, and renal tubule necrosis may follow 36-48 hours after exposure

Absorption: Oral: ~30%

Distribution: V_d: 2 L/kg; found extensively in red blood cells, kidney, liver, and lungs

Protein binding: 95% to ceruloplasmin: 5% to albumin

Half-life: 26 days

Elimination: Urine: 4%; bile and feces: 80%

Reference Range Serum copper concentrations average 1 mg/L in normal patients, and 2 mg/L in pregnant patients (10.5-23 μmol/L); serum copper concentrations >5 mg/mL are usually accompanied by signs of toxicity; whole blood copper concentrations correlate more closely with toxicity, but are usually not available; normal urinary copper excretion: 33 mcg/L (602 mcg/L in Wilson's disease); normal hair level: 17.7 ppm copper in first 3 cm of proximal end of scalp hair and ~11.9 ppm copper in pubic hair

Overdosage/Treatment
Decontamination: **Oral**: Lavage within 1 hour cautiously, but because of gastrointestinal ulceration and erosion, **do not** induce emesis. Activated charcoal does not bind copper. **Dermal**: Prompt thorough scrubbing of all affected areas with soap and water **Inhalation**: Remove from exposure, give supplemental oxygen, and treat wheezing. **Ocular**: Irrigation with copious tepid water or saline

Supportive therapy: Airway management, treatment of wheezing, humidified oxygen administration, and close monitoring for renal compromise. BAL (dimercaprol) (1 to 5 mg/kg/m) or penicillamine. Penicillamine dose is 1 to 2 grams daily (20 to 30 mg/kg) in 4 divided doses should be considered for massive ingestions, persistent symptomatology, or persistently elevated serum copper concentrations. BAL may be useful; penicillamine may be used in patients who will tolerate oral therapy. Trientine might be an effective copper chelator in an overdose setting, although it has not been studied for this use. Monitor for hemolysis.

Shock: Treat blood loss aggressively with I.V. fluids and vasopressors such as dopamine or norepinephrine. Consider endoscopy to rule out corrosive gastrointestinal injury and blood loss.

Enhancement of elimination: Dialysis or hemoperfusion has not been demonstrated to increase the elimination of copper. Adding albumin to dialysate may enhance the removal of copper sulphate by means of peritoneal dialysis.

Antidote(s)
- Dimercaprol [ANTIDOTE]
- DOPamine [ANTIDOTE]
- Edetate Calcium Disodium [ANTIDOTE]
- Norepinephrine [ANTIDOTE]
- Penicillamine [ANTIDOTE]
- Trientine [ANTIDOTE]

Diagnostic Procedures
- Creatinine, Serum
- Electrolytes, Blood
- Methemoglobin, Blood
- Urea Nitrogen, Blood

Additional Information

Metal fume fever has been reported at copper dust concentrations of 0.075-0.12 mg/m^3. Copper salts were previously used as medicinal agents. Exposure may also follow the use of older vending machines, and brass or copper cooking or drinking vessels. Copper metal is radiopaque, but copper salts are not; elemental copper is poorly absorbed orally, but dusts or fumes may cause pneumonitis and metal fume fever. Copper salts may be irritating to the gastrointestinal tract, and may possess other toxicities due to salts such as arsenate or cyanide. Anhydrous compounds may produce thermal injury following contact with water or mucous membranes. Most U.S. coins contain 75% copper; diethyldithiocarbonate (intraocular use) is not useful to prevent ocular opacification due to copper nitrate.

How supplied: Elemental copper as solid metal (coin, etc); powdered copper; copper salt powder and granules; liquid for spraying (with or without petroleum distillate, organochlorine, or carbamate)

Diethyldithiocarbamate (intraocular use) is not useful to prevent ocular opacification due to copper nitrate.

Nut and nut products (especially unsalted pecans) contain the highest amount of copper (0.067-1.245 mg of copper per 100 g/nut). Most U.S. coins contain 75% copper.

Average daily intake of copper by inhalation: 600 mcg. Average daily intake of copper through drinking water: 0.15 mg. Average daily intake is ~1-2 mg. Mean copper content of cigarette tobacco: 24.7 ppm (only 0.2% of this copper passes through mainstream smoke)

Soil copper concentration: ~50 ppm; Atmospheric copper concentration: 5-200 ng/m^3. Airborne copper concentration is 8-12 ng/m^3 in indoor atmosphere (increased with use of kerosene-based space heaters). Water copper concentration: <100 mcg/L. Seawater contains <5 ppb of copper.

Taste threshold of copper in water: 1-5 mg/L. Discoloration (blue/green) in water: >5 mg/L.

ACGIH TLV: 1 mg/m^3 (dusts/mists), 0.2 mg/m^3 (fumes); PEL-TWA: 1 mg/m^3 (dusts/mists), 0.1 mg/m^3 (fumes)

See table.

Agricultural Sources of Copper Contamination in Soils

Source	Concentration (ppm dry weight)*
Sewage sludges	50-3300
Phosphate fertilizers	1-300
Limestones	2-125
Nitrogen fertilizers	<1-15
Manure	2-60
Pesticides (percent)	12-50

*Equivalent to mg/kg-dry weight

Reference: Breckenridge RP and Crockett AB, "Determination of Background Concentrations of Inorganics in Soils and Sediments at Hazardous Waste Sites," *EPA Engineering Forum Issue*, 1995, EPA/540/S096/500. Available at: http://www.epa.gov/tio/tsp/download/bckgrnd.pdf.

Specific References

Agency for Toxic Substances and Disease Registry (ATSDR), 2002. Toxicological Profile for Copper (Draft for Public Comment). Atlanta, GA: U.S. Department of Health and Human Services, Public Health Service. Available at: http://www.atsdr.cdc.gov/toxprofiles/tp132.html.

Cech I, Smolensky MH, Afshar M, et al, "Lead and Copper in Drinking Water Fountains – Information for Physicians," *South Med J*, 2006, 99(2):137-42.

Gorter RW, Butorac M, and Cobian EP, "Examination of the Cutaneous Absorption of Copper After the Use of Copper-Containing Ointments," *Am J Ther*, 2004, 11(6):453-8.

Kvietkauskaite R, Dringeliene A, Marevicius A, et al, "Original Research: Effect of Low Copper Exposure on the Antioxidant System and Some Immune Parameters," *Vet Hum Toxicol*, 2004, 46(4):169-72.

Ortolani EL, Antonelli AC, and de Souza Sarkis JE, "Acute Sheep Poisoning from a Copper Sulfate Footbath," *Vet Hum Toxicol*, 2004, 46(6):315-8.

Ortolani EL, Machado CH, and Sucupira MC, "Assessment of Some Clinical and Laboratory Variables for Early Diagnosis of Cumulative Copper Poisoning in Sheep," *Vet Hum Toxicol*, 2003, 45(6):289-93.

Yang CC, Wu ML, and Deng JF, "Prolonged Hemolysis and Methemoglobinemia Following Organic Copper Fungicide Ingestion," *Vet Hum Toxicol*, 2004, 46(6):321-3.

Coumaphos

CAS Number 56-72-4

UN Number 2783

U.S. Brand Names Asuntol®; Baymix®; Co-Ral® Animal Insecticide; Co-Ral®; Meldane®; Muscatox®; Resitox®

Synonyms Bayer-21199; Coumafos

Use Used as a topical ectoparasiticide for livestock

Mechanism of Toxic Action Irreversible inhibition of acetylcholinesterase and plasma cholinesterase, resulting in excess accumulation of acetylcholine at muscarinic and nicotinic receptors, and in the central nervous system

Adverse Reactions Central nervous system: Cognitive dysfunction, hypothermia

Signs and Symptoms of Overdose Abdominal pain, agitation, asystole, AV block, bradycardia, bronchorrhea, coma, confusion, cranial nerve palsies, decreased hemoglobin, decreased platelet count, decreased red blood cell count, diaphragmatic paralysis, dysarthria, excessive sweating, fecal and urinary incontinence, generalized asthenia, headache, heart block, hypotension, hypertension, lacrimation, metabolic acidosis and hyperglycemia (severe intoxication), miosis (unreactive to light), mydriasis (rarely), nausea, pallor, pulmonary edema, respiratory depression, salivation, seizures, skeletal muscle fasciculation and flaccid paralysis, QT prolongation, tachycardia, tachypnea, vomiting

An "intermediate syndrome" of limb asthenia and respiratory paralysis has been reported to occur between 24 and 96 hours postorganophosphate exposure, and is independent of the acute cholinergic crisis. Late paresthesia characterized by stocking and glove paresthesia, anesthesia, and asthenia is infrequently observed weeks to months following acute exposure to certain organophosphates.

Warnings/Precautions Risk of aspiration pneumonitis exists with agents having a hydrocarbon vehicle; severe laryngeal irritation and violent coughing may result from exposure to dusting powders; exposure to dusting powders and insecticide granules may cause contact dermatitis

Overdosage/Treatment

Decontamination: Isolation, bagging, and disposal of all contaminated clothing and other articles. All emergency medical workers and hospital staff should follow appropriate precautions regarding exposure to hazardous material including the use of protective clothing, masks, goggles, and respiratory equipment.

Oral: Activated charcoal can be administered either orally or via a nasogastric tube. **Do not** induce emesis because of danger of sudden respiratory compromise, alterations in mental status, seizures, coma, and possible aspiration of hydrocarbon vehicles. **Do not** give a cathartic.

Dermal: Prompt thorough scrubbing of all affected areas with soap and water, including hair and nails; 5% bleach can be used

Ocular: Irrigation with copious tepid sterile water or saline

Supportive therapy: Airway management, ventilatory assistance, humidified oxygen administration, and close monitoring for sudden respiratory failure

Enhancement of elimination: Dialysis and hemoperfusion are not indicated due to effectiveness of the prescribed antidotal treatment and large volumes of distribution of organophosphates.

Antidote:

Atropine: Administration should be guided by respiratory status, starting at 2-5 mg I.V. every 5-10 minutes as needed, and should be titrated to the resolution of excess pulmonary secretions. Frequent administration of large doses (cumulative doses >100 mg) may be necessary in massive exposures.

Glycopyrrolate: May be administered if atropine is unavailable (200-400 mcg I.V. or I.M., or ~$^1/_2$ the dose of atropine).

2-PAM: For more significant exposures (ie, exposures requiring large doses of atropine, or with recurring symptoms, or exposures to more lipid soluble agents), administration should follow: 1-2 g I.V. over 10-30 minutes, repeated in 1 hour if asthenia recurs, then every 4-12 hours for recurring symptoms.

Antidote(s)
- Atropine [ANTIDOTE]
- Pralidoxime [ANTIDOTE]

Additional Information Very high mortality rate when ingested (17% to 31%).

The intermediate syndrome is not related to delayed neuropathy.

QT$_c$ prolongation on ECG in the setting of organophosphate poisoning is associated with a high incidence of respiratory failure and mortality.

Heat stable; a colorless (or tan) combustible crystalline solid with a slight sulfur odor and insoluble in water.

Creosote

Related Information
- Toxins Which Should Be Lavaged with Solutions Other Than Water

CAS Number 8001-58-9 (coal tar); 8021-39-4 (wood)

U.S. Brand Names Sakresote® 100 (Coal Tar Creosote)

Synonyms Coal Tar Creosote (Creosote Oil, Brick Oil); Wood Creosote (Beechwood Creosote)

Use
Wood creosote: Disinfectant, carbonate, laxative, and expectorant (rarely used in U.S.)

Coal tar creosote: Carbonization of coal (bituminous) to produce natural gas (coking procedure); also used as a timber preservative

Mechanism of Toxic Action Mucosal irritant

Adverse Reactions
Cardiovascular: Increased diastolic pressure, hypertension, hyperemia

Dermatologic: Dermal burns/irritation, phototoxic, photosensitivity

Gastrointestinal: Oropharyngeal ulceration, esophageal corrosion

Hepatic: Hepatic degeneration

Ocular: Keratoconjunctivitis, photophobia

Renal: Albuminuria, renal failure

Signs and Symptoms of Overdose Anuria, dizziness, dyspnea, light-headedness, myoclonus, nasal irritation on inhalation

Toxicodynamics/Kinetics
Absorption: Dermal absorption may occur

Metabolism: Hepatic to 1-hydroxypyrene

Reference Range Workers of coal tar creosote excrete from 1-40 mcg of creosote/g creatinine in urine

Overdosage/Treatment
Decontamination: **Oral**: **Do not** induce emesis. Lavage (within 1 hour) with olive oils may be effective. Activated charcoal (not castor oil) should be given. **Ocular**: Copious irrigation with saline should be performed.

Supportive therapy: Inhalation: Give 100% humidified oxygen.

Enhancement of elimination: Charcoal hemoperfusion may be effective; hemodialysis is not effective.

Additional Information Fatal oral dose of coal tar creosote: Children: 1-2 g; Adults: 7 g

Coal tar creosote is possibly related to increased incidence of bladder cancer, squamous papilloma, and carcinomas. Phototoxicity of coal tar creosote may be enhanced with tetracycline.

Cresols

CAS Number 108-39-4 (meta); 1319-77-3; 95-48-7 (ortho)

UN Number 2022; 2076

Synonyms Cresylic Acid; Hydroxytoluene; Methylphenol; Tar Acids

Use Organic acid which occurs naturally in mammals and plants (Easter lily, jasmine, camphor, eucalyptus); also found as a byproduct of natural fires (volcano lightening), through the combustion of petroleum fuels, wood, or coal (fly-ash); ortho cresol has been used as an antiseptic; a metabolic breakdown product of toluene

Mechanism of Toxic Action Mucosal irritant and a central nervous system depressant

Adverse Reactions
Cardiovascular: Premature ventricular contractions, tachycardia, sinus tachycardia, cerebral edema

Dermatologic: Dermal burns

Gastrointestinal: Oropharyngeal burns, hemorrhagic pancreatitis

Hematologic: Methemoglobinemia, intravascular hemolysis, Heinz body anemia

Hepatic: Fatty degeneration

Ocular: Lacrimation, corneal burns, optic atrophy

Renal: Hematuria, eosinophilic necrosis, renal failure

Respiratory: Necrosis of bronchial epithelium, pulmonary edema

Signs and Symptoms of Overdose Abdominal pain, aspiration, coma, cough with bloody sputum, drowsiness, dyspnea, facial paralysis, hypoactivity, seizures, tremor, vomiting

Toxicodynamics/Kinetics
Absorption: Dermal: May be absorbed (fatalities can occur)

Elimination: Renal

Reference Range Para-cresol concentration in urine normally averages ~90 mg/L (range: 20-200 mg/L); serum cresol level >90 mg/L associated with lethality

Overdosage/Treatment
Decontamination: **Oral:** Dilute with water or milk; activated charcoal may be useful. **Do not** induce emesis. **Dermal:** Wash copiously with soap and water. **Ocular:** Irrigate copiously with saline.

Supportive therapy: Convulsions can be treated with a benzodiazepine or phenobarbital. Significant methemoglobinemia should be treated with methylene blue.

Antidote(s)
- Methylene Blue [ANTIDOTE]

Diagnostic Procedures
- Methemoglobin, Blood

Additional Information
Lethal oral dose: 2 g/kg. Lethal dermal dose: 2 g/kg

Individuals with glucose-6-phosphate deficiency may be at higher risk for methemoglobin formation. Toxicity may be enhanced when a patient is exposed concomitantly to oxidizing compounds (ie, hydroquinone). Cigarette smokers may inhale as much as 3 mcg/day of cresols. Not to be used for dermal disinfection

Cyanide

Related Information
- Donor Victims of Poisoning in Whom Transplantation of Organs Occurred
- Laetrile®

CAS Number 57-12-5

UN Number 1588

Synonyms Carbon Nitride Ion

Commonly Found In Gold and silver ore extraction, electroplating, fumigant, stainless steel manufacture, petroleum refining, rodenticide; plant sources include amygdalin glycodes (such as peach pits), cassava, linium, prunus, sorghum, and bamboo sprouts; also a byproduct of nitroprusside and succinonitrile along with laetrile

Mechanism of Toxic Action Forms a stable complex with ferric ion of cytochrome oxidase enzymes inhibiting cellular respiration (at cytochrome aa$_3$); then converted to thiocyanate (less toxic form) by rhodanase enzyme. Cyanide can also cause lipid peroxidation in the brain due to inhibition of antioxidant enzymes.

Adverse Reactions
Cardiovascular: Myocardial depression, hypotension, sinus bradycardia, angina, chest pain, congestive heart failure, sinus tachycardia, vasodilation

Central nervous system: CNS stimulation followed by CNS depression, extrapyramidal reactions, bilateral putaminal involvement

Endocrine & metabolic: Goiter, hypothyroidism

Gastrointestinal: Bitter almond, burning taste

Neuromuscular & skeletal: Rhabdomyolysis

Ocular: Blurred vision

Respiratory: Respiratory depression

Signs and Symptoms of Overdose Agitation, apnea, bitter almond breath, coma, cyanosis, dizziness, flushing, headache, hyperventilation, hypothermia, hypotension, metabolic acidosis, mydriasis, myoglobinuria, nausea, nystagmus, pruritus, pulmonary edema, ototoxicity, seizures, skin irritation, tachycardia followed by bradycardia, tachypnea, tinnitus, vomiting

Admission Criteria/Prognosis All symptomatic patients should probably be admitted to an intensive care unit for 1-2 days; asymptomatic patients should be observed for at least 2 hours and then can be discharged; survival after 4 hours (in an acute exposure) is usually associated with recovery

Toxicodynamics/Kinetics
Absorption: By inhalation (58% to 77%), oral (~50%), dermally, and ocular

Distribution: V$_d$: 0.4 L/kg

Metabolism: Hepatic by rhodanese or 3-mercaptopyruvate to thiocyanate; also combines with hydroxocobalamin to form cyanocobalamin (vitamin B$_{12}$)

Half-life: 0.7-2.1 hours

Elimination: Excreted through the lungs and the kidneys

Reference Range
Whole blood levels: Smoker: ≤0.5 mg/L

Flushing and tachycardia seen at 0.5-1.0 mg/L; obtundation at 1.0-2.5 mg/L

Coma and death occur at >2.5 mg/L

Plasma cyanide: Normal: 4-5 mcg/L; Asymptomatic (with metabolic acidosis): 80 mcg/L; Death: >260 mcg/L

Red blood cell cyanide: Normal: <26 mcg/L; Metabolic acidosis: 1040 mcg/L; Symptomatic: 5200 mcg/L; Fatal: >10,400 mcg/L

Note: A plasma lactate concentration >8 mM/L is 94% sensitive and 70% specific for a blood cyanide level >1 mg/L (40 μmol/L).

Mean urine cyanide level of 37 mg/L (range 0.4-230 mg/L) associated with fatal poisoning

Overdosage/Treatment
Decontamination: Basic poison management (lavage within 1 hour/ activated charcoal). Emesis is contraindicated due to the rapid course of neurologic symptoms. Give 100% oxygen.

Supportive therapy: Give sodium bicarbonate for acidosis. Cyanide antidote kit (amyl nitrite, sodium nitrite followed by sodium thiosulfate) was the primary therapeutic modality. Hydroxocobalamin (5 grams IV., repeat as necessary in adults) is the current therapy. Methemoglobin formation due to nitrites occurs with a target methemoglobin level of ~20%, although clinical responses do occur at levels of 5%.

Enhancement of elimination: Hemodialysis and charcoal hemoperfusion have been utilized. Hyperbaric oxygen may also be utilized, although its efficacy is uncertain.

Antidote(s)
- Amyl Nitrite [ANTIDOTE]
- Cyanide Antidote Kit [ANTIDOTE]
- Hydroxocobalamin [ANTIDOTE]
- Oxygen (Hyperbaric) [ANTIDOTE]
- Sodium Nitrite [ANTIDOTE]
- Sodium Thiosulfate [ANTIDOTE]

Diagnostic Procedures
- Anion Gap, Blood
- Cyanide, Blood
- Electrolytes, Blood
- Methemoglobin, Blood
- Thiocyanate, Blood or Urine

Additional Information
Fatal dose of cyanide: 200-300 mg (adult)

Fatal dose (hydrogen cyanide): **Dermal:** 100 mg/kg. **Inhalation** for <1 hour: 110-135 ppm. **Oral:** 0.6-1.5 mg/kg

Toxic inhalation concentration of cyanide is 10 ppm.

Bitter almond odor, zinc cyanide is odorless. Up to 60% of the population may be unable to smell cyanide. Parkinsonism has been noted after ingestion of sodium or potassium cyanide. Hydroxocobalamin and dicobalt-EDTA are used for chelation in Europe.

The ratio of red blood cell to plasma cyanide concentrations is 60:1.

Residence time in atmosphere of hydrogen cyanide: 2 years. In natural rivers half-life of cyanide is 10-24 days.

Daily intake of hydrogen cyanide by inhalation: ~3.8 mcg; through drinking water: 0.4-0.7 mcg. Allowable daily intake: ~0.6 mg

Fruit juice typically contains from 1.9-5.3 mg/L of hydrogen cyanide while apricot pits contain 89-2,170 mg/kg (wet weight). Inhaled smoke from cigarettes contains from 10-400 mcg/cigarette, while sidestream smoke usually runs <27% of mainstream smoke concentrations. Average cyanide emission rate in automobiles varies from 11-14 mg/mile in cars; catalytic converters can reduce cyanide emissions by 90%.

Dermal exposure of 10% sodium cyanide to a large body surface area will cause symptoms within 20 minutes

A 5 g dose of hydroxocobalamin appears to bind all cyanide ions in patients with initial cyanide levels up to 40 µmol/L

Plasma lactate (half-life ~4 hours in treated cyanide poisoning) may be useful in determining treatment efficacy in cyanide poisoning

ACGIH-TLV-TWA: 5 mg/m^3; IDLH: 50 mg/m^3; PEL-TWA: 5 mg/m^3

For listing of cyanogenic plants: See table.

Cyanogenic Plants

Plant	Amount of Hydrogen Cyanide Released	Maximum Amygdalin Content (in the seeds or pits)
Apricot seeds	0.1-4.1 mg/g	8%
Peach seeds	0.4-2.6 mg/g	6%
Apple seeds	0.61 mg/g	
Bitter almond seeds	0.9-4.9 mg/g	5%
Cassava (whole root)	0.4 mg/g	
Cassava (dried root)	2.45 mg/g	
Sorghum whole plant (immature)	2.5 mg/g	
Amygdalin	59.1 mg/g	
Cotoneaster	15-185 ppm	
Plum		2.5%

Specific References

Bromley J, Hughes BG, Leong DC, et al, "Life-Threatening Interaction Between Complementary Medicines: Cyanide Toxicity Following Ingestion of Amygdalin and Vitamin C," *Ann Pharmacother*, 2005, 39(9):1566-9.

DesLouriers CA, Burda AM, and Wahl M, "Hydroxocobalamin as a Cyanide Antidote," *KeePosted*, 2004, 23-7,

Dumas P, Gingras G, and LeBlanc A, "Isotope Dilution-Mass Spectrometry Determination of Blood Cyanide by Headspace Gas Chromatography," *J Anal Toxicol*, 2005, 29:71-3.

Horton DK, Berkowitz Z, and Kaye WE, "Secondary Contamination of ED Personnel from Hazardous Materials Events, 1995-2001," *Am J Emerg Med*, 2003, 21(3):199-204.

Hung YM, Hung SY, Chou KJ, et al, "Acute Poisoning of Yam Bean Seeds: Clinical Manifestation Mimicking Acute Cyanide Intoxication," *J Toxicol Clin Toxicol*, 2004, 42(5):725.

Kales SN and Christiani DC, "Acute Chemical Emergencies," *N Engl J Med*, 2004, 350(8):800-8.

McFee RB, Leikin JB, and Kiernan K, "Preparing for an Era of Weapons of Mass Destruction (WMD)—Are We There Yet? Why We Should All Be Concerned. Part II," *Vet Hum Toxicol*, 2004, 46(6):347-51.

McGeorge F, Pham Cuong J, Huang D, et al, "Hemodyamic Effects of Cyanide Toxicity," *Acad Emerg Med*, 2003, 10:519b-20b.

Megarbane B, Delahaye A, Goldgran-Toledano D, et al, "Antidotal Treatment of Cyanide Poisoning," *J Chin Med Assoc*, 2003, 66(4):193-203 (review).

Rella JG, Marcus S, and Wagner BJ, "Rapid Cyanide Detection Using the Cyantesmo® Kit," *J Toxicol Clin Toxicol*, 2004, 42(6):897-900.

Rella JG, Marcus S, and Wagner BJ, "Rapid Cyanide Detection Using the Cyantesmo® Kit," *Clin Toxicol (Phila)*, 2005, 43:687.

Renard C, Borron SW, Renandeau C, et al, "The Diagnostic Value of Biological Markers of Cellular Hypoxia in Cyanide Poisoning in a Rat Model," *Clin Toxicol (Phila)*, 2005, 43:686.

Stanford CF, Ries NL, Bogdan GM, et al, "Do Hospitals in the 50 Largest Cities of the United States Carry Sufficient Supply of the Cyanide Antidote Kit?" *Clin Toxicol (Phila)*, 2005, 43:713.

Stefanidou M and Athanaselis S, "Toxicological Aspects of Fire," *Vet Hum Toxicol*, 2004, 46(4):196-8.

von Landenberg F, Stonerook M, Judge K, et al, "Efficacy of Hydroxocobalamin in a Canine Model of Cyanide Poisoning: A Pilot Study," *Clin Toxicol (Phila)*, 2005, 43:692.

Yeoh MJ and Braitberg G, "Carbon Monoxide and Cyanide Poisoning in Fire Related Deaths in Victoria, Australia," *J Toxicol Clin Toxicol*, 2004, 42(6):855-63.

Cyclohexyl Nitrite

Related Information
- Nitrites

U.S. Brand Names D and E®

Use Principle abuse potential in male homosexuals used to facilitate anal intercourse

Mechanism of Toxic Action Vasodilitation/smooth muscle relaxation

Signs and Symptoms of Overdose Toxicity in rodents noted primarily anemia and leukopenia at doses of 100 ppm; hypotonia and methemoglobinemia are possible.

Overdosage/Treatment

Decontamination: Basic poison management; methylene blue for symptomatic methemoglobinemia

Supportive therapy: Hyperbaric oxygen may be of use, though controlled human data are lacking.

Additional Information Estimated dose of inhalation by abuse: 2200±200 ppm

DDD

Related Information
- DDT
- Toxins Which Should Be Lavaged with Solutions Other Than Water

CAS Number 72-54-8

U.S. Brand Names Dilene®; Rothane®

Synonyms 1,1-Bis(4-Chlorophenyl)-2; 2-Dichloroethane; TDE

Use Primarily as a pesticide; one form (ortho, para DDD) was used as a medicinal agent for the treatment of adrenal gland carcinoma

Mechanism of Toxic Action Organochlorine agent, interferes with sodium, potassium, and calcium ion movement along neuronal membranes; may be related to serotonin deficiency in the brain

Adverse Reactions Not well described in humans, but probably very similar to DDT; nervous system would appear to be target organ

Toxicodynamics/Kinetics

Absorption: Inhalation, oral, and dermal

Metabolism: Hepatic to 1,1-bis(parachlorophenyl) ethane (DDNU)

Elimination: Renal

Overdosage/Treatment

Decontamination: **Oral:Do not** induce emesis. Lavage within 1 hour (with water or mannitol)/activated charcoal is effective. **Do not** use an oil-based cathartic in that absorption may increase. **Dermal:** Wash with soap and water. **Ocular:** Irrigate copiously with saline.

Supportive therapy: Seizures may be treated with a benzodiazepine, phenobarbital, or phenytoin. Avoid catecholamines.

Enhancement of elimination: Multiple dosing of activated charcoal or cholestyramine (4 g every 8 hours) may be effective after recent oral exposure.

Additional Information Metabolite of DDT; degrades slowly by solar radiation in the atmosphere to carbon dioxide and hydrochloric acid

DDT

Related Information
- DDD

CAS Number 50-29-3

UN Number 2761

U.S. Brand Names Anofex®; Chlorophenothane®; Detoxan®; Dicophane®; Genitox® Pentachlorin®

Synonyms 4,4′ DDT; Dichlorodiphenyltrichloroethane

Use Primarily as an insecticide on cotton, peanut, and soybean crops; not imported into the U.S. since 1972; contaminant of dicofol

Mechanism of Toxic Action Organochlorine agent, interferes with sodium, potassium, and calcium ion movement along neuronal membranes; may be related to serotonin deficiency in the brain; estrogenic action has been described

Adverse Reactions

Cardiovascular: Tachycardia, Raynaud's phenomenon, sinus tachycardia

Central nervous system: Headache, dizziness, seizures can occur at oral doses >16 mg/kg, anxiety, delirium

Dermatologic: Sclerodermatous changes on hands have been described

Endocrine & metabolic: Hypomagnesemia

Gastrointestinal: Nausea noted at oral doses of 6 mg/kg; vomiting noted at a dose of 10 mg/kg; stomatitis

Hematologic: Aplastic anemia, thrombocytopenia

Hepatic: Liver enzymes (elevated) can occur, centrilobular hepatic necrosis

Neuromuscular & skeletal: Tremors, myoclonus

Ocular: Opsoclonus, optic neuropathy, neuritis (retrobulbar), visual evoked potential abnormalities

Miscellaneous: Diaphoresis, breast cancer

Toxicodynamics/Kinetics

Absorption: Through inhalation, oral, and dermal exposure

Distribution: Concentrated in fat

Metabolism: Hepatic to 2,2-bis(parachlorophenyl) acetic acid (DDA)

Elimination: Urine (feces at high doses)

Reference Range DDT blood levels in asymptomatic individuals not occupationally exposed to DDT was <15 mcg/L (0.04 µmol/L); in those individuals occupationally exposed, average blood DDT level was 57 mcg/L (0.16 µmol/L); average daily intake of 18 mg by occupational exposure results in DDA urine levels of ~1.27 mg/L (3.59 µmol/L)

Overdosage/Treatment

Decontamination: **Oral:Do not** induce emesis. Lavage within 1 hour (with water or mannitol)/activated charcoal is effective. **Do not** use an oil-based cathartic in that absorption may increase. **Dermal:** Wash with soap and water. **Ocular:** Irrigate copiously with saline.

Supportive therapy: Seizures may be treated with a benzodiazepine, phenobarbital, or phenytoin. Avoid catecholamines.

Enhancement of elimination: Multiple dosing of activated charcoal or cholestyramine (4 g every 8 hours) may be effective after recent oral exposure.

Additional Information Carcinogenic in animals (primarily liver)

Atmospheric half-life: 2 days (to carbon dioxide and hydrochloric acid). Soil half-life: 2-15 years

Estimated dietary intake of DDT in the U.S. (per person): 1970: 240 mcg; 1974: 8 mcg; 1980: 2.4 mcg; 1981: 2.2 mcg

Acceptable daily DDT intake established by WHO: 20 mcg/kg; root and leafy vegetables have highest amount of DDT (0.4-0.6 ppb)

PEL-TWA (skin designation): 1 mg/m³; TLV-TWA: 1 mg/m³

Specific References

al-Saleh I, Shinwari N, Basile P, et al, "DDT and Its Metabolites in Breast Milk from Two Regions in Saudi Arabia," *J Occup Environ Med*, 2003, 45(4):410-27.

Cohn BA, Cirillo PM, Wolff MS, et al, "DDT and DDE Exposure in Mothers and Time to Pregnancy in Daughters," *Lancet*, 2003, 361(9376):2205-6.

Eskenazi B, Marks AR, Bradman A, et al, "In Utero Exposure to Dichlorodiphenyltrichloroethane (DDT) and Dichlorodiphenyldichloroethylene (DDE) and Neurodevelopment Among Young Mexican American Children," *Pediatrics*, 2006, 118(1):233-41.

Wang RY and Needham LL, "Levels of Persistent Organic Chemicals in Human Milk at Two U.S. Locations," *J Toxicol Clin Toxicol*, 2004, 42(5):806.

Demeton-S-Methyl

Applies to Meta-Systox

CAS Number 919-86-8

UN Number 3018

Use Pesticide

Mechanism of Toxic Action Irreversible inhibition of acetylcholinesterase and plasma cholinesterase, resulting in excess accumulation of acetylcholine at muscarinic and nicotinic receptors, and in the central nervous system. Delayed presentation of toxicity.

Adverse Reactions

Cardiovascular: **Hyperdynamic** (~18% to 21%) or hypodynamic (~7% to 10%) states, tachycardia, hypertension, QT prolongation, sinus bradycardia, sinus tachycardia

Central nervous system: Depression, seizures, hyperactivity, cognitive dysfunction, hypothermia, opisthotonos

Endocrine & metabolic: Hypokalemia

Gastrointestinal: Pancreatitis (after ingestion of 1.5 mg/kg), diarrhea

Genitourinary: Urinary incontinence

Neuromuscular & skeletal: Weakness (delayed paralysis, delayed paresthesia), rhabdomyolysis

Ocular: Miosis

Respiratory: Pulmonary edema, respiratory depression

Miscellaneous: Flu-like symptoms (especially with chronic exposure), diaphoresis

Signs and Symptoms of Overdose

Abdominal pain, agitation, asystole, AV block, bradycardia, bronchorrhea, coma, confusion, cranial nerve palsies, decreased hemoglobin, decreased platelet count, decreased red blood cell count, dementia, diaphragmatic paralysis, dysarthria, excessive sweating, fecal and urinary incontinence, generalized asthenia, headache, heart block, hypertension, hypotension, lacrimation, metabolic acidosis and hyperglycemia (severe intoxication), miosis (unreactive to light), mydriasis (rarely), nausea, nystagmus, pallor, pulmonary edema, QT prolongation, respiratory depression, salivation, seizures, skeletal muscle fasciculation and flaccid paralysis, tachycardia, tachypnea, vomiting

An "intermediate syndrome" of limb asthenia and respiratory paralysis has been reported to occur between 24 and 96 hours postorganophosphate exposure and is independent of the acute cholinergic crisis. Late paresthesia characterized by stocking and glove paresthesia, anesthesia and asthenia is infrequently observed weeks to months following acute exposure to certain organophosphates.

Admission Criteria/Prognosis Any symptomatic patient or an asymptomatic patient following a severe exposure should be admitted probably into an intensive care unit; asymptomatic patients following a moderate exposure can be discharged after 8 hours of observation

Overdosage/Treatment

Decontamination: Isolation, bagging, and disposal of all contaminated clothing and other articles. All emergency medical workers and hospital staff should follow appropriate precautions regarding exposure to hazardous material including the use of protective clothing, masks, goggles, and respiratory equipment. Gastric lavage with water, 5% sodium bicarbonate or 2% potassium permanganate can be considered within 1 hour of ingestion. **Do not** use a cathartic with activated charcoal.

Oral: Activated charcoal can be administered either orally or via a nasogastric tube. **Do not** induce emesis because of danger of sudden respiratory compromise, alterations in mental status, seizures, coma, and possible aspiration of hydrocarbon vehicles.

Dermal: Prompt thorough scrubbing of all affected areas with soap and water, including hair and nails; 5% bleach can be used

Ocular: Irrigation with copious tepid sterile water or saline

Supportive therapy: Airway management, ventilatory assistance, humidified oxygen administration, and close monitoring for sudden respiratory failure

Antidote:

Atropine: Administration should be guided by respiratory status, starting at 2-5 mg I.V. every 5-10 minutes as needed, and should be titrated to the resolution of excess pulmonary secretions. Frequent administration of large doses (cumulative doses >100 mg) may be necessary in massive exposures.

Glycopyrrolate: May be administered if atropine is unavailable (200-400 mcg I.M. or I.V. initially, or ~¹/₂ the dose of atropine).

2-PAM: For more significant exposures (ie, exposures requiring large doses of atropine, or with recurring symptoms, or exposures to more lipid soluble agents), administration should follow: 1-2 g I.V. over 10-30 minutes, repeated in 1 hour if asthenia recurs, then every 4-12 hours for recurring symptoms.

Obidoxime: 4-6 mg/kg of obidoxime repeated every 4-6 hours may be given instead of 2-PAM

Diazepam is effective in reducing muscle fasciculations or treating seizure.

Enhancement of elimination: Dialysis and hemoperfusion are not indicated due to effectiveness of the prescribed antidotal treatment and large volumes of distribution of organophosphates.

Denatonium Benzoate

CAS Number 3734-33-6; 86398-53-0

U.S. Brand Names Bitrex®; Bitter Safe®

Use An alcohol denaturant (in toilet preparations) which is used as a bittering taste agent in household automotive or industrial compounds; used for nail-biting/thumb-sucking deterrent

Mechanism of Toxic Action Recognition of bitter taste by oral taste cells may be due to intracellular calcium rise leading to neurotransmitter release

Adverse Reactions

Cardiovascular: Chest pain, angina

Dermatologic: Urticaria, dermal irritation can occur at concentrations >500 ppm

Gastrointestinal: Vomiting

Respiratory: Bronchospasm

Admission Criteria/Prognosis If not symptomatic following 4 hours observation (postexposure), the patient may be discharged

Overdosage/Treatment Decontamination: **Oral:** Essentially no therapy is required when used as a food or industrial additive. If >1 g is ingested, emesis with ipecac within 30 minutes or lavage (within 1 hour) and activated charcoal can be administered. **Ocular:** Irrigate copiously with saline.

Additional Information Lethal dose: Animals: ~600 mg/kg. Taste threshold: 10 ppb. Bitter taste: 10 ppm (0.001%). Usually found in powder or granular form; in industrial solutions may be found with ethylene glycol (25%) or ethyl alcohol (21.45%)

Specific References

Mullins ME and Zane Horowitz B, "Was It Necessary to Add Bitrex (Denatonium Benzoate) to Automotive Products?" *Vet Hum Toxicol*, 2004, 46(3):150-2.

Diazinon

CAS Number 333-41-5

UN Number 2783

U.S. Brand Names Alfa-Tox®; Bazinon®; Diazol®; Gardentox®; Knox-Out®; Spectracide®

Synonyms O,O-Diethyl O-2-Isopropyl-4-Methyl-6-Pyrimidinyl Thiophosphate

Use Marketed as insecticide granules, dusting agent, or spray liquid with or without petroleum derivative as a solvent

Mechanism of Toxic Action Irreversible inhibition of acetylcholinesterase and plasma cholinesterase, resulting in excess accumulation of acetylcholine at muscarinic and nicotinic receptors, and in the central nervous system. High lipid solubility which can result in delayed presentation of toxicity.

Adverse Reactions

Cardiovascular: **Hyperdynamic** (~18% to 21%) or hypodynamic (~7% to 10%) states, tachycardia, hypertension, QT prolongation, sinus bradycardia, sinus tachycardia

Central nervous system: Depression, seizures, hyperactivity, cognitive dysfunction, hypothermia

Endocrine & metabolic: Hypokalemia

Gastrointestinal: Pancreatitis (after ingestion of 1.5 mg/kg), diarrhea

Genitourinary: Urinary incontinence

Neuromuscular & skeletal: Weakness (delayed), paralysis, delayed paresthesia, rhabdomyolysis

Ocular: Miosis

Respiratory: Pulmonary edema, respiratory depression

Miscellaneous: Flu-like symptoms (especially with chronic exposure), diaphoresis, intermediate syndrome

Signs and Symptoms of Overdose Abdominal pain, agitation, asystole, AV block, bradycardia, bronchorrhea, coma, confusion, cranial nerve palsies, decreased hemoglobin, decreased platelet count, decreased red blood cell count, dementia, diaphragmatic paralysis, dysarthria, excessive sweating, fecal and urinary incontinence, generalized asthenia, headache, heart block, hypertension, hypotension, lacrimation, metabolic acidosis and hyperglycemia (severe intoxication), miosis (unreactive to light), mydriasis (rarely), nausea, nystagmus, pallor, pulmonary edema, QT prolongation, respiratory depression, salivation, seizures, skeletal muscle fasciculation and flaccid paralysis, tachycardia, tachypnea, vomiting

An "intermediate syndrome" of limb asthenia and respiratory paralysis has been reported to occur between 24 and 96 hours postorganophosphate exposure and is independent of the acute cholinergic crisis. Late paresthesia characterized by stocking and glove paresthesia, anesthesia and asthenia is infrequently observed weeks to months following acute exposure to certain organophosphates.

Admission Criteria/Prognosis Any symptomatic patient or an asymptomatic patient following a severe exposure should be admitted probably into an intensive care unit; asymptomatic patients following a moderate exposure can be discharged after 8 hours of observation

Toxicodynamics/Kinetics

Absorption: Readily through gastrointestinal (~85%), dermal (3% to 4%), or inhalation

Metabolism: Rapidly metabolized to weakly active compounds through hepatic hydrolysis and other pathways

Half-life: 15 hours

Elimination: Metabolites are excreted in urine

Warnings/Precautions Significant dermal absorption may occur across intact skin; risk of aspiration pneumonitis exists following oral exposure to agents having a hydrocarbon vehicle; severe laryngeal irritation and violent coughing may result from exposure to dusting powders; exposure to dusting powders and insecticide granules may cause contact dermatitis

Reference Range

Peak plasma diazinon levels in symptomatic patients (who survived) ranged from 0.1-1.7 mg/L

Mild poisoning: Serum cholinesterase: 20% to 50% of normal

Moderate poisoning: Serum cholinesterase: 10% to 20% of normal

Severe poisoning (respiratory distress and coma): Serum cholinesterase: <10%

Overdosage/Treatment

Decontamination: Isolation, bagging, and disposal of all contaminated clothing and other articles. All emergency medical workers and hospital staff should follow appropriate precautions regarding exposure to hazardous material including the use of protective clothing, masks, goggles, and respiratory equipment. Gastric lavage with water, 5% sodium bicarbonate or 2% potassium permanganate can be considered within 1 hour of ingestion; **do not** use cathartic with activated charcoal.

Dermal: Prompt thorough scrubbing of all affected areas with soap and water, including hair and nails; 5% bleach can be used

Oral: Activated charcoal can be administered either orally or via a nasogastric tube. **Do not** induce emesis because of danger of sudden respiratory compromise, alterations in mental status, seizures, coma, and possible aspiration of hydrocarbon vehicles.

Ocular: Irrigation with copious tepid sterile water or saline

Supportive therapy: Airway management, ventilatory assistance, humidified oxygen administration, and close monitoring for sudden respiratory failure

Antidote:

Atropine: Administration should be guided by respiratory status, starting at 2-5 mg I.V. every 5-10 minutes as needed, and should be titrated to the resolution of excess pulmonary secretions. Frequent administration of large doses (cumulative doses >100 mg) may be necessary in massive exposures.

Glycopyrrolate: May be administered if atropine is unavailable (200-400 mcg I.M. or I.V. initially, or ~1/2 the dose of atropine).

2-PAM: For more significant exposures (ie, exposures requiring large doses of atropine, or with recurring symptoms, or exposures to more lipid soluble agents), administration should follow: 1-2 g I.V. over 10-30 minutes, repeated in 1 hour if asthenia recurs, then every 4-12 hours for recurring symptoms

Enhancement of elimination: Dialysis and hemoperfusion are not indicated due to effectiveness of the prescribed antidotal treatment and large volumes of distribution of organophosphates.

Antidote(s)

- Atropine [ANTIDOTE]
- Pralidoxime [ANTIDOTE]

Diagnostic Procedures

- Creatinine, Serum
- Pseudocholinesterase, Serum

Drug Interaction Paralysis is potentiated by neuromuscular blockade (ie, pancuronium, vecuronium, succinylcholine, atracurium, doxacurium, mivacurium); inhibition of serum esterase prolongs the half-life of succinylcholine, cocaine, and other ester anesthetics; cholinergic toxicity is potentiated by cholinesterase inhibitors such as physostigmine

Additional Information Oral ingestion of 294 mg/kg of a 10% diazinon formulation associated with fatality; diazinon may prolong the effects of succinylcholine

Red blood cell cholinesterase and serum pseudocholinesterase may be depressed following acute or chronic organophosphate exposure; RBC cholinesterase is typically not analyzed by in-house laboratories, and is usually not available for consideration during acute management. Pseudocholinesterase levels may be rapidly available from some in-house laboratories, but are not as reliable a marker of organophosphate exposure because of variability secondary to variant genotypes, hepatic disease, oral estrogen use, or malnutrition. Because of this variability, true indication of suppression of either of these enzymes can only be estimated through comparison to pre-exposure values; these enzymes may be useful in measuring a patient's recovery postexposure, especially if the recovery is not progressing as expected.

The intermediate syndrome is not related to delayed neuropathy.

QT_c prolongation on ECG in the setting of organophosphate poisoning is associated with a high incidence of respiratory failure and mortality.

Yellow to brown liquid; vapor pressure: 0.00014 mm Hg at 20°C; thermal breakdown products include nitrogen and sulfur oxides

Water solubility: 40 ppm. Water half-life: 3 days to 7.7 weeks (shorter in acidic conditions)

Mean atmospheric diazinon levels in urban areas: 2.1 ng/m^3

ACGIH TLV: 0.1 mg/m^3; PEL-TWA: 0.1 mg/m^3

Other information concerning pesticide exposures is available through the EPA-funded National Pesticide Telecommunications Network: 1-800-858-7378 (weekdays, 8 AM to 6 PM, Central Standard time)

Specific References

Cho JH, Jeong SH and Yun HI, "Changes of Urinary and Blood Porphyrin Profiles by Exposure to PCBs, Lead or Diazinon in Rats," *Vet Hum Toxicol*, 2003, 45(4):193-8.

Dahlgren JG, Takhar HS, Ruffalo CA, et al, "Health Effects of Diazinon on a Family," *J Toxicol Clin Toxicol*, 2004, 42(5):579-91.

Knaak JB, Dary CC, Power F, et al, "Physicochemical and Biological Data for the Development of Predictive Organophosphorus Pesticide QSARs and PBPK/PD Models for Human Risk Assessment," *Crit Rev Toxicol*, 2004, 34(2):143-207.

Morrissey BF, Harter LC, Cropley JM, et al, "Residential Phaseout of Chlorpyrifos and Diazinon: Reductions in Reported Human Exposure Cases in Washington State," *J Toxicol Clin Toxicol*, 2004, 42(5):806-7.

Nesime Y, Lokman B, Akif IM, et al, "Acute Pesticide Poisoning Related Deaths in Turkey," *Vet Hum Toxicol*, 2004, 46(6):342-4.

Thompson B, Coronado GD, Grossman JE, et al, "Pesticide Take-Home Pathway Among Children of Agricultural Workers: Study Design, Methods, and Baseline Findings," *J Occup Environ Med*, 2003, 45(1):42-53.

Tutudaki M and Tsatsakis AM, "Pesticide Hair Analysis: Development of a GC-NCI-MS Method to Assess Chronic Exposure to Diazinon in Rats," *J Anal Toxicol*, 2005, 29(8):805-9.

Dibenzoyl Peroxide

CAS Number 94-36-0

UN Number 2085; 2086; 2087; 2088; 2089; 2090

Synonyms Benzoyl Peroxide; Lucidol

Use In concentrations of 5% to 10% topically for the treatment of acne, ulcers, bed sores, and pyoderma gangrenosum

Mechanism of Toxic Action Allergen for skin sensitization, enhances platelet aggregation

Adverse Reactions

Cardiovascular: Sinus bradycardia

Dermatologic: Dermal irritation, immunologic contact urticaria

Gastrointestinal: Irritation of throat

Hematologic: Can cause platelet aggregation (vitamin E may be of some use in preventing platelet aggregation)

Ocular: Eye irritation

Respiratory: Irritation of nose

Miscellaneous: May be a tumor promoter

Signs and Symptoms of Overdose Conjunctivitis, erythema, skin edema

Toxicodynamics/Kinetics

Absorption: Not well absorbed

Elimination: Metabolized to and excreted as benzoic acid (95%)

Overdosage/Treatment Decontamination: **Oral:** Dilution with 4-8 oz of milk or water. **Inhalation:** Give 100% humidified oxygen. **Dermal:** Irrigate with soap and water.

Additional Information Odorless gas, flammable and explosive. TLV-TWA: 5 mg/m^3; IDLH: 1000 mg/m^3; PEL-TWA: 5 mg/m^3

Diborane

CAS Number 19287-45-7

UN Number 1911

Synonyms Boroethane; Boron Hydride

Use Doping agent in semiconductors; strong reducing agent; used in rubber manufacture and rocket fuels

Mechanism of Toxic Action Pulmonary irritant (upper airway); a colorless gas

Adverse Reactions

Cardiovascular: Chest tightness

Central nervous system: Headache, chills, dizziness, fever

Gastrointestinal: Nausea

Neuromuscular & skeletal: Tremor, paresthesia

Respiratory: Cough, bronchospasm, tachypnea, pneumonitis, pulmonary edema

Overdosage/Treatment Decontamination: **Inhalation:** Administer 100% humidified oxygen.

Additional Information Hydrolyzes rapidly in water to hydrogen and boric acid; very flammable and may autoignite. Specific gravity: 0.21. Odor threshold (rotten egg): 2-4 ppm. IDLH: 40 ppm; TLV: 0.1 ppm

Dibromochloromethane

Related Information

- Adipose Tissue Ranges of Toxins
- Bromoform

CAS Number 124-48-1

Synonyms Chlorodibromomethane

Use Inadvertently generated during water chlorination process (usually <5 mcg/L; median: 1.2 mcg/L)

Mechanism of Toxic Action CNS depressant

Adverse Reactions No human data; hepatitis; hepatotoxic (centrilobular necrosis) in animal models; a central nervous system depressant with little long lasting behavioral effect

Toxicodynamics/Kinetics

Absorption: Absorbed by inhalation and oral routes

Metabolism: Hepatic oxidation

Elimination: Pulmonary

Overdosage/Treatment

Decontamination (oral overdose): Lavage (within 1 hour)/activated charcoal

Supportive therapy: Although human overdose experience is virtually nonexistent over the past 90 years, respiratory support appears to be a crucial modality. Naloxone may be of some benefit; otherwise, treat as for bromides.

Additional Information Not flammable; a colorless to pale yellow liquid. Mean ambient air chlorodibromomethane urban values: 3.8 ppt. Average daily dose: <1 mcg/kg. PEL-TWA: 0.5 ppm

Dichloronaphthoquinone

Applies to Disinfectant (Vegetable Seeds); Fungicide (Foliage/Textile); Herbicide (Aquatic)

CAS Number 117-80-6

U.S. Brand Names Algistat®; Compound 605®; Phygon®

Synonyms Dichlone; Quintar; Sanquinon

Use Vegetable seed disinfectant; foliage/textile fungicide; aquatic herbicide

Adverse Reactions

Dermatologic: Dermal irritation

Gastrointestinal: Nausea, vomiting

Ocular: Conjunctivitis

Signs and Symptoms of Overdose Coma, vomiting

Toxicodynamics/Kinetics Absorption: Poor from the GI tract

Overdosage/Treatment

Decontamination: Lavage (within 1 hour)/charcoal. Irrigate skin with soap and water. Irrigate eyes with saline with a Morgan lens.

Supportive therapy: Endoscopy for oral ingestion to evaluate gastrointestinal mucosal injury

Additional Information Heating dichloronaphthoquinone can emit chloride fumes.

Dichlorphenamide

Pronunciation (dye klor FEN a mide)

CAS Number 120-97-8

U.S. Brand Names Daranide®

Synonyms Diclofenamide

Use Adjunct in treatment of open-angle glaucoma and perioperative treatment for angle-closure glaucoma; also has been used to treat muscle weakness in patients with hypokalemic periodic paralysis resistant to acetazolamide

Mechanism of Action A nonbacteriostatic sulfonamide that inhibits carbonic anhydrase resulting in renal excretion of sodium potassium, bicarbonate, and water

Adverse Reactions

Central nervous system: **Tiredness, malaise**, CNS depression, disorientation, drowsiness, fever, **fatigue**, depression

Dermatologic: Rash, urticaria, erythema multiforme, toxic epidermal necrolysis

Endocrine & metabolic: Hyperchloremic metabolic acidosis, hypokalemia, elevated blood glucose

Gastrointestinal: **Diarrhea, anorexia, metallic taste**, GI irritation, xerostomia, black stools

Genitourinary: Dysuria, **increased urination**

Hematologic: Blood dyscrasias, bone marrow suppression

Neuromuscular & skeletal: Paresthesias

Ocular: Myopia

Renal: Renal calculi, polyuria

Toxicodynamics/Kinetics

Onset of action: 0.1-5 hours

Peak effect: 2-4 hours

Duration: 6-12 hours

Distribution: Wide volume of distribution

Dosage

Oral:

Adults: 100-200 mg to start followed by 100 mg every 12 hours until desired response is obtained; maintenance dose: 25-50 mg 1-3 times/day

Hypokalemic periodic paralysis: 50 mg 2 twice daily for 1 week then 50 mg 3 times/day

Contraindications Hypersensitivity to dichlorphenamide or any component of the formulation; severe pulmonary obstruction; severe renal impairment

Warnings Chemical similarities are present among sulfonamides, sulfonylureas, carbonic anhydrase inhibitors, thiazides, and loop diuretics (except ethacrynic acid). In patients with allergy to one of these compounds, a risk of cross-reaction exists; avoid use when previous reaction has been severe.

Dosage Forms Tablet: 50 mg

Overdosage/Treatment

Decontamination: Lavage (within 1 hour)/activated charcoal

Enhancement of elimination: Hemodialysis may remove as much as 30% of dose if performed prior to significant distribution

Test Interactions ↑ chloride (S); ↓ potassium; false-positive urinary protein

Drug Interactions Increased lithium excretion and altered excretion of other drugs by alkalinization of the urine

Pregnancy Risk Factor C

Nursing Implications May cause drowsiness, institute safety measures

Additional Information More potent than acetazolamide

Dichlorvos

Applies to SD 1750

CAS Number 11095-17-3; 11096-21-2; 116788-91-1; 12772-40-6; 55819-32-4; 62-73-7; 62139-95-1; 95828-55-0

UN Number 2783

U.S. Brand Names Astrobot®; Atgard®; Canogard®; Duo-Kill®

Synonyms DDVP

Use Organophosphate insecticide (which is a breakdown product of trichlorfon); usually used to control insects in warehouses (tobacco, mushroom, animal shelters) and also is an active ingredient in flea collars for dogs and cats

Mechanism of Toxic Action Irreversible inhibition of acetylcholinesterase and plasma cholinesterase, resulting in excess accumulation of acetylcholine at muscarinic and nicotinic receptors, and in the central nervous system

Adverse Reactions

Cardiovascular: **Hyperdynamic** (~18% to 21%) or hypodynamic (~7% to 10%) states; edema, QT prolongation

Central nervous system: Depression, seizures, hyperactivity, cognitive dysfunction, hypothermia

Genitourinary: Urinary incontinence

Neuromuscular & skeletal: Weakness (delayed), paralysis, delayed paresthesia, polyneuropathy, Horner's syndrome

Respiratory: Respiratory depression

Miscellaneous: Flu-like symptoms (especially with chronic exposure)

Signs and Symptoms of Overdose

Abdominal pain, agitation, asystole, bronchorrhea, AV block, bradycardia, coma, confusion, cranial nerve palsies, decreased hemoglobin, decreased platelet count, decreased red blood cell count, diaphragmatic paralysis, dysarthria, excessive sweating, fecal and urinary incontinence, generalized asthenia, headache, heart block, hypertension, hypotension, lacrimation, metabolic acidosis and hyperglycemia (severe intoxication), miosis (unreactive to light), mydriasis (rarely), nausea, pallor, pulmonary edema, QT prolongation, respiratory depression, salivation, seizures, skeletal muscle fasciculation and flaccid paralysis, tachycardia, tachypnea, vomiting

An "intermediate syndrome" of limb asthenia and respiratory paralysis has been reported to occur between 24-96 hours postorganophosphate exposure, and is independent of the acute cholinergic crisis; late paresthesia characterized by stocking and glove paresthesia, anesthesia, and asthenia is infrequently observed weeks to months following acute exposure to certain organophosphates; symptoms may be delayed for 3 hours

Admission Criteria/Prognosis Any symptomatic patient or an asymptomatic patient following a severe exposure should be admitted probably into an intensive care unit; asymptomatic patients following a moderate exposure can be discharged after 8 hours of observation

Toxicodynamics/Kinetics

Absorption: Rapid

Half-life: 8-20 minutes

Elimination: 27% eliminated as CO_2 in lungs; 9% in urine

Overdosage/Treatment

Decontamination: Isolation, bagging, and disposal of all contaminated clothing and other articles. All emergency medical workers and hospital staff should follow appropriate precautions regarding exposure to hazardous material including the use of protective clothing, masks, goggles, and respiratory equipment. Gastric lavage with water, 5% sodium bicarbonate or 2% potassium permanganate can be considered within 1 hour of ingestion. **Do not** use a cathartic with activated charcoal.

Oral: Activated charcoal can be administered either orally or via a nasogastric tube. **Do not** induce emesis because of danger of sudden respiratory compromise, alterations in mental status, seizures, coma, and possible aspiration of hydrocarbon vehicles.

Dermal: Prompt thorough scrubbing of all affected areas with soap and water, including hair and nails; 5% bleach can be used

Ocular: Irrigation with copious tepid sterile water or saline

Supportive therapy: Airway management, ventilatory assistance, humidified oxygen administration, and close monitoring for sudden respiratory failure. Asoxime chloride or HI-6 (an experimental oxime) has been used effectively in reactivating red blood cell cholinesterase (at a dose of 500 mg dissolved in 3 mL of distilled water, I.M. 4 times/day for 2-7 days) in 60 patients with dichlorvos poisoning. Therapeutic serum level of HI-6: ~4 mcg/mL; it may act synergistically when given with atropine; total dosage of HI-6 ranged from 4-14 g; no adverse symptoms were noted.

Antidote:

Atropine: Administration should be guided by respiratory status, starting at 2-5 mg I.V. every 5-10 minutes as needed, and should be titrated to the resolution of excess pulmonary secretions. Frequent administration of large doses (cumulative doses >100 mg) may be necessary in massive exposures

Glycopyrrolate: May be administered if atropine is unavailable (200-400 mcg I.M. or I.V. initially, or ~1/2 the dose of atropine).

2-PAM: For more significant exposures (ie, exposures requiring large doses of atropine, or with recurring symptoms, or exposures to more lipid soluble agents), administration should follow: 1-2 g I.V. over 10-30 minutes, repeated in 1 hour if asthenia recurs, then every 4-12 hours for recurring symptoms.

Enhancement of elimination: Dialysis and hemoperfusion are not indicated due to effectiveness of the prescribed antidotal treatment and large volumes of distribution of organophosphates.

Antidote(s)
- Atropine [ANTIDOTE]
- Pralidoxime [ANTIDOTE]

Additional Information

Toxic dose: 300 mg/kg. Lethal oral dose: 400 mg/kg

Red blood cell cholinesterase, and serum pseudocholinesterase may be depressed following acute or chronic organophosphate exposure; RBC cholinesterase is typically not analyzed by in-house laboratories, and is usually not available for consideration during acute management. Pseudocholinesterase levels may be rapidly available from some in-house laboratories, but are not as reliable a marker of organophosphate exposure because of variability secondary to variant genotypes, hepatic disease, oral estrogen use, or malnutrition. Because of this variability, true indication of suppression of either of these enzymes can only be estimated through comparison to pre-exposure values; these enzymes may be useful in measuring a patient's recovery postexposure, especially if the recovery is not progressing as expected.

Threshold dose that would produce reduction of plasma cholinesterase (but not red blood cell cholinesterase) is ~0.03 mg/kg/day by inhalation (0.006 mg/kg/day in patients with liver disease) and 0.02 mg/kg/day by oral ingestion

QT_c prolongation on ECG in the setting of organophosphate poisoning is associated with a high incidence of respiratory failure and mortality.

Emits a sulfur (garlic) odor at airborne concentrations >1 ppb.

The intermediate syndrome is not related to delayed neuropathy.

Colorless to amber liquid; does not bioaccumulate in the human body

Estimated atmospheric half-life: 2-320 days. Soil half-life: 10-17 days.

Specific gravity: 1.415

TLV-TWA: 0.9 mg/m^3 (skin)

Malathion may potentiate the toxicity of dichlorvos.

Other information concerning pesticide exposures is available through the EPA-funded National Pesticide Telecommunications Network: 1-800-858-7378 (weekdays, 8 AM to 6 PM, Central Standard time)

Specific References

Arima H, Sobue K, So M, et al, "Transient and Reversible Parkinsonism After Acute Organophosphate Poisoning," *J Toxicol Clin Toxicol*, 2003, 41(1):67-70.

Bird SB, Dickson EW, Gaspari RJ, et al, "Brain Functional MRI After Acute Organophosphate Poisoning," *Acad Emerg Med*, 2004, 11(5):473.

Bird SB, Gaspari RJ, and Dickson EW, "Early Death Due to Severe Organophosphate Poisoning Is a Centrally Mediated Process," *Acad Emerg Med*, 2003, 10(4):295-8.

Bird SB, Gaspari RJ, Lee WJ, et al, "Diphenhydramine as a Protective Agent in Severe Organophosphate Poisoning," *Acad Emerg Med*, 2002, 9(5):357-8.

Bird SB, Gaspari RJ, Lee WJ, et al, "Early Death Due to Severe Organophosphate Poisoning Is a Centrally-Mediated Process," *Acad Emerg Med*, 2002, 9(5):485.

Brahmi N, Gueye PN, Thabet H, et al, "Extrapyramidal Syndrome as a Delayed and Reversible Complication of Acute Dichlorvos Organophosphate Poisoning," *Vet Hum Toxicol*, 46(4):187-88.

Bryant SM, Wills BK, Rhee J, et al, "Intramuscular Ophthalmic Homatropine vs Atropine to Prevent Lethality in Rats with Dichlorvos Poisoning," *Clin Toxicol (Phila)*, 2005, 43:694.

Bryant SM, Wills BK, Rhee JW, et al, "Intramuscular Ophthalmic Homatropine vs Atropine to Prevent Lethality in Rats with Dichlorvos Poisoning," *J Med Toxicol*, 2006, 2(4):156-59.

Gaspari RJ and Paydarfar D, "Respiratory Failure Following Acute Organophosphate Poisoning Is Not Vagally Mediated," *Acad Emerg Med*, 2006, 13(5):S179.

Guloglu C, Aldemir M, Orak M, et al, "Dichlorvos Poisoning After Intramuscular Injection," *Am J Emerg Med*, 2004, 22(4):328-30.

Lee EY, Gil HW, Yang JO, et al, "A Case of Horner's Polyneuropathy Due to Dichlorvos Intoxication," *Clin Toxicol*, 2006, 44:197-9.

Schaeffer TH, Hung OL, and Shih RD, "Comparison of Diphenhydramine, Glycopyrrolate, and Atropine in the Treatment of Organophosphate-Poisoned Mice," *J Toxicol Clin Toxicol*, 2004, 42(5):797-8.

Sivilotti MLA, Bird SB, Lo CT, et al, "Multiple Centrally-Acting Antidotes Protect Against Severe Organophosphate Toxicity," *Acad Emerg Med*, 2006, 13:359-64.

Dicrotophos

CAS Number 141-66-2

U.S. Brand Names Bidrin®; Ektofos®

Synonyms Dimethyl *cis*-2-Dimethylcarbamoyl-1-Methylvinyl Phosphate

Use Marketed as insecticide granules, dusting agent, or spray liquid with or without petroleum derivative as a solvent

Mechanism of Toxic Action Potent, irreversible inhibition of acetylcholinesterase and plasma cholinesterase, resulting in excess accumulation of acetylcholine at muscarinic and nicotinic receptors, and in the central nervous system

Adverse Reactions

Cardiovascular: **Hyperdynamic** (~18% to 21%) or hypodynamic (~7% to 10%) states, QT prolongation, sinus bradycardia, sinus tachycardia

Central nervous system: Depression, seizures, hyperactivity, cognitive dysfunction, hypothermia

Genitourinary: Urinary incontinence

Neuromuscular & skeletal: Weakness (delayed), paralysis, delayed paresthesia

Respiratory: Pulmonary edema, respiratory depression

Miscellaneous: Flu-like symptoms (especially with chronic exposure)

Signs and Symptoms of Overdose Abdominal pain, agitation, asystole, AV block, bradycardia, bronchorrhea, coma, confusion, cranial nerve palsies, decreased hemoglobin, decreased platelet count, decreased red blood cell count, diaphragmatic paralysis, dysarthria, fecal and urinary incontinence, excessive sweating, generalized asthenia, headache, heart block, hypertension, hypotension, lacrimation, metabolic acidosis and hyperglycemia (severe intoxication), miosis (unreactive to light), mydriasis (rarely), nausea, pallor, pulmonary edema, QT prolongation, salivation, seizures, skeletal muscle fasciculation and flaccid paralysis, tachycardia, tachypnea, respiratory depression, vomiting

An "intermediate syndrome" of limb asthenia and respiratory paralysis has been reported to occur between 24 and 96 hours postorganophosphate exposure, and is independent of the acute cholinergic crisis. Late paresthesia characterized by stocking and glove paresthesia, anesthesia, and asthenia is infrequently observed weeks to months following acute exposure to certain organophosphates

Toxicodynamics/Kinetics

Absorption: Readily through oral, dermal, or respiratory exposure

Metabolism: Rapidly metabolized to weakly active compounds through hepatic hydrolysis and other pathways

Elimination: Metabolites are excreted in urine

Warnings/Precautions Significant absorption through intact skin may occur; risk of aspiration pneumonitis exists with agents having a hydrocarbon vehicle; severe laryngeal irritation and violent coughing may result from exposure to dusting powders; exposure to dusting powders and insecticide granules may cause contact dermatitis

Overdosage/Treatment

Decontamination: Isolation, bagging, and disposal of all contaminated clothing and other articles. All emergency medical workers and hospital staff should follow appropriate precautions regarding exposure to hazardous material including the use of protective clothing, masks, goggles, and respiratory equipment

Oral: Activated charcoal can be administered either orally or via a nasogastric tube. **Do not** induce emesis because of danger of sudden respiratory compromise, alterations in mental status, seizures, coma, and possible aspiration of hydrocarbon vehicles. **Do not** give a cathartic.

Dermal: Prompt thorough scrubbing of all affected areas with soap and water, including hair and nails; 5% bleach may be used

Ocular: Irrigation with copious tepid sterile water or saline

Supportive therapy: Airway management, ventilatory assistance, humidified oxygen administration, and close monitoring for sudden respiratory failure

Enhancement of elimination: Dialysis and hemoperfusion are not indicated due to effectiveness of the prescribed treatment and large volumes of distribution of organophosphates.

Antidote:

Atropine: Administration should be guided by respiratory status, starting at 2-5 mg I.V. every 5-10 minutes as needed, and should be titrated to the resolution of excess pulmonary secretions. Frequent administration of large doses (cumulative doses >100 mg) may be necessary in massive exposures.

Glycopyrrolate: May be administered if atropine is unavailable (200-400 mcg I.M. or I.V. initially, or ~$^1/_2$ the dose of atropine).

2-PAM: For more significant exposures (ie, exposures requiring large doses of atropine, or with recurring symptoms, or exposures to more lipid soluble agents), administration should follow: 1-2 g I.V. over 10-30 minutes, repeated in 1 hour if asthenia recurs, then every 4-12 hours for recurring symptoms.

Antidote(s)
- Atropine [ANTIDOTE]
- Pralidoxime [ANTIDOTE]

Diagnostic Procedures
- Creatinine, Serum
- Pseudocholinesterase, Serum

Drug Interaction Paralysis is potentiated by neuromuscular blockade (ie, pancuronium, vecuronium, succinylcholine, atracurium, doxacurium, mivacurium); inhibition of serum esterase prolongs the half-life of succinylcholine, cocaine, and other ester anesthetics; cholinergic toxicity is potentiated by cholinesterase inhibitors such as physostigmine

Additional Information Brown liquid with mild ester odor; red blood cell cholinesterase, and serum pseudocholinesterase may be depressed following acute or chronic organophosphate exposure; RBC cholinesterase is typically not analyzed by in-house laboratories, and is usually not available for consideration during acute management. Pseudocholinesterase levels may be rapidly available from some in-house laboratories, but are not as reliable a marker of organophosphate exposure because of variability secondary to variant genotypes, hepatic disease, oral estrogen use, or malnutrition. Because of this variability, true indication of suppression of either of these enzymes can only be estimated through comparison to pre-exposure values; these enzymes may be useful in measuring a patient's recovery postexposure, especially if the recovery is not progressing as expected.

The intermediate syndrome is not related to delayed neuropathy.

QT_c prolongation on ECG in the setting of organophosphate poisoning is associated with a high incidence of respiratory failure and mortality.

ACGIH TLV: 0.25 mg/m^3; PEL-TWA: 0.25 mg/m^3

Other information concerning pesticide exposures is available through the EPA-funded National Pesticide Telecommunications Network: 1-800-858-7378 (weekdays, 8 AM to 6 PM, Central Standard time)

Dieldrin

Related Information
- Adipose Tissue Ranges of Toxins
- Aldrin

CAS Number 60-57-1

U.S. Brand Names Alvit®; Dieldrix®; Octalox®; Quintox®; Red Shield®

Synonyms HEOD

Use Termiticide; banned by EPA in 1970s

Mechanism of Toxic Action Organochlorine agent which may be a competitive inhibitor of the inhibitory neurotransmitter GABA at the GABA A receptor

Adverse Reactions

Cardiovascular: Tachycardia, hypertension, sinus tachycardia

Central nervous system: Convulsions, headache, dizziness, seizures

Dermatologic: Contact dermatitis

Gastrointestinal: Nausea, vomiting, anorexia

Hematologic: Hemolysis

Hepatic: Elevated liver enzymes

Neuromuscular & skeletal: Muscle twitching

Ocular: Nystagmus, optic neuropathy, scotoma, visual evoked potential abnormalities

Miscellaneous: May increase serum cholesterol levels

Toxicodynamics/Kinetics

Absorption: Absorbed by oral and dermal routes

Distribution: V_d: 13-69 L/kg

Metabolism: By epoxide hydrase to 6,7-trans-dihydroxydihydroaldrin glucuronide; aldrin dicarboxylic acid; also metabolized to pentachloroketone (Klein's metabolite) and 9-hydroxydieldrin glucuronide

Half-life: 2-12 months

Elimination: Feces

Overdosage/Treatment

Decontamination: **Oral:** Activated charcoal. **Dermal:** Soap and water wash. **Ocular:** Irrigate with saline.

Supportive therapy: Beta-adrenergic blocking agents may be used for tachycardia or hypertension. Benzodiazepines, phenobarbital, or phenytoin can be used for seizures.

Enhancement of elimination: Multiple dosing of activated charcoal may be effective.

Additional Information Lethal dose: Oral: 71 mg/kg. Highest dietary intake is from garden fruits (0.0021 mcg/day), fish, poultry, and meat (0.0012 mcg/day). Odor threshold: 0.047 mg/kg. Estimated atmospheric lifetime: 1 day

Diethyl Phthalate

Related Information
- Adipose Tissue Ranges of Toxins

CAS Number 84-66-2

U.S. Brand Names Anozol®; Neantine®; Palatinol® A; Phthalol®; Placidol® E; Solvanol®

Synonyms DEP; Ethyl Phthalate

Use Plasticizer (photographic applications, toothbrushes, toys, tool handles) and in cosmetics (nail polish, hair spray, perfume, bath products)

Mechanism of Toxic Action Irritant

Adverse Reactions Dermatologic: Dermal irritant, allergic contact dermatitis

Toxicodynamics/Kinetics Absorption: Slightly through intact human skin

Overdosage/Treatment Decontamination: **Dermal:** Wash with soap and water. **Ocular:** Irrigate copiously with water.

Diethylene Glycol

CAS Number 111-46-6

Synonyms Diglycol; Ethylene Diglycol; Glycol Ether

Commonly Found In Industrial solvents and antifreeze; softening agent in cellophane; in silver sulfadiazine; A Plasticizer

Mechanism of Toxic Action Central nervous system depression and nephrotoxicity with intravascular hemolysis, mechanism unknown

Adverse Reactions

Hepatic: Hepatotoxicity

Renal: Renal tubular necrosis (acute); renal failure due to bilateral cortical necrosis (onset 2 to 6 days)

Signs and Symptoms of Overdose Coma and pulmonary edema can develop; metabolic acidosis is less common than with ethylene glycol; diarrhea, drowsiness, feces discoloration (black), hepatotoxicity, jaundice, leukocytosis, porphyria, tachypnea; Onset may be delayed for 1-2 days

Toxicodynamics/Kinetics

Absorption: Small amount may be absorbed dermally; not absorbed by inhalation

Metabolism: Oxidized by alcohol dehydrogenase and aldehyde dehydrogenase to 2-hydroxyethoxy-acetaldehyde and then to 2-hydroxy-ethoxyacetic acid (2-HEAA)

Half-life: 3 hours

Elimination: 70% excreted unchanged; major metabolite is (2-hydroxyethoxy) acetic acid

Overdosage/Treatment

Decontamination: **Do not** induce emesis; lavage (within 2 hours/activated charcoal)

Supportive therapy: Ethanol therapy may be theoretically useful to block conversion to toxic metabolites, but there is no human experience. Treat acidosis with I.V. sodium bicarbonate (1-2 mEq/kg). 4-Methylpyrazole (10 mg/kg body weight, I.V.) over a 1-hour period and repeated in 2 hours has been helpful in one case.

Enhancement of elimination: Hemodialysis for severe metabolic disturbance or renal failure

Antidote(s)
- Sodium Bicarbonate [ANTIDOTE]

Diagnostic Procedures
- Osmolality, Serum

Additional Information Diethylene glycol is colorless and odorless but has a sweet taste; more toxic than ethylene glycol. A radiopaque compound with rapid absorption. Can cause centrilobular necrosis of the liver. Average amount of diethylene glycol in PEG: 4.3 mcg/mL; average amount consumed in a patient is ~11 mg.

Specific References

Alfred S, Coleman P, Harris D, et al, "Delayed Neurologic Sequelae Resulting from Epidemic Diethylene Glycol Poisoning," *Clin Toxicol (Phila)*, 2005, 43(3):155-9.

Casas R, Ruck B, and Marcus S, "A Case of Diethylene Glycol Ingestion Treated Successfully with Blocking Therapy and Dialysis," *Clin Toxicol (Phila)*, 2005, 43:741.

Marraffa JM, Holland MG, Stork CM, et al, "Multi-Organ Effects After Intentional Diethylene Glycol Ingestion," *Clin Toxicol (Phila)*, 2005, 43:690.

Diethylene Glycol Monobutyl Ether

CAS Number 112-34-5

Synonyms Butoxyethoxy Ethanol; Butyl Carbitol; Butyl Digol; Butyl Diicinol

Use Low foaming cleaning agent; solvent for cellulose nitrate; oil, dye, rubber, soap, and printing industry

Mechanism of Toxic Action A monoalkyl ether of diethylene glycol can cause mild mucosal irritation with some nephrotoxic potential

Signs and Symptoms of Overdose Conjunctivitis, cyanosis, dermal erythema on contact, increased intraocular pressure, renal failure, tachypnea, uremia

Admission Criteria/Prognosis Admit any symptomatic patient or any ingestion >2 mL/kg

Toxicodynamics/Kinetics Absorption: Some dermal absorption can occur (0.035 mg/cm²/hour)

Monitoring Parameters Renal function: Arterial blood gas

Overdosage/Treatment

Decontamination: **Oral:** Emesis within 30 minutes or lavage with ingestions >2 mL/kg within 2 hours of ingestion; activated charcoal may be effective. **Dermal:** Wash with soap and water. **Inhalation:** Give 100% humidified oxygen. **Ocular:** Irrigate copiously with saline.

Supportive therapy: Ethanol treatment should **not** be utilized.

Additional Information Rise in intraocular pressure is usually transient in animal studies (lasting <1 hour). Ocular toxicity is probably dose related with the threshold for production of keratitis and conjunctivitis at 25% and 10% concentration, respectively. A colorless, odorless liquid with a specific gravity of 0.95; miscible in water and oils; flammable. IDLH: 700 ppm; OSHA: PEL: 1 ppm

Diisopropylmethylphosphonate

CAS Number 1445-75-6

Synonyms DIMP

Use A byproduct (2% to 3%) in the manufacture process of the nerve gas sarin (GB); used in the military as a stimulant in chemical warfare training

Mechanism of Toxic Action Essentially unknown; while this agent is an organophosphate compound, acetylcholinesterase inhibition is minimal; central nervous system toxicity is major effect in animal studies

Adverse Reactions

No human data available

Central nervous system: Ataxia noted in animal studies

Ocular: Eye irritation

Toxicodynamics/Kinetics

Absorption: Orally and somewhat dermally (7% in animal studies)

Metabolism: Hydrolysis to isopropyl methylphosphonic acid and methylphosphonic acid (does not accumulate in the body)

Elimination: Renal

Overdosage/Treatment

Decontamination: **Oral:** Lavage/activated charcoal. **Dermal:** Remove contaminated clothing, wash skin with soap and water. **Ocular:** Irrigate eyes with saline.

Supportive therapy: It is unclear whether treatment with atropine/pralidoxime would be helpful.

Enhanced elimination: Hemoperfusion with a grafted butyl-XAD-4 sorbent may be most efficacious.

Additional Information Colorless liquid with a boiling point of 174°C; density: 0.976 g/mL. Slightly soluble in water; negligible human exposure due to vaporization from surface water; degrades slowly in the environment. Was manufactured as a byproduct of sarin at the Rocky Mountain Arsenal (RMA) near Denver, Colorado from 1953-1957.

Dimethyl Phthalate

Related Information
- Di-n-Butyl Phthalate

CAS Number 131-11-3

Synonyms Avolin

Use Insect repellent

Mechanism of Toxic Action Mucosal irritant

Adverse Reactions

Ocular: Eye pain

Respiratory: Oropharyngeal burning

Overdosage/Treatment Decontamination: **Oral:** Lavage (within 1 hour)/activated charcoal. **Dermal:** Wash exposed area with soap and water. **Ocular:** Irrigate with water or saline. **Inhalation:** Administer 100% humidified oxygen.

Additional Information Oral LD$_{50}$ in rats: 2400 mg/kg. Dibutylphthalate is more resistant to laundering removal in fabrics than dimethyl phthalate.

Dimethylnitrosamine

CAS Number 62-75-9

Synonyms DMN; DMNA; NDMA; Nitrous Dimethylamine

Use Formerly used as a solvent in the production of rubbers, plastics, rocket fuels and lubricants, this agent may be found as an environmental pollutant and in nitrate-cured meats

Mechanism of Toxic Action As a potent methylating agent; this compound is hepatotoxic and liver or renal carcinogen (in animals)

Adverse Reactions

Cardiovascular: Cerebral edema

Central nervous system: Fever (oral exposure), seizures, headache, malaise

Gastrointestinal: Prolonged vomiting (for up to 2 days), GI hemorrhage

Hematologic: Coagulopathy, thrombocytopenia

Hepatic: Icterus, hepatomegaly, hepatic necrosis, centrilobular necrosis, ascites, hepatic fibrosis

Ocular: Photophobia, conjunctivitis, uveitis

Respiratory: Pulmonary edema, pulmonary hemorrhage

Admission Criteria/Prognosis Admit any ingestion >10 mg/kg or any symptomatic patient

Toxicodynamics/Kinetics

Absorption: Oral, dermal and inhalation

Metabolism: Hepatic to metabolites which may be carcinogenic (methyl carbonium ion)

Monitoring Parameters PT, PTT, liver function tests, CBC, chest x-ray

Overdosage/Treatment

Decontamination: **Oral:Do not** induce emesis. Lavage (within 1 hour)/ activated charcoal. **Dermal:** Remove clothing, wash skin with soap and water. **Inhalation:** Administer 100% humidified oxygen. **Ocular:** Irrigate copiously with water or saline.

Supportive therapy: Benzodiazepines can be initially used for seizures. Phenytoin or phenobarbital can be used for refractory seizures.

Additional Information Potential lethal oral dose: Child: 30 mg/kg; Adult: 1.8 g. A yellow, oily liquid; pretreatment with ethanol may increase hepatotoxicity.

Di-n-Butyl Phthalate

Related Information
- Dimethyl Phthalate

Applies to Caswell No 292; Glow-in-the-Dark Products; Insect Repellent; Plasticizer; Solvent

CAS Number 84-74-2

UN Number 9095

U.S. Brand Names Staflex® DBP; Uniflex® DBP

Synonyms Butylphthalate; DBP; Dibutyl Ester; Dibutyl Phthalate

Use Plasticizer for polyvinyl chloride; insect repellent, also used as a solvent for perfume oils; concrete additive; in plastisol formulations for carpets; a solvent for nail polish; found in glow-in-the-dark wands and necklaces

Mechanism of Toxic Action Uncouples oxidative phosphorylation

Adverse Reactions

Cardiovascular: Hypertension

Central nervous system: Dizziness, coma, polyneuritis

Dermatologic: Allergic dermatitis

Gastrointestinal: Nausea

Ocular: Keratitis, photophobia, lacrimation

Renal: Nephritis

Signs and Symptoms of Overdose Asthenia, dizziness (after a 10 g ingestion), lacrimation, ocular irritation, photophobia, spasms

Admission Criteria/Prognosis Admit any symptomatic patient

Toxicodynamics/Kinetics

Absorption: Inhalation: Well absorbed. Dermal: Absorbed slowly through intact skin (0.07 mcg/cm^2/hour)

Metabolism: Hepatic hydrolysis to phthalic acid and butanol

Overdosage/Treatment Decontamination: **Oral:** Dilute with water; lavage (within 1 hour)/activated charcoal. **Dermal:** Wash exposed area with soap and water. **Inhalation:** Administer 100% oxygen. **Ocular:** Irrigate with water or saline.

Additional Information Seasonal peak exposure for glow compound is July. Bitter taste. Specific gravity: 1.05. TLV-TWA: 5 mg/m^3; IDLH: 9,300 mg/m^3

Dinitrocresol

CAS Number 497-56-3; 534-52-1; 609-93-8; 616-73-9

UN Number 1598

U.S. Brand Names Antinonnin®; Detal®; Dinitrol®; Ditrosol®; Elgetol®; Selinon®; Sinox®; Victoria Orange®

Synonyms DNC; DNOC; DNPC

Use Contact herbicide (for broad leaf weeds); insecticide useful against locusts; fungicide; unapproved for weight reduction earlier this century

Mechanism of Toxic Action Uncouples oxidative phosphorylation

Adverse Reactions

Cardiovascular: Tachycardia, sinus tachycardia

Central nervous system: Lethargy, seizures, headaches, hyperthermia

Dermatologic: Yellow stains on skin, rash, mild dermal irritant, fingernail discoloration (yellow)

Gastrointestinal: Nausea

Neuromuscular & skeletal: Acrodynia

Ocular: Cataracts

Respiratory: Tachypnea, dyspnea

Miscellaneous: Diaphoresis

Toxicodynamics/Kinetics

Absorption: Inhalation, oral (40%), and by dermal routes

Metabolism: Hepatic

Half-life: 5-6 days

Reference Range Serum dinitrocresol (ortho) level of 1000 mcg/mL associated with fatality; toxic blood levels if exposed to >30 ppm

Overdosage/Treatment

Decontamination: **Oral:Do not** induce emesis; lavage (within 1 hour)/ activated charcoal. Castor oil (nonpurgative dose) may reduce absorption by almost 50%. **Dermal:** Wash with soap and water. **Ocular:** Irrigate with copious amounts of saline.

Supportive therapy: Benzodiazepine for seizure control; chlorpromazine (high doses), salicylates, barbiturates, or anticholinergic agents can potentiate toxicity of dinitrocresol. Reduce body temperature by means of sponge baths or lavage with cold solutions. Haloperidol use (in competing with binding sites) is experimental. Ten mL of a 2.5% solution (I.V.) of sodium methyl thiouracil has been claimed to reduce the metabolic rate induced by dinitrocresol, although this is unproven.

Enhancement of elimination: Dialysis or forced diuresis is not helpful.

Additional Information Toxic oral dose: >0.75 mg/kg/day. After death, rigor mortis develops rapidly.

Dinitrophenols

CAS Number 25550-58-7; 329-71-5; 51-28-5; 573-56-8; 577-71-9; 586-11-8; 66-56-8

UN Number 1320; 1599

Use In synthesis of dyes and organic chemicals; pesticide, herbicide, fungicide, and acaricide; pH reagent; potassium and ammonium ion detection; wood preservative; World War I explosive agent; had been used against lice; also used in weight control (100 mg 3 times/day) in the 1930s

Mechanism of Toxic Action Uncouples oxidative phosphorylation

Adverse Reactions

Cardiovascular: Tachycardia, shock

Central nervous system: Lethargy, seizures, headache, fever, hyperthermia, coma, sedation

Dermatologic: Yellow stains on skin, rash, mild dermal irritant

Endocrine & metabolic: Acidosis

Gastrointestinal: Nausea, vomiting, feces discoloration (yellow), hypogeusia, salt hypogeusia

Hematologic: Neutropenia, hemolytic anemia, methemoglobinemia (by 2,4 dinitrophenol only), agranulocytosis, aplastic anemia

Hepatic: Hepatic injury, jaundice

Neuromuscular & skeletal: Peripheral neuritis, neuropathy (peripheral)

Ocular: Cataracts, increased intraocular pressure, nystagmus, blurred vision

Renal: Oliguria, renal failure

Respiratory: Tachypnea, dyspnea, hyperventilation

Miscellaneous: Diaphoresis

Admission Criteria/Prognosis Any patient with change in mental status, cardiopulmonary complaints, or methemoglobin levels >30% should be admitted; asymptomatic patients with methemoglobin levels <30% may be considered for discharge after 6 hours of observation and if methemoglobin levels fall to <15% or oral dose over 3 mg/kg

Toxicodynamics/Kinetics

Absorption: Dermal and oral routes

Metabolism: Hepatic to aminonitrophenols

Half-life: 5-14 days

Elimination: Hepatic

Reference Range

Blood dinitrophenol level >10 mcg/mL associated with toxicity; blood dinitrophenol levels >28 mcg/mL associated with fatality

Postmortem Blood Dinitrophenol level of 48 mg/L associated with fatality. Toxicity associated with serum and urine DNP levels of 11 and 37 mg/L, respectively

Overdosage/Treatment

Decontamination: **Oral:Do not** induce emesis; lavage (within 1 hour)/ activated charcoal. Castor oil (nonpurgative dose) may reduce absorption by almost 50%. **Dermal:** Wash with soap and water. **Ocular:** Irrigate with copious amounts of saline.

Supportive therapy: Benzodiazepine for seizure control. Chlorpromazine (high doses), salicylates, barbiturates, or anticholinergic agents can potentiate the toxicity of dinitrocresol. Reduce body temperature by means of sponge baths, ice packs, or lavage with cold solutions. Haloperidol use (in competing with binding sites) is experimental. Ten mL of a 2.5% solution (intravenous) of sodium methyl thiouracil has been claimed to reduce the metabolic rate induced by dinitrocresol, although this is unproven. Methemoglobinemia can be treated with methylene blue. Dantrolene can be used to treat hyperthermia.

Enhancement of elimination: Dialysis or forced diuresis is not helpful.

Additional Information Toxic oral dose: 3-5 mg/kg. Atmospheric half-life: Probably exceeds 1 month; does not accumulate in the body; fatal dose: 1 g

Specific References

Hsiao AL, Santucci KA, Seo-Mayer P, et al, "Pediatric Fatality Following Ingestion of Dinitrophenol: Postmortem Identification of a Dietary Supplement," *Clin Toxicol (Phila)*, 2005, 43(4):281-5.

Miranda EJ, McIntyre IM, Parker DR, et al, "Two Deaths Attributed to the Use of 2,4-Dinitrophenol," *J Anal Tox*, 2006, 30:219-22.

Politi L, Vignali C and Polettini A, "LC-MS-MS Analysis of 2,4-Dinitrophenol and Its Phase I and II Metabolites in a Case of Fatal Poisoning," *J Anal Toxicol*, 2007, 31:55-61.

Di-n-Octylphthalate

CAS Number 117-84-0

U.S. Brand Names Celluflux DOP®; Dinopol NOP®; Polycizer 162®; PX-138®; Vinicizer 85®

Synonyms DNOP; DOP; Phthalic Acid, Dioctyl Ester

Use Colorless, odorless chemical primarily used as a plasticizer in plastics and PVC resin production; active ingredient in pesticides and can be found in electrical capacitor fluid and plastisols for carpetback coating

Mechanism of Toxic Action Hepatotoxin which causes centrilobular necrosis and accumulation of fat; loss of glycogen has also been noted

Adverse Reactions No human health effects noted, while this agent is a skin and eye irritant, the liver appears to be the target organ of toxicity with centrilobular fat accumulation and glycogen loss; can also serve as a promoter that results in hepatic adenomas and carcinomas

Toxicodynamics/Kinetics

Absorption: Primarily oral; not significantly absorbed by dermal or inhalation route

Metabolism: Hepatic hydrolysis to mono-n-octylphthalate beta oxidation then occurs to form phthalate monoesters

Half-life: 20 minutes (I.V. administration)

Elimination: Renal

Monitoring Parameters Liver function tests, glucose

Overdosage/Treatment Decontamination: **Oral:** Dilute with milk or water; activated charcoal can be utilized. **Dermal:** Wash with soap and water. **Ocular:** Copious irrigation with saline.

Additional Information Lethal oral dose: ~0.5-15 g/kg. Levels of di-n-octylphthalate in drinking water: <0.5 ppb. Atmospheric half-life: 4.5-4.8 hours. TLV-TWA: 5 mg/m^3

Dioxathion

CAS Number 78-34-2

U.S. Brand Names Delnatex®; Delnav®; Deltic®

Use Marketed as insecticide granules, dusting agent, or spray liquid with or without petroleum derivative as a solvent

Mechanism of Toxic Action Irreversible inhibition of acetylcholinesterase and plasma cholinesterase, resulting in excess accumulation of acetylcholine at muscarinic and nicotinic receptors, and in the central nervous system

Adverse Reactions

Cardiovascular: **Hyperdynamic** (~18% to 21%) or hypodynamic (~7% to 10%) states, QT prolongation, sinus bradycardia, sinus tachycardia

Central nervous system: Depression, seizures, hyperactivity, cognitive dysfunction, hypothermia

Genitourinary: Urinary incontinence

Neuromuscular & skeletal: Weakness (delayed), paralysis, delayed paresthesia

Respiratory: Pulmonary edema, respiratory depression

Miscellaneous: Flu-like symptoms (especially with chronic exposure)

Signs and Symptoms of Overdose Abdominal pain, agitation, asystole, AV block, bradycardia, bronchorrhea, coma, confusion, cranial nerve palsies, decreased hemoglobin, decreased platelet count, decreased red blood cell count, diaphragmatic paralysis, dysarthria, excessive sweating, fecal and urinary incontinence, generalized asthenia, headache, heart block, hypertension, hypotension, lacrimation, metabolic acidosis and hyperglycemia (severe intoxication), miosis (unreactive to light), mydriasis (rarely), nausea, pallor, pulmonary edema, QT prolongation, respiratory depression, salivation, seizures, skeletal muscle fasciculation and flaccid paralysis, tachycardia, tachypnea, vomiting

An "intermediate syndrome" of limb asthenia and respiratory paralysis has been reported to occur between 24 and 96 hours postorganophosphate exposure, and is independent of the acute cholinergic crisis. Late paresthesia characterized by stocking and glove paresthesia, anesthesia, and asthenia is infrequently observed weeks to months following acute exposure to certain organophosphates.

Toxicodynamics/Kinetics

Absorption: Readily through oral, dermal, or respiratory exposure

Metabolism: Rapidly metabolized to weakly active compounds through hepatic hydrolysis and other pathways

Elimination: Metabolites are excreted in urine

Warnings/Precautions Risk of aspiration pneumonitis exists with agents having a hydrocarbon vehicle; severe laryngeal irritation and violent coughing may result from exposure to dusting powders; exposure to dusting powders and insecticide granules may cause contact dermatitis

Overdosage/Treatment

Decontamination: Isolation, bagging, and disposal of all contaminated clothing and other articles. All emergency medical workers and hospital staff should follow appropriate precautions regarding exposure to hazardous material including the use of protective clothing, masks, goggles, and respiratory equipment.

Oral: Activated charcoal can be administered either orally or via a nasogastric tube. **Do not** induce emesis because of danger of sudden respiratory compromise, alterations in mental status, seizures, coma, and possible aspiration of hydrocarbon vehicles. **Do not** give a cathartic

Dermal: Prompt thorough scrubbing of all affected areas with soap and water, including hair and nails; 5% bleach can be used

Ocular: Irrigation with copious tepid sterile water or saline.

Supportive therapy: Airway management, ventilatory assistance, humidified oxygen administration, and close monitoring for sudden respiratory failure

Enhancement of elimination: Dialysis and hemoperfusion are not indicated due to effectiveness of the prescribed treatment and large volumes of distribution of organophosphates.

Antidote:

Atropine: Administration should be guided by respiratory status, starting at 2-5 mg I.V. every 5-10 minutes as needed, and should be titrated to the resolution of excess pulmonary secretions. Frequent administration of large doses (cumulative doses > 100 mg) may be necessary in massive exposures.

Glycopyrrolate: May be administered if atropine is unavailable (200-400 mcg I.V. or I.M. initially, or ~$^1/_2$ the dose of atropine).

2-PAM: For more significant exposures (ie, exposures requiring large doses of atropine, or with recurring symptoms, or exposures to more lipid soluble agents), administration should follow: 1-2 g I.V. over 10-30 minutes, repeated in 1 hour if asthenia recurs, then every 4-12 hours for recurring symptoms.

Antidote(s)
- Atropine [ANTIDOTE]
- Pralidoxime [ANTIDOTE]

Diagnostic Procedures
- Creatinine, Serum
- Pseudocholinesterase, Serum

Drug Interaction Paralysis is potentiated by neuromuscular blockade (ie, pancuronium, vecuronium, succinylcholine, atracurium, doxacurium, mivacurium); inhibition of serum esterase prolongs the half-life of succinylcholine, cocaine, and other ester anesthetics; cholinergic toxicity is potentiated by cholinesterase inhibitors such as physostigmine

Additional Information

Poorly volatile amber liquid; thermal degradation products include sulfur oxides; red blood cell cholinesterase, and serum pseudocholinesterase may be depressed following acute or chronic organophosphate exposure; RBC cholinesterase is typically not analyzed by in-house laboratories, and is usually not available for consideration during acute management. Pseudocholinesterase levels may be rapidly available from some in-house laboratories, but are not as reliable a marker of organophosphate exposure because of variability secondary to variant genotypes, hepatic disease, oral estrogen use, or malnutrition. Because of this variability, true indication of suppression of either of these enzymes can only be estimated through comparison to pre-exposure values; these enzymes may be useful in measuring a patient's recovery postexposure, especially if the recovery is not progressing as expected. The intermediate syndrome is not related to delayed neuropathy.

QT$_c$ prolongation on ECG in the setting of organophosphate poisoning is associated with a high incidence of respiratory failure and mortality.

ACGIH TLV: 0.2 mg/m^3; PEL-TWA: 0.2 mg/m^3

Other information concerning pesticide exposures is available through the EPA-funded National Pesticide Telecommunications Network: 1-800-858-7378 (weekdays, 8 AM to 6 PM, Central Standard time)

Diquat Dibromide

Related Information
- Paraquat

Applies to Herbicide

CAS Number 2764-72-9; 85-00-7

Commonly Found In Ethylene bipyridylium

Mechanism of Toxic Action Similar to paraquat, diquat is a potent redox cycler, which through a hydroxyl radical, can cause oxidative stress (through depletion of NADPH) and lipid peroxidation; can result in brainstem (particularly pons) infarction

Adverse Reactions

Dermatologic: Fingernail dystrophy, fingernail discoloration (brown)

Gastrointestinal: Third spacing of gastrointestinal fluid; paralytic ileus

Neuromuscular & skeletal: Rhabdomyolysis

Ocular: Cataract

Renal: Renal failure, proximal tubular degeneration, proteinuria

Respiratory: Pulmonary fibrosis less likely to occur than with paraquat, epistaxis

Signs and Symptoms of Overdose

Coma, dermal burns, fingernail loss, drowsiness (72-96 hours postingestion), hypotension, Mees' lines, paralytic ileus, parkinsonism, seizures

Oliguria/Anuria usually begins within 2-3 days post ingestion with ingestions (oral) exceeding one gram. Renal function improves within 7 to 10 days.

Admission Criteria/Prognosis Patients with known or suspected exposures should be admitted

Overdosage/Treatment

Decontamination: **Oral:** Emesis (within 30 minutes)/lavage (within 1 hour) with activated charcoal: 15%; Fuller's earth; or 7% bentonite (Bentonite/Fuller's earth dosage: Children <12 years of age: 2 g/kg; Adults: 100-150 g). Sodium polystyrene sulfonate may also be effective. **Dermal:** Flush skin with copious amounts of water.

Supportive therapy: Do not utilize oxygen in that it may promote pulmonary fibrosis, although this is not as likely to occur as in paraquat. Monitor for hypercalcemia if Fuller's earth is used. Morphine sulfate can be used for pain control.

Enhancement of elimination: Multiple dosing of activated charcoal, Fuller's earth (100-150 g in adults or 2 g/kg in children), or bentonite may be given every 2-4 hours. Charcoal hemoperfusion for prolonged periods of time (up to 10 hours) may be helpful if instituted within 4 hours. Forced diuresis is not helpful.

Additional Information

Minimal lethal dose: 20 mL of a 20% solution (6-12 g)

A 60 g diquat ingestion resulting in a diquat serum level of 64 mcg/mL was fatal with marked renal tubular damage on autopsy. Does not produce pulmonary fibrosis. Dithionate test: 1 part urine, 0.5 part sodium dithionate in NaOH: Deep blue color indicates presence of paraquat or diquat

Disulfoton

CAS Number 298-04-4

UN Number 2783

U.S. Brand Names Di-Syston®; Dimax®; Dithiosystox®; Solvirex®

Synonyms Ethylthiodemeton; Thiodemeton

Use Crop systemic organophosphate insecticide and acaricide; useful for mosquito abatement

Mechanism of Toxic Action Highly toxic organophosphate agent which causes irreversible inhibition of acetylcholinesterase and plasma cholinesterase, resulting in excess accumulation of acetylcholine at muscarinic and nicotinic receptors, and in the central nervous system

Adverse Reactions

Cardiovascular: **Hyperdynamic** (~18% to 21%) or hypodynamic (~7% to 10%) states, tachycardia, hypertension, QT prolongation, sinus bradycardia, sinus tachycardia

Central nervous system: Depression, seizures, hyperactivity, cognitive dysfunction, hypothermia

Endocrine & metabolic: Hypokalemia

Gastrointestinal: Pancreatitis (after ingestion of 1.5 mg/kg), diarrhea

Genitourinary: Urinary incontinence

Neuromuscular & skeletal: Weakness (delayed), paralysis, delayed paresthesia

Ocular: Can cause myopia in children, miosis

Respiratory: Pulmonary edema, respiratory depression

Miscellaneous: Flu-like symptoms (especially with chronic exposure), diaphoresis

Signs and Symptoms of Overdose Abdominal pain, agitation, asystole, AV block, bradycardia, bronchorrhea, coma, confusion, cranial nerve palsies, decreased hemoglobin, decreased platelet count, decreased red blood cell count, diaphragmatic paralysis, dysarthria, excessive sweating, fecal and urinary incontinence, generalized asthenia, headache, heart block, hypertension, hypotension, lacrimation, metabolic acidosis and hyperglycemia (severe intoxication), miosis (unreactive to light), mydriasis (rarely), nausea, pallor, pulmonary edema, QT prolongation, respiratory depression, salivation, seizures, skeletal muscle fasciculation and flaccid paralysis, tachycardia, tachypnea, vomiting

An "intermediate syndrome" of limb asthenia and respiratory paralysis has been reported to occur between 24 and 96 hours postorganophosphate exposure and is independent of the acute cholinergic crisis. Late paresthesia characterized by stocking and glove paresthesia, anesthesia and asthenia is infrequently observed weeks to months following acute exposure to certain organophosphates.

Toxicodynamics/Kinetics

Absorption: Easily absorbed orally and possibly dermally

Metabolism: To phosphorothiolate sulfone (active metabolite)

Warnings/Precautions Risk of aspiration pneumonitis exists following oral exposure to agents having a hydrocarbon vehicle; severe laryngeal irritation and violent coughing may result from exposure to dusting powders; exposure to dusting powders and insecticide granules may cause contact dermatitis

Reference Range Blood disulfoton level of 1.45 nmol/g associated with fatality; peak plasma phosphorodithioate sulfone concentration of 1322 ng/mL 56 hours postingestion resulted in severe toxicity, but survival levels may rebound in first 2-3 days

Overdosage/Treatment

Decontamination: Isolation, bagging, and disposal of all contaminated clothing and other articles. All emergency medical workers and hospital staff should follow appropriate precautions regarding exposure to hazardous material including the use of protective clothing, masks, goggles, and respiratory equipment. Gastric lavage with water, 5% sodium bicarbonate or 2% potassium permanganate can be considered within 1 hour of ingestion. **Do not** use a cathartic with activated charcoal.

Oral: Activated charcoal can be administered either orally or via a nasogastric tube. **Do not** induce emesis because of danger of sudden respiratory compromise, alterations in mental status, seizures, coma, and possible aspiration of hydrocarbon vehicles. Prolonged or repetitive gastric lavage (with activated charcoal) may be beneficial to prevent rebound of plasma levels due to delayed absorption.

Dermal: Prompt thorough scrubbing of all affected areas with soap and water, including hair and nails; 5% bleach can be used

Ocular: Irrigation with copious tepid sterile water or saline

Supportive therapy: Airway management, ventilatory assistance, humidified oxygen administration, and close monitoring for sudden respiratory failure

Antidote:

Atropine: Administration should be guided by respiratory status, starting at 2-5 mg I.V. every 5-10 minutes as needed, and should be titrated to the resolution of excess pulmonary secretions. Frequent administration of large doses (cumulative doses >100 mg) may be necessary in massive exposures.

Glycopyrrolate: May be administered if atropine is unavailable (200-400 mcg I.M. or I.V. initially, or ~$\frac{1}{2}$ the dose of atropine).

2-PAM: For more significant exposures (ie, exposures requiring large doses of atropine, or with recurring symptoms, or exposures to more lipid soluble agents), administration should follow: 1-2 g I.V. over 10-30 minutes, repeated in 1 hour if asthenia recurs, then every 4-12 hours for recurring symptoms.

Enhancement of elimination: Dialysis and hemoperfusion are not indicated due to effectiveness of the prescribed antidotal treatment and large volumes of distribution of organophosphates. Due to enterohepatic recirculation, multiple dosing of activated charcoal may be effective.

Antidote(s)
- Atropine [ANTIDOTE]
- Pralidoxime [ANTIDOTE]

Diagnostic Procedures
- Creatinine, Serum
- Pseudocholinesterase, Serum

Additional Information Lethal adult dose: 500 mg

Not carcinogenic; cross tolerance with chlorpyrifos noted in rodents

The intermediate syndrome is not related to delayed neuropathy.

QT_c prolongation on ECG in the setting of organophosphate poisoning is associated with a high incidence of respiratory failure and mortality.

Diuron

CAS Number 330-54-1

Commonly Found In Dailon®; Diater®; Di-On®; Direx 4L®; Diurex®; Diurol®; Rout®

Mechanism of Toxic Action Inhibitor of plant photosynthesis, a urea substituted herbicide

Signs and Symptoms of Overdose Can cause methemoglobinemia

Admission Criteria/Prognosis Any patient with change in mental status, cardiopulmonary complaints, or methemoglobin levels >30% should be admitted; asymptomatic patients with methemoglobin levels <30% may be considered for discharge after 6 hours of observation and if methemoglobin levels fall to <15%

Toxicodynamics/Kinetics

Metabolism: To 1-(3,4-dichlorophenyl)-3-methyl urea and to 1-(3,4-dichlorophenyl) urea

Elimination: Urine

Reference Range Maximum tolerated dose: 38 mg/kg

Overdosage/Treatment Supportive therapy: Methylene blue 1-2 mg/kg/dose if methemoglobinemia is noted

Antidote(s)
- Methylene Blue [ANTIDOTE]

Additional Information Available as a 80% powder/40% suspension in water; or can be combined with bramacil or sodium metaborate

Endosulfan

CAS Number 1031-07-8; 115-29-7; 33213-65-9

UN Number 2761

U.S. Brand Names Beosit®; Endocide®; Endosulphan®; Malix®; Thifor®; Thiodan®; Thionex®

Synonyms Hoe-2671

Use Crop pesticide usually applied before harvest on tobacco and fruit trees; used as a wood preservative

Mechanism of Toxic Action No mechanism proven although decrease of brain acetylcholinesterase, serotonin, norepinephrine has been hypothesized; also acts as a GABA antagonist; chlorinated hydrocarbon (sulfurous acid ester)

Adverse Reactions

Cardiovascular: Tachycardia, cyanosis, edema, sinus tachycardia

Central nervous system: Seizures, dizziness, confusion, loss of consciousness, agitation, ataxia

Endocrine & metabolic: Metabolic acidosis, hyperglycemia

Gastrointestinal: Nausea, vomiting, diarrhea

Hematologic: Thrombocytopenia, leukocytosis

Neuromuscular & skeletal: Tremors

Ocular: Miosis

Renal: Tubular necrosis (acute)

Respiratory: Dyspnea, pulmonary edema

Signs and Symptoms of Overdose Rhabdomyolysis, seizures

Toxicodynamics/Kinetics

Absorption: By inhalation, oral (65%) and dermal (25%) routes

Distribution: V_d: Alpha-endosulfan: 43,740 L; beta-endosulfan: 260,600

Metabolism: Hepatic to endosulfan lactone, hydroxyether, and ether

Half-life: Alpha-endosulfan: 24 hours; beta-endosulfan: 60 hours

Elimination: Primarily fecal

Reference Range Blood and urine endosulfan sulfate levels following a 260 mg/kg ingestion, resulting in a fatality, were 874 mcg/L and 1 mcg/L, respectively.

Overdosage/Treatment

Decontamination: **Do not** induce emesis. Lavage (within 1 hour)/ activated charcoal or cholestyramine; **do not** use an oil-based cathartic.

Supportive therapy: Diazepam or phenobarbital for seizure control

Enhancement of elimination: Multiple dosing of activated charcoal or cholestyramine (4 g every 8 hours) may be useful in increasing clearance.

Additional Information Ethanol may enhance toxicity.

Specific References

Mor F and Ozmen O, "Acute Endosulfan Poisoning in Cattle," *Vet Hum Toxicol*, 2003, 45(6):323-4.

Oktay C, Goksu E, Bozdemir N, et al, "Unintentional Toxicity Due to Endosulfan: A Case Report of Two Patients and Characteristics of Endosulfan Toxicity," *Vet Hum Toxicol*, 2003, 45(6):318-20.

Endothall

CAS Number 145-73-3

Commonly Found In Endothall; Aquathol; Hydout; Hydrothol 47; Tri-Endothall; Niagrathal; 3,6-Endoxohexahydrophthalic Acid

Mechanism of Toxic Action Water herbicide (organic acid)

Signs and Symptoms of Overdose Mucous membrane and skin irritation; can cause abdominal pain, acidosis, anuria, disseminated intravascular coagulation, diarrhea, hematemesis, hypotension

Toxicodynamics/Kinetics Absorption: Dermal: Slight

Reference Range Postmortem blood level of 1 mg/dL documented

Overdosage/Treatment

Decontamination: **Oral:** Activated charcoal; dilute with 4-8 oz of milk or water; lavage or emesis is contraindicated. **Dermal:** Flush skin with soap and water. **Ocular:** Flush eyes with water or saline.

Supportive therapy: Avoid adrenergic amines.

Additional Information Minimum lethal dose: 130 mg/kg; 7 g ingestion can be lethal. Emits acrid fumes when heated.

Endrin

Related Information

- Adipose Tissue Ranges of Toxins

CAS Number 53494-70-5; 72-20-8; 7421-93-4

UN Number 2811

U.S. Brand Names Delta-keto® 153; Hexadrin®; Medrin®

Use Chlorinated hydrocarbon pesticide, rodenticide, and avicide used on tobacco, apple trees, cotton, sugar cane, and grain; not used in U.S. since 1986

Mechanism of Toxic Action Interferes with normal flux of sodium and potassium ions over axonal membrane

Adverse Reactions

Cardiovascular: Hypotension, shock

Central nervous system: Seizures, dizziness, hyperthermia

Gastrointestinal: Nausea, vomiting, hypersalivation

Hematologic: Thrombocytopenia

Neuromuscular & skeletal: Tremors

Otic: Temporary deafness

Respiratory: Respiratory depression

Toxicodynamics/Kinetics

Absorption: By inhalation, oral, and dermal (1.5%) routes

Metabolism: Hepatic oxidation and hydroxylation occurs to 12-hydroxyedrin and 12-ketoedrin

Elimination: Urine

Reference Range Blood endrin level of 0.05 mg/L associated with seizures

Overdosage/Treatment

Decontamination: **Do not** induce emesis. Lavage (within 1 hour)/ activated charcoal or cholestyramine; **do not** use an oil-based cathartic.

Supportive therapy: Diazepam or phenytoin may be used for seizure control. Try to avoid catecholamines as arrhythmias can be induced. Assisted ventilation with succinylcholine (0.5-1 mg/minute for 1 day) for seizure control may be necessary. Atropine can be used to control bronchial secretions.

Enhancement of elimination: Multiple dosing of activated charcoal or cholestyramine (4 g every 8 hours) may be useful in increasing clearance.

Additional Information Fatal oral dose: 12 g (100 mg/kg). Seizurgenic oral dose: 0.25 mg/kg

IDLH: 200 mg/m^3

Endrin concentration in foods (contaminated flour) >150 ppm can cause seizures upon ingestion.

Milk or ethanol can increase toxicity of endrin by enhancing its absorption; onset of seizures is usually within 4 hours postingestion; bioaccumulation does not occur

Epichlorohydrin

CAS Number 106-89-8

UN Number 2023

Synonyms 1-Chloro-2,3-Epoxypropane; Chloromethyloxirane; ECH; Oxirane

Use Used in Epoxy production; also used in insecticide, agricultural chemicals; elastomers and as a solvent in rubber, paper and paint industries. It is a curing agent.

Mechanism of Toxic Action Mucosal irritant at air concentrations >10 ppm; also is a contact allergen

Adverse Reactions

Cardiovascular: Facial edema

Dermatologic: Dermal burns, blisters

Gastrointestinal: Nausea, vomiting, abdominal pain

Hepatic: Hepatomegaly

Ocular: Eye irritation (at concentrations >20 ppm), blepharospasm, eyelid or corneal edema

Renal: Renal lesions (at concentrations >100 ppm)

Respiratory: Rhinorrhea, cough, pneumonitis, possible incidence of lung cancer (increased)

Toxicodynamics/Kinetics Absorption: Inhalation, dermal, or GI routes

Overdosage/Treatment Decontamination: **Dermal:** Wash carefully with soap and water. Dermal reaction may be delayed for several hours. Epichlorhydrin can penetrate leather or rubber, therefore, these clothing items need to be discarded. **Inhalation:** Administer 100% humidified oxygen. **Ocular:** Irrigate copiously.

Additional Information Causes dose-dependent decrease in sperm motility and decrease male (but not female) fertility in animals; possibly mutagenic. TLV-TWA: 2 ppm; OSHA: PEL-TWA (transitional limit): 5 ppm. Odor threshold (chloroform like): 10 ppm; IDLH: 75 ppm.

Ether

Pronunciation (EE ther)

CAS Number 60-29-7

UN Number 1155

Synonyms Diethyl Ether; Ethyl Oxide

Use Anesthetic/industrial solvent in manufacture of synthetic dyes and plastics

Mechanism of Toxic Action Dermal/mucosal irritant

Signs and Symptoms of Overdose Anorexia, bradycardia, CNS depression, coma, conjunctivitis, cough, dermal ulcers, dizziness, euphoria, headache, hepatotoxicity, hyperglycemia (2.9 mg % per ounce of ether), hypothermia, laryngeal spasm, nephritis, proteinuria, respiratory depression, salivation, seizures, slurred speech, visual/auditory hallucinations, vomiting

Toxicodynamics/Kinetics

Absorption: Well absorbed by inhalation and oral routes; not well absorbed dermally

Metabolism: Primarily to carbon dioxide and acetaldehyde

Elimination: Primary pulmonary (87%)

Dosage Forms Liquid: 4 oz, 8 oz

Reference Range

Analgesic level: Arterial blood ether level of 100-500 mg/L

Anesthetic level: Arterial blood ether level between 500-1500 mg/L

Estimated blood level at 400 ppm: ~18 mg/L

Overdosage/Treatment

Decontamination: **Oral:** Dilute with 4-8 ounces of milk or water. **Dermal:** Wash with soap and water. **Inhalation:** Administer 100% humidified oxygen. **Ocular:** Irrigate with copious amounts of normal saline.

Supportive therapy: Benzodiazepine can be used to treat seizures. Barbiturates or phenytoin/fosphenytoin can be used as a secondary agent.

Additional Information Lethal oral dose: 1 ounce

A colorless, liquid with an aromatic odor; highly flammable. Specific gravity: 0.7. Boiling point: 35°C. TLV-TWA: 400; IDLH: 19,000

Effect/standards (ether concentration ppm): Range of odor detection: 0.8-1920. Mucosal irritation: 200. Dizziness: 2000. Surgical anesthesia induction: 100,000-150,000. Fatal: >100,000

Ethion

Applies to Bladan; Ethanox; Nialate; Rodocide
CAS Number 563-12-2
Use An organothiophosphate pesticide used as an acaricide on fruit trees, fiber crops, nut trees, forage crops, and vegetables; also used as a topically applied pesticide agent on livestock
Mechanism of Toxic Action Irreversible inhibition of acetylcholinesterase and plasma cholinesterase, resulting in excess accumulation of acetylcholine at muscarinic and nicotinic receptors, and in the central nervous system
Adverse Reactions
Cardiovascular: **Hyperdynamic** (18% to 21%) or hypodynamic (~7% to 10%) states, tachycardia, hypertension, QT prolongation, sinus bradycardia, sinus tachycardia
Central nervous system: Depression, seizures, hyperactivity, cognitive dysfunction, hypothermia
Endocrine & metabolic: Hypokalemia
Gastrointestinal: Diarrhea
Genitourinary: Urinary incontinence
Neuromuscular & skeletal: Weakness (delayed), paralysis, delayed paresthesia
Ocular: Can cause myopia in children, miosis
Respiratory: Pulmonary edema, respiratory depression
Miscellaneous: Flu-like symptoms (especially with chronic exposure), diaphoresis
Signs and Symptoms of Overdose
Abdominal pain, agitation, asystole, AV block, bradycardia, bronchorrhea, coma, confusion, cranial nerve palsies, decreased hemoglobin, decreased platelet count, decreased red blood cell count, diaphragmatic paralysis, dysarthria, excessive sweating, fecal and urinary incontinence, generalized asthenia, headache, heart block, hypertension, hypotension, lacrimation, metabolic acidosis and hyperglycemia (severe intoxication), miosis (unreactive to light), mydriasis (rarely), nausea, pallor, pulmonary edema, QT prolongation, respiratory depression, salivation, seizures, skeletal muscle fasciculation and flaccid paralysis, tachycardia, tachypnea, vomiting
An "intermediate syndrome" of limb asthenia and respiratory paralysis has been reported to occur between 24 and 96 hours postorganophosphate exposure and is independent of the acute cholinergic crisis. Late paresthesia characterized by stocking and glove paresthesia, anesthesia and asthenia is infrequently observed weeks to months following acute exposure to certain organophosphates.
Toxicodynamics/Kinetics
Absorption: Rapid by oral and dermal routes
Metabolism: Desulfurated by hepatic enzymes to active form (ethion monooxon)
Overdosage/Treatment
Decontamination: Isolation, bagging, and disposal of all contaminated clothing and other articles. All emergency medical workers and hospital staff should follow appropriate precautions regarding exposure to hazardous material including the use of protective clothing, masks, goggles, and respiratory equipment.
Oral: Activated charcoal can be administered either orally or via a nasogastric tube. **Do not** induce emesis because of danger of sudden respiratory compromise, alterations in mental status, seizures, coma, and possible aspiration of hydrocarbon vehicles. **Do not** give a cathartic.
Dermal: Prompt thorough scrubbing of all affected areas with soap and water, including hair and nails; 5% bleach can be used
Ocular: Irrigation with copious tepid sterile water or saline
Supportive therapy: Airway management, ventilatory assistance, humidified oxygen administration, and close monitoring for sudden respiratory failure
Enhancement of elimination: Dialysis and hemoperfusion are not indicated due to effectiveness of the prescribed treatment and large volumes of distribution of organophosphates.
Antidote:
Atropine: Administration should be guided by respiratory status, starting at 2-5 mg I.V. every 5-10 minutes as needed, and should be titrated to the resolution of excess pulmonary secretions. Frequent administration of large doses (cumulative doses >100 mg) may be necessary in massive exposures.
Glycopyrrolate: May be administered if atropine is unavailable (200-400 mcg I.M. or I.V. initially, or ~1/2 the dose of atropine).
2-PAM: For more significant exposures (ie, exposures requiring large doses of atropine, or with recurring symptoms, or exposures to more lipid soluble agents), administration should follow: 1-2 g I.V. over 10-30 minutes, repeated in 1 hour if asthenia recurs, then every 4-12 hours for recurrent symptoms.

Additional Information Lethal oral dose is ~15 mg/kg. Exposure limit (TWA) of skin: 0.4 mg/m^3. A white or amber liquid with a sulfur odor. Atmospheric half-life: 40 minutes. Aerobic soil half-life: 69-102 days

Ethyl Acetate

CAS Number 141-78-6
UN Number 1173
Synonyms Acetic Acid; Ethyl Ester; Vinegar Naphtha
Use A solvent utilized in the lacquer industry and in artificial fruit essences
Mechanism of Toxic Action Mild mucosal irritant
Signs and Symptoms of Overdose Conjunctivitis, nose/throat irritation (at concentrations >400 ppm), eczema
Toxicodynamics/Kinetics
Metabolism: Hydrolysis to acetic acid and ethanol
Half-life: 10 minutes
Overdosage/Treatment Decontamination: **Oral:** Lavage within 1 hour/ activated charcoal **Dermal:** Wash skin with water. **Inhalation:** 100% humidified oxygen should be utilized. **Ocular:** Irrigate with copious amounts of water or saline for at least 15 minutes.
Additional Information IDLH: 10,000 ppm; TLV-TWA: 400 ppm; Odor threshold: 1 ppm (ether-like)

Ethyl Mercaptan

CAS Number 75-08-1
UN Number 2363
Synonyms Ethyl Sulfhydrate; Ethyl Thioalcohol
Use A product of vinous fermentation and petroleum products, it is used as an odorant for natural gas; also used in production of fungicides, plastics, and insecticides
Mechanism of Toxic Action Mucosal irritant which can cause CNS depression; may inhibit mitochondrial electron transport
Adverse Reactions
Central nervous system: Fatigue, lethargy, coma
Gastrointestinal: Oropharyngeal irritation, nausea
Respiratory: Nasal irritation, respiratory depression
Admission Criteria/Prognosis Admit any patient with neurologic symptomatology or known exposure >500 ppm
Toxicodynamics/Kinetics
Absorption: Inhalation and oral routes
Metabolism: Hepatic oxidation
Elimination: Renal
Monitoring Parameters Chest x-ray, arterial blood gases, liver and renal function tests
Reference Range Blood ethyl mercaptan levels in rats of ~200 nanomoles/mL associated with reversible coma
Overdosage/Treatment Decontamination: **Oral: Do not** lavage or induce emesis. Activated charcoal may be used. **Dermal:** Wash area with soap and water. **Inhalation:** Administer 100% humidified oxygen. **Ocular:** Irrigate with water or saline.
Additional Information Symptoms can occur at exposures >4 ppm; a colorless to yellow liquid with a garlic- or leek-like odor. Odor threshold: 0.26-0.97 ppb. Specific gravity: 0.8

Ethyl Methacrylate

CAS Number 97-63-2
UN Number 2277
Use In manufacture of plastics, building and furniture, dental plates
Mechanism of Toxic Action Mucosal/irritant; TLV-5 ppm.
Adverse Reactions
Central nervous system: Dizziness, lethargy
Dermatologic: Allergic contact dermatitis
Gastrointestinal: Oropharyngeal irritation
Neuromuscular & skeletal: Tremors
Ocular: Eye irritant
Respiratory: Nasal irritation
Overdosage/Treatment Decontamination: **Oral:** Activated charcoal. **Dermal:** Wash exposed area with soap and water. **Ocular:** Irrigate with saline or water.

Ethylbenzene

Related Information
● Adipose Tissue Ranges of Toxins
Applies to Degreaser; Paint Thinner; Solvent (Asphalt, Fuels, Naphtha)
CAS Number 100-41-4
UN Number 1175
Synonyms EB; Ethylbenzol; Phenylethane
Use Solvent which is found in asphalt, fuels, and naphtha; used in the products of styrene and other organic chemicals; used in paint thinners and as a degreaser

Mechanism of Toxic Action Aromatic hydrocarbon with mucosal irritant effects; central nervous system depression can occur at very high concentrations

Adverse Reactions

Central nervous system: Dizziness at levels >2000 ppm

Dermatologic: Dermal irritant at levels of 200 ppm

Hematologic: Anemia (long-term exposure)

Hepatic: Hepatotoxicity

Ocular: Eye irritation with lacrimation at levels >1000 ppm

Respiratory: Upper respiratory tract irritation at levels >2000 ppm

Toxicodynamics/Kinetics

Absorption: Rapid from inhalation (57%) and skin (rate of 20-33 mg/cm²/hour)

Metabolism: Hepatic to mandelic acid and phenylglyoxylated acid

Elimination: Renal

Reference Range Ethylbenzene blood levels of 61 mcg/L associated with anemia; at 100 ppm exposure of ethylbenzene, it has been estimated that urine phenylglyoxylic acid and mandelic acid concentrations would be 95 mg/L and 395 mg/L, respectively

Overdosage/Treatment

Decontamination: **Do not** induce emesis or lavage due to risk of aspiration pneumonia. Activated charcoal can adsorb benzene.

Supportive therapy: Benzodiazepines for seizure control; avoid use of catecholamines due to risk of ventricular arrhythmia

Additional Information Not associated with cancer; carbon monoxide and ethanol inhibit metabolism of ethylbenzene in rodents; does not bioaccumulate. Minimal uptake of fluorescein on ocular exposure; BEI (urinary mandelic acid) at the end of shift at the end of work week: 2 g/L or 1.5 g/g creatinine. Frequently found in ground water at hazardous waste sites (average concentration: 0.65 ppm). IDLH: 2000 ppm; TLV-PEL: 100 ppm

Ethylene Dichloride

Applies to Fumigant; Solvent

CAS Number 107-06-2

UN Number 1184

Synonyms 1,2-Bichlorethane; 1,2-Dichloroethane (1,2-DCE); Borer Sol; Brocide; DCE; Dutch Oil; EDC; Freon 150; Glycol Dichlorid

Use Fat solvent; soil fumigant

Mechanism of Toxic Action CNS depression; also can cause increased myocardial irritability and mucosal injury; glutathione depletion may occur

Adverse Reactions

Cardiovascular: Cardiovascular failure, fibrillation (ventricular), arrhythmias (ventricular)

Central nervous system: CNS depression, delirium, headache, dizziness

Endocrine & metabolic: Hypercalcemia (late finding)

Hepatic: Elevated liver enzymes, fatty degeneration

Renal: Tubular necrosis (acute)

Respiratory: Pulmonary edema, respiratory failure

Signs and Symptoms of Overdose Abdominal pain, asthenia, corneal lesions, diarrhea, dizziness, dyspnea, headache, throat burning, tremor, vomiting

Toxicodynamics/Kinetics

Absorption: Well absorbed dermally, through lung (90%) and GI tract (90%)

Metabolism: Hepatic (saturated at oral dose of 25 mg/kg orally or 50 ppm by inhalation)

Elimination: Through lungs

Reference Range Oral dose of 25 mg/kg or inhalation dose >150 ppm correspond to blood level of 5-10 mcg/mL

Overdosage/Treatment

Decontamination: **Oral:** Emesis is contraindicated; dilute with milk or water. **Dermal:** Wash exposed areas with soap and water. **Ocular:** Irrigate with saline.

Supportive therapy: Supplemental oxygen. Benzodiazepines can be used for seizure control. Phenytoin or barbiturates can be used for refractory seizures. Although not formally studied, administration of N-acetylcysteine may replenish glutathione and may decrease pulmonary injury.

Additional Information Fatalities have occurred at doses of 30-70 g. Pleasant odor. Odor threshold: 50-100 ppm. Specific gravity: 1.26. TLV-TWA: 10 ppm; IDLH: 1000 ppm; PEL-TWA: 50 ppm

Ethylene Glycol

Applies to Antifreeze; Coolant

CAS Number 107-21-1

Synonyms Ethylene Alcohol; Ethylene Dihydrate; Glycol Alcohol; Mono-ethylene Glycol

Use Automotive radiator antifreeze and coolants, solvent

Mechanism of Toxic Action Metabolized into glycolic acid and oxalate via the alcohol dehydrogenase pathway (ADH), thus producing profound metabolic acidosis

Adverse Reactions

Cardiovascular: Myocarditis, QT prolongation, sinus tachycardia

Central nervous system: Ataxia, anisocoria, coma, cranial nerve palsies, cranial nerve dysfunction (6th nerve), seizures, headache, slurred speech

Endocrine & metabolic: Hypocalcemia, metabolic acidosis, osmolal gap

Gastrointestinal: Feces discoloration (black)

Hematologic: Leukemoid reaction, porphyria

Neuromuscular & skeletal: Hyperreflexia, rhabdomyolysis

Ocular: Diplopia, mydriasis, nystagmus, optic neuropathy

Renal: Myoglobinuria, renal tubular damage progressing to renal insufficiency

Respiratory: Hyperventilation, respiratory irritation/cough on inhalation

Miscellaneous: Breast cancer

Signs and Symptoms of Overdose

Similar to methanol ingestion, ethylene glycol can initially result in inebriation. Ethylene glycol toxicity can be divided into three stages:

Stage I (30 minutes to 12 hours after ingestion): Inebriation, ataxia, and metabolic acidosis with resulting respiratory compensation (Kussmaul's breathing), seizures, hypocalcemia, cranial nerve palsies, calcium oxaluria (4-8 hours after ingestion), and myoclonus. Coma can occur, and death is usually due to cerebral edema during this stage.

Stage II (12-36 hours after ingestion): Respiratory status deteriorates with tachypnea, tachycardia, cyanosis, dyspnea, and pulmonary edema with developing cardiomegaly. Death is usually due to cardiovascular causes or bronchopneumonia during this stage.

Stage III (36-72 hours after ingestion): Renal failure dominates this phase, with acute tubular necrosis, hematuria, oliguria, albuminuria, or anuria occurring. Noncardiogenic pulmonary edema may occur in this stage.

Admission Criteria/Prognosis Any symptomatic patient, acidosis, any patient with suspected ingestion, or serum ethylene glycol levels >10 mg/dL 2 hours postexposure should be admitted

Toxicodynamics/Kinetics

Absorption: Oral: Rapid. Inhalation: Not well absorbed, unless aerosilized; inhalation of aerosilized ethylene glycol usually results in a blood ethylene glycol level <30 mg/dL; repiratory irration can occur at air levels >50 ppm; dermal: negligible through intact skin

Distribution: V_d: 0.83 L/kg; glycolate: 0.55 L/kg

Metabolism: Liver with principle toxic metabolites including glycolic acid (96%) and oxalic acid (2.3%). See figure.

Metabolic Pathway for Oxidation of Ethylene Glycol*

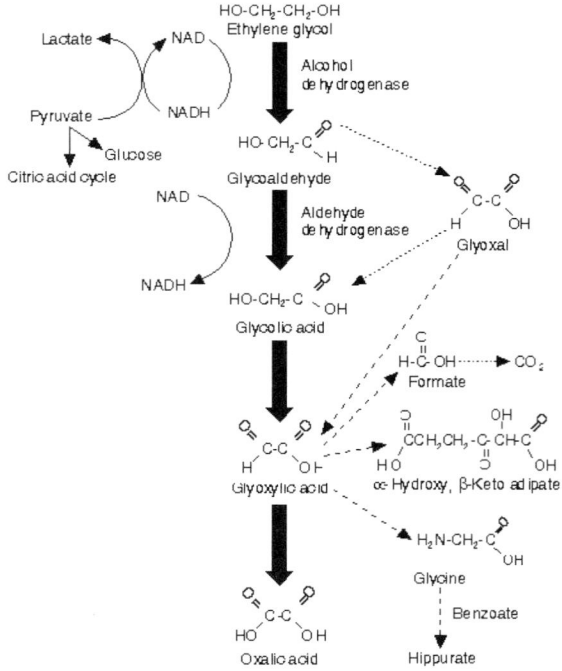

Adapted from the U.S. Department of Health and Human Services, "Technical Report for Ethylene Glycol/Propylene Glycol," Agency for Toxic Substances and Disease Registry, May 1993.

Half-life: Elimination:
No ethanol therapy: 3 hours. During ethanol therapy: 17 hours. During ethanol therapy and hemodialysis: $2^1/_2$ hours. During 4-MP therapy: 19.7 hours. During 4-MP therapy and hemodialysis: 3.5 hours. Glycolate: 10 hours (endogenous). $2^1/_2$ hours (during hemodialysis)
Elimination: Renal clearance: 3.2 mL/kg/minute

Reference Range
Highest survivable serum ethylene glycol level: 2361 mg/dL (after ingestion of 3 L ethylene glycol in an adult)
Toxic: Plasma level: 20 mg/dL
Fatal: Levels >85 mg/dL
Mean urine ethylene glycol concentration of 5700 mg/L (range 600-10,800 mg/L) associated with fatal poisoning

Overdosage/Treatment
Decontamination: **Oral:** Avoid emesis with ipecac. Activated charcoal is not effective at a 5:1 ratio (charcoal:toxin). Higher doses of activated charcoal may be needed, but this is of unproven benefit. **Dermal:** Wash with soap and water. **Ocular:** Irrigate copiously with saline.

Supportive therapy: Ethanol or 4-methylpyrazole therapy should be initiated at ethylene glycol level 20 mg/dL, severe acidosis or electrolyte abnormality present, or renal failure. Treat acidosis with I.V. sodium bicarbonate. Administer thiamine and pyridoxine, 100 mg once a day for 2 days for both drugs. Calcium chloride or calcium gluconate can be given for hypocalcemia. 4-MP is a specific antagonist of alcohol dehydrogenase and can be used instead of ethanol therapy.

Enhancement of elimination: Hemodialysis should be considered if ethylene glycol level is >20 mg/dL or if metabolic acidosis is present. Continuous arteriovenous or venovenous hemodiafiltration may be useful. The hemodialysis clearance of glycolate with a blood flow rate of 250-400 mL/minute is ~170 mL/minute.

Antidote(s)
- Alcohol, Ethyl [ANTIDOTE]
- Fomepizole [ANTIDOTE]
- Pyridoxine [ANTIDOTE]
- Sodium Bicarbonate [ANTIDOTE]

Diagnostic Procedures
- Anion Gap, Blood
- Crystals, Urine
- Electrolytes, Blood
- Osmolality, Serum
- Osmolality, Urine

Test Interactions Falsely increased whole blood lactate levels may occur with certain enzymatic analyzers due to interference with glycolate

Additional Information
Lethal dose: 100 mL (1.5 mL/kg). Lowest survival pH reported was 6.46 in an ethylene glycol toxic patient (no neurologic sequelae).
Specific gravity: 1.12 g/mL; odor threshold: 62.5 mg/m^3
Sweet tasting liquid. Atmospheric half-life: 24-50 hours. Water half-life: 3-5 days
Contribution of a serum concentration level of 100 mg/dL to elevation of osmolar gap: 16
Existence of propionic acid through inborn errors of metabolism can give a false-positive ethylene glycol level

Specific References
Caravati EM, Erdman AR, Christianson G, et al, "Ethylene Glycol Exposure: An Evidence-Based Consensus Guideline for Out-of-Hospital Management," *Clin Toxicol*, 2005, 43(5):327-45.

Cragin LS, Geller RJ, and Morgan BW, "Intentional Ethylene Glycol Poisonings Increase After Extensive Media Coverage of Alleged Antifreeze Murders," *Clin Toxicol (Phila)*, 2005, 43:717.

DesLauriers C, Mazor S, Metz J, et al, "Toxic Alcohol Evaluation of Pediatric Patients Is Often Incomplete," *J Toxicol Clin Toxicol*, 2004, 42(5):719.

DeWitt C, Palmer R, Phillips S, et al, "False-Positive Ethylene Glycol Level," *J Toxicol Clin Toxicol*, 2003, 41(5):736.

Froberg K, Dorion RP, and McMartin KE, "The Role of Calcium Oxalate Crystal Deposition in Cerebral Vessels During Ethylene Glycol Poisoning," *Clin Toxicol*, 2006, 44(3):315-8.

Goicoa A, Barreiro A, Pena ML, et al, "Atypical Presentation of Long-Term Ethylene Glycol Poisoning in a German Shepherd Dog," *Vet Hum Toxicol*, 2003, 45(4):207-9.

Greene SL, Dargan PI, Shiew CM, et al, "AACT Recommendations for Antidotal Treatment of Ethylene Glycol Poisoning: Do We Have Enough Information?" *Clin Toxicol (Phila)*, 2005, 43:740.

Haroz R, Salzman MS, and Greenberg MI, "Hyperammonemia: A Possible Marker for Methanol and Ethylene Glycol Intoxication," *Clin Toxicol (Phila)*, 2005, 43:689.

Koga Y, Purssell RA, and Lynd LD, "The Irrationality of the Present Use of the Osmole Gap: Applicable Physical Chemistry Principles and Recommendations to Improve the Validity of Current Practices," *Toxicol Rev*, 2004, 23(3):203-11.

Laoang J, Brooks DE, Akhtar J, et al, "Hyperosmolality: Another Indication for Hemodialysis Following Ethylene Glycol Poisoning," *J Toxicol Clin Toxicol*, 2004, 42(5):720.

Lepik KJ, Purssell RA, Levy AR, et al, "Adverse Reactions to Hemodialysis in 72 Cases of Toxic Alcohol Poisoning," *Clin Toxicol (Phila)*, 2005, 43:676.

Lepik KJ, Purssell RA, Levy AR, et al, "Adverse Reactions to Ethanol Antidote for Toxic Alcohol Poisoning: A Multi-Center Retrospective Review," *Clin Toxicol (Phila)*, 2005, 43:675.

Loh CH, Shih TS, Hsieh AT, et al, "Hepatic Effects in Workers Exposed to 2-Methoxy Ethanol," *J Occup Environ Med*, 2004, 46(7):707-13.

Marraffa JM, Stork CM, and Cantor R, "Risk for Long-Term Nephrotoxicity After Ethylene Glycol Poisoning," *J Toxicol Clin Toxicol*, 2004, 42(5):737.

McMartin KE and Guo C, "Inhibition of Cellular Toxicity of Oxalate by EDTA and Citrate," *J Toxicol Clin Toxicol*, 2003, 41(5):694.

McStay CM and Gordon PE, "Urine Fluorescence in Ethylene Glycol Poisoning," *N Engl J Med*, 2007, 356:6-12.

Michael JB and Sztajnkrycer MD, "Deadly Pediatric Poisons: Nine Common Agents That Kill at Low Doses," *Emerg Med Clin N Am*, 2004, 22:1019-50.

Morgan DL, Cooney NL, Cooney DR, et al, "Recent Changes in the Treatment of Toxic Alcohol Ingestions," *Clin Toxicol (Phila)*, 2005, 43:670.

Mullins ME and Zane Horowitz B, "Was it Necessary to Add Bitrex (Denatonium Benzoate) to Automotive Products?" *Vet Hum Toxicol*, 2004, 46(3):150-2.

Mycyk MB and Aks SE, "A Visual Schematic for Clarifying the Temporal Relationship Between the Anion and Osmol Gaps in Toxic Alcohol Poisoning," *Am J Emerg Med*, 2003, 21(4):333-5.

Pizon AF and Brooks DE, "Hyperosmolality: Another Indication for Hemodialysis Following Acute Ethylene Glycol Poisoning," *Clin Toxicol*, 2006, 44:181-3.

Rottinghaus D, Bryant S, and Harchelroad FP, "Survival After Ethylene Glycol Overdose with Blood pH of 6.54," *J Toxicol Clin Toxicol*, 2003, 41(5):674.

Shiew CM, Dargan PI, Greene SL, et al, "An Economic Analysis: Is Fomepizole Really More Expensive Than Ethanol for the Treatment of Ethylene Glycol Poisoning?" *Clin Toxicol (Phila)*, 2005, 43:690.

Shiew CM, Dargan PI, Greene SL, et al, "Survey of Ethanol Assay Availability in the UK: Can We Cope with Ethylene Glycol/Methanol Poisoning?" *Clin Toxicol (Phila)*, 2005, 43:742.

Spivak LA and Horowitz BA, "Treatment of Severe Ethylene Glycol Poisoning Without Dialysis," *Clin Toxicol (Phila)*, 2005, 43:691.

Takayesu JK, Bazari H, and Linshaw M, "Case Records of the Massachusetts General Hospital. Case 7-2006: A 47-Year-Old Man with Altered Mental Status and Acute Renal Failure," *N Engl J Med*, 2006, 354(10):1065-72.

Tilson C and McCurdy H, "Recent Experiences with Incidences of Ethylene Glycol Poisoning in the State of Georgia," *J Anal Toxicol*, 2003, 27:198.

Woo MY, Greenway DC, Nadler SP, et al, "Artifactual Elevation of Lactate in Ethylene Glycol Poisoning," *J Emerg Med*, 2003, 25(3):289-93.

Ethylene Oxide

Applies to Brake Fluids; Cosmetics; Detergents; Ethylene Glycol (Production); Fumigant; Inks; Plasticizers
CAS Number 75-21-8
UN Number 1040
U.S. Brand Names Anprolene®; Oxyfume®
Synonyms Dihydrooxirene; Dimethylane Oxide; E+O; Merpol; Oxidoethane; Oxirane; T-Gas
Use Gas sterilization agent (can inactivate all organisms); used in the production of ethylene glycol, cosmetics, detergents, inks, brake fluids, plasticizers, fumigant
Mechanism of Toxic Action Alkylating agent; irritant
Adverse Reactions
Cardiovascular: Cardiovascular collapse, sinus bradycardia
Central nervous system: CNS depression, axonopathy (peripheral)
Gastrointestinal: Mucous membrane irritation
Hematologic: Methemoglobinemia
Neuromuscular & skeletal: Motor and sensory neuropathy, peripheral neuropathy
Respiratory: Asthma, bronchospasm, reactive airways disease syndrome
Miscellaneous: Cutaneous T-cell lymphoma
Signs and Symptoms of Overdose Bradycardia, coma, conjunctivitis, contact dermatitis, cough, dermal burns, dizziness, dyspnea, headache, myoclonus, nystagmus, polyneuropathy, possible increased risk for leukemia or gastric cancer, pulmonary edema, seizures, vomiting
Admission Criteria/Prognosis Any symptomatic patient 12 hours postexposure should be admitted; any patient with bronchospasm or pulmonary edema should be admitted

Toxicodynamics/Kinetics

Absorption: Orally and by inhalation

Metabolism: Hepatic; two pathways: hydrolysis to ethylene glycol and glutathione conjugation to mercapturic acid

Overdosage/Treatment Decontamination: Basic poison management; **do not** induce emesis. Irrigate skin with high pressure water.

Additional Information

A blister agent

It has been estimated that 270,000 U.S. workers are potentially exposed to ethylene oxide, most in the health care industry.

Air levels in a hospital sterilizing unit: 0.1-7.8 ppm

Ether-like odor. Odor threshold: 430 ppm (air); 140 mg/L (water). Atmospheric half-life: 69-149 days. Water half-life: 9-14 days. TLV-TWA: 1 ppm; IDLH: 800 ppm; PEL-TWA: 1 ppm

Specific References

Finch CK and Lobo BL, "Acute Inhalant-Induced Neurotoxicity with Delayed Recovery," *Ann Pharmacother*, 2005, 39(1):169-72.

Fensulfothion

CAS Number 115-90-2

U.S. Brand Names Dansit®

Use Marketed as insecticide granules, dusting agent, or spray liquid with or without petroleum derivative as a solvent

Mechanism of Toxic Action Potent, irreversible inhibition of acetylcholinesterase and plasma cholinesterase, resulting in excess accumulation of acetylcholine at muscarinic and nicotinic receptors, and in the central nervous system

Adverse Reactions

Cardiovascular: **Hyperdynamic** (~18% to 21%) or hypodynamic (~7% to 10%) states, QT prolongation, sinus bradycardia, sinus tachycardia

Central nervous system: Depression, seizures, hyperactivity, cognitive dysfunction, hypothermia

Genitourinary: Urinary incontinence

Neuromuscular & skeletal: Weakness (delayed), paralysis, delayed paresthesia

Respiratory: Pulmonary edema, respiratory depression

Miscellaneous: Flu-like symptoms (especially with chronic exposure)

Signs and Symptoms of Overdose

Abdominal pain, agitation, asystole, AV block, bradycardia, bronchorrhea, coma, confusion, cranial nerve palsies, decreased hemoglobin, decreased platelet count, decreased red blood cell count, diaphragmatic paralysis, dysarthria, excessive sweating, fecal and urinary incontinence, generalized asthenia, headache, heart block, hypertension, hypotension, lacrimation, metabolic acidosis and hyperglycemia (severe intoxication), miosis (unreactive to light), mydriasis (rarely), nausea, pallor, pulmonary edema, respiratory depression, salivation, seizures, skeletal muscle fasciculation and flaccid paralysis, QT prolongation, tachycardia, tachypnea, vomiting

An "intermediate syndrome" of limb asthenia and respiratory paralysis has been reported to occur between 24 and 96 hours postorganophosphate exposure, and is independent of the acute cholinergic crisis. Late paresthesia characterized by stocking and glove paresthesia, anesthesia, and asthenia is infrequently observed weeks to months following acute exposure to certain organophosphates.

Admission Criteria/Prognosis Any symptomatic patient or an asymptomatic patient following a severe exposure should be admitted probably into an intensive care unit; asymptomatic patients following a moderate exposure can be discharged after 8 hours of observation

Toxicodynamics/Kinetics

Absorption: Readily through oral, dermal, or respiratory exposure

Metabolism: Rapidly metabolized to weakly active compounds through hepatic hydrolysis and other pathways

Elimination: Metabolites are excreted in urine

Warnings/Precautions Risk of aspiration pneumonitis exists with agents having a hydrocarbon vehicle; severe laryngeal irritation and violent coughing may result from exposure to dusting powders; exposure to dusting powders and insecticide granules may cause contact dermatitis

Overdosage/Treatment

Decontamination: Isolation, bagging, and disposal of all contaminated clothing and other articles. All emergency medical workers and hospital staff should follow appropriate precautions regarding exposure to hazardous material including the use of protective clothing, masks, goggles, and respiratory equipment.

Oral: Activated charcoal can be administered either orally or via a nasogastric tube. **Do not** induce emesis because of danger of sudden respiratory compromise, alterations in mental status, seizures, coma, and possible aspiration of hydrocarbon vehicles. **Do not** give a cathartic.

Dermal: Prompt thorough scrubbing of all affected areas with soap and water, including hair and nails; 5% bleach can be used

Ocular: Irrigation with copious tepid sterile water or saline

Supportive therapy: Airway management, ventilatory assistance, humidified oxygen administration, and close monitoring for sudden respiratory failure

Antidote:

Atropine: Administration should be guided by respiratory status, starting at 2-5 mg I.V. every 5-10 minutes as needed, and should be titrated to the resolution of excess pulmonary secretions. Frequent administration of large doses (cumulative doses >100 mg) may be necessary in massive exposures.

Glycopyrrolate: May be administered if atropine is unavailable (200-400 mcg I.V. or I.M. initially, or ~$^1/_2$ the dose of atropine).

2-PAM: For more significant exposures (ie, exposures requiring large doses of atropine, or with recurring symptoms, or exposures to more lipid soluble agents), administration should follow: 1-2 g I.V. over 10-30 minutes, repeated in 1 hour if asthenia recurs, then every 4-12 hours for recurring symptoms.

Enhancement of elimination: Dialysis and hemoperfusion are not indicated due to effectiveness of the prescribed antidotal treatment and large volumes of distribution of organophosphates.

Antidote(s)

- Atropine [ANTIDOTE]
- Pralidoxime [ANTIDOTE]

Diagnostic Procedures

- Creatinine, Serum
- Pseudocholinesterase, Serum

Drug Interaction Paralysis is potentiated by neuromuscular blockade (ie, pancuronium, vecuronium, succinylcholine, atracurium, doxacurium, mivacurium); inhibition of serum esterase prolongs the half-life of succinylcholine, cocaine, and other ester anesthetics; cholinergic toxicity is potentiated by cholinesterase inhibitors such as physostigmine

Additional Information

Red blood cell cholinesterase, and serum pseudocholinesterase may be depressed following acute or chronic organophosphate exposure; RBC cholinesterase is typically not analyzed by in-house laboratories, and is usually not available for consideration during acute management. Pseudocholinesterase levels may be rapidly available from some in-house laboratories, but are not as reliable a marker of organophosphate exposure because of variability secondary to variant genotypes, hepatic disease, oral estrogen use, or malnutrition. Because of this variability, true indication of suppression of either of these enzymes can only be estimated through comparison to pre-exposure values; these enzymes may be useful in measuring a patient's recovery postexposure, especially if the recovery is not progressing as expected.

The intermediate syndrome is not related to delayed neuropathy.

QT_c prolongation on ECG in the setting of organophosphate poisoning is associated with a high incidence of respiratory failure and mortality.

Yellow/tan viscous/oily liquid with a garlic odor; noncombustible, with a vapor pressure of 0.00003 mm Hg at 20°C

ACGIH TLV: 0.2 mg/m³; PEL-TWA: 0.2 mg/m³

Other information concerning pesticide exposures is available through the EPA-funded National Pesticide Telecommunications Network: 1-800-858-7378 (weekdays, 8 AM to 6 PM, Central Standard time)

Fenthion

CAS Number 55-38-9

U.S. Brand Names Baytex®; Entex®; Lysoff®; Spotton®; Tiguvon®

Use Marketed as insecticide granules, dusting agent, or spray liquid with or without petroleum derivative as a solvent

Mechanism of Toxic Action Irreversible inhibition of acetylcholinesterase and plasma cholinesterase, resulting in excess accumulation of acetylcholine at muscarinic and nicotinic receptors, and in the central nervous system

Adverse Reactions

Cardiovascular: **Hyperdynamic** (~18% to 21%) or hypodynamic (~7% to 10%) states, QT prolongation, sinus bradycardia, sinus tachycardia

Central nervous system: Depression, seizures, hyperactivity, extrapyramidal symptoms (dystonia, resting tremor, choreoathetosis) can develop from 4-40 days postexposure, cognitive dysfunction, hypothermia

Genitourinary: Urinary incontinence

Neuromuscular & skeletal: Weakness (delayed), paralysis, delayed paresthesia

Respiratory: Pulmonary edema, respiratory depression

Miscellaneous: Flu-like symptoms (especially with chronic exposure), intermediate syndrome

Signs and Symptoms of Overdose

Abdominal pain, agitation, asystole, AV block, bradycardia, bronchorrhea, coma, confusion, cranial nerve palsies, decreased hemoglobin, decreased platelet count, decreased red blood cell count, diaphragmatic paralysis, dysarthria, excessive sweating, fecal and urinary incontinence, generalized asthenia, headache, heart block, hypertension, hypotension, lacrimation, metabolic acidosis and hyperglycemia (severe intoxication), miosis (unreactive to light), mydriasis (rarely), nausea, pallor, pulmonary edema, QT prolongation, respiratory depression, salivation, seizures, skeletal muscle fasciculation and flaccid paralysis, tachycardia, tachypnea, vomiting

An "intermediate syndrome" of limb asthenia and respiratory paralysis has been reported to occur between 24 and 96 hours postorganophosphate exposure, and is independent of the acute cholinergic crisis. Late paresthesia characterized by stocking and glove paresthesia, anesthesia, and asthenia is infrequently observed weeks to months following acute exposure to certain organophosphates. Symptomatology may be delayed over 12 hours due to high lipid solubility.

Admission Criteria/Prognosis Observe for 96 hours

Toxicodynamics/Kinetics

Absorption: Readily through oral, dermal, or respiratory exposure

Metabolism: Rapidly metabolized to weakly active compounds through hepatic hydrolysis and other pathways

Elimination: Metabolites are excreted in urine

Warnings/Precautions Rapid dermal absorption may occur across intact skin; toxicity may be prolonged due to the high lipid solubility exhibited by fenthion; a risk of aspiration pneumonitis exists following oral exposure to agents having a hydrocarbon vehicle; severe laryngeal irritation and violent coughing may result from exposure to dusting powders; exposure to dusting powders and insecticide granules may cause contact dermatitis

Reference Range Postmortem blood fenthion level of 3.8 mcg/mL

Overdosage/Treatment

Decontamination: Isolation, bagging, and disposal of all contaminated clothing and other articles. All emergency medical workers and hospital staff should follow appropriate precautions regarding exposure to hazardous material including the use of protective clothing, masks, goggles, and respiratory equipment.

Dermal: Prompt thorough scrubbing of all affected areas with soap and water, including hair and nails; 5% bleach can be used

Oral: Activated charcoal can be administered either orally or via a nasogastric tube. **Do not** induce emesis because of danger of sudden respiratory compromise, alterations in mental status, seizures, coma, and possible aspiration of hydrocarbon vehicles. **Do not** give a cathartic.

Ocular: Irrigation with copious tepid sterile water or saline

Supportive therapy: Airway management, ventilatory assistance, humidified oxygen administration, and close monitoring for sudden respiratory failure; pralidoxime may be required to be given for a longer period of time (4-6 days; 22 days in 1 report)

Enhancement of elimination: Dialysis and hemoperfusion are not indicated due to effectiveness of the prescribed treatment and large volumes of distribution of organophosphates.

Antidote:

Atropine: Administration should be guided by respiratory status, starting at 2-5 mg I.V. every 5-10 minutes as needed, and should be titrated to the resolution of excess pulmonary secretions. Frequent administration of large doses (cumulative doses >100 mg) may be necessary in massive exposures.

Glycopyrrolate: May be administered if atropine is unavailable (200-400 mcg I.V. or I.M. initially, or $\sim^1/_2$ the dose of atropine)

2-PAM: For more significant exposures (ie, exposures requiring large doses of atropine, or with recurring symptoms, or exposures to more lipid soluble agents), administration should follow: 1-2 g I.V. over 10-30 minutes, repeated in 1 hour if asthenia recurs, then every 4-12 hours for recurring symptoms.

Antidote(s)

- Atropine [ANTIDOTE]
- Pralidoxime [ANTIDOTE]

Diagnostic Procedures

- Creatinine, Serum
- Pseudocholinesterase, Serum

Drug Interaction Paralysis is potentiated by neuromuscular blockade (ie, pancuronium, vecuronium, succinylcholine, atracurium, doxacurium, mivacurium); inhibition of serum esterase prolongs the half-life of succinylcholine, cocaine, and other ester anesthetics; cholinergic toxicity is potentiated by cholinesterase inhibitors such as physostigmine

Additional Information

Red blood cell cholinesterase and serum pseudocholinesterase may be depressed following acute or chronic organophosphate exposure; RBC cholinesterase is typically not analyzed by in-house laboratories, and is usually not available for consideration during acute management. Pseudocholinesterase levels may be rapidly available from some in-house laboratories, but are not as reliable a marker of organophosphate exposure because of variability secondary to variant genotypes, hepatic disease, oral estrogen use, or malnutrition. Because of this variability, true indication of suppression of either of these enzymes can only be estimated through comparison to pre-exposure values; these enzymes may be useful in measuring a patient's recovery postexposure, especially if the recovery is not progressing as expected. While muscarinic signs may not be marked, neurologic paralysis can occur within 72 hours; respiratory paralysis can last for a mean time of 132 hours.

Fenthion is very lipid soluble with peak intensity of symptoms occurring in 30-96 hour postexposure.

The intermediate syndrome is not related to delayed neuropathy.

QT_c prolongation on ECG in the setting of organophosphate poisoning is associated with a high incidence of respiratory failure and mortality.

Yellow to tan viscous liquid with a mild garlic odor

Vapor pressure: 0.00003 mm Hg at 20°C

ACGIH TLV: 0.2 mg/m^3; PEL-TWA: 0.2 mg/m^3

Other information concerning pesticide exposures is available through the EPA-funded National Pesticide Telecommunications Network: 1-800-858-7378 (weekdays, 8 AM to 6 PM, Central Standard time)

Specific References

Eddleston M, Eyer P, Worek F, et al, "Differences Between Organophosphorus Insecticides in Human Self-Poisoning: A Prospective Cohort Study," *Lancet*, 2005, 366(9495):1452-9.

Fipronil

CAS Number 120068-37-3

U.S. Brand Names Regent 50 SC®

Use Broad spectrum pesticide for use against crop infestation (rice, cotton); against locusts/grasshoppers, human head lice, cockroaches, ants, fleas/ticks on domestic animals; usually available as a 4.95 solution in propylene glycol; an ectoparasiticide (topical) in veterinary practice

Mechanism of Toxic Action An N-phenyl-pyrazole which blocks gamma-aminobutyric acid (GABA) induced rapid chloride currents in neurons. Affinity of fipronil for insects' receptors is about 1000 fold as compared to human receptors.

Signs and Symptoms of Overdose Ocular irritation, drowsiness, seizures are possible (28%); dermal irritation, dizziness, nausea, vomiting, diaphoresis, agitation; symptoms usually resolve in 12 hours

Toxicodynamics/Kinetics

Absorption (oral): Rapid

Metabolism: To active sulfone metabolites. Photoconversion to a desulfinyl compound can occur.

Reference Range Serum fipronil level of 1600 mcg/L associated with seizure

Overdosage/Treatment

Decontamination: Oral: Lavage within 1 hour / activated charcoal

Supportive therapy: Diazepam (10-15 mg I.V. in adults) is effective in termination of seizures; phenytoin is not likely to be beneficial

Additional Information Clear, slightly yellow liquid with almond or ester odor

Specific References

Fung HT, Chan KK, Ching WM, et al, "A Case of Accidental Ingestion of Ant Bait Containing Fipronil," *J Toxicol Clin Toxicol*, 2003, 41(3):245-8.

Mohammed F, Senarathna L, Percy A, et al, "Acute Human Self-Poisoning with the N-Phenylpyrazole Insecticide Fipronil - A GABA-A-Gated Chloride Channel Blocker," *J Toxicol Clin Toxicol*, 2004, 42(7):955-63.

Formaldehyde

Applies to Adhesive; Disinfectant (Hemodialysis Machines); Electrical Insulation; Embalming; Fireproofing; Glue; Lacquer; Tannery Products

CAS Number 50-00-0

UN Number 1198 (solution); 2209 (formalin)

Synonyms Fannoform; Formic Aldehyde, Formalin; Fyde; Hoch; Methanol; Morbicid; Paraform; Trioxane; Veracur

Use Embalming, fireproofing, glues/adhesives, lacquers, electrical insulation, tannery products; disinfectant use is limited to hemodialysis machines

Mechanism of Toxic Action Covalently binds to proteins and causes cell necrosis; mucous membrane irritant; synthesized by methanol oxidation.

Adverse Reactions

Cardiovascular: Cardiovascular collapse, hypotension

Central nervous system: CNS depression, panic attacks

Dermatologic: Contact dermatitis, dermal irritation, nonimmunologic contact urticaria, immunologic contact urticaria, airborne contact dermatitis

Endocrine & metabolic: Metabolic acidosis

Gastrointestinal: Coagulation necrosis on ingestion, vomiting, diarrhea, feces discoloration (black), throat irritation

Ocular: Visual evoked potential abnormalities

Renal: Nephritis, renal failure

Respiratory: Wheezing, tachypnea, bronchospasm, sinonasal cancer, asthma

Miscellaneous: Aneuploidy induction, cutaneous T-cell lymphoma

Signs and Symptoms of Overdose Ataxia, coma, cough, dizziness, drowsiness, dyspnea, tachypnea, gastritis, wheezing (at levels as low as 0.1 ppm), epistaxis, hyposmia, sore throat (over 5 ppm), anosmia, laryngospasm, ocular irritation (at 2 ppm), urticaria, pustuovesicular lesions, brownish skin and discoloration

Admission Criteria/Prognosis Development of metabolic acidosis or bronchospasm within 6 hours postexposure should constitute admission; asymptomatic patients may be discharged after 6 hours of observation; any patient with cardiopulmonary symptoms developing 6-12 hours postexposure should probably be admitted into an intensive care unit; survival after 2 days postexposure usually results in recovery

Toxicodynamics/Kinetics

Absorption: Well absorbed from the GI tract and by inhalation; to a lesser extent, absorbed through the skin. Dermal absorption is ~5%. Absorption from nasal portion of respiratory tract is near 100%.

Metabolism: Rapidly (within 1.5 minutes) to formic acid which is then metabolized to carbon dioxide and water

Half-life: Formate: 1.5 hours; formaldehyde: 3.3 hours

Reference Range Blood formaldehyde levels of 4.8 mg/L and 11 mg/L associated with fatality due to ingestion

Overdosage/Treatment

Decontamination: Basic poison management. Lavage within 1 hour; **do not** induce emesis; dilute with water.

Oral: Activated charcoal may be useful.

Inhalation: Administer 100% humidified oxygen

Ocular: Irrigate with copious amounts of saline.

Supportive therapy: Correct acidosis with sodium bicarbonate (1-2 mEq/kg I.V.); endoscopy to evaluate mucosal injury. Bronchospasm can be treated with beta-agonist therapy.

Enhancement of elimination: Consider hemodialysis if acidosis develops or if methanol is elevated due to formalin exposure.

Antidote(s)

● Sodium Bicarbonate [ANTIDOTE]

Diagnostic Procedures

● Anion Gap, Blood

● Electrolytes, Blood

Additional Information Implicated in squamous cell carcinoma of the nasopharynx (probable human carcinogen)

Ingestion of 30 mL (of a 37% solution) may cause fatalities. See table.

Indoor Concentrations of Formaldehyde in U.S. Homes

Building Type	Concentration (ppm)		
	Number	Range	Mean
With UFFI*	>1200	0.01-3.4	0.05-0.12
Without UFFI*	131	0.01-0.17	0.025-0.07
Compliant			
Mobile homes	>500	0.00-4.2	0.1-0.9
Non-compliant			
Conventional, randomly selected	560	<0.005-0.48	0.027-0.091
Mobile homes, randomly selected	~1,200	<0.01-2.9	0.091-0.62
By age			
Mobile homes			
New	260	–	0.86
Older, occupied	–	–	0.25
Conventional homes			
0-5 years	18	–	0.08
5-15 years	11	–	0.04
>15 years	11	–	0.03
Overall	40	<0.02-0.4	0.06

*UFFI = Urea formaldehyde foam insulation

Reference: U.S. Department of Health and Human Services, "Toxicological Profile for Formaldehyde," Agency for Toxic Substancers and Disease Registry, September 1997.

Odor threshold in water: 50 ppm. Odor threshold in air: 0.5-1 ppm. Taste threshold: 50 ppm. TLV-TWA: 1 ppm; IDLH: 20 ppm; PEL-TWA: 3 ppm. Airborne concentrations >2 ppm can cause mucosal irritation, while concentratons >50 ppm will cause serious injury within 10 minutes. Formalin contains 37% formaldehyde and 12% to 15% methanol

Potential Human Exposure to Formaldehyde

Source of Formaldehyde	(mg/day)
Air	
Outdoor air (10% of time)	0.02
Indoor air	
Home (65% of time)	
Conventional	0.5-2.0
Prefabricated (chipboard)	1-10

Table (Continued)

Source of Formaldehyde	(mg/day)
Workplace (25% of time)	
Without occupational exposure	0.2-0.8
With 1 mg/m^3 occupational exposure	5
Food (formaldehyde not in free form)	1-10
Environmental tobacco smoke (10% to 25% of total indoor exposure)	0.1-1
Smoking (20 cigarettes/day)	1

Reference: ATSDR and Fishbein L, "Exposure from Occupational Versus Other Sources," *Scand J Work Environ Health*, 1992, 18(1):5-16.

Atmospheric half-life: 19 hours in clean air; 9-10 hours in polluted air

Ambient urban formaldehyde air levels range from 5.5-67.7 ppb

Pulmonary function tests are recommended in patients with reactive airways dysfunction following formaldehyde inhalation

Dermal exposures >2% concentration can cause skin irritation

Dissolves easily in water

Metabolic Pathways of Formaldehyde Biotransformation

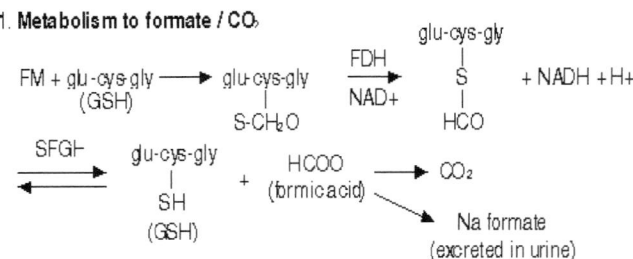

1. Metabolism to formate / CO$_2$

2. Binding to tetrahydrofolate (TH$_4$)

3. Nonenymatic reactions with sulfhydryl groups and urea

4. DNA and protein cross-linking

FM = formaldehyde, TH$_4$ = tetra hydrofolate, DNA = deoxyribonucleic acid, GSH = glutathione, NAD+ = nicotinomide adenosine dinucleotide, SFGH = S-formyl glutathione hydrolase, FDH = formaldehyde dehydrogenase.

From 'Toxicological Profile for Formaldehyde,' U.S. Department of Health and Human Services, Agency for Toxic Substances and Disease Registry, September 1997.

Specific References

Darkazally N, Judge BS, and Rusyniak DE, "Early Hemodialysis in Acute Formalin Ingestion," *J Toxicol Clin Toxicol*, 2003, 41(5):665.

Golden R, Pyatt D, and Shields PG, "Formaldehyde as a Potential Human Leukemogen: An Assessment of Biological Plausibility," *Crit Rev Toxicol*, 2006, 36:135-53.

O'Brien PJ, Siraki AG, and Shangari N, "Aldehyde Sources, Metabolism, Molecular Toxicity Mechanisms, and Possible Effects on Human Health," *Crit Rev Toxicol*, 2005, 35:609-62.

Yanagawa Y, Kuneko N, Hatanaka K, et al, "A Case of Attempted Suicide from Ingestion of Formalin," *Clin Toxicol*, 2007, 45(1):72-76.

Freon

Applies to Fire Extinguishers; Propellant; Refrigerant

Synonyms Dichlorodifluoromethane; Difluoroethane (Freon 152); Fluorinated Hydrocarbons; Halon

Use Refrigerant and in fire extinguishers/propellant

Mechanism of Toxic Action Can cause cold injury to surface on contact, sensitizer of myocardium to catecholamines

Adverse Reactions

Cardiovascular: Myocardial depression, arrhythmias, sinus bradycardia, congestive heart failure

Dermatologic: Contact dermatitis

Respiratory: Pulmonary edema, bronchoconstriction, asthma

Signs and Symptoms of Overdose Ataxia, bradycardia, coma, conjunctivitis, diarrhea, dizziness, drowsiness, dyspnea, hemoptysis, seizures, slurred speech, tremor

Toxicodynamics/Kinetics

Absorption: Immediate

Half-life: 75 minutes

Reference Range Postmortem blood levels of chlorodifluoromethane (Freon 22) and trichlorofluoromethane (Freon 11) of 71 mg/L and 63 mg/L, respectively, have been associated with fatality.

Overdosage/Treatment Decontamination: Basic poison management; avoid emesis; avoid catecholamines

Additional Information Odor of "fresh cut grass;" levels peak almost immediately after inhalation; heating may produce phosgene

Specific References

Delgado JH and Waksman JC, "Polymer Fume Fever-Like Syndrome Due to Hairspray Inhalation," *Vet Hum Toxicol*, 2004, 46(5):266-7.

Kubota T and Miyata A, "Acute Inhalational Exposure to Chlorodifluoromethane (Freon-22): A Report of 43 Cases," *Clin Toxicol (Phila)*, 2005, 43(4):305-8.

Furfural

CAS Number 98-01-1

UN Number 1199

Synonyms Furol; Quakeral

Use A heterocyclic aldehyde commonly used as a solvent in butadiene/aromatic compound extractions, and in manufacture of ant poisons, food products, and fuels (found in cocoa, tea, coffee, beer, wine, bread, and milk)

Mechanism of Toxic Action A dermal and mucosal irritant which can cause CNS depression

Signs and Symptoms of Overdose Conjunctivitis, excessive lacrimation, headache, nasal irritation, and throat irritation can occur at air concentrations of 2-14 ppm. Dermal exposure can cause eczema, pain, and irritation. Inhalation exposure can cause cough, shortness of breath, and sore throat.

Toxicodynamics/Kinetics

Metabolism: Hepatic oxidation to furoic acid

Half-life: 2-2.5 hours

Elimination: Renal

Reference Range Normal amount of urinary furoic acid: 15 mmol/mol creatinine (15 mg/g creatinine). Biological exposure index (BEI): 200 mmol/mol creatinine (200 mg/g creatinine) at end of work shift.

Overdosage/Treatment Decontamination: **Dermal**: Wash with water. **Inhalation**: Administer 100% humidified oxygen. **Ocular**: Irrigate with saline. **Oral**: Dilute wtih 4-8 ounces of milk and water. Activated charcoal may be useful.

Additional Information A colorless oily liquid. A 60 mg oral ingestion can cause headache. Atmospheric half-life is 0.44 days. No significant bioconcentration.

Specific References

Tan ZB, Tonks CE, O'Donnell GE, et al, "An Improved HPLC Analysis of the Metabolite Furoic Acid in the Urine of Workers Occupationally Exposed to Furfural," *J Anal Toxicol*, 2003, 27(1):43-6.

Gasoline

Related Information
- Benzene
- Lead
- Methyl Tert-Butyl Ether
- Toluene Diisocyanate

CAS Number 8006-61-9

UN Number 1203; 1257

Synonyms Mogas; Motor Fuel; Motor Spirit; Natural Gasoline; Petrol

Use Fuel for internal combustion engines

Mechanism of Toxic Action A volatile hydrocarbon with central nervous system depressant and arrhythmogenic effects

Adverse Reactions

Cardiovascular: Sinus bradycardia

Central nervous system: Panic attacks with inhalation

Neuromuscular & skeletal: Rhabdomyolysis

Renal: Alpha 2u-globulin nephropathy

Signs and Symptoms of Overdose

Death from ingestion is usually due to aspiration. Symptoms occur at 1000 ppm after 1 hour; ataxia, confusion, delirium dysarthria, euphoria, hallucinations (visual, auditory and tactile), headache, mania, tremor, vertigo

Inhalation: Arrhythmia, ataxia, dizziness, drowsiness, hallucinations, insomnia, intra-alveolar hemorrhage, muscle cramps, myoclonus, nausea, paresthesias, pulmonary edema, vomiting

Ingestion: Aspiration, belching, disseminated intravascular coagulation can occur, elevated hepatic enzymes, hematuria, hemolysis, hypotension, oliguria, pulmonary congestion

Admission Criteria/Prognosis Patients who develop tachypnea, cyanosis, dyspnea, CNS depression, tachycardia, or fever within 8 hours of exposure should be admitted; asymptomatic patients can be discharged after 8 hours observation

Toxicodynamics/Kinetics

Protein binding: None

Half-life: 17 hours

Elimination: Pulmonary/renal

Reference Range Urine phenol level (for benzene measurement) >40 mg/L is consistent with gasoline exposure in gasoline pump workers; blood 2 methylpentane level >50 mg/L has been associated with fatality Postmortem Gasoline concentration in heart blood and vitreous humor of 22.3 and 1 mg/L respectively, associated with fatal inhalation of motorcycle exhaust.

Overdosage/Treatment

Decontamination: **Do not** induce emesis or lavage due to risk of aspiration pneumonia. Activated charcoal can adsorb benzene.

Dermal: Wash with soap and water

Supportive therapy: Benzodiazepines for seizure control; avoid use of catecholamines due to risk of ventricular arrhythmia; treat burns with standard burn therapy; monitor for carbon monoxide

Aggressive airway management; intubation if pulmonary response is worrisome and/or loss of consciousness/CNS symptoms suggest potential loss of airway protection

For inhalaton injuries, nebulized budesonide (0.5 mg every 12 hours for 4 days - pediatric dose) may be helpful

Diagnostic Procedures
- Lead, Urine

Additional Information

Boiling point : 104-401°F

Highly lipid soluble; gasoline contains a mixture of benzene (0.5%-2.5%), toluene, xylene, ethyl benzene, and possible lead (tetraethyl lead); other additives include ethylene dichloride and ethylene dibromide; lead poisoning is unusual from inhalation of gasoline containing tetraethyl lead

Odor threshold of gasoline: 0.25 ppm. Lethal inhalation concentration: 5000 ppm. Lethal ingestion concentration: 5 g/kg (12 oz)

Ambient level of gasoline at service stations is usually <100 ppm

OSHA - PEL-TWA: 300 ppm; TLV-TWA: 300 ppm

Lead in agriculture gasoline use should be phased out in 1995; goal of phase I toxic reduction is 15% and phase II toxic reduction is 20% to 22%; see table.

Aviation gasoline has a lead concentration of 1.28 grams per liter (as opposed to unleaded gasoline which has 0.03 grams per liter of lead).

Aviation gasoline is 24% toulene and 75% aliphatic hydrocarbon.

Automotive Gasoline				
Fuel Parameter	Conventional Gasoline (prior to 1995)	Reformulated Gasoline		
		Phase I (1995-1999)	Phase II (2000-)	California
Reid vapor pressure (psi)	8.7/7.8	8.0/7.1	6.7	6.8
Sulfur (ppm)	339	305	140	30
Oxygen (w%)*	<0.5	2.1	2.1	2
Aromatics (vol%)	32	27	25	22
Olefins (vol%)	13	12	12	4
E200 (%)†	41	49	49	49
E300 (%)‡	83	87	87	91
Benzene (vol%)	1.5	0.95	0.95	0.8

*Increased oxygen percentage obtained by addition of ethanol or methanol.

†Of fuel evaporated at 200°F.

‡Of fuel evaporated at 300°F.

Specific gravity for gasoline is 0.75-0.8

A 1% solution of gasoline (inhaled) can produce symptoms within 5 minutes; 15-20 breaths of gasoline can result in intoxication for as long as 6 hours; Canada has replaced lead with methylcyclopentadrenyl manganese tricarbonyl (MMT) which can produce manganese toxicity

Specific References

Byard RW, Chivell WC, and Gilbert JD, "Unusual Facial Markings and Lethal Mechanisms in a Series of Gasoline Inhalation Deaths," *Am J Forensic Med Pathol*, 2003, 24(3):298-302.

Gurkan F and Bosnak M, "Use of Nebulized Budesonide in Two Critical Patients with Hydrocarbon Intoxication," *Am J Ther*, 2005, 12(4):366-7.

Hesterberg TW, Bunn WB, McClellan RO, et al, "Carcinogenicity Studies of Diesel Engine Exhausts in Laboratory Animals: A Review of Past Studies and a Discussion of Future Research Needs," *Crit Rev Toxicol*, 2005, 35:379-411.

Klein KR, White SR, Herzog P, et al, "Demand for PCC Services 'Surged' During the 2003 Blackout," *J Toxicol Clin Toxicol*, 2004, 42(5):814-5.

Martinez MA and Ballesteros S, "Investigation of Fatalities Due to Acute Gasoline Poisoning," *J Anal Toxicol*, 2006, 30:154-5.

Martinez MA and Ballesteros S, "Suicidal Inhalation of Motor Bike Exhaust: Adding New Data to the Literature about the Contribution of Gasoline in the Cause of Death," *J Anal Toxicol*, 2006, (30):697-702.

Takamiya M, Niitsu H, Saigusa K, et al, "A Case of Acute Gasoline Intoxication at the Scene of Washing a Petrol Tank," *Leg Med*, 2003, 5(3):165-9.

Glufosinate

Applies to Herbicide
U.S. Brand Names Basta®
Synonyms GLA
Use Herbicide (plant inhibitor of glutamine synthetase); replaces paraquat in use
Mechanism of Toxic Action Related to glutamic acid; can excite amino acid in the central nervous system
Signs and Symptoms of Overdose May be delayed for up to 38 hours. Amnesia, ataxia, coma, dysarthria, edema, fever, hypotension, lethargy, leukocytosis, nystagmus, oral ulcers, seizures, tremor
Admission Criteria/Prognosis Admit any asymptomatic ingestion of Basta® >1 mL/kg for at least 48 hours
Toxicodynamics/Kinetics
Absorption, oral: 30%
Distribution: V_d: ~2 L/kg
Elimination: Renal (clearance: 83 mL/minute)
Overdosage/Treatment
Decontamination: Do not use ipecac or induce vomiting. Lavage within 1 hour of ingestion; activated charcoal should be used.
Supportive therapy: Benzodiazepines should be used to treat seizures.
Enhancement of elimination: Hemodialysis may be useful (clearance by hemodialysis is ~50 mL/minute).
Additional Information Lethal dose: 3 mL/kg; Toxic oral dose: 1.6 mL/kg. Basta® is 18.5% glufosinate.

Glutaraldehyde

CAS Number 111-30-8
Synonyms 1,5,-Pentanedial; Glutaral; GTA
Use An aliphatic dialdehyde as a biocide/disinfectant; often used as a sterilizing agent in medical facilities and as a histological fixative; also used in embalming solutions; used topically in a 2% to 10% solution to treat warts, hyperhidrosis, and onychomycosis (#2 aldehyde used in the U.S.)
Mechanism of Toxic Action A contact irritant and sensitizer
Adverse Reactions
Cardiovascular: Chest pain, tachycardia
Central nervous system: Headache, dizziness, ataxia
Neuromuscular & skeletal: Muscle twitching
Ocular: Conjunctivitis, corneal opacity
Respiratory: Nasal irritation, bronchospasm, asthma
Overdosage/Treatment
Decontamination: **Dermal**: Irrigate with copious amounts of water. **Inhalation**: Administer 100% humidified oxygen. **Ocular**: Irrigate with saline.
Supportive Care: Treat bronchospasm with standard therapy. (Beta-2 agonists)
Additional Information TLV: 0.05 ppm; odor threshold: 0.04 ppm; ocular/respiratory irritant at 0.3 ppm; rubber gloves are not protective; ocular injury (in animal studies) occurred at glutaraldehyde concentrations >1%; dermal injury (in rabbits) occurred at 5% concentration
Oily liquid/not flammable

Glycol Ethers

Applies to Anti-icing Agents; Leather Treatment Products; Solvent (Industrial); Varnish Remover
Synonyms Alkylene Oxide Adducts; Cellosolves
Use In the production of photoresists of the microelectronic industry, industrial solvents, varnish removers, leather treatment products, anti-icing agents
Mechanism of Toxic Action Hemolysis, bone marrow depression by metabolites by interfering with RNA and DNA synthesis
Adverse Reactions
Cardiovascular: Sinus tachycardia, arrhythmias (ventricular)
Central nervous system: Encephalopathy, coma
Hematologic: Bone marrow suppression, hemolytic anemia
Hepatic: Fatty degeneration of the liver (methyl ether)
Renal: Tubular necrosis (acute), renal failure
Signs and Symptoms of Overdose Ataxia, coma, confusion, drowsiness, headache, hemorrhagic gastritis, hyperventilation, hypocalcemia, hypokalemia, hypotension, metabolic acidosis, tachycardia (ventricular), tremor; symptoms may be delayed up to 18 hours
Toxicodynamics/Kinetics
Absorption: Readily through the skin, lungs, and GI tract
Elimination: Oxidized by alcohol dehydrogenase and excreted in urine
Overdosage/Treatment
Decontamination: Lavage (within 1 hour)/ activated charcoal
Supportive therapy: Treat acidosis with sodium bicarbonate. Ethanol administration may be of some use.
Enhancement of elimination: Hemodialysis is useful for renal failure or acid abnormalities.
Antidote(s)
• Sodium Bicarbonate [ANTIDOTE]
Diagnostic Procedures
• Crystals, Urine
• Electrolytes, Blood
Additional Information Minimum lethal dose: 8 mL (methoxyethanol)
Mild ethereal odor
Order of toxicity: Methoxyethanol > ethoxyethanol > butoxyethanol; may give a positive ethylene glycol level on laboratory testing
Diagnostic effects caused by glycol ethers include hypocalcemia (methyl ether), hypokalemia (methyl ether and butyl ether), pancytopenia, metabolic acidosis with high anion gap, and oxalate crystals may be seen in urine; does not affect osmolar gap

Glyphosate

Applies to Herbicide
CAS Number 1071-83-6
U.S. Brand Names Bronco®; Glifonox®; Glycel®; Glyphotox®; Kleen-up®; Network®; Rodeo®; Roundup®; Weedoff®
Synonyms N-(Phosphonomethyl) glycine; GlySH
Use Herbicide
Mechanism of Toxic Action The surfactant (polyoxyethyleneamine) may cause uncoupling of oxidative phosphorylation (although this mechanism is in question); additionally is a mucosal irritant and a myocardial depressant
Signs and Symptoms of Overdose Acute tubular necrosis (10%), anuria, bronchospasm, cough, diarrhea, drowsiness, dysphagia, dyspnea, vomiting, esophagitis, excessive hematemesis, gastritis, hematuria, hypotension, hyperkalemia, leukocytosis (average 14,300 cells/mm³), metabolic acidosis (78% of cases), noncardiogenic pulmonary edema (5% to 13%), nystagmus, oliguria, oral mucosal ulceration, piloerection, respiratory failure, salivation, hemolysis
Toxicodynamics/Kinetics
Absorption: May be absorbed dermally (<2%)
Half-life: 2-3 hours
Elimination: Renal
Monitoring Parameters CBC, arterial blood gases, electrolytes
Reference Range
Serum glyphosate levels >1000 ppm associated with severe symptoms
Urine glyphosate concentration of 11,200 mg/L associated with fatal poisoning
Overdosage/Treatment
Decontamination: Lavage (within 1 hour)/activated charcoal; **do not** induce emesis; may dilute with milk or water
Supportive therapy: Primarily supportive; do not give pralidoxime; sodium bicarbonate can be given for metabolic acidosis
Enhanced elimination: No evidence that forced diuresis is effective; early use of hemodialysis may be useful to treat acidosis or other metabolic abnormalities
Additional Information
Minimal lethal dose: 60 mL (in an 84-year-old man)
Patients >40 years who ingest >150 mL are at highest risk for death

Specific References

Bradberry SM, Proudfoot AT, and Vale JA, "Glyphosate Poisoning," *Toxicol Rev*, 2004, 23(3):159-67.

Hori Y, Fujisawa M, Shimada K, et al, "Determination of the Herbicide Glyphosate and Its Metabolite in Biological Specimens by Gas Chromatography-Mass Spectrometry: A Case of Poisoning by Round-up® Herbicide," *J Anal Toxicol*, 2003, 27(3):162-6.

Horswell J and Dickson S, "Use of Biosensors to Screen Urine Samples for Potentially Toxic Chemicals," *J Anal Toxicol*, 2003, 27(6):372-6.

Matteucci MJ and Clark RF, "Glyphosate Surfactant Herbicide-Induced Acute Renal Failure," *Clin Toxicol (Phila)*, 2005, 43:726.

Mehler LN, Comment on "An Analysis of Glyphosate Data from the California Environmental Protection Agency Pesticide Illness Surveillance Program," *J Toxicol Clin Toxicol*, 2003, 41(7):1039-40.

Moon JM, Young IM, and Chun BJ, "Can Early Hemodialysis Affect the Outcome of the Ingestion of Glyphosate Herbicide?" *Clin Toxicol*, 2006, 44(3):329-32.

Helium

CAS Number 7440-59-7

UN Number 1046

Synonyms He

Use Often used as an inhalant of misuse; also may be a byproduct in welding; a balloon filler heating medium; used in neon signs and mixed-gas sea diving

Mechanism of Toxic Action Can cause arterial gas embolism

Signs and Symptoms of Overdose Blurriness, clonus, coma, nausea, dizziness, headache, limb weakness, neck pain, paresthesia, seizures (all symptoms of cerebral gas embolism); can cause dermal burns upon skin contact. Laryngeal changes can occur.

Admission Criteria/Prognosis Admit any patient with neurologic symptoms or signs of pneumothorax

Overdosage/Treatment

Decontamination: Inhalation: Humidified 100% oxygen

Supportive therapy: Hyperbaric oxygen may be useful if signs of arterial gas embolism develop.

Antidote(s)

- Oxygen (Hyperbaric) [ANTIDOTE]

Additional Information Liquid helium is a colorless, tasteless, odorless liquid which is easily vaporized. Atmospheric concentrations >20 mg/dL can cause symptoms. Heliox is 20% oxygen and 80% helium, used in patients with airway disease and decompression illness. Specific gravity: 0.15. Vapor density: 0.14

Specific References

Gallagher KE, Smith DM, and Mellen PF, "Suicidal Asphyxiation by Using Pure Helium Gas: Case Report, Review, and Discussion of the Influence of the Internet," *Am J Forensic Med Pathol*, 2003, 24(4):361-3.

Poklis JL, Garside D, and Winecker RE, "A Qualitative Method for the Detection of Helium in Postmortem Blood and Tissues," *J Anal Toxicol*, 2006, 30:137.

Heptachlor

Related Information

- Adipose Tissue Ranges of Toxins
- Chlordane

CAS Number 1024-57-3; 76-44-8

U.S. Brand Names Drinox®; Heptagran®; Heptamul®; Soleptax®; Termide®; Velsicol 104®

Use While it had been used as a dermal insecticide and for control of crop pests and termites, its use has been sharply curtailed in the U.S. by the EPA since 1988; primarily currently used as a termiticide for domestic use and in fire ant control in power transformers

Mechanism of Toxic Action In the cyclodiene class of organochlorine pesticides; interferes with axonal transmembrane flux of sodium and potassium; also inhibits oxidative phosphorylation

Adverse Reactions

Cardiovascular: Raynaud's phenomenon

Dermatologic: Scleroderma

Gastrointestinal: Nausea, vomiting

Hematologic: Thrombocytopenia

Neuromuscular & skeletal: Tremors

Ocular: Mydriasis

Toxicodynamics/Kinetics

Absorption: Oral

Metabolism: Hepatic epoxidation to heptachlor epoxide and oxychlordane

Reference Range Dairy farm workers exposed to hepachlor from raw milk (levels up to 89 ppm) had elevated blood heptachlor epoxide levels (0.84±1.0 ppb) and oxychlordane levels (0.71±0.8 ppb). U.S. sampling of adipose tissue averages ~0.1 ppm (FDA "action level").

Overdosage/Treatment

Decontamination: **Oral:** Lavage (within 1 hour)/activated charcoal or cholestyramine; **do not** administer milk or cream as it can enhance absorption. **Dermal:** Wash with soap and water; avoid oils as they can enhance absorption. **Inhalation:** Administer 100% humidified oxygen.

Enhancement of elimination: Multiple dosing of activated charcoal or cholestyramine may be effective.

Additional Information Usually found in conjunction with chlordane exposure. Heptachlor can be formed as a chlordane metabolite. Some association with leukemia noted; can cause sclerodermatous changes of the hands. Leather clothing absorbs heptachlor. Odor threshold: 0.3 mg/m³. TLV-TWA: 0.5 mg/m³; IDLH: 100 mg/m³

Hexabromobiphenyl

Related Information

- Polychlorinated Biphenyls

CAS Number 36355-01-8; 59536-65-1; 67774-32-7

Synonyms Firemaster BP-6; Firemaster FF-1

Use Fire retardant in thermoplastics for use in motor housing, electrical products, and auto upholstery; not imported or produced in the U.S. since 1979

Mechanism of Toxic Action Binds to a cellular receptor (Ah receptor) which alters protein and enzyme synthesis

Adverse Reactions Similar to polychlorinated biphenyl agents; halogen acne, hypothyroidism, impairment of memory upon inhalation; elevated liver function test results and hepatomegaly have been noted after oral ingestion; hepatocellular carcinomas have been noted in animal models

Toxicodynamics/Kinetics

Absorption: By dermal contact, oral, or inhalation routes

Protein binding: 80%

Metabolism: Hepatic debromination and hydroxylation

Elimination: Fecal and urinary routes

Reference Range General population adipose tissue concentration: Ranges from 1.0-2.0 mcg/kg; baseline serum level of polybrominated biphenyls: ~0.2 mcg/L

Overdosage/Treatment Decontamination: **Oral:** Lavage (within 1 hour)/activated charcoal or cholestyramine. **Dermal:** Wash with soap and water. **Ocular:** Irrigate with saline.

Additional Information Exposure can occur via ingestion of contaminated food; one such episode occurred in Michigan involving contaminated feed from polybrominated biphenyls (PBB) in May 1973; dairy products were involved. While spray drying of milk reduced PBB levels in milk, there was no effect when pasteurization, aging of cheese, or freeze drying occurred; pressure cooking meat also reduces meat PBB content. Atmospheric half-life: 182 days

Hexachlorobenzene

Related Information

- Cholestyramine Resin [ANTIDOTE]
- Edetate Calcium Disodium [ANTIDOTE]
- Pentachlorophenol

Applies to Seed Treatment

CAS Number 118-74-1

UN Number 2729

U.S. Brand Names Amatin®; Anti-Carie®; Bent-Cure®; Bent-No-More®; No Bent®; Sanocide®

Synonyms HCB; Perchlorobenzene; Phenyl Perchloryl

Use Waste product of perchlorethylene used for seed treatment

Mechanism of Toxic Action Induction of porphyria can occur by inhibition of the enzyme uroporphyrinogen decarboxylase and increased d-ALA-synthetase, thus increasing uroporphyrin III levels; lipid peroxidation and mitochondrial inhibition can also occur

Adverse Reactions

In children, diarrhea, fever, pink skin papules are noted; hypochromic anemia

Central nervous system: Hypothermia

Dermatologic: Skin blisters, epidermolysis, increased pigmentation, porphyria cutanea tarda syndrome ("pink sore disease") from estimated ingestion of 0.05-0.2 g/day; scleroderma

Endocrine & metabolic: Thyromegaly

Gastrointestinal: Anorexia

Genitourinary: Urine discoloration (port wine)

Hematologic: Porphyria

Hepatic: Hepatomegaly, centrilobular hepatic necrosis

Neuromuscular & skeletal: Hand atrophy, muscle weakness, paresthesia in children

Respiratory: Pulmonary irritant

Signs and Symptoms of Overdose Alopecia, ataxia, hirsutism, hyperthermia, porphyria

Toxicodynamics/Kinetics

Distribution: Very lipophilic; found in breast milk

Metabolism: Hepatic to pentachlorophenol, pentachlorobenzene, and tetrachlorobenzene

Half-life: 60 days

Reference Range Whole blood hexachlorobenzene levels of 0.41 ppb not associated with adverse health effects

Overdosage/Treatment

Decontamination: Lavage (within 1 hour)/activated charcoal

Supportive therapy: Avoid sunlight. Calcium disodium ethyl-enediamine-tetraacetic acid (EDTA) at 1.5 g I.V. for 5 days or 500 mg to 1.5 g/day orally has been shown to be useful. Barbiturates should be used for seizure control.

Enhancement of elimination: Multiple dosing of activated charcoal or cholestyramine may be effective.

Additional Information Increased death rate in children with maternal hexachlorobenzene-induced porphyria during first 2 years of life, probably through contaminated breast milk. Little CNS toxicity. Insoluble in water. Atmospheric half-life: 90 days. Soil half-life: 3-6 years Pentachlorophenol can increase toxicity (porphyringenicity) of hexachlorobenzene.

Hexachlorobutadiene

Related Information

- Adipose Tissue Ranges of Toxins

Applies to Fumigant; Solvent (Rubber, Lubricants, Chlorofluorocarbons)

CAS Number 87-68-3

UN Number 2279

Synonyms Dolen-Pur; Perchlorobutadiene

Use Solvent in the manufacture of rubber, lubricants, and chlorofluoro-carbons; fumigant; fluid in gyroscopes

Mechanism of Toxic Action Cysteine metabolite causes uncoupling of oxidative phosphorylation and inhibition of cytochrome oxidase activity and electron transport in the mitochondria

Adverse Reactions Increased serum bile acids with chronic inhalation exposure (0.005-0.02 ppm)

Toxicodynamics/Kinetics

Absorption: After inhalation

Metabolism: Conjugation with glutathione (toxic metabolite)

Elimination: Biliary

Reference Range Range noted in human adipose tissue 0.8-8.0 mcg/kg wet weight

Overdosage/Treatment

Decontamination: Lavage (within 1 hour)/activated charcoal; **do not** use oil-based cathartic

Supportive therapy: In animal studies, probenecid decreased levels of mercapturic acid derivative and decreased renal toxicity.

Enhancement of elimination: Due to enterohepatic recirculation, multiple dosing of activated charcoal may be effective.

Additional Information Range of urban ambient air hexachlorobuta-diene levels: 2-11 ppt. Drinking water contains <3 ppt; not found in sewage samples. PEL-TWA: 0.02 ppm; TLV-TWA: 0.02 ppm

Hexachlorocyclopentadiene

Applies to C-56; HRS1655

CAS Number 77-47-4

UN Number 2646

U.S. Brand Names Graphlox

Synonyms HCCPD; Perchlorocyclopentadiene

Use Key chemical intermediate in chlorinated pesticides (present up to 1% as a contaminant), in manufacture of flame retardants, nonflammable resins, and dyes

Mechanism of Toxic Action A mucosal irritant which is directly toxic at the cellular level

Signs and Symptoms of Overdose Abdominal cramps, dermal irritation, elevation of hepatic enzymes, headache (may last up to 6 weeks), lacrimation, nasal irritation (at levels >1 ppm), nausea, ocular irritation, proteinuria (usually resolves in 3 weeks); may increase risk of urogenital infection in females

Toxicodynamics/Kinetics Absorption: By lung, dermal, and GI routes

Overdosage/Treatment

Decontamination: **Oral:** Dilute with milk or water. **Dermal:** Wash with soap and water. **Inhalation:** Remove from environment and administer humidified oxygen.

Enhancement of elimination: Hemodialysis or hemoperfusion is unlikely to be of any benefit.

Additional Information Readily absorbed by soil and sediment. Atmospheric half-life: <1 day. Water half-life: <5 minutes. OSHA: PEL-TWA: 0.1 ppm; TLV-TWA: 0.01 ppm

Hexachloroethane

CAS Number 67-72-1

UN Number 9037

U.S. Brand Names Avlothane®; Distokal®; Distopan®; Egitol®; Phenohep®

Synonyms Carbon Hexachloride; HCE; Perchloroethane

Use Moth repellent; antihelmintic agent in sheep; used in the military in smoke screens and pyrotechnic devices

Mechanism of Toxic Action Mucosal irritant; this chlorinated hydro-carbon can cause a tubular nephropathy and hepatic toxicity through free radical-induced lipid peroxidation

Adverse Reactions No systemic adverse effects described in humans although there is one report of a liver tumor associated with a 6-year hexachloroethane exposure; liver and kidneys are target organs for pathology in animals; neurotoxicity (ataxia and tremor) has also been noted; not fetotoxic in rodent models; blepharospasm, lacrimation, and photophobia noted to fume exposure; alpha 2u-globulin nephropathy

Toxicodynamics/Kinetics

Absorption: Limited from inhalation or dermal routes. Oral absorption: 50% to 88%

Metabolism: Hepatic to tetrachloroethane and pentachloroethane

Overdosage/Treatment

Decontamination: **Oral:Do not** induce emesis. Lavage (within 1 hour)/activated charcoal; **do not** administer milk or cream in that it can increase absorption. **Dermal:** Remove contaminated clothing; wash with soap and water. **Ocular:** Irrigate copiously with saline.

Supportive therapy: Although there is no experience in this toxicity, N-acetylcysteine may have a theoretical role in reducing hepatotoxic effects.

Enhancement of elimination: Although there is no experience in this toxicity, hemodialysis may play a role in enhancing elimination of hexachloroethane in patients developing renal failure.

Additional Information Hexachloroethane is a metabolite of carbon tetrachloride. Odor threshold: Air: 0.015 ppm (camphoraceous); water: 0.01 mg/L. Background air level in northern hemisphere: 5-7 ppt. Water half-life: 1 year. TLV-TWA: 1 ppm

Hexamethylene Diisocyanate

CAS Number 822-06-0

UN Number 2281

U.S. Brand Names Desmodur H; Mondur HX

Synonyms HDI; HMDI

Use Production of plastics, synthetic rubber, varnishes, lacquers, paints (hardener in automobile and airline paint), wire insulation, polyurethane foam and glues

Mechanism of Toxic Action Respiratory tract irritant which can induce bronchospasm

Adverse Reactions

Cardiovascular: Chest tightness, cor pulmonale

Central nervous system: Fever, headache, fatigue

Hematologic: Leukocytosis

Respiratory: Bronchospasm, wheezing, cough, bronchitis, laryngitis, nasal irritation, dyspnea

Admission Criteria/Prognosis Admit any symptomatic patient; asymptomatic patients may be discharged after 6 hours of observation

Toxicodynamics/Kinetics

Absorption: By dermal, inhalation and oral routes

Metabolism: 1,6-hexamethylene diamine (HDA)

Half-life (HDA): 1.2 hours

Elimination: Renal

Monitoring Parameters Arterial blood gas, chest x-ray

Overdosage/Treatment

Decontamination: **Dermal:** Flush skin with soap and water. Isopropyl alcohol can also be used to help decontaminate intact skin. **Inhalation:** Administer 100% humidified oxygen. **Ocular:** Irrigate with saline.

Supportive therapy: For treatment of bronchoconstriction, administer inhaled beta-agonist agents.

Additional Information Concentrations >0.02 ppm can cause severe respiratory symptoms.

Pale yellow liquid with a pungent odor. Density: ~1.05 g/mL. Odor threshold in air: 0.001-0.02 ppm. Atmospheric half-life: 2 days. Rapidly hydrolyzed in water (water half-life: 10 minutes). TLV-TWA: 0.005 ppm

Hexane

CAS Number 110-54-3

UN Number 1208

Synonyms Dipropyl; Hexyl Hydride; Skellysolve B

Commonly Found In Production of glues, adhesives, paints, shoes, and furniture; component of crude oil

Mechanism of Toxic Action Metabolite 2,5-hexanedione is neurotoxic; 2-methyl pentone leads to hexone

Adverse Reactions
Cardiovascular: Tachycardia, sinus tachycardia
Central nervous system: CNS depression, axonopathy
Ocular: Visual evoked potential abnormalities
Respiratory: Respiratory depression

Signs and Symptoms of Overdose Blurred vision, dyspnea, lacrimation, muscle cramps, ototoxicity, upper airway irritation, tinnitus, peripheral sensorimotor neuropathy; muscle wasting/atrophy (peripheral muscles are affected first). Exposure to 500 ppm of hexane over several months can lead to peripheral neuropathy.

Admission Criteria/Prognosis Symptomatic patients or patients with abnormal chest x-rays should be admitted

Toxicodynamics/Kinetics
Absorption: Through the skin (within 30 minutes), GI tract, and lungs
Metabolism: To 2,5-hexanedione
Half-life: 1.5-2 hours
Elimination: Excreted renally

Reference Range Urine concentration of 2,5-hexanedione should be <5 mg/L; background blood hexane concentrations in unexposed adults range from 0.02-7.7 mcg/L (average: 0.6 mcg/L); it has been estimated that ~3 mg hexanedione per gram creatinine corresponds to inhalation daily exposure of 50 ppm of hexane

Overdosage/Treatment Decontamination: **Oral:** Lavage within 1 hour; dilute with 4-8 oz of milk or water. **Dermal:** Wash skin with soap and water. **Inhalation:** Administer 100% humidified oxygen.

Drug Interaction Acetone may potentiate neurotoxicity of hexane

Additional Information
Parkinsonism may occur with chronic exposure, along with a sensory polyneuropathy and memory deficits.

A colorless liquid with a faint odor; insoluble in water. Odor threshold: 0.0064 mg/L in water and 130 ppm in air. Estimated half-life in pond water: 2.7 hours to 6.8 days. TLV-TWA: 50 ppm

Ambient atmospheric hexane levels in urban areas: 1.6-5.5 ppb; hexane comprises ~2% of volatile organic compounds in urban air from combustible sources

HMX

Related Information
• RDX

Applies to Plastic Explosives; Rocket Fuel Propellant
CAS Number 2691-41-0
UN Number 0226
Synonyms Cyclotetramethylenetetranitramine; High Melting Explosive; Octogen

Use Explosive polynitramine which is primarily used in nuclear devices to implode fissionable material; also used as a solid rocket fuel propellant and in plastic explosives; also used to implode fissionable materials in nuclear devices to achieve critical mass; primarily produced in the U.S. at the Holston Army Ammunition Plant in Kingsport, Tennessee

Mechanism of Toxic Action Essentially not known but may involve its toxic metabolites nitrite, hydrazines, and formaldehyde

Adverse Reactions No documented adverse effects to exposure in humans have been described; in animals, this toxin appears to act as a neurological stimulant at oral doses over 1500 mg/kg; methemoglobinemia, mild skin irritation

Signs and Symptoms of Overdose Seizures

Toxicodynamics/Kinetics
Absorption: Oral: Poor (<5% in animals); peak absorption: 6-10 hours
Metabolism: To nitrites and then nitroreduction to hydrazines
Elimination: Renal, expired air, fecal (primarily oral ingestion)

Reference Range Measured blood octogen level of 2.5 mg/L associated with seizure

Overdosage/Treatment
Decontamination: **Oral:** Emesis (within 30 minutes) or lavage (within 1 hour); activated charcoal may help reduce absorption. **Dermal:** Wash with soap and water. **Do not** use oils since they may increase absorption. **Ocular:** Irrigate with saline.

Supportive therapy: Methylene blue for symptomatic methemoglobinemia or methemoglobin levels >30%; benzodiazepines/phenobarbital for seizures

Additional Information
Colorless, odorless, solid crystals

Explodes at high temperatures (over 279°C); not usually found in air; essentially insoluble in water (5 mL/L at 25°C). Photolytic half-life in water: 1-70 days

EPA lifetime drinking water standard: 400 mcg/L

Specific References
Testud F, Descotes J, and LeMeur B, "Acute Occupational Poisoning by Octogen: First Case Report," *Clin Toxicol*, 2006, 44:189-90.

Hydrazine

Applies to Corrosion Inhibitor; Laboratory Reagent; Mirrors (Silvering); Pesticides; Pharmaceutical Agents (Production); Photography; Rocket Fuel; Scavenging Agent for Oxygen; Soldering Flux
CAS Number 302-01-2
UN Number 2029; 2030
U.S. Brand Names Levoxin®; Oxytreat 35®; Zerox®
Synonyms Anhydrous Hydrazine; Diamide; Diamine

Use Commonly used as a rocket fuel, laboratory reagent, soldering flux, photography, silvering of mirrors and inhibitor of corrosion; also used in preparation of pharmaceutical agents, pesticides, and as a scavenging agent for oxygen; had been used (unapproved) as medication for sickle cell disease and cancer

Mechanism of Toxic Action Hydrazines are direct cellular toxins which also produce a pyridoxine deficiency by binding to vitamin B_6 derivatives and thus inhibiting reactions that require vitamin B_6 as a cofactor

Adverse Reactions
Cardiovascular: Hypotension (due to myocardial depression), fibrillation (atrial), shock, flutter (atrial), congestive heart failure, facial edema
Central nervous system: Fever, coma, headache, ataxia, seizures
Dermatologic: Dermal irritant, eczema, photosensitivity. Burns (>2.5% concentration)
Gastrointestinal: Anorexia, vomiting, nausea, salivation
Genitourinary: Renal failure
Hematologic: Hemolysis, methemoglobinemia (monomethylhydrazine)
Hepatic: Hepatotoxicity (fatty degeneration), hepatic failure
Neuromuscular & skeletal: Arthralgia, tremor
Ocular: Eye irritation, nystagmus, mydriasis
Respiratory: Dyspnea, pulmonary edema, rhinitis, cough
Miscellaneous: Cutaneous T-cell lymphoma, periarteritis nodosa, systemic lupus erythematosus

Admission Criteria/Prognosis Any patient with change in mental status, cardiopulmonary complaints, or methemoglobin levels >30% should be admitted; asymptomatic patients with methemoglobin levels <30% may be considered for discharge after 6 hours of observation and if methemoglobin levels fall to <15%

Toxicodynamics/Kinetics
Absorption: By oral, inhalation, and dermal routes
Half-life: 2 hours
Metabolism: Hepatic to acetyl hydrazine, diacetyl hydrazine, and pyruvate hydrazine (through binding with ketoacids)
Elimination: Renal

Overdosage/Treatment
Dermal: Irrigate with water
Decontamination: **Oral:** Do **not** induce emesis; lavage (within 1 hour)/ activated charcoal. **Ocular:** Hydrazine hydrate is a strong corrosive alkali agent, need to irrigate copiously with saline
Supportive therapy: Pyridoxine hydrochloride (25 mg/kg I.V.) may be antidotal for coma or seizures. Methylene blue can be used for symptomatic methemoglobinemia due to monomethylhydrazine.
Enhancement of elimination: Force urine diuresis (with the addition of mannitol); may increase the clearance of hydrazine

Antidote(s)
• Methylene Blue [ANTIDOTE]
• Pyridoxine [ANTIDOTE]

Additional Information Symptoms may be delayed for 14 hours following skin exposure. Weak ammonia odor threshold: 3.7 ppm (ammonia gas odor). Water and atmospheric half-life: <2 hours. TLV-TWA: 0.1 ppm; IDLH: 80 ppm: Does not react to water.

Specific References
Keyes DC, Shepherd G, Borys D, et al, "Space Shuttle Columbia Disaster: Utilization of Poison Centers," *J Toxicol Clin Toxicol*, 2003, 41(5):688.

Hydrogen Chloride

Applies to Rubber; Vinyl Chloride
CAS Number 7647-01-0
UN Number 1050; 1789
Synonyms Chlorohydric Acid; Hydrochloride; Muriatic Acid; Spirits of Salt
Use In the manufacture of vinyl chloride and rubber; a combustible product of vinyl chloride (PVC); Metal/toilet bowl cleaner
Mechanism of Toxic Action Corrosive through strong acidity to the skin, eyes, nose, respiratory and GI tract; primarily local effects through denatured enzymes, minimal systemic effects; high water solubility leading to upper airway edema

Adverse Reactions
Inhalation:
Cardiovascular: Chest pain, angina, tachycardia
Central nervous system: Chills, hyperthermia, fever
Nasal: Irritation, ulceration, epistaxis
Ocular: Corneal injury, conjunctivitis
Respiratory: Laryngeal spasms, noncardiogenic pulmonary edema (may be delayed for 24-72 hours), reactive airways disease syndrome, cough

Signs and Symptoms of Overdose By inhalation: tachycardia, laryngospasm, hyperchloremic metabolic acidosis, chest tightness, choking sensation, conjunctivitis, cough, dermal burns, dizziness, dyspnea, headache, hemoptysis, nasal ulcerations, nausea

Admission Criteria/Prognosis Patients with cardiopulmonary symptoms should be admitted

Toxicodynamics/Kinetics

Absorption: Not absorbed

Metabolism: Ionized to hydronium and chloride ions

Reference Range Postmortem results of fatality due to hydrogen chloride ingestion are very low blood pH (<5) within 24 hours after death, and elevated Cl⁻ concentration in heart blood (about 200 nmol/L) and gastric contents (about 700 mmol/L - normal value about 100 mmol/L)

Overdosage/Treatment

Decontamination: **Dermal:** Remove contaminated clothing. Wash area with copious amounts of soap and water. **Ocular:** Remove contact lenses; irrigate with saline or water for at least 20 minutes

Supportive therapy: Give 100% humidified oxygen. Treat wheezing with inhaled beta agonists. Corticosteroids may be helpful. I.V. fluids should be administered cautiously to avoid a net positive fluid balance. Dopamine or norepinephrine are vasopressors of choice. Partial liquid ventilation may be useful. Dermal burns can be treated with standard therapy. Inverse-ratio ventilation using lower tidal volume mechanical ventilation (6 mL/kg) and plateau pressures of 30 cm water may decrease mortality. While positive end expiratory pressures should be considered, oxygen toxicity should be monitored. Use of perfluorocarbon partial liquid ventilation and exogenous surfactant in chemical-induced ARDS is investigational.

Additional Information Pungent odor; clear, colorless. Odor threshold: 1-5 ppm. TLV-ceiling: 5 ppm; IDLH: 100 ppm

Throat irritation at 5 ppm. Amounts over 1000 ppm can be fatal within afew minutes. Plant toxicity at 100 ppm

Metal: Incompatible with zinc

pH of 1 N solution is 0.1

Specific References

Hsieh CH and Lin GT, "Corrosive Injury from Arterial Injection of Hydrochloric Acid," *Am J Emerg Med*, 2005, 23(3):394-6.

Yoshitome K, Miyaishi S, Ishihaw T, et al, "Distribution of Orally-Ingested Hydrochloric Acid in the Thoraco-Abdominal Cavity After Death," *J Anal Toxicol*, 2006, 30:278-80.

Hydrogen Fluoride

Related Information

- Ammonium Bifluoride

Applies to Computer Screen (Production); Etching (Glass/Porcelain); Fluorescent Bulbs (Production)

CAS Number 7664-39-3

UN Number 1052; 1786; 1790

Synonyms Fluohydric Acid; Hydrofluoric Acid

Commonly Found In Automotive cleaning products; production of integrated circuits

Use In etching and cleaning of glass and porcelain; produce computer screen, fluorescent bulbs; refine high octane gasoline

Mechanism of Toxic Action Corrosive, produces heat when exposed to water; binds calcium, potassium, and magnesium; dissociates in tissue to free H⁺ and F⁻ ions; fluoride anion inhibits Na⁺/K⁺ ATPase enzyme

Adverse Reactions

Cardiovascular: Fibrillation (ventricular)

Dermatologic: Dermal burns, onycholysis

Gastrointestinal: Vomiting (with ingestion)

Respiratory: Pneumonitis, hemorrhagic pulmonary edema, reactive airways disease syndrome

Signs and Symptoms of Overdose Bone pain, blistering, burns, diarrhea (22%), pain, pulmonary edema, nausea (22%), skin erythema, vomiting (with ingestion)

Admission Criteria/Prognosis Patients with >1% total body surface area burns, abnormal serum calcium levels, or who do not respond to treatment should probably be admitted; if pain occurs within 1 hour of exposure, patient should probably be admitted; survival after 4 days postexposure usually results in recovery. Note: QT interval may be prolonged for as long as 60 hours. Any ingestion should be admitted.

Toxicodynamics/Kinetics

Onset of action: Immediate corrosive effects although symptoms may be delayed 12-24 hours

Absorption: Inhalation and dermal routes

Half-life: 2-9 hours

Elimination: Renal

Reference Range Normal plasma fluoride levels are <0.1 mcg/L; highest survivable fluoride level after 10 g HF ingestion was 38.4 mg/L

Overdosage/Treatment

Decontamination:

Oral: Dilute with 250 mL of milk or water. Emesis is contraindicated. As first aid, affected extremity can be irrigated with water and bathed in

an iced solution of 25% magnesium sulfate. Give 300 mL of magnesium citrate orally for oral ingestion. Give 20 mL 10% calcium gluconate I.V. for oral ingestion. Magnesium sulfate may also be given I.V. (**do not** use calcium chloride for injection). The total I.V. calcium dose is ~1 g of calcium for each gram of fluoride ingested. Monitor serum calcium every 30 minutes until calcium normalizes. A 2.5% calcium gluconate gel can also be utilized.

Dermal: Remove all contaminated clothing; irrigate with copious amounts of water.

Inhalation: Give 100% oxygen. Nebulized calcium gluconate (4 mL of a 2.5% solution mixed in normal saline and delivered with 100% oxygen as a nebulized treatment) for inhalation exposures, or infiltrate with subcutaneous injection of 0.5 mL of 10% calcium gluconate, or 10% magnesium sulfate with a 30-gauge needle not greater than 0.5 mL/cm².

Ocular: Irrigate with normal saline. **Do not** give calcium gluconate subconjunctivally. Irrigation with 1% calcium gluconate may be also used, but does not appear to have any significant advantage over irrigation with normal saline. Treat for 2 days with topical antibiotics, cycloplegics and corticosteroids.

Supportive therapy: Arterial infusion of dilute calcium concentrations for distal extremity burns may be useful. Suggested dose is 10 mL of 10% calcium gluconate diluted in 50 mL of D₅W infused over a 4-hour period with a pump. Do not infuse magnesium through arterial cannula.

Enhancement of elimination: Hemodialysis may be used to remove fluoride anions.

Antidote(s)

- Amyl Nitrite [ANTIDOTE]
- Calcium Gluconate [ANTIDOTE]
- Magnesium Sulfate [ANTIDOTE]

Diagnostic Procedures

- Electrolytes, Blood

Additional Information

Fatal ingested dose: 1.5 g or 20 mg/kg.

Minimum lethal exposure: 1.5 g (20 mg/kg orally) or 2.5% to 22% total body surface area third degree burns

Concentrations >20% will result in burns becoming apparent within hours. It may take up to 1 day for burns to be apparent following topical exposure to concentrations <20%.

There were 33,795 hydrofluoric acid exposures called into U.S. Poison Centers with 26 deaths reported (1983-8).

Solution: Colorless. Odor threshold: 0.03 mg/m³. TLV-ceiling: 3 ppm; IDLH: 20 ppm; PEL-TWA: 3 ppm

Latex gloves are not protective; as little as 7 mL of anhydrous topical hydrogen fluoride can cause profound hypocalcemia; a 2.5% total body surface burn can be fatal due to electrolyte imbalance

To make calcium gel for dermal exposure to hydrogen fluoride, 3.5 g of calcium gluconate can be added to 5 oz tube of a surgical lubricant (water soluble such as K-Y® Jelly); alternatively can be ground into a fine powder and added to 20 mL of surgical lubricant (water soluble such as K-Y® Jelly), resulting in a 32.5% slurry. Calcium chloride should not be used for these purposes.

A commercial 2.5% calcium gluconate gel (as "H-F Antidote Gel") is available in 25 g tubes from Pharmascience, Inc, Montreal, Quebec, Canada (514-340-1114); in U.S. at 175 Rano St. Buffalo, NY, 14207 (1-800-207-4477).

Specific References

Björnhagen V, Höjer J, Karlson-Stiber C, et al, "Hydrofluoric Acid-Induced Burns and Life-Threatening Systemic Poisoning - Favorable Outcome After Hemodialysis," *J Toxicol Clin Toxicol*, 2003, 41(6):855-60.

Cordero SC, Goodhue WW, Splichal EM, et al, "A Fatality Due to Ingestion of Hydrofluoric Acid," *J Anal Toxicol*, 2004, 28(3):211-3.

Hall AH, Blomet J, Mathieu L, "Topical Treatments for Hydrofluoric Acid Burns: A Blind Controlled Experimental Study," *J Toxicol Clin Toxicol*, 2003, 41(7):1031-2.

Heard K and Delgado J, "Oral Decontamination with Calcium or Magnesium Salts Does Not Improve Survival Following Hydrofluoric Acid Ingestion," *J Toxicol Clin Toxicol*, 2003, 41(6):789-92.

Holstege C, Baer A, and Brady WJ, "The Electrocardiographic Toxidrome: The ECG Presentation of Hydrofluoric Acid Ingestion," *Am J Emerg Med*, 2003, 23(2):171-6.

Soderberg K, Kuusinen P, Mathieu L, et al, "An Improved Method for Emergent Decontamination of Ocular and Dermal Hydrofluoric Acid Splashes," *Vet Hum Toxicol*, 2004, 46(4):216-8.

Hydrogen Sulfide

Related Information

- Asphalt
- Calcium Polysulfide
- Sulfhemoglobin

Applies to Brewing; Farming; Glue; Lithography; Rayon (Manufacture); Tanning

CAS Number 7783-06-4

UN Number 1053

Synonyms Hepatic Gas; Hydrosulfuric Acid; Sewer Gas; Stink Damp; Sulfureted Hydrogen

Commonly Found In Volcanoes, manure

Use In farming, brewing, tanning, glue making, lithography, rayon manufacture

Mechanism of Toxic Action Inhibition of cytochrome oxidase; irritant

Adverse Reactions

Cardiovascular: Sinus bradycardia

Central nervous system: CNS depression, subacute encephalopathy, amnesia

Dermatologic: Dermal irritation

Neuromuscular & skeletal: Myoglobinuria

Ocular: Color vision abnormalities

Respiratory: Pulmonary edema, respiratory depression, hyperventilation

Signs and Symptoms of Overdose Conjunctivitis, cough, dementia, dyspnea, extrapyramidal symptoms, hypertension, hyposmia, hypothermia, lacrimation, myoglobinuria, nausea, vomiting. Higher concentrations may cause bradycardia, coma, confusion, dizziness, headache, hypotension, paresthesia, rotten egg breath, seizures.

Admission Criteria/Prognosis Symptomatic patients 4 hours postexposure should be admitted; survival after 4 hours is usually associated with recovery

Toxicodynamics/Kinetics

Absorption: Readily as a systemic toxicant through the lungs and GI tract

Metabolism: To thiosulfate

Elimination: Oxidized by hemoglobin and liver and renally excreted

Monitoring Parameters Albuminuria and hematuria; methemoglobin if giving nitrite therapy; sulfhemoglobin levels are of no use

Reference Range Normal whole blood sulfide: <0.05 mg/L; >0.9 mg/L has been correlated with death; serum thiosulfate >1.3 mcg/mL associated with toxicity; serum thiosulate level >12 mcg/mL associated with immediate fatality; normal levels of thiosulfate: blood: not detectable; urine: <8 mcg/mL

Overdosage/Treatment

Supportive therapy: 100% humidified oxygen; hyperbaric oxygen if symptoms do not improve with supplemental oxygen. Amyl nitrate and sodium nitrite (10 mg/kg up to 300 mg) can be given within 15 minutes of exposure (monitor for methemoglobinemia). Do not give sodium thiosulfate. **Dermal:** Wash surfaces with soap and water.

Enhancement of elimination: For infants, consider exchange transfusion.

Antidote(s)

- Oxygen (Hyperbaric) [ANTIDOTE]
- Sodium Nitrite [ANTIDOTE]

Diagnostic Procedures

- Lactic Acid, Blood
- Methemoglobin, Blood
- Urinalysis

Additional Information

Air levels >800 ppm can be fatal; overall mortality: 2% to 6%.

Neurologic sequelae of survivors include intention tremor, amnesia, ataxia

Measurement of sulfhemoglobin or sulfmethemoglobin levels are not clinically useful in hydrogen sulfide poisoning.

Produced by decaying organic matter; colorless; rotten egg odor at levels of 0.0047 ppm; note that olfactory fatigue occurs at 100-150 ppm

Occupations at risk for hydrogen sulfide poisoning: Agriculture (liquid manure systems); fishing; brewers; leather industry (tanning); glue making; rubber volcanization; geologists; nuclear reactor technicians (heavy water production); natural gas/petroleum/oil (exploration, refining, or transport); felt/artificial silk production; abattoirs; chemist (purification and preparation of phosphorus barium sulfur/sesquisulfide carbonate; organic sulfur); sulfur dye production (brown, black, blue); beet sugar factory; lithography; fertilizer production; sausage production; industrial paper plants (Kraft process); mining (coal, lead, gypsum, sulfur); sewer construction; well/tunnel digging; septic tank cleaning, industrial waste disposal; caisson work; metal smelting; roofing asphalt; pesticide production; rayon production (viscose process). See table.

Hydrogen Sulfide Dose–Effect Relationship

PPM	Response
0.05	Taste threshold
0.005 to 0.25	Odor threshold
5 to 10	Odor is obvious/muscle fatigability
50 to 150	Ocular irritation
80 to 100	Mild symptoms (nausea, vomiting, salivation, lacrimation)
100 to 150	Olfactory nerve paralysis/fatal to birds and guinea pigs
150 to 300	Blepharospasm, blurred vision
250 to 500	Pulmonary edema/bronchopneumonia
50 to 500	Respiratory irritant
500	Central nervous system depression within 30 minutes

Table (*Continued*)

PPM	Response
800 to 1000	Lethal level, coma or respiratory arrest within 30 minutes
Over 1000	One single breath can cause coma or respiratory arrest
Work Place Standards	
10	TLV-TWA
15	STEL
300	IDLH
Short-Term Inhalation Limits	
200	10 minutes
100	30 minutes
50	60 minutes

Specific References

Almeida AF, Nation PN, and Guidotti TL, "Pretreatment of H$_2$S 'Knockdown': A Rat Model," *J Occup Environ Med*, 2004, 46(9):1000.

Dougherty T, Greene T, Lafferty K, et al, "Delayed Cardiac Death from Hydrogen Sulfide Exposure," *J Toxicol Clin Toxicol*, 2004, 42(5):808.

Nikkanen HE and Burns MM, "Severe Hydrogen Sulfide Exposure in a Working Adolescent," *Pediatrics*, 2004, 113(4):927-9.

Schwartz M and Geller R, "Toxic Chemical Release: A Fatal H$_2$S Exposure with Multiple Secondary Casualties," *J Toxicol Clin Toxicol*, 2004, 42(5):803-4.

Imazapyr

Applies to Assault; Chopper; Contain; HerbicideArsenal; Pivot

Use An imidazolinone herbicide which blocks the biosynthesis of valine, leucine, and isoleucine through inhibition of the plant enzyme acetohydroxy acid synthetase

Mechanism of Toxic Action Can cause GI irritation upon ingestion or pulmonary injury from aspiration; it is a weak acid

Signs and Symptoms of Overdose Abdominal pain, coma, elevated bilirubin, fever, hypotension, leukocytosis, liver dysfunction, metabolic acidosis, oral ulcers, renal dysfunction, respiratory distress, stool incontinence, urine incontinence, vomiting

Admission Criteria/Prognosis Admit any ingestion over a mouthful

Overdosage/Treatment

Decontamination: **Oral:** Activated charcoal with cathartic for any ingestion over a mouthful. **Ocular:** Irrigate with copious amounts of saline.

Supportive therapy: Metabolic acidosis should be treated with 1-2 mEq/kg of sodium bicarbonate I.V.

Additional Information Slight odor of acetic acid

Isofenphos

CAS Number 25311-71-1

U.S. Brand Names Amaze®; Oftanol®

Use Insecticide

Mechanism of Toxic Action Irreversible inhibition of acetylcholinesterase and plasma cholinesterase, resulting in excess accumulation of acetylcholine at muscarinic and nicotinic receptors, and in the central nervous system

Signs and Symptoms of Overdose Bradycardia, bronchorrhea, bronchospasm, diaphoresis, mental confusion, miosis, and salivation usually start within 6 hours of symptoms and may persist for 2 weeks.

Toxicodynamics/Kinetics

Distribution: V$_d$: 3.3 L/kg (central compartment); 6.3 L/kg (at steady state)

Half-life: ~2-3 days

Clearance: 0.86 L/kg/day

Reference Range Following an injected (I.M.) dose of 21.15 mg/kg, peak plasma isofenphos concentration: 2.25 mg/L and associated with severe muscarinic and nicotinic symptoms

Overdosage/Treatment

Decontamination: Isolation, bagging, and disposal of all contaminated clothing and other articles. All emergency medical workers and hospital staff should follow appropriate precautions regarding exposure to hazardous material including the use of protective clothing, masks, goggles, and respiratory equipment.

Oral: Activated charcoal can be administered either orally or via a nasogastric tube. **Do not** induce emesis because of danger of sudden respiratory compromise, alterations in mental status, seizures, coma, and possible aspiration of hydrocarbon vehicles. **Do not** give a cathartic.

Dermal: Prompt thorough scrubbing of all affected areas with soap and water, including hair and nails; 5% bleach can be used

Ocular: Irrigation with copious tepid sterile water or saline

Supportive therapy: Airway management, ventilatory assistance, humidified oxygen administration, and close monitoring for sudden respiratory failure

Enhancement of elimination: Dialysis and hemoperfusion are not indicated due to the effectiveness of the prescribed treatment and large volumes of distribution of organophosphates.

Antidote:

Atropine: Administration should be guided by respiratory status, starting at 2-5 mg I.V. every 5-10 minutes as needed, and should be titrated to the resolution of excess pulmonary secretions. Frequent administration of large doses (cumulative doses > 100 mg) may be necessary in massive exposures.

Glycopyrrolate: May be administered if atropine is unavailable (200-400 mcg I.M. or I.V. initially, or $\sim^1/_2$ the dose of atropine).

2-PAM: For more significant exposures (ie, exposures requiring large doses of atropine, or with recurring symptoms, or exposures to more lipid soluble agents), administration should follow: 1-2 g I.V. over 10-30 minutes, repeated in 1 hour if asthenia recurs, then every 4-12 hours for recurring symptoms.

Antidote(s)
- Atropine [ANTIDOTE]
- Pralidoxime [ANTIDOTE]

Diagnostic Procedures
- Creatinine, Serum
- Pseudocholinesterase, Serum

Isopropyl Alcohol

Applies to Rubbing Alcohol
CAS Number 67-63-0
UN Number 1219
Synonyms Alcojel; Chromar; Dimethyl Carbinol; Isopropanol; Propol; "Blue Heaven"
Commonly Found In Rubbing alcohol (usually 70% concentration), secondary propyl alcohol, solvents in perfumes, paint thinners, cleaners, disinfectants, racing fuels
Mechanism of Toxic Action Metabolized by alcohol dehydrogenase to acetone which contributes to central nervous system depression
Adverse Reactions
Cardiovascular: Congestive heart failure, sinus tachycardia, Reye's-like syndrome
Central nervous system: Ataxia, depression, drowsiness, headache
Dermatologic: Immunologic contact urticaria
Hepatic: Impaired gluconeogenesis
Neuromuscular & skeletal: Areflexia
Miscellaneous: Acute traumatic compartment syndrome
Signs and Symptoms of Overdose Aplastic anemia, coma, feces discoloration (black), hemolytic anemia, hyperglycemia, hypoglycemia, hypotension due to myocardial depression, hypothermia, lethargy, myoglobinuria, porphyria, rhabdomyolysis, tachycardia, vomiting
Admission Criteria/Prognosis Ingestion of > 15 mL of 70% alcohol (3 swallows) in an infant (~ 1.5 mL/kg) is an indication for admission; any symptomatic patient (within 3 hours postexposure) or with a serum isopropyl alcohol level > 100 mg/dL or with ketosis should probably be admitted
Toxicodynamics/Kinetics
Absorption: Rapid from GI tract or by inhalation; little absorption through intact skin
Distribution: V_d: 0.5-0.7 L/kg
Metabolism: In the liver; 15% metabolized to acetone; acetone is present in serum within 1 hour and in urine within 3 hours of ingestion
Half-life: Isopropyl alcohol: 1-3 hours. Acetone: 17-24 hours
Peak plasma level: 1 hour postingestion
Elimination: Excreted renally, 25% to 50% unchanged
Reference Range
Toxic: > 50 mg/dL
Serum level > 128 mg/dL associated with profound lethargy; death can also occur at this level, but usually occurs at levels > 200 mg/dL if no medical supportive care is available
Overdosage/Treatment
Decontamination: Activated charcoal may be useful when used in a charcoal solvent ratio of 20:1. **Do not** induce emesis with ipecac.
Enhancement of elimination: Hemodialysis in those patients who do not respond to supportive therapy or whose levels exceed 400 mg/dL. Hemodialysis can clear 137 mL/minute of isopropanol and 165 mL/minute of acetone. Peritoneal dialysis offers no clear benefit.
Diagnostic Procedures
- Glucose, Random
- Osmolality, Serum
- Osmolality, Urine

Test Interactions Acetone and acetoacetate may result in false elevation of serum creatinine at serum acetone levels > 40 mg/dL; serum creatinine rises 1 mg/dL for every 100 mg/dL of acetone
Additional Information Lethal dose: Adults: 240 mL. Serious illness may occur with ingestion of 10 mL; twice as lethal as ethanol. No long-

term sequelae; can cause skin burns when used topically on premature infants. Spirituous odor but a clean colorless liquid; bitter taste. Contribution of a serum concentration level of 100 mg/dL to elevation of osmolar gap: 17. Specific gravity: 0.79 g/mL; IDLH: 20,000 ppm; TLV-TWA: 400 ppm; Odor threshold: 90 mg/mm^3
Specific References
Emadi A and Coberly L, "Intoxication of a Hospitalized Patient with an Isopropanol-Based Hard Sanitizer," *N Engl J Med*, 2007, 356:5:530-1.
Martin TL and Lalonde BR, "Isopropanol: A Putrefactive Product in Deaths Due to Drowning," *J Anal Toxicol*, 2003, 27:199.
Trullas JC, Aguilo S, Castro P, et al, "Life-Threatening Isopropyl Alcohol Intoxication: Is Hemodialysis Really Necessary?" *Vet Hum Toxicol*, 2004, 282-3.
Wood JN, Calello DP, Carney J, et al, "Transplacental Isopropanol Intoxication: A Report," *Clin Toxicol (Phila)*, 2005, 43:669.

Jet Fuel-4

Related Information
- Stoddard Solvent

Applies to MIL-T-5624-L-Amd 1
CAS Number 50815-00-4
UN Number 1863
Synonyms Jet Fuel: JP-4; JP-4
Use Aviation turbine fuel used by the U.S. military (constitutes 85% of turbine fuel used by Department of Defense)
Mechanism of Toxic Action A mixture of alkanes (43%), cycloalkanes (11%), alkylbenzenes (12%), and naphthalenes (2%) which can cause CNS depression
Adverse Reactions
Central nervous system: Neurologic: headache, dizziness, polyneuropathy (on long-term exposure), ataxia, panic attacks
Dermatologic: Dermal irritant
Gastrointestinal: Nausea
Neuromuscular & skeletal: Weakness (at inhalation levels between 3000-7000 ppm)
Renal: Alpha$_2\mu$-globulin nephropathy
Admission Criteria/Prognosis Patients who develop tachypnea, cyanosis, dyspnea, CNS depression, tachycardia, or fever within 8 hours of exposure should be admitted; asymptomatic patients can be discharged after 8 hours observation
Overdosage/Treatment
Decontamination: **Oral: Do not** induce emesis or lavage due to risk of aspiration pneumonia. Activated charcoal can adsorb benzene. **Dermal:** Wash with soap and water. **Inhalation:** Administer 100% humidified oxygen. **Ocular:** Flush with saline or water for at least 15 minutes.
Supportive therapy: Benzodiazepines for seizure control; avoid use of catecholamines due to risk of ventricular arrhythmia
Additional Information Odor threshold: 1 ppm; PEL-TWA: 400 ppm
Specific References
Wright BR, "Hydrocarbon Fuels," *Forensic Examiner*, 2004, 13(2):16-9.

Jet Fuel-5/Jet Fuel-8

CAS Number 70892-10-3; 8008-20-6
UN Number 1223
Synonyms Aviation Kerosene; JP-5; JP-8; Nato F-34; NATO F-44
Use Aviation fuel with higher kerosene content than Jet Fuel-4. Jet Fuel-5 is used by the United States Navy for use aboard aircraft carriers and also used on surface ships. Jet Fuel-8 is used by the United States Air Force and NATO forces.
Mechanism of Toxic Action Kerosene-based organic solvent causing CNS depression and bronchoconstriction by acting on the vagus nerve and inhibiting acetylcholinesterase
Adverse Reactions
Cardiovascular: Palpitations, hypertension (mild), tachycardia, cardiomegaly
Central nervous system: Ataxia, concentration difficulties, headache, dizziness, fatigue, fever, coma
Dermatologic: Blisters, erythema, peeling skin, pruritus
Gastrointestinal: Nausea, anorexia, vomiting
Hematologic: Leukocytosis
Ocular: Eye irritation
Renal: Alpha 2u-globulin nephropathy
Respiratory: Aspiration pneumonia, bronchitis, cough, dyspnea, tachypnea, bronchoconstriction, pulmonary edema, pneumothorax, lipoidal pneumonia
Miscellaneous: Neurasthenia
Admission Criteria/Prognosis Admit any symptomatic patient; fever may be a prognostic sign for pulmonary involvement; any patient with fever, abnormal chest x-ray, dyspnea, history of spontaneous emesis, or mixed ingestion should be admitted; ingestions > 1 mL/kg and/or any symptomatic patient 6 hours postexposure should be considered for admission

Toxicodynamics/Kinetics Absorption: By inhalation, oral and dermal routes

Monitoring Parameters Arterial blood gases, chest x-ray (2 hours after ingestion), prothrombin time, liver function tests

Overdosage/Treatment

Decontamination:

Oral: Do not consider gastric emptying if the amount ingested is <100 mL. While some studies suggest ipecac-induced emesis in the alert patient, gastric lavage with airway protection may also be used. Activated charcoal may be useful (although human data is lacking). Saline-based cathartics may be used.

Dermal: Flush skin with soap and water; if blisters develop, use sterile water.

Inhalation: Administer 100% humidified oxygen.

Ocular: Irrigate with saline.

Supportive therapy: Selective beta$_2$ agonists (inhaled) can be used to treat bronchospasm. Antibiotics or corticosteroids are not useful (prophylactically) in treating pneumonitis. Extracorporeal membrane oxygenation can be considered if respiratory failure occurs.

Drug Interaction Asbestos may increase toxicity of kerosene based fuels

Additional Information Both jet fuels are clear liquids with kerosene-like odor. Benzene content: <0.02%. Odor threshold: 0.08 ppm. Density: ~0.8 kg/L. Aromatic content of JP-8: 14.5% to 18.8%.

Specific References

Rhodes AG, LeMasters GK, Lockey JE, et al, "The Effects of Jet Fuel on Immune Cells of Fuel System Maintenance Workers," *J Occup Environ Med*, 2003, 45(1):79-86.

Wright BR, "Hydrocarbon Fuels," *Forensic Examiner*, 2004, 13(2):16-9.

Kerosene

Related Information

- Jet Fuel-5/Jet Fuel-8

Applies to Mobil Oil Cooling System Cleaner

CAS Number 70892-10-3; 8008-20-6

UN Number 1223

U.S. Brand Names Deobase®

Synonyms Coal Oil; Fuel Oil Number 1; Kerosine; Range Oil; Straight Run Kerosene

Use Originally produced for jet fuel engine; domestic heating; illuminating fuel; a vehicle in pesticides and lighter fluid; solvent in paints

Mechanism of Toxic Action A product of straight-run distillation of crude petroleum, kerosene is a hydrocarbon with low viscosity and low volatility which can produce a pneumonitis upon aspiration

Adverse Reactions

Cardiovascular: Tachycardia, cardiomegaly, cyanosis, chest pain

Central nervous system: Fatigue, sleep disturbances, dizziness, headache, coma, fever, irritability, ataxia, cognitive dysfunction

Dermatologic: Erythema, bullae, pruritus, blisters, acne, eczema

Gastrointestinal: Vomiting, hematemesis, abdominal pain

Hematologic: **Leukocytosis** (37% to 80%)

Hepatic: Hepatotoxicity, cirrhosis

Respiratory: Pneumonitis, aspiration pneumonia, pleural effusion, lipoidal pneumonia, pneumothorax, emphysema, cough, dyspnea

Admission Criteria/Prognosis Any patient with fever, abnormal chest x-ray, dyspnea, history of spontaneous emesis, or mixed ingestion should be admitted; ingestions >1 mL/kg and/or any symptomatic patient 6 hours postexposure should be considered for admission

Toxicodynamics/Kinetics Absorption: Dermal, oral and inhalation absorption can occur

Monitoring Parameters Arterial blood gases, chest x-ray (2 hours after ingestion), prothrombin time, liver function tests

Overdosage/Treatment

Decontamination:

Oral: Very controversial; certainly it is generally agreed that in ingestions of small amounts (<30 mL in children), no gastrointestinal decontamination should occur.

Due to the relative lack of CNS toxicity of kerosene, it is probably not efficacious to perform gastric evacuation for a pure kerosene ingestion. If a toxic additive (ie, benzene, insecticide, heavy metal, etc) is ingested, emesis with syrup of ipecac within 30 minutes (in an alert individual who has not vomited), or gastric lavage within 1 hour, may be performed. Activated charcoal is probably of some use. Avoid use of mineral oil cathartics.

Dermal: Wash liberally with soap and water.

Ocular: Irrigate eyes copiously with saline or water.

Supportive therapy: Prophylactic administration of antibiotics and/or corticosteroids does **not** appear to be useful. Avoid catecholamine use due to the risk of precipitating cardiac arrhythmia.

Respiratory failure: Extracorporeal membrane oxygenation can be considered.

Drug Interaction May increase sedative properties of hexobarbital

Additional Information

Minimum lethal oral dose: 1890 mg/kg

Toxic inhalation dosage: 0.1-0.2 mL. Maximum tolerated oral exposure: 1700 mg/kg.

Oral ingestion of 10-30 mL can result in pulmonary complications in 2% to 3% of individuals.

Hypoprothrombinemia may be the earliest laboratory indicator for liver dysfunction.

Note that use of kerosene space heaters can result in increased emission rates of carbon monoxide (average of 7.4 ppm).

Specific gravity: 0.8. Odor threshold: 0.08-1 ppm

Specific References

Tagwireyi D, Ball DE, and Nhachi CB, "Toxicoepidemiology in Zimbabwe: Admissions Resulting from Exposure to Parafin (Kerosene)," *Clin Toxicol*, 2006, 44:103-7.

Yu IT, Lee NL, Zhang XH, et al, "Occupational Exposure to Mixtures of Organic Solvents Increases the Risk of Neurological Symptoms Among Printing Workers in Hong Kong," *J Occup Environ Med*, 2004, 46(4):323-30.

Kratom

Scientific Name *Mitragyna speciosa*

Use As an opium substitute; the tree is native to Thailand and Malaysia. Used as a tea, or the leaves can be chewed or smoked. Typical tea dose is 10-15 g.

Mechanism of Toxic Action Contains mitragynine, an indole alkaloid that is similar to psilocybin and is a μ- and Δ-subtype receptor agonist (about 10% of the action of morphine)

Signs and Symptoms of Overdose Coma, vertigo, lethargy, tremors, nausea, vomiting, can be a stimulant (at doses of mitragynine >50 mg), miosis, constipation, doses >25 g of kraton leaves can be toxic.

Overdosage/Treatment Supportive care: Supportive care is mainstay of therapy. Mild withdrawal syndrome with chronic use may occur.

Pregnancy Implications Effects not known

Additional Information Alkaloids resemble yohimbine; illegal in Australia, Cambodia, Malaysia, Myanmar, and Thailand. Exhibits psychoactive properties; typical effects last for 2-6 hours

Specific References

Matsumoto K, Horie S, Ishikawa H, et al, "Antinociceptive Effect of 7-Hydroxymitragynine in Mice: Discovery of an Orally Active Opioid Analgesic from the Thai Medicinal Herb *Mitragyna speciosa*," *Life Sci*, 2004, 74:2143-55.

Lead

CAS Number 10031-22-8; 10101-63-0; 13424-46-9; 13814-96-5; 301-04-2; 7439-92-1; 7758-95-4; 7758-97-6

UN Number 1616; 2291; 2811

Use Lead is available in 19 inorganic and 2 organic compounds; common sources (especially for children) are air, water, soil, and leaded paint chips. Use of tap water (as "first-drawn" or with excessive boiling or stored in lead-based kettles) in reconstituting infant formulas for infants; additional sources/uses include leaded foreign bodies such as bullet fragments, numerous imported Asian products, herbal/folk remedies, Mexican remedies for "empacho" and home abortifacients; recreational sources include lead-based cosmetics, contamination of illicitly distilled alcohols or illicit intravenous drug products, leaded gasoline "sniffing", and even chewing colored plastic wires.

Mechanism of Toxic Action

Lead's effects are mediated by its ability to complex sulfhydryl groups and other ligands, in enzyme systems throughout the body

Alkyl lead is moderately irritating. Hemoglobin biosythesis is affected by inhibition of Delta aminolevolnic acid synthetase and dehydrase, Copropurphyrinogen decarboxylase and Ferrochelatase thus leading to increase, in porotoporphyrine. Red Blood cell survival time is shortened. Renal lesions in proximale tubule and loop of Henle occur leading to renal insufficiency. Degenerative changes in motorneurons (axons) and encephalopathic changes in nervous system are target sites

Adverse Reactions

Lead toxicity occurs in the acute, acute-on-chronic, or chronic settings secondary to environmental, occupational, intentional, or recreational activities. Acute exposures are commonly associated with symptoms of malaise, nausea, vomiting, myoclonus, metallic taste, fasciculations, abdominal pain; severe exposures can result in encephalopathy, and death; chronic exposures manifest with neuropsychiatric symptoms, anemia, renal dysfunction/chronic failure, hypertension, arthralgias, teratogenesis, and impotence. See chart.

Effects of Inorganic Lead on Children and Adults-- Lowest Observable Adverse Effect Levels

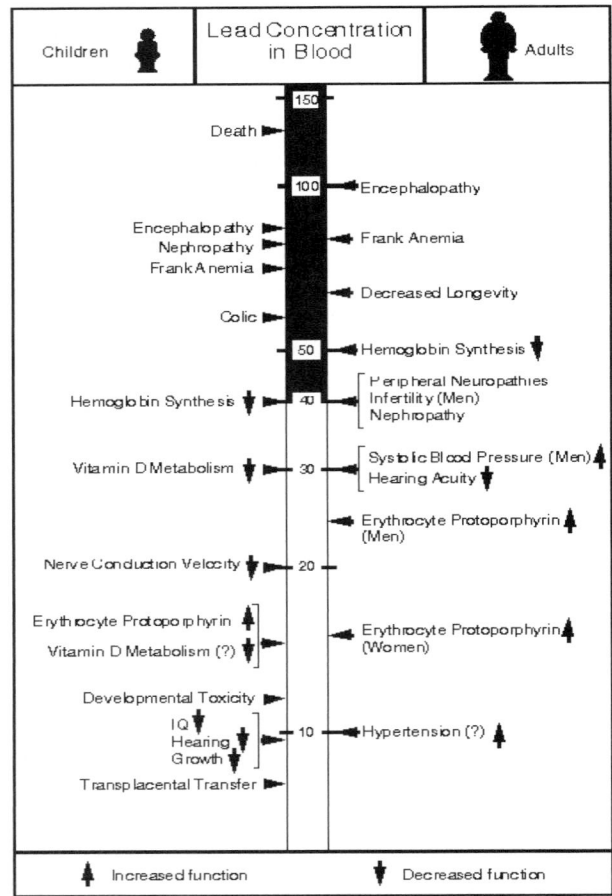

| Children | Lead Concentration in Blood | Adults |

150 — Death
100 — Encephalopathy
Encephalopathy, Nephropathy, Frank Anemia — Frank Anemia
Colic — Decreased Longevity
50 — Hemoglobin Synthesis
Hemoglobin Synthesis — 40 — Peripheral Neuropathies, Infertility (Men), Nephropathy
Vitamin D Metabolism — 30 — Systolic Blood Pressure (Men), Hearing Acuity
Erythrocyte Protoporphyrin (Men)
Nerve Conduction Velocity — 20
Erythrocyte Protoporphyrin, Vitamin D Metabolism (?) — Erythrocyte Protoporphyrin (Women)
Developmental Toxicity
IQ, Hearing, Growth — 10 — Hypertension (?)
Transplacental Transfer

▲ Increased function   ▼ Decreased function

Note that blood levels are usually > 40 μg/dL when anemia is recognized (ie, an apparently normal CBC does not rule out plumbism).

Adapted from U.S. Department of Health and Human Services, Royce SE and Needleman HL, eds, "Case Studies in Environmental Medicine: Lead Toxicity," Agency for Toxic Substances and Disease

Cardiovascular: Sinus bradycardia, cardiomyopathy, cardiomegaly, vasoconstriction, Reye's-like syndrome

Central nervous system: Ataxia, encephalopathy, headache, learning disabilities, drowsiness, dementia, mood and/or mental status changes, seizures, memory disturbance, catatonia, CNS depression, depression, psychosis, fever, hyperthermia, aggressive behavior

Endocrine & metabolic: Growth suppression, syndrome of inappropriate antidiuretic hormone, hypermineralization

Gastrointestinal: Abdominal pain, colic, constipation, nausea, vomiting, sweet taste

Hematologic: Anemia (at lead levels >40 mcg/dL), hemolysis

Hepatic: Hepatitis

Neuromuscular & skeletal: Arthralgia, paresthesia, rhabdomyolysis

Ocular: Blurred vision, diplopia, optic neuropathy, color vision abnormalities, visual evoked potential abnormalities

Renal: Proteinuria, hematuria, chronic renal failure due to interstitial nephritis, acute tubular necrosis, renal cell cancer

Signs and Symptoms of Overdose

Mild toxicity: Drowsiness, irritability, mild fatigue, myalgia or paresthesia, occasional abdominal discomfort

Moderate toxicity: Arthralgia, constipation, deafness, difficulty concentrating, diffuse abdominal pain, general fatigue, headache, muscular exhaustibility, tremor, vomiting, weight loss

Severe toxicity: Blindness, colic (intermittent, severe abdominal cramps), cranial nerve palsies, encephalopathy (may abruptly lead to seizures, changes in consciousness, coma, and death), lead line (blue-black) on gingival tissue, paresis or paralysis

Admission Criteria/Prognosis Any symptomatic patient, or blood lead level >60 mcg/dL, or free erythrocyte porphyrin level >7 times normal (>35 mcg/dL), or radiopacities in gastrointestinal tract on KUB, should be admitted; mortality in patients with lead encephalopathy approaches 25% with 50% of survivors exhibiting permanent neurological deficits

Toxicodynamics/Kinetics

Absorption: Pulmonary absorption is 30% to 85%; gastric absorption is 5% to 15% in adults and up to 40% in children; gastric absorption can increase to 50% in the presence of calcium, iron, and zinc deficiencies and is also increased in pregnancy

Distribution: Three compartment model predominantly stored in bones (90%), lead is also found in brain, kidney, and liver tissue; blood lead (<1% body stores) is 95% intracellular

Half-life: blood: 28-36 days; soft Tissues: 30-40 days

Elimination: Elimination rates between the three compartments vary from ~40 days for blood and soft tissues to 20-30 years for bone stores; blood contains about 4% of total body burden of lead

Monitoring Parameters Lead concentrations, erythrocyte protoporphyrin, KUB, potassium x-ray fluorescence, CBC, creatinine, electrolytes, CNS effects

Warnings/Precautions After chelation, especially in chronic toxicity, redistribution of lead into blood and soft tissues leads to a "rebound" in lead concentrations; also failure to remove the patient from the source(s) of lead will prevent adequate response to chelation therapy

Reference Range

Asymptomatic and whole blood lead concentrations of >10-25 mcg/dL is an indication for the initiation of community prevention programs, 25-50 mcg/dL with positive LMT is an indication for EDTA, >45 mcg/dL is an indication for succimer, and >50 mcg/dL is an indication for BAL and EDTA; lead mobilization test (LMT); this test is performed by administering 500 mg/m^2 of CaNa$_2$-ethylenediaminetetracetic acid (EDTA) and then collecting urine for 8 hours; a positive result is defined as determining a ratio of urinary lead/dose EDTA >0.6 or a total urinary excretion of >200 mcg of lead

Inhibition of hemoglobin Synthesis is reflected by an Erythrocyte protoporphyrin blood level over 35 ug/dl, and may lag in respect to lead exposure by up to six weeks

See chart for the CDC's action level for blood lead in children.

Centers for Disease Control's Action Level for Lead Over Past 35 Years

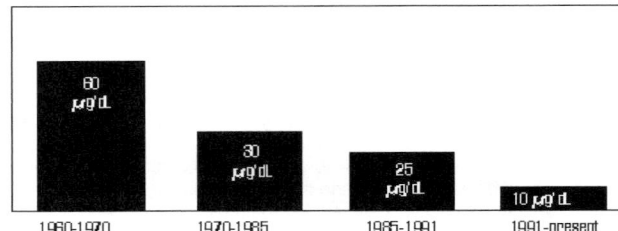

| 1960-1970 | 1970-1985 | 1985-1991 | 1991-present |

60 μg/dL   30 μg/dL   25 μg/dL   10 μg/dL

Adapted from Health and Human Services, "Case Studies in Environmental Medicine: Lead Toxicity," Agency for Toxic Substances and Disease Registry, June 1990.

Number of Workers with Elevated Blood Levels (BLLs) by Industry Adult Blood Lead Epidemiology and Surveillance (ABLES) Program*, 2002

Industry (Standard Industrial Classification [SIC])	≥25 mcg/dL	≥40 mcg/dL
Manufacture of storage batteries (SIC 3691)	1494	141
Painting, paperhanging, and decorating (SIC 1721)	863	236
Mining of lead and zinc ores (SIC 1031)	522	70
Secondary smelting (SIC 3341)	384	63
Wholesale distribution of electrical apparatus and equipment, wiring supplies, and construction materials (SIC 5063)	351	55
Manufacture of primary batteries (SIC 3692)	209	15
Bridge tunnel and elevated highway construction (SIC 1622)	149	16
Special trade contractors (eg, lead abatement workers) (SIC 1799)	144	33
Primary smelting (SIC 3339)	121	17
Auto repair shops (eg, radiator repair) (SIC 7539)	106	24

*A total of 27 of 35 ABLES states reported; eight states (Alabama, Arizona, Georgia, Kentucky, North Carolina, Pennsylvania, Rhode Island, and Wyoming) did not track BLLs by SIC code.

Rate* of Adult Blood Lead Levels ≥25 mcg/dL, By State - Adult Blood Lead Epidemiology and Surveillance Program†, United States, 2002

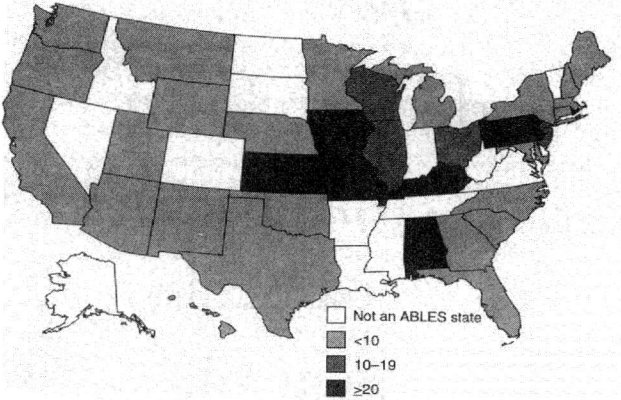

Not an ABLES state
<10
10–19
≥20

* Per 100,000 employed persons aged ≥16 years, according to the Bureau of Labor Statistics' Current Population Survey.

† Alabama, Arizona, California, Connecticut, Florida, Georgia, Hawaii, Illinois, Iowa, Kansas, Kentucky, Maine, Maryland, Massachusetts, Michigan, Minnesota, Missouri, Montana, Nebraska, New Hampshire, New Jersey, New Mexico, New York, North Carolina, Ohio, Oklahoma, Oregon, Pennsylvania, Rhode Island, South Carolina, Texas, Utah, Washington, Wisconsin, and Wyoming.

Average State Rate* of Adult Blood Lead Levels (BLLs), By Year Adult Blood Lead Epidemiology and Surveillance Program†, United States, 1994-2002

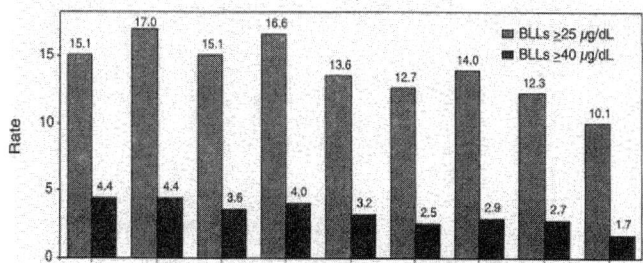

Year (no. states reporting)

* Per 100,000 employed persons aged ≥16 years, according to the Bureau of Labor Statistics' Current Population Survey. The average is determined by First calculating individual state rates for each year, and then calculating the average.

† Alabama, Arizona, California, Connecticut, Florida, Georgia, Hawaii, Illinois, Iowa, Kansas, Kentucky, Maine, Maryland, Massachusetts, Michigan, Minnesota, Missouri, Montana, Nebraska, New Hampshire, New Jersey, New Mexico, New York, North Carolina, Ohio, Oklahoma, Oregon, Pennsylvania, Rhode Island, South Carolina, Texas, Utah, Washington, Wisconsin, and Wyoming.

Overdosage/Treatment

Decontamination: Prehospital ipecac within 30 minutes, otherwise gastric lavage within 1 hour or whole bowel irrigation (especially if abdominal radiograph is positive for lead ingestion)

Antidotes:

BAL indicated for: Any encephalopathic patient for at least one 5-day treatment course; any other symptomatic patient for at least one 3-day treatment course; any asymptomatic patient with a lead concentration of 70 mcg/dL

EDTA indicated for: Any patient receiving BAL at least 4 hours after the initial BAL dose; as single agent, for any asymptomatic patient with a lead concentration of >45 mcg/dL; any patient with lead concentrations between 25-55 mcg/dL with the lead mobilization test

Succimer indicated for: Asymptomatic patients with blood lead concentrations >45 mcg/dL; encephalopathic patients with contraindications to BAL therapy

Penicillamine indicated for: Any patient unable to receive or tolerate BAL, EDTA, and succimer

Supportive: Seizures should be treated with diazepam: Children: 0.1-0.3 mg/kg slowly; Adults: Up to 10 mg I.V.. may repeat if necessary. For cerebral edema, controlled ventilation (keeping CO_2 arterial pressure between 25-30 mm Hg) along with an osmotic diuretic (ie, mannitol) may be helpful. Urine output should be maintained at 1-2 mL/kg/hour, but forced diuresis should not be utilized.

Enhancement of elimination: Succimer: Lead complex is hemodialyzable, there is no other effective use for elimination enhancement

procedures in lead poisoning. When hemodialysis is combined with chelation with EDTA, the plasma half-life of lead decreases from 9-6 hours to 9 hours, as compared with EDTA chelation alone. Exchange transfusion may be helpful in patients with acute elevation of lead levels (>100 mcg/dL).

Antidote(s)
- Dimercaprol [ANTIDOTE]
- Edetate Calcium Disodium [ANTIDOTE]
- Penicillamine [ANTIDOTE]
- Succimer [ANTIDOTE]
- Unithiol [ANTIDOTE]

Diagnostic Procedures
- Heavy Metal Screen, Blood
- Lead, Blood
- Lead, Urine

Pregnancy Implications The adverse effect on fetal neuro-development due to fetal lead exposure is most pronounced during the first trimester.

Additional Information

Long-term lead exposure can lead to renal impairment and hypertension in middle-aged men. Suggestion of an association between gliomas and occupational lead exposure (blood lead levels >1.4 µmol/L) has recently been noted. Lead appears to decrease erythropoietin production.

Three hallmarks of lead-induced immunotoxicity

1. Suppression of the Th1-dependent delayed-type hypersensitivity response as well as production of Th1 cytokines
2. Elevate production of IgE antibodies
3. Macrophage modulation into increased production of proinflammatory cytokines

Tibial x-ray fluorescence (XRF) provides an estimate of cumulative lead exposure.

Urinary N-acetyl-3-D-glucosamidase activity may be a sensitive but nonspecific marker for lead-induced renal tubular damage. Equation for calculating blood lead levels from a single route of exposure is:

Lead concentration (mcg/dL = daily exposure of lead (mcg) × fractional absorption divided by 3.3)

Between 1976 and 1999, mean blood lead levels in pediatric patients (younger than 6 years of age) have decreased from 13 mcg/dL (0.66 µmol/L) to 2.0 mcg/dL (0.15 µmol/L). Prevalence of blood lead levels >10 mcg/dL (0.48 µmol/L) in non-Hispanic Blacks is estimated to be 21.9% for those living in housing built before 1946 and 13.7% for those residing in housing built between 1946-73.

1 mcg/dL = 0.0483 µmol/L

In 1991, 9% of children in the U.S. had blood lead levels ≥10 mcg/dL.

Lead intoxication has been observed in children but rarely in adults in a residential setting. The following table shows the average daily intake of lead over a 10-year span in children and adults. See table.

Daily Average Intake of Lead* (mcg lead/day)

Age	Year					
	1980	1982	1984	1986	1988	1990
6-11 mo	~ 34	20	16.7	10	5	3.8
2 y						
female	No data	No data	No data	No data	No data	No data
male	~ 45	25.1	23	12.8	5	4.3
14-16 y						
female	No data	No data	28.7	15.2	6.1	6.1
male	No data	No data	40.9	21.8	8.2	8.5
25-30 y						
female	No data	32	28.7	14.8	7.9	6.7
male	84	45.2	40.9	21.2	10	8.5
60-65 y						
female	No data	No data	30.4	15.6	No data	2.2
male	No data	No data	37.6	19.1	No data	8.1

*Adapted from U.S. Department of Health and Human Services, *Toxicological Profile for Lead, TP 92/12*, Agency for Toxic Substances and Diseases Registry, April, 1993.

The following table shows the average daily intakes of lead for adults, based on an analysis of 27 market basket samples taken nationwide for a 1980-82 Total Diet Study.

Food Group	Average Adult Intake (mcg/d)
Dairy products	4.54
Meat, fish, and poultry	4.09
Grain and cereal products	9.84
Potatoes	1.39

Table (Continued)

Food Group	Average Adult Intake (mcg/d)
Leafy vegetables	0.94
Legume vegetables	9.18
Root vegetables	1.39
Garden fruits	4.44
Fruits	10
Oils and fats	1.23
Sugar and adjuncts	2.34
Beverages	6.86
Total lead intake per day	56.5

Lead has been detected in a variety of foods; typical concentrations of lead in various foods are listed in the table.

Food Group	Concentration (mcg/g)
Dairy products	0.003-0.083
Meat, fish, and poultry	0.002-0.159
Grain and cereal products	0.002-0.136
Vegetables	0.005-0.649
Fruit and fruit juices	0.005-0.223
Oils, fats, and shortenings	0.002-0.028
Sugar and adjuncts	0.006-0.073
Beverages	0.002-0.041 (mcg/L)

PEL-TWA: 0.05 mg/m^3

Action level in drinking water: 0.015 mg/L

Action level for home water lead amounts are 15 ppb for first draw water and 5 ppb for purged-line water (water that has run for at least 1 minute)

In Illinois, 2231 cases of adult lead poisoning were reported in 1994 (up 43% from 1993). Overall in the United States, an estimated 900,000 workers are exposed to lead on the job.

Sources of lead exposure:

Occupational: Auto repairers, battery manufacturers, bridge reconstruction workers, construction workers, gas station attendants, glass manufacturers, lead miners, lead smelters and refiners, plastic manufacturers, plumbers, pipe fitters, policemen, printers, rubber product manufacturers, shipbuilders, steel welders or cutters

Environmental: Ceramicware, lead containing paint, leaded gasoline, plumbing leachate, soil/dust near lead industries, roadways, lead painted homes

Hobbies & related activities: Car or boat repair, glazed pottery making, home remodeling, lead soldering (eg, electronics), painting, preparing lead shot, fishing sinkers, stained glass making, target shooting at firing ranges; pool cue chalk may contain more than 500 ppm of lead

Substance use: Cosmetics, folk remedies, gasoline "huffing", health foods, moonshine whiskey

OSHA requires removal of any adult employee with blood lead levels ≥50 mcg/dL

OSHA Interim Final Standard for Lead in Construction (permissible lead exposure limit) is 50 mcg/m^3

Current CDC recommendations for allowable lead concentration: Surface paint: ≤.06% lead; Household soil and dust: <1000 ppm lead; Tap water: <15 ppm lead; Household floor dust: 200 mcg/sq ft; Household window sill dust: 500 mcg/sq ft; Household window well dust: 800 mcg/sq ft

Some types of imported plastic miniblinds contain as much as 2,874 mcg/sq ft (Federal Housing and Urban Development Child-Safety limit is 500 mcg/sq ft of window sill); other sources for lead include imported (from China) crayons, bulk water tanks, wrappers from certain brands of Mexican candy, pool cue chalk and folk-remedy powders (ie, azarcon, greta)

Lead dust can be removed by scrubbing with water plus a phosphate detergent or powdered dishwasher detergent. Vacuuming lead dust should be performed with a high efficiency particle arresting (HEPA) vacuum cleaner. Since lead is more soluble in acidic solutions, vinegar can cause leaching of lead from leaded containers or bottles.

The Environmental Protection Agency lowered the amount of lead used in gasoline from 1.1 g of lead/gallon to 0.1 g of lead/gallon in 1985. In 1996, a total ban of lead in gasoline went into effect.

Adulterants, including lead, have been noted in Asian traditional or folk medicines. Folk remedies and cosmetics from East Indian, Pakistani, Chinese, and Latin American cultures that have contained lead include alarcon, alkohl, azarcon, bali goli, coral, gliasard, greta, kohl, "Koo Sar Pills", liga, pay-loo-ah, rueda, and surma. Other sources of lead ingestion have included contaminated ground paprika, ayurvedic metal-mineral tonics, Deshi Dewa (a fertility drug), hai gen fen (clamshell powder) added to tea, and pigment used in plastic wire insulation.

Observational data suggests a 2-3 point IQ decrease with a serum lead increase from 10 to 20 mcg/dL in children; however, there appears to be no cognitive, behavioral, or neuropsychological improvement after 3 years of succimer therapy in chronic lead exposure with serum lead <45 mcg/dL.

Mean time for blood lead to decline has been linearly related to the peak in blood lead. The linear relationship was described by the following equation: time (# of months required to achieve a blood lead <10 mcg/dL) = 0.845 times peak lead.

Estimated Prevalence[1] of Children Aged 1-5 Years with Blood Lead Levels (BLLs) ≥10 mcg/dL[2] – United States, 1976-1980, 1988-1991, 1991-1994, and 1999-2000

Survey	Prevalence of BLLs ≥10 mcg/dL		Children with BLLs ≥10 mcg/dL	
	(%)	(95% CI[3])	No.	(95% CI)
1976-1980	88.2	(83.8-92.6)	13,500,000	(12,800,000-14,100,000)
1988-1991	8.6[4]	(4.8-12.4)	1,700,000	(960,000-2,477,000)
1991-1994	4.4	(2.9-6.6)	890,000	(590,000-1,330,000)
1999-2000	2.2[5]	(1.0-4.3)	434,000[5]	(189,000-846,000)

Source: National Health and Nutrition Examination Surveys (NHANES).

Note: In 1991, NHANES III Phase 1 was completed and Phase 2 was begun.

[1]Estimated number of children 1-5 years of age with BLLs ≥10 mcg/dL divided by estimated population of children 1-5 years of age.

[2]CDC has determined BLL ≥10 mcg/dL is a level of concern.

[3]Confidence interval.

[4]Estimate differs slightly from that published previously because of updates in coding and weighting of survey data.

[5]Data for 1999-2000 are highly variable (relative standard error >30%).

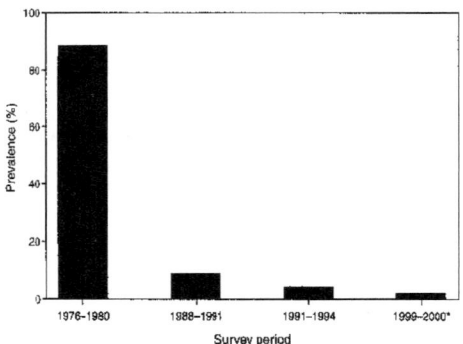

Blood Lead Levels ≥10 µg/dL Among Children 1-5 Years — United States, 1976-1980, 1988-1991, 1991-1994, and 1999-2000[1]

[1]Data for 1999-2000 are highly variable (relative standard error >30%).
Source: National Health and Nutrition Examination Surveys (NHANES).
Note: In 1991, NHANES III Phase 1 was completed and Phase 2 was begun.
Adapted from Meyer PA, Pivetz T, Dignam TA, et al, "Surveillance for Elevated Blood Lead Levels Among Children - United States, 1997-2001," *MMWR Surveill Summ*, 2003, 52(10):1-21.

Specific References

American Academy of Pediatrics Committee on Environmental Health, "Lead Exposure in Children: Prevention, Detection, and Management," *Pediatrics*, 2005, 116(4):1036-46.

Bellinger DC, "Lead," *Pediatrics*, 2004, 113(4 Suppl):1016-22.

Berkowitz, S, Tarrago, R, "Acute Brain Herniation from Lead Toxicity," *Pediatrics*, 2006, 118(6):2548-9.

Cech I, Smolensky MH, Afshar M, et al, "Lead and Copper in Drinking Water Fountains – Information for Physicians," *South Med J*, 2006, 99(2):137-42.

Centers for Disease Control and Prevention, "Adult Blood Lead Epidemiology and Surveillance - United States, 2002," *MMWR Morb Mortal Wkly Rep*, 2004, 53(26):578-82.

Centers for Disease Control and Prevention, "Blood Lead Levels in Residents of Homes with Elevated Lead in Tap Water - District of Columbia, 2004," *MMWR Morb Mortal Wkly Rep*, 2004, 53(12):268-270.

Centers for Disease Control and Prevention, "Death of a Child After Ingestion of a Metallic Charm - Minnesota, 2006," *MMWR Morb Mortal Wkly Rep*, 2006, 55(12):340-1.

Centers for Disease Control and Prevention (CDC), "Lead Exposure from Indoor Firing Ranges Among Students on Shooting Teams–Alaska, 2002-2004," *MMWR Morb Mortal Wkly Rep*, 2005, 54(23):577-9.

Centers for Disease Control and Prevention, "Lead Poisoning Associated with Ayurvedic Medications - Five States, 2000-2003," *MMWR Morb Mortal Wkly Rep*, 2004, 53(26):582-4.

Centers for Disease Control and Prevention, "Lead Poisoning from Ingestion of a Toy Necklace - Oregon, 2003," *MMWR Morb Mortal Wkly Rep*, 2004, 53(23):509-11.

Centers for Disease Control and Prevention, "Surveillance for Elevated Blood Lead Levels Among Children - United States, 1997-2001," *MMWR Morb Mortal Wkly Rep*, 2003, 52(SS-10):1-21.

Chalupka S, "Tainted Water on Tap," *Am J Nurs*, 2005, 105(11):40-52; quiz 53 (review).

Chan GM, Hoffman RS, and Nelson LS, "Get the Lead Out," *Ann Emerg Med*, 2004, 44(5):551-2.

Coon T, Miller M, Shirazi F, et al, "Lead Toxicity in a 14-Year-Old Female with Retained Bullet Fragments," *Pediatrics*, 2006, 117(1):227-30.

Counter SA, Buchanan LH, and Ortega F, "Current Pediatric and Maternal Lead Levels in Blood and Breast Milk in Andean Inhabitants of a Lead-Glazing Enclave," *J Occup Environ Med* 2004, 46(9):967-73.

Dargan PI, Greene SL, House IM, et al, "Two Cases of Lead Poisoning from Ayurvedic Medicine: The Tip of the Iceberg?" *Clin Toxicol (Phila)*. 2005, 43:652.

Dey S and Dwivedi S, "Lead in Blood of Urban Indian Horses," *Vet Hum Toxicol*, 2004, 46(4):194-5.

Diefert RR and Piepenbrink MS, "Lead and Immune Function," *Crit Rev Toxicol*, 2006, 36:359-85.

Dorsey CD, Lee BK, Bolla KI, et al, "Comparison of Patella Lead with Blood Lead and Tibia Lead and Their Associations with Neurobehavioral Test Scores," *J Occ Environ Med*, 2006, 48(5):489-96.

Eisenberg J and Greenberg M, "Lead Dust Transport from Firing Ranges on the Footwear of Recreational Shooters - a Pilot Study," *J Toxicol Clin Toxicol*, 2003, 41(5):729-30.

Ellis LT and Schwartz BS, "Association of Blood Lead and Patella Lead with Blood Pressure and Lack of Effect Modification by VDR and ALAD Genotypes," *J Occup Environ Med*, 2004, 46(9):999.

Falk H, "International Environmental Health for the Pediatrician: Case Study of Lead Poisoning," *Pediatrics*, 2003, 112(1 Pt 2):259-64.

Ferguson JD, Holstege CP, Wolf CE, et al, "Analysis of Moonshine for Contaminants," *Acad Emerg Med*, 2003, 10:511.

Goldstein RA, McKay CA, Burke E, et al, "Management of Acute Pediatric Lead Paint Chip Ingestion," *J Toxicol Clin Toxicol*, 2003, 41(5):691.

Gorter RW, Butorac M, and Cobian EP, "Cutaneous Resorption of Lead After External Use of Lead-Containing Ointments in Volunteers with Healthy Skin," *Am J Ther*, 2005, 12(1):17-21.

Graziano J, Slavkovich V, Liu XH, et al, "A Prospective Study of Prenatal and Childhood Lead Exposure and Erythropoietin Production," *J Occup Environ Med*, 2004, 46(9):924-9.

Guest R, Halluska M, Hendrickson R, et al, "Stroke and Environmental Lead Exposure in Adults: Is There an Association?" *J Toxicol Clin Toxicol*, 2003, 41(5):732.

Guilarte TR, Toscano CD, McGlothan JL, et al, "Environmental Enrichment Reverses Cognitive and Molecular Deficits Induced by Developmental Lead Exposure," *Ann Neurol*, 2003, 53:50-6.

Gustausson P and Gerhardsson L, "Intoxication from an Accidentally Ingested Lead Shot Retained in the Gastrointestinal Tract," *Environ Health Perspect*, 2005, 113:491-3.

Haroz R, Qahwash O, Kralick FA, et al, "Intraoperative Lead Levels During Surgical Removal of Retained Bullet Fragments," *Clin Toxicol (Phila)*, 2005, 43:756.

Hu H, Téllez-Rojo, MM, Bellinger D, et al, "Fetal Lead Exposure at Each Stage of Pregnancy as a Predictor of Infant Mental Development," *Environ Health Perspective*, 2006, 114:1730-5.

Kaul PP, Sing U, Singh N, et al, "Intrauterine Lead Exposure in Pre-Eclamptic Pregnancies," *J Toxicol Clin Toxicol*, 2004, 42(5):802.

Kondrashov VS, "Cosmonauts and Lead: Resorption and Increased Blood Lead Levels During Long Tterm Space Flight," *J Med Toxicol*, 2006, 2(4):172-3.

Krause E, Nussle P, Santana D, et al, "Arsenic and Lead Soil Contamination near a Heavy Metal Refinery in the Andes Mountains," *J Toxicol Clin Toxicol*, 2003, 41(5):739.

Krause E, Nussle P, Santana D, et al, "Blood Lead Levels in People Living Near a Heavy Metal Refinery: A Cause for Concern and Further Study," *J Toxicol Clin Toxicol*, 2003, 41(5):740.

Lemos RA, Driemeier D, Guimaraes EB, et al, "Lead Poisoning in Cattle Grazing Pasture Contaminated by Industrial Waste," *Vet Hum Toxicol*, 2004, 46(6):326-8.

Li GJ, Zhang LL, Lu L, et al, "Occupational Exposure to Welding Fume Among Welders: Alterations of Manganese, Iron, Zinc, Copper, and Lead in Body Fluids and the Oxidative Stress Status," *J Occup Environ Med*, 2004, 46:241-8.

Lin JL, Lin-Tan DT, Hsu KH, et al, "Environmental Lead Exposure and Progression of Chronic Renal Diseases in Patients Without Diabetes," *N Engl J Med*, 2003, 348(4):277-86.

Lustberg ME, Schwartz BS, Lee BK, et al, "The G(894)-T(894) Polymorphism in the Gene for Endothelial Nitric Oxide Synthase and Blood Pressure in Lead-exposed Workers from Korea," *J Occup Environ Med*, 2004, 46(6):584-90.

Miranda ML, Kim D, Hull AP, et al, "Changes in Blood Lead Levels Associated with Use of Chloramines in Water Treatment Systems," *Environ Health Perspect*, 2007, 115:221-5.

Morgan BW, Parramore CS, and Ethridge M, "Lead Contaminated Moonshine: A Report of Bureau of Alcohol, Tobacco and Firearms Analyzed Samples," *Vet Hum Toxicol*, 2004, 46(2):89-90.

Mycyk MB and Leikin JB, "Combined Exchange Transfusion and Chelation Therapy for Neonatal Lead Poisoning," *Ann Pharmacother*, 2004, 38(5):821-4.

Nash D, Magder L, Lustberg M, et al, "Blood Lead, Blood Pressure, and Hypertension in Perimenopausal and Postmenopausal Women," *JAMA*, 2003, 289(12):1523-32.

Onisko N, Daubert GP, White SR, et al, "Is Total Urinary Lead Excretion by Children During Chelation Predicted by Optimally Time 24-Hour Urine Aliquots?" *Clin Toxicol (Phila)*, 2005, 43:776.

Ozmen O and Mor F, "Acute Lead Intoxication in Cattle Housed in an Old Battery Factory," *Vet Hum Toxicol*, 2004, 46(5):255-6.

Paopairochanakorn C, Grzybowski M, White SR, et al, "Efficacy of DMSA and CaNa$_2$EDTA Versus BAL and CaNa$_2$EDTA in Asymptomatic Children with Lead Poisoning," *J Toxicol Clin Toxicol*, 2003, 41(5):721-2.

Park SK, Schwartz J., Weisskopf M, et al, "Low-Level Lead Exposure, Metabolic Syndrome, and Heart Rute Variability: The VA Normative Aging Study," *Environ Health Perspect*, 2006, 114:1718-24.

Piper D, Krantz A, Bryant SM, et al, "Acute Ceramic Glaze Ingestion Resulting in Lead Poisoning," *J Toxicol Clin Toxicol*, 2003, 41(5):656.

Rosenman KD, Sims A, Luo Z, et al, "Occurrence of Lead-Related Symptoms Below the Current Occupational Safety and Health Act Allowable Blood Lead Levels," *J Occup Environ Med*, 2003, 45(5): 546-55.

Sawyer TS, Oller LK, and Lowry JA, "Lead Poisoning Misdiagnosed as Acute Intermittent Porphyria," *J Toxicol Clin Toxicol*, 2004, 42(5):814.

Schier JG, Hoffman RS, and Nelson LS, "Lead-Tainted Herbal Remedy Used for Developmental Delay," *J Toxicol Clin Toxicol*, 2003, 41(5):739.

Schober SE, Mirel LB, Graubard BI, et al, "Blood Lead Levels and Death from All Causes, Cardiovascular Disease, and Cancer: Results from the NHANES III Mortality Study," *Environ Health Perspect 2006*, 114:1538-41.

Schwab LT, Roberts JR, and Reigart JR, "Inaccuracy in Parental Reporting of the Age of Their Home for Lead-Screening Purposes," *Arch Pediatr Adolesc Med*, 2003, 157(6):584-6.

Schwarz KA and Alsop JA, "Pediatric Ingestion of Seven Lead Bullets Successfully Treated with Outpatient Whole Bowel Irrigation," *Clin Toxicol (Phila)*, 2005, 43:680.

Shalan MG, Mostafa MS, Hassouna MM, et al, "Amelioration of Lead Toxicity with Vitamin C and Silymarin Supplementation," *J Toxicol Clin Toxicol*, 2004, 42(5):798.

Soldin OP, Pezzullo JC, Hanak B, et al, "Changing Trends in the Epidemiology of Pediatric Lead Exposure: Interrelationship of Blood Lead and ZPP Concentrations and a Comparison to the US Population," *Ther Drug Monit*, 2003, 25(4):415-20.

Temple KJ and Aaron CK, "Marked Elevation in Blood Lead Levels in a Pediatric Patient Without Evidence of Encephalopathy," *Clin Toxicol (Phila)*, 2005, 43:758.

Theppeang K, Schwartz BS, Lee B, et al, "Associations of Patella Lead with Polymorphisms in the Vitamin D Receptor, Delta-Aminolevulinic Acid Dehydratase and Endothelial Nitric Oxide Synthase Genes," *J Occup Environ Med*, 2004, 46(6):528-37.

U.S. Preventive Services Task Force, "Screening for Elevated Lead Levels in Children and Pregnant Women," *Pediatrics* 2006, 118(6): 2514-8.

Vassilev ZP, Marcus SM, Ayyanathan K, et al, "Case of Elevated Blood Lead in a South Asian Family That Has Used Sindoor for Food Coloring," *Clin Toxicol (Phila)*, 2005, 43(4):301-3.

Wanananukul W, Sura T, Salaitanawatwong P, et al, "A Study of the Genetic Polymorphism of Delta Aminolevulinic Dehydratase (ALAD) in Thai Lead Exposure Workers," *J Toxicol Clin Toxicol*, 2003, 41(5): 716-7.

Yassin AS, Martonik JF, and Davidson JL, "Blood Lead Levels in U.S. Workers, 1988-1994," *J Occup Environ Med*, 2004, 46(7):720-8.

Zadnik T, "Lead in Topsoil, Hay, Silage, and Blood of Cows from Farms near a Former Lead Mine and Current Smelting Plant Before and After Installation of Filters," *Vet Hum Toxicol*, 2004, 46(5):337-9.

Lewisite

Related Information
- Arsenic

CAS Number 541-25-3

Synonyms Chlorovinyl Arsine Dichloride

Use First synthesized in U.S. in 1918 for vesicant warfare. It is ten times more volatile than mustard gas and is often mixed with sulfur mustard (U.S. stockpiles are scheduled to be destroyed by April, 2007).

Mechanism of Toxic Action Dermal exposure results in increased capillary permeability and localized edema, thus enhancing absorption. Combines with thiol groups to cause local toxicity.

Signs and Symptoms of Overdose Hypotension, tachycardia, hypothermia, ocular burns, conjunctivitis, miosis, lacrimation, noncardiogenic pulmonary edema (usually associated with plural effusion), cough, dyspnea, tachypnea, weakness, nausea, vomiting, salivation, hypovolemia, hemolytic anemia (**no** bone marrow depression), dermal burns, blisters, erythema (within 30 minutes), skin edema

Overdosage/Treatment

Decontamination: **Inhalation:** Administer 100% humidified oxygen; remove from source. **Ocular:** Remove contact lenses, irrigate with tepid water or saline for at least 20 minutes. A 5% ophthalmologic compounded ointment or solution may be helpful if given within minutes of exposure. **Dermal:** Decontaminate immediately with 5% solution of sodium hypochlorite; use soap and water if bleach is not available. A 5% topical dimercaprol ointment or solution may prevent vesicant effects.

Supportive therapy: Monitor serum/24-hour urine arsenic levels. Indications for chelation include: cough with dyspnea or signs of pulmonary edema, >1% total body surface area of dermal burn, or ≥5% of body surface in which there is skin damage or erythema noted within 30 minutes of exposure. Chelation should be continued until 24-hour urinary arsenic excretion falls under 50 mcg/L. Chelators include 2,3-dimercapto-1-propanesulfonic acid, succimer, or dimercaprol.

Antidote(s)
- Dimercaprol [ANTIDOTE]
- Succimer [ANTIDOTE]
- Unithiol [ANTIDOTE]

Additional Information An oily liquid with a geranium odor

150 mg/m^3/minute causes 1% mortality

Dermal absorption: As little as 0.5 mL can cause systemic effects (2 mL can be lethal). Vesication can occur with 14 mcg exposure.

All plants die at levels over 50 mg/L. Atmospheric half-life: 1.2 days; water half-life: 5-10 days

Environmental persistence: Shorter in hot climates

Specific References

Lindsay CD, Hambrook JL, Brown RF, et al, "Examination of Changes in Connective Tissue Macromolecular Components of Large White Pig Skin Following Application of Lewisite Vapour," *J Appl Toxicol*, 2004, 24(1):37-46.

Limonene

CAS Number 138-86-3

UN Number 2052

Synonyms Cinene; Dipentene

Use Manufacture of resins, solvent, flavoring agent; in perfumes, stabilizer for aerosols; used medicinally in Japan to dissolve gallstones; found in citrus dill and pine oils

Mechanism of Toxic Action Dermal irritant/sensitizing agent

Signs and Symptoms of Overdose Aspiration may lead to lipoid pneumonia; contact dermatitis, dermal irritation, oliguria, proteinuria, pruritus

Toxicodynamics/Kinetics

Absorption: Oral/dermal routes

Elimination: Renal (~90%). Fecal (~10%)

Monitoring Parameters Urine analysis/chest x-ray

Overdosage/Treatment

Decontamination: **Oral: Do not** induce emesis. Lavage can be performed within 1 hour, with activated charcoal. Dilute oral ingestions with 4-8 ounces of milk or water (in children up to 15 mL/kg). **Dermal:** Wash with soap and water. **Inhalation:** Treat with 100% humidified oxygen.

Supportive therapy: Topical corticosteroids with systemic antihistamines can be used to treat dermal irritation.

Additional Information Lethal dose: Oral: 0.5-5 g/kg. Colorless liquid with lemon-like odor. Odor threshold: 10 ppb. Specific gravity: 0.84.

Lysergic Acid Diethylamide

Related Information
- Highlights of Recent Reports (2006) on Substance Abuse and Mental Health

CAS Number 50-37-3

Synonyms LSD

Impairment Potential Yes. Blood LSD level >0.002 mg/L has been associated with cognitive dysfunction. (Baselt RC and Cravey RH, *Disposition of Toxic Drugs and Chemicals in Man*, 4th ed, Foster City, CA: Chemical Toxicology Institute, 1995, 436.)

Mechanism of Action Agonist at 5-hydroxytryptamine presynaptic receptor in midbrain

Mechanism of Toxic Action Agonist at 5-hydroxytryptamine presynaptic receptor in the midbrain

Adverse Reactions

Cardiovascular: Sinus tachycardia

Central nervous system: Palinopsia, dysphoria, memory disturbance, psychosis

Ocular: Color vision abnormalities

Signs and Symptoms of Overdose Ataxia, coma, delirium, diarrhea, euphoria, fear, fever, flushing, hallucinations (auditory and visual), hyperglycemia, hyperreflexia, hyperthermia, hypertonia, lacrimation, leukocytosis, mydriasis, nausea, neuroleptic malignant syndrome, psychosis, respiratory arrest, rhabdomyolysis, seizures, sweating, tachycardia, tachypnea, tremors, vision color changes (increased color perception), vomiting

Admission Criteria/Prognosis Persistent psychotic/confused behavior

Pharmacodynamics/Kinetics

Onset of action: 20-90 minutes (10 minutes I.V.)

Duration: 6-8 hours

Distribution: V$_d$: 0.28 L/kg

Protein binding: 90%

Metabolism: To 2-oxylysergic acid diethylamide

Half-life: 3-5 hours

Toxicodynamics/Kinetics

Onset of action: 20-90 minutes (10 minutes I.V.)

Duration: 6-8 hours

Distribution: V$_d$: 0.28 L/kg

Protein binding: 90%

Metabolism: To 2-oxylysergic acid diethylamide

Half-life: 3-5 hours

Reference Range Dose of 500 mcg orally resulted in peak plasma levels of 4.2 ng/mL

Overdosage/Treatment

Decontamination: Activated charcoal with oral ingestion

Supportive therapy: Dantrolene (25 mg 3 times/day) should be given for neuroleptic malignant syndrome. Diazepam or lorazepam can be used for agitation. Haloperidol can be given for hallucinations. L-5-hydroxy-tryptophan with carbidopa (25 mg 4 times/day) may improve LSD-induced psychosis.

Diagnostic Procedures
- Lysergic Acid Diethylamine Level

Drug Interaction When combined with lithium and fluoxetine, can cause seizures; sertraline or paroxetine can incite occurrence of LSD flashback episodes (primarily visual); LSD, like panic attacks and visual disorders, can be exacerbated by risperidone; reserpine enhances LSD effect; chronic monoamine oxidase inhibitor use; allopurinol and fluoxetine inhibits LSD effect

Drug Interactions When combined with lithium and fluoxetine, can cause seizures; sertraline or paroxetine can incite occurrence of LSD flashback episodes (primarily visual); LSD, like panic attacks and visual disorders, can be exacerbated by risperidone; reserpine enhances LSD effect; chronic monoamine oxidase inhibitor use; allopurinol and fluoxetine inhibits LSD effect

Pregnancy Implications Can cause uterine contractions; effects on fetus is unknown, although increased incidence of limb defects and ocular abnormalities

Additional Information

Lethal dose: 0.2-1 mg/kg. Hallucinogenic dose: Oral: 100-750 mcg; I.V.: 50-500 mcg.

May be given as sugar cube, on filter or blotting paper, as a tablet or capsule; flashbacks may be induced by alcohol or selective serotonin reuptake inhibitory (SSRI) drugs; urine may be positive for up to 120 hours by radioimmunoassay; odorless, colorless, tasteless

Oregon has the highest rate of LSD users: 4.9% in high school and 2.5% of eighth graders report current use. LSD is the second most commonly used drug (second to marijuana) by United States military personnel with 0.6% and 1.5% reporting its use within the past month and year respectively in 1995.

Mid-Year 2000 Emergency Department Drug Abuse Warning Network (DAWN) data: **Note**: LSD is sometimes used in combination with other drugs; therefore, one Emergency Department (ED) episode can include mentions of one or more drugs.

  * During the first half of 2000, there were 2096 ED mentions of LSD, which is not significantly different than the 2427 mentions for the first half of 1999.

Specific References

Burnley BT and George S, "The Development and Application of a Gas Chromatography-Mass Spectrometric (GC-MS) Assay to Determine the Presence of 2-Oxo-3-Hydroxy-LSD in Urine," *J Anal Toxicol*, 2003, 27(4):249-52.

Horn CK, Klette KL, and Stout PR, "LC-MS Analysis of 2-Oxo-3-Hydroxy LSD from Urine Using a Speedisk® Positive-Pressure Processor with Cerex® PolyChrom™ CLIN II Columns," *J Anal Toxicol*, 2003, 27: 459-63.

Libong D, Bouchonnet S, and Ricordel I, "A Selective and Sensitive Method for Quantitation of Lysergic Acid Diethylamide (LSD) in Whole Blood by Gas Chromatography-Ion Trap Tandem Mass Spectrometry," *J Anal Toxicol*, 2003, 27(1):24-9.

Wiegand RF, Klette KL, Stout PR, et al, "Comparison of EMIT® II, CEDIA®, and DPC® RIA Assays for the Detection of Lysergic Acid Diethylamide in Forensic Urine Samples," *J Anal Toxicol*, 2003, 27:191.

Malathion

Related Information
- Donor Victims of Poisoning in Whom Transplantation of Organs Occurred

CAS Number 121-75-5

UN Number 2783

U.S. Brand Names Carbofos®; Compound 4049®; Cython®; Fosfothion®; Mercaptothion®; Ovide®

Synonyms O,O-Dimethyldithiophosphate Diethylmercaptosuccinate

Use Marketed as insecticide granules, powder or dusting agent, or spray liquid concentrate with or without petroleum derivative as a solvent

Mechanism of Toxic Action Irreversible inhibition of acetylcholinesterase and plasma cholinesterase, resulting in excess accumulation of acetylcholine at muscarinic and nicotinic receptors, and in the central nervous system

Adverse Reactions
Cardiovascular: **Hyperdynamic** or **hypodynamic** states, QT prolongation, Raynaud's phenomenon, sinus bradycardia, sinus tachycardia, torsade de pointes

Central nervous system: Depression, seizures, hyperactivity, cognitive dysfunction, hypothermia, extrapyramidal reactions

Dermatologic: Scleroderma

Endocrine & metabolic: Diabetes insipidus, hypernatremia

Gastrointestinal: Pancreatitis

Genitourinary: Urinary incontinence

Neuromuscular & skeletal: Weakness (delayed), paralysis, sclerodermatous changes accompanied by Raynaud's phenomena, delayed paresthesia

Respiratory: Pulmonary edema, respiratory depression

Miscellaneous: Flu-like symptoms (especially with chronic exposure), intermediate syndrome

Signs and Symptoms of Overdose
Abdominal pain, agitation, asystole, AV block, bradycardia, bronchorrhea, coma, confusion, cranial nerve palsies, decreased hemoglobin, decreased platelet count, decreased red blood cell count, dementia, diaphragmatic paralysis, dysarthria, excessive sweating, fecal and urinary incontinence, garlic-like breath, generalized asthenia, headache, heart block, hypertension, hypotension, lacrimation, metabolic acidosis and hyperglycemia (severe intoxication), miosis (unreactive to light), mydriasis (rarely), nausea, pallor, pulmonary edema, QT prolongation, respiratory depression, salivation, seizures, skeletal muscle fasciculation and flaccid paralysis, tachycardia, tachypnea, vomiting

An "intermediate syndrome" of limb asthenia and respiratory paralysis has been reported to occur between 24 and 96 hours postorganophosphate exposure, and is independent of the acute cholinergic crisis. Late paresthesia characterized by stocking and glove paresthesia, anesthesia, and asthenia is infrequently observed weeks to months following acute exposure to certain organophosphates.

Admission Criteria/Prognosis Any symptomatic patient or an asymptomatic patient following a severe exposure should be admitted probably into an intensive care unit; asymptomatic patients following a moderate exposure can be discharged after 8 hours of observation

Toxicodynamics/Kinetics
Absorption: Readily through oral, dermal, or respiratory exposure

Metabolism: Rapid to weakly active compounds through hepatic hydrolysis and other pathways

Half-life: 2.9 hours

Elimination: Metabolites excreted in urine

Administration Refer to Dosing.

Contraindications Hypersensitivity to malathion or any component of the formulation; use in neonates and/or infants

Warnings
For topical use only; avoid contact with eyes. Lotion is flammable; do not expose to open flames; patients should avoid electric heat sources (eg, hair dryers, curling irons). Safety and efficacy in children <6 years of age have not been established.

Significant dermal absorption may occur across intact skin; risk of aspiration pneumonitis exists following oral exposure to agents having a hydrocarbon vehicle; severe laryngeal irritation and violent coughing may result from exposure to dusting powders; exposure to dusting powders and insecticide granules may cause contact dermatitis

Dosing Forms Lotion: 0.5% (59 mL)

Dosage Forms Lotion: 0.5% (59 mL) [contains isopropyl alcohol 78%]

Reference Range
A 1.8 g ingestion with undetectable pseudocholinesterase resulted in a serum malathion level of 0.35 mg/L 2 hours postingestion.

Mild poisoning: Serum cholinesterase is 20% to 50% of normal;

Moderate poisoning: Serum cholinesterase is 10% to 20% of normal

Severe poisoning (respiratory distress and coma): Serum cholinesterase is <10%

Fatal malathion blood levels range from 0.3-1880 mg/L

Overdosage/Treatment
Decontamination: Isolation, bagging, and disposal of all contaminated clothing and other articles. All emergency medical workers and hospital staff should follow appropriate precautions regarding exposure to hazardous material including the use of protective clothing, masks, goggles, and respiratory equipment.

Oral: Activated charcoal can be administered either orally or via a nasogastric tube. **Do not** induce emesis because of danger of sudden respiratory compromise, alterations in mental status, seizures, coma, and possible aspiration of hydrocarbon vehicles. **Do not** give a cathartic.

Dermal: Prompt thorough scrubbing of all affected areas with soap and water, including hair and nails; 5% bleach can be used

Ocular: Irrigation with copious tepid sterile water or saline

Supportive therapy: Airway management, ventilatory assistance, humidified oxygen administration, and close monitoring for sudden respiratory failure

Enhancement of elimination: Dialysis and hemoperfusion are not indicated due to effectiveness of the prescribed treatment and large volumes of distribution of organophosphates.

Antidote:
Atropine: Administration should be guided by respiratory status, starting at 2-5 mg I.V. every 5-10 minutes as needed, and should be titrated to the resolution of excess pulmonary secretions. Frequent administration of large doses (cumulative doses >100 mg) may be necessary in massive exposures.

Glycopyrrolate: May be administered if atropine is unavailable (200-400 mcg I.M. or I.V. initially. or ~$^1/_2$ the dose of atropine).

2-PAM: For more significant exposures (ie, exposures requiring large doses of atropine, or with recurring symptoms, or exposures to more lipid soluble agents), administration should follow: 1-2 g I.V. over 10-30 minutes, repeated in 1 hour if asthenia recurs, then every 4-12 hours for recurring symptoms.

Antidote(s)
- Atropine [ANTIDOTE]
- Pralidoxime [ANTIDOTE]

Diagnostic Procedures
- Creatinine, Serum
- Pseudocholinesterase, Serum

Drug Interaction Paralysis is potentiated by neuromuscular blockade (ie, pancuronium, vecuronium, succinylcholine, atracurium, doxacurium, mivacurium); inhibition of serum esterase prolongs the half-life of succinylcholine, cocaine, and other ester anesthetics; cholinergic toxicity is potentiated by cholinesterase inhibitors such as physostigmine

Pregnancy Risk Factor B

Pregnancy Implications No evidence of teratogenicity in animal models. There are no adequate and well-controlled studies in pregnant women. Use (or handle) during pregnancy only if clearly needed.

Additional Information
Red blood cell cholinesterase and serum pseudocholinesterase may be depressed following acute or chronic organophosphate exposure. RBC cholinesterase is typically not analyzed by in-house laboratories, and is usually not available for consideration during acute management. Pseudocholinesterase levels may be rapidly available from some in-house laboratories, but are not as reliable a marker of organophosphate exposure because of variability secondary to variant genotypes, hepatic disease, oral estrogen use, or malnutrition. Because of this variability, true indication of suppression of either of these enzymes can only be estimated through comparison to pre-exposure values; these enzymes may be useful in measuring a patient's recovery postexposure, especially if the recovery is not progressing as expected.

QT$_c$ prolongation on ECG in the setting of organophosphate poisoning is associated with a high incidence of respiratory failure and mortality.

The intermediate syndrome is not related to delayed neuropathy.

Colorless to brown liquid with foul, skunk-like odor; thermal degradation products include sulfur and phosphorus oxides

Water solubility: 143 ppm. Vapor pressure: 0.00004 mm Hg at 20°C.

ACGIH TLV: 10 mg/m^3; PEL-TWA: 10 mg/m^3 (total dust); 5 mg/m^3 (respirable fraction of dust); IDLH: 5000 mg/m^3

Other information concerning pesticide exposures is available through the EPA-funded National Pesticide Telecommunications Network: 1-800-858-7378

Specific References

Bentur Y, Raikhlin-Eisenkraft B, and Singer P, "Beneficial Late Administration of Obidoxime in Malathion Poisoning," *Vet Hum Toxicol*, 2003, 45(1):33-5.

Butera R, Locatelli C, Barretta S, et al, "Secondary Exposure to Malathion in Emergency Department Health-Care Workers," *J Toxicol Clin Toxicol*, 2002, 40(3):386-7.

Centers for Disease Control and Prevention, "Surveillance for Acute Insecticide-Related Illness Associated with Mosquito-Control Efforts - Nine States, 1999-2002," *MMWR Morb Mortal Wkly Rep*, 2003, 52(27):629-34.

Horton DK, Berkowitz Z, and Kaye WE, "Secondary Contamination of ED Personnel from Hazardous Materials Events, 1995-2001," *Am J Emerg Med*, 2003, 21(3):199-204.

O'Sullivan BC, Lafleur J, Fridal K, et al, "The Effect of Pesticide Spraying on the Rate and Severity of ED Asthma," *Am J Emerg Med*, 2005, 23(4):463-7.

Manganese

Related Information

- Adipose Tissue Ranges of Toxins

CAS Number 1313-13-1; 1317-34-6; 14024-58-9; 6156-78-1; 7439-96-5; 7773-01-5; 7785-87-7

UN Number 1490

U.S. Brand Names Mangimin [OTC]

Synonyms Manganese Chloride; Manganese Sulfate

Commonly Found In Elemental manganese metal, and as the following salts: acetate, chloride, dioxide, and sulfate; found in fertilizer, welding rods, ceramics, electrical coils, matches, animal food additives

Mechanism of Action Cofactor in many enzyme systems, stimulates synthesis of cholesterol and fatty acids in liver, and influences mucopolysaccharide synthesis

Mechanism of Toxic Action Catalyses dopamine depletion and free radical production within the central nervous system; results in diffuse cortical and cerebellar degeneration

Adverse Reactions

Central nervous system: Parkinson-like syndrome, nervousness, dementia, ataxia, irritability, "manganese psychosis", memory disturbance, metal fume fever, CNS depression, depression, psychosis, extrapyramidal reactions

Genitourinary: Impotence

Hematologic: Methemoglobinemia

Neuromuscular & skeletal: Bradykinesia, gait instability, chorea (extrapyramidal)

Ocular: Visual evoked potential abnormalities

Otic: Ototoxicity

Respiratory: Pleuritis, pneumonia

Signs and Symptoms of Overdose Symptoms correlate with duration of exposure, either acute or chronic. Acute exposure primarily results in respiratory symptoms such as cough, pleuritis, pneumonia, and in GI irritation and pancreatitis. Chronic exposure primarily results in CNS symptoms such as nervousness, irritability, Parkinson-like symptoms, nystagmus, tremor, fasciculations, slurred speech, feces discoloration (dark brown); diminished libido, "manganese psychosis" (*Locura manganical*), limb asthenia, and insomnia may persist for several months.

Pharmacodynamics/Kinetics

Absorption: Oral: Poor (3% to 4%)

Distribution: Concentrated in mitochondria of pituitary gland, pancreas, liver, kidney, and bone

Excretion: Bile (primarily); urine (negligible)

Monitoring Parameters Periodic manganese plasma level

Administration

Solution for injection: Do not administer I.M. or by direct I.V. injection; acidic pH of the solution may cause tissue irritations and it is hypotonic

Contraindications High manganese levels; severe liver dysfunction or cholestasis (conjugated bilirubin >2 mg/dL) due to reduced biliary excretion

Warnings Manganese chloride solution for injection contains aluminum; use caution with impaired renal function and in premature infants. Use caution with hepatic impairment.

Dosage Forms

Injection, solution, as chloride [preservative free]: 0.1 mg/mL (10 mL) [contains aluminum ≤100 mcg/mL]

Injection, solution, as sulfate: 0.1 mg/mL (10 mL)

Tablet, as aspartate: 93 mg [equivalent to elemental manganese 25 mg]

Tablet, as gluconate: 5.7 mg [as elemental manganese]; 550 mg [equivalent to elemental manganese 30 mg]; 600 mg [equivalent to elemental manganese 50 mg]

Tablet, chelated: 50 mg [as elemental manganese]

Mangimin: 10 mg [as elemental manganese]

Reference Range Typical normal ranges in adults: CSF: 0.4-1.2 mcg/100 mL. Serum: 0.9-2.9 mcg/L. Whole blood: 4-15 mcg/L. Urine: <10 mcg/L.

Overdosage/Treatment

Decontamination:

Oral: Since most symptomatic exposures are chronic, emesis with ipecac within 30 minutes or gastric lavage within 1 hour may be used to eliminate large acute ingestions. Chronically exposed patients may become obtunded or may develop acute respiratory symptoms, and should not receive lavage or ipecac. Single dose activated charcoal will not adsorb manganese but is useful for coingestants.

Dermal: Prompt thorough scrubbing of all affected areas with soap and water

Ocular: Irrigation with copious tepid water or saline

Inhalation: Remove patient from source of exposure

Supportive therapy: Airway management, ventilatory assistance, humidified oxygen administration; and close monitoring for renal compromise, respiratory decompensation, or further convulsive activity

Chelation: EDTA therapy instituted early in manganese intoxication is most promising. BAL and succimer have not demonstrated utility in chronic toxicity.

Intention tremor: Trihexyphenidil 1-5 mg/day orally in divided doses

Anti-Parkinson's therapy: Improvement in neurologic toxicity may result with using anti-Parkinson's therapy of levodopa 3.5-12 g/day orally, or levodopa/carbidopa (Sinemet®) 100 mg/25 mg 2-3 times/day orally, up to 6 tablets/day for 8 weeks.

Antidote(s)

- Charcoal [ANTIDOTE]
- Edetate Calcium Disodium [ANTIDOTE]

Diagnostic Procedures

- Creatinine, Serum
- Electrolytes, Blood
- Glucose, Random
- Magnetic Resonance Scan, Brain
- Urea Nitrogen, Blood

Pregnancy Risk Factor C

Pregnancy Implications Mn crosses the placenta but does not accumulate in the fetus.

Lactation Enters breast milk/compatible

Additional Information

Urine or plasma concentrations of manganese do not correlate with severity of symptoms. Toxicity following ingestion of inorganic salts is unlikely because of poor gastrointestinal absorption; neurologic manifestations may be permanently established after 1-2 years of chronic exposure. Magnetic resonance imaging may be useful for manganese encephalopathy (T_1 weighted imaging).

Foods with the highest amount of manganese concentrations are nuts and nut products (18-47 ppm); average amount of ingestion of manganese from food: 3.8 mg/day; average cup of tea may contain from 0.4-1.3 mg of manganese; legumes may contain from 2-7 ppm of manganese

Manganese toxic patients have a tendency to fall backwards, to not have a prominent tremor, and do not respond well to dopaminomimetic medication as opposed to idiopathic parkinsonism patients.

Safe infant daily dose: 0.7-1 mg

Mean level in drinking water: 4-32 mcg/L

Average ambient atmospheric manganese levels: Urban: 33 ng/m^3; Nonurban: 5 ng/m^3

Concentration in soil: 40-900 mg/kg. Atmospheric half-life (in sunlight): 15 seconds

TLV-TWA: Dust: 5 mg/m^3; Fumes: 1 mg/m^3; IDLH: 10,000 mg/m^3; PEL-TWA: 1 mg/m^3 (fumes)

Specific References

Aschner M, Erikson KM, and Dorman DC, "Manganese Dosimetry: Species Differences and Implications for Neurotoxicity," *Crit Rev Toxicol*, 2005, 35(1):1-32.

Bouchard M, Laforest F, Vandelac L, et al, "Hair Manganese and Hyperactive Behaviors: Pilot Study of School-Age Children Exposed through Tap Water," *Environ Health Perspective*, 2007, 115:122-7.

Crossgrove J and Zheng W, "Manganese Toxicity upon Overexposure," *NMR Biomed*, 2004, 17:544-53.

Fruzek JP, Hansen J, Cohen S, et al, "A Cohort Study of Parkinson's Disease and Other Neurodegenerative Disorders in Danish Welders," *J Occup Environ Med*, 2005, 47:466-72.

Jiang YM, Mo XA, Du FQ, et al, "Effective Treatment of Manganese-Induced Occupational Parkinsonism with *p*-Aminosalicylic Acid: A Case of 17-Year Follow-Up Study," *J Occup Environ Med*, 2006, 48(6):644-9.

Li GJ, Zhang LL, Lu L, et al, "Occupational Exposure to Welding Fume Among Welders: Alterations of Manganese, Iron, Zinc, Copper, and Lead in Body Fluids and the Oxidative Stress Status," *J Occup Environ Med*, 2004, 46:241-8.

Missy P, Lanhers MC, Grignon Y, et al, "*In vitro* and *in vivo* Studies on Chelation of Manganese," *Hum Experiment Toxicol*, 2000, 19:448-56.

Ohtake T, Negishi K, Okamoto K, et al, "Manganese-Induced Parkinsonism in a Patient Undergoing Maintenance Hemodialysis," *Am J Kidney Dis*, 2005, 46(4):749-53.

Mercury

Related Information
- Dimercaprol [ANTIDOTE]
- Mercury Levels in Commercial Fish and Shellfish
- Toxins Which Should Be Lavaged with Solutions Other Than Water

CAS Number 7439-97-6

UN Number 1629; 2024; 2025; 2809

Commonly Found In
Inorganic mercury salts; organic mercury; elemental mercury; found in thimerosal, fireworks, button batteries

Used by amalgam makers, jewelers, paint manufacturers, laboratorians, taxidermists, embalmers, dye makers, fur processors, photographers, electroplaters

Mechanism of Toxic Action
Causes cell membrane damage; elemental and organic mercury are CNS toxins; inorganic is a corrosive; organic mercury causes teratogenicity; high-binding affinity of divalent cation form of mercury to thiol or sulfhydryl protein groups occur

Adverse Reactions
Cardiovascular: Hypertension, tachycardia, hypotension, cranial nerve palsies, cardiomyopathy, cardiomegaly, palpitations, QT prolongation, sinus tachycardia, arrhythmias (ventricular), vasoconstriction

Central nervous system: Dementia, hyperthermia, encephalopathy, ataxia, Jarisch-Herxheimer reaction, CNS depression

Dermatologic: Dermal granuloma, skin granuloma, systemic contact dermatitis, exanthem

Gastrointestinal: Salivation, metallic taste

Hematologic: Thrombocytopenia, eosinophilia

Neuromuscular & skeletal: Tremor, myoclonus, neuritis, rhabdomyolysis

Ocular: Nystagmus, diplopia, photophobia, visual evoked potential abnormalities

Otic: Deafness

Renal: Glomerulonephritis

Respiratory: Hyposmia

Miscellaneous: Toxic shock-like syndrome

Signs and Symptoms of Overdose
Elemental mercury is poorly absorbed orally, with minimal adverse effects. Inhalation acutely can cause chemical pneumonitis, gingivostomatitis, and noncardiogenic pulmonary edema. Chronic exposure to mercury vapor causes acrodynia, alopecia, fasciculations, fatigue, hematuria, insomnia, leukocytosis, memory loss, proteinuria, tremor

Inorganic mercury: After oral administration: Abdominal pain, ATN, GI bleeding, GI irritation, possible CNS toxicity, renal failure, shock

Organic mercury: CNS toxicity including ataxia, dysarthria, hearing and visual loss, paresthesias; gastrointestinal distress

Admission Criteria/Prognosis
Significant exposure to mercury vapor, inorganic mercury, or organic mercury compounds usually requires admission; ingestion of small amounts of elemental mercury usually does not require admission; alkyl mercury inhalation exposure (chronic) may result in residual central nervous system impairments

Toxicodynamics/Kinetics
Absorption: Elemental mercury is poorly absorbed orally and well absorbed by inhalation while inorganic and organic mercury are well absorbed orally; metallic mercury is minimally absorbed dermally (0.024 ng of mercury absorbed per cm^2 of skin)

Distribution: Elemental to CNS, kidney, liver, and heart; inorganic mercury concentrates in the kidney; organic mercury (alkyl mercury groups) distributes throughout the body while methylmercury concentrates in blood and CNS

Metabolism: Metallic/inorganic mercury: Oxidized to an inorganic divalent form in the red blood cells (note that ethanol can inhibit this step)

Half-life:
Elemental and inorganic: 40-60 days. Organic: 70 days; organic converted to divalent cation form in tissues

Elimination: Metallic: Urine, feces, and lung. Inorganic: Urine, feces. Organic: Primarily feces

Reference Range
Urinary and whole blood levels can be obtained; urinary values are normally <10 mcg/L and whole blood <20 mcg/L; geometric mean blood mercury levels are 0.3 mcg/L for children 1-5 years of age and 1.2 mcg/L for women 16-49 years of age. Whole blood levels >50 mcg/L are usually associated with gastroenteritis and acute tubular necrosis. Urinary levels for organic mercury are not useful since 90% is eliminated through bile in the feces. Urinary mercury levels >56 mcg/L can result in neurotoxic effects (due to elemental mercury), although neurologic signs are not usually manifested until urinary mercury levels exceed 100 mcg/L.

Note that hair mercury analysis measures organic (not organic or elemental mercury) methyl mercury exposures only. Reference range for unexposed individuals is <1 mcg/g.

Overdosage/Treatment
Decontamination:
Oral: Lavage if ingested within 1 hour. Charcoal has been shown to decrease inorganic mercury absorption in rats and should be used. Milk or egg white may also be useful to bind mercury, as is 5% sodium formaldehyde or a 2% to 5% sodium bicarbonate solution. Whole bowel irrigation with GoLYTELY® may be beneficial if abdominal x-ray shows evidence of mercury. **Do not** induce emesis for inorganic mercury ingestions as this agent has corrosive properties.

Inhalation: Patients should be monitored for pulmonary edema and pneumonitis; give oxygen if necessary.

Dermal: Wash with tincture of green soap and water.

Ocular: Copious irrigation with saline

Supportive therapy: D-penicillamine can be administered orally in 4 divided doses totaling 20-30 mg/kg (250 mg 4 times/day in adults) if prolonged therapy is required, especially for short-chain alkyl organic mercury compounds. Another less toxic form of penicillamine, N-acetyl-penicillamine (from Aldrich Chemical Co, Milwaukee, WI), is a specific chelator for mercury. Both are also effective for long-chain alkyl, aryl mercurials, or for treatment of acrodynia. 2,3-Dimercaptopropane sulphonate (DMPS or unithiol) is also useful to enhance mercury elimination.

Elemental mercury: Oral DMSA (succimer) 10 mg/kg every 8 hours for 5 days, then 10 mg/kg every 12 hours for 2 or more weeks, will enhance urinary mercury excretion.

Inorganic mercury: BAL 5 mg/kg deep I.M. initially, then 2.5 mg/kg every 12 hours for 10 days. If given within the first 2 hours, BAL may prevent renal toxicity. **Do not give BAL I.V.**.

Organic mercury: Oral DMSA (succimer) with dosing as above for methyl mercury exposure. BAL is contraindicated.

BAL is not recommended for elemental and organic mercury poisoning since BAL may cause redistribution of mercury to the brain, which is the primary target organ in these poisonings.

Enhancement of elimination: Generally ineffective. BAL, mercury complex is dialyzable and is useful in patients with renal failure; it does not enhance elimination in those with good renal function. Some clinical improvement with increased clearance has been noted after exchange transfusion.

Organic mercury: Oral neostigmine may improve motor strength in chronic methyl mercury exposure.

Antidote(s)
- Succimer [ANTIDOTE]
- Unithiol [ANTIDOTE]

Diagnostic Procedures
- Mercury, Blood
- Mercury, Urine
- Urinalysis

Drug Interaction
BAL forms toxic metabolites with cadmium, iron, selenium, and uranium; BAL may cause interference with iodine accumulation in the thyroid

Additional Information
BAL should be administered deep I.M.; **do not give I.V.**. See table.

Estimated Average Daily Intake and Retention of Total Mercury and Mercury Compounds in the General Population

Source of Exposure	Elemental Mercury Vapor	Inorganic Mercury Compounds	Methylmercury
Air	0.030 (0.024)	0.002 (0.001)	0.008 (0.0064)
Food			
Fish	0	0.600 (0.042)	2.4 (2.3)
Non-fish	0	3.6 (0.25)	0
Drinking water	0	0.050 (0.0035)	0
Dental amalgams	3.8-21 (3-17)	0	0
Total	3.9-21 (3-17)	4.3 (0.3)	2.41 (2.31)

Note: Values given are the estimated average daily intake (in mcg/day) for adults in the general population who are not occupationally exposed to mercury; the figures in parentheses represent the estimated amount retained in the body of an adult.

Source: *WHO* 1990, 1991.

Reference: "Toxicological Profile for Mercury," U.S. Department of Health and Human Services, Agency for Toxic Substances and Disease Registry, March 1999.

Estimated Number of Workers Potentially Exposed to Mercury and Various Mercury Compounds in the Workplace

Mercury Compounds	Number of Workers	Number of Female Workers
Mercury (metallic)	71,933	23,826
Mercury chloride	45,492	18,717
Mercury acetate	6063	2770
Mercuric sulfide	98	—
Phenylmercuric acetate	28,347	5150
Methylmercuric chloride	14	5

Source: RTECS 1998.
Reference: "Toxicological Profile for Mercury," U.S. Department of Health and Human Services, Agency for Toxic Substances and Disease Registry, March 1999.

EPA maximum mercury exposure limit: 0.1 mcg/kg/day

Ambient atmospheric mercury levels range from 10-20 ng/m^3. Surface water levels: <5 ng/L. Soil levels: 20-625 ng/g

IDLH: Mercury vapor: 28 mg/m^3

Alkyl mercury compounds: 10 mg/m^3

WHO guideline for drinking water: 1 mcg/L; EPA standard mercury limit for drinking water: 2 mcg/L; FDA standard limit for bottled water: 2 mcg/L

Resident air mercury level limit (ATSDR): 0.05 mcg/m^3

Permissible tolerable weekly intake: 5 mcg/kg

Mean mercury levels in fish: ~0.4 mcg/g. See Mercury Concentrations in the Top 10 Types of Fish Consumed by the U.S. Population and Fish and Shellfish with Much Lower Mercury Levels

Other foods: ~0.004 mcg/g

Cigarette smoke: ~0.004 mcg/cigarette

Estimated daily intake of mercury from air: 0.2 mcg; from drinking water: 0.1 mcg

Residence atmospheric time of elemental mercury: 6-24 months

Average methyl mercury content in tuna: 0.17 ppm

Chinese herbal balls may contain from 7.8-621.3 mg of mercury and from 0.1-36.6 mg of arsenic

Latex gloves are of no protection with mercury. Suggested hand protection is use of a flexible, plastic laminate glove worn under a heavy duty neoprene outer glove.

Accidental soft tissue deposition of liquid mercury from a thermometer results in little to no toxicity and usually does not require chelation

What to do if elemental (metallic) mercury spills in your home: Mercury spills should be considered a hazardous material incident. If any amount greater than that from a small thermometer is spilled (or if mercury from a fever thermometer is spilled on a porous surface), call your local environmental health department, local board of health, poison control center, or your physician, even if no one has symptoms. Do not attempt to clean the spills by yourself or with a vacuum cleaner, or to remove mercury from carpeting or a porous (eg, furniture or unfinished wood) surface. Discard contaminated carpeting and rugs. Open windows to ventilate and evacuate the area until professionally assessed and cleaned. If a small amount (eg, from a fever thermometer) is spilled on a nonporous (eg, tile or wood) surface follow the instructions below:

- Remove all gold jewelry.
- Using an index card or stiff paper, gather the droplets together into a glass jar with a tight lid or a "Ziplock" plastic bag. Masking, cellophane, or duct tape may be helpful in removing mercury.
- Avoid skin contact.
- Contact your local health department as to proper disposal.
- Provide additional ventilation for the affected area for 2 days.
- Ordinary gloves are of no protection in handling mercury and thereby preventing poisoning. Flexible laminated gloves worn under heavy duty neoprene outer gloves afford adequate hand protection.

Elemental Mercury can volatilize at temperatures over 88°F. Density of elemental mercury is 13.5 g/ml, in water and 6.93 (vapor density) in air. Air Elemental mercury concentrations are usually less than 0.001 mg/m^3 in relation to broken mercury based thermometers or thermostats.

Specific References

Abbaslou P and Zaman T, "A Child with Elemental Mercury Poisoning and Unusual Brain MRI Findings," Clin Toxicol (Phila), 2006, 44(1): 85-8.

Aposhian HV, Morgan DL, Queen HL, et al, "Vitamin C, Glutathione, or Lipoic Acid Did Not Decrease Brain or Kidney Mercury in Rats Exposed to Mercury Vapor," J Toxicol Clin Toxicol, 2003, 41(4):339-47.

Azizz-Baumgartner E, Luber G, Jones R, et al, "Mercury Exposure Assessment in a Nevada Middle School - 2004," J Toxicol Clin Toxicol, 2004, 42(5):808-9.

Baltarowich L, Boyle B, Smolinske S, et al, "Mercury Excretion in Sweat," J Toxicol Clin Toxicol, 2004, 42(5):825.

Bellinger DC, Trachtenberg F, Barregard L, et al,. "Neuropsychological and Renal Effects of Dental Amalgam in Children: A Randomized Clinical Trial," JAMA, 2006, 295(15):1775-83.

Button G and Vicas I, "Household Mercury (Hg) Spills: Variation in Poison Centers (PC): Has Anything Changed?" J Toxicol Clin Toxicol, 2003, 41(5):696.

Casavanat MJ, Hunter A, Maloy R, et al, "Collaboration of Multiple Agencies in the Management of a Home Mercury Spill," J Toxicol Clin Toxicol, 2003, 41(5):731.

Centers for Disease Control and Prevention (CDC), "Measuring Exposure to an Elemental Mercury Spill–Dakota County, Minnesota, 2004," MMWR Morb Mortal Wkly Rep, 2005, 18;54(6):146-9.

Centers for Disease Control and Prevention (CDC), "Mercury Exposure – Kentucky, 2004," MMWR Morb Mortal Wkly Rep, 2005, 54(32):797-9.

Clarkson TW, Magos L, and Myers GJ, "The Toxicology of Mercury - Current Exposures and Clinical Manifestations," N Engl J Med, 2003, 349(18):1731-7.

Counter SA, "Neurophysiological Anomalies in Brainstem Responses of Mercury-Exposed Children of Andean Gold Miners," J Occup Environ Med, 2003, 45(1):87-95.

Davidson PW, Myers GJ, and Weiss B, "Mercury Exposure and Child Development Outcomes," Pediatrics, 2004, 113(4 Suppl):1023-9.

Dellinger J, Gerstenberger S, Dewailly E, et al, "Whole Blood and Hair Mercury Concentrations in Upper Great Lakes Fish Eaters: Total and Inorganic Mercury," J Toxicol Clin Toxicol, 2003, 41(5):723.

Dellinger J, Hudson J, Krabbenhoft D, et al, "Pacific Volcanoes, Mercury Contaminated Fish, and Polynesiam Taboos," Clin Toxicol, 2005, 43(6):595-6.

DeRouen TA, Martin MD, Leroux BG, et al, "Neurobehavioral Effects of Dental Amalgam in Children: A Randomized Clinical Trial," JAMA, 2006, 295(15):1784-92.

Eyer F, Felgenhauer N, Pfab R, et al, "Neither DMPS nor DMSA is Effective in Quantitative Elimination of Elemental Mercury After Intentional IV Injection, Clin Toxicol, 2006, 44:395-7.

Gaffney W, Caraccio TR, and McGuigan MA, "Availability of Mercury in High Schools and Awareness of Clean-Up Procedures by School Nurses," Clin Toxicol (Phila), 2005, 43:702.

Ginsburg BY, Greller HA, Freyberg C, et al, "Mercury Absorption Following Elemental Mercury Ingestion," Clin Toxicol (Phila), 2005, 43:749.

Gordon AT, "Short-Term Elemental Mercury Exposures at Three Arizona Schools: Public Health Lessons Learned," J Toxicol Clin Toxicol, 2004, 42(2):179-87.

Gray T, Baker B, Lintner C, et al, "Chronic Consumption of Fish Associated with Mercury Toxicity," J Toxicol Clin Toxicol, 2004, 42(5):807-8.

Haas NS, Shih R, and Gochfeld M, "A Patient with Postoperative Mercury Contamination of the Peritoneum," J Toxicol Clin Toxicol, 2003, 41(2):175-80.

Ho BS, Lin JL, Huang CC, et al, "Mercury Vapor Inhalation from Chinese Red (Cinnabar)," J Toxicol Clin Toxicol, 2003, 41(1):75-8.

Kurt TL, "ACMT Position Statement: The IOM Report on Thimerosal and Autism," J Med Toxicol, 2006, 2(4):170-1.

Latshaw MW, Glass T, Parsons P, et al, "Predictors of Blood Mercury Levels in Older Urban Residents," J Occup Environ Med, 2006, 48:715-22.

Lech T and Goszcz H, "Poisoning from Aspiration of Elemental Mercury," Clin Toxicol, 2006, 44(3):333-6.

Lykissa E, Gonzalez C, Kaffity I, et al, "ICP-MS Uncovers Life Threatening Mercury + Cadmium Intoxication with Negative GC-MS and LC-MS Blood Screens for Rat Poison," J Anal Toxicol, 2003, 27:177.

Madsen KM, Lauritsen MB, Pedersen CB, et al, "Thimerosal and the Occurrence of Autism: Negative Ecological Evidence from Danish Population-Based Data," Pediatrics, 2003, 112(3 Pt 1):604-6.

Mohan S, Tiller M, van der Voet G, et al, "Mercury Exposure of Mothers and Newborns in Surinam: A Pilot Study," Clin Toxicol (Phila), 2005, 43(2):101-4.

Montuori P, Jover E, Diez S, et al, "Mercury Speciation in the Hair of Preschool Children Living near a Chlor-Alkali Plant," Sci Total Environ, 2006, [epub ahead of print].

Naũagas KA, O'Connor AD, Potts ME, et al, "Conservative Management of Elemental Mercury Sequestration in the Appendix," J Toxicol Clin Toxicol, 2003, 41(5):662.

Needleman HL, "Mercury in Dental Amalgam - A Neurotoxic Risk?," JAMA, 2006, 295(15):1731-860.

Nehls-Lowe H, Stanton M, and Stremski E, "Air Sampling and Urine Analysis Following Decontamination of an Elemental Mercury (Hg) Spill in a High School Chemistry Lab," J Toxicol Clin Toxicol, 2004, 42(5):825.

Nenov VD, Marinov P, Sabeva J, et al, "Current Applications of Plasmapheresis in Clinical Toxicology," Nephrol Dial Transplant, 2003, 18(Suppl 5):v56-8.

Petrovski D, Naumovski J, Pereska Z, et al, "Clinical Outcomes in Inorganic Mercury Salts Ingestions," *J Toxicol Clin Toxicol*, 2003, 41(5):738.

Spiller HA, Thoroughman D, and Kaelin C, "Mercury Contamination in a Rural Setting," *Clin Toxicol (Phila)*, 2005, 43:719.

Tarabar AF and Su M, "Mercury and Cadmium Toxicity in a Haitian Voodoo Minister That Resulted in Acute Renal Failure," *J Toxicol Clin Toxicol*, 2003, 41(5):741.

Xue F, Holzman C, Rahbar MH, et al, "Maternal Fish Consumption Mercury Levels, and Risk of Preterm Delivery," *Environ Health Perspect*, 2007, 115:42-7

Metal Fume Fever

Related Information
- Zinc Oxide

Synonyms Brass Chills; Braz's Disease; Copper Fever; Fume Fever; Metal Shakes; Monday Morning Fever; Welding Fume Fever; Zinc Shakes

Commonly Found In Produced when inhaling metal oxides such as zinc oxide, copper, brass, cadmium, tin, iron, nickel, manganese, aluminum, antimony, arsenic, lead, silver, selenium, chromium, cobalt, magnesium; encountered with welding or torch cutting

Mechanism of Toxic Action May have a direct respiratory tract effect resulting in chemotaxis of leukocytes with pyrogen and chemotactic factor release. May be a form of hypersensitivity pneumonitis.

Adverse Reactions
Respiratory and gastrointestinal symptoms ~5 hours postexposure
Respiratory: Asthma (zinc/cobalt exposure)
Hematology: Leukocytosis

Signs and Symptoms of Overdose Usually occur 3-12 hours after exposure. Sudden onset of abdominal pain, blurred vision, dyspnea, flushing, headache, metallic taste, mild fever (<104°F or 40°C), myalgia, nausea, nonproductive cough, pleuritic chest pain, sore throat, tachypnea, sweating, thirst, vomiting; usually does not last for over 48 hours. Chest radiographs are usually normal.

Admission Criteria/Prognosis Abnormal chest x-ray, cardiopulmonary symptomatic patients not resolving 8 hours postexposure should be admitted

Toxicodynamics/Kinetics Absorption: Primary route is inhalation

Reference Range Zinc levels >2 mg/L are above normal

Overdosage/Treatment Supportive therapy: Humidified oxygen; chelation is not effective. The course is usually benign; symptoms usually resolve in 1-2 days. Antacids can be used to treat GI symptoms. Chest x-rays are unlikely to be abnormal (except with exposure to zinc oxide fumes). Leukocytosis of 12,000-16,000 cells/mm^3 is common. Glucocorticoid administration is of uncertain benefit and can be considered in patients with pulmonary infiltrates.

Diagnostic Procedures
- Heavy Metal Screen, Blood

Metaldehyde

CAS Number 108-62-3; 9002-91-9

UN Number 1332

U.S. Brand Names Halizan®; Meta-Fuel®; Metason®; Slug Death®; Slugit® Pellets

Use A molluscicide (in pellet form); snail/slug bait, heating fuel, ingredient in fire lighters

Mechanism of Toxic Action Acyclic tetramer of acetaldehyde with direct effects on neurotransmitters (ie, decreases gamma-aminobutyric acid, noradrenaline, 5-hydroxytrytamine); mucosal irritant

Adverse Reactions
Cardiovascular: Hypotension, flushing
Central nervous system: Lethargy, seizures, ataxia, coma, fever, confusion, opisthotonos, hyperthermia
Dermatologic: Pruritus
Endocrine & metabolic: Metabolic acids
Gastrointestinal: Salivation, nausea, diarrhea, abdominal pain, vomiting
Ocular: Mydriasis
Neuromuscular & skeletal: Tremors, hypertonia
Respiratory: Bronchial secretions, cough

Signs and Symptoms of Overdose Hyperthermia, mydriasis, conjunctivitis, hypotension, drowsiness, seizures, nausea, vomiting, abdominal pain, diarrhea, coma, headache, epistaxis, metabolic acidosis, thrombocytopenia, rhabdomyolysis, dermatitis, tachycardia

Toxicodynamics/Kinetics
Onset of action: Usually within 3 hours
Metabolism: Hydrolyzed in the stomach (by gastric acid) to acetaldehyde
Half-life: 27 hours

Reference Range Serum acetaldehyde level of 1 mg/dL (and urine metaldehyde level of 3 mg/dL) associated with seizures and acidosis

Overdosage/Treatment
Decontamination: Lavage (within 2 hours)/activated charcoal

Supportive therapy: Seizures should be treated with benzodiazepine, phenobarbital, or phenytoin; sodium bicarbonate for acidosis. Movement disorders can be treated with diphenhydramine (1 mg/kg up to 50 mg).
Enhancement of elimination: Diuresis or hemodialysis is not expected to be useful.

Drug Interaction May have synergistic toxic effects with ethanol

Additional Information
Tasteless white crystalline substrate; minimal lethal dose: Children: 4 g; fatal dose (oral): ~100 mg/g
Adverse reactions often related to dose ingested:
<50 mg/kg: Spasms, tachycardia, nausea
50-100 mg/kg: Ataxia, hypertonia
100-200 mg/kg: Seizures, tremor
>400 mg/kg: Coma, death
Memory loss may occur and last for several months.
Usual concentration in U.S. is <4%; but in Europe, metaldehyde concentration in molluscicides may approach 50%
Very flammable

Specific References
Shih CC, Chang SS, Chan YL, et al, "Acute Methaldehyde Poisoning in Taiwan," *Vet Hum Toxicol*, 2004, 46(3):140-3.

Methacrylates

CAS Number 80-62-6

Synonyms Methacrylate Monomer; Methyl Ester of Methacrylic Acid; Methyl Methacrylate Monomer; MMA; Monocite Methacrylate Monomer; Pegalan

Use In bone cements; artificial fingernail extender

Mechanism of Toxic Action Not well known

Adverse Reactions Moderate irritant and sensitizer, once polymerized becomes inert and nontoxic; vasodilation and transient hypotension have been reported following use as a bone cement; direct cardiotoxicity has been noted; oral ingestion can produce vomiting, GI ulceration

Signs and Symptoms of Overdose Allergic dermatitis, headache and irritability, hepatic metabolism disturbances. Occupational asthma has been associated with various methyl methacrylates.

Toxicodynamics/Kinetics Metabolism: Possible in liver and hydroxylated to an alcohol, then oxidized to aldehyde and deformulated to pyruvic acid where it enters Kreb cycle

Overdosage/Treatment
Decontamination: Lavage (within 1 hour)/activated charcoal
Supportive therapy: Parenteral nutrition for severe gastrointestinal burns

Additional Information
How supplied: Bone cement, medicinal spray adhesives, or nonirritant bandage, solvent, dental ceramic filler or cement, surgical implants; to coat contact lenses, the polymer is a constituent of plexiglass, lucite and Perspex
Monomer has an acrid odor until polymerizes; the colorless liquid form has a fruity smell; may polymerize and cause an exothermic reaction

Methane

CAS Number 74-82-8

UN Number 1971

Synonyms Fire Damp; Marsh Gas; Methyl Hydride; Natural Gas (85% Methane)

Commonly Found In Sludge digestion; produced through natural breakdown of sewage; raw material for hydrogen, ammonia, or acetylene production; found in mining industry

Mechanism of Toxic Action Asphyxiant - Displaces oxygen from the atmosphere

Adverse Reactions
Cardiovascular: Sinus tachycardia
Respiratory: Hypoxia, hyperventilation; no direct lung damage

Signs and Symptoms of Overdose Blurred or decreased vision, CNS depression, cough, tachycardia, tachypnea, unconsciousness

Overdosage/Treatment Supportive therapy: 100% humidified oxygen

Additional Information Death can occur at 75% concentration. Colorless, odorless. TLV-TWA: No limits as long as sufficient atmospheric oxygen is available. Usually when asphyxiant is 33% of atmosphere, symptoms will develop. Methane is flammable at concentrations of 5%.

Methanol

Related Information
- Donor Victims of Poisoning in Whom Transplantation of Organs Occurred

Applies to Antifreeze (Gas Line); Antifreeze (Windshield Washer); Gasoline Additive; Paint Remover

CAS Number 67-56-1

UN Number 1230

Synonyms Carbinol; Methyl Alcohol; Wood Alcohol; Wood Naphtha

Commonly Found In Industrial and household solvent

Use Fuel, paint remover; also an additive to gasoline; used in gas line antifreeze, windshield washer antifreeze

Mechanism of Toxic Action Slowly metabolized to formaldehyde and then converted rapidly to formic acid which accounts for the acidosis and ocular toxicity

Adverse Reactions

Cardiovascular: Sinus bradycardia

Central nervous system: Bilateral putaminal involvement

Endocrine & metabolic: Anion gap metabolic acidosis (lactic acidosis)

Neuromuscular & skeletal: Rhabdomyolysis

Ocular: Visual abnormalities, blindness with edematous optic disk, photophobia, optic neuropathy

Renal: Hematuria, osmolal gap

Signs and Symptoms of Overdose Symptoms may not occur for 6-30 hours. Blurred vision or diplopia progressing to blindness in ~33% of patients; bilateral basal ganglia lesions, bradycardia, coma, dementia, dyspnea, extrapyramidal symptoms, feces discoloration (black), headache, hemorrhage, hyperventilation, hypomagnesemia, hypophosphatemia, hypotension, porphyria, metabolic acidosis, myoglobinuria, nystagmus, ototoxicity, parkinsonism, paresthesia, renal failure, tinnitus, seizures, visual changes

Admission Criteria/Prognosis Any symptomatic patient, acidosis, any patient with suspected ingestion, ingestion of >4 mL of 100% methanol or peak serum methanol levels >20 mg/dL should be admitted

Toxicodynamics/Kinetics

Specific gravity: 0.79 g/mL

Absorption: Dermally (enhanced with gasoline mixtures), by inhalation (58%), and through the GI tract (~100%)

Distribution: V_d: 0.6 L/kg

Protein binding: 0%

Metabolism: Slowly in the liver by alcohol dehydrogenase to formaldehyde and then to formic acid. See figure.

Methanol Metabolism to Toxic Intermediates—Formaldehyde and Formic Acid (Formate)

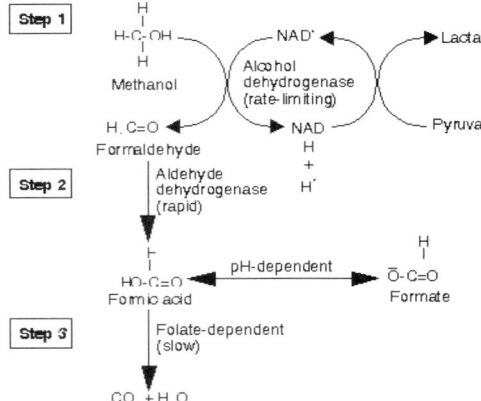

Discovery of methanol's metabolic pathway has led to several practical treatments; among them are the therapeutic administration of ethanol and folic acid. Alcohol dehydrogenase, the enzyme responsible for the first step of methanol metabolism, has an approximately nine fold greater affinity for ethanol than for methanol. Administration of ethanol blocks the oxidation of methanol, preventing the lethal synthesis of formaldehyde and formic acid and increasing the amount of methanol that is eliminated unchanged (now approximately equal amounts in urine and exhaled breath). Administration of folic acid and its analogues, which affect Step 3, enhances the conversion of toxic formic acid to carbon dioxide and water.

Adapted from Shusterman D and Osterloh JD, "Methanol Toxicity," *Case Studies in Environmental Medicine*, U.S. Department of Health and Human Services, Agency for Toxic Substances and Disease Registry, July 1992.

Peak serum concentration: Within 1 hour; found in higher concentrations in ocular and cerebrospinal fluids

Half-life, elimination: 8-28 hours (8 mg/dL/hour); with hemodialysis: 2 hours; 50 hours in the presence of ethanol

During 4-MP therapy: 54.4 hours. During 4-MP therapy and hemodialysis: 2.8 hours

Elimination: ~3% excreted unchanged renally and 12% by the lungs; ~22% of the drug is normally excreted in 4 hours

Reference Range

Blood methanol level >50 mg/dL is associated with severe toxicity; minimal lethal level without treatment: 80 mg/dL; baseline methanol level from endogenous and dietary sources: <0.15 mg/dL

Central nervous system toxicity usually appears at blood methanol level of 20 mg/dL; ocular symptoms occur at 100 mg/dL; fatality can occur at blood methanol level >150 mg/dL; serum formate level >20 mg/dL is consistent with ocular symptoms and metabolic acidosis

Endogenous serum formate concentrations: 0.6-1.6 mg/L; inhalation of methanol at concentrations of 200 ppm for 4 hours (or roughly 4 mg/kg) can result in peak serum and urine methanol levels of 6.5 mg/L and 0.9 mg every 4 hours, respectively

Overdosage/Treatment

Decontamination: Lavage (within 1 hour)/activated charcoal with cathartic in a 5:1 ratio (charcoal:methanol); higher doses of activated charcoal may be needed, but this is of unproven benefit. **Do not** induce emesis by ipecac if initiated longer than 30 minutes after ingestion.

Dermal: Wash with soap and water.

Ocular: Irrigate copiously with saline.

Supportive therapy: Treat acidosis with sodium bicarbonate (I.V.). Leucovorin calcium, 1 mg/kg up to 50 mg, followed by folic acid, 1 mg/kg up to 50 mg (every 4 hours), should be given in symptomatic patients. Folic acid, at the same dose, may be given alone in asymptomatic patients. Treat acidosis aggressively with I.V. sodium bicarbonate. Ethanol therapy should be initiated if the methanol level is >20 mg/dL, the patient has anion-gap acidosis, or other symptoms develop. 4-MP is a specific antagonist of alcohol dehydrogenase and can be used instead of ethanol therapy.

Enhancement of elimination: Hemodialysis (with ethanol) should be utilized for methanol levels >20 mg/dL or if metabolic acidosis is present, if any visual impairment is present, or if adult consumption exceeds 40 mL. Clearance of methanol by hemodialysis is estimated to be 98-176 mL/minute.

The following pototcol has been used in India to treat vision loss due to methanol

- 1 gram intravenous methylprednisolone in 500 ml of ringers lactate infused slowly over 2 hours daily for 3 days followed by oral prednisolone (40 mg) daily for 14 days. Oral steroids were tapened over 4 to 6 weeks
- Oral cyclendelate (400 mg) once daily for six weeks
- Intramuscular hydroxycobalamine (1.5 ml) once daily for one week
- Oral pentoxyphylline (400 mg) once daily for six weeks

Antidote(s)

- Alcohol, Ethyl [ANTIDOTE]
- Folic Acid [ANTIDOTE]
- Fomepizole [ANTIDOTE]
- Leucovorin [ANTIDOTE]
- Sodium Bicarbonate [ANTIDOTE]

Diagnostic Procedures

- Anion Gap, Blood
- Electrolytes, Blood
- Magnetic Resonance Scan, Brain
- Osmolality, Serum
- Osmolality, Urine

Drug Interaction Methanol poisoning and heparin can increase risk for cerebral hemorrhage

Additional Information Minimum oral lethal exposure: ~50 mL with blindness occurring at 10 mL

Methanol has one-third the intoxicating effect of ethanol; discontinue ethanol therapy if methanol level is <10 mg/dL, or acidosis or central nervous system abnormalities have resolved.

Parkinson syndrome has been described. Headaches can occur at air methanol levels in the range of 200-375 ppm.

Bilateral basal ganglion lesions along with symmetrical putamen necrosis may be noted on CT scan or MRI

Reduction of serum pH and development of acidosis may take 6-8 hours.

Contribution of a serum concentration level of 100 mg/dL to elevation of osmolar gap: 31

Dose of methanol that will saturate the folate pathway is ~210 mg/kg.

Methanol content in fruits, vegetables, and fruit juices can approach 140 mg/L; in fermented beverages it can be up to 1.5 g/L; since ~10% of ingested aspartame is converted to methanol in the intestine, a 12-ounce can of carbonated soda (containing 200 mg of aspartame) can produce ~20 mg of methanol; estimated daily methanol ingestion from noncarbonated drinks: 0.3-1.1 mg/kg

Odor threshold: 100-250 ppm. TLV-TWA: 200 ppm

Specific References

Avella J, Briglia E, Harleman G, et al. "Percutaneous Absorption and Distribution of Methanol in a Homicide," *J Anal Toxicol*, 2006, 30:162.

Bebarta V, Heard K, Delgado J, et al, "Lack of Toxicity or Significantly Elevated Formate Levels Following Inhalational Abuse of Methanol Containing Solvents," *J Toxicol Clin Toxicol*, 2003, 41(5):674.

Belson M and Morgan BW, "Methanol Toxicity in a Newborn," *J Toxicol Clin Toxicol*, 2004, 42(5):673-7.

DesLauriers C, Mazor S, Metz J, et al, "Toxic Alcohol Evaluation of Pediatric Patients is Often Incomplete," *J Toxicol Clin Toxicol*, 2004, 42(5):719.

Elwell RJ, Darouian P, Bailie GR, et al, "Delayed Absorption and Postdialysis Rebound in a Case of Acute Methanol Poisoning," *Am J Emerg Med*, 2004, 22(2):126-7.

Ernstgard L, Shibata E, and Johanson G, "Uptake and Disposition of Inhaled Methanol Vapor in Humans," *Toxicol Sci*, 2005, 88(1):30-8.

Haroz R, Salzman MS, and Greenberg MI, "Hyperammonemia: A Possible Marker for Methanol and Ethylene Glycol Intoxication," *Clin Toxicol (Phila)*, 2005, 43:689.

Hernandez MA, Holanda MS, Tejerina EE, et al, "Methanol Poisoning and Heparin: A Dangerous Couple?" *Am J Emer Med*, 2004, 22(7):620-1.

Holstege CP, Ferguson JD, Wolf CE, et al, "Analysis of Moonshine for Contaminants," *J Toxicol Clin Toxicol*, 2004, 42(5):597-601.

Hovda KE, Froyshov S, Gudmundsdottir H, et al, "Fomepizole May Change Indication for Hemodialysis in Methanol Poisoning: Prospective Study in Seven Cases," *Clin Nephrol*, 2005, 64(3):190-7.

Hovda KE, Urdal P, and Jacobsen D, "Increased Serum Formate in the Diagnosis of Methanol Poisoning," *J Anal Toxicol*, 2005, 29:586-9.

Hunduri OH, Hovda KE, Jacobsen D, "Use of the Osmolal Gap to Guide the Start and Duration of Dialysis in Methanol Poisoning," *Scandinavian Journal of Urology and Nephrology*, 2006, 40(1): 70-4.

Koga Y, Purssell RA, and Lynd LD, "The Irrationality of the Present Use of the Osmole Gap: Applicable Physical Chemistry Principles and Recommendations to Improve the Validity of Current Practices," *Toxicol Rev*, 2004, 23(3):203-11.

Kostic MA and Dart RC, "Rethinking the Toxic Methanol Level," *J Toxicol Clin Toxicol*, 2003, 41(6):793-800.

Lepik KJ, Purssell RA, Levy AR, et al, "Adverse Reactions to Ethanol Antidote for Toxic Alcohol Poisoning: A Multi-Center Retrospective Review," *Clin Toxicol (Phila)*, 2005, 43:675.

Lepik KJ, Purssell RA, Levy AR, et al, "Adverse Reactions to Hemodialysis in 72 Cases of Toxic Alcohol Poisoning," *Clin Toxicol (Phila)*, 2005, 43:676.

Levy P, Hexdall A, Gordon P, et al, "Methanol Contamination of Romanian Home-Distilled Alcohol," *J Toxicol Clin Toxicol*, 2003, 41(1):23-8.

Lushine KA, Harris CR, and Holger JS, "Methanol Ingestion: Prevention of Toxic Sequelae After Massive Ingestion," *J Emerg Med*, 2003, 24(4): 433-6.

Morgan DL, Cooney NL, Cooney DR, et al, "Recent Changes in the Treatment of Toxic Alcohol Ingestions," *Clin Toxicol (Phila)*, 2005, 43:670.

Manoj S, Imran S, Akbar S, "Intravenous Methyl Prednisolone could Salvage Vision in Methyl Alcohol Patients," *Indian J of Ophthalmology*, 2006, 54(1):68-9.

Megarbane B, Borron SW, Baud FJ, "Current Recommendations for Treatment of Severe Toxic Alcohol Poisonings," *Intensive Care Medicine*, 2005, 31(2):189-95.

Mycyk MB and Aks SE, "A Visual Schematic for Clarifying the Temporal Relationship Between the Anion and Osmol Gaps in Toxic Alcohol Poisoning," *Am J Emerg Med*, 2003, 21(4):333-5.

Mycyk MB and Leikin JB, "Antidote Review: Fomepizole for Methanol Poisoning," *Am J Ther*, 2003, 10(1):68-70.

Prinz S, Tiefenbach B, Kobow M, et al, "Formation of Methanol and Formate in Wistar Rats After Oral Administration of Methylated Rapeseed Oil: A Fuel for Lamps," *Clin Toxicol*, 2006, 44:115-9.

Purssell RA, Lynd LD, and Koga Y, "The Use of the Osmole Gap as a Screening Test for the Presence of Exogenous Substances," *Toxicol Rev*, 2004, 23(3):189-202.

Rathi M, Sakhuja V, Jha V, "Visual Blurring and Metabolic Acidosis After Ingestion of Bootlegged Alcohol," *Hemodial Int*, 2006, 10(1):8-14.

Schaeffer S, McGoodwin L, and Riley M, "Inhalation Abuse of Methanol-Containing Carburetor Cleaners," *J Toxicol Clin Toxicol*, 2003, 41(5):654.

Schier JG, Shapiro WB, Howland MA, et al, "Role of Continuous Arteriovenous Hemodialysis (CAVHD) in Methanol Poisoning," *J Toxicol Clin Toxicol*, 2003, 41(5):743.

Shiew CM, Dargan PI, Greene SL, et al, "Survey of Ethanol Assay Availability in the UK: Can We Cope with Ethylene Glycol/Methanol Poisoning?" *Clin Toxicol (Phila)*, 2005, 43:742.

Skopp G, Schmitt G, and Potsch L, "Plasma-to-Blood Ratios of Congener Analytes," *J Anal Toxicol*, 2005, 29:145-6.

Stremski E, Kostecki E, and Gummin D, "Delayed Presentation of Methanol Ingestion Leading to Cerebral Herniation and Fatality in Three of Four Severe Cases," *J Toxicol Clin Toxicol*, 2003, 41(5):643.

Suchard JR, "Intra-Subject Variability of the Baseline Serum Osmolal Gap," *Clin Toxicol (Phila)*, 2005, 43:689.

Velez LI, Kulstad E, Shepherd G, et al, "Inhalational Methanol Toxicity in Pregnancy Treated Twice with Fomepizole," *Vet Hum Toxicol*, 2003, 45(1):28-30.

Wiener SW, Ravikumar PR, Cotter B, et al, "Variability in Methanol Content Among Solid Fuel Products," *J Toxicol Clin Toxicol*, 2004, 42(5):796-7.

Methidathion

CAS Number 950-37-8

U.S. Brand Names Sumonil®; Supracide®; Ultracide®

Use Marketed as insecticide granules, dusting agent, or spray liquid with or without petroleum derivative as a solvent

Mechanism of Toxic Action Potent, irreversible inhibition of acetylcholinesterase and plasma cholinesterase, resulting in excess accumulation of acetylcholine at muscarinic and nicotinic receptors, and in the central nervous system

Adverse Reactions

Cardiovascular: **Hyperdynamic** (~18% to 21%) or hypodynamic (~7% to 10%) states, QT prolongation, sinus bradycardia, sinus tachycardia

Central nervous system: Depression, seizures, hyperactivity, cognitive dysfunction, hypothermia

Genitourinary: Urinary incontinence

Neuromuscular & skeletal: Weakness (delayed), paralysis, delayed paresthesia

Respiratory: Pulmonary edema, respiratory depression

Miscellaneous: Flu-like symptoms (especially with chronic exposure)

Signs and Symptoms of Overdose Abdominal pain, agitation, asystole, AV block, bradycardia, bronchorrhea, coma, confusion, cranial nerve palsies, decreased hemoglobin, decreased platelet count, decreased red blood cell count, diaphragmatic paralysis, dysarthria, excessive sweating, fecal and urinary incontinence, generalized asthenia, headache, heart block, hypertension, hypotension, lacrimation, metabolic acidosis and hyperglycemia (severe intoxication), miosis (unreactive to light), mydriasis (rarely), nausea, pallor, pulmonary edema, QT prolongation, respiratory depression, salivation, seizures, skeletal muscle fasciculation and flaccid paralysis, tachycardia, tachypnea, vomiting

An "intermediate syndrome" of limb asthenia and respiratory paralysis has been reported to occur between 24 and 96 hours postorganophosphate exposure, and is independent of the acute cholinergic crisis. Late paresthesia characterized by stocking and glove paresthesia, anesthesia, and asthenia is infrequently observed weeks to months following acute exposure to certain organophosphates.

Toxicodynamics/Kinetics

Absorption: Readily through oral, dermal, or respiratory exposure

Metabolism: Rapidly metabolized to weakly active compounds through hepatic hydrolysis and other pathways

Elimination: Metabolites are excreted in urine

Warnings/Precautions Risk of aspiration pneumonitis exists with agents having a hydrocarbon vehicle; severe laryngeal irritation and violent coughing may result from exposure to dusting powders; exposure to dusting powders and insecticide granules may cause contact dermatitis

Overdosage/Treatment

Decontamination: Isolation, bagging, and disposal of all contaminated clothing and other articles. All emergency medical workers and hospital staff should follow appropriate precautions regarding exposure to hazardous material including the use of protective clothing, masks, goggles, and respiratory equipment.

Oral: Activated charcoal can be administered either orally or via a nasogastric tube. **Do not** induce emesis because of danger of sudden respiratory compromise, alterations in mental status, seizures, coma, and possible aspiration of hydrocarbon vehicles. **Do not** give a cathartic.

Dermal: Prompt thorough scrubbing of all affected areas with soap and water, including hair and nails; 5% bleach can be used

Ocular: Irrigation with copious tepid sterile water or saline

Supportive therapy: Airway management, ventilatory assistance, humidified oxygen administration, and close monitoring for sudden respiratory failure

Enhancement of elimination: Dialysis and hemoperfusion are not indicated due to effectiveness of the prescribed antidotal treatment and large volumes of distribution of organophosphates.

Antidote:

Atropine: Administration should be guided by respiratory status, starting at 2-5 mg I.V. every 5-10 minutes as needed, and should be titrated to the resolution of excess pulmonary secretions. Frequent administration of large doses (cumulative doses > 100 mg) may be necessary in massive exposures.

Glycopyrrolate: May be administered if atropine is unavailable (200-400 mcg I.V. or I.M. initially, or ~$1/2$ the dose of atropine).

2-PAM: For more significant exposures (ie, exposures requiring large doses of atropine, or with recurring symptoms, or exposures to more lipid soluble agents), administration should follow: 1-2 g I.V. over 10-30 minutes, repeated in 1 hour if asthenia recurs, then every 4-12 hours for recurring symptoms.

Antidote(s)
- Atropine [ANTIDOTE]
- Pralidoxime [ANTIDOTE]

Diagnostic Procedures
- Creatinine, Serum
- Pseudocholinesterase, Serum

Drug Interaction Paralysis is potentiated by neuromuscular blockade (ie, pancuronium, vecuronium, succinylcholine, atracurium, doxacurium, mivacurium); inhibition of serum esterase prolongs the half-life of succinylcholine, cocaine, and other ester anesthetics; cholinergic toxicity is potentiated by cholinesterase inhibitors such as physostigmine

Additional Information

Red blood cell cholinesterase, and serum pseudocholinesterase may be depressed following acute or chronic organophosphate exposure; RBC cholinesterase is typically not analyzed by in-house laboratories, and is usually not available for consideration during acute management. Pseudocholinesterase levels may be rapidly available from some in-house laboratories, but are not as reliable a marker of organophosphate exposure because of variability secondary to variant genotypes, hepatic disease, oral estrogen use, or malnutrition. Because of this variability, true indication of suppression of either of these enzymes can only be estimated through comparison to pre-exposure values; these enzymes may be useful in measuring a patient's recovery postexposure, especially if the recovery is not progressing as expected.

The intermediate syndrome is not related to delayed neuropathy.

QT_c prolongation on ECG in the setting of organophosphate poisoning is associated with a high incidence of respiratory failure and mortality.

Other information concerning pesticide exposures is available through the EPA-funded National Pesticide Telecommunications Network: 1-800-858-7378 (weekdays, 8 AM to 6 PM, Central Standard time)

Methiocarb

CAS Number 2032-65-7
U.S. Brand Names Draza®; Mesurol®
Synonyms 3,5-Dimethyl-4-Methylthiophenyl N-Methylcarbamate
Use Marketed as an insecticide dusting powder or a colorless spray liquid
Mechanism of Toxic Action Reversible inhibition of acetylcholinesterase and plasma cholinesterase, resulting in excess accumulation of acetylcholine at muscarinic and nicotinic receptors, and in the central nervous system

Adverse Reactions

Cardiovascular: **Hyperdynamic** (~18% to 21%) or hypodynamic (~7% to 10%) states, QT prolongation, edema, sinus bradycardia, sinus tachycardia

Central nervous system: Toxicity is limited because carbamates do not significantly cross the blood-brain barrier; CNS changes occur with most severe intoxications, hyperactivity, cognitive dysfunction, hypothermia

Endocrine & metabolism: Hypoglycemia

Genitourinary: Urinary incontinence

Neuromuscular & skeletal: Weakness, paralysis

Ocular: Diplopia

Respiratory: Cough, respiratory depression

Miscellaneous: Flu-like symptoms (especially with chronic exposure)

Signs and Symptoms of Overdose Abdominal pain, agitation, asystole, AV block, bradycardia, bronchorrhea, coma, confusion, cranial nerve palsies, decreased hemoglobin, decreased platelet count, decreased red blood cell count, diaphragmatic paralysis, dysarthria, excessive sweating, fecal and urinary incontinence, generalized asthenia, headache, heart block, hypertension, hypotension, lacrimation, metabolic acidosis and hyperglycemia (severe intoxication), miosis (unreactive to light), mydriasis (rarely), nausea, pallor, pulmonary edema, QT prolongation, respiratory depression, salivation, seizures, skeletal muscle fasciculation and flaccid paralysis, tachycardia, tachypnea, vomiting

Toxicodynamics/Kinetics

Absorption: Readily through oral, dermal, or respiratory exposure

Metabolism: Rapidly metabolized to weakly active compounds through hepatic hydrolysis and other pathways

Elimination: Metabolites are excreted in urine

Warnings/Precautions Risk of aspiration pneumonitis exists following oral exposure to agents having a hydrocarbon vehicle; severe laryngeal irritation and violent coughing may result from exposure to dusting powders; exposure to dusting powders and insecticide granules may cause contact dermatitis

Overdosage/Treatment

Decontamination: Isolation, bagging, and disposal of all contaminated clothing and other articles. All emergency medical workers and hospital staff should follow appropriate precautions regarding exposure to hazardous material including the use of protective clothing, masks, goggles, and respiratory equipment.

Oral: Activated charcoal can be administered either orally or via a nasogastric tube. **Do not** induce emesis because of danger of sudden respiratory compromise, alterations in mental status, seizures, coma, and possible aspiration of hydrocarbon vehicles. **Do not** give a cathartic.

Dermal: Prompt thorough scrubbing of all affected areas with soap and water, including hair and nails; 5% bleach may be effective

Ocular: Irrigation with copious tepid sterile water or saline

Supportive therapy: Airway management, ventilatory assistance, humidified oxygen administration, and close monitoring for sudden respiratory failure

Antidote:

Atropine: Administration should be guided by respiratory status, starting at 2-5 mg I.V. every 5-10 minutes as needed, and should be titrated to the resolution of excess pulmonary secretions. Frequent administration of large doses (cumulative doses >100 mg) may be necessary in massive exposures.

Glycopyrrolate: May be administered if atropine is unavailable (200-400 mcg I.V. or I.M. initially, or ~$^1/_2$ the dose of atropine).

2-PAM: Although not specifically indicated, 2-PAM may be considered in the following situations:

Life-threatening symptoms such as respiratory paralysis

Continued excessive atropine requirements

Concomitant organophosphate and carbamate exposure

Enhancement of elimination: Dialysis and hemoperfusion are not indicated due to effectiveness of the prescribed antidotal treatment and large volumes of distribution of carbamates

Antidote(s)

● Atropine [ANTIDOTE]

Diagnostic Procedures

● Creatinine, Serum

● Pseudocholinesterase, Serum

Drug Interaction Paralysis is potentiated by neuromuscular blockade (ie, pancuronium, vecuronium, succinylcholine, atracurium, doxacurium, mivacurium); inhibition of serum esterase prolongs the half-life of succinylcholine, cocaine, and other ester anesthetics; cholinergic toxicity is potentiated by cholinesterase inhibitors such as physostigmine

Additional Information

Red blood cell cholinesterase, and serum pseudocholinesterase may be depressed following acute or chronic organophosphate exposure and are theoretically useful for differentiating between carbamate and organophosphate exposures; RBC cholinesterase is typically not analyzed by in-house laboratories, and is usually not available for consideration during acute management. Pseudocholinesterase levels may be rapidly available from some in-house laboratories, but are not as reliable a marker of organophosphate exposure because of variability secondary to variant genotypes, hepatic disease, oral estrogen use, or malnutrition, thus they may not be useful in ruling out carbamate exposure.

The intermediate syndrome is not related to delayed neuropathy.

QT_c prolongation on ECG in the setting of organophosphate poisoning is associated with a high incidence of respiratory failure and mortality.

Other information concerning pesticide exposures is available through the EPA-funded National Pesticide Telecommunications Network: 1-800-858-7378 (weekdays, 8 AM to 6 PM, Central Standard time)

Methomyl

CAS Number 16752-77-5
U.S. Brand Names Lannate®; Lanox®; Nudrin®
Use Marketed as an insecticide dusting agent
Mechanism of Toxic Action Potent, reversible inhibition of acetylcholinesterase and plasma cholinesterase, resulting in excess accumulation of acetylcholine at muscarinic and nicotinic receptors, and in the central nervous system

Adverse Reactions

Cardiovascular: **Hyperdynamic** (~18% to 21%) or hypodynamic (~7% to 10%) states, QT prolongation, sinus bradycardia, sinus tachycardia

Central nervous system: Toxicity is limited because carbamates do not significantly cross the blood-brain barrier; CNS changes occur with most severe intoxications, paresthesia, hyperactivity, cognitive dysfunction, hypothermia

Genitourinary: Urinary incontinence

Neuromuscular & skeletal: Weakness, paralysis

Respiratory: Pulmonary edema, respiratory depression

Miscellaneous: Flu-like symptoms (especially with chronic exposure)

Signs and Symptoms of Overdose Abdominal pain, agitation, asystole, AV block, bradycardia, bronchorrhea, coma, confusion, cranial nerve palsies, decreased hemoglobin, decreased platelet count, decreased red blood cell count, diaphragmatic paralysis, dysarthria, excessive sweating, fecal and urinary incontinence, generalized asthenia, headache, heart block, hypertension, hypotension, lacrimation, metabolic acidosis and hyperglycemia (severe intoxication), miosis (unreactive to light), mydriasis (rarely), nausea, pallor, pulmonary edema, QT prolongation, respiratory depression, salivation, seizures, skeletal muscle fasciculation and flaccid paralysis, tachycardia, tachypnea, vomiting

An "intermediate syndrome" of limb asthenia and respiratory paralysis has been reported to occur between 24 and 96 hours postorganophosphate exposure, and is independent of the acute cholinergic crisis. Late paresthesia characterized by stocking and glove paresthesia, anesthesia, and asthenia is infrequently observed weeks to months following acute exposure to certain organophosphates.

Toxicodynamics/Kinetics

Absorption: Readily through oral, dermal, or respiratory exposure

Metabolism: Rapidly metabolized to weakly active compounds through hepatic hydrolysis and other pathways

Elimination: Metabolites are excreted in urine

Warnings/Precautions Severe laryngeal irritation and violent coughing may result from exposure to dusting powders; exposure to dusting powders and insecticide granules may cause contact dermatitis

Overdosage/Treatment

Decontamination: Isolation, bagging, and disposal of all contaminated clothing and other articles. All emergency medical workers and hospital staff should follow appropriate precautions regarding exposure to hazardous material including the use of protective clothing, masks, goggles, and respiratory equipment.

Oral: Activated charcoal can be administered either orally or via a nasogastric tube. **Do not** induce emesis because of danger of sudden respiratory compromise, alterations in mental status, seizures, coma, and possible aspiration of hydrocarbon vehicles. **Do not** give a cathartic.

Dermal: Prompt thorough scrubbing of all affected areas with soap and water, including hair and nails; 5% bleach can be used

Ocular: Irrigation with copious tepid sterile water or saline

Supportive therapy: Airway management, ventilatory assistance, humidified oxygen administration, and close monitoring for sudden respiratory failure

Antidote:

Atropine: Administration should be guided by respiratory status, starting at 2-5 mg I.V. every 5-10 minutes as needed, and should be titrated to the resolution of excess pulmonary secretions. Frequent administration of large doses (cumulative doses >100 mg) may be necessary in massive exposures.

Glycopyrrolate: May be administered if atropine is unavailable (200-400 mcg I.M. or I.V. initially, or ~$1/2$ the dose of atropine).

2-PAM: Although not specifically indicated, 2-PAM may be considered in the following situations:

Life-threatening symptoms such as respiratory paralysis

Continued excessive atropine requirements especially nicotinic symptoms

Concomitant organophosphate and carbamate exposure

Enhancement of elimination: Dialysis and hemoperfusion are not indicated due to effectiveness of the prescribed antidotal treatment and large volumes of distribution of carbamates.

Antidote(s)
- Atropine [ANTIDOTE]

Diagnostic Procedures
- Creatinine, Serum
- Pseudocholinesterase, Serum

Drug Interaction Paralysis is potentiated by neuromuscular blockade (ie, pancuronium, vecuronium, succinylcholine, atracurium, doxacurium, mivacurium); inhibition of serum esterase prolongs the half-life of succinylcholine, cocaine, and other ester anesthetics; cholinergic toxicity is potentiated by cholinesterase inhibitors such as physostigmine

Additional Information

Red blood cell cholinesterase, and serum pseudocholinesterase may be depressed following acute or chronic organophosphate exposure; RBC cholinesterase is typically not analyzed by in-house laboratories, and is usually not available for consideration during acute management. Pseudocholinesterase levels may be rapidly available from some in-house laboratories, but are not as reliable a marker of organophosphate exposure because of variability secondary to variant genotypes, hepatic disease, oral estrogen use, or malnutrition, thus they may not be useful in ruling out carbamate exposure.

The intermediate syndrome is not related to delayed neuropathy.

QT_c prolongation on ECG in the setting of organophosphate poisoning is associated with a high incidence of respiratory failure and mortality.

Possesses a slight sulfur odor

Thermal breakdown products include nitrogen oxides and sulfur oxides.

ACGIH TLV: 2.5 mg/m³; PEL-TWA: 2.5 mg/m³

Vapor pressure: 0.00005 mm Hg at 20°C

Other information concerning pesticide exposures is available through the EPA-funded National Pesticide Telecommunications Network: 1-800-858-7378 (weekdays, 8 AM to 6 PM, Central Standard time)

Specific References

Tsai MJ, Wu SN, Cheng HA, et al, "An Outbreak of Food-Borne Illness Due to Methomyl Contamination," *J Toxicol Clin Toxicol*, 2003, 41(7):969-73.

Methoxychlor

CAS Number 72-43-5

UN Number 2761

U.S. Brand Names Marlate®; Methoxcide®; Metox®; Metron®; Prentox®

Synonyms DMDT; Methoxy-DDT

Use Essentially has replaced DDT (dichlorodiphenyltrichloroethane); methoxychlor is an effective insecticide used on crops, stored grain, livestock, pets, garbage containers, and sewage areas; also used in aerial operations regarding mosquito abatement

Mechanism of Toxic Action Metabolites of methoxychlor essentially act as estrogen analogues; also may deactivate the sodium channel after neuronal activation thus leading to neuronal hyperexcitability

Adverse Reactions While no systemic adverse effects have been attributed solely to methoxychlor to date, the central nervous system and reproductive system (as an estrogen analogue) have been target organs in animal studies

Toxicodynamics/Kinetics

Metabolism: Hepatic demethylation to metabolites conjugated to glucuronic acid

Elimination: Primarily fecal

Reference Range Serum methoxychlor level of 0.67 mcg/mL associated with hypotension in a suicide attempt.

Overdosage/Treatment

Decontamination: **Oral:** Lavage (within 1 hour)/activated charcoal; **do not** use oil-based cathartics in that increased absorption of methoxychlor may result. **Dermal:** Remove contaminated clothing; wash with soap and water. **Ocular:** Copious irrigation with saline

Supportive therapy: Benzodiazepines or phenobarbital can be used for seizure control.

Enhancement of elimination: Due to its high lipid solubility and low rate of enterohepatic recirculation (5% to 10%), multiple dosing of activated charcoal is not expected to be effective.

Additional Information

Lethal oral dose of methoxychlor is ~6400 mg/kg

No adverse effects noted in human volunteers ingesting 2 mg/kg/day for 8 weeks

Average daily intake is estimated to be from 0.15 mcg in infants to 0.28 mcg in adults.

TLV-TWA: 10 mg/m². Odor threshold in water: 4.7 ppm (fruity).

Half-life: Atmospheric: 1-11 hours. Water: 1 year. Soil: 30-100 days.

Methyl Bromide

Applies to Fire Extinguishers; Fumigant (Insects)

CAS Number 74-83-9

UN Number 1062

U.S. Brand Names Embafume®; Terabol®

Synonyms Bercema; Bromomethane; Monobromomethane

Use Degreasing wool, extracting oils, insect fumigant, fire extinguishers

Mechanism of Toxic Action Intense vesicant; alkylating agent/sulfhydryl enzyme inhibitors

Adverse Reactions

Cardiovascular: Myocardial irritability, Reye's-like syndrome, hypotension

Central nervous system: CNS depression, extrapyramidal signs, cerebellar ataxia, headache, confusion, seizures, psychosis, amnesia

Dermatologic: Skin necrosis, blister

Hepatic: Liver injury, hepatomegaly, centrilobular necrosis

Neuromuscular & skeletal: tremors, axonopathy, myoclonus

Ocular: Blurred vision, diplopia, mydriasis

Renal: Nephritis, oliguria, albuminuria

Respiratory: Pulmonary edema, pulmonary hemorrhage

Miscellaneous: Potentially carcinogenic

Signs and Symptoms of Overdose Acetone breath, anorexia, coma, dermal burns, distal neuritis, dizziness, drowsiness, dyspnea, focusing difficulty, headache, hyperthermia, hyposmia, loss of ankle reflexes, myoclonus, nausea, nystagmus, seizures, vomiting

Admission Criteria/Prognosis Symptomatic patients 12 hours post-exposure should be admitted; while survival after 3 days is usually associated with recovery, central nervous system abnormalities may persist for months

Toxicodynamics/Kinetics

Absorption: By inhalation or through the skin

Metabolism: Hepatic, metabolites to methanol and bromide ion

Half-life: Probably <1 hour

Reference Range Serum bromide levels >5 mg/100 mL require worker removal from the contaminated environment; levels >15 mg/100 mL are associated with toxicity. Serum bromide level of 27 mg/dL and urine bromide level of 6.2 mg/dL were related to fatality.

Overdosage/Treatment

Decontamination: Basic poison management; **do not** induce vomiting; dilute with 4-8 oz of milk or water. For inhalation, give 100% humidified oxygen.

Supportive therapy: Benzodiazepines or phenobarbital can be used for seizure control, if seizures are unresponsive to these agents, thiopental anesthesia should be considered. Use of N-acetylcysteine for dermal exposure to "chelate" unbound methyl bromide is experimental and may worsen clinical effects. Fosphenytoin can be used to treat seizures, vasopressors such as dopamine and phenylephrine can also be used.

Enhancement of elimination: Hemodialysis can increase clearance of bromide.

Antidote(s)
- Dimercaprol [ANTIDOTE]

Additional Information Permanent neurological sequelae include depression, paralysis, ataxia, myoclonus. Colorless, odorless gas; burning taste. Readily penetrates leather. Average daily inhalation dose in U.S. urban areas: 4.5-24.5 mcg/adult. TLV-TWA: 5 ppm; IDLH: 250 ppm; PEL-TWA: 5 ppm

Methyl Ethyl Ketone

Applies to Aluminum Foil (Manufacture); Drugs of Abuse (Production); Solvent; Synthetic Leather (Manufacture)

CAS Number 78-93-3

UN Number 1193; 1232

U.S. Brand Names Meetco®

Synonyms 2-Butanone; 2-Oxobutane; Ethyl Methyl Ketone; MEK; Methyl Acetone

Use In production of drugs of abuse; used as a solvent for coatings, adhesives, magnetic tapes, printing inks, paint remover, vinyl films, polystyrene, polyurethane; also used in manufacture of aluminum foil and synthetic leather

Mechanism of Toxic Action Mucosal irritant and central nervous system depressant

Adverse Reactions
Cardiovascular: Hypotension, tachycardia
Central nervous system: Headache at 300 ppm; coma, dizziness, fatigue, panic attacks
Dermatologic: Urticaria, immunologic contact urticaria
Endocrine & metabolic: Metabolic acidosis, hyperglycemia
Hematologic: Methemoglobinemia
Gastrointestinal: Nausea
Neuromuscular & skeletal: Paresthesia
Ocular: Eye irritant at 200 ppm; can cause conjunctival irritation, mydriasis
Respiratory: Irritant at 100 ppm; hyperventilation

Toxicodynamics/Kinetics
Absorption: Inhalation: 41% to 56%
Protein binding: 0%
Metabolism: Hepatic to 3-hydroxy-2-butanone and 2,3-butanediol
Half-life: 49-96 minutes
Elimination: Lungs

Reference Range Plasma 2-butanone level of 95 mg/100 mL consistent with coma in an oral ingestion

Overdosage/Treatment
Decontamination: **Do not** use ipecac. Lavage (preferably with a cuffed endotracheal tube in place to prevent aspiration) for large ingestions within 2 hours; activated charcoal may be useful.
Supportive therapy: Sodium bicarbonate for acidosis

Additional Information Colorless liquid with acetone odor. Odor threshold: <10 ppm. OSHA-PEL: 200 ppm. OSHA-STEL: 300 ppm. BEI: 2 mg MEK/L.

Methyl Ethyl Ketone Peroxide

Applies to Curing Agent for Plastics and Fiberglass Resins; Hardener for Plastics and Fiberglass Resins

CAS Number 1338-23-4

UN Number 2550

Synonyms 2-Butanone Peroxide; MEK Peroxide; MEKP

Use As a hardener and curing agent for plastics and fiberglass resins

Mechanism of Toxic Action Free radical formation with lipid peroxidation; caustic agent which can also cause glutathione depletion; a strong oxidizer

Adverse Reactions
Cardiovascular: Myocarditis
Central nervous system: Coma
Dermatologic: Eczema
Gastrointestinal: Vomiting
Hematologic: Coagulopathy, leukocytosis
Ocular: Irritation (at concentrations >3%)
Respiratory: Pneumonitis, stridor

Admission Criteria/Prognosis Admit any ingestion >10 mL

Overdosage/Treatment
Decontamination: **Oral**: Avoid emesis or lavage. **Dermal**: Irrigate with soap and water. **Ocular**: Irrigate with copious amounts of saline
Supportive therapy: Early upper gastrointestinal endoscopy is suggested but not studied
Acetylcysteine at I.V. doses of 140 mg/kg loading followed by 70 mg/kg every 4 hours for 12 doses may be hepatoprotective

Additional Information Ingestion of >50 mL is toxic. A colorless liquid with an acetone-like odor, often available in a 40% to 60% solution with dimethyl phthalate; often stored in refrigerators

Specific References
Maloney GE, Pallasch EM, Ahkter S, et al, "Methyl Ethyl Ketone Peroxide Ingestion in a Toddler Treated with N-Acetylcysteine," *Clin Toxicol (Phila)*, 2005, 43:658.

Methyl Isocyanate

Related Information
- Methylene Diisocyanate
- Toluene Diisocyanate

CAS Number 624-83-9

UN Number 2480

Synonyms Isocyanate; Isocyanatomethane; MIC

Use Intermediate agent in the production of carbaryl (Sevin®, a carbamate pesticide) and herbicides. Etiologic agent of inadvertent release in 1984 in Bhopal, India.

Mechanism of Toxic Action Mucosal irritant; reacts with water to form exothermic reaction; hydrolyzes to form methylamine and CO_2. MIC is a more potent irritant than other forms of isocyanates. May also result in an allergic response.

Adverse Reactions
Cardiovascular: Chest pain, angina
Central nervous system: Fatigue, vertigo, ataxia, anxiety
Dermal: Erythema, edema
Gastrointestinal: Vomiting, throat irritation
Ocular: Burning eyes, lacrimation, blepharospasm, photophobia, corneal ulceration, punctate keratopathy, lid edema, corneal irritation may persist for one year postexposure
Neuromuscular & skeletal: Muscle weakness, tremor
Renal: Acidosis (renal tubular)
Respiratory: Cough, dyspnea, bronchospasm (persists for 3-7 days), wheezing, interstitial edema, bronchiolitis

Toxicodynamics/Kinetics Absorption: By inhalation and dermal routes

Reference Range Leukocytosis, lymphocytosis and elevated erythrocyte sedimentation rate noted; blood carboxyhemoglobin, methemoglobin, and thiocyanate levels may be high, but this may be due to contaminants

Overdosage/Treatment
Decontamination:
Inhalation: Give 100% humidified oxygen.
Ocular: Remove contact lenses; irrigation with copious amount of water or saline
Supportive therapy: Beta agonist agents with theophylline may be helpful; steroids (prednisone or high-dose inhaled beclomethasone) may be useful. Thiosulfate does not appear to be helpful and cyanide antidotal therapy should not be utilized. Inverse-ratio ventilation using lower tidal volume mechanical ventilation (6 mL/kg) and plateau pressures of 30 cm water may decrease mortality. While positive end expiratory pressures should be considered, oxygen toxicity should be monitored. Use of perfluorocarbon partial liquid ventilation and exogenous surfactant in chemical-induced ARDS is investigational.
Experience after Bhopal, India 1984 exposure of 865 pregnancies revealed that 43% did not result in a live birth and an infant death rate of 14%. MIC can cross placental barrier; skeletal malformations noted in rodent studies.

Additional Information
Mucous membrane irritant threshold: 0.2 ppm. Unbearable exposure: 21 ppm; respiratory response is likely at an air concentration of >0.5 ppm
Very flammable. TLV-TWA: 0.02 ppm. Odor threshold: 2 ppm
Toxic agent responsible for 3,828 deaths in December 1984 in Bhopal, India
Pyrolysis decomposition products include hydrogen cyanide and carbon dioxide; MDI is more toxic when heated
Involved in the recall of >8 billion cigarettes by the Philip Morris Co in May 1995 due to contaminated plasticizer compound in the cigarette filter

Specific References
Ranjan N, Sarangi S, Padmanabhan VT, et al, "Methyl Isocyanate Exposure and Growth Patterns of Adolescents in Bhopal," *JAMA*, 2003, 290(14):1856-7.

Methyl Mercaptan

Applies to Jet Fuel; Odorless Hazardous Gases (Agent to Add Odor); Pesticides; Plastics

CAS Number 74-93-1

UN Number 1064

Synonyms Methanethiol; Thiomethanol; Thiomethyl Alcohol

Use Production of jet fuel, pesticides, and plastics; used as an agent to add odor to odorless hazardous gases (not natural gas)

Mechanism of Toxic Action Can cause oxidative stress to red blood cell membranes (especially in patients with glucose-6-phosphate dehydrogenase deficiency) thus resulting in hemolysis

Adverse Reactions
Cardiovascular: Tachycardia, hypertension, sinus tachycardia
Central nervous system: Seizures, coma, headache, dizziness
Hematologic: Hemolytic anemia, methemoglobinemia, anemia
Ocular: Eye irritation
Renal: Diuresis
Miscellaneous: Mucosal irritation

Admission Criteria/Prognosis Any patient with change in mental status, cardiopulmonary complaints, or methemoglobin levels >30% should be admitted; asymptomatic patients with methemoglobin levels <30% may be considered for discharge after 6 hours of observation and if methemoglobin levels fall to <15%

Toxicodynamics/Kinetics

Absorption: By inhalation

Metabolism: To dimethyl sulfide

Elimination: Primarily by lungs

Overdosage/Treatment

Decontamination: **Dermal:** Wash with soap and water. **Inhalation:** Give 100% humidified oxygen. **Ocular:** Irrigate copiously with saline.

Supportive therapy: Treat symptomatic methemoglobinemia with methylene blue (monitor closely in G6PD-deficient patients). Promote an alkaline diuresis to avoid adverse renal effects of hemolysis. Diazepam or lorazepam can be initially used to treat seizures. Refractory seizures can be treated with phenytoin or phenobarbital. Hypertensive emergencies can be treated with nitroprusside (0.1-5 mcg/kg/minute up to 10 mcg/kg/minute). Labetalol or hydralazine can be used for hypertensive urgencies.

Antidote(s)

● Methylene Blue [ANTIDOTE]

Diagnostic Procedures

● Methemoglobin, Blood

Additional Information Flammable gas which can be explosive; a reduced sulfur gas from pulp air emissions. Gas specific gravity: 1.66. Very soluble in water. Odor threshold: 1.6 ppb (rotten cabbage). TLV-TWA: 0.5 ppm; IDLH: 400 ppm. Atmospheric half-life: 0.2-30 hours

Methyl Tert-Butyl Ether

Related Information

● Gasoline

CAS Number 1634-04-4

UN Number 2398

Synonyms MBE; MTBE; Tert-Butyl Methyl Ether

Use Reformulated gasoline; pharmaceutical agent to dissolve gallstones through an intraductal route via a thistle catheter; to increase octane (up to 15%) and reduce levels of carbon monoxide emissions; oxygenate agent in motor gasoline

Investigational: Cholesterol gallstones

Mechanism of Toxic Action Lipophilic, volatile solvent which acts as a central nervous system depressant (through changes in neuronal membrane fluidity)

Adverse Reactions

Central nervous system: Headache, dizziness, sedation, ataxia, coma

Gastrointestinal: Nausea, vomiting

Hematologic: Hemolysis

Ocular: Eye irritation, lacrimation

Respiratory: Coughing, nasal irritation

Admission Criteria/Prognosis Patients who develop tachypnea, cyanosis, dyspnea, CNS depression, tachycardia, or fever within 8 hours of exposure should be admitted; asymptomatic patients can be discharged after 8 hours observation

Toxicodynamics/Kinetics

Absorption: Inhalation (2.4%), orally, and dermally

Metabolism: Hepatic to tert-butanol, formaldehyde, methanol, and carbon dioxide

Half-life (rodents): 1-2 hours

Elimination: Lungs, feces, and urine

Monitoring Parameters Liver function tests, chest x-ray

Reference Range

Median blood levels of MTBE: Commuters: 0.1 mcg/L; Car repairers: 2.0 mcg/L (tert-butanol: 15 mcg/L); Gas station attendants: 15.0 mcg/L (tert-butanol: 75 mcg/L)

Healthy volunteers exposed for 1 hour at 1.7 ppm: 17.0 mcg/L

After intracystic administration, mean tert-butanol blood levels were 0.04 mg/mL and 0.02-0.03 mg/mL in urine

Overdosage/Treatment

Decontamination: **Oral:Do not** induce emesis. Activated charcoal is not recommended since it is poorly absorbed to activated charcoal; dilute with milk or water. **Dermal:** Wash with soap and water. **Ocular:** Copious irrigation with saline. **Inhalation:** 100% humidified oxygen

Not genotoxic; no specific toxicity to reproduction and development

Additional Information

Intraductal dose of MTBE for treatment of gallstones: 1-15 mL (up to 140 mL) instilled 3-6 times/minute and then reaspirated.

Methanol is only detected in trace amounts and is not considered to be a major problem.

Odor threshold in water: 680 ppb. Atmospheric lifetime: 4 days. Ambient water level of MTBE: 15-81 mcg/L. Median level of MTBE in snow samples (near Denver): 0.05 mcg/L. Workplace environmental exposure level (8-hour weighted average): 100 ppm

Maximum permissible concentration of MTBE in Europe: 15%

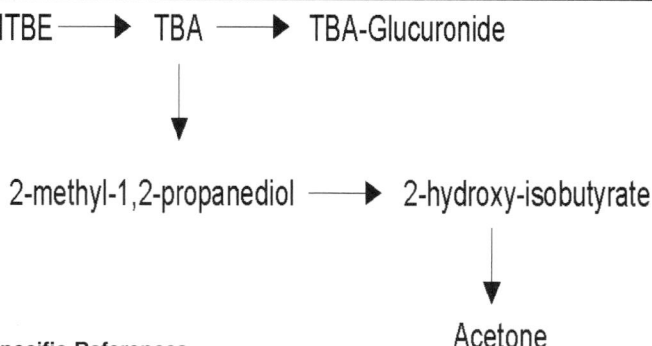

Specific References

McGregor D, "Methyl Tertiary-Butyl Ether: Studies for Potential Human Health Hazards," *Crit Rev Toxicol*, 2006, 36:319-58.

Methylene Chloride

CAS Number 75-09-2

UN Number 1593

Synonyms Dichloromethane; Freon 30; Methane Dichloride

Commonly Found In Paint and varnish removers, fire extinguishers, and fumigants

Mechanism of Toxic Action Solvent-induced depression/carbon monoxide effects

Adverse Reactions

Central nervous system: Anesthesia, headache (5000 ppm), decreased hearing (300 ppm), syncope, memory disturbance, chest pain, lightheadedness (500 ppm), hyperthermia, erythema (mild burns), dry scaling, dyspnea, lethargy, seizures, fatigue, corneal vorns, nausea, vomiting

Renal: Tubular necrosis (acute)

Signs and Symptoms of Overdose Dermal burns, dizziness, dyspnea, encephalopathy, eye irritation, lightheadedness, skin irritation, tremor

Admission Criteria/Prognosis Oral ingestions >0.5 mL/kg, carboxyhemoglobin level >5% in nonsmokers, or symptomatic patients should be admitted

Toxicodynamics/Kinetics

Absorption: Inhalation (70% to 75%), oral (98% within 20 minutes), and dermal

Metabolism: Converted hepatically to carbon monoxide (30%) and carbon dioxide (70%)

Half-life: 40 minutes

Elimination: Primarily pulmonary (carbon monoxide/carbon dioxide)

Monitoring Parameters Laboratory data for surveillance would include complete blood count, liver function tests, post-shift carboxyhemoglobin, pulmonary function testing, and electrocardiogram

Reference Range

Blood levels of 2 mg/L correlate with exposure of 200 ppm; carboxyhemoglobin levels in nonsmokers are usually in the range of 8% to 20% postexposure

Fatal methylene chloride urine levels range from 2-160 mg/L

Overdosage/Treatment

Decontamination: Basic poison management. Dermal/occular: Irrigate with copious amounts of saline or water

Supportive therapy: 100% humidified oxygen; hyperbaric oxygen has been advocated for patients with neurological abnormalities; monitor carboxyhemoglobin levels

Diagnostic Procedures

● Carboxyhemoglobin, Blood

Additional Information Minimum lethal oral dose: 0.5-5.0 mL/kg; acute oral lethal dose: 375 mg/kg; acute air concentration exposure for lethality: 50,000 ppm

Colorless fluid, pleasant odor; not flammable or explosive

Adverse health effects on newborns may occur at methylene chloride levels of >565 mg/L in drinking water.

Mean concentrations in drinking water: Usually <1 mcg/L. Odor threshold (sweet): Water: 9.1 ppm; air: 160-620 ppm. Atmospheric half-life: 100-500 days. TLV-TWA: 50 ppm; IDLH: 5000 ppm; PEL-TWA: 500 ppm

Ambient atmospheric concentrations of methylene chloride in U.S. urban areas range from 0.8-6.7 ppt; in rural/suburban areas, the range is from 0.18-2.1 ppt. Hair spray can cause levels as high as 50 ppm (TWA: 0.17 ppm) of methylene chloride.

Upon heating of methylene chloride to decomposition, phosgene gas may be liberated.

Specific References

Hoffer E, Tabak A, Scherb I, et al, "Monitoring of Occupational Exposure to Methylene Chloride: Sampling Protocol and Stability of Urine Samples," *J Anal Toxicol*, 2005, 29(8):794-8.

Methylene Dianiline

Applies to Corrosive Inhibitor; Hardening Agent (Epoxy Resin); Polyurethane (Curing Agent); Polyurethane Foam (Production)

CAS Number 101-77-9

UN Number 2651

U.S. Brand Names Ancamine TL; Epicure DDM; Tonox

Synonyms 4,4-Methylene Dianiline; DDM; MDA

Use Curing agent for polyurethane; corrosive inhibitor; used in preparation of A_{30} dyes; production of 4-4'-methenedianiline diisocyanate and other polymeric isocyanates which are used in polyurethane foam, isocyanate resins and elastomer; also used in production of epoxy-resin hardening agents

Mechanism of Toxic Action Contact allergen, hepatotoxin; possibly carcinogenic in humans (urinary tract)

Adverse Reactions

Central nervous system: Psychosis

Dermatologic: Erythema multiforme

Hematologic: Eosinophilia

Hepatic: Toxic hepatitis ("Epping jaundice"), cholestasis

Ocular: Optic neuritis

Respiratory: Bronchoconstriction

Signs and Symptoms of Overdose Dyspnea, epigastric pain, hepatomegaly, jaundice, myalgia, nausea, ocular irritation, visual dysfunction; yellow discoloration of skin, fingernails, and hair

Toxicodynamics/Kinetics

Absorption: Dermal (13%), inhalation and oral

Metabolism: Hepatic oxidation to N-hydroxymethylenedianiline

Half-life: 9-19 hours

Elimination: Renal (primarily) and feces

Reference Range Can be measured in urine to a detection level of 2 mcg/L

Overdosage/Treatment

Decontamination: **Oral:** Ipecac or lavage within 1 hour; activated charcoal. **Dermal:** Flush with soap and water. **Ocular:** Irrigate with saline.

Supportive therapy: Beta agonists (nebulized) can be utilized for bronchoconstriction.

Additional Information Faint amine-like odor; irritating at levels of 1 ppm. Specific gravity: 1.1; not volatile in water. Atmospheric half-life: 1.6 hours. TLV-TWA: 0.1 ppm. Causative agent in "epping jaundice" due to flour contamination in Epping, England in 1965.

Specific References

Stout PR, Horn CK, and Klette KL, "Rapid Simultaneous Determination of Amphetamine (AMP); Methamphetamine; 3,4-Methylenedioxyamphetamine (MDA); 3,4-Methylenedioxymethamphetamine (MDMA); and 3,4-Methylenedioxyethylamphetamine (MDEA) in Urine by Solid-Phase Extraction and GC-MS: A Method Optimized for High-Volume Laboratories," *J Anal Toxicol*, 2003, 27:190.

Methylene Diisocyanate

Related Information

• Methyl Isocyanate

• Toluene Diisocyanate

CAS Number 101-68-8

UN Number 2487; 2489

Synonyms MDI; Methylene Bisphenyl Isocyanate

Use Production of rigid polyurethane foams and plastics

Mechanism of Toxic Action A respiratory irritant and pulmonary sensitizer

Adverse Reactions Respiratory: Asthma, reactive airways dysfunction syndrome

Signs and Symptoms of Overdose Abdominal pain, bronchospasm, chest pain, conjunctivitis, cough, dyspnea, eye irritation, headache, vomiting

Overdosage/Treatment

Decontamination: **Oral:** Do **not** induce emesis; dilute with milk or water. **Dermal:** Wash with soap and water. **Inhalation:** Administer 100% humidified oxygen. **Ocular:** Irrigate with copious amounts of saline.

Supportive therapy: Bronchodilators can be used for bronchospasm.

Additional Information Light yellow to white crystals. Specific gravity: 1.19. TLV-TWA: 0.005 ppm; IDLH: 10 ppm. Magna Dry Incorporated, Henison, MI 42428 (616) 457-6664 can be contacted regarding emergency information of MDI.

Methylparathion

CAS Number 298-00-0

UN Number 3017

U.S. Brand Names A-Gro®; Azofos®; Bladan-M®; Dalf®; E601®, ME-Parathion®; Metapon®; Nitrox®; Penncap-M®; Wofatox®

Synonyms Cotton Poison

Use Insecticide which is applied to crops, cotton, soybeans, and fruit trees; approved for outdoor use only. See tables.

Incidents of Illegal Domestic Indoor Use of Methyl Parathion			
Year	Location	Number of Residences Involved	Estimated Cost of Clean-up
1984	Tunica, Mississippi	1*	—
1994	Lorain County, Ohio	232	$20 million
1995	Detroit, Michigan	4	$1 million
1996	Jackson County, Mississippi	2600	$50 million
1997	Cook County, Illinois	680	$20 million
1997	Texas City, Texas	7	—

* Two deaths (children)

Action Level for Residential Relocation	
Age (years)	Urinary Methylparathion Level (parts per billion)
0-1 (and pregnant women)	>50
1-16	>300
>16	>600

All urine levels are creatinine adjusted.

Relocation rate in previous episodes ranges from 4% to 12%.

From Environmental Protection Agency, 1997.

Mechanism of Toxic Action Potent, irreversible inhibition of acetylcholinesterase and plasma cholinesterase, resulting in excess accumulation of acetylcholine at muscarinic and nicotinic receptors, and in the central nervous system; this is in the class of a phosphorthioate organophosphate; high lipid solubility which can result in delayed toxicity

Adverse Reactions

Cardiovascular: **Hyperdynamic** (~18% to 21%) or hypodynamic (~7% to 10%) states, QT prolongation, AV block

Central nervous system: Depression, seizures, hyperactivity, cognitive dysfunction, hypothermia

Endocrine & metabolic: Hypoglycemia

Genitourinary: Urinary incontinence

Neuromuscular & skeletal: Weakness (delayed), paralysis, delayed paresthesia, rhabdomyolysis

Ocular: Ptosis

Respiratory: Pulmonary edema, respiratory depression

Miscellaneous: Flu-like symptoms (especially with chronic exposure), intermediate syndrome

Admission Criteria/Prognosis Any symptomatic patient or an asymptomatic patient following a severe exposure should be admitted probably into an intensive care unit; asymptomatic patients following a moderate exposure can be discharged after 8 hours of observation

Toxicodynamics/Kinetics

Absorption: Inhalation, oral, and dermal routes

Metabolism: Enzymatic hydrolysis to dimethylphosphoric acid and 4-nitrophenol

Elimination: Renal

Reference Range

Mild poisoning: Serum cholinesterase is 20% to 50% of normal

Moderate poisoning: Serum cholinesterase is 10% to 20% of normal

Severe poisoning (respiratory distress and coma): Serum cholinesterase is <10%

Overdosage/Treatment

Decontamination: Isolation, bagging, and disposal of all contaminated clothing and other articles. All emergency medical workers and hospital staff should follow appropriate precautions regarding exposure to hazardous material including the use of protective clothing, masks, goggles, and respiratory equipment.

Oral: Activated charcoal can be administered either orally or via a nasogastric tube. **Do not** induce emesis because of danger of sudden respiratory compromise, alterations in mental status, seizures, coma, and possible aspiration of hydrocarbon vehicles.

Dermal: Prompt thorough scrubbing of all affected areas with soap and water, including hair and nails; 5% bleach can also be used

Ocular: Irrigation with copious tepid sterile water or saline

Supportive therapy: Airway management, ventilatory assistance, humidified oxygen administration, and close monitoring for sudden respiratory failure

Enhancement of elimination: Dialysis and hemoperfusion are not indicated due to effectiveness of the prescribed antidotal treatment and large volumes of distribution of organophosphates.

Antidote:
Atropine: Administration should be guided by respiratory status, starting at 2-5 mg I.V. every 5-10 minutes as needed, and should be titrated to the resolution of excess pulmonary secretions. Frequent administration of large doses (cumulative doses >100 mg) may be necessary in massive exposures.
Glycopyrrolate: May be administered if atropine is unavailable (200-400 mcg I.V. or I.M.)
2-PAM: For more significant exposures (ie, exposures requiring large doses of atropine, or with recurring symptoms, or exposures to more lipid soluble agents), administration should follow: 1-2 g I.V. over 10-30 minutes, repeated in 1 hour if asthenia recurs, then every 4-12 hours for recurring symptoms.

Additional Information
Estimated lethal dose: Oral: Adults: 5-50 mg/kg (7 drops to 1 teaspoon)
No neurologic effect at oral daily doses of up to 19 mg
Depression of cholinesterase can occur with daily dosage >0.43 mg/kg.
The intermediate syndrome is not related to delayed neuropathy.
QT_c prolongation on ECG in the setting of organophosphate poisoning is associated with a high incidence of respiratory failure and mortality.
Toxicity is lower than that of parathion
Estimated daily intake in adults: **Inhalation:** In agricultural areas: 0.1-2.6 mcg. **Ingestion:** Food: 0.01-2 mcg; Drinking water: 0.4 mcg
Soil half-life (degrades faster in nonsterile soil): Aerobic: 64 days; Anaerobic: 7 days. Odor threshold: 0.012 ppm (rotten egg). Water half-life: pH <8: 72-89 days (40°C); pH >8: 4 days (40°C)
Can leave a yellow stain following spraying
As of mid-July 1997, approximately 4500 premises have been reported sprayed with methylparathion; 18,000 people have been affected, including 10,000 children and 2300 people have been relocated until their homes can be cleaned up. The U.S. Environmental Protection Agency (EPA) estimates that the cost of this problem as of July 1997 is $200 million. Incidents of indoor methylparathion use continue to be reported, the most recent in Texas City, Texas, in May 1997. For more information, or to obtain the "ATSDR Methyl Parathion Expert Panel Report," contact Leslie Campbell, MS at ATSDR, DHEP, 1600 Clifton Road, NE, MS E33, Atlanta, GA 30333; telephone: (404)639-6205; fax: (404)639-6208; e-mail: lca2@cdc.gov

Specific References
Cox RD, "Comparison of Urinary Paranitrophenol and Plasma/RBC Cholinesterase Measurements in the Evaluation of Domestic Methyl-parathion Exposure," *J Toxicol Clin Toxicol*, 2003, 41(5):736-7.
Cox RD, Kolb JC, Galli RL, et al, "Evaluation of Potential Adverse Health Effects Resulting from Chronic Domestic Exposure to the Organophosphate Insecticide Methyl Parathion," *Clin Toxicol (Phila)*, 2005, 43(4):243-53.
Jayashanker G, Srivastava AK, Afzal M, et al, "Detection of Methyl Parathion in Suicide Cases in India," *J Anal Toxicol*, 2006, 30:164.

Metobromuron

Applies to Herbicide
U.S. Brand Names Galex®; Patoran®
Synonyms 3-(Para-Bromophenyl)-L-Methoxyl-L-Methylurea
Use Herbicide used in control of grasses and broadleaf weeds
Mechanism of Toxic Action A substituted phenylurea herbicide which can cause methemoglobinemia due to its aniline derivative.
Adverse Reactions
Cardiovascular: Cyanosis, hemolysis
Central nervous system: Dizziness
Endocrine & metabolic: Metabolic acidosis
Gastrointestinal: Vomiting
Hematologic: Methemoglobinemia (may be late onset)
Admission Criteria/Prognosis Monitor for methemoglobinemia in any ingestion, for 24 hours
Toxicodynamics/Kinetics
Metabolism: Hydrolysis pathway yielding toxic aniline metabolites (4-bromoanaline, bromoacetanilide, bromophenylurea)
Elimination: Renal
Reference Range Peak serum and urine levels following an adult ingestion of 250 mL (50% metobromuron) were 4.9 mg/L and 0.6 mg/L respectively, 17 hours postingestion.
Overdosage/Treatment
Decontamination: Lavage within 2 hours any ingestion; activated charcoal can be given
Supportive therapy: I.V. methylene blue (1% concentration: 1.5-2 mg/L) should be given for symptomatic patients or methemoglobin levels >30%. Administer 100% oxygen therapy.
Antidote(s)
● Methylene Blue [ANTIDOTE]

Mineral-Based Crankcase Oil

CAS Number 8002-05-9
UN Number 1267; 1270
Synonyms API 79-7; Automotive Motor Oil; Base Engine Oil; Marine Diesel Oil; Petroleum
Use Supplemental fuel in engines, steam boilers, and domestic oil burners; incorporated into asphalt and as a dust suppressant on rural roads
Mechanism of Toxic Action Mixture of low and high molecular weight hydrocarbons (aliphatic, aromatic, naphthenic, and paraffinic); sulfur, oxygen, nitrogen compounds, and metals (lead, zinc, cadmium, nickel) may be present
Adverse Reactions
Central nervous system: Headache
Dermatologic: Rash
Gastrointestinal: Stomatitis
Neuromuscular & skeletal: Tremors
Ocular: Eye irritation at levels of 18.9 mg/m^3
Admission Criteria/Prognosis Patients who develop tachypnea, cyanosis, dyspnea, CNS depression, tachycardia, or fever within 8 hours of exposure should be admitted; asymptomatic patients can be discharged after 8 hours observation
Toxicodynamics/Kinetics
Absorption: Some dermally
Elimination: Primarily fecal
Overdosage/Treatment Decontamination: **Oral:** Dilute with water. **Dermal:** Wash skin with water and mild green (lipophilic) soap. **Ocular:** Copious irrigation with normal saline
Additional Information Monitor for toxicity of lead or molybdenum in used oil.
Oil from engines emitted directly with auto exhaust at concentrations of 0.1-0.3 L/1000 km
Lead levels on road surfaces treated with this compound are over 5 times higher than background lead levels (209 mg/kg vs 39 mg/kg respectively).
Hydrocarbon levels at the surface of treated roads range from 5880-13,441 mg/kg.
Background concentration of hydrocarbons in road soil near industrial area is ~856 mcg/g; near highways it is 265 mcg/g

Mirex

Related Information
● Adipose Tissue Ranges of Toxins
CAS Number 2385-85-5
U.S. Brand Names Dechlorane® 4070; Ferriamicide®
Synonyms Fire Ant Bait
Use Primarily an insecticide to control fire ants and Western harvester ants; control leaf cutters, mealy bugs, and yellow jackets; historical use (until 1972) as a fire retardant
Mechanism of Toxic Action In animal models, mirex induces liver growth possibly mediated by corticosterone
Adverse Reactions None described in humans; target organ in animal models for toxicity is liver and thyroid
Toxicodynamics/Kinetics
Metabolism: Not metabolized
Half-life: >1 year
Elimination: Primarily fecal and through breast milk
Reference Range Mirex blood levels in asymptomatic unexposed individuals should be <0.04 ng/g whole blood
Overdosage/Treatment
Decontamination: **Oral:** Lavage within 1 hour/activated charcoal or cholestyramine. **Dermal:** Flush skin with soap and water.
Supportive therapy: Propranolol may be effective in treatment of tremors. Phenobarbital can be used for seizure control.
Enhancement of elimination: Although data are lacking, cholestyramine resin (4 g every 8 hours) may be effective.
Additional Information Water half-life: 48 hours; virtually insoluble in water. Soil half-life: 10 years. FDA action level for fish: 0.1 ppm.

Molybdenum

CAS Number 7439-98-7
Synonyms Mo
Use A byproduct of uranium mining, molybdenum is used in metallurgy; molybdenum trioxide is a corrosive inhibitor as is zinc molybdate; molybdenite is used as a lubricant
Mechanism of Toxic Action An essential component of several enzymes (aldehyde oxidase, xanthine oxidase, and sulfite oxidase) which catalyze oxidation-reduction reactions. It is an upper respiratory tract irritant and in animals the formation of trithiomolybate may disturb copper metabolism.

Signs and Symptoms of Overdose Anorexia, arthralgias, diarrhea, fatigue, gout (hyperuricemia), headache, and low copper levels have occurred with chronic exposure. Pneumoconiosis can occur.

Toxicodynamics/Kinetics
Absorption: Oral: 50% to 93%
Elimination: Renal (high copper and sulfates appear to enhance renal elimination)

Monitoring Parameters Uric acid, copper, renal/liver function tests

Reference Range Normal population range: Whole blood: <5 ng/mL; urine: 10-124 mcg/L

Overdosage/Treatment Decontamination: **Oral:** Emesis or lavage within 2 hours for ingestions >100 mg. Activated charcoal is of unknown utility. **Dermal:** Wash skin with soap and water. **Inhalation:** Administer 100% humidified oxygen.

Additional Information Average dietary intake: 0.1-0.5 mg/day
Ambient air concentrations: Urban: 0.01-0.03 mcg/m^3. Rural: 0.001-0.0032 mcg/m^3. From coal fly ash: 7-160 mg/kg.
Soil average concentration: 1-2 mg/kg. Sewage sludge: 1-40 mg/kg. Water: <3 mcg/L

Monosodium Methanarsenate

Applies to Arsenic
CAS Number 2163-80-6
Synonyms Arsonate Liquid; MSMA
Use Pesticide / herbicide
Signs and Symptoms of Overdose Agranulocytosis, alopecia, blindness, cough, encephalopathy, fasciculations, fever, garlic-like breath, hematuria, hemolytic anemia, hypotension, lacrimation, leukopenia, Mees' lines (on nail beds; forms at 4-6 weeks postexposure), myoglobinuria, neuritis, nystagmus, pancytopenia, paresthesia, radiopacity, seizures, stocking-glove sensory neuropathy, sweating, tachycardia, torsade de pointes, tremor

Reference Range
Urine concentrations in nonexposed individuals ≤50 mcg/L; hair concentrations detectable 30 hours postingestion; urine ≥100 mcg/L is suggestive for chronic exposure; blood not usually helpful, although blood arsenic levels >1000 mcg/L are usually associated with fatality; background blood arsenic level is usually <1 mcg/L
Mean urine concentration of arsenic 0.2 mg/L associated with fatal poisoning

Overdosage/Treatment
Decontamination:
Oral: Lavage (within 1 hour)/activated charcoal. Aluminum hydroxide may prevent absorption of pentavalent arsenic compounds (due to its phosphate-binding abilities), although this has not been investigated in humans. Whole bowel irrigation is effective.
Dermal: Remove contaminated clothing; wash with soap and water.
Ocular: Copious irrigation with saline
Supportive therapy: Succimer (at standard doses to treat lead poisoning) is probably the treatment of choice. 2,3-Dimercaptopropane sulphonate (DMPS or unithiol) is also useful to enhance this metal's elimination at a dose of 100 mg 3 times/day orally for 5 days. 2,3-Dimercaptopropane-sulphonate (DMPS), a water soluble derivative of dimercaprol, has been recently demonstrated to prevent polyneuropathy when started within 48 hours of exposure at a dose of 5 mg/kg I.V. every 4 hours for 24 hours, and then 400 mg orally every 4 hours for 5-7 days. BAL should be utilized for severe acute exposures except for arsine gas. Penicillamine provides long-term therapy or alternatives to BAL.
Enhanced elimination: Hemodialysis clearance of arsenic ranges from 76-87 mL/minute; the clinical utility of this modality is unknown. No studies have been performed regarding hemodialysis with metal-chelate compound. Clearance of arsenic through hemodialysis is estimated to range from 76-87 mL/minute. Due to tissue binding of arsenic, this is not felt to be a useful modality for removal of arsenic. No current studies exist on the use of chelation with extracorporeal removal methods.

Additional Information Probably more hepatotoxic and ototoxic than inorganic arsenic
Monitor audiometry
Lethal dose is probably about 1700 mg/kg

Specific References
DeCapitani EM, Vieira RJ, Madureira PR, et al, "Auditory Neurotoxicity and Hepatotoxicity After MSMA (Monosodium Methanarsenate) High Dose Oral Intake," *J Tox Clin Tox*, 2005, 43:287-9.

Morpholine

CAS Number 110-91-8; 147-90-0
UN Number 1760; 2054
U.S. Brand Names Deposal®; Retarcyl®
Synonyms Diethylene Imidoxide; Diethylene Oxide
Use
A corrosion inhibitor and solvent for resins, waxing and dyes; used also as an emulsifier, plasticizer, antioxidant, and insecticide
Morpholine salicylate: Therapeutically for musculoskeletal disorders

Mechanism of Toxic Action Mucosal irritants; an alkaline caustic agent (pH ~11)

Signs and Symptoms of Overdose Conjunctivitis, corneal edema, cough and nasal irritation (after 1.5 minute exposure at 1200 ppm), dermal irritation at concentrations >25%, foggy blue-grey vision with halos surrounding lights after vapor exposure (glaucopsia), pharyngitis

Admission Criteria/Prognosis Patients with persistent pulmonary symptoms 6-8 hours after exposure or known exposures at concentrations >1000 ppm should be considered for hospital admission

Toxicodynamics/Kinetics
Absorption: Via dermal/oral routes
Protein binding: None
Half-life: 2-5 hours in animal studies
Elimination: Renal

Monitoring Parameters Chest x-ray, liver/renal function test

Overdosage/Treatment Decontamination: **Oral:** Dilute with water within 1 hour postexposure. **Dermal:** Wash with soap and water. **Inhalation:** Administer 100% oxygen. **Ocular:** Irrigate copiously with saline for at least 30 minutes.

Additional Information Colorless liquid (with an amine-like odor). Specific gravity 1.002, with a vapor density at 38°C of 1.1. Odor threshold (in air): 0.01 ppm. Odor threshold (in water): 0.2 mg/L. Taste threshold (in water): 0.2 mg/L. TLV: 20 ppm, PEL-STEL 30 ppm; IDLH: 8000 ppm

Mustard Gas

CAS Number 505-60-2
Synonyms Bis(2-Chloroethyl) Sulfide; Distilled Mustard; HD; MG; S-Mustard; Yperite
Use Primarily of historical use during World War I as a vesicant chemical warfare agent; most recently used for this purpose during the Iran-Iraq War in the 1980s; derivative of this chemical has been used as an antineoplastic agent (an alkylating agent - nitrogen mustard)
Mechanism of Toxic Action Dermal, ocular, and respiratory corrosive agent; this agent combines with DNA thus preventing cell replication

Adverse Reactions
Children may have a shorter time for symptom onset with more severe skin lesions.
Central nervous system: Fever
Dermatologic: Erythema and pruritus; may be delayed for up to 8 hours, then ulceration, dermal burns, and blisters can result
Gastrointestinal: Vomiting, nausea, diarrhea, anorexia
Hematologic: Bone marrow suppression, pancytopenia; leukopenia usually occurs 7-10 days postexposure; eosinophilia can be seen in children
Ocular: Lacrimation, photophobia, blepharospasm, ocular irritation, opacification, blindness
Respiratory: Dyspnea, cough (usual onset is 1-12 hours postexposure)

Toxicodynamics/Kinetics
Absorption: Lungs or skin (at a rate of 1-4 mcg/cm^2/minute); 20% absorption rate dermally
Metabolism: Hepatic through hydrolysis and glutathione pathways
Elimination: Renal accounts for ~21% of excretion

Reference Range Urine thiodiglycol levels >30 ng/mL 12 days postexposure associated with severe ocular and skin lesions

Overdosage/Treatment
Decontamination: **Note:** Penetrates wood, leather, rubber, and paints; decontamination must occur within 2 minutes.
Oral: Activated charcoal or 150 mL of 2% sodium thiosulfate orally
Dermal: Remove all contaminated clothing. Towels soaked in 0.2% chloramine-T in water (Dakin solution) placed over wounds for the first 2 hours may be helpful. Wash with soap and water (not hot). Can wash with dilute (0.5%) hypochlorite, then neutralize with 2.5% sodium thiosulfate. If no water is available, dry decontamination with Fuller's earth can be utilized. Treat wounds as burns with use of 1% silver sulfadiazine (twice daily). Leave small blisters (<1 cm) intact; unroof larger blisters and irrigate.
Ocular: Copious irrigation with saline (neutralize with 2.5% solution of sodium thiosulfate); remove contact lenses
Respiratory: Administer 100% oxygen. A nebulized mist of 2.5% sodium thiosulfate may be helpful as a neutralizing agent if given within 15 minutes of exposure.
Supportive therapy: N-acetylcysteine 4 times/day (up to 150 mg/kg), along with ascorbic acid (3 g), thienamycin (2 g twice daily), L-carnitine (3 g), and sodium thiosulfate (3-12.5 g/day), has been used to ameliorate effects, but it is unproven in its efficacy. For ocular exposure, topical antibiotics, mydriatics, and possibly corticosteroids can be utilized. Vaseline® placed on eyelid edges may prevent lids from adhering. For dermal burns, topical antibiotics with systemic analgesics are the mainstay of therapy. Do not overhydrate the patient. Do not fluid resuscitate as in thermal burns. Colony stimulating factor may be helpful in treating leukopenia. Prednisone (60-125 mg/day) orally can be helpful in treating pulmonary toxicity. Bronchospasm should be treated with beta$_2$ adrenergic agonist agents.

Additional Information Toxic dermal dose: 0.1% solution

Fair skinned individuals are more at risk for adverse dermal effects than dark skinned individuals.

Total white blood cell count <200 is a harbinger for fatality. No mustard can be isolated in blister fluid.

Higher wind speeds, higher temperature and humidity increase the atmospheric vaporization rate; may persist in soil for weeks

Combat zones atmospheric concentration of mustard gas during WWI was estimated to be from 3-5 ppm; case fatality rate: 2% to 4%.

Since mustard gas binds rapidly and avidly to tissue proteins, decontamination must begin immediately, and increasing elimination of absorbed chemical is difficult.

Specific References

Barr JR, Driskell WJ, Aston LS, et al, "Quantitation of Metabolites of the Nerve Agents Sarin, Soman, Cyclohexylsarin, VX, and Russian VX in Human Urine Using Isotope-Dilution Gas Chromatography-Tandem Mass Spectrometry," *J Anal Toxicol*, 2004, 28(5):372-8.

Boyer AE, Ash D, Barr DB, et al, "Quantitation of the Sulfur Mustard Metabolites 1,1'-Sulfonylbis[2-(methylthio)ethane] and Thiodiglycol in Urine Using Isotope-dilution Gas Chromatography-Tandem Mass Spectrometry," *J Anal Toxicol*, 2004, 28(5):327-32.

Byers CE, Holloway ER, Korte WD, et al, "Gas Chromatographic-Mass Spectrometric Determination of British Anti-Lewisite in Plasma," *J Anal Toxicol*, 2004, 28(5):384-9.

Capacio BR, Smith JR, DeLion MT, et al, "Monitoring Sulfur Mustard Exposure by Gas Chromatography-Mass Spectrometry Analysis of Thiodiglycol Cleaved from Blood Proteins," *J Anal Toxicol*, 2004, 28(5):306-10.

Degenhardt CE, Pleijsier K, van der Schans MJ, et al, "Improvements of the Fluoride Reactivation Method for the Verification of Nerve Agent Exposure," *J Anal Toxicol*, 2004, 28(5):364-71.

Jakubowski EM, McGuire JM, Evans RA, et al, "Quantitation of Fluoride Ion Released Sarin in Red Blood Cell Samples by Gas Chromatography-Chemical Ionization Mass Spectrometry Using Isotope Dilution and Large-Volume Injection," *J Anal Toxicol*, 2004, 28(5):357-63.

Kales SN and Christiani DC, "Acute Chemical Emergencies," *N Engl J Med*, 2004, 350(8):800-8.

Khateri S, Ghanei M, Keshavarz S, et al, "Incidence of Lung, Eye, and Skin Lesions as Late Complications in 34,000 Iranians with Wartime Exposure to Mustard Agent," *J Occup Environ Med*, 2003, 45(11):1136-43.

Khateri S, Ghanei M, Soroush MR, et al, "Effects of Mustard Gas Exposure in Pediatric Patients (Long-Term Health Status of Mustard-Exposed Children, 14 Years After Chemical Bombardment of Sardasht)," *J Toxicol Clin Toxicol*, 2003, 41(5):733.

Lemire SW, Barr JR, Ashley DL, et al, "Quantitation of Biomarkers of Exposure to Nitrogen Mustards in Urine from Rats Dosed with Nitrogen Mustards and from an Unexposed Human Population," *J Anal Toxicol*, 2004, 28(5):320-6.

Noort D, Fidder A, Benschop HP, et al, "Procedure for Monitoring Exposure to Sulfur Mustard Based on Modified Edman Degradation of Globin," *J Anal Toxicol*, 2004, 28(5):311-5.

Noort D, Fidder A, Hulst AG, et al, "Retrospective Detection of Exposure to Sulfur Mustard: Improvements on an Assay for Liquid Chromatography-tandem Mass Spectrometry Analysis of Albumin-Sulfur Mustard Adducts," *J Anal Toxicol*, 2004, 28(5):333-8.

Read RW and Black RM, "Analysis of Beta-Lyase Metabolites of Sulfur Mustard in Urine by Electrospray Liquid Chromatography-Tandem Mass Spectrometry," *J Anal Toxicol*, 2004, 28(5):346-51.

Read RW and Black RM, "Analysis of the Sulfur Mustard Metabolite 1,1'-Sulfonylbis[2-S-(N-Acetylcysteinyl)ethane] in Urine by Negative Ion Electrospray Liquid Chromatography-Tandem Mass Spectrometry," *J Anal Toxicol*, 2004, 28(5):352-6.

Smith JR, "Analysis of the Enantiomers of VX Using Normal-Phase Chiral Liquid Chromatography with Atmospheric Pressure Chemical Ionization-Mass Spectrometry," *J Anal Toxicol*, 2004, 28(5):390-2.

Thomason JW, Rice TW, and Milstone AP, "Bronchiolitis Obliterans in a Survivor of a Chemical Weapons Attack," *JAMA*, 2003, 290(5):598-9.

van der Schans GP, Mars-Groenendijk R, de Jong LPA, et al, "Standard Operating Procedure for Immunuslotblot Assay for Analysis of DNA/Sulfur Mustard Adducts in Human Blood and Skin," *J Anal Toxicol*, 2004, 28(5):316-9.

Young CL, Ash D, Driskell WJ, et al, "A Rapid, Sensitive Method for the Quantitation of Specific Metabolites of Sulfur Mustard in Human Urine Using Isotope-Dilution Gas Chromatography-Tandem Mass Spectrometry," *J Anal Toxicol*, 2004, 28(5):339-45.

N,N-Dimethyl-P-Toluidine

CAS Number 99-97-8

Use Found in solutions used in production of artificial fingernails solution

Mechanism of Toxic Action Methemoglobin producer through active metabolite

Signs and Symptoms of Overdose Acetone breath, cyanosis, drooling, Heinz body formation (formation of methemoglobinemia takes 2-3 hours), methemoglobinemia

Toxicodynamics/Kinetics Metabolism: Probably to paramethylphenyl hydroxylamine (active producer of methemoglobin)

Monitoring Parameters Methemoglobin

Reference Range Ingestion of 6 mg/kg resulted in methemoglobinemia of 43%

Overdosage/Treatment

Decontamination: Emesis within 30 minutes, lavage (within 1 hour)/activated charcoal. Remove patient from inhalation and administer 100% humidified air. Exposed skin and eyes should be irrigated with water.

Supportive therapy: Methemoglobinemia: Treat symptomatic patients or if level is >20%, administer 100% oxygen. If required, methylene blue: 1-2 mg/kg/dose I.V. over a few minutes; may repeat in 4 hours if needed. Doses >15 mg/kg may cause hemolysis. High doses of methylene blue may precipitate Heinz body formation and hemolysis. Transfusion of PRBCs may be needed. Treatment for myoglobinuria may require urine alkalinization and maintenance of adequate urinary output to prevent renal damage.

Antidote(s)

- Methylene Blue [ANTIDOTE]

Naphthalene

Related Information

- Adipose Tissue Ranges of Toxins

CAS Number 91-20-3

UN Number 1334; 2304

Synonyms Camphor Tar; Moth Balls; Moth Flakes; Naphthalin; Naphthene; White Tar

Use Moth repellents, toilet bowel deodorizers, in scintillation counters, in the manufacture of phallic anhydride, naphthol, hydrogenated naphthalenes, and halogenated naphthalenes; formerly used as an antihelmintic

Mechanism of Toxic Action Hemolysis caused by oxidation products of naphthalene; in patients with G6PD deficiency, metabolites cause instability of erythrocyte glutathione

Adverse Reactions

Cardiovascular: Sinus tachycardia

Hematologic: Glucose-6-phosphate dehydrogenase deficiency-induced hemolytic anemia

Signs and Symptoms of Overdose Anemia, coma, drowsiness, fever, headache, hematuria, hemolysis, hyperkalemia, methemoglobinemia, restlessness, seizures, urine discoloration (black) and vomiting may develop in severe intoxications. Tachycardia or hypotension may also occur. Hepatocellular injury is rare, but may occur in 3-5 days after exposure.

Admission Criteria/Prognosis Consider admission if ingestion of more than one mothball has occurred and patient is symptomatic, if CBC or urinalysis is abnormal, or if the patient has a previous hematological condition (ie, G6PD deficiency); any patient with change in mental status, cardiopulmonary complaints, or methemoglobin levels >30% should be admitted; asymptomatic patients with methemoglobin levels <30% may be considered for discharge after 6 hours of observation and if methemoglobin levels fall to <15%

Toxicodynamics/Kinetics

Absorption: Dermal: Also enhanced by oil. Inhalation: Rapid. Oral: Erratic; soluble in oil so coadministration will enhance absorption

Metabolism: Through liver; oxidation to naphthol and naphthoquinone; glutathione conjugated to thioethers are also noted

Elimination: Excreted in kidney as a 1,4-naphthoquinone metabolite over a 2-week period; fecal excretion accounts for <10%

Reference Range Adipose tissue levels up to 63 mcg/kg have been detected in asymptomatic individuals

Overdosage/Treatment

Decontamination: **Oral:** Emesis or lavage within 2 hours; activated charcoal. Avoid milk for 2-3 hours in that absorption may increase. **Dermal:** Wash with soap and water; avoid oil-based compounds. **Ocular:** Copious irrigation with saline

Supportive therapy: Alkaline diuresis may be needed if hemolysis occurs (use Ringer's lactate or I.V. sodium bicarbonate to keep urine pH >7.5). Mannitol or furosemide may be required to promote urine flow. Methylene blue: 1-2 mg/kg of 1% if the patient is symptomatic or has a methemoglobin level >30%. Transfusion for severe anemia. Dialysis has been used for supportive care. Exchange transfusion has been used for supportive care, but is not routinely recommended.

For inhalation injuries, nebulized budesonide (0.5 mg every 12 hours for 4 days - pediatric dose) was found to be helpful

Antidote(s)

- Methylene Blue [ANTIDOTE]

Additional Information Detection and quantitation of naphthalene and metabolites through TLC, HPLC, gas chromatography with mass spectrometry, and high resolution proton magnetic resonance. CBC with smear to detect for schistocytes and cell fragments, BUN, creatinine, electrolytes, methemoglobin, urinalysis (check for hemoglobinuria), G6PD, LFTs; urine may be sent for 1-naphthol.

See table.

Distinguishing Characteristics of Mothballs

	PDB	Naphtha	Camphor
Physical	Wet and oily	Dry	
Water	Sink	Sink	Float
4 oz water + 3 heaping tsp salt	Sink	Float	Float
Drop of turpentine	Soluble	Moderately soluble	
Heating	Green color	No color	

PDB = paradichlorobenzene.
Naphtha = naphthalene.

Odor threshold: Water: 0.021 mg/L. Air: 0.44 mg/m^3

Water half-life (photolysis): 71 hours (surface water); 550 days (deep water >5 meters)

Ambient atmospheric concentration in U.S.: ~1 ppm

PEL-TWA: 10 ppm (50 mg/m^3); TLV-TWA: 10 ppm (52 mg/m^3); IDLH: 500 ppm

In drinking water, concentrations as high as 1.5 mcg/L have been noted.

Average daily intake of naphthalene is ~19 mcg by inhalation and 0.002-4 mcg from drinking water.

Specific References

Gurkan F and Bosnak M, "Use of Nebulized Budesonide in Two Critical Patients with Hydrocarbon Intoxication," *Am J Ther*, 2005, 12(4):366-7.

Ikegami Y, Hasegawa A, Tase C,et al, "Delayed Massive Hemoptysis Complicated with Aspiration of Organophosphorus Compound," *Am J Emerg Med*, 2003, 21(6):509-11.

N-Butyl Chloride

Applies to Butylchloride; Sergeants Capsules
CAS Number 109-69-3
UN Number 1127
Synonyms 1-Chlorobutane
Use Veterinary antinematodal agent (for ascarids and hookworms)
Mechanism of Toxic Action Dermal irritant; weak central nervous system depressant
Signs and Symptoms of Overdose Skin irritation (human data lacking)
Overdosage/Treatment Decontamination: **Dermal:** Irrigate with soap and water. **Gastric:** Do not induce emesis; dilute with milk or water. **Ocular:** Irrigate with normal saline. **Respiratory:** Administer 100% humidified oxygen.
Additional Information LD$_{50}$ in rats: 2.67 g/kg by oral ingestion and ~8000 ppm by inhalation
No evidence for carcinogenicity
Colorless liquid with a pungent odor; usually found in capsule form.
Moderately explosive; when heated, can decompose to hydrochloric acid and phosgene
Density: 0.88. Vapor density: 3.2. Boiling point: 78°C

Nerve Agents

Related Information

• Diisopropylmethylphosphonate

CAS Number 107-44-8 (sarin); 50782-69-9 (VX); 77-81-6 (tabun); 96-64-0 (soman)
Synonyms Sarin (GB or Isopropyl Methylphosphonofluoridate); Soman (GD or Pinacolyl Methylphosphonofluoridate); Tabun (Ethyl N-Dimethylphophoramidocyanidate or GA); VX (Methylphosphonothioic Acid S-(2-(bis(1-Methyl-Ethyl)Amino)Ethyl) o-Ethyl Ester or V)
Use Chemical warfare weapon
Mechanism of Toxic Action Similar to organophosphate agent; inhibits the enzyme acetylcholinesterase thus resulting in acetylcholine excess at the neuronal synapse; may penetrate blood brain barrier and thus affect GABA transmission
Adverse Reactions

Cardiovascular: Sinus bradycardia
Central nervous system: Insomnia, fatigue, memory loss, seizures (soman), ataxia, coma, headache
Gastrointestinal: Diarrhea, nausea
Ocular: Lacrimation, miosis (may take 40-50 days for pupillary response to normalize)
Respiratory: Rhinorrhea; death is usually due to respiratory failure, cough

Miscellaneous: Excess muscarinic activity (bronchial secretion, salivation, diaphoresis, miosis, bronchospasm, bradycardia) and nicotinic activity (muscle twitching, weakness, paralysis)

Admission Criteria/Prognosis Patients who are asymptomatic 18 hours postexposure can be discharged; there are no delayed effects

Toxicodynamics/Kinetics

Onset of action: Inhalation (except for VX): Within 5 minutes. Dermal: 1 hour
Half-time: Aging of sarin-acetylcholine complex: 5 hours. Aging of soman-acetylcholine complex: 2 minutes. Aging of VX-acetylcholine complex: 1-2 days
Metabolism of VX: VX hydrolysis → EMP + DAET; DAET + S-adenosyl-L-methione (through thiol-s-methyl transferase) → DAEMS + S-adenosyl-L-homocysteine

Reference Range

Cholinesterase activity <10% of normal is consistent with severe poisoning
Serum DAEMS and EMPA levels 1 hour following a fatal VX dermal exposure was 143 ng/mL and 1.25 mcg/mL, respectively.

Overdosage/Treatment

Decontamination: **Dermal:** Remove all contaminated clothing. Wash with 1% to 5% hypochlorite solution (household bleach) followed by copious water irrigation. If bleach is not available, a gentle blotting with an alkaline soap can be used. Dilute ammonia may be helpful for VX exposure. **Inhalation:** Administer 100% humidified oxygen. **Ocular:** Irrigate with saline.
Supportive therapy: Atropine is the mainstay of treatment with doses from 10-20 mg cumulatively over the first 2-3 hours usually required. This should be titrated to bronchial secretions and not to ocular signs. Pralidoxime should be administered (1-2 g I.V. over 10 minutes, repeat in 1 hour if weakness occurs, then every 4-12 hours as needed). Pralidoxime should be used within 3 hours post-sarin exposure; may not be useful for soman or tabun. Obidoxime may be effective for tabun, sarin, or GF at an initial I.M. or slow I.V. infusion of 250 mg; may be repeated every 2 hours up to 750 mg total dose. Homatropine can be utilized to treat miosis which may last for weeks postexposure. Diazepam or midazolam has been an effective anticonvulsant in primate models. Since aging is longer for tabun or VX, pralidoxime may be particularly useful; administer oxygen. Seizures often respond to atropine or pralidoxime. For refractory seizures, diazepam can be used. In fact, 5-10 mg of diazepam is often given as pretreatment in severely affected patients. Hemodialysis/hemoperfusion has been noted to increase cholinesterase levels and improve clinical symptomatology in one patient. Asoxime chloride may be useful when used with atropine for treatment of sarin, soman, and GF exposure.

Antidote(s)

• Asoxime Chloride [ANTIDOTE]
• Atropine [ANTIDOTE]
• Obidoxime Chloride [ANTIDOTE]
• Pralidoxime [ANTIDOTE]
• Pyridostigmine [ANTIDOTE]

Additional Information

Lethal dermal dose (70 kg adult): Sarin: 1.7 g. Tabun: 1 g. Soman: 100 mg; VX: 6 mg
Acute sarin exposure may cause a delayed effect on the vestibulocerebellar system with females being more sensitive than males.
G agents are volatile and are both an inhalation and dermal threat. VX exhibits low volatility (like motor oil) and is primarily a dermal threat while also an inhalation threat.
Sarin has been implicated in the Tokyo subway terrorist incident occurring in March, 1995. It has been estimated that 800 kg of sarin will cause heavy casualties over 1 square mile area. Sarin is 4000 times more potent than parathion. Lethal inhaled dose of tabun, sarin, and soman is ~1 mg; VX has highest lethality in dermal applications (as an oily liquid) rather than through inhalation; while sarin and tabun may cause a delayed neuropathy, VX is not known to cause a delayed neuropathy. Emergency medical ambulances in New York City now stock up to 52 mg of atropine; this is up from 4 mg which was a typical ambulance stock of atropine before the March, 1995 Tokyo subway sarin attack.
In the sarin subway attack in Tokyo (March 20, 1995), of the 5510 cases there were 12 deaths and 17 patients requiring ventilatory support.
Rescuers should wear protective masks (ie, charcoal filter of self-contained breathing apparatus) with heavy rubber gloves.
Pretreatment with pyridostigmine bromide (30 mg orally every 8 hours) may be effective (especially for soman).
For maximum control limits: See table.

Maximum Agent Control Limits

	Workplace (8 h in mg/m^3)	General Population (72 h TWA mg/m^3)
Sarin and tabun	1×10^{-5}	3×10^{-3}
VX	1×10^{-4}	3×10^{-6}

Contaminated equipment an be washed with 10% hypochlorite solution. These agents are 4-6 times denser than air and thus remain close to the ground; they are soluble in water, but hydrolyze in alkaline solutions (see Treatment). Contaminated vegetation with VX can cause toxic effects upon ingestion.

Butyrylcholinesterase can sequester tabun, soman, VX, and sarin within 5 seconds in a rodent model. Human data is lacking.

Specific References

Buckley NA, Roberts D, and Eddleston M, "Overcoming Apathy in Research on Organophosphate Poisoning," *BMJ*, 2004, 329(7476): 1231-3 (review).

Burda AM, Pallasch E, Metz J, et al, "Comparison of Pre-9/11 and Post-9/11 Rates of Nerve Agent Antidote Stocking in Metropolitan Hospitals," *J Toxicol Clin Toxicol*, 2003, 41(5):715.

Kuca K and Jun D, "Reactivation of Sarin-inhibited Pig Brain Acetylcholinesterase Using Oxime Antidotes," *J Med Toxicol*, 2006, 2(4):141-144.

Lee EC, "Clinical Manifestations of Sarin Nerve Gas Exposure," *JAMA*, 2003, 290(5):659-62.

Lynch EL and Thomas TL, "Pediatric Considerations in Chemical Exposures: Are We Prepared?" *Pediatr Emerg Care*, 2004, 20(3): 198-208.

Nechiporenko SP and Zatsepin EP, "A Study to Establish an Efficient Means for Delivering Antidotal Therapy at Nerve Agent Destruction Facilities," *J Toxicol Clin Toxicol*, 2003, 41(5):723.

Rotenberg JS and Newmark J, "Nerve Agent Attacks on Children: Diagnosis and Management," *Pediatrics*, 2003, 112(3 Pt 1):648-58.

Wei G, Chang A, and Hamilton RJ, "Nerve Agent Antidote Kits Enable Nurses to Treat More Mass-Casualty Patients than Multidose Vials," *Acad Emerg Med*, 2006, 13(5):S177.

Yanagisawa N, Morita H, and Nakajima T, "Sarin Experiences in Japan: Acute Toxicity and Long-Term Effects," *J Neurol Sci*, 2006, 249:76-85.

Nickel

Related Information
- Nickel Carbonyl

CAS Number 7440-02-0

UN Number 2881;1325

Synonyms Carbonyl Nickel Powder; Nickel Sponge; Raney Alloy; Raney Nickel

Mechanism of Toxic Action In nickel refiners, nickel is a respiratory tract carcinogen

Adverse Reactions

Nickel carbonyl is much more toxic than nickel metal or alloys; dermal reactions to nickel carbonyl are rare

Cardiovascular: Cardiomyopathy

Central nervous system: Dizziness, headache

Dermatologic: Eczema

Gastrointestinal: Diarrhea, metallic taste, nausea, vomiting

Hematologic: Leukocytosis

Hepatic: Elevated bilirubin, elevated transaminases (SGPT)

Neuromuscular & skeletal: Weakness

Respiratory: Asthma, cough, dyspnea, hoarseness, nasal carcinomas, pulmonary edema

Miscellaneous: Cutaneous T-cell lymphoma

Signs and Symptoms of Overdose CNS stimulation followed by cold clammy skin, contact dermatitis (nickel itch), coma, cough, diarrhea, dyspnea, ECG changes, erythrocytosis, giddiness, hematuria, hyposmia, hypothermia, impaired thermoregulation, leukocytosis, metallic taste, nasal carcinoma, nausea, seizures, sleeplessness, sore throat, transient increase in ALT and bilirubin, urticaria, vomiting

Admission Criteria/Prognosis Admit any symptomatic patient or ingestion >500 mg

Toxicodynamics/Kinetics

Absorption: Inhalation: 35%. Oral: 1% to 27% (reduced by food). Dermal: Nickel sulfate: 55% to 77%

Distribution: Nickel carbonyl crosses the alveolar membrane and dissociates to nickel and carbon monoxide; wide volume of distribution

Protein binding: 59%

Half-life: 11-60 hours

Elimination: Excreted primarily in urine; oral ingestion results in a large amount excreted through gastrointestinal tract

Warnings/Precautions Do not use DDC for divalent nickel poisoning.

Reference Range Normal blood levels: 1.1-4.6 mcg/L; serum nickel concentrations >8 mcg/L are associated with excessive exposure; normal urine level is ~50 mcg/L; an 8-hour urine level of <100 mcg/L associated with mild exposure, 100-500 mcg/L associated with moderate exposure, and >500 mcg/L associated with severe exposure

Overdosage/Treatment

Decontamination: **Oral:** Dilute with milk. **Dermal:** Wash with soap and water. **Inhalation:** Give 100% humidified oxygen. **Ocular:** Copious irrigation with saline.

Supportive therapy: To treat moderate to severe nickel exposures (urine nickel concentrations over 100 mcg per L): Oral diethyldithiocarbamate (DDC) 50 mg/kg is administered during first 24 hours. On suceeding days, oral DDC is administered every 8 hours until the patient is asymptomatic (and the urine nickle is under 50 mcg/L). DDC may be given intravenously by adding ten ml of a sterile phosphate buffer solution (500 mg/dl) to one grams of powdered DDC contained in a sterile ampule. DDC I.V. is then administered at a dose of 25 to 100 mg/kg over the first 24 hours, and as outlined above on succeeding days.

Enhancement of elimination: Forced saline diuresis can decrease half-life of nickel sulfate and nickel chloride by >50%

Antidote(s)
- Diethyldithiocarbamate Trihydrate [ANTIDOTE]

Diagnostic Procedures
- Nickel, Urine

Additional Information

Fatal dose of elemental nickel: ~2 g. 30 minute exposure of 30 ppm airbourne concentration is potentially fatal.

Oral ingestion of 73 mg of elemental nickel can produce toxic symptoms.

Skin application of 1:10,000 dose of nickel salts can elicit a sensitivity reaction.

Cigarette smoking accounts for 2-12 mcg of nickel inhaled per cigarette pack.

Baking powder (13.4 ppm), orange pekoe tea (7.6 ppm), buckwheat (6.5 ppm), and cocoa (5 ppm) contain the highest amount of nickel.

Most U.S. coins contain ~25% nickel.

Range of atmospheric nickel concentration in urban U.S. areas: 1-328 ng/m^3. In rural areas, the range is 0.6-78 ng/m^3.

Average daily intake of nickel from food: ~168 mcg; from drinking water: ~2 mcg; from inhalation: 0.1-1 mcg

Range of nickel in drinking water: 3-7 mcg/L. Range of nickel in soil: 5-500 ppm

TWA-TLV: 15 mcg/m^3

Specific References

Lippmann M, Ito K, Hwarg J-S, et al "Cardiovascular Effects of Nickel in Ambient Air," *Environment Health Pespect*, 2006, 114:1662-9.

Nickel Carbonyl

Related Information
- Nickel
- Nickel Carbonyl

CAS Number 13463-39-3

UN Number 1259

Synonyms Nickel Tetracarbonile

Use Catalyst in petroleum and rubber industries; used in electroplating; formed as an intermediate (by a reaction with carbon monoxide) in nickel ore purification

Mechanism of Toxic Action Inhibits ribonucleic acid synthesis; mucosal irritant

Adverse Reactions

Symptoms may be delayed 12-24 hours

Cardiovascular: Tachycardia, bradycardia, QT prolongation, chest pain, myocarditis, cyanosis (may be a delayed effect), sinus bradycardia, angina, sinus tachycardia

Central nervous system: Headache, dizziness, delirium, hyperthermia, chills, seizures, low grade fever, neurasthenic syndrome

Dermatologic: Dermal burns

Gastrointestinal: Nausea, vomiting, diarrhea (2-3 days postexposure), stomach pains, sore throat

Hematologic: Leukocytosis

Hepatic: Elevated liver enzymes

Neuromuscular & skeletal: Weakness

Renal: Proteinuria

Respiratory: Pulmonary edema, dyspnea, interstitial pneumonitis may be delayed from 12 hours to 5 days postexposure and may last for 1 month, tachypnea, asthma, cough, bronchospasm, interstitial fibrosis

Miscellaneous: Diaphoresis

Admission Criteria/Prognosis Any symptomatic patients; any patient with a urinary nickel level >100 mcg/L; or inhalation of >2 ppm (essentially if one can detect the odor of this agent for 30 minutes, the patient should be admitted)

Toxicodynamics/Kinetics

Absorption: By inhalation

Metabolism: Metabolized to carbon monoxide and nickel

Elimination: Urine

Monitoring Parameters Carboxyhemoglobin levels, urinary nickel levels, chest x-ray, arterial blood gases

Reference Range Normal blood levels: 1.1-4.6 mcg/L; an 8-hour urine level of <100 mcg/L associated with mild exposure, 100-500 mcg/L associated with moderate exposure, and >500 mcg/L associated with severe exposure

Overdosage/Treatment

Decontamination: **Dermal:** Wash with soap and water. **Inhalation:** Give 100% humidified oxygen. **Ocular:** Copious irrigation with saline

Supportive therapy: Diethyldithiocarbamate (DDC) is the preferred chelating agent.

Indication for treatment of sodium DDC is 8-hour postexposure urine nickel concentration >100 mcg Ni/L. Benzodiazepines can be used to treat seizures. Disulfiram can enhance the elimination of nickel and has been used to treat nickel dermatitis. Disulfiram (250-750 mg every 8 hours or half the DDC dose) is second-choice therapy to diethyldithiocarbamate. Oxygen, bronchodilators, and steroids (for adrenocortical insufficiency) may be required. The dose of DDC is 35-45 mg DDC/kg orally over the first day, followed by 400 mg every 8 hours until the patient is symptom free. I.V. dose is 12.5 mg DDC/kg.

Enhancement of elimination: Forced saline diuresis can decrease half-life.

Antidote(s)

- Diethyldithiocarbamate Trihydrate [ANTIDOTE]

Diagnostic Procedures

- Nickel, Urine

Additional Information

Lethal air concentration: 3-30 ppm at 30 minutes. Symptoms can occur at 2 ppm.

Potentially carcinogenic (nasal and lung cancer)

Nickel carbonyl is the most toxic of nickel compounds. nickel carbonyl is formed when nickel is in contact with carbon monoxide. Toxicity from nickel carbonyl results from inhalation, whereas toxicity from Ni^{2+} results from oral/parenteral exposure. In nickel carbonyl poisoning, after the acute symptoms subside, delayed pulmonary, cardiac, and neurologic symptoms occur after 1-5 days.

Cigarette smoke contains ~3.5 ppm of nickel carbonyl

Colorless gas with a "sooty" or musty odor with an odor threshold of 1 ppm; heavier than air (vapor density is almost 6); highly explosive

Nitrates

Related Information

- Propylene Glycol Dinitrate

Applies to Cold Packs

UN Number 1477; 3218

Commonly Found In Munition and explosives (dynamite is 60% nitrates); may be found in well water; certain plants (datura, solanum, sorghum species)

Use Ammonium nitrates are in cold packs

Mechanism of Toxic Action Accelerates atherosclerosis

Adverse Reactions

Cardiovascular: Hypotension, tachycardia, fibrillation (atrial), bigeminy; nitrate withdrawal syndrome includes vasodilatory effects (flushing, headaches), flutter (atrial), angina, chest pain, sinus tachycardia, arrhythmias (ventricular)

Gastrointestinal: Gastritis, feces discoloration (black)

Hematologic: Methemoglobinemia

Miscellaneous: Can produce sulfhemoglobin

Signs and Symptoms of Overdose Fatigue, headaches, hematuria, nausea, vomiting, dyspnea within 2 hours; coma, cyanosis, and pallor may develop later

Toxicodynamics/Kinetics

Absorption: Oral: Well absorbed; not absorbed through intact skin

Metabolism: By gastrointestinal bacteria to nitrites

Elimination: Renal

Reference Range Mean urine nitrate level: 41-56 mcg/mL; normal plasma nitrate level: ~37 μmol/L; normal saliva nitrate level: 5-10 mg/L

Overdosage/Treatment

Decontamination: **Do not** induce emesis for ammonium nitrate ingestion; methylene blue (1-2 mg/kg per dose) for elevated methemoglobin as needed every 4 hours

Oral: Dilute with 4-8 ounces of milk or water; activated charcoal may be useful for oral decontamination

Ocular: Irrigate eyes with normal saline.

Enhanced elimination: Although formal studies are lacking, hyperbaric oxygen may be useful in severe exposures. Exchange transfusion may be useful.

Antidote(s)

- Methylene Blue [ANTIDOTE]

Diagnostic Procedures

- Methemoglobin, Blood
- Sulfhemoglobin

Test Interactions May result in a low measured oxygen saturation, resulting in an oxygen saturation gap

Additional Information Toxic dose: 5 mg/kg/day (chronically)

Can penetrate gloves

It appears that age and serum creatinine levels are inversely associated with development of vascular headache due to nitrates. Risk for headache decreases by ~40% for a 10 year increase in age and is 5 times less likely in patients with serum creatinine levels >133 μmol/L as opposed to levels <97 μmol/L.

EPA standard for nitrate in drinking water: 10 mg/L, 9% of household wells nationally exceed this value.

Nitrites

Applies to Corrosive Inhibition; Cyanide Antidote Kits; Dyes; Fabrics; Linen; Photography

UN Number 2627

Synonyms Poppers; Snappers; Thrust

Commonly Found In Inhalation abuse of volatile nitrates

Use In cyanide antidote kits; used in the manufacture of dyes, fabrics, and linen; photography; corrosive inhibition

Mechanism of Toxic Action Peripheral vasodilation; produces methemoglobin; is an oxidizing agent

Adverse Reactions

Cardiovascular: Paradoxical bradycardia, hypotension, sinus bradycardia, vasodilation

Hematologic: Methemoglobinemia followed by hemolysis

Ocular: Visual disturbances

Respiratory: Tachypnea

Miscellaneous: Infants, pregnant women, and patients with malignancy may be especially sensitive

Signs and Symptoms of Overdose Abdominal pain, blurred vision, cyanosis, diarrhea, dyspnea, flushing, headache, lightheadedness (postural), nausea, seizures, skin irritation, vomiting

Admission Criteria/Prognosis Any patient with change in mental status, cardiopulmonary complaints, or methemoglobin levels >30% should be admitted; asymptomatic patients with methemoglobin levels <30% may be considered for discharge after 6 hours of observation and if methemoglobin levels fall to <15%

Toxicodynamics/Kinetics

Absorption: May be by inhalation, ingestion or dermal routes

Metabolism: 60% metabolized - most to ammonia

Elimination: Excreted renally (40% unchanged)

Monitoring Parameters Obtain methemoglobin levels - cyanosis may occur at levels >20%

Reference Range Fatal nitrite serum range: 0.5-350 mg/L

Overdosage/Treatment

Decontamination: Basic poison management; methylene blue for symptomatic methemoglobinemia

Supportive therapy: Hyperbaric oxygen may be of use, though controlled human data are lacking.

Antidote(s)

- Methylene Blue [ANTIDOTE]

Diagnostic Procedures

- Methemoglobin, Blood

Additional Information Ingestion of 10 mL of isobutyl or amyl nitrate may be toxic. Oral ingestion produces more rapid methemoglobin than inhalation. May be toxic at >0.4 mg/kg

Specific References

Ringling S, Boo T, and Bottei E, "Methemoglobinemia from Nitrite-Contaminated Punch," *J Toxicol Clin Toxicol*, 2003, 41(5):730-1.

Nitrobenzene

Applies to Caswell No 66

CAS Number 98-95-3

UN Number 1662

Synonyms Nitrobenzol Oil of Mirbane

Use Production of aniline, cellulose ethers, and acetaminophen; perfume agent in soaps; solvent in shoe dyes (preservative) and floor polishes

Mechanism of Toxic Action Binds to hemoglobin which results in methemoglobin formation; resembles aniline in its action

Adverse Reactions

Cardiovascular: Tachycardia, hypotension, shock, sinus tachycardia, cyanosis

Central nervous system: Headache, coma, seizures, dizziness

Dermatologic: Skin discoloration (blue-black)

Gastrointestinal: Nausea

Genitourinary: Urine discoloration (dark)

Hematologic: Methemoglobin formation (postexposure from 30 minutes to 12 hours), hemolytic anemia

Hepatic: Hepatomegaly, elevated liver function test results

Neuromuscular & skeletal: Paresthesia

Ocular: Retrobulbar neuritis, optic neuropathy

Respiratory: Respiratory failure, bitter almond breath, apnea

Admission Criteria/Prognosis Any patient with change in mental status, cardiopulmonary complaints, or methemoglobin levels >30% should be admitted; asymptomatic patients with methemoglobin levels <30% may be considered for discharge after 6 hours of observation and if methemoglobin levels fall to <15%

Toxicodynamics/Kinetics

Absorption: Inhalation: 80% to 87%. Oral, dermal: ~50%

Half-life: 84 hours (of metabolites)

Metabolism: Primarily intestinal reduction to nitrosobenzene, phenylhydroxylamine, and aniline

Elimination: Primarily renal (within first 2 hours) in the forms of para-aminophenol and para-nitrophenol (most toxic metabolite)

Overdosage/Treatment

Decontamination: **Oral:** Lavage (within 1 hour)/activated charcoal. **Dermal:** Wash with soap and water. **Ocular:** Irrigate copiously with saline.

Supportive therapy: Treat symptomatic methemoglobinemia with methylene blue. Seizures can be treated with benzodiazepines or phenobarbital.

Enhancement of elimination: Exchange transfusion has been utilized in an adult for 6 hours, to reduce severe methemoglobinemia from 65% to 25% levels.

Additional Information

Fatal oral dose: 1 g

Higher airborne concentrations of nitrobenzene (up to 0.1 ppb) are noted in summer than in winter. Methemoglobinemia can develop after exposure of 3-6 ppm for several hours.

Odor threshold (almond-like): Water: 0.11 mg/L. Air: 0.092 mg/m^3. PEL-TWA: 1 ppm; TLV-TWA: 1 ppm; IDLH: 200 ppm. Atmospheric half-life: 6 months to 6 years

Specific References

Chang AS, Morgan BW, Birkholz DA, et al, "A Case Report and Laboratory Analysis of Fatal Methemoglobinemia After Ingestion of Nitrobenzene," *Clin Toxicol (Phila)*, 2005, 43:746.

Martinez MA, Ballesteros S, Almarza E, et al, "Acute Nitrobenzene Poisoning with Severe Associated Methemoglobinemia: Identification in Whole Blood by GC-FID and GC-MS," *J Anal Toxicol*, 2003, 27(4):221-5.

Nitroethane

CAS Number 79-24-3

UN Number 2842

Use Industrial solvent found in artificial nail removers

Mechanism of Toxic Action A mucosal irritant which can produce methemoglobinemia in 6-12 hours postexposure; a potent oxidizing agent

Signs and Symptoms of Overdose Cyanosis, dyspnea, methemoglobinemia

Admission Criteria/Prognosis Observe any ingestion for 24 hours

Toxicodynamics/Kinetics

Half-life: 6 hours

Metabolism: To nitrite by the liver and GI tract

Overdosage/Treatment

Decontamination: **Oral:** Do not induce emesis. **Inhalation:** Administer 100% humidified oxygen.

Supportive therapy: Methylene blue (1-2 mg/kg/dose I.V.) for symptomatic methemoglobinemia

Antidote(s)

• Methylene Blue [ANTIDOTE]

Diagnostic Procedures

• Methemoglobin, Blood

Additional Information A colorless liquid with a fruity odor. IDLH: 1000 ppm

Nitrofen

CAS Number 1836-75-7

U.S. Brand Names Mezotox®; Niclofen®; Nip®; Nitrochlor®; Tokkorn® Trixilin®; Tok®

Synonyms Nitrofene

Mechanism of Toxic Action A diphenyl ether which can cause photobleaching and has phytotoxic effects by interfering with ATP synthesis

Signs and Symptoms of Overdose Diarrhea, dizziness, headache, nausea, vomiting; eye, skin, and lung irritation

Overdosage/Treatment Decontamination: Remove contaminated clothing (especially leather); wash thoroughly with soap and water. Irrigate eyes with normal saline for ocular exposure.

Nitrogen Dioxide

CAS Number 10102-44-0

UN Number 1067

Synonyms Nitrogen Peroxide

Commonly Found In Exhaust from metal cleaning, electric arc welding

Use Found in grain storage silos (levels as high as 2000 ppm), encountered in welding, production of fuels

Mechanism of Toxic Action Pulmonary lipid auto-oxidation and free radical reactions with proliferation of pulmonary Type II cells

Adverse Reactions

Cardiovascular: Weak, rapid pulse; cardiovascular collapse

Central nervous system: Hyperthermia

Dermatologic: Hair discoloration

Gastrointestinal: Acid taste

Respiratory: Pulmonary edema, asphyxia, asthma, bronchospasm

Signs and Symptoms of Overdose Bronchiolitis obliterans (may develop 2-6 weeks postexposure), bronchospasm, cough, dyspnea, fever, leukocytosis, methemoglobin (possible), ocular irritation, pulmonary edema (may be delayed for 30 hours)

Admission Criteria/Prognosis Admit all patients with pulmonary symptomatology

Toxicodynamics/Kinetics

Absorption: Through the lungs

Metabolism: Reacts in pulmonary tract to form nitric acid

Monitoring Parameters Arterial blood gas, methemoglobin, chest x-ray

Overdosage/Treatment

Decontamination: Inhalation: Administer 100% humidified oxygen.

Supportive therapy: Directed at the pulmonary system. Although it has been advocated to give corticosteroids early on (ie, 1 g of methylprednisolone), no data from controlled trials are available. Hyperbaric oxygen was detrimental in one animal model. Ascorbic acid (1 g orally) or deferoxamine has been proposed for respiratory protection, although these modalities have not been studied in humans. Symptomatic methemoglobinemia should be treated with methylene blue.

Antidote(s)

• Methylene Blue [ANTIDOTE]

Diagnostic Procedures

• Methemoglobin, Blood

Additional Information

Death: 100 ppm.

Mucous membrane irritation: 13 ppm. Pulmonary irritation: 25 ppm (at 1 hour). Pulmonary edema: 50-100 ppm (at 1 hour)

A reddish-brown gas which is formed by nitrates in corn, hay, or alfalfa by anaerobic fermentation; concentrations in silos: 200-2000 ppm of nitrogen dioxide

Poorly water soluble. Specific gravity: 1.45 (liquid); 1.58 (gas). Odor threshold: 1-5 ppm. IDLH: 50 ppm; TLV-TWA: 3 ppm.

Specific References

Nitschke M, Pilutto LS, Attewell RG, et al, , "A Cohort Study of Indoor Nitrogen Dioxide and House Dust Mite Exposure in Asthmatic Children," *J Occup Environ Med*, 2006, 48:462-9.

Witten A, Solomon C, Abbritti E, et al, "Effects of Nitrogen Dioxide on Allergic Airway Responses in Subjects with Asthma," *J Occup Environ med*, 2005, 47:1250-9.

Nitromethane

CAS Number 75-52-5

UN Number 1261

Use Constituent found in fuels for model aircraft engines and dragsters; solvent also used for rocket fuel; component in fuel-based fires

Mechanism of Toxic Action A lipid soluble solvent with relatively low toxicity; animal studies reveal sciatic nerve degeneration; a mild irritant

Signs and Symptoms of Overdose Bronchospasm, cough, local eye or dermal irritation, Parkinson-like motor dysfunction (chronic exposure)

Overdosage/Treatment

Decontamination: **Dermal:** Wash skin with soap and water. **Inhalation:** Administer 100% humidified oxygen. **Ocular:** Irrigate eyes with water.

Supportive therapy: Inhaled sympathomimetic bronchodilators should be used to treat bronchospasm.

Test Interactions Will produce false elevation of serum creatinine by the Jaffé-based assay; a nitromethane serum concentration of 5 μmol/L (which will result in minimal symptoms) can result in a serum creatinine of ~18 mg/dL.

Additional Information A colorless oily liquid with a fruity odor. Solution pH: 6.1. IDLH: 1000 ppm; PEL-TWA: 100 ppm. Odor threshold: <200 ppm

Specific References

Cook MD and Clark RF, "Creatinine Elevation Associated with Nitromethane Exposure: The Experience of One Poison Control System," *Clin Toxicol (Phila)*, 2005, 43:697.

Mell HK, Lintner CP, and Sztajnkrycer MD, "Artifactually Elevated Serum Creatinine Determination After Nitromethane Ingestion," *Clin Toxicol (Phila)*, 2005, 43:660.

Nitrophenol

Applies to Dye Stuffs and Pigments (Production); Fungicide; Laboratory Reagent

CAS Number 100-02-7 (4-Nitrophenol); 88-75-5 (2-Nitrophenol)

UN Number 1663

U.S. Brand Names Atonik®

Use Primarily as a laboratory reagent, fungicide, and in production of dye stuffs and pigments; 4-nitrophenol is a metabolite of nitrobenzene

Mechanism of Toxic Action Formation of methemoglobinemia

Adverse Reactions No experience in humans; animals develop methemoglobinemia; stomatitis is also noted; skin discoloration (blue-black) hyperthermia may occur

Toxicodynamics/Kinetics

Absorption: Probably by inhalation, oral, or dermal exposure

Metabolism: Hepatic to glucuronide or sulfate conjugates

Elimination: Renal within 48 hours

Reference Range Urinary 4-nitrophenol levels in general population is <10 mcg/L; may also be noted in nitrobenzene, methyl, or ethyl parathione exposures

Overdosage/Treatment

Decontamination: **Oral:** Lavage (within 1 hour)/activated charcoal. **Dermal:** Wash with soap and water. **Ocular:** Irrigate with saline.

Supportive therapy: Methylene blue for symptomatic methemoglobinemia. Treat hyperthermia with sponge baths, ice pack and cool oral fluids. Avoid salicylates and atropine.

Additional Information 4-nitrophenol is more toxic than 2-nitrophenol. Vehicular exhaust contains 3.1 ppb of 2-nitrophenol. Atmospheric half-life: 18 days. Water half-life (photolysis): 1-13 days (longer with high pH)

Nitrophenolurea

Synonyms PNU; Pyriminil; Vacor

Mechanism of Toxic Action Interferes with nicotinamide metabolism resulting in pancreatic beta-cell destruction

Adverse Reactions

Cardiovascular: Chest pain, shock

Central nervous system: Neuropathic, chills

Endocrine & metabolic: Diabetes mellitus, hyperinsulinemia

Neuromuscular & skeletal: Peripheral neuropathy

Signs and Symptoms of Overdose GI irritation, hyperglycemia with or without ketoacidosis, hypotension

Admission Criteria/Prognosis Any patient with change in mental status, cardiopulmonary complaints, or methemoglobin levels >30% should be admitted; asymptomatic patients with methemoglobin levels <30% may be considered for discharge after 6 hours of observation and if methemoglobin levels fall to <15%

Overdosage/Treatment

Decontamination: Emesis within 30 minutes or lavage within 1 hour, followed by oral activated charcoal

Supportive therapy: Nicotinamide (also known as niacinamide) (I.M., I.V.): 500 mg loading dose followed by doses of 100-200 mg I.M. or I.V. every 4 hours for 48 hours. Orally, patient may take 100 mg nicotinamide 3-5 times/day for 2 weeks; children can be given half the adult dose. Insulin may be needed for hyperglycemia.

Supportive therapy: Diabetes: Insulin and fluids

Diagnostic Procedures

• Anion Gap, Blood

Additional Information Withdrawn in U.S. as general use pesticide in 1979; smells like peanuts; yellow color appears like cornmeal

Nitrous Oxide

Applies to Anesthetic; Foaming Agent; Rocket Fuel

CAS Number 10024-97-2

UN Number 1020

Synonyms Factitious Air; Laughing Gas; Nitrogen Monoxide; Whippet

Use As an anesthetic, foaming agent, and rocket fuel

Mechanism of Action General CNS depressant action; may act similarly as inhalant general anesthetics by stabilizing axonal membranes to partially inhibit action potentials leading to sedation; may partially act on opiate receptor systems to cause mild analgesia; central sympathetic stimulating action supports blood pressure, systemic vascular resistance, and cardiac output; it does not depress carbon dioxide drive to breath. Nitrous oxide increases cerebral blood flow and intracranial pressure while decreasing hepatic and renal blood flow; has analgesic action similar to morphine.

Mechanism of Toxic Action Asphyxiant; oxidizes cobalt in vitamin B_{12}; partial agonist of opioid receptors

Adverse Reactions

Cardiovascular: Hypotension, arrhythmias, AV dissociation, cerebral edema

Central nervous system: CNS depression, ataxia

Hematologic: Bone marrow suppression, methemoglobin formation, aplastic anemia (chronic use)

Neuromuscular & skeletal: Neuropathy (peripheral), myeloneuropathies

Miscellaneous: Potential carcinogen

Signs and Symptoms of Overdose Agranulocytosis, dizziness, dyspnea, euphoria, headache, leukopenia, mood disorder, neuritis, nausea and vomiting (rarely); possible pneumothorax by barotrauma

Pharmacodynamics/Kinetics

Onset of action: Inhalation: 2-5 minutes

Absorption: Rapid via lungs; blood/gas partition coefficient is 0.47

Metabolism: Body: <0.004%

Excretion: Primarily exhaled gases; skin (minimal amounts)

Contraindications Hypersensitivity to nitrous oxide or any component of the formulation; nitrous oxide should not be administered without oxygen; should not be given to patients after a full meal

Warnings Nausea and vomiting occurs postoperatively in ~15% of patients. Prolonged use may produce bone marrow suppression and/or neurologic dysfunction. Oxygen should be briefly administered during emergence from prolonged anesthesia with nitrous oxide to prevent diffusion hypoxia. Patients with vitamin B_{12} deficiency (pernicious anemia) and those with other nutritional deficiencies (alcoholics) are at increased risk of developing neurologic disease and bone marrow suppression with exposure to nitrous oxide. May be addictive.

Dosing Forms Supplied in blue cylinders

Dosage Forms Supplied in blue cylinders

Reference Range Arterial blood nitrous oxide concentrations associated with surgical anesthesia range from 170-220 mL/L

Overdosage/Treatment Supportive therapy: Give 100% humidified oxygen. Hyperventilation and 20% mannitol for cerebral edema; dexamethasone may be useful. Naloxone may reverse analgesic action; avoid epinephrine. Treat symptomatic methemoglobinemia with methylene blue. Replace vitamin B_{12} as needed for chronic exposures. Do not administer hyperbaric oxygen. Pretreatment with methylcobalamin (5 mg I.V.) 2 hours postanesthesia induction and folinic acid (15 mg I.V.) at end of anesthesia has been hematoprotective.

Antidote(s)

• Methylene Blue [ANTIDOTE]

• Naloxone [ANTIDOTE]

Drug Interactions No data reported

Pregnancy Risk Factor No data reported

Additional Information Minimal toxic dose by inhalation: 24 mg/kg over 2 hours. Chronic inhalation may result in pancytopenia. Colorless, sweet odor. TLV-TWA: 50 ppm. Nitrous oxide cylinders are painted blue.

N-Methyl-2-Pyrrolidone

CAS Number 872-50-4

Synonyms M-Pyrol; Methylpyrrolidone; NMP

Use A dipolar solvent used in microelectronics (cleaning of silicon chips, deflashing); in petroleum industry (natural gas, acetylene and toluene recovery); paint strippers (replacing methylene chloride); and in wire coating operations

Mechanism of Toxic Action A cyclic amide with mucosal irritant properties; can cause encephalopathy; also is a weak acetylcholinesterase inhibitor

Adverse Reactions

Headaches and eye irritation at air levels as low as 0.7 ppm for 30-minute exposure

Dermatologic: Contact dermatitis, pruritus, vesicular dermal eruptions

Toxicodynamics/Kinetics

Absorption: Dermal and inhalation routes

Metabolism: Hepatic hydrolysis

Elimination: Renal

Overdosage/Treatment Decontamination: **Dermal:** Flush with soap and water. **Ocular:** Irrigate copiously with saline.

Additional Information Colorless liquid with a mild odor; can penetrate latex gloves. Density: 1.027. Vapor density: 3.4

N-Nitrosodiphenylamine

Applies to TJB

CAS Number 86-30-6

U.S. Brand Names Curetard A®; Delac J®; Naugard TJB®; Redax®; Retarder J®; Vulcatard A®

Synonyms Diphenylnitrosamine; NDPA; NDPHA

Use Retardant (to prevent premature volcanization of rubber) in rubber processing industry

Mechanism of Toxic Action DNA adduct formation in bladder may be the mechanism for urinary bladder cancer

Adverse Reactions No human toxic effects described; toxic effects in animals appear to be carcinogenesis (bladder) and skin ulcerations on dermal contact (0.1 mL of 0.1% solution for 20 weeks); nephrotoxicity has also been noted; does not bioaccumulate

Toxicodynamics/Kinetics

Absorption: Oral and dermal

Metabolism: Hepatic denitrosation to diphenylamine and nitric oxide

Elimination: Primarily renal within 2 days

Overdosage/Treatment Decontamination: **Oral:** Lavage (within 1 hour)/activated charcoal. **Dermal:** Wash with soap and water. **Ocular:** Irrigate with saline.

Additional Information Soluble in water (40 mg/L). Atmospheric half-life: ~7 hours.

Adding wheat straw in soil to increase microbial activity reduces soil residence time from 30 days to 10 days. Tire chemical factories may have workplace air levels as high as 6 ppm (47 mcg/m^3).

Osmium

CAS Number 20816-12-0
UN Number 2471
Synonyms Osmic Acid; Osmium Tetroxide; Parosmic Acid
Mechanism of Toxic Action Direct irritant to mucous membranes, skin, eyes
Adverse Reactions Eyes, nose, throat, neurologic, gastrointestinal, dermatologic
Signs and Symptoms of Overdose Angina, chest pain, conjunctivitis, cough, dermatitis, headache, pulmonary edema, respiratory tract irritation, rhinitis, visual changes, wheezing
Toxicodynamics/Kinetics No human ingestions reported
Overdosage/Treatment
Decontamination: Remove patient from toxic environment, administer 100% humidified oxygen. Provide ventilatory assistance if needed. Decontaminate skin and eyes with water.
Supportive therapy: Treat wheezing with bronchodilators. The role of steroids is equivocal in the prevention of pulmonary edema.
Additional Information Concentration of 0.1 mg/m^3 associated with ocular irritation. Direct contact may cause green-black discoloration of skin. No harmful effects at 0.001 mg/m^3 for 6 hours (ACGIH 1986). TCLO (human): 133 mcg/m^3 lacrimation; 1 ppm = 10 mg/m^3. TLV-TWA: 0.002 ppm; TLV-STEL: 0.0006 ppm; OSHA PEL-TWA: 0.002 mg/m^3

Palladium

CAS Number 7440-05-3
Mechanism of Toxic Action Colloidal palladium hydroxides cause RBC hemolysis; chronic intoxication results in malignant lung tumor and decreased growth
Adverse Reactions
Dermatologic: Dermal irritant, dermatitis
Respiratory: Inhalation: Wheezing, asthma
Signs and Symptoms of Overdose Classic signs/symptoms of allergic reaction; cough, eczema, eosinophilia, dyspnea, lymphocytosis, rash, rhinorrhea, urticaria, wheezing
Toxicodynamics/Kinetics Absorption: Poor from gastrointestinal tract
Reference Range No TLV recommended
Overdosage/Treatment
Decontamination: Irrigation
Supportive therapy: Beta agonists can be used for wheezing.
Additional Information Causes black discoloration at site of injection; water soluble

Para-Dichlorobenzene

Applies to Fumigant (Mold/Mildew); Moth Repellent; Pesticide; Toilet Deodorant
CAS Number 106-46-7
UN Number 1592
U.S. Brand Names Paracide®; Paradow; Paramoth; Santochlor
Synonyms 1,4-Dichlorobenzene; Dichloricide; PDB
Use Toilet/refuse deodorant; mold and mildew fumigant; moth repellent; diaper pail repellent; pesticide (for tree boring insects and ants); control blue mold in tobacco seed beds
Mechanism of Toxic Action Mucosal irritant due to necrosis of tissue proteins by epoxide intermediates which are nephrotoxic and hepatotoxic by promoting cellular degeneration and vacuolation
Adverse Reactions
Central nervous system: Cerebellar ataxia
Dermatologic: Allergic purpura, dermal burns, skin edema, hyperpigmentation
Hematological: Hemolysis/methemoglobin formation (especially in children), granuloma development
Hepatic: Hepatitis and hepatic necrosis with cirrhosis
Ocular: Eye irritation (at 80-160 ppm)
Renal: Glomerulonephritis, alpha 2u-globulin nephropathy
Signs and Symptoms of Overdose Acute hemolytic anemia, ataxia, cirrhosis, diarrhea, dyspnea, headache, hepatic necrosis, jaundice, methemoglobinemia, nausea, oral burning, petechiae, pulmonary granulomas (upon inhalation), purpura, slurred speech, vomiting
Toxicodynamics/Kinetics
Absorption: By dermal routes, and: Inhalation: 20%. Oral: 100%
Metabolism: Hepatic: Oxidation to 2,5-dichlorophenol and 2,3-dichloroquinol
Elimination: Renal and biliary
Monitoring Parameters Methemoglobin level, CBC, liver function test
Reference Range Urine 2,5-dichlorophenol level range of 90-100 mg/L associated with air para-dichlorobenzene levels of 33 ppm; mean urinary 2,5-dichlorophenol in nonoccupationally exposed subjects is 2 mg/L; whole blood paradichlorobenzene levels averaging 10 mcg/L associated with Tokyo residents; mean blood level of 1,4-dichlorobenzene is 3.2 ng/L in nonsmokers and 2.2 ng/L in smokers.

Overdosage/Treatment
Decontamination: **Oral**: Emesis within 30 minutes (>5 g ingestion) or lavage (within 1 hour) in conjunction with activated charcoal may be utilized. **Do not** dilute with milk. **Dermal**: Wash with soap and water; remove contaminated clothing. **Ocular**: Irrigate with saline.
Supportive therapy: Treat symptomatic methemoglobinemia (or methemoglobinemia >30%) with methylene blue.
Antidote(s)
• Methylene Blue [ANTIDOTE]
Diagnostic Procedures
• Methemoglobin, Blood
Additional Information
A nasal irritant at air levels >50 ppm.
Strongly radiopaque aromatic odor with an odor threshold of 0.2 ppm in air and 0.01 mg/L in water.
Average adult exposure: 35 mcg/day by inhalation and 0.2 mcg/day through drinking water
For drinking water, median dichlorobenzene levels are ∼0.03 ppb; mean soil level is ∼0.4 ppb.
Milk or fatty foods promote oral absorption.
Soft drink and milk samples contained 0.1 mcg/kg (ppb), while butter, margarine, peanut butter, flour, and pastry mix contained concentrations of 1.3-2.7 mcg/kg, 12.2-14.5 mcg/kg, 7.3 mcg/kg, and 22 mcg/kg (ppb), respectively.
PEL-TWA: 77 ppm; IDLH: 1000 ppm
Mean indoor air dichlorobenzene concentration is ∼4 ppb.

Levels of 1,4-dichlorobenzene Detected in Workplace Air

Occupation	Concentration (ppm)	
	Maximum	Range
Monochlorobenzene manufacturing plant	8.3	5.48-8.63
Abrasive-wheel plant	16.43	7.97-16.43
Mothball manufacturing plant	24.90	8.96-24.90
Chlorobenzene manufacturing plant	33.86	23.90-33.86
1,4-Dichlorobenzene manufacturing plant	548	11.95-548
Monochlorobenzene and dichlorobenzene manufacturing plant	722	—

Source: IARC 1982
Reference: U.S. Department of Health and Human Services, *Toxicological Profile for 1,4-Dichlorobenzene*, Agency for Toxic Substances and Disease Registry, December, 1998.

Paramethoxyamphetamine

Synonyms 4-Methoxyamphetamine; PMA
Impairment Potential Blood PMA levels >0.09 mg/L are associated with driving impairment
Use A recreational hallucinogen found primarily in Australia and Western Europe
Mechanism of Toxic Action A methoxylated phenethylamine with sympathomimetic actions
Admission Criteria/Prognosis Admit any patient with elevated temperature or ingestion >100 mg.
Toxicodynamics/Kinetics
Metabolism: Hepatic demethylation to 4-hydroxyamphetamine
Elimination: Urine
Dosing Forms
Capsule: 80 mg, 90 mg
Tablet: 50 mg, 60 mg, 90 mg
Reference Range
Hallucinogenic effects seen with PMA blood levels: 0.4 mg/L
Toxic effects seen with PMA levels: >0.5 mg/L
Fatality associated with levels >1 mg/L
Overdosage/Treatment
Decontamination: Gastric decontamination should be considered for any ingestion >100 mg; lavage within 1 hour; activated charcoal should be given.
Supportive therapy: Severe hyponatremia (serum sodium <120 mM/L) can be treated with either continuous infusion of 0.9% normal saline or 3% normal saline at 50 mL/hour, with furosemide 40 mg twice daily. Seizures should be treated with a benzodiazepine or barbiturate. Hyperthermia should be aggressively treated with cooling blankets, ice packs, and cooling fans. The role of chlorpromazine, cyproheptadine, dantrolene, or beta-adrenergic blockers is uncertain in treating hyperthermia. Ventricular arrhythmias may respond to lidocaine. Benzodiazepines can be given for agitation. Nitroprusside or phentolamine can be given for hypertensive emergency. Hypotension should be treated with crystalloid fluids. Hypertension can be treated with an alpha-

blocker (phentolamine) and beta-adrenergic blocker. Esmolol may be useful in treating tachyarrhythmias.

Additional Information Hallucinogenic dose: 50 mg

Specific References

Caldicott DG, Edwards NA, Kruys A, et al, "Dancing with 'Death': P-Methoxyamphetamine Overdose and Its Acute Management," *J Toxicol Clin Toxicol*, 2003, 41(2):143-54.

Dams R, De Letter EA, Mortier KA, et al, "Fatality Due to Combined Use of the Designer Drugs MDMA and PMA: A Distribution Study," *J Anal Toxicol*, 2003, 27(5):318-22.

Johansen SS, Hansen AC, Muller IB, et al, "Three Fatal Cases of PMA and PMMA Poisoning in Denmark," *J Anal Toxicol*, 2003, 27(4):253-6.

Kalasinsky K, Dixon M, and Kish S, "PMA Overdose Case: Examination of Blood, Brain, and Hair," *J Anal Toxicol*, 2003, 27:199.

Paraphenylenediamine

CAS Number 106-50-3; 624-18-0

UN Number 1673

Synonyms Paradiaminobenzene; PPD; "Blackstones"

Use Black dye used on fur or as a hair dye, photographic developer, and as a chemical intermediate in the production of polyparaphenylene terephthalamide

Mechanism of Toxic Action Aniline derivative; can cause muscle necrosis through free radical production; ~4% of individuals can develop allergic reactions

Adverse Reactions

Cardiovascular: Hypotension, shock, facial edema, myocarditis

Central nervous system: Vertigo

Dermatologic: Erythema multiforme, skin necrosis, hyperkeratosis

Gastrointestinal: Vomiting, abdominal pain

Hematologic: Methemoglobinemia

Hepatic: Hepatic necrosis

Neuromuscular & skeletal: Tremor, rhabdomyolysis

Ocular: Lacrimation, exophthalmos, proptosis, iritis, optic neuritis, cataract, conjunctival erythema

Renal: Acute tubular necrosis, oliguria, proximal tubular degeneration

Respiratory: Dyspnea, bronchospasm, wheezing

Miscellaneous: Laryngeal edema, anaphylaxis

Toxicodynamics/Kinetics Absorption: Orally; <1% absorbed by dermal route

Monitoring Parameters Urinalysis, CPK, renal function tests

Overdosage/Treatment

Decontamination: **Oral: Do not** administer ipecac for oral ingestion; activated charcoal can be administered. **Dermal:** Wash with soap and water. **Ocular:** Irrigate copiously with saline.

Supportive therapy: Intravenous fluid hydration and diuretics should be given for treatment of myoglobinuria. Standard antianaphylaxis therapy can be administered.

Additional Information

Ingestion of 1.8 g associated with acute renal failure in an adult

White to light purple crystals. IDLH: 25 mg/m³; TLV-TWA: 0.1 mg/m³

Cosmetic use is common in Sudan, India, Israel, Pakistan, and Morocco, but is not permitted in the U.S.

Paraquat

Related Information

- Diquat Dibromide
- Toxins Which Should Be Lavaged with Solutions Other Than Water

Applies to Herbicide

CAS Number 1910-42-5; 2074-50-2; 4685-14-7

Synonyms 1,1′-Dimethyl-4,4′-Dipyridilium Ion; Dimethyl Viologen; Gamoxone; PP-148; PP-190

Commonly Found In Crisquat; Dextrone; Dexuron; Esgran; Goldquat 276; Gramoxone; Hebaxon; Osaquat Super; Sweep

Mechanism of Toxic Action

Usually in a 20% solution; a quaternary nitrogen compound which can produce photobleaching by destroying plant cellular membrane; can also inhibit photosynthesis; pulmonary toxicity involves xanthine oxidase

Adverse Reactions

Cardiovascular: Vasodilatation

Central nervous system: No acute neurological signs, hyperthermia

Dermatologic: Dermal irritation, fingernail atrophy, fingernail loss, Mees' lines, fingernail discoloration (brown), fingernail dystrophy, burns, blisters

Gastrointestinal: Nausea, vomiting, GI ulceration, pancreatitis, dysphagia

Hematologic: Hemolytic anemia

Hepatic: Centrilobular hepatic necrosis

Neuromuscular & skeletal: Rhabdomyolysis

Ocular: Corneal edema (by ocular contact)

Renal: Myoglobinuria

Respiratory: Cough, pulmonary fibrosis, nasal bleeding with inhalation, acute respiratory distress syndrome

Signs and Symptoms of Overdose

Group I, mild poisoning (<20 mg/kg): Diarrhea, nausea, vomiting

Group II, moderate poisoning (20-40 mg/kg): Diarrhea, pulmonary fibrosis, immediate vomiting, renal/hepatic failure - death in 2 weeks

Group III, severe poisoning (>40 mg/kg): Diarrhea, immediate vomiting, oropharyngeal ulceration with cardiac, respiratory, hepatic, and renal failure - death usually within 1-4 days

Admission Criteria/Prognosis Patients with known or suspected exposures should be admitted

Toxicodynamics/Kinetics

Absorption: Dermal absorption can occur through skin that is not intact.

Oral absorption: 30%

Distribution: V_d: 1.2-1.6 L/kg

Half-life: 12-120 hours

Elimination: Renal

Reference Range Severity index of paraquat poisoning (SIPP) is determined by multiplying the elapsed time (hours) from ingestion to arrival, by the serum paraquat level (in mg/L). A value >10 is indicative of a fatality. Plasma level of 3 mg/L associated with death

Overdosage/Treatment

Decontamination: Emesis (within 30 minutes)/lavage (within 1 hour) with activated charcoal, Fuller's earth (15%), or 7% bentonite (dose of Fuller's Earth or Bentonite: Children <12 years: 2 g/kg; Adults: 100-150 g). Sodium polystyrene sulfonate may also be effective.

Ocular: Irrigate with saline or water for at least 15 minutes

Dermal: Remove contaminated clothing and wash skin with copious amounts of soap and water. Skin damage may be delayed for 1-3 days. Systemic toxicity is rare from dermal exposure.

Supportive therapy:

Vomiting can be controlled with ondansetron 8 mg (5 mg/m³ in children) by slow I.V. injection or I.V. infusion over 15 minutes

Do not utilize oxygen in that it may promote pulmonary fibrosis. Monitor for hypercalcemia if Fuller's earth is used. Inhaled nitric oxide (at 25 ppm) has been used to treat ARDS. Nitric oxide inhalation (10-20 ppm) via BiPAP has been used successfully in case reports. Vitamin C (4000 mg/day) and vitamin E (250 mg/day), dexamethasone, cyclophosphamide, and acetylcysteine have been used to treat lung toxicity, but are of unproven benefit. As antioxidants, deferoxamine (100 mg/kg over 24 hours) and acetylcysteine (loading dose: 150 mg/kg then 300 mg/kg/day for 3 weeks) with hemodialysis (6 hours) have been utilized successfully in a massive paraquat ingestion (maximum serum paraquat level of 28 mcg/mL). High-dose cyclophosphamide (15 mg/kg I.V. the first day followed by 10 mg/kg on day two, 7 mg/kg on days 3-5 and 5 mg/kg daily until total dose is 4 g or leukocyte count is <3000/mm³), along with dexamethasone (1.5 mg/kg daily for first 4 days followed by 1 mg/kg on days 5-7 and 24 mg/day thereafter), has been used to increase survival in mild to severe paraquat poisoning, when used in conjunction with basic poison management. Morphine sulphate can be used for pain control. S-carboxymethylcysteine (20 mg/kg orally four times per day for 2-3 weeks) has been used, in conjunction with general supportive measures, successfully as an antioxidant.

Enhancement of elimination: Multiple dosing of activated charcoal, Fuller's earth (100-150 g in adults or 2 g/kg in children), or bentonite may be given every 2-4 hours. Charcoal hemoperfusion for prolonged periods of time (up to 10 hours) may be helpful if instituted within 10 hours. Forced diuresis is not helpful. Hemoperfusion clearance is estimated to be 57-156 mL/minute. Continuous arteriovenous hemodialysis/hemoperfusion (CAVHD-HP) can also result in nondetectable serum paraquat levels (without rebound) within 2-3 days after treatment. Paraquat clearance with CAVHD ranges from 730-2,145 mL/minute.

Diagnostic Procedures

- Paraquat, Blood

Additional Information Faint ammonia-like odor. Not well absorbed through intact skin but prolonged contact can cause systemic toxicity. Restrictive pulmonary dysfunction is a long-term sequelae following acute paraquat exposure. Dithionate test: 1 part urine, 0.5 part sodium dithionate in 1N NaOH: deep blue color indicates presence of paraquat or diquat. For additional information contact Syngenta: (800) 327-8633.

Specific References

Chomchai S and Chomchai C, "Treatment of Moderate to Severe Paraquat Poisoning with Vincristine and Dexamethasone," *J Toxicol Clin Toxicol*, 2003, 41(5):659.

Cope RB and Oncken A, "Fatal Paraquat Posioning in Seven Portland, Oregon Dogs," *Vet Hum Toxicol*, 2004, 46(5):258-9.

Goldberger BA, Merves ML, MacDougall KN, et al, "Paraquat in Exhumed Remains by Gas Chromatography-Mass Spectrometry," *J Anal Toxicol*, 2006, 30:135.

Hsu HH, Chang CT, and Lin JL, "Intravenous Paraquat Poisoning-Induced Multiple Organ Failure and Fatality - A Report of Two Cases," *J Toxicol Clin Toxicol*, 2003, 41(1):87-90.

Huang NC, Hung YM, Lin SL, et al, "Further Evidence of the Usefulness of Acute Physiology and Chronic Health Evaluation II Scoring System in Acute Paraquat Poisoning," *Clin Toxicol*, 2006, 44:99-102.

Hung YM, "Evaluation of Disease Severity Following Acute Paraquat Poisoning by Apache II Scores," *J Toxicol Clin Toxicol*, 2003, 41(5): 657.

Imbenotte M, Azaroual N, Cartigny B, et al, "Detection and Quantitation of Xenobiotics in Biological Fluids by 1H NMR Spectroscopy," *J Toxicol Clin Toxicol*, 2003, 41(7):955-62.

Jenq CC, Wu CD, and Lin JL, "Mother and Fetus Both Survive from Severe Paraquat Intoxication," *Clin Toxicol (Phila)*, 2005, 43(4):291-5.

Kim K, Suh G, Kwak Y, et al, "Hemoperfusion Using a Portable Dual Pulsatile Extracorporeal Life Support on Paraquat Intoxication," *Ann Emerg Med*, 2004, 44:S91.

Lin NC, Lin JL, Lin-Tan DT, et al, "Combined Initial Cyclophosphamide with Repeated Methylprednisolone Pulse Therapy for Severe Paraquat Poisoning from Dermal Exposure," *J Toxicol Clin Toxicol*, 2003, 41(6):877-81.

Lugo-Vallin N, Maradei-Irastorza I, Pascuzzo-Lima C, et al, "Thirty-five Cases of S-Carboxymethylcysteine Use in Paraquat Poisoning," *Vet Hum Toxicol*, 2003, 45(1):45-7.

Richardson JR, Quan Y, Sherer TB, et al, "Paraquat Neurotoxicity is Distinct from That of MPTP and Rotenone," *Toxicol Sci*, 2005, 88(1):193-201.

Wills BK, Aks SE, Maloney GE, et al, "The Effect of Amifostine, a Cytoprotective Agent, on Parquat Toxicity in Mice," *Clin Toxicol (Phila)*, 2005, 43:695.

Parathion

CAS Number 56-38-2
UN Number 2783; 2784
U.S. Brand Names Bay E-605®; Bladan F®; Orthophos®
Synonyms Ethyl Parathion; O,O-Diethyl O-p-Nitrophenyl Phosphorothioate
Mechanism of Toxic Action Potent, irreversible inhibition of acetylcholinesterase and plasma cholinesterase, resulting in excess accumulation of acetylcholine at muscarinic and nicotinic receptors, and in the central nervous system

Adverse Reactions
Cardiovascular: **Hyperdynamic** (~18% to 21%) or hypodynamic (~7% to 10%) states, edema, QT prolongation, Raynaud's phenomenon, sinus bradycardia, sinus tachycardia, torsade de pointes
Central nervous system: Depression, seizures, hyperactivity, cognitive dysfunction, hypothermia, extrapyramidal reactions
Dermatologic: Scleroderma
Endocrine & metabolic: Parotitis
Gastrointestinal: Pancreatitis
Genitourinary: Urinary incontinence
Neuromuscular & skeletal: Weakness (delayed), paralysis, delayed paresthesia, rhabdomyolysis, peripheral neuropathy
Ocular: Visual evoked potential abnormalities
Miscellaneous: Flu-like symptoms (especially with chronic exposure); intermediate syndrome

Signs and Symptoms of Overdose
Abdominal pain, agitation, AV block, asystole, bradycardia, bronchorrhea, coma, confusion, cranial nerve palsies, decreased hemoglobin, decreased platelet count, decreased red blood cell count, dementia, diaphragmatic paralysis, dysarthria, excessive sweating, fecal and urinary incontinence, garlic-like breath, generalized asthenia, headache, heart block, hypertension, hypotension, lacrimation, metabolic acidosis and hyperglycemia (severe intoxication), miosis (unreactive to light), mydriasis (rarely), nausea, nystagmus, pallor, pulmonary edema, QT prolongation, respiratory depression, salivation, seizures, skeletal muscle fasciculation and flaccid paralysis, tachycardia, tachypnea, vomiting

An "intermediate syndrome" of limb asthenia and respiratory paralysis has been reported to occur between 24 and 96 hours postorganophosphate exposure, and is independent of the acute cholinergic crisis. Late paresthesia characterized by stocking and glove paresthesia, anesthesia, and asthenia is infrequently observed weeks to months following acute exposure to certain organophosphates.

Admission Criteria/Prognosis Any symptomatic patient or an asymptomatic patient following a severe exposure should be admitted probably into an intensive care unit; asymptomatic patients following a moderate exposure can be discharged after 8 hours of observation

Toxicodynamics/Kinetics
Absorption: Readily through oral, dermal, or respiratory exposure
Metabolism: Rapidly metabolized to weakly active compounds through hepatic hydrolysis and other pathways
Elimination: Metabolites are excreted in urine as p-nitrophenol

Warnings/Precautions Risk of aspiration pneumonitis exists with agents having a hydrocarbon vehicle; severe laryngeal irritation and violent coughing may result from exposure to dusting powders; exposure to dusting powders and insecticide granules may cause contact dermatitis

Reference Range
Serum parathion levels in asymptomatic occupationally exposed worker range from 0.004-0.2 mg/L; urine p-nitrophenol levels in these individuals ranged from 0.4-13.2 mg/L; no correlation in cholinesterase (plasma or red blood cell) noted
Mild poisoning: Serum cholinesterase is 20% to 50% of normal;
Moderate poisoning: Serum cholinesterase is 10% to 20% of normal
Severe poisoning (respiratory distress and coma): Serum cholinesterase is <10%
Fatal parathion blood levels range from 0.5-34 mcg/mL; postmortem fat tissue parathion level: 6.5 mg/kg

Overdosage/Treatment
Decontamination: Isolation, bagging, and disposal of all contaminated clothing and other articles. All emergency medical workers and hospital staff should follow appropriate precautions regarding exposure to hazardous material including the use of protective clothing, masks, goggles, and respiratory equipment
Oral: Activated charcoal (without cathartic) can be administered either orally or via a nasogastric tube. **Do not** induce emesis because of danger of sudden respiratory compromise, alterations in mental status, seizures, coma, and possible aspiration of hydrocarbon vehicles.
Dermal: Prompt thorough scrubbing of all affected areas with soap and water, including hair and nails; 5% bleach can be used
Ocular: Irrigation with copious tepid sterile water or saline
Supportive therapy: Airway management, ventilatory assistance, humidified oxygen administration, and close monitoring for sudden respiratory failure; asoxime chloride may be useful when used with atropine
Enhancement of elimination: Exchange transfusion in adults: 500-2000 mL may be useful in severe poisoning. While hemodialysis has **not** been shown to be useful, charcoal hemoperfusion has produced a clearance of 59% of the blood flow. While parathion in itself is not dialyzable, its toxic metabolite paroxon can be removed by hemodialysis. Parathion and paroxon are also removable by hemoperfusion, although the clinical utility of these methods requires further investigation.
Antidote:
Atropine: Administration should be guided by respiratory status, starting at 2-5 mg I.V. every 5-10 minutes as needed, and should be titrated to the resolution of excess pulmonary secretions. Frequent administration of large doses (cumulative doses >100 mg) may be necessary in massive exposures.
Glycopyrrolate: May be administered if atropine is unavailable (200-400 mcg I.V. or I.M. initially, or ~$^1/_2$ the dose of atropine).
2-PAM: For more significant exposures (ie, exposures requiring large doses of atropine, or with recurring symptoms, or exposures to more lipid soluble agents), administration should follow: 1-2 g I.V. over 10-30 minutes, repeated in 1 hour if asthenia recurs, then every 4-12 hours for recurring symptoms.
Obidoxime: Adults: 250 mg I.V. bolus (slow) followed by continuous I.V. infusion at 750 mg/24 hours.

Antidote(s)
- Asoxime Chloride [ANTIDOTE]
- Atropine [ANTIDOTE]
- Pralidoxime [ANTIDOTE]

Diagnostic Procedures
- Creatinine, Serum
- Pesticide Screen, Chlorinated
- Pesticide Screen, Organophosphate
- Pseudocholinesterase, Serum

Drug Interaction Paralysis is potentiated by neuromuscular blockade (ie, pancuronium, vecuronium, succinylcholine, atracurium, doxacurium, mivacurium); inhibition of serum esterase prolongs the half-life of succinylcholine, cocaine, and other ester anesthetics; cholinergic toxicity is potentiated by cholinesterase inhibitors such as physostigmine

Additional Information
Lethal oral dose: Adults: 25 g;
Yellow to brown liquid with a garlic odor; thermal degradation products include sulfur, nitrogen, and phosphorus oxides; red blood cell cholinesterase, and serum pseudocholinesterase may be depressed following acute or chronic organophosphate exposure; RBC cholinesterase is typically not analyzed by in-house laboratories, and is usually not available for consideration during acute management. Pseudocholinesterase levels may be rapidly available from some in-house laboratories, but are not as reliable a marker of organophosphate exposure because of variability secondary to variant genotypes, hepatic disease, oral estrogen use, or malnutrition. Because of this variability, true indication of suppression of either of these enzymes can only be estimated through comparison to pre-exposure values; these enzymes may be useful in measuring a patient's recovery postexposure, especially if the recovery is not progressing as expected.
The intermediate syndrome is not related to delayed neuropathy.
Reactive when combined with endrin.
QT_c prolongation on ECG in the setting of organophosphate poisoning is associated with a high incidence of respiratory failure and mortality.
Water solubility: 12 ppm. Odor threshold: 0.04 ppm. Vapor pressure: 0.0004 mm Hg at 20°C

ACGIH TLV: 0.1 mg/m³; PEL-TWA: 0.1 mg/m³ IDLH: 20 mg/m³

Other information concerning pesticide exposures is available through the EPA-funded National Pesticide Telecommunications Network: 1-800-858-7378 (weekdays, 8 AM to 6 PM, Central Standard time)

Specific References

Beseler C and Stallones L, "Safety Practices, Neurological Symptoms, and Pesticide Poisoning," *J Occup Environ Med*, 2003, 45(10):1079-86.

Eyer F, Meischner V, Kiderlen D, et al, "Human Parathion Poisoning: A Toxicokinetic Analysis," *Toxicol Rev*, 2003, 22(3):143-63.

Gokel Y, Gulalp B, and Acikalin A, "Parotitis Due to Organophosphate Intoxication," *J Toxicol Clin Toxicol*, 2002, 40(5):563-5.

Pentaborane

CAS Number 19624-22-7
UN Number 1380
Synonyms Dihydropentaborane
Use Rocket propellant; reducing agents; gasoline additive
Mechanism of Toxic Action May deplete monoamine neurotransmitters in the central nervous system (inhibition of norepinephrine, dopamine and serotonin metabolism)

Adverse Reactions

Cardiovascular: Hypotension, tachycardia, fibrillation (atrial), flutter (atrial), sinus tachycardia, cerebral edema

Central nervous system: Hyperthermia, seizures, coma, increased intracranial pressure, opisthotonos, headache, hallucinations, dizziness, memory deficits, confusion, impaired concentration

Endocrine & metabolic: Increased serum transaminase levels, metabolic acidosis

Gastrointestinal: Garlic-like breath

Hepatic: Liver necrosis, fatty liver degeneration

Ocular: Cortical blindness

Neuromuscular & skeletal: Quadriplegia, tremor, muscle spasm

Renal: Myoglobinuria

Miscellaneous: Hiccups

Toxicodynamics/Kinetics Absorption: Oral, inhalation or dermal
Overdosage/Treatment

Decontamination: **Oral: Do not** induce emesis; lavage (within 1 hour)/ activated charcoal may be useful. **Dermal:** Use cool water. An exothermic reaction may develop, therefore, monitor for dermal burns. A 3% aqueous ammonia solution can also be used to complex the borane. **Inhalation:** Administer 100% oxygen. **Ocular:** Irrigate with saline or water.

Supportive therapy: Benzodiazepines can be used to treat seizures. Phenobarbital or phenytoin can be used to treat refractory seizures. Sodium bicarbonate (1-2 mEq/kg) can be used to treat acidosis.

Additional Information Colorless liquid with garlic-like odor. Can ignite spontaneously in air. Specific gravity: 0.61. Odor threshold: 0.8 ppm. TLV: 0.005 ppm; IDLH: 3 ppm

Pentachlorophenol

Applies to Disinfectant; Fungicide; Herbicide; Termiticide; Wood Preservative
CAS Number 87-86-5
UN Number 3155
U.S. Brand Names Chlon®; Dowicide® 7; Dura Treet® II; Fungifen®; Lauxtol®; Penta Ready®; Permasan®; Santophen® 20; Woodtreat®
Synonyms PCP; Penchlorol
Use Termiticide, fungicide, herbicide, and disinfectant; primarily used as a wood preservative, 0.1% concentration; restricted use pesticide
Mechanism of Toxic Action Uncouples oxidative phosphorylation; hexachlorobenzene, pentachlorobenzene, and hexachlorocyclobenzene all metabolize to pentachlorophenol

Adverse Reactions

Cardiovascular: Tachycardia, sinus tachycardia

Central nervous system: Seizures, hyperthermia

Dermatologic: Alopecia, urticaria

Endocrine & metabolic: Acidosis, polydipsia

Gastrointestinal: Nausea, vomiting

Hematologic: Hemolysis, aplastic anemia

Hepatic: Hepatotoxicity with elevated liver function test results

Neuromuscular & skeletal: Tremors, muscle spasms

Ocular: Mydriasis, retrobulbar neuritis

Renal: Nephrotoxicity (reduced glomerular filtration rate and tubular function)

Respiratory: Hyperventilation, pulmonary irritation

Miscellaneous: Dermal and ocular irritant (at levels in air >0.1 ppm), intense thirst, diaphoresis

Admission Criteria/Prognosis Symptomatic patients, urine pentachlorophenol levels >36 ppm, acidosis, hyperthermia, or electrolyte abnormalities should be admitted

Toxicodynamics/Kinetics

Absorption: Dermal: 62% in oil-based solution and 16% in aqueous based. Inhalation: 76% to 88%. Oral: Within 1.3 hours

Distribution: V_d: 0.35 L/kg

Protein binding: 99% in animal models

Metabolism: Hepatic conjugation to form a glucuronide and oxidative dechlorination to form tetrachloro-para-hydroquinone (TCHQ)

Half-life: 13-19 days (ethanol solution); 30 hours (sodium salt)

Elimination: Renal (~78% as pentachlorophenol and 12% as pentachlorophenol glucuronide)

Reference Range

Mean blood pentachlorophenol level in patients with neurological symptoms: 22 mcg/L (range: 4-60 mcg/L); people living in log homes can have 10 times the blood levels than general population (420 ppb vs 40 ppb, respectively); adipose tissue levels in general population: 26.3 mcg/kg; baseline urine pentachlorophenol level in general population: 3.4 ppb; for residents of log homes: 69 ppb; mean urinary daily excretion of pentachlorophenol: ~4.3 nmol

Mean pentachlorophenol urine level of 153 mg/L (range 28-520 mg/L) associated with fatal poisoning

Overdosage/Treatment

Decontamination: **Oral:** Lavage within 1 hour of exposure. Cholestyramine can be effective in adsorbing this agent. **Dermal:** Remove all contaminated clothing; wash with soap and water. **Ocular:** Copious irrigation with saline

Supportive: Cool with external methods. Avoid use of aspirin or atropine. Diazepam can be used for muscle spasm.

Enhancement of elimination: Exchange transfusion may be effective in infants. Due to enterohepatic recirculation, multiple dosing of cholestyramine (4 g every 8 hours) may be effective. Dialysis, forced diuresis, or hemoperfusion is not useful. Plasmapheresis may be useful.

Additional Information

Lethal oral dose: 1 g (~17 mg/kg); profound rigor mortis can be observed immediately after death

Concentrations >10% can cause dermal irritation

Usually contaminated with chlorinated dibenzo-para-dioxins.

WHO guideline for drinking water is 10 mcg/L.

Dairy products, grains, and cereals have highest levels of this agent

Daily dietary intake: ~1.5 mg. Daily drinking water intake: 0.02-24 mcg

Inhalation exposure of general U.S. population: 12-136 mcg/day; residents of log homes: 140-157 mcg/day due primarily to treated logs (although this agent is no longer used for this purpose); sealers decrease this concentration significantly

Soil samples within one foot of treated utility poles: 3-654 ppm

PEL-TWA (skin): 0.5 mg/m³; IDLH: 150 mg/m³. Half-life in soil: 2-4 weeks

Year-End 1999 Emergency Department Drug Abuse Warning Network (DAWN) data: Emergency Department mentions for PCP/PCP combinations remained relatively stable between 1998 (4033 mentions) and 1999 (4969 mentions). Mentions of PCP/PCP combinations in 1999 were 6% lower than in 1992 (5282 mentions).

Specific References

Proudfoot AT, "Pentachlorophenol Poisoning," *Toxicol Rev*, 2003, 22(1):3-11.

Pepper Spray

CAS Number 404-86-4 (capsaicin)
Use Riot control; active ingredient in tear gas
Mechanism of Toxic Action Lacrimator - irritation due to the active halogen group reacting with sulfhydryl groups; contains the mucosal irritant oleoresin of capsicum (which stimulates pain fibers) in a 1% to 10% concentration.

Adverse Reactions

Dermatologic: Vesiculation of skin (rare)

Ocular: **Ocular burning (56%)**, blepharospasms, cataract, **conjunctival irritation (44%), lacrimation (16%)**, corneal abrasion

Respiratory: Bronchospasm (may be delayed for 36 hours), pulmonary edema (may be delayed for 24 hours)

Overdosage/Treatment

Decontamination: Move patient to fresh air and monitor for wheezing. Personnel should avoid contaminating themselves. Wash skin with soap and water. Avoid rubbing of eyes as it may prolong effect. Copious irrigation is needed.

Supportive therapy: Solution of antacid (magnesium hydroxide - aluminum hydroxide - simethicone) gently blotted topically over exposed facial areas (avoiding eyes) may help resolve symptoms.

Additional Information Exists as a white solid
Specific References

Swami RH, Judge BS, and Furbee RB, "Accidental Ingestion of Cayenne Pepper Sauce Requiring Prolonged Ventilatory Support," *J Toxicol Clin Toxicol*, 2003, 41(5):653.

Petroleum Distillates - Naphtha

CAS Number 8030-30-6
UN Number 2553
Synonyms Benzin; Painters' Naphtha; Petroleum Spirit; White Spirit

Commonly Found In Coal tar, solvent for oils, lacquers, paints, rubber cement

Mechanism of Toxic Action Aspiration pneumonia related to low viscosity agents

Adverse Reactions

Central nervous system: CNS depression

Gastrointestinal: Irritant of mucous membranes

Hematologic: Methemoglobinemia

Respiratory: Aspiration pneumonitis

Miscellaneous: Intravenous administration produces fever and local tissue damage

Signs and Symptoms of Overdose Unlikely to produce systemic signs. Cough (persistent), dermatitis, dizziness, dyspnea, erythema, fever, headache, hematuria, hemoptysis, nausea

Admission Criteria/Prognosis Patients who develop tachypnea, cyanosis, dyspnea, CNS depression, tachycardia, or fever within 8 hours of exposure should be admitted; asymptomatic patients can be discharged after 8 hours observation

Toxicodynamics/Kinetics Absorption: Not well absorbed in the GI tract

Overdosage/Treatment

Supportive therapy: Pulsed corticosteroid therapy (1000 mg/day of I.V. hydrocortisone for 3 days with a 7-week gradual taper) may lead to improvement of naphtha-induced adult respiratory distress syndrome

Decontamination: **Do not** induce emesis or lavage; basic poison management; avoid positive net fluid balance; avoid catecholamines due to sensitivity of myocardium

Additional Information IDLH: 10,000 ppm; PEL-TWA: 500 ppm

Phencyclidine

CAS Number 77-10-1; 956-90-1

Synonyms PCP

Impairment Potential Yes. Blood phencyclidine levels >0.007 mg/L are associated with driving impairment (Baselt RC and Cravey RH, *Disposition of Toxic Drugs and Chemicals in Man*, 4th ed, Foster City, CA: Chemical Toxicology Institute, 1995, 602.)

Mechanism of Action Related to ketamine, PCP is an arylcyclohexylamine which stimulates alpha-adrenergic receptors

Adverse Reactions

Cardiovascular: Tachycardia, pericardial effusion/pericarditis, sinus tachycardia

Central nervous system: Violent behavior, aggressive behavior; psychosis, paranoia, hallucinations, ataxia, synesthesia, dysphoria, sympathetic storm

Endocrine & metabolic: Hypoglycemia

Gastrointestinal: Vomiting

Hepatic: Aminotransferase level elevation (asymptomatic)

Ocular: Nystagmus, lacrimation, mydriasis (miosis in children)

Signs and Symptoms of Overdose Coma, delirium, depression, encephalopathy, fasciculations, fear, fever, headache, hyperacusis, hypertension, hyperthermia, hyperuricemia, hypoglycemia, hypothermia, impotence, insomnia, lacrimation, mania, myoclonus, myoglobinuria, myopathy, ptosis, respiratory depression, rhabdomyolysis, seizures, sweating, tachycardia

Admission Criteria/Prognosis Patients with blood phencyclidine level >30 ng/mL; transient apnea, catatonia, severe psychosis, rhabdomyolysis; sustained adrenergic signs may require admission

Pharmacodynamics/Kinetics

Distribution: V_d: 6.2 L/kg

Protein binding: 60% to 70%

Metabolism: Hepatic via oxidative hydroxylation

Half-life elimination: 1 hour; Overdose: 17.6 hours

Excretion: Urine (33 mL/minute)

Dosage Joints are 100-400 mg PCP by weight; tablets are ~5 mg

Reference Range

Serum levels: Catatonia and excitation: 20-30 ng/mL; myoclonus and coma: 30-100 ng/mL; hypotension, seizures, fatalities: >100 ng/mL

Urinary levels do not correlate with clinical symptoms

In the postmortem state, anatomical site concentration differences (ie, postmortem redistribution) may occur.

Overdosage/Treatment

Decontamination: Activated charcoal for oral ingestions

Supportive therapy: Benzodiazepine for agitation; haloperidol (5 mg I.M.) improves psychotic symptoms; rhabdomyolysis can be treated with I.V. hydration, alkalinization, and mannitol; lorazepam or diazepam can be used to calm and sedate the patient

Enhanced elimination: Continuous gastric suction (due to gastric secretion of PCP) may increase elimination and should be considered in the comatose patient; multiple dosing of activated charcoal may be effective

Test Interactions Adulteration with bleach can cause false-negative urine immunoassays; doxylamine may result in a false-positive urine gas chromatographic test; dextromethorphan, diphenhydramine, or high doses of thioridazine may result in a false-positive immunoassay screen;

ketamine is not expected to result in a positive immunoassay on most systems

Drug Interactions

Substrate of CYP3A4 (major); **Inhibits** CYP3A4 (weak)

CYP3A4 inhibitors: May increase the levels/effects of phencyclidine. Example inhibitors include azole antifungals, clarithromycin, diclofenac, doxycycline, erythromycin, imatinib, isoniazid, nefazodone, nicardipine, propofol, protease inhibitors, quinidine, telithromycin, and verapamil.

Pregnancy Implications Neonatal irritability, hypertonia, tremors

Additional Information Mid-Year 2000 Emergency Department Drug Abuse Warning Network (DAWN) data: **Note:** Phencyclidine is sometimes used in combination with other drugs; therefore, one Emergency Department (ED) episode can include mentions of one or more drugs.

- In the first half of 2000, there were 3153 ED mentions of PCP/PCP combinations, which was 49% greater than in the first half of 1999. The number of PCP/PCP combination mentions, which began to decline in 1996, has since leveled off.

Specific References

Bond GR, Steele PE, and Uges DR, "Massive Venlafaxine Overdose Resulted in a False Positive Abbott AxSYM® Urine Immunoassay for Phencyclidine," *J Toxicol Clin Toxicol*, 2003, 41(7):999-1002.

Gordon AM and Logan BK, "Phencyclidine Findings in Drivers in Washington State," *J Anal Toxicol*, 2004, 28:280-1.

Pestaner JP and Southall PE, "Sudden Death During Arrest and Phencyclidine Intoxication," *Am J Forensic Med Pathol*, 2003, 24(2):119-22.

Phenibut

CAS Number 35568-37-7

Synonyms Beta-phenyl-gamma-aminobutyric Acid HCl; Fenibut; Phenylgam

Use Neuropsychotropic drug developed in Russia in the 1960s; has anxiolytic effects; usually ingested as a powder

Mechanism of Action A beta-phenyl derivative of the inhibitory central nervous sytem neuromediator GABA with GABA(A) and GABA(B) agonist effects. Also stimulates dopamine receptors.

Adverse Reactions Sedation, lethargy

Dosage About 250 mg 3 times/day

Overdosage/Treatment

Decontamination: Oral activated charcoal may be useful within 1 hour of ingestion

Supportive care: Naloxone is not effective; flumazenil has unknown effectiveness; respiratory depression and cardiac effects are minimal

Specific References

Lapin I, "Phenibut (Beta-phenyl-GABA): A Tranquilizer and Nootropic Drug," *CNS Drug Rev*, 2001, 7(4):471-81.

Phenmedipham

Applies to Weed Control (Sugar Beets)

CAS Number 13684-63-4

U.S. Brand Names Betanal®; EP-452; Fenmedifam®; Kemifan®; Spin-Aid®

Synonyms Methyl-3-Metatolycarbamoloxyphenyl Carbamate

Use Control weeds of sugar beet crops

Mechanism of Toxic Action Inhibitor of photosynthesis

Signs and Symptoms of Overdose Bullous dermatitis, photosensitivity reaction

Overdosage/Treatment Decontamination: Remove contaminated clothing (especially leather); wash thoroughly with soap and water. Irrigate eyes with normal saline for ocular exposure.

Additional Information Does not affect cholinesterase; leather absorbs phenmedipham

Phosdrin

CAS Number 7786-34-7

UN Number 2783

U.S. Brand Names Mevinphos®; Phosdrin®

Use Insecticide

Mechanism of Toxic Action Highly toxic organophosphate agent which causes irreversible inhibition of acetylcholinesterase and plasma cholinesterase, resulting in excess accumulation of acetylcholine at muscarinic and nicotinic receptors, and in the central nervous system

Adverse Reactions

Cardiovascular: **Hyperdynamic** (~18% to 21%) or hypodynamic (~7% to 10%) states, tachycardia, hypertension, edema

Central nervous system: Depression, seizures, hyperactivity

Endocrine & metabolic: Hypokalemia

Gastrointestinal: Pancreatitis, diarrhea

Genitourinary: Urinary incontinence

Neuromuscular & skeletal: Weakness, paralysis, paresthesia (delayed)

Ocular: Can cause myopia in children, miosis, vertical nystagmus

Miscellaneous: Flu-like symptoms (especially with chronic exposure), diaphoresis

Signs and Symptoms of Overdose

Abdominal pain, agitation, asystole, AV block, bradycardia, bronchorrhea, coma, confusion, cranial nerve palsies, decreased hemoglobin, decreased platelet count, decreased red blood cell count, diaphragmatic paralysis, dysarthria, excessive sweating, fecal and urinary incontinence, generalized asthenia, headache, heart block, hyperamylasemia, hypertension, hypotension, lacrimation, metabolic acidosis and hyperglycemia (severe intoxication), miosis (unreactive to light), mydriasis (rarely), nausea, pallor, pulmonary edema, QT prolongation, respiratory depression, salivation, seizures, skeletal muscle fasciculation and flaccid paralysis, tachycardia, tachypnea, vomiting

An "intermediate syndrome" of limb asthenia and respiratory paralysis has been reported to occur between 24 and 96 hours postorganophosphate exposure and is independent of the acute cholinergic crisis. Late paresthesia characterized by stocking and glove paresthesia, anesthesia and asthenia is infrequently observed weeks to months following acute exposure to certain organophosphates.

Admission Criteria/Prognosis Patients will usually be symptomatic within 2 hours of ingestion; admit any adult ingestion >5 mg or any symptomatic patient

Toxicodynamics/Kinetics

Onset: Within 2 hours

Absorption: GI: Dermal-toxic, dermal: 14 mg/kg

Elimination: Renal (as dimethylphosphate)

Reference Range Postmortem blood and urine levels after a successful suicide attempt (dose unknown): 360 ppm and 8 ppm, respectively; urine dimethylphosphate levels in a mildly symptomatic patient: 2 ppm

Overdosage/Treatment

Decontamination: Isolation, bagging, and disposal of all contaminated clothing and other articles. All emergency medical workers and hospital staff should follow appropriate precautions regarding exposure to hazardous material including the use of protective clothing, masks, goggles, and respiratory equipment. Gastric lavage with water, 5% sodium bicarbonate or 2% potassium permanganate can be considered within 1 hour of ingestion. **Do not** use a cathartic with activated charcoal.

Oral: Activated charcoal can be administered either orally or via a nasogastric tube. **Do not** induce emesis because of danger of sudden respiratory compromise, alterations in mental status, seizures, coma, and possible aspiration of hydrocarbon vehicles. Prolonged or repetitive gastric lavage (with activated charcoal) may be beneficial to prevent rebound of plasma levels due to delayed absorption. **Do not** give a cathartic.

Dermal: Prompt thorough scrubbing of all affected areas with soap and water, including hair and nails; 5% bleach can also be used

Ocular: Irrigation with copious tepid sterile water or saline

Supportive therapy: Airway management, ventilatory assistance, humidified oxygen administration, and close monitoring for sudden respiratory failure

Antidote:

Atropine: Administration should be guided by respiratory status, starting at 2-5 mg I.V. every 5-10 minutes as needed, and should be titrated to the resolution of excess pulmonary secretions. Frequent administration of large doses (cumulative doses >100 mg) may be necessary in massive exposures.

Glycopyrrolate: May be administered if atropine is unavailable (200-400 mcg I.V. or I.M. initially, or ~$^1/_2$ the dose of atropine).

2-PAM: For more significant exposures (ie, exposures requiring large doses of atropine, or with recurring symptoms, or exposures to more lipid soluble agents), administration should follow: 1-2 g I.V. over 10-30 minutes, repeated in 1 hour if asthenia recurs, then every 4-12 hours for recurring symptoms.

Enhancement of elimination: Dialysis and hemoperfusion are not indicated due to effectiveness of the prescribed antidotal treatment and large volumes of distribution of organophosphates. Due to enterohepatic recirculation, multiple dosing of activated charcoal may be effective.

Antidote(s)
- Atropine [ANTIDOTE]
- Pralidoxime [ANTIDOTE]

Additional Information Toxic daily dose (which can result in reduced red cell cholinesterase): ~1.5 mg. A pale yellow to orange liquid with little odor. Specific gravity: 1.25. TLV: 0.1 mg/m^3. Associated solvent: Hexyleneglycol

---

Phosgene

Applies to Dyes, Aniline (Manufacture); Insecticides (Manufacture); Plastics (Manufacture)

CAS Number 75-44-5

UN Number 1076

Synonyms Agent CG; Carbon Oxychloride; Carbonic Dichloride; Carbonyl Chloride; Chloroformyl Chloride; Diphosgene; Phosgen

Use In the manufacture of isocyanates, aniline dyes, plastics, and insecticides. Initially prepared in 1812, but used extensively in World War I gas warfare (approximately 1.3 million victims and 90,000 fatalities); product of combustion of volatile chlorine compounds

Mechanism of Toxic Action Direct cytotoxicity through diamide formation which crosslink cell components. Reacts readily with hydroxyl, sulfhydryl, and ammonia groups found in albumin, amino acids, and vitamins; pulmonary irritant with low water solubility thus primarily affecting lung parenchyma on inhalation (delayed alveolar injury)

Adverse Reactions

Cardiovascular: Hypotension, bradycardia, sinus bradycardia, angina, Raynaud's phenomenon, leukocytosis

Endocrine & metabolic: Hypovolemia

Hematologic: Methemoglobinemia, leukocytosis (atypical lymphocytosis), hemolysis (>200 ppm)

Ocular: Conjunctivitis, corneal opacification

Respiratory: Respiratory distress, pulmonary edema ("pink foam"), acute respiratory distress syndrome, tachypnea, dyspnea

Signs and Symptoms of Overdose Asthenia, chest pain, cough, dermal burns, dyspnea, headache, hemoptysis, nausea, ocular irritation, throat burning, vomiting; pulmonary edema within 1-2 hours (high dose), 4-6 hours (moderate dose), 8-24 hours (low dose)

Admission Criteria/Prognosis Patients with known or suspected phosgene exposure >25 ppm/minute, should be observed for at least 12 hours. Patients with development of bronchospasm or pulmonary edema should probably be admitted into an intensive care unit. Survival after 48 hours is usually associated with recovery.

Toxicodynamics/Kinetics Metabolism: Hydrolyzes slowly to produce carbon dioxide and hydrochloric acids

Overdosage/Treatment

Decontamination: **Oral:** Lavage within 1 hour. Irrigate exposed areas. Steroids may be helpful. **Do not** use diuretics. **Dermal:** Remove contaminated clothing. Irrigate copiously with saline or water (especially with diphosgene exposure). **Respiratory:** Administer 100% humidified oxygen. **Ocular:** Irrigate with saline

Supportive therapy: Bedrest; monitor and treat for pulmonary edema. Support of pulmonary function is the mainstay of therapy with mechanical ventilation and positive end-expiratory pressure. The use of nebulized sodium bicarbonate, leukotriene-receptor antagonists, ibuprofen, methylprednisolone, cyclophosphamide, colchicine, and N-acetylcysteine (I.V. or nebulized) has met with some success in experimental models, but is of uncertain clinical benefit. Even so, if exposure to over 50 ppm of phosgene is considered, suggested regimen for pulmonary edema prophylaxis include: ibuprofen 800 mg P.O., methylprednisolone 1 g I.V. or dexamethasone phosphate 10 mg by aerosol, aminophylline 5 mg/kg I.V. or P.O. followed by 1 mg/kg every 8-12 hours to achieve serum aminophylline level of 10-20 mcg/mL, terbutaline 0.25 mg SubQ, N-acetylcysteine 10-20 mL of a 20% solution by aerosolization, oxygen as needed. Use of parenteral prednisolone (1 g I.V.), aerosolized dexamethasone, and theophylline may be useful, but has not been studied in humans. Prophylactic administration of prednisolone (250 mg I.V.), ibuprofen, or N-acetylcysteine (20 mL of a 20% solution) has also not been clinically demonstrated to prevent pulmonary edema. Inverse-ratio ventilation using lower tidal volume mechanical ventilation (6 mL/kg) and plateau pressures of 30 cm water may decrease mortality. While positive end expiratory pressures should be considered, oxygen toxicity should be monitored. Use of perfluorocarbon partial liquid ventilation and exogenous surfactant in chemical-induced ARDS is investigational.

Diagnostic Procedures
- Electrolytes, Blood
- Pulse Oximetry

Additional Information

Vapor contact of >3 ppm phosgene with wet skin may lead to erythema. Phosgene levels >330 ppm/minute can be fatal. Prolonged exposure at 3 ppm for 3 hours can be fatal. Levels >4 ppm can cause ocular irritation and 5 ppm can cause cough. Liquid phosgene is a frostbite hazard.

Pulmonary edema developing within 4 hours is a bad prognosis; usually it will develop within 4-8 hours postexposure. Olfactory paralysis may occur after a short time of initial exposure. Blindness may occur. On chest x-ray, blurred enlargement of hilar area may be the earliest finding. Rescuer contamination possibility from affected patients is low.

Colorless gas; latent period may last 3 days. Estimated worldwide production is >5 billion pounds. Odor threshold: 0.5 ppm. At low doses, it has a freshly mowed grass odor; higher doses give a pungent odor. Vapor density: >4. TLV-TWA: 0.1 ppm; IDLH: 2 ppm; PEL-TWA: 0.1 ppm

Soluble in water; rapidly hydrolyzed in water to hydrochloric acid and carbon dioxide. Does not bioconcentrate.

Environmental half-life of phosgene in soil and water: 3 minutes to 1 hour

Clinically resembles: Chlorine

Environmental persistence: Low; air concentrations are reduced by rain or fog

Specific References

Kales SN and Christiani DC, "Acute Chemical Emergencies," *N Engl J Med*, 2004, 350(8):800-8.

Phosphine

Related Information
- Aluminum Phosphide
- Zinc Phosphide

Applies to Grain Fumigation; Rat Poison

CAS Number 7803-51-2

UN Number 2199

Synonyms Delicia; Detia Gas EX-B; Hydrogen Phosphide; PH3; Phosphoreted Hydrogen; Phosphorus Trihydride

Use Silicon crystal treatment in semiconductor industry, contaminant in acetylene, grain fumigation, and rat poisons. Produced by reaction of hydrogen with metal phosphides.

Mechanism of Toxic Action Protoplasmic toxicity inhibits cytochrome C oxidase pathway primarily in myocardium

Adverse Reactions
Cardiovascular: Tachycardia, cardiovascular collapse, hypotension, flutter (atrial), angina, sinus tachycardia, arrhythmias (ventricular), chest tightness
Central nervous system: Panic attacks, coma, seizures, dizziness
Hepatic: Hepatic toxicity (late)
Neuromuscular & skeletal: Rhabdomyolysis, intention tremor
Renal: Oliguria, renal failure
Respiratory: Pulmonary edema, shortness of breath, dyspnea

Signs and Symptoms of Overdose Abdominal pain, ataxia, cardiac arrhythmia, chest pain, cough, diplopia, dizziness, drowsiness, dyspnea, fibrillation (atrial), garlic-like breath, irritability, jaundice, seizures, tachycardia (ventricular), tremor, vomiting, diarrhea

Admission Criteria/Prognosis
Mild exposure: Asymptomatic individuals can be discharged after 6 hours of observation
Serious exposure: Patients should be observed for pulmonary edema or liver damage for 72 hours; survival after 4 days is usually associated with recovery

Toxicodynamics/Kinetics Onset of action: Rapid, within 3 hours of exposure

Reference Range Blood and urine phosphorus levels are not reliable

Overdosage/Treatment
Decontamination: Inhalation: Oxygenation; if ingested, lavage within 1 hour with 1:10,000 dilution of potassium permanganate to reduce availability of phosphine; activated charcoal may be useful
Supportive therapy: Calcium gluconate and magnesium sulfate may be useful for cardiac arrhythmia. Magnesium sulphate may be particularly useful at a dose of 3 g (continuous I.V. infusion) over 3 hours followed by 6 g/day for the next 3-5 days; may be unresponsive to vasopressin. Inverse-ratio ventilation using lower tidal volume mechanical ventilation (6 mL/kg) and plateau pressures of 30 cm water may decrease mortality. While positive end expiratory pressures should be considered, oxygen toxicity should be monitored. Use of perfluorocarbon partial liquid ventilation and exogenous surfactant in chemical-induced ARDS is investigational.
Enhancement of elimination: Hemodialysis may be useful in cases of renal damage.

Antidote(s)
- Calcium Gluconate [ANTIDOTE]
- Magnesium Sulfate [ANTIDOTE]

Additional Information Adult deaths have been described with ingestion of 4 g of zinc phosphide or 500 mg aluminum phosphide. Colorless gas; flammable; garlic odor. Odor (garlic) threshold: 2 ppm. IDLH: 50 ppm

Specific References
Lauterbach M, Solak E, Kaes J, et al, "Epidemiology of Hydrogen Phosphide Exposures in Humans Reported to the Poison Center in Mainz, Germany, 1983-2003," *Clin Toxicol*, 2005, 43:575-81.

Pine Oil

Related Information
- Turpentine Oil

CAS Number 8002-09-3

UN Number 1272

Synonyms Unipine; Yurmor Pine Oil

Use Disinfectant/cleaning agent

Mechanism of Toxic Action CNS depression and mucosal irritation

Adverse Reactions
Cardiovascular: Bradycardia, hypotension, syncope
Central nervous system: Fever, ataxia, coma, headache
Dermatologic: Nonimmunologic contact urticaria
Gastrointestinal: Nausea, vomiting, diarrhea
Renal: Anuria, renal failure, myoglobinuria
Respiratory: Tachypnea, coughing, aspiration pneumonitis, dyspnea

Admission Criteria/Prognosis Admit ingestions of >20% solution or any symptomatic individual 6 hours postingestion

Toxicodynamics/Kinetics
Absorption: Gastrointestinal
Elimination: Pulmonary (violet-like odor)

Monitoring Parameters Arterial blood gas, renal function, chest x-ray, urine analysis

Reference Range Postmortem levels of 1-α-terpineol following an ingestion of ~100 mL of Pine-Sol® were: Blood: 11.2 mg/L; urine: 5.76 mg/L; gastric: 15.3 g/L. Postmortem acetone concentrations were: Blood: 25 mg/dL; vitreous humor: 31 mg/dL; urine: 33 mg/dL; and gastric: 28 mg/dL. Postmortem concentrations of isopropanol were <10 mg/dL in the blood, vitreous humor, urine, and gastric contents.

Overdosage/Treatment
Decontamination: **Oral:** May be considered if the patient presentation is within 1 hour of ingestion. Emesis in the alert patient may be the preferred method for gastric decontamination, in that, pulmonary complications appear to be less frequent as compared to gastric lavage. Activated charcoal can be used although there is no data on its effectiveness. **Dermal:** Wash with soap and water. **Ocular:** Irrigate copiously with saline.
Supportive therapy: Hypotension: Crystalloid fluid bolus (10-20 mL/kg) with placement in Trendelenburg position should be utilized. Dopamine or norepinephrine can be used as vasopressors.
Enhanced elimination: Exchange transfusion (over a 3 hour period) helped improve the CNS respiratory depression in one pediatric patient.

Additional Information
Fatal dose: 0.5 ounces (14 g) of pure pine oil (or 75 mL of a 20% solution) in a child, 8 ounces in an adult
Ingestions of pine oil solutions <20% result in minimal symptomatology. Monitor for coingestants (ie, isopropyl alcohol).
Respiratory odor is that of violets. Specific gravity: 9
Pine oil is a mixture of terpene alcohols; Pine-Sol® may contain from 15% to 35% pine oil.

Platinum

CAS Number 7440-06-4

Synonyms Liquid Bright Platinum; Platin; Platinum Black; Platinum Sponge

Adverse Reactions
Eyes, nose, respiratory, dermatologic, immunologic contact urticaria
Central nervous system: Axonopathy
Respiratory: Asthma

Signs and Symptoms of Overdose Classic signs/symptoms of allergic reaction; cough, dyspnea, eczema, eosinophilia, lymphocytosis, neuritis, rash, rhinorrhea, urticaria, wheezing

Toxicodynamics/Kinetics
Absorption: Oral: Poor. Inhalation: Readily absorbed
Distribution: To soft tissue
Protein binding: 90% to 95%
Half-life: 59-73 hours

Overdosage/Treatment
Decontamination: Irrigation
Supportive therapy: Beta agonists can be used for wheezing

Diagnostic Procedures
- Platinum, Blood
- Platinum, Urine

Additional Information Platinum metal is biologically inert. Parenteral administration of platinum salts in an animal model produces seizures, coma, and death. Simple platinum salts are toxic to the gastrointestinal tract. Complex platinum salts are toxic to the nervous system. An allergic response to complex platinum salts is known as platinosis. TLV-TWA metallic platinum dust: 1 mg/m^3; for soluble platinum salts: 0.002 mg/m^3

Plutonium

Applies to Nuclear Weapons

CAS Number 7440-07-5

UN Number 2918

Synonyms Plutonium Metal; Plutonium-236 Isotope; Plutonium-237 Isotope; Plutonium-238 Isotope; Plutonium-239 Isotope; Plutonium-240 Isotope; Plutonium-241 Isotope; Plutonium-242 Isotope; Plutonium-243 Isotope; Pu

Use Primarily in the production of nuclear weapons (plutonium-239 isotope); also used as a heat source for thermoelectric power devices (plutonium-238 isotope) (especially the breeder type of reactor)

Adverse Reactions
Dermatologic: Dermal burns
Local: Causes tissue necrosis on contact

Toxicodynamics/Kinetics
Absorption: By inhalation (especially more soluble forms of plutonium such as plutonium citrate or plutonium nitrate); very limited absorption by oral or dermal routes (0.0002% per hour of plutonium nitrate)
Distribution: Highest concentration after inhalation in tracheobronchial lymph nodes and liver
Half-life: 180-200 years
Elimination: By feces and urine

Overdosage/Treatment

Decontamination: Remove contaminated clothing; isolate all run-off.

Dermal: Irrigate with water; scrub gently with soft sponge or brush (avoid abrading skin). A 50% powdered detergent solution followed by a 5% sodium hypochlorite solution can be used for persistent contamination.

Ocular: Wash copiously with saline.

Supportive therapy: DTPA (diethylenetriamine pentacetic acid) which is available from the Radiation Emergency Assistance Center (865-576-1004) is an effective chelator. The calcium salt should be used as follows: 1 g of Ca^{++} DTPA diluted in 250 mL of 5% dextrose in water should be infused over a 1- to $1^1/_2$-hour time period daily for 5 days. $CaNa_2$ EDTA (calcium Versenate®) can also be used, but is less effective. DTPA should be used for dermal exposure with open wounds as well as inhalation or oral ingestion.

Antidote(s)

- Diethylene Triamine Penta-Acetic Acid [ANTIDOTE]

Additional Information Carcinogenic in animals (squamous cell).

Decontamination should be monitored by use of a Geiger-Mueller counter.

Cigarettes can accentuate plutonium toxicity.

Odorless and tasteless. Physical half-life: 24,900 years

Background radiation to an individual in U.S. is estimated to be 360 mrem (2.6 mSv).

Specific References

Dainiak N, Waselenko JK, Armitage JO, et al, "The Hematologist and Radiation Casualties," *Hematology (Am Soc Hematol Educ Program)*, 2003, 473-96 (review).

Khokhryakov VF, Suslova KG, Kudryavtseva TI, et al, "Relative Role of Plutonium Excretion with Urine and Feces from Human Body," *Health Phys*, 2004, 86(5):523-7.

Polychlorinated Biphenyls

Related Information

- Adipose Tissue Ranges of Toxins
- Polychlorinated Dibenzofurans

CAS Number 11096-82-5; 11097-69-1; 11100-14-4; 11104-28-2; 11141-16-5; 12672-29-6; 12674-11-2; 12737-87-0; 1336-36-3; 37317-41-2; 37324-23-5; 53469-21-9

UN Number 2315

Synonyms Aroclor; Chlorbipheny; Clophen; Fenclor; Kanechlor; PCB; Phenochlor

Use Was used (up until 1979) as a coolant in capacitors and transformers; also had been used as a lubricant for gas turbine engines

Mechanism of Toxic Action Binds to a cellular receptor (Ah receptor) which alters protein and enzyme synthesis

Adverse Reactions

Central nervous system: Headache, fatigue

Dermatologic: Hyperpigmentation, chloracne, orbital swelling, pruritus, fingernail dystrophy, acne

Endocrine & metabolic: Elevated serum triglycerides, Hashimoto's disease, Graves' disease, autoimmune thyroid disease, thyroiditis

Gastrointestinal: Nausea, vomiting, diarrhea

Hepatic: Hepatitis

Neuromuscular & skeletal: Peripheral neuropathy

Miscellaneous: Hyperthyroxinemia (with normal TSH levels) have been noted; clearly carcinogenic in animals (hepatocellular), not well described in humans

Toxicodynamics/Kinetics

Absorption: By inhalation (80%), oral, and dermal (15% to 56%)

Distribution: Accumulates in fat

Metabolism: Hepatic hydroxylation and conjugation with glucuronic acid; as rate of chlorination of biphenyl rings increases, metabolic rate decreases

Half-life: 4 months to 2 years

Elimination: Primarily fecal

Reference Range

Blood level of general unexposed population: ~20 ppb; in adipose tissue: 1-2 ppm

Geometric means of serum PCB levels found among the general population (serum PBCs in humans):

- Occupational exposure to PCBs (workers): 12.0-119.0 ppb
- Nonoccupational exposure and eating PCB-contaminated fish: 2.1-56.0 ppb
- Nonoccupational exposure and not eating PCB-contaminated fish: 0.9-15.0 ppb

Note: PCB production is banned or sharply curtailed throughout the world; therefore, the above levels are steadily decreasing

Overdosage/Treatment Decontamination: Oral: Lavage (within 1 hour)/ activated charcoal. Dermal: Remove contaminated clothing; wash with soap and water. Acetone can also be used for dermal washing.

Inhalation: Administer 100% humidified oxygen.

Additional Information

Toxic oral dose: 500 mg

Low water solubility inducer of hepatic microsomal enzymes

Usually mixed with chlorine; high food concentration is in fish (almost 1 ppm)

Average daily intake of PCB by inhalation: ~100 ng; by drinking water: <200 ng

Tropospheric water half-life: 3.5-83.2 days. Water half-life: 27-82 days

Urban atmospheric concentrations of PCB in the U.S. range from 0.5-30 ng/m^3 (mean: 5-10 ng/m^3).

Lake Michigan average PCB level: 1.8 ng/L; Lake Huron: 0.5 ng/L

Specific References

Charlier C, Dubois N, Cucchiaro S, et al, "Analysis of Polychlorinated Biphenyl Residues in Human Plasma by Gas Chromatography-Mass Spectrometry," *J Anal Toxicol*, 2003, 27(2):74-7.

Hsu PC, Huang W, Yao WJ, et al, "Sperm Changes in Men Exposed to Polychlorinated Biphenyls and Dibenzofurans," *JAMA*, 2003, 289(22):2943-4.

Langer P, Kocan A, Tajtakova M, et al, "Possible Effects of Polychlorinated Biphenyls and Organochlorinated Pesticides on the Thyroid After Long-Term Exposure to Heavy Environmental Pollution," *J Occup Environ Med*, 2003, 45(5):526-32.

Wang RY and Needham LL, "Levels of Polychlorinated Dibenzo-P-Dioxins (PCDDs), Polychlorinated Dibenzofurans (PCDFs), and Polychlorinated Biphenyls (PCBs) in Human Milk at Two U.S. Locations," *J Toxicol Clin Toxicol*, 2003, 41(5):730.

Polychlorinated Dibenzofurans

Related Information

- Polychlorinated Biphenyls

CAS Number 39001-02-0; 51207-31-9; 55673-89-7; 57117-31-4; 57117-35-8; 57117-37-0; 57117-41-6; 57117-44-9; 60851-34-5; 67517-48-0; 67562-39-4; 69698-58-4; 70648-25-8; 70648-26-9; 72918-21-9; 75627-02-0

Synonyms Chlorodibenzofurans; Dibenzo-p-Dioxins; PCDF

Use No commercial use; primarily produced as byproducts during the production of polychlorinated biphenyl agents (PCBs) (ie, Agent Orange), polychlorinated phenols, herbicides, and chlorine bleaching at paper and pulp mills; formed from the photolysis of PCBs and from PCB transformer fires or incineration

Mechanism of Toxic Action Binds to a cellular receptor (Ah receptor) which alters protein and enzyme synthesis

Adverse Reactions

Central nervous system: Headache

Dermatologic: Dermal changes include comedo formatting, hyperpigmentation, hyperkeratosis, acneform eruptions on face, head, and trunk

Endocrine & metabolic: Elevated serum triglycerides

Gastrointestinal: **Vomiting** (25% on oral exposure), **diarrhea** (18%)

Genitourinary: Increased urinary excretion of uroporphyrin

Hematologic: Normocytic anemia, leukocytosis

Neuromuscular & skeletal: Limb neuralgia, neuropathy (peripheral), paresthesia

Toxicodynamics/Kinetics

Absorption: Through ingestion, inhalation, or dermal routes

Metabolism: Hepatic hydroxylation followed by glucuronidation

Half-life: >7 years of 2,3,7,8-tetrachlorodibenzoparadioxin

Elimination: Feces

Reference Range Whole blood level of total PCDFs in occupationally exposed individuals is over double that of nonexposed subjects (103 ppt vs 47 ppt, respectively)

Overdosage/Treatment

Decontamination: **Oral:** Lavage (within 1 hour)/activated charcoal. **Dermal:** Remove contaminated clothing; wash with soap and water. **Ocular:** Irrigate copiously with saline.

Enhancement of elimination: Multiple dosing of cholestyramine (4 g 3 times/day) has been inconclusive.

Additional Information Carcinogenic in mice models at doses of 0.5-2 mcg/kg/week.

Possible increased risk of soft tissue sarcoma

These chemicals are solid at room temperature.

2,3,7,8-substituted PCDFs seem to be the most hepatotoxic agent of CDF; tetra-CDF, penta-CDF, and hexa-CDF have skin tumor promoter activity

Tropospheric lifetime of PCDFs: 1.9-39 days (higher chlorinated congeners have longer lifetimes)

Foods (especially meat and shellfish) account for the highest amount of CDF ingested daily.

Inhalation accounts for only 3% of total daily CDF intake.

Specific References

Gupta A, Schecter A, Aragaki CC, et al, "Dioxin Exposure and Benign Prostatic Hyperplasia," *J Occup Environ Med*, 2006, 48:708-14.

Polycyclic Aromatic Hydrocarbons

CAS Number 120-12-7; 129-00-0; 191-24-2; 192-97-2; 193-39-5; 205-82-3; 205-99-2; 206-44-0; 207-08-9; 208-96-8; 218-01-9; 50-32-8; 53-70-3; 56-55-3; 83-32-9; 85-01-8; 86-73-7

Synonyms Acenaphthylene; Anthracene; Benzo[a]pyrene (BaP); Benzo[b]fluoranthene; Benzo[e]pyrene; Benzo[ghi]perylene; Benzo[j]fluoranthene; Benzo[k]fluoranthene; Benz[a]anthracene; Chrysene; Dibenz[a,h]anthracene; Dihydroacenapthylene; Fluoranthene; Fluorene; PAH; Phenanthrene; Polycyclic Organic Matter; POM; Pyrene

Commonly Found In Tobacco smoke, tar oil, automobile exhaust, flue gases, smoked foods, coke production

Use In rubber industry as a plasticizer; anthracene is used in dye production

Mechanism of Toxic Action Fused benzene ring compounds (usually 3 rings) which bind to DNA (especially diol-epoxide metabolites) leading to tumor initiation; can also cause decrease in brain dopamine and norepinephrine in the corpus striatum and hypothalamus

Adverse Reactions

Gastrointestinal: Anthracene laxatives can cause melanosis of colon and rectum

Miscellaneous: Lung (upon inhalation) and skin cancers can occur

Dermatologic: Warts can occur upon dermal exposure as can pemphigus vulgaris

Endocrine & metabolic: Ovotoxic

Benzo(a)anthracene, benzo(b)fluoranthene, benzo(k)fluoranthene, benzo(a)pyrene, chrysene, and indeno(1,2,3-c,d)pyrene are considered a probable human carcinogen (EPA classification B_2)

Respiratory: Upper airway irritation, Decreased pulmonary function

Admission Criteria/Prognosis Patients who develop tachypnea, cyanosis, dyspnea, CNS depression, tachycardia, or fever within 8 hours of exposure should be admitted; asymptomatic patients can be discharged after 8 hours observation

Toxicodynamics/Kinetics

Absorption: Orally, by inhalation, and dermal exposure

Metabolism: Hepatic, epoxidation and epoxide conversion to Arene oxides, phenols, and quinones

Elimination: Renal

Overdosage/Treatment Decontamination: Oral: Do not induce emesis; activated charcoal may be useful. Dermal: Wash with soap and water. **Ocular:** Copious irrigation with saline

Additional Information

Soluble in organic solvents; relatively insoluble in water

Skin carcinogen in animals

Retinoids, dietary plant phenols (ie, tannic acid) and N-acetylcysteine (NAC) may be effective in animal models in antagonizing the tumorigenic effect of benzo(a)pyrene.

Formed after incomplete pyrolysis of fossil fuel; furnaces, coal refuse fires, and coke production account for a large amount of emissions; formed when tars and mineral oils are heated.

Smoking three packs of cigarettes daily can increase exposure of PAH to 6-15 mcg/day.

Spinach, tea, meat, and fish have the highest amount of PAH levels.

Daily intake of carcinogenic PAHs by an adults is estimated to be 1-5 mcg (6-9 mcg for individuals ingesting a large amount of meat).

Inhalation daily dose is estimated to be 0.2 mcg/day.

Drinking water is estimated to contribute 0.006 mcg/day of PAHs.

Surface water concentrations of BaP range from 0.6-114 ng/L.

Atmospheric half-life: Usually ~1 month. Soil half-life: 2 days to 2 months

Polyethylene Glycol - Low Molecular Weight

Related Information

● Polyethylene Glycol - High Molecular Weight [ANTIDOTE]

CAS Number 19005-08-7; 25322-68-3

Synonyms Aklapol; PEG-200, PEG-400, PEG-600

Use A liquid found as vehicles in cosmetics, topical medications and hair products; also found in Lava Lamps® (PEG-200)

Mechanism of Toxic Action Proximal renal tubular necrosis can develop; hypercalcemia may be relatable to increased parathyroid hormone secretion

Signs and Symptoms of Overdose Azotemia, coma, contact dermatitis, hypercalcemia, hyperosmolarity, metabolic acidosis (anion gap), oliguria, renal failure. Topical use can cause systemic effects, especially in burn patients.

Monitoring Parameters Osmolarity, pH, calcium, creatinine

Overdosage/Treatment

Decontamination: Dermal: Wash with soap and water.

Supportive therapy: Treat acidosis with sodium bicarbonate (1-2 mEq/kg).

Enhanced elimination: Six hours of dialysis were useful in one case of accidental intoxication. It is unclear whether dialysis enhanced elimination or was used to support deteriorating renal status.

Additional Information When heated, fumes can be irritating.

Specific References

Shih RD, Laird D, Ruck B, et al, "Completion of Whole Bowel Irrigation in PCC Overdose Patients," *J Toxicol Clin Toxicol*, 2003, 41(5):672.

Potassium Permanganate

Related Information

● Manganese

CAS Number 7722-64-7

UN Number 1490

U.S. Brand Names Permatasico; Permitabs

Synonyms Chameleon Mineral; Condy's Crystals; $KMnO_4$

Use Bleaching agent, dyeing wood, chemistry reagent, photography, purifying water; also used in illegal fireworks production. Used as a topical bactericidal agent at concentrations of 0.01% (1:10,000 solution).

Mechanism of Toxic Action Solutions >1:5000 concentration are irritating; an oxidizing agent with alkaline caustic effects; systemic injury is due to oxidative injury by free radicals

Signs and Symptoms of Overdose Brownish discoloration of mucous membranes, cough, esophageal stricture, GI hemorrhage, hemorrhagic pancreatitis, ocular irritation, stridor, vomiting

Admission Criteria/Prognosis Admit any patient with gastrointestinal symptoms

Toxicodynamics/Kinetics Absorption: Poor

Dosage Forms Solution, topical: 0.1% [1 mg/mL = 1:1000]; 0.02% [0.2 mg/mL = 1:5000]; 0.01% [0.1 mg/mL = 1:10,000]

Overdosage/Treatment

Decontamination: **Oral:** Activated charcoal may be useful. Dilute with milk or water. **Ocular:** Irrigate with saline or 5% to 10% ascorbic acid solution to dissolve manganese oxide deposits. (Dissolve 550 mg tablet of ascorbic acid in 25 mL of 0.9% NaCl and irrigate the eyes.)

Supportive therapy: Consider esophagogastroscopy within 1 day for esophageal injury.

Additional Information Fatal oral dose is 10 g

For phosphides and yellow or white phosphorous ingestion, a 1:5000 solution is given orally to convert phosphorous to nontoxic oxides followed by activated charcoal and mineral oil cathartic.

On contact with water, it forms potassium hydroxide, oxygen, and manganese dioxide.

Specific References

Johnson TB and Cassidy DD, "Unintentional Ingestion of Potassium Permanganate," *Pediatr Emerg Care*, 2004, 20(3):185-7.

Profenofos

CAS Number 41198-08-7

U.S. Brand Names Curacron®; Polycron®; Selecron®

Synonyms O-(4-Bromo-2-Chlorophenyl)-O-Ethyl-S-Propylphosparathioate

Use Marketed as insecticide granules, dusting agent, or spray liquid with or without petroleum derivative as a solvent

Mechanism of Toxic Action Irreversible inhibition of acetylcholinesterase and plasma cholinesterase, resulting in excess accumulation of acetylcholine at muscarinic and nicotinic receptors, and in the central nervous system

Adverse Reactions

Cardiovascular: **Hyperdynamic** (~18% to 21%) or hypodynamic (~7% to 10%) states, QT prolongation, sinus bradycardia, sinus tachycardia

Central nervous system: Depression, seizures, hyperactivity, cognitive dysfunction, hypothermia

Genitourinary: Urinary incontinence

Neuromuscular & skeletal: Weakness (delayed), paralysis, delayed paresthesia

Respiratory: Pulmonary edema, respiratory depression

Miscellaneous: Flu-like symptoms (especially with chronic exposure)

Signs and Symptoms of Overdose Abdominal pain, agitation, asystole, AV block, bradycardia, bronchorrhea, coma, confusion, cranial nerve palsies, decreased hemoglobin, decreased platelet count, decreased red blood cell count, diaphragmatic paralysis, dysarthria, excessive sweating, fecal and urinary incontinence, generalized asthenia, headache, heart block, hypertension, hypotension, lacrimation, metabolic acidosis and hyperglycemia (severe intoxication), miosis (unreactive to light), mydriasis (rarely), nausea, pallor, pulmonary edema, QT prolongation, respiratory depression, salivation, seizures, skeletal muscle fasciculation and flaccid paralysis, tachycardia, tachypnea, vomiting

An "intermediate syndrome" of limb asthenia and respiratory paralysis has been reported to occur between 24 and 96 hours postorganophosphate exposure, and is independent of the acute cholinergic crisis. Late paresthesia characterized by stocking and glove paresthesia, anesthesia, and asthenia is infrequently observed weeks to months following acute exposure to certain organophosphates.

Toxicodynamics/Kinetics

Absorption: Readily through oral, dermal, or respiratory exposure

Metabolism: Rapidly metabolized to weakly active compounds through hepatic hydrolysis and other pathways

Elimination: Metabolites are excreted in urine

Warnings/Precautions Risk of aspiration pneumonitis exists with agents having a hydrocarbon vehicle; severe laryngeal irritation and violent coughing may result from exposure to dusting powders; exposure to dusting powders and insecticide granules may cause contact dermatitis

Reference Range Postmortem whole blood and urine profenofos concentration following suicide ingestion: 1200 ng/mL and 350 ng/mL, respectively

Overdosage/Treatment

Decontamination: Isolation, bagging, and disposal of all contaminated clothing and other articles. All emergency medical workers and hospital staff should follow appropriate precautions regarding exposure to hazardous material including the use of protective clothing, masks, goggles, and respiratory equipment.

Oral: Activated charcoal (without cathartic) can be administered either orally or via a nasogastric tube. **Do not** induce emesis because of danger of sudden respiratory compromise, alterations in mental status, seizures, coma, and possible aspiration of hydrocarbon vehicles.

Dermal: Prompt thorough scrubbing of all affected areas with soap and water, including hair and nails; 5% bleach can be used

Ocular: Irrigation with copious tepid sterile water or saline

Supportive therapy: Airway management, ventilatory assistance, humidified oxygen administration, and close monitoring for sudden respiratory failure

Enhancement of elimination: Dialysis and hemoperfusion are not indicated due to effectiveness of the prescribed treatment and large volumes of distribution of organophosphates.

Antidote:

Atropine: Administration should be guided by respiratory status, starting at 2-5 mg I.V. every 5-10 minutes as needed, and should be titrated to the resolution of excess pulmonary secretions. Frequent administration of large doses (cumulative doses >100 mg) may be necessary in massive exposures.

Glycopyrrolate: May be administered if atropine is unavailable (200-400 mcg I.V. or I.M. initially, or ~$^1/_2$ the dose of atropine).

2-PAM: For more significant exposures (ie, exposures requiring large doses of atropine, or with recurring symptoms, or exposures to more lipid soluble agents), administration should follow: 1-2 g I.V. over 10-30 minutes, repeated in 1 hour if asthenia recurs, then every 4-12 hours for recurring symptoms.

Antidote(s)

- Atropine [ANTIDOTE]
- Pralidoxime [ANTIDOTE]

Diagnostic Procedures

- Creatinine, Serum
- Pseudocholinesterase, Serum

Drug Interaction Paralysis is potentiated by neuromuscular blockade (ie, pancuronium, vecuronium, succinylcholine, atracurium, doxacurium, mivacurium); inhibition of serum esterase prolongs the half-life of succinylcholine, cocaine, and other ester anesthetics; cholinergic toxicity is potentiated by cholinesterase inhibitors such as physostigmine

Additional Information Red blood cell cholinesterase, and serum pseudocholinesterase may be depressed following acute or chronic organophosphate exposure; RBC cholinesterase is typically not analyzed by in-house laboratories, and is usually not available for consideration during acute management. Pseudocholinesterase levels may be rapidly available from some in-house laboratories, but are not as reliable a marker of organophosphate exposure because of variability secondary to variant genotypes, hepatic disease, oral estrogen use, or malnutrition. Because of this variability, true indication of suppression of either of these enzymes can only be estimated through comparison to pre-exposure values; these enzymes may be useful in measuring a patient's recovery postexposure, especially if the recovery is not progressing as expected.

The intermediate syndrome is not related to delayed neuropathy.

QT_c prolongation on ECG in the setting of organophosphate poisoning is associated with a high incidence of respiratory failure and mortality.

Other information concerning pesticide exposures is available through the EPA-funded National Pesticide Telecommunications Network: 1-800-858-7378 (weekdays, 8 AM to 6 PM, Central Standard time)

Propane

Applies to Ethylene (Manufacture)

CAS Number 74-98-6

UN Number 1978

Synonyms Dimethylmethane; Propyl Hydride

Commonly Found In Component in fuels, solvent

Use In the manufacture of ethylene

Mechanism of Toxic Action Displaces oxygen resulting in hypoxia

Adverse Reactions

Cardiovascular: Tachycardia, myocardial ischemia, angina, sinus tachycardia

Central nervous system: Coma

Neuromuscular & skeletal: Rhabdomyolysis

Ocular: Decreased visual acuity

Respiratory: Tachypnea

Signs and Symptoms of Overdose Chest pain, cyanosis, dizziness, dyspnea, headache, seizures

Reference Range Postmortem blood propane level of 2.8 mg/L associated with fatality from inhalant abuse

Overdosage/Treatment Supportive therapy: Oxygen therapy - 100% humidified oxygen

Additional Information Colorless gas; petroleum-like odor; heavier than air; may form a vapor cloud as a result from refrigeration effect of liquified propane. IDLH: 20,000 ppm

Propoxur

CAS Number 114-26-1

U.S. Brand Names Baygon®; Isocarb®

Synonyms N-Methyl-2-Isopropoxyphenylcarbamate

Use Marketed as insecticide granules, dusting agent, or spray liquid with or without petroleum derivative as a solvent

Mechanism of Toxic Action Reversible inhibition of acetylcholinesterase and plasma cholinesterase, resulting in excess accumulation of acetylcholine at muscarinic and nicotinic receptors, and in the central nervous system

Adverse Reactions

Cardiovascular: **Hyperdynamic** (~18% to 21%) or hypodynamic (~7% to 10%) states, QT prolongation, edema, sinus bradycardia, sinus tachycardia, arrhythmias (ventricular)

Central nervous system: Toxicity is limited because carbamates do not significantly cross the blood-brain barrier; CNS changes occur with most severe intoxications; hyperactivity

Endocrine & metabolism: Hypoglycemia

Genitourinary: Urinary incontinence

Neuromuscular & skeletal: Weakness, paralysis

Ocular: Diplopia

Respiratory: Cough, respiratory depression

Miscellaneous: Flu-like symptoms (especially with chronic exposure)

Signs and Symptoms of Overdose Abdominal pain, agitation, asystole, AV block, bradycardia, bronchorrhea, coma, confusion, cranial nerve palsies, decreased hemoglobin, decreased platelet count, decreased red blood cell count, diaphragmatic paralysis, dysarthria, excessive sweating, fecal and urinary incontinence, generalized asthenia, headache, heart block, hypertension, hypotension, lacrimation, metabolic acidosis and hyperglycemia (severe intoxication), miosis (unreactive to light), mydriasis (rarely), nausea, pallor, pulmonary edema, QT prolongation, respiratory depression, salivation, seizures, skeletal muscle fasciculation and flaccid paralysis, tachycardia, tachypnea, vomiting. Disseminated intravascular coagulation has been reported following massive exposure.

Toxicodynamics/Kinetics

Absorption: Readily through oral, dermal, or respiratory exposure

Metabolism: Rapidly metabolized to weakly active compounds through hepatic hydrolysis and other pathways, and may undergo enterohepatic recirculation

Elimination: Metabolites are excreted in urine

Warnings/Precautions Risk of aspiration pneumonitis exists following oral exposure to agents having a hydrocarbon vehicle; severe laryngeal irritation and violent coughing may result from exposure to dusting powders; exposure to dusting powders and insecticide granules may cause contact dermatitis

Overdosage/Treatment

Decontamination: Isolation, bagging, and disposal of all contaminated clothing and other articles. All emergency medical workers and hospital staff should follow appropriate precautions regarding exposure to hazardous material including the use of protective clothing, masks, goggles, and respiratory equipment.

Oral: Activated charcoal can be administered either orally or via a nasogastric tube. **Do not** induce emesis because of danger of sudden respiratory compromise, alterations in mental status, seizures, coma, and possible aspiration of hydrocarbon vehicles. **Do not** give a cathartic.

Dermal: Prompt thorough scrubbing of all affected areas with soap and water, including hair and nails; 5% bleach can be used

Ocular: Irrigation with copious tepid sterile water or saline

Supportive therapy: Airway management, ventilatory assistance, humidified oxygen administration, and close monitoring for sudden respiratory failure

Antidote:

Atropine: Administration should be guided by respiratory status, starting at 2-5 mg I.V. every 5-10 minutes as needed, and should be titrated to the resolution of excess pulmonary secretions. Frequent administration of large doses (cumulative doses >100 mg) may be necessary in massive exposures.

Glycopyrrolate: May be administered if atropine is unavailable (200-400 mcg I.V. or I.M. initially, or ~$^1/_2$ the dose of atropine).

2-PAM: Although not specifically indicated, 2-PAM may be considered in the following situations:

Life-threatening symptoms such as respiratory paralysis

Continued excessive atropine requirements

Concomitant organophosphate and carbamate exposure

Enhancement of elimination: Dialysis and hemoperfusion are not indicated due to effectiveness of the prescribed antidotal treatment and large volumes of distribution of carbamates.

Antidote(s)
- Atropine [ANTIDOTE]

Diagnostic Procedures
- Creatinine, Serum
- Pseudocholinesterase, Serum

Drug Interaction Paralysis is potentiated by neuromuscular blockade (ie, pancuronium, vecuronium, succinylcholine, atracurium, doxacurium, mivacurium); inhibition of serum esterase prolongs the half-life of succinylcholine, cocaine, and other ester anesthetics; cholinergic toxicity is potentiated by cholinesterase inhibitors such as physostigmine

Additional Information

Red blood cell cholinesterase, and serum pseudocholinesterase may be depressed following acute or chronic organophosphate exposure and are theoretically useful for differentiating between carbamate and organophosphate exposures; RBC cholinesterase is typically not analyzed by in-house laboratories, and is usually not available for consideration during acute management. Pseudocholinesterase levels may be rapidly available from some in-house laboratories, but are not as reliable a marker of organophosphate exposure because of variability secondary to variant genotypes, hepatic disease, oral estrogen use, or malnutrition, thus they may not be useful in ruling out carbamate exposure.

Other information concerning pesticide exposures is available through the EPA-funded National Pesticide Telecommunications Network: 1-800-858-7378 (weekdays, 8 AM to 6 PM, Central Standard time)

Specific References

Ramagri S, Kosanam H, and Prakas PK, "Stability Study of Propoxur (Baygon) in Whole Blood and Urine Stored at Varying Temperature Conditions," *J Anal Toxicol*, 2006, 30:313-6.

Propylene Glycol

Pronunciation (PROE pi leen GLYE kole)

Applies to Antifreeze; Cosmetics; De-icer; Silver Sulfadiazine Cream, Topical; Solvent (Pharmaceuticals)

CAS Number 57-55-6

Synonyms Methyl Glycol; PG 12; Propane-1,2-Diol; Trimethyl Glycol

Use In cosmetics and as a solvent in pharmaceuticals; also used as a de-icer; automobile radiator antifreeze; found in intravenous preparations of Ativan®, Apresoline®, Bactrim™, Dilantin®, Brevibloc®, Lanoxin®, Librium®, MVI-12®, phenobarbital, Tridil®, and Valium.® Also found in topical silver sulfadiazine cream.

Mechanism of Toxic Action Metabolized to lactic acid, pyruvic acid, acetic acid, and propionaldehyde

Adverse Reactions

Cardiovascular: Bradycardia, arrhythmias (ventricular), arrhythmias, shock, sinus bradycardia

Endocrine & metabolic: Hypoglycemia, lactic acidosis, hyperosmolality, acidosis

Hematologic: Hemolysis, anemia

Renal: Renal failure

Signs and Symptoms of Overdose CNS depression, feces discoloration (black), hypotension, lacrimation, porphyria, seizures, stupor

Toxicodynamics/Kinetics

Distribution: V_d: 0.55 L/kg

Metabolism: To lactic acid and pyruvic acid

Half-life: Adults: 2-5 hours

Peak serum concentration: 1 hour postingestion

Elimination: 12% to 45% excreted unchanged renally; total body elimination: 0.1 L/kg/hour

Dosage Forms Liquid: 10%, 100%

Reference Range Propylene glycol level (mg/dL): 84.6 + (7.8 × osmolar gap in mOsm/kg); serum level of 6-1000 mg/L has been noted following intravenous administration; serum propylene glycol level >177 mg/L can result in anion gap lactic acidosis

Overdosage/Treatment

Decontamination: **Do not** use ipecac.

Supportive therapy: Sodium bicarbonate (I.V.) for metabolic acidosis; ethanol therapy is not useful

Enhancement of elimination: Hemodialysis may be effective.

Antidote(s)
- Sodium Bicarbonate [ANTIDOTE]

Diagnostic Procedures
- Glucose, Random
- Lactic Acid, Blood
- Osmolality, Serum

Drug Interaction May cause a transient neutralization of heparin.

Additional Information

60 mL of propylene glycol can cause stupor in infants

Patients with burns over 35% of total body surface area are at risk for propylene glycol toxicity if silver sulfadiazine is used.

Clear, colorless, and odorless; ~$^1/_3$ as intoxicating as ethanol

Added to foods at concentrations up to 15% in food seasoning

Density: 1.036 g/mL. Atmospheric half-life: 20-32 hours. Water half-life 1.3-2.3 years

How supplied: Liquid: 10%, 100% Emergency information can be obtained from Dow Chemical Company (Midland, Michigan) (517) 636-4400 or 800-258-2436.

Specific References

Bouchard NC, Abou Rjaili, Choufani D, et al, "Severe Lactic Acidemia and Systemic Toxicity Following Oral Propylene Glycol Ingestion: A Role for Fomepizole and Hemodialysis," *Clin Toxicol (Phila)*, 2005, 43:740.

Doty JD and Sahn SA, "An Unusual Case of Poisoning," *South Med J*, 2003, 96(9):923-5.

Jorens PG, Demey HE, Schepens PJ, et al, "Unusual D-Lactic Acid Acidosis from Propylene Glycol Metabolism in Overdose," *J Toxicol Clin Toxicol*, 2004, 42(2):163-9.

Neale BW, Mesler EL, Young M, et al, "Propylene Glycol-Induced Lactic Acidosis in a Patient with Normal Renal Function: A Proposed Mechanism and Monitoring Recommendations," *Ann Pharmacother*, 2005, 39(10):1732-6.

Propylene Glycol Dinitrate

CAS Number 106602-80-6 (Otto Fuel II); 6423-43-4

Synonyms Isopropylene Dinitrate; Methyl Nitroglycol; PGDN

Use Nitrated ester primarily used as a propellant in Oto Fuel II (a liquid monopropellant used by the U.S. Navy in torpedoes and other weapons); has been used in explosives

Adverse Reactions

Central nervous system: Ataxia at air levels of 1.5 ppm; headaches; dizziness at levels of 0.5 ppm

Gastrointestinal: Nausea at levels of 0.5 ppm

Hematologic: Methemoglobin levels as high as 24% noted in rodents exposed to 200 ppm for 4 hours

Toxicodynamics/Kinetics

Absorption: Inhalation and dermal

Metabolism: Broken down in erythrocytes to nitrate

Elimination: Urinary

Monitoring Parameters Methemoglobin

Reference Range Blood propylene glycol dinitrate level of 5 ppb noted after 3.2 hours exposure to 1.5 ppm air concentration

Overdosage/Treatment

Decontamination: **Oral:** Dilute with milk or water. Activated charcoal may be given. **Dermal:** Wash with soap and water. **Inhalation:** Administer 100% oxygen. **Ocular:** Irrigate with saline.

Supportive therapy: Methylene blue for symptomatic methemoglobinemia

Antidote(s)
- Methylene Blue [ANTIDOTE]

Additional Information Highly explosive agent. Slightly soluble in water (1.3 g/L) and does not persist in water for more than a few days; near U.S. torpedo facilities, air levels of propylene glycol dinitrate range from 0-2.2 ppm. PEL-TWA: 0.05 ppm. TLV-TWA (skin designation): 0.05 ppm

Pyrethrins

CAS Number 121-20-0; 121-21-1; 121-29-9; 25402-06-6; 52645-53-1; 8003-34-7

U.S. Brand Names A-200™ Pyrinate [OTC]; Alfadex®; RID® [OTC]; Tisit® [OTC]

Synonyms *Chrysanthemum cinerareaefolium*; Ambush; Buhach; BW-21-Z; Cinerin; Cyclopropanecarboxylic Acid; Dalmation-Insect Flowers; Dalmation-Insect Powder; Ectiban; Firmotox; FMX 33297; Insect Powder; Jasmolin; Permethrin; Permetrina (Portuguese); Persian-Insect Powder; Pounce; Pyrethrum Esters; Trieste Flowers

Commonly Found In Pyrethrins include pyrethrum extract and the pyrethrum esters: cinerin I and II, jasmolin I and II, and pyrethrin I and II; semisynthetic derivatives (pyrethroids) include allethrin, barthrin, bioallethrin, bioresmethrin, cyclethrin, cypermethrin, decamethrin, dimethrin, fenvalerate, flucythrinate, permethrin, phenothrin, and resmethrin; preparations often contain a synergist which increases stability and insecticidal activity, such as N-isobutyldecylenamidepiperonyl butoxide, piperonyl cyclonene, n-octyl sulfoxide of isosafrole, n-propylisome, and sesamex; sprays often formulated in petroleum solvent bases, such as kerosene and naphtha, which are generally more hazardous than the pyrethrins

Use Treatment of *Pediculus humanus* infestations; primarily used for indoor insect control

Mechanism of Toxic Action Delay closure of sodium channel by holding activation gate in the open position, producing a prolonged sodium current during the end of depolarization; sodium tail currents are more prolonged with pyrethroids with an alpha-cyano group (eg, cypermethrin, fenvalerate, flucythrinate) than with other pyrethroids. Derived from flowers that belong to the chrysanthemum family. The mechanism of action on the neuronal membranes of lice is similar to that of DDT. Piperonyl butoxide is usually added to pyrethrin to enhance the product's activity by decreasing the metabolism of pyrethrins in arthropods.

Adverse Reactions

Cardiovascular: Chest pain, angina

Central nervous system: Axonopathy

Dermatologic: Pruritus, erythema

Local: Burning, stinging

Respiratory: Oropharyngeal irritation, wheezing, sneezing, rhinitis, hypersensitivity pneumonitis, bronchospasm, asthma

Signs and Symptoms of Overdose Generally of very low order of toxicity in man due to low bioavailability and high first-pass metabolism. Pyrethrins are potent sensitizers, therefore, the most common complications are hypersensitivity reactions including anaphylactic shock, asthma; erythematous, vesicular, papular bullous contact dermatitis (occurs in 50% of those sensitive to ragweed, sometimes with eosinophilia); and wheezing. Asthenia, dizziness, headache, nausea, and vomiting are commonly seen with oral ingestions. Other symptoms that may occur include chest pain, cough, pneumonitis, pulmonary edema, and seizures. Ingestion of massive quantities or concentrated formulations may cause ataxia, cardiopulmonary arrest, CNS stimulation, and tremor. Hypersensitivity reactions (dyspnea, sneezing, wheezing), nasal congestion, rhinorrhea, and scratchy throat may be seen with inhalational exposure. Corneal abrasions may occur with eye exposure. Paresthesia and erythema are common following dermal exposure. In general, pyrethroids or synthetic derivatives are neither cutaneous sensitizers nor irritants and are less toxic than natural pyrethrins; however, they may cause paresthesias following dermal exposure. Synergists appear to be of even lower toxicity, based on experiments with laboratory mammals, despite their ability to enhance insecticidal activity. However, it has been postulated that they might have the potential to inhibit the microsomal enzyme metabolism of pyrethrins and perhaps increase their toxicity in man.

Admission Criteria/Prognosis Symptomatic patients 6 hours postexposure

Toxicodynamics/Kinetics

Onset of action: ~30 minutes

Absorption: Rapid; pyrethrins and pyrethroids are believed to be poorly absorbed through intact skin

Distribution: Through body tissues and brain

Metabolism: Rapid, however pathways of metabolism are somewhat controversial; pyrethrins I and II are metabolized rapidly by hydrolysis to chrysanthemumic acid and an alcohol, which is oxidized to the aldehyde and acid or conjugated with glucuronide; more recent evidence in rats indicates that the principal metabolites are oxidation products; pyrethroids are primarily metabolized by ester hydrolysis

Elimination: Slowly excreted in bile and urine and may remain detectable in body tissues for up to 3 weeks after ingestion

Monitoring Parameters Seizures, respiratory distress, and hypersensitivity reactions

Dosing Forms

All in combination with piperonyl butoxide

Gel, topical: 0.3% (30 g)

Liquid, topical: 0.2% (60 mL, 120 mL); 0.3% (60 mL, 118 mL, 120 mL, 177 mL, 237 mL, 240 mL)

Shampoo, topical: 0.3% (59 mL, 60 mL, 118 mL, 120 mL, 240 mL); 0.33% (120 mL)

Reference Range Pyrethrin plasma levels are not clinically useful; peak permethrin blood concentration of 868 ng/mL following ingestion of 600 mL of 20% permethrin emulsion resulted in GI irritation and little neurotoxicity

Overdosage/Treatment

Decontamination: Usually sufficient for most causal exposures. For oral ingestions, gastric emptying should be performed with lavage (within 1 hour), avoiding syrup of ipecac/emesis due to risk of seizures. Follow with administration of activated charcoal. The principal concern with most solutions and sprays is the hydrocarbon solvent. For preparations containing a hydrocarbon, refer to the appropriate monograph. Avoid administration of fats and oils, which increase intestinal absorption of pyrethrins. Diazepam or lorazepam for seizures; atropine may be effective for diarrhea. Irrigate eye exposures promptly with copious amounts of water. Wash contaminated skin promptly with copious amounts of soap and water.

Supportive therapy: Topical oil of vitamin E, (every 4 hours lightly applied), may relieve paresthesias; symptomatic and supportive treatment for allergic reactions; epinephrine or diphenhydramine for allergic reactions; nebulized bronchodilators for wheezing

Additional Information For external use only

Avoid touching eyes, mouth, or other mucous membranes; contact physician if irritation occurs or if condition does not improve in 2-3 days; patients with allergy to ragweed may develop cross-allergy to pyrethrins; avoid if known hypersensitivity to pyrethrins

IDLH: 5000 mg/m³; TLV-TWA: 5 mg/m³; PEC-TWA: 5 mg/m³

How supplied: **Gel, topical:** 0.3% (30 g, 480 g); **Liquid, topical:** 0.18% (60 mL); 0.2% (60 mL, 120 mL); 0.3% (60 mL, 120 mL, 240 mL); **Shampoo:** 0.3% (60 mL, 118 mL); 0.33% (60 mL, 120 mL)

Specific References

Lovecchio F and Knight J, "Injection of Pyrethroids Without Significant Sequelae," *Am J Emerg Med*, 2005, 23(3):406.

Naumovski J, Krenzelok EP, Bozinovska C, et al, "Transaminase Elevation in Pyrethroid Intoxications," *J Toxicol Clin Toxicol*, 2003, 41(5):652.

Ramesh A and Ravi PE, "Negative Ion Chemical Ionization-Gas Chromatographic-Mass Spectrometric Determination of Residues of Different Pyrethroid Insecticides in Whole Blood and Serum," *J Anal Toxicol*, 2004, 28(8):660-6.

Sudakin DL, "Pyrethroid Insecticides: Advances and Challenges in Biomonitoring," *Clin Toxicol (Phila)*, 2006, 44(1):31-7.

Pyridine

CAS Number 110-86-1

UN Number 1282

Synonyms Azabenzine; Azine

Use Primarily in production of pesticides, herbicides, antihistamines, steroids, sulfa antibiotics, water repellents, dyes, paint, and rubber; flavoring agent and as an agent to denature alcohol

Mechanism of Toxic Action Lipid peroxidation of the brain can occur

Adverse Reactions

Cardiovascular: Tachycardia, sinus tachycardia

Central nervous system: Lethargy, headaches, slurred speech, insomnia, fatigue

Dermatologic: Dermatitis

Gastrointestinal: Nausea, vomiting

Hematologic: Methemoglobinemia

Hepatic: Cirrhosis

Ocular: Visual evoked potential abnormalities

Respiratory: Tachypnea

Admission Criteria/Prognosis Any patient with change in mental status, cardiopulmonary complaints, or methemoglobin levels >30% should be admitted; asymptomatic patients with methemoglobin levels <30% may be considered for discharge after 6 hours of observation and if methemoglobin levels fall to <15%

Toxicodynamics/Kinetics

Absorption: with oral ingestion

Metabolism: Hepatic to N-methylpyridinium

Elimination: Renal

Overdosage/Treatment Decontamination: **Oral:** Lavage (within 1 hour)/ activated charcoal; **do not** induce emesis. **Dermal:** Wash with soap and water. **Ocular:** Irrigate with saline.

Additional Information Lethal dose: 125 mL

Central nervous symptoms can occur with exposures of 6-12 ppm; inhibits metabolism of benzene; not usually detected in ambient air

Yearly total pyridine intake: ~500 mg

Odor threshold: Air: 0.17 ppm; water: 0.95 mg/L. Atmospheric half-life: 23-46 days. Water half-life: 1.2 years. Soil half-life: 3 days. PEL-TWA: 5 ppm; TLV-TWA: 5 ppm; IDLH: 3600 ppm

Pyrimidifen

Synonyms 5-chloro-N-(2-[4-(2-ethoxyethyl)-2,3-dimethylphenoxy]ethyl)-6-ethylpyridimin-4- amine

Use An acaricide and insecticide first synthesized in Japan; used against fruit/vegetable mites

Mechanism of Toxic Action Similar structure to organochlorine agents with central nervous system effects (primarily depression)

Signs and Symptoms of Overdose Mydriasis, coma, apnea, hypotension, hypothermia, metabolic acidosis, hyperkalemia, hepatitis, acute renal failure

Overdosage/Treatment

Decontamination: Oral: Lavage within 1 hour/activated charcoal

Supportive therapy: Metabolic acidosis can be treated with 1-2 mEq/kg. Hypotension can be treated with crystalloid fluids; dopamine or norepinephrine are vasopressors of choice

Additional Information 40 mL of a 10% solution ingested orally is fatal

Specific References
Eisinger M and Almog Y, "Pyrimidifen Intoxication," *Ann Emerg Med*, 2003, 42(2):289-91.

Radium

Related Information
● Radon
CAS Number 7440-14-4
Synonyms Radium-223; Radium-224; Radium-226; Radium-228
Use Radiation source in treating neoplasms
Adverse Reactions
Hematologic: Leukopenia
Hepatic: Cirrhosis
Ocular: Cataracts
Miscellaneous: Sarcoma
Toxicodynamics/Kinetics
Absorption: Inhalation and oral (~20%)
Elimination: Primarily fecal
Overdosage/Treatment Decontamination: **Dermal:** Wash with soap and water. Monitor with a Geiger-Mueller counter. **Ocular:** Irrigate with saline.
Additional Information
Lethal dose: Oral: 56 uCi/kg (2.074 kBq/kg)
Bone sarcomas, breast cancer, and liver cancer have been associated with radium exposure; chronic myeloid leukemia also noted
Malignancy can occur at a dose of 1.03 uCi/kg (38 kBq/kg)
Residence atmosphere time: 1-10 days
Radium-223: Decay mode: Alpha; Soil half-life: 11 days
Radium-224: Decay mode: Alpha; Soil half-life: 4 days
Radium-226: Decay mode: Alpha; Soil half-life: 1620 years
Radium-228: Decay mode: Beta; Soil half-life: 6 years
Specific References
Koenig KL, Goans RE, Hatchett RJ, et al, "Medical Treatment of Radiological Casualties: Current Concepts," *Ann Emerg Med*, 2005, 45(6):643-52.
Lloyd RD, Taylor GN, and Miller SC, "Does Low Dose Internal Radiation Increase Lifespan?" *Health Phys*, 2004, 86(6):629-32.

Radon

Related Information
● Radium
CAS Number 10043-92-2; 14859-67-7
Synonyms Radon 222; Rn
Use Product of natural decay of uranium which is then converted to radium 222 and finally as a sixth decay product as uranium 238; miners can be exposed in uranium or phosphate mines; also used as a gas tracer in detecting leaks and in the study of atmospheric transport; building materials made of vanadium or concrete produced from phosphate slag may have elevated radon content. See figure.

Sources of Radon and Common Entry Points

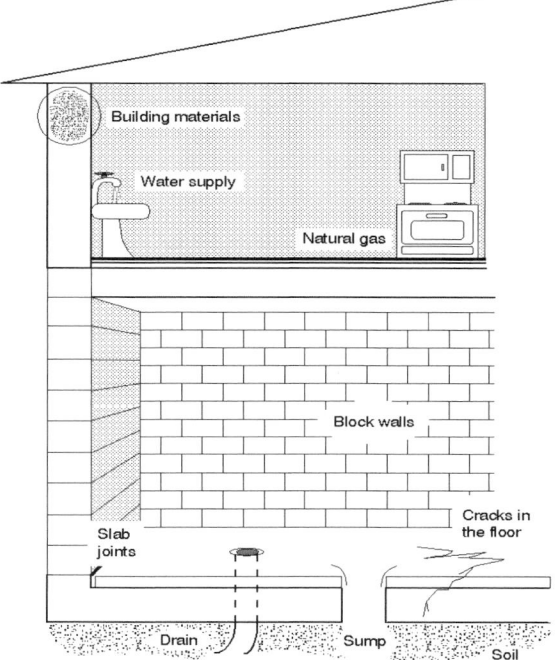

Mechanism of Toxic Action Attaches to bronchial epithelium which can lead to malignant transformation
Adverse Reactions
Dermal: Radiation recall dermatitis
Ocular: Cataracts
Renal: Nephritis
Respiratory: Emphysema, pulmonary fibrosis at high doses
Miscellaneous: Lung cancer (additive effect with smoking)
Toxicodynamics/Kinetics
Absorption: Inhalation: 30% to 40%. Oral: 90%. Dermal: 5%
Half-life: Air: 4 days. Lungs: 6-60 hours. Fat: 21-130 minutes. Oral ingestion: 18-180 minutes
Metabolism: Radon daughters include polonium 218, lead 214, bismuth 214, and polonium 214; does not undergo biological metabolism
Elimination: Exhalation primarily
Overdosage/Treatment
Decontamination: Affected homes may require subslab depressurization. Open windows can reduce indoor radon levels by 50% to 70%. See figure.

Subslab Depressurization

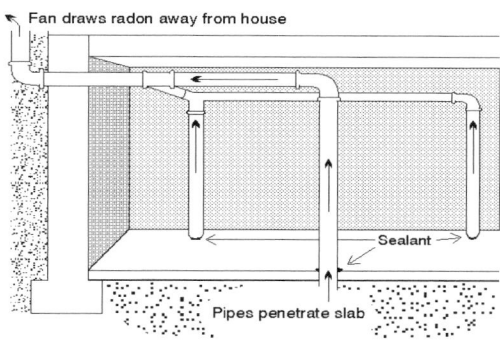

Supportive therapy: Cataracts and lung carcinoma are treated with standard therapies. Affected individuals should stop smoking.
Additional Information Radon is odorless, inert, and colorless. For radioactive properties: See table.

Radioactive Properties of ^{222}Radon and Its Daughter Products				
		Radiation Energies (MeV)		
Radionu-clide	**Half-life**	α	β	γ
^{222} Radon	3.8 days	5.49	–	–
^{218} Polonium	3.1 min	6.00	–	–
^{214} Lead	26.8 min	–	0.67 0.73	0.30 0.35
^{214} Bismuth	19.9 min	–	1.51 1.54 3.27	0.61 1.12 1.76
^{214} Polonium	164 μsec	7.60	–	0.8
^{210} Lead	22.3 yr	–	0.016 0.06	0.05
^{210} Bismuth	5 d	–	1.16	–
^{210} Polonium	138 d	5.31	–	–
^{206} Lead	No half-life; stable element			

Adapted from: Shlein B, *The Health Physics and Radiological Health Handbook*, Scinta; Silver Spring, MD, 1992

Ambient, outdoor air concentration: 0.2-0.7 pCi/L. EPA action level: 4 pCi/L (0.02 working level of radon); levels exceeding the EPA action level may be present in ~25% of homes in the U.S. Average radon 222 concentration in groundwater: 200-600 pCi/L (7-22 Bq/L). For risk assessment: See tables.

Radon Risk if You Smoke

Radon Level	If 1000 people who smoked were exposed to this level over a lifetime...	The risk of cancer from radon exposure compares to...	What to Do: Stop smoking and...
20 pCi/L	About 135 people could get lung cancer	100 times the risk of drowning	Fix your home
10 pCi/L	About 71 people could get lung cancer	100 times the risk of dying in a home fire	Fix your home
8 pCi/L	About 57 people could get lung cancer		Fix your home
4 pCi/L	About 29 people could get lung cancer	100 times the risk of dying in an airplane crash	Fix your home
2 pCi/L	About 15 people could get lung cancer	2 times the risk of dying in a car crash	Consider fixing between 2 and 4 pCi/L
1.3 pCi/L	About 9 people could get lung cancer	(Average indoor radon level)	(Reducing radon levels below 2 pCi/L is difficult)
0.4 pCi/L	About 3 people could get lung cancer	(Average outdoor radon level)	

U.S. Department of Health and Human Services, "Radon Toxicity," *Case Studies in Environmental Medicine,* Agency for Toxic Substances and Disease Registry, September, 1992.
Note: If you are a former smoker, your risk may be lower.

Radon Risk if You Have Never Smoked

Radon Level	If 1000 people who never smoked were exposed to this level over a lifetime...	The risk of cancer from radon exposure compares to...	What to Do:
20 pCi/L	About 8 people could get lung cancer	The risk of being killed in a violent crime	Fix your home
10 pCi/L	About 4 people could get lung cancer		Fix your home
8 pCi/L	About 3 people could get lung cancer	10 times the risk of dying in an airplane crash	Fix your home
4 pCi/L	About 2 people could get lung cancer	The risk of drowning	Fix your home
2 pCi/L	About 1 person could get lung cancer	The risk of dying in a home fire	Consider fixing between 2 and 4 pCi/L
1.3 pCi/L	<1 person could get lung cancer	(Average indoor radon level)	(Reducing radon levels below 2 pCi/L is difficult)
0.4 pCi/L	<1 person could get lung cancer	(Average outdoor radon level)	

U.S. Department of Health and Human Services, "Radon Toxicity," *Case Studies in Environmental Medicine,* Agency for Toxic Substances and Disease Registry, September, 1992.
Note: If you are a former smoker, your risk may be higher.

Specific References

Norris MJ, Guiseppe VE, and Hess CT, "Waterborne Radon in Seven Maine Schools," *Health Phys*, 2004, 86(5):528-35.

Pawel DJ and Puskin JS, "The U.S. Environmental Protection Agency's Assessment of Risks from Indoor Radon," *Health Phys*, 2004, 87(1):68-74.

RDX

Applies to Composition C-4
CAS Number 121-82-4
Synonyms Cyclonite; Hexogen; Hexolite; PBX
Use Class A explosive; nitrate compound used in plastic explosives, fireworks, and as a detonator; rodenticide
Mechanism of Toxic Action Causes fatty degeneration of liver; seizure mechanism of action is unknown
Adverse Reactions
Cardiovascular: Tachycardia, sinus tachycardia
Central nervous system: Seizures, irritability, amnesia, confusion, hyperthermia
Dermatologic: Dermal irritant
Gastrointestinal: Nausea, vomiting
Hematologic: Anemia
Hepatic: Hepatic steatosis
Neuromuscular & skeletal: Muscle twitching, myoclonus
Renal: Hematuria
Miscellaneous: Liver tumors (adenomas and carcinomas) produced in rodent models
Toxicodynamics/Kinetics
Absorption: Oral (slowly) and inhalation; not readily absorbed by dermal route
Distribution: V_d: 2.2 L/kg
Half-life: 15 hours
Elimination: Feces (primarily) and urine
Reference Range Serum RDX level of 10.7 mg/L associated with seizures
Overdosage/Treatment
Decontamination: **Oral:** Activated charcoal may be used; gastric lavage within 5 hours. **Dermal:** Wash hands with soap and water. **Inhalation:** Humidified 100% oxygen. **Ocular:** Irrigate with saline.
Supportive therapy: Seizures can be treated with benzodiazepines or phenobarbital. Clonazepam is also an effective anticonvulsant.
Additional Information
Toxic oral dose: 15 mL
Oral dose of 85 mg/kg has caused seizures in a child; symptoms can occur with ingested daily dose of 0.1 mg/kg; can produce a "high" similar to ethanol
Atmospheric half-life: 1.5 hours. Water half-life: 9-13 hours (by photolysis). PEL-TWA: 1.5 mg/m^3 (skin designation). TLV-TWA: 1.5 mg/m^3 (skin designation)

Rhodium

CAS Number 7440-16-6
Mechanism of Toxic Action Some reaction with rhodium and DNA/RNA is apparent; it is not known what the clinical implication of this is
Adverse Reactions Likely that soluble rhodium is toxic, but there is no human literature to support this; mice have shown both respiratory and CNS depression; immunologic contact urticaria
Signs and Symptoms of Overdose Mild ocular irritation, urticaria
Toxicodynamics/Kinetics Absorption: Elemental rhodium is poorly soluble and minimally absorbed; organic rhodium and rhodium trichloride are more readily absorbed
Reference Range No established toxic levels; TWA (metal): 1 mg/m^3; TWA (insoluble compound): 1 mg/m^3; TWA (soluble compound): 0.01 mg/m^3
Overdosage/Treatment Decontamination: Irrigate eyes with normal saline using a Morgan's lens.

Ruthenium

CAS Number 7440-18-8
Signs and Symptoms of Overdose Fumes may be injurious to eyes and lungs.
Reference Range No TLV recommended
Overdosage/Treatment
Decontamination: Irrigate eyes with normal saline using a Morgan's lens.
Supportive therapy: Humidified oxygen for fume exposure

Selenious Acid

CAS Number 7783-00-8
Synonyms Selenous Acid, Monohydrated Selenium Dioxide
Commonly Found In Component of compound for gun blueing agent, reagent for alkaloids
Mechanism of Toxic Action Inhibition of sulfhydryl-containing enzymes
Adverse Reactions
Cardiovascular: Hypertension, tachycardia, cardiomyopathy, sinus tachycardia
Central nervous system: Convulsions
Dermatologic: Alopecia

Gastrointestinal: Pharyngeal edema, intestinal distention, hypersalivation, garlic odor, vomiting, watery diarrhea, burns to the esophagus, pharyngeal, and gastrointestinal tract

Neuromuscular & skeletal: Myopathy

Signs and Symptoms of Overdose Dermal irritation, diarrhea, garlic breath odor, hypersalivation, muscle spasms, seizures, vomiting

Toxicodynamics/Kinetics

Absorption: Inhalation: 97%. Ingestion: 87%. Dermal: 9% to 27% in rodent studies

Half-life: 1.2 days

Elimination: 50% excreted renally

Monitoring Parameters Thrombocytopenia, leukocytosis, metabolic acidosis, hyperglycemia, transient elevation of hepatic enzymes

Reference Range

Normal range: Urine: 7.0-160.0 mcg/L; Blood: 100.0-340.0 mcg/L; Serum: 86.0-125.0 mcg/L

Toxic range: Urine: >400.0 mcg/L; Postmortem serum level of 18.4 mg/L and urine level of 2.11 mg/L described in one case report

Overdosage/Treatment

Decontamination: Emesis is contraindicated; basic poison management with lavage (within 1 hour)/activated charcoal

Supportive therapy: British Anti-Lewisite (BAL), calcium sodium EDTA, D-penicillamine are contraindicated since they can increase renal injury

Diagnostic Procedures

- Glucose, Random

Additional Information Ingestion of 15 mL of 2% solution has been fatal in a 2 year old; 30-60 mL fatal in adults. Garlic odor; vapors are pink; bitter taste. Odor threshold: 0.002 mg/m^3. TLV-TWA: 0.2 mg/m^3 IDLH: 100 mg/m^3; PEL-TWA: 0.2 mg/m^3

Selenium

CAS Number 7782-49-2

UN Number 2658

U.S. Brand Names Selenicaps [OTC]; Selenimin [OTC]; Selepen®

Synonyms Selenate

Use Blasting caps, rectifiers, photoelectric cells, nutritional food additive for poultry and livestock

Mechanism of Action Part of glutathione peroxidase which protects cell components from oxidative damage due to peroxidases produced in cellular metabolism

Adverse Reactions Eyes, nose, throat, cardiovascular, respiratory, neurologic, gastrointestinal, hepatic, genitourinary, dermatologic, alopecia, blind staggers

Signs and Symptoms of Overdose CNS depression → coma, eye redness, fatty degeneration of liver, fingernail loss, garlic-like breath, hair discoloration (red), hyposmia, increased LFTs, metal fume fever, metallic taste, myoglobinuria, nasal irritation, nausea, paresthesia, photocontact dermatitis, prolonged QT, pruritus, pulmonary edema, salivation, sore throat, thrombocytopenia, tremor, T-wave flattening → inversion, tubular degeneration, vomiting

Admission Criteria/Prognosis Admit any patient exhibiting gastrointestinal or pulmonary effects, or with a serum selenium level >1000 ng/mL

Pharmacodynamics/Kinetics

Absorption: Orally (80%) and by inhalation

Distribution: To all soft tissue, especially liver and kidney

Protein binding: 95%

Half-life: 12-41 hours

Excretion: Urine, feces, lungs, skin

Contraindications Hypersensitivity to selenium or any component of the formulation

Dosage Forms

Capsule (Selenicaps): 200 mcg [sugar, starch, wheat, yeast, gluten free]

Injection, solution: 40 mcg/mL (10 mL)

Selepen®: 40 mcg/mL (10 mL, 30 mL) [30 mL size contains benzyl alcohol]

Tablet: 50 mcg, 100 mcg, 200 mcg

Selenimin: 50 mcg, 125 mcg, 200 mcg

Tablet, timed release: 200 mcg

Reference Range

Normal range:

Serum: 95-165 ng/mL; serum levels >1000 ng/mL are associated with gastrointestinal toxicity, while serum selenium levels >2000 ng/mL may be lethal

Urine: 15-150 mcg/L

Overdosage/Treatment

Decontamination: **Oral:** Emesis is contraindicated; basic poison management with lavage (within 1 hour)/activated charcoal. **Dermal:** Remove contaminated clothing; wash with soap and water. **Ocular:** Irrigate with saline.

Supportive therapy: British Anti-Lewisite (BAL), calcium sodium EDTA, D-penicillamine are contraindicated since they can increase renal injury;

humidified oxygen for fume exposure; ascorbic acid can increase toxic effects and should be avoided

Diagnostic Procedures

- Selenium, Serum
- Selenium, Urine

Drug Interactions No data reported

Pregnancy Risk Factor C

Additional Information

Fatal dose: Children: 15 mL (2% selenious acid); Adults: 30 mL

Serum selenium levels are significantly lower (24 ng/mL versus 39 ng/mL in control patients) in chronic alcohol abuse patients

Soluble selenites, selenates, and organic selenium compounds are more toxic than the insoluble (ie, selenium sulfide)

24-hour urine level: <30 mcg/L

Average hair levels in U.S.: 0-0.5 ppm Average air concentrations: 0.1-10 ng/m^3. Average seawater selenium: 0.04-0.12 mcg/L

Average concentration in earth's crust: 0.05-0.09 mg/kg; highest concentrations are found in volcanic rocks in Western and Midwest U.S. and may be as high as 120 mg/kg; coal contains 2 mg/kg, while crude petroleum contains as high as 950 mg/kg

Daily intake: ~0.07-0.15 mg

Raw beef kidney (average 1.7 mg selenium/kg weight), swordfish (2.8 mg/kg), and Brazilian nuts (14.7 mg/kg) are foods containing highest amount of selenium. Selenium content in milk: <2 ppm. Selenium content in marlin: <4.3 ppm

TLV-TWA: 0.2 mg/m^3

Specific References

Fessler AJ, Moller G, Talcott PA, et al, "Selenium Toxicity in Sheep Grazing Reclaimed Phosphate Mining Sites," *Vet Hum Toxicol*, 2003, 45(6):294-8.

Spiller HA and Pfeifer E, "Selenium Toxicity: Two Fatal Cases," *J Anal Toxicol*, 2006, 30:155.

Selenium Dioxide

CAS Number 7746-08-4

UN Number 2811

Synonyms Selenium Oxide

Commonly Found In Gun-blueing solution

Use Catalyst in production of organic compounds

Mechanism of Toxic Action Inhibition of sulfhydryl-containing enzymes; selenium is a component of glutathione peroxidase enzyme

Adverse Reactions

Central nervous system: Coma

Neuromuscular & skeletal: Rhabdomyolysis

Respiratory: Wheezing

Miscellaneous: Fingernails, teeth, and hair may stain red

Signs and Symptoms of Overdose Cough, dermal burns, dizziness, dyspnea, fever, gagging, headache, sternal pain, tachypnea, throat irritation, transient loss of consciousness

Toxicodynamics/Kinetics Absorption: Inhalation: Well absorbed

Reference Range Normal range: Serum: 95-165 ng/mL; Urine: 15-150 mcg/L

Overdosage/Treatment

Decontamination: Oxygenation; 10% ointment of sodium thiosulfate may be useful. British Anti-Lewisite (BAL) is contraindicated.

Dermal: Remove contaminated clothing; wash with soap and water.

Ocular: Irrigate with saline.

Supportive therapy: British Anti-Lewisite (BAL), calcium sodium EDTA, D-penicillamine are contraindicated since they can increase renal injury. Ascorbic acid can increase toxic effects and should be avoided.

Silver

CAS Number 7440-22-4

Synonyms Argentum; Shell Silver; Silber

Use Primarily in photography and electronic products (ie, batteries); coinage use was discontinued in 1970

Mechanism of Toxic Action Silver has a strong affinity for sulfhydryl groups and proteins; systemic toxicity is rare due to rapid binding to proteins; argyria is a blue-gray discoloration of skin, mucous membrane, and eye which results from silver deposition

Adverse Reactions HEENT, respiratory, photocontact dermatitis, sinus bradycardia

Signs and Symptoms of Overdose Blue-gray discoloration of conjunctiva, cornea, and lens; abdominal pain, bradycardia, bronchitis, cough, feces discoloration (black), hypertension, hyposmia, nail bed pigmentation, proteinuria, skin burns, throat irritation, wheezing

Admission Criteria/Prognosis Adult ingestions >3 g (or 1 g of elemental silver by injection) should be considered for admission

Toxicodynamics/Kinetics

Absorption: Oral (10% to 20%); absorption from the respiratory tract and gastrointestinal tract occurs with soluble silver salts; complex salts are dermally absorbed; burn patients absorb silver from silver sulfadiazine

Distribution: Widely distributed
Half-life, biological: Human lung: ~1 day
Elimination: Primarily excreted through bile

Reference Range
Normal blood levels: Undetectable
Mean blood silver levels: 0.11 mcg/mL documented in workers of a photographic materials manufacturer exposed to 0.001-0.1 mg/m^3 of silver

Overdosage/Treatment
Decontamination: **Do not** induce emesis. Activated charcoal may be utilized.
Supportive therapy: Wheezing can be treated with nebulized beta-agonist agents.

Diagnostic Procedures
- Silver, Serum
- Silver, Urine

Additional Information
Lethal dose: Silver nitrate: Oral: 10 g; Colloidal metal solution: I.V.: 50 g; Toxic dose: Silver nitrate: Oral: 2 g
Argyria is the development of a slate gray or blue gray irreversible pigmentation of skin due to deposition of silver sulfide in the dermis; argyria generally occurs after injection of 1 g of elemental silver or ingestion of 3.8 g;
Average dietary intake of silver: 70-88 mcg with drinking water providing ~20 mcg of silver
Permissible amount of silver in bottled water: 0.05 mg/L
Background water silver levels: ~0.2 mcg/L in freshwater and 0.25 mcg/L in salt water
Background atmospheric silver levels: <1 ng/m^3
Average silver concentration in earth's crust: 0.1 ppm
Shellfish (particularly oysters) may contain as much as 5.5 mg/kg of silver
Cigarettes contain from 0.2 mg/kg (nonfilter) to 0.3 mg/kg (filter) of silver
OSHA TWA: 0.01 mg/m^3. PEL-TWA: 0.01 mg/m^3

Specific References
Vukmir RB, "Abdominal Pain in a Child Associated with Dental Amalgam Ingestion," *Am J Emerg Med*, 2005, 23(3):391-3.

Sodium Azide

CAS Number 12136-89-9; 26628-22-8
UN Number 1687
Synonyms Azium; Azomide
Use Shell detonators in explosive industry; found as principle agent (350-600 g) for providing nitrogen for the rapid expansion (in 0.05 seconds) of automobile air bags; preservative for laboratory reagents (concentration ~1 mg/mL); nematocide; herbicide
Mechanism of Toxic Action Mucosal irritant; may inhibit oxidative phosphorylation; can cause vasodilitation
Adverse Reactions
Cardiovascular: Asystole, hypotension, initial bradycardia followed by tachycardia, chest pain, arrhythmias (atrial/ventricular), myocardial depression, congestive heart failure, vasodilation, cardiopathy
Central nervous system: Hypothermia, hyperthermia, headache, agitation, seizures, coma
Dermatologic: Dermal burns
Endocrine & metabolic: Polydipsia, metabolic acidosis
Gastrointestinal: Diarrhea, nausea, vomiting, abdominal cramps
Hematologic: Leukocytosis
Neuromuscular & skeletal: Weakness, hyporeflexia, paresthesia
Ocular: Photophobia, lacrimation, keratitis, corneal burn, mydriasis
Respiratory: Hyperventilation, tachypnea, dyspnea, pulmonary edema
Miscellaneous: Diaphoresis
Admission Criteria/Prognosis Admit any ingestion >40 mg in adults or any symptomatic patient 2 hours postexposure; any patient with metabolic acidosis should be admitted
Toxicodynamics/Kinetics
Absorption: Inhalation, dermal or ingestion
Metabolism: Converted to nitric oxide
Monitoring Parameters Arterial blood gas, ECG, creatine phosphokinase, electrolytes, chest x-ray
Reference Range Postmortem blood levels (following ingestion of sodium azide): 8-262 mg/L
Overdosage/Treatment
Decontamination: **Oral:** Activated charcoal. **Dermal:** Flush with water. **Inhalation:** Administer 100% humidified oxygen. **Ocular:** Copious irrigation with saline or water
Supportive therapy: I.V. sodium bicarbonate (1-3 mEq/kg) for acidosis; phenobarbital is probably the most effective agent to treat seizures. Hypotension can be treated with crystalloid solution (10-20 mL/kg) and placement in Trendelenburg position. Vasopressors (dopamine or norepinephrine) can be used for resistant cases. The use of sodium nitrite or hyperbaric oxygen is of theoretical benefit, with human data lacking in efficacy.

Enhancement of elimination: Extracorporeal removal is of no benefit. Exchange transfusion does not appear to be beneficial.

Additional Information
Fatal oral dose: 13 mg/kg
Oral dose of 0.5 mcg/kg can result in reduction of blood pressure; positive ferric chloride (10% to 20%) test of gastric aspirate can occur (red precipitate)
Rescuer can become mildly toxic (headache, nausea) from expired air or gastric aspirate of sodium azide toxic patients (due to hydrazoic acid)
Odorless, colorless, highly explosive. Specific gravity: 1.846. TLV-ceiling: 0.11 ppm
Byproducts of sodium azide detonation include sodium hydroxide and nitrogen.
Other chemical constituents in automobile air bags include 2,4-dinitrotoluene, boron, potassium nitrate, nitrocellulose and cupric oxide

Specific References
Cooper H and Thomas T, "Ocular Injuries Related to Airbag Use," *Am J Emerg Med*, 2004, 22(2):135-7.
Duma SM, Rath AL, Jernigan MV, et al, "The Effects of Depowered Airbags on Eye Injuries in Frontal Automobile Crashes," *Am J Emerg Med*, 2005, 23(1):13-9.
Martin TG and Robertson WO, "Laboratory Workplace Coffee Tampering with Sodium Azide," *J Toxicol Clin Toxicol*, 2004, 42(5):748-9.
Nordt SP, Molloy M, Ryan J, et al, "Burns from Automobile Airbags," *J Emerg Med*, 2003, 25(2):201-2.

Sodium Hypochlorite

Related Information
- Calcium Hypochlorite
- Chlorine

Applies to Bleach
CAS Number 8007-59-8
UN Number 1791
Synonyms Carrel-Dakin Solution; Clorox; Hypochlorous Acid; Sodium Salt
Commonly Found In Bleach, disinfectants, deodorizers, water purifiers
Mechanism of Toxic Action Corrosive - oxidizing agent directly related to concentration of chlorine; the pH of household bleach: 10.8-11.4
Adverse Reactions
Cardiovascular: Hypotension, bradycardia, cardiac arrest, chest pain, shock, sinus bradycardia, angina
Dermatologic: Dermal burns, blistering, onycholysis
Gastrointestinal: Esophageal perforation
Hematologic: Hemolysis, anemia
Ocular: Photophobia, blepharospasm, conjunctival edema and pain
Respiratory: Aspiration
Signs and Symptoms of Overdose Chest pain, dyspnea, erythema, hypernatremia, local edema, pain, sore throat, vomiting
Admission Criteria/Prognosis Admit any patient with change in mental status.
Toxicodynamics/Kinetics Metabolism: In the stomach, acid solution forms hypochlorous acid and HCl
Monitoring Parameters Produces high osmolal gap (I.V. use). May cause hypernatremia and hyperchloremia.
Overdosage/Treatment
Decontamination: **Do not** induce vomiting. **Do not** use gastric lavage; dilute with milk or water. Irrigate eyes and skin with saline. Early endoscopy may be useful for oral ingestions; **do not** neutralize.
Oral: Endoscopy is usually not required with a 3% to 6% solution ingestion. **Dermal:** Rinse with water. **Ocular:** Irrigate copiously with water, or saline.
Supportive therapy: Ocular: Topical mydriatic agents (ie, 1% atropine twice daily) and topical antibiotics with topical steroids (1% prednisolone tapered over 10 days) can be used.
Dexamethasone (1 mg/kg/day) should be considered for management of airway edema.
Diagnostic Procedures
- Electrolytes, Blood
- Osmolality, Serum
Additional Information Odor of liquid bleach. Chloramine gas is liberated when ammonia and bleach are mixed. Chlorine gas is emitted when sodium hypochlorite decomposes in a fire.

Sodium Monofluoroacetate

Related Information
- Toxins Which Should Be Lavaged with Solutions Other Than Water
CAS Number 62-74-8
UN Number 2629
U.S. Brand Names Compound 1080®
Synonyms Fluoroacetic Acid (Sodium Salt); SMFA; Sodium Fluoroacetate
Use Rodenticide (banned in U.S. in 1972); used for coyote control in Mexico; possible agroterrorism agent

Mechanism of Toxic Action Metabolized to fluorocitrate which then blocks Kreb cycle metabolism by inhibiting the mitochondrial enzyme aconitase

Adverse Reactions

Cardiovascular: Prolonged QT intervals on ECG, fibrillation (ventricular), hypotension, arrhythmias (ventricular)

Central nervous system: Auditory hallucinations, seizures, tetany, coma, ataxia

Endocrine & metabolic: Hypocalcemia

Gastrointestinal: Vomiting, salivation

Hepatic: Hepatic necrosis

Neuromuscular & skeletal: Paresthesia, hypertonicity, carpopedal spasms

Ocular: Nystagmus

Renal: Renal failure (acute)

Respiratory: Hemorrhagic pulmonary edema, hyperventilation

Signs and Symptoms of Overdose Typically begin 30-90 minutes after exposure; coma, hallucinations, hypotension, muscle spasms, mydriasis, myoglobinuria, paresthesia, seizures, sinus tachycardia, stupor. Late findings include renal and/or hepatic necrosis.

Admission Criteria/Prognosis Any symptomatic patient, any electrolyte abnormalities, acidosis, or suspected ingestions >2 mg/kg should be considered for admission into an intensive care unit; poor prognostic signs include hypotension, metabolic acidosis, increased serum creatinine and ventricular tachycardia development

Toxicodynamics/Kinetics Absorption: Through gastrointestinal tract and lungs; dermal absorption does not appear to occur if skin is intact

Reference Range

Autopsy urinary levels of 368 mg/L associated with lethality 17 hours after exposure to 465 mg of sodium fluoroacetate

Mean urinary sodium monofluoroacetate level of 368 mg/L associated with fatal poisoning

Overdosage/Treatment

Decontamination: Lavage within 1 hour with magnesium sulfate or activated charcoal. Dermal: Remove contaminated clothing and irrigate skin with soap and water.

Supportive therapy: Treat seizures with phenobarbital or diazepam, intravenous calcium (10-20 mL of 10% calcium chloride in adults or 10-20 mL/kg in children); or 0.1-0.2 mL/kg of 10% calcium gluconate up to 20 mL should be given for evidence of hypocalcium (prolonged QT interval, tetany). Mephentermine may be more effective than levarterenol in treating hypotension. Digitalis can be utilized in pulmonary edema. Procainamide may be useful for ventricular arrhythmias. Glycerol monoacetate effective in animals; clinical use not as promising. Acetamide (500 mL of 10% solution in D_5W infused over 30 minutes every 4 hours) or ethanol use is also controversial (to inhibit the conversion of fluoroacetate to fluorocitrate). Acetamide or ethanol therapy has been used in experimental models, but this modality has not been substantiated in humans.

Enhancement of elimination: Multiple dose of activated charcoal may be effective

Diagnostic Procedures
- Glucose, Random

Additional Information

Approximately 2-10 mg/kg is fatal.

A white, odorless powder usually associated with a blue dye; initially developed for chemical warfare

Vinegar taste only when in solution; water soluble. When heated, toxic sodium oxide and fluoride fumes are emitted.

Ethanol treatment may aggravate hypokalemia.

Fluoroacetamide is less toxic; trifluoroacetic acid used in high performance liquid chromatography is an irritant and can be dermally absorbed, but is not as toxic

IDLH: 2.5 mg/m^3

STEL: 0.15 mg/^{3}

Specific References

Höjer J, Hung HT, Du NT, et al, "An Outbreak of Severe Rodenticide Poisoning in North Vietnam Caused by Illegal Fluoroacetate," *J Toxicol Clin Toxicol*, 2003, 41(5):646.

Sodium Oleate

Applies to Oleate

CAS Number 143-19-1

Synonyms Olate Flakes

Use Insecticide; also used topically in hemorrhoidal therapy

Mechanism of Toxic Action An anionic surfactant which can result in localized injury. Lung exposure can result in activation of coagulation and thus creation of microemboli.

Signs and Symptoms of Overdose Oral ingestion: Hypoxia, leukocytosis, pneumonitis, tachypnea

Admission Criteria/Prognosis Admit any symptomatic patient

Overdosage/Treatment

Decontamination: No gastric decontamination required

Supportive therapy: High-dose glucocorticosteroids may be helpful to prevent lung injury. High-frequency jet ventilation and PEEP may be required.

Stoddard Solvent

CAS Number 8030-30-6; 8052-41-3

UN Number 1255; 1256; 1271; 2553

U.S. Brand Names Texsolve S®; Varsol 1®

Synonyms Dry Cleaning Safety Solvent (used in 15% of plants); Spotting Naphtha; White Spirits

Use Petroleum solvent which is used as a paint thinner, printing ink, adhesive, in liquid photocopier toners, degreaser used in dry cleaning plants

Mechanism of Toxic Action Mixture of hydrocarbons (alkanes, cycloalkanes, and aromatics), this solvent can cause central nervous system depression and cerebral atrophy and axonal prenodal swellings

Adverse Reactions

Central nervous system: Dizziness, headache, ataxia, memory disturbance

Gastrointestinal: Nausea

Hematologic: Methemoglobinemia

Hepatic: Elevated liver function test results

Ocular: Eye irritation

Renal: Glomerulonephritis, nephritis

Admission Criteria/Prognosis Patients who develop tachypnea, cyanosis, dyspnea, CNS depression, tachycardia, or fever within 8 hours of exposure should be admitted; asymptomatic patients can be discharged after 8 hours observation

Toxicodynamics/Kinetics

Absorption: From lungs, orally, and dermally

Distribution: V_d: 10-11 L/kg

Metabolism: Hepatic to dimethylbenzoic acid

Elimination: Urine/feces (clearance: 263 mL/minute)

Reference Range Mean blood level after an exposure (airborne) of 600 mg/m^3 for 5 days (6 hours/day): ~2-2.5 mg/L

Overdosage/Treatment Decontamination: **Oral:** Dilute with water. **Dermal:** Wash with soap and water. **Ocular:** Irrigate with saline.

Additional Information Odor threshold: 0.9 ppm. Insoluble in water. TLV-TWA: 100 ppm; PEL-TWA: 100 ppm

Strychnine

Related Information
- Toxins Which Should Be Lavaged with Solutions Other Than Water

CAS Number 509-42-2; 57-24-9; 60-41-3; 60491-10-3; 66-32-1

UN Number 1692

U.S. Brand Names Certox®; Dolco Mouse Ceral®; Kwik-kil®; Mouse-Rid®; Mouse-Tox®; Pied Piper Mouse Seed®; Ro-Dex®

Synonyms *Strychnos ignatii*; *Strychnos nux-vomica*; *Strychnos tiente*

Use Rodenticide; also used as an adulterant in production of illicit cocaine, heroin, and amphetamine; an antiquated antidote historically used in analeptic treatment for barbiturate overdose; unapproved use for non-ketotic hyperglycinemia and sleep apnea (100 mcg/kg)

Mechanism of Toxic Action Strychnine competitively antagonizes the inhibitory action of glycine at the postsynaptic receptors in the spinal cord; this loss of postsynaptic inhibition results in excessive motor neuron activity; binding within the CNS may also be responsible for exaggerated responses to visual, auditory, and tactile stimulation

Adverse Reactions

Cardiovascular: Sinus tachycardia

Central nervous system: Anxiety and seizures without loss of consciousness, dysesthesia

Endocrine & metabolic: Hypokalemia

Gastrointestinal: Dysphagia, bitter taste

Neuromuscular & skeletal: Rigidity, muscle cramps, hypertonicity, trismus

Ocular: Nystagmus

Respiratory: Tachypnea, apnea, respiratory paralysis

Miscellaneous: Hypersensitivity to external stimuli

Signs and Symptoms of Overdose Acidosis, agitation and anxiety (followed by excessive muscular activity and hypertonicity), apnea and cyanosis, death (from respiratory and cardiac arrest), fasciculations; hypertension, hypomagnesemia, tachypnea, and hyperthermia accompanying muscular activity; hypertonicity, leukocytosis, limb rigidity, metabolic acidosis, neck and back stiffness, opisthotonos, prodromal syndrome of muscular cramps and pain, respiratory paralysis, rhabdomyolysis and myoglobinuria, risus sardonicus (sardonic grinning), seizures (during which patients remain awake and lucid), tachycardia, trismus

Admission Criteria/Prognosis Any symptomatic patient should probably be admitted into an intensive care unit; asymptomatic patients 6-8 hours after a suspected exposure can be discharged; asymptomatic patients 4- to 6-hours postingestion may be discharged

849

Toxicodynamics/Kinetics

Onset of symptoms: Oral: 15-30 minutes. Intranasal, parenteral: <5 minutes

Absorption: Complete and rapid absorption following oral or parenteral exposure; readily absorbed through intact skin and mucosal surfaces

Distribution: V_d: 13 L/kg; rapid tissue distribution

Metabolism: Hepatic microsomal oxidation through P450 pathways; evidence of saturable metabolism at higher concentrations with V_{max} = 3.7 mg/kg/hour and K_m = 1.46 mg/L

Half-life: 10 hours; half-life in overdose: 10-16 hours

Elimination: ~10% to 20% excreted unchanged in liver within 24 hours

Warnings/Precautions

Any external visual, auditory, or tactile stimuli may precipitate muscle hyperactivity and seizures; minimize any external stimuli

Reference Range

Postmortem levels following a fatal exposure of strychnine were: Concentrations in subclavian blood: 1.82 mg/mL; inferior vena cava blood: 3.32 mg/mL; urine: 3.35 mg/mL; bile: 11.4 mg/mL; liver: 98.6 mg/kg: lung: 12.3 mg/kg; spleen: 11.8 mg/kg; brain: 2.42 mg/kg; skeletal muscle: 2.32 mg/kg. Dermal exposure (~1 cupfull) results in plasma and urine strychnine levels of 196 ng/mL and 6850 ng/mL, respectively.

Overdosage/Treatment

Decontamination:

Oral: **Do not** induce emesis because of danger of sudden respiratory compromise or aspiration following seizures or muscle spasms. Gastric lavage should be approached cautiously and only after aggressive control of muscular dysphoria. Activated charcoal should be administered as soon as possible. The efficacy of repeated-dose activated charcoal has not been documented.

Dermal exposure: Prompt thorough scrubbing of all affected areas with soap and water

Ocular exposure: Irrigation with copious tepid water or saline

Supportive therapy: Airway management, ventilatory assistance, and humidified oxygen administration

Hyperthermia: Treat with cooling blankets, cool water sponging, and cold water lavage. Antipyretics are not effective.

Rhabdomyolysis: Vigorously hydrate to a urine output of 100-200 mL/hour

Metabolic acidosis: Treat with sodium bicarbonate.

Hyperkalemia: Consider insulin and sodium polystyrene sulfonate for significant hyperkalemia. Also consider urinary alkalinization or parenteral mannitol administration of 0.5-1 g/kg I.V. every 4-6 hours to enhance elimination.

Convulsions: Minimize external stimuli and treat with benzodiazepines or barbiturates. Consider neuromuscular blockade with pancuronium and barbiturate coma with status epilepticus. Diazepam is the anticonvulsant of choice.

Enhancement of elimination: Rapid metabolism and early onset and resolution of symptoms reduce the utility of dialysis or hemoperfusion.

Antidote(s)

- Charcoal [ANTIDOTE]
- Mannitol [ANTIDOTE]
- Sodium Bicarbonate [ANTIDOTE]

Additional Information

Lethal dose: Children: 15 mg; Adults: 50 mg

Has a bitter taste

Any exposure to strychnine should be considered potentially life-threatening.

Intensive care unit admission criteria include seizures, acidosis, and hypoxia. Observation care unit admission criteria include evidence of hyperreflexia or neuromuscular irritability, hypertension or tachycardia, that persists longer than 4 hours for onset.

Patients who remain asymptomatic for at least 6 hours, or who become asymptomatic and remain so for at least 6 hours, may be considered for medical clearance.

How supplied: Powder/tablets (veterinary)

Specific References

Barroso M, Gallardo E, Margalho C, et al, "Determination of Strychnine in Human Blood Using Solid-Phase Extraction and GC-EI-MS," *J Anal Toxicol*, 2005, 29(5):383-6.

Cantrell FL, "Look What I Found! - Poison Hunting on eBay®," *Clin Toxicol*, 2005, 43(5):375-9.

Lindsey T, O'Hara J, Irvine R, et al, "Strychnine Overdose Following Ingestion of Gopher Bait," *J Anal Toxicol*, 2004, 28(2):135-7.

Moltz E, Marshall S, Andrenyak D, et al, "Strychnine Poisoning Following Ingestion of a Chinese Herbal Liniment," *Clin Toxicol (Phila)*. 2005, 43:645.

Shadnia S, Moiensadat M, and Abdollahi M, "A Case of Acute Strychnine Poisoning," *Vet Hum Toxicol*, 2004, 46(2):76-7.

Wang Z, Zhao J, Xing J, et al, "Analysis of Strychnine and Brucine in Postmortem Specimens by RP-HPLC: A Case Report of Fatal Intoxication," *J Anal Toxicol*, 2004, 28(2):141-4.

Styrene

Related Information

- Adipose Tissue Ranges of Toxins

CAS Number 100-42-5

UN Number 2055

Synonyms Cinnamene; Ethenylbenzene; Phenylethylene; Vinylbenzene

Use Production of polystyrene plastics for use in insulation or fiberglass materials

Mechanism of Toxic Action Essentially unknown; may cause increase in brain serotonin and noradrenaline levels; can cause central nervous system depression

Adverse Reactions

Central nervous system: Air styrene levels >30 ppm can cause changes in EEG and psychomotor changes, cognitive dysfunction

Gastrointestinal: Nausea (at 376 ppm after 1 hour), metallic taste, stomatitis, sore throat

Neuromuscular & skeletal: Neuropathy (peripheral)

Ocular: Eye irritation (at 376 ppm after 1 hour exposure), rotatory nystagmus, neuritis (retrobulbar), optic neuropathy, visual evoked potential abnormalities

Otic: Ototoxicity (decreased hearing at middle/high frequencies)

Respiratory: Rhinorrhea, bronchospasm, cough, aspiration, asthma

Toxicodynamics/Kinetics

Absorption: Inhalation: 63%. Oral/dermal: Limited with absorption rate being 1 mcg/cm^2/minute or ~0.1% to 2% of inhalation absorption amount

Distribution: V_d: 1.2-1.7 L/kg Adipose tissue

Metabolism: Hepatic to hippuric acid, mandelic acid (MA) and phenyl-glyoxylic acid (PGA)

Elimination: Urine as MA (57%), PGA (33%), and hippuric acid (8%)

Half-life: 2-4 days

Reference Range

Workers exposed to TWA levels of inhalation of styrene (biological exposure indices or BEI): Before shift: 0.02 mg/L; End shift: 1 mg/L

Urine levels of MA (1 g/L) and PGA (250 mcg/L); urine level of AA of 0.8 g/L has been associated with some central nervous system depression

An exposure of 80 ppm of styrene has been associated with a blood styrene level of ~1 mcg/mL; general population blood styrene level: 0.4 mcg/L; fat levels range from 8-350 ng/g

Central nervous system effects can occur at blood styrene levels >2.4 mg/L.

Overdosage/Treatment

Decontamination: **Oral:** Dilute with water; **do not** induce emesis. Activated charcoal may be effective. **Dermal:** Remove contaminated clothing; wash with soap and water. **Ocular:** Irrigate with saline.

Supportive therapy: Inhaled beta agonist agents may be used for bronchospasm.

Additional Information

Dissolves rubber and corrodes copper

Increased cholinesterase activity noted

Relationship between workplace styrene air levels and urine MA concentration is expressed as: ln (styrene air concentration in PPM equals - 3.4915 + 1.0568) times ln (urinary MA level in mg/L)

Indoor air exposure daily of styrene: 14-151 mcg. Exposure from drinking water: 0-0.5 mcg/day. Exposure from food: ~30 mcg/day. Urban ambient air styrene levels: 0.6-21 mcg/m^3

Half-life in groundwater: 6 weeks to 7.5 months. Atmospheric half-life: 0.5-17 hours. Atmospheric half-life by photolysis: 50 years

Styrene is found in cigarette smoke at the level of 18 mcg/cigarette

PEL-TWA: 50 ppm; TLV-TWA: 50 ppm; IDLH: 700 ppm

Specific References

Delzell E, Sathiakumar N, Graff J, et al, "Styrene and Ischemic Heart Disease Mortality Among Synthetic Rubber Industry Workers," *J Occup Environ Med*, 2005, 47:1235-43.

Sliwinska-Kowalska M, Zamyslowska-Szmytke E, Szymczak W, et al, "Ototoxic Effects of Occupational Exposure to Styrene and Co-Exposure to Styrene and Noise," *J Occup Environ Med*, 2003, 45(1):15-24.

Sulfur Dioxide

Applies to Bleach (Production); Solvent (Petroleum Manufacture); "Acid Rain" (Component)

CAS Number 7446-09-5

UN Number 1079

Synonyms Sulfur Oxide; Sulfurous Anhydride

Commonly Found In Disinfectant, fumigant, food preservative, Portland cement manufacture, antioxidant; air pollutant near smelters; associated with kerosene space heaters

Use In the manufacture of sulfites, thiosulfates, and sulfonation of oils. Also used in production of sulfuric acid; used in bleach production and as a solvent in petroleum manufacture. A component of "acid rain".

Mechanism of Toxic Action Irritation to mucous membranes, highly soluble. Upon inhalation can cause increased airway resistance due to bronchoconstriction; impairs mucociliary clearance in the lungs.

Adverse Reactions

Cardiovascular: Angina, tachycardia

Dermatologic: Immunologic contact urticaria

Ocular: Eye irritation with corneal injury (at 10 ppm)

Gastrointestinal: Nausea and vomiting (at 40 ppm)

Respiratory: Upper respiratory tract edema and obstruction, pulmonary edema, bronchoconstriction, reactive airways disease syndrome, hyposmia, cough, bronchiolitis obliterans

Signs and Symptoms of Overdose Caustic dermal burns, chest pain, choking sensation, cough, cyanosis, dyspnea, lacrimation, rhinorrhea

Toxicodynamics/Kinetics

Metabolism: with ambient air, it is oxidized to sulfur trioxide then hydrated to sulfuric acid by sulfite oxidase

Elimination: Excreted in urine as inorganic sulfate

Reference Range Sulfhemoglobin formation has been associated with exposure; levels of 6% to 12% associated with death

Overdosage/Treatment

Decontamination: Oxygenation/respiratory support: 100% humidified oxygen. Irrigate eyes with saline water.

Supportive therapy: Aerosolized sodium bicarbonate (5%) may alleviate respiratory mucous membrane irritation (although this is not proven); beta-adrenergic agents for wheezing. Zafirlukast (20 mg orally) inhibits sulfur dioxide-induced bronchoconstriction (at sulfur dioxide concentrations of $\sim$3 ppm) in patients with asthma. Cromolyn sodium may be useful.

Diagnostic Procedures

- Sulfhemoglobin

Additional Information Bronchoconstriction may progress to reactive airway disease. Colorless; sulfur odor. Odor threshold: 1 ppm. TLV-TWA: 2 ppm. IDLH: 100 ppm. For ambient air concentrations and levels found in foods and vegetables: See tables.

Ambient Air Concentrations of Sulfur Dioxide in Different Parts of the World *

Location	Sulfur Dioxide Concentrations (mcg/m^3)	Year
Rural New York	3.38-7.44 (0.0013-0.0028 ppm)	1984-6
Pennsylvania	26-31 (0.01-0.012 ppm)	1983
Rural Pennsylvania	3-131 (0.0011-0.05 ppm)	1984
Bermuda	0-1.67 (0-0.0006 ppm)	1982-3
Coastal Delaware	13.4 (0.005 ppm)	1985
Bermuda (mid-ocean)	0.7 (0.00027 ppm)	1985
Northwest Territories, Canada	0.33-0.69 (0.00013-0.00026 ppm)	1981 (Nov-Dec)
Northwest Territories, Canada	2.3-4.3 (0.00088-0.0016 ppm)	1982 (Feb)
Ontario, Canada	8.4-16.2 (0.0032-0.0062 ppm)	1982
Ontario, Canada	0.1-62.8 (0.024 ppm)	1984
Near H$_2$SO$_4$ producer, United Kingdom	0.5-120 (0.002-0.046 ppm)	1981

*IARC

Adapted from: U.S. Department of Health and Human Services, *Toxicological Profile for Sulfur Dioxide*, Agency for Toxic Substances and Disease Registry, September 1997.

Levels of Sulfur Dioxide in Various Foods and Beverages*

Food/Beverage	Concentration of Sulfur Dioxide (ppm)
Cherries	24
Garlic, dried	121
Leek, dried soup mix	7
Onions, canned, boiled	4
Onions, dried	60
Onions, dried soup mix	10-30
Onions, fresh	17
Soya bean protein, nonsulfited	20
Soya bean protein, sulfited	80-120
Wine, "burgundy"	150
Wine, white	14

*IARC

Adapted from: U.S. Department of Health and Human Services, *Toxicological Profile for Sulfur Dioxide*, Agency for Toxic Substances and Disease Registry, September 1997.

Sulfur Trioxide

Related Information

- Sulfuric Acid

Applies to Sulfan

CAS Number 7446-11-9

UN Number 1829

Synonyms Sulfur Oxide

Use Intermediate in production of sulfuric acid and explosives; an oxidizing agent

Mechanism of Toxic Action Mucosal irritation

Signs and Symptoms of Overdose Bronchospasm, cough, dizziness, nasal irritation, pleuritic chest pain, wheezing

Toxicodynamics/Kinetics Metabolism: Forms with water in the respiratory tract to form sulfuric acid and heat

Reference Range Normal sulfate concentration range in blood is 0.8-1.2 mg/dL

Overdosage/Treatment

Decontamination: Inhalation: Administer 100% humidified oxygen.

Supportive therapy: Nebulized beta-agonists should be used to treat bronchospasm.

Additional Information A clear, colorless acidic liquid which is not flammable

Sulfuric Acid

Applies to Dyes (Manufacture); Explosives (Manufacture); Fertilizer Production (Phosphate); Metal Cleaning; Ore Processing; Paper Pulp; Petroleum (Manufacture); Toilet Bowl Cleaners

CAS Number 7664-93-9; 8014-95-7 (oleum)

UN Number 1830; 1831; 1832

Synonyms Battery Acid; Dihydrogen Sulfate; Oil of Vitriol; Oleum (Fuming Sulfuric Acid); Sulfur Acid; Sulphine Acid; Vitriol Brown Oil

Commonly Found In Automotive batteries; used in fur and leather industries; component in smog; major component in acid rain; formed from sulfur trioxide and water

Use In the manufacture of acetic acid, hydrochloric acid, hydrolysis of cellulose; used for metal cleaning; primarily used in phosphate fertilizer production; it is also used in the manufacture of dyes, explosives, petroleum, paper pulp, ore processing. Toilet bowl cleaners (which contain sodium bisulfite) produce sulfuric acid upon contact with water.

Mechanism of Toxic Action Acid oxidizer; corrosive to the skin, eyes, mucous membranes, gastrointestinal and respiratory tracts; chars tissue by removing water

Adverse Reactions

Cardiovascular: Shock, vascular collapse, chest pain, angina

Central nervous system: Headache

Gastrointestinal: Gastritis, throat irritation

Ocular: Lacrimation, iritis, cataracts, glaucoma

Renal: Renal failure

Respiratory: Tachypnea, bronchoconstriction, ARDS, laryngeal edema, cough, dyspnea

Signs and Symptoms of Overdose Choking, corneal burns, cough, discoloration of teeth, dyspnea, hemoptysis/hematemesis. Esophageal/gastric burns are rare, but ingestion of 15-50 mL (of a 26.4 to 35.4 normal solution) can cause severe gastroesophageal burns and gastric perforation. Dermal contact with >10% concentration is caustic. Dermal contact at >50% total body surface area can be fatal as dermal burns with coagulative necrosis develop. Corneal exposure at concentrations >1.25% can result in severe ocular damage.

Admission Criteria/Prognosis Admit any symptomatic patient, or dermal contact >30% total body surface area over extremities or trunk

Toxicodynamics/Kinetics

Absorption: Can be absorbed

Metabolism: Dissociates into hydronium and sulfate

Elimination: Renal (as sulfate)

Reference Range Normal blood sulfate concentration range: 0.8-1.2 mg/dL

Overdosage/Treatment

Decontamination: **Do not** induce emesis. Treat inhalation injuries with supplemental oxygen. Activated charcoal is not effective. Dilute with cold milk, cornstarch, or large amounts of cold water; endoscopy for severe mouth burns

Ocular: Irrigate copiously with saline (preferred over water due to less heat production). Irrigation may need to last for 3 hours. Continue to irrigate until runoff exhibits a neutral pH. Topical mydriatics and antibiotics may be useful.

Dermal: Irrigate affected area with copious amounts of water. Remove jewelry and clothing

Enhancement of elimination: Hemodialysis if renal failure develops

Additional Information

Lethal dose: 135 mg/kg

Clear, colorless gas; odorless except when heating (choking odor)

Reacts violently with water or alcohol; will corrode or dissolve metals

Miscible in water
pH of a 1N solution: 0.3; 0.1N: 1.2; 0.01N: 2.1
Vapor density: 3.4
TLV-TWA: 1 mg/m^3
TLV-STEL: 3 mg/m^3
IDLH: 80 mg/m^3
PEL-TWA: 1 mg/m^3
Background sulfate levels in North American lakes are 20-40 ueq/L, although eastern North American lakes can have concentrations as high as 100 ueq/L.

Sulfuryl Fluoride

CAS Number 2699-79-8
UN Number 2191
U.S. Brand Names Vikane®
Synonyms Sulfonyl Fluoride; Sulfur Difluoride; Sulfuric Oxyfluoride
Use Fumigant insecticide against drywood termites; also used in organic synthesis and produced by heating barium diflurosilicate
Mechanism of Toxic Action Mucosal irritant; direct content in its liquified form can cause a frostbite injury; systemic fluorosis can occur
Adverse Reactions
Cardiovascular: Tachycardia (supraventricular), hypotension
Central nervous system: Seizures, cognitive dysfunction, irritability
Dermatologic: Pruritus, dermatitis congelations
Gastrointestinal: Vomiting, nausea, anorexia, abdominal cramps
Neuromuscular & skeletal: Weakness, paresthesia, carpopedal spasm
Ocular: Eye irritation
Renal: Proteinuria, azotemia
Respiratory: Pharyngeal irritation, dyspnea, cough, pulmonary edema, bronchospasm, nasal irritation
Miscellaneous: Frostbite
Admission Criteria/Prognosis Admit any patient who is symptomatic 6 hours postexposure
Toxicodynamics/Kinetics Absorption: Inhalation
Monitoring Parameters Chest x-ray, fluoride level, calcium level, ECG
Reference Range Serum fluoride level of 0.5 mg/L associated with fatality; serum fluoride level >0.1 mg/L is consistent with exposure
Overdosage/Treatment
Decontamination: **Inhalation:** Give 100% humidified oxygen. **Ocular:** Irrigate copiously with saline. **Dermal:** Wash the area with soap and water.
Supportive therapy: Frostbite can be treated with standard therapy. Hypocalcemia can be treated with calcium (0.5-1 g). Hypotension can be treated with isotonic fluids and placement in Trendelenburg position. Dopamine or norepinephrine can be used for refractory hypotension. Benzodiazepines or barbiturates can be used for seizure control.
Additional Information Odorless, colorless, nonflammable gas which is heavier than air (density: 3.72 g/L). TLV-TWA: 5 ppm; TLV-STEL: 10 ppm; IDLH: 1000 ppm

Terbufos

CAS Number 13071-79-9
U.S. Brand Names Counter®
Synonyms Phosphorodithiotic Acid S-((Tert-Butylthio)methyl) O,O-Diethyl Ester
Use Commonly marketed as insecticide granules, or spray liquid with or without petroleum derivative as a solvent
Mechanism of Toxic Action Potent, irreversible inhibition of acetylcholinesterase and plasma cholinesterase, resulting in excess accumulation of acetylcholine at muscarinic and nicotinic receptors, and in the central nervous system
Adverse Reactions
Cardiovascular: **Hyperdynamic** (~18% to 21%) or hypodynamic (~7% to 10%) states, QT prolongation, sinus bradycardia, sinus tachycardia
Central nervous system: Depression, seizures, hyperactivity, cognitive dysfunction, hypothermia
Genitourinary: Urinary incontinence
Neuromuscular & skeletal: Weakness (delayed), paralysis, delayed paresthesia
Respiratory: Pulmonary edema, respiratory depression
Miscellaneous: Flu-like symptoms (especially with chronic exposure)
Signs and Symptoms of Overdose
Abdominal pain, agitation, asystole, AV block, bradycardia, bronchorrhea, coma, confusion, cranial nerve palsies, decreased hemoglobin, decreased platelet count, decreased red blood cell count, diaphragmatic paralysis, dysarthria, excessive sweating, fecal and urinary incontinence, generalized asthenia, headache, heart block, hypertension, hypotension, lacrimation, metabolic acidosis and hyperglycemia (severe intoxication), miosis (unreactive to light), mydriasis (rarely), nausea, pallor, pulmonary edema, QT prolongation, respiratory depression, salivation, seizures, skeletal muscle fasciculation and flaccid paralysis, tachycardia, tachypnea, vomiting

An "intermediate syndrome" of limb asthenia and respiratory paralysis has been reported to occur between 24 and 96 hours postorganophosphate exposure and is independent of the acute cholinergic crisis. Late paresthesia characterized by stocking and glove paresthesia, anesthesia and asthenia is infrequently observed weeks to months following acute exposure to certain organophosphates.
Toxicodynamics/Kinetics
Absorption: Readily through oral, dermal, or respiratory exposure
Metabolism: Rapidly metabolized to weakly active compounds through hepatic hydrolysis and other pathways
Elimination: Metabolites are excreted in urine
Warnings/Precautions Risk of aspiration pneumonitis exists with agents having a hydrocarbon vehicle; severe laryngeal irritation and violent coughing may result from exposure to dusting powders; exposure to dusting powders and insecticide granules may cause contact dermatitis
Overdosage/Treatment
Decontamination: Isolation, bagging, and disposal of all contaminated clothing and other articles. All emergency medical workers and hospital staff should follow appropriate precautions regarding exposure to hazardous material including the use of protective clothing, masks, goggles, and respiratory equipment.
    Dermal: Prompt thorough scrubbing of all affected areas with soap and water, including hair and nails; 5% bleach can be used
    Oral: Activated charcoal (without cathartic) can be administered either orally or via a nasogastric tube. **Do not** induce emesis because of danger of sudden respiratory compromise, alterations in mental status, seizures, coma, and possible aspiration of hydrocarbon vehicles.
    Ocular: Irrigation with copious tepid sterile water or saline
Supportive therapy: Airway management, ventilatory assistance, humidified oxygen administration, and close monitoring for sudden respiratory failure
Enhancement of elimination: Dialysis and hemoperfusion are not indicated due to effectiveness of the prescribed antidotal treatment and large volumes of distribution of organophosphates.
Antidote:
    Atropine: Administration should be guided by respiratory status, starting at 2-5 mg I.V. every 5-10 minutes as needed, and should be titrated to the resolution of excess pulmonary secretions. Frequent administration of large doses (cumulative doses >100 mg) may be necessary in massive exposures.
    Glycopyrrolate: May be administered if atropine is unavailable (200-400 mcg I.V. or I.M. initially, or ~$^1/_2$ the dose of atropine)
    2-PAM: For more significant exposures (ie, exposures requiring large doses of atropine, or with recurring symptoms, or exposures to more lipid soluble agents), administration should follow: 1-2 g I.V. over 10-30 minutes, repeated in 1 hour if asthenia recurs, then every 4-12 hours for recurring symptoms.
Antidote(s)
• Atropine [ANTIDOTE]
• Pralidoxime [ANTIDOTE]
Diagnostic Procedures
• Creatinine, Serum
• Pseudocholinesterase, Serum
Drug Interaction Paralysis is potentiated by neuromuscular blockade (ie, pancuronium, vecuronium, succinylcholine, atracurium, doxacurium, mivacurium); inhibition of serum esterase prolongs the half-life of succinylcholine, cocaine, and other ester anesthetics; cholinergic toxicity is potentiated by cholinesterase inhibitors such as physostigmine
Additional Information
Red blood cell cholinesterase and serum pseudocholinesterase may be depressed following acute or chronic organophosphate exposure; RBC cholinesterase is typically not analyzed by in-house laboratories, and is usually not available for consideration during acute management. Pseudocholinesterase levels may be rapidly available from some in-house laboratories, but are not as reliable a marker of organophosphate exposure because of variability secondary to variant genotypes, hepatic disease, oral estrogen use, or malnutrition. Because of this variability, true indication of suppression of either of these enzymes can only be estimated through comparison to pre-exposure values; these enzymes may be useful in measuring a patient's recovery postexposure, especially if the recovery is not progressing as expected.
The intermediate syndrome is not related to delayed neuropathy.
QT$_c$ prolongation on ECG in the setting of organophosphate poisoning is associated with a high incidence of respiratory failure and mortality.
Water solubility: 6 ppm
Other information concerning pesticide exposures is available through the EPA-funded National Pesticide Telecommunications Network: 1-800-858-7378 (weekdays, 8 AM to 6 PM, Central Standard time)

Tetrachloroethane

CAS Number 79-34-5
UN Number 1702
U.S. Brand Names Bonoform®; Cellon®; Westron®

Synonyms 1,1,2,2-Tetrachloroethane; Acetylene Tetrachloride

Use Primarily as a solvent in metal cleaning procedures, paint removers, varnishes, photographic films, and oil or fat extractant; production of trichloroethylene, tetrachloroethylene, and 1,2-dichloroethylene

Mechanism of Toxic Action Central nervous system depression; direct effect on neuronal membrane and hepatotoxic effects can occur through lipid peroxidation

Adverse Reactions

Cardiovascular: Hypotension

Central nervous system: Confusion, delirium, coma

Gastrointestinal: Nausea, vomiting, anorexia (gastrointestinal effects seen with exposure levels of 116 ppm for 10-30 minutes), diarrhea

Hematologic: Leukocytosis

Hepatic: Fatty degeneration of liver, centrilobular hepatic necrosis

Ocular: Lacrimation, eye irritation

Miscellaneous: Cutaneous T-cell lymphoma

Admission Criteria/Prognosis Patients who develop tachypnea, cyanosis, dyspnea, CNS depression, tachycardia, or fever within 8 hours of exposure should be admitted; asymptomatic patients can be discharged after 8 hours observation

Toxicodynamics/Kinetics

Absorption: Through inhalation (97%), oral, and dermal routes

Metabolism: Hepatic to glyoxylic acid and oxyalic acid, tetrachloroethylene is also a metabolite

Elimination: Through lungs, feces, and urine

Reference Range Toxic effects are predicted to occur at blood tetrachloroethane levels >1.1 ng/mL (1.1 ppt)

Overdosage/Treatment Decontamination: **Oral:** Dilute with milk. **Dermal:** Remove contaminated clothing; wash with soap and water. **Ocular:** Irrigate with saline or water.

Additional Information

Minimal lethal dose: Oral: 357 mg/kg; Toxic dose (causing coma): Oral: 100 mg/kg

Nonflammable. Odor threshold: Air: 3-5 ppm (chloroform-like); water: 0.5 ppm. PEL-TWA: 1 ppm; TLV-TWA (skin): 1 ppm; IDLH: 150 ppm. Atmospheric half-life: >800 days. Atmospheric concentrations in U.S. (urban/suburban): Mean level: 5.4 ppt; drinking water: <0.5 ppb

Specific References

Clewell HJ, Gentry PR, Kester JE, et al, "Evaluation of Physiologically Based Pharmacokinetic Models in Risk Assessment: An Example with Perchloroethylene," *Crit Rev Toxicol*, 2005, 35(5):413-33.

Tetrachloroethylene

Applies to Degreaser; Dry Cleaning (Fabrics); Freon (Manufacture)

CAS Number 127-18-4

UN Number 1897

Synonyms 1,1,2,2-Tetrachloroethylene; PCE®; Perchlor; Perclene; Tetra

Use In textile industry for dry cleaning fabric; degreasing; used in the manufacture of freons, anthelmintic for animals

Mechanism of Toxic Action CNS depressant, irritant; probable human carcinogen

Adverse Reactions

Central nervous system: CNS depression

Ocular: Eye irritation at air levels >1000 ppm, visual evoked potential abnormalities

Respiratory: Irritation, respiratory depression

Signs and Symptoms of Overdose Ataxia, conjunctival injection, cough, dermatitis, epistaxis, euphoria, headache, hepatomegaly, irritability, nausea, short-term memory deficiency, sweating

Toxicodynamics/Kinetics

Absorption: Well absorbed in the lungs and GI tract; not well absorbed dermally; highly lipid soluble

Distribution: V_d: 8.2 L/kg

Half-life: Oral: 144 hours. Inhalation: 33-72 hours. In adipose tissues: 72 hours

Metabolism: In the liver to trichloroacetic acid and trichloroethanol

Elimination: 80% excreted through the lungs, metabolites excreted renally

Reference Range Tetrachloroethylene serum level of 100 mcg/dL and trichloroacetic acid levels in urine of 7 mg/L correlate with weekly exposure of 50 ppm; BEI of 1 mg/L; an oral ingestion of 12-16g in a 6-year-old boy resulted in a blood tetrachloroethylene level of 21 mcg/dL 1-hour postingestion; mean blood concentration of tetrachloroethylene following 50 ppm exposure 8 hours daily, 5 days weekly: Estimated to range from 1.6-2.3 mg/L; urine levels would be ~19 mg/L

Overdosage/Treatment

Decontamination: **Dermal:** Remove contaminated clothing; wash with soap and water. **Inhalation:** Give 100% humidified oxygen. **Ocular:** Irrigate with saline.

Supportive therapy: Controlled hyperventilation (volume 10 L/minute) may be useful. Epinephrine may predispose the patient to cardiac arrhythmia.

Additional Information

Clear, colorless; fruity odor of chloroform; radiopaque. Odor threshold: 5-50 ppm. TLV-TWA: 50 ppm. Symptoms occur at 75 ppm.

Estimated daily intake: Inhalation: 41-204 mcg; Drinking water: 0.6-6 mcg

Ambient atmospheric urban concentrations: ~0.8 ppb

Drinking water tetrachloroethylene: 0.3-3 ppb

Dairy products contain 0.3-13 mcg/kg; beverages average 2-3 mcg/kg

Water half-life at pH 7 (25°C): ~9 months (by hydrolysis). Atmospheric half-life: 96-251 days

Air tetrachloroethylene levels: Cars: Up to 300 ppm. Homes: 3-480 ppm. Dry cleaning operations: 0-1200 ppm. Retained on clothes after dry cleaning: 1-3.7 kg

For duration and effect of inhaling vapors: See table.

Dose-Response Relationship for Humans Inhaling Tetrachlorothylene Vapors

Levels in Air	Duration of Exposure	Effect on Nervous System
50 ppm		Odor threshold
100 ppm	7 h	Headache, drowsiness
200 ppm	2 h	Dizziness, uncoordination
600 ppm	10 min	Dizziness, loss of inhibitions
1000 ppm	1-2 min	Marked dizziness, intolerable eye and respiratory tract irritation
1500 ppm	30 min	Coma

U.S. Department of Health and Human Services, "Hospital Emergency Departments: A Planning Guide for the Management of Contaminated Patients," *Managing Hazardous Materials Incidents,* Agency for Toxic Substances and Diseases Registry, 1995, 2:796.

Specific References

Lomax RB, Ridgway P, and Meldrum M, "Does Occupational Exposure to Organic Solvents Affect Colour Discrimination?" *Toxicol Rev*, 2004, 23(2):91-121 (review).

Tetraethyl Pyrophosphate

CAS Number 107-49-3

UN Number 3018

U.S. Brand Names Fosvex®; Grisol®; Hexamite®; Tetron®

Synonyms TEPP

Use Marketed as insecticide spray liquid with or without petroleum derivative as a solvent

Mechanism of Toxic Action Potent, irreversible inhibition of acetylcholinesterase and plasma cholinesterase, resulting in excess accumulation of acetylcholine at muscarinic and nicotinic receptors, and in the central nervous system

Adverse Reactions

Cardiovascular: **Hyperdynamic** (~18% to 21%) or hypodynamic (~7% to 10%) states, QT prolongation, sinus bradycardia, sinus tachycardia

Central nervous system: Depression, seizures, hyperactivity, cognitive dysfunction, hypothermia

Genitourinary: Urinary incontinence

Neuromuscular & skeletal: Weakness (delayed), paralysis, delayed paresthesia

Respiratory: Pulmonary edema, respiratory depression

Miscellaneous: Flu-like symptoms (especially with chronic exposure)

Signs and Symptoms of Overdose Abdominal pain, agitation, asystole, AV block, bradycardia, bronchorrhea, coma, confusion, cranial nerve palsies, decreased hemoglobin, decreased platelet count, decreased red blood cell count, diaphragmatic paralysis, dysarthria, excessive sweating, fecal and urinary incontinence, generalized asthenia, headache, heart block, hypertension, hypotension, lacrimation, metabolic acidosis and hyperglycemia (severe intoxication), miosis (unreactive to light), mydriasis (rarely), nausea, pallor, pulmonary edema, QT prolongation, respiratory depression, salivation, seizures, skeletal muscle fasciculation and flaccid paralysis, tachycardia, tachypnea, vomiting

An "intermediate syndrome" of limb asthenia and respiratory paralysis has been reported to occur between 24 and 96 hours postorganophosphate exposure and is independent of the acute cholinergic crisis. Late paresthesia characterized by stocking and glove paresthesia, anesthesia and asthenia is infrequently observed weeks to months following acute exposure to certain organophosphates.

Toxicodynamics/Kinetics

Absorption: Readily through oral, dermal, or respiratory exposure

Metabolism: Rapidly metabolized to weakly active compounds through hepatic hydrolysis and other pathways

Elimination: Metabolites are excreted in urine

Warnings/Precautions Risk of aspiration pneumonitis exists with agents having a hydrocarbon vehicle; severe laryngeal irritation and violent coughing may result from exposure to dusting powders; exposure to dusting powders and insecticide granules may cause contact dermatitis

Overdosage/Treatment

Decontamination: Isolation, bagging, and disposal of all contaminated clothing and other articles. All emergency medical workers and hospital staff should follow appropriate precautions regarding exposure to hazardous material, including the use of protective clothing, masks, goggles, and respiratory equipment.

Oral: Activated charcoal can be administered either orally or via a nasogastric tube. **Do not** induce emesis because of danger of sudden respiratory compromise, alterations in mental status, seizures, coma, and possible aspiration of hydrocarbon vehicles. **Do not** give a cathartic.

Dermal: Prompt thorough scrubbing of all affected areas with soap and water, including hair and nails; 5% bleach can be used

Ocular: Irrigation with copious tepid sterile water or saline

Supportive therapy: Airway management, ventilatory assistance, humidified oxygen administration, and close monitoring for sudden respiratory failure

Enhancement of elimination: Dialysis and hemoperfusion are not indicated due to effectiveness of the prescribed antidotal treatment and large volumes of distribution of organophosphates.

Antidote:

Atropine: Administration should be guided by respiratory status, starting at 2-5 mg I.V. every 5-10 minutes as needed, and should be titrated to the resolution of excess pulmonary secretions. Frequent administration of large doses (cumulative doses >100 mg) may be necessary in massive exposures.

Glycopyrrolate: May be administered if atropine is unavailable (200-400 mcg I.V. or I.M. initially, or ~$^1/_2$ the dose of atropine).

2-PAM: For more significant exposures (ie, exposures requiring large doses of atropine, or with recurring symptoms, or exposures to more lipid soluble agents), administration should follow: 1-2 g I.V. over 10-30 minutes, repeated in 1 hour if asthenia recurs, then every 4-12 hours for recurring symptoms

Antidote(s)

- Atropine [ANTIDOTE]
- Pralidoxime [ANTIDOTE]

Diagnostic Procedures

- Creatinine, Serum
- Pseudocholinesterase, Serum

Drug Interaction Paralysis is potentiated by neuromuscular blockade (ie, pancuronium, vecuronium, succinylcholine, atracurium, doxacurium, mivacurium); inhibition of serum esterase prolongs the half-life of succinylcholine, cocaine, and other ester anesthetics; cholinergic toxicity is potentiated by cholinesterase inhibitors such as physostigmine

Additional Information Red blood cell cholinesterase and serum pseudocholinesterase may be depressed following acute or chronic organophosphate exposure; RBC cholinesterase is typically not analyzed by in-house laboratories, and is usually not available for consideration during acute management. Pseudocholinesterase levels may be rapidly available from some in-house laboratories, but are not as reliable a marker of organophosphate exposure because of variability secondary to variant genotypes, hepatic disease, oral estrogen use, or malnutrition. Because of this variability, true indication of suppression of either of these enzymes can only be estimated through comparison to pre-exposure values; these enzymes may be useful in measuring a patient's recovery postexposure, especially if the recovery is not progressing as expected.

The intermediate syndrome is not related to delayed neuropathy.

QT_c prolongation on ECG in the setting of organophosphate poisoning is associated with a high incidence of respiratory failure and mortality.

Colorless/light amber liquid with faint fruity odor; noncombustible; slowly hydrolyses in water and is therefore environmentally persistent; thermal breakdown products include phosphoric acid;

ACGIH TLV: 0.0004 ppm; IDLH: 10 mg/m³

Other information concerning pesticide exposures is available through the EPA-funded National Pesticide Telecommunications Network: 1-800-858-7378 (weekdays, 8 AM to 6 PM, Central Standard time)

Tetrahydrofuran

Applies to Audio and Video Tapes; Glue; Ink; Paint; Solvent to Dissolve Plastic (Polyvinyl Chloride, Polyurethane, Epoxy); Varnish

CAS Number 109-99-9

UN Number 2056

Synonyms Butylene Oxide; THF

Use Solvent used to dissolve several types of plastic (polyvinyl chloride, polyurethanes, epoxy); also used in processing of glue, paint, varnish, ink; used in production of audio and video tapes

Mechanism of Toxic Action A mild respiratory irritant with general anesthetic-like effects; a possible precursor to gamma hydroxybutyric acid (GHB); has been described in one bacterium (*Rhodoccus ruber*) and case report (see Reference Range and Specific References)

Signs and Symptoms of Overdose Blurred vision, chest pain, coma, conjunctivitis, cough, dermatitis (at liquid concentrations >20%), dizzi-

ness, elevated hepatic enzymes, headache, hypotension, mydriasis, nausea, tinnitus

Reference Range Following an oral ingestion with resultant deep coma, serum and urine tetrahydrofuran were reported as 813 mg/L (11.3 mM/L) and 850 mg/L (11.8 mM/L), respectively. Serum and urine gamma hydroxybutyric acid levels in this patient were 239 mg/L (2.3 mM/L) and 2977 mg/L (28.6 mM/L), respectively.

Overdosage/Treatment

Decontamination: **Dermal:** Wash with soap and water. **Oral:** Dilute with milk or water. **Inhalation:** Administer 100% humidified oxygen. **Ocular:** Irrigate with copious amounts of saline.

Supportive therapy: Care is supportive; ventilatory support may be required. Hypotension can be treated initially with isotonic saline (I.V.) at 10-20 mL/kg with Trendelenburg positioning. Dopamine or norepinephrine can be utilized for refractory hypotension.

Additional Information TLV-TWA: 220 ppm; IDLH: 20,000 ppm; odor threshold (ether-like odor): 20-50 ppm; coma producing at 25,000 ppm

Tetramethylammonium Hydroxide

CAS Number 75-59-2

Synonyms TMA

Commonly Found In Snails (*Neptunea* species) - found in salivary glands

Mechanism of Toxic Action A ganglionic blocker; direct action on nicotinic/muscarinic receptors on postganglionic nerves in smooth muscle, cardiac muscle, and exocrine glands through an increase of intracellular sodium ions which causes increase in neuronal membrane potential and reduced ganglionic excitability. Similar mode of action as nicotine.

Signs and Symptoms of Overdose Temporary blindness, diplopia, photophobia, lacrimation, blurred vision, hypotension, dizziness, headache, seizures, apnea, nausea, vomiting, paralytic ileus, dry mouth, urticaria

Toxicodynamics/Kinetics

Oral absorption: Rapid

Protein binding: Low

Half-life: One hour

Elimination: Renal (95%)

Overdosage/Treatment

Decontamination: Oral: Activated charcoal

Supportive therapy: Seizures can be treated with benzodiazepines or phenobarbital. Hypotension can be treated with crystalloid infusion (10-20 mL/kg) intravenously and Trendelenburg placement. Dopamine or norepinephrine can be given if hypotension is refractory. Symptoms usually short-lived.

Additional Information Lethal dose is ~3-4 mg/kg

Tetramethylenedisulfotetramine

CAS Number 80-12-6

Synonyms Tetramine; TETS

Use Rodenticide (found in China)

Mechanism of Toxic Action Noncompetitive gamma-aminobutyric acid (GABA) antagonist through neuronal chloride channel blockade

Signs and Symptoms of Overdose Tachycardia, seizures (generalized), coma, mydriasis. Onset of symptoms may be 30 minutes to 13 hours

Overdosage/Treatment

Decontamination: Activated charcoal; lavage within 1 hour

Supportive therapy: Lorazepam/phenobarbital needed for seizure control. Succinylcholine (1 mg/kg) may be required. Pyridoxine (70 mg/kg) has been used with uncertain benefit.

Additional Information Oral human LD_{50}: 100 mcg/kg; white powder 100 times more toxic than potassium cyanide

Specific References

Barrueto F Jr, Furdyna PM, Hoffman RS, et al, "Status Epilepticus from an Illegally Imported Chinese Rodenticide: Tetramine," *J Toxicol Clin Toxicol*, 2003, 41(7):991-4.

Tetryl

CAS Number 479-45-8

UN Number 0208

Synonyms CE; N-Methyl-N,2,4,6-Tetranitroaniline; Nitramine; Tetralite; Tetril

Use Primarily as a military explosive (detonator and primer)

Mechanism of Toxic Action Essentially unknown; can cause an allergic reaction

Adverse Reactions

Central nervous system: Fatigue, headache, irritability

Dermatologic: Yellow staining of skin, rash, urticaria, skin discoloration (brown-yellow) upon exposure to sunlight

Gastrointestinal: Nausea, vomiting, abdominal pain, anorexia, stomatitis

Hematologic: Leukocytosis

Hepatic: Liver failure, jaundice
Ocular: Conjunctivitis
Respiratory: Bronchospasm, cough, epistaxis, sneezing

Toxicodynamics/Kinetics
Absorption: By inhalation, dermal, and oral routes
Metabolism: Hepatic to picramic acid
Elimination: Probably renal

Overdosage/Treatment
Decontamination: **Dermal:** Wash with soap and water. Calamine lotion or zinc oxide may be used to treat dermatitis. **Ocular:** Irrigate with saline. Supportive therapy: Epistaxis can be treated with local therapy.

Additional Information Odorless but highly explosive; colorless but becomes yellow when exposed to light. Atmospheric half-life: 11 days. Water half-life: 302 days (lower at higher pH). Soil half-life: 1.2 weeks. PEL-TWA (skin designation): 1.5 mg/m^3

Thallium Sulfate

Related Information
• Toxins Which Should Be Lavaged with Solutions Other Than Water

CAS Number 7440-28-0

Use Primarily in semiconduction industry in manufacture of switches and closures; radiopharmaceutical agent banned by the EPA as a pesticide in 1972

Mechanism of Toxic Action Thallium distributes intracellularly like potassium; it is a cellular toxin; inhibits mitochondrial oxidative phosphorylation, disrupts protein synthesis, alters heme metabolism

Adverse Reactions Neurologic, dysphagia, cardiac, hepatic, renal, dermatologic, gastrointestinal, pulmonary, salivation, chorea (extrapyramidal), xerostomia, sinus bradycardia, QRS prolongation, sinus tachycardia

Signs and Symptoms of Overdose Alopecia, ataxia, bradycardia, cardiac arrhythmias, cerebral edema, coma, degeneration of central and peripheral nervous systems, tremor, delirium, dementia, disorientation, drowsiness, fatty infiltration, feces discoloration (black), fever (poor prognostic sign), garlic-like breath, gastroenteritis, hyperesthesia of palm and sole, lacrimation, liver necrosis, Mees' lines, metallic taste, motor/sensory neuropathy, mydriasis, nausea, nephritis, optic neuropathy, paresthesia, pulmonary edema, seizures, tachycardia, vomiting. GI symptoms occur within 1 day. Neurological symptoms occur 4-6 days postingestion.

Admission Criteria/Prognosis Any symptomatic patient or development of hypocalcemia should be admitted; suspected ingestions should also be admitted

Toxicodynamics/Kinetics
Absorption: Through skin and gastrointestinal tract
Distribution: V$_d$: 1-5 L/kg; following intoxication, highest concentration found in kidney and urine with lesser amounts in intestine, thyroid, testes, pancreas, skin, bone, spleen
Half-life: 2-4 days
Elimination: Large amount excreted in urine within first 24 hours after which fecal elimination predominates

Reference Range Blood levels >30 mcg/L are indicative of thallium exposure; toxicity associated urine levels >20 mcg/L. Serum thallium and cerebrospinal fluid levels of 8700 mcg/L and 1200 mcg/L, respectively, have been associated with fatality. Unexposed individuals will have Blood and urine thallium levels less than 2 ug/L (9.78 nmole/c) and 5 ug/L (24.5 nmole/L), respectively.

Overdosage/Treatment
Decontamination:
Oral: Lavage (with 1% sodium iodine to convert thallium sulfate to thallium iodine) is preferable over ipecac. Activated charcoal or polystyrene sulfonate may be effective. Prussian blue (not commercially available for therapeutic use and not FDA approved) exchanges thallium for potassium and is fecally excreted; dosage: 250 mg/kg orally in 4 divided doses; continue therapy until thallium urinary level falls to <0.5 mcg/24 hours. Acetylcysteine treatment is investigational.
Dermal: Remove contaminated clothing; wash with soap and water.
Ocular: Irrigate with saline.
Enhancement of elimination: Multiple dosing of activated charcoal may be effective. Potassium chloride has been recommended in the past to increase elimination (when given after 48-72 hours), but may result in increased CNS toxicity. Forced saline diuresis (500 mL/hour of urine output) is recommended. Hemodialysis or hemoperfusion may theoretically be effective, but has not been demonstrated to be beneficial in humans. Furosemide can enhance urinary thallium excretion in animal models.

Additional Information
Estimated lethal dose: Humans: 10-12 mg/kg
Odorless, tasteless, radiopaque
Chelating agents are not effective. Dithiocarb worsens symptoms by causing central redistribution of thallium. Monitor for hypocalcemia in the acute phase. Assay blood by flame atomic absorption.
The water soluble salts of thallium (sulfate, acetate, malonate, and carbonate) are more toxic than the sulfide and iodide (less water soluble).
Estimated daily thallium intake in a 70 kg adult: Drinking water: 2 mcg; Food: 5 mcg; Inhalation: 3.4 ng

Thallium is present in concentrations of 0.024 mcg/g of cigarettes and 0.06-0.17 mcg/g in cigar stubs
Thallium contaminated heroin has been documented in France.
Average ambient urban air concentration of thallium: 0.04 ng/m^3; thallium is present in earth's crust at concentrations of 0.3-0.7 ppm
PEL-TWA: 0.1 mg/m^3; TLV-TWA: 0.1 mg/m^3; IDLH: 20 mg/m^3

Specific References
Cumpston KL, Burk M, Burda A, et al, "Darkness on the Edge of Town: A Rural Family Maliciously Poisoned by Thallium," *J Toxicol Clin Toxicol*, 2003, 41(5):739.

Hoffman RS, "Thallium Toxicity and the Role of Prussian Blue in Therapy," *Toxicol Rev*, 2003, 22(1):29-40.

Mercurio-Zappala M, Hardej D, Hoffman RS, et al, "Diethyldithiocarbamate (DDC) Exacerbates Thallium Toxicity in Rat Hippocampal Astrocytes (RHA)," *J Toxicol Clin Toxicol*, 2004, 42(5):741.

Mercurio-Zappala M, Hardej D, Hoffman RS, et al, "Using Cell Culture to Assess Thallium Neurotoxicity: A Preliminary Study," *J Toxicol Clin Toxicol*, 2004, 42(5):826.

Rusyniak DE, Kao LW, Nanagas KA, et al, "Dimercaptosuccinic Acid and Prussian Blue in the Treatment of Acute Thallium Poisoning in Rats," *J Toxicol Clin Toxicol*, 2003, 41(2):137-42.

Sharma AN, Nelson LS, and Hoffman RS, "Cerebrospinal Fluid Analysis in Fatal Thallium Poisoning: Evidence for Delayed Distribution into the Central Nervous System," *Am J Forensic Med Pathol*, 2004, 25(2):156-8.

Thiram

Applies to Foliage Disinfectant; Latex; Rubber Accelerator; Seed Disinfectant

CAS Number 137-26-8

U.S. Brand Names Arasan®; Pomarsol®; Puralin®; Rezifilm®; Spotrete®; Tersan-75®; Thiurad®; Tuads®; Tulisan®

Synonyms Tetramethyl Thiuram Disulfide; Thirame; Thiuram

Use Foliage disinfectant for fruits, mushrooms; rubber accelerator (volcanizing agent); seed disinfectant; a component of latex

Mechanism of Toxic Action Antioxidant and bisdithiocarbamate; inhibits the enzyme acetaldehyde dehydrogenase

Adverse Reactions
Dermatologic: Dermal irritation, eczema
Endocrine & metabolic: Disulfiram-like reaction with ethanol may occur
Ocular: Conjunctivitis
Respiratory: Sneezing, rhinitis, cough

Signs and Symptoms of Overdose Cholinergic symptoms do not occur. Ataxia, confusion, diarrhea, dizziness, drowsiness, nausea, paralysis, vomiting

Toxicodynamics/Kinetics Metabolism: To carbon disulfide

Overdosage/Treatment
Decontamination: Lavage (within 1 hour)/activated charcoal for ingestion; irrigate for skin exposure
Supportive therapy: Oxygen for antabuse-like reaction; crystalloid solution for hypotension

Drug Interaction Disulfiram-like reaction with ethanol may occur

Additional Information No effect on cholinesterase; acceptable daily intake: 5 mcg/kg affects acetylaldehyde dehydrogenase for 10-14 days; ~10 times as potent as disulfiram

Thorium

CAS Number 7440-29-1

UN Number 2975

Synonyms Pyrophoric; Thorium 232

Use Refractory applications, welding electrodes, lamp mantles, and in nuclear weapon production, portable gas lighters

Mechanism of Toxic Action Most toxic effects are through alpha-radiation effects

Adverse Reactions
Hematologic: Aplastic anemia, leukopenia, anemia
Hepatic: Elevated liver function test results
Miscellaneous: Increased incidence of pancreatic cancers and hematopoietic tissue malignancies

Toxicodynamics/Kinetics
Absorption: By inhalation (5%); limited absorption by oral route (0.02% to 1%)
Distribution: Bone and soft tissue
Half-life: 2.6 years
Elimination: Feces

Reference Range
General population blood level in the United Kingdom: 2.4 mcg/L
Background urine level: <0.001 mcg/L

Overdosage/Treatment
Decontamination: Remove contaminated clothing; isolate all run-off.
Dermal: Irrigate with water; scrub gently with a soft sponge or brush (avoid abrading skin). A 50% powdered detergent solution followed by a

5% sodium hypochlorite solution can be used for persistent contamination.

Ocular: Wash copiously with saline.

Supportive therapy: DTPA (diethylenetriamine pentacetic acid), which is available from the Radiation Emergency Assistance Center (615-576-1004), is an effective chelator. The calcium salt should be used as follows: 1 g of calcium DTPA diluted in 250 mL of 5% dextrose in water should be infused over a 1- to 1.5-hour time period daily for 5 days. CaNa$_2$ EDTA (calcium Versenate®) can also be used, but is less effective. DTPA should be used for dermal exposure with open wounds as well as inhalation or oral ingestion.

Additional Information

Thorotrast is a colloid consisting of thorium-232 dioxide (25%) and dextran used as an I.V. contrast agent up to 1955. Granulomas, blood disorders, and hemangiosarcoma of the liver have been associated with its use (after a delay of 20 years).

Estimated daily intake in U.S.: <0.02 pCi Sesame seeds are foods with highest thorium concentration (0.01 pCi/g wet weight). Thorium 232 rarely exceeds 0.1 pCi/L in natural waters. In soil the average soil concentration is 6 mcg/g.

Tin

Related Information

• Adipose Tissue Ranges of Toxins

CAS Number 18282-10-5 (Stannic Oxide); 683-18-1 (Dibutyltin Chloride); 7440-31-5; 7772-99-8 (Stannous Chloride)

UN Number 1759 (Stannous Chloride)

Synonyms Mat Powder; Sn; Tin Flake

Use Primarily in the manufacture of containers (particularly aerosol cans); used to coat copper wire and as a soldering agent. Tributyltin salts are used as fungicides on ships.

Mechanism of Toxic Action Possible toxic mechanism may involve uncoupling of oxidative phosphorylation; mucosal irritant

Adverse Reactions

Inorganic tin:

> Dermatologic: Dermal irritation
> Gastrointestinal: Nausea, vomiting, diarrhea
> Respiratory: Pneumoconiosis
> Miscellaneous: Mucosal irritation

Organic tin:

> Central nervous system: Headache, disorientation, dizziness, seizures, polyneuropathy, dementia, vascular encephalopathy, photophobia
> Dermatologic: Dermal burns on contact with phenyltin
> Gastrointestinal: Stomatitis
> Hepatic: Fatty degeneration of liver
> Ocular: Photophobia, nystagmus, diplopia, visual evoked potential abnormalities
> Otic: Tinnitus, ototoxicity
> Neuromuscular & skeletal: Hyporeflexia
> Renal: Renal tubule injury
> Respiratory: Respiratory depression

Toxicodynamics/Kinetics

Absorption: Inorganic tin is not readily absorbed by any route; organic tin is readily absorbed by inhalation, dermal, and oral routes

Half-life: 4-400 days

Elimination: Feces and urine

Reference Range General population adipose tissue level: 8.7-15 mcg/g; normal mean urine tin concentration: 17 mcg/mL; average blood tin level: ~0.14 mg/L

Overdosage/Treatment

Decontamination: **Oral:** Dilute with water. **Dermal:** Wash with soap and water. **Ocular:** Irrigate with saline.

Supportive therapy: Chelation therapy is not effective.

Additional Information

Toxic oral dose: Triethyltin: 70 mg (>8 days)

Radiopaque; a cause of metal fume fever

Half-life in water: >89 days (photolysis)

Ambient air concentrations of tin in U.S. cities: <0.8 mcg/m^3

Mean soil background tin levels in U.S.: 0.89 mg tin/kg soil. Inorganic metal tin: 2 mg/m^3. Organic tin (skin exposure): 0.1 mg/m^3

TLV-TWA:

Canned food may contain from 1.8-500 mg/kg with all-lacquered cans having lower tin concentrations.

Estimated daily intake of tin in U.S. by an adult: 4 mg from food and 0.003 mg by inhalation (virtually none from drinking water)

Specific References

Dopp E, Hartmann LM, Florea AM, et al, "Environmental Distribution, Analysis, and Toxicity of Organometal(loid) Compounds," *Crit Rev Toxicol*, 2004, 34(3):301-33 (review).

Titanium

CAS Number 7550-45-0

UN Number 1838

Synonyms Titanic Chloride; Titanium Tetrachloride; Titanocene; "Tickle"

Use Production of iridescent glass and artificial pearls; production of inorganic titanium compounds; has been used by the military as a smoke-producing screen

Mechanism of Toxic Action Respiratory irritant

Adverse Reactions Respiratory, eye, nose, throat, gastrointestinal, temperature regulation, dermatologic (including dermal burns), fever

Signs and Symptoms of Overdose Irritation of mouth, nose, and throat; chemical pneumonitis; pulmonary edema; edema of pharynx and vocal cord; stenosis of larynx, trachea, upper bronchia; vomiting. Eye exposure may result in cataract, suppurative conjunctivitis, and keratitis. Burns of the GI tract may lead to strictures and fever.

Toxicodynamics/Kinetics

Absorption: Oral: ~3%

Elimination: In urine

Reference Range Normal urine concentration: 10 mcg/L

Overdosage/Treatment

Decontamination:

> Oral: **Do not** evacuate gastric contents. Following oral exposure, dilute with water or milk. **Do not** use a neutralizing solution because of exothermic reaction.
> Dermal: **Do not** immediately wash with water. First dry wipe (with towels or gauze, before irrigating with water to prevent hydrochloric acid burns), whereupon a yellow or white granular deposit will be noted. At this point, wash the deposit off with cool water. Dermal burns can be treated by traditional methods.
> Ocular: Wipe eyelids preliminarily with a dry cloth or gauze, then irrigate copiously with water (3-4 L over 20 minutes). **Do not** use neutralizing solutions.

Supportive therapy: The utility of corticosteroids is unclear in the prevention and treatment of noncardiogenic pulmonary edema.

Additional Information Colorless, fuming liquid; soluble in cold water; has a penetrating acid odor. Titanium tetrachloride in the presence of moisture decomposes to hydrochloric acid and titanium dioxide; heat is liberated. Titanium forms four oxides: titanium monoxide, titanium trioxide, titanium dioxide, and titanium trioxide. ACGIH TLV: 10 mg/m^3; OSHA TWA: 15 mg/m^3 dust

Specific References

Fryzek JP, Chadda B, Marano D, et al, "A Cohort Mortality Study Among Titanium Dioxide Manufacturing Workers in the United States," *J Occup Environ Med*, 2003, 45(4):400-9.

Toluene

Related Information

• Adipose Tissue Ranges of Toxins
• Methyl Isocyanate
• Methylene Diisocyanate

CAS Number 108-88-3

UN Number 1294

Synonyms Methyl Benzene; Tolu-Sol

Impairment Potential Exposure to >500 ppm toluene or blood toluene level >1 mg/L can result in impairment

Commonly Found In Glues, paint removers, pesticides, degreasers

Mechanism of Toxic Action Three mechanisms proposed: Alters lipid structure of cell membranes; Alters membrane-bound enzyme or receptor-site specificity; Toxic metabolite modifies function of cell microsomal proteins and RNA

Adverse Reactions

Cardiovascular: Angina, cardiomyopathy, cardiomegaly, bradycardia, syncope

Central nervous system: CNS depression following early CNS stimulation, panic attacks, memory disturbance, dizziness, leukoencephalopathy

Endocrine & metabolic: Adrenal insufficiency due to bilateral adrenal hemorrhage

Hepatic: Transient liver injury, aminotransferase level elevation (asymptomatic)

Neuromuscular & skeletal: Rhabdomyolysis, muscle weakness (usually spares central and respiratory muscles), quadriparesis

Ocular: Visual evoked potential abnormalities

Renal: Renal tubular acidosis type IV, renal tubular acidosis type I

Respiratory: Bronchitis, wheezing, pulmonary edema

Signs and Symptoms of Overdose Asthenia, bradycardia, burns, chorea (extrapyramidal), dementia, euphoria, eye irritation, fatigue, hypokalemia, irritability, memory loss, metabolic acidosis, mydriasis, myoglobinuria, nonoliguric renal failure, ototoxicity, skin irritation, tachycardia, tinnitus, vomiting

Admission Criteria/Prognosis Symptomatic patients (or patients who ingested toluene) should be admitted; asymptomatic patients can be discharged after 6-12 hours of observation; survival after 3 days postacute exposure is usually associated with recovery; any patient with cardiopulmonary complaints should be admitted; asymptomatic patients 8 hours postexposure can be discharged; survival after 1 day postexposure is usually associated with recovery. Patients exposed to known air concentration of toluene levels >500 ppm should be admitted.

Toxicodynamics/Kinetics
Absorption: Readily by inhalation (within 30 minutes) or ingestion (within 2 hours); slowly by dermal route (14-23 mg/cm^2/hour); accumulates in adipose tissue

Metabolism: Hepatic to hippuric acid (60% to 70%), benzoyl glucuronide (10% to 20%), and ortho or para cresol (<1%)

Half-life: 3 days

Elimination: Hippuric acid excreted in urine, 20% excreted through the lungs, unchanged

Monitoring Parameters Monitor for benzene contamination

Reference Range Determined by measurement of urine hippuric acid. Average urine hippuric acid level in nonexposed individuals is ~0.8 g/L; for individuals exposed to 200 ppm toluene, average urinary hippuric acid level is ~6 g/L. Blood toluene levels of 1.0-2.5 mg/L are associated with intoxication. Coma and death occur at levels of 2.5-10.0 mg/L. Blood toluene BEI is 1.0 mg/L. S-benzyl-N-acetyl-L-cysteine can be measured by HPLC and GC/MS at a lower urinary detection limit of 0.01 mg/L. Median *S-p*-toluylmercapturic acid urinary level following exposure is 63 ppm toluene is 20 mcg/L.

Overdosage/Treatment
Decontamination: **Oral:** Emesis is contraindicated. Lavage is not to be used unless there is a large ingestion. **Dermal:** Wash with soap and water **Inhalation:** Administer 100% humidified oxygen. **Ocular:** Irrigate with saline.

Supportive therapy: Avoid epinephrine because of myocardial sensitization. Avoid haloperidol which can further deplete dopamine concentration of the brain. Avoid aspirin due to increased ototoxicity and decreased toluene clearance. Prednisone or aerosolized beclomethasone may prevent bronchospasm in TDI-sensitized patients, while atropine or cromolyn do not appear to exhibit a protective effect. Theophylline may have only a partial effect. Amantadine hydrochloride (100 mg daily, increased after 2 weeks to 100 mg twice daily) has been use successfully in treating cerebellar and visual dysfunction.

Diagnostic Procedures
• Electrolytes, Blood

Additional Information
Lethal oral dose: 625 mg/kg

Colorless liquid, sweet odor. Odor threshold: 0.4-2 ppm. Specific gravity: 1.22. Urinary BEI of o-cresol: 1 mg/g creatinine. Atmospheric half-life: 10-104 hours. Soil half-life: 1-7 days. TLV-TWA: 100 ppm; PEL-TWA: 200 ppm

The largest source of airborne emissions is through combustion of gasoline (5% to 7% toluene by weight).

Levels in drinking water are usually <3 mcg/L. Drinking water contributes 0.3-0.5 mcg/day of toluene exposure.

Estimated daily dose by inhalation: 300 mcg. Cigarette smoking can cause a daily increase in toluene inhalation of 1000 mcg.

Mean toluene level in ambient air: 2.8 ppb in urban areas; 0.4 ppb in rural areas

Median level of toluene found in snow samples (near Denver, Colorado): 0.05 mcg/L. See table.

Median Toulene Levels in Ambient Air

Sampling Location	Number of Samples	Daily mean (ppb)	Concentration (mcg/m^3)
Remote	225	0.049	0.18
Rural	248	0.35	1.3
Suburban	958	0.195	0.731
Urban	2519	2.883	10.81
Source dominated	104	6.314	23.67
Indoor	101	8.4	31.5
Workplace	80	0.865	3.24

Reference: U.S. Department of Health and Human Services, "Toxicological Profile for Toulene," Agency for Toxic Substances and Disease Registry, August 1998.

Metabolism of Toluene in Humans and Animals

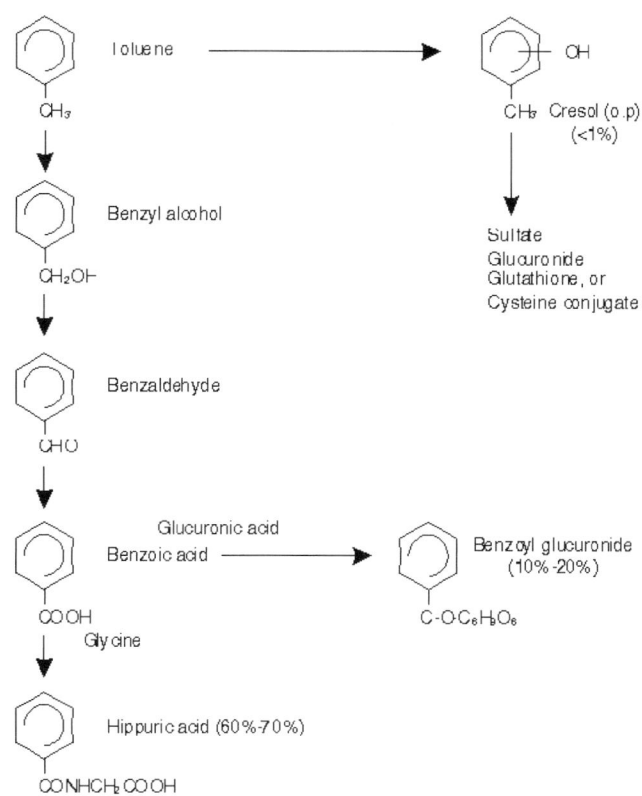

From "Toxicological Profile for Toluene," U.S. Department of Health and Human Services, Agency for Toxic Substances and Disease Registry, August 1998.

Specific References

Al-Ghamdi SS, Raftery MJ, and Yaqoob MM, "Organic Solvent-Induced Proximal Tubular Cell Toxicity via Caspase-3 Activation," *J Toxicol Clin Toxicol*, 2003, 41(7):941-5.

Chou JS, Lim YC, Ma YC, et al, "Measurement of Benzylmercapturic Acid in Human Urine by Liquid Chromatography-Electrospray Ionization-Tandem Quadrupole Mass Spectrometry," *J Anal Toxicol*, 2006, 30:306-12.

Doty RL, Cometto-Muñiz JE, Jalowayski AA, et al, "Assessment of Upper Respiratory Tract and Ocular Irritative Effects of Volatile Chemicals in Humans," *Crit Rev Toxicol*, 2004, 34(2):85-142.

Haut MW, Kuwabara H, Ducatman AM, et al, "Corpus Callosum Volume in Railroad Workers with Chronic Exposure to Solvents," *J Occup Environ Med*, 2006, 48(6):615-24.

Lomax RB, Ridgway P, and Meldrum M, "Does Occupational Exposure to Organic Solvents Affect Colour Discrimination?" *Toxicol Rev*, 2004, 23(2):91-121 (review).

Ramon MF, Ballesteros S, Martinez-Arrieta R, et al, "Volatile Substance and Other Drug Abuse Inhalation in Spain," *J Toxicol Clin Toxicol*, 2003, 41(7):931-6.

Toluene Diisocyanate

Related Information
• Hexamethylene Diisocyanate

Applies to Elastomers (Manufacture); Polyurethane Foams (Manufacture)

CAS Number 584-84-9

UN Number 2078

Synonyms Meta-Toluene Diisocyanate; TDI

Use In the manufacture of polyurethane foams, elastomers

Mechanism of Toxic Action Irritation to mucous membranes/sensitizer as an allergen

Adverse Reactions
Cardiovascular: Chest pain, angina, cor pulmonale

Central nervous system: Panic attacks, headache, insomnia, euphoria, ataxia, memory loss

Respiratory: Respiratory irritation and sensitization, wheezing, hemorrhagic alveolitis, reactive airways disease syndrome, pulmonary hemorrhage, asthma

Signs and Symptoms of Overdose Ataxia, burning of nose and throat, chest pain, choking, cough, decreased libido, dyspnea, euphoria, eye irritation, hemoptysis, impotence, nausea, nystagmus, retrosternal chest pain, vomiting

Toxicodynamics/Kinetics
Metabolism: May be metabolized to 2,4-toluene diamine (a carcinogen)
Elimination: Renal

Reference Range Air level exposure of ~0.005 ppm can result in a 6-8 hour urine level of 8.6 mcg/L

Overdosage/Treatment Decontamination: Emesis is contraindicated. **Oral:** Dilute with milk or water; basic poison management. **Inhalation:** Give supplemental oxygen, bronchodilators

Additional Information
Asthma and chronic bronchitis are long-term sequelae. Acute pulmonary pathology will be evident within 8 hours. While solid tumor formation has been associated with TDI exposure in rodents, NIOSH considers TDI to be a potential human carcinogen.

There is a potential for secondary contamination after liquid exposure; no risk for secondary (ie, from victims) contamination exposure.

Fruity, pungent odor; TDI reacts with water to form carbon dioxide and polyureas; it is essentially insoluble in water. Odor threshold: 2 ppm. TLV-TWA: 0.005 ppm; IDLH: 10 ppm

Toxaphene

CAS Number 8001-35-2
UN Number 2761
U.S. Brand Names Agricide Maggot Killer®; Alltox®; Camphofene®; Geniphene®; Huilex®; Motox®; Penphene®; Phenatox®; Phenicide®; Tox-Sol®; Toxakil®
Synonyms Campheclor; Chlorinated Camphene
Use Chlorinated hydrocarbon insecticide used on livestock to control lice, flies, ticks, mange, and mites; used in treating flowering plants; not used on agricultural commodities as of 1993
Mechanism of Toxic Action Blocks GABA-regulated chloride ionophore of the neuronal synapse
Adverse Reactions
Gastrointestinal: Salivation
Neuromuscular & skeletal: Rhabdomyolysis
Signs and Symptoms of Overdose Ataxia, elevated liver function tests, hyperthermia, nausea, respiratory failure, seizures, tremor
Toxicodynamics/Kinetics
Absorption: Oral and dermal
Metabolism: Hepatic dechlorination, oxidation, and dehydrodechlorination
Elimination: Urine and feces
Overdosage/Treatment
Decontamination: **Oral: Do not** induce emesis; lavage (within 1 hour)/ activated charcoal. **Dermal:** Remove contaminated clothing (especially leather); wash with soap and water. **Inhalation:** Administer 100% humidified oxygen. **Ocular:** Irrigate copiously with saline.
Supportive therapy: Benzodiazepines, phenobarbital, or phenytoin may be used for seizure control. Avoid catecholamine in that it may increase myocardial irritability and result in ventricular arrhythmias.
Enhancement of elimination: Multiple dosing of activated charcoal or cholestyramine may be effective. Hemodialysis or hemoperfusion is not likely to be beneficial.
Drug Interaction May decrease effect of warfarin
Additional Information
Minimum lethal dose: Oral: 2-7 g. Seizurgenic dose: Oral: 10 mg/kg. Toxic dose: Dermal: 660 mg/kg
Adrenal-based corticosteroid synthesis may be decreased; contains 67% to 69% chlorine
Average dietary intake for an adult: <0.01 mcg/kg/day, Average inhalation exposure: ~0.0004-0.0033 mcg/day
Atmospheric residence time: 46-70 days. Water half-life: >10 years
PEL-TWA: 0.5 mg/m^3; TLV-TWA: 0.5 mg/m^3

Tributyl Phosphate

Related Information
• Adipose Tissue Ranges of Toxins
CAS Number 126-73-8
Synonyms TBP
Use Antifoaming agent; hydraulic fluid; plasticizer; solvent for uranium extraction
Mechanism of Toxic Action Vapors (especially hot) are irritants; weak cholinesterase inhibition
Adverse Reactions
Central nervous system: Headache
Dermatologic: Dermatitis
Gastrointestinal: Nausea
Ocular: Eye irritation
Respiratory: Cough

Admission Criteria/Prognosis Admit any patient with systemic symptomatology or ingestion >100 mL
Monitoring Parameters Cholinesterase levels
Overdosage/Treatment
Decontamination: **Oral:** For amounts >100 mL, emesis with ipecac can be considered if performed within 30 minutes of ingestion. Activated charcoal may be useful. **Inhalation:** Administer 100% humidified oxygen.
Supportive therapy: If muscarinic symptoms develop, use of atropine may be helpful. Nicotinic signs should be treated with pralidoxime or obidoxime.
Antidote(s)
• Atropine [ANTIDOTE]
• Obidoxime Chloride [ANTIDOTE]
• Pralidoxime [ANTIDOTE]
Additional Information Symptoms of respiratory irritation can occur for 6-hour exposures >123 ppm. Specific gravity: 0.976. IDLH: 1300 mg/m^3

Trichloroethane

CAS Number 71-55-6
UN Number 2831
Synonyms CF 2; Methyl Chloroform; Strobane; TCA; TCE
Impairment Potential Exposure to air trichloroethane levels >1000 ppm can result in impairment.
Commonly Found In Cleaning solvent, lubricant, ink, typewriter correction fluid; also is frequently used in an abused setting ("bagging")
Mechanism of Toxic Action CNS depression, rapid anesthetic action
Adverse Reactions
Cardiovascular: Hypotension, cardiovascular collapse, fibrillation (ventricular), shock, arrhythmias (ventricular)
Central nervous system: Anesthesia, axonopathy (peripheral)
Hematologic: Methemoglobinemia
Neuromuscular & skeletal: Neuropathy (peripheral), paresthesias
Ocular: Eye irritation
Respiratory: Pulmonary edema, respiratory depression, eosinophilic pneumonia
Signs and Symptoms of Overdose Acetone breath, agitation, ataxia, coma, diarrhea, diplopia, dizziness, drowsiness, erythema, hallucinations, nausea, seizures, vomiting
Toxicodynamics/Kinetics
Absorption: Rapid dermally, through inhalation, or through ingestion
Metabolism: Hepatic (<10%) to trichloroacetic acid
Half-life: 53 hours
Elimination: Primarily by the lungs (91%)
Reference Range Fatal serum levels range from 1.7-42.0 mg/L of trichloroethane concentration. Blood level of 1.4 mg/L consistent with exposure of 250 ppm for $^1/_2$ hour.
Overdosage/Treatment
Decontamination: **Oral:** Emesis is contraindicated; dilute with milk. **Dermal:** Wash with soap and water; isopropyl alcohol can be used. **Inhalation:** Administer 100% humidified oxygen. **Ocular:** Irrigate with saline.
Supportive therapy: Propranolol may be beneficial for tachycardia. Avoid catecholamines as they can sensitize the myocardium. Calcium gluconate or phenylephrine has been useful to treat hypotension in the dog model.
Drug Interaction Alcohol-Disulfiram like reaction (Degreaser's Flush): Initiated within 30 minutes of alcohol ingestion; Peaks in one hour and then resolves in one hour. Flushing starts on the nose and cheeks.
Additional Information
Levels of 1000 ppm will cause ataxia.
BEI of urinary trichloroacetic acid is 10 mcg/L
Estimated daily intake: 50-1000 mg by all routes of exposure
Door spray lubricants, VCR cleaners, typewriter correction fluid, and nonacid drain cleaners have the highest amount of 1,1,1-trichloroethane.
Foods with the highest levels include allspice (16,000 ppb), celery seed (909 ppb), and pickling spice (549 ppb).
Pleasant odor. Odor threshold: 120-500 ppm. Atmospheric half-life: 2.7-6 years. Soil half-life (aerobic degradation): ~1 week. Urban atmospheric concentration in U.S.: 0.1-1 ppb. TLV-TWA: 350 ppm; PEL-TWA: 350 ppm
Specific References
DiCarlo MA, "Household Products: A Review," *Vet Hum Toxicol*, 2003, 45(5):256-61.

Trichloroethylene

Applies to Adhesives; degreaser (Industrial); fire retardant; lacquer; solvents (house cleaning); typewriter correction fluid
CAS Number 79-01-6
UN Number 1710
Synonyms Acetylene Trichloride; TRI; trichloren; trilene

Use Industrial degreaser, fire retardant, lacquer/adhesive, house cleaning solvent, typewriter correction fluid

Mechanism of Toxic Action CNS depressant; may induce peroxisome proliferation

Adverse Reactions

Cardiovascular: Fibrillation (ventricular), bradycardia, Raynaud's phenomenon, sinus bradycardia, arrhythmias (ventricular)

Central nervous system: CNS depression

Hepatic: Hepatitis, centrilobular hepatic necrosis, aminotransferase level elevation (asymptomatic)

Ocular: Diplopia, blurred vision progressing to blindness, optic neuropathy

Renal: Tubular necrosis (acute)

Respiratory: Pulmonary edema, respiratory depression

Miscellaneous: Aneuploidy induction, trigeminal neuro-pathy

Signs and Symptoms of Overdose Ataxia, bradycardia, cranial nerve palsies, cyanosis, dementia, dizziness, dyspnea, fatigue, headache, impotence, loss of taste, mydriasis, nystagmus, resting tremor, salivation, seizures, slurred speech, vomiting

Admission Criteria/Prognosis Patients (regardless of radiological signs) should be admitted if they are symptomatic 6 hours postexposure; survival after 6 hours usually associated with recovery

Toxicodynamics/Kinetics

Absorption: Rapid by ingestion and inhalation; minimal dermal exposure

Metabolism: In the liver; fat soluble

Half-life: 30-38 hours

Elimination: Excreted in urine, feces, and lung (16%)

Reference Range Blood concentrations of 5.0-10.0 mg/dL related to anesthetic action; levels of 0.3-11.0 mg/dL are associated with fatalities; blood level of 0.1 mg/dL is consistent with exposure of 100 ppm

Overdosage/Treatment

Decontamination: Dermal: Wash with soap and water. Ocular: Irrigate with saline. Oral:Do not induce emesis; activated charcoal may be used.

Supportive therapy: Avoid catecholamines in that they may sensitize the myocardium. Propranolol may be useful for treatment.

Drug Interaction Alcohol - Disulfiram like reaction (Degreaser's Flush): Initiated within 30 minutes of alcohol ingestion; peaks in one hour and then resolves in one hour. Flushing starts on the nose and cheeks.

Additional Information

Toxic ingestion: 0.5 mL/kg

Degreaser's flush occurs in workers who ingest ethanol following exposure to trichloroethylene.

Chloroform odor. Odor threshold: 20 ppm. TLV-TWA: 50 ppm; PEL-TWA: 100 ppm

BEI of urinary trichloroacetic acid: 100 mg/g creatinine

Atmospheric half-life: 6.8 days. Ambient atmospheric levels in urban areas: 0.46 ppb.

Average air intake: 11-33 mcg/day. Average intake through drinking water: 2-20 mcg/day

Trichloroethylene Subregistry: Je Anne Burg PhD, Agency for Toxic Substances and Disease Registry, 1600 Clifton Road, NE, Mailstop E 31, Atlanta, GA 30333: (404) 639-6202

Specific References

Chalupka S, "Tainted Water on Tap," *Am J Nurs*, 2005, 105(11):40-52; quiz 53 (review).

Harper AA, Maher TJ, Quang LS, et al, "Enhancement by Disulfiram on Trichloroethylene-Induced Neurobehavioral Toxicity in a Murine System," *J Toxicol Clin Toxicol*, 2004, 42(5):752-3.

Harper AA, Maher TJ, Quang LS, et al, "Modulation of Murine CYPE2E1 Activity by Disulfiram on Trichloroethylene-Induced Neurotoxicity - A Pilot Study," *J Toxicol Clin Toxicol*, 2004, 42(5):753.

Iavicoli I, Marinaccio A, and Carelli G, "Effects of Occupational Trichloroethylene Exposure on Cytokine Levels in Workers," *J Occup Environ Med*, 2005, 47(5):453-7.

Triethylene Glycol

Applies to Brake Fluid

CAS Number 112-27-6

Synonyms Glycdonitrile; TEG

Use Found in brake fluid

Mechanism of Toxic Action A short chain polyethylene glycol which can break down into organic acids through an alcohol dehydrogenase pathway. It is unclear whether ethylene glycol or its metabolites are produced by this pathway.

Signs and Symptoms of Overdose Coma, metabolic acidosis

Antidotes

Sodium bicarbonate fomepizole

Admission Criteria/Prognosis Admit any ingestion

Overdosage/Treatment

Decontamination: Oral: Activated charcoal should be administered. Dermal: Irrigate with soap and water

Supportive therapy: Intravenous sodium bicarbonate should be used to treat acidosis. Ethanol administration or fomepizole should be given as

an inhibitor of alcohol dehydrogenase. Thiamine, pyridoxine, and folinic acid can also be administered.

Enhancement of elimination: Although no formal studies exist, the low molecular weight and high water solubility of TEG makes this a candidate for hemodialysis removal.

Trimellitic Anhydride

CAS Number 552-30-7

Synonyms Anhidrotrimellitic Acid; TMA; TMAN

Use Curing agent for epoxy; used in manufacture of plastics and paints; used as anticorrosive surface

Mechanism of Toxic Action Causes four clinical respiratory illnesses, three of which are immunologically mediated upon inhalation (1) IgE-mediated allergic rhinitis with bronchospasm; (2) a late respiratory systemic syndrome with cough, dyspnea, fever, and arthralgias occurring 4-12 hours postexposure; (3) hemoptysis, dyspnea and cough leading to restrictive lung disease and respiratory failure often termed "pulmonary disease-anemia syndrome"; and (4) respiratory irritation from high-dose exposure

Adverse Reactions

Central nervous system: Fever

Dermatologic: Contact dermatitis

Hematologic: Hemolytic anemia

Neuromuscular & skeletal: Myalgia, arthralgia

Respiratory: Pulmonary hemorrhage, hemorrhagic alveolitis, allergic rhinitis, cough, bronchospasm, dyspnea, pneumonitis, pulmonary edema, asthma

Admission Criteria/Prognosis Symptomatic patients should be admitted; asymptomatic exposures may be discharged after 12-hour observation postexposure

Monitoring Parameters Arterial blood gas, chest x-ray

Overdosage/Treatment Supportive therapy: Administer 100% humidified oxygen. Bronchodilators and beta agonist agents can be useful. Corticosteroids are of uncertain benefit.

Additional Information Levels of IgE antibody activity to trimellityl human serum albumin may be elevated. Usually found as crystals with a melting point of 162°C. OSHA 8-hour TWA: 0.005 ppm. Soluble in either and acetone.

Tungsten

CAS Number 7440-33-7

Use Found in light filaments, heating elements, welding electrodes, electron tubes, ceramics, cutting tools. Mostly used in the form of tungsten carbide. Also used in heat shields, arc lamps, electrodes, and gyroscopes

Mechanism of Toxic Action Irritant - may generate hydroxyl radicals in lungs contributing to pulmonary fibrosis

Signs and Symptoms of Overdose Pulmonary fibrosis, ocular/nasal irritation, cough, dyspnea, memory deficits, seizures, headache, coma, renal insufficiency, acute tubular necrosis, skin irritation; nausea, metabolic acidosis, hyperkalemia (oral ingestion)

Toxicodynamics/Kinetics Elimination: Renal

Reference Range General population: Blood tungsten level: 1-6 mcg/L; urine tungsten level: <0.085 mcg/L; hair tungsten level: 16 ppb

Overdosage/Treatment

Decontamination:

Inhalation: Administer 100% humidified oxygen

Ocular: Copiously irrigate with saline or water

Oral: Lavage within 1 hour of oral ingestion

Supportive therapy: Seizures can be treated with benzodiazepines

Drug Interaction May enhance pulmonary toxicity of cobalt

Additional Information

Most common valence is +6; highest melting point of all metals (3,410°C)

Concentration of tungsten:

Ambient air: <10 ng/m^3

Surface soil: 0.68-2.7 mg/kg dry weight

Sea water: 0.1 mcg/L

Usual dietary intake: ~49 mcg/day

Occupational exposure: See table.

Occupations with Potential Tungsten Exposure	
Alloy makers	Melting, pouring, casting workers
Carbonyl workers	Metal sprayers
Ceramic workers	Ore-refining and foundry workers
Cemented tungsten carbide workers	Paint and pigment makers
Cement makers	Papermakers
Dyemakers	Penpoint makers

Dyers	Petroleum refinery workers
Flameproofers	Photographic developers
High-speed tool steelworkers	Spark-plug makers
Incandescent-lamp makers	Textile dryers
Industrial chemical synthesizers	Tool grinders
Inkmakers	Tungsten and molybdenum miners
Lamp-filament makers	Waterproofing makers
Lubricant makers	Welders

"Occupational Exposure to Tungsten and Cemented Carbide," *NIOSH*, 1977, 21-171.

Specific References

U.S. Department of Health and Human Services, *Toxicological Profile for Tungsten*, Syracuse Research Corp, 2003.

Turpentine Oil

Related Information
- Limonene
- Pine Oil

CAS Number 8006-64-2; 9005-90-7
UN Number 1299
U.S. Brand Names Ozothine®
Synonyms Gum Spirits; Spirits of Turpentine
Commonly Found In Oleoresin solvent, paint vehicle, deodorizer fragrance, rubefacient
Mechanism of Toxic Action CNS depressant, irritant to mucous membranes; high volatility with low viscosity

Adverse Reactions
Cardiovascular: Tachycardia, sinus tachycardia
Central nervous system: Ataxia, coma, fever, insomnia, dizziness, seizures (can occur after ingestions >200 mL), headache (inhalation >750 ppm for several hours)
Dermatologic: Contact dermatitis, erythema, blister, urticaria, nonimmunologic contact urticaria, airborne contact dermatitis
Gastrointestinal: Hemorrhagic gastritis, diarrhea
Genitourinary: Hemorrhagic cystitis, dysuria
Ocular: Conjunctivitis, blepharospasm, mydriasis, eye irritation is perceptible at 175 ppm
Renal: Glomerulonephritis, hematuria, albuminuria
Respiratory: Pulmonary edema, aspiration pneumonitis, wheezing, coughing, dyspnea
Miscellaneous: Hypersensitivity reactions in 2.6% of population

Signs and Symptoms of Overdose Aspiration, chills, cough, dyspnea, eye pain, fever, seizures, vomiting
Admission Criteria/Prognosis Patients who develop tachypnea, cyanosis, dyspnea, CNS depression, tachycardia, or fever within 8 hours of exposure should be admitted; asymptomatic patients can be discharged after 8 hours observation; admit if the patient is symptomatic 6 hours postingestion or if pediatric ingestion is >5 mL

Toxicodynamics/Kinetics
Absorption: Well absorbed through the GI tract, by inhalation, and dermally; high fat solubility
Metabolism: In the liver
Elimination: Renally and through the lungs

Reference Range Blood and urine turpentine level after a severe adult overdose was 28 mcg/mL and 15 mcg/mL, respectively

Overdosage/Treatment
Decontamination: Emesis is indicated only for large ingestions and within 30 minutes of ingestion. Lavage only after the patient is intubated. Activated charcoal is useful. Steroids are not beneficial. Seizures can be treated with a benzodiazepine. Phenobarbital or phenytoin can be used for refractory seizures. **Ocular:** Irrigate copiously with saline.
Enhanced elimination: Hemoperfusion may be useful if utilized very early in the hospital course.

Additional Information
Minimum lethal dose: Children: 15 mL; Adults: 140 mL
Pungent odor, although an odor of violets may be noted in overdose settings; urinary odor is that of violets. Combustible. TLV-TWA: 100 ppm; IDLH: 1900 ppm; PEL-TWA: 100 ppm
Density: 0.9, constituents; terpenes and camphenes, and 3-carene
Usual amount of turpentine oil used in food or beverage flavoring: ~20 ppm

Uranium

CAS Number 7440-61-1
UN Number 2979
Use Primarily in nuclear power plants, radiation shielding material, x-ray targets, gyro compasses, and in large incandescent lamps; mordant in silk and wood industry

Mechanism of Toxic Action Uranyl ion complexes with bicarbonate and produces acute renal proximal tubular damage/failure
Adverse Reactions
Renal: Renal tubular damage with a dose >0.1 mg/kg, acute tubular necrosis
Miscellaneous: Possible increase in skin cancer rate
Signs and Symptoms of Overdose Albuminuria, elevated BUN, pulmonary edema, weight loss, wheezing
Toxicodynamics/Kinetics
Absorption: Uranyl ion is rapidly absorbed from gastrointestinal tract
Distribution: Lung retains insoluble salts following inhalation
Half-life: 1500 days
Elimination: 66% renal excretion within 24 hours
Reference Range Average uranium concentration in N.Y. human blood donors: 0.14 mcg uranium/kg wet weight of both whole blood and red blood cells; a urinary uranium concentration of >100 mcg/L is indicative of recent uranium exposure
Overdosage/Treatment
Decontamination: Irrigate with soap and water. Waste should be kept in separate receptacles. Use a Geiger-Mueller meter to survey the extent of contamination.
Supportive therapy: Give 1-3 mEq/kg of I.V. sodium bicarbonate to cause a forced alkaline diuresis which can be nephroprotective. Chelating agents such as sodium 4,5-dihydroxybenzene-1,3-disulphonate (Tiron®) or diethylamine-tetramine pentaacetic acid (DTPA) are of uncertain efficacy.

Additional Information
Soluble uranium compound is known as uranyl ion. Radon decays and forms radon daughters (isotopes of lead, bismuth, and polonium). The radon daughters attach to dust particles and are inhaled by uranium miners. Uranium tetrafluoride and uranyl fluoride are hydrolyzed to HF. Can call U.S. Department of Energy Regional Coordinating Office at 615-576-1004.
Average daily intake from food and water: 1 mcg
Estimated intake due to drinking water: 0.6-2 pCi/day (0.02-0.07 Bq/day)
Rock levels of uranium range from 0.5-4.7 mcg/g
Soil levels average ~1.8 mcg/g in the U.S.
Atmospheric half-life of uranyl fluoride: 35 minutes
Root crops (potatoes, parsnips, turnips) have the highest uranium levels, and thus dietary daily uranium intake may range from 3.3-4.2 mcg
Essentially insoluble in water

Average Uranium Concentrations in Drinking Water for States Where Concentration Exceeds 1pCi/L

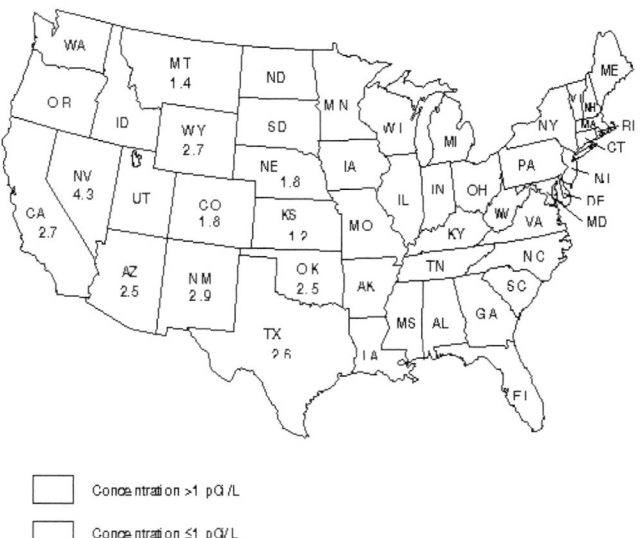

	Concentration >1 pCi/L
	Concentration ≤1 pCi/L

Source: NCRP 198 4b

Department of Energy
Major Offices, Facilities, and Laboratories

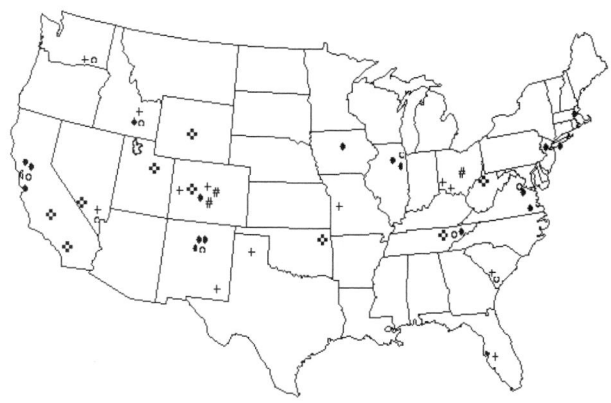

Operations Offices (o)
Oakland CA
Idaho Falls ID
Chicago IL
Las Vegas NV
Albuquerque NM
Savannah SC
Oak Ridge TN
Richland WA

Laboratories / National Laboratories (♦)
Lawrence Berkeley Natl Lab, Berkeley CA
Lawrence Livermore Natl Lab, Berkeley CA
Stanford Linear Accelerator, Menlo Park CA
Natl Renewable Energy Lab, Golden CO
Idaho National Energy and Env Lab, ID
Fermi Natl Accelerator Lab, Batavia IL
Argonne Natl Lab, Argonne IL
Ames Lab, Ames IA
MIT Bates Lab, Cambridge MA
Princeton Plasma Physics Lab, NJ
Inhalation Toxicology Res Inst, Albuquerque NM

Los Alamos Natl Lab, Los Alamos NM
Sandia Natl Labs, Albuquerque NM
Livermore CA
Brookhaven Natl Lab, Brookhaven NY
Oak Ridge Natl Lab, Oak Ridge TN
T Jefferson Natl Accelerator, Newport News VA
Pacific Northwest Natl Lab, Richland WA

Special Purpose Offices (❖)
Energy Technology Eng Ctr, LA, CA
Naval Petroleum Reserves 1&2, Kern Co, CA
Naval Oil Shale Reserves 1&3, Rifle CO
Yucca Mountain Project, NV
Natl Petroleum Technology Office, Tulsa OK
Federal Energy Technology Centers, Pittsburg PA, Morgantown WV
Oak Ridge Inst for Science & Education, TN
Naval Oil Shale Reserve 2, Vernal UT
Naval Petroleum Reserve 3, Casper WY

Facilities (+)
Grand Junction CO
Rocky Flats CO
Pinellas FL
Idaho Falls ID
Kansas City Plant, Kansas City MO
Las Vegas NV
Waste Isolation Pilot Plant, Carlsbad NM
Fernald Env Management Project, Cincinnati OH
Miamisburg Environmental Management Project, OH
Savannah River SC
Oak Ridge Reservation, Oak Ridge TN
Pantex Plant, Amarillo TX
Hanford WA

Field Offices (#)
Rocky Flats CO
Golden CO
Ohio (4 sites in OH, 1 site in New York)

See table.

| Concentrations of Uranium in Some Foods ||
Food	Uranium Concentration (ng/g raw weight)
Whole grain products	1.45*
Potatoes	2.66-2.92*; 15-18†
Carrots	7.7†
Root vegetables	0.94-1.20*
Cabbage	4.7†
Meat	0.58-1.32*; 20†
Poultry	0.14-0.42*
Beef	14†
Beef liver	26†
Beef kidney	70†
Eggs	0.23*; 9.6†
Dairy products	0.08-0.31*
Cow milk	4†
Milk	1-2†
Fresh fish	0.43-0.85*; 11†
Shellfish	9.5-31.0*
Welsh onion	69†
Flour	0.25-0.68*
Wheat bread	19†
Baked products	1.32-1.5*; 12†

Table   (*Continued*)

| Concentrations of Uranium in Some Foods ||
Food	Uranium Concentration (ng/g raw weight)
Polished rice	1.43-6.0*; 15†
Macaroni	0.4-0.63*
Tea	5†
Coffee	6†
Parsley	60†
Red pepper	5†
Mustard	0.2†
Table salt	40†
Canned vegetables	0.09-0.18*
Fruit juices	0.04-0.12*
Canned fruits	0.18-0.29*
Fresh fruits	0.71-1.29*
Dried beans	1.5-3.67*
Fresh vegetables	0.52-0.92*

From: U.S. Department of Health and Human Services, "Toxicological Profile for Uranium," Agency for Toxic Substances and Disease Registry, September 1999.
*Reference: National Council on Radiation Protection and Measurements
†Reference: Environmental Protection Agency

Specific References

Archer VE, Coons T, Saccomanno G, et al, "Latency and the Lung Cancer Epidemic Among United States Uranium Miners," *Health Phys*, 2004, 87(5):480-9.

Dainiak N, Waselenko JK, Armitage JO, et al, "The Hematologist and Radiation Casualties," *Hematology (Am Soc Hematol Educ Program)*, 2003, 473-96 (review).

DeVol TA and Woodruff RL Jr, "Uranium in Hot Water Tanks: A Source of TENORM," *Health Phys*, 2004, 87(6):659-63.

Iyengar GV, Kawamura H, Dang HS, et al, "Contents of Cesium, Iodine, Strontium, Thorium, and Uranium in Selected Human Organs of Adult Asian Population," *Health Phys*, 2004, 87(2):151-9.

McDiarmid MA, Squibb K, and Engelhardt SM, "Biologic Monitoring for Urinary Uranium in Gulf War I Veterans," *Health Phys*, 2004, 87(1):51-6.

Vanadium

Related Information
- Adipose Tissue Ranges of Toxins

CAS Number 7440-62-2

UN Number 3285

Use Primarily as an alloying agent in steel; jet engine manufacture; pesticide production, inks, dyes and pigments

Mechanism of Toxic Action Vanadium reduces alveolar macrophage viability; this may account for vanadium's respiratory irritant effect; vanadium also causes redistribution of iron, chromium, copper, manganese, and zinc; it also has positive inotropic effects on the heart

Adverse Reactions
HEENT, cardiovascular, respiratory, neurologic, gastrointestinal, dermatologic, salivation
Respiratory: Asthma

Signs and Symptoms of Overdose Abdominal pain, black stools, CNS depression, dermatitis, diarrhea, dry mouth, epistaxis, green tongue, headache, metallic taste, occupational asthma, ocular irritation, peripheral vasoconstriction (of lungs, spleen, kidney, intestine) pulmonary edema, rhinitis, tracheitis

Toxicodynamics/Kinetics
Absorption: Primarily through inhalation; oral and dermal absorption is poor
Distribution: Although vanadium is found throughout tissues, majority is found in fat
Elimination: Excreted in both urine and feces

Reference Range Normal urine levels: <8 mcg/24 hours; total body burden considered to be safe in U.S.: 0.5 mg/L; normal serum vanadium levels: 1-2 mcg/L

Overdosage/Treatment
Decontamination: **Oral:** Lavage within 1 hour, followed by dilution with milk or water; give a cathartic. **Dermal:** Wash with soap and water. **Ocular:** Irrigate with saline.
Enhancement of elimination: BAL is not useful. Deferoxamine mesylate or ethylene diamine tetracetate has had some success in animal models.

Additional Information Toxic dose of ammonium metavanadate is 10 g.

Pentavalent vanadium is more toxic than other forms; the parenteral form is most toxic, followed by inhalation and oral; U.S. coal can contain as much as 10 g/kg of vanadium

Drinking water concentrations: Average 4.3 mcg/L

Daily adult intake by inhalation: ~ 1 mcg

Atmospheric residence time: 1 day

Mean vanadium content in urban areas is ~11 ng/m^3

Vanadium concentration in earth's crust: 150 mg/kg; Average content in U.S. soil: 200 mg/kg

Food items with highest levels include ground parsley (1800 ng/g), freeze-dried spinach (533-840 ng/g), wild mushrooms (50-2000 ng/g), and oysters (450 ng/g)

ACGIH TLV: 0.05 mg/m^3 respirable dust or fumes; OSHA TWA: 0.5 mg/m^3 dust, 0.1 mg/m^3 fumes

Air content of Bahrain (during burning of oil fields of Kuwait in 1991): 11-42 ng/m^3

Vinyl Acetate

CAS Number 108-05-4

UN Number 1301

U.S. Brand Names VAC®; VYAC®; Zeset T®

Synonyms 1-Acetoxy-Ethylene; Acetic Acid; Ethanoic Acid; Ethenyl Ester; Vinyl Ethanoate

Use Production of polyvinyl acetate (adhesives, wood gluing, paints) and polyvinyl alcohol (adhesives, textiles, automobile glass)

Mechanism of Toxic Action Primarily a respiratory irritant

Adverse Reactions

Cardiovascular: Chest pain, angina

Central nervous system: Insomnia, dizziness

Dermatologic: Dermatitis, blisters

Gastrointestinal: Throat irritation, mucous membrane irritation

Hepatic: Elevated liver function test results

Neuromuscular & skeletal: Neuropathy (peripheral)

Ocular: Eye irritation

Respiratory: Cough, hoarseness, bronchospasm

Miscellaneous: Polyneuritis

Toxicodynamics/Kinetics

Absorption: Probably through inhalation, oral, and dermal routes

Metabolism: Plasma and liver esterases hydrolyze vinyl acetate to acetaldehyde and acetic acid along with carbon dioxide

Overdosage/Treatment Decontamination: **Oral:** Dilute with milk or water. **Dermal:** Wash with soap and water. **Inhalation:** Administer 100% humidified oxygen. **Ocular:** Irrigate with saline.

Additional Information Irritation can occur at air concentrations >20 ppm. Odor threshold: 0.12 ppm. Half-life in water: 7.3 days. Atmospheric half-life: 4-6.5 hours. Amount of vinyl acetate in a cigarette: 400 ng. TLV-TWA: 10 ppm.

Vinyl Chloride

Applies to Methylchloroform (Production); Polyvinyl Chloride (Production); Refrigerant

CAS Number 75-01-4

UN Number 1086

Synonyms Chloroethylene; Ethylene Monochloride

Commonly Found In Adhesives, propellants

Use As a refrigerant, used in production of methylchloroform and in manufacture of polyvinyl chloride (PVC)

Mechanism of Toxic Action Dermal exposure to escaping pressurized gas may cause injury or frostbite due to rapid evaporation; narcotic properties; metabolite (chloroethylene epoxide) is toxic; human carcinogen - angiosarcoma of the liver

Adverse Reactions

Cardiovascular: Fibrillation (ventricular), Raynaud's phenomenon, arrhythmias (ventricular)

Central nervous system: CNS depression

Neuromuscular & skeletal: Peripheral neuropathy

Respiratory: Respiratory irritation, respiratory depression

Signs and Symptoms of Overdose Arthralgia, ataxia, dyspnea, epigastric pain, euphoria, fatigue, fingernail clubbing, headache, hepatomegaly, loss of libido, ocular irritation, seizures. Inhalation of high concentrations may result in narcotic-like CNS and apnea. Chronic exposure may result in hepatic angiosarcoma. Cancers of the brain, liver, and lung have also been documented. In addition, chronic exposure may result in "vinyl chloride disease" which consists of a scleroderma-like condition of the connective tissue of the fingers and thickening of the dermis, acro-osteolysis, and Raynaud's-type phenomenon. Thrombocytopenia may also occur.

Admission Criteria/Prognosis Any patient with central nervous system or respiratory abnormalities should be admitted

Toxicodynamics/Kinetics

Absorption: Inhalation or dermal exposure; 42% retained in the lungs; concentrated in the liver and kidneys

Metabolism: In the liver, thiodiglycolic acid is the major metabolite

Elimination: Excreted renally

Reference Range Urine thiodiglycolic acid level of 0.3-4.0 mg/L may indicate recent exposure

Overdosage/Treatment

Decontamination: **Oral: Do not** induce emesis; lavage/activated charcoal

Dermal: Remove and discard all contaminated clothing as hazardous waste. Wash exposed areas twice with soap and water and rinse well. Wash water should be contained and appropriately discarded. **Ocular:** Irrigate with saline.

Supportive therapy: Symptomatic and supportive care are the mainstay of treatment. Administer 100% humidified oxygen as needed. Frostbite should be treated with rapid rewarming in a 42°C water bath.

Additional Information

Liver and renal function tests should be performed and repeated annually. Rescue and treatment personnel should take care not to become exposed; this may include self-contained breathing apparatus, chemical protective gloves and goggles, and fluorocarbon rubber protective clothing.

Colorless, pleasant sweet ether odor. Odor threshold: 260 ppm. TLV-TWA: 5 ppm. Atmospheric half-life: 1.2-1.8 days. Cigarette smoke contains 5.6-27 ng/cigarette. Daily intake by an average U.S. adult by inhalation, ingestion, or dermal route is essentially zero

Specific References

Bolt HM, "Vinyl Chloride - A Classical Industrial Toxicant of New Interest," *Clinical Reviews in Toxicology,* 2005, 35:307-23.

Hsiao TJ, Wang JD, Yang PM, et al, "Liver Fibrosis in Asymptomatic Polyvinyl Chloride Workers," *J Occup Environ Med,* 2004, 46(9):967.

Lewis R and Rempala G, "A Case-Cohort Study of Angiosarcoma of the Liver and Brain Cancer at a Polymer Production Plant," *J Occup Environ Med,* 2003, 45(5):538-45.

Wong RH, Chen PC, Wang JD, et al, "Interaction of Vinyl Chloride Monomer Exposure and Hepatitis B Viral Infection on Liver Cancer," *J Occup Environ Med,* 2003, 45(4):379-83.

White Phosphorus

CAS Number 12185-10-3; 7723-14-0

UN Number 1381 (dry or in water); 2447 (molten)

Synonyms Phosphorus Tetramen; Red Phosphorus; Yellow Phosphorus

Commonly Found In Phosphorus sesquisulfide, phosphine gas

Use Fertilizers, roach poisons, rodenticides, water treatment; used in military as ammunition in motor/artillery shells

Mechanism of Toxic Action Damages endoplasmic reticulum; inhibits fatty acid oxidation

Adverse Reactions

Cardiovascular: Hypotension, tachycardia, fibrillation (atrial), flutter (atrial), sinus tachycardia

Central nervous system: Lethargy, irritability, coma, hyperthermia

Dermatologic: Dermal burns

Endocrine & metabolic: Hypoglycemia can occur on chronic exposure

Gastrointestinal: GI Irritant, vomiting, abdominal cramps

Hematologic: Anemia, leukopenia, hemolysis

Hepatic: Degeneration and hepatic necrosis

Neuromuscular & skeletal: Degeneration and osteoporosis, fasciculations, asterixis, hemiplegia

Renal: Tubular necrosis (acute) and cortical necrosis

Respiratory: Cough on inhalation, tachypnea, dyspnea

Miscellaneous: "Phossy jaw" (degeneration and necrosis of soft tissue and teeth in oral cavity resulting in life-threatening infections); fatty deposition of muscles and liver, decreases in serum calcium, potassium, and sodium; liver/renal toxicity along with cerebral edema may occur after 5-10 days

Signs and Symptoms of Overdose Breath odor, coma, dermal burns, flatulence, GI irritation, hypocalcemia, luminescent stool, seizures; vomiting followed by asymptomatic phase of <12 hours to 3 days with subsequent signs/symptoms of hepatic or renal failure. Chronic exposure (5+ years) results in osteoporosis and bone degeneration, commonly of jaw ("phossy jaw"), and feces discoloration (black).

Admission Criteria/Prognosis Any patient with ingestion of white or yellow phosphorus should probably be admitted

Toxicodynamics/Kinetics

Absorption: By oral routes; yellow phosphorus well absorbed dermally and orally; phosphine gas absorbable in lungs; red phosphorus nonabsorbable

Metabolism: Oxidation and hydrolysis to hypophosphites

Elimination: Urine and feces

Reference Range Normal serum phosphate concentrations: 3.0-4.5 mg/100 mL

Overdosage/Treatment

Decontamination:

Oral: **Do not** induce emesis. Lavage within 2-3 hours with 1:5000 to 1:10,000 potassium permanganate or water. Activated charcoal may be used.

Dermal: Remove contaminated clothing; brush off phosphorus from skin and then continuously irrigate skin with water. Apply saline soaked dressings to the affected area. Avoid any lipid-based ointments. Phosphorus will fluoresce under a Wood's lamp. Remove visualized phosphorus particles with metal forceps or a WaterPik® appliance. A 1% copper sulfate solution or silver nitrate has been advocated to aid in decontamination of dermal burns, although its use is controversial. Burns may give off odor or smoke.

Inhalation: Administer 100% humidified oxygen

Ocular: Irrigate with saline for at least 15 minutes. Following saline irrigation, several drops of 3% copper sulfate solution (applied within 15 minutes) can be given to help prevent ocular burns and then remove particles mechanically.

Supportive therapy: Treat dermal burns in traditional method. Watch for secondary infections. Monitor calcium and glucose levels. Steroids are of no benefit in preventing liver injury. Morphine sulfate can be used to treat pain. Monitor fluids as third spacing and fluid loss can occur with GI or dermal injury. N-acetylcysteine may reduce hepatic toxicity when given early postexposure:

Dose regimen: 150 mg/kg in 200 mL D_5W over 15 minutes, then 50 mg/kg in 500 mL D_5W for 4 hours, then 100 mg/kg in 1000 mL D_5W for 16 hours has been utilized. Monitor for hypocalcemia.

Enhancement of elimination: Mineral oil (100 mL in adults or 1.5 mL/kg in children < 12 years of age) can be used as a cathartic. Exchange transfusion may be helpful.

Additional Information Lethal oral dose: 1 mg/kg (yellow phosphorus)

Garlic breath odor and luminescent vomitus, flatus, or stool is pathognomonic although not frequent.

Vomiting can occur after oral ingestion of 2-23 mg/kg.

Note that phosphine gas may emanate from emesis, lavage fluid, and feces from affected patients. Thus, the patient's room should be well ventilated.

Red phosphorus is not soluble and essentially not absorbed through the gastrointestinal tract and is, therefore, considered nontoxic.

Phosphine gas has a garlic odor.

Gas release occurs in industrial use or with moisture contamination of aluminum or zinc phosphide rodenticides.

Match phosphorus content is essentially nontoxic. Match toxicities are secondary to potassium chlorate content.

Atmospheric half-life: 5 minutes

PEL-TWA: 0.1 mg/m³; TLV-TWA: 0.1 mg/m³

Xylene

Related Information
- Amitraz

Applies to Glue; Paint; Polymers

CAS Number 106-42-3; 108-38-3; 1330-20-7; 95-47-6

UN Number 1307

Synonyms Dimethyl Benzene; Methyltoluene; Violet 3; Xylol

Impairment Potential Acute exposures > 300 ppm or blood xylene levels > 3 mg/L are consistent with impairment.

Use In histology laboratories (M-xylene), manufacture of polymers, glues, paints, and as a vehicle for pesticides

Mechanism of Toxic Action Anesthetic at high doses (> 5000 ppm)

Adverse Reactions

Central nervous system: CNS depression

Dermatologic: Scleroderma

Endocrine & metabolic: Sexual dysfunction

Hepatic: Liver necrosis

Renal: Hematuria

Respiratory: Irritation to upper airway

Signs and Symptoms of Overdose CNS depression, cough, dementia, dizziness, fatigue, headache, nausea, nystagmus, ocular irritation, skin irritation, syncope, throat burning

Admission Criteria/Prognosis Symptomatic patients should be admitted; asymptomatic patients can be discharged after 6-12 hours observation

Toxicodynamics/Kinetics

Absorption: By inhalation, dermally, or through the GI tract

Protein binding: 90%

Metabolism: In the liver

Half-life: 20-30 hours

Elimination: 2,4-Xylenol and methyl hippuric acid are excreted renally; xylene is protein bound

Reference Range BEI of methyl hippuric acid (urine) is 1.5 g/g creatinine; blood level of 1 mg/L is consistent with exposure of 100 ppm

Overdosage/Treatment

Decontamination: **Oral: Do not** induce emesis; dilute with milk or water. **Dermal:** Wash with soap and water. **Ocular:** Irrigate with saline.

Supportive therapy: Avoid use of catecholamines since they may exacerbate myocardial irritability.

Diagnostic Procedures
- Electrolytes, Blood

Additional Information Lethal oral dose: 15 mL

Patients may be more sensitive to ethanol.

Aspirin or ethanol can produce a false-positive urine test result for hippuric acid.

Air xylene concentrations > 10,000 ppm can result in unconsciousness and death.

Xylene may be present in the gas phase delivery in cigarettes at a concentration of up to 20 mcg/cigarette.

Sweet odor. Odor threshold: 0.05 ppm

Average daily intake by inhalation: ~353 mcg. Average daily intake through drinking water: ~39.4 mcg/kg/day. Average amount in drinking water: ~2 mcg/L.

Soil half-life: 1-2 days (photo-oxidation). Water half-life (by biodegradation) 10.3 days; by volatilization: 5.6 hours. TLV-TWA: 100 ppm; PEL-TWA: 100 ppm. Median urban atmospheric level: 7.2 ppb. Atmospheric half-life: 0.5-1 day.

Specific References

Al-Ghamdi SS, Raftery MJ, and Yaqoob MM, "Organic Solvent-Induced Proximal Tubular Cell Toxicity via Caspase-3 Activation," *J Toxicol Clin Toxicol*, 2003, 41(7):941-5.

Meggs WJ, "Neuropsychologic Impairment, MRI Abnormalities, and Solvent Abuse," *J Toxicol Clin Toxicol*, 2003, 41(2):209-10.

Mottaleb MA, Brumley WC, Pyle SM, et al, "Determination of a Bound Musk Xylene Metabolite in Carp Hemoglobin as a Biomarker of Exposure by Gas Chromatography-Mass Spectrometry Using Selected Ion Monitoring," *J Anal Toxicol*, 2004, 28:581-6.

Yilmaz HL and Yildizdas DR, "Amitraz Poisoning, An Emerging Problem: Epidemiology, Clinical Features, Management, and Preventive Strategies," *Arch Dis Child*, 2003, 88(2):130-4.

Zinc Phosphide

Related Information
- Phosphine
- White Phosphorus

CAS Number 1314-84-7; 39342-49-9

UN Number 1714

Synonyms Blue-Ox®; Kil-Rat®; Mous-Con®; Ratol; Rumetan®; Stutox; Zinc Tox

Use Rodenticide

Mechanism of Toxic Action Liberates phosphine gas when ingested; phosphine (which is a cytochrome C oxidase inhibitor) acts rapidly to cause gastrointestinal and pulmonary irritation

Adverse Reactions

Central nervous system: Headache, fatigue, ataxia

Endocrine & metabolic: Metabolic acidosis, hypocalcemia

Gastrointestinal: Nausea, vomiting

Hepatic: Centrilobular necrosis (hepatic), jaundice

Neuromuscular & skeletal: Paresthesias, intention tremor

Ocular: Diplopia

Respiratory: Pulmonary edema, cough, dyspnea

Admission Criteria/Prognosis Admit any exposure for 48-72 hours to monitor respiratory status; ingestions > 1 g should be admitted

Reference Range 180 g of the rodenticide ingestion resulted in a zinc serum level of ~6 ppm

Overdosage/Treatment

Decontamination:

Oral: Very controversial; if the patient has not vomited, emesis can be induced with syrup of ipecac within 30 minutes of ingestion. Although several cases which recovered involved gastric lavage, it should be noted that water can assist in liberating phosphine gas. A 5% sodium bicarbonate solution has been advocated to limit acid hydrolysis of zinc phosphide, but this modality has not been studied in humans.

Dermal: Brush/scrape off the flakes from the skin and then wash skin copiously

Inhalation: Use 100% humidified oxygen.

Supportive therapy: Intravenous crystalloid fluid hydration with sodium bicarbonate (1-2 mEq/kg) to treat acidosis; pulmonary edema should be aggressively treated; mechanical ventilation may be necessary. Monitor and treat for hypocalcemia. Morphine sulfate can be used to treat pain.

Enhancement of elimination: Mineral oil (Adults: 100 mL; Children < 12 years: 1.5 mL/kg) may be of some benefit in treating ingested zinc phosphide.

Additional Information Lethal dose may be as little as 4 g, although survival of ingestions up to 100 g has occurred. Symptoms may occur at 10 ppm. Monitor for phosphine gas from GI fluids of affected patients; keep patient's room well ventilated. Rotten fish odor at 1-3 ppm. Less corrosive than white phosphorus

Specific References

Mohanty MK, Kumar V, Bastia BK, et al, "An Analysis of Poisoning Deaths in Manipal, India," *Vet Hum Toxicol*, 2004, 46(4):208-9.

SECTION III
BIOLOGICAL AGENTS

GENERAL CONSIDERATIONS REGARDING EXPOSURES TO BIOLOGICAL AGENTS

Anthony M. Burda, RPh, CSPI, DABAT and Carol Ann DesLauriers, PharmD, CSPI

Some of the most interesting and challenging poisonings for the toxicologist or specialist in poison information are exposures to biological agents. Included in this category are a myriad of naturally occurring chemical toxins, alkaloids, venoms, and microbial contaminants. Representative sources for these biologicals are plants, fungi (mushrooms), spoiled or tainted food (food contamination), venomous fish (fish stings), insect/spider bites and stings, and reptile/snake envenomations.

The incidence and significance of biological intoxications can be illustrated through data extracted from the 2004 annual report of the American Associations of Poison Control Centers Toxic Exposure Surveillance System (TESS). See following table. Data reported to TESS in 2004 were compiled from 62 poison control centers.

Frequency and Outcomes of Human Exposures to Biologicals						
Biological	2004 Exposures	No Effect	Minor Effect	Moderate Effect	Major Effect	Death
Fish stings	2,814	84	739	252	7	0
Food contamination	69,915	5,672	12,537	2,517	82	1
Insect/spider bites/stings	79,020	1,133	18,101	4,577	138	2
Mammal bites	6,653	296	1,613	312	6	0
Mushroom ingestion	8,601	3,769	1,094	848	59	5
Plant exposures	74,811	14,982	6,278	1,442	80	5
Snake and other reptile bites	8,313	293	3,011	1,793	187	3
Other/unknown bite or envenomation	463	5	145	43	2	0
Total	250,590	26,234	43,518	11,784	561	16

Adapted from Watson WA, Litovitz TL, Rodgers GC Jr, et al, "2004 Annual Report of the American Association of Poison Control Centers Toxic Exposure Surveillance System," *Am J Emerg Med*, 2005, 23(5):589-666.

Out of 2,438,644 human exposure cases in 2004, 250,590 involved poisonings with biological agents. Therefore, it is significant to note that 10.3 percent of all poisoning episodes handled by clinicians involved a substance in this group. Accordingly, it is incumbent upon physicians and poison control center specialists to be familiar with toxicity and treatment approaches.

Although the incidence of these poisonings is high, morbidity and mortality are low. Only 5 percent of the outcomes reported had a moderate or major outcome. Fatalities were rare with only 16 reported deaths. This figure accounts for only 1.35 percent of the 1,183 fatal cases reported to TESS in 2004.

It should also be pointed out that TESS data is largely comprised of ingestions of small quantities of both toxic and nontoxic specimens by pediatric patients. For instance, a large number of pediatric "tastes" of nontoxic houseplants (eg, spider plant, jade, etc.) far outnumber the more serious poisonings such as the adult foraging for mushrooms for food.

There are at least five important considerations for the clinician managing an exposure involving a biological substance: identification of the poison, quantification of the dose, lack of specific laboratory analysis, lack of specific antidotes, and use of nonmedical consultants. Although these potential problems may add to the complexities of patient management, they are by no means insurmountable. Patient management may be enhanced when available resources are combined with consultations with the nearest regional poison control center and skilled toxicologist. The designated regional poison control center can be reached via the toll-free national hot line,1-800-222-1222.

Identification of the Poison

In many cases of unintentional poisoning or intentional overdose, the identification of the offending medication or chemical can be determined with little difficulty. An accurate patient or family history, over-the-counter and prescription bottles retrieved from the scene, ingredient listings on containers, or a material safety data sheet (MSDS) on file at the work site can provide immediate identification of the substance(s) involved.

When triaging exposures involving biological agents, however, the above methods of identification may be of little or no value. Plants, mushrooms, spiders and snakes are not conveniently tagged with their unique botanical, mycological, or zoological nomenclature. Accurate identification may hinge on a combination of piecing together a fragmented exposure history, recognizing a constellation of signs and symptoms as a particular toxidrome, and/or utilizing the expertise of a nonhealthcare professional such as a botanist or mycologist.

Consider the problem of substance identification inherent in each of the following scenarios:

- A small child arrives home to admit he/she "ate a small handful of those little red berries on a bush out in the prairie."
- A mother calls to state that her toddler ingested a few bites of a household plant she can best describe as "green and has leaves."
- The weekend trail hiker clad in shorts and sandals who arrives in the ED after being bitten by a snake but was too stunned to recall any pertinent identifying characteristics.
- The amateur mushroom picker who experiences cramping, vomiting, and diarrhea one hour after consuming his gatherings with no intact specimens which would allow you to compare the mushrooms to ones pictured in reference manuals or online.
- An adult who presents with a necrotic lesion on the leg several days after being bitten or stung by an unknown insect while sleeping in a basement apartment.
- An otherwise healthy adult complains of gastritis and malaise after dining out at a restaurant buffet. Suspected causes may include, but not be limited to, *Salmonella* in poultry, a seafood toxin, *Staphylococcus* in a creamed dressing, a food additive, or preservative, *Clostridium perfringens* in a gravy, or a drug-alcohol interaction.

Quantification of a Dose

In most cases of exposure to biological agents, the exact dose of the offending agent may never be known. Marked variation exists inter- and intra-species, between geographic or structural location, and even seasonally. Under these circumstances, the severity of the event is best judged by the nature and extent of the signs, symptoms, or laboratory abnormalities.

The following are a few examples:

- It may be well documented that a small child ingested exactly six unripe Black Nightshade (*Solanum nigrum*) berries. It is unknown how many milligrams of solanine alkaloid comprised the actual ingested dose.
- In some instances of exposure, the dose involved may be zero. For instance, a person may show fang marks as proof of a rattlesnake bite yet show no local or systemic toxicity, since approximately 20 percent of all snake bites are described as "dry bites."
- With regard to food-borne microbial toxins, quantification may be performed in some laboratories (ie, public health departments). This process is slow, not routinely ordered, and is of little clinical value in treating individual cases of food poisoning.
- Individual susceptibility may play a major role in determining a response to a given dose of biological agent. For example, several people may be exposed to dusts and pollens of the common chrysanthemum flowers (*Chrysanthemum morifolium*). However, only one may require ED treatment to correct bronchospasm and wheezing secondary to hypersensitivity to the naturally occurring pyrethrum in the plant.

Nonspecificity of Laboratory Analysis

When a patient exposed to a biological agent presents to a healthcare facility, rapid laboratory analysis to identify and quantify the agent is not readily available. In these cases, treatment plans will be influenced by exposure history, clinical presentation, and other laboratory indices. These considerations taken together will give a much clearer picture of the severity of the exposure and development of a reasonable patient plan.

Examples where nonspecific laboratory tests are valuable in the monitoring and management of patients exposed to biological agents are:

- Serial serum potassium measurements and continuous EKG monitoring in ingestions of Oleander (*Nerium oleander*), a cardiac glycoside—containing plant
- Frequent coagulation profiles and CBCs following Crotalinae snake envenomation
- Frequent liver and kidney function tests following ingestion of death cap (*Amanita phalloides*), a cyclopeptide-containing mushroom
- A stat CBC, electrolytes, and urinalysis in evaluating a debilitated food poison patient
- Platelet count, PT, PTT, BUN, and creatinine in suspected bites of the brown recluse (*Loxosceles reclusa*) spider

Few Specific Antidotes

Few specific antidotes exist to treat exposures to biological agents. In a vast majority of these cases, close observation and conservative symptomatic and supportive care are the mainstays of therapy.

A majority of exposures to biologicals, especially those originating from the home environment, can be safely handled with calm reassurance and simple over-the-counter remedies such as:

- The BRATT diet with glucose/electrolyte solutions for mild food poisoning cases
- Application of ice and antipruritics (eg, diphenhydramine, hydrocortisone, or benzocaine) for non-venomous insect bites and stings
- Antiseptics and wound care for nonpoisonous snake bites
- Home observation and telephone follow-up for ingestion of mouthful amounts of lawn mushrooms
- Antihistamines (eg, diphenhydramine) may ameliorate mild histamine reactions (flushing, pruritus, headache, and palpitations) associated with scombroid fish poisoning

A few notable antidotes for biologic toxins do exist. Their use is generally reserved for serious and life-threatening poisoning incidents. Examples of these antidotes are:

- Rattlesnake or pit viper (polyvalent Crotalidae; polyvalent immune fab, Crofab®) antivenin
- Eastern coral snake (*Micrurus fulvius*) antivenin (Note: No antivenin for Arizona coral snake [*Micruoides euryxantus*])
- Black widow spider (*Latrodectus mactans*) antivenin
- Botulism (trivalent types A, B, and E) for botulism (*Clostridium botulinum*)
- Physostigmine for severe anticholinergic complications from Jimson Weed (*Datura stramonium*) or Deadly Nightshade (*Atropa belladonna*)
- Pyridoxine for neurologic symptoms due to ingestion of monomethyl hydrazine mushrooms like the false morel (*Gyromitra esculenta*)
- Atropine to reverse cholinergic symptoms due to ingestion of muscarine-containing mushrooms like the Inocybe
- Digoxin-specific Fab fragments to reverse toxicity associated with Oleander (*Nerium oleander*) and Foxglove (*Digitalis purpurea*) plant poisoning
- Although more of an infectious disease issue, various antimicrobial agents may be indicated for specific illnesses attributed to food-borne pathogens (eg, sulfamethoxazole/trimethoprim in cases of shigellosis and ampicillin with gentamicin for severe cases of listeriosis).

Hospital pharmacies affiliated with regional poison control centers may serve as antidote depots. Rarely used antidotes such as antivenin along with guidelines for their usage are available on a 24-hour basis. If a particular pharmaceutical is not stored in the center, referrals for emergency access from other sources such as pharmaceutical companies, zoos or aquariums can be quickly made.

Need for Nonmedical Consultants

In providing optimal care to the patient poisoned by more commonly encountered medications and chemicals, the clinician may call upon the services of a number of other medical consultants. Biological intoxications are unique in that identification of the toxic specimen may require consultation with nonmedical professionals. Accordingly, these professionals and scientists are located in diverse nonhealthcare facility settings such as museums, zoos, aquariums, arboretums, botanical gardens, greenhouses, florist shops, universities, cooperative extension services, and mycological societies.

Consider the indispensable value of the expertise rendered by a nonmedical consultant in the following scenarios:

- a herpetologist to identify an unknown snake
- a mycologist to identify an unknown mushroom
- an entomologist for insect identification
- a botanist to identify an unknown wild plant specimen
- a florist or horticulturist to identify an unknown household plant

Regional poison control centers often maintain updated consultant files and are an excellent source for these referrals. To expedite the identification of specimens, consultants may rely on the Internet through digital imaging and e-mail.

Until such time as the biological specimen is identified precisely, the poison control center can formulate a management strategy. The treatment regimen can then be modified once the accurate identification of the substance is made.

MANAGEMENT OF PLANT EXPOSURES

Edward P. Krenzelok, PharmD, FAACT, DABAT and Terry D. Jacobsen, PhD, FLS

The toxicity of some plants has been recognized and feared for millennia. Historically, plant toxins have played important roles in ancient medicine and politics. As testimony, the Ebers Papyrus, which has origins to 1600 BC, contains hundreds of prescriptions and concoctions, many containing toxic plants as the primary ingredients. The infamous death of Socrates in 399 BC is attributed to ingestion of a beverage laced with poison hemlock.[1] Ancient Romans allegedly assassinated political adversaries through the use of poisonous plants. History has painted a nefarious picture of various plants, and when considered with the gross distortions about the toxicity of some botanicals, plant exposures are often regarded as being indiscriminately associated with significant morbidity and mortality. However, plant exposures are associated only rarely with a fatal outcome - only 19 fatalities in nearly one million reported plant exposures![2]

Plant exposures, as reported to poison information centers, are common, accounting for 4.4% of all exposures. Following are the 15 most common human exposures.[3]

The 15 Most Common Human Exposures

1. Analgesics
2. Cleaning substances
3. Cosmetics and personal care products
4. Sedatives/hypnotics/antipsychotics
5. Foreign bodies
6. Topicals
7. Cough and cold preparations
8. Antidepressants
9. Pesticides
10. Bites/envenomations
11. Plants
12. Alcohols
13. Cardiovascular drugs
14. Antihistamines
15. Food products, food poisoning

Plants are ubiquitous, being found both indoors and outdoors. Their presence in every aspect of society influences the large number of exposures reported to poison information centers. Furthermore, their beautiful foliage, enticing berries, and mystical qualities attract both young children and adults. Young children sample their environment due to curiosity and excessive hand-to-mouth activity, resulting in the ingestion of a plant. Adults are intrigued by the use of plants, especially herbs, as alternatives to traditional medicine. (See Herbal Agents section.) Additionally, adults may boldly sample the roots or other parts of unidentified plants as food sources. The majority of exposures involve children younger than 6 years of age.

The following list identifies the most common plant exposures.[4] The presence of a plant on this list does not suggest that it is associated with significant toxicity. However, to paraphrase Paracelsus, "everything is poisonous, only the amount differentiates a poison from a remedy," and this idiom should be considered in the evaluation of each plant exposure. It is most important not to become complacent with plant exposures, since a limited number of plants are associated with significant morbidity and rare, but sobering mortality. A discussion of outcomes and toxicity following exposure to common plants is included, as well as a discussion of plants that are likely to produce adverse outcomes.

The 20 Most Common Plant Exposures in the U.S.[3]

1. Peace lily (*Spathiphyllum* spp)
2. Holly (*Ilex* spp)
3. Philodendron (*Philodendron* spp)
4. Poinsettia (*Euphorbia pulcherrima*)
5. Pokeweed, inkberry (*Phytolacca americana*)

6. Poison ivy (*Toxicodendron radicans*)
7. Rubber tree, weeping fig (*Ficus* spp)
8. Nightshade, Jerusalem cherry (*Solanum* spp)
9. Apple, crabapple (plant parts) (*Malus* spp)
10. Christmas cactus (*Schlumbergera bridgesii*)
11. Jade plant (*Crassula* spp)
12. Oleander (*Nerium oleander*)
13. Pothos, devil's ivy (*Epipremnum aureum*)
14. Chrysanthemum (*Chrysanthemum*) spp
15. Caladium (*Caladium* spp)
16. Dumbcane (*Dieffenbachia* spp)
17. English ivy (*Hedera helix*)
18. Cactus (*Cactus* spp)
19. Dandelion (*Taraxacum officinale*)
20. Lilyturf (*Liriope muscari*)

Most plant exposures that involve the ingestion route are not associated with the development of any symptoms. A review of 768,284 plant ingestions revealed that only 6.9% of patients became symptomatic.[5] The most common symptom group categories were:

Gastrointestinal	63.7%	Respiratory	3.9%
Dermatological	16.9%	Cardiovascular	2.0%
Neurological	5.0%	Other	4.5%
Ophthalmological	4.0%		

Pitfalls

There are numerous pitfalls that challenge the clinician who is concerned about potential plant toxicity or is treating acute toxicity from exposure to plants.

Many of the frightening stories about the precipitous demise of individuals who consumed water from a vase that contained lily of the valley, roasted wieners on oleander sticks, consumed apple seeds, swallowed a poinsettia leaf, etc, are unsubstantiated. However, these myths have been perpetuated in "authoritative" textbooks, leading to undue concern, aggressive therapy, and inappropriate hospitalization.

Proper identification of a plant is the key to prognosis, therapy, and preventing unnecessary treatment. However, identification of the botanical is often difficult. The patient who attempts to describe a plant over the telephone is rarely successful, unless the clinician has exceptional knowledge about the flora of a particular region. Even having an actual sample of the plant (often dried and traumatized) in the office or emergency department presents a significant identification challenge. There are several ways to resolve the issue if a sample is available. Place the plant sample in water (if possible) to restore its natural appearance. The local floral shop or nursery may be able to assist in the identification. Consider sending a fax or pdf of the plant leaves to a poison information center. County agricultural agents are an excellent resource, especially for the identification of outdoor plants. Those fortunate enough to have botanists available at a local university may have an arrangement to assist in the identification of plants. However, if a patient is asymptomatic and there is no implication that the plant may be very toxic, such as water or poison hemlock, ultimate identification is unnecessary and only expends resources unnecessarily.

Ideally, each cultivated plant should be labeled with its botanical name. For example, *Euphorbia pulcherrima* is the botanical name for poinsettia, which is also known as the Christmas flower and Christmas star. Knowing the botanical name will direct the poison center specialist or the botanist to the correct toxicology information. Common names are often regional and a single common name may be associated with several different botanical species, leading to the other dissemination of incorrect information. To further confound the identification process, hundreds of imported exotic plants are available commercially. The botanical name may not be known and the same plant may have numerous common names.

Treatment

The majority of plant exposures can be managed with the proverbial "glass of milk for the child and a tincture of reassurance for the parent." Few exposures will require gastrointestinal decontamination or the use of a pharmacological antagonist such as digoxin immune Fab or physostigmine. Therefore, the general management of plant exposures will be addressed in this section since it is applicable to most plant exposures and specific antidotal therapy will be discussed only as necessary.

Most plant exposures are ingestions and terminating further exposure to the plant will limit the potential for toxicity. Careful removal of clothing that may be contaminated with poison ivy or other plant residue can prevent the development of problems. Removing any visible plant debris from the victim's (usually a child) mouth is adequate intervention in most patients. While there is no evidence to support the use of oral irrigation or dilution with a beverage, they are customary therapies. Dilution with cool fluids may relieve the irritating sensation or disagreeable taste associated with some plants. The placebo effect of dilution should not be overlooked. Similarly, perioral and other dermal exposures may respond to gentle cleansing with soap and water. Rashes and dermatitis may develop and the use of nonprescription hydrocortisone-containing lotion, ointment, or cream may have palliative effects.

The majority of plant ingestions are accidental, involving exposure to small amounts. This makes the use of gastrointestinal decontamination unnecessary. Additionally, several other factors make the use of gastro-intestinal decontamination of limited value. Of primary importance is the fact that gastrointestinal decontamination procedures have not been proven to have any impact on morbidity and mortality of the poisoned patient ("AACT/EAPCCT Position Statements on Gastrointestinal Decontamination," *J Toxicol Clin Toxicol*, 1997, 35:695-762). Secondly, the intentional ingestion of plants for abuse purposes or self-harm are the incidents that have the highest morbidity. Like most intentional poisonings, there is a significant delay in the time from the ingestion to when treatment is sought. Delays decrease the efficacy of gastrointestinal decontamination. Activated charcoal must come in contact with the toxin to be absorbed. It is unlikely that toxins distal to the stomach can be "caught" by activated charcoal. Therefore, most therapy is supportive care to manage the occasional adverse sequelae that may develop.

Ipecac-Induced Emesis

Ipecac Syrup. Induced emesis has no role to play in the management of toxic plant ingestions. There are no available data that demonstrate a reduction in poisoning morbidity or mortality from the induction of emesis.[6,7] If morbidity or mortality are anticipated, immediate referral to an emergency department is advised.

Gastric Lavage

Gastric lavage has no demonstrated utility in the management of plant exposures. The delay from ingestion to decontamination therapy may result in gastric emptying, moving the toxic plant from the stomach to the small intestine, and making it nonretrievable. Plant debris may consist of large fragments which are too large for removal via the gastric lavage tube. This is especially true in the pediatric population, where small bore lavage tubes are used. However, there are no data which demonstrate the effectiveness of gastric lavage in the management of plant poisonings.[8]

Activated Charcoal

Many alkaloids and derivatives are known to be adsorbed by activated charcoal. If a plant toxin is adsorbed by activated charcoal, its absorption will be reduced and subsequent toxicity limited or eliminated. However, activated charcoal efficacy is limited by the delay in the institution of therapy. Activated charcoal must come in contact with the toxin to be effective. It does not have the ability to "catch" the toxic plant unless the toxic components of the plant are subject to enterohepatic circulation or enteroenteric secretion. These characteristics have not been elucidated for most plants; therefore, multiple dose activated charcoal therapy is of hypothetical use only. If activated charcoal is used to manage a patient with actual or potential plant poisoning, 25-50 g may be administered as aqueous activated charcoal to children and 50-100 g to adults. Be cognizant that commercial activated charcoal products are slurries and not suspensions. Therefore, the products must be agitated vigorously for at least 30 seconds prior to administration. The container should be rinsed repetitively with small amounts of water to ensure that the entire contents of the container have been administered. Only aqueous activated charcoal should be used. Products that contain a fixed dose of sorbitol are especially hazardous to very young children and should not be used in children or adults.[9,10]

Cathartics

Cathartics used alone or in combination with activated charcoal have no role in the management of plant poisoning exposures or in any type of poisoning case.[11]

Whole Bowel Irrigation

There may be some limited value of whole bowel irrigation in the management of patients who have ingested large quantities of plant material, especially seeds which may not have rapid bioavailability. Beyond such special circumstances, whole bowel irrigation has little utility in the treatment of plant ingestion patients.[12]

Common Plant Exposures

- **Philodendron species** (heartleaf philodendron, parlor ivy) and **Dieffenbachia species** (Dumbcane, mother-in-law's tongue)
  Philodendron and *Dieffenbachia* species account for approximately 10% of the reported plant exposures and are members of the family Araceae.[13] As such, they share common toxins and accordingly, common manifestations of toxicity.[14]
  The sap and morphological parts (stems, leaves, etc) of the plant contain calcium oxalate crystals, aromatic amines, alkaloids, and proteolytic enzymes.[15] When a portion of the plant is chewed by a curious child, toxicity may be induced both mechanically and chemically. Raphides of calcium oxalate may be fired into oral mucosa when idioblasts are physically disrupted via chewing.[15,16] The mechanical injury of tissues allows the secondary entry of irritants such as proteolytic enzymes. The net effect is irritation and inflammation.[15-18] Hence, the common name "Dumbcane" for *Dieffenbachia* reflects the acute oral inflammation (inability to speak = dumb) which may occur after biting into the "cane" or stalk of the *Dieffenbachia*.
  There is documented support of a cause:effect relationship between exposure to *Philodendron/Dieffenbachia* species and toxicity.[14-20] However, the villainous reputation of these plants is greatly exaggerated and not justified. A review of nearly 97,000 exposures to *Philodendron/Dieffenbachia* species demonstrated clearly that moderate and major toxicity were rare.[13] Overall, *Philodendron* exposures are associated with a lower incidence of adverse effects.[4] This may be secondary to the presence of less calcium oxalate or there may be differences which are related to chemical constituents and proteolytic enzymes. Minor irritation may occur in up to 10.5% of *Philodendron* exposure patients and 24.5% of those exposed to *Dieffenbachia* species, but it is rare for the irritation to justify referral to an emergency department.[4] *Epipremnum aureum* (pothos, devil's ivy, golden pothos) is also a member of the family Araceae and often confused with the *Philodendron*. It should be considered to have the same toxic principles.
  There is no merit to using gastrointestinal decontamination procedures unless an inordinate amount of plant material has been ingested as in an intentional event. Most importantly, any visible plant debris should be removed from the oral pharynx. Dilution with a cold beverage is used customarily and may soothe irritation in symptomatic patients. Symptomatic patients may also respond to sucking on ice or a popsicle.

- **Euphorbia pulcherrima** (Poinsettia, Christmas flower, Christmas star)
  A 1920 publication by JF Rock in a Hawaiian journal catapulted *Euphorbia pulcherrima*, most commonly referred to as the poinsettia, into the limelight as being one of the most poisonous plants in the world.[21] Allegedly, a 2-year-old child had a fatal outcome after ingesting a portion of a poinsettia plant. Botanical and medical texts used this unconfirmed incident to perpetuate the poinsettia as a sinister plant. The lay press and even the Food and Drug Administration sensationalized the poinsettia as a botanical villain with statements like "one poinsettia leaf can kill a child."[22] However, neither animal studies nor human case reports have substantiated the claims of significant morbidity and mortality – exonerating the poinsettia from being labeled as a truly poisonous plant in the category with water and poison hemlock. Research conducted in animals where poinsettia doses of up to 50 g/kg were ingested failed to reveal significant toxicity.[23-25] This is supported by the analysis of 22,793 human exposures where there were no fatalities and only 3% of patients developed minor toxicity.[22] The latex sap which exudes from damaged leaves may produce dermal irritation.[26] Dermal exposures to poinsettia may produce a slightly higher incidence of irritation than that experienced by individuals who have oral exposures or ingestions.[22]

The ingestion of poinsettia does not require gastrointestinal decontamination and removal of plant debris from the mouth is adequate intervention. Skin irritation, although uncommon and usually minor, may be prevented by washing the exposed area(s) with soap and water.

- **Capsicum annuum** (pepper, chili pepper, hot pepper, Christmas pepper, cayenne, jalapeño)

  There are very few plants which produce acute toxicity. *Capsicum annuum* is one of the exceptions and is associated with very common manifestations – extreme irritation to the skin, mucous membranes, and even the gastrointestinal tract due to peristaltic effects. The generic name is aptly attributed to and is derived from a Greek word meaning "I bite."[27] While peppers of the *Capsicum* genus are used primarily in Southwestern and Mexican-style cooking, they must not be confused with the table pepper which is a spice derived from the berry of *Piper nigrum* and not related phytogenetically.[27]

  The peppers in genus *Capsicum* contain capsaicin which is extremely irritating. As testimony to its irritant properties, the oleoresin extracted from *Capsicum* is the major ingredient in "pepper gas," which is used for personal protection and by law enforcement officials as a way to immobilize temporarily an assailant by spraying the pepper gas into the eyes. Handling peppers can produce discomforting irritation which is often spread to the face, eyes, and mouth via the hands. Children are especially vulnerable since they may develop dermal irritation resulting in crying, which leads to ocular irritation as the child wipes tears from her eyes. While the dermal irritation may be intense, the development of blisters is rare.

  There are many suggested panaceas to remedy the intense irritation – most of which are of little or no value. Multiple washing of the skin with soap and warm water is probably the best intervention. Immersion of the affected skin in cold water may provide short-term relief, but does not remove the source of the problem.[28] The use of a vinegar/water solution has been proposed, but not supported enthusiastically.[29] Soaking the affected skin in vegetable oil is thought to provide relief of longer duration than the sole use of cold water.[28] Severe dermal pain may necessitate the use of topical anesthetics to ameliorate the discomfort.[30] Prolonged ocular irrigation may provide some relief in patients with eye exposures.

- **Ilex species** (holly, English holly, European holly, Christmas holly, American holly, emetic holly)

  American holly *(Ilex opaca)* and English holly *(Ilex aquifolium)* are outdoor plants that have green rigid leaves and bright red berries. These colorful plants are common components of Christmas holiday centerpieces and other decorations. The bright red berries are enticing to small children and result in a high incidence of holiday exposures.

  Holly was once thought to be highly toxic, rivaling some of the most poisonous plants. Ilicin and saponins may produce gastrointestinal irritation, but the profound toxicity which included central nervous system depression and life-threatening hematemesis appears to be without foundation.[31] In one series assessing the toxicity of 21,675 *Ilex* species exposures, only 4.4% of the patients developed minor symptoms and 0.11% had moderate effects.[32] There were neither major sequelae nor fatalities. The ingestion of multiple berries does not usually produce toxic manifestations unless the berries are chewed, resulting in nausea, vomiting, cramping, and diarrhea.[31] Since the leaf tips are spine-like, mechanical irritation may develop. One member of the genus, *Ilex vomitoria*, as its botanical name suggests, has potent emetic properties. It is differentiated easily from American and English hollies since it has a different leaf structure and the berries are usually yellow. Exposures to this species are uncommon.

  Most exposures require no intervention. However, patients, especially children, who ingest a large quantity of berries may benefit from the use of activated charcoal. While unlikely to occur, excessive emesis or diarrhea may necessitate fluid and electrolyte replacement.

- **Crassula argentea** (jade plant, dwarf rubber plant, rubber plant, cauliflower ears)

  This is a very popular houseplant and there is no documented evidence that it is associated with toxicity. However, the size and semirigid nature of the leaves make the ingestion of this plant a possible esophageal or airway obstruction hazard in small children.

- **Ficus species** (fig, weeping fig)

  Several *Ficus* species are common houseplants. In general, they should be considered to be relatively nontoxic. Some species of the genus may exude a sap that is capable of causing dermatitis. However, this is a rare manifestation. Washing affected areas with soap and water should provide adequate intervention for dermal exposures.

- **_Toxicodendron_ species** (poison ivy, poison oak, poison sumac)

Poison ivy is probably the most well-known of all poisonous plants. Its notoriety is well-attested to by the tens of thousands who experience its classic toxic effect – dermatitis. Although the toxicity of poison ivy is appreciated universally, most people are unable to identify the plant, which is characterized by a three leaf cluster. Further complicating the identification process is the ability of poison ivy to grow as a climbing, woody, opportunistic vine or as a shrub of varying proportions.

Like _Capsicum annuum_, poison ivy and the other _Toxicodendron_ species are associated with a high incidence of toxicity following exposure. Unlike _Capsicum_ species, the toxicity is delayed for periods of hours up to 2 weeks and not everyone develops a sensitivity reaction after exposure. Examination of nearly 19,000 exposures to _Toxicodendron_ species revealed that at least 70% of individuals who reported their exposure to a poison center became symptomatic.[4] The pruritic, erythematous, and vesicular rash which develops is caused by a phenolic oily resin. The resin persists even in dead foliage and vines. Burning dead plant material, which contains a _Toxicodendron_ species, volatilizes the resin and makes it bioavailable for inhalation and extensive dermal exposure.

Most individuals are not aware of the exposure until they become symptomatic. Therefore, dermal decontamination is of little or no value unless the exposure is repetitive by wearing clothing that has been contaminated with the sensitizing resin. The resin fixes rapidly to the skin and washing with soap and water may be of value only if instituted within the first 5-10 minutes after exposure. Barrier creams are thought to be of little or no value. The use of cool compresses and topical steroids may relieve the symptoms. Patients with extensive dermatitis or systemic involvement may have a dramatic response to oral or parenteral corticosteroids. The use of oral antihistamines may relieve the pruritus. Barrier creams are available commercially and may help to prevent an exposure and the resultant dermatitis.

- **_Phytolacca_ species** (poke, pokeweed, pokeberry, scoke, inkberry, pigeonberry, poke salet)

This genus contains the well-known species _Phytolacca americana_, commonly referred to as poke. The toxic principles are triterpene saponins and a variety of mitogens.[33] This plant is considered to be a delicacy. The young leaves and stems are soaked in salt water and then undergo successive cookings, each time in fresh water.[33] Allegedly, this eliminates the toxins, which is a matter of some contention.

Contrary to popular opinion, most patients do not become symptomatic after a modest exposure to poke. Analysis of 17,773 reported poke exposures yielded minor toxic effects in 5.8% and moderate toxicity in 0.4%.[4] No major toxic effects were reported and there were no fatalities. The primary manifestations of ingestion are gastrointestinal effects, which may include abdominal cramping, nausea, vomiting, and diarrhea. Fluid and electrolyte imbalance may occur if vomiting and diarrhea are severe. Headache may develop and the symptom complex can persist for 48 hours.

There is not concurrence as to what constitutes a toxic exposure to poke. The ingestion of small amounts is unlikely to be associated with toxic effects. Soap and water decontamination should be considered for dermal exposures.

- **_Brassaia actinophylla_** (schefflera, umbrella plant, umbrella tree, Australian ivy palm, queens umbrella tree)

This plant is known commonly as the schefflera or umbrella tree. The exact nomenclature status of schefflera is in flux and it may appear in the literature or on plant labels as either _Schefflera actinophylla_ or _Brassaia actinophylla_. It is native to Australia, but it thrives as a houseplant. Along with _Euphorbia pulcherrima_, _Crassula argentea_, and _Ficus_ species, this plant should be considered to be relatively nontoxic.

Brassaia actinophylla contains a small amount of calcium oxalate in its leaves.[34] However, this should not be regarded as being a clinically significant amount. Although rare, contact dermatitis has been reported.[35]

The ingestion of a small amount of this plant should be regarded as a nontoxic exposure. Dermatitis is a rare event, but simple decontamination with soap and water may eliminate that possibility.

Selected Plants with Known Morbidity and Mortality

As illustrated by the most common plant exposures, most plant exposures are not associated with significant toxicity. However, there are a notable few that have the potential to produce significant toxicity, even death. Most patients who suffer severe toxicity or who have a fatal outcome are those who ingested large amounts of plant material intentionally for substance abuse or with suicidal intent. The ingestion of a small amount by a child is not usually associated with any morbidity.

- ***Datura* species** (jimson weed, Jamestown weed, angel's trumpet, moon flower, thornapple, stinkweed, La Reina del la Noche)

  Datura stramonium and *Datura meteloides* are commonly referred to as jimson weed. All parts of jimson weed contain the belladonna tropine alkaloids, such as atropine, hyoscyamine, and scopolamine. Jimson weed, especially the seeds, is abused for the psychoactive effects of the belladonna alkaloids. Hallucinogenic effects are sought, but the anticholinergic toxidrome (tachycardia, fever, dry mouth, confusion, etc) also develops when hallucinogenic amounts are used. The majority of abusers are 17-18 years of age and most recover with conservative therapy.[2,36,37] Gastrointestinal decontamination is of little value since the patient rarely presents for therapy until becoming symptomatic, suggesting that substantial absorption has occurred. Patients with severe anticholinergic poisoning may require the administration of the cholinesterase inhibitor physostigmine.[36] However, physostigmine should not be used prophylactically or injudiciously since it is not without its own toxic effects. A retrospective study of 17 individuals who were self-poisoned by jimson weed revealed that neither the administration of physostigmine nor the use of gastric lavage decreased the need for intensive care or the duration of hospitalization.[37,38]

- **Lethal hemlocks** (water hemlock, poison hemlock)

  Conium maculatum (poison hemlock) and *Cicuta maculata* (water hemlock) were responsible for 7 of the 19 plant-related fatalities that occurred from 1985-1994.[2] This is a relatively high fatality rate since the total number of reported exposures was only 582.[2] Most of the fatalities are the result of improper identification of these plants. The roots are mistaken as being wild carrots or parsnips and when consumed in sufficient quantity, grave toxicity develops.

  Conium maculatum contains coniine which is a peripheral neurotoxin that produces curare-like effects on neuromuscular junctions and nicotinic effects on autonomic ganglia.[39-42] The toxidrome consists of ascending skeletal muscle hypotonia or flaccidity that can progress to paralysis of the respiratory musculature. Initial effects may include sialorrhea, nausea, vomiting, abdominal cramps, and diarrhea followed by gastrointestinal hypotonia and dry mouth.[41]

  The toxicity from *Cicuta maculata* ingestion is attributed to cicutoxin. The toxic effects of cicutoxin are more morbidly impressive and violent than those from coniine.[42-46] Early muscarinic effects are localized to the gastrointestinal tract.[44,46] Systemic muscarinic effects (bronchial secretions) leading to respiratory distress may occur. However, pathognomonic of severe cicutoxin poisoning are violent multiple major motor seizures.[42-46] The symptoms may begin within 30 minutes after ingestion.[46]

  Gastrointestinal decontamination with activated charcoal may be beneficial in patients with recent ingestions. Otherwise, the cornerstone of therapy is aggressive supportive care.

- ***Nerium oleander*** (oleander, rosebay, rose laurel)

  Nerium oleander is the subject of considerable folklore concerning fatal poisoning in children who ingested hot dogs cooked on an oleander branch. This report surfaces frequently and results in profound anxiety among those who treat oleander exposures. While that anecdote has not been confirmed, there are numerous reports that describe oleander poisoning in humans.[47-51] *Nerium oleander* contains cardiac glycosides, similar in pharmacological activity to digitalis glycosides. However, nearly all of the serious cases involved the intentional ingestion of *Nerium oleander* as an herbal tea for medicinal use or for self-harm.[47-49] Symptoms typical of digitalis poisoning that may develop include gastrointestinal, cardiac arrhythmias, and hyperkalemia. The unintentional ingestion of a small amount by a child does not mandate gastrointestinal decontamination. Large ingestions, usually intentional, may necessitate the use of aggressive gastrointestinal decontamination. Serious oleander poisoning may respond to the use of digoxin immune Fab, since the oleander and digitalis glycosides are similar structurally.[50,51] *Nerium oleander* should not be confused with *Thevetia peruviana*, commonly referred to as yellow oleander. *Thevetia peruviana* has been associated with serious cardiovascular toxicity and numerous fatalities. While it is cultivated in North America, it is not a common North American oleander.

Footnotes

1. Ober WB, "Did Socrates Die of Hemlock Poisoning?" *NY St J Med*, 1977, 254-8.

2. Krenzelok EP, Jacobsen TD, and Aronis JM, "Hemlock Ingestions: The Most Deadly Plant Exposures," *J Toxicol Clin Toxicol*, 1996, 34:601-2.

3. Watson WA, Litovitz TL, Rodgers GC, et al, "2004 Annual Report of the American Association of Poison Control Centers," *Am J Emerg Med*, 2005, 23:589-666.

4. Krenzelok EP, Jacobsen TD, and Aronis JM, "Plant Exposures: A Profile of the Most Common Species," *Vet Hum Toxicol*, 1996, 38:289-98.

5. Mrvos R, Krenzelok EP, and Jacobsen TD, "Toxidromes Associated With the Most Common Plant Ingestions," *Vet Hum Toxicol*, 2001, 43:366-9.

6. Krenzelok EP, "Ipecac Syrup-Induced Emesis... No Evidence of Benefit," *Clin Toxicol*, 2005, 434:11-2.

7. Manoguerra AS, Krenzelok EP, McGuigan M, et al, "AACT/EAPCCT Position Paper: Ipecac Syrup," *Clin Toxicol*, 2004, 42:133-43.

8. Kulig K and Vale JA, "AACT/EAPCCT Position Paper: Gastric Lavage," *Clin Toxicol*, 2004, 42:933-44.

9. Krenzelok EP, Vale JA, Chyka PA, et al, "AACT/EAPCCT Position Paper: Single-Dose Activated Charcoal," *Clin Toxicol*, 2005, 43:61-87.

10. Vale JA, Krenzelok EP, and Barceloux DG, "Position Statement and Practice Guidelines on the Use of Multi-Dose Activated Charcoal in the Treatment of Acute Poisoning," *Clin Toxicol*, 1999, 37:731-51.

11. Bateman DN, Barceloux DG, McGuigan M, et al, "Position Paper: Cathartics," *Clin Toxicol*, 2004, 42:243-53.

12. Lheureux P and Tenenbein MT, "Position Paper: Whole Bowel Irrigation," *Clin Toxicol*, 2004, 42:843-54.

13. Krenzelok EP, Jacobsen TD, and Aronis JM, "A Review of 96,695 *Dieffenbachia* and *Philodendron* Exposures," *J Toxicol Clin Toxicol*, 1996, 34:601.

14. Mrvos R, Dean BS, and Krenzelok EP, " *Philodendron/Dieffenbachia* Ingestions: Are They a Problem?" *J Toxicol Clin Toxicol*, 1991, 29:485-91.

15. Kuball B, Lugnier AAAAJ, and Anton R., "Study of *Dieffenbachia*-Induced Edema in a Mouse and Rat Hindpaw: Respective Role of Oxalate Needles and Trypsin-Like Protease," *Toxicol Appl Pharmacol*, 1981, 58:444-51.

16. Seet B, Chan WK, and Ang CL, "Crystalline Keratopathy from *Dieffenbachia* Plant Sap," *Brit J Ophthal*, 1995, 79:98-9.

17. Gardner DG, "Injury to the Oral Mucous Membranes Caused by the Common Houseplant, *Dieffenbachia*," *Oral Surg Med Oral Pathol*, 1994, 78:31-3.

18. Pamies RJ, Powell R, Herold AH, et al, "The *Dieffenbachia* Plant," *J Florida Med Assoc*, 1992, 79:760-1.

19. McIntire MS, Guest JR, and Porterfield JF, "*Philodendron*, An Infant Death," *J Toxicol Clin Toxicol*, 1990, 28:177-83.

20. Pedaci L, Krenzelok EP, Jacobsen TD, et al, "Dieffenbachia Species Exposures: An Evidence-Based Assessment of Symptom Presentation," *Vet Human Toxicol*, 1999, 41:335-8.

21. Rock JF, "The Poisonous Plants of Hawaii," *Hawaiian Forest Agric*, 1920, 17:61.

22. Krenzelok EP, Jacobsen TD, and Aronis JM, "Poinsettia Exposures Have Good Outcomes... Just As We Thought," *Am J Emerg Med*, 1996, 14:671-4.

23. Stone RP and Collins WJ, "*Euphorbia pulcherrima:* Toxicity to Rats," *Toxicon*, 1971, 9:301-2.

24. Winek CL, Butala J, Shanor SP, et al, "Toxicology of Poinsettia," *J Toxicol Clin Toxicol*, 1978, 13:27-45.

25. Runyon R, "Toxicity of Fresh Poinsettia *(Euphorbia pulcherrima)* to Sprague-Dawley Rats," *J Toxicol Clin Toxicol*, 1980, 16:167-73.

26. D'Arcy W, "Severe Contact Dermatitis From Poinsettia," *Arch Dermatol*, 1974, 109:909-10.

27. Jacobsen TD and Krenzelok EP, "Botanical Villains? Common Plant Exposures, Part II," *Family Pract Recertif*, 1992, 14:108-18,21.

28. Jones LA, Tandberg D, and Troutman WG, "Household Treatment for 'Chile Burns' of the Hands," *J Toxicol Clin Toxicol*, 1987, 25:483-91.

29. Vogl TP, "Treatment of Human Hand," *N Engl J Med*, 1982, 306:178.

30. Robieux I, Kumar R, Rhadakrishnan S, et al, "The Feasibility of Using EMLA Cream in Pediatric Outpatient Clinics," *Can J Hosp Pharm*, 1990, 43:235.

31. Rodrigues TD, Johnson PN, and Jeffre LP, "Holly Berry Ingestion: Case Report," *Vet Hum Toxicol*, 1984, 26:157-8.

32. Jacobsen TD and Krenzelok EP, "Botanical Villains? Common Plant Exposures, Part I," *Family Pract Recertif*, 1992, 14:74-5, 79-80, 85-6.

33. Jacobsen TD and Krenzelok EP, "Botanical Villains? Common Plant Exposures, Part III," *Family Pract Recertif*, 1992, 14:22-3, 27-8, 31-2, 34, 37-8.

34. Stowe CM, Fangmann G, and Trampel D, "Schefflera Toxicosis in a Dog," *J Am Vet Med Assoc*, 1975, 167-74.

35. Mitchell JC, "Allergic Contact Dermatitis from *Hedera helix* and *Brassaia actinophylla* (Araliaceae)," *Contact Dermatitis*, 1981, 7:158-9.

36. Klein-Schwartz W and Oderda GM, "Jimsonweed Intoxication in Adolescents and Young Adults," *Am J Dis Child*, 1984, 138:737-9.

37. Rodgers GC and von Kanel RL, "Conservative Treatment of Jimsonweed Ingestions," *Vet Hum Toxicol*, 1993, 35:32-3.

38. Salem P, Shih R, Sierzenski P, et al, "Effect of Physostigmine and Gastric Lavage on a Datura Stramonium–Induced Anticholinergic Poisoning Epidemic ," *Am J Emerg Med*, 2003, 21:316-7.

39. Krenzelok EP, Jacobsen TD, and Aronis JM, "Hemlock Ingestions: The Most Deadly Plant Exposures," *J Toxicol Clin Toxicol*, 1996, 34:601-2.

40. Scatizzi A, Di Maggio A, Rizzi D, et al, "Acute Renal Failure Due to Tubular Necrosis Caused by Wildfowl-Mediated Hemlock Poisoning," *Renal Failure*, 1993, 15:93-6.

41. Rizzi D, Basile C, Di Maggio A, et al, "Clinical Spectrum of Accidental Hemlock Poisoning: Neurotoxic Manifestations, Rhabdomyolsis, and Acute Tubular Necrosis," *Nephrol Dial Transplant*, 1991, 6:939-44.

42. Landers D, Seppi K, and Blauer W, "Seizures and Death on a White River Float Trip," *West J Med*, 1985, 142:637-40.

43. Mutter L, "Poisoning by Western Water Hemlock," *Can J Public Health*, 1976, 67:386.

44. Starreveld E and Hope CE, "Cicutoxin Poisoning (Water Hemlock)," *Neurology*, 1975, 25:730-4.

45. Mitchell MI and Rutledge PA, "Hemlock Water Dropwort Poisoning - A Review," *J Toxicol Clin Toxicol*, 1978, 12:417-26.

46. Applefeld JJ and Caplan ES, "A Case of Water Hemlock Poisoning," *J Am Coll Emerg Phys*, 1979, 8:401-3.

47. Krenzelok EP, Jacobsen TD, and Aronis JM, "The Outcome of *Nerium oleander* Exposures," *Acad Emerg Med*, 1997, 4:449.

48. Driggers DA, Solbrig R, Steiner JF, et al, "Acute Oleander Poisoning - A Suicide Attempt in a Geriatric," *West J Med*, 1989, 151:660-2.

49. Haynes BE, Bessen HA, and Wightman WD, "Oleander Tea: Herbal Draught of Death." *Ann Emerg Med*, 1985, 14:350-3.

50. Shumaik GM, Wu AW, and Ping AC, "Oleander Poisoning: Treatment with Digoxin-Specific Fab Antibody Fragments," *Ann Emerg Med*, 1988, 17:732-5.

51. Safaadi F, Levy I, Amitai Y, et al, "Beneficial Effect of Digoxin-Specific Fab Antibody Fragments in Oleander Intoxication," *Arch Intern Med*, 1995, 155:2121-5.

Ackee Fruit Food Poisoning

Scientific Name *Blighiu sapida*
Commonly Found In
Unripe ackee fruit in Jamaica (introduced in 1778), West Africa, Central America, South Florida, southern California, and Hawaii
Mechanism of Toxic Action Contains hypoglycin A and B which are CNS depressants and inhibit fatty acid oxidation; incubation period: 6-48 hours (can be as short as 2 hours)
Signs and Symptoms of Overdose Symptoms may be delayed 6-48 hours (can be as short as 2 hours); overdose can lead to seizures(31%) and coma; hypokalemia may occur; hypothermia, hypoglycemia (19%), vomiting (97%), loss of consciousness (43%)
Admission Criteria/Prognosis Patients with dehydration (who cannot take fluids orally), immunocompromised patients, severe disturbance in electrolytes or acid-base status, or patients at extreme in terms of age group should be considered for admission. Asymptomatic patients may be discharged after 6 hours of observation.
Overdosage/Treatment
Decontamination: Do not utilize ipecac; activated charcoal may be useful
Supportive therapy: Intravenous fluids/electrolyte replacement including glucose
Treat seizures with benzodiazepines.
In a single report, methylene blue (to stimulate hepatic gluconeogenesis) along with riboflavin have been used to treat encephalopathy.
Antidote(s)
- Dextrose [ANTIDOTE]
Diagnostic Procedures
- Electrolytes, Blood
- Glucose, Random
Additional Information
Also known as "Jamaican vomiting sickness"; incidence in the Caribbean is estimated at 1:1000 persons/year; ingestion usually occurs at breakfast or lunch
Hypoglycin is water soluble. A pear-shaped fruit with a leathery, straw-colored to brightly red capsule with a bright yellow inner coating; emanates from a 40 foot tree. It is the unripe fruit and seeds that are most toxic. The unripe fruit is toxic even if cooked. The fruit first appears in the trees in winter (December to March).
Specific References
Joskow R, Belson M, Vesper H, et al, "Ackee Fruit Poisoning: An Outbreak Investigation in Haiti 2000-2001, and Review of the Literature," *Clin Toxicol*, 2006, 44:267-73.

Acorns

Scientific Name *Quercus* species
Mechanism of Toxic Action Contains tannic acid, an astringent that precipitates proteins; at least partially metabolized to gallic acid
Signs and Symptoms of Overdose Abdominal pain, bloody diarrhea, constipation, hemorrhagic colitis, possible kidney and liver damage, nausea, vomiting
Toxicodynamics/Kinetics Absorption: Peak absorption of tannic acid solutions has been reported as 2-3 hours
Overdosage/Treatment
Decontamination: Induction of vomiting is controversial, vomiting may be appropriate for large ingestions; activated charcoal and cathartics may also be of value
Supportive therapy: As needed
Additional Information Toxic dose in humans has not been established

Aloe

Pronunciation (AL oh)
Scientific Name *Aloe vera*
Synonyms Aloe Vera
Uses For topical use only; irritant dermatitis, minor burns, roentgen dermatitis
Mechanism of Toxic Action
Contains barbaloin (a glycoside of anthraquinone origin); also contains tannins, emodin, and volatile oils, as well as bradykinase (a protease inhibitor)
Adverse Reactions
Central nervous system: Catharsis
Dermatologic: Contact dermatitis (allergic)
Endocrine & metabolic: Hypokalemia
Gastrointestinal: Diarrhea, abdominal cramps
Renal: Albuminuria, proteinuria, hematuria (may cause red discoloration of urine)
Contraindications Known hypersensitivity to aloe
Warnings Do not use in eyes
Dosage Forms Gel: 4 oz
Overdosage/Treatment Supportive care: Replace gastrointestinal fluid with I.V. or oral fluids

Pregnancy Risk Factor C
Specific References
Lee A, Chui PT, Aun CS, et al, "Possible Interaction Between Sevoflurane and Aloe Vera," *Ann Pharmacother*, 2004, 38(10):1651-4.

Amaryllis

Related Information
- Star-of-Bethlehem (*Hippobroma longiflora*)
- Star-of-Bethlehem (*Ornithogalum pyrenaicum*)
Mechanism of Toxic Action Contains lycorine (an *Amaryllidaceae* alkaloid), a centrally acting emetic
Adverse Reactions Dermatologic: May cause dermatitis
Signs and Symptoms of Overdose Symptoms develop soon after oral ingestion (within 30 minutes) and resolve within 3 hours (according to one report); abdominal pain, diarrhea, nausea, salivation, vomiting
Overdosage/Treatment Decontamination: Ipecac relatively contraindicated, may be useful, if given soon after ingestion; vomiting has not occurred with ingestion of more than one bulb; activated charcoal with cathartic/lavage (within 1 hour) may be beneficial depending on amount ingested and time elapsed since ingestion
Additional Information All parts contain alkaloid. Toxic part: Bulb is most toxic

Angel's Trumpet

Scientific Name *Brugmansia sauvelen*; *Datura sauveolens*
Uses As a hallucinogen; often brewed as tea
Mechanism of Toxic Action Contains as much as 0.65 mg scopalamine and 0.2 mg atropine in each blossom, thus producing central anticholinergic activity; also contains hycosamine. All parts of the plant are toxic.
Adverse Reactions
Cardiovascular: Tachycardia
Central nervous system: Hyperthermia, agitation, coma, delirium, hallucination (auditory and visual)
Gastrointestinal: Xerostomia
Genitourinary: Urinary retention
Neuromuscular & skeletal: Hyperreflexia, seizures, clonus
Ocular: Mydriasis
Signs and Symptoms of Overdose Paralysis or seizures noted after ingestion of >6 flowers (a lethal dose). Symptoms usually develop within 10 minutes after tea ingestion and 3 hours after leaf ingestion. Tea from ~5 flowers can produce symptoms within 1 hour. Hallucinations may last for 4 days. Mydriasis may last for several days. Usual recovery time: 48-72 hours.
Overdosage/Treatment
Decontamination: Oral: Lavage within 2 hours if >3 flowers are ingested. Activated charcoal may be useful.
Supportive therapy: Physostigmine (1-4 mg I.V.) has been used in life-threatening cases.
Additional Information Indigenous to South America, Australia, and Florida. A perennial shrub or small tree up to 15 feet tall, with white, pendulous, trumpet-shaped flowers up to 1 foot long. Found as an ornamental bush in low elevations in the tropics.
Specific References
Centers for Disease Control and Prevention (CDC), "Suspected Moonflower Intoxication - Ohio, 2002," *MMWR Morb Mortal Wkly Rep*, 2003, 52(33):788-91.

Anthrax

Scientific Name *Bacillus anthracis*
Commonly Found In A disease of herbivores (sheep, goats, cattle, pigs); primarily found in Africa and Asia; also may be a biological warfare agent
Mechanism of Toxic Action A gram-positive sporulating rod which contains a lethal toxin (a metalloprotease) and an edema toxin (which inhibits phagocytosis). The lethal toxin also causes lysis of macrophages and induces release of tumor necrosis factor and interleukin 1.
Signs and Symptoms of Overdose Three forms:
Cutaneous anthrax: Spores gain entry through broken skin. Disease develops 2-5 days postexposure. Starts as a nonpainful papule which over 1-2 days becomes vesicular with localized surrounding edema. The vesicle generally ruptures in 1 week, thereby creating an ulcer which progresses to a black eschar. The eschar falls off in ~2-3 weeks. Fever, headache, and painful lymphadenopathy may also occur. Fatality rate for cutaneous anthrax is 5% to 20% in untreated patients and 1% in treated patients. Systemic manifestation may occur in 5% to 20% of patients.
Gastrointestinal anthrax: Spore-contaminated meat is ingested and invasion in the terminal ileum or cecum can occur. Disease manifests itself in 2-5 days with severe abdominal pain, bloody vomitus and stools (melena), massive ascites, and copious, watery diarrhea. Oropharynx ulcers and lymphadenopathy (cervical) may develop.

Inhalation: Inhaled spores are taken up by macrophages and transported to hilar and mediastinal lymph nodes where germination occurs. Incubation is 1-6 days. Low-grade fever, nonproductive cough, diaphoresis, and myalgias initially occur followed abruptly by respiratory distress, bacteremia, sepsis, shock, and death. Chest x-ray typically reveals widened mediastinum and pleural effusions. Meningitis with subarachnoid hemorrhage may also occur in up to 50% of patients.

Admission Criteria/Prognosis Any inhalation or gastrointestinal exposure or symptomatic patient.

Overdosage/Treatment
Decontamination:

Dermal: Thoroughly wash exposed skin and clothing with soap and water.

Gastrointestinal or inhalation exposure: High-dose intravenous penicillin G (4 million units every 4 hours) is the drug of choice. Alternative agents include ciprofloxacin (400 mg I.V. every 12 hours) or doxycycline (100 mg every 12 hours). Antibiotics should be given for 60 days; pediatric dosage is 20-30 mg/kg of ciprofloxacin I.V. divided into two daily doses not to exceed 1 g/day. For children <45 kg, 2.2 mg/kg doxycycline I.V. every 12 hours can also be used. For children younger than 12 years of age, penicillin G 50,000 units/kg I.V. every 6 hours is optimal therapy if strain is susceptible. Early mechanical ventilation, vasopressors, and correcting electrolyte imbalances can help improve survival.

Cutaneous anthrax can be treated with oral antibiotics (fluoroquinolones, tetracycline, or amoxicillin) for 2 months. Short courses of prophylactic antibiotics delay but do not prevent disease.

Contained Casualty Setting Inhalational Anthrax - Recommended Therapy:
Children:

Initial I.V. therapy[1]:

Ciprofloxacin 10-15 mg/kg every 12 hours. **Note**: Oral ciprofloxacin may be acceptable, if I.V. ciprofloxacin is not available, because it is rapidly and well-absorbed from the GI tract without substantial first-pass metabolism loss. After oral dosing, maximum serum concentration is attained in 1-2 hours, except in the presence of vomiting or ileus. Maximum dose should not exceed 1 g/day.

or

Doxycycline: **Note**: Doxycycline may be less optimal in suspected meningitis due to poor CNS penetration. Serious infections (eg, Rocky Mountain spotted fever) in young children should be treated with tetracyclines (American Academy of Pediatrics recommendation).

>8 years (>45 kg): 100 mg every 12 hours
>8 years (≤45 kg): 2.2 mg/kg every 12 hours
≤8 years: 2.2 mg/kg every 12 hours

and

1-2 additional microbials: [2]

Duration: Initial: I.V.:[3]

Ciprofloxacin 10-15 mg/kg every 12 hours (dosage should not exceed 1 g/day),

or

Doxycycline:

>8 years (>45 kg): 100 mg twice daily
>8 years (≤45 kg): 2.2 mg/kg twice daily
≤8 years: 2.2 mg/kg twice daily
Continue oral and I.V. treatment for 60 days due to potentially persistent spores following aerosol exposure.

Adults:

Initial I.V. therapy[1]: Ciprofloxacin 400 mg every 12 hours, **or**, doxycycline, 100 mg every 12 hours (doxycycline may be less optimal with suspected meningitis, due to poor CNS penetration), **and**, 1-2 additional antimicrobials.[2]

Duration: Initial: I.V.[3]: Ciprofloxacin 500 mg twice daily **or** doxycycline 100 mg twice daily. Continue oral and I.V. treatment for 60 days due to potentially persistent spores following aerosol exposure.

Pregnant women[4]: Same for nonpregnant Adults

Initial I.V. therapy: Same as Adults.

Duration: I.V. treatment initially before switching to oral antimicrobial therapy when clinically appropriate (ciprofloxacin and doxycycline should be considered essential first-line therapy). Oral regimens are the same as Adults.[3]

Immunocompromised individuals: Same as Children and Adults.

[1] For patients with severe edema and for meningitis (based on experience with bacterial meningitis of other etiologies) steroids may be considered as adjunct therapy.

[2] Other agents with *in vitro* activity include rifampin, vancomycin, penicillin, ampicillin, chloramphenicol, imipenem, clindamycin, and clarithromycin. Penicillin and ampicillin should not be used alone due to possible constitutive and inducible β-lactamases in *Bacillus anthracis*. Infectious disease consult is advised.

[3] Initial I.V. therapy may be adjusted based upon the clinical course, prior to switching to oral antimicrobial therapy when appropriate (1-2 antimicrobial agents may be adequate with clinical improvement).

[4] Tetracyclines may be indicated for life-threatening illness (even in pregnant women). Adverse effects on developing teeth and bones are dose-related; thus, doxycycline may be used briefly (7-14 days) before 6 months of gestation. A high death rate from infection outweighs the risk associated with the antimicrobial agent.

Mass Casualty Setting or Postexposure Prophylaxis Inhalational Anthrax - Recommended Therapy: (Some of the following recommendations are not FDA approved, but are based on *in vitro* and animal studies.)
Oral:

Children:

Initial[1]: Ciprofloxacin 20-30 mg/kg/day in 2 daily doses; do not exceed 1 g/day.

Alternative (if proven susceptible strain):

Weight ≥20 kg: Amoxicillin 500 mg every 8 hours[3]
Weight <20 kg: Amoxicillin 40 mg/kg in 3 doses ever 8 hours[3]

Adults:

Initial[1]: Ciprofloxacin 500 mg every 12 hours

Alternative (if proven susceptible strain):

Doxycycline 100 mg every 12 hours. Based on *in vitro* studies, tetracycline 500 mg every 6 hours could be substituted; the fluoroquinolones gatifloxacin and moxifloxacin have mechanisms of action consistent with ciprofloxacin and could be substituted.
Amoxicillin 500 mg every 8 hours[3]

Duration: 60 days after exposure

Pregnant women:

Initial[1]: Ciprofloxacin 500 mg every 12 hours

Alternative (if proven susceptible strain): Amoxicillin 500 mg every 8 hours[3]

Duration: 60 days after exposure

Immunosuppressed individuals: Same as for Children and Adults

[1] Ofloxacin 400 mg orally every 12 hours or levofloxacin 500 mg orally every 24 hours could be substituted for ciprofloxacin (based on *in vitro* studies).

[2] If use of ciprofloxacin is precluded (eg, adverse reactions, antibiotic susceptibility testing, or exhausted drug supply), doxycycline adult dosage (for weight >45 kg) can be used. For children weighing <45 kg, doxycycline 2.5 mg/kg orally every 12 hours can be used.

[3] Amoxicillin is suitable for postexposure prophylaxis only after 10-14 days of fluoroquinolone or doxycycline treatment and only if these two classes of medications are contraindicated (eg, pregnancy, lactation, intolerance to other antibiotics, age <18 years) per CDC recommendations.

Cutaneous Anthrax Associated with Bioterrorism - Recommended Therapy[1]:
Oral:

Children: **Note**: Young children should be treated with tetracyclines for serious infections (eg, Rocky Mountain spotted fever), according to the American Academy of Pediatrics.

Initial[2]:

Ciprofloxacin 10-15 mg/kg every 12 hours; do not exceed 1 g/day

or

Doxycycline:

>8 years (>45 kg): 100 mg every 12 hours
>8 years (≤45 kg): 2.2 mg/kg every 12 hours
≤8 years: 2.2 mg/kg every 12 hours
Duration: 60 days[3]

Adults:

Initial[2]: Ciprofloxacin 500 mg twice daily **or** doxycycline 100 mg twice daily
Duration: 60 days[3]

Pregnant women:

Initial[2,4]: Ciprofloxacin 500 mg twice daily **or** doxycycline 100 mg twice daily.
Duration: 60 days[3]

Immunocompromised individuals: Same as Children and Adults.

[1] Signs of systemic involvement, extensive edema, or head/neck lesions require I.V. therapy and a multidrug approach. See Contained Casualty Setting - Recommended Therapy.

[2] First-line therapy should be ciprofloxacin or doxycycline. If fluoroquinolone or tetracycline class drugs cannot be taken, amoxicillin can be substituted: Children: Amoxicillin 80 mg/kg orally divided into 3 doses at 8-hour increments can be used for completion of therapy following clinical improvement. Adults: Amoxicillin 500 mg orally 3 times a day. The need to achieve appropriate minimum inhibitory drug concentration is the basis for oral amoxicillin dosage.

[3] Sixty days is recommended for bioterrorism-related attacks due to the likelihood of aerosolized *Bacillus anthracis* exposure (previous guidelines suggest 7-10 days of treatment for cutaneous anthrax).

[4] Tetracyclines or ciprofloxacin may be indicated for life-threatening illness, though they are not recommended during pregnancy. Adverse effects on developing teeth and bones are dose-related; thus, doxycycline could be used briefly (7-14 days) before 6 months of gestation.

Additional Information
Can be cleared to work in research laboratory 3 weeks after 3rd anthrax vaccine dose (0.5 mL SubQ) with annual booster dose after 18 months

Toxic dose: Inhalation: 4000-80,000 spores

Industrial processing of animal hair accounted for 153 (65%) of 236 anthrax cases reported to the CDC from 1955-1999. While most of these cases were cutaneous anthrax, 10% were inhalation anthrax.

Methods to prevent inhalation anthrax from animal hide/hair exposure:

Work with hides that are tanned or treated (air drying does not destroy *B anthracis* spores)

Regular hand washing with soap and warm water

Wearing durable protective gloves

Working in a well-ventilated workplace

Spores can be inactivated by heating hides to an internal temperature of 158°F (70°C) or placement in boiling water for over 30 minutes

Remove clothing before leaving workplace and launder

Clean workplace with high-efficiency particulate air vacuum

Avoid vigorous shaking or beating hides

Diagnosis of Inhalational Anthrax:

Sudden appearance of several cases of severe acute febrile illness with fulminant course and death; or acute febrile illness in those identified as at-risk following a specific attack.

Widened mediastinum, infiltrates, and pleural effusion on chest radiograph. Hyperdense hilar and mediastinal nodes, mediastinal edema, infiltrates, and pleural effusion on chest CT scan. Hemorrhagic pleural effusions on thoracentesis.

Gram-positive bacilli on peripheral blood smear. Growth of large Gram-positive bacilli with preliminary identification of *Bacillus* species on blood culture.

Pathology findings of hemorrhagic mediastinitis, hemorrhagic thoracic lymphadenitis, and hemorrhagic meningitis. DFA stain of infected tissues.

Anthrax vaccine adsorbed (AVA) product (obtained from Michigan Department of Public Health) is given at 0, 2, and 4 weeks and 6, 12, and 18 months with yearly boosters (at a dose of 0.5 mL subcutaneously). Two doses may be protective against inhalation exposure. Overall efficacy for cutaneous anthrax is 92.5%. Protective masks should be capable of filtering 1-5 µm particles (U.S. military current M17 and M40 gas masks). Standard blood cultures can grow out organisms in 6-24 hours.

Interim Guidelines for Evacuation and Personal Decontamination of Workers After a Positive Autonomous Detection System (ADS) Signal Indicates Presence of a Biologic Agent	
Worker Category	**Evacuation / Decontamination Procedures**
Group 1. Workers who did not enter the production area containing the ADS device during the sampling and testing period (eg, 1.5 hours) before the positive ADS signal and who were not in an area that shares a heating, ventilating, and air conditioning (HVAC) system with the production area experiencing the positive signal	Evacuate; no special decontamination steps are needed
Group 2. All workers who were present in the production area containing the ADS device during the sampling and testing period before the positive ADS signal or who were in an area that shares an HVAC system with the production area experiencing the positive signal.	• Evacuate immediately • Remove potentially contaminated outer garments at the site • Wash all areas of skin (eg, face, arms, hands, and legs) exposed at the time of the positive ADS signal with mild soap and copious amounts of warm water • Use replacement outer garments and shoes
Group 3. Workers identified in advance as particularly at risk of exposure to a higher concentration of deposited spores as a result of direct physical contact with aerosol-generating equipment	• Evacuate immediately • Remove potentially contaminated garments at the site • Take a shower at the site to wash all areas of exposed and unexposed skin with mild soap and warm water • Use replacement outer garments, underwear, and shoes

Adapted from Meehan PJ, Rosenstein NE, Gillen M, et al, "Responding to Detection of Aerosolized *Bacillus anthracis* by Autonomous Detection Systems in the Workplace," *MMWR*, 2004, 53(RR07):1-12.

Patients who progress to the fulminant phase have a mortality rate of 97% (regardless of the treatment they receive).

Specific References

American Medical Association; American Nurses Association-American Nurses Foundation; Centers for Disease Control and Prevention; Center for Food Safety and Applied Nutrition, Food and Drug Administration; Food Safety and Inspection Service, US Department of Agriculture, "Diagnosis and Management of Foodborne Illnesses: A Primer for Physicians and Other Health Care Professionals," *MMWR Recomm Rep*, 2004, 53(RR-4):1-33.

Beatty ME, Ashford DA, Griffin PM, et al, "Gastrointestinal Anthrax: Review of the Literature," *Arch Intern Med*, 2003, 163(20):2527-31.

Ben-Noun LL, "Figs - The Earliest Known Ancient Drug for Cutaneous Anthrax," *Ann Pharmacother*, 2003, 37(2):297-300.

Blank S, Moskin LC, and Zucker JR, "An Ounce of Prevention is a Ton of Work: Mass Antibiotic Prophylaxis for Anthrax, New York City, 2001," *Emerg Infect Dis*, 2003, 9(6):615-22.

Bottei EM, "It's Ricin and VX and Anthrax. Oops, Our Bad—It's Baking Powder," *J Toxicol Clin Toxicol*, 2004, 42(5):794.

Cantrell FL and Carlson T, "Impact of Biological/Chemical Terrorism on Poison Centers," *J Toxicol Clin Toxicol*, 2003, 41(5):681.

Centers for Disease Control, "Inhalation Anthrax Associated with Dried Animal Hides - Pennsylvania and New York City," *MMWR*, 2006, 55(10):280-2.

Crupi RS, Asnis DS, Lee CC, et al, "Meeting the Challenge of Bioterrorism: Lessons Learned from West Nile Virus and Anthrax," *Am J Emerg Med*, 2003, 21(1):77-9.

Fine AM, Wong JB, Fraser HS, et al, "Is It Influenza or Anthrax? A Decision Analytic Approach to the Treatment of Patients with Influenza-Like Illnesses," *Ann Emerg Med*, 2004, 43(3):318-28.

Forrester MB and Stanley SK, "Calls About Anthrax to the Texas Poison Center Network in Relation to the Anthrax Bioterrorism Attack in 2001," *Vet Hum Toxicol*, 2003, 45(5):247-8.

Gundry CS, "Four Common Myths about Chemical and Biological Terrorism," *Inside Homeland security*, 2007, 5(1):8-13.

Hupert N, Bearman GM, Mushlin AI, et al, "Accuracy of Screening for Inhalational Anthrax After a Bioterrorist Attack," *Ann Intern Med*, 2003, 139(5 Pt 1):337-45.

Holty JC, Bravata DM, Liu H, et al, "Systematic Review: A Century of Inhalational Anthrax Cases from 1900 to 2005," *Ann Intern Med*, 2006, 144:270-80.

Muniz AE, "Lymphocytic Vasculitis Associated with the Anthrax Vaccine: Case Report and Review of Anthrax Vaccination," *J Emerg Med*, 2003, 25(3):271-6.

Partridge R, Alexander J, Lawrence T, et al, "Medical Counterbioterrorism: The Response to Provide Anthrax Prophylaxis to New York City US Postal Service Employees," *Ann Emerg Med*, 2003, 41(4):441-6.

Roche K, McKay CA, and Bayer MJ, "Hospital Antidote Stocking Subsequent to the 2001 Terror Acts," *J Toxicol Clin Toxicol*, 2003, 41(5):719.

Rusnak J, Boudreau E, Bozue J, et al, "An Unusual Inhalational Exposure to *Bacillus anthracis* in a Research Laboratory," *J Toxicol Clin Toxicol*, 2004, 46(4):313-4.

Rusnak JM, Kortepeter MG, Aldis J, et al, "Experience in the Medical Management of Potential Laboratory Exposures to Agents of Bioterrorism on the Basis of Risk Assessment at the United States Army Medical Research Institute of Infectious Diseases (USAMRIID)," *J Occup Environ Med*, 2004, 46(8):801-11.

Rusnak JM, Kortepeter MG, Hawley RG, et al, "Management Guidelines for Laboratory Exposures to Agents of Bioterrorism," *J Occup Environ Med*, 2004, 46(8):791-800.

Schultz CH, "Chinese Curses, Anthrax, and the Risk of Bioterrorism," *Ann Emerg Med*, 2004, 43(3):329-32.

Sikka R, Khalid M, Chae E, et al, "Impact of the Anthrax Bioterrorism Incidents of 2001 on Antibiotic Utilization," *Ann Emerg Med*, 2004, 44:S92.

Sox HC, "A Triage Algorithm for Inhalational Anthrax," *Ann Intern Med*, 2003, 139(5 Pt 1):379-81.

Sternbach G, "The History of Anthrax," *J Emerg Med*, 2003, 24(4):463-7.

Subbarao IA, Johnson C, Bond WF, et al, "Creation and Pilot Testing of the Advanced Bioterrorism Triage Card," *Ann Emerg Med*, 2004, 44:S93.

Wills BK, Leikin J, Weidner K, et al, "Analysis of Suspicious Powders in Northern Illinois Following the Post 9/11 Anthrax Scare," *Clin Toxicol (Phila)*, 2005, 43:696.

Apple

Scientific Name *Malus sylvestris*

Mechanism of Toxic Action Fruit contains up to 17% pectin and pectic acids; seeds contain amygdalin which is a cyanogenic glycoside

Adverse Reactions Dermatologic: Immunologic contact urticaria

Signs and Symptoms of Overdose Apple seed ingestion: Acidosis, anorexia, ataxia, coma, cyanosis, dizziness, hypotension, tachypnea, vomiting (may be the initial symptom), weakness

Admission Criteria/Prognosis Admit any ingestion >50 seeds

Overdosage/Treatment

Decontamination: Lavage (within 1 hour)/activated charcoal with cathartic; **do not** induce emesis; a 25% solution of sodium thiosulfate (300 mL in adults) can be instilled in the stomach following lavage

Supportive therapy: Administer high flow oxygen; cyanide antidote kit should be administered for symptomatic or acidotic patients; sodium bicarbonate (1-2 mEq/kg) should be administered to treat acidosis

Antidote(s)

- Cyanide Antidote Kit [ANTIDOTE]

Additional Information A deciduous tree with white or pink flowers; apple seeds contain $\sim$0.61 mg of hydrogen cyanide per gram of seed (Average lethal dose of cyanide: Oral: Adult: $\sim$50 mg).

Apricot

Scientific Name *Prunus armeniaca*

Mechanism of Toxic Action Amygdalin (a cyanogenic glycoside) is hydrolyzed in the gut to release hydrocyanic acid, cellular hypoxia occurs after absorption and complexation with cytochrome oxidase

Adverse Reactions

Cardiovascular: Cyanosis

Central nervous system: Lethargy, drowsiness, headache, coma, seizures

Gastrointestinal: Abdominal pain, vomiting

Neuromuscular & skeletal: Paralysis

Respiratory: Dyspnea

Miscellaneous: Diaphoresis

Signs and Symptoms of Overdose Symptoms delayed 30 minutes to 2 hours or longer due to hydrolysis preferentially occurring in alkaline duodenum, plus intestinal flora hydrolyzing amygdalin

Admission Criteria/Prognosis All symptomatic patients should probably be admitted to an intensive care unit for 1-2 days; asymptomatic patients should be observed for at least 2 hours and then can be discharged; survival after 4 hours (in an acute exposure) is usually associated with recovery

Overdosage/Treatment

Decontamination: Basic poison management; vomiting is contraindicated due to rapid course of the neurologic symptoms; give 100% oxygen

Supportive therapy: Give sodium bicarbonate for acidosis; cyanide antidote kit should be used for patients symptomatic from cyanide toxicity

Enhancement of elimination: Hemodialysis and charcoal hemoperfusion have been utilized; hyperbaric oxygen may also be utilized; hydroxocobalamin and dicobalt-EDTA used for chelation in Europe

Antidote(s)

- Cyanide Antidote Kit [ANTIDOTE]

Diagnostic Procedures

- Anion Gap, Blood
- Cyanide, Blood
- Electrolytes, Blood
- Methemoglobin, Blood

Additional Information Toxic dose: 1-2 pits likely nontoxic; toxicity unusual with accidental ingestion. Amygdalin is also found in leaves, flowers, bark, seeds; young leaves have highest concentration; intact pit does not release chemical; apricot most toxic within species. Cyanide content in apricot kernels ranges from 0.122-4.09 mg/g.

Aristolochic Acid

CAS Number 313-67-7; 61117-05-3

Commonly Found In Herbal preparations (Aristolochia Fang Chi) and in plants in the family Aristolochia, a perennial herb which grows in forests. The dried rhizome and roots are the active parts. The herbal products have been use in Europe for weight reduction.

Mechanism of Toxic Action The alkaloids aristolochic acid I and aristolochic acid II can produce acute tubular necrosis and are carcinogenic/mutagenic through metabolite binding [7-(deoxyadenosine-N^{6}0yl)-aristolactam I DNA adduct] in the renal system.

Signs and Symptoms of Overdose Mean period of usage for development of renal toxicity is 13.3 months. Hypertension, interstitial renal (cortical) fibrosis (also called Chinese herb nephropathy and possibly Balkan nephropathy), metabolic acidosis (with renal failure), reversible hepatitis, tachycardia, urothelial carcinoma

Admission Criteria/Prognosis Admit any patient with renal or electrolyte abnormalities.

Overdosage/Treatment Supportive therapy: Treat acidosis with intravenous sodium bicarbonate (1-2 mEq/kg). Prednisolone 1 mg/kg for 1 month tapering off 0.1 mg/kg every 2 weeks may slow progression of renal disease. Avoid alkalinizing the urine, since renal toxicity may increase.

Additional Information Fatal acute I.V. dose: 2 mg/kg

Arizona Bark Scorpion

Scientific Name *Centruroides sculpturatus*

Mechanism of Toxic Action Neurotoxin which is heat stable; neurotoxin increases sodium transfer

Adverse Reactions

Cardiovascular: **Sinus tachycardia** (92%), arrhythmias (ventricular); sudden death (7%)

Respiratory: Bronchospasm, laryngospasm, pulmonary edema (especially in children)

Signs and Symptoms of Overdose Abnormal ocular movements (33% to 58%), agitation (5% to 59%), ataxia, AV block, blurred vision, dysphagia (4% to 33%), fasciculations, hyperglycemia, hypersalivation (21% to 35%), hyperreflexia, hypertension (33%), hyperthermia, myoclonus, pain, pain at site of bite (19% to 70%), paresthesia (8% to 53%), restlessness, salivation, seizures, slurred speech, stridor, sweating, tachycardia, tachypnea, vomiting

Grading for *Centruroides sculpturatus* envenomation:

Grade I: Local pain and/or paresthesia

Grade II: Pain and/or paresthesias remote from envenomation site with local signs present

Grade III: Either cranial nerve or somatic skeletal neuromuscular dysfunction

Grade IV: Both cranial nerve and somatic skeletal neuromuscular dysfunction

Admission Criteria/Prognosis Admit symptomatic patients; rapid progression within 4 hours indicates poor prognosis; survival after 2 days usually associated with recovery

Toxicodynamics/Kinetics Onset of symptoms: Within 1 hour

Overdosage/Treatment

Decontamination: Pressure tourniquet (50-70 mm Hg) to slow systemic absorption on affected limb; apply cold packs to bite area

Supportive therapy: Antivenom from goat serum (I.V.); propranolol or phentolamine can be used for hypertension; bradycardia can respond to atropine. Steroids are probably not useful. Prazosin (0.125 mg in children and 0.5 mg in adults) may also be useful in treating hypertension. Seizures can initially be treated with benzodiazepines; phenobarbital can be utilized for refractory seizures. Hyperthermia can be treated with tepid water sponge bathing and acetaminophen. For grade III or IV envenomations, a midazolam bolus of 0.3 mg/kg (maximum 2 mg in children) followed by, if necessary, a continuous I.V. infusion of 0.1 to 0.3 mg/kg/hour, can be used for treatment. Atropine can be used to treat excessive oral secretions. Prazosin (1 mg every 6 hours) can assist in resolution of significant sympathetic symptoms (ie, hypertension).

Antivenin is available from the Good Samaritan Poison Center in Phoenix, Arizona (602-253-3334); available in Arizona only.

Antidote(s)

- Centruroides Scorpion Venom Antisera [ANTIDOTE]

Drug Interaction Avoid phenothiazines in that they can lower the seizure threshold

Additional Information Antivenom dose is one vial; give second vial at 1 hour if symptoms not improved; allergic effects can occur. An arthropod with two body segments and eight legs. The long, segmented abdomen terminates into a curved tail (the stinging apparatus). Claw-like pincers anteriorly are characteristic features.

Specific References

Bouaziz M, Bahloul M, Hergafi L, et al, "Factors Associated with Pulmonary Edema in Severe Scorpion Sting Patients - A Multivariate Analysis of 428 Cases," *Clin Toxicol*, 2006, 44(3):293-300.

Koseoglu Z and Koseoglu A, "Use of Prazosin in the Treatment of Scorpion Envenomation," *Am J Ther*, 2006, 13(3):285-7.

LoVecchio F and McBride C, "Scorpion Envenomations in Young Children in Central Arizona," *J Toxicol Clin Toxicol*, 2003, 41(7):937-40.

Asparagus (Berries and Young Shoots)

Scientific Name *Asparagus officinalis*

Adverse Reactions

Dermatologic: Pruritus, vesiculation

Gastrointestinal: GI irritation, GI upset

Signs and Symptoms of Overdose Allergic dermatitis after repeated exposure; berries may cause GI irritation

Overdosage/Treatment

Decontamination: Wash thoroughly

Supportive therapy: Treat symptoms

Atlantic Mussel Food Poisoning

Commonly Found In Shellfish, mussels

Mechanism of Toxic Action Toxin involves domoic acid structurally similar to glutamate which can cause neuronal necrosis in the amygdaloid nucleus and hippocampus; incubation period: 5 hours

Adverse Reactions Central nervous system: Memory disturbances

Signs and Symptoms of Overdose Bronchorrhea, diarrhea, facial grimacing, nausea, short-term memory loss. Long-term anterograde memory loss (10%), GI cramping, vomiting. Onset of GI signs ranges from 15 minutes to 38 hours; onset of neurological signs occurs within 2 days. Can cause headache, hypotension, myoclonus, piloerection, and seizures

Admission Criteria/Prognosis Patients with dehydration (who cannot take fluids orally), immunocompromised patients, severe disturbance in electrolytes or acid-base status, or patients at extreme in terms of age group should be considered for admission

Overdosage/Treatment

Decontamination: Avoid ipecac; activated charcoal with cathartic may be used; lavage (with isotonic bicarbonate solution) within 1 hour may be useful

Supportive therapy: Diazepam or phenobarbital is useful for seizures, fluids for hypotension

Test Interactions Can result in elevated serum creatinine

Additional Information Toxic Dose: Probably >60 mg orally. Heat stable toxin which is not destroyed by cooking; neurologic symptoms may be more pronounced in the elderly; domoic acid activates glutamate receptors thus causing seizures; mortality rate: 2%. Found in North Atlantic, Pacific coast, and Gulf of Mexico; Canadian standards for domoic acid in mussels is 20 mcg/100 g of tissue

Azalea

Related Information

- Rhododendron

Scientific Name *Rhododendron nudiflorum*

Mechanism of Toxic Action Contains grayanotoxin which binds to a subset of sodium channels causing structural modifications which cause slow opening of these channels which leads to cell depolarization

Adverse Reactions Cardiovascular: Sinus bradycardia

Signs and Symptoms of Overdose Asthenia, bradycardia, dermatitis, hypotension, nausea, oral numbness or burning, paresthesia, sweating, seizures, transient blindness, visual changes, vomiting

Overdosage/Treatment

Decontamination: Avoid ipecac, vagal stimulation increases toxicity; lavage (within 1 hour)/activated charcoal with cathartic

Supportive therapy: Atropine for bradycardia, I.V. fluids should be sufficient for hypotension

Antidote(s)

- Atropine [ANTIDOTE]

Additional Information Three whole leaves or flowers likely nontoxic; consider decontamination if more. Toxicity is unpredictable, variable among rhododendron types. Toxic part: Whole plant is toxic, especially foliage; contaminated honey may cause systemic symptoms

Bacillus cereus Food Poisoning (Type I and II)

Commonly Found In Fried rice (Type I), cereals (Type II), vegetables (Type II), milk (Type II), meat (Type II), turkey (Type II)

Mechanism of Toxic Action

Type I: Heat and pH stable toxin; incubation period: 1-6 hours (emetic form)

Type II: Heat labile enterotoxin; incubation period: 10-12 hours (diarrheal form)

Signs and Symptoms of Overdose Fever is uncommon

Type I: Vomiting is prominent, abdominal cramps and diarrhea can occur

Type II: Watery diarrhea, abdominal cramps; can cause more volume depletion than Type I

Admission Criteria/Prognosis Patients with dehydration (who cannot take fluids orally), immunocompromised patients, severe disturbance in electrolytes or acid-base status, or patients at extreme in terms of age group should be considered for admission

Overdosage/Treatment *Bacillus cereus* food poisoning does not respond to antimicrobial therapy. Attention should instead be focused on supportive measures such as hydration and electrolyte balance. Clinically significant infections with this organism should be treated with vancomycin intravenously. Unlike other *Bacillus* species (eg, *Bacillus alvei*, *B. subtilis*, *B. circulans*, etc), *Bacillus cereus* is often resistant to beta-lactam antibiotics such as the penicillins and cephalosporins. Vancomycin should be used until the antimicrobial susceptibility pattern is finalized; limited data suggests the addition of an aminoglycoside to vancomycin may have some minor benefit in serious infections. Due to high biliary levels of the emetic toxin, multiple dosing of activated charcoal may be effective.

Diagnostic Procedures

- Electrolytes, Blood
- Stool Culture

Additional Information

Microbiology: *Bacillus cereus* is an aerobic, gram-positive bacillus associated with a variety of disease states including food poisoning, ocular infections, bacteremia, and septicemia. *Bacillus cereus* is a spore-forming aerobe which stains gram-positive or gram-variable. It grows readily on standard laboratory media and does not need special culturing techniques.

Epidemiology: *Bacillus cereus* is ubiquitous in the environment, growing readily in such diverse areas as soil, water, vegetables, decaying matter, and dust. In certain individuals, it can be part of the normal

human flora, explaining in part its tendency to colonize surgical wounds and serious burn injuries. The needles and syringes of heroin addicts in the United States have also been found to be contaminated with this bacterium. *Bacillus cereus* food poisoning, caused by ingestion of a toxin elaborated by this organism, has been reported from several countries around the world, including the United States and Canada.

Clinical Syndromes:

- **The "emetic form" of *Bacillus cereus* food poisoning:** This results from the ingestion of a preformed toxin produced by this organism. Nausea, vomiting, and abdominal cramping usually occur soon (1-6 hours) following the ingestion of contaminated foods. In particular, this emetic toxin has been associated with fried rice served in Chinese food restaurants. The spores of *B. cereus* can survive the process of boiling rice followed by quick frying. Fulminant liver failure has been described.
- **The "diarrheal form" of *Bacillus cereus* food poisoning:** This results from ingestion of a different, heat-labile enterotoxin. The incubation period is longer than for the emetic form, usually more than 9 hours. Profuse watery diarrhea is the predominant symptom, along with abdominal cramping.

Diagnosis: *Bacillus cereus* is readily identified in the laboratory from cultures of blood and other sterile body fluids. In cases of suspected *Bacillus* food poisoning, the implicated foods should be cultured for this organism. There is little benefit in culturing the patient's stool since GI tract colonization is not uncommon. As mentioned previously, isolation of *Bacillus cereus* from the blood need not be treated in every case, and clinical judgment is required.

Baneberries

Scientific Name *Actaea alba*; *Actaea arguta*; *Actaea pachypoda*; *Actaea rubra*

Mechanism of Toxic Action GI is unclear; dermatitis is contact type; protoanemonin reacts with SH groups and inactivates enzymes

Adverse Reactions

Cardiovascular: Sinus tachycardia

Dermatologic: Dermatitis and vesiculation may occur

Ocular: Conjunctivitis

Signs and Symptoms of Overdose Bloody diarrhea, circulatory failure, confusion, dizziness, dysuria, gastroenteritis, headache, hematuria, oral irritation, seizures, tachycardia, visual hallucinations

Admission Criteria/Prognosis Patients who are persistently symptomatic three hours postexposure should be admitted

Toxicodynamics/Kinetics

Onset of effect: Oral: Within 30 minutes

Duration: Dermal: May take several weeks to resolve. Oral: Within 3 hours

Overdosage/Treatment

Decontamination: Ipecac relatively contraindicated due to rapid onset of symptoms, lavage within 1 hour recommended in large ingestion; activated charcoal with cathartic may be beneficial; **do not** give cathartic if diarrhea has developed

Supportive therapy: Maintain hydration and electrolyte balance; hydration also decreases protoanemonin concentration in urine; for dermal, wash thoroughly; antihistamine and corticosteroid therapy as indicated; monitor fluid and electrolyte status

Additional Information Oral symptoms of pain and burning usually limit potential for systemic toxicity. Toxic part: Root, berries, and sap

Bird of Paradise

Mechanism of Toxic Action Seeds contain tannins, leaves may contain hydrocyanic acid

Signs and Symptoms of Overdose Diarrhea, dizziness, drowsiness, GI irritation, vomiting

Toxicodynamics/Kinetics

Onset of effect: Within 30 minutes

Duration: Within 24 hours

Overdosage/Treatment

Decontamination: Emesis within 30 minutes or lavage within 1 hour recommended if asymptomatic and more than small amount ingested

Supportive therapy: Fluid and electrolyte replacement as needed

Additional Information Toxic dose: Ingestion of 5 seed pods has caused poisoning. Not a cyanide risk. Toxic part: Seeds, pods, leaves, and roots

Black Locust

Scientific Name *Robinia pseudoacacia*

Mechanism of Toxic Action Ricin, a toxalbumin inhibits protein synthesis

Adverse Reactions In addition to vomiting and diarrhea, late phase toxicity due to cytotoxic effects on liver, CNS, kidney, and adrenal system

Signs and Symptoms of Overdose Acutely causes irritation to oropharynx, esophagus, and GI tract; may cause hemorrhage and tissue sloughing

Toxicodynamics/Kinetics Acute effects occur within 8 hours; late phase complications delayed by 2-5 days possibly with asymptomatic phase in between

Overdosage/Treatment
Decontamination: Activated charcoal may be useful; consider using osmotic cathartic despite hyperactive bowel as decreased exposure to mucosa may be beneficial, follow fluid and electrolyte status closely if symptomatic; if symptomatic, maintain high urine flow; consider alkalinization to prevent hemoglobin crystallization in severe poisonings; guaiac emesis, stool, follow fluid and electrolyte status; check hematologic parameters in severe poisoning, hepatic enzymes

Additional Information Toxicity may occur with as little as one bean. Toxicity is variable; related to variations within plants and GI absorption, seed has hard coat; rupture makes toxin available; symptomatic patients should be hospitalized; asymptomatic patients that have received early thorough decontamination may be observed at home. Honey locust is nontoxic. Toxic part: Bark, seeds, and leaves are toxic

Black Mustard

Related Information
● Black Pepper

Scientific Name *Brassica nigra*

Uses Often used as a spice or seasoning agent; it is currently illegally sold in the U.S. as a mustard oil. Also used as a folk remedy for upset stomach.

Mechanism of Toxic Action Contains ~1% sinigrin (a thioglycoside) which is converted upon contact with water to isothiocyanate, a volatile compound which is a severe irritant.

Signs and Symptoms of Overdose Adult respiratory distress syndrome, airway edema, aspiration, cough, dyspnea, hypoxemia, irritant contact dermatitis, pneumonitis

Overdosage/Treatment
Dermal: Irrigate with soap and water.
Supportive: Pulmonary support may be necessary (supplemental oxygen, intubation, ventilator, inhaled beta$_2$-agonists).

Black Nightshade

Related Information
● Deadly Nightshade

Scientific Name *Solanum americanum*; *Solanum nigrum*

Mechanism of Toxic Action Contains toxic alkaloids; some plants may also contain alpha-cholinergic alkaloids

Adverse Reactions Central nervous system: Psychosis

Signs and Symptoms of Overdose Anticholinergic effects may or may not be present to varying degrees; asthenia, diarrhea, drowsiness, fever, headache, hallucinations, nausea, sweating, visual changes, vomiting

Toxicodynamics/Kinetics Toxicity occurs within 2-24 hours, diarrhea may last 3-6 days, anticholinergic effects may delay GI emptying and produce delayed effects

Overdosage/Treatment
Decontamination: Ipecac if vomiting has not already occurred, lavage (within 1 hour) and/or charcoal may be beneficial if the patient presents symptomatic
Supportive therapy: Maintain fluid and electrolyte balance as necessary, support vital signs; physostigmine will reverse anticholinergic toxicity that may be associated with exposure; intravenous physostigmine can be useful in treating anticholinergic toxicity

Antidote(s)
● Physostigmine [ANTIDOTE]

Drug Interaction Solanine poorly absorbed, delayed decontamination may be effective

Additional Information Toxic dose: 2-3 green berries or 6 red or black berries should not cause significant toxicity (fatal dose reported as: 200 berries). Toxicity may be mistaken for food poisoning; plants may also contain varying amounts of anticholinergic alkaloids. Toxic part: Green or yellow berries more toxic than red or black

Black Pepper

Related Information
● Black Mustard

Scientific Name *Piper nigrum*

Uses Spice/seasoning agent

Mechanism of Toxic Action Dried, unripe fruit contains 5% to 9% piperine (a volatile oil) which is a potent irritant.

Signs and Symptoms of Overdose Adult respiratory distress syndrome, airway edema, aspiration, cough, diaphoresis, dyspnea, hypoxemia, pneumonitis

Overdosage/Treatment
Decontamination: **Inhalation:** Administer 100% humidified oxygen.
Ocular: Irrigate with saline

Additional Information A vine native to southern India and Sri Lanka.

Black Widow Spider

Scientific Name *Latrodectus mactans*

Mechanism of Toxic Action Contains a highly neurotoxic venom which destroys cholinergic and adrenergic nerve terminals; also increases calcium permeability of the nerve terminal, thus resulting in acetylcholine release

Adverse Reactions
Cardiovascular: Hypertension, myocarditis
Dermatologic: Target lesions, erythema, edema, toxic epidermal necrolysis, urticarial rash
Genitourinary: Priapism, urinary retention
Hematologic: Leukocytosis
Neuromuscular & skeletal: Fasciculations, muscle weakness, paresthesia, peripheral neuropathy
Ocular: Ptosis
Renal: Pyuria, proteinuria, microscopic hematuria
Respiratory: Respiratory arrest
Miscellaneous: Lymphadenopathy, diaphoresis

Signs and Symptoms of Overdose
The initial bite may be sharply painful or unrecognized; possible papule or punctum on exam, with surrounding skin slightly erythematous and indurated. Within 30-60 minutes of the bite, however, involuntary spasm and rigidity affect the large muscle groups of the abdomen and limbs. Abdominal pain (15% to 50%), dyspnea, fever (10% to 15%), headaches (5% to 25%), hyperreflexia, hypersalivation, nausea, ptosis, tachypnea, tachycardia, vomiting
Abdominal rigidity without specific tenderness is characteristic of envenomation. Mortality rate is ~5% (patients in the extremes of age groups or individuals with pre-existing hypertension are especially susceptible). Death is usually due to cardiovascular collapse.

Admission Criteria/Prognosis Admit any patient in respiratory distress; with cardiovascular symptoms (including hypertension); protracted pain; pediatric or elderly patients, pregnancy or cardiac history. Hospitalization is usually required for known black widow spider bite. Recovery usually occurs within 1 week; fatalities are exceedingly rare.

Overdosage/Treatment
Decontamination: Wound care including tetanus prophylaxis; pain and muscle spasm may be managed initially with calcium gluconate 10% solution at 10 mL/dose; may start calcium infusion; mean calcium dose is 1.4 g
Antivenin is available and should be reserved for cases involving respiratory arrest, seizures, uncontrolled hypertension, or pregnancy; usual therapeutic dose: I.V. infusion: 1-2 vials. Monitor for anaphylactoid reactions due to horse serum protein in the antivenom. Pretreatment with SubQ epinephrine 1:1000 (0.01 mL/kg or 0.01 mg/kg; maximum: 0.3 mL) is suggested.
Treatment dose of antivenom: I.V.: 2.5 mL (1 vial) in 50-100 mL of D$_5$W or normal saline infused over ~20-30 minutes
Administration of a second vial is considered for individuals who weigh >40 kg or for patients who do not respond to the first dose within 1 hour.
Supportive therapy: Alternative muscle relaxants including methocarbamol or benzodiazepines do not appear to be as effective as calcium for pain control

Antidote(s)
● Antivenin (Latrodectus mactans) [ANTIDOTE]
● Calcium Gluconate [ANTIDOTE]

Additional Information The *Lactrodectus* species is found in the entire North American continent although it prefers warmer climates. It avoids human dwellings and is most often located in corners of buildings, gardens, ground cover, trash piles, stables, outdoor toilets and woodpiles. The female (10-18 mm in size and 4 times larger than the male) is responsible for all envenomations. The venom gland contains ~0.2 mg of venom. The spider exhibits a shiny black color with a red hour glass appearance on the abdomen of the female. Its bite usually occurs on the extremities, with leg bites usually resulting in abdominal pain.

Specific References
Forrester MB and Stanley SK, "Black Widow Spider and Brown Recluse Spider Bites in Texas from 1998 Through 2002," *Vet Hum Toxicol*, 2003, 45(5):270-3.
Gonzales VA, Vazquez IM, Robles GD, et al, "Measuring Pain Intensity in Patients with Latrodectism: The Visual Analog Scale (VAS)," *Clin Toxicol (Phila)*, 2005, 43:707.
Hoover NG and Fortenberry JD, "Use of Antivenin to Treat Priapism After a Black Widow Spider Bite," *Pediatrics*, 2004, 114(1):e128-9.
Isbister GK, Graudins A, White J, et al, "Antivenom Treatment in Arachnidism," *J Toxicol Clin Toxicol*, 2003, 41(3):291-300.
Isbister GK and Gray MR, "Effects of Envenoming by Comb-Footed Spiders of the Genera *Steatoda* and *Achaearanea* (Family Theridiidae: Araneae) in Australia," *J Toxicol Clin Toxicol*, 2003, 41(6):809-19.
Pneumatikos IA, Galiatsou E, Goe D, et al, "Acute Fatal Toxic Myocarditis After Black Widow Spider Envenomation," *Ann Emerg Med*, 2003, 41(1):158.

Rogers JJ, Stanford C, and Dart RC, "The Use of Visual Analog Pain Scales in Black Widow Spider Envenomation," *J Anal Toxicol*, 2006, 2(1):46-7.

Bleeding Heart

Scientific Name *Dicentra spectabilis*
Mechanism of Toxic Action Isoquinoline-type alkaloids may cause dermatitis
Signs and Symptoms of Overdose Burning sensation, erythema, pruritus
Overdosage/Treatment
Decontamination: Dermal: Wash thoroughly
Supportive therapy: Antihistamines and corticosteroids as needed
Additional Information Do not confuse with nontoxic hemorrhage heart vine; systemic toxicity not seen in humans. Toxic part: All parts are toxic; foliage and roots are most toxic

Blue-Ringed Octopus

Mechanism of Toxic Action Bite - envenomation; autonomic ganglia blockade; maculotoxin (tetrodotoxin)
Adverse Reactions
Central nervous system: Ataxia, perioral and intra-oral anesthesia
Neuromuscular & skeletal: Flaccid muscular paralysis, paresthesia
Respiratory: Respiratory depression
Signs and Symptoms of Overdose Aphonia, blurred vision, burning sensation, coma, local ischemia, numbness, pain, paresthesia, respiratory collapse, slurred speech
Admission Criteria/Prognosis All patients should be observed at least 12-24 hours
Overdosage/Treatment
Decontamination: No antivenin
Supportive therapy: Symptomatic and supportive; for serious envenomations, be prepared to provide artificial ventilation, wound care
Additional Information Range: Waters off the coast of Australia

Boston Ivy

Scientific Name *Parthenocissus tricuspidata*
Mechanism of Toxic Action Leaves are toxic and contain soluble and insoluble oxalates
Signs and Symptoms of Overdose
Dermal: Irritation, pain, swelling; may also cause dermatitis
Ocular: Sap may cause corneal abrasion, lacrimation, pain, photophobia
Oral: Diarrhea, dysphonia, edema, salivation, vomiting
Miscellaneous: Hypocalcemia, renal injury due to calcium oxalate precipitation
Overdosage/Treatment
Decontamination: Oral: Dilute; ipecac/lavage/activated charcoal not likely necessary; milk/water to dilute
Supportive therapy: For treatment of soluble oxalates, which may cause systemic oxalate toxicity, keep well hydrated, monitor renal function, fluid/electrolytes; hypocalcemia may occur which can be treated with calcium gluconate, monitor urine for crystals; treat other symptoms supportively

Box Jellyfish

Related Information
- Jellyfish
- Sea Wasp

Scientific Name *Carybdea rastonii* (Jimble); *Chironex fleckeri*; *Chiropsalmus marsupialis*; *Chiropsalmus quadrigatus*; *Chiropsalmus quadrumanus*; *Scyphozoa* Class
Mechanism of Toxic Action Sting, venom; lethal fraction and lethal hemolytic-dermatonecrotic fraction. The neurotoxin may cause an influx of calcium ion into the cell.
Adverse Reactions
Cardiovascular: Hypotension, cardiovascular collapse, vasoconstriction
Dermatologic: Vesicular dermal eruption; pruritus; edema. Red-brown to purple flare pattern. Skin blisters can develop within 6 hours. Skin necrosis can develop in 12-18 hours.
Central nervous system: CNS depression, coma
Local: Wheal
Musculoskeletal: Muscle spasm, cramps
Ocular: Conjunctivitis, corneal ulcer, iritis, chemosis
Respiratory: Wheezing, pulmonary edema, respiratory depression/collapse
Signs and Symptoms of Overdose Symptoms usually do not develop for 6-12 hours; atrioventricular block, cardiovascular collapse, coma, erythema, hypotension, laryngeal edema, nausea, pain, respiratory depression, vomiting. An annular or ladder-like pattern of small papular or wheal-like eruptions may suggest a box jellyfish sting.

Overdosage/Treatment
Decontamination: Rapidly assess airway; support with artificial ventilation, if necessary; immediately rinse with seawater, should then prevent further envenomation by applying acetic acid 5% (vinegar) to any tentacles still adhering to tissue; if acetic acid is not available, use isopropyl alcohol 40% to 70% or finally may use aluminum sulfate; following dermal decontamination, shave the area with a scalpel, then repeat local decontamination therapy. Ocular exposures are to be decontaminated by water irrigation only. **Do not** rub affected area. Wear gloves during decontamination. Meat tenderizers have been used, however, they are not preferred decontamination measures and should not have prolonged contact times (>10 minutes). Do not use fresh water, in that, nematocyst firing may occur. Nematocysts can be removed by using sticky tape. Cold packs can be applied to the affected area.
Supportive therapy: Give intravenous fluids (isotonic saline) to treat hypotension
Antivenin should be administered I.V. diluted 1:5 with isotonic crystalloid; dose equals 1 ampul or 20,000 units over 5 minutes; if administered I.M., use 3 ampuls or 60,000 units
Antivenin available in Australia through Commonwealth Serum Laboratories, Melbourne.
Additional Information Most venomous of all sea creatures; appears as a gelatinous umbrella with multiple long tentacles. The stinging apparatus is located at the outer surface of the tentacles or near its tubular mouth. Stings from tentacles >5 meters result in severe symptoms; use of verapamil is still controversial. Range: Found chiefly in the waters off Northern Queensland, Australia; may be found in the open ocean
Specific Reference
Currie BJ, "Marine Antivenoms," *J Toxicol Clin Toxicol*, 2003, 41(3):301-8.

Box Thorn

Scientific Name *Lycium halimifolium*
Mechanism of Toxic Action The whole plant may contain atropine and other anticholinergic compounds
Adverse Reactions Cardiovascular: Sinus tachycardia
Signs and Symptoms of Overdose Constipation, delirium, dry mouth, mydriasis, tachycardia
Overdosage/Treatment
Decontamination: Ipecac (within 30 minutes)/lavage (within 1 hour), activated charcoal, cathartic may be considered in large ingestions
Supportive therapy: Propranolol may be used for tachyarrhythmias
Antidote(s)
- Physostigmine [ANTIDOTE]

Breynia officinalis

Mechanism of Toxic Action Can cause direct liver toxicity and is a mucosal irritant
Adverse Reactions
Ingestion:
Cardiovascular: Hypertension
Central nervous system: Vertigo, headache, numbness, fatigue
Gastrointestinal: Vomiting, diarrhea, bloody diarrhea, gastritis
Hepatic: Hepatomegaly, hepatitis
Renal: Hematuria
Overdosage/Treatment
Decontamination: Activated charcoal
Supportive therapy: Monitor liver function tests; administer H_2 blocking agents to treat gastritis
Additional Information Often marketed as a herbal drug under the proprietary name "Chi R Yun," which has been used to treat venereal diseases, growth retardation, and heart failure. Hepatotoxicity usually occurs within 1 day of ingestion and lasts for 2-4 weeks.

Brown Recluse Spider

Scientific Name *Loxosceles reclusa*
Mechanism of Toxic Action Toxin has sphingomyelinase activity which has lytic action on red blood cells
Signs and Symptoms of Overdose Mild erythema and pruritus can progress to severe skin ulceration. Systemic findings occur at 1-3 days and can include: Anemia, dark urine, fever, hemolysis, hemolytic anemia, hypotension, myalgias, myopathy, nausea, severe vomiting, thrombocytopenia. The bite site may have a "halo" appearance with a small pustule surrounded by pallor. The wound can become necrotic in 3 days. Death may be related to disseminated intravascular coagulation or renal failure.
Admission Criteria/Prognosis Hospitalization usually not required acutely; necrotic lesions may require hospitalization 2-3 days postexposure; patients with rapidly expanding lesions or evidence of hemolysis should be admitted
Overdosage/Treatment Supportive therapy: Elevate affected limb; antihistamine may be given for pruritus; dexamethasone (4 mg I.M. 4 times/day)

can be helpful if given early in the course; dapsone (50-200 mg orally divided into twice daily dosing) or colchicine (1.2 mg orally, then 0.6 mg every 2 hours for 2 days, then 0.6 mg every 4 hours for 2 days) may be helpful to avoid cutaneous necrosis; ice packs may relieve pain/heat may exacerbate pain; hyperbaric oxygen has been used (2-6 days postbite) in order to improve necrotic lesions. Hyperbaric oxygen if used within 48 hours may reduce skin necrosis. A recent rabbit study did not reveal any benefit of hyperbaric oxygen, dapsone, or cyproheptadine in the treatment of brown recluse spider envenomation. Nitro-patches applied over the bite site for 12 hours may be helpful in reducing pain and skin necrosis, although it must be noted that this method is unproven and has not been formally studied.

Antidote(s)
- Oxygen (Hyperbaric) [ANTIDOTE]

Additional Information Bites usually occur at night; dorsal cephalothorax has characteristic fiddle-shaped marking. Range: South/Southwestern U.S., Illinois, Iowa, Ohio, not found in Pacific northwest; necrotic arachnidism is likely due to *Tegenaria agrestis* bites

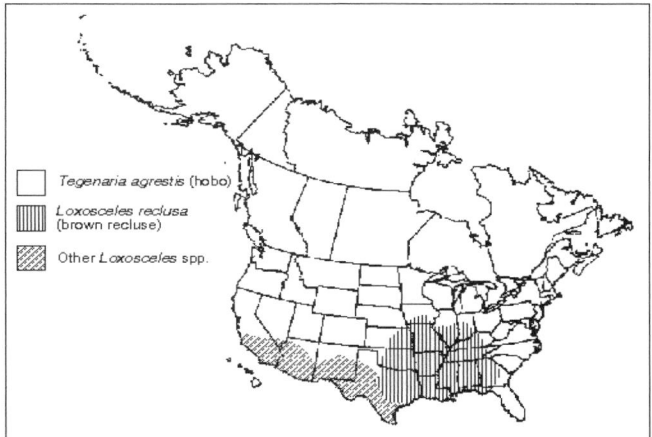

Key:
- ☐ *Tegenaria agrestis* (hobo)
- ▥ *Loxosceles reclusa* (brown recluse)
- ▨ Other *Loxosceles* spp.

From "Necrotic Arachnidism," *MMWR Morb Mortal Wkly Rep*, 1996, 45(21):435.

Specific References

Atilla R, Cevik AA, Atilla OD, et al, "Clinical Course of a Loxosceles Spider Bite in Turkey," *Vet Hum Toxicol*, 2004, 46(6):306-8.

Bryant SM and Pittman LM, "Dapsone Use in *Loxosceles Reclusa* Envenomation: Is There an Indication?" *Am J Emerg Med*, 2003, 21(1):89-90.

Forrester MB and Stanley SK, "Black Widow Spider and Brown Recluse Spider Bites in Texas from 1998 Through 2002," *Vet Hum Toxicol*, 2003, 45(5):270-3.

Hogan CJ, Barbaro KC, and Winkel K, "Loxoscelism: Old Obstacles, New Directions," *Ann Emerg Med*, 2004, 44(6):608-24.

Hostetler MA, Dribben W, Wilson DB, et al, "Sudden Unexplained Hemolysis Occurring in an Infant Due to Presumed Loxosceles Envenomation," *J Emerg Med*, 2003, 25(3):277-82.

Isbister GK, Graudins A, White J, et al, "Antivenom Treatment in Arachnidism," *J Toxicol Clin Toxicol*, 2003, 41(3):291-300.

Vetter RS and Bush SP, "Additional Considerations in Presumptive Brown Recluse Spider Bites and Dapsone Therapy," *Am J Emerg Med*, 2004, 22(6):494-5.

Buckeye

Scientific Name *Aesculus californica*; *Aesculus glabra*; *Aesculus parviflora*

Mechanism of Toxic Action Contains aesculin which is a mixture of saponins and is cytotoxic

Signs and Symptoms of Overdose Diarrhea, oral irritation, vomiting. Repeat exposure or large amounts in small children may also produce ataxia, CNS depression, muscle asthenia, myoclonus, and paralysis.

Overdosage/Treatment
Decontamination: 1-2 berries: Activated charcoal alone may be more beneficial than vomiting since effects of ipecac are similar to toxicity; more than 1-2 berries may cause more severe GI effects and systemic effects, therefore, use of ipecac may be worthwhile to prevent more serious effects; cathartics should be avoided

Supportive therapy: Maintain proper electrolyte and fluid balance, support cardiac and respiratory function if necessary; monitor fluid and electrolytes

Additional Information Toxic dose: 1-2 seeds may cause gastroenteritis only; repeat exposures allow saponin absorption through irritated mucous membranes. Aesculin content in seeds varies with growth and peaks in mid-July to mid-August. Toxic part: Young leaves, flowers, and bark are most toxic

Buffalo Pea

Scientific Name *Thermopsis montana*; *Thermopsis rhombifolia*

Mechanism of Toxic Action Flowers and seeds contain quinololizidine alkaloids

Signs and Symptoms of Overdose Abdominal cramping, dizziness, headache, nausea, oral irritation, tachycardia, tremors, vomiting

Admission Criteria/Prognosis Patients who are asymptomatic 10 hours postingestion can be discharged home

Overdosage/Treatment
Decontamination: Lavage within 1 hour; activated charcoal can be given
Supportive therapy: Rehydration with I.V. crystalloid solution

Additional Information Found in Western Canada; seed ingestions may exhibit a longer delay of symptoms; flower ingestions become symptomatic within 3 hours

Bufotenine

CAS Number 487-93-4

Commonly Found In Skin glands (parotid glands) of toads (*Bufo alvarius*, Colorado river toad) and *Bufo marinus* (cane toad); in the seeds and leaves of *Piptadenia peregrina* and *Piptadenia macrocarpa*; found in the Chinese preparation Yixin Wan, Kyushin, and Lu-Shen Wan; also found in the mushrooms *Amanita citrina*, *Amanita porphyria*, and *Amanita tomentella*

Mechanism of Toxic Action Indole alkaloid with serotonergic activity; also inhibits sodium, potassium, and muscle ATPase activity in muscle similar to digoxin

Signs and Symptoms of Overdose Cardiac arrhythmias similar to digitalis toxicity, dyspnea, hypokalemia, salivation, seizures

Admission Criteria/Prognosis Asymptomatic patients with normal electrocardiogram and electrolytes can be discharged after a 12-hour observation; any symptomatic patient should be admitted to a cardiac monitor bed

Reference Range Serum digoxin levels as high as 3.9 ng/mL have been described

Overdosage/Treatment
Decontamination: Activated charcoal with cathartic may be effective in ingestions; mucous membranes should be flushed with water

Supportive therapy: Diazepam or lorazepam may be utilized for agitation or seizures; phenobarbital is also effective for seizures; although it is unproven in a clinical setting, digoxin specific Fab antibodies can be considered if a toxic arrhythmia develops (5-10 vials); atropine can be utilized for bradyarrhythmias while phenytoin can be used for ventricular arrhythmias

Enhancement of elimination: Multiple dosing of activated charcoal may be effective

Antidote(s)
- Digoxin Immune Fab [ANTIDOTE]

Test Interactions Cross reacts to give a positive digoxin reading in immunoreactive assays; cardioactive steroids of the bufadienolide class may cross react with polyclonal digoxin immunoassays

Additional Information Hyperkalemia can be a prognostic sign in overdose situations. Usual mechanism of abuse is through licking the skin of the toad, although "toad smoking" and ingestions have occurred; the Colorado river toad is found in the Sonoran desert of Northern Mexico along with southern California and Arizona; while the toads primarily live underground, they do emerge during the rainy season in midsummer; not centrally active at oral doses of 50 mg or I.V. doses of 20 mg or I.M. doses of 40 mg; 100 kg of *Amanita citrina* contains only 7 g of bufotenine. Adverse reactions to bufotenin should be reported to FDA's Med Watch Program: (800)332-1088.

Bushmaster

Scientific Name *Lachesis mutus*

Signs and Symptoms of Overdose Coagulopathy

Overdosage/Treatment
Decontamination: Rapid transport to medical facility; immobilize area; if negative pressure suction device is available, this may be used; **do not** incise the wound; constriction band may be applied, not a tourniquet; ABC assessment, physical exam; mark extent of local edema with skin-marking pen

Supportive therapy: Repeat lab testing every 3-4 hours for first 12 hours; I.V. fluids, tetanus prophylaxis and analgesics may need to be given; antibiotics may be indicated for infected wound sites; antivenin indicated for moderate to severe envenomation

Antidote: Wyeth crotalid polyvalent antivenin: Treat moderate to severe envenomations with increments of 5-10 vials at a time; skin test per manufacturer's instructions; if positive, may prophylax with H_1- and H_2-histamine receptor blockers; give until local injury has stopped and coagulopathy is reversed; complications include allergic reaction, anaphylaxis, and delayed serum sickness

Antidote(s)
- Antivenin (Crotalidae) Polyvalent [ANTIDOTE]

Additional Information Largest American poisonous snake (length to 12 feet); unlike other pit vipers, lays eggs from which young are hatched

Buttercup

Scientific Name *Ranunculus aquatilis*
Mechanism of Toxic Action Contains protoanemonin, which reacts with SH groups to produce irritation and vesication, excreted unchanged in urine
Signs and Symptoms of Overdose Abdominal cramps, blistering, bloody diarrhea, contact dermatitis, pain and swelling, potential for renal irritation or damage if a large enough amount is ingested, salivation, vomiting, ulceration
Toxicodynamics/Kinetics Significant dermal symptoms may take several weeks to resolve
Overdosage/Treatment
Decontamination: Avoid use of ipecac or cathartics, consider lavage (within 1 hour) and/or activated charcoal with large ingestion to prevent systemic absorption and possibility of subsequent renal irritation
Supportive therapy: Maintain fluid and electrolytes, maintain adequate urine flow in large overdose; monitor symptomatic patients for fluid or electrolyte deficiencies
Additional Information Toxic dose: Not established, but overdose producing systemic effects is unlikely due to painful skin contact. Plant is most toxic during flowering stage. Toxic part: Sap

Caterpillars

Commonly Found In Larvae of *Lepidoptera* (moths and butterflies)
Mechanism of Toxic Action Caterpillar spines and spicules can cause an urticarial dermatitis; stings by *Lonomia obliqua* and *Lonomia achelous* may cause a hemorrhagic syndrome (melena, hematuria, ecchymosis); coagulopathy may last 1 month
Adverse Reactions
Central nervous system: Fever, malaise, headache, seizures (*Megalopyge opercularis* exposures)
Dermatologic: Erythema, urticaria, pruritus, vesiculation (*Megalopyge lanata*), erythema multiforme (*Euproctis chrysorrhoea*), nonimmunologic contact urticaria, vesicular dermal eruptions
Gastrointestinal: Vomiting (after oral ingestion)
Hematologic: Eosinophilia
Neuromuscular & skeletal: Pain (Puss caterpillar can cause severe pain)
Ocular: Eye irritation, photophobia, uveitis, keratoconjunctivitis, lacrimation
Respiratory: Rhinorrhea, bronchitis, dyspnea, bronchospasm
Overdosage/Treatment
Decontamination: **Oral:** Dilute with milk or water. **Dermal:** Apply and strip (with adhesive tape or facial peel) at sting site promptly; spicules can be washed out with running water or can be removed manually with a forceps; intermittent ice application may reduce pain. **Ocular:** Irrigate with water
Supportive therapy: Local symptoms can be treated with a potent topical steroid to a small area over a 2- to 3-day period (ie, Temovate® cream 0.05%, Ultravate™ cream 0.05% or Diprolene® ointment 0.05%); severe cases can be treated with an antihistamine (terfenadine 60 mg 3 times/day) or anti-inflammatory agents (tolmetin sodium 400 mg 3 times/day); codeine, meperidine or oxymorphone can be used to treat severe pain; calcium gluconate (10 mL of a 10% solution, I.V.) has been useful to treat pain in a small series of patients
Additional Information Hand and feet are primarily envenomation sites; 61% of patients will experience symptoms for over 24 hours; peak incidence of *Megalopyge opercularis* stings is in the autumn

Caladium

Mechanism of Toxic Action Contains insoluble calcium oxalate crystals which cause mechanical injury
Signs and Symptoms of Overdose Ocular: Contact with sap may produce corneal abrasion, lacrimation, pain, photophobia, and deposition of calcium oxalate crystals on corneal epithelium
Oral: Dysphonia, irritation, pain, swelling, vomiting
Toxicodynamics/Kinetics Irritation is immediate
Overdosage/Treatment
Decontamination: **Oral:** Dilute; ipecac/lavage/activated charcoal/cathartic not likely necessary; milk/water to rinse crystals. **Dermal:** Wash thoroughly. **Ocular:** Irrigate with tepid water for 15 minutes
Supportive therapy: Cool compresses may minimize pain and swelling
Additional Information Contact with sap or mouthful ingestions may produce symptoms. Ice or popsicles may help oral irritation, especially in children. Toxic part: Whole plant including sap

Calla

Scientific Name *Zantedeschia aethiopica*
Mechanism of Toxic Action Contains insoluble calcium oxalate crystals which cause mechanical irritation

Signs and Symptoms of Overdose
Oral: Diarrhea, dysphonia, edema, salivation, vomiting
Dermal: Irritation, pain, swelling
Ocular: Sap may cause corneal abrasion, lacrimation, pain, and photophobia; oxalate crystals may be deposited on cornea; may also cause dermatitis
Toxicodynamics/Kinetics Rapid onset of local symptoms
Overdosage/Treatment
Decontamination: **Dermal:** Wash thoroughly. **Ocular:** Irrigate. **Oral:** Dilute; ipecac/lavage/activated charcoal with cathartic not likely necessary; milk/water to rinse crystals
Supportive therapy: Cool compresses may minimize pain and swelling
Additional Information Symptoms dependent on liberation of oxalate crystals or contact with sap, dried plant will not liberate crystals; wide variation in potential for toxicity between plants; treat symptoms. Toxic part: Whole plant

Campylobacter jejuni Food Poisoning

Commonly Found In Poultry, meat, dairy products
Mechanism of Toxic Action Heat labile enterotoxin; incubation period: 1-7 days
Adverse Reactions Central nervous system: Guillain-Barré syndrome (within 3 months of infection - median 9 days)
Signs and Symptoms of Overdose Abdominal pain, bloody diarrhea, cramping, diarrhea, feces discoloration (red), fever, malaise, vomiting
Admission Criteria/Prognosis Patients with dehydration (who cannot take fluids orally), immunocompromised patients, severe disturbance in electrolytes or acid-base status, or patients at extreme in terms of age group should be considered for admission
Overdosage/Treatment The organism is sensitive *in vitro* to many common antimicrobial agents including erythromycin, ciprofloxacin, tetracyclines, aminoglycosides, and others. Ampicillin or penicillin should usually be avoided, and the susceptibility to co-trimoxazole is variable. Most patients with *Campylobacter* enteritis do not require antibiotics; they recover quickly without sequelae. Antimicrobial therapy should be targeted towards the more acutely ill patient. Limited clinical trials suggest that the following groups may benefit from the prompt use of antibiotics: children with severe dysentery, adults with severe bloody diarrhea and fever, individuals with worsening symptoms when seeking medical attention, and prolonged diarrhea (>1 week). Treatment with antibiotics does not prolong the fecal carriage of *C. jejuni* (as opposed to *Salmonella*). The drug of choice is erythromycin. For the toxic patient, combination therapy may be useful, but consultation should be made with an Infectious Disease specialist.
Diagnostic Procedures
• Stool Culture
Additional Information
Febrile seizures may occur in children; meningitis or endocarditis may occur as may Guillain-Barré syndrome
Microbiology:
Campylobacter jejuni is a curved, gram-negative bacillus which is the most common cause of bacterial diarrhea in the United States; on Gram's stain, *Campylobacter jejuni* appears as a curved, comma-shaped, gram-negative rod which often has a distinctive "seagull wing" appearance
Campylobacter jejuni is a microaerophilic organism and fails to grow under routine aerobic and anaerobic conditions. The laboratory should be informed that *C. jejuni* is suspected clinically and a special request made for *Campylobacter* culture. A 5% to 10% oxygen, 5% to 10% carbon dioxide, and 80% to 90% nitrogen atmosphere is generally used to facilitate growth.
Epidemiology: Infection with this agent occurs worldwide. With >2 million cases per year in the U.S., *Campylobacter*-induced enteritis is more common than *Salmonella* and *Shigella* combined. The organism is found in the gastrointestinal flora of a number of wild and domestic animals, most notably in chickens. Transmission to humans generally occurs by consumption of the meat or milk of an infected animal, consumption of water contaminated with the feces of infected animals (eg, mountain streams), or fecal-oral transmission from an infected human or household pet. Undercooked chicken is notorious for transmission of *C. jejuni*, accounting for >50% of the cases of campylobacteriosis. Outbreaks have been linked to unpasteurized goat's cheese, clams, and untreated stream water in Wyoming. Infection occurs year-round but is most common in the summer months.
Clinical Syndromes:
• **Acute enteritis:** The organism can cause destructive, ulcerative changes in the mucosal surfaces of the small intestine (especially jejunum and distal ileum) and colon. Invasion of the organism causes inflammation of the lamina propria, bowel wall edema, and crypt abscesses. Patients initially present with nonspecific symptoms such as fever, headache, and myalgias. One to 2 days later, there is crampy abdominal pain and diarrhea. The quality and severity of the diarrhea is variable (although usually mild), and stools may be frequent and watery

or visibly bloody. Most cases resolve spontaneously without antimicrobial therapy within 1 week. Less commonly, a fulminant acute colitis may occur. Again, a nonspecific prodrome of fever and malaise precedes any gastrointestinal complaints. However, the diarrhea which follows is voluminous and bloody with large amounts of mucus. Tenesmus is common and further suggests involvement of the colon. Fevers can reach 40°C and occasionally the patient can appear in extremis. This syndrome may be confused with bacillary dysentery from *Shigella* species, severe salmonellosis, or even the initial presentation of inflammatory bowel disease (particularly if it is in a young adult). Toxic megacolon may complicate the hospital course.

• **Appendicitis-like syndrome:** Occasionally, *C. jejuni* can cause right lower quadrant pain mimicking appendicitis, without diarrhea. This "pseudoappendicitis" has been seen in association with other enteric pathogens including *Yersinia enterocolitica*.

• **Bacteremia:** This is an unusual finding in *C. jejuni* infection (even when the patient is febrile), unlike *Campylobacter fetus* which is commonly recovered from the blood. Blood cultures may turn positive several days after a mild diarrheal illness has already resolved; in such cases, antibiotic therapy is usually unnecessary. In other cases, bacteremia may be sustained, particularly in immunocompromised hosts, and this may suggest a deep focus of infection. Infectious disease consultation is appropriate in such cases since prolonged antimicrobial therapy may be necessary.

• **Septic abortion:** *C. jejuni* infection in the pregnant female may lead to this complication. However, *Campylobacter* bacteremia during pregnancy does not automatically justify a therapeutic abortion since the outcome is not uniformly poor.

Diagnosis: *Campylobacter jejuni* should be suspected in any case of acute gastroenteritis or fulminant colitis. The findings of fecal leukocytes and occult blood in the stool are suggestive of campylobacteriosis and other gastrointestinal infections such as those caused by *Salmonella* sp, *Shigella* sp, enteroinvasive *E. coli*, enterohemorrhagic *E. coli* (0157:H7), Crohn's disease or ulcerative colitis, and others. The diagnosis is confirmed by a positive stool culture for *C. jejuni* or positive blood cultures for the organism.

Cashew

Scientific Name *Anacardium occidentale*

Mechanism of Toxic Action Shell contains anacardic acid, cardol, anacardol, irritants that can precipitate type IV cell-mediated allergic reaction (allergic contact dermatitis)

Signs and Symptoms of Overdose Dermatitis, nausea, vomiting

Toxicodynamics/Kinetics
Onset of effect: Variable, but effects usually seen within 24-48 hours
Peak dermal effect: After 3-5 days

Overdosage/Treatment
Decontamination: Soap and water washing likely ineffective unless done within 5-15 minutes after exposure
Supportive therapy: Cool compresses or showers, Burow's solution, topical/oral steroids

Additional Information Raw nut should not be eaten; may cause dermatitis in persons sensitized to toxicodendron species. Toxic part: Shell contains toxin

Castor Bean

Scientific Name *Ricinus communis*

Mechanism of Toxic Action Contains ricin: A toxalbumin which inhibits protein metabolism and DNA synthesis; can cause agglutination of defibrinated blood *in vitro*

Signs and Symptoms of Overdose Latent symptom period may be as long as 8 hours; abdominal burning, anaphylaxis, bronchospasm, contact dermatitis, diarrhea, elevation of hepatic enzymes and serum creatinine can occur, fever, hematuria, hypotension, GI hemorrhage, GI irritation, general weakness may manifest, miosis and urticaria may manifest, nausea, oropharyngeal burning, seizures, shivering, tachycardia, thirst, vomiting

Admission Criteria/Prognosis Any symptomatic patient should be admitted. Asymptomatic patients may be discharged after an 8- to 10-hour observation.

Toxicodynamics/Kinetics
Absorption: Poorly absorbed orally; can be absorbed by inhalation
Half-life: 48 hours
Elimination: Renal

Monitoring Parameters CBC, liver and renal function, blood sugar

Reference Range Following adult ingestion of 30 beans, plasma and urine ricin levels were 1.5 mcg/L and 0.3 mcg/L, respectively

Overdosage/Treatment
Decontamination: **Oral:** Emesis or lavage within 1 hour with ingestions of 1 castor bean/10 kg body weight. Activated charcoal can be used without a cathartic. **Dermal:** Wash with soap and water. **Inhalation:** Give 100% humidified oxygen. **Ocular:** Copious irrigation with saline for at least 20 minutes

Supportive: Replace fluid/electrolyte loss; suggest alkalinization of urine to prevent hemoglobin agglutination in kidney
Enhanced elimination: Hemodialysis is not useful

Additional Information
By injection, ricin can be quite toxic with: Estimated lethal dose: Humans: 1 mg/kg; Animals: 0.0001 mg/kg. Lethal dose: Oral: ~5-8 seeds.
Chewing the seeds increases the toxic potential with lethality occurring after a 1- or 2-seed ingestion. Ricin is not dialyzable, but is water soluble and heat labile. Seeds and foliage are toxic parts of the plant. Due to ricin's insolubility in oil, castor oil is not toxic and can be used as a laxative or a lubricant in industry. The plant is found in southern United States, Guam, and Hawaii. The bean's hard coat must be ruptured for toxicity to occur. Hepatic/adrenal/renal toxicity may occur after 2-5 days postexposure. As of 1996, 15 deaths in 839 case reports have been documented (most occurring before 1945).

Cathinone

Related Information
• Methcathinone

CAS Number 71031-15-7

Mechanism of Toxic Action Derived from the leaves of the *Catha edulis* (Khat) plant (an evergreen bush which grows up to 5 meters in Eastern Africa at high altitudes); this stimulant possesses local anesthetic, anorectic, and neuromuscular junction blocking activities; may have some monoamine oxidase inhibition properties; similar in action to cocaine or amphetamines

Adverse Reactions
Cardiovascular: Tachycardia, hypertension, palpitations, flushing
Central nervous system: Fever, insomnia, headache, mania, visual/auditory hallucinations, euphoria, psychosis, paranoia, hyperthermia
Gastrointestinal: Xerostomia, anorexia, constipation
Genitourinary: Urinary retention, impotence
Neuromuscular & skeletal: Tremors, rhabdomyolysis
Ocular: Mydriasis
Respiratory: Tachypnea, dyspnea
Miscellaneous: Diaphoresis

Toxicodynamics/Kinetics
Onset of action: 20 minutes
Duration of action: 2 hours
Metabolism: To norephedrine and norpseudoephedrine
Elimination: Renal

Overdosage/Treatment
Decontamination: Lavage (within 1 hour)/activated charcoal with cathartic
Supportive therapy: Agitation can be treated with chlorpromazine, benzodiazepines, or haloperidol; ventricular arrhythmias can be treated with lidocaine, procaine, or bretylium; hyperthermia can be treated with standard cooling techniques (avoid salicylates)
Enhancement of elimination: Multiple dosing of activated charcoal may be effective; although acid diuresis may enhance its elimination, this modality is not recommended due to its danger in exacerbating renal failure due to rhabdomyolysis

Test Interactions May result in false-positive urinary amphetamine or phenylpropanolamine radioimmunoassay test

Additional Information
Toxic dose: Khat (0.1% to 0.3% cathinone): 100-200 g Anorexiant: 15-60 mg.
Khat is usually utilized by chewing the leaves and swallowing its juice; red khat has a higher cathinone content than white khat; khat addiction can be treated with bromocriptine mesylate (1.25 mg every 6 hours as an initial dose); for medicinal purposes (as an anorexiant): 15-60 mg

Century Plant

Scientific Name *Agave americana*

Mechanism of Toxic Action Contains insoluble calcium oxalate crystals which cause mechanical irritation; may also cause dermatitis

Signs and Symptoms of Overdose
Oral: Dysphonia, diarrhea, edema, salivation, vomiting
Dermal: Irritation, pain, swelling
Ocular: Sap may cause corneal abrasion, lacrimation, pain, and photophobia; oxalate crystals may be deposited on cornea; may also cause dermatitis

Toxicodynamics/Kinetics Onset of action: Rapid onset of local symptoms due to oxalate; dermatitis reaction may develop within a few hours

Overdosage/Treatment
Decontamination: **Oral:** Dilute; ipecac/lavage/activated charcoal with cathartic not likely necessary. **Dermal:** Wash thoroughly; antihistamines/steroids may be useful. **Ocular:** Irrigate
Supportive therapy: Cool compresses may minimize pain and swelling

Additional Information Toxic part: Sap, although other parts may be also (especially thorns)

Cherry

Scientific Name *Prunus serotina*

Mechanism of Toxic Action Contains amygdalin, a cyanogenic glycoside hydrolyzed to hydrocyanic acid in the gut, complexes with cytochrome oxidase to produce cellular hypoxia after absorption

Signs and Symptoms of Overdose Abdominal pain, coma, cyanosis, drowsiness, dyspnea, headache, lethargy, paralysis, seizures, sweating, vomiting

Overdosage/Treatment

Decontamination: Basic poison management; vomiting is contraindicated due to rapid course of the neurologic symptoms; give 100% oxygen

Supportive therapy: Give sodium bicarbonate for acidosis; cyanide antidote kit should be used for patients symptomatic from cyanide toxicity

Enhancement of elimination: Hemodialysis and charcoal hemoperfusion have been utilized; hyperbaric oxygen may also be utilized; hydroxocobalamin and dicobalt-EDTA used for chelation in Europe

Additional Information Toxic dose: 1-2 pits likely nontoxic, toxicity uncommon after accidental ingestion. Intact pit does not release CN

Chicken Soup

Scientific Name *Gallus domesticus* (in a broth)

Uses Food product; has been advocated to treat emaciation, upper respiratory tract infections, leprosy, asthma, and for aircraft-fuel (sodium chloride)

Mechanism of Toxic Action High sodium content

Adverse Reactions Gastrointestinal: Salty taste

Signs and Symptoms of Overdose Coma, dehydration, delirium, hyperchlorhydria, hypernatremia, hyperosmolarity, tachycardia

Overdosage/Treatment

Decontamination: Gastric: Activated charcoal probably is not useful; Ocular: Irrigate copiously with water

Supportive therapy: For hypernatremia, give 30-50 mEq/L of sodium (half chloride, half bicarbonate) by slow I.V. infusion; prepare solution by adding 15-25 mEq/L sodium chloride (2.5 mEq/mL) and 15-25 mEq sodium bicarbonate (1 mEq/mL) to 1 liter D_5W; administer at a rate of $2/3$ maintenance with a goal of achieving normal serum sodium at 24-36 hours after initiating treatment; seizures may occur if serum sodium is lowered too quickly; seizures can be treated with lorazepam or diazepam 0.1-0.25 mg/kg; hypernatremia is resolved through the use of diuretics and free water replacement

Enhancement of elimination: Peritoneal dialysis should be considered in infants who are salt poisoned; hemodialysis should be considered in patients who are refractory to other therapies on in patients with renal impairment

Additional Information Should **not** be given in large amounts to infants or the elderly. Contains sodium cytarabine hexa-methyl-acetyl lututric tetrazolamine (schmaltz). Some broths may contain from 200-250 mEq/L sodium. A therapeutic effect has been documented for the common cold by one study (Saketkhoo, et al) which demonstrated an increased nasal mucous velocity following hot chicken soup ingestion. The Campbell's® Low Sodium Chicken Noodle soup contains ~1.5 mg of sodium per serving ounce of soup (2.17 mEq/L) and ~1 mEq of potassium per ounce. Patients with significant renal impairment should reduce their portion or further dilute low-sodium formulations of chicken soup. Monitoring parameters: Sodium serum osmolarity

Christmas Cherry

Scientific Name *Solanum pseudocapsicum*

Mechanism of Toxic Action Contains solanocapsine, an alkaloid related to salanine that is structurally similar to a cardiac glycoside and has irritant effect similar to saponins

Adverse Reactions

Cardiovascular: Sinus bradycardia

Central nervous system: Psychosis

Signs and Symptoms of Overdose Bradycardia, diarrhea, drowsiness, headache, hypotension, nausea, vomiting

Toxicodynamics/Kinetics Effects expected within 2-24 hours

Overdosage/Treatment

Decontamination: If necessary due to large ingestion, use ipecac (within 30 minutes) if soon after ingestion; otherwise, consider activated charcoal with cathartic or lavage within 1 hour

Supportive therapy: Maintain proper fluid and electrolyte balance

Additional Information Toxic dose: Unclear, but large amount likely necessary for toxicity. Potential for solamine toxicity but no cases on record

Christmas Rose

Mechanism of Toxic Action Primary toxicity relates to proteoanemonin which reacts with SH groups to produce vesicant action; also contains saponins that act as irritants

Signs and Symptoms of Overdose Abdominal pain, bloody diarrhea, oral numbness, seizures, vomiting

Toxicodynamics/Kinetics Significant dermal symptoms may take several weeks to resolve

Overdosage/Treatment

Decontamination: Avoid use of ipecac or cathartics, consider lavage within 1 hour and/or activated charcoal with large ingestion to prevent systemic absorption and possibility of subsequent renal irritation

Supportive therapy: Maintain fluid and electrolytes, maintain adequate urine flow in large overdose; monitor symptomatic patients for fluid or electrolyte deficiencies

Additional Information Small amounts likely to produce symptoms; Family: Buttercup; Toxic part: Entire plant; digitalis toxicity; varies within the species and is not seen in *Helleborus niger*

Chrysanthemum

Scientific Name *Chrysanthemum*

Adverse Reactions Dermatologic: Photoallergy

Signs and Symptoms of Overdose Allergic dermatitis, pruritus, erythema, hives, localized edema

Overdosage/Treatment

Decontamination: Wash skin with soap and water

Supportive therapy: Oral or topical corticosteroids or diphenhydramine may be beneficial

Additional Information Ingestion of large amounts of flowers may cause pyrethrin-type toxicity

Ciguatera Food Poisoning

Related Information

- Neurotoxic Shellfish Poisoning

Commonly Found In Amberjack, barracuda, dolphin, eel, emperor fish, red snapper, sea bass, surgeon fish in Caribbean or South Pacific oceans

Mechanism of Toxic Action Due to ingestion of dinoflagellates, ciguatoxin accumulates in larger fish; affects membranes and ionic flux of nervous tissue. Ciguatoxin is a lipid soluble toxin which modulates sodium ion entry in neuronal tissue, thus producing sustained depolarization. Other toxins include maitotoxin (a hemolysin) and palytoxin (which inhibits sodium-potassium ATPase, thus resulting in muscle contractions and rhabdomyolysis).

Adverse Reactions

Dermatologic: Pruritus

Gastrointestinal: Nausea, vomiting, diarrhea, abdominal cramping

Genitourinary: Balanitis, dyspareunia

Neuromuscular & skeletal: Peripheral neuropathy, cold allodynia

Signs and Symptoms of Overdose Three phases:

Phase I (1-6 hours postingestion): Abdominal pain, gastrointestinal symptoms, headache, nausea, vomiting, watery diarrhea

Phase II (6-12 hours postingestion): Neurologic symptoms: Adynamic ileus, extremity paresthesias, heat-cold reversal. Blurred vision, metallic taste, myalgia, pruritus, and sinus bradycardia are also common.

Phase III (>12 hours postingestion): Ataxia, dysesthesia, hypotension, hypothermia, weakness; respiratory complications are rare

Admission Criteria/Prognosis Admit if there is significant volume loss; neurologic symptoms (within 24 hours postingestion), or bradycardia occurs; patients with dehydration (who cannot take fluids orally), immunocompromised patients, severe disturbance in electrolytes or acid-base status, or patients at extreme in terms of age group should be considered for admission

Overdosage/Treatment

Decontamination: Activated charcoal (a cathartic is usually not required); avoid magnesium containing cathartics

Supportive therapy: Atropine is useful for bradycardia (sinus); amitriptyline (25 mg twice daily), nifedipine, or mannitol (1 g/kg over 30-45 minutes) has been used for paresthesias with some effect; fluid/electrolyte replacement; atropine can be utilized for treatment of symptomatic hypotension; crystalloid fluids are initial therapy for hypotension; dopamine is a vasopressor of choice if necessary; gabapentin (400 mg 3 times/day, orally) may be helpful in treating pruritus and dysesthesia

Antidote(s)

- Mannitol [ANTIDOTE]

Diagnostic Procedures

- Electrolytes, Blood

Additional Information Ciguatoxin is odorless and tasteless. Minimum pathogenic dose of ciguatoxin: 0.6 ng/kg; stable in heat and gastric acid. Can be transmitted through sexual intercourse. May occur in farm-raised salmon. Mortality rate: 0.1%. Duration of acute GI symptoms: 8.5 hours.

Specific References

Bentur Y and Spanier E, "Evaluation of Ciguatoxin on the Eastern Mediterranean Coast," *J Toxicol Clin Toxicol*, 2004, 42(5):754.

Perkins RA and Morgan SS, "Poisoning, Envenomation, and Trauma from Marine Creatures," *Am Fam Physician*, 2004, 69(4):885-90.

Claviceps purpurea

Commonly Found In A contaminant fungus (ascomycete) which is found in rye, wheat, barley, oats, and bluegrasses; etiologic agent for "St Anthony's Fire." See Mycotoxins

Mechanism of Toxic Action Contains an ergot/alkaloid; additional substances this fungus can produce include histamine, tyramine, isoamylamine, acetylcholine, acetaldehyde, and tryptophan

Adverse Reactions Central nervous system: Psychosis

Signs and Symptoms of Overdose Dysphoria, gangrene, hallucinations, headache, paresthesias, seizures, vasospasm

Overdosage/Treatment

Decontamination: Lavage (within 1 hour)/activated charcoal

Supportive therapy: Seizures can be treated with benzodiazepines initially; phenobarbital or phenytoin can be used for refractory seizures; treatment is symptomatic with captopril, nifedipine, prazosin, vasodilators (nitroprusside) or nitroglycerin for hypertension; phentolamine can also be used; diazepam can be utilized for seizures; heparin, dextran, or corticosteroids can be used for hypercoagulable state; hyperbaric oxygen can be used as an adjunct to treat localized tissue hypoxia. Hyperbaric oxygen can be used to treat peripheral ischemia. Cyproheptadine (orally 4 mg 3 times/day) can be used to reverse ergot-induced vasoconstriction.

Additional Information This mold can invade rye ovaries producing a dark, purplish mass called a sclerotium. Found during warm, rainy weather in the summer and ingested in bread. LSD can be synthesized from one of its ergot alkaloids (ergometrine). Current standards require that <0.3% of grain be contaminated.

Clostridium botulinum Food Poisoning

Related Information
- Antitoxin Botulinin Types A, B, and E [ANTIDOTE]
- Botulinum Toxin Type A
- Botulism, Diagnostic Procedure
- Heroin
- Stool Culture

Commonly Found In Food poisoning: Poorly preserved meat, sausage, fruit, or vegetables (type A or B), marine products (type E), liver pate, venison jerky (type F); black tar heroin-intravenous drug abusers (wound botulism)

Mechanism of Toxic Action An anaerobic, spore-forming, gram-positive bacteria; ingestion of the toxin or wound contamination are likely routes of exposure; a heat labile neurotoxin which causes irreversible neuromuscular blockade and prevents acetylcholine release; the spores are heat-resistant

Signs and Symptoms of Overdose Symptoms may be delayed 12-36 hours. GI symptoms are usually absent in wound botulism. Adynamic ileus, aspiration, blurred vision, constipation followed by descending paralysis and respiratory failure, cranial nerve palsies, dry mouth, dry skin, dysphagia, fasciculations, hyporeflexia, mydriasis, ptosis, slurred speech

Admission Criteria/Prognosis Any suspected exposure or symptomatic patient should be admitted; patients with neurologic toxicity or respiratory failure should be admitted into intensive care unit

Overdosage/Treatment

Decontamination: **Do not** induce vomiting, lavage (within 1 hour) with activated charcoal (sorbitol as a cathartic) may be useful to remove spores if there is a known ingestion; activated charcoal avidly bind to *C. botulinum*, type A neurotoxin. Avoid magnesium-based cathartics since magnesium may enhance neurotoxicity.

Supportive therapy: Primarily respiratory: Mechanical ventilation may be necessary; "tensilon test" up to 10 mg of edrophonium I.V. over 5 minutes; may show improvement in muscle strength in botulism; guanidine (15-50 mg/kg/day orally) may be given (although its use is not proven). Trivalent (A, B, E) (Liosiero) antitoxin should precede administration; give 2 mL of antitoxin diluted in 100 mL of 0.9% saline over 30 minutes; 10 mL of antitoxin may be given in another 2-4 hours, then at 12- to 24-hour intervals as necessary. Sensitivity skin testing should proceed antitoxin administration. Give 20 mL of antitoxin diluted in 100 mL of 0.9% saline over 30 minutes intravenously. 10 mL of antitoxin may be given in another 2-4 hours, then at 12- to 24-hour intervals as necessary. 4-Aminopyridine (0.5 mg/kg I.V. bolus; 0.25 mg/kg/hour continuous infusion I.V.) may improve peripheral strength but not respiratory parameters. Avoid magnesium since it may enhance the action of the toxin. Trivalent (ABE) antitoxin is usually most effective if administered within 24 hours. Usually, only one vial dose is necessary.

Antidote(s)
- Antitoxin Botulinin Types A, B, and E [ANTIDOTE]

Diagnostic Procedures
- Botulism, Diagnostic Procedure

Additional Information

Lethal dose: Humans: 1 pg/kg

Stools or gastric contents may be contagious; infantile botulism has been related to honey ingestion; symptoms may be delayed for 1 week.

Antitoxin can be obtained from the CDC (404-639-3753 [days], 404-639-2888 [nights]).

Electromyogram shows decreased evoked action potential at 2 Hz/sec and an increased evoked action potential at 50 Hz/sec; up to 15% of affected individuals will have normal electromyograms

Thirty-four cases of foodborne botulism have been reported to the CDC in 1994. Boiling food for 10 minutes (>100°C) destroys the toxin; cooked foods should not be kept at room temperature (4°C to 60°C) for longer than 4 hours; recent cases have been associated with commercial pot pies, home-canned foods, asparagus, green beans, peppers, and onions sauteed in margarine.

Twenty-five cases of wound botulism reported in 1995 (23 of them in California, almost all due to intravenous drug injection).

Injection of "black tar" heroin (which has been the predominant form of heroin in the western United States during the 1990's either intramuscularly or subcutaneously) is the primary risk factor for development of wound botulism (46 cases in California from 1988 to 1995).

Type A toxin has the highest case fatality rate; overall fatality rate for foodborne botulism is 5% to 10%; for wound botulism it is 15%

Epidemiology, diagnosis, treatment, prevention, and reporting of infant (intestinal) botulism (*MMWR*, 2003, 52(2):23)

Epidemiology
- Intestinal botulism is the most common form of human botulism reported in the United States; approximately 100 cases are reported annually.
- The majority of cases occur among infants aged ≤6 months; intestinal botulism is seen rarely in adults.
- The majority of cases are caused by botulinum toxin types A and B.
- The case-fatality rate of hospitalized patients is <1%
- Although ingesting honey is a known risk factor, the source of spores for the majority of cases is unknown.
- Ingestion of *Clostridium botulinum* spores, which exist worldwide in the soil and dust, is believed to be the principal route of exposure.

Clinical findings
- Reporting symptoms range from constipation and mild lethargy to hypotonia and respiratory insufficiency.
- Symptoms in infants aged ≤12 months include constipation, lethargy, poor feeding, weak cry, bulbar palsies (eg, ptosis, expressionless face, and difficulty swallowing), and failure to thrive.
- Presenting symptoms might be followed by progressive weakness, impaired respiration, and sometimes death.
- Differential diagnosis includes sepsis, dehydration, Werdnig-Hoffman disease, Guillain-Barré syndrome, myasthenia gravis, drug or toxin ingestions, metabolic disorders, and meningoencephalitis or myelitis.

Laboratory testing
- Laboratory confirmation requires detection of 1) botulinum toxin in stool or serum by using mouse neutralization assay or 2) isolation of toxigenic *C. botulinum* (or related clostridia) in the feces by using stool enrichment culture techniques.
- To avoid delay, treatment should be administered without awaiting laboratory confirmation.

Prevention and reporting
- Avoid feeding honey to infants aged ≤12 months.
- Report all cases to local and state health departments.

Epidemiology, diagnosis, treatment, and prevention of foodborne botulism (*MMWR*, 2003, 52(2):25)

Epidemiology
- Caused by eating foods contaminated with preformed toxins of *Clostridium botulinum*
- Home-canned foods and raw or fermented Alaska Native dishes commonly associated with illness
- During 1973-1998, a total of 814 cases and an annual median of 24 cases (range: 14-94 cases) of foodborne botulism reported in the United States; 236 (29%) in Alaska.
- Humans affected by toxin types A, B, E, and rarely F; type E intoxication associated exclusively with eating marine animals
- Classified as a category A terrorism agent

Clinical findings
- Cranial nerve palsies
- Symmetrically descending flaccid voluntary muscle weakness possibly progressing to respiratory compromise
- Normal body temperature
- Normal sensory nerve examination findings
- Intact mental status despite groggy appearance
- Differential diagnosis includes Guillain-Barré syndrome, myasthenia gravis, stroke, drug overdose, and other entities

Laboratory findings
- Normal cerebrospinal fluid values
- Specific electromyography (EMG) findings including:
  - normal motor conduction velocities
  - normal sensory nerve amplitudes and latencies
  - decreased evoked muscle action potential
  - facilitation following rapid repetitive nerve stimulation

- Standard mouse bioassay positive for toxin from clinical specimens and/or suspect food; requires up to 4 days for final results

Recommended treatment

- Prompt administration of polyvalent equine-source antitoxin:
  - can decrease the progression of paralysis and severity of illness
  - will not reverse existing paralysis
  - available in the United States only through the public health system
- Place suspect cases in an intensive care setting
- Monitor for respiratory function deterioration every 4 hours using forced vital capacity testing.
- Provide mechanical ventilation if necessary

Prevention and control

- Boil raw or fermented Alaska Native dishes and home-canned foods $\geq$ 10 minutes before eating.
- Follow recommended home-canning procedures.
- Notify state health department immediately of suspected cases.

Environmental conditions that facilitate spore growth and germination include pH < 4.6 anaerobic conditions, low salt or sugar content, and temperatures over 4°C (39.2°F)

Symptoms and Physical Findings in Patients with Types A and B Foodborne Botulism

	Percentage of Patients Developing Symptoms or Signs		Significant Difference (p < 0.05)
	Type A	Type B	
Symptoms			
Neurologic Symptoms			
Dysphagia	96	97	0
Dry mouth	9683	97100	00
Diplopia	90	92	0
Dysarthria	100	69	+
Upper extremity weakness	86	64	0
Lower extremity weakness	76	64	0
Blurred vision	100	42	+
Dyspnea	91	34	+
Paresthesia	20	12	0
Gastrointestinal Symptoms			
Constipation	73	73	0
Nausea	73	57	0
Vomiting	70	50	0
Abdominal cramps	33	45	0
Diarrhea	35	8	+
Miscellaneous Symptoms			
Fatigue	92	69	0
Sore throat	75	39	+
Dizziness	86	30	+
Physical Findings			
Cranial Nerve Examination			
Ptosis	96	55	+
Hypoactive gag	81	54	0
Ophthalmoplegia	87	46	+
Facial palsy	84	48	+
Tongue weakness	91	31	+
Pupils fixed or dilated	33	56	0
Nystagmus	44	4	+
Ataxia	24	13	0
Extremity Power			
Upper	91	62	+
Lower	82	59	0
Deep Tendon Reflexes			
Hypoactive or absent	54	29	0
Hyperactive	12	0	0
Altered Sensorium	12	7	0

Adapted from Hughes, et al, "Clinical Features of Types A and B Foodborne Botulism," *Ann Intern Med*, 1981, 95:442-5.

Fermented tofu (soybean curd) may be a media for Botulism Type A. Between 1958 to 1989 home-fermented bean products accounted for 63% of the 2000 cases of food borne botulism in China.

Specific References

Arnon SS, Schecter R, Maslank SE, et al, "Human Botulism Immune Globulin for the Treatment of Infant Botulism," *N Engl J Med*, 2006, 354:462-71.

Horowitz BZ, "Polar Poisons: Did Botulism Doom the Franklin Expedition?" *J Toxicol Clin Toxicol*, 2003, 41(6):841-7.

CDC: Brief Report: Food Borne Botulism from Home-Prepared Fermented Tofu-California, 2006," *MMWR*, 2007, 56(05):96-7.

CDC: "Infant Botulism - New York City, 2001-2002," *MMWR Morb Mortal Wkly Rep*, 2003, 52(2):21-4.

CDC: "Outbreak of Botulism Type E Associated with Eating a Beached Whale - Western Alaska, July 2002," *MMWR Morb Mortal Wkly Rep*, 2003, 52(2): 24-6.

Robinson RF and Nahata MC, "Management of Botulism," *Ann Pharmacother*, 2003, 37(1):127-31.

Clostridium perfringens Poisoning

Related Information

- Botulism, Diagnostic Procedure
- Electrolytes, Blood
- Stool Culture

Commonly Found In Meat, poultry, dairy products, fruits, vegetables, meat-based gravies (food poisoning)

Mechanism of Toxic Action Anaerobic, gram-positive, spore-forming organism; 12 toxins have been associated with toxin A and C causing disease in humans. Enterotoxin causes fluid secretion; incubation period: 12-24 hours; rarely lasts more than 1 day.

Signs and Symptoms of Overdose Abdominal cramps, diarrhea, myocarditis, myopathy; vomiting and fever are rare

Admission Criteria/Prognosis Patients with dehydration (who cannot take fluids orally), immunocompromised patients, severe disturbance in electrolytes or acid-base status, or patients at extreme in terms of age group should be considered for admission

Overdosage/Treatment In general, the treatment of clostridial infection is high-dose penicillin G, to which the organism has remained susceptible. For skin and soft tissue infections, the extent of infection determines the need for surgical debridement. When wounds are simply colonized with clostridia, neither antibiotics nor surgery are indicated. Localized soft tissue infections can often be managed by surgical debridement alone, without antibiotics. When systemic symptoms are present and there is extension of infection into deeper tissues, antibiotics and surgical intervention are required. In fulminant cases of gas gangrene with myonecrosis, immediate surgical intervention (debridement, amputation) is the primary treatment of choice, and antibiotics have little effect. Hyperbaric oxygen with surgery and antibiotic therapy may reduce mortality.

Diagnostic Procedures

- Botulism, Diagnostic Procedure

Additional Information

Heat labile; destroyed by cooking at 100°C

Microbiology: *Clostridium perfringens* is an anaerobic gram-positive rod; occasionally it can appear gram-negative or gram-variable. It is a spore-forming organism, but the spores are not usually seen on Gram's stain. It has been termed "aerotolerant" because of its ability to survive when exposed to oxygen for limited periods of time.

The organism produces 12 toxins active in tissues and several enterotoxins which cause severe diarrhea; four toxins can be lethal. The toxins separate the species into five types, A-E.

- Alpha toxin: A lecithinase which damages cell membranes. It is produced by *C. perfringens* type A. It is the major factor causing tissue damage in *C. perfringens*-induced gas gangrene (myonecrosis). The toxin is a phospholipase which hydrolyzes phosphatidylcholine and sphingomyelin and leads to increased vascular permeability, myocardial depression, hypotension, bradycardia, and shock.
- Enterotoxin: Produced mainly by *C. perfringens* type A but also by types C and D. This toxin is responsible for the diarrheal syndromes classically ascribed to this organism. The enterotoxin binds to intestinal epithelial cells after the human ingests food contaminated with *C. perfringens*. The small bowel (ileum) is primarily involved. The toxin inhibits glucose transport and causes protein loss.
- Beta toxin: Produced by *C. perfringens* type B and C. This toxin causes enteritis necroticans or pigbel. This disease is seen in New Guinea where some natives ingest massive amounts of pork at feasts after first gorging on sweet potatoes. The sweet potatoes have protease inhibitors which prevent the person from degrading the beta toxin which is ingested in the contaminated pork.

Epidemiology: *C. perfringens* is ubiquitous in the environment, being found in soil and decaying vegetation. The organism has been isolated from nearly every soil sample ever examined except in the sand of the

Sahara desert. In the human, *C. perfringens* is common in the human GI tract. In one study, it was found in 28 of 40 adults. It can also be commonly recovered from many mammals including cats, dogs, whales, and others. About 1000 cases of gas gangrene occur yearly in the United States.

Clinical Syndromes:

The organism can be pathogenic, commensal, or symbiotic. Important diseases caused by *C. perfringens* include the following:

• **Food poisoning:** *C. perfringens* is one of the most common causes of food poisoning in the United States. Foods commonly contaminated with *C. perfringens* are meat, poultry, and meat products such as gravies, hash, and stew. Human disease is caused by ingestion of heat-labile toxin; the highest risk comes from meats which are partially cooked, cooled, then reheated. Spores present in the food germinate during the reheating process. Symptoms include watery diarrhea and abdominal cramps, which occur about 12 hours after the meal; fever is generally not part of this illness. Vomiting is unusual. Duration of symptoms is about 24 hours; the diagnosis is made by culturing the stools and, for epidemiological purposes, the food.

• **Pigbel:** See description under Microbiology above. This follows massive ingestion of contaminated pork and sweet potatoes. Incubation period is 24 hours. There is intense abdominal pain, bloody diarrhea, vomiting, shock, and intestinal perforation in some cases; a vaccine is available for travelers.

• **Gas gangrene:** Usually seen near wounds, swelling, crepitus, bullae, can advance at a rate of 2 cm/hour. Nontraumatic gas gangrene has a strong association with underlying malignancy (most often colorectal)

Diagnosis:

The diagnosis of infection by *C. perfringens* begins with a high index of suspicion when a patient presents with one of the clinical syndromes described above. One important caveat is that the laboratory isolation of *C. perfringens* from a necrotic wound does not necessarily imply disease from this organism; many wounds can be colonized. In the right clinical setting, however, a positive *C. perfringens* culture and a compatible clinical presentation are highly suggestive of disease caused by this agent. Gram's stain preparations of wound material, uterine tissue, cervical discharge, muscle tissues, and other relevant materials should be made; a predominance of gram-positive rods should bring anaerobic infection, including *C. perfringens*, to mind.

In patients with clostridial septicemia, accompanying abnormalities may be a clue to clostridial disease before culture confirmation is made. Patients may have disseminated intravascular coagulation with a brisk hemolysis, hemoglobinuria, and proteinuria. X-rays of diseased areas may reveal the presence of gas in muscle or soft tissue; this is suggestive of clostridial infection, although other anaerobes (and aerobes) can cause gas formation. If clostridial myonecrosis is suspected, a muscle biopsy usually performed at the time of tissue debridement, can be diagnostic.

The classic presentation of infant botulism is hypotonia (floppy baby syndrome), constipation, difficulty in feeding, and a weak cry. Some cases of sudden death syndrome have been traced to ingesting honey containing *C. botulinum*. Both *C. botulinum* and *C. butyricum* have been identified as species capable of toxin production. Autointoxication may occur from toxin production during organism growth in tissue, the intestinal tract in both adults and infants, and in wounds.

Cobras

Scientific Name *Boulengerina annulata* (Banded Water Cobra); *Dendraspis* species; *Naja kaouthia* (Asiatic Cobra); *Naja naja arabicus* (Arabian Cobra); *Naja naja naja* (Indian Cobra, Asian Cobra); *Naja nigricollis* (African Spitting Cobra); *Naja nivea* (Cape Cobra)

Mechanism of Toxic Action Venom: Antitoxins that are neuromuscular depolarizing agents; also may contain phospholipases and cardiotoxins

Adverse Reactions

Cardiovascular: Hypotension, cardiovascular collapse, local edema

Central nervous system: Coma, seizures, hyperthermia

Local: Tissue necrosis

Neuromuscular & skeletal: Paresthesias, paralysis

Ocular: Eye pain, conjunctivitis, blindness, corneal injury (with spitting cobra spit), ptosis, ophthalmoplegia

Signs and Symptoms of Overdose Coagulopathy

Admission Criteria/Prognosis All patients should be admitted (probably into an intensive care unit); admit all leg bites; asymptomatic arm/hand bites may be observed for 6 hours and then discharged

Overdosage/Treatment

Decontamination: Rapid transport to medical facility; immobilize area; if negative pressure suction device is available, this may be used; **do not** incise the wound; constriction band may be applied, not a tourniquet; ABC assessment, physical exam; mark extent of local edema with skin-marking pen

Supportive therapy: Repeat lab testing every 3-4 hours for first 12 hours; I.V. fluids, tetanus prophylaxis and analgesics may need to be given; antibiotics may be indicated for infected wound sites; antivenin indicated for moderate to severe envenomation; neurologic findings may respond to intravenous edrophonium (10 mg for adults following pretreatment with 0.6 mg of atropine to block the muscarinic acetylcholine effects). The patient may then be treated with a longer-acting anticholinesterase agent such as neostigmine methyl sulfate (0.5 mg I.V. or SQ in adults) every 20 minutes. Alternatively, neostigmine methyl sulfate (0.5 mg I.V. or SQ every 20 minutes) has been used to reverse neurotoxicity due to an Asiatic Cobra bite. Thai Red Cross Asiatic Cobra antivenin (up to 600 mL) may be needed to treat neurotoxicity due to Asiatic Cobra bites. For antidote, in U.S., contact nearest regional poison center for availability. France, India, and South Africa are international sources for antivenin.

Additional Information Family: Elapidae; neck flares to form characteristic hood

Colubrids

Scientific Name *Dispholidus typhus*; *Thelotornis kirtlandi*

Signs and Symptoms of Overdose Venoms may cause fatality; venom of *Dispholidus typhus* may contain a prothrombin-activating enzyme that can cause a prolonged coagulation defect; coagulopathy

Overdosage/Treatment Supportive therapy: Monitor blood counts and replace with blood products as necessary; monitor for occult hemorrhage

Additional Information Family: Colubridae; *Opisthoglypha* (grooved fangs under eyes). Range: (Boomslang): African rain forest, southern African rain forest; *Thelotornis kirtlandi* (Bird Snake): central and southern African rain forest. Adults average 4-6 feet in length

Cone Shells

Scientific Name *Conus aulicus*; *Conus geographus*; *Conus gloriamaris*; *Conus omaria*; *Conus strictus*; *Conus textile*; *Conus tulipa*

Mechanism of Toxic Action Venom; neurotoxin (may have a curare effect)

Adverse Reactions

Cardiovascular: Cardiac failure, cerebral edema

Central nervous system: Coma

Hematologic: Disseminated intravascular coagulation

Respiratory: Respiratory arrest

Signs and Symptoms of Overdose Aphonia, blurred vision, burning sensation, coma, local ischemia, pain, numbness, paresthesia, respiratory collapse, slurred speech

Overdosage/Treatment

Decontamination: Place involved area in hot water (110°F to 115°F) to relieve pain; tetanus toxoid and immune globulin should be administered if not current; no antivenin available

Additional Information Range: Shallow Indo-Pacific waters

Copperhead Snake

Scientific Name *Agkistrodon contortrix*

Mechanism of Toxic Action Venom; quality and potency vary among species; composition: 90% water with 5-15 enzymes, 3-12 nonenzymatic proteins, as well as other unidentified substances

Signs and Symptoms of Overdose

Local signs: Bullae, edema, erythema, ecchymosis, hemorrhage, lymphangitis, tenderness, and (rarely) compartment syndrome.

Systemic signs: Asthenia, chills, CNS depression, coagulopathy, fasciculations, hypotension, nausea, paresthesia, sweating, vomiting Coagulopathies can occur including hypofibrinogenemia, increased PT and PTT, and thrombocytopenia. Hematuria, hemoconcentration, hypoproteinemia, hypotension, lactic acidosis, proteinuria, and shock are also potential complications.

Admission Criteria/Prognosis Patients with evidence of snakebite should be observed for 6-12 hours; if there are no systemic abnormalities (such as coagulopathy) or rapidly expanding edema, patient can be discharged

Overdosage/Treatment

Decontamination: Immobilize the area, rapid transport to medical facility. Use negative pressure device to remove venom if available, **do not** incise the wound; constriction band may be applied, **not** a tourniquet

Wyeth crotalid polyvalent antivenin; treat moderate to severe envenomations with increments of 5-10 vials at a time; skin test per manufacturer's instructions; if positive skin test develops, may prophylax with H$_1$- and H$_2$-receptor blockers; give until local injury has stopped and coagulopathy is reversed; complications include allergic reactions, anaphylaxis, and delayed serum sickness

Supportive therapy: ABC assessment, physical exam; mark the extent of local edema with skin marking pen; repeat CBC, platelets, PT, PTT, fibrinogen, CPK, UA every 3-4 hours for at least first 12 hours; I.V. fluids, tetanus prophylaxis, and analgesics may be given as needed;

treat infected wounds with antibiotics. Snakes' mouths contain primarily gram-negative and anaerobic organisms.

Antidote(s)

- Antivenin (Crotalidae) Polyvalent [ANTIDOTE]

Additional Information Family: Crotalidae (Pit Viper). Range: Eastern U.S. to southern Texas. Distinguishing characteristics: Facial pits, vertical elliptical pupils, triangular head, single row of subcaudal scales. Case fatality rate: 0.01%; usually there is a relative benign course and antivenon is not required.

Specific References

Caravati EM, "Copperhead Bites and Crotalidae Polyvalent Immune Fab (Ovine): Routine Use Requires Evidence of Improved Outcomes," *Ann Emerg Med*, 2004, 43(2):207-8.

Spiller HA and Bosse GM, "Prospective Study of Morbidity Associated with Snakebite Envenomation," *J Toxicol Clin Toxicol*, 2003, 41(2): 125-30.

Thorson A, Lavonas EJ, Rouse AM, et al, "Copperhead Envenomations in the Carolinas," *J Toxicol Clin Toxicol*, 2003, 41(1):29-35.

Corn Lily (Veratrum)

Scientific Name *Veratrum californicum*

Mechanism of Toxic Action Contains veratrum alkaloids which act on nerve cells lowering the stimulus threshold, thus resulting in repetitive nerve firing after a single stimulus

Adverse Reactions Cardiovascular: Sinus bradycardia

Signs and Symptoms of Overdose Abdominal pain, blurred vision, bradycardia, confusion, hypertension (uncommon), hypotension, mydriasis, nausea, sweating, oral burning, vomiting, vertigo. These alkaloids produce different effects in various nerve groups depending on their baseline stimulus threshold (afferent vagal fibers of coronary sinus and left ventricle are most affected).

Toxicodynamics/Kinetics

Onset: Within 30 minutes to 4 hours

Duration: 12-15 hours

Overdosage/Treatment

Decontamination: Avoid ipecac due to vagal stimulation, potentiating rapid onset of symptoms; activated charcoal with cathartic may be useful, but might not be tolerated if the patient is vomiting

Supportive therapy: Atropine for bradycardia, hypotension may require I.V. fluids or vasopressors

Additional Information Toxic dose: Unclear; likely 1-2 bulbs in a child. Grows to 4 feet. Range: Western U.S. Toxic part: All. Monitoring parameters: Monitor fluid and electrolyte status in symptomatic patients; ECG monitoring in severely symptomatic patients.

Specific References

Rottinghaus D, Kurta D, Krenzelok EP, et al, "Pontine Stroke After Acute White Hellebore Poisoning," *J Toxicol Clin Toxicol*, 2003, 41(5):721.

Crotalidae

Related Information

- Rattlesnakes

Scientific Name *Agkistrodon contortrix* (Copperhead); *Agkistrodon piscivorus* (Cottonmouth); *Sistrurus catenatus* (Pygmy Rattler, Massasauga)

Mechanism of Toxic Action Venom, quality and potency vary among species; composition is 90% water with 5-15 enzymes, 3-12 nonenzymatic proteins, as well as other unidentified substances

Adverse Reactions

Gastrointestinal: Metallic taste

Neuromuscular & skeletal: Rhabdomyolysis

Signs and Symptoms of Overdose Systemic: Asthenia, chills, CNS depression, fasciculations, hypotension, orolingual edema, paresthesia, nausea, sweating, vomiting. Coagulopathy can occur including hypofibrinogenemia, increased PT and PTT, and thrombocytopenia. Hematuria, hemoconcentration, hypoproteinemia, lactic acidosis, myopathy, proteinuria, and shock are also potential complications

Local: Bullae, ecchymosis (ascending), edema, erythema, hemorrhage, lymphangitis, tenderness, and (rarely) compartment syndrome

Admission Criteria/Prognosis Admit all leg bites. Patients with evidence of snakebite should be observed for 12 hours; if there are no systemic abnormalities (such as coagulopathy) or edema, patient can be discharged

Overdosage/Treatment

Decontamination: Rapid transport to medical facility; wash the site with soap and water; immobilize and keep it lower than the heart; if negative pressure suction device is available, this may be used; **do not** incise the wound; do not apply tourniquet or ice. ABC assessment, physical exam; mark extent of local edema with skin-marking pen

Supportive therapy: Repeat lab testing every 3-4 hours for first 12 hours; I.V. fluids, tetanus prophylaxis and analgesics may need to be given; antibiotics may be indicated for infected wound sites; antivenin indicated for moderate to severe envenomation. Fasciotomy should be considered if the compartment pressure remains elevated after

infusion of at least 20 vials of antivenin and before the patient has signs or symptoms of compartment syndrome (pressures >30 mm Hg despite limb elevation) for 12 hours.

Antidote:

Wyeth crotalid polyvalent antivenin: Treat moderate to severe envenomations with increments of 5-10 vials at a time; skin test per manufacturer's instructions; prophylax with H_1- and H_2- histamine receptor blockers; give until local injury has stopped or coagulopathy is reversed; complications include allergic reaction, anaphylaxis, and delayed serum sickness

Newer affinity-purified, mixed monospecific crotalid antivenom ovine Fab antivenom is being developed by Protherics, Inc. (Nashville, TN); each vial contains 750 mg Fab and 90 mg NaCl and is reconstituted in 10 mL of normal saline; initial dose: 4 vials diluted in normal saline (250 mL) administered over 60 minutes I.V. See Antivenin (Crotalidae) Polyvalent [ANTIDOTE] for further dosing details.

Antidote(s)

- Antivenin (Crotalidae) Polyvalent [ANTIDOTE]
- Antivenin, Polyvalent Crotalid (Ovine) Fab [ANTIDOTE]

Additional Information Distinguishing characteristics: Facial pits, vertical elliptical pupils, triangular head, single row of subcaudal scales; 6-12 foot brown/tan snake with dark rhomboid markings. Range: Indigenous to Central and South America. Case fatality rate is as high as 14% in some case series. Copperhead exposure is unlikely to require antivenin therapy.

Specific References

Cham G, Pan JC, Lim F, et al, "Effects of Topical Heparin, Antivenom, Tetracycline and Dexamethasone Treatment in Corneal Injury Resulting from the Venom of the Black Spitting Cobra (*Naja sumatrana*), in a Rabbit Model," *Clin Toxicol*, 2006, 44:287-92.

Clements EA, Riley BD, and Judge BS, "Severe Coaguloopathy from Envenomation by an Eastern Massassauga Rattlesnake (*Sistrurus catenatus*) Successfully Treated with Crofab™," *J Toxicol Clin Toxicol*, 2004, 42(5):743-4.

de Haro L and Pommier P, "Envenomation: A Real Risk of Keeping Exotic House Pets," *Vet Hum Toxicol*, 2003, 45(4):214-6.

Feng S and Stephan M, "What a Bite - Review of Snakebites in Children," *Clin Toxicol (Phila)*, 2005, 43:712.

German BT, "Systemic Effects of Crotalid Envenomation Mislabeled as Anaphylaxis," *Ann Emerg Med*, 2005, 45(1):101; author reply 101-2.

German BT, Hack JB, Brewer KL, et al, "Efficacy of a Pressure-Immobilization Bandage in Delaying the Onset of Systemic Toxicity in a Porcine Model of Eastern Coral Snake (*Micrurus fulvius*) Envenomation," *Ann Emerg Med*, 2004, 44:S90.

Holstege CP and Singletary EM, "Images in Emergency Medicine: Skin Damage Following Application of Suction Device for Snakebite," *Ann Emerg Med*, 2006, 48(1):105, 113.

Lalloo DG and Theakston RD, "Snake Antivenoms," *J Toxicol Clin Toxicol*, 2003, 41(3):277-90; 317-27.

Lavonas EJ, Gerardo CJ, O'Malley G, et al, "Initial Experience with Crotalidae Polyvalent Immune Fab (Ovine) Antivenom in the Treatment of Copperhead Snakebite," *Ann Emerg Med*, 2004, 43(2):200-6.

Meier KH, Tsukaoka BT, and Dudyala V, "Anaphylaxis During Crofab™ Administration," *J Toxicol Clin Toxicol*, 2003, 41(5):671.

Offerman SR, Barry JD, Richardson WH, et al, "Subcutaneous Injection of Crotaline Fab Antivenom for the Treatment of Rattlesnake Envenomation in a Porcine Model," *J Toxicol Clin Toxicol*, 2003, 41(5):692.

Palmer RB, Mackessy SP, and Dart RC, "Does CROFAB Bind All Components in Crotaline Venoms?" *J Toxicol Clin Toxicol*, 2004, 42(5):740-1.

Singletary EM, Rochman AS, Bodmer JC, et al, "Envenomations," *Med Clin North Am*, 2005, 89(6):1195-224 (review).

Stanford CF, Olsen D, Bogdan GM, et al, "Complications of Crotaline Antivenom Therapy in the United States," *Clin Toxicol (Phila)*, 2005, 43:708.

Crown of Thorns

Related Information

- Milkbush

Scientific Name *Euphorbia milii*; *Euphorbia*

Mechanism of Toxic Action Contact dermatitis

Signs and Symptoms of Overdose Blistering, erythema, irritation, potentially severe ocular pain, swelling, temporary blindness ulceration, vesication

Toxicodynamics/Kinetics Symptoms are delayed 2-8 hours with peak effects at 8-24 hours; blisters heal in several days; ocular symptoms may take a month to resolve

Overdosage/Treatment

Decontamination: **Oral**: Dilute with milk or water. **Dermal**: Wash thoroughly with soap and water. **Ocular**: Irrigate with copious tepid water or saline

Supportive therapy: Antibiotics if infected, oral corticosteroids may be useful for severe reactions; no antidote; antihistamines are not likely to be beneficial

Additional Information Toxicity varies within species; blisters should heal without scarring

Cycad Nut

Scientific Name *Cycas circinalis*

Mechanism of Toxic Action Contains cyasin (methylazoxymethanol), an aglycone which is a hepatocarcinogen and colonic tumorigen through means of methylation

Adverse Reactions

Neuromuscular & skeletal: Amyotropic lateral sclerosis

Hepatic: Hepatitis, hepatic necrosis

Toxicodynamics/Kinetics Metabolism: Gut hydrolysis to methylazoxymethanol (MAM), a potent hepatocarcinogen and colonic tumorigen

Overdosage/Treatment Decontamination: Ipecac within 30 minutes or lavage (within 1 hour)/activated charcoal with cathartic

Additional Information Cycads had been used for food; detoxification occurs by cutting stems and seeds into small pieces, soaking in water for several days, drying and grinding into flour

Cyclospora cayetanenis Food Poisoning

Commonly Found In Reptiles, myriapods, insectivores, raspberries, strawberries, contaminated water, raw vegetables, cow manure

Mechanism of Toxic Action A coccidian parasitic agent which can cause protracted watery diarrhea of uncertain mechanism

Adverse Reactions

Central nervous system: Low grade fever, headache, fatigue

Gastrointestinal: One day prodrome of anorexia, malaise, explosive watery diarrhea, nausea, severe abdominal cramping and vomiting; while diarrhea may remit and relapse over a 4-day cycle, the duration of illness lasts a mean time of 43 days

Overdosage/Treatment Supportive therapy: Fluid replacement is the mainstay of therapy; antibiotic treatment consists of a 7-day course of oral trimethoprim (TMP)-sulfamethoxazole (SMX); 160 mg TMP plus 800 mg SMX twice daily for adults and 5 mg/kg TMP plus 25 mg/kg SMX twice daily for children

Additional Information Seasonal peak is from April to June; cyanobacteria (blue-green algae) with variable acid-fast staining properties; previously called cyanobacterium-like body; under light microscopy, these organisms appear as a cluster of nonrefractile 8-10 μm spheres with a thick cell wall and an absence of a nucleus but presence of dark granules in cytoplasma; under ultraviolet light, these organisms autofluoresce; incubation period is one week; transmission is by fecal-oral route; suspected cases should be reported to the CDC's Division of Parasitic Diseases (770) 488-7760; may be found in developing countries (Nepal, Haiti), Mexico and in AIDS patients; midwestern outbreak in summer of 1996 relatable to contaminated raspberries and strawberries

Daffodil

Scientific Name *Narcissus pseudo-narcissus*

Mechanism of Toxic Action Contains lycorine alkaloid

Signs and Symptoms of Overdose Humans: Abdominal pain, allergic and contact dermatitis, nausea, vomiting

Toxicodynamics/Kinetics All parts of plant are toxic, especially the bulb; contains crinine, narcissine, lycorine, and other

Overdosage/Treatment

Decontamination: Ipecac relatively contraindicated; may be useful, if given soon after ingestion; vomiting has not occurred with ingestion of more than one bulb; activated charcoal with cathartic/lavage (within 1 hour) may be beneficial depending on amount ingested and time elapsed since ingestion

Supportive therapy: Wash skin extremely thoroughly with soap and water

Additional Information Toxic dose: Not established. Bulbs have been mistaken for onions. Toxic part: All parts contain alkaloid, bulb is most toxic

Daphne

Scientific Name *Daphne mezereum*

Mechanism of Toxic Action Contains mezerein (in the bark) and daphne toxin which are extremely irritating; seeds contain acrid resin; drying does not decrease toxicity

Adverse Reactions

Cardiovascular: Shock, facial edema

Central nervous system: Fever, headache, delirium, seizures, lethargy

Dermatologic: Blisters

Gastrointestinal: Nausea, vomiting, abdominal pain, watery diarrhea, dysphagia

Hematologic: Hematuria, proteinuria

Neuromuscular & skeletal: Muscle twitching

Miscellaneous: Thirst

Signs and Symptoms of Overdose Diarrhea, inflammation, mild to severe dermal irritation (which may include pruritus, edema, erythema, vesiculation), nausea, ocular irritation, possible severe gastroenteritis, possible temporary blindness, vomiting

Toxicodynamics/Kinetics Few reports of exposure available, unclear; dermal symptoms may be immediate or delayed by several hours and resolve within 4-7 days

Absorption: Orally and through intact skin

Overdosage/Treatment

Decontamination: **Oral:** Ipecac relatively contraindicated, may be useful if given soon after ingestion if the patient is asymptomatic, activated charcoal with cathartic may be of benefit, lavage within 1 hour may be beneficial in large overdose or in asymptomatic patients presenting later. **Dermal:** Wash thoroughly even if asymptomatic. **Ocular:** Irrigate copiously with saline.

Supportive therapy: Monitor fluid and electrolyte balance in patients with vomiting and diarrhea; seizures can be treated with benzodiazepines, phenobarbital, or phenytoin

Oral: Maintain proper fluid and electrolyte balance in symptomatic patients

Dermal: Antihistamines and steroids have not clearly been beneficial

Ocular: Supportive care

Additional Information Toxic dose: A single berry or leaf may produce symptoms; 2-3 may be fatal in a child; 12 may cause significant toxicity in an adult. Family: Thymelaeaceae. Range: Common hedge of United States, Eastern Canada, and Europe. Toxic part: Whole plant is poisonous. About 4-5 feet in height; leaves are elliptic and vivid green; flowers are lilac purple or while and about 1 cm in length; fruits are scarlet or yellow.

Deadly Nightshade

Related Information

- Black Nightshade
- Woody Nightshade

Scientific Name *Solanum dulcamara*

Mechanism of Toxic Action Contains toxic alkaloids, solanine most significant structurally similar to cardioglycoside, causes hemolytic and hemorrhagic damage to GI tract similar to saponins; some plants may also contain alpha-cholinergic alkaloids

Adverse Reactions Central nervous system: Psychosis

Signs and Symptoms of Overdose Anticholinergic effects (may or may not be present to varying degrees), asthenia, diarrhea, drowsiness, fever, hallucinations, headache, nausea, seizures, sweating, vomiting, visual changes

Toxicodynamics/Kinetics Toxicity occurs within 2-24 hours, diarrhea may last 3-6 days, anticholinergic effects may delay GI emptying and produce delayed effects

Overdosage/Treatment

Decontamination: Ipecac within 30 minutes if vomiting has not already occurred, lavage (within 1 hour) and/or charcoal may be beneficial if the patient presents symptomatic

Supportive therapy: Maintain fluid and electrolyte balance as necessary, support vital signs; physostigmine will reverse anticholinergic toxicity that may be associated with exposure

Antidote(s)

- Physostigmine [ANTIDOTE]

Additional Information Toxic dose: 2-3 green berries or 6 red or black berries should not cause significant toxicity (fatal dose: 200 berries). Toxic part: All parts of plant contain solanine and are regarded as toxic. Peak plasma and urine atropine levels 10 hours after ingestion of 6 raw berries and 200 g of cooked berries (and associated with coma) were 217 mcg/L and 3092 mcg/L respectively

Death Camas

Scientific Name *Zigadenus nuttallii*; *Zigadenus paniculatus*; *Zigadenus venenosus*

Mechanism of Toxic Action Contains an alkaloid (zygacine) of the veratrum group which increases muscle and nerve excitability; younger plants are more toxic

Adverse Reactions Cardiovascular: Sinus bradycardia

Signs and Symptoms of Overdose Ataxia, bradycardia, diarrhea, hyperactive deep tendon reflexes, coma, hypotension, muscle fasciculation, muscle spasticity, respiratory depression, vomiting, nausea, abdominal pain, dizziness, flushing, headache, hematemesis

Overdosage/Treatment

Decontamination: Gastric lavage within 2 hours; activated charcoal

Supportive therapy: While bradycardia may respond to atropine, hypotension will not; give isotonic saline I.V. and supplement with vasopressors (dopamine or norepinephrine) as needed; recovery usually noted within 2 days

895

Additional Information A common plant of the lily family often confused with sego lilies or wild onion; leaves are V-shaped; yellow flowers appear in summer; 1-2 bulbs (10-15 g) can produce symptoms. Range: Found in the dry soil of the Western U.S.

Specific References

Peterson MC and Rasmussen GJ, "Intoxication with Foothill Camas (*Zigadenus paniculatus*)," *J Toxicol Clin Toxicol*, 2003, 41(1):63-5.

Delphinium

Adverse Reactions Cardiovascular: Sinus bradycardia, sinus tachycardia, arrhythmias (ventricular)

Signs and Symptoms of Overdose No reports of human toxicity. May contain alkaloids with effects similar to monkshood; tingling and burning of fingers, lips, toes and tongue are seen first; then sweats, hypothermia, chills, paresthesia, numbness, dry mouth; later: arrhythmias (supraventricular), bradycardia, diarrhea, hypotension, pain, paralysis, seizures, ventricular fibrillation

Overdosage/Treatment

Decontamination: Ipecac is questionable due to inducing rapid onset of symptoms; lavage within 1 hour may be beneficial, activated charcoal with cathartic

Supportive therapy: Fluid and electrolyte replacement; arrhythmias are relatively refractory to drug therapy

Additional Information Range: Found in central U.S.

Devil's Ivy

Scientific Name *Epipremnum aureum*

Mechanism of Toxic Action Contains insoluble calcium oxalate crystals which cause mechanical irritation; also may cause irritant dermatitis

Signs and Symptoms of Overdose Sap may cause ocular pain, lacrimation, photophobia, corneal abrasion; oxalate crystals may be deposited on cornea; dermal pain, irritation, and swelling; edema, diarrhea, dysphonia, salivation, vomiting

Toxicodynamics/Kinetics Rapid onset of local symptoms

Overdosage/Treatment

Decontamination: **Oral**: Dilute; ipecac/lavage/activated charcoal not likely necessary. **Dermal**: Wash thoroughly. **Ocular**: Irrigate

Supportive therapy: **Oral**: Ice cream may provide some relief. **Dermal/ocular**: Cool compresses may minimize pain.

Additional Information Symptoms dependent on liberation of oxalate crystals or contact with sap; dried plant will not liberate crystals; insoluble calcium oxalates will not cause systemic symptoms. Toxic part: Whole plant

Dieffenbachia

Mechanism of Toxic Action Contains insoluble calcium oxalate crystals which cause mechanical irritation; may also cause irritation through an unclear enzymatic process.

Signs and Symptoms of Overdose Dermal pain, diarrhea, dysphonia, edema, irritation, salivation, swelling, vomiting; oxalate crystals may be deposited on cornea; sap may cause corneal abrasion, lacrimation, ocular pain, photophobia; may cause dermatitis

Admission Criteria/Prognosis Admit any ingestion >3 g (of the leaf) or evidence of upper airway obstruction

Toxicodynamics/Kinetics Rapid onset of local symptoms

Overdosage/Treatment

Decontamination: Dermal: Wash thoroughly; Ocular: Irrigate; Oral: Dilute; ipecac/lavage/activated charcoal not likely necessary; oral irritation can be treated with ice or a popsicle

Supportive therapy: Cool compresses may minimize pain and swelling; dexamethasone ophthalmic ointment can be used for eye exposure

Additional Information

Lethal dose: Oral: 3 g.

Symptoms are dependent on liberation of oxalate crystals or contact with sap; dried plant will not liberate crystals; wide variation in potential for toxicity between plants. Treat symptoms. Insoluble calcium oxalate will not cause systemic symptoms; ingestion of stems or stalk may cause upper airway obstruction. Toxic part: Whole plant

Specific References

Burda A, Wahl M, Fischbein C, et al, "Atypical Poisonings with Botanicals Raise Suspicion of Malicious Activity," *Vet Hum Toxicol*, 2004, 46(6):341.

Cumpston KL, Vogel SN, Leikin JB, et al, "Acute Airway Compromise After Brief Exposure to a *Dieffenbachia* Plant," *J Emerg Med*, 2003, 25(4): 391-7.

Loretti AP, da Silva Ilha MR, and Ribeiro RE, "Accidental Fatal Poisoning of a Dog by *Dieffenbachia picta* (Dumb Cane)," *Vet Hum Toxicol*, 2003, 45(5):233-9.

Watson JT, Jones RC, Siston AM, et al, "An Outbreak of Food-Borne Illness Associated with Plant Material Containing Raphides - Chicago, 2003," *J Toxicol Clin Toxicol*, 2003, 41(5):728.

Watson JT, Jones RC, Siston AM, et al, "Outbreak of Food-borne Illness Associated with Plant Material Containing Raphides," *Clin Toxicol (Phila)*. 2005, 43(1):17-21.

Elapids

Scientific Name *Micrurus euryxanthus*; *Micrurus fulvius*

Mechanism of Toxic Action Neurotoxin - average amount of dry venom injected: 2-6 mg; significant envenomations occur in 60% of cases

Signs and Symptoms of Overdose Western coral snake: Local injury Eastern coral snake: Asthenia (within 1-2 hours), coagulopathy, diplopia, fasciculations, nausea, paresthesias, vomiting; complete paralysis within 36 hours may occur

Admission Criteria/Prognosis All patients should be admitted (probably into an intensive care unit)

Overdosage/Treatment

Decontamination: Incision and suction can be performed within 30 minutes (1 hour if a tourniquet is in place); wide excision and suction should be reserved for severe envenomations on the trunk

Supportive therapy: Antivenin should be administered as soon as possible for Eastern coral snake envenomation (usual dose: 4-6 vials); horse-derived antivenin is available (Wyeth)

Antidote(s)

● Antivenin (Micrurus fulvius) [ANTIDOTE]

Additional Information Family: Elapidae. Range: Western coral snake is found in Arizona and New Mexico, while Eastern coral snake is found in North Carolina, Florida, and the gulf states; average length is 16-28 inches

Antivenin has been given on affected extremity distal to a blood pressure cuff (inflated to block arterial flow) while massaging the extremity to the blood pressure cuff (similar to the Bier-block anesthetic technique)

Specific References

Borys DJ, Tobleman WR, Stanford RD, et al, "Is Antivenin Required for All Texas Coral Snake (*Micrurus fulvius tenere*) Envenomations?" *Clin Toxicol (Phila)*, 2005, 43:709.

de Roodt AR, Paniagua-Solis JF, Dolab JA, et al, "Effectiveness of Two Common Antivenoms for North, Central, and South American *Micrurus* Envenomations," *J Toxicol Clin Toxicol*, 2004, 42(2):171-8.

Stanford RD, Borys DJ, Morgan DL, et al, "Red on Yellow Kill a Fellow, But Not in Texas: Five Years of Texas Coral Snake (*Micrurus fulvius tenere*) Envenomations," *Clin Toxicol (Phila)*, 2005, 43:707.

Elderberry

Scientific Name *Sambucus*

Mechanism of Toxic Action Laxative effect unclear; also contains cyanogenic glycoside

Signs and Symptoms of Overdose Diarrhea, nausea; effects of cyanogenic glycoside include abdominal pain, coma, cyanosis, drowsiness, dyspnea, headache, seizures, sweating, vomiting

Overdosage/Treatment

Decontamination: Ipecac (within 30 minutes) recommended in ingestions of leaves, roots, bark, unripe fruit; activated charcoal with cathartic may be useful; **do not** give cathartic if diarrhea has developed

Supportive therapy: Maintain fluid and electrolyte balance

Additional Information Toxic dose: Unclear; variable. Ripe fruit is edible when cooked; raw fruit may cause nausea or diarrhea if eaten in large amounts; leaves, roots, bark, unripe fruit may cause more severe diarrhea, although roots, stems, and leaves contain cyanogenic glycosides; there are no documented reports of cyanide toxicity. Range: Native to Western U.S. and Canada

English Ivy

Scientific Name *Hedera helix*

Mechanism of Toxic Action Falcarinol which is an irritant and sensitizer, is a potent alkylating agent; polyacetylenes cause direct contact irritation

Signs and Symptoms of Overdose Irritant contact dermatitis is the most common finding. Linear and streaked vesicles may be seen. Ingestion may cause ataxia, burning sensation in the throat, coma, diarrhea, difficulty breathing, mydriasis, nausea, rash, and vomiting.

Overdosage/Treatment

Decontamination: Oral: Corticosteroids are used to treat the irritant dermatitis, but the reaction may not subside for 3-4 weeks

Supportive therapy: Systemic symptoms require symptomatic and supportive treatment

Additional Information Low concentrations of falcarinol have been found to be irritating; specific amounts of plant material required to produce systemic symptoms are unknown, but poisonings are rare. Range: Native to Europe; commonly found throughout the U.S. and southern Canada. Toxic part: All of the plant, especially leaves and berries

Escherichia coli Food Poisoning

Commonly Found In Contaminated water

Mechanism of Toxic Action Can produce heat labile and heat stable enterotoxins. Enteropathogenic *E. coli* and enterohemorrhagic *E. coli* (serogroup 0157) produce Shiga toxin; incubation period: 1-3 days. Enterohemorrhagic *E. coli* produces hemorrhagic colitis and hemolytic uremia syndrome.

Adverse Reactions Hematologic: Hemolytic/uremic syndrome

Signs and Symptoms of Overdose Watery diarrhea (enterotoxin); fever and vomiting are unlikely

Admission Criteria/Prognosis Patients with dehydration (who cannot take fluids orally), immunocompromised patients, severe disturbance in electrolytes or acid-base status, or patients at extreme in terms of age group should be considered for admission

Overdosage/Treatment Supportive therapy: While fluoroquinolones are effective for empiric treatment in adults with severe acute diarrhea, antibiotics should be avoided if initial infection with enterohemorrhagic *E. coli* is suspected, especially in children. Thus, the stool culture should be used to guide therapy. Fluid/electrolyte replacement is the mainstay of therapy. Antimotility agents should **not** be used.

Diagnostic Procedures

- Stool Culture

Additional Information

Can cause necrotizing enterocolitis in the newborn or weanling diarrhea (in poor sanitation areas)

Escherichia coli, enterohemorrhagic:

Microbiology: Enterohemorrhagic *E. coli* causes a distinct form of hemorrhagic colitis in humans. Like other *E. coli* strains, enterohemorrhagic *E. coli* is a facultative, gram-negative bacillus. The most common serotype is 0157:H7; essentially all published information regarding enterohemorrhagic *E. coli* refers only to this serotype.

Epidemiology:

In 1982, the first large-scale outbreak of *E. coli* 0157:H7 colitis was described. Multiple cases of severe bloody diarrhea were found to be epidemiologically linked to ingestion of contaminated hamburger meat. Since then, the organism has been recognized as an important cause of bloody diarrhea and the hemolytic uremic syndrome. Over 12 major outbreaks have been reported, along with numerous sporadic cases. The majority of cases have been traced to contaminated ground beef, although other potential sources have been cited, including unpasteurized milk, apple cider, municipal water, and roast beef. The organism inhabits the GI tract of some healthy cattle and is thought to contaminate meat during slaughter and the processing of ground beef ("internal contamination"). If the ground beef is undercooked, the organism remains viable; undercooking of hamburger patties has proven important in several outbreaks.

In 1993, a well-publicized multistate outbreak of *E. coli* 0157:H7 took place in the Western United States (Washington, California, Idaho, and Nevada). Over 500 infections and four deaths were documented. The vast majority of cases were ultimately linked to contaminated hamburger meat from a particular restaurant chain. Further investigation by the Centers for Disease Control identified several slaughter plants in the United States and one in Canada as the probable source. Thousands of contaminated patties not yet consumed were discovered. In March, 1994, the USDA Food Safety and Inspection Service recommended that all raw meat should be cooked thoroughly, with an increase in the internal temperature for cooked hamburgers to 155°F.

A 2-year nationwide surveillance study by the Centers for Disease Control has found *E. coli* 0157:H7 to be the most commonly identified pathogen associated with bloody diarrhea. In many parts of the U.S., *E. coli* 0157:H7 is the second most common cause of bacterial diarrhea.

Acquisition of disease is usually by ingestion of contaminated food, but person-to-person transmission has been documented, especially in day care centers. Children and elderly individuals are at highest risk for severe infections. Simple and careful hand washing essentially eliminates the probability of person-to-person transmission.

Case fatality rates in elderly patients range from 3% to 36%. Incidence of *E. coli* 0157:H7 in all cases of diarrhea range from 0.6% to 2.4% (highest in children <5 years of age; lower for persons 50-59 years of age). Progression to hemorrhagic colitis with *E. coli* 0157:H7 is 38% to 61%.

Clinical Syndromes:

- **Hemorrhagic colitis:** *E. coli* 0157:H7 causes a bloody diarrhea associated with abdominal cramps. Pathologically, there is no invasion or inflammation of the intestinal mucosa, and thus fever is often absent. The diarrhea is caused by Shiga-like toxins. In most cases, the illness resolves within 7 days, but death can occur in the elderly.

- **Hemolytic uremic syndrome:** ~5% to 10% of patients with *E. coli* 0157:H7 diarrhea develop a syndrome characterized by acute renal failure, thrombocytopenia, and evidence of hemolysis on a peripheral blood smear. Children are at high risk for this syndrome, with ~15% of children developing hemolytic-uremic syndrome soon after diarrhea. Ten percent of children with this syndrome present with a generalized seizure. The patient may be toxic-appearing, and the presentation may be confused with a variety of diseases including sepsis with disseminated intravascular coagulation, vasculitis, thrombotic thrombocytopenia purpura, and others. The estimated mortality is 3% to 5%.

Diagnosis:

Enterohemorrhagic *E. coli* should be strongly considered in any patient presenting with bloody diarrhea, whether or not hemolytic uremic syndrome is present. It is likely that many sporadic cases of *E. coli* 0157:H7 diarrhea occur in the community and go unrecognized for two reasons: many clinicians do not order stool cultures for stable patients with diarrhea; many microbiology laboratories do not routinely culture stools for *E. coli* 0157:H7 unless there is a specific order from the physician.

Diagnosis is confirmed by isolation of *E. coli* 0157:H7 from stool specimens and subsequent serological confirmation. This requires special media in the microbiology laboratory (sorbitol-MacConkey medium). Other methods for the rapid detection of this organism are currently under study.

Escherichia coli, nonenterohemorrhagic:

Microbiology: *Escherichia coli* is a lactose-positive, gram-negative, facultative bacillus with variable motility. A member of the Enterobacteriaceae family, *E. coli* is probably the most widely studied free-living organism. Most *E. coli* are nonpigmented, produce lysine decarboxylase, utilize acetate as a carbon source, and hydrolyze tryptophan to indole. Serologic typing is based on three surface antigens (O, H, K). The lipopolysaccharide of the cell wall is known as endotoxin and is a factor in sepsis and septic shock in infected individuals.

Epidemiology: *E. coli*, as well as other Enterobacteriaceae, are normal colonizers of the human and animal gastrointestinal tract. It is often considered an opportunistic pathogen in hospitalized or debilitated patients but is the most common cause of urinary tract infections among "normal" hosts.

Diagnosis: *E. coli* infection diagnosis can be made by identification through Gram's stain and culture in patients with relevant clinical syndromes. No special media or conditions are necessary to grow this organism. *E. coli* should always be one of several suspected organisms in patients with peritonitis.

Escherichia coli 0157:H7 causes an estimated 20,000 cases of diarrhea in the U.S. of which 6% result in the hemolytic-uremic syndrome. As of March, 1995, 33 states have enacted legislation designating *E. coli* 0157:H7 infection as a reportable disease.

From January 1, 1993 through September 14, 1995, there were a total of 63 outbreaks of *E. coli* 0157:H7 in 32 states; 40% of these outbreaks were related to ground beef

USDA Meat and Poultry Hotline for *E. coli* 0157:H7 and 0111:H2 exposures: (800) 535-4555.

Specific Reference

Bruce MG, Curtis MB, Payne MM, et al, "Lake-Associated Outbreak of *Escherichia coli* O157:H7 in Clark County, Washington, August 1999," *Arch Pediatr Adolesc Med*, 2003, 157(10):1016-21.

Eucalyptus Oil

Scientific Name *Eucalyptus globulus*

U.S. Brand Names Bosisto's® Eucalyptus Spray; Eucalyptamint®; Gelodurat®

Uses A volatile oil often used as a liniment; taken orally for treatment of cough or catarrh

Mechanism of Toxic Action Contains as much as 70% of the substance citronellal which is an irritant. Obtained from the leaves and terminal branches of the Eucalyptus (Myrtaceae) dives or Eucalyptus radiata.

Adverse Reactions

Central nervous system: Fever, dizziness, ataxia

Dermatologic: Contact dermatitis (allergic and irritant)

Gastrointestinal: Nausea, vomiting, diarrhea

Respiratory: Bronchospasm, cough, tachypnea, lipoid pneumonia

Signs and Symptoms of Overdose Apnea, coma, cyanosis, hyporeflexia, miosis, pulmonary edema, respiratory depression, seizures, slurred speech, tachycardia

Toxicodynamics/Kinetics Elimination: Lungs/GI tract

Overdosage/Treatment

Decontamination: Lavage (within 1 hour) if any amount is ingested; **do not** induce emesis; activated charcoal with cathartic can be used

Supportive therapy: Benzodiazepines are initial choice for seizure control; phenytoin or phenobarbital can be used for refractory seizures

Enhanced elimination: Hemodialysis (with peritoneal dialysis and with mannitol) has been used successfully in one case

Additional Information
Toxic dosage:
Fatal dose: ~3.5 mL
Liniments: Concentrations as high as 25% eucalyptus oil
Therapeutic: Oral: ~0.5 mL/dose
Specific gravity: 0.9;
Camphor-like odor; after ingestion, the patient's breath may continue to elicit this odor for as long as 2 weeks; oil solution can cause a lipoid pneumonia

Fir Club Moss

Scientific Name *Lycopodium selego*
Mechanism of Toxic Action Contains huperzine A, an alkaloid agent with significant inhibition of acetylchoinesterase; contains 3.6 µmol of huperzine A per gram of dried plant
Signs and Symptoms of Overdose Vomiting and diarrhea usually develop within 1.5 hours. Dizziness, extremity cramps, hypertension, and slurred speech can occur. Five grams of the dried substance can cause the above symptoms. Symptoms usually abate in 2-3 days; mild hypokalemia may develop.
Reference Range Ingestion of 4 µmol of huperzine A will yield a peak plasma concentration of 35 mM/L at 80 minutes. A plasma level of 78 mM/L results in approximately a 56% inhibition of acetylcholinesterase.
Overdosage/Treatment
Decontamination: Activated charcoal within 1 hour of ingestion may be useful.
Supportive therapy: Monitor electrolytes. Atropine may be useful in treating cholinergic symptoms.
Additional Information A small (<30 cm) creeping evergreen found in temperate climates; these plants resemble pine with needle-like leaves.

Fire Ants

Scientific Name *Solenopsis invicta; Solenopsis richteri*
Mechanism of Toxic Action Venom (average amount injection: 0.04-0.11 µL), piperidine alkaloids causing histamine release and necrosis in human skin; similar toxin to the brown recluse spider; also contains phospholipase and hyaluronidase
Adverse Reactions
Cardiovascular: Sinus tachycardia
Miscellaneous: Allergic reaction symptoms; anaphylaxis in 0.6% to 1% of stings
Signs and Symptoms of Overdose Characteristic signs include edema, erythema, pain, and wheal formation at the sting site. Dyspnea, fever (for 1-2 days), hypertension, nausea, tachycardia, and seizures may occur. Classic allergic reaction symptoms may be seen. A 2-3 mm sterile pustule may be noted (occasionally this may be hemorrhagic). Pustules may last 3-8 days.
Overdosage/Treatment Supportive therapy: Urticaria can be treated with epinephrine and antihistamines (H_1- and H_2-blocking agents); oral corticosteroids can be given; local pain can be treated with local injections of lidocaine
Antidote(s)
• Epinephrine [ANTIDOTE]
Additional Information Family: Formicidae. Range: southern U.S.; native to South America; attracted to electric current. Infestations found as far north as Virginia Beach, Virginia. In Eastern Tennessee, 7% of the ant population survived during the winter of 1993-4. There are ~3000 bites reported annually in the U.S.; ~2% of fire ant bites result in severe consequences.

Fire-Bellied Toad

Scientific Name *Bombina bombina*
Uses Found in aquariums as pets
Mechanism of Toxic Action Contains bombesin (a cardiovascular toxin which can cause increased blood pressure and smooth muscle stimulation) and bombinine (which can cause hemolysis) which can be secreted from venom glands on the skin
Adverse Reactions
Central nervous system: Lethargy
Dermatologic: Hives, dermal irritation
Gastrointestinal: Oral irritation
Ocular: Irritation, eyelid edema, miosis
Admission Criteria/Prognosis Admit any patient with systemic toxicity
Overdosage/Treatment
Decontamination: **Oral**: Emesis within 30 minutes of ingestion, or lavage within 1 hour of ingestion; activated charcoal with cathartic. **Dermal**: Wash with soap and water. **Ocular**: Irrigate with saline.
Supportive therapy: Systemic allergic symptoms can be treated with diphenhydramine.

Additional Information Native to Eastern Europe and Western Asia; ocular symptoms usually resolve within 1 day; dorsal side of toad is green with black splotches; ventral is black with red splotches

Fire Coral

Scientific Name *Hydrozoa millepor*
Mechanism of Toxic Action Nematocysts bear tentacles which cause intense local reaction
Signs and Symptoms of Overdose Burning and pain; rash and erythema may also occur. Abdominal pain, chills, and fever occur less commonly. Severe abrasions can result from sharp exoskeletons. Full thickness skin burns may result. Rubbing the affected area worsens the envenomation. Blisters can be seen within 6 hours. Symptom resolution occurs within 1 week.
Overdosage/Treatment
Decontamination: Soak affected area in hot water (110°F to 115°F); sea water rather than freshwater is preferred. Coral cuts should be cleansed (with acetic acid 5% or isopropyl alcohol 40% to 70%) and debrided. **Do not** rub affected area.
Supportive therapy: Treat rash with epinephrine and antihistamines; dermatitis can be treated with a topical steroid cream
Additional Information Family: Milleporidae; *Millepora alcicornis*: Found in Caribbean; *Millepora dichotoma*: Found in Red Sea, Pacific

Flowering Maple

Scientific Name *Abutilon Hybridum*
Adverse Reactions
Dermatologic: May cause dermatitis
Miscellaneous: Allergic skin reactions have been reported
Overdosage/Treatment
Decontamination: Wash skin with soap and water
Supportive: Mild cases can be treated with antihistamines (with or without epinephrine)

Four-O'Clock

Scientific Name *Mirabilis jalapa*
Signs and Symptoms of Overdose Handling the roots or seeds may result in dermatitis. Ingestion may cause abdominal pain, diarrhea, nausea, and vomiting. Smoking or eating the seeds is rumored to result in hallucinogenic effects.
Overdosage/Treatment Decontamination: Charcoal may be of value, one dose of cathartic may be considered if symptoms have not begun
Additional Information Toxic dose: Not established; Toxin: Trigonelline; Range: Native to Mexico and Central and South America, cultivated throughout the U.S.; Toxic part: Roots and seeds

Foxglove

CAS Number 17575-20-1
Scientific Name *Digitalis purpurea*
Mechanism of Toxic Action Leaves and seeds contain digitalis glycosides which inhibit the sodium - potassium ATPase pump, causing decreased intracellular potassium and increased intracytoplasmic calcium
Adverse Reactions Cardiovascular: Sinus bradycardia
Signs and Symptoms of Overdose GI effects (nausea and vomiting) usually precede cardiovascular effects by several hours. Asystole, AV block, bradycardia, decreased QT interval and prolonged P-R interval, fibrillation (atrial), flutter (atrial), heart block (first, second, and third degree), hypotension, ventricular arrhythmias. Contact dermatitis, delirium, dizziness, confusion, fatigue, headache, hyperkalemia and seeing yellow halos have also been reported.
Admission Criteria/Prognosis Asymptomatic patients with normal electrocardiogram and electrolytes can be discharged after a 12-hour observation; any symptomatic patient should be admitted to a cardiac monitor bed; unintentional ingestions rarely require admission
Toxicodynamics/Kinetics Upper limit of peak toxicity: 12 hours; all symptomatic patients should be observed for a minimum of 24 hours
Reference Range Serum concentration of digitalis glycosides following a nonfatal adult overdose was: gitoxin 13.1 ng/mL: digitoxin 112.6 ng/mL, digitoxigenin 3.3 ng/mL, and digitoxigenin mono-digitoxoside 8.9 ng/mL. Peak urinary levels were reached at 30 hours postingestion.
Overdosage/Treatment
Decontamination: Lavage within 1 hour and multidose activated charcoal with cathartic enhance total body clearance of digitalis; whole bowel irrigation is also beneficial in removing plant debris from the GI tract and is recommended for ingestions of large amounts of plant material
Supportive therapy: Monitor cardiac status and serum potassium levels; bradycardia will frequently respond to atropine; phenytoin is the recommended treatment for ventricular arrhythmias because it will also improve conduction through the AV node; lidocaine can also be used to treat ventricular arrhythmias, but will not have an effect on AV

conduction; other antiarrhythmics which have been used in arrhythmias resistant to the above therapy include magnesium, amiodarone, and bretylium; a pacemaker should be considered for bradycardia and AV nodal blocks resistant to medical management

Antidote: Digoxin immune Fab has been shown to interact with several different plant cardiac glycosides and may be beneficial in cases resistant to conventional treatment; indications for its use include ventricular arrhythmias resistant to conventional treatment, severe bradycardia and/or second or third degree heart block resistant to atropine and phenytoin

Antidote(s)
- Digoxin Immune Fab [ANTIDOTE]

Diagnostic Procedures
- Digitoxin, Blood

Additional Information

One cup of foxglove tea produced junctional rhythm with a heart rate the 40s with frequent PVCs, in an adult.

In accidental ingestion in children, ipecac and home observation are recommended for ingestion of one leaf or less. If more than one leaf is ingested, decontamination and observation in the emergency room are recommended.

Persons taking digoxin, beta-blockers, and calcium channel blockers are more susceptible to the toxin. Digitoxin assay has been shown to cross-react with the digitalis glycoside and thus may be beneficial in documenting ingestion; however, serum levels and toxicity do not necessarily correlate.

Family: Schrophulariaceae; Range: Native to Europe, but commonly found in the U.S. Toxin: Digitalis, digitoxin, cardiac glycosides

Specific References

Ciancaglini PP, Vence T, Benitez JG, et al, "Foxglove Salad Ingestion," *Clin Toxicol (Phila)*, 2005, 43:761.

Francisella tularenis

Mechanism of Toxic Action A nonmotile, aerobic gram-negative coccobacillus which can cause infections via dermal, gastrointestinal, and pulmonary routes. As little as 10 organisms can result in infection. Causes focal suppurative necrosis of tissue, resulting in granulomatous reactions. Target organs include lungs, lymph nodes, spleen, liver, and kidney. Two strains exist: Type A (highly virulent in humans) and Type B.

Adverse Reactions Miscellaneous: Mononucleosis-like syndrome

Signs and Symptoms of Overdose

Abrupt onset with high fever, headache, low backache, rigors, and sore throat. Other associated symptoms include dry cough, dyspnea, hemoptysis, pleuritic chest pain, and tachypnea. Radiological studies reveal peribronchial infiltrates leading to hilar adenopathy, multilobar pneumonia, and pleural effusion. Extrapulmonary symptoms include anorexia, diarrhea, diaphoresis, nausea, vomiting, and weakness. Type A infection fatality rate may be as high as 60% in untreated pneumonia, although in the U.S., the fatality rate is <2%. Type B strains are rarely fatal. Incubation is ~3-5 days.

Ulceroglandular tularemia results from handling a contaminated carcass, or after an arthropod bite. A local cutaneous papule forms which then ulcerates within 2-3 days. Regional adenopathy then develops.

Oropharyngeal tularemia results from drinking contaminated water or eating contaminated food. Stomatitis develops with exudative pharyngitis and pronounced cervical or retropharyngeal adenopathy. See tables.

Working Group Consensus Recommendations for Treatment of Patients with Tularemia in a Contained Casualty Setting*

Contained Casualty Recommended Therapy	
Adults	
Preferred choices	
	Streptomycin, 1 g I.M. twice daily
	Gentamicin, 5 mg/kg I.M. or I.V. once daily†
Alternative choices	
	Doxycycline, 100 mg I.V. twice daily
	Chloramphenicol, 15 mg/kg I.V. 4 times/day†
	Ciprofloxacin, 400 mg I.V. twice daily†
Children	
Preferred choices	
	Streptomycin, 15 mg/kg I.M. twice daily (should not exceed 2 g/day)
	Gentamicin, 2.5 mg/kg I.M. or I.V. 3 times/day†

Table (Continued)

Contained Casualty Recommended Therapy	
Alternative choices	
	Doxycycline; if weight ≥45 kg, 100 mg I.V. twice daily; if weight <45 kg, 2.2 mg/kg I.V. twice daily
	Chloramphenicol, 15 mg/kg I.V. 4 times/day†
	Ciprofloxacin, 15 mg/kg I.V. twice daily†‡
Pregnant Women	
Preferred choices	
	Gentamicin, 5 mg/kg I.M. or I.V. once daily†
	Streptomycin, 1 g I.M. twice daily
Alternative choices	
	Doxycycline, 100 mg I.V. twice daily
	Ciprofloxacin, 400 mg I.V. twice daily†

*Treatment with streptomycin, gentamicin, or ciprofloxacin should be continued for 10 days; treatment with doxycycline or chloramphenicol should be continued for 14-21 days. Persons beginning treatment with intramuscular (I.M.) or intravenous (I.V.) doxycycline, ciprofloxacin, or chloramphenicol can switch to oral antibiotic administration when clinically indicated.
†Not a U.S. Food and Drug Administration-approved use.
‡Ciprofloxacin dosage should not exceed 1 g/day in children
Adapted from Dennis DT, Inglesby TV, Henderson DA, et al, "Tularemia as a Biological Weapon: Medical and Public Health Management," *JAMA*, 2001, 285(21):2763-73.

Working Group Consensus Recommendations for Treatment of Patients with Tularemia in a Mass Casualty Setting and for Postexposure Prophylaxis*

Mass Casualty Recommended Therapy	
Adults	
Preferred choices	
	Doxycycline, 100 mg orally twice daily
	Ciprofloxacin, 500 mg orally twice daily†
Children	
Preferred choices	
	Doxycycline; if ≥45 kg, give 100 mg orally twice daily; if <45 kg, give 2.2 mg/kg orally twice daily
	Ciprofloxacin, 15 mg/kg orally twice daily†‡
Pregnant Women	
Preferred choices	
	Ciprofloxacin, 500 mg orally twice daily†
	Doxycycline, 100 mg orally twice daily

*One antibiotic appropriate for patient age, should be chosen from among alternatives. The duration of all recommended therapies in this table is 14 days.
†Not a U.S. Food and Drug Administration-approved use.
‡Ciprofloxacin dosage should not exceed 1 g/day in children
Adapted from Dennis DT, Inglesby TV, Henderson DA, et al, "Tularemia as a Biological Weapon: Medical and Public Health Management," *JAMA*, 2001, 285(21):2763-73.

Additional Information

A potential biological weapon. Natural reservoirs for infection include small mammals (eg, mice, water rats, squirrels, rabbits) which are infected through tick, fly, or mosquito bites. Tularemia is found in the U.S. and Eurasia. Most cases in the U.S. are located in rural areas of south central and western states. Adults involved in hunting, trapping, butchering, and farming are at particular risk. Most cases occur between June and September. Information on diagnostic testing of specimens can be obtained from state public health laboratories and the

Division of Vector-Borne Infectious Diseases: CDC, Fort Collins, Colorado [(970) 221-6400; e-mail: dvbid@cdc.gov].

Human-to-human transmission is lacking. In the event of a laboratory spill, decontaminate by spraying the suspected contaminate with a 10% bleach solution (one part bleach to nine parts water). After 10 minutes, clean the area with a 70% solution of isopropyl alcohol. Soapy water can be used to irrigate the remaining solution. Standard levels of chlorine in water usually protect against waterborne infection.

Correlates of protective immunity appear ~2 weeks following natural infection or vaccination. Given the short incubation period of tularemia and incomplete protection of current vaccination against inhalational tularemia, vaccination is not recommended for postexposure prophylaxis. The Working Group recommends use of the live vaccine strain only for laboratory personnel routinely working with *F. tularensis*.

Can be cleared to work in research lab after any positive skin reaction at site following live vaccine administration with seroconversion.

Specific References

Rusnak JM, Kortepeter MG, Aldis J, et al, "Experience in the Medical Management of Potential Laboratory Exposures to Agents of Bioterrorism on the Basis of Risk Assessment at the United States Army Medical Research Institute of Infectious Diseases (USAMRIID)," *J Occup Environ Med*, 2004, 46(8):801-11.

Rusnak JM, Kortepeter MG, Hawley RG, et al, "Management Guidelines for Laboratory Exposures to Agents of Bioterrorism," *J Occup Environ Med*, 2004, 46(8):791-800.

Funnel Web Spider

Related Information
- Tarantulas

Scientific Name *Atrax robustus* (Southern Australia); *Hadronyche formidabilus* (New South Wales); *Trechona venosa* (South America)

Mechanism of Toxic Action Venom contains a potent neurotoxin (atraxotoxin) which causes neurotransmitter release (acetylcholine, norepinephrine and epinephrine) at the motor end plate through the autonomic nervous system; hypertension is caused by vasoconstriction; robustoxin can cause dyspnea and muscle fasciculations

Signs and Symptoms of Overdose Two phases:

Phase I (minutes following envenomation): Localized piloerection with widespread muscle fasciculations (first noted in facial, lingual and intercostal regions). Over the next 20 minutes muscle fasciculations may become generalized. From 5-30 minutes severe hypertension, tachycardia, hyperthermia, and coma with increased intracranial pressure develop. Diaphoresis, diarrhea, elevated creatine phosphokinase levels, lacrimation, metabolic acidosis, muscle writhing, salivation, and trismus also are noted. Death within 30 minutes may be due to laryngeal spasm, apnea, or pulmonary edema.

Phase II (1-2 hours after envenomation): Cholinergic crisis abates (and patient may regain consciousness). In severe cases, hypotension may ensue with pulmonary edema and apnea.

Admission Criteria/Prognosis Admit any symptomatic patient; asymptomatic patients 4 hours postbite may be discharged

Overdosage/Treatment

Decontamination: Since the venom travels primarily through lymphatics, the affected limb should be immobilized with crepe bandage tourniqueting; proximal pneumatic tourniquets may also be useful as is a Sawyer negative pressure suction device

Supportive therapy: Atropine should be used to control bronchorrhea and salivation; esmolol or propranolol can be used for hypertension or tachycardia; a purified IgG antivenom of rabbit origin is the mainstay of treatment and should be considered in any patient with muscle fasciculations, salivation, lacrimation, piloerection, hypertension, dyspnea, or mental status changes; developed by Commonwealth Serum Laboratories in Australia in 1980, it is given intravenously 2 ampules (100 mg) every 15 minutes until symptoms improve; pretreatment should occur with an antihistamine and 100 mg of hydrocortisone sodium succinate; no skin testing is needed

Antidote(s)
- Atropine [ANTIDOTE]

Additional Information These large spiders (up to 5 cm) prefer cool moist regions and can inhabit burrows under rocks or logs (*Atrax*), be tree dwelling (*Hadronyche*) or be sedentary living in holes or plants (*Trechona*)

Giant Elephants Ear

Scientific Name *Alocasia macrorrhiza*

Mechanism of Toxic Action Calcium oxalate (which is distributed throughout the entire plant and can cause local mucosal swelling) and a saphotoxin (which can result in gastroenteritis or neurotoxicity).

Signs and Symptoms of Overdose Develop almost immediately: Abdominal pain, dysarthria, dysphagia, dysphonia, excess salivation, hypocalcemia, lip swelling, ocular irritation, oral cavity numbness, oral

cavity ulcers, sore throat. All symptoms (except for oral cavity numbness) resolve within one week.

Admission Criteria/Prognosis Admit any patient with abdominal pain or airway compromise. Monitor for renal failure and hypocalcemia. Admit any patient ingesting more than three mouthfuls.

Overdosage/Treatment Supportive therapy: Ingestions should be treated with the patient drinking 120-240 mL of ice water. Oral gargling with Xylocaine® can reduce oral pain. Monitor for hypocalcemia and renal failure.

Additional Information A plant native to Southwest Asia and Northern Australia, found along costal wetlands and valleys. Has been used to treat snake and insect bites by either topical application or drinking the plant's juice with vinegar and ginger juice.

Gila Monster

Related Information
- Mexican Beaded Lizard

Scientific Name *Heloderma cinctum*; *Heloderma suspectum*

Mechanism of Toxic Action Venom contains hyaluronidase gilatoxin, helothermine, phospholipase A, kallikrein, and serotonin; venom is proteolytic with minimal tissue breakdown seen

Adverse Reactions

Cardiovascular: Sinus tachycardia

Hematologic: Coagulopathy

Miscellaneous: Anaphylaxis

Signs and Symptoms of Overdose Exophthalmus, tachypnea, thrombocytopenia, tinnitus. Generalized asthenia, hypotension, localized erythema and edema, leukocytosis, nausea, regional lympadenopathy, sweating, tachycardia, and vomiting may occur. Localized pain may be severe.

Admission Criteria/Prognosis Admit if symptomatic for systemic reaction after 6 hours postexposure; mortality: ~5% (children), ~1% (adults)

Overdosage/Treatment

Decontamination: Avoid breaking off teeth when removing lizard; flame, cold water immersion, and handheld cast spreaders can assist in disengaging lizard

Supportive therapy: Local wound care with broad spectrum antibiotics should be administered; monitor tetanus immunization status; patient should be observed for at least 6 hours for systemic reactions; antivenom therapy (through the Poisonous Animal Research Laboratory at Arizona State University or the Venom Poisoning Center at the University of Southern California) is experimental

Additional Information Lethal dose: 5-8 mg. Endemic in the southwestern United States, these lizards are 30-50 cm long; usually docile but will bite and hang on tenaciously when provoked; teeth may break and be left in the wound (teeth are not radiopaque); venom glands are located in lower anterior jaw; 30% of bites have no venom injected; *Heloderma horridum* (the beaded lizard) found in Mexico has a similar type of venom; submerging the animal in cold water may subdue the lizard thus allowing for disengagement; a handheld cast spreader can also be used to disengage the reptile's mandible

Specific Reference

Morgan BW, Lee C, Damiano L, et al, "Reptile Envenomation 20-Year Mortality as Reported by US Medical Examiners," *South Med J*, 2004, 97(7):642-4.

Golden Chain Tree

Mechanism of Toxic Action Contains cytisine which has effects similar to nicotine

Adverse Reactions

Cardiovascular: Sinus tachycardia

Gastrointestinal: Constipation

Genitourinary: Urinary retention

Signs and Symptoms of Overdose Asthenia, ataxia, drowsiness, headache, hypotension, mydriasis, nausea, pallor, paralysis, seizures, tachycardia, vomiting

Admission Criteria/Prognosis Symptomatic patients 4-6 hours postexposure should be admitted

Toxicodynamics/Kinetics Onset of symptoms: Within 15 minutes to 4 hours

Overdosage/Treatment

Decontamination: Ipecac relatively contraindicated because of risk of seizures occurring rapidly with large ingestion; lavage (within 1 hour)/ activated charcoal with cathartic if large amounts ingested

Supportive care: Maintain respiration and blood pressure in symptomatic patient; urinary retention may respond to bethanechol

Additional Information Small tree (grows to 30 feet high). Range: Found in southern U.S. Toxic part: All parts toxic, no reports of toxic exposure to this plant exist in the U.S.; however, British literature reports poisonings

Grass Spider

Scientific Name *Agelenopsis aperta*
Mechanism of Toxic Action Unknown; can cause local tissue necrosis.
Signs and Symptoms of Overdose Ataxia, disorientation, headache, lethargy, myalgia, pallor. Local lesions are ~1.5 cm in diameter and are black-blue in color with a white center, appearing within 30 minutes. Local lesions may last for ~1 week.
Overdosage/Treatment Supportive therapy: Oral antibiotics should be considered such as dicloxacillin (250 mg 4 times/day). Analgesics (ibuprofen or acetaminophen) can be used for pain control.
Additional Information The spider is native to the western United States. It is 13-18 mm long with eight eyes and two brown longitudinal stripes on its tan cephalothorax. Its abdomen is long with an undulating pattern of brown and tannish coloring on the dorsal aspect. It also contains two long spinnerets posterior to the abdomen.

Green Lynx Spider

Mechanism of Toxic Action Venom is "squirted" from the oral cavity (at a range of 40 cm); envenomation can also occur through bites; venom is thought to be proteolytic
Signs and Symptoms of Overdose Sharp pain at bite site, erythema, pruritus. Symptoms usually resolve within 48 hours. Conjunctivitis can occur with ocular envenomation. Wound necrosis usually does not occur.
Overdosage/Treatment Supportive therapy: Local wound care (with tetanus prophylaxis) is all that is usually required; antibiotics are usually not necessary. If ocular envenomation occurs, copious irrigation of the affected eye with saline or water is suggested.
Additional Information A bright green spider with long, spiny-haired legs, usually found in grass or on plants in the southern U.S. and central Mexico. Most envenomations occur in the fall.

Hawaiian Baby Woodrose

Scientific Name *Argyreia nervosa*
Impairment Potential Can occur if >3 seeds are ingested
Mechanism of Toxic Action Related to LSD; contains ergoline alkaloids (ergine/isoergine) in the seeds, which exhibit indole alkaloid effects similar to LSD
Adverse Reactions
Cardiovascular: Tachycardia
Central nervous system: Paranoia, agitation, psychosis (which can start ~5 hours postingestion)
Gastrointestinal: Nausea, vomiting
Hematologic: Leukocytosis
Ocular: Visual hallucinations
Overdosage/Treatment
Decontamination: Oral: If >3 seeds are ingested, activated charcoal can be given; lavage (within 1 hour) may be useful
Supportive therapy: Benzodiazepine can be given to treat agitation
Additional Information A tropical woody vine with rose-colored flowers and thick black seeds; found in Hawaii, Florida, southern California, and India

Hobo Spider

Scientific Name *Tegenaria agrestis*
Mechanism of Toxic Action Arachnotoxins have hemolytic properties
Signs and Symptoms of Overdose While the bite of the hobo spider may initially be painless, induration (with surrounding erythema) may occur within 30 minutes. Blisters can develop in 15-35 hours. Following blister rupture (with exudative fluid), eschar with underlying necrosis and eventual sloughing can occur. Lesions become fully necrotic in ~50% of cases and can take 45 days to fully heal (with scar formation). Deeper bites may take up to 3 years to heal. Systemic symptoms can occur as early as 30 minutes postbite. Severe headache, anorexia, nausea, dizziness, lethargy, dry mouth, and generalized weakness initially occur and can be followed by fever, visual disturbances, memory loss, hallucinations and vomiting. Severe systemic reactions such as aplastic anemia, thrombocytopenia, pancytopenia, and profuse secretory diarrhea are rare but can be fatal.

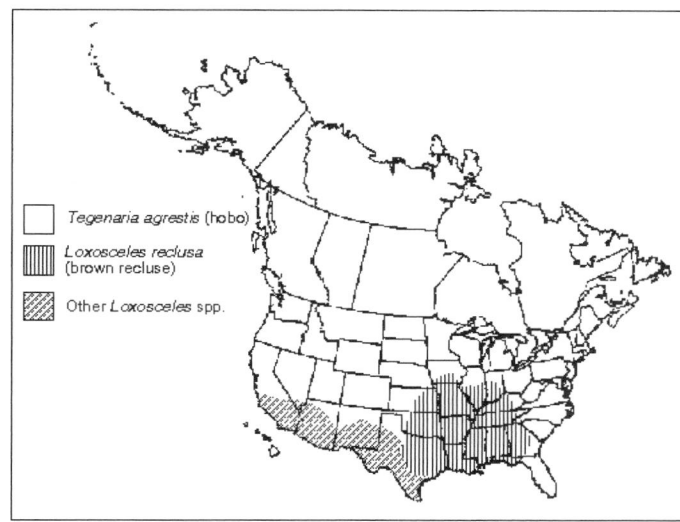

From "Necrotic Arachnidism," *MMWR Morb Mortal Wkly Rep*, 1996, 45(21):435.

Overdosage/Treatment Supportive therapy: Oral diphenhydramine with alternating local applications of heat and ice can be utilized; severe hematologic abnormalities (other than leukocytosis) may respond to systemic corticosteroids; while surgical repair may be necessary, it should not be initiated until primary necrotizing process is completed; in severe cases with rapidly progressive necrosis, dapsone (50-200 mg/day in twice daily dosing) or colchicine (1.2 mg orally followed by 0.6 mg every 2 hours for 2 days then 0.6 mg every 4 hours for 2 days) may be useful; hyperbaric oxygen can be considered for necrotic lesions progressing to skin sloughing
Additional Information A large (7-14 mm body length: 27-45 mm leg span) brown spider with gray markings which can move quickly (1 meter/second); it is found in dark moist areas on ground or basement levels (ie, wood piles, crawl spaces) and are abundant from midsummer to fall; found in central Utah, Alaskan panhandle, southwest Canada, Washington, Oregon and Idaho; bites may be confused with brown recluse spiders
Specific Reference
Vetter RS and Isbister GK, "Do Hobo Spider Bites Cause Dermonecrotic Injuries?" *Ann Emerg Med*, 2004, 44(6):605-7.

Holly

Scientific Name *Ilex aquifolium*; *Ilex opaca*; *Ilex vomitoria*
Uses Native Americans used the plant as an emetic and cardiac stimulant
Mechanism of Toxic Action Irritation of the gastrointestinal tract
Signs and Symptoms of Overdose Diarrhea, nausea, and vomiting
Overdosage/Treatment
Decontamination: Charcoal may be of value; one dose of cathartic may be given if symptoms have not begun; gastric decontamination emesis with ipecac within 30 minutes or lavage within 1 hour for ingestions over six berries (especially if the berries are chewed)
Supportive therapy: Replace fluids and electrolytes as needed to prevent dehydration
Additional Information Toxic dose: Not well established; apparently berries must be eaten in quantity to produce toxic symptoms. Range: Found throughout the eastern and southern U.S. Toxin: Ilexanthin, ilex acid, tannic acid, ilicin. Toxic part: Berries are toxic in quantity

Hyacinth

Scientific Name *Hyacinthus orientalis*
Signs and Symptoms of Overdose Predominantly include diarrhea, GI irritation, nausea, stomach cramps, and vomiting. Contact dermatitis has been reported. May cause rhinitis or trigger an asthma attack in sensitive individuals.
Overdosage/Treatment Supportive therapy: Maintain fluid and electrolyte balance as needed
Additional Information Toxic dose: Not well quantified; symptoms have been reported after small ingestions. Range: Common garden plant throughout U.S.. Toxin: Thought to be narcissine-like alkaloids. Toxic part: Bulb

Hydrangea

Scientific Name *Hydrangea arborescens*; *Hydrangea paniculata*
Mechanism of Toxic Action Amygdalin (a cyanogenic glycoside) is hydrolyzed in the gut to release hydrocyanic acid; cellular hypoxia occurs after absorption and complexation with cytochrome oxidase

Signs and Symptoms of Overdose Reported poisonings have shown hydrangea to cause nausea and gastroenteritis; may also cause contact dermatitis

Admission Criteria/Prognosis All symptomatic patients should probably be admitted to an intensive care unit for 1-2 days; asymptomatic patients should be observed for at least 2 hours and then can be discharged; survival after 4 hours (in an acute exposure) is usually associated with recovery

Overdosage/Treatment
Decontamination: Activated charcoal with cathartic may be beneficial; lavage within 1 hour would be indicated if the patient exhibited cyanogenic effects

Supportive therapy: Maintain fluid and electrolyte balance; give sodium bicarbonate for acidosis; treat as cyanide exposure if acidosis is present.

Antidote(s)
- Cyanide Antidote Kit [ANTIDOTE]

Diagnostic Procedures
- Anion Gap, Blood
- Electrolytes, Blood
- Methemoglobin, Blood

Additional Information No cases of cyanogenic toxicity on record. Toxic part: Buds, flowers, and leaves

Hydroids (Coral)

Mechanism of Toxic Action Nematocysts cause intense local reaction

Signs and Symptoms of Overdose Stings produce a painful stinging sensation. Abdominal pain, fever, diarrhea have occurred rarely. Rash and erythema are likely for free-floating Portuguese Man-of-War, orange-striped jellyfish, and the stinging Medusa. May cause generalized symptoms including arthralgia, coagulopathy, intense local pain (electric shock-like), myalgias, and lymphadenopathy with asthenia, fever, and headache.

Overdosage/Treatment Supportive therapy: Epinephrine or antihistamines can be used for rash; muscle spasms can be treated with calcium gluconate I.V.; coral cuts should be cleansed and debrided; dermatitis can be treated with a topical corticosteroid cream. Meat tenderizer solution neutralizes protein toxin and thus can be sprinkled over wound of Portuguese Man-of-War; irrigate with sea water (not fresh water); apply 5% acetic acid or 40% to 70% isopropyl alcohol to inactivate nematocysts; diluted ammonia hydroxide may also be used; remove remaining nematocysts by shaving the area.

Additional Information Exoskeleton of calcium carbonate; an encrustation. Family: Hydrozoa; *Millepora* (Florida Keys and Caribbean). Phylum: Coelenterata Range: Found attached to rocks in shallow water in temperate zones

Hymenoptera

Related Information
- Fire Ants

Scientific Name *Apoidea* (Honey Bee); *Formicidae* (Fire Ant); *Myrmecia* (Jumper Ant, primarily located in Australia); *Politinae* (Wasp); *Vespoidea* (Yellow Jacket, Hornet)

Mechanism of Toxic Action The venom contains multiple allergens (phospholipase, hyaluronidase, acid phosphatase, etc) which can result in an IgE mediated anaphylactic reaction. Mast cell degranulating peptides are also found and can cause histamine release from mast cells.

Signs and Symptoms of Overdose
Multiple stings can result in systemic reactions. Anaphylactic reactions can occur immediately and are characterized by chest tightness, chills, dyspnea, hypotension, laryngeal edema, tachycardia, stridor, and urticaria.

Hepatic necrosis, hemolysis, proteinuria, renal failure and thrombocytopenia have been noted following multiple bee or hornet stings. Local dermal effects have included angioedema, erythema, localized pain, pruritus, and swelling (>10 cm). Serum sickness (with arthralgia) may occur along with rhabdomyolysis.

Admission Criteria/Prognosis Admit any patient with systemic symptomatology or with more than 50 stings.

Overdosage/Treatment
Decontamination: Remove the stinger and venom apparatus as soon as possible. Irrigate the area as soon as possible with soap and water.

Supportive therapy: Anaphylaxis should be treated with standard measures (ie, epinephrine, antihistamines, vasopressors, and corticosteroids). Methylprednisolone 1-2 mg/kg I.V. every 6 hours should be considered. Serum sickness can be treated with corticosteroids; urticaria often improves with SubQ administration of epinephrine (1:1000) or an antihistamine. Monitor for rhabdomyolysis in severe and multiple stings.

Antidote(s)
- Epinephrine [ANTIDOTE]

Drug Interaction Use of calcium channel blockers, beta adrenergic blockers, or nonsteroidal anti-inflammatory drugs may increase the severity of Hymenoptera stings.

Additional Information The African honey bees (*Apis mellifera scutellata*) have been migrating north from Latin America since 1956. As opposed to the European honey bees (*Apis mellifera*), African honey bees (also known as "killer bees") exhibit more aggressive behavior with multiplicity of stings and a larger reaction distance (1091 yards for the African honey bee as compared to <30 yards for the European bee). Thus, a healthy adult can usually outrun these bees since they do not usually pursue farther than the above distances. The individual should run with mouth and nose covered. Spraying the bees with soapy water can help immobilize the insect. Anaphylactic emergency treatment kits containing epinephrine should be readily available to individuals with a history of anaphylaxis. Venom immunotherapy can be considered for individuals with a history of anaphylaxis or life-threatening systemic reaction. Patients with a history of dermal reactions are usually not candidates for venom immunotherapy.

Specific References

Ashley JR, Otero H, and Aboulafia DM, "Bee Envenomation: A Rare Cause of Thrombotic Thrombocytopenic Purpura," *South Med J*, 2003, 96(6):588-91.

Balit CR, Isbister GK, and Buckley NA, "Randomized Controlled Trial of Topical Aspirin in the Treatment of Bee and Wasp Stings," *J Toxicol Clin Toxicol*, 2003, 41(6):801-8.

Betten DP, Richardson WH, Tong TC, et al, "Massive Honey Bee Envenomation-induced Rhabdomyolysis in an Adolescent," *Pediatrics*. 2006, 117(1):231-5.

Lin CC, Chang MY, and Lin JL, "Hornet Sting Induced Systemic Allergic Reaction and Large Local Reaction with Bulle Formation and Rhabdomyolysis," *J Toxicol Clin Toxicol*, 2003, 41(7):1009-11.

Stefanidou M, Athanaselis S, and Koutselinis A, "The Toxicology of Honey Bee Poisoning," *Vet Hum Toxicol*, 2003, 45(5):261-5.

Indian Tobacco

Related Information
- Star-of-Bethlehem (*Ornithogalum pyrenaicum*)
- Star-of-Bethlehem (*Ornithogalum umbellatum*)

Scientific Name *Lobelia inflata*

Uses Variety of purposes over the years; the extract has been used as an emetic; lobeline sulfate has been used as an aid to stop smoking

Mechanism of Toxic Action Contains lobeline alkaloids which have nicotinic-like action and other piperidine alkaloids

Adverse Reactions Cardiovascular: Sinus bradycardia

Signs and Symptoms of Overdose Abdominal pain, bradycardia, coma, diarrhea, euphoria, hypertension, nausea, paralysis, vomiting, seizures, tremor; dermatitis has also been reported

Overdosage/Treatment Decontamination: Emesis within 30 minutes or lavage within 1 hour may be useful in large, recent ingestions if the patient has not started vomiting; activated charcoal with cathartic should be administered; seizures should be managed by benzodiazepines

Additional Information
Lobeline content may vary; specific toxic amounts of plant material is unknown; most poisonings have been from herbal preparations

Other related toxic species are *Lobelia cardinalis*, *Lobelia siphilitica*, and *Lobelia berlandieri*; *Eriogonum umbellatum* is also known as Indian tobacco and is considered nontoxic

Family: Campanulaceae; Range: Grows extensively throughout the U.S.; Toxic part: All parts, especially roots and seeds; Toxic dose: 50 mg of dried herb; poisoning is more transient than that of nicotine

Iris

Scientific Name *Iris germanica*

Mechanism of Toxic Action Resinous substance irisin which acts as an irritant

Signs and Symptoms of Overdose Abdominal pain, burning sensation in mouth and throat, diarrhea, nausea, vomiting. Dermal contact may result in burning sensation and dermatitis.

Overdosage/Treatment Decontamination: Gastrointestinal decontamination may be of value in large recent ingestions

Supportive therapy: Replace fluids and electrolytes as necessary

Additional Information Toxic dose: Specific quantities have not been determined. There are many species of iris with similar toxicities. Family: Iridaceae. Range: Common garden flower cultivated throughout the U.S. Toxic part: Mainly the bulb, but possibly all parts

Jack-in-the-Pulpit

Scientific Name *Arisaema triphyllum*

Mechanism of Toxic Action Entire plant contains calcium oxalate crystals which cause oral irritation, swelling, pain, and slurred speech; large ingestions necessary for systemic toxicity are unlikely to occur due to oral irritation seen with ingestion

Signs and Symptoms of Overdose
Dermal: Irritation, pain, swelling

Ocular: Sap may cause corneal abrasion, lacrimation, pain, photophobia; may also cause dermatitis; oxalate crystals may be deposited on cornea
Oral: Diarrhea, dysphonia, edema, salivation, vomiting

Overdosage/Treatment
Decontamination: **Oral**: Dilute; ipecac/lavage/activated charcoal not likely necessary; milk/water to rinse crystals. **Dermal**: Wash thoroughly. **Ocular**: Irrigate with tepid water for 15 minutes.
Supportive therapy: Cool compresses may minimize pain and swelling

Additional Information Toxin: Calcium oxalate crystals

Jatropha Multifida

Synonyms Coral Plan; Physic Nut
Use Oil used in West Africa to treat parasitic conditions and rheumatism.
Mechanism of Toxic Action Plant contains curcin (a toxalbumin - a proteolytic enzyme that inhibits the 60S ribosomal subunit) and a purgative oil that resembles ricinoleic acid in castor oil. Toxins found in seeds/fruit/sap.
Adverse Reactions Miosis, leukocytosis, vomiting (protracted), lethargy. As few as one seed can cause intoxication in children.
Overdosage/Treatment
Decontamination: Oral: Activated charcoal; Dermal: Wash with soap and water
Supportive care: Intravenous rehydration with crystalloid solutions
Additional Information Native to tropical Americas, West Africa, and Australia. A decorative garden plant with sweet flavored fruit.
Specific References
Koltin D, Uziel Y, Schneidermann D, et al, "A Case of Jatropha Multifida Poisoning Resembling Organophosphate Intoxication," *Clin Toxicol*, 2006, 44:337-8.

Jellyfish

Related Information
● Box Jellyfish
Scientific Name *Aurelia aurita*; *Carybdea alata*
Mechanism of Toxic Action Stings; venoms from nematocysts contain antigenic polypeptides and enzymes (DNAase, histamine); prostaglandin-induced vasodilitation can occur
Adverse Reactions
Severe stings may include hematuria, syncope, paralysis, renal insufficiency, hypotension, cardiorespiratory failure
Central nervous system: Fever, chills
Dermatologic: Nonimmunologic contact urticaria
Neuromuscular & skeletal: Muscle spasms
Signs and Symptoms of Overdose Anaphylactic shock (rare), ataxia, burning, diaphoresis, headache, nausea, pain, rash (usually a linear flagellate pattern of small, papular erythematous eruptions), regional lymph node involvement, skin ulceration, urticaria
Overdosage/Treatment
Decontamination: Wear gloves during decontamination. **Do not** rub affected area. Hot fresh water (40°C to 41°C) immersion of the affected area within 30 minutes may be effective in decreasing pain due to Hawaiian box jellyfish (*Carybdea alata*) stings. Immediately rinse with seawater. Prevent further envenomation by applying acetic acid 5% (vinegar) to any tentacles still adhering to tissue. If acetic acid is not available, use isopropyl alcohol 40% to 70%; or finally, may use aluminum sulfate. Remove tentacles with a gloved hand or forceps. Meat tenderizers have been used; however, they are not preferred for decontamination and should not have prolonged contact time (>10 minutes). Shave envenomated area after initial treatment, then repeat local decontamination therapy. Ocular exposures are to be decontaminated by water irrigation only.
Supportive therapy: Local symptoms persisting after the initial treatment may be treated with antihistamines, local anesthetics, or steroid lotion; tetanus prophylaxis should be given according to patient's immunization status. Refractory hyperpigmentation can be treated with topical hydroquinone bleaches. Anaphylaxis should be treated with standard therapy.
Additional Information Largest jellyfish in the Arctic Lion's Mane whose tentacles can reach >100 feet in length. Dead jellyfish can release toxins. Class: Scyphozoa. Range: All oceans
Specific Reference
Armoni M, Ohali M, and Hay E, "Severe Dyspnea Due to Jellyfish Envenomation," *Pediatr Emerg Care*, 2003, 19(2):84-86.

Jequirity Bean

Scientific Name *Abrus precatorius*
Mechanism of Toxic Action Abrin, a toxalbumin, inhibits protein synthesis
Signs and Symptoms of Overdose Acutely causes irritation to esophagus, GI tract, and oropharynx; may cause hemorrhage and tissue sloughing. Acute demylination encephalitis.

Toxicodynamics/Kinetics Acute effects occur within 8 hours; late phase complications delayed by 2-5 days possibly with asymptomatic phase in between
Overdosage/Treatment Decontamination: Activated charcoal may be useful; consider using osmotic cathartic despite hyperactive bowel as decreased exposure to mucosa may be beneficial, follow fluid and electrolyte status closely if symptomatic; if symptomatic, maintain urine flow; consider alkalinization to prevent hemoglobin crystallization in severe poisonings; guaiac vomiting, stool, follow fluid and electrolyte status; check hematologic parameters in severe poisoning, hepatic enzymes
Additional Information Toxicity may occur with as little as one bean. Scarlet bean-shaped seed with a black spot where attached inside pod; used in necklaces and as good luck charms; toxicity will not occur unless seed coat is broken; toxicity is variable; related to variations within plants and GI absorption, seed has hard coat; rupture makes toxin available; symptomatic patients should be hospitalized; asymptomatic patients that have received early thorough decontamination may be observed at home; has been used as an abortifacient; Toxic part: Bark, seeds, and leaves
Specific References
Dickers KJ, Bradberry SM, Rice P, et al, "Abrin Poisoning," *Toxicol Rev*, 2003, 22(3):137-42.
Sahni V, Agarwal SK, Singh NP, Sikdar S, "Acute Demyelinating Encephalitis After Jequirity Pea Ingestion (Abrus Precatorius)," *Clin Toxicol*, 2007, 45 (1):77-9.

Jimson Weed

Scientific Name *Datura stramonium*
Impairment Potential Yes
Mechanism of Toxic Action The whole plant, especially the foliage and seeds, contains anticholinergic compounds like atropine, hyoscyamine, and scopolamine; seeds contain highest amount of atropine (0.1 mg atropine per seed); ~50-100 seeds may cause severe intoxication and hallucinations. **Note:** Seeds are often ingested for their deliriant effect.
Adverse Reactions
Cardiovascular: Sinus tachycardia
Central nervous system: Memory disturbances, psychosis, fever, hyperthermia
Signs and Symptoms of Overdose Usually occur within 1 hour and may last for 2 days: Auditory hallucinations, decreased bowel sounds, delirium, disorientation, dizziness, hypertension, mydriasis, nausea, pruritus, seizures, tachycardia, urinary retention, visual hallucinations, vomiting. Hallucinations usually resolve within 18 hours. Mydriasis can persist for several days.
Toxicodynamics/Kinetics May decrease GI motility and, therefore, slow absorption
Overdosage/Treatment
Decontamination: Due to decreased GI motility, lavage may be useful unless the patient is symptomatic with anticholinergic toxidrome
Supportive therapy: Physostigmine may be useful to treat life-threatening anticholinergic symptoms; physostigmine should not be used in this ingestion if tricyclic antidepressants are a suspected coingestant due to the potential for seizures; propranolol can be used to help in treating cardiovascular complications; benzodiazepines should be used for treatment of agitation
Additional Information Toxin: Anticholinergic compounds; $^2/_3$ of exposures occur from August through November; manifestations of anticholinergic poisoning usually resolve within 3 days; not sold as an herbal dietary supplement in U.S. The 50-100 brown-black seeds in the fruit pods each contain ~0.05-0.1 mg of atropine.
Specific References
Bania TC, Chu J, Bailes D, et al, "Jimsonweed (*Datura stramonium*) Seed Extract as a Protective Agent in Severe Organophosphate Poisoning," *Acad Emerg Med*, 2003, 10:511b-12b.
Bania TC, Chu J, Bailes D, et al, "Jimson Weed Extract as a Protective Agent in Severe Organophosphate Toxicity," *Acad Emerg Med*, 2004, 11:335-8.
Bania TC, Chu J, Smith J, et al, "Mechanism of Protective Effects of *Datura stramonium* in Organophosphate Poisoning," *Acad Emerg Med*, 2003, 10:518a.
Bania TC, Chu J, Stobach A, et al, "Gastric Pretreatment with Jimsonweed Does Not Increase Survival in Severe Organophosphate Toxicity," *Acad Emerg Med*, 2004, 11(5):471.
Boumba VA, Mitselou A, and Vougiouklakis T, "Fatal Poisoning from Ingestion of *Datura stramonium* Seeds," *Vet Hum Toxicol*, 2004, 46(2):81-2.

Jonquil

Scientific Name *Narcissus jonquilla*
Mechanism of Toxic Action Contains lycorine (an *Amaryllidaceae* alkaloid) a centrally acting emetic

Signs and Symptoms of Overdose Usually abdominal pain, diarrhea, nausea, salivation, and vomiting. Symptoms develop soon after oral ingestion (within 30 minutes) and resolve within 3 hours (according to one report).

Overdosage/Treatment Decontamination: Ipecac relatively contraindicated; activated charcoal with cathartic/lavage within 1 hour may be beneficial depending on amount ingested and time elapsed since ingestion

Additional Information Toxic dose: Not established. Colchicine-like effects seen at ingestions >5 mg/kg. Toxic part: All parts contain alkaloid; bulb is most toxic

Juniper Tar

Scientific Name *Juniperus oxycedrus*

Uses Sebhorrhea, eczema, psoriasis (topical use)

Mechanism of Toxic Action Has keratolytic, antipruritic, and antimicrobial effects *in vitro* due to the extracts (methanol, dichloromethane) which can inhibit histamine, serotonin, acetylcholine, and anti-inflammatory response; contains ehteric oils, triepene, and phenols

Adverse Reactions Ocular: Conjunctivitis (on contact)

Signs and Symptoms of Overdose Oral: Fever, headache, myalgias, nausea, vomiting, cough, hypotension, gingival erosions, leukocytosis, polyuria, renal insuficiency, hematuria, proteinuria, thrombocytopenia, tachycardia

Dosage

Ointments are in the 1% to 5R range

Shampoos are in the 4% to 20% range

Overdosage/Treatment

Decontamination: Lavage/activated charcoal within 2 hours of ingestion

Supportive therapy: Crystalloid intravenous fluids for hypotension; dopamine (10 mcg/kg/minute) can be vasopressor of choice

Additional Information Evergreen tree which grows in Europe, Asia (specifically Turkey), and North America. Destructive distillation of wood of the plant is used to prepare the oil. The oil is dark with a tar-like odor and bitter taste.

Specific References

Koruk St, Ozyilkan E, Kaya P, et al, "Juniper Tar Poisoning," *Clin Tox*, 2005, 1:47-9.

King Cobra

Scientific Name *Ophiophagus hannah*

Mechanism of Toxic Action Venom contains polypeptides which cause a postsynaptic neuromuscular block along with possessing hemorrhagic activity.

Signs and Symptoms of Overdose Usually occur within 6 hours: Abdominal pain, cranial nerve palsies, dysarthria, dysphagia with increased secretions, facial muscle weakness, headache, hypotension (in ~5% to 10% of cases), leukocytosis, nausea, ptosis, tachycardia, vomiting. Neurological symptoms may progress to coagulopathy (increased prothrombin time), coma, confusion, flaccid paralysis, hyporeflexia, and lethargy. Local tissue necrosis from the bite may be delayed 2-4 days.

Admission Criteria/Prognosis Transport any bite to the hospital. Asymptomatic individuals may be discharged at 6 hours postbite with close follow-up.

Overdosage/Treatment Supportive therapy: Monitor respiratory status. Cholinesterase inhibitors are ineffective. Specific antivenin is available: Thai Red Cross king cobra antivenin (Bangkok, Thailand) may be found at zoological parks. Skin testing may be required. After a negative skin test, infuse intravenously 15 vials (150 mL) of reconstituted antivenin diluted in 850 mL of 0.9% normal saline over a 2-hour period. Australian tiger snake antivenin is a second choice if king cobra antivenin is not available. Mechanical ventilation may be required.

Diagnostic Procedures

- Prothrombin Time

Additional Information Largest poisonous snake (~7-13 feet long), found in Southeast Asia and India. Ninety-four percent of bites result in envenomation. When biting, these snakes hold tightly to the victim and chew the tissue while envenomation occurs. It has a large occipital shield with a narrow hood. Adults are brown or greenish-yellow with a darker tail.

Lantana

Scientific Name *Lantana camara*

Adverse Reactions Central nervous system: Delirium

Signs and Symptoms of Overdose Ataxia, coma, cyanosis, death, diarrhea, drowsiness, dyspnea, mydriasis, photophobia, vomiting

Overdosage/Treatment Decontamination: If the patient is not already vomiting, then vomiting or lavage (within 1 hour) should be initiated following ingestion of green berries, not ripe berries or leaves, followed by activated charcoal with cathartic

Drug Interaction Thujone-containing and gamolenic-acid containing herbs can lower the seizure threshold leading to increased anticonvulsant dosage requirements.

Additional Information Toxic dose: Specific quantities are unknown, any amount of unripe (green) berries should be considered potentially hazardous; animal toxicity from grazing on leaves is well known. Family: Verbenaceae; Toxin: Leaves contain triterpenes, lantadene A or B; toxic component of berry is unknown. Range: Tropical plant found in Florida and Texas. Toxic part: Unripe berries, toxicity of other parts is unknown

Leeches

Scientific Name *Hirudo medicinalis*

U.S. Brand Names Exhirud®

Uses Blood evacuation; used in skin graft repair, breast reconstruction, periorbital hematomas, digital reimplantations, ring avulsion injuries; useful in areas where there is good arterial flow but no venous outflow

Mechanism of Toxic Action Contains several anticoagulants in its salivary glands including hirudin, hementin, hyaluronidase, lodellins, eglins, cathepsin G, subtilisin, and fibrinases

Adverse Reactions

Dermatologic: Ecchymosis

Hematologic: Hemorrhage, anemia

Local: Wound infection, scarring at wound site

Toxicodynamics/Kinetics Elimination: Hirudin: Renal

Overdosage/Treatment

Decontamination: **Pharyngeal**: Gargle with salt water or vinegar. **Dermal**: **Do not** pull leech off since its jaws may break off resulting in an ulcer or wound infection; salt, salt water, or vinegar can aid in topical leech removal

Supportive therapy: Wound infection rate is ~20%; wound infections can be treated with amoxicillin (with or without clavulanic acid) or cefuroxime; tetanus prophylaxis should be performed; localized hemorrhage can be controlled with firm pressure

Additional Information

A black freshwater annelid, 25-40 mm in length.

A leech can ingest ~5-15 mL of blood; leeches should never be reused; therapy is usually 3-7 days. Localized wound hemorrhage may continue for up to one day. Contraindications include hemorrhagic diathesis, croup, and erysipelas.

Leeches may be vectors for *Aeromonas hydrophila* and *Trypanosoma cruzi*. Erysipelas and puerperal fevers have been known to be transmitted by leeches.

Disposal: Place leeches in a container of 70% isopropyl alcohol for 5 minutes, then dispose per infectious waste protocol.

Medicinal leeches may be obtained from: Leeches USA, 300 Shames Dr, Westbury, NY 11590: (516) 333-2570 or (800) 645-3569

Emergency delivery: (800) 488-4400, ext 2475

Lepidoptera

Scientific Name *Megalopyge opercularis*

Mechanism of Toxic Action Toxin found on spines that break off into skin - "passive stinging"; irritant; may also contain histamine

Signs and Symptoms of Overdose Blindness, coughing can occur on inhalation, dyspnea, fever, headache, lymphadenopathy (lepidopterism), muscle cramps, pain at injury site, paralysis, pruritus, rash, seizures, vomiting

Overdosage/Treatment

Decontamination: Wash skin with warm water, hairs or broken spines can be removed by applying and then peeling Scotch® tape on the surface of the skin

Supportive therapy: Antihistamines/analgesics

Lice

Scientific Name *Pediculus humanus*; *Phthirus pubis*

Mechanism of Toxic Action Requires human blood to survive; an ectoparasite

Signs and Symptoms of Overdose Erythema, pruritus. Secondary impetiginization can occur. Small macules may be seen in *Phthirus pubis* (maculae ceruleae).

Overdosage/Treatment

General principles of treating pediculosis include discarding or carefully laundering clothing, discarding infested combs or hats, and laundering bedsheets. In general, clothes and bedsheets can be effectively decontaminated by dry cleaning or by machine washing and drying in a hot cycle. Secondary bacterial infections of the skin are common and generally respond to antibiotics effective against *Staphylococcus aureus* (dicloxacillin, erythromycin, and others). Pruritus is typically quite severe and may be alleviated by hydroxyzine (Atarax®), diphenhydramine (Benadryl®), and/or topical steroid creams.

Treatment guidelines:

- Pediculosis corporis: Since the louse resides mainly in the creases of clothes and not on the host, the infection can often be eradicated by delousing contaminated items and maintaining careful hygiene.
- Pediculosis capitis: Several agents are effective: 1% lindane (Kwell®) shampoo to the scalp, pyrethrin liquid (RID), or permethrin creme rinse (Nix™) These insecticides are probably equal in efficacy. Only lindane requires a prescription. **Caution:** Lindane has been associated with seizures and other nervous system toxicities. However, the risk of serious adverse effects during treatment for pediculosis is small due to its minimal systemic absorption. Nevertheless, lindane should be avoided in pregnancy and in lactating women.
- Pediculosis pubis: The treatment recommendations are the same as for *P. capitis*. In addition, sexual partners should be identified and treated in the same manner. Pediculosis involving the eyelashes should **not** be treated with insecticides. Instead, occlusive ophthalmic ointment should be applied to the eyelashes twice daily for at least 8 days in an attempt to smother the parasites.

Patients should be seen in follow-up if symptoms persist 1 week after treatment. A second application may be necessary. Some clinicians routinely instruct patients to reapply the insecticide at the 1 week point.

Diagnostic Procedures
- Arthropod Identification

Additional Information Transmitted through body contact. Family: Anoplura; *Pediculus humanus corporis* (head louse, body louse); *Phthirus pubis* (crab louse)

Microbiology: Human lice are ectoparasites and thus tend to live on or in the skin of the host. They belong to the insect class *Hexapoda*. There are three species important in human infection. *Pediculus humanus* var. *corporis* is the human body louse, *Pediculus humanus* var. *capitis* is the human head louse, and *Phthirus pubis* is the crab louse. The body and head louse have similar appearances and are ~4 mm long. The pubic louse is much wider and has a crab-like appearance from which its name is derived; the eggs adhere to human hair and to clothing, and are termed nits.

Epidemiology: Humans are the reservoir for lice. Infestations have been described worldwide especially in areas of overcrowding. The incubation period is ~1-4 weeks following exposure. Individuals are communicable until all the lice and eggs have been treated and destroyed. Pediculosis capitis is a particular problem with school-aged children, where the practice of sharing combs or brushes facilitates epidemic transmission. All socioeconomic backgrounds are at risk for head lice. In contrast, pediculosis corporis is seen mainly in areas of poor sanitation. The body louse resides almost exclusively in soiled clothing, rather than the skin, and only leaves the clothing for a blood meal from the host. Pediculosis corporis also transmits the rickettsial infection epidemic typhus, as well as several others. *Phthirus pubis* is usually sexually transmitted, although spreading via infested bedding or clothing can occur.

Clinical Syndromes:
- **Pediculosis corporis:** Typically, the patient complains of severe pruritus, and small, erythematous papules are found on the body. Often extensive self-induced excoriations across the trunk are noted. If left untreated for long periods, hyperpigmentation and scarring may occur, called "vagabond's disease."
- **Pediculosis capitis:** The most common presentation is intractable scalp pruritus. On examination there may be evidence of secondary bacterial infection of the scalp from excoriations. At times, an "id reaction" occurs, characterized by a dramatic skin eruption over the arms and trunk, felt to be a hypersensitivity reaction.
- **Phthirus pubis:** Most patients present with pruritus in the region of the pubic hairs, but other areas may be involved including the eyelashes and hairs in the axilla; secondary bacterial infections are less common.

Diagnosis: The diagnosis of pediculosis is often suspected when an individual presents with severe pruritus. On some occasions, the patient may have identified lice themselves or have had a recent contact history. The diagnosis is confirmed by finding lice (1-4 mm long, depending on species) and/or the "nits" (usually 1 mm or less, attached to hairs).

Lily-of-the-Valley

Scientific Name *Convallaria majalis*

Mechanism of Toxic Action Whole plant contains cardiac glycosides convallamatian and convallarin

Adverse Reactions Cardiovascular: Sinus bradycardia

Signs and Symptoms of Overdose GI effects (nausea and vomiting) usually precede cardiovascular effects by several hours. Asystole, AV block, bradycardia, confusion, contact dermatitis, dizziness, fatigue, fibrillation (atrial), flutter (atrial), decreased QT interval and prolonged P-R interval, heart block (first, second, and third degree), headache,

hypotension, ventricular arrhythmias; seeing yellow halos and hyperkalemia have also been reported

Admission Criteria/Prognosis Asymptomatic patients with normal electrocardiogram and electrolytes can be discharged after a 12-hour observation; any symptomatic patient should be admitted to a cardiac monitor bed

Overdosage/Treatment

Decontamination: Lavage within 1 hour and multidose activated charcoal enhance total body clearance of digitalis; whole bowel irrigation is also beneficial in removing plant debris from the GI tract and is recommended for ingestions of large amounts of plant material

Supportive therapy: Monitor cardiac status and serum potassium levels; bradycardia will frequently respond to atropine; phenytoin is the recommended treatment for ventricular arrhythmias because it will also improve conduction through the AV node; lidocaine can also be used to treat ventricular arrhythmias, but will not have an effect on AV conduction; other antiarrhythmics which have been used in arrhythmias resistant to the above therapy include magnesium, amiodarone, and bretylium; a pacemaker should be considered for bradycardia and AV nodal blocks resistant to medical management

Digoxin immune Fab has been shown to interact with several different plant cardiac glycosides and may be beneficial in cases resistant to conventional treatment; indications for its use include ventricular arrhythmias resistant to conventional treatment, severe bradycardia, and/or second or third degree heart block resistant to atropine and phenytoin

Antidote(s)
- Digoxin Immune Fab [ANTIDOTE]

Additional Information Toxin: Cardiac glycosides

Lionfish

Scientific Name *Pterosis volitans*

Adverse Reactions Cardiovascular: Sinus bradycardia, sinus tachycardia

Signs and Symptoms of Overdose Burning, pain, swelling in wound; erythema, nausea, numbness, paresthesia, or vomiting which lasts 8-12 hours. Systemic symptoms are rare and include abdominal cramps, bradycardia, dyspnea, headache, hypotension, tachycardia, sweating, syncope

Overdosage/Treatment

Decontamination: Soak affected limb in hot water for 30-90 minutes (110°F to 115°F); provides relief in 94% of patients; antivenin is rarely needed (may be available in seaquariums)

Supportive therapy: Digital nerve block with 0.25% bupivacaine can help reduce pain from digital bites

Additional Information Venom has vasodilatory effect. Range: Found in Pacific/Indian Oceans; bottom-dwelling fish

Listeria monocytogenes Food Poisoning

Commonly Found In Unpasteurized milk, feta cheese, undercooked chicken

Mechanism of Toxic Action

Listeria monocytogenes is a gram-positive bacillus which causes sporadic cases of meningoencephalitis, neonatal infection, septicemia, and several less common syndromes; it is a leading cause of meningitis in immunocompromised individuals, especially renal transplant patients.

The organism is an aerobic, gram-positive rod which does not produce spores. At times it may assume a more coccoid appearance on Gram's stain of clinical samples (eg, cerebrospinal fluid) and may thus be mistaken for gram-positive cocci such as *Streptococcus pneumoniae*. *Listeria* can also be confused morphologically with the more commonly seen *Corynebacterium* species, which are also gram-positive bacilli (but are often contaminants). *Listeria* is primarily an intracellular pathogen, and tends to reside within mononuclear phagocytes of the host. This feature is thought to contribute to its pathogenicity, since the organism can spread from cell to cell in a somewhat protected fashion.

When *Listeria monocytogenes* meningitis is suspected, the clinician should try to submit at least 10 mL of cerebrospinal fluid for bacterial culture, since only a few *Listeria* organisms may be present. The organism generally grows well on most routine media used in the laboratory, and special requests for selective or enrichment cultures for *Listeria* are usually not necessary. It is important that the clinician does not automatically dismiss a report of a "gram-positive rod" isolated from multiple blood or a sterile body site as a contaminant, particularly in an immunocompromised host in whom *Listeria* infection is possible.

Adverse Reactions Cardiovascular: Pericardial effusion/pericarditis

Signs and Symptoms of Overdose Foodborne listeriosis: A prodromal illness of fever with nausea, vomiting, headache, or backache may precede the clinical syndrome (refer to Additional Information) by as long as one week.

Admission Criteria/Prognosis Patients with dehydration (who cannot take fluids orally), immunocompromised patients, severe disturbance in electrolytes or acid-base status, or patients at extreme in terms of age group should be considered for admission

Overdosage/Treatment Supportive therapy: No randomized comparison trials have been performed to determine the drug(s) of choice for listeriosis. *In vitro* data show the organism is susceptible to many antibiotics. The most clinical experience has been limited to penicillin and ampicillin, and they are probably equivalent. Occasionally, penicillin-resistant strains of *Listeria* have been reported, and thus results of susceptibility testing should be followed up on. There is some *in vitro* evidence to suggest the combination of penicillin (or ampicillin) with an aminoglycoside may be synergistic against *Listeria*, and this combination has been used in serious, life-threatening infections; trimethoprim-sulfamethoxazole may also be effective. Cephalosporins do not reliably cover this organism and should not be used for cases of *Listeria* meningitis. Consultation with an infectious disease specialist is appropriate in complicated cases or in the patient with a penicillin allergy.

Additional Information

Incidence of listeriosis has decreased by 44% in the U.S. from 1989 to 1993.

Epidemiology: The epidemiology of listeriosis can be important in certain cases, since clinical presentations may be nonspecific. The precise prevalence of human infection is unclear, but the attack rate appears to be increasing (perhaps due to better reporting or laboratory recognition). Asymptomatic carriage of *Listeria* in stools is relatively frequent; some studies suggest a fecal excretion rate of 1% or more in healthy humans. Humans may be exposed to *Listeria* by one of several routes: consumption of contaminated food, direct exposure to infected animals, or exposure to environmental reservoirs (soil, water, etc).

Cases of listeriosis tend to be sporadic and difficult to predict. Most infections occur in the summer months and are more common in urban than rural settings, despite its reputation as a zoonotic infection. Often, the source of the *Listeria* remains unknown. Increasing attention has been given to foodborne transmission, particularly in the setting of a traceable outbreak. Mexican-style cheese, coleslaw, undercooked chicken, hot dogs, dairy products, and other foods have caused outbreaks. The ability of the organism to survive (and even multiply) during refrigeration probably contributes to food-related transmission.

Infection with *Listeria* usually occurs in definable groups in the community. Cell mediated immunity is critically important in defense against *Listeria*, whereas neutropenia is not clearly a risk factor. Those at highest risk include patients with solid organ transplants, malignancies (particularly lymphoma), and patients receiving corticosteroids. Pregnant females, neonates, and alcoholics are additional groups at risk for infection. Interestingly, listeriosis does not appear to be a common pathogen in patients with AIDS, despite the deficiencies in T-cell function. Although uncommon, serious infections with *Listeria* have been described in otherwise healthy individuals.

Diagnosis: Except for granulomatosis infantiseptica, the clinical presentations of listeriosis are not unique and microbiological confirmation is necessary. Depending on the clinical site of infection, specimens of blood and body fluids should be sent, as described above. Agglutination studies for antibodies directed against *L. monocytogenes* have little value. Stool culture or serologic testing is not useful.

Clinical Syndromes:

● **Adult meningoencephalitis:** *Listeria* is the most common cause of community-acquired meningitis in immunosuppressed individuals. *Listeria* meningitis can be quite variable in its presentation and can range from a subacute course to a rapid and fulminant one. In some cases the diagnosis may be quite difficult when high fevers and nuchal rigidity are absent. There are no pathognomonic features of *Listeria* meningitis which allow diagnosis on clinical grounds alone. CSF chemical analysis is variable and frequently nondiagnostic. The degree of CSF pleocytosis can range from several cells to $>12,000$ cells/mm^3. Differential cell counts vary from nearly 100% polymorphonuclear cells to 100% mononuclear cells. Often a modest elevation of CSF protein is seen, along with a minor decrease in CSF glucose. The differential diagnosis of a subacute meningitis in an immunosuppressed host must also include *Cryptococcus neoformans*. The finding of focal brain lesions by CT scan or MRI broadens the differential to include toxoplasmosis, *Nocardia asteroides*, bacterial brain abscess, fungal meningitis, and others. Meningoencephalitis has also been sporadically reported in otherwise healthy individuals and should be considered in the differential diagnosis of any community-acquired meningitis.

● **Meningoencephalitis of the neonate:** This is a "late-onset" neonatal disease, occurring several days to weeks postpartum. As with adult cases, isolated neonatal meningitis from *Listeria* can be variable in its presentation. Fever may be low grade or absent, and irritability and failure to thrive may be the only clues. CSF findings in the neonate are similar to those in the adult. It is important to review the Gram's stain of CSF carefully to avoid confusing *Listeria* with Group B streptococci, a common cause of neonatal meningitis.

● **Cerebritis:** This form of nonmeningeal central nervous system infection is gaining increased recognition. Patients may complain of fever, cephalgia, and hemiparesis. This form of listeriosis may be mistaken for a stroke, vasculitis, brain tumor, or abscess. CT and MRI scans suggest focal inflammation without a discrete abscess or ring enhancement. Cerebrospinal fluid is usually normal and CSF cultures are negative for *Listeria*. The diagnosis is usually made when *Listeria* is isolated from blood cultures.

● **Listeriosis in pregnancy:** Unfortunately, this is often difficult to diagnose, since the woman may be asymptomatic or complain of only a mild fever and malaise. Other symptoms variably present include diarrhea and flank pain. The differential diagnosis is usually broad and listeriosis may be mistaken for pyelonephritis, lower urinary tract infection, and viral syndromes (eg, influenza). Blood cultures may be positive and should be performed. Complications include premature delivery, septic abortion, and *in utero* fetal infection.

● **Granulomatosis infantiseptica:** This unique, transplacentally acquired infection is severe and often lethal. It is an "early onset" neonatal infection apparent within hours of birth. Typically, the infants are seriously ill. There are widespread abscesses involving visceral organs such as the liver, spleen, lungs, intestinal tract, and brain. The lesions are usually abscesses with polymorphonuclear leukocytes, but granulomas have also been seen (referred to as "miliary granulomatosis"). Dark papular skin lesions may be present on the trunk and lower extremities, suggesting the diagnosis. Gram's stain and culture of meconium, amniotic fluid, conjunctival exudates, CSF, throat, blood, or skin lesions frequently are positive for *L. monocytogenes*. Antibiotic therapy should be started immediately if this diagnosis is suspected, since death may occur if treatment is withheld until cultures are finalized.

● **Septicemia:** *Listeria* can be isolated from the blood in adults and neonates who present from the community with nonspecific fever and chills. Bacteremias are more likely in profoundly immunosuppressed hosts but have been seen in alcoholics, diabetics, pregnancy, and normal healthy individuals. The clinical presentation can be indistinguishable from gram-negative sepsis, with high fevers and hypotension (so-called "typhoidal listeremia"). On rare occasion, the diagnosis is suggested by the finding of a monocytosis on the peripheral blood smear, but blood cultures remain the highest yield.

● **Miscellaneous:** Endocarditis, ocular infections, lymphadenitis, osteomyelitis, brain abscess, peritonitis, and other focal infections have been rarely reported.

Lupine

Scientific Name *Lupinus* species

Mechanism of Toxic Action All parts of the plants, especially the ripe seeds, contain quinolizidine alkaloids, lupanine, and some piperidine compounds; different species have varying concentrations of these alkaloids, and therefore, produce various effects; not all species are toxic; toxin is inactivated if the plant is dried

Adverse Reactions Cardiovascular: Sinus tachycardia

Signs and Symptoms of Overdose Asthenia, coma, difficulty breathing, frothing of the mouth, jaundice, loss of motor control, mydriasis, myoclonus, nervousness, PVCs, seizures, tachycardia. Amyotrophy and spasticity have been reported from chronic ingestions. Death generally occurs from respiratory paralysis.

Toxicodynamics/Kinetics Onset of symptoms: Within 1 hour, but can be delayed up to one day

Overdosage/Treatment

Decontamination: Ipecac is probably not necessary in accidental ingestions and relatively contraindicated in large ingestions; lavage within 1 hour and activated charcoal with cathartic are probably beneficial for large ingestions

Supportive therapy: Required with particular attention to respiratory status

Additional Information Accidental ingestion of one plant leaf or a few seeds should be considered basically nontoxic; ingestion of 3 g of seeds per month for 8 years was associated with amyotrophy and spasticity; ingestion of 500 mL of water used to "debitter" lupine seeds resulted in mydriasis, tachycardia, PVCs, and urinary retention which resolved in 48 hours. Toxin: Lupinine

Mango

Scientific Name *Mangifera indica*

Mechanism of Toxic Action Shell contains anacardic acid, cardol, anacardol, irritants that can precipitate type IV cell-mediated allergic reaction (allergic contact dermatitis)

Signs and Symptoms of Overdose Dermatitis, nausea, orange skin discoloration, vomiting

Toxicodynamics/Kinetics Onset of effect: Variable, but effects usually seen within 24-48 hours

Peak effect: After 3-5 days

Overdosage/Treatment

Decontamination: Soap and water washing likely ineffective unless done within 5-15 minutes after exposure

Supportive therapy: Cool compresses or showers, Burow's solution, topical/oral steroids

Additional Information An evergreen found in India and most of the tropics (cultivated for its fruit); remove skin before eating; fruit weighs 4-5 lbs; indigenous on Indian subcontinent. May cause dermatitis in persons previously exposed to *Toxicoderon* (genus) plants. Toxic part: Fruit skin, sap, and shell

Marijuana (Cannabis)

Related Information
- Highlights of Recent Reports (2006) on Substance Abuse and Mental Health

CAS Number 8063-14-7

Scientific Name *Cannabis sativa*

Impairment Potential Yes; Mean detection time for marijuana metabolites using a 100 ng/mL urinary cutoff by immunoassay is about 24 hours. Delta-9-THC plasma levels as low as 2 ng/mL (or whole blood levels of 1.1 ng/mL) is consistent with recent usage and probably impairment. Studies have demonstrated that 94% of drivers with plasma delta-9-THC levels over 25 ng/mL have failed standard roadside sobriety testing. Pilots exposed to marijuana demonstrated impaired flying skills as long as 24 hours postexposure.

Mechanism of Toxic Action Antiemetic for therapeutic uses/hallucinogen; derived from the hemp plant, *Cannabis sativa* (which contains 2% to 6% tetrahydrocannabinol and which is psychotropically active in the (-) enantiomeric form); affects serotonin release along with increasing catecholaminergic effect while inhibiting parasympathetic effects

Adverse Reactions
Cardiovascular: Dose-related tachycardia, sinus tachycardia, postural hypotension (may last for 2 hours), ventricular tachycardia

Central nervous system: Irritability, disorientation, euphoria, short-term memory disturbance, distortion of time and space, dysphoria, hyperthermia, synesthesia, hypothermia, psychosis

Dermatologic: Urticaria, pruritus, exanthem

Gastrointestinal: Constipation

Genitourinary: Urinary retention, impotence

Neuromuscular & skeletal: Trismus, fine tremor

Ocular: Lateral gaze nystagmus, mydriasis, injected conjunctival vessels

Respiratory: Bronchial irritation

Miscellaneous: Thirst

Signs and Symptoms of Overdose
I.V. administration can cause diarrhea, nausea, vomiting, fevers and can progress in 12 hours to cyanosis, hypotension, renal failure, thrombocytopenia, rhabdomyolysis.

Mild cannabis intoxication (10 g/month): Fatigue, impaired recall, perceptual alterations, relaxation, sense of well being

Moderate intoxication (30 g/month): Depersonalization, memory deficits, mood swings

Excessive intoxication (60 g/month): Delusions, hallucinations, impaired coordination, paranoia, slurred speech

Admission Criteria/Prognosis Any patient who has injected a cannabinoid (need to monitor for azotemia, thrombocytopenia, and rhabdomyolysis), will require admission; severe psychotic episodes or hyperthermia will require admission

Toxicodynamics/Kinetics
Onset of action: Inhalation: 6-12 minutes; Oral: 30-120 minutes

Duration of acute effect: 0.5-3 hours

Absorption: Smoking: 18% to 50%; Ingestion: 5% to 20%

Distribution: V_d: 10 L/kg; increases with chronic use

Metabolism: Major metabolite is 11-hydroxy-tetrahydrocannabinol

Protein binding: 97% to 99%

Half-life: 28 hours (first-time users); 56 hours (chronic users)

Elimination: Feces (30% to 35%); renal (15% to 20%)

Reference Range
Following single use of marijuana (by an infrequent user): Serum concentration of $\triangle^9$-tetrahydrocannabinol (THC) peaks in 10 minutes and falls below 5 ng/mL (or 2.75 ng/mL of whole blood) within 3 hours and to below 1 ng/mL (or 0.55 ng/mL of whole blood) within 6 hours.

The carboxylic acid metabolite, 11-nor-9-carboxy-$\triangle^9$-tetrahydrocannabinol (THCA) peaks in about 2.5 hours after a single use and can persist above 2 ng/mL (plasma) for more than 3 days.

One puff of marijuana cigarette yields a plasma THC concentration of 7.0 ng/mL (1.75% THC cigarette) to 18.1 ng/mL (3.55% THC cigarette); mean peak salivary levels correspond to 864 ng/mL (1.75% THC) to 4167 ng/mL (3.55% THC); bleach may cause a 14% to 45% decrease in THC concentration in urine immunoassay results; THC plasma levels of 7-29 ng/mL can result in production of 50% of maximal subjective high effect

Overdosage/Treatment
Decontamination: Ingestion: Lavage oral ingestion (within 1 hour)/activated charcoal with cathartic

Supportive therapy: Benzodiazepines for agitation; hypotension can be treated with Trendelenburg/crystalloid infusion; tachycardia can be treated with beta-blockers

Test Interactions Alkaline/acidic urine (or dilute urine) may cause false-negative urinary immunoassay tests; Visine® adulteration may also cause false-negative tests; bleach may cause a 14% to 45% decrease in THC concentration in urine immunoassays; urine drug screen is positive for 6 days with one-time use; may be positive for weeks with chronic use. When Pyridium® chlorochromate ("Urine Luck") adulterant is added to urine (at pH of 5-7), ~58% to 100% of THC-acid is lost, resulting in a possible false-negative assay. There have been reports of false-positive urine immunoassay screening tests for tetrahydrocannabinol (THC) in patients receiving pantoprazole.

Drug Interaction Attenuation of drowsiness can occur with concomitant administration of CNS depressants; pretreatment with indomethacin may cause attenuation of the euphoria with decreased cardiac effects; cocaine, atropine along with tricyclic antidepressants may cause additive increase in heart rate; disulfiram may produce hypomanic state; may cause additive increase in blood pressure when given with amphetamines

Additional Information
Lethal dose: 30 mg/kg.

One "joint" weighs 0.5-1 g with an average THC content of 1% to 2% (5-20 mg); hash oil contains 30% to 50% THC; hashish is 3% to 6% THC; toxic dose is 15 mg/kg THC;

Decreases intraocular pressure; can cause bronchodilatation; therapeutic uses include prevention of nausea (oral THC dose of 5-15 mg/m^2), and appetite suppression; higher THC levels are associated with higher puff amount and higher potency; levels are not associated with how long puffs are held. THC levels can range from 33 ng/mL (with a 30 mL puff, 1.75% THC) to 167 ng/mL (90 mL puff, 3.55% THC concentration). Potential for medicinal uses of cannabinoids include to alleviate chemotherapy-induced nausea and vomiting, lowering intraocular pressure, antiseizure medication, muscle relaxation in spastic disorders, appetite stimulation, relief of phantom limb pain, menstrual cramps, and migraine therapy.

First-time use of cannabis can precipitate an acute psychotic episode persisting for several months, with no previous psychiatric history. Decreases intraocular pressure; can cause bronchodilatation; therapeutic uses include prevention of nausea (oral THC dose of 5-15 mg/m^2), and appetite suppression; higher THC levels are associated with higher puff amount and higher potency; levels are not associated with how long puffs are held. THC levels can range from 33 ng/mL (with a 30 mL puff, 1.75% THC) to 167 ng/mL (90 mL puff, 3.55% THC concentration). Potential for medicinal uses of cannabinoids include to alleviate chemotherapy-induced nausea and vomiting, lowering intraocular pressure, antiseizure medication, muscle relaxation in spastic disorders, appetite stimulation, relief of phantom limb pain, menstrual cramps, and migraine therapy.

According to the Drug Abuse Warning Network (DAWN)
- Marijuana was estimated to be involved in 215, 665 emergency department visits in 2004.
- Marijuana was found in 8% of visits related to suicide attempts and 15% seeking detox visits.
- Marijuana was also involved in 15% of ED visits involving malicious poisoning.
- Marijuana rates of ED use was highest for patients aged 18 to 24 years old.
- Marijuana and alcohol combination use accounted for 33, 954 ED visits.

Specific References
Augsburger M, Donze N, Menetrey A, et al, "Concentration of Drugs in Blood of Suspected Impaired Drivers," *Forensic Sci Int*, 2005, 153(1):11-5.

Burns TL and Ineck JR, "Cannabinoid Analgesia as a Potential New Therapeutic Option in the Treatment of Chronic Pain," *Ann Pharmacother*, 2006, 40(2):251-60.

Compton WM, Grant BF, Colliver JD, et al, "Prevalence of Marijuana Use Disorders in the United States: 1991-1992 and 2001-2002," *JAMA*, 2004, 291(17):2114-21.

Day D, Kuntz D, and Feldman M, "THCA Detection in Oral Fluid down to 10 pg/mL," *J Anal Toxicol*, 2006, 30:148.

Day D, Kuntz DJ, Feldman M, and Presley L, "Detection of THCA in Oral Fluid by GC-MS-MS," *J Anal Toxicol*, 2006, (30):645-50.

Fergusson DM, Poulton R, Smith PF, et al, "Cannabis and Psychosis," *BMJ*, 2006, 332(7534):172-5 (review).

Galloway JH, El-Kadiki A, Forrest AR, et al, "Analysis of Samples for $\triangle^9$-Tetrahydrocannabinol: A Possible Analytical Problem," *J Anal Toxicol*, 2006, 30:142.

Geller T, Loftis L, and Brink DS, "Cerebellar Infarction in Adolescent Males Associated with Acute Marijuana Use," *Pediatrics*, 2004, 113(4):e365-70.

Gustafson RA, Kim I, Stout PR, et al, "Urinary Pharmacokinetics of 11-Nor-9-Carboxy-Delta-9-Tetrahydrocannabinol After Controlled Oral Delta-9-Tetrahydrocannabinol Administration," *J Anal Toxicol*, 2004, 28:160-7.

Gustafson RA, Stout P, Klette K, "Controlled Oral $\triangle$-Tetrahydrocannabinol Administration: Detection Rates and Times in Urine by CEDIA®,

Syva® EMIT II, Microgenics® DRI and GC-MS," *J Anal Toxicol*, 2004, 28:283.

Henquet C, Krabbendam L, Spauwen J, et al, "Prospective Cohort Study of Cannabis Use, Predisposition for Psychosis, and Psychotic Symptoms in Young People," *BMJ*, 2005, 330(7481):11-4.

Hewavitharana AK, Golding G, Tempany G, et al, "Quantitative GCEthMS Analysis of D9-Tetrahydrocannabinol in Fiber Hemp Varieties," *J Anal Toxicol*, 2005, 29(4):258-61.

"High Times," *The Economist*, 2001, 360(8232):1-16.

Honey D, Mazarr-Proo S, Benski L, et al, "Marijuana and Driving: A Retrospective Study of New Mexico Drivers," *J Anal Toxicol*, 2006, 30:141-2.

Huestis MA and Cone EJ, "Relationship of Delta⁹-Tetrahydrocannabinol Concentrations in Oral Fluid and Plasma After Controlled Administration of Smoked Cannabis," *J Anal Toxicol*, 2004, 28(6):394-9.

Huestis MA, Zigbuo E, Heishman SJ, et al, "Determination of Time of Last Exposure Following Controlled Smoking of Multiple Marijuana Cigarettes," *J Anal Toxicol*, 2003, 27(3):197.

Jamerson MH, McCue JJ, and Klette KL, "Urine pH, Container Composition, and Exposure Time Influence Adsorptive Loss of 11-nor-△⁹-Tetrahydrocannabinol-9-Carboxylic Acid," *J Anal Toxicol*, 2005, 29:627-31.

Jamerson MH, McCue JJ, and Klette KL, "Urine pH, Container Composition, and Exposure Time Influence Adsorptive Loss of 11-nor-△⁹-Tetrahydrocannabinol-9-Carboxylic Acid," *J Anal Toxicol*, 2006, 30:128.

Jamerson MH, Welton RM, Morris-Kukoski CL, et al, "Rapid Quantification of Urinary 11-nor-△⁹-Tetrahydrocannabinol-9-Carboxylic Acid Using Fast Gas Chromatography-Mass Spectrometry," *J Anal Toxicol*, 2006, 30:151-2.

Janczyk P, Donaldson CW, and Gwaltney S, "Two Hundred and Thirteen Cases of Marijuana Toxicoses in Dogs," *Vet Hum Toxicol*, 2004, 46(1):19-21.

Joffe A, American Academy of Pediatrics Committee on Substance Abuse, American Academy of Pediatrics Committee on Adolescence, "Legalization of Marijuana: Potential Impact on Youth," *Pediatrics*, 2004, 113(6):1825-6.

Kauert GF, Iwersen-Bergmann S, and Toesnnes SW, "Assay of △⁹-tetrahydrocannabinol (THC) in Oral Fluid Evaluation of the OraSure Oral Specimen Collection Device," *J Anal Toxicol*, 2006, 30:274-7.

Kintz P, Bernhard W, Villain M, et al, "Detection of Cannabis Use in Drivers with the Drugwipe Device and by GC-MS After Intercept® Device Collection," *J Anal Toxicol*, 2005, 29:724-33.

Laumon B, Gadegbeku B, Martin JL, et al, "Cannabis Intoxication and Fatal Road Crashes in France: Population Based Case-Control Study," *BMJ*, 2006, 331(7529):1371.

Lavins ES, Lavins BD, and Jenkins AJ, "Cannabis (Marijuana) Contamination of United States and Foreign Paper Currency," *J Anal Toxicol*, 2004, 28(6):439-42.

Lin DL and Lin RL, "Distribution of 11-Nor-9-Carboxy-△⁹-Tetrahydrocannabinol in Traffic Fatality Cases," *J Anal Toxicol*, 2005, 29:58-61.

Lynskey MT, Heath AC, Bucholz KK, et al, "Escalation of Drug Use in Early-Onset Cannabis Users vs Co-Twin Controls," *JAMA*, 2003, 289(4):427-33.

Mallaret M, Dail Bo-Rohrer D, and Dematteis, M, "Adverse Effects of Marijuana," *Rev prat*, 2005, 15:55(1):41-9.

Mathew RJ, Wilson WH, and Davis R, "Postural Syncope After Marijuana: A Transcranial Doppler Study of the Hemodynamics," *Pharmacol Biochem Behav*, 2003, 75(2):309-18.

Menetrey A, Augsburger M, Favrat B, et al, "Assessment of Driving Capability Through the Use of Clinical and Psychomotor Tests in Relation to Blood Cannabinoids Levels Following Oral Administration of 20 mg Dronabinol or of a Cannabis Decoction Made with 20 or 60 mg Delta9-THC," *J Anal Toxicol*, 2005, 29(5):327-38.

Moore C, Rana S, Coulter C, et al, "Application of Two-Dimensional Gas Chromatography with Electron Capture Chenical Ionization Mass Spectrometry to Detection of 11-nor-△⁹-Tetrahydrocannabinol-9-Carboxylic Acid (THC-COOH) in Hair," *J Anal Toxicol*, 2006, 30:171-7.

Moore C, Rana S, Feyerherm F, et al, "Application of Two-Dimensional Gas Chromatography to the Detection of 11-nor-△⁹-Tetra-Hydrocannabinol-9-Carboxylic Acid (THC-COOH) in Hair," *J Anal Toxicol*, 2006, 30:147.

Mura P, Kintz P, Dumestre V, et al, "THC Can Be Detected in Brain While Absent in Blood," *J Anal Toxicol*, 2005, 29(8):842-3.

Nadulski T, Sporkert F, Schnelle M, et al, "Simultaneous and Sensitive Analysis of THC, 11-OH-THC, THC-COOH, CBD, and CBN by GC-MS in Plasma After Oral Application of Small Doses of THC and Cannabis Extract," *J Anal Toxicol*, 2005, 29(8):782-9

Nebro W, Gustafson RA, Moolchan ET, et al, "Comparison of △-Tetrahydrocannabinol, 11-Hydroxy-Tetrahydrocannabinol and 11-Nor-9-Carboxy-Tetrahydrocannabinol Concentrations in Human Plasma Following *Escherichia coli* β-Glucuronidase Hydrolysis," *J Anal Toxicol*, 2004, 28:291.

Niedbala RS, Kardos KW, Fritch DF, et al, "Passive Cannabis Smoke Exposure and Oral Fluid Testing. II: Two Studies of Extreme Cannabis Smoke Exposure in a Motor Vehicle," *J Anal Toxicol*, 2005, 29:607-15.

Niedbala RS, Kardos KW, Salamone S, et al, "Passive Cannabis Smoke Exposure and Oral Fluid Testing," *J Anal Toxicol*, 2004, 28:546-52.

Pacifici R, Zuccaro P, Pichini S, et al, "Modulation of the Immune System in Cannabis Users," *JAMA*, 2003, 289(15):1929-31.

Paul BD and Jacobs A, "Effects of Oxidizing Adulterants on Detection of 11-Nor-Delta-9-THC-9-Carboxylic Acid in Urine," *J Anal Toxicol*, 2003, 27:191.

Pedersen-Bjergaard U, Reubsaet JL, Nielsen SL, et al, "Psychoactive Drugs, Alcohol, and Severe Hypoglycemia in Insulin-Treated Diabetes: Analysis of 141 Cases," *Am J Med*, 2005, 118(3):307-10.

Pfannkoch EA, Whitecavage JA, Bramlett R, et al, "Feasibility of Extraction and Quantitation of △⁹-Tetrayhydrocannabinol in Body Fluids by Stir Bar Sorptive Extraction (SBSE) and Fast GC-MS," *J Anal Toxicol*, 2006, 30:141.

Pragst F and Nadulski T, "Cut-Off for THC in Hair in Context of Driving Ability," *Annale de Toxicologie Analytique*, 2005, 17(4):237-43.

Raes E and Verstraete AG, "Usefulness of Roadside Urine Drug Screening in Drivers Suspected of Driving Under the Influence of Drugs (DUID)," *J Anal Toxicol*, 2005, 29:632-42.

Rezkalla SH, Sharma P, and Kloner RA, "Coronary No-Flow and Ventricular Tachycardia Associated with Habitual Marijuana Use," *Ann Emerg Med*, 2003, 42(3):365-9.

Runkle JL, Lowe RH, Abraham TT, et al, "Optimization of Glucuronide Hydrolysis for Improved Recovery of 11-Hydroxy-△⁹-Tetrahydrocannabinol in Urine," *J Anal Toxicol*, 2006, 30:143.

Sasaki TA and Boehme D, "LC-MS-MS Analysis of THC and Its Metabolites," *J Anal Toxicol*, 2006, 30:163.

Scurlock RD, Ohlson GB, and Worthen DK, "The Detection of △⁹-Tetrahydrocannabinol (THC) and 11-nor-△⁹-Tetrahydrocannabinol (THCA) in Whole Blood Using Two-Dimensional Gas Chromatography and EI-Mass Spectrometry," *J Anal Toxicol*, 2006, 30:262-6.

Setter CR, Brown WC, Kuntz DJ, et al, "Comparison of Commercially Available ELISA Kits for the Analysis of THC-COOH in Hair," *J Anal Toxicol*, 2004, 28:285.

Skopp G and Potsch L, "An Investigation of the Stability of Free and Glucuronidated 11-nor-△⁹-Tetrahydrocannabinol-9-Carboxylic Acid in Authentic Urine Samples," *J Anal Toxicol*, 2004, 28(1):35-40.

Smeal SJ, Wilkins DG, Rollins DE, "The Incorporation of △⁹-Tetrahydrocannabinol and Its Metabolite, 11-Nor-9-Carboxy-△⁹-Tetrahydrocannabinol, Into Hair," *J Anal Toxicol*, 2006, 30:139-40.

Swank JL, Smith RK, and Marinetti L, "The Detection of △-Tetrahydrocannabinol in Whole Blood, Plasma, and Liver Homogenates and the Detection of 11-nor-△-Tetrahydrocannabinol-9-Carboxylic Acid in Urine Using Disposable Pipette Extraction," *J Anal Toxicol*, 2004, 28:297-8.

Wolf CE and Poklis A, "Evaluation of a Modified Emit® Immunoassay for Screening Fresh and Aged Whole Blood Specimens for the Detection of Marijuana Constituents," *J Anal Toxicol*, 2006, 30:143.

Woolard R, Nirenberg TD, Becker B, et al, "Marijuana Use and Prior Injury Among Injured Problem Drinkers," *Acad Emerg Med*, 2003, 10(1):43-51.

Zumwalt M, Fandino A, Vollmer M, et al, "Detection of Carboxy-THC in Hair Using a Novel Nanoscale LC-MC-MC Technique," *J Anal Toxicol*, 2006, 30:147.

Marsh Marigold

Scientific Name *Caltha palustris*

Mechanism of Toxic Action Contains protoanemonin, which reacts with SH groups to produce irritation and vesication; chemical is excreted unchanged in urine

Signs and Symptoms of Overdose Abdominal cramps, blistering, bloody diarrhea, contact dermatitis, hematemesis, pain and swelling, salivation, and ulceration. Potential for renal irritation or damage if a sufficient amount is ingested.

Toxicodynamics/Kinetics Significant dermal symptoms may take several weeks to resolve

Overdosage/Treatment

Decontamination: Avoid use of ipecac or cathartics, consider lavage (within 1 hour) and/or activated charcoal with large ingestion to prevent systemic absorption and possibility of subsequent renal irritation

Supportive therapy: Maintain fluid and electrolytes, maintain adequate urine flow in large overdose; monitor symptomatic patients for fluid or electrolyte deficiencies

Additional Information Toxic dose: Not established, but overdose producing systemic effects is unlikely due to painful skin contact. Toxic part: All parts are toxic, young plants prior to flowering probably not toxic

Mayapple

Scientific Name *Podophyllum peltatum*

Uses Podophyllum has been used for treatment of venereal warts; podophyllotoxin appears to have anticancer activity

Mechanism of Toxic Action Podophyllum and podophyllotoxin block cell division in the metaphase; they have a direct effect on mitochondria and are spindle poisons

Adverse Reactions

Cardiovascular: Sinus tachycardia

Endocrine & metabolic: Abortifacient

Signs and Symptoms of Overdose Severe diarrhea, nausea, and vomiting are typical early toxic manifestations. Dyspnea, hypotension, tachypnea, and tachycardia are frequently seen. Ataxia, coma, dizziness, drowsiness, paralysis, paresthesia, and stupor have been reported. Agranulocytopenia, death, granulocytopenia, leukopenia, liver injury, neutropenia, oliguria, renal failure, and thrombocytopenia have all been reported. Hypokalemia and metabolic alkalosis have been reported from chronically using podophyllum as a purgative. Conjunctivitis, keratitis, and ulcerative skin lesions have been reported in workers handling the powdered rhizome.

Toxicodynamics/Kinetics Absorption: Well absorbed both orally and dermally

Overdosage/Treatment

Decontamination: Lavage (within 1 hour) may be useful in patients with large ingestions that have not developed vomiting yet; activated charcoal with cathartic should be administered

Elimination: Hemodialysis is ineffective in removing podophyllum but may be required in patients experiencing renal failure

Additional Information Toxic dose: Not well established, 350 mg of podophyllum has been reported to cause death. European Mandrake (*Mandragora officinarum*) is unrelated to Mayapple or American Mandrake. Family: Podophyllaceae (formerly *Berberidaceae*). Toxin: Podophyllin resin, podophyllotoxin. Range: Florida to Texas, north to western Quebec, southern Ontario, and Minnesota. Toxic part: Leaves, roots, and unripe fruit; ripe fruit is edible

Mescaline

Related Information

- Peyote

CAS Number 54-04-6

Scientific Name *Lophophora williamsii*

Mechanism of Toxic Action Hallucinogenic methoxylated amphetamine stimulating both serotonin and dopamine receptors in the central nervous system

Adverse Reactions

Cardiovascular: Sinus bradycardia, angina

Endocrine & metabolic: Hyperprolactinemia

Signs and Symptoms of Overdose Ataxia, bradycardia, chest pain, coma, dizziness, fever, flashbacks, flushing, hallucinations, headache, hyperreflexia, hypertension, mydriasis, myoglobinuria, psychosis, rhabdomyolysis, sweating, tachypnea, tremor, vomiting

Admission Criteria/Prognosis Patients who are asymptomatic after 4 hours postexposure may be discharged

Toxicodynamics/Kinetics

Duration of effect: Psychic effects last 6-12 hours

Protein binding: No binding

Metabolism: Hepatic to inactive metabolites

Half-life: 6 hours

Elimination: Renal (55% to 60% unchanged)

Reference Range Hallucinogenic effects occur at blood levels of mescaline of 1.5-14.8 mcg/mL; peak blood level after an oral 500 mg dose: 3.8 mg/mL at 2 hours postingestion and 1.5 mg/L at 7 hours postingestion; after a 5 mg/kg intravenous dose, peak blood mescaline level was 14.8 mcg/mL 15 minutes postdose.

Overdosage/Treatment

Decontamination: Lavage (within 1 hour)/activated charcoal with cathartic

Supportive therapy: Benzodiazepines are useful for agitation; haloperidol or chlorpromazine can be used if psychiatric symptoms are not responsive to benzodiazepines; do not use phenothiazines for treatment of flashback

Drug Interaction Flashbacks may be exacerbated by phenothiazines

Additional Information Hallucinogenic dose: Oral: 5 mg/kg. Active ingredient in the peyote cactus (*Lophophora williamsii*). Available as whole dried cactus tops ("buttons"); peyote contains 1% to 6% mescaline; each "button" contains ~45 mg of mescaline. Range: Found in the Southwestern U.S. and Mexico

Specific References

Henry JL, Epley J, and Rohrig TP, "The Analysis and Distribution of Mescaline in Postmortem Tissues," *J Anal Toxicol*, 2003, 27(6): 381-2.

Methcathinone

Related Information

- Cathinone

CAS Number 71031-15-7

Mechanism of Toxic Action Related to cathinone (khat) found naturally in *Catha edulis*; found primarily in production of clandestine labs in Washington, Illinois, Missouri, and upper Michigan peninsula; derived from ephedrine with amphetamine-like actions; causes release of dopamine from caudate nucleus

Adverse Reactions Cardiovascular: Sinus tachycardia

Signs and Symptoms of Overdose Abdominal pain, agitation, anorexia, auditory hallucinations, back pain, constipation, fever, headache, hypertension (dose related), leukocytosis, myoglobinuria, paranoia, rhabdomyolysis, slurred speech, sweating, tachycardia (dose-related), tremor, visual hallucinations

Toxicodynamics/Kinetics Metabolism: To ephedrine and phenylpropanolamine (norephedrine)

Reference Range Reference levels of methcathinone in symptomatic individuals were measured at 56 ng/mL and 78 ng/mL

Overdosage/Treatment

Decontamination: GI lavage (within 1 hour)/activated charcoal with cathartic or phenothiazines

Supportive therapy: Benzodiazepines for agitation

Test Interactions Does not result in positive amphetamine on urine immunoassays

Additional Information Toxic Dose: Estimated to be 80-250 mg by intranasal use (can be used I.V.); typical daily dose: 500-1000 mg. Ephedrine, pseudoephedrine, and phenylpropanone may turn up positive in drug testing in that these chemicals are used in the production of methcathinone

Mexican Beaded Lizard

Related Information

- Gila Monster

Mechanism of Toxic Action Venom is secreted from glands which are located at the posterior edge of the lower jaw and then released into the wound upon mastication. The venom contains hyaluronidase, phospholipase A2, proteolytic enzymes, serotonin, N-benzoyl-L-arginine ethyl ester hydrolase, exendin-4, helothermine, and gilatoxin. Helothermine may have calcium channel blocking properties; gilatoxin is a presynaptic neurotoxin without any hemotoxic effects. Effective envenomation rate in bites is approximately 70%.

Signs and Symptoms of Overdose Anaphylaxis, severe pain, local wound edema, erythema, nausea, vomiting, anxiety, hypotension, tachycardia, diaphoresis, leukocytosis, dizziness, lymphangitis, angioedema

Overdosage/Treatment

Decontamination: Methods to disengage the lizard include pulling the lizard by its tail, prying the jaws open with sticks or metallic objects, or pouring noxious substances down its mouth. Irrigate wound with copious amounts of water.

Supportive therapy: Anaphylaxis can be treated with standard therapy; pain can be treated with opioids. Symptoms usually resolve within one day.

Additional Information The Mexican beaded lizard is native to arid, rocky regions of southwestern Mexico and Guatemala. The lizards are slow moving, nocturnal creatures growing to lengths of 1 meter and weighing 2 kg. The tough dorsal skin is comprised of large, blackish bead-like scales with yellow spots. Normally docile, these lizards are tenacious biters when provoked. The more prolonged the attachment time, the more severe envenomation. Anaphylaxis can occur upon repeated envenomation.

Specific Reference

Cantrell FL, "Envenomation by the Mexican Beaded Lizard: A Case Report," *J Toxicol Clin Toxicol*, 2003, 41(3):241-4.

Milkbush

Related Information

- Crown of Thorns

Scientific Name *Euphorbia*

Signs and Symptoms of Overdose Entire plant can cause an irritant dermatitis; gastroenteritis (nausea, vomiting, diarrhea) can develop upon ingestion. Keratoconjunctivitis and iritis can also develop upon ocular contact.

Overdosage/Treatment

Decontamination: Lavage (within 1 hour)/activated charcoal with sorbitol

Dermal: Wash with soap and water

Supportive therapy: Replace fluid loss with saline and electrolytes as needed antihistamines and/or corticosteroids can be utilized for severe dermal reactions

Mistletoe

Scientific Name *Phoradendron flavescens*; *Phoradendron macrophyllum*; *Phoradendron rubrum*; *Phoradendron serotinum*; *Phoradendron tomentosum*; *Viscum album*

Adverse Reactions
Cardiovascular: Sinus bradycardia, myocardial depression, congestive heart failure, angina, orthostatic hypotension
Central nervous system: Chills, fever, headache

Signs and Symptoms of Overdose Abdominal pain, diarrhea, nausea, and vomiting may be seen. Ataxia, bradycardia, cardiovascular collapse, hypotension, and seizures have all been reported.

Admission Criteria/Prognosis Any patient asymptomatic 6 hours postingestion can be discharged home; admit any ingestion >20 berries or 5 leaves

Overdosage/Treatment
Decontamination: Ipecac (within 30 minutes) or lavage (within 1 hour) may be of value in recent, large ingestions (over 3 berries or 2 leaves) where vomiting has not yet occurred; activated charcoal should be administered; because of the probable diarrhea from substantial mistletoe ingestion, activated charcoal should be given as a water slurry
Supportive therapy: Replace fluids and electrolytes as needed; benzodiazepine can be given for seizure control

Additional Information
Toxic dose: Specific quantities are unknown; it is generally thought that ingestion of more than 2-3 berries is required for poisoning; most serious poisonings are from ingestion of teas or extracts of mistletoe
Family: Loranthaceae; Toxin: Phoratoxin and viscotoxin; Range: All mistletoes are parasitic plants and typically grow on deciduous trees such as oak; *P. rubrum* grows only on mahogany trees; in the U.S., *Viscum album* is found only in California. Toxic part: All parts are considered toxic except for the berries of *Viscum album*

Mites

Scientific Name *Arachnida*; *Demodex folliculorum*; *Sarcoptes scabiei*; *Trombicula irritans*

Signs and Symptoms of Overdose Pruritic erythematous papules, eczematous eruption, erythema multiforme, fever

Overdosage/Treatment Supportive therapy: For scabies: All infested cohabitants should be treated simultaneously to avoid reinfection. Bed linens and clothing worn within 2 days should be washed and dried on hot settings or stored in tightly sealed plastic bags for one week. Permethrin (5% cream) should be applied topically and left on for 8-12 hours. Retreatment can occur in one week. Lindane (1% lotion) is an alternative treatment; it can be applied and left topically for 8 hours and then washed off. Retreatment can occur in one week. Lindane should not be used on nonintact skin or immediately after bathing or in patients with neurological or hepatic diseases. Additionally, neither permethrin should be used in young infants, pregnant or nursing mothers. For infants, pregnant or nursing mothers, precipitated sulfur (6%) in petrolatum can be applied for 3 consecutive nights. A recently described alternative therapy for patients older than 5 years of age: ivermectin: 200 mcg/kg as a single dose in healthy patients or 200 mcg/kg one time dose (repeating as necessary in two weeks) in HIV-infected patients. Pruritus or eczema can be treated with topical steroids. Oral antihistamines and topical steroid cream (ie, fluocinonide cream) for relief of pruritus

Additional Information
May transmit rickettsial pox, murine typhus, Q fever, tularemia, plague; the follicle mite (*Demodex folliculorum*) may be implicated in Kawasaki syndrome; Family: Acarina

Microbiology: *Sarcoptes scabiei*, or the human mite, is the causative agent of scabies, a common parasitic infestation of the skin *Sarcoptes scabiei* is an ectoparasite of humans belonging to the class *Arachnida*. It tends to form skin "burrows" several millimeters wide within the stratum corneum of the epidermis. The fertilized female deposits its eggs in these skin burrows, and the larvae exit after several days to become adults weeks later. The adult is ~0.3 mm long.

Epidemiology: Scabies is distributed world wide. The incidence in the U.S. has been increasing since the 1970s. The reservoir resides in humans, although animal mites can sometimes cause brief human disease. Transmission is person to person by direct contact. Occasionally, transmission may occur when there is contact with heavily contaminated clothing or bedsheets. The incubation period varies from several days to weeks. Infected individuals remain communicable until all the ova and mites are eradicated from the skin.

Clinical Syndromes:
- **Human scabies:** Patients present with intense itching, usually in the interdigital web spaces, along the "belt line," the genital region, the periumbilical area, and also on the wrists, elbows, knees, and feet. Additional areas are common in children, including the hands and face. On physical examination, the characteristic burrows may be seen, appearing linear and several millimeters wide, often in the interdigital spaces. Atypical presentations of scabies may occur, including vesicles

and bullae in infants, eczema, and rash. A variant known as "nodular scabies" has been described in which there are small, brown, intensely pruritic nodules usually on the penis and scrotum. An unusual manifestation of severe scabies called "Norwegian scabies" has been seen in immunocompromised individuals and patients with Down syndrome. The skin is diffusely scaling and thickened as a result of infestation of thousands of mites. Secondary bacterial infections of the skin may occur in all forms of scabies.
- **Animal scabies:** This is due to *Sarcoptes scabiei* var. *Canis*, carried on some dogs; the clinical presentation is similar to human scabies although burrows are not present

Diagnosis: Infestation with scabies is often suspected when an individual presents with pruritic papules, or an otherwise compatible clinical history. Some patients may present because of a recent history of contact. It should be noted that scabies often imitates other skin lesions, and thus a broad differential diagnosis should be entertained if the linear burrows are not demonstrated. Other diagnostic considerations include impetigo, insect bites, drug eruptions, varicella, eczema, and others.

The linear burrows of the mite can be further demonstrated by applying blue ink over a possible burrow. The ink is drawn into the defect and when excess ink is wiped off with an alcohol pad, the ink within the burrow remains. This and other suspicious areas should be covered with oil, the area should be scraped with a sterile blade, the scrapings should be placed into oil on a microscope slide, and the preparation should be examined with a microscope.

To decrease mite allergen measurements below sensitization level, the following interventions may be helpful:
- Remove carpeting from floors
- Replace upholstered furniture with leather or vinyl covered furniture
- Reduce indoor humidity level
- Hot dry steam cleaning followed by vacuuming carpeting or upholstered furniture if present

Monkshood

Scientific Name *Aconitum napellus*; *Aconitum uncinatum*

Mechanism of Toxic Action Aconite has a vagal action on the heart and also a more direct action on the heart muscle; death usually occurs; 2 hours to respiratory failure or heart failure usually 1-6 hours but can be from minutes to 4 days

Adverse Reactions
Cardiovascular: Torsade de pointes, sinus bradycardia, sinus tachycardia, tachycardia (supraventricular), arrhythmias (ventricular)
Central nervous system: Lack of CNS depression
Miscellaneous: Poor prognosis

Signs and Symptoms of Overdose Symptoms occur in 10-20 minutes. Tingling and burning of fingers, lips, toes, and tongue are seen first. Then chills, dry mouth, hypothermia, numbness, paresthesia, and sweating occur. Arrhythmias (supraventricular), bradycardia, diarrhea, hypotension, pain, paralysis, seizures, and ventricular fibrillation occur later. Vaguely mediated bradycardia (which may be associated with AV block) is found in 10% to 20% of fatal poisonings.

Overdosage/Treatment
Decontamination: Ipecac use is contraindicated due to inducing rapid onset of symptoms; lavage within 1 hour may be beneficial, activated charcoal with cathartic
Supportive therapy: Fluid and electrolyte replacement; arrhythmias are relatively refractory to drug therapy; I.V. magnesium sulfate can be used to treat ventricular dysrhythmia; bradycardia can be treated with atropine
Enhancement of elimination: Charcoal hemoperfusion can help reverse ventricular arrhythmias.

Additional Information Fatal dose: 2 g. Fatalities have occurred with ingestion of 2-4 g of root. Estimated lethal dose of plant: 1 g. Toxin: Aconitine. Toxic part: All parts, especially seeds and roots. Monitoring parameters: Cardiac rhythm

Specific References
Lin CC, Chan TY, and Deng JF, "Clinical Features and Management of Herb-Induced Aconitine Poisoning," *Ann Emerg Med*, 2004, 43(5):574-9.
Moritz F, Compagnon P, Kaiszczak IG, et al, "Severe Acute Poisoning with Homemade *Aconitum napellus* Capsules: Toxicokinetic and Clinical Data," *Clin Toxicol*, 2006, 43:873-6.
Smith SW, Shah RR, Hunt JL, et al, "Bidirectional Ventricular Tachycardia Resulting from Herbal Aconite Poisoning," *Ann Emerg Med*, 2005, 45(1):100-1.

Monosodium Glutamate Food Poisoning

CAS Number 142-47-2

Commonly Found In Chinese food, sausage, canned soup, Accent®

Signs and Symptoms of Overdose Angina, angioedema, burning sensation, chest pain, flushing, headache, hypokalemia, paresthesia, syncope, tremor, and wheezing occur within 30 minutes postingestion and may last for 1-3 hours. GI symptoms are minimal.

Admission Criteria/Prognosis Patients with dehydration (who cannot take fluids orally), immunocompromised patients, severe disturbance in electrolytes or acid-base status, or patients at extreme in terms of age group should be considered for admission

Overdosage/Treatment Supportive therapy: Diphenhydramine may be useful, usually self-limited

Diagnostic Procedures
- Electrolytes, Blood

Additional Information Salty or sweet to taste; soluble in water; used as a flavor enhancer. Intravenous doses can cause hypokalemia or alkalosis; absorption is most rapid in a fasting state. Patients with severe, poorly controlled asthma are predisposed to an adverse reaction. The symptom complex can occur in healthy individuals within 20 minutes after ingestion of 3 g of monosodium glutamate on an empty stomach. Symptoms usually last <1 hour. A typical serving of glutamate-treated food contains <0.5 mg of monosodium glutamate.

Moonseed

Scientific Name *Menispermum canadense*

Signs and Symptoms of Overdose Reportedly a stimulant action similar to water hemlock; seizures are the major concern

Overdosage/Treatment Decontamination: Activated charcoal with cathartic may be of value in recent ingestions; manage seizures with diazepam or lorazepam

Additional Information Family: Menispermaceae. A woody, smooth vine which can grow up to 12 feet. Toxin: Dauricine and other isoquinoline alkaloids. Range: Found in the eastern U.S. Toxic part: Probably the whole plant, but especially the fruit

Morning Glory

CAS Number 2390-99-0; 2889-26-1; 478-94-4; 548-43-6; 602-85-7

Scientific Name *Ipomoea purpurea*; *Rivea corymbosa*

Mechanism of Toxic Action Source of lysergic acid amide which is ~10% as potent as lysergic acid diethylamide (LSD)

Adverse Reactions
Cardiovascular: Shock, sinus tachycardia
Central nervous system: CNS depression, memory loss, psychosis, delirium, dysphoria, memory disturbance
Ocular: Vision color changes (increased color perception)
Miscellaneous: Synesthesia

Signs and Symptoms of Overdose Anxiety, depersonalization, depression, diarrhea, drowsiness, flushing, hypotension, mydriasis, tachycardia

Overdosage/Treatment
Decontamination: Activated charcoal with cathartic with oral ingestion
Supportive therapy: Dantrolene (25 mg 2-4 times/day) should be given for neuroleptic malignant syndrome; diazepam or lorazepam can be used for agitation; haloperidol can be given for hallucinations

Additional Information Toxic dose: 300 seeds contain the equivalent of 200-300 mcg of LSD. Often a contaminant in soy bean crops.

Mosquitoes

Scientific Name *Anopheles freeborni*; *Anopheles quadrimaculatus*

Signs and Symptoms of Overdose Anaphylactic reaction, urticarial reaction (rash)

Overdosage/Treatment Supportive therapy: Local application of calamine lotion or aluminum acetate (Burow's solution); allergic reactions can be treated with standard therapy; parenteral corticosteroids can also be given for severe systemic symptoms; cetirizine (5-10 mg orally) can reduce wheal/flare response by 50%

Additional Information Order: Diptera. Family: Culicidae. Vectors for filariasis. Anopheline (*A. quadrimaculatus* and *A. freeborni*) are the vectors for malaria (*Plasmodium*); N,N-diethyl-m-toluamides or DEET is an effective repellent.

Mountain Laurel

Scientific Name *Kalmia latifolia*; *Kalmia*

Mechanism of Toxic Action Contains grayanotoxin which binds to a subset of sodium channels causing structural modifications, thereby causing slow opening of these channels which leads to cell depolarization

Adverse Reactions Cardiovascular: Sinus bradycardia

Signs and Symptoms of Overdose Asthenia, bradycardia, dermatitis, hypotension, nausea, oral numbness or burning, paresthesia, seizures, sweating, transient blindness, visual changes, vomiting

Overdosage/Treatment
Decontamination: Avoid ipecac, vagal stimulation increases toxicity; lavage (within 1 hour)/activated charcoal with cathartic
Supportive therapy: Atropine for bradycardia, I.V. fluids should be sufficient for hypotension

Additional Information Three whole leaves or flowers likely nontoxic; consider decontamination if more; toxicity is unpredictable, variable among azalea types. Toxic part: Leaves and honey

Mushrooms, Toxic (Group 1) Cyclopeptides

CAS Number 17466-45-4; 21150-22-1; 21150-23-2; 23109-05-9; 28227-92-1; 39412-56-1

Scientific Name *Amanita bisporigera*; *Amanita ocreata*; *Amanita phalloides*; *Amanita suballiacea*; *Amanita tenuifolia*; *Amanita verna*; *Amanita virosa*; *Conocybe filaris*; *Galerina autumnalis*; *Galerina marginatus*; *Galerina speciosissimus*; *Lepiota clypeolarioides*; *Lepiota helveola*; *Lepiota rufescens*

Mechanism of Toxic Action
Contains the cyclopeptides phallotoxins, amatoxins, and virotoxins. Only amatoxins are considered important in human poisoning and cause liver necrosis through inhibition of RNA polymerase II.

Adverse Reactions
Three phases: I: Gastroenteritis: up to 24 hours postingestion (incubation is 8-12 hours); II: Remission: up to 72 hours postingestion; III: Hepatic/renal effects: 3-6 days postingestion
Cardiovascular: Hypotension, cardiomyopathy
Central nervous system: Encephalopathy, coma, seizures
Gastrointestinal: Nausea, vomiting, colicky abdominal pain, hepatitis, pancreatitis
Hematologic: Coagulopathy
Hepatic: Hepatic failure (fulminant), chronic active hepatitis may be long-term sequelae
Renal: Renal failure, acute tubular necrosis

Admission Criteria/Prognosis All suspected ingestions should be admitted; probably in an intensive care unit

Toxicodynamics/Kinetics
Absorption: Phallotoxin not well absorbed though the gastrointestinal tract
Distribution: V_d: 160-290 mL/kg
Protein binding: Not protein bound
Elimination: Excreted in urine, feces, and bile; enterohepatic recirculation may occur

Reference Range There is no correlation of symptoms or outcome to concentration of amatoxin in serum

Overdosage/Treatment
Decontamination: Lavage (within 1 hour)/activated charcoal with cathartic
Supportive Therapy: I.V. fluids, lactulose, neomycin for hepatic failure; vitamin K and fresh frozen plasma may be needed to treat coagulopathy
Proposed antidotes: High dose Penicillin G (300,000-1,000,000 units/kg/day), silymarin, cimetidine 300 mg I.V. every 8 hours, thioctic acid and N-acetylcysteine (efficacy of each has been questioned). Silymarin and thiotic acid are not commercially available in the United States. Dose of silymarin (Silibinin): I.V.: 5 mg/kg I.V. infusion over 1 hour followed by 20 mg/kg/day by continuous infusion for 6 days. N-acetylcysteine therapy or silybin dihemisuccinate appear to be the most effective therapy
Extracorporeal liver assistance methods utilizing an albumin dialysate (molecular absorbent recycling system or MARS) has been utilized to remove protein-bound and water soluble substances in patients with liver failure and grade III or IV hepatic encephalopathy in Europe. Successful results with avoidance of orthotopic hepatic transplantation have been noted with patients exposed to *Amanita phalloides*. It has been safely utilized in children as young as seven years old. Complications include decreases in platelet counts (by 15%) and prolongation of activated prothrombin time (by 21%). Blood pressure, hemoglobin, white blood cell count, electrolytes, transaminases, and albumin levels do not appear to be significantly affected. Refer to Specific References.
Other proposed treatments: Charcoal hemoperfusion within 24 hours of ingestion (efficacy is controversial). **Orthotopic liver transplant has been successful and may be necessary in the most severe cases.** Multiple dosing of activated charcoal may be useful.

Antidote(s)
- Silymarin [ANTIDOTE]

Test Interactions
Monitor for hypochloronatremia and hypokalemia during gastroenteritis phase. Insulin, calcitonin, and parathyroid hormone levels are increased. Serum thyroxine levels are decreased. Hypoglycemia may also develop.

Additional Information
Estimated lethal dose: 0.1 mg/kg; one *Amanita* cap may be lethal in an adult
Amanita species are diagnosed by having a white spore print, gills that do not reach the stem, the presence of a volva (see figure), and often, but not always, an annulus (see figure). *Lepiota* species display these same features, but they always lack a volva. *Galerina* and *Conocybe* species have brown to rusty brown spore prints. The species listed above have an annulus but no volva. Differentiation and correct identification for small brown fungi are based on microscopic examination of spores and other features. Amatoxins are extremely stable

compounds, resistant to heat, drying, freezing, and not degraded enzymatically. The Meixner/Wieland test can be used to detect the presence of amatoxins. Squeeze one drop of juice from a fresh mushroom cap onto newsprint or filter paper (circle spot with a pencil to locate). Let dry at room temperature and out of sunlight. Apply one drop of concentrated hydrochloric acid. A change to a blue color will indicate the presence of amatoxins; compare to a control spot (without mushroom juice). *Amanita phalloides* ingestion may account for up to 90% of mushroom-related deaths worldwide with a fatality rate of 20% to 30%. Fatality is associated with large dose, short latency period before onset of symptoms, severe coagulopathy, and age younger than 10 years. See figure.

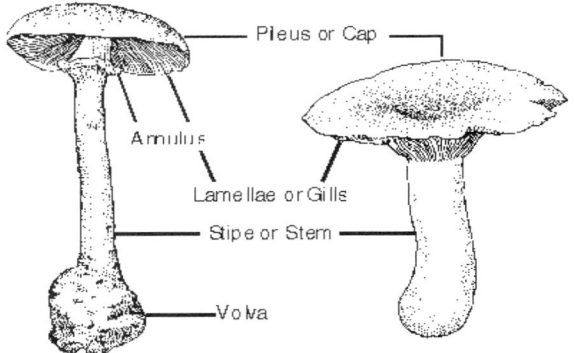

Specific References

Butera R, Locatelli C, Coccini T, et al, "Diagnostic Accuracy of Urinary Amanitin in Suspected Mushroom Poisoning: A Pilot Study," *J Toxicol Clin Toxicol*, 2004, 42(6):901-12.

Catalina MV, Nunez O, Ponferrada A, et al, "Liver Failure Due to Mushroom Poisoning: Clinical Course and New Treatment Perspectives," *Gastroenterol Hepatol*, 2003, 26(7):417-20.

Covic A, Goldsmith DJ, Gusbeth-Tatomir P, et al, "Successful Use of Molecular Absorbent Regenerating System (MARS) Dialysis for the Treatment of Fulminant Hepatic Failure in Children Accidentally Poisoned by Toxic Mushroom Ingestion," *Liver Int*, 2003, 23(Suppl 3):21-7.

Faybik P, Hetz H, Baker A, et al, "Extracorporeal Albumin Dialysis in Patients with *Amanita phalloides* Poisoning," *Liver Int*, 2003, 23(Suppl 3):28-33.

Friesen M, Pringle A, Callan B, et al, "*Amanita phalloides* Heads North," *Clin Toxicol (Phila)*, 2005, 43:761.

Koivusalo AM, Yildirim Y, Vakkuri A, et al, "Experience with Albumin Dialysis in Five Patients with Severe Overdoses of Paracetamol," *Acta Anaesthesiol Scand*, 2003, 47(9):1145-50.

Mrvos R, Swanson-Biearman B, and Krenzelok EP, "Backyard Mushroom Ingestions: No Gastrointestinal Decontamination - No Effect," *J Toxicol Clin Toxicol*, 2004, 42(5):801-2.

Petkovska L, Pereska Z, Naumovski J, et al, "Aminotransferases as Markers in *Amanita phalloides* Poisonings," *J Toxicol Clin Toxicol*, 2003, 41(5):720.

Roche K, Webster C, Sangalli B, et al, "A Poison Center's Management of Mushroom Exposures: An 8-Year Retrospective Study," *J Toxicol Clin Toxicol*, 2004, 42(5):800-1.

Satora L, "Nonspecific Mushroom Poisoning," *Vet Hum Toxicol*, 2004, 46(4):224 (letter).

Unluoglu I, Cevik AA, Bor O, et al, "Mushroom Poisonings in Children in Central Anatolia," *Vet Hum Toxicol*, 2004, 46(3):134-7.

Wills B, Haller N, Peter D, et al, "Cytoprotective Effects of Intraperitoneal Amifostine on α-Amanitin Toxicity in Mice," *Acad Emerg Med*, 2003, 10:521a.

Wills BK, Haller NA, Peter D, et al, "Use of Amifostine, A Novel Cytoprotective, in Alpha-Amanitin Poisoning," *Clin Toxicol (Phila)*, 2005, 43(4):261-7.

Mushrooms, Toxic (Group 2) Monomethylhydrazines

CAS Number 16568-02-8; 60-34-4; 69349-96-8

Scientific Name *Gyromitra ambigua*; *Gyromitra brunnea*; *Gyromitra caroliniana*; *Gyromitra esculenta*; *Gyromitra fastigiata*; *Gyromitra gigas*; *Gyromitra infula*; *Helvella* species, *Sarcosphaera crasa*; *Peziza* species

Uses Monomethylhydrazine is used as rocket fuel; it is a strong reducing agent in industry (DOT/UN: 1244) and a corrosive inhibitor

Mechanism of Toxic Action Gyromitrin present in the mushroom is hydrolyzed upon digestion to N-methyl-N-formylhydrazine (MFH) and monomethylhydrazine (MMH); MMH is an inhibitor of coenzyme pyridoxyl

phosphate and gamma-aminobutyric acid in the CNS; MFH is believed to deplete hepatic cytochrome P450

Adverse Reactions

Central nervous system: Seizures, coma, dizziness, delirium, fever

Gastrointestinal: Nausea, vomiting, abdominal pain, cramps, watery diarrhea

Hematologic: Hemolytic anemia

Hepatic: Hepatitis, jaundice

Renal: Nephritis may develop in 1-2 days

Admission Criteria/Prognosis All suspected ingestions should be admitted

Toxicodynamics/Kinetics

Absorption: May also occur via inhalation of fumes while cooking, MMH can be absorbed through intact skin

Metabolism: 25% metabolized to monomethylhydrazine

Overdosage/Treatment

Decontamination: Lavage (within 1 hour)/activated charcoal with cathartic

Supportive therapy: I.V. fluids

Antidotal therapy: Pyridoxine 25 mg/kg I.V. for seizures

Antidote(s)

● Methylene Blue [ANTIDOTE]

● Pyridoxine [ANTIDOTE]

Diagnostic Procedures

● Glucose, Random

Drug Interaction Phenobarbital may have an enhanced effect due to interference of hepatic metabolism

Additional Information

Lethal dose: Children: 10-30 mg/kg; Adults: 20-50 mg/kg

These species are not typical mushroom shaped; *Gyromitra* and *Helvella* species are stalked with a brain-shaped or saddle-shaped swollen "cap" on top, respectively; species of *Peziza* are typical cup fungi; *Sarcoscypha crasa* starts out spherical and then splits open to form a star-shaped cup; all of these species are usually found on the ground and are most commonly encountered in the spring; there is wide variation in individual susceptibility to poisoning by gyromitrins, estimated tolerance up to 35 mcg/kg of gyromitrin; toxins are heat labile, however, parboiling does not guarantee edibility and toxicity may occur from inhaling vapors

---

Mushrooms, Toxic (Group 3) Cholinergic

CAS Number 2552-55-8 (ibotenic acid); 2763-96-4 (muscimol)

Scientific Name *Clitocybe dealbata*; *Clitocybe dilatata*; *Clitocybe morbifera*; *Clitocybe rivulosa*; *Inocybe fastigiata*; *Inocybe geophylla*; *Inocybe lacera*; *Inocybe mapipes*; *Inocybe mixtilis*; *Inocybe pantouillardi*; *Inocybe pudica*; *Inocybe sororia*; *Inocybe subdestricta*; *Mycena pura*

Mechanism of Toxic Action Contains the compound muscarine which is structurally similar to acetylcholine and produces symptoms of cholinergic excess; muscarine is not degraded by acetylcholinesterase enzyme

Adverse Reactions

Cardiovascular: Bradycardia, hypotension, hypertension, arrhythmias

Central nervous system: Delirium, dizziness, ataxia, somnolence, seizures, psychosis, euphoria, residual headaches, fever, coma, visual hallucinations, hyperthermia

Gastrointestinal: Vomiting, watery diarrhea, salivation

Neuromuscular & skeletal: Myoclonus

Ocular: Miosis, lacrimation, teichopsia

Miscellaneous: Diaphoresis

Admission Criteria/Prognosis Can observe for 6-8 hours; if symptomatic, admission is suggested; ingestions >20 mushrooms will probably require admission

Toxicodynamics/Kinetics

Onset of action: Within 30 minutes

Duration: Variable, dose-related

Overdosage/Treatment Decontamination: Lavage (within 1 hour)/activated charcoal with cathartic; I.V. hydration with isotonic saline; atropine 1-2 mg I.V. in adults or 0.05 mg/kg in children, only if significant signs of cholinergic crisis are present; benzodiazepines are indicated for treating seizures

Diagnostic Procedures

● Electrolytes, Blood

Additional Information

Estimated lethal dose: Muscarine: 40-180 mg; Toxic dose: Fresh mushrooms: ~100 g or less

These species of *Clitocybe* usually grow in grassy areas or along roadways. They are whitish in color, have white spores, and have gills that often run part way down the stem. The common name for *Inocybe* is fiber head because of the distinctive fibers that radiate from the center of the cap and run to the margin. Species of *Inocybe* have a clay brown spore print and often have a spermatic odor.

Specific References

Saviuc P, Dematteis M, Mezin P, et al, "Toxicity of the *Clitocybe amoenolens* Mushroom in the Rat," *Vet Hum Toxicol*, 2003, 45(4):180-2.

Mushrooms, Toxic (Group 4) [Antabuse®]

Scientific Name *Coprinus atramentarius*

Mechanism of Toxic Action The metabolite of coprine, 1-aminocyclo-propanol, inhibits aldehyde dehydrogenase and thus produces an antabuse-like reaction when consumed with alcohol

Adverse Reactions

Cardiovascular: Flushing, cardiovascular collapse, myocardial infarction, chest pain

Central nervous system: Dizziness, headache, seizures

Gastrointestinal: Nausea, vomiting, metallic taste

Hepatic: Hepatitis

Neuromuscular & skeletal: Paresthesia

Ocular: Retrobulbar neuritis, nystagmus

Respiratory: Dyspnea

Miscellaneous: Diaphoresis

Admission Criteria/Prognosis Admit if there are ECG changes or persistent symptoms

Toxicodynamics/Kinetics

Onset of action: 0.5-2 hours

Duration of action: 4-6 hours

Duration of effects: 3-6 hours

Sensitivity to alcohol may last up to 72 hours

Overdosage/Treatment Decontamination: Lavage (within 1 hour)/activated charcoal; management of disulfiram reaction: Institute support measures to restore blood pressure (pressors and fluids); monitor for hypokalemia; metoclopramide or prochlorperazine can be used for vomiting; dopamine is **not** useful to treat disulfiram-ethanol induced hypotension; norepinephrine is the preferred agent; use of 4-methylpyr-azole is investigational

Antidote(s)

- Norepinephrine [ANTIDOTE]

Drug Interaction INH, metronidazole, phenytoin, alcohol, warfarin, diazepam, chlordiazepoxide; can cause elevation of theophylline

Additional Information Toxic dose: Hallucinogenic: 10-20 mg of psilo-cin. *Coprinus atramentarius* is one of the inky-caps which are characterized by having fruit bodies that undergo autodigestion; it usually grows in clusters in grassy areas; it gives a black spore print; approximately less than 1100th the potency of LSD

Mushrooms, Toxic (Group 5) Anticholinergic

CAS Number 2552-55-8 (ibotenic acid); 2763-96-4 (muscimol)

Scientific Name *Amanita cothurnata*; *Amanita crenulata*; *Amanita frostiana*; *Amanita gemmata*; *Amanita muscaria*; *Amanita pantherina*

Mechanism of Toxic Action Inebriation syndrome is due primarily to the toxin ibotenic acid and its decarboxylation product, muscimol; ibotenic acid is structurally related to the excitatory neurotransmitter glutamic acid while muscimol is related to the inhibitory neurotransmitter GABA; combined action of both toxins may explain the initial excitation and inebriation followed by the prolonged coma-like sleep seen with poisoning by Group V mushrooms

Adverse Reactions

Cardiovascular: Tachycardia, hypotension

Central nervous system: Delirium, dizziness, ataxia, somnolence, seizures, psychosis, euphoria, residual headaches, fever, coma, hyperthermia, visual hallucinations

Gastrointestinal: Vomiting (rare), xerostomia

Neuromuscular & skeletal: Myoclonus, fasciculations

Ocular: Mydriasis

Renal: Renal failure (within 1 week of ingestion)

Admission Criteria/Prognosis Can observe for 6-8 hours; if symptomatic, admission is suggested; ingestion of more than two mushrooms will probably require admission

Toxicodynamics/Kinetics

Onset of action: 1 hour

Duration of action: 24 hours

Overdosage/Treatment

Decontamination: Lavage (within 1 hour)/activated charcoal

Supportive therapy: Diazepam can be utilized for delirium and for seizures; physostigmine should only be used for life-threatening anticholinergic crisis (0.5-2 mg I.V. over a 5 minute period); hemodialysis if renal failure develops

Antidote(s)

- Physostigmine [ANTIDOTE]

Additional Information

Toxic dose: Ibotenic acid: 30-60 mg; Muscimol: 6 mg. Sensory derangement can be produced at a dose of 2-4 mushrooms; maximum survivable ingestion: 20 mushrooms

Amanita muscaria contains only trace amounts of muscarine and is not considered part of Group III; *Amanita* species are diagnosed by having a white spore print, gills that do not reach the stem, the presence of a volva, and often, but not always, an annulus. See figure in Mushrooms,

Toxic (Group I) Cyclopeptides; do not confuse any of these with the *Amanita* species containing Group I toxins.

Mushrooms, Toxic (Group 6) Psychedelic

CAS Number 520-52-5; 520-53-6

Scientific Name *Conocybe cyanopus*; *Conocybe smithii*; *Gymnopilus aeruginosa*; *Gymnopilus luteus*; *Gymnopilus spectabilis*; *Gymnopilus validipes*; *Panaeolus campanatuus*; *Panaeolus foenisecii*; *Panaeolus sphinctrinus*; *Panaeolus subbalteatus*; *Pluteus salicinus*; *Psilocybe baeocystis*; *Psilocybe caerulescens*; *Psilocybe caerulipes*; *Psilocybe cubensis*; *Psilocybe cyanescens*; *Psilocybe pelliculosa*; *Psilocybe semilanceolata*; *Psilocybe strictipes*; *Psilocybe stuntzii*; *Stropharia semiglobata*

Mechanism of Toxic Action Contains psilocybin and psilocin which are indole alkaloids similar to LSD, possible serotonin antagonists

Adverse Reactions

Cardiovascular: Tachycardia, flushing, hypertension, sinus tachycardia, Wolff-Parkinson-White syndrome

Central nervous system: Ataxia, chills, headache, dizziness, fever, seizures, visual hallucinogens (colored patterns, impaired distance perception), psychosis, leukoencephalopathy

Gastrointestinal: Vomiting

Genitourinary: Urinary incontinence

Hematologic: Methemoglobinemia

Neuromuscular & skeletal: Myalgias, paresthesias, hyperkinesis, rigors, weakness

Ocular: Mydriasis

Admission Criteria/Prognosis Admit if fever/seizures occur; any patient with change in mental status, cardiopulmonary complaints, or methemoglobin levels >30% should be admitted; asymptomatic patients with methemoglobin levels <30% may be considered for discharge after 6 hours of observation and if methemoglobin levels fall to <15%

Toxicodynamics/Kinetics

Onset of action: Within 20 minutes

Duration: 6-15 hours

Absorption: Oral: 50%

Metabolism: Hepatic

Elimination: Renal

Overdosage/Treatment Decontamination: Lavage (within 1 hour)/activated charcoal with cathartic

Supportive therapy: Diazepam for panic attacks; chlorpromazine may be useful for treatment of hallucinations; flashback may occur 4 months later

Additional Information

Roughly 5-6 dried mushroom caps may produce hallucinations, perceptual changes at 6-12 mg psilocybin, true hallucinations at >12 mg psilocybin

The base of the stem of most of these species turns blue to blue-green when handled; many of these species are small and brown to dark colored and as such are easy to confuse with other species including the deadly toxic Group I species *Conocybe filaris* (Deadly *Conocybe*); most species in these genera are not hallucinogenic.

Specific References

Grieshaber AF, Moore KA, and Levine B, "The Detection of Psilocin in Human Urine," *J Forensic Sci*, 2001, 46(3):627-30.

Gross ST, "Psychotropic Drugs in Developmental Mushrooms: A Case Study Review," *J Forensic Sci*, 2002, 47(6):1298-302.

Kunz MW, Rauber-Lüthy CH, Meier PJ, et al, "Acute Poisoning with Hallucinogenic Psilocybe Mushrooms in Switzerland," *J Toxicol Clin Toxicol*, 2000, 38(2):233-4.

Tiscione NB and Miller MI, "Psilocin Identified in a DUID Investigation," *J Anal Toxicol*, 2006, 30:342-3..

Mushrooms, Toxic (Group 7) Gastrointestinal Irritants

Scientific Name *Agaricus arvensis*; *Agaricus hondensis*; *Agaricus placomyces*; *Agaricus silvicola*; *Agaricus xanthodermus*; *Amanita brunnescens*; *Amanita chlorinosma*; *Amanita flavoconia*; *Amanita flavorubescens*; *Amanita frostiana*; *Amanita parcivolvata*; *Boletus luridus*; *Boletus pulcherrimus*; *Boletus satanus*; *Boletus sensibilis*; *Chlorophyllum molybdites*; *Entoloma* species; *Gomphus floccosa*; *Gomphus kauffmani*; *Hebeloma crustuliniforme*; *Hebeloma fastibile*; *Hebeloma mesophaeum*; *Hebeloma sinapizans*; *Helvella* species; *Hypholoma fasciculare*; *Lactarius chrysorheus*; *Lactarius glaucescens*; *Lactarius helvus*; *Lactarius repraesentaneus*; *Lactarius rufus*; *Lactarius scrobiculatus*; *Lactarius torminosus*; *Lactarius uvidus*; *Lepiota clypeolaria*; *Lepiota cristata*; *Lepiota lutea*; *Lepiota naucina*; *Omphalotus olearius*; *Paxillus involutus*; *Ramaria formosa*; *Ramaria gelatinosa*; *Russula emetica*; *Scleroderma citrinum*; *Tricholoma* species; *Tylopilus felleus*; *Verpa bohemica*

Mechanism of Toxic Action Gastrointestinal irritants, diverse toxins, most mechanisms have not been identified

Adverse Reactions

Cardiovascular: Pallor

Central nervous system: Fatigue, drowsiness, headache (*Entoloma lividum*), chills

Gastrointestinal (within 3 hours): Nausea, vomiting, watery diarrhea progressing to bloody diarrhea, abdominal pain

Neuromuscular & skeletal: Myalgias

Overdosage/Treatment

Decontamination: Activated charcoal

Supportive therapy: Isotonic fluids for rehydration; symptoms usually resolve within 24 hours

Additional Information Species listed as having Group VII toxins are numerous and diverse ranging from mushrooms to coral fungi to puffballs; the Jack O'Lantern (*Omphalotus olearius*) is commonly ingested due to a superficial similarity to the choice edible chanterelle; *Chlorophyllum molybdites* (Green-spored *Lepiota*) is another commonly ingested toxic mushroom; it is large, white, and grows commonly in lawns throughout the United States; it can be identified by the green tinted gills and green spore print.

Mushrooms, Toxic (Group 8) Renal Toxic

CAS Number 37338-80-0

Scientific Name *Cortinarius atrovirens*; *Cortinarius gentilis*; *Cortinarius orellanoides*; *Cortinarius orellanus*; *Cortinarius rainierensis*; *Cortinarius splendens*; *Cortinarius vitellinus*

Mechanism of Toxic Action Contains orelline and orellanine which can cause interstitial nephritis, renal tubular damage

Adverse Reactions

Central nervous system: Chills, headaches

Dermatologic: **Skin rash** (12%)

Gastrointestinal: Nausea, vomiting, **diarrhea** (20%), anorexia, constipation

Neuromuscular & skeletal: Myalgias, **paresthesias** (15%)

Otic: Ototoxicity, tinnitus

Renal: Oliguria, **renal failure** (30% to 46%) can be delayed in onset up to weeks after exposure, **polyuria** (30%)

Miscellaneous: Coldness, cold feeling, intense thirst

Toxicodynamics/Kinetics Onset of action: Delay of symptoms may occur as long as 17 days later but usually occur 24-36 hours postingestion

Overdosage/Treatment

Decontamination: Lavage (within 1 hour)/activated charcoal

Supportive therapy: Isotonic fluids for rehydration; renal transplant may be required for renal failure; forced diuresis is not effective; furosemide may increase renal dysfunction

Enhanced elimination: Hemodialysis or charcoal hemoperfusion should be started as soon as possible to prevent renal failure

Drug Interaction Increased toxicity may occur with phenobarbital or furosemide

Additional Information Lethal dose: Fresh mushrooms or 3-10 caps: 100-200 g/kg

Cortinarius gentilis (Deadly Cort) and *Cortinarius rainierensis* have been found in the western United States but, to our knowledge, poisonings due to these fungi are unknown in the United States. May be present (orellanine) in renal biopsy materials.

Mushrooms, Toxic (Group 9) Renal Toxic

Scientific Name *Amanita smithiana*

Mechanism of Toxic Action

Contains the nephrotoxic compounds allenic norleucine and chlorocrotylglycine

Adverse Reactions Gastrointestinal side effects (nausea, vomiting, and diarrhea), along with dizziness and diaphoresis, usually occur within $^1/_2$-12 hours. Oliguric renal failure associated with renal tubular necrosis usually occurs within 2-5 days postingestion. Other side effects include blurred vision, elevated liver function tests, pruritus, and metabolic acidosis associated with the renal failure.

Overdosage/Treatment

Decontamination: Although no formal studies exist, activated charcoal (1 g/kg) could be given to prevent absorption within 1 hour of ingestion

Supportive therapy: Treatment is entirely supportive; monitor electrolytes; renal failure may require hemodialysis for several weeks before resolution.

Additional Information *Amanita smithiana* is a large white mushroom with a 5-12.5 cm wide cap, a 10-20 cm stem, and a 1-3 cm thick bulb. It is found primarily in the Pacific Northwest and resembles the matsutake mushroom (*Tricholoma magnivalere*). Unlike the matsutake mushroom, *Amanita smithiana* is odorless.

Mushrooms, Toxic (Group 10)

Scientific Name *Amanita smithiana*

Synonyms Smith's amarita

Mechanism of Toxic Action Can cause renal toxicity through the chemicals amino-hexadienoic acid and chlorocrotyl glycine which can result in renal tubular acidosis and necrosis

Adverse Reactions

Onset of nausea and vomiting may be delayed for as long as 12 hours.

Ocular: Blurred vision

Central nervous system: Anxiety, dizziness

Gastrointestinal: Nausea, vomiting, diarrhea, abdominal pain

Hepatic: Elevated transaminase level

Renal: Acute renal failure, oliguria, anura can occur 4 to 6 days post ingestion. Renal Tubular acidosis.

Dermal: Diaphoresis, Pruritis.

Overdosage/Treatment

Decontamination: Although no formal studies exist, activated charcoal (1 g/kg) could be given to prevent absorption within 1 hour of ingestion

Supportive therapy: Treatment is entirely supportive; monitor electrolytes; renal failure may require hemodialysis for several weeks before resolution.

Additional Information Commonly found in the Pacific Northwest, it usually appears in the full. *Amanita smithiana* has an ivory colored, convex cap up to 1.8 cm in diameter with felt-like brownish patches.

Mustard Tree

Scientific Name *Nicotiana glauca*

Mechanism of Toxic Action All parts of the plant contain nicotine and are considered toxic

Adverse Reactions Cardiovascular: Sinus bradycardia, sinus tachycardia

Signs and Symptoms of Overdose Low doses can cause asthenia, headache, nausea, oral irritation, sweating, thirst, and vomiting. Higher doses can cause CNS stimulation followed by depression, confusion, hallucinations, hypertension, hyperthermia, seizures, and tachycardia followed by bradycardia, hypotension, and an irregular pulse.

Admission Criteria/Prognosis Symptomatic patients or patients with tachycardia or hypertension 4 hours postexposure should be admitted; survival after 4 hours is usually associated with complete recovery

Overdosage/Treatment

Decontamination: **Oral**: Emesis not recommended due to potential for seizures. Lavage within 1 hour with 1:10,000 potassium permanganate (100 mg/L) is recommended in ingestions after control of seizures; activated charcoal with cathartic use in acute ingestions not well established. **Dermal**: Wash area well with cool water and dry; soap (especially alkaline soaps) may increase absorption; remove any remaining transdermal systems; nicotine will continue to be absorbed several hours after removal due to depot in skin

Supportive therapy: Control seizures with benzodiazepines; if continuous, use phenytoin or phenobarbital; atropine can be utilized for cholinergic toxicity while phentolamine can be used for hypertension

Enhancement of elimination: Hemodialysis/hemoperfusion of unknown value; multiple doses of activated charcoal may be effective; while acidifying the urine may enhance elimination, this modality is not recommended due to inherent dangers; would proceed with forced diuresis

Additional Information Range: Arizona, Texas, Mexico, California, Hawaii

Needlefish

Scientific Name *Tylosurus crocodilus*

Mechanism of Toxic Action Penetrating bite injury not involving envenomation.

Adverse Reactions

Local: Wound edema, erythema; vascular injury with compartment syndrome may occur. Secondary infections (myositis or cellulitis) may be caused by *Vibrio* species.

Miscellaneous: Radiopaque

Admission Criteria/Prognosis Admit any nonextremity bite or bite with suspected vascular injury.

Overdosage/Treatment Supportive therapy: Apply direct pressure over wound if vascular injury is suspected. Obtain x-ray of affected area (the beak of the needlefish is radiopaque). Wound exploration may be necessary to remove fragments. If a joint is involved, arthroscopy should be considered. Vigorously irrigate all wounds. Tetanus prophylaxis (if not up to date) should be given. Appropriate intravenous antibiotics include ciprofloxacin, imipenem-cilastatin, cefoperazone, cefotaxime, ceftazidime, gentamicin, or trimethoprim-sulfamethoxazole. Oral antibiotics which are appropriate include trimethoprim-sulfamethoxazole, ciprofloxacin, or doxycycline.

Additional Information A blue-green surface fish found in all oceans of the subtropical or tropical regions; this fish may grow to ~5 feet long with its beak accounting for ~25% of its length. May leap out of the water at high speeds in the direction of light.

Nephthytis

Scientific Name *Syngonium podophyllum*; *Syngonium*

Mechanism of Toxic Action Contains insoluble calcium oxalate crystals which cause mechanical irritation; may also cause irritation through an unclear enzymatic process

Signs and Symptoms of Overdose

Dermal: Dermatitis, irritation, pain, swelling

Ocular: Sap may cause corneal abrasion, lacrimation, pain, photophobia; oxalate crystals may be deposited on cornea; may also cause dermatitis

Oral: Diarrhea, dysphonia, edema, salivation, vomiting

Toxicodynamics/Kinetics Rapid onset of local symptoms

Overdosage/Treatment

Decontamination: **Oral:** Dilute; ipecac/lavage/activated charcoal not likely necessary. **Dermal:** Wash thoroughly. **Ocular:** Irrigate

Supportive therapy: Cool compresses may minimize pain and swelling

Additional Information Toxic part: Whole plant contains calcium oxalate crystals

Neurotoxic Shellfish Poisoning

Related Information

- Ciguatera Food Poisoning
- Paralytic Shellfish Poisoning

Commonly Found In Mussels, shellfish (bivalves)

Mechanism of Toxic Action Shellfish ingestion of the toxic dinoflagellate *Ptychodiscus brevis*, produces the neurotoxin brevetoxin; additionally, the dinoflagellate *Ptychodiscus veneficum* can cause this illness. Brevetoxins are a muscarinic agonist.

Signs and Symptoms of Overdose Abdominal pain, ataxia, bradycardia (lasting up to 12 hours), coma, confusion, diarrhea, dizziness, dysphagia, headache, hyporeflexia, lacrimation, myalgia, mydriasis, paresthesia, pruritus, reversal of hot/cold temperature, rhinorrhea, seizures, sneezing, tremor. Bronchospasm and cough can occur from aerosolized *P. brevis* particles.

Admission Criteria/Prognosis All symptomatic patients should be admitted

Overdosage/Treatment

Decontamination: Dermal: Wash with soap and water; lavage (within 1 hour)/activated charcoal (avoid magnesium cathartics)

Supportive therapy: Although no human studies exist, atropine has been useful in treating bronchospasm, rhinorrhea, lacrimation, and salivation in animal studies. Thus ipratropium bromide may be efficacious in treating bronchospasm. Seizures can be treated with benzodiazepines; refractory seizures can be treated with barbiturates or phenytoin. Hypotension can be treated with intravenous fluids or vasopressors.

Additional Information Incubation period: ~3 hours (range: 15 minutes to 18 hours). Duration of illness: ~17 hours (range: 1-72 hours). Heat stable, lipid soluble toxin; may be a cause of red tides. Usually found off of Florida in the Gulf of Mexico.

Oak

Scientific Name *Quercus*

Signs and Symptoms of Overdose Abdominal pain, bloody diarrhea, constipation, nausea, possible kidney and liver damage, vomiting

Overdosage/Treatment

Decontamination: Induction of vomiting is controversial, vomiting may be appropriate for large ingestions; activated charcoal and cathartics may also be of value

Supportive therapy: As needed

Octopus

Scientific Name *Octopus bairdi*

Mechanism of Toxic Action Bite - envenomation

Adverse Reactions Local: Erythema

Signs and Symptoms of Overdose Aphonia, blurred vision, burning sensation, cardiovascular collapse, coma, local ischemia, numbness, pain, paresthesia, slurred speech

Admission Criteria/Prognosis All patients should be observed at least 12-24 hours

Overdosage/Treatment Symptomatic/supportive/wound care; no antidote available; Hypotension should be treated with standard therapy; if unresponsive to standard therapy, norepinephrine or phenylephrine infusion may be required.

Additional Information Octopus bites are rare, but can result in severe envenomations if due to blue-ringed octopus. Range: Warm/shallow waters including rock pools in the intertidal zones

Oleander

Scientific Name *Nerium odorum*; *Nerium oleander*

Mechanism of Toxic Action Entire plant contains cardiac glycosides oleandrin, oleandroside, and neriin

Adverse Reactions Cardiovascular: Sinus bradycardia

Signs and Symptoms of Overdose GI effects (nausea and vomiting) usually precede cardiovascular effects by several hours. Asystole, AV block, bradycardia, confusion, contact dermatitis, decreased QT interval and prolonged P-R interval, delirium, dizziness, fatigue, fibrillation (atrial),

flutter (atrial), headache, heart block (first, second, and third degree), hyperkalemia, hypotension, seeing yellow halos, ventricular arrhythmias

Admission Criteria/Prognosis Asymptomatic patients with normal electrocardiogram and electrolytes can be discharged after a 12-hour observation; any symptomatic patient should be admitted to a cardiac monitor bed

Reference Range Postmortem concentrations following suicide by water extraction of oleander: Heart blood: 9.8 ng/ml; Cerebrospinal fluid: 10.1 ng/mL

Overdosage/Treatment

Decontamination: Lavage within 1 hour and multidose activated charcoal enhance total body clearance of digitalis; whole bowel irrigation is also beneficial in removing plant debris from the GI tract and is recommended for ingestions of large amounts of plant material

Supportive therapy: Monitor cardiac status and serum potassium levels; bradycardia will frequently respond to atropine; phenytoin is the recommended treatment for ventricular arrhythmias because it will also improve conduction through the AV node; lidocaine can also be used to treat ventricular arrhythmias, but will not have an effect on AV conduction; other antiarrhythmics which have been used in arrhythmias resistant to the above therapy include magnesium, amiodarone, and bretylium; a pacemaker should be considered for bradycardia and AV nodal blocks resistant to medical management

Enhancement of elimination: Multiple-dose activated charcoal is effective in reducing deaths and life-threatening arrhythmias after yellow oleander poisoning.

Antidote: Digoxin immune Fab has been shown to interact with several different plant cardiac glycosides and may be beneficial in cases resistant to conventional treatment; indications for its use include ventricular arrhythmias resistant to conventional treatment, severe bradycardia and/or second or third degree heart block resistant to atropine and phenytoin

Antidote(s)

- Digoxin Immune Fab [ANTIDOTE]

Additional Information Variable toxicity of leaves depending on growing conditions and time of year; seven leaves have produced bradycardia, nausea, vomiting, and abdominal cramps. Toxin: Cardiac glycosides. Oleander poisoning can occur from smoke inhalation from burning oleander leaves.

Specific References

Barrueto F, Kirrare BM, Cotter BW, et al, "Cardioactive Steroid Poisoning: A Comparison of Plant- and Animal-Derived Compounds," *J Med Toxicol*, 2006, 2(4):152-5.

Dasgupta A, Cao S, and Wells A, "Activated Charcoal is Effective but Equilibrium Dialysis is Ineffective in Removing Oleander Leaf Extract and Oleandrin from Human Serum: Monitoring the Effect by Measuring Apparent Digoxin Concentration," *Ther Drug Monit*, 2003, 25(3):323-30.

de Silva HA, Fonseka MM, Pathmeswaran A, et al, "Multiple-Dose Activated Charcoal for Treatment of Yellow Oleander Poisoning: A Single-Blind, Randomised, Placebo-Controlled Trial," *Lancet*, 2003, 361(9373):1935-8.

Downer J, Craigmill A and Holstege D, "Toxic Potential of Oleander Derived Compost and Vegetables Grown with Oleander Soil Amendments," *Vet Hum Toxicol*, 2003, 45(4):219-21.

Eddleston M and Persson H, "Acute Plant Poisoning and Antitoxin Antibodies," *J Toxicol Clin Toxicol*, 2003, 41(3):309-15.

Suchard JR and Janssen MU, "Negligible Oleandrin Content of Hot Dogs Cooked on Nerium Oleander Skewers," *Clin Toxicol (Phila)*, 2005, 43:760.

Oriental Hornet

Scientific Name *Vespa orientalis* (*Hymenoptera* sp.)

Mechanism of Toxic Action Venom contains acetylcholine, histamine, serotonin, catecholamines, kinins, and phospholipases

Signs and Symptoms of Overdose Acute tubular necrosis, anaphylaxis, anuria, coagulopathy, dyspnea, fever, hemolysis, hepatotoxicity, hypoglycemia, hyporeflexia, hypotension, rhabdomyolysis, seizures, thrombocytopenia

Overdosage/Treatment Supportive therapy: Treat anaphylaxis with epinephrine, antihistamines, and corticosteroids; hypotension can be treated with I.V. crystalloid fluid and vasopressor agents

Additional Information Lethal dose: Mice: 2.5 mg/kg. Hemolysis is due to orientotoxin and phospholipase A_2 and is usually manifested within 12 hours of envenomations

Ostrich Fern

Scientific Name *Matteuccia struthiopteris*; *Onoclea struthiopteris*; *Pteretis struthiopteris*

Mechanism of Toxic Action Essentially unknown; may contain a heat-labile toxin that can cause gastroenteritis

Signs and Symptoms of Overdose Usually begin within 12 hours of ingestion (incubation mean: 6 hours); abdominal pain, diarrhea, headache, nausea, vomiting. Symptoms usually last ∼1 day.

Overdosage/Treatment Supportive therapy: Primarily symptomatic; replace fluid loss either orally or with intravenous hydration

Additional Information Spring vegetable; large fern with oblong shaped leaves found along rivers, streams, and coastal waters; usually nontoxic, but a gastroenteritis syndrome has recently been described; recommendation is to boil the plant for 15 minutes or steam for 10-12 minutes before eating. Range: Eastern North America

Pansy

Scientific Name *Viola* species

Mechanism of Toxic Action Myosin and glucosides produce a cathartic effect, but large ingestions are required

Signs and Symptoms of Overdose Diarrhea, nausea, vomiting

Overdosage/Treatment Supportive therapy: Fluid replacement is seldom required; treat symptomatically

Additional Information Toxin: Seeds contain myosin and glucosides

Paralytic Shellfish Poisoning

Related Information
- Neurotoxic Shellfish Poisoning

Commonly Found In Alaskan butterclam, sea scallop, Californian sea mussel, Australian xanthid crab, butterclams, oysters, rock scallop, Washington clam

Mechanism of Toxic Action Consumption of toxic dinoflagellate (protistans) by the shellfish (bivalve mollusks) can then concentrate the neurotoxin (saxitoxin, neosaxitoxin, gonyautoxin); these neurotoxins can block neuromuscular transmission by blocking ionic permeability of neurons to sodium. Additional vasodilitation can occur.

Adverse Reactions Cardiovascular: Sinus tachycardia

Signs and Symptoms of Overdose Aphonia, ataxia, blindness (temporary), diarrhea, dizziness, dysphagia, dyspnea, headache, hypotension, incoherent speech, nystagmus, ophthalmoplegia, paralysis, paresthesias, respiratory failure, salivation, tachycardia, tongue/lip numbness, trismus. Death is usually due to respiratory paralysis within 12 hours. Sensation of loose teeth can occur, as can diaphoresis.

Admission Criteria/Prognosis All symptomatic patients should be admitted; asymptomatic patients can be discharged following 8 hours observation postexposure

Toxicodynamics/Kinetics
Absorption: Oral: Well absorbed
Elimination: Renal

Overdosage/Treatment
Decontamination: Oral: Lavage with water or 2% sodium bicarbonate within 2 hours of exposure; activated charcoal can be utilized with cathartics (but avoid magnesium-based cathartics)
Supportive therapy: Hypotension can be treated with intravenous fluids and vasopressors
Enhanced elimination: Hemodialysis has been utilized with uneven results; cannot be recommended for routine use

Test Interactions Elevation of creatine kinase (MB) not related to severity of poisoning

Drug Interaction Ethyl alcohol may increase toxicity of this agent

Additional Information
Lethal dose: ∼0.5 mg (or ∼80 mcg of pure toxin/100 g of tissue); Toxic oral dose: ∼0.2 mg
Presence of blooms indicates that >20,000 organisms exist in 1 mL of water, and it is possible that blooms may reach 40 million/mL. Typically, time of onset is from May to November.
The toxin is acid and heat stable and stored in the liver, gills, and siphons of the shellfish. Onset can occur in ∼30 minutes. Children may be more sensitive to neurotoxin than adults
Saxitoxin from the dinoflagellate *Pyrodinium bahamense* have been found in the Southern (*Sphoeroides nephelus*), checkered (Sphoeroides testudineus) and bandtail (*sphoeroides spengleri*) puffer fish in the Western Atlantic. Saxitoxins were detected in skin, muscle and viscera at concentrations up to 22, 104 micrograms of saxitox in equivalents per 100 grams tissue in the ovaries (action level is 80 micrograms of saxitoxin equivalents per 100 grams of tissue).

Specific Reference
Landsberi JH, Hall, S, Johannessen JN et al, "Saxitoxin Puffer Fish Poisoning in the United States with the First Report of *Pyrodinium bahamense* as the Potative Toxin Source," *Environ Health Perspect*, 2006, 114:1502-7.

Pasteurella multocida

Signs and Symptoms of Overdose
Animal bite-wound infections: Patients who have *Pasteurella* inoculated via a bite wound develop rapid onset of local pain, erythema, and edema. This may occur within hours of the bite or may be delayed by several days. Common sites include the upper extremities (in particular, hands), legs, and the head and neck region. An important complication is the development of regional lymphadenopathy. Occasionally, *Pasteurella* infection may be the cause of lymph node enlargement of unknown etiology; such patients should be questioned about seemingly minor animal scratches as well. Bite-wound infections are often limited to soft tissue cellulitis or focal abscesses. At times, the course may be complicated by tenosynovitis and osteomyelitis, which can be particularly difficult to treat when involving the hand. Note that the specific entity known as "cat scratch disease" is not caused by *Pasteurella multocida*. The exact cause of this lymphadenopathy syndrome is still being debated.

Upper and lower respiratory infections: This unusual presentation of *Pasteurella* infection may be seen in patients who have had a significant exposure to animals but lack a history of an animal bite. *Pasteurella* has been implicated as a rare cause of bronchitis, sinusitis, and pneumonia in both healthy individuals and in those with underlying chronic bronchitis.

Infection in the immunocompromised host: Serious and life-threatening *Pasteurella* infections have been reported in patients with underlying malignancies, organ transplantations, and HIV infection.

Miscellaneous infections: Meningitis, arthritis, peritonitis (particularly patients undergoing peritoneal dialysis), corneal ulcers, ophthalmitis, and urinary tract infections are rarely reported.

Overdosage/Treatment Supportive therapy: Drug of choice for pasteurellosis is penicillin. If the infection is minor and limited to soft tissue, a trial of oral penicillin may be attempted (eg, penicillin V, 500 mg orally every 6 hours). If the infection is more serious, parenteral penicillin should be used. This includes deep wound infections of the extremities, osteomyelitis, septic arthritis, tenosynovitis, and pneumonia. Consultation with an infectious disease specialist may be useful in complicated cases, where therapy may be prolonged and surgical debridement necessary. Other antimicrobial agents are probably effective, but the clinical experience is more limited: tetracycline, ampicillin, possibly ciprofloxacin, and the cephalosporins. Infectious disease consultation may be helpful for therapy with alternative agents.

Additional Information
Microbiology: *Pasteurella multocida* is a gram-negative rod which is primarily a pathogen in wild and domestic animals, but is also capable of causing sporadic human diseases such as animal bite infection, osteomyelitis, pneumonia, and sepsis. *P. multocida* is an aerobic, gram-negative coccobacillus which does not form spores. It belongs to the family Pasteurellaceae and is thus related to *Haemophilus* species. There are six distinct species of *Pasteurella*, but the most common to cause human disease is *Pasteurella multocida*. Special requests for identification for this organism are helpful for the microbiology laboratory but are usually not necessary; the organism grows readily on several standard culture media such as blood agar or chocolate agar.

Epidemiology:
P. multocida is a normal commensal of the oropharynx and the GI tract of several kinds of animals. However, it is only rarely recovered from the respiratory tract of humans, and has been found to be part of the normal oral flora only in individuals with significant animal contact (eg, veterinarians). The frequency of recovery of this organism from a healthy animal depends on the particular animal species, as follows: cats, 50% to 75%; dogs, 10% to 60%; pigs, 50%; and rats, 15%.
Pasteurella has been reported in all age groups. Human infection usually occurs following an animal bite or scratch. One study found that up to 17% of patients being treated in an emergency room for an animal bite ultimately developed a *Pasteurella* infection. Cat scratches or bites cause the majority of *Pasteurella* infections (∼65% of cases). Dog bites are responsible for ∼35% of cases. A smaller number of cases of *Pasteurella* infections is due to animal exposures without a clear history of an animal bite or scratch; the patient tends to be frequently exposed to animals (such as a veterinarian, livestock handler, pet shop worker), and the infections are generally in the respiratory tract, although cases of intra-abdominal infection have also been described. A small percentage of patients are infected with *P. multocida* without any significant animal exposure.

Diagnosis: *P. multocida* infection should be included in the differential diagnosis of any wound infection following an animal bite or deep scratch. The diagnosis strongly suggests if the onset of local inflammation is within 3-24 hours of the bite, and if the animal involved was a cat. Longer periods of incubation are more suggestive of streptococcal or staphylococcal infection, although certainly cases of pasteurellosis may have a delayed onset. The diagnosis is more difficult for nonbite *Pasteurella* infections; the clinician must carefully inquire about unusual or prolonged animal exposures in the workplace and at home.

Peach

Scientific Name *Prunus persica* species
Mechanism of Toxic Action Amygdalin (a cyanogenic glycoside) is hydrolyzed in the gut to release hydrocyanic acid; cellular hypoxia occurs after absorption and complexation with cytochrome oxidase
Signs and Symptoms of Overdose Symptoms may be delayed 30 minutes to 2 hours or longer due to hydrolysis preferentially occurring in alkaline duodenum, plus intestinal flora hydrolyzing amygdalin
Admission Criteria/Prognosis All symptomatic patients should probably be admitted to an intensive care unit for 1-2 days; asymptomatic patients should be observed for at least 2 hours and then can be discharged; survival after 4 hours (in an acute exposure) is usually associated with recovery
Overdosage/Treatment
Decontamination: Basic poison management; vomiting is contraindicated due to rapid course of the neurologic symptoms. Give 100% oxygen.
Supportive therapy: Give sodium bicarbonate for acidosis
Enhancement of elimination: Hemodialysis and charcoal hemoperfusion have been utilized; hyperbaric oxygen may also be utilized; hydroxocobalamin and dicobalt-EDTA used for chelation in Europe
Antidote(s)
- Cyanide Antidote Kit [ANTIDOTE]

Diagnostic Procedures
- Anion Gap, Blood
- Electrolytes, Blood
- Methemoglobin, Blood

Additional Information Toxic dose: 1-2 pits likely nontoxic; toxicity unusual with accidental ingestion. Intact pit does not release chemical; apricot most toxic within the genus; peach leaves (in Australia) may have a cyanide content as high as 66 mg per 100 g of leaves. Toxic part: Amygdalin is found in leaves, flowers, bark, seeds; young leaves have highest concentration.

Peony (Common)

Scientific Name *Paeonia* species
Mechanism of Toxic Action Toxin is located in plant's roots and the site of action is unknown
Signs and Symptoms of Overdose Contact dermatitis with dermal exposure. Oral exposure based on rat data: Low dose (62.5 mg/kg) produces a diuretic effect; medium dose (125-500 mg/kg) produces anti-inflammatory activity and decreased GI secretions; high dose (>500 mg/kg) causes CNS depression
Toxicodynamics/Kinetics
Absorption: Rapid
Half-life: 30 minutes
Overdosage/Treatment
Topical steroids are probably beneficial for contact dermatitis
Decontamination: Ipecac is of questionable benefit due to the rapid absorption and onset of action; activated charcoal with sorbitol will aid in clearance of the toxin
Supportive therapy: Respiratory support is most critical intervention; maintain fluid and electrolyte replacement during diuretic phase, however, electrolyte depletion is not as severe as with hydrochlorothiazide
Additional Information Minimal clinical symptoms are expected with accidental plant ingestion; clinically significant doses may be seen in ingestions of many Oriental medicines which contain this ingredient; paeonol 250 mg/kg is about as effective of a diuretic as hydrochlorothiazide 10 mg/kg; LD_{50} (based on rat data): 3430 mg/kg. Toxin: Paeonol. Monitor electrolytes during the diuretic phase.

Peyote

Related Information
- Mescaline

Scientific Name *Lophophora williamsii*
Mechanism of Toxic Action Mescaline - structurally similar to amphetamines producing CNS and sympathetic stimulation and hallucinations
Signs and Symptoms of Overdose Anxiety, asthenia, ataxia, blurred vision, dizziness, drowsiness, fever, flashbacks, flushing, hallucinations (visual, auditory), headache, hunger, hypertension, increased pulse, increased respiratory rate, mydriasis, nausea and vomiting preceding hallucinations, paranoia, polyuria, salivation, suicide, tremor
Admission Criteria/Prognosis Patients who are asymptomatic after 4 hours postexposure may be discharged
Toxicodynamics/Kinetics
Urine, blood levels not correlated with clinical effects
Duration of action: >6 hours
Overdosage/Treatment
Decontamination: Ipecac may cause increased agitation especially in paranoid individuals and is unlikely to be of benefit once clinical symptoms present; activated charcoal with cathartic preferred

Supportive therapy: Symptoms may need to be treated with benzodiazepines and/or haloperidol/chlorpromazine; flashbacks may be worsened by phenothiazines; no deaths reported from overdosage of mescaline/peyote
Additional Information Toxic dose: Typically, 300-500 mg or 6-12 peyote "buttons". May be contaminated; consider coingestants; "microdots" may also contain LSD; ~1/2000 the potency of LSD and ~1/20 the potency of psilocybin

Pfiesteria piscicida

Mechanism of Toxic Action
A dinoflagellate found in sediment of primary freshwater (salinity <15,000 ppm) with an unidentifiable toxin (lipid/water soluble) that appears to affect frontal and inferior temporal cortical brain areas.
Portal of entry: Dermal or pulmonary
Signs and Symptoms of Overdose Conjunctivitis, burning sensation, cough, bronchospasm, and sore throat are the immediate symptoms noted on contact. Within 3 hours, myalgia, generalized headache, pruritus, and memory impairment (decreased concentration ability) along with peripheral neuropathy can occur. Nausea, vomiting, secretory diarrhea, vesicular/papular rash, and abdominal cramps can occur within 24 hours. Persistent effects include rash (up to 2 months), memory loss (up to 6 months), bronchospasm, and diarrhea.
Overdosage/Treatment Supportive therapy: Symptomatic care. Diphenhydramine (up to 1 mg/kg every 4-6 hours I.V. or P.O.) can assist in pruritus and headache treatment. Cholestyramine (4 grams 3 times/day for 3 days) may decrease loose stools.
Additional Information
Person-to-person or fish-to-person transmission does not occur. Associated with fish kills and ulcers on fish. Found in coastal areas near the mouth of a river.

Pfiesteria hotlines:
Maryland: 888-584-3100
Virginia: 888-238-6154
North Carolina: 888-823-6915

For further information contact:
Dr. R. Shoemaker
P.O. Box 25
500 Market St.
Pocomoke, Maryland 21851
Phone: 410-957-1550

Philodendron

Scientific Name *Philodendron*
Mechanism of Toxic Action Entire plant contains calcium oxalate crystals which cause oral irritation, swelling, pain, and slurred speech; large ingestions necessary for systemic toxicity are unlikely to occur due to oral irritation seen with ingestion
Signs and Symptoms of Overdose Oral irritation, pain, slurred speech, swelling, vomiting
Overdosage/Treatment
Decontamination: Emesis within 30 minutes or lavage (within 1 hour)/activated charcoal not usually necessary unless massive ingestion is suspected; dilution may be beneficial; milk/water to rinse crystals; oral irritation can be treated with ice or a popsicle
Supportive therapy: I.V. hydration may be needed
Additional Information Fatal dose due to oxalates is estimated to be 700 g of leaves (5 g of oxalate). Toxin: Calcium oxalate crystals concentration is <1%.

Pit Vipers

Commonly Found In Genera *Crotalus* (rattlesnake), *Agkistrodon* (copperhead, cottonmouth), *Sistrurus* (pygmy rattler, massasauga)
Mechanism of Toxic Action Venom; quality and potency vary among species; composition: 90% water with 5-15 enzymes, 3-12 nonenzymatic proteins, as well as other unidentified substances
Signs and Symptoms of Overdose
Local: Bullae, ecchymosis, edema, erythema, hemorrhage, lymphangitis, tenderness, compartment syndrome (rarely)
Systemic: Asthenia, chills, CNS depression, fasciculations, hypotension, nausea, paresthesia, sweating, vomiting
Coagulopathy including hypofibrinogenemia, increased PT and PTT, and thrombocytopenia can occur. Hematuria, hemoconcentration, hypoproteinemia, hypotension, lactic acidosis, proteinuria, and shock are potential complications.
Overdosage/Treatment
Decontamination: Rapid transport to medical facility; immobilize area; if negative pressure suction device is available, this may be used; **do not** incise the wound; constriction band may be applied, **not** a tourniquet

- Wyeth crotalid polyvalent antivenin; treat moderate to severe envenomations with increments of 5-10 vials at a time; skin test per manufacturer's instructions; if positive skin test develops, may prophylax with H_1- and H_2-receptor blockers; give until local injury has stopped and coagulopathy is reversed; complications include allergic reactions, anaphylaxis, and delayed serum sickness

Supportive therapy: ABC assessment, physical exam; mark the extent of local edema with skin marking pen; repeat CBC, platelets, PT, PTT, fibrinogen, CPK, urinalysis every 3-4 hours for at least first 12 hours; I.V. fluids, tetanus prophylaxis, and analgesics may be given as needed; treat infected wounds with antibiotics. Snakes' oral cavity contain primarily gram-negative and anaerobic organisms.

Antidote(s)
- Antivenin (Crotalidae) Polyvalent [ANTIDOTE]

Additional Information
Family: Viperidae; subfamily: Crotalidae

Distinguishing characteristics: Facial pits, vertical elliptical pupils, triangular head, single row of subcaudal scales. All poisonous serpents except coral snakes belong to this group; copperheads, cottonmouths, and rattlesnakes are members

Antivenin has been given on affected extremity distal to a blood pressure cuff (inflated to block arterial flow) while massaging the extremity to the blood pressure cuff (similar to the Bier-block anesthetic technique). Monitor coagulation parameters for at least 2 days

Poinsettia

Related Information
- Star-of-Bethlehem (*Ornithogalum pyrenaicum*)
- Star-of-Bethlehem (*Ornithogalum umbellatum*)

Scientific Name *Euphorbia pulcherrima*

Signs and Symptoms of Overdose Frequently believed to be a toxic (even lethal) plant, the poinsettia has little toxicity. Nausea, vomiting, and skin irritation are rarely reported to Poison Control Centers. Gastrointestinal symptoms are mild, self-limited, and seldom require fluid replacement. Estimates, based on animal data, have indicated that a 50-pound child would have to ingest 500-600 leaves to cause symptoms.

Overdosage/Treatment Wash off patient if irritation is experienced; dilute with water, milk, or juice for ingestions

Additional Information Family: Euphorbiaceae. Toxin: Acrid principle, not fully defined chemically. Range: Tropical plant widely distributed as a Christmas decoration

Poison Hemlock

Scientific Name *Conium maculatum*

Mechanism of Toxic Action Coniine toxicity resembles that of nicotine; there is initial stimulation of autonomic ganglia, followed by depression

Adverse Reactions Cardiovascular: Sinus bradycardia, sinus tachycardia

Signs and Symptoms of Overdose Apnea, ataxia, burning sensation in the throat, coma, disconjugate gaze, miosis, myoglobinuria, nausea, paralysis of skeletal muscles, renal failure, respiratory paralysis, rhabdomyolysis, seizures, slurred speech, tachycardia followed by bradycardia, vomiting

Overdosage/Treatment
Decontamination: Lavage within 1 hour may be performed; administer activated charcoal with cathartic

Supportive therapy: Be prepared to support respirations; provide symptomatic and supportive treatment; manage seizures with diazepam or lorazepam

Additional Information Reportedly used by the Greeks to execute Socrates; human toxicity has been reported from eating birds that feed on poison hemlock. Family: Umbelliferae. Range: Found in the Eastern U.S., the West coast, and the Rocky Mountains. Toxin: Coniine. Toxic part: Whole plant

Specific References
Labay L, McMullin M, Diamond F, et al, "Analysis of Coniine in Blood and Gastric in a Poison Hemlock Death," *J Anal Toxicol*, 2006, 30:134.

Poison Ivy

Scientific Name *Rhus radicans*; *Toxicodendron radicans*

Mechanism of Toxic Action Contains urushiol; shell contains anacardic acid, cardol, anacardol, irritants that can precipitate type IV cell-mediated allergic reaction (allergic contact dermatitis)

Signs and Symptoms of Overdose Dermatitis, proteinuria

Admission Criteria/Prognosis Patient with disabling symptoms (who are immunocompromised) should be admitted. Ingestion of over 2-3 berries should have gastric decontamination and admission

Toxicodynamics/Kinetics
Onset of effect: Variable, but effects usually seen within 24-48 hours
Peak effect: After 3-5 days

Overdosage/Treatment
Decontamination: **Dermal**: Soap and water washing likely ineffective unless done within 5-15 minutes after exposure; wash clothes thoroughly; clean fingernails **Ocular**: Irrigate copiously for 15-20 minutes with saline/topical use of steroids may be useful

Supportive therapy: Cool compresses or showers, Burow's solution, topical/oral steroids; oral prednisone should be used (and tapered) over a 2-3 week course. Frequent soapless showers several times daily with warm but not hot water may be useful. Oral antihistamines can be useful. Steroid creams which may be useful include hydrocortisone creams (>0.5%), desoximetasone cream (0.25% - do not use on face or intertriginous areas), fluocinonide (0.05%), or triamcinolone cream (0.025% or 0.1%); all applied 3 times daily. Only use a thin film in children due to possible adrenal reaction.

Additional Information
Exudate in blisters is sterile.

Toxic part: Sap of entire plant is toxic

Bentoquatam (5%), when applied topically 15 minutes prior to potential exposure, may prevent development of rash due to poison ivy, poison oak, or poison sumac; do not use if rash has developed.

Topical agents used for relief of pruritus with varying efficacy include baking soda paste; Calamine® lotion; ice; jewelweed (*Impatiens capens*), crushed leaf or liquid extracts; gumweed (*Grindelia squarrosa* or *Grindelia robusta*) - alcohol-based tincture; oak and willow bark (*Quercus*; *Salix*) - added to bath; plantain (*Plantago*); chickweed (*Stellaria media*); witch hazel lotion; green clay powder

Specific References
Davila A, Laurora M, Fulton J, et al, "A New Topical Agent, Zanfel, Ameliorates Urushiol-Induced Toxicodendron Allergic Contact Dermatitis," *Ann Emerg Med*, 2003, 42(4):S98.

Poison Lily

Scientific Name *Veratrum viride*

Mechanism of Toxic Action Contains alkaloids which modulate the sodium channel of cardiac tissue, thus increasing sodium conductivity

Signs and Symptoms of Overdose Symptoms usually occur within 1 hour and consist of a bitter/sharp taste followed by nausea, vomiting, diaphoresis, and confusion. Cardiovascular signs include bradycardia, hypotension, bundle branch block, and myocardial ischemia. Numbness and decreased bowel sounds with miosis can develop. Peaked T waves may be seen on ECG.

Overdosage/Treatment
Decontamination: Activated charcoal without a cathartic within 1 hour postingestion

Supportive therapy: Monitor for hypotension; crystalloid fluids and vasopressor support may be required for treatment. Atropine is useful in treating bradycardia. Resolution of symptoms usually occurs within 48 hours.

Additional Information Commonly mistaken for leeks or skunk cabbage

Poison Oak

Scientific Name *Rhus quercifolium*; *Toxicodendron quercifolium*

Mechanism of Toxic Action Contains urushiol; shell contains anacardic acid, cardol, anacardol, irritants that can precipitate type IV cell-mediated allergic reaction (allergic contact dermatitis)

Signs and Symptoms of Overdose Dermatitis

Admission Criteria/Prognosis Patient with disabling symptoms (who are immunocompromised) should be admitted. Ingestion of over 2-3 berries should have gastric decontamination and admission

Toxicodynamics/Kinetics Onset of effect: Variable, but effects usually seen within 24-48 hours
Peak effect: After 3-5 days

Overdosage/Treatment
Decontamination: **Dermal**: Soap and water washing likely ineffective unless done within 5-15 minutes after exposure; clean fingernails; wash clothes thoroughly. Topical use of steroids may be useful. **Ocular**: Irrigate copiously for 15-20 minutes with saline.

Supportive therapy: Cool compresses or showers, Burow's solution, topical/oral steroids; oral prednisone should be used (and tapered) over a 2-3 week course. Oral antihistamines can be useful. Steroid creams which may be useful include hydrocortisone creams (>0.5%), desoximetasone cream (0.25% - do not use on face or intertriginous areas), fluocinonide (0.05%), or triamcinolone cream (0.025% or 0.1%); all applied 3 times daily. Only use a thin film in children due to possible adrenal reaction. Frequent soapless showers several times daily (with warm but not hot water) may be useful.

Additional Information
Exudate in blisters is sterile.

Toxic part: Sap of entire plant is toxic

Bentoquatam (5%), when applied topically 15 minutes prior to potential exposure, may prevent development of rash due to poison ivy, poison oak, or poison sumac; do not use if rash has developed.

Topical agents used for relief of pruritus with varying efficacy include baking soda paste; Calamine® lotion; ice; jewelweed (*Impatiens capens*), crushed leaf or liquid extracts; gumweed (*Grindelia squarrosa* or *Grindelia robusta*) - alcohol-based tincture; oak and willow bark (*Quercus*; *Salix*) - added to bath; plantain (*Plantago*); chickweed (*Stellaria media*); witch hazel lotion; green clay powder

Poison Sumac

Scientific Name *Rhus vernix*; *Toxicodendron vernix*

Mechanism of Toxic Action Contains urushiol, shell contains anacardic acid, cardol, anacardol, irritants that can precipitate type IV cell-mediated allergic reaction (allergic contact dermatitis)

Signs and Symptoms of Overdose Dermatitis

Admission Criteria/Prognosis Patient with disabling symptoms (who are immunocompromised) should be admitted. Ingestion of over 2-3 berries should have gastric decontamination and admission.

Toxicodynamics/Kinetics Onset of effect: Variable, but effects usually seen within 24-48 hours
Peak effect: After 3-5 days

Overdosage/Treatment
Decontamination: **Dermal**: Soap and water washing likely ineffective unless done within 5-15 minutes after exposure; clean fingernails; topical steroids may be useful; wash clothes thoroughly. **Ocular**: Irrigate copiously for 15-20 minutes with saline.
Supportive therapy: Cool compresses or showers, Burow's solution, topical/oral steroids; oral prednisone should be used (and tapered) over a 2-3 week course. Oral antihistamines can be useful. Steroid creams which may be useful include hydrocortisone creams (>0.5%), desoximetasone cream (0.25% do not use on face or intertriginous areas), fluocinonide (0.05%) or triamcinolone cream (0.025% or 0.1%); all applied 3 times daily. Only use a thin film in children due to possible adrenal reaction. Frequent soapless showers several times daily (with warm but not hot water) may be useful.

Additional Information
Exudate in blisters is sterile.
Toxic part: Sap of entire plant is toxic
Bentoquatam (5%), when applied topically 15 minutes prior to potential exposure, may prevent development of rash due to poison ivy, poison oak, or poison sumac; do not use if rash has developed.
Topical agents used for relief of pruritus with varying efficacy include baking soda paste; Calamine® lotion; ice; jewelweed (*Impatiens capens*), crushed leaf or liquid extracts; gumweed (*Grindelia squarrosa* or *Grindelia robusta*) - alcohol-based tincture; oak and willow bark (*Quercus*; *Salix*) - added to bath; plantain (*Plantago*); chickweed (*Stellaria media*); witch hazel lotion; green clay powder

Pokeweed

Scientific Name *Phytolacca americana*

Uses In folk medicine for rheumatism, arthritis, ringworm, and purgative, etc

Adverse Reactions
Cardiovascular: Mobitz type 1 heart block
Miscellaneous: Increased plasma cells

Signs and Symptoms of Overdose Symptoms usually occur within 6 hours. Abdominal pain, AV block, death, diarrhea, dyspnea, lymphocytosis, nausea, seizures, vomiting

Overdosage/Treatment
Decontamination: **Oral**: Administer activated charcoal (in aqueous slurry) for recent ingestions. **Dermal**: Wash with soap and water
Supportive therapy: Replace fluids and electrolytes as needed. Symptoms usually resolve within 1 day.

Additional Information Young leaves may be rendered nontoxic if boiled, rinsed, and boiled again; berries also appear to be edible if cooked. Grows up to 10 feet. Family: Phytolaccaceae. Toxin: Triterpene saponins, pokeweed mitogen. Range: Eastern half of the U.S., California, and Hawaii. Toxic part: Whole plant, especially the root

Portuguese Man-of-War

Scientific Name *Physalia pelagica*; *Physalia utriculus*

Commonly Found In Atlantic Portuguese Man-of-War (*Physalia physalis*); Pacific Portuguese Man-of-War (*Physalia utriculus*)

Signs and Symptoms of Overdose Maculopapular rash with intense pain; may progress to hyperpigmented vesicles and pustules. Systemic reaction includes asthenia, muscle spasms, nausea, pain, paresthesia, and vomiting. In rare cases, respiratory and cardiovascular depression may occur. Systemic effects are more common with the Atlantic Portuguese Man-of-War. Symptoms may last for up to 48 hours.

Overdosage/Treatment
Decontamination: Immobilize area to avoid further discharge of nematocysts; inactivate nematocysts with alcohol or vinegar (5% acetic acid); remove remaining tentacles by applying flour or shave cream and scraping with a sharp instrument

Supportive therapy: Pain control, oral antihistamine, local anesthetics, steroid cream, and tetanus prophylaxis as indicated; systemic effects may require respiratory and circulatory support

Additional Information Invertebrate, contains a nitrogen and carbon monoxide flotation device which functions as a sail similar to a Portuguese admiral's hat; venom consists of a protein neurotoxin

Potato (Leaves, Stems, Tubercles)

Scientific Name *Solanum tuberosum*

Mechanism of Toxic Action Contains toxic alkaloids, solanine most significant structurally similar to cardioglycoside, causes hemolytic and hemorrhagic damage to GI tract similar to saponins; some plants may also contain alpha-cholinergic alkaloids

Adverse Reactions Central nervous system: Psychosis

Signs and Symptoms of Overdose Asthenia, diarrhea, drowsiness, fever, hallucinations, headache, nausea, sweating, vomiting, visual changes. Anticholinergic effects may or may not be present to varying degrees.

Toxicodynamics/Kinetics Unclear

Overdosage/Treatment
Decontamination: Ipecac (within 30 minutes) if vomiting has not already occurred, lavage (within 1 hour) and/or charcoal may be beneficial if the patient presents symptomatic
Supportive therapy: Maintain fluid and electrolyte balance as necessary, support vital signs; physostigmine will reverse anticholinergic toxicity that may be associated with exposure

Antidote(s)
• Physostigmine [ANTIDOTE]

Additional Information Toxic dose: Variable. Mature, properly stored tuber is edible; green foliage, immature tuber, improperly stored tuber (exposed to light) may be toxic

Privet (Berries and Leaves)

Scientific Name *Ligustrum vulgare*

Signs and Symptoms of Overdose Symptoms develop shortly after ingestion and include abdominal tenderness, diarrhea, GI irritation, nausea, vomiting

Overdosage/Treatment
Decontamination: Emesis/lavage usually not necessary due to vomiting which commonly occurs when the plant is ingested
Supportive therapy: Replace fluid/electrolyte losses

Additional Information Toxin: Ligon glycosides, saponins, and secoiridoid bitter agents; gastroenteritis may last for 2-3 days; a small deciduous shrub with lanceolated leaves found in eastern U.S.

Puss Caterpillar

Scientific Name *Megalopyge opercularis* (in Texas, North Carolina); *Lagoa crisputu* (Oklahoma)

Commonly Found In Southern U.S.

Mechanism of Toxic Action Spines/hairs can penetrate the skin and inject toxins than can exhibit proteolytic activity

Signs and Symptoms of Overdose Immediate, intense local pain on contact followed by, within one hour, erythema and vesicles. Blister development may occur within 48 hours. Pruritis may also occur.

Overdosage/Treatment
Decontamination: Dermal - Immediate application of adhesive tape to site may be effective in removing spines. Avoid scatching or rubbing area.
Supportive therapy: Topical corticosteroid preparations may be effective. Opioid agents typically not effective for pain control

Rabies Virus

Related Information
• Animal and Human Bites Guidelines

Mechanism of Toxic Action
Rabies virus is a bullet-shaped single-stranded RNA virus which belongs to the family Rhabdoviridae. A number of important viral proteins have been identified such as viral polymerase, nucleocapsid protein, glycoprotein, and others. Some of these proteins have been used to develop specific diagnostic monoclonal antibodies. Rabies virus can be isolated under the proper conditions in tissue culture. During active rabies infection, the virus can be cultured from a variety of human (and animal) tissues including saliva, brain tissue, respiratory secretions, and urine; the virus is most easily recovered from brain tissue.
The virus is highly neurotropic. When a human is inoculated with rabies virus, the viral glycoprotein attaches to the plasma membrane of cells, possibly the nicotinic acetylcholine receptor. The virus then replicates in skeletal muscle, and when the titer is high enough, it invades nearby sensory and motor nerves and enters the nervous system. It travels along the axon at speeds up to 20 mm/day and eventually reaches the spinal cord. From there, dissemination through the central nervous

system occurs rapidly and encephalitis ensues. Other peripheral nerves become involved; the organism can be recovered from the saliva due to infection of nerves in the salivary glands.

Adverse Reactions Central nervous system: Cranial nerve palsies, aerophobia, hydrophobia

Signs and Symptoms of Overdose Clinical rabies: There is a variable period of incubation before the onset of symptoms (4 days to 19 years), but most cases occur within 1 year of exposure (usually 1-3 months). The initial prodrome of rabies is nonspecific with malaise, fatigue, and fever. In many patients, there may be pain at the initial exposure site. After ~10 days, the patient enters an acute neurologic phase, characterized by bizarre behavior, hyperactivity, and confusion. Photophobia, aniso-coria, areflexia, and paresthesia may be noted. A small stimulus can elicit short periods of thrashing, biting, and other behaviors. Many patients will display hydrophobia (fear of water); there is often severe laryngos-pasm and choking when trying to drink water. This will progress to paralysis, which dominates the clinical picture for some days. Patients typically lapse into coma and develop respiratory failure or arrhythmias, leading to death in most cases, despite full support in intensive care units. Occasional cases of recovery from rabies have been reported.

Overdosage/Treatment

Supportive therapy: Wound treatment and the administration of both RIG and vaccine (for previously unvaccinated persons) are essential components of rabies postexposure prophylaxis. Postexposure prophylaxis should begin immediately for persons bitten by animals suspected or proven to be rabid. A greater than 1-year incubation period has been reported in humans. Therefore, if the clinical signs of rabies are not present, postexposure prophylaxis is indicated regardless of the length of delay when a documented or likely exposure has occurred.

Clinical management consists of supportive care and neuroprotective measures, including a drug-induced coma and ventilator support. Intravenous ribavirin has been used under an investigational protocol.

Coma induction with ketamine (2 mg/kg/hour) with midazolam (1-3.5 mg/kg/hour) to suppress background EEG has shown to be helpful. Ribavirin (33 mg/kg load followed by 16 mg/kg every 6 hours); amantadine (200 mg/day) has also been used.

Based on studies done in Germany and Iran, the World Health Organization, in 1997, recommended a regimen of RIG and six doses of HDCV over a 90-day period. Used this way, the vaccine was found to be safe and effective in protecting persons bitten by animals proven to be rabid, and produced excellent antibody response in all recipients. U.S. studies by the CDC documented that a regimen of one dose of RIG and five doses of HDCV over a 28-day period was safe and produced an excellent antibody response in all recipients. RVA and PCEC clinical trials have demonstrated immunogenicity equivalent to that of HDCV.

Important measures for preventing rabies include immediate and thorough washing of all bite wounds and scratches with soap and water and a virucidal agent (eg, povidone-iodine solution) irrigation. In animal studies, the likelihood of rabies has been shown to be markedly reduced with thorough wound cleansing alone, without other postexposure prophylaxis.

There is currently no treatment for rabies once it has become clinically established. Mortality approaches 100%. Thus, the main treatment issues involve rabies prevention, particularly postexposure prophylaxis. The physician deciding whether or not to initiate rabies treatment (rabies vaccine, rabies immunoglobulin) must answer the following questions: Has a significant exposure occurred, and what is the risk that an animal is rabid?

A significant exposure includes the following.
- An animal bite, defined as penetration of the person's skin by teeth with contamination of the wound with saliva
- Contamination of the mucous membranes with saliva or other potentially infectious tissue from an infected animal
- Certain nonbite exposures, including contamination of scratches, scrapes, wounds, or mucous membranes with saliva or other infectious tissues. The risk of rabies after nonbite exposures is extremely rare, although scattered cases have been reported.

Petting a rabid animal or contacting its blood or body fluids is not an exposure. If it appears that a significant exposure has taken place, the physician must determine whether or not the animal was rabid. As outlined by Fishbein and Robinson, this depends on the percentage of animals found to be rabid in the species in the particular geographical area.

Group 1: Rabies is endemic in animal species involved in exposure. This includes:
- bats - anywhere in the United States (3% to 20% positive for rabies); almost 50% of the rabies cases in the U.S. since 1980 were associated with bat vectors
- terrestrial animals - skunks, raccoons, foxes in areas of United States where rabies is endemic
- dogs in developing countries
- dogs in the United States along the Mexican border.
- For Group 1 exposure, treatment should be initiated for both bite and nonbite exposures.

Group 2: Rabies is not endemic in species involved, but is endemic in other wild animals in the area. The risk of rabies is ~10 times lower in these animals compared with the predominant species. These animals include:
- wild carnivores such as wolves, bobcats, bears, and groundhogs. Up to 20% may have rabies. Bite exposures from these should be treated. Nonbite exposures should either be treated or the local health department consulted.
- rodents (squirrels, hamsters, guinea pigs, gerbils, rats, mice) have a low incidence of rabies, 0.01%. Bite exposures should not be treated (or in exceptional cases, the local health department could be consulted). Nonbite exposures should not be treated.
- dogs and cats - in the United States, the risk of rabies in dogs is less than 1% (except along the Mexican border) in areas where rabies is common in other land animals. In addition, dogs almost always show signs of clinical rabies shortly after the virus is present in saliva. Bite exposure should not be treated if a healthy dog (or cat) is captured; the animal should be observed for 10 days. If the animal develops signs of rabies, treatment in the human should be commenced immediately. If the animal is a stray, it should be sacrificed immediately and the head removed and shipped to an appropriate laboratory. Treatment is delayed pending laboratory testing. The same approach is recommended for nonbite exposures.

Group 3: Rabies is not endemic in the animal species involved in the exposure and is uncommon in other wild animals in the region. This includes most domestic cats and dogs and wild land animals in Idaho, Washington, Utah, Nevada, and Colorado, where the proportion of rabid animals is very low. For bite or nonbite exposures from Group 3 animals, either consult the local health department or do not treat.

Postexposure treatment consists of:
- Vigorous wound cleaning - this has been shown to decrease the risk of rabies.
- Administration or rabies vaccine, either human diploid-cell rabies vaccine or rabies vaccine adsorbed. For persons not previously vaccinated, rabies vaccine should be given 1 mL I.M. on days 0, 3, 7, 14, and 28. Abbreviated regimens have been described. For persons previously vaccinated, the rabies vaccine should be given 1 mL I.M. on days 0 and 3.
- Administration of rabies immunoglobulin. For persons not previously vaccinated, this should be given at 20 int. units/kg of body weight. If possible, one-half the dose should be injected locally near the original wound and the rest given I.M. (using a new needle). For persons previously vaccinated, rabies immunoglobulin is not recommended.

Diagnostic Procedures
- Rabies Identification

Additional Information

Bats remain an important reservoir of rabies and cause sporadic cases. Risk of rabies after a bite by a rabid animal is ~50 times that of the risk after scratches.

During 1980-2000, a total of 26 (74%) of rabies-virus variants obtained from patients in the United States were associated with insectivorous bats, most commonly silver-haired and Eastern pipestrelle bats, including a variant from a fatal case of rabies reported in Wisconsin in 2000.

Human rabies is distinctly unusual in the U.S. although it is still problematic in some areas worldwide; in large part, this is due to the control of canine rabies in this country. Of the rabies cases reported since 1960, the great majority involved males <16 years of age or >50 years of age. Most cases in the U.S. are now reported from the following groups:
- U.S. travelers to foreign countries who sustain a dog bite in a rabies-endemic region
- persons bitten by wild animals in the U.S.
- persons with unknown exposure history

A few cases of "nonbite rabies" have been reported and include:
- laboratory exposure to rabies virus (aerosolized virus)
- rabies contracted from corneal transplant from an infected donor (6 cases)
- inhalation of aerosolized virus in caves with high concentrations of bat secretions (rare)
- contact of virus on mucous membranes, scratches, or eyes (rare)

Diagnosis: Currently, there are no tests available to detect rabies prior to the development of symptoms. The virus is felt to be immunologically "protected" in the muscle cells or nerve cells near the inoculation site, and antibody production occurs late in infection. Rabies encephalitis may be difficult to distinguish from other forms of viral encephalitis. Laboratory tests available include:
- rabies neutralizing antibody
- rabies viral culture of saliva, cerebrospinal fluid, urine, respiratory secretions
- brain biopsy - specimens may be submitted for rabies viral culture; immunofluorescent rabies antibody staining of brain cells; and pathologic examination for Negri bodies, which are cytoplasmic inclusions characteristic of rabies encephalitis seen in 20% to 30% of cases

Caribbean islands in which there is a risk of rabies infections (particularly in rural areas) include Cuba, Dominican Republic, Grenada, Haiti, Puerto Rico, Trinidad, and Tobago

Mean duration between initial presentation and death: ~16 days

Rabies is transmitted in the saliva of infected mammals. The virus enters the host's central nervous system causing encephalomyelitis that is almost always fatal. Due to a marked decrease of rabies cases among domestic animals in the U.S. in the 1940s and 1950s, indigenously acquired rabies among humans substantially decreased. From 1980-1997, 95-247 cases were reported each year among dogs, and only two human cases were reported each year on average, in which rabies was attributable to variants of the virus associated with indigenous dogs. Therefore, in the U.S. the likelihood of human exposure to a rabid domestic animal has greatly decreased. But during the same period, 12 human rabies cases were attributed to rabies virus variants, associated with dogs from outside the U.S. Thus, in areas where canine rabies is still endemic, international travelers have an increased risk of exposure to rabies.

Rabies among wildlife (eg, raccoons, skunks, bats) has become more prevalent since the 1950s, accounting for >85% of all reported cases of animal rabies since 1976. Rabies occurs throughout the continental U.S. among wildlife with only Hawaii remaining consistently rabies-free. The most important potential source of infection for humans and domestic animals in the U.S. is wildlife. Twenty-one (58%) of the 36 human cases of rabies diagnosed in the U.S. since 1980 have been associated with bat variants. In most other countries including most of Asia, Africa, and Latin America, dogs are still the major species with rabies, and the most common source of rabies among humans. From 1980 through 1997, of the 36 human rabies deaths reported to the Centers for Disease Control and Prevention (CDC), 12 (33%) appear to have been related to rabid animals outside the U.S.

Every year approximately 16,000-39,000 persons receive postexposure prophylaxis, even though rabies among humans is rare in the U.S. The risk of infection must be accurately assessed in order to appropriately manage potential human exposure to rabies. Administering postexposure rabies prophylaxis is medically urgent, and though not a medical emergency, decisions must not be delayed.

Safety, immunogenicity, and efficacy data of active and passive rabies comes from both human and animal studies. Extensive field experience from many areas of the world indicates that postexposure prophylaxis combining wound treatment, passive immunization, and vaccination is uniformly effective when appropriately applied; though controlled human trials have not been performed. Rabies has occasionally developed among humans, however, when key elements of rabies postexposure prophylaxis were omitted or incorrectly administered. See tables.

Rabies Biologics – United States, 1999

Human Rabies Vaccine	Product Name	Manufacturer
Human diploid cell vaccine (HDCV)		Pasteur-Merieux Serum et Vaccins, Connaught Laboratories, Inc Phone: (800) VACCINE or 822-2463
• Intramuscular	Imovax® Rabies	
• Intradermal	Imovax® Rabies I.D.	
Rabies vaccine adsorbed (RVA)	Rabies Vaccine Adsorbed (RVA)	BioPort Corporation Phone: (517) 335-8120
• Intramuscular		
Purified chick embryo cell vaccine (PCEC)	RabAvert™	Chiron Corporation Phone: (800) CHIRON8 (244-7668)
• Intramuscular		
Rabies immune globulin (RIG)	Imogam® Rabies-HT	Pasteur-Merieux Serum et Vaccins, Connaught Laboratories, Inc Phone: (800) VACCINE or 822-2463
	BayRab™	Bayer Corporation Pharmaceutical Division Phone: (800) 288-8370

Adapted from "Human Rabies Prevention – United States, 1999. Recommendations of the Advisory Committee on Immunization Practices (ACIP)," *MMWR Morb Mort Wkly Rep*, 1999, 48(RR-1):1-13.

Rabies Pre-exposure Prophylaxis Guide – United States, 1999

Risk Category	Nature of Risk	Typical Populations	Pre-exposure Recommendations
Continuous	Virus present continuously, often in high concentrations. Specific exposures likely to go unrecognized. Bite, nonbite, or aerosol exposure.	Rabies research laboratory workers;* rabies biologics production workers.	Primary course. Serologic testing every 6 months; booster vaccination if antibody titer is below acceptable level.†
Frequent	Exposure usually episodic, with source recognized, but exposure also might be unrecognized. Bite, nonbite, or aerosol exposure.	Rabies diagnostic lab workers,* spelunkers, veterinarians and staff, and animal-control and wildlife workers in rabies-enzootic areas.	Primary course. Serologic testing every 2 years; booster vaccination if antibody titer is below acceptable level.†
Infrequent (greater than population at large)	Exposure nearly always episodic with source recognized. Bite or nonbite exposure.	Veterinarians and animal-control and wildlife workers in areas with low rabies rates. Veterinary students. Travelers visiting areas where rabies is enzootic and immediate access to appropriate medical care including biologics is limited.	Primary course. No serologic testing or booster vaccination.
Rare (population at large)	Exposure always episodic with source recognized. Bite or nonbite exposure.	U.S. population at large, including persons in rabies-epizootic areas.	No vaccination necessary.

*Judgment of relative risk and extra monitoring of vaccination status of laboratory workers is the responsibility of the laboratory supervisor.
†Minimum acceptable antibody level is complete virus neutralization at a 1:5 serum dilution by the rapid fluorescent focus inhibition test. A booster dose should be administered if the titer falls below this level.
Adapted from "Human Rabies Prevention – United States, 1999. Recommendations of the Advisory Committee on Immunization Practices (ACIP)," *MMWR Morb Mort Wkly Rep*, 1999, 48(RR-1):1-21.

Rabies Postexposure Prophylaxis Guide – United States, 1999

Animal Type	Evaluation and Disposition of Animal	Postexposure Prophylaxis Recommendations
Dogs, cats, and ferrets	Healthy and available for 10 days observation	Persons should not begin prophylaxis unless animal develops clinical signs of rabies.*
	Rabid or suspected rabid	Immediately vaccinate.
	Unknown (eg, escaped)	Consult public health officials.
Skunks, raccoons, foxes, and most other carnivores; bats	Regarded as rabid unless animal proven negative by laboratory tests†	Consider immediate vaccination.

Table *(Continued)*

Animal Type	Evaluation and Disposition of Animal	Postexposure Prophylaxis Recommendations
Livestock, small rodents, lagomorphs (rabbits and hares), large rodents (woodchucks and beavers), and other mammals	Consider individually.	Consult public health officials. Bites of squirrels, hamsters, guinea pigs, gerbils, chipmunks, rats, mice, other small rodents, rabbits, and hares almost never require antirabies postexposure prophylaxis.

*During the 10-day observation period, begin postexposure prophylaxis at the first sign of rabies in a dog, cat, or ferret that has bitten someone. If the animal exhibits clinical signs of rabies, it should be euthanized immediately and tested.
†The animal should be euthanized and tested as soon as possible. Holding for observation is not recommended. Discontinue vaccine if immunofluorescence test results of the animal are negative.
Adapted from "Human Rabies Prevention – United States, 1999. Recommendations of the Advisory Committee on Immunization Practices (ACIP)," *MMWR Morb Mort Wkly Rep*, 1999, 48(RR-1):1-21.

Rabies Pre-exposure Prophylaxis Schedule – United States, 1999

Type of Vaccination	Route	Regimen
Primary	Intramuscular	HDCV, PCEC, or RVA; 1 mL (deltoid area), one each on days 0,* 7, and 21 or 28
	Intradermal	HDCV; 0.1 mL, one each on days 0,* 7, and 21 or 28
Booster	Intramuscular	HDCV, PCEC, or RVA; 1 mL (deltoid area), day 0* only
	Intradermal	HDCV; 0.1 mL, day 0* only

HDCV = human diploid cell vaccine; PCEC = purified chick embryo cell vaccine; RVA = rabies vaccine adsorbed.
* Day 0 is the day the first dose of vaccine is administered.
Adapted from "Human Rabies Prevention – United States, 1999. Recommendations of the Advisory Committee on Immunization Practices (ACIP)," *MMWR Morb Mort Wkly Rep*, 1999, 48(RR-1):1-21.

Rabies Postexposure Prophylaxis Schedule – United States, 1999

Vaccination Status	Treatment	Regimen*
Not previously vaccinated	Wound cleansing	All postexposure treatment should begin with immediate thorough cleansing of all wounds with soap and water. If available, a virucidal agent such as a povidone-iodine solution should be used to irrigate the wounds.
	RIG	Administer 20 int. units/kg body weight. If anatomically feasible, **the full dose** should be infiltrated around the wound(s) and any remaining volume should be administered I.M. at an anatomical site distant from vaccine administration. Also, RIG should not be administered in the same syringe as vaccine. Because RIG might partially suppress active production of antibody, no more than the recommended dose should be given.

Table *(Continued)*

Vaccination Status	Treatment	Regimen*
	Vaccine	HDCV, RVA, or PCEC 1 mL, I.M. (deltoid area†), one each on days 0‡, 3, 7, 14, and 28.
Previously vaccinated§	Wound cleansing	All postexposure treatment should begin with immediate thorough cleansing of all wounds with soap and water, If available, a virucidal agent such as a povidone-iodine solution should be used to irrigate the wounds.
	RIG	RIG should **not** be administered.
	Vaccine	HDCV, RVA, or PCEC 1 mL, I.M. (deltoid area†), one each on days 0‡ and 3.

HDCV = human diploid cell vaccine; PCEC = purified chick embryo cell vaccine; RVA = rabies vaccine adsorbed. I.M. = intramuscular.
*These regimens are applicable for all age groups, including children.
†The deltoid area is the only acceptable site of vaccination for adults and older children. For younger children, the outer aspect of the thigh may be used. Vaccine should never be administered in the gluteal area.
‡Day 0 is the day the first dose of vaccine is administered.
§Any person with a history of pre-exposure vaccination with HDCV, RVA or PCEC; prior postexposure prophylaxis with HDCV, RVA, or PCEC; or previous vaccination with any other type of rabies vaccine and a documented history of antibody response to the prior vaccination.
Adapted from "Human Rabies Prevention – United States, 1999. Recommendations of the Advisory Committee on Immunization Practices (ACIP)," *MMWR Morb Mort Wkly Rep*, 1999, 48(RR-1):1-21.

Cell Culture Rabies Vaccines Widely Available Outside the United States

Purified chick embryo cell vaccine (PCEC)	Rabipur®
Purified vero cell rabies vaccine (PVRV)	Verorab™ Imovax® Rabies Vero TRC Verorab™
Human diploid cell vaccine (HDCV)	Rabivac™
Purified duck embryo vaccine (PDEV)	Lyssavac N™

Adapted from "Human Rabies Prevention – United States, 1999. Recommendations of the Advisory Committee on Immunization Practices (ACIP)," *MMWR Morb Mort Wkly Rep*, 1999, 48(RR-1):1-21.

When chloroquine phosphate was routinely used for malaria prophylaxis, it was discovered that the drug decreased the antibody response to concomitantly administered HDCV rabies vaccine. Therefore, HDCV should not be administered intradermally to a person who is traveling to malaria-endemic countries while the person is receiving one of the chloroquine-related antimalarials. In this situation, I.M. administration of three doses of 0.1 mL of rabies vaccine for pre-exposure prophylaxis provides a sufficient margin of safety.

Animal rabies epidemiology and evaluation of involved species:

Bats: Bats are increasingly implicated as important wildlife reservoirs for variants of rabies virus transmitted to humans. Rabid bats have been documented in 49 continental states. Recent epidemiologic data suggest that transmission of rabies virus can occur from minor, seemingly unimportant, or unrecognized bat bites. Inaccurate recall of exposure history and the limited injury inflicted by a bat bite (in contrast to lesions caused by terrestrial carnivores) could limit the ability of healthcare providers to determine the risk for rabies resulting from a bat encounter. Human and domestic animal contact with bats should be minimized, bats should not be kept as pets, and untrained and unvaccinated persons should never handle bats.

In all potential exposures of humans to bats, the bat should be safely collected (if possible) and submitted for rabies diagnosis. Human postexposure rabies prophylaxis is recommended with bite, scratch, or mucous membrane exposure to a bat, unless the bat is available for testing and is negative for evidence of rabies. When there is reasonable probability that a bite, scratch, or mucous membrane exposure has occurred, even if not apparent, postexposure prophylaxis might be appropriate.

On the basis of available, but sometimes conflicting information from the 21 reported bat-associated cases of human rabies since 1980, in 1-2 cases a bite was reported and in 10-12 cases no bite was detected, though apparent contact occurred. In 7-10 cases no bat exposure was reported, but an undetected or unreported bat bite remains the most plausible hypothesis. Clustering of bat-associated human cases within the same household has never been reported. Consequently, when direct contact between a human and bat has occurred, postexposure prophylaxis should be considered unless the exposed person can be certain a bite, scratch, or mucous membrane exposure did not occur.

When a bat is found indoors and there is no history of contact with a human, postexposure prophylaxis must be balanced between its likely effectiveness and the apparent low risk such exposures present. In this case, for persons who were in the same room as the bat and who might be unaware that direct contact occurred (eg, a mentally disabled or intoxicated person, a sleeping person who awakens and finds a bat in the room, or an adult who witnesses a bat in the room of a previously unattended child) and rabies cannot be ruled out by testing the bat, postexposure prophylaxis can be considered. However, postexposure prophylaxis for other household members would not be warranted.

Wild terrestrial carnivores: Terrestrial animals most often infected with rabies are raccoons, skunks, foxes, and coyotes. Possible exposure must be considered for all bites by such wildlife. After patients are exposed to wildlife, postexposure prophylaxis should be initiated as soon as possible, unless the animal has already been tested and shown not to be rabid. Postexposure prophylaxis can be stopped if already initiated, when subsequent immunofluorescence testing shows the exposing animal was not rabid. Since signs of rabies cannot be reliably interpreted among wildlife, any such animal that exposes a person should be immediately euthanized (avoiding unnecessary damage to the head) and the brain submitted for rabies testing. If testing results are negative by immunofluorescence, the saliva can be assumed to be virus-free, and postexposure prophylaxis is not required for the person bitten.

Other wild animals: Small rodents (eg, squirrels, hamsters, guinea pigs, gerbils, chipmunks, rats, mice) and lagomorphs (including rabbits and hares) are almost never found to be infected with rabies and have not been known to transmit rabies to humans. In areas of the country where raccoon rabies was enzootic, woodchucks accounted for 93% of the 371 cases reported to the CDC from 1990-1996. Consultation with the state or local health department should be made before deciding to initiate antirabies postexposure prophylaxis. Wild animal hybrids, the offspring of wild animals crossbred to domestic dogs and cats, are considered wild animals by the the National Association of State and Public Health Veterinarians (NASPHV) and the Council of State and Territorial Epidemiologists (CSTE). These animals should be euthanized and tested rather than confined and observed when they bite humans, because the period of rabies virus shedding is unknown. Neither wild animals nor wild animal hybrids should be kept as pets. Animals kept in the U.S. Department of Agriculture-licensed research facilities or accredited zoological parks should be evaluated on a case-by-case basis.

Domestic dogs, cats, and ferrets: Because the likelihood of rabies in domestic animals varies by region, the need for postexposure prophylaxis also varies. Rabies among dogs (in the continental U.S.) is reported most commonly along the United States/Mexico border and sporadically in areas with enzootic wildlife rabies in the U.S. More rabid cats than dogs were reported in the U.S. during most of the 1990s. Of these cases, the majority were associated with the epizootic of rabies among raccoons in the eastern U.S. Fewer cat vaccination laws, fewer leash laws, and the roaming habits of cats may contribute to the large number of rabies-infected cats. Dogs are the major vectors of rabies in developing countries and exposures to dogs in such countries represent an increased risk of rabies transmission. Ferrets are now considered in the category with dogs and cats, rather than in the category of wild terrestrial carnivores due to new information about rabies pathogenesis and viral shedding patterns in ferrets. Healthy domestic cats, dogs, or ferrets that bite a person can be confined and observed for 10 days. Any illness in the animal during confinement or before release should be evaluated by a veterinarian and immediately reported to the public health department. If signs suggestive of rabies develop, the animal should be euthanized and its refrigerated head sent for examination to a qualified laboratory. If the animal is a stray or unwanted, it should be observed for 10 days or euthanized immediately and submitted for rabies examination.

Specific References

Centers for Disease Control and Prevention (CDC), "Human Rabies – Mississippi, 2005," *MMWR Morb Mortal Wkly Rep*, 2006, 55(8):207-8.

Centers for Disease Control and Prevention (CDC), "Investigation of Rabies Infections in Organ Donor and Transplant Recipients – Alabama, Arkansas, Oklahoma, and Texas, 2004," *MMWR Morb Mortal Wkly Rep*, 2004, 53(26):586-9.

Centers for Disease Control and Prevention (CDC), "Recovery of a Patient from Clinical Rabies–Wisconsin, 2004," *MMWR Morb Mortal Wkly Rep*, 2004, 53(50):1171-3.

Centers for Disease Control and Prevention, "Human Death Associated with Bat Rabies - California, 2003," *MMWR Morb Mortal Wkly Rep*, 2004, 53(2):33-5.

Centers for Disease Control and Prevention, "Human Rabies - Iowa, 2002," *MMWR Morb Mortal Wkly Rep*, 2003, 52(3):47-8.

Jackson AC, "Recovery from Rabies," *N Engl J Med*, 2005, 352(24):2549-50.

Mrvos R and Krenzelok EP, "Accidental Exposure to Oral Rabies Vaccine," *Clin Toxicol (Phila)*, 2005, 43:724.

Sheikh KA, Ramos-Alvarez M, Jackson AC, et al, "Overlap of Pathology in Paralytic Rabies and Axonal Guillain-Barre Syndrome," *Ann Neurol*, 2005, 57(5):768-72.

Willoughby RE Jr, Tieves KS, Hoffman GM, et al, "Survival After Treatment of Rabies with Induction of Coma," *N Engl J Med*, 2005, 16;352(24):2508-14.

Rapeseed Oil

Uses Liniment (in place of olive oil), edible oil (in place of soybean oil), soaps

Mechanism of Toxic Action A vegetable oil expressed from the seeds of *Brassica napus* (*Brassica campestris*), contains isothiocyanates (3-butenyl isothiocyate and erucic acid); can contain several irritant oils; 5-vinyloxazolidinethione can stimulate growth of the thyroid gland

Adverse Reactions

Cardiovascular: Pulmonary hypertension

Hepatic: Hepatic necrosis, cholestatic jaundice

Respiratory: Pneumonitis

Signs and Symptoms of Overdose Goitrogenic (can stimulate growth of the thyroid gland). Toxic oil syndrome (which is very similar to eosinophilia-myalgia syndrome) has been related to an aniline-like contaminant (3-phenylaminoalanine) in rapeseed oil used for cooking in Spain (in 1981). Symptoms (lasting 5-20 days) consisted of non-necrotizing vasculitis, pneumonitis, pruritic maculopapular exanthema, cutaneous leukocytoclastic vasculitis, or erythema multiforme. Eosinophilia, liver function abnormalities, and ANA levels may remain elevated for 4 months. Ten percent of patients developed cutaneous brown or yellow papules in 5 or 6 months. Other manifestations include pneumonitis, pulmonary hypertension, scleroderma-like features, or esophageal motility abnormalities. More than 19,000 people were affected (with at least 340 deaths) in Spain in 1981. Hepatic necrosis and cholestatic jaundice can also develop, with a mortality rate of this veno-occlusive injury approaching 20%.

Overdosage/Treatment Decontamination: Gastric: No need to decontaminate after ingestions of rapeseed oil with low (ie, under 2%) content of erucic acid; otherwise treatment is entirely supportive

Additional Information Level of erucic acid below 2% used in edible foods or oils (except infant formula), and as stabilizer in peanut butter, or emulsifier in shortenings of cake mixes. At this amount of erucic acid, ingestion essentially is not toxic. Monitoring parameters: Thyroid function test, liver function test, eosinophil count

Rattlesnakes

Related Information

• Crotalidae

Scientific Name *Crotalus adamanteus*; *Crotalus atrox*; *Crotalus horridus*; *Crotalus lepidus*; *Crotalus molossus*; *Crotalus scutulatus*; *Crotalus viridis*; *Sistrurus catenatus*; *Sistrurus miliarius*

Mechanism of Toxic Action Venom; quality and potency vary among species; composition: 90% water with 5-15 enzymes, 3-12 nonenzymatic proteins, as well as other unidentified substances

Signs and Symptoms of Overdose Local signs include bullae, compartment syndrome (rarely), ecchymosis, edema, erythema, hemorrhage, lymphangitis, and tenderness. Systemic signs and symptoms include asthenia, chills, CNS depression, fasciculations, hyperthermia, hypotension, nausea, paresthesia, sweating, and vomiting. Coagulopathy can occur including hypofibrinogenemia, increased PT and PTT, and thrombocytopenia. Hematuria, hemoconcentration, hypotension, hypoproteinemia, lactic acidosis, proteinuria, and shock are also potential complications. Neurotoxic effects of Mojave rattlesnake venom may be delayed in onset.

Admission Criteria/Prognosis Patients with evidence of snakebite should be observed for 6-12 hours; if there are no systemic abnormalities (such as coagulopathy) or rapidly expanding edema, patient can be discharged; patients with bites due to Mojave rattlesnake (*Crotalus lepidus lepidus*) should be admitted to monitor respiratory and neurologic status

Overdosage/Treatment

Decontamination: Rapid transport to medical facility; immobilize area; if negative pressure suction device is available, this may be used; **do not** incise the wound; constriction band may be applied, **not** a tourniquet

• Wyeth crotalid polyvalent antivenin: treat moderate to severe envenomations with increments of 5-10 vials at a time; skin test per manufacturer's instructions; if positive skin test develops, may prophylax with H_1- and H_2-receptor blockers; give until local injury has stopped and coagulopathy is reversed; complications include allergic reactions, anaphylaxis, and delayed serum sickness

• Newer affinity-purified, mixed monospecific crotalid antivenom ovine Fab antivenom is being developed by Therapeutics Antibodies, Inc. (Nashville, TN); each vial contains 750 mg Fab and 90 mg NaCl and is reconstituted in 10 mL of normal saline; initial dose: 4 vials diluted in normal saline (250 mL) administered over 60 minutes I.V.; a second dose of 4 vials can be given if clinical signs or laboratory parameters worsen

Supportive therapy: ABC assessment, physical exam; mark the extent of local edema with skin marking pen; repeat CBC, platelets, PT, PTT, fibrinogen, CPK, UA every 3-4 hours for at least first 12 hours; I.V. fluids, tetanus prophylaxis, and analgesics may be given as needed; treat infected wounds with antibiotics. Snakes' mouths contain primarily gram-negative and anaerobic organisms. Ocular exposure from rattlesnake "spitting" can be treated with ocular irrigation of normal saline.

Antidote(s)

• Antivenin (Crotalidae) Polyvalent [ANTIDOTE]
• Antivenin, Polyvalent Crotalid (Ovine) Fab [ANTIDOTE]

Additional Information
Family: Crotalidae (Pit Viper): Banded Rock Rattlesnake: *Crotalus lepidus klauberi*; Black-Tailed Rattlesnake: *Crotalus molossus molossus*; Canebrake Rattlesnake: *Crotalus horridus atricaudatus*; Carolina Pygmy Rattlesnake: *Sistrurus miliarius miliarius*; Dusky Pygmy Rattlesnake: *Sistrurus miliarius barbouri*; Eastern Diamondback Rattlesnake: *Crotalus adamanteus*; Eastern Massasauga: *Sistrurus catenatus catenatus*; Mojave Rattlesnake: *Crotalus scutulatus scutulatus*; Mottled Rock Rattlesnake: *Crotalus lepidus lepidus*; Prairie Rattlesnake: *Crotalus viridis viridis*; Timber Rattlesnake: *Crotalus horridus horridus*; Western Diamondback Rattlesnake: *Crotalus atrox*; Western Massasauga: *Sistrurus catenatus tergeminus*; Western Pygmy Rattlesnake: *Sistrurus miliarius streckeri*

Specific References
Blair HW, Ramsey RP, and Morgan SL, "Intravenous Injection of Rattlesnake Venom," *J Toxicol Clin Toxicol*, 2003, 41(5):701.

Bush SP, Green SM, Laack TA, et al, "Pressure Immobilization Delays Mortality and Increases Intracompartmental Pressure After Artificial Intramuscular Rattlesnake Envenomation in a Porcine Model," *Ann Emerg Med*, 2004, 44(6):599-604.

Camilleri C, Offerman S, Gosselin R, et al, "Conservative Management of Delayed, Multicomponent Coagulopathy Following Rattlesnake Envenomation," *Clin Toxicol (Phila)*, 2005, 43(3):201-6.

Cantrell FL, Barry J, and Breckenridge H, "Ocular Exposure to Rattlesnake Venom," *J Toxicol Clin Toxicol*, 2003, 41(5):605-6.

Dart RC, "Can Steel Heal a Compartment Syndrome Caused by Rattlesnake Venom?" *Ann Emerg Med*, 2004, 44(2):105-7.

Feng S and Stephan M, "What a Bite - Review of Snakebites in Children," *Clin Toxicol (Phila)*, 2005, 43:712.

Klemens J, LoVecchio F, Thole D, et al, "Long-Term Outcomes Following Rattlesnake Envenomations: A Preliminary Study," *J Toxicol Clin Toxicol*, 2003, 41(5):699.

Schaper A, de Haro L, Desel H, et al, "Rattlesnake Bites in Europe - Experiences from Southeastern France and Northern Germany," *J Toxicol Clin Toxicol*, 2004, 42(5):635-41.

Vohra RB, Cantrell FL, and Williams SR, "Fasciculations After Rattlesnake Envenomation Are Not a Seasonal Phenomenon: A Statewide Retrospective Study," *Clin Toxicol (Phila)*, 2005, 43:710.

Vohra RB, Williams SR, and Cantrell FL, "Non-Bite Exposures to Rattlesnakes: A Retrospective Statewide Poison Center Study," *Clin Toxicol (Phila)*, 2005, 43:708.

Red-back Spider

Applies to Black Widow Spider
Scientific Name *Latrodectus hasseltii*
Mechanism of Toxic Action Venom contains alpha-latrotoxin, a polypeptide which acts on the neuromuscular junction to cause release of norepinehrine and acetylcholic with resultant neuromediation blockade. Red-back spiders found in Australia often result in more severe envenomations than black widow spider bites.

Signs and Symptoms of Overdose Median duration of effect: 2 hours; local pain (20%), erythema, localized diaphoresis, irritability, hypertension, paresthesias (6% to 10% occuring within 2 hours and peaking in 24 hours); local muscular pain, edema, nausea, vomiting; muscle pain begins within 2 hours of envenomation; fasiculations, tachycardia (50%), fever (15%), hyperreflexia (15% to 30%), salivation, leukocytosis

Overdosage/Treatment
Decontamination: Skin: Wash with soap and water

Supportive therapy: Morphine (Adults: 2-10 mg in adults I.V. or Children: 0.1 mg/kg I.V.) is effective for pain control; dizepam or methocarbamol

---

can be given as a muscle relaxant. For severe systemic signs, high-risk patients or pain resistant to opiates, antivenom can be given. *Latrodectus hasseltii* antivenom is effective in 94% of cases; dose is 1-2 vials I.M. or slow I.V. (diluted in 40-100 mL of normal saline). Monitor for allergic reaction or serum sickness. *Latrodectus mactans* antivenom can be given in place of *Latrodectus hasseltii* antivenom at a dose of 1 vial (2.5 mL) of antivenom in 50-100 mL of D_5W or normal saline given I.V. over 20-30 minutes. The antivenom may also be given I.M. in the anterolateral thigh. No specific therapy for parasthesias.

Additional Information Adult female is 10-15 mm with leg span of 30 mm; black body with characteristic red or orange stripe on upper abdomen and red hourglass shape on underside. Found in open country area, rubbish, wood heaps, and under bark of dead trees in Australia/New Zealand.

Specific References
Isbister GK, "Prospective Cohort Study of Definite Spider Bites in Australian Children," *J Paediatr Child Health*. 2004, 40(7):360-4.

Trethewy CE, Bolisetty S, and Wheaton G, "Red-back Spider Envenomation in Children in Central Australia," *Emerg Med (Fremantle)*, 2003, 15(2):170-5.

Reduviids

Scientific Name *Triatoma sanguisuga*
Signs and Symptoms of Overdose Multiple, essentially painless bites. Dermal lesions may be papular, vesicular, or a rash. Lymphangitis, nausea, and vomiting may also occur. Laryngeal and oropharyngeal edema may occur in sensitive individuals.

Overdosage/Treatment Supportive therapy: Ice to area decreases edema and pain; antihistamine may be useful for rash, lesions

Additional Information Family: Reduviidae. Characteristics: Almost 1 inch in length, *Triatoma sanguisuga* is dark brown with orange markings along the posterior two-thirds of its body. Range: Located on the Pacific coast; habits are nocturnal; generally found in South America. *Triatoma* species are the vectors (through insect waste material) of Chagas' disease by transmission of *Trypanosoma cruzi*

Rhododendron

Related Information
• Azalea

Scientific Name *Rhododendron*
Mechanism of Toxic Action Contains grayanotoxin which binds to a subset of sodium channels causing structural modifications which cause slow opening of these channels which leads to cell depolarization

Adverse Reactions
Cardiovascular: Sinus bradycardia
Gastrointestinal: Abdominal cramps, nausea

Signs and Symptoms of Overdose Asthenia, ataxia, AV block, bradycardia, dermatitis, hypotension, nausea, oral numbness or burning, paresthesia, seizures, sweating, transient blindness and visual changes, vomiting

Overdosage/Treatment
Decontamination: Avoid ipecac, vagal stimulation increases toxicity; lavage (within 1 hour)/activated charcoal with cathartic

Supportive therapy: Atropine for bradycardia, I.V. fluids should be sufficient for hypotension

Antidote(s)
• Atropine [ANTIDOTE]

Additional Information Three whole leaves or flowers likely nontoxic; consider decontamination if more; toxicity is unpredictable, variable among rhododendron types. Toxic part: Whole plant, especially foliage. Contaminated honey may cause systemic symptoms

---

Rubber Vine

Scientific Name *Cryptostegia grandiflora*
Mechanism of Toxic Action All parts of the plant contain potentially cardioactive substances

Adverse Reactions Cardiovascular: Sinus bradycardia

Signs and Symptoms of Overdose Gastrointestinal irritation likely only; potential to cause digitalis-like toxicity including arrhythmias, bradycardia, dizziness, gastrointestinal upset, hypotension, vomiting

Admission Criteria/Prognosis Asymptomatic patients with normal electrocardiogram and electrolytes can be discharged after a 12-hour observation; any symptomatic patient should be admitted to a cardiac monitor bed

Overdosage/Treatment
Decontamination: Lavage (within 1 hour) and multidose activated charcoal enhance total body clearance of digitalis; whole bowel irrigation is also beneficial in removing plant debris from the GI tract and is recommended for ingestions of large amounts of plant material

Supportive therapy: Monitor cardiac status and serum potassium levels; bradycardia will frequently respond to atropine; phenytoin is the recommended treatment for ventricular arrhythmias because it will also improve conduction through the AV node; lidocaine can also be used to treat ventricular arrhythmias, but will not have an effect on AV conduction; other antiarrhythmics which have been used in arrhythmias resistant to the above therapy include magnesium, amiodarone, and bretylium; a pacemaker should be considered for bradycardia and AV nodal blocks resistant to medical management

Antidote: Digoxin immune Fab has been shown to interact with several different plant cardiac glycosides and may be beneficial in cases resistant to conventional treatment; indications for its use include ventricular arrhythmias resistant to conventional treatment, severe bradycardia and/or second or third degree heart block resistant to atropine and phenytoin

Antidote(s)
- Digoxin Immune Fab [ANTIDOTE]

Additional Information Cases of death from these plants have been reported in India; GI irritant. Toxin: Cardiac glycoside

Salmonella Food Poisoning

Commonly Found In Unpasteurized milk, raw eggs, meat (poultry), pet turtles, pet chicks

Mechanism of Toxic Action Gram-negative rod which is invasive to the intestines (endotoxin); incubation period: ~8 hours postingestion

Adverse Reactions

Cardiovascular: Pericardial effusion/pericarditis, QT prolongation, sinus tachycardia

Endocrine & metabolic: Hypokalemia

Signs and Symptoms of Overdose May last 3-5 days. Asthenia, bloody diarrhea, fever, GI cramping, headache, green loose stools, photophobia, myocarditis, vomiting

Admission Criteria/Prognosis Patients with dehydration (who cannot take fluids orally), immunocompromised patients, severe disturbance in electrolytes or acid-base status, or patients at extreme in terms of age group should be considered for admission

Overdosage/Treatment

Note: *Salmonella* species resistant to multiple antimicrobials are increasing in frequency. *In vitro* susceptibility studies should be performed, particularly in severe cases. Treatment guidelines vary with the type of syndrome, as follows:

- **Enterocolitis:** The majority of cases are self-resolving and do not need antibiotics. Clinical trials have demonstrated that a variety of antibiotics fail to influence the course of mild infections and may prolong excretion of the organisms. For severe cases, or in the immunosuppressed host, a number of antibiotics are usually effective including ampicillin, chloramphenicol, co-trimoxazole, and third-generation cephalosporins.

- **Typhoid fever:** Cases should be treated promptly. Chloramphenicol and ampicillin are effective and have been the most extensively studied. Recent studies show that ciprofloxacin is highly active. Third-generation cephalosporins and co-trimoxazole are useful in organisms that are resistant to standard agents.

- **Bacteremia:** Ampicillin, chloramphenicol, co-trimoxazole, and third-generation cephalosporins are all effective. However, chloramphenicol should be avoided in endocarditis or mycotic aneurysms. Ciprofloxacin is effective in treating recurrent *Salmonella* bacteremia in AIDS.

- **Chronic carriage:** Ampicillin or amoxicillin for 6 weeks, although relapses are common; if there is underlying gallbladder disease, cholecystectomy may be an option with repeated relapses; ciprofloxacin may also be effective

Diagnostic Procedures
- Electrolytes, Blood
- Stool Culture

Additional Information

Outbreaks occur most commonly in summer months; *Salmonella enteritidis* is the most common in the U.S.; killed by heat (72°C); can cause carrier state, septic arthritis

Microbiology: *Salmonella* species are gram-negative bacilli which are important causes of bacterial gastroenteritis, septicemia, and a nonspecific febrile illness called typhoid fever. Unfortunately, the classification system for the different *Salmonella* species is complex and confusing to most clinicians. Over 2000 separate serotypes have been identified; and, in the past and currently, each is named as if it was a species. Most experts agree that there are 7 distinct subgroups of *Salmonella* (1, 2, 3a, 3b, 4, 5, and 6), each of which contain many serotypes ("species"). The main pathogens in humans are serotypes, *S. choleraesuis*, *S. typhi*, and *S. paratyphi*, (all in subgroup 1).

Salmonella is an aerobic gram-negative bacillus in the family Enterobacteriaceae. It is almost always associated with disease when isolated from humans, and is not considered part of the normal human flora. As with other members of this family, *Salmonella* carries the endotoxin lipopolysaccharide on its outer membrane, which is released upon cell lysis.

Epidemiology: It is estimated that ~3 million new cases of salmonellosis occur each year. *Salmonella* species are found worldwide. Many are easily recovered from animals such as chickens, birds, livestock, rodents, and reptiles (turtles). Some serotypes cause disease almost exclusively in man (*S. typhi*) while others are primarily seen in animals but can cause severe disease when infecting humans (*S. choleraesuis*). Transmission is via ingestion of contaminated materials, particularly raw fruits and vegetables, oysters and other shellfish, and contaminated water. Eggs, poultry, and other dairy products are important sources. Outbreaks have been described in the summer months where children consume contaminated egg salad. Other outbreaks have been associated with pet turtles, other pets, marijuana, and rarely food handlers. The incubation period is ~1-3 weeks. The period of communicability lasts until all *Salmonella* have been eradicated from the stool or urine. Reptile-associated salmonellosis (lizards, snakes, turtles, and especially Iguanas), can be quite hazardous to pregnant women, children <5 years of age, or immunocompromised patients. The Centers for Disease Control have recommended that reptiles should not be kept in child care centers and may not be appropriate pets in the above patient categories. Individuals should always wash hands after handling reptiles or reptile cages and reptiles should be kept out of food preparation areas.

Clinical infection is favored when there is a high inoculum of bacteria in the ingested food, since experimental models suggest that 10^6 bacteria are needed for clinical disease. Contaminated food improperly refrigerated will allow such multiplication. Host factors are important; and disease is more likely in immunocompromised individuals, sickle cell disease, or achlorhydria (gastric acid decreases the viable bacterial inoculum). Although salmonellosis can occur at any age, children are most commonly infected.

Clinical Syndromes: The following are the major syndromes associated with salmonellosis; it should be emphasized that these syndromes are often overlapping

- **Gastroenteritis:** The most common manifestation of *Salmonella* infection. After ingestion of contaminated food, the bacteria are absorbed in the terminal portion of the small intestine. The organisms then penetrate into the lamina propria of the ileocecal area. Following this, there is reticuloendothelial hypertrophy with usually a brisk host immune response. As the organisms multiply in the lymphoid follicles, polymorphonuclear leukocytes attempt to limit the infection. There is release of prostaglandins and other mediators which stimulate cyclic AMP. This results in intestinal fluid secretion which is nonbloody. Clinically, the patient complains of nausea, vomiting, and diarrhea from several hours to several days after consumption of contaminated food. Other symptoms include fever, malaise, muscle aches, and abdominal pain. Symptoms usually resolve from several days to 1 week, even without antibiotics.

- **Typhoid fever:** Also known as enteric fever, this febrile illness is caused classically by *S. typhi*. Following ingestion of the bacteria, the organisms pass into the ileocecal area where intraluminal multiplication occurs. There is a mononuclear host cell response, but the organisms remain viable within the macrophages. The bacteria are carried to the organs of the reticuloendothelial system (spleen, liver, bone marrow) by the macrophages; and clinical signs of infection become apparent. Patients complain of insidious onset of fever, myalgias, headache, malaise, and constipation, corresponding to this phase of bacteremia. A pulse-temperature dissociation may be present. A characteristic rash may be seen in ~50% of patients, called "rose spots", which are 2-4 mm pink maculopapular lesions that blanch with pressure, usually on the trunk. Symptoms last for 1 or more weeks. During this time, bacteria multiply in the mesenteric lymphoid tissue; and these areas eventually exhibit necrosis and hemorrhage. There are microperforations of the abdominal wall. *Salmonella* spreads from the liver through the gallbladder and eventually back into the intestines. This phase of intestinal reinfection is characterized by prominent GI symptoms including diarrhea. Overall, fatality with treatment is <2%. A similar, but milder syndrome, can occur with *S. paratyphi*, called paratyphoid fever.

- **Chronic carrier state:** Following infection with *S. typhi*, up to 5% of patients will excrete the bacteria for over 1 year. Such patients are termed chronic carriers and are asymptomatic. Millions of viable bacteria are present in the biliary tree and are shed into the bile and into the feces. Urinary carriage can also occur, particularly in patients who are co-infected with *Schistosoma haematobium*. The chronic carrier state is less important for other *Salmonella* species, where the carriage rate is <1%.

Diagnosis: Laboratory confirmation is generally required, since the major syndromes are seldom distinctive enough to be diagnosed solely on clinical criteria. *Salmonella* grows readily on most media under standard aerobic conditions. Cultures from blood, joint aspirations, and cerebrospinal fluid can be plated on routine media. Specimens which are likely to contain other organisms, such as stool or sputum, require selective media; and the laboratory should be appropriately notified. Recovery of *Salmonella* from the stool is the most common means of establishing the diagnosis, and enrichment media are available to maximize the yield. Other laboratory findings may suggest salmonellosis, including a profound leukopenia often seen with typhoid fever.

Recent antimicrobial therapy may render blood and stool cultures negative. In such cases, proctoscopy with biopsy and culture of ulcerations may establish the diagnosis in the enterocolitis syndrome. Serologic tests are not particularly useful in this instance. When typhoid fever is suspected but the patient has already received antimicrobial agents, bone marrow biopsies as well as skin biopsies of any rose spots may yield *Salmonella typhi* in culture. Serologic studies are more helpful in diagnosing typhoid fever, but >50% of patients will fail to show the expected rise in agglutinins against the typhoid O antigen.

Prevalence of *Salmonella* in raw beef carcasses is 1% and in ground beef is 5% to 7%. From 1976 through 1994, rates of isolation of *Salmonella* serotype enteritidis in the United States increased from 0.5-3.9/ thousand population. During and through 1985, there were 582 *Salmonella* enterides outbreaks involving 24,058 cases, 2290 hospitalizations and 70 deaths. 12% of all outbreaks (but 90% of all deaths) in the United States from 1985-91 occurred in hospitals or nursing homes.

Recommendations for preventing *Salmonella* serotype enteritidis (SE) infections associated with eggs (*MMWR* Morb Mortal Wkly Rep, 2003):

For egg producers:
- Flock-based SE-control programs that include routine microbiological testing should be adopted and implemented by industry nationwide.

For retail and food service establishments and institutional settings:
- In retail and food service establishments, pasteurized egg products or pasteurized in-shell eggs are recommended in place of pooled eggs or raw or undercooked shell eggs. If used, raw shell eggs should be fully cooked. If shell eggs are served undercooked, a consumer advisory should be posted in accordance with the Food Code.
- In hospitals, nursing homes, adult or childcare facilities, and senior centers, pasteurized egg products or pasteurized in-shell eggs should be used in place of pooled eggs or raw or undercooked eggs.
- Eggs should be purchased or received from a distributor refrigerated, and stored refrigerated at ≤45°F (≤7°C) at all times.

For egg consumers:
- Consumption of raw or undercooked eggs should be avoided, especially by young children, elderly persons, and persons with weakened immune systems or debilitating illness.
- Eggs should be cooked until both the white and the yolk are firm and eaten promptly after cooking.
- Hands, cooking utensils, and food-preparation surfaces should be washed with soap and water after contact with raw eggs.
- Eggs should be purchased or received from a retail store or distributor refrigerated, and stored refrigerated at ≤45°F (≤7°C) at all times.

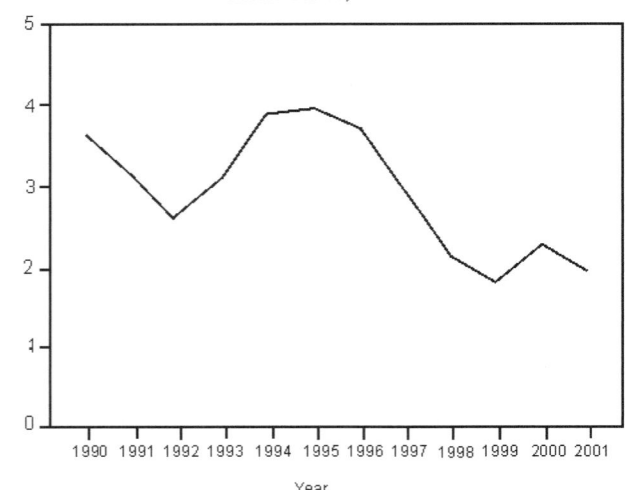

Isolation Rate* of *Salmonella* Serotype Enteritidis (SE), by Year United States, 1990-2001

*Per 100,000 population

Specific References

American Medical Association; American Nurses Association-American Nurses Foundation; Centers for Disease Control and Prevention; Center for Food Safety and Applied Nutrition, Food and Drug Administration; Food Safety and Inspection Service, US Department of Agriculture, "Diagnosis and Management of Foodborne Illnesses: A Primer for Physicians and Other Health Care Professionals," *MMWR Recomm Rep*, 2004, 53(RR-4):1-33.

Centers for Disease Control and Prevention (CDC), "Outbreaks of *Salmonella,* Infections Associated with Eating Roma Tomatoes – United States and Canada, 2004," *MMWR Morb Mortal Wkly Rep*, 2005, 8;54(13):325-8.

Frenzen PD, "Deaths Due to Unknown Foodborne Agents," *Emerg Infect Dis* [serial on the Internet] 2004 [9/07/04]. Available from http:// www.cdc.gov/ncidod/EID/vol10no9/03-0403.htm.

"Outbreaks of *Salmonella* Serotype Enteritidis Infection Associated with Eating Shell Eggs - United States, 1999-2001," *MMWR Morb Mortal Wkly Rep*, 2003, 51(51-52):1149-52.

Rosti L and Gastaldi G, "Chronic Salmonellosis and Cinnamon," *Pediatrics*, 2005, 116(4):1057.

Sand Brier

Scientific Name *Solanum carolinense*
Mechanism of Toxic Action Whole plant contains solanine, a gastrointestinal irritant; spines or prickles can cause local ocular damage
Adverse Reactions Central nervous system: Psychosis
Signs and Symptoms of Overdose Ingestion: Diaphoresis, diarrhea (within 2-24 hours, lasting up to 6 days), fever, nausea, vomiting; headache and salivation may also occur
Overdosage/Treatment
Decontamination: Lavage (within 1 hour)/activated charcoal
Supportive therapy: Monitor and replace electrolytes
Additional Information A perennial weed which can grow to 3 feet having creeping rhizomes, loose clusters of white or bluish, five-lobed flowers, and yellow berries; found in sandy soil, gardens and fields from New England to Nebraska and southern U.S.

Schefflera

Scientific Name *Brassaia actinophylla*
Adverse Reactions Dermatologic: Minimal risk of contact dermatitis
Overdosage/Treatment Oral prednisone can help relieve vesiculobullous eruptions; minimally toxic
Additional Information Does not include umbrella tree of *Musanga* genus. Toxin: Falcarinol. An evergreen native to Australia, can grow to 40 feet high.

Scombroid Food Poisoning

Commonly Found In Skipjack, mackerel, bluefish, mahi-mahi, salmon, Japanese saury, kingfish, tuna (usually poorly refrigerated). See table.

Fish Implicated in Scombroid Fish Poisoning

Scientific Name		Common Name
Family	**Genus and Species**	
Scombridae	*Thunnus thunnus*	Northern bluefin tuna
	Euthynnus peiamia	Skipjack tuna
	E. affinis	Kawskawa
	Auxis thazard	Frigate tuna
	Sarda sarda	Atlantic bonito
	Scomber scombrus	Atlantic mackerel
	Scomber japonicus	Chub of Pacific mackerel
	Rastrelliger kanagurta	Long-jawed mackerel, Indian mackerel
	Grammatorcymus bicarinatus	Double-lined mackerel, scaly kingfish
	Scomberomous cavalla	King mackerel
Scomberesocidae	*Scomberesox*	Altantic saury
	Cololabis saira	Pacific saury
Xiphiidae	*Xiphias gladius*	Swordfish
	Tetrapurus audax	Striped marlin fish
Istiophoridae	*Istiophorus latypterus*	Indo-Pacific sailfish
	Makaira mazara	Indo-Pacific blue marlin
Pomatomidae	*Scombrops boops*	Japanese bluefish
	Pomatomus saltatrix	Bluefish
Coryphaenidae	*Coryphaena hippurus*	Dolphin fish, mahi-mahi
Cerangidae	*Trachurus japonicus*	Horse mackerel
	Seriola colburni	Pacific amberjack
	Decapierus muroadsi	Amberstripe
Cluperidae	*Clupea pallasi*	Pacific herring
	Herklotsichthys zunasi	Japanese scaled sardine
	Sardinops melanotistictus	Japanese pilchard
	Sardina pilchardus	European pilchard
	Sardinella aurita or *S. lemura*	Round sardinella
	Amblygaster sirrn	Spotted sardinella

Table	(Continued)	
Scientific Name		**Common Name**
Family	**Genus and Species**	
Dorosomatinae	*Clupanodon thrissa*	
Engraulidae	*Engraulis encrasicholus*	European anchovy
	Centengraulis mysticentus	Anchoveta
Arripidae	*Arripia*	Australian salmon, Kahawai
Salmonidae	*Oncorhynchus*	Salmon, trout
Syndoatidae	*Harpadon neherens*	Bombay duck

From Wu M-L, Yang C-C, Yang G-Y, et al, "Scombroid Fish Poisoning: An Overlooked Marine Food Poisoning," *Vet Hum Toxicol*, 1997, 39(4):237, with permission.

Mechanism of Toxic Action Histidine found in fish musculature causes clinical syndrome; onset develops within 1 hour (often with 10 minutes); resolves within 36 hours

Signs and Symptoms of Overdose Erythematous flushing, facial edema, headache, nausea, palpitations, pruritus, slurred speech, vomiting, watery diarrhea (explosive), wheezing. See table.

Symptoms and Signs of 48 Cases of Scombroid Fish Poisoning

Symptoms or Signs	Number of Cases (%)	Onset time (minutes, range, and median)
Dizziness	28 (58.3)	15-240 (100)
Diarrhea	23 (47.9)	5-480 (180)
Hot flush	22 (45.8)	5-210 (60)
Headache	19 (39.6)	5-290 (80)
Weakness	18 (37.5)	15-180 (75)
Abdominal cramps	14 (29.2)	5-200 (75)
Nausea	15 (31.3)	5-60 (37)
Pruritis	12 (25.0)	30-205 (75)
Palpitation	10 (20.8)	15-210 (85)
Chest tightness	9 (18.8)	25-210 (90)
Conjunctiva hyperemia	10 (20.8)	5-120 (75)
Swelling of lips and face	6 (12.5)	25-85 (50)
Skin rash	8 (16.7)	45-85 (50)
Numbness of mouth, tongue	6 (12.5)	5-50 (5)
Blurred vision	6 (12.5)	15-75 (45)
Dyspnea	5 (10.4)	25-120 (25)
Vomiting	3 (6.3)	120 (120)
Anxiety	3 (6.3)	25 (25)
Chill	3 (6.3)	75-120 (85)
Burning throat	2 (4.2)	55 (55)
Rhinorrhea	1 (2.1)	

From Wu M-L, Yang C-C, Yang G-Y, et al, "Scombroid Fish Poisoning: An Overlooked Marine Food Poisoning," *Vet Hum Toxicol*, 1997, 39(4):238.

Admission Criteria/Prognosis Admit if symptoms persist after 6 hours of observation, if bronchospasm, hypotension, or urticaria occur, or if neurologic symptoms occur; symptoms usually resolve in 36 hours; patients with dehydration (who cannot take fluids orally), immunocompromised patients, severe disturbance in electrolytes or acid-base status, or patients at extreme in terms of 6:14R age group should be considered for admission

Overdosage/Treatment Supportive therapy: Fluids for dehydration; diphenhydramine (25-50 mg) with cimetidine (300 mg) or ranitidine (50 mg) can cause resolution of symptoms; angioedema/bronchospasm can be treated with beta agonists (under 15°C)

Additional Information Heat stable; refrigeration prevents scombroid poisoning; fish may have a peppery taste; can cause elevated blood and urine histamine levels; cultures are not useful; isoniazid may exacerbate symptoms

Specific References
Thundiyil JF, Murphy NG, Tan JH, et al, "Scombroid-Induced Myocardial Ischemia," *J Toxicol Clin Toxicol*, 2004, 42(5):727.

Scorpion Fish

Scientific Name *Synaceja horrida*
Mechanism of Toxic Action Fish contains spines covered with integumentary sheaths from which venom is released through grooves on the spine as it travels from glands located at the base; venom is composed of high-molecular weight, heat labile, nondialyzable proteins; potency between the scorpion fish and other species is similar; the difference in clinical presentation may lie in the amount and way in which the venom is delivered; venom is a muscle toxin affecting cardiac, involuntary, and skeletal muscles
Adverse Reactions Cardiovascular: Sinus bradycardia, sinus tachycardia, arrhythmias (ventricular)
Signs and Symptoms of Overdose
Severity depends on the number of stings, species, amount of venom, patient age and health. Severe pain peaks in 60-90 minutes and lasts 6-12 hours, up to 24 hours. The wound may become cyanotic and ischemic and with edema, erythema, warmth, and vesicle formation.
Systemic signs and symptoms include abdominal pain, anxiety, arthritis, AV block, bradycardia, CHF, delirium, diarrhea, dyspnea, fasciculations, fever, headache, hypertension, hypotension, lymphangitis, nausea, pallor, paralysis, paresthesia, pericardial effusion, pericarditis, rash, respiratory distress, seizures, sweating, syncope, tachycardia, tremor, ventricular fibrillation, and vomiting. Death usually occurs within the first 6-8 hours from respiratory paralysis.
Admission Criteria/Prognosis Asymptomatic patients should be observed for 8-12 hours and if the patient remains asymptomatic, may be safely discharged
Overdosage/Treatment
Decontamination: Immerse wound in hot water (110 to 115°F) to tolerance to inactivate heat labile components of the venom for 30-90 minutes as needed for pain relief, repeat if pain reoccurs; remove pieces of spine from wound; surgical removal of the spines may be necessary
Supportive therapy: Local pain may be treated with tissue infiltration with lidocaine; systemic symptoms should be treated with supportive care (fluids for hypotension). Drain and unroof blisters.
Antidote: Antivenin for stonefish envenomations does exist (Commonwealth Serum Laboratories, Melbourne, Australia); bites from other members of the Scorpaenidae family usually do not require this antivenin
Additional Information Family: Scorpaenidae; three groups separated by different genera based on the venom apparatus; *Pterois* (zebrafish, turkeyfish, lionfish, butterfly cod); *Scorpaena* (scorpion fish, sculpin); *Synanceja* (stonefish). Range: Bottom dwellers found in shallow water, bays, and among coral reef and rocky coastlines; camouflaged by their shape and color; found in tropical and sometimes temperate oceans
Specific References
Bahloul M, Ben Hamida C, Chtourou K, et al, "Evidence of Myocardial Ischaemia in Severe Scorpion Envenomation. Myocardial Perfusion Scintigraphy Study," *Intensive Care Med*, 2004, 30(3):461-7.
Forrester MB and Stanley SK, "Epidemiology of Scorpion Envenomations in Texas," *Vet Hum Toxicol*, 2004, 46(4):219-20.
LoVecchio F and McBride C, "Scorpion Envenomations in Young Children in Central Arizona," *J Toxicol Clin Toxicol*, 2003, 41(7):937-40.

Scotch Broom

Scientific Name *Cytisus*; *Genista scoparia*; *Sarothamnus scoparius*; *Spartium scoparium*
Mechanism of Toxic Action Contains cytisine which has effects similar to nicotine
Adverse Reactions Cardiovascular: Sinus tachycardia
Signs and Symptoms of Overdose Asthenia, ataxia, drowsiness, headache, hypotension, mydriasis, nausea, pallor, paralysis, possible dermatitis, seizures, tachycardia, vomiting
Toxicodynamics/Kinetics Onset of symptoms: Within 15 minutes to 4 hours
Overdosage/Treatment
Decontamination: Ipecac relatively contraindicated because of risk of seizures occurring rapidly with large ingestion; lavage (within 1 hour)/activated charcoal with cathartic if large amounts ingested
Supportive care: Maintain respiration and blood pressure in symptomatic patient

Sea Anemones

Scientific Name *Actinia* species; *Actinodendron* species; *Adamsia* species; *Anemonia* species; *Anthea* species; *Anthoptreura* species; *Chondylactis* species; *Physobrachia* species; *Rhodactis howesii*; *Sagartia* species; *Stichactis* species; *Triactis* species
Mechanism of Toxic Action Hemolysis through phospholipase A activity; thalassin, congestin, hypnotoxin; toxic proteins: equinatoxin, possible potassium channel blockers, sodium channel blockers, cytolysin activity

Signs and Symptoms of Overdose

Dermal sting: Abdominal pain, burning, chills, fever, headache, malaise, myalgias, necrosis, thirst, ulceration, vomiting. Hepatic failure may occur from the sting of the genus *Chondylactis*.

Ingestion of *R. howesii*: Agitated hemolysis can also be seen with coelenterate venoms

Overdosage/Treatment

Decontamination: If ingested, gastric decontamination including charcoal/lavage within 1 hour; irrigate if eye exposure; hot water generally recommended, though heat will denature

Supportive therapy: Pain control, wound care, antihistamines (oral and topical), topical steroids

Toxin neutralization:

- Dilute ammonium hydroxide, sodium bicarbonate, olive oil, sugar, ethyl alcohol with varying success
- Irrigate with sea water and then topical acetic acid 5% (vinegar) recommended; shave area

Antidote: No specific antidote; antihistamines (oral and topical), topical steroids

Additional Information Phylum: Coelenterata; Class: Anthozoa: *Rhodactis howesii* (brown or green anemone)

Sea Cucumber

Scientific Name *Actinopya agassizi*; *Neothyone gibbosa*

Mechanism of Toxic Action Contains a potent triterpenoid tetraglycoside called holothurin in its body walls which has hemolytic and cytolytic properties

Adverse Reactions

Cardiovascular: Edema

Dermatologic: Contact dermatitis, pruritus, erythema, dermal granuloma

Ocular: Blindness (can cause severe eye irritation with blindness if there is eye contact)

Overdosage/Treatment

Decontamination: **Dermal**: Immerse wound in hot water (110°F to 115°F) for 30-90 minutes; decontaminate with 5% acetic acid (vinegar) or 40% to 70% isopropyl alcohol **Ocular** Anesthetize with proparacaine (0.5%) and irrigate with 100-250 mL of normal saline

Supportive: Ocular: Cycloplegics and corticosteroid ophthalmic solutions can be used

Additional Information Found in Gulf of California, Bahamian sea; this sausage-shaped bottom feeder with a white/purple body can be found in shallow or deep waters

Specific References

Robinson R, Nahata M, Mahan J, et al, "Potential Heavy Metal Exposure from Tiger Tail Cucumber (*Holothuria thomas*) Envenomation," *Vet Hum Toxicol*, 2004, 46(4):225 (letter).

Sea Urchins

Scientific Name *Arbacia punctulata*

Mechanism of Toxic Action The venom apparatus (pedicellaria) is located in the spines and is attached to the stalks; venom contains steroid glycosides, hemolysins, proteases, serotonin and cholinergic substances; some Pacific urchins (Tripneustes) contain neurotoxic substances; detached venom apparatus can remain active for several hours

Adverse Reactions

Central nervous system: Guillain-Barré syndrome

Hematologic: Dermal granuloma

Neuromuscular & skeletal: Bulbar palsy

Miscellaneous: Delayed hypersensitivity (local edema) may occur at 2-4 weeks postexposure.

Signs and Symptoms of Overdose

Burning, hypersensitivity hepatitis, myalgias, pain, redness, stinging, swelling. Guillain-Barré syndrome with hyporeflexia, meningoencephalitis, and bulbar polyneuritis has been reported. Dermal granulomas and paralysis have also been reported.

Overdosage/Treatment

Decontamination: Remove spines if possible. Use hot water soaks (<113°F for 30-90 minutes). Surgical removal may be necessary, especially if located in or near a joint.

Supportive therapy: 2-hour infections, tetanus; all pedicellaria must be removed; the venom apparatus is opaque on soft tissue radiographs; removal may require microsurgical techniques; antibiotics and tetanus should be considered; intralesional injection of triamcinolone hexacetonide (5 mg/mL) can be used to treat granulomas; spines are quite brittle and will usually be extruded within 3 days. Prednisone (20 mg/day orally for 5 days) can be given for delayed hypersensitivity reactions.

Antidote: No specific antidote

Additional Information Egg-shaped or globular echinoderm found on rocky or sandy bottoms; slow moving and nocturnal in habits

Specific References

Morocco A, "Sea Urchin Envenomation," *Clin Toxicol (Phila)*, 2005, 43(2):119-20.

Wu ML, Chou SL, Huang TY, et al, "Sea-Urchin Envenomation," *Vet Hum Toxicol*, 2003, 45(6):307-9.

Sea Wasp

Related Information

- Box Jellyfish

Scientific Name *Chironex fleckeri*

Commonly Found In Australia *Chiropsalmus quadrigatus* - Philippines

Signs and Symptoms of Overdose Edema, erythema, pain, necrosis, vesiculation. Systemic effects include myocardial and respiratory depression, nausea, and vomiting. Fatality can occur within 1 minute of exposure.

Overdosage/Treatment

Decontamination: Sheep antivenins, fluids, vasopressors, antiarrhythmics as needed; immobilize affected area, inactivate nematocysts with alcohol or vinegar; immediately rinse with seawater, should then prevent further envenomation by applying acetic acid 5% (vinegar) to any tentacles still adhering to tissue; if acetic acid is not available, use isopropyl alcohol 40% to 70% or finally may use aluminum sulfate; shave envenomated area after initial treatment, then repeat local decontamination therapy. Ocular exposures are to be decontaminated by water irrigation only. **Do not** rub affected area. Wear gloves during decontamination. Meat tenderizers have been used, however they are not preferred decontamination measures and should not have prolonged contact times (>10 minutes).

Sheep antivenin (Commonwealth Serum Laboratories, Melbourne, Australia): Dose: I.V.: 20,000 units (1 vial) over 5 minutes after skin testing

Additional Information Invertebrate, most venomous sea creature

Sedum

Signs and Symptoms of Overdose There is no evidence that the plant is toxic when taken internally. Some species have produced contact dermatitis.

Overdosage/Treatment

Decontamination: Wash, irrigate

Supportive therapy: Corticosteroids or antihistamines may be used

Shamrock

Scientific Name *Oxalis hedysaroides*

Mechanism of Toxic Action Contains soluble and insoluble oxalates; soluble oxalates may cause damage to the kidney, brain, liver, or heart

Signs and Symptoms of Overdose Dermatitis, hypocalcemia, hypocalcemic arrhythmia, metabolic acidosis, renal damage, tetany

Toxicodynamics/Kinetics Onset: Within 2-12 hours

Overdosage/Treatment

Decontamination: Dilute; ipecac/lavage/activated charcoal not likely necessary; milk/water to dilute crystals

Supportive therapy: For treatment of soluble oxalates, which may cause systemic oxalate toxicity, keep well hydrated, monitor renal function, fluid/electrolytes; hypocalcemia may occur which can be treated with calcium gluconate, monitor urine for crystals; treat other symptoms supportively

Additional Information Toxic dose: Unclear, but unlikely due to large amount necessary. Family: Oxalidaceae

Shellfish Food Poisoning

Commonly Found In Shellfish, blue mussel

Mechanism of Toxic Action May contain either clinophysistoxin (okadaic acid), pectenotoxin, or yessotoxin which can cause fluid secretion in the intestines; incubation period: 4-12 hours postingestion

Signs and Symptoms of Overdose Abdominal cramping, chills, diarrhea, fasciculations, nausea, slurred speech, vomiting

Admission Criteria/Prognosis Patients with dehydration (who cannot take fluids orally), immunocompromised patients, severe disturbance in electrolytes or acid-base status, or patients at extreme in terms of age group should be considered for admission

Overdosage/Treatment

Decontamination: **Do not** use ipecac or laxatives; activated charcoal is of little use; lavage with isotonic bicarbonate solution may make shellfish toxin less potent

Supportive therapy: Fluid and electrolyte replacement therapy

Diagnostic Procedures

- Electrolytes, Blood

Additional Information Heat stable toxin

Shigella Food Poisoning

Scientific Name *Shigella sonnei*

Commonly Found In Potatoes, milk products, tossed salad, meat salad, stewed apples, raw oysters

Mechanism of Toxic Action Can produce an enterotoxin along with a Shiga toxin (*S. dysenteriae*) which stimulates fluid secretion from the intestines; intestinally invasive gram-negative bacteria; incubation period: 1-3 days postingestion

Adverse Reactions Hematologic: Hemolytic/uremic syndrome

Signs and Symptoms of Overdose Feces discoloration (yellow/green); watery, mucoid, bloody diarrhea. Possible cough, dementia, high fever, nausea, and vomiting, seizures in children

Admission Criteria/Prognosis Patients with dehydration (who cannot take fluids orally), immunocompromised patients, severe disturbance in electrolytes or acid-base status, or patients at extreme in terms of age group should be considered for admission

Overdosage/Treatment Most cases of *Shigella* dysentery are self-resolving. Some have suggested that antibiotics be reserved for severe cases, but this does not eliminate the reservoir for infection in the community. Antibiotics have been shown to shorten the period of excretion of the organism in the feces as well as decreasing morbidity. The antibiotic of choice is co-trimoxazole for both children and adults. Ciprofloxacin (500 mg twice daily for 5 days) or azithromycin (500 mg orally on day 1 then, 250 mg once daily for 4 days) is also effective. However, some strains are resistant to trimethoprim, particularly in Africa and Southeast Asia, and *in vitro* susceptibility testing should be performed on all isolates. The quinolones have been effective for shigellosis in clinical trials and are useful alternatives. Antimotility agents such as opiates, paregoric, and diphenoxylate (Lomotil®) should be avoided, because of the potential for worsening the dysentery and for predisposing to toxic megacolon.

Diagnostic Procedures
- Electrolytes, Blood
- Stool Culture

Test Interactions WBCs have a marked shift to the left (bandemia)

Additional Information
Outbreaks occur most commonly in the summer; large amount of fecal leukocytes (polymorphonuclear) are noted; monitor electrolytes

Microbiology: *Shigella* species are gram-negative rods which cause a severe diarrheal syndrome, called shigellosis or bacillary dysentery. *Shigella* species belong to the family Enterobacteriaceae, and are, for all practical purposes, biochemically and genetically identical to *E. coli*. Four species of *Shigella* have been identified: *S. dysenteriae*, *S. flexneri*, *S. boydii*, and *S. sonnei*; there are approximately 40 serotypes.
- *Shigella sonnei* is most common in the industrial world and accounts for ~64% of the cases in the United States. *S. flexneri* is seen primarily in underdeveloped countries. Shigellosis can be seen following ingestion of as few as 200 organisms.

Epidemiology: Infection with *Shigella* sp is primarily a problem in the pediatric population, with most infections in the 1- to 4-year age group. Outbreaks of epidemic proportions have been described in day care centers and nurseries. The reservoir for the bacteria is in humans. Transmission is by direct or indirect fecal-oral transmission from patient or carrier; hand transmission is important. Less commonly, transmission occurs by consumption of contaminated water, milk, and food. The organism is able to produce outbreaks in areas of poor sanitation, in part due to the low number of organisms required to produce disease. Shigellosis is the most communicable of the bacterial diarrheas.

Clinical Syndromes: *Shigella* species invade the intestinal mucosa wherein they multiply and cause local tissue damage. The organisms rarely penetrate beyond the mucosa and thus the isolation in blood cultures is unusual, even with the toxic patient. Mucosal ulcerations are common. Some strains are known to elaborate a toxin (the Shiga-toxin), which contributes to mucosal destruction and probably causes the watery diarrhea seen initially.
- **Dysentery:** Initially, the patient complains of acute onset of fever, abdominal cramping, and large volumes of very watery diarrhea. This phase is enterotoxin mediated and reflects small bowel involvement. Within 24-48 hours, the fever resolves but the diarrhea turns frankly bloody, with mucus and pus in the stools as well. Fecal urgency and tenesmus are common. This phase reflects direct colonic invasion. This two-phased "descending infection" is suggestive of dysentery. Diarrhea and abdominal pain are almost universally present, but the other symptoms may be absent. Physical examination is variable and patients may be comfortable or frankly toxic. Rectal examination is often painful due to friable and inflamed rectal mucosa. The course may be complicated from dehydration from diarrhea and vomiting, particularly in the elderly and in infants. Normally, the infection is self limited and resolves within ~1 week even without antibiotics. Complications are unusual and include febrile seizures (particularly in infants), septicemia, and the hemolytic uremic syndrome (usually from the Shiga-toxin from *S. dysenteriae* 1).
- **Reactive arthritis:** Following dysentery from *Shigella*, a postinfectious arthropathy resembling Reiter's syndrome has been described, particularly in patients who are HLA-B27 positive

Diagnosis: Dysentery from *Shigella* should be suspected in any patient presenting with fever and bloody diarrhea. A history of a "descending infection" as described above is further suggestive. However, the differential diagnosis of fever with bloody diarrhea is broad and includes salmonellosis, *Campylobacter* enteritis, infection with *E. coli* 0157:H7, and inflammatory bowel disease. The WBC count may show either a leukocytosis, leukopenia, or be normal.

There are two important laboratory tests indicated in suspected cases.
- Stool exam for fecal leukocytes: Numerous white blood cells will be present during the colonic phase of the infection. Note that this is not diagnostic for *Shigella* infections; it indicates that the colonic mucosa is inflamed, from whatever cause. The finding of sheets of fecal leukocytes on smear narrows the differential diagnosis of infectious diarrheas considerably.
- Stool culture for *Shigella*: Recovery of the organism from stool is more easily performed early in the illness when the concentration in the stool is highest. Samples should be brought to the laboratory as soon as possible to maximize viability, and specific culture for *Shigella* sp should be requested.

Specific References
American Medical Association; American Nurses Association-American Nurses Foundation; Centers for Disease Control and Prevention; Center for Food Safety and Applied Nutrition, Food and Drug Administration; Food Safety and Inspection Service, US Department of Agriculture, "Diagnosis and Management of Foodborne Illnesses: A Primer for Physicians and Other Health Care Professionals," *MMWR Recomm Rep*, 2004, 53(RR-4):1-33.

Squill

Scientific Name *Scilla maritima*; *Urginea maritima*

Mechanism of Toxic Action Contains scillaren-A, scillaren-B, glucoscillaren A, scillaridin A, and scilliroside which are cardiac glycosides

Adverse Reactions
Cardiovascular: Arrhythmias (ventricular), bradycardia, sinus bradycardia, vasodilation
Central nervous system: Seizures
Endocrine & metabolic: Hyperkalemia, hypothyroidism
Gastrointestinal: Nausea, vomiting, diarrhea

Admission Criteria/Prognosis Asymptomatic patients with normal electrocardiogram and electrolytes can be discharged after a 12-hour observation; any symptomatic patient should be admitted to a cardiac monitor bed

Overdosage/Treatment
Decontamination: Lavage (within 1 hour) and multidose activated charcoal enhance total body clearance of digitalis; whole bowel irrigation is also beneficial in removing plant debris from the GI tract and is recommended for ingestions of large amounts of plant material
Supportive therapy: Monitor cardiac status and serum potassium levels; bradycardia will frequently respond to atropine; phenytoin is the recommended treatment for ventricular arrhythmias because it will also improve conduction through the AV node; lidocaine can also be used to treat ventricular arrhythmias, but will not have an effect on AV conduction; other antiarrhythmics which have been used in arrhythmias resistant to the above therapy include magnesium, amiodarone, and bretylium; a pacemaker should be considered for bradycardia and AV nodal blocks resistant to medical management
Antidote: Digoxin immune Fab has been shown to interact with several different plant cardiac glycosides and may be beneficial in cases resistant to conventional treatment; indications for its use include ventricular arrhythmias resistant to conventional treatment, severe bradycardia and/or second or third degree heart block resistant to atropine and phenytoin

Antidote(s)
- Digoxin Immune Fab [ANTIDOTE]

Test Interactions Serum digoxin level can be detectable by enzyme immunoassay method

Additional Information Bulbs (which resemble onions) can weigh as much as 2 mg and often are used as a folk remedy. Range: Eastern Mediterranean and South Africa

Squirting Cucumber

Scientific Name *Ecballium elaterium*

Mechanism of Toxic Action Irritant; contains alkaloid resins and glycosides; also a purgative and has anti-inflammatory effects

Adverse Reactions Cardiovascular: Sinus tachycardia

Signs and Symptoms of Overdose Diarrhea, dyspnea, facial edema, laryngeal edema, mucosal irritation, neurotoxicity, renal failure, tachycardia, vomiting

Overdosage/Treatment Supportive therapy: Corticosteroids can be used for edema; hemodialysis can be utilized for renal failure; epinephrine (0.3 mg I.V.) can be used to treat uvular angioedema

Additional Information Region: Endemic to the Mediterranean region; has been used medicinally in Crete and Greece for constipation, rheumatic diseases, and sinusitis, although a death has recently been reported by its use for sinusitis through aspiration; similar toxins also found in colocynth (bitter apple). Toxic part: All parts of the plant are toxic, especially the ovoid green fruit.

Staphylococcus Food Poisoning

Scientific Name *Staphylococcus aureus*

Commonly Found In Ham, pork, poultry, potato salad, egg salad, and foods stored at room temperature

Mechanism of Toxic Action Heat stable enterotoxin; incubation period: 1-6 hours

Adverse Reactions
Cardiovascular: Myocarditis
Miscellaneous: Toxic shock-like syndrome

Signs and Symptoms of Overdose Abdominal pain, diarrhea (associated with upper GI signs), low-grade fever, nausea, vomiting

Admission Criteria/Prognosis Patients with dehydration (who cannot take fluids orally), immunocompromised patients, severe disturbance in electrolytes or acid-base status, or patients at extreme in terms of age group should be considered for admission

Overdosage/Treatment Supportive therapy: Fluid/electrolyte replacement; usual duration of illness is 20 hours.

Diagnostic Procedures
• Electrolytes, Blood
• Stool Culture

Additional Information
Microbiology: *Staphylococcus* derives its name from the Greek word staphyle meaning "bunch of grapes". On Gram's stain, staphylococci are gram-positive cocci, 0.7-1.2 μm, nonspore forming, occurring singly, in pairs, in short 4-5 cocci chains or clusters. Staphylococci grow rapidly both as an aerobe and anaerobe on blood agar. The colonies are sharply defined, smooth, and 1-4 mm in diameter. Staphylococci are catalase-positive and differ from micrococci by the following: anaerobic acid production from glucose, sensitivity <200 mg/mL lysostaphin, and production of acid from glycerol in the presence of 0.4 mg/mL erythromycin.

• *Staphylococcus aureus* may have a golden pigmentation secondary to carotenoid and produce β-hemolysis on horse, sheep, or human blood agar after an incubation of 24-48 hours. *Staphylococcus epidermidis* and coagulase-negative staph (CNS) are often used interchangeably but recognize that there are over 30 species of CNS of which *S. epidermidis* is the most common. It is important to distinguish three clinically relevant species: *S. aureus*, *S. epidermidis*, and *S. saprophyticus*.

Clinical Syndromes:
Food poisoning: Usually caused by ingestion of heat stable enterotoxin B; second most common cause of acute food poisoning. May occur by person-to-person transmission. Incubation 2-6 hours after ingestion of toxin contained in custard-filled bakery goods, canned foods, processed meats, potato salads, and ice cream. Patients present with acute salivation, nausea, vomiting progressing to abdominal cramps, and watery, nonbloody diarrhea (risk of dehydration).

Diagnosis: Diagnosis is made by Gram's stain and culture with sensitivities of appropriate site. Semiquantitation roll technique by Dennis Maki in which catheter is rolled over surface of blood agar plate is useful in suggesting a true intravascular catheter sepsis when both blood culture grows MSSE and count >15 colonies on blood agar plate.

Star-of-Bethlehem (*Hippobroma longiflora*)

CAS Number 134-63-4; 90-69-7

Scientific Name *Hippobroma longiflora*; *Isotoma longiflora*; *Laurentia longiflora*

Mechanism of Toxic Action All parts of the plant, especially seed capsules and roots, contain the toxin diphenyl lobelidiol; this toxin produces primary stimulation and secondary depression of autonomic ganglia; also acts as a central stimulant, affecting medullary centers for respiration and vomiting; high concentrations have a curare-like effect

Adverse Reactions Cardiovascular: Sinus bradycardia

Signs and Symptoms of Overdose Low doses cause abdominal pain, dermatitis, diarrhea, hypothermia, increased salivation, metallic taste, nausea, sweating, tachypnea, and vomiting. High doses cause bradycardia, coma, hypertension, paralysis, and seizures.

Admission Criteria/Prognosis Asymptomatic patients with normal electrocardiogram and electrolytes can be discharged after a 12-hour observation; any symptomatic patient should be admitted to a cardiac monitor bed

Toxicodynamics/Kinetics
Onset of symptoms: Following SubQ injection, within minutes
Absorption: Well absorbed orally, cutaneously, and by inhalation

Overdosage/Treatment
Decontamination: Ipecac is generally not necessary for houseplant ingestions; ipecac is controversial for other preparations which contain lobeline, but probably not advisable secondary to the rapid onset of symptoms and the possibility of seizures; lavage (within 1 hour) and activated charcoal with cathartic are the treatment of choice for symptomatic patients
Supportive therapy: Respiratory status and seizures

Additional Information
Toxic dose: In cats: 0.4-4 mg/kg: Nausea, vomiting; 60 mg/kg: Convulsions and death; 80 mg/kg: Respiratory paralysis; toxicity is very unlikely with the houseplants which are available; dried material has little activity; lobeline is used in many homeopathic medicines (antiasthmatic, spasmolytics, and emetics); toxicity is possible from these preparations due to the narrow therapeutic margin

Family: Lobeliaceae. Range: Native to the tropics, but found throughout the West Indies, Hawaii, and Guam. Toxin: Lobeline

Star-of-Bethlehem (*Ornithogalum pyrenaicum*)

Related Information
• Amaryllis
• Indian Tobacco
• Poinsettia

Scientific Name *Ornithogalum pyrenaicum*

Mechanism of Toxic Action All parts of the plant, especially the bulb, contain the digitalis-like glycosides convallatoxin and convalloside

Adverse Reactions Cardiovascular: Sinus bradycardia

Signs and Symptoms of Overdose GI effects (nausea and vomiting) usually precede cardiovascular effects by several hours. Asystole, AV block, bradycardia, heart block (first, second, and third degree), decreased QT interval and prolonged P-R interval, fibrillation (atrial), flutter (atrial), hypotension, ventricular arrhythmias. Confusion, contact dermatitis, dizziness, fatigue, headache, hyperkalemia, and seeing yellow halos have also been reported.

Overdosage/Treatment
Decontamination: Lavage (within 1 hour) and multidose activated charcoal enhance total body clearance of digitalis; whole bowel irrigation is also beneficial in removing plant debris from the GI tract and is recommended for ingestions of large amounts of plant material
Supportive therapy: Monitor cardiac status and serum potassium levels; bradycardia will frequently respond to atropine; phenytoin is the recommended treatment for ventricular arrhythmias because it will also improve conduction through the AV node; lidocaine can also be used to treat ventricular arrhythmias, but will not have an effect on AV conduction; other antiarrhythmics which have been used in arrhythmias resistant to the above therapy include magnesium, amiodarone, and bretylium; a pacemaker should be considered for bradycardia and AV nodal blocks resistant to medical management
Antidote: Digoxin immune Fab has been shown to interact with several different plant cardiac glycosides and may be beneficial in cases resistant to conventional treatment; indications for its use include ventricular arrhythmias resistant to conventional treatment, severe bradycardia and/or second or third degree heart block resistant to atropine and phenytoin

Antidote(s)
• Digoxin Immune Fab [ANTIDOTE]

Additional Information Toxin: Cardiac glycoside

Star-of-Bethlehem (*Ornithogalum umbellatum*)

Related Information
• Amaryllis
• Indian Tobacco
• Poinsettia

Scientific Name *Ornithogalum umbellatum*

Mechanism of Toxic Action All parts of the plant, especially the bulb, contain digitalis-like glycosides similar to those seen in Lily-of-the-Valley

Adverse Reactions Cardiovascular: Sinus bradycardia

Signs and Symptoms of Overdose GI effects (nausea and vomiting) usually precede cardiovascular effects by several hours. Asystole, AV block, bradycardia, confusion, contact dermatitis, decreased QT interval and prolonged P-R interval, dizziness, fatigue, fibrillation (atrial), flutter (atrial), headache, heart block (first, second, and third degree) hyperkalemia, hypotension, ventricular arrhythmias, and seeing yellow halos have also been reported.

Overdosage/Treatment
Decontamination: Lavage (within 1 hour) and multidose activated charcoal enhance total body clearance of digitalis; whole bowel irrigation is also beneficial in removing plant debris from the GI tract and is recommended for ingestions of large amounts of plant material
Supportive therapy: Monitor cardiac status and serum potassium levels; bradycardia will frequently respond to atropine; phenytoin is the recommended treatment for ventricular arrhythmias because it will also improve conduction through the AV node; lidocaine can also be used to treat ventricular arrhythmias, but will not have an effect on AV conduction; other antiarrhythmics which have been used in arrhythmias resistant to the above therapy include magnesium, amiodarone, and bretylium; a pacemaker should be considered for bradycardia and AV nodal blocks resistant to medical management
Antidote: Digoxin immune Fab has been shown to interact with several different plant cardiac glycosides and may be beneficial in cases

resistant to conventional treatment; indications for its use include ventricular arrhythmias resistant to conventional treatment, severe bradycardia and/or second or third degree heart block resistant to atropine and phenytoin

Antidote(s)
- Digoxin Immune Fab [ANTIDOTE]

Additional Information Toxin: Cardiac glycosides

Starfish

Scientific Name *Acanthaster planci*

Mechanism of Toxic Action *Acanthaster planci* is the only venomous starfish; it contains toxic saponins and histamine-like substances in its spine surfaces; other venom components include phospholipase A_2; some starfish contain tetrodotoxin

Adverse Reactions

Cardiovascular: Edema

Central nervous system: Dizziness

Dermatologic: Wounds can be quite painful and pruritic with copious bleeding; dermal symptoms usually resolve within 3 hours; retained spinal fragments can result in dermal granuloma

Gastrointestinal: Vomiting (~1-hour postinjury), nausea

Hematologic: Dermal granuloma

Neuromuscular & skeletal: Paresthesia

Overdosage/Treatment

Decontamination: **Dermal:** Immerse wound in hot water (110°F to 115°F) for 30-90 minutes; **do not** scald the wound; cold water, vinegar soak, or aluminum acetate soaks can be used for local pain relief; irrigate site of puncture wound; obtain soft tissue radiograph if there is a possibility of retained spine. **Ocular:** Irrigate copiously with saline

Supportive therapy: Steroid creams, antihistamines or topical solutions such as calamine with 0.5% menthol can be used to treat dermatitis

Additional Information Crown-of-Thorns Starfish is found in Gulf of California, Pacific and Indian oceans, and Red Sea; a stellate echinoderm with thorny spines held erect by muscle tissue, the starfish are usually bottom dwellers and attain sizes up to 70 cm in diameter; the spines may grow up to 6 cm

Starfruit Food Poisoning

Scientific Name *Averrhoa carambola*

Commonly Found In Southern China, Taiwan, India, Pacific Islands, Australia, Central America, Caribbean Islands, Brazil, Phillipines, tropical West Africa, and southern Florida

Mechanism of Toxic Action Unknown, possibly a metabolite

Signs and Symptoms of Overdose Intractable hiccups, nausea, vomiting, asthenia, insomnia, confusion, agitation, numbness, paresthesias, seizures, coma, death when ingested by chronic renal failure dialysis-dependent patients. Symptoms typically occur 2-4 hours after consumption. Oxalic acid nephropathy reported in patients without underlying renal disease.

Admission Criteria/Prognosis All dialysis-dependent patients with suspected starfruit intoxication should be admitted and referred for urgent hemodialysis. Deaths reported in patients treated by either intermittent peritoneal or hemodialysis, especially after altered consciousness has occurred.

Overdosage/Treatment

Decontamination: Activated charcoal may be useful

Supportive therapy: Treat accordingly, however, patients have generally been responsive to daily hemodialysis therapy only. Hiccups have not responded to phenothiazines or metoclopramide; seizures have persisted and worsened despite phenytoin and barbiturates. Treat seizures with benzodiazepines. Continuous renal replacement therapies also appear effective.

Additional Information As many as 80% of dialysis-dependent patients consuming starfruit may develop hiccups. One case series had 7 deaths in 32 dialysis-dependent patients. Symptoms have rebounded/reoccurred within a few hours after individual dialysis sessions.

Specific References

Neto MM, da Costa JAC, Cairasco NG, et al, "Intoxication by Starfruit (*Averrhoa carambola*) in 32 Uremic Patients: Treatment and Outcome," *Nephrol Dial Transplant*, 2003, 18:120-5.

Stinging Catfish

Scientific Name *Heteropneutes fossilis*

Synonyms Celu Neenu; Pla Sheet

Mechanism of Toxic Action A venomous freshwater catfish found in Asia and India and a popular aquarium fish in Eastern Europe. Venom causes inflammatory reactions and venom glands are located near the pectoral and dorsal fins of the male.

Signs and Symptoms of Overdose Dermal erythema, edema, local wound necrosis, tachycardia, weakness, hypotension, nausea, vomiting,

paresthesias, dizziness, local pain, numbness. Symptoms are virtually immediate.

Overdosage/Treatment Supportive: Major focus is on symptomatic care. Wound can be immersed in hot water (45°C or 113°F) for about 45 minutes to inactivate the toxin - irrigate with fresh water and remove foreign material. Consider delayed surgical closure (if possible). Hypotension can be treated with isotonic saline (10-20 mL/kg) and Trendelenberg position. Dopamine or norepinephrine can be used as vasopressors. There is no antivenom.

Additional Information Fish can reach up to 70 cm in length

Specific References

Satora L, Pach J, Targosz D, et al, "Stinging Catfish Poisoning," *Clin Tox (Phila)*, 2005, 43:893-4.

Stonefish

Scientific Name *Synanceja horrida*

Mechanism of Toxic Action Fish contains spines covered with integumentary sheaths from which venom is released through grooves on the spine as it travels from glands located at the base; venom is composed of high-molecular weight, heat labile, nondialyzable proteins; potency between the scorpion fish and other species are similar, the difference in clinical presentation may lie in the amount and way in which the venom is delivered; venom is a muscle toxin affecting cardiac, involuntary, and skeletal muscles

Adverse Reactions Cardiovascular: Sinus bradycardia, sinus tachycardia, arrhythmias (ventricular)

Signs and Symptoms of Overdose

Severity depends on the number of stings, species, amount of venom, and patient age and health. Severe pain peaks in 60-90 minutes and lasts 6-12 hours, up to 24 hours. The wound may become cyanotic and ischemic with edema, erythema, warmth, and vesicle formation.

Systemic signs and symptoms include abdominal pain, anxiety, arthritis, AV block, bradycardia, CHF, delirium, diarrhea, fever, headache, hypertension, hypotension, lymphangitis, nausea, pallor, paralysis, pericardial effusion/pericarditis, peripheral neuropathies, rash, respiratory distress, seizures, sweating, syncope, tachycardia, tremor, ventricular fibrillation, and vomiting. Death usually occurs within the first 6-8 hours from respiratory paralysis.

Overdosage/Treatment

Decontamination: Immerse wound in hot water to tolerance to inactivate heat labile components of the venom for 30-90 minutes as needed for pain relief, repeat if pain reoccurs; remove pieces of spine from wound; surgical removal of the spines may be necessary

Supportive therapy: Local pain may be treated with tissue infiltration with lidocaine; systemic symptoms should be treated with supportive care (fluids for hypotension)

Antidote: Antivenin for stonefish envenomations does exist (Commonwealth Serum Laboratories, Melbourne, Australia); bites from other members of the Scorpaenidae family usually do not require this antivenin

Antivenin is available in 2 mL vials; made of hyperimmune horse serum; 10 mg of dried antivenin neutralized by 1 mL; dilute in 50-100 mL normal saline and give slow I.V.; skin test before administration; adverse reactions include anaphylaxis and serum sickness; available from Sea World, San Diego (619-222-6363, ext 2201); Sea World, Aurora, OH (216-562-8101); and Steinhart Aquarium, San Francisco, CA (415-770-7171).

Additional Information Family: Scorpaenidae; three groups separated by different genera based on the venom apparatus: *Pterois* (zebrafish, turkeyfish, lionfish, butterfly cod); *Scorpaena* (scorpion fish, sculpin); *Synanceja* (stonefish). Range: Found in shallow waters, very motionless, near rocks, coral, or buried in sand

Specific References

Currie BJ, "Marine Antivenoms," *J Toxicol Clin Toxicol*, 2003, 41(3):301-8.

Streptococcus Food Poisoning

Commonly Found In Eggs/dairy products, steamed lobster, meat, sausage

Mechanism of Toxic Action Groups A, D, or G *Streptococcus* onset: 1-4 days postingestion

Adverse Reactions

Cardiovascular: Pericardial effusion/pericarditis

Miscellaneous: Toxic shock-like syndrome

Signs and Symptoms of Overdose Asthenia, diarrhea, enlarged cervical adenopathy, fever, headache, myalgia, pyoderma, sore throat, vomiting

Admission Criteria/Prognosis Patients with dehydration (who cannot take fluids orally), immunocompromised patients, severe disturbance in electrolytes or acid-base status, or patients at extreme in terms of age group should be considered for admission

Overdosage/Treatment Supportive therapy: Fluid/electrolyte therapy; penicillin may prevent secondary attacks

Diagnostic Procedures
- Electrolytes, Blood

Additional Information Heat sensitive

Striped Blister Beetles

CAS Number 56-25-7
Scientific Name Epicauta species (*Meloidae*)
Mechanism of Toxic Action Cantharidin causing a dermatitis manifesting several hours postexposure; average concentration: 2.6% to 4.3%
Adverse Reactions
Dermatologic: Blisters, vesiculobullae
Ocular: Conjunctivitis
Renal: Nephritis, renal failure
Signs and Symptoms of Overdose Blisters, vesiculobullae (usually painless when broken or rubbed)
Overdosage/Treatment
Decontamination: Wash skin with soap and water
Supportive therapy: Steroid cream may be helpful to decrease inflammation
Additional Information Range: Eastern U.S., Nova Scotia, Saskatchewan

Sulfite Food Poisoning

CAS Number 10196-04-0; 10257-55-3; 4429-42-9; 7446-09-5; 7631-90-5; 7757-74-6; 7757-83-7; 7790-56-9
Commonly Found In Sausages, fruits, vegetables, wine, beer, soft drinks, bronchodilator aerosols, injectable preparation of metoclopramide, epinephrine, aminophylline, photography, metal lubricants, lidocaine, dexamethasone, phenylephrine, isoproterenol, dopamine
Mechanism of Toxic Action Preservative in food as an antioxidant; can cause type I hypersensitivity reaction due to a cholinergic reflex mechanism. Onset of symptoms: Within 1 hour
Adverse Reactions Cardiovascular: Sinus tachycardia
Signs and Symptoms of Overdose Abdominal cramps, flushing, hand eczema, hypotension, nausea, rash, seizures, sweating, tachycardia, vomiting, watery diarrhea, wheezing
Admission Criteria/Prognosis Patients with dehydration (who cannot take fluids orally), immunocompromised patients, severe disturbance in electrolytes or acid-base status, or patients at extreme in terms of age group should be considered for admission
Overdosage/Treatment
Decontamination: Avoid ipecac; dilute with 4-8 oz of milk or water
Supportive therapy: Fluid/electrolyte replacement; epinephrine or diphenhydramine for allergic manifestations
Antidote(s)
- Epinephrine [ANTIDOTE]
Diagnostic Procedures
- Electrolytes, Blood
Additional Information Primary route of exposure is by ingestion, inhalation, or intravenous; minimum dose for CNS toxicity is 6 mg/kg

Sweet Pea

Scientific Name *Lathyrus odoratus*
Adverse Reactions Cardiovascular: Sinus bradycardia
Signs and Symptoms of Overdose Bradycardia, paralysis, respiratory depression, seizures
Overdosage/Treatment
Large quantities must be ingested chronically to result in toxicity
Exclude *Lathyrus* peas from the diet
Symptomatic and supportive treatment
Additional Information Toxin: Beta-aminopropionitrite. Range: Found throughout the U.S. Toxic part: All parts, particularly the seeds

Tabernanthe iboga Baillon

Mechanism of Toxic Action African shrub which contains ibogaine (or igobine) which is an indole alkaloid that acts as an interruption of psychostimulant or opiate addiction; decreases extracellular dopamine levels
Adverse Reactions Central nervous system: Chewing roots can cause excitement, confusion, hallucinations
Toxicodynamics/Kinetics
Distribution (in primate model): 7 L/kg;
Metabolism: To noribogaine in liver by demethylation
Bioavailability (in primate model): 8%
Overdosage/Treatment Decontamination: Oral: Activated charcoal
Additional Information Can potentiate analgesic effect of morphine; after a 25 mg/kg dose, peak serum ibogaine concentration is almost 200 ng/mL (peak noribogaine level: 600 ng/mL); brand name of ibogaine: Endabuse® (NIH - 10567)

Tarantulas

Related Information
- Funnel Web Spider
Scientific Name *Aphonopelma* species; *Bothriocyrtum* species; *Dugesiella henzi*; *Pamphobeteus* species; *Theraphosa blondi*; *Ummidia* species
Mechanism of Toxic Action Venom contains hyaluronidase, nucleotides and polyamines (spermine); local histamine release can occur at site of bites or contact with the spider's hair
Signs and Symptoms of Overdose Local dermal reaction consists of erythema and edema. Wound necrosis usually does not occur. Urticaria is usually caused by penetration of barbed hairs into the skin. Pruritus can last for weeks. Lymphangitis and paresthesias can occur.
Overdosage/Treatment
Decontamination: Barbed hairs can be removed by adhesive or cellophane tape followed by irrigation of skin with normal saline
Supportive therapy: Topical or systemic corticosteroids with oral antihistamines can be used to treat pruritus
Additional Information A large (up to 10 cm), slow jumping spider found in tropical (Western desert U.S.) areas; bites are rarely encountered; hairs often used in "itching powder" in novelty stores
Specific Reference
Seifert SA, "Sunburst Tarantula (*Pterinochilus murinus*) Envenomation," *J Toxicol Clin Toxicol*, 2003, 41(5):700.

Tartrazine Food Poisoning

CAS Number 1934-21-0
Mechanism of Toxic Action Coloring agent in foods can cause hypersensitivity reactions (not IgE-related); incubation period: 30 minutes
Signs and Symptoms of Overdose Can last several hours; anaphylaxis, angioedema, rash, wheezing
Admission Criteria/Prognosis Patients with dehydration (who cannot take fluids orally), immunocompromised patients, severe disturbance in electrolytes or acid-base status, or patients at extreme in terms of age group should be considered for admission
Overdosage/Treatment Supportive therapy: Epinephrine/diphenhydramine for allergic manifestations; intravenous crystalloid with electrolyte replacement for dehydration
Antidote(s)
- Epinephrine [ANTIDOTE]
Additional Information 8% to 15% of affected individuals are intolerant of salicylates

Tetrodotoxin Food Poisoning

Commonly Found In Pufferfish, blow fish, botete, tambores, swell fish, *Taricha* newt, blue-ringed octopus, Atelopus frogs, xanthid crab, starfish, and fugu, ocean sunfishes, porcupine fishes
Mechanism of Toxic Action A neurotoxin on the motor axons and skeletal muscle tissue (inhibits sodium conductance of nerve cells); incubation time: 10 minutes to 3 hours postingestion
Adverse Reactions
Cardiovascular: **Hypertension** (24%), hypotension, sinus bradycardia
Neuromuscular & skeletal: Peripheral neuropathy
Ocular: Miosis (4%) may last for 24 hours followed by mydriasis
Signs and Symptoms of Overdose Asthenia, ataxia, blurred vision, dysarthria, dysphagia, dyspnea, fasciculation, headache, hypothermia, hypotension following apnea, lacrimation, mydriasis, paralysis, salivation, seizures, slurred speech, sweating, tingling of the lips, vomiting, watery diarrhea. Respiratory depression can occur within 2 hours as can paralysis. Fatality rate is 60%. Death is usually due to respiratory paralysis and can occur within 6-24 hours.
Admission Criteria/Prognosis All patients should be observed at least 12-24 hours
Toxicodynamics/Kinetics
Half-life: ~3 hours
Elimination: Urine
Overdosage/Treatment
Decontamination: Lavage (within 1 hour) with 2% bicarbonate solution/activated charcoal with laxative; avoid ipecac
Supportive therapy: Fluids, norepinephrine (8-12 mcg/minute in adults, 0.1-0.2 mcg/kg/minute in children) for hypotension; atropine is useful for bradycardia; mechanical ventilation may be required for respiratory support; early intubation is of vital importance in severe tetrodotoxin toxicity
Additional Information Fatal dose: 10 mcg/kg (200,000 mouse units of tetrodotoxin). Can produce total paralysis with fixed mydriasis; when pronouncing patients dead, caution is advised; not heat labile; heat stable, water soluble toxin; mean time to onset of symptoms: 2 hours; duration of symptoms: 22 hours to 5 days.
Specific References
Hayashida M, Hayakawa H, Wada K, et al, "Sensitive Determination of Tetrodotoxin Using Column-Switching Liquid Chromatography-Mass

Spectrometry with Electrospray Ionization in Mouse Serum," *J Anal Toxicol*, 2004, 28(1):46-9.

How CK, Chern CH, Huang YC, et al, "Tetrodotoxin Poisoning," *Am J Emerg Med*, 2003, 21(1):51-4.

Tobacco

Scientific Name *Nicotiana tabacum*

Mechanism of Toxic Action All parts of the plant contain the toxin nicotine which stimulates motor endplates, ganglionic sites, and smooth muscles by a direct acetylcholine-like action

Adverse Reactions

Cardiovascular: Sinus bradycardia, sinus tachycardia

Respiratory: Eosinophilic pneumonia

Signs and Symptoms of Overdose Low doses can cause asthenia, headache, nausea, oral irritation, sweating, thirst, and vomiting. Higher doses can cause confusion, hallucinations, CNS stimulation followed by CNS depression, hypertension, hyperthermia, seizures; and tachycardia followed by hypotension, bradycardia, and an irregular pulse.

Admission Criteria/Prognosis Symptomatic patients or patients with tachycardia or hypertension 4 hours postexposure should be admitted; survival after 4 hours is usually associated with complete recovery

Toxicodynamics/Kinetics

Onset of action: 15-60 minutes

Duration: 3-12 hours

Absorption: Well absorbed by all routes

Half-life: 0.8-2.2 hours

Overdosage/Treatment

Decontamination: Ipecac is contraindicated due to the risk of seizures; lavage (within 1 hour) and multidose activated charcoal may enhance total body clearance of nicotine

Supportive therapy: Seizures usually respond to diazepam or lorazepam; hypotension generally resolves with I.V. fluids

Additional Information Human fatalities have been seen at 0.8 mg/kg of nicotine, but depend largely on the extent of spontaneous vomiting. Toxin: Nicotine

Tomato (Leaves and Stems)

Scientific Name *Lycopersicon lycopersicum*; *Lycopersicon*; *Solanum*

Mechanism of Toxic Action Contains toxic alkaloids, solanine most significant structurally similar to cardioglycoside, causes hemolytic and hemorrhagic damage to GI tract similar to saponins; some plants may also contain alpha-cholinergic alkaloids

Signs and Symptoms of Overdose Asthenia, diarrhea, drowsiness, fever, hallucinations, headache, nausea, sweating, visual changes, vomiting. Anticholinergic effects may or may not be present to varying degrees.

Toxicodynamics/Kinetics Toxicity occurs within 2-24 hours, diarrhea may last 3-6 days, anticholinergic effects may delay GI emptying and produce delayed effects

Overdosage/Treatment

Decontamination: Ipecac (within 30 minutes) if vomiting has not already occurred, lavage (within 1 hour) and/or charcoal may be beneficial if the patient presents symptomatic

Supportive therapy: Maintain fluid and electrolyte balance as necessary, support vital signs; physostigmine will reverse anticholinergic toxicity that may be associated with exposure

Antidote(s)

- Physostigmine [ANTIDOTE]

Additional Information Toxic dose: Unclear, toxicity reported in livestock. Toxic part: Green fruit and entire plant excluding ripe fruit potentially toxic

Trichinella spiralis Food Poisoning

Commonly Found In Dogs, swine, cats, rats, bear meat, pork

Mechanism of Toxic Action Ingestion of *Trichinella* cysts which will eventually produce mucosal invasive larvae; incubation period: ~1 week

Signs and Symptoms of Overdose Abdominal cramps, cranial nerve palsies, fever, headache, malaise, myalgia, periorbital edema, rash

Admission Criteria/Prognosis Patients with dehydration (who cannot take fluids orally), immunocompromised patients, severe disturbance in electrolytes or acid-base status, or patients at extreme in terms of age group should be considered for admission

Overdosage/Treatment

Decontamination: Majority of symptomatic patients need supportive care only as infection is self-limited. Benzimidazole carbonates may be given. Mebendazole 200-400 mg 3 times/day for 3 days followed by 400-500 mg 3 times/day for 10 days is active against both invasive and encystment stages. Mebendazole does not cross the blood-brain barrier. Thiabendazole 25 mg/kg twice daily for 7 days is indicated to eliminate gut-dwelling adult worms. It is not effective against larval stages in tissue. Not well tolerated secondary to increased GI side

effects. Albendazole is still under investigation. Steroids (prednisone 40-60 mg/day) may reduce inflammation and are recommended in serious infections.

Overall prognosis is related to severity and intensity of initial infection as well as effectiveness of antiparasitic agents, anti-inflammatory agents, patient's immune status, and whether any end-organ damage was rendered. Mortality related to pulmonary, cardiac, and CNS involvement.

All patients traveling outside the United States should receive pre-travel counseling. Smoking, microwaving, and freezing are not reliable means of eliminating trichinosis.

Diagnostic Procedures

- Electrolytes, Blood

Additional Information

Dissemination to striated muscles can occur in the second week; can cause myocarditis or meningitis. Prevalent on both coasts in the U.S., Australia, and the Pacific islands.

Microbiology: *Trichinella spiralis*, a nematode, is the infectious agent of human trichinosis. The adult male worm measures 1.5 mm in length and the adult female measures 2-4 mm; the average lifespan is 4 months. Identification is made by demonstration of the characteristic encapsulated larvae in biopsy specimens of infected muscles. The cyst wall is derived from the host cell muscle; the larva may incite an inflammatory reaction characterized by surrounding lymphocytes and eosinophils and eventual larval calcification.

Epidemiology: *Trichinella* is found worldwide except Australia and several Pacific islands. Trichinosis results from consumption of undercooked pork, unsanitary cooking practices and contaminated meats; its reservoirs include pigs, horses, bears, and arctic mammals. The three subspecies reflect three sylvatic cycles - arctic, temperate, and tropical.

The incidence in the U.S. continues to decline probably because of increased public awareness, commercial freezing, and legislature prohibiting feeding of raw garbage to swine. From 1982-1986, approximately 57 cases per year were reported with three associated deaths. From 1987-1990, 206 cases were reported to the CDC. Most of the cases reported in the U.S. are associated with improperly cooked game animals and travel to Mexico, Asia, and other endemic areas.

Trichinosis results from ingestion of encysted larvae in the contaminated meat. The acid-pepsin environment in the stomach digest the cyst wall, releasing the infectious larvae which burrow and attach to the mucosa at the base of the villi. Over a 6- to 10-day period, the larvae molt four times to become sexually mature adult worms which attach to the duodenal and jejunal mucosa producing between 200-1500 larvae over the next 2 weeks. The newborn or first-stage larvae penetrate the gut mucosa into the lamina propria. An immunologic reaction partially mediated by IgE-mast cell system results in release of vasoactive substances that promote intestinal motility and secretion (diarrhea). The larvae then migrate into the draining lymphatics and blood vessels and have a high predilection to invade muscles of increased use and blood flow (ie, diaphragm, extraocular muscles, masseters, tongue, deltoids, and gastrocnemius). Once penetrated into the skeletal muscle, the larvae elicit a host inflammatory response which surrounds the larvae and creates granulomas and calcifications; only larvae that encyst mature. Larvae may remain viable and infective for many years even in calcified cysts.

The severity of the symptoms is directly related to the larvae load. Patients usually remain asymptomatic with 1-10 larvae per gram muscle, and systemic illness occurs with 50-100 larvae per gram.

Clinical Syndromes:

- **Asymptomatic:** 90% to 95% infections are asymptomatic
- **Self-limited:** 1-2 weeks after ingestion, patients experience enteric phase associated with nonbloody diarrhea and abdominal cramps. Approximately 2-4 weeks later, patients experience fever, intense myalgia especially extraocular and masseters, periorbital edema, conjunctivitis, headache, and/or subconjunctival and subungual petechia. 90% will have peripheral eosinophilia which peaks at 3-4 weeks. Absence of eosinophilia is a poor prognostic sign; ~50% will have elevated CK and LDH enzymes.
- **Arctic trichinosis:** Described in Northern Canada and Alaska in which patients have eaten contaminated walruses or seals. Associated with diarrhea lasting up to 14 weeks, mild and transitory myalgia without fever, peripheral eosinophilia, and no pathogens isolated in stools to explain etiology.
- **Myocarditis:** Incidence of ~5% of symptomatic patients. Typically occurs 3 weeks after larvae migration and presents with tachycardia and chest pain mimicking infarction. Patients have myocardium invasion without encystment; ECG reveals benign, reversible nonspecific ECG changes. May develop nonspecific inflammatory myocarditis predominantly eosinophilic and sometimes associated with pericarditis. Fewer than 0.1% patients die from cardiac complications (ie, congestive heart failure).
- **Pulmonary:** Up to 6% symptomatic patients may develop cough and dyspnea on exertion presumed secondary to larvae migration associated with infiltrates, hemorrhage, and allergic granulomatous reactions

● **CNS:** Prevalence of 10% to 24% in symptomatic patients. In the first 2 weeks when larvae migration is maximal, can result in CNS invasion which appears as meningoencephalitis with delirium and confusion. Larvae encystment may result in focal neurological deficits, anal/urinary sphincter dysfunction, cranial nerve palsies especially VI and VII, seizures, dizziness, anisocoria, tinnitus, diminished auditory acuity, or ataxia. Papilledema, hemianopia, aphasia, and paresis have been reported. CNS and peripheral nerve deficits generally resolve in 4-6 months but may persist up to 10 years. May also cause eosinophilic meningitis. CT scan is usually normal but may see multiple nodular or ring enhancing lesions 3-8 mm and calcification. EEG reveals nonspecific abnormalities consistent with diffuse encephalopathy.

Diagnosis: CDC case definition must fit one of two criteria:

● Positive muscle biopsy or positive serology titer in a patient with clinical symptoms compatible with trichinosis including eosinophilia, fever, myalgias, or periorbital edema

● In an outbreak (at least one person must fit above criteria), must have either a positive serology titer or clinical symptoms compatible with trichinosis in a person who shared the implicated meat source IgM and IgE serology tests are helpful in distinguishing active from previous infection

Tulip

Scientific Name *Tulipa*
Mechanism of Toxic Action Allergic dermatitis
Signs and Symptoms of Overdose Blistering, brittle nails, crusting, fissuring, hyperkeratosis, rash (possibly with associated erythema). Tingling sensation of fingers may be an early indication of symptoms. Symptoms are not necessarily restricted to the area of direct exposure. Dust may produce symptoms.
Toxicodynamics/Kinetics Dermal reaction may be delayed 12 hours
Overdosage/Treatment
Decontamination: Dermal: Wash thoroughly
Supportive therapy: Corticosteroids or antihistamines may be useful for allergic reactions

Tung Nut

Scientific Name *Aleurites fordii*
Commonly Found In Southeastern U.S., Cuba, Taiwan, China, Japan, India, Central Asia
Mechanism of Toxic Action A deciduous tree (15-40 feet tall) in which all parts of the plant (especially the hard seeds) are toxic; contains several constituents (pentosan, phorbol, triolein) which are mucosal irritants; the seeds can be confused for chestnuts or walnuts and may have a peanut-like odor; tung oil is extracted from the seeds
Signs and Symptoms of Overdose Abdominal pain, anorexia, chills, diarrhea, dizziness, dyspnea, elevated liver function tests, fever, headache, hyperglycemia, hyperthermia, leukocytosis, muscle weakness, seizures, sore throat, tachypnea, tremor, urinary retention, vomiting. Tung oil poisonings are more likely to produce systemic effects (fever, dyspnea, seizures), while tung nut toxicity is more likely to produce acute gastrointestinal complaints.
Admission Criteria/Prognosis Admit any seed ingestion or any patient symptomatic 4 hours postingestion.
Overdosage/Treatment
Decontamination: Oral: Activated charcoal
Supportive therapy: Monitor fluid/electrolyte status; replace as needed
Additional Information Ingestion of 1 seed may be toxic. Not sold as dietary supplement; upon heating, tung oil vapors can result in an allergic contact dermatitis; tung oil has been prescribed (in herbal medicine) for erysipelas, scabies, and to treat constipation; onset of symptoms is usually within 4 hours; commonly found in U.S., Cuba, Taiwan, China, Japan, India, Central Asia

Turkey Fish

Mechanism of Toxic Action Fish contains spines covered with integumentary sheaths from which venom is released through grooves on the spine as it travels from glands located at the base; venom is composed of high-molecular weight, heat labile, nondialyzable proteins; potency between the scorpion fish and other species are similar, the difference in clinical presentation may lie in the amount and way in which the venom is delivered; venom is a muscle toxin affecting cardiac, involuntary, and skeletal muscles
Adverse Reactions Cardiovascular: Sinus bradycardia, sinus tachycardia, arrhythmias (ventricular)
Signs and Symptoms of Overdose
Severity depends on the number of stings, species, amount of venom, and the patient's age and health. Severe pain peaks in 60-90 minutes and lasts 6-12 hours, up to 24 hours. The wound may become ischemic and cyanotic with edema, erythema, vesicle formation, and warmth.

Systemic signs and symptoms may include abdominal pain, anxiety, arthritis, AV block, bradycardia, CHF, delirium, diarrhea, fever, headache, hypertension, hypotension, lymphangitis, nausea, pallor, paralysis, paresthesia, pericardial effusion/pericarditis, rash, respiratory distress, seizures, sweating, syncope, tachycardia, tremor, ventricular fibrillation, vomiting. Death usually occurs within the first 6-8 hours from respiratory paralysis.
Overdosage/Treatment
Decontamination: Immerse wound in hot water to tolerance to inactivate heat labile components of the venom for 30-40 minutes; remove pieces of spine from wound; surgical removal of the spines may be necessary
Supportive therapy: Local pain may be treated with tissue infiltration with lidocaine; systemic symptoms should be treated with supportive care (fluids for hypotension)
Antidote: Antivenin for stonefish envenomations does exist (Commonwealth Serum Laboratories, Melbourne, Australia); bites from other members of the Scorpaenidae family usually do not require this antivenin
Additional Information Family: Scorpaenidae; three groups separated by different genera based on the venom apparatus: *Pterois* (zebrafish, turkeyfish, lionfish, butterfly cod); *Scorpaena* (scorpion fish, sculpin); *Synanceja* (stonefish). Range: Very beautiful coral reef fish found in Asia; usually single or paired in shallow water; contains vertical dark stripes with lengths up to 35 inches

Tyramine Hydrochloride Food Poisoning

CAS Number 51-67-2; 60-19-5
Commonly Found In Cheeses (especially aged cheeses), yeast extracts, spoiled (decaying) meats, pickled herring, smoked fish, alcohol-containing beverages, broad bean pods (fava beans)
Mechanism of Toxic Action Can precipitate the release of norepinephrine
Adverse Reactions Hepatic: G6PD deficiency-induced hemolytic anemia
Signs and Symptoms of Overdose Headache, hypertension, hypotension, mydriasis, palpitations, possible intracerebral hemorrhage, sweating, vertigo
Admission Criteria/Prognosis Patients with dehydration (who cannot take fluids orally), immunocompromised patients, severe disturbance in electrolytes or acid-base status, or patients at extreme in terms of age group should be considered for admission
Overdosage/Treatment Supportive therapy: Phentolamine mesylate to treat hypertensive crises (I.V.: 2.5-5 mg; titrate as necessary)
Additional Information Should not consume tyramine-containing foods within 14 days of MAO ingestion; can cause hypertensive crisis when given with MAO inhibitors or amphetamines; when given in combination with chlorpromazine, hypotension can result. Tyramine hydrochloride is not noted in cottage cheese or cream cheese. Milk and cream are also safe; cooking does not inactivate tyramine.

Upas Tree

Scientific Name *Antiaris toxicaria*
Uses In poison darts (from blowpipe), spears, and arrows
Mechanism of Toxic Action Contains cardiac glycoside and dihydrochalcone (antiarone) derivatives; also is a mucosal irritant
Signs and Symptoms of Overdose Arrhythmias, coma, dermal burns, elevated creatine kinase, esophageal ulceration, mouth ulceration, myoglobinuria, oliguric renal failure, rhabdomyolysis
Overdosage/Treatment
Decontamination: Oral: Lavage (within 1 hour)/activated charcoal with cathartic
Supportive therapy: Although data are lacking, since this agent has digoxin-like effects, an approach similar to digoxin overdose management (including digoxin-specific Fab fragments) may be helpful
Additional Information Found in tropical Asia and Africa, a tall tree which grows up to 250 feet with oblong leaves and pear shaped purple or red fruit; the latex of this plant may be mixed with other plant extracts, arsenic or snake venom in order to increase toxicity; although there are case reports of death due to ingestion, usually this route of entry is not toxic to a healthy adult. Similar toxicity to *Antiaris africana*. Monitor electrolytes, ECG, and creatinine kinase.

Vibrio cholerae and *Vibrio parahaemolyticus* Food Poisoning

Commonly Found In Uncooked shellfish and raw seafood
Mechanism of Toxic Action *Vibrio parahaemolyticus* and *Vibrio cholerae* are motile, gram-negative rods; *V. parahaemolyticus* produces Shiga toxin; *V. cholerae* produces cholera toxin (an enterotoxin) which inhibits absorption and enhances intestinal secretion; incubation period: 12-14 hours

Adverse Reactions Endocrine & metabolic: Hypokalemia

Signs and Symptoms of Overdose Grayish, watery diarrhea [rice-water stools] (profuse); fluid losses may exceed 1 L/hour

Admission Criteria/Prognosis Patients with dehydration (who cannot take fluids orally), immunocompromised patients, severe disturbance in electrolytes or acid-base status, or patients at extreme in terms of age group should be considered for admission

Overdosage/Treatment

Vibrio cholerae: Early and rapid replacement of fluid and electrolytes can decrease the mortality to <1%. Oral rehydration is usually successful, but in severe cases, intravenous replacement is required. When fluid and electrolyte imbalances are corrected, cholera is a short, self-limiting disease lasting a few days. According to the *MMWR*, doxycycline, tetracycline, co-trimoxazole, erythromycin, and furazolidone have all demonstrated effectiveness in decreasing the diarrhea and bacterial shedding in this disease. The usual recommendation is doxycycline 300 mg as a single dose for adults, and co-trimoxazole 5 mg/kg as trimethoprim, twice daily for 3 days. Single dose azithromycin (20 mg/kg P.O.; maximum dose: 1 g) is also effective.

Vibrio parahaemolyticus: Tetracycline: 500 mg 4 times/day for 5 days

Supportive therapy: Cholera: Azithromycin at a single oral 1 g dose can shorten the duration of diarrhea.

Diagnostic Procedures

- Electrolytes, Blood
- Stool Culture

Additional Information

Immunity with cholera vaccines is relatively short-lived; can cause hypokalemia; toxin is heat labile; in 1993-94, a total of 69 cholera cases were reported to the CDC with 65 cases (94%) being associated with foreign travel

Microbiology:

Vibrio cholerae is an oxidase-positive, fermentative, gram-negative rod that can have a comma-shaped appearance on initial isolation. *V. cholerae* can be subdivided by the production of endotoxin and agglutination in 0-1 antisera with the nomenclature of *V. cholerae* 0-1, atypical or nontoxigenic 0-1, or non-0-1. The serogroup 0-1 can further be subdivided into the El Tor and classic cholera biotypes which can be further subdivided into a variety of serotypes. The major virulence factor of *V. cholerae* is the extracellular enterotoxin produced by the 0-1 strain, although nontoxin-producing organisms have been implicated in some outbreaks.

V. cholerae is a facultative anaerobe which grows best at a pH of 7.0 and at a wide temperature range (18°C to 37°C). *Vibrio* species can be differentiated from other gram-negative bacilli by their sensitivity to 0129 and may be speciated by a variety of biochemical tests.

Epidemiology:

Cholera is usually spread and transmitted by contamination of water and food by infected feces. Person-to-person transmission is less common due to the large organism load necessary for infection. Asymptomatic carriers play a minor role in cholera outbreaks. Outbreaks may be seasonally dependent based on either temperature or rainfall. Transmission by food can be eliminated by thorough cooking; adequate sanitation is the best means of cholera prevention.

There have been several pandemics of cholera reported since 1817, originating in Bengal and subsequently spreading to a variety of geographic locations, responsible for hundreds of thousands of deaths. The latest pandemic originated in Indonesia in 1961 and moved to the Western hemisphere. In 1991, a cholera outbreak in Peru and 20 other countries in the Western hemisphere accounted for >600,000 cases with 5000 deaths caused by El Tor 0-1.

Clinical Syndromes: After a 2- to 5-day incubation period, classic cholera is characterized by an abrupt onset of vomiting and profuse watery diarrhea with flecks of mucus (rice water stool). Fluid losses can be significant (up to 20 L/day). Hypovolemic shock and metabolic acidosis can cause death within a few hours of onset, especially in children. Mortality, in untreated cases, is as high as 60%. Milder forms of the disease also occur, especially with the non-0-1 cholera.

Diagnosis: Organisms can be identified by darkfield microscopy showing large numbers of comma-shaped organisms with significant motility. However, this test is relatively insensitive and is nonspecific. Thiosulfate-citrate-bile salt-sucrose agar (TCBS) or alkaline peptone broth are used to facilitate growth and identification. Positive identification depends on serologic and biochemical testing.

Specific References

Centers for Disease Control and Prevention (CDC), "Vibrio illnesses After Hurricane Katrina – Multiple States, August-September 2005," *MMWR Morb Mortal Wkly Rep*, 2005, 54(37):928-31.

Guerrant RL, "Cholera - Still Teaching Hard Lessons," *N Engl J Med*, 2006, 354(23):2500-2.

Saha D, Karim MM, Khan WA, et al, "Single-Dose Azithromycin for the Treatment of Cholera in Adults," *N Engl J Med*, 2006, 354(23):2452-62.

Vibrio vulnificus

Commonly Found In Ingestion of raw oysters and clams; stingray exposure; handling of raw shellfish. Found in highest concentrations between April and October in warm salt water.

Mechanism of Toxic Action A gram-negative bacteria that possesses a hemolytic and cytotoxic toxin. Also produces protease, collagenase, and phospholipases.

Signs and Symptoms of Overdose

Three distinct syndromes occur:

Primary septicemia: Following ingestion, fever (103°F to 104°F) and chills occur first followed by nausea, vomiting, anorexia, and diarrhea (in less than one-half of affected patients). Dramatic skin eruptions can occur beginning as hemorrhagic bullae on the trunk and extremities, progressing to necrotic ulcers. Necrotic fasciitis, myositis, and gangrene can also occur. Hypotension develops with 12 hours of ingestion and is associated with a 90% mortality. Median incubation time is 28 hours.

Gastroenteritis following ingestion is usually self-limited and associated with vomiting, abdominal cramps, and watery diarrhea.

By handling affected salt water shellfish, wound infections can occur with associated skin lacerations, puncture wounds, or abrasions. Penetrating stingray or crab-bite injuries may also cause wound infections. Initially, swelling and erythema with intense pain occur at the site of infection, followed by fluid-filled bullae with surrounding erythema and edema. Septicemia or gas gangrene may develop.

Admission Criteria/Prognosis Admit any symptomatic patient.

Overdosage/Treatment Supportive therapy: Intravenous fluids should be used to treat hypotension. Septicemia or wound infection can be treated with tetracycline (or intravenous doxycycline) with ceftazidime. Aminoglycosides may also be effective as is chloramphenicol. Surgical debridement or even limb amputation may be required for wound infection.

Additional Information Between 1989 and 1996, 149 serious illnesses resulting in 75 deaths from *Vibrio vulnificus* have been documented by the CDC. Individuals at high risk for septicemia include those patients with liver disease, alcoholism, hemochromatosis, or compromised immune status. Preventive measures include boiling live oysters in water for 3-5 minutes after the shells open or steaming live oysters for 4-9 minutes. Shucked oysters or clams should be boiled for at least 3 minutes (or until edges curl), or fried in oil for at least 3 minutes at 375°F for 10 minutes, or broiled 3 inches from heat for 3 minutes, or baked at 450°F for 10 minutes.

Vietnamese Centipede

Scientific Name *Scolopendra subspinipes*

Mechanism of Toxic Action Venom may contain bioactive compounds which may contain proteases, immunoreactive agents, and cytolytic agents.

Signs and Symptoms of Overdose Local signs: Burning, edema, lymphadenitis, pain, transient bleeding, skin erythema. There are few systemic signs.

Overdosage/Treatment Local wound care is the mainstay of treatment. Diphenhydramine may reduce localized edema. Prophylactic antibiotics are not necessary.

Additional Information Large centipede (23 cm in length), often acquired as pets.

Specific References

Balit CR, Harvey MS, Waldock JM, et al, "Prospective Study of Centipede Bites in Australia," *J Toxicol Clin Toxicol*, 2004, 42(1):41-8.

Bouchard NC, Chan GM, and Hoffman RS, "Vietnamese Centipede Envenomation," *Vet Hum Toxicol*, 2004, 46(6):312-3.

Forrester MB, "Epidemiology of Centipede Exposures Reported to Poison Centers, 1998-2004," *Clin Toxicol (Phila)*, 2005, 43:710.

Water Hemlock

Scientific Name *Cicuta bulbifera*; *Cicuta douglasii*; *Cicuta maculata*

Mechanism of Toxic Action Conatins the toxin cicutoxin which is located throughout the plant but especially in its root. Circutoxin is seizurgenic possibly through stimulation of central nervous system cholinergic pathways.

Adverse Reactions

Cardiovascular: Sinus tachycardia

Central nervous system: Memory disturbance (of short-term memory) may last for 1 week, seizures within 1 hour

Gastrointestinal: GI symptoms occur within 30 minutes

Signs and Symptoms of Overdose Acidosis, death, diarrhea, hypotension, mydriasis, myoglobinuria, nausea, renal failure, rhabdomyolysis, seizures, tachycardia, vomiting

Overdosage/Treatment

Decontamination: Activated charcoal with cathartic for recent ingestions

Supportive therapy: Provide symptomatic and supportive therapy; manage seizures with diazepam or lorazepam; recurring seizures may need barbiturate or phenytoin treatment, general anesthesia may be required for seizure control; sodium bicarbonate can be given for acidosis

Enhancement of elimination: Hemodialysis was useful in one case report

Additional Information Fatal dose: 1 square inch piece of root may be fatal upon ingestion. Family: Umbelliferae. Toxin: Cicutoxin. Toxic part: Whole plant, especially the root. Range: *Cicuta douglasii* is found in swamps in Western U.S. and Alaska; *Cicuta maculata* and *Cicuta bulbifera* are common in the Eastern U.S.; all are deadly.

Whelk Poisoning

Scientific Name *Neptunea antiqua*; *Neptunea arthritica*; Buccinum; Fusitriton

Uses Commonly used as fish bait

Mechanism of Toxic Action Contains tetramine (an automatic ganglionic blocker which is a curare-like substance) in the salivary gland of the red whelk

Adverse Reactions

Symptoms usually resolve within 1 day

Central nervous system: Dizziness, headache, ataxia

Dermatologic: Urticaria

Gastrointestinal: Nausea, constipation, vomiting, xerostomia

Neuromuscular & skeletal: Muscle paralysis, muscle twitching, weakness

Ocular: Blurred vision, photophobia

Overdosage/Treatment

Decontamination: **Do not** induce emesis

Supportive therapy: Replace fluids; can treat urticaria with antihistamines

Additional Information No fatalities known; found in Britain and Japan. Whelks are brightly colored mollusks found on rocks, sand or gravel. Intoxication can occur in the raw, cooked or canned state. Concentration of tetramine is highest during the summer.

White Chameleon

Scientific Name *Atractylis gummifera*

Mechanism of Toxic Action A thistle-like plant found in the dry areas of the Mediterranean (Tunisia, Morocco, Italy), it is often confused with wild artichoke. Major toxicity is from rhizome ingestion which are oxidative phosphorylation inhibitors (the glycosides atractyloside and carboxyatractyloside).

Signs and Symptoms of Overdose Tachypnea, hypothermia, hypotension, metabolic acidosis, hyperkalemia, tachycardia, headache, abdominal pain, vomiting, mydriasis, hematemesis, diarrhea, hyporeflexia, hepatic failure, hepatic necrosis (due to prolonged ischemia), renal failure, coagulopathy, leukocytosis (80%), hypoglycemia (93% of children)

Overdosage/Treatment

Decontamination: Oral: Activated charcoal/lavage within 2 hours. Dermal: Wash skin with soap and water

Supportive therapy: Treat hypotension with 10-20 mL/kg of isotonic I.V. fluids and place in Trendelenburg position; dopamine/norepinephrine are vasopressors of choice

Additional Information One root/root extract may be toxic

Specific References

Hamouda C, Hedhili A, Ben Salah N, et al, "A Review of Acute Poisoning from Atractylis Gummifera L," *Vet Hum Toxicol*, 2004, 46(3):144-6.

Wild Cucumber

Scientific Name *Echinocystis oregana*; *Marah oreganus*

Mechanism of Toxic Action Contains cucurbitacin which is a cytotoxic substance

Signs and Symptoms of Overdose Abdominal pain, cyanosis, DIC, hypotension, leg cramps, mydriasis

Toxicodynamics/Kinetics Symptoms can occur within 9 hours

Overdosage/Treatment Supportive therapy: Treat hypotension with fluids, colloids, and pressor solutions

Additional Information Ovoid fruit found on a perennial vine; similar spiny pods as Jimson weed. Range: Usually located in Western North America

Wild Hops

Scientific Name *Bryonia*

Mechanism of Toxic Action Contains bryonin, bryonidin, bryonicine and bryoamarid glycosides in the berries and rootstock which are irritants

Adverse Reactions

Dermatologic: Contact dermatitis

Gastrointestinal: Vomiting, diarrhea, abdominal pain

Overdosage/Treatment Decontamination: Lavage (within 1 hour)/activated charcoal with cathartic

Additional Information A perennial climbing plant with yellow-green flowers and scarlet pea-sized berries; berries are quite toxic with 40 berries and 15 berries being a fatal dose in an adult and child, respectively

Wild Mustard

Scientific Name *Brassica* species

Signs and Symptoms of Overdose Contact dermatitis, nausea, vomiting

Overdosage/Treatment

Decontamination: Dermal: Decontaminate area, remove any foreign bodies which remain, topical steroids may be of benefit

Supportive therapy:

Dermal: Observe for any signs of infection

Oral: Supportive care and fluid replacement is seldom required

Additional Information No specific cases of human toxicity have been reported. Family: Cruciferae. Range: Seen over much of the temperate zones of the U.S. Toxin: Hairs of the plant can cause mechanical injury, and seeds contain GI irritants.

Wisteria

Scientific Name *Wisteria*

Mechanism of Toxic Action Contains glycosides which cause GI upset

Signs and Symptoms of Overdose Abdominal pain, fluid loss, minimal diarrhea, oral burning, nausea, shock, vomiting

Toxicodynamics/Kinetics Unclear, but duration reported to be 24 hours

Overdosage/Treatment

Decontamination: Oral: Activated charcoal with cathartic may be beneficial

Supportive therapy: Maintain fluid and electrolyte balance

Additional Information Toxic dose: Two seeds or pods can be toxic. Toxic part: All, pods and seeds mostly; symptoms resolve within 1-2 days

Woody Nightshade

Scientific Name *Solanum dulcamara*

Mechanism of Toxic Action Contains the toxic glycoalkaloid solanine (in all parts of the plant) which can inhibit cholinesterase activity, irritate gastrointestinal mucosal membranes and exhibits weak cardiac glycoside activity

Adverse Reactions

Cardiovascular: Bradycardia

Central nervous system: Fever, headache, CNS depression, delirium

Gastrointestinal: Nausea, vomiting

Hematologic: Increased white blood cell count

Ocular: Mydriasis

Neuromuscular & skeletal: Weakness, tremor

Respiratory: Apnea

Miscellaneous: Diaphoresis

Admission Criteria/Prognosis Admit ingestions >10 berries

Toxicodynamics/Kinetics

Peak GI absorption: 12 hours

Half-life: 11 hours

Elimination: Renal

Overdosage/Treatment

Decontamination: Do **not** induce emesis; lavage within 6-8 hours/activated charcoal with cathartic

Supportive therapy: Physostigmine can be utilized for anticholinergic crisis; monitor fluids/electrolytes

Antidote(s)

● Physostigmine [ANTIDOTE]

Additional Information A weed that is found in northern and eastern United States and Canada; usually a shrub or slender vine with red berries, purple flowers and often heart-shaped leaves; bitter tasting

Yellow Sac Spider

Scientific Name *Chiracanthium* sp

Mechanism of Toxic Action Unknown; spider may hold on very tightly causing mechanical damage along with dermal irritation

Signs and Symptoms of Overdose Pruritic, erythematous wheal and dull pain occur at bite site within 30 minutes. Eschar formation can develop within 24 hours. Abdominal cramps, headache, lymphadenopathy, and nausea can develop.

Overdosage/Treatment Supportive therapy: Oral antihistamines can be utilized; cool compresses, limb elevation and immobilization with analgesics are suggested; monitor for secondary infections

Additional Information Body size: 7-16 mm with long slender hairy legs (total diameter 30 mm); dorsal abdomen can have a median longitudinal stripe; most bites occur in autumn; found in New England, Hawaii, eastern U.S. and Utah; very tenacious; often must be removed from bite area

Yersinia enterocolitica Food Poisoning

Commonly Found In Milk, tofu

Mechanism of Toxic Action *Yersinia enterocolitica* is a gram-negative bacillus which is invasive and produces a heat stable toxin; incubation period: 1 to 3 days

Adverse Reactions Gastrointestinal: Appendicitis

Signs and Symptoms of Overdose Abdominal pain (may resemble appendicitis), arthritis, diarrhea, erythema nodosum, fever, mesenteric lymphadenitis

Admission Criteria/Prognosis Patients with dehydration (who cannot take fluids orally), immunocompromised patients, severe disturbance in electrolytes or acid-base status, or patients at extreme in terms of age group should be considered for admission

Overdosage/Treatment Many cases of enterocolitis and mesenteric adenitis secondary to *Yersinia* are self-resolving, and the role of antibiotics is unclear. Patients with *Yersinia* septicemia, however, definitely require antibiotic therapy since the mortality approaches 50%. The organism is susceptible *in vitro* to a number of agents, including third-generation cephalosporins, ciprofloxacin, piperacillin, co-trimoxazole, and aminoglycosides. Most isolates are resistant to penicillin, ampicillin, and first-generation cephalosporins. The optimal drug regimen *in vivo* has not been defined in the literature. For serious infections it seems reasonable to treat initially with a combination (eg, third-generation cephalosporin and aminoglycoside) until the patient has stabilized.

Diagnostic Procedures
- Electrolytes, Blood

Additional Information
Infection rate is increased with prolonged (>36 hours) deferoxamine use

Microbiology: *Yersinia enterocolitica* is a gram-negative bacillus named for the French bacteriologist Alexander Yersin, who discovered *Yersinia pestis* (the cause of plague) in 1894. *Y. enterocolitica* is an unusual cause of enterocolitis, terminal ileitis mimicking acute appendicitis, and septicemia. The organism is an aerobic gram-negative rod, nonlactose fermenting, which is motile at 25°C. It is unusual in that it grows better at somewhat cooler temperatures than do other pathogenic gram-negative rods (25°C to 32°C); it also is able to grow well at 4°C, which is the basis for CEM.

Epidemiology: *Yersinia enterocolitica* is endemic in many animals which serve as reservoirs (cattle, pigs, dogs, cats, and others). The usual route of human infection is via ingestion of contaminated food, milk, and water. There have been three major foodborne epidemics in the United States:
- June 1982, outbreak in several states linked to consumption of milk pasteurized at a plant in Memphis, Tennessee; 172 positive cultures from cases in Tennessee, Arkansas, and Mississippi, where patients presented with diarrhea, fever, and abdominal pain; it also included 24 cases of extraintestinal infections including throat, blood, urinary tract, central nervous system, and wounds
- 1976, contaminated chocolate milk in New York state
- 1982, contaminated tofu in Washington state

Clinical Syndromes:
- **Enterocolitis:** *Yersinia enterocolitica* is a rare cause of enterocolitis. The severity of symptoms can be quite variable and can range from mild fever, diarrhea and abdominal pain, to fulminant colitis with spiking fevers and rectal hemorrhage.
- **Mesenteric adenopathy with or without terminal ileitis:** This form of *Yersinia* infection is known to mimic acute appendicitis. Patients present with right lower quadrant pain, fever, and leukocytosis. Upon laparotomy, the appendix is normal; but enlarged mesenteric lymph nodes are palpable and when cultured will yield the organism. This has been described primarily in adolescents, although cases have been reported in adults.
- **Polyarthritis:** This has been described as the sole manifestation of *Yersinia enterocolitica* infection or as a secondary manifestation of gastrointestinal infection. Well documented cases have been described in Scandinavia, where up to 30% of cases develop erythema nodosum; and 10% to 30% develop polyarthritis (especially associated with HLA-B27 haplotype). *Yersinia* antigens have recently been found in synovial fluid cells from patients suffering from reactive arthritis following *Yersinia* infection.
- **Liver abscess:** *Yersinia* is a rare, but reported cause of liver abscess in the absence of typical enterocolitis symptoms
- **Ascending infection of an extremity:** Recently cases of infections of the hand and upper extremity due to *Yersinia enterocolitica* have been described. These infections occurred in adults preparing contaminated chitterlings (pig intestines) with local inoculation into the hand via small cuts.
- **Septicemia:** *Yersinia* is an unusual cause of community-acquired septicemia, but may occur following ingestion of heavily contaminated food. Risk factors for septicemia are cirrhosis, malignancy, diabetes mellitus, and patients with iron overload syndromes (such as hemachromatosis, frequent blood transfusions). Typically, there is fever, myalgias, confusion, and possibly hypotension. Symptoms of enter-

ocolitis, such as diarrhea and abdominal pain, may be completely absent, adding to the diagnostic confusion; elevated liver enzymes and muscle enzymes may occur; blood cultures are often positive for the organism.
- **Miscellaneous:** Other manifestations of *Yersinia* infection include osteomyelitis, meningitis, pharyngitis (without enterocolitis), intra-abdominal abscess

Diagnosis: In the absence of an outbreak, the diagnosis of enterocolitis due to *Yersinia* is difficult to make on clinical grounds alone. Thus, laboratory confirmation is important in most cases. Appropriate specimens for culture include stool, blood, lymph node, pharyngeal exudates, ascites fluid, and cerebrospinal fluid. Joint aspiration fluid may be sent for *Yersinia* culture in the appropriate clinical setting (ie, reactive polyarthritis following a diarrheal illness), but the yield is extremely low. The laboratory should be notified if a stool specimen is being examined for *Yersinia*; serologic tests for specific antibody production to *Yersinia enterocolitica* are available in some laboratories.

Yersinia pestis

Mechanism of Toxic Action An enzootic infection of rodents found in every continent (except Australia and Antarctica); most U.S. cases are found in the western U.S.; an anaerobic nonmotile, gram-negative coccobacillus usually transmitted by a flea bite (although it can be transmitted by domestic cats). The organism migrates through the lymphatic system resulting in lymph node destruction. Primary pneumonic plague occurs through inhalation of bacilli with symptoms occurring within 6 days of exposure. Symptoms of bubonic plague include fever, chills, tender lymphadenopathy, and buboes. The lesions are 1-10 cm in diameter, painful, warm, and are located in the groin, axilla, or neck region. Symptoms usually begin within 8 days after being infected. Septicemia, gangrene of acral regions, and disseminated intravascular coagulation can occur. A secondary pneumonic plague due to hematogenous spread of the bacilli can occur, with symptoms of dyspnea, cough, and hemoptysis.

Signs and Symptoms of Overdose Pneumonic and plague: Abdominal pain (17%), aminotransferase elevation, ARDS (50% mortality), azotemia, bronchopneumonia, chest pain, cough, cyanosis, delirium, diarrhea (28%), dyspnea, epistaxis, fever, headache, hemoptysis, hypotension, leukocytosis, lobar consolidation, lymphadenopathy, malaise, meningitis, myalgias, nausea (34%), purpura, seizures, shortness of breath, splenomegaly, tachycardia, tachypnea, vomiting (39%)

Overdosage/Treatment
Any person with a fever of 38.5°C or higher, should begin prophylactic antibiotic therapy during a pneumonic plague epidemic; any infected patient should be isolated for the first 2 days of antibiotic therapy until clinical improvement occurs; respiratory droplet precautions should be utilized; exudates or discharge should be handled with rubber gloves; seizures can be treated with a benzodiazepine or phenobarbital

Supportive therapy: See table.

Recommendations for Treatment of Patients With Pneumonic Plague		
Patient Category	**Recommended Therapy**	
		Contained Casualty Setting*
Adults	Preferred	Streptomycin 1 g I.M. twice daily Gentamicin, 5 mg/kg I.M. or I.V. once daily or 2 mg/kg loading dose followed by 1.7 mg/kg I.M. or I.V. 3 times/day[†]
	Alternative	Doxycycline, 100 mg I.V. twice daily or 200 mg I.V. once daily Ciprofloxacin, 400 mg I.V. twice daily[‡] Chloramphenicol, 25 mg/kg I.V. 4 times/day[§]
Children	Preferred	Streptomycin, 15 mg/kg I.M. twice daily (maximum daily dose, 2 g) Gentamicin, 2.5 mg/kg I.M. or I.V. 3 times/day[†]
	Alternative	Doxycycline: If ≥45 kg, give adult dosage; if <45 kg, give 2.2 mg/kg I.V. twice daily (maximum, 200 mg/day) Ciprofloxacin, 15 mg/kg I.V. twice daily[‡] Chloramphenicol, 25 mg/kg I.V. 4 times/day[§]

Table *(Continued)*

Patient Category	Recommended Therapy	
	Contained Casualty Setting*	
Pregnant women	Preferred	Gentamicin, 5 mg/kg I.M. or I.V. once daily or 2 mg/kg loading dose followed by 1.7 mg/kg I.M. or I.V. 3 times/day[†]
	Alternative	Doxycycline, 100 mg I.V. twice daily or 200 mg I.V. once daily Ciprofloxacin, 400 mg I.V. twice daily[‡]
Patient Category	**Mass Casualty Setting and Postexposure Prophylaxis•**	
Adults	Preferred	Doxycycline, 100 mg orally twice daily** Ciprofloxacin, 500 mg orally twice daily[‡]
	Alternative	Chloramphenicol, 25 mg/kg orally 4 times/day[§°]
Children[¶]	Preferred	Doxycycline**: If ≥45 kg, give adult dosage; if <45 kg, then give 2.2 mg/kg orally twice daily Ciprofloxacin, 20 mg/kg orally twice daily
	Alternative	Chloramphenicol, 25 mg/kg orally 4 times/day[§]
Pregnant women#	Preferred	Doxycycline, 100 mg orally twice daily** Ciprofloxacin, 500 mg orally twice daily
	Alternative	Chloramphenicol, 25 mg/kg orally 4 times/day[§°]

*These are consensus recommendations of the Working Group on Civilian Biodefense and are not necessarily approved by the FDA. One antimicrobial agent should be selected; therapy should be continued for 10 days; oral therapy should be substituted when the patient's condition improves.

I.M. = intramuscular; I.V. = intravenous.

[†]Aminoglycosides must be adjusted according to renal function. Evidence suggests that gentamicin 5 mg/kg I.M. or I.V. once daily, would be efficacious in children, although this is not yet widely accepted in clinical practice. Neonates up to 1 week of age and premature infants should receive gentamicin, 2.5 mg/kg I.V. twice daily.

[‡]Other fluoroquinolones can be substituted at doses appropriate for age. Ciprofloxacin dosage should not exceed 1 g/day in children.

[§]Concentration should be maintained between 5 and 20 mcg/mL. Concentrations >25mcg/mL can cause reversible bone marrow suppression.

[¶]In children, ciprofloxacin dose should not exceed 1 g/day, chloramphenicol should not exceed 4 g/day. Children younger than 2 years of age should not receive chloramphenicol.

#In neonates, gentamicin loading dose of 4 mg/kg should be given initially.

•Duration of treatment of plague in mass casualty setting is 10 days. Duration of postexposure prophylaxis to prevent plague infection is 7 days.

°Children younger than 2 years of age should not receive chloramphenicol. Oral formulation available only outside the U.S.

**Tetracycline could be substituted for doxycycline

Additional Information
An aerosol of plague bacillus could remain viable for up to 1 hour at a distance of 10 kilometers

Mortality: 50% to 60% for untreated bubonic plague; 100% for untreated septicemia, or 10% to 20% in treated cases of pneumonic plague

Largest number of reported cases in Tanzania, Viet Nam and Zaire

Additional information can be obtained from the Center for Disease Control's plague center in Fort Collins, Colorado: (970) 221-6450

Specific References
Drancourt M, Roux V, Dang LV, et al, "Genotyping, Orientalis-Like *Yersinia pestis*, and Plague Pandemics," *Emerg Infect Dis*, [serial on the Internet], 2004, [9/7/04]. Available from http://www.cdc.gov/ncidod/EID/vol10no9/03-0933.htm.

Rusnak JM, Kortepeter MG, Aldis J, et al, "Experience in the Medical Management of Potential Laboratory Exposures to Agents of Bioterrorism on the Basis of Risk Assessment at the United States Army Medical Research Institute of Infectious Diseases (USAMRIID)," *J Occup Environ Med*, 2004, 46(8):801-11.

Rusnak JM, Kortepeter MG, Hawley RG, et al, "Management Guidelines for Laboratory Exposures to Agents of Bioterrorism," *J Occup Environ Med*, 2004, 46(8):791-800.

Yew

Scientific Name *Taxus* species

Mechanism of Toxic Action All parts of the plant are toxic except the red fleshy aril; the toxin appears to inhibit sodium and calcium current in cardiac cells causing a block of the distal portion of the conduction tissue of the heart; the hard seed coat is resistant to digestive enzymes and is nontoxic unless chewed or broken

Adverse Reactions Cardiovascular: Sinus bradycardia, sinus tachycardia, arrhythmias (ventricular)

Signs and Symptoms of Overdose Abdominal pain, asthenia, AV block, cardiac arrhythmias (sinus bradycardia, ventricular tachycardia, ventricular fibrillation, heart block), coma, contact dermatitis, cyanotic lips, dizziness, headache, hypokalemia, hypotension, mydriasis, nausea, pale complexion, respiratory distress/arrest, seizures, tachycardia, vomiting. Death is usually secondary to arrhythmias, circulatory collapse, or respiratory failure.

Admission Criteria/Prognosis Asymptomatic patients with normal electrocardiogram and electrolytes can be discharged after a 12-hour observation; any symptomatic patient should be admitted to a cardiac monitor bed; patients who are symptomatic 3 hours postexposure should be admitted

Toxicodynamics/Kinetics Onset of symptoms: Generally within 1-3 hours; in large ingestions, cardiovascular collapse can occur within 30 minutes

Reference Range Postmortem 3,5-dimethoxyphenol blood and bile levels of 21 ng/mL and 104 ng/mL, respectively, were noted in a male who died of yew toxicity.

Overdosage/Treatment
Decontamination: Ipecac is contraindicated secondary to rapid onset of symptoms; lavage is of questionable benefit, due to the large size of the seeds, unless the seeds are chewed well; activated charcoal with sorbitol is recommended; **do not** consider gastric decontamination if fewer than 6 berries are ingested; whole bowel irrigation is beneficial for ingestions of large amounts of plant material

Supportive therapy: Hypotension can be resistant to dopamine and dobutamine, and may require norepinephrine; bradycardia and complete heart block has on occasion been resistant to atropine; external pacing and/or digoxin immune Fab may be of benefit; monitor electrolytes; anaphylactoid reactions should be treated with epinephrine, antihistamines and fluids. Dysrhythmias with widened QRS complex should be treated with I.V. sodium bicarbonate.

Antidote(s)
- Digoxin Immune Fab [ANTIDOTE]
- Norepinephrine [ANTIDOTE]

Additional Information
Literature suggests that <6 berries produce minimal symptoms, and ingestion of 150 leaves can produce death within 5 hours; LD_{50} in mice and rats is ~20 mg/kg. Red aril is not toxic; ingestion of 150 yew leaves has been fatal; ingestion of intact berries may cause only mild GI symptoms.

Family: Taxaceae. Range: The Yew genus occurs in many areas of the world, however in the U.S., it is located deep in the woods of Western North Carolina to the North Central and Northeastern U.S. Toxin: Taxine

Specific References
Cope RB, Camp C, and Lohr CV, "Fatal Yew (*Taxus* sp) Poisoning in Willamette Valley, Oregon Horses," *Vet Hum Toxicol*, 2004, 46(5):279-81.

Weaver JD and Brown DL, "Incubation of European Yew (*Taxus baccata*) with White-tailed Deer (*Odocoileus virginianus*) Rumen Fluid Reduces Taxine A Concentrations," *Vet Hum Toxicol*, 2004, 46(6):300-2.

SECTION IV
HERBAL AGENTS

Achyranthes Aspera

Synonyms Abora; Mnyoli; Muyon; Nara

Uses Chinese folk medicine used as an antipyretic/anti-inflammatory agent and diuretic. Also used for treatment of constipation, malaria, bronchitis, and sprains.

Mechanism of Toxic Action Contains saponins which are cardiotoxic by inhibition of cyclic adenosine 3′, 5′ monophosphate (CAMP) phosphodiesterase; also exhibits muscaric acetylcholine inhibition; contains achyranthine

Signs and Symptoms of Overdose Hypotension, coma, bradycardia, hypoactive bowel sounds

Admission Criteria/Prognosis Admit ingestion over 1000 mL of decoction or any symptomatic patient.

Overdosage/Treatment
Decontamination: Oral: Lavage within 1 hour/activated charcoal
Supportive therapy: Hypotension can be treated with intravenous crystalloid solutions. Dopamine (8-12 mcg/kg/minute) can be used as a vasopressor.

Additional Information A perennial herb 1.5-5 feet tall found in Africa. Single green to pink ovate flower with small (2.5-3 mm) fruit; lance-shaped leaves

Specific References
Han ST and Un CC, "Cardiac Toxicity Caused by Achyranthes Aspera," *Vet Hum Toxicol*, 2003, 45(4):212-3.

Ajuga Nipponensis Makino

Use Antitussive, expectorant, diuretic, anti-inflammatory, hepatoprotection

Mechanism of Action Contains cyasterone and ajugasterone which may exhibit inhibitory effects on TPA-induced tumor promotion; may be nephrotoxic

Signs and Symptoms of Overdose Vomiting, diarrhea, anorexia, renal failure, hyponatremia, oliguria, weakness

Dosage Possibly toxic dosage: 30 g of fresh plant mixed in 100 g of water

Overdosage/Treatment
Oral:
Decontamination: Activated charcoal is of unknown efficacy
Supportive care: Monitor electrolytes/renal status

Additional Information Usually found North and West of Taiwan; leaves are oval shaped (3-7 cm long) with white petal blossoms in summer and autumn; grows in sandy soil near the sea

Specific References
Liao SC, Chiu TF, Chen JC, et al, "Ajuga Nipponensis Makino Poisoning," *Clin Toxicol*, 2005, 43(6):583-5.

Arnica Flower

Scientific Name *Arnica chamissonis*; *Arnica latfolia*; *Arnica montana*

Synonyms Leopard's Bane; Mountain Snuff; Mountain Tobacco

Uses For external topical use in treatment of minor trauma (bruises, contusions, hematomas). Not to be taken for internal use.

Mechanism of Toxic Action Contains several flavonoid glycosides and sesquiterpene lactones along with coumarins (scopoletin and umbelliferone) and volatile oils. The sesquiterpene lactones exhibit a slight anti-inflammatory and analgesic effect.

Adverse Reactions Dermatologic: Contact dermatitis, eczema

Signs and Symptoms of Overdose A 1 oz ingestion can cause mucous membrane irritation which can result in abdominal pain, vomiting, and diarrhea. Dyspnea and cardiac arrest can occur.

Dosage Ointment: Apply topically, not more than 25% tincture or more than 15% "arnica oil". Do not use for prolonged therapy or on damaged skin. One suggested dose is use of 1 tablespoon of arnica tincture in 500 mL of cold water applied to the affected area several times daily. A patch test may be necessary to denote allergy to arnica.

Overdosage/Treatment Oral: If >1 oz is ingested, gastric lavage followed by activated charcoal should be given; otherwise, dilute with water. **Dermal, topical:** Irrigate with soap and water.

Additional Information A perennial bright daisy-like flower which grows up to 2 feet in Europe and Southern Russia.

Autumn Crocus

Related Information
- Colchicine

CAS Number 64-86-8

Scientific Name *Colchicum autumnale*

Synonyms Fall Crocus; Meadow Crocus; Meadow Saffron; Mysteria; Wonderbulb

Uses Colchicine has been used for centuries to treat gout and rheumatism

Mechanism of Toxic Action Inhibits cell division by blocking spindle formation and inhibiting mitosis; cells with high turnover rates are most affected

Adverse Reactions
Central nervous system: Hyperthermia, sedation
Dermatologic: Skin alterations and alopecia (with prolonged use)
Gastrointestinal: Diarrhea, nausea, vomiting, abdominal pain
Hematologic: Leukopenia, agranulocytosis and aplastic anemia (with prolonged use)
Neuromuscular & skeletal: Myopathy (with prolonged use)

Signs and Symptoms of Overdose
1st phase: 2-24 hours postexposure: Abdominal pain, electrolyte abnormalities, hypotension, nausea, vomiting and diarrhea resulting in hypovolemia; peripheral leukocytosis has been reported
2nd phase: 1-7 days postexposure: Bone marrow depression, coagulopathy, multisystem failure, mental status changes, oliguric renal failure, paresthesia, proteinuria, pulmonary edema, respiratory failure, sudden asystole
3rd phase: 7 or more days: Alopecia and rebound leukocytosis

Toxicodynamics/Kinetics
Absorption: Rapid with peak levels occurring in 30 minutes to 2 hours
Distribution: V_d: 2 L/kg; distributed within 30 minutes; deacetylated in the liver and both colchicine and its metabolites undergo enterohepatic recirculation
Protein binding: Weak, 10% to 30%

Dosage
As little as 7-8 mg of colchicine have resulted in fatalities; ingestion of 12 flowers of *Colchicum autumnale* has caused death; colchicine ingestions ≥ 0.5 mg/kg are associated with severe poisoning and death
Per Commission E: Therapeutic dosage for acute gout attack: Initial: Oral: 1 mg colchicine, followed by 0.5-1.5 mg every 1-2 hours until pain subsides; total daily dosage must not exceed 8 mg colchicine

Overdosage/Treatment
Decontamination: Lavage (within 1 hour) may be indicated if performed prior to the onset of symptoms; multiple dose activated charcoal should be of value; one dose of a cathartic may be used if administered prior to the onset of symptoms; due to the delay in the onset of toxicity, asymptomatic patients should be observed for at least 12 hours
Supportive therapy: Aggressive supportive therapy may be required in symptomatic patients; this includes fluid and electrolyte replacement and respiratory support. Hypotension unresponsive to fluids should be treated with dopamine or norepinephrine.
Enhancement of elimination: Hemodialysis and exchange transfusions have not been useful and are not recommended

Antidote(s)
- DOPamine [ANTIDOTE]
- Epinephrine [ANTIDOTE]

Test Interactions Colchicine decreases serum cholesterol levels; may interfere with some urine steroid tests

Drug Interaction None known with this plant (as per Commission E); colchicine therapy can increase cyclosporine levels

Pregnancy Risk Factor Contraindicated by Commission E

Additional Information Nasal insufflation can result in toxicity. Toxic parts: Entire plant. Colchicine concentrations range from 0.1% in the flowers to 0.8% in the seeds. Family: Liliaceae; Toxin: Colchicine and related alkaloids. Range: Native to Europe, widely cultivated in the U.S. Not sold in U.S. herb/dietary supplement market; use is pharmaceutical only for production of colchicine

Specific References
Gabrscek L, Lesnicar G, Krivec B, et al, "Accidental Poisoning with Autumn Crocus," *J Toxicol Clin Toxicol*, 2004, 42(1):85-8.

Ayahuasca

Scientific Name *Banisteriopsis* species

Synonyms Caapi; Daime; Hoasca; Lagé; Yajé

Use Religious purposes in South America (as a sacrament)

Mechanism of Action Derived from the woody vine *Banisteriopsis caapi*; this tea contains harmala alkaloids which reversibly inhibit monoamine oxidase type-A; contains N,N dimethyltryptamine (DMT) which acts as a psychotrope; the leaves of the plant *Psychotria viridia* may also be added to the tea

Adverse Reactions Central nervous system: Hallucinations

Toxicodynamics/Kinetics Peak plasma levels (DMT): Oral: 60 minutes: I.V.: 2 minutes

Dosage 2 mL/kg of the tea

Overdosage/Treatment
Decontamination: **Do not** induce emesis; lavage within 60 minutes/ activated charcoal with cathartic
Supportive therapy: Benzodiazepines may be useful for sedation

Drug Interactions Although this interaction has not been described, use of this tea with specific serotonin reuptake inhibitors may precipitate the serotonin syndrome

Additional Information Average levels of DMT and tetrahydroharmine following a dose of 2 mL/kg: ~15.8 ng/mL and 90.8 ng/mL respectively

Betel Nut

Scientific Name *Areca catechu*
U.S. Brand Names Sting (Tantric Corporation)
Synonyms Quids
Uses Often chewed with betel leaves and lime slake for mood elevation. Used in India, Pakistan, Bangladesh, China, New Guinea, Sri Lanka, Singapore, Thailand, and Taiwan. Also used for pain control, as a masticatory.
Mechanism of Toxic Action Contains six reduced pyridine alkaloids which may be carcinogenic. Also, the unroasted betel nut contains arecoline which is a cholinergic agent. Roasting the betel nut converts arecoline to arecaidine which is far less toxic. CNS depression may occur by inhibiting uptake of gamma-aminobutyric acid.
Adverse Reactions
Cardiovascular: **Palpitations** (45% to 50%), tachycardia (within 6 minutes of use; lasts ~17 minutes), hypotension; supraventricular tachycardia has been described
Central nervous system: **Dizziness** (70%)
Gastrointestinal: Oral cancer, vomiting, leukoplakia (chronic use), dark brown staining of teeth
Ocular: Miosis, blurred vision
Renal: Milk alkali syndrome
Respiratory: Wheezing, bronchoconstriction, dyspnea; pulmonary edema with high dosage
Miscellaneous: Diaphoresis (on first use)
Dosage Less than three nuts are usually chewed in combination with slaked lime, tobacco, clove, or cinnamon.
Overdosage/Treatment
Decontamination: Lavage within 1 hour. Activated charcoal can be given.
Supportive therapy: For bronchoconstriction, aerosolized beta-agonists with steroids and ipratropium should be given. Supraventricular tachycardia has been treated with verapamil (1-5 mg I.V.). Diazepam (5 mg I.V.) can be used for agitation.
Drug Interaction Use with alcohol may accentuate cardiac abnormalities.
Additional Information Betel nut is the ripe seed of the palm tree *Areca catechu*. An estimated 600 million people worldwide (15% of the world's population) use it daily. The *Areca* palm tree grows up to 100 feet tall with a thin (6 inch) trunk; native to Malaysia, the fruit of this tree is about the size and shape of a hen's egg.
Specific References
Kumar M, Kannan A, and Upreti RK, "Effect of Betel/Areca Nut (*Areca catechu*) Extracts on Intestinal Epithelial Cell Lining," *Vet Hum Toxicol*, 2000, 42(5):257-60.

Bilberry

Scientific Name *Vaccinium myrtillus*
U.S. Brand Names Alcodin®; Antocin®; Difrarel®; Largitor®; Myrataven®; Myrticol®; Retinol®; Tegens®
Synonyms Bog Bilberries; Myrtillus; Whortleberries
Uses In herbal medicine, dried fruits are used as a diuretic and astringent; also used to treat diarrhea; antiulcer effect may also prevent cataracts or macular degeneration
Mechanism of Toxic Action Anthocyanidin pigment increases gastric mucosal release of prostaglandin E2
Signs and Symptoms of Overdose Hypotension (secondary to vaso-dilatation)
Dosage Oral: 240-480 mg extract standardized to 25% anthocyanosides in 2-3 doses
Overdosage/Treatment Decontamination: Oral: Dilute with milk or water; activated charcoal with cathartic may be used
Additional Information See Commission E; blue/blackberries are edible and have a sweet taste; a European plant whose leaves are utilized in teas

Black Cohosh

Scientific Name *Cimcifuga racemosa*
U.S. Brand Names Remifemin (an ethanolic extract of the rhizome)
Uses Alleviate perimenopausal and postmenopausal symptoms; also used for premenstrual discomfort and dysmenorrhea
Mechanism of Toxic Action Contains triterpene glycosides which exhibit estrogenic effects and suppression of luteinizing hormone with no effect on follicle-stimulating hormone or prolactin. Also contains isoflavone and formononetin, which may bind to estrogen receptors.
Adverse Reactions
Cardiovascular: Plants have been known to cause bradycardia and hypotension
Central nervous system: Dizziness, tremor
Endocrine & metabolic: Abortifacient
Gastrointestinal: GI discomfort (7%)
Dosage Each 20 mg of Remifemin contains 1 mg of triterpene 27-deoxyacetin. Current dosage is 20 mg Remifemin twice daily for menopausal symptoms.

Overdosage/Treatment Decontamination: Ipecac or lavage within 1 hour of any ingestion >200 mg of extract. Activated charcoal is of unknown utility.
Drug Interaction May augment antiproliferative effect of tamoxifen.
Additional Information Tall upright perennial herb (3-8 feet tall), native to eastern United States. Roots and leaves are most toxic parts. Fruit is ovoid with flat seeds.
Specific References
Hernández MG and Pluchino S, "*Cimicifuga racemosa* for the Treatment of Hot Flashes in Women Surviving Breast Cancer," *Maturitas*, 2003, 44(Suppl 1):S59-65.

Buckthorn Bark

Related Information
- Cascara Sagrada
- Senna

Scientific Name *Rhamnus alnifolia*; *Rhamnus cathartica*; *Rhamnus frangula*
APHA Botanical Safety Rating System Class 2b, 2c, 2d
Synonyms Alder Buckthorn; Arrow Wood; Berry Alder; Black Dogwood; Frangula; Hart's Horn; Maythorn; Persian Berry; Purging Buckthorn
Uses Laxative
Mechanism of Toxic Action Contains frangulin, an anthraquinone which stimulates the colon
Adverse Reactions
Per Commission E:
Endocrine & metabolic: Long-term use/abuse can cause electrolyte imbalance
Gastrointestinal: In single incidents, cramp-like discomforts of gastrointestinal tract requiring a reduction in dosage
Signs and Symptoms of Overdose Abortifacient; could potentially cause kidney damage with a large enough ingestion; abdominal pain, cramping, diarrhea, nausea, vomiting
Toxicodynamics/Kinetics Onset is likely soon after ingestion
Dosage 1 g; mild intoxication upon ingestion of berries by children; apparently ingestion of ~20 berries or chewing the fresh bark is necessary to induce pronounced symptoms;
Per Commission E: 20-30 mg hydroxyanthracene derivatives, calculated as glycofrangulin A
Warnings Use of two stimulating laxatives longer than recommended can cause intestinal sluggishness per Commission E
Overdosage/Treatment
Decontamination: Ipecac/cathartic not recommended, activated charcoal/lavage (within 1 hour) may be useful
Supportive therapy: Treat any fluid or electrolyte imbalance
Drug Interaction Per Commission E: Potentiation of cardiac glycosides (with long-term use) is possible due to loss in potassium; effect on anti-arrhythmics is possible; potassium deficiency can be increased by simultaneous application of thiazide diuretics, corticosteroids, and licorice root
Additional Information May color alkaline urine red; do not confuse with hematuria; bark should be aged 1 year in order to decrease harsh laxative action; berry (fruit) also used in Germany. Toxic parts: Fruit, leaves, and bark

Cascara Sagrada

Related Information
- Buckthorn Bark
- Senna

CAS Number 8015-89-2; 8047-27-6
Scientific Name *Rhamnus purshiana*
APHA Botanical Safety Rating System Class 2b, 2c, 2d
U.S. Brand Names Brevilax®; Colamin®; Legapas® 100; Péristaline®; Sagrada-Lax®
Uses Laxative
Mechanism of Toxic Action Contains anthraquinone glycosides (>8%) called cascarosides A, B, C and D which can increase colonic motility
Adverse Reactions
Central nervous system: Dizziness
Per Commission E:
Endocrine & metabolic: Long-term use/abuse can cause electrolyte imbalance
Gastrointestinal: In single incidents, cramp-like discomforts of GI tract requiring a reduction in dosage
Toxicodynamics/Kinetics
Onset of laxative effect: 6-8 hours
Metabolism: Hydrolyzed by colonic bacteria to active ingredients
Dosage Oral:
Bitter cascara, fluid extract: 1 mL
Aromatic cascara sagrada: 5 mL
Cascara sagrada extract (tablet): 325 mg at bedtime
Powdered bark (capsule): 1 g ($^1/_2$ teaspoon)
Per Commission E: 20-30 mg hydroxyanthracene derivatives, calculated as glycofrangulin A

Overdosage/Treatment Decontamination: **Do not** induce emesis; lavage (within 1 hour)/activated charcoal can be used

Drug Interaction Per Commission E: Potentiation of cardiac glycosides (with long-term use) is possible due to loss in potassium; effect on antiarrhythmics is possible; potassium deficiency can be increased by simultaneous application of thiazide diuretics, corticosteroids, and licorice root

Pregnancy Risk Factor C

Additional Information A deciduous tree (grows to 12 feet) native to Pacific Northwest with small green flowers (in clusters); like buckthorn, the bark should be aged 1 year to decrease the harsh laxative effects

Catnip

Scientific Name *Nepata cataria*

Synonyms Cat's Play; Cataria; Catmint; Catnep; Catrup; Catswort; Field Balm; Nip

Uses Antidiarrheal, antipyretic, carminutive, menstrual cramps, sedative. Used for colic in infants (as an enema). Also used to treat migraine. Tea has a diuretic effect.

Mechanism of Toxic Action Contains nepetalactone (80% to 95%) and tannin substances which may cause central nervous system stimulation and hallucinations.

Signs and Symptoms of Overdose Headache, malaise, vomiting. Symptoms usually last a few hours.

Dosage Tea: Two teaspoons of ground or dried forms mixed in 1 L of water to prepare tea; can drink 2-3 cups/day.

Tincture: 0.5-1 teaspoon up to 3 times/day

Overdosage/Treatment

Decontamination: Oral activated charcoal may be effective.

Supportive therapy: Symptomatic treatment: Diazepam (0.1-0.3 mg/kg in children or 10 mg in adults) may be used to treat hallucinations.

Additional Information Native in Europe. Active agents are found in the aerial parts of this 1 meter tall perennial plant with 2-8 cm leaves. Not recommended in Commission E. Dried leaves have also been smoked as a "joint" or in a pipe. Mint-like odor.

Chamomile

Scientific Name *Anthemis nobilis*; *Chamaemelum nobile*; *Chamomilla recutita*; *Matricaria chamomilla*; *Matricaria recutita L.*

APHA Botanical Safety Rating System Class 1

Synonyms *Matricaria chamomilla*; *Matricarta recutita*

Uses Topical anti-inflammatory agent; the tea (which may contain 10% to 15% of the volatile oil) has been used for indigestion and its hypnotic properties; used to flavor cigarette tobacco

Mechanism of Action

Pharmacologic activities include antispasmodic, anti-inflammatory, antiulcer, and antibacterial effects; a sedative effect has also been documented

While the toxicity of its main chemical constituent (Bisabolol) is low, the tea is essentially prepared from various allergens (ie, pollen-laden flower heads) which can cause hypersensitivity reactions especially in atopic individuals; contains various flavonoids (apigenin, herniarin)

Adverse Reactions

Only 5-7 cases have been reported in California, 100 years of the medical literature, associated with those with severe ragweed allergies

Dermatologic: Contact dermatitis, immunologic contact urticaria

Gastrointestinal: Vomiting (from dried flowering heads)

Miscellaneous: Anaphylaxis

Dosage

Tea: ±150 mL H_2O poured of heaping tablespoon (±3 g) of herb, covered and steeped 5-10 minutes; tea used 3-4 times/day for G.I. upset

Contraindications Known hypersensitivity to *Asteraceae/Compositae* family

Dosage Forms Ointment:

Reference Range Peak blood level of herniarin: ~35 ng/mL ~1 hour after an oral dose of 40 mL

Overdosage/Treatment Supportive therapy: Treat allergic reactions with standard therapy (ie, epinephrine, antihistamines, vasopressors if required)

Drug Interactions

May increase effect of coumarin-type anticoagulants at high dosages

Tannin-containing herbs can cause a decrease in iron absorption.

Pregnancy Implications Excessive use should be avoided due to potential teratogenicity

Additional Information See Commission E; cross sensitivity may occur in individuals allergic to ragweed pollens, asters or chrysanthemums

Chaparral

Scientific Name *Larrea tridentata*

APHA Botanical Safety Rating System

Class 2d; not to be used in large amounts by persons with pre-existing kidney disease and liver conditions (eg, hepatitis and cirrhosis)

Synonyms *Larrea tridentata*; Creosote bush; Greasewood; Hediodilla

Use Herbal medicine to treat acne, bowel cramps, analgesic agent and to "retard aging" (not substantiated)

Mechanism of Action Contains a potent antioxidant (nordihydroguaiaretic acid or NDGA) which inhibits lipoxygenase and cyclo-oxygenase pathways

Adverse Reactions

Dermatologic: Contact dermatitis

Gastrointestinal: Anorexia

Hematologic: Coagulopathy

Hepatic: Lobular necrosis, jaundice, aminotransferase level elevation (asymptomatic)

Miscellaneous: Necrosis

Overdosage/Treatment

Decontamination: Ipecac within 30 minutes or lavage (within 1 hour)/ activated charcoal with cathartic

Supportive therapy: Orthotopic liver transplantation may be required to treat liver failure

Additional Information A branched bush or shrub that is olive green and can grow to a height of 9 feet in the desert regions of Southwestern U.S. and Mexico. Approximately 200 tons of chaparral were sold in the U.S. for use as teas and herbal dietary supplements in the 20 years from 1973-1993, according to informal herb industry estimates. Few adverse reactions were reported during this period. A medical review by three physicians of patient records obtained from FDA regarding hepatitis associated with chaparral ingestion could not definitively conclude that chaparral was the causative agent. Idiosyncratic reactions were suggested.

Chaste Tree

Scientific Name *Vitex agnus-castus*

APHA Botanical Safety Rating System Class 2b; may counteract the effectiveness of birth control pills

Synonyms *Vitex agnus-castus*

Uses In herbal medicine, it is used in treatment of menstrual disorders, premenstrual syndrome and mastodynia

Mechanism of Action The fruit (actually a drupe) contains triterpenoids which may have dopaminergic properties, thus decreasing prolactin secretion

Adverse Reactions

Dermatologic: Pruritus, rash, hives, urticaria

Endocrine & metabolic: Decreased prolactin level

Dosage As a concentrated alcoholic extract: ~20 mg/day

Per Commission E: Average daily dose: 3 g herb or equivalent preparations

Overdosage/Treatment

Decontamination: Lavage (within 1 hour)/activated charcoal with cathartic

Supportive therapy: Antihistamines can be used to treat pruritus although there is no data on this modality

Drug Interactions None known per Commission E but may counteract the effectiveness of birth control pills

Additional Information A small deciduous multitrunk tree which can grow up to 25 feet; native to Mediterranean region with flowers blooming in summer; the dried ripe fruit (which is brown/black with a pepperish flavor or aroma) contains the active chemical ingredients

Cleistanthus Collinus

Synonyms Oduvan

Uses Extract of crushed leaves used as a cattle/fish poison or abortifacient

Mechanism of Toxic Action Toxic constituents are dyphyllin and its glycosides (cleistanthin A and cleistanthin B) and collinusin which are irritants. Can induce DNA damage or apoptosis and may reduce or inhibit thiol/thiol-containing enzymes (specifically lactate dehydrogenase or cholinesterase). May cause glutathione depletion.

Signs and Symptoms of Overdose Leukocytosis, hypokalemia (72%), renal failure (30%), weakness, prolonged QT_c interval, inverted T waves, premature ventricular complexes, respiratory failure, elevated hepatic transaminases, hypotension, metabolic acidosis (high anion gap), hyperchloremia, coagulopathy, proteinuria, alkaline urinary pH, ptosis, mydriasis, hyporeflexia

Overdosage/Treatment

Decontamination: Lavage within 2 hours/activated charcoal

Supportive therapy: Hypotension can be treated with intravenous crystalloids. Vasopressor of choice is dopamine or norepinephrine. Monitor and replace potassium as needed. Sodium bicarbonate (1-2 mEq/kg) to treat acidosis. N-acetylcysteine may be of hepatoprotective benefit.

Additional Information A plant found in India, Malaysia, and Africa

Specific References

Eswarappa S, Chakraborty AR, Palatty BU, et al, "Cleistanthus Collinus Poisoning: Case Reports and Review of the Literature," *J Toxicol Clin Toxicol*, 2003, 41(4):369-72.

Clove

Scientific Name *Caryophyllus aromaticus*; *Eugenia caryophyllata Syzygium aromaticum*

APHA Botanical Safety Rating System Class 1 (clove bud not oil)

Synonyms Caryoph; Eugenol; Oil of Cloves; Pentogen (clove oil); Tropical Myrtle

Use

Applied topically to alleviate toothache

Carminative; flavoring agent; clove oil contains 85% to 92% eugenol which is effective as a local anesthetic and anesthetic in dentistry; soap fragrance

Mechanism of Toxic Action Eugenol acts similarly to other phenol agents by inhibiting prostaglandin synthesis and causing depression of pain receptors; can also cause uncoupling of oxidative phosphorylation

Adverse Reactions

Dermatologic: Dermatitis, urticaria

Endocrine & metabolic: Hypoglycemia, metabolic acidosis

Gastrointestinal: Vomiting

Hematologic: Disseminated intravascular coagulation

Hepatic: Hepatotoxicity

Ocular: Lacrimation

Renal: Proteinuria

Respiratory: Pulmonary edema (when injected)

Miscellaneous: Anaphylaxis, anhidrosis

Clove cigarettes:

Gastrointestinal: Sore throat

Respiratory: Bronchospasm, hemoptysis, pulmonary edema, epistaxis, bronchiectasis, pleural effusion

Toxicodynamics/Kinetics Metabolism: Hepatic

Dosage

Clove oil:

Oral: Toxic dose: Infant: 15 mL (500 mg/kg of eugenol); oil is not used therapeutically in concentrations >0.06%

Therapeutic: 1-2 drops on tooth cavity not more than 4 times/day

Warnings Per Commission E: Oil:

Oral: Alcoholism, anticoagulants, hemophilia, kidney disease, paracetamol, prostatic cancer, SLE

Dermal: Hypersensitive, diseased or damaged skin, all children <2 years of age

Oil in concentrated form may irritate mucous membranes

Dosage Forms Liquid: 3.75 mL

Overdosage/Treatment

Decontamination:

Oral: Dilute with milk or water; activated charcoal with cathartic may be given; endoscopy may be required within 1 day of ingestion to assess local gastrointestinal mucosal injury

Ocular: Irrigate copiously with saline

Supportive therapy: Anaphylaxis should be treated with epinephrine, diphenhydramine and corticosteroids; beta-adrenergic agonist agents can be used for bronchospasm; while the use of N-acetylcysteine has been proposed (due to the common metabolic pathways of acetaminophen and eugenol), this modality has not been studied in humans; disseminated intravascular coagulopathy (DIC) can be treated with vitamin K, fresh frozen plasma, heparin and factor VII with protein C, and antithrombin III

Additional Information The clove tree grows to ~30 feet and is found in warm climates in the Molucca Islands. The stems, buds and leaves can yield clove oil. Acceptable daily oral intake of eugenol: 2.5 mg/kg. Level of clove in foods does not exceed 0.236%. Clove cigarettes ("Kreteks") contain 60% tobacco and 40% ground clove. The primary components of clove cigarette smoke include eugenol (13 mg), beta-caryophyllene (1.2 mg), eugenol acetate (0.7 mg), alpha-humulene (0.16 mg), and caryophyllene-epoxide (<0.1 mg).

Specific References

Eisen JS, Koren G, Juurlink DN, et al, "N-Acetylcysteine for the Treatment of Clove Oil–Induced Fulminant Hepatic Failure," *J Toxicol Clin Toxicol*, 2004, 42(1):89-92.

Coltsfoot

Scientific Name *Tussilago farfara*

Synonyms Cough Plant; Coughwort; Horse Foot; Horse Hoof

Uses Coughs/bronchial congestion/respiratory infections; antitussive agent banned in Canada

Mechanism of Toxic Action Contains pyrrolizidine alkaloid senkirkine (0.015%) which is a hepatic carcinogen. While young preblooming flowers contain the highest amount of this agent, senkirkine is also found in its leaves. May also suppress platelet activating factor (or PAF).

Adverse Reactions While toxicity has not been described in humans, hepatic veno-occlusive disease and hemangioendothelial sarcoma of the liver has been described in laboratory rodents. Classified by the FDA as a herb of undefined safety.

Dosage Per Commission E: 4 g, 5 g, or 6 g of drug (dried herb) daily; not to exceed 10 mcg pyrrolizidine alkaloids with 1,2 unsaturated necine structure including their N-oxides. Not longer than 4-6 weeks per year.

Overdosage/Treatment Decontamination: Ipecac within 30 minutes or lavage (within 1 hour)/activated charcoal with cathartic; be aggressive in gastric decontamination in children

Additional Information A low, woolly perennial herb with solitary terminal yellow flowers and basal leaves which appear after flowering. Plant is native in Europe but found in northern U.S. and southern Canada. Flowers and leaves have been used for herbal medicine, particularly in Europe. Monitor liver function tests.

Comfrey

Scientific Name *Symphytum officinale*

APHA Botanical Safety Rating System

Class 2a: *Symphytum uplandicum* (Russian Comfrey): External use only, except under supervision of a qualified expert

Class 2a, 2b, 2c: *Symphytum officinale* (Common Comfrey)

U.S. Brand Names Traumaplant®

Synonyms Blackwort; Bruisewort; Bum Plant; Green Drink; Knitbone; Russian Comfrey; Slippery Root

Uses External use in herbal medicine for wound healing

Mechanism of Toxic Action Contains hepatotoxic pyrrolizidine alkaloids with the highest concentration occurring in the root

Adverse Reactions Hepatic: Hepatotoxicity, hepatic veno-occlusive disease, hepatic necrosis, ascites, jaundice

Dosage Per Commission E: External use should not exceed 100 mcg/day equivalent of pyrrolizidine alkaloid content with 1,2-unsaturated necine structure, including their N-oxides

Overdosage/Treatment Decontamination: Ipecac within 30 minutes or lavage within 1 hour; activated charcoal with cathartic

Additional Information A perennial with bell-shaped yellow or rose flowers (~1 cm long); plant grows to a height of 3 feet in moist grasslands; liver damage is dose dependent; causes liver and pancreatic tumors in animals. Unfortunately, the comfrey products (made from roots and/or leaves) sold in U.S. are not assayed for PA content, as they are in Germany. The American Herbal Products Association has voluntarily restricted its members from selling comfrey for internal use.

Cottonseed

Synonyms *Gossypium*; Gossypol; Mian Hua Gam

Uses Has been used as a male antifertility agent in China at doses from 75-100 mg twice monthly (~3 g/year). Spermatogenesis usually normalizes after 3 months postdiscontinuation, although the inhibition of spermatogenesis may be long-term in 20% of males.

Mechanism of Toxic Action Cottonseed (family: Malvaceae) contains from 0.1% to 6.6% gossyphol (a yellowish binaphthol compound) which is a nonsteroidal agent that inhibits human sperm motility and production, by inhibition of the gonadal enzyme lactate dehydrogenase X. There are no hormonal abnormalities noted, with testicular mitochondria being the target organ.

Signs and Symptoms of Overdose Amenorrhea, anorexia; azoospermia, oligospermia; doses >2 g may cause diarrhea and heart failure; fatigue (13%) and decreased libido (7%) have been observed; hypokalemia can occur due to renal potassium loss

Admission Criteria/Prognosis Admit any ingestion >1 g

Toxicodynamics/Kinetics Half-life: 286 hours

Monitoring Parameters Serum potassium

Reference Range Peak plasma gossypol level 5 hours after a 20 mg oral dose: ~996 ng/mL

Overdosage/Treatment

Decontamination: Any ingestion >20 mg in adults: Ipecac or lavage within 1 hour

Supportive therapy: Monitor serum potassium; potassium supplementation may be necessary

Drug Interaction May enhance the androgenic effect of methyltestosterone; hypokalemia may be exacerbated when gossypol is given with diuretic agents

Creatine Monohydrate

Synonyms Methyl Guanidine-Acetic Acid

Uses Reportedly can increase performance in short-duration, high-intensity, repetitive (isokinetic) muscle actions (ie, weightlifting, rowing); not useful for endurance

Mechanism of Toxic Action

Reportedly increases adenosine triphosphate levels by acting as a substrate for creatine kinase.

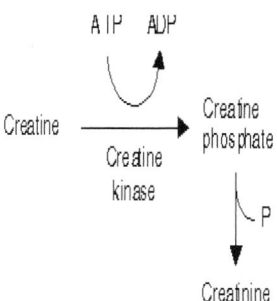

May also enhance actin/myosin production in muscles.

Adverse Reactions

Endocrine & metabolic: Water retention

Gastrointestinal: Weight gain (up to 5 lb), abdominal cramps, diarrhea

Neuromuscular & skeletal: Myalgia

Renal: Renal dysfunction, proteinuria

Toxicodynamics/Kinetics Elimination: In urine as creatinine

Dosage Loading dose of 5 g 4 times/day (0.3 g/kg) for 5-9 days followed by a maintenance dose of 2-5 g/day for up to 8 weeks

Overdosage/Treatment Decontamination: No reports of acute adverse effects in overdosage situation. Suggest gastric decontamination (ipecac or lavage) for ingestions >1 g/kg. Monitor BUN.

Test Interactions No effect on serum creatinine, although BUN increase may be seen; CPK may be elevated

Additional Information Total body creatine pool is 120 g (95% in skeletal muscle). Average daily dietary intake is 1 g/day. Red meat, tuna, cod, salmon, herring, beef, and pork have the highest amount of creatine. 1 kg of raw steak contains almost 4 g of creatine. Endogenous creatine (~2 g/day) is synthesized in the liver, kidneys, and pancreas from glycine, arginine, and methionine.

Specific References

Bohnhorst B, Geuting T, Peter CS, et al, "Randomized, Controlled Trial of Oral Creatine Supplementation (Not Effective) for Apnea of Prematurity," *Pediatrics*, 2004, 113(4):e303-7.

Gomez J, American Academy of Pediatrics Committee on Sports Medicine and Fitness, "Use of Performance-Enhancing Substances," *Pediatrics*, 2005, 115(4):1103-6.

Haller CA, Meier KH, and Olson KR, "Seizures Reported in Association with Use of Dietary Supplements," *Clin Toxicol (Phila)*, 2005, 43(1):23-30 (review).

Pline KA and Smith CL, "The Effect of Creatine Intake on Renal Function," *Ann Pharmacother*, 2005, 39(6):1093-6.

Echinacea

Scientific Name *Echinacea angustifolia*; *Echinacea pallida*; *Echinacea purpurea*

APHA Botanical Safety Rating System Class 1

U.S. Brand Names Echinaguard®; Echinase®; Super Echinacea®

Synonyms *Echinacea angustifolia*; American Coneflower; Black Sampson; Black Susans; Comb Flower; Coneflower; Indian Head; Purple Coneflower; Scurvy Root; Scury Root, American Coneflower; Snakeroot

Use Prophylaxis and treatment of cold and flu; also used as an immunostimulant in herbal medicine; used to treat minor upper respiratory tract infections, urinary tract infections, wound/skin infections, arthritis, vaginal yeast infections

Mechanism of Action Contains a caffeic acid glycoside named echinacoside (0.1% concentration) which is bactericidal. Other caffeic acid glycosides and isolutylamides associated with the plant can cause immune stimulation by increasing leukocyte phagocytosis and promoting T-cell activation. Also has an antihyaluronidase and anti-inflammatory activity; constituents have been associated with antitumor, antispasmodic effects

Adverse Reactions

Central nervous system: Fever

Gastrointestinal: Tingling sensation of tongue, nausea, vomiting

Hematologic: Leukocytosis

Miscellaneous: Allergic reactions (rarely)

Per Commission E: None known for oral and external use

Dosage

Capsule/tablet or tea form: 500 mg to 2 g 3 times/day

May be applied topically

Continuous use should not exceed 8 weeks

Per Commission E: Expressed juice (of fresh herb): 6-9 mL/day

Contraindications Autoimmune diseases, such as collagen vascular disease (Lupus, RA), multiple sclerosis; allergy to sunflowers, daisies, ragweed; tuberculosis, HIV, AIDS, pregnancy, breast-feeding; parenteral administration only contraindicated per Commission E; oral use of Echinacea not contraindicated during pregnancy by Commission E

Overdosage/Treatment Supportive therapy: Can treat allergic manifestations with an antihistamine

Drug Interactions

Theoretically may alter response to immunosuppressive therapy

Avoid using with other hepatotoxic agents (anabolic steroids, amiodarone, methotrexate, or ketoconazole)

Additional Information Commission E only approves *E. purpurea* fresh juice from leaves and herb, and *E. pallida* root preparations; persons allergic to sunflowers may display cross-allergy potential with this herb; a perennial daisy-like flowering plant 2-5 feet high usually found in the midwest and southeastern United States; contraindications in tuberculosis, leukocytosis, collagen vascular disease, multiple sclerosis, tachyphylaxis can occur if used >8 weeks

Specific References

Cohen HA, Varsano I, Kahan E, et al, "Effectiveness of an Herbal Preparation Containing Echinacea, Propolis, and Vitamin C in Preventing Respiratory Tract Infections in Children: A Randomized, Double-Blind, Placebo-Controlled, Multicenter Study," *Arch Pediatr Adolesc Med*, 2004, 158(3):217-21.

Kligler B, "Echinacea," *Am Fam Physician*, 2003, 67(1):77-80.

Lanski SL, Greenwald M, Perkins A, et al, "Herbal Therapy Use in a Pediatric Emergency Department Population: Expect the Unexpected," *Pediatrics*, 2003, 111:981-5.

Taylor JA, Weber W, Standish L, et al, "Efficacy and Safety of *Echinacea* in Treating Upper Respiratory Tract Infections in Children: A Randomized Controlled Trial," *JAMA*, 2003, 290(21):2824-30.

Turner RB, Bauer R, Woelkart K, et al, "An Evaluation of *Echinacea angustifolia* in Experimental Rhinovirus Infections," *N Engl J Med*, 2005, 28;353(4):341-8.

Ephedra

Related Information

• Ephedrine

Scientific Name Consists of dried young branches of *Ephedra sinica*, *Ephedra equisetina*, and *Ephedra gerardiana*

APHA Botanical Safety Rating System Class 2b, 2c, 2d; contraindicated in anorexia, bulimia, glaucoma, and persons with thyroid imbalance; not recommended for long-term use

U.S. Brand Names Cloud 9; Ultimate Xphoria

Synonyms *Ephedra sinica*; Joint Fir; Ma-Huang; Mormon Tea; Poptillo; Sea Grape; Squaw Tea; Teamsters' Tea; Yellow Horse

Use Herbal medicinal uses include treatment for asthma, bronchitis, edema, arthritis, headache, fever, urticaria; also used for weight reduction and for euphoria

Mechanism of Action An alpha- and beta-adrenergic stimulant; most species contain ephedrine and/or pseudoephedrine although *E. nevadensis* may not contain any ephedrine; tannin contributes to its bitter taste

Adverse Reactions

Cardiovascular: Hypertension, cardiomyopathy, vasculitis, cardiomegaly, palpitations, vasoconstriction, tachycardia, myocarditis

Central nervous system: CNS-stimulating effects, **nervousness**, anxiety, fear, psychosis, tension, agitation, excitation, **restlessness**, irritability, **insomnia**, auditory and visual hallucinations, sympathetic storm, headache

Endocrine & metabolic: Hypokalemia

Gastrointestinal: Nausea, anorexia

Hepatic: Aminotransferase level elevation (asymptomatic)

Neuromuscular & skeletal: Tremors, weakness

Signs and Symptoms of Overdose CNS depression, depression, dry skin, dysrhythmias, insomnia, mydriasis, respiratory alkalosis, respiratory depression, seizures, vomiting

Dosage

E. sinica extracts (with 10% alkaloid content): 125-250 mg 3 times/day

As a tea: Steepening 1 heaping teaspoon in 240 mL of boiling water for 10 minutes (equivalent to 15-30 mg of ephedrine)

Per Commission E: Single dose: Herb preparation corresponds to 15-30 mg total alkaloid (calculation as ephedrine)

Contraindications Per Commission E: Anxiety, restlessness, hypertension, glaucoma, impaired cerebral circulation, prostate adenoma with residual urine accumulation, pheochromocytoma, thyrotoxicosis

Warnings AHPA warning as of March 1994 for ephedra product labels: "Seek advice from 2 healthcare professionals prior to use if you are pregnant or nursing, or if you have high blood pressure, heart or thyroid disease, diabetes, difficulty in urination due to prostate enlargement, or if taking 2 MAO inhibitors or any other prescription drug. Reduce or discontinue use if nervousness, tremor, sleeplessness, loss of appetite, or nausea occur. Not intended for use by persons <18 years of age. Keep out of reach of children."

Reference Range Therapeutic serum level of ephedrine: 0.04-0.08 mcg/mL

Overdosage/Treatment

Decontamination: Lavage (within 1 hour)/activated charcoal with cathartic Supportive therapy: There is no specific antidote for ephedrine intoxication and the bulk of the treatment is supportive. Hyperactivity and agitation usually respond to reduced sensory input, however with extreme agitation haloperidol (2-5 mg I.M. for adults) may be required. Hyperthermia is best treated with external cooling measures, or when severe or unresponsive, muscle paralysis with pancuronium may be needed. Hypertension is usually transient and generally does not require treatment unless severe. For diastolic blood pressures >110 mm Hg, a nitroprusside infusion should be initiated. Seizures usually respond to diazepam or lorazepam I.V. and/or phenytoin maintenance regimens.

Drug Interactions Per Commission E: May potentiate with MAO inhibitors in combination with cardiac glycosides or halothane; arrhythmias; with guanethidine: Enhancement of sympathomimetic effect; with MAO inhibitors: Potentiates sympathomimetic effect of ephedrine

Pregnancy Risk Factor Contraindicated

Additional Information Erect evergreen shrubs growing up to 6 feet in height with rounded flowers blooming in early spring; while the fruits are nearly alkaloid free, the green stems and twigs contain the highest amount of ephedrine and pseudoephedrine; Mormon tea (*Ephedra nevadensis*) contains large amount of tannin, no ephedrine (but possibly t-norpseudoephedrine, a CNS stimulant) and can produce a mild diuresis along with constipation; in fact North and Central American ephedra species lack sympathomimetic alkaloids

Specific References

Clark BM and Schofiled BSI, "Dilated Cardiomyopathy and Acute Liver Injury Associated with Combined Use of Ephedra, Gamma-Hydroxybutyrate and Anabolic Steroids," *Pharmacotherapy*, 2005, 25(5): 756-61.

Haller C, Duan M, Benowitz NL, et al, "Concentrations of Ephedra Alkaloids and Caffeine in Commercial Dietary Supplements," *J Anal Toxicol*, 2004, 28:145-51.

Haller CA, Meier KH, and Olson KR, "Seizures Reported in Association with Use of Dietary Supplements," *Clin Toxicol (Phila)*, 2005, 43(1):23-30 (review).

Holstege CP, Mitchell K, Barlotta K, et al, "Toxicity and Drug Interactions Associated with Herbal Products: Ephedra and St. John's Wort," *Med Clin North Am*, 2005, 89(6):1225-57 (review).

Jacob P, Haller CA, Duan M, et al, "Determination of Ephedra Alkaloid and Caffeine Concentrations in Dietary Supplements and Biological Fluids," *J Anal Toxicol*, 2004, 28:152-9.

Levisky JA, Karch SB, Bowerman DL, et al, "False-Positive RIA for Methamphetamine Following Ingestion of an Ephedra-Derived Herbal Product," *J Anal Toxicol*, 2003, 27(2):123-4.

McBride BF, Karapanos AK, Krudysz A, et al, "Electrocardiographic and Hemodynamic Effects of a Multicomponent Dietary Supplement Containing Ephedra and Caffeine: A Randomized Controlled Trial," *JAMA*, 2004, 291(2):216-21.

Meier KH, Haller CA, and Olson KR, "A Review of Seizures Reported to the FDA in Association with Use of Dietary Supplements," *J Toxicol Clin Toxicol*, 2003, 41(5):659.

Naik SD and Freudenberger RS, "Ephedra-Associated Cardiomyopathy," *Ann Pharmacother*, 2004, 38(3):400-3.

Peters CM, O'Neill JO, Young JB, et al, "Is There An Association Between Ephedra and Heart Failure? A Case Series," *J Card Fail*, 2005, 11(1):9-11.

Shekelle PG, Hardy ML, Morton SC, et al, "Efficacy and Safety of Ephedra and Ephedrine for Weight Loss and Athletic Performance: A Meta-Analysis," *JAMA*, 2003, 289(12):1537-45.

Sweet BV, Gay WE, Leady MA, et al, "Usefulness of Herbal and Dietary Supplement References," *Ann Pharmacother*, 2003, 37(4):494-9.

Woolf AD, "Herbal Remedies and Children: Do They Work? Are They Harmful?" *Pediatrics*, 2003, 112(1 Pt 2):240-6.

Woolf A, Watson W, Smolinske S, et al, "Severe Toxic Reactions to Ephedra: National Trends from 1993-2002," *J Toxicol Clin Toxicol*, 2003, 41(5):727.

Feverfew

Scientific Name *Chrysanthemum parthenium*; *Tanacetum parthenium*
APHA Botanical Safety Rating System Class 2b
U.S. Brand Names Feverfew Herb®; Partenelle®
Synonyms *Tanacetum parthenium*; Altamisa; Bachelor's Buttons; Chamomile Grande; Chrysanthememmatricaire; European Feverfew; Feather-Fully; Featherfew; Featherfoil; Febrifuge Plant; Feddygen Fenyw; Flirt-root; Grande Chamomile; Midsummer Daisy; Mutterkraut; Nosebleed; Santa Maria; Vetter-Voo; Wild Chamomile; Wild Quinine
Use Prophylaxis and treatment of migraine headaches; used to treat menstrual complaints and fever

Mechanism of Action Active ingredient is parthenolide ($\approx$0.2% concentration), a sesquiterpene which is a serotonin antagonist; also, the plant may be an inhibitor of prostaglandin synthesis and platelet aggregation; has spasmolytic effect on cerebral blood vessels; other anti-inflammatory effects, antimicrobial, antifungal

Adverse Reactions

Dermatologic: Contact dermatitis

Gastrointestinal: **Mouth ulcerations**, swelling of tongue

Signs and Symptoms of Overdose Abdominal pain, loss of taste, nausea, vomiting

Dosage

125 mg of a preparation standardized to 0.2% parthenolide (250 mcg)

Dried aerial parts: Oral: 50-200 mg

Tincture: (1:5, 25% ethanol): 5-20 drops

Contraindications Pregnancy, breast-feeding; children <2 years of age; allergies to feverfew and other members of the Asteraceae, daisy, ragweed, chamomile

Overdosage/Treatment

Decontamination: **Oral: Do not** induce emesis; dilute with milk or water **Dermal:** Wash skin with soap and water

Supportive therapy: Treat contact dermatitis with diphenhydramine and/or steroids

Drug Interactions Use with caution in patients taking aspirin or anticoagulants due to increased potential for bleeding; tannin-containing herbs can cause a decrease in iron absorption; nonsteroidal anti-inflammatory drugs may reduce the effectiveness of feverfew

Additional Information

Not reviewed by Commission E; a perennial bush which grows up to 3 feet tall with daisy-like yellow or white flowers; leaves are bitter tasting; contraindications in pregnancy and children <2 years of age

This herbal preparation should be discontinued for 2-3 weeks prior to surgery.

Garcinia cambogia

U.S. Brand Names Citrin®
Synonyms HCA
Uses Rheumatism; purgative; potential for weight loss and appetite control
Mechanism of Toxic Action Contains an organic acid known as (-) hydroxy citric acid (HCA) which inhibits lipogenesis and increases production of glycogen; also may be an appetite suppressant
Signs and Symptoms of Overdose None known
Dosage 250-800 mg of HCA/day
Overdosage/Treatment Decontamination: Oral: Lavage within 1 hour; activated charcoal
Additional Information Fruit of the evergreen tree *G. cambogia* and *G. indica* found in southern Asia; usually associated with chromium; additional information can be obtained by calling America's Finest, Inc, 3481 Old Conejo Road (#101), Newbury Park, CA 91320 (1-800-350-3305)

Garlic

CAS Number 8008-99-9
Scientific Name *Allium sativum*
APHA Botanical Safety Rating System Class 2c; GI upset in sensitive persons
U.S. Brand Names Carisano®; Cirkulin®; Garlicin®; Garlimega®; Garlique®; Ilja Rogoff®; Kwai®; Kyolic®; PureGar®; Sapec®
Synonyms *Allium savitum*; Ajo; Chives; Comphor of the Poor; Nectar of the Gods; Poor Mans Treacle; Rustic Treacle; Shallots; Stinking Rose; Taisan
Use Herbal medicine used for lowering LDL cholesterol and triglycerides, and raising HDL cholesterol; protection against atherosclerosis, hypertension, antiseptic agent; may lower blood glucose and decrease thrombosis; potential anti-inflammatory and antitumor effects
Mechanism of Action Garlic bulbs contain alliin, a parent to the substance allicin (after the bulb is ground), which is odoriferous and may have some antioxidant activity; ajoene (a byproduct of allicin) has potent platelet inhibition effects; garlic can also decrease LDL cholesterol levels and increase fibrinolytic activity
Adverse Reactions

Cardiovascular: Prolonged prothrombin time

Dermatologic: Skin blistering, eczema, systemic contact dermatitis, immunologic contact urticaria

Gastrointestinal: Gastrointestinal upset and changes in intestinal flora (in rare cases) per Commission E

Ocular: Lacrimation

Respiratory: Asthma (upon inhalation of garlic dust)

Miscellaneous: Allergic reactions (in rare cases); change in odor of skin and breath per Commission E

Signs and Symptoms of Overdose Burning sensation of mouth, dizziness, hematoma, leukocytosis, lightheadedness, nausea, sweating. At doses >50 g daily anorexia, diarrhea, vomiting, and menorrhagia may develop.

Toxicodynamics/Kinetics

Half-life: N-acetyl-S-allyl-L-cysteine: 6 hours

Elimination: Pulmonary and renal

Dosage Average daily dose for cardiovascular benefits: ~0.25-1 g/kg or 1-4 cloves daily in an 80 kg individual in divided doses

Toxic dose: >5 cloves or >25 mL of extract can cause gastrointestinal symptoms

Reference Range Urinary N-acetyl-S-allyl-L-cysteine following ingestion of 600 mg of fresh garlic totals ~0.4 mg

Overdosage/Treatment Decontamination: **Oral:** Ipecac within 30 minutes or lavage within 1 hour acute ingestions >25 mL of garlic extract; dilute with milk or water; activated charcoal may prevent absorption. **Ocular:** Irrigate with saline

Drug Interactions Iodine uptake may be reduced with garlic ingestion; can exacerbate bleeding in patients taking aspirin or anticoagulant agents; may increase risk of hypoglycemia, may increase response to antihypertensives

Pregnancy Implications Avoid use in pregnancy/lactation

Additional Information See Commission E; ~1% as active as penicillin as an antibiotic; number one over-the-counter drug in Germany

Specific References

Delgoda R and Westlake AC, "Herbal Interactions Involving Cytochrome P450 Enzymes: A Mini Review," *Toxicol Rev*, 2004, 23(4):239-49.

Schneider B, Hanisch J, and Weiser M, "Complementary Medicine Prescription Patterns in Germany," *Ann Pharmacother*, 2004, 38(3):502-7.

Germander

Scientific Name *Teucrium chamaedrys*

APHA Botanical Safety Rating System Class 3

Synonyms *Teucrium chamaedrys*; Wall Germander

Use In folk medicine to treat obesity

Mechanism of Action Hepatotoxic; possibly through cytochrome P-450 isozymes by reactive intermediates (epoxides) that are detoxified by glutathione; contains polyphenol derivatives, diterpenes, flavonoids, and tannins

Adverse Reactions Hepatic: Jaundice, elevated liver function test results, hepatic necrosis (centrilobular), aminotransferase level elevation (asymptomatic)

Dosage Daily dose: 600 mg to 1.62 g

Monitoring Parameters Liver function tests

Dosage Forms Capsules: 200-275 mg (no longer marketed)

Herbal teas: ≈1 g/bag of germander (no longer marketed)

Overdosage/Treatment

Decontamination: Ipecac within 30 minutes or lavage (within 1 hour)/ activated charcoal with cathartic

Supportive therapy: Although there are no human or animal data, due to the fact that glutathione depletion can result in increased hepatotoxicity in mice, there exists a rational to use N-acetylcysteine

Additional Information Not reviewed by Commission E; not generally sold in the United States, mainly in Europe; plant is found in Eastern Europe and Mediterranean; dexamethasone or clotrimazole may increase hepatotoxicity; hepatotoxicity usually presents 3-18 hours after ingestion; blossoms are used in folk medicine in Europe, not in U.S.

Germanium

Synonyms Ge

Uses Health food supplement in Japan; thought to exhibit immunomodulating effects (organogermanium compounds)

Mechanism of Toxic Action Organic germanium compounds and germanium oxide can cause lactic acidosis and renal dysfunction (tubular epithelial cell injury with lipofuscin granule accumulation) usually after long-term use (>5 g).

Signs and Symptoms of Overdose Anorexia, fatigue, hepatic failure, lactic acidosis, muscular pain, nephritis, neuropathy, paresthesia, pulmonary edema, vomiting, weight loss

Toxicodynamics/Kinetics

Absorption: Rapid, from the GI tract

Elimination: Renal

Reference Range Normal serum Ge level is ~0.005 mcg/mL. Normal urinary Ge level is <1 mcg/g creatinine.

Overdosage/Treatment

Decontamination: Oral: Emesis within 30 minutes or lavage within 1 hour any ingestion.

Supportive therapy: Monitor renal status; note that urinalysis is likely to be unremarkable. Prednisone is unlikely to be beneficial in treating muscle or renal dysfunction. Monitor BUN and creatinine.

Additional Information Usual daily ingestion is ~1 mg in foods rich in germanium (oat and barley)

Ginger

Scientific Name *Zingiber officinale*

APHA Botanical Safety Rating System Class 1

U.S. Brand Names Travel Sickness®; Travellers®; Zintona®

Synonyms *Zingiber officinale*

Use In herbal medicine as a digestive aid; for treatment of nausea (antiemetic) and motion sickness; also used as a menstruation promoter in Chinese herbal medicine; headaches, colds and flu; ginger oil is used as a flavoring agent in beverages and mouthwashes; may be useful in some forms of arthritis

Mechanism of Action Unknown; may increase GI motility and thus block nausea feedback from the GI tract; appears to decrease prostaglandin synthesis; may have cardiotonic activity; may inhibit platelet aggregation

Adverse Reactions Gastrointestinal: Increased salivation

Signs and Symptoms of Overdose Possible CNS depression with large doses

Dosage

For preventing motion sickness or digestive aid: 1-4 g/day (250 mg of ginger root powder 4 times/day)

Per Commission E: 2-4 g/day or equivalent preparations

Contraindications Gallstones per Commission E

Overdosage/Treatment Decontamination: Lavage (within 1 hour)/activated charcoal with cathartic

Drug Interactions May alter response to cardiotonic, hypoglycemia, anticoagulant, antiplatelet agents; avoid concomitant use with warfarin.

Pregnancy Risk Factor No administration for morning sickness during pregnancy per Commission E; however, two-peer reviewed revision of the literature does not justify this caution; Commission E made its cautions based on animal studies and *in vitro* mutagenicity studies (2) on one compound, gingerol. Indian and Chinese women use large amounts of ginger routinely in their diet during pregnancy with no ill effects on pregnancy or fetus.

Pregnancy Implications No administration for morning sickness during pregnancy per Commission E; however, two-peer reviewed revision of the literature does not justify this caution; Commission E made its cautions based on animal studies and *in vitro* mutagenicity studies (2) on 1 compound, gingerol. Indian and Chinese women use large amounts of ginger routinely in their diet during pregnancy with no ill effects on pregnancy or fetus. High doses may be abortifacient.

Additional Information Density of ginger oil is ~0.9; ginger is a perennial plant with green-purple flowers similar to orchids which grows in India, the Orient, and Jamaica; 8 oz of ginger ale contains ~1 g of ginger; ginger tea (1 cup) contains ~250 mg of ginger

Specific References

Boone SA and Shields KM, "Treating Pregnancy-Related Nausea and Vomiting with Ginger," *Ann Pharmacother*, 2005, 39(10):1710-3.

Ginkgo biloba

Scientific Name Ginkgoaceae (family)

APHA Botanical Safety Rating System Class 1

U.S. Brand Names Ginkoba®

Synonyms BN-52063; EGb; GBE; Ginkgold; Ginkgopower; Ginkogink; Kaveri; Kew Tree; Maidenhair Tree; Oriental Plum Tree; Rökan; Silver Apricot; Superginkgo; Tanakan; Tanakene; Tebonin; Tramisal; Valverde; Vasan; Vital

Use

Dilates blood vessels; plant/leaf extract has been used in Europe for intermittent claudication, arterial insufficiency, and cerebral vascular disease (dementia); tinnitus, visual disorders, traumatic brain injury, vertigo of vascular origin

Per Commission E: Demential syndromes including memory deficits, etc (tinnitus, headache); depressive emotional conditions, primary degenerative dementia, vascular dementia, or both

Investigational: Asthma, impotence (male)

Mechanism of Action Inhibits platelet aggregation; *Gginkgo biloba* leaf extract contains terpenoids and flavonoids which can allegedly inactivate oxygen-free radicals causing vasodilatation and antagonize effects of platelet activating factor (PAF); fruit pulp contains ginkolic acids which are allergens (seeds are not sensitizing)

Adverse Reactions

Cardiovascular: Palpitations, bilateral subdural hematomas

Central nervous system: Headache (very seldom per Commission E), dizziness, seizures (in children), restlessness, subarachnoid hemorrhage

Dermatologic: Urticaria, cheilitis

Gastrointestinal: Nausea, diarrhea, vomiting, stomatitis, proctitis; very seldom stomach or intestinal upsets (per Commission E)

Ocular: Hyphema

Miscellaneous: Allergic skin reactions (very seldom per Commission E)

Admission Criteria/Prognosis Admit any ingestion with neurologic abnormalities or ingestions >2 pieces of fruit

Toxicodynamics/Kinetics
Onset of CNS effects: 1 hour
Peak absorption: 2-3 hours
Duration of action: 7 hours
Bioavailability: 70% to 100%
Half-life: Ginkgolide A: 4 hours; Ginkgolide B: 10.6 hours; Bilobalide: 3.2 hours

Dosage Usual dosage: ~40 mg 3 times/day with meals; 60 mg twice daily depending on indication; maximum dose: 360 mg/day
Cerebral ischemia: 120 mg/day in 2-3 divided doses (24% flavonoid-glycoside extract, 6% terpene glycosides)

Contraindications Pregnancy, patients with clotting disorders; hypersensitivity to *Ginkgo biloba* preparations per Commission E

Reference Range Peak plasma concentration of flavonol-glycoside following a 300 mg oral dose: ~150 ng/mL. The serum concentration of 4-metoxypyridoxine was 360 ng/mL following ingestion of 60 roasted ginko seeds in a 2-year-old female with seizures.

Overdosage/Treatment
Decontamination: **Dermal:** Washing skin within 10 minutes may prevent dermal allergic contact dermatitis; remove all clothing. **Oral:** Lavage (within 1 hour)/activated charcoal (laxative not needed)
Supportive therapy: Although human data are lacking, since the central nervous system effects may be due to 4-*o*-methylpyridoxine (an antipyridoxine compound), pyridoxine may be useful after ingestion of ginkgo seeds or kernels in children; topical corticosteroids can be used for skin reactions

Drug Interactions Due to effects on PAF, use with caution in patients receiving anticoagulants or platelet inhibitors; may diminish the effectiveness of anticonvulsants

Additional Information Beneficial effects for cerebral ischemia in the elderly occur after one month of use
Grown on plantations, leaves are extracted with organic solvent (acetone) to a potency of 24% flavonoids and 6% terpenoids. Can increase alpha waves and decrease slow potentials in EEG. An Oriental deciduous tree with plum-like fruits (in autumn) and flowers in spring. May reach a height of 125' (20' girth) and is found in U.S., Europe, China, and Japan. Cross reactivity for contact dermatitis due to the fruit pulp exists with poison ivy and poison oak; the dermatological symptoms may last for 10 days. Inner bark is used as a whitish brown cloth dye. Leaf extract has been used in herbal medicine to treat dementia, chronic tinnitus, vertigo, cochlear deafness, and impotence.
Reference range: Maximum plasma level of gingkolide A and gingkolide B after an 80 mg oral dose: 15 mg/mL and 4 mg/mL, respectively; maximum plasma level of bilobalide after a 120 mg oral dose: ~18.8 mg/mL
Ginkgo biloba may reverse genital anesthesia and diminished sexual desire induced by fluoxetine.
This herbal preparation should be discontinued for 2-3 weeks prior to surgery.

Specific References
Bal Dit Sollier C, Caplain H, and Drouet L, "No Alteration in Platelet Function of Coagulation Induced by EGb761 in a Controlled Study," *Clin Lab Haematol*, 2003, 25(4):251-3.
Bressler R, "Herb-drug Interactions: Interactions Between *Ginkgo biloba* and Prescription Medications," *Geriatrics*, 2005, 60(4):30-3 (review).
Delgoda R and Westlake AC, "Herbal Interactions Involving Cytochrome P450 Enzymes: A Mini Review," *Toxicol Rev*, 2004, 23(4):239-49.
Kalus JS, Piotrowski AA, Fortier CR, et al, "Hemodynamic and Electrocardiographic Effects of Short-Term *Ginkgo biloba*," *Ann Pharmacother*, 2003, 37(3):345-9.
Kupiec T and Raj V, "Fatal Seizures Due to Potential Herb-Drug Interactions with *Ginkgo biloba*," *J Anal Toxicol*, 2005, 29:755-8.
Markowitz JS, Donovan JL, DeVane CL, et al, "Common Herbal Supplements Did Not Produce False-Positive Results on Urine Drug Screens Analyzed by Enzyme Immunoassay," *J Anal Toxicol*, 2004, 28:272-3.
Mauro VF, Mauro LS, Kleshinski JF, et al, "Impact of *Ginkgo biloba* on the Pharmacokinetics of Digoxin," *Am J Ther*, 2003, 10(4):247-51.
Quaranta L, Bettelli S, Uva MG, et al, "Effect of *Ginkgo biloba* Extract on Pre-existing Visual Field Damage in Normal Tension Glaucoma," *Ophthalmology*, 2003, 110(2):359-62
Wolsko PM, Solondz DK, Phillips RS, et al. "Lack of Herbal Supplement Characterization in Published Randomized Controlled Trials," *Am J Med*, 2005, 118(10):1087-93 (review).

Ginseng

Scientific Name *Panax* ginseng
APHA Botanical Safety Rating System Class 2d; contraindicated in hypertension
U.S. Brand Names Bio-Star®; Ginsana®; Ginsun®; Neo Ginsana®
Synonyms *P. quinquefolium* L.; *P. trifolius* L.; Korean Ginseng; Ninjin; Panax; Pannag

Use A popular ingredient in herbal teas; has been advocated for its antistress and adaptogenic effects although these effects have not been scientifically confirmed, there's much "suggestive" scientific literature

Mechanism of Action The active agent (ginsenosides) may have CNS stimulant and estrogen-like effect, anti-inflammatory, antiplatelet; used as an adaptogen; may lower cholesterol; not effective as an aphrodesiac

Adverse Reactions
Cardiovascular: Tachycardia, hypertension, sinus tachycardia
Central nervous system: Nervousness, agitation, mania, cerebral arteritis
Dermatologic: Stevens-Johnson syndrome
Endocrine & metabolic: Hypoglycemia, metrorrhagia
Hematologic: Lymphocytosis

Signs and Symptoms of Overdose Ginseng abuse syndrome (noted in patients ingesting 3-15 g/day for up to 2 years) is characterized by morning edema, euphoria, diarrhea, insomnia, nervousness, and skin eruptions.

Dosage Herbal tea: Usually ~1.75 g; 0.5-2 g/day
Per Commission E: 1-2 g of dried root or equivalent preparations

Monitoring Parameters Blood sugar, blood pressure

Contraindications Estrogen-receptor positive breast cancer

Dosage Forms
Capsule: 100 mg
Liquid: 140 mg/15 mL

Overdosage/Treatment Decontamination: Usually decontamination is not required for ingestions under 3 g; lavage (within 1 hour)/activated charcoal can be utilized

Drug Interactions
May decrease effects of loop diuretics (furosemide); theoretically may increase effect of antiplatelet agents, anticoagulants, hypoglycemics, and hypotensive agents
May cause increase in INR when given with warfarin. Avoid aspirin or anticoagulant use due to the antiplatelet effect of *P. ginseng*. Mania can occur when given with phenelzine. Siberian ginseng has been reported to cause elevated digoxin levels when given with digoxin. Insomnia, headaches, irritability, and tremulousness have been reported after simultaneous administration of ginseng and phenelzine.

Pregnancy Implications Not recommended in pregnancy or breast-feeding

Additional Information In U.S., the root crop of ginseng is obtained from *Panax quinquefolius* L (American ginseng) or *Panax trifolius* L (Dwarf ginseng). The plants are found in woody areas and are ~3 feet tall with yellow-green flowers and red/yellow fruits (from June to July). Additional information can be obtained from: Ginseng Board of Wisconsin, 16-H Menard Plaza, Wausau, Wisconsin 54401; (715)845-7300
Capsules: 100-200 mg ginseng claimed per capsule (0.4-23.2 mg of ginsenoside noted per capsule). Most brands contain <8% concentration of ginsenoside/capsule. Contraindicated in diabetes and hypertension. Vaginal administration can cause serious vaginal hemorrhage.

Specific References
Delgoda R and Westlake AC, "Herbal Interactions Involving Cytochrome P450 Enzymes: A Mini Review," *Toxicol Rev*, 2004, 23(4):239-49.
Myles D, "Saving Wild Ginseng, Golden Seal, and Other Native Plants from Mountain Top Removal," *Herbalgram*, 2007, 73: 50-55
Palanisamy A, Haller C, Olson KR, "Photosensitivity Reaction in a Woman Using an Herbal Supplement Containing Ginseng, Goldenseal, and Bee Pollen," *J Toxicol Clin Toxicol*, 2003, 41(6):865-7.
Xin C, Liu J, Li X, et al, "Extraction of 20(S)-Ginsenoside Rg₂ from Cultured *Panax notoginseng* Cells *in vitro* Stimulates Human Umbilical Cord Vein Endothelial Cell Proliferation," *Am J Ther*, 2006, 13(3):205-10.

Golden Seal

Scientific Name *Hydrastis canadensis*
APHA Botanical Safety Rating System Class 2b
Synonyms *Hydrastis canadensis*; Eye Balm; Eye Root; Indian Eye: Orange Root; Jaundice Root; Tumeric Root; Yellow Indian Paint; Yellow Root
Use Gastrointestinal and peripheral vascular activity; also used in sterile eye washes, as a mouthwash, laxative, hemorrhoids, and to stop postpartum hemorrhage. Efficacy not established in clinical studies; has been used to treat mucosal inflammation/gastritis
Mechanism of Action Contains the alkaloids hydrastine (4%) and berberine (6%), which at higher doses can cause vasoconstriction, hypertension, and mucosal irritation; berberine can produce hypotension
Signs and Symptoms of Overdose Brown discoloration of urine, diarrhea, hypotension, mydriasis, nausea, paresthesias, respiratory depression, seizures, uterine contractions, vomiting
Toxicodynamics/Kinetics
Absorption: Oral
Elimination: Renal
Dosage
Solid form: Usual dosage: 5-10 grains
Tea: Prepared from 6 g (10 mL) of the herb in 240 mL of water
Contraindications Pregnancy, breast-feeding

Overdosage/Treatment

Decontamination: Activated charcoal with cathartic

Supportive therapy: Benzodiazepines can be utilized for seizure control

Test Interactions Can produce a false-negative for urinary cannabinoids by immunoassay

Drug Interactions May interfere with vitamin B absorption

Additional Information Not reviewed by Commission E; a perennial with green-white flowers and dark red berries (from April to May) that is found from Vermont to Arkansas

Specific References

Myles D, "Saving wild Ginseng, Goldenseal, and Other Native Plants from Mountain Top Removal" *Herbalgram*, 2007, 73: 50-55

Palanisamy A, Haller C, Olson KR, "Photosensitivity Reaction in a Woman Using an Herbal Supplement Containing Ginseng, Goldenseal, and Bee Pollen," *J Toxicol Clin Toxicol*, 2003, 41(6):865-7.

Hawthorn

Scientific Name *Crataegus laevigata*; *Crataegus monogyna*; *Crataegus oxyacantha*

APHA Botanical Safety Rating System Class 1

U.S. Brand Names Arterio-K®; Basticrat®; Born®; Cardiplant®; Cordapur®; Coronal®; Cratamed®; Naranocor®; Regulacor®

Synonyms *Crataegus laevigata*; *Crataegus monogyna*; *Crataegus oxyacantha*; *Crataegus pinnatifida*; Blackthorn; English Hawthorn; Haw; Maybush; Thorn Plum; Whitehorn

Use In herbal medicine to treat cardiovascular abnormalities (arrhythmia, angina), increased cardiac output, increased contractility of heart muscle; also used as a sedative

Mechanism of Action Contains flavonoids, catechin, and epicatechin which may be cardioprotective and have vasodilatory properties; shown to dilate coronary vessels

Signs and Symptoms of Overdose CNS depression, hypotension, syncope

Dosage

Tincture: 1 teaspoon twice daily for up to several weeks

Tea: 2 teaspoons of crushed leaves or fruit per cup of boiling water

Daily dose of total flavonoids: ~10 mg

Per Commission E: 160-900 mg native water-ethanol extract (ethanol 45% v/v or methanol 70% v/v, drug-extract ratio: 4-7:1, with defined flavonoid or procyanidin content), corresponding to 30-168.7 mg procyanidins, calculated as epicatechin, or 3.5-19.8 mg flavonoids, calculated as hyperoside in accordance with DAB 10 [German pharmacopoeia #10] in 2 or 3 individual doses; duration of administration: 6 weeks minimum

Contraindications Pregnancy and breast-feeding

Overdosage/Treatment

Decontamination: Lavage (within 1 hour)/activated charcoal with cathartic

Supportive therapy: Treat hypotension with I.V. crystalloid infusion and placement in Trendelenburg position; vasopressor agents can be used in refractory cases

Drug Interactions Antihypertensives (effect enhanced), digoxin; effects with Viagra® unknown

Pregnancy Implications Do not use

Additional Information A small deciduous tree which can grow up to 25'; its white, strongly aromatic flowers bloom in mid to late spring; tincture has a bitter taste

Hops

Scientific Name *Humulus lupulus*

APHA Botanical Safety Rating System Class 2d; some writers advise against use in depression

Synonyms *Humulus lupulus*; Common Hops; European Hops; Lupulin

Use

In herbal medicine as a sleep aid (sometimes combined with valerian root)

Per Commission E: Mood disturbances such as restlessness and anxiety, sleep disturbances

Mechanism of Action Contains several bitter acids (lupulone, myrcene, humulone) which may have antimicrobial activity, inhibit smooth muscle activity, and exhibit CNS depression; probable dermal irritant

Adverse Reactions None known relating to herb (as per Commission E); Dermatologic: Contact dermatitis (upon exposure to extracts)

Dosage Per Commission E: Single dose: 0.5 g

Overdosage/Treatment Decontamination: **Oral**: **Do not** induce emesis; lavage (within 1 hour)/activated charcoal with cathartic. **Dermal**: Wash with soap and water

Additional Information A perennial, climbing vine with heights up to 25 feet found in Germany and Pacific Northwest; loses most of its activity (85%) after 9 months of storage; not to be confused with Wild Hops (*Bryonia*)

Horse Chestnuts

CAS Number 11072-93-8; 531-75-9; 6805-41-0

Scientific Name *Aesculus hippocastanum*

U.S. Brand Names Aescorin N; Aescuven; Feparil; Flogencyl; Plissamur; Rexiluven S; Réparil; Tecura; Vasotonin; Venoplant; Venostasin

Uses In herbal medicine for treatment of chronic venous insufficiency (varicose veins); I.V. use in Europe to prevent postoperative edema

Mechanism of Toxic Action Contains aesculin, a saponin glycoside with diuretic effects and can reduce lysosomal enzyme activity; also increases venous tone

Adverse Reactions

Per Commission E:

Dermatologic: Pruritus

Gastrointestinal: Nausea, and gastric complaints may occur in isolated cases after oral intake

Signs and Symptoms of Overdose Abdominal pain, cramping, diarrhea, mydriasis, nausea, twitching, vomiting. Could potentially cause kidney damage with a large enough ingestion. Fever (in children), headache, and vomiting can occur after ingesting a single seed. Anaphylaxis and renal failure have been reported following I.V. administration.

Toxicodynamics/Kinetics

Onset: Soon after ingestion

Absorption: Oral: Poor

Protein binding: 50% (in frogs)

Dosage Mild intoxication upon ingestion of berries by children; apparently ingestion of ~20 berries or chewing the fresh bark is necessary to induce pronounced symptoms

Aescin:

Oral: Initial: 90-150 mg

Maintenance daily dose: 35-70 mg

Maximum I.V. dose: 20 mg

Per Commission E: Aescin (escin): 100 mg corresponds to 250-312.5 mg extract twice daily in delayed release form

Reference Range Peak plasma concentration of beta-aesculin after oral ingestion of 300 mg of extract: ~30 ng/mL

Overdosage/Treatment

Decontamination: Ipecac/cathartic not recommended, activated charcoal/lavage (within 1 hour) may be useful; dilute with milk or water; activated charcoal or lavage if 3 or more seeds are ingested

Supportive therapy: Treat any fluid or electrolyte imbalance

Additional Information May color alkaline urine red; do not confuse with hematuria; bitter taste; a large deciduous tree with fruit containing 1-6 seeds and predominantly white flowers found in U.S., Canada, and southeastern Europe

Toxic parts: Fruit, leaves, and bark are poisonous

Kava

CAS Number 495-85-2; 500-62-9; 500-64-1

Scientific Name *Piper methysticum*

APHA Botanical Safety Rating System Class 2d; caution required when driving or when operating other equipment; simultaneous consumption with alcohol or barbiturates may potentiate inebriation

U.S. Brand Names Herbal Ecstacy 2; Herbal Ecstacy; Kavosporal Forte

Synonyms *Piper methysticum*; Awa; Kev; Kew; Tonga

Impairment Potential Yes

Use Conditions of nervous anxiety, stress, and restlessness per Commission E; used for sleep inducement and to reduce anxiety

Mechanism of Action Contains alpha-pyrones in root extracts; may possess central dopaminergic antagonistic properties

Adverse Reactions Central nervous system: Euphoria

Signs and Symptoms of Overdose Ataxia, deafness, extrapyramidal effects, sedation, yellow skin discoloration

Dosage Per Commission E: Herb and preparations equivalent to 60-120 mg kava pyrones

Contraindications Per Commission E: Pregnancy, breast-feeding, endogenous depression. "Extended continuous intake can cause a temporary yellow discoloration of skin, hair and nails. In this case, further application must be discontinued. In rare cases, allergic skin reactions occur. Also, accommodative disturbances (eg, enlargement of the pupils and disturbances of the oculomotor equilibrium) have been described."

Overdosage/Treatment

Decontamination: Lavage (within 1 hour)/activated charcoal with cathartic

Supportive therapy: Can treat extrapyramidal reactions with benztropine and/or diphenhydramine

Drug Interactions Coma can occur from concomitant administration of kava and alprazolam; may potentiate alcohol or CNS depressants, barbiturates, psychopharmacological agents

Pregnancy Risk Factor Contraindicated per Commission E

Pregnancy Implications Do not use

Additional Information Social and ceremonial drink in South Pacific islands; has medicinal use as a G.U. antiseptic, antipyretic, diuretic, local anesthetic, and muscle relaxant agent; shrubs can grow 8-20 feet tall with green stems and rounded fruit; characteristic yellow discoloration rash resembles pellagra, but does not respond to nicotinamide

Kava lactones detected in urine by gas chromatography/mass spectrometry following ingestion of 450 g of commercial kava: Dihydrokawain, kawain, desmethoxyyangonin, tetrahydroyangonin, dihydromethysticin, 11-methoxytetrahydroyangonin, yangonin, methysticin, dehydromethysticin

Specific References

Clough AR, Bailie RS, and Currie B, "Liver Function Test Abnormalities in Users of Aqueous Kava Extracts," *J Toxicol Clin Toxicol*, 2003, 41(6):821-9.

Delgoda R and Westlake AC, "Herbal Interactions Involving Cytochrome P450 Enzymes: A Mini Review," *Toxicol Rev*, 2004, 23(4):239-49.

Dennehy CE, Tsourounis C, and Miller AE, "Evaluation of Herbal Dietary Supplements Marketed on the Internet for Recreational Use," *Ann Pharmacother*, 2005, 39(10):1634-9.

Humberston CL, Akhtar J, and Krenzelok EP, "Acute Hepatitis Induced by Kava Kava," *J Toxicol Clin Toxicol*, 2003, 41(2):109-13.

Schmidt, M, "Quality Criteria for Kava," *Herbalgram*, 2007, 73:44-49.

Kombucha

Synonyms Kargasok "Tea"; Kombucha Mushroom; Kombucha Tea; Kwassan; Manchurian Tea; Manchurian "Fungus"; T'Chai from the Sea; Teekwass; "Fungus" Japonica

Uses Folk/herbal remedy used to relieve arthritis; treat insomnia, hypertension, ache; stimulate hair growth; used by AIDS patients to stimulate the immune (T-cell) system (all these actions are unproven); other claims include elimination of wrinkles and cleansing the gallbladder; has been used in alternative medicine for HIV therapy although its use has markedly decreased

Mechanism of Toxic Action Unknown bacterial products may affect gut's bacterial flora

Adverse Reactions

Central nervous system: Coma

Dermatologic: Erythematous rash

Endocrine & metabolic: Severe metabolic acidosis

Gastrointestinal: Anorexia

Hepatic: Hepatotoxicity, hepatitis, hepatomegaly

Hematologic: Thrombocytopenia, disseminated intravascular coagulopathy

Respiratory: Cough (nonproductive)

Signs and Symptoms of Overdose Abdominal cramping, allergic symptoms, anorexia, chest pain, cough, elevated prothrombin time, erythematous rash, hepatomegaly, hepatotoxicity (usually resolves within a month), nausea, thrombocytopenia

Dosage 4-8 ounces/day

Overdosage/Treatment Decontamination: Lavage (within 1 hour)/activated charcoal with cathartic

Supportive therapy: Symptoms are usually self limited

Additional Information

Due to acidic nature of the tea (pH is ~1.8), it should not be prepared or stored in ceramic or lead crystal containers. During fermentation process, ethanol (up to 1.5%), ethyl acetate, acetic acid, lactic acid, glucuronic acid, heparin, hyaluronic acid, chondroitin sulfate acid, mukoitin sulfate, or lactic acid may be produced. Found as a gray, flat patty (3" in diameter) which is fermented in black tea and sugar. A 6" wide gray fungus that is often ingested in sugared tea after fermentation; production of 0.5% alcohol, glucuronic acid, hyaluronic acid, chondroitin sulfate acid, usnic acid, mukoitin sulfate, heparin, lactic acid along with *Acetobacter ketogenum* and *Pichia fermentans* has been associated with the tea; not a fungus but a fungal symbiot that is a 6" patty which has been used in Asia and Europe as an unproven therapeutic agent for rheumatism, intestinal disorders, and premenstrual syndrome.

Usually referred to as a mushroom, several species of yeast and bacteria are held together by a thin membrane. Some species associated with the Kombucha colony include *S. ludwigii*, *S. pombe*, *Bacterium xylinum*, *Acetobacter ketogenum*, *S. gluconicum*, *B. xylinoides*, *B. katogenum*, *Pichia fermentans*, and *Torula* sp, *Saccharomyces cerevisiae*, and *Candida valida*. In addition, contamination with *Aspergillus* may be present.

Laetrile®

Related Information

- Amyl Nitrite [ANTIDOTE]
- Cyanide

CAS Number 1332-94-1; 29883-15-6

Synonyms Amygdalin; Vitamin B$_{12}$; Vitamin B$_{17}$

Uses While it has been used for cancer therapy, it is ineffective and no known medicinal or nutritional value exists.

Mechanism of Toxic Action Releases cyanide within the GI tract through enzymatic degradation by betaglucosidase or emulsion; intrave-

nous laetrile does not result in cyanide exposure; synthesized from Amygdalin (mandelonitrile beta-d-gentiobioside)

Signs and Symptoms of Overdose Coma, headache, hypotension, metabolic acidosis, seizures, tachycardia, tachypnea, vomiting

Reference Range 500 mg 3 times/day results in blood cyanide level of 2.1 mcg/mL

Overdosage/Treatment

Decontamination: Basic poison management (lavage within 1 hour/activated charcoal with cathartic); emesis is contraindicated due to rapid course of the neurologic symptoms; give 100% oxygen

Supportive therapy: Give sodium bicarbonate for acidosis; cyanide antidote kit (amyl nitrate, sodium nitrate followed by sodium thiosulfate)

Enhancement of elimination: Hemodialysis and charcoal hemoperfusion have been utilized; hyperbaric oxygen may also be utilized; hydroxocobalamin, dicobalt-EDTA, and 4-dimethylaminophenol used for chelation in Europe

Antidote(s)

- Cyanide Antidote Kit [ANTIDOTE]
- Hydroxocobalamin [ANTIDOTE]
- Oxygen (Hyperbaric) [ANTIDOTE]
- Sodium Nitrite [ANTIDOTE]
- Sodium Thiosulfate [ANTIDOTE]

Additional Information Usual commercial source is from the kernel of *Prunus armeniaca*. A 500 mg laetrile tablet may contain between 5-51 mg of hydrogen cyanide per gram.

Lemon Grass Oil

Scientific Name *Andropogon citratus*; *Cymbopogon citratus*

APHA Botanical Safety Rating System Class 2b (herb)

Synonyms Capim-Cidrao; Guatemala Lemongrass; Lemongrass; Madagascar Lemongrass

Use Perfumes; flavoring agent; used also as a hypotensive and carminative in folk medicine

Mechanism of Action Major active ingredient is citral which is an irritant and has sedative effect (by decreasing neuronal activity)

Signs and Symptoms of Overdose Allergic contact dermatitis, CNS depression at high doses, mucosal irritation, skin irritation with citral concentrations >8%

Admission Criteria/Prognosis Admit any ingestion >1 mL/kg

Toxicodynamics/Kinetics

Absorption: Rapidly absorbed orally, can be absorbed dermally

Metabolism: Hepatic

Elimination: Renal

Dosage Acceptable daily intake for food: 500 mcg of citral

Overdosage/Treatment Decontamination: **Oral**: Dilute with milk or water. **Dermal**: Wash with cool water (warm water may increase severity of reactions). **Ocular**: Irrigate copiously with saline

Additional Information Not widely used in U.S. market as an herbal dietary supplement; plant is a perennial grass native to Ceylon and Southern India

Licorice

Scientific Name *Glycyrrhiza glabra*; *Glycyrrhiza lepidota*; *Glycyrrhiza uralensis*

APHA Botanical Safety Rating System Class 2b, 2c, 2d; not for prolonged use or in high doses except under supervision of 2 qualified health practitioners; contraindicated for diabetes and in hypertension, liver disorders, severe kidney insufficiency, and hypokalemia; may potentiate potassium depletion of thiazide diuretics and stimulant laxatives, and cardiac glycosides and cortisol

U.S. Brand Names DGL Licorice

Synonyms *G. palidiflora*; *G. uralensis*; *Glycyrrhiza glabra*; Glycocome; Lakriment Neu; Liquorice; Sweet Root; Ulgastrin Neo

Use

Foodstuff in chewing gum, chewing tobacco, cough preparations

Per Commission E: Catarrhs of the upper respiratory tract and gastric/duodenal ulcers

Mechanism of Action From the root of the plants *Glycyrrhiza glabra*, *Glycyrrhiza lepidota*, *Glycyrrhiza uralensis*; the toxic component is glycyrrhizic acid which inhibits enzymes in the degradation of mineralocorticoid hormones (aldosterone); also may act as a mineralocorticoid; inhibits steroid dehydrogenase and release enzymes

Adverse Reactions

Cardiovascular: Hypertension, edema

Central nervous system: Headache, seizures, tetany

Endocrine & metabolic: Amenorrhea, hyponatremia, hypokalemia, hypomagnesemia

Neuromuscular & skeletal: Myopathy, carpopedal spasms, rhabdomyolysis

Ocular: Bilateral ptosis

Renal: Myoglobinuria

Per Commission E: On prolonged use and with higher doses, mineral corticoid effects may occur in the form of sodium and water retention and potassium loss, accompanied by hypertension, edema, and hypokalemia, and in rare cases, myoglobinuria

Toxicodynamics/Kinetics
Metabolism: Glycyrrhizic acid is converted to glycyrrhetic acid
Half-life: Glycyrrhizic acid: 5 hours
Elimination: Fecal: 53% to 61%

Dosage 100 g (equivalent to 700 mg of glycyrrhizinic acid) of licorice found in 2-4 licorice twists; toxic effect can be seen if ingested daily (2-3 twists) for 2-4 weeks

Per Commission E: 5-15 g root/day, equivalent to 200-600 mg glycyrrhizin; succus liquiritiae (juice): 0.5-1 g for catarrhs of upper respiratory tract; 1.5-3 g for gastric/duodenal ulcers; equivalent preparations

Contraindications Per Commission E: Cholestatic liver disorders, liver cirrhosis, hypertonia, hypokalemia, severe kidney insufficiency, pregnancy

Reference Range Peak plasma concentration of glycyrrhetic acid after 100 mg oral dose: ~0.2 mcg/mL

Overdosage/Treatment Supportive therapy: Fluid/electrolyte (especially potassium) replacement; spironolactone (1 g/day in divided doses) also may be useful in reversing electrolyte abnormalities; tetany can be treated with magnesium sulfate

Drug Interactions
Attenuated effect of strychnine, tetrodoxine, nicotine, cocaine, barbiturates, pilocarpine, urethane, epinephrine, and ephedrine through glucuronic-like conjugation action; traditional emmenagogue; increases progesterone and cortisol half-life; concomitant use of furosemide can exacerbate hypokalemia
Per Commission E: Potassium loss due to other drugs (eg, thiazide diuretics), can be increased; with potassium loss, sensitivity to digitalis glycosides increases

Pregnancy Risk Factor Contraindicated per Commission E

Additional Information Syndrome of pseudoprimary hyperaldosteronism is a complication of chronic licorice ingestion; serum potassium as low as 0.9 mM/L has been noted; licorice ingestion can result in serum testosterone decreases and an increase in serum 17-hydroxy-progesterone
Reference range: Ingestions of 2-4 licorice twists daily (100 g of licorice) for 2-4 weeks can result in a plasma glycyrrhetic acid level of up to 480 ng/mL; renin, antidiuretic hormone, aldosterone, potassium levels fall; elevated prolactin levels may occur. Daily use of 20-40 g can result in severe hypokalemia.

Specific References
Cinatl J, Morgenstern B, Bauer G, et al, "Glycyrrhizin, An Active Component of Liquorice Roots, and Replication of SARS-Associated Coronavirus," *Lancet*, 2003, 361(9374):2045-6.
Delgoda R and Westlake AC, "Herbal Interactions Involving Cytochrome P450 Enzymes: A Mini Review," *Toxicol Rev*, 2004, 23(4):239-49.

Lobelia

Scientific Name *Lobelia inflata*
APHA Botanical Safety Rating System Class 2b, 2d; may cause nausea and vomiting; not to be taken in large doses; dose-dependent cardioactivity has been observed
U.S. Brand Names Bantron Smoking Deterrent Tablets; Lobatox; Lobidram Computabs; Nikoban; Refrane; Stop Smoke
Synonyms *Lobela inflata*; Bladder-Pod; Emetic Herb; Eye-Bright; Indian Tobacco; Kinnikinnik; Lobelia Herb; Low Belia; Puke Weed; Wild Tobacco
Use In herbal medicine as an expectorant, relief of muscle spasms; also incorporated (in doses of 2-4 mg) in tablets/lozenges or chewing gum to aid in smoking cessation
Mechanism of Action Plant contains ≈0.48% of pyridine-derived alkaloids (lobeline, lobelanine, lobelanidine); Lobeline acts similarly to nicotine as a stimulant with ≈5% to 20% of its potency
Signs and Symptoms of Overdose Abdominal pain, coma, dermal irritation, diaphoresis, euphoria, hypertension, hypothermia, nausea, paralysis, respiratory depression, salivation, seizures, tachycardia, vomiting
Toxicodynamics/Kinetics Absorption: Orally, dermally, and through inhalation
Dosage Toxic dose:
Dried herb: 50 mg
Lobelia, tincture: 1 mL
Lobeline: 8 mg
Toxic daily dose: >20 mg
Therapeutic dose:
Lobeline hydrochloride:
SubQ: 10 mg (up to 20 mg/day)
I.V.: 3 mg (maximum daily dose: 20 mg)
Lobeline sulfate: 2-4 mg
Overdosage/Treatment
Decontamination:
Oral: **Do not** induce emesis; lavage (within 1 hour)/ingestions >8 mg of lobeline, 50 mg of dried herb or 1 mL of tincture of lobelia; activated charcoal with cathartic can then be used

Occular: Irrigate with saline copiously
Dermal: Wash with soap and water
Supportive therapy: Seizures can be treated with benzodiazepines; phenobarbital or phenytoin can be used for refractory seizures; hypotension can be treated with intravenous fluid bolus (10-20 mL/kg) and placement in Trendelenburg position; dopamine or norepinephrine can be used for refractory cases
Additional Information Not reviewed by Commission E; found in eastern North America with small, pale blue flowers; acrid/bitter taste; can cause euphoria; an annual weed which grows by roadsides and in open woods; irritating odor

Margosa Oil

Synonyms Azadirachta
Use A folk remedy in India, Japan, and Southeast Asia; antihelminthic, insecticidal, or analgesic agent; an extract from the dried stem bark and tree leaves of *Azadirachta indica* (Neem tree)
Mechanism of Action Irritant: CNS stimulant; toxin (an unsaturated hydroxy-aldehyde) appears to be heat stable
Adverse Reactions
Cardiovascular: Reye's-like syndrome, cerebral edema
Central nervous system: Lethargy, seizures, coma
Endocrine & metabolic: Metabolic acidosis
Gastrointestinal: Vomiting (15 minutes to 4 hours)
Hematology: Leukocytosis
Hepatic: Steatosis of the liver
Neuromuscular & skeletal: Tremor
Respiratory: Tachypnea, dyspnea
Overdosage/Treatment
Decontamination: **Do not** induce emesis; lavage within 1 hour (if spontaneous emesis has not already occurred), activated charcoal with cathartic
Supportive therapy: Benzodiazepines have been used to treat seizures; paraldehyde has also been used to terminate seizures; mannitol and/or dexamethasone should be used to treat cerebral edema
Additional Information Not generally available in U.S. market; not listed with Commission E; some Neem extracts are used as ingredients in imported (from India) toothpastes and in natural cosmetics, but **not** as a dietary supplement for oral consumption

Maté

Scientific Name *Ilex paraguariensis*
APHA Botanical Safety Rating System Class 2d; not recommended for excessive or long-term use
Synonyms *Ilex paraguariensis*; Jesuit's Tea; Paraguay Tea; St Bartholomew's Tea
Use
Herbal medicine as a depurative, stimulant, and diuretic
Per Commission E: Physical fatigue
Mechanism of Action Plant contains caffetanin; leaves contain rutin, alpha-amyrin, trigonelline, choline and ursolic acid; teas contain caffeine; may also contain belladonna alkaloids as a contamination
Adverse Reactions
Cardiovascular: Tachycardia
Central nervous system: Fever, disorientation
Dermatologic: Flushed skin
Gastrointestinal: Xerostomia
Genitourinary: Urinary retention
Ocular: Mydriasis
Miscellaneous: Incidence of esophageal cancer and bladder cancer increased when used with tobacco (in chronic users)
Dosage One cup of maté (6 ounces) is equivalent to 25-50 mg of caffeine
Per Commission E: Daily dose: 3 g of drug (dried herb); equivalent preparations
Overdosage/Treatment
Decontamination: Lavage (within 1 hour)/activated charcoal with cathartic
Supportive therapy: Physostigmine (0.5 mg in children, up to 4 mg in adult as a total dose) has been used to treat severe anticholinergic toxicity due to ingestion of Paraguay tea contaminated with anticholinergic agents. This modality should not be used for treating effects of caffeine exposure.
Additional Information A climbing evergreen shrub which can grow to 20 feet; native to South American countries; greenish white flowers with small deep red berries; leaves contain as much as 2% caffeine along with theophylline (0.05%); teas should be used with caution in patients with elevated blood pressure, diabetes, or ulcer disease

Melaleuca Oil

CAS Number 8022-72-8
Scientific Name *Melaleuca alternifolia*
U.S. Brand Names Amber Gold; Dessert Essence

Synonyms Australian Tree Oil; Tea Tree Oil; Ti-Tree Oil

Use Marketed as having fungicidal, bactericidal properties; also used as a topical dermal agent for burns

Mechanism of Action Consists of plant terpenes, pinenes, and cineole, derived from the *Melaleuca alternifolia* tree, the colorless or pale yellow oil can cause CNS depression

Signs and Symptoms of Overdose Aspiration pneumonitis, ataxia, CNS depression, lethargy

Admission Criteria/Prognosis Admit any patient who is symptomatic 5 hours postexposure

Toxicodynamics/Kinetics Metabolism: Hepatic

Dosage Minimal toxic dose: Infant: <10 mL

Monitoring Parameters Pulse oximetry

Overdosage/Treatment Decontamination: Activated charcoal with cathartic

Additional Information

Oral: Mildly toxic. Dermal: Very mild irritant; no dermal sensitization; no phototoxicity

Found in New South Wales (Australia) on the north coast in swampy lowlands, this paper-bark tree can grow up to 20 feet high; the tree may also be found in southern U.S. (Florida), Spain, or Portugal; nutmeg odor; has been used to treat acne vulgaris, athlete's foot, and vaginitis

Specific References

Morris MC, Donoghue A, Markowitz JA, et al, "Ingestion of Tea Tree Oil (Melaleuca Oil) by a 4-Year-Old Boy," *Pediatr Emerg Care*, 2003, 19(3):169-171.

Nettles

Scientific Name *Urtica dioica*; *Urtica parviflora*; *Urtica urens*

APHA Botanical Safety Rating System Class 1 (leaf)

Synonyms Stinging Nettles

Uses Root extracts used in herbal medicine for treatment of urinary difficulties due to enlarged prostate (prostate adenoma stages 1 and 11); leaf extracts have been used topically for rheumatic disorders

Mechanism of Toxic Action Unknown; the hairs on stems and leaves contain dermal irritants (histamine, acetylcholine, and 5-hydroxytryptamine); also may have a diuretic action

Adverse Reactions

Dermatologic: Dermal irritation/stinging may last up to 12 hours; burning sensation, contact urticaria, nonimmunologic contact urticaria

Neuromuscular & skeletal: Paresthesias

Dosage Prostatic hypertrophy: 4-6 g/day or as a fluid extract from roots: 5 mL every 8 hours for 6 months

Leaf: 8-12 g/day

Overdosage/Treatment

Decontamination: **Dermal**: Wash with soap and water. **Oral**: Ipecac within 30 minutes or lavage (within 1 hour)/activated charcoal with cathartic

Supportive therapy: Topical steroids or systemic antihistamines may be useful to treat dermal irritation; brush and wash exposed clothing

Additional Information A perennial plant which has stems which can grow to 6 feet; the stems and leaves contain the toxic bristles or stinging hairs; fresh tender shoots do not cause stinging sensation; also boiling or drying can eliminate the stinging sensation; small, greenish flowers bloom from June through September; young roots are edible when cooked and contain significant amounts of carotene and vitamin C; contraindications in pregnancy

---

Nutmeg

Scientific Name *Myristica fragrans*

APHA Botanical Safety Rating System Class 2b; Class 3; **Note**: Classification and concerns are based on therapeutic use, not relevant to consumption as a spice

Use In folk medicine for delayed menses

Mechanism of Action One theory for nutmeg's pharmacologic properties is that myristicin and elemicin are metabolized to psychoactive amphetamine derivatives, MMDA (3-methoxy-4,5 dimethylenedioxyamphetamine) and TMA (3,4,5-trimethoxyamphetamine); geraniol is a potent emetic

Adverse Reactions

Cardiovascular: Sinus tachycardia

Endocrine & metabolic: Abortion

Signs and Symptoms of Overdose The most prominent effects of significant ingestions include hallucinations, nausea, and profound vomiting. Dry skin, feeling of impending doom, hypotension, hypothermia, miosis, mydriasis, and tachycardia may also be seen. Symptoms may be delayed up to 8 hours after ingestion.

Dosage It is estimated that 2 tablespoons of ground nutmeg will produce toxicity; however, amounts may vary depending on the content of volatile oil. See Additional Information

Overdosage/Treatment

Decontamination: Administer activated charcoal with cathartic for recent substantial ingestions

Supportive therapy: Symptomatic and supportive treatment as needed

Drug Interactions

Decreased effect of antihypertensives

Increased toxicity with disulfiram (possible seizures, delirium), fluoxetine (and other serotonin active agents), TCAs (cardiovascular instability), meperidine (cardiovascular instability), phenothiazine (hyperpyretic crisis), levodopa, sympathomimetics (hyperpyretic crisis), barbiturates, Rauwolfia alkaloids (eg, reserpine), dextroamphetamine (psychoses), foods containing tyramine (hypertension, headache, seizures); theophylline/caffeine (hyperthermia), cyclobenzaprine (fever/seizures)

Potentiation of hypoglycemia with oral hypoglycemic agents

Serotonin syndrome (shivering, muscle rigidity, salivation, agitation, and hyperthermia) can occur with concomitant administration of venlafaxine and tranylcypromine

Pregnancy Implications Nutmeg ingestion has been reported to increase fetal heart rate

Additional Information

Toxic dose: 1-3 nutmegs can cause toxic symptoms

Toxic parts: Volatile oil in seed and seed coat appears to be responsible for pharmacologic effects

Nutmeg is the seed of *Myristica fragrans*; the spice mace is from the seed coat of *Myristica fragrans*

Family: Myristicaceae

Toxin: Myristicin, elemicin, geraniol

Range: Grows in India, Ceylon, and Grenada

Passion Flower

Scientific Name *Passiflora incarnata*

U.S. Brand Names Sedacalm®

Synonyms *Passiflora* spp; Apricot Vine; Maypop; Passion Vine

Use Mild insomnia, neuralgia, anxiety; sedative (Wolfman, 1994; Speroni, 1988)

Mechanism of Action

The constituents, maltol and ethylmaltol, have been shown to produce central nervous system sedation and a reduction in spontaneous motor activity (low doses) in laboratory animals. In humans, passion flower may be effective when used in combination with other sedative and antianxiety herbs such as valerian. These effects may be due to synergism, but also may be due to the potential binding of passion flower constituents to benzodiazepine receptors *in vivo*.

Contains flavonoids (vitexin, isvitexin, apigenin, schaftoside, isoschaftoside, and swertisin) and harmane alkaloids (concentration <0.01%) which may affect neurotransmitter metabolism and exhibit a motility inhibiting effect on smooth muscle in animal studies (as per Commission E).

Adverse Reactions

Cardiovascular: Bradycardia, ventricular bigeminy, ventricular tachycardia, prolonged QT interval, U waves on ECG

Central nervous system: Lethargy

Dermatologic: Urticaria

Gastrointestinal: Nausea, vomiting

Respiratory: IgE mediated occupational asthma, rhinitis

Admission Criteria/Prognosis Admit any ingestion >1 g/kg or any symptomatic patient.

Dosage Sedacalm®: 500 mg to 1 g, 3 times/day; up to 8 g daily of active drug has been recommended

Contraindications Based on pharmacological effects, may cause drowsiness; use caution when driving an automobile or operating heavy machinery. Use with caution in individuals taking antianxiety agents, antidepressants, hypnotics, or sedatives. Reported in animal studies to increase sleeping time induced by hexobarbital (Aoyagi, 1974).

Warnings Use all herbal supplements with extreme caution in children <2 years of age and in pregnancy or lactation. Some herbs are contraindicated in pregnancy or lactation; make sure to observe warnings. Use with caution in individuals on medication and with pre-existing medical conditions. Always review for potential herb-drug interactions (HDIs) and other warnings. Large and prolonged doses may increase the potential for adverse effects. Herbs may cause transient adverse effects such as nausea, vomiting, and GI distress due to a variety of chemical constituents. Caution should be used in individuals having known allergies to plants.

Overdosage/Treatment

Decontamination: Lavage within 1 hour/activated charcoal without cathartic

Supportive therapy: Antiemetics and crystalloid I.V. fluids can be utilized for dehydration

Drug Interactions Anxiolytics, antidepressants, barbiturates, sedatives

Additional Information A perennial climbing vine with large (5-9 cm) white, blue, purple, or pale red flowers and a yellow oval fruit. The woody stem may be as long as 10 meters in length. The plant is usually found in the Southeast U.S. and South America.

Specific References

Wolfman C, Viola H, Paladini A, et al, "Possible Anxiolytic Effects of Chrysin, A Central Benzodiazepine Receptor Ligand Isolated from *Passiflora coerulea*," *Pharmacol Biochem Behav*, 1994 47(1):1-4

Pennyroyal Oil

CAS Number 8007-44-1
APHA Botanical Safety Rating System
Class 2b
Synonyms *Mentha pulegium*; Pulegium Oil
Use Insect repellent; inducing delayed menses, rubefacient; is used primarily by natural health advocates (not FDA approved for stated use)
Mechanism of Action Derived from the herbs European pennyroyal (*Mentha pulegium*) and American pennyroyal (*Hedeoma pulegioides*); contain several monoterpenes, one of which (pulegone) is hepatotoxic by causing depletion of glutathione
Adverse Reactions
Cardiovascular: Hypotension
Central nervous system: Confusion, delirium, agitation, hallucinations (auditory and visual), seizures (within 3 hours)
Endocrine & metabolic: Abortifacient, menstrual bleeding
Gastrointestinal: Nausea, vomiting, abdominal pain
Hematologic: Hemolytic anemia, disseminated intravascular coagulation
Hepatic: Hepatic failure, centrilobular necrosis
Renal: Renal failure, hematuria, acute tubular necrosis
Respiratory: Epistaxis
Admission Criteria/Prognosis Patients can be discharged home if asymptomatic 4 hours postingestion; admit any adult ingestion >5 mL
Toxicodynamics/Kinetics
Absorption: Oral: Good
Metabolism: Hepatic to menthofuran (toxic metabolite)
Half-life: 2.2 hours (animals)
Dosage Oil dose used for above purposes: 0.12-0.6 mL
Reference Range Menthofuran serum levels of 10 ng/mL and 41 ng/mL associated with multiple organ failure in infants
Overdosage/Treatment
Decontamination: Due to aspiration risk, **do not** induce emesis; lavage (within 1 hour) is recommended; activated charcoal (with cathartic) may be useful
Supportive therapy: N-acetylcysteine (loading dose: 140 mg/kg, then 70 mg/kg every 4 hours) should be administered within the first few hours postingestion for ingestions >10 mL; benzodiazepines can be used for seizures
Additional Information Fatal dose: 15 mL. Not reviewed by Commission E; mint-like odor; pulegone may deplete glutathione stores in the liver; a yellow oil; hepatotoxicity has occurred after drinking teas from the herb; should not be taken internally; postmortem pulegone and menthofuran levels in a fatality were 18 ng/mL and 1 ng/mL respectively; a menthofuran level of 40 ng/mL obtained 10 hours postingestion associated with mild toxicity
Specific References
Mullen WH, Camarata G, Bergman K, et al, "First Use of IV N-Acetylcysteine in a Pennyroyal Oil Poisoning," *Clin Toxicol (Phila)*, 2005, 43:763.
Sztajnkrycer MD, Otten EJ, Bond GR, et al, "Mitigation of Pennyroyal Oil Hepatotoxicity in the Mouse," *Acad Emerg Med*, 2003, 10(10):1024-8.

Peppermint Oil

CAS Number 8006-90-4
Scientific Name *Mentha piperita*
APHA Botanical Safety Rating System Class 1 (leaf); oil not listed
U.S. Brand Names China Maze; Cholaktol; Citaethol; Colpermin; Kiminto; Mentacur; Mintec
Uses
Fragrant/flavoring agent; this volatile oil is also used in herbal medicine as a spasmolytic (for upper GI tract/bile duct); for irritable bowel syndrome; antibacterial agent; treatment for nausea and dyspepsia; none of these uses are FDA approved
Per Commission E: External use: Myalgia and neuralgia
Mechanism of Toxic Action The oil contains menthol (29% to 48%), menthone (20% to 31%), and methyl acetate (3% to 10%) along with small quantities of eucalyptol and azulene; may have spasmolytic activity on smooth muscles
Adverse Reactions
Cardiovascular: Flushing
Central nervous system: Headache
Dermatologic: Contact dermatitis, urticaria, erythematous
Signs and Symptoms of Overdose Menthol is the major toxic constituent. Abdominal pain, ataxia, atrial fibrillation, bradycardia, coma, dizziness, lethargy, nausea, skin rash, tremor, vomiting, vertigo
Admission Criteria/Prognosis Admit adult ingestions >1 g of peppermint oil

Toxicodynamics/Kinetics
Absorption: Rapid
Metabolism (menthol): To menthol glucuronide
Dosage
Peppermint oil: 0.2-0.4 mL 3 times/day
Peppermint spirit (10% peppermint oil and 15% peppermint leaf extract): 1 mL (20 drops) with water
Toxic dose: 0.3 g (12 drops of pure oil)
Per Commission E:
Daily internal dose: 6-12 drops
Irritable colon: Single dose: 0.2 mL
Enterically coated form, daily dose: 0.6 mL
Inhalation: 3-4 drops in hot H_2O
External: Semisolid preparations: 5% to 20%
Aqueous-alcohol preparations: 5% to 10%
Nasal ointments: 1% to 5% oil
Reference Range Peak urinary total menthol content following ingestion of 0.6 mL of peppermint oil: ~117 mg
Overdosage/Treatment
Decontamination:
Oral: Lavage (within 1 hour)/activated charcoal with cathartic; **do not** induce emesis
Ocular: Irrigate copiously with saline or water
Supportive therapy: Symptomatic bradycardia can be treated with atropine (although this has not been formally studied)
Additional Information Peppermint plant is a perennial with purple/lilac-colored flowers and yields up to 1% volatile oil; do not give to children; contraindications in pregnancy, cholecystitis, and hepatic damage

Polygonum multiflorum

Synonyms Chinese Cornbind; Fo-Ti; He Shou-Wu
Use Tuberous root (raw or processed) used for vertigo, insomnia, constipation
Mechanism of Action Contains 2 anthraquinones (emodin and physcin) which may cause catharsis and a toxic hepatitis
Adverse Reactions
Cardiovascular: Palpitations
Central nervous system: Dizziness, fever
Dermatologic: Erythema, rash, pruritus, photosensitivity
Gastrointestinal: Nausea, diarrhea
Hepatic: Hepatitis, jaundice
Ocular: Blurred vision
Respiratory: Tachypnea
Overdosage/Treatment Supportive therapy: Hepatitis can resolve within 3 weeks upon discontinuation of drug; antihistamines can be used for pruritus
Additional Information A climbing evergreen plant native in Japan

Propolis

Synonyms Bee Glue; Bee Propolis; Hive Dross
Uses Has been advocated as an anti-inflammatory agent, antibacterial agent (for treatment of tuberculosis), treatment for gastric or duodenal ulcers, superficial dermal infections
Mechanism of Toxic Action A natural resin obtained from the buds of conifers or poplar trees; collected and used by honey bees to seal their hives; most of the anti-inflammatory properties seem to be due to its flavonoid pigments; aqueous extract of propolis can inhibit the enzyme dihydrofolate reductase; a dermal sensitizing agent; has been known to cause hypersensitivity reactions; contains flavonoids, phenolic acids, hydrogen peroxide, and pollen (5%); a component of honey; a known free radical scavenger
Signs and Symptoms of Overdose No systemic toxicity seen; local dermatitis, erythema, and pruritus may occur; oral ulceration/mucositis can occur with lozenges
Overdosage/Treatment
Decontamination: Dermal: Wash with soap and water
Supportive therapy: Topical corticosteroids with diphenhydramine can be used to treat propolis-induced dermatitis
Specific References
Cohen HA, Varsano I, Kahan E, et al, "Effectiveness of an Herbal Preparation Containing Echinacea, Propolis, and Vitamin C in Preventing Respiratory Tract Infections in Children: A Randomized, Double-Blind, Placebo-Controlled, Multicenter Study," *Arch Pediatr Adolesc Med*, 2004, 158(3):217-21.

Psoralea Corylifolia

Synonyms Babchi; Boh-Gol-Zhee; Pa-Go-Zhee
Use Folk remedy prevalent in Far East Asia for management of osteoporosis, osteomalacia, bone fractures; also has been used to treat psoriasis and vitiligo. Usually dried mature seeds or leaves are used daily, often in tea-form.

Mechanism of Action Seeds contain psoralen, isosoralen, and psoralidin which are potent cell growth inhibitors; leaves contain genistein - a phytoestrogen

Signs and Symptoms of Overdose Photodermatitis (from seeds), cholestatic hepatitis, jaundice, elevated transaminase

Overdosage/Treatment

Oral:

Decontamination: Activated charcoal is of uncertain benefit

Supportive care: Monitor liver function tests

Additional Information Native to India; herbaceous plant of the leyominosae family with pea-like flowers

Specific References

Nam SW, Baek JT, Lee DS, et al, "A Case of Acute Cholestatic Hepatitis Associated with the Seeds of Psoralea Corylifolia (Boh-Gol-Zhee)," *Clin Toxicol*, 2005, 43(6):589-91.

Pygeum africanum

U.S. Brand Names Tadenan

Uses Treatment of mild to moderate benign prostatic hyperplasia

Mechanism of Toxic Action Contains beta-sitosterol (a phytosterol) which competes with androgens, thus decreasing intraprostatic prostaglandin levels. The pentacyclic triterpenes also reduce inflammation and edema through inhibition of glycosyl-transferase activity. Androgen synthesis in the prostate is also inhibited by ferulic acid esters of fatty alcohols.

Adverse Reactions Gastrointestinal: GI upset

Dosage Oral: 50 mg twice daily (tablets); maximum daily dose: 200 mg

Overdosage/Treatment Decontamination: Gastric decontamination should probably occur for ingestions >500 mg. Lavage within 1 hour and/or activated charcoal should be used.

Additional Information Found in the bark of the evergreen African prune tree. Commonly used as a second-line agent if *Serenoa repens* (saw palmetto) is unsuccessful. Not evaluated by Commission E.

Reishi Mushroom

Scientific Name *Ganoderma lucidum*

Uses Antineoplastic/immune stimulant agent in herbal medicine

Mechanism of Toxic Action Contains ganoderan B which can induce hepatic enzymes and increase plasma insulin levels

Adverse Reactions

Central nervous system: Dizziness

Dermatologic: Dermatitis, pruritus

Gastrointestinal: Diarrhea

Neuromuscular & skeletal: Bone pain

Overdosage/Treatment Decontamination: Lavage (within 1 hour)/activated charcoal with cathartic

Supportive therapy: Oral antihistamines can be used to treat pruritus

Additional Information Contraindications with hemophilia (due to high adenosine content); an edible brown mushroom found on California hardwoods

Rhubarb

Scientific Name *Rheum officinale*; *Rheum palmatum*; *Rheum rhaponticum*

APHA Botanical Safety Rating System Class 2b, 2d; contraindicated in intestinal obstruction, abdominal pain of unknown origin, or any inflammatory condition of the intestines (appendicitis, colitis, Crohn's disease, irritable bowel, etc), and in children <12; not for long-term use in excess of 8-10 days; individuals with a history of kidney stones should use cautiously

Uses Stimulant laxative; constipation (per Commission E)

Mechanism of Toxic Action Leaves are toxic and contain soluble and insoluble oxalates; contains soluble and insoluble sodium and potassium oxalates

Adverse Reactions

Per Commission E:

Endocrine & metabolic: Disturbances of electrolyte balance, especially potassium deficiency in long-term use/abuse; potassium deficiency can lead to disorders of cardiac function especially with cardiac glycosides, diuretics, and corticoadrenal steroids

Gastrointestinal: Cramp-like discomforts of gastrointestinal tract in single incidents; pseudomelanosis coli in long-term use/abuse

Renal: Albuminuria, hematuria in long-term use/abuse

Signs and Symptoms of Overdose Dermal pain, dermatitis, diarrhea, dysphonia, edema, feces discoloration (yellow-green), hypocalcemia, irritation, oxalate crystals may be deposited on cornea, renal injury (due to calcium oxalate precipitation), salivation, seizures, swelling, vomiting. Sap may cause corneal abrasion, lacrimation, ocular pain, photophobia

Dosage Per Commission E: 20-30 mg hydroxyanthracene derivatives/day calculated as Rhein

Warnings Per Commission E: Use of stimulant laxatives for longer than recommended short-term application can cause an increase in intestinal sluggishness

Overdosage/Treatment

Decontamination: Oral: Dilute; ipecac/lavage/activated charcoal not likely necessary; milk/water to rinse crystals

Supportive therapy: For treatment of soluble oxalates, which may cause systemic oxalate toxicity, keep well hydrated, monitor renal function, fluid/electrolytes; hypocalcemia may occur which can be treated with calcium gluconate, monitor urine for crystals; treat other symptoms supportively

Drug Interaction Per Commission E: Long-term use/abuse, due to loss in potassium, an increase in effectiveness of cardiac glycosides and an effect on antiarrhythmics is possible. Potassium deficiency can be increased by simultaneous application of thiazide diuretics, corticoadrenal steroids or licorice root.

Rue

Scientific Name *Ruta graveolens*

APHA Botanical Safety Rating System Class 2b, 2d; contraindicated in poor kidney function; avoid prolonged exposure to sunlight

Synonyms Common Rue; Garden Rue; German Rue; Herb-of-Grace

Use Antispasmodic, abortifacient, emmenagogue, topical insect repellent

Mechanism of Action Contains the alkaloids, arborine, and arborinine; also contains rutamarin (a coumarin); antispasmodic effect on gastrointestinal smooth muscle; may inhibit implantation of fertilized cells in uterus; the furocoumarins found on fresh leaves can cause a photosensitivity reaction

Adverse Reactions

Per Commission E:

Dermatologic: Oil can cause contact dermatitis; phototoxic reactions causing dermatoses have been noted

Hepatic: Severe liver damage

Renal: Proteinuria, hematuria

Therapeutic dosages can have these effects:

Central nervous system: Melancholic moods, sleep disorders, tiredness, dizziness

Neuromuscular & skeletal: Spasms

Juice of fresh leaves can lead to:

Cardiovascular: Low pulse

Central nervous system: Fainting, sleepiness

Endocrine & metabolic: Abortion

Gastrointestinal: Painful irritations of stomach and intestines, swelling of the tongue

Miscellaneous: Clammy skin

Signs and Symptoms of Overdose Topical administration of fresh leaves can cause dermal erythema, blistering, and photosensitization. Volatile oil may be an irritant and can cause hepatic and renal abnormalities. Nausea and vomiting upon ingestion

Overdosage/Treatment Decontamination: **Oral**: Lavage (within 1 hour)/ activated charcoal with cathartic **Dermal**: Wash with soap and water; avoid sunlight

Pregnancy Risk Factor Contraindicated

Additional Information Fatal dose: ~100 mL of the oil or 4 ounces of fresh leaves.

See Commission E; rue oil is used as an abortifacient; it is a pale yellow oil (density: 0.8) which is not water soluble; the plant (which is native to Europe but found worldwide) is an evergreen shrub which can grow to 2-3 feet with yellow flowers blooming in summer

Sabah Vegetable

Scientific Name *Sauropus albicans*; *Sauropus androgynus*

U.S. Brand Names Defat® (in U.S.)

Synonyms Asin-Asin; Checkor Manis; Weight Reduction Vegetable

Commonly Found In Malaysia, Thailand, India, Taiwan; shrub-like plant which can grow up to 1.5 m high

Use Has been used (at a daily dose of 150 g) for weight reduction and vision protection

Mechanism of Action Fresh leaves contain papaverine alkaloid (580 mg/100 g of leaves); papaverine inhibits cellular respiration, is a mild calcium antagonist and vasodilator

Adverse Reactions

Cardiovascular: Palpitations, prolonged QT interval, torsade de pointes, chest tightness

Central nervous system: Insomnia, anxiety, fatigue, dizziness

Dermatologic: Rashes

Endocrine & metabolic: Hypokalemia

Gastrointestinal: Anorexia

Neuromuscular & skeletal: Tremor

Respiratory: Dyspnea, hypoxia, cough, tachypnea, obstructive lung disease, bronchiolitis obliterans (may all develop after 4 months of use), wheezing and rales may also occur

Overdosage/Treatment

Decontamination: Ipecac (within 30 minutes)/activated charcoal with cathartic is useful

Supportive therapy: Lorazepam or diazepam 10-20 mg (0.25-0.4 mg/kg for children) is helpful for seizures; I.V. fluids and alpha-adrenergic pressors should be used for hypotension; sodium bicarbonate (1 mEq/kg) is useful to treat acidosis

Enhanced elimination: Multiple dosing of activated charcoal may be useful

Additional Information Not sold in U.S. market; commonly found in Malaysia, Thailand, India, Taiwan; shrub-like plant which can grow up to 1.5 meters high

Sassafras Oil

CAS Number 8006-80-2

Scientific Name *Sassafras albidum*

APHA Botanical Safety Rating System Class 2d (leaf, root); not for long-term use; do not exceed recommended dosage

Synonyms *Sassafras albidum*; Oleum Sassafras

Use Banned by FDA in food since 1960; has been used as a mild counterirritant on the skin (ie, for lice or insect bites); should not be ingested

Mechanism of Action Contains safrole (up to 80%) which inhibits liver microsomal enzymes; its metabolite may cause hepatic tumors

Adverse Reactions

(Primarily related to sassafras oil and safrole)

Cardiovascular: Tachycardia, flushing, hypotension, sinus tachycardia

Central nervous system: Anxiety, hallucinations, vertigo, aphasia

Dermatologic: Contact dermatitis

Gastrointestinal: Vomiting

Hepatic: Fatty changes of the liver, hepatic necrosis

Ocular: Mydriasis

Miscellaneous: Diaphoresis

Little documentation of adverse effects due to ingestion of herbal tea

Toxicodynamics/Kinetics

Absorption: Safrole is absorbed orally

Metabolism: Hepatic to 1-hydroxysafrole (possible carcinogenic metabolite)

Elimination: Renal primarily

Dosage Sassafras tea can contain as much as 200 mg (3 mg/kg) of safrole

Overdosage/Treatment

Decontamination: Emesis (within 30 minutes) can be considered for ingestion >5 mL if airway is protected; activated charcoal with cathartic can be used

Supportive therapy: Hypotension can be treated with intravenous crystalloid (10-20 mL/kg) and placement in Trendelenburg position; dopamine or norepinephrine can be used for refractory cases

Additional Information Lethal dose: ~5 mL; Toxic dose: Humans: 0.66 mg/kg based on rodent studies. A yellow liquid which may also contain eugenol, pinene, and d-camphor; specific gravity: 1.07; not reviewed by Commission E

Saw Palmetto

Scientific Name *Serenoa repens*

APHA Botanical Safety Rating System Class 1

U.S. Brand Names Prostactive

Synonyms *Sabal serrulata*; *Sabaslis serrulatae*; *Serenoa repens*; American Dwarf Palm Tree; Cabbage Palm; Palmetto Scrub; Sabal Palmetto; Sabel

Use

In herbal medicine, plant extracts have been used to manage prostatic enlargement (benign prostate hyperplasia only)

Per Commission E: Urination problems in benign prostatic hyperplasia stages 1 & 2

Mechanism of Action Liposterolic extract of the berries may inhibit the enzymes 5α-reductase, along with cyclo-oxygenase and 5-lipoxygenase, thus exhibiting antiandrogen and anti-inflammatory effects; does not reduce prostatic enlargement but may help increase urinary flow (not FDA approved)

Adverse Reactions

Central nervous system: Headache

Endocrine & metabolic: Gynecomastia

Gastrointestinal: Stomach problems (in rare cases) per Commission E

Signs and Symptoms of Overdose Diarrhea

Toxicodynamics/Kinetics Absorption: Oral: Low

Dosage

Daily dose: ~320 mg; tea products are not utilized

Per Commission E: 1-2 g fruits/berries daily or 320 mg standardized extract; lipophilic ingredients extracted with lipophilic solvents (hexane or ethanol 90% v/v)

Contraindications Pregnancy and breast-feeding

Warnings Per Commission E: Relieves only the difficulties associated with enlarged prostate without reducing the enlargement; consult a physician at regular intervals

Overdosage/Treatment

Decontamination: Ipecac within 30 minutes or lavage (within 1 hour)/activated charcoal with cathartic

Pregnancy Implications Do not use

Additional Information A fan palm plant growing up to 10' tall on the southern Atlantic coast; the red to brownish black berries, when ripe, are used in herbal medicine; this product has no effect on PSA or testosterone levels

Specific References

Markowitz JS, Donovan JL, DeVane CL, et al, "Common Herbal Supplements Did Not Produce False-Positive Results on Urine Drug Screens Analyzed by Enzyme Immunoassay," *J Anal Toxicol*, 2004, 28:272-3.

Wolsko PM, Solondz DK, Phillips RS, et al. "Lack of Herbal Supplement Characterization in Published Randomized Controlled Trials," *Am J Med*, 2005, 118(10):1087-93 (review).

Senna

Related Information

- Buckthorn Bark
- Cascara Sagrada

CAS Number 128-57-4; 52730-36-6; 52730-37-7; 8013-11-4; 81-27-6

Scientific Name *Cassia acutifolia*; *Cassia angustifolia*; *Cassia senna*

U.S. Brand Names Senlax®; Sennakot®; Sennocol®; X-Prep®

Synonyms Alexandrine Senna; Tinnevelley Senna

Use Short-term treatment of constipation; evacuate the colon for bowel or rectal examinations

Mechanism of Toxic Action Contains up to 3% anthraquinone glycosides which can cause colonic stimulation

Adverse Reactions

Cardiovascular: Palpitations

Central nervous system: Tetany, dizziness

Dermatologic: Finger clubbing (reversible)

Endocrine & metabolic: Hypokalemia

Gastrointestinal:Vomiting (with fresh plant leaves or pods), diarrhea, abdominal cramping, nausea, melanosis coli (reversible), cachexia

Genitourinary: Red discoloration in alkaline urine (yellow-brown in acidic urine)

Hepatic: Hepatitis, aminotransferase level elevation (asymptomatic)

Renal: Oliguria, proteinuria

Respiratory: Dyspnea

Per Commission E:

Endocrine & metabolic: Long-term use/abuse can cause electrolyte imbalance

Gastrointestinal: In single incidents, cramp-like discomforts of gastrointestinal tract requiring a reduction in dosage

Toxicodynamics/Kinetics

Onset of action: Oral: 6-8 hours; Suppository: 0.5-2 hours

Metabolism: Hydrolyzed by bacteria in the colon thus releasing active sennosides

Elimination: Urine and feces

Dosage Sennosides:

Children >6 years: 20 mg at bedtime

Adults: 20-40 mg with water at bedtime

Senna granules: 2.5-5 mL (163-326 mg) at bedtime; maximum dose: 10 mL (652 mg)/day

Senna tablets:

Children >60 pounds: 1 tablet (187 mg) at bedtime; maximum daily dose: 2 tablets

Adults: 1-2 tablets (187-374 mg) at bedtime; maximum daily dose: 4 tablets (Note: Extra strength senna tablets contain 374 mg each)

Senna syrup:

Children

1 month to 1 year: 1.25-2.5 mL (55-109 mg) at bedtime up to 5 mL/day

1-5 years: 2.5-5 mL (109-218 mg) at bedtime, up to 10 mL/day

5-15 years: 5-10 mL (218-436 mg) at bedtime, up to 20 mL/day

Adults: 10-15 mL (436-654 mg); maximum daily dose: 30 mL (1308 mg)

Senna suppositories:

Children >60 pounds: $^1/_2$ suppository (326 mg)

Adults: 1 suppository (652 mg) at bedtime; can repeat in 2 hours

Tea: $^1/_2$ to 2 teaspoons of leaves (0.5-4 g of the herb)

Administration Oral: Once daily doses should be taken at bedtime. Granules may be eaten plain, sprinkled on food, or mixed in liquids

Contraindications Per Commission E: Intestinal obstruction, acute intestinal inflammation (eg, Crohn's disease), colitis ulcerosa, appendicitis, abdominal pain of unknown origin; pregnancy

Warnings Not recommended for over-the-counter (OTC) use in patients experiencing stomach pain, nausea, vomiting, or a sudden change in bowel movements which lasts >2 weeks. Not recommended for OTC use in children <2 years of age.

Dosage Forms
[DSC] = Discontinued product
Granules (Senokot®): Sennosides 15 mg/teaspoon (60 g, 180 g, 360 g) [cocoa flavor] [DSC]
Liquid:
  Senexon: Sennosides 8.8 mg/5 mL (240 mL)
  X-Prep®: Sennosides 8.8 mg/5 mL (75 mL) [alcohol free; contains sugar 50 g/75 mL; available individually or in a kit] [DSC]
Liquid concentrate (Fletcher's® Castoria®): Senna concentrate 33.3 mg/mL (75 mL) [alcohol free; contains sodium benzoate; root beer flavor]
Syrup (Uni-Senna): Sennosides 8.8 mg/5 mL (240 mL) [contains alcohol; butterscotch flavor]
Tablet: Sennosides 8.6 mg, 15 mg, 25 mg
  ex-lax®: Sennosides USP 15 mg
  ex-lax® Maximum Strength: Sennosides USP 25 mg
  Perdiem® Overnight Relief: Sennosides USP 15 mg
  Sennatural™, Senokot®, Senexon®, Senna-Gen®, Uni-Senna: Sennosides 8.6 mg
Tablet, chewable:
  ex-lax®: Sennosides USP 15 mg [chocolate flavor]
  Evac-U-Gen: Sennosides 10 mg

Reference Range Total rhein plasma concentration does not exceed 160 ng/mL after therapeutic dosing

Overdosage/Treatment Decontamination: **Do not** induce emesis; lavage (within 1 hour)/activated charcoal can be used

Drug Interaction Per Commission E: Potentiation of cardiac glycosides (with long-term use) is possible due to loss in potassium; effect on anti-arrhythmics is possible; potassium deficiency can be increased by simultaneous application of thiazide diuretics, corticosteroids, and licorice root

Pregnancy Risk Factor C

Nursing Implications May discolor urine or feces; monitor I & O

Additional Information Both leaf and fruits ("pods") are use; avoid prolonged use; may increase potency and toxicity of digitalis; the plant is found in North Africa and India; a low branching shrub with large yellow leaves on the top of the plant are harvested; hypersensitivity to the ingredients; contraindications in fecal impaction, bowel obstruction, and abdominal pain

Specific References
Spiller HA, Winter ML, Weber JA, et al, "Skin Breakdown and Blisters from Senna-Containing Laxatives in Young Children," *Ann Pharmacother*, 2003, 37(5):636-9.
Vanderperren B, Rizzo M, Angenot L, et al, "Acute Liver Failure with Renal Impairment Related to the Abuse of Senna Anthraquinone Glycosides," *Ann Pharmacother*, 2005, 39(7):1353-7.

St John's Wort

CAS Number 548-04-9 (hypericin)
Scientific Name *Hypericum perforatum*
APHA Botanical Safety Rating System Class 2d; may potentiate pharmaceutical MAO inhibitors
U.S. Brand Names Esbericum®; Hyperforat®; Lophakomp-Hypericum®; Millepertuis®; Neuroplant®; Psychotonin M®; VIMRxgn
Synonyms *Hypercium perforatum*; Amber Touch-and-Feel; Goatweed; Klamath Weed; Rosin Rose

Use
Mild to moderate depression; also used traditionally for treatment of stress, anxiety, insomnia; used topically for vitiligo; also a popular drug for AIDS patients due to possible antiretroviral activity; used topically for wound healing
Per Commission E: Psychovegetative disorders, depressive moods, anxiety and/or nervous unrest; oily preparations for dyspeptic complaints; oily preparations externally for treatment of post-therapy of acute and contused injuries, myalgia, first degree burns

Mechanism of Action Active ingredients are xanthones flavonoids (hypericin) which can act as monoamine oxidase inhibitors, although *in vitro* activity is minimal; majority of activity appears to be related to GABA modulation; may be related to dopamine, serotonin norepinephrine modulation also

Adverse Reactions
Cardiovascular: Sinus tachycardia
Central nervous system: Hypomania
Dermatologic: Photosensitization is possible, especially in fair-skinned persons (per Commission E)
Gastrointestinal: Stomach pains, abdominal pain
Miscellaneous: Allergic reactions (0.5%)

Signs and Symptoms of Overdose Diarrhea, drowsiness, fever, hypertension, nausea, photosensitivity, pruritus, rash, tachycardia

Dosage
Tincture: ¼ to 1 teaspoon up to 3 times/day
Topical: Crushed leaves and flowers are applied to affected area after cleansing with soap and water

Per Commission E: 2-4 g drug (dried herb) or 0.2-1 mg of total hypericin in other forms of drug application

Contraindications Endogenous depression, pregnancy, children <2 years of age (not confirmed in animal models, *in vitro* only).

Reference Range Hypericin serum level of 4 ng/mL obtained 8 hours after ingestion of 1 mg extract of hypericin

Overdosage/Treatment
Decontamination: Lavage (within 1 hour)/activated charcoal with cathartic
Supportive therapy: Agitation, tachycardia, and hypertension can be treated with a benzodiazepine

Drug Interactions Avoid amphetamines or other stimulants; use with caution in patients taking MAO inhibitors, levodopa, and 5-hydroxytryptophan; avoid tyramine-containing foods due to presence of hypercin although human data of this potential drug interaction is lacking; tannin-containing herbs can cause a decrease in iron absorption; may enhance the side effects of narcotics and selective serotonin reuptake inhibitors; may increase side effects of ethanol and melatonin. Photosensitivity may be particularly aggravated with tetracycline or chlorpromazine use. St John's wort may induce hepatic enzymes, thus enhancing theophylline clearance. Concomitant administration with protease inhibitors may result in decreased plasma levels of the protease inhibitor; similar effects can be seen with cyclosporine and non-nucleoside reverse transcriptase inhibitors. Hypericum (St John's wort) extract reduces the bioavailability of digoxin by 25%. Concomitant administration of St John's Wort and paroxetine can result in serotonin syndrome. St John's wort *(Hypericum)* appears to induce CYP3A enzymes and has lead to 57% reductions in indinavir AUCs and 81% reductions in trough serum concentrations, which may lead to treatment failures. St John's wort may decrease atorvastatin levels.

Pregnancy Implications Do not use
VIMRxgn is a synthetic hypericin for HIV treatment; leaves and tops of *Hypericum perforatum* plant used in herbal medicine. St John's wort is a perennial that reaches 2 feet tall with the aroma similar to turpentine; golden yellow flowers bloom in early summer. Young plant is almost as toxic as the mature plant. Hypericin inhibits both type A and type B monoamine oxidase; contraindications in endogenous depression, pregnancy, children <2 years of age (not confirmed in animal models, *in vitro* only). This herbal preparation should be discontinued for 2-3 weeks prior to surgery.
Hypericum extract ZE, 250 mg twice daily, appears to be as effective as imipramine, 75 mg twice daily, for treatment of mild to moderate depression for 6 weeks.

Specific References
Bell EC, Ravis WR, Lloyd KB, Stokes TJ, "Effects of St. John's Wort Supplementation on Ibuprofen," *Pharmacokinetics*.
Brazier NC and Levine MA, "Drug-Herb Interaction Among Commonly Used Conventional Medicines: A Compendium for Health Care Professionals," *Am J Ther*, 2003, 10(3):163-9.
Bryant SM and Kolodchak J, "Serotonin Syndrome Resulting from an Herbal Detox Cocktail," *AJEM*, 2004, 22(7):626-6.
Dean AJ, Moses GM, and Vernon JM, "Suspected Withdrawal Syndrome After Cessation of St. John's Wort," *Ann Pharmacother*, 2003, 37(1):151.
Holstege CP, Mitchell K, Barlotta K, et al, "Toxicity and Drug Interactions Associated with Herbal Products: Ephedra and St. John's Wort," *Med Clin North Am*, 2005, 89(6):1225-57 (review).
Markowitz JS, Donovan JL, DeVane CL, et al, "Effect of St John's Wort on Drug Metabolism by Induction of Cytochrome P450 3A4 Enzyme," *JAMA*, 2003, 290(11):1500-4.
Pfrunder A, Schiesser M, Gerber S, et al, "Interaction of St John's Wort with Low-Dose Oral Contraceptive Therapy: A Randomized Controlled Trial," *Br J Clin Pharmacol*, 2003, 56(6):683-90.
Woolf AD, "Herbal Remedies and Children: Do They Work? Are They Harmful?" *Pediatrics*, 2003, 112(1 Pt 2):240-6.

Ting Kung Teng

Scientific Name *Erycibe henryi prain*
Synonyms Bao Gong Teng
Use Stems/roots are used to treat arthritis/musculoskeletal symptoms; eye drops are used to treat glaucoma in China
Mechanism of Action A member of the morning glory family (convolulaceae), this plant is a shrub which grows at low elevations in Taiwan, Southern China, and Southern Japan. Contains EhP which are tropane alkaloids (scopoletin and scopoline) which exhibit muscarinic, cholinergic, and sedative effects.
Signs and Symptoms of Overdose Onset is usually within 10 minutes; vomiting, diarrhea, dizziness, lacrimation, hypersalivation, diaphoresis, weakness, rhinorrhea, ventricular tachycardia, miosis, bradycardia, hypotension, hypothermia
Overdosage/Treatment
Decontamination: Activated charcoal may be useful
Supportive: Treatment is primarily supportive; atropine can be used to treat symptomatic bradycardia; lidocaine or amiodarone can be used to

treat ventricular arrhythmias - cardioversion (electrical) may be necessary

Additional Information Therapaeutic dose for arthritis: 3-8 g; oral doses >27 g can produce severe symptoms

Specific References
Huang HH, Yen DH, Wu ML, et al, "Acute *Erycibe henryi prain* (Ting Kung Teng) Poisoning," *Clin Tox,* 2006, 44:71-5.

Valerian

CAS Number 8057-49-6
Scientific Name *Valeriana officinalis*
APHA Botanical Safety Rating System Class 1
U.S. Brand Names Nervex®; Neurol®; Orasedon®; Sanox-N®; Ticalma®; Valerian Root; Valerianaheel®; Valmane®
Synonyms *Valeriana edulis*; *Valeriana wallichi*; Garden Heliotrope; Jacob's Ladder; Phu; Radix Valerianae; Radix; Red Valerian
Use
Herbal medicine use as a sleep-promoting agent and minor tranquilizer (similar to benzodiazepines); used in anxiety, panic attacks, intestinal cramps, headaches
Per Commission E: Restlessness, sleep disorders based on nervous conditions
Mechanism of Action Most pharmacologic activity located in fresh root or dried rhizome; the plant contains essential oils (valerenic acid and valenol, valepotriates, and alkaloids <0.2% concentration) which may affect neurotransmitter levels (serotonin, GABA, and norepinephrine); also has antispasmodic properties
Signs and Symptoms of Overdose Abdominal cramping, blurred vision, fatigue, fine tremor, headache, mydriasis. Intravenous exposure can cause hypocalcemia, hypokalemia, hypophosphatemia, hypotension, lethargy, and piloerection. Contact with the plant can cause contact dermatitis. Hepatotoxicity (probably due to an idiosyncratic hypersensitivity) has been noted.
Admission Criteria/Prognosis Admit any intravenous exposure or any adult oral ingestion >20 g
Dosage Up to 1 g at night
Per Commission E:
Tea: 2-3 g of drug per cup of H_2O for tea; once to several times/day
Tincture: $^1/_2$ to 1 teaspoon (1-3 mL) once to several times/day
Extracts: Equal to 2-3 g of drug
Overdosage/Treatment
Decontamination: Lavage (within 1 hour)/activated charcoal with cathartic
Supportive therapy: Hypotension can be treated with I.V. crystalloid therapy
Drug Interactions Not synergistic with alcohol; potentiation of other CNS depressants is possible
Additional Information *Valeriana officinalis* is a perennial plant that can reach 5 feet in height with tiny white or pink flowers. It is found in Europe, Canada, and Northern U.S. Preparations may contain multiple components.

Specific References
Wiener SW, Hoffman RS, and Nelson LS, "Withdrawal Symptoms After Valerian Cessation," *J Toxicol Clin Toxicol*, 2003, 41(5):721.

Wormwood

CAS Number 471-15-8; 546-80-5
Scientific Name *Artemisia absinthium*
APHA Botanical Safety Rating System Class 2b, 2c, 2d; not for long-term use; do not exceed recommended dose
Synonyms *Artemisia absinthium*; Absinthium; Assenzio; Bitter Wormwood; Losna; Mugwort; Pelin; Qinghaosu Extract; Wormseed
Use
Homeopathic medicine, used as an anthelmintic, bitter tonic, hair tonic, sedative, flavoring agent (in vermouth)
Per Commission E: Loss of appetite, dyspepsia, biliary dyskinesia
Mechanism of Action Contains Thujone (a volatile oil of tenpene structure), which binds to the same neuronal receptors as tetrahydrocannabinol; can inhibit porphyrin synthesis; also contains absinthin (bittering agent) and santonica (anthelmintic for roundworms)
Signs and Symptoms of Overdose "Absinthism": Anorexia, color vision disturbance, coma, contact dermatitis (from flowers), delirium, diaphoresis, diarrhea, dysphoria, euphoria, giddiness, headache, mania, memory impairment, paranoia, psychosis, respiratory depression, seizures (>15 g ingestion), thirst, tremors, vertigo, visual hallucinations, vomiting
Toxicodynamics/Kinetics Metabolism: (Thujone) Hepatic (oxidative metabolism)
Dosage Tea: 2-3 g/day
Overdosage/Treatment
Decontamination: Lavage (within 1 hour)/activated charcoal with cathartic
Supportive therapy: Seizures can be managed with a benzodiazepine or barbiturate; psychiatric abnormalities can be managed with a benzodiazepine or neuroleptic agent
Drug Interaction Thujone-containing and gamolenic acid-containing herbs can lower the seizure threshold leading to increased anticonvulsant dosage requirements.
Pregnancy Implications Avoid
Additional Information
Not popular in the U.S.; taste threshold (Absinthin): 1 part in 70,000: A shrub with small green-yellow flowers from July through September. Grows naturally in Europe but found in Northeastern and North Central U.S. Wormwood extract has been used in absinth, an emerald green bitter liquor banned in Europe and U.S. Absinth has been thought to cause Vincent van Gogh's psychosis. The tea uses dried leaves and flowering tops.
Per Commission E: In toxic doses, thujone, the active component of the oil, acts as a convulsant poison. Thus, essential oil must not be used except in combinations.

SECTION V

ANTIDOTES AND DRUGS USED IN TOXICOLOGY

POISON ANTIDOTE PREPAREDNESS IN HOSPITALS

Anthony Burda, RPh, Illinois Poison Center

Michael Wahl, MD, Advocate Illinois Masonic Medical Center & Illinois Poison Center

Christina Hantsch, MD, Loyola University Medical Center & Illinois Poison Center

The quantities of medications listed in the IPC's (Illinois Poison Center's) antidote list are suggested guidelines; the amounts may be adjusted based on factors such as anticipated usage in the hospital's local area, the nearest alternate sources of antidotes, the distance to tertiary care institutions, etc. Keep in mind that some antidotes (eg, the cyanide antidote kit) must be immediately available on-site when a patient arrives at a hospital. Inadequate antidote preparedness may lead to increased morbidity or mortality.

All healthcare professionals should become familiar with regional poison control center poison prevention and treatment services. Staffed by pharmacists, nurses, physicians, and poison specialists, poison centers are available 24 hours a day, 7 days a week to all residents and health professionals of each state for consultation on the treatment of poisonings, medication interactions, occupational exposures, hazardous material incidents, envenomations, and other poison-related concerns.

The following statement can be attributed to Darryl S. Rich, PharmD, JCAHO Associate Director, Home Care Accreditation Services.

"The Joint Commission, in moving towards a functional and nondepartmental approach to its standard manuals, no longer has such a specific standard related to antidotes. However, there are two standards that would apply to the need for a pharmacy to maintain a supply of common antidotes in stock. Standard TX 3.1. The organization identified an appropriate selection of medications available for prescribing and ordering. This standard specifically required hospitals to develop criteria for the selection of products maintained in stock by the pharmacy. Those criteria must address patient need, given the diseases and conditions treated by the hospital and its emergency room.

The second relevant standard is TX 3.5.5. Emergency medications are consistently available, controlled, and secure in the pharmacy and patient care areas. Although this standard usually refers to the control and security of medications in emergency medication carts on the patient units, it can be used if appropriately selected antidotes (which the Joint Commission considers emergency medications) are not readily available.

Thus, from TX 3.1, it is incumbent upon the medical staff and the pharmacy, through its Pharmacy and Therapeutics Committee or other medical staff committee responsible for formulary selection, to select which antidotes the pharmacy should stock. Under standard TX 3.5.5, the pharmacy must then make sure the selected antidotes are readily available."

Illinois Poison Center Antidote List			
Uses and Suggested Minimum Stock Quantities for Various Poison Antidotes Used for Treatment of Poisonings Illinois Poison Center 24-Hour Hotline: 1-800-942-5969			
Antidote	**Poison/Drug/Toxin**	**Suggested Minimum Stock Quantity**	**Rationale/Comments**
N-Acetylcysteine (Mucomyst®)	Acetaminophen Carbon tetrachloride Other hepatotoxins	600 mL in 10 mL or 30 mL vials of 20% solution	Acetaminophen is the most common drug involved in intentional and un-intentional poisonings. This amount (600 mL/120 g) provides enough antidote to treat an adult for an entire 3-day course of therapy, or enough to treat 3 adults for 24 hours. Several vials may be stocked in the ED to provide a loading dose and the remaining vials in the pharmacy for the q4h maintenance doses.

Illinois Poison Center Antidote List (*Continued*)

Antidote	Poison/Drug/Toxin	Suggested Minimum Stock Quantity	Rationale/Comments
Amyl nitrite, sodium nitrite, and sodium thiosulfate (cyanide antidote kit)	Acetonitrile Acrylonitrile Bromates (thiosulfate only) Chlorates (thiosulfate only) Cyanide (eg, HCN, KCN and NaCN) Cyanogenic glycoside natural sources (eg, apricot pits and peach pits) Hydrogen sulfide (nitrites only) Laetrile Nitroprusside (thiosulfate only) Smoke inhalation (combustion of synthetic materials)	One to two kits	Stock one kit in the ED. Consider also stocking one kit in the pharmacy. **Note:** This has a short shelf-life of 18 months.
Antivenin, Crotalidae polyvalent	Pit viper envenomation (eg, rattlesnakes, cottonmouths, and copperheads)	Ten vials	Stock in pharmacy. Advised in geographic areas with endemic populations of copperhead, water moccasin, or eastern massasauga rattlesnakes. In low-risk areas, know nearest alternate source of antivenin. **Note:** 20-40 vials or more may be needed for moderate to severe envenomations. The antivenin must be administered in a critical care setting since it is an equine-derived product.
Antivenin, Crotalidae polyvalent Immune Fab - Ovine (CroFab®)	Pit viper envenomation (eg, rattlesnakes, cottonmouths, and copperheads)	Four to six vials	Stock in pharmacy. Recently FDA-approved product that is a possible alternate to equine product. May have lower risk of hypersensitivity reaction than equine product. Average dose in premarketing trials was 12 vials, but more may be needed. **Note:** Store in refrigerator. See equine antivenin also.
Antivenin, *Latrodectus mactans* (black widow spider)	Black widow spider envenomation	Zero to one vial	*Latrodectus* envenomations are very rare in Illinois. This product is only used for severe envenomations. Antivenin must be given in a critical care setting since it is an equine-derived product. Know the nearest source of antidote. **Note:** Product must be refrigerated at all times.
Atropine sulfate	α_2-agonists (eg, clonidine, guanabenz, and guanfacine) Antimyasthenic agents (eg, pyridostigmine) Bradyarrhythmia-producing agents (eg, beta-blockers, calcium channel blockers, and digitalis glycosides) Cholinergic agonists (eg, bethanechol) Organophosphate and carbamate insecticides Muscarine-containing mushrooms (eg, Clitocybe and Inocybe) Nerve agents (eg, sarin, soman, tabun, and VX) Tacrine	Total 100-150 mg Available in various formulations: 0.4 mg/mL (1 mL, 0.4 mg ampuls) 0.4 mg/mL (20 mL, 8 mg vials) 0.1 mg/mL (10 mL, 1 mg ampuls)	The product should be immediately available in the ED. Some may also be stored in the pharmacy or other hospital sites, but should be easily mobilized if a severely poisoned patient needs treatment. **Note:** Product is necessary for adequate preparedness for a weapon of mass destruction (WMD) incident.
Calcium chloride and Calcium gluconate	Beta-blockers Black widow spider (*Latrodectus mactans*) envenomation Calcium channel blockers Fluoride salts (eg, NaF) Hydrofluoric acid (HF) Hyperkalemia (not digoxin-induced) Hypermagnesemia	10% calcium chloride: fifteen 10 mL vials 10% calcium gluconate: five 10 mL vials	Stock in ED. More may be stocked in pharmacy. Many ampuls of calcium chloride may be necessary in life-threatening calcium channel blocker or hydrofluoric acid poisoning.
Calcium disodium EDTA (Versenate®)	Lead Zinc salts (eg, zinc chloride)	One 5 mL amp (200 mg/mL)	Stock in pharmacy. One vial provides one day of therapy for a child. More may be needed in lead endemic areas.

Illinois Poison Center Antidote List   (*Continued*)

Antidote	Poison/Drug/Toxin	Suggested Minimum Stock Quantity	Rationale/Comments
Deferoxamine mesylate (Desferal®)	Iron	Twelve 500 mg vials	Stock in pharmacy. **Note:** Per package insert, the maximum daily dose is 6 g (12 vials). However, this dose may be exceeded in serious poisonings.
Digoxin immune fab (Digibind®)	Cardiac glycoside-containing plants (eg, foxglove and oleander) Digitoxin Digoxin	Ten vials	Stock in ED or pharmacy. This amount (10 vials) may be given to a digoxin-poisoned patient in whom the digoxin level is unknown. This amount would effectively neutralize a steady-state digoxin level of 14.2 ng/mL in a 70 kg patient. More may be necessary in severe intoxications. Know nearest source of additional supply.
Dimercaprol (BAL in Oil®)	Arsenic Copper Gold Lead Mercury	Two 3 mL ampuls (100 mg/mL)	Stock in pharmacy. This amount provides two doses of 3-5 mg/kg/dose given q4h to treat one seriously poisoned adult or provides enough to treat a 15 kg child for 24 hours.
Ethanol	Ethylene glycol Methanol	4 L of 10% ethanol in D $_5$W and 1 pint of 95% ethanol	Stock in pharmacy. This amount (4 L) provides enough to treat an adult (70 kg) with a loading dose followed by a maintenance infusion for 12 hours during dialysis. **Note:** Ethanol is unnecessary if fomepizole is stocked.
Flumazenil (Romazicon®)	Benzodiazepines Zolpidem	Total 1 mg: two 5 mL vials (0.1 mg/mL)	Suggested minimum is for ED stocking. Due to risk of seizures, use with extreme caution, if at all, in poisoned patients. More may be stocked in the pharmacy for use in reversal of conscious sedation.
Folic acid Folinic acid (leucovorin)	Methanol Methotrexate, trimetrexate Pyrimethamine Trimethoprim	Folic acid: three 50 mg vials Folinic acid: one 50 mg vial	Stock in pharmacy. For methanol-poisoned patients with an acidosis, give 50 mg folinic acid initially, then 50 mg of folic acid q4h for six doses.
Fomepizole (Antizol®)	Ethylene glycol Methanol	One 1.5 g vial **Note:** Available in a kit of four 1.5 g vials	Stock in pharmacy. Know where nearest alternate supply is located. One vial will provide at least one initial adult dose. Hospitals with critical care and hemodialysis capabilities may consider stocking one kit of four vials (enough to treat one patient for up to several days). **Note:** Product has a two-year shelf life; however, the manufacturer will replace expired product at no cost.
Glucagon	Beta-blockers Calcium channel blockers Hypoglycemia Hypoglycemic agents	Fifty 1 mg vials	Stock 20 mg in ED and remainder in pharmacy. This amount provides approximately 5-10 hours of high-dose therapy in life-threatening beta-blocker or calcium channel blocker poisoning.
Hyperbaric oxygen (HBO)	Carbon monoxide Carbon tetrachloride Cyanide Hydrogen sulfide Methemoglobinemia Brown recluse spider (*Loxosceles reclusus*) envenomation	Post the location and phone number of nearest HBO chamber.	Consult the regional poison control center to determine if HBO treatment is indicated.
Methylene blue	Methemoglobin-inducing agents including aniline, butyl nitrite, nitrates, nitrites, dapsone, dinitrophenol, local anesthetics (eg, benzocaine), metoclopramide, monomethylhydrazine-containing mushrooms (eg, *Gyromitra*), naphthalene, nitrobenzene, phenazopyridine	Three 10 mL ampuls 3 (10 mg/mL)	Stock in pharmacy. This amount provides 3 doses of 1-2 mg/kg (0.1-0.2 mL/kg).

Illinois Poison Center Antidote List   (*Continued*)

Antidote	Poison/Drug/Toxin	Suggested Minimum Stock Quantity	Rationale/Comments
Nalmefene (Revex®) Naloxone (Narcan®)	α_2 agonists (eg, clonidine, guanabenz, and guanfacine) Angiotensin converting enzyme (ACE) inhibitors Coma of unknown cause Imidazoline decongestants (eg, oxymetazoline and tetrahydrozoline) Opioids (eg, codeine, dextromethorphan, diphenoxylate, fentanyl, heroin, meperidine, morphine, and propoxyphene) Tramadol Valproic acid	Nalmefene: None required Naloxone: Total 40 mg, any combination of 0.4 mg, 1 mg, and 2 mg ampuls	Stock 20 mg naloxone in the ED and 20 mg elsewhere in the institution. **Note:** Nalmefene has a longer duration of action but it offers no therapeutic advantage over a naloxone infusion.
D-Penicillamine (Cuprimine®)	Arsenic Copper Mercury	None required as an antidote. Available in bottles of 100 capsules (125 mg or 250 mg/capsule)	D-Penicillamine is no longer considered the drug of choice for heavy metal poisonings. It may be stocked in the pharmacy for other indications such as Wilson's disease or rheumatoid arthritis.
Physostigmine salicylate (Antilirium®)	Anticholinergic alkaloid-containing plants (eg, deadly nightshade and jimson weed) Antihistamines Atropine and other anticholinergic agents Intrathecal baclofen	Two 2 mL ampuls (1 mg/mL)	Stock in ED or pharmacy. Usual adult dose is 1-2 mg slow I.V. push. **Note:** Duration of effect is 30-60 minutes.
Phytonadione (vitamin K$_1$) (AquaMEPHYTON®, Mephyton®)	Indanedione derivatives Long-acting anticoagulant rodenticides (eg, brodifacoum and bromadiolone) Warfarin	Two 0.5 mL ampuls (2 mg/mL) and two 5 mL ampuls (10 mg/mL)	Stock in pharmacy. **Note:** Menadione (vitamin K$_3$, Synkavite®) is ineffective and cannot be stocked as a substitute.
Pralidoxime chloride (2-PAM) (Protopam®)	Antimyasthenic agents (eg, pyridostigmine) Nerve agents (eg, sarin, soman, tabun and VX) Organophosphate insecticides Tacrine	Six 1 g vials	Stock in ED or pharmacy. **Note:** Serious intoxications may require 500 mg/h (12 g/day). Product is necessary for adequate preparedness for a weapon of mass destruction (WMD) incident.
Protamine sulfate	Enoxaparin Heparin	Variable, consider recommendation of hospital P&T Committee Available as 5 mL ampuls (10 mg/mL) and 25 mL vials (250 mg/25 mL)	Stock in pharmacy.
Pyridoxine hydrochloride (vitamin B$_6$)	Acrylamide Ethylene glycol Hydrazine Isoniazid (INH) Monomethylhydrazine-containing mushrooms (eg, Gyromitra)	Four 30 mL vials (100 mg/mL 3 g/vial) or ten 10 mL vials (100 mg/mL, 1 g/vial)	Stock in ED or pharmacy. Usual dose is 1 g pyridoxine HCl for each g of INH ingested. If amount ingested is unknown, give 5 g of pyridoxine. Repeat dose if seizures are uncontrolled. Know nearest source of additional supply.
Sodium bicarbonate	Chlorine gas Hyperkalemia Serum alkalinization: Agents producing a quinidine-like effect as noted by widened QRS complex on EKG (eg, amantadine, carbamazepine, chloroquine, cocaine, diphenhydramine, flecainide, propoxyphene, tricyclic antidepressants, quinidine, and related agents) Urine alkalinization: Weakly acidic agents (eg, chlorophenoxy herbicides, chlorpropamide, phenobarbital, and salicylates	Twenty 50 mEq vials	Stock 10 vials in the ED and 10 vials elsewhere in the hospital.
Succimer (Chemet®)	Arsenic Lead Mercury	One bottle of 100 capsules (100 mg/capsule)	Stock in pharmacy. FDA approved only for pediatric lead poisoning; however it has shown efficacy for other heavy metal poisonings.

©Illinois Poison Center

Acetylcysteine

Pronunciation (a se teel SIS teen)

CAS Number 19542-74-6 (Acetylcysteine Sodium); 616-91-1

U.S. Brand Names Acetadote®; Mucomyst®

Synonyms *N*-Acetyl-L-cysteine; *N*-Acetylcysteine; Acetylcysteine Sodium; Mercapturic Acid; Mucomyst; NAC

Impairment Potential bypass

Use

Antidote for acute acetaminophen toxicity; for hepatic failure/encephalopathy following delayed presentation (>24 hours) of an acute acetaminophen overdose; has been used in alternative medicine to treat HIV infection; possibly beneficial as a free radical scavenger for any significant acute hepatotoxic exposures.

Acute acetaminophen ingestions:

>7.5 g ingested in an adult or >200 mg/kg in a child if no serum acetaminophen level is available

Serum acetaminophen 4-hour level >150 mcg/mL

Evidence of hepatotoxicity or measurable acetaminophen levels >24 hours postacute ingestion

Unknown quantity ingested and >24 hours has elapsed since time of ingestion or unable to obtain serum acetaminophen levels within 12 hours of ingestion

Repeated supratherapeutic dosing: Initial serum acetaminophen level >10 mcg/mL or with evidence of hepatotoxicity

Unlabeled/Investigational Use Prevention of radiocontrast-induced renal dysfunction (oral, I.V.); distal intestinal obstruction syndrome (DIOS, previously referred to as meconium ileus equivalent)

Mechanism of Action An antioxidant; exerts mucolytic action through its free sulfhydryl group which opens up the disulfide bonds in the mucoproteins thus lowering the viscosity. The exact mechanism of action in acetaminophen toxicity is unknown. It may act by maintaining or restoring glutathione levels or by acting as an alternative substrate for conjugation with the toxic metabolite.

Adverse Reactions

Inhalation: Frequency not defined.

Central nervous system: Drowsiness, chills, fever

Gastrointestinal: Vomiting, nausea, stomatitis

Local: Irritation, stickiness on face following nebulization

Respiratory: Bronchospasm, rhinorrhea, hemoptysis

Miscellaneous: Acquired sensitization (rare), clamminess, unpleasant odor during administration

Intravenous:

Cardiovascular: Angioedema, vasodilation, hypotension, tachycardia, syncope, chest tightness, flushing (15%)

Central nervous system: Dysphoria

Dermatologic: Urticaria (14%), rash, facial erythema, palmar erythema, pruritus (3%), pruritus with rash and vasodilation

Gastrointestinal: Vomiting (<1% to 10%), nausea (1% to 10%), dyspepsia

Neuromuscular & skeletal: Gait disturbance

Ocular: Eye pain

Otic: Ear pain

Respiratory: Bronchospasm (9%), cough, dyspnea pharyngitis, rhinorrhea, rhonchi, throat tightness,

Miscellaneous: Anaphylactoid reactions (2% to 10%; reported as severe in 1% or moderate in 10% of patients within 15 minutes of first infusion; mild to moderate in 6% to 7% of patients after 60 minutes); diaphoresis

Pharmacodynamics/Kinetics

Onset of action: Inhalation: 5-10 minutes

Duration: Inhalation: >1 hour

Distribution: 0.47 L/kg

Protein binding, plasma: 83%

Half-life elimination:

Reduced acetylcysteine: 2 hours

Total acetylcysteine: Adults: 5.5 hours; Newborns: 11 hours

Time to peak, plasma: Oral: 1-2 hours

Excretion: Urine

Dosage

Acetaminophen poisoning: Children and Adults:

Oral: 140 mg/kg; followed by 17 doses of 70 mg/kg every 4 hours; repeat dose if emesis occurs within 1 hour of administration; therapy should continue until all doses are administered even though the acetaminophen plasma level has dropped below the toxic range

I.V. (Acetadote®): Loading dose: 150 mg/kg over 60 minutes. Loading dose is followed by 2 additional infusions: Initial maintenance dose of 50 mg/kg infused over 4 hours, followed by a second maintenance dose of 100 mg/kg infused over 16 hours. To avoid fluid overload in patients <40 kg and those requiring fluid restriction, decrease volume of D₅W proportionally. Total dosage: 300 mg/kg administered over 21 hours.

Note: If commercial I.V. form is unavailable, the following dose has been reported for I.V. administration using solution for oral inhalation (unlabeled): Loading dose: 140 mg/kg, followed by 70 mg/kg every 4 hours, for a total of 13 doses (loading dose and 48 hours of treatment); infuse each dose over 1 hour through a 0.2 micron Millipore filter (in-line).

Experts suggest that the duration of acetylcysteine administration may vary depending upon serial acetaminophen levels and liver function tests obtained during treatment. In general, patients without measurable acetaminophen levels and without significant LFT elevations (>3 times the ULN) can safely stop acetylcysteine after ≤24 hours of treatment. The patients who still have detectable levels of acetaminophen, and/or LFT elevations (>1000 units/L) continue to benefit from addition acetylcysteine administration

THREE-BAG Method Dosage Guide by Weight, Patients <40 kg

Body Weight		LOADING Dose		SECOND Dose		THIRD Dose	
(kg)	(lb)	Aceta-dote (mL)	5% Dex-trose (mL)	Aceta-dote (mL)	5% Dex-trose (mL)	Aceta-dote (mL)	5% Dex-trose (mL)
30	66	22.5	100	7.5	250	15	500
25	55	18.75	100	6.25	250	12.5	500
20	44	15	60	5	140	10	280
15	33	11.25	45	3.75	105	7.5	210
10	22	7.5	30	2.5	70	5	140

Adjuvant therapy in respiratory conditions (such as phosgene): **Note:** Patients should receive an aerosolized bronchodilator 10-15 minutes prior to acetylcysteine.

Inhalation, nebulization (face mask, mouth piece, tracheostomy): Acetylcysteine 10% and 20% solution (Mucomyst®) (dilute 20% solution with sodium chloride or sterile water for inhalation); 10% solution may be used undiluted

Infants: 1-2 mL of 20% solution or 2-4 mL 10% solution until nebulized given 3-4 times/day

Children and Adults: 3-5 mL of 20% solution or 6-10 mL of 10% solution until nebulized given 3-4 times/day for about 20 minutes; dosing range: 1-10 mL of 20% solution or 2-20 mL of 10% solution every 2-6 hours

Inhalation, nebulization (tent, croupette): Children and Adults: Dose must be individualized; may require up to 300 mL solution/treatment

Direct instillation: Adults:

Into tracheostomy: 1-2 mL of 10% to 20% solution every 1-4 hours

Through percutaneous intrathecal catheter: 1-2 mL of 20% or 2-4 mL of 10% solution every 1-4 hours via syringe attached to catheter

Diagnostic bronchogram: Nebulization or intrathecal: Adults: 1-2 mL of 20% solution or 2-4 mL of 10% solution administered 2-3 times prior to procedure

Prevention of radiocontrast-induced renal dysfunction (unlabeled use): Adults: Oral: 600 mg twice daily for 2 days (beginning the day before the procedure); may be given as powder in capsules, some centers use solution (diluted in cola beverage or juice). Hydrate patient with saline concurrently.

Treatment of phosgene inhalation (investigational): Children and Adults: 10-20 mL of a 20% solution by aerosolization

Stability

Solution for injection (Acetadote®): Store vials at room temperature, 20°C to 25°C (68°F to 77°F); following reconstitution with D₅W, solution is stable for 24 hours at room temperature

Acetadote®: Discard unused portion

Loading dose: Dilute 150 mg/kg in D₅W 200 mL

Initial maintenance dose: Dilute 50 mg/kg in D₅W 500 mL

Second maintenance dose: Dilute 100 mg/kg in D₅W 1000 mL

Solution for inhalation (Mucomyst®): Store unopened vials at room temperature; once opened, store under refrigeration and use within 96 hours. The 20% solution may be diluted with sodium chloride or sterile water; the 10% solution may be used undiluted. A color change may occur in opened vials (light purple) and does not affect the safety or efficacy.

Intravenous administration of solution for inhalation (unlabeled route): Using D₅W, dilute acetylcysteine 20% oral solution to a 3% solution.

Acetadote® is compatible with 5% dextrose, 1/2 normal saline (0.45% sodium chloride injection), and water for injection.

Monitoring Parameters Acetylcysteine overdose: AST, ALT, bilirubin, PT, serum creatinine, BUN, serum glucose and electrolytes. Acetylcysteine levels at ~4 hours post-ingestion (~8 hours if extended release acetaminophen), and 4-6 hours later to assess for possible hepatotoxicity.

Administration

Inhalation: Acetylcysteine is incompatible with tetracyclines, erythromycin, amphotericin B, iodized oil, chymotrypsin, trypsin, and hydrogen peroxide. Administer separately. Intermittent aerosol treatments are commonly given when patient arises, before meals, and just before retiring at bedtime.

Oral: For treatment of acetaminophen overdosage, administer orally as a 5% solution. Dilute the 20% solution 1:3 with a cola, orange juice, or other soft drink. Use within 1 hour of preparation. Unpleasant odor becomes less noticeable as treatment progresses. If patient vomits within 1 hour of dose, readminister.

I.V.: Intravenous formulation (Acetadote®): Administer loading dose of 150 mg/kg over 60 minutes, followed by two separate maintenance infusions: 50 mg/kg over 4 hours followed by 100 mg/kg over 16 hours. If not using commercially available I.V. formulation, use a 0.2-μ millipore filter (in-line).

Contraindications
Hypersensitivity to acetylcysteine or any component of the formulation

Warnings

Inhalation: Since increased bronchial secretions may develop after inhalation, percussion, postural drainage, and suctioning should follow. If bronchospasm occurs, administer a bronchodilator; discontinue acetylcysteine if bronchospasm progresses.

Intravenous: Acute flushing and erythema have been reported; usually occurs within 30-60 minutes and may resolve spontaneously. Serious anaphylactoid reactions have also been reported. Acetylcysteine infusion may be interrupted until treatment of allergic symptoms is initiated; the infusion can then be carefully restarted. Treatment for anaphylactic reactions should be immediately available. Use caution with asthma or history of bronchospasm.

Acetaminophen overdose: The modified Rumack-Matthew nomogram allows for stratification of patients into risk categories based on the relationship between the serum acetaminophen level and time after ingestion. There are several situations where the nomogram is of limited use. Serum acetaminophen levels obtained prior to 4-hour postingestion are not interpretable; patients presenting late may have undetectable serum concentrations, but have received a lethal dose. The nomogram is less predictive in a chronic ingestion or in an overdose with an extended release product. Acetylcysteine should be administered for any signs of hepatotoxicity even if acetaminophen serum level is low or undetectable. The nomogram also does not take into account patients at higher risk of acetaminophen toxicity (eg, alcoholics, malnourished patients).

Dosage Forms

Injection, solution:

Acetadote®: 20% [200 mg/mL] (30 mL) [contains disodium edetate]
Solution, inhalation/oral: 10% [100 mg/mL] (4 mL, 10 mL, 30 mL); 20% [200 mg/mL] (4 mL, 10 mL, 30 mL)

Reference Range
Determine acetaminophen level as soon as possible, ideally at least 4 hours after ingestion; toxic concentration with possible hepatotoxicity >150 mcg/mL (probably hepatotoxicity >200 mcg/mL) at 4 hours or 50 mcg/mL at 12 hours; serum N-acetylcysteine level is ~500 mg/L 15 minutes after a loading dose of 150 mg/kg. An I.V. dose of 150 mg/kg results in an approximate serum N-acetylcysteine level of 554 mg/L. Peak plasma N-acetylcysteine level in the I.V. protocol is approximately 6-35 times higher than in the oral protocol.

Test Interaction
Intravenous N-Acetylcystein can decrease clothing factors within the first hour of administration thus increasing Prothrombin time; usually resolved in 16 hours

Drug Interactions
Adsorbed orally by activated charcoal; clinical significance is minimal, though, once a pure acetaminophen ingestion requiring N-acetylcysteine is established; further charcoal dosing is unnecessary once the appropriate initial charcoal dose is achieved (5-10 g:g acetaminophen)

Pregnancy Risk Factor
B

Pregnancy Implications
Based on limited reports using acetylcysteine to treat acetaminophen overdose in pregnant women, acetylcysteine has been shown to cross the placenta in a limited manner and may provide protective levels in the fetus

Lactation
Excretion in breast milk unknown/use caution

Nursing Implications
Assess patient for nausea, vomiting, and skin rash following oral administration for treatment of acetaminophen poisoning; intermittent aerosol treatments are commonly given when patient arises, before meals, and just before retiring at bedtime

Additional Information
Rate of adverse effects from intravenous N-acetylcysteine is 11% to 14% Acetadote® may turn from an essentially colorless liquid to a slight pink or purple color once the stopper is punctured. Acetadote® is a hyperosmolar solution.

Specific References

Asif A, Garces G, Preston RA, et al, "Current Trials of Interventions to Prevent Radiocontrast-Induced Nephropathy," *Am J Ther*, 2005, 12(2):127-32.

Asif A, Preston RA, and Roth D, "Radiocontrast-Induced Nephropathy," *Am J Ther*, 2003, 10(2):137-47.

Betten DP, Burner EF, Williams SR, et al, "A Retrospective Evaluation of Shortened Course Oral N-Acetylcysteine for the Treatment of Acute Acetaminophen Poisoning," *Clin Toxicol (Phila)*, 2005, 43:671.

Betten DP, Cantrell FL, Thomas S, et al, "A Prospective Evaluation of Shortened Course Oral N-Acetylcysteine for the Treatment of Acute Acetaminophen Poisoning," *Clin Toxicol (Phila)*, 2005, 43:681.

Bailey B, Blais R, and Letarte A, "Status Epilepticus After a Massive Intravenous N-Acetylcysteine Overdose Leading to Intracranial Hypertension and Death," *Ann Emerg Med*, 2004, 44:401-6.

Birck R, Krzossok S, Markowetz F, et al, "Acetylcysteine for Prevention of Contrast Nephropathy: Meta-Analysis," *Lancet*, 2003, 362(9384):598-603.

Bird SB, Mazzola JL, Brush DE, et al, "A Prospective Evaluation of Abbreviated Oral N-Acetylcysteine (NAC) Therapy for Acetaminophen Poisoning," *Acad Emerg Med*, 2003, 10:521.

Burns KE, Chu MW, Novick RJ, et al, "Perioperative N-Acetylcysteine to Prevent Renal Dysfunction in High-Risk Patients Undergoing CABG Surgery: A Randomized Controlled Trial," *JAMA*, 2005, 20;294(3):342-50.

Dandoy CE, Crouch BI, and Caravati EM, "Masking the Smell and Taste of Acetylcysteine (NAC): What Is the Best Option?" *Clin Toxicol (Phila)*, 2005, 43:672.

Desai A, Kadleck D, Hufford L, et al, "N-Acetylcysteine Use in Ischemic Hepatitis," *Am J Ther*, 2006, 13(1):80-3.

Dribben WH, Porto SM, and Jeffords BK, "Stability and Microbiology of Inhalant N-Acetylcysteine Used as an Intravenous Solution for the Treatment of Acetaminophen Poisoning," *Ann Emerg Med*, 2003, 42(1):9-13.

Feng S and Stephan M, "Inhalational Intravenous N-Acetylcysteine (Inh IVNAC) Use in Children for Acetaminophen Toxicity," *Clin Toxicol (Phila)*, 2005, 43:678.

Fukumoto M, Fukushima R, Soma K, et al, "*In vitro* Evaluation of Concomitant Use of Activated Charcoal and N-Acetylcysteine," *J Toxicol Clin Toxicol*, 2004, 42(5):752.

Gurbuz AK, Ozel AM, Ozturk R, et al, "Effect of N-Acetyl Cysteine on *Helicobacter pylori*," *South Med J*, 2005, 98(11):1095-7.

Lindgren K, Lattrez J, Nguyen C, et al, "Intravenous N-Acetylcysteine (NAC) Protocols Recommended by North American Poison Centers," *J Toxicol Clin Toxicol*, 2004, 42(5):733.

Maloney GE, Pallasch EM, Ahkter S, et al, "Methyl Ethyl Ketone Peroxide Ingestion in a Toddler Treated with N-Acetylcysteine," *Clin Toxicol (Phila)*, 2005, 43:658.

Marenzi G, Assanelli E, Marana I, et al, "N-Acetylcysteine and Contrast-Induced Nephropathy in Primary Angioplasty," *N Engl J Med*, 2006, 354(26):2773-82.

Merl W, Koutsogiannis Z, Kerr D, et al, "How Safe is Intravenous N-Acetylcysteine for the Treatment of Acetaminophen Toxicity?" *Acad Emerg Med*, 2006, 13(5):S176-7.

Mullins ME, Schmidt RU Jr, and Jang TB, "What is the Rate of Adverse Events with Intravenous Versus Oral N-Acetylcysteine in Pediatric Patients?" *Ann Emerg Med*, 2004, 44(5):547-8.

Ritter C, Andrades ME, Reinke A, et al, "Treatment with N-Acetylcysteine Plus Deferoxamine Protects Rats Against Oxidative Stress and Improves Survival in Sepsis," *Crit Care Med*, 2004, 32(2):342-9.

Schmidt P, Parg D, Nykamp D et al, "N-Acetylcystein and Sodium Bicarbonate Versus N-Acetylcysteine and Standard Hydration for the Prevention of Radio Contrast Induced Nephropathy Following Coronary Angiography," *Ann of Pharmacol*, 2006, 41(1):46-50.

Schmidt R, Jang T, Schmidt L, "Comparison of Pediatric Use of IV and Oral N-Acetylcysteine," *J Toxicol Clin Toxicol*, 2003, 41(5):675.

Sivilotti ML, Yarema MC, Juurlink DN, et al, "A Risk Quantification Instrument for Acute Acetaminophen Overdose Patients Treated with N-Acetylcysteine," *Ann Emerg Med*, 2005, 46(3):263-71.

Sklar GE and Subramaniam M, "Acetylcysteine Treatment for Non-Acetaminophen-Induced Acute Liver Failure," *Ann Pharmacother*, 2004, 38(3):498-500.

Spapen HD, Diltoer MW, Nguyen DN, et al, "Effects of N-Acetylcysteine on Microalbuminuria and Organ Failure in Acute Severe Sepsis: Results of a Pilot Study," *Chest*, 2005, 127(4):1413-9.

Tsai CL, Chang WT, and Fang CC, "Acetaminophen Half-Life as a Reference in Choosing Shorter Oral N-Acetylcysteine Therapy for the Overdosed Patients," *J Toxicol Clin Toxicol*, 2003, 41(5):725.

Wasserman GS and Garg U, "Intravenous Administration of N-Acetylcysteine: Interference with Coagulopathy Testing," *Ann Emerg Med*, 2004, 44(5):546-7.

Alcohol, Ethyl

Pronunciation (AL koe hol, ETH il)

Related Information
- Ethyl Alcohol

U.S. Brand Names Lavacol® [OTC]

Synonyms Alcohol, Absolute; Alcohol, Dehydrated; Ethanol; Ethyl Alcohol EtOH

Impairment Potential Yes. See Ethyl Alcohol

Commonly Includes Whiskey; Vodka

Use Antidotal therapy for methanol and ethylene glycol intoxication

Unlabeled/Investigational Use Antidote for ethylene glycol overdose; antidote for methanol overdose; treatment of fat occlusion of central venous catheters

Mechanism of Action Competitive antagonism with methanol and ethylene glycol as substrate alcohol dehydrogenase; the interaction thereby results in decreased formation of toxic metabolites and metabolic acidosis

Adverse Reactions

Cardiovascular: Postural hypotension, palpitations, hypotension (orthostatic), syncope

Central nervous system: Inebriation, sedation, coma, memory loss

Endocrine & metabolic: Hypoglycemia, osmolal gap, breast cancer, hyperprolactinemia

Gastrointestinal: Nausea, vomiting, gastritis

Neuromuscular & skeletal: Osteoporosis

Ocular: Ptosis

Respiratory: Respiratory sedation, apnea

Signs and Symptoms of Overdose See Ethyl Alcohol

Pharmacodynamics/Kinetics

Absorption: Oral: Rapid

Distribution: V_d: 0.6-0.7 L/kg; decreased in women

Metabolism: Hepatic (90% to 98%) to acetaldehyde or acetate

Half-life elimination: Rate: 15-20 mg/dL/hour (range: 10-34 mg/dL/hour); increased in alcoholics

Excretion: Kidneys and lungs (~2% unchanged)

Dosage

Oral: Loading dose: 1 g/kg (may be diluted in juice), then for maintenance: 0.1 g/kg/hour (in nondrinkers) or 0.2 g/kg/hour (in a chronic drinker); on dialysis, double the maintenance dose

I.V.: Administer 750 mg/kg as a loading dose, followed by 100-150 mg/hour; increase to 175-200 mg/kg in chronic alcoholics, or during hemodialysis; see table.

Ethyl Alcohol Dosage

	5% I.V.	10% I.V.	50% P.O.
Loading	15 mL/kg	7.5 mL/kg	1.5 mL/kg
Maintenance	2-4 mL/kg	1-2 mL/kg	0.2-0.4 mL/kg/hr
Maintenance during hemodialysis	4-7 mL/kg	2-3.5 mL/kg	0.4-0.7 mL/kg/hr

Monitoring Parameters Respiration rate, blood pressure

Administration

Oral: Ethylene glycol or methanol poisoning: Dilute ethyl alcohol to 20% solution and administer hourly via NG tube. Oral treatment is not recommended outside of a hospital setting.

I.V.: Ethylene glycol or methanol poisoning: Administer as a 10% solution in D_5W. Initial dose should be administered over 1 hour.

Treatment of occluded central venous catheter: Instill a 70% solution with a volume equal to the internal volume of the catheter. Assess patency at 30-60 minutes (or per institutional protocol).

Intraneural: Separate needles should be used for each of multiple injections or sites to prevent residual alcohol deposition at sites not intended for tissue destruction. Inject slowly after determining proper placement of needle. Since dehydrated alcohol is hypobaric when compared with spinal fluid, proper positioning of the patient is essential to control localization of injections into the subarachnoid space.

Contraindications Hypersensitivity to ethyl alcohol or any component of the formulation; seizure disorder and diabetic coma; subarachnoid injection of dehydrated alcohol in patients receiving anticoagulants; pregnancy

Warnings

Ethyl alcohol is a flammable liquid and should be kept cool and away from any heat source. Proper positioning of the patient for neurolytic administration is essential to control localization of the injection of dehydrated alcohol (which is hypobaric) into the subarachnoid space; avoid extravasation. Not for SubQ administration. Do not administer simultaneously with blood due to the possibility of pseudoagglutination or hemolysis; may potentiate severe hypoprothrombic bleeding. Clinical evaluation and periodic lab determinations, including serum ethanol levels, are necessary to monitor effectiveness, changes in electrolyte concentrations, and acid-base balance (when used as an antidote).

Use with caution in patients with diabetes (ethyl alcohol decreases blood sugar), hepatic impairment, patients with gout, shock, following cranial surgery, and in anticipated postpartum hemorrhage. Monitor blood glucose closely, particularly in children as treatment of ingestions is associated with hypoglycemia. Avoid extravasation during I.V. administration. Water intoxication can occur with high infusion rates using I.V. products. Ethyl alcohol passes freely into breast milk at a level approximately equivalent to maternal serum level; minimize dermal exposure of ethyl alcohol in infants as significant systemic absorption and toxicity can occur.

Dosage Forms

Foam, topical:
Epi-Clenz™: 62% (240 mL, 480 mL) [instant hand sanitizer; contains aloe vera and vitamin E]

Gel, topical:
Epi-Clenz™: 70% (45 mL, 120 mL, 480 mL) [instant hand sanitizer; contains aloe vera and vitamin E]
GelRite: 67% (120 mL, 480 mL, 800 mL) [instant hand sanitizer; contains vitamin E)
Gel-Stat™: 62% (120 mL, 480 mL) [instant hand sanitizer]
Isagel®: 60% (59 mL, 118 mL, 621 mL, 800 mL) [instant hand sanitizer]
Prevacare®: 60% (120 mL, 240 mL, 960 mL, 1200 mL, 1500 mL) [instant hand sanitizer]
Protection Plus®: 62% (800 mL) [instant hand sanitizer]
Purell®: 62% (15 mL, 30 mL, 59 mL, 120 mL, 236 mL, 250 mL, 360 mL, 500 mL, 800 mL,1000 mL, 2000 mL) [instant hand sanitizer; contains moisturizers and vitamin E]
Purell® Moisture Therapy: 62% (75 mL) [instant hand sanitizer]
Purell® with Aloe: 62% (15 mL, 59 mL, 236 mL, 360 mL, 800 mL, 1000 mL, 2000 mL) [instant hand sanitizer; contains aloe and tartrazine]

Infusion [in D_5W, dehydrated]: Alcohol 5% (1000 mL)

Injection, solution [dehydrated]: 98% (1 mL, 5 mL)

Liquid, topical [denatured]: 70% (3840 mL)
Lavacol®: 70% (473 mL)

Lotion, topical:
Purell® 2 in 1: 62% (60 mL, 360 mL, 1000 mL) [instant hand sanitizer]

Towelettes, topical:
Isagel®: 60% (50s, 300s) [instant hand sanitizer]
Purell®: 62% (24s, 35s, 175s) [instant hand sanitizer]

Pregnancy Risk Factor D/X (prolonged use or high doses at term)

Pregnancy Implications Use only if the potential benefits outweigh the risks; ethanol crosses the placenta readily and enters fetal circulation

Lactation Enters breast milk/use caution (AAP rates "compatible")

Nursing Implications Patients receiving ethanol by infusion or mouth, may become obtunded and inebriated; they should be cared for in a carefully monitored environment

Specific References

Al-Sanouri I, Dikin M, and Soubani AO, "Critical Care Aspects of Alcohol Abuse," *South Med J*, 2005, 98(3):372-81 (review).

Astley SJ, *Diagnostic Guide for Fetal Alcohol Spectrum Disorders: The 4-Digit Diagnostic Code*, 3rd ed, Seattle, WA: University of Washington Publication Services, 2004.

Bertrand J, Floyd LL, Weber MK, et al, *Fetal Alcohol Syndrome Guidelines for Referral and Diagnosis*, Atlanta, GA: US Department of Health and Human Services, CDC, 2004.

Bertrand J, Floyd LL, Weber MK, et al, "Guidelines for Identifying and Referring Persons with Fetal Alcohol Syndrome," *MMWR Recomm Rep*, 2005, 54(RR-11):1-14

Burd L, Klug MG, Martsolf JT, et al, "Fetal Alcohol Syndrome: Neuropsychiatric Phenomics," *Neurotoxicol Teratol*, 2003, 25(6):697-705.

Eldridge DL, Stoeckle MM, Holstege CP, et al, "Elevated Troponin Level and ST Wave Depression Secondary to Disulfiram-Like Reaction Resulting from Suspected Deficit in Ethanol Metabolism," *Clin Toxicol*, 2005, 43:640.

Johnson RD, Lewis RJ, Angier MK, et al, "The Formation of Ethanol in Postmortem Tissues," *U.S. Department of Transportation*, Final Report, 2004.

Johnson RD, Lewis RJ, Canfield DV, et al, "Accurate Assignment of Ethanol Origin in Postmortem Urine: Liquid Chromatographic-Mass Spectrometric Determination of Serotonin Metabolites," *J Chromatogr B Analyt Technol Biomed Life Sci*, 2004, 805(2):223-34.

Kelly CA, Upex A, and Bateman DN, "Comparison of Consciousness Level Assessment in the Poisoned Patient Using the Alert/Verbal/Painful/Unresponsive Scale and the Glasgow Coma Scale," *Ann Emerg Med*, 2004, 44(2):108-13.

Kristoffersen L, Skuterud B, Larssen BR, et al, "Fast Quantification of Ethanol in Whole Blood Specimens by the Enzymatic Alcohol Dehydrogenase Method, Optimization by Experimental Design," *J Anal Toxicol*, 2005, 29:66-9.

Moriya F and Hashimoto Y, "Postmortem Production of Ethanol and N-Propanol in the Brain of Drowned Persons," *Am J Forensic Med Pathol*, 2004, 25(2):131-3.

Roccella M and Testa D, "Fetal Alcohol Syndrome in Developmental Age: Neuropsychiatric Aspects," *Minerva Pediatr*, 2003, 55(1):63-9, 69-74.

Roy M, Bailey B, Chalut D, et al, "What Are the Adverse Effects of Ethanol Used as an Antidote in the Treatment of Suspected Methanol Poisoning in Children?" *J Toxicol Clin Toxicol*, 2003, 41(2):155-61.

Suchard J, "Osmotic Activity of Ethanol in Fresh Whole Blood," *J Toxicol Clin Toxicol*, 2004, 42(5):751.

Amifostine

Pronunciation (am i FOS teen)
Related Information
- Cisplatin
- Cyclophosphamide

CAS Number 20537-88-6; 63717-27-1
U.S. Brand Names Ethyol®
Synonyms Ethiofos; Gammaphos; WR-2721; YM-08310
Use Reduce the incidence of moderate to severe xerostomia in patients undergoing postoperative radiation treatment for head and neck cancer, where the radiation port includes a substantial portion of the parotid glands. Reduce the cumulative renal toxicity associated with repeated administration of cisplatin in patients with advanced ovarian cancer or nonsmall cell lung cancer.
Mechanism of Action Organic thiophosphate compound which acts as a free radical scavenger agent; can be nephroprotective from alkylating agent effects; radioprotectant and can cause hypocalcemia through inhibition of bone resorption and parathyroid hormone secretion
Adverse Reactions
Cardiovascular: **Hypotension** (related to dose and infusion rates), **flushing**, cardiac arrest
Central nervous system: Drowsiness, sedation, fever, **chills, dizziness, somnolence**
Dermatologic: Exfoliative dermatitis, toxicoderma
Endocrine & metabolic: Hypocalcemia, hypomagnesemia
Gastrointestinal: **Nausea, vomiting** (may be severe)
Respiratory: **Sneezing**
Miscellaneous: **Feeling of warmth/coldness**, hiccups
Pharmacodynamics/Kinetics
Distribution: V_d: 3.5 L
Metabolism: Hepatic dephosphorylation to two metabolites (active-free thiol and disulfide)
Half-life elimination: 8-9 minutes
Excretion: Urine
Clearance, plasma: 2.17 L/minute
Dosage
Adults:
Cisplatin-induced renal toxicity, reduction: I.V.: 740-910 mg/m^2 once daily 30 minutes prior to cytotoxic therapy
Note: Doses >740 mg/m^2 are associated with a higher incidence of hypotension and may require interruption of therapy or dose modification for subsequent cycles. For 910 mg/m^2 doses, the manufacturer suggests the following blood pressure-based adjustment schedule:
The infusion of amifostine should be interrupted if the systolic blood pressure decreases significantly from baseline, as defined below:
Decrease of 20 mm Hg if baseline systolic blood pressure <100
Decrease of 25 mm Hg if baseline systolic blood pressure 100-119
Decrease of 30 mm Hg if baseline systolic blood pressure 120-139
Decrease of 40 mm Hg if baseline systolic blood pressure 140-179
Decrease of 50 mm Hg if baseline systolic blood pressure ≥180
If the blood pressure returns to normal within 5 minutes (assisted by fluid administration and postural management) and the patient is asymptomatic, the infusion may be restarted so that the full dose of amifostine may be administered. If the full dose of amifostine cannot be administered, the dose of amifostine for subsequent cycles should be 740 mg/m^2.
Xerostomia from head and neck cancer, reduction:
I.V.: 200mg/m^2/day during radiation therapy **or**
SubQ: 500 mg/day during radiation therapy
Stability Store intact vials of lyophilized powder at room temperature (20°C to 25°C/68°F to 77°F). Reconstitute with 9.7 mL of sterile 0.9% sodium chloride. The reconstituted solution (500 mg/10 mL) is chemically stable for up to 5 hours at room temperature (25°C) or up to 24 hours under refrigeration (2°C to 8°C). Amifostine should be further diluted in 0.9% sodium chloride to a concentration of 5-40 mg/mL; diluted solutions (5-40 mg/mL) are stable for up to 5 hours at room temperature (25°C) or up to 24 hours under refrigeration (2°C to 8°C). For SubQ administration, reconstitute with 2.4 mL NS or SWFI.
Monitoring Parameters Blood pressure should be monitored every 5 minutes during the infusion
Administration I.V.: Administer over 3-15 minutes; administration as a longer infusion is associated with a higher incidence of side effects
Contraindications Hypersensitivity to amifostine, aminothiol compounds, or any component of the formulation
Warnings
Patients who are hypotensive or dehydrated should not receive amifostine. Interrupt antihypertensive therapy for 24 hours before amifostine. Patients who cannot safely stop their antihypertensives 24 hours before amifostine should not receive it. Patients should be adequately hydrated prior to amifostine infusion and kept in a supine position during the infusion. Blood pressure should be monitored every 5 minutes during the infusion. If hypotension requiring interruption of therapy occurs, patients should be placed in the Trendelenburg position and given an infusion of normal saline using a separate I.V. line; subsequent infusions may require a dose reduction. Use caution in patients with cardiovascular and cerebrovascular disease and any other patients in whom the adverse effects of hypotension and nausea/vomiting may have serious adverse events.
It is recommended that antiemetic medication, including dexamethasone 20 mg I.V. and a serotonin 5-HT$_3$ receptor antagonist be administered prior to and in conjunction with amifostine. Rare hypersensitivity reactions, including anaphylaxis and severe cutaneous reaction, have been reported with a higher frequency in patients receiving amifostine as a radioprotectant. Discontinue if allergic reaction occurs; do not rechallenge.
Reports of clinically-relevant hypocalcemia are rare, but serum calcium levels should be monitored in patients at risk of hypocalcemia, such as those with nephrotic syndrome. Safety and efficacy in children have not been established.
Dosage Forms
Injection, powder for reconstitution:
Ethyol®: 500 mg
Reference Range Peak serum amifostine after an I.V. dose of 150 mg/m^2 ranges from 100-900 µmol/L
Overdosage/Treatment Supportive therapy: Keep patient well hydrated; monitor renal status, calcium, and magnesium
Antidote(s)
- Cisplatin
- Cyclophosphamide

Drug Interactions Antihypertensives: May potentiate the hypotensive effects of amifostine.
Pregnancy Risk Factor C
Pregnancy Implications Animal studies have demonstrated embryotoxicity. There are no adequate and well-controlled studies in pregnant women.
Lactation Excretion in breast milk unknown/not recommended

Amyl Nitrite

Pronunciation (AM il NYE trite)
Related Information
- Cyanide Antidote Kit [ANTIDOTE]

CAS Number 110-46-3; 463-04-7
Synonyms Isoamyl Nitrite
Impairment Potential Yes
Use Coronary vasodilator in angina pectoris; an adjunct in treatment of cyanide poisoning; also used to produce changes in the intensity of heart murmurs
Mechanism of Action Vasodilator (vascular smooth muscle relaxant)
Adverse Reactions
Cardiovascular: Postural hypotension, cutaneous flushing of head, neck, and clavicular area, palpitations, tachycardia, sinus tachycardia, vasodilation
Central nervous system: Headache, incoherent speech
Dermatologic: Contact dermatitis
Gastrointestinal: Nausea, colitis, vomiting
Genitourinary: Penile erection is enhanced, retarded ejaculation
Hematologic: Heinz body hemolysis/hemolytic anemia, methemoglobinemia followed by hemolysis
Ocular: Increased intraocular pressure, blurred vision, yellow vision
Respiratory: Tracheobronchitis
Signs and Symptoms of Overdose Ataxia, bradycardia, coma, cyanosis, dyspnea, methemoglobinemia (may be followed by hemolysis), stupor, tachycardia, hypotension due to vasodilitation
Admission Criteria/Prognosis Any patient with change in mental status, cardiopulmonary complaints, or methemoglobin levels >30% should be admitted; asymptomatic patients with methemoglobin levels <30% may be considered for discharge after 6 hours of observation and if methemoglobin levels fall to <15%
Pharmacodynamics/Kinetics
Onset of action: Angina: Within 30 seconds
Duration: 3-15 minutes
Dosage 1-6 inhalations from one capsule are usually sufficient to produce the desired effect
Stability Store in cool place, protect from light; insoluble in water; inflammable
Monitoring Parameters Monitor blood pressure during therapy
Administration Administer nasally. Patient should not be sitting. Crush ampul in woven covering between fingers and then hold under patient's nostrils.
Contraindications Hypersensitivity to nitrates; severe anemia; head injury; angle-closure glaucoma; postural hypotension; head trauma or cerebral hemorrhage; pregnancy
Warnings Use with caution in patients with increased intracranial pressure, low systolic blood pressure, and coronary artery disease.
Dosage Forms Vapor for inhalation [crushable covered glass capsules]: Amyl nitrite USP (0.3 mL)

Drug Interactions
Ethanol taken with amyl nitrite may have additive side effects.
Sildenafil: Avoid concurrent use of sildenafil; severe reactions may result.
Pregnancy Risk Factor X
Lactation Excretion in breast milk unknown/not recommended
Nursing Implications Administer by nasal inhalation; patient should be sitting; crush ampul in woven covering between fingers and then hold under patient's nostrils

Angiotensin Amide

CAS Number 11128-99-7; 53-73-6
Use Has been used to treat hypotension; may be antidotal for angiotensin-converting enzyme inhibitor overdose. May possibly be useful in treating hypotension due to amiodarone.
Mechanism of Action Related to the peptide angiotensin II, this pressor agent increases peripheral resistance of peripheral blood vessels (splanchnic, renal, cutaneous).
Adverse Reactions Cardiovascular: Hypertension, bradycardia (reflex)
Dosage Hypotension: Continuous intravenous infusion: 1-10 mg of drug in 1 liter of 0.9% sodium chloride or 5% glucose. Titrate to desired blood pressure. Doses up to 18 mcg/minute have been used, but most patients will respond to doses of 3-10 mcg/minute.

Antitoxin Botulinin Types A, B, and E

Use Prophylaxis or active treatment of individuals who have eaten food known or strongly suspected of being infected with *Clostridium botulinum*
Adverse Reactions
Cardiovascular: Tachycardia, cardiovascular collapse, flushing, cyanosis, sinus tachycardia
Dermatologic: Urticaria
Ocular: **Dry eyes, lagophthalmos, ptosis, photophobia, vertical deviation**
Respiratory: Wheezing, bronchospasm, apnea
Miscellaneous: Signs or symptoms of anaphylaxis (typically occur within 20-60 minutes); serum sickness may occur within 14 days of administration and is more likely to follow a repeat injection of equine serum; hypersensitivity
Stability Excessive agitation or shaking of the reconstituted vial may cause foaming, which may lead to denaturation of the antivenin
Monitoring Parameters Resolution of symptoms of botulism, or emergence of symptoms of sensitivity to the antitoxin
Administration Administer 1-2 vials slowly I.V. in a 1:10 dilution with 0.9% normal saline (may also give a dose of 1 vial I.M.), and then subsequent doses every 2-4 hours I.V. based on clinical findings. Avoid magnesium since it may enhance the action of the toxin. Trivalent (ABE) antitoxin is usually most effective if administered within 24 hours. Usually, only one vial dose is necessary.
Pregnancy Risk Factor C
Pregnancy Implications Use only if the potential benefits outweigh the risks; it is not known if botulinum antitoxin antibodies cross the placenta

Antivenin (Crotalidae) Polyvalent

Pronunciation (an tee VEN in (kroe TAL ih die) pol i VAY lent)
U.S. Brand Names Antivenin Polyvalent [Equine]; CroFab™ [Ovine]
Synonyms Crotalidae Antivenin; Crotaline Antivenin, Polyvalent; North and South American Antisnake-Bite Serum; Pit Viper Antivenin; Snake (Pit Vipers) Antivenin
Use Neutralization of venoms of North and South American crotalids: rattlesnake, massauga, cantil, copperhead, cottonmouth, water moccasins, fer-de-lance, bushmaster
Mechanism of Action Enhances venom elimination but has no effect on local tissue injury
Adverse Reactions
Cardiovascular: Chest pain, hypotension
Central nervous system: Chills, nervousness
Dermatologic: Cellulitis, bruising, pruritus, rash, urticaria
Gastrointestinal: Anorexia, nausea
Hematologic: Coagulation disorder, thrombocytopenia
Neuromuscular & skeletal: Back pain, circumoral paresthesia, general paresthesia, myalgia
Respiratory: Asthma, cough, dyspnea, sputum increased, wheezing
Miscellaneous: Allergic reaction, serum sickness, subcutaneous nodule, wound infection
Pharmacodynamics/Kinetics
Half-life elimination: Antivenin polyvalent (ovine): 12-23 hours (based on limited data)
Time to peak: Antivenin polyvalent (equine): I.M.: ≥8 hours
Dosage
Children and Adults: Crotalid envenomation:
Antivenin polyvalent (equine): I.M., I.V.: Initial sensitivity test: 0.02-0.03 mL of a 1:10 dilution of normal horse serum or antivenin given

intracutaneously; also give a control test using normal saline in the opposite extremity. A positive reaction occurs within 5-30 minutes. A negative reaction does not rule out the possibility of an immediate or delayed reaction with treatment.
Minimal envenomation: 50-100 mL (5-10 vials)
Moderate envenomation: 100-200 mL (10-20 vials)
Severe envenomation: >200 mL (≥20 vials)
Note: The entire initial dose of antivenin should be administered as soon as possible to be most effective (within 6 hours after the bite). I.V. is the preferred route of administration. When administered I.V., infuse the initial 5-10 mL dilution over 3-5 minutes while carefully observing the patient for signs and symptoms of sensitivity reactions. If no reaction occurs, continue infusion at a safe I.V. fluid delivery rate. Additional doses of antivenin are based on clinical response to the initial dose. If swelling continues to progress, symptoms increase in severity, hypotension occurs, or decrease in hematocrit appears, an additional 10-50 mL (1-5 vials) should be administered.
Antivenin polyvalent (ovine): Skin testing is not indicated. If it is necessary to give I.M., administer in the buttocks; avoid if possible.
I.V.: Minimal or moderate envenomation:
Initial dose: 4-6 vials, dependent upon patient response. Treatment should begin within 6 hours of snakebite; monitor for 1 hour following infusion. Repeat with an additional 4-6 vials if control is not achieved with initial dose. Continue to treat with 4- to 6-vial doses until complete arrest of local manifestations, coagulation tests, and systemic signs are normal. Administer I.V. over 60 minutes at a rate of 25-50 mL/hour for the first 10 minutes. If no allergic reaction is observed, increase rate to 250 mL/hour. Monitor closely
Maintenance dose: Once control is achieved, administer 2 vials every 6 hours for up to 18 hours (3 doses); optimal dosing past 18 hours has not been established; however, treatment may be continued if deemed necessary based on the patient's condition.
Stability
Antivenin polyvalent (equine): Store in refrigerator, avoid temperatures >37°C. For I.V. infusion; reconstitute each vial with 10 mL of bacteriostatic water for injection, provided with the antivenin; mix by gentle swirling; use within 48 hours. To prepare for I.V. use, further prepare a 1:1-1:10 dilution of reconstituted antivenin in normal saline or D₅W; use within 24 hours
Antivenin polyvalent (ovine): Store between 2°C to 8°C (36°F to 46°F); do not freeze. Reconstitute each vial with 10 mL sterile water and mix by gentle swirling. Further dilute total dose in 250 mL NS; use within 4 hours of reconstitution
Monitoring Parameters Vital signs; hematocrit, hemoglobin, platelet count (multiple times daily); prothrombin time, clot retraction, bleeding and coagulation times, BUN, electrolytes, bilirubin, size of bitten area (repeat every 15-30 minutes); intake and output, signs and symptoms of anaphylaxis/allergy
Administration
I.M.: Antivenin polyvalent (equine): May be used in cases of minimal envenomation; I.V. route is preferred. Administer into a large muscle mass, preferably the gluteal area. Avoid nerve trunks. Do not inject into finger or toe.
I.V.:
Antivenin polyvalent (equine): Infuse the initial 5-10 mL dilution over 3-5 minutes while carefully observing the patient for signs and symptoms of sensitivity reactions. If no reaction occurs, continue infusion at a safe I.V. fluid delivery rate. Total dose should be administered as soon as possible.
Antivenin polyvalent (ovine): Administer I.V. over 60 minutes at a rate of 25-50 mL/hour for the first 10 minutes. If no allergic reaction is observed, increase rate to 250 mL/hour. Monitor closely Epinephrine and diphenhydramine should be available during the infusion. Decreasing the rate of infusion may help control some adverse effects. Do not inject into finger or toe.
Contraindications Hypersensitivity to any component of the formulation, unless the benefits outweigh the risks and appropriate management for anaphylaxis is available
Warnings Should be used within 4-6 hours of snakebite to prevent clinical deterioration and development of coagulation abnormalities. Coagulation abnormalities are due directly to snake venom interference with the coagulation cascade. Recurrent coagulopathy occurs in approximately 50% of patients and may persist for 1-2 weeks or more. Patients should be monitored for at least 1 week and evaluated for other, pre-existing conditions associated with bleeding disorders. In severe rattlesnake bites, a decrease in platelets may occur, lasting hours to several days, and whole blood transfusions may not be effective treatment. Anaphylaxis and anaphylactoid reactions are possible due to animal proteins in the antivenin. Patients should also be monitored for delayed allergic reactions or serum sickness. Antivenin polyvalent (equine) contains phenol, thimerosal, and is made from horse serum. A skin test for horse-serum sensitivity should be done prior to treatment. Antivenin polyvalent (ovine) is processed with papain and may cause hypersensitivity reactions in patients allergic to papaya, other papaya extracts, papain, chymopapain,

or the pineapple enzyme bromelain. There may also be cross allergy with dust mite and latex allergens. Antivenin polyvalent (ovine) also contains thimerosal and is made from sheep plasma.

Dosage Forms

Injection, powder for reconstitution:

Antivenin (Crotalidae) polyvalent [equine]: Derived from *Crotalus adamanteus*, *C. atrox*, *C. durissus terrificus*, and *Bothrops atrox* snake venoms [equine origin; contains phenol and thimerosal; packaged with diluent and normal horse serum for sensitivity testing]

CroFab™ [ovine]: Derived from *Crotalus adamanteus*, *C. atrox*, *C. scutulatus*, and *Agkistrodon piscivorus* snake venoms [ovine origin; contains thimerosal; manufactured with papain]

Drug Interactions No drug interaction studies have been conducted

Pregnancy Risk Factor C

Pregnancy Implications Reproduction studies have not been conducted. Products contain thimerosal, which may be associated with neurological and renal toxicities in the fetus and very young children.

Lactation Excretion in breast milk unknown/use caution

Nursing Implications

Administer at a slower rate initially; monitor for signs and symptoms of sensitivity reactions. Reactions to antivenin may occur anytime during treatment and for weeks after administration.

Antivenin polyvalent (equine): Antivenin may be administered I.M. for minimal envenomation. I.V. administration of antivenin is preferred for moderate to severe envenomation or in the presence of shock; do not inject into a finger or toe

Specific References

Baer AB, Kirk MA, Eldridge DL, et al, "Profound Thrombocytopenia Induced by *Crotalus Horridus* Envenomation Unresponsive to Crofab," *J Toxicol Clin Toxicol*, 2004, 42(5):810.

Bebarta V and Dart R, "Effectiveness of Delayed Use of Crotalidae Polyvalent Immune Fab (Ovine) Antivenom," *J Toxicol Clin Toxicol*, 2003, 41(5):702.

Goto CS, Gutglass DJ, Richardson WH, et al, "Pediatric Rattlesnake Envenomation with Neurotoxicity Refractory to Treatment with Crotaline Fab Antivenom," *J Toxicol Clin Toxicol*, 2003, 41(5):702.

Pizon AF, Riley BD, LoVecchio F, et al, "Safety and Efficacy of CroFab in Pediatric Crotaline Envenomations," *Acad Emerg Med*, 2006, 13(5):S178-9.

Richardson WH, Barry JD, Tong TC, et al, "Rattlesnake Envenomation to the Face of an Infant," *J Toxicol Clin Toxicol*, 2003, 41(5):700-1.

Richardson WH 3rd, Tanen DA, Tong TC, et al, "Crotalidae Polyvalent Immune Fab (Ovine) Antivenom is Effective in the Neutralization of South American Viperidae Venoms in a Murine Model," *Ann Emerg Med*, 2005, 45(6):595-602.

Schier JG, Wiener SW, Touger M, et al, "Efficacy of Crotalidae Polyvalent Antivenin for the Treatment of Hognosed Viper (*Porthidium nasutum*) Envenomation," *Ann Emerg Med*, 2003, 41(3):391-5.

Stanford CF, Olsen D, Bogdan GM, et al, "Complications of Crotaline Antivenom Therapy in the United States," *Clin Toxicol (Phila)*, 2005, 43:708.

Tanen DA, Danish DC, and Clark RF, "Crotalidae Polyvalent Immune Fab Antivenom Limits the Decrease in Perfusion Pressure of the Anterior Leg Compartment in a Porcine Crotaline Envenomation Model," *Ann Emerg Med*, 2003, 41(3):384-90.

Antivenin (*Latrodectus mactans*)

Pronunciation (an tee VEN in lak tro DUK tus MAK tans)

Synonyms Black Widow Spider Species Antivenin (*Latrodectus mactans*)

Use Symptoms of envenomation by the black widow spider (*Latrodectus mactans*) including severe hypertension or pain refractory to analgesia, calcium, or sedation; and/or abdominal muscle spasm in pregnancy, threatened spontaneous abortion or early onset labor; also patients in respiratory distress; patients with cardiac disease; pediatric patients or the elderly

Mechanism of Action Refined, concentrated, and lyophilized preparation of serum globulins from horses immunized with black widow spider (*Latrodectus mactans*) venom

Adverse Reactions

Cardiovascular: Tachycardia, cardiovascular collapse, flushing, cyanosis, sinus tachycardia

Dermatologic: Urticaria

Respiratory: Wheezing, bronchospasm, apnea

Miscellaneous: Other signs or symptoms of anaphylaxis (typically occur within 20-60 minutes); serum sickness may occur within 14 days of administration, and is more likely to follow a repeat injection of equine serum

Signs and Symptoms of Overdose Localized diaphoresis at site of bite

Stability Excessive agitation or shaking of the reconstituted vial may cause foaming, which may lead to denaturation of the antivenin

Monitoring Parameters Resolution of symptoms of *L. mactans* intoxication or emergence of symptoms of sensitivity to the antivenin

Administration Administer a test dose: 0.01-0.02 mL of reconstituted antivenom diluted 1:10, administered SubQ. Resuscitation equipment should be readily available. After one test dose, give 1 vial I.V. diluted in normal saline (50-100 mL) infused over ~20-30 minutes; pretreatment with epinephrine or with an antihistamine may prevent allergic reactions; may repeat with a second dose if the patient weighs >40 kg or if there is no response

Warnings Carefully review allergies and history of exposure to products containing horse serum. History of atopic sensitivity to horses may increase risk of immediate sensitivity reactions. A skin or conjunctival test should be performed prior to use in all patients. A desensitization protocol is available if sensitivity tests are mildly or questionably positive to reduce risk of immediate severe hypersensitivity reaction. Desensitization should be performed only when antivenin administration would be lifesaving. In otherwise healthy adults (16-60 years), use of antivenin may be deferred and other treatments may be considered. Epinephrine 1:1000 should be readily available.

Dosage Forms Injection, powder for reconstitution: 6000 antivenin units [equine origin; contains thimerosal; packaged with diluent and normal horse serum for sensitivity testing]

Pregnancy Risk Factor C

Pregnancy Implications Use only if the potential benefits outweigh risks; it is not known if *L. mactans* antivenin antibodies cross the placenta

Lactation Excretion in breast milk unknown/use caution

Nursing Implications Patient should be closely monitored for symptoms of hypersensitivity or anaphylaxis during skin or eye testing, desensitization, drug administration, and for 24 hours following administration

Antivenin (*Micrurus fulvius*)

Pronunciation (an tee VEN in mye KRU rus FUL vee us)

Synonyms North American Coral Snake Antivenin

Use Envenomation by the eastern coral snake (*Micrurus fulvius fulvius*) or the Texas coral snake (*M. fulvius tenere*); antivenin therapy should be instituted as soon as the biting snake is identified as *M. fulvius fulvius* or *M. fulvius tenere*, because systemic symptoms may be impossible to reverse at a later time

Mechanism of Action Refined, concentrated, and lyophilized preparation of serum globulins from horses immunized with eastern coral snake (*M. fulvius fulvius*) venom

Adverse Reactions

Cardiovascular: Shock, facial edema

Central nervous system: Apprehension

Dermatologic: Urticaria

Neuromuscular & skeletal: Peripheral neuritis, muscle weakness

Miscellaneous: Anaphylaxis, serum sickness

Dosage I.V.: Children and Adults: 3-5 vials by slow injection (dependent on severity of signs/symptoms; some patients may need more than 10 vials)

Stability Prior to reconstitution, store at 2°C to 8°C (36°F to 46°F); do not freeze. Dilute each vial with SWFI 10 mL. Vial contains a vacuum which will pull the diluent in, point diluent stream at the center of the lyophilized pellet. If diluent runs down side of vial, the pellet will float and adhere to vial stopper. Swirl gently, do not shake, for 1 minute then repeat every 5 minutes. Reconstitution takes ~30 minutes/vial. Color of final solution may vary from clear to slight yellow or green.

Excessive agitation or shaking of the reconstituted vial may cause foaming, which may lead to denaturation of the antivenin

Monitoring Parameters Resolution of symptoms of *M. fulvius* intoxication or emergence of symptoms of sensitivity to the antivenin; also monitor respiratory function and oxygenation, as well as the urine for hemoglobinuria

Administration Similar scheme as per antivenin for Crotalidae; usually less amount of vials need to be administered; average dose: 4-6 vials; rarely more than 10 vials are necessary; can treat allergic reactions with antihistamines and corticosteroids

Contraindications Concomitant use with opioid analgesics or other respiratory depressants; history of anaphylaxis to equine-derived serum is a relative contraindication

Warnings When administering this agent, have ready access to drugs and equipment for resuscitation. Use caution with asthma, hay fever, urticaria, equine allergy, prior injections with equine serum. Perform skin test prior to administration. The absence of a skin hypersensitivity reaction does not exclude anaphylaxis or hypersensitivity following antivenin administration. False-negative rate for skin testing is 10% with similar agents. Conversely, hypersensitivity is not an absolute contraindication in a significantly envenomated patient. Delayed serum sickness may occur even with a negative allergic history and absence of reaction to skin test.

Dosage Forms Injection, powder for reconstitution: Derived from *Micrurus fulvius* venom [equine origin; contains phenol and thimerosal; packaged with diluent] [DSC]

Drug Interactions

Beta-blockers: May increase severity of anaphylaxis.

Opioid analgesics: Use of morphine and other narcotics which depress respiration are contraindicated.

Sedatives: Use with extreme caution.

Pregnancy Risk Factor C

Pregnancy Implications Use only if the potential benefits outweigh risks; it is not known if *M. fulvius* antivenin antibodies cross out the placenta

Nursing Implications Patient should be closely monitored for symptoms of hypersensitivity or anaphylaxis during skin or eye testing, desensitization, drug administration, and for 24 hours following administration

Specific References

de Roodt AR, Paniagua-Solis JF, Dolab JA, et al, "Effectiveness of Two Common Antivenoms for North, Central, and South American *Micrurus* Envenomations," *J Toxicol Clin Toxicol*, 2004, 42(2):171-8.

German BT, Hack JB, Brewer K, et al, "Pressure-Immobilization Bandages Delay Toxicity in a Porcine Model of Eastern Coral Snake (*Micrurus fulvius fulvius*) Envenomation," *Ann Emerg Med*, 2005, 45(6):603-8.

Wisniewski MS, Hill RE, Havey JM, et al, "Australian Tiger Snake (*Notechis scutatus*) and Mexican Coral Snake (*Micruris species*) Antivenoms Prevent Death from United States Coral Snake (*Micrurus fulvius fulvius*) Venom in a Mouse Model," *J Toxicol Clin Toxicol*, 2003, 41(1):7-10.

Antivenin, Polyvalent Crotalidae (Ovine) Fab

U.S. Brand Name CroFab®

Use Neutralization of venoms of North American crotalid (minimal to moderate severity)

Mechanism of Action ~5.2 times as potent as Wyeth antivenin in neutralization of venom with reversal of venom-induced platelet aggregation; may reverse neurotoxicity

Adverse Reactions

Miscellaneous: Serum sickness (1 in 42 patients)

Dermal: Urticaria, rash

Pharmacodynamics/Kinetics

Half life: (Total Fab): 12 to 23 hours

Dosage Initial dose: 4 to 6 vials infused IV over 60 minutes. Infuse initial dose slowly over the first ten minutes at a 25 to 50 ml/hour rate. Repeat, if necessary, until initial control is achieved (complete arrest of local manifestations and normalization of coagulation test results and systemic signs). After initial control is achieved, give two vials I.V. every six hours for up to 18 hours. Follow up dose of two vials may be given as deemed necessary. In clinical trials, a medium dose of 12 vials was used. No skin testing is required.

Monitoring Parameters Prothrombin time, platelet count, fibrinogen concentration

Contraindications Hypersensitivity to papaga or papain (weigh benefits to risks)

Reference Range Total Fab following injection of 6 vials: 740 mg/L

Pregnancy Risk Factor C

Additional Information Distributed by Fougera (www.fougera.com): Phone 800-645-9833 Reconstitute with 250 ml of 0.9% sodium chloride (4 to 6 vials).

Specific Reference

Kravitz J and Gerardo CJ,, "Copperhead Snakebite Treated with Crotalidae Polyvalent Immune Fab (Ovine) Antivenom in Third Trimester Pregnancy," *Clin Toxicol*, 2006, 44(3):353-4.

Asoxime Chloride

Related Information
- Obidoxime Chloride [ANTIDOTE]
- Pralidoxime [ANTIDOTE]

CAS Number 34433-31-3

Unlabeled/Investigational Use

Investigational: Has been used in dichlorvos and dimethoate poisoning; rodent experiments indicate that it may be effective in tabun, sarin, VX soman or GF exposure with atropine used as a pretreatment

Mechanism of Action A cholinesterase reactivator; may be more effective for the diethoxy group of organophosphates than the dimethoxy type; may be effective in treating VX, sarin, soman, or GF-type nerve gas

Dosage Nerve gas or parathion exposure: 500 mg diluted in 3 mL of distilled water intramuscularly 4 times/day for 2-7 days; total dosage range: 4-14 g

Reference Range Therapeutic serum HI-6 level is ~4 mcg/mL

Antidote(s)
- Obidoxime Chloride [ANTIDOTE]
- Pralidoxime [ANTIDOTE]

Atropine

Pronunciation (A troe peen)

CAS Number 51-55-8; 55-48-1; 5908-99-6

U.S. Brand Names AtroPen®; Atropine-Care®; Isopto® Atropine; Sal-Tropine™

Synonyms Atropine Sulfate

Use

Injection: Preoperative medication to inhibit salivation and secretions; treatment of symptomatic sinus bradycardia; AV block (nodal level); ventricular asystole; antidote for nerve agents, organophosphate pesticide poisoning; anticholinesterase, cholinergic medication poisoning, and muscarinic symptoms of mushroom poisoning (*Clitocybe*, *Inocybe*)

Ophthalmic: Produce mydriasis and cycloplegia for examination of the retina and optic disc and accurate measurement of refractive errors; uveitis

Oral: Inhibit salivation and secretions

Unlabeled/Investigational Use Pulseless electric activity, asystole, neuromuscular blockade reversal; treatment of nerve agent toxicity (chemical warfare) in combination with pralidoxime

Mechanism of Action Blocks the action of acetylcholine at parasympathetic sites in smooth muscle, secretory glands, and the central muscarinic receptors; increases cardiac output, dries secretions, antagonizes histamine and serotonin

Adverse Reactions

Severity and frequency of adverse reactions are dose related and vary greatly; listed reactions are limited to significant and/or life-threatening.

Cardiovascular: Arrhythmia, flushing, hypotension, palpitation, tachycardia

Central nervous system: Ataxia, coma, delirium, disorientation, dizziness, drowsiness, excitement, fever, hallucinations, headache, insomnia, nervousness, weakness

Dermatologic: Anhidrosis, urticaria, rash, scarlatiniform rash

Gastrointestinal: Bloating, constipation, delayed gastric emptying, loss of taste, nausea, paralytic ileus, vomiting, xerostomia

Genitourinary: Urinary hesitancy, urinary retention

Ocular: Angle-closure glaucoma, blurred vision, cycloplegia, dry eyes, mydriasis, ocular tension increased

Respiratory: Dyspnea, laryngospasm, pulmonary edema

Miscellaneous: Anaphylaxis

Signs and Symptoms of Overdose Ataxia, blurred vision, coma, dilated unreactive pupils, diminished or absent bowel sounds, dryness of mucous membranes, flushing, foul breath, hallucinations (lilliputian), hypertension, hyperthermia, ileus, increased respiratory rate, ototoxicity (deafness), seizures, swallowing difficulty, tachycardia, tinnitus, urinary retention

Pharmacodynamics/Kinetics

Onset of action: I.V.: Rapid

Absorption: Complete

Distribution: Widely throughout the body; crosses placenta; trace amounts enter breast milk; crosses blood-brain barrier

Metabolism: Hepatic

Half-life elimination: 2-3 hours

Excretion: Urine (30% to 50% as unchanged drug and metabolites)

Dosage

Neonates, Infants, and Children: Doses <0.1 mg have been associated with paradoxical bradycardia.

Inhibit salivation and secretions (preanesthesia): Oral, I.M., I.V., SubQ:

<5 kg: 0.02 mg/kg/dose 30-60 minutes preop then every 4-6 hours as needed. Use of a minimum dosage of 0.1 mg in neonates <5 kg will result in dosages >0.02 mg/kg. There is no documented minimum dosage in this age group.

>5 kg: 0.01-0.02 mg/kg/dose to a maximum 0.4 mg/dose 30-60 minutes preop; minimum dose: 0.1 mg

Alternate dosing:

3-7 kg (7-16 lb): 0.1 mg

8-11 kg (17-24 lb): 0.15 mg

11-18 kg (24-40 lb): 0.2 mg

18-29 kg (40-65 lb): 0.3 mg

>30 kg (>65 lb): 0.4 mg

Bradycardia: I.V., intratracheal: 0.02 mg/kg, minimum dose 0.1 mg, maximum single dose: 0.5 mg in children and 1 mg in adolescents; may repeat in 5-minute intervals to a maximum total dose of 1 mg in children or 2 mg in adolescents. (**Note:** For intratracheal administration, the dosage must be diluted with normal saline to a total volume of 1-5 mL). When treating bradycardia in neonates, reserve use for those patients unresponsive to improved oxygenation and epinephrine.

Children: Organophosphate or carbamate poisoning:

I.V.: 0.03-0.05 mg/kg every 10-20 minutes until atropine effect, then every 1-4 hours for at least 24 hours

I.M. (AtroPen®): Mild symptoms: Administer dose listed below as soon as exposure is known or suspected. If severe symptoms develop after first dose, 2 additional doses should be repeated in 10 minutes; do not administer more than 3 doses. Severe symptoms: Immediately administer 3 doses as follows:

<6.8 kg (15 lbs): Use of **AtroPen®** formulation not recommended; administer atropine 0.05 mg/kg

6.8-18 kg (15-40 lbs): 0.5 mg/dose

18-41 kg (40-90 lbs): 1 mg/dose

>41 kg (>90 lbs): 2 mg/dose

Adults (doses <0.5 mg have been associated with paradoxical bradycardia):

Asystole or pulseless electrical activity: I.V.: 1 mg; repeat in 3-5 minutes if asystole persists; total dose of 0.04 mg/kg; may give intratracheally in 10 mL NS (intratracheal dose should be 2-2.5 times the I.V. dose)

Inhibit salivation and secretions (preanesthesia):

I.M., I.V., SubQ: 0.4-0.6 mg 30-60 minutes preop and repeat every 4-6 hours as needed

Oral: 0.4 mg, may repeat every 4-6 hours

Bradycardia: I.V.: 0.5-1 mg every 5 minutes, not to exceed a total of 3 mg or 0.04 mg/kg; may give intratracheally in 10 mL NS (intratracheal dose should be 2-2.5 times the I.V. dose)

Neuromuscular blockade reversal: I.V.: 25-30 mcg/kg 60 seconds before neostigmine or 7-10 mcg/kg in combination with edrophonium

Organophosphate or carbamate poisoning:

I.V.: 2 mg, followed by 2 mg every 15 minutes until adequate atropinization has occurred; initial doses of up to 6 mg may be used in life-threatening cases. Total daily doses as high as 100 mg daily have been reported.

I.M. (AtroPen®): Mild symptoms: Administer 2 mg as soon as exposure is known or suspected. If severe symptoms develop after first dose, 2 additional doses should be repeated in 10 minutes; do not administer more than 3 doses. Severe symptoms: Immediately administer three 2 mg doses.

Mydriasis, cycloplegia (preprocedure): Ophthalmic (1% solution): Instill 1-2 drops 1 hour before procedure.

Uveitis: Ophthalmic:

1% solution: Instill 1-2 drops 4 times/day

Ointment: Apply a small amount in the conjunctival sac up to 3 times/day; compress the lacrimal sac by digital pressure for 1-3 minutes after instillation

Stability Store injection at controlled room temperature of 15°C to 30°C (59°F to 86°F); avoid freezing. In addition, AtroPen® should be protected from light.

Monitoring Parameters Heart rate, blood pressure, pulse, mental status; intravenous administration requires a cardiac monitor

Administration

I.M.: AtroPen®: Administer to outer thigh. May be given through clothing as long as pockets at the injection site are empty. Hold auto-injector in place for 10 seconds following injection; massage the injection site.

I.V.: Administer undiluted by rapid I.V. injection; slow injection may result in paradoxical bradycardia.

Contraindications Hypersensitivity to atropine or any component of the formulation; narrow-angle glaucoma; adhesions between the iris and lens; tachycardia; obstructive GI disease; paralytic ileus; intestinal atony of the elderly or debilitated patient; severe ulcerative colitis; toxic megacolon complicating ulcerative colitis; hepatic disease; obstructive uropathy; renal disease; myasthenia gravis (unless used to treat side effects of acetylcholinesterase inhibitor); asthma; thyrotoxicosis; Mobitz type II block

Warnings

Heat prostration can occur in the presence of a high environmental temperature. Psychosis can occur in sensitive individuals. The elderly may be sensitive to side effects. Use caution in patients with myocardial ischemia. Use caution in hyperthyroidism, autonomic neuropathy, BPH, CHF, tachyarrhythmias, hypertension, and hiatal hernia associated with reflux esophagitis. Use with caution in children with spastic paralysis.

AtroPen®: There are no absolute contraindications for the use of atropine in organophosphate poisonings, however, use caution in those patients where the use of atropine would be otherwise contraindicated. Formulation for use by trained personnel only.

Dosage Forms

Injection, solution, as sulfate: 0.05 mg/mL (5 mL); 0.1 mg/mL (5 mL, 10 mL); 0.4 mg/mL (0.5 mL, 1 mL, 20 mL); 0.5 mg/mL (1 mL); 1 mg/mL (1 mL)

AtroPen® [prefilled autoinjector]: 0.5 mg/0.7 mL (0.7 mL); 1 mg/0.7 mL (0.7 mL); 2 mg/0.7 mL (0.7 mL)

Ointment, ophthalmic, as sulfate: 1% (3.5 g)

Solution, ophthalmic, as sulfate: 1% (5 mL, 15 mL)

Atropine-Care®: 1% (2 mL)

Isopto® Atropine: 1% (5 mL, 15 mL)

Tablet, as sulfate (Sal-Tropine™): 0.4 mg

Reference Range Therapeutic range: 3-25 ng/mL. Peak serum atropine level after a 1 mg I.V. dose: ~0.003 mg/L (within 30 minutes of administration); blood level (postmortem) of 0.2 mg/L and urine level of 1.5 mg/L associated with fatality; peak plasma and urine atropine levels 10 hours after ingestion of 6 raw nightshade berries and 200 g of cooked berries (and associated with coma) were 217 mcg/L and 3092 mcg/L, respectively

Drug Interactions

Drugs with anticholinergic activity (including phenothiazines and TCAs) may increase anticholinergic effects when used concurrently.

Sympathomimetic amines may cause tachyarrhythmias; avoid concurrent use.

Pregnancy Risk Factor C

Pregnancy Implications Crosses the placenta

Lactation Enters breast milk (trace amounts)/use caution (AAP rates "compatible")

Nursing Implications Give by rapid I.V. injection since slow infusion may cause a paradoxical bradycardia; may give intratracheal in 1 mg/10 mL dilution only

Additional Information Expired atropine products have been shown to have significant potency and may be an option in mass casualty events.

Specific References

Asari Y, Kamijyo Y, and Soma K, "Changes in the Hemodynamic State of Patients with Acute Lethal Organophosphate Poisoning," *Vet Hum Toxicol*, 2004, 46(1):5-9.

Bryant SM, Wills BK, Rhee J, et al, "Intramuscular Ophthalmic Homatropine vs Atropine to Prevent Lethality in Rats with Dichlorvos Poisoning," *Clin Toxicol (Phila)*, 2005, 43:694.

Corner B, "Intravenous Atropine Treatment in Infantile Hypertrophic Pyloric Stenosis," *Arch Dis Child*, 2003, 88(1):87; author reply 87.

Dix J, Weber RJ, Frye RF, et al, "Stability of Atropine Sulfate Prepared for Mass Chemical Terrorism," *J Toxicol Clin Toxicol*, 2003, 41(6):771-5.

Eddleston M, Buckley NA, Checketts H, et al, "Speed of Initial Atropinisation in Significant Organophosphorus Pesticide Poisoning - A Systematic Comparison of Recommended Regimens," *J Toxicol Clin Toxicol*, 2004, 42(6):865-75.

Geller RJ, Lopez GP, Cutler S, et al, "Atropine Availability as an Antidote for Nerve Agent Casualties: Validated Rapid Reformulation of High-Concentration Atropine from Bulk Powder," *Ann Emerg Med*, 2003, 41(4):453-6.

Kalkan S, Ergur BU, Akgun A, et al, "Efficacy of an Adenosine A_1 Receptor Agonist Compared with Atropine and Pralidoxime in a Rat Model of Organophosphate Poisoning," *Clin Toxicol (Phila)*, 2005, 43:694.

Kozak RJ, Siegel S, and Kuzma J, "Rapid Atropine Synthesis for the Treatment of Massive Nerve Agent Exposure," *Ann Emerg Med*, 2003, 41(5):685-8.

Mordel A, Bar Haim S, Bulkobstein M, et al, "Pediatric Trimedoxime (TMB4) and Atropine Poisoning," *J Toxicol Clin Toxicol*, 2003, 41(5):660.

Schier JG, PR Ravikumar, Nelson LS, et al, "Preparing for Chemical Terrorism: Stability of Injectable Atropine Sulfate," *Acad Emerg Med*, 2004, 11(4):329-34.

Seifert SA, Caravati EM, and Crouch DJ, "Atropine Overdose from a Suppository Compounding Error," *J Toxicol Clin Toxicol*, 2003, 41(5):648.

Tomassoni AJ and Simone KE, "Development and Use of a Decentralized Antidote Stockpile in a Rural State," *J Toxicol Clin Toxicol*, 2004, 42(5):824-5.

Bromocriptine

Pronunciation (broe moe KRIP teen)

CAS Number 22260-51-1; 25614-03-3

U.S. Brand Names Parlodel®

Synonyms Bromocriptine Mesylate

Use

Amenorrhea with or without galactorrhea; infertility or hypogonadism; prolactin-secreting adenomas; acromegaly; Parkinson's disease

A previous indication for prevention of postpartum lactation was withdrawn voluntarily by Sandoz Pharmaceuticals Corporation

Has been used to decrease drug craving following discontinuation of cocaine abuse

Unlabeled/Investigational Use Neuroleptic malignant syndrome

Mechanism of Action Semisynthetic ergot alkaloid derivative with direct dopaminergic agonist activity at striatal receptors

Adverse Reactions

Cardiovascular: Hypertension then hypotension, syncope, hypertensive crisis, cerebral infarction, hypotension (orthostatic), acrocyanosis, Raynaud's phenomenon, shock, sinus bradycardia, arrhythmias (ventricular), vasoconstriction, vasculitis, pericarditis, postpartum intracranial hemorrhage

Central nervous system: Headache, dizziness, insomnia, auditory and visual hallucinations, seizures, extrapyramidal symptoms, cognitive dysfunction, hallucinations, lightheadedness, mania, meningitis, night terrors, paranoia, psychosis, gustatory hallucinations, hypothermia, paresthesia

Dermatologic: Alopecia, scleroderma, exanthema, urticaria, purpura

Endocrine & metabolic: Hyponatremia, hypoprolactinemia

Gastrointestinal: Nausea, vomiting, abdominal cramps, anorexia, xerostomia

Genitourinary: Retroperitoneal fibrosis, impotence, clitoral hypertrophy

Hematologic: Leukopenia, coagulopathy, thrombocytopenia

Neuromuscular & skeletal: Clonus, myoclonus, erythromelalgia, chorea (extrapyramidal), dyskinesias

Ocular: Myopia

Otic: Ototoxicity

Renal: Renal insufficiency

Respiratory: Pleuropulmonary fibrosis, pleural effusion, rhinorrhea, hyposmia

Pharmacodynamics/Kinetics
Bioavailability: 28%
Protein binding: 90% to 96%
Metabolism: Primarily hepatic
Half-life elimination: Biphasic: Initial: 6-8 hours; Terminal: 50 hours
Time to peak, serum: 1-2 hours
Excretion: Feces; urine (2% to 6% as unchanged drug)

Dosage
Oral: Adults:
Parkinsonism: 1.25 mg 2 times/day, increased by 2.5 mg/day in 2- to 4-week intervals (usual dose range is 30-90 mg/day in 3 divided doses), though elderly patients can usually be managed on lower doses
Neuroleptic malignant syndrome: 2.5-5 mg 3 times/day
Hyperprolactinemia: 2.5 mg 2-3 times/day
Acromegaly: Initial: 1.25-2.5 mg increasing as necessary every 3-7 days; usual dose: 20-30 mg/day
Prolactin-secreting adenomas: Initial: 1.25-2.5 mg/day; daily range 2.5-10 mg.

Dosing adjustment in hepatic impairment: No guidelines are available, however, may be necessary

Monitoring Parameters Monitor blood pressure closely as well as hepatic, hematopoietic, and cardiovascular function

Contraindications Hypersensitivity to bromocriptine, ergot alkaloids, or any component of the formulation; ergot alkaloids are contraindicated with potent inhibitors of CYP3A4 (includes protease inhibitors, azole antifungals, and some macrolide antibiotics); uncontrolled hypertension; severe ischemic heart disease or peripheral vascular disorders; pregnancy (risk to benefit evaluation must be performed in women who become pregnant during treatment for acromegaly, prolactinoma, or Parkinson's disease - hypertension during treatment should generally result in efforts to withdraw)

Warnings
Complete evaluation of pituitary function should be completed prior to initiation of treatment. Use caution in patients with impaired renal or hepatic function, a history of peptic ulcer disease, dementia, psychosis, or cardiovascular disease (myocardial infarction, arrhythmia). Symptomatic hypotension may occur in a significant number of patients. In addition, hypertension, seizures, MI, and stroke have been rarely associated with bromocriptine therapy. Severe headache or visual changes may precede events. The onset of reactions may be immediate or delayed (often may occur in the second week of therapy).

Concurrent antihypertensives or drugs which may alter blood pressure should be used with caution. Concurrent use with levodopa has been associated with an increased risk of hallucinations. Consider dosage reduction and/or discontinuation in patients with hallucinations. Hallucinations may require weeks to months before resolution.

In the treatment of acromegaly, discontinuation is recommended if tumor expansion occurs during therapy. Digital vasospasm (cold sensitive) may occur in some patients with acromegaly; may require dosage reduction. Patients who receive bromocriptine during and immediately following pregnancy as a continuation of previous therapy (eg, acromegaly) should be closely monitored for cardiovascular effects. Should not be used post-partum in women with coronary artery disease or other cardiovascular disease. Use of bromocriptine to control or prevent lactation or in patients with uncontrolled hypertension is not recommended.

Monitoring and careful evaluation of visual changes during the treatment of hyperprolactinemia is recommended to differentiate between tumor shrinkage and traction on the optic chiasm; rapidly progressing visual field loss requires neurosurgical consultation. Discontinuation of bromocriptine in patients with macroadenomas has been associated with rapid regrowth of tumor and increased prolactin serum levels. Pleural and retroperitoneal fibrosis have been reported with prolonged daily use. Cardiac valvular fibrosis has also been associated with ergot alkaloids. Safety and effectiveness in patients <15 years of age (for pituitary adenoma) have not been established.

Dosage Forms
Capsule, as mesylate: 5 mg
  Parlodel®: 5 mg
Tablet, as mesylate: 2.5 mg
  Parlodel®: 2.5 mg

Reference Range Peak plasma level of 24.6 ng/mL achieved after a dose of 100 mg

Test Interactions Bromocriptine may increase BUN, serum AST, serum ALT, serum CPK, alkaline phosphatase, and serum uric acid; may interfere with TSH assay resulting in falsely low TSH levels

Drug Interactions
Substrate of CYP3A4 (major); **Inhibits** CYP1A2 (weak), 3A4 (weak)
Alpha agonists/sympathomimetics: May enhance the adverse/toxic effect of bromocriptine, including increased blood pressure, ventricular arrhythmias, and seizures. Monitor. **Note:** The use of epinephrine in combination local anethetics should pose no clinical concern.

Antihypertensives: Concurrent use with bromocriptine may increase the risk of hypotension and/or orthostasis. Use caution.
Antifungals, azole derivatives (itraconazole, ketoconazole) increase levels of ergot alkaloids by inhibiting CYP3A4 metabolism, resulting in toxicity; concomitant use is contraindicated.
Antipsychotics: May diminish the effects of bromocriptine (due to dopamine antagonism); these combinations should generally be avoided.
CYP3A4 inhibitors: May increase the levels/effects of bromocriptine. Example inhibitors include azole antifungals, clarithromycin, diclofenac, doxycycline, erythromycin, imatinib, isoniazid, nefazodone, nicardipine, propofol, protease inhibitors, quinidine, telithromycin, and verapamil.
Levodopa: Concurrent use may increase the risk of hallucinations. Dosage reduction may be required.
Macrolide antibiotics: Erythromycin, clarithromycin, and troleandomycin may increase levels of ergot alkaloids by inhibiting CYP3A4 metabolism, resulting in toxicity (ischemia, vasospasm); concomitant use is contraindicated.
MAO inhibitors: The serotonergic effects of ergot derivatives may be increased by MAO inhibitors. Monitor for signs and symptoms of serotonin syndrome.
Metoclopramide: May diminish the effects of bromocriptine (due to dopamine antagonism); concurrent therapy should generally be avoided.
Protease inhibitors (ritonavir, amprenavir, indinavir, nelfinavir, and saquinavir) increase blood levels of ergot alkaloids by inhibiting CYP3A4 metabolism, acute ergot toxicity has been reported; concomitant use is contraindicated.
Serotonin agonists: Concurrent use with bromocriptine may increase the risk of serotonin syndrome (includes buspirone, SSRIs, TCAs, nefazodone, sumatriptan, and trazodone).
Sibutramine: May cause serotonin syndrome; concurrent use with ergot alkaloids is contraindicated.
Telithromycin: May increase levels of ergot alkaloids by inhibiting CYP3A4 metabolism, resulting in toxicity (ischemia, vasospasm); concomitant use is contraindicated.

Pregnancy Risk Factor B
Pregnancy Implications No evidence of teratogenicity or fetal toxicity in animal studies. Bromocriptine is used for ovulation induction in women with hyperprolactinemia. In general, therapy should be discontinued if pregnancy is confirmed unless needed for treatment of macroprolactinoma. Data collected from women taking bromocriptine during pregnancy suggest the incidence of birth defects is not increased with use. However, the majority of women discontinued use within 8 weeks of pregnancy. Women not seeking pregnancy should be advised to use appropriate contraception.
Lactation Enters breast milk/contraindicated
Nursing Implications Raise bed rails and institute safety measures; aid patient with ambulation; may cause postural hypotension and drowsiness

Budesonide

Pronunciation (byoo DES oh nide)
U.S. Brand Names Entocort™ EC; Pulmicort Respules®; Pulmicort Turbuhaler®; Rhinocort® Aqua®
Use
Intranasal: Children ≥6 years of age and Adults: Management of symptoms of seasonal or perennial rhinitis
Nebulization: Children 12 months to 8 years: Maintenance and prophylactic treatment of asthma; may be useful for hydrocarbon inhalation injuries
Oral capsule: Treatment of active Crohn's disease (mild to moderate) involving the ileum and/or ascending colon
Oral inhalation: Maintenance and prophylactic treatment of asthma; includes patients who require corticosteroids and those who may benefit from systemic dose reduction/elimination
Mechanism of Action Controls the rate of protein synthesis, depresses the migration of polymorphonuclear leukocytes, fibroblasts, reverses capillary permeability, and lysosomal stabilization at the cellular level to prevent or control inflammation
Adverse Reactions
Reaction severity varies by dose and duration; not all adverse reactions have been reported with each dosage form.
>10%:
  Central nervous system: Oral capsule: Headache (up to 21%)
  Gastrointestinal: Oral capsule: Nausea (up to 11%)
  Respiratory: Respiratory infection, rhinitis, dysphonia
  Miscellaneous: Symptoms of HPA axis suppression and/or hypercorticism (acne, easy bruising, fat redistribution, striae, edema) may occur in >10% of patients following administration of dosage forms which result in higher systemic exposure (ie, oral capsule), but may be less frequent than rates observed with comparator drugs (prednisolone). These symptoms may be rare (<1%)

following administration via methods which result in lower exposures (topical).

1% to 10%:

Cardiovascular: Syncope, edema, hypertension

Central nervous system: Chest pain, dysphonia, emotional lability, fatigue, fever, insomnia, migraine, nervousness, pain, dizziness, vertigo

Dermatologic: Bruising, contact dermatitis, eczema, pruritus, pustular rash, rash

Endocrine & metabolic: Hypokalemia, adrenal insufficiency

Gastrointestinal: Abdominal pain, anorexia, diarrhea, dry mouth, dyspepsia, gastroenteritis, oral candidiasis, taste perversion, vomiting, weight gain, flatulence, oral candidiasis (4% to 13%)

Hematologic: Cervical lymphadenopathy, purpura, leukocytosis

Neuromuscular & skeletal: Arthralgia, fracture, hyperkinesis, hypertonia, myalgia, neck pain, weakness, paresthesia, back pain

Ocular: Conjunctivitis, eye infection, cataracts

Otic: Earache, ear infection, external ear infection

Respiratory: Bronchitis, bronchospasm, cough, epistaxis, nasal irritation, pharyngitis, sinusitis, stridor

Miscellaneous: Allergic reaction, flu-like syndrome, herpes simplex, infection, moniliasis, viral infection, voice alteration, weight gain, 22% elevation of HDL cholesterol

<1%: Aggressive reactions, alopecia, angioedema, avascular necrosis of the femoral head, depression, dyspnea, hoarseness, hypersensitivity reactions (immediate and delayed; include rash, contact dermatitis, angioedema, bronchospasm), intermenstrual bleeding, irritability, nasal septum perforation, osteoporosis, psychosis, somnolence

Postmarketing and/or case reports: Growth suppression, benign intracranial hypertension

Pharmacodynamics/Kinetics

Onset of action: Respules®: 2-8 days; Rhinocort® Aqua®: ~10 hours; Turbuhaler®: 24 hours

Duration: Asthma: 12-24 hours

Peak effect: Respules®: 4-6 weeks; Rhinocort® Aqua®: ~2 weeks; Turbuhaler®: 1-2 weeks

Absorption: Capsule: Rapid and complete

Dermal absorption: 1% to 3%

Distribution: 2.2-3.9 L/kg

Protein binding: 85% to 90%

Metabolism: Hepatic via CYP3A4 to two metabolites: 16 alpha-hydroxyprednisolone and 6 beta-hydroxybudesonide; minor activity

Bioavailability: Limited by high first-pass effect; Capsule: 9% to 21%; Respules®: 6%; Turbuhaler®: 6% to 13%; Nasal: 34%

Half-life elimination: 2-3.6 hours

Time to peak: Capsule: 30-600 minutes (variable in Crohn's disease); Respules®: 10-30 minutes; Turbuhaler®: 1-2 hours; Nasal: 1 hour

Excretion: Urine (60%) and feces as metabolites

Total body clearance: 0.9-1.8 L/minute

Dosage

Nasal inhalation: (Rhinocort® Aqua®): Children ≥6 years and Adults: 64 mcg/day as a single 32 mcg spray in each nostril. Some patients who do not achieve adequate control may benefit from increased dosage. A reduced dosage may be effective after initial control is achieved.

Maximum dose: Children <12 years: 128 mcg/day; Adults: 256 mcg/day

Nebulization: Children 12 months to 8 years: Pulmicort Respules®: Titrate to lowest effective dose once patient is stable; start at 0.25 mg/day or use as follows:

Hydrocarbon inhalation injuries: 0.5 mg every 12 hours for 4 days

Previous therapy of bronchodilators alone: 0.5 mg/day administered as a single dose or divided twice daily (maximum daily dose: 0.5 mg)

Previous therapy of inhaled corticosteroids: 0.5 mg/day administered as a single dose or divided twice daily (maximum daily dose: 1 mg)

Previous therapy of oral corticosteroids: 1 mg/day administered as a single dose or divided twice daily (maximum daily dose: 1 mg)

Oral inhalation:

Children ≥6 years:

Previous therapy of bronchodilators alone: 200 mcg twice initially which may be increased up to 400 mcg twice daily

Previous therapy of inhaled corticosteroids: 200 mcg twice initially which may be increased up to 400 mcg twice daily

Previous therapy of oral corticosteroids: The highest recommended dose in children is 400 mcg twice daily

Adults:

Previous therapy of bronchodilators alone: 200-400 mcg twice initially which may be increased up to 400 mcg twice daily

Previous therapy of inhaled corticosteroids: 200-400 mcg twice initially which may be increased up to 800 mcg twice daily

Previous therapy of oral corticosteroids: 400-800 mcg twice daily which may be increased up to 800 mcg twice daily

NIH Guidelines (NIH, 1997) (give in divided doses twice daily):

Children:

"Low" dose: 100-200 mcg/day

"Medium" dose: 200-400 mcg/day (1-2 inhalations/day)

"High" dose: >400 mcg/day (>2 inhalation/day)

Adults:

"Low" dose: 200-400 mcg/day (1-2 inhalations/day)

"Medium" dose: 400-600 mcg/day (2-3 inhalations/day)

"High" dose: >600 mcg/day (>3 inhalation/day)

Oral: Adults: Crohn's disease: 9 mg once daily in the morning; safety and efficacy have not been established for therapy duration >8 weeks; recurring episodes may be treated with a repeat 8-week course of treatment

Note: Treatment may be tapered to 6 mg once daily for 2 weeks prior to complete cessation. Patients receiving CYP3A4 inhibitors should be monitored closely for signs and symptoms of hypercorticism; dosage reduction may be required.

Dosage adjustment in hepatic impairment: Monitor closely for signs and symptoms of hypercorticism; dosage reduction may be required.

Stability

Nebulizer: Store upright at 20°C to 25°C (68°F to 77°F) and protect from light. Do not refrigerate or freeze. Once aluminum package is opened, solution should be used within 2 weeks. Continue to protect from light.

Nasal inhaler: Store with valve up at 15°C to 30°C (59°F to 86°F). Use within 6 months after opening aluminum pouch. Protect from high humidity.

Nasal spray: Store with valve up at 20°C to 25°C (68°F to 77°F) and protect from light. Do not freeze.

Monitoring Parameters Monitor growth in pediatric patients.

Administration

Inhalation: Inhaler should be shaken well immediately prior to use; while activating inhaler, deep breathe for 3-5 seconds, hold breath for ~10 seconds and allow ≥1 minute between inhalations. Rinse mouth with water after use to reduce aftertaste and incidence of candidiasis.

Nebulization: Shake well before using. Use Pulmicort Respules® with jet nebulizer connected to an air compressor; administer with mouthpiece or facemask. Do not use ultrasonic nebulizer. Do not mix with other medications in nebulizer. Rinse mouth following treatments to decrease risk of oral candidiasis (wash face if using face mask).

Oral capsule: Capsule should be swallowed whole; do not crush or chew.

Contraindications

Hypersensitivity to budesonide or any component of the formulation

Inhalation: Contraindicated in primary treatment of status asthmaticus, acute episodes of asthma; not for relief of acute bronchospasm

Warnings

May cause hypercorticism and/or suppression of hypothalamic-pituitary-adrenal (HPA) axis, particularly in younger children or in patients receiving high doses for prolonged periods. Particular care is required when patients are transferred from systemic corticosteroids to products with lower systemic bioavailability (ie, inhalation). May lead to possible adrenal insufficiency or withdrawal from steroids, including an increase in allergic symptoms. Patients receiving prolonged therapy ≥20 mg per day of prednisone (or equivalent) may be most susceptible. Aerosol steroids do **not** provide the systemic steroid needed to treat patients having trauma, surgery, or infections.

Controlled clinical studies have shown that orally-inhaled and intranasal corticosteroids may cause a reduction in growth velocity in pediatric patients. (In studies of orally-inhaled corticosteroids, the mean reduction in growth velocity was approximately 1 centimeter per year [range 0.3-1.8 cm per year] and appears to be related to dose and duration of exposure.) To minimize the systemic effects of orally-inhaled and intranasal corticosteroids, each patient should be titrated to the lowest effective dose. Growth should be routinely monitored in pediatric patients.

May suppress the immune system; patients may be more susceptible to infection. Use with caution in patients with systemic infections or ocular herpes simplex. Avoid exposure to chickenpox and measles. Corticosteroids should be used with caution in patients with diabetes, hypertension, osteoporosis, peptic ulcer, glaucoma, cataracts, or tuberculosis. Use caution in hepatic impairment. Enteric-coated capsules should not be crushed or chewed.

Dosage Forms

[CAN] = Canadian brand name

Capsule, enteric coated (Entocort® EC): 3 mg

Powder for oral inhalation:

Pulmicort Turbuhaler®: 200 mcg/inhalation (104 g) [delivers ~160 mcg/inhalation; 200 metered doses]

Pulmicort Turbuhaler® [CAN]: 100 mcg/inhalation [delivers 200 metered doses]; 200 mcg/inhalation [delivers 200 metered doses]; 400 mcg/inhalation [delivers 200 metered doses] [not available in the U.S.]

Suspension, intranasal [spray] (Rhinocort® Aqua®): 32 mcg/inhalation (8.6 g) [120 metered doses]

Suspension for nebulization (Pulmicort Respules®): 0.25 mg/2 mL (30s), 0.5 mg/2 mL (30s)

Reference Range Plasma budesonide level of 5 nmol/L obtained within 5 hours of a 9 mg oral dose

Overdosage/Treatment

Acute overdosage does not require any treatment.

Inhaled formulations: Symptoms of overdose include irritation and burning of the nasal mucosa, sneezing, intranasal and pharyngeal *Candida* infections, nasal ulceration, epistaxis, rhinorrhea, nasal stuffiness, headache.

When consumed in excessive quantities, over 3 weeks, systemic hypercorticism and adrenal suppression may occur, in those cases discontinuation and withdrawal of the corticosteroid should be done judiciously. Treatment should be symptomatic and supportive; monitor electrolytes

Drug Interactions

Substrate of CYP3A4 (major)

Cimetidine: Decreased clearance and increased bioavailability of budesonide.

CYP3A4 inhibitors: Serum level and/or toxicity of budesonide may be increased; this effect was shown with ketoconazole, but not erythromycin. Other potential inhibitors include amiodarone, cimetidine, clarithromycin, delavirdine, diltiazem, dirithromycin, disulfiram, fluoxetine, fluvoxamine, grapefruit juice, indinavir, itraconazole, ketoconazole, nefazodone, nevirapine, propoxyphene, quinupristin-dalfopristin, ritonavir, saquinavir, telithromycin, verapamil, zafirlukast, and zileuton.

Proton pump inhibitors (omeprazole, pantoprazole, rabeprazole): Theoretically, alteration of gastric pH may affect the rate of dissolution of enteric-coated capsules. Administration with omeprazole did not alter kinetics of budesonide capsules.

Salmeterol: The addition of salmeterol has been demonstrated to improve response to inhaled corticosteroids (as compared to increasing steroid dosage).

Pregnancy Risk Factor C/B (Pulmicort Respules® and Turbuhaler®, Rhinocort® Aqua®)

Pregnancy Implications Use only if potential benefit to the mother outweighs the possible risk to the fetus. Studies of pregnant women using inhaled budesonide have not demonstrated an increased risk of abnormalities. Hypoadrenalism has been reported in infants.

Lactation Enters breast milk/use caution

Specific References

Gurkan F and Bosnak M, "Use of Nebulized Budesonide in Two Critical Patients with Hydrocarbon Intoxication," *Am J Ther*, 2005, 12(4):366-7.

Calcium Chloride

Pronunciation (KAL see um KLOR ide)

CAS Number 10035-04-8; 10043-52-4; 7774-34-7

Use Cardiac resuscitation when epinephrine fails to improve myocardial contractions, cardiac disturbances of hyperkalemia, hypocalcemia or calcium channel blocking agent toxicity; also used for fluoride, hydrogen fluoride, ethylene glycol, magnesium sulfate, oxalate, and possibly for black widow spider bites

Unlabeled/Investigational Use Calcium channel blocker overdose

Mechanism of Action Moderates nerve and muscle performance via action potential excitation threshold regulation

Mechanism of Toxic Action Moderates nerve and muscle performance via action potential excitation threshold regulation

Adverse Reactions

Cardiovascular: Vasodilation, hypotension, bradycardia, cardiac arrhythmias, fibrillation (ventricular), syncope, shock, sinus bradycardia, arrhythmias (ventricular),

Central nervous system: Lethargy, coma

Dermatologic: Erythema

Endocrine & metabolic: Hypomagnesemia, hypercalcemia

Gastrointestinal: Elevated serum amylase

Local: Tissue necrosis (more irritant than calcium gluconate), extravasation injury

Neuromuscular & skeletal: Muscle weakness

Renal: Hypercalciuria

Signs and Symptoms of Overdose Coma, lethargy, nausea, vomiting

Pharmacodynamics/Kinetics

Distribution: Crosses placenta; enters breast milk

Excretion: Primarily feces (as unabsorbed calcium); urine (20%)

Dosage

I.V. (calcium chloride is 3 times as potent as calcium gluconate):

Cardiac arrest in the presence of hyperkalemia or hypocalcemia, magnesium toxicity, or calcium antagonist toxicity:

Infants and Children: 10-30 mg/kg; may repeat in 5-10 minutes if necessary

Adults: 10 mL/dose every 10-20 minutes

Hypocalcemia:

Infants and Children: 10-20 mg/kg/dose, repeat every 4-6 hours if needed

Adults: 500 mg to 1 g at 1- to 3-day intervals

Hydrofluoric acid burns: Intra-arterial infusion: 10 mL of 10% calcium chloride in 40 mL of normal saline over 4 hours

Tetany:

Neonates: 2.4 mEq/kg/day

Infants and Children: 10 mg/kg over 5-10 minutes; may repeat after 6 hours or follow with an infusion with a maximum dose of 200 mg/kg/day

Adults: 1 g over 10-30 minutes; may repeat after 6 hours

Electrical-mechanical dissociation:

Due to propranolol: 1 g

Due to disopyramide: 1-3 g

Reversal of neuromuscular blockade due to polymixin antibiotics and anesthetic agents: I.V.: 1 g

Hypocalcemia secondary to citrated blood transfusion give 0.45 mEq **elemental** calcium for each 100 mL citrated blood infused

Stability Admixture incompatibilities: Carbonates, phosphates, sulfates, tartrates

Monitoring Parameters ECG

Administration Generally, I.V. infusion rates should not exceed 0.7-1.5 mEq/minute (0.5-1 mL/minute); stop the infusion if the patient complains of pain or discomfort; do not inject calcium chloride I.M. or administer SubQ since severe necrosis and sloughing may occur. Do not use scalp vein or small hand or foot veins for I.V. administration. Warm to body temperature; administer slowly, do not exceed 1 mL/minute (inject into ventricular cavity - not myocardium).

Contraindications In ventricular fibrillation during cardiac resuscitation, hypercalcemia, and in patients with risk of digitalis toxicity, renal or cardiac disease; not recommended in treatment of asystole and electromechanical dissociation; patients with suspected digoxin toxicity

Warnings Avoid too rapid I.V. administration (<1 mL/minute) and extravasation. Use with caution in digitalized patients, respiratory failure, or acidosis. Hypercalcemia may occur in patients with renal failure, and frequent determination of serum calcium is necessary. Avoid metabolic acidosis (ie, administer only 2-3 days then change to another calcium salt).

Dosage Forms Injection, solution [preservative free]: 10% [100 mg/mL] (10 mL) [equivalent to elemental calcium 27.2 mg/mL, calcium 1.36 mEq/mL]

Reference Range Serum 9-10.4 mg/dL; due to a poor correlation between the serum ionized calcium (free) and total serum calcium, particularly in states of low albumin or acid/base imbalances, direct measurement of ionized calcium is recommended. In low albumin states, the corrected **total** serum calcium may be estimated by this equation (assuming a normal albumin of 4 g/dL); corrected total calcium = total serum calcium + 0.8 (4- measured serum albumin).

Overdosage/Treatment

Supportive therapy: Can be used to treat electromechanical dissociation caused by atenolol overdose

Following withdrawal of the drug, treatment consists of bedrest, liberal intake of fluids, reduced calcium intake, and cathartic administration. Severe hypercalcemia requires I.V. hydration and forced diuresis. Urine output should be monitored and maintained at >3 mL/kg/hour. I.V. saline and natriuretic agents (eg, furosemide) can quickly and significantly increase excretion of calcium.

Test Interactions Increases calcium (S); decreases magnesium

Drug Interactions

Calcium channel blockers (eg, verapamil) effects may be diminished; monitor response.

Levothyroxine: Calcium carbonate (and possibly other calcium salts) may decrease T_4 absorption; separate dose from levothyroxine by at least 4 hours.

Thiazide diuretics can cause hypercalcemia; monitor response.

May potentiate digoxin toxicity. High doses of calcium with thiazide diuretics may result in milk-alkali syndrome and hypercalcemia.

Pregnancy Risk Factor C

Pregnancy Implications Crosses the placenta

Nursing Implications Monitor ECG if calcium is infused faster than 2.5 mEq/minute (occasionally necessary in treating hyperkalemia)

Extravasation: Give hyaluronidase (1:10 dilution of a 150 unit vial in saline equivalent to 15 units/mL) SubQ in multiple (usually about 5) injections of 0.2 mL each to help increase absorption

Specific References

Main BW, Clark JO, Tucker TJ, et al, "Attenuation of Tillmicosin Cardiotoxicity with Calcium Chloride Infusion in Conscious Beagle Dogs," *Clin Toxicol (Phila)*, 2005, 43:695.

Van Deusen SK, Birkhahn RH, and Gaeta TJ, "Treatment of Hyperkalemia in a Patient with Unrecognized Digitalis Toxicity," *J Toxicol Clin Toxicol*, 2003, 41(4):373-6.

Calcium Gluconate

Pronunciation (KAL see um GLOO koe nate)

CAS Number 18016-24-5; 299-28-5

Use Treatment and prevention of hypocalcemia, treatment of tetany, cardiac disturbances of hyperkalemia, cardiac resuscitation when epinephrine fails to improve myocardial contractions, hypocalcemia, calcium channel blocker toxicity, black widow spider bites

Unlabeled/Investigational Use Hydrofluoric acid (HF) burns; calcium channel blocker overdose

Mechanism of Action Moderates nerve and muscle performance via action potential excitation threshold regulation

Adverse Reactions

Cardiovascular: Vasodilation, hypotension, bradycardia, cardiac arrhythmias, fibrillation (ventricular), syncope, sinus bradycardia, arrhythmias (ventricular)

Central nervous system: Lethargy, coma, mental confusion, mania

Dermatologic: Erythema

Endocrine & metabolic: Hypomagnesemia, hypercalcemia

Gastrointestinal: Elevated serum amylase

Local: Tissue necrosis, extravasation injury

Neuromuscular & skeletal: Muscle weakness

Ocular: Corneal calcification

Renal: Hypercalciuria

Signs and Symptoms of Overdose Coma, lethargy, nausea, vomiting

Pharmacodynamics/Kinetics

Absorption: Requires vitamin D; calcium is absorbed in soluble, ionized form; solubility of calcium is increased in an acid environment

Distribution: Primarily in bones and teeth; crosses placenta; enters breast milk

Protein binding: Primarily albumin

Excretion: Primarily feces (as unabsorbed calcium); urine (20%)

Dosage

Dosage is in terms of **elemental** calcium

Dietary Reference Intake:

0-6 months: 210 mg/day

7-12 months: 270 mg/day

1-3 years: 500 mg/day

4-8 years: 800 mg/day

Adults, Male/Female:

9-18 years: 1300 mg/day

19-50 years: 1000 mg/day

≥51 years: 1200 mg/day

Female: Pregnancy: Same as for Adults, Male/Female

Female: Lactating: Same as for Adults, Male/Female

Dosage expressed in terms of **calcium gluconate**

Hypocalcemia: I.V.:

Neonates: 200-800 mg/kg/day as a continuous infusion or in 4 divided doses

Infants and Children: 200-500 mg/kg/day as a continuous infusion or in 4 divided doses

Adults: 2-15 g/24 hours as a continuous infusion or in divided doses

Hypocalcemia: Oral:

Children: 200-500 mg/kg/day divided every 6 hours

Adults: 500 mg to 2 g 2-4 times/day

Osteoporosis/bone loss: Oral: 1000-1500 mg in divided doses/day

Hypocalcemia secondary to citrated blood infusion: I.V.: Give 0.45 mEq **elemental** calcium for each 100 mL citrated blood infused

Hypocalcemic tetany: I.V.:

Neonates: 100-200 mg/kg/dose, may follow with 500 mg/kg/day in 3-4 divided doses or as an infusion

Infants and Children: 100-200 mg/kg/dose (0.5-0.7 mEq/kg/dose) over 5-10 minutes; may repeat every 6-8 hours **or** follow with an infusion of 500 mg/kg/day

Adults: 1-3 g (4.5-16 mEq) may be administered until therapeutic response occurs

Calcium antagonist toxicity, magnesium intoxication, or cardiac arrest in the presence of hyperkalemia or hypocalcemia: Calcium chloride is recommended calcium salt: I.V.:

Infants and Children: 60-100 mg/kg/dose (maximum: 3 g/dose)

Adults: 500-800 mg; maximum: 3 g/dose

Maintenance electrolyte requirements for total parenteral nutrition: I.V.: Daily requirements: Adults: 8-16 mEq/1000 kcal/24 hours

Dosing adjustment in renal impairment: Cl_{cr} <25 mL/minute: Dosage adjustments may be necessary depending on the serum calcium levels

Stability

Do not refrigerate solutions; IVPB solutions/I.V. infusion solutions are stable for 24 hours at room temperature

Standard diluent: 1 g/100 mL D_5W or NS; 2 g/100 mL D_5W or NS

Maximum concentration in parenteral nutrition solutions is variable depending upon concentration and solubility (consult detailed reference).

Incompatible with sodium bicarbonate, carbonates, phosphates, sulfates, and tartrates

Stable in D_5LR, D_5NS, D_5W, $D_{10}W$, $D_{20}W$, LR, NS; **incompatible** in fat emulsion 10%

Y-site administration: Incompatible with amphotericin B cholesteryl sulfate complex, fluconazole, indomethacin

Compatibility in syringe: Incompatible with metoclopramide

Compatibility when admixed: Incompatible with amphotericin B, cefamandole, cefazolin, clindamycin, dobutamine, floxacillin, methylprednisolone sodium succinate

Monitoring Parameters Serum calcium

Administration I.M. injections should be administered in the gluteal region in adults, usually in volumes <5 mL; avoid I.M. injections in children and adults with muscle mass wasting; do not use scalp veins or small hand or foot veins for I.V. administration; generally, I.V. infusion rates should not exceed 0.7-1.5 mEq/minute (1.5-3.3 mL/minute); stop the infusion if the patient complains of pain or discomfort. Warm to body temperature; administer slowly, usually no faster than 1.5-3.3 mL/minute, do not inject into the myocardium when using calcium during advanced cardiac life support. Topical therapy for hydrofluoric acid exposures with 2.5% gel applied to affected area every 4 hours as needed. 2.5% gel can be prepared by mixing 5 oz of KY Jelly or Surgilube® with 25 mL of 10% calcium gluconate.

Contraindications Ventricular fibrillation during cardiac resuscitation; digitalis toxicity or suspected digoxin toxicity; hypercalcemia

Warnings Injection solution is for I.V. use only; do not inject SubQ or I.M. Avoid too rapid I.V. administration and avoid extravasation. Use with caution in digitalized patients, severe hyperphosphatemia, respiratory failure, or acidosis. May produce cardiac arrest. Hypercalcemia may occur in patients with renal failure; frequent determination of serum calcium is necessary. Use caution with renal disease. Solutions may contain aluminum; toxic levels may occur following prolonged administration in premature neonates or patients with renal dysfunction.

Dosage Forms

Injection, solution [preservative free]: 10% [100 mg/mL] (10 mL, 50 mL, 100 mL, 200 mL) [equivalent to elemental calcium 9 mg/mL; calcium 0.46 mEq/mL]

Powder: 347 mg/tablespoonful (480 g)

Tablet: 500 mg [equivalent to elemental calcium 45 mg]; 650 mg [equivalent to elemental calcium 58.5 mg]; 975 mg [equivalent to elemental calcium 87.75 mg]

Reference Range Serum: 9.0-10.4 mg/dL; due to a poor correlation between the serum ionized calcium (free) and total serum calcium, particularly in states of low albumin or acid/base imbalances, direct measurement of ionized calcium is recommended. If ionized calcium is unavailable, in low albumin states, the corrected **total** serum calcium may be estimated by this equation (assuming a normal albumin of 4 g/dL); corrected total calcium = total serum calcium + 0.8(4 - measured serum albumin).

Overdosage/Treatment Acute single ingestions of calcium salts may produce mild gastrointestinal distress, but hypercalcemia or other toxic manifestations are extremely unlikely. Treatment is supportive.

Test Interactions ↑ calcium (S); ↓ magnesium

Drug Interactions

Bisphosphonate derivatives: Absorption may be decreased by calcium salts.

Calcium channel blockers (eg, verapamil) effects may be diminished; monitor response.

Digoxin: May potentiate digoxin toxicity.

Dobutamine: Calcium salts may diminish the therapeutic effect of dobutamine.

Levothyroxine: Calcium carbonate (and possibly other calcium salts) may decrease T_4 absorption; separate dose from levothyroxine by at least 4 hours.

Phosphate supplements: Calcium salts may decrease the absorption of phosphate supplements.

Quinolone antibiotics: Calcium salts may decrease the absorption of quinolone antibiotics with oral administration of both agents.

Thiazide diuretics: Thiazide diuretics may decrease the excretion of calcium salts. Continued concomitant use can also result in metabolic alkalosis.

Pregnancy Risk Factor C

Pregnancy Implications Crosses the placenta

Lactation Enters breast milk

Centruroides Scorpion Venom Antisera

Use Severe *Centruroides* scorpion envenomation (grade IV)

Mechanism of Action Made by lyophilizing micron-filtered hypersensitized goat serum

Adverse Reactions

Cardiovascular: Sinus tachycardia

Gastrointestinal: Pancreatitis

Miscellaneous: Delayed **allergic reactions** (58%) include rash, urticaria, serum sickness

Dosage One vial I.V.; give second vial I.V. in 1 hour if symptoms not improved; do not administer I.M.

Overdosage/Treatment Supportive therapy: Midazolam (by continuous I.V. infusion) can be given to treat agitation and involuntary motor activity.

Specific References

Babu KM, Ganetsky M, Sheroff AD, et al, "A Deathstalker Scorpion Envenomation in Rhode Island," *Clin Toxicol (Phila)*, 2005, 43:710.

Riley BD, LaVecchio F, and Pizo AF, "Lack of Scorpion Antivenom Leads to Increased Pediatric ICU Admissions," *Ann Emerg Med*, 2006, 47(4):398-9.

Charcoal

Pronunciation (CHAR kole)

CAS Number 16291-96-6

U.S. Brand Names Actidose-Aqua® [OTC]; Actidose® with Sorbitol [OTC]; CharcoAid G® [OTC]; Charcoal Plus® DS [OTC]; Charcocaps® [OTC]; EZ-Char™ [OTC]; Kerr Insta-Char® [OTC]; Liqui-Char® [OTC] [DSC]

Synonyms Activated Carbon; Activated Charcoal; Adsorbent Charcoal; Liquid Antidote; Medicinal Carbon; Medicinal Charcoal

Use Emergency treatment in poisoning by drugs and chemicals; repetitive doses for gastrointestinal dialysis for drug overdose and in uremia to adsorb various waste products; hyperbilirubinemia; has been used as an aid in the diagnosis of colouterine fistula

Mechanism of Action Adsorbs toxic substances or irritants, thus inhibiting GI absorption and for selected drugs increasing clearance by interfering with enterohepatic recycling or dialysis across intestinal vascular membranes; adsorbs intestinal gas; the addition of sorbitol results in hyperosmotic laxative action causing catharsis

Adverse Reactions

Gastrointestinal: **Vomiting** 6%-15% with charcoal alone, 16%-56% with sorbitol; **diarrhea with sorbitol, constipation**, intestinal obstruction can occur (only with multiple dosing of activated charcoal), **stools will turn black**

Ocular: Corneal abrasions (2 cases)

Respiratory: Aspiration usually does not cause major problems in adults, but can cause tracheal obstruction in infants; very rarely, aspiration pneumonitis (8 case reports; 3 fatalities) more likely with ingestions treated with multiple doses

Pharmacodynamics/Kinetics Excretion: Feces (as charcoal)

Dosage

Oral: Ideally, achieving a 10 g charcoal:1 g toxin dose is the desired outcome

Acute poisoning: Single dose: Charcoal with sorbitol (**Note:** Check product label for sorbitol content):

Children and Adults: At least 5-10 times the weight of the ingested poison and other coingestants on a g:g ratio; minimum dose is probably 15-30 g; in young children sorbitol dose should not exceed 1.5 g/kg/day

Adults: 30-100 g

Charcoal in water: Same as above, but sorbitol should be added in appropriate daily doses

Single dose:

Infants and Children 1-12 years: 15-30 g

Adults: 30-100 g

Multiple dose (use only one appropriate dose of cathartic daily):

Infants <1 year: 15-30 g every 4-6 hours

Children 1-12 years: 20-25 g every 2 hours until clinical observations and serum drug concentration have returned to a subtherapeutic range or the development of absent bowel sounds or ileus

Adults: 20-25 g every 2 hours

Stability Adsorbs gases from air, store in closed container

Administration Flavoring agents (eg, chocolate) and sorbitol can enhance charcoal's palatability. If treatment includes ipecac syrup, induce vomiting prior to administration of charcoal. Often given with a laxative or cathartic; check for presence of bowel sounds before administration.

Contraindications Intestinal obstruction; GI tract not anatomically intact; patients at risk of hemorrhage or GI perforation; if use would increase risk and severity of aspiration; not effective for cyanide, mineral acids, caustic alkalis, organic solvents, iron, ethanol, methanol poisoning, lithium; do not use charcoal with sorbitol in patients with fructose intolerance; charcoal with sorbitol not recommended in children <1 year of age

Warnings When using ipecac with charcoal, induce vomiting with ipecac before administering activated charcoal since charcoal adsorbs ipecac syrup. Charcoal may cause vomiting which is hazardous in petroleum distillate and caustic ingestions. If charcoal in sorbitol is administered, doses should be limited to prevent excessive fluid and electrolyte losses. Use caution with decreased peristalsis. Most effective when administered within 1 hour of ingestion for most ingestions. May absorb maintenance medicatons too.

Dosage Forms

[DSC] = Discontinued product

Capsule, activated (Char-Caps, Charcocaps®): 260 mg

Granules, activated (CharcoAid G®): 15 g (120 mL) [DSC]

Liquid, activated:

Actidose-Aqua®: 15 g (72 mL); 25 g (120 mL); 50 g (240 mL)

Kerr Insta-Char®: 25 g (120 mL) [cherry flavor]; 50 g (240 mL) [unflavored or cherry flavor]

Liquid, activated [with sorbitol]:

Actidose® with Sorbitol: 25 g (120 mL); 50 g (240 mL)

Kerr Insta-Char®: 25 g (120 mL); 50 g (240 mL) [cherry flavor]

Pellets, activated (EZ-Char™): 25 g

Powder for suspension, activated: 30 g, 240 g

Tablets, activated (Charcoal Plus® DS): 250 mg

Drug Interactions Do not administer concomitantly with syrup of ipecac.

Pregnancy Risk Factor C

Lactation Does not enter breast milk/compatible

Nursing Implications Instruct patient to drink slowly, rapid administration appears to increase frequency of vomiting; for persistent vomiting, activated charcoal can be administered as a continuous enteral infusion at doses of 10-25 g/hour; fluid volume and sorbitol dosing must be reviewed carefully; concentrated slurries may clog airway; stools will turn black; vigorous shaking of the product is suggested

Specific References

Arnold TC, Zhang S, Xiao F, et al, "Pressure-Controlled Ventilation Attenuates Lung Microvascular Injury in a Rat Model of Activated Charcoal Aspiration," *J Toxicol Clin Toxicol*, 2003, 41(2):119-24.

Bailey DN and Briggs JR, "The Effect of Ethanol and pH on the Adsorption of Drugs from Simulated Gastric Fluid Onto Activated Charcoal," *Ther Drug Monit*, 2003, 25(3):310-3.

Bonner AB, Liebelt EL, Williamson E, et al, "Does the Addition of Chocolate Milk Reduce the Adsorption Capacity of Orally Administered Activated Charcoal for GI Decontamination of Acetaminophen Ingestion?" *Clin Toxicol (Phila)*, 2005, 43:672.

Chyka PA, Seger D, Krenzelok EP, et al, American Academy of Clinical Toxicology; European Association of Poisons Centres and Clinical Toxicologists, "Position Paper: Single-Dose Activated Charcoal," *Clin Toxicol (Phila)*, 2005, 43(2):61-87 (review).

Cope RB, "A Screening Study of Xylitol Binding *in vitro* to Activated Charcoal," *Vet Hum Toxicol*, 2004, 46(6):336-7.

Dawson A, "Superactivated Charcoal," *Am J Emerg Med*, 2004, 22(6):496.

Dorrington CL, Johnson DW, Brant R, "The Frequency of Complications Associated with the Use of Multiple-Dose Activated Charcoal," *Ann Emerg Med*, 2003, 41(3):370-7.

Eroglu A, Kucuktulu U, Erciyes N, et al, "Multiple Dose-Activated Charcoal as a Cause of Acute Appendicitis," *J Toxicol Clin Toxicol*, 2003, 41(1):71-3.

Hack JB, Meggs WJ, and Gilliland MGB, "Activated Charcoal Aspiration: Death in a Dose," *Clin Toxicol (Phila)*, 2005, 43:679.

Heard K, "Gastrointestinal Decontamination," *Med Clin N Am*, 2005, 89(6):1067-78 (review).

Hoegberg LC, Christophersen AB, Christensen HR, et al, "Comparison of the Adsorption Capacities of an Activated-charcoal–Yogurt Mixture Versus Activated-Charcoal–Water Slurry *in vivo* and *in vitro*," *Clin Toxicol (Phila)*, 2005, 43(4):269-75.

Hoffman RJ, Hahn I, Shen JM, et al, "In Vitro Charcoal Binding of Staphylococcal Enterotoxin B," *Clin Toxicol (Phila)*, 2005, 43:675.

Justice HM, Knapp BJ, Pianalto DA, et al, "Failure of Emergency Medical Services Providers to Administer Activated Charcoal Add to Emergency Delay," *Acad Emerg Med*, 2006, 13(5):S180.

LoVecchio F, Bermudez J, Shriki J, et al, "Aspiration Pnuemonia Rarely Occurs with Single-Dose Activated Charcoal," *J Toxicol Clin Toxicol*, 2004, 42(5):812.

LoVecchio F, Shriki J, Innes K, et al, "It is Rarely Feasible to Administer Charcoal Within One Hour of Acute Overdose," *J Toxicol Clin Toxicol*, 2004, 42(5):812.

McKinney PE, Wares JB, and Crandall C, "Delays to Activated Charcoal in the ED: Why Bother?" *J Toxicol Clin Toxicol*, 2003, 41(5):644.

Seger D, "Single-Dose Activated Charcoal-Backup and Reassess," *J Toxicol Clin Toxicol*, 2004, 42(1):101-10.

Wiegand TJ, Wu, L, and Dempsey DA, "Algorithm for Activated Charcoal (AC) Use for Ingestion," *Clin Toxicol (Phila)*, 2005, 43:673.

Wilson L, Van Bebber SL, Kearney TE, et al, "Cost-Effectiveness of Promotion by Poison Centers of Activated Charcoal in the Home," *J Toxicol Clin Toxicol*, 2003, 41(5):681.

Wilson L, Van Bebber SL, Kearney TE, et al, "Policies and Experience of US Poison Centers with Home Administration of Single-Dose Activated Charcoal," *J Toxicol Clin Toxicol*, 2003, 41(5):682.

Cholestyramine Resin

Pronunciation (koe LES teer a meen REZ in)

CAS Number 11041-12-6

U.S. Brand Names Prevalite®; Questran® Light; Questran®

Use Adjunct in the management of primary hypercholesterolemia; pruritus associated with elevated levels of bile acids; diarrhea associated with excess fecal bile acids, tropical diarrhea; binding toxicologic agents, such as digitoxin, possibly phenobarbital, warfarin, lindane, lithium lorazepam, methotrexate, chlordecone; pseudomembraneous colitis (*Clostridium difficile*), oxaluria

Mechanism of Action Forms a nonabsorbable complex with bile acids in the intestine, releasing chloride ions in the process; inhibits enterohepatic reuptake of intestinal bile salts and thereby increases the fecal loss of bile salt-bound low density lipoprotein cholesterol; an anion-exchange resin (chloride form)

Adverse Reactions

Dermatologic: Rash, irritation of perianal area, skin

Endocrine & metabolic: Hyperchloremic acidosis, hypoprothrombinemia, hypernatremia from free water loss due to diarrhea

Gastrointestinal: Constipation, nausea, vomiting, abdominal distention and pain, malabsorption of fat-soluble vitamins, fecal impaction, steatorrhea, tongue irritation

Genitourinary: Increased urinary calcium excretion

Hepatic: Elevation of alkaline phosphatase and liver function test results

Signs and Symptoms of Overdose Gastrointestinal obstruction/concretion

Pharmacodynamics/Kinetics

Onset of action: Peak effect: 21 days

Absorption: None

Excretion: Feces (as insoluble complex with bile acids)

Dosage

Oral (dosages are expressed in terms of anhydrous resin):

Children: 240 mg/kg/day in 3 divided doses; need to titrate dose depending on indication

Adults: 4 g 1-2 times/day to a maximum of 24 g/day and 6 doses/day

Dialysis: Not removed by hemo- or peritoneal dialysis; supplemental doses not necessary with dialysis or continuous arteriovenous or venovenous hemofiltration

Stability Store powder at controlled room temperature of 15°C to 30°C (59°F to 86°F). Mix contents of 1 packet or 1 level scoop of powder with 4-6 oz of beverage. Allow to stand 1-2 minutes prior to mixing. May also be mixed with highly-fluid soups, cereals, applesauce, etc. Suspension may be used for up to 48 hours after refrigeration.

Administration Administer with water or pulpy fruit

Contraindications Hypersensitivity to bile acid sequestering resins or any component of the formulation; complete biliary obstruction; bowel obstruction

Warnings Not to be taken simultaneously with many other medicines (decreased absorption). Treat any diseases contributing to hypercholesterolemia first. May interfere with fat-soluble vitamins (A, D, E, K) and folic acid. Chronic use may be associated with bleeding problems (especially in high doses). May produce or exacerbate constipation problems. Fecal impaction may occur. Hemorrhoids may be worsened.

Dosage Forms

Powder for oral suspension: 4 g of resin/5 g of powder (5 g packets, 210 g can) [contains phenylalanine 14 mg/5 g]; 4 g of resin/5.7 g of powder (5.7 g packets, 240 g can) [light formulation]; 4 g of resin/9 g of powder (9 g packets, 378 g can)

Prevalite®: 4 g of resin/5.5 g of powder (5.5 g packets, 231 g can) [contains phenylalanine 14.1 mg/5.5 g; orange flavor]

Questran®: 4 g of resin/9 g of powder (9 g packets, 378 g can)

Questran® Light: 4 g of resin/6.4 g of powder (5 g packets, 268 g can) [contains phenylalanine 28.1 mg/6.4 g]

Test Interactions ↑ prothrombin time (S); ↓ cholesterol (S), iron (B)

Drug Interactions

Cholestyramine can reduce the absorption of numerous medications when used concurrently. Give other medications 1 hour before or 4-6 hours after giving cholestyramine. Medications which may be affected include HMG-CoA reductase inhibitors, thiazide diuretics, propranolol (and potentially other beta-blockers), corticosteroids, thyroid hormones, digoxin, valproic acid, NSAIDs, loop diuretics, sulfonylureas, troglitazone (and potentially other agents in this class).

Warfarin and other oral anticoagulants: Hypoprothrombinemic effects may be reduced by cholestyramine. Separate administration times (as detailed above) and monitor INR closely when initiating or discontinuing.

Pregnancy Risk Factor C

Pregnancy Implications Cholestyramine is not absorbed systemically, but may interfere with vitamin absorption; therefore, regular prenatal supplementation may not be adequate. There are no studies in pregnant women; use with caution.

Lactation Does not enter breast milk/use caution

Nursing Implications Do not administer the powder in its dry form; just prior to administration, mix with fluid or with applesauce; administer warfarin at least 1-2 hours prior to, or 6 hours after cholestyramine because cholestyramine may bind warfarin and decrease its total absorption. (Note: Cholestyramine itself may cause hypoprothrombinemia in patients with impaired enterohepatic circulation.)

Specific References

Balagani R, Wills B, amd Leikin JB, "Cholestyramine Improves Tropical-Related Diarrhea," *Am J Ther*, 2006, 13(3):281-2.

White CM, Kalus JS, Caron MF, et al, "Cholestyramine Ointment Used on an Infant for Severe Buttocks Rash Resistant to Standard Therapeutic Modalities," *J Pharm Technol*, 2003, 19:11-3.

Cyanide Antidote Kit

Pronunciation (SOW dee um NYE trite, SOW dee um thye oh SUL fate, & AM il NYE trite)

U.S. Brand Names Cyanide Antidote Package

Synonyms Amyl Nitrite, Sodium Thiosulfate, and Sodium Nitrite; Cyanide Antidote Kit; Sodium Thiosulfate, Sodium Nitrite, and Amyl Nitrite

Use Treatment of cyanide poisoning

Dosage For cyanide poisoning, a 0.3 mL ampul of amyl nitrite is crushed every minute and vapor inhaled for 15-30 seconds until an I.V. sodium nitrite infusion is available. Following administration of 300 mg I.V. sodium nitrite, inject 12.5 g sodium thiosulfate I.V. (over ~10 minutes), if needed; injection of both may be repeated at $^1/_2$ the original dose.

Administration Sodium nitrite should be administered at a rate of 2.5-5 mL/minute.

Contraindications Hypersensitivity to amyl nitrite, sodium nitrite, nitrates, sodium thiosulfate, or any component of the formulation; severe anemia, pregnancy (amyl nitrite)

Warnings When cyanide poisoning is related to smoke inhalation, if possible, the patient should be in a hyperbaric chamber before the kit is administered; the methemoglobin initially produced by sodium nitrite injection may otherwise exacerbate concomitant carbon monoxide poisoning that has already severely diminished oxygen-carrying capacity in red cells

Dosage Forms

Kit [each kit contains] (Cyanide Antidote Package):

Injection, solution:

Sodium nitrite 300 mg/10 mL (2)

Sodium thiosulfate 12.5 g/50 mL (2)

Inhalant: Amyl nitrite 0.3 mL (12)

[kit also includes disposable syringes, stomach tube, tourniquet, and instructions]

Drug Interactions Sodium nitrite antagonizes acetylcholine, epinephrine, and histamine effects; sodium nitrite potentiates hypotensive effects and/or anticholinergic effects of tricyclic antidepressants, antihistamines, and meperidine and related CNS depressants; ethanol increases the toxicity of amyl nitrite

Pregnancy Risk Factor C (sodium thiosulfate and sodium nitrite); X (amyl nitrite)

Deferiprone

CAS Number 30652-11-0

Unlabeled/Investigational Use

Investigational: Prevention of chronic iron overload in patients with transfusion-dependent beta-thalassemia

Mechanism of Action Orally active iron chelator

Adverse Reactions

Cardiovascular: Vasculitis

Hematologic: Bone marrow suppression, thrombocytopenia, leukopenia

Neuromuscular & skeletal: Arthritis, arthralgia

Dosage Oral: 75-100 mg/kg/day in 3 divided doses

Reference Range Oral dose of 25 mg/kg produces a peak plasma level of 14-17 mcg/mL

Test Interactions ↓ serum ferritin; ↑ urinary excretion of iron

Deferoxamine

Pronunciation (de fer OKS a meen)

CAS Number 138-14-7; 1950-39-6; 70-51-9

U.S. Brand Names Desferal®

Synonyms Deferoxamine Mesylate

Use Acute iron intoxication when serum iron is >450-500 mcg/dL or when clinical signs of significant iron toxicity exist; chronic iron overload secondary to multiple transfusions; iron overload secondary to congenital anemias; hemochromatosis

Unlabeled/Investigational Use Removal of corneal rust rings following surgical removal of foreign bodies; diagnosis or treatment of aluminum induced toxicity associated with chronic kidney disease (CKD)

Mechanism of Action Complexes with trivalent ions (ferric ions) to form ferrioxamine, which is removed by the kidneys

Adverse Reactions

Cardiovascular: Flushing, hypotension, tachycardia, shock, edema, sinus tachycardia

Central nervous system: Fever, seizures

Dermatologic: Erythema, urticaria, pruritus, rash, cutaneous wheal formation

Endocrine & metabolic: Growth suppression

Gastrointestinal: Abdominal discomfort, diarrhea, appendicitis

Genitourinary: Dysuria, urine discoloration (pink)

Local: Pain and induration at injection site

Neuromuscular & skeletal: Leg cramps, exacerbation of myasthenia gravis

Ocular: Blurred vision, cataract, visual field defects, night blindness, macular edema, retinopathy

Otic: Hearing loss, tinnitus

Renal: Renal insufficiency

Miscellaneous: Anaphylaxis, possible risk of fungal and *Y. enterocolitica* infections (increased); *Yersinia*, Zygomycetes and *Aeromonas hydrophila* infection have been associated with deferoxamine administration;

phycomycosis; thrombocytopenia, toxicity, fibrosis and edema at high doses (over 24 hours) - restrictive lung pathology has been noted

Signs and Symptoms of Overdose Seizures

Pharmacodynamics/Kinetics
Absorption: I.M.: Erratic
Metabolism: Hepatic; binds with iron to form ferrioxamine
Half-life elimination: Parent drug: 6.1 hours; Ferrioxamine: 5.8 hours
Excretion: Urine (as unchanged drug and ferrioxamine)

Dosage
Oral use is probably not effective; 100 mg DFO binds ~10 mg iron and 4.1 mg of aluminum
Children:
Acute iron intoxication:
I.M.: 90 mg/kg/dose every 8 hours
I.V.: 10-15 mg/kg/hour (up to 35 mg/kg/hour with caution in severe poisoning); in nonpoisoning settings, maximum dose
Chronic iron overload:
I.V.: 15 mg/kg/hour
SubQ: 20-40 mg/kg/day over 8-12 hours
Aluminum-induced bone disease (unlabeled use): 20-40 mg/kg every hemodialysis treatment, frequency dependent on clinical status of the patient
Dialysis patients for general aluminum toxicity (levels >60 mcg/dL): 40-80 mg/kg I.V. once weekly prior to dialysis with a dose reduction to 20-60 mg/kg with a postive response
Adults:
Acute iron intoxication:
I.M.: 1 g stat, then 0.5 g every 4 hours for two doses, then 0.5 g every 4-12 hours up to 6 g/day
I.V.: 15 mg/kg/hour, up to 6-8 g/day; maximum given 16 g/day without side effects
Chronic iron overload:
I.M.: 0.5-1 g every day
SubQ: 1-2 g every day over 8-24 hours

Stability Protect from light; reconstituted solutions (sterile water) may be stored at room temperature for 7 days

Monitoring Parameters Serum iron, total iron-binding capacity; ophthalmologic exam (fundoscopy, slit-lamp exam) and audiometry with chronic therapy

Administration
I.V.: Urticaria, hypotension, and shock have occurred following rapid I.V. administration; limiting infusion rate to 15mg/kg/hour may help avoid infusion-related adverse effects.
Acute iron toxicity: The manufacturer states that the I.M. route is preferred; however, the I.V. route is generally preferred in patients with severe toxicity (ie, patients in shock). For the first 1000 mg, infuse at 15 mg/kg/hour (although rates up to 40-50 mg/kg/hour have been given in patients with massive iron intoxication). Subsequent doses may be given over 4-12 hours; maximum I.V. rate (per manufacturer): 15 mg/kg/hour.
Diagnosis or treatment of aluminum induced toxicity with CKD: Administer dose over 1 hour
SubQ: When administered for chronic iron overload, daily dose should be given over 8-24 hours using portable pump.

Contraindications Hypersensitivity to deferoxamine or any component of the formulation; patients with severe renal disease and anuria, primary hemochromatosis

Warnings Use with caution in patients with pyelonephritis; may increase susceptibility to *Yersinia enterocolitica*. Ocular and auditory disturbances and growth retardation (children only), have been reported following prolonged administration. Has been associated with adult respiratory distress syndrome (ARDS) following excessively high-dose treatment of acute intoxication. Caution must be used in performing tasks which require alertness (eg, operating machinery or driving). Patients should be informed that urine may have a reddish color.

Dosage Forms Injection, powder for reconstitution, as mesylate: 500 mg, 2 g

Test Interactions May interfere with colorimetric iron assays, along with total iron binding capacity

Drug Interactions
Prochlorperazine: Concurrent use may cause loss of consciousness or coma.
Vitamin C: Concomitant treatment with vitamin C (>500 mg/day) has been associated with cardiac impairment

Pregnancy Risk Factor C

Pregnancy Implications Do not withhold chelation treatment for iron overdose solely due to pregnancy; has caused fetal skeletal abnormalities in animal models but is probably safe to use in the gravid patient

Lactation Excretion in breast milk unknown/use caution

Nursing Implications Iron chelate colors urine salmon pink, which is concentration and pH dependent; I.M. is preferred route; maximum I.V. rate is 35 mg/kg/hour; incompatible with heparin

Specific References
Prasannan L, Flynn JT, Levine JE, et al, "Acute Renal Failure Following Deferoxamine Overdose," *Pediatr Nephrol*, 2003, 18(3):283-5.

Dexrazoxane

Pronunciation (deks ray ZOKS ane)
CAS Number 24584-09-6
U.S. Brand Names Zinecard®
Synonyms ICRF-187
Use Reduction of the incidence and severity of cardiomyopathy associated with doxorubicin administration in women with metastatic breast cancer who have received a cumulative doxorubicin dose of 300 mg/m^2 and who would benefit from continuing therapy with doxorubicin. It is not recommended for use with the initiation of doxorubicin therapy.

Mechanism of Action Derivative of EDTA; potent intracellular chelating agent. The mechanism of cardioprotectant activity is not fully understood. Appears to be converted intracellularly to a ring-opened chelating agent that interferes with iron-mediated oxygen free radical generation thought to be responsible, in part, for anthracycline-induced cardiomyopathy.

Adverse Reactions
Dermatologic: Alopecia, urticaria, recall skin reaction, extravasation
Endocrine & metabolic: Serum amylase increased, serum calcium decreased, serum triglycerides increased
Gastrointestinal: Nausea, vomiting (mild)
Hematologic: Myelosuppression, **neutropenia**, thrombocytopenia
Hepatic: AST/ALT increased, bilirubin increased

Pharmacodynamics/Kinetics
Distribution: V_d: 22-22.4 L/m^2
Protein binding: None
Half-life elimination: 2.1-2.5 hours
Excretion: Urine (42%)
Clearance, renal: 3.35 L/hour/m^2; Plasma: 6.25-7.88 L/hour/m^2

Dosage
Adults: I.V.: A 10:1 ratio of dexrazoxane:doxorubicin (500 mg/m^2 dexrazoxane: 50 mg/m^2 doxorubicin)
Dosage adjustment in hepatic impairment: Since doxorubicin dosage is reduced in hyperbilirubinemia, a proportional reduction in dexrazoxane dosage is recommended (maintain ratio of 10:1).

Stability
Store intact vials at controlled room temperature (15°C to 30°C/59°F to 86°F). Reconstituted and diluted solutions are stable for 6 hours at controlled room temperature or under refrigeration (2°C to 8°C/36°F to 46°F).
Must be reconstituted with 0.167 Molar (M/6) sodium lactate injection to a concentration of 10 mg dexrazoxane/mL sodium lactate. Reconstituted dexrazoxane solution may be diluted with either 0.9% sodium chloride injection or 5% dextrose injection to a concentration of 1.3-5 mg/mL in intravenous infusion bags.

Monitoring Parameters Since dexrazoxane will always be used with cytotoxic drugs, and since it may add to the myelosuppressive effects of cytotoxic drugs, frequent complete blood counts are recommended

Administration Administer by slow I.V. push or rapid (5-15 minutes) I.V. infusion from a bag. Administer doxorubicin within 30 minutes after beginning the infusion with dexrazoxane.

Contraindications Hypersensitivity to dexrazoxane or any component of the formulation; use with chemotherapy regimens that do not contain an anthracycline

Warnings Hazardous agent; use appropriate precautions for handling and disposal. Dexrazoxane may add to the myelosuppression caused by chemotherapeutic agents. Dexrazoxane does not eliminate the potential for anthracycline-induced cardiac toxicity. Carefully monitor cardiac function. Dosage adjustment required for moderate or severe renal insufficiency. Safety and efficacy in pediatric patients have not been established.

Dosage Forms Injection, powder for reconstitution: 250 mg, 500 mg [10 mg/mL when reconstituted]

Reference Range Peak plasma dexrazoxane level after a 500 mg/m^2 infusion: 36.5 mcg/mL

Test Interactions ↑ serum amylase (without evidence for pancreatitis); ↑ serum iron, ↓ serum zinc

Pregnancy Risk Factor C

Pregnancy Implications Avoid use in pregnant women unless the potential benefit justifies the potential risk to the fetus

Lactation Excretion in breast milk unknown/not recommended

Dextran 1

Pronunciation (DEKS tran won)
CAS Number 9004-54-0
U.S. Brand Names Promit®
Use Prophylaxis of serious anaphylactic reactions to I.V. infusion of dextran in a dose-dependent manner; can prevent clot formation due to ergotism

Mechanism of Action Binds to dextran-reactive immunoglobulin without bridge formation and no formation of large immune complexes

Mechanism of Toxic Action Produces plasma volume expansion by virtue of its highly colloidal starch structure, similar to albumin

Adverse Reactions

Cardiovascular: Mild hypotension, bradycardia, tightness of chest, chest pain, shock, sinus bradycardia, angina

Central nervous system: Fever

Dermatologic: Urticaria

Gastrointestinal: Nausea, vomiting

Hematologic: Coagulopathy

Neuromuscular & skeletal: Arthralgia

Renal: Renal failure

Respiratory: Wheezing, nasal congestion

Miscellaneous: Anaphylaxis

Signs and Symptoms of Overdose Bradycardia, hypotension

Dosage

I.V. (time between dextran 1 and dextran solution should not exceed 15 minutes):

Children: 0.3 mL/kg 1-2 minutes before I.V. infusion of dextran

Adults: 20 mL 1-2 minutes before I.V. infusion of dextran

Administration Infuse over 1 minute.

Contraindications Hypersensitivity to dextrans or any component of the formulation; **dextran** contraindicated

Warnings Severe hypotension and bradycardia can occur. If any reaction occurs, do not administer dextran. Mild dextran-induced anaphylactic reactions are not prevented.

Dosage Forms Injection, solution: 150 mg/mL (20 mL)

Pregnancy Risk Factor C

Lactation Excretion in breast milk unknown

Nursing Implications Do not dilute or admix with dextrans

Dextrose

CAS Number 50-99-7; 5996-10-1

Use Patients with altered mental status due to hypoglycemia

Mechanism of Action A carbohydrate substrate for aerobic metabolism

Adverse Reactions

Central nervous system: Confusion, has been associated with worsening of ischemic strokes

Endocrine & metabolic: Hypokalemia, hyperglycemia, hypomagnesemia, hypophosphatemia

Gastrointestinal: Sweet taste

Local: Vein irritation, thrombophlebitis, extravasation injury

Respiratory: Pulmonary edema

Miscellaneous: Hyperosmolar solution which can cause a Volkmann's contraction of an extremity if extravasation occurs

Dosage

Dextrose 50% solution (parenteral administration)

Children: Dilute to 10% to 25% and give 2-4 mL/kg body weight

"Rule of 50" for Providing 0.5 g of Dextrose Intravenously in Pediatric Patients with Sulfonylurea-induced Hypoglycemia	
Dextrose Concentration of I.V. Fluid	Volume to be Administered
10%	5 mL/kg
25%	2 mL/kg
50%	1 mL/kg

Adults: 50-100 mL

Use caution in elderly patients, starting at the low end of the dosing range, reflecting the greater frequency of decreased hepatic, renal, or cardiac function, and of concomitant disease or other drug therapy.

Monitoring Parameters Serum glucose

Test Interactions May cause false elevation of serum creatinine through interference with laboratory determination

Specific References

Calello DP, Kelly A, and Osterhoudt KC, "Case Files of the Medical Toxicology Fellowship Training Program at the Children's Hospital of Philadelphia: A Pediatric Exploratory Sulfonylurea Ingestion," *J Med Toxicol*, 2006, 2(1):19-24.

McGee D, Chen A, and de Garavilla L, "Dextrose Is Absorbed by Rectum in Hypoglycemic Rats," *J Emerg Med*, 2003, 24(3):253-7.

Diethyldithiocarbamate Trihydrate

CAS Number 148-18-5

Synonyms DDC

Unlabeled/Investigational Use

Investigational: Chelating agent for nickel; a metabolite of disulfiram, it has also been used to treat thallium poisoning, but is not effective; shown to be active against HIV *in vitro*

Mechanism of Action Binds to nickel; the nickel-diethyldithiocarbamate complex is lipophilic thus enhancing its elimination

Adverse Reactions Gastrointestinal: Nausea

Dosage

Mild or doubtful nickel exposure (urine nickel <100 mcg/L): Oral: 2 g in divided doses (every 4 hours)

Severe nickel exposure urine (levels 100-500 mcg/L): adult dose Oral: Initial: 2 g with 1 g sodium bicarbonate, then 1 g at 4 hours, 600 mg at 8 hours, 400 mg at 16 hours, and 400 mg every 8 hours thereafter until urine Ni is <50 mcg/L

Alternatively, 35-45 mg/kg/day on day one, then 400 mg every 8 hours until symptoms are resolved or urine nickel levels are <50 mcg/L;

Urine nickel levels >500 mcg/L: Give 25-100 mg/kg/day (I:V)

DDC may be given intravenously by adding ten ml of a sterile phosphate buffer solution to one gram of powdered DDC contained in a sterile ampule IV DDC 25-100 mg/kg is administered over the first 24 hours as described above.

How supplied: One gram sterile powder ampule.

Diethylene Triamine Penta-Acetic Acid

CAS Number 67-43-6

Use Chelating absorbed multivalent radioisotopes of the actinide series (plutonium, neptunium, americium) as well as cesium and actinide; may be useful for uranium, curium, californium, cerium, yttrium, lanthanum, scandium, promethium, niobium, manganese, thorium, lutetium, zirconium, and zinc; on IND status

Mechanism of Action Chelation for multivalent radioisotopes

Adverse Reactions

Central nervous system: Chills, fever

Dermal: Pruritus

Gastrointestinal: Transient nausea, vomiting, diarrhea

Neuromuscular & skeletal: Muscle cramps in first day of therapy

Renal: Nephrotoxicity

Miscellaneous: Ca-DTPA may cause zinc depletion leading to transient anosmia

Dosage 1 g of the calcium salt diluted in 250 mL of 5% dextrose in water infused over 60-90 minutes; may be repeated daily for 5 days; zinc salt can be used for pregnant patients; may be aerosolized through nebulization

Stability Store in cool environment and away from sunlight

Monitoring Parameters Urine analysis, radioassay, renal function and blood counts during therapy, pulse and blood pressure

Pregnancy Risk Factor C (Zn-DTPA); D (Ca-DTPA)

Digoxin Immune Fab

U.S. Brand Names Digibind®; DigiFab™

Synonyms Antidigoxin Fab Fragments, Ovine

Use Treatment of life-threatening or potentially life-threatening digoxin intoxication, including:

- Acute digoxin ingestion (ie, >10 mg in adults or >4 mg in children)
- Acute digoxin serum level > 15 ng/ml
- Empiric diagnosis for undiagnosed bradycardia, ventricular arrhythmics or bradyarrhythmia unresponsive to atropine
- Chronic ingestions leading to steady-state digoxin concentrations > 6 ng/mL in adults or >4 ng/mL in children
- Manifestations of digoxin toxicity due to overdose (life-threatening ventricular arrhythmias, progressive bradycardia, second- or third-degree heart block not responsive to atropine, serum potassium >5 mEq/L in adults or >6 mEq/L in children)

Useful in treating delirium due to digitalis; also effective for oleander, Squill, Yellow oleander, Doghane, Bufo toads, Lily of the Valley, Purple Foxglove, foxglove lanatoside C ingestions

Mechanism of Action Binds with molecules of digoxin or digitoxin and is then excreted by the kidneys and removed from the body; promotes egress of free intracellular digoxin into extracellular fluid whereupon it is rapidly bound; prevents reassociation to membrane receptors

Adverse Reactions Allergic reactions (very rare), hypokalemia, phlebitis, postural hypotension, serum sickness. Cardiovascular effects (due to withdrawal of digitalis) include exacerbation of low cardiac output states and congestive heart failure, rapid ventricular response in patients with atrial fibrillation.

Pharmacodynamics/Kinetics

Onset of action: I.V.: Improvement in 2-30 minutes for toxicity

Half-life elimination: 15-20 hours; prolonged with renal impairment

Excretion: Urine; undetectable amounts within 5-7 days

Dosage

See package insert. To determine the dose of digoxin immune Fab, first determine the total body load of digoxin (TBL) as follows (using either an approximation of the amount ingested or a postdistribution serum digoxin concentration):

TBL of digoxin (in mg) = C (in ng/mL) $\times$ 5.6 $\times$ body weight (in kg)/1000 or TBL = mg of digoxin ingested (as tablets or elixir) $\times$ 0.8; C = postdistribution digoxin concentration (taken minimally 6 hours after ingestion)

Dose of digoxin immune Fab (in mg) I.V. = TBL × 66.7 or dose of digoxin immune Fab (in number of 38 mg vials) = [C of digoxin (in ng/mL) × body weight (in kg)]/100

If neither ingestion amount or serum level is known: Adult dosage is 20 vials (760 mg) I.V. infusion; see tables.

Approximate Digibind® Dose for Reversal of a Single Large Digoxin Overdose

Number of Digoxin Tablets or Capsules Ingested*	Dose of Digibind® # of Vials
25	10
50	20
75	30
100	40
150	60
200	80

*0.25 mg tablets with 80% bioavability of 0.2 mg Lanoxicaps®capsules with 100% bioavailability

Adult Dose Estimates of Digibind® (in # of Vials) from Steady-State Serum Digoxin Concentration

Patient Weight (kg)	Serum Digoxin Concentration (ng/mL)						
	1	2	4	8	12	16	20
40	0.5 v	1 v	2 v	3 v	5 v	7 v	8 v
60	0.5 v	1 v	3 v	5 v	7 v	10 v	12 v
70	1 v	2 v	3 v	6 v	9 v	11 v	14 v
80	1 v	2 v	3 v	7 v	10 v	13 v	16 v
100	1 v	2 v	4 v	8 v	12 v	16 v	20 v

v = vials.

Infants and Small Children Dose Estimates of Digibind® (in mg) from Serum DigoxinConcentration

Patient Weight (kg)	Serum Digoxin Concentration (ng/mL)						
	1	2	4	8	12	16	20
1	0.4 mg*	1 mg*	1.5 mg*	3 mg*	5 mg	6 mg	8 mg
3	1 mg*	2 mg*	5 mg	9 mg	14 mg	18 mg	23 mg
5	2 mg*	4 mg	8 mg	15 mg	23 mg	30 mg	38 mg
10	4 mg	8 mg	15 mg	30 mg	46 mg	61 mg	76 mg
20	8 mg	15 mg	30 mg	61 mg	91 mg	122 mg	152 mg

*Dilution of reconstituted vial to 1 mg/mL may be desirable.

Stability Should be refrigerated (2°C to 8°C). Reconstitute by adding 4 mL sterile water, resulting in 10 mg/mL for I.V. infusion. The reconstituted solution may be further diluted with NS to a convenient volume (eg, 1 mg/mL). Reconstituted solutions should be used within 4 hours if refrigerated. For very small doses, vial can be reconstituted by adding an additional 36 mL of sterile isotonic saline, to achieve a final concentration of 1 mg/mL.

Monitoring Parameters Serum potassium, serum digoxin concentration prior to first dose of digoxin immune Fab; **digoxin levels will greatly increase with digoxin immune Fab use and are not an accurate determination of body stores**; standard digoxin concentration measurements may be misleading until Fab fragments are eliminated from the body. Patients with renal failure should be monitored for a prolonged period for reintoxication with digoxin following the rerelease of bound digoxin into the blood.

Administration Continuous I.V. infusion over 15-30 minutes is preferred; digoxin immune Fab is reconstituted by adding 4 mL sterile water, resulting in 10 mg/mL for I.V. infusion, the reconstituted solution may be further diluted with NS to a convenient volume (eg, 1 mg/mL).

Contraindications Hypersensitivity to sheep products or any component of the formulation

Warnings Suicidal attempts often involve multiple drugs. Consider other drug toxicities as well. Hypersensitivity reactions can occur. Epinephrine should be immediately available. Serum potassium levels should be monitored, especially during the first few hours after administration. Total serum digoxin concentrations will rise precipitously following administration of this drug (has no clinical meaning - avoid monitoring serum concentrations). If digoxin was being used to treat CHF then may see exacerbation of symptoms as digoxin level is reduced. Use with caution in renal failure (experience limited) - the complex will be removed from the body more slowly. Monitor for reoccurrence of digoxin toxicity. Has reversed thrombocytopenia induced by digoxin. Failure of response to adequate treatment may call diagnosis of digitalis toxicity into question. Digoxin immune Fab is processed with papain and may cause hypersensitivity reactions in patients allergic to papaya, other papaya extracts, papain, chymopapain, or the pineapple enzyme bromelain. There may also be cross allergy with dust mite and latex allergens.

Dosage Forms Injection, powder for reconstitution:
Digibind®: 38 mg
DigiFab™: 40 mg

Reference Range Digoxin toxic concentration: >2.0 ng/mL

Test Interactions ↑ digoxin 50-fold; ↓ potassium; may ↓ glucose in patients with low glycogen stores

Drug Interactions Digoxin: Following administration of digoxin immune Fab, serum digoxin levels are markedly increased due to bound complexes (may be clinically misleading, since bound complex cannot interact with receptors).

Pregnancy Risk Factor C

Pregnancy Implications Animal reproduction studies have not been conducted. Safety and efficacy in pregnant women have not been established. Use during pregnancy only if clearly needed.

Lactation Excretion in breast milk unknown/use caution

Nursing Implications Continuous I.V. infusion over 15-30 minutes is preferred; digoxin immune Fab is reconstituted by adding 4 mL sterile water, resulting in 10 mg/mL for I.V. infusion, the reconstituted solution may be further diluted with normal saline to a convenient volume (eg, 1 mg/mL)

Specific References
Barrueto F Jr, Hirsch ON, Mercurio-Zappalla M, et al, "Efficacy of Digibind Versus Digifab in Binding Cinobufotalin," J Toxicol Clin Toxicol, 2003, 41(5):726-7.

Barrueto F Jr, Jortani SA, Valdes R Jr, et al, "Cardioactive Steroid Poisoning from an Herbal Cleansing Preparation," Ann Emerg Med, 2003, 41(3):396-9.

Eddleston M, Senarathna L, Mohamed F, et al, "Deaths Due to Absence of an Affordable Antitoxin for Plant Poisoning," Lancet, 2003, 362(9389):1041-4.

Kirrane BM, Barrueto F Jr, Hoffman RS, et al, "A Retrospective Analysis of Cardioactive Steroid Poisoning," J Toxicol Clin Toxicol, 2003, 41(5):716.

Dimercaprol

Pronunciation (dye mer KAP role)

Related Information
● Unithiol [ANTIDOTE]

CAS Number 59-52-9

U.S. Brand Names BAL in Oil®

Synonyms BAL; British Anti-Lewisite; Dithioglycerol

Use Antidote to gold, arsenic, mercury, methyl bromide, methyl iodide, or trivalent antimony poisoning; adjunct to edetate calcium disodium in lead poisoning; possibly effective for bismuth, polonium, chromium, copper, nickel, tungsten, or zinc

Mechanism of Action Sulfhydryl group combines with ions of various heavy metals to form relatively stable, nontoxic, soluble chelates which are excreted in bile and urine

Adverse Reactions
Cardiovascular: **Hypertension, tachycardia**, chest pain, angina, sinus tachycardia
Central nervous system: Nervousness, fever, headache, seizures, **convulsions**
Gastrointestinal: Vomiting, nausea, salivation
Hematologic: Transient neutropenia, glucose-6-phosphate dehydrogenase deficiency-induced hemolytic anemia
Local: Pain at injection site
Ocular: Blepharospasm
Renal: Nephrotoxicity
Respiratory: Rhinorrhea
Miscellaneous: Burning sensation of the lips, mouth, throat, eyes, diaphoresis

Pharmacodynamics/Kinetics
Distribution: To all tissues including the brain
Metabolism: Rapidly hepatic to inactive metabolites
Time to peak, serum: 0.5-1 hour
Excretion: Urine

Dosage

Children and Adults:

I.M.:

Mild arsenic and gold poisoning: 2.5 mg/kg/dose every 6 hours for 2 days, then every 12 hours on the third day, and once daily thereafter for 10 days

Severe arsenic and gold poisoning: 3 mg/kg/dose every 4 hours for 2 days then every 6 hours on the third day, then every 12 hours thereafter for 10 days

Mercury poisoning: Initial: 5 mg/kg followed by 2.5 mg/kg/dose 1-2 times/day for 10 days

Lead poisoning (use with edetate calcium disodium):

Mild: 3-5 mg/kg/dose every 4 hours for 2 days, then 2.5-3 mg/kg/dose every 6 hours for 2 days, then 2.5-3 mg/kg/dose every 12 hours for 1 week

Severe: 4 mg/kg/dose every 4 hours for 5-7 days

Acute encephalopathy: Initial: 4 mg/kg/dose, then every 4 hours

Topical dermal/ocular dose for Lewisite exposure: <20% solution

Administration Administer deep I.M. only; keep urine alkaline to protect renal function

Contraindications Hepatic insufficiency (unless due to arsenic poisoning); do not use on iron, cadmium, or selenium poisoning

Warnings Potentially a nephrotoxic drug, use with caution in patients with oliguria or glucose 6-phosphate dehydrogenase deficiency; keep urine alkaline to protect kidneys; administer all injections deep I.M. at different sites

Dosage Forms Injection, oil: 100 mg/mL (3 mL) [contains benzyl benzoate and peanut oil]

Test Interactions May ↓ Iodine I-131 thyroid uptake values

Drug Interactions Toxic complexes with iron, cadmium, selenium, or uranium

Pregnancy Risk Factor C

Pregnancy Implications C

Nursing Implications Administer deep I.M. only; urine should be kept alkaline

Specific References

Vilensky JA and Redman K, "British Anti-Lewisite (Dimercaprol): An Amazing History," *Ann Emerg Med*, 2003, 41(3):378-83.

DOBUTamine

CAS Number 49745-95-1

U.S. Brand Names Dobutrex®

Synonyms Dobutamine Hydrochloride

Use Short-term management of patients with cardiac decompensation; useful for hypotension induced by tricyclic antidepressants, beta-adrenergic blockers, doxazosin, calcium channel blockers, or sedative-hypnotic toxicity

Unlabeled/Investigational Use Positive inotropic agent for use in myocardial dysfunction of sepsis

Mechanism of Action Stimulates $beta_1$-adrenergic receptors, causing increased contractility and heart rate, with little effect on $beta_2$- or alpha-receptors

Adverse Reactions

Symptoms can occur for up to 2 hours

Cardiovascular: **Ectopic beats, chest pain, angina,** tachycardia, fibrillation (atrial), hypertension, **palpitations, elevated blood pressure;** in higher doses, **tachycardia (ventricular)** or **cardiac arrhythmias** may be seen; patients with fibrillation (atrial) or flutter (atrial) are at risk of developing a rapid ventricular response; syncope, sinus tachycardia, arrhythmias (ventricular)

Central nervous system: Headache, fever, hyperthermia

Endocrine & metabolic: Hypokalemia

Gastrointestinal: Nausea, vomiting

Genitourinary: Urinary incontinence

Hematologic: Coagulopathy, platelet inhibition

Local: Extravasation injury

Neuromuscular & skeletal: Leg cramps (mild), neuropathy (peripheral), paresthesia, tingling sensation

Respiratory: Dyspnea, tachypnea

Signs and Symptoms of Overdose Fatigue, nervousness

Pharmacodynamics/Kinetics

Onset of action: I.V.: 1-10 minutes

Peak effect: 10-20 minutes

Metabolism: In tissues and hepatically to inactive metabolites

Half-life elimination: 2 minutes

Excretion: Urine (as metabolites)

Dosage

I.V. infusion:

Neonates and Children: 2.5-15 mcg/kg/minute, titrate to desired response

Adults: 2.5-15 mcg/kg/minute; maximum: 40 mcg/kg/minute, titrate to desired response. See table.

Dobutamine

Creatinine Clearance (mL/min)	Dosage Interval
30-40	q8h
15-30	q12h
<15	q24h

Maximum I.V. dose: 40 mcg/kg/minute

Maximum survivable dose on record: 130 mcg/kg/minute for 30 minutes. See table.

Infusion Rates of Various Dilutions of Dobutamine

Desired Delivery Rate (mcg/kg/min)	Infusion Rate (mL/kg/min)	
	500 mcg/mL*	1000 mcg/mL†
2.5	0.005	0.0025
5.0	0.01	0.005
7.5	0.015	0.0075
10.0	0.02	0.01
12.5	0.025	0.0125
15.0	0.03	0.015

*500 mg per liter or 250 mg per 500 mL of diluent.

†1000 mg per liter or 250 mg per 250 mL of diluent.

Stability Remix solution every 24 hours; incompatible with sodium bicarbonate solutions; store reconstituted solution under refrigeration for 48 hours or 6 hours at room temperature; pink discoloration of solution indicates slight oxidation but **no** significant loss of potency

Monitoring Parameters Blood pressure, ECG, heart rate, CVP, RAP, MAP, urine output; if pulmonary artery catheter is in place, monitor CI, PCWP, and SVR; also monitor serum potassium

Administration Use infusion device to control rate of flow; administer into large vein. Do not administer through same I.V. line as heparin, hydrocortisone sodium succinate, cefazolin, or penicillin.

To prepare for infusion:

$$\frac{6 \times \text{weight (Kg)} \times \text{desired dose (mcg/kg/min)}}{\text{I.V. infusion rate (mL/h)}} = \frac{\text{mg drug to be added to}}{\text{10 mL of I.V.fluid}}$$

Contraindications Hypersensitivity to dobutamine or sulfites (some contain sodium metabisulfate), or any component of the formulation; idiopathic hypertrophic subaortic stenosis (IHSS)

Warnings May increase heart rate. Patients with atrial fibrillation may experience an increase in ventricular response. An increase in blood pressure is more common, but occasionally a patient may become hypotensive. May exacerbate ventricular ectopy. If needed, correct hypovolemia first to optimize hemodynamics. Ineffective in the presence of mechanical obstruction such as severe aortic stenosis. Use caution post-MI (can increase myocardial oxygen demand). Use cautiously in the elderly starting at lower end of the dosage range.

Dosage Forms

Infusion, as hydrochloride [premixed in dextrose]: 1 mg/mL (250 mL, 500 mL); 2 mg/mL (250 mL); 4 mg/mL (250 mL)

Injection, solution, as hydrochloride: 12.5 mg/mL (20 mL, 40 mL, 100 mL) [contains sodium bisulfite]

Test Interactions Dobutamine (and to a lesser extent dopamine) can cause profound negative interference with the enzymatic method for serum creatinine determination, producing a false depression of serum creatinine

Drug Interactions

Beta-blockers (nonselective ones) may increase hypertensive effect; avoid concurrent use.

Cocaine may cause malignant arrhythmias; avoid concurrent use.

Guanethidine can increase the pressor response; be aware of the patient's drug regimen.

MAO inhibitors potentiate hypertension and hypertensive crisis; avoid concurrent use.

Methyldopa can increase the pressor response; be aware of patient's drug regimen.

Reserpine increases the pressor response; be aware of patient's drug regimen.

TCAs increase the pressor response; be aware of patient's drug regimen.

Pregnancy Risk Factor B

Pregnancy Implications B

Lactation Excretion in breast milk unknown

Nursing Implications

Alkaline solutions (sodium bicarbonate); do not give through same I.V. line as heparin, hydrocortisone sodium succinate, cefazolin, or penicillin; administer into large vein; use infusion device to control rate of flow

982

Extravasation: Use phentolamine as antidote; mix 5 mg with 9 mL of normal saline; inject a small amount of this dilution into extravasated area; blanching should reverse immediately. Monitor site; if blanching should recur, additional injections of phentolamine may be needed.

DOPamine

Pronunciation (DOE pa meen)
CAS Number 51-61-6; 62-31-7
Synonyms Dopamine Hydrochloride; Intropin
Use Adjunct in the treatment of shock which persists after adequate fluid volume replacement; dose-related inotropic and vasopressor effects; stimulates dopaminergic, beta- and alpha-receptors
Unlabeled/Investigational Use Symptomatic bradycardia or heart block unresponsive to atropine or pacing
Mechanism of Action Stimulates both adrenergic and dopaminergic receptors, lower doses are mainly dopaminergic stimulating and produces renal and mesenteric vasodilation, higher doses also are both dopaminergic and beta$_1$-adrenergic and produces cardiac stimulation and renal vasodilation, large doses stimulate alpha-adrenergic receptors. A metabolic precursor to norepinephrine.
Adverse Reactions
Cardiovascular: **Ectopic heartbeats, tachycardia, vasoconstriction, hypotension, cardiac conduction abnormalities, widened QRS complex**, bradycardia, hypertension, **arrhythmias (ventricular)**, gangrene of the extremities (with high doses for prolonged periods or even with low doses in patients with occlusive vascular disease), **palpitations**, facial flushing, fibrillation (atrial), flutter (atrial), sinus bradycardia, pulmonary hypertension, sinus tachycardia, tachycardia (supraventricular)
Central nervous system: Anxiety, **headache**, dizziness,
Endocrine & metabolic: Hypoprolactinemia
Gastrointestinal: **Nausea, vomiting**, decreased esophageal sphincter tone
Genitourinary: Decreased urine output
Local: Extravasation injury
Neuromuscular & skeletal: Piloerection
Ocular: Mydriasis
Renal: Azotemia
Respiratory: **Dyspnea**
Signs and Symptoms of Overdose Fixed and dilated pupils, tachycardia, severe hypertension
Pharmacodynamics/Kinetics
Children: Dopamine has exhibited nonlinear kinetics in children; with medication changes, may not achieve steady-state for ~1 hour rather than 20 minutes
Onset of action: Adults: 5 minutes
Duration: Adults: <10 minutes
Metabolism: Renal, hepatic, plasma; 75% to inactive metabolites by monoamine oxidase and 25% to norepinephrine
Half-life elimination: 2 minutes
Excretion: Urine (as metabolites)
Clearance: Neonates: Varies and appears to be age related; clearance is more prolonged with combined hepatic and renal dysfunction
Dosage
I.V. infusion:
Neonates: 1-20 mcg/kg/minute continuous infusion, titrate to desired response
Children: 1-20 mcg/kg/minute, maximum: 50 mcg/kg/minute continuous infusion, titrate to desired response
Adults: 1-5 mcg/kg/minute up to 50 mcg/kg/minute, titrate to desired response; infusion may be increased by 1-4 mcg/kg/minute at 10- to 30-minute intervals until optimal response is obtained
If dosages >20-30 mcg/kg/minute are needed, a more direct-acting pressor may be more beneficial (ie, epinephrine, norepinephrine)
The hemodynamic effects of dopamine are dose-dependent:
Low-dose: 1-5 mcg/kg/minute, increased renal blood flow and urine output
Intermediate-dose: 5-15 mcg/kg/minute, increased renal blood flow, heart rate, cardiac contractility, and cardiac output
High-dose: >15 mcg/kg/minute, alpha-adrenergic effects begin to predominate, vasoconstriction, increased blood pressure
Stability Protect from light; solutions that are darker than slightly yellow should not be used; incompatible with alkaline solutions or iron salts; compatible when coadministered with dobutamine, epinephrine, isoproterenol, and lidocaine
Monitoring Parameters Blood pressure, ECG, heart rate, CVP, RAP, MAP, urine output; if pulmonary artery catheter is in place, monitor CI, PCWP, SVR, and PVR
Administration
Administer into large vein to prevent the possibility of extravasation; use infusion device to control rate of flow; due to short half-life, withdrawal of the drug is often the only necessary treatment

Extravasation: Use phentolamine as antidote; mix 5 mg with 9 mL of normal saline; inject a small amount of this dilution into extravasated area; blanching should reverse immediately. Monitor site; if blanching should recur, additional injections of phentolamine may be needed.
Contraindications Hypersensitivity to sulfites (commercial preparation contains sodium bisulfite); pheochromocytoma; ventricular fibrillation
Warnings Use with caution in patients with cardiovascular disease or cardiac arrhythmias or patients with occlusive vascular disease. Correct hypovolemia and electrolytes when used in hemodynamic support. May cause increases in HR and arrhythmia. Avoid infiltration - may cause severe tissue necrosis. Use with caution in post-MI patients.
Dosage Forms
Infusion, as hydrochloride [premixed in D$_5$W]: 0.8 mg/mL (250 mL, 500 mL); 1.6 mg/mL (250 mL, 500 mL); 3.2 mg/mL (250 mL)
Injection, solution, as hydrochloride: 40 mg/mL (5 mL, 10 mL); 80 mg/mL (5 mL); 160 mg/mL (5 mL) [contains sodium metabisulfite]
Test Interactions Dobutamine (and to a lesser extent dopamine) can cause profound negative interference with the enzymatic method for serum creatinine determination, producing a false depression of serum creatinine; may interfere with TSH assay resulting in falsely low TSH levels
Drug Interactions
Beta-blockers (nonselective ones) may increase hypertensive effect; avoid concurrent use.
Cocaine may cause malignant arrhythmias; avoid concurrent use.
Guanethidine's hypotensive effects may only be partially reversed; may need to use a direct-acting sympathomimetic.
MAO inhibitors potentiate hypertension and hypertensive crisis; avoid concurrent use.
Methyldopa can increase the pressor response; be aware of patient's drug regimen.
Reserpine increases the pressor response; be aware of patient's drug regimen.
TCAs increase the pressor response; be aware of patient's drug regimen.
Pregnancy Risk Factor C
Pregnancy Implications Not known if it crosses the placenta
Lactation Excretion in breast milk unknown
Nursing Implications
Monitor continuously for free flow
Extravasation: Use phentolamine as antidote; mix 5 mg with 9 mL of normal saline; inject a small amount of this dilution into extravasated area; blanching should reverse immediately. Monitor site; if blanching should recur, additional injections of phentolamine may be needed. If phentolamine is not available, topical nitroglycerin paste or subcutaneous administration of terbutaline (at a 1:1 to 1:10 dilution) may be effective alternative treatment.
Specific References
Friedrich JO, Adhikari N, Herridge MS, et al, "Meta-Analysis: Low-Dose Dopamine Increases Urine Output But Does Not Prevent Renal Dysfunction or Death," *Ann Intern Med*, 2005, 142(7):510-24 (review).
Holmes CL and Walley KR, "Bad Medicine: Low-Dose Dopamine in the ICU," *Chest*, 2003, 123(4):1266-75.

Edetate Calcium Disodium

Pronunciation (ED e tate KAL see um dye SOW dee um)
CAS Number 23411-34-9; 62-33-9
U.S. Brand Names Calcium Disodium Versenate®
Synonyms CaEDTA ; Calcium Disodium Edetate; Calcium EDTA; EDTA (Calcium Disodium)
Use Treatment of acute and chronic lead, manganese, scandium, lanthanum, plutonium, or zinc poisoning; may aid in the diagnosis of lead poisoning
Unlabeled/Investigational Use
Investigational: Cholelitholytic agent (through biliary duct infusion) for pigment bile duct stones
Mechanism of Action Calcium is displaced by divalent and trivalent heavy metals, forming a nonionizing soluble complex that is excreted in urine.
Adverse Reactions
Cardiovascular: Hypotension, arrhythmias, ECG changes
Central nervous system: Fever, headache, chills
Dermatologic: Skin lesions, cheilosis
Endocrine & metabolic: Hypercalcemia, zinc deficiency
Gastrointestinal: GI upset, anorexia, nausea, vomiting
Hematologic: Transient marrow suppression, anemia
Hepatic: Mild increase in liver function test results
Local: Pain at injection site following I.M. injection, thrombophlebitis following I.V. infusion (at concentration >5 mg/mL)
Neuromuscular & skeletal: Arthralgia, tremor, numbness, paresthesia
Ocular: Lacrimation
Renal: Renal tubular necrosis, proteinuria, microscopic hematuria
Respiratory: Sneezing, nasal congestion
Miscellaneous: Zinc depletion

Pharmacodynamics/Kinetics
Onset of action: Chelation of lead: I.V.: 1 hour
Absorption: I.M., SubQ: Well absorbed
Distribution: Into extracellular fluid; minimal CSF penetration
Half-life elimination, plasma: I.M.: 1.5 hours; I.V.: 20 minutes
Excretion: Urine (as metal chelates or unchanged drug); decreased GFR decreases elimination

Dosage
Several regimens have been recommended:
Diagnosis of lead poisoning: Mobilization test (not recommended by AAP guidelines): I.M., I.V.:
Children: 500 mg/m^2/dose, (maximum dose: 1 g) as a single dose or divided into 2 doses
Adults: 500 mg/m^2/dose
Treatment of lead poisoning: Children and Adults (each regimen is specific for route):
Symptoms of lead encephalopathy and/or blood lead level >70 mcg/dL: Treat 5 days; give first dose after, then given in conjunction with dimercaprol; wait a minimum of 2 days with no treatment before considering a repeat course:
I.M.: 250 mg/m^2/dose every 4 hours
I.V.: 50 mg/kg/day as 24-hour continuous I.V. infusion **or** 1-1.5 g/m^2 I.V. as either an 8- to 24-hour infusion or divided into 2 doses every 12 hours
Symptomatic lead poisoning **without** encephalopathy **or** asymptomatic with blood lead level >70 mcg/dL: Treat 3-5 days; treatment with dimercaprol is recommended until the blood lead level concentration <50 mcg/dL:
I.M.: 167 mg/m^2 every 4 hours
I.V.: 1 g/m^2 as an 8- to 24-hour infusion or divided every 12 hours
Asymptomatic **children** with blood lead level 45-69 mcg/dL: I.V.: 25 mg/kg/day for 5 days as an 8- to 24-hour infusion or divided into 2 doses every 12 hours
Depending upon the blood lead level, additional courses may be necessary; repeat at least 2-4 days and preferably 2-4 weeks apart
Adults with lead nephropathy: An alternative dosing regimen reflecting the reduction in renal clearance is based upon the serum creatinine. Refer to the following:
Dose of Ca EDTA based on serum creatinine:
S_{cr} ≤2 mg/dL: 1 g/m^2/day for 5 days*
S_{cr} 2-3 mg/dL: 500 mg/m^2/day for 5 days*
S_{cr} 3-4 mg/dL: 500 mg/m^2/dose every 48 hours for 3 doses*
S_{cr} >4 mg/dL: 500 mg/m^2/week*
*Repeat these regimens monthly until lead excretion is reduced toward normal.

Stability Dilute with 0.9% sodium chloride or D$_5$W; physically **incompatible** with D$_{10}$W, lactated Ringer's, Ringer's

Monitoring Parameters BUN, creatinine, urinalysis, I & O, and ECG during therapy; intravenous administration requires a cardiac monitor, blood and urine lead concentrations

Administration For intermittent I.V. infusion, administer the dose I.V. over at least 1 hour in asymptomatic patients, 2 hours in symptomatic patients; for I.V. continuous infusion, dilute to 2-4 mg/mL in D$_5$W or normal saline and infuse over at least 8 hours, usually over 12-24 hours; for I.M. injection, 1 mL of 1% procaine hydrochloride may be added to each mL of EDTA calcium to minimize pain at injection site

Contraindications Severe renal disease, anuria

Warnings
[U.S. Boxed Warning]: Use with extreme caution in patients with lead encephalopathy and cerebral edema. In these patients, I.V. infusion has been associated with lethal increase in intracranial pressure; I.M. injection is preferred.
Edetate calcium disodium is potentially nephrotoxic; renal tubular acidosis and fatal nephrosis may occur, especially with high doses; ECG changes may occur during therapy; do not exceed recommended daily dose. If anuria, increasing proteinuria, or hematuria occurs during therapy, discontinue calcium EDTA. Minimize nephrotoxicity by adequate hydration, establishment of good urine output, avoidance of excessive doses, and limitation of continuous administration to ≤5 days.
Exercise caution in the ordering, dispensing, and administration of this EDTA product. Edetate calcium disodium (CaEDTA) may be confused with edetate disodium (Na$_2$EDTA). CDC recommends that edetate disodium should never be used for chelation therapy in children. Fatal hypocalcemia may result if edetate disodium is used for chelation therapy instead of edetate calcium disodium.

Dosage Forms Injection, solution: 200 mg/mL (5 mL)

Test Interactions If calcium EDTA is given as a continuous I.V. infusion, stop the infusion for at least 1 hour before blood is drawn for lead concentration, to avoid a falsely elevated value.

Drug Interactions Decreased effect: Do not use simultaneously with zinc insulin preparations; do not mix in the same syringe with dimercaprol

Pregnancy Risk Factor B

Edetate Disodium

Pronunciation (ED e tate dye SOW dee um)
CAS Number 139-33-3; 150-38-9; 6381-92-6
U.S. Brand Names Endrate®
Synonyms Edathamil Disodium; EDTA (Disodium); Na2EDTA ; Sodium Edetate
Use Emergency treatment of hypercalcemia; also used as contact lens cleaner; also used as a 0.05 molar topical solution for alkali ocular exposure due to calcium hydroxide (lime) from motor or cement exposures; also chelates lead, copper, manganese, zinc, lanthanum, plutonium, scandium, or yttrium; useful in treating extravasation due to mithramycin
Mechanism of Action Chelates with divalent or trivalent metals to form a soluble complex that is then eliminated in urine

Adverse Reactions
Cardiovascular: Arrhythmias, transient hypotension, shock, vasculitis, pericardial effusion/pericarditis
Central nervous system: Seizures, fever, headache, chills
Dermatologic: Skin eruptions, exfoliative dermatitis, dermatitis, skin lesions
Endocrine & metabolic: Hypocalcemic tetany, hypomagnesemia, hypokalemia
Gastrointestinal: Nausea, vomiting, abdominal cramps, diarrhea
Genitourinary: Urinary frequency
Hematologic: Anemia
Local: Pain at the site of injection, thrombophlebitis
Neuromuscular & skeletal: Back pain, muscle cramps, paresthesia, myalgia, leg cramps
Renal: Nephrotoxicity, acute tubular necrosis
Respiratory: Death from respiratory arrest, respiratory failure, sneezing
Miscellaneous: Yawning

Pharmacodynamics/Kinetics
Metabolism: None
Half-life elimination: 20-60 minutes
Time to peak: I.V.: 24-48 hours
Excretion: Following chelation: Urine (95%); chelates within 24-48 hours

Dosage
Hypercalcemia: I.V.:
Children: 40-70 mg/kg/day slow infusion over 3-4 hours or more to a maximum of 3 g/24 hours; administer for 5 days and allow 5 days between courses of therapy
Adults: 50 mg/kg/day over 3 or more hours to a maximum of 3 g/24 hours; a suggested regimen of 5 days followed by 2 days without drug and repeated courses up to 15 total doses
Mithramycin extravasation: 150 mg of sodium edetate either through offending I.V. catheter of through multiple SubQ injections; apply ice to affected area

Monitoring Parameters Cardiac function (ECG monitoring); blood pressure during infusion; renal function should be assessed before and during therapy; monitor calcium, magnesium, and potassium levels; cardiac monitor required

Administration Must be diluted before use in 500 mL D$_5$W or normal saline to <30 mg/mL

Contraindications Severe renal failure or anuria

Warnings
Use of this drug is recommended only when the severity of the clinical condition justifies the aggressive measures associated with this type of therapy. Use with caution in patients with renal dysfunction, intracranial lesions, seizure disorders, coronary or peripheral vascular disease.
Exercise caution in the ordering, dispensing, and administration of this EDTA product. Edetate disodium (Na$_2$EDTA) may be confused with edetate calcium disodium (CaEDTA). CDC recommends that edetate disodium should never be used for chelation therapy in children. Fatal hypocalcemia may result if edetate disodium is used for chelation therapy instead of edetate calcium disodium.

Dosage Forms Injection, solution: 150 mg/mL (20 mL)
Drug Interactions Increased effect of insulin (edetate disodium may decrease blood glucose concentrations and reduce insulin requirements in diabetic patients treated with insulin)
Pregnancy Risk Factor C
Nursing Implications Avoid extravasation; patient should remain supine for a short period after infusion

Epinephrine

Pronunciation (ep i NEF rin)
Related Information
● Insect Sting Kit [ANTIDOTE]
CAS Number 51-43-4
U.S. Brand Names Adrenalin®; Epifrin®; EpiPen® Jr; EpiPen®; Primatene® Mist [OTC]
Synonyms Adrenaline; Epinephrine Bitartrate; Epinephrine Hydrochloride; Racepinephrine

Use Bronchospasms, anaphylactic reactions, bradycardia, cardiac arrest, management of open-angle (chronic simple) glaucoma, hypotension, allergic reactions to antivenin, specifically improved mortality secondary to chloroquine overdose

Unlabeled/Investigational Use ACLS guidelines: Ventricular fibrillation (VF) or pulseless ventricular tachycardia (VT) unresponsive to initial defibrillatory shocks; pulseless electrical activity, asystole, hypotension unresponsive to volume resuscitation; symptomatic bradycardia or hypotension unresponsive to atropine or pacing; inotropic support

Mechanism of Action Stimulates alpha-adrenergic, β_1- and β_2-adrenergic receptors; small doses can causes vasodilation via β_2 vascular receptors; decreases production of aqueous humor and increases aqueous outflow; dilates the pupil by contracting the dilator muscle

Adverse Reactions

Cardiovascular: Pallor, **tachycardia**, hypertension, increased myocardial oxygen consumption, cardiac arrhythmias, sudden death, chest pain, superior mesenteric artery thrombosis, shock, ventricular arrhythmias, cardiomyopathy, cardiomegaly, angina, palpitations, sinus tachycardia, tachycardia (supraventricular), tachycardia (ventricular, bidirectional), vasoconstriction, **pounding heartbeat**

Central nervous system: Anxiety, headache, sympathetic storm, **nervousness, restlessness**

Dermatologic: Exfoliative dermatitis, alopecia, urticaria, exanthem

Endocrine & metabolic: Lactic acidosis, hyperglycemia, hypophosphatemia, hyperkalemia, hypokalemia

Gastrointestinal: Nausea, intestinal ischemia, xerostomia

Genitourinary: Acute urinary retention in patients with bladder outflow obstruction

Local: Tissue ischemia and necrosis with extravasation

Neuromuscular & skeletal: Weakness

Ocular: Precipitation of or exacerbation of narrow-angle glaucoma, vision color changes (green tinge)

Renal: Decreased renal and splanchnic blood flow

Miscellaneous: Allergic reactions, fixed drug eruption

Signs and Symptoms of Overdose Cardiac arrhythmias, hyperglycemia, hypertension (which may result in subarachnoid hemorrhage and hemiplegia), metabolic acidosis, pulmonary edema, renal failure, tachycardia (ventricular, bidirectional), unusually large pupils

Pharmacodynamics/Kinetics

Onset of action: Bronchodilation: SubQ: ~5-10 minutes; Inhalation: ~1 minute

Distribution: Crosses placenta

Metabolism: Taken up into the adrenergic neuron and metabolized by monoamine oxidase and catechol-o-methyltransferase; circulating drug hepatically metabolized

Excretion: Urine (as inactive metabolites, metanephrine, and sulfate and hydroxy derivatives of mandelic acid, small amounts as unchanged drug)

Dosage

Neonates: Cardiac arrest: I.V.: 0.01-0.03 mg/kg (0.1-0.3 mL/kg of **1:10,000** solution) every 3-5 minutes as needed. Although I.V. route is preferred, may consider administration of doses up to 0.1 mg/kg through the endotracheal tube until I.V. access established; dilute intratracheal doses to 1-2 mL with normal saline.

Infants and Children:

Asystole/pulseless arrest, bradycardia, VT/VF (after failed defibrillations):

I.V., I.O.: 0.01 mg/kg (0.1 mL/kg of **1:10,000** solution) every 3-5 minutes as needed (maximum: 1 mg)

Intratracheal: 0.1 mg/kg (0.1 mL/kg of **1:1000** solution) every 3-5 minutes (maximum: 10 mg)

Continuous I.V. infusion: 0.1-1 mcg/kg/; doses <0.3 mcg/kg/minute generally produce β-adrenergic effects and higher doses generally produce α-adrenergic vasoconstriction; titrate dosage to desired effect

Bronchodilator: SubQ: 0.01 mg/kg (0.01 mL/kg of **1:1000**) (single doses not to exceed 0.5 mg) every 20 minutes for 3 doses

Nebulization: 1-3 inhalations up to every 3 hours using solution prepared with 10 drops of 1:100

Children <4 years: S2® (racepinephrine, OTC labeling): Croup: 0.05 mL/kg (max 0.5 mL/dose); dilute in NS 3 mL. Administer over ~15 minutes; do not administer more frequently than every 2 hours.

Inhalation: Children ≥4 years: Primatene® Mist: Refer to Adults dosing.

Decongestant: Children ≥6 years: Refer to Adults dosing

Hypersensitivity reaction:

SubQ, I.V.: 0.01 mg/kg every 20 minutes; larger doses or continuous infusion may be needed for some anaphylactic reactions

SubQ, I.M.:

15-30 kg: Twinject™: 0.15 mg (for self-administration following severe allergic reactions to insect stings, food, etc)

>30 kg: Refer to Adults dosing

I.M.:

<30 kg: Epipen® Jr: 0.15 mg (for self-administration following severe allergic reactions to insect stings, food, etc)

>30 kg: Refer to Adults dosing

Adults:

Asystole/pulseless arrest, bradycardia, VT/VF:

I.V., I.O.: 1 mg every 3-5 minutes; if this approach fails, higher doses of epinephrine (up to 0.2 mg/kg) may be indicated for treatment of specific problems (eg, beta-blocker or calcium channel blocker overdose)

Intratracheal: Administer 2-2.5 mg for VF or pulseless VT if I.V./I.O. access is delayed or cannot be established; dilute in 5-10 mL NS or distilled water. **Note:** Absorption is greater with distilled water, but causes more adverse effects on PaO_2.

Bradycardia (symptomatic) or hypotension (not responsive to atropine or pacing): I.V. infusion: 2-10 mcg/minute; titrate to desired effect

Bronchodilator:

SubQ: 0.3-0.5 mg **(1:1000)** every 20 minutes for 3 doses

Nebulization: 1-3 inhalations up to every 3 hours using solution prepared with 10 drops of the **1:100** product

S2® (racepinephrine, OTC labeling): 0.5 mL (~10 drops). Dose may be repeated not more frequently than very 3-4 hours if needed. Solution should be diluted if using jet nebulizer.

Inhalation: Primatene® Mist (OTC labeling): One inhalation, wait at least 1 minute; if relieved, may use once more. Do not use again for at least 3 hours.

Decongestant: Intranasal: Apply 1:1000 locally as drops or spray or with sterile swab

Hypersensitivity reaction:

I.M., SubQ: 0.3-0.5 mg (1:1000) every 15-20 minutes if condition requires (I.M route is preferred)

>30 kg: Twinject™: 0.3 mg (for self-administration following severe allergic reactions to insect stings, food, etc)

I.M.: >30 kg: Epipen®: 0.3 mg (for self-administration following severe allergic reactions to insect stings, food, etc)

I.V.: 0.1 mg (1:10,000) over 5 minutes. May infuse at 1-4 mcg/minute to prevent the need to repeat injections frequently.

Stability Protect from light, oxidation turns drug pink, then a brown color; solutions should not be used if they are discolored or contain a precipitate; stability of injection of parenteral admixture at room temperature and refrigeration: 24 hours; unstable in alkaline solution; do not use D_5W as a diluent; D_5W is incompatible with epinephrine

Monitoring Parameters Pulmonary function, heart rate, blood pressure, site of infusion for blanching, extravasation; cardiac monitor and blood pressure monitor required

Administration Central line administration only; intravenous infusions require an infusion pump

Endotracheal: Doses (2-2.5 times the I.V. dose) should be diluted to 10 mL with NS or distilled water prior to administration

Epinephrine can be administered SubQ, I.M., I.V., or intracardiac injection I.M. administration into the buttocks should be avoided

Preparation of adult I.V. infusion: Dilute 1 mg in 250 mL of D_5W or NS (4 mcg/mL); administer at an initial rate of 1 mcg/minute and increase to desired effects; at 20 mcg/minute pure alpha effects occur

1 mcg/minute: 15 mL/hour

2 mcg/minute: 30 mL/hour

3 mcg/minute: 45 mL/hour, etc

Extravasation management:

Initial care:

Treatment of digital epinephrine autoinjector injuries is primarily supportive.

Warm soaks and warm compresses are the mainstay of treatment.

If symptoms persist or worsen after 1-2 hours of conservative management, consider using an antidotal therapy.

Antidotal therapy:

Phentolamine: Mix 5 mg with 9 mL of NS. Inject a small amount of this dilution into extravasated area using a 24- to 27 gauge needle. Blanching should reverse immediately. Monitor site. If blanching should recur, additional injections of phentolamine may be needed (not to exceed a total volume of 10 mL).

Terbutaline: Create a 1 mg/mL solution of terbutaline to normal saline (1:1 dilution). Use a 24- to 27-gauge needle to inject the terbutaline subcutaneously in affected area; response is usually immediate; repeat as necessary.

Nitroglycerin paste: Apply paste to affected portion of the digit until clinical improvement is noted.

Disposition of extravasation:

Most patients who present with digital injections of an epinephrine autoinjector have a mild and self-limited clinical course. If an antidotal therapy is used, observation for ~1 hour is recommended. If the presentation has worsened or not improved during that time, consider repeating the initial therapy or trying an alternate treatment modality.

Contraindications Hypersensitivity to epinephrine or any component of the formulation; cardiac arrhythmias; angle-closure glaucoma

Warnings Use with caution in elderly patients, patients with diabetes mellitus, cardiovascular diseases (angina, tachycardia, myocardial infarction), thyroid disease, or cerebral arteriosclerosis, Parkinson's; some products contain sulfites as preservatives. Rapid I.V. infusion may cause death from cerebrovascular hemorrhage or cardiac arrhythmias. Oral inhalation of epinephrine is **not** the preferred route of administration. Avoid topical application where reduced perfusion could lead to ischemic tissue damage (eg, penis, ears, digits).

Dosage Forms
Aerosol for oral inhalation:
  Primatene® Mist: 0.22 mg/inhalation (15 mL, 22.5 mL) [contains CFCs]
Injection, solution [prefilled auto injector]:
  EpiPen®: 0.3 mg/0.3 mL [1:1000] (2 mL) [contains sodium metabisulfite; available as single unit or in double-unit pack with training unit]
  EpiPen® Jr: 0.15 mg/0.3 mL [1:2000] (2 mL) [contains sodium metabisulfite; available as single unit or in double-unit pack with training unit]
  Twinject™: 0.15 mg/0.15 mL [1:1000] (1.1 mL) [contains sodium bisulfite; two 0.15 mg doses per injector]; 0.3 mg/0.3 mL [1:1000] (1.1 mL) [contains sodium bisulfite; two 0.3 mg doses per injector]
Injection, solution, as hydrochloride: 0.1 mg/mL [1:10,000] (10 mL); 1 mg/mL [1:1000] (1 mL) [products may contain sodium metabisulfite]
  Adrenalin®: 1 mg/mL [1:1000] (1 mL, 30 mL) [contains sodium bisulfite]
Solution for oral inhalation, as hydrochloride:
  Adrenalin®: 1% [10 mg/mL, 1:100] (7.5 mL) [contains sodium bisulfite]
Solution for oral inhalation [racepinephrine]:
  S2®: 2.25% (0.5 mL, 15 mL) [as d-epinephrine 1.125% and l-epinephrine 1.125%; contains metabisulfites]
Solution, topical [racepinephrine]:
  Raphon: 2.25% (15 mL) [as d-epinephrine 1.125% and l-epinephrine 1.125%; contains metabisulfites]

Reference Range Therapeutic: 31-95 pg/mL (SI: 170-520 pmol/L); norepinephrine level of 438 pg/mL associated with myocardial ischemia in children

Test Interactions ↑ bilirubin (S), catecholamines (U), glucose, uric acid (S)

Drug Interactions Increased toxicity: Increased cardiac irritability if administered concurrently with halogenated inhalational anesthetics, beta-blocking agents, alpha-blocking agents

Pregnancy Risk Factor C

Pregnancy Implications Crosses the placenta

Lactation Excretion in breast milk unknown

Nursing Implications
Protect from light; oxidation turns dark pink, then brown - solutions should not be used if they are discolored or contain a precipitate. Epinephrine is unstable in alkaline solution.
Extravasation: Use phentolamine as antidote; mix 5 mg with 9 mL of normal saline; inject a small amount of this dilution into extravasated area; blanching should reverse immediately. Monitor site; if blanching should recur, additional injections of phentolamine may be needed. If phentolamine is not available, topical nitroglycerin paste or subcutaneous administration of terbutaline (at a 1:1 to 1:10 dilution) may be effective alternative treatment.

Specific References
Anchor J and Settipane RA, "Appropriate Use of Epinephrine in Anaphylaxis," *Am J Emerg Med*, 2004, 22(6):488-90.
Bond GR, "Seizure, Dysrhythmia, and Cardiac Arrest Following I.V. Tetracaine/Epinephrine Solution in Two Neonates," *J Toxicol Clin Toxicol*, 2004, 42(5):744.
Hartling L, Wiebe N, Russell K, et al, "A Meta-Analysis of Randomized Controlled Trials Evaluating the Efficacy of Epinephrine for the Treatment of Acute Viral Bronchiolitis," *Arch Pediatr Adolesc Med*, 2003, 157(10):957-64.
Lin RY, Curry A, Pitsios VI, et al, "Cardiovascular Responses in Patients with Acute Allergic Reactions Treated with Parenteral Epinephrine," *Am J Emerg Med*, 2005, 23(3):266-72.
McIntyre CL, Sheetz AH, Carroll CR, et al, "Administration of Epinephrine for Life-Threatening Allergic Reactions in School Settings," *Pediatrics*, 2005, 116(5):1134-40.
Putland M, Kerr D, and Kelly AM, "Adverse Events Associated with the Use of Intravenous Epinephrine in Emergency Department Patients Presenting with Severe Asthma," *Ann Emerg Med*, 2006, 47(6):559-63.
Roberts D, Colbert R, Anderson S, et al, "Fatal Myositis Associated with Epinephrine Auto-Injector," *J Toxicol Clin Toxicol*, 2004, 42(5):733.
Silverberg M, Manoach S, "Accidental Self-Administration of Epinephrine with an Auto-Injector," *Clinical toxicology*, 2007, 45: 83-4.
Smith D, Riel J, Tilles I, et al, "Intravenous Epinephrine in Life-Threatening Asthma," *Ann Emerg Med*, 2003, 41(5):706-11.
Vecchio FL and VanTran T, "Allergic Reactions from Insect Bites," *AJEM*, 22(7):631.
Wyer PC, Perera P, Jin Z, et al, "Vasopressin or Epinephrine for Out-of-Hospital Cardiac Arrest," *Ann Emerg Med*, 2006, 48:86-97.

Filgrastim

U.S. Brand Names Neupogen®

Synonyms G-CSF; Granulocyte Colony Stimulating Factor

Use Stimulation of granulocyte production in patients with malignancies, including myeloid malignancies; receiving myelosuppressive therapy associated with a significant risk of neutropenia; severe chronic neutropenia (SCN); receiving bone marrow transplantation (BMT); undergoing peripheral blood progenitor cell (PBPC) collection useful for colchicine toxicity or radiation

Mechanism of Action Stimulates the production, maturation, and activation of neutrophils, G-CSF activates neutrophils to increase both their migration and cytotoxicity. See table.

Comparative Effects — G-CSF vs GM-CSF		
Proliferation/Differentiation	G-CSF (Filgrastim)	GM-CSF (Sargramostim)
Neutrophils	Yes	Yes
Eosinophils	No	Yes
Macrophages	No	Yes
Neutrophil migration	Enhanced	Inhibited

Adverse Reactions
Cardiovascular: Chest pain, transient arrhythmia (supraventricular), pericardial effusion/pericarditis, ventricular arrhythmias, angina, tachycardia (supraventricular)
Central nervous system: **Fever**, headache, **neutropenic fever**
Dermatologic: **Alopecia**, skin rash, neutrophilic dermatosis (Sweet's syndrome), exacerbation of acne, psoriasis, angioneurotic edema, cutaneous vasculitis
Endocrine & metabolic: Fluid retention, hypothyroidism
Gastrointestinal: **Nausea, vomiting, diarrhea**, anorexia, stomatitis, constipation, **mucositis, splenomegaly**, sore throat
Hematologic: Leukocytosis, thrombocytopenia
Local: Pain at injection site, thrombophlebitis
Neuromuscular & skeletal: **Skeletal pain**, weakness
Ocular: Iritis, photophobia
Renal: Renal vasculitis
Respiratory: Dyspnea, cough, eosinophilic pneumonia
Miscellaneous: Anaphylactic reaction, lymphoma

Pharmacodynamics/Kinetics
Onset of action: ~24 hours; plateaus in 3-5 days
Duration: ANC decreases by 50% within 2 days after discontinuing filgrastim; white counts return to the normal range in 4-7 days; peak plasma levels can be maintained for up to 12 hours
Absorption: SubQ: 100%
Distribution: V_d: 150 mL/kg; no evidence of drug accumulation over a 11- to 20-day period
Metabolism: Systemically degraded
Half-life elimination: 1.8-3.5 hours
Time to peak, serum: SubQ: 2-6 hours

Dosage
Refer to individual protocols.
Dosing, even in morbidly obese patients, should be based on actual body weight. Rounding doses to the nearest vial size often enhances patient convenience and reduces costs without compromising clinical response.
Myelosuppressive therapy: 5 mcg/kg/day - doses may be increased by 5 mcg/kg according to the duration and severity of the neutropenia.
Bone marrow transplantation: 5-10 mcg/kg/day - doses may be increased by 5 mcg/kg according to the duration and severity of neutropenia; recommended steps based on neutrophil response:
  When ANC >1000/mm³ for 3 consecutive days: Reduce filgrastim dose to 5 mcg/kg/day
  If ANC remains >1000/mm³ for 3 more consecutive days: Discontinue filgrastim
  If ANC decreases to <1000/mm³: Resume at 5 mcg/kg/day
  If ANC decreases <1000/mm³ during the 5 mcg/kg/day dose, increase filgrastim to 10 mcg/kg/day and follow the above steps
Peripheral blood progenitor cell (PBPC) collection: 10 mcg/kg/day **or** 5-8 mcg/kg twice daily in donors. The optimal timing and duration of growth factor stimulation has not been determined.
Severe chronic neutropenia:
  Congenital: 6 mcg/kg twice daily
  Idiopathic/cyclic: 5 mcg/kg/day
Colchicine overdose: Daily doses of 300 mg SubQ for 5 days has been used in adults
Not removed by hemodialysis

Stability
Store at 2°C to 8°C (36°F to 46°F); do not expose to freezing or dry ice. Prior to administration, filgrastim may be allowed to be at room

temperature for a maximum of 24 hours. It may be diluted in dextrose 5% in water to a concentration ≥15 mcg/mL for I.V. infusion administration. Minimum concentration is 15 mcg/mL; concentrations <15 mcg/mL require addition of albumin (1 mL of 5%) to the bag to prevent absorption. This diluted solution is stable for 7 days under refrigeration or at room temperature. **Filgrastim is incompatible with 0.9% sodium chloride (normal saline).**

Standard diluent: ≥375 mcg/25 mL D$_5$W

Monitoring Parameters CBC and platelet count should be obtained twice weekly. Leukocytosis (white blood cell counts ≥100,000/mm^3) has been observed in ~2% of patients receiving G-CSF at doses >5 mcg/kg/day. Monitor platelets and hematocrit regularly.

Administration

The UHC Colony-Stimulating Factors Expert Panel has made the following clinical and administrative recommendations:

Clinical:

Very few data are available to support the therapeutic interchangeability of G-CSF and GM-CSF. On the basis of the panel's clinical experience and in the absence of conclusive data, interchangeability is acceptable in limited situations, as indicated in the UHC CSF guidelines.

For most indications, an ANC of <500 × 10^6 cells/L can be recommended as a starting point for the initiation of therapy. Stopping CSF therapy is based on a biologic endpoint, and the panel felt that CSF therapy could be discontinued in most patients at an ANC ≥5000 × 10^6 cells/L, depending on the expected nadir of chemotherapy. Several panel members suggested an ANC endpoint to CSF therapy at 2000 × 10^6 cells/L.

Food and Drug Administration labeling recommends daily dosing of G-CSF at 5 mcg/kg, but panel members felt that doses as low as 2 mcg/kg might be effective for some indications. Daily doses of >10 mcg/kg were considered not appropriate for any chemotherapy regimens. Overall, CSF dosing on the basis of patient weight has not been well studied.

In general, patients should not receive CSFs with their first cycle of cancer chemotherapy. Patients who have previously demonstrated febrile neutropenia following chemotherapy or have had a previous positive response to CSF therapy following chemotherapy would be appropriate for CSF therapy.

Certain chemotherapeutic regimens may warrant CSF use for every patient. These clinical situations should be determined at each UHC member institution. Some examples cited by the panel include patients in the following categories: adult acute lymphocytic leukemia, induction therapy; previously radiated Hodgkin's disease; previous pelvic radiation; adjuvant breast cancer chemotherapy (to avoid any treatment delays caused by neutropenia); and AIDS lymphoma treatment with myelosuppressive chemotherapy.

Administrative:

CSF guidelines developed by an institution for inpatient use should apply to the outpatient setting

Several examples of strategies for CSF cost-containment were offered by the panel, including requiring blood count results prior to dispensing CSF doses; strictly enforced inpatient and outpatient use guidelines; institutional reimbursement precertification for CSF patients; accessing pharmaceutical company reimbursement assistance/indigent programs; forming biotechnology review committees; and dosing based on vial size, rather than on a mcg/kg basis, using the smallest clinically acceptable vial size

Contraindications Hypersensitivity to filgrastim, *E. coli*-derived proteins, or any component of the formulation

Warnings

Do not use filgrastim in the period 24 hours before to 24 hours after administration of cytotoxic chemotherapy because of the potential sensitivity of rapidly dividing myeloid cells to cytotoxic chemotherapy. Precaution should be exercised in the usage of filgrastim in any malignancy with myeloid characteristics. Filgrastim can potentially act as a growth factor for any tumor type, particularly myeloid malignancies. Tumors of nonhematopoietic origin may have surface receptors for filgrastim. Safety and efficacy have not been established with patients receiving radiation therapy, or with chemotherapy associated with delayed myelosuppression (eg, nitrosoureas, mitomycin C).

Allergic-type reactions have occurred with first or later doses. Reactions tended to occur more frequently with intravenous administration and within 30 minutes of infusion. Rare cases of splenic rupture or adult respiratory distress syndrome have been reported in association with filgrastim; patients must be instructed to report left upper quadrant pain or shoulder tip pain or respiratory distress. Use caution in patients with sickle cell diseases; sickle cell crises have been reported following filgrastim therapy.

Dosage Forms

Injection, solution [preservative free]: 300 mcg/mL (1 mL, 1.6 mL) [vial; contains sodium 0.035 mg/mL and sorbitol]

Injection, solution [preservative free]: 600 mcg/mL (0.5 mL, 0.8 mL) [prefilled Singleject® syringe; contains sodium 0.035 mg/mL and sorbitol]

Reference Range Peak plasma level as high as 600 ng/mL achieved after I.V. doses of 3-60 mcg/kg

Test Interactions ↑ uric acid, lactate dehydrogenase, alkaline phosphatase; may ↓ cholesterol

Pregnancy Risk Factor C

Pregnancy Implications Animal studies have demonstrated adverse effects and fetal loss. Filgrastim has been shown to cross the placenta in humans. There are no adequate and well-controlled studies in pregnant women. Use only if potential benefit to mother justifies risk to the fetus.

Lactation Excretion in breast milk unknown/use caution

Nursing Implications Do not mix with sodium chloride solutions

---

Flumazenil

CAS Number 78755-81-4

U.S. Brand Names Romazicon®

Use Benzodiazepine antagonist - reverses sedative effects of benzodiazepines used in general anesthesia; for management of benzodiazepine or zolpidem overdose; flumazenil does **not** antagonize the CNS effects of other GABA agonists (such as ethanol, barbiturates, or general anesthetics), **does not** reverse narcotics; may be useful for baclofen, carbamazepine, chloral hydrate, and zopiclone overdoses; chlorzoxazone overdose; gabapentin-induced coma; may be used to reverse paradoxical reactions to benzodiazepines in children; possible antidotal effect by flumazenil in zaleplon-induced coma and bluish-green urine; has been reported to reverse antihistamine-induced coma

Mechanism of Action Antagonizes the effect of benzodiazepines on the GABA/benzodiazepine receptor complex, including synergistic effects with the other GABA agonists.

Adverse Reactions

Cardiovascular: Cardiac arrhythmias, bradycardia, tachycardia, chest pain, hypertension, extrasystoles (ventricular), altered blood pressure (increases and decreases), AV block, sinus bradycardia, angina, sinus tachycardia, arrhythmias (ventricular), junctional tachycardia, ventricular tachycardia

Central nervous system: Convulsions (more common in patients with tricyclic antidepressant overdoses), fatigue, **dizziness/vertigo**, amnesia, delirium, dysphoria, fear, headache, agitation, emotional lability, anxiety, nervousness, malaise, abnormal crying, euphoria, CNS depression, somnolence

Endocrine & metabolic: Hot flashes

Gastrointestinal: **Nausea, vomiting**, xerostomia

Local: Pain at injection site

Neuromuscular & skeletal: Tremors, weakness

Ocular: Blurred vision, vision disorders

Otic: Abnormal hearing

Respiratory: Dyspnea, hyperventilation

Miscellaneous: Withdrawal syndrome, hiccups, diaphoresis (increased), cold sensation, shivering

Pharmacodynamics/Kinetics

Onset of action: 1-3 minutes; 80% response within 3 minutes
Peak effect: 6-10 minutes

Duration: Resedation: ~1 hour; duration related to dose given and benzodiazepine plasma concentrations; reversal effects of flumazenil may wear off before effects of benzodiazepine

Distribution: Initial V$_d$: 0.5 L/kg; V$_{dss}$ 0.77-1.6 L/kg

Protein binding: 40% to 50%

Metabolism: Hepatic; dependent upon hepatic blood flow

Half-life elimination: Adults: Alpha: 7-15 minutes; Terminal: 41-79 minutes

Excretion: Feces; urine (0.2% as unchanged drug)

Dosage

Children and Adults: I.V.: See table.

Flumazenil	
Pediatric Dosage (further studies needed)	
Pediatric dosage for **reversal of conscious sedation and general anesthesia:**	
Initial dose	0.01 mg/kg over 15 seconds (maximum: 0.2 mg)
Repeat doses (maximum: 4 doses)	0.005-0.01 mg/kg (maximum: 0.2 mg) repeated at 1-minute intervals
Maximum total cumulative dose	1 mg or 0.05 mg/kg (whichever is lower)
Adult Dosage	
Adult dosage for **reversal of conscious sedation and general anesthesia:**	
Initial dose	0.2 mg intravenously over 15 seconds

Table (Continued)

Adult Dosage	
Repeat doses	If desired level of consciousness is not obtained, 0.2 mg may be repeated at 1-minute intervals.
Maximum total cumulative dose	1 mg (usual dose: 0.6-1 mg) **In the event of resedation:** Repeat doses may be given at 20-minute intervals with maximum of 1 mg/dose and 3 mg/hour.
Adult dosage for **suspected benzodiazepine overdose:**	
Initial dose	0.2 mg intravenously over 30 seconds; if the desired level of consciousness is not obtained, 0.3 mg can be given over 30 seconds
Repeat doses	0.5 mg over 30 seconds repeated at 1-minute intervals
Maximum total cumulative dose	3 mg (usual dose 1-3 mg) Patients with a partial response at 3 mg may require additional titration up to a total dose of 5 mg. If a patient has not responded 5 minutes after cumulative dose of 5 mg, the major cause of sedation is not likely due to benzodiazepines. **In the event of resedation:** May repeat doses at 20-minute intervals with maximum of 1 mg/dose and 3 mg/hour.

Resedation: Repeated doses may be given at 20-minute intervals as needed; repeat treatment doses of 1 mg (at a rate of 0.5 mg/minute) should be given at any time and no more than 3 mg should be given in any hour. After intoxication with high doses of benzodiazepines, the duration of a single dose of flumazenil is not expected to exceed 1 hour; if desired, the period of wakefulness may be prolonged with repeated low intravenous doses of flumazenil, or by an infusion of 0.1-0.4 mg/hour. Most patients with benzodiazepine overdose will respond to a cumulative dose of 1-3 mg and doses >3 mg do not reliably produce additional effects. Rarely, patients with a partial response at 3 mg may require additional titration up to a total dose of 5 mg. **If a patient has not responded 5 minutes after receiving a cumulative dose of 5 mg, the major cause of sedation is not likely to be due to benzodiazepines.**

Elderly: No differences in safety or efficacy have been reported. However, increased sensitivity may occur in some elderly patients.

Dosing in renal impairment: Not significantly affected by renal failure ($Cl_{cr} < 10$ mL/minute) or hemodialysis beginning 1 hour after drug administration

Dosing in hepatic impairment: Initial dose of flumazenil used for initial reversal of benzodiazepine effects is not changed; however, subsequent doses in liver disease patients should be reduced in size or frequency

Stability Store at 15°C to 30°C (59°F to 86°F). For I.V. use only; **compatible** with D_5W, lactated Ringer's, or normal saline; once drawn up in the syringe or mixed with solution use within 24 hours; discard any unused solution after 24 hours

Monitoring Parameters Monitor patients for return of sedation or respiratory depression

Administration I.V.: Administer in freely-running I.V. into large vein. Inject over 15 seconds for conscious sedation and general anesthesia and over 30 seconds for overdose.

Contraindications Hypersensitivity to flumazenil, benzodiazepines, or any component of the formulation; patients given benzodiazepines for control of potentially life-threatening conditions (eg, control of intracranial pressure or status epilepticus); patients who are showing signs of serious cyclic-antidepressant overdosage

Warnings [U.S. Boxed Warning]: Benzodiazepine reversal may result in seizures in some patients. Patients who may develop seizures include patients on benzodiazepines for long-term sedation, tricyclic antidepressant overdose patients, concurrent major sedative-hypnotic drug withdrawal, recent therapy with repeated doses of parenteral benzodiazepines, myoclonic jerking or seizure activity prior to flumazenil administration. Flumazenil does not reverse respiratory depression/hypoventilation or cardiac depression. Resedation occurs more frequently in patients where a large single dose or cumulative dose of a benzodiazepine is administered along with a neuromuscular blocking agent and multiple anesthetic agents. Flumazenil should be used with caution in the intensive care unit because of increased risk of unrecognized benzodiazepine dependence in such settings. Should not be used to diagnose benzodiazepine-induced sedation. Reverse neuromuscular blockade before considering use. Flumazenil does not antagonize the CNS effects of other GABA agonists (such as ethanol, barbiturates, or general anesthetics); nor does it reverse narcotics. Use with caution in patients with a history of panic disorder; may provoke panic attacks. Use caution in drug and ethanol-dependent patients; these patients may also be dependent on benzodiazepines. Not recommended for treatment of benzodiazepine dependence. Use with caution in head injury patients. Use caution in patients with mixed drug overdoses; toxic effects of other drugs taken may emerge once benzodiazepine effects are reversed. Flumazenil does not consistently reverse amnesia; patient may not recall verbal instructions after procedure. Use caution in severe hepatic dysfunction and in patients relying on a benzodiazepine for seizure control. Safety and efficacy have not been established in children >1 year of age.

Dosage Forms Injection, solution: 0.1 mg/mL (5 mL, 10 mL) [contains edetate sodium]

Reference Range Plasma flumazenil levels between 10-20 mcg/L for 1-2 hours reverse benzodiazepine-induced CNS depression; average peak flumazenil blood level of 66 ng/mL achieved within 1 minute of administering 1 mg of flumazenil endotracheally

Drug Interactions Nonbenzodiazepine hypnotics (zaleplon, zolpidem, zopiclone): Flumazenil reverses the effects of these hypnotics.

Pregnancy Risk Factor C

Pregnancy Implications Teratogenic effects were not seen in animal studies. Embryocidal effects were seen at large doses. There are no adequate or well-controlled studies in pregnant women. Use only if clearly needed.

Lactation Excretion in breast milk unknown/use caution

Nursing Implications Parenteral: For I.V. use only; administer via freely running I.V. infusion into larger vein to decrease chance of pain, phlebitis

Specific References

Butler TC, Rosen RM, Wallace AL, et al, "Flumazenil and Dialysis for Gabapentin-Induced Coma," *Ann Pharmacother*, 2003, 37(1):74-6.

Kent DA, Elko CJ, Gibson J, et al, "Use of Flumazenil for Lorazepam-Induced Paradoxical Reactions in Children," *J Toxicol Clin Toxicol*, 2003, 41(5):666.

Lassaletta A, Martino R, Gonzalez-Santiago P, et al, "Reversal of an Antihistamine-Induced Coma with Flumazenil," *Pediatr Emerg Care*, 2004, 20(5):319-20.

Ondo WG and Hunter C, "Flumazenil, a GABA Antagonist, May Improve Features of Parkinson's Disease," *Mov Disord*, 2003, 18(6):683-5.

Satz WA, Lee DC, Greene T, et al, "Does Flumazenil Prolong GHB Poisoning?" *J Toxicol Clin Toxicol*, 2003, 41(5):747.

Seger DL, "Flumazenil - Treatment or Toxin?" *J Toxicol Clin Toxicol*, 2004, 42(2):209-16.

Folic Acid

Pronunciation (FOE lik AS id)

CAS Number 59-30-3; 6484-89-5

Synonyms Folacin; Folate; Pteroylglutamic Acid

Use Treatment of megaloblastic and macrocytic anemias due to folate deficiency; used in methanol toxicity, methotrexate toxicity, chronic alcoholism

Mechanism of Action Necessary for normal erythropoiesis

Adverse Reactions

Central nervous system: Irritability, difficulty sleeping, confusion, insomnia, hyperthermia, fever

Dermatologic: Pruritus

Gastrointestinal: GI upset, bitter taste, flatulence

Miscellaneous: Hypersensitivity reactions, anaphylactic shock, zinc depletion, anaphylaxis

Pharmacodynamics/Kinetics

Onset of effect: Peak effect: Oral: 0.5-1 hour

Absorption: Proximal part of small intestine

Dosage

Oral, I.M., I.V., SubQ:

Minimal daily requirement: 50 mcg; pregnant/critically ill: 100-200 mcg

Infants: 0.1 mg/day

Children: Initial: 1 mg/day

Deficiency: 0.5-1 mg/day

Maintenance dose:

<4 years: Up to 0.3 mg/day

>4 years: 0.4 mg/day

Adults: Initial: 1 mg/day

Deficiency: 1-3 mg/day

Maintenance dose: 0.5 mg/day

Pregnant and lactating women: 0.8 mg/day

Stability Incompatible with oxidizing and reducing agents and heavy metal ions

Monitoring Parameters Hemoglobin

Administration Oral, but may also be administered by deep I.M., SubQ, or I.V. injection; a diluted solution for oral or for parenteral administration may be prepared by diluting 1 mL of folic acid injection (5 mg/mL), with 49 mL sterile water for injection; resulting solution is 0.1 mg folic acid/1 mL

Contraindications Hypersensitivity to folic acid or any component of the formulation

Warnings Not appropriate for monotherapy with pernicious, aplastic, or normocytic anemias when anemia is present with vitamin D deficiency. Doses >0.1 mg/day may obscure pernicious anemia with continuing irreversible nerve damage progression. Resistance to treatment may occur with depressed hematopoiesis, alcoholism, deficiencies of other vitamins. Injection contains benzyl alcohol (1.5%) as preservative (use care in administration to neonates).

Dosage Forms
Injection, solution, as sodium folate: 5 mg/mL (10 mL) [contains benzyl alcohol]
Tablet: 0.4 mg, 0.8 mg, 1 mg

Reference Range Therapeutic: 0.005-0.015 mcg/mL

Test Interactions Falsely low serum concentrations may occur with the *Lactobacillus casei* assay method in patients on anti-infective (ie, tetracycline) therapy

Drug Interactions
Phenytoin: Folic acid may decrease phenytoin concentrations
Raltitrexed: Folic acid may diminish the therapeutic effect of raltitrexed

Pregnancy Risk Factor A/C (dose exceeding RDA recommendation)

Pregnancy Implications 400 mcg/day needed to prevent neural tube defects (spina bifida)

Lactation Enters breast milk/compatible

Nursing Implications Oral, but may also be administered by deep I.M., SubQ, or I.V. injection; a diluted solution for oral or for parenteral administration may be prepared by diluting 1 mL of folic acid injection (5 mg/mL), with 49 mL sterile water for injection; resulting solution is 0.1 mg folic acid per 1 mL

Fomepizole

Pronunciation (foe ME pi zole)

CAS Number 7554-65-6

U.S. Brand Names Antizol®

Synonyms 4-Methylpyrazole; 4-MP

Use FDA approved for ethylene glycol and methanol toxicity

Unlabeled/Investigational Use Known or suspected propylene glycol toxicity

Mechanism of Action Complexes and inactivates alcohol dehydrogenase competitively, thus preventing formation of the toxic metabolites of the alcohols

Adverse Reactions
Central nervous system: **Headache**, dizziness
Dermatologic: Rash
Gastrointestinal: **Dose-related nausea**, metallic taste
Hematologic: Eosinophilia
Hepatic: Transient increases in liver transaminases (possibly due to underlying ingestion)
Ocular: Nystagmus, vertical nystagmus

Pharmacodynamics/Kinetics
Onset of effect: Peak effect: Maximum: 1.5-2 hours
Absorption: Oral: Readily absorbed
Distribution: V_d: 0.6-1.02 L/kg; rapidly into total body water
Protein binding: Negligible
Metabolism: Hepatic to 4-carboxypyrazole (80% to 85% of dose), 4-hydroxymethylpyrazole, and their N-glucuronide conjugates; following multiple doses, induces its own metabolism via CYP oxidases after 30-40 hours
Half-life elimination: Has not been calculated; varies with dose
Excretion: Urine (1% to 3.5% as unchanged drug and metabolites)

Dosage
Oral: 15 mg/kg followed by 5 mg/kg in 12 hours and then 10 mg/kg every 12 hours until levels of toxin are not present
One other protocol (from France) suggests an infusion of 10-20 mg/kg before dialysis and intravenous infusion of 1-1.5 mg/kg/hour during hemodialysis
Loading dose of 15 mg/kg I.V. followed by 10 mg/kg I.V. every 12 hours for 48 hours, then 15 mg/kg every 12 hours until methanol or ethylene glycol levels are <20 mg/dL; supplemental doses required during dialysis
Dosing in patients requiring hemodialysis:
Dose at the beginning of hemodialysis. If <6 hours since last dose, do not administer dose; if ≥6 hours since last dose, administer next scheduled dose.
Dosing during hemodialysis: every 4 hours
Dosing at the time hemodialysis is **completed**:
Time between last dose and the end of hemodialysis:
<1 hour: Do not administer dose at the end of hemodialysis
1-3 hours: Administer $1/2$ of next scheduled dose
>3 hours: Administer next scheduled dose
Maintenance dosing **off** hemodialysis: Give next scheduled dose 12 hours from last dose administered

Stability Store vials at room temperature. Antizol® diluted in 0.9% sodium chloride injection or 5% dextrose injection is stable for at least 48 hours when stored refrigerated or at room temperature. After dilution, do not use beyond 24 hours.

Monitoring Parameters Fomepizole plasma levels should be monitored; response to fomepizole; monitor plasma/urinary ethylene glycol or methanol levels, urinary oxalate (ethylene glycol), plasma/urinary osmolality, renal/hepatic function, serum electrolytes, arterial blood gases; anion and osmolar gaps, resolution of clinical signs and symptoms of ethylene glycol or methanol intoxication

Administration Antizol® solidifies at temperatures <25°C (<77°F). If the Antizol® solution has become solid in the vial, the solution should be liquefied by running the vial under warm water or by holding in the hand. Solidification does not affect the efficacy, safety, or stability of Antizol®. Using sterile technique, the appropriate dose of Antizol® should be drawn from the vial with a syringe and injected into at least 100 mL of sterile 0.9% sodium chloride injection or dextrose 5% injection. Mix well. The entire contents of the resulting solution should be infused over 30 minutes. Antizol®, like all parenteral products, should be inspected visually for particulate matter prior to administration, whenever solution and container permit.

Contraindications Documented serious hypersensitivity reaction to fomepizole or other pyrazoles; hypersensitivity to any component of the formulation

Warnings Should not be given undiluted or by bolus injection; fomepizole is metabolized in the liver and excreted in the urine, use caution with hepatic or renal impairment; hemodialysis should be used in patients with renal failure, significant or worsening metabolic acidosis, or ethylene glycol/methanol levels ≥50 mg/dL; monitor and manage adverse events of intoxication (respiratory distress syndrome, visual disturbances, hypocalcemia); safety and efficacy in pediatric patients have not been established

Dosage Forms Injection, solution [preservative free]: 1 g/mL (1.5 mL)

Reference Range Serum fomepizole concentrations >15 mg/L provide complete inhibition of alcohol dehydrogenase

Pregnancy Risk Factor C

Pregnancy Implications Reproduction studies have not been conducted; use in pregnant women only if the benefits clearly outweigh the risks.

Lactation Excretion in breast milk unknown/not recommended

Specific References
Gracia R, Guo C, and McMartin K, "Fomepizole Concentrations in Rat Fetal Tissue," *J Toxicol Clin Toxicol*, 2004, 42(5):714.
Gracia R, Latimer B, Guo C, et al, "Determination of Fomepizole Concentrations in Tissue," *J Toxicol Clin Toxicol*, 2004, 42(5):751.
Hovda KE, Andersson KS, Urdal P, et al, "Methanol and Formate Kinetics During Treatment with Fomepizole," *Clin Toxicol (Phila)*, 2005, 43(4):221-7.
Kostic MA, Heard K, Palmer RB, et al, "A Pilot Study of Fomepizole for the Treatment of Acute Diethylene Glycol Poisoning," *J Toxicol Clin Toxicol*, 2004, 42(5):713.
Marraffa JM, Stork CM, Howland MA, et al, "Pharmacokinetics of Intravenous (IV) Fomepizole Versus Oral (PO) Fomepizole in Healthy Human Volunteers: Preliminary Results," *J Toxicol Clin Toxicol*, 2004, 42(5):747.
Marraffa JM, Stork CM, and Medicis JJ, "Cost-Effectiveness of Fomepizole Versus Ethanol in the Management of Acute Ethylene Glycol Exposure," *Clin Toxicol (Phila)*, 2005, 43:691.
Mycyk MB, DesLauriers C, Metz J, et al, "Compliance with Poison Center Fomepizole Recommendations is Suboptimal in Cases of Toxic Alcohol Poisoning," *Am J Therapeutics*, 2006, 13:485-9.
Mycyk MB, Willis B, Mazor S, et al, "Fomepizole Use Is Often Suboptimal in Cases of Toxic Alcohol Poisoning," *Ann Emerg Med*, 2004, 44:S89.
Quang LS, Sandasivan S, and Maher TJ, "4-MP Blocks 1,4-BD Neuroprotection in Rodent Stroke," *J Toxicol Clin Toxicol*, 2004, 42(5):755-6.
Ries NL, Dart RC. "New Developments in Antidotes," *Med Clin North Am*, 2005, 89(6):1379-97 (review).
Wallemacq PE, Vanbinst R, Haufroid V, et al, "Plasma and Tissue Determination of 4-Methylpyrazole for Pharmacokinetic Analysis in Acute Adult and Pediatric Methanol/Ethylene Glycol Poisoning," *Ther Drug Monit*, 2004, 26(3):258-62.

Glucagon

Pronunciation (GLOO ka gon)

CAS Number 16941-32-5

U.S. Brand Names GlucaGen® Diagnostic Kit; GlucaGen®; Glucagon Diagnostic Kit; Glucagon Emergency Kit

Synonyms Glucagon Hydrochloride

Use
Hypoglycemia; diagnostic aid in the radiologic examination of GI tract when a hypotonic state is needed; useful in esophageal food impaction, cardiogenic shock
Investigational: Nebulized for asthma

Unlabeled/Investigational Use Used with some success as a cardiac stimulant in management of severe cases of beta-adrenergic or calcium channel blocking agent, calcium channel blocker, or oral hypoglycemia overdosage; may be useful in treating hypotension due to imipramine toxicity; noninsulin-dependent diabetes mellitus; also used in allergic reactions

Mechanism of Action Stimulates adenylate cyclase to produce increased cyclic AMP, which promotes hepatic glycogenolysis and gluconeogenesis, causing a raise in blood glucose levels

Adverse Reactions

Frequency not defined.

Cardiovascular: Hypotension (up to 2 hours after GI procedures), hypertension, tachycardia

Gastrointestinal: Nausea, vomiting (high incidence with rapid administration of high doses)

Miscellaneous: Hypersensitivity reactions, anaphylaxis

Signs and Symptoms of Overdose Allergic reactions, dizziness, hyperglycemia, hypertension, hypokalemia, hypotension, nausea, weakness, vomiting

Pharmacodynamics/Kinetics

Onset of action: Peak effect: Blood glucose levels: Parenteral:

I.V.: 5-20 minutes

I.M.: 30 minutes

SubQ: 30-45 minutes

Duration: Hyperglycemia: 60-90 minutes

Metabolism: Primarily hepatic; some inactivation occurring renally and in plasma

Half-life elimination, plasma: 3-10 minutes

Dosage

Allergic reactions: I.V.:

Children: 0.03-0.1 mg/kg/dose up to 1 mg; repeat every 5-20 minutes

Adults: 1 mg; repeat every 5 minutes; can give up to 5 mg/dose; for infusion, can titrate at a rate of 1-5 mg/hour

Hypoglycemia or insulin shock therapy: I.M., I.V., SubQ:

Neonates: 0.3 mg/kg/dose; maximum: 1 mg/dose

Children: 0.025-0.1 mg/kg/dose, not to exceed 1 mg/dose, repeated in 20 minutes as needed

Adults: 0.5-1 mg, may repeat in 20 minutes as needed

Cardiotoxic agent toxicity: I.V.: 0.05 mg/kg (up to 10 mg) over 1 minute, then continuous infusion of 2-5 mg/hour in 5% dextrose

Diagnostic aid: Adults: I.M., I.V.: 0.25-2 mg 10 minutes prior to procedure

Facilitate passage of foreign bodies from distal esophagus into stomach: I.V.: 0.5-1 mg over 30 seconds, may be repeated

Nebulized for asthma: 2 mg diluted in 3 mL of saline

Stability Prior to reconstitution, store at controlled room temperature of 20°C to 25° (69°F to 77°F); do not freeze. Reconstitute powder for injection by adding 1 mL of sterile diluent to a vial containing 1 unit of the drug, to provide solutions containing 1 mg of glucagon/mL. Gently roll vial to dissolve. If dose to be administered is <2 mg of the drug, then use only the diluent provided by the manufacturer. If >2 mg, use sterile water for injection. Use immediately after reconstitution. May be kept at 5°C for up to 48 hours if necessary.

Monitoring Parameters Blood pressure, blood glucose, heart rate

Administration I.V.: Bolus may be associated with nausea and vomiting. Continuous infusions may be used in beta-blocker overdose/toxicity.

Contraindications Hypersensitivity to glucagon or any component of the formulation; insulinoma; pheochromocytoma

Warnings Use caution with prolonged fasting, starvation, adrenal insufficiency or chronic hypoglycemia; levels of glucose stores in liver may be decreased. Following response to therapy, oral carbohydrates should be administered to prevent hypoglycemia.

Dosage Forms

Injection, powder for reconstitution, as hydrochloride:

GlucaGen® 1 mg [equivalent to 1 unit; contains lactose 107 mg]

GlucaGen® Diagnostic Kit: 1 mg [equivalent to 1 unit; contains lactose 107 mg; packaged with sterile water]

GlucaGen® HypoKit™: 1 mg [equivalent to 1 unit; contains lactose 107 mg; packaged with prefilled syringe containing sterile water]

Glucagon®: 1 mg [equivalent to 1 unit; contains lactose 49 mg]

Glucagon Diagnostic Kit, Glucagon Emergency Kit: 1 mg [equivalent to 1 unit; contains lactose 49 mg; packaged with diluent syringe containing glycerin 12 mg/mL and water for injection]

Reference Range Normal range: 50-60 pg/mL

Drug Interactions Oral anticoagulant: Hypoprothrombinemic effects may be increased possibly with bleeding; effect seen with glucagon doses of 50 mg administered over 1-2 days

Pregnancy Risk Factor B

Lactation Excretion in breast milk unknown/compatible

Specific References

Bailey B, "Glucagon in Beta-Blocker and Calcium Channel Blocker Overdoses: A Systematic Review," *J Toxicol Clin Toxicol*, 2003, 41(5):595-602.

Holger JS, Engebretsen KM, Obetz CL, et al, "A Comparison of Vasopressin and Glucagon in Beta-Blocker Induced Toxicity," *Clin Toxicol (Phila)*, 2006, 44(1):45-51.

Wax PM, Erdman AR, Chyka PA, et al, "Beta-Blocker Ingestion: An Evidence-Based Consensus Guideline for Out-of-Hospital Management," *Clin Toxicol (Phila)*, 2005, 43(3):131-46.

Glycopyrrolate

Pronunciation (glye koe PYE roe late)

U.S. Brand Names Robinul® Forte; Robinul®

Synonyms Glycopyrronium Bromide

Use Vagal-mediated bradycardia, gastric secretion reduction; also used as a adjunct to relieve GI tract spasms, as an antisialagogue agent, adjunct in anesthesia, to reverse effects of nondepolarizing muscle relaxants

Unlabeled/Investigational Use

Investigational: Asthma

May be helpful in treating organophosphate poisoning; gustatory sweating (Frey syndrome)

Mechanism of Action Quaternary ammonium anticholinergic agent 5 times as potent as atropine with fewer cardiovascular or CNS side effects

Adverse Reactions

Cardiovascular: Palpitations, tachycardia

Central nervous system: Headache, insomnia, dizziness, fever

Dermatologic: **Dry skin**

Gastrointestinal: **Xerostomia, dry throat, constipation**, loss of taste perception

Genitourinary: Impotence

Local: **Irritation at injection site**

Ocular: Mydriasis (after large doses)

Neuromuscular & skeletal: Weakness

Respiratory: **Dry nose**

Miscellaneous: **Diaphoresis (decreased)**

Pharmacodynamics/Kinetics

Onset of action: Oral: 50 minutes; I.M.: 15-30 minutes; I.V.: ~1 minute

Peak effect: Oral: ~1 hour; I.M.: 30-45 minutes

Duration: Vagal effect: 2-3 hours; Inhibition of salivation: Up to 7 hours; Anticholinergic: Oral: 8-12 hours

Absorption: Oral: Poor and erratic

Distribution: V_d: 0.2-0.62 L/kg

Metabolism: Hepatic (minimal)

Bioavailability: ~10%

Half-life elimination: Infants: 22-130 minutes; Children 19-99 minutes; Adults: ~30-75 minutes

Excretion: Urine (as unchanged drug, I.M.: 80%, I.V.: 85%); bile (as unchanged drug)

Dosage

Children:

Reduction of secretions (preanesthetic):

Oral: 40-100 mcg/kg/dose 3-4 times/day

I.M., I.V.: 4-10 mcg/kg/dose every 3-4 hours; maximum: 0.2 mg/dose or 0.8 mg/24 hours

Intraoperative: I.V.: 4 mcg/kg not to exceed 0.1 mg; repeat at 2- to 3-minute intervals as needed

Preoperative: I.M.:

<2 years: 4.4-8.8 mcg/kg 30-60 minutes before procedure

>2 years: 4.4 mcg/kg 30-60 minutes before procedure

Children and Adults: Reverse neuromuscular blockade: I.V.: 0.2 mg for each 1 mg of neostigmine or 5 mg of pyridostigmine administered or 5-15 mcg/kg glycopyrrolate with 25-70 mcg/kg of neostigmine or 0.1-0.3 mg/kg of pyridostigmine (agents usually administered simultaneously, but glycopyrrolate may be administered first if bradycardia is present)

Adults:

Reduction of secretions:

Intraoperative: I.V.: 0.1 mg repeated as needed at 2- to 3-minute intervals

Preoperative: I.M.: 4.4 mcg/kg 30-60 minutes before procedure

Peptic ulcer:

Oral: 1-2 mg 2-3 times/day

I.M., I.V.: 0.1-0.2 mg 3-4 times/day

Monitoring Parameters Heart rate; anticholinergic effects; bowel sounds

Administration For I.V. administration, glycopyrrolate may also be administered via the tubing of a running I.V. infusion of a compatible solution; may be administered in the same syringe with neostigmine or pyridostigmine.

Contraindications Hypersensitivity to glycopyrrolate or any component of the formulation; severe ulcerative colitis, toxic megacolon complicating ulcerative colitis, paralytic ileus, obstructive disease of GI tract, intestinal atony in the elderly or debilitated patient; unstable cardiovascular status in acute hemorrhage; narrow-angle glaucoma; acute hemorrhage; tachycardia; obstructive uropathy; myasthenia gravis

Warnings Use caution in elderly, patients with autonomic neuropathy, hepatic or renal disease, ulcerative colitis (may precipitate/aggravate toxic megacolon), hyperthyroidism, CAD, CHF, arrhythmias, tachycardia, BPH, or hiatal hernia with reflux. Use of anticholinergics in gastric ulcer treatment may cause a delay in gastric emptying due to antral statis. Caution should be used in individuals demonstrating decreased pigmentation (skin and iris coloration, dark versus light) since there has been some evidence that these individuals have an enhanced sensitivity to the anticholinergic response. May cause drowsiness, eye sensitivity to light, or blurred vision; caution should be used when performing tasks which require mental alertness, such as driving. The risk of heat stroke with this medication may be increased during exercise or hot weather. Infants, patients with Down syndrome, and children with spastic paralysis or brain damage may be hypersensitive to antimuscarine effects. Product packaging may contain latex. Injection contains benzyl alcohol (associated with gasping syndrome in neonates). Not recommended for use in children <12 years of age for the management of peptic ulcer or <16 years for preanesthetic use.

Dosage Forms
Injection, solution (Robinul®): 0.2 mg/mL (1 mL, 2 mL, 5 mL, 20 mL) [contains benzyl alcohol]
Tablet:
 Robinul®: 1 mg
 Robinul® Forte: 2 mg

Reference Range Peak plasma glycopyrrolate level was ~6.3 ng/mL 10 minutes after intramuscular injection of 6 mcg/kg

Drug Interactions
Anticholinergic agents: Effects of other anticholinergic agents or medications with anticholinergic activity may be increased by glycopyrrolate.
Potassium chloride: Severity of potassium chloride-induced gastrointestinal lesions (when potassium is given in a wax matrix formulation, eg, Klor-Con®) may be increased by glycopyrrolate.
Pramlinitide: May enhance the anticholinergic effects of anticholinergics. These effects are specific to the GI tract.

Pregnancy Risk Factor B

Pregnancy Implications No teratogenic effects; in normal doses (4 mcg/kg), does not appear to affect fetal heart rate

Lactation Excretion in breast milk unknown/use caution

Specific Reference
Sivilotti ML, Bird SB, Lo JC, et al, "Multiple Centrally-Acting Antidotes Protect Against Severe Organophosphate Toxicity," *Clin Toxicol (Phila)*, 2005, 43:693.

Hydroxocobalamin

Pronunciation (hye droks oh koe BAL a min)

U.S. Brand Names Cyanokit®

CAS Number 13422-52-1

Synonyms Vitamin B$_{12}$

Use Treatment of pernicious anemia, vitamin B$_{12}$ deficiency, increased B$_{12}$ requirements due to pregnancy, thyrotoxicosis, hemorrhage, malignancy, liver or kidney disease

Unlabeled/Investigational Use Neuropathies, multiple sclerosis

Mechanism of Action Coenzyme for various metabolic functions, including fat and carbohydrate metabolism and protein synthesis, used in cell replication and hematopoiesis. Also binds to cyanide ion preferentially than iron in cytochrome oxidase.

Adverse Reactions
Cardiovascular: Transient hypertension and tachycardia
Dermatologic: Itching, urticaria, erythema, pink discoloration to skin/mucous membranes (at doses >4 g, resolves in 1-2 days)
Endocrine & metabolic: Hypokalemia
Gastrointestinal: Diarrhea, feces discoloration (red), nausea
Genitourinary: Urine discoloration (pink/deep red)
Hematologic: Polycythemia
Local: Pain at injection site, erythema, rash
Respiratory: Pulmonary edema
Miscellaneous: Anaphylactoid reactions

Pharmacodynamics/Kinetics
Distribution: V$_d$: 0.2-0.3 L/kg
Half-life: 1.6-5.4 hours
Elimination: Renal (clearance: ~0.31 L/hour): Cyanide exposure: 37%; Normal subjects: 62%

Dosage
Vitamin B$_{12}$ deficiency: I.M.:
 Children: 1-5 mg given in single doses of 100 mcg over 2 or more weeks, followed by 30-50 mcg/month
 Adults: 30 mcg/day for 5-10 days, followed by 100-200 mcg/month
Cyanide toxicity starting dose is 5 grams in adults (two 2.5 gram vials) administered by intravenous infusion over 15 minutes. A second close of five grams I.V. may be given depending on the response and clinical situation. The recommended diluent is 0.9% sodium chloride

Administration Administer I.M. only; may require coadministration of folic acid

Contraindications None

Warnings Some products contain benzoyl alcohol; avoid use in premature infants; an intradermal test dose should be performed for hypersensitivity; use only if oral supplementation not possible or when treating pernicious anemia. Hypersensitivity to cyanocobalamin or any component of the formulation, cobalt; patients with hereditary optic nerve atrophy

Dosage Forms Substantial increases in blood pressure may occur

Reference Range Normal vitamin B$_{12}$ plasma level: 200-800 pg/mL; peak serum level after a 5 g dose: ~300 µmol/L

Test Interaction May result in artificial increases in serum creatinine, bilirubin, triglycerides, cholesterol, total protein, glucose, albumin, alkaline phosphatase, hemoglobin, basophils and urine pH. May artificially decrease ALT and anylase.

Drug Interactions Incompatable with diazepam, dobutamine, dopamine, fentanyl, nitroglycerin, pentoburbital, propofol and thiopental.

Pregnancy Risk Factor How supplied: 2.5 grams vials pregnancy category C

Lactation Enters breast milk/compatible

Nursing Implications Administer I.M. only; may require coadministration of folic acid

Additional Information Suspected adverse effects can be reported to Dey L.P. (800-429-7751) or FDA at 1-800-FDA-1088.

Specific References
DesLouriers CA, Burda AM, and Wahl M, "Hydroxocobalamin as a Cyanide Antidote," *Am J Ther*, 2006, 13:161-5.
Fortin WL, Waroux S, Ruttimann M, et al, "Hydroxocobalamin for Poisoning Caused by Ingestion of Potassium Cyanide: A Case Study," *Clin Toxicol (Phila)*, 2005, 43:731.
Weng TI, Fang CC, Lin SM, et al, "Elevated Plasma Cyanide Level After Hydroxocobalamin Infusion for Cyanide Poisoning," *Am J Emerg Med*, 2004, 22(6):492-3.

Insect Sting Kit

Pronunciation (ep i NEF rin & klor fen IR a meen)

U.S. Brand Names Ana-Kit®

Synonyms Insect Sting Kit

Use Anaphylaxis; emergency treatment of insect bites or stings (ie, yellow jacket, honeybee, hornet, wasp, deerfly, kissing bug) by the sensitive patient when self-treatment may occur within minutes of insect sting or exposure to an allergenic substance

Dosage
Children and Adults:
Epinephrine:
 <2 years: 0.05-0.1 mL
 2-6 years: 0.15 mL
 6-12 years: 0.2 mL
 >12 years : 0.3 mL
Chlorpheniramine:
 <6 years: 1 tablet
 6-12 years: 2 tablets
 >12 years: 4 tablets

Stability Protect from light, store at room temperature, prevent from freezing

Dosage Forms Kit: Epinephrine hydrochloride 1:1000 [prefilled syringe, delivers two 0.3 mL doses; contains sodium bisulfite] (1 mL), chlorpheniramine maleate chewable tablet 2 mg (4), sterile alcohol pads [isopropyl alcohol 70%] (2), tourniquet (1)

Antidote(s)
• Epinephrine [ANTIDOTE]

Drug Interactions
Chlorpheniramine: **Substrate** of CYP2D6 (minor), 3A4 (major); **Inhibits** CYP2D6 (weak)
Also see individual agents.

Pregnancy Implications Refer to Epinephrine monograph.

Nursing Implications Not intended for I.V. use (I.M. or SubQ only)

Ipecac Syrup

Pronunciation (IP e kak SIR up)

CAS Number 8012-96-2

Synonyms Syrup of Ipecac

Use Formerly used for the treatment of acute oral drug overdosage and in certain poisonings; now largely abandoned for routine use; potential value in treating cellular poisons without antidotes or supportive care options

Mechanism of Action Irritates the gastric mucosa and stimulates the medullary chemoreceptor trigger zone to induce vomiting

Adverse Reactions
Cardiovascular: Cardiotoxicity, tachycardia, heart block, congestive heart failure, pericardial effusion/pericarditis, hypotension, prolongation of QT interval, shock, flutter (atrial), cardiomegaly, myocardial depression, myocarditis, sinus tachycardia
Central nervous system: Lethargy, hypotonia
Dermatologic: Stevens-Johnson syndrome
Gastrointestinal: Protracted vomiting, diarrhea, gastric rupture, Mallory-Weiss tear, hemorrhagic colitis
Hepatic: Hepatomegaly, elevated liver enzymes
Neuromuscular & skeletal: Myopathy, myalgia, tremor
Respiratory: Pneumomediastinum

Signs and Symptoms of Overdose Cardiomyopathy, diarrhea, fibrillation (atrial), hypotension, persistent vomiting

Pharmacodynamics/Kinetics

Onset of action: 15-30 minutes

Duration: 20-25 minutes; 60 minutes in some cases

Absorption: Significant amounts, mainly when it does not produce emesis

Excretion: Urine; emetine (alkaloid component) may be detected in urine 60 days after excess dose or chronic use

Dosage

Oral:

Children:

6-12 months: 5-10 mL followed by 10-20 mL/kg of water; repeat dose one time if vomiting does not occur within 20 minutes

1-12 years: 15 mL followed by 10-20 mL/kg of water; repeat dose one time if vomiting does not occur within 20 minutes

Adults: 15-30 mL followed by 200-300 mL of water; repeat dose one time if vomiting does not occur within 20 minutes

Administration Do **not** administer to unconscious patients. Patients should be kept active and moving following administration of ipecac. If vomiting does not occur after second dose, gastric lavage may be considered to remove ingested substance.

Contraindications Hypersensitivity to ipecac or any component of the formulation; do not use in unconscious patients; patients with no gag reflex; following ingestion of strong bases, acids, or volatile oils; when seizures are likely

Warnings Do not confuse ipecac syrup with ipecac fluid extract, which is 14 times more potent; use with caution in patients with cardiovascular disease and bulimics; may not be effective in antiemetic overdose

Dosage Forms Syrup: 70 mg/mL (30 mL) [contains alcohol]

Reference Range Blood emetine level within hours of a 30 mL oral dose: 0-75 mcg/L

Drug Interactions

Decreased effect: Activated charcoal, milk, carbonated beverages

Increased toxicity: Phenothiazines (chlorpromazine has been associated with serious dystonic reactions)

Pregnancy Risk Factor C

Lactation Excretion in breast milk unknown/use caution

Nursing Implications Do **not** administer to unconscious patients; if vomiting does not occur after second dose, gastric lavage may be considered to remove ingested substance

Specific References

Garrison J, Shepherd G, Huddleston WL, et al, "Evaluation of the Time Frame for Home Ipecac Syrup Use When Not Kept in the Home," *J Toxicol Clin Toxicol* 2003, 41(3):217-21.

Manoguerra AS, Cobaugh DJ, Guidelines for the Management of Poisoning Consensus Panel, "Guideline on the Use of Ipecac Syrup in the Out-of-Hospital Management of Ingested Poisons," *Clin Toxicol (Phila)*, 2005, 43(1):1-10 (review).

"Position Paper: Ipecac Syrup," *J Toxicol Clin Toxicol*, 2004, 42(2):133-43 (review).

Isoproterenol

Pronunciation (eye soe proe TER e nole)

CAS Number 299-95-6; 51-30-9; 6700-39-6; 7683-59-2

U.S. Brand Names Isuprel®

Synonyms Isoproterenol Hydrochloride

Use Ventricular arrhythmias due to AV nodal block; hemodynamically compromised bradyarrhythmias or atropine- and dopamine-resistant bradyarrhythmias (when transcutaneous/venous pacing is not available); temporary use in third-degree AV block until pacemaker insertion

Unlabeled/Investigational Use Pharmacologic overdrive pacing for torsade de pointes; diagnostic aid (vasovagal syncope)

Mechanism of Action Relaxes bronchial smooth muscle by action on β_2-receptors; causes increased heart rate and contractility by action on β_1-receptors

Adverse Reactions

Cardiovascular: Premature ventricular beats, bradycardia, hypertension, hypotension, chest pain, palpitations, tachycardia, ventricular arrhythmias, myocardial infarction size increased

Central nervous system: Headache, nervousness, restlessness

Endocrine & metabolic: Serum glucose increased, serum potassium decreased, hypokalemia

Gastrointestinal: Nausea, vomiting

Respiratory: Dyspnea

Signs and Symptoms of Overdose Tachycardia, tremor, hypertension, hypotension, angina, and seizures. Hypokalemia also may occur. Cardiac arrest and death may be associated with abuse of beta-agonist bronchodilators.

Pharmacodynamics/Kinetics

Onset of action: Bronchodilation: I.V.: Immediate

Duration: I.V.: 10-15 minutes

Metabolism: Via conjugation in many tissues including hepatic and pulmonary

Half-life elimination: 2.5-5 minutes

Excretion: Urine (primarily as sulfate conjugates)

Dosage

I.V.: Cardiac arrhythmias:

Children: Initial: 0.1 mcg/kg/minute (usual effective dose 0.2-2 mcg/kg/minute)

Adults: Initial: 2 mcg/minute; titrate to patient response (2-10 mcg/minute)

Stability Do not use discolored solutions; limit exposure to heat, light or air; stability of parenteral admixture at room temperature (25°C) and at refrigeration temperature (4°C): 24 hours; **incompatible** when mixed with aminophylline, furosemide; **incompatible** with alkaline solutions

Monitoring Parameters ECG, heart rate, respiratory rate, arterial blood gas, arterial blood pressure, CVP; serum glucose, serum potassium, serum magnesium

Administration I.V. infusion administration requires the use of an infusion pump. To prepare infusion: See formula.

6 × weight (kg) × desired dose (mcg/kg/min)

I.V. infusion rate (mL/h) = mg of drug added to 100 mL I.V. fluid

Contraindications Hypersensitivity to sulfites or isoproterenol, any component of the formulation, or other sympathomimetic amines; angina, pre-existing cardiac arrhythmias (ventricular); tachycardia or AV block caused by cardiac glycoside intoxication

Warnings Use with extreme caution; not currently a treatment of choice; use with caution in elderly patients, diabetics, renal or cardiovascular disease, seizure disorder, or hyperthyroidism; excessive or prolonged use may result in decreased effectiveness.

Dosage Forms Injection, solution, as hydrochloride: 0.02 mg/mL (10 mL); 0.2 mg/mL (1:5000) (1 mL, 5 mL) [contains sodium metabisulfite]

Reference Range Peak plasma isoproterenol level of 0.0004 mg/L achieved after an I.V. injection of 0.063 mcg/kg postmortem level of 0.1 mg/L noted following a death in an asthmatic patient relatable to isoproterenol use

Overdosage/Treatment Treatment includes immediate discontinuation and symptomatic and supportive therapies. Cautious use of beta-adrenergic blocking agents may be considered in severe cases.

Drug Interactions Increased toxicity: Sympathomimetic agents may cause headaches and elevate blood pressure; general anesthetics may cause arrhythmias

Pregnancy Risk Factor C

Lactation Excretion in breast milk unknown

Nursing Implications Give around-the-clock to promote less variation in peak and trough serum levels

Leucovorin

CAS Number 1492-18-8; 41926-89-3; 58-05-9

Synonyms 5-Formyl Tetrahydrofolate; Calcium Leucovorin; Citrovorum Factor; Folinic Acid; Leucovorin Calcium

Use Antidote for folic acid antagonists (methotrexate, trimethoprim, pyrimethamine); treatment of megaloblastic anemias when folate is deficient as in infancy, sprue, pregnancy, and nutritional deficiency when oral folate therapy is not possible; in combination with fluorouracil in the treatment of colon cancer

Mechanism of Action Reduced form of folic acid, but does not require a reduction reaction by an enzyme for activation, allows for purine and thymidine synthesis, a necessity for normal erythropoiesis

Adverse Reactions

Frequency not defined.

Dermatologic: Rash, pruritus, erythema, urticaria

Hematologic: Thrombocytosis

Respiratory: Wheezing

Miscellaneous: Anaphylactoid reactions

Signs and Symptoms of Overdose ECG changes

Pharmacodynamics/Kinetics

Onset of action: Oral: ~30 minutes; I.V.: ~5 minutes

Absorption: Oral, I.M.: Rapid and well absorbed

Metabolism: Intestinal mucosa and hepatically to 5-methyl-tetrahydrofolate (5MTHF; active)

Bioavailability: 31% following 200 mg dose; 98% following doses ≤25 mg

Half-life elimination: Leucovorin: 15 minutes; 5MTHF: 33-35 minutes

Excretion: Urine (80% to 90%); feces (5% to 8%)

Dosage

Children and Adults:

Adjunctive therapy with antimicrobial agents (pyrimethamine): Oral: 2-15 mg/day for 3 days or until blood counts are normal or 5 mg every 3 days; doses of 6 mg/day are needed for patients with platelet counts <100,000/mm³

Rescue dose: I.V.: 10 mg/m² to start, then 10 mg/m² every 6 hours orally for 72 hours; if serum creatinine 24 hours after methotrexate is elevated 50% or more **or** the serum MTX concentration is $>5 \times 10^{-6}$ M, increase dose to 100 mg/m^2/dose every 3 hours until serum methotrexate level is $< 1 \times 10^{-8}$ M. See graph.

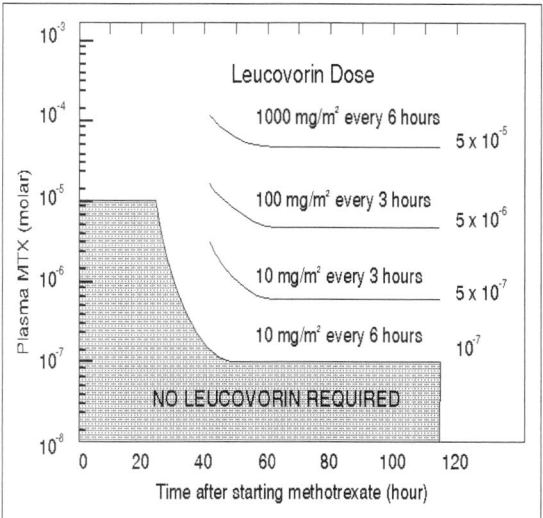

Investigational: Post I.T. methotrexate: Oral, I.V.: 12 mg/m^2 as a single dose; post high-dose methotrexate: 100-1000 mg/m^2/dose until the serum methotrexate level is $< 1 \times 10^{-7}$ M; with 5FU: Oral: 500 mg/m^2/day divided into 4 doses for 5 days

Methanol poisoning: 1 mg/kg; may repeat in 4 hours; further therapy should be with folic acid (secondary to cost and availability)

Plasma MTX concentration as a therapeutic guide to high-dose MTX therapy with leucovorin factor rescue. Leucovorin is continued until the plasma MTX level is $< 1 \times 10^{-7}$ M. Each dose of leucovorin is increased if the plasma MTX concentration is excessively high, according to the guidelines. With 4- to 6-hour high-dose MTX infusions, plasma drug values $> 5 \times 10^{-5}$ and 10^{-6} M at 24 and 48 hours after starting the infusion, respectively, are often predictive of delayed MTX clearance. See graph.

The drug should be given parenterally instead of orally in patients with GI toxicity, nausea, vomiting, and when individual doses are > 25 mg.

Stability Store at room temperature; protect from light. Leucovorin should be reconstituted with SWFI, bacteriostatic NS, BWFI, NS, or D$_5$W. Reconstituted solution is chemically stable for 7 days; reconstitutions with bacteriostatic water for injection, U.S.P., must be used within 7 days. Parenteral admixture is stable for 24 hours stored at room temperature (25°C) and for 4 days when stored under refrigeration (4°C).

Monitoring Parameters

Plasma methotrexate concentration as a therapeutic guide to high-dose methotrexate therapy with leucovorin factor rescue. Leucovorin is continued until the plasma methotrexate level < 0.05 μmol/mL.

With 4- to 6-hour high-dose methotrexate infusions, plasma drug values in excess of 50 and 1 μmol at 24 and 48 hours after starting the infusion, respectively, are often predictive of delayed methotrexate clearance

Administration Refer to individual protocols. Leucovorin should not be administered concurrently with methotrexate. It is commonly initiated 24 hours after the start of methotrexate. Toxicity to normal tissues may be irreversible if leucovorin is not initiated by ~40 hours after the start of methotrexate. As a rescue after folate antagonists, leucovorin may be administered by I.V. bolus injection, I.M. injection, or orally. Doses > 25 mg should be administered parenterally. In combination with fluorouracil, leucovorin is given before or concurrent with fluorouracil. Leucovorin is usually administered by I.V. bolus injection or short (10-15 minutes) I.V. infusion. Other administration schedules have been used; refer to individual protocols.

Contraindications Hypersensitivity to leucovorin or any component of the formulation; pernicious anemia or vitamin B$_{12}$-deficient megaloblastic anemias

Dosage Forms

Injection, powder for reconstitution, as calcium: 50 mg, 100 mg, 200 mg, 350 mg, 500 mg

Injection, solution, as calcium: 10 mg/mL (50 mL)

Tablet, as calcium: 5 mg, 10 mg, 15 mg, 25 mg

Drug Interactions May decrease efficacy of co-trimoxazole against *Pneumocystis carinii* pneumonitis

Pregnancy Risk Factor C

Lactation Enters breast milk/compatible

Nursing Implications I.V. infusion should not exceed 160 mg of leucovorin per minute

Levocarnitine

CAS Number 541-15-1

U.S. Brand Names Carnitor®

Synonyms L-Carnitine

Use

Orphan drug:

Oral: Primary systemic carnitine deficiency; acute and chronic treatment of patients with an inborn error of metabolism which results in secondary carnitine deficiency

I.V.: Acute and chronic treatment of patients with an inborn error of metabolism which results in secondary carnitine deficiency; prevention and treatment of carnitine deficiency in patients with end-stage renal disease who are undergoing hemodialysis.

Also used to treat hepatotoxicity due to valproic acid overdose/toxicity See Overdosage/Treatment in Valproic Acid and Derivatives

Mechanism of Action Involved in fatty acid transport from the cytosol to mitochondria where upon lipid catabolism occurs

Adverse Reactions

Gastrointestinal: Nausea, vomiting, abdominal cramps, diarrhea (dose related)

Neuromuscular & skeletal: Myasthenia

Pharmacodynamics/Kinetics

Metabolism: Hepatic (limited with moderate renal impairment), to trimethylamine (TMA) and trimethylamine N-oxide (TMAO)

Bioavailability: Oral: ~10% to 20%

Half-life elimination: 17.4 hours

Time to peak: Oral: 3.3 hours

Excretion: Urine (76%, 4% to 9% as unchanged drug); feces ($< 1\%$)

Dosage

Oral:

Infants/Children: Initial: 50 mg/kg/day; titrate to 50-100 mg/kg/day in divided doses with a maximum dose of 3 g/day

Adults: 990 mg (oral tablets) 2-3 times/day or 1-3 g/day (oral solution)

I.V.:

Metabolic disorders: 50 mg/kg as a slow 2- to 3-minute I.V. bolus or by I.V. infusion

Severe metabolic crisis:

A loading dose of 50 mg/kg over 2-3 minutes followed by an equivalent dose over the following 24 hours administered as every 3 hours or every 4 hours (never less than every 6 hours either by infusion or by intravenous injection)

All subsequent daily doses are recommended to be in the range of 50 mg/kg or as therapy may require

The highest dose administered has been 300 mg/kg

It is recommended that a plasma carnitine concentration be obtained prior to beginning parenteral therapy accompanied by weekly and monthly monitoring

ESRD patients on hemodialysis:

Predialysis levocarnitine concentrations below normal (40-50 μmol/L): 10-20 mg/kg dry body weight as a slow 2- to 3-minute bolus after each dialysis session

Dosage adjustments should be guided by predialysis trough levocarnitine concentrations and downward dose adjustments (to 5 mg/kg after dialysis) may be made as early as every 3rd or 4th week of therapy

Note: Safety and efficacy of oral carnitine have not been established in ESRD. Chronic administration of high oral doses to patients with severely compromised renal function or ESRD patients on dialysis may result in accumulation of metabolites.

For treatment of valproic acid induced hyperammonemia: Clinically ill: 100 mg/kg IV (up to six grams) over 30 min then 15 mg/kg over 30 min 94 hours; clinically well: 100 mg/kg/day divided 96 hr up to 3 grams per day

Monitoring Parameters Plasma concentrations should be obtained prior to beginning parenteral therapy, and should be monitored weekly to monthly. In metabolic disorders: monitor blood chemistry, vital signs, and plasma carnitine levels (maintain between 35-60 μmol/L). In ESRD patients on dialysis: Plasma levels below the normal range should prompt initiation of therapy. Monitor predialysis (trough) plasma carnitine levels.

Administration

Oral: Solution may be dissolved in either drink or liquid food, and should be consumed slowly. Doses should be spaced every 3-4 hours throughout the day, preferably during or following meals.

I.V.:

Hemodialysis patients: Injection should be administered over 2-3 minutes into the venous return line after each dialysis session.

Carnitine deficiency: Administer as a bolus dose over 2-3 minutes or by infusion. Doses should be administered every 3-6 hours

Warnings Caution in patients with seizure disorders or in those at risk of seizures (CNS mass or medications which may lower seizure threshold). Both new-onset seizure activity as well as an increased frequency of seizures has been observed. Safety and efficacy of oral carnitine have not been established in ESRD. Chronic administration of high oral doses to patients with severely compromised renal function or ESRD patients on dialysis may result in accumulation of potentially toxic metabolites.

Dosage Forms
Capsule: 250 mg
Injection, solution: 200 mg/mL (5 mL, 12.5 mL)
  Carnitor®: 200 mg/mL (5 mL)
Solution, oral: 100 mg/mL (118 mL)
  Carnitor®: 100 mg/mL (118 mL) [cherry flavor]
Tablet: 330 mg, 500 mg
  Carnitor®: 330 mg

Reference Range Normal endogenous serum levocarnitine level is 57 μmol/L for obese men, 50 μmol/L for men who are not obese, 46 μmol/L for obese women and 39 μmol/L for women who are not obese. A plasma free carnitine level below 20 μmol/L represents a deficient state. Human breast milk contains levocarnitine concentrations of 50-100 nmol/L.

Pregnancy Risk Factor B

Pregnancy Implications No adequate or well controlled studies in pregnant women. However, carnitine is a naturally occurring substance in mammalian metabolism. In breast-feeding women, use must be weighed against the potential exposure of the infant to increased carnitine intake.

Lactation Excretion in breast milk unknown/use caution

Specific References
Caraccio TR and Mofenson HC, "Carnitine," *J Toxicol Clin Toxicol*, 2003, 41(6):897.
Kumaran S, Deepak B, Naveen B, et al, "Effects of Levocarnitine on Mitochondrial Antioxidant Systems and Oxidative Stress in Aged Rats," *Drugs R D*, 2003, 4(3):141-7.58

Mafenide

Pronunciation (MA fe nide)
CAS Number 13009-99-9; 138-39-6
U.S. Brand Names Sulfamylon®
Synonyms Mafenide Acetate

Use
Adjunct in the treatment of second- and third-degree burns to prevent septicemia caused by susceptible organisms such as *Pseudomonas aeruginosa*; vesicant exposure

Orphan drug: Prevention of graft loss of meshed autografts on excised burn wounds

Mechanism of Action Interferes with bacterial folic acid synthesis through competitive inhibition of para-aminobenzoic acid

Adverse Reactions
Frequency not defined.
Cardiovascular: Facial edema
Central nervous system: Pain
Dermatologic: Rash, erythema, pruritus
Endocrine & metabolic: Hyperchloremia, metabolic acidosis
Hematologic: Porphyria, bone marrow suppression, hemolytic anemia, bleeding, methemoglobinemia (in 2 pediatric patients)
Local: Burning sensation, excoriation
Respiratory: Hyperventilation, tachypnea, dyspnea
Miscellaneous: Hypersensitivity

Pharmacodynamics/Kinetics
Absorption: Diffuses through devascularized areas and is rapidly absorbed from burned surface
Metabolism: To para-carboxybenze sulfonamide, a carbonic anhydrase inhibitor
Time to peak, serum: 2-4 hours
Excretion: Urine (as metabolites)

Dosage Children and Adults: Topical: Apply once or twice daily with a sterile gloved hand; apply to a thickness of approximately 16 mm; the burned area should be covered with cream at all times

Stability
Mafenide 5% topical solution preparation:
  Dissolve the 50 g mafenide acetate (Sulfamylon®) packet in 200 mL of either sterile water for irrigation or sterile saline for irrigation (minimum solubility of 50 g of mafenide is in 200 mL of either solution)
  Sterilize this solution by pushing through a 0.22 micron filter
  Further dissolve this 200 mL of sterile Sulfamylon® solution in 800 mL of the initial diluent (either sterile water for irrigation or normal saline for irrigation)
  This solution is stable and sterile for a total of 48 hours at room temperature

Note: Mafenide acetate topical solution **cannot** be mixed with nystatin due to reduced activity of mafenide

Note: Pilot *in vitro* studies: Silvadene® and Furacin® cream combined with nystatin cream were equally effective against the microorganisms as were the individual drugs. However, Sulfamylon® cream combined with nystatin lost its antimicrobial capability. [*J Burn Care Rehabil* 1989, 109:508-11.]

Monitoring Parameters Acid base balance

Contraindications Hypersensitivity to mafenide, sulfites, or any component of the formulation

Warnings Use with caution in patients with renal impairment and in patients with G6PD deficiency; prolonged use may result in superinfection

Dosage Forms
Cream, topical, as acetate: 85 mg/g (60 g, 120 g, 454 g) [contains sodium metabisulfite]
Powder, for topical solution: 5% (5s) [50 g/packet]

Reference Range After topical use, maximum serum mafenide levels range from 0.05 to 1.7 mmol/L after 2- to 4-hour exposure

Drug Interactions No data reported

Pregnancy Risk Factor C

Lactation Excretion in breast milk unknown

Nursing Implications For external use only; monitor acid base balance

Magnesium Citrate

Pronunciation (mag NEE zhum SIT rate)
CAS Number 3344-18-1
Synonyms Citrate of Magnesia

Use Evacuates bowel prior to certain surgical and diagnostic procedures

Mechanism of Action A saline cathartic which promotes bowel evacuation by causing osmotic retention of fluid which distends the colon with increased peristaltic activity

Adverse Reactions
Cardiovascular: Hypotension, shock, QRS prolongation, vasodilation
Gastrointestinal: Abdominal cramps, diarrhea, gas formation; vomiting (frequency of 17% at doses >233 mg/kg)
Endocrine & metabolic: Hypermagnesemia
Renal: Renal failure
Respiratory: Respiratory depression

Signs and Symptoms of Overdose Diarrhea, nausea, vomiting. Serious, potentially life-threatening electrolyte disturbances may occur with long-term use or overdosage. **Serum level** >**12 mEq/L** may be fatal. **Serum level** ∼**10 mEq/L** may cause complete heart block.

Pharmacodynamics/Kinetics
Absorption: Oral: 15% to 30%
Excretion: Urine

Dosage
Cathartic: Oral:
Children:
  <6 years: 0.5 mL/kg up to a maximum of 200 mL repeated every 4-6 hours until stools are clear
  6-12 years: $^1/_3$ to $^1/_2$ bottle
Adults ≥12 years: $^1/_2$ to 1 full bottle as needed

Administration To increase palatability, chill the solution prior to administration.

Contraindications Renal failure, appendicitis, abdominal pain, intestinal impaction, obstruction or perforation, diabetes mellitus, complications in gastrointestinal tract, patients with colostomy or ileostomy, ulcerative colitis or diverticulitis

Warnings Use with caution in patients with impaired renal function, especially if Cl_{cr}<30 mL/minute (accumulation of magnesium which may lead to magnesium intoxication). Use caution in patients receiving a cardiac glycoside; may increase the AV-blocking effects. Use with caution in patients with lithium administration; use with caution with neuromuscular-blocking agents, and CNS depressants.

Dosage Forms
Solution, oral: 290 mg/5 mL (300 mL) [cherry and lemon flavors]
Tablet: 100 mg [as elemental magnesium]

Reference Range Normal urine level: 1-6 mM/L. Serum magnesium: Children: 1.5-1.9 mg/dL ∼1.2-1.6 mEq/L; Adults: 2.2-2.8 mg/dL ∼1.8-2.3 mEq/L

Test Interactions ↑ magnesium; ↓ protein, calcium (S), ↓ potassium (S)

Pregnancy Risk Factor B

Nursing Implications To increase palatability, manufacturer suggests chilling the solution prior to administration

Specific Reference
Dribben WH, Farber NB, and Olney JW, "High-Dose Magnesium Induces Apoptotic Neurodegeneration in the Developing Mouse Brain," *J Toxicol Clin Toxicol*, 2003, 41(5):749.

Magnesium Sulfate

Pronunciation (mag NEE zhum SUL fate)
CAS Number 10034-99-8; 7487-88-9
Synonyms Epsom Salts; MgSO₄ (error-prone abbreviation)

Use Treatment and prevention of hypomagnesemia; seizure prevention in severe pre-eclampsia or eclampsia, pediatric acute nephritis; short-term treatment torsade de pointes; treatment of cardiac arrhythmias (VT/VF) caused by hypomagnesemia; short-term treatment of constipation or soaking aid; useful for digitalis toxicity, chronic alcoholism, injection for hydrofluoric acid burns

Mechanism of Action Essential in the synthesis of adenosine triphosphate (ATP) and other enzymes involved in muscle contractility and neuronal transmissions; promotes bowel evacuation by causing osmotic retention of fluid which distends the colon with increased peristaltic activity when taken orally; parenterally, decreases acetylcholine in motor nerve terminals and acts on myocardium by slowing rate of S-A node impulse formation and prolonging conduction time

Adverse Reactions
Adverse effects with parenteral $MgSO_4$ therapy are related to the magnesium serum level
Serum magnesium levels >3 mg/dL:
    Central nervous system: CNS depression
    Gastrointestinal: Diarrhea
Serum magnesium >5 mg/dL:
    Cardiovascular: Flushing
    Central nervous system: Somnolence
    Gastrointestinal: Diarrhea
    Neuromuscular & skeletal: Depressed deep tendon reflexes, myalgia, blocked peripheral neuromuscular transmission leading to anticonvulsant effects
Serum magnesium >12 mg/dL:
    Cardiovascular: Complete heart block
    Endocrine & metabolic: Hypercalcemia, hypernatremia
    Gastrointestinal: Diarrhea
    Respiratory: Respiratory paralysis

Signs and Symptoms of Overdose Coma, diuresis, ECG changes, fibrillation (atrial), flushing, flutter (atrial), heart block, hyporeflexia, hypotension, hypothermia, lethargy, muscle weakness, nausea, QRS prolongation, respiratory depression, vomiting

Pharmacodynamics/Kinetics
Onset of action: Oral: Cathartic: 1-2 hours; I.M.: 1 hour; I.V.: Immediate
Duration: I.M.: 3-4 hours; I.V.: 30 minutes
Absorption: Oral: Inversely proportional to amount ingested; 40% to 60% under controlled dietary conditions; 15% to 36% at higher doses
Distribution: Bone (50% to 60%); extracellular fluid (1% to 2%)
Protein binding: 30%, to albumin
Excretion: Urine (as magnesium)

Dosage
The recommended dietary allowance (RDA) of magnesium is 4.5 mg/kg which is a total daily allowance of 350-400 mg for adult men and 280-300 mg for adult women. During pregnancy the RDA is 300 mg and during lactation the RDA is 355 mg. Average daily intakes of dietary magnesium have declined in recent years due to processing of food. The latest estimate of the average American dietary intake was 349 mg/day. Dose represented as $MgSO_4$ unless stated otherwise.
Note: Serum magnesium is poor reflection of repletional status as the majority of magnesium is intracellular; serum levels may be transiently normal for a few hours after a dose is given, therefore, aim for consistently high normal serum levels in patients with normal renal function for most efficient repletion
Hypomagnesemia:
    Neonates: I.V.: 25-50 mg/kg/dose (0.2-0.4 mEq/kg/dose) every 8-12 hours for 2-3 doses
    Children: I.M., I.V.: 25-50 mg/kg/dose (0.2-0.4 mEq/kg/dose) every 4-6 hours for 3-4 doses, maximum single dose: 2000 mg (16 mEq), may repeat if hypomagnesemia persists (higher dosage up to 100 mg/kg/dose $MgSO_4$ I.V. has been used); maintenance: I.V.: 30-60 mg/kg/day (0.25-0.5 mEq/kg/day)
    Adults:
        Oral: 3 g every 6 hours for 4 doses as needed
        I.M., I.V.: 1 g every 6 hours for 4 doses; for severe hypomagnesemia: 8-12 g $MgSO_4$/day in divided doses has been used
Management of seizures and hypertension: Children: I.M., I.V.: 20-100 mg/kg/dose every 4-6 hours as needed; in severe cases doses as high as 200 mg/kg/dose have been used
Eclampsia, pre-eclampsia: Adults:
    I.M.: 1-4 g every 4 hours
    I.V.: Initial: 4 g, then switch to I.M. or 1-4 g/hour by continuous infusion
    Note: Maximum dose not to exceed 30-40 g/day; maximum rate of infusion: 1-2 g/hour
Life-threatening arrhythmia: I.V.: 1-2 g (8-16 mEq) in 100 mL D_5W, administered over 5-60 minutes followed by an infusion of 0.5-1 g/hour, **or**
    1-6 g administered over several minutes, followed by (in some cases) I.V. infusion of 3-20 mg/minute for 5-48 hours (depending on patient response and serum magnesium levels)
Maintenance electrolyte requirements:
    Daily requirements: 0.2-0.5 mEq/kg/24 hours or 3-10 mEq/1000 kcal/24 hours
    Maximum: 8-16 mEq/24 hours
Cathartic: Oral:
    Children:
        2-5 years: 2.5-5 g/kg/day in a single or divided doses
        6-11 years: 5-10 g/day in a single or divided doses
    Children ≥12 years and Adults: 10-30 g/day in a single or divided doses

Soaking aid: Topical: Adults: Dissolve 2 capfuls of powder per gallon of warm water

Dosing adjustment/comments in renal impairment: Cl_{cr}<25 mL/minute: Do not administer or monitor serum magnesium levels carefully. See guidelines below.

Magnesium Replacement Guidelines
Normal magnesium serum concentrations (MDACC):
Children: 1.5-1.5 mg/dL (1.2-1.6 mEq/L)
Adults: 1.5-2.5 mg/dL (1.2-2.0 mEq/L)
If serum magnesium is <1.5 mg/dL (<1.2 mEq/L), repletion should be considered.
    Note: Serum magnesium is a poor reflection of repletional status as the majority of magnesium is intracellular; serum levels may be transiently normal for a few hours after a dose is given; therefore, aim for consistently high normal serum levels in patients with normal renal function for most efficient repletion.
Magnesium formulations:
    Magnesium gluconate 500 mg tablet (2.5 mEq/tablet)
    Magnesium hydroxide (MOM) (13.7 mEq/5 mL)
    Magnesium chloride 535 mg tablet (5.2 mEq/tablet)
    Magnesium oxide 420 mg (20.8 mEq/capsule)
    Magnesium citrate liquid (3.85-4.71 mEq/5 mL)
    Mylanta®-II (13.7 mEq/5 mL)
    Maalox® Plus (6.9 mEq/5 mL)
Oral magnesium supplementation:
    Oral magnesium is generally not adequate for repletion in patients with serum magnesium concentrations <1.5 mg/dL (<1.2 mEq/L).
    Magnesium chloride 535 mg/tablet = 5.2 mEq/tablet given 2 tablets 3 times/day for 5-7 days.
May need **more** if renal function is good or absorptive capacity is poor. May need **less** if renal function deteriorates. Reassess to determine maintenance dose, if necessary, at 0.35-0.45 mEq/kg/day.
Intravenous repletion (available as 50% solution, 2 mL vials = 1 g or 8 mEq)
    Asymptomatic or serum concentration >1.2 mg/dL (>1.0 mEq/L)
        <50 kg 16-32 mEq/day infused over 24 hours for 5-7 days
        >50 kg 24-40 mEq/day infused over 24 hours for 5-7 days
    Symptomatic or serum concentration <1.2 mg/dL (<1.0 mEq/L)
        <50 kg 24-40 mEq/day infused over 24 hours for 5-7 days
        >50 kg 32-48 mEq/day infused over 24 hours for 5-7 days
Maximal rate of infusion: 2 g/hour to avoid hypotension. Doses of 4 g/hour have been given in emergencies (eclampsia, seizures).
Optimally, should add magnesium to I.V. fluids, but bolus doses are also effective. Monitor renal function and for hypocalcemia. Patients exhibiting hypokalemia should receive concomitant potassium replacement therapy.
Follow-up monitoring:
    Serum magnesium will equilibrate over 2-4 days with intracellular concentrations. Therefore, caution should be exercised in interpreting serum levels immediately after boluses.

Stability
Refrigeration of intact ampuls may result in precipitation or crystallization. Parenteral admixture is stable at room temperature (25°C) for 60 days. I.V. is **incompatible** when mixed with fat emulsion (flocculation), calcium gluceptate, clindamycin, dobutamine, hydrocortisone (same syringe), nafcillin, polymyxin B, procaine hydrochloride, tetracyclines, thiopental.

Monitoring Parameters Monitor blood pressure when administering $MgSO_4$ I.V.; serum magnesium levels should be monitored to avoid overdose; monitor for diarrhea; monitor for arrhythmias, hypotension, respiratory and CNS depression during rapid I.V. administration

Administration
Oral: Dissolve powder in $1/2$ glass of water; may add lemon juice to improve taste
Injection: May be administered I.M. or I.V.
    I.M.: A 25% or 50% concentration may be used for adults and a 20% solution is recommended for children
    I.V.: Magnesium may be administered IVP, IVPB or I.V.; when giving I.V. push, must dilute first and should not be given any faster than 150 mg/minute. Hypotension and asystole may occur with rapid administration.
        Maximal rate of infusion: 2 g/hour to avoid hypotension; doses of 4 g/hour have been given in emergencies (eclampsia, seizures); optimally, should add magnesium to I.V. fluids, but bolus doses are also effective
Topical: Dissolve 2 cups of powder per gallon of warm water to use as a soaking aid. To make a compress, dissolve 2 cups of powder per 2 cups of hot water and use a towel to apply as a wet dressing.

Contraindications Hypersensitivity to any component of the formulation; heart block; myocardial damage

Warnings
Use with caution in patients with impaired renal function, hepatitis, or Addison's disease (accumulation of magnesium may lead to magnesium intoxication). Monitor serum magnesium level, respiratory rate, deep tendon reflex, renal function when magnesium sulfate is

administered parenterally. Use with extreme caution in patients with myasthenia gravis or other neuromuscular disease.

Constipation (self-medication, OTC use): For occasional use only; serious side effects may occur with prolonged use. For use only under the supervision of a healthcare provider in patients with kidney dysfunction, or with a sudden change in bowel habits which persist for >2 weeks. Do not use if abdominal pain, nausea, or vomiting are present.

Dosage Forms
Infusion [premixed in D_5W]: 10 mg/mL (100 mL); 20 mg/mL (500 mL, 1000 mL)

Infusion [premixed in water for injection]: 40 mg/mL (100 mL, 500 mL, 1000 mL); 80 mg/mL (50 mL)

Injection, solution: 125 mg/mL (8 mL); 500 mg/mL (2 mL, 5 mL, 10 mL, 20 mL, 50 mL)

Powder: Magnesium sulfate USP (480 g, 1810 g, 1920 g)

Reference Range
Serum magnesium:
Children: 1.5-1.9 mg/dL ~1.2-1.6 mEq/L
Adults: 2.2-2.8 mg/dL ~1.8-2.3 mEq/L
Cardiotoxic effects: >12 mg/dL
Muscle paralysis: >15 mg/dL

Test Interactions
Analytical interference by calcium salts can result in false depression of magnesium levels.

Drug Interactions
Calcium channel blockers: Calcium channel blockers may enhance the adverse/toxic effect of magnesium salts. Magnesium salts may enhance the hypotensive effect of calcium channel blockers.

Neuromuscular-blocking agents: Magnesium salts may enhance the neuromuscular-blocking effect of neuromuscular-blocking agents. Only of concern in patients with increased serum magnesium concentrations.

Pregnancy Risk Factor B
Pregnancy Implications
No harmful effects regarding breast-feeding; hypermagnesemia can lead to neonatal intrauterine growth retardation, CNS respiratory depression

Lactation
Enters breast milk/compatible

Nursing Implications
Monitor arrhythmias, hypotension, diarrhea, respiratory and CNS depression during rapid I.V. administration; monitor serum magnesium level to avoid overdosages

Specific References
Ali A, Walentik C, Mantych GJ, et al, "Iatrogenic Acute Hypermagnesemia After Total Parenteral Nutrition Infusion Mimicking Septic Shock Syndrome: Two Case Reports," *Pediatrics Electronic Pages*, 2003, 112(1):e70-72 [online].

Belfort MA, Anthony J, Saade GR, et al, "A Comparison of Magnesium Sulfate and Nimodipine for the Prevention of Eclampsia," *N Engl J Med*, 2003, 348(4):304-11.

"Do Women with Pre-Eclampsia, and Their Babies, Benefit from Magnesium Sulphate? The Magpie Trial: A Randomised Placebo-Controlled Tria: The Magpie Trial Collaborative Group," *Lancet*, 359(9321):1877-90.

Hughes R, Goldkorn A, Masoli M, et al, "Use of Isotonic Nebulised Magnesium Sulphate as an Adjuvant to Salbutamol in Treatment of Severe Asthma in Adults: Randomised Placebo-Controlled Trial," *Lancet*, 2003, 361(9375):2114-7.

Lewis-Younger C, Speranza V, and Gaar G, "Temporary Paralysis Resulting from Medical Error," *J Toxicol Clin Toxicol*, 2004, 42(5):732.

Livingston JC, Livingston LW, Ramsey R, et al, "Magnesium Sulfate in Women with Mild Pre-Eclampsia: A Randomized Controlled Trial," *Obstet Gynecol*, 2003, 101(2):217-20.

Shadnia SH, Rahimi M, Abdi M, et al, "Benefits of Magnesium Sulfate in the Management of Acute Human Poisoning by Organophosphorus Insecticides," *Clin Toxicol (Phila)*, 2005, 43:677.

Mannitol

Pronunciation
(MAN i tole)

CAS Number
69-65-8

U.S. Brand Names
Osmitrol®; Resectisol®

Synonyms
D-Mannitol

Use
Reduction of increased intracranial pressure associated with cerebral edema; promotion of diuresis in the prevention and/or treatment of oliguria or anuria due to acute renal failure; reduction of increased intraocular pressure; promoting urinary excretion of toxic substances (lithium); used for ciguatera poisoning

Mechanism of Action
Increases the osmotic pressure of glomerular filtrate, which inhibits tubular reabsorption of water and electrolytes and increases urinary output

Adverse Reactions
Cardiovascular: Circulatory overload, diuresis, congestive heart failure, angina

Central nervous system: Convulsions/seizures, **headache**

Dermatologic: Urticaria

Endocrine & metabolic: Fluid and electrolyte imbalance, water intoxication, hypernatremia, dehydration and hypovolemia secondary to rapid diuresis, hyponatremia

Gastrointestinal: Xerostomia, diarrhea (oral ingestion), colonic perforation (oral ingestion), **nausea, vomiting**

Local: Tissue necrosis

Ocular: Blurred vision

Renal: Focal osmotic nephrosis of proximal convoluted tubules, **polyuria**

Respiratory: Pulmonary edema

Miscellaneous: Allergic reactions, osmolal gap

Signs and Symptoms of Overdose
Cardiovascular collapse, chest pain, chills, headache, hypotension, ototoxicity (deafness), polyuria, renal failure, tinnitus. Pulmonary edema has occurred after a dose of 400 g over 2.5 hours; can cause diarrhea when taken orally.

Pharmacodynamics/Kinetics
Onset of action: Diuresis: Injection: 1-3 hours; Reduction in intracranial pressure: ~15-30 minutes

Duration: Reduction in intracranial pressure: 1.5-6 hours

Distribution: Remains confined to extracellular space (except in extreme concentrations); does not penetrate the blood-brain barrier (generally, penetration is low)

Metabolism: Minimally hepatic to glycogen

Half-life elimination: 1.1-1.6 hours

Excretion: Primarily urine (as unchanged drug)

Dosage
I.V.:

Children:
Test dose (to assess adequate renal function): 200 mg/kg over 3-5 minutes to produce a urine flow of at least 1 mL/kg/hour for 1-3 hours
Initial: 0.5-1 g/kg
Maintenance: 0.25-0.5 g/kg/hour given every 4-6 hours

Adults:
Test dose: 12.5 g (200 mg/kg) over 3-5 minutes to produce a urine flow of at least 30-50 mL of urine per hour over the next 2-3 hours
Initial: 0.5-1 g/kg
Maintenance: 0.25-0.5 g/kg every 4-6 hours; usual adult dose: 20-200 g/24 hours
Intracranial pressure: Cerebral edema: 1.5-2 g/kg/dose I.V. as a 15% to 20% solution over ≥30 minutes; maintain serum osmolality 310-320 mOsm/kg
Preoperative for neurosurgery: 1.5-2 g/kg administered 1-1.5 hours prior to surgery
Transurethral irrigation: Use urogenital solution as required for irrigation

Stability
Should be stored at room temperature (15°C to 30°C) and protected from freezing; crystallization may occur at low temperatures; do not use solutions that contain crystals, heating in a hot water bath and vigorous shaking may be utilized for resolubilization; cool solutions to body temperature before using

Monitoring Parameters
Renal function, daily fluid I & O, serum electrolytes, serum and urine osmolality; for treatment of elevated intracranial pressure, maintain serum osmolality 310-320 mOsm/kg

Administration
Inspect for crystals prior to administration. If crystals present redissolve by warming solution. Use filter-type administration set; in-line 5-micron filter set should always be used for mannitol infusion with concentrations ≥20%; administer test dose (for oliguria) I.V. push over 3-5 minutes; avoid extravasation; for cerebral edema or elevated ICP, administer over 20-30 minutes; crenation and agglutination of red blood cells may occur if administered with whole blood.

Contraindications
Hypersensitivity to mannitol or any component or the formulation; severe renal disease (anuria); severe dehydration; active intracranial bleeding except during craniotomy; progressive heart failure, pulmonary congestion, or renal dysfunction after mannitol administration; severe pulmonary edema or congestion

Warnings
Should not be administered until adequacy of renal function and urine flow is established;use 1-2 test doses to assess renal response. Diuretic effects may mask and intensify underlying dehydration; excessive loss of water and electrolytes may lead to imbalances and aggravate pre-existing hyponatremia. May cause renal dysfunction especially with high doses; use caution in patients taking other nephrotoxic agents, with sepsis or pre-existing renal disease. To minimize adverse renal effects, adjust to keep serum osmolality less than 320 mOsm/L. Discontinue if evidence of acute tubular necrosis.

In patients being treated for cerebral edema, mannitol may accumulate in the brain (causing rebound increases in intracranial pressure) if circulating for long periods of time as with continuous infusion; intermittent boluses preferred. Cardiovascular status should also be evaluated; do not administer electrolyte-free mannitol solutions with blood. If hypotension occurs monitor cerebral perfusion pressure to insure adequate.

Dosage Forms
Injection, solution: 5% [50 mg/mL] (1000 mL); 10% [100 mg/mL] (500 mL, 1000 mL); 15% [150 mg/mL] (500 mL); 20% [200 mg/mL] (150 mL, 250 mL, 500 mL); 25% [250 mg/mL] (50 mL)

Osmitrol®: 5% [50 mg/mL] (1000 mL); 10% [100 mg/mL] (500 mL, 1000 mL); 15% [150 mg/mL] (500 mL); 20% [200 mg/mL] (250 mL, 500 mL)

Solution, urogenital (Resectisol®): 5% [50 mg/mL] (2000 mL, 4000 mL)

Test Interactions ↑ or ↓ inorganic phosphorus (B); lowers serum sodium; causes false-positive ethylene glycol

Drug Interactions Lithium toxicity (with diuretic-induced hyponatremia)

Pregnancy Risk Factor C

Pregnancy Implications Reproduction studies have not been conducted.

Lactation Excretion in breast milk unknown/use caution

Nursing Implications In-line 5-micron filter set should always be used for mannitol infusion with concentrations of 20% or greater; avoid extravasation; crenation and agglutination of red blood cells may occur if administered with whole blood; appears to be compatible with furosemide

Specific References

Chen WH, Kao YF, and Hsu MC, "Detrusor Hyporeflexia Presents as an Early Manifestation in Encephalitis," *Am J Emerg Med*, 2005, 23(4):583-5.

Eroglu A and Uzunlar H, "Forearm Compartment Syndrome After Intravenous Mannitol Extravasation in a Carbosulfan Poisoning Patient," *J Toxicol Clin Toxicol*, 2004, 42(5):649-52.

Mesna

Pronunciation (MES na)

CAS Number 19767-45-4

U.S. Brand Names Mesnex®

Synonyms Sodium 2-Mercaptoethane Sulfonate

Use Orphan drug: Prevention of hemorrhagic cystitis induced by ifosfamide

Unlabeled/Investigational Use Prevention of hemorrhagic cystitis induced by cyclophosphamide

Mechanism of Action In blood, mesna is oxidized to dimesna which in turn is reduced in the kidney back to mesna, supplying a free thiol group which binds to and inactivates acrolein, the urotoxic metabolite of ifosfamide and cyclophosphamide

Adverse Reactions

It is difficult to distinguish reactions from those caused by concomitant chemotherapy.

Cardiovascular: Tachycardia

Gastrointestinal: **Bad taste in mouth with oral administration (100%), vomiting** (secondary to the bad taste after oral administration, or with high I.V. doses)

Hematologic: Decreased platelet count

Local: Injection site reaction

Neuromuscular & skeletal: Limb pain, myalgia

Respiratory: Tachypnea

Miscellaneous: Anaphylaxis, hypersensitivity

Pharmacodynamics/Kinetics

Distribution: No tissue penetration

Protein binding: 69% to 75%

Metabolism: Rapidly oxidized intravascularly to mesna disulfide; mesna disulfide is reduced in renal tubules back to mesna following glomerular filtration.

Bioavailability: Oral: 45% to 79%

Half-life elimination: Parent drug: 24 minutes; Mesna disulfide: 72 minutes

Time to peak, plasma: 2-3 hours

Excretion: Urine; as unchanged drug (18% to 26%) and metabolites

Dosage

Children and Adults (refer to individual protocols):

I.V.: Recommended dose is 60% of the ifosfamide dose given in 3 divided doses (0, 4, and 8 hours after the start of ifosfamide)

Alternative I.V. regimens include 80% of the ifosfamide dose given in 4 divided doses (0, 3, 6, and 9 hours after the start of ifosfamide) and continuous infusions

I.V./Oral: Recommended dose is 100% of the ifosfamide dose, given as 20% of the ifosfamide dose I.V. at hour 0, followed by 40% of the ifosfamide dose given orally 2 and 6 hours after start of ifosfamide

Stability Store intact vials and tablets at controlled room temperature of 20°C to 25°C (68°F to 77°F). Opened multidose vials may be stored and used for up to 8 days after opening. Dilute injection in 50-1000 mL D_5W, NS, or lactated Ringer's for infusion. Solutions in D_5W or lactated Ringer's are stable for at least 48 hours at room temperature. Solutions in NS are stable for at least 24 hours at room temperature. Solutions in plastic syringes are stable for 9 days under refrigeration, or at room or body temperature. Stability in syringes decreases if air is in the filled syringe. Solutions of mesna and ifosfamide in lactated Ringer's are stable for 7 days in a PVC ambulatory infusion pump reservoir. Mesna injection is stable for at least 7 days when diluted 1:2 or 1:5 with grape- and orange-flavored syrups or 11:1 to 1:100 in carbonated beverages for oral administration.

Monitoring Parameters Urinalysis

Administration

Oral: Administer orally in tablet formulation or parenteral solution diluted in water, milk, juice, or carbonated beverages; patients who vomit within 2 hours of taking oral mesna should repeat the dose or receive I.V. mesna

I.V.: Administer by short (15-30 minutes) infusion or continuous (24 hour) infusion

Contraindications Hypersensitivity to mesna or other thiol compounds, or any component of the formulation

Warnings Examine morning urine specimen for hematuria prior to ifosfamide or cyclophosphamide treatment; if hematuria (>50 RBC/HPF) develops, reduce the ifosfamide/cyclophosphamide dose or discontinue the drug; will not prevent or alleviate other toxicities associated with ifosfamide or cyclophosphamide and will not prevent hemorrhagic cystitis in all patients. Allergic reactions have been reported; patients with autoimmune disorders may be at increased risk. Symptoms ranged from mild hypersensitivity to systemic anaphylactic reactions. I.V. formulation contains benzyl alcohol; do not use in neonates or infants.

Dosage Forms

Injection, solution: 100 mg/mL (10 mL) [contains benzyl alcohol]

Tablet: 400 mg

Test Interactions False-positive urinary ketones with Multistix® or Labstix®

Drug Interactions Decreased effect: Warfarin: Questionable alterations in coagulation control

Pregnancy Risk Factor B

Pregnancy Implications Teratogenic effects were not observed in animal studies. There are no adequate and well-controlled studies in pregnant women. Use during pregnancy only if clearly needed.

Lactation Excretion in breast milk unknown/not recommended

Nursing Implications Used in conjunction with ifosfamide; examine morning urine specimen for hematuria prior to ifosfamide or cyclophosphamide treatment; if hematuria develops, reduce the ifosfamide/cyclophosphamide dose or discontinue the drug

Methylene Blue

Pronunciation (METH i leen bloo)

CAS Number 61-73-4; 7220-79-3

U.S. Brand Names Urolene Blue®

Use Antidote for drug-induced methemoglobinemia, indicator dye, chronic urolithiasis; bacteriostatic genitourinary antiseptic

Unlabeled/Investigational Use Has been used topically (0.1% solutions) in conjunction with polychromatic light to photoinactivate viruses such as herpes simplex; has been used alone or in combination with vitamin C for the management of chronic urolithiasis; also has been suggested to treat ackee fruit encephalopathy.

Mechanism of Action Weak germicide; in low concentrations, hastens the conversion of methemoglobin to hemoglobin; has opposite effect at high concentrations by converting ferrous iron of reduced hemoglobin to ferric iron to form methemoglobin; in cyanide toxicity, it combines with cyanide to form cyanmethemoglobin preventing the interference of cyanide with the cytochrome system; indicated for symptomatic methemoglobinemia (usually when methemoglobin levels are >20%)

Adverse Reactions

Cardiovascular: Hypotension, cyanosis, large I.V. doses have been associated with precordial pain

Central nervous system: Dizziness/vertigo, mental confusion, headache, fever/pyrexia at doses of 7 mg/kg

Dermatologic: Stains skin a bluish color at doses >80 mg/kg

Gastrointestinal: Nausea, vomiting, abdominal pain at doses of 7 mg/kg; **fecal discoloration (blue-green)**

Genitourinary: Bladder irritation, dysuria, **urine discoloration (blue or green)**

Hematologic: Formation of methemoglobin, hemolytic anemia in patients with glucose-6-phosphate dehydrogenase deficiency, hemolytic anemia

Local: Extravasation injury

Neuromuscular & skeletal: Hyperreflexia

Ocular: Vision color changes (blue tinge)

Miscellaneous: Diaphoresis

Signs and Symptoms of Overdose Feces discoloration (black; blue), jaundice, urine discoloration (blue; blue-green; green; green-yellow; yellow-brown). Doses >20 mg/kg can cause hemolysis and hypotension.

Pharmacodynamics/Kinetics

Absorption: Oral: 53% to 97%

Excretion: Urine and feces

Dosage

Children: NADPH-methemoglobin reductase deficiency: Oral: 1-1.5 mg/kg/day (maximum: 4 mg/kg/day) given with 5-8 mg/kg/day of ascorbic acid

Children and Adults: Methemoglobinemia: I.V.: 1-2 mg/kg or 25-50 mg/m² over several minutes; may be repeated in 1 hour if necessary; use the higher dose if methemoglobin levels exceed 60%

Adults:

Genitourinary antiseptic: Oral: 55-130 mg 3 times/day with a full glass of water (maximum: 300 mg/day)

Monitoring Parameters Hemoglobin, methemoglobin concentrations should drop within 1 hour

Administration Administer I.V. undiluted by direct I.V. injection over several minutes.

Contraindications Hypersensitivity to methylene blue or any component of the formulation; intraspinal injection; renal insufficiency; pregnancy (injected intra-amniotically)

Warnings Do not inject SubQ or intrathecally; use with caution in young patients and in patients with G6PD deficiency; continued use can cause profound anemia

Dosage Forms

Injection, solution: 10 mg/mL (1 mL, 10 mL)

Tablet (Urolene Blue®): 65 mg

Test Interactions Can reduce arterial lactate concentration in septic shock

Pregnancy Risk Factor C/D (injected intra-amniotically)

Nursing Implications Inject over several minutes to avoid high concentration; SubQ injection may cause necrotic abscess; may be diluted with normal saline

Specific References

Bradberry SM, "Occupational Methaemoglobinaemia: Mechanisms of Production, Features, Diagnosis, and Management Including the Use of Methylene Blue," *Toxicol Rev*, 2003, 22(1):13-27.

Clifton J 2nd and Leikin JB, "Methylene Blue," *Am J Ther*, 2003, 10(4):289-91.

Gaudette NF and Lodge JW, "Determination of Methylene Blue and Leucomethylene Blue in Male and Female Fischer 344 Rat Urine and B6C3F$_1$ Mouse Urine," *J Anal Toxicol*, 2005, 29:28-33.

Sivilotti ML, "Oxidant Stress and Haemolysis of the Human Erythrocyte," *Toxicol Rev*, 2004, 23(3):169-88.

Nalmefene

Pronunciation (NAL me feen)

CAS Number 55096-26-9; 58895-64-0

U.S. Brand Names Revex®

Synonyms Nalmefene Hydrochloride

Use Reversal of adverse opiate effects

Unlabeled/Investigational Use May be useful for pruritus

Mechanism of Action Derivative of naltrexone with opioid antagonist effects; does not produce opiate agonist effects

Adverse Reactions

Cardiovascular: Hypotension, tachycardia, hypertension, shock, sinus bradycardia, sinus tachycardia

Central nervous system: Dizziness, fatigue, fever, headache, chills

Gastrointestinal: **Nausea**, vomiting

Neuromuscular & skeletal: Paresthesia

Respiratory: Pulmonary edema

Pharmacodynamics/Kinetics

Onset of action: I.M., SubQ: 5-15 minutes

Distribution: V_d: 8.6 L/kg; rapid

Protein binding: 45%

Metabolism: Hepatic via glucuronide conjugation to metabolites with little or no activity

Bioavailability: I.M., SubQ: 100%

Half-life elimination: 10.8 hours

Time to peak, serum: Serum: I.M.: 2.3 hours; I.V.: <2 minutes; SubQ: 1.5 hours

Excretion: Feces (17%); urine (<5% as unchanged drug)

Clearance: 0.8 L/hour/kg

Dosage

Reversal of postoperative opioid depression: Blue labeled product (100 mcg/mL): Titrate to reverse the undesired effects of opioids; initial dose for nonopioid dependent patients: 0.25 mcg/kg followed by 0.25 mcg/kg incremental doses at 2- to 5-minute intervals; after a total dose >1 mcg/kg, further therapeutic response is unlikely

Management of known/suspected opioid overdose: Green labeled product (1000 mcg/mL): Initial dose: 0.5 mg/70 kg; may repeat with 1 mg/70 kg in 2-5 minutes; further increase beyond a total dose of 1.5 mg/70 kg will not likely result in improved response and may result in cardiovascular stress and precipitated withdrawal syndrome. (If opioid dependency is suspected, administer a challenge dose of 0.1 mg/70 kg; if no withdrawal symptoms are observed in 2 minutes, the recommended doses can be administered.)

Note: If recurrence of respiratory depression is noted, dose may again be titrated to clinical effect using incremental doses.

Note: If I.V. access is lost or not readily obtainable, a single SubQ or I.M. dose of 1 mg may be effective in 5-15 minutes.

Dosing adjustment in renal or hepatic impairment: Not necessary with single uses, however, slow administration (over 60 seconds) of incremental doses is recommended to minimize hypertension and dizziness

Monitoring Parameters Symptoms of withdrawal; signs/symptoms of respiratory depression; pain

Administration Check dosage strength carefully before use to avoid error. Slow administration (over 60 seconds) of incremental doses is recommended to minimize hypertension and dizziness in renal patients. Dilute drug (1:1) with diluent and use smaller doses in patients known to be at increased cardiovascular risk. May be administered via I.M. or SubQ routes if I.V. access is not feasible. A single SubQ or I.M. dose of 1 mg may be effective in 5-15 minutes.

Contraindications Hypersensitivity to nalmefene, naltrexone, or any component of the formulation

Warnings May induce symptoms of acute withdrawal in opioid-dependent patients; recurrence of respiratory depression is possible if the opioid involved is long-acting; observe patients until there is no reasonable risk of recurrent respiratory depression. Safety and efficacy have not been established in children. Avoid abrupt reversal of opioid effects in patients of high cardiovascular risk or who have received potentially cardiotoxic drugs. Pulmonary edema and cardiovascular instability, including ventricular fibrillation, have been reported in association with abrupt reversal with other narcotic antagonists. Animal studies indicate nalmefene may not completely reverse buprenorphine-induced respiratory depression. Use caution with renal impairment.

Dosage Forms

Injection, solution:

Revex®: 100 mcg/mL (1 mL) [blue label]; 1 mg/mL (2 mL) [green label]

Reference Range Therapeutic plasma level: 0.5 ng/mL

Drug Interactions

Flumazenil: May increase the risk of toxicity with flumazenil. An increased risk of seizures has been associated with flumazenil and nalmefene coadministration

Narcotic analgesics: Decreased effect of narcotic analgesics; may precipitate acute withdrawal reaction in physically dependent patients

Pregnancy Risk Factor B

Pregnancy Implications Animal studies have not demonstrated fetal harm or fertility impairment. There are no adequate and well-controlled studies in pregnant women. Use only if clearly needed.

Lactation Excretion in breast milk unknown/use caution

Nursing Implications Check dosage strength carefully before use to avoid error (labeling is color-coded; postoperative reversal - blue, overdose management - green); monitor patients for signs of withdrawal, especially those physically dependent who are in pain or at high cardiovascular risk

Specific Reference

Fang WB, Andrenyak DM, Moody DE, et al, "Determination of Nalmefene in Plasma by High-Performance Liquid Chromatography-Electrospray Ionization-Tandem Mass Spectrometry," *J Anal Toxicol*, 2004, 28:298-9.

Naloxone

CAS Number 357-08-4; 465-65-6; 51481-60-8

U.S. Brand Names Narcan®

Synonyms *N*-allylnoroxymorphine Hydrochloride; Naloxone Hydrochloride

Use Reverses CNS and respiratory depression in suspected narcotic/opiate overdose; neonatal opiate depression; coma of unknown etiology

Unlabeled/Investigational Use

Investigational: Shock, alcohol ingestion; pruritus due to cholestasis; also useful in clonidine, camylofin, valproic acid, and captopril overdose; may be useful in reversing cardiac depression due to dextropropoxyphene

Mechanism of Action Competes and displaces narcotics at narcotic/opiate receptor sites

Adverse Reactions

Cardiovascular: Hypertension (may be significant), hypotension, tachycardia, arrhythmias (ventricular), shock, sinus tachycardia

Central nervous system: Insomnia, irritability, anxiety, narcotic withdrawal, psychosis, dysphoria

Dermatologic: Rash

Gastrointestinal: Nausea, vomiting

Genitourinary: Urinary urgency

Hematologic: Coagulopathy

Ocular: Blurred vision

Respiratory: Pulmonary edema has been described

Miscellaneous: Diaphoresis

Signs and Symptoms of Overdose Agitation, anxiety, anorexia, bradycardia, diaphoresis (at 2-4 mg/kg), focal seizures, hypotension, irritability, laryngospasm, nausea

Pharmacodynamics/Kinetics

Onset of action: Endotracheal, I.M., SubQ: 2-5 minutes; I.V.: ~2 minutes

Duration: 20-60 minutes; since shorter than that of most opioids, repeated doses are usually needed

Distribution: Crosses placenta

Metabolism: Primarily hepatic via glucuronidation

Half-life elimination: Neonates: 1.2-3 hours; Adults: 1-1.5 hours

Excretion: Urine (as metabolites)

Dosage

I.M., I.V. (preferred), intratracheal, SubQ:

Postanesthesia narcotic reversal: Infants and Children: 0.01 mg/kg; may repeat every 2-3 minutes, as needed based on response

Opiate intoxication:
Children:
Birth (including premature infants) to 5 years or <20 kg: 0.1 mg/kg; repeat every 2-3 minutes if needed; may need to repeat doses every 20-60 minutes
>5 years or ≥20 kg: 2 mg/dose; if no response, repeat every 2-3 minutes; may need to repeat doses every 20-60 minutes
Children and Adults: Continuous infusion: I.V.: If continuous infusion is required, calculate dosage/hour based on effective intermittent dose used and duration of adequate response seen, titrate dose 0.04-0.16 mg/kg/hour for 2-5 days in children, adult dose typically 0.25-6.25 mg/hour (short-term infusions as high as 2.4 mg/kg/hour have been tolerated in adults during treatment for septic shock); alternatively, continuous infusion utilizes $^2/_3$ of the initial naloxone bolus on an hourly basis; add 10 times this dose to each liter of D_5W and infuse at a rate of 100 mL/hour; $^1/_2$ of the initial bolus dose should be readministered 15 minutes after initiation of the continuous infusion to prevent a drop in naloxone levels; increase infusion rate as needed to assure adequate ventilation; 2 mg naloxone in 3 mL saline can be delivered via nebulization
Narcotic overdose: Adults: I.V.: 0.4-2 mg every 2-3 minutes as needed; may need to repeat doses every 20-60 minutes, if no response is observed after 10 mg, question the diagnosis. **Note:** Use 0.1-0.2 mg increments in patients who are opioid dependent and in postoperative patients to avoid large cardiovascular changes.

Stability Protect from light; stable in 0.9% sodium chloride and D_5W at 4 mcg/mL for 24 hours; do not mix with alkaline solutions

Monitoring Parameters Respiratory rate, heart rate, blood pressure

Administration
Intratracheal: Dilute to 1-2 mL with normal saline
I.V. push: Administer over 30 seconds as undiluted preparation
I.V. continuous infusion: Dilute to 4 mcg/mL in D_5W or normal saline

Contraindications Hypersensitivity to naloxone or any component of the formulation

Warnings Due to an association between naloxone and acute pulmonary edema, use with caution in patients with cardiovascular disease or in patients receiving medications with potential adverse cardiovascular effects (eg, hypotension, pulmonary edema or arrhythmias). Excessive dosages should be avoided after use of opiates in surgery. Abrupt postoperative reversal may result in nausea, vomiting, sweating, tachycardia, hypertension, seizures, and other cardiovascular events (including pulmonary edema and arrhythmias). May precipitate withdrawal symptoms in patients addicted to opiates, including pain, hypertension, sweating, agitation, irritability; in neonates: shrill cry, failure to feed. Recurrence of respiratory depression is possible if the opioid involved is long-acting; observe patients until there is no reasonable risk of recurrent respiratory depression.

Dosage Forms
[DSC] = Discontinued product
Injection, solution, as hydrochloride: 0.4 mg/mL (1 mL, 10 mL)
Narcan®: 0.4 mg/mL (1 mL) [DSC]

Reference Range Plasma naloxone levels at 2 and 5 minutes after a 0.4 mg I.V. dose: 0.01 mg/L and 0.004 mg/L, respectively

Test Interactions Will not give a false-positive enzymatic urine screen for opiates

Drug Interactions Narcotic analgesics: Decreased effect of narcotic analgesics; may precipitate acute withdrawal reaction in physically dependent patients

Pregnancy Risk Factor B

Pregnancy Implications Consider benefit to the mother and the risk to the fetus before administering to a pregnant woman who is known or suspected to be opioid dependent. May precipitate withdrawal in both the mother and fetus.

Lactation Excretion in breast milk unknown/not recommended

Nursing Implications The use of neonatal naloxone is no longer recommended because unacceptable fluid volumes will result, especially to small neonates; the 0.4 mg/mL preparation is available and can be accurately dosed with appropriately sized syringes (1 mL)

Specific References
American Heart Association, ECC Committee, Subcommittees, and Task Forces, "Toxicology in ECC," *Circulation*, 2005, 112(Suppl 1):IV126-IV132.
Greenwald PW, Provataris J, Coffey J, et al, "Low-Dose Naloxone Does Not Improve Morphine-Induced Nausea, Vomiting, or Pruritus," *Am J Emerg Med*, 2005, 23(1):35-9.
Hasan RA, Benko AS, Nolan BM, et al, "Cardiorespiratory Effects of Naloxone in Children," *Ann Pharmacother*, 2003, 37(11):1587-92.
Mycyk MB, Szyszko AL, and Aks SE, "Nebulized Naloxone Gently and Effectively Reverses Methadone Intoxication," *J Emerg Med*, 2003, 24(2):185-7.
Sporer KA, Kral AH, "Prescription Naloxone: A Novel Approach to Heroin Overdose Prevention," *Ann Emerg Med*, 2007, 49:172-177.

Neostigmine

Pronunciation (nee oh STIG meen)
CAS Number 114-80-7; 51-60-5; 59-99-4
U.S. Brand Names Prostigmin®
Synonyms Neostigmine Bromide; Neostigmine Methylsulfate
Use Second-line agent for envenomation by Asian snakes or intoxication with tetradotoxin exposures if edrophonium supplies are depleted; reversal of the effects of nondepolarizing neuromuscular blocking agents after surgery

Mechanism of Action Inhibits destruction of acetylcholine by acetylcholinesterase which facilitates transmission of impulses across myoneural junction

Adverse Reactions
Cardiovascular: Bradycardia, hypotension, bradyarrhythmias, asystole (maximum effect: 90 minutes), chest pain, sinus bradycardia, angina
Central nervous system: Restlessness, agitation, seizures, slurred speech, headache, coma, ataxia
Gastrointestinal: **Hyperperistalsis, nausea, vomiting, salivation, stomach cramps, diarrhea**, defecation
Neuromuscular & skeletal: Tremors, fasciculations, weakness
Ocular: Miosis, lacrimation, nystagmus
Respiratory: Bronchoconstriction, increased bronchial secretion
Miscellaneous: **Diaphoresis**, radiopaque

Signs and Symptoms of Overdose Blurred vision, bradycardia, excessive sweating, muscle weakness, nausea, tachypnea, tearing and salivation, vomiting

Pharmacodynamics/Kinetics
Onset of action: I.M.: 20-30 minutes; I.V.: 1-20 minutes
Duration: I.M.: 2.5-4 hours; I.V.: 1-2 hours
Absorption: Oral: Poor, <2%
Metabolism: Hepatic
Half-life elimination: Normal renal function: 0.5-2.1 hours; End-stage renal disease: Prolonged
Excretion: Urine (50% as unchanged drug)

Dosage
Myasthenia gravis: Diagnosis: I.M.:
Children: 0.04 mg/kg as a single dose
Adults: 0.02 mg/kg as a single dose
Myasthenia gravis: Treatment:
Children:
Oral: 2 mg/kg/day divided every 3-4 hours
I.M., I.V., SubQ: 0.01-0.04 mg/kg every 2-4 hours
Adults:
Oral: 15 mg/dose every 3-4 hours
I.M., I.V., SubQ: 0.5-2.5 mg every 1-3 hours
Reversal of nondepolarizing neuromuscular blockade after surgery in conjunction with atropine or glycopyrrolate: I.V.:
Infants: 0.025-0.1 mg/kg/dose
Children: 0.025-0.08 mg/kg/dose
Adults: 0.5-2.5 mg; total dose not to exceed 5 mg
Bladder atony: Adults: I.M., SubQ:
Prevention: 0.25 mg every 4-6 hours for 2-3 days
Treatment: 0.5-1 mg every 3 hours for 5 doses after bladder has emptied

Monitoring Parameters Respiratory status/muscle weakness
Administration May be administered undiluted by slow I.V. injection over several minutes
Contraindications Hypersensitivity to neostigmine, bromides, or any component of the formulation; GI or GU obstruction
Warnings Does **not** antagonize and may prolong the phase I block of depolarizing muscle relaxants (eg, succinylcholine); use with caution in patients with epilepsy, asthma, bradycardia, hyperthyroidism, cardiac arrhythmias, or peptic ulcer; adequate facilities should be available for cardiopulmonary resuscitation when testing and adjusting dose for myasthenia gravis; have atropine and epinephrine ready to treat hypersensitivity reactions; overdosage may result in cholinergic crisis, this must be distinguished from myasthenic crisis; anticholinesterase insensitivity can develop for brief or prolonged periods

Dosage Forms
Injection, solution, as methylsulfate: 0.5 mg/mL (1 mL, 10 mL); 1 mg/mL (10 mL)
Tablet, as bromide: 15 mg

Test Interactions ↑ aminotransferase [ALT (SGPT)/AST (SGOT)] (S), amylase (S)

Drug Interactions
Anticholinergics: Effects may be reduced with cholinesterase inhibitors; atropine antagonizes the muscarinic effects of cholinesterase inhibitors
Beta-blockers without ISA: Activity may increase risk of bradycardia
Calcium channel blockers (diltiazem or verapamil): May increase risk of bradycardia
Cholinergic agonists: Effects may be increased with cholinesterase inhibitors

Corticosteroids: May see increased muscle weakness and decreased response to anticholinesterases shortly after onset of corticosteroid therapy in the treatment of myasthenia gravis. Deterioration in muscle strength, including severe muscular depression, has been documented in patients with myasthenia gravis while receiving corticosteroids and anticholinesterases.

Digoxin: Increased risk of bradycardia with concurrent use

Neuromuscular blockers: Depolarizing neuromuscular blocking agents effects may be increased with cholinesterase inhibitors; nondepolarizing agents are antagonized by cholinesterase inhibitors

Pregnancy Risk Factor C

Pregnancy Implications Does not cross placental barrier except with large doses

Lactation Excretion in breast milk unknown/not recommended

Nursing Implications In the diagnosis of myasthenia gravis, all anticholinesterase medications should be discontinued for at least 8 hours before administering neostigmine

Norepinephrine

Pronunciation (nor ep i NEF rin)

CAS Number 51-40-1; 51-41-2; 6981-49-5

U.S. Brand Names Levophed®

Synonyms Levarterenol Bitartrate; Noradrenaline Acid Tartrate; Noradrenaline; Norepinephrine Bitartrate

Use Treatment of shock which persists after adequate fluid volume replacement; useful for hypotension induced by tricyclic antidepressants, disulfiram-ethanol interaction, phenothiazine antidysrhythmic agents

Mechanism of Action Stimulates beta$_1$-adrenergic receptors and alpha-adrenergic receptors causing increased contractility and heart rate as well as vasoconstriction, thereby increasing systemic blood pressure and coronary blood flow

Adverse Reactions

Cardiovascular: Cardiac arrhythmias, palpitations, bradycardia, tachycardia, hypertension, chest pain, superior mesenteric artery thrombosis, pallor, ischemic necrosis and sloughing of superficial tissue after extravasation, sinus bradycardia, cardiomyopathy, cardiomegaly, angina, sinus tachycardia, vasoconstriction

Central nervous system: Anxiety, fear, headache

Gastrointestinal: Vomiting

Genitourinary: Uterine contractions

Local: Organ ischemia (due to vasoconstriction of renal and mesenteric arteries)

Ocular: Photophobia, nystagmus

Respiratory: Respiratory distress

Miscellaneous: Diaphoresis

Signs and Symptoms of Overdose Cerebral hemorrhage, hypotension, seizures, sweating

Pharmacodynamics/Kinetics

Onset of action: I.V.: Very rapid-acting

Duration: Limited

Metabolism: Via catechol-o-methyltransferase (COMT) and monoamine oxidase (MAO)

Excretion: Urine (84% to 96% as inactive metabolites)

Dosage

I.V. infusion (dose stated in terms of norepinephrine base):

Children: Initial: 0.05-0.1 mcg/kg/minute, titrate to desired effect

Rate (mL/hour) = dose (mcg/kg/minute) × weight (kg) × 60 minutes/hour divided by concentration (mcg/mL)

Adults: 8-12 mcg/minute as an infusion; initiate at 4 mcg/minute and titrate to desired response

Note: Dose stated in terms of norepinephrine base

Rate of infusion: 4 mg in 500 mL D$_5$W

2 mcg/minute = 15 mL/hour
4 mcg/minute = 30 mL/hour
6 mcg/minute = 45 mL/hour
8 mcg/minute = 60 mL/hour
10 mcg/minute = 75 mL/hour
12 mcg/minute = 90 mL/hour
14 mcg/minute = 105 mL/hour
16 mcg/minute = 120 mL/hour
18 mcg/minute = 135 mL/hour
20 mcg/minute = 150 mL/hour

Stability

Readily oxidized; protect from light. Do not use if brown coloration. Stable in D$_5$NS, D$_5$W, LR; may dilute with D$_5$W or D$_5$NS, but not recommended to dilute in normal saline; not stable in alkaline solutions. Stability of parenteral admixture at room temperature (25°C) is 24 hours.

Y-site administration: Incompatible with insulin (regular), thiopental

Compatibility when admixed: Incompatible with aminophylline, amobarbital, chlorothiazide, chlorpheniramine, pentobarbital, phenobarbital, phenytoin, sodium bicarbonate, streptomycin, thiopental

Monitoring Parameters Blood pressure, heart rate, urine output, peripheral perfusion

Administration Administer into large vein to avoid the potential for extravasation; potent drug, must be diluted prior to use. Rate (mL/hour) = dose (mcg/kg/minute) × weight (kg) × 60 minutes/hour divided by concentration (mcg/mL)

To prepare for infusion:

$$\frac{6 \times \text{weight (Kg)} \times \text{desired dose (mcg/kg/min)}}{\text{I.V. infusion rate (mL/h)}} = \begin{array}{l}\text{mg drug to be added to} \\ \text{10 mL of I.V. fluid}\end{array}$$

Contraindications Hypersensitivity to norepinephrine, bisulfites (contains metabisulfite), or any component of the formulation; hypotension from hypovolemia except as an emergency measure to maintain coronary and cerebral perfusion until volume could be replaced; mesenteric or peripheral vascular thrombosis unless it is a lifesaving procedure; during anesthesia with cyclopropane or halothane anesthesia (risk of ventricular arrhythmias)

Warnings Assure adequate circulatory volume to minimize need for vasoconstrictors. Avoid hypertension; monitor blood pressure closely and adjust infusion rate. Avoid extravasation; infuse into a large vein if possible. Avoid infusion into leg veins. Watch I.V. site closely. **[U.S. Boxed Warning]: If extravasation occurs, infiltrate the area with diluted phentolamine (5-10 mg in 10-15 mL of saline) with a fine hypodermic needle. Phentolamine should be administered as soon as possible after extravasation is noted.**

Dosage Forms Injection, solution, as bitartrate: 1 mg/mL (4 mL) [contains sodium metabisulfite]

Reference Range 24-hour urine catecholamine level: <100 mcg; normal plasma basal norepinephrine level: 100-447 pg/mL

Drug Interactions

Beta-blockers (nonselective ones) may increase hypertensive effect; avoid concurrent use.

Cocaine may cause malignant arrhythmias; avoid concurrent use.

Guanethidine can increase the pressor response; be aware of the patient's drug regimen.

MAO inhibitors potentiate hypertension and hypertensive crisis; avoid concurrent use.

Methyldopa can increase the pressor response; be aware of patient's drug regimen.

Reserpine increases the pressor response; be aware of patient's drug regimen.

TCAs increase the pressor response; be aware of patient's drug regimen.

Pregnancy Risk Factor C

Pregnancy Implications Crosses the placenta

Lactation Excretion in breast milk unknown

Nursing Implications

Central line administration required; do not administer NaHCO$_3$ through an I.V. line containing norepinephrine; administer into large vein to avoid the potential for extravasation; potent drug, must be diluted prior to use

Extravasation: Use phentolamine as antidote; mix 5 mg with 9 mL of NS; inject a small amount of this dilution into extravasated area; blanching should reverse immediately. Monitor site; if blanching should recur, additional injections of phentolamine may be needed.

Obidoxime Chloride

Related Information

- Asoxime Chloride [ANTIDOTE]
- Pralidoxime [ANTIDOTE]

CAS Number 114-90-9; 7683-36-5

Use A cholinesterase activator similar to pralidoxime; used primarily in Europe for organophosphate poisoning and sarin or tabun nerve gas toxicity

Mechanism of Action A quaternary oxime which reactivates cholinesterase; used in conjunction with atropine; less toxic than pralidoxime; has weak anticholinergic activity

Adverse Reactions

Cardiovascular: Hypertension, tachycardia at doses >5 mg/kg

Gastrointestinal: Nausea, vomiting, diarrhea, xerostomia

Hepatic: Transient rise in liver enzymes

Local: Pain at injection site

Neuromuscular & skeletal: Paresthesia

Ocular: Diplopia, blurred vision

Miscellaneous: Menthol-like aftertaste, "hot-feeling"

Dosage

Children: 4-8 mg/kg not to exceed 250 mg

Adults:

I.M. or slow I.V.: Initial: 250 mg, may be repeated once or twice at 2-hour intervals; maximum daily dose: 750 mg; a 5-day course can be considered for moderate to severe exposure

Continuous infusion: About 0.5 mg/kg/hour up to a maximum dose of 750 mg daily

Reference Range Therapeutic blood level: 4 mg/L

Specific References

Bentur Y, Raikhlin-Eisenkraft B, and Singer P, "Beneficial Late Administration of Obidoxime in Malathion Poisoning," *Vet Hum Toxicol*, 2003, 45(1):33-5.

Eyer P, "The Role of Oximes in the Management of Organophosphorus Pesticide Poisoning," *Toxicol Rev*, 2003, 22(3):165-90.

Thierman H, Worek F, Szinicz L, et al, "Effectiveness of Obidoxime in Organophosphate Poisoning," *J Toxicol Clin Toxicol*, 2003, 41(5):677.

Octreotide

Pronunciation (ok TREE oh tide)

CAS Number 79517-01-4; 83150-76-9

U.S. Brand Names Sandostatin LAR®; Sandostatin®

Synonyms NSC-671663; Octreotide Acetate

Use Useful in treating hypoglycemia due to sulfonylurea ingestion; variceal hemorrhage, acromegaly, carcinoid syndrome, vasoactive intestinal peptide tumors, pancreatic and enteric fistulas, secretory diarrhea; radiation-induced diarrhea; treatment of L-asparaginase induced pancreatitis

Unlabeled/Investigational Use AIDS-associated secretory diarrhea (including *Cryptosporidiosis*), control of bleeding of esophageal varices, breast cancer, cryptosporidiosis, Cushing's syndrome (ectopic), cystoid macular edema, insulinomas, small bowel fistulas, pancreatic tumors, gastrinoma, postgastrectomy dumping syndrome, chemotherapy-induced diarrhea, graft-versus-host disease (GVHD) induced diarrhea, Zollinger-Ellison syndrome, congenital hyperinsulinism

Mechanism of Action An octapeptide analogue of somatostatin which inhibits growth hormone secretion and insulin secretion

Adverse Reactions

Adverse reactions vary by route of administration. Frequency of cardiac, endocrine, and gastrointestinal adverse reactions were generally higher in acromegalics.

>16%:

Cardiovascular: Sinus bradycardia (19% to 25%), chest pain (16% to 20%)

Central nervous system: Fatigue (1% to 20%), malaise (16% to 20%), dizziness (5% to 20%), headache (6% to 20%), fever (16% to 20%)

Endocrine & metabolic: Hyperglycemia (2% to 27%)

Gastrointestinal: Diarrhea (5% to 61%), abdominal discomfort (5% to 61%), flatulence (<10% to 38%), constipation (9% to 21%), nausea (5% to 61%), cholelithiasis (27%; length of therapy dependent), biliary duct dilatation (12%), biliary sludge (24%; length of therapy dependent), loose stools (5% to 61%), vomiting (4% to 21%)

Hematologic: Antibodies to octreotide (up to 25%; no efficacy change)

Local: Injection pain (2% to 50%; dose- and formulation-related)

Neuromuscular & skeletal: Backache (1% to 20%), arthropathy (16% to 20%)

Respiratory: Dyspnea (16% to 20%), upper respiratory infection (16% to 20%)

Miscellaneous: Flu symptoms (1% to 20%)

5% to 15%:

Cardiovascular: Conduction abnormalities (9% to 10%), arrhythmia (3% to 9%), hypertension, palpitations, peripheral edema

Central nervous system: Anxiety, confusion, depression, hypoesthesia, insomnia, vertigo

Dermatologic: Pruritus, rash

Endocrine & metabolic: Hypothyroidism (2% to 12%), goiter (2% to 8%)

Gastrointestinal: Abdominal pain, anorexia, cramping, dehydration, discomfort, hemorrhoids, tenesmus (4% to 6%), dyspepsia (4% to 6%), steatorrhea (4% to 6%), feces discoloration (4% to 6%), weight loss

Genitourinary: UTI

Hematologic: Anemia

Hepatic: Hepatitis

Neuromuscular & skeletal: Arthralgia, leg cramps, myalgia, paresthesia, rigors, weakness

Otic: ear ache, otitis media

Renal: renal calculus

Respiratory: coughing, pharyngitis, sinusitis, rhinitis

Miscellaneous: Allergy, diaphoresis

1% to 4%:

Cardiovascular: Angina, cardiac failure, cerebral vascular disorder, edema, flushing, hematoma, phlebitis, tachycardia

Central nervous system: Abnormal gait, amnesia, dysphonia, hallucinations, nervousness, neuralgia, neuropathy, somnolence, tremor, vertigo

Dermatologic: Acne, alopecia, bruising, cellulitis, urticaria

Endocrine & metabolic: Hypoglycemia (2% to 4%), hypokalemia, hypoproteinemia, gout, cachexia, menstrual irregularities, breast pain, impotence, hyperkalemia

Gastrointestinal: Colitis, diverticulitis, dysphagia, fat malabsorption, gastritis, gastroenteritis, gingivitis, glossitis, melena, rectal bleeding, stomatitis, taste perversion, xerostomia

Genitourinary: Incontinence

Hematologic: Epistaxis

Hepatic: Ascites, jaundice

Local: Injection hematoma

Neuromuscular & skeletal: Hyperkinesia, hypertonia, joint pain

Ocular: Blurred vision, visual disturbance

Otic: Tinnitus

Renal: Albuminuria, renal abscess

Respiratory: Bronchitis, pleural effusion, pneumonia, pulmonary embolism

Miscellaneous: Bacterial infection, cold symptoms, moniliasis

<1%: Abdomen enlarged, anaphylactic shock, anaphylactoid reaction, aneurysm, aphasia, appendicitis, arthritis, atrial fibrillation, basal cell carcinoma, Bell's palsy, breast carcinoma, burning eyes, cardiac arrest, CHF, CK increased, creatinine increased, deafness, diabetes insipidus, diabetes mellitus, facial edema, fatty liver, galactorrhea, gallbladder polyp, gallstones, GI hemorrhage, glaucoma, gynecomastia, hematuria, hemiparesis, hepatitis, hyperesthesia, hypertensive reaction, hypoadrenalism, intestinal obstruction, intracranial hemorrhage, iron deficiency, ischemia, joint effusion, lactation, leg cramps, LFTs increased, libido decreased, malignant hyperpyrexia, MI, migraine, muscle cramping, nephrolithiasis, orthostatic hypotension, pancreatitis, paranoia, paresis, peptic ulcer, petechiae, pituitary apoplexy, pneumothorax, pulmonary hypertension, pulmonary nodule, Raynaud's syndrome, renal insufficiency, retinal vein thrombosis, rhinorrhea, scotoma, seizure, status asthmaticus, suicide attempt, throat discomfort, thrombocytopenia, thrombophlebitis, thrombosis, vaginitis, visual field defect, wheal/erythema

Pharmacodynamics/Kinetics

Duration: SubQ: 6-12 hours

Absorption: SubQ: Rapid

Distribution: V_d: 14 L (13-30 L in acromegaly)

Protein binding: 65%, mainly to lipoprotein (41% in acromegaly)

Metabolism: Extensively hepatic

Bioavailability: SubQ: 100%; I.M: 60% to 63% of SubQ dose

Half-life elimination: 1.7-1.9 hours; up to 3.7 hours with cirrhosis

Time to peak, plasma: SubQ: 0.4 hours (0.7 hours acromegaly); I.M.: 1 hour

Excretion: Urine (32%)

Dosage

Infants and Children:

Secretory diarrhea (unlabeled use): I.V., SubQ: Doses of 1-10 mcg/kg every 12 hours have been used in children beginning at the low end of the range and increasing by 0.3 mcg/kg/dose at 3-day intervals. Suppression of growth hormone (animal data) is of concern when used as long-term therapy.

Congenital hyperinsulinism (unlabeled use): SubQ: Doses of 3-40 mcg/kg/day have been used

Adults: SubQ, I.V.: Initial: 50 mcg 2 to 4 times/day and titrate dose based on patient tolerance, response, and indication

For sulfonylurea overdose: Adults 50 to 100 mcg SQ every 6 hours; Children; 1 to 1.5 mcg per kg every 6 hours SQ.

Carcinoid: Initial 2 weeks: 100-600 mcg/day in 2-4 divided doses; usual range 50-1500 mcg/day

VIPomas: Initial 2 weeks: 200-300 mcg/day in 2-4 divided doses; usual range 150-750 mcg/day

Diarrhea (unlabeled use): Initial: I.V.: 50-100 mcg every 8 hours; increase by 100 mcg/dose at 48-hour intervals; maximum dose: 500 mcg every 8 hours

Esophageal varices bleeding (unlabeled use): I.V. bolus: 25-50 mcg followed by continuous I.V. infusion of 25-50 mcg/hour

Acromegaly: Initial: SubQ: 50 mcg 3 times/day; titrate to achieve growth hormone levels <5 ng/mL or IGF-I (somatomedin C) levels <1.9 U/mL in males and <2.2 U/mL in females; usual effective dose 100 mcg 3 times/day; range 300-1500 mcg/day

Note: Should be withdrawn yearly for a 4-week interval (8 weeks for depot injection) in patients who have received irradiation. Resume if levels increase and signs/symptoms recur.

Acromegaly, carcinoid tumors, and VIPomas (depot injection): Patients must be stabilized on subcutaneous octreotide for at least 2 weeks before switching to the long-acting depot: Upon switch: 20 mg I.M. intragluteally every 4 weeks for 2-3 months, then the dose may be modified based upon response. Patients receiving depot injection for carcinoid tumor or VIPoma should continue to receive their SubQ injections for the first 2 weeks at the same dose in order to maintain therapeutic levels.

Dosage adjustment for acromegaly: After 3 months of depot injections the dosage may be continued or modified as follows:

GH ≤2.5 ng/mL, IGF-1 is normal, symptoms controlled: Maintain octreotide LAR® at 20 mg I.M. every 4 weeks

GH >2.5 ng/mL, IGF-1 is elevated, and/or symptoms uncontrolled: Increase octreotide LAR® to 30 mg I.M. every 4 weeks

GH ≤ 1 ng/mL, IGF-1 is normal, symptoms controlled: Reduce octreotide LAR® to 10 mg I.M. every 4 weeks

Note: Patients not adequately controlled may increase dose to 40 mg every 4 weeks. Dosages >40 mg are not recommended

Dosage adjustment for carcinoid tumors and VIPomas: After 2 months of depot injections the dosage may be continued or modified as follows:

Increase to 30 mg I.M. every 4 weeks if symptoms are inadequately controlled

Decrease to 10 mg I.M. every 4 weeks, for a trial period, if initially responsive to 20 mg dose

Dosage >30 mg is not recommended

Elderly: Elimination half-life is increased by 46% and clearance is decreased by 26%; dose adjustment may be required.

Dosage adjustment in renal impairment: Severe renal failure requiring dialysis: Clearance is reduced by $\sim 50\%$; specific dosing guidelines not available

Monitoring Parameters

Acromegaly: Growth hormone, somatomedin C (IGF-1)

Carcinoid: 5-HIAA, plasma serotonin and plasma substance P

VIPomas: Vasoactive intestinal peptide

Chronic therapy: Thyroid function (baseline and periodic), vitamin B_{12} level, blood glucose, cardiac function (heart rate, EKG)

Administration

Regular injection formulation (do not use if solution contains particles or is discolored): Administer SubQ or I.V.; I.V. administration may be IVP, IVPB, or continuous I.V. infusion:

IVP should be administered undiluted over 3 minutes

IVPB should be administered over 15-30 minutes

Continuous I.V. infusion rates have ranged from 25-50 mcg/hour for the treatment of esophageal variceal bleeding

Depot injection: Administer I.M. intragluteal (avoid deltoid administration); alternate gluteal injection sites to avoid irritation. Do not administer Sandostatin LAR® intravenously or subcutaneously; must be administered immediately after mixing.

Contraindications Hypersensitivity to octreotide or any component of the formulation

Warnings May impair gall bladder function; monitor patients for cholelithiasis. Use with caution in patients with renal impairment. Somatostatin analogs may affect glucose regulation; in type I diabetes, severe hypoglycemia may occur; in type II diabetes or nondiabetic patients, hyperglycemia may occur. Insulin and other hypoglycemic medication requirements may change. Bradycardia, conduction abnormalities, and arrhythmia have been observed in acromegalic patients; use caution with CHF or concomitant medications that alter heart rate or rhythm. May alter absorption of dietary fats; monitor for pancreatitis. Chronic treatment has been associated with abnormal Schillings test; monitor vitamin B_{12} levels. Tumors which secrete growth hormone may increase in size; monitor. Suppresses secretion of TSH; monitor for hypothyroidism.

Dosage Forms

Injection, microspheres for suspension, as acetate [depot formulation]:

Sandostatin LAR®: 10 mg, 20 mg, 30 mg [with diluent and syringe]

Injection, solution, as acetate: 0.2 mg/mL (5 mL); 1 mg/mL (5 mL)

Sandostatin®: 0.2 mg/mL (5 mL); 1 mg/mL (5 mL)

Injection, solution, as acetate [preservative free]: 0.05 mg/mL (1 mL); 0.1 mg/mL (1 mL); 0.5 mg/mL (1 mL)

Sandostatin®: 0.05 mg/mL (1 mL); 0.1 mg/mL (1 mL); 0.5 mg/mL (1 mL)

Reference Range Peak plasma octreotide after 200 mcg I.V. and SubQ doses: ~ 27.8 ng/mL and 10.6 ng/mL, respectively

Test Interactions May interfere with the TSH assay, resulting in falsely low TSH levels

Drug Interactions

Bromocriptine: Bioavailability of bromocriptine may be increased by octreotide.

Cyclosporine: Case reports of transplant rejection due to reduction of serum cyclosporine levels when cyclosporine was given orally in conjunction with a somatostatin analogue.

QT_c-prolonging agents: Octreotide may enhance the adverse/toxic effects of other QT_c-prolonging agents. Use with caution; monitor.

Pregnancy Risk Factor B

Pregnancy Implications Teratogenic effects were not reported in animal studies. Octreotide crosses the human placenta; data concerning use in pregnancy is limited.

Lactation Excretion in breast milk unknown/use caution

Specific References

Al-Zubairy SA and Al-Jazairi AS, "Octreotide as a Therapeutic Option for Management of Chylothorax," *Ann Pharmacother*, 2003, 37(5):679-82.

Calello DP, Osterhoudt KC, Henretig FM, et al, "Octreotide for Pediatric Sulfonylurea Overdose: Review of 5 Cases," *Clin Toxicol (Phila)*, 2005, 43:671.

Curtis JA and Greenberg MI, "Bradycardia and Hyperkalemia Associated with Octreotide Administration," *Clin Toxicol*, 44:498.

Fansano CJ, O'Malley GF, and Dominic PF, "A Prospective Trial of Octreotide vs Placebo in Recurrent Sulfonylurea-Associated Hypoglycemia," *Acad Emerg Med*, 2006, 13(5):S180.

Fernandez-Real JM, Recasaens M, and Rucart W, "Octreotide-Induced Manic Episodes in a Patient with Acromegaly," *Ann Int Med*, 2006, 144(9):704.

Green RS and Palatnick W, "Effectiveness of Octreotide in a Case of Refractory Sulfonylurea-Induced Hypoglycemia," *J Emerg Med*, 2003, 25(3):283-7.

Kent DA, Main BA, and Friesen MS, "Use of Octreotide in Sulfonylurea Poisoning in a Child," *J Toxicol Clin Toxicol*, 2003, 41(5):669.

Ries NL, Dart RC. "New Developments in Antidotes," *Med Clin North Am*, 2005, 89(6):1379-97 (review).

Oxygen (Hyperbaric)

Use Carbon monoxide, carbon tetrachloride, cyanide, hydrocarbon, hydrogen sulfide, methylene chloride, mushroom (*Amanita* toxin), brown recluse spider bite, chloroform; also decompression sickness, air emboli, and anaerobic infections

Unlabeled/Investigational Use May also be useful in methemoglobinemia; treatment of helium-induced embolism; to treat ergotamine-induced peripheral ischemia; useful for necrotic arachnidism caused by Lampona cylindrata (spider found in Australia); radiation-related bone and soft tissue complications (osteoradionecrosis); gas gangrene

Mechanism of Action Displaces carbon monoxide from binding sites and increases elimination rate; also alleviates cerebral edema and CO-induced peroxidation

Adverse Reactions

Ocular: Temporary visual deficits, vision color changes (increased color perception), retinal vessel narrowing

Otic: Otic discomfort, ruptured tympanic membranes

Miscellaneous: Barotrauma to CNS or lung and seizures are reported with prolonged durations (greater than those used for CO poisoning)

Dosage 2.5-3 atmospheres

Reference Range Concentrations of CO $>30\%$ in nonpregnant patients or $>20\%$ in pregnant patients are indications for treatment

Pregnancy Risk Factor No data reported

Pregnancy Implications Well tolerated in the treatment of carbon monoxide and indicated for the treatment of pregnant patients when symptomatic or with carboxyhemoglobin levels $>20\%$

Specific References

Domachevsky L, Adir Y, Grupper M, et al, "Hyperbaric Oxygen in the Treatment of Carbon Monoxide Poisoning," *Clin Toxicol (Phila)*, 2005, 43(3):181-8 (review).

Judge BS and Brown MD. "Evidence-Based Emergency Medicine/Systematic Review Abstract: To Dive or Not To Dive? Use of Hyperbaric Oxygen Therapy to Prevent Neurologic Sequelae in Patients Acutely Poisoned with Carbon Monoxide," *Ann Emerg Med*, 2005, 46(5):462-4.

Workman WT "Hyperbaric Oxygen Therapy: A High Risk Procedure? An Update," *Undersea Hyperb Med*, 2006, 33(4):310-11.

Workman WT "Hyperbaric Oxygen Therapy: A High Risk Procedure? An Update II," *Undersea Hyperb Med*, 2006, 33(6):473.

Penicillamine

Pronunciation (pen i SIL a meen)

CAS Number 2219-30-9; 52-67-5; 59-53-0

U.S. Brand Names Cuprimine®; Depen®

Synonyms D-3-Mercaptovaline; D-Penicillamine; β,β-Dimethylcysteine

Use Treatment of Wilson's disease, cystinuria, adjunct in the treatment of rheumatoid arthritis

Unlabeled/Investigational Use Lead, mercury, copper, arsenic, and possibly gold poisoning (**Note:** Oral succimer [DMSA] is preferable for lead or mercury poisoning)

Mechanism of Action Chelates with lead, copper, mercury, iron, and other heavy metals to form stable, soluble complexes that are excreted in urine; depresses circulating IgM rheumatoid factor, depresses T-cell but not B-cell activity; combines with cystine to form a compound which is more soluble, thus cystine calculi are prevented

Adverse Reactions

Cardiovascular: Edema of the feet, or lower legs; periarteritis nodosa, AV block, facial edema, vasculitis

Central nervous system: **Fever**, seizures, chills, tiredness, dysphoria, dysosmia, Guillain-Barré syndrome, sedation, extrapyramidal reactions, agitation, anxiety, dystonia, mental disorders

Dermatologic: **Rash**, pemphigus, increased friability of the skin, hirsutism, epidural necrolysis, **hives, itching**, psoriasiform eruptions, fingernail discoloration (yellow), fingernail dystrophy, lichenoid eruptions, scleroderma, seborrheic dermatitis, skin discoloration (yellow), **urticaria**, vitiligo, bullous pemphigoid, exfoliative dermatitis, alopecia, toxic epidermal necrolysis, xerosis, purpura, erythema nodosum, exanthem, cutaneous vasculitis

Endocrine & metabolic: Iron deficiency, gynecomastia, hyperglycemia, insulin antibody formation, Hashimoto's disease, Graves' disease, autoimmune thyroid disease, thyroiditis, thymoma, breast enlargement (3-18 months)

Gastrointestinal: Oral lesions, diarrhea, colitis, nausea, vomiting, **hypogeusia**, anorexia, weight gain, sore throat, metallic taste, altered taste, stomatitis, salt hypogeusia, aphthous stomatitis

Genitourinary: Bloody and cloudy urine

Hematologic: Leukopenia, thrombocytopenia (12% to 27% in patients with rheumatoid arthritis), eosinophilia, aplastic anemia, hemolytic anemia, lymphopenia, sideroblastic anemia, neutropenia, agranulocytosis

Hepatic: Hepatic dysfunction

Neuromuscular & skeletal: **Arthralgia**, myasthenia gravis, polymyositis (dermatomyositis), myositis, weakness, peripheral sensory and motor neuropathies, myasthenic syndrome, dysarthria, myalgia, tremor

Ocular: Optic neuritis, ptosis, diplopia, retinopathy, photophobia, ophthalmoplegia

Otic: Tinnitus

Renal: Nephrotic syndrome, renal vasculitis, hematuria, glomerulonephritis, Goodpasture-like syndrome, albuminuria

Respiratory: Obliterative bronchiolitis, pulmonary fibrosis, interstitial pneumonitis, coughing or wheezing, rhinitis, pleural effusion, alveolar hemorrhage, pulmonary hemorrhage, bronchiolitis obliterans organizing pneumonia, asthma, eosinophilic pneumonia, pulmonary vasculitis

Miscellaneous: Lymphadenopathy, allergic reactions, SLE-like syndrome, white spots on lips or mouth, elevated antineutrophilic cytoplasmic antibodies (ANCA)

Signs and Symptoms of Overdose Acrodynia, agitation, dysphagia, hemoptysis, hypertrichosis, nausea, seizures, vomiting

Pharmacodynamics/Kinetics

Onset of action: Rheumatoid arthritis: 2-3 months; Wilson's disease: 1-3 months

Absorption: 40% to 70%

Protein binding: 80% to albumin

Metabolism: Hepatic (small amounts)

Half-life elimination: 1.7-3.2 hours

Time to peak, serum: ~2 hours

Excretion: Urine (30% to 60% as unchanged drug)

Dosage

Oral:

Rheumatoid arthritis:

Children: Initial: 3 mg/kg/day ($\leq$250 mg/day) for 3 months, then 6 mg/kg/day ($\leq$500 mg/day) in divided doses twice daily for 3 months to a maximum of 10 mg/kg/day in 3-4 divided doses

Adults: 125-250 mg/day, may increase dose at 1- to 3-month intervals up to 1-1.5 g/day

Wilson's disease (doses titrated to maintain urinary copper excretion >1 mg/day):

Infants <6 months: 250 mg/dose once daily

Children <12 years: 250 mg/dose 2-3 times/day

Adults: 250 mg 4 times/day

Cystinuria:

Children: 30 mg/kg/day in 4 divided doses

Adults: 1-4 g/day in divided doses every 6 hours

Lead poisoning (unlabeled use): In acute poisoning, continue until blood lead level is <15 mcg/dL; may also be used in other heavy metal poisoning:

Children: 25-35 mg/kg/day, administered in 3-4 divided doses; initiating treatment at 25% of this dose and gradually increasing to the full dose over 2-3 weeks may minimize adverse reactions

Adults: 250-500 mg/dose every 8-12 hours

Primary biliary cirrhosis: 250 mg/day to start, increase by 250 mg every 2 weeks up to a maintenance dose of 1 g/day, usually given 250 mg 4 times/day

Arsenic poisoning: Children: 100 mg/kg/day in divided doses every 6 hours for 5 days; maximum: 1 g/day

Dosing adjustment/comments in renal impairment: Cl_{cr} <50 mL/minute: Avoid use

Stability Store in tight, well-closed containers

Monitoring Parameters

Urinalysis, CBC with differential, platelet count (twice weekly); weekly measurements of urinary and blood concentration of the intoxicating metal is indicated (3 months has been tolerated). In Wilson's disease, liver function tests should be monitored every 3 months during the first year of treatment.

CBC: WBC <3500/mm^3, neutrophils <2000/mm^3 or monocytes >500/mm^3 indicate need to stop therapy immediately; quantitative 24-hour urine protein at 1- to 2-week intervals initially (first 2-3 months); urinalysis, LFTs occasionally; platelet counts <100,000/mm^3 indicate need to stop therapy until numbers of platelets increase

Administration

For patients who cannot swallow, contents of capsules may be administered in 15-30 mL of chilled puréed fruit or fruit juice. Give on an empty stomach (1 hour before meals and at bedtime).

Cystinuria: If administering 4 equal doses is not feasible, administer the larger dose at bedtime.

Rheumatoid arthritis: Doses $\leq$500 mg/day may be given as a single dose; >500 mg administer in divided doses

Contraindications Hypersensitivity to penicillamine or any component of the formulation; renal insufficiency (in patients with rheumatoid arthritis); patients with previous penicillamine-related aplastic anemia or agranulocytosis; breast-feeding; pregnancy (in patients with rheumatoid arthritis)

Warnings Cross-sensitivity with penicillin is possible; therefore, should be used cautiously in patients with a history of penicillin allergy. Once instituted for Wilson's disease or cystinuria, continue treatment on a daily basis; interruptions of even a few days have been followed by hypersensitivity with reinstitution of therapy. Penicillamine has been associated with fatalities due to agranulocytosis, aplastic anemia, thrombocytopenia, Goodpasture's syndrome, and myasthenia gravis. **[U.S. Boxed Warning]: Patients should be warned to report promptly any symptoms suggesting toxicity (fever, sore throat, chills, bruising, or bleeding);** approximately 33% of patients will experience an allergic reaction; toxicity may be dose related, use caution in the elderly. Use caution with other hematopoietic-depressant drugs (eg, gold, immunosuppressants, antimalarials, phenylbutazone); hematologic and renal adverse reactions are similar. Proteinuria or hematuria may develop; monitor for membranous glomerulopathy which can lead to nephrotic syndrome. In rheumatoid arthritis patients, discontinue if gross hematuria or persistent microscopic hematuria develop. Monitor liver function tests periodically due to rare reports of intrahepatic cholestasis or toxic hepatitis. **[U.S. Boxed Warning]: Should be administered under the close supervision of a physician familiar with the toxicity and dosage considerations.**

Dosage Forms

[DSC] = Discontinued product

Capsule (Cuprimine®): 125 mg [DSC], 250 mg

Tablet (Depen®): 250 mg

Test Interactions Positive ANA

Drug Interactions

Antacids: May decrease the effects of penicillamine.

Digoxin: Penicillamine may decrease the levels of digoxin; monitor.

Iron salts: May decrease the effects of penicillamine.

Pregnancy Risk Factor D

Pregnancy Implications Correlated with cutis laxa in neonates

Lactation Excretion in breast milk unknown/contraindicated

Nursing Implications For patients who cannot swallow, contents of capsules may be administered in 15-30 mL of chilled puréed fruit or fruit juice; patients should be warned to report promptly any symptoms suggesting toxicity

Phentolamine

Pronunciation (fen TOLE a meen)

CAS Number 65-28-1

U.S. Brand Names Regitine®

Synonyms Phentolamine Mesylate; Regitine [DSC]

Use Diagnosis of pheochromocytoma and treatment of hypertension associated with pheochromocytoma or other forms of hypertension caused by excess sympathomimetic amines; as treatment of dermal necrosis after extravasation of drugs with alpha-adrenergic effects (norepinephrine, dopamine, epinephrine); may reverse cocaine-induced coronary artery vasoconstriction.

Unlabeled/Investigational Use Treatment of pralidoxime-induced hypertension

Mechanism of Action Competitively blocks alpha-adrenergic receptors to produce brief antagonism of circulating epinephrine and norepinephrine to reduce hypertension caused by these catecholamines; no inotropic activity

Adverse Reactions

Cardiovascular: **Reflex tachycardia, anginal pain**, myocardial infarction, **hypotension (orthostatic), tachycardia**, chest pain, facial flushing, pulmonary hypertension, sinus tachycardia, vasodilation

Central nervous system: Fainting, severe headache

Endocrine & metabolic: Hypocalcemia, can precipitate disulfiram-like reaction with ethanol

Gastrointestinal: **Nausea, abdominal pain, diarrhea, vomiting, exacerbation of peptic ulcer**, decreased esophageal sphincter tone

Genitourinary: Priapism with injection into corpus cavernosum

Neuromuscular & skeletal: Weakness

Respiratory: **Nasal congestion**

Pharmacodynamics/Kinetics

Onset of action: I.M.: 15-20 minutes; I.V.: Immediate

Duration: I.M.: 30-45 minutes; I.V.: 15-30 minutes

Metabolism: Hepatic

Half-life elimination: 19 minutes

Excretion: Urine (10% as unchanged drug)

Dosage

Treatment of alpha-adrenergic drug extravasation: SubQ:

Children: 0.1-0.2 mg/kg diluted in 10 mL 0.9% sodium chloride infiltrated into area of extravasation within 12 hours

Adults: Infiltrate area with small amount of solution made by diluting 5-10 mg in 10 mL 0.9% sodium chloride within 12 hours of extravasation; do not exceed 0.1-0.2 mg/kg or 5 mg total

If dose is effective, normal skin color should return to the blanched area within 1 hour

Diagnosis of pheochromocytoma: I.M., I.V.:

Children: 0.05-0.1 mg/kg/dose, maximum single dose: 5 mg

Adults: 5 mg

Surgery for pheochromocytoma: Hypertension: I.M., I.V.:

Children: 0.05-0.1 mg/kg/dose given 1-2 hours before procedure; repeat as needed every 2-4 hours until hypertension is controlled; maximum single dose: 5 mg

Adults: 5 mg given 1-2 hours before procedure and repeated as needed every 2-4 hours

Hypertensive crisis: Adults: 5-20 mg

Treatment of pralidoxime-induced hypertension (unlabeled use): I.V.:

Children: 1 mg

Adults and Elderly: 5 mg

Reverse cocaine-induced cardiac vasoconstriction: Titrate in 1 mg doses

Treatment of opioid-induced acute gastroparesis: 0.5 mg/kg I.V. over sixty minutes

Stability Reconstituted solution is stable for 48 hours at room temperature and 1 week when refrigerated

Monitoring Parameters Blood pressure, heart rate; area of infiltration

Administration Treatment of extravasation: Infiltrate area of extravasation with multiple small injections; use 27- or 30-gauge needles and change needle between each skin entry

Contraindications Hypersensitivity to phentolamine or any component of the formulation; renal impairment; coronary or cerebral arteriosclerosis; concurrent use with phosphodiesterase-5 (PDE-5) inhibitors including sildenafil (>25 mg), tadalafil, or vardenafil

Warnings Myocardial infarction, cerebrovascular spasm and cerebrovascular occlusion have occurred following administration. Use with caution in patients with gastritis or peptic ulcer, tachycardia, or a history of cardiac arrhythmias.

Dosage Forms Injection, powder for reconstitution, as mesylate: 5 mg

Test Interactions ↑ LFTs, rarely

Drug Interactions

Epinephrine, ephedrine: Effects may be decreased.

Ethanol: Increased toxicity (disulfiram reaction).

Sildenafil, tadalafil, vardenafil: Blood pressure-lowering effects are additive. Use of tadalafil or vardenafil is contraindicated by the manufacturer. Use sildenafil with extreme caution (dose ≤25 mg).

Pregnancy Risk Factor C

Lactation Excretion in breast milk unknown

Nursing Implications Infiltrate the area of dopamine extravasation with multiple small injections using only 27- or 30-gauge needles and changing the needle between each skin entry; take care not to cause so much swelling of the extremity or digit that a compartment syndrome occurs; monitor patient for orthostasis; assist with ambulation

Specific Reference

Philips WJ, Tollefson B, Johnson A et al, "Relief of Acute Pain in Chronic Idiopathic Gastroparesis with Intravenous Phentolamine," *Ann Pharmacol*, 2006, 40(11):2032-6.

Physostigmine

Pronunciation (fye zoe STIG meen)

Related Information

● Toxins Which Should Be Lavaged with Solutions Other Than Water

CAS Number 57-47-6; 57-64-7; 64-47-1

U.S. Brand Names Antilirium®

Synonyms Eserine Salicylate; Physostigmine Salicylate; Physostigmine Sulfate

Use Second-line agent for envenomation of Asian snakes or intoxication with tetradotoxin exposures if edrophonium supplies are depleted; reverse toxic CNS effects caused by anticholinergic drugs; controversial role for baclofen, and tricyclic antidepressant toxicity

Mechanism of Action Inhibits destruction of acetylcholine by acetylcholinesterase which facilitates transmission of impulses across myoneural junction

Adverse Reactions

Cardiovascular: Palpitations, bradycardia

Central nervous system: Restlessness, nervousness, hallucinations, seizures

Gastrointestinal: Nausea, salivation, diarrhea, stomach pains

Genitourinary: Frequent urge to urinate

Neuromuscular & skeletal: Muscle twitching

Ocular: Lacrimation, miosis

Respiratory: Dyspnea, bronchospasm, respiratory paralysis, pulmonary edema

Miscellaneous: Diaphoresis

Signs and Symptoms of Overdose Blurred vision, excessive sweating, fasciculations, hallucinations, hypertension, laryngospasm, muscle weakness, nausea, seizures, tearing and salivation, vomiting

Pharmacodynamics/Kinetics

Onset of action: ~5 minutes

Duration: 0.5-5 hours

Absorption: I.M., SubQ: Readily absorbed

Distribution: Crosses blood-brain barrier readily and reverses both central and peripheral anticholinergic effects

Metabolism: Hepatic and via hydrolysis by cholinesterases

Half-life elimination: 15-40 minutes

Dosage

Children: Anticholinergic drug overdose: Reserve for life-threatening situations only: I.V.: 0.01-0.03 mg/kg/dose (maximum: 0.5 mg/minute); may repeat after 5-10 minutes to a maximum total dose of 2 mg or until response occurs or adverse cholinergic effects occur

Adults: Anticholinergic drug overdose:

I.M., I.V., SubQ: 0.5-2 mg to start, repeat every 20 minutes until response occurs or adverse effect occurs

Repeat 1-4 mg every 30-60 minutes as life-threatening signs (arrhythmias, seizures, deep coma) recur; maximum I.V. rate: 1 mg/minute

Stability Do not use solution if cloudy or dark brown

Monitoring Parameters Heart rate, respiratory rate

Administration Injection: Infuse slowly I.V. at a maximum rate of 0.5 mg/minute in children or 1 mg/minute in adults. Too rapid administration (I.V. rate not to exceed 1 mg/minute) can cause bradycardia, hypersalivation leading to respiratory difficulties and seizures.

Contraindications Hypersensitivity to physostigmine or any component of the formulation; GI or GU obstruction; physostigmine therapy of drug intoxications should be used with extreme caution in patients with asthma, gangrene, severe cardiovascular disease, or mechanical obstruction of the GI tract or urogenital tract. In these patients, physostigmine should be used only to treat life-threatening conditions.

Warnings Use with caution in patients with epilepsy, asthma, diabetes, gangrene, cardiovascular disease, bradycardia. Discontinue if excessive salivation or emesis, frequent urination or diarrhea occur. Reduce dosage if excessive sweating or nausea occurs. Administer I.V. slowly or at a controlled rate not faster than 1 mg/minute. Due to the possibility of hypersensitivity or overdose/cholinergic crisis, atropine should be readily available; not intended as a first-line agent for anticholinergic toxicity or Parkinson's disease.

Dosage Forms Injection, solution, as salicylate: 1 mg/mL (2 mL) [contains benzyl alcohol and sodium metabisulfite]

Reference Range Fifteen minutes after a 2 mg oral dose of physostigmine salicylate, plasma level was reported as 1.03 ng/mL

Test Interactions ↑ aminotransferase [ALT (SGPT)/AST (SGOT)] (S), amylase (S); ↑ serum cortisol, prolactin, and epinephrine levels

Drug Interactions Increased toxicity: Bethanechol, methacholine, succinylcholine may increase neuromuscular blockade with systemic administration

Pregnancy Risk Factor C

Lactation Excretion in breast milk unknown

Specific References

Bania TC, Chu J, O'Neil M, et al, "Effects of Physostigmine Following Cessation of Chronic GHB Administration in Mice," *Acad Emerg Med*, 2003, 10:518.

Brown DV, Heller F, and Barkin R, "Anticholinergic Syndrome After Anesthesia: A Case Report and Review," *Am J Ther*, 2004, 11(2):144-53.

Ganetsky M, Babu KM, Lian IE, et al, "Case Series of Physostigmine for Olanzapine and Quetiapine-Induced Anticholinergic Syndrome," *Clin Toxicol (Phila)*, 2005, 43:674.

Schneir AB, Offerman SR, Ly BT, et al, "Complications of Diagnostic Physostigmine Administration to Emergency Department Patients," *Ann Emerg Med*, 2003, 42(1):14-9.

Suchard JR, "Assessing Physostigmine's Contraindication in Cyclic Antidepressant Ingestions," *J Emerg Med*, 2003, 25(2):185-91.

Watts D and Wax P, "Physostigmine Administration for Quetiapine Toxicity," *J Toxicol Clin Toxicol*, 2003, 41(5):646.

Zvosec DL, Smith SW, and Litonjua MR, "Physostigmine for Gamma Hydroxybutyrate Coma: Lack of Efficacy and Adverse Events in 5 Patients," *Clin Toxicol (Phila)*, 2005, 43:674.

Phytonadione

Pronunciation (fye toe na DYE one)

CAS Number 84-80-0

U.S. Brand Names AquaMEPHYTON® [DSC]; Mephyton®

Synonyms Methylphytyl Napthoquinone; Phylloquinone; Phytomenadione; Vitamin K₁

Use Prevention and treatment of hypoprothrombinemia caused by drug-induced or anticoagulant-induced vitamin K deficiency, hemorrhagic disease of the newborn; phytonadione is more effective and is preferred to other vitamin K preparations in the presence of impending hemorrhage; oral absorption depends on the presence of bile salts

Mechanism of Action Promotes liver synthesis of clotting factors (II, VII, IX, X)

Adverse Reactions

Cardiovascular: Acrocyanosis

Dermatologic: Scleroderma, eczematous dermatitis (following subcutaneous administration)

Gastrointestinal: GI upset

Local: Pain, swelling, tenderness at injection site

Miscellaneous: Acrosclerosis

Signs and Symptoms of Overdose Hemiplegia

Pharmacodynamics/Kinetics

Onset of action: Increased coagulation factors: Oral: 6-10 hours; I.V.: 1-2 hours

Peak effect: INR values return to normal: Oral: 24-48 hours; I.V.: 12-14 hours. Half life is 2 hours

Absorption: Oral: From intestines in presence of bile; SubQ: Variable

Metabolism: Rapidly hepatic

Excretion: Urine and feces

Dosage

SubQ is the preferred (per manufacturer) parenteral route; I.V. route should be restricted for emergency use only

Minimum daily requirement: Not well established

Infants: 1-5 mcg/kg/day

Adults: 0.03 mcg/kg/day

Hemorrhagic disease of the newborn:

Prophylaxis: I.M.: 0.5-1 mg within 1 hour of birth

Treatment: I.M., SubQ: 1-2 mg/dose/day

Oral anticoagulant overdose:

Infants and Children:

No bleeding, rapid reversal needed, patient **will require** further oral anticoagulant therapy: SubQ, I.V.: 0.5-2 mg

No bleeding, rapid reversal needed, patient **will not require** further oral anticoagulant therapy: SubQ, I.V.: 2-5 mg

Significant bleeding, not life-threatening: SubQ, I.V.: 0.5-2 mg

Significant bleeding, life-threatening: I.V.: 5 mg over 10-20 minutes

Adults: Oral, I.V., SubQ: 1-10 mg/dose depending on degree of INR elevation

Serious bleeding or major overdose: 10 mg I.V. (slow infusion); may repeat every 12 hours (have required doses up to 25 mg)

Vitamin K deficiency: Due to drugs, malabsorption, or decreased synthesis of vitamin K

Infants and Children:

Oral: 2.5-5 mg/24 hours

I.M., I.V., SubQ: 1-2 mg/dose as a single dose

Adults:

Oral: 5-25 mg/24 hours

I.M., I.V., SubQ: 10 mg

For Rodenticide (long-acting anti-coagulants) (oral): 15 to 600 mg per day divided every 6 to 12 hours. If INR > 5, Begin with an oral dose of fifty mg and then titrate with 9 to 12 hours dosing. May require weeks to months of therapy.

Stability Protect injection from light at all times; may be autoclaved

Monitoring Parameters PT

Administration I.V. administration: Dilute in normal saline, D$_5$W or D$_5$NS and infuse slowly; rate of infusion should not exceed 1 mg/minute. **This route should be used only if administration by another route is not feasible.** The parenteral preparation has been administered orally to neonates. I.V. administration should not exceed 1 mg/minute; for I.V. infusion, dilute in PF (preservative free) D$_5$W or normal saline.

Contraindications Hypersensitivity to phytonadione or any component of the formulation

Warnings

Allergic reactions (injectable): [U.S. Boxed Warning]: **Severe reactions resembling hypersensitivity (eg, anaphylaxis) reactions have occurred rarely during or immediately after I.V. administration (even with proper dilution and rate of administration).** Allergic reactions have also occurred with I.M. and SubQ injections.

Route: Oral administration is the safest and requires the presence of bile salts for absorption. In obstructive jaundice or with biliary fistulas, concurrent administration of bile salts would be necessary for proper absorption. Manufacturers recommend the SubQ route over other parenteral routes, however, SubQ is less predictable when compared to the oral route, and efficacy may be delayed. The American College of Chest Physicians recommends the I.V. route in patients with serious or life-threatening bleeding secondary to use of vitamin K antagonists such as warfarin. The I.V. route should be restricted to emergency situations only where oral phytonadione cannot be used. Efficacy (eg, control of bleeding, decrease in INR) is delayed regardless of route of administration; patient management may require other treatments in the interim.

Reversing anticoagulant induced hypoprothrombinemia: Administer a dose that will quickly lower the INR into a safe range without causing resistance to warfarin. High phytonadione doses may lead to warfarin resistance for at least one week.

Newborns: Use caution in newborns, especially premature infants; hemolysis, jaundice, and hyperbilirubinemia have been reported with larger than recommended doses. Some dosage forms contain benzyl alcohol which has been associated with "gasping syndrome" in premature infants.

Hypoprothrombinemia caused by liver disease: If initial doses do not reverse coagulopathy, then higher doses are unlikely to have any effect. **Note:** Ineffective in hereditary hypoprothrombinemia.

Renal dysfunction: Use caution with renal dysfunction (including premature infants). Injectable products may contain aluminum; may result in toxic levels following prolonged administration.

Dosage Forms

Injection, aqueous colloidal: 2 mg/mL (0.5 mL); 10 mg/mL (1 mL) [contains benzyl alcohol]

Tablet: 5 mg

Reference Range Normal range: 0.09-2.12 mcg/L

Drug Interactions

Coumarin derivatives: Phytonadione may diminish the anticoagulant effect; monitor INR.

Orlistat: Phytonadione (oral) may not be properly absorbed when administered concurrently; separate doses by at least 2 hours.

Pregnancy Risk Factor C

Lactation Enters breast milk/use caution (APP rates "compatible")

Nursing Implications I.V. administration: Dilute in normal saline, D$_5$W or D$_5$NS and infuse slowly; rate of infusion should not exceed 1 mg/minute. **This route should be used only if administration by another route is not feasible.** The parenteral preparation has been administered orally to neonates. I.V. administration should not exceed 1 mg/minute; for I.V. infusion, dilute in PF (preservative free) D$_5$W or normal saline.

Additional Information Coagulation factors increase within 3 to 6 hours after I.V. administration and 6 to 12 hours after oral administration.

Specific References

Lubetsky A, Yonath H, Olchovsky D, et al, "Comparison of Oral vs Intravenous Phytonadione (Vitamin K$_1$) in Patients with Excessive Anticoagulation: A Prospective Randomized Controlled Study," *Arch Intern Med*, 2003, 163(20):2469-73.

Tegzes JH, Scaglione JM, Muller AA, et al, "Vitamin K1 for Them All? A Multicenter Review of Treatment of Brodifacoum Ingestion in Animals," *J Toxicol Clin Toxicol*, 2004, 42(5):799.

Wjasow C and McNamara R, "Anaphylaxis After Low Dose Intravenous Vitamin K," *J Emerg Med*, 2003, 24(2):169-72.

Polyethylene Glycol - High Molecular Weight

Pronunciation (pol i ETH i leen GLY kol ee LEK troe lite soe LOO shun)

CAS Number 25322-68-3

U.S. Brand Names Colyte®; GoLYTELY®; MiraLax™; NuLytely®; Tri-Lyte™

Synonyms Electrolyte Lavage Solution

Use Whole bowel irrigation in acute overdoses of iron, zinc sulfate, lead oxide, lithium, ampicillin, heavy metals, "body packers", sustained release medications; also used in bowel cleansing procedures

Mechanism of Action Nonabsorbable agent which increases bowel osmotic pressure

Adverse Reactions

Cardiovascular: Ectopy (ventricular)

Central nervous system: Coma

Dermatologic: Nonimmunologic contact urticaria, systemic contact dermatitis, immunologic contact urticaria

Endocrine & metabolic: Metabolic acidosis, hypercalcemia

Gastrointestinal: **Nausea**, diarrhea, **abdominal fullness, bloating**, vomiting, taste disturbance

Pharmacodynamics/Kinetics Onset of effect: Oral: ~1-2 hours

Dosage

For gastrointestinal decontamination:

Oral: Children and Adults: 15-60 mL/kg/hour until clear rectal effluent appears; rate nearly universally requires a naso- or orogastric tube

Nasogastric tube: Administer through a #12 French nasogastric tube with head of bed elevated at least 45°

Children: 9 months to 6 years: 500 mL/hour

Children: 6-12 years: 1000 mL/hour

Adolescents and Adults: 1500-2000 mL/hour

If emesis occurs, decrease infusion rate by 50% for up to 1 hour and then return to the original rate. Metoclopramide can be utilized as an antiemetic and promotility agent (10 mg I.V. initial dose, with 10 mg I.V. in 8 hours with erythromycin 250 mg I.V.)

Monitoring Parameters Electrolytes, serum glucose, BUN, urine osmolality; children <2 years of age should be monitored for hypoglycemia, dehydration, hypokalemia

Administration Oral: Rapid drinking of each portion is preferred to drinking small amounts continuously. Do not add flavorings as additional ingredients before use. Chilled solution often more palatable.

Contraindications Hypersensitivity to polyethylene glycol or any component of the formulation; gastrointestinal obstruction, gastric retention, bowel perforation, toxic colitis, megacolon

Warnings Do not add flavorings as additional ingredients before use; observe unconscious or semiconscious patients with impaired gag reflex or those who are otherwise prone to regurgitation or aspiration during administration; use with caution in ulcerative colitis, caution against the use of hot loop polypectomy. Evaluate patients with symptoms of bowel obstruction (nausea, vomiting, abdominal pain or distension) prior to use.

Dosage Forms
Powder, for oral solution: PEG 3350 240 g, sodium sulfate 22.72 g, sodium bicarbonate 6.72 g, sodium chloride 5.84 g, and potassium chloride 2.98 g (4000 mL)
Colyte®:
PEG 3350 240 g, sodium sulfate 22.72 g, sodium bicarbonate 6.72 g, sodium chloride 5.84 g, and potassium chloride 2.98 g (4000 mL) [available with citrus berry, lemon lime, cherry, and pineapple flavor packets]
PEG 3350 227.1 g, sodium sulfate 21.5 g, sodium bicarbonate 6.36 g, sodium chloride 5.53 g, and potassium chloride 2.82 g (4000 mL) [regular and pineapple flavor]
GoLytely®:
Disposable jug: PEG 3350 236 g, sodium sulfate 22.74 g, sodium bicarbonate 6.74 g, sodium chloride 5.86 g, and potassium chloride 2.97 g (4000 mL) [regular and pineapple flavor]
Packets: PEG 3350 227.1 g, sodium sulfate 21.5 g, sodium bicarbonate 6.36 g, sodium chloride 5.53 g, and potassium chloride 2.82 g (4000 mL) [regular flavor]
NuLytely®: PEG 3350 420 g, sodium bicarbonate 5.72 g, sodium chloride 11.2 g, and potassium chloride 1.48 (4000 mL) [cherry, lemon-lime, and orange flavors]
TriLyte™: PEG 3350 420 g, sodium bicarbonate 5.72 g, sodium chloride 11.2 g, and potassium chloride 1.48 (4000 mL) [supplied with flavor packets]

Drug Interactions Oral medications should not be administered within 1 hour of start of therapy

Pregnancy Risk Factor C

Pregnancy Implications Reproduction studies have not been conducted in animals or in humans.

Lactation Excretion in breast milk unknown/use caution

Specific References
Bell EA and Wall GC, "Pediatric Constipation Therapy Using Guidelines and Polyethylene Glycol 3350," *Ann Pharmacother*, 2004, 38(4):686-93. Epub 2004 Feb 27.
Farmer JW, Chan SB, Beranek G, et al, "Whole Bowel Irrigation for Contraband Bodypackers: A Case Series," *Ann Emerg Med*, 2000, 36(4):585.
Guzman DD, Teoh D, Velez LI, et al, "Accidental Intravenous Infusion of Golytely® in a 4-Year-Old Female," *J Toxicol Clin Toxicol*, 2002, 40(3):361-2.
Ly BT, Schneir AB, Williams SR, et al, "Effect of Whole Bowel Irrigation on the Pharmacokinetics of Tylenol Extended Relief," *Acad Emerg Med*, 2002, 9(5):529.
Narsinghani U, Chadha M, Farrar H, et al, "Life-Threatening Respiratory Failure Following Accidental Infusion of Polyethylene Glycol Electrolyte Solution into the Lung," *J Toxicol Clin Toxicol*, 2001, 39(1):105-7.
"Position Paper: Whole Bowel Irrigation," *J Toxicol Clin Toxicol*, 2004, 42(6):843-54 (review); erratum in *J Toxicol Clin Toxicol*, 2004, 42(7):1000.
Rivera W, Velez LI, Guzman DD, et al, "Unintentional Intravenous Infusion of Golytely in a 4-year-old Girl," *Ann Pharmacother*, 2004, 38(7-8):1183-5.
Shih RD, Laird D, Ruck B, et al, "Completion of Whole Bowel Irrigation in PCC Overdose Patients," *J Toxicol Clin Toxicol*, 2003, 41(5):672.
Shih RD, Laird D, Ruck B, et al, "Completion of Whole Bowel Irrigation in Emergency Department Overdose Patients," *Ann Emerg Med*, 2004, 44:S91.
Tuckler V, Cramm K, Martinez J, et al, "Accidental Large Intravenous Infusion of Golytely®," *J Toxicol Clin Toxicol*, 2002, 40(5):687-8.

Potassium Iodide

Pronunciation (poe TASS ee um EYE oh dide)
CAS Number 7681-11-0
U.S. Brand Names Iosat™ [OTC]; Pima®; SSKI®
Synonyms KI
Use Block thyroidal uptake of radioactive isotopes of iodine in a radiation emergency
Unlabeled/Investigational Use Lymphocutaneous and cutaneous sporotrichosis
Mechanism of Action Inhibits uptake of I-131 by thyroid

Adverse Reactions
Central nervous system: Fever, headache
Dermatologic: Urticaria, acne, angioedema, cutaneous hemorrhage
Endocrine & metabolic: Goiter with hypothyroidism, parotitis
Gastrointestinal: Metallic taste, GI upset, soreness of teeth and gums
Hematologic: Eosinophilia, hemorrhage (mucosal)
Neuromuscular & skeletal: Arthralgia
Respiratory: Rhinitis
Miscellaneous: Lymph node enlargement

Signs and Symptoms of Overdose Angioedema, laryngeal edema

Pharmacodynamics/Kinetics
Onset of action: Hyperthyroidism: 24-48 hours
Peak effect: 10-15 days after continuous therapy
Duration: Radioactive iodine exposure: ~24 hours

Dosage
Oral:
Adults: RDA: 150 mcg (iodide)
Expectorant:
Children (Pima®):
<3 years: 162 mg 3 times day
>3 years: 325 mg 3 times/day
Adults:
Pima®: 325-650 mg 3 times/day
SSKI®: 300-600 mg 3-4 times/day
Preoperative thyroidectomy: Children and Adults: 50-250 mg (1-5 drops SSKI®) 3 times/day **or** 0.1-0.3 mL (3-5 drops) of strong iodine (Lugol's solution) 3 times/day; administer for 10 days before surgery
Radiation protectant to radioactive isotopes of iodine (Pima®):
Children:
Infants up to 1 year: 65 mg once daily for 10 days; start 24 hours prior to exposure
>1 year: 130 mg once daily for 10 days; start 24 hours prior to exposure
Adults: 195 mg once daily for 10 days; start 24 hours prior to exposure
To reduce risk of thyroid cancer following nuclear accident (dosing should continue until risk of exposure has passed or other measures are implemented):
Children (see adult dose for children >68 kg):
Infants <1 month: 16 mg once daily
1 month to 3 years: 32 mg once daily
3-18 years: 65 mg once daily
Children >68 kg and Adults (including pregnant/lactating women): 130 mg once daily
Thyrotoxic crisis:
Infants <1 year: 150-250 mg (3-5 drops SSKI®) 3 times/day
Children and Adults: 300-500 mg (6-10 drops SSKI®) 3 times/day or 1 mL strong iodine (Lugol's solution) 3 times/day
Sporotrichosis (cutaneous, lymphocutaneous): Adults: Oral: Initial: 5 drops (SSKI®) 3 times/day; increase to 40-50 drops (SSKI®) 3 times/day as tolerated for 3-6 months
Note: Ineffective for disseminated sporotrichosis.

Stability Store in tight, light-resistant containers at temperature <40°C; freezing should be avoided

Monitoring Parameters Thyroid function tests, signs/symptoms of hyperthyroidism

Administration
Pima®: When used as an expectorant, take each dose with at least 4-6 ounces of water
SSKI®: Dilute in a glassful of water, fruit juice or milk. Take with food to decrease gastric irritation

Contraindications Hypersensitivity to iodine or any component of the formulation; hyperkalemia; pulmonary edema; impaired renal function; hyperthyroidism; iodine-induced goiter; dermatitis herpetiformis; hypocomplementemic vasculitis

Warnings Prolonged use can lead to hypothyroidism; cystic fibrosis patients have an exaggerated response; can cause acne flare-ups, can cause dermatitis; use with caution in patients with a history of thyroid disease, Addison's disease, cardiac disease, myotonia congenita, tuberculosis, acute bronchitis

Dosage Forms
Solution, oral:
SSKI®: 1 g/mL (30 mL, 240 mL) [contains sodium thiosulfate]
ThyroShield™: 65 mg/mL (30 mL) [black raspberry flavor]
Syrup (Pima®): 325 mg/5 mL (473 mL) [equivalent to iodide 249 mg/5 mL; black raspberry flavor]
Tablet:
Iosat™: 130 mg
ThyroSafe™: 65 mg [equivalent to iodine 50 mg]

Test Interactions Thyroid function tests

Drug Interactions
ACE inhibitors: Concurrent use may lead to hyperkalemia, cardiac arrhythmias or cardiac arrest.
Diuretics, potassium-sparing: Concurrent use may lead to hyperkalemia, cardiac arrhythmias, or cardiac arrest.
Lithium: May cause additive hypothyroid effects.

Potassium (and potassium-containing products): Concurrent use may lead to hyperkalemia, cardiac arrhythmias, or cardiac arrest.
Pregnancy Risk Factor D
Pregnancy Implications Crosses the placenta
Lactation Enters breast milk/use caution (AAP rates "compatible")

Pralidoxime

Pronunciation (pra li DOKS eem)
Related Information
● Obidoxime Chloride [ANTIDOTE]
CAS Number 51-15-0
U.S. Brand Names Protopam®
Synonyms 2-PAM; 2-Pyridine Aldoxime Methochloride; Pralidoxime Chloride
Use Reverse muscle paralysis caused by toxic exposure to organophosphate anticholinesterase pesticides and chemicals; control of overdose of anticholinesterase medications used to treat myasthenia gravis (ambenonium, neostigmine, pyridostigmine). Not usually useful for cabamate poisoning
Unlabeled/Investigational Use
May be effective for tacrine toxicity; treatment of nerve agent toxicity (chemical warfare) in combination with atropine
Not generally indicated for carbamate ingestions, although recent reports have shown a benefit in reversing nicotinic symptoms refractory to atropine; questionable efficacy for selected organophosphates (ciodrin, dimefox, dimethoate, methyl diazinon, phorate, schaadan, weesyn)
Mechanism of Action Reactivates cholinesterase that had been inactivated by phosphorylation due to exposure to organophosphate pesticides by displacing the enzyme from its nicotinic receptor sites; most effective if given within 24 hours of exposure; has greater impact on reversing nicotinic effects versus muscarinic
Adverse Reactions
Cardiovascular: Tachycardia, hypertension
Central nervous system: Dizziness, headache, drowsiness
Dermatologic: Rash
Gastrointestinal: Nausea
Hepatic: Transient increases in ALT, AST
Local: Pain at injection site after I.M. administration
Neuromuscular & skeletal: Muscle rigidity, weakness
Ocular: Accommodation impaired, blurred vision, diplopia
Renal: Renal function decreased
Respiratory: Hyperventilation, laryngospasm
Signs and Symptoms of Overdose Blurred vision, dizziness, nausea, tachycardia, vertigo
Pharmacodynamics/Kinetics
Protein binding: None
Metabolism: Hepatic
Half-life elimination: 74-77 minutes
Time to peak, serum: I.V.: 5-15 minutes
Excretion: Urine (80% to 90% as metabolites and unchanged drug)
Dosage
Organic phosphorus poisoning (use in conjunction with atropine; atropine effects should be established before pralidoxime is administered): I.V. (may be given I.M. or SubQ if I.V. is not feasible):
Children: 20-50 mg/kg/dose; repeat in 1-2 hours if muscle weakness has not been relieved, then at 8- to 12-hour intervals if cholinergic signs recur
Adults: 1-2 g; repeat in 1 hour if muscle weakness has not been relieved, then at 8- to 12-hour intervals if cholinergic signs recur. When the poison has been ingested, continued absorption from the lower bowel may require additional doses; patients should be titrated as long as signs of poisoning recur; dosing may need repeated every 3-8 hours.
Treatment of acetylcholinesterase inhibitor toxicity: Adults: I.V.: Initial: 1-2 g followed by increments of 250 mg every 5 minutes until response is observed
Elderly: Refer to Adults dosing; dosing should be cautious, considering possibility of decreased hepatic, renal, or cardiac function
Dosing adjustment in renal impairment: Dose should be reduced
Monitoring Parameters Heart rate, respiratory rate, blood pressure, continuous ECG; cardiac monitor and blood pressure monitor required for I.V. administration
Administration I.V.: Infuse over 15-30 minutes at a rate not to exceed 200 mg/minute; may administer I.M. or SubQ if I.V. is not accessible. If a more concentrated 5% solution is used, infuse over at least 5 minutes.
Contraindications Hypersensitivity to pralidoxime or any component of the formulation; poisonings due to phosphorus, inorganic phosphates, or organic phosphates without anticholinesterase activity; poisonings due to pesticides or carbamate class (may increase toxicity of carbaryl)
Warnings Use with caution in patients with myasthenia gravis; dosage modification required in patients with impaired renal function; use with caution in patients receiving theophylline, succinylcholine, phenothiazines, respiratory depressants (eg, narcotics, barbiturates).

Dosage Forms Injection, powder for reconstitution, as chloride: 1 g
Reference Range Pralidoxime concentration of 4 mcg/mL therapeutic *in vitro*; pralidoxime plasma level >14 mcg/mL is associated with side effects (ie, dizziness and blurred vision)
Drug Interactions
Decreased effect: Atropine, although often used concurrently with pralidoxime to offset muscarinic stimulation, these effects can occur earlier than anticipated
Increased effect: Barbiturates (potentiated)
Increased toxicity: Use with aminophylline, morphine, theophylline, and succinylcholine is contraindicated; use with reserpine and phenothiazines should be avoided in patients with organophosphate poisoning
Pregnancy Risk Factor C
Lactation Excretion in breast milk unknown/not recommended
Additional Information Intramuscular pralidoxime can be drawn from autoinjectors and be used for intravenous therapy.
Specific References
Bouchard NC, Mercurio-Zappala M, Abrey EM, et al, "Expired 2-PAM Effectively Reverses Cholinergic Crisis in Humans," *J Toxicol Clin Toxicol*, 2004, 42(5):742.
Burillo-Putze G, Hoffman RS, Howland MA, et al, "Late Administration of Pralidoxime in Organophosphate (Fenitrothion) Poisoning," *Am J Emerg Med*, 2004, 22(4):327-8.
Corvino TF, Nahata MC, Angelos MG, et al, "Availability, Stability, and Sterility of Pralidoxime for Mass Casualty Use," *Ann Emerg Med*, 2006, 47(3):272-7.
Eyer P, "The Role of Oximes in the Management of Organophosphorus Pesticide Poisoning," *Toxicol Rev*, 2003, 22(3):165-90.
Pannbacker RG and Oehme FW, "Pralidoxime Hydrolysis of Thiocholine Esters," *Vet Hum Toxicol*, 2003, 45(1):39-41.
Roh HK, Um WH, and Kin JS, "Prolonged Treatment with 2-PAM in a Large Amount of Organophosphate Insecticide Intoxication," *Clin Toxicol (Phila)*, 2005, 43:738.
Wolowich WR, Weisman RS, Cacace JL, et al, "The Stabiity of Pralidoxime Solution After Discharge from a Mark-1 Autoinjector," *J Toxicol Clin Toxicol*, 2004, 42(5):715.

Protamine Sulfate

CAS Number 9009-65-8; 9012-00-4
Use Treatment of heparin, dalteparin, enoxaparin overdosage; neutralize heparin during surgery or dialysis procedures
Unlabeled/Investigational Use Treatment of low molecular weight heparin (LMWH) overdose
Mechanism of Action Weak anticoagulant; combines with strongly acidic heparin to form a stable complex (salt) neutralizing the anticoagulant activity of both drugs: Derived from male salmon gonads.
Adverse Reactions
Cardiovascular: Hypotension, cyanosis, bradycardia, flushing, syncope, sinus bradycardia, vasodilation
Central nervous system: Lassitude
Dermatologic: Urticaria
Gastrointestinal: Nausea, vomiting
Hematologic: Thrombocytopenia, bleeding, coagulopathy, leukopenia
Neuromuscular & skeletal: Numbness
Respiratory: Wheezing, dyspnea, pulmonary edema, pulmonary hypertension
Miscellaneous: Hypersensitivity reactions (anaphylaxis and anaphylactic shock)
Signs and Symptoms of Overdose Hypertension; may cause hemorrhage
Pharmacodynamics/Kinetics Onset of action: I.V.: Heparin neutralization: ~5 minutes
Dosage
Heparin neutralization: I.V.: Protamine dosage is determined by the dosage of heparin; 1 mg of protamine neutralizes 90 USP units of heparin (lung) and 115 USP units of heparin (intestinal); maximum dose: 50 mg
Heparin overdosage, following intravenous administration: I.V.: Since blood heparin concentrations decrease rapidly after administration, adjust the protamine dosage depending upon the duration of time since heparin administration as follows: See table.

Time Elapsed	Dose of Protamine (mg) to Neutralize 100 units of Heparin
Immediate	1-1.5
30-60 min	0.5-0.75
>2 h	0.25-0.375

Heparin overdosage, following SubQ injection: I.V.: 1-1.5 mg protamine per 100 units heparin; this may be done by a portion of the dose (eg, 25-50 mg) given slowly I.V. followed by the remaining portion as a continuous infusion over 8-16 hours (the expected absorption time of the SubQ heparin dose)

LMWH overdose (unlabeled use): **Note:** Anti-factor Xa activity never completely neutralized (maximum: ~60% to 75%)

Enoxaparin: 1 mg protamine for each mg of enoxaparin; if PTT prolonged 2-4 hours after first dose, consider additional dose of 0.5 mg for each mg of enoxaparin.

Dalteparin or tinzaparin: 1 mg protamine for each 100 anti-Xa int. unit of dalteparin or tinzaparin; if PTT prolonged 2-4 hours after first dose, consider additional dose of 0.5 mg for each 100 anti-Xa int. unit of dalteparin or tinzaparin.

Note: Excessive protamine doses may worsen bleeding potential.

Stability Refrigerate, avoid freezing; remains stable for at least 2 weeks at room temperature; **incompatible** with cephalosporins and penicillins; preservative-free formulation does not require refrigeration. Reconstitute vial with 5 mL sterile water; if using protamine in neonates, reconstitute with preservative-free sterile water for injection; resulting solution equals 10 mg/mL.

Monitoring Parameters Coagulation test, aPTT or ACT, cardiac monitor and blood pressure monitor required during administration

Administration For I.V. use only; **incompatible** with cephalosporins and penicillins; administer slow IVP (50 mg over 10 minutes); rapid I.V. infusion causes hypotension; resulting solution equals 10 mg/mL; inject without further dilution over 1-3 minutes; maximum of 50 mg in any 10-minute period

Contraindications Hypersensitivity to protamine or any component of the formulation

Warnings May not be totally effective in some patients following cardiac surgery despite adequate doses; may cause hypersensitivity reaction in patients with a history of allergy to fish (have epinephrine 1:1000 available) and in patients sensitized to protamine (via protamine zinc insulin); too rapid administration can cause severe hypotensive and anaphylactoid-like reactions. Heparin rebound associated with anticoagulation and bleeding has been reported to occur occasionally; symptoms typically occur 8-9 hours after protamine administration, but may occur as long as 18 hours later.

Dosage Forms Injection, solution, as sulfate [preservative free]: 10 mg/mL (5 mL, 25 mL)

Reference Range Protamine plasma levels of 0.02-0.5 mg/mL are associated with prolonged activated partial thromboplastin time and prothrombin time

Pregnancy Risk Factor C - Generally safe

Lactation Excretion in breast milk unknown

Additional Information Lepirudin, Desirudin and Bivalirudin are not reversed by protamine

Pyridostigmine

Pronunciation (peer id oh STIG meen)
CAS Number 101-26-8
U.S. Brand Names Mestinon® Timespan®; Mestinon®
Synonyms Pyridostigmine Bromide
Use Second-line agent for envenomation by Asian snakes or intoxication with tetradotoxin exposures if edrophonium supplies are depleted; reversal of the effects of nondepolarizing neuromuscular blocking agents after surgery; pretreatment for chemical warfare agents (ie, Soman nerve gas), thus making the use of atropine and pralidoxime more effective; symptomatic treatment of myasthenia gravis
Mechanism of Action Inhibits destruction of acetylcholine by acetylcholinesterase which facilitates transmission of impulses across myoneural junction

Adverse Reactions
Cardiovascular: Arrhythmias (especially bradycardia), hypotension, tachycardia, AV block, nodal rhythm, nonspecific ECG changes, cardiac arrest, syncope, flushing
Central nervous system: Convulsions, dysarthria, dysphonia, dizziness, loss of consciousness, drowsiness, headache
Dermatologic: Skin rash, thrombophlebitis (I.V.), urticaria
Gastrointestinal: Hyperperistalsis, nausea, vomiting, salivation, diarrhea, stomach cramps, dysphagia, flatulence, abdominal pain
Genitourinary: Urinary urgency
Neuromuscular & skeletal: Weakness, fasciculations, muscle cramps, spasms, arthralgias, myalgia
Ocular: Small pupils, lacrimation, amblyopia
Respiratory: Increased bronchial secretions, laryngospasm, bronchiolar constriction, respiratory muscle paralysis, dyspnea, respiratory depression, respiratory arrest, bronchospasm
Miscellaneous: Diaphoresis (increased), anaphylaxis, allergic reactions

Signs and Symptoms of Overdose Blurred vision, excessive sweating, muscle weakness, nausea, salivation, tearing, vomiting

Pharmacodynamics/Kinetics
Onset of action: Oral, I.M.: 15-30 minutes; I.V. injection: 2-5 minutes
Duration: Oral: Up to 6-8 hours (due to slow absorption); I.V.: 2-3 hours
Absorption: Oral: Very poor

Distribution: 19 ± 12 L
Metabolism: Hepatic
Bioavailability: 10% to 20%
Half-life elimination: 1-2 hours; Renal failure: ≤6 hours
Excretion: Urine (80% to 90% as unchanged drug)

Dosage
Myasthenia gravis:
Oral:
Children: 7 mg/kg/24 hours divided into 5-6 doses
Adults: Highly individualized dosing ranges: 60-1500 mg/day, usually 600 mg/day divided into 5-6 doses, spaced to provide maximum relief
Sustained release formulation: Highly individualized dosing ranges: 180-540 mg once or twice daily (doses separated by at least 6 hours); **Note:** Most clinicians reserve sustained release dosage form for bedtime dose only.
I.M., slow I.V. push:
Children: 0.05-0.15 mg/kg/dose
Adults: To supplement oral dosage pre- and postoperatively during labor and postpartum, during myasthenic crisis, or when oral therapy is impractical: ~1/30th of oral dose; observe patient closely for cholinergic reactions
or
I.V. infusion: Initial: 2 mg/hour with gradual titration in increments of 0.5-1 mg/hour, up to a maximum rate of 4 mg/hour
Pretreatment for Soman nerve gas exposure (military use): Oral: Adults: 30 mg every 8 hours beginning several hours prior to exposure; discontinue at first sign of nerve agent exposure, then begin atropine and pralidoxime
Reversal of nondepolarizing muscle relaxants:
Note: Atropine sulfate (0.6-1.2 mg) I.V. immediately prior to pyridostigmine to minimize side effects: I.V.:
Children: Dosing range: 0.1-0.25 mg/kg/dose*
Adults: 0.1-0.25 mg/kg/dose; 10-20 mg is usually sufficient*
*Full recovery usually occurs ≤15 minutes, but ≥30 minutes may be required

Dosage adjustment in renal dysfunction: Lower dosages may be required due to prolonged elimination; no specific recommendations have been published

Stability
Injection: Protect from light.
Tablet:
30 mg: Store under refrigeration at 2°C to 8°C (36°F to 46°F) and protect from light; stable at room temperature for up to 3 months
Mestinon®: Store at 25°C (77°F); protect from moisture

Monitoring Parameters Observe for cholinergic reactions, particularly when administered I.V.

Administration Do **not** crush sustained release tablet.

Contraindications Hypersensitivity to pyridostigmine, bromides, or any component of the formulation; GI or GU obstruction

Warnings Use with caution in patients with epilepsy, asthma, bradycardia, hyperthyroidism, cardiac arrhythmias, or peptic ulcer; adequate facilities should be available for cardiopulmonary resuscitation when testing and adjusting dose for myasthenia gravis; have atropine and epinephrine ready to treat hypersensitivity reactions; overdosage may result in cholinergic crisis, this must be distinguished from myasthenic crisis; anticholinesterase insensitivity can develop for brief or prolonged periods. Safety and efficacy in pediatric patients have not been established.
Regonol® injection contains 1% benzyl alcohol as the preservative (not intended for use in newborns).

Dosage Forms
Injection, solution, as bromide:
Mestinon®: 5 mg/mL (2 mL)
Regonol®: 5 mg/mL (2 mL) [contains benzyl alcohol]
Syrup, as bromide (Mestinon®): 60 mg/5 mL (480 mL) [raspberry flavor; contains alcohol 5%, sodium benzoate]
Tablet, as bromide (Mestinon®): 60 mg
Tablet, sustained release, as bromide (Mestinon® Timespan®): 180 mg

Test Interactions ↑ aminotransferase [ALT (SGPT)/AST (SGOT)] (S), amylase (S)

Drug Interactions
Aminoglycosides (gentamicin, kanamycin, neomycin, streptomycin): Use of high parenteral doses may intensify/prolong neuromuscular blockade, or lead to resistance of neuromuscular blockade reversal, especially if used with other nondepolarizing neuromuscular-blocking drugs.
Antibiotics (bacitracin, colistin, polymyxin B, sodium colistimethate, tetracycline): Use of high parenteral doses may intensify/prolong neuromuscular blockade, or lead to resistance of neuromuscular blockade reversal, especially if used with other nondepolarizing neuromuscular-blocking drugs.
Beta blockers: Pyridostigmine and beta-blockers may both cause bradycardia and hypotension, effect may be additive; monitor.
Depolarizing neuromuscular-blocking agents (succinylcholine): Increased neuromuscular blocking effect with concomitant use.

Edrophonium: Increased toxicity with concomitant use.

Magnesium: Patients with elevated serum magnesium concentrations may experience enhanced neuromuscular blockage with blocking agents. The reversing effect of pyridostigmine may be compensated.

Quinidine: Recurrent paralysis may occur when quinidine is administered with nondepolarizing neuromuscular-blocking drugs. This may complicate attempts to reverse blockade with pyridostigmine.

Quinolone antibiotics (ciprofloxacin, norfloxacin): Case reports suggest these drugs may exhibit neuromuscular-blocking effects (especially in some patients with myasthenia gravis); monitor.

Pregnancy Risk Factor C

Pregnancy Implications Safety has not been established for use during pregnancy. The potential benefit to the mother should outweigh the potential risk to the fetus. When pyridostigmine is needed in myasthenic mothers, giving dose parenterally 1 hour before completion of the second stage of labor may facilitate delivery and protect the neonate during the immediate postnatal state.

Lactation Enters breast milk/compatible

Nursing Implications Observe for cholinergic reactions, particularly when administered I.V.

Pyridoxine

Pronunciation (peer i DOKS een)

CAS Number 58-56-0; 65-23-6

U.S. Brand Names Aminoxin® [OTC]

Synonyms Pyridoxine Hydrochloride; Vitamin B_6

Use Prevents and treats vitamin B_6 deficiency, pyridoxine-dependent seizures in infants, adjunct to treatment of acute toxicity from acrylamide, isoniazid, cycloserine, penicillamine, altretamine, or hydrazine overdose; optic neuritis due to isoniazid or chloramphenicol; hydrazine-containing mushrooms (*Gyromitra*)

Unlabeled/Investigational Use Useful for primary oxaluria; questionable and unproven use in carbon disulfide toxicity; has been used subcutaneously to treat mitomycin C extravasation; seizures due to ginko seed ingestion

Mechanism of Action Precursor to pyridoxal, which functions in the metabolism of proteins, carbohydrates, and fats; pyridoxal also aids in the release of liver and muscle stored glycogen, inhibits lactation

Adverse Reactions

Central nervous system: Sensory neuropathy (after chronic administration of large doses), seizures (following I.V. administration of very large doses), headache, hypotonia, memory disturbance

Dermatologic: Photosensitivity, bullous lesions, palmar-plantar erythrodysesthesia syndrome

Endocrine & metabolic: Decreased serum folic acid concentration

Gastrointestinal: Nausea

Hepatic: Elevated AST

Local: Burning or stinging at injection site

Neuromuscular & skeletal: Paresthesia

Respiratory: Respiratory distress

Miscellaneous: Allergic reactions have been reported; may suppress lactation at doses >600 mg/day

Signs and Symptoms of Overdose Ataxia, lethargy, seizures, sensory neuropathy

Pharmacodynamics/Kinetics

Absorption: Enteral, parenteral: Well absorbed

Metabolism: Via 4-pyridoxic acid (active form) and other metabolites

Half-life elimination: 15-20 days

Excretion: Urine

Dosage

Neuropathy may occur at doses >2 g/day.

Acute hydrazine toxicity (treatment): A pyridoxine dose of 25 mg/kg in divided doses I.M./I.V. has been used.

Acute isoniazid toxicity (treatment of seizures and/or coma): A dose of pyridoxine hydrochloride equal to the amount of INH ingested can be given I.M./I.V. in divided doses together with other anticonvulsants; can give as much as 1 g/kg in adults or 250 mg/kg in children

Dietary deficiency: Oral:

Children: 5-10 mg/24 hours for 3 weeks

Adults: 10-20 mg/day for 3 weeks

Drug-induced neuritis (eg, isoniazid, hydralazine, penicillamine, cycloserine): Oral:

Children: 10-50 mg/24 hours; prophylaxis: 1-2 mg/kg/24 hours

Adults: 100-200 mg/24 hours; prophylaxis: 10-100 mg/24 hours

Ginko seed ingestion (seizure treatment and prevention): I.V.: 2 mg/kg

Mitomycin C extravasation: SubQ: Inject (100 mg/mL- 75-300 mg total) around affected area - dilute one to threefold

Pyridoxine-dependent Infants:

Oral: 2-100 mg/day

I.M., I.V.: 10-100 mg

Nausea and vomiting during pregnancy: 25-30 mg daily

Stability Protect from light

Administration Burning may occur at the injection site after I.M. or SubQ administration; seizures have occurred following I.V. administration of very large doses

Contraindications Hypersensitivity to pyridoxine or any component of the formulation

Warnings Dependence and withdrawal may occur with doses >200 mg/day

Dosage Forms

Capsule, as hydrochloride: 250 mg

Injection, solution, as hydrochloride: 100 mg/mL (1 mL)

Tablet, as hydrochloride: 25 mg, 50 mg, 100 mg, 200 mg, 250 mg, 500 mg

Tablet, enteric coated, as hydrochloride (Aminoxin®): 20 mg

Reference Range

A broad normal range is ~25-80 ng/mL (SI: 122-389 nmol/L)

HPLC method for pyridoxal phosphate normal range: 3.5-18 ng/mL (SI: 17-88 nmol/L)

Peak serum level following 1 g: I.V. infusion: 9.97 ng/µL; I.V. bolus: 44.6 ng/µL; Oral: 15.75 ng/µL

Test Interactions Urobilinogen

Drug Interactions Decreased serum levels of levodopa, phenobarbital, and phenytoin

Pregnancy Risk Factor A/C (dose exceeding RDA recommendation)

Pregnancy Implications Seizures in an infant following *in utero* exposure

Lactation Enters breast milk/compatible

Nursing Implications Burning may occur at the injection site after I.M. or SubQ administration; seizures have occurred following I.V. administration of very large doses

Serpacwa [Antidote]

Use Topical agent serving as protectant (physical barrier) to urushiol and methyl nicotinate (surrogates for chemical warfare agents); currently indicated only for military personnel wearing mission-oriented protective posture (MOPP) gear; it should be applied only when chemical warfare is imminent and not for training purposes

Mechanism of Action Contains a 50:50 mixture of perfluoroakylpolyether and polytetrafluoroethylene which acts as a physical barrier to agents

Adverse Reactions Miscellaneous: Flu-like syndrome

Dosage Apply to skin by hand until there is a barely noticeable white film layer. One-third of the packet should be applied evenly around wrists, neck, and boot tops (of the lower leg); remaining two-thirds of the packet should be applied evenly to axillae, groin, and waist. Prior to application, use a dry towel or cloth to remove perspiration, insect repellant, camouflage paint or dirt from skin.

Pregnancy Risk Factor C

Silver Sulfadiazine

Pronunciation (SIL ver sul fa DYE a zeen)

CAS Number 22199-08-2

U.S. Brand Names Silvadene®; SSD® AF; SSD®; Thermazene®

Use Prevention and treatment of infection in second and third degree burns; vesicant exposure

Mechanism of Action Acts upon the bacterial cell wall and cell membrane. Bactericidal for many gram-negative and gram-positive bacteria and is effective against yeast. Active against *Pseudomonas aeruginosa*, *Pseudomonas maltophilia*, *Enterobacter* species, *Klebsiella* species, *Serratia* species, *Escherichia coli*, *Proteus mirabilis*, *Morganella morganii*, *Providencia rettgeri*, *Proteus vulgaris*, *Providencia* species, *Citrobacter* species, *Acinetobacter calcoaceticus*, *Staphylococcus aureus*, *Staphylococcus epidermidis*, *Enterococcus* species, *Candida albicans*, *Corynebacterium diphtheriae*, and *Clostridium perfringens*

Adverse Reactions

Frequency not defined.

Dermatologic: Itching, rash, erythema multiforme, discoloration of skin, photosensitivity

Hematologic: Hemolytic anemia, leukopenia (usually transient), agranulocytosis, aplastic anemia

Hepatic: Hepatitis

Renal: Interstitial nephritis, crystalluria

Miscellaneous: Allergic reactions may be related to sulfa component, hyperthermia

Pharmacodynamics/Kinetics

Absorption: Significant percutaneous absorption of silver sulfadiazine can occur especially when applied to extensive burns

Half-life elimination: 10 hours; prolonged with renal impairment

Time to peak, serum: 3-11 days of continuous therapy

Excretion: Urine (~50% as unchanged drug)

Dosage Children and Adults: Topical: Apply once or twice daily with a sterile-gloved hand; apply to a thickness of $^1/_{16}$"; burned area should be covered with cream at all times

Stability Silvadene® cream will occasionally darken either in the jar or after application to the skin. This color change results from a light catalyzed reaction which is a common characteristic of all silver salts. A similar analogy is the oxidation of silverware. The product of this color change reaction is silver oxide which ranges in color from gray to black. Silver oxide has rarely been associated with permanent skin discoloration. Additionally, the antimicrobial activity of the product is not substantially diminished because the color change reaction involves such a small amount of the active drug and is largely a surface phenomenon.

Monitoring Parameters Serum electrolytes, urinalysis, renal function tests, CBC in patients with extensive burns on long-term treatment

Administration Apply with a sterile-gloved hand. Apply to a thickness $^1/_{16}$". Burned area should be covered with cream at all times.

Contraindications Hypersensitivity to silver sulfadiazine or any component of the formulation; premature infants or neonates <2 months of age (sulfonamides may displace bilirubin and cause kernicterus); pregnancy (approaching or at term)

Warnings Use with caution in patients with G6PD deficiency, renal impairment, or history of allergy to other sulfonamides; sulfadiazine may accumulate in patients with impaired hepatic or renal function; fungal superinfection may occur; use of analgesic might be needed before application; systemic absorption is significant and adverse reactions may occur

Dosage Forms
Cream, topical: 1% (25 g, 50 mg, 85 g, 400 g)
Silvadene®, Thermazene®: 1% (20 g, 50 g, 85 g, 400 g, 1000 g)
SSD®: 1% (25 g, 50 g, 85 g, 400 g)
SSD® AF: 1% (50 g, 400 g)

Drug Interactions Decreased effect: Topical proteolytic enzymes are inactivated

Pregnancy Risk Factor B

Lactation For external use

Specific Reference
Ronen G, Cohen AD, Bogdanov-Berezovsky A, et al, "A Randomized Controlled Trial of Silver Sulfadiazine, Biafine, and Saline-Soaked Gauze in the Treatment of Superficial Partial-Thickness Burn Wounds in Pigs," *Acad Emerg Med*, 2004, 11:339-342.

Silymarin

CAS Number 22888-70-6; 65666-07-1

Unlabeled/Investigational Use Used in Europe for treatment of mushroom-induced hepatic disorders (not FDA approved in U.S.) caused by Group I mushrooms and organic solvents

Mechanism of Action Hepatotropic: May prevent amatoxin penetration into hepatocytes

Adverse Reactions
Dermatologic: Rashes
Gastrointestinal: Laxative effects, colicky abdominal pain, fluid diarrhea, vomiting
Neuromuscular & skeletal: Weakness
Miscellaneous: Allergic reactions, diaphoresis

Dosage
Oral: 140 mg 2-3 times/day
I.V.: 20-80 mg/kg/day in 4 divided doses (over a 2-hour period for each infusion)

Sodium Bicarbonate

Pronunciation (SOW dee um bye KAR bun ate)

CAS Number 144-55-8

U.S. Brand Names Brioschi® [OTC]; Neut®

Synonyms Baking Soda; NaHCO₃; Sodium Acid Carbonate; Sodium Hydrogen Carbonate

Use Management of metabolic acidosis; antacid; alkalinize urine; severe diarrhea; can reverse QRS prolongation in antidepressant overdose, cocaine, and propoxyphene; cardiac conduction defects due to quinidine-like action of cardiotoxic drugs; increases protein binding of tricyclic antidepressants

Unlabeled/Investigational Use Nebulized sodium bicarbonate is useful to treat chlorine gas exposure; also used to prevent rhabdomyolysis-induced renal failure; useful in extravasation injury due to carmustine; metformin-induced lactic acidosis

Mechanism of Action Dissociates to provide bicarbonate ion which neutralizes hydrogen ion concentration and raises blood and urinary pH

Adverse Reactions
Cardiovascular: Edema, cerebral hemorrhage (especially with rapid injection of the hyperosmotic NaHCO₃ solution in infants)
Endocrine & metabolic: Metabolic alkalosis, hypernatremia, hypokalemia, hypocalcemia, intracranial acidosis, increased affinity of hemoglobin for oxygen-reduced pH in myocardia
Gastrointestinal: **Gastric distention, flatulence may occur with oral administration,** gastric rupture
Local: Tissue necrosis, ulceration after I.V. extravasation

Signs and Symptoms of Overdose Confusion, cyanosis, hypocalcemia, hypokalemia, hypokalemic/hypochloremic metabolic alkalosis, hypernatremia, muscle cramps, nausea, pulmonary edema, seizures, tetany, weakness

Pharmacodynamics/Kinetics
Onset of action: Oral: Rapid; I.V.: 15 minutes
Duration: Oral: 8-10 minutes; I.V.: 1-2 hours
Absorption: Oral: Well absorbed
Excretion: Urine (<1%)

Dosage
Cardiac arrest: **Routine use of NaHCO₃ is not recommended and should be given only after adequate alveolar ventilation has been established and effective cardiac compressions are provided**
Infants and Children: I.V.: 0.5-1 mEq/kg/dose repeated every 10 minutes or as indicated by arterial blood gases; rate of infusion should not exceed 10 mEq/minute; neonates and children <2 years of age should receive 4.2% (0.5 mEq/mL) solution
Adults: I.V.: Initial: 1 mEq/kg/dose one time; maintenance: 0.5 mEq/kg/dose every 10 minutes or as indicated by arterial blood gases
Metabolic acidosis: Infants, Children, and Adults: Dosage should be based on the following formula if blood gases and pH measurements are available:
HCO₃⁻ (mEq) = 0.3 × weight (kg) × base deficit (mEq/L)
Administer $^1/_2$ dose initially, then remaining $^1/_2$ dose over the next 24 hours; monitor pH, serum HCO₃⁻, and clinical status
Note: If acid-base status is not available: Dose for older Children and Adults: 2-5 mEq/kg I.V. infusion over 4-8 hours; subsequent doses should be based on patient's acid-base status
Chronic renal failure: Oral: Initiate when plasma HCO₃⁻ <15 mEq/L
Children: 1-3 mEq/kg/day
Adults: Start with 20-36 mEq/day in divided doses, titrate to bicarbonate level of 18-20 mEq/L
Hyperkalemia: Adults: I.V.: 1 mEq/kg over 5 minutes
Renal tubular acidosis: Oral:
Distal:
Children: 2-3 mEq/kg/day
Adults: 0.5-2 mEq/kg/day in 4-5 divided doses
Proximal: Children and Adults: Initial: 5-10 mEq/kg/day; maintenance: Increase as required to maintain serum bicarbonate in the normal range
Urine alkalinization: Oral:
Children: 1-10 mEq (84-840 mg)/kg/day in divided doses every 4-6 hours; dose should be titrated to desired urinary pH
Adults: Initial: 48 mEq (4 g), then 12-24 mEq (1-2 g) every 4 hours; dose should be titrated to desired urinary pH; doses up to 16 g/day (200 mEq) in patients <60 years and 8 g (100 mEq) in patients >60 years
Antacid: Adults: Oral: 325 mg to 2 g 1-4 times/day

Stability Store injection at room temperature; protect from heat and from freezing; use only clear solutions; do not mix NaHCO₃ with calcium salts, catecholamines, atropine

Monitoring Parameters Serum electrolytes including calcium, urinary pH, arterial blood gases (if indicated)

Administration For I.V. administration to infants, use the 0.5 mEq/mL solution or dilute the 1 mEq/mL solution 1:1 with **sterile water**; for direct I.V. infusion in emergencies, administer slowly (maximum rate in infants: 10 mEq/minute); for infusion, dilute to a maximum concentration of 0.5 mEq/mL in dextrose solution and infuse over 2 hours (maximum rate of administration: 1 mEq/kg/hour)

Contraindications Alkalosis, hypernatremia, severe pulmonary edema, hypocalcemia, unknown abdominal pain

Warnings Rapid administration in neonates and children <2 years of age has led to hypernatremia, decreased CSF pressure and intracranial hemorrhage. **Use of I.V. NaHCO₃ should be reserved for documented metabolic acidosis and for hyperkalemia-induced cardiac arrest.** Routine use in cardiac arrest is not recommended. Avoid extravasation, tissue necrosis can occur due to the hypertonicity of NaHCO₃. May cause sodium retention especially if renal function is impaired; not to be used in treatment of peptic ulcer; use with caution in patients with CHF, edema, cirrhosis, or renal failure. Not the antacid of choice for the elderly because of sodium content and potential for systemic alkalosis.

Dosage Forms
Granules, effervescent (Brioschi®): 2.69 g/packet (6 g) [unit-dose packets; contains sodium 770 mg/packet; lemon flavor]; 2.69 g/capful (120 g, 240 g) [contains sodium 770 mg/capful; lemon flavor]
Infusion [premixed in sterile water]: 5% (500 mL)
Injection, solution:
4.2% [42 mg/mL = 5 mEq/10 mL] (10 mL)
7.5% [75 mg/mL = 8.92 mEq/10 mL] (50 mL)
8.4% [84 mg/mL = 10 mEq/10 mL] (10 mL, 50 mL)
Neut®: 4% [40 mg/mL = 2.4 mEq/5 mL] (5 mL)
Powder: Sodium bicarbonate USP (120 g, 480 g) [contains sodium 30 mEq per $^1/_2$ teaspoon]
Tablet: 325 mg [3.8 mEq]; 650 mg [7.6 mEq]

Reference Range Therapeutic (sodium): 135-145 mEq/L (SI: 135-145 mM/L)

Drug Interactions
Decreased effect/levels of lithium, chlorpropamide, methotrexate, tetracyclines, and salicylates due to urinary alkalinization
Increased toxicity/levels of amphetamines, anorexiants, mecamylamine, ephedrine, pseudoephedrine, flecainide, quinidine, quinine due to urinary alkalinization

Pregnancy Risk Factor C

Lactation Enters breast milk/compatible

Nursing Implications Advise patient of milk-alkali syndrome if use is long-term; observe for extravasation when giving I.V.; incompatible with acids, acidic salts, alkaloid salts, calcium salts, catecholamines, atropine

Specific References
Balali-Mood M, Ayati MH, and Ali-Akbarian H. "Effect of High Doses of Sodium Bicarbonate in Acute Organophosphorous Pesticide Poisoning," *Clin Toxicol*, 2005, 43(6):571-4.
Cronin KA, Caraccio T, and McGuigan M, "A Survey of US Poison Center Directors on the Treatment of Tricyclic Antidepressant Overdose with Cardiotoxicity," *J Toxicol Clin Toxicol*, 2003, 41(5):670.
Sharma AN, Hexdall AH, Chang EK, et al, "Diphenhydramine-Induced Wide Complex Dysrhythmia Responds to Treatment with Sodium Bicarbonate," *Am J Emerg Med*, 2003, 21(3):212-5.

Sodium Nitrite

Pronunciation (SOW dee um NYE trite)

Related Information
• Cyanide Antidote Kit [ANTIDOTE]

CAS Number 7632-00-0

Use Cyanide toxicity in conjunction with amyl nitrite pearls and sodium thiosulfate

Unlabeled/Investigational Use May be of use in hydrogen sulfide poisoning

Mechanism of Action Vasodilation and methemoglobin producer

Adverse Reactions
Cardiovascular: Tachycardia, hypotension from vasodilation, syncope, cyanosis, flushing, sinus tachycardia
Central nervous system: Headache
Gastrointestinal: Nausea, vomiting
Miscellaneous: Forms methemoglobin

Signs and Symptoms of Overdose Cardiovascular collapse, coma, hemolysis/hemolytic anemia, seizures

Admission Criteria/Prognosis Any patient with change in mental status, cardiopulmonary complaints, or methemoglobin levels >30% should be admitted; asymptomatic patients with methemoglobin levels <30% may be considered for discharge after 6 hours of observation and if methemoglobin levels fall to <15%

Dosage
Cyanide toxicity:
Children (without anemia): 4.5-10 mg/kg (0.15-0.33 mL/kg of a 3% solution up to 10 mL)
Adults: 300 mg (10 mL of a 3% solution)
Acceptable daily intake: 0.4 mg/kg

Monitoring Parameters Methemoglobin levels

Warnings Sodium nitrite and amyl nitrite in excessive doses induce methemoglobinemia

Dosage Forms Injection: 300 mg/10 mL

Reference Range Sodium nitrite levels associated with fatalities range from 0.5-350 mg/L

Antidote(s)
• Cyanide Antidote Kit [ANTIDOTE]

Sodium Polystyrene Sulfonate

Pronunciation (SOW dee um pol ee STYE reen SUL fon ate)

Related Information
• Adipose Tissue Ranges of Toxins

CAS Number 25704-18-1; 9003-59-2

U.S. Brand Names Kayexalate®; Kionex™; SPS®

Use Treatment of hyperkalemia; gastric decontamination for lithium

Mechanism of Action Removes potassium by exchanging sodium ions for potassium ions in the intestine before the resin is passed from the body

Adverse Reactions
Frequency not defined.
Endocrine & metabolic: Hypernatremia, hypokalemia, hypocalcemia, hypomagnesemia
Gastrointestinal: Anorexia, colonic necrosis (rare), constipation, fecal impaction, intestinal obstruction (due to concretions in association with aluminum hydroxide), nausea, vomiting

Pharmacodynamics/Kinetics
Onset of action: 2-24 hours
Absorption: None
Excretion: Completely feces (primarily as potassium polystyrene sulfonate)

Dosage Hyperkalemia:
Children:
Oral: 1 g/kg/dose every 6 hours
Rectal: 1 g/kg/dose every 2-6 hours (In small children and infants, employ lower doses by using the practical exchange ratio of 1 mEq K$^+$/g of resin as the basis for calculation)
Adults:
Oral: 15 g (60 mL) 1-4 times/day
Rectal: 30-50 g every 6 hours
Instructions for sodium polystyrene sulfonate enema:
Insert the tubing into the rectum ~20 cm. Administer a body-temperature tap water enema (250-500 mL) to remove any feces in the rectum and sigmoid colon.
Shake the sodium polystyrene sulfonate suspension well and mix 2:1 with tap water in the enema bucket prior to administration (ie, 60 mL sodium polystyrene sulfonate and 30 mL water).
Reinsert the enema tube into the rectum ~20 cm and administer the prescribed sodium polystyrene sulfonate dose (usual range, 15-60 g), then remove the tube.
Make sure the enema is retained for several hours, to allow exchange of sodium for potassium ions. If leakage occurs, elevate the patient's hips with pillows.
Reinsert the tube to 20 cm and administer cleansing enema(s) of body-temperature tap water (250-1000 mL) to flush any remaining sodium polystyrene sulfonate enema out of the colon to remove potassium ions and prevent adverse reactions.
For additional information, call your pharmacist or the drug information center.

Stability Store prepared suspensions at 15°C to 30°C (59°F to 86°F); store repackaged product in refrigerator and use within 14 days; freshly prepared suspensions should be used within 24 hours; do not heat resin suspension

Monitoring Parameters Exchange capacity is 1 mEq/g *in vivo*, and *in vitro* capacity is 3.1 mEq/g, therefore, a wide range of exchange capacity exists such that close monitoring of serum electrolytes (potassium, sodium, calcium, magnesium) is necessary; ECG

Administrations
Oral: Administer oral (or NG) as ~25% sorbitol solution; never mix in orange juice. Chilling the oral mixture will increase palatability.
Rectal: Enema route is less effective than oral administration. Administer cleansing enema first. Retain enema in colon for at least 30-60 minutes and for several hours, if possible. Enema should be followed by irrigation with normal saline to prevent necrosis.

Contraindications Hypersensitivity to sodium polystyrene sulfonate or any component of the formulation; hypernatremia, hypokalemia, obstructive bowel disease

Warnings Use with caution in patients with severe CHF, hypertension, edema, or renal failure; avoid using the commercially available liquid product in neonates due to the preservative content; large oral doses may cause fecal impaction (especially in elderly); enema will reduce the serum potassium faster than oral administration, but the oral route will result in a greater reduction over several hours.

Dosage Forms
Powder for suspension, oral/rectal:
Kayexalate®: 15 g/4 level teaspoons (480 g) [contains sodium 100 mg (4.1 mEq)/g]
Kionex™: 15 g/4 level teaspoons (454 g) [contains sodium 100 mg (4.1 mEq)/g]
Suspension, oral/rectal: 15 g/60 mL (60 mL, 120 mL, 200 mL, 500 mL) [contains sodium 1500 mg (65 mEq)/60 mL, sorbitol, and alcohol 0.1%; cherry/caramel flavor]
SPS®: 15 g/60 mL (60 mL, 120 mL, 480 mL) [contains alcohol 0.3%, sodium 1500 mg (65 mEq)/60 mL, and sorbitol; cherry flavor]

Reference Range Serum potassium: Adults: 3.5-5.2 mEq/L

Test Interactions ↑ sodium; ↓ potassium (S), calcium (S), magnesium (S)

Drug Interactions Systemic alkalosis and seizure has occurred after cation-exchange resins were administered with nonabsorbable cation-donating antacids and laxatives (eg, magnesium hydroxide, aluminum carbonate). Digitalis toxicity may occur with hypokalemia.

Pregnancy Risk Factor C

Lactation Excretion in breast milk unknown/use caution

Nursing Implications Administer oral (or NG) as ~25% sorbitol solution, never mix in orange juice; enema route is less effective than oral administration; retain enema in colon for at least 30-60 minutes and for several hours, if possible. Repeated oral doses can lead to sorbitol-induced electrolyte abnormalities.

Sodium Thiosulfate

Pronunciation (SOW dee um thye oh SUL fate)

Related Information
• Sodium Nitrite [ANTIDOTE]

CAS Number 10102-17-7; 7772-98-7

U.S. Brand Names Versiclear™

Synonyms Disodium Thiosulfate Pentahydrate; Pentahydrate; Sodium Hyposulfate; Sodium Thiosulphate; Thiosulfuric Acid Disodium Salt

Use Alone or with sodium nitrite or amyl nitrite (or hydroxocobalamin) in cyanide poisoning; to reduce the risk of nephrotoxicity associated with cisplatin therapy; topically in the treatment of tinea versicolor; an inorganic reducing agent used as a fixative bleaching of bone; used in manufacture of leather; for selenium dioxide burns; can reduce cisplatin nephrotoxicity; oral lavage use (1% to 5%) for use in gastric decontamination for iodine exposure, can be used for mechlorethamine extravasation along with actinomycin D and mitomycin C; may be useful in chlorate salt toxicity and bromate toxicity; may be used alone in smoke inhalations and to reduce the toxicity of sodium nitroprusside

Unlabeled/Investigational Use Management of I.V. extravasation

Mechanism of Action

Cyanide toxicity: Increases the rate of detoxification of cyanide by the enzyme rhodanese by providing an extra sulfur

Cisplatin toxicity: Complexes with cisplatin to form a compound that is nontoxic to either normal or cancerous cells

Adverse Reactions

Cardiovascular: Hypotension

Central nervous system: Coma, CNS depression secondary to thiocyanate intoxication, psychosis, confusion

Dermatologic: Contact dermatitis, local irritation

Gastrointestinal: Diarrhea (following large oral doses)

Neuromuscular & skeletal: Weakness

Otic: Tinnitus

Pharmacodynamics/Kinetics

Absorption: Oral: Poor

Distribution: Extracellular fluid

Half-life elimination: 0.65 hour

Excretion: Urine (28.5% as unchanged drug)

Dosage

Cyanide and nitroprusside antidote: I.V.:

Children <25 kg: 50 mg/kg after receiving 4.5-10 mg/kg sodium nitrite; a half dose of each may be repeated if necessary

Children >25 kg and Adults: 12.5 g after 300 mg of sodium nitrite; a half dose of each may be repeated if necessary

Cyanide poisoning: I.V.: Dose should be based on determination as with nitrite, at rate of 2.5-5 mL/minute to maximum of 50 mL.

Variation of sodium nitrite and sodium thiosulfate dose, based on hemoglobin concentration*:

Cisplatin rescue should be given before or during cisplatin administration: I.V. infusion (in sterile water): 12 g/m^2 over 6 hours or 9 g/m^2 I.V. push followed by 1.2 g/m^2 continuous infusion for 6 hours

Arsenic poisoning: I.V.: 1 mL first day, 2 mL second day, 3 mL third day, 4 mL fourth day, 5 mL on alternate days thereafter

Children and Adults:

Topical: 20% to 25% solution: Apply a thin layer to affected areas twice daily

SubQ: Drug extravasation (unlabeled use):

2% solution: Infiltrate SubQ into the affected area

1/6 M (~4%) solution: 5-10 mL infused through I.V. line and SubQ into the affected area

Stability Explosive when titrated with chlorates, nitrates, or permanganates

Monitoring Parameters Monitor for signs of thiocyanate toxicity

Administration

I.V.: Inject slowly, over at least 10 minutes; rapid administration may cause hypotension.

Topical: Do not apply to or near eyes.

Contraindications Hypersensitivity to sodium thiosulfate or any component of the formulation

Warnings Safety in pregnancy has not been established; discontinue topical use if irritation or sensitivity occurs; rapid I.V. infusion has caused transient hypotension and ECG changes in dogs; can increase risk of thiocyanate intoxication

Dosage Forms

Injection, solution [preservative free]: 100 mg/mL (10 mL); 250 mg/mL (50 mL)

Lotion: Sodium thiosulfate 25% and salicylic acid 1% (120 mL) [contains isopropyl alcohol 10%]

Reference Range Serum levels of 11.13±1.1 mg/L are normal in adults; levels may be decreased to 5-8 mg/L in postoperative coronary artery bypass graft patients; levels may be elevated up to 22 mg/L in patients kept NPO for 1-3 weeks

Antidote(s)

● Sodium Nitrite [ANTIDOTE]

Pregnancy Risk Factor C

Pregnancy Implications Safety has not been established in pregnant women. Use only when potential benefit to the mother outweighs the possible risk to the fetus.

Nursing Implications Given I.V. as slow I.V. push only over 10 minutes

Specific Reference

Matteucci MJ, Reed WJ, and Tanen DA, "Sodium Thiosulfate Fails to Reduce Nitrite-Induced Methemoglobinemia *In Vitro*," *Acad Emerg Med*, 2003, 10(4):299-302.

Sorbitol

Pronunciation (SOR bi tole)

CAS Number 50-70-4

Use Genitourinary irrigant in transurethral prostatic resection or other transurethral resection or other transurethral surgical procedures; diuretic; humectant; sweetening agent; hyperosmotic laxative; facilitate the passage of sodium polystyrene sulfonate through the intestinal tract

Mechanism of Action Polyalcoholic sugar with osmotic cathartic actions

Adverse Reactions

Cardiovascular: Edema

Central nervous system: Fever, hyperthermia

Endocrine & metabolic: Fluid and electrolyte losses, hypernatremia, lactic acidosis

Gastrointestinal: Diarrhea, nausea, vomiting, abdominal discomfort, xerostomia

Signs and Symptoms of Overdose Diarrhea, fluid and electrolyte loss, hyperglycemia, hypernatremia, nausea

Pharmacodynamics/Kinetics

Onset of action: 0.25-1 hour

Absorption: Oral, rectal: Poor

Metabolism: Primarily hepatic to fructose

Dosage

Hyperosmotic laxative (as single dose, at infrequent intervals):

Children 2-11 years:

Oral: 2 mL/kg (as 70% solution)

Rectal enema: 30-60 mL as 25% to 30% solution

Children >12 years and Adults:

Oral: 30-150 mL (as 70% solution)

Rectal enema: 120 mL as 25% to 30% solution

Adjunct to sodium polystyrene sulfonate: 15 mL as 70% solution orally until diarrhea occurs (10-20 mL/2 hours) or 20-100 mL as an oral vehicle for the sodium polystyrene sulfonate resin

When administered with charcoal:

Oral:

Children: 4.3 mL/kg of 35% sorbitol with activated charcoal/day

Adults: 4.3 mL/kg of 70% sorbitol with activated charcoal/day

Topical: 3% to 3.3% as transurethral surgical procedure irrigation

Monitoring Parameters Monitor for fluid overload and/or electrolyte disturbances following large volumes; changes may be delayed due to slow absorption

Contraindications Anuria

Warnings Use with caution in patients with severe cardiopulmonary or renal impairment and in patients unable to metabolize sorbitol; large volumes may result in fluid overload and/or electrolyte changes

Dosage Forms

Solution, genitourinary irrigation: 3% (3000 mL, 5000 mL); 3.3% (2000 mL, 4000 mL)

Solution, oral: 70% (30 mL, 480 mL, 3840 mL)

Pregnancy Risk Factor C

Lactation Excretion in breast milk unknown

Nursing Implications Do not use unless solution is clear

Specific Reference

Adams BK, Mann MD, Aboo A, et al, "The Effects of Sorbitol on Gastric Emptying Half-Times and Small Intestinal Transit After Drug Overdose," *Am J Emerg Med*, 2006, 24(1):130-2.

Succimer

Pronunciation (SUKS si mer)

Related Information

● Unithiol [ANTIDOTE]

CAS Number 304-55-2

U.S. Brand Names Chemet®

Synonyms DMSA

Use Orphan drug: Treatment of lead poisoning in children with blood levels >45 mcg/dL. It is not indicated for prophylaxis of lead poisoning in a lead-containing environment. Following oral administration, succimer is generally well tolerated and produces a linear dose-dependent reduction in serum lead concentrations. This agent appears to offer advantages over existing lead chelating agents; also has been used for arsenic and mercury poisoning; also used in children with blood lead levels <45 mcg/dL; also useful for mercury and arsenic toxicity

Mechanism of Action Succimer is an analog of dimercaprol. It forms water soluble chelates with heavy metals which are subsequently excreted renally. Initial data have shown encouraging results in the treatment of mercury and arsenic poisoning. Succimer binds heavy metals; however, the chemical form of these chelates is not known.

Adverse Reactions

The most common events attributable to succimer have been observed in ~10% of patients treated

Central nervous system: **Fever**

Dermatologic: Rash

Gastrointestinal: **Nausea, vomiting, diarrhea, appetite loss, metallic taste**, sulfurous odor to breath, **hemorrhoidal symptoms**, hemorrhoids, sulfurous odor to flatulence

Genitourinary: Sulfurous odor to urine, dysuria

Hematologic: Thrombocytosis, eosinophilia, neutropenia (transient)

Hepatic: Elevation of AST, ALT, alkaline phosphatase, and serum cholesterol

Neuromuscular & skeletal: **Back pain**

Respiratory: Rhinitis

Miscellaneous: Flu-like symptoms

Signs and Symptoms of Overdose Anorexia, GI bleeding, hepatotoxicity, nephritis, renal tubular necrosis, respiratory depression, vomiting

Pharmacodynamics/Kinetics

Absorption: Rapid but incomplete

Metabolism: Rapidly and extensively to mixed succimer cysteine disulfides

Half-life elimination: 2 days

Time to peak, serum: ~1-2 hours

Excretion: Urine (~25%) with peak urinary excretion between 2-4 hours (90% as mixed succimer-cysteine disulfide conjugates, 10% as unchanged drug); feces (as unabsorbed drug)

Dosage Children and Adults: Oral: 10 mg/kg/dose every 8 hours for 5 days followed by 10 mg/kg/dose every 12 hours for 14 days

Dosing adjustment in renal/hepatic impairment: Administer with caution and monitor closely

Concomitant iron therapy has been reported in a small number of children without the formation of a toxic complex with iron (as seen with dimercaprol); courses of therapy may be repeated if indicated by weekly monitoring of blood lead levels; lead levels should be stabilized <15 mcg/dL; 2 weeks between courses is recommended unless more timely treatment is indicated by lead levels

Monitoring Parameters Blood lead levels, serum aminotransferases

Contraindications Hypersensitivity to succimer or any component of the formulation

Warnings Caution in patients with renal or hepatic impairment; adequate hydration should be maintained during therapy

Dosage Forms Capsule: 100 mg

Antidote(s)

- Unithiol [ANTIDOTE]

Test Interactions False-positive ketones (U) using nitroprusside methods, falsely elevated serum CPK; falsely decreased uric acid

Drug Interactions Not recommended for concomitant administration with edetate calcium disodium or penicillamine

Pregnancy Risk Factor C

Pregnancy Implications No evidence for mutagenicity

Nursing Implications Adequately hydrate patients; rapid rebound of serum lead levels can occur; monitor closely

Specific Reference

Rencova J, Volf V, Jones MM, Singh PK, "Mobilization and Detoxification of Polonium-210 in Ratio by 2,3-Dinercaptosuccinic Acid and Its Derivatives," *Int J Radiat Biol*, 2000, 76(10):1409-15.

Thrombopoietin

Unlabeled/Investigational Use Investigational: Thrombocytopenia relatable to cytotoxic drugs or cancer; may be useful in treating drug-induced thrombocytopenia not due to immunological destruction

Mechanism of Action Promotes the proliferation and maturation of megakaryocyte progenitors into platelet-producing megakaryocytes; a ligand for the C-Mpl receptor on megakaryocytes

Adverse Reactions

Cardiovascular: Thrombosis is a theoretical concern

Central nervous system: Mild headache has been described although not temporarily related

Dosage I.V.: 0.3-1 mcg/kg/day for up to 10 days; alternatively, a single dose of 0.3-2.4 mcg/kg 3 weeks before chemotherapy has been used; all doses are intravenous

Reference Range Peak serum thrombopoietin level after a 2.4 mcg/kg dose: ~50 ng/mL; endogenous serum thrombopoietin levels range from 0.096-0.24 ng/mL

Tricyclic Antidepressant Antibody Fragments

Synonyms TCA-Fab

Use Tricyclic antidepressant cardiac toxicity (investigational)

Mechanism of Action Binds to tricyclic antidepressant agents in overdose patients by redistributing the antidepressant from tissue to serum. In animals, TCA-Fab reversed hypotension, shortened QRS duration, and improved survival.

Adverse Reactions Mild bronchospasm, cough

Dosage

Investigational: I.V.: Two protocols:

Low dose: 1 g over 30 minutes; if cardiac toxicity (defined as QRS >100 msec or if terminal deflection of the QRS in lead aVR amplitude was >3 mm), then infuse 2 g over 30 minutes; if cardiac toxicity remains: 4 g over 60 minutes

High dose: 2 g over 30 minutes; if cardiac toxicity remains then 4 g over 60 minutes; if cardiac toxicity remains: 8 g over 120 minutes

Additional Information Manufactured by Protherics, Inc, Brentwood, TN (615) 963-4528 or (615) 327-1027

Specific Reference

Heard K, Dart RC, Bogdan G, et al, "A Preliminary Study of Tricyclic Antidepressant (TCA) Ovine Fab for TCA Toxicity," *Clin Toxicol*, 2006, 44:75-81.

Trientine

Pronunciation (TRYE en teen)

CAS Number 112-24-3; 38260-01-4

U.S. Brand Names Syprine®

Synonyms Trientine Hydrochloride

Use Treatment of Wilson's disease in patients intolerant to penicillamine; possible use in copper poisoning

Mechanism of Action Trientine hydrochloride is an oral chelating agent structurally dissimilar from penicillamine and other available chelating agents; an effective oral chelator of copper used to induce adequate cupriuresis

Adverse Reactions

Central nervous system: Malaise

Dermatologic: Tenderness, thickening and fissuring of skin

Endocrine & metabolic: Iron deficiency

Gastrointestinal: Heartburn, diarrhea, abdominal pain, stomach pains

Neuromuscular & skeletal: Muscle pain and cramps, leg cramps

Miscellaneous: Systemic lupus erythematosus, zinc depletion

Dosage Oral (administer on an empty stomach):

Children <12 years: 500-750 mg/day in divided doses 2-4 times/day; maximum: 1.5 g/day

Adults: 750-1250 mg/day in divided doses 2-4 times/day; maximum daily dose: 2 g

Monitoring Parameters Iron levels

Administration Do not chew capsule, swallow whole followed by a full glass of water; notify physician of any fever or skin changes; any skin exposed to the contents of a capsule should be promptly washed with water

Contraindications Hypersensitivity to trientine or any component of the formulation; rheumatoid arthritis, biliary cirrhosis, cystinuria

Warnings May cause iron-deficiency anemia; monitor closely; use with caution in patients with reactive airway disease

Dosage Forms Capsule, as hydrochloride: 250 mg

Drug Interactions Decreased effect with iron and possibly other mineral supplements

Pregnancy Risk Factor C

Trimedoxime Bromide

CAS Number 56-97-3

Synonyms TMB4; Dioxime

Mechanism of Action Acetylcholinesterase reactivator which is a bispyridium oxime which appears to be particularly effective for tabun and minimally effective for soman.

Adverse Reactions

To TMB$_4$: Headache, paresthesia, sensation of warmth, respiratory depression and hypotension at doses >30 mg/kg

To autoinjectors: Local effects (pain, swelling) in 23%; systemic effects of atropinization in 18%

Dosage

As autoinjector (injected into thigh) combined with atropine:

Children <2 years (blue-colored): 0.5 mg atropine/20 mg TMB$_4$

Children 3-10 years and adults >60 years (rose-colored): 1 mg atropine/40 mg TMB$_4$

Children and Adults 10-60 years (yellow-colored): 2 mg atropine/80 mg TMB$_4$

Stability Stable at a pH of 3

Specific References

Kassa J, Kuca K, and Cabul J, "A Comparison of the Potency of Trimedoxime and Other Currently Available Oximes to Reactivate Tabun-Inhibited Acetylcholinesterase and Eliminate Acute Toxic Effects of Tabun," *Biomed Pap Med Fac Palacky Olomouc Czech Republic*, 2005, 149(2):419-23.

Kozer E, Mordel A, Haim SB, et al, "Pediatric Poisoning from Trimedoxime (TMB$_4$) and Atropine Autoinjectors," *J Pediatr*, 2005, 146:41-4.

Unithiol

CAS Number 4076-02-2
Use May be effective for Wilson's disease
Unlabeled/Investigational Use
  Investigational in the U.S.: Antidote for arsenic, bismuth, lead, zinc, mercury (inorganic and organic), chromium, antimony, and cobalt
Mechanism of Action A water soluble chemical analogue of dimercaprol
Adverse Reactions
  Dermatologic: Macular erythematous rash
  Cardiovascular: Hypotension at high doses
  Gastrointestinal: Nausea, vomiting
  Hematologic: Leukopenia
Dosage
  Oral:
    Antimony: Children: 50-100 mg 3 times/day

Arsenic: Mild poisoning: 200 mg orally 3 times/day; severe poisoning: 200 mg I.V. or 400 mg orally initially, then 100-200 mg I.V., or 200-400 mg orally every 2 hours; taper dose slowly
Bismuth: 250 mg every 4 hours I.V., then 250 mg orally 3 times/day for 14 days
Metal chelation: 100 mg 3 times/day for 5 days
Wilson's disease: 200 mg 2 times/day
Dosing scheme for mercury intoxication: I.V.: 250 mg every 4 hours for 48 hours, followed by 250 mg every 6 hours for the succeeding 48 hours, and then 250 mg every 8 hours thereafter; if no gastrointestinal lesions are present, conversion to oral route of administration can occur; following 96 hours of administration, 300 mg 3 times/day can be given orally; continue treatment until mercury levels in blood and urine fall below 100 mcg/L and 300 mcg/L, respectively. Neurological improvement has occurred following three 5-day courses of 30 mg/kg/day.
Pregnancy Implications Not embryotoxic

SECTION VI

DIAGNOSTIC TESTS/PROCEDURES

DRUG TESTING IN THE 21ST CENTURY

Drug Use and Abuse in the U.S.A.

Christine M. Moore, PhD

The number of people who currently use or admit to having used an illicit drug continues to increase.

A survey by the Drug Abuse Warning Network (DAWN) estimates that for the latter two quarters of 2003, cocaine was involved in 125,921 emergency room visits (approximately 1/5 of all drug-related visits); marijuana was involved in 79,663; heroin in 47,604; stimulants, including the amphetamines, were involved in over 40,000 cases, and other illicit drugs such as phencyclidine (PCP), Ecstasy, and GHB were much less frequently encountered.[1]

In 2004, adolescents accounted for approximately 15,000 emergency department visits where drugs were involved in suicide attempts. Antidepressants and other psychotherapeutic drugs were present in over 40% of the cases.[2]

The increasing number and type of illicit and prescription drugs being encountered, continues to challenge drug testing laboratories.

Objectives And Guidelines For Drug Testing

Analysis of body fluids is a necessary step in determining whether or not an individual has ingested illegal or prescription drugs. It is important to note that at this time, the amount of drug in urine does not give any direct information about the amount of drug ingested, the route of ingestion, the degree of impairment, or the extent of drug dependence of the individual. However, studies and research are ongoing to provide as much interpretive data as possible.

Some questions need to be considered before the implementation of any drug testing program and these include:

- Which drugs should be included in the test?
- How sensitive should the screening procedure be?
- How sensitive and specific should the confirmation be?
- Is an adequate chain-of-custody present?
- How will the results be used?

In 1986, the National Institute on Drug Abuse (NIDA), which is now known as the Substance Abuse and Mental Health Services Administration (SAMHSA), addressed some of these issues and developed urine drug testing proficiency guidelines leading to laboratory certification.[3] This was revised December 19, 2000, in order to take effect on August 1, 2001. The guidelines provide for accurate analysis of urine samples by proficiency testing followed by satisfactory laboratory inspections carried out by qualified personnel. Laboratories are required to adhere to Good Laboratory Practice (GLP) as well as establish defensible sample handling (chain-of-custody), reporting, and data reviewing.

The guidelines require the screening and confirmation capability to the levels shown in Table 1 for cocaine metabolite (benzoylecgonine), opiates (codeine and morphine), phencyclidine (PCP), marijuana metabolite (THC-COOH), and amphetamines (amphetamine and methamphetamine).

Table 1. Federal Drug Test Panel		
	Initial (Screening) Cutoff (ng/mL)	Confirmatory (GC/MS) Cutoff (ng/mL)
Marijuana metabolites	50	15*
Cocaine metabolites	300	150†
Opiate metabolites	2000¶	
Morphine		2000¶
Codeine		2000
6-Acetylmorphine		10‡
Phencyclidine	25	25

Table 1. Federal Drug Test Panel (*Continued*)

	Initial (Screening) Cutoff (ng/mL)	Confirmatory (GC/MS) Cutoff (ng/mL)
Amphetamines	1000	
Amphetamine		500
Methamphetamine		500

*Assayed as 11-nor-delta-9-THC-9-carboxylic acid (a THC metabolite).
†Assayed as benzoylecgonine (a cocaine metabolite).
‡Test for 6-AM when the morphine concentration exceeds 2000 ng/mL.
¶4000 for Department of Defense employees.

A positive result for methamphetamine is only reported if amphetamine is also present at a concentration >200 ng/mL. The reasoning behind this is that the *l*-methamphetamine isomer, which is present in the Vicks inhaler, does not metabolize to amphetamine as efficiently as the illegal *d*-methamphetamine isomer, and, therefore, concentrations >200 ng/mL of amphetamine should not be present if a Vicks inhaler only is used.

More recently, the cut-off for opiate screening was changed to 2000 ng/mL and requires that 6-acetyl morphine (6-AM) be present in the confirmatory test in order for a positive result to be reported. The change is to help medical review officers interpret opiate positive results and attempt to eliminate positives caused by, for example, the ingestion of poppy seed bagels or muffins.

New guidelines for the testing of adulterants in urine specimens were also recently approved.

Other agencies such as the Centers for Disease Control, the American Association of Clinical Chemistry, and the American Society of Bioanalysts have administered drug testing programs. The College of American Pathologists (CAP) continues to run and monitor regular proficiency testing services for laboratories involved in drug analysis.[4]

Alternative Specimens For Drug Testing

Urine

Urine is the most common specimen chosen for drug analysis and is the only matrix to which the NIDA guidelines apply at this time. NIDA (SAMHSA) approved laboratories are **not** certified to carry out drug analysis in plasma, serum, blood, meconium, amniotic fluid, hair, or any other tissue or fluid.

Urine is chosen for many reasons:
- it is easy to collect.
- large volumes can often be collected.
- drugs and metabolites are often present in higher concentrations than in other body fluids.
- it is easier to analyze than other fluids or tissues.
- drugs and metabolites are usually stable in frozen urine allowing long-term storage of positive samples.

Urine, however, can be easily adulterated since observed specimen collection is not a common practice. Additionally, most drugs are only present in urine for 2-3 days after ingestion, so only recent drug use will be detected.

Blood, Plasma, and Serum

Blood is considered to be an invasive sample to take for routine drug testing; therefore, it is usually only used in forensic cases as requested at autopsy. It is a difficult specimen with which to work, particularly if hemolyzed.

In December 2004, SAMHSA released proposed guidelines for the use of sweat, oral fluid, and hair for workplace testing. At this time, the final guidelines have not been released, but the proposed cut-off concentrations and drug testing profile are shown in Table 2.[5]

Table 2. Proposed Cut-Off Concentrations and Drug Testing Profile for Federal Workplace Drug Testing						
Drug	Sweat (ng/sweat patch)		Oral Fluid (ng/mL)		Hair (pg/mg)	
	Screen	Confirmation	Screen	Confirmation	Screen	Confirmation
Cocaine & metabolites	25	25	20	8	500	Cocaine 500 BZE, NC, CE: 50
Opiates	25	25	40 6-AM = 4	40 6-AM = 4	200	200
Phencyclidine	20	20	10	10	300	300
Amphetamines	25	25	50	50	500	300
Marijuana & metabolites	4	1	4	2	1	0.05
BZE = benzoylecgonine; NC = norcocaine; CE = cocaethylene						
Amphetamines include amphetamine, methamphetamine, MDMA, MDA, and MDEA						
Opiates include codeine, morphine, and 6-acetylmorphine (6-AM)						

Sweat

The presence of alcohol, as well as a number of drugs, in sweat has been reported. The collection of sweat from various parts of the body can be difficult and unequal, since sweat production depends on temperature, adrenaline level, and degree of physical activity. About 50% of the body's sweat is produced by the torso, with about 25% produced by the head and legs.

However, there are many reports of drugs being detected in sweat and these include methadone, phencyclidine, amphetamine, phenobarbital, morphine, and cocaine.[6] Most drugs take 4-6 hours to appear in sweat, the exception being alcohol which takes 2-4 hours. The Food and Drug Administration has approved wearing the "sweat-patch"® for 7-day monitoring of drug abstinence, such as in parolees.

Lactate concentration is being investigated as a method of normalization of drug concentrations in sweat so that individual results can be compared and interpreted.

Advantages to this type of testing include noninvasive sample collection (the patch is worn on the back, biceps, or chest), ability to carry out normal activities, including swimming and showering, without removing the patch, and the ability to tell if a patch has been removed and reapplied, so preventing adulteration.[7] The predominant species found in sweat are parent compounds, not drug metabolites. Analysis of duplicate patches in controlled studies have reported that intrasubject variability is low but intersubject variability is high.

Oral Fluid (Saliva)

Saliva is considered a possible alternative specimen to urine for drug testing because it is an easy and a noninvasive sample to collect. Additionally, it offers an advantage over urine testing if impairment determination is required. Generally drug concentrations in saliva are lower than those found in urine or plasma and the major compound detected is the parent drug, not the metabolites. Initially, oral, intranasal, or smoking drugs may produce high concentrations in saliva for a few hours. However, later, the concentration of drug in saliva is thought to reflect free drug fraction in blood.

Drug excretion in saliva depends on pH and salivary flow, leading to highly variable saliva/plasma ratios for drugs of abuse. It is important to note that most collection devices sequester "oral fluid," not strictly saliva, which accounts for some of the variability of drug testing results experienced with this sample matrix. Disadvantages to saliva testing are mainly associated with the collection of the sample, in that often the actual amount of oral fluid collected is not known, and compared to urine, there is a much smaller volume available for testing.

A comprehensive review of saliva testing for drugs of abuse, which includes information on alcohol, amphetamines, barbiturates, benzodiazepines, caffeine, cocaine, inhalants, LSD, marijuana, opioids, phencyclidine, and tobacco products, is available.[8]

Hair

Hair has been used as an alternative to urine over the last few years. Hair is a noninvasive specimen and can give historical information on drug use which urine cannot. Additionally, it is easy to transport and store. Disadvantages to hair analysis include the determination of drug use versus environmental exposure; potential color bias; and effect of bleaching, coloring, and other hair treatments on the analytical results.[9-11]

Meconium and Amniotic Fluid

Drug-, alcohol-, and tobacco-exposed babies suffer from a variety of adverse effects at birth including low birth weight and head size, and in later life, possible learning disabilities.[12,13]

Pediatricians and nurses are now requesting the analysis of neonatal meconium rather than urine. Studies show meconium to be a better indicator of drug use during pregnancy than urine.[14,15] As previously discussed, the half-life of drugs and metabolites in urine only allows fairly recent use of a drug to be detected. Meconium begins to form after about 16 weeks of gestation and is cumulative thereafter. Testing is widely available in commercial laboratories, hospitals, and as ELISA procedures become more prevalent, the screening of meconium for a wide variety of drugs is a simple process.

Amniotic fluid, umbilical cord, and cord blood have also been suggested as alternative samples. Amniotic fluid is present throughout gestation and is constantly diluted due to fetal urination. Fetal swallowing of amniotic fluid may also contribute to the recirculation of drug metabolites through the baby.[16,17]

Techniques in Drug Testing

Drug Screening

The technology of drug screening has greatly improved. Screening tests are designed for maximum sensitivity at the expense of selectivity. It is important, however, that screening tests do not give false-negative results since this terminates the testing process. False-positives at this stage are acceptable because all presumptive positive samples are re-extracted and analyzed by a confirmatory technique.

Thin-Layer Chromatography (TLC)

TLC is an old, but still widely used, technique for the separation and identification of drugs. Essentially, the drug is extracted from urine and concentrated onto a silica plate. The plate is then placed in a solvent tank of chosen polarity. As the solvent rises up the plate, it "elutes" the drugs and carries them to various distances depending upon the affinity of the drug for the plate and for the solvent (or mobile phase). The plate is then sprayed with suitable reagents which allow the drugs to be identified by color and specific positioning relative to drug standards.[18]

The technique is cheap and relatively simple, and there are many choices of stationary and mobile phases making complex separations possible.

Disadvantages include interpretation due to interference from endogenous substances. Also, the technique involves lengthy extraction and concentration steps, difficulties in saving data (spots on plates fade with time and photographic representations do not reproduce colors well), and a need for operator experience and skill in spotting and spraying plates. However, TLC is not very specific and results require further confirmation.

Immunoassays

Immunoassay techniques are now the most widely used screening procedures in drug testing. Popular versions of these tests include radioimmunoassay (RIA), enzyme-multiplied immunoassay technique (EMIT), enzyme-linked immunosorbent assay (ELISA), and fluorescence polarization immunoassay (FPIA).

These techniques use antibodies specific to the drug being assayed and a labeled form of the same drug. The label itself may be a radioactive isotope (RIA), an active enzyme (EMIT and ELISA), or a fluorescent label (FPIA) which is incorporated synthetically. A fixed quantity of antibody and labeled drug is added to the test sample. The binding sites on the antibody attract both labeled drug and the unlabeled drug in the sample. The amount of labeled drug bound is inversely proportional to the number of unlabeled drug molecules present.

In RIA, a radioactively labeled drug competes for the same antibody binding site as the unlabeled drug. The analytical measurement of bound radioactivity determines the amount of unlabeled drug in the sample. This method is used to detect opiates, cannabinoids, benzoylecgonine, amphetamines, and phencyclidine, as well as more esoteric drugs such as fentanyl and LSD, although the sensitivity of ELISA screens and their wide availability have largely replaced RIA screening procedures.

In EMIT and FPIA testing, the analytical measurement is of an optically detected change such as UV absorption, fluorescence, or luminescence. These systems avoid the use of radioactive isotopes but also have reduced sensitivity when compared to RIA, because the optical signal is measured in the presence of the original biological fluid.

The application of these types of assays to forensic drug testing has recently been described.[19-21]

Additional antibody kits are also available expanding the use of these systems to include methadone, benzodiazepines, methaqualone, and barbiturates. Advantages include high sensitivity, no extraction steps, and applicability to large numbers of samples.

All immunoassay tests are susceptible to false-positive results due to cross-reactivity of the antibodies with legal or prescription drugs. Several publications on the effect of poppy seed intake on opiate assays have been reported.[22-23]

Potential cross reactants to immunoassays are included with manufacturer package inserts when kits are purchased for use.

Table 3. Usual Maximum Concentrations of Street Drugs Due to Passive Inhalation	
	Urinary Concentration (unless otherwise noted)
Marijuana (all metabolites)	
Small, unventilated room	
4 cigarettes	12 ng/mL
16 cigarettes (acid metabolite)	30 ng/mL
Car	14 ng/mL
Cocaine benzoylecgonine (from volatilized cocaine freebase)	14 ng/mL
Phencyclidine (serum sample)	129 ng/mL
References:	
Baselt RC, Yoshikawa DM, and Chang JY, "Passive Inhalation of Cocaine," *Clin Chem*, 1991, 2150-61.	
Cone EJ, "Marijuana Effects and Urinalysis After Passive Inhalation and Oral Ingestion. In Research Findings on Smoking Abused Substances," Chiang CN and Hawks RL, eds, NIDA Res Monograph, 1990, 99:88-96.	
Cone EJ, Yousefnejad D, Hillsgrove MJ, et al,"Passive Inhalation of Cocaine," *J Anal Toxicol*, 1995, 19:399-411.	
ElSohly MA and Jones AB, "Drug Testing in the Workplace: Could a Positive Test for One of the Mandated Drugs be for the Reasons Other than Illicit Use of the Drug?" *J Anal Toxicol*, 1995, 19:450-8.	
Schwartz RH and Einhorn A, "PCP Intoxication in Seven Young Children," *Pediatr Emerg Care*, 1986, 2:238-41.	

Drug Confirmations

High Performance Liquid Chromatography (HPLC)

HPLC allows the separation of nonvolatile substances from each other or from other components of an extraction residue. When a mixture of substances is injected onto the column, each component is partitioned between the stationary phase (column) and the liquid (mobile) phase. Molecules with greater affinity for the column spend more time in that phase and, therefore, take longer to reach the detector. The time taken from injection to the peak maximum is known as the retention time. The detector responds in direct proportion to the concentration of material passing through it, hence peak heights and areas shown on the chromatogram are directly related to the concentration of each analyte.

HPLC shows good sensitivity and high specificity depending upon the detection system used. The most common detectors utilize absorption of UV light by the drug. A diode array detector will allow a full UV spectrum of the analyte to be obtained. This can be compared to a standard spectrum of the drug, and identification is then based both on retention time and UV spectra. Most instruments also include the facility to obtain first and second derivative spectra to provide an additional means of identification. Postcolumn reactions for increased sensitivity have also been described.[24]

HPLC is relatively inexpensive and can be used for confirmations.

Gas Chromatography (GC)

Gas chromatography is also a method of separating substances of analytical interest. It is one of the most sensitive techniques available for detecting drugs in body fluids. The separation is carried out on an analytical column containing a stationary phase (liquid or solid, depending on temperature) which is maintained at a given temperature inside an oven. The whole GC system comprises six components: gas supply and flow controllers, injector, oven, column, detector, and recording device. In drug testing, GC capillary (rather than packed) columns are commonly used. A compound is identified by matching its retention time (the time between injection and peak maximum) with that of a drug standard under the same conditions (gas flow rate, temperature, column length, etc).

GC equipment is now relatively inexpensive and experienced personnel are required to run and maintain instruments and interpret chromatograms. Additionally, while GC is fairly specific, its use with nonspecific detectors such as flame ionization (FID), nitrogen-phosphorus (NPD), or electron capture (ECD) does not absolutely identify a compound.

Gas Chromatography/Mass Spectrometry (GC/MS)

GC/MS is the most widely used technique for confirmatory procedures following initial screening assays. It is the so-called gold standard of forensic and drug testing work. The use of GC with a mass spectrometric detection system is forensically defensible as an absolute identification procedure.

When a molecule is injected into the chromatographic system, it is separated from other components of the extraction residue on the basis of its degree of affinity for and interaction with the stationary phase. Upon elution from the chromatographic column, it is bombarded with electrons which cause it to break apart. The fragments produced are separated on the basis of their mass to charge ratio. Under the same conditions, a molecule will fragment in exactly the same way every time, producing the same spectrum. This spectrum or "fingerprint" can then be compared to that of a drug standard for absolute identification.

Figure 2

    a. GC/MS Chromatogram
         Drug test mixture containing cocaine (retention time 5.8 minutes)

    b. GC/MS Spectrum
         Spectrum of peak at 5.8 minutes

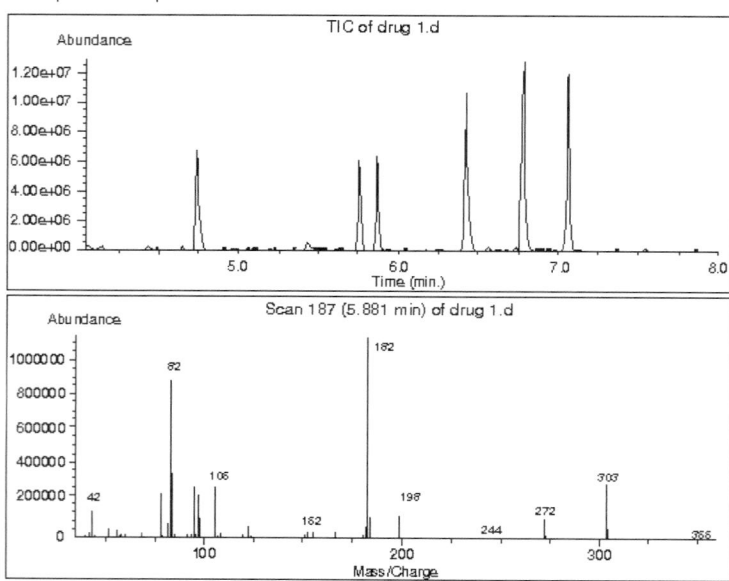

GC/MS is a relatively expensive technique but is necessary in every laboratory which is carrying out confirmatory testing for drugs of metabolites in biological fluids.[25,26] Experienced operators and interpreters are also needed in order to produce good data. For even more sensitive analyses, an additional gas chromatograph can be added giving two-dimensional gas chromatography (GC/GC/MS); or an additional mass spectrometer giving a triple quadrople spectrometric system (GC/MS/MS).

Gas Chromatography-Fourier Transform Infrared Spectrophotometry

GC-FTIR is also a forensically acceptable and defensible technique. It is more expensive and less common than GC/MS because it is more difficult to interpret the spectra, requiring skilled and experienced operators and reviewers.

Liquid Chromatography - Mass Spectrometry - Mass Spectrometry (LC/MS/MS)

LC/MS/MS is becoming increasingly used in forensic and drug testing laboratories. The use of liquid chromatography eliminates the need for derivatization of the molecule, which is often required in gas chromatographic procedures. Additionally, run times are short, allowing more samples to be analyzed in less time.[27,28]

LC/MS/MS equipment is expensive and does require skilled operators.

Future Trends

Potency of Illicit Drugs and Pharmaceuticals

- **LSD**
  The recent resurgence of lysergic acid diethylamide (LSD) as a drug of choice poses particular problems for the physician in diagnosis and the analyst in determination. The amounts ingested in order to produce the desired effect are extremely low and, therefore, very difficult to detect in biological specimens. There are no FPIA kits readily available to screen for LSD; but ELISA and RIA methods are commonly used as screening procedures. For confirmation, some papers have suggested using electron impact GC/MS (the most common approach) but it is likely that the sensitivity of GC/MS/MS systems will be required, or chemical ionization procedures.[29] Such techniques are somewhat complicated and not currently used in the majority of routine hospital laboratories.

- **Fentanyl**
  Fentanyl (N-phenyl-N-[1-(2-phenylethyl)-4-piperidinyl] (propanamide)) is a potent, fast-acting, synthetic narcotic analgesic. Its potency is considered to be 100-200 times that of morphine, but its effects are shorter. It was developed as an intravenous anesthetic, marketed in the U.S.A. as Sublimaze® and as Innovar® when used with droperidol. However, a number of fentanyl analogues are also available, specifically alphamethylfentanyl (twice the potency of fentanyl), sufentanil, carfentanil, alfentanil, thienylfentanyl, lofentanil, 3-methylfentanyl, and p-fluorofentanyl. These are mostly sold for surgical and veterinary purposes but have appeared on the street as "designer drugs," "synthetic heroin," and "China White."
  Most of the screening for these drugs is currently carried out using ELISA technology.[30] Confirmation is by GC/MS and the levels present are detectable using electron impact GC/MS.

- **Benzodiazepines**
  Potent benzodiazepines, such as alprazolam, flunitrazepam, and triazolam, are administered at very low doses. Detection of the parent drug in biological fluids is extremely difficult and the majority of laboratories search for metabolites. Benzodiazepine immunoassays do cross react well with some metabolites as well as parent drugs, but the confirmation procedures become more difficult. Different modes of detection are usually employed such as negative or positive ion chemical ionization GC/MS or LC/MS/MS.

- **MDMA, MDEA**
  The European "designer drugs," MDMA and MDEA are being encountered more frequently in the U.S.A. MDMA, its metabolite MDA, and MDEA have been included in the SAMHSA guidelines for drug testing laboratories.

- **Synthetic Opiates**
  According to the DEA, the most highly abused prescription drugs in the U.S. today are opioid painkillers (eg, hydrocodone, oxycodone). OxyContin®, which was first marketed in 1996, is a 12-hour time-release formulation of oxycodone, which is also the active ingredient in Percocet® and Percodan®. OxyContin® allows patients to take fewer pills over a longer time for increased relief from pain, but its abuse potential is enormous. Similarly, Vicodin® (hydrocodone), which is often prescribed following major surgery, has a high abuse potential.

- **Anabolic Steroids**
  The use of anabolic steroids among teenagers and young adults is becoming increasingly popular, particularly in those involved in sports requiring great strength such as weight lifting and body building. All anabolic steroids are derivatives of the male hormone testosterone and all are intended for "tissue building" and increasing masculinizing effects.

Over 100 anabolic steroids are widely available in oral or injectable form. They are used for many medical reasons including the treatment of some breast cancers, growth promotion, and delayed puberty. Reported psychological side effects associated with their use include aggression, psychosis, and changes in libido.

In 1974, they were added to the list of doping agents banned by the International Olympic Committee (IOC). Extensive metabolic pathways, as well as natural occurrence, makes the detection of these substances difficult. However, athletic drug testing laboratories are routinely able to detect many of the anabolic steroids in urine samples by using gas chromatography/mass spectrometry (GC/MS) methods. Other drug classes which have become widely abused include GHB, ketamine, and antidepressants such as sertraline and fluoxetine. Drug testing laboratories will be required to expand their drug profiles as more and more new drugs are used and abused.

Conclusions

- It is important to be aware of the limitations of screening and confirmatory drug testing techniques. Even though GC/MS instrumentation is expensive, it is the cheapest way to absolutely identify the contents of a biological sample, ensuring the analysis is forensically defensible.

- Drug levels do not give any information about possible drug abuse or dependence, route or amount of drug ingestion, or (with the possible exception of blood and saliva) the degree of impairment. It is recommended that readers familiarize themselves with metabolic routes and pharmacokinetics of the drugs in question.

- Urine is still the most commonly tested biological fluid although the search continues for a noninvasive, adulterant-free sample which will provide a history of drug use.

- The increasing potency of new drugs and pharmaceuticals, as well as the increasing number of drugs, will place new demands on the laboratory. A wider range of immunoassay kits with better sensitivity and specificity will be required, as will increasingly sensitive confirmation instrumentation.

Footnotes

1. DAWN Report Interim National Emergency Department Estimates (2003).
2. The New DAWN Report 6 (2006).
3. Part II Department of Transportation: Procedures for Transportation Workplace Drug and Alcohol Testing Programs; Final Rule. 49 CFR, Part 40, *Fed Reg*, 2000, 65(244):79462-576.
4. Substance-Abuse Testing Committee, "Critical Issues in Urinalysis of Abused Substances," *Clin Chem*, 1988, 34(3):605-32.
5. Department of Health and Human Services. Substance Abuse and Mental Health Services Administration. Proposed Revisions to Mandatory Guidelines for Federal Workplace Drug Testing Programs, *Fed Reg*, 2004, 69(71):19673-732.
6. Cone EJ, Hillsgrove MJ, Jenkins AJ, et al, "Sweat Testing for Heroin, Cocaine, and Metabolites," *J Anal Toxicol*, 1994, 18(6):298-305.
7. Burns M and Baselt RC, "Monitoring Drug Use With a Sweat Patch: An Experiment with Cocaine," *J Anal Toxicol*, 1995, 19(1):41-8.
8. Cone EJ, "Saliva Testing for Drugs of Abuse," *Ann N Y Acad Sci*, 1993, 694:91-127.
9. Cone EJ, "Testing Human Hair for Drugs of Abuse. Individual Dose and Time Profiles of Morphine and Codeine in Plasma, Saliva, Urine, and Beard Compared to Drug-Induced Effects on Pupils and Behavior," *J Anal Toxicol*, 1990, 14(1):1-7.
10. Hold K, Wilkins D, Rollins D, et al, "Simultaneous Quantitation of Cocaine, Opiates, and Their Metabolites in Human Hair by Positive Ion Chemical Ionization Gas Chromatography-Mass Spectrometry," *J Chromatogr Sci*, 1998, 36:125-30.
11. Strano-Rossi S, Bermejo-Barrera A, and Chiarotti M, "Segmental Hair Analysis for Cocaine and Heroin Abuse Determination," *Forens Sci Int*, 1995, 70:211-6.
12. Singer LT, Salvator A, Arendt R, et al, "Effects of Cocaine/Polydrug Exposure and Maternal Psychological Distress on Infant Birth Outcomes," *Neurotoxicol Teratol*, 2002, 24(2):127-35.
13. Dusick AM, Covert RF, Schreiber MD, et al, "Risk of Intracranial Hemorrhage and Other Adverse Outcomes After Cocaine Exposure in a Cohort of 323 Very Low Birth Weight Infants," *J Pediatr*, 1993, 122(3):438-45.
14. Ostrea EM, Jr, Brady MJ, Parks PM, et al, "Drug Screening of Meconium in Infants of Drug Dependent Mothers: An Alternative to Urine Testing," *J Pediatr*, 1989, 115(3):474-7.

15. Browne SP, Tebbett IR, Moore CM, et al, "Analysis of Meconium for Cocaine in Neonates," *J Chromatogr*, 1992, 575(1):158-61.

16. Moore CM, Brown S, Negrusz A, et al, "Determination of Cocaine and Its Major Metabolite Benzoylecgonine, in Amniotic Fluid, Umbilical Cord Blood, Umbilical Cord Tissue, and Neonatal Urine: A Case Study," *J Anal Toxicol*, 1993, 17(1):62.

17. Jain L, Meyer W, Moore C, et al, "Detection of Fetal Cocaine Exposure by Analysis of Amniotic Fluid," *Obstet Gynecol*, 1993, 81(5 Pt 1):787-90.

18. Schmidt M and Bracher F, "A Convenient TLC Method for the Identification of Local Anesthetics," *Pharmazie*, 2006, 61(1):15-7.

19. Kerrigan S and Phillips WJ, Jr, "Comparison of ELISAs for Opiates, Methamphetamine, Cocaine Metabolite, Benzodiazepines, Phencyclidine, and Cannabinoids in Whole Blood and Urine," *Clin Chem*, 2001, 47(3):540-7.

20. Kroener L, Musshoff F, and Madea B, "Evaluation of Immunochemical Drug Screenings of Whole Blood Samples: A Retrospective Optimization of Cutoff Levels After Confirmation-Analysis on GC-MS and HPLC-DAD," *J Anal Toxicol*, 2003, 27(4):205-12.

21. Hino Y, Ojanpera L, Rasanen I, et al, "Performance of Immunoassays in Screening for Opiates, Cannabinoids, and Amphetamines in Post-Mortem Blood," *Forens Sci Int*, 2003, 131(2-3):148-55.

22. Rohrig T and Moore C, "The Determination of Morphine in Urine and Oral Fluid Following Ingestion of Poppy Seeds," *J Anal Toxicol*, 2003, 27(7):449-52.

23. Thevis M, Opfermann G, and Schanzer W, "Urinary Concentrations of Morphine and Codeine After Consumption of Poppy Seeds," *J Anal Toxicol*, 2003, 27(1):53-6.

24. Roy IM, Jefferies TM, Threadgill MD, et al, "Analysis of Cocaine, Benzoylecgonine, Ecgonine Methyl Ester, Ethylcocaine, and Norcocaine in Human Urine Using HPLC With Post-Column Ion-pair Extraction and Fluorescence Detection," *J Pharm Biomed Anal*, 1992, 10(10-12):943-8.

25. Klette KL, Jamerson MH, and Morris-Kukoski CL, "Rapid Simultaneous Determination of Amphetamine, Methamphetamine, 3,4-Methylenedioxyamphetamine, 3,4-Methylenedioxymethamphetamine, and 3,4-Methylenedioxyethylamphetamine in Urine by Fast Chromatography-Mass Spectrometry," *J Anal Toxicol*, 2005, 29(7):669-74.

26. Jamerson MH, Welton RM, Morris-Kukoski CL, et al, "Rapid Quantification of Urinary 11-nor-δ9-Tetrahydrocannabinol-9-Carboxylic Acid Using Fast Gas Chromatography-Mass Spectrometry," *J Anal Toxicol*, 2005, 29(7):664-8.

27. Edinboro LE, Backer RC, and Poklis A, "Direct Analysis of Opiates in Urine by Liquid Chromatography-Tandem Mass Spectrometry," *J Anal Toxicol*, 2005, 29(7):704-10.

28. Herrin GL, McCurdy HH, and Wall WH, "Investigation of an LC-MS-MS (QTrap) Method for the Rapid Screening and Identification of Drugs in Postmortem Toxicology Whole Blood Samples," *J Anal Toxicol*, 2005, 29(7):599-606.

29. Reuschel SA, Eades D, and Foltz R, "Recent Advances in Chromatographic and Mass Spectrometric Methods for Determination of LSD and Its Metabolites in Physiological Specimens," *J Chromatogr B Biomed Sci Applns*, 1999, 733(1-2)145-59.

30. Makowski GS, Richter JJ, Moore RE, et al, "An Enzyme-Linked Immunosorbent Assay for Urinary Screening of Fentanyl Citrate Abuse," *Ann Clin Lan Sci*, 1995, 25(2):169-78.

31. Drummer OH, "Drug Testing in Oral Fluid," *Clin Biochem Rev*, 2006, 27(3):147-159.

32. Walsh JM, Crouch DJ, Danaceau JP, et al, "Evaluation of Ten Oral Fluid Point of Collection Drug-Testing Devices," *J Anal Toxicol*, 2007, 31(1):44-54.

Acetaminophen, Serum

Synonyms Anacin-3® Level, Blood; Datril® Level, Blood; Liquiprin® Level, Blood; Panadol® Level, Blood; Panex® Level, Blood; Paracetamol Level, Blood; Phenaphen® Level, Blood; Tempra® Level, Blood; Tylenol® Level, Blood

Uses Therapeutic monitoring; evaluate acetaminophen toxicity

Reference Range Acetaminophen, serum: 20-110 mcg/mL (SI: 43-240 μmol)

Abstract Acetaminophen is an analgesic-antipyretic widely used as a replacement for aspirin. It is frequently seen in the deliberate overdose situation.

Specimen Blood

Volume 10 mL

Minimum Volume 3 mL

Container Red top tube

Critical Values Toxic: > 150 mcg/mL (SI: > 990 μmol/L) (within 4 hours); > 50 mcg/mL (SI: > 330 μmol/L) (within 12 hours)

Methodology UV spectrophotometry, immunoassay, gas-liquid chromatography (GLC), or high performance liquid chromatography (HPLC)

Additional Information

Hydrochlorothiazide may cause false increase in acetaminophen assay by HPLC method.

Phenols (from throat lozenges) can cause a false elevation of acetaminophen by the ortho-cresol method. Conversely, N-acetylcysteine can falsely lower acetaminophen level by the ortho-cresol method.

Salicylates and methyl salicylate can cause an increase of serum acetaminophen level of 10% by spectrochemical method. Each rise of 1 mg/dL of creatinine can cause a 30 mg/L rise of acetaminophen. Cephalosporins and sulfonamides can also falsely elevate serum acetaminophen level by HPLC.

Specific References

Song W and Dou C, "One-Step Immunoassay for Acetaminophen and Salicylate in Serum, Plasma, and Whole Blood," *J Anal Toxicol*, 2003, 27(6):366-71.

Acetylcholinesterase, Red Blood Cell

Related Information

- Pseudocholinesterase, Serum

Synonyms Acetylcholinesterase, RBC; Cholinesterase, Erythrocytic; Erythrocyte Cholinesterase; Red Cell Cholinesterase; True Cholinesterase

Uses Erythrocyte cholinesterase is measured to diagnose organophosphate and carbamate toxicity and to detect atypical forms of the enzyme. Cholinesterase is irreversibly inhibited by organophosphate insecticides and reversibly inhibited by carbamate insecticides. Serum or plasma pseudocholinesterase is a better measure of acute toxicity, while erythrocyte levels are better for chronic exposure. (Serum level returns to normal prior to normalizing of red cell level.) Acetylcholinesterase is increased in amniotic fluid in cases of neural tube defect. Persons with an atypical form of the enzyme (with low enzyme activity) exhibit prolonged apnea following the use of certain suxamethonium-type muscle relaxants in anesthesia (succinylcholine sensitivity - AA phenotype). These atypical forms may be detected by the use of fluoride or dibucaine inhibition. In amniotic fluid, it is used for the evaluation of neural tube defects in conjunction with alpha-fetoprotein.

Reference Range Not well established, varies with method, age, sex, and use of oral contraceptives. Normally absent in amniotic fluid. Usual range in healthy individuals: 4000-12,000 unit/L. While neonatal levels are initially low, adult levels are achieved after 2 months of age. Mild poisoning usually results in acetylcholinesterase levels 20% to 50% of normals; moderate poisoning results in a depression to 10% to 20% of normal, while severe poisoning results in a depression of <10% of normal.

Specimen Blood

Minimum Volume 2 mL whole blood

Container Green top (heparin) tube or heparinized capillary tubes

Storage Instructions Stable at 4°C to 25°C for 1 week only.

Limitations Values decrease as erythrocytes become senescent.

Methodology Methods are based on determination of result (rate) of hydrolysis of an ester catalyzed by the enzyme acetylcholinesterase and include colorimetry, fluorometry, spectrophotometry based systems. Polyacrylamide gel electrophoresis is used for the qualitative demonstration of acetylcholinesterase in amniotic fluid. Screening methods are available.

Additional Information

The cholinesterase activity in human red cells is highly but not exclusively specific for acetylcholine. It is referred to as true or specific cholinesterase. Cholinesterase activity present in the serum/plasma hydrolyses both choline and aliphatic esters, has a broader range of esterolytic activity and is referred to as "pseudo-" or "nonspecific" cholinesterase. It hydrolyses acetylcholine only slowly. The systematic name for acetylcholinesterase is acetylcholine acetylhydrolase. Systematic name for cholinesterase (serum/plasma) is acylcholine acylhydrolase. The different nature of the cholinesterases was first described in 1940.

The plasma enzyme is synthesized by the liver, the red cell enzyme during erythropoiesis.

Cholinesterase activity is low at birth and higher in adult males than females. The enzyme is a large complex protein. There is evidence that it has a multiple subunit structure, four peptide chains that form two dimers. Because of the many constituent amino acids, many molecular variants are possible. The RBC level is **increased** in hemolytic states such as the thalassemias, spherocytosis, hemoglobin SS, and acquired hemolytic anemias. It is **decreased** in paroxysmal nocturnal hemoglobinuria and in relapse of megaloblastic anemia. (It returns to normal with therapy.)

Potent inhibitors of cholinesterase may present important clinical toxicological problems. Systemic insecticides (eg, organophosphates or carbamates) are examples. Both RBC acetylcholinesterase and plasma cholinesterase are usually inhibited. The effect on the plasma enzyme is more marked, however, and serum levels are usually utilized in diagnosis and assessment of recovery. Recovery is best determined by looking for a plateau in erythrocyte cholinesterase activity. Toxic potency may vary, plasma versus red cell cholinesterase, such that in some cases erythrocyte levels may be needed for diagnosis and/or monitoring. If there is suspicion that a decrease in cholinesterase activity may not relate to the inhibitor effect of an organophosphate then red cell level of acetylcholinesterase should be obtained. If both serum and RBC levels are significantly decreased, findings are those of exogenous toxic effect.

True cholinesterase (acetylcholinesterase-RBC cholinesterase) is not normally present in amniotic fluid. The presence of acetylcholinesterase activity and increased levels of alpha-fetoprotein in amniotic fluid is presumptive evidence of an open neural tube defect (eg, anencephaly, open spina bifida, or omphalocele) in the fetus.

Activated Partial Thromboplastin Time

Applies to Antiaggregating Agents; Heparin Inhibitors; Heparin; Low Molecular Weight; Protamine Sulfate; Thrombin Clotting Time Heparin Assay

Synonyms APTT; Partial Thromboplastin Time, Activated; PTT

Uses Evaluate intrinsic coagulation system; useful in monitoring heparin therapy; aid in screening for presence of classical hemophilia A and B; congenital deficiencies of factors II, V, VIII, IX, X, XI, and XII; dysfibrinogenemia; disseminated intravascular coagulation; liver failure; congenital hypofibrinogenemia; vitamin K deficiency; congenital deficiency of Fitzgerald factor; congenital deficiency of prekallikrein (Fletcher factor)

Contraindicating Factors Specimen obtained less than 3 hours after dose of heparin

Reference Range 25-39 seconds, usually stated to be within 10 seconds of control. Healthy premature newborns have prolonged coagulation test screening results (eg, PT, PTT, TT) which return to normal adult values at ~6 months of age. Healthy prematures, however, do not develop spontaneous hemorrhage or thrombotic complications because of a balance between procoagulants and inhibitors. A plasma heparin level of 0.4 units/mL results in changes of APTT of 11-57 seconds while a mean dose of heparin of 13.9 units/kg/hour can double the APTT. The normal range in childhood (ages 1-16) is similar to that in adults.

Test Commonly Includes Patient time and control time

Abstract The activated partial thromboplastin time (APTT) is a readily available low cost screening test. The test procedure is usually automated, batch processing is efficient, and the turnaround time is reasonably rapid in the individual or stat mode. The test finds application in screening for intrinsic factor deficiencies and for monitoring of heparin anticoagulation.

Patient Preparation Draw specimen 1 hour before next dose of heparin if heparin is being given by intermittent injection; not applicable to patients on continuous heparin infusion therapy. Do not draw from an arm with a heparin lock or heparinized catheter.

Specimen Plasma

Minimum Volume 4.5 mL

Container Blue top (sodium citrate) tube

Collection Routine venipuncture. If multiple tests are being drawn, draw coagulation studies last. If only a PTT is being drawn, draw 1-2 mL into another Vacutainer®, discard, and then collect the PTT (two-tube or two-syringe technique). This collection procedure avoids contamination of the specimen with tissue thromboplastins. Transport the specimen to the Hematology Laboratory as soon as possible.

Storage Instructions Keep refrigerated.

Causes for Rejection Tube not full; specimen hemolyzed; specimen clotted; specimen received more than 2 hours after collection; specimen improperly labeled; specimen contaminated by anticoagulant, effect of which is not being measured

Possible Panic Range > 70 seconds

Methodology Methods involve addition of a contact activator (eg, Celite, kaolin, microsilicate, elagic acid). Plasma sample is added to activator and incubated at 37°C, usually for 5 minutes. Thromboplastin preparation is added, mixed, and with addition of $CaCl_2$, a timer is started. A variety of automated instruments have been designed to perform this test, often with the capability of also performing the prothrombin time test. A variety of instruments and reagents are used in the field resulting in many combinations, most monitored by the College of American Pathologists survey process.

Additional Information

Hemolysis significantly shortens the activated partial thromboplastin time in normal but not in abnormal persons. The APTT may be normal in persons with mild hereditary bleeding disorders. About 30% of normal concentration of factors V, VIII, IX, X, XI, and XII will maintain a rate of thrombin formation sufficient to produce a normal APTT. Fibrinogen level, if <80 mg/dL, may result in an abnormal APTT. If Fletcher or Fitzgerald factors are <5% of normal the APTT may be abnormal. A prolonged APTT can be caused by inherited factor deficiency (I, II, V, VIII-XII), Fletcher or Fitzgerald, Coumadin® type therapy, liver disease, circulating anticoagulant (heparin, lupus anticoagulant, fibrin breakdown products), specific factor inhibitor (rheumatoid arthritis, penicillin reaction, occasional hemophiliacs), or intravascular coagulation.

The results of the College of American Pathologists surveys indicate that the source and type of heparinized specimen is important to consider when interpreting APTT test results. Different reagent/instrument combinations effect the APTT response to heparin. Sensitivity is most influenced by the APTT reagent used while precision is most effected by the instrument utilized.

Control of heparin therapy: Heparin is an acidic mucopolysaccharide that inhibits all of the active serine proteases (IIa, Xa, IXa, XIa, and XIIa). It has a strong negative charge and a circulating half-life of only a few hours. It is stable for 24 hours in a 5% dextrose solution. Elimination is largely by the kidney so that heparin must be used cautiously in patients with impaired glomerular filtration.

Administration, dosage: Heparin is best administered intravenously, intermittently, or better as continuous infusion in a dosage of 400-500 units/kg body weight/day divided into every 6-hour dosage (so that 100-125 units/kg body weight is given each 6 hours). Laboratory monitoring can be accomplished using the Lee-White clotting time, APTT, activated clotting time (ACT) or heparin assay. Dosage is adjusted to maintain the coagulation test result at about two times the control or "normal" level (APTT target range 60-85 seconds or APTT ratio which is equivalent to a heparin level by antifactor Xa assay of 0.3-0.7 units/mL).

There are three levels of heparin therapy: low dose, moderate dose, and large dose. Low dose refers to small amounts of heparin (10,000-20,000 units/day) given subcutaneously and useful in the prophylaxis against venous thrombosis (selected patients). Measurable change in APTT does not usually occur. See review by Hirsh and Levine listed in references. Moderate dose implies full anticoagulation, requires 20,000-60,000 units/day, the APTT is adjusted to 1.5 to 2 times the control, and the regimen is applied to patients without active thromboembolic disease. Large dose heparin therapy utilizes dosage levels of 60,000-100,000 units/day during the first 24-48 hours and then reverting to 30,000-45,000 units/day. Large dose therapy is for patients with active thromboembolic disease.

Heparin should not be given intramuscularly (risk of hematoma formation). There is a trend to favor subcutaneous administration in the initial treatment of deep vein thrombosis. In support of this trend are studies claiming efficacy and safety, and procedural simplification allowing outpatient or home therapy.

Complications: Not all individuals respond ideally or predictably to heparin. One must investigate the causes and management of aberrant cases.

Drugs which antagonize the action of heparin include streptomycin, erythromycin, gentamicin, chlorpromazine, ascorbic acid, antihistamines, and digitalis.

Untoward effects of heparin include development of osteoporosis with fractures (doses of 20,000 units/day over 6 months), anti-inflammatory effect, and inhibition of antidiuretic effect resulting in diuresis. Unusual reactions include anaphylaxis and erythematous reactions (species specific), alopecia, urticaria, headache, and bronchospasm. There may be significant morbidity (including amputation of extremities) and mortality associated with heparin induced platelet aggregation and resultant new thrombosis and thrombocytopenia.

Heparin-induced thrombocytopenia: Pretherapeutic laboratory evaluation may be desirable. Abnormalities in platelet count, whole blood clotting time, activated PTT, or antithrombin III may indicate that the patient has a predisposition to an unusual heparin response. Heparin-induced thrombocytopenia appears to have immune etiology and occurs in the presence of either an IgG or IgM heparin dependent platelet aggregating antibody. These patients have a measurable abnormal response to ADP, heparin and ADP, and heparin alone in the platelet aggregation procedure when thrombocytopenia is present.

The **progressive thromboembolic syndrome** appears to be always associated with thrombocytopenia. Monitoring of the heparinized patient has been recommended and includes daily physical examination for evidence of further thrombosis and periodic platelet counts, the need for which is determined clinically. Evidence of new thrombosis or decrease

in platelet count to <100,000/mm³ should be further investigated with aggregation studies to see if an abnormal response to platelet aggregation is present. The platelet abnormality quickly reverses when heparin is discontinued. Added beneficial therapy includes antiaggregating agents such as dextran (Rheomacrodex®) I.V., 25 mL/hour; acetylsalicylic acid; dipyridamole; and Coumadin®. Iloprost® has been utilized to prevent heparin-induced thrombocytopenia during open heart surgery.

The table summarizes the relation of three coagulation tests that have been and can be utilized to adjust the heparin anticoagulant effect. See table.

Heparin Anticoagulant Effect		
Test	Usual Normal Control Results	Anticoagulant Range (Heparin Level 0.2-0.4 units/mL)
Lee-White clotting time	8-15 min	20-30 min
Activated clotting time	70-120 sec	180-240 sec
Activated PTT	25-39 sec	60-80 sec
(About twice the normal control value)		

Early studies suggested that thrombi do not propagate when the heparin level is such as to prolong the Lee and White (L&W) clotting time to twice that of a normal control. The level of heparin required or desirable, however, varies on an individual basis depending on the severity of the thrombotic process, the potential bleeding risk, variations in the heparin preparation - varying polymer length, sulfonation of polymers, medications that inactivate or inhibit heparin (antihistamines, digitalis, nicotine, penicillin, tetracyclines, phenothiazines and protamine), poor coordination in timing the dose and collection of specimens, antithrombin III level, platelet factor IV level, and fibrinogen level. If the latter factors are in normal range, heparin level of 0.3 units/mL of plasma is required to result in a Lee-White clotting time of twice the normal control. Heparin level of 0.6 units/mL (3 times normal Lee-White clotting time) may result in clinical bleeding. Therapeutic range is usually attained with heparin level of 0.2-0.4 units/mL. Heparin dose of 100-125 units/kg body weight given at six hourly intervals bolus I.V. or SubQ or 400-500 units/kg body weight/day as constant infusion will usually provide effective anticoagulation.

Monitoring: The activated clotting time (ACT) and the activated plasma thromboplastin time (APTT) are most commonly used to monitor heparin therapy.

Low molecular weight heparin (LMWH): Standard heparin is composed of sulfated mucopolysaccharides, heterogeneous fragments of different molecular weights. LMWH is less heterogeneous, consists of fragments with high and low affinity for AT III but LMWH use is associated with decreased antithrombin activity while anti-Xa activity is largely preserved. There is evidence that LMWH is able to protect against thromboembolic events while the risk of hemorrhage is reduced. Conventional tests used in monitoring of standard heparin treatment (eg, APTT, TT, ACT) are not affected by LMWH at the doses usually employed. Laboratory control of the use of LMWH is, therefore, not applicable. Heparin-induced thrombocytopenia is usually seen, however, some 7-12 days after LMWH therapy begins so that periodic platelet counts are recommended.

Lupus anticoagulant: Patients with a prolonged APTT not corrected by mixing with normal plasma but with no family or clinical/surgical history of bleeding are (in screening situations) most commonly due to a phospholipid (lupus type) anticoagulant. College of American Pathologists surveys (1986 and 1987) found significant difference in the sensitivity of different APTT reagents to the presence of lupus anticoagulants. The difference in reagent responsiveness can affect the apparent factor activity and also the dilutional effect on mixing patient with normal plasma samples, thus impairing the ability to differentiate a lupus anticoagulant from a specific factor inhibitor.

Alcohol, Semiquantitative, Urine

Synonyms Ethyl Alcohol, Urine; Urine Alcohol Level; Urine Ethanol

Reference Range Negative

Test Commonly Includes Ethyl alcohol for medical purpose only, not for legal use. Assay also measures methyl alcohol, isopropyl alcohol, and paraldehyde. Results reported as ethanol unless another alcohol is requested.

Specimen Random urine

Volume 15 mL

Minimum Volume 1 mL

Container Plastic urine container

Collection Freshly voided random urine

Methodology Dichromate diffusion

Additional Information The average urine/blood ratio is 1.35 in the postabsorptive state.

Alcohol, Serum

Synonyms Ethanol, Blood; Ethyl Alcohol, Blood; EtOH

Uses Quantitation of alcohol level for medical or legal purposes; screen unconscious patients; used to diagnose alcohol intoxication and determine appropriate therapy; screen for alcoholism and monitor ethanol treatment for methanol intoxication. Must be tested as possible cause of coma of unknown etiology since alcohol intoxication may mimic diabetic coma, cerebral trauma, and drug overdose.

Reference Range Blood: negative. In most laboratories, values <10 mg/dL (SI: <2.0 mM/L) are considered negative. Signs of intoxication can be observed at levels of 30-100 mg/dL (SI: 6.6-21.7 mM/L).

Patient Preparation While it should be noted that the possibility of an isopropyl-based swab significantly interfering with an ethanol-based assay is negligible, this aspect may be challenged in court, and therefore it may be best to avoid this argument by using a nonalcohol-based swab. Hexachlorophene-based, iodine-based, or mercury-based antiseptics not containing alcohol may be used.

Specimen Blood

Volume 5 mL

Minimum Volume 2 mL serum or plasma

Container Red top tube; gray top (sodium fluoride) tube is recommended for medicolegal specimens and prolonged storage.

Collection **Do not prepare venipuncture site with an alcohol swab for forensic samples.** When police agencies bring an individual in for blood alcohol levels, medical and laboratory people should at all times be aware of their state statutes.

Storage Instructions Refrigerate in a tightly stoppered tube.

Special Instructions Concentrations of ethanol are 12% to 18% higher in serum and plasma versus whole blood. For forensic purposes, only whole blood values are used.

Critical Values Fatal concentration is usually considered to be >400 mg/dL (SI: >86.8 mM/L). Whole blood levels of 300 mg/dL (SI: 65.1 mM/L) are associated with coma. In most states, whole blood levels ≥80 mg/dL are considered evidence of impairment for driving.

Possible Panic Range ≥300 mg/dL (SI: ≥65.1 mM/L)

Limitations Certain other alcohols (in high concentration) can interfere with enzymatic methods. The rate of dehydrogenation of isopropanol (2-propanol) is 6% and that of n-propanol (1-propanol) is 36% that of ethanol. Methanol does not interfere. Gas chromatography is the most specific methodology because it can separate, identify, and quantitate each type of alcohol present. Freezing point osmometry and enzymatic analysis can together determine the presence of volatile intoxicants and can determine causes of metabolic intoxication.

Methodology Enzymatic analysis (alcohol dehydrogenase), freezing point osmometry, gas chromatography (GC)

Additional Information Elevated serum lactate and lactate dehydrogenase levels may interfere with enzymatic ethanol assays. Lactate dehydrogenase and lactate can cause false positive serum ethanol screen (by EMIT) in postmortem state. Postmortem urinary lactate dehydrogenase levels (>592 units/L) and lactate levels (>12 mm) and proteinuria can lead to false positive results on drugs of abuse screening by enzyme-multiplied immunoassay techniques (EMIT)

Specific References

Fabbri A, Marchesini G, Dente M, et al, "A Positive Blood Alcohol Concentration is the Main Predictor of Recurrent Motor Vehicle Crash," *Ann Emerg Med*, 2005, 46(2):161-7.

Kristiansen J and Petersen HW, "An Uncertainty Budget for the Measurement of Ethanol in Blood by Headspace Gas Chromatography," *J Anal Toxicol*, 2004, 28(6):456-63.

Kristoffersen L and Smith-Kielland A, "An Automated Alcohol Dehydrogenase Method for Ethanol Quantification in Urine and Whole Blood," *J Anal Toxicol*, 2005, 29(5):387-9.

Zittel DB and Hardin GG, "Comparison of Blood Ethanol Concentrations in Samples Simultaneously Collected Into Expired and Unexpired Venipuncture Tubes," *J Anal Toxicol*, 2006, 30:317-8.

Aluminum, Serum

Uses

Monitor patients for prior and ongoing exposure to aluminum. Patients at risk include:

- infants on parenteral fluids, particularly parenteral nutrition
- burn patients through administration of intravenous albumin, particularly with coexisting renal failure
- adult and pediatric patients with chronic renal failure, who accumulate aluminum readily from medications and dialysate
- adult parenteral nutrition patients (less so, recently)
- patients with industrial exposure

Monitor dialysate and water to prepare dialysate to prevent aluminum toxicity in dialysis patients. Research use: investigation of amyotrophic lateral sclerosis (in Guam) and Alzheimer's disease.

Reference Range Serum (normal patient): 0-10 ng/mL (SI: 0-0.37 μmol/L) (may vary with laboratory); serum (dialysis patients): up to 40 ng/mL

(SI: <1.48 μmol/L) without apparent acute effects, >100 ng/mL (SI: >3.7 μmol/L) possible CNS toxicity, >200 ng/mL (SI: >7.4 μmol/L) probable multisystem toxicity; urine: 0-32 ng/day (SI: 0-1.2 μmol/day); dialysate: <0.01 mg/L (AAMI standards)

Specimen Blood, dialysis fluid, urine, cerebrospinal fluid

Volume 5 mL

Container Special metal-free Sherwood Monoject™ trace element blood collection tube #8881-307006 for serum separation; acid-washed plastic vials for other samples.

Collection Use B-D #5175 20-gauge stainless steel needle, or Terumo or Abbot butterfly needle. Draw any trace metal tube prior to any other type of blood sample to prevent contamination of needle by regular rubber stoppers.

Causes for Rejection Contamination by aluminum contact, dust, or ordinary collection tubes or stoppers. Urine must not be contaminated by stool.

Special Instructions The patient should take no aluminum containing antacids or medicines (such as Basaljel®, Gelusil®, Maalox®, Amphojel®, Sucralfate) for 24 hours prior to blood test.

Limitations Serum levels rise and fall after each dose of aluminum-containing phosphate binder or sucralfate. If renal function is normal, renal clearance of aluminum is prompt with urine levels rising quickly after a course of aluminum-containing antacid is begun and elevated levels persisting for over a week. Urine levels rise after a dose of desferrioxamine given for any reason. The degree of rise in serum aluminum after desferrioxamine is regarded as reflecting total body aluminum burden.

Methodology Atomic absorption (AA), inductively coupled plasma atomic emission spectrometry

Additional Information Serum aluminum correlates with encephalopathy; red cell aluminum correlates with microcytic anemia; and bone aluminum correlates with aluminum bone disease.

Amphetamines, Qualitative, Urine

Related Information

- Drug Testing in the 21st Century
- Methamphetamines, Urine

Synonyms Bennies; Crystal; Dexies; Ice; Speed; Uppers

Uses Drug abuse evaluation; toxicity assessment

Reference Range Negative (less than cutoff)

Test Commonly Includes Amphetamine, methamphetamine

Test Interactions Spurious positive amphetamine urinary immunoassay screen can result from trazodone therapy.

Abstract Amphetamine and methamphetamine are major drugs of abuse. They have limited medical use and are DEA schedule II drugs.

Specimen Random urine

Volume 50-60 mL

Minimum Volume 5 mL

Container Plastic urine container

Collection If forensic, observe precautions.

Storage Instructions Refrigerate

Causes for Rejection If forensic, failure to meet temperature requirements and/or tests for unusual urine dilution (specific gravity or creatinine) or alteration

Special Instructions If forensic, use chain-of-custody form.

Critical Values Cutoff: screen: 1000 ng/mL; confirmation: 500 ng/mL

Limitations Some over-the-counter cold and antiallergy medications may cross react in certain immunoassay screens; confirmation by a different, more sensitive method (eg, GC/MS) is necessary. Clobenzorex hydrochlorate (an anoretic) can give a positive urine result for amphetamine by immunoassay and GC/MS. A labetalol metabolite (3-amino-1-phenylbutane or APB) may cause a false-positive result with amphetamine/methamphetamine by thin layer chromatography or immunoassay. Mexiletine may give a false-positive test for amphetamine by urinary fluorescence polarization assay.

Methodology Screen: fluorescence polarization immunoassay (FPIA), radioimmunoassay (RIA), enzyme immunoassay (EIA), gas chromatography (GC), thin-layer chromatography (TLC), high performance liquid chromatography (HPLC); confirmation: gas chromatography/mass spectrometry (GC/MS)

Additional Information For the amphetamine class, the material detected is the parent drug. Alum (25 g/L) can elicit a false-negative urinary assay for methamphetamine; urine will be acidic in these cases.

Specific References

Chen HJ, Liang CL, Lu K, et al, "Rapidly Growing Internal Carotid Artery Aneurysm After Amphetamine Abuse: Case Report," *Am J Forensic Med Pathol*, 2003, 24(1):32-4.

Cody JT, Valtier S, and Nelson SL, "Amphetamine Enantiomer Excretion Profile Following Administration of Adderall," *J Anal Toxicol*, 2003, 27:485-92.

Cody JT, Valtier S, and Nelson SL, "Amphetamine Excretion Profile Following Multidose Administration of Mixed Salt Amphetamine Preparation," *J Anal Toxicol*, 2004, 28:563-74.

Greenhill B, Valtier S, and Cody JT, "Enantiomer Profile of Amphetamine and Methamphetamine Derived from Famprofazone," *J Anal Toxicol*, 2003, 27(3):189.

Huang MK, Dai YS, Lee CH, et al, "Performance Characteristics of DRI, CEDIA, and REMEDi Systems for Preliminary Tests of Amphetamines and Opiates in Human Urine," *J Anal Toxicol*, 2006, 30:61-70.

Hung MJ, Kuo LT, and Cherng WJ, "Amphetamine-Related Acute Myocardial Infarction Due to Coronary Artery Spasm," *Int J Clin Pract*, 2003, 57(1):62-4.

Kraemer T, Roditis SK, Peters FT, et al, "Amphetamine Concentrations in Human Urine Following Single-Dose Administration of the Calcium Antagonist Prenylamine-Studies Using Fluorescence Polarization Immunoassay (FPIA) and GC-MS," *J Anal Toxicol*, 2003, 27(2):68-73.

Mobini Far HR, Torabi F, Danielsson B, et al, "ELISA on a Microchip with a Photodiode for Detection of Amphetamine in Plasma and Urine," *J Anal Toxicol*, 2005, 29(8):790-3.

Moore C, Feldman M, Harrison E, et al, "Analysis of Amphetamines in Hair, Oral Fluid, and Urine," *Annale de Toxicologie Analytique*, 2005, 17(4):229-36.

Nyström I, Trygg T, Woxler P, et al, "Quantitation of *R*-(-)- and *S*-(+)-Amphetamine in Hair and Blood by Gas Chromatogrpahy-Mass Spectrometry: An Application to Compliance Monitoring in Adult-Attenton Deficit Hyperactivity Disorder Treatment," *J Anal Toxicol*, 2005, 29:682-8.

Paul BD, Jemionek J, Lesser D, et al, "Enantiomeric Separation and Quantitation of ($\pm$)-Amphetamine, ($\pm$)-Methamphetamine, ($\pm$)-MDA, ($\pm$)-MDMA, and ($\pm$)-MDEA in Urine Specimens by GC-EI-MS After Derivatization with (R)-(-)- or (S)-(+)-alpha-Methoxy-alpha-(Trifluoromethy)phenylacetyl Chloride (MTPA)," *J Anal Toxicol*, 2004, 28(6):449-55.

Rodriguez AT, Valtier S, and Cody JT, "Metabolic Profile of Famprofazone Following Multidose Administration," *J Anal Toxicol*, 2004, 28(6):432-8.

Stanaszek R and Piekoszewski W, "Simultaneous Determination of Eight Underivatized Amphetamines in Hair by High-Performance Liquid Chromatography-Atmospheric Pressure Chemical Ionization Mass Spectrometry (HPLC-APCI-MS)," *J Anal Toxicol*, 2004, 28(2):77-85.

Stout PR, Klette KL, and Wiegand R, "Comparison and Evaluation of DRI® Methamphetamine, DRI® Ecstasy, Abuscreen® ONLINE Amphetamine, and a Modified Abuscreen® ONLINE Amphetamine Screening Immunoassays for the Detection of Amphetamine (AMP), Methamphetamine (MTH), 3,4-Methylenedioxyamphetamine (MDA), and 3,4-Methylenedioxymethamphetamine (MDMA) in Human Urine," *J Anal Toxicol*, 2003, 27(5):265-9.

Verstraete AG and Heyden FV, "Comparison of the Sensitivity and Specificity of Six Immunoassays for the Detection of Amphetamines in Urine," *J Anal Toxicol*, 2005, 29(5):359-64.

Wood M, De Boeck G, Samyn N, et al, "Development of a Rapid and Sensitive Method for the Quantitation of Amphetamines in Human Plasma and Oral Fluid by LC-MS-MS," *J Anal Toxicol*, 2003, 27(2):78-87.

Anion Gap, Blood

Applies to Urinary Anion Gap

Synonyms Electrolyte Gap; Gap; Ion Gap

Uses

Extensively used for quality control in the laboratory, the widest clinical application of the anion gap is in the diagnosis of types of metabolic acidosis. Unmeasured cations include calcium and magnesium. Unmeasured anions include protein, PO_4^{3-}, SO_4^{2-}, and organic acids. Organic acidosis includes lactic acidosis and ketoacidosis.

A marked elevation of anion gap, >30 mM/L, bears a strong implication of metabolic acidosis. Increased anion gaps are found in states such as renal failure and toxic ingestions. A >30 mM/L gap increase commonly is secondary to lactic acidosis or ketoacidosis, but can also be caused by rhabdomyolysis or nonketotic hyperglycemic coma.

In diabetic ketoacidosis, plasma glucose is high, often much >300 mg/dL (SI: >16.7 mM/L), pH is <7.3, and ketones are found in blood and urine. Increased serum osmolality and increased calculated osmolality (osmolar gap) are found, and serum sodium is often decreased.

In alcoholic ketoacidosis glucose may be increased, normal or low, but a high alcohol level may be found, and amylase and uric acid may be increased.

Reference Range 6-16 mM/L (SI: 6-16 mM/L); slight differences may be established in different laboratories. Until recently electrolytes were done mostly by flame photometry. As ion-selective electrodes have come into wider use, reference ranges for anion gap will probably change.

Test Commonly Includes A calculation from electrolytes, sodium, potassium, HCO_3^-, and chloride to ascertain quantities of unmeasured cations and anions

Abstract The anion gap is useful in evaluation of patients with acid-base abnormalities. The sum of anions and cations must be equal in the blood.

Specimen Blood

Container Red top tube

Limitations Minor differences in formula are used by different laboratories. A spurious increase may follow excessive exposure of the sample to room air, as well as, underfilling the Vacutainer® tube. Some gaps remain unexplained. Not all metabolic abnormalities are detected by abnormal gaps (eg, isopropanol ingestion is accompanied by normal gap, but ketone bodies are positive). There are a number of causes of normal anion gap acidosis associated with hyperchloremia. Anion gap is unsuitable as a quick screen for lactic acidosis. Still useful, the anion gap should not replace assay for lactate, creatinine, ketone bodies, or osmolality. In one study, only 66% of patients with an anion gap of 20-29 mM/L could be proven to have an organic acidosis.

Methodology Calculation: $(Na^+ + K^+) \sim (Cl^- + HCO_3^-)$ or $Na^+ \sim (Cl^- + HCO_3^-)$ = anion gap; actually determined by the difference between concentrations of anions and cations.

Additional Information

Anion gap represents approximately the sum of the unmeasured anions, charges of which, with chloride and HCO_3^-, balance sodium. (Measured anions are chloride and bicarbonate. Measured cations are sodium.)

Anion gap high ("unmeasured anions"): with **pH high:** extracellular volume contraction; massive transfusion (with renal failure and/or volume contraction); carbenicillin, penicillin (large doses), salts of organic acids such as citrate. With **pH low:** uremia: most common cause; abnormal anion gap in uremia is usually seen only when creatinine is >4.0 mg/dL (SI: >354 μmol/L). Uremic acidosis is rare without hyperphosphatemia. Nonketotic hyperglycemic coma and rhabdomyolysis may cause high anion gap metabolic acidosis. Lactic acidosis and diabetic or alcoholic ketoacidosis characteristically fall into this group. With **normal osmolal gap:** salicylate and paraldehyde toxicity; with **increased osmolal gap:** methanol and ethylene glycol toxicity.

High anion gap metabolic acidosis without elevated lactic acid or acetone; consider: ketoacidosis with negative or slightly positive "acetone" if the patient is hypoxic and/or has alcoholic ketoacidosis, such ketoacidosis may be life-threatening; salicylate toxicity; methanol toxicity (paint thinners); ethylene glycol toxicity (antifreeze) - urinary sediment contains abundant calcium oxalate and/or hippurate crystals; paraldehyde intoxication (may have positive ketone reactions); toluene toxicity (transmission fluid, paint thinner inhalation or sniffing).

Anion gap low: Caused by retained unmeasured anions. The most common cause is hypoalbuminemia (eg, in nephrosis, cirrhosis), dilution, hypernatremia, very marked hypercalcemia, very severe hypermagnesemia, IgG myeloma and polyclonal gamma globulin increases - hyperviscosity with certain lab instruments, lithium toxicity, bromism (low anion gap may not be present). Decreased anion gap with spurious hyperchloremia and with hyponatremia is reported in hyperlipidemia. Dilution of extracellular fluid may cause a decreased gap. The finding of a low anion gap is perceived as an unreliable diagnostic parameter and may indicate potential laboratory error.

Normal anion gap may occur with **metabolic acidosis,** causes have been published. They include diarrhea, renal tubular acidosis, hyperalimentation, ureteroileostomy, ureterosigmoidostomy, external drainage of pancreaticobiliary fluids, NH_4Cl and other drugs.

The urinary anion gap is used in the diagnosis of hyperchloremic metabolic acidosis and evaluation of renal potassium wasting.

Antibiotic Level, Serum

Synonyms Antimicrobial Assay

Uses Evaluate adequacy of serum antibiotic level; detect toxic levels

Reference Range Therapeutic range depends on agent being tested for, and minimal inhibitory concentration of drug against organism. Selected ranges in mcg/mL are presented as a guide only. See table.

Antibiotic Level, Serum				
Drug	**Peak**		**Trough**	
	mcg/mL	SI: μmol/L	mcg/mL	SI: μmol/L
Amikacin	15-25	26-43	<10	<17
Chloramphenicol	25	77		
Flucytosine	100	775		
Gentamicin	4-10	8-21	<2	<4
Netilmicin	4-8	8.0-17.0	1-2	0.7-1.4
Streptomycin	5-20	9-34	<5	<9
Tobramycin	4-10	8-21	<2	<4
Trimethoprim	≥5	17		
Sulfamethoxazole	≥100	395		
Vancomycin	20-40	13.6-27.2	5-10	3.4-6.8

Selected ranges in mcg/mL are presented as a guide only.

Abstract Assays for antimicrobial agents in serum are performed for two primary reasons: 1. to ensure therapeutic levels, and 2. to monitor for potentially toxic levels. In most situations, it is not necessary to monitor antimicrobial levels because serum levels are relatively predictable based on dosing; *in vitro* susceptibility testing uses those predictable levels to determine clinical efficacy. Similarly, toxicity is not always related to serum levels. It may be more appropriate to monitor for toxicity by following determinants of hematologic, renal, or hepatic function. In certain situations however (eg, aminoglycoside antibiotics which have a narrow therapeutic range and a high potential for toxicity), it is essential to follow serum levels.

Specimen Serum

Container Red top tube or serum separator tube

Sampling Time Peak: 30 minutes after 30 minute I.V. infusion; 1 hour after I.M. dose. Trough: immediately prior to next dose.

Collection Keep frozen if not assayed immediately.

Causes for Rejection Incomplete clinical information (eg, specific antimicrobial, dosage and schedule, other concurrent antimicrobials)

Limitations May not be technically possible in a patient taking more than one antibiotic

Methodology Bioassay: cephalosporins, clindamycin, erythromycin, metronidazole, penicillins, polymyxin, tetracycline, trimethoprim. High performance liquid chromatography: chloramphenicol, flucytosine, mezlocillin. Fluorescence polarization immunoassay (FPIA): amikacin, gentamicin, tobramycin, kanamycin, streptomycin, vancomycin, neomycin, netilmicin.

Additional Information With the increasing availability of *in vitro* sensitivity testing expressed as the minimal inhibitory or bactericidal concentration of an antibiotic, measurement of serum levels of these drugs has taken on practical clinical importance. This is especially true for agents with narrow therapeutic ranges and significant toxicity. It should be remembered, however, that in most patients, cure of infection depends on numerous host factors as well as on antibiotics. Therefore, antibiotic levels should not be relied on as the sole guide to therapy.

Arsenic, Blood

Related Information
- Heavy Metal Screen, Blood

Uses Blood arsenic is for diagnosis of acute poisoning only

Reference Range <5 mcg/dL (SI: <93.5 nmol/g)

Abstract Arsenic is a toxic heavy metal. The largest source of human exposure is arsenic in food resulting from broad use of arsenical pesticides.

Specimen Blood

Volume 30 mL

Minimum Volume 10 mL

Container Trace metal-free container

Causes for Rejection Containers not metal-free

Critical Values Lethal oral dose: Acute: 2-10 mg/kg; chronic: 1 mg/kg/day. Chronic poisoning: 10-50 mcg/dL (SI: 133.5-667.5 nmol/g). Acute poisoning: >60 mcg/dL (SI: >801 nmol/g)

Limitations Short half-life in blood

Methodology Electrothermal atomic absorption spectrometry (AA)

Additional Information Heparinized whole blood and serum have been used for arsenic determination. Blood levels of arsenic have a short half-life and are useful only within a few days of exposure. Urine arsenic concentration is a better measure of arsenic poisoning. In addition to pesticides, rodenticides, weed killers, paint, and wood preservatives contain arsenic.

Arsenic, Hair, Nails

Synonyms Arsenic, Hair; Arsenic, Nails

Uses Diagnose chronic arsenic intoxication

Reference Range Hair: up to 65 mcg/100 g (SI: 8.7 nmol/g); nail: 90-180 mcg/100 g (SI: 12-24 nmol/g)

Abstract This is a toxic heavy metal that is incorporated into hair and nails. Its presence there in abnormal concentrations is a sign of chronic poisoning.

Specimen Clean hair or nails

Volume 0.5 g

Container Clean envelope or heavy metal-free screw top plastic container

Collection Extreme care is necessary to avoid surface contamination; pubic hair is preferable as are toenails.

Special Instructions Hair should be clean, free of oil and tonic; clip close. Nails should be thoroughly washed, dried, and clipped close to cuticle.

Critical Values Values >100 mcg/100 g (SI: >13.4 nmol/g) of hair are considered toxic

Limitations Curly hair may pose problems in dating. Not useful for diagnosing acute toxicity. Urine arsenic concentration is a better indication of recent exposure.

Methodology Electrothermal atomic absorption spectrometry (AA), neutron activation analysis

Additional Information Arsenic accumulates in bones, hair, and nails and is used to detect chronic exposure, since arsenic is laid down in keratin soon after ingestion. Arsenic binds to protein sulfhydryl groups. Variations in arsenic hair levels may be due to geographic location and exposure to industrial waste and drinking water.

Specific References

Goulle JP, Mahieu L, and Kintz P, "The Murder Weapon Was Found in the Hair!" *Annale de Toxicologie Analytique*, 2005, 17(4):243-6.

Arsenic, Urine

Related Information
- Heavy Metal Screen, Urine

Applies to Arsenic, Gastric Content

Synonyms As, Quantitative, Urine

Uses Evaluate recent exposure to arsenic, arsenic toxicity

Reference Range Ranges for urine inorganic arsenic levels can be variable among different laboratories. A general guideline is given: normal: 0-50 mcg/L (SI: 0-0.65 μmol/L); chronic industrial exposure: >100 mcg/L (SI: >1.3 μmol/L). The 24-hour urinary excretion rate should be <50 mcg/24 hours.

Abstract This toxic heavy metal appears in urine, and its excretion rate is used to determine toxicity.

Specimen 24-hour urine

Volume Entire collection

Container Acid-washed plastic container, no preservative

Collection Collect a 24-hour urine specimen, on ice, with care to avoid specimen contact with metal. Container must be securely closed and properly labeled.

Storage Instructions Refrigerate

Causes for Rejection Specimen not collected on ice, specimen in contact with metal during collection

Critical Values Toxic: >850 mcg/L (SI: >11.3 μmol/L) (inorganic)

Methodology Atomic absorption spectrometry (AA)

Additional Information 25 mL acidified gastric washing is acceptable for arsenic analysis; gastric content normally contains no arsenic. Random urine samples are acceptable. Refrain from eating seafood for 1 week prior to 24-hour urine collection. Following a seafood meal, spot urinary arsenic levels peak at 24 hours and decrease to below detectable limits at 7 days.

Arthropod Identification

Applies to *Cimex* Identification; *Ixodes dammini* Identification; *Pediculus humanus* Identification; *Phthirus pubis* Identification; *Sarcoptes scabiei* Skin Scrapings Identification; Bed Bugs Identification; Body Lice Identification; Crab Lice Identification; Deer Tick Identification; Flea Identification; Head Lice Identification; Lice Identification; Mite Identification; Nits Identification; Pubic Lice Identification; Skin Scrapings for *Sarcoptes scabiei* Identification; Tick Identification

Synonyms Ectoparasite Identification; Insect Identification

Uses Identify arthropods affecting humans; establish the presence of ectoparasite infestation

Reference Range No arthropod identified

Specimen Gross arthropod, skin scrapings

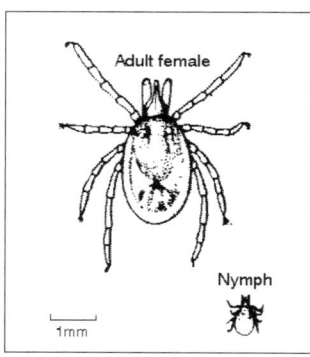

Deer tick (*Ixodes dammini*)

Container Screw cap tube or screw cap jar

Collection Arthropods (gross) are to be submitted in alcohol (70%) or formaldehyde in tube or container with secure closure. To establish the diagnosis of scabies, skin scrapings may be collected with a scalpel and a drop of mineral oil. The liquid may be examined directly or alternatively the organism may be teased away from its burrow or papule with a needle or scalpel.

Storage Instructions Room temperature, fill the container with preservative as completely as possible to avoid damage to the specimen by air bubbles in the container

Methodology Macroscopic evaluation

Barbiturates, Qualitative, Urine

Applies to Amobarbital, Urine; Butalbital, Urine; Mephobarbital, Urine; Pentobarbital, Urine; Secobarbital, Urine

Uses Urine drugs of abuse testing, pre-employment screens, random drug testing

Reference Range Less than cutoff

Test Commonly Includes Identification and confirmation of barbiturates in urine

Abstract This test is usually used to detect barbiturate as a drug of abuse.

Specimen Random urine

Volume 20 mL

Minimum Volume 10 mL

Container Plastic urine container

Collection If forensic, observe precautions

Storage Instructions Refrigerate

Causes for Rejection If forensic, failure to meet temperature requirements or test for unusual urine dilution

Special Instructions Chain-of-custody documentation required for samples submitted for pre-employment, random employee testing, and forensic purposes.

Critical Values Cutoff: screen: 300 ng/mL, confirmation: 300 ng/mL

Limitations Short- and intermediate-acting barbiturates can be detected in urine 24-72 hours following ingestion, longer-acting drugs up to 7 days.

Methodology Enzyme immunoassay (EIA), gas chromatography/mass spectrometry (GC/MS)

Additional Information Withdrawal symptoms from any barbiturate may be severe and may include convulsions. The presence of barbiturates in urine is presumptively positive at a level >300 ng/mL using secobarbital as a standard and can indicate prescribed or abused intake of this class of drugs. The presence of these drugs should be confirmed. 10 mL of Donnatal® elixir does **not** cause a positive urinary barbiturate assay.

Barbiturates, Quantitative, Blood

Applies to Amobarbital; Aprobarbital; Blue Angels; Butalbital; Red Devils; Talbutal; Yellow Jackets

U.S. Brand Names Alurate®; Amytal®; Butisol Sodium®; Fiorinal®; Lotusate®; Luminal®; Nembutal®

Uses Evaluate barbiturate toxicity, drug abuse, therapeutic levels; if barbiturates are suspected in a drug overdose, determination of long-, medium-, or short-acting may influence treatment.

Reference Range Negative. Therapeutic: short-acting (secobarbital): 1-5 mcg/mL (SI: 4.2-21.0 μmol/L); intermediate-acting (amobarbital): 5-15 mcg/mL (SI: 22-66 μmol/L); long-acting (phenobarbital): 15-40 mcg/mL (SI: 65-172 μmol/L); for seizure control, phenobarbital therapeutic levels: 10-30 mcg/mL (SI: 43-129 μmol/L)

Test Commonly Includes Quantitation of barbiturates present in blood

Abstract Measurement of barbiturates as a class is usually used for drug-of-abuse testing or as evidence for toxicity.

Specimen Blood

Volume 7 mL

Minimum Volume 5 mL plasma or serum

Container Lavender top (EDTA) tube, green top (heparin) tube, red top tube; avoid serum separator tube for pentobarbital.

Critical Values Toxic: short-acting: >10 mcg/mL (SI: >43 μmol/L); intermediate-acting: >20 mcg/mL (SI: >86 μmol/L); long-acting: >40 mcg/mL (SI: >172 μmol/L)

Limitations Only barbiturates will be identified and quantitated; individual agents cannot be identified by screening tests, particularly if there has been a mixed ingestion

Methodology Gas chromatography (GC), high performance liquid chromatography (HPLC), immunoassay

Additional Information To monitor therapeutic phenobarbital level: See Phenobarbital, Blood. The implication of any concentration is more serious for short-acting barbiturates than for phenobarbital. The toxic or lethal blood level varies with many factors and cannot be stated with certainty. Lethal blood levels determined at autopsy may be as low as 60 mcg/mL (SI: 258 μmol/L) for long-acting (barbital and phenobarbital) and 10 mcg/mL (SI: 43 μmol/L) for intermediate- and short-acting barbiturates (amobarbital, butabarbital, butalbital, pentobarbital, secobarbital). In presence of alcohol or other depressant drugs, the lethal concentrations may be lower. Addicts, however, may tolerate with no ill effect levels which would be acutely toxic to a nonaddicted individual. Except for barbital, all barbiturates are primarily transformed by the liver. Only barbital is dependent mainly on renal excretion for termination of its pharmacological action. Individual barbiturates can be identified and separated from each other by HPLC.

Benzodiazepines, Qualitative, Urine

Synonyms Tranquilizers (Valium®, Librium®, etc)

Uses Drug abuse evaluation; toxicity assessment

Reference Range None present unless prescribed. When used as drug-of-abuse screen, negative (less than cutoff).

Abstract This group of drugs is used as antianxiety agents (tranquilizers). They are used by more Americans than any other single prescription drug.

Specimen Random urine

Volume 50 mL

Minimum Volume 10 mL

Container Clean plastic urine container

Storage Instructions Refrigerate or freeze if not analyzing immediately

Critical Values Cutoff: screen: 300 ng/mL (as oxazepam); confirmation: 200 ng/mL

Methodology Immunoassay, thin-layer chromatography (TLC), high performance liquid chromatography (HPLC), gas chromatography (GC), gas chromatography/mass spectrometry (GC/MS)

Additional Information Urine should be screened for benzodiazepines in suspected overdose cases, or as part of an abused drug program. These drugs have a relatively low potential for abuse. They are, however, frequently found with other drugs in emergency room drug screens. Immunoassay screens detect a broad range of drugs and their metabolites in this class using either oxazepam or nordiazepam as positive controls. Using the latter, the test is more specific and more sensitive for detecting flurazepam. Positive screen results (usually >300 ng/mL of urine metabolites) should be confirmed by an alternate technique. High concentrations of fenoprofen, flurbiprofen, indomethacin, ketoprofen, and tolmetin may give a false-positive result by a TDx assay. Oxaprozin may interfere with urinary benzodiazepine result immunoassay methods. Flunitrazepam is detected in urine by GC/MS but not by EMIT assay techniques. Sertraline may cause a false-positive urinary benzodiazepine assay using the original cloned enzyme donor immunoassay system.

Brand name prescription medications that can result in a positive urinary immunoassay:

- Librium®
- Paxipam®
- Tranxene®
- Valium®
- Verstran®
- Restoril®
- Serax®
- Tranxene®
- Verstran®
- Restoril®
- Xarax®
- Klonipin® (In overdose only)

Specific References

Chaplinsky L, Powell K, Coy D, et al, "A Comparison of Confirmatory Methods for the Quantitation of Benzodiazepines in Whole Blood or Urine," *J Anal Toxicol*, 2006, 30:129.

Dahn TD, Downs T, and Terrell AR, "The Analysis of Benzodiazepines in Urine Using Sold-Phase Extraction and LC-MS," *J Anal Toxicol*, 2006, 30:144.

Hegstad S, Oiestad EL, Johansen U, et al, "Determination of Benzodiazepines in Human Urine Using Solid-Phase Extraction and High-Performance Liquid Chromatography-Electrospray Ionization Tandem Mass Spectrometry," *J Anal Toxicol*, 2005, 30:31-43.

Juhascik M, Le NL, Tomlinson K, et al, "Development of an Analytical Approach to the Specimens Collected from Victims of Sexual Assault," *J Anal Toxicol*, 2004, 28(6):400-10.

Klette KL, Wiegand RF, Horn CK, et al, "Urine Benzodiazepine Screening Using Roche Online KIMS Immunoassay with Beta-Glucuronidase Hydrolysis and Confirmation by Gas Chromatography-Mass Spectrometry," *J Anal Toxicol*, 2005, 29(3):193-200.

Kurisaki E, Hayashida M, Nihira M, et al, "Diagnostic Performance of Triage™ for Benzodiazepines: Urine Analysis of the Dose of Therapeutic Cases," *J Anal Toxicol*, 2005, 29:539-44.

Musselman J and Solanky A, "Extraction of Benzodiazepines Using the Cerex Polychrom Clin II SPE Cartridges in Blood and Urine and Analysis by GC-MS in Selective Ion Monitoring (SIM) Mode," *J Anal Toxicol*, 2006, 30:142.

Vena J, Wu A, and McKay CM, "What Constitutes Confirmatory Testing for Drugs of Abuse? A Case Study of Benzodiazepine False-Positive Immunoassay with Significant Social and Clinical Consequences," *J Toxicol Clin Toxicol*, 2004, 42(5):760-1.

Bishydroxycoumarin, Blood

Synonyms Dicumarol Level, Blood

Uses Evaluate toxicity. It is helpful when surreptitious ingestion is suspected or when a possible medication error is involved. It should **not** be used for TDM.

Reference Range 20-30 mcg/mL
Specimen Blood
Volume 10 mL
Collection Blood must be accurately added to special tube.
Storage Instructions Transport specimen to the laboratory immediately. Do not store.
Causes for Rejection Excessive delay in transport, improper specimen collection
Critical Values Toxic: >70 mcg/mL
Limitations This test does not quantitate warfarin and should not be used to monitor any other anticoagulant. Warfarin may be ordered separately.
Additional Information This test should be ordered only if the patient's prothrombin time is prolonged. It is not as useful for TDM as the prothrombin time.

Botulism, Diagnostic Procedure

Related Information
- Clostridium botulinum Food Poisoning
- Clostridium perfringens Poisoning

Synonyms *Clostridium botulinum* Toxin Identification Procedure; Infant Botulism, Toxin Identification
Use Diagnose infant botulism, classic botulism in adults
Contraindications Due to the difficulty in performance of the diagnostic test and because of the extensive epidemiological studies initiated upon receipt of the specimen, State Department of Health Laboratories require specific clinical symptomatology for infant botulism and therefore should be consulted early to optimize handling of the suspect case.
Reference Range No toxin identified, no *Clostridium botulinum* isolated
Abstract A neurotoxin, botulin, may be produced by *C. botulinum* in foods which have been improperly preserved. Characteristics of this type of food poisoning include vomiting and abdominal pain, disturbances of vision, motor function and secretion, mydriasis, ptosis, dry mouth, and cough.
Specimen Vomitus, serum, stool, gastric aspirates, cerebrospinal fluid or autopsy tissue; food samples
Volume 50 g vomitus or feces, gastric washings, cerebrospinal fluid or autopsy tissue, 15-20 mL serum; infant botulism: 25 g feces
Container Sterile wide-mouth, leakproof, screw-cap jar; red top tube
Storage Instructions Keep refrigerated at 4°C except for unopened food samples.
Special Instructions The laboratory must be notified prior to obtaining specimen in order to prepare for transport of the specimen to the State Health Laboratory or Center for Disease Control.
Limitations The toxin from *C. botulinum* binds almost irreversibly to individual nerve terminals; thus, serum and cerebrospinal fluid specimens may yield false-negative results. Can detect as little as 0.03 ng of botulinum toxicity.
Methodology Toxin neutralization test in mice
Specific References

Armada M, Love S, Barrett E, et al, "Foodborne Botulism in a Six-Month-Old Infant Caused by Home-Canned Baby Food," *Ann Emerg Med*, 2003, 42(2):226-9.

Fox CK, Keet CA, and Strober JB, "Recent Advances in Infant Botulism," *Pediatr Neurol*, 2005, 32(3):149-54.

Richardson WH, Frei SS, and Williams SR, "A Case of Type F Botulism in Southern California," *J Toxicol Clin Toxicol*, 2003, 41(5):653.

Thompson JA, Filloux FM, Van Orman CB, et al, "Infant Botulism in the Age of Botulism Immune Globulin," *Neurology*, 2005, 64(12):2029-32.

Bromide, Serum

Uses Evaluate bromide toxicity. This test is seldom ordered.
Reference Range Therapeutic: 750-1500 mcg/mL (SI: 9.4-18.7 mM/L)
Abstract Inorganic bromide salts were formerly used as antiepileptics. They are no longer available as nonprescription items in the United States.
Specimen Blood
Volume 5 mL
Minimum Volume 3 mL serum
Container Red top tube
Critical Values Toxic: >1500 mcg/dL (SI: >18.7 mM/L)
Limitations Patients on iodide therapy will have falsely elevated serum bromide levels. A high level of bromide in the serum will falsely elevate the chloride level.
Methodology Reaction of bromide in a protein-free filtrate with gold chloride
Additional Information In order to convert mg/dL to mEq/L (the same units in which serum or plasma chlorides are reported), multiply the bromide values in mg/dL by 0.125. Both chloride and bromide react identically to titrimetric chloride methods (chloridometer). Many ion selective chloride electrodes give a response to bromide which is double that for chloride. A reported "chloride" value will equal the true sum of chloride and bromide. Bromism may be suspected in the presence of a

history of ingestion of proprietary bromide preparations, fever, skin rash, and neurologic symptoms.

Butabarbital, Quantitative

Related Information
- Barbiturates, Quantitative, Blood

Synonyms Buticaps®; Butisol Sodium®
Uses Monitor therapeutic drug level; evaluate toxicity
Contraindicating Factors Presence of other barbiturates
Reference Range Therapeutic: mildly sedated 3-25 mcg/mL
Specimen Blood
Volume 7 mL
Minimum Volume 0.5 mL serum
Container Red top tube
Collection Collect specimen immediately prior to next dose unless specified otherwise by physician. Put time of last dose on requisition, if it is available.
Critical Values Toxic: mildly comatose 20-40 mcg/mL; severely comatose >40 mcg/mL
Limitations Can only be performed if the patient is not taking other barbiturates
Methodology Enzyme immunoassay (EIA)

Cadmium, Blood

Related Information
- Heavy Metal Screen, Blood

Synonyms Cd, Blood
Uses Evaluate cadmium toxicity in industrial exposure to cadmium fumes or cadmium ingestion
Reference Range Whole blood: <1 mcg/L
Abstract This toxic heavy metal is used in industry in alloys and metal platings
Specimen Whole blood
Volume Entire specimen
Container Metal-free tube
Collection Blood must be collected into metal-free tubes with a plastic syringe.
Causes for Rejection Specimen allowed to contact metal
Special Instructions Requisition must state date and time urine collection started and date and time collection finished.
Possible Panic Range Levels >10 mcg/L (SI: >88.97 μmol/L) in whole blood probably reflect excessive exposure.
Methodology Flameless atomic absorption spectrophotometry (AA); electrothermal atomization atomic absorption
Additional Information Inhalation of cadmium fumes produces an acute pneumonitis. Long-term exposure may lead to emphysema (with decreased α_1-antitrypsin). Increased cadmium is reported to be associated with hypertension and (perhaps) prostatic cancer. Cadmium ingestion may result from contact of acid foods with metal containers. There is exposure of the general populace to cadmium from food, water, and air contamination. Because of slow excretion and constant exposure cadmium values increase with age. Body cadmium elimination half-life may be as long as 30 years. Chronic cadmium exposure can cause proteinuria and a degree of renal insufficiency.

Cadmium, Hair

Synonyms Cd, Hair
Uses Evaluate chronic cadmium toxicity; hair analysis can reflect chronic cadmium poisoning for long-term exposure.
Specimen Hair
Container Envelope or plastic Petri dish
Collection Clip lock of hair at nape of neck extending to a distance of 20 mm. Place in an envelope or plastic Petri dish.
Limitations Hair analysis does not reflect cadmium concentration in the body at the time the sample is collected, but at some prior time.
Methodology Flameless atomic absorption spectrophotometry (AA)

Cadmium, Urine

Related Information
- Heavy Metal Screen, Urine

Synonyms Cd, Urine
Uses Evaluate cadmium toxicity in industrial exposure to cadmium fumes or cadmium ingestion
Reference Range Nonexposed: 0-20 mcg/L; exposed: 10-580 mcg/L
Patient Preparation Patient should be instructed to use a plastic bedpan or urinal if necessary.
Specimen Random urine
Volume Entire collection
Minimum Volume 100 mL aliquot

Container Plastic urine container
Collection Freshly voided random urine
Storage Instructions Keep specimen on ice or refrigerate.
Causes for Rejection Specimen allowed to contact metal, specimen not kept chilled

Cannabinoid Confirmation

Uses Confirm positive screen result by an alternate, specific method
Reference Range Levels >10 ng/mL reported as confirmed positive
Test Commonly Includes Confirmation of positive screen test; measurement of THC-9-carboxy metabolite by gas chromatography/mass spectrometry.
Specimen Random urine
Volume 50 mL aliquot
Minimum Volume 25 mL
Container Plastic urine container
Collection Freshly voided random urine
Storage Instructions Refrigerate or freeze specimen.
Limitations Limit of detection for THC-9-carboxy metabolite is 10 ng/mL.
Methodology Gas chromatography/mass spectrometry (GC/MS)
Specific Reference
Mitchell vs Mr. Hood Meadows Oreg Oregon Court of Appeals 0005-05389; A116119, October 6, 2004

Cannabinoids, Qualitative

Synonyms 11-Nor-9-Carboxy-Delta-9-Tetrahydrocannabinol; Cannabis; Carboxy THC; Grass; Hashish; Hemp; Herb and Al; Marijuana; Pot; THC (Delta-9-Tetrahydrocannabinol); Weed
Uses Drug abuse evaluation; toxicity assessment
Reference Range Negative (less than cutoff)
Test Interactions
Gemfibrozil can cause a false positive urinary assay for cannabinoids utilizing the OnTraK TestCup method (Roche Diagnostic Systems, Inc). When Pyridium® chlorochromate ("Urine Luck") adulterant is added to urine (at pH of 5-7), ~58% to 100% of THC-acid is lost, resulting in a possible false-negative assay.
Pantoprazole may cause a false positive cannabinoid urinary immunoassay.
Abstract The main active ingredient of marijuana (cannabinoids) is tetrahydrocannabinol (THC). It is metabolized to THC-carboxylic acid which is detected in the urine. The name comes from the source of marijuana, the plant *Cannabis sativa*. It is a DEA schedule I drug and a widely used drug of abuse.
Specimen Random urine
Volume 20 mL
Minimum Volume 10 mL
Container Plastic urine container
Collection For employee screening or forensic purpose, use precautions during collection.
Causes for Rejection Evidence of urine dilution or alteration
Special Instructions If forensic, use chain-of-custody protocol and form.
Critical Values Cutoff: screen (NIDA): 50 ng/mL. Some laboratories use 100 ng/mL and a few use 20 ng/mL; confirmation: 15 ng/mL.
Limitations Cannabinoids are rapidly metabolized from blood. Urine is the best specimen for screening although blood (serum or plasma) and saliva have been used. Cannabinoids can adhere to plastic.
Methodology Enzyme immunoassay (EIA), fluorescence polarization immunoassay (FPIA), thin-layer chromatography (TLC), gas chromatography/mass spectrometry (GC/MS)
Additional Information
While exceptionally long urinary detection times have been reported in heavy, chronic marijuana users during abstinence (up to 6 weeks); few controlled studies exist on the excretory temporal patterns of marijuana metabolites. Urinary detection times (at a 50 ng/mL cutoff) after smoking a single 1.75% or 3.55% THC cigarette range from 8.4-26 hours and 31-57 hours by immunoassay, respectively. Longer detection times for the last positive urine at the 20 ng/mL cutoff immunoassay is ~51 hours (at 1.75% THC) and 93 hours (at 3.55% THC). While detection times at the 100 ng/mL cutoff may range from 12-33 hours, rapid storage of THC metabolites in body fat occurs after use. These substances are then released from storage sites slowly over time.
A marijuana cigarette is made form the dried particles of the plant, *Cannabis sativa*. The immediate effects of smoking marijuana include a faster heartbeat and pulse rate, bloodshot eyes, and a dry mouth and throat. The drug can impair or reduce short-term memory, alter sense of time, and reduce the ability to do things which require concentration, swift reactions and coordination, such as driving and operating machinery.
While positive urine FPIA screen virtually will not occur due to passive inhalation at a cutoff of 100 ng/mL, there may be positive EMIT screen in children at threshold of 10 ng/mL.
Driving experiments show that marijuana affects a wide range of skills needed for safe driving. Thinking and reflexes are slowed, making it hard for drivers to respond to sudden unexpected events. Furthermore, a driver's ability to "track" through curves, brake quickly, and maintain speed and proper distance between vehicles is affected. Research shows that these skills are impaired for at least 4-6 hours after smoking a single marijuana cigarette. If a driver drinks alcohol along with using marijuana, the risks of a vehicular collision greatly increase.
Small amounts of hypochlorite (household bleach: 8-64 µL/mL of urine) can cause a significant decrease in cannabinoid urine level as measured by immunoassay and GC/MS
Tolmetin may give false-negative results by Emit® assay.
Ingestion of Seedy Sweetie® snack bars (produced by Hungry Bear Hemp Foods, Eugene, Oregon) which contains pressed hemp seeds, can cause a positive urine assay for THC at 11 hours.
Delta 9-tetrahydrocannabinol plasma concentrations are roughly double that of whole blood because delta 9-tetrahydrocannabinol is protein bound and thus concentrated in plasma.
Identification of 11-nor-$\triangle^9$-THCV-9-COOH in a urine specimen indicates the use or ingestion of cannabis-related product(s) and would not explain the sole use of Marinol®.

Specific References
Brewer W and Clelland B, "Improved Rapid and Sensitive Analysis of THC and Metabolites in Whole Blood by Disposable Pipette Extraction," *J Anal Toxicol*, 2003, 27:177.
Coles R, Clements TT, Nelson GJ, et al, "Simultaneous Analysis of the Delta^9-THC Metabolites 11-nor-9-Carboxy-Delta^9-THC and 11-Hydroxy-Delta^9-THC in Meconium by GC-MS," *J Anal Toxicol*, 2005, 29:522-7.
De Cock KJ, Delbeke FT, De Boer D, et al, "Quantitation of 11- nor-$\triangle^9$-Tetrahydrocannabinol-9-Carboxylic Acid with GC-MS in Urine Collected for Doping Analysis," *J Anal Toxicol*, 2003, 27(2):106-9.
Mura P, Raul SB, Dumestre V, et al, "Comparison of Blood and Brain Cannabinoids Concentrations in 11 Human Cases: Consequences on Traffic Safety," *J Anal Toxicol*, 2005, 29:446.
Nadulski T, Pragst F, Stadelmann AM, et al, "Prospective Study About the Effect of Cannabidiol (CBD) on the Pharmacokinetics of Delta-9-Tetrahydrocannabinol (THC) After Oral Application of 10 mg THC and 5.4 mg CBD in Cannabis Extract," *J Anal Toxicol*, 2005, 29:446.
Svendsen KB, Jensen TS, and Bach FW, "Does the Cannabinoid Dronabinol Reduce Central Pain in Multiple Sclerosis? Randomised Double Blind Placebo Controlled Crossover Trial," *BMJ*, 2004, 329(7460):253.

Carbamazepine, Blood

Related Information
• Carbamazepine-10,11-Epoxide
Applies to P450 System Inhibitor
Synonyms Tegretol®
Uses Monitor for compliance, efficacy, or possible toxicity
Contraindicating Factors Half-life of warfarin is shortened; monoamine oxidase inhibitors not recommended.
Reference Range 4-12 mcg/mL (SI: 17-51 µmol/L). Low level: The most common cause of a low level is noncompliance. The addition of anticonvulsants which induce the P450 system, such as phenytoin, primidone, and phenobarbital, may decrease carbamazepine levels without causing seizures. (The P450 system is a liver enzymatic system which degrades drugs.) The withdrawal of phenytoin from the regimen of a patient on carbamazepine may lower the level and cause seizures. Because of autoinduction of metabolism, patients in the first 2 months of therapy may have diminishing levels and be at risk for seizures. Occasionally, patients may have toxicity when levels are within the reference range. High level: Drugs which inhibit the P450 system, including isoniazid, fluoxetine, propoxyphene, verapamil, and stiripentol can cause a precipitous rise in carbamazepine levels and clinical toxicity, usually within 48 hours. Danazol may cause a delayed toxicity. The addition of cimetidine, erythromycin, lithium, triacetyloleandomycin, and valproic acid also can cause toxicity.
Abstract Carbamazepine is a first-line antiepileptic drug for generalized and partial seizures. It is used for control of pain in trigeminal neuralgia and in treatment of bipolar affective disorder.
Patient Preparation Levels should be drawn before next oral dose with patient at steady-state.
Specimen Blood
Volume 5 mL
Minimum Volume 1 mL serum
Container Red top tube
Sampling Time A consistent sampling time, ideally a trough level, should be used to monitor patients on chronic therapy.
Critical Values Toxic: >20 mcg/mL
Possible Panic Range Central nervous system toxicity occurs progressively with levels near or above high end of reference range.
Limitations See Carbamazepine-10,11-Epoxide listing.
Methodology Enzyme immunoassay (EIA), gas-liquid chromatography (GLC), high performance liquid chromatography (HPLC)

Additional Information

Indications for measurement of a serum antiepileptic drug level include:

- within 6 hours of a seizure
- suspected dose-related drug toxicity
- suspected patient noncompliance

Additional indications for serum drug assay during steady state conditions (after 6 days for phenytoin, 3 days for carbamazepine, 3 days for valproic acid, 20 days for phenobarbital) include:

- baseline measurement after starting antiepileptic drug therapy
- control measurement after a change in dosage regimen
- addition of a second drug with a potential interaction with the antiepileptic drug (ie, a second antiepileptic drug, warfarin, isoniazid, or rifampicin)
- change in patient's hepatic or gastrointestinal function

Carbamazepine, Free

Synonyms Tegretol®, Free

Reference Range Therapeutic free: 1.6-2.4 mcg/mL; therapeutic total: 6.0-12.0 mcg/mL

Test Commonly Includes Free and total carbamazepine

Specimen Blood

Volume 2 mL

Minimum Volume 1 mL

Container Red top tube

Collection Draw just prior to next dose.

Methodology Ultrafiltrate assayed by fluorescence polarization immunoassay (FPIA)

Carbamazepine-10,11-Epoxide

Related Information

- Carbamazepine, Blood

Synonyms Carbamazepine Metabolite

Reference Range 0.8-3.2 mg/L. High level: In patients on chronic carbamazepine therapy, the addition of valpromide or progabide produces clinical toxicity with high levels of metabolite and normal levels of parent compound.

Test Commonly Includes Carbamazepine and carbamazepine-10,11-epoxide

Abstract Occasional cases of carbamazepine toxicity occur with normal levels of carbamazepine due to accumulation of the active metabolite, 10,11-epoxide.

Specimen Blood

Volume 7 mL

Minimum Volume 1 mL serum

Container Red top tube

Limitations Valproic acid, a compound chemically related to valpromide, may increase the epoxide/carbamazepine ratio by eliminating excretion of the epoxide. Since most cases of fatal valproate hepatotoxicity occur in young children on multiple anticonvulsants, the combination of valproate and carbamazepine is not recommended. Phenytoin may also increase the ratio of epoxide/parent compound.

Methodology High performance liquid chromatography (HPLC), fluorescence polarization immunoassay (FPIA); enzyme multiplied immunoassay (EMIT)

Additional Information Carbamazepine-10,11-epoxide has been shown to be pharmacologically active in animals.

Carboxyhemoglobin, Blood

Synonyms Carbon Monoxide Level, Blood; CO, Blood; COHb, Blood

Uses Determine the extent of carbon monoxide poisoning, toxicity; check the effect of smoking on the patient; work up headache, irritability, nausea, vomiting, vertigo, dyspnea, collapse, coma, convulsions; work up persons exposed to fires and smoke inhalation

Reference Range Nonsmokers: <3%; smokers: 1-2 packs/day: 4% to 5%, >2 packs/day: 8% to 9%. Carboxyhemoglobin in the **newborn** may run 10% to 12%. Carbon monoxide hemoglobin in the newborn, together with decreased efficiency of the infant's respiratory system, may, and does lead to higher levels of carboxyhemoglobin. Venous and arterial samples are equivalent.

Test Commonly Includes COHb is sometimes included in blood gases but may be ordered as a separate test.

Patient Preparation In suspected carbon monoxide poisoning, the specimen should be collected immediately.

Specimen Blood

Minimum Volume 1 mL whole blood

Container Green top (heparin) tube or lavender top (EDTA) tube, depending upon laboratory

Sampling Time Draw before the patient is started on oxygen, if possible.

Collection Keep tube capped

Storage Instructions Refrigerate immediately after collection. Do not remove cap. Carboxyhemoglobin is stable 4 months in filled, well-capped tube.

Critical Values Toxic concentration: 20%; lethal: >40%

Possible Panic Range Disturbance of judgment, headache, and dizziness occur at 10% to 30%; coma at 50% to 60%; fatality occurs at ≥60%, and rapid death at 80%.

Limitations Carbon monoxide levels are of limited value in screening for smoking, since it is cleared rapidly. The half-life of carboxyhemoglobin in individuals with normal cardiopulmonary function is 1-2 hours on 100% oxygen. Urinary nicotine, if available, is preferable as a screening test for tobacco use. Arterial blood gases may be of limited value in treatment decisions for carbon monoxide poisoning. Pulse oximetry is of no use. Fetal hemoglobin (in neonates younger than 3 months of age) may interfere with carboxyhemoglobin determination by causing a falsely elevated carboxyhemoglobin level in direct proportion to fetal hemoglobin levels.

Methodology Spectrophotometric, gas-liquid chromatography (GLC), pulse oximetry

Additional Information Carboxyhemoglobin is useful in judging the extent of carbon monoxide toxicity and in considering the effect of smoking on the patient. A direct correlation has been claimed between CO level and symptoms of atherosclerotic diseases, intermittent claudication, angina, and myocardial infarction. Exposure may occur not only from smoking, but also from garage exposure and from various engines. This test may be included when blood gases are ordered, when there is sufficient sample, and when such instrumentation is available.

A danger of missed diagnosis of CO intoxication is continued exposure of the patient and others to a toxic environment. The cherry red color of CO poisoning is not consistently seen. CO intoxication may contribute to the risk of myocardial infarction.

A strong correlation is present between carboxyhemoglobin levels and psychometric testing abnormalities. Psychometric testing measures actual neurologic disability and may therefore better define carboxyhemoglobin poisoning severity than blood CO level. The half-life with O_2 administration is 80 minutes. With O_2 at 3 atmospheres, the half-life is 24 minutes.

Also elevated in methylene chloride intoxications due to endogenous hepatic metabolism to carbon monoxide.

Fetal hemoglobin interferes with COHb determination by falsely elevating COHb in direct proportion to fetal hemoglobin. Interpretation of COHb levels in infants younger than 90 days must consider the clinical relevance of this interference.

Specific References

Chee KJ, Suner S, Partridge RA, et al, "Noninvasive Carboxyhemoglobin Monitoring: Screening Emergency Department Patients for Carbon Monoxide Exposure," *Acad Emerg Med*, 2006, 13(5):S177.

Chang SJ, Shih TS, Chou TC, et al, "Electrocardiographic Abnormality for Workers Exposed to Carbon Disulfide at a Viscose Rayon Plant," *J Occup Environ Med*, 2006, 48:394-9.

Lewis RJ, Johnson RD, and Canfield DV, "An Accurate Method for the Determination of Carboxyhemoglobin in Postmortem Blood Using GC-TCD," *J Anal Toxicol*, 2004, 28(1):59-62.

Chain-of-Custody Protocol

Applies to Medical Legal Specimens

Synonyms Specimen Chain-of-Custody Protocol

Uses Chain-of-custody is a legal term that describes a method to maintain sample integrity in the collection, handling, and storage of urine samples.

Reference Range Normal: all seals intact and Chain-of-Custody form completed.

Abstract A procedure to ensure sample integrity from collection through transport, receipt, sampling, and analysis. It is associated with a chain-of-custody form.

Causes for Rejection Sample cup or bag containing sample cup not sealed

Additional Information The chain-of-custody protocol is a clerical and custodial service offered by the laboratory to document specimen transfer and provide for extended specimen storage. A written record of specimen transfer from patient, to analyst, to storage and disposal is maintained on all specimens covered by chain-of-custody. All drug screens, blood alcohols, or any other tests that have medicolegal significance should be accompanied by Chain-of-Custody form and a written release form. (Department of Transportation collections or any collection involving Medical Review officers.)

Cholinesterase Inhibitors, Quantitative, Serum

Synonyms Carbamates, Quantitative, Serum

Uses Evaluate exposure to organophosphate and carbamate insecticides; preoperative screening of patients who are at risk for prolonged paralysis following surgical choline administration during anesthesia

Reference Range 559-1493 units/L

Test Commonly Includes Neostigmine, pyridostigmine, physostigmine
Specimen Blood
Volume 15 mL
Minimum Volume 2 mL serum
Container Red top tube
Collection Routine venipuncture
Limitations May be decreased in a number of advanced chronic diseases.
Methodology UV spectrophotometry
Additional Information Organophosphate and carbamate insecticides inhibit both serum and erythrocyte cholinesterase. Serum cholinesterase falls and returns to normal more rapidly than erythrocyte levels. Decreases in activity are best evaluated by comparison to baseline levels established before exposure. Patients with atypical variants of serum cholinesterase, which are autosomal recessively inherited, may be unable to effectively hydrolyze certain muscle relaxants such as succinylcholine, which may be administered during anesthesia, resulting in prolonged paralysis. Most patients with such variants will have low plasma cholinesterase activity and resistance to dibucaine inhibition.
Specific References
Guven M, Sungur M, Eser B, et al, "The Effects of Fresh Frozen Plasma on Cholinesterase Levels and Outcomes in Patients with Organophosphate Poisoning," *J Toxicol Clin Toxicol*, 2004, 42(5):617-23.

Chromium, Serum

Related Information
- Chromium, Urine

Synonyms Cr, Serum
Uses Evaluate suspected chromium toxicity or exposure; follow patients receiving chromium in their parenteral nutrition; evaluate acquired glucose intolerance in refeeding programs, or in parenteral or enteral nutrition; evaluate insulin resistance in the nonseptic patient during parenteral nutrition
Reference Range 0.05-0.15 ng/mL (SI: 1-3 nmol/L). Some laboratories report much higher "normals" because the methods they use or the collection technique is not adequate to prevent substantial contamination. If a laboratory reports "<1 ng/mL" or some similar figure without a lower level for normal, the value can be relied upon to discover toxic states, perhaps, but not deficiency states. Serum levels of 10 ng/mL correspond to short-term atmospheric exposure limit of 0.1 mg/m^3 of chromium trioxide. Serum levels even higher would be expected in acute systemic toxicity. Almost a twofold diurnal variation is noted in serum chromium levels, with the level highest in the morning and falling after each meal as insulin levels rise. Serum chromium levels are ~60% of normal in diabetic patients, which overlaps the normal range.
Patient Preparation The patient should be fasting for basal level.
Specimen Blood
Container Special metal-free, Sherwood Monoject™ trace element blood collection tube #8881-307006
Sampling Time In the nocturnal total parenteral nutrition patient, the sample will be drawn "fasting" in the afternoon, before the nocturnal solution is started for the evening.
Collection Follow specific instructions of laboratory to which sample will be submitted. Contact with steel, dust, ordinary glassware, or plastic is to be avoided. Draw blood through indwelling plastic intracath needle. Some siliconized stainless steel needles have also been found to be acceptable as is the B-D #5175 20-gauge stainless steel needle, or the Terumo or Abbot butterfly needles. Draw trace metal sample prior to any other blood samples. Remove serum with an all-plastic pipette (no internal metal parts) and store serum in plastic vial. Leeching plastic containers in 10% nitric acid for 48 hours removes trace metal contamination if special purpose vials are not available. The containers are then rinsed three times with twice distilled water and air dried in a dust-free environment prior to use.
Storage Instructions Some reference laboratories request specimens to be frozen and sent on dry ice.
Causes for Rejection Improper collection or storage with contact by steel, dust, or ordinary Vacutainer® tubes
Limitations Extreme attention to detail is needed to achieve reliable results; for many laboratories even now a high serum metal level more often reflects sample contamination rather than excess chromium exposure.
Methodology Any reported levels in biological materials prior to ~1979 are suspect, as the available methods did not have the sensitivity to separate normal values from the "blank." Reported levels were tenfold or more too high. Accurate and independently verified values have been reported with:

- stable isotope dilution, isotope ratio mass spectroscopy
- graphite furnace atomic absorption spectroscopy

All pipettes must have plastic tips and no exposed internal metal parts. Work is done in the laboratory under a laminar flow class 100 work station, free from exposed stainless steel to avoid airborne contamination. This is essential to reduce contamination sufficiently to detect "normal levels" in human serum or urine. Even with these precautions, different laboratories report different normal values.
Additional Information Iron competitively inhibits the binding of chromium III to transferrin. Iron overloaded patients with hemochromatosis poorly retain a radioactive tracer dose of chromium III. It has been suggested that chromium deficiency at a cellular level may play a role in the development of diabetes in hemochromatosis.

Chromium, Urine

Related Information
- Chromium, Serum

Synonyms Cr, Urine
Uses Evaluate industrial exposure, suspected toxicity; or in conjunction with serum levels, to attempt to detect suspected chromium deficiency, especially in a recent onset of glucose intolerance
Reference Range <1.8 mcg/L. Levels vary with the laboratory and have declined with improved methods of avoiding contamination. Levels two- to threefold above this may reflect supplementation or excess losses. Levels elevated tenfold and higher have been seen in exposed asymptomatic tannery workers. Spot levels of chromium in urine of 30 ng/g creatinine correspond to the short-term atmospheric exposure limit of 0.1 mg/m^3 of chromium trioxide in industrial exposure situations.
Abstract Urine chromium levels are extremely low, and until recently, not reliable. Urine chromium assay is used to look for chromium toxicity in cases of potential exposure. As testing becomes more reliable, new applications of the test will arise to determine chromium III nutritional adequacy or deficiency states. There are also potential uses in the follow-up of patients with mild glucose intolerance. See listing, Chromium, Serum for signs and symptoms of toxicity and deficiency states, and for additional references.
Specimen 24-hour urine
Container Plastic metal-free container. To prepare, leech 48 hours in 10% nitric acid and wash with distilled water that has had no contact with metal. Dry in quiet air in a metal-free environment.
Collection Care must be taken to avoid contact with metal. Use plastic urinal, prepared as above. Stool contamination must be avoided.
Causes for Rejection Improper collection, contact with metal, ordinary containers, or stool contamination
Limitations Levels are so low in normal people (on the order of one part in 10 billion in urine) that many laboratories are not able to detect the lower limit of normal, and thus report "less than" some set level as being normal. Thus, for many laboratories, the test can only be used to detect toxicity. Contamination of the specimen may result in a tenfold or more increase in urine concentration being reported, making potential contamination the major limiting factor in the test.
Methodology Atomic absorption (AA) or neutron activation
Additional Information As improved methods have progressively reduced the lower level of detection, urine chromium levels have been found to be related to glucose metabolism. Recent studies have demonstrated the metabolic relationships between serum insulin, serum glucose, and serum chromium III in the fasting and postprandial states and the relationship of the postprandial state to urine chromium concentration. Briefly, diabetic patients lose threefold more chromium in the urine than nondiabetics, and despite increased intestinal absorption, diabetic patients on ordinary diets develop and maintain lower serum levels. Chromium loss is not specifically related to micro- or macro-albuminuria and precedes the onset of diabetic nephropathy. Urine chromium rises threefold 40 minutes after a carbohydrate meal and more so with carbohydrates that stimulate higher insulin levels. Serum levels fall after a meal, more so than can be explained by urine loss. Thus, glucose stimulates insulin to take chromium to a cellular location, which favors increased renal excretion.

Cobalt, Serum

Related Information
- Heavy Metal Screen, Blood

Synonyms Co, Blood
Uses Evaluate cobalt toxicity, nutritional status
Reference Range 0.4-1.2 mcg/100 mL
Specimen Blood
Minimum Volume 7 mL
Container Red top tube
Storage Instructions Refrigerate serum.

Cobalt, Urine

Related Information
- Heavy Metal Screen, Urine

Synonyms Co, Urine
Uses Evaluate cobalt toxicity
Reference Range Diet dependent, normals not well established but estimated to be ~2.2 mcg/mL

Patient Preparation Patient should be instructed to use a plastic bedpan or urinal if necessary.
Specimen 24-hour urine
Volume Entire collection
Minimum Volume 100 mL
Container Plastic urine container, no preservative
Collection Instruct the patient to void at 8 AM and discard the specimen. Then collect all urine including the final specimen voided at the end of the 24-hour collection period (ie, 8 AM the next morning). Avoid contact with metal during collection. Screw the lid on securely. Transport the specimen promptly to the laboratory. Container **must** be labeled with patient's full name, room number, date and time collection started, and date and time collection finished.
Special Instructions Requisition **must** state date and time collection started and date and time collection finished.

Cocaine (Cocaine Metabolite), Qualitative

Synonyms Coke; Crack; Snow
Uses Evaluate cocaine use
Reference Range Negative (less than cutoff)
Test Commonly Includes Cocaine is detected in urine as its metabolite, benzoylecgonine
Abstract A prominent metabolite of cocaine is benzoylecgonine, which is the substance measured in urine to detect the presence of cocaine. Cocaine is a heavily abused drug which has legitimate medical uses in some ENT procedures.
Specimen Urine
Volume 50 mL
Minimum Volume 10 mL
Container Plastic urine container
Collection If forensic, observe precautions concerning surreptitious dilution or alteration.
Storage Instructions Refrigerate; optimal storage conditions for urine specimens with cocaine and benzoylecgonine are at 18°C and a pH of 5.0; unsilanized glass is a favorable container material
Causes for Rejection If forensic, failure to meet temperature requirements immediately after collection and/or tests for unusual dilution (specific gravity, urine creatinine) or alteration.
Special Instructions If forensic, use chain-of-custody protocol and form.
Critical Values Cutoff: screen: 300 ng/mL; confirmation: 150 ng/mL
Methodology Screen: immunoassay, fluorescence polarization immunoassay (FPIA), thin-layer chromatography (TLC); confirmation: gas chromatography/mass spectrometry (GC/MS)
Additional Information
Positive urine screen due to passive inhalation of cocaine virtually will not occur at cutoff of 300 ng/mL by FPIA, but is possible in children if test by EMIT with a cutoff of 30 ng/mL. Absorption of at least 1 mg of cocaine is usually necessary to produce a cocaine positive urine screen.
Ecgonine urinary levels >50 ng/mL can increase sensitivity of cocaine assays. Urine cocaine metabolites levels may be elevated after a series of sauna treatments. The metabolite anhydroecgonine methyl ester is considered to be a marker for "crack" cocaine use (urine concentration ranges from 5-1477 ng/mL).
Benzoylecgonine to cocaine urinary quantitative ratios less than 100:1 are indicative of cocaine exposure less than ten hours before collection. Serum Benzoylecgonine to cocaine quantitative ratios less than one are indicative of cocaine exposure within two hours of collection Benzoylecgonine can be produced by metabolism of cocaethylene. Pyrolytic cocaine products include anhydroecgonine, anhydroecgonine methyl ester, methylecgonidine and Ecgonidine (the latter two from crack smokers). Purity of illicit cocaine is 80 to 97%.

Specific References
Cardona PS, Chaturvedi AK, Soper JW, Canfield DV "Simultaneous Analyses of Cocaine, Coca- and Pyrolytic Products," *Forensic Sci Int*, 2006, 157(1):46-56.
Cone EJ, Sampson-Cone AH, Darwin WD, et al, "Urine Testing for Cocaine Abuse: Metabolic and Excretion Patterns Following Different Routes of Administration and Methods for Detection of False-Negative Results," *J Anal Toxicol*, 2003, 27:386-92.
Kolbrich EA, Barnes AJ, Gorelick DA, et al, "Major and Minor Metabolites of Cocaine in Human Plasma Following Controlled Subcutaneous Cocain Administration," *J Anal Toxicol*, 2006, 30(8):501-10.
Shults TF, "Key Cocaine Metabolites and Their Toxicological Significance: A Guide to Medical Review Officers," *MRO Alert*, 2006, 17(10): 6-9.

Codeine, Urine

Related Information
• Opiates, Qualitative, Urine
Uses Evaluate codeine toxicity; detect drug-of-abuse
Reference Range Negative (below cutoff)
Test Commonly Includes Part of opiate screen

Abstract Codeine occurs naturally in opium but is produced commercially by 3-O-methylation of morphine. It is used as a narcotic analgesic. It is present in numerous proprietary preparations combined with non-narcotic analgesics and antihistamines. It is a drug of abuse.
Specimen Random urine
Volume 20 mL
Minimum Volume 10 mL
Container Plastic urine container
Storage Instructions Refrigerate
Special Instructions If forensic, use precautions in collection and Chain-of-Custody form.
Critical Values Cutoff: screen: 300 ng/mL (for drug-of-abuse screen), confirmation: 300 ng/mL
Methodology Enzyme immunoassay (EIA); thin-layer chromatography (TLC)
Additional Information
Urine codeine/morphine ratio is usually >1.0 during first the 24 hours postingestion, decreases <1.0 from 24-30 hours and usually only morphine is detectable after 30 hours. Poppy seed ingestion can result in urine codeine levels as high as 4.5 mg/L and urine morphine levels as high as 0.2 mg/L; urine drug screen remains positive for 2-4 days. Hydrocodone is a minor metabolite of codeine and could be excreted in urinary concentrations as high as 5% of parent codeine compound.

Computed Transaxial Tomography, Head Studies

Synonyms Brain, CT; Head Studies, CT
Uses Evaluate known/suspected primary or secondary neoplasm, cystic lesions, hydrocephalus, head trauma, seizure disorder, multiple sclerosis, atrophy, Alzheimer's disease, normal pressure hydrocephalus, Parkinson's disease, dementia, depression, organic brain syndrome, etc
Contraindicating Factors Assuming a cooperative or quiescent patient, there are no absolute contraindications to a CT scan of the head. A decision must be taken, however, as to whether the study is to be done with or without intravenous contrast material. While each case must be assessed individually, the following broad guidelines may be helpful. Those studies indicated by virtue of a recent infarct, cerebrovascular accident or stroke, or those being done for assessment of atrophy, Alzheimer's disease, normal pressure hydrocephalus, Parkinson's disease, hydrocephalus, evaluation of an intraventricular shunt, assessment of ventricular size, subdural hematoma, or suspected dementia are examined without contrast material. Patients for whom the indication is headache, psychiatric condition (such as anorexia or bulimia), tumor follow-up, rule out tumor, rule out metastasis, multiple sclerosis, seizure disorders, depression, and organic brain syndrome are generally studied with contrast material. Patients in whom the indication is one of infection, abscess, meningitis, transient ischemic attack, arteriovenous malformation, remote subdural hematoma, or who have recently undergone a craniotomy and are being studied for postoperative evaluation are best studied with and without contrast material. Patients with a known diagnosis of plasmacytoma or multiple myeloma should not receive intravenous contrast material. Patients with compromised renal function may or may not benefit from intravenous contrast material. A recent serum creatinine and BUN will be helpful in deciding whether or not the latter group of patients receive contrast material.
Test Commonly Includes CT scan of the brain
Patient Preparation The examination should be ordered and a requisition with information pertaining to the reason for the request and the clinical history should be completed by the referring physician. If there is the slightest possibility that intravenous contrast material will be administered, the patient's oral intake should be limited to liquids for at least 4 hours prior to the examination. Care must be taken to ensure the patient does not become dehydrated and medications should not be interrupted. A recent serum creatinine is requested on patients with pre-existing renal disease, diabetes mellitus, significant atherosclerotic disease, and advancing age (60 years and older). Agitated patients and children may require sedation prior to the examination. In these cases, an order for the appropriate sedative and dose should be recently recorded within the patient's chart. Sedatives should be administered by a physician within the Radiology Department.
Additional Information
Causes of basal ganglia calcification on CT scan include carbon monoxide and lead. Cerebral and/or cerebellar atrophy is caused by chronic alcoholism and chronic toulene exposure. Focal necrosis of the basal ganglia can result from carbon monoxide, cyanide, hydrogen sulfide, or methyl alcohol.
Brain changes in carbon monoxide poisoning include diffuse cerebral edema and low density changes of the globus pallidus and subcortical white matter within 6 hours of exposure. Cerebral edema is also seen in toxic alcohol exposure. Methanol poisoning can produce frontal lobe, basal ganglion, and putaminal hemorrhages or infarcts, while ethylene glycol exposure produces abnormalities of the basal ganglia, pons, temporal lobe, and cerebellum. Cerebellar edema may be noted in severe lead exposure (especially in pediatric patients). Diffuse cerebral

edema is also noted in patients with sodium valproate or pentachlorophenol exposure. Cerebral atrophy has been documented after methyl mercury exposure, chronic ethanol use; podophyllin, glucocorticoid exposure; phenytoin, lithium, toluene, amphetamine, or radiation therapy. Changes compatible with pseudotumor cerebri or benign intracranial hypertension include vitamin A poisoning; glucocorticoid, tetracycline, levothyroxine, lithium, or estrogen use.

CO-Oximetry Arterial

Synonyms Arterial CO-Oximetry

Uses Evaluate fractional components of hemoglobin in arterial blood; evaluate the extent of carbon monoxide poisoning

Reference Range Calculated THb: 12% to 15%; % COHb: ≤ 1.5 nonsmokers, 1.5-5 smokers; % MetHb: 0.4-1.5; vol % O_2: 15-23

Test Commonly Includes % carboxyhemoglobin (COHb), % methemoglobin (MetHb), % O_2Hb = oxyhemoglobin and O_2 saturation, total hemoglobin (THb), and volume % O_2 = O_2 content

Patient Preparation The patient should be supine and relaxed

Specimen Arterial blood

Volume 2 mL

Minimum Volume 0.5 mL

Container Preheparinized sampler, heparinized syringe, heparinized capillary tube, or lavender top (EDTA) tube

Collection Specimen drawn into air-free heparinized syringe with stopper. All specimens should be on ice and brought to the laboratory immediately. For capillary collection the skin area to be punctured should be warmed a full 10 minutes. The puncture should be deep enough to allow a free flow of blood. Blood is then collected in heparinized capillary tubes, which should be filled as much as possible, capped and mixed well. All specimens must be labeled with the patient's name and hospital number. Indicate on the requisition mode of oxygen delivery or room air if applicable. Also indicate capillary specimen type (heel or digital) if applicable.

Storage Instructions Place specimen in ice water.

Causes for Rejection Specimen not received on ice, air bubbles or clots in syringe

Special Instructions Requisition must indicate source (ie, arterial) and time sample was drawn.

Limitations Arterial punctures may be extremely difficult in some individuals

Methodology CO-Oximeter™, spectrophotometry

Additional Information Patients on methylene blue or sulfhemoglobin may have erroneous results due to spectral interferences.

Coproporphyrin Screen, Urine

Uses Evaluate porphyrias, including those involving deficiencies of enzymes which are needed for heme synthesis and chemical porphyrias

Reference Range Negative

Specimen Random urine

Volume 10 mL

Minimum Volume 5 mL

Container Plastic urine container wrapped in aluminum foil

Storage Instructions Transport specimen within 1 hour. Protect from light.

Causes for Rejection Excessive delay in transport, specimen not protected from light

Limitations Certain drugs may cause interference

Additional Information Porphyrins are the byproducts of porphyrinogens. Accumulations of either cause porphyrias, which are characterized by increased excretion of porphyrins, porphyrinogens, or their precursors. The following conditions result in an increase of coproporphyrins: congenital erythropoietic porphyria, acute intermittent porphyria (mild increases), hereditary coproporphyria (markedly increased), and lead poisoning.

Creatinine, Serum

Uses

The most common clinical renal function test, providing a rough approximation of glomerular filtration.

Causes of high creatinine include renal diseases and insufficiency with decreased glomerular filtration (uremia or azotemia if severe); urinary tract obstruction; reduced renal blood flow including congestive heart failure, shock and dehydration; rhabdomyolysis causes high serum creatinine, which may be elevated out of proportion to BUN, or to the reduction in renal function.

Causes of low creatinine include small stature, debilitation, decreased muscle mass, some complex cases of severe hepatic disease. In advanced liver disease, low creatinine may result from decreased hepatic production of creatinine and inadequate dietary protein as well as reduced muscle mass.

Index of fetal maturity in amniotic fluid analysis.

Reference Range Children: 1-5 years: 0.3-0.5 mg/dL (SI: 27-44 μmol/L), 5-10 years: 0.5-0.8 mg/dL (SI: 44-71 μmol/L); adults: male: up to 1.2 mg/dL (SI: 106 μmol/L), female: up to 1.1 mg/dL (SI: 97 μmol/L). Variation between sources for serum creatinine normal ranges is perhaps greater than for many other important tests. There are slight differences between the sexes with males higher, since the range relates to the amount of muscle mass present. The glomerular filtration rate increases in pregnancy; thus, serum creatinine should be slightly less during that period. In older patients, decrease of muscle mass must be considered in interpretation of results; the elderly have reduced creatinine generation. Similarly, other patients may have creatinine levels in which muscle abnormalities must be considered, including long-term corticosteroid therapy, hyperthyroidism, muscular dystrophy and paralysis, and dermatomyositis and polymyositis.

Patient Preparation Fasting may be desirable. Certain cephalosporins, especially cefoxitin, cause misleading (high) results.

Specimen Blood

Volume 10 mL

Minimum Volume 1 mL serum

Container Red top tube

Collection Pediatrics: Blood drawn from heelstick.

Causes for Rejection Hemolysis

Limitations

With reduced renal blood flow, creatinine rises less quickly than urea nitrogen. Concentration of creatinine only becomes abnormal when $\sim^1/_2$ or more of the nephrons have stopped functioning in chronic progressive renal disease.

Increased serum creatinine results may occur from noncreatinine substances, including meat ingestion, glucose, pyruvate, uric acid, fructose, guanidine, ketonemia (acetoacetate), hydantoin, ascorbic acid, and numerous cephalosporin antibiotics, especially cefoxitin. Cefoxitin and cefepime interfere with the Jaffé method causing a false elevation. Cefoxitin levels fall in patients with normal kidney function, such that a sample can be drawn 2 hours after a dose but preferably, 4 hours or more afterwards. With severe renal disease, creatinine is not reliable in the presence of cefoxitin therapy. There is less interference reported from the cephalosporins cephalothin, cephaloridine, cephadrile sodium, and cephaloglycin dihydrate. Cefazolin and cefamandole may cause increased colorimetric values. Cephapirin and moxalactam are described as not causing interference. Differences in the interference of such cephalosporins between assay systems are published. Cefoxitin and cefpirome interfere with the Jaffé method causing a false elevation. Levodopa, methyldopa, nitromethane, and trimethoprim may increase serum creatinine levels. Lipemia, hemolysis, and bilirubin may interfere. High creatinine in serum has been reported with methanol intoxication. An antifungal drug, 5-flucytosine, and glucose interfere with the imidohydrolase method.

Tagamet® interferes with creatinine excretion in the renal tubule, causing a rise in creatinine without reduction in renal function. It may also cause an allergic nephritis with reduced renal function. Other drugs which interfere with the tubular secretion of creatine include probenecid, triamterene, amiloride, and spironolactone.

Moderate variation of results exists between chemistry analyzer systems.

Serum creatinine is only a crude guide to the progress of renal disease. Moderate changes in the glomerular filtration rate (GFR) may not be detected by serum creatinine levels. Levey et al and others emphasize that the serum creatinine does **not** provide an adequate estimate of GFR. A fraction of urine creatinine is from tubular secretion. Such tubular secretion increases with declining renal function.

Methodology Alkaline picrate (Jaffé reaction), o-nitrobenzaldehyde (Sakaguchi reaction), imidohydrolase (Ektachem®). Many interference problems are still unresolved in the Jaffé reaction.

Additional Information

Serum creatinine level is proportional to lean body muscle mass. It is unaffected by most diet or activity and is freely filtered by the glomerulus. Both BUN and creatinine are often ordered to follow renal problems. Creatinine overall is the more reliable index, but each has pitfalls. As creatinine increases in chronic renal failure, the hematocrit decreases, total carbon dioxide and bicarbonate fall, and serum phosphate and BUN increase. When serum creatinine increases postoperatively, a group of patients may be identified who are at risk for more severe renal failure. Creatinine clearances have a role in such investigations. Serum creatinine has a role in determination of dosages of some drugs (eg, the aminoglycosides and digoxin), especially in elderly subjects.

Dobutamine (and to a lesser extent dopamine) can produce a profound negative interference with the enzymatic method for serum creatinine determination thus producing a false depression of serum creatinine

Cryptosporidium Diagnostic Procedures, Stool

Synonyms Acid-Fast Stain, Modified, *Cryptosporidium*

Uses A part of the differential work-up of diarrhea, particularly in immunocompromised hosts and suspected AIDS patients; establish the diagnosis of cryptosporidiosis by demonstration of the oocysts. A recent outbreak in healthy individuals from a contaminated water supply was noted. May be useful in treatment of cryptosporidial diarrhea

Reference Range Negative

Test Commonly Includes Examination of stool for the presence of *Cryptosporidium* by phase contrast microscopy and/or modified acid-fast stain, or fluorescent labeled antibody

Abstract *Cryptosporidium*, a parasite, may cause severe diarrhea, predominantly in immunocompromised individuals.

Specimen Fresh stool; stool preserved with 10% formalin or sodium acetate-acetic acid formalin preservative

Container Plastic stool container

Collection Transport fresh specimen to the laboratory promptly following collection. Specimen on outside of container poses excessive risk of contamination to laboratory personnel.

Special Instructions Procedures for the detection of *Cryptosporidium* in humans have recently become available in most clinical laboratories. Consult the laboratory regarding availability of the procedure and specific specimen collection instructions before collecting the specimen.

Limitations *Cryptosporidium* is not detected by standard methods used to examine stool specimens for other ova and parasites; special stains are required for its detection, and in many laboratories, must be specifically requested. The organisms are most readily demonstrated in concentrated diarrheal stools. Forms of *Blastocystis hominis* may cause confusion if Giemsa stain is used. Most recommended procedures cannot be performed on polyvinyl alcohol (PVA) preserved specimens.

Methodology Phase contrast microscopy after sucrose floatation concentration technique (Sheather's); modified acid-fast stain on air-dried, methanol-fixed smears (decolorization with 1% H_2SO_4). Auramine and carbol-fuchsin stain is used by some laboratories for screening. A technique utilizing formalin-ethyl acetate and floatation over hypertonic saline is reported to enhance detection of *Cryptosporidium* oocysts. Fluorescent-labeled IgG monoclonal anti-*Cryptosporidium* antibodies are commercially available.

Additional Information *Cryptosporidium* (similar to *Isospora belli*) is a coccidian parasite of the intestines and respiratory tract of many animals including mice, sheep, snakes, turkeys, chickens, cows, monkeys, and domestic cats. The first reported human case occurred in 1976. The prevalence of cryptosporidial infection in the U.S. is estimated to be 2.6%. It is a cause of severe and chronic diarrhea in patients with hypogammaglobulinemia and the acquired immune deficiency syndrome. Diarrhea lasts an average of 10 days. The organism is widely recognized as a disease of the immunocompromised patient, however, it can also cause disease in immunocompetent subjects. Animal contact, travel to endemic areas, living in a rural environment, and day care attendance by toddlers have been recognized as risk factors for the development of cryptosporidiosis. Perinatal infection has been reported. Children are more prone to develop infection than are adults. In these patients, the disease is a self-limited gastroenteritis, but in immunocompromised patients, a profound enteropathy results. A seasonal variation in incidence exists with the highest frequency reported in summer and autumn. The organism can be demonstrated in biopsies of small bowel and colon, adherent to surface of the epithelial cells (Giemsa stain) and by demonstration in feces by floatation with modified acid-fast stain (cold Kinyoun stain) or smear. Most therapeutic regimens for cryptosporidiosis are not successful unless immunosuppression is reversed. Enteric precautions should be taken. Transmission of *Cryptosporidium* can occur via swimming pools; *Cryptosporidium* oocysts are chloride-resistant. Nitazoxanide is undergoing phase II clinical testing at Cornell Medical Center in New York City.

Crystals, Urine

Related Information
- Urinalysis

Synonyms Urine Crystals

Uses Diagnose metabolic disorders, calculus formation, regulation of medication

Diagnostic Procedures
- Urinalysis

Test Commonly Includes Test is part of a routine urinalysis; includes checking for uric acid, cystine, tyrosine, leucine, cholesterol, sulfa, oxalate, and phosphate crystals

Specimen Random urine, catheterized urine

Volume 12 mL

Minimum Volume 2 mL

Container Plastic urine container, tightly capped

Storage Instructions Refrigerate specimen if test cannot be performed immediately.

Causes for Rejection Quantity not sufficient, improperly labeled specimen, specimen not brought to the laboratory within 1 hour of collection

Methodology Microscopic examination

Additional Information

Crystalluria is uncommon despite maximal concentrations in warm, fresh urine because of the normal presence of crystal inhibitors, the lack of

available nidus, and the time factor. When properly observed in fresh urine, crystals are diagnostically useful for a physician evaluating microhematuria, nephrolithiasis, or toxin ingestion.

In abundance, calcium oxalate and/or hippurate crystals may suggest ethylene glycol ingestion (can be accompanied by neurological abnormalities, appearance of drunkenness, hypertension, and a high anion gap acidosis).

Calcium magnesium ammonium phosphate may be present in massive quantities in alkaline urine. They usually are associated with urine infected by urea splitting bacteria which cause "infection," or "triple phosphate" stones.

Tyrosine and leucine crystals are found in acid urine, indicating abnormal metabolism. These crystals occur together in acute yellow atrophy and in other destructive diseases of the liver.

Crystals may also provide a clue to the composition of renal stones not yet passed.

Cyanide, Blood

Synonyms CN⁻; Hydrocyanic Acid; Potassium or Sodium Cyanide

Uses Establish the diagnosis of cyanide poisoning

Reference Range

Whole blood levels: Smoker: ≤ 0.5 mg/L

Flushing and tachycardia seen at 0.5-1.0 mg/L; obtundation at 1.0-2.5 mg/L

Coma and death occur at >2.5 mg/L

Plasma cyanide:

    Normal: 4-5 mcg/L

    Asymptomatic (with metabolic acidosis): 80 mcg/L

    Death: >260 mcg/L

Red blood cell cyanide:

    Normal: <26 mcg/L

    Metabolic acidosis: 1040 mcg/L

    Symptomatic: 5200 mcg/L

    Fatal: $>10,400$ mcg/L

Abstract This highly toxic substance is one of the oldest poisons known. It binds to cytochrome oxidase and prevents cellular respiration.

Specimen Blood

Volume 10 mL

Minimum Volume 7 mL whole blood or 5 mL serum

Container Lavender top (EDTA) tube or red top tube

Storage Instructions Fill tube to capacity and keep tightly closed; analyze as soon as possible. Refrigerate whole blood, gastric contents or tissue.

Critical Values In whole blood, values >2.5 mcg/mL are potentially fatal although subjects with higher values have survived.

Possible Panic Range Toxic: >1.0 mcg/mL (SI: >77 μmol/L); >2.0 mcg/mL (SI: >115 μmol/L) is lethal

Methodology Conway diffusion, color reaction, ion specific potentiometry

Additional Information

Whole blood cyanide determination by acidification usually provides an overestimation of levels by ~70%; it is most correlated with thiocyanate levels. Most accurate tissue cyanide levels concentration are reflected by plasma cyanide levels. Ratio of red blood cell to plasma cyanide concentration is 60:1. Signs or symptoms due to thiocyanate toxicity usually do not occur at plasma or serum levels <100 mg/L.

A 5 g dose of hydroxocobalamin appears to bind all cyanide ions in patients with initial cyanide levels up to 40 μmol/L

Plasma lactate (half-life ~4 hours in treated cyanide poisoning) may be useful in determining treatment efficacy in cyanide poisoning

Cyclosporine, Blood

Applies to Cyclosporine A

Synonyms Sandimmune®

Uses Monitor blood level in management of immunosuppression of organ transplant recipients

Reference Range RIA: immediately following transplant: 150-250 ng/mL (SI: 125-210 nmol/L) (plasma levels), 450-750 ng/mL (SI: 374-624 nmol/L) (whole blood levels). Maintenance levels months after transplant: 50-150 ng/mL (SI: 40-125 nmol/L) (plasma levels), 150-450 ng/mL (SI: 125-375 nmol/L) (whole blood levels). Reference ranges are method dependent and specimen dependent.

Abstract This drug is widely used as an immunosuppressant, especially after organ transplants.

Specimen Whole blood, plasma, or serum

Container Lavender top (EDTA) tube (whole blood), green top (heparin) tube (plasma), red top tube (serum)

Sampling Time Trough levels should be obtained 12-18 hours after oral dose (chronic usage), 12 hours after intravenous dose, or immediately prior to next dose.

Limitations Results are method dependent - some measure multiple metabolites as well as parent drug. It is not yet clearly established whether whole blood or plasma/serum levels are clinically most appropriate. Single assays are not as informative as a series over time.

Methodology
Radioimmunoassay (RIA), high performance liquid chromatography (HPLC), fluorescence polarization immunoassay (FPIA)

Additional Information
Monitoring of blood levels is imperative because the pharmacokinetics of cyclosporine are not only complex, but vary over time in the same patient; thus, blood levels cannot be well predicted from dosing schedules. Furthermore, this drug has a narrow therapeutic window and significant toxicity at levels above that range.

Renal toxicity with eventual renal failure is the most severe complication. Other assays to assess renal function (ie, BUN, creatinine clearance) should be ordered along with cyclosporine level, since toxicity may begin even with "acceptable" blood levels. Other toxicities include hypertension, convulsions, tremors, pulmonary edema, and an increased risk of lymphoma.

Because results will vary depending on whether the assay is done on whole blood or serum/plasma and on the method and cyclosporine antibody employed (monospecific or polyspecific), it is best for a given patient's specimens to be analyzed at a single laboratory to eliminate as many assay-dependent variables as possible. If switching of laboratories is unavoidable, it is advisable to have a few specimens run in parallel in the second laboratory prior to changing.

The clinical use of cyclosporine is difficult and requires experience and judgment. A drug blood level is only one of many pieces in the puzzle of transplant medicine.

Digitoxin, Blood

Synonyms Crystodigin®; Digitalis; Lanotoxin®; Purodigin®
Uses Therapeutic monitoring; toxicity assessment
Contraindicating Factors Patient on **digoxin**; recent radioactive tracer
Reference Range Therapeutic: 18-22 ng/mL (SI: 23-28 nmol/L)
Abstract One of a group of plant glycosides used in the treatment of congestive heart failure, digitoxin is infrequently used compared to digoxin. It must not be confused with digoxin when serum levels are ordered.
Specimen Blood
Minimum Volume 3 mL serum
Container Red top tube
Sampling Time 6-12 hours after dose
Storage Instructions Separate serum and store in refrigerator.
Critical Values Levels >35 ng/mL (SI: >46 nmol/L) are associated with clinical toxicity in 80% of patients.
Limitations Do not order digitoxin level on a patient receiving digoxin. Digitoxin is not commonly used. Digoxin immune Fab can increase digitoxin levels by assay.
Methodology Radioimmunoassay (RIA), gas-liquid chromatography (GLC), high performance liquid chromatography (HPLC)
Additional Information
Optimal sampling time after dosage is 6 hours. Optimal resampling time after change in dosage is 48-96 hours. Be sure the patient is not on digoxin instead of digitoxin. There is cross reactivity between the two drugs and the levels reported will not be valid, and in fact could be misleading and catastrophic. Digitalis leaf has both digoxin and digitoxin as active components. Digitoxin is the best test for evaluation of toxicity in a patient taking digitalis leaf, but neither test is truly satisfactory. There is considerable overlap in the upper therapeutic ranges with levels which may be toxic. **Digitoxin levels must be correlated with clinical and other chemical data.** Numerous factors modify the effect of cardiac glycosides, including serum potassium, calcium, magnesium, and cardiac blood flow.
Specific References
Van Deusen SK, Birkhahn RH, and Gaeta TJ, "Treatment of Hyperkalemia in a Patient with Unrecognized Digitalis Toxicity," *J Toxicol Clin Toxicol*, 2003, 41(4):373-6.
Walson PD, "Comment on Treatment of Hyperkalemia in a Patient with Unrecognized Digitalis Toxicity," *J Toxicol Clin Toxicol*, 2004, 42(1):119.

Digoxin, Blood

Synonyms Digacin® Level, Blood; Digoxosodium Level, Blood; Lanoxin® Level, Blood
Uses Cardiac glycoside
Reference Range Therapeutic: 0.5-2.0 ng/mL
Specimen Blood
Container Red top tube
Critical Values Toxic effects: Serum: >2.0 ng/mL
Possible Panic Range Fatalities: 1.5-300.0 ng/mL
Limitations Digoxin immune Fab fragments can interfere with assay. Endogenous digoxin-like immunoreactive substances (DLIS) may cause artificial elevation of serum digoxin level. Chinese toad venom used in

medicinals also cross-reacts with FPIA technique. Cardioactive steroids of the bufadienolide class may cross react with polygonal digoxin immunoassays. Large doses of uzara root or Siberian ginseng may interfere with the digoxin assay.
Methodology High performance liquid chromatography (HPLC), radioimmunoassay (RIA); fluorescence polarization immunoassay with ultra filtration (FPIA-UF) accurately measures free digoxin in the presence of immune Fab fragments
Additional Information
Cardioactive steroids of the bufadienolide class may cross react with polyclonal digoxin immunoassays. Serum digoxin concentrations determined by the ACA immunoassay method (DuPont) may overestimate (by 0.3-1.1 ng/mL) digoxin levels in patients with renal, liver or diabetic disease.
The Digoxin immunoreactive substance (DLIS) is rarely above 2 ng/ml. It is elevated in pregnency, neonates, renal/liver insufficiency, congestive heart failure and hypothermia. Digoxin levels may be falsely elevated due to elevated bilirobin, or spironolactone administration.

Electrolytes, Blood

Synonyms Plasma Electrolytes; Serum Electrolytes
Uses Monitor electrolyte status; screen water balance; diagnose respiratory and metabolic acid-base balance; evaluate hydrational status, diarrhea, dehydration, ketoacidosis in diabetes mellitus and other disorders; evaluate alcoholism and other toxicity states
Test Commonly Includes Sodium, potassium, chloride; often total CO_2, but in some laboratories pH and pCO_2 are measured and bicarbonate (HCO_3) and CO_2T are calculated. Anion gap is reported with electrolytes by some laboratories.
Specimen Blood
Volume 10 mL
Minimum Volume 3 mL serum or plasma
Container Red top tube or green top (heparin) tube
Collection Best to collect without tourniquet if possible. Do **not** allow patient to clench-unclench his/her hand.
Storage Instructions Do not freeze.
Limitations Hemolysis and prolonged contact of serum with cells produces elevation of potassium. The usual order for "electrolytes" does not include magnesium, osmolality, phosphorus, or lactic acid.
Methodology Ion-selective electrodes (ISE) or flame photometry are used for sodium and potassium. Sodium and potassium may also be measured by inductively-coupled plasma emission spectrometry.
Additional Information May be performed on heparinized plasma but not on EDTA plasma. Knowledge of pertinent clinical criteria allows for more cost effective ordering of blood electrolytes in patients in whom the information will be clinically significant. The anion gap, calculated $Na^+ \sim (Cl^\sim + HCO_3{}^\sim)$, provides useful information for interpreting acid-base disorders and may be useful for establishing a differential diagnosis in some conditions.
Specific Reference
Rosenson J, Smolin C, Spurer KA. et al, "Patterns of Ecstasy Associated Hyponatremia in California," *Ann Emerg Med*, 2007, 49:164-171.

Electrolytes, Urine

Related Information
• Osmolality, Urine
Synonyms Urine Electrolytes
Uses Monitor kidney function, fluid and electrolyte balance, water balance, acid-base balance; evaluate electrolyte composition of urine, correlation with renin and aldosterone studies. Urine sodium levels are appropriate in patients with volume depletion, with acute oliguria, and with decreased plasma sodium. Urine potassium levels are needed in work-up of hypokalemia of unknown etiology (eg, possible Conn's syndrome (primary aldosteronism), adrenal hyperplasia, Bartter's syndrome, renal tubular acidosis, Fanconi syndrome). Urine chloride is helpful to work up metabolic alkalosis in patients who are not on diuretics; assess dietary salt restriction. Urine electrolytes are used in work-up with aldosterone and renin assays.
Reference Range There is a large diurnal variation in range for spot samples. Na/K ratio: 0.90-3.88; borderline Na/K ratio: 0.3-6.0.
Test Commonly Includes Sodium, potassium, and chloride on random or timed collections. Osmolality must be ordered as such.
Specimen Random, 12-, or 24-hour urine
Volume 10 mL
Container Clean urine container
Collection Specify whether random or timed collection.
Causes for Rejection Blood in urine
Special Instructions Urine osmolality may be ordered with urine electrolytes, usually it must be specifically ordered.
Additional Information If a 24-hour timed specimen is collected, other tests which may be ordered simultaneously include Protein, Quantitative, 24-hour Urine and/or Creatinine Clearance, (all of which can be collected

together). Aldosterone and other adrenocortical steroids enhance reabsorption of sodium and promote excretion of potassium. In subjects with hyponatremia, normal blood volume, and urine Na and Cl >40 mM/L, the differential diagnosis includes hypothyroidism and the syndrome of inappropriate secretion of antidiuretic hormone. Fetal (amniotic fluid) electrolytes are not predictive of ultimate renal function.

Ethylene Glycol, Blood

Applies to Antifreeze
Synonyms 1,2-Ethanediol
Uses Detect and quantitate ingestion of ethylene glycol
Reference Range Negative
Test Commonly Includes Propylene glycol
Abstract A commercial chemical used as a radiator antifreeze and for commercial chemical synthesis.
Specimen Blood
Container Red top tube or green top (heparin) tube
Possible Panic Range Levels at 0.2 g/L indicate toxicity.
Methodology Gas-liquid chromatography (GLC), photometry, fluorometry, enzymatic assay (automated)
Additional Information Existence of propionic acid through inborn errors of metabolism can give a false-positive ethylene glycol level. Glycerol, elevated triglycerides, and propylene glycol can falsely elevate serum ethylene glycol level.

Ethyl Glucuronide (Urine)

Related Information
- Ethyl Sulfate (Urine)

Synonyms EtG
Use Monitor alcohol use or dependence
Reference Range Usual cutoff ranges from 0.1 to 1 mg/L in commercial labs
Abstract Ethyl glucuronide is produced by a phase 2 conjugation reaction with glucuronic acid and is excreted in the urine. This assay is often combined with measurement of urinary ethyl sulfate (EtS).
Specimen 10 mL urine
Methodology Specific direct electrospray liquid chromatographic-mass spectrometric method performed in the negative ion mode
Additional Information Can be measured up to 80 hours postingestion. False-positive results can result due to fermentation following sample collection. Urinary tract infections with *Escherichia coli* can result in false-negative results due to bacterial hydrolysis. Incidental exposure to mouthwash containing 12% ethanol (while gargling) can result in urinary ethyl glucuronide levels over 50 ng/ml.

Specific References
Bih C, Mitra S, Bodepudi V, et al, "Development of a Homogeneous Enzyme Immunoassay for the Detection of Ethyl Glucuronide in Urine and Its Evaluation on the MGC 240 Analyzer," *J Anal Toxicol*, 2006, 30:146.

Constantino A, Di Gregorio EJ, Korn W, et al, "The Effect of the Use of Mouthwash on Ethylglucuronide Concentrations in Urine," *J Anal Toxicol*, 2006, 30:659-62.

Helander A and Beck O, "Ethyl Sulfate: A Metabolite of Ethanol in Humans and a Potential Biomarker of Acute Alcohol Intake," *Clin Chem*, 2005, 29(5):270-4.

Helander A and Beck O, "Mass Spectrometric Identification of Ethyl Sulfate as an Ethanol Metabolite in Humans," *Clin Chem*, 2004, 50(5):936-7.

Helander A and Dahl H "Urinary Tract Infection: A Risk Factor for False-negative Urinary Ethyl Glucuronide But Not Ethyl Sulfate in the Detection of Recent Alcohol Consumption," *Clin Chem*, 2005, 51(9):1728-30.

Kaushik R, Levine B, and LaCourse WR, "An Improved Method to Determine Ethyl Glucuronide in Urine Using Reversed-Phase HPLC and Pulsed Electrochemical Detection," *J Anal Toxicol*, 2006, 30:151.

Rohrig TP, Huber C, Goodson L, Ross W, "Detection of Ethylglucuronide in Urine Following Application of Germ-X," *J Anal Toxicol*, 2006, 30:703-4.

Ethyl Sulfate (Urine)

Related Information
- Ethyl Glucuronide (Urine)

Synonyms EtS
Use Monitor alcohol use or dependence
Reference Range Usual cutoff is 100 ng/mL
Abstract Ethanol undergoes sulfate conjugation through the actions of sulfotransferase to produce ethyl sulfate (EtS), which is excreted in the first 24 hours. Often combined with measurement of urinary ethyl glucuronide (EtG).
Specimen 10 mL urine

Methodology Specific direct electrospray liquid chromatographic-mass spectrometric method performed in the negative ion mode
Additional Information Unlike ethyl glucuronide, there appears to be little effect with urinary tract infections and false negatives. Can be measured up to about 36 hours postingestion (shorter window of detection than EtG)

Specific References
Helander A and Beck O, "Ethyl Sulfate: A Metabolite of Ethanol in Humans and a Potential Biomarker of Acute Alcohol Intake," *Clin Chem*, 2005, 29(5):270-4.

Helander A and Beck O, "Mass Spectrometric Identification of Ethyl Sulfate as an Ethanol Metabolite in Humans," *Clin Chem*, 2004, 50(5):936-7.

Helander A and Dahl H "Urinary Tract Infection: A Risk Factor for False-negative Urinary Ethyl Glucuronide But Not Ethyl Sulfate in the Detection of Recent Alcohol Consumption," *Clin Chem*, 2005, 51(9):1728-30.

Glucose, Random

Uses Evaluate carbohydrate metabolism, acidosis and ketoacidosis, dehydration; work up alcoholism, or apparent alcoholism; work-up of coma, neuroglycopenia. Hypoglycemia if present should be investigated with insulin levels as well. For the diagnosis of diabetes mellitus in nonpregnant adult subjects, random glucose >200 mg/dL (SI: >11.1 mM/L) is required. Other criteria exist. Determination of blood glucose on admission in patients who have had an out-of-hospital cardiac arrest can serve as a predictor of neurologic recovery. Higher levels are indicative of more severe brain ischemia and difficult resuscitation. In pregnant women, a value >105 mg/dL usually prompts further investigation.
Reference Range Dependent on time and content of last meal. Glucose of >200 mg/dL (SI: >11.1 mM/L) in a nonstressed, ambulatory subject supports the diagnosis of diabetes mellitus. Values in term neonates are published.
Specimen Blood
Volume 10 mL
Minimum Volume 5 mL plasma or serum
Container Gray top (sodium fluoride) tube preferred; red top tube acceptable
Collection Pediatrics: Draw blood from heelstick.
Causes for Rejection Blood stored overnight on clot
Possible Panic Range Neonates: <40 mg/dL (SI: <2.2 mM/L); adults: male: <50 mg/dL (SI: <2.8 mM/L), >400 mg/dL (SI: >22.2 mM/L); adults female: <40 mg/dL (SI: <2.2 mM/L), >400 mg/dL (SI: >22.2 mM/L)
Limitations Glucose will decrease in samples left on the clot and in tubes other than fluoride prior to analysis. Acetaminophen can cause a false elevation of serum glucose when the neocuprine method is utilized.
Methodology Hexokinase, glucose oxidase, oxygen rate, ortho-toluidine
Additional Information

Recall that **blood glucose** values are not equivalent to **plasma glucose**. If glucose is >400 mg/dL (SI: >22.2 mM/L), an acetone (ketone body) examination probably should be done. A fasting and a 2-hour postprandial specimen is preferable to a random specimen for evaluation of possible diabetes mellitus. The incidence of hypoglycemia in hospitalized patients appears to be significant, but may be better controlled if frequent monitoring of glucose levels is employed. Wider utilization of bedside glucose testing may allow for closer patient monitoring, but the establishment of uniform quality control procedures is necessary to ensure valid results from this type of testing. Evaluation of glycated hemoglobin and self-monitoring of blood glucose are two relatively new means of assessing glycemia which have become widely available.

May cause a false elevation of serum creatinine through interference with laboratory determination

Tumors which induce hypoglycemia: Pancreatic islet-cell tumor (insulinoma); fibrosarcomas; mesotheliomas; leiomyosarcomas; hemangiopericytomas; gastric carcinoma; pancreatic exocrine carcinoma; lung carcinoma; cervical carcinoma (small-cell)

Specific References
Abarbanell NR. "Is Prehospital Blood Glucose Measurement Necessary in Suspected Cerebrovascular Accident Patients?" *Am J Emerg Med*, 2005, 23(7):823-7.

Jee SH, Ohrr H, Sull JW, et al, "Fasting Serum Glucose Level and Cancer Risk in Korean Men and Women," *JAMA*, 2005, 293(2):194-202.

Gold Level

Synonyms Aurothioglucose; Chrysotherapy; Gold Sodium Thiomalate; Myochrysine®; Solganal®
Reference Range Normal: 0-0.1 mcg/mL (SI: 0-0.5 µmol/L); therapeutic: 1.0-3.0 mcg/mL (SI: 5.1-15.2 µmol/L); urine <0.1 mcg/24 hours
Abstract Gold is used as a treatment for rheumatoid arthritis, but its value is being questioned.
Specimen Blood, urine

Volume 7 mL blood or entire collection urine

Container Red top tube for blood, acid-washed polyethylene container for urine

Limitations Blood levels do not correlate with therapeutic or toxic effects. No relationship between serum gold levels and efficacy is established. Serum gold concentrations have not been helpful in monitoring adverse reactions. A relationship is not recognized between urinary gold and response to therapy. Hair and nail gold concentrations have not been helpful.

Methodology Atomic absorption spectrometry (AA)

Additional Information Complex gold compounds are used in the treatment of severe, progressive rheumatoid arthritis which is not controlled by other medical therapy. It is also used selectively for juvenile rheumatoid arthritis and for psoriatic arthritis affecting peripheral joints. The mechanism of action is not clear, but may be due to reticuloendothelial system blockade, and/or effects on lymphocyte proliferation and antibody production. Gold toxicity may be manifested by dermatitis, pruritus, stomatitis, metallic taste, eosinophilia, leukopenia, anemia, thrombocytopenia, hematuria, proteinuria, nephrosis, and bone marrow suppression, among other possible effects.

Heavy Metal Screen, Blood

Synonyms Metals, Blood; Poisonous Metals, Blood; Toxic Metals, Blood

Uses Screen for heavy metal poisoning

Reference Range Varies with metal detected.

Test Commonly Includes Antimony, arsenic, bismuth, boron, cadmium, cobalt, copper, lead, mercury, selenium, tellurium, thallium, zinc

Abstract Used principally to detect arsenic, cadmium, mercury, and lead poisoning.

Specimen Whole blood (EDTA) plus serum

Volume 20 mL

Container Special metal-free tube and red top tube

Storage Instructions Refrigerate: do not spin down.

Special Instructions Check with laboratory performing the assay to determine what elements will be detected and for any special instructions.

Methodology Atomic absorption spectrometry (AA)

Heavy Metal Screen, Urine

Applies to Heavy Metal Screen, Hair

Synonyms Metal Screen; Metals, Toxic; Poisonous Metals, Urine; Toxic Metals, Urine

Uses Screen for heavy metal poisoning and toxic exposure; urine lead analysis is useful for organic lead exposure and to monitor chelation. Blood is preferred for inorganic lead exposure monitoring.

Reference Range Arsenic: <50 mcg/L; lead: <80 mcg/L; mercury: <20 mcg/L; nickel: <25 mcg/L; cadmium: <10 mcg/L

Test Commonly Includes Arsenic, mercury, lead (could also include nickel and cadmium)

Abstract Used to detect arsenic, mercury, lead, and cadmium poisoning

Specimen 24-hour urine

Volume Entire collection

Minimum Volume 150 mL aliquot

Container Plastic, acid-washed urine container (preferably polyethylene), no preservative, 20-25 mL 6N HCl (low metal content)

Collection 24-hour collection

Storage Instructions Refrigerate

Special Instructions Include volume of urine

Limitations

Hair analysis is not useful for lead exposure; should be used for arsenic and mercury poisoning or exposure, especially if one is interested in determining chronic exposure. Hair should be clean, free of oil, and clipped (0.5 g for As; 2 g for Hg) as close as possible.

Recent ingestion of seafood can cause misleading increases of urine arsenic.

Methodology Atomic absorption spectrometry (AA)

Iron and Total Iron Binding Capacity/Transferrin

Synonyms Fe and TIBC; Iron Binding Capacity; Iron Profile; TIBC; Total Iron Binding Capacity

Uses Differential diagnosis of anemia, especially with hypochromia and/or low MCV. The **percent saturation** sometimes is more helpful than is the iron result to estimate iron stores and iron deficiency anemia. Evaluate thalassemia and possible sideroblastic anemia; work up hemochromatosis, in which iron is increased and iron saturation is high. Decrease in iron level after performance of a Schilling test supports the diagnosis of vitamin B_{12} deficiency, *vide infra*. Evaluate iron poisoning (toxicity) and overload in renal dialysis patients or patients with transfusion dependent anemias. Use of TIBC in iron toxicity may be less useful than previously believed. TIBC or transferrin is a useful index of nutritional status, but is not useful for evaluating iron poisoning.

Uncomplicated iron deficiency: Serum transferrin (and TIBC) high, serum iron low, saturation low. Usual causes of depleted iron stores include blood loss, inadequate dietary iron. RBCs in moderately severe iron deficiency are hypochromic and microcytic. The red cell distribution width increases and MCV decreases. Stainable marrow iron is absent. Serum ferritin decrease is the earliest indicator of iron deficiency if inflammation is absent.

Anemia of chronic disease: Serum transferrin (and TIBC) low to normal, serum iron low, saturation low or normal. Transferrin decreases with many inflammatory diseases. With chronic disease there is a block in movement to and utilization of iron by marrow. This leads to low serum iron and decreased erythropoiesis. Examples include acute and chronic infections, malignancy, and renal failure.

Sideroblastic anemia: Serum transferrin (and TIBC) normal to low, serum iron normal to high, saturation high.

Hemolytic anemias: Serum transferrin (and TIBC) normal to low, serum iron high, saturation high.

Hemochromatosis: Serum transferrin (and TIBC) slightly low, serum iron high, saturation very high.

Protein depletion: Serum transferrin (and TIBC) may be low, serum iron normal or low (if the patient is also iron deficient). This may occur as a result of malnutrition, liver disease, renal disease (eg, nephrosis) or other entities.

Liver disease: Serum transferrin variable; with acute viral hepatitis, high along with serum iron and ferritin. With chronic liver disease (eg, cirrhosis), transferrin may be low. Patients who have cirrhosis and portacaval shunting have saturated TIBC/transferrin as well as high ferritin.

Chronic dialysis for renal failure: Monitor iron levels in patients undergoing dialysis. To follow treatment of iron overload with deferoxamine or with regimen of recombinant human erythropoietin and phlebotomy.

Contraindicating Factors Parenteral iron before sample is drawn will cause misleading high iron results. Recent blood transfusion may have only a small positive effect on iron.

Reference Range A variety of approaches to the estimation of serum iron, TIBC, and transferrin are in use. Expect normal ranges to vary between laboratories as they are in part method dependent. Iron: 75-175 mcg/dL (SI: 13.4-31.3 μmol/L) for adult males; slightly lower (5% to 10%) values for adult females. Iron binding capacity: 250-350 mcg/dL (SI: 45-63 μmol/L). Percent saturation (transferrin saturation): 20% to 50%. TIBC is a chemical approximation of transferrin. Quantitative assays for transferrin are widely available. A mathematical relationship between TIBC and transferrin can be derived, depending on methodology, in which transferrin can be measured, then TIBC calculated.

Test Commonly Includes Serum iron, total iron binding capacity and/or transferrin, percent of saturation

Patient Preparation Specimen should be drawn fasting in the morning (circadian rhythm affects iron; levels are lower in the evening). Sample should be drawn before the patient is given therapeutic iron or blood transfusion. Iron determinations on patients who have had blood transfusions should be delayed several days.

Specimen Blood

Volume 10 mL

Minimum Volume 7 mL serum

Container Red top tube

Sampling Time Morning; marked daily variation occurs

Collection Serum iron levels are 30% higher in the morning and blood levels should be determined on fasting AM samples. Blood should be drawn before other specimens which require anticoagulated tubes. Separate serum from cells as soon as possible.

Storage Instructions Stable 1 week at 4°C

Limitations Except for iron poisoning, a serum iron without TIBC or transferrin is of limited value. Ferritin levels are also useful for iron deficiency. Low iron level may not indicate iron deficiency in acute infection with leukocytosis. Low iron levels may be misleading in chronic infection, inflammation, and malignancy; high ferritin levels occur in many such states. TIBC and transferrin are increased in patients on oral contraceptives, with normal saturation. Gross hemolysis may interfere with serum iron.

Methodology Ferrozine, bathophenanthroline (iron); nephelometry (transferrin); $MgCO_3$ column, other methods (TIBC); atomic absorption (iron, TIBC), anodal stripping; inductively coupled plasma atomic emission spectroscopy

Additional Information

Serum iron is **increased** in hemosiderosis, hemolytic anemias especially thalassemia, sideroachrestic anemias, hepatitis, acute hepatic necrosis, hemochromatosis, and with inappropriate iron therapy. Iron may reach high levels with iron poisoning. Levels as high as 16,700 mcg/dL have been survivable. Some patients who receive multiple transfusions (eg, some hemolytic anemias, thalassemia, renal dialysis patients) will have increased serum iron levels. Patients receiving chloramphenicol, estrogens, and methyldopa can have elevated iron levels.

Serum iron is **decreased** with insufficient dietary iron, chronic blood loss (including the hemolytic anemias, paroxysmal nocturnal hemoglobinuria), inadequate absorption of iron and impaired release of iron stores as in inflammation, infection, and chronic diseases. Cholestyramine and colchicine can cause a decrease in serum iron. Deferoxamine may interfere with colorimetric iron and total iron binding capacity assays. The combination of low iron, high TIBC and/or transferrin, and low saturation indicates iron deficiency. Without all of these findings together, iron deficiency is unproven. Low ferritin supports the diagnosis of iron deficiency. **Detection of iron deficiency may lead to detection of adenocarcinoma of GI tract, a point which cannot be overemphasized.** In recovery from pernicious anemia, especially just after B$_{12}$ dose, iron levels are low. In fact, the drop in serum iron 1 to several days after the Schilling test flushing dose of vitamin B$_{12}$ may be more useful in diagnosis than the radioactivity of the 24-hour urine collection. Serum iron is reported to drop with acute infarct of myocardium.

TIBC is increased in iron-deficiency, use of oral contraceptives, and in pregnancy. It is falsely increased with deferoxamine treatment. It is not useful in managing iron poisoning.

TIBC decreased in hypoproteinemia from many causes, and in a number of inflammatory states. Also, chloramphenicol and corticotropin can decrease TIBC.

Increased saturation occurs with HLA-related (classical) hemochromatosis before ferritin is greatly increased, and also with iron overload (eg, cirrhosis and portacaval shunt), in hemolytic anemias, and with iron therapy. Saturation >70% in females, >80% in males is described as prerequisite for parenchymal loading. However, sample contamination and the vagaries of fluctuation in serum iron levels can make such criteria misleading on occasion.

The serum ferritin is a more sensitive test than the serum iron or TIBC for iron deficiency and for iron overload. When all these tests are used together, as is often necessary, they usually can distinguish between iron deficiency anemia and the anemia of chronic disease. The best and most reliable evaluation of total body iron stores is by bone marrow aspiration and biopsy. The best evaluation of iron deficiency in childhood (unless lead toxicity is suspected) is free erythrocyte porphyrins. With recombinant erythropoietin therapy serum iron, transferrin saturation, and ferritin levels decline due to rapid utilization by stimulated erythropoiesis with resultant decrease in storage iron.

Lactic Acid, Blood

Applies to Biotin; Phenformin
Synonyms Blood Lactate; Lactate, Blood
Uses Suspect lactic acidosis when unexplained anion gap metabolic acidosis is encountered, especially if azotemia or ketoacidosis are not present. Evaluate metabolic acidosis, regional or diffuse tissue hypoperfusion, hypoxia, shock, congestive heart failure, dehydration, complicated postoperative state, ketoacidosis or nonketotic acidosis in diabetes mellitus, patients with infections, inflammatory states, postictal state, certain myopathies, acute leukemia and other neoplasia, enzyme defects, glycogen storage disease (type I), thiamine deficiency, and hepatic failure. A spontaneous form of lactic acidosis occurs. It is a prognostic index in particular clinical settings, especially in critically ill patients in shock. A relationship to renal disease also exists. With skin rash, seizures, alopecia, ataxia, keratoconjunctivitis, and lactic acidosis in children, consider defective biotin metabolism. Phenformin, ethanol, methanol, and salicylate and ethylene glycol poisoning may cause lactic acidosis. Acetaminophen toxicity causes lactic acidosis, sometimes with hypoglycemia. Cyanide, isoniazid, and propylene glycol are among the causes of lactic acidosis. Lactic acidosis may be due to inborn errors of metabolism.

Contraindicating Factors Lack of acidosis is **not** a contraindication for this test.

Reference Range Plasma values: venous: 4.5-19.8 mg/dL (SI: 0.5-2.2 mM/L); arterial: 4.5-14.4 mg/dL (SI: 0.5-1.6 mM/L)

Abstract Hypoperfusion is the most common cause of lactic acidosis, and hyperlactacidemia may be the only marker of tissue hypoperfusion.

Specimen Whole blood, arterial or venous, or plasma
Volume 7 mL
Minimum Volume 4 mL whole blood
Container Gray top (sodium fluoride) tube
Collection Avoid hand-clenching and use of a tourniquet. A tourniquet or a patient clenching and unclenching his/her hand will lead to build-up of potassium and lactic acid from the hand muscles. Commonly needed with or as stat follow-up to venous or arterial pH. Serial determinations are often valuable. Send specimen on ice.
Storage Instructions Centrifuge immediately and take off plasma (unless laboratory uses a whole blood method). Keep plasma on ice or at 2°C to 8°C, analyze promptly. A recent study of blood handling techniques and their effect on lactate concentration has been published.
Causes for Rejection Specimen not received on ice

Special Instructions Keep tube on ice until delivered to the laboratory. Tube must be in laboratory within 15 minutes of being drawn.
Possible Panic Range ≥45.0 mg/dL
Limitations Gross hemolysis depresses results. Intravenous injections or infusions which modify acid-base balance, may cause alterations in lactate levels. Epinephrine and exercise elevate lactate, as may I.V. sodium bicarbonate, glucose, and hyperventilation. False low values with a high LD (LDH) value. Normal L-lactate occurs with high D-lactate in D-lactic acidosis. Metabolic acidosis following bypass for obesity, related to altered gastrointestinal flora, is a feature of subjects who develop mental changes as well, in whom D-lactate is the causative anion.
Methodology Enzymatic; other methods include gas chromatography (GC)
Additional Information Phosphorus is sometimes significantly abnormal in lactic acidosis. Creatinine is higher in ketoacidosis than in lactic acidosis, by interference produced by acetoacetic acid on creatinine. Causes of lactic acidosis (usually <45 mg/dL (SI: <5.0 mM/L)) include carbohydrate infusions, exercise, diabetic ketosis, alcohol. Causes of lactic acidosis (>45 mg/dL) include shock (in which lactic acidosis may occur early, before fall in blood pressure, decrease in urine output), hypoxia (including congestive failure, severe anemia, hypotension) and malignancies. Severe lactic acidosis can develop in minutes. Lactic acidosis can accompany dehydration. Blood lactate concentration correlates negatively with survival in patients with acute myocardial infarction, with persistent elevation, >36 mg/dL (SI: >4.0 mM/L) for more than 12 hours, being associated with poor prognosis. At a given bicarbonate level, the average pCO$_2$ is lower in lactic acidosis than in diabetic ketoacidosis. Lactic acid determination is generally indicated if anion gap is >20 mM/L and if pH is <7.25 and the pCO$_2$ is not elevated. The measurement of lactate levels may be indicated in the clinical setting of metabolic acidosis. Serum salicylate, ethanol level, and osmolality may be helpful. Spontaneous lactic acidosis may be fatal. Protocols are available for measurement of lactate in cord blood. Plasma lactate (half-life ~4 hours in treated cyanide poisoning) may be useful in determining treatment efficacy in cyanide poisoning. The presence of high urine concentrations of lactate dehydrogenase, lactic acid, and protein may cause a false-positive urinary immunoassay of amphetamines, barbiturates, opiates, cocaine metabolite, propoxyphene, benzodiazepines, and ethanol (urine and serum); and low serum phenytoin (high LDH in blood).

Lead, Blood

Related Information
- Heavy Metal Screen, Blood

Applies to Delta Aminolevulinic Acid Dehydratase
Synonyms Pb, Blood
Uses Evaluate lead toxicity, poisoning
Reference Range <10 mcg/dL (whole blood) (SI: <0.97 μmol/L). See accompanying CDC chart for evaluating blood lead concentrations in children.

CDC Classification of Blood Lead in Children		
Class	Blood Lead Level* (mcg/dL)	Comment
I	<10	Not lead-poisoned
IIA	10-14	Rescreen frequently and consider prevention activities
IIB	15-19	Institute nutritional and educational interventions
III	20-44	Evaluate environment and consider chelation therapy
IV	45-69	Institute environmental intervention and chelation therapy
V	>69	A medical emergency

*Due to possible contamination during collection, elevated levels should be confirmed with a second specimen before action is instituted.

Abstract Blood lead concentrations are used to detect recent lead exposure. Does not necessarily measure lead body burden from chronic exposure in the past.
Specimen Whole blood
Volume 10 mL
Container Special lead-free tube with heparin
Storage Instructions Do not separate red cells.
Special Instructions Avoid contact with leaded glass during collection
Possible Panic Range >80 mcg/dL (SI: >3.86 μmol/L) in acute lead poisoning; toxicity at lower levels in chronic poisoning
Limitations Lead poisoning is not ruled out by normal blood levels; clinical findings and heme synthetic enzymes must also be evaluated.

Methodology Electrothermal atomic absorption spectrometry (AA), photometry, anodic stripping voltammeter

Additional Information Great care is required to avoid contamination in the collection of specimens for lead analysis. Lead can be measured in tissue and urine. Another test that may be used to evaluate lead intoxication is **free erythrocyte protoporphyrin (FEP)**. FEP concentrations >35 mcg/dL are consistent with undue absorption of lead. However, FEP is also elevated in iron deficiency, sickle cell anemia, and chronic infection. **Erythrocyte zinc protoporphyrin** is a more specific indicator of lead toxicity and, therefore, superior to FEP. Normal values for erythrocyte zinc protoporphyrin are <100 ng/dL. Inhibition of erythrocyte **delta aminolevulinic acid dehydratase** is a very sensitive measure of lead toxicity. However, a blood lead assay is the definitive test for recent acute exposure if sample collection is meticulous. Blood lead concentrations are evidence of **recent** exposure but do not indicate the body burden from past exposure. Capillary tube collections of fingerstick blood provides adequate samples for atomic absorption spectrophotometry; false-positive rates per this method (19%) are comparable to conventional venous blood sampling (13%).

Specific References

Centers for Disease Control and Prevention (CDC), "Blood Lead Levels– United States, 1999-2002," *MMWR Morb Mortal Wkly Rep*, 2005, 27;54(20):513-6.

Kemper AR, Cohn LM, Fant KE, et al, "Follow-up Testing Among Children with Elevated Screening Blood Lead Levels," *JAMA*, 2005, 11;293(18):2232-7.

Lahn M, Sing W, Nazario S, et al, "Increased Blood Lead Levels in Severe Smoke Inhalation," *Am J Emerg Med*, 2003, 21(6):458-60.

Yassin AS, Martonik JF, and Davidson JL, "Blood Lead Levels in U.S. Workers, 1988-1994," *J Occup Environ Med*, 2004, 46(7):720-8.

Lead, Urine

Related Information

• Heavy Metal Screen, Urine

Applies to Lead Excretion Ratio

Synonyms Pb, Urine

Uses Evaluate lead toxicity and chelation therapy

Reference Range ≤80 mcg/24 hours (SI: ≤0.39 µmol/day)

Abstract This test is used to assess lead body burden (lead mobilization test), not to diagnose lead poisoning.

Patient Preparation Patient should be instructed to use a specially cleaned plastic urinal or bedpan

Specimen Random or 24-hour urine

Volume 50 mL random, entire 24-hour collection

Container Plastic (preferably polyethylene) acid-washed urine container

Storage Instructions Record total volume. Acidify to pH 2 with concentrated HCl or add 20 mL 6N HCl to the 24-hour volume.

Causes for Rejection Specimen allowed to contact glass or metal, specimen not collected in acid-washed containers

Special Instructions Indicate if a chelating agent has been administered

Possible Panic Range >125 mcg/24 hours (SI: >0.60 µmol/day) is considered excessive and associated with toxicity; values of 80-125 mcg/24 hours (SI: 0.39-0.60 µmol/day) are inconclusive

Methodology Electrothermal atomic absorption (AA)

Additional Information Lead is poorly excreted and is found in lower concentrations in urine versus blood. Urine is not the specimen for screening potential toxicity. Urine lead mobilization tests (postchelation therapy) are good indicators of lead body burden. A lead mobilization test is carried out by giving Ca EDTA and measuring the lead excreted in the next 24-hour urine. The lead excretion ratio (LER) is calculated by dividing the amount of lead excreted (in mcg/24 hours) by the amount of Ca EDTA given (in mg). A ratio >0.60 is considered positive for the LER. Unstimulated urinary excretion at rates >0.19 mcg lead/mg creatinine may also be used to indicate need for chelation therapy.

Lidocaine, Blood

Applies to GX; MEGX

Synonyms Lignocaine; Xylocaine®

Uses Monitor therapeutic drug level. Lidocaine is used especially in acute arrhythmias.

Reference Range Therapeutic: 1.5-5.0 mcg/mL (SI: 6.4-21.4 µmol/L), up to 6.0 mcg/mL (SI: 25.6 µmol/L) if necessary.

Abstract Lidocaine is a local anesthetic which more recently has been used as an antiarrhythmic. The most active metabolite is MEGX.

Specimen Blood

Volume 10 mL

Container Red top tube, green top (heparin) tube, or lavender top (EDTA) tube

Sampling Time Draw specimens 12 hours after initiating therapy for arrhythmia prophylaxis, then every 24 hours thereafter. Obtain specimens every 12 hours when cardiac or hepatic insufficiency exists.

Collection Avoid collection tubes with stoppers containing the plasticizer, TBEP.

Possible Panic Range At levels >6.0 mcg/mL (SI: >25.6 µmol/L), there may be seizure activity.

Limitations Cross reactions with other drugs occur. Certain blood collection tubes have been shown to lead to falsely low results. See Collection.

Methodology Enzyme immunoassay (EIA), gas-liquid chromatography (GLC), high performance liquid chromatography (HPLC)

Additional Information Time to reach steady-state by I.V. is 6-12 hours. In most cases, a relatively constant plasma level may be maintained by slow intravenous infusion administered over a period of 6-10 hours. Blood levels are also elevated by impaired cardiac or hepatic function. The drug is metabolized by the liver to two active metabolites, monoethylglycinexylidide (MEGX) and glycinexylidide (GX). Both accumulate and MEGX most likely contributes to toxicity.

Lithium, Blood

Synonyms Eskalith®; Lithonate®

Uses Monitor therapeutic drug level; evaluate coma

Reference Range Therapeutic: 0.6-1.2 mEq/L (SI: 0.6-1.2 mM/L), for acute mania; 0.8-1.0 mEq/L (SI: 0.8-1.0 mM/L) for protection against future episodes in most patients with bipolar disorder. A higher rate of relapse is described in subjects who are maintained at levels <0.4 mEq/L (SI: 0.4 mM/L).

Abstract Lithium is used in the treatment of depression and particularly for manic-depressive psychosis. It should be monitored.

Specimen Blood

Volume 7 mL

Minimum Volume 2 mL serum

Container Red top tube

Collection Collect at a standard time from last dose, 6-12 hours is recommended.

Storage Instructions Refrigerate a minimum of 2 mL serum. Serum specimens are stable for 24 hours at room temperature. Separate serum immediately.

Causes for Rejection Specimen collected in tube containing lithium heparin, hemolysis

Possible Panic Range Toxic: >1.5 mEq/L (SI: >1.5 mM/L). Toxicity can become serious when levels rise to levels ≥2.0 mEq/L (SI: ≥2.0 mM/L). Levels >4.0 mEq/L (SI: >4.0 mM/L) are associated with coma, death. A narrow therapeutic index exists for lithium.

Limitations Lithium toxicity can occur with normal serum lithium levels. Thiazides can cause significant rise in serum lithium.

Methodology Flame photometry, atomic absorption spectrophotometry (AA), ion-selective electrode (ISE)

Additional Information Speckled green top tubes (Becton-Dickinson) which contain lithium heparin as an anticoagulant can increase plasma lithium levels by ~1.5 mEq/L (1.5 mM/L). Benzamide, quinidine, and procainamide can result in falsely elevated serum lithium levels by spectrochemical assays.

Lithium RBC/Plasma Ratio

Reference Range RBC lithium: 0.10-0.40 mEq/L; plasma lithium; 1.00-1.50 mEq/L; RBC plasma/ratio: none defined

Test Commonly Includes Plasma lithium, RBC lithium, and RBCs/plasma ratio

Specimen Blood

Volume 10 mL

Minimum Volume 2 mL

Container Lavender top (EDTA) tube

Storage Instructions Do not refrigerate.

Causes for Rejection Gross hemolysis, clotted specimen

Methodology Atomic absorption spectrophotometry (AA)

Lung Scan, Ventilation

Applies to Quantitative Ventilation Lung Scan; Ventilation-Perfusion Lung Scan

Synonyms Aerosol Lung Scan; Radionuclide Ventilation Lung Scan; Ventilation Lung Scan; Xenon Lung Scan

Uses The primary indication for lung ventilation and perfusion imaging is the detection of acute pulmonary emboli. These procedures together provide an accurate noninvasive screening test both for the detection of emboli and for documentation of resolution during and after therapy. Lung ventilation imaging is also helpful in quantifying regional pulmonary ventilation in patients with severe obstructive lung disease or who are being considered for lung resection surgery. Useful for acute toxic inhalation; retention of xenon indicative of parenchymal lung damage.

Reference Range

Homogeneous distribution of activity throughout the lungs

Test Commonly Includes The patient inhales a radioactive gas or nebulized aerosol and multiple images of the lungs are then acquired to assess lung ventilation. **Special note:** This procedure is almost always combined with a lung perfusion scan to detect a characteristic pattern of segmental perfusion deficits with normal corresponding regional ventilation that is the hallmark of pulmonary emboli.

Patient Preparation Patient should have all RIA blood work performed, or at least drawn, prior to injection of any radioactive material. The patient does not need to be fasting or NPO for this procedure. The patient should have a routine chest radiograph performed within 12 hours prior to imaging or receive one immediately after. Notify the Nuclear Medicine Department if patients require high flow oxygen or respirator assistance.

Causes for Rejection Other recent Nuclear Medicine procedure may interfere. If uncertain, call the Nuclear Medicine Department.

Special Instructions

Requisition must state the current patient diagnosis in order to select the most appropriate radiopharmaceutical and/or imaging technique. The duration of the procedure is 30 minutes to 1 hour. For radiopharmaceuticals: See table.

Radiopharmaceuticals for Lung Ventilation Imaging

Agent	Isotope Half-life	Timing vs Perfusion Scan	Advantages	Disadvantages
^{99m}Tc DTPA aerosol	6 hours	Before	Multiple views of ventilation	Turbulent air flow can cause patchy distribution; no washout phase
^{133}Xe gas*	5 days	Before	Single view with equilibrium and washout phases	Requires good single-breath effort; single view (usually posterior)
^{127}Xe gas	36 days	After	Single view with equilibrium and washout phases; may be performed after perfusion scan	
^{81m}Kr gas	13 seconds	During	Multiple views of ventilation; no gas trap required	Nonavailability on 24-hour basis; expense

*Used to detect inhalation injuries

Limitations Patients must be able to cooperate in performing this test. They will be required to breathe through a mouthpiece, remain still for approximately 15 minutes, (usually in the supine position) and if xenon gas is used, hold their breath for 10 seconds or longer. The procedure is somewhat nonspecific in the presence of underlying lung conditions such as pneumonia or chronic obstructive disease. A same day chest radiograph is necessary for review and comparison with scan findings.

Additional Information Patients on high flow oxygen or respirator assistance can undergo ventilation scans with radioactive aerosols using special nebulizer adaptors.

Lysergic Acid Diethylamine Level

Synonyms LSD
Uses Evaluate LSD toxicity; confirm suspected overdose or abuse
Reference Range
None detected
Urine, LSD: Department of Defense cutoff concentration: 200 pg/mL (will be positive for ~24 hours after a single LSD street dose)
Specimen Blood or urine
Volume 10 mL blood, 10 mL urine
Container Royal blue top tube, plastic urine container
Limitations Ambroxol brompheniramine, fentanyl, haloperidol, imipramine, methylphenidate, metoclopramide, or sertraline can result in a false-positve immunoassay urinary screen.
Methodology Gas chromatography/mass spectrometry (GC/MS)
Additional Information Lysergic acid diethylamine, LSD, is a synthetic hallucinogen that acts on multiple sites in the CNS. Ingestion of this drug may result in sensory distortions, hallucinations, delusions, euphoria or dysphoria, dizziness, and paresthesia. Prolonged use may lead to psychological dependence and significant hazards such as panic, serious depression, paranoid behavior, and a persistent psychotic state.

Magnetic Resonance Scan, Brain

Applies to Magnetic Resonance Scan, Head
Synonyms Brain MRI; Head MRI
Uses Diagnose intracranial abnormalities including tumors, ischemia, infection, multiple sclerosis or any abnormalities relating to the brain or calvarium. MRI is an excellent modality for assessment of congenital brain abnormalities or relating to the status of brain maturation in the pediatric population. May reveal deposition of iron, copper, and manganese. Also useful for carbon monoxide, methanol, and barium.

Contraindicating Factors Patients weighing more than 300 lb and patients unable to squeeze into the magnet cannot undergo MRI. An absolute contraindication for MRI is a cardiac pacemaker. Relative contraindications to magnetic resonance imaging include intracranial aneurysm clips, cochlear implants, insulin infusion and chemotherapy pumps, neurocutaneous stimulators and prosthetic heart valves, depending on date of manufacture and metallurgical composition. Please consult MRI physician if questions arise. Patients who have metallic foreign bodies within the eye or who have undergone recent surgery within the last 6 weeks requiring placement of a vascular surgical clip, should also not undergo MRI. The safety of MRI in pregnant patients has not been determined. In such cases, prior consultation with the MRI physician is required. Generally, patients who have undergone recent surgery not requiring vascular clips or who have had coronary artery bypass surgery in the past may undergo MRI. Patients who have shrapnel wounds or orthopedic prostheses can generally safely undergo MRI unless the metallic device is in the anatomic region to be scanned which results in degradation of the images. Patients with surgically implanted intravascular vena cava filters to prevent pulmonary embolism can usually be scanned if the device has been in place for at least 6 weeks. Patients requiring life support equipment including ventilators require special preparation. Please contact MRI physician ahead of time. Central venous lines, Swan-Ganz catheters, and nasogastric (NG) tubes usually present no problems. If the patient is positive when screened for metallic devices and you are uncertain of their significance, the MRI radiologist will provide additional information to assist you.

Patient Preparation Inpatient: Patient must be able to lie quietly while the scan is performed. The patient should be screened for metallic devices by nursing personnel. (See Contraindications.) This includes metal introduced into the patient either surgically or by trauma. All metallic objects must be removed from the patient including jewelry or any other metal objects which may be in the patient's bedding. Please remove dentures or other dental appliances. I.V.s which contain no metal are fine, but infusion pumps must be removed. Oxygen tanks and metallic backboards may come with the patient but will be removed prior to the patient entering the magnet room. Oxygen may be provided in the magnet room. Trauma, ICU, or CCU patients should be accompanied by a nurse. If the patient is restless, combative, or claustrophobic, proper sedation may be administered on the floor prior to the MRI, or at the MRI Center. Consult the MRI radiologists with questions on proper sedation. Outpatient: The patient should be screened for metallic devices. (See Contraindications.) If a question exists as to the patient's suitability for MRI, the MRI radiologist will assist you with your questions. If the patient is claustrophobic, oral or parenteral sedation may be necessary. If so, the patient should be accompanied by another adult to provide transportation home after the examination.

Limitations Generally, the greatest limitation of magnetic resonance imaging results from the patient's fear of the procedure. The patient must remain quiet and still for several scans, each lasting from several minutes to 10 minutes in length. Total examination time is usually 30-45 minutes and occasionally up to 1 hour. If the patient is restless during the examination, motion artifacts will be present on the images limiting their diagnostic value. If the patient is claustrophobic, mild oral sedation or occasionally parenteral sedation may be needed. Also the patient can be accompanied by a family member or friend during the examination which helps calm the patient's anxiety in many cases. Patients requiring life support equipment such as ventilators require special preparation.

Methodology Unlike most conventional radiologic procedures, magnetic resonance imaging does not utilize ionizing radiation, but relies upon radio frequency or radio signals induced within the patient by the magnetic field to obtain images. There are no known biologic effects secondary to the magnetic fields currently used in clinical MRI. Prior to the scan, the patient will be asked to remove all metallic objects from their person, including loose change, hair pins, earrings, belts, etc. This is for safety reasons as the strong magnetic field could result in these and any other metal objects becoming projectiles resulting in injury to the patient or MRI personnel. Also the patient should not carry a purse or wallet into the magnet room, as the magnetic field can permanently erase bank cards or credit cards. The magnet is open on both ends and music can be played for the patient if desired. Fresh air is constantly circulated through the magnet room and the patient is continually monitored by the MRI technologist. An intercom system is provided for communication between

Table 1. Geometric Means (GMs) and Selected Percentiles of Total Blood Mercury (Hg) Concentrations (μg/L) for Women Aged 16-49 Years and Children Aged 1-5 Years, by Selected Variables - National Health and Nutrition Examination Survey, United States, 1999-2002.

Variable	No.	GM	(95% CI*)	5th	(95% CI)	10th	(95% CI)	25th	(95% CI)
Women									
Race/Ethnicity									
Mexican American	1106	0.74	(0.64-0.84)	0.10	(0.08-0.15)	0.17	(0.12-0.23)	0.34	(0.27-0.45)
White, non-Hispanic	1377	0.87	(0.75-0.99)	0.09	(0.08-0.10)	0.15	(0.13-0.18)	0.37	(0.34-0.45)
Black, non-Hispanic	794	1.18	(1.00-1.36)	0.17	(0.12-0.25)	0.30	(0.24-0.38)	0.60	(0.55-0.73)
Age group (yrs)									
16-29	2004	0.68	(0.60-0.76)	0.08	(0.07-0.09)	0.11	(0.09-0.14)	0.29	(0.25-0.37)
30-49	1633	1.10	(0.97-1.24)	0.13	(0.10-0.16)	0.24	(0.20-0.29)	0.52	(0.45-0.60)
Pregnancy Status									
Pregnant	629	0.75	(0.60-0.76)	0.08	(...†-0.10)	0.10	(0.08-0.20)	0.32	(0.24-0.44)
Not pregnant	2976	0.94	(0.84-1.04)	0.10	(0.09-0.11)	0.18	(0.15-0.21)	0.41	(0.38-0.47)
Total	**3637**	**0.92**	**(0.82-1.02)**	**0.09**	**(0.09-0.11)**	**0.17**	**(0.15-0.20)**	**0.40**	**(0.36-0.47)**
ChildrenRace/Ethnicity									
Mexican American	526	0.35	(0.30-0.40)	...		0.08	(...-0.09)	0.13	0.10-0.16)
White, non-Hispanic	447	0.29	(0.24-0.33)	...		0.07	(...-0.08)	0.09	(0.09-0.10)
Black, non-Hispanic	424	0.50	(0.44-0.57)	0.08	(...-0.10)	0.10	(0.09-0.13)	0.22	(0.18-0.26)
Total	**1577**	**0.33**	**(0.30-0.37)**	...		**0.07**	**(...-0.08)**	**0.10**	**(0.09-0.12)**

*Confidence interval.
†Below the limits of detection.

the patient and the technologist. For MRI of the brain, a special coil surrounds, but does not touch the patient's head. The patient will be asked to remain very still while scans are being obtained. In certain cases, an MRI contrast agent, Gadopentetate Dimeglumine (Magnevist®) may be necessary to increase the diagnostic accuracy of the MRI examination. This is administered intravenously, via an antecubital vein in a small volume (less than 20 mL). This contrast agent may be used in patients who are allergic to conventional iodinated contrast agents such as is used in IVPs or CT examination without difficulty. There are very few contraindications to its use. (See Contraindications.)

Additional Information
In some cases, an MRI contrast agent (Magnevist®) may be needed to increase the diagnostic accuracy of the MRI. This contrast agent can be administered to patients with a previous history of allergies to conventional iodinated x-ray agents as it contains no iodine. Contraindications to its use include previous allergy to the contrast agent itself, renal failure, certain types of anemia, and Wilson's disease. The contrast agent is generally very safe and increases the diagnostic efficacy of the MRI.

Bilateral putaminal injury (with hemorrhage and necrosis) can be noted in methanol poisoning; hyperintense signal on T_1 weighted images in lenticular and caudate indicative of chronic manganese poisoning. Hypersignal intensities on T_2 weighted images in the basal ganglia noted with barium poisoning. Carbon monoxide poisoning may be demonstrated by globus pallidi lesions with endematous changes. Organic solvents, hexachlorophene, triethyltin and toluene can cause selective myelin damage. Furthermore, chronic toluene sniffing can cause cerebral, cerebellar and brainstem atrophy detectable by MRI. Bromate poisoning can cause small high intensity spots on T_2 bilaterally in the frontal white matter. Increased signal density near the fourth ventricle noted following metronidazole (>60 g) ingestion.

Meconium Drug Screen

Synonyms Drug Screen, Meconium
Uses Drugs of abuse screen (amphetamines, opiates, cocaine, marijuana, phencyclidine)
Specimen 1 g first meconium
Container Small plastic vial with cap
Collection Sample must be first specimen, second accepted but less desirable
Storage Instructions Refrigerate
Causes for Rejection Specimen later than the second meconium, specimen mixed with stool
Methodology Fluorescent polarization immunoassay (FPIA) confirmed by gas chromatography/mass spectrometry (GC/MS) is the most effective assay method.
Additional Information
Can detect maternal drug usage during the final 20 weeks of gestation. May detect three times higher rate of drugs of abuse then maternal urinary screening at time of birth. Cocaethylene can also be detected.

In an adequate meconium specimen, a total fatty acid ethyl ester concentration >10,000 ng/g may indicate that the newborn has been exposed to significant amounts of alcohol during pregnancy.

Specific References
Coles R, Kushir MM, Nelson GJ, "Simultaneous Determination of Codeine, Morphine, Hydrocodone, Hydromorphone, Oxycodone, and 6-Acetylmorphine in Urine, Serum, Plasma, Whole Blood and Meconium by LC-MS-MS," *J Anal Tox*, 2007, 31(1):1-14.
Moore C, Jones J, Lewis D, et al, "Prevalence of Fatty Acid Ethyl Esters in Meconium Specimens," *Clin chem*, 2005, 49(1):133-6.

Mercury, Blood

Related Information
- Heavy Metal Screen, Blood
- Mercury, Urine
Applies to Mercury Analysis, Hair
Synonyms Hg, Blood
Uses Evaluate for mercury toxicity, neurological findings related to organic mercurials, inhalation of mercury vapors
Reference Range 0.020-0.080 mcg/mL (SI: 0.10-0.80 μmol/L)
Abstract This metal is toxic in any of its three forms: elemental, inorganic, and organic. The mode of entry into the body varies among the three forms.
Specimen Whole blood
Volume 7 mL
Container Special metal-free EDTA tube
Special Instructions Whole blood is analyzed.
Possible Panic Range >0.10 mcg/mL
Limitations Methyl mercury must be measured in whole blood or erythrocytes.
Methodology Electrothermal atomic absorption (AA), gold electrode deposition, gas chromatography (GC)
Additional Information See table
Specific References
Centers for Disease Control and Prevention (CDC), "Blood Mercury Levels in Young Children and Childbearing-Aged Women – United States, 1999-2002," *MMWR Morb Mortal Wkly Rep*, 2004, 5;53(43):1018-20.

Mercury, Urine

Related Information
- Heavy Metal Screen, Urine
- Mercury, Blood
Synonyms Hg, Urine
Uses Inorganic mercury toxicity is best evaluated by urine mercury levels.
Reference Range 10-50 mcg/24 hours (SI: 0.05-0.25 μmol/day); urinary mercury levels >56 mcg/L can result in neurotoxic effects (due to elemental mercury)

Table 1. *(Continued)* **Geometric Means (GMs) and Selected Percentiles of Total Blood Mercury (Hg) Concentrations (µg/L) for Women Aged 16-49 Years and Children Aged 1-5 Years, by Selected Variables - National Health and Nutrition Examination Survey, United States, 1999-2002.**

Variable	50th	(95% CI)	75th	(95% CI)	90th	(95% CI)	95th	(95% CI)
Women								
Race/Ethnicity								
Mexican American	0.73	(0.67-0.83)	1.27	(1.16-1.48)	2.38	(2.05-2.95)	3.60	(3.03-6.48)
White, non-Hispanic	0.81	(0.75-0.92)	1.69	(1.51-2.15)	3.73	(2.84-5.14)	6.17	(4.64-9.30)
Black, non-Hispanic	1.15	(1.05-1.41)	2.12	(1.86-2.70)	3.89	(3.24-5.03)	5.54	(4.27-11.08)
Age group (yrs)								
16-29	0.64	(0.55-0.77)	1.34	(1.24-1.54)	2.58	(2.28-3.13)	3.87	(3.32-7.80)
30-49	1.02	(0.91-1.19)	2.10	(1.79-2.69)	4.56	(3.74-5.76)	6.97	(5.73-11.62)
Pregnancy Status								
Pregnant	0.73	(0.63-0.97)	1.50	(1.38-1.90)	3.11	(2.14-4.79)	4.86	(3.00-8.02)
Not pregnant	0.88	(0.80-1.00)	1.83	(1.65-2.11)	3.93	(3.26-4.93)	6.11	(5.12-10.90)
Total	**0.86**	**(0.80-0.98)**	**1.81**	**(1.62-2.16)**	**3.89**	**(3.20-4.88)**	**6.04**	**(5.08-10.74)**
ChildrenRace/Ethnicity								
Mexican American	0.28	(0.24-0.33)	0.63	(0.56-0.81)	1.36	(1.05-1.57)	1.85	(1.60-2.66)
White, non-Hispanic	0.20	(0.17-0.25)	0.49	(0.38-0.63)	1.15	(0.80-1.49)	1.78	(1.18-2.69)
Black, non-Hispanic	0.47	(0.40-0.58)	0.88	(0.78-1.02)	1.54	(1.31-2.04)	2.37	(1.75-3.64)
Total	**0.26**	**(0.23-0.29)**	**0.61**	**(0.56-0.70)**	**1.29**	**(1.08-1.69)**	**2.21**	**(1.80-3.66)**

*Confidence interval.
†Below the limits of detection.

Abstract This metal is toxic in elemental, inorganic, and organic forms. Urine mercury is used for evaluation of inorganic and possibly elemental forms.
Specimen 24-hour urine
Volume Entire collection
Minimum Volume 50 mL aliquot
Container Plastic (preferably polyethylene) acid-washed container, no preservative
Storage Instructions Store in special metal-free container
Possible Panic Range > 100 mcg/24 hours (SI: > 0.50 µmol/day)
Limitations Organic mercury is found mostly in red cells; see Mercury, Blood listing. Urine mercury would not be useful for organic mercury poisoning.
Methodology Electrothermal atomic absorption (AA), gold electrode deposition, gas chromatography (GC)
Additional Information Industrial and agricultural exposure includes inhalation of vapor and ingestion.

Methadone, Urine

Synonyms Dolophine®
Uses Evaluate toxicity; detect drugs of abuse
Reference Range Negative (less than cutoff); when used therapeutically for pain, plasma levels are in the range of 0.05-0.10 mcg/mL
Abstract This drug is a synthetic opiate agonist used during World War II as a morphine substitute. It is used for detoxification of opiate addicts. It is a drug of abuse.
Specimen Urine
Volume 50 mL
Minimum Volume 20 mL
Container Plastic urine container
Storage Instructions Refrigerate
Special Instructions If forensic, use chain-of-custody protocol and form.
Critical Values Cutoff for screening: 0.30 mcg/mL; confirmation: 0.20 mcg/mL
Methodology Thin-layer chromatography (TLC) and enzyme immunoassay (EIA) for screening; gas chromatography/mass spectrometry (GC/MS) for confirmation
Additional Information Patients on methadone maintenance protocols will test above cutoff in urine drug screens. False-positive results with methadone or opiate enzyme immunoassay may occur with diphenhydramine or doxylamine.

Methamphetamines, Urine

Related Information
- Amphetamines, Qualitative, Urine
Applies to Chlorpromazine; d-Methamphetamine; l-Methamphetamine; MDMA; Methylenedioxymethamphetamine; Phentermine; Phenylpropanolamine; Pseudoephedrine; Ranitidine

Synonyms Desoxyn® Level, Urine; Doe, Urine; Methedrine® Level, Urine; Speed, Urine; "Crystal" Level, Urine
Uses Evaluate for drug abuse; assess toxicity
Reference Range Negative (less than cutoff)
Test Commonly Includes Amphetamine
Abstract The D-isomer of this drug is used therapeutically as an anorectic agent and for treatment of hyperactive children. It is also a drug of abuse.
Specimen Random urine
Volume 50 mL
Minimum Volume 5 mL
Container Plastic urine container
Collection If forensic, observe precautions.
Storage Instructions Refrigerate
Causes for Rejection If forensic, failure to meet temperature check and reasonable urine creatinine concentration
Special Instructions If forensic, use chain-of-custody protocol and form.
Critical Values Cutoff: screen: 1000 ng/mL; confirmation: 500 ng/mL
Limitations Screening test may give false-positives with common cold and antiallergy medications. Qualitative results only (positive or negative). A labetalol metabolite (3-amino-1-phenylbutane or APB) may cause a false-positive result with amphetamine/methamphetamine by thin-layer chromatography or immunoassay.
Methodology Screening: enzyme immunoassay (EIA), fluorescence polarization immunoassay (FPIA), thin-layer chromatography (TLC); confirmation: gas chromatography/mass spectrometry (GC/MS), gas-liquid chromatography (GLC), high performance liquid chromatography (HPLC)
Additional Information
The most abused drug in this class is d-methamphetamine. The optical isomer, l-methamphetamine, has less pronounced central effects and is used as a nasal decongestant in Vicks Inhaler® (legal, over-the-counter). Amphetamine isomers are present in Dexedrine® and Benzedrine®. These drugs are self-administered orally, I.V., or by smoking. Half-life is 10-20 hours and it can be detected in urine within 3 hours of use. The parent drugs are the substances detected by the screening tests. Over-the-counter medication for colds and allergies (Contac®, Dimetapp®, Sine-Off®, Sudafed®) contain phenylpropanolamine or pseudoephedrine which give a positive EIA screening test when the polyclonal antibody is used. This antibody also detects methylenedioxymethamphetamine (MDMA), a controlled substance classed as an hallucinogen and "designer" drug. With the monoclonal EIA test, the above medications are not detected, but phentermine (Adipex®, Fastin®), ranitidine (Zantac®), and chlorpromazine (Thorazine®) give a positive test. Confirmation by GC/MS rules out these false-positives. In order to rule out the false-positive given by l-methamphetamine (legal nasal decongestant), a chiral column or procedure, which separates the "l" and "d" isomers, must be used in the GC/MS confirmation. Famprofazone (which metabolizes to methamphetamine and amphetamine) can give a positive immunoassay and GC/MS assay for methamphetamine for up to 56 hours.
Alum (25 g/L) can elicit a false-negative urinary assay for methamphetamine - urine will be acidic in these cases

Methanol, Blood

Related Information
- Volatile Screen

Synonyms Methyl Alcohol; Wood Alcohol
Uses Determine methanol toxicity
Reference Range Normal: <0.005%
Specimen Blood
Volume 14 mL
Minimum Volume 5 mL serum or plasma
Container Red top tube or gray top (sodium fluoride) tube
Collection Routine venipuncture
Special Instructions Note if methanol ingested.
Critical Values Toxic: >0.02%; lethal: >0.04%
Methodology Gas-liquid chromatography (GLC)

Methaqualone Level

Synonyms Lude®
Uses Evaluate for toxicity; evaluate for drug abuse
Reference Range Urine: negative (less than cutoff); serum: 1-5 mcg/mL (SI: 4-20 nmol/L)
Abstract This drug is a sedative-hypnotic but is currently a DEA schedule II drug. It is a drug of abuse.
Specimen Blood, urine
Volume 5 mL
Container Red top tube, plastic urine container
Special Instructions If forensic, use chain-of-custody protocol and form.
Critical Values Cutoff for urine: screen: 300 ng/mL; confirmation: 200 ng/mL
Possible Panic Range Serum values >8 mcg/mL (SI: >32 nmol/L) associated with unconsciousness; toxic: >10 mcg/mL (SI: >40 nmol/L)
Methodology Immunoassay, gas-liquid chromatography (GLC), UV spectrophotometry, fluorometry
Additional Information Methaqualone is a common drug of abuse, and "street" preparations may be adulterated with other pharmacoactive substances. It is extensively metabolized and screening methods must detect metabolites. Enzyme-multiplied immunoassay technique (EMIT) detects four of the most common metabolites.

Methemoglobin, Blood

Applies to Cytochrome b₅ Reductase
Synonyms MetHb; NADH-MetHb Reductase
Uses Evaluate cyanosis, especially in the presence of normal arterial gases; evaluate polycythemia and hemoglobinopathies; work up dyspnea and headache; work up "poppers" and "sniffers"; evaluate drug or chemical toxicity, since most instances of methemoglobinemia are so acquired; monitor patients on high dose nitrate therapy; measurement in CSF may detect small cerebral and subdural hematomas.
Reference Range Up to 1.5% of total hemoglobin. Smokers have a slightly higher percent methemoglobin than do nonsmokers.
Abstract This pigment is hemoglobin in which the iron is in the trivalent state. It cannot act as an oxygen carrier.
Specimen Blood
Volume 5 mL
Minimum Volume 1 mL whole blood
Container Green top (heparin) tube
Storage Instructions Keep tube on ice. pH dependent. Should be run within 8 hours, or false-negatives may occur. Run as promptly as possible after draw. Studies have shown up to 10% drop in 4 hours, up to 16% drop in 8 hours, in samples kept on ice. Such studies have not been extensive. May be drawn into sodium fluoride-containing tubes and immediately frozen at 0°C to -4°C prior to analysis.
Possible Panic Range Headache and other symptoms occur at levels >30%. Methemoglobinemia can be fatal, particularly >70% saturation levels.
Limitations Sulfhemoglobin, methylene blue, and Evans blue dye may interfere. Methemoglobin exhibits pH sensitivity.
Methodology Spectrophotometry; Hb M variants are best detected by electrophoresis because spectrophotometry is unreliable due to their abnormal ferrihemoglobin spectra.
Additional Information Methemoglobin is an inactive, oxidized form of hemoglobin resulting in decreased oxygen-carrying capacity of blood. Concentrations of methemoglobin of >10% to 15% of hemoglobin will cause cyanosis. Sulfhemoglobin will interfere with methemoglobin determined by the above method. Methemoglobinemia may be hereditary or acquired. Polycythemia is occasionally present as a compensatory mechanism. Elevations of methemoglobin lead to dyspnea and headache, and can be lethal. Most instances of methemoglobinemia are acquired, from drugs and chemicals. Nitro and amino groups are especially involved, eg, aniline and derivatives, nitrites, nitroglycerin, nitrate salts in burn patients, dapsone (perhaps the most common cause of drug-induced methemoglobinemia), acetophenetidin, phenacetin and

some sulfonamides, chlorates, quinones, large doses of ferrous sulfate, and many other drugs and some intestinal bacteria. Well water containing nitrate is the most common cause of methemoglobinemia in the newborn. Methemoglobinemia has been reported after exposure to automobile exhaust fumes.

Hereditary methemoglobinemia is uncommon. It may be due to a deficiency of red cell NADH-methemoglobin reductase (diaphorase, also termed cytochrome b₅ reductase), which has an autosomal recessive mode of inheritance. It may also be the result of presence of certain hemoglobinopathies, members of the Hb M family including Hb M Saskatoon, Boston, Iwate, Hyde Park, and Milwaukee. These have autosomal dominant mode of inheritance and may be associated with clinical cyanosis. Hb Seattle and other hemoglobinopathies also show increase in the in vitro rate of methemoglobin formation. A recently identified new hemoglobin variant, Hb Warsaw, is also characterized by elevated blood levels of methemoglobin.

A study of postmortem methemoglobin levels showed a range of 0.8% to 57% in individuals who, clinically, should have had normal antemortem concentrations. There was no correlation with antemortem circumstances, autopsy findings, or interval of time from death to autopsy. Chocolate brown color to arterial blood indicates methemoglobin concentration is >10%. Brown skin color, tachycardia, and tachypnea occur with levels >30%.

Lipemia will give falsely elevated methemoglobin levels.
Specific Reference
Linz AJ, Greeham RK, and Fallon LF, Jr , "Methemoglobinemia: An Industrial Outbreak Among Rubber Molding Workers," J Occup Environ Med, 2006, 48:523-8.

Methsuximide, Blood

Synonyms Celontin® Level, Blood
Uses Monitor therapeutic drug level
Reference Range Methsuximide: 0.1-1.4 mcg/mL; normethsuximide: 10-40 mcg/mL
Test Commonly Includes Methsuximide and active metabolite normethsuximide
Specimen Blood
Volume 15 mL
Minimum Volume 4 mL serum
Container Red top tube
Collection Collect specimen immediately prior to next dose unless specified otherwise.
Storage Instructions Separate serum and refrigerate.
Critical Values Toxic: normethsuximide: >40 mcg/mL
Additional Information Methsuximide is a succinimide derivative used to control absence (petit mal) seizures and as an adjunct in refractory, partial complex seizures. Its actions are similar to those of ethosuximide. Methsuximide is rapidly absorbed and metabolized to its active form, N-desmethylmethsuximide. It is this metabolite that probably accounts for the anticonvulsant action. Peak levels are achieved in 1-3 hours and the plasma half-life is 2-4 hours. Adverse effects include eosinophilia, leukopenia, monocytosis, pancytopenia, Stevens-Johnson syndrome, nervousness, headaches, mental confusion, and nausea and vomiting.

Mexiletine, Blood

Synonyms Mexitil®
Uses Therapeutic monitoring; toxicity assessment
Reference Range Therapeutic 0.75-2.00 mcg/mL (SI: 4-9 µmol/L)
Abstract Mexiletine is an antiarrhythmic used to treat ventricular arrhythmia.
Specimen Blood
Container Red top tube
Sampling Time Draw 2-4 hours after last dose for peak level. Draw immediately prior to next dose for trough level.
Possible Panic Range >2.00 mcg/mL (SI: >9 µmol/L)
Methodology Fluorometry, high performance liquid chromatography (HPLC), gas chromatography (GC)
Additional Information Mexiletine is a class I antiarrhythmic approved for treatment of ventricular arrhythmias. It has no active metabolites. Toxic effects include dizziness, vomiting, confusion, tremor, bradycardia, and hypotension. Metabolism of mexiletine is accelerated by rifampin, phenobarbital, and phenytoin and retarded by cimetidine and ketoconazole. Half-life is 10-14 hours and is urine pH dependent. Acidic urine accelerates elimination.

Morphine, Urine

Synonyms Heroin Metabolite, Urine
Uses Evaluate toxicity or detect drug of abuse. Heroin is metabolized to morphine, therefore morphine detection may suggest heroin use. To **prove** heroin use, 6-O-acetylmorphine must be identified in the urine.
Reference Range Negative (less than cutoff)

Test Commonly Includes Codeine, heroin, hydromorphone (Dilaudid®), morphine, and morphine glucuronide

Abstract This drug is widely used therapeutically as an analgesic. Morphine itself is not an extensively used drug of abuse but two derivatives, heroin and codeine, are.

Specimen Urine

Volume 50 mL

Minimum Volume 20 mL

Container Plastic urine container

Storage Instructions Refrigerate

Special Instructions If forensic, use chain-of-custody protocol and form.

Critical Values Cutoff: screen (total opiates): 300 ng/mL; confirmatory: 300 ng/mL

Methodology Immunoassays, gas-liquid chromatography (GLC), high performance liquid chromatography-electrochemical detection (HPLC-ECD)

Additional Information

Urine codeine/morphine ratio usually exceeds 1.0 during the first 24 hours postingestion, decreases <1.0 from 24-30 hours and usually only morphine is detectable after 30 hours. Poppy seed ingestion can result in urine codeine levels as high as 4.5 mg/L and urine morphine levels as high as 0.2 mg/L; urine opiate levels due to poppy seeds will not exceed 15,000 ng/mL; urine drug screen remains positive for 2-4 days.

Poppy seed use can be ruled out as a cause for a urinary morphine screen when codeine levels exceed 300 ng/mL; morphine to codeine ratio is <2 and high levels of morphine (>1000 ng/mL) are detected without codeine being present

Nickel, Urine

Related Information
• Heavy Metal Screen, Urine

Synonyms Ni, Urine

Uses Evaluate nickel toxicity

Reference Range ≤25 mcg/L; fatality can occur at urinary nickel concentrations >500 mcg/L; moderate toxicity occurs at urine nickel concentration of 100-500 mcg/L; mild toxicity occurs at urine nickel concentrations of 60-100 mcg/L

Patient Preparation Instruct patient to use plastic urinal or bedpan if necessary.

Specimen 24-hour urine

Volume Entire collection

Minimum Volume 100 mL

Container Plastic container, kept on ice

Collection Instruct the patient to void at 8 AM and discard the specimen. Then collect all urine including the final specimen voided at the end of the 24-hour collection period (ie, 8 AM the next morning). Avoid contact with metal during specimen collection. Screw the lid on securely. Transport the specimen promptly to the laboratory. Container **must** be labeled with patient's full name, room number, date and time collection started, and date and time collection finished.

Storage Instructions Keep on ice or refrigerate. Laboratory will measure urine volume and remove 120 mL aliquot.

Causes for Rejection Specimen in contact with metal

Special Instructions Requisition **must** state date and time collection started and date and time collection finished.

Nicotine Level

Synonyms 3-(1-Methylpyrrolidine-2-yl)pyridine

Reference Range Plasma nicotine levels peak rapidly after each cigarette (from 0.03-0.05 mg/L); moderate accumulation over a longer time period. In pipe smokers, average plasma levels average 0.004 mg/L; nicotine gum chewers (2 mg size) average 0.012 mg/L. Plasma concentrations of cotinine in children living with smokers are four times higher than those in children from nonsmoking environments.

Specimen Blood

Critical Values Lethal dose: 40 mg. Dermal exposure has usually caused nonfatal poisoning. Postmortem blood concentrations: 11-600 mg/L; postmortem urine concentrations: 17-58 mg/L.

Methodology Spectrophotometry, thin-layer chromatography (TLC), high performance liquid chromatography (HPLC), fluorescence polarization immunoassay (FPIA), gas chromatography (GC); confirmation: gas chromatography/mass spectrometry (GC/MS)

Additional Information Nicotine is extensively transformed to inactive metabolites (eg, cotinine). Cotinine is further oxidized to hydroxycotinine. Other metabolites include nornicotine and nicotine-1'-N-oxide. Plasma half-life of nicotine in cigarette smokers: 0.5-2 hours (average 40 minutes); cotinine: 6-16 hours (average 11 hours). Twenty-four hours after nicotine dosing, 5% to 10% is excreted unchanged in urine, 10% as cotinine, and 4% as other metabolites. Excretion is decreased if the urine is alkaline.

Nortriptyline, Blood

Synonyms Aventyl®; Pamelor®

Uses Monitor therapeutic drug level; evaluate toxicity

Reference Range Therapeutic: 50-150 ng/mL

Abstract This is a tricyclic antidepressant.

Specimen Blood

Volume 7 mL

Minimum Volume 3 mL serum

Container Red top tube

Collection Collect specimen immediately prior to next dose unless specified otherwise.

Storage Instructions Separate serum and refrigerate.

Critical Values Toxic: >500 ng/mL

Limitations Results not valid if receiving imipramine or desipramine

Methodology High performance liquid chromatography (HPLC)

Additional Information Nortriptyline, a tricyclic antidepressant, is a derivative and metabolite of amitriptyline and is used to treat endogenous depression. The half-life of nortriptyline is 20-80 hours. Nortriptyline may be associated with cholestasis and cholestatic jaundice. Hematological consequences include agranulocytosis, purpura, and thrombocytopenia. Other side effects include a host of GI, endocrinologic, allergic, anticholinergic, cardiovascular, and neurologic disorders. Red cell levels of metabolites may be a more sensitive indicator of myocardial toxicity.

Opiates, Qualitative, Urine

Related Information
• Codeine, Urine

Applies to Heroin; Narcotics; Poppy Seeds

Uses Evaluate drug abuse; assess toxicity

Reference Range Negative (less than cutoff)

Test Commonly Includes Morphine, codeine, hydrocodone (Hycodan®), hydromorphone (Dilaudid®)

Abstract The qualitative detection of urine opiates is used almost exclusively to show presence of drugs of abuse in this class. Morphine and codeine are used therapeutically for pain.

Specimen Random urine

Volume 50-60 mL

Container Plastic urine container

Collection If forensic, observe precautions.

Storage Instructions Refrigerate

Special Instructions If forensic, use chain-of-custody protocol and form.

Critical Values Cutoff: screen: 300 ng/mL; confirmation: 300 ng/mL of specific opiates

Limitations In most immunoassays a number of narcotic drugs can cross react to give a positive screen. Every effort should be made to confirm, by an analytically different and more sensitive method, all presumptive, positive opiate screens. Hydromorphone, hydrocodone, oxymorphone, and oxycodone usually will test negative after 48 hours by gas chromatography-mass spectrometric methods. EMIT immunoassays may not detect oxymorphone. Hydromorphone, hydrocodone, and oxycodone may become negative by immunoassay after one day. See Test Commonly Includes. Rifampicin can cause false-positive urine assay of opiates by kinetic interaction of microparticle in solution (KIMS) method up to a concentration of 0.9 mcg/mL.

Methodology Screening: immunoassay, thin-layer chromatography (TLC), high performance liquid chromatography (HPLC), gas chromatography (GC); confirmation: gas chromatography/mass spectrometry (GC/MS)

Additional Information

A qualitative urine screen for opiates is performed in suspected overdose cases or as part of a drugs-of-abuse program. The test is most sensitive for morphine and codeine, but other drugs will cross react in an immunoassay and give positive results (eg, hydrocodone, hydromorphone). All presumptive positive assays should be confirmed, preferably by GC/MS. Morphine is a prescribed drug for pain relief, a metabolite of heroin, a metabolite of codeine, and a constituent of poppy seeds. Its presence in urine, even after confirmation, must be interpreted very carefully. Ingestion of poppy seeds (bagels, Danish) can cause positive opiate screens at a 300 ng/mL cutoff. The intake of heroin by the user can only be proved by the detection of 6-o-acetylmorphine by the urine confirmatory test.

Levofloxacin, ofloxacin, and perfloxacin can lead to a false-positive opiate immunoassay result.

Tolmetin can give false-negative results by Emit® assay. False-positive results with methadone or opiate enzyme immunoassay may occur with diphenhydramine or doxylamine.

Opiate concentrations in poppy seeds range from 0.1-3.8 mcg/g for codeine, 5.1-106 mcg/g for morphine, and 0.3-14 mcg/g for thebaine; analysis for thebaine may be a direct marker for poppy seed use. Urinary opiate concentrations >15,000 ng/mL are not due to poppy seed ingestion.

Usual 6-monoacetyl morphine (6-MAM) cutoff is 10 ng/mL. A 12 mg intravenous dose of heroin will give a detection time of 6-MAM and a

2000 ng/mL opiate urinary cutoff of 2.3-7.5 hours and 5.9-13.5 hours, respectively.

Specific References

Edinboro LE, Backer RC, and Poklis A, "Direct Analysis of Opiates in Urine by Liquid Chromatography-Tandem Mass Spectrometry," *J Anal Toxicol*, 2005, 29:704-14.

Huang MK, Dai YS, Lee CH, et al, "Performance Characteristics of DRI, CEDIA, and REMEDi Systems for Preliminary Tests of Amphetamines and Opiates in Human Urine," *J Anal Toxicol*, 2006, 30:61-70.

Monforte JR, Backer R, and Poklis A, "Evaluation of the Abbott AxSYN Opiate Immunoassay with Modified Cut-off Calibrations of 100 ng/mL and 50 ng/mL for the Detection of Opiates in Urine," *J Anal Toxicol*, 2006, 30:129.

Rohrig TP and Moore C, "The Determination of Morphine in Urine and Oral Fluid Following Ingestion of Poppy Seeds," *J Anal Toxicol*, 2003, 27:449-52.

Osmolality, Serum

Applies to Osmolal Gap

Synonyms Serum Osmolality

Uses Evaluate electrolyte and water balance, hyperosmolar status and hydration status, dehydration, acid-base balance, seizures; evaluate antidiuretic hormone function, liver disease, hyperosmolar coma. Osmolality measures the concentration of particles in solution. Freezing point depression serum osmolality with calculated osmolal gap, is useful in screening for and approximating the serum concentrations of certain low molecular weight toxins, such as ethanol, ethylene glycol, isopropanol, and methanol, especially as a rapid approximation for emergent situations. See Limitations.

High serum osmolality may result from hypernatremia, dehydration, hyperglycemia, mannitol therapy, azotemia, ingestion of ethanol, methanol, ethylene glycol. Thus, osmolality has a role in toxicology and in coma evaluation. Very low birth weight infants may have elevated serum osmolality for the first week of life.

Low serum osmolality may be secondary to overhydration, hyponatremia, syndrome of inappropriate antidiuretic hormone secretion (SIADH) with carcinoma of lung and other entities. Chlorpropamide use can also result in a low serum osmolality.

Causes of hyperosmolality, hypo-osmolality, and of factors affecting ADH are published. Serum osmolality measurements do not measure the fraction of serum that is water. Osmolality measurement by freezing point depression is also indifferent to permeability of solutes to cell membranes.

Reference Range 275-295 mOsm/kg (SI: 275-295 mM/kg) H_2O. Some consider normal to be 280-290 mOsm/kg (SI: 280-290 mM/kg) H_2O and others within 270-310 mOsm/kg (SI: 270-310 mM/kg) H_2O.

Abstract The osmolality of a solution is defined as the number of molecules or ions (particles) in a solution of water. Osmolality is independent of particle size or charge. Nonpolar solutions yield one molecule (eg, glucose) while polar solutions yield multiples of the number of ions solubilized (eg, sodium chloride yields two ions while magnesium chloride yields three ions).

Specimen Blood

Volume 7 mL

Minimum Volume 4 mL serum

Container Red top tube

Collection Pediatrics: Blood drawn from heelstick

Storage Instructions Refrigerate or freeze serum if not run within 4 hours.

Possible Panic Range <265 mOsm/kg (SI: <265 mM/kg), >320 mOsm/kg (SI: >320 mM/kg). Result of 385 mOsm/kg (SI: 385 mM/kg) relates to stupor in hyperglycemia. Values 400-420 mOsm/kg (SI: 400-420 mM/kg) can relate to grand mal seizures. Values >420 mOsm/kg (SI: >420 mM/kg) may be lethal.

Limitations When vapor pressure osmometry is used, volatile solutes (eg, alcohols and glycols) may remain in the vapor phase and not be detected.

Methodology Freezing point depression (more often used) or vapor pressure. (Do not use for toxicologic determination.)

Additional Information Measured osmolality is usually more than calculated osmolality. If measured osmolality is >15 mOsm/kg (SI: >15 mM/kg) greater than calculated, consider methanol, ethylene glycol, or ethanol ingestion or other toxicity; shock; or trauma. Elevated serum osmolality with normal sodium suggests possible hyperglycemia, uremia, or alcoholism. Both serum and urine values and calculated osmolality (see previous listing) are sometimes needed. Although lactic acidosis theoretically should not contribute to the osmolal gap, increases in the osmolal gap in lactic acidosis have been reported. Drugs including thiazide diuretics, steroids, cimetidine, and others have been implicated in the development of hyperosmolar hyperglycemic nonketotic coma. Slight elevation of serum osmolality over expected values have been reported in the elderly. After overnight dehydration, urine/serum ratio is usually ≥3.

Osmolality, Urine

Related Information
- Electrolytes, Urine

Applies to Osmolal Gap, Urine; U/P Ratio

Synonyms Urine Osmolality

Uses Evaluate concentrating ability of the kidneys (eg, in acute and chronic renal failure); evaluate electrolyte and water balance; used in work-up for renal disease, syndrome of inappropriate antidiuretic hormone secretion (SIADH), and diabetes insipidus; may be used with urinalysis when patient has had radiopaque substances, has glycosuria or proteinuria; evaluate dehydration, amyloidosis; estimate urine ammonium concentrations using the urine osmolal gap and detect increased osmolality due to the presence of unusual molecules. Osmolality is desirable in examination of neonatal urine when protein or glucose are present.

Reference Range Random urine: neonates: 75-300 mOsm/kg (SI: 75-300 mM/kg); children and adults: 250-900 mOsm/kg (SI: 250-900 mM/kg). Normal range of serum sodium (mM/L) to osmolality (mOsm/kg) ratio is 0.43-0.50. Patients with normal renal function after 14-hour restriction of fluids should be able to concentrate to >800 mOsm/kg (SI: >800 mM/kg); <400 mOsm/kg (SI: <400 mM/kg) is interpreted by Weisberg as severe renal impairment. Prolonged dehydration may be dangerous for some patients.

Abstract Osmolality is a definitive measure of urine concentration.

Specimen Random urine or timed specimen

Volume Entire collection

Minimum Volume 5 mL

Container Clean urine container

Storage Instructions Refrigerate during collection and storage.

Possible Panic Range <100 mOsm/kg (SI: <100 mM/kg) in overhydration, >800 mOsm/kg (SI: >800 mM/kg) in dehydration

Limitations Serum osmolality is often needed to interpret urine osmolality.

Methodology Freezing point depression

Oxazepam, Serum

Synonyms Serax®

Uses Monitor therapeutic drug level; evaluate toxicity

Reference Range 0.2-1.4 mcg/mL (SI: 0.7-4.9 µmol/L)

Abstract Oxazepam is a benzodiazepine used as an antianxiety agent. It is an active metabolite of several other benzodiazepines that are used therapeutically.

Specimen Blood

Volume 15 mL

Minimum Volume 5 mL serum

Container Red top tube

Sampling Time Collect specimen immediately prior to next dose unless specified otherwise.

Storage Instructions Separate serum and refrigerate.

Possible Panic Range <2.0 mcg/mL

Methodology High performance liquid chromatography (HPLC)

Additional Information Oxazepam, a benzodiazepine derivative, is related to chlordiazepoxide and shares many of its qualities. It does, however, have a shorter duration of action and causes fewer adverse effects. It is rapidly eliminated by urinary excretion as a glucuronide conjugate. Oxazepam is used to manage tension and anxiety and to aid in the control of acute withdrawal symptoms in chronic alcoholism. Peak plasma levels are achieved in 2-3 hours and the half-life is 5-15 hours. Adverse effects are mild and infrequent. They include drowsiness, vertigo, ataxia, headache, tremor, slurred speech, nausea, hypotension, and leukopenia. Simultaneous alcohol ingestion potentiates some of the effects of benzodiazepines.

Paraquat, Blood

Uses Evaluate exposure to paraquat

Reference Range <0.25 mcg/mL

Specimen Blood

Volume 14 mL

Minimum Volume 10 mL whole blood

Container Two gray top (sodium fluoride) tubes

Perphenazine, Blood

Synonyms Chlorpiprazine; Trilafon®

Uses Monitor therapeutic drug level; evaluate toxicity

Reference Range 0.004-0.064 mg/L

Test Commonly Includes Chlorpromazine, mesoridazine, perphenazine, prochlorperazine, promazine, promethazine, thioridazine

Specimen Blood

Volume 10 mL

Minimum Volume 3 mL serum
Container Red top tube
Storage Instructions Refrigerate serum.
Possible Panic Range 3 mg/L
Methodology High performance liquid chromatography (HPLC), gas chromatography (GC)
Additional Information Perphenazine, a piperazine phenothiazine, is used to manage the manifestations of psychotic disorders. It is also used to control hiccups, nausea and vomiting, and violent retching during surgery. Adverse effects include convulsions, xerostomia, nasal congestion, tachycardia, bradycardia, hypotension, and photosensitivity.

Pesticide Screen, Chlorinated

Uses Screen aids in identification or confirmation of exposure to common polychlorinated hydrocarbon compounds used as pesticidal sprays or dusts.
Reference Range None detected
Test Commonly Includes Aldrin, chlordane, DDT, dieldrin, heptachlor, lindane, methoxychlor
Specimen Urine, blood, or gastric contents
Volume 100 mL urine, 20 mL whole blood, 50 mL gastric contents
Container Two royal blue top (heparin) tubes
Special Instructions Requisition must state date and time of specimen collection. Specify suspected pesticide. Specify if quantitation of a positive screen result is desired.

Pesticide Screen, Organophosphate

Uses Screen aids in identification or confirmation of exposure to common organophosphate compounds used as pesticidal sprays or dusts
Reference Range None detected
Test Commonly Includes Diazinon; Dicapthon; Malathion; Parathion; Trichlorfon; Dichloron
Specimen Urine, blood, or gastric contents
Volume 100 mL urine, 20 mL whole blood, 50 mL gastric contents
Container Two royal blue top (heparin) tubes
Special Instructions Requisition must state date and time of specimen collection. Specify suspected pesticide. Specify if quantitation of a positive screen result is desired.

pH, Urine

Uses Urine pH is a crude measure of the acid-base balance of the body. It may be helpful in determining subtle presence of distal renal tubular disease or pyelonephritis. Urine pH is useful for identifying crystals in urine and determining predisposition to form a given type of stone. See table. When an accurate pH assessment of acid-base status and renal response is desired, the urine should be collected under circumstances more controlled than is usual. Attention is given to the time of day, the fasting status of the patient, and transfer of sample so as to prevent degaussing of sample or growth of bacteria; rapid analysis by pH meter rather than dipstick is indicated. Usually simultaneous serum pH is then also ordered. See table.

Conditions Associated with Acid Urine	Conditions Associated with Alkaline Urine	
Metabolic acidosis	Respiratory alkalosis	Postprandial alkaline tide (1 hour after meal)
Diabetes mellitus		
Diarrhea	Metabolic alkalosis	Fanconi syndrome and Milkman's syndrome (increased urinary loss of bicarbonate)
Starvation	Urea-splitting bacteria (*Proteus* sp)	
Respiratory acidosis	Vegetable diet	Alkali therapy (citrate, bicarbonate)
Emphysema	Gastric suction and vomiting	
Sleep		
Renal failure with lack of NH$_3$ buffer	Diuretic therapy	

Reference Range 4.5-7.8; normal kidneys can produce urine with pH from 4.5-8.2, but with ordinary diet, urine pH is ~6.0. Urine becomes more alkaline after meals and is most acidic fasting in the morning.
Test Commonly Includes pH is part of a routine urinalysis.
Specimen Random urine
Volume 5 mL
Minimum Volume 2 mL
Container Plastic urine container
Storage Instructions If the specimen cannot be processed promptly, it should be refrigerated.
Causes for Rejection Improper labeling, specimen not refrigerated
Limitations On standing urine becomes alkaline due to the action of urea splitting bacteria (*Proteus* sp).

Methodology Dipstick double indicator principle (methyl red and bromthymol blue) which gives a broad range of colors covering the urinary pH range 5-9 ±0.5 pH units. A pH meter is the back-up and most accurate method.
Additional Information Dietary factors affect urine pH. Alkaline urine is observed in persons who eat large quantities of citrus fruit and vegetables. Acid urine is observed with high meat intake. Pyridium® metabolites may mask the pH reaction. Urine pH >6.5 indicates presence of bicarbonate while pH <5.5 indicates absence of bicarbonate. Consistently acid urine, pH <5.5, is associated with xanthine, cystine, and uric acid stones. Calcium oxalate and apatite stones are not associated with any particular disturbance of urine pH. Alkaline urine (pH >7) is associated with calcium carbonate, calcium phosphate, and especially magnesium ammonium phosphate stones. In conjunction with serum pH and bicarbonate levels, urine pH may be applied to the study of renal tubular acidification.

Phencyclidine, Qualitative, Urine

Synonyms Angel Dust; Elephant Tranquilizers; Hog; Killer Weed; PCP; Peace Pills; Rocket Fuel
Uses Evaluate presence of phencyclidine, drug abuse, PCP toxicity; determine phencyclidine involvement in unexplained psychoses
Reference Range Negative (less than cutoff)
Abstract This is a widely used drug of abuse which was formerly sold as a veterinary tranquilizer. All legal manufacture and sale has been stopped. It is classified by DEA as a Schedule II controlled substance.
Specimen Random urine
Volume 100 mL
Minimum Volume 5 mL
Container Plastic urine container
Collection If forensic, observe precautions.
Special Instructions If forensic, use chain-of-custody protocol and form.
Critical Values Cutoff: screen: 25 ng/mL; confirmation: 25 ng/mL (SI: 100 nmol/L)
Methodology Immunoassay, thin-layer chromatography (TLC), gas chromatography (GC), gas chromatography/mass spectrometry (GC/MS). Immunoassays are very specific and detect PCP at 25 ng/mL
Additional Information
Phencyclidine is most often called "angel dust." It was first developed as an anesthetic in the 1950s. It was taken off the market for human use because it sometimes caused hallucinations. PCP is available in a number of forms. It can be a pure white crystal-like powder, a tablet or capsule, and it can be swallowed, smoked (alone or with marijuana), sniffed, or injected. Although PCP is illegal, it is easily manufactured.
Effects depend on how much of the drug is taken, the way it is used, and the individual. Small amounts act as a stimulant, speeding up body functions. For many users, PCP changes how they see their own bodies and things around them. Speech, muscle coordination, and vision are affected; sense of touch and pain are dulled; and body movements are slowed. Time seems to "space out." Effects include increased heart rate and blood pressure, flushing, sweating, dizziness, and numbness. When large doses are taken, effects include drowsiness, convulsions, and coma. Taking large amounts of PCP can also cause death from repeated convulsions, heart and lung failure, or ruptured blood vessels in the brain. PCP can be detected for 7 days after administration; 2-4 weeks in chronic users. Half-life is 7-46 hours.
Dextromethorphan, diphenhydramine, and high doses of thioridazine can give a false-positive on an immunoassay screen; ketamine is not expected to give a positive immunoassay.

Phencyclidine, Quantitative, Serum

Synonyms Angel Dust; Hog; Killer Weed; PCP; Rocket Fuel; Sernyl®
Uses Detect drug abuse; evaluate toxicity
Specimen Blood
Volume 10 mL
Minimum Volume 3 mL serum
Container Gray top (sodium fluoride) tube
Additional Information
Phencyclidine, most often called "angel dust," is available in a number of forms. It can be a pure white crystal-like powder, a tablet or capsule, and it can be swallowed, smoked (alone or with marijuana), sniffed, or injected. Although PCP is illegal, it is easily manufactured and is a legitimate veterinary tranquilizer.
Effects depend on how much of the drug is taken, the way it is used, and the individual. Small amounts act as a stimulant, speeding up body functions. For many users, PCP changes how they see their own bodies and things around them. Speech, muscle coordination and vision are affected; sense of touch and pain are dulled; and body movements are slowed. Time seems to "space out." Effects include increased heart rate and blood pressure, flushing, sweating, dizziness, and numbness. When large doses are taken effects include drowsiness, convulsions, and

coma. Taking large amounts of PCP can also cause death from repeated convulsions, heart and lung failure or ruptured blood vessels in the brain. Dextromethorphan can give a false-positive on an immunoassay screen; ketamine is not expected to give a positive immunoassay. Serum PCP levels: Catatonia and excitation: 20-30 ng/mL; myoclonus and coma: 30-100 ng/mL; hypotension, seizures, fatalities: >100 ng/mL

Phenobarbital, Blood

Related Information
● Barbiturates, Quantitative, Blood

Synonyms Gardenal®; Luminal®; Phenemal; Phenemalum; Phenobarb; Phenobarbitone; Stental Extentabs®

Uses Monitor patients for compliance, efficacy, and possible toxicity. Mephobarbital and primidone are metabolized to phenobarbital and, therefore, patients taking these drugs will have detectable levels of phenobarbital on therapeutic monitoring.

Reference Range Infants and children: 15-30 mcg/mL (SI: 65-129 µmol/L); adults: 20-40 mcg/mL (SI: 86-172 µmol/L). Low level: Most common cause is noncompliance. Other causes include drug interactions, including antipsychotic medication, chloramphenicol, acetazolamide, and phenytoin. Some patients are fast metabolizers, such as infants and children. High level: addition of valproic acid to regimen inhibits phenobarbital metabolism (parahydroxylation) and should be accompanied by a cut in phenobarbital dosage. Newborns, unlike older infants, have very long half-lives which may be associated with high levels.

Abstract Phenobarbital is indicated for generalized tonic-clonic and partial seizures.

Specimen Blood

Volume 7 mL

Minimum Volume 1 mL serum or plasma

Container Red top tube, green top (heparin) tube, or lavender top (EDTA) tube

Sampling Time Consistent sampling time is desirable but less important than for other anticonvulsants due to its long half-life.

Critical Values Toxic: >40 mcg/mL (SI: >172 µmol/L) but if given intravenously, life-threatening side effects can occur with much lower levels, and patients should be monitored. Toxic effects are mostly neurologic. Adults present with lethargy and coma; children may present with irritability or hyperactivity.

Methodology Enzyme immunoassay (EIA), gas-liquid chromatography (GLC), high performance liquid chromatography (HPLC)

Additional Information
Indications for measurement of a serum antiepileptic drug level include:
● within 6 hours of a seizure
● suspected dose-related drug toxicity
● suspected patient noncompliance
Additional indications for serum drug assay during steady state conditions (after 6 days for phenytoin, 3 days for carbamazepine, 3 days for valproic acid, 20 days for phenobarbital) include:
● baseline measurement after starting antiepileptic drug therapy
● control measurement after a change in dosage regimen
● addition of a second drug with a potential interaction with the antiepileptic drug (ie, a second antiepileptic drug, warfarin, isoniazid or rifampicin)
● change in patient's hepatic or gastrointestinal function

Phenobarbital, Free, Blood

Uses Monitor therapeutic drug level; evaluate toxicity

Reference Range Therapeutic free: 7.5-20.0 mcg/mL; therapeutic total: 15-40 mcg/mL

Test Commonly Includes Total and free phenobarbital

Specimen Blood

Volume 2 mL

Minimum Volume Two plain Microtainer™ tubes

Container Red top tube

Collection Draw just prior to the next dose.

Critical Values Toxic total: >60 mcg/mL

Methodology Ultrafiltrate assayed by fluorescence polarization immunoassay (FPIA) or enzyme immunoassay (EIA)

Phenytoin, Blood

Synonyms Dilantin® Level, Blood; Diphenylhydantoin Level, Blood

Uses Monitor for compliance, efficacy, and possible toxicity

Reference Range 10-20 mcg/mL (SI: 40-79 µmol/L). Patients treated for status epilepticus should have levels at or slightly above the upper limit of range. Low level: The most common cause of a low level is noncompliance. Absorption problems are most important in young infants (younger than 3 months) or occasionally in patients given phenobarbital, charcoal, or antacids at the same time as the phenytoin. Pediatric and some adult patients (fast metabolizers), who have breakthrough seizures at the end of the day, require more than once daily dosing. Some

formulations other than Kapseals® may require more than once daily dosing, and changing formulations can cause changes in levels. Pregnancy or intercurrent illness such as mononucleosis can cause subtherapeutic levels with seizures. The addition of carbamazepine to a patient taking phenytoin can lower or raise phenytoin level but usually does not cause seizures. Disulfiram administration can increase phenytoin metabolism, lower levels, and may cause seizures. Patients can have lower than expected values if intravenous formulations are given with fluids containing glucose, which precipitates in solution with phenytoin. High levels: In patients chronically controlled on phenytoin who become clinically toxic without a change in dose, toxicity can be brought on by a change in formulation, drug interaction, or intercurrent infection. Drugs which can precipitate phenytoin toxicity include chloramphenicol, tricyclic antidepressants, fluconazole, and levodopa. Small dose changes or changes in formulation (including change from one brand to another or to a generic) can cause large changes in antiepileptic drug (AED) levels and toxicity, because phenytoin manifests zero-order kinetics.

Abstract Phenytoin is effective for generalized tonic-clonic and partial seizures.

Specimen Blood, saliva

Volume 7 mL

Minimum Volume 1 mL serum or plasma; 1 mL saliva

Container Red top tube or lavender top (EDTA) tube

Sampling Time In monitoring patients maintained on chronic therapy, a trough level or consistent sampling time should be used.

Possible Panic Range Toxicity may manifest progressively at >30 mcg/mL (SI: >120 µmol/L) with ataxia, dizziness, nystagmus, and diplopia. Patients can have life-threatening complications with I.V. administration with normal levels; such patients should be placed on a cardiac monitor during I.V. administration.

Methodology Routine: Enzyme-multiplied immunoassay technique (EMIT), enzyme-linked immunosorbent assay (ELISA), and fluorescence polarization immunoassay (FPIA). For physician's office testing, apoenzyme reactive immunoassay (ARIS; Ames Seralyzer®) is rapid, accurate, and may become increasingly important.

Additional Information
Indications for measurement of a serum antiepileptic drug level include:
● within 6 hours of a seizure
● suspected dose-related drug toxicity
● suspected patient noncompliance
Additional indications for serum drug assay during steady state conditions (after 6 days for phenytoin, 3 days for carbamazepine, 3 days for valproic acid, 20 days for phenobarbital) include:
● baseline measurement after starting antiepileptic drug therapy
● control measurement after a change in dosage regimen
● addition of a second drug with a potential interaction with the antiepileptic drug (ie, a second antiepileptic drug, warfarin, isoniazid or rifampicin)
● change in patient's hepatic or gastrointestinal function
Oxaprozin may result in false elevation of phenytoin blood levels if performed by fluorescence polarization immunoassay.

Platinum, Blood

Synonyms Pt, Blood

Uses Evaluate platinum toxicity, usually from the use of cis-platinum for cancer chemotherapy and occasionally from industrial exposure

Specimen Blood

Volume 10 mL

Minimum Volume 1 mL serum or plasma

Container Red top tube or green top (sodium heparin) tube

Storage Instructions Refrigerate specimen. Do not separate.

Methodology Flameless atomic absorption spectrophotometry (AA)

Additional Information Since normal biological fluids are free from detectable platinum, quantitation enables direct correlation between exposure and distribution in the body.

Platinum, Urine

Synonyms Pt, Urine

Uses Monitor platinum excretion during chemotherapy or industrial exposure

Specimen Random urine

Volume 100 mL

Minimum Volume 5 mL

Container Plastic urine container

Storage Instructions Refrigerate.

Methodology Flameless atomic absorption spectrophotometry (AA), high performance liquid chromatography (HPLC), voltametry

Additional Information Since normal biological fluids are free from detectable platinum, quantitation enables direct correlation between exposure and distribution in the body.

Primidone, Blood

Applies to Metabolites of Primidone; PEMA; Phenylethylmalonamide
Synonyms Majsolin®; Mylepsin®; Mysoline®; Prysolin®
Uses Monitor efficacy, compliance, and possible toxicity
Reference Range Children younger than 5 years of age: 7-10 mcg/mL (SI: 32-46 μmol/L); adults: 5-12 mcg/mL. Phenobarbital concentration can also be used to guide dosing.
Test Commonly Includes Phenobarbital, PEMA
Abstract Primidone is indicated for generalized tonic-clonic and partial seizures.
Specimen Blood
Volume 5 mL
Minimum Volume 2 mL serum or plasma
Container Red top tube, green top (heparin) tube, or lavender top (EDTA) tube
Sampling Time Trough or consistent sampling time. Levels of phenobarbital and PEMA can be measured simultaneously.
Critical Values At levels >12 mcg/mL (SI: >55 μmol/L) primidone produces CNS depression, vertigo, visual disturbances, areflexia, somnolence, and lethargy. Clinical toxicity correlates with primidone rather than metabolite concentrations. In overdosage, a biphasic peak may be seen with highest toxicity a few hours after ingestion and again 48 hours afterwards. Crystalluria is a feature of overdosage.
Possible Panic Range >12 mcg/mL (SI: >55 μmol/L)
Methodology Enzyme immunoassay (EIA), gas-liquid chromatography (GLC), high performance liquid chromatography (HPLC)
Additional Information Since phenobarbital requires a longer interval (48 hours) to achieve therapeutic blood levels than primidone, checking both levels can be used to determine chronic compliance. The phenobarbital/primidone ratio normally is 2.5, can be higher (4.3 mean) in patients on other anticonvulsants (phenytoin, carbamazepine) and lower than normal among patients discontinued from those medicines or who are chronically noncompliant. Primidone decreases the effects of oral anticoagulants.

Propranolol, Blood

Synonyms Inderal®
Uses Monitor therapeutic drug level in patients with cardiac arrhythmias, angina pectoris, and hypertension; evaluate for potential toxicity
Reference Range Therapeutic: 50-100 ng/mL (SI: 190-390 nmol/L) at end of dose interval
Abstract A relatively short-acting beta blocker. Propranolol is used as an antiarrhythmic and antihypertensive.
Specimen Blood
Volume 5 mL
Container Red top tube
Sampling Time Trough: immediately prior to next dose
Special Instructions The stoppers of some blood collection tubes contain TBEP plasticizers that affect drug distribution in sample. Check with local laboratory.
Possible Panic Range >1000 ng/mL (SI: >3860 nmol/L)
Methodology Fluorometry, fluorescence polarization immunoassay (FPIA), enzyme immunoassay (EIA), gas-liquid chromatography (GLC), high performance liquid chromatography (HPLC)

Prothrombin Time

Related Information
● Heparin
Applies to Coumarins; Heparin; INR; International Normalized Ratio; PT Ratio
Synonyms Protime; PT
Uses Evaluate extrinsic coagulation system; aid in screening for congenital deficiencies of factors II, V, VII, X; dysfibrinogenemia, afibrinogenemia (complete); heparin effect, coumarin or warfarin effect; liver failure; disseminated intravascular coagulation (DIC); and screen for vitamin K deficiency
Reference Range 10-13 seconds. Healthy premature newborns have prolonged coagulation test screening results (eg, PT, APTT, TT) which return to normal adult values at about 6 months of age. Healthy prematures, however, do not develop spontaneous hemorrhage or thrombotic complications because of a balance between procoagulants and inhibitors. The normal range in childhood (ages 1-16) is similar to that in adults. For factors affecting PT response: See tables.

The Following Factors, Alone or in Combination, May Be Responsible for Increased PT Response

Endogenous Factors		
Cancer	Elevated temperature	Poor nutritional state
Collagen disease	Hepatic disorders	Steatorrhea
Congestive heart failure	Infectious hepatitis, jaundice	Vitamin K deficiency
Diarrhea	Hyperthyroidism	
Exogenous Factors		
Acetaminophen	Dong quai (dang qui)	Nortriptyline
Alcohol*	Enoxacin	Nonsteroidal anti-inflammatory drugs
Allopurinol	Ethacrynic acid	Omeprazole
Aminosalicylic acid	Fenofibrate	Pentoxifylline
Amiodarone HCl	Fenoprofen	Phenobarbital*
Amprenavir	Fluconazole	Phenylbutazone
Anabolic steroids	5-Fluorouracil	Phenytoin*
Ancrod	Fluvoxamine	Piroxicam
Anesthetics, inhalation	Fluoxetine	Ponalrestat
Azithromycin	Fluvastatin	Proguanil
Bezabifrate	Glucagon	Propafenone
Boldo-Fenugreek	Green tea	Protriptyline
Bromelains	Gemcitabine	Quetiapine
Broxuridine	Hepatotoxic drugs	Quinidine
Celecoxib	Ibuprofen	Quinine
Chenodiol	Ifosfamide	Interferon alpha
Chloral hydrate*	Indomethacin	Rifampin*
Chlorpropamide	Influenza virus vaccine	Ritonavir
Chymotrypsin	Interferon alpha	Salicylates
Cimetidine (rarely)	Isoniazid	Saquinavir
Clofibrate	Itraconazole	Stanozolol
Coumadin® overdose	Ketoconazole	Sulfinpyrazone
COX-2 inhibitors	Levamisole	Sulindac
Cyclophosphamide*	Lovastatin	Sulofenur
Cyclosporine	Levonorgestrel	Tamoxifen
Danazol	Mefenamic acid	Thyroid drugs
Danshen	Methyldopa	Ticlopidine*
Delaviridine	Methylphenidate	Tramadol
Dextran	Miconazole	Triclofas
Dextrothyroxine	Mitotane	Troglitazone
Diazoxide	Monoamine oxidase inhibitors	Tolterodine
Diflusinal	Moricizine hydrochloride*	Trastuzumab
Digibind®	Nabumetone	Valproic acid
Dipyridamole	Nalidixic acid	Vitamin A
Diuretics*	Naproxen	Vitamin E (>400 IU daily)
Disulfiram	Narcotics, prolonged	Zafirlukast
Antibiotics:		
Carbenicillin	Fluoroquinolones	Quinolones (Ciprofloxacin)
Cephalosporins (2nd & 3rd generations)	Macrolides (Norfloxacin)	Sulfonamides
Chloramphenicol	Metronidazole	Tetracycline
Cloxacillin	Ofloxacin	Trimethoprim/sulfamethoxazole
Erythromycin	Piroxicam	Nafcillin*
Other factors affecting blood elements which may modify hemostasis:		
Dietary deficiencies	Prolonged hot weather	Unreliable PT determinations

*Increased and decreased PT responses have been reported. INRs are unreliable in patients with lupus anticoagulant.

The Following Factors, Alone or in Combination, May Be Responsible for Decreased PT Response

Endogenous Factors		
Edema	Hyperlipemia	Hypothyroidism
Hereditary Coumadin® resistance		

Exogenous Factors		
Adrenocortical steroids	Diuretics	Paraldehyde
Alcohol*	Estrogens	Phenytoin
Aminoglutethimide	Ethychlorvynol	Primidone
Antacids	Etretinate	Raloxifene
Antihistamines	Furosemide	Ranitidine*
Azathioprine	Glutethimide	Rifampin
Barbiturates	Griseofulvin	Ritonavir
Carbamazepine	Haloperidol	Secobarbital
Chloral hydrate*	Meprobamate	Sulcralfate
Chlordiazepoxide	Mesalamine	Sulfasalazine
Cholestyramine	Mitotaine	Toxaphene
Coumadin® underdosage	Moricizine hydrochloride*	Trazodone
Cyclophosphamide	Nafcillin	Vitamin C
Disopyramide	Oral contraceptives	Vitamin K

Also:	
Diet high in vitamin K	Unreliable PT determinations

*Increased and decreased PT responses have been reported.

Test Commonly Includes Patient time and control time

Abstract A simple, low cost test useful for the evaluation of the extrinsic system of coagulation as it is sensitive to reduced levels (or activity) of factors II, V, VII, and fibrinogen. It is the time, in seconds, required for clot formation after addition of calcium and thromboplastin to the patient's citrated plasma. A common application is monitoring the effect of warfarin type anticoagulation.

Specimen Plasma

Minimum Volume 4.5 mL

Container Blue top (sodium citrate) tube

Collection Routine venipuncture. If multiple tests are being drawn, draw coagulation studies last. If only a prothrombin time is being drawn, two-syringe collection technique is recommended to avoid contamination of the specimen with tissue thromboplastins.

Storage Instructions Plasma should be separated from cells as soon as possible and refrigerated if testing cannot be immediately performed. Testing should be performed within 4 hours.

Causes for Rejection Tube not full; specimen clotted; specimen hemolyzed, lipemic, or icteric (possible interference with photo-optical clot detection); specimen received more than 3-4 hours after collection

Special Instructions Transport specimen to the Hematology Laboratory as soon as possible.

Possible Panic Range Nonanticoagulated: >20 seconds; anticoagulated: >three times control

Limitations Prothrombin times drawn less than 2 hours after heparin administration will be prolonged. The prothrombin time determination is sensitive to the ratio of plasma to citrate anticoagulant. That is, if enough blood is not added to the liquid citrate-containing tube when the specimen is drawn (tube usually contains 0.5 mL of 3.2% or 3.8% sodium citrate), a falsely elevated prothrombin time may result. The minimum amount of blood in the tube necessary to a reliable PT is not readily predictable. **The citrate tube for PT/PTT must be completely filled.**

Methodology The clotting time of citrate anticoagulated plasma is determined after the addition of an optimum concentration of calcium and an excess of thromboplastin. Clot detection is by manual (tilt tube visual) or, more commonly, by an automated device for fibrin clot detection, electrode, electro-optical or other method. The result is always reported with that obtained on a commercial normal control plasma run at the same time. Attempts in recent years to standardize prothrombin time results has led to reporting of the "international normalized ratio" (INR). See comments under Additional Information concerning INR and International Sensitivity Index (ISI). Chromogenic assays for determination of prothrombin have been developed. If the PT is prolonged repeat testing using half patient and half normal control plasma will identify presence of a circulating anticoagulant (prolonged PT will not correct).

Additional Information

Antibiotic therapy and prolonged prothrombin time: Biochemical mechanisms have been defined that support results of clinical studies indicating that broad-spectrum antibiotics, in particular second- and third-generation cephalosporins exert a hypoprothrombinemic effect. Destruction of menaquinone-producing GI bacteria and/or interference with prothrombin synthesis by N-methyl-thio-tetrazole side chains has resulted in recommendations that prophylactic use of vitamin K be considered.

Control of coumarin derivative therapy: Long-term anticoagulant therapy usually involves the use of a coumarin derivative (eg, Coumadin®). The prothrombin time (PT) provides for "control" of the dosage. The attempt is to impede thrombus formation without the threat of morbidity or mortality from hemorrhage. In the past this goal has been approached by administering a Coumadin® dosage that prolongs the PT to twice that of a normal control plasma. More recently, this practice has been considered to result in overanticoagulation when using warfarin derivatives (Coumadin®, dicumarol, Tramexan®).

As the result of a series of conferences on antithrombotic therapy held in 1985, 1989, 1992, and most recently in 1995 (Fourth American College of Chest Physicians (ACCP) Consensus Conference on Antithrombotic Therapy), the earlier recommendation that the intensity of warfarin therapy be reduced (for most indications) has found support in the result of subsequent clinical trials. The ACCP recommends use of the INR for monitoring oral (warfarin-coumarin derivative) therapy. INR of 2.0-3.0 is recommended for all conditions with the exception of patients anticoagulated for thrombotic complications of mechanical heart valves for which an INR of 2.5-3.5 is recommended.

Warfarin anticoagulant effect occurs gradually. Without a loading dose, 7.5 mg/day of warfarin anticoagulant will produce desired therapeutic effect in 5-7 days. With a loading dose of 10-15 mg the anticoagulant effect can be achieved in some 3 days but with greater risk of bleeding. When warfarin compounds are discontinued the PT will require 2-4 days to return to normal. If oral vitamin K is given PT returns to normal within ~24 hours. The overanticoagulated state can be quickly reversed by giving vitamin K by subcutaneous injection or by slow intravenous infusion.

Onset of prothrombin time prolongation following first-time warfarin use is within 12-24 hours. A one-time warfarin dose of 0.5 mg/kg will result in a prothrombin time of 18-30 seconds in children following heart valve surgery.

Warfarin therapy can be started soon after the onset of heparin therapy in patients with venous thromboembolic disease with resultant savings in hospitalization costs. A 1-year course of warfarin therapy may be needed for patients with prior deep vein thrombosis and indefinite treatment if there have been over two previous episodes.

The variability in sensitivity of thromboplastins with resultant lack of between laboratory comparability in results of PT testing provided stimulus for standardization. In 1983, the International Normalized Ratio (INR) system was adopted by the International Committee for Standardization in Haematology, International Committee on Thrombosis and Haemostasis (ISCH/ICTH). This system is based on the first World Health Organization (WHO) primary international reference preparation of thromboplastin. The system is centered about the concept of the International Sensitivity Index (ISI). The ISI represents the responsiveness of a thromboplastin to the reduction in vitamin K-dependent factors. The ISI is derived by calibrating a thromboplastin reagent with the WHO reference preparation. Use is made of a linear relation between the logarithm of the prothrombin time ratio of the reference material and that of the test thromboplastin. INR=(PT ratio)^{ISI}, where the PT ratio = patient PT/mean normal PT. The "mean normal PT" should be the geometric, as opposed to the arithmetic, mean PT. It is important to avoid large biases in determining the reference mean. Theoretically, the INR is the PT ratio that would result if the WHO reference thromboplastin had been used in performing the test.

Recombinant human tissue factor (rTF), with very low ISI of 1.0 ± 0.1, has been developed. rTF reagents are more sensitive to lower levels of factors II, VII, IX, and X. Thromboplastin reagents are not equivalent. Results from use of rTF reagents are not comparable to those obtained with mammalian thromboplastins when testing oral anticoagulated patients. Commercial availability and use of rTF reagents may allow for accurate and uniform reporting of PT results as INR.

The prothrombin time has been shown to lack sensitivity (in its current form) as a monitor for the anticoagulant effect of recombinant hirudin (originally an anticoagulant from the medicinal leech *Hirudo medicinalis*).

Protoporphyrin, Free Erythrocyte

Synonyms FEP; Free Erythrocyte Protoporphyrin; Protoporphyrins, Fractionation, Erythrocytes; RBC Protoporphyrin

Uses Differential diagnosis of disorders of heme production versus diseases of globin synthesis. FEP is increased in lead poisoning, protoporphyria, in iron deficiency, anemia of chronic disease and with some sideroblastic anemias. FEP levels are also reported increased in entities characterized by marked increase in erythropoiesis, such as severe hemolytic anemias. Thus, FEP is useful in work-up of the microcytic anemias. FEP is increased with lead poisoning but not in acute intermittent porphyria. FEP is reported normal with presumed alpha thalassemia trait, hemoglobin H, beta thalassemia trait, and hemoglobin E.

Reference Range Depends on method; ascertain ranges for individual testing laboratory. The FEP is considered unreliable in infants younger than 6 months of age. Pediatric upper limit is 50 mcg/dL (SI: 0.89 μmol/L) RBC. Adults: male: <30 mcg/dL (SI: <0.53 μmol/L), female: <40 mcg/dL (SI: <0.71 μmol/L) by hematofluorometer; 11-45 (SI: 0.20-0.80 μmol/L) for adult men and 19-52 (SI: 0.34-0.92 μmol/L) for adult women by Piomelli FEP expressed as mcg/dL blood.

Abstract Free erythrocyte protoporphyrin expresses the amount of nonheme protoporphyrin in red cells.

Specimen Whole blood (test done on washed erythrocytes)

Volume 7 mL

Minimum Volume 1 mL whole blood

Container Lavender top (EDTA) tube or green top (heparin) tube

Collection Pediatrics: Blood drawn from heelstick for capillary.

Storage Instructions Stable 3 weeks at 4°C. Do not freeze.

Special Instructions Current hematocrit must be measured or specified.

Possible Panic Range >190 mcg/dL (SI: >3.38 μmol/L)

Limitations Fluorescent substances in plasma may interfere with hematofluorometer results. Elevated FEPs should be verified by retesting washed RBCs or by microextraction. Skin contamination may lead to false elevations. Both this test and blood lead are needed for full evaluation.

Methodology Hematofluorometer, extraction method, and high performance liquid chromatography (HPLC). The hematofluorometer measures porphyrins unbound in erythrocytes. With iron deficiency and diminished heme synthesis, free porphyrin accumulates in the red blood cell.

Additional Information "Free" protoporphyrin is not complexed, nonheme protoporphyrin. **Lead poisoning** is characterized by elevated plasma and urine delta aminolevulinic acid and increased urinary coproporphyrin. Urinary porphobilinogen and uroporphyrin are normal to slightly increased. Free erythrocyte protoporphyrin is a sensitive test for lead toxicity or chronic exposure, **although, a careful study based on receiver operator curves showed that erythrocyte protoporphyrin levels should not be used as a screening test for lead poisoning in children.** The diagnosis of lead exposure or poisoning includes consideration of environmental exposure, as well as symptoms and abnormal erythrocyte protoporphyrin. FEP is given as 92-288 mcg/dL (SI: 1.63-5.12 μmol/L) RBC in level II increased lead absorption, with higher FEP results in level III. Increased lead absorption is reported in the presence of iron deficiency. Increased erythrocyte protoporphyrin exists as free protoporphyrin in protoporphyria, not as a zinc chelate, in contrast to lead poisoning and iron deficiency. These two compounds, zinc protoporphyrin and metal free protoporphyrin, can be distinguished from each other by spectrophotofluorometry.

Protoporphyrin, Zinc, Blood

Synonyms Zinc Protoporphyrin; ZPP

Uses Evaluate iron deficiency, especially nonanemic iron deficiency. ZPP is superior to hemoglobin in identifying female blood donors with nonanemic iron deficiency.

Reference Range 17-77 mcg/dL (SI: 0.27-1.23 μmol/L). Results may be obtained as ZPP/heme ratio; reference range: 30-80 μmol/mol heme.

Abstract Zinc protoporphyrin measurement may be a useful adjunct in the diagnosis of nonanemic iron deficiency but is not useful in screening programs for lead intoxication.

Specimen Whole blood

Volume 3 mL

Minimum Volume 1 mL whole blood

Container Lavender top (EDTA) tube, green top (heparin) tube

Collection Routine venipuncture

Storage Instructions Do not centrifuge. Refrigerate and protect from light. Stable 1 week at 4°C.

Causes for Rejection Specimen not protected from light, specimen improperly collected, hemolysis, icterus

Critical Values >100 mcg/dL (SI: >1.6 μmol/L)

Limitations Zinc protoporphyrin may also be increased in lead poisoning, anemia of chronic disease, and erythropoietic protoporphyria. ZPP should **not** be used to screen or diagnose lead poisoning.

Methodology Hematofluorometry (front-face); if washed erythrocytes are used, the assay becomes more specific and sensitive

Additional Information Zinc protoporphyrin levels increase as blood lead levels increase. Various authorities caution using ZPP as a screening test for lead poisoning. The Center for Disease Control has lowered the cutoff level for lead intoxication in children younger than 6 years of age to **10 mcg/dL (SI: 0.48 μmol/L)**, and this level is so low that **ZPP is not useful** in this context because it is insensitive to such a lead level. Therefore, it is mandatory to measure lead levels in any screening program, rather than ZPP. ZPP appears only in new RBCs and remains for the life of the RBC; therefore, ZPP does not increase until several weeks after the onset of lead exposure and remains high long after exposure to lead. It is a reasonable indicator of total body burden of lead and remains a useful adjunct to the diagnosis of iron deficiency, particularly in nonanemic or questionably anemic patients. It reflects iron depletion in the bone marrow.

Protriptyline, Blood

Synonyms Vivactil®

Uses Monitor therapeutic drug level; evaluate toxicity

Reference Range Therapeutic: 70-250 ng/mL

Specimen Blood

Volume 20 mL

Minimum Volume 4 mL serum

Container Red top serum separator tube preferred, plain red top tube acceptable

Storage Instructions Freeze serum.

Critical Values Toxic: >500 ng/mL

Methodology Gas-liquid chromatography (GLC)

Additional Information Protriptyline, a tricyclic antidepressant, is used to treat endogenous depression. The drug is very similar to imipramine in actions, limitations, and interactions. The half-life is 54-98 hours and peak serum levels are reached in 24-30 hours. Adverse reactions include CNS stimulation, tachycardia, and strong anticholinergic activity. Orthostatic hypotension frequently occurs.

Pseudocholinesterase, Serum

Related Information
- Acetylcholinesterase, Red Blood Cell

Synonyms Cholinesterase, Serum; PCE®; Plasma Cholinesterase

Uses

Screen preoperative patients for succinylcholine (suxamethonium) anesthetic sensitivity, genetic or secondary to insecticide exposure, in appropriate circumstances. Prevent or evaluate prolonged anesthetic effect, prolonged apnea, after surgery. Very small amounts (0.04-0.06 mg/kg) of succinylcholine are needed to obtain 90% of neuromuscular blockade in patients with low levels of plasma cholinesterase activity.

Monitor organophosphorous or carbamate insecticide poisoning, in which level is decreased; establish patient's baseline value before exposure. Indications include such pesticide exposure, especially with miosis, blurred vision, muscle weakness, twitching, and fasciculation, bradycardia, nausea, diarrhea, vomiting, salivation, sweating, pulmonary edema, arrhythmias, and convulsions. The value of assessing risk status in persons exposed to organophosphate insecticides on the basis of plasma cholinesterase levels alone has been called into question. Are normal levels indicative of no exposure or of a genetic variant with or without exposure? There are interpretive problems with low or high values.

Family studies may be done when an individual with a genetically abnormal type is documented by serum pseudocholinesterase deficiency and, ideally, confirmed by phenotyping.

Contraindicating Factors Not useful to screen for toxicity from chlorinated insecticides.

Reference Range Low in infancy, then increasing in early childhood. Ranges vary between methods and laboratories.

Antidote(s)
- Acetylcholinesterase, Red Blood Cell

Abstract Two types of cholinesterase are found in blood: "true" cholinesterase (acetylcholinesterase) in red cells and "pseudocholinesterase" (acylcholine acylhydrolase) in serum (plasma).

Specimen Blood

Volume 7 mL

Minimum Volume 1 mL serum

Container Red top tube

Storage Instructions Cholinesterase is stable in separated serum for 80 days at room temperature and 3 years at -20°C. However, specimens submitted to evaluate possible pesticide toxicity should be collected on ice, separated in a refrigerated centrifuge, and frozen until analyzed.

Possible Panic Range Less than lower limit of normal

Limitations Serum pseudocholinesterase may be decreased in patients on estrogens and oral contraceptives. Fluoride interferes. Pseudocholinesterase is low also in some instances of liver disease, including decompensated cirrhosis, hepatitis, metastatic carcinoma, CHF, and in malnutrition, but not sufficiently consistently enough to be a useful clinical test for such disorders. Genetic atypical enzyme does not explain every instance of prolonged postsurgical apnea. Red cell cholinesterase is more useful for chronic insecticide exposure. Carbamate-poisoned persons can appear to have near normal or normal levels of pseudocholinesterase. Plasma cholinesterase is lower and red blood cell cholinesterase higher in pregnant women than in nonpregnant women. Thus, a low red blood cell cholinesterase in pregnant women is more consistent with a possible overexposure to anticholinesterases than a low plasma cholinesterase.

Methodology Colorimetry, kinetic enzyme utilizing different substrates, fluorometry

Additional Information

Low serum cholinesterase activity may relate to exposure to insecticides or to one of a number of variant genotypes. Dibucaine and fluoride numbers are useful to phenotype such homozygous and heterozygous individuals, who are genetically sensitive to succinylcholine.

One patient in 1500 is susceptible to succinyldicholine anesthetic mishap. Plasmapheresis has been noted to decrease the level of plasma cholinesterase. Patients with abnormally low cholinesterase activity after transfusion of blood or plasma will experience temporary augmentation of enzyme level. In estimating the duration of this enhanced activity, measures of plasma cholinesterase half-life have been utilized. The true half-life value has, however, been uncertain. A half-life value determined by measuring the rate of disappearance after intravenous injection of human cholinesterase has provided an average value of 11 days.

A low level of activity of pseudocholinesterase has been demonstrated in cerebrospinal fluid, at $\sim$1/20 to 1/100 the activity present in the corresponding plasma. With clinical conditions characterized by bleeding into the CSF, pseudocholinesterase activity increases 25% to 50% that of plasma.

Patients with a variety of carcinomas have been reported to accumulate an embryonic type of cholinesterase activity in their sera. Such novel cholinesterase activity was found only in the sera of patients undergoing antitumor therapy (eg, chemotherapy or radiation therapy and/or hormone therapy).

Increase in acetylcholinesterase activity, notably, in an acetylcholinesterase to butyrylcholine esterase ratio (histochemical study, not as measured in serum) has provided discriminatory diagnostic value in some cases of Hirschsprung's disease.

Pulse Oximetry

Applies to Ear Oximetry; Finger Oximetry

Synonyms CPAP Titration; Desaturation Oximetry; Oxygen Titration Test; Photoplethysmography

Uses Determine an estimate of the level of arterial oxygenation at rest and in the presence of positive and negative intervention. These include exercise, sleep, and during procedures such as surgery, bronchoscopy, ventilator assist/support therapy, etc.

Contraindicating Factors Not to be used in the presence of flammable anesthetics. Contraindications for exercise may be found in the section on cardiopulmonary exercise testing.

Reference Range

Normal adult oxyhemoglobin saturation is >95%. Drops in oxyhemoglobin are usually the result of cardiac, pulmonary, or combined cardiopulmonary disease. Significant declines (>5%) during exercise or sleep are abnormal.

Test Commonly Includes Report generally includes baseline heart rate and functional O_2 saturation, heart rate and lowest functional O_2 saturation during whatever event may be taking place: exercise, sleep or therapeutic intervention such as nasal CPAP or oxygen therapy.

Patient Preparation Fingernail polish should be removed with acetone. Permanent or disposable sensors should be applied according to the manufacturer's instructions. When finger probes are used, the patient should be instructed not to grip treadmill rail or handlebars tightly to avoid reduction of circulation to the digits. Preparation depends on the type of test being performed. Exercise patients should wear loose comfortable clothing. Patients should refrain from smoking 24 hours prior to test to avoid functional versus fractional O_2 saturation discrepancy that occurs with elevated carboxyhemoglobin levels. If possible, an arterial blood gas should be drawn and pH, pCO_2, pO_2, hemoglobin, oxyhemoglobin (O_2Hb%), carboxyhemoglobin (COHb%) and methemoglobin (metHb%) should be measured. Draw the heparinized arterial blood sample while the pulse oximetry sensor is in place and is stable. Correlation of oxyhemoglobin (O_2Hb%) (measured by blood oximetry) and SpO_2% (measured by pulse oximetry) should be made. The discrepancy between the O_2Hb% - SpO_2% should be used to determine the endpoint of the maneuver inducing arterial desaturation. For example, if the pulse oximeter displays a SpO_2 reading of 93% and a simultaneously obtained arterial blood sample shows an O_2Hb% of 91%, 2% should be subtracted from subsequent SpO_2 measurements during exercise for a more valid estimate of arterial oxygen saturation. This adjustment should also be made to determine the therapeutic endpoint when titrating supplemental oxygen therapy at rest, during sleep, or exercise.

Specimen Spectrophotometric measurement is made by passing light at two specific wavelengths through a pulsing capillary bed (finger, toe, bridge of nose, and ear are the most common sites for sensor placement). Light collection on the other side of the site is proportional to the amount of oxyhemoglobin present in the arterial capillary bed relative to the amount of hemoglobin available for binding with oxygen (exclusive of the dyshemoglobins: carboxyhemoglobin and methemoglobin).

Causes for Rejection Unstable readings secondary to any cause: external light, poor peripheral circulation, or skin pigmentation are common causes.

Special Instructions Poor collateral circulation may be compensated for by warming the hands with warm towels. Fluctuation $\pm$1% is acceptable. Range of fluctuation should be noted.

Possible Panic Range Values <90% indicate the need for oxygen therapy. Values <85% are require immediate attention. If available, add the measured carboxyhemoglobin and methemoglobin to the values listed to adjust for nonfunctioning dyshemoglobins.

Limitations Test does not measure or take into consideration total hemoglobin or the dyshemoglobins, carboxyhemoglobin, and methemoglobin. May overestimate total oxygen delivery (oxygen content) if not correlated with blood oximetry. Not accurate in the presence of poor peripheral circulation. Accuracy at most units is $\pm$2%, standard deviation is usually 1%. Pulse oximetry underestimates arterial blood saturation by 1.3%.

Additional Information

Guidelines for reimbursement of home oxygen therapy state that a resting arterial pO_2 <55 torr or a resting oxygen saturation (SpO_2%) <88% with evidence of improvement with oxygen therapy qualify a patient for continuous oxygen therapy reimbursement. Guidelines for reimbursement for nocturnal and exercise oxygen therapy state that O_2 saturations during exercise or sleep that fall to <88% that improve with oxygen therapy will be reimbursed. Because of the limitations of pulse oximetry, decisions regarding discontinuing oxygen therapy should **not** be made on the basis of pulse oximetry alone. Assessment of the PaO_2 by arterial blood gas and/or O_2Hb% by arterial blood oximetry should be done before such decisions are made. Room air pulse oximetry reading $\geq$97% virtually rules out hypoxemia and may also rule out moderate hypercapnia. Pulse oximetry is accurate to an arterial blood flow as low as 4% of baseline. Pulse oximetry has been used for evaluating and monitoring digital vascular flow. Oxygen digital saturation readings >95% are consistent with viable replanted digits while digital saturations <85% can be seen in venous occlusion. Pulse oximetry may underestimate oxygenation in patients with sickle cell crisis. Accurate determinations of oxygen saturation can be made with pulse oximetry after individuals were given hemoglobin-based oxygen carrier 201 (a glutaraldehyde-polymerized bovine hemoglobin)

There is growing use of **transcutaneous pulse oximetry** to determine oxygen saturation, particularly in premature and in critically ill newborns and children. This noninvasive technique avoids the rigors of arterial puncture, necessity of subsequent proper sample handling, and can provide continual monitoring. This technique has generally been found reliable and useful in monitoring adequacy of oxygenation, effectiveness of resuscitative efforts, detection of development of prolonged periods of decreased SO_2 in neonates, and monitoring preterm infant's response to physical therapy. Pulse oximetry has also been applied to detection of hyperoxemia in newborns but has low specificity. Limitations of pulse oximetry have included overestimation of SO_2 at values $\leq$65%, and variation from *in vitro* determined SO_2 in samples with >50% fetal hemoglobin as compared with samples having <25% fetal hemoglobin. Furthermore, it is not useful in carbon monoxide or methemoglobin intoxication because false elevations of saturation may occur. A study of pulse oximeter determined oxygen saturation in pregnant patients and their newborns has found that SO_2 in neonates is commonly $\leq$90% within 10 minutes after birth and may not always be indicative of pathologic hypoxia. Specialized devices (eg, balloon-tipped, thermodilution, fiberoptic, pulmonary arterial catheter) have been developed for the intraoperative monitoring of mixed venous oxygen saturation.

Specific References

Boychuk RB, Yamamoto LG, DeMesa CJ, et al, "Correlation of Initial Emergency Department Pulse Oximetry Values in Asthma Severity Classes (Steps) with the Risk of Hospitalization," *Am J Emerg Med*, 2006, 24(1):48-52.

Chan MM, Chan MM, and Chan ED, "What is the Effect of Fingernail Polish on Pulse Oximetry?" *Chest*, 2003, 123(6):2163-4.

Getti R, Gallmard X, Abderrahim N, et al, "Pulse Oximetry in the Emergency Department," *Acad Emerg Med*, 2006, 13(5):S166.

Lopez BL, Cogen JF, Kerkula L, et al, "Pulse Oximetry in the Adult ED Patient with Sickle Cell," *Am J Emerg Med*, 2005, 23(4):429-32.

Stemp LI and Ramsay MA, "Pulse Oximetry in the Detection of Hypercapnia," *Am J Emerg Med*, 2006, 24(1):136-7.

Witting MD, Hsu S, and Granja CA, "The Sensitivity of Room-Air Pulse Oximetry in the Detection of Hypercapnia," *Am J Emerg Med*, 2005, 23(4):497-500.

Rabies Identification

Related Information

- Animal and Human Bites Guidelines

Uses Diagnose rabies; evaluate animal bites

Contraindicating Factors Formalin fixation precludes fluorescent antibody application

Reference Range Serum levels >1000 ng/mL are associated with GI toxicity, while serum selenium levels >2000 ng/mL may be lethal

Test Commonly Includes Examination of animal brain for Negri bodies or inoculation of mice with suspension of brain tissue

Specimen Head of large animal or entire small animal suspected of rabies. Use gloves and mask when handling an animal carcass suspected of rabies.

Container Sealed container

Storage Instructions Ideally, animal brain should be examined in the fresh state. Transport using wet ice or place in absorbent material, then in two plastic bags, or, place half the brain in 50% glycerol, half in 10% formalin, depending on instructions from state laboratory. Local state laboratory must be consulted. Rabies virus may also be demonstrated by immunofluorescence in skin biopsies of patients suspected of having rabies (*vide infra*).

Causes for Rejection Unlabeled or improperly packaged specimen

Limitations Negri bodies are found in ~90% of rabid animals.

Methodology Fluorescent antibody examination (but Negri bodies can be seen in H & E)

Additional Information

Antemortem rabies virus has been isolated from human saliva, brain tissues, CSF, urine sediment, and tracheal secretions. Rabies virus may also be demonstrated by immunofluorescent rabies antibody staining of skin biopsy tissue. The most reliable and reproducible of the immunofluorescent studies that can aid in patient diagnosis is biopsy of the neck skin. A 6-8 mm full thickness wedge or punch biopsy specimen from the neck containing as many hair follicles as possible should be sampled, snap frozen, and shipped frozen at -70°C to a reference laboratory. Consult with reference laboratory for shipping instructions. False-negative results do occur especially after the development of neutralizing antibodies.

Rabies immune globulin (RIG) may be obtained through Connaught Laboratories (800-822-2463) or through Miles Pharmaceutical Division (203-937-2242 or 800-288-8371); RIG has been tested negative for HCV-RNA

Salicylate, Blood

Applies to Methyl Salicylate; Oil of Wintergreen

Synonyms Acetylsalicylic Acid, Blood; ASA, Blood; Aspirin, Blood; Salicylic Acid, Blood

Uses Monitor therapeutic drug level; evaluate aspirin toxicity

Reference Range Therapeutic: <10 mg/dL (SI: <0.72 mM/L) for analgesic; 15-20 mg/dL (SI: 1.09-1.45 mM/L) for anti-inflammatory

Abstract This is the active product produced from aspirin (acetylsalicylic acid) in the body. It is an analgesic, antipyretic, and anti-inflammatory drug.

Specimen Blood

Volume 7 mL

Minimum Volume 2 mL serum or plasma

Container Red top tube or lavender top (EDTA) tube

Possible Panic Range Mild toxicity: 30 mg/dL (SI: 2.17 mM/L) (tinnitus, dizziness); severe toxicity: >80 mg/dL (SI: >3.62 mM/L) (CNS effects)

Limitations Bilirubin (at concentrations of 5-20 mg/dL) has been shown to depress salicylate results by 1-5 mg/dL. Sodium azide will increase results significantly; anticoagulants interfere. Diflunisal and salazosulfapyridine, may give falsely positive blood salicylate levels by some assays.

Methodology Photometry, fluorometry, high performance liquid chromatography (HPLC), gas-liquid chromatography (GLC)

Additional Information Optimal sampling time after dosage is 2-6 hours. Serum half-life is 2-3 hours on low dose therapy, 15-30 hours on high dose treatment. Optimal resampling time after change in dosage is 6 hours. In patients on chronic therapy, small dose changes may produce disproportionate changes in serum level. Use of antacids, which increase renal excretion, can lower serum levels. Steady-state concentrations for an individual patient are not adequately predicted from nomograms or standard dose schedules. In salicylate poisoning the following symptoms may occur: initial alkalosis followed by acidosis in the blood, ketosis, and possible elevated plasma glucose. Glucose should be measured when levels >25 mg/dL (SI: >1.81 mM/L) are detected. Salicylate can be done on urine or gastric juice. Salicylate hepatitis, usually at blood levels of 20-25 mg/dL (1.45-1.81 mM/L), occurs. Salicylates are believed to play a role in the hepatonecrosis of Reye's syndrome in children. They are no longer recommended for use in children.

Selenium, Serum

Related Information

• Heavy Metal Screen, Blood

Synonyms Se, Serum

Uses Monitor selenium nutritional status in long-term parenteral nutrition. Studies have indicated no factor or factors that can accurately predict serum selenium levels to preclude need for measurement. May be used diagnostically in cardiomyopathy of unknown cause, especially where nutritional factors are suspected.

Reference Range Serum: 95-165 ng/mL. Approximately 40% higher for whole blood. Serum reflects recent intake; red cells reflect more remote intake. Whole blood therefore reflects an average of recent and remote intake of selenium. (Selenium-dependent glutathione peroxidase activity reflects selenium available for enzyme synthesis - see below.) Levels are depressed in HIV infection, critical illness, kwashiorkor, inflammatory bowel disease, renal failure, hemodialysis status, low protein diet, phenylketonuria, maple syrup urine disease, (possibly all in part related to poor protein intake), low birth weight, and premature infants with inadequate selenium intake. Levels are increased mostly with the use of glucocorticoids. Levels >500 ng/mL are associated with toxicity. Serum levels >1000 ng/mL are associated with gastrointestinal toxicity while serum selenium levels >2000 ng/mL may be lethal.

Abstract The essential nature of selenium in human nutrition is beyond dispute. The element is part of the enzyme that converts T_4 to the active thyroid hormone T_3. It is also part of selenium-dependant glutathione peroxidase, an important antioxidant in blood and tissue. Multiple cases of selenium deficiency have been reported, mostly among patients given parenteral nutrition with no added selenium. Deficiency also occurs endemically in places where soil selenium is low, and low levels are thus present throughout the food chain. Endemic cretinism, Balkan nephropathy, Keschan disease (endemic dilated cardiomyopathy), and Kashin-Bek disease (endemic deforming osteoarthritis) are probably all caused by endemic selenium deficiency conditioning the host to poorly tolerate an additional environmental stress (cretinism: iodine deficiency; the others: unknown local toxins). Simple deficiency is marked by whitening of the nailbeds, erythrocyte macrocytosis, cardiomyopathy, painful weak muscles, skin and hair depigmentation, and elevations of transaminase and creatinine kinase. The cardiomyopathy may be mild and asymptomatic or fulminant and fatal. Selenium toxicity can occur endemically, again due to high soil levels, or through accidental or industrial exposure. Symptoms include garlic breath, odor, thick brittle fingernails, dry brittle hair, red swollen skin of the hands and feet, and nervous system abnormalities of numbness, convulsions, or paralysis.

Specimen Blood

Container Sherwood Monoject™ trace element blood collection tube #8881-307006 or #8881-307022 with EDTA for whole blood

Collection Draw blood through B-D #5175 stainless steel needle into special trace metal vacuum tube. Centrifuge and pour serum into special plastic metal-free vial for transport.

Limitations

Some controversy exists regarding the "best" marker for selenium status. Since selenium as selenomethionine is incorporated nonspecifically into protein, serum and whole blood selenium concentration increases with increasing selenium intake to different degrees depending on inorganic or organic sources of selenium. Glutathione peroxidase activity is more sensitive to deficiency but the test is not well standardized and therefore not reproducible from laboratory to laboratory. Hair selenium may be contaminated by selenium-containing shampoo. Serum selenium level correlates best with intake and therefore with both deficiency and toxicity states, but a wide range of serum levels is compatible with apparent good health.

Methodology Atomic absorption, fluorometric methods

Additional Information Selenium is excreted in feces from the bile, in sweat and skin losses, and the remaining 50% to 70% in the urine. Significant breath losses occur only in toxic states. Dosages in renal failure need not be modified. The deficiency syndrome may be rapidly induced under surgery or other stress after a long asymptomatic phase. Serum selenium levels are significantly lower (24 ng/mL versus 39 ng/mL in control patients) in chronic alcohol abuse patients.

Selenium, Urine

Synonyms Se, Urine

Uses Monitor nutritional therapy, especially parenteral nutrition; monitor potential toxic exposure

Reference Range Levels <15 mcg/L or >150 mcg/L probably represent unusually low or high intake without necessarily representing illness. Values vary widely and in apparently healthy U.S. citizens they have been reported to vary from 7 mcg/L (24-hour sample) to 231 mcg/L. Intake is partly determined by local soil content of selenium and use of local vegetables as food. Healthy persons in New Guinea have been reported with levels as low as 0.9 mcg/L but similar patients have rapidly developed symptomatic selenium deficiency when placed on total parenteral nutrition lacking selenium. Urine levels of 7 mcg/L have been reported from China in areas where selenium deficiency is symptomatic. Levels >880 mcg/L have been seen in chronic selenosis and >600 mcg/L during the first 24 hours after acute selenium intoxication. Levels >500 mcg/L probably represent toxicity. See the comprehensive review by Robberecht and Deelstra. Some authors or laboratories report as mcg/day.

Abstract Urine selenium is used in conjunction with serum selenium to assess selenium nutrition or potential toxic exposure. Like any other 24-hour urine collection of an essential element, this reflects recent intake, assuming the patient is in selenium balance. In the case of selenium, skin and stool losses are significant and amount to 30% to 50% of total losses; nevertheless, urine losses often represent overflow losses and can help indicate whether recent intake has been adequate or possibly toxic. When selenium intake is low to normal, less than approximately 140 mcg/day, 24-hour urine may not reflect the 24-hour intake of the previous day. This is especially true when the body stores are low and selenium is retained to fill body stores. At higher levels of intake, the 24-hour urine is well correlated with intake and can be used as evidence of excess intake, adequate intake, or prior toxic exposure. Twenty-four hour urine selenium reflects recent intake. When selenium supplementation normalizes serum selenium and whole blood selenium, and then selenium supplementation is stopped, urine selenium falls back toward baseline much faster than blood or serum levels. Urine selenium has recently been found to be correlated with 24-hour urine urea in critically ill patients. This probably reflects catabolism of protein and release of body stores of selenium, though details of the selenium intake of the patients (proportional to protein intake in tube-fed patients) were not provided.

Specimen 24-hour urine

Container Acid-washed plastic urine container

Collection Avoid contamination by hair since some patients use selenium-containing shampoos.

Limitations Selenomethionine is incorporated into body protein nonspecifically as methionine, so it is not as quickly excreted in the urine as inorganic selenium (selenite). Thus, the form of selenium ingested will affect short-term balance estimates. Spot urine selenium is of little value, as urine selenium goes up after each meal related to selenium intake and probably other factors, and dilution in spot urine samples varies.

Methodology Fluorometry, atomic absorption (AA)

Additional Information In addition to serum and urine levels of selenium, red cell glutathione peroxidase can be monitored as an example of the activity of a seleno-enzyme. Levels will be depressed in deficiency but will not monitor toxicity.

Sertraline, Blood

Synonyms Zoloft®

Uses Antidepressant used when undesirable side effects noted with Prozac®; therapeutic monitoring and toxicity assessment

Reference Range Postmortem blood sertraline levels >1.5 mg/L may indicate that this drug was the cause of death; therapeutic clinical trials: sertraline: 0.03-0.19 mg/L

Abstract Antidepressant with fewer adverse side effects than Prozac®; metabolizes to desmethylsertraline which has 10% of the activity of sertraline

Specimen Blood

Volume 5 mL

Minimum Volume 1 mL serum or plasma

Container Red top tube

Methodology High performance liquid chromatography (HPLC), gas chromatography (GC), gas chromatography/mass spectrometry (GC/MS)

Silver, Serum

Synonyms Ag, Blood

Uses Evaluate silver toxicity

Reference Range Nondetectable

Specimen Blood

Volume 5 mL

Container Red top tube

Silver, Urine

Synonyms Ag, Urine

Uses Evaluate silver toxicity

Reference Range Negative

Patient Preparation Patient should be instructed to use a plastic urinal or bedpan is necessary.

Specimen 24-hour urine

Volume Entire collection

Minimum Volume 100 mL aliquot

Container Plastic urine container, no preservative

Collection Instruct the patient to void at 8 AM and discard the specimen. Then collect all urine including the final specimen voided at the end of the 24-hour collection period (ie, 8 AM the next morning). Avoid contact with

metal during collection. Screw the lid on securely. Transport the specimen promptly to the laboratory. Container **must** be labeled with patient's full name, room number, date and time collection started, and date and time collection finished.

Storage Instructions Keep on ice or refrigerate. Laboratory will measure urine volume and remove 120 mL aliquot.

Causes for Rejection Specimen allowed to contact metal

Special Instructions Requisition **must** state date and time collection started and date and time collection finished.

Stool Culture

Applies to Rectal Swab Culture; Routine Culture, Rectal Swab

Synonyms Enteric Pathogens Culture, Routine; Stool for Culture

Uses
Screen for common bacterial pathogenic organisms in the stool; diagnose typhoid fever, enteric fever, bacillary dysentery, *Salmonella* infection.
Indications for stool culture include: bloody diarrhea; fever; tenesmus; severe or persistent symptoms; recent travel to a third world country; known exposure to a bacterial agent; presence of fecal leukocytes

Contraindicating Factors A rectal swab culture is not as effective as a stool culture for detection of the carrier state.

Reference Range Negative for *Salmonella*, *Shigella*, and *Campylobacter*. In endemic areas the isolation of a pathogen may not indicate the cause or only cause of diarrhea.

Test Commonly Includes Screening culture for *Salmonella*, *Shigella*, *Helicobacter*, and, if requested, *Staphylococcus*.

Specimen Fresh random stool, rectal swab

Volume 5 mL

Container Plastic stool container, Culturette®

Collection
If stool is collected in a clean bedpan, it must not be contaminated with urine, residual soap, or disinfectants. Swabs of lesions of the rectal wall during proctoscopy or sigmoidoscopy are preferred.
Rectal swab: Insert the swab past the anal sphincter, move the swab circumferentially around the rectum. Allow 15-30 seconds for organisms to adsorb onto the swab. Withdraw swab, place in Culturette® tube, and crush media compartment.

Storage Instructions Refrigerate if the specimen cannot be processed promptly.

Causes for Rejection Because of risk to laboratory personnel, specimens sent on diaper or tissue paper, specimen contaminating outside of transport container may not be acceptable to the laboratory. Specimen containing interfering substances (eg, castor oil, bismuth, Metamucil®, barium), specimens delayed in transit and those contaminated with urine may not have optimal yield.

Special Instructions The laboratory should be informed of the specific pathogen suspected if not *Salmonella*, *Shigella*, or *Campylobacter*.

Limitations *Yersinia* species and *Vibrio* species may not be isolated unless specifically requested.

Methodology Aerobic culture on selective media

Additional Information Stool cultures on patients hospitalized ≥3 days **are not productive and should not be ordered** unless special circumstances exist.
In enteric fever caused by *Salmonella typhi*, *S. choleraesuis*, or *S. enteritidis*, blood culture may be positive before stool cultures, and blood cultures are indicated early. Diarrhea is common in patients with the acquired immunodeficiency syndrome (AIDS). Diarrhea in AIDS is frequently caused by the classic bacterial pathogens; however, parasitic infestation is also common with *Giardia* and *Cryptosporidium*. Rectal swabs are useful for the diagnosis of *Neisseria gonorrhoeae* and *Chlamydia* infections.
In acute or subacute diarrhea, three common syndromes are recognized: gastroenteritis, enteritis, and colitis (dysenteric syndrome). With colitis, patients have fecal urgency and tenesmus. Stool are frequently small in volume and contain blood, mucus, and leukocytes. External hemorrhoids are common and painful. Diarrhea of small bowel origin is indicated by the passage of few large volume stools. This is due to accumulation of fluid in the large bowel before passage. Leukocytes indicate colonic inflammation rather than a specific pathogen. Bacterial diarrhea may be present in the absence of fecal leukocytes and fecal leukocytes may be present in the absence of bacterial or parasitic agents (ie, idiopathic inflammatory bowel disease). See table. Although most bacterial diarrhea is transient (1-30 days) cases of persistent symptoms (10 months) have been reported. The etiologic agent in the reported case was *Shigella flexneri* diagnosed by culture of rectal swab. In infants younger than 1 year of age, a history of blood in the stool, more than 10 stools in 24 hours, and temperature greater than 39°C have a high probability of having bacterial diarrhea. See table.

Diarrhea Syndromes Classified by Predominant Features

Syndrome (anatomic site)	Features	Characteristic Etiologies
Gastroenteritis (stomach)	Vomiting	Rotavirus
		Norwalk virus
		Staphylococcal food poisoning
		Bacillus cereus food poisoning
Enteritis (small bowel)	Watery diarrhea Large-volume stools, few in number	Enterotoxigenic *Escherichia coli*
		Vibrio cholerae
		Any enteric microbe
		Inflammatory bowel disease
Dysentery, colitis (colon)	Small-volume stools containing blood and/or mucus and many leukocytes	*Shigella*
		Campylobacter
		Salmonella
		Invasive *E. coli*
		Plesiomonas shigelloides
		Aeromonas hydrophila
		Vibrio parahaemolyticus
		Clostridium difficile
		Entamoeba histolytica
		Inflammatory bowel disease

Strychnine, Quantitative

Uses Evaluate toxicity
Specimen Blood
Volume 15 mL
Minimum Volume 5 mL serum
Container Red top tube
Critical Values Toxic: >2.0 mcg/mL

Sulfhemoglobin

Uses Evaluate cyanosis
Reference Range None detectable
Specimen Blood
Volume 10 mL
Minimum Volume 1 mL whole blood
Container Amber top tube
Storage Instructions Maintain specimen at room temperature.
Methodology Spectrophotometry
Additional Information The term sulfhemoglobin refers to a poorly characterized hemoglobin derivative which can be produced *in vitro* from the action of hydrogen sulfide on hemoglobin. Sulfhemoglobinemia may occur in association with the administration of various drugs, including sulfonamides, phenacetin, metoclopramide, and acetanilide but has been reported also in the absence of exposure to drugs or toxins. The symptoms are few but the cyanosis is intense even though the concentration is seldom >10%. Once formed, sulfhemoglobin is stable and cannot be reduced back to hemoglobin. It disappears as the red cells become senescent and are destroyed. Measurement of sulfhemoglobin or sulfmethemoglobin levels are not clinically useful in hydrogen sulfide poisoning.

Thallium, Urine or Blood

Related Information
• Heavy Metal Screen, Blood
Uses Diagnose thallium toxicity in patients exposed to insecticides and rat poisons
Reference Range Urine: <10 mcg/24 hours; serum: <10 ng/mL (SI: <49 nmol/L)
Abstract Thallium salts are components of insecticides and rodenticides.
Patient Preparation The patient should be instructed to use a plastic bedpan or urinal if necessary
Specimen 24-hour urine, blood
Volume Entire collection
Container Plastic urine container, red top tube
Causes for Rejection Specimen allowed to contact metal
Methodology Atomic absorption spectrometry (AA)

Theophylline, Blood

Synonyms Aminophylline; Elixophyllin®; Slo-Phyllin®; Sustaire®; Theo-Dur®; Theolair™; Theospan®
Uses Monitor therapeutic drug level; detect noncompliance and subtherapeutic levels; attempt to predict theophylline toxicity if possible
Reference Range Therapeutic: 10-20 mcg/mL (SI: 56-111 µmol/L)
Abstract Theophylline is an antiasthmatic which is frequently monitored.
Specimen Blood
Volume 7 mL
Minimum Volume 3 mL serum
Container Red top tube
Sampling Time Measure **trough** (just before the next dose) and **peak**. Ideally, to measure peak serum theophylline **no** missed doses for previous 48 hours; blood drawn at 2 hours after most recent dose for rapid dissolution preparations; 4-6 hours after sustained release preparations.
Storage Instructions Refrigerate (do not freeze) a minimum of 0.5 mL serum.
Causes for Rejection Stored specimen not refrigerated
Possible Panic Range >20 mcg/mL (SI: >111 µmol/L); neonates: >10 mcg/mL (SI: >56 µmol/L); high probability of seizures when levels are >40 mcg/mL.
Methodology Enzyme immunoassay (EIA), high performance liquid chromatography (HPLC), gas chromatography (GC)
Additional Information Blood levels should be interpreted in light of the patient's clinical status and use of other medications. Acetazolamide can cause falsely elevated serum theophylline level by HPLC method.

Thiocyanate, Blood or Urine

Applies to Nitroprusside
U.S. Brand Names Nipride®
Synonyms Ethyl and Methyl Thiocyanate (Thanite® and Lethane®); Potassium Thiocyanate (KCN)
Uses Evaluate thiocyanate toxicity, nitroprusside poisoning, smoking. Toxic manifestations are psychotic behavior, agitation, and convulsions.
Reference Range Serum, therapeutic: 1-4 mcg/mL (SI: 0.02-0.07 mM/L), smokers: 3-12 mcg/mL (SI: 0.05-0.21 mM/L); urine: 1-4 mg/24 hours, smokers: 7-17 mg/24 hours
Abstract Thiocyanate is a metabolite of the antihypertensive drug, nitroprusside. It is also a product of cyanide metabolism.
Specimen Blood, urine
Volume 7 mL
Container Red top tube, lavender top (EDTA) tube, plastic urine container
Possible Panic Range Serum: >35 mcg/mL (SI: >0.60 mM/L); 200 mcg/mL (SI: 3.44 mM/L) is lethal
Limitations Because of rapid metabolism of the drug, results are usually meaningless in the clinical setting by the time they are reported.
Methodology Photometry/chromatography
Additional Information Thiocyanate is a major metabolite of cyanide produced in the liver by the enzyme rhodanase. Thiocyanate is present in healthy subjects. It is a component of cigarette smoke, and it can arise from the drug nitroprusside.

Thioridazine, Quantitative

Applies to Phenothiazines
Synonyms Mellaril®
Uses Monitor therapeutic drug level; evaluate toxicity
Reference Range <1 mcg/mL
Specimen Blood
Volume 15 mL
Minimum Volume 5 mL
Container Three yellow top (ACD) tubes
Collection Collect specimen immediately prior to next dose unless specified otherwise.
Storage Instructions Separate and refrigerate.
Critical Values 2 mcg/mL
Additional Information Thioridazine, a piperidine phenothiazine, is used to manage the manifestations of psychotic disorders, depressive neurosis, alcohol withdrawal, dementia in the elderly, and attention deficit disorders in children. Thioridazine shares many characteristics with chlorpromazine, but ECG changes and retinal pigmentation is more common than with chlorpromazine. Extrapyramidal effects are rare, and sedation and anticholinergic effects are more pronounced. The half-life is 26-36 hours. Adverse effects include anxiety, extrapyramidal reactions, pseudoparkinsonian signs and symptoms, seizures, hypotension, tachycardia and arrhythmias, agranulocytosis, leukopenia, amenorrhea, galactorrhea, and gynecomastia.

Thiothixene, Blood

Synonyms Navane®
Reference Range Therapeutic: 10-40 ng/mL
Specimen Blood
Volume 10 mL
Minimum Volume 3 mL serum
Container Red top tube
Storage Instructions Refrigerate serum.
Possible Panic Range >200 ng/mL
Methodology High performance liquid chromatography (HPLC)
Additional Information Thiothixene, a thioxanthene derivative, is used to manage psychotic disorders. It is similar pharmacologically and chemically to chlorprothixene and the piperazine phenothiazines. Therapeutic effects are achieved 1-6 hours after an I.M. injection and the half-life is 34 hours. Adverse effects include anticholinergic effects, tachycardia, hypotension, and ECG changes, drowsiness, insomnia, seizures, nonreversible tardive dyskinesia, gynecomastia, amenorrhea, and transient leukopenia.

Toxicology Drug Screen, Blood

Related Information
- Toxicology Drug Screen, Urine

Applies to Comatose Profile
Synonyms Drug Screen, Comprehensive Panel or Analysis
Uses Monitor toxic/overdose situations; most desirable to analyze in conjunction with urine toxicology testing; used to quantitate drug identified qualitatively in urine
Test Commonly Includes Amobarbital, butabarbital, butalbital, chlordiazepoxide, diazepam, ethchlorvynol, glutethimide, meprobamate, methaqualone, pentobarbital, phenobarbital, secobarbital, ethanol, methanol, acetone, isopropanol, acetaminophen, phenytoin, salicylates, tricyclics, other drugs could also be analyzed.
Abstract This toxicology screen is carried out by performing individual quantitative tests for each drug. Many times urine qualitative screening is faster and more useful in toxicologic emergencies but both may be needed. Recent introduction of systems such as the Remedi® make an automated approach to this screen possible.
Specimen Blood
Volume 10 mL
Minimum Volume 5 mL serum or plasma
Container Red top tube or lavender top (EDTA) tube; do **not** collect blood in heparinized tubes.
Causes for Rejection Specimen collected in heparinized tube
Limitations Evidence for presence of a drug/drug metabolite (screening, qualitative) in the case of most groups of therapeutic agents and drugs of abuse will be found in urine rather than serum. See Toxicology Drug Screen, Urine. **All agents identified in a screening test should be confirmed with a specific test.**
Methodology Immunoassay, thin-layer chromatography (TLC), gas chromatography (GC), high performance liquid chromatography (HPLC), colorimetry, spectrophotometry
Additional Information If only documentation of exposure to toxic drugs or drugs of abuse is desired, a urine drug screen is the most economical approach. See listing for Toxicology Drug Screen, Urine. When Toxicology Drug Screen, Blood is ordered, the individual drugs are quantitated in serum. When Toxicology Drug Screen, Urine is ordered, qualitative identification is carried out.

Toxicology Drug Screen, Gastric

Synonyms Gastric Aspirate, Drug Screen
Uses Detect drug abuse; evaluate toxicity
Reference Range None detected
Test Commonly Includes Amobarbital, amphetamine, butabarbital, codeine, heroin (as morphine), meperidine, methadone, methamphetamine, pentobarbital, phencyclidine (PCP), phenobarbital, phenothiazines, propoxyphene, quinine, secobarbital
Specimen Gastric aspirate
Volume 50 mL
Minimum Volume 30 mL
Container Plastic urine container
Special Instructions Specify the drug or drugs suspected.
Methodology Thin-layer chromatography (TLC)

Toxicology Drug Screen, Urine

Related Information
- Toxicology Drug Screen, Blood

Applies to Narcotics Drug Screen, Urine
Synonyms Abuse Screen; DAU-10; DAU; Drug Screen, Comprehensive Panel or Analysis, Urine; Pre-employment Drug Screen
Uses Screen for drug of abuse, drug overdose/toxicity alone, or in conjunction with serum/plasma testing

Reference Range None detected or negative (less than cutoff for drugs of abuse)
Test Commonly Includes A variety of qualitative screens are in use. Sensitivity and specificity vary and are method dependent. Screens should detect drugs (qualitatively) in the following classes: amphetamines, analgesics, anticonvulsants, antidepressants, antihistamines, cardiacs, narcotics, sedative/hypnotics, tranquilizers, volatiles, and drugs of abuse. Screens for common classes of abused drugs: Amphetamines, barbiturates, benzodiazepines, cannabinoids, cocaine, methadone, methaqualone, opiates, phencyclidine, propoxyphene. In some laboratories, urine ethanol is included.
Abstract This is a qualitative screen which, in the case of thin-layer chromatography or automated high performance liquid chromatography, can detect any of several hundred drugs. The usual drug-of-abuse screening panel consists of the 10 drugs listed above under "test includes".
Specimen Random urine.
Volume 50-100 mL
Minimum Volume 50 mL
Container Plastic urine container
Collection If forensic, observe precautions.
Storage Instructions Keep refrigerated
Causes for Rejection If forensic, failure to meet temperature requirements and tests for unusual urine dilution or alteration
Special Instructions Specify the drug or drugs suspected; if forensic, use chain-of-custody protocol and form
Limitations Test provides **only** qualitative detection of drugs, unless laboratory automatically confirms and quantitates drugs detected as a part of the "screening" procedure. Quantitation of urine drug levels is usually not included and is not recommended because urine levels are time and clearance dependent and are not directly related to toxic symptoms seen clinically. Some drugs and/or metabolites are not detected or optimally detected in urine, again relating to method. Serum may be preferable because of clinical, and at times technical/kinetic, factors (eg, barbiturates, phenytoin). Sensitivity is of the order of 0.5-1.0 mcg/mL for TLC of urine. Some substances should be quantitated in blood or serum (eg, iron overdose, methanol, acetaminophen, salicylate, carbon monoxide, ethanol, digoxin, lithium, theophylline, and methemoglobin). Ofloxacin can cause the EMIT II drug screen to become positive for opiates.

In a nonclinical setting (eg, pre-employment drug screening, etc), the sample should be collected under chain-of-custody, and all positive screens must be confirmed by a different, more sensitive method, preferably GC/MS. The transportation industry [Department of Transportation (DOT)] tests certain employees by screening for five classes of drugs only (amphetamines, cannabinoids, cocaine, opiates, phencyclidine) and confirms all positive results with GC/MS. National Institute on Drug Abuse (NIDA) certification required to perform tests for DOT. (See Federal Register 49(40), December 19, 2000 at www.dot.gov/ost/dapc.) Chain-of-custody protocol must be followed for these specimens. Any agent identified in a screening test **should be confirmed** by a test specific for that drug (usually GC/MS).
Methodology A variety of methods or combination of methods are in fairly common use and include thin-layer chromatography (TLC), colorimetry/spectrophotometry, enzyme immunoassay technique (EIA), enzyme-multiplied immunoassay technique (EMIT), gas chromatography (GC), gas chromatography/mass spectrometry (GC/MS), high performance liquid chromatography (HPLC).
Additional Information

Some toxins (eg, metals, volatiles, gaseous compounds) may require specific methodology (eg, atomic absorption spectrophotometry, gas chromatography). Lactate dehydrogenase and lactate can cause false-positive serum ethanol screen (by EMIT) in the postmortem state. Postmortem urinary lactate dehydrogenase levels (>592 units/L) and lactate levels (>12 mM) and proteinuria can lead to false positive results on drugs of abuse screening by enzyme-multiplied immunoassay techniques (EMIT) and are unlikely to be of clinical significance in living samples. Aspirin or bleach can cause a reduction of immunoassay signal.

Causes of false positive tricyclic antidepressant urine drug screens include cyclobenzaprine, diphenhydramine, cyproheptadine, carbamazepine, thioridazine, and quetiapine.

Mean confirmation rates for initial urinary immunoassay are for:

	Range
Cocaine metabolite	98.1% (91.1 to 99.9%)
Opiates	30.2% (17.3 to 55.9%)
Phencyclidine	69.7% (51.6 to 91%)
Marijuana metabolite	91% (73 to 98.8%)
Amphetamine	
Screened once	51.9% (37.4 to 77.8%)
Screened twice	82.8% (81.3 to 84.3%)

Specific References
ACOEM: MRO update: Immunoassay Confirmation Rates. Nov/Dec 2004: 3-4.
Bjornaas MA, Hovda KE, Mikalsen H, et al, "Clinical vs Laboratory Identification of Drugs of Abuse in Patients Admitted for Acute Poisoning," *Clin Toxicol*, 2006, 44:127-34.

Brazwell E, Crossey M, Racz M, et al, "Urine Adulterant Test for Oxidants Yields Positive Results from Microbial-Contaminated Urine," *J Anal Toxicol*, 2004, 28(8):692-3.

Burrows DL, Nicolaides A, Rice PJ, et al, "Papain: A Novel Urine Adulterant," *J Anal Toxicol*, 2005, 29(5):275-395.

Feldman M, Kuntz D, Botelho K, et al, "Evaluation of Roche Diagnostics ONLINE® DAT II, A New Generation of Assays for the Detection of Drugs of Abuse," *J Anal Toxicol*, 2004, 28:593-8.

Gantverg A, Feldman M, Kuntz D, et al, "Simultaneous Screening of 26 Drugs in Urine by Liquid Chromatogrpahy-Tandem Mass Spectrometry," *J Anal Toxicol*, 2006, 30:130.

Maloney G and Casavant MJ, "The Utility of Comprehensive Send-Out Toxicology Screening in Pediatric Emergency Department Patients," *J Toxicol Clin Toxicol*, 2004, 42(5):747.

Maloney G, Casavant MJ, and Marcon M, "Send-Out Comprehensive Toxicology Screens Increase Length of Stay Without Affecting Disposition," *J Toxicol Clin Toxicol*, 2004, 42(5):746-7.

Ojanpera I, Pelander A, Laks S, et al, "Application of Accurate Mass Measurement to Urine Drug Screening," *J Anal Toxicol*, 2005, 29:34-40.

Paul BD, "Six Spectroscopic Methods for Detection of Oxidants in Urine: Implication in Differentiation of Normal and Adulterated Urine," *J Anal Toxicol*, 2004, 28:599-608.

Schaff JE, Montgomery MA, and Morris-Kukoski CL, "Validation of Commercial ELISA Immunoassay Kits Beyond Manufacturer Specifications," *J Anal Toxicol*, 2006, 30:131.

Sutheimer CA, et al, "Confirmation Rates of Initial Drug Assays in a Group of HHS-Certified Laboratories", January 1 to December 31, 2003-II. Non-Regulated Specimens Joint Meeting of the Society of Forensic Toxicologists and the International Association of Forensic Toxicologists Washington, DC 2004.

Toxicology Studies, Not Specifically Listed

Synonyms Drug Analysis, Not Specifically Listed; Drug Levels, Not Specifically Listed
Uses Confirm toxicity due to a specific drug; detect drug abuse
Contraindicating Factors Suspect drug identity doubtful or unknown
Reference Range None detected
Specimen Blood, urine, gastric washings
Volume 30 mL blood, 100 mL urine, 100 mL gastric washings
Minimum Volume As much of specified volume as possible
Container Gray top (sodium fluoride) tube, plastic urine container, 100 mL plastic gastric washing bottle
Special Instructions Specify the drug or drugs suspected.
Limitations Analysis will be limited to those drugs specifically requested. Toxicologic screening for drugs is extremely expensive and seldom results in modification of the patients therapy. The potential effect of the data obtained on the patients course and therapy should be carefully considered before the studies are requested.

Toxicology, Steroid Drug Screen, Urine

Synonyms Steroid Drug Screen, Urine
Uses Detect anabolic steroid use in athletes
Test Commonly Includes Anabolic steroids screen and testosterone/epitestosterone ratio; confirmation of positive results is available.
Patient Preparation Sample collection should be observed and specimen chain of custody should be documented.
Specimen Random urine
Volume 100 mL
Minimum Volume 50 mL
Container Glass bottle
Collection Freshly voided random urine
Special Instructions Specify the drug or drugs suspected.
Methodology Chromatography

Toxicology, Stimulant Panel, Urine

Synonyms Urine Stimulant Drug Screen
Uses Detect drug abuse; evaluate toxicity
Reference Range None detected
Test Commonly Includes Qualitative identification of D-amphetamine, methamphetamine, phentermine, phenmetrazine, phenylpropanolamine, cocaine, phencyclidine
Specimen Random urine
Volume 30 mL
Minimum Volume 20 mL
Container Plastic urine container
Collection Freshly voided random urine
Special Instructions Specify the drug or drugs suspected.
Limitations This test provides **only** qualitative detection of drugs. Quantitation of urine drug levels is not included and is not recommended because urine levels are time and clearance dependent and are not directly related to toxic symptoms seen clinically.
Methodology Enzyme immunoassay (EIA), gas chromatography (GC)

Toxicology, Opiates Drug Screen, Urine with Confirmation

Uses Detect drug abuse; evaluate toxicity
Test Commonly Includes Codeine, Darvon®, Demerol®, Dolophine®, heroin, meperidine, methadone, morphine, oxycodone, pentazocine, Percodan®, propoxyphene, Talwin®
Specimen Random urine
Volume 50 mL
Minimum Volume 10 mL aliquot
Container Plastic urine container
Collection Freshly voided random urine
Storage Instructions Refrigerate
Special Instructions Specify the drug or drugs suspected.
Critical Values Toxic propoxyphene: 0.4-14.0 mcg/mL
Limitations This test provides **only** qualitative detection of drugs. Quantitation of urine drug levels is not included and is not recommended because urine levels are time and clearance dependent and are not directly related to toxic symptoms seen clinically.
Methodology Thin-layer chromatography (TLC) and enzyme immunoassay (EIA), gas chromatography (GC) for confirmation
Additional Information
Opiates in general are a group of drugs (commonly referred to as narcotics) which are used medically to relieve pain, but which also have a high potential for abuse.

A qualitative urine screen for opiates is performed in suspected overdose cases or as part of a drug of abuse program. The test is most sensitive for morphine and codeine but other drugs will cross react in an immunoassay and give positive results (eg, hydrocodone, hydromorphone). All presumptive positive assays are confirmed by GC/MS. Morphine is a prescribed drug for pain relief, a metabolite of heroin, a metabolite of codeine and a constituent of poppy seeds. Its presence in urine, even after confirmation must be interpreted very carefully.

Opiates tend to relax the user. When the opiates are injected, the user feels an immediate "rush." Other initial and unpleasant effects include restlessness, nausea, and vomiting. The user may go "on the nod," going back and forth from feeling alert to drowsy. With very large doses, the user cannot be awakened, pupils become smaller, and the skin becomes cold, moist, and bluish in color. Furthermore, breathing slows down and death may occur. Clearance may be slower in geriatric patients.

Trazodone, Blood

Synonyms Desyrel® Level, Blood
Uses Therapeutic monitoring; toxicity assessment
Reference Range Therapeutic: 0.5-2.5 mcg/mL (SI: 1-6 µmol/L)
Abstract This drug is an antidepressant chemically unrelated to the tricyclic or tetracyclic antidepressants.
Specimen Blood
Container Red top tube or green top (heparin) tube
Sampling Time Trough: just before next dose
Critical Values >2.5 mcg/mL (SI: >6 µmol/L)
Possible Panic Range 4 mcg/mL (SI: 10 µmol/L)
Methodology High performance liquid chromatography (HPLC), gas chromatography (GC)
Additional Information Trazodone is a structurally unique antidepressant that is pharmacologically different from other drugs of this class. The toxicities observed in tricyclic overdose (neuro- and cardiotoxicity and respiratory depression) are not seen with trazodone. Chronic toxicity is very low with trazodone although it does have unique side effects including akathisia, allergic reactions, chest pain, delayed urine flow, early and delayed menses, hypersalivation and hypomania, among others. The half-life of trazodone is 4-7 hours, peak plasma concentrations with average daily dosing is reached in 2-4 hours.

Tricyclic Antidepressants, Blood

Related Information
● Donor Victims of Poisoning in Whom Transplantation of Organs Occurred
Synonyms Antidepressants; TAD; TCA; Tetracyclic Antidepressants
Uses Therapeutic monitoring; toxicity assessment
Contraindicating Factors Patient taking more than one tricyclic antidepressant, patient taking phenothiazines or monoamine oxidase inhibitors
Reference Range
Therapeutic:
● amitriptyline: 100-250 ng/mL (SI: 360-900 nmol/L)
● amoxapine: 50-400 ng/mL
● desipramine: 150-300 ng/mL (SI: 563-1126 nmol/L)
● doxepin: 100-200 ng/mL (SI: 360-720 nmol/L)
● imipramine: 75-250 ng/mL (SI: 279-890 nmol/L)

- maprotiline: 150-400 ng/mL (SI: 541-1442 nmol/L)
- nortriptyline: 50-150 ng/mL (SI: 190-570 nmol/L)
- protriptyline: 50-150 ng/mL (SI: 190-570 nmol/L)
- trazodone: 300-1600 ng/mL

Abstract Drugs in this class are widely used as antidepressants. They are frequently involved in suicidal ingestion and responsible for a large percentage of drug-related deaths.

Specimen Blood

Volume 7 mL

Container Red top tube, green top (heparin) tube; avoid serum separator tubes and the plasticizer, TBEP.

Sampling Time Steady-state specimen after 1 week of dose schedule; draw specimen 12 hours after the last dose.

Storage Instructions Remove serum within 2 hours of drawing; refrigerate or freeze if not analyzed immediately.

Special Instructions Order individual drug level or tricyclic overdose screen

Possible Panic Range >500 ng/mL; toxicity observed at ≥300 ng/mL

Limitations Immunoassays for tricyclic antidepressants (toxic overdose) do not distinguish between parent compounds and active metabolites. Immunoassays are available for amitriptyline, nortriptyline, desipramine, and imipramine. Drug-drug interactions occur; hydrocortisone, neuroleptics, methylphenidate, cimetidine, and oral contraceptives produce higher levels by inhibiting metabolism of tricyclics by the liver. Barbiturates, chloral hydrate, and glutethimide lower plasma tricyclic levels by stimulating liver microsomal activity. Cigarette smoking also lowers steady-state plasma levels, apparently by a similar hepatic enzyme induction mechanism. Red blood cell metabolite assays may be a more sensitive biomarker for cardiac conduction disturbances.

Methodology Immunoassay, gas chromatography (GC), gas chromatography/mass spectrometry (GC/MS), high performance liquid chromatography (HPLC)

Additional Information
Tricyclic antidepressants (TADs) are metabolized to secondary active compounds. These agents are useful in treating clinical depression, and enuresis (imipramine). However, they show a narrow therapeutic window, and great individual variations in blood levels associated with dosage. Blacks usually have 50% greater blood level than whites for same dose schedule. Symptoms of overdose may mimic those of condition for which agent was prescribed. The most important of the more serious or toxic effects of TADs is cardiotoxicity. Arrhythmias and conduction defects with precipitation of congestive heart failure and possibly myocardial infarction are common at combined levels >1000 ng/mL. Widening of the QRS interval to >100 msec is highly suggestive of a TAD overdose.

Tricyclic antidepressant drugs represent a frequent and serious problem in both unintentional and intentional overdosage. Reports of poor correlations between plasma levels and toxic clinical manifestations indicate that QRS duration >100 msec may provide the most reliable indicator of toxicity. It has been reported that levels of parent to metabolite (P/M) ratios >2 are associated with acute overdosage. In contrast, P/M ratios <2 are more consistent with high steady-state plasma levels following "therapeutic" dosages although plasma levels or other clinical evidence of toxicity may be present. Variations in blood levels between doses are comparatively small. Peak levels occur 4-8 hours after oral ingestion. A level dose of medication should be prescribed for at least 2 weeks to obtain steady plasma levels. Monitoring of tricyclic antidepressant plasma levels is useful in a number of situations. Older patients may develop higher steady-state plasma levels than younger individuals. In geriatric patients conventional doses may lead to toxic levels. Toxic plasma levels of tricyclic drugs may be dangerous in cardiac disease patients. Recommended lower and higher plasma levels for the different tricyclic drugs are evolving and are discussed in the literature.

Thyroxine, Blood

Synonyms T$_4$ (RIA); T$_4$ by EIA; T$_4$; Tetraiodothyronine; Thyroxine by RIA

Uses Best general thyroid function screening test. **Decreased** in hypothyroidism, in genetically decreased TBG, and in the third stage of (painful) subacute thyroiditis; **increased** with hyperthyroidism, with subacute thyroiditis in its first stage, with thyrotoxicosis due to Graves' disease, with increased TBG (pregnancy, genetically increased TBG, acute intermittent porphyria, primary biliary cirrhosis), thyrotoxicosis factitia, and occasionally in euthyroid patients with familial dysalbuminemic hyperthyroxinemia. Used to diagnose T$_4$ thyrotoxicosis.

Primary hypothyroidism (hypometabolism) is caused by Hashimoto's thyroiditis, idiopathic myxedema, prior radioactive iodine therapy for hyperthyroidism, prior thyroid surgery, endemic goiter and other entities. Congenital causes include enzyme blocks and agenesis. Causes of **secondary hypothyroidism** include primary pituitary disease (eg, postpartum pituitary necrosis (Sheehan's syndrome) and pituitary tumors). The expression "myxedema" indicates advanced clinical hypothyroidism, with dermal mucopolysaccharide deposits. Comprehensive lists of causes of hypothyroidism are published. A diagnosis of primary hypothyroidism should be confirmed by a TSH assay.

Graves' disease is classical thyrotoxicosis (hypermetabolism) caused by an immune or autoimmune disorder. Other causes of **hyperthyroidism** include toxic multinodular or uninodular goiter, phases of thyroiditis and a number of uncommon to rare entities, which cause increased T$_4$. Tabulations of causes of hyperthyroidism are widely available.

T$_4$ and other tests are used to investigate goiter, an expression for thyroid enlargement, which may be found with hypothyroidism, euthyroidism, or hyperthyroidism.

Reference Range
Pediatrics: Cord T$_4$ and values in the first few weeks are much higher, falling over the first months and years; 10 years and older: approximately 5.8-11.0 mcg/dL (SI: 75-142 nmol/L), varying somewhat between laboratories. Borderline low is ≤4.5-5.7 mcg/dL (SI: ≤58-73 nmol/L); low is ≤4.4 mcg/dL (SI: ≤57 nmol/L); results <2.5 mcg/dL (SI: <32 nmol/L) are strong evidence for hypothyroidism.

Approximate adult normal range is given by Ingbar as 4.0-12.0 mcg/dL (SI: 51-154 nmol/L) and by Larsen as 5.0-11.0 mcg/dL (SI: 64-142 nmol/L); borderline high is 11.1-13.0 mcg/dL (SI: 143-167 nmol/L); high is ≥13.1 mcg/dL (SI: ≥169 nmol/L). High is sometimes given as ≥8-10 mcg/dL (SI: ≥103-129 nmol/L). Normal range is increased in women on birth control pills, owing to increased TBG. Free thyroxine index will still be within the normal range. Normal range in pregnancy: approximately 5.5-16.0 mcg/dL (SI: 71-206 nmol/L).

Drug Interactions Decreased serum concentration with concomitant ritonavir

Abstract Thyroxine (T$_4$) is the major secretory product of the thyroid gland. It is carried through the blood bound (in equilibrium) to thyroxine binding globulin (TBG), prealbumin, and albumin. T$_4$ secretion is stimulated by thyroid stimulating hormone (TSH).

Patient Preparation Avoid radioisotope administration prior to collection of specimen.

Specimen Blood

Volume 7 mL

Minimum Volume 1 mL serum

Container Red top tube

Storage Instructions Separate serum within 48 hours and refrigerate. Separated serum stable 1 week at 25°C.

Possible Panic Range At values <2.0 mcg/dL (SI: <26 nmol/L), myxedema coma is possible. At values >20.0 mcg/dL (SI: >257 nmol/L), thyroid storm is possible.

Limitations
T$_4$ may be increased with excess intake of iodine or or with surreptitious use of thyroxine. T$_4$ levels may be abnormal in the presence of systemic nonthyroidal disease. Alterations in binding capacity or quantity of TBG may increase or decrease total thyroxine without causing symptoms. A common cause of elevated T$_4$ in nonthyroidal disease is said to be liver disease.

Serum thyroxine and free thyroxine (FT$_4$) are increased in familial dysalbuminemic hyperthyroxinemia, a euthyroid syndrome in which an abnormal binding site has affinity for thyroxine. The T$_3$ is usually normal in this entity, as is T$_3$ uptake. Thus, T$_3$ uptake is commonly ordered with T$_4$. T$_4$ is less sensitive than TSH in the diagnosis of hypothyroidism.

Euthyroid hyperthyroxinemia has been reviewed. It is an expression used as a collective term for nonthyroidal diseases and states which increase thyroxine levels with normal thyroid tissue and metabolism. In addition to thyroid hormone binding globulin changes and drug related phenomena, peripheral resistance to thyroid hormones and increases related to medical and acute psychiatric illness are described. Hyperemesis gravidarum and hyponatremia may cause euthyroid hyperthyroxinemia. Extensive tabulations of thyroid tests and some causes of changes in them have been published.

Anti-T$_4$ antibodies may exist, interfering with T$_4$ and free T$_4$ determinations. Heparin can cause false readings by interfering with assays.

Methodology Radioimmunoassay (RIA), enzyme-linked immunosorbent assay (ELISA), fluorescence polarization immunoassay (FPIA), chemiluminescence assay (CIA)

Additional Information
The combination of the serum T$_4$ and T$_3$ uptake as an assessment of TBG, helps to determine whether an abnormal T$_4$ value is due to alterations in serum thyroxine binding globulin or to changes of thyroid hormone levels. Deviations of both tests in the same direction usually indicate that an abnormal T$_4$ is due to abnormalities in thyroid hormone. Deviations of the two tests in opposite directions provide evidence that an abnormal T$_4$ may relate to alterations in TBG. See table.

Thyroid Tests with Disease and Varying TBG

Diagnosis	T$_4$	FT$_4$ (or FT$_4$ I)	TSH
Normal	Normal	Normal	Normal
Hyperthyroid	Increased	Increased	Decreased
Hypothyroid	Decreased	Decreased	Increased
Increased TBG	Increased	Normal	Normal
Decreased TBG	Decreased	Normal	Normal

Causes of increased TBG binding include neonatal state, molar and conventional pregnancy, estrogens, oral contraceptives, heroin, methadone, 5-fluorouracil, clofibrate, infectious hepatitis, chronic active hepatitis, and primary biliary cirrhosis, acute intermittent porphyria, lymphoma, and hereditary TBG increase.

Causes of decreased TBG binding include abnormal protein states. These include nephrotic syndrome, androgens, anabolic steroids, prednisone, acromegaly, liver or other systemic illness, severe stress, and hereditary TBG deficiency. Salicylates and diphenylhydantoin may lower T_4 significantly. Amiodarone may cause increased thyroxine levels and can cause hypothyroidism or hyperthyroidism.

Lithium carbonate may cause goiter with or without hypothyroidism.

Carbamazepine (Tegretol®) is reported to cause decreased values in thyroid function tests.

This brief review must point out that clinical interpretation of patients' signs and symptoms has primary significance. Definitive treatment based on insufficient laboratory tests is condemned.

The sensitive TSH assay has been advocated as a single screening test for thyroid disease. Such proposals are controversial; others find it difficult to accept one test as adequate for screening and warn that a single test cannot adequately, in all settings, reflect thyroid status. An inverse relationship exists between thyroxine and TSH. While the former represents thyroid hormone concentration, the latter is a test of thyroid regulation.

Agents that interfere with the TSH assay resulting in falsely low TSH levels include dopamine, levodopa, bromocriptine, dexamethasone (>0.5 mg/day), hydrocortisone (>100 mg/day), octreotide, and amphetamines.

Agents that produce falsely elevated TSH values (usually <10 units/L) include metoclopramide (>1 mg/kg), amiodarone, and iodinated radiographic contrast media (ipodate, iopanic acid, tyropanoate).

Agents which cause a falsely increased free thyroxine level include intravenous furosemide (>80 mg/day), salicylates (>2 g/day), salsalate (>1.5 g/day), diclofenac, naproxen, I.V. heparin (producing a five-fold increase in free thyroxine), amiodarone, and iodinated contrast media.

Agents which produce sustained reductions of both free thyroxine and free triiodothyronine levels include phenytoin and carbamazepine - at therapeutic levels.

Specific Reference

Lo DK, Szeto CC, and Chan TY, "Mild Symptoms of Toxicity Following Deliberate Ingestion of Thyroxine," *Vet Hum Toxicol*, 2004, 46(4):192-3.

Urea Nitrogen, Blood

Synonyms Blood Urea Nitrogen; BUN

Uses

High BUN occurs in chronic glomerulonephritis, pyelonephritis, and other causes of chronic renal disease; with acute renal failure, decreased renal perfusion (prerenal azotemia) as in shock. With urinary tract obstruction BUN increases (postrenal azotemia), for example as caused by neoplastic infiltration of the ureters, hyperplasia, or carcinoma of the prostate. BUN is useful to follow hemodialysis and other therapy. "Uremia" was defined by Luke as an expression of a constellation of signs and symptoms in patients with severe azotemia secondary to acute or chronic renal failure. Causes of increased BUN include severe congestive heart failure, increased protein catabolism, tetracyclines with diuretic use, hyperalimentation, ketoacidosis, and dehydration as in diabetes mellitus, but even moderate dehydration can cause BUN to increase. Corticosteroids tend to increase BUN by causing increased protein catabolism. Bleeding from the GI tract is an important cause of high urea nitrogen, commonly accompanied by elevation of BUN/creatinine ratio. Nephrotoxic drugs must be considered. Chloral hydrate or chloramphenicol can cause false elevation. Steroids and tetracycline can stimulate a catabolic response resulting in high BUN without renal impairment.

Borderline high values may occur after recent ingestion of high protein meal and muscle wasting may cause an elevation as well.

With creatinine, BUN is used to monitor patients on dialysis.

Low BUN occurs in late normal pregnancy, decreased protein intake, with intravenous fluids, with some antibiotics, and in severe liver damage.

As described by DeCaux et al in 1980, in the syndrome of inappropriate secretion of antidiuretic hormone (SIADH), findings include hyponatremia with serum or plasma sodium ≤128 mM/L, serum hypo-osmolality, <260 mOsm/kg, with urine osmolality >300 mOsm/kg (SI: >300 mM/kg) with low BUN. Such findings occur in situations in which patients are overhydrated. Clinical findings included absence of edema or evidence of heart, liver, thyroid, renal or adrenal disease. Hypouricemia, with uric acid levels in 16 of 17 patients <4 mg/dL (SI: <238 μmol/L), is reported with the syndrome of inappropriate secretion of antidiuretic hormone. SIADH can be seen with higher serum sodiums and higher osmolalities. Urine osmolality is greater than serum osmolality in SIADH. Chloramphenicol or streptomycin can cause false depression.

Osmolality (mOsm/kg H_2O) may be calculated as follows: Osmolality = [Na^+ (mM/L) × 2] + urea N (mg/dL)/2.8 + glucose (mg/dL)/18.

Reference Range Birth to 1 year: 4-16 mg/dL (SI: 1.4-5.7 mM/L); 1-40 years: 5-20 mg/dL (SI: 1.8-7.1 mM/L); gradual slight increase subsequently occurs >40 years of age.

Abstract Urea nitrogen reflects the ratio between urea **production** and **clearance**. Increased BUN may be due to increased production or decreased excretion. Although we commonly use the expression "BUN," most laboratories use serum, occasionally plasma but never whole blood.

Specimen Blood

Volume 10 mL

Minimum Volume 3 mL serum or plasma

Container Red top tube. Avoid fluoride and sodium citrate tubes if urease reaction is used and ammonium heparin tubes when conductometric method is used. EDTA is suitable as well as lithium heparin for young children.

Collection Pediatrics: Blood drawn from heelstick for capillary (lithium heparin tube)

Storage Instructions Stable 1 day at room temperature, 3 days at 4°C to 8°C, and 3 months at ~20°C.

Possible Panic Range BUN >100 mg/dL (SI: >35.7 mM/L) has been used in the definition of uremia.

Limitations Uremia is best evaluated with creatinine as well as urea nitrogen. In both prerenal and postrenal azotemia, for instance, BUN is apt to be increased somewhat more than is creatinine. In chronic progressive renal disease, ~75% of renal parenchyma must be damaged or destroyed before azotemia develops. BUN lacks sensitivity and specificity, but still remains a useful test.

Methodology Diacetyl monoxime; urease, Berthelot reaction; rate conductivity

Additional Information Although creatinine is generally considered a more specific test to evaluate renal function, they are commonly used together. Luke points out that clinical renal failure is variable between individual patients. Drug effects have been summarized.

Urinalysis

Applies to Casts, Urine

Synonyms UA

Uses Screen for abnormalities of urine; diagnose and manage renal diseases, urinary tract infection, urinary tract neoplasms, systemic diseases, and inflammatory or neoplastic diseases adjacent to the urinary tract

Reference Range

Crystals are interpreted by the physician. Warm, freshly voided urine sediment from normal subjects almost never contains crystals, despite maximal concentration. Xanthine, cystine, and uric acid crystal (and stone) formation is favored by a consistently acid urine (pH <5.5-6). Calcium oxalate and apatite stones are associated with no particular disturbance of urine pH. Calcium carbonate, calcium phosphate, and especially magnesium ammonium phosphate stones are associated with pH >7. Urine pH >7.5 may briefly follow meals (alkaline tide) but more commonly indicate systemic alkali intake ($NaHCO_3$, etc) or urine infected by bacteria which split urea to ammonia. See table.

Urinalysis	
Test	**Reference Range**
Specific gravity	1.003-1.029
pH	4.5-7.8
Protein	Negative
Glucose	Negative
Ketones	Negative
Bilirubin	Negative
Occult blood	Negative
Leukocyte esterase	Negative
Nitrite	Negative
Urobilinogen	0.1-1.0 EU/dL
WBCs	0-4/hpf
RBCs	male: 0-3/hpf female: 0-5/hpf
Casts	0-4/lpf hyaline
Bacteria	Negative

hpf = high power field
lpf = low power field
EU = Ehrlich units

Diagnostic Procedures

- Crystals, Urine

Test Commonly Includes Opacity, color, appearance, specific gravity, pH, protein, glucose, occult blood, ketones, bilirubin, and in some laboratories, urobilinogen and microscopic examination of urine sediment. Some laboratories include screening for leukocyte esterase and nitrite and do not perform a microscopic examination unless one of the chemical screening (macroscopic) tests is abnormal or unless a specific request for microscopic examination is made.

Abstract The examination of urine is one of the oldest practices in medicine. A carefully performed urinalysis still provides a wealth of information about the patient, both in terms of differential diagnosis, and by exclusion of many conditions when the urinalysis is "normal."

Patient Preparation Instructions should be given in method of collection. Both males and females need instruction in cleansing the urethral meatus. "Midstream collections" are performed by initiating urination into the toilet, then bringing the collection device into the urine stream to catch the midportion of the void.

Specimen Urine

Volume 5 mL

Minimum Volume 2 mL

Container Plastic urine container

Collection A voided specimen is usually suitable. If the specimen is likely to be contaminated by vaginal discharge or hemorrhage, a clean catch specimen is desirable. If the specimen is collected by catheter, it should be so labeled. The timing of urine collection will vary with the purpose of the test. To check for casts or renal concentration ability, a first voided morning specimen may be preferred. For screening purposes, this is also the best time, as a later and more dilute specimen may make small increases in protein, RBC, or WBC excretion harder to detect. The upright position increases protein excretion by hemodynamic factors. Midmorning urine is likely to give the highest albumin excretion, but early morning urine is best when attempting to detect Bence Jones protein.

Storage Instructions Transport specimen to the laboratory as soon as possible after collection. If the specimen cannot be processed immediately by the laboratory it should be refrigerated. Refrigeration preserves formed elements in the urine, but may precipitate crystals not originally present.

Causes for Rejection Specimen delayed in transport, fecal contamination, decomposition, or bacterial overgrowth

Possible Panic Range The presence of massive amounts of oxalate crystals in fresh urine should be reported promptly to the physician, as this finding may represent ethylene glycol intoxication.

Limitations Insufficient volume, less than 2 mL, may limit the extent of procedures performed. Metabolites of Pyridium® may interfere with the dipstick reactions by producing color interference. High vitamin C intake may cause an underestimate of glucosuria, or a false-negative nitrate test. Survival of WBCs is decreased by low osmolality, alkalinity, and lack of refrigeration. Formed elements in the urine including casts disintegrate rapidly, therefore the specimen should be analyzed as soon as possible after collection. Specific gravity is affected by glucosuria, mannitol infusion, or prior administration of iodinated contrast material for radiologic studies (IVP dye). Some brands of test strips give a "trace positive" protein indication if not stored in dry atmosphere (cap of test strip bottle not on tight). Ambient humidity exposure of the test strips over time also causes some reduction of sensitivity for occult blood and nitrate and increased sensitivity for glucose (false-positive). This can be detected by using tap water as a negative control. False-positive tests for protein can also be due to contamination of the urine by an ammonium-containing cleansing solution.

Methodology The chemical portion of the urinalysis is done by test strip, with confirming chemical method for protein (sulfosalicylic acid precipitation).

Additional Information

MICROSCOPY:

Crystalluria is frequently observed in urine specimens stored at room temperature or refrigerated. Such crystals are diagnostically useful when observed in warm, fresh urine by a physician evaluating microhematuria, nephrolithiasis, or toxin ingestion.

In abundance, **calcium oxalate** and/or **hippurate crystals** may suggest ethylene glycol ingestion (especially if known to be accompanied by neurological abnormalities, appearance of drunkenness, hypertension, and a high anion gap acidosis.) Urine is usually supersaturated in calcium oxalate, often in calcium phosphate, and acid urine is often saturated in uric acid. Yet crystalluria is uncommon (in warm, fresh urine) because of the normal presence of crystal inhibitors, the lack of available nidus, and the time factor. When properly observed in fresh urine, crystals may provide a clue to the composition of renal stones even not yet passed, the nidus for such stones, or, as such, have been associated with microhematuria.

Uric acid crystals are reddish brown, rectangular, rhomboidal, or flower-like structures of narrow rectangular petals. **Ammonium urates,** in alkaline urine, are irregular blobs and crescents, sometimes resembling fragmented red cell shapes.

Calcium oxalate crystals are fairly uniform small double pyramids, base to base, which under the microscope look like little crosses on a square.

Calcium phosphate crystallizes in urine as flowers of narrow rectangular needles.

Cystine crystals, uniquely in urine, form large irregular hexagonal plates, which may dissolve if alkalinized. They occur only in the urine of subjects with cystinuria.

Calcium magnesium ammonium phosphate, or "triple phosphate," forms unique "coffin lid" angularly domed rectangles which may be present in massive quantities in alkaline urine. They usually are associated with urine infected by urea splitting bacteria which cause "infection," or "triple phosphate" stones.

Leukocyturia may indicate inflammatory disease in the genitourinary tract, including bacterial infection, glomerulonephritis, chemical injury, autoimmune diseases, or inflammatory disease adjacent to the urinary tract such as appendicitis or diverticulitis.

White cell casts indicate the renal origin of leukocytes, and are most frequently found in acute pyelonephritis. White cell casts are also found in glomerulonephritis such as lupus nephritis, and in acute and chronic interstitial nephritis. When nuclei degenerate, such leukocyte casts resemble renal tubular casts.

Red cell casts indicate renal origin of hematuria and suggest glomerulonephritis, including lupus nephritis. Red cell casts may also be found in subacute bacterial endocarditis, renal infarct, vasculitis, Goodpasture's syndrome, sickle cell disease, and in malignant hypertension. Degenerated red cell casts may be called "**hemoglobin casts**". Orange to red casts may be found with myoglobinuria as well.

Dysmorphic red cells are observed in glomerulonephritis. "Dysmorphic" red cells refer to heterogeneous sizes, hypochromia, distorted irregular outlines and frequently small blobs extruding from the cell membrane. Phase contrast microscopy best demonstrates RBC and WBC morphology. Nonglomerular urinary red blood cells resemble peripheral circulating red blood cells. Schramek et al have used the presence or absence of dysmorphic red cells to direct the degree of work-up for hematuria and for follow-up.

Crenated RBCs provide no implication regarding RBC source.

Dark brown or smoky urine suggests a renal source of hematuria.

A **pink or red urine** suggests an extrarenal source.

Hyaline casts occur in physiologic states (eg, after exercise) and many types of renal diseases. They are best seen in phase contrast microscopy or with reduced illumination.

Renal tubular (epithelial) casts are most suggestive of tubular injury, as in acute tubular necrosis. They are also found in other disorders, including eclampsia, heavy metal poisoning, ethylene glycol intoxication, and acute allograft rejection.

Granular casts: Very finely granulated casts may be found after exercise and in a variety of glomerular and tubulointerstitial diseases.; coarse granular casts are abnormal and are present in a wide variety of renal diseases.

"**Dirty brown**" **granular casts** are typical of acute tubular necrosis.

Waxy casts are found especially in chronic renal diseases, and are associated with chronic renal failure; they occur in diabetic nephropathy, malignant hypertension, and glomerulonephritis, among other conditions. They are named for their waxy or glossy appearance. They often appear brittle and cracked.

Fatty casts are generally found in the nephrotic syndromes, diabetic nephropathy, other forms of chronic renal diseases, and glomerulonephritis. The fat droplets originate in renal tubular cells when they exceed their capacity to reabsorb protein of glomerular origin. Their inclusions have the features and significance of oval fat bodies.

Broad casts originate from dilated, chronically damaged tubules or the collecting ducts. They can be granular or waxy. **Broad waxy casts** are called "renal failure casts."

Spermatozoa may be seen in male urine related to recent or retrograde ejaculation. In female urine, the presence of spermatozoa may provide evidence of vaginal contamination following recent intercourse.

Automation of the urinalysis is routine in many laboratories. Some authors wish to abandon microscopic evaluation of the urine, which is not easily automated, on urine samples testing "normal" by dipstick screening. A urine sample that is normal to inspection and dipstick will be normal to microscopic exam 95% of the time.

One instrument for automating the entire urinalysis, the Yellow IRIS®, includes a module that automates the microscopic sediment exam. This has been found to be more consistent than the manual method for routine urinalysis and has increased the number of abnormal urines detected.

Valproic Acid, Blood

Synonyms Depakene® Level, Blood; Depakote® (Enteric-Coated Divalproex Sodium), Blood; Depamide® Level, Blood; Epilim® Level, Blood; Ergenyl® Level, Blood

Uses Monitor for compliance, efficacy, and possible toxicity

Reference Range 50-100 mcg/mL (SI: 350-690 µmol/L). Low levels: The most important cause is noncompliance. Phenytoin, phenobarbital, primidone, and carbamazepine decrease the half-life of valproic acid.

High levels: Carbamazepine and phenytoin can increase the level of valproic acid.

Abstract Valproic acid is a first-line anticonvulsant for absence seizures. It is useful for many other seizure types, including primary generalized tonic-clonic, myoclonic, atonic, and mixed seizures. It is the drug of choice for mixed absence and generalized seizures and for the epileptic syndromes of juvenile myoclonic epilepsy and generalized tonic-clonic seizures on awakening.

Specimen Blood

Volume 5 mL

Minimum Volume 3 mL serum or plasma

Container Red top tube or green top (heparin) tube

Sampling Time Trough values drawn just before next dose or consistent sampling time in chronic monitoring

Critical Values Toxic concentration >200 mcg/mL (SI: >1390 μmol/L). Seizure control may improve at levels >100 mcg/mL (SI: >690 μmol/L), but toxicity may occur at levels of 100-150 mcg/mL (SI: 690-1040 μmol/L).

Limitations Since valproic acid is highly bound, drugs that compete for protein binding sites can increase the amount of free valproic acid (biologically active fraction). These include dicumarol, high dose salicylates, and phenylbutazone. If toxicity is suspected, a free valproic acid level should be obtained.

Methodology Enzyme immunoassay (EIA), gas-liquid chromatography (GLC), high performance liquid chromatography (HPLC)

Additional Information Indications for measurement of a serum antiepileptic drug level include:
- within 6 hours of a seizure
- suspected dose-related drug toxicity
- suspected patient noncompliance

Additional indications for serum drug assay during steady state conditions (after 6 days for phenytoin, 3 days for carbamazepine, 3 days for valproic acid, 20 days for phenobarbital) include:
- baseline measurement after starting antiepileptic drug therapy
- control measurement after a change in dosage regimen
- addition of a second drug with a potential interaction with the antiepileptic drug (ie, a second antiepileptic drug, warfarin, isoniazid or rifampicin)
- change in patient's hepatic or gastrointestinal function

Vancomycin Level

Synonyms Vancocin®

Uses Monitor therapeutic levels and potential toxicities, particularly in patients with impaired renal function and in patients also being treated with aminoglycoside antibiotics

Reference Range Therapeutic concentration: peak: 20-40 mcg/mL (SI: 14.0-27.0 μmol/L) (depends in part on minimum inhibitory concentration of organism being treated); trough: 5-10 mcg/mL (SI: 3.4-6.8 μmol/L)

Abstract Vancomycin is an antimicrobial agent with potent activity against most gram-positive bacteria. Its use has occasionally been associated with nephrotoxicity and/or ototoxicity, though the frequency of these toxicities has decreased as vancomycin preparations have become more purified.

Specimen Blood, body fluid

Volume 10 mL blood or 2 mL body fluid

Container Red top tube, sterile fluid container

Sampling Time Peak: 30 minutes following dose; trough: immediately prior to next dose

Storage Instructions Separate serum using aseptic technique and place in freezer

Causes for Rejection Specimen more than 4 hours old

Possible Panic Range Toxic: >80 mcg/mL (SI: >54.0 μmol/L)

Methodology High performance liquid chromatography (HPLC), gas-liquid chromatography (GLC), immunoassay

Additional Information Ototoxicity is seen primarily in patients with extremely high serum concentrations (80-100 mcg/mL) and rarely occurs when serum concentrations are maintained at ≤30 mcg/mL. Both oto- and nephrotoxicity is enhanced by concurrent administration of aminoglycosides.

Volatile Screen

Applies to Acetone; Ethanol

Synonyms Toxicology, Volatiles

Uses Evaluate methanol and isopropanol toxicity, and alcohol drug abuse

Reference Range None detected

Test Commonly Includes Determination of volatiles by GLC including acetone, ethanol, isopropanol, and methanol. Note: Ethylene glycol in not considered to be a volatile alcohol.

Abstract This screening profile measures ethanol and other possible volatiles.

Specimen Blood, urine, gastric fluid

Volume 7 mL blood, 25 mL urine, 25 mL gastric washing

Minimum Volume 3 mL serum or plasma

Container Red top tube, gray top (sodium fluoride) tube; tightly stoppered container for urine and gastric fluid

Collection All containers should be tightly stoppered and transported on ice. The gray (oxalate/fluoride) tube top is recommended for medicolegal collections and if storage is prolonged. Sodium fluoride (50 mg) can be added as a preservative to urine and gastric samples. Other anticoagulants (eg, heparin EDTA) are acceptable.

Causes for Rejection Specimen leakage

Possible Panic Range Blood: acetone, methanol, isopropanol >500 mcg/mL (SI: acetone: >8610 μmol/L, methanol: >15.6 mM/L, isopropanol: >8.32 mM/L), ethanol: >2000 mcg/mL (SI: >43.4 mM/L); urine: acetone, methanol, isopropanol >500 mcg/mL (SI: acetone: >8610 μmol/L, methanol: >15.6 mM/L, isopropanol: 8.32 mM/L), ethanol: >1600 mcg/mL (SI: >34.7 mM/L)

Methodology Gas-liquid chromatography (GLC)

Warfarin, Blood

Applies to Anticoagulants, Oral

Synonyms Athrombin-K®; Coumadin®; Panwarfin®

Uses Therapeutic monitoring; toxicity assessment

Reference Range Therapeutic: 2-5 mcg/mL (SI: 6.5-16.2 μmol/L); free warfarin level: 5-23 ng/mL

Abstract Warfarin is an oral anticoagulant. Serum warfarin concentrations are seldom used to manage therapy; rather, typically, prothrombin time is used.

Specimen Blood

Volume 7 mL

Container Red top tube, lavender top (EDTA) tube

Possible Panic Range Toxic: >10 mcg/mL (SI: >32.4 μmol/L)

Limitations This test **does not** measure bishydroxycoumarin and should not be used to monitor this drug.

Methodology High performance liquid chromatography (HPLC), gas-liquid chromatography (GLC), UV spectrophotometry

Zalcitabine, Blood or Urine

Synonyms DDC

Uses AIDS therapy; therapeutic monitoring

Reference Range <10 ng/mL

Specimen Blood, urine

Volume 5 mL

Limitations Only used in combination with zidovudine; not approved for use in children; if used concurrently with drugs causing renal clearance problems, do so with caution

Methodology Radioimmunoassy (RIA), gas chromatography/mass spectrometry (GC/MS), high performance liquid chromatography (HPLC)

Additional Information Potential toxicities include congestive heart failure, cardiomyopathy. No liver metabolites have been identified in humans; half-life: 8.5 hours.

Zidovudine, Blood

Synonyms Azidothymidine; AZT; Retrovir®

Uses Not established for routine clinical use. Monitoring should probably be limited to studies on pharmacokinetics and efficacy of antiretroviral therapy.

Reference Range Not established

Abstract Azidothymidine (AZT) is the first FDA approved drug for the treatment of human immunodeficiency virus (HIV) infection, the cause of AIDS. The drug is a competitive inhibitor of HIV reverse transcriptase; it is incorporated into the viral DNA in place of thymidine and interrupts viral replication because the DNA can no longer elongate.

Specimen Blood

Minimum Volume Volume needed is method dependent (0.1-1 mL serum or plasma)

Container Red top tube preferred, green top (heparin) tube acceptable

Sampling Time Trough level, just before next dose

Causes for Rejection Incorrect specimen sampling time

Methodology High performance liquid chromatography (HPLC), radioimmunoassay (RIA), fluorescence polarization immunoassay (FPIA)

Additional Information Zidovudine is usually administered at a total daily dose of 500 mg (100 mg orally, every 4 hours while the patient is awake); optimal dosing, however, has not been established. Peak serum concentrations are attained within 30-40 minutes after ingestion. The drug has a half-life of approximately 1 hour; the main metabolite is a glucuronide derivative with no antiviral activity that is excreted by the kidneys. The major toxicity associated with zidovudine use is hematologic suppression which may manifest as anemia, leukopenia, and/or granulocytopenia. Monitoring hematologic parameters is the most reasonable approach toward evaluating toxicity; serum levels currently contribute little to evaluating toxic effects of zidovudine. Coadministration of probenecid results in increased serum levels due to competition for glucuronidation pathways. Hepatic and renal failure increases serum levels.

APPENDIX

UNINTENTIONAL POISONING DEATHS—UNITED STATES, 1999–2004

Reprinted from *MMWR*, February 9, 2007/56/05; 93–96

In 2004, poisoning was second only to motor-vehicle crashes as a cause of death from unintentional injury in the United States[1]. Nearly all poisoning deaths in the United States are attributed to drugs, and most drug poisonings result from the abuse of prescription and illegal drugs[2]. Previous reports have indicated a substantial increase in unintentional poisoning mortality during the 1980s and 1990s[2,3]. To further examine this trend, CDC analyzed the most current data from the National Vital Statistics System. This report summarizes the results of that analysis, which determined that poisoning mortality rates in the United States increased each year from 1999 to 2004, rising 62.5% during the 5-year period. The largest increases were among females (103.0%), whites (75.8%), persons living in the southern United States (113.6%), and persons aged 15–24 years (113.3%). Larger rate increases occurred in states with mostly rural populations. Rates for drug poisoning deaths increased 68.3%, and mortality rates for poisonings by other substances increased 1.3%. The largest increases were in the "other and unspecified," psychotherapeutic, and narcotic drug categories. The results suggest that more aggressive regulatory, educational, and treatment measures are necessary to address the increase in fatal drug overdoses.

Mortality data for 2004 were collected from the National Vital Statistics System[1]. Unintentional poisoning deaths that occurred during 1999–2004 were defined as those with underlying cause-of-death codes X40–X49 from the *International Classification of Diseases, Tenth Revision* (ICD-10). This category included overdoses of illegal drugs and legal drugs taken for nonmedical reasons, poisoning from legal drugs taken in error or at the wrong dose, and poisoning from other substances (e.g., alcohol, pesticides, or carbon monoxide). Adverse effects of legal drugs taken in the proper doses and as directed are coded elsewhere in ICD-10 and were not included in this analysis. Rates were age adjusted to the 2000 U.S. Census population using bridged-race[4] population figures. Information on the percentage of the population that was rural, defined as the percentage living in census blocks below a certain population density, was derived from U.S. Census data for 2000[5].

The number of unintentional poisoning deaths increased from 12,186 in 1999 to 20,950 in 2004. The annual age-adjusted rate increased 62.5%, from 4.4 per 100,000 population in 1999 to 7.1 in 2004. The increase among females, from 2.3 to 4.7 per 100,000 population (103.0%), was twice the increase among males, from 6.5 to 9.5 per 100,000 population (47.1%) (Table 1). Among males, rates among whites, American Indians/ Alaska Natives, and Asians/Pacific Islanders all increased approximately 50%. Rates among black males were highest in 1999 but did not increase. Among females, rates among whites more than doubled, whereas nonwhites had smaller increases or decreased. Overall, rates increased 75.8% among whites, 55.8% among American Indians/Alaska Natives, 27.4% among Asians/Pacific Islanders, and 11.2% among blacks. Rates among non-Hispanics increased more than rates among Hispanics for both sexes. Among all sex and racial/ ethnic groups, the largest increase (136.5%) was among non-Hispanic white females. Among all age groups, the largest increase occurred among persons aged 15–24 years (113.3%). In 2004, the highest rates were among persons aged 35–54 years, who accounted for 59.6% of all poisoning deaths that year.

From 1999 to 2004, rates increased by less than one third in the Northeast and West but more than doubled in the South and nearly doubled in the Midwest.[6] Delaware, Maryland, New York, and Rhode Island had decreases in rates, and California had the smallest increase (4.0%) (Figure). States with the largest relative increases were West Virginia (550%), Oklahoma (226%), Maine (210%), Montana (195%), and Arkansas (195%). Increases of 100% or more occurred in 23 states: 11.8% (two of 17) of states[7] in the most urban tertile, 41.2% (seven of 17) of those in the middle tertile, and 82.4% (14 of 17) of those in the most rural tertile (extended Mantel-Haenszel chi-square for linear trend across the tertiles = 15.4, p < 0.001).

The increase in poisoning mortality occurred almost exclusively among persons whose deaths were coded as unintentional drug poisoning (X40–X44), for which the rate increased 68.3% (Table 2). The rate for poisoning deaths attributed to other substances (X45–X49) increased 1.3%. By 2004, drug poisoning accounted for 19,838 deaths, 94.7% of all unintentional poisoning deaths. Among types of drug poisoning, the greatest increases were in the "other and unspecified" drug, psychotherapeutic drug, and "narcotic and hallucinogen" drug categories.

Reported by: *L Paulozzi, MD, Div of Unintentional Injury Prevention; J Annest, PhD, Office of Statistics and Programming, National Center for Injury Prevention and Control, CDC.*

TABLE 1. Unintentional poisoning mortality rates,* by selected characteristics — United States, 1999 and 2004

Characteristic	1999	2004	Rate change (%)
Sex and race/ethnicity			
Males	6.5	9.5	47.1
White	6.3	10.0	58.6
Hispanic	*8.5*	*7.1*	*-16.3*
Non-Hispanic	*6.0*	*10.7*	*79.0*
Black	9.8	9.9	1.0
American Indian/Alaska Native	6.7	10.6	57.5
Asian/Pacific Islander	1.1	1.7	50.5
Females	2.3	4.7	103.0
White	2.3	5.0	121.8
Hispanic	*1.7*	*2.4*	*40.8*
Non-Hispanic	*2.3*	*5.4*	*136.5*
Black	3.2	4.5	40.3
American Indian/Alaska Native	4.3	6.6	54.8
Asian/Pacific Islander	0.6	0.5	-10.3
Age group (yrs)			
0–14	0.1	0.1	0.0
15–24	2.5	5.3	113.3
25–34	5.9	9.1	54.8
35–44	10.1	14.5	43.8
45–54	7.8	14.5	87.0
55–64	2.8	5.4	91.1
65–74	1.6	2.3	39.3
≥75	2.5	2.7	7.2
Region†			
Northeast	4.5	5.9	31.7
Midwest	3.3	6.1	85.5
South	3.7	7.9	113.6
West	6.4	7.9	22.7
Total	**4.4**	**7.1**	**62.5**

* Age-adjusted rates per 100,000 population.
† *Northeast*: Connecticut, Maine, Massachusetts, New Hampshire, New Jersey, New York, Pennsylvania, Rhode Island, and Vermont; *Midwest*: Illinois, Indiana, Iowa, Kansas, Michigan, Minnesota, Missouri, Nebraska, North Dakota, Ohio, South Dakota, and Wisconsin; *South*: Alabama, Arkansas, Delaware, District of Columbia, Florida, Georgia, Kentucky, Louisiana, Maryland, Mississippi, North Carolina, Oklahoma, South Carolina, Tennessee, Texas, Virginia, and West Virginia; *West*: Alaska, Arizona, California, Colorado, Hawaii, Idaho, Montana, Nevada, New Mexico, Oregon, Utah, Washington, and Wyoming.

Editorial Note

Unintentional drug poisoning mortality rates increased substantially in the United States during 1999–2004. Previous studies, using multiple cause-of-death data, have indicated that the trend described in this report can be attributed primarily to increasing numbers of deaths associated with prescription opioid analgesics (e.g., oxycodone) and secondarily to increasing numbers of overdoses of cocaine and prescription

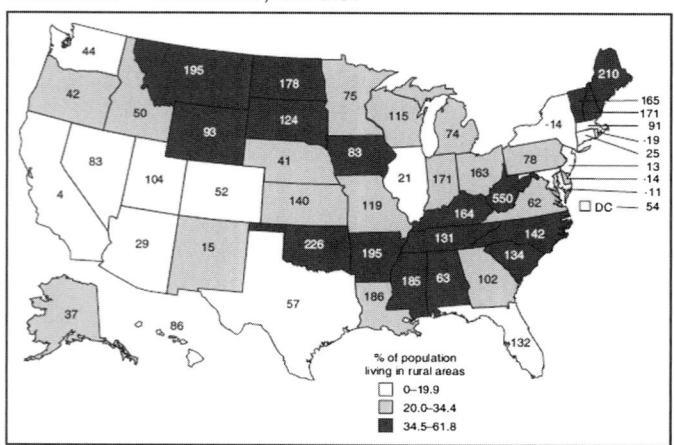

FIGURE. Percentage change in unintentional poisoning mortality rates,* by rural status of state† — United States, 1999–2004

* Age-adjusted rates per 100,000 population.
† Defined as the percentage of the population living in census blocks below a certain population density, based on U.S. Census data for 2000 (4).

TABLE 2. Number of deaths and mortality rates* attributed to unintentional poisoning, by type of substance – United States, 1999 and 2004

Type of substance	ICD-10[†] code	1999 No.	1999 Rate	2004 No.	2004 Rate	Rate change (%)
Drugs	X40–X44	11,155	4.0	19,838	6.7	68.3
Nonopioid analgesics[§]	X40	168	0.1	212	0.1	18.1
Psychotherapeutic drugs[¶]	X41	671	0.2	1,300	0.4	83.5
Narcotics and hallucinogens**	X42	6,009	2.1	9,789	3.3	64.6
Other drugs acting on the central nervous system	X43	21	0.0	22	0.0	-0.5
Other and unspecified drugs[††]	X44	4,286	1.5	8,506	2.9	87.3
Other substances	X45–X49	1,031	0.4	1,112	0.4	1.3
Alcohol	X45	320	0.1	358	0.1	6.0
Organic solvents and halogenated hydrocarbons	X46	63	0.0	67	0.0	2.0
Carbon monoxide and other gases	X47	534	0.2	562	0.2	-1.7
Pesticides	X48	12	—[§§]	3	—[§§]	—[§§]
Other and unspecified chemicals[¶¶]	X49	102	0.0	122	0.0	10.6
Total	**X40–X49**	**12,186**	**4.4**	**20,950**	**7.1**	**62.5**

* Age-adjusted rates per 100,000 population.

† *International Classification of Diseases. Tenth Revision.*

§ Includes painkillers such as aspirin and acetaminophen and other antipyretic or antirheumatic drugs, both prescription and over-the-counter drugs.

¶ Includes antepileptic, sedative-hypnotic, antidepressant, antipsychotic, and other psychotherapeutic drugs.

** Includes heroin opioid analgesics (e.g., oxycodone), and cocaine.

†† Category used to classify deaths attributed to drugs from more than one of the other categories (e.g., deaths attributed to both an opioid analgesic and a sedative) and deaths attributed simply to "drug overdose."

§§ Rates based on fewer than 20 deaths are not included.

¶¶ Includes corrosives, metals, plants, and detergents.

psychotherapeutic drugs (e.g., sedatives), and cannot be attributed to heroin, methamphetamines, or other illegal drugs[3,8].

The mortality increases might be the result of greater use and abuse of potentially lethal prescription drugs in recent years, behaviors that are more common among whites than nonwhites[9,10]. The substantial increase in deaths among persons aged 15–24 years is consistent with substantial recent increases in recreational prescription drug and cocaine use among adolescents and young adults[11].

Studies by state health agencies have reported recent increases in prescription-drug–poisoning mortality in rural communities[2,13], despite historically higher rates in urban areas. The South and Midwest regions, which had the largest relative and absolute increases among regions in this study, are the most rural regions of the country[5]. Further research is needed to determine how differences in drug use, drug-abuse–control measures, and demographic characteristics (e.g., race/ethnicity) contribute to this pattern.

The findings in this report are subject to at least three limitations. First, mortality coding assigns the underlying cause of death to broad drug categories rather than to specific drugs. Second, death certificates do not reveal the circumstances of drug use. Third, determining the intent of a person who took a drug is often difficult for a coroner or medical examiner and might result in misclassification; some of these deaths might have been suicides, although not classified as such, and some deaths categorized as suicides or of undetermined intent might have been unintentional and therefore not analyzed in this study. The extent of this error is not known.

Effective response to increasing fatal drug overdoses requires strengthening regulatory measures to reduce unsafe use of drugs, increasing physician awareness regarding appropriate pharmacologic treatment of pain and psychiatric problems, supporting best practices for treating drug dependence, and potentially modifying prescription drugs to reduce their potential for abuse. State agencies that manage prescription-monitoring programs should use such systems to proactively identify 1) patients who abuse drugs and fill multiple prescriptions from different health-care providers and 2) providers whose prescribing practices are outside the standards of appropriate medical care. Both federal and state prevention measures should be evaluated periodically to determine their effectiveness.

Footnotes

1. CDC. Web-based Injury Statistics Query and Reporting System (WISQARS) [Online]. Available at http://www.cdc.gov/ncipc/wisqars.

2. Paulozzi LJ, Ballesteros MF, Stevens JA, "Recent Trends in Mortality from Unintentional Injury in the United States," *J Safety Res*, 2006, 37:277–83.

3. Paulozzi LJ, Budnitz DS, Xi Y, "Increasing Deaths from Opioid Analgesics in the United States," *Pharmacoepidemiol Drug Safety*, 2006, 15:618–27.

4. Information about bridged-race categories is available at http://www.cdc.gov/nchs/about/major/dvs/popbridge/popbridge.htm.

5. US Department of Commerce, Census Bureau. 2000 Census: summary file 3, table P.5 urban and rural. Available at http://www.nemw.org/poprural.htm.

6. *Northeast*: Connecticut, Maine, Massachusetts, New Hampshire, New Jersey, New York, Pennsylvania, Rhode Island, and Vermont; *Midwest*: Illinois, Indiana, Iowa, Kansas, Michigan, Minnesota, Missouri, Nebraska, North Dakota, Ohio, South Dakota, and Wisconsin; *South*: Alabama, Arkansas, Delaware, District of Columbia, Florida, Georgia, Kentucky, Louisiana, Maryland, Mississippi, North Carolina, Oklahoma, South Carolina, Tennessee, Texas, Virginia, and West Virginia; *West*: Alaska, Arizona, California, Colorado, Hawaii, Idaho, Montana, Nevada, New Mexico, Oregon, Utah, Washington, and Wyoming.

7. Includes the District of Columbia.

8. Fingerhut LA. Increases in methadone-related deaths: 1999–2004. Health E-Stats. Hyattsville, MD: National Center for Health Statistics; 2006. Available at http://www.cdc.gov/nchs/products/pubs/pubd/hestats/methadone1999-04/methadone1999-04.htm.

9. Simoni-Wastila L, "The Use of Abusable Prescription Drugs: The Role of Gender," *J Womens Health Gend Based Med*, 2000, 9:289–97.

10. Simoni-Wastila L, Ritter G, Strickler G, "Gender and Other Factors Associated with the Nonmedical Use of Abusable Prescription Drugs," *Subst Use Misuse*, 2004, 39:1–23.

11. US Department of Health and Human Services, Substance Abuse and Mental Health Services Administration Office of Applied Studies. Results from the 2005 National Survey on Drug Use and Health: national findings. Rockville, MD: Substance Abuse and Mental Health Services Administration; 2006. Available at http://www.oas.samhsa.gov/nsduh/2k5nsduh/2k5results.htm.

12. CDC, "Increase in Poisoning Deaths Caused by Non-Illicit Drugs–Utah, 1991–2003," *MMWR*, 2005, 54:33–6.

13. CDC, "Unintentional Deaths from Drug Poisoning by Urbanization of Area–New Mexico, 1994–2003," *MMWR*, 2005, 54:870–3.

5-HYDROXYTRYPTAMINE (5-HT)

Pharmacotherapeutic Agents Acting on Reuptake and Metabolism of 5-HT*

5-HT Reuptake Inhibitors	5-HT Inhibitors/Depletors Intracellular Granular Uptake and Storage	5-HT Metabolic Inhibitors
Antidepressants SSRIs Paroxetine Citalopram Sertraline Fluvoxamine Fluoxetine Others Clomipramine Venlafaxine Amitriptyline Imipramine Nortriptyline Desipramine Nefazodone Doxepin Protriptyline Amphetamine Anorexiant/antidepressant Sibutramine (5-HT$_{2a/2c}$) Trazodone Bupropion (also for smoking cessation) Analgesic (centrally acting) Tramadol Local anesthetic Cocaine	Antihypertensive Reserpine (initially) Anorexiants Dexfenfluramine dl-Fenfluramine Analgesic (centrally acting) Meperidine (pethidine) Cough suppressant Dextromethorphan (DM)	MAOIs (used in psychiatry) Moclobemide Phenelzine (hydrazine) Isocarboxazid (hydrazine) Tranylcypromine (nonhydrazine) Anti-Parkinson's treatment Selegiline (deprenyl)

*Potency of reuptake inhibitors (Ki value based), listed from most potency to least potency.

Adapted with permission from Barkin RL, Schwer WA, and Barkin SJ, "Recognition and Management of Depression in Primary Care: A Focus on the Elderly. A Pharmacotherapeutic Overview of the Selection Process Among the Traditional and New Antidepressants," *Am J Therap*, 1999, 7:216.

Pharmacotherapeutic Agents That Act as Serotonin (5-HT)Receptor Antagonists

Nonselective 5-HT	5-HT$_{1A}$	5-HT$_{1B}$	5-HT$_{2A}$	
Neuroleptic/antiemetic Chlorpromazine Other migraine treatment and H$_1$ receptor antagonists Oxetorone Pizotifen	β-Adrenergic blockade Pindolol Propranolol Neuroleptics Quetiapine	β-Adrenergic blockade Pindolol Propranolol	Antidepressants Amoxapine Ketanserin Maprotiline Mirtazapine Nefazodone Ritanserin Trazodone Neuroleptics Clozapine Fluphenazine Haloperidol Loxapine Olanzapine Quetiapine Risperidone	Migraine treatment Dihydroergotamine (DHE) Methysergide Ergotamine H$_1$ receptor antagonist Cyproheptadine H$_2$ receptor antagonist

5-HT$_{2C}$	5-HT$_3$	5-HT$_6$	5-HT$_7$	
Migraine prophylaxis Methysergide Other mCPP Neuroleptics Clozapine Olanzapine Quetiapine Risperidone Sertindole Antidepressants Amoxapine Mirtazapine Ritanserin	Antiemetics Dolasetron Granisetron Itasetron Metoclopramide Ondansetron Renzapride Trimethobenzamide Tropisetron Antidepressants Mirtazepine	Neuroleptics Clozapine Antidepressants Amoxapine	Neuroleptics Clozapine Fluphenazine Loxapine Pimozide Risperidone	

Adapted with permission from Barkin RL, Schwer WA, and Barkin SJ, "Recognition and Management of Depression in Primary Care: A Focus on the Elderly. A Pharmacotherapeutic Overview of the Selection Process Among the Traditional and New Antidepressants," *Am J Therap*, 1999, 7:217.

Pharmacotherapeutic Agents Modulating 5-HT by Various Mechanisms

5-HT Release Inhibition	5-HT Inhibition	5-HT Release Facilitators	5-HT Precursor
Calcium channel blockers Nifedipine Verapamil	Anticonvulsants Lamotrigine	Psychostimulants Amphetamine Methamphetamine Mood stabilizers Lithium carbonate Anorexiants Dexfenfluramine dl-Fenfluramine Local anesthetics Cocaine Anti-Parkinson's Levodopa Antidepressants Mirtazapine	Postanoxic intention myoclonus L-5 hydroxytryptophan (L-5-HTP) Oral amino acid/hypnotic/antidepressant L-tryptophan

Adapted with permission from Barkin RL, Schwer WA, and Barkin SJ, "Recognition and Management of Depression in Primary Care: A Focus on the Elderly. A Pharmacotherapeutic Overview of the Selection Process Among the Traditional and New Antidepressants," *Am J Therap*, 1999, 7:218.

Pharmacotherapeutic Agents Providing 5-HT Receptor Agonism

Nonselective 5-HT	5-HT$_{1A}$	5-HT$_{1B/1D}$	5-HT$_2$	5-HT$_4$
Hallucinogens Dimethyltryptamine (bufotenine) Lysergic acid diethylamide (LSD) Mescaline (Peyote) Psilocybin Mood stabilizers Lithium	Migraine therapy (abortive) Ergotamine Triptans Anxiolytics Buspirone	Migraine therapy (abortive) Dihydroergotamine (DHE) Ergotamine Methysergide (partial) Triptans Sumatriptan Zolmitriptan Naratriptan Rizitriptan Alniditan Eletriptan Presynaptic α_2-adrenergic blockers Yohimbine	Hallucinogens (substance of abuse) Phencyclidine (PCP) Lysergic acid diethylamide (LSD)	Gastrointestinal prokinetic agents Cisapride

Adapted with permission from Barkin RL, Schwer WA, and Barkin SJ, "Recognition and Management of Depression in Primary Care: A Focus on the Elderly. A Pharmacotherapeutic Overview of the Selection Process Among the Traditional and New Antidepressants," *Am J Therap*, 1999, 7:218.

ACUTE INTERMITTENT PORPHYRIA, HEREDITARY COPROPORPHYRIA, AND VARIEGATE PORPHYRIA, CATEGORIES OF SAFE AND UNSAFE DRUGS/CHEMICALS

Unsafe	Safe
Alcohol	Acetaminophen
Barbiturates	Acetazolamide
Carbamazepine	Aspirin
Carisoprodol	Atropine
Chloramphenical	Bromides
Chlordiazepoxide	Glucocorticoids
Clemastine	Halothane
Clorazepute	Insulin
Danazol	Isoflurane
Dapsone	Narcotic analgesics
Diclofenac	Penicillin and derivatives
Ergots	Phenothiazines
Ethchlorvynol	Streptomycin
Glutethimide	
Griseofulvin	
Hydralazine	
Hydroxyzine	
Lead	
Mephenytoin	
Meprobamate	
Methyldopa	
Methyprylon	
Nifedipine	
Phenytoin	
Pyrazolones	
Rifampin	
Succinimides	
Sulfonamide antibiotics	
Synthetic estrogens and progestins	
Tolbotamide	
Valproic acid	
Verapamil	

GLUCOSE-6-PHOSPHATE DEHYDROGENASE DEFICIENCY

Drugs/Chemicals Which Can Induce Hemolysis in Patients With Glucose-6-Phosphate Dehydrogenase Deficiency

Acetanilid

Aluminum phosphide

Aspirin*

Copper (?)

Doxorubicin

Fava beans

Furazolidone

Isosorbide dinitrate

Methylene blue

Nalidixic acid

Niridazole

Nitrofurantoin

Phenazopyridine

Primaquine

Probenecid (?)

Silver sulfadiazine

Sulfamethoxazole

2,4,6-Trinitrotoluene

*Hemolysis is usually due to infection and fever; red blood cell survival may be shortened in patients with hereditary nonspherocytic hemolytic anemia due to G6PD deficiency.

References

Anderson KE, Bloomer JR, Bonkovsky HL et al., "Recommendations for the Diagnosis and Treatment of the Acute Porphyrias," *Ann Intern Med.*, 2005, 142(6):439-50.

Beutler E, "Glucose-6-Phosphate Dehydrogenase Deficiency," *N Engl J Med*, 1991, 324(3):169-74.

ADDICTION TREATMENTS

Acamprosate (Campral®)	Maintenance of alcohol abstinence: 666 mg 3 times/day; 333 mg 3 times/day in patients with Cl_{cr} 30-50 mL/minute.
Buprenorphine (Buprenex®, Subutex®)	Opioid dependence: Induction: 12-16 mg/day; maintenance: 4-24 mg/day; target dose: 16 mg/day.
Buprenorphine and Naloxone (Suboxone®)	Opioid dependence: Induction: Not recommended; maintenance: 4-24 mg/day; target dose: 16 mg/day.
Bupropion SR (Zyban®)	Smoking cessation: Initiate at 150 mg every morning for 3 days. If tolerated, increase to 150 mg twice daily on day 4 of dosing. Should be an interval of at least 8 hours between successive doses. Target quit date after at least 1 week of treatment. Trial may be up to 12 weeks. Contraindicated in patients with seizures, anorexia, or bulimia.
Clonidine (Catapres®)	Alcohol, nicotine, opioid withdrawal: Initiate 0.1 mg 2-3 times/day.
Disulfiram (Antabuse®)	Management of chronic alcoholism: 125-500 mg/day; patients must be free of alcohol for at least 12 hours prior to initiation. Contraindicated with metronidazole and alcohol (including cough syrups).
Levomethadyl (Orlaam®)	Narcotic dependence: Initiate at 20-40 mg 3 times/week.
Methadone (Dolophine®)	Narcotic dependence: 15-60 mg every 6-8 hours; can only be initiated in approved treatment programs.
Naltrexone (ReVia®)	Alcohol and narcotic dependence: Initiate 25-50 mg/day; patient should be free of opioid for 7-10 days prior to initiation.
Nicotine gum	Smoking cessation: 1-2 pieces/hour; maximum: 30 pieces/day (2 mg/piece). If high tobacco use, give DS (4 mg/piece); maximum: 20/day.
Nicotine nasal spray	Smoking cessation: 1 spray in each nostril once or twice per hour; maximum: 80 sprays.
Nicotine patches	Smoking cessation: One patch daily for 8 weeks.

ADIPOSE TISSUE RANGES OF TOXINS

General Population (Background)

Beta-hexachlorocyclohexane	ND* to 570 ng/g
Boron	ND
Bromoform	ND
Chlorobenzene	1-9 ng/g
Chloroform	ND to 580 ng/g
Cobalt	0.035-0.078 mg/kg
Di-(2-ethylhexyl)phthalate	ND to 850 ng/g
Diethyl phthalate	ND to 0.65 mcg/g
Dibromochloromethane	ND
1,4-Dichlorobenzene	12-500 ng/g
Dieldrin	ND to 4100 ng/g
Di-N-octylphthalate	ND to 850 ng/g
Endrin	ND
Ethylbenzene	ND to 280 ng/g
Heptachlor epoxide	ND to 310 ng/g
1,2,3,4,6,7,8-Heptachlorodibenzofurans	21 ppt
Hexachlorobenzene	12-1300 ng/g
Hexachlorobutadiene	0.8-8 mcg/kg
1,2,3,4,7,8-Hexachlorodibenzofurans	9.3 ppt
1,2,3,6,7,8-Hexachlorodibenzofurans	5.4 ppt
2,3,4,6,7,8-Hexachlorodibenzofurans	1.8 ppt
Manganese	0.07 mcg/g
Mirex	ND to 41 ng/g
Naphthalene	ND to 63 ng/g
Octachlorodibenzofurans	60 ppt
Oxychlordane	90-120 ng/g
2,3,4,7,8-Pentachlorodibenzofurans	40 ppt
Phenanthrene	ND to 24 ng/g
Polybrominated biphenyls (in Michigan)	15-12,820 mcg/kg
Polychlorinated biphenyl (PCB)	14-1700 ng/g
Polycyclic aromatic hydrocarbons (PAH)	ND
Styrene	8-350 ng/g
2,3,7,8-Tetrachlorodibenzofurans	9.1 ppt
Tin	8.7-15 mcg/g
Toluene	ND to 250 ng/g
Tributyl phosphate	ND to 120 ng/g
1,1,1-Trichloroethane	ND to 830 ng/g
1,1,2-Trichloroethane	ND
Vanadium	0.7 ng/g

*ND = not detected.
Reference: U.S. Department of Health and Human Services, Toxicology Profile Series, ATSDR.

AGENTS FOR TREATMENT OF EXTRAPYRAMIDAL SYMPTOMS

A variety of agents exist for treatment of extrapyramidal symptoms (EPS) associated with the use of antipsychotic agents. See the Antiparkinsonian Agents Comparison Chart. These include anticholinergic agents, dopaminergic agents, levodopa, beta-blockers, clonidine, and benzodiazepines. Ideally, prevention of EPS should be attempted with lowest effective dosing of conventional antipsychotics or use of the newer atypical antipsychotics.

Anticholinergic drugs may be used to treat all forms of acute EPS and are generally considered first-line agents for these drug-induced syndromes. Anticholinergic agents are believed to work by normalizing the dopaminergic-cholinergic balance in the corpus striatum, although a clear understanding of exactly how this may occur remains lacking.

Anticholinergic medication should begin with benztropine 1-2 mg/day or an equivalent dosage of an alternative anticholinergic. For severe, painful, or potentially dangerous EPS, such as dysarthria or laryngospasm, anticholinergic medication may be given I.V. or I.M. I.V. anticholinergic (eg, benztropine 2 mg or diphenhydramine 50 mg) relieves EPS within 2-3 minutes, while I.M. administration requires 15-30 minutes for symptom relief. Individuals with a history of acute EPS should be given prophylactic anticholinergic medication. Additionally, clinicians may consider prophylactic anticholinergic medication for individuals with high risk for EPS (eg, young males on higher doses of high-potency conventional antipsychotic).

Geriatric patients generally require lower doses of anticholinergic drug. Adverse effects associated with anticholinergic medication include constipation, urinary retention, tachycardia, and blurred vision. Intraocular pressure may be increased, posing some danger for patients with narrow-angle glaucoma. In addition, some individuals, particularly elderly patients, may develop a delirium-like presentation associated with anticholinergics that is characterized by disorientation, hallucinations, behavioral lability, and cognitive impairment. Occasionally, patients may abuse anticholinergics.

Patients on anticholinergic medication should be reassessed on a regular basis to determine continued need for medication. A significant number of patients on antipsychotic medication exhibit spontaneous reduction or resolution of EPS during continued antipsychotic medication therapy, particularly during the first 3 months of treatment. Therefore, after this time period, one should consider tapering anticholinergic agent.

Dopaminergic agents, such as amantadine and levodopa, have also been reported to be useful in management of EPS. Amantadine has been reported to be beneficial in acute dystonia, akathisia, and drug-induced parkinsonism. As with anticholinergics, amantadine is believed to work by normalizing dopamine-acetylcholine balance in the striatum. Dosing of 100-400 mg/day in a once or twice daily pattern is usually used. Adverse effects with amantadine include orthostasis, peripheral edema, and a skin reaction called livedo reticularis (venous marbleization of the skin, usually lower extremities). Also, worsening of psychosis or delirium have been reported. Generally, amantadine should only be utilized after failure of anticholinergic agents. Levodopa is far less commonly used due to concern regarding worsening of psychotic illness.

Beta-blocking drugs (eg, propranolol, atenolol, pindolol) may be useful in EPS. Beta-blockers appear to be most effective in treating akathisia. Patients on beta-blockers may experience hypotension or bradycardia, thus, blood pressure and pulse should be monitored during initial drug titration.

Clonidine is another agent that may be effective in akathisia. Usual dosage for akathisia is 0.2-0.8 mg/day. As with beta-blockers, hypotension may occur, and blood pressure should be monitored during initial titration. Clonidine should generally be tried after failure of beta-blockers to control akathisia.

Benzodiazepines may also be useful in improving symptoms of dystonia and akathisia, although they are generally less effective than anticholinergic medications. Lorazepam, clonazepam, and diazepam have been most often utilized, generally at dosages of diazepam $\leq$40 mg/day, or its equivalent.

ALLERGIC REACTIONS

An allergic drug reaction can be considered an adverse effect involving immunologic mechanisms. True allergic reactions are much less common than nonallergic responses such as side effects and drug-drug interactions. As a result, it is important to carefully evaluate patients who present with allergies to drugs. Patients frequently state an allergy to a drug when the reaction was a predictable side effect (eg, nausea/vomiting with codeine). If a patient presents a history of one or more of the following signs or symptoms after drug administration, an allergic reaction should be assumed until proven otherwise: skin manifestations (pruritus with hives or flushing), facial or oral swelling, shortness of breath, choking, wheezing, and vascular collapse. In this situation, an alternate agent should be selected.

Classification of Allergic Reactions

Allergic reactions can be classified using the Coombs and Gell Classification System into one of four immunopathologic categories (types I through IV). The following table summarizes the key characteristics of each type of reaction.

Type	Characteristics	Usual Onset	Examples
I - Anaphylactic (IgE mediated)	Requires the presence of IgE specific for drug antigen or other allergen; allergen binds to IgE on basophils and mast cells resulting in release of inflammatory mediators (eg, histamine, serotonin, proteases, bradykinin generating factor, eosinophil chemotactic factors, neutrophil chemotactic factor, leukotrienes, prostaglandins, thromboxanes)	Within 30 minutes	Immediate penicillin reaction Immediate latex reaction Blood products Vaccines Dextran Polypeptide hormones
II - Cytotoxic	Destruction of host cells; cell-associated antigen initiates cytolysis by antigen-specific antibody (IgG or IgM); most often involves blood elements (eg, erythrocytes, leukocytes, platelets)	Usually 5-12 hours	Penicillin, quinidine, phenylbutazone, thiouracils, sulfonamides, methyldopa
III - Immune complex	Antigen-antibody complexes form and deposit on blood vessel walls and activate complement. Result is a serum-sickness-like syndrome.	3-8 hours	Serum sickness; may be caused by penicillins, sulfonamides, I.V. contrast media, hydantoins
IV - Cell mediated (delayed)	Antigens cause activation of lymphocytes (T cells), which release inflammatory mediators	24-48 hours	Graft rejection Latex contact dermatitis Tuberculin reaction

Modified from DiPiro JT and Stafford CT, "Allergic and Pseudoallergic Drug Reactions," *Pharmacotherapy: A Pathophysiologic Approach*, 3rd ed, Stamford CT: Appleton and Lange, 1997, 1675-88.

Anesthesia-Related Agents Associated with Allergy

Certain agents are most often responsible for allergic reactions in surgical patients. These include neuromuscular blocking agents, latex, colloids, hypnotics, antibiotics, benzodiazepines, opioids, local anesthetics, I.V. contrast media, and blood products. The antibiotics most commonly associated with allergic reactions are the sulfonamides, penicillins, and cephalosporins. Propofol contains soybean oil and egg yolk components; in patients with allergies to these items, propofol should be avoided. The ester-type local anesthetics can produce allergic reactions secondary to the metabolite para-aminobenzoic acid. The methylparaben preservative in amide-type local anesthetics may also produce an allergic reaction in patients sensitive to para-aminobenzoic acid. Sulfites, which are used as preservatives in various drug products, can produce pulmonary complications in patients, occurring more frequently in asthmatics. Cross allergenicity exists between shellfish/seafood and protamine and I.V. contrast media; care should be taken when using these agents in patients with these types of allergies. Special consideration should be given to a patient who presents a personal or family history of allergy to halothane or succinylcholine as this may actually represent an occurrence of malignant hyperthermia.

Anaphylaxis

Anaphylaxis is the most severe form of allergic reaction. It can present as an acute, life-threatening reaction with multiple organ system involvement or it can be more localized in appearance. It has been estimated that 1 in every 2700 hospitalized patients experience drug-induced anaphylaxis. When antibodies are not involved in the process, the reaction is termed anaphylactoid. It is not possible through clinical observation to distinguish between anaphylactic and anaphylactoid reactions. Life-threatening reactions are more likely to occur in patients with a history of allergy, atopy, or asthma. Although these patients are frequently pretreated with corticosteroids, there is no evidence to suggest this practice is effective for preventing true anaphylactic reactions. In a survey examining the incidence of intraoperative anaphylaxis, 70.2% were due to neuromuscular blocking agents, 12.5% due to latex, 4.6% due to colloids, 3.6% due to hypnotics, 2.6% due to antibiotics, 2% due to benzodiazepines, 1.7% due to opioids, 0.7% due to local anesthetics, and 2.8% due to other agents.

Pathophysiology

Anaphylaxis is initiated by an antigen binding to IgE antibodies; however, prior exposure to the antigen or a substance with a similar structure is first required to sensitize the patient to the antigen. The binding of the antigen to the IgE antibodies on the surface of basophils and mast cells causes release of histamine and the chemotactic factors of anaphylaxis. Other chemical mediators (leukotrienes, prostaglandins, kinins) are also released in response to cellular activation. The liberated mediators produce bronchospasm, upper airway edema, vasodilation, increased capillary permeability, and urticaria. The effects of multiple mediators on the heart and peripheral vasculature cause the cardiovascular collapse seen during anaphylaxis. Antigenic challenge in a sensitized individual usually produces immediate clinical manifestations of anaphylaxis; however, the onset may be delayed by up to 30 minutes. The reaction can vary in severity, from minor clinical changes to acute cardiopulmonary collapse.

Signs/Symptoms of Anaphylactic Reaction

The following table lists the signs and symptoms that may indicate an anaphylactic reaction during anesthesia.

Systems	Symptoms	Signs
Cutaneous	Itching, burning	Urticaria (hives), flushing, periorbital edema, perioral edema
Respiratory	Dyspnea, chest tightness	Coughing, wheezing, sneezing, laryngeal edema, decreased pulmonary compliance, pulmonary edema, acute respiratory distress, bronchospasm
Cardiovascular	Dizziness, malaise, retrosternal oppression	Disorientation, diaphoresis, loss of consciousness, hypotension, tachycardia, dysrhythmias, decreased systemic vascular resistance, pulmonary hypertension, cardiovascular collapse

Modified from Levy JH, *Anaphylactic Reactions in Anesthesia and Intensive Care*, Stoneham, Butterworth-Heinemann, 1992.

Treatment of Anaphylactic Reaction

Treatment of a severe, life-threatening anaphylactic reaction must be immediate. Initial therapy comprises: 1) stoping administration of precipitating drug; 2) maintaining airway with 100% oxygen; 3) discontinuing all anesthetic agents; 4) intravascular volume expansion with crystalloid solution; and 5) epinephrine administration. Secondary therapy consists of administration of antihistamines (eg, diphenhydramine), catecholamine infusions (eg, norepinephrine, epinephrine, inhaled bronchodilators (eg, albuterol) for bronchospasm, corticosteroids (eg, hydrocortisone, methylprednisolone, dexamethasone), and sodium bicarbonate. Patients should be admitted to an ICU for 24 hours following an anaphylactic reaction because of the possibility of recurrent "late-phase" reactions.

Latex Allergy

The incidence of latex allergy is increasing. This increase has been suggested to be due in part to the implementation of universal precautions by the CDC in 1987 secondary to the AIDS epidemic. **Because of the increased incidence of latex allergy, all patients should be asked about allergic responses to latex products.** For example, patients should be questioned about the presence of swelling or itching of the hands or other areas after contact with rubber gloves, condoms, diaphragms, toys, or other rubber products and about itching or swelling of the lips or mouth after dental exams, blowing up balloons, or after eating bananas, chestnuts, and avocados.

It is important today for health care institutions to have a comprehensive plan (including a perioperative component) in place for dealing with the latex allergic patient.

Hypersensitivity Reactions Caused by Latex

Latex-containing products can produce type I and type IV hypersensitivity reactions.

The type I hypersensitivity reaction is the true "allergic" reaction seen with latex products. Proteins found in the latex promote the production of an antibody of the IgE class which attaches to basophils and mast cells. When the antigen (protein) is encountered again, histamine and other physiologically active mediators are released from mast cells and basophils. The clinical manifestations can include single or multiple system involvement, be mild or severe, and range from itching to edema and from mild hypotension to shock. It has been estimated that 10% of the true anaphylactic reactions during anesthesia are due to latex allergy. These reactions are usually seen 5-30 minutes after induction of anesthesia and start of surgery.

In the type IV reaction, a contact dermatitis is seen. The preservatives, stabilizers, accelerators, and antioxidants used in the latex manufacturing process serve as the antigens for T-cell lymphocytes. The dermatitis produced can be uncomfortable but is not life-threatening.

Routes of Exposure to Latex Proteins

It is important to consider the route of exposure of the latex protein in allergic patients as this can be a determinant of the type of reaction produced. The following table summarizes major routes of exposure.

Type of Exposure	Reaction
Direct skin contact	Localized or generalized urticaria
Mucous membrane	Rhinitis, conjunctivitis, stomatitis, angioedema; severe anaphylactic reactions and death reported
Inhalation of airborne starch-protein particles	Wheezing, bronchospasm, reduced lung compliance, episodes of desaturation and/or severe hypoxemia
Intravascular absorption of water soluble latex particles from surgical gloves	Sudden tachycardia, severe hypotension, cardiorespiratory collapse

High-Risk Patients

Several groups have been identified as "high-risk" for allergic reactions to latex. Special consideration should be given these individuals.

Healthcare providers. Latex allergy has been reported to be 7.5% for physicians, 5.6% for nurses, and 13.7% for dental personnel. The overall incidence for hospital employees is 1.3% (versus 0.08% for the general population).

Spina bifida patients/patients with congenital urologic abnormalities. An 18% to 40% incidence of latex allergy has been reported for spina bifida patients. These patients are routinely exposed to latex-containing urinary catheters.

Workers in rubber industry. A 10% incidence of latex allergy has been reported.

Patients with a history of atopy. In patients with latex allergy, there is a 35% to 83% incidence of atopy. Patients report allergies to rubber gloves, balloons, and various fruits and foods. Cross-reactivity has been reported with bananas, avocados, kiwis, celery, and chestnuts.

Treatment of Anaphylactic Reaction

Management of an anaphylactic reaction which is thought to be due to latex allergy is similar to that described earlier. In addition, all latex products should be removed from the surgical field, surgeons must switch to nonlatex gloves, and latex-free tubing should be used for I.V. administration. Further, tests to determine if latex allergy was the cause of the reaction should be performed (eg, RAST, AlaSTAT).

Perioperative Management of a Latex Allergic Patient

No evidence exists to demonstrate that prophylaxis before surgery prevents latex-induced anaphylactic reactions. In spite of this, prophylaxis has been used in patients with a positive history of allergy; one suggested regimen uses diphenhydramine P.O. or I.V. every 6 hours at 13, 7, and 1 hour before surgery, prednisone P.O. every 6 hours at 13, 7, and 1 hours before surgery (hydrocortisone I.V. may be substituted), and ranitidine P.O. or I.V. every 12 hours at 13 and 1 hours before surgery. This regimen is continued for 12 hours after surgery.

The key to perioperative management of the latex allergic patient is to provide a latex-free environment. To accomplish this, the following actions should be taken:

Substitute all items with nonlatex alternatives when possible; if there is a question concerning the latex content of a product, the manufacturer should be called

Gloves made of neoprene or other polymers should be used

Latex-based adhesives should be eliminated

Stopcocks should be used for drug administration instead of injection ports on I.V. tubing

Syringes not containing rubber tips on the plunger should be used

Drug products in glass ampuls should be used whenever possible; if a vial must be used, utilize a vial stopper remover so the stopper does not have to be punctured, and

To reduce exposure to aerosolized glove powder which is a known carrier of latex proteins, schedule the surgery as the first case of the day; some institutions have reserved an OR suite for latex allergic patients.

Testing for Latex Allergy

Testing for latex allergy is recommended for high-risk patients. Both *in vitro* and *in vivo* tests are available as seen in the following table.

Test	Type	Description
Skin prick	*in vivo*	Sensitive method to confirm IgE-mediated latex hypersensitivity; correlates well with clinical presence of allergy; high sensitivity (100%), high specificity (99%)
Patch	*in vivo*	Test for type IV hypersensitivity reaction; test performed with 1 inch square of rubber glove; skin observed for contact dermatitis after 48 hours
Radioallergosorbent (RAST)	*in vitro*	Performed on the serum of patients with natural latex as the antigen; used to detect and quantify allergen specific IgE in patient's serum; positive RAST response correlates strongly with *in vivo* allergic response; sensitivity 67% to 82%
AlaSTAT	*in vitro*	Enzyme-linked immunometric assay used to measure latex-specific IgE antibodies; raw natural rubber latex used as source material for AlaSTAT latex allergens; sensitivity 94%, specificity 81%

References and Recommended Reading

DiPiro JT and Stafford CT, "Allergic and Pseudoallergic Drug Reactions," *Pharmacotherapy: A Pathophysiologic Approach*, 3rd ed, Stamford, CT: Appleton and Lange, 1997, 1675-88.

Hamid RK, "Latex Allergy: Diagnosis, Management and Safe Equipment," *Refresher Courses in Anesthesiology*, 1996, 24:85-96.

Holzman RS, "Latex Allergy: An Emerging Operating Room Problem," *Anesth Analg*, 1993, 76(3):635-41.

Levy JH, "Allergy and Anesthesia," Paper presented at the ASA 1996 Annual Refresher Course Lectures, New Orleans, LA, 1996 Oct 20.

Mostello LA, "The Clinical Significance and Management of Latex Allergy," Paper presented at the ASA 1996 Annual Refresher Course Lectures, New Orleans, LA, 1996 Oct 20.

Senst BL and Johnson RA, "Latex Allergy," *Am J Health Syst Pharm*, 1997, 54:1071-5.

Steelman VM, "Latex Allergy Precautions: A Research-Based Protocol:" *Nurs Clin North Am*, 1995, 30(3):475-93.

AMINOGLYCOSIDE DOSING AND MONITORING

All aminoglycoside therapy should be individualized for specific patients in specific clinical situation. The following are guidelines for initiating therapy.

1. Loading dose based on estimated ideal body weight (IBW). **All patients require a loading dose independent of renal function.**

Agent	Dose
Gentamicin	2 mg/kg
Tobramycin	2 mg/kg
Amikacin	7.5 mg/kg

Significantly higher loading doses may be required in severely ill intensive care unit patients.

2. Initial maintenance doses as a percent of loading dose according to desired dosing interval and creatinine clearance (Cl_{cr}):

Male Cl_{cr} (mL/min) = $\dfrac{(140-age) \times IBW}{72 \times serum\ creatinine}$

Female = 0.85 x Cl_{cr} males

Cl_{cr}	Dosing Interval (h)		
(mL/min)	8	12	24
90	84%	—	—
80	80%	—	—
70	76%	88%	—
60	—	84%	—
50	—	79%	—
40	—	72%	92%
30	—	—	86%
25	—	—	81%
20	—	—	75%

Patients >65 years of age should not receive initial aminoglycoside maintenance dosing more often than every 12 hours.

3. Serum concentration monitoring

- Serum concentration monitoring is necessary for **safe** and **effective** therapy, particularly in patients with serious infections and those with risk factors for toxicity.
- Peak serum concentrations should be drawn 30 minutes after the completion of a 30-minute infusion. Trough serum concentrations should be drawn within 30 minutes prior to the administered dose.
- Serum concentrations should be drawn after 5 half-lives, usually around the third dose or thereafter.

4. Desired measured serum concentrations

	Peak (mcg/mL)	Trough (mcg/mL)
Gentamicin	6-10	0.5-2.0
Tobramycin	6-10	0.5-2.0
Amikacin	20-30	<5

5. For patients receiving hemodialysis:
- administer the **same** loading dose
- administer $^2/_3$ of the loading dose after each dialysis

- **serum concentrations must be monitored**
- watch for ototoxicity from accumulation of drug
- For individual clinical situations the prescribing physician should feel free to consult Infectious Disease, the Pharmacology Service, or the Pharmacy.

"Once Daily" Aminoglycosides

High dose, "once daily" aminoglycoside therapy for treatment of gram-negative bacterial infections has been studied and remains controversial. The pharmacodynamics of aminoglycosides reveal dose-dependent killing which suggests an efficacy advantage of "high" peak serum concentrations. It is also suggested that allowing troughs to fall to unmeasurable levels decreases the risk of nephrotoxicity without detriment to efficacy. Because of a theoretical saturation of tubular cell uptake of aminoglycosides, decreasing the number of times the drug is administered in a particular time period may play a role in minimizing the risk of nephrotoxicity. Ototoxicity has not been sufficiently formally evaluated through audiometry or vestibular testing comparing "once daily" to standard therapy. Over 100 letters, commentaries, studies, and reviews have been published on the topic of "once daily" aminoglycosides with varying dosing regimens, monitoring parameters, inclusion and exclusion criteria, and results (most of which have been favorable for the "once daily" regimens). The caveats of this simplified method of dosing are several, including assurance that creatinine clearances be calculated, that all patients are not candidates and should not be considered for this regimen, and that "once daily" is a semantic misnomer.

Because of the controversial nature of this method, it is beyond the scope of this book to present significant detail and dosing regimen recommendations. Considerable experience with two methods warrants mention. The Hartford Hospital has experience with over 2000 patients utilizing a 7 mg/kg dose, a dosing scheme for various creatinine clearance estimates, and a serum concentration monitoring nomogram.[1] Providence Medical Center utilizes a 5 mg/kg dosing regimen but only in patients with excellent renal function; serum concentrations are monitored 4-6 hours prior to the dose administered.[2] Two excellent reviews discuss the majority of studies and controversies regarding these dosing techniques.[3,4] An editorial accompanies one of the reviews and is worth examination.[5]

"Once daily" dosing may be a safe and effective method of providing aminoglycoside therapy to a large number of patients who require these efficacious yet toxic agents. As with any method of aminoglycoside administration, dosing must be individualized and the caveats of the method considered.

Footnotes

1. Nicolau DP, Freeman CD, Belliveau PP, et al, "Experience with a Once-Daily Aminoglycoside Program Administered to 2,184 Patients," *Antimicrob Agents Chemother*, 1995, 39:650-5.
2. Gilbert DN, "Once-Daily Aminoglycoside Therapy," *Antimicrob Agents Chemother*, 1991, 35:399-405.
3. Preston SL and Briceland LL, "Single Daily Dosing of Aminoglycosides," *Pharmacotherapy*, 1995, 15:297-316.
4. Bates RD and Nahata MC, "Once-Daily Administration of Aminoglycosides," *Ann Pharmacother*, 1994, 28:757-66.
5. Rotschafer JC and Rybak MJ, "Single Daily Dosing of Aminoglycosides: A Commentary," *Ann Pharmacother*, 1994, 28:797-801.

Aminoglycoside Penetration Into Various Tissues	
Site	**Extent of Distribution**
Eye	Poor
CNS	Poor (<25%)
Pleural	Excellent
Bronchial secretions	Poor
Sputum	Fair (10%-50%)
Pulmonary tissue	Excellent
Ascitic fluid	Variable (43%-132%)
Peritoneal fluid	Poor
Bile	Variable (25%-90%)

Aminoglycoside Penetration Into Various Tissues *(Continued)*

Site	Extent of Distribution
Bile with obstruction	Poor
Synovial fluid	Excellent
Bone	Poor
Prostate	Poor
Urine	Excellent
Renal tissue	Excellent

Adapted from Neu HC, "Pharmacology of Aminoglycosides," *The Aminoglycosides*, Whelton E and Neu HC, eds, New York, NY: Marcel Dekker, Inc, 1981.

ANGIOTENSIN AGENTS

ACE Inhibitors: Comparison of Indications and Adult Dosages

Drug	Hypertension	CHF	Renal Dysfunction	Dialyzable	Strengths (mg)
Benazepril (Lotensin®)	10-40 mg/day	Not FDA approved	$Cl_{cr} < 30$ mL/min: 5 mg/day initially Maximum: 40 mg/day	Yes	Tablets 5, 10, 20, 40
Captopril (Capoten®)	25-100 mg/day bid-tid	6.25-100 mg tid Maximum: 450 mg/day	Cl_{cr} 10-50 mL/min: 75% of usual dose $Cl_{cr} < 10$ mL/min: 50% of usual dose	Yes	Tablets 12.5, 25, 50, 100
Enalapril (Vasotec®)	2.5-40 mg/day qd-bid	2.5-20 mg bid Maximum: 20 mg bid	Cl_{cr} 30-80 mL/min: 5 mg/day initially $Cl_{cr} < 30$ mL/min: 2.5 mg/day initially	Yes	Tablets 2.5, 5, 10, 20
Enalaprilat[1]	0.625 mg, 1.25 mg, 2.5 mg q6h Maximum: 5 mg q6h	Not FDA approved	$Cl_{cr} < 30$ mL/min: 0.625 mg q6h	Yes	2.5 mg/2 mL vial
Fosinopril (Monopril®)	10-40 mg/day	10-40 mg/day	No dosage reduction necessary	Not well dialyzed	Tablets 10, 20, 40
Lisinopril (Prinivil®, Zestril®)	10-40 mg/day Maximum: 40 mg/day	5-40 mg/day	Cl_{cr} 10-30 mL/min: 5 mg/day initially $Cl_{cr} < 10$ mL/min: 2.5 mg/day initially	Yes	Tablets 2.5, 5, 10, 20, 30, 40
Moexipril (Univasc®)	7.5-30 mg/day qd-bid Maximum: 30 mg/day	LV dysfunction (post-MI): 7.5-30 mg/day	$Cl_{cr} < 40$ mL/min: 3.75 mg/day initially Maximum: 15 mg/day	Unknown	Tablets 7.5, 15
Perindopril (Aceon®)	4-8 mg/day	4-8 mg/day Maximum: 16 mg/day	Cl_{cr} 30-60 mL/min: 2 mg/day Cl_{cr} 15-29 mL/min: 2 mg qod $Cl_{cr} < 15$ mL/min: 2 mg on dialysis days	Yes	Tablets 2, 4, 8
Quinapril (Accupril®)	10-40 mg/day qd-bid	5-20 mg bid	Cl_{cr} 30-60 mL/min: 5 mg/day initially $Cl_{cr} < 10$-30 mL/min: 2.5 mg/day initially	Not well dialyzed	Tablets 5, 10, 20, 40
Ramipril (Altace®)	2.5-20 mg/day qd-bid	2.5-10 mg/day	$Cl_{cr} < 40$ mL/min: 25% of normal dose	Unknown	Capsules 1.25, 2.5, 5, 10
Trandolapril (Mavik®)	1-4 mg/day Maximum: 8 mg/day qd-bid	LV dysfunction (post-MI): 1-4 mg/day	$Cl_{cr} < 30$ mL/min: 0.5 mg/day initially	No	Tablets 1, 2, 4

Dosage is based on 70 kg adult with normal hepatic and renal function.
[1]Enalaprilat is the only available ACE inhibitor in a parenteral formulation.

Angiotensin II Receptor Blockers: Comparison of Indications and Adult Dosages

Drug	Hypertension	CHF	Renal Dysfunction	Dialyzable	Strengths (mg)
Candesartan (Atacand®)	8-32 mg/day	Target: 32 mg once daily	No dosage adjustment necessary	No	Tablets 4, 8, 16, 32
Eprosartan (Teveten®)	400-800 mg/day qd-bid	Not FDA approved	No dosage adjustment necessary	Unknown	Tablets 400, 600
Irbesartan (Avapro®)	150-300 mg/day	Not FDA approved	No dosage reduction necessary	No	Tablets 75, 150, 300
Losartan (Cozaar®)	25-100 mg qd or bid	Not FDA approved	No dosage adjustment necessary	No	Tablets 25, 50, 100
Olmesartan (Benicar®)	20-40 mg/day	Not FDA approved	No dosage adjustment necessary	Unknown	Tablets 5, 20, 40
Telmisartan (Micardis®)	20-80 mg/day	Not FDA approved	No dosage reduction necessary	No	Tablets 20, 40, 80
Valsartan (Diovan®)	80-320 mg/day	Target: 160 mg bid	Decrease dose only if $Cl_{cr} < 10$ mL/minute	No	Tablets 40, 80, 160, 320

Dosage is based on 70 kg adult with normal hepatic and renal function.

ACE Inhibitors: Comparative Pharmacokinetics

Drug	Prodrug	Absorption (%)	Serum $t_{1/2}$ (h) Normal Renal Function	Serum Protein Binding (%)	Elimination	Onset of BP Lowering Action (h)	Peak BP Lowering Effects (h)	Duration of BP Lowering Effects (h)
Benazepril	Yes	37		~97	Renal (32%), biliary (~12%)	1	2-4	24
Benazeprilat			10-11 (effective)	~95				
Captopril	No	60-75 (fasting)	1.9 (elimination)	25-30	Renal	0.25-0.5	1-1.5	~6
Enalapril	Yes	55-75	2	50-60	Renal (60%-80%), fecal	1	4-6	12-24
Enalaprilat			11 (effective)					
Fosinopril		36			Renal (~50%), biliary (~50%)	1		24
Fosinoprilat			12 (effective)	>99				
Moexipril	Yes		1	90	Fecal (53%), renal (8%)		1-2	>24
Moexiprilat			2-10	50				
Perindopril	Yes		1.5-3	60	Renal		3-7	
Perindoprilat			3-10 (effective)	10-20				
Quinapril	Yes	>60	0.8	97	Renal (~60%) as metabolite, fecal	1	2-4	24
Quinaprilat			2					
Ramipril	Yes	50-60	1-2	73	Renal (60%), fecal (40%)	1-2	3-6	24
Ramiprilat			13-17 (effective)	56				
Trandolapril	Yes		6	80	Renal (33%), fecal (66%)	1-2	6	≥24
Trandolaprilat			10	65-94				

Angiotensin II Receptor Blockers: Comparative Pharmacokinetics

	Candesartan (Atacand®)	Eprosartan (Teveten®)	Irbesartan (Avapro®)	Losartan (Cozaar®)	Olmesartan (Benicar®)	Telmisartan (Micardis®)	Valsartan (Diovan®)
Prodrug	Yes[1]	No	No	Yes[2]	Yes	No	No
Time to peak	3-4 h	1-2 h	1.5-2	1 h / 3-4 h[2]	1-2 h	0.5-1 h	2-4 h
Bioavailability	15%	13%	60%-80%	33%	26%	42%-58%	25%
Food – area-under-the-curve	No effect	No effect	No effect	9%-10%	No effect	9.6%-20%	9%-40%
Elimination half-life	9 h	5-9 h	11-15 h	1.5-2 h / 6-9 h[2]	13 h	24 h	6 h
Elimination altered in renal dysfunction	Yes[3]	No	No	No	Yes	No	No
Precautions in severe renal dysfunction	Yes	Yes	Yes	Yes	Yes	Yes	Yes
Elimination altered in hepatic dysfunction	No	No	No	Yes	Yes	Yes	Yes
Precautions in hepatic dysfunction	No	Yes	No	No	No	Yes	No
Protein binding	>99%	98%	90%	~99%	99%	>99.5%	95%

[1]Candesartan cilexetil: Active metabolite candesartan.
[2]Losartan: Active metabolite E-3174.
[3]Dosage adjustments are not necessary.

ANIMAL AND HUMAN BITES GUIDELINES

Bite Wound Antibiotic Regimens

	Dog Bite	Cat Bite	Human Bite
Prophylactic Antibiotics			
Prophylaxis	No routine prophylaxis, consider if involves face or hand, or immuno-suppressed or asplenic patients	Routine prophylaxis	Routine prophylaxis
Prophylactic antibiotic	Amoxicillin	Amoxicillin	Amoxicillin
Penicillin allergy	Doxycycline if >10 y or co-trimoxazole	Doxycycline if >10 y or co-trimoxazole	Doxycycline if >10 y or erythromycin and cephalexin*
Outpatient Oral Antibiotic Treatment (mild to moderate infection)			
Established infection	Amoxicillin and clavulanic acid	Amoxicillin and clavulanic acid	Amoxicillin and clavulanic acid
Penicillin allergy (mild infection only)	Doxycycline if >10 y	Doxycycline if >10 y	Cephalexin* or clindamycin
Outpatient Parenteral Antibiotic Treatment (moderate infections – single drug regimens)			
	Ceftriaxone	Ceftriaxone	Cefotetan
Inpatient Parenteral Antibiotic Treatment			
Established infection	Ampicillin + cefazolin	Ampicillin + cefazolin	Ampicillin + clindamycin
Penicillin allergy	Cefazolin*	Ceftriaxone*	Cefotetan* or imipenem
Duration of Prophylactic and Treatment Regimens			
Prophylaxis: 5 days			
Treatment: 10-14 days			
*Contraindicated if history of immediate hypersensitivity reaction (anaphylaxis) to penicillin.			

References

Richardson M, "The Management of Animal and Human Bite Wounds," *Nurs Times*, 2006, 102(3):34-36.

Taplitz RA, "Managing Bite Wounds: Currently Recommended Antibiotics for Treatment and Prophylaxis," *Postgrad Med*, 2004, 116(2):49-59.

ANTACID DRUG INTERACTIONS

Drug	Antacid				
	Al Salts	Ca Salts	Mg Salts	NaHCO₃	Mg/Al
Allopurinol	↓				
Anorexiants				↑	
Atorvastatin	↓		↓		
Benzodiazepines	↑		↓	↓	↓
Calcitriol			x*		x*
Captopril					↓
Cimetidine	↓		↓		↓
Corticosteroids	↓		↓		↓
Digoxin	↓		↓		
Flecainide				↑	
Indomethacin	↓		↓		↓
Iron	↓	↓	↓	↓	↓
Isoniazid	↓				
Itraconazole	↓	↓	↓	↓	↓
Ketoconazole	↓	↓	↓	↓	↓
Levodopa					↑
Lithium				↓	
Mycophenolate	↓		↓		
Naproxen	↑		↑	↓	↑
Nitrofurantoin			↓		
Penicillamine	↓		↓		↓
Phenothiazines	↓		↓		↓
Phenytoin		↓			↓
Quinidine		↑	↑		↑
Quinolones	↓	↓	↓		↓
Ranitidine	↓				↓
Rofecoxib	—	↓	—	—	↓
Salicylates				↓	↓
Sodium polystyrene sulfonate	x†		x†		x†
Sulfonylureas				↑	
Sympathomimetics				↑	
Tetracyclines	↓	↓	↓	↓	↓
Tolmetin				x‡	

Pharmacologic effect increased (↑) or decreased (↓) by antacids.
*Concomitant use in patients on chronic renal dialysis may lead to hypermagnesemia.
†Concomitant use may cause metabolic alkalosis in patients with renal failure.
‡Concomitant use not recommended by manufacturer.

ANTIARRHYTHMIC DRUGS

Vaughan Williams Classification of Antiarrhythmic Drugs Based on Cardiac Effects				
Class	**Drug(s)**	**Conduction Velocity[1]**	**Refractory Period**	**Automaticity**
I	Moricizine	↓	↓	↓ (0 on SA node)
Ia	Disopyramide Procainamide Quinidine	↓	↑	↓
Ib	Lidocaine Mexiletine Tocainide	0/↓	↓	↓
Ic	Flecainide Propafenone[2]	↓↓	0	↓
II	Beta-blockers	0	0	↓
III	Amiodarone Bretylium Dofetilide Ibutilide Sotalol [2]	0	↑↑	0
IV	Diltiazem Verapamil[3]	↓	↑	↓

[1]Variables for normal tissue models in ventricular tissue.
[2]Also has type II, beta-blocking action.
[3]Variables for SA and AV nodal tissue only.

Vaughan Williams Classification of Antiarrhythmic Agents and Their Indications/Adverse Effects				
Class	**Drug(s)**	**Indication**	**Route of Administration**	**Adverse Effects**
I	Moricizine	VT	P.O.	Dizziness, nausea, rash, seizures
Ia	Disopyramide	AF, VT	P.O.	Anticholinergic effects, CHF
	Procainamide	AF, VT, WPW	P.O./I.V.	GI, CNS, lupus, fever, hematological, anticholinergic effects
	Quinidine	AF, PSVT, VT, WPW	P.O./I.V.	Hypotension, GI, thrombocytopenia, cinchonism
Ib	Lidocaine	VT, VF, PVC	I.V.	CNS, GI
	Mexiletine	VT	P.O.	GI, CNS
	Tocainide	VT	P.O.	GI, CNS, pulmonary, agranulocytosis
Ic	Flecainide	VT	P.O.	CHF, GI, CNS, blurred vision
	Propafenone	VT	P.O.	GI, blurred vision, dizziness
II	Esmolol	VT, SVT	I.V.	CHF, CNS, lupus-like syndrome, hypotension, bradycardia, bronchospasm
	Propranolol	SVT, VT, PVC, digoxin toxicity	P.O./I.V.	CHF, bradycardia, hypotension, CNS, fatigue
III	Amiodarone	VT	P.O.	CNS, GI, thyroid, pulmonary fibrosis, liver, corneal deposits
	Bretylium	VT, VF	I.V.	GI, orthostatic hypotension, CNS
	Dofetilide	AF	P.O.	Headache, dizziness, VT, torsade de pointes
	Ibutilide	AF	I.V.	Torsade de pointes, hypotension, branch bundle block, AV block, nausea, headache
	Sotalol	AF, VT	P.O.	Bradycardia, hypotension, CHF, CNS, fatigue
IV	Diltiazem	AF, PSVT	P.O./I.V.	Hypotension, GI, liver
	Verapamil	AF, PSVT	P.O./I.V.	Hypotension, CHF, bradycardia, vertigo, constipation
Miscellaneous	Adenosine	SVT, PSVT	I.V.	Flushing, dizziness, bradycardia, syncope
	Digoxin	AF, PSVT	P.O./I.V.	GI, CNS, arrhythmias
	Magnesium	VT, VF	I.V.	Hypotension, CNS, hypothermia, myocardial depression

AF = atrial fibrillation; PSVT = paroxysmal supraventricular tachycardia; VT = ventricular tachycardia; WPW = Wolf-Parkinson-White arrhythmias; VF = ventricular fibrillation; SVT = supraventricular tachycardia; PVC = premature ventricular contraction.

Comparative Pharmacokinetic Properties of Antiarrhythmic Agents

Class	Drug(s)	Bioavailability (%)	Primary Route of Elimination	Volume of Distribution (L/kg)	Protein Binding (%)	Half-Life	Therapeutic Range (mcg/mL)
I	Moricizine	34-38	Hepatic	6-11	92-95	1-6 h	—
Ia	Disopyramide	70-95	Hepatic/Renal	0.8-2	50-80	4-8 h	2-6
	Procainamide	75-95	Hepatic/Renal	1.5-3	10-20	2.5-5 h	4-15
	Quinidine	70-80	Hepatic	2-3.5	80-90	5-9 h	2-6
Ib	Lidocaine	20-40	Hepatic	1-2	65-75	60-180 min	1.5-5
	Mexiletine	80-95	Hepatic	5-12	60-75	6-12 h	0.75-2
	Tocainide	90-95	Hepatic	1.5-3	10-30	12-15 h	4-10
Ic	Flecainide	90-95	Hepatic/Renal	8-10	35-45	12-30 h	0.3-2.5
	Propafenone[1]	11-39	Hepatic	2.5-4	85-95	12-32 h 2-10 h	—
II	Esmolol			Refer to Beta-Blocker Comparison Chart			
	Propranolol			Refer to Beta-Blocker Comparison Chart			
III	Amiodarone	22-28	Hepatic	70-150	95-97	15-100 d	1-2.5
	Bretylium	15-20	Renal	4-8	Negligible	5-10 h	0.5-2
	Dofetilide	>90%	Renal	3 L/kg	60-70	10 h	—
	Ibutilide	NA	Hepatic	11	40	2-12 h	—
	Sotalol	90-95	Renal	1.6-2.4	Negligible	12-15 h	—
IV	Diltiazem	80-90	Hepatic/Renal	1.7	77-85	4-6 h	0.05-0.2
	Verapamil	20-40	Hepatic	1.5-5	95-99	4-12 h	>50 ng/mL

[1]**Top** numbers reflect **poor** metabolizers and **bottom** numbers reflect **extensive** metabolizers.

ANTICHOLINERGIC EFFECTS OF COMMON PSYCHOTROPICS

Drug	Atropine Equivalence Factor*	Common Daily Dose (mg)	Atropine Equivalent (mg/dose)
ANTICHOLINERGICS			
Benztropine	0.849	2	1.70
Diphenhydramine	0.011	50	0.55
Trihexyphenidyl	0.828	5	4.14
NEUROLEPTICS			
Chlorpromazine	0.030	500	15.00
Clozapine	0.125	500	62.50
Fluphenazine	0.001	25	0.03
Haloperidol	0.000	20	0.00
Loxapine	0.005	150	0.75
Mesoridazine	0.025	150	3.75
Molindone	0.000	150	0.00
Perphenazine	0.001	32	0.03
Thioridazine	0.104	300	31.20
Thiothixene	0.001	40	0.04
Trifluoperazine	0.003	25	0.08
ANTIDEPRESSANTS			
Amitriptyline	0.121	150	18.15
Amoxapine	0.002	150	0.30
Desipramine	0.011	150	1.65
Doxepin	0.026	150	3.90
Fluoxetine	0.001	20	0.02
Imipramine	0.024	150	3.60
Maprotiline	0.004	150	0.60
Nortriptyline	0.015	75	1.13
Trazodone	0.000	100	0.00

*Anticholinergic effects of 1 mg of drug in equivalent mg of atropine.

ANTIDEPRESSANT AGENTS

Comparison of Usual Dosage, Mechanism of Action, and Adverse Effects

Drug	Initial Dose	Usual Dosage (mg/d)	Dosage Forms	Adverse Effects						Comments
				ACH	Drowsiness	Orthostatic Hypotension	Conduction Abnormalities	GI Distress	Weight Gain	
Tricyclic Antidepressants and Related Compounds[1]										
Amitriptyline (Elavil®, Vanatrip®)	25-75 mg qhs	100-300	T, I	4+	4+	3+	3+	1	4+	Also used in chronic pain, migraine, and as a hypnotic; contraindicated with cisapride
Amoxapine	50 mg bid	100-400	T	2+	2+	2+	2+	0	2+	May cause extrapyramidal symptom (EPS)
Clomipramine[2] (Anafranil®)	25-75 mg qhs	100-250	C	4+	4+	2+	3+	1+	4+	Approved for OCD
Desipramine (Norpramin®)	25-75 mg qhs	100-300	T	1+	2+	2+	2+	0	1+	Blood levels useful for therapeutic monitoring
Doxepin (Sinequan®, Zonalon®)	25-75 mg qhs	100-300	C, L	3+	4+	2+	2+	0	4+	
Imipramine (Tofranil®, Tofranil-PM®)	25-75 mg qhs	100-300	T, C	3+	3+	4+	3+	1+	4+	Blood levels useful for therapeutic monitoring
Maprotiline (Ludiomil®)	25-75 mg qhs	100-225	T	2+	3+	2+	2+	0	2+	
Nortriptyline (Aventyl®, Pamelor®)	25-50 mg qhs	50-150	C, L	2+	2+	1+	2+	0	1+	Blood levels useful for therapeutic monitoring
Protriptyline (Vivactil®)	15 mg qAM	15-60	T	2+	1+	2+	3+	1+	1+	
Trimipramine (Surmontil®)	25-75 mg qhs	100-300	C	4+	4+	3+	3+	0	4+	
Selective Serotonin Reuptake Inhibitors[3]										
Citalopram (Celexa™)	20 mg qAM	20-60	T	0	0	0	0	3+[4]	1+	
Escitalopram (Lexapro™)	10 mg qAM	10-20	T	0	0	0	0	3+	1+	S-enantiomer of citalopram
Fluoxetine (Prozac®, Prozac® Weekly™, Sarafem™)	10-20 mg qAM	20-80	C, L, T	0	0	0	0	3+[4]	1+	CYP2B6 and 2D6 inhibitor
Fluvoxamine (Luvox®)[2]	50 mg qhs	100-300	T	0	0	0	0	3+[4]	1+	Contraindicated with pimozide, thioridazine, mesoridazine, CYP1A2, 2B6, 2C19, and 3A4 inhibitors
Paroxetine (Paxil®, Paxil® CR™)	10-20 mg qAM	20-50	T, L	1+	1+	0	0	3+[4]	2+	CYP2B6 and 2D6 inhibitor

Comparison of Usual Dosage, Mechanism of Action, and Adverse Effects (*Continued*)

Drug	Initial Dose	Usual Dosage (mg/d)	Dosage Forms	Adverse Effects						Comments
				ACH	Drowsiness	Orthostatic Hypotension	Conduction Abnormalities	GI Distress	Weight Gain	
Sertraline (Zoloft®)	25-50 mg qAM	50-200	T	0	0	0	0	3+[4]	1+	CYP2B6 and 2C19 inhibitor
Dopamine-Reuptake Blocking Compounds										
Bupropion (Wellbutrin®, Wellbutrin SR®, Wellbutrin XL™, Zyban®)	100 mg bid-tid IR[5] 150 mg qAM-bid SR[6]	300-450[7]	T	0	0	0	1+/0	1+	0	Contraindicated with seizures, bulimia, and anorexia; low incidence of sexual dysfunction IR: A 6-h interval between doses preferred SR: An 8-h interval between doses preferred
Serotonin / Norepinephrine Reuptake Inhibitors[8]										
Duloxetine (Cymbalta®)	40-60 mg/d	40-60	C	1+	1+	0	1+	3+	0	Useful for stress incontinence and chronic pain
Venlafaxine (Effexor®, Effexor® XR)	25 mg bid-tid IR 37.5 mg qd XR	75-375	T	1+	1+	0	1+	3+[4]	0	High-dose is useful to treat refractory depression; frequency of hypertension increases with dosage >225 mg/d
5HT2 Receptor Antagonist Properties										
Nefazodone (Serzone®)	100 mg bid	300-600	T	1+	1+	2+	1+	1+	0	Contraindicated with carbamazepine, pimozide, astemizole, cisapride, and terfenadine; caution with triazolam and alprazolam; low incidence of sexual dysfunction
Trazodone (Desyrel®)	50 mg tid	150-600	T	0	4+	3+	1+	1+	2+	
Noradrenergic Antagonist										
Mirtazapine (Remeron®, Remeron® SolTab™)	15 mg qhs	15-45	T	1+	3+	1+	1+	0	3+	Dose >15 mg/d less sedating, low incidence of sexual dysfunction

Comparison of Usual Dosage, Mechanism of Action, and Adverse Effects *(Continued)*

Drug	Initial Dose	Usual Dosage (mg/d)	Dosage Forms	Adverse Effects							Comments
				ACH	Drowsiness	Orthostatic Hypotension	Conduction Abnormalities	GI Distress	Weight Gain	
Monoamine Oxidase Inhibitors										
Isocarboxazid (Marplan®)	10 mg tid	10-30	T	2+	2+	2+	1+	1+	2+	Diet must be low in tyramine; contraindicated with sympathomimetics and other antidepressants
Phenelzine (Nardil®)	15 mg tid	15-90	T	2+	2+	2+	0	1+	3+	
Tranylcypromine (Parnate®)	10 mg bid	10-60	T	2+	1+	2+	1+	1+	2+	

ACH = anticholinergic effects (dry mouth, blurred vision, urinary retention, constipation); 0 - 4+ = absent or rare - relatively common. T = tablet, L = liquid, I = injectable, C = capsule; IR = immediate release, SR = sustained release.

[1]**Important note:** A 1-week supply taken all at once in a patient receiving the maximum dose can be fatal.

[2]Not approved by FDA for depression. Approved for OCD.

[3]Flat dose response curve, headache, nausea, and sexual dysfunction are common side effects for SSRIs.

[4]Nausea is usually mild and transient.

[5]IR: 100 mg bid, may be increased to 100 mg tid no sooner than 3 days after beginning therapy.

[6]SR: 150 mg qAM, may be increased to 150 mg bid as early as day 4 of dosing.

[7]To minimize seizure risk, do not exceed IR 150 mg/dose or SR 200 mg/dose.

[8]Do not use with sibutramine; relatively safe in overdose.

ANTIDEPRESSANT RECEPTOR PROFILE

Generic Name (Brand Name)	NE-T	5HT-T	DA-T	M_1	H_1	α_1
Amitriptyline	34.5	4.33	3200	**17.9**	1.1	27
Amoxapine	16.1	58.5	4350	1000	25	50
Bupropion (Wellbutrin®; Wellbutrin SR®; Wellbutrin XL™; Zyban®)	52,600	9100	526	40,000	6200	4550
Citalopram (Celexa™)	4000	1.16	28,000	2200	476	1890
Clomipramine (Anafranil®)	37	0.28	2200	**37**	31.2	38.5
Desipramine (Norpramin®)	**0.83**	17.5	3200	196	110	130
Doxepin (Prudoxin™; Sinequan®; Zonalon®)	29.4	66.7	12,200	83	**0.24**	23.8
Escitalopram (Lexapro™)	7841	1.10	27,410	1242	1973	3870
Fluoxetine (Prozac®; Prozac® Weekly™; Sarafem™)	244	**0.81**	3600	2000	6250	5900
Fluvoxamine	1300	2.22	9100	24,000	>100,000	7700
Imipramine (Tofranil®; Tofranil-PM®)	37	1.41	8300	91	11	90.9
Maprotiline	11.1	5900	1000	560	2.0	90.9
Mirtazapine (Remeron®; Remeron SolTab®)	4760	100,000	100,000	670	**0.14**	500
Nefazodone (Serzone®)	60	200	360	11,000	21.3	25.6
Nortriptyline (Aventyl® HCl; Pamelor®)	4.35	18.5	1140	149	10	58.8
Paroxetine (Paxil®; Paxil CR™)	40	**0.13**	500	108	22,000	>100,000
Protriptyline (Vivactil®)	1.40	19.6	2130	**25**	25	130
Sertraline (Zoloft®)	417	**0.29**	**25**	625	24,000	370
Trazodone (Desyrel®)	8300	160	7140	>100,000	345	35.7
Trimipramine (Surmontil®)	2400	1500	10,000	58.8	0.27	23.8
Venlafaxine (Effexor®; Effexor® XR)	1060	9.10	9100	>100,000	>100,000	>100,000

Note: NE-T = norepinephrine transporter; 5HT-T = serotonin transporter; DA-T = dopamine transporter; M_1 = muscarinic$_1$ receptor; H_1 = histamine H_1 receptor; α_1 = alpha$_1$ receptor

ANTIMIGRAINE DRUGS: 5-HT1 RECEPTOR AGONISTS

Pharmacokinetic Differences

Pharmacokinetic Parameter	Almotriptan (Axert™)	Eletriptan (Relpax®)	Frovatriptan (Frova®)	Naratriptan (Amerge®)	Rizatriptan (Maxalt®, Maxalt-MLT®)		Sumatriptan (Imitrex®)			Zolmitriptan (Zomig®, Zomig-ZMT™)	
	Oral (6.25 mg)	Tablets	Oral	Oral	Tablets	Disintegrating Tablets	SubQ (6 mg)	Oral (100 mg)	Nasal (20 mg)	Oral (5 mg)	Oral (10 mg)
Onset	<60 min	<2 h	<2 h	30 min	~30 min	~30 min	10 min	30-60 min	<60 min	0.5-1 h	
Duration	Short	Short	Long	Long	Short	Short	Short	Short	Short	Short	
Time to peak serum concentration (h)	1-3	1.5-2	2-4	2-4	1-1.5	1.6-2.5	5-20	1.5-2.5	1	1.5	2-3.5
Average bioavailability (%)	70	50	20-30	70	45	—	97	15	17	40-46	46-49
Volume of distribution (L)	180-200	138	210-280	170	110-140	110-140	170	170	NA	—	402
Half-life (h)	3-4	4	26	6	2-3	2-3	2	2-2.5[1]	2	2.8-3.4	2.5-3.7
Fraction excreted unchanged in urine (%)	40	—	32	50	14	14	22	3	3	8	8

[1]With extended dosing, the half-life extends to 7 hours.

ANTIPARKINSONIAN AGENTS

Drug	Formulation	Dosage Range (mg/d)	Relative Oral Potency
Anticholinergic			
Benztropine (Cogentin®[1])	Tablet: 0.5 mg, 1 mg, 2 mg	1-6	2
	Injection: 1 mg/mL (2 mL ampul)		
Biperiden (Akineton®)	Tablet: 2 mg	2-8	2
	Injection: 5 mg/mL (1 mL ampul)		
Orphenadrine (Norflex™)	Tablet: 100 mg	50-400	50
	Tablet, sustained release: 100 mg		
	Injection: 30 mg/mL (2 mL, 10 mL)		
Antihistaminic			
Diphenhydramine (Benadryl®[1])	Capsule: 25 mg, 50 mg	25-300	25
	Elixir: 12.5 mg/5 mL (4 oz, 8 oz, 16 oz bottle)		
	Injection: 10 mg/mL (10 mL, 30 mL); 50 mg/mL (1 mL, 10 mL)		
	Syrup: 12.5 mg/5 mL		
	Tablet: 25 mg, 50 mg		
Procyclidine (Kemadrin®)	Tablet: 5 mg	7.5-20	5
Trihexyphenidyl (Artane®[1])	Capsule: 5 mg	2-15	5
	Tablet: 2 mg, 5 mg		
	Elixir: 2 mg/5 mL		
Dopaminergic			
Amantadine (Symmetrel®[1])	Tablet: 100 mg	100-400	N/A
	Syrup: 50 mg/5 mL (16 oz bottle)		
Apomorphine (Apokyn™)	Injection: 10 mg/mL (2 mL ampuls; 3 mL cartridges)	1-6	N/A

[1]Available in generic form.

ANTIPSYCHOTIC AGENTS

Antipsychotic Agent	Dosage Forms	I.M./P.O. Potency	Equiv. Dosages (approx) (mg)	Usual Adult Daily Maint. Dose (mg)	Sedation (Incidence)	Extrapyramidal Side Effects	Anticholinergic Side Effects	Orthostatic Hypotension	Comments
Aripiprazole (Abilify™)	Soln, tab		4	10-30	Low	Very low	Very low	Very low	Low weight gain; activating
Chlorpromazine (Thorazine® [DSC])	Conc, inj, supp, syr, tab	4:1	100	200-1000	High	Moderate	Moderate	Moderate / high	
Clozapine (Clozaril®)	Tab		100	75-900	High	Very low	High	High	~1% incidence of agranulocytosis; weekly-biweekly CBC required; potential for weight gain, lipid abnormalities, and diabetes
Fluphenazine (Permitil®, Prolixin®, Prolixin Decanoate®, Prolixin Enanthate®)	Conc, elix, inj, tab	2:1	2	0.5-20	Low	High	Low	Low	
Haloperidol (Haldol®, Haldol® Decanoate)	Conc, inj, tab	2:1	2	0.5-20	Low	High	Low	Low	
Loxapine (Loxitane®, Loxitane® C, Loxitane® I.M.)	Cap, conc, inj		10	25-250	Moderate	Moderate	Low	Low	
Mesoridazine (Serentil®)	Inj, liq, tab	3:1	50	30-400	High	Low	High	Moderate	Prolongs QTc; use only in treatment of refractory illness
Molindone (Moban®)	Conc, tab		15	15-225	Low	Moderate	Low	Low	May cause less weight gain
Olanzapine (Zyprexa®, Zyprexa® Zydis®)	Inj, tab, tab (oral-disintegrating)		4	5-20	Moderate / high	Low	Moderate	Moderate	Potential for weight gain, lipid abnormalities, diabetes
Perphenazine (Trilafon®)	Conc, inj, tab		10	16-64	Low	Moderate	Low	Low	
Pimozide (Orap™)	Tab		2	1-20	Moderate	High	Moderate	Low	Contraindicated with CYP3A inhibitors
Quetiapine (Seroquel®)	Tab		125	50-800	Moderate / high	Very low	Moderate	Moderate	Moderate weight gain; potential for lipid abnormalities; diabetes
Risperidone (Risperdal®)	Inj, soln, tab, tab (oral-disintegrating)		1	0.5-6	Low / moderate	Low	Very low	Moderate	Low to moderate weight gain; potential for diabetes
Thioridazine (Mellaril®)	Conc, tab		100	200-800	High	Low	High	Moderate / high	May cause irreversible retinitis pigmentosa at doses >800 mg/d; prolongs QTc; use only in treatment of refractory illness
Thiothixene (Navane®)	Cap, conc, powder for inj	4:1	4	5-40	Low	High	Low	Low / moderate	
Trifluoperazine (Stelazine® [DSC])	Conc, inj, tab		5	2-40	Low	High	Low	Low	
Ziprasidone (Geodon®)	Cap, powder for inj	2:1	40	40-160	Low / moderate	Low	Very low	Low / moderate	Low weight gain; contraindicated with QTc-prolonging agents

ANTIRETROVIRAL AGENTS

Single Agent Nucleoside Reverse Transcriptase Inhibitors					
Generic Name (Brand Name)	Dosage Form	Normal Dosing	Renal Dosing Adjustment	Hepatic Dosing Adjustment	Selected Adverse Reactions
Single Agent NRTIs (Nucleoside Reverse Transcriptase Inhibitors)					
Abacavir (Ziagen®)	Tablet: 300 mg Solution, oral: 20 mg/mL (240 mL)	300 mg bid or 600 mg daily	None necessary	No recommendation	Hypersensitivity syndrome (fever, fatigue, GI symptoms, ± rash); **do not restart abacavir in patients who have experienced this**; GI symptoms
Didanosine (ddI) (Videx®)	Tablet, chewable: 25 mg, 50 mg, 100 mg, 150 mg, 200 mg Capsule, sustained release: 125 mg, 200 mg, 250 mg, 400 mg	≥60 kg: 200 mg bid or 400 mg daily <60 kg: 125 mg bid or 250 mg daily (take on empty stomach)	≥60 kg: 100-200 mg/day <60 kg: 75-150 mg/day (adjust for $Cl_{cr} <60$) Renal adjustment varies by dosage form and renal function. Consult additional references/product labeling.	No recommendation	Peripheral neuropathy, pancreatitis, abdominal pain, nausea, diarrhea, retinal depigmentation, anxiety, insomnia
Emtricitabine (Emtriva®)	Capsule: 200 mg Solution, oral: 10 mg/mL (170 mL)	Capsule: 200 mg daily Solution: 240 mg daily	Capsule: Cl_{cr} 30-49: 200 mg q48h Cl_{cr} 15-29: 200 q72h $Cl_{cr} <15$ (including hemodialysis [HD] patients): 200 mg q96h Solution: Cl_{cr} 30-49: 120 mg q24h Cl_{cr} 15-29: 80 mg q24h $Cl_{cr} <15$ (including hemodialysis [HD] patients): 60 mg q24h	No recommendation	Headache, dizziness, insomnia, diarrhea, rash, hyperpigmentation of palms/soles
Lamivudine (3TC) (Epivir®, Epivir-HBV®)	Epivir®: Tablet: 150 mg, 300 mg Solution, oral: 10 mg/mL (240 mL) Epivir-HBV®: Tablet: 100 mg Solution, oral: 5 mg/mL (240 mL)	150 mg bid or 300 mg daily	Cl_{cr} 30-49: 150 mg qd Cl_{cr} 15-29: 150 mg first dose, then 100 mg qd Cl_{cr} 5-14: 150 mg first dose, then 50 mg qd $Cl_{cr} <5$ or HD: 50 mg first dose, then 25 mg qd	No recommendation	Headache, insomnia, nausea, vomiting, diarrhea, abdominal pain, myalgia, arthralgia, pancreatitis in children
Stavudine (d4T) (Zerit®)	Capsule: 15 mg, 20 mg, 30 mg, 40 mg Solution, oral: 1 mg/mL (200 mL)	≥60 kg: 40 mg bid <60 kg: 30 mg bid	≥60 kg: Cl_{cr} 26-50: 20 mg bid Cl_{cr} 10-25: 20 mg daily <60 kg: Cl_{cr} 26-50: 15 mg bid Cl_{cr} 10-25 or HD: 15 mg daily	No recommendation	Peripheral neuropathy, headache, abdominal or back pain, asthenia, nausea, vomiting, diarrhea, myalgia, anxiety, depression, pancreatitis, lipodystrophy, hyperlipidemia, hepatotoxicity (less frequently)
Tenofovir (Viread®)	Tablet: 300 mg	300 mg daily	Cl_{cr} 30-49: 300 mg q48h Cl_{cr} 10-29: 300 mg twice a week ESRD or HD: 300 mg once a week	No recommendation	Nausea, vomiting, diarrhea
Zalcitabine (ddC) (Hivid®)	Tablet: 0.375 mg, 0.75 mg	0.75 mg q8h	Cl_{cr} 10-40: 0.75 mg bid $Cl_{cr} <10$: 0.75 mg qd	No recommendation	Peripheral neuropathy, oral/esophageal ulceration, rash, nausea, vomiting, diarrhea, abdominal pain, myalgia, pancreatitis
Zidovudine (AZT) (Retrovir®)	Tablet: 300 mg Capsule: 100 mg Syrup: 50 mg/5 mL (240 mL) Injection: 10 mg/mL (20 mL)	300 mg bid or 200 mg tid	ESRD: 100 mg q6-8h	No recommendation	Anemia, neutropenia, thrombocytopenia, headache, nausea, vomiting, myopathy, hepatitis, hyperpigmentation of nails

Combination Nucleoside Reverse Transcriptase Inhibitors			
Generic Name (Brand Name)	Dosage Form	Normal Dosing	Renal / Hepatic Dosing / Adverse Reactions
Combination NRTIs (Nucleoside Reverse Transcriptase Inhibitors)			
Abacavir + lamivudine (Epzicom™)	Tablet: 600 mg abacavir + 300 mg lamivudine	1 tablet daily	See individual agents
Abacavir + lamivudine + zidovudine (Trizivir®)	Tablet: 300 mg abacavir + 150 mg lamivudine + 300 mg zidovudine	1 tablet bid	
Emtricitabine + tenofovir (Truvada®)	Tablet: 200 mg emtricitabine and 300 mg tenofovir	1 tablet daily	
Zidovudine + lamivudine (Combivir®)	Tablet: 300 mg zidovudine and 150 mg lamivudine	1 tablet bid (see lamivudine for dose adjustment)	

Non-nucleoside Reverse Transcriptase Inhibitors					
Generic Name (Brand Name)	Dosage Form	Normal Dosing	Renal Dosing Adjustment	Hepatic Dosing Adjustment	Selected Adverse Reactions
NNRTIs (Non-nucleoside Reverse Transcriptase Inhibitors)					
Delavirdine (Rescriptor®)	Tablet: 100 mg, 200 mg	400 mg tid	None necessary	No recommendation; use caution	Rash, abnormal liver function tests
Efavirenz (Sustiva®)	Capsule: 50 mg, 100 mg, 200 mg Tablet: 600 mg	600 mg qd (take on empty stomach)	None necessary	No recommendation; use caution	Dizziness, psychiatric symptoms (hallucinations, confusion, depersonalization, others), agitation, vivid dreams, rash, GI intolerance
Nevirapine (Viramune®)	Tablet: 200 mg Suspension, oral: 50 mg/5 mL (240 mL)	200 mg qd for 14 days, then 200 mg bid	None necessary	Avoid use in mild to moderate hepatic impairment	Rash (severe), abnormal liver function tests, fever, nausea, headache

Protease Inhibitors					
Generic Name (Brand Name)	Dosage Form	Normal Dosing	Renal Dosing Adjustment	Hepatic Dosing[1] Adjustment	Selected Adverse Reactions
PIs (Protease Inhibitors)					
Amprenavir (Agenerase®)	Capsule: 50 mg Solution, oral: 15 mg/mL (240 mL) (contains propylene glycol 550 mg/mL)	Capsule: 1200 mg bid Solution: 1400 mg bid (Avoid high fat meal)	Capsule: None necessary Solution: Contra-indicated	C-P 5-8: 450 mg bid C-P 9-12: 300 mg bid	Rash (life-threatening), paresthesias (perioral), depression, nausea, diarrhea, vomiting, hyperglycemia (and sometimes diabetes), dyslipidemia including fat redistribution ("buffalo hump," "protease paunch"), hyperlipidemia, hypercholesterolemia
Atazanavir (Reyataz®)	Capsule: 100 mg, 150 mg, 200 mg	400 mg daily (take with food)	None necessary	C-P 7-9: 300 mg daily C-P >9: Not recommended	Headache, nausea, increased bilirubin, lipodystrophy, hyperglycemia, increased P-R interval
Fosamprenavir (Lexiva™)	Tablet: 700 mg	1400 mg bid (1400 mg/day with ritonavir)	None necessary	C-P 5-8: 700 mg bid C-P 9-12: Not recommended	Rash, increased LFTs

Protease Inhibitors *(Continued)*

Generic Name (Brand Name)	Dosage Form	Normal Dosing	Renal Dosing Adjustment	Hepatic Dosing[1] Adjustment	Selected Adverse Reactions
Indinavir (Crixivan®)	Capsule: 100 mg, 200 mg, 333 mg, 400 mg	800 mg q8h with water	None necessary	Mild to moderate hepatic insufficiency due to cirrhosis: 600 mg q8h	Hyperbilirubinemia, nephrolithiasis, elevated AST/ALT, abdominal pain, nausea, vomiting, diarrhea, taste perversion, hyperglycemia (and sometimes diabetes), dyslipidemia including fat redistribution ("buffalo hump," "protease paunch"), hyperlipidemia, hypercholesterolemia
Lopinavir and ritonavir (Kaletra®)	Capsule: Lopinavir 133.3 mg and ritonavir 33.3 mg Solution, oral: Lopinavir 80 mg and ritonavir 20 mg/mL (contains 42% ethanol)	3 capsules or 5 mL bid (take with food) or if treatment naive: 6 capsules or 10 mL daily Once daily dosing and using with efavirenz or nevirapine: 4 capsules or 6.7 mL bid	None necessary	No recommendation; use caution	GI intolerance (eg, nausea, vomiting, abdominal pain, and diarrhea, with incidence increased with daily dosing), asthenia, circumoral and peripheral paresthesia, taste perversion, headache, hyperglycemia (and sometimes diabetes), dyslipidemia including fat redistribution ("buffalo hump," "protease paunch"), hyperlipidemia, hypercholesterolemia
Nelfinavir (Viracept®)	Tablet: 250 mg, 625 mg Powder, oral: 50 mg/g	750 mg tid or 1250 mg bid (take with food)	None necessary	No recommendation; use caution	Diarrhea, nausea, hyperglycemia (and sometimes diabetes), dyslipidemia including fat redistribution ("buffalo hump," "protease paunch"), hyperlipidemia, hypercholesterolemia
Ritonavir (Norvir®)	Capsule: 100 mg Solution, oral: 80 mg/mL (240 mL)	600 mg bid (take with food)	None necessary	No adjustment for mild impairment; use caution in moderate to severe impairment	Asthenia, nausea, diarrhea, vomiting, anorexia, abdominal pain, circumoral and peripheral paresthesia, taste perversion, headache, hyperglycemia (and sometimes diabetes), dyslipidemia including fat redistribution ("buffalo hump," "protease paunch"), hyperlipidemia, hypercholesterolemia
Saquinavir (Invirase®, Fortovase® [DSC])	Hard gelatin capsule (hgc): 200 mg Tablet: 500 mg Soft gelatin capsule: 200 mg	1200 mg tid (hgc only) or 1000 mg bid (with ritonavir) (take with food)	None necessary	No recommendation; use caution	Diarrhea, abdominal discomfort, nausea, headache, hyperglycemia (and sometimes diabetes), dyslipidemia including fat redistribution ("buffalo hump," "protease paunch"), hyperlipidemia, hypercholesterolemia
Tipranavir (Aptivus®)	Gelatin capsule: 250 mg	500 mg (with ritonavir 200 mg) bid (take with high-fat meal)	None necessary	No recommendation; use caution in mild impairment. Contraindicated with moderate to severe (C-P ≥5)	Diarrhea, skin rash, hyperglycemia, fat redistribution ("buffalo hump," "protease paunch"), dyslipidemia, increased bleeding time, increased LFTs, hepatitis and hepatic decompensation

[1]Hepatic impairment as defined by the Child-Pugh (C-P) classification.

Fusion Inhibitor					
Generic Name (Brand Name)	Dosage Form	Normal Dosing	Renal Dosing Adjustment	Hepatic Dosing Adjustment	Selected Adverse Reactions
Enfuvirtide (Fuzeon™)	Injection (lyophilized powder): 90 mg/mL	90 mg SubQ bid	None necessary	No recommendation; use caution	Injection site reaction, bacterial pneumonia, hypersensitivity

Protease Inhibitor (PI) Drug Interactions

Antiretroviral Agent	Interacting Agent	Severity[1]	Additional Comments
General, may apply to all PIs and combinations (except where noted)	Antacids	C/D	May reduce the serum levels of PI by decreasing absorption; administer PI 2 hours before or 1 hour after antacids.
	Amiodarone	X	PIs may decrease metabolism of amiodarone, leading to increased serum levels and life-threatening adverse effects; **concomitant use contraindicated.**
	Calcium channel blockers	D	PIs may decrease metabolism of these agents; 50% dose reduction of diltiazem recommended if used with atazanavir; no interaction identified with tipranavir.
	Phenytoin, phenobarbital	C	May decrease serum levels/effectiveness of PI through increased metabolism; additionally, increased carbamazepine levels may occur with concomitant ritonavir.
	Carbamazepine	D	
	Cimetidine, azole antifungals	C	May increase serum levels/effects of PI; limited data with azoles, but reduced dosage of antifungal agent may be necessary (see individual product information).
	Midazolam, triazolam	D	An increase in benzodiazepine serum levels may occur resulting in significant oversedation when administered with PI; avoid combination.
	Clarithromycin	D	PIs may increase the serum levels/toxic effects; due to risk of QT_c prolongation with clarithromycin, dose adjustment of clarithromycin may be necessary (see individual product information).
	Corticosteroids, orally inhaled (fluticasone, budesonide)	D	Serum levels may be increased by PI (with or without ritonavir boost) resulting in decreased serum cortisol, HPA axis suppression; concurrent use of ritonavir boosted PI not recommended; no interactions identified with tipranavir.
	Delavirdine	D	Delavirdine may increase the levels/toxicities of various protease inhibitors, particularly nelfinavir, ritonavir, and saquinavir. Conversely, PIs may decrease the serum levels of delavirdine, leading to loss of virologic response and possible resistance to delavirdine. **Concomitant use is not recommended.**
	Ergot alkaloids (eg, dihydro-ergotamine, ergotamine, ergonovine, methylergonovine); pimozide	X	Serum levels/toxicity may be increased by PI; serious and/or life-threatening reactions may occur; **concurrent use is contraindicated.**
	Digoxin, eplerenone, nefazodone, fentanyl	C	PIs may increase serum levels/toxicity.
	Efavirenz, H_2 antagonists, nevirapine	D	Serum levels of PIs may be reduced. Avoid concurrent use if possible; if coadministering with antihistamine agents, separate dosing by at least 12 hours.
	HMG-CoA reductase inhibitors	D	PIs may increase serum levels of HMG-CoA reductase inhibitors, increasing the risk of myopathy. Concurrent use of lovastatin or simvastatin with PIs are not recommended. Atorvastatin may be used with careful monitoring, in the lowest dose possible. Fluvastatin and pravastatin may have lowest risk.
	Immunosuppressants (eg, cyclosporine, sirolimus, tacrolimus)	C/D	PIs may increase the serum levels of these agents; monitor levels.
	Indinavir	D	Concurrent use may increase the risk of hyperbilirubinemia; **concurrent administration is not recommended.**
	Irinotecan	C/D	PIs may increase irinotecan levels via inhibition of metabolism through UGT1A1 leading to severe toxicity; **concurrent use, particularly with atazanavir, is not recommended.**
	Lidocaine (systemic)	C/D	Serum levels/toxicity may be increased by PI; serious and/or life-threatening reactions may occur. Monitor serum levels of lidocaine.

Protease Inhibitor (PI) Drug Interactions   *(Continued)*

Antiretroviral Agent	Interacting Agent	Severity[1]	Additional Comments
	Oral contraceptives	D	With concomitant PI therapy, serum levels of estradiol/norethindrone may be increased (atazanavir, amprenavir, indinavir) or decreased (ritonavir, nelfinavir); alternate forms of (nonhormonal) contraception are recommended.
	Methadone	C	Effect of methadone may be increased or reduced; caution advised when initiating or changing dosages of concomitant therapy (dosage adjustment of methadone may be required). No interaction identified with indinavir or atazanavir.
	Phosphodiesterase-5 (PDE-5) enzyme inhibitors (sildenafil, tadalafil, vardenafil)	D	Serum levels/toxicity may be increased by PI; do not exceed doses of 25 mg sildenafil in 48 hours, 10 mg tadalafil in a 72-hour period, or 2.5 mg vardenafil in 24 hours.
	Quinidine	X	Serum levels/toxicity may be increased by PI; serious and/or life-threatening reactions may occur. Monitor serum levels of quinidine.
	Protease inhibitors	D	May decrease the metabolism, via inhibition of CYP isoenzymes, of other protease inhibitors. See individual product information for recommended dosing adjustments.
	Rifamycin derivatives	D/X	An increase in rifabutin plasma AUC (>200%) has been observed when coadministered with several PIs. Concurrent decreases in serum levels of PIs have also been observed, which may lead to loss of virologic response and resistance. See individual product information for recommended dosing adjustments; **concurrent use with rifampin is contraindicated.**
	St John's wort (*Hypericum perforatum*)	X	May reduce trough serum levels of PI, which may lead to treatment failures. **Concurrent use is contraindicated.**
	Theophylline	C	May decrease serum levels/effects of theophylline; monitor.
	Trazodone	D	Serum levels/effects may be increased; use caution and reduce trazodone dose.
	Tricyclic antidepressants	C	Serum levels/toxicity may be increased by PIs.
PIs: Specific Agents			
Amprenavir/fosamprenavir	Disulfiram	X	Concurrent use with amprenavir **oral solution** is contraindicated due to risk of propylene glycol toxicity.
	Metronidazole	X	Concurrent use with amprenavir **oral solution** is contraindicated due to risk of propylene glycol toxicity.
	H$_2$ antagonists (eg, ranitidine)	D	May decrease absorption of amprenavir; consider boosting with ritonavir; separate dosing by 12 hours.
	Methadone	C	Effect of PI may be diminished (consider alternative antiretroviral). In addition, the effect of methadone may be reduced (dosage increase may be required).
	Ritonavir	D	The serum levels of amprenavir may be increased. With ritonavir, the risk of cholesterol/triglyceride elevations may be increased; specific dosing has been recommended for both agents. Concurrent use of amprenavir oral solution with ritonavir oral solution is not recommended (due to competition for metabolic elimination between propylene glycol and ethanol in these formulations).
Atazanavir	Clarithromycin	D	Clarithromycin AUC increased 94% with atazanavir; reduce clarithromycin dose by 50%.
	Efavirenz	D	Serum levels of atazanavir are significantly reduced by efavirenz. If coadministration is desirable, atazanavir 300 mg plus ritonavir 100 mg may be administered with efavirenz 600 mg as a single daily dose (with a meal). Atazanavir should not be administered with efavirenz alone.
	Indinavir	D	Increased risk of hyperbilirubinemia; avoid concurrent use.

1103

Protease Inhibitor (PI) Drug Interactions *(Continued)*

Antiretroviral Agent	Interacting Agent	Severity[1]	Additional Comments
	Didanosine	D	May reduce the serum levels of atazanavir by decreasing absorption; administer PI 2 hours before or 1 hour after didanosine.
	H₂ antagonists (eg, ranitidine), proton pump inhibitors	D	May decrease absorption of atazanavir; separate dosing by 12 hours; concurrent use of proton pump inhibitors not recommended.
	Tenofovir	C	May decrease serum levels of atazanavir, resulting in a loss of virologic response and/or resistance to atazanavir. Atazanavir increases tenofovir concentrations. Atazanavir-specific dosing recommendations are provided by the manufacturer. Atazanavir should not be coadministered with tenofovir **without** ritonavir.
Indinavir	Amlodipine	D	Amlodipine AUC increased 90% by indinavir/ritonavir; monitor BP closely.
	Atazanavir	D	Increased risk of hyperbilirubinemia; avoid concurrent use.
	Didanosine	D	May reduce the serum levels of indinavir by decreasing absorption; administer PI 2 hours before or 1 hour after didanosine.
Ritonavir or antiretroviral combinations with ritonavir	Carbamazepine	D	Serum levels of carbamazepine may be increased; monitor anticonvulsant levels.
	Clarithromycin	D	Clarithromycin levels increased 77%; adjust dosage as for moderate-to-severe renal impairment.
	Desipramine	C	Desipramine AUC increased 145% with concurrent ritonavir.
	Flecainide, propafenone, thioridazine	X	May increase serum levels/toxicity leading to arrhythmia.
	Methadone	C	Methadone AUC decreased 53%; monitor for possible withdrawal symptoms and adjust methadone dose as necessary.
	Voriconazole	X	May reduce serum levels of voriconazole leading to treatment failure.
	Disulfiram	X	Due to risk of acetaldehyde accumulation, **concurrent use with lopinavir/ritonavir** *oral solution* **is contraindicated**.
	Alfuzosin	D	May increase serum levels/effects of alfuzosin; **concurrent use with ritonavir is contraindicated**.
	Trazodone	C	May increase serum levels/effects of trazodone.
Saquinavir	Tipranavir	D	Saquinavir AUC decreased 67% when given (with ritonavir) in combination with tipranavir/ritonavir; concurrent use should be avoided.
Tipranavir/ritonavir	Abacavir	D	May decrease the serum levels of abacavir 35% to 44%; dosing adjustment for concomitant therapy not available.
	Zidovudine	D	May decrease the serum levels of zidovudine 30% to 43%; dosing adjustment for concomitant therapy not available.
	Loperamide	C	May decrease the serum levels of loperamide 51%.
	Disulfiram	X	Due to risk of acetaldehyde accumulation, **concurrent use with tipranavir/ritonavir** *oral solution* **is not recommended**.
	Didanosine	D	May reduce the serum levels of tipranavir by decreasing absorption; if coadministering, recommend using enteric coated form of didanosine and separate dosing by 2 hours.
	Saquinavir	D	Saquinavir AUC decreased 67% when given (with ritonavir) in combination with tipranavir/ritonavir; concurrent use should be avoided.

[1]Severity rating: C = monitor therapy; D = consider therapy modification; X = avoid combination.

Non-nucleoside Reverse Transcriptase Inhibitor (NNRTI) Drug Interactions

Antiretroviral Agent	Interacting Agent	Severity[1]	Additional Comments
General, may apply to all NNRTIs (except where noted)	Voriconazole	D	NNRTIs may reduce serum levels of voriconazole leading to treatment failure.
	Rifamycin derivatives	D/X	May decrease serum levels of NNRTIs; **contraindicated with delavirdine**; avoid combination with nevirapine; increase dose of efavirenz to 800 mg/day if used concomitantly.
	Protease inhibitors	D	Metabolism of PIs may increase (efavirenz, nevirapine) or decrease (delavirdine) with concomitant therapy; use caution and monitor.
	St John's wort	X	May decrease serum levels of NNRTIs.
	Enzyme-inducing anticonvulsants (eg, phenytoin, phenobarbital, carbamazepine)	D/X	May decrease serum levels/effectiveness of NNRTIs; monitor levels; these agents specifically **contraindicated with delavirdine**.
	Dapsone	C/D	Efavirenz and nevirapine may decrease the levels/effectiveness of dapsone; delavirdine may increase dapsone levels/toxicity.

NNRTIs: Specific Agent Interactions

Delavirdine, efavirenz	HMG-CoA reductase inhibitors	C/D	May significantly increase statin levels; avoid concomitant use of delavirdine with simvastatin or atorvastatin; reduce statin dose with efavirenz.
	Methadone	D	May decrease serum levels/effects of methadone; adjust opiate dose as necessary.
	Cisapride	C/D	May increase serum levels of cisapride, increasing the risk of arrhythmias; avoid concomitant use.
	Midazolam, triazolam, (alprazolam)	D	An increase in serum levels may occur resulting in significant oversedation when administered with NNRTIs; avoid combination. Alprazolam not recommended for use with delavirdine.
	Ergot alkaloids (eg, dihydroergotamine, ergotamine, ergonovine, methylergonovine)	X	Serum levels/toxicity or ergotamine derivatives may be increased; serious and/or life-threatening reactions may occur; **concurrent use is contraindicated**.
	Warfarin	C/D	May increase the levels/effects of warfarin; monitor INR.
Nevirapine	Clarithromycin	C	Nevirapine may decrease the levels/effectiveness of clarithromycin.
	Oral contraceptives	C	May decrease levels/effects of estradiol; recommend alternate forms of contraception.
	Fluconazole	D	May increase nevirapine AUC 100%; monitor for increased risk of hepatotoxicity.
Delavirdine	Antacids	C	Antacids may decrease absorption; separate dosing by 1 hour.
	Clarithromycin	D	Delavirdine and clarithromycin levels may be increased with concomitant use; adjust clarithromycin dose for renal failure and monitor for toxicity if used with delavirdine.
	H$_2$ antagonists, proton pump inhibitors	D	Coadministration not recommended.
	Phosphodiesterase-5 (PDE-5) enzyme inhibitors (sildenafil, tadalafil, vardenafil)	D	Serum levels/toxicity may be increased by atazanavir; do not exceed doses of 25 mg sildenafil in 48 hours, 10 mg tadalafil in a 72-hour period, or 2.5 mg vardenafil in 24 hours.
Efavirenz	Atazanavir	D	May decrease the serum level of atazanavir; manufacturer recommends dosing adjustment of atazanavir 300 mg/day (with ritonavir 100 mg/day) if used with efavirenz.
	Clarithromycin	C	Efavirenz may decrease the levels/effectiveness of clarithromycin.
	Oral contraceptives	C	May increase levels/effects of estradiol; recommend alternate forms of contraception.

[1] Severity rating: C = monitor therapy; D = consider therapy modification; X = avoid combination.

Nucleoside Reverse Transcriptase Inhibitor (NRTI) Drug Interactions

Antiretroviral Agent	Interacting Agent	Severity[1]	Additional Comments
General, may apply to all NRTIs (except where noted)	Ribavirin	D	Coadministration may increase exposure to the NRTI and/or its active metabolite(s), increasing the risk or severity of toxicities such as hepatotoxicity, pancreatitis, lactic acidosis, or peripheral neuropathy. Concurrent use should be avoided. No data available with ribavirin + tenofovir combination.
	Ganciclovir-valganciclovir	D	May increase NRTI levels, and the risk of hematology toxicity (eg, pancytopenia); concomitant use with didanosine or zidovudine not recommended; stavudine and zalcitabine appear to be safe alternatives.

NRTIs: Specific Agent Interactions			
Didanosine (ddI)	Quinolones, itraconazole, ketoconazole, dapsone, tetracyclines, ganciclovir-valganciclovir, atazanavir, indinavir	D	Buffered formulations of didanosine (tablets, pediatric oral solution) may decrease absorption of these medications; separate dosing by 2 hours (recommended that quinolones be given 6 hours after didanosine).
	Tipranavir/ritonavir	C	Concurrent administration may result in decreased serum levels of both ddI and tipranavir/ritonavir; if coadministering, use enteric coated form of didanosine and separate dosing by 2 hours.
	Allopurinol	D	May increase didanosine concentration; avoid concurrent use.
	Hydroxyurea	D	May precipitate didanosine-induced pancreatitis if added to therapy; concomitant use is not recommended.
	Methadone	C	May decrease buffered didanosine AUC by −63%; monitor and consider dose adjustment.
	Tenofovir, stavudine	D	Coadministration may increase exposure to didanosine and/or its active metabolite increasing the risk or severity of didanosine toxicities, including pancreatitis, hyperglycemia, lactic acidosis, and peripheral neuropathy. Some patients have experienced reduced CD4 cell counts and/or decreased virologic response; specific dosing adjustment of ddI with tenofovir is recommended; suspend therapy if signs or symptoms of toxicity are noted.
	Zalcitabine	D	Increased risk of peripheral neuropathy.
Stavudine	Didanosine	D	Risk of pancreatitis may be increased with concurrent use. Cases of fatal lactic acidosis have been reported with this combination when used during pregnancy; use only if clearly needed.
	Doxorubicin, zidovudine, ribavirin	D	May inhibit intracellular phosphorylation of stavudine reducing efficacy; concomitant use not recommended.
	Zalcitabine	D	May increase risk of peripheral neuropathy; concurrent use not recommended.
	Zidovudine	D	Zidovudine may decrease the antiviral activity of stavudine (based on *in vitro* data). Avoid concurrent use.
Tenofovir	Atazanavir	C	Tenofovir may decrease serum levels of atazanavir, resulting in a loss of virologic response and/or resistance to atazanavir. Atazanavir-specific dosing recommendations (use with ritonavir) are provided by the manufacturer.
	Didanosine	D	Concomitant use of tenofovir with didanosine has been noted to increase exposure to didanosine and/or its active metabolite, potentially increasing the risk of pancreatitis, hyperglycemia, peripheral neuropathy, or lactic acidosis. Some patients have experienced reduced CD4 cell counts and/or decreased virologic response. Specific dosing adjustment is recommended. Use caution and monitor closely. Suspend therapy if signs/symptoms of toxicity are present.

Nucleoside Reverse Transcriptase Inhibitor (NRTI) Drug Interactions *(Continued)*

Antiretroviral Agent	Interacting Agent	Severity[1]	Additional Comments
	Protease inhibitors	C	Tenofovir may decrease the serum levels/effectiveness of protease inhibitors; conversely, PIs may increase the levels/toxicity of tenofovir.
	Cidofovir, acyclovir-valacyclovir, ganciclovir-valganciclovir	C	Concomitant use of the agents with tenofovir may lead to accumulation of both due to competition for active tubular secretion.
Zidovudine	Bone marrow suppressants/cytotoxic agents (eg, adriamycin, dapsone, flucytosine, vincristine, vinblastine)	D	Concomitant use may increase risk of hematologic toxicity.
	Ganciclovir-valganciclovir, interferon alfa	D	Concomitant use may increase risk of hematologic toxicities; monitor hemoglobin, hematocrit, and white blood cell count with differential frequently; dose reduction or interruption of either agent may be needed.
	Lamivudine	C	Plasma levels of zidovudine are increased by −39% with concomitant use.
	Methadone	C	May increase serum levels/effects of zidovudine; monitor for toxicities.
	Probenecid	C	Probenecid may increase zidovudine levels. Myalgia, malaise, and/or fever and maculopapular rash have been reported with concomitant use.
	Ribavirin	D	May inhibit intracellular phosphorylation of zidovudine reducing efficacy; concomitant use not recommended.
	Rifamycin derivatives, tipranavir/ritonavir	D	May decrease the levels/effects of zidovudine; no interaction with rifabutin noted; dose adjustment for tipranavir/ritonavir + zidovudine have not been established.
	Stavudine	D	Zidovudine may decrease the antiviral activity of stavudine (based on *in vitro* data). Avoid concurrent use.
	Valproic acid	C	Valproic acid may increase plasma levels of zidovudine; monitor for possible increase in side effects (AUC increased by 80%).
Zalcitabine	Nephrotoxic drugs (eg, amphotericin, foscarnet, cimetidine, probenecid, aminoglycosides)	C	May potentiate the risk of developing peripheral neuropathy or other toxicities associated with zalcitabine by interfering with the renal elimination of zalcitabine.
	Didanosine, stavudine	D	May increase risk of peripheral neuropathy; concurrent use not recommended.
	Lamivudine	D	May decrease the therapeutic efficacy of zalcitabine by inhibiting intracellular phosphorylation of zalcitabine; concomitant use not recommended.
Lamivudine	Trimethoprim (and other drugs excreted by organic cation transport)	C	May increase serum levels/effects of lamivudine by competing for active tubular secretion.
	Zalcitabine	D	Intracellular phosphorylation of lamivudine and zalcitabine may be inhibited if used together; concomitant use should be avoided.
	Zidovudine	C	Plasma levels of zidovudine are increased by −39% with concomitant use.

[1]Severity rating: C = monitor therapy; D = consider therapy modification; X = avoid combination.

Drugs That Should Not Be Used with Protease Inhibitors

Drug Category	Indinavir	Ritonavir[1]	Saquinavir[2]	Nelfinavir	Alternatives
Analgesics	None	Piroxicam, propoxyphene	None	None	ASA, oxycodone, acetaminophen
Cardiac	None	Amiodarone, encainide, flecainide, propafenone, quinidine	None	None	Limited experience
Antimycobacterial	Rifampin	Rifabutin[3]	Rifampin, rifabutin	Rifampin	For rifabutin (as alternative for MAI treatment): clarithromycin, ethambutol (treatment, not prophylaxis), or azithromycin
Calcium channel blocker	None	Bepridil	None	None	Limited experience
Antihistamine	Astemizole	Astemizole	Astemizole	Astemizole	Loratadine
Gastrointestinal	Cisapride	Cisapride	Cisapride	Cisapride	Limited experience
Antidepressant	None	Bupropion	None	None	Fluoxetine, desipramine
Neuroleptic	None	Clozapine, pimozide	None	None	Limited experience
Psychotropic	Midazolam, triazolam	Clorazepate, diazepam, estazolam, flurazepam, midazolam, triazolam, zolpidem	Midazolam, triazolam	Midazolam, triazolam	Temazepam, lorazepam
Ergot alkaloid (vasoconstrictor)		Dihydroergotamine (D.H.E. 45), ergotamine[4] (various forms)		Dihydroergotamine (D.H.E. 45), ergotamine[4] (various forms)	

[1]The contraindicated drugs listed are based on theoretical considerations. Thus, drugs with low therapeutic indices yet with suspected major metabolic contribution from CYP3A, CYP2D6, or unknown pathways are included in this table. Actual interactions may or may not occur in patients.

[2]Given as Invirase® or Fortovase® [DSC].

[3]Reduce rifabutin dose to one-fourth of the standard dose.

[4]This is likely a class effect.

ASSESSMENT OF LIVER FUNCTION

Child-Pugh Score			
Component	Score Given for Observed Findings		
	1	2	3
Encephalopathy grade[1]	None	1-2	3-4
Ascites	None	Mild or controlled by diuretics	Moderate or refractory despite diuretics
Albumin (g/dL)	>3.5	2.8-3.5	<2.8
Total bilirubin (mg/dL)	<2 (<34 micromoles/L)	2-3 (34-50 micromoles/L)	>3 (>50 micromoles/L)
or			
Modified total bilirubin[2]	<4	4-7	>7
Prothrombin time (seconds prolonged)	<4	4-6	>6
or			
INR	<1.7	1.7-2.3	>2.3

[1]Encephalopathy grades:

Grade 0: Normal consciousness, personality, neurological examination, electroencephalogram

Grade 1: Restless, sleep disturbed, irritable/agitated, tremor, impaired handwriting, 5 cps waves

Grade 2: Lethargic, time-disoriented, inappropriate, asterixis, ataxia, slow triphasic waves

Grade 3: Somnolent, stuporous, place-disoriented, hyperactive reflexes, rigidity, slower waves

Grade 4: Unrousable coma, no personality/behavior, decerebrate, slow 2-3 cps delta activity

Alternative encephalopathy grades:

Grade 1: Mild confusion, anxiety, restlessness, fine tremor, slowed coordination

Grade 2: Drowsiness, disorientation, asterixis

Grade 3: Somnolent but rousable, marked confusion, incomprehensible speech, incontinent, hyperventilation

Grade 4: Coma, decerebrate posturing, flaccidity

[2]Modified total bilirubin used to score patients who have Gilbert's syndrome or who are taking indinavir.

Child-Pugh Classification

Class A (mild hepatic impairment): Score 5-6

Class B (moderate hepatic impairment): Score 7-9

Class C (severe hepatic impairment): Score 10-15

References

Centers for Disease Control and Prevention, "Report of the NIH Panel to Define Principles of Therapy of HIV Infection and Guidelines for the Use of Antiretroviral Agents in HIV-Infected Adults and Adolescents," March 23, 2004, located at (URL) http://www.aidsinfo.nih.gov.

U.S. Department of Health and Human Services, Food and Drug Administration, "Guidance for Industry, Pharmacokinetics in Patients with Impaired Hepatic Function: Study Design, Data Analysis, and Impact on Dosing and Labeling," May 2003, located at (URL) http://www.fda.gov/cder/guidance/3625fnl.pdf.

ATYPICAL ANTIPSYCHOTICS

Drug	DR EPS	PROL	TD[1]	ACH	SZ	OH	LFTs	SED	WT GAIN	NMS	AGRAN	TX REFR	Lipid	DM	QTc
Aripiprazole (Abilify™)	No	No	Uncommon	Very low	Low	Low	Low	Low	Very low	?	?	Maybe	Very low	Very low	Low
Clozapine (Clozaril®)	No	No	Uncommon	High	DD	High	Low	High	High	Yes	Yes	Yes	High	High	Low
Risperidone (Risperdal®)	Yes	Yes	Uncommon	Very low	Low	Moderate	Low	Low	Low/ Moderate	Yes	Yes[2]	Maybe	Low	Low/ Moderate	Low
Olanzapine (Zyprexa®, Zyprexa® Zydis®)	Yes	Yes	Uncommon	Moderate	Low	Low/ Moderate	Low/ Moderate	Moderate	High	Yes	Yes[2]	Maybe	High	High	Low
Quetiapine (Seroquel®)	No	No	Uncommon	Moderate	Low	Moderate	Low/ Moderate	Moderate	Moderate	Yes	Yes[2]	No	Moderate	Low/ Moderate	Low
Ziprasidone (Geodon®)	Yes	Yes	Uncommon	Very low	Low	Low/ Moderate	Low	Low	Very low	Yes	?	No	Very low	Very low	Moderate[3]

Note: Atypical antipsychotics are defined as 1) decrease or no EPS at doses producing antipsychotic effect; 2) minimum or no increase in prolactin; 3) decrease in both positive and negative symptoms of schizophrenia.

[1]Rate of TD ~ $^{1}/_{5}$ that seen with conventional antipsychotics

[2]Case reports.

[3]Dose related within 40-160 mg dosage range.

DR EPS = dose related extrapyramidal symptoms.

PROL = prolactin elevation (may cause amenorrhea, galactorrhea, gynecomastia, impotence).

TD = tardive dyskinesia.

ACH = anticholinergic side effects (dry mouth, blurred vision, constipation, urinary hesitancy).

SZ = seizures.

OH = orthostatic hypotension (blood pressure drops upon standing).

LFTs = increased liver function test results.

SED = sedation.

WT GAIN = weight gain.

NMS = neuroleptic malignant syndrome.

AGRAN = agranulocytosis (without white blood cells to fight infection).

TX REFR = efficacy in treatment refractory schizophrenia.

Lipid = lipid abnormalities; cholesterol and/or triglyceride elevations.

DM = diabetes (based on case reports).

QTc = QTc prolongation.

DD = dose dependent.

AVERAGE WEIGHTS AND SURFACE AREAS

Average Weight and Surface Area of Preterm Infants, Term Infants, and Children		
Age	**Average Weight (kg)[1]**	**Approximate Surface Area (m^2)**
Weeks Gestation		
26	0.9-1	0.1
30	1.3-1.5	0.12
32	1.6-2	0.15
38	2.9-3	0.2
40 (term infant at birth)	3.1-4	0.25
Months		
3	5	0.29
6	7	0.38
9	8	0.42
Years		
1	10	0.49
2	12	0.55
3	15	0.64
4	17	0.74
5	18	0.76
6	20	0.82
7	23	0.90
8	25	0.95
9	28	1.06
10	33	1.18
11	35	1.23
12	40	1.34
Adults	70	1.73

[1]Weights from age 3 months and older are rounded off to the nearest kilogram.

AVERAGES AND CONVERSIONS

Apothecary-Metric Conversions

Metric Abbreviations					
L	=	liter	kg	=	kilogram
mL	=	milliliter	g	=	gram
m	=	meter	mg	=	milligram
cm	=	centimeter	µg/mcg	=	microgram
			ng	=	nanogram

Exact Equivalents					
1 gram (g)	=	15.43 grains	0.1 mg	=	1/600 gr
1 milliliter (mL)	=	16.23 minims	0.12 mg	=	1/500 gr
1 minim	=	0.06 milliliter	0.15 mg	=	1/400 gr
1 grain (gr)	=	64.8 milligrams	0.2 mg	=	1/300 gr
1 ounce (oz)	=	31.1 grams	0.3 mg	=	1/200 gr
1 fluid ounce	=	29.57 milliliters	0.4 mg	=	1/150 gr
1 pint (pt)	=	473.2 milliliters	0.5 mg	=	1/120 gr
1 ounce (oz)	=	28.35 grams	0.6 mg	=	1/100 gr
1 pound (lb)	=	453.6 grams	0.8 mg	=	1/80 gr
1 kilogram (kg)	=	2.2 pounds	1 mg	=	1/65 gr
1 quart (qt)	=	946.4 milliliters			

Approximate Equivalents*					
Liquids			Solids		
1 teaspoonful	=	5 mL	$^1/_4$ grain	=	15 mg
1 tablespoonful	=	15 mL	$^1/_2$ grain	=	30 mg
1 fluid ounce	=	30 mL	1 grain	=	60 mg
15 minims	=	1 mL	$1^1/_2$ grains	=	100 mg
			5 grains	=	300 mg
			10 grains	=	600 mg
			1 ounce	=	30 g

*Use exact equivalents for compounding and calculations requiring a high degree of accuracy.

Pounds-Kilograms Conversion

1 pound = 0.45359 kilograms

1 kilogram = 2.2 pounds

Temperature Conversion

Celsius to Fahrenheit = (°C × 9/5) + 32 = °F

Fahrenheit to Celsius = (°F − 32) × 5/9 = °C

°C	=	°F	°C	=	°F	°C	=	°F
100.0		212.0	39.0		102.2	36.8		98.2
50.0		122.0	38.8		101.8	36.6		97.9
41.0		105.8	38.6		101.5	36.4		97.5
40.8		105.4	38.4		101.1	36.2		97.2
40.6		105.1	38.2		100.8	36.0		96.8
40.4		104.7	38.0		100.4	35.8		96.4
40.2		104.4	37.8		100.1	35.6		96.1
40.0		104.0	37.6		99.7	35.4		95.7
39.8		103.6	37.4		99.3	35.2		95.4
39.6		103.3	37.2		99.0	35.0		95.0
39.4		102.9	37.0		98.6	0		32.0
39.2		102.6						

Millimole and Milliequivalent Calculations

Definitions		
mole	=	gram molecular weight of a substance (aka molar weight)
millimole (mM)	=	milligram molecular weight of a substance (a millimole is 1/1000 of a mole)
equivalent weight	=	gram weight of a substance which will combine with or replace 1 gram (1 mole) of hydrogen; an equivalent weight can be determined by dividing the molar weight of a substance by its ionic valence
milliequivalent (mEq)	=	milligram weight of a substance which will combine with or replace 1 milligram (1 millimole) of hydrogen (a milliequivalent is 1/1000 of an equivalent)

Calculations		
moles	=	$\dfrac{\text{weight of a substance (grams)}}{\text{molecular weight of that substance (grams)}}$
millimoles	=	$\dfrac{\text{weight of a substance (milligrams)}}{\text{molecular weight of that substance (milligrams)}}$
equivalents	=	moles × valence of ion
milliequivalents	=	millimoles × valence of ion
moles	=	$\dfrac{\text{equivalents}}{\text{valence of ion}}$
millimoles	=	$\dfrac{\text{milliequivalents}}{\text{valence of ion}}$
millimoles	=	moles × 1000
milliequivalents	=	equivalents × 1000

Note: Use of equivalents and milliequivalents is valid only for those substances which have fixed ionic valences (eg, sodium, potassium, calcium, chlorine, magnesium bromine, etc). For substances with variable ionic valences (eg, phosphorous), a reliable equivalent value cannot be determined. In these instances, one should calculate millimoles (which are fixed and reliable) rather than milliequivalents.

Milliequivalent Conversions

To convert mg/100 mL to mEq/L the following formula may be used:

$$\frac{(mg/100\ mL) \times 10 \times valence}{atomic\ weight} = mEq/L$$

To convert mEq/L to mg/100 mL the following formula may be used:

$$\frac{(mEq/L) \times atomic\ weight}{10 \times valence} = mg/100\ mL$$

To convert mEq/L to volume of percent of a gas the following formula may be used:

$$\frac{(mEq/L) \times 22.4}{10} = volume\ percent$$

Milliequivalents for Selected Ions

Approximate Milliequivalents — Weights of Selected Ions		
Salt	mEq/g Salt	mg Salt/mEq
Calcium carbonate [$CaCO_3$]	20	50
Calcium chloride [$CaCl_2 \cdot 2H_2O$]	14	74
Calcium gluceptate [$Ca(C_7H_{13}O_8)_2$]	4	245
Calcium gluconate [$Ca(C_6H_{11}O_7)_2 \cdot H_2O$]	5	224
Calcium lactate [$Ca(C_3H_5O_3)_2 \cdot 5H_2O$]	7	154
Magnesium gluconate [$Mg(C_6H_{11}O_7)_2 \cdot H_2O$]	5	216
Magnesium oxide [MgO]	50	20
Magnesium sulfate [$MgSO_4$]	17	60
Magnesium sulfate [$MgSO_4 \cdot 7H_2O$]	8	123
Potassium acetate [$K(C_2H_3O_2)$]	10	98
Potassium chloride [KCl]	13	75
Potassium citrate [$K_3(C_6H_5O_7) \cdot H_2O$]	9	108
Potassium iodide [KI]	6	166
Sodium acetate [$Na(C_2H_3O_2)$]	12	82
Sodium acetate [$Na(C_2H_3O_2) \cdot 3H_2O$]	7	136
Sodium bicarbonate [$NaHCO_3$]	12	84
Sodium chloride [$NaCl$]	17	58
Sodium citrate [$Na_3(C_6H_5O_7) \cdot 2H_2O$]	10	98
Sodium iodine [NaI]	7	150
Sodium lactate [$Na(C_3H_5O_3)$]	9	112
Zinc sulfate [$ZnSO_4 \cdot 7H_2O$]	7	144

Valences and Atomic Weights of Selected Ions

Substance	Electrolyte	Valence	Molecular Wt
Calcium	Ca^{++}	2	40
Chloride	Cl^-	1	35.5
Magnesium	Mg^{++}	2	24
Phosphate	HPO_4^{--} (80%)	1.8	96[1]
pH = 7.4	$H_2PO_4^-$ (20%)	1.8	96[1]
Potassium	K^+	1	39
Sodium	Na^+	1	23
Sulfate	SO_4^{--}	2	96[1]

[1]The molecular weight of phosphorus only is 31, and sulfur only is 32.

AVERAGE WEIGHTS AND SURFACE AREAS

Average Weight and Surface Area of Preterm Infants, Term Infants, and Children

Age	Average Weight (kg)[1]	Approximate Surface Area (m²)
Weeks Gestation		
26	0.9-1	0.1
30	1.3-1.5	0.12
32	1.6-2	0.15
38	2.9-3	0.2
40 (term infant at birth)	3.1-4	0.25
Months		
3	5	0.29
6	7	0.38
9	8	0.42
Years		
1	10	0.49
2	12	0.55
3	15	0.64
4	17	0.74
5	18	0.76
6	20	0.82
7	23	0.90
8	25	0.95
9	28	1.06
10	33	1.18
11	35	1.23
12	40	1.34
Adults	70	1.73

[1]Weights from age 3 months and older are rounded off to the nearest kilogram.

Body Surface Area of Adults and Children

Calculating Body Surface Area in Children

In a child of average size, find weight and corresponding surface area on the boxed scale to the left; or, use the nomogram to the right. Lay a straightedge on the correct height and weight points for the child, then read the intersecting point on the surface area scale.

FOR CHILDREN OF NORMAL HEIGHT AND WEIGHT

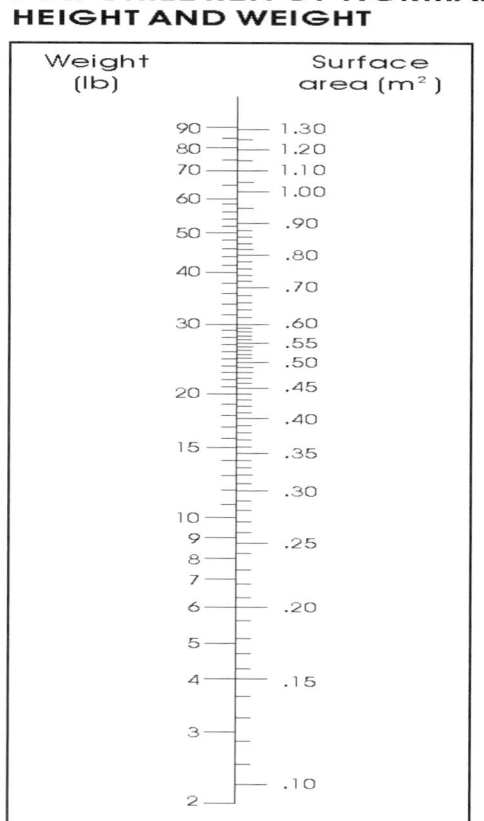

NOMOGRAM

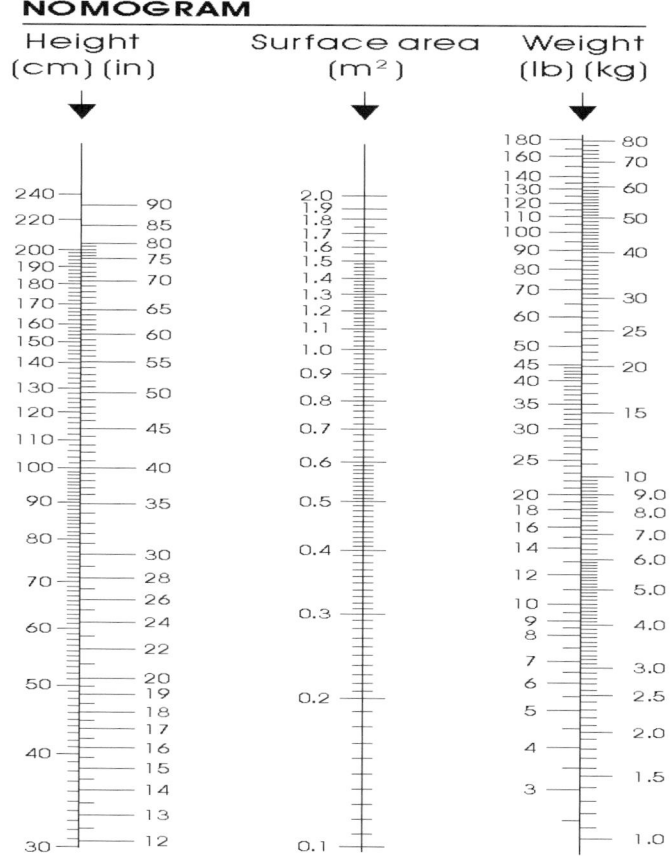

BODY SURFACE AREA FORMULA
(Adult and Pediatric)

$$BSA\ (m^2) = \sqrt{\frac{ht\ (in)\ x\ wt\ (lb)}{3131}} \quad \text{or, in metric: } BSA\ (m^2) = \sqrt{\frac{ht\ (cm)\ x\ wt\ (kg)}{3600}}$$

References

Lam TK and Leung DT, "More on Simplified Calculation of Body Surface Area," *N Engl J Med*, 1988, 318(17):1130 (letter).

Mosteller RD, "Simplified Calculation of Body Surface Area," *N Engl J Med*, 1987, 317(17):1098 (letter).

BENZODIAZEPINES

Agent	Dosage Forms	Approximate Equivalent Dose (mg)	Peak Blood Levels (oral) (h)	Protein Binding (%)	Volume of Distribution (L/kg)	Major Active Metabolite	Half-Life (parent) (h)	Half-Life[1] (metabolite) (h)	Usual Initial Dose	Adult Oral Dosage Range
Anxiolytic										
Alprazolam (Alprazolam Intensol®, Xanax®)	Sol, tab	0.5	1-2	80	0.9-1.2	No	12-15	—	0.25-0.5 tid	0.75-4 mg/d
Chlordiazepoxide (Librium®)	Cap, powder for inj	10	2-4	90-98	0.3	Yes	5-30	24-96	5-25 mg tid-qid	15-100 mg/d
Diazepam (Diastat® Rectal Delivery System, Diazepam Intensol®, Valium®)	Gel, inj, sol, tab	5	0.5-2	98	1.1	Yes	20-80	50-100	2-10 mg bid-qid	4-40 mg/d
Lorazepam (Ativan®)[2]	Inj, sol, tab	1	1-6	88-92	1.3	No	10-20	—	0.5-2 mg tid-qid	2-4 mg/d
Oxazepam (Serax®)	Cap, tab	15-30	2-4	86-99	0.6-2	No	5-20	—	10-30 mg tid-qid	30-120 mg/d
Sedative/Hypnotic										
Estazolam (ProSom®)	Tab	0.3	2	93	—	No	10-24	—	1 mg qhs	1-2 mg
Flurazepam (Dalmane®)	Cap	5	0.5-2	97	—	Yes	Not significant	40-114	15 mg qhs	15-60 mg
Quazepam (Doral®)	Tab	5	2	95	5	Yes	25-41	28-114	15 mg qhs	7.5-15 mg
Temazepam (Restoril®)	Cap	5	2-3	96	1.4	No	10-40	—	15-30 mg qhs	15-30 mg
Triazolam (Halcion®)	Tab	0.1	1	89-94	0.8-1.3	No	2.3	—	0.125-0.25 qhs	0.125-0.25 mg
Miscellaneous										
Clonazepam (Klonopin®)	Tab	0.25-0.5	1-2	86	1.8-4	No	18-50 h	—	0.5 mg tid	1.5-20 mg/d
Clorazepate (Tranxene®)	Cap, tab	7.5	1-2	80-95	—	Yes	Not significant	50-100 h	7.5-15 mg bid-qid	15-60 mg
Midazolam	Inj	—	0.4-0.7[3]	95	0.8-6.6	No	2-5 h	—	NA	NA

[1]Significant metabolite.

[2]Reliable bioavailability when given I.M.

[3]I.V. only.

NA = not available.

BETA-BLOCKERS

Agent	Adrenergic Receptor Blocking Activity	Lipid Solubility	Protein Bound (%)	Half-Life (h)	Bioavailability (%)	Primary (Secondary) Route of Elimination	Indications	Usual Dosage
Acebutolol (Sectral®)	β_1	Low	15-25	3-4	40, 7-fold[1]	Hepatic (renal)	Hypertension, arrhythmias	P.O.: 400-1200 mg/d
Atenolol (Tenormin®)	β_1	Low	<5-10	6-9[2]	50-60, 4-fold[1]	Renal (hepatic)	Hypertension, angina pectoris, acute MI	P.O.: 50-200 mg/d; I.V.: 5 mg × 2 doses
Betaxolol (Kerlone®)	β_1	Low	50-55	14-22	84-94	Hepatic (renal)	Hypertension	P.O.: 10-20 mg/d
Bisoprolol (Zebeta®)	β_1	Low	26-33	9-12	80	Renal (hepatic)	Hypertension, heart failure	P.O.: 2.5-5 mg
Carteolol (Cartrol®)	β_1 β_2	Low	20-30	6	80-85	Renal	Hypertension	P.O.: 2.5-10 mg/d
Carvedilol (Coreg®)	β_1 β_2 α_1	ND	98	7-10	25-35	Bile into feces	Hypertension, heart failure (mild to severe)	P.O.: 6.25 mg twice daily
Esmolol (Brevibloc®)	β_1	Low	55	0.15	NA, 5-fold[1]	Red blood cell	Supraventricular tachycardia, sinus tachycardia	I.V. infusion: 25-300 mcg/kg/min
Labetalol (Trandate®)	α_1 β_1 β_2	Moderate	50	5.5-8	18-30, 10-fold[1]	Renal (hepatic)	Hypertension	P.O.: 200-2400 mg/d; I.V.: 20-80 mg at 10-min intervals up to a maximum of 300 mg or continuous infusion of 2 mg/min
Metoprolol (Lopressor®, Toprol-XL®)	β_1	Moderate	10-12	3-7	50, 10-fold[1] (Toprol XL®: 77)	Hepatic/renal	Hypertension, angina pectoris, acute MI, heart failure (mild to moderate; XL formulation only)	P.O.: 100-450 mg/d; I.V.: Post-MI 15 mg; Angina: 15 mg then 2-5 mg/hour; Arrhythmias: 0.2 mg/kg
Nadolol (Corgard®)	β_1 β_2	Low	25-30	20-24	30, 5- to 8-fold[1]	Renal	Hypertension, angina pectoris	P.O.: 40-320 mg/d
Penbutolol (Levatol®)	β_1 β_2	High	80-98	5	100	Hepatic (renal)	Hypertension	P.O.: 20-80 mg/d
Pindolol	β_1 β_2	Moderate	57	3-4[2]	90, 4-fold[1]	Hepatic (renal)	Hypertension	P.O.: 20-60 mg/d
Propranolol (Inderal®, various)	β_1 β_2	High	90	3-5[2]	30, 20-fold[1]	Hepatic	Hypertension, angina pectoris, arrhythmias	P.O.: 40-480 mg/d; I.V.: Reflex tachycardia 1-10 mg
Propranolol long-acting (Inderal-LA®)	β_1 β_2	High	90	9-18	20- to 30-fold[1]	Hepatic	Hypertrophic subaortic stenosis, prophylaxis (post-MI)	P.O.: 180-240 mg/d
Sotalol (Betapace®, Betapace AF®, Sorine®)	β_1 β_2	Low	0	12	90-100	Renal	Ventricular arrhythmias/tachyarrhythmias	P.O.: 160-320 mg/d
Timolol (Blocadren®)	β_1 β_2	Low to moderate	<10	4	75, 7-fold[1]	Hepatic (renal)	Hypertension, prophylaxis (post-MI)	P.O.: 20-60 mg/d; P.O.: 20 mg/d

Dosage is based on 70 kg adult with normal hepatic and renal function.

Note: All beta$_1$-selective agents will inhibit beta$_2$ receptors at higher doses.

[1]Interpatient variations in plasma levels.

[2]Half-life increased to 16-27 hours in creatinine clearance of 15-35 mL/minute and >27 hours in creatinine clearance <15 mL/minute.

BLOOD LEVEL SAMPLING TIME GUIDELINES

Drug	Infusion Time	Therapeutic Range	When to Draw Levels
Amikacin sulfate			
I.V.	30 min	Peak: 20-30 mcg/mL	Peak: 30 min after end of 30 min infusion
		Trough: <10 mcg/mL	Trough: Within 30 min before next dose
I.M.			Peak: 1 h after I.M. injection
			Trough: Within 30 min before next dose
Carbamazepine		4-12 mcg/mL	Just before next dose
Chloramphenicol			
I.V.	30 min	Peak: 15-25 mcg/mL	Peak: 90 min after end of 30 min infusion
			Trough: Just before next dose
P.O.			Peak: 2 h post-P.O. dose
Cyclosporine			
I.V./P.O.		BMT 100-200 ng/mL	Just before next dose
		Liver transplant: 200-300 ng/mL	
		Renal transplant 100-200 ng/mL	
Digoxin			
I.V./P.O.		Age and disease related: 0.8-2 ng/mL	6 h postdose to just before next dose
Ethosuximide			
P.O.		40-100 mcg/mL	Just before next dose
Flucytosine			
P.O.		25-100 mcg/mL	Peak: 2 h postdose after at least 4 d of therapy
Fosphenytoin (measure phenytoin levels)			
I.V.		Phenytoin: 10-20 mcg/mL	Peak: 2 h after end of an infusion
I.M.			Peak: 4 h after I.M. injection
Gentamicin			
I.V.	30 min	Peak: 4-10 mcg/mL	Peak: 30 min after end of 30 min infusion
		Trough: 0.5-2 mcg/mL	Trough: Within 30 min before next dose
I.M.			Peak: 1 h after I.M. injection
			Trough: Within 30 min before next dose
Phenobarbital		15-40 mcg/mL	Trough: Just before next dose
Phenytoin			
P.O., I.V.		10-20 mcg/mL	Trough: Just before next dose
I.V.			Post-load/Peak: 1 h after end of infusion
Theophylline			
I.V. bolus	30 min	10-20 mcg/mL	Peak: 30 min after end of 30 min infusion
Continuous infusion			16-24 h after the start or change in a constant I.V. infusion
P.O. liquid, fast-release tablet (Somophyllin®, Slo-Phyllin® liquid & tablet)			Peak: 1 h postdose Trough: Just before next dose
P.O. slow-release (Theo-Dur®, Slo-Phyllin® GC, Slo-bid®)			Peak: 4 h postdose Trough: Just before next dose

(*Continued*)

Drug	Infusion Time	Therapeutic Range	When to Draw Levels
Tobramycin			
I.V.	30 min	Peak: 4-10 mcg/mL	Peak: 30 min after end of 30 min infusion
		Trough: 0.5-2 mcg/mL	Trough: Within 30 min before next dose
I.M.			Peak: 1 h post-I.M. injection
			Trough: Within 30 min before next dose
Trimethoprim			
I.V., dose 20 mg/kg	60 min	Peak: 5-10 mcg/mL	Peak: 30 min after end of 60 min infusion
I.V., dose 8-10 mg/kg		Peak 1-3 mcg/mL	
P.O.			Peak: 1 h postdose
Valproic acid			
P.O.		50-100 mcg/mL	Trough: Just before next dose
Vancomycin	60 min	Peak: 25-40 mcg/mL	Peak: 20-30 min after end of 60 min infusion[1]
		Trough: 5-15 mcg/mL	Trough: Within 30 min before next dose

Note: In any ingestion, blood level sampling should occur on presentation and repeated soon after (1-2 hours) to determine if significant ongoing absorption is occuring.

[1]Some institutions may draw vancomycin peak 1 hour after 1-hour infusion and accept the lower range of therapeutic.

BREAST-FEEDING - TOXINS/DRUGS TO AVOID

Toxins/Drugs to Be Avoided During Breast-Feeding

Acebutolol
Aloe (*Aloe vera*)
Alprazolam
Amantadine
5-Aminosalicylic acid
Amiodarone
Amphetamine
Anthraquinones (laxatives)
Antineoplastic agents*
Atenolol
Atropine
Azathioprine
Basil (*Oaknum basillcum*)
Betaxolol
Bismuth subsalicylate
Bromides (>5 g/day)
Bromisovalerylurea
Bromocriptine
Buckthorn bark and berry
Buflomedill
Calciferol
Carisoprodol
Cascara sagrada
Chloral hydrate
Chloramphenicol
Chlordane
Chlordiazepoxide
Chlorpromazine
Chlorthalidone
Chromium
Chocolate (>16 oz/day)
Cimetidine
Clemastine
Clofazimine
Clonidine
Cocaine
Colchicine
Coltsfoot leaf
Copper-64 (50 hours)
Cyclophosphamide
Cyclosporine
Cyproheptadine
Danazol
Danthron
Dexfenfluramine
Dexrazoxane
Diazepam

Dieldrin
Dihydrotachysterol
Diphenhydramine
Diuretics
Donepezil
Doxepin
Doxorubicin
Dyphylline
Ergonovine
Ergotamine
Ethanol
Ethylene dichloride
Famciclovir (Penciclovir)
Fenfluramine
Fluconazole
Fluorescein
Fluoxetine
Gallium-67 (14 days*)†
Gold salts
Guanfacine
Heptachlor
Heroin
Hexachlorobenzene
Hexachlorophene
Hydroxyurea
Indian snakeroot (*Rauwolfia serpentina*)
Indium-111 isotope (20 hours*)
Iodides (especially potassium iodide)
Iodine-123 (36 hours*)
Iodine-125 (12 days*)†
Iodine-131 (14 days*)†
Isoniazid
Ivermectin
Lamotrigine
Lead (venous blood lead levels >35 mcg/dL)
Lindane
Lithium
Lovastatin
Marijuana (dronabinol)
Maté (Paraguay tea)
Meperidine
Mepindolol
Meprobamate
Mercaptopurine
Methimazole
Methotrexate
Methylmercury

Metoclopramide

Metronidazole (discontinue breast-feeding for 1 day)

Mifepristone

Minocycline

Moricizine

Nadolol

Nefazodone

Nicergoline

Nicotine

Olanzapine

Opiates

Organochlorines

Oxcodone

Oxprenolol

Perchloroethylene

Petasite root

Phencyclidine

Phenindione

Phenobarbital

Phenolphthalein

Piperazine

Piroxicam

Polychlorinated/polybrominated biphenyls

Povidone-iodine

Prazepam

Prednisone (>20 mg/day)

Primidone

Proguanil

Propofol

Quetiapine

Quinolone antibiotics

Radioactive diagnostic and therapeutic agents

Ranitidine

Reserpine

Retinoids

Rhubarb root

Riluzole

Salicylate (>1 g)

Selegiline

Senna (*Cassia senna*)

Sodium isotope (4 days*)

Sotalol

Strontium chloride (Sr 89)

Sulfasalazine

Technetium-99m (1-3 days†)

Tetrachloroethylene

Tetracycline

Theophylline

Thiouracil

Tilidine

Timolol

Tinidazole (discontinue breast-feeding for 1 day)

Tolbutamide

Tocainide

Zipeprol

*Antineoplastic agents, in general, with the possible exception of azathioprine (75-100 mg/day) with close infant monitoring.

†Duration of radioactivity excretion in breast milk.

Breast-feeding should be discontinued if the following radioisotopes are utilized: ^{131}I-HSA, ^{125}I-HSA, ^{125}I-fibrinogen, Na-^{131}I, ^{67}Ga-citrate, ^{75}Se-methionine, sodium ^{32}P phosphate, and chromic ^{32}P phosphate.

References

Ito S, "Drug Therapy for Breast-Feeding Women," *New Engl J Med*, 2000, 343(2):118-26; American Academy of Pediatrics, Committee on Drugs, "Transfer of Drugs and Other Chemicals Into Human Milk," *Pediatrics*, 2001, 108(3):776-89; Corley RA, Mast TJ, Carney EW, et al, "Evaluation of Physiologically Based Models of Pregnancy and Lactation for Their Application in Children's Health Risk Assessments," *Crit Rev Toxicol*, 2003, 33(2):137-211.

BREAST-FEEDING AND DRUGS

Prior to recommending or prescribing medications to a lactating woman, the following should be considered:

Is drug therapy necessary?

Can drug exposure to the infant be minimized? (Using a different route of administration, timing of the dose in relation to breast-feeding, length of therapy, using breast milk stored prior to treatment, etc)

The infant's age and health status (her own ability to metabolize the medication)

The pharmacokinetics of the drug

Will the drug interact with a medication the infant is prescribed?

If medications must be used, pick the safest drug possible.

In situations where the only drug available may have adverse effects in the nursing infant, consider measuring the infant's blood levels.

The tables presented below have been adapted from the American Academy of Pediatrics Committee on Drugs report, "Transfer of Drugs and Other Chemicals Into Human Milk," September, 2001. It should not be inferred that if a medication is not in the tables it is considered safe for administration to a lactating woman; only that published reports concerning their use were not available at the time the report was published.

Table 1. Cytotoxic Drugs	
Cyclophosphamide	Doxorubicin
Cyclosporine	Methotrexate

These are medications thought to interfere with cellular metabolism in the nursing infant. Immune suppression may be possible; effects on growth or carcinogenesis are not known. In addition, doxorubicin is concentrated in human milk; methotrexate is associated with neutropenia in the nursing infant.

Table 2. Drugs of Abuse	
Amphetamine	Marijuana
Cocaine	Phencyclidine
Heroin	

Drugs of abuse are not only dangerous to the nursing infant, but also to the mother. Women should be encouraged to avoid their use completely. Effects to the infant reported with amphetamine use in the mother include irritability and poor sleeping; it is also a substance that is concentrated in human milk. Cocaine may cause irritability, vomiting, diarrhea, tremors, or seizures in the infant. Heroin may also cause tremors as well as restlessness, vomiting, and poor feeding.

Nicotine, which was previously on this list, is associated with decreased milk production, decreased weight gain in the infant, and possible increased respiratory illness in the infant. Although there are still questions outstanding regarding smoking and breast-feeding, women should be counseled on the possible effects to their infants and offered aid to smoking cessation if appropriate.

Table 3. Radioactive Compounds That Require Temporary Cessation of Breast-Feeding	
Drug	**Recommended Time for Cessation of Breast-Feeding**
Copper 64 (^{64}Cu)	Radioactivity in milk present at 50 h
Gallium 67 (^{67}Ga)	Radioactivity in milk present for 2 wk
Indium 111 (^{111}In)	Very small amount present at 20 h
Iodine 123 (^{123}I)	Radioactivity in milk present up to 36 h
Iodine 125 (^{125}I)	Radioactivity in milk present for 12 d
Iodine 131 (^{131}I)	Radioactivity in milk present 2-14 d, depending on study

Table 3. Radioactive Compounds That Require Temporary Cessation of Breast-Feeding (*Continued*)

Drug	Recommended Time for Cessation of Breast-Feeding
Iodine[131]	If used for thyroid cancer, high radioactivity may prolong exposure to infant
Radioactive sodium	Radioactivity in milk present 96 h
Technetium-99m (^{99m}Tc), ^{99m}Tc macroaggregates, ^{99m}Tc O4	Radioactivity in milk present 15 h to 3 d

Consider pumping and storing milk prior to study for use during the radioactive period. Pumping should continue after the study to maintain milk production; however, this milk should be discarded until radioactivity is gone. Notify nuclear medicine physician prior to study that the mother is breast-feeding; a short-acting radionuclide may be appropriate. Contact Radiology Department after testing is complete to screen milk samples before resuming feeding.

Table 4a. Psychotropic Drugs Whose Effect on Nursing Infants is Unknown But May Be of Concern

Antianxiety	Antidepressant	Antipsychotic
Alprazolam	Amitriptyline	Chlorpromazine
Diazepam	Amoxapine	Clozapine[1]
Lorazepam	Bupropion	Haloperidol
Midazolam	Clomipramine	Mesoridazine
Perphenazine	Desipramine	Trifluoperazine
Prazepam[1]	Doxepin	
Quazepam	Fluoxetine	
Temazepam	Fluvoxamine	
	Imipramine	
	Nortriptyline	
	Paroxetine	
	Sertraline[1]	
	Trazodone	

[1]Drug is concentrated in human milk.

Psychotropic medications usually appear in the breast milk in low concentrations. Although adverse effects in the infant may be limited to a few case reports, the long half-life of these medications and their metabolites should be considered. In addition, measurable amounts may be found in the infant's plasma and also brain tissue. Long-term effects are not known. Colic, irritability, feeding and sleep disorders, and slow weight gain are effects reported with fluoxetine. Chlorpromazine may cause galactorrhea in the mother, while drowsiness and lethargy have been reported in the nursing infant. A decline in developmental scores has been reported with chlorpromazine and haloperidol.

Table 4b. Additional Drugs Whose Effect on Nursing Infants is Unknown But May Be of Concern

Drug	Reported Effect in Nursing Infant
Amiodarone	Hypothyroidism
Chloramphenicol	Idiosyncratic bone marrow suppression
Clofazimine	Increase in skin pigmentation; high transfer of mother's dose to infant is possible
Lamotrigine	Therapeutic serum concentrations in infant
Metoclopramide[1]	
Metronidazole	
Tinidazole	

[1]Drug is concentrated in human milk.

No adverse effects to the infant have been reported for metoclopramide; however, it should be recognized that it is a dopaminergic agent. Metronidazole and tinidazole are *in vitro* mutagenic agents. In cases where single dose therapy is appropriate for the mother, breast-feeding may be discontinued for 12-24 hours to allow excretion of the medication.

Table 5. Drugs That Have Been Associated With Significant Effects on Some Nursing Infants and Should Be Given to Nursing Mothers With Caution[1]	
Drug	**Reported Effect**
Acebutolol	Hypotension, bradycardia, tachypnea
5-Aminosalicylic acid	Diarrhea (one case)
Atenolol	Cyanosis, bradycardia
Bromocriptine	Suppresses lactation; may be hazardous to the mother
Aspirin (salicylates)	Metabolic acidosis (one case)
Clemastine	Drowsiness, irritability, refusal to feed, high-pitched cry, neck stiffness (one case)
Ergotamine	Vomiting, diarrhea, convulsions (doses used in migraine medications)
Lithium	One-third to one-half therapeutic blood concentration in infants
Phenindone	Anticoagulant; increased prothrombin and partial thromboplastin time in one infant; not used in the United States
Phenobarbital	Sedation; infantile spasms after weaning from milk-containing phenobarbital, methemoglobinemia (one case)
Primidone	Sedation, feeding problems
Sulfasalazine (salicylazosulfapyri-dine)	Bloody diarrhea (one case)

[1]Blood concentration in the infant may be of clinical importance; measure when possible.

References

American Academy of Pediatrics Committee on Drugs, "Transfer of Drugs and Other Chemicals into Human Milk," *Pediatrics*, 2001, 108(3): 776-89.

2000 Red Book: *Report of the Committee on Infectious Diseases*, 25th ed, Elk Grove Village, IL: American Academy of Pediatrics, 2000, 98-104.

BRONCHODILATORS

Comparison of Inhaled Sympathomimetic Bronchodilators			
Drug	**Adrenergic Receptor**	**Onset (min)**	**Duration Activity (h)**
Albuterol (Proventil®)	$\beta_1 < \beta_2$	<5	3-8
Epinephrine (various)	α and β_1 and β_2	1-5	1-3
Formoterol (Foradil®)	$\beta_1 < \beta_2$	3-5	12
Isoetharine (various)	$\beta_1 < \beta_2$	<5	1-3
Isoproterenol (Isuprel®)	β_1 and β_2	2-5	0.5-2
Levalbuterol (Xopenex®)	$\beta_1 < \beta_2$	10-17	5-6
Metaproterenol (Alupent®)	$\beta_1 < \beta_2$	5-30	2-6
Pirbuterol (Maxair™)	$\beta_1 < \beta_2$	<5	5
Salmeterol (Serevent®)	$\beta_1 < \beta_2$	5-14	12
Terbutaline (Brethine®)	$\beta_1 < \beta_2$	5-30	3-6

CALCIUM CHANNEL BLOCKERS

Comparative Pharmacokinetics								
Agent	Bioavailability (%)	Protein Binding (%)	Onset of BP Effect (min)	Duration of BP Effect (h)	Half-Life (h)	Volume of Distribution	Route of Metabolism	Route of Excretion
Dihydropyridines								
Amlodipine (Norvasc®)	64-90	93-98	30-50	24	30-50	21 L/kg	Hepatic; inactive metabolites	Urine; 10% as parent
Felodipine (Plendil®)	20	>99	2-5 h	24	11-16	10 L/kg	Hepatic; CYP3A4 substrate (major); inactive metabolites; extensive first pass	Urine (70%; as metabolites); feces 10%
Isradipine (DynaCirc® [DSC]) (immediate release)	15-24	95	20	>12	8	3 L/kg	Hepatic; CYP3A4 substrate (major); inactive metabolites; extensive first pass	Urine as metabolites
Nicardipine (Cardene®) (immediate release)	35	>95	30	≤8	2-4		Hepatic; CYP3A4 substrate (major); saturable first pass	Urine (60%; as metabolites); feces 35%
Nifedipine (Procardia®) (immediate release)	40-77	92-98	Within 20		2-5		Hepatic; CYP3A4 substrate (major); inactive metabolites	Urine as metabolites
Nimodipine (Nimotop®)	13	>95	ND	4-6	1-2		Hepatic; CYP3A4 substrate (major); metabolites inactive or less active than parent; extensive first pass	Urine (50%; as metabolites); feces 32%
Nisoldipine (Sular®)	5	>99	ND	6-12	7-12		Hepatic; CYP3A4 substrate (major); 1 active metabolite (10% of parent); extensive first pass	Urine as metabolites
Phenylalkylamines								
Verapamil (Calan®) (immediate release)	20-35	90	30	6-8	4.5-12		Hepatic; CYP3A4 substrate (major); 1 active metabolite (20% of parent); extensive first pass	Urine (70%; 3%-4% as unchanged drug); feces 16%
Benzothiazepines								
Diltiazem (Cardizem®) (immediate release)	~40	70-80	30-60	6-8	3-4.5	3-13 L/kg	Hepatic; CYP3A4 substrate (major); 1 major metabolite (20%-50% of parent); extensive first pass	Urine as metabolites

CHRONIC RENAL FAILURE

In chronic renal failure, there is a progressive loss of nephron function. Depending upon the extent of loss, signs, symptoms, and biochemical abnormalities may or may not be present. Signs of renal failure (eg, nocturia) begin to appear when the number of functioning nephrons decreases to 10% to 40%. This stage of renal failure is referred to as renal insufficiency. Patients at this stage have little or no renal reserve; the ability to metabolize and excrete certain drugs is impaired as is the ability to eliminate large quantities of protein catabolic products. Serum creatinine (Cr) and blood urea nitrogen (BUN) are increased. The loss of approximately 95% of functioning nephrons results in the uremic syndrome. Acid-base, hematologic, and electrolyte abnormalities (hyperkalemia, hyponatremia, hypercalcemia, hypocalcemia, hypermagnesemia, hyperphosphatemia) are routinely seen, as is fluid overload, which can result in CHF, hypertension, and left ventricular hypertrophy. Hyperkalemia is an important consideration because of its ability to precipitate fatal cardiac arrhythmias. Gastrointestinal disorders (eg, nausea, vomiting, anorexia, GI bleeding), chronic anemia, and an altered immune system are also present.

Effect on Drug Disposition

Bioavailability

Several factors affect drug absorption in renal failure patients. Absorption of drugs can be decreased in uremic patients who have nausea, vomiting, diarrhea, gastritis, and pancreatitis. Uremia can result in an increase in gastric pH, thereby reducing the bioavailability of drugs requiring an acidic medium for absorption. An increase in gastric pH can also occur secondary to antacid use, which is often needed by renal failure patients. Antacids bind to other drugs, reducing their absorption. Gastric emptying time, gastric mobility, and intestinal motility can be decreased in the uremic patient, which can influence drug absorption.

Protein Binding

A drug's effect is produced by its free or unbound fraction. In renal failure patients, protein binding is reduced, which increases the amount of unbound drug. For example, this is seen with acidic drugs normally bound to albumin; since albumin is frequently decreased in renal failure, a greater free fraction of drug is seen. This effect is most important for drugs with high protein binding (>80%), such as phenytoin and valproic acid . The increase in free fraction can increase clearance of phenytoin since it is a low extraction ratio drug. Increased free drug can also result from the displacement of acidic drugs from albumin binding sites by acidic by-products seen in uremia and as a result of conformational changes in albumin which reduce the number/ affinity of binding sites for drugs. Decreased tissue protein binding of digoxin decreases its volume of distribution, necessitating smaller loading digoxin loading doses in renal failure.

Metabolism

Renal failure significantly impacts on drug metabolism in a number of organs. The kidney houses the renal cytochrome P450 system, which contributes to the metabolism of a number of drugs. Renal failure has been demonstrated to potentially increase, decrease, or have no effect on drug metabolism. Renal failure can also impact on drugs, which are metabolized by the liver to active metabolites. If these metabolites are renally eliminated, they accumulate in renal failure leading to increased activity and/or adverse effects. Meperidine (normeperidine), morphine (morphine-6-glucuronide), procainamide (N-acetylprocainamide), and allopurinol (oxypurinol) are four examples of such drugs. Dosages of these drugs should be carefully titrated in renal failure patients, and potential toxic effects should be monitored.

Elimination

The degree of renal impairment and the percentage of drug normally excreted unchanged in the urine will determine the impact of renal failure on elimination. Drugs are eliminated by the kidney via either filtration or active secretion. Molecular size and protein binding will determine a drug's filterability; low protein bound and small drugs are filtered more easily. Renal secretion is dependent on the anionic and cationic pathways. Depending on the cause of the renal disease, alterations in secretion and filtration can occur independently of each other. Estimates of GFR such as creatinine clearance are generally used to estimate renal function. But estimates of GFR may not predict alterations in clearance due to tubular dysfunction and altered secretion. Therefore close monitoring for efficacy and toxicity of renally eliminated drugs is necessary even when appropriate dosage alterations based on estimates of creatinine clearance have been performed.

Renal Dosing

Individualized drug dosage regimens for patients with renal failure generally utilize a correlation between creatinine clearance and drug clearance. Creatinine clearance is best estimated from a stable serum creatinine in patients with normal muscle mass and weight. A number of equations to estimate creatinine clearance are available. Multiple methods of renal dosage modification may be available, and they generally include increasing the interval or decreasing the dose. Both of these methods maintain the same steady state serum concentrations. Increasing the interval maintains similar peaks and troughs as usual dosing. Decreasing the dose results in lower peaks and higher troughs. This method is useful for antibiotics such as cephalosporins where the lack of postantibiotic effect necessitates maintenance of serum concentrations above the MIC.

Drug Dosing in Renal Replacement Therapy

Drug removal by hemodialysis is impacted by numerous drug-related factors. Molecular weight less than 500 daltons is generally associated with drug removal by traditional hemodialysis methods. However, hi-flux filters can remove drugs of 5,000 daltons or greater. Water soluble drugs are more likely to be removed than drugs of poor solubility in aqueous media. Protein binding is an additional significant factor, since only free drug is available to diffuse across the semi-permeable membrane. Volume of distribution also correlates well, as drugs with smaller volumes of distribution are more likely to come in contact with the semi-permeable membrane and are more significantly dialyzed than drugs with large volumes of distribution that are largely distributed to tissue.

Characteristics of the dialysis procedure also impact on the amount of drug removed. A variety of dialysis filters of various compositions are available. Significant differences in drug clearances with different dialysis membranes and filters have been described. In addition, blood and dialysate flow rates vary along with the length of the dialysis session. Therefore, drug clearances can vary significantly based on the specific dialysis prescription.

The need for supplemental dosing after dialysis is based on the relative amount of drug removed by a typical dialysis session. When >25% to 30% of a dose is removed by a typical 4-hour dialysis session, it is generally recommended that a supplemental dose be administered. Use of hi-flux membranes may necessitate more aggressive supplementation, especially for some drugs that are not removed by typical procedures (eg, vancomycin). Given the multitude of factors impacting the potential amount of drug removed, close monitoring for efficacy and toxicity is necessary.

Preoperative Evaluation of the Chronic Renal Failure Patient

Assessment of renal function should be part of the comprehensive preoperative evaluation of the chronic renal failure patient. Tests are used in an attempt to quantify renal function and include BUN, serum creatinine, measured creatinine clearance, and estimated creatinine clearance. The following table lists the advantages and disadvantages for each test as well as their normal values.

Test	Normal Values	Advantages/Disadvantages
BUN	8-20 mg/dL	- Rapid, inexact estimate of creatinine clearance
		- BUN is increased by high protein intake, blood in GI tract, accelerated catabolism
		- Hepatic dysfunction decreases BUN concentration
		- Reabsorption of urea is greater when urinary flow is low
Cr (serum creatinine)	0.5-1.2 mg/dL	- Rapid, inexact estimate of creatinine clearance
		- Creatinine is produced at a lower rate in elderly and in females; levels may fail to accurately reflect degree of nephron loss
		- Patients with muscle wasting from chronic disease may have low serum creatinine levels
		- Heavily muscled patients or acutely catabolic patients may have higher than normal serum creatinine levels secondary to more rapid muscle breakdown

Test	Normal Values	Advantages/Disadvantages
(Continued)		
C$_{cr}$ (measured)	120 mL/minute	- Best overall indicator of GFR
		- Must accurately record urinary volume
		- Hydration can influence GFR determination
C$_{cr}$ (estimated)	120 mL/ minute	- Superior to BUN or serum creatinine for quantification of renal reserve
		- Same disadvantages as serum creatinine

Urinalysis assesses urinary pH as well as the presence of hematuria, pyuria, cellular casts, and proteinuria. The patient's cardiovascular status, hemoglobin concentration, and adequacy of dialysis therapy should also be assessed.

Intraoperative Management of the Chronic Renal Failure Patient

Monitoring

Intraoperative monitoring should include blood pressure, heart rate, EKG, oxygen saturation (via pulse oximeter), carbon dioxide (via capnometry), and degree of neuromuscular blockade (via a peripheral nerve stimulator). Invasive cardiovascular monitoring should be performed as needed.

Fluid Management

Fluid management must take into consideration the chronic renal failure patient's inability to excrete excess sodium and water. In those patients not requiring hemodialysis, a urine output >0.5 mL/kg/hour can usually be maintained by administration of a balanced salt solution at a rate of 3-5 mL/kg/hour. If necessary, the patient can be dialyzed postoperatively if intravascular volume is increased to an unsatisfactory level intraoperatively.

Selection of Anesthetic Agents

A knowledge of drug action in renal failure is important in determining an appropriate drug regimen (drug and dose). The reader is referred to the drugs' individual monographs to determine dosing in renal failure. Several examples follow.

I.V. anesthetic agents. Thiopental is highly bound to plasma proteins. Since protein binding is reduced in renal failure, a larger fraction of unbound thiopental is available. Further, a greater proportion of thiopental is found in the nonionized, unbound form secondary to the acidic pH seen in renal failure. Finally, uremia alters the blood-brain barrier, which results in an increased sensitivity to thiopental. Because of these factors, a lower induction dose of thiopental is needed for uremic patients.

Induction doses of ketamine and benzodiazepines require less reduction since they are less protein-bound than thiopental. Normal benzodiazepine doses, however, may show an exaggerated response in debilitated renal failure patients. Ketamine, because of its ability to increase blood pressure and cardiac output, may worsen the hypertension seen with renal failure.

Morphine's elimination half-life and clearance are not changed in renal failure. As already alluded to, its glucuronide metabolite accumulates in renal failure and can cause prolonged respiratory depression The synthetic opioids, fentanyl , sufentanil , and alfentanil are hepatically metabolized with their metabolites renally excreted. The rapid tissue redistribution seen with these agents after small doses should result in a short duration of action in both normal and renal failure patients. Sufentanil does, however, have an active metabolite which can accumulate in chronic renal failure patients. Remifentanil , because of its metabolism by nonspecific esterases in blood and tissue, is not affected by renal failure. Dosing remains the same as in normal patients.

Inhalational agents. The major route of elimination of these agents is via the lungs, not the kidneys. Metabolism of some of these agents can result in renally excreted metabolites. Enflurane and sevoflurane are metabolized to inorganic fluoride, which can accumulate in renal failure patients. Sevoflurane is currently not recommended for use in patients with a serum creatinine >1.5 mg/dL. An advantage of the volatile inhalation agents is that they produce neuromuscular blockade, which can reduce the dose of neuromuscular blocking agent required.

Neuromuscular blocking agents. The depolarizing neuromuscular blocking agent succinylcholine causes a transient increase in serum potassium of approximately 0.5-1 mEq/L. This may become a problem in uremic patients who have an elevated serum potassium; the increase may be enough to produce cardiac arrhythmias. Plasma cholinesterase levels are sufficient in renal failure patients so that no clinically significant prolongation of succinylcholine's effect should be expected.

The elimination of nondepolarizing neuromuscular blocking agents is dependent to varying degrees on renal excretion. The following table lists the elimination profiles of the commercially available nondepolarizing agents. The elimination half-lives of agents primarily eliminated renally are increased in patients with renal failure. Atracurium and cisatracurium, because of their primarily nonrenal elimination, are ideal agents to use in renal failure patients. Both pancuronium and vecuronium have active metabolites that can accumulate in renal failure. One of atracurium's metabolites, laudanosine, can also accumulate in renal failure. Laudanosine has no neuromuscular blocking activity but has been shown to cause CNS excitation in animals; this effect has not been demonstrated in humans.

Agent	Renal	Hepatic	Biliary	Plasma
Atracurium	<5%	—	—	Hofmann elimination
				Ester hydrolysis
Cisatracurium	R/H <20%	R/H <20%	—	Hofmann elimination
Doxacurium	80% to 100%	—	Yes	—
Gallamine	95% to 100%	—	<1%	—
Mivacurium	<10%	—	Minor	Plasma cholinesterase
Pancuronium	60% to 80%	15% to 40%	5% to 10%	—
Rocuronium	30%	—	50%	—
Vecuronium	30%	20% to 30%	40% to 75%	—

R/H = renal/hepatic metabolism.

Renal failure increases the duration of action of the anticholinesterase agents (neostigmine, pyridostigmine, edrophonium) commonly used to reverse the residual effects of neuromuscular blockade by 100% or more (secondary to their elimination primarily by the kidneys). This makes the possibility of recurarization unlikely. Other factors which influence reversal of neuromuscular blockade in the renal failure patient include acid-base status, electrolyte levels, concomitant use of potentiating drugs (eg, aminoglycosides), and temperature.

Postoperative Management of the Chronic Renal Failure Patient

Hypertension is frequently seen in the postoperative period. Vasodilators (eg, fenoldopam and hydralazine) may be useful as initial therapy. Nitroprusside can be used transiently, but large doses or prolonged use could be associated with thiocyanate toxicity in renal failure. If hypervolemia is the cause, dialysis can be used to remove excess fluid if it is an option. Supplemental oxygen should be considered if anemia is present, continuous monitoring of the EKG is warranted if arrhythmias are a concern in a hyperkalemic patient, and caution should be used when administering opioids for pain secondary to the potential for CNS depression and hypoventilation.

References and Recommended Reading

Matzke GR and Frye RF, "Drug Therapy Individualization for Patients with Renal Insufficiency," *Pharmacotherapy: A Pathophysiologic Approach*, DiPiro JT, Talbert RL, Yess GC, et al, eds, 5th ed, Stamford, CT: Appleton and Lange, 2002, 939-52.

Monk TG and Weldon BC, "The Renal System and Anesthesia for Urologic Surgery," *Clinical Anesthesia*, Barash PG, Cullen BF, Stoelting RK, eds, 3rd ed, Philadelphia, PA: Lippincott Williams & Wilkins, 1996, 945-73.

Quan DJ and Aweeka FT, "Dosing of Drugs in Renal Failure," *Applied Therapeutics: The Clinical Use of Drugs*, Young LY and Koda-Kimble MA, eds, 8th ed, Vancouver, WA: Applied Therapeutics Inc, 2004, 32(1)-(26).

Stoelting RK and Dierdorf SF, "Renal Disease," *Anesthesia and Co-Existing Disease*, 3rd ed, New York, NY: Churchill Livingstone, 1993, 289-312.

CIGARETTE SMOKING AND EFFECTS ON DRUGS/TOXINS

Drug	Effect
Amitriptyline	Possible decrease in tricyclic antidepressant drug levels due to increased hepatic metabolism
Arsenic	Possible increase in lung cancer
Asbestos	Increased risk of lung cancer (not mesothelioma)
Ascorbic acid	Increased recommended dietary allowance (to 100 mg/day)
Beta carotene	Increased risk of lung cancer
Byssinosis	Risk factor in textile workers
Caffeine	Increases metabolism by 56%
Chlordiazepoxide	Larger dose required to achieve sedative effects
Chlorpromazine	Decreases serum concentrations by 24%
Chlorzepate	Decreased area under the curve (AUC)
Chromium (hexavalent)	Increased risk of lung cancer
Cocaine	Enhances (additively) cocaine-induced vasoconstriction in areas of atherosclerosis
Codeine	Induced glucuronidation of codeine
Cotton dust	Exacerbation of respiratory effects of byssinosis
Desipramine	Possible decrease in tricyclic antidepressant drug levels due to increased hepatic metabolism
Diazepam	Larger dose required to achieve sedative effects
Diesel exhaust	Possible added effect for lung cancer
Estradiol	Increases 2-hydroxylation
Estrogen	Increased risk of cardiovascular events
Ethyl alcohol	Increased risk for oral and esophageal cancer; delayed gastric emptying
Flecainide	Reduction of serum flecainide levels (by possibly increasing hepatic metabolism)
Fluvoxamine	Increased metabolism of fluvoxamine by 25%; lower serum concentrations of fluvoxamine
Haloperidol	Increases clearance by 44% and decreases serum levels by 70%
Heparin	Shorter heparin half-life
Imipramine	Possible decrease in tricyclic antidepressant drug levels due to increased hepatic metabolism
Insulin	Decreased subcutaneous absorption; heavy smokers may require a 15% to 30% increase in insulin dosage compared to nonsmokers; possible decrease in tricyclic antidepressant drug levels due to increased hepatic metabolism
Leflunomide	Increases drug plasma clearance by 38%
Lidocaine	Decreased oral bioavailability with increased oral clearance
Lisinopril	Improves both receptor mediated and tonic nitric-oxide release
Mexiletine	Increases oral clearance by 25% with decreased half-life by 36%
Mineral oil (cutting oil) mists	Synergistic effect of reduced lung function and chronic cough
Mustard gas	Possible increase in lung cancer
Neuroleptics	Increased risk for tardive dyskinesia
Nicotine	Increased metabolism
Nortriptyline	Possible decrease in tricyclic antidepressant drug levels due to increased hepatic metabolism
Olanzapine	Increases clearance by 98%
Pentazocine	Decreased analgesic effect
Phenacetin	Increased metabolism
Propoxyphene	Decreased analgesic effect
Propranolol	Decreased therapeutic effect
Radiation	Possible increased risk of lung cancer
Radon	Increased risk of lung cancer
Riluzole	Clearance decreased from 32% to 36% in smokers

Drug	Effect
	(Continued)
Ritonavir	Decreased ritonavir levels
Sertraline	Nausea, dizziness, and flushing
Silica	Possible increased risk of lung cancer
Tacrine	Increases tacrine clearance and decreases tacrine half-life by 50%; mean plasma tacrine levels are decreased three-fold
Theophylline	Decreased theophylline levels with decreased effect; decreases half-life by 63% and increases V_d by 31%
Uranium	Probable increase in lung cancer
Vinyl acetate	Enhanced respiratory impairment
Warfarin	Increases warfarin clearance by 13% - no effect on prothrombin time

From Schein JR, "Cigarette Smoking and Clinically Significant Drug Interactions", *Ann Pharmacother,* 1995, 29:1129-48.

Pinkofsky HB, Stone KD, and Reeves RR, "Serotonin, Cigarettes, and Nausea," *J Clin Psychopharm,* 1997, 17:492.

Spigset O, Carleborg L, Hedenmalm K, et al, "Effect of Cigarette Smoking on Fluvoxamine Pharmacokinetics in Humans," *Clin Pharmacol Ther,* 1995, 58:399-403.

Zevin S and Benowitz NL, "Drug Interactions with Tobacco Smoking," *Clin Pharmacokinet,* 1999, 36(6)425-38.

Conditions Associated With Environmental Tobacco Smoke (ETS)

Infants (50% of all infants exposed to ETS)
- Behavior problems
- Otitis media (38% higher rate)
- Elevated blood pressure
- Bronchiolitis/bronchitis
- Pneumonia (double the risk)
- Decreased stature
- Inflammatory bowel disease
- Delayed dental maturation
- Increased lipoprotein concentration
- Meningococcal disease
- Sinusitis (risk is 50% greater)
- Sudden infant death syndrome (threefold risk)

Adolescents
- Asthma (49% more exacerbations with delayed recovery)
- Asthma in children with parental atopy and ETS (odds ratio 2.68)
- Almost 9% greater ratio of total cholesterol to HDL cholesterol and almost 7% greater ratio of total cholesterol to LDL cholesterol
- Increased clearance of theophylline in asthmatic children
- Increased rates of leukemia, lymphoma, and lung cancer

Adults
- Lung cancer (3000-5000 cases annually)
- Increase in arteriosclerosis (50,000 deaths annually)
- Increased incidence of chronic obstructive pulmonary disease
- Increases risk of death from coronary artery disease in "never smokers" by about 5%

Pets
- Increased risk of malignancy in dogs
- Double the risk of lymphoma in cats

CLINICAL SYNDROMES ASSOCIATED WITH FOOD-BORNE DISEASES

Clinical Syndromes	Incubation Period (h)	Causes	Commonly Associated Vehicles
Nausea and vomiting	<1-6	*Staphylococcus aureus* (preformed toxins, A, B, C, D, E)	Ham, poultry, cream-filled pastries, potato and egg salad, mushrooms
		Bacillus cereus (emetic toxin)	Fried rice, pork
		Heavy metals (copper, tin, cadmium, zinc)	Acidic beverages
Histamine response and gastrointestinal (GI) tract	<1	Histamine (scombroid)	Fish (bluefish, bonito, mackerel, mahi-mahi, tuna)
Neurologic, including paresthesia and GI tract	0-6	Tetrodotoxin, ciguatera	Puffer fish
			Fish (amberjack, barracuda, grouper, snapper)
		Paralytic compounds	Shellfish (clams, mussels, oysters, scallops, other mollusks)
		Neurotoxic compounds	Shellfish
		Domoic acid	Mussels
		Monosodium glutamate	Chinese food
Neurologic and GI tract manifestations	0-2	Mushroom toxins (early onset)	Mushrooms
Moderate-to-severe abdominal cramps and watery diarrhea	8-16	*B. cereus* enterotoxin	Beef, pork, chicken, vanilla sauce
		Clostridium perfringens enterotoxin	Beef, poultry, gravy
	16-48	Caliciviruses	Shellfish, salads, ice
		Enterotoxigenic *Escherichia coli*	Fruits, vegetables
		Vibrio cholerae 01 and 0139	Shellfish
		V. cholerae non-01	Shellfish
Diarrhea, fever, abdominal cramps, blood and mucus in stools	16-72	*Salmonella*	Poultry, pork, eggs, dairy products including ice cream, vegetables, fruit
		Shigella	Egg salad, vegetables
		Campylobacter jejuni	Poultry, raw milk
		Invasive *E. coli*	
		Yersinia enterocolitica	Pork chitterlings, tofu, raw milk
		Vibrio parahaemolyticus	Fish, shellfish
Bloody diarrhea, abdominal cramps	72-120	Enterohemorrhagic *E. coli*	Beef (hamburger), raw milk, roast beef, salami, salad dressings
Methemoglobin poisoning	6-12	Mushrooms (late onset)	Mushrooms
Hepatorenal failure	6-24	Mushrooms (late onset)	Mushrooms
Gastrointestinal then blurred vision, dry mouth, dysarthria, diplopia, descending paralysis	18-36	*Clostridium botulinum*	Canned vegetables, fruits and fish, salted fish, bottled garlic
Extraintestinal manifestations	Varied	Brainerd disease	Unpasteurized milk
		Brucella	Cheese, raw milk
		Group A *Streptococcus*	Egg and potato salad
		Listeria monocytogenes	Cheese, raw milk, hot dogs, cole slaw, cold cuts
		Trichinella spiralis	Pork
		Vibrio vulnificus	Shellfish

Adapted from "Report of the Committee on Infectious Diseases," *1997 Red Book®*, 24th ed.

COMPATIBILITY OF MEDICATIONS MIXED IN A SYRINGE

	Atropine	Chlorpromazine	Codeine	Diphenhydramine	Droperidol	Fentanyl	Glycopyrrolate	Hydroxyzine	Meperidine	Metoclopramide	Midazolam	Morphine	Pentazocine	Pentobarbital†	Prochlorperazine	Promazine	Promethazine	Trimethobenzamide
Atropine		C	•	C	C	C	C	C	C	C	C	C	C	C	C	C	C	•
Chlorpromazine	C		•	C	C	C	C	C	C	C	C	C	C	X	C	C	C	•
Codeine	•	•		•	•	•	C	C	•	•	•	•	•	X	•	•	•	•
Diphenhydramine	C	C	•		C	C	C	C	C	C	C	C	C	X	C	C	C	•
Droperidol	C	C	•	C		C	C	C	C	C	C	C	C	X	C	C	C	•
Fentanyl	C	C	•	C	C		C	C	C	C	C	C	C	X	C	C	C	•
Glycopyrrolate	C	C	C	C	C	C		C	C	•	C	C	X	X	C	C	C	C
Hydroxyzine	C	C	C	C	C	C	C		C	C	C	C	C	X	C	C	C	•
Meperidine	C	C	•	C	C	C	C	C		C	C	X	C	X	C	C	C	•
Metoclopramide	C	C	•	C	C	C	•	C	C		C	C	C	•	C	C	C	•
Midazolam	C	C	•	C	C	C	C	C	C	C		C	•	X	X	C	C	C
Morphine	C	C	•	C	C	C	C	C	C	C	C		C	X	C*	C	C	•
Pentazocine	C	C	•	C	C	C	C	C	C	C	•	C		X	C	C	C	C
Pentobarbital†	C	X	X	X	X	X	X	X	X	•	X	X	X		X	X	X	•
Prochlorperazine	C	C	•	C	C	C	C	C	C	C	X	C*	C	X		C	C	•
Promazine	C	C	•	C	C	C	C	C	C	C	C	C	C	X	C		C	•
Promethazine	C	C	•	C	C	C	C	C	C	C	C	C	C	X	C	C		•
Trimethobenzamide	•	•	•	•	•	•	C	•	•	•	C	•	C	•	•	•	•	

C = Physically compatible if used within 15 minutes after mixing in a syringe
X = Incompatible
• = No documented information
C* = Potential incompatibility produced by certain manufacturers
† = Compatibility profile is characteristic of most barbiturate salts, such as

The following combinations have been found to be compatible:
    atropine / meperidine / promethazine
    atropine / meperidine / hydroxyzine
    meperidine / promethazine / chlorpromazine

The following drugs should not be mixed with any other drugs in the same syringe:
    diazepam, chlordiazepoxide

CONTRAINDICATIONS AND PRECAUTIONS TO COMMONLY USED VACCINES

Vaccine	Contraindications	Precautions[1]	Vaccines Can Be Administered
General for all vaccines, including diphtheria and tetanus toxoids and acellular pertussis vaccine (DTaP); pediatric diphtheria-tetanus toxoid (DT); adult tetanus-diphtheria toxoid (Td); inactivated poliovirus vaccine (IPV); measles-mumps-rubella vaccine (MMR); *Haemophilus influenzae* type b vaccine (Hib); hepatitis A vaccine; hepatitis B vaccine; varicella vaccine; pneumococcal conjugate vaccine (PCV); influenza vaccine; and pneumococcal polysaccharide vaccine (PPV)	• Serious allergic reaction (eg, anaphylaxis) after a previous vaccine dose • Serious allergic reaction (eg, anaphylaxis) to a vaccine component	• Moderate or severe acute illnesses with or without a fever	• Mild acute illness with or without fever • Mild to moderate local reaction (ie, swelling, redness, soreness); low-grade or moderate fever after previous dose • Lack of previous physical examination in well-appearing person • Current antimicrobial therapy • Convalescent phase of illnesses • Premature birth (hepatitis B vaccine is an exception in certain circumstances)[2] • Recent exposure to an infectious disease • History of penicillin allergy, other nonvaccine allergies, receiving allergen extract immunotherapy • Temperature <40.5°C, fussiness or mild drowsiness after a previous dose of diphtheria toxoid-tetanus toxoid-pertussis vaccine (DTP)/DTaP • Family history of seizures[3] • Family history of sudden infant death syndrome • Family history of an adverse event after DTP or DTaP administration • Stable neurologic conditions (eg, cerebral palsy, well-controlled convulsions, developmental delay)
DTaP	• Severe allergic reaction after a previous dose or to a vaccine component • Encephalopathy (eg, coma, decreased level of consciousness, prolonged seizures) within 7 days of administration of previous dose of DTP or DTaP • Progressive neurologic disorder, including infantile spasms, uncontrolled epilepsy, progressive encephalopathy; defer DTaP until neurologic status clarified and stabilized	• Fever >40.5°C ≤48 hours after vaccination with a previous dose of DTP or DTaP • Collapse or shock-like state (ie, hypotonic hyporesponsive episode) ≤48 hours after receiving a previous dose of DTP/DTaP • Seizure ≤3 days of receiving a previous dose of DTP/DTaP[3] • Persistent, inconsolable crying lasting ≥3 hours, ≤48 hours after receiving a previous dose of DTP/DTaP • Moderate or severe acute illness with or without fever	Same as above
DT, Td	• Severe allergic reaction after a previous dose or to a vaccine component	• Guillain-Barré syndrome ≤6 weeks after previous dose of tetanus toxoid-containing vaccine • Moderate or severe acute illness with or without fever	Same as above
IPV	• Severe allergic reaction to previous dose or vaccine component	• Pregnancy • Moderate or severe acute illness with or without fever	—
MMR[4]	• Severe allergic reaction after a previous dose or to a vaccine component • Pregnancy • Known severe immunodeficiency (eg, hematologic and solid tumors; congenital immunodeficiency; long-term immunosuppressive therapy;[5] or severely symptomatic human immunodeficiency virus [HIV] infection)	• Recent (≤11 months) receipt of antibody-containing blood product (specific interval depends on product) • History of thrombocytopenia or thrombocytopenic purpura • Moderate or severe acute illness with or without fever	• Positive tuberculin skin test • Simultaneous TB skin testing[6] • Breast-feeding • Pregnancy of recipient's mother or other close or household contact • Recipient is child-bearing-age female • Immunodeficient family member or household contact • Asymptomatic or mildly symptomatic HIV infection • Allergy to eggs

(*Continued*)

Vaccine	Contraindications	Precautions[1]	Vaccines Can Be Administered
Hib	• Severe allergic reaction after a previous dose or to a vaccine component • Age <6 weeks	• Moderate or severe acute illness with or without fever	—
Hepatitis B	• Severe allergic reaction after a previous dose or to a vaccine component	• Infant weighing <2000 g[2] • Moderate or severe acute illness with or without fever	• Pregnancy • Autoimmune disease (eg, systemic lupus erythematosis or rheumatoid arthritis)
Hepatitis A	• Severe allergic reaction after a previous dose or to a vaccine component	• Pregnancy • Moderate or severe acute illness with or without fever	—
Varicella	• Severe allergic reaction after a previous dose or to a vaccine component • Substantial suppression of cellular immunity • Pregnancy	• Recent ($\leq$11 months) receipt of antibody containing blood product (specific interval depends on product) • Moderate or severe acute illness with or without fever	• Pregnancy of recipient's mother or other close or household contact • Immunodeficient family member or household contact[7] • Asymptomatic or mildly symptomatic HIV infection • Humoral immunodeficiency (eg, agammaglobulinemia)
PCV	• Severe allergic reaction after a previous dose or to a vaccine component	• Moderate or severe acute illness with or without fever	—
Influenza	• Severe allergic reaction to previous dose or vaccine component, including egg protein	• Moderate or severe acute illness with or without fever	• Nonsevere (eg, contact) allergy to latex or thimerosal • Concurrent administration of Coumadin® or aminophylline
PPV	• Severe allergic reaction after a previous dose or to a vaccine component	• Moderate or severe acute illness with or without fever	—

[1]Events or conditions listed as precautions should be reviewed carefully. Benefits and risks of administering a specific vaccine to a person under these circumstances should be considered. If the risk from the vaccine is believed to outweigh the benefit, the vaccine should not be administered. If the benefit of vaccination is believed to outweigh the risk, the vaccine should be administered. Whether and when to administer DTaP to children with proven or suspected underlying neurologic disorders should be decided on a case-by-case basis.

[2]Hepatitis B vaccination should be deferred for infants weighing <2000 g if the mother is documented to be hepatitis B surface antigen (Hb $_s$Ag)-negative at the time of the infant's birth. Vaccination can commence at chronological age 1 month. For infants born to (Hb $_s$Ag)-positive women, hepatitis B immunoglobulin and hepatitis B vaccine should be administered at or soon after birth regardless of weight.

[3]Acetaminophen or other appropriate antipyretic can be administered to children with a personal or family history of seizures at the time of DTaP vaccination and every 4-6 hours for 24 hours thereafter to reduce the possibility of postvaccination fever (source: American Academy of Pediatrics, Pickering LK, ed, "Active Immunization," *2000 Red Book® Report of the Committee on Infectious Diseases*, 25th ed, Elk Grove Village, IL: American Academy of Pediatrics, 2000).

[4]MMR and varicella vaccines can be administered on the same day. If not administered on the same day, these vaccines should be separated by $\geq$28 days.

[5]Substantially immunosuppressive steroid dose is considered to be $\geq$2 weeks of daily receipt of 20 mg or 2 mg/kg body weight of prednisone or equivalent.

[6]Measles vaccination can suppress tuberculin reactivity temporarily. Measles-containing vaccine can be administered on the same day as tuberculin skin testing. If testing cannot be performed until after the day of MMR vaccination, the test should be postponed for $\geq$4 weeks after the vaccination. If an urgent need exists to skin test, do so with the understanding that reactivity might be reduced by the vaccine.

[7]If a vaccine experiences a presumed vaccine-related rash 7-25 days after vaccination, avoid direct contact with immunocompromised persons for the duration of the rash.

Adapted from "Recommendations and Reports," *MMWR Morb Mortal Wkly Rep*, 2002, 51(RR-2):9-10.

CONTRAST MEDIA REACTIONS, PREMEDICATION FOR PROPHYLAXIS

American College of Radiology Guidelines for Use of Nonionic Contrast Media

It is estimated that approximately 5% to 10% of patients will experience adverse reactions to administration of contrast dye (less for nonionic contrast). In approximately 1000-2000 administrations, a life-threatening reaction will occur.

A variety of premedication regimens have been proposed, both for pretreatment of "at risk" patients who require contrast media and before the routine administration of the intravenous high osmolar contrast media. Such regimens have been shown in clinical trials to decrease the frequency of all forms of contrast medium reactions. Pretreatment with a 2-dose regimen of methylprednisolone 32 mg, 12 and 2 hours prior to intravenous administration of HOCM (ionic), has been shown to decrease mild, moderate, and severe reactions in patients at increased risk and perhaps in patients without risk factors. Logistical and feasibility problems may preclude adequate premedication with this or any regimen for all patients. It is unclear at this time that steroid pretreatment prior to administration of ionic contrast media reduces the incidence of reactions to the same extent or less than that achieved with the use of nonionic contrast media alone. Information about the efficacy of nonionic contrast media combined with a premedication strategy, including steroids, is preliminary or not yet currently available. For high-risk patients (ie, previous contrast reactors), the combination of a pretreatment regimen with nonionic contrast media has empirical merit and may warrant consideration. Oral administration of steroids appears preferable to intravascular routes, and the drug may be prednisone or methylprednisolone. Supplemental administration of H_1 and H_2 antihistamine therapies, orally or intravenously, may reduce the frequency of urticaria, angioedema, and respiratory symptoms. Additionally, ephedrine administration has been suggested to decrease the frequency of contrast reactions, but caution is advised in patients with cardiac disease, hypertension, or hyperthyroidism. No premedication strategy should be a substitute for the ABC approach to preadministration preparedness listed above. Contrast reactions do occur despite any and all premedication prophylaxis. The incidence can be decreased, however, in some categories of "at risk" patients receiving high osmolar contrast media plus a medication regimen. For patients with previous contrast medium reactions, there is a slight chance that recurrence may be more severe or the same as the prior reaction; however, it is more likely that there will be no recurrence.

A General Premedication Regimen

Methylprednisolone	32 mg orally 12 and 2 hours prior to procedure
Diphenhydramine	50 mg orally 1 hour prior to the procedure

An Alternative Premedication Regimen

Prednisone	50 mg orally 13, 7, and 1 hour before the procedure
Diphenhydramine	50 mg orally 1 hour before the procedure
Ephedrine	25 mg orally 1 hour before the procedure (except when contraindicated)

Unlabeled Use (Nephroprotective)

N-acetylcysteine, P.O.	600 mg orally twice daily on the day before and the day of the scan in addition to hydration with 0.45% saline intravenously

Indications For Nonionic Contrast

Previous reaction to contrast – premedicate[1]
Known allergy to iodine or shellfish
Asthma, especially if on medication
Myocardial instability or CHF

Risk for aspiration or severe nausea and vomiting
Difficulty communicating or inability to give history
Patients taking beta-blockers
Small children at risk for electrolyte imbalance or extravasation
Renal failure with diabetes, sickle cell disease, or myeloma
At physician or patient request

[1]If life-threatening reactions (throat swelling, laryngeal edema, etc), consider omitting the intravenous contrast.

CONTROLLED SUBSTANCES: USES AND EFFECTS

Drugs (Trade or Other Names)	Medical Uses	Physical Dependence	Psychological Dependence	Tolerance	Duration (h)	Usual Method	Possible Effects	Effects of Overdose	Withdrawal Syndrome
Anabolic Steroids									
Testosterone (cypionate, enanthate) (C-V) (Depo®-Testosterone, Delatestryl®)	Hypogonadism	Unknown	Unknown	Unknown	14-28 d	Injected	Virilization, acne, testicular atrophy, gynecomastia, aggressive behavior, edema	Unknown	Possible depression
Nandrolone (decanoate, phenpropionate) (C-III) (Nortestosterone, Durabolin, Deca-Durabolin®, Deca)	Anemia, breast cancer	Unknown	Unknown	Unknown	14-21 d	Injected			
Oxymetholone (C-III) (Anadrol®-50)	Anemia	Unknown	Unknown	Unknown	24	Oral			
Cannabis									
Marijuana (C-I) (Pot, Acapulco gold, grass, reefer, sinsemilla, Thai sticks)	None	Unknown	Moderate	Yes	2-4	Smoked, oral	Euphoria, relaxed inhibitions, increased appetite, disorientation	Fatigue, paranoia, possible psychosis	Occasional reports of insomnia, hyperactivity, decreased appetite
Tetrahydrocannabinol (C-I, II) (THC, Marinol®)	Antinauseant	Unknown	Moderate	Yes	2-4	Smoked, oral			
Hashish and hashish oil (C-I) (Hash, hash oil)	None	Unknown	Moderate	Yes	2-4	Smoked, oral			
Depressants									
Chloral hydrate (C-IV) (Noctec, Somnos, Felsules)	Hypnotic	Moderate	Moderate	Yes	5-8	Oral	Slurred speech, disorientation, drunken behavior without odor of alcohol	Shallow respiration, clammy skin, dilated pupils, weak and rapid pulse, coma, possible death	Anxiety, insomnia, tremors, delirium, convulsions, possible death
Barbiturates (C-II, III, IV) (Amytal®, Fiorinal®, Nembutal®, Seconal™, Tuinal®, phenobarbital, pentobarbital)	Anesthetic, anticonvulsant, sedative, hypnotic, veterinary euthanasia agent	High-moderate	High-moderate	Yes	1-16	Oral, injected			
Benzodiazepines (C-IV) (Ativan®, Dalmane®, diazepam, Librium®, Xanax®, Serax®, Valium®, Tranxene®, Verstran, Versed®, Halcion®, Paxipam®, Restoril®)	Antianxiety, sedative, anticonvulsant, hypnotic	Low	Low	Yes	4-8	Oral, injected			
Glutethimide (C-II) (Doriden)	Sedative, hypnotic	High	Moderate	Yes	4-8	Oral			
Other depressants (C-I, II, III, IV) (Equanil®, Miltown®, Noludar, Placidyl®, Valmid, methaqualone)	Antianxiety, sedative, hypnotic	Moderate	Moderate	Yes	4-8	Oral			

(Continued)

Drugs (Trade or Other Names)	Medical Uses	Physical Dependence	Psychological Dependence	Tolerance	Duration (h)	Usual Method	Possible Effects	Effects of Overdose	Withdrawal Syndrome
Hallucinogens									
LSD (C-I) (Acid, microdot)	None	None	Unknown	Yes	8-12	Oral	Illusions and hallucinations, altered perception of time and distance	Longer, more intense "trip" episodes, psychosis, possible death	Unknown
Mescaline and peyote (C-I) (Mescal, buttons, cactus)	None	None	Unknown	Yes	8-12	Oral			
Amphetamine variants (C-I) (2,5-DMA, STP, MDA, MDMA, ecstasy, DOM, DOB)	None	Unknown	Unknown	Yes	Variable	Oral, injected			
Phencyclidine and analogs (C-I, II) (PCE, PCPy, TCP, PCP, hog, loveboat, angel dust)	None	Unknown	High	Yes	Days	Oral, smoked			
Other hallucinogens (C-I) (Bufotenine, ibogaine, DMT, DET, psilocybin, psilocyn)	None	None	Unknown	Possible	Variable	Smoked, oral, injected, sniffed			
Narcotics									
Heroin (C-I) (Diacetylmorphine, horse, smack)	None in U.S; analgesic, antitussive	High	High	Yes	3-6	Injected, sniffed, smoked	Euphoria, drowsiness, respiratory depression, constricted pupils, nausea	Slow and shallow breathing, clammy skin, convulsions, coma, possible death	Watery eyes, runny nose, yawning, lose of appetite, irritability, tremors, panic, cramps, nausea, chills and sweating
Morphine (C-II) (Duramorph®, MS-Contin®, Roxanol™, Oramorph SR™)	Analgesic	High	High	Yes	3-6	Oral, smoked, injected			
Codeine (C-II, III, V) (Tylenol® w/codeine, Empirin® w/codeine, Robitussin® A-C, Fiorinal® w/codeine, APAP w/codeine)	Analgesic, antitussive	Moderate	Moderate	Yes	3-6	Oral, injected			
Hydrocodone (C-II, III) (Tussionex®, Vicodin®, Hycodan®, Lorcet®)	Analgesic, antitussive	High	High	Yes	3-6	Oral			
Hydromorphone (C-II) (Dilaudid®)	Analgesic	High	High	Yes	3-6	Oral, injected			
Oxycodone (C-II) (Percodan®, Percocet®, Tylox®, Roxicet®, Roxicodone™)	Analgesic	High	High	Yes	4-5	Oral			
Methadone and LAAM (C-I, II) (Dolophine®, methadone, levo-alpha-acetylmethadol, levomethadyl acetate)	Analgesic, treatment of dependence	High	High	Yes	12-72	Oral, injected			

(Continued)

Drugs (Trade or Other Names)	Medical Uses	Physical Dependence	Psychological Dependence	Tolerance	Duration (h)	Usual Method	Possible Effects	Effects of Overdose	Withdrawal Syndrome
Fentanyl and analogs (C-I, II) (Innovar, Sublimaze®, Alfenta®, Sufenta®, Duragesic®)	Analgesic, adjunct to anesthesia, anesthetic	High	High	Yes	0.1-72	Injected, transdermal patch			
Other narcotics (C-II, III, IV, V) (Percodan®, Percocet®, Tylox®, opium, Darvon®, Talwin®,[1] buprenorphine, meperidine (pethidine), Demerol®)	Analgesic, antidiarrheal	High-low	High-low	Yes	Variable	Oral, injected			
Stimulants									
Cocaine[2] (C-II) (Coke, flake, snow, crack)	Local anesthetic	Possible	High	Yes	1-2	Sniffed, smoked, injected	Increased alertness, excitation, euphoria, increased pulse rate and blood pressure, insomnia, loss of appetite	Agitation, increased body temperature, hallucinations, convulsions, possible death	Apathy, long periods of sleep, irritability, depression, disorientation
Amphetamine/methamphetamine (C-II) (Biphetamine, Desoxyn®, Dexedrine®, Obetrol, ice)	Attention deficit disorder, narcolepsy, weight control	Possible	High	Yes	2-4	Oral, injected, smoked			
Methylphenidate (C-II) (Ritalin®)	Attention deficit disorder, narcolepsy	Possible	High	Yes	2-4	Oral, injected			
Other stimulants (C-I, II, III, IV) (Adipex®, Didrex®, Ionamin®, Melfiat®, Plegine, Captagon, Sanorex®, Tenuate®, Tepanil, Prelu-2®, Preludin)	Weight control	Possible	High	Yes	2-4	Oral, injected			

[1]Not designated a narcotic under the CSA.

[2]Designated a narcotic under the CSA.

Adapted from U.S. Department of Justice, Drug Enforcement Administration, *Drugs of Abuse*, 1996.

COPPER CONTENT OF HUMAN TISSUES AND BODY FLUIDS

Tissue	Mean Content (mcg/g dry weight)	
	Normal	Wilson's Disease
Adrenal	7.4	17.6
Aorta	6.7	—
Bone	4.2	—
Brain	—	—
Caudate nucleus	—	212
Cerebellum	—	261
Frontal lobe cortex	—	118
Globus pallidus	—	255
Putamen	—	314
Cornea	—	92.9
Erythrocytes (per 100 mL packed red blood cells)	23.1	—
Hair	89.1	—
Heart	16.5	12.7
Kidney	14.9	96.2
Leukocytes (per 109 cells)	0.9	—
Liver	25.5	584
Lung	9.5	15.5
Muscle	5.4	25.9
Nail	18.1	—
Ovary	8.1	5.2
Pancreas	7.4	4.2
Placenta	13.5	—
Prostate	6.5	—
Skin	2	5.2
Spleen	6.8	5.6
Stomach and intestines	12.6	22.9
Thymus	6.7	—
Thyroid	6.1	—
Uterus	8.4	—
Aqueous humor	12.4	—
Bile (common duct)	1050	173
Cerebrospinal fluid	27.8	—
Gastric juice	28.1	—
Pancreatic juice	28.4	—
Plasma, Wilson's disease		—
Saliva	50	—
Serum		
Female	120	—
Male	109	—
Newborn	36	—
Sweat		
Female	148	—

(Continued)		
Tissue	**Mean Content (mcg/g dry weight)**	
	Normal	**Wilson's Disease**
Male	55	—
Tissue		
Synovial fluid	21	—
Urine (24-hour)	18	—

Source: Georgopoulos, et al (2001); Scheinberg (1979); Sternlieb and Scheinberg (1977)

Adapted from: Agency for Toxic Substances and Disease Registry (ATSDR). 2002. Toxicological Profile for Copper (Draft for Public Comment). Atlanta, GA: U.S. Department of Health and Human Services, Public Health Service. Available at: http://www.atsdr.cdc.gov/toxprofiles/tp132.html.

COPPER CONTENT OF SELECTED FOODS

Food Description	mg/kg*	
	Mean	S.D.†
Fruit Juices		
Apple juice, bottled	0	0.1
Grape juice, bottled	0	0.1
Grapefruit juice, from frozen	0.3	0.1
Orange juice, from frozen	0.3	0.1
Pineapple juice, from frozen	0.4	0.1
Prune juice	0.1	0.1
Tomato juice, bottle	0.6	0.1
Dairy Products		
American, processed cheese		
Cheddar cheese	0.3	0.2
Chocolate milk, fluid	0.3	0.2
Cottage cheese, 4% milkfat	0	0
Cream cheese	0	0
Eggs, boiled/fried	0.6	0.1
Eggs, scrambled	0.5	0.1
Half & half	0	0
Lowfat (2%) milk, fluid	0	0
Skim milk	0	0
Sour cream	0	0
Swiss cheese	0.4	0.4
Whole milk	0	0
Milk, poultry, and seafood		
Beef chuck roast, baked	1.0	0.1
Beef steak, loin, pan-cooked	1.0	0.2
Bologna, sliced	0.4	0.2
Chicken breast, roasted	0.3	0.1
Chicken, fried (breast, leg)	0.7	0.1
Frankfurters, beef, boiled	0.4	0.1
Ground beef, pan-cooked	0.8	0.1
Haddock, pan-cooked	0.06	0.13
Ham, baked	0.6	0.2
Ham luncheon meat, sliced	0.5	0.1
Lamb chop, pan-cooked	1.4	0.2
Liver, beef, fried	123	57
Pork bacon, pan-cooked	1.2	0.4
Pork chop, pan-cooked	0.8	0.2
Pork roast	0.8	0.1
Pork sausage, pan-cooked	0.8	0.1
Quarter-pound hamburger	0.9	0.1
Salami, sliced	1.0	0.2
Salmon, steaks or filets, fresh	0.5	0.1
Shrimp, boiled	2.3	0.6

(*Continued*)

Food Description	mg/kg*	
	Mean	S.D.†
Tuna, canned in oil	0.5	0.1
Turkey breast, roasted	0.4	0.1
Veal cutlet, pan-cooked	1.0	0.3
Legumes, nuts, and nut products		
Kidney beans, dry, boiled	2.7	0.5
Mixed nuts, no peanuts, dry	15.5	2.6
Peanut butter, smooth	5.2	0.6
Peanuts, dry roasted	5.8	0.6
Pinto beans, dry, boiled	2.4	0.2
Pork and beans, canned	1.8	0.2
Fats, oils, condiments, snacks, and sweets		
Butter, regular (salted)	0	0
Corn chips	1.0	0.2
Fruit flavor sherbert	0	0.1
Gelatin dessert, any flavor	0	0
Honey	0	0
Jelly, any flavor	0	0.1
Margarine, stick, regular	0	0
Mayonnaise, regular, bottled	0	0
Olive/safflower oil	0	0
Popcorn, popped in oil	1.7	0.4
Potato chips	2.8	0.8
Pretzels, hard, salted, any	1.6	0.2
Vanilla ice cream	0.06	0.24
Whole sugar, ganulated	0	0
Beverages		
Coffee, from ground	0	0
Cola carbonated beverage	0	0
Tea, from tea bag	0	0
Breads		
Bagel, plain	1.3	0.2
Cracked wheat bread	1.8	0.2
English muffin, plain, toasted	1.3	0.1
Graham crackers	1.5	0.3
Rye bread	1.5	0.2
Saltine crackers	1.4	0.1
White bread	1.1	0.2
White roll	1.3	0.2
Whole wheat bread	2.3	0.3
Cereal, rice, and pasta		
Corn flakes	0.5	0.1
Crisped rice cereal	2.0	0.2

(*Continued*)

Food Description	mg/kg*	
	Mean	**S.D.†**
Egg noodles, boiled	1.0	0.2
Granola cereal	3.0	0.4
Macaroni, boiled	0.9	0.1
Oatmeal, quick (1-3 minutes)	0.7	0.1
Oatring cereal	3.3	0.4
Raisin bran cereal	4.4	0.4
Shredded wheat cereal	3.7	0.5
Wheat cereal, farina, quick	0.3	0.3
White rice, cooked	0.7	0.1
Vegetables		
Asparagus, fresh/frozen	1.0	0.2
Beets, fresh/frozen, boiled	0.7	0.2
Black olives	1.4	0.4
Broccoli, fresh/frozen, boiled	0.2	0.1
Brussels sprouts, fresh/frozen	0.4	0.1
Cabbage, fresh, boiled	0	0
Carrot, fresh, boiled	0.3	0.2
Cauliflower, fresh/frozen	0	0
Celery	0	0.1
Collards, fresh/frozen boiled	0.5	0.4
Corn, fresh/frozen, boiled	0.3	0.2
Cream style corn, canned	0.1	0.2
Cucumber, raw	0.2	0.2
Eggplant, fresh, boiled	0.5	0.2
Green beans, fresh/frozen	0.5	0.3
Green peas, fresh/frozen	1.0	0.2
Green pepper, raw	0.7	0.3
Iceberg lettuce, raw	0.2	0.2
Lima beans, immature, frozen	1.5	0.2
Mixed vegetables, frozen	0.6	0.2
Mushrooms, raw	2.4	0.6
Okra, resh/frozen, boiled	0.8	0.3
Onion, mature, raw	0.4	0.1
Peas, mature, dry, boiled	2.3	0.3
Spinach, fresh/frozen, boiled	0.8	0.3
Summer squash, fresh/frozen	0.5	0.1
Sweet potato, fresh, baked	1.4	0.4
Tomato, red, raw	0.5	0.2
Tomato sauce, plain, bottled	1.2	0.4
Tomato, stewed, canned	0.7	0.2
Turnip, fresh/frozen, boiled	0	0.1
White potato, baked with skin	1.0	0.4

(*Continued*)

Food Description	mg/kg*	
	Mean	S.D.†
White potato, boiled without	0.6	0.2
Winter squash, fresh/frozen		
Fruits		
Apple, red, raw	0.2	0.2
Applesauce, bottled	0.2	0.1
Apricot, raw	0.8	0.3
Avocado, raw	2.2	0.6
Banana, raw	1.1	0.2
Cantaloupe, raw	0.3	0.1
Fruit cocktail, canned in heavy	0.5	0.1
Grapefruit, raw	0.3	0.1
Grapes, red/green, seedless	1.1	0.6
Orange, raw	0.4	0.1
Peach, canned in light/medium	0.3	0.2
Peach, raw	0.7	0.2
Pear, canned in light syrup	0.4	0.1
Pear, raw	0.8	0.1
Pineapple, canned in juice	0.5	0.1
Plums, raw	0.6	0.1
Prunes, dried	2.9	0.3
Raisins, dried	3.3	0.4
Strawberries, raw	0.5	0.3
Watermelon, raw	00.4	0.1

*Data excerpted from the U.S. FDAT Total Diet Study on element results. Washington, D.C. (2001).

†S.D. = Standard Deviation

Adapted from Agency for Toxic Substances and Disease Registry (ATSDR). 2002. Toxicological Profile for Copper (Draft for Public Comment). Atlanta, GA: U.S. Department of Health and Human Services, Public Health Service. Available at: http://www.atsdr.cdc.gov/toxprofiles/tp132.html.

CORTICOSTEROIDS

							Half-life	
Glucocorticoid	Pregnancy Category	Approximate Equivalent Dose (mg)	Routes of Administration	Relative Anti-inflammatory Potency	Relative Mineralocorti-coid Potency	Protein Binding (%)	Plasma (min)	Biologic (h)
Short-Acting								
Cortisone	D	25	P.O., I.M.	0.8	2	90	30	8-12
Hydrocortisone	C	20	I.M., I.V.	1	2	90	80-118	8-12
Intermediate-Acting								
Methylpredni-solone[1]	—	4	P.O., I.M., I.V.	5	0	—	78-188	18-36
Prednisolone	B	5	P.O., I.M., I.V., intra-articular, intradermal, soft tissue injection	4	1	90-95	115-212	18-36
Prednisone	B	5	P.O.	4	1	70	60	18-36
Triamcinolone[1]	C	4	P.O., I.M., intra-articular, intradermal, in-trasynovial, soft tissue injection	5	0	—	200+	18-36
Long-Acting								
Betamethasone	C	0.6-0.75	P.O., I.M., intra-articular, intradermal, in-trasynovial, soft tissue injection	25	0	64	300+	36-54
Dexametha-sone	C	0.75	P.O., I.M., I.V., intra-articular, intradermal, soft tissue injection	25-30	0	—	110-210	36-54
Mineralocorticoids								
Fludrocortisone	C	—	P.O.	10	125	42	210+	18-36

[1]May contain propylene glycol as an excipient in injectable forms.

Guidelines For Selection and Use of Topical Corticosteroids

The quantity prescribed and the frequency of refills should be monitored to reduce the risk of adrenal suppression. In general, short courses of high-potency agents are preferable to prolonged use of low potency. After control is achieved, control should be maintained with a low-potency preparation.

Low-to-medium potency agents are usually effective for treating thin, acute, inflammatory skin lesions, whereas high or super-potent agents are often required for treating chronic, hyperkeratotic, or lichenified lesions.

Since the stratum corneum is thin on the face and intertriginous areas, low-potency agents are preferred but a higher potency agent may be used for 2 weeks.

Because the palms and soles have a thick stratum corneum, high or super-potent agents are frequently required.

Low-potency agents are preferred for infants and the elderly. Infants have a high body surface area to weight ratio; elderly patients have thin, fragile skin.

The vehicle in which the topical corticosteroid is formulated influences the absorption and potency of the drug. Ointment bases are preferred for thick, lichenified lesions; they enhance penetration of the drug. Creams are preferred for acute and subacute dermatoses; they may be used on moist skin areas or intertriginous areas. Solutions, gels, and sprays are preferred for the scalp or for areas where a nonoil-based vehicle is needed.

In general, super-potent agents should not be used for longer than 2-3 weeks unless the lesion is limited to a small body area. Medium-to-high potency agents usually cause only rare adverse effects when treatment is limited to 3 months or less and use on the face and intertriginous areas are avoided. If long-term treatment is needed, intermittent vs continued treatment is recommended.

Most preparations are applied once or twice daily. More frequent application may be necessary for the palms or soles because the preparation is easily removed by normal activity and penetration is poor due to a thick stratum corneum. Every-other-day or weekend-only application may be effective for treating some chronic conditions.

Corticosteroids, Topical		
Steroid		**Vehicle**
Very High Potency		
0.05%	Betamethasone dipropionate, augmented	Lotion, ointment
0.05%	Clobetasol propionate	Cream, foam, gel, lotion, ointment, shampoo, spray
0.05%	Diflorasone diacetate	Ointment
0.05%	Halobetasol propionate	Cream, ointment
High Potency		
0.1%	Amcinonide	Cream, ointment, lotion
0.05%	Betamethasone dipropionate, augmented	Cream
0.05%	Betamethasone dipropionate	Cream, ointment
0.1%	Betamethasone valerate	Ointment
0.05%	Desoximetasone	Gel
0.25%	Desoximetasone	Cream, ointment
0.05%	Diflorasone diacetate	Cream, ointment
0.05%	Fluocinonide	Cream, ointment, gel
0.1%	Halcinonide	Cream, ointment
0.5%	Triamcinolone acetonide	Cream
Intermediate Potency		
0.05%	Betamethasone dipropionate	Lotion
0.1%	Betamethasone valerate	Cream
0.1%	Clocortolone pivalate	Cream
0.05%	Desoximetasone	Cream
0.025%	Fluocinolone acetonide	Cream, ointment
0.05%	Flurandrenolide	Cream, ointment, lotion, tape
0.005%	Fluticasone propionate	Ointment
0.05%	Fluticasone propionate	Cream
0.1%	Hydrocortisone butyrate[1]	Ointment, solution
0.2%	Hydrocortisone valerate[1]	Cream, ointment
0.1%	Mometasone furoate[1]	Cream, ointment, lotion
0.1%	Prednicarbate	Cream, ointment
0.025%	Triamcinolone acetonide	Cream, ointment, lotion
0.1%	Triamcinolone acetonide	Cream, ointment, lotion
Low Potency		
0.05%	Alclometasone dipropionate[1]	Cream, ointment
0.05%	Desonide	Cream
0.01%	Fluocinolone acetonide	Cream, solution
0.5%	Hydrocortisone[1]	Cream, ointment, lotion

Corticosteroids, Topical (*Continued*)

Steroid		Vehicle
0.5%	Hydrocortisone acetate[1]	Cream, ointment
1%	Hydrocortisone acetate[1]	Cream, ointment
1%	Hydrocortisone[1]	Cream, ointment, lotion, solution
2.5%	Hydrocortisone[1]	Cream, ointment, lotion

[1]Not fluorinated.

DISCOLORATION OF FECES DUE TO TOXINS

Black

Acetazolamide
Aconitine
Alcohols
Alkalies
Aluminum hydroxide
Aminophylline
Aminopyrine
Aminosalicylic acid
Amphetamine
Amphotericin
Amyl alcohol
Anticoagulants
Arsenic
Aspirin
Barium
Benzene
Betamethasone
Bismuth
Bismuth sodium thioglycollate
Blackberries
Boric acid
Bromides
Carmine
Charcoal
Chloramphenicol
Chlorophenothane
Chlorpropamide
Chocolate
Cinchophen
Clindamycin
Copper
Corticosteroids
Cortisone
Cyclophosphamide
Cytarabine
Dicumarol
Digitalis
Dipyrone
Dithiazanine iodine
Ethacrynic acid
Fenoprofen
Ferrous salts
Floxuridine
Fluorides
Fluorouracil
Fluroxene
Formaldehyde
Halothane

Heparin
Hetacilline
Histamine
Huckleberries
Hydralazine
Hydrocortisone
Hypochlorites
Ibufenac
Ibuprofen
Indomethacin
Iodine drugs
Iron salts
Isopropanol
Lead
Levarterenol
Levodopa
Lincomycin
Lipomul
Manganese
Mefenamic acid
Melphalan
Mercury
Methylprednisolone
Methotrexate
Methylene blue
Nitrates
Novobiocin
Oxalate
Oxyphenbutazone
Paraldehyde
Paramethadione
Paramethasone
Phenacetin
Phenolphthalein
Phenylbutazone
Phenylephrine
Phosphorous
Potassium salts
Prednisolone
Procarbazine
Pyrazolones
Pyrvinium
Reserpine
Salicylates
Silver
Sulfonamides
Sulthiame
Tetracycline
Thallium

Theophylline
Thioglycollamate
Thiotepa
Triamcinolone
Trimethadione
Warfarin

Blue

Boric acid (ingested)
Chloramphenicol
Diathiazine
Manganese dioxide
Methylene blue

Blue-Green

Boric acid

Clay/Putty

Barium
Carbon tetrachloride
Cocoa
Kerosene

Dark Brown

Cocoa
Dexamethasone
Manganese dioxide
Mercurous chloride

Gray

Cocoa
Colchicine
Dithiazanine

Green

Beets
Dithiazanine iodine
Indocyanine green
Indomethacin
Iron
Medroxyprogesterone
Mercurous chloride
Spinach

Greenish Gray

Oral antibiotics
Oxyphenbutazone
Phenylbutazone

Light Brown

Anticoagulants
Milk

Orange-Red

Phenazopyridine
Pyrivinium
Rifampin

Pink

Anticoagulants
Aspirin
Heparin
Manganese dioxide
Oxyphenbutazone
Phenylbutazone
Salicylates

Red

Anticoagulants
Aspirin
Barium
Beets
Blackberries
Carmine
Cocoa
Hematoxylin
Heparin

Hydroxocobalamin
Lead
Oxyphenbutazone
Phenolphthalein
Phenylbutazone
Pyrvinium pamoate
Salicylates
Sulfobromopthalein
Tetracycline syrup
Tomatoes (undigested)

Red-Brown

Clofazimine palmitate
Hematoxylin
Oxyphenbutazone
Phenylbutazone
Rifampin

Tan

Mercury

Tarry

Ergot preparations
Ibuprofen

Salicylates
Warfarin

White/Speckling

Aluminum hydroxide
Antibiotics (oral)
Barium
Indocyanine green

Yellow

Acetanilid
Mercurous chloride
Milk
Rhubarb
Santonin
Senna

Yellow-Green

1,8-Dihydroxyanthraquinone
Gold
Mercurous chloride
Rhubarb
Santonin
Senna

Adapted from Drugdex® — Drug Consults, Micromedex, vol 109, Denver, CO: Rocky Mountain Drug Consultation Center, August, 2001, and Knoben JE and Anderson PO, *Handbook of Clinical Drug Data*, 7th ed, Hamilton, IL: Drug Intelligence Publication, 1993, 22.

DISCOLORATION OF URINE DUE TO TOXINS

Amber

Trinitrotoluene

Black

Cascara
Co-trimoxazole
Cresols
Fava bean
Ferrous salts
Hydroquinone
Iron dextran
Levodopa
Methocarbamol
Methyldopa
Naphthalene
Pamaquine
Phenacetin
Phenols
Pyrogallol
Quinine
Rhubarb
Sulfonamides
Thymol

Blue

Anthraquinone
Arbutin
Azuresin
Carbolic acid
DeWitt's pills
Dithiazanine iodide
Evans blue
Indigo blue
Indigo carmine
Methocarbamol
Methylene blue
Mitoxantrone
Nitrofurans
Resorcinol
Tetrahydronaphthalene
Thymol
Tolonium
Triamterene (pale)

Blue-Green

Amitriptyline
Anthraquinone
Arbutin
Azuresin
Blutene

Boric acid
Carbolic acid
DeWitt's pills
Dithiazanine iodide
Doan's® pills
Indigo blue
Indigo carmine
Magnesium salicylate
Methylene blue
Propofol
Resorcinol
Tetrahydronaphthalene
Thymol
Tolonium

Brown

Aminopyrine
Aniline
Anthraquinone dyes
Cascara
Chloroquine
Cinchophen
Cresols
Danthron
Dipyrone
Eosin dyes
Furazolidone
Furoxone®
Hydroquinone
Levodopa
Methocarbamol
Methyldopa
Metronidazole
Naphthalene
Nitrofurans
Nitrofurantoin
Pamaquin
Phenacetin
Phenols
Phenylhydrazine
Primaquine
Pyrogallol
Quinine
Rifabutin
Rifampin
Rhubarb
Riboflavin
Senna
Sodium diatrizoate
Sulfonamides

Tannins
Thymol

Brown-Black

Erythrityl tetranitrate
Isosorbide mono/dinitrate
Methocabomol
Methyldopa
Metronidazole
Nitrates
Nitrofuran
Phenacetin
Povidone iodine
Quinine
Senna

Brown-Green

Hydroquinone

Dark

p-Aminosalicylic acid
Analine
Cadmium
Cascara
Chlorobenzenes
Chloronaphthalene
Dacium
Ferrous salts
Furazolidone
Furoxone®
Hydroquinone
Iron sorbitex
Levodopa
Metronidazole
Naphthol
Nitridazol
Nitrites
Nitrobenzene
Para-aminosalicylic acid
Phenacetin
Phenol
Phenyl salicylate
Primaquine
Propofol
Pyrogallol
Quinine
Resorcinol
Rhubarb
Riboflavin
Senna

Thymol
Trinitrophenol
Trinitrotoluene

Fluorescent

Acriflavine (green)
Ethylene glycol
Merbromin (pink)
Triamterene (pale blue)

Green

Acriflavine
Amitriptyline
Anthraquinone
Antipyrine
Arbutin
Azuresin
Bromeform
Carbolic acid
Creosote
DeWitt's pills
Guaiacol
Hydroquinone
Indigo blue
Indigo carmine
Indomethacin
Methocarbamol
Methylene blue
Mitoxantrone
Nitrofurans
Phenols
Phenyl salicylate
Pyrogallo
Propofol
Resorcinol
Santonin
Suprofen
Tetrahydronaphthalene
Thymol

Green-Yellow

Bromoform
DeWitt's pills
Methylene blue

Milky

Chloroguanide
Phosphates
Urates

Orange

Anisindione
Canthaxanthines

Chlorzoxazone
Chrysophanic acid
Dihydroergotamine mesylate
Diphenadione
Entacapone
Ethoxazene
Heparin sodium
Monnose
Paprika
Phenazopyridine
Phenindione
Rifabutin
Rifampin
Rhubarb
Riboflavin
Salicylazosulfapyridine
Sulfasalazine
Warfarin

Orange-Brown

Furazolidone
Ethoxazene

Orange-Red

Anisindione
Chlorzoxazone
Doxidan with PSP
Ethoxazene
Phenazopyridine
Phenindione
Rifampin
Warfarin

Orange-Yellow

Fluorescein sodium
Riboflavin
Rifampin
Sulfasalazine

Pale

Chlorosis

Pink

Aminopyrine
Anisindione
Anthraquinone dyes
Aspirin
Benorilate
Cascara
Chrysophanic acid
Cinchophen
Danthron
Deferoxamine

1,8-Dihydroxyanthraquinone
Dipyrone
Emodin
Eosin dyes
Ethoxazine
Merbromin
Methyldopa
Phenazopyridone
Phenindione
Phenolphthalein
Phenothiazines
Phensuximide
Phenytoin
Porphyrins
Salicylates
Santonin
Senna
Serenium
Thiazolsulfone
Urates

Purple

Phenophthalein

Red

Acetanilid
Aminopyrine
Aniline
Anthraquinone
Antipyrine
Beets
Blackberries
Blood
Cardiografin
Cascara
Chlorpromazine
Chrysarobin
Chrysophanic acid
Cinchophen
Danthson
Daunorubicin
Deferoxamine mesylate
Dihydroergotamine mesylate
1,8-Dihydroxyanthraquinone
Dimethyl sulfoxide
Dipyrone
DMSO
Doxorubicin
Emodin
Eosin dyes
Ethoxazene
Fava bean

Fuscin
Heparin
Ibuprofen
Idarubicin
Logwood
Methyldopa
Naphthalene
Oxamniquine
Oxyphenbutazone
Phenacetin
Phenazopyridine
Phenolphthalein
Phenothiazines
Phensuximide
Phenylbutazone
Phenytoin
Porphyphenazone
Rhodamine
Riboflavin
Rifampin
Santonin
Senna
Selenium
Sulfonal
Thiazolsulfone
Tolcapone
Trinitrotoluene
Trional
Urates
Uroerythrin

Red-Brown

Aloin
Aminopyrine
Anisindione
Antipyrine
Beets
Benzene
Carbon tetrachloride
Cascara
Chrysarobin
Chrysophanic acid
Clofazimine palmitate
Danthron
Deferoxamine
1,8-Dihydroxyanthraquinone
Dinitrophenol
Dipyrone
Emodin
Fava bean

Lead
Mercury
Methyldopa
Oxyphenbutazone
Pamaquine
Phenacetin
Phenazopyridine
Phenolphthalein
Phenothiazines
Phensuximide
Phenylbutazone
Phenytoin
Picric acid
Propaphenazone
Quinine
Rhubarb
Santonin
Senna
Urates

Red-Purple

Chlorzoxazone
Ibuprofen
Methemoglobin
Phenacetin
Phenol sulfonphtaleine
Senna

Red-Yellow

Urates

Rust

Acetanilid
Acriflavine
Aloin
Bromoform
Carrots
Cascara
Chloroquine
Furazolidone
Furoxone®
Metronidazole
Nitrofurantoin
Pamaquine
Phenacetin
Picric acid
Pyrogallol
Quinacrine
Rhubarb
Riboflavin
Santonin

Senna
Sulfonal
Sulfonamides
Trinitrophenol
Trional
Urates

Yellow

Acetanilid
Acriflavine
5-Aminoacridine
Bromoform
Carrots
Nitrofurantoin
Phenacetin
Picric acid
Pyrogallol
Quinacrine
Riboflavin
Santonin
Sulfasalazine
Sulfonal
Trinitrophenol
Trional

Yellow, Bright

Flavine

Yellow-Brown

Aloin
Aminosalicylate acid
Cascara
Chloroquine
DeWitt's pills
Flurazolidone
Methylene blue
Metronidazole
Nitrofurantoin
Pamaquine
Primaquine
Quinacrine
Rhubarb
Senna
Sulfonamides

Yellow-Pink

Aloin
Cascara
Rhubarb
Senna
Urates

Changes color in contact with hypochlorite: methyldopa (black or red), levodopa (dark), aminosalicylic acid (red).

Adapted from Drugdex® — Drug Consults, Micromedex, vol 109, Rocky Mountain Drug Consultation Center, Denver, CO: August, 2001; and Knoben JE and Anderson PO, *Handbook of Clinical Drug Data*, 7th ed, Hamilton, IL: Drug Intelligence Publication, 1993, 23-4.

DONOR VICTIMS OF POISONING IN WHOM TRANSPLANTATION OF ORGANS OCCURRED

Toxin	Organs Transplanted
Acetaminophen	Heart, cornea, kidney, pancreas (islet cells)
Barbiturate	Liver, heart, kidney
Benzodiazepines	Kidney, heart, liver
Brodifacoum	Kidney, liver, heart
Carbamazepine	Heart
Carbon monoxide	Heart, liver, kidney, lung, pancreas
Cocaine	Kidney, liver
Cyanide	Corneal, skin, bone, heart, liver, kidney, pancreas
Digitalis	Heart
Ethanol	Heart, kidney
Hemlock (*Conium maculatum*)	Liver, kidney, pancreas
Insulin	Kidney, heart, pancreas (islet cells)
Lead	Liver
Malathion	Kidney, liver
Methanol	Kidney, liver, heart, lung
Methaqualone	Liver
2,3 methylenedioxymethamphetamine (Ecstasy)	Heart, lung, kidney, liver, pancreas
Tricyclic antidepressants	Kidney, liver
Venlafaxine	Heart

Guidelines Published for Optimal Time to Transplant From Poisoned Organ Donor for Certain Selected Toxins	
Toxin	**Optimal Time for Transplant**
Ethylene glycol Methanol	Acidosis corrected; serum level < 0.5 g/L
Cyanide	Shock corrected; serum level < 8 µmol/L

References

Bentley MJ, Mullen JC, Lopushinsky, SR, et al, "Successful Cardiac Transplantation with Methanol or Carbon Monoxide-Poisoned Donors," *Ann Thorac Surg,*, 2001, 71(4):1194-7.

Caballero F, Lopez-Naviada A, Gomex M, et al, "Successful Transplantation of Organs from a Donor Who Died from Acute Cocaine Intoxication," *Clin Transplant*, 2003, 17(2):89-92.

Dribben W, Capiello H, and Kirk M, "Successful Organ Procurement and Transplantation from a Victim of Malathion Poisoning," *J Toxicol Clin Toxicol*, 1999, 37(5):665.

Dribben WH and Kirk MA, "Organ Procurement and Successful Transplantation After Malathion Poisoning," *J Toxicol Clin Toxicol*, 2001, 39(6):633-6.

Foster PF, McFadden R, Trevino R, et al, "Successful Transplantation of Donor Organs from a Hemlock Poisoning Victim," *Transplantation*, 2003, 76(5):874-6.

Hantson P, "Organ Procurement After Poisoning," *Presse Med*, 2004, 33(13):871-80.

Hantson P, Mahieu P, Hassoun A, et al, "Outcome Following Organ Removal from Poisoned Donors in Brain Death Status: A Report of 12 Cases and Review of Literature," *J Toxicol Clin Toxicol*, 1995, 33(6):709-12.

Hantson P, Vekemans MC, Laterre PF, et al, "Heart Donation After Fatal Acetaminophen Poisoning," *J Toxicol Clin Toxicol*, 1997, 35(3):325-6.

Leikin JB, Heyn-Lamb R, Aks S, et al, "The Toxic Patient as a Potential Organ Donor," *Am J Emerg Med*, 1994, 12:151-4.

Lopez-Navidad A, Caballero F, Gonzalez-Segura C, et al, "Short- and Long-Term Success of Organs Tranplanted from Acute Methanol Poisoned Donors," *Clin Transplant*, 2002, 16(3):151-62.

Luckraz H, Tsui SS, Parameshwar J, et al, "Improved Outcome with Organs from Carbon Monoxide Poisoned Donors for Intrathoracic Transplantation," *Ann Thorac Surg*, 2001, 72(3):709-13.

Mueller PD and Prairie LD, "Recipient Graft Survival After Organ Donation by Poisoned Victims," *Vet Hum Toxicol*, 1994, 36:365.

Roberts JR, Bain M, Klachko MN, et al, "Successful Heart Transplantation from a Victim of Carbon Monoxide Poisoning," *Ann Emerg Med*, 1995, 26:652-5.

Seifert S, Holstege CP, Furbee RB, et al, "Organ Procurement After Brodifacoum Poisoning," *J Toxicol Clin Toxicol*, 1998, 36(5):463-4.

Tenderich G, Dagge A, Schulz U, et al, "Successful Use of Cardiac Allograft from Serotonin Antagonist Intoxication," *Transplantation*, 2001, 72(3):529.

Wood DM, Dargan PI, and Jones AL, "Poisoned Patients as Potential Organ Donors: Postal Survey of Transplant Centres and Intensive Care Units," *Crit Care*, 2003, 7(2):147-54.

DRUGS THAT CAUSE XEROSTOMIA

>10%	1% to 10%	Undocumented Incidence
Acitretin	Acrivastine and pseudoephedrine	Angel's trumpet
Adinazolam	Albuterol	Barium
Alizapride	Alfuzosin	Black henbane
Alprazolam	Amantadine hydrochloride	Box thorn
Amitriptyline hydrochloride	Ambroxol	Cestrum nocturnum
Amoxapine	Amphetamine sulfate	Chloroform
Anisotropine methylbromide	Angel's trumpet	*Clostridium botulinum* food poisoning
Atropine sulfate	Astemizole	*Datura fastuosa*
Belladonna and opium	Barium	*Datura innoxia* mill
Benztropine mesylate	Beclomethasone dipropionate	*Datura metel* L.
Botulinum A toxin	Bepridil hydrochloride	Deadly nightshade
Bupropion	Bitolterol mesylate	Delphinium
Chlordiazepoxide	Black henbane	Jimson weed
Clidinium bromide	Box thorn	*Lantana camera*
Citalopram	Bromfenac	*Lycium halimifolium*
Clomipramine hydrochloride	Brompheniramine maleate	Monkshood
Clonazepam	Budesonide	Mushrooms (Group V)
Clonidine	Buspirone	*Solandra* species of plants
Clorazepate dipotassium	Carbinoxamine and pseudoephedrine	Thallium
Clovoxamine	Cestrum nocturnum	Vanadium
Cyclobenzaprine	Chloroform	
Desipramine hydrochloride	Chlorpheniramine maleate	
Dexfenfluramine	Cifenline	
Dexmedetomidine	Clemastine fumarate	
Diazepam	*Clostridium botulinum* food poisoning	
Dicyclomine hydrochloride	Clozapine	
Diethylpropion	Cromolyn sodium	
Diphenoxylate and atropine	Cyproheptadine hydrochloride	
Doxepin hydrochloride	*Datura fastuosa*	
Ergotamine	*Datura innoxia* mill	
Estazolam	*Datura metel* L.	
Fenoldopam	Deadly nightshade	
Fentanyl	Delphinium	
Flavoxate	Dexchlorpheniramine maleate	
Fluoxetine	Dextroamphetamine sulfate	
Flurazepam hydrochloride	Didanosine	
Glycopyrrolate	Dimenhydrinate	
Guanabenz acetate	Diphenhydramine hydrochloride	
Guanfacine hydrochloride	Disopyramide phosphate	
Hyoscine N-butylbromide	Doxazosin	
Hyoscyamine sulfate	Dronabinol	
Imipramine	Ephedrine sulfate	
Interferon alfa-2a	Etretinate	
Interferon alfa-2b	Flumazenil	

(*Continued*)

>10%	1% to 10%	Undocumented Incidence
Interferon alfa-N3	Fluvoxamine	
Ipratropium bromide	Formoterol	
Isoproterenol	Gabapentin	
Isotretinoin	Ganciclovir	
Ketobemidone	Guaifenesin and codeine	
Lofepramine	Guanadrel sulfate	
Loratadine	Guanethidine sulfate	
Lorazepam	Halazepam	
Loxapine	Hydroxyzine	
Maprotiline hydrochloride	Hyoscyamine, atropine, scopolamine, and phenobarbital	
Methscopolamine bromide	Isoetharine	
Mirtazapine	Isoniazide	
Molindone hydrochloride	Jimson weed	
Moxonidine	Ketorolac	
Nabilone	*Lantana camera*	
Nefazodone	Levocabastine hydrochloride	
Nomifensine	Levodopa	
Oxybutynin chloride	Levodopa and carbidopa	
Oxazepam	Levorphanol tartrate	
Paroxetine	Lofexidine	
Phenelzine sulfate	Loratadine	
Pirenzepine	*Lycium halimifolium*	
Pirmenol	Meclizine hydrochloride	
Pizotifen hydrogen maleate	Meperidine hydrochloride	
Prochlorperazine	Methadone hydrochloride	
Propafenone hydrochloride	Methamphetamine hydrochloride	
Protriptyline hydrochloride	Methyldopa	
Quazepam	Metoclopramide	
Remoxipride	Mexiletine	
Reserpine	Monkshood	
Scopolamine (transdermal)	Morphine sulfate	
Selegiline hydrochloride	Mushrooms (Group V)	
Temazepam	Nabumetone	
Terodiline	Nisoldipine	
Tetrahydrocannabinols	Nortriptyline hydrochloride	
Thiethylperazine maleate	Ondansetron	
Thioridazine	Oxycodone and acetaminophen	
Tizanidine	Oxycodone and aspirin	
Tramadol	Penbutolol	
Trazodone	Pentazocine	
Trihexyphenidyl hydrochloride	Phenylpropanolamine hydrochloride	
Trimipramine maleate	Pirbuterol	
Tripelennamine	Pizotyline	

(Continued)		
>10%	1% to 10%	Undocumented Incidence
Trospium (I.V. doses >1 mg)	Prazosin hydrochloride	
Venlafaxine	Promethazine hydrochloride	
Zotepine	Propoxyphene	
Zuclopenthixol	Pseudoephedrine	
	Quazepam	
	Rimantadine	
	Risperidone	
	Ritonavir	
	Sertraline hydrochloride	
	Solandra species of plants	
	Terazosin	
	Terbutaline sulfate	
	Terfenadine	
	Thallium	
	Vanadium	

DRUGS USED IN ADDICTION TREATMENT

Bupropion SR	Smoking cessation:
(Zyban®)	Initiate at 150 mg every morning for 3 days.
	If tolerated, increase to 150 mg twice daily on day 4 of dosing. Should be an interval of at least 8 hours between successive doses. Target quit date after at least 1 week of treatment. Trial may be up to 12 weeks. Contraindicated in patients with seizures, anorexia, or bulimia.
Clonidine	Alcohol, nicotine, opioid withdrawal:
(Catapres®)	Initiate 0.1 mg 2-3times/day; transdermal patch: 0.2 mg, patch change weekly for 3-10 weeks
Disulfiram	Sobriety:
(Antabuse®)	125-500 mg/day; patients must be free of alcohol for at least 12 hours prior to initiation. Contraindicated with metronidazole and alcohol (including cough syrups).
Doxepin	Smoking cessation:
(Adapin® or Sinequan®)	50 mg daily for 3 days
	100 mg daily for days 4-6
	150 mg daily for days 7-21
Levomethadyl	Narcotic dependence:
(ORLAAM®)	Initiate at 20-40 mg 3 times/week
Methadone	Narcotic dependence:
(Dolophine®)	15-60 mg every 6-8 hours; can only be initiated in approved treatment programs
Naltrexone	Alcohol and narcotic dependence:
(ReVia®)	Initiate 25-50 mg/day; patientshould be free of opioid for 7-10 days prior to initiation
Nicotine gum	Smoking cessation:
	1-2 pieces/hour; maximum: 30 pieces/day (2 mg/piece). If high tobacco use, give DS (4 mg/piece); maximum: 20/day
Nicotine nasal spray	Smoking cessation:
	1 spray in each nostril (0.5 mg per inhalation) once or twice per hour; maximum: 80 sprays
Nicotine patches	Smoking cessation:
	One patch daily (7-22 mg) for 8 weeks; initiate patch on the quit date
Nortriptyline tablets	Smoking cessation: Maximum dose of 75-100 mg daily; treat for 8-12 weeks
(Aventyl® or Pamelor®)	

Drugs/Toxins Sexually Transmitted

Transmission via Reproductive Fluids	Intimate Contact Transmission
Cephalosproins	Ambrette
Ciguatera	Benzethonium chloride
Penicillins	Benzoyl peroxide
Steroids	Clotrimazole
Sulfas (men)	Nickel
	Nitrates
	Nitrofuratel
	Penicillamine

(*Continued*)	
Transmission via Reproductive Fluids	**Intimate Contact Transmission**
	Peru balsam
	Poison oak
	Propylene glycol
	Sulfas (men & women)
	Thioridazine

DRUGS/TOXINS THAT CAN RESULT IN COMA

Drug/Toxin	Serum Level Conventional Units
Acebutolol	20 mg/L
Acetaminophen	300 mcg/mL
Acetone	500 mg/L
Amitriptyline	2 mg/L
Amobarbital	43 mg/L
Baclofen	1 mg/L
Barbital	160 mg/L
Bromides	2000 mcg/mL
Butabarbital	39 mg/L
Caffeine	100 mg/L
Carbamazepine	18 mg/L
Carboxyhemoglobin	30%
Carisoprodol	30 mg/L
Cetrizine	2 mg/L
Chloral hydrate (trichloroethanol)	20 mg/L
Chloralose	3 mg/L
Chlordiazepoxide	20 mg/L
Chlormethiazole	7 mg/L
Chlormezanone	60 mg/L
Chloroquine	1 mg/L
Chlorpromazine	0.5 mg/L
Chlorprothixene	0.8 mg/L
Cimetidine	10 mg/L
Clonazepam	0.07 mg/L
Clonidine	2 mcg/L
Clozapine	2 mg/L
Codeine	5 mg/L
Diazepam	20 mg/L
Diethyltoluamide (DEET)	50 mg/L
Digoxin	4 ng/L
Dothiepin	1 mg/L
Doxepin	0.4 mg/L
Ethanol	300 mg/dL
Ethchlorvynol	50 mg/L
Ethylene glycol	50 mg/dL
Gamma-hydroxybutyrate	100 mg/L
Glutethimide	10 mg/L
Iron	500 mcg/dL
Isoniazid	20 mg/L
Lead	100 mcg/dL
Levetiracetam	400 mcg/mL
Lidocaine	5 mcg/mL
Lithium	3 mEq/L

Drug/Toxin	Serum Level Conventional Units
(Continued)	
Lorazepam	0.3 mg/L
Loxapine	0.7 mg/L
Meprobamate	60 mg/L
Mephobarbital	40 mg/L
Methanol	100 mg/dL
Methaqualone	8 mg/L
Methemoglobin	20%
Methyprylon	50 mg/L
Nomifensine	10 mg/L
Olanzapine	100 mcg/L
Orphenadrine	3 mg/L
Phenobarbital	65 mg/L
Phenytoin	40 mg/L
Propoxyphene	1 mg/L
Quetiapine	13 mg/L
Quinine	12 mcg/mL
Salicylates	100 mg/dL
Secobarbital	7 mg/L
Theophylline	40 mg/L
Tetrahydrocannabinol	180 mcg/L
Toluene	10 mg/L
Tramadol	2000 mcg/L
Tranylcypromine	1 mg/L
Triazolam	31 mcg/L
Valproic acid	500 mg/L
Venlafaxine	6 mg/L
Zopiclone	300 μL

EMERGENCY DRUG DOSAGES, ADULT

Drug and Strength	Recommended I.V. Doses	Comments and Preparation for Infusion
Adenosine 3 mg/mL	Adult: 6 mg bolus I.V. followed by 12 mg	May repeat the 12 mg dose
Aminophylline 500 mg/20 mL	Load 5.6 mg/kg then infusion at 0.4-0.8 mg/kg/h IBW or less based upon patient status	Give ½ loading dose if previous theophylline on board and no signs of toxicity. Give load slowly in 50-100 mL over 30-60 minutes. Max rate 25 mg/min. Can antagonize adenosine
Amiodarone	Supraventricular tachycardia: 2.5-5 mg/kg (over 3-5 minutes) Ventricular arrhythmia: 150 mg over 10 minutes; then 360 mg over 6 hours followed by 540 mg over next 18 hours	Maintenance infusion after first 24 hours: 0.5 mg/minute; boluses of 150 mg over 10 minutes may be given for breakthrough episodes
Atropine 1 mg/10 mL 1 mg/1 mL	0.5 mg increments I.V. push up to 2 mg max. May give ET	Initial slowing of rate with small doses (<0.4 mg)
Bretylium 500 mg/10 mL	For resistant ventricular fibrillation or ventricular tachycardia 5 mg/kg I.V. push. If ineffective in 10 minutes and after 1 or more DC shocks, give 10 mg/kg. May repeat to maximum of 30 mg/kg total. If effective begin drip at 1-2 mg/min	Rapid I.V. infusion may cause nausea and vomiting. May cause transient HTN, PVCs, or other arrhythmia. Hypotension is most frequent side effect. May accumulate in renal failure. Not recommended in digitalis toxicity. Initial response may take up to 60 minutes in ventricular tachycardia. Infusion: mix 1 g/500 mL = 2 mg/mL
Calcium salts Ca chloride 5 mL = 7 mEq (1.3 mEq/mL) Ca gluconate 10 mL = 5 mEq (0.5 mEq/mL)	0.5-1 g I.V.	May repeat every 10 minutes. Give cautiously in digitalis toxicity. Inactivated by blood products. Precipitates with sodium bicarbonate. Current ACLS guidelines do not recommend routine administration
Dexamethasone 20 mg/5 mL	Variable Cerebral edema: 10 mg I.V. initially	I.V. push over 30 seconds
Dextrose 25 g/50 mL	50 mL I.V. push for hypoglycemia	
Diazepam 10 mg/2 mL	Initially 5-10 mg. May repeat prn	Max 5 mg/min I.V. push; propylene glycol solvent. Cardiorespiratory toxicity with rapid administration
Digoxin 0.5 mg/2 mL	0.125-0.5 mg I.V.	Give slowly 0.25 mg/min; propylene glycol solvent. I.V. push may increase systemic vascular resistance
Diphenhydramine 50 mg/mL	Max 100 mg I.V. over 60 seconds	I.V. administration with epinephrine for anaphylaxis; or for drug-induced extrapyramidal reactions
Dobutamine 250 mg/vial	Infusion only. Initial infusion 2.5-10 mcg/kg/min	Increases cardiac output and heart rate. Titrate to patient's response. Recommend close hemodynamic monitoring. Mix 500 mg in 500 mL = 1000 mcg/mL
Dopamine 400 mg/5 mL 800 mg/5 mL	Infusion only 1-5 mcg/kg/min: ↑ renal blood flow only 5-10 mcg/kg/min: ↑ CO, ↑ HR, ↑ RBF >10 mcg/kg/min: ↑ CO, ↑ HR, ↓ RBF >20 mcg/kg/min: ↑ CO, ↑ HR, ↑ SVR, ↓ RBF Above are approximate ranges only	Infusion: 400 mg in 250 mL = 1600 mcg/mL (double strength); titrate to BP. Increasing dose increases potential for tachyarrhythmia. Not effective for ethanol-disulfiram–induced hypotension
Epinephrine 1:10,000 10 mL 1:1000 30 mL	0.5-1 mg push every 5 min; may give intracardiac or in ET tube. Initial infusion 1-4 mcg/min	Stimulates heart, increases BP, and coarsens ventricular fibrillation. Infusion: 2 mg in 500 mL = 4 mcg/mL; titrate to BP. Avoid in solvent exposures
Esmolol 250 mg/mL	Loading dose 500 mcg/kg/min for 1 minute	50-300 mcg/kg/min
Furosemide 40 mg/4 mL 100 mg/10 mL	Variable	Initiate at 20-40 mg I.V. push over 1-2 minutes. Larger doses, maximum rate = 500 mg over 30 minutes diluted. Rapid administration may lead to ototoxicity
Heparin 1000 units/mL	80 units/kg IBW I.V. push for PE or DVT. Start constant infusion – 15-20 units/kg IBW/h. Varies with age and clinical status	Caution in elderly patients or patients with bleeding potential. If patient weight is less than IBW, then base dose on actual weight
Hydrocortisone 1 g	Variable dosing Shock: 50 mg/kg I.V. initially	If dose >500 mg, give over several minutes

(Continued)

Drug and Strength	Recommended I.V. Doses	Comments and Preparation for Infusion
Inamrinone	75 mg/kg over 3 minutes	2-10 mcg/kg/min. Effective against calcium channel blocker–induced hypotension. Do not mix in dextrose
Isoproterenol 1 mg/5 mL 0.2 mg/mL	Infusion initial 1-4 mcg/min I.V. push initial 0.02-0.04 mg May repeat with up to 0.2 mg every 5 minutes. May use 0.1 mg I.V. push to counter 1 mg I.V. propranolol	Used in complete heart block prior to pacer. May cause tachyarrhythmias. May have varied effect on BP Infusion: mix 2 mg in 500 mL =4 mcg/mL; titrate to BP I.V. push: dilute 1 mg of 1:5000 with 9 mL of NS = 0.02 mg/mL
Lidocaine 100 mg/5 mL 2 g/50 mL	Initial 0.5-1 mg/kg I.V. push – may give ET. May repeat 0.5-1.0 mg/kg every 10 min to maximum load. Begin infusion at 1-4 mg/min	Infusion: mix 2 g in 500 mL = 4 mg/mL Maximum load: 200-300 mg over 1 h Severe adverse effects include respiratory depression, seizures, psychosis, and arrhythmias. May exacerbate cocaine-induced seizures
Metaraminol 100 mg/10 mL	0.1-5.0 mg I.V. push. Initial infusion = 0.1-0.4 mg/min	Mix 100 mg/500 mL = 0.2 mg/mL; titrate to BP. For direct I.V. push, dilute 1 mg (0.1 mL) in 9.9 mL NS (0.1 mg/mL). Direct/indirect-acting alpha adrenergic agonist
Methylprednisolone 1 g	Variable	100-1000 mg given over 5-minute period
Midazolam	0.4-0.6 mcg/kg/min	1-12 mcg/kg/min infusion
Naloxone 0.4 mg/mL	0.4 mg to 2 mg I.V. push, may repeat every 2 - 3 minutes, as needed	Short-acting, may need to repeat frequently. If no response after 10 mg total, re-evaluate diagnosis of narcotic overdose
Nitroglycerin	0.5-10 mcg/kg/min infusion	In glass container with special "Nitro" tubing
Nitroprusside	0.5-10 mcg/kg/min infusion	Protect from light
Norepinephrine 4 mg/4 mL	Infusion only: initial 1-4 mcg/min	Infusion: mix 8 mg in 500 mL = 16 mcg/mL; titrate to BP. Infiltration causes tissue necrosis (reverse with 5-10 mg Regitine® I.V. around infiltrated site)
Phenytoin 100 mg/2 mL	Load: 15 mg/kg IBW to maximum 1 g. Maximum rate 50 mg/min I.V. push	Reduce if phenytoin on board already. Useful in digoxin or tricyclic antidepressant toxic arrhythmias. Propylene glycol solvent can cause cardiotoxicity with rapid infusion. Must infuse with NS or ½ NS. Not soluble in D_5W
Potassium chloride 40 mEq/20 mL	Recommend infusion only. Usual maximum by infusion 10-40 mEq/h for short periods	Rates >10 mEq/h require EKG monitoring. Too rapid I.V. infusion may cause heart block or asystole. I.V. push not recommended
Procainamide 100 mg/mL 1000 mg/2 mL	Maximum 50 mg/min up to total of 1 g. Initial infusion 2-6 mg/min	Reduce loading dose if procainamide on board already. Infusion: mix 2 g in 500 mL = 4 mg/mL. Do not use in tricyclic-induced ventricular arrhythmia
Propranolol 1 mg/mL	Maximum 1 mg/min up to total dose 5 mg	Beta blocker. Decreases AV conduction. Adverse reactions: heart block, hypotension, heart failure, and bronchospasm (may be reversed with isoproterenol). Caution in patients with verapamil on board
Sodium bicarbonate 50 mEq/50 mL	Initially 1 mEq/kg then 0.5 mEq/kg every 10 minutes. For tricyclic induced ventricular arrhythmia, dose is 1-3 mEq/kg	Indicated only in hypoxemic arrest. Excessive amounts lead to alkalosis, hyperosmolality. Doses should be determined by repeat ABGs
Terbutaline	2 mcg/kg I.V. over 5 minutes. Infusion is 0.1-2 mcg/kg/min	
Verapamil 5 mg/2 mL	2.5-10 mg slow I.V. push initial. May repeat dose every 15-30 minutes	Give over 3 minutes in older patients. Caution in patients with beta blocker or digitalis on board. Contraindicated in patients with second or third degree AV block, sick sinus syndrome, or shock. Hypotension may be controlled with metaraminol

EMERGENCY DRUG DOSAGES, PEDIATRIC

Drug	Dose
Adenosine	40-50 mcg/kg. Increase by 40 mcg/kg increments to conversion.
Albumin 5% injection	5-10 mL/kg, may repeat in 15 min
Atropine injection 0.1 mg/mL	0.02 mg/kg q 5 min (min = 0.1 mg) Max total dose: 0.04 mg/kg or 2 mg, whichever is smaller
Bretylium injection 50 mg/mL	1st dose: 5 mg/kg 2nd dose: 10 mg/kg q 15-30 min Max total dose: 30 mg/kg
Calcium chloride injection 100 mg/mL	0.2-0.5 mL/kg q 10 min **Note:** Role in resuscitation questionable, should only be used when hyper kalemia, hypermagnesemia, hypocalcemia, or calcium channel blocker toxicity is present
Dextrose 50% injection 0.5 g/mL	0.5 g/kg or (2 mL/kg of dextrose 25%) **Warning:** Dilute to a 25% solution before administration
Diazepam 10 mg/2 mL	0.2-0.5 mg/kg
Dobutamine injection 12.5 mg/mL	I.V. infusion: 2.5-20 mcg/kg/min
Dopamine injection 40 mg/mL	I.V. infusion: 2.5-20 mcg/kg/min
Epinephrine injection 1:10,000	0.01-0.02 mg/kg q 5 min Max dose: 0.5-1 mg I.V. infusion: 0.1-1.5 mcg/kg/min
Furosemide injection	0.5-1 mg/kg as needed
Isoproterenol injection 0.2 mg/mL	I.V. infusion: 0.05-1 mcg/kg/min (rarely >0.5 mcg/kg/min)
Lidocaine injection 10 mg/mL	0.5-1 mg/kg loading dose (total dose not greater than 3 mg/kg) I.V. infusion: 20-50 mcg/kg/min
Naloxone injection 0.4 mg/mL or 1 mg/mL	Birth to 5 y or 20 kg: 0.1 mg/kg/dose >5 y or 20 kg: 2 mg/dose May repeat doses q 2-3 minutes
Propranolol 1 mg/mL	0.1 mg/kg slowly May repeat in 2 minutes
Sodium bicarbonate injection 1 mEq/mL or 0.5 mEq/mL	1 mEq/kg x 1 may repeat with 0.5 mEq/kg **Warning:** Use only the 0.5 mEq/mL solution for neonates or dilute 1 mEq/mL solution 1:1 with sterile water for injection. **Note:** $NaHCO_3$ should be used based on documented metabolic acidosis. Routine use in cardiac arrest is not recommended.
Terbutaline	2 mcg/kg over 5 minutes Infusion is 0.1-2 mcg/kg/min
Verapamil	0.1-0.2 mg/kg up to 5 mg

ENHANCEMENT OF ELIMINATION OF TOXINS

Toxins Eliminated by Multiple Dosing of Activated Charcoal

Acetaminophen

Amitriptyline

Atrazine (?)

Baclofen (?)

Bupropion (?)

Carbamazepine

Chlordecone

Cyclosporine

Dapsone

Dextropropoxyphene

Diazepam (desmethyldiazepam)

Digitoxin

Digoxin (with renal impairment)

Disopyramide

Glutethimide

Maprotiline

Meprobamate

Methotrexate

Methyprylon

Nadolol

Nortriptyline

Phencyclidine (?)

Phenobarbital

Phenylbutazone

Phenytoin (?)

Piroxicam

Propoxyphene

Propranolol (?)

Salicylates (?)

Theophylline

Valproic acid

Vancomycin (?)

The following agents have been studied and have not been demonstrated to result in enhanced elimination.

Amiodarone

Chlorpropamide

Imipramine

Tobramycin

Toxins Eliminated by Forced Saline Diuresis

Barium

Bromides

Chromium

Cimetidine (?)

Cis-platinum

Cyclophosphamide

Hydrazine

Iodide

Iodine

Isoniazid (?)

Meprobamate

Methyl iodide

Mushrooms (Group I)

Nickel

Potassium chloroplatinite

Thallium

Valproic acid (?)

Toxins Eliminated by Alkaline Diuresis

2,4-D-chlorophenoxyacetic acid

Barbital (serum levels >10 mg/dL)

Chlorpropamide

Fluoride

Iopanoic acid (?)

Isoniazid (?)

Mephobarbital

Methotrexate

2-Methyl-4-chlorophenoxyacetic acid (MCPA)

Orellanine (?)

Phenobarbital

Primidone

Quinolones antibiotic

Salicylates

Sulfisoxazole

Uranium

Drugs and Toxins Removed by Hemodialysis

Acetaminophen

Acetazolamide

Acyclovir

Alkyl phosphate

Allopurinol

Aluminum

Amanita phalloides (?)

Amantadine (?)

Amikacin

Ammonia

Ammonium chloride

Amobarbital

Amoxicillin

Amphetamine

Ampicillin

Anilines

Antimony (Pentavalent) (?)

Arsenic (?)

Atenolol

Azathioprine

Azlocillin

Aztreonam

Bacitracin (?)

Barbital

Boric acid

Bretylium

Bromides

Bromisoval

Butalbital

Calcium

Captopril (?)

Carbamazepine

Carbenicillin

Carbromal

Carisoprodol

Cefaclor

Cefamandole

Cefazolin

Cefotaxime

Cefoxitin

Ceftazidime

Cephalexin

Cephaloridine

Cephalothin

Cephapirin

Cephradine

Chloral hydrate

Chloramphenicol (?)

Chlordiazepoxide (?)

Chloride

Chlorpropamide

Chromic acid

Chromium

Cimetidine (?)

Ciprofloxacin (?)

Colistin

Cyclobarbital

Cyclophosphamide

Cycloserine

Dapsone

Demeton-S-methyl sulfoxide

Dextropropoxyphene

Diethyl pentenamide

Dimethoate

Dinitro-ortho-cresol

Diquat

Disopyramide

Enalapril (?)

Ergotamine

Erythromycin

Ethambutol

Ethanol

Ethchlorvynol (?)

Ethinamate

Ethosuximide (?)

Ethylene glycol

Eucalyptus oil

Famciclovir (Penciclovir)

Famotidine (?)

Flucytosine

Fluoride

Fluoridem chlorate

5-Fluorouracil (?)

Folic acid

Formaldehyde

Foscarnet sodium

Fosfomycin

Gabapentin

Gallamine triethiodide

Ganciclovir

Gentamicin

Glufosinate ammonium

Glutethimide (?)

Glycol ethers

Hydrazine (?)

Hydrochlorothiazide

Imipenem/Cilastatin

Iodides

Isoniazid

Isopropanol

Kanamycin

Ketoprofen

Lead (with EDTA)

Linezolid

Lithium

Magnesium

Mannitol

Meprobamate

Meropenem

Metal-chelate compounds

Metformin (?)

Methanol

Methaqualone

Methotrexate

Methyldopa

Methylprednisolone (?)

Methylprylone

4-Methylpyrazole

Metronidazole

Mezlocillin

Monochloroacetic acid

Nadolol

Nafcillin

Neomycin

Netilmicin

Nitrates

Nitrite

Orellanine (?)

Ouabain (?)

Oxalic acid

Paraldehyde

Paraquat (?)

Pargyline

Penicillin G

Pentobarbital

Phenelzine (?)

Phenobarbital

Phosphate

Phosphoric acid

Piperacillin

Potassium chloride

Potassium dichromate

Practolol

Prednisone (?)

Primidone

Procainamide

Propoxyphene

Quinalbital

Quinidine

Ranitidine (?)

Rifabutin

Salicylates

Secobarbital (?)

Sodium chlorate

Sodium chloride

Sodium citrate

Sotalol

Streptomycin

Strychnine

Succimer (?)

Sulfamethoxazole

Sulfisoxazole

Tetracycline (?)

Thallium

Theophylline

Thiocyanates

Ticarcillin

Tobramycin

Tocainide

Topiramate

Tranylcypromine sulfate (?)

Trimethoprim

Valproic acid (?)

Vancomycin

Verapamil (?)

Vidarabine

Drugs and Toxins Removed by Hemoperfusion (Charcoal)

Aconitine

Amanita phalloides (?)

Atenolol (?)

Bromisoval

Bromoethylbutyramide

Caffeine

Carbamazepine

Carbon tetrachloride (?)

Carbromal

Chloral hydrate (trichloroethanol)

Chloramphenicol

Chlorfenvinphos (?)

Chlorpropamide

Cibenzoline succinate

Clonidine

Colchicine (?)

Creosote (?)

Dapsone

Demeton-S-methyl sulfoxide

Diltiazem (?)

Dimethoate

Disopyramide

Ethchlorvynol

Ethylene oxide

Glutethimide

Levothyroxine (?)

Lindane

Liotrix

Meprobamate

Methaqualone

Methotrexate

Methsuximide

Methyprylon (?)

Metoprolol (?)

Nadolol (?)

Orellanine (?)

Oxalic acid (?)

Paraquat

Parathion (?)

Pentamidine

Phenelzine (?)

Phenobarbital

Phenol

Phenytoin

Podophyllin (?)

Procainamide (?)

Quinidine (?)

Rifabutin (?)

Sotalol (?)

Thallium

Thyroglobulin/Thyroid hormone

Theophylline

Valproic acid

Verapamil (?)

ESTIMATED ALUMINUM CONCENTRATIONS OF SELECTED FOODS

Foods	Aluminum Concentration (mcg/g)
Beverages (mg/L)	
Fruit juices (eg, orange, reconstituted lemon, peach)	0.043-4.130
Soft drinks (eg, ginger ale, diet cola)	0.103-2.084
Cola, carbonated	0.1
Alcoholic beverages (eg, beer, wine, wine coolers, champagne)	0.067-3.20
Beer, canned	0.07
Spirits (eg, brandy, vodka, whiskey)	0.148-0.635
Hot water–extracted, tea bags	0.424-2.931
Herbal teas (1% extract)	0.14-1.065
Tea, steeped	4.3
Instant coffee (1% solution)	0.02-0.581
Whole coffee (3% extract)	0.235-1.163
Animal Products	
Beef, cooked*	0.2†
Cheese (eg, Swiss, cheddar, bleu)	3.83-14.10
Cheese, cheddar	0.2
Cheese, cottage, creamed	0.1
Cheese, processed	297†
Chicken, with skin, cooked*	0.7
Egg	0.107
Eggs, scrambled	2.865
Eggs, cooked*	0.1
Fish (cod), cooked*	0.4
Fish, salmon	5.44
Fish, herring	0.127
Ham, cooked*	1.2
Milk, whole	0.06
Milk (skim, whole, and powdered)	0.102-1.409
Salami	1.1
Yoghurt, plain low-fat	1.1
Fruits	
Apple	0.1
Banana, fresh	0.05
Grapes	0.5†
Orange juice, frozen reconstituted	0.06
Peaches	0.4†
Raisins, dried	3.1
Strawberries, fresh	2.2
Grains	
Biscuits, baking powder, refrigerated	16.3
Bread, white	3
Bread, white	0.351

(Continued)

Foods	Aluminum Concentration (mcg/g)
Bread, pumpernickel	13.2
Bread, whole wheat	5.4
Cereal (eg, Post Raisin Bran®, Malt-O-Meal Wheat Cereal®)	0.040-29.33
Corn chips	1.2
Cornbread, homemade	400
Muffin, blueberry	128
Oatmeal, cooked	0.7
Oats	2.21-4.18
Rice, cooked*	1.7
Rice, yellow, Rice-a-Roni®	1.97
Spaghetti, cooked	0.4
Vegetables & Legumes	
Asparagus	4.4†
Beans, green, cooked*	3.4
Beans, navy, boiled	2.1
Cabbage, raw	0.1
Cauliflower, cooked	0.2
Corn	0.1
Cucumber, fresh, pared	0.1
Lettuce	0.6
Lettuce	7.16
Peanut butter	5.8
Peanut butter, natural	6.29
Peas, frozen, Pict Sweet®	1.64
Peas, green, cooked	1.9
Potatoes, unpeeled, boiled*	0.1
Potatoes, unpeeled, baked	2.4
Potato, red	3.63
Potato, sweet	1.01
Spinach, cooked*	25.2†
Tomatoes, cooked*	0.1
Herbs & Spices	
Basil	3082†
Celery seed	465†
Cinnamon	82†
Oregano	600†
Pepper, black	143†
Thyme	750†
Other Food Products	
Baking powder	2300†
Candy, milk chocolate	6.8
Chocolate cookie, Oreo®	12.7
Cocoa	45

(*Continued*)

Foods	Aluminum Concentration (mcg/g)
Cream substitute, powdered	139
Nondairy creamer	25.7-94.3
Pickles with A1 additives	39.2†
Pickles	0.126-9.97
Salad dressing, Kraft Miracle Whip®	3.7
Salt with A1 additives	164†
Salt	31.3-36.6
Soup	0.032-3.6

*Food reported to not be stored or cooked in aluminum pans, trays, or foil

†Value is an average of several values reported in the reference

Reference:
  U. S. Department of Health and Human Services, "Toxicological Profile for Aluminum," Agency for Toxic Substances and Disease Registry, September 1997.

FOOD-DRUG INTERACTIONS, KEY SUMMARY

Drug	Food	Interaction
Acetaminophen	Watercress	Decreased levels of oxidative metabolites (mercapturate) of acetaminophen
	High pectin	Delayed absorption
Amoxicillin	Any	Decreased absorption
Ampicillin		
Aspirin		
Azithromycin		
Captopril		
Cephalexin (suspension)		
Chlorpromazine		
Didanosine		
Erythromycin stearate		
Fosfomycin		
Isoniazid		
Ketoconazole		
Levodopa		
Lincomycin		
Mercaptopurine		
Methotrexate		
Methyldopa		
Nafcillin		
Nefazodone		
Penicillamine		
Penicillin G and V		
Phenobarbital		
Propantheline		
Rifampin (150 mg)		
Riluzole		
Tetracycline		
Valproic acid		
Valsartan		
Zidovudine		
Aspirin	Any	Delayed absorption
Atenolol		
Cefaclor		
Cephalexin (capsule)		
Cephradine		
Cimetidine		
Glipizide		
Ibuprofen		
Metronidazole		
Piroxicam		
Potassium (tablet)		
Quinidine		

Drug	Food	Interaction
Sulfonamides (suspension)		
Tacrine		
Warfarin		
Alpha-tocopherol	Any	Increased absorption
Carbamazepine		
Cefuroxime		
Chlorothiazide		
Hydralazine		
Hydrochlorothiazide		
Labetalol		
Lithium		
Mebendazole		
Metroprolol		
Nitrofurantoin		
Phenytoin		
Propoxyphene		
Propranolol		
Riboflavin		
Spironolactone		
Cyclosporine	Many	Decreased absorption
Acitretin	Dietary fat	Increased absorption
Albendazole		
Atovaquone		
Beta-caortene		
Cyclosporine		
Diazepam		
Dicumarol		
Etretinate		
Griseofulvin		
Halofantrine		
Isotretinoin		
Mefenamic acid		
Phenytoin		
Vitamin A		
Vitamin D		
Vitamin E		
Vitamin K		
Ziprasidone		
Biphosphonates (ie, etidronate, alendronate, tiludronate)	Foods with high mineral content (ie, milk)	Reduced absorption
Griseofulvin	High-fat meal	Faster absorption; increased serum levels by 50%
Misoprostol		Reduced peak by delaying absorption
Digoxin		Reduced absorption
Pilocarpine (tablets)		Reduced absorption

(*Continued*)

Drug	Food	Interaction
Zidovudine		Reduced absorption
Amiodarone	Grapefruit juice (narigen)	Amiodarone metabolism is inhibited with grapefruit juice
Atorvastatin		Increased serum atorvastatin acid and atorvastatin lactone levels
Carbamazepine		Increased absorption; increased oral bioavailability
Cisapride		
Cyclosporine		
Felodipine		
Nifedipine		
Nisoldipine		
Nimlodipine		
Nitrendipine		
Saquinivir		
Verapamil		
Caffeine		Possibly prolongs caffeine's half-life
Coumarin		Delayed urinary excretion of 7-hydroxy-coumarin
Losartan		Increased half-life and decreased area under the curve of the metabolite
Lovastain		Increases lovastatin and metabolite concentrations
Midazolam (oral)		Delayed absorption; increased bioavailability
Sildenafil		Increases bioavailability and tends to delay sildenafil absorption
Quinidine		Delayed absorption of quinidine; inhibits metabolism of quinidine
Ziprasidone		May increase serum concentration of ziprasidone
Terfenadine	Any	Increases terfenadine bioavailability (can increase QT interval on EKG); increased absorption
Erythromycin stearate		Increased or decreased absorption
Furosemide		Decreased rate of absorption, potentially decreasing effect
Mercaptopurine	Any	Decreased bioavailability by 30%
Isoniazid	Tuna, mackerel, salmon (dark meat fish)	Increased risk for scromboid fish poisoning
Levodopa	High-protein diet	Decreased absorption
Digoxin	High fiber meal	Decreased absorption
Lovastatin		
Lithium	Sodium	Enhanced elimination requiring higher doses
Methyldopa	Iron	Reduced absorption
MAO inhibitors (isocarboxazid, phenelzine, procarbazine, tranylcypromine)	High-protein foods that have undergone aging, fermentation, pickling, or smoking; aged cheeses, red wines, pods of broad beans and fava beans; bananas, raisins, avocados; caffeine-containing beverages, beer, ale, and chocolate	Elevated blood pressure
Phenobarbital	High doses of vitamin B_6 (pyridoxine) and folic acid	Decreased absorption
Phenytoin		
Levodopa	Vitamin B_6 (pyridoxine)	Reduces blood level

(*Continued*)

Drug	Food	Interaction
Diprafenone	Any	Increased bioavailability
Hydralazine		
Metoprolol		
Felodipine		
Nitrofurantoin		
Propranolol		
Phenobarbital	Charcoal-broiled foods	Increased metabolism requiring higher doses
Theophylline		
Phenytoin		
Warfarin		
Ketoconazole	Acidic beverages (pH <2.5, [Coca-Cola Classic®]	Increased absorption
Phenytoin	Most foods	Absorption increased by 25%
	Pudding	Absorption decreased by 50%
Quinolones (eg, ciprofloxacin)	Iron, calcium, aluminum, zinc, magnesium (eg, dairy products)	Decreased absorption
Quinidine	High salt (>400 mEq/day)	Increased first-pass hepatic elimination
Warfarin	Diets rich in vitamin K such as cauliflower, spinach, broccoli, turnip greens, liver, beans, rice, pork, fish, and some cheeses	Antagonism of effect
ACE inhibitors	Potassium-containing salt substitutes	Increased serum potassium level
Warfarin	Cranberry juice	INR instability

Adapted from Saltiel E, "Food-Drug Interactions," *New Developments in Medicine & Drug Therapy*, Glenview, IL: Physicians & Scientists Publishing Co, Inc, 1994, 3(4):61.

D'Arcy PF, "Nutrient-Drug Interactions," *Adv Drug React Toxicol Rev*, 1995, 14:233-54.

Gauthier I and Malone M, "Drug-Food Interactions in Hospitalized Patients: Methods of Prevention," *Drug Safety*, 1998, 18(6):383-93.

Parnetti L and Lowenthal DT, "How to Recognize and Prevent Dangerous Food-Drug Interactions," *J Crit Illness*, 1998, 13(2):126-33.

GASTROINTESTINAL CANCER RISKS FROM ASBESTOS

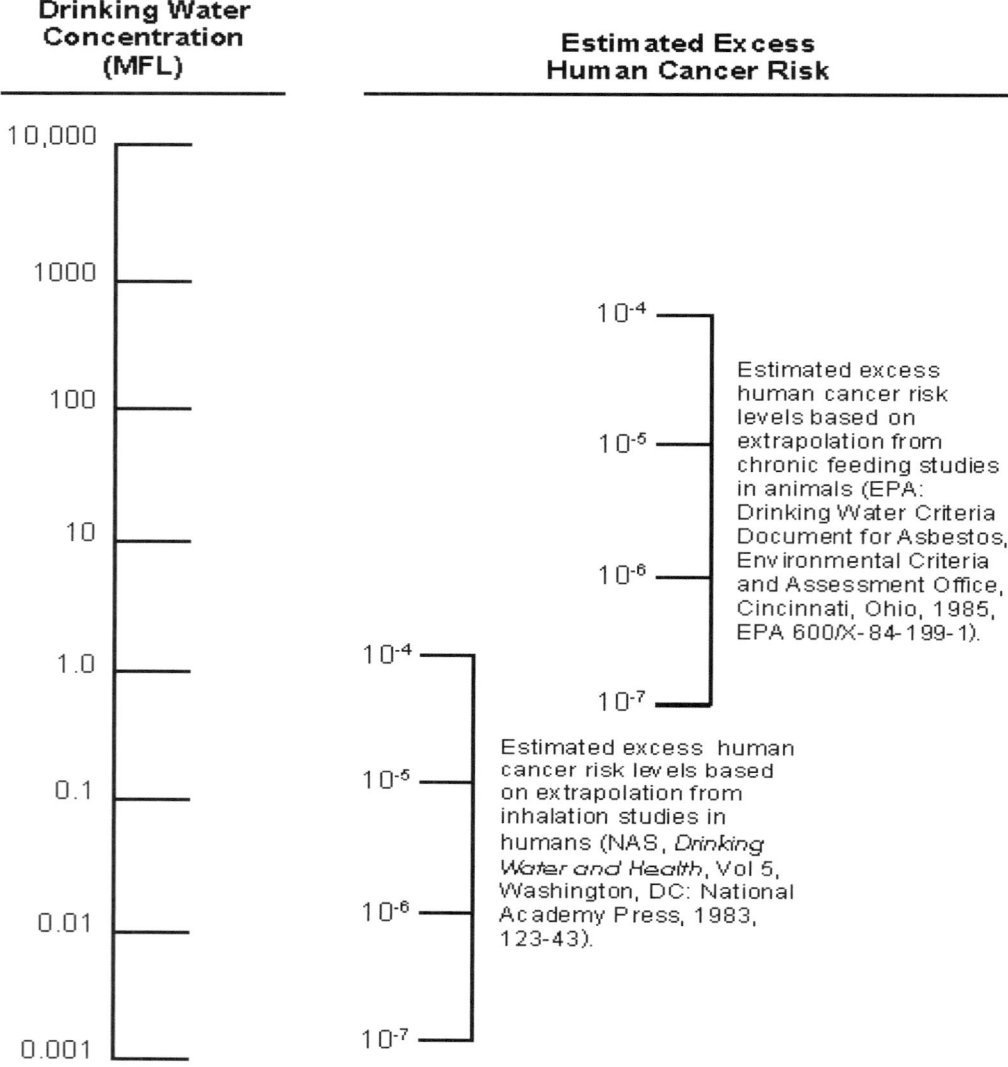

Summary of Calculated Gastrointestinal Cancer Risks From Ingestion of Asbestos

Drinking Water Concentration (MFL)

Estimated Excess Human Cancer Risk

Estimated excess human cancer risk levels based on extrapolation from chronic feeding studies in animals (EPA: Drinking Water Criteria Document for Asbestos, Environmental Criteria and Assessment Office, Cincinnati, Ohio, 1985, EPA 600/X-84-199-1).

Estimated excess human cancer risk levels based on extrapolation from inhalation studies in humans (NAS, *Drinking Water and Health*, Vol 5, Washington, DC: National Academy Press, 1983, 123-43).

Since there are no human studies in which ingestion of a known amount of asbestos can be associated with a clear increase in gastrointestinal cancer risk, NAS (1983) extrapolated date on gastrointestinal risk from epidemiological studies of workers exposed to asbestos by inhalation. These calculations indicated that lifetime ingestion of 1.1×10^6 TEM fibers/liter of water corresponded to an excess gastrointestinal cancer risk of 10^{-4} (NAS 1983).

In order to present this risk estimate in this figure, the concentration of 1.1×10^6 f/L was converted to a dose of 3.1×10^4 f/kg/day (assuming ingestion of 2 L/day by a 70 kg adult), and this was converted to a dose of 1.6×10^{-5} mg/kg/day by multiplying by a factor of 5.0×10^{-10} mg/TEM fiber (NRC, *Asbestiform Fibers: Nonoccupational Health Risks*, Washington, DC: National Academy Press, 1984.

From "Toxicological Profile for Asbestos," U.S. Department of Health and Human Services, Agency for Toxic Substances and Disease Registry, August, 1995.

HABITUAL, TOXIC, AND LETHAL CONCENTRATIONS (MG/L) OF 103 DRUGS OF ABUSE

Drug	Habitual/Therapeutic			Toxic			Lethal/Postmortem		
	Whole Blood	Serum/ Plasma	Urine	Whole Blood	Serum/ Plasma	Urine	Whole Blood	Serum/ Plasma	Urine
Alfentanil		0.1-0.4§			0.1				
Alprazolam		0.01-0.05			0.075		0.1	0.1	
Amphetamine		0.02-0.15	1-5		0.2	25	0.5	0.5	25-700
Barbiturates									
Long acting		5-20			10		50		
Intermediate acting		0.3-10.0			20		30		
Short acting		0.1-8.0			10		20		
Benzoylecgonine		0-0.1	0-5				1		15
Bromazepam		0.08-0.20			0.3		5	1	
Buprenorphine		0.001-0.005	0.001			0.02			
Buspirone		0.001-0.004							
Butabarbital		1-15	4-17		10-20		30	30	
Butalbital		1-5		8.5	10		26	25	51
Butaperazine		0-0.5							
Caffeine		2-10	0-10		15	15	80	80	25
Chlordiazepoxide		0.4-2.0			3	1	20		8
Demoxepam*									
Nordiazepam*									
Oxazepam*									
Clobazam		0.1-0.6							
Norclobazam*									
Clonazepam		0.01-0.08			0.1				
Clorazepate		0.02-1.00			2				
Nordiazepam*									
Oxazepam*									
Clotiazepam		0.1-0.7							
Clozapine		0.1-0.5			0.6		4.5	3	11
Cocaine		0-0.3	0-10		0.5		1	1	35
Benzoylecgonine*									
Codeine	0.03-0.10	0.01-0.10	5-20		0.2	25	1.6	1.8	50
Cotinine		0.01-0.35#				1			5
Cyclobarbitone		2-10			10			20	
Demoxepam		0.50-0.74			1		2.7		
Desalkylflurazepam		0.01-0.15			0.2				
Desmethyldiazepam (see Nordiazepam)									
Desmethylmaprotiline		0.1-0.4			0.75				
Dextromethorphan		0.01-0.04			0.1		3	3	
Dextromoramide		0.09			0.11		0.15		
Dextropropoxyphen	0.05-0.40	0.05-0.50			0.6	2-20	2	2	20
Norpropoxyphen*									

	Habitual/Therapeutic			Toxic			Lethal/Postmortem		
Drug	Whole Blood	Serum/ Plasma	Urine	Whole Blood	Serum/ Plasma	Urine	Whole Blood	Serum/ Plasma	Urine
Diacetylmorphine (Heroin) (see Morphine)									
Diazepam	0.5	0.1-1.5		5	1.5-15.0**		10	20	
Nordiazepam*									
Oxazepam*									
Temazepam*									
Diclofenac		0.5-3.0			60‡				
Dihydrocodeine		0.03-0.25			0.3-1.0		0.8	2	
Ecstasy (see MDMA)									
Ephedrine		0.02-0.10	2-30		1		5†		547†
Ethambutol		2-5			6				
Ethanol	1.5-30.0			1000			4000		5000
Fenclofenac		87							
Fenfluramine		0.04-0.15	1-30	1	0.3	50	6.5	6	90
Fenoprofen		5-60					710		
Fentanyl		0.001-0.002			0.003		0.003	0.017	0.005-0.090
Flunitrazepam		0.001-0.015			0.05				
Fluoxetine		0.1-0.5					6†	2	
Norfluoxetine*									
Flurazepam		0.002-0.100			0.2	2	0.5	0.8	
Desalkylflurazepam*									
Heroin (see Morphine)									
Hexobarbital		1-5			8			50	
Hydrocodone		0.01-0.10			0.1		0.2		
Hydromorphone		0.001-0.030	0.1-1		0.1	1-5	0.1		8
Ketazolam		0.001-0.010							
Nordiazepam*									
Levomepromazine	0.08†	0.005-0.150			0.4		8†	0.4	
Levomethadone (see 1-Methadone)									
Levorphanol		0.007-0.020			0.1	1-5	2.7		2.3†
Loprazolam		0.005-0.010							
Lorazepam		0.02-0.25			0.3		0.5		
Lormetazepam		0.001-0.025							
LSD		0.001	0.001		0.002	0.002-0.030	0.005	0.005	
MA (see Methamphetamine)									
Maprotiline	0.05-0.55	0.03-0.20			0.3		1.3	1	4-25
Desmethylmaprotiline*									
MDA		0-0.4	0-10		1.5‡	50‡	6	4	50-175
MDMA		0-0.35	0-17		0.5 × 6.5‡		0.6	0.42† 1.26†	
MDA*									
Medazepam	0.01-0.17	0.01-0.15			0.6				
Nordiazepam*									

(Continued)

Drug	Habitual/Therapeutic			Toxic			Lethal/Postmortem		
	Whole Blood	Serum/ Plasma	Urine	Whole Blood	Serum/ Plasma	Urine	Whole Blood	Serum/ Plasma	Urine
Meperidine		0.1-0.5	1-10		0.5	25	1	2	25-150
Norpethidine*									
Mephenesin		3-10							
Meprobamate	3-26	5-15	25-100		10-25		43	120	200
Metaclazepam		0.05-0.20							
Methaqualone	0.4	0.4-4.0		2	4-10	0.5	5	30	17†
1,d-Methadone	0.03-0.30	0.05-0.75††	0.2		1	1	0.4	4.5	4.78†
1-Methadone		0.04-0.30			0.5			1	
Methamphetamine		0.01-0.05	0.5-4.0		0.2	25	0.23	10	28
Methoxyamphetamine		0-0.2	0-5		0.3	5	0.3		10
Methylamphetamine (see Methamphetamine)									
Methylenedioxyamphetamine (see MDA)									
Methylenedioxymethylamphetamine (see MDMA)									
Methylfentanyl	0.001						0.002		5-150
Methylphenidate		0.01-0.06	0.1-1.0		0.5	1-40	2.8	2.3	
Midazolam		0.04-0.10			1				
Morphine	0-0.1	0-0.1	0-0.5		0.1	0.5	0.2	0.1	5
Naloxone		0.01-0.03							
Naltrexone		0.01-0.03							
Naproxen		20-50			400				
Nicotine‡‡		0.01-0.04# 0.001-0.006¶	0.1-3.0# 0.07¶		1		5	5	17
Cotinine*									
Nitrazepam		0.03-0.10			0.2		1	5	1-10
Norclobazam		2-4							
Nordiazepam		0.1-1.7			1.5-2.0	1-10			
Norfluoxetine		0.15-0.50					5†		
Norpethidine					0.5				
Norpropoxyphen		0.2-1.4			2	20-200	2		40-200
Oxazepam		0.1-1.4			2			3	
Oxycodone		0.005-0.100	0.2-2.0		0.2	1-5	5	5	
Pemoline		1-7							
Pentazocine	0.03-0.15	0.01-0.20	1	0.5	1	3	3	3	3-10
Pentobarbital		1-5	0.5-1.8	8	10		15	15	15-50
Pethidine (see Meperidine)									
Phencyclidine		0.01-0.20	0.04	0.02	0.1-0.8	0.4	0.3	0.5	5
Phenformin		0.1-0.5			0.6		3		
Phenobarbital	6-30	10-25	4-20	30	15-30		50	60	40
Phentermine		0.03-0.10	5-25	0.2	0.9	50	1		70
Phenylephrine		0.03-0.35							
Pindolol		0.015-0.080			0.7			0.01†	

(*Continued*)

Drug	Habitual/Therapeutic			Toxic			Lethal/Postmortem		
	Whole Blood	Serum/ Plasma	Urine	Whole Blood	Serum/ Plasma	Urine	Whole Blood	Serum/ Plasma	Urine
Prazepam		0.05-0.20			1-5				
Nordiazepam*									
Propoxyphen (see Dextropropoxyphen)									
Pseudoephedrine		0.5-0.7	4-50				19	20	100
Quazepam		0.01-0.15							
Sulpiride		0.03-0.60							
Temazepam		0.02-0.80			1		0.8	8	
Tetrahydrocannabinol (see THC)									
Tetrazepam		0.05-0.60							
THC									
Smoker of hashish		0.004-0.200	0.05-0.25				0.002		
Passive smoker		0.001-0.007	0.02-0.08						
Tiapride		1-2							
Tilidine		0.05-0.15						1.7†	
XTC (see MDMA)									
Zolpidem	0.2	0.03-0.20			0.5		1†		
Zomepirac		0.1-4.0					153		
Zopiclone		0.01-0.05			0.05		1.4		

*Metabolite, shown under the original product and listed in alphabetical order, where concentrations are given.

†Isolated case.

‡Serious toxic effects from large single doses.

§Level in surgical anesthesia.

#Level in smokers.

¶Level in nonsmokers.

**Drowsiness/coma.

††Therapeutic level in plasma: up to 0.3 as analgesic, and 0.20-0.75 in a methadone program for addicts. Toxic levels are higher in addicts as with other drugs of abuse.

‡‡Nicotine, transdermal in smokers: 0.004-0.030 mg/L.

HEMATOLOGIC ADVERSE EFFECTS OF DRUGS

Drug	Red Cell Aplasia	Thrombocytopenia	Neutropenia	Pancytopenia	Hemolysis
Acetazolamide		+	+	+	
Allopurinol			+		
Amiodarone	+				
Amphotericin B				+	
Amrinone		++			
Asparaginase		+++	+++	+++	++
Barbiturates		+		+	
Benzocaine					++
Captopril			++		+
Carbamazepine	++	+++	++	+	+
Cephalosporins			+		++
Chloramphenicol		+	++	+++	
Chlordiazepoxide			+	+	
Chloroquine		+			
Chlorothiazides		++			
Chlorpropamide	+	++	+	++	+
Chlortetracycline				+	
Chlorthalidone			+		
Cimetidine		+	++	+	
Clozapine		++	+++		
Codeine		+			
Colchicine				+	
Cyclophosphamide		+++	+++	+++	+
Dapsone					+++
Desipramine		++			
Digitalis		+			
Digitoxin		++			
Erythromycin		+			
Estrogen		+		+	
Ethacrynic acid			+		
Fluorouracil		+++	+++	+++	+
Furosemide		+	+		
Gold salts	+	+++	+++	+++	
Heparin		++		+	
Ibuprofen			+		+
Imipramine			++		

(Continued)

Drug	Red Cell Aplasia	Thrombocytopenia	Neutropenia	Pancytopenia	Hemolysis
Indomethacin		+	++	+	
Isoniazid		+		+	
Isosorbide dinitrate					+
Levodopa					++
Meperidine		+			
Meprobamate		+	+	+	
Methimazole			++		
Methyldopa		++			+++
Methotrexate		+++	+++	+++	++
Methylene blue					+
Metronidazole			+		
Nalidixic acid					+
Naproxen				+	
Nitrofurantoin			++		+
Nitroglycerine		+			
Penicillamine		++	+		
Penicillins		+	++	+	+++
Phenazopyridine					+++
Phenothiazines		+	++	+++	+
Phenylbutazone		+	++	+++	+
Phenytoin		++	++	++	+
Potassium iodide		+			
Prednisone		+			
Primaquine					+++
Procainamide			+		
Procarbazine		+	++	++	+
Propylthiouracil		+	++	+	+
Quinidine		+++	+		
Quinine		+++	+		
Reserpine		+			
Rifampicin		++	+		+++
Spironolactone			+		
Streptomycin		+		+	
Sulfamethoxazole with trimethoprim			+		
Sulfonamides	+	++	++	++	++
Sulindac	+	+	+	+	

(*Continued*)

Drug	Red Cell Aplasia	Thrombocytopenia	Neutropenia	Pancytopenia	Hemolysis
Tetracyclines		+			+
Thioridazine			++		
Tolbutamide		++	+	++	
Triamterene					+
Valproate	+	+++	++	++	
Vancomycin			+		

+ = rare or single reports.

++ = occasional reports.

+++ = substantial number of reports.

Adapted from D'Arcy PF and Griffin JP, eds, *Iatrogenic Diseases*, New York, NY: Oxford University Press, 1986, 128-30.

HERB - DRUG INTERACTIONS/CAUTIONS

Herb	Drug Interaction / Caution
Acidophilus/bifidobacterium	Antibiotics (oral)
Activated charcoal	Vitamins or oral medications may be adsorbed
Alfalfa	Do not use with lupus due to amino acid L-canavanine; causes pancytopenia at high doses; warfarin (alfalfa contains a large amount of vitamin K)
Aloe vera	Caution in pregnancy, may cause uterine contractions; digoxin, diuretics (hypokalemia)
Ashwagandha	May cause sedation and other CNS effects
Asparagus root	Causes diuresis
Barberry	Normal metabolism of vitamin B may be altered with high doses
Birch	If taking a diuretic, drink plenty of fluids
Black cohosh	Estrogen-like component; pregnant and nursing women should probably avoid this herb; also women with estrogen-dependent cancer and women who are taking birth control pills or estrogen supplements after menopause; caution also in people taking sedatives or blood pressure medications
Black haw	Do not give to children <6 years of age (salicin content) with flu or chickenpox due to potential Reye's syndrome; do not take if allergic to aspirin
Black pepper (*Piper nigrum*)	Antiasthmatic drugs (decreases metabolism)
Black tea	May inhibit body's utilization of thiamine
Blessed thistle	Do not use with gastritis, ulcers, or hyperacidity since herb stimulates gastric juices
Blood root	Large doses can cause nausea, vomiting, CNS sedation, low BP, shock, coma, and death
Broom (*Cytisus scoparius*)	MAO inhibitors lead to sudden blood pressure changes
Bugleweed (*Lycopus virginicus*)	May interfere with nuclear imaging studies of the thyroid gland (thyroid uptake scan)
Cat's claw (*Uncaria tomentosa*)	Avoid in organ transplant patients or patients on ulcer medications, antiplatelet drugs, NSAIDs, anticoagulants, immunosuppressive therapy, intravenous immunoglobulin therapy
Chaste tree berry (*Vitex agnus-castus*)	Interferes with actions of oral contraceptives, HRT, and other endocrine therapies; may interfere with metabolism of dopamine-receptor antagonists
Chicory (*Cichorium intybus*)	Avoid with gallstones due to bile-stimulating properties
Chlorella (*Chlorella vulgaris*)	Contains significant amounts of vitamin K
Chromium picolinate	Picolinic acid causes notable changes in brain chemicals (serotonin, dopamine, norepinephrine); do not use if patient has behavioral disorders or diabetes
Cinnabar root (*Salviae multorrhizae*)	Warfarin (increases INR)
Deadly nightshade (*Atropa belladonna*)	Contains atropine
Dong quai	Warfarin (increases INR), estrogens, oral contraceptives, photosensitizing drugs, histamine replacement therapy, anticoagulants, antiplatelet drugs, antihypertensives
Echinacea	Caution with other immunosuppressive therapies; stimulates TNF and interferons
Evening primrose oil	May lower seizure threshold; do not combine with anticonvulsants or phenothiazines
Fennel	Do not use in women who have had breast cancer or who have been told not to take birth control pills
Fenugreek	Practice moderation in patients on diabetes drugs, MAO inhibitors, cardiovascular agents, hormonal medicines, or warfarin due to the many components of fenugreek
Feverfew	Antiplatelets, anticoagulants, NSAIDs
Forskolin, coleonol	This herb lowers blood pressure (vasodilator) and is a bronchodilator and increases the contractility of the heart, inhibits platelet aggregation, and increases gastric acid secretion
Foxglove	Digitalis-containing herb
Garlic	Blood sugar-lowering medications, warfarin, and aspirin at medicinal doses of garlic
Ginger	May inhibit platelet aggregation by inhibiting thromboxane synthetase at large doses; *in vitro* and animal studies indicate that ginger may interfere with diabetics; has anticoagulant effect, so avoid in medicinal amounts in patients on warfarin or heart medicines
Ginkgo biloba	Warfarin (ginkgo decreases blood clotting rate); NSAIDs, MAO inhibitors
Ginseng	Blood sugar-lowering medications (additive effects) and other stimulants
Ginseng (American, Korean)	Furosemide (decreases efficacy)

(*Continued*)

Herb	Drug Interaction / Caution
Ginseng (Siberian)	Digoxin (increases digoxin level)
Glucomannan	Diabetics (herb delays absorption of glucose from intestines, decreasing mean fasting sugar levels)
Goldenrod	Diuretics (additive properties)
Gymnema	Blood sugar-lowering medications (additive effects)
Hawthorn	Digoxin or other heart medications (herb dilates coronary vessels and other blood vessels, also inotropic)
Hibiscus	Chloroquine (reduced effectiveness of chloroquine)
Hops	Those with estrogen-dependent breast cancer should not take hops (contains estrogen-like chemicals); patients with depression (accentuate symptoms); alcohol or sedative (additive effects)
Horehound	May cause arrhythmias at high doses
Horseradish	In medicinal amounts with thyroid medications
Kava	CNS depressants (additive effects, eg, alcohol, barbiturates, etc); benzodiazepines
Kelp	Thyroid medications (additive effects or opposite effects by negative feedback); kelp contains a high amount of sodium
Labrador tea	Plant has narcotic properties, possible additive effects with other CNS depressants
Lemon balm	Do not use with Graves disease since it inhibits certain thyroid hormones
Licorice	Acts as a corticosteroid at high doses (about 1.5 lbs candy in 9 days) which can lead to hypertension, edema, hypernatremia, and hypokalemia (pseudoaldosteronism); do not use in persons with hypertension, glaucoma, diabetes, kidney or liver disease, or those on hormonal therapy; may interact with digitalis (due to hypokalemia)
Lobelia	Contains lobeline which has nicotinic activity; may mask withdrawal symptoms from nicotine; it can act as a polarizing neuromuscular blocker
Lovage	Is a diuretic
Ma huang	MAO inhibitors, digoxin, beta-blockers, methyldopa, caffeine, theophylline, decongestants (increases toxicity)
Marshmallow	May delay absorption of other drugs taken at the same time; may interfere with treatments of lowering blood sugar
Meadowsweet	Contains salicylates
Melatonin	Acts as contraceptive at high doses; antidepressants (decreases efficacy)
Mistletoe	May interfere with medications for blood pressure, depression, and heart disease
L-phenylalanine	MAO inhibitors
Pleurisy root	Digoxin (plant contains cardiac glycosides); also contains estrogen-like compounds; may alter amine concentrations in the brain and interact with antidepressants
Prickly ash (Northern)	Contains coumarin-like compounds
Prickly ash (Southern)	Contains neuromuscular blockers
Psyllium	Digoxin (decreases absorption)
Quassia	High doses may complicate heart or blood-thinning treatments (quassia may be inotropic)
Red clover	May have estrogen-like actions; avoid when taking birth control pills, HRT, people with heart disease or at risk for blood clots, patients who suffer from estrogen-dependent cancer; do not take with warfarin
Red pepper	May increase liver metabolism of other medications and may interfere with high blood pressure medications or MAO inhibitors
Rhubarb, Chinese	Do not use with digoxin (enhanced effects)
St John's wort	Indinavir, cyclosporine, SSRIs or any antidepressants, tetracycline (increases sun sensitivity); digoxin (decreases digoxin concentration); may also interact with diltiazem, nicardipine, verapamil, etoposide, paclitaxel, vinblastine, vincristine, glucocorticoids, cyclosporine, dextromethorphan, ephedrine, lithium, meperidine, pseudoephedrine, selegiline, yohimbine, ACE inhibitors (serotonin syndrome, hypertension, possible exacerbation of allergic reaction)
Saw palmetto	Acts an antiandrogen; do not take with prostate medicines or HRT
Squill	Digoxin or persons with potassium deficiency; also not with quinidine, calcium, laxatives, saluretics, prednisone (long-term)

(*Continued*)

Herb	Drug Interaction / Caution
Tonka bean	Contains coumarin, interacts with warfarin
Vervain	Avoid large amounts of herb with blood pressure medications or HRT
Wild Oregon grape	High doses may alter metabolism of vitamin B
Wild yam	May interfere with hormone precursors
Wintergreen	Warfarin, increased bleeding
Sweet woodruff	Contains coumarin
Yarrow	Interferes with anticoagulants and blood pressure medications
Yohimbe	Do not consume tyramine-rich foods; do not take with nasal decongestants, PPA-containing diet aids, antidepressants, or mood-altering drugs

HERBS

Hemostatic Herbs (Coagulants)

Agrimony (*Agrimony eupatoria* or *Agrimony procera*)

Bai Ji (*Bletilla striata*)

Ce Bai Ye (*Biota orientalis*)

Duan Xue Liu (*Clinopodium polycephalum* or *Clinopodium chinense*)

Goldenseal (*Hydrastis canadensis*)

Huai Hua or Huai Mi (*Sophora japonica*)

Ji Cai (*Capsella bursa-pastoris*)

Jing Tin San Qui (*Sedum aizoon*)

Juan Bai (*Selaginella tamariscina*)

Ma Han Lian (*Eclipta prostrata*)

Mistletoe (*Viscum album*)

Oregon grape root (*Mahonia aquifolium*)

Periwinkle (*Vinca minor*)

Qian Cao (*Rubis cordifolia*)

Senecio herb (*Senecio nemorensis*)

Shepherd's purse (*Capsella bursa-pastoris*)

Shu Liang (*Dioscorea cirrhosa*)

Su Mu (*Caesalpinia sappan*)

Tie Shu (*Cycas revoluta*)

Tu Tai Huang (*Rhumex patientia*)

Witch hazel* (leaf and bark) (*Hamamelis virginiana*)

Xiao Ji (*Cephalanoplos segetum* or *Cephalanoplos setasum*)

Yarrow (*Achillea millefolium*)

Zi Ju Cua (*Callicarpa macrophylla, Callicarpa pedunculata*, or *Callicarpa dichotoma*)

*Approved herb by Kommission E Monograph.

Herbs to Avoid Prior to Surgery (Due to Anticoagulant Activity)

Alfalfa (*Medicago sativa*)

American ginseng (*Panax quinquefolius*)

Angelica (*Angelica archangelica*)

Aniseed (*Pimpinella anisum*)

Arnica (*Arnica montana*)

Asafoetida (*Ferula asafoetida, Ferula foetida*)

Bilberry (*Vaccinum myrtillus*)

Bromelain (pineapple stem) (*Anas cosmosus*)

Cayenne (*Capsicum annuum*)

Celery (*Apium graveolens*)

Chamomile

English (*Anthemis nobilis*)

German (*Matricaria recutita*)

Roman (*Chamaemilum nobile*)

Clove (*Syzygium aromaticum*)

Coleus or forskolin (*Coleus forskohlii*)

Danshen (*Salvia miltiorrhiza*)

Dong Quai (*Angelica sinensis*)

Fenugreek (*Trigonella foenum-graecum*)

Feverfew (*Tanacetum parthenium*)

Flaxseed oil (*Linum usitatissimum*)

Fo-Ti (*Polygonum multiflorum*)

Fucus (*Fucus vesiculosus*)

Garlic (*Allium sativum*)

Ginger (*Zingiber officinale*)

Ginkgo (*Ginkgo biloba*)

Green tea (*Camellia sinesis*)

Horse chestnut (*Aesculus hippocastanum*)

Horseradish (*Armoacia rusticana*)

Licorice (*Glycyrrhiza glabra*)

Meadowsweet (*Filipendula ulmaria*)

Motherwort (*Leonurus cardiaca*)

Onion (*Allium cepa*)

Poplar (*Populus* sp)

Prickley ash

Northern (*Zanthoxylum americanum*)

Southern (*Zanthoxylum clava-herculis*)

Quassia (*Quassia amara, Picrasma excelsa*)

Red clover (*Trifolium pratense*)

Turmeric (*Curcuma longa*)

Willowbark (*Salix* sp)

LABORATORY DETECTION OF DRUGS

Agent	Time Detectable in Urine[1] by Immunoassay
Amobarbital	2-4 d
Amphetamine	2-4 d
Butalbital	2-4 d
Cannabinoids	
Occasional use	2-7 d
Regular use	Up to 30 d
Cocaine (benzoylecgonine)	12-96 h
Codeine	2-4 d
Chlordiazepoxide	Up to 30 d
Diazepam	Up to 30 d
Dilaudid®	2-4 d
Ethanol	12-24 h
Heroin (morphine)	2-4 d
Hydromorphone	2-4 d
Librium®	30 d
Methamphetamine	2-4 d
Methaqualone	2-4 d
Morphine	2-4 d
Pentobarbital	2-4 d
Phencyclidine (PCP)	
Occasional use	2-7 d
Regular use	Up to 30 d
Phenobarbital	Up to 30 d
Quaalude®	2-4 d
Secobarbital	2-4 d
Valium®	30 d

[1]The periods of detection for the various abused drugs listed above should be taken as estimates since the actual figures will vary due to metabolism, user, laboratory, and excretion.

Reference: Chang JY, "Drug Testing and Interpretation of Results," *Pharmchem Newsletter*, 1989, 17:1.

LAXATIVES

Classification and Properties of Laxatives					
Laxative	Onset of Action	Site of Action	Mechanism of Action	Adverse Effects	Toxicologic Perspective for Gastric Decontamination
Bulk-Producing					
Methylcellulose psyllium (Metamucil®) Malt soup extract (Maltsupex®)	12-24 h (up to 72 h)	Small and large intestine	Holds water in stool; mechanical distention; malt soup extract reduces fecal pH; peristalsis is stimulated reflexly	No systemic effects	Not useful for gastric decontamination
Irritant/Stimulant					
Senna (Senokot®)	6-10 h	Colon	Direct action on intestinal mucosa; stimulate myenteric plexus; alter water and electrolyte secretion (especially potassium)	Chronic use can cause hepatitis	Not useful for gastric decontamination
Bisacodyl (Dulcolax®) tablets, suppositories	6-12 h (oral) 0.25-1 h (rectal)			Chronic use can cause atonic colon; do not use suppositories in patients with hemorrhoids	
Castor oil (ricinoleic acid)	2-6 h	Small intestine		May induce labor	May reduce the absorption of dinitrocresol by 50% (non-purgative dose). Not useful for routine gastric decontamination. May increase absorption of organochlorine agents
Cascara aromatic fluid extract	6-10 h	Colon		Can alter water and electrolyte secretion	
Lubricant					
Mineral oil (Agoral®)	6-8 h	Colon	Lubricates intestine; retards colonic absorption of fecal water	Lipoid pneumonia may occur with aspiration	May increase absorption of organochlorine agents. Not recommended for children <6 years due to aspiration risk. Not useful for gastric decontamination (except in phosphorus exposure)
Miscellaneous and Combination Laxatives					
Glycerin suppository	0.25-0.5 h	Colon	Hyperosmotic action	Local irritation, hyperosmotic action	Not useful for gastric decontamination
Lactulose (Cephulac®)	24-48 h	Colon	Delivers osmotically active molecules to colon		
Docusate/casanthranol (Peri-Colace®)	8-12 h	Small and large intestine	Casanthranol — mild stimulant; docusate — stool softener		
Osmotic					
Sorbitol (70%)	1-1.5 h	Small and large intestine	Increase intraluminal water volume — can stimulate peristalsis	Vomiting, hypernatremic dehydration at high doses	Dose 0.5-3 g/kg (0.5 g/kg in children <1 year; up to 50 g of a 35% solution) Not to be used more than once daily in combination with multiple dosing of activated charcoal. Increases elimination by about 30% when used with charcoal for decontamination
Combination macrogols with polyethylene glycol/sodium sulphate (GoLYTELY®)	1 h	Small and large intestine	Increases osmotic pressure	Vomiting may occur (related to rate of administration); do not give in presence of GI obstruction, bowel perforation, toxic megacolon, clinically significant gastrointestinal hemorrhage, ileus, unprotected compromised airway, hemodynamic instability, or uncontrolled intractable vomiting	Drug of choice for whole bowel irrigation. Dose is: children: 9 months to 6 years: 500 mL/hour, 6-12 years: 1000 mL/hour; adolescents and adults: 1500-2000 mL/hour. Elevate head of bed to 45°. If emesis occurs, decrease infusion rate by 50% for up to 1 hour, then return to original rate

Classification and Properties of Laxatives (Continued)

Laxative	Onset of Action	Site of Action	Mechanism of Action	Adverse Effects	Toxicologic Perspective for Gastric Decontamination
Saline					
Magnesium citrate (Citroma®)	0.5-3 h	Small and large intestine	Attract/retain water in intestinal lumen increasing intraluminal pressure; cholecystokinin release (magnesium cathartics)	Vomiting at doses exceeding 233 mg/kg	300 mL magnesium citrate should be given for oral hydrofluoric acid ingestion. Dose for decontamination of a 10% magnesium citrate solution is 250 mL for adults or about 4 mL/kg for children
Magnesium hydroxide (Milk of Magnesia)				Do not use in renal failure	Dose for decontamination: 4 mL/kg - 300 mL/dose 250 mL/kg - 30 g Do not use if botulism is suspected
Magnesium sulfate (Epsom salts)				Hypermagnesemia with multiple doses (99 mg or 8.1 mEq of magnesium/g). Vomiting at doses >250 mg/kg may occur.	Calcium gluconate (1 mL/kg of a 10% solution) can be given for magnesium intoxication Dose for gastric decontamination: 250 mg/kg (pediatric); 20-30 g (adult)
Sodium phosphate/ biphosphate enema (Fleet® Enema)	2-15 min	Colon		Can cause hypocalcemia	Do not use in children. Contraindicated in ethylene glycol ingestions
Sodium sulfate	0.5-3 h	Small and large intestine		Do not use in patient with congestive heart failure; hypernatremia may develop	Useful for barium ingestions to convert to nonabsorbable barium sulfate. Dose 250 mg/kg (pediatric); 15-20 g (adult)
Surfactants/Stool Softener					
Docusate (Colace®)	24-72 h	Small and large intestine	Detergent activity; facilitates admixture of fat and water to soften stool	Excreted in breast milk and bile	Due to slow onset, not used in gastric decontamination

MANAGEMENT OF DRUG EXTRAVASATIONS

Vesicant: An agent that causes tissue destruction.	
Irritant: An agent that causes aching, tightness, and phlebitis with or without inflammation.	
Extravasation: Unintentional leakage of fluid out of a blood vessel into surrounding tissue.	
Vesicant extravasation: Leakage of a drug that causes pain, necrosis, or tissue sloughing.	
Delayed extravasation: Symptoms occur 48 hours, or later, after drug administration.	
Flare: Local, nonpainful, possibly allergic reaction often accompanied by reddening along the vein.	

A potential, and potentially highly morbid, complication of drug therapy is soft tissue damage caused by leakage of the drug solution out of the vein. A variety of complications, including erythema, ulceration, pain, tissue sloughing, and necrosis are possible. This problem is not unique to antineoplastic therapy; a variety of drugs have been reported to cause tissue damage if extravasated. See table.

Vesicant Agents			
Hyperosmotic Agents (>280 mOsmol/L)	**Ischemia Inducers**	**Direct Cellular Toxins**	
		Nonantineoplastic Agents	**Antineoplastic Agents**
Calcium chloride (>10%)	Aminophylline	Chlordiazepoxide	Amsacrine[1]
Calcium gluconate	Dobutamine	Diazepam	Dactinomycin
Calcium gluceptate	Dopamine	Digoxin	Daunorubicin
Contrast media	Epinephrine	Ethanol	Doxorubicin
Crystalline amino acids (4.25%)	Esmolol	Nafcillin	Epirubicin
Dextrose (>10%)	Metaraminol	Nitroglycerin	Esorubicin[1]
Mannitol (>5%)	Metoprolol	Phenytoin	Idarubicin
Potassium acetate (>2 mEq/mL)	Norepinephrine	Propylene glycol	Mechlorethamine
Potassium chloride (>2 mEq/mL)	Phenylephrine	Sodium thiopental	Mitomycin
Sodium bicarbonate (≥8.4%)	Vasopressin	Tetracycline	Streptozocin (?)
Sodium chloride (>1%)			Valrubicin
Thiopentone			Vinblastine
Urea (30%)			Vincristine
			Vindesine[1]
			Vinorelbine

In addition to the known vesicants, a number of other antineoplastic agents, not generally considered to be vesicants, have been associated with isolated reports of tissue damage following extravasation.

Agents Associated With Occasional Extravasation Reactions

Aclarubicin[1]
Arsenic trioxide
Bleomycin
Carboplatin ≥10 mg/mL
Carmustine
Cisplatin
Cyclophosphamide
Dacarbazine
Daunorubicin citrate (liposomal)
Dexrazoxane

Docetaxel
Doxorubicin (liposomal)
Etoposide
Floxuridine
Fluorouracil
Gemcitabine
Gemtuzumab
Ifosfamide
Irinotecan
Menogaril[1]

Mitoxantrone	Teniposide
Oxaliplatin	Topotecan
Paclitaxel	

[1]Not commercially available in the U.S.

The actual incidence of drug extravasations is unknown. Some of the uncertainty stems from varying definitions of incidence. Incidence rates have been reported based on total number of drug doses administered, number of vesicant doses administered, number of treatments, number of patients treated with vesicants, and total number of patients treated. Most estimates place the incidence of extravasations with cytotoxic agents in the range of 0.6% to 6%.

The optimal treatment of drug extravasations is uncertain. A variety of antidotes have been proposed; however, objective clinical evidence to support these recommendations frequently is not available. There are no well-done randomized prospective trials of potential treatments. Controlled clinical trials are not feasible, limiting efforts to identify optimal management of these reactions. Extant reports are based on animal models, anecdotal cases, and/or small uncontrolled series of patients. Many of the existing reports, both animal and human, used more than one therapeutic intervention simultaneously, adding to the difficulty of identifying the efficacy of any single approach.

The best "treatment" for extravasation reactions is prevention. Although it is not possible to prevent all accidents, a few simple precautions can minimize the risk to the patient. The vein used should be a large, intact vessel with good blood flow. To minimize the risk of dislodging the catheter, veins in the hands and in the vicinity of joints (eg, antecubital) should be avoided. Veins in the forearm (ie, the basilic, cephalic, and median antebrachial, basilic and cephalic) are usually good options for peripheral infusions. Prior to drug administration, the patency of the I.V. line should be verified. The line should be flushed with 5-10 mL of a saline or dextrose solution and should be flushed with I.V. fluids every 2-3 minutes between a bolus injection and again at the end of administration, and the drug(s) infused through the side of a free-flowing isotonic saline or dextrose infusion.

A frequently recommended precaution against drug extravasation is the use of a central venous catheter. Use of a central line has several advantages, including high patient satisfaction, reliable venous access, high flow rates, and rapid dilution of the drug. A wide variety of devices are readily available. Many institutions encourage or require use of a vascular access device for administration of vesicant agents.

Despite their benefit, central lines are not an absolute solution. Vascular access devices are subject to a number of complications. The catheter tip may not be properly positioned in the superior vena cava/right atrium, or may migrate out of position. Additionally, these catheters require routine care to maintain patency and avoid infections. Finally, extravasation of drugs from venous access devices is possible. Misplacement/ migration of the catheter tip, improper placement of the needle in accessing injection ports, and cuts, punctures, or rupture of the catheter itself have all been reported. Reports of extravasation from central catheters range from 0.3% to 50%, and are similar to extravasation rates reported from peripheral lines.

When a drug extravasation does occur, a variety of immediate actions have been recommended. Although there is considerable uncertainty regarding the value of some potential treatments, a few initial steps seem to be generally accepted.

1. **Stop the infusion.** At the first suspicion of infiltration, the drug infusion should be stopped. If infiltration is not certain, the line can be tested by attempting to aspirate blood, and careful infusion of a few milliliters of saline or dextrose solution.

2. **Do NOT remove the catheter/needle.** The infiltrated catheter should not be removed immediately. It should be left in place to facilitate aspiration of fluid from the extravasation site with a small (1-3 mL) syringe, and, if appropriate, administration of an antidote directly into the extravasation site.

3. **Aspirate fluid.** To the extent possible, the extravasated drug solution should be removed from the subcutaneous tissues.

4. **Do NOT flush the line.** Flooding the infiltration site with saline or dextrose in an attempt to dilute the drug solution generally is not recommended. Rather than minimizing damage, such a procedure may have the opposite effect by distributing the vesicant solution over a wider area.

5. **Remove the catheter/needle.** If an antidote is not going to be injected into the extravasation site, the infiltrated catheter should be removed. If an antidote is to be injected into the area, it should be injected through the catheter to ensure delivery of the antidote to the infiltration site. When this has been accomplished, the catheter should then be removed. Consider photographing the area to monitor at 1 day, 1 week, and every week thereafter.

Two issues for which there is less consensus are the application of heat or cold, and the use of various antidotes. A variety of recommendations exist for each of these concerns; there is no consensus concerning the proper approach.

Cold. Intermittent cooling of the area of infiltration results in vasoconstriction, which tends to restrict the spread of the drug. It may also inhibit the local effects of some drugs (eg, anthracyclines). Application of cold is usually recommended as immediate treatment for most drug extravasations, except the vinca alkaloids. In one report of antineoplastic drug extravasation treatment, almost 90% of the extravasations treated only with topical cold required no further therapy.

The largest single published series of antineoplastic drug extravasations was 175 patients reported by Larson in 1985. This series includes some of the more commonly used vesicants, including the anthracyclines, mechlorethamine, mitomycin, and the vinca alkaloids. For 119 patients, local application of cold (15 minutes four times a day for 3 days) and close observation was the sole treatment. The remaining 56 patients received a variety of antidotes. In 89% of the patients treated with cold alone, the extravasation resolved without further treatment. Of the patients treated by other methods, only 53% resolved without further treatment.

Helpful as it may be, Larson's report does have some limitations. Agents such as the epipodophyllotoxins and taxanes which are occasionally associated with soft tissue damage were not included, nor were extravasations of nonantineoplastic agents mentioned. The report included infiltrations of the vinca alkaloids, even though the literature recommends use of heat to treat these. Also, except for doxorubicin extravasations in the group treated with ice and observation, responses for the individual drugs were not indicated. In this group, 72% of the doxorubicin extravasations resolved completely.

Heat. Application of heat results in a localized vasodilation and increased blood flow. Increased circulation is believed to facilitate removal of the drug from the area of infiltration. The data supporting use of heat are less convincing than for cold. One report of the application of heat for nonantineoplastic drug extravasations suggested application of heat increased the risk of skin maceration and necrosis. Most data are from animal studies, with relatively few human case reports. Animal models indicate application of heat exacerbates the damage from anthracycline extravasations. No large series of extravasations managed with the application of heat has been published. Heat is generally recommended for treatment for vinca alkaloid extravasations; a few reports recommend it for treatment of amino acid solutions, aminophylline, calcium, contrast media, dextrose, mannitol, nafcillin, paclitaxel, phenytoin, podophyllotoxin, potassium, and vinca alkaloid infiltrations. There are conflicting reports on the initial management of paclitaxel infiltrations.

For some agents, such as cisplatin, epipodophyllotoxins, mechlorethamine, and paclitaxel, there are conflicting recommendations. Some reports recommend application of cold, others recommend heat. At least one report suggests neither cold nor heat is effective for paclitaxel extravasations.

Antidotes

A very wide variety of agents have been reported as possible antidotes for extravasated drugs, with no consensus on their proper use. For a number of reasons, evaluation of the various reports is difficult.

1. **Mechanism of action.** For many drugs, the underlying mechanism responsible for the tissue damage is not certain. For some of the antidotes, the purported mechanism of action of the antidote is also unclear.
2. **Controlled trials.** Prospective, randomized controlled trials are not practical. Information concerning treatment of extravasations is based almost exclusively on animal models, anecdotal reports, and small, uncontrolled studies.
3. **Outcome definitions.** Published reports use a number of different end-points and outcomes to define efficacy of a given treatment.
4. **Confounding factors.** A number of confounding factors exist which make assessment of various antidotes difficult. Among these are:
   a. *Response to nonpharmacologic therapy.* Application of heat or cold alone, especially the latter, appears to have a significant protective effect.
   b. *Multiple therapies.* A number of reports used more than one therapeutic modality to treat drug extravasations. In many cases, cold or heat is applied along with the antidote. In some cases, more than one antidote is used, sometimes in conjunction with heat or cold. Use of multiple approaches further complicates the determination of the possible effect of a particular antidote, or the additive effect of various combinations.

c. *Variable applications.* For some proposed antidotes, a wide variety of different doses, concentrations, methods of application, and duration of therapy have been reported, making determination of the optimal treatment regimen difficult.

Agents Used as Antidotes

Albumin	Hyyperbaric oxygen
Antihistamines	Iron dextran
Antioxidants	Isoproterenol
Beta-adrenergics	Nitroglycerin paste
Carnitine	Phentolamine
Corticosteroids[1]	Radical dimer
Dexrazoxane	Saline
Dextranomer	Sodium bicarbonate
Dimethyl sulfoxide (99%)	Sodium hypochlorite
Dopamine	Sodium thiosulfate[1]
Fluorescein	Terbutaline
Hyaluronidase[1]	Vitamin E

[1]Listed in the package insert of at least one agent.

Sodium bicarbonate. An 8.4% solution of sodium bicarbonate was briefly recommended for treatment of anthracycline extravasations. The recommendation was based on a case report of its use in a single patient. The proposed mechanism of action was that the high pH of the bicarbonate solution would break the glycosidic bond of the anthracycline, thereby inactivating it. Follow-up studies in a variety of animal models failed to confirm the original report. Also, the concentrated sodium bicarbonate may itself be a vesicant. At present, most reviews and guidelines discourage its use for treating extravasations.

Corticosteroids. Steroids are most commonly used to treat anthracycline extravasations. Hydrocortisone is the steroid most frequently recommended, although dexamethasone has also been used. It is suggested that steroids reduce local inflammation from the extravasated drug. Such activity has not been confirmed; nor has it been demonstrated that the tissue damage from drug infiltrations is the result of an inflammatory process. Interpretation of steroid efficacy is complicated by the multiple doses, routes of administration, duration of therapy, and outcome measurements used. Reports of animal trials offer little additional information, being plagued by many of the limitations of the clinical case reports. The official labeling of only one of the three suppliers of doxorubicin includes a steroid as part of the treatment for drug extravasations. The product labeling from two doxorubicin suppliers (as well as the suppliers of daunorubicin, idarubicin, and liposome-encapsulated daunorubicin and doxorubicin) do not mention corticosteroids to treat drug infiltrations. Most reports question the efficacy of steroids for treatment of drug extravasations; they are not recommended by most guidelines.

Dexrazoxane. Dexrazoxane, a derivative of EDTA, is an intracellular chelating agent often used as a cardioprotective agent in patients receiving anthracycline therapy. It is believed that dexrazoxane's cardioprotective effect is a result by chelating iron following intracellular hydrolysis. Dexrazoxane is not an effective chelator itself, but is hydrolyzed intracellularly to an open-ring chelator form, which complexes with iron, other heavy metals, and doxorubicin complexes to inhibit the generation of free radicals. It has been postulated that dexrazoxane's chelating effect, or its ability to inhibit topoisomerase II, may be useful in preventing tissue damage from anthracycline infiltrations. There have been individual case reports of dexrazoxane being used to reduce tissue damage after extravasation of doxorubicin and epirubicin. Tests in mice suggest it might also be effective for treatment of daunorubicin and idarubicin.

Dimethyl sulfoxide (DMSO). A number of reports have suggested application of DMSO is an effective treatment for infiltrations of a number of different drugs. It is believed DMSO's protective effect is due to its ability to act as a free radical scavenger (one theory suggests tissue damage from vesicants, particularly anthracyclines, is due to formation of hydroxyl free radicals). Results in animal models have been equivocal, with some reports indicating DMSO is beneficial, and some showing little or no effect. Clinical reports of its use are extremely difficult to interpret due to variations in DMSO concentration, number of applications/day, duration of therapy, and concomitant treatments. A number of different treatments, including cold, steroids, vitamin E, and sodium bicarbonate have been used in conjunction with DMSO. Also, most reports that suggest DMSO is effective in preventing tissue damage used DMSO concentrations >90%, which is not available for clinical use in the United States.

A further complication to interpretation of DMSO's efficacy is that some series included infiltrations of agents not generally considered to be vesicants. The largest clinical series included infiltrations in 75 patients; but only 31 of the extravasations involved vesicants (doxorubicin, epirubicin, or mitomycin). The remaining incidents involved drugs not usually associated with tissue damage (cisplatin, ifosfamide, and mitoxantrone). Application of 99% DMSO for 7 days and cold for 3 days resulted in a 93.5% success rate in the patients with vesicant extravasations. Only two patients (6.5%) had complications requiring further therapy. Whether the addition of DMSO represented a real improvement over cold alone is difficult to assess.

Hyaluronidase. Hyaluronidase is an enzyme that destroys hyaluronic acid, an essential component of connective tissue. This results in increased permeability of the tissue, facilitating diffusion and absorption of fluids. It is postulated that increasing the diffusion of extravasated fluids results in more rapid absorption, thereby limiting tissue damage. In individual case reports, hyaluronidase has been reported effective in preventing tissue damage from a wide variety of agents, including amino acid solutions, aminophylline, calcium, contrast media, dextrose, mannitol, nafcillin, phenytoin, potassium, and vinca alkaloids. Other reports suggest it might also be useful in managing extravasations of epipodophyllotoxins and taxanes, although not all guidelines recommend its use for these agents.

Phentolamine. Phentolamine is an alpha$_1$ adrenergic antagonist which produces peripheral vasodilation. It has been reported to reduce tissue necrosis following extravasation of pressor (vasoconstrictor) agents such as dobutamine, dopamine, epinephrine and norepinephrine.

Sodium thiosulfate. A freshly prepared $^1/_6$ M ($\sim$4%) solution of sodium thiosulfate has been recommended for treatment of mechlorethamine and cisplatin infiltrations. A 2% solution has been recommended for doxorubicin, epirubicin, mitomycin, and vinblastine extravasations. This recommendation is based on *in vitro* data demonstrating an interaction between sodium thiosulfate and cisplatin, dacarbazine, and mechlorethamine; and very limited animal data on thiosulfate's ability to inactivate dacarbazine and mechlorethamine. At present, no clinical reports of its efficacy for treating cisplatin or dacarbazine extravasations have been published. Since cisplatin and dacarbazine are generally not considered to be vesicants, the use of thiosulfate to treat infiltrations of these drugs may not be required.

The use of sodium thiosulfate to treat mechlorethamine infiltrations is based almost exclusively on the *in vitro* and animal data. A single case report of successful thiosulfate treatment of an accidental intramuscular mechlorethamine injection has been published. Thus far, no reports of thiosulfate treatment of mechlorethamine infiltrations have been published.

One study of thiosulfate therapy of antineoplastic drug extravasations has been published. In a series of 63 patients with extravasation of doxorubicin, epirubicin, mitomycin, or vinblastine, 31 were treated with subcutaneous hydrocortisone and topical dexamethasone. The remaining 32 patients received subcutaneous injection of a 2% thiosulfate solution in addition to the subcutaneous and topical steroids. No patient in either group developed skin ulceration or required surgery; but the patients who received the thiosulfate healed in about half the time as the patients who received only the steroid therapy.

Reported Treatment Regimens for Drug Extravasations

Treatment	Dose	Route	Duration	Concomitant Therapy	Used to Treat	Preparation	Administration
Cold[1]	15 min qid	Topical	3-4 days	None	All agents[2]	N/A	N/A
Heat[1]	15 min on; 15 min off	Topical	1 day	None	Vinca alkaloids	N/A	N/A
Heat[1]	NS	Topical	NS	None	Epipodophyllotoxins, taxanes[3]	N/A	N/A
Dexrazoxane (within 5 hours of extravasation)	1000 mg/m^2 500 mg/m^2	I.V.	Days 1 and 2 Day 3	Cold	Daunorubicin, doxorubicin, epirubicin, idarubicin	NS	NS
Dexrazoxane	1000 mg	I.V.	Day 1	Cold, DMSO, topical hydrocortisone	Epirubicin	NS	NS
Dexamethasone	4 mg	SubQ, I.D.	One time	Cold	Daunorubicin, doxorubicin	NS	Inject into several sites surrounding the area of extravasation
Dimethyl sulfoxide[4]	50%-99% q2-4h	Topical	3 days	Dexamethasone 8 mg I.D.	Doxorubicin	N/A	N/A
Dimethyl sulfoxide[4]	70% q3-4h	Topical	10 days	Sodium bicarbonate SubQ, dexamethasone 4 mg SubQ	Daunorubicin	N/A	N/A
Dimethyl sulfoxide[4]	90% q12h	Topical	2 days	Vitamin E 10% topical	Doxorubicin, esorubicin, mitomycin	N/A	N/A
Dimethyl sulfoxide[4]	99% q8h for up to 1 week	Topical	1 week	Cold for 3 days	Doxorubicin, mitomycin, mitoxantrone	N/A	Apply 4 drops/10 cm^2 of skin surface over an area twice the size of the extravasation; allow to air dry without dressings
Dimethyl sulfoxide[4]	99% q2-4h	Topical	3 days	None	Doxorubicin	N/A	N/A
Dimethyl sulfoxide[4]	99% q6-24h	Topical	14 days	None	Doxorubicin, daunorubicin	N/A	N/A
Dimethyl sulfoxide[4]	99% q6-8h	SubQ	Until resolution	None	Mitomycin	N/A	N/A
Hyaluronidase[1]	15 units	SubQ	One time	Heat	Amino acid solutions, aminophylline, calcium, contrast media[5], dextrose, mannitol, nafcillin, phenytoin, potassium, vinca alkaloids	Reconstitute vial with NS to a concentration of 150 units/mL. Dilute 0.1 mL (15 units) with 0.9 mL NS for a final concentration of 15 units/mL	4-5 injections (0.2 mL) into area of extravasation
Hyaluronidase[1]	150 units	SubQ	One time	Heat	Amino acid solutions, aminophylline, calcium, contrast media[5], dextrose, mannitol, nafcillin, phenytoin, potassium, vinca alkaloids	Reconstitute with 1 mL NS	5-10 injections (0.5-1 mL) into area of extravasation

Reported Treatment Regimens for Drug Extravasations (*Continued*)

Treatment	Dose	Route	Duration	Concomitant Therapy	Used to Treat	Preparation	Administration
Hyaluronidase[1]	250 units	SubQ	One time	None	Amino acid solutions, aminophylline, calcium, contrast media[5], dextrose, mannitol, nafcillin, phenytoin, potassium, vinca alkaloids	Reconstitute with 6 mL NS	Inject directly through the original needle; **OR** 6 SubQ injections into area of extravasation
Hydrocortisone	50-200 mg	I.V., SubQ, I.D.	NS	Cold	All agents *except vinca alkaloids*	NS	Inject into several sites surrounding the area of extravasation
Hydrocortisone	500 mg	SubQ	One time	Betamethasone and gentamicin ointment q12h for 2 days, then qd	Doxorubicin, epirubicin, vinblastine, mitomycin	500 mg in 10 mL NS	Inject at 1 cm intervals around the area of extravasation
Nitroglycerin paste	NS	Topical	NS	NS	Vasopressors (dobutamine, dopamine, epinephrine, norepinephrine, phenylephrine)	N/A	N/A
Phentolamine	5 mg	SubQ	1 day	None	Vasopressors (dobutamine, dopamine, epinephrine, norepinephrine, phenylephrine)	Mix 5 mg with 9 mL NS	Inject a small amount into extravasated area. Blanching should reverse immediately. If blanching should recur, additional injections may be needed
Sodium thiosulfate[1,5]	2%	SubQ	One time	Hydrocortisone 500 mg SubQ, betamethasone and gentamicin ointment q12h for 2 days, then qd	Doxorubicin, epirubicin, vinblastine, mitomycin	NS	Inject at 1 cm intervals around the area of extravasation
Sodium thiosulfate[1]	$\frac{1}{6}$ M (~4%)	I.V., SubQ	One time	Ice or heat	Mechlorethamine, cisplatin	Mix 4 mL of 10% sodium thiosulfate with 6 mL sterile water	Inject 2 mL for each 1 mg of mechlorethamine or 100 mg of cisplatin
Terbutaline	1 mg	SubQ	NS	NS	Vasopressors (dobutamine, dopamine, epinephrine, norepinephrine, phenylephrine)	NS	NS

N/A = Not applicable; NS = Not specified; I.V. = Intravenous; SubQ = Subcutaneous; I.D. = Intradermal.

[1]Listed in the package insert of at least one product.

[2]Most guidelines discourage application of cold to treat infiltrations of vinca alkaloids. Some reports discourage its use to treat infiltrations of epipodophyllotoxins and/or taxanes.

[3]There are conflicting data on the efficacy of heat or cold for infiltrations of epipodophyllotoxins and taxanes. Each approach has been reported to be effective, harmful, and of no discernable effect.

[4]DMSO concentrations >50% are not available for human use in the U.S.

[5]Large extravasations only.

Selected Readings

Bertelli G, "Prevention and Management of Extravasation of Cytotoxic Drugs," *Drug Safety*, 1995, 12(4): 245-55.

Boyle DM and Engelking C, "Vesicant Extravasation: Myths and Realities," *Oncol Nurs Forum*, 1995, 22(1):57-67.

deLemo ML and Walliser S, "Management of Extravasation of Exaliplatin," *J Oncol Pharm Pract*, 2005, 11(4):159-62.

Ener RA, Meglathery SB, and Styler M, "Extravasation of Systemic Hemato-Oncological Therpaies," *Ann Oncol*, 2004, 15:858-62.

Goolsby TV and Lombardo FA, "Extravasation of Chemotherapeutic Agents: Prevention and Treatment," *Semin Oncol*, 2006, 33(1):139-43.

Kurul S, Saip P, and Aydin T, "Totally Implantable Venous-Access Ports: Local Problems and Extravasation Injury," *Lancet Oncol*, 2002, 3(11):684-92.

Larson DL, "What Is the Appropriate Management of Tissue Extravasation by Antitumor Agents?" *J Plast Reconstr Surg*, 1985, 75(3):397-402.

Larson DL, "Treatment of Tissue Extravasation by Antitumor Agents," *Cancer*, 1982, 49(9):1796-9.

Larson DL, "Alterations in Wound Healing Secondary to Infusion Injury," *Clin Plast Surg*, 1990, 17(3): 509-17.

Luke E, "Mitoxantrone-Induced Extravasation," *Oncol Nurs Forum*, 2005, 32(1):27-9.

MacCara ME, "Extravasation: A Hazard of Intravenous Therapy," *Drug Intell Clin Pharm*, 1983, 17(10):713-7.

Salameh Y and Shoufani A, "Full-Thickness Skin Necrosis After Arginine Extravasation - A Case Report and Review of the Literature," *J Pediatr Surg*, 2004, 39(4):e9-11.

Schrijvers DL, "Extravasation: A Dreaded Complication of Chemotherapy," *Ann Oncol*, 2003, 14(Suppl 3): iii26-30.

Schulmeister L and Camp-Sorrell D, "Chemotherapy Extravasation from Implanted Ports," *Oncol Nurs Forum*, 2000, 27(3):531-8.

Tran DE QH and Finlayson RJ, "Use of Stellate Ganglion Block to Salvage an Ischemic Hand Caused by the Extravasation of Vasopressors," *Reg Anesth Pain Med*, 2005, 30(4):405-8.

MATERNAL-FETAL TOXICOLOGY

Drugs and Chemicals Proven to Be Teratogenic in Humans

Drug/Chemical	Fetal Adverse Effects	Relative Risk for Teratogenicity	Clinical Intervention
Alcohol	**Fetal alcohol syndrome:** Mental retardation, microcephaly, poor coordination, hypotonia, hyperactivity, short upturned nose, micrognathia or retrognathia (infancy) or prognathia (adolescence), short palpebral fissures, hypoplastic philtrum, thinned upper lips, microphthalmia, antenatal/postnatal growth retardation, occasional pathologies of eyes, mouth, heart, kidneys, gonads, skin, muscle, and skeleton	In alcoholic women consuming >2 g/kg/d ethanol over first trimester: 2- to 3-fold higher risk for congenital malformations (about 10%)	To calculate accurate dose of alcohol: **Prospective:** To discontinue exposure; if woman is alcoholic, refer to addiction center **During pregnancy:** To alleviate fears in mild or occasional drinkers who may terminate pregnancy based on unrealistic perception of risk, level 2 ultrasound to rule out visible malformation
Alkylating agents (busulfan, chlorambucil, cyclophosphamide, mechlorethamine)	Growth retardation, cleft palate, microphthalmia hypoplastic ovaries, cloudy corneas, agenesis of kidney, malformations of digits, cardiac defects, multiple other anomalies	Based on case reports, between 10% and 50% of cases were malformed for different drugs. It is possible that adverse outcome was overrepresented	Level 2 ultrasound to rule out visible malformations. Supplement folic acid to women receiving antifolates (eg, methotrexate)
Antimetabolite agents (aminopterin azauridine, cytarabine, 5-FU, 6-MP, methotrexate)	Hydrocephalus, meningoencephalocele, anencephaly, malformed skull, cerebral hypoplasia, growth retardation, eye and ear malformations, malformed nose and cleft palate, malformed extremities and fingers **Aminopterin syndrome:** Cranial dysostosis, hydrocephalus, hypertelorism, anomalies of external ear, micrognathia, posterior cleft palate	Based on case reports 7%-75% of cases were malformed. It is possible that adverse outcome was overrepresented	Level 2 ultrasound to rule out visible malformations
Carbamazepine	Increased risk for neural tube defects (NTDs)	NTDs estimated at 1% with carbamazepine	Periconceptional folate; maternal and/or amniotic α-fetoprotein; ultrasound to rule out NTD
Carbon monoxide	Cerebral atrophy, mental retardation, microcephaly, convulsions, spastic disorders, intrauterine or postnatal death	Based on case reports, when mother is severely poisoned, high risk for neurological sequelae; no increased risk in mild accidental exposures	Measure maternal carboxyhemoglobin levels. Treat with 100% oxygen for 5 hours after maternal carboxyhemoglobin returns to normal because fetal equilibration takes longer If hyperbaric chamber available, should be used, as elimination half-life of CO is more rapid Fetal monitoring by an obstetrician; sonographic follow-up
Coumadin®	**Fetal warfarin syndrome:** Nasal hypoplasia, chondrodysplasia punctata, branchydactyly, skull defects, abnormal ears, malformed eyes, CNS malformations, microcephaly, hydrocephalus, skeletal deformities, mental retardation, optic atrophy, spasticity, Dandy Walker malformations	16% of exposed fetuses have malformation; another 3% hemorrhages; 8% stillbirths	**Prospective:** Switch to heparin for the first trimester. Deliver by a cesarean section. Women should be followed up in a high-risk perinatal unit
Diethylstilbestrol (DES)	**Female offspring:** Clear cell vaginal or cervical adenocarcinoma in young female adults exposed in utero (before 18th week); irregular menses (oligomenorrhea), reduced pregnancy rates, increased rate of preterm deliveries, increased perinatal mortality and spontaneous abortion **Male offspring:** Cysts of epididymis, cryptorchidism, hypogonadism, diminished spermatogenesis	Exposure before 18 weeks of gestation: ≤1.4/1000 of exposed female with carcinoma. Congenital morphological changes in vaginal epithelium in 39% of exposures	**Diagnosis:** Direct observation of mucosa and Shiller's test **Treatment:** Mechanical excision or destruction in relatively confined area. Surgery and radiotherapy for diffused tumor

Drugs and Chemicals Proven to Be Teratogenic in Humans (*Continued*)

Drug/Chemical	Fetal Adverse Effects	Relative Risk for Teratogenicity	Clinical Intervention
Lead	Lower scores in developmental tests	Higher risk when maternal lead is >10 mcg/dL	**Maternal lead levels >10 mcg/dL:** Investigate for possible source of contamination **Levels >25 mcg/dL:** Consider chelation
Lithium carbonate	Possibly higher risk for Ebstein's anomaly; no detectable higher risk for other malformations		Women who need lithium should continue therapy, with sonographic follow-up. Patients may need higher doses because of increased clearance rate.
Methyl mercury, mercuric sulfide	Microcephaly, eye malformations, cerebral palsy, mental retardation, malocclusion of teeth	Women of affected babies consumed 9-27 ppm mercury; greater risk when ingested at 6-8 gestational months. Relative risk was not elucidated, but 13/220 babies born in Minamata, Japan, at time of contamination had severe disease	Good correlation between mercury concentrations in maternal hair follicles and neurological outcome of the fetus. Hair mercury content >50 ppm was used successfully as a cut point for termination In acute poisoning, the fetus is 4-10 times more sensitive than the adult to methylmercury toxicity
PCBs	**Stillbirth** **Signs at birth:** White eye discharge, 30% (32/108); teeth present, 8.7% (11/127); irritated/swollen gums, 11% (11/99); hyperpigmentation ("cola" staining), 42.5% (54/127); deformed/small nails, 24.6% (30/122); acne, 12.8% (16/125) **Subsequent history:** Bronchitis or pneumonia, 27.2% (30/124); chipped or broken teeth, 35.5% (38/107); hair loss, 12.2% (14/115); acne scars, 9.6% (11/115); generalized itching, 27.8% (32/1150) **Developmental:** Do not meet milestones; lower scores than unexposed controls; evidence of CNS damage	4%-20% (6/159-8/39)	These figures, which are from cases poisoned by high consumption of PCB-contaminated rice oil, cannot be extrapolated to cases in which maternal poisoning has not been verified Women working near PCBs (eg, hydroelectric facilities) should use effective protection
Penicillamine	Skin hyperelastosis	Few case reports; risk unknown	
Phenytoin	**Fetal hydantoin syndrome:** Low nasal bridge, inner epicanthal folds, ptosis, strabismus, hypertelorism, low set or abnormal ears, wide mouth, large fontanels, anomalies and hypoplasia of distal phalanges and nails, skeletal abnormalities, microcephaly and mental retardation, growth deficiency, neuroblastoma, cardiac defects, cleft palate/lip	5%-10% of typical syndrome; about 30% of partial picture Relative risk of 7 for offspring IQ ≤84	Neurologist should consider changing to other medications. Keep phenytoin concentrations at lower effective levels. Level 2 ultrasound to rule out visible malformations, vitamin K to neonate. Epilepsy itself increases teratogenic risk
Systemic retinoids (isotretinoin, etretinate)	Spontaneous abortions; deformities of cranium, ears, face, heart, limbs, liver; hydrocephalus, microcephalus, heart defects. Cognitive defects even without dysmorphology	For isotretinoin: 38% risk. 80% of malformation are CNS	Treated women should have an effective method of contraception. Pregnancy termination. If diagnosed too late, sonographic follow-up to rule out confirmed malformations
Tetracycline	Yellow, gray-brown, or brown staining of deciduous teeth, destruction of enamel	From 4 months of gestation and on, occurs in 50% of fetuses exposed to tetracycline; 12.5% to oxytetracycline	If exposure before 14-16 weeks of gestation, no known risk
Thalidomide	Limb phocomelia, amelia, hypoplasia, congenital heart defects, renal malformations, cryptorchidism, abducens paralysis, deafness, microtia, anotia	About 20% risk when exposure to drug occurs in days 34-50 of gestation	Thalidomide is an effective drug for some forms of leprosy. Treated women should have an effective mode of contraception

Drugs and Chemicals Proven to Be Teratogenic in Humans (*Continued*)

Drug/Chemical	Fetal Adverse Effects	Relative Risk for Teratogenicity	Clinical Intervention
Trimethadione	**Fetal trimethadione syndrome:** Intrauterine growth retardation, cardiac anomalies, microcephaly, cleft palate and lip, abnormal ears, dysmorphic face, mental retardation, tracheoesophageal fistula, postnatal death	Based on case reports: 83% risk; 32% infantile or neonatal death	No need for this antiepileptic to date
Valproic acid	Lumbosacral spina bifida with meningomyelocele; CNS defects, microcephaly, cardiac defects	1.2% risk of neural tube defects	Level 2 ultrasound and maternal α-fetoproteins or amniocentesis to rule out neural tube defects. Epilepsy itself increases teratogenic risk

Reprinted with permission from "Drugs and Chemicals Proven to Be Teratogenic in Humans," *Maternal-Fetal Toxicology: A Clinician's Guide*, 2nd ed, Koren G, ed, New York, NY: Marcel Dekker, Inc, 1994, 37-43.

MERCURY LEVELS IN COMMERCIAL FISH AND SHELLFISH

Fish and Shellfish With Lower Levels of Mercury						
Species	Mercury Concentration (PPM)					No. of Samples
	Mean	Median	STDEV	Min	Max	
Anchovies	0.043	N/A	N/A	ND	0.340	40
Butterfish	0.058	N/A	N/A	ND	0.360	89
Catfish	0.049	ND	0.084	ND	0.314	23
Clam*	ND	ND	ND	ND	ND	6
Cod	0.095	0.087	0.080	ND	0.420	39
Crab (includes blue, king, and snow)	0.060	0.030	0.112	ND	0.610	63
Crawfish	0.033	0.035	0.012	ND	0.051	44
Croaker Atlantic (Atlantic)	0.072	0.073	0.036	0.013	0.148	35
Flatfish* (includes flounder, plaice, and sole)	0.045	0.035	0.049	ND	0.180	23
Haddock (Atlantic)	0.031	0.041	0.021	ND	0.041	4
Hake	0.014	ND	0.021	ND	0.048	9
Herring	0.044	N/A	N/A	ND	0.135	38
Jacksmelt	0.108	0.060	0.115	0.040	0.500	16
Lobster (Spiny)	0.09	0.14	Standard deviation data generated for new data 2004 or later only	ND	0.27	9
Mackeral Atlantic (N. Atlantic)	0.050	N/A	N/A	0.020	0.160	80
Mackeral Chub (Pacific)	0.088	N/A	N/A	0.030	0.190	30
Mullet	0.046	N/A	N/A	ND	0.130	191
Oyster	0.013	ND	0.042	ND	0.250	38
Perch Ocean*	ND	ND	ND	ND	0.030	6
Pollock	0.041	ND	0.106	ND	0.780	62
Salmon (canned)*	ND	ND	ND	ND	ND	23
Salmon (fresh/frozen)*	0.014	ND	0.041	ND	0.190	34
Sardine	0.016	0.013	0.007	0.004	0.035	29
Scallop	0.050	N/A	N/A	ND	0.220	66
Shad American	0.065	N/A	N/A	ND	0.220	59
Shrimp*	ND	ND	ND	ND	0.050	24
Squid	0.070	N/A	N/A	ND	0.400	200
Tilapia*	0.010	ND	0.023	ND	0.070	9
Trout (freshwater)	0.072	0.025	0.143	ND	0.678	34
Tuna (canned, light)	0.118	0.075	0.119	ND	0.852	347
Whitefish	0.069	0.054	0.067	ND	0.310	28
Whiting	ND	ND	Standard deviation data generated for new data 2004 or later only	ND	ND	2

Mercury was measured as total mercury except for species (*) when only methylmercury was analyzed.

ND: Mercury concentration below detection level (Level of Detection (LOD) = 0.01 ppm).

N/A: Data not available.

Source of data: FDA Monitoring Program, 1990-2004; Hall, RA, Zook, EG, and Meaburn, GM, "National Marine Fisheries Service Survey of Trace Elements in the Fishery Resource" 1978; Ache, BW, "The Occurrence of Mercy in the Fishery Resources of the Gulf of Mexico," 2000.

Mercury Levels of Other Fish and Shellfish

Species	Mercury Concentration (PPM)					No. of Samples
	Mean	Median	STDEV	Min	Max	
Bass (Saltwater, black, striped) (includes sea bass, striped bass, and rockfish)	0.219	0.130	0.227	ND	0.960	47
Bass Chilean	0.386	0.303	0.364	0.085	2.180	40
Bluefish	0.337	0.303	0.127	0.139	0.634	52
Buffalofish	0.19	0.14	Standard deviation data generated for new data 2004 or later only	0.05	0.43	4
Carp	0.14	0.14	Standard deviation data generated for new data 2004 or later only	0.01	0.27	2
Croaker White (Pacific)	0.287	0.280	0.069	0.180	0.410	15
Grouper (all species)	0.465	0.410	0.293	0.053	1.205	43
Halibut	0.252	0.200	0.233	ND	1.520	46
Lobster (Northern/American)	0.310	N/A	N/A	0.050	1.310	88
Lobster (species unknown)	0.169	0.182	0.089	ND	0.309	16
Mackeral Spanish (Gulf of Mexico)	0.454	N/A	N/A	0.070	1.560	66
Mackeral Spanish (So Atlantic)	0.182	N/A	N/A	0.050	0.730	43
Marlin*	0.485	0.390	0.237	0.100	0.920	16
Monkfish	0.180	N/A	N/A	0.020	1.020	81
Orange Roughy	0.554	0.563	0.148	0.296	0.855	49
Perch (freshwater)	0.14	0.15	Standard deviation data generated for new data 2004 or later only	ND	0.31	5
Sablefish	0.220	N/A	N/A	ND	0.700	102
Scorpionfish	0.286	N/A	N/A	0.020	1.345	78
Sheepshead	0.128	N/A	N/A	0.020	0.625	59
Skate	0.137	N/A	N/A	0.040	0.360	56
Snapper	0.189	0.114	0.274	ND	1.366	43
Tilefish (Atlantic)	0.144	0.099	0.122	0.042	0.533	32
Tuna (canned, albacore)	0.353	0.339	0.126	ND	0.853	399
Tuna (fresh/frozen, all)	0.383	0.322	0.269	ND	1.300	228
Tuna (fresh/frozen, bigeye)	0.639	0.560	0.184	0.410	1.040	13
Tuna (fresh/frozen, skipjack)	0.205	N/A	0.078	0.205	0.260	2
Tuna (fresh/frozen, yellowfin)	0.325	0.270	0.220	ND	1.079	87
Tuna (fresh/frozen, species unknwon)	0.414	0.339	0.316	ND	1.300	100
Weakfish (sea trout)	0.256	0.168	0.226	ND	0.744	39

Mercury was measured as total mercury except for species (*) when only methylmercury was analyzed.

ND: Mercury concentration below detection level (Level of Detection (LOD) = 0.01 ppm).

N/A: Data not available.

Source of data: FDA Monitoring Program, 1990-2004; Hall, RA, Zook, EG, and Meaburn, GM, "National Marine Fisheries Service Survey of Trace Elements in the Fishery Resource" 1978; Ache, BW, "The Occurrence of Mercy in the Fishery Resources of the Gulf of Mexico," 2000.

FDA RECOMMENDATIONS FOR CONSUMPTION OF FISH

Pregnant women and women of childbearing age should avoid consumption of:

- shark
- king mackerel
- swordfish
- tilefish

Children and nursing mothers should limit consumption to no more than ~7 ounces (one serving) per week of:

- shark
- swordfish
- other fish containing more than 1 ppm of mercury

For other types of commercially obtained fish (ie, tuna), the FDA has advised that consumption by children and pregnant women be kept at less than 12 ounces weekly. For fish caught through local rivers or streams and no local advice is given, ingestion of up to 6 ounces per week is considered "safe."

FDA advisory limit for methylmercury in commercial fish is 1 ppm (1 mcg/g).

References

http://www.cfsan.fda.gov/~dms/admehg.html

http://www.epa.gov.ost/fish

http://www.fda.gov/oc/opacom/mehgadvisory1208.html

Further information can be accessed by calling 1-888-SAFESEAFOOD.

Goldman LR and Shannon MW, Technical Report: "Mercury in the Environment: Implications for Pediatricians," *Pediatrics*, 2001, 108(1):197-205.

MILLIEQUIVALENT FOR SELECTED IONS

Approximate Milliequivalents — Weights of Selected Ions

Salt	mEq/g Salt	mg Salt/mEq
Calcium carbonate ($CaCO_3$)	20	50
Calcium chloride ($CaCl_2 \cdot 2H_2O$)	14	73
Calcium gluconate (Ca gluconate$_2 \cdot 1H_2O$)	4	224
Calcium lactate (Ca lactate$_2 \cdot 5H_2O$)	6	154
Magnesium sulfate ($MgSO_4$)	16	60
Magnesium sulfate ($MgSO_4 \cdot 7H_2O$)	8	123
Potassium acetate (K acetate)	10	98
Potassium chloride (KCl)	13	75
Potassium citrate (K_3 citrate $\cdot 1H_2O$)	9	108
Potassium iodide (KI)	6	166
Sodium bicarbonate ($NaHCO_3$)	12	84
Sodium chloride (NaCl)	17	58
Sodium citrate (Na_3 citrate $\cdot 2H_2O$)	10	98
Sodium iodide (NaI)	7	150
Sodium lactate (Na lactate)	9	112
Zinc sulfate ($ZnSO_4 \cdot 7H_2O$)	7	144

Valences and Approximate Weights of Selected Ions

Substance	Electrolyte	Valence	Ionic Wt
Calcium	Ca^{++}	2	40
Chloride	Cl^-	1	35.5
Magnesium	Mg^{++}	2	24
Phosphate	PO_4^{3-}	3	95[1]
	HPO_4^{2-}	2	96
	$H_2PO_4^-$	1	97
Potassium	K^+	1	39
Sodium	Na^+	1	23
Sulfate	SO_4^{2-}	2	96[1]

[1]The atomic weight of phosphorus is 31, and of sulfur is 32.

NARCOTIC ANALGESIC PHARMACOKINETIC PROFILE

I.V. administration is most reliable and rapid; I.M. or SubQ use may cause delayed absorption and peak effect, especially with impaired tissue perfusion. Many agents undergo a significant first-pass effect. All are metabolized by the liver and excreted primarily in urine. Meperidine is metabolized to normeperidine, a metabolite with significant pharmacologic activity. The half-life of normeperidine is 15-30 hours and accumulates with chronic dosing, especially in patients with renal dysfunction. The accumulation of this metabolite may lead to CNS excitation (eg, tremors, twitches, seizures).

Drug	Onset (min)	Peak (h)	Duration* (h)	t½ (h)	Equianalgesic Doses† I.M. (mg)	Equianalgesic Doses† Oral (mg)	Volume of Distribution (L/kg)	Protein Binding (%)
Alfentanil	Immediate	ND	ND	1.2‡	ND	NA	0.6-1	92
Codeine	30-60	1-1.5	4-6	3	120	200	3.5	7
Diamorphine	5-10	0.5-1.2	3-4	0.05-1.5	3-5	60	25	40
Fentanyl	7-8	ND	1-2	1.5-6	0.1	NA	4	80-86
Hydrocodone	ND	0.5-2	4-8	3.3-4.5	ND	15-20	—	—
Hydromorphone	15-30	0.5-1	4-5	2-3	1.5	7.5	1.2	—
Levorphanol	10-30	0.5-1	6-8	12-16	2	4	—	—
Meperidine	10-45	0.5-1	2-4	3-4††	75	300	3.1-5	55-75
Meptazinol	30	0.5-1	2-3	2	140	ND	2-3	23-27
Methadone	30-60	0.5-1	4-6§	15-30	10	20	3.6	80-89
Morphine	15-60¶	0.5-1	3-7	1.5-2	10	60	3-4	35
Oxycodone, P.O.	15-30	1	3-6	2-5	NA	30	—	—
Oxymorphone	5-10	0.5-1	3-6	ND	1	10#	—	—
Propoxyphene, P.O.	30-60	2-2.5	4-6	15+	ND	130*/200**	12-26	78
Sufentanil	1.3-3‡	ND	0.5-1	2.5	0.02	NA	2.9	93
Tilidine	15-30	0.5	4-6	5	100	150	3.71	—

ND = no data available. NA = not applicable.

*After I.V. administration, peak effects may be more pronounced but duration is shorter. Duration of action may be longer with the oral route.

†Based on acute, short-term use. Chronic administration may alter pharmacokinetics and decrease the oral:parenteral dose ratio. The morphine oral:parenteral ratio decreases to 1.5-2.5:1 upon chronic dosing.

‡Data based on I.V. administration.

§Duration and half-life increase with repeated use due to cumulative effects.

¶Data based on intrathecal or epidural administration.

#Rectal.

*HCl salt.

**Napsylate salt.

††Normeperidine (active metabolite) has a half-life of 14-21 hours.

+Norpropoxyphene (active metabolite) has a half-life of 30-36 hours.

NEUROMUSCULAR-BLOCKING AGENTS

Suggested Dosing Guidelines for the Use of Neuromuscular Blocking Agents in the Intensive Care Unit		
Agent	**Intermittent Injection**	**Continuous Infusion**
Short Duration		
Mivacurium (Mivacron®)	0.15-0.25 mg/kg followed by 0.1 mg/kg every 15 minutes	1-15 mcg/kg/min
Intermediate Duration		
Atracurium (Tracrium®)	0.4-0.5 mg/kg every 25-35 minutes	0.4-1 mg/kg/h
Cisatracurium (Nimbex®)	0.15-0.2 mg/kg every 40-60 minutes	0.03-0.6 mg/kg/h
Rocuronium (Zemuron®)	0.6 mg/kg every 30 minutes	0.6 mg/kg/h
Vecuronium	0.1 mg/kg every 35-45 minutes	0.05-0.1 mg/kg/h
Long Duration		
Doxacurium (Nuromax®)	0.025 mg/kg every 2-3 hours	0.015-0.045 mg/kg/h
Pancuronium	0.1 mg/kg every 90-100 minutes	0.05-0.1 mg/kg/h

Pharmacokinetic and Pharmacodynamic Properties of Neuromuscular Blocking Agents								
Agent	**Clearance (mL/kg/min)**	**V_{dss} (L/kg)**	**Half-life (min)**	**ED95[1] (mg/kg)**	**Initial Adult Dose[2,3] (mg/kg)**	**Onset (min)**	**Clinical Duration of Action of Initial Dose (min)**	**Administration as an Intraoperative Infusion (mcg/kg/min)**
Ultra-Short Duration								
Succinylcholine	Unknown	Unknown	Unknown	0.2	1-1.5	0.5-1	4-8	10-100
Short Duration								
Mivacurium	50-100[2]	0.2	2[4]	0.07	0.15-0.25	1.5-3	12-20	1-15
Intermediate Duration								
Atracurium	5-7	0.2	20	0.2	0.4-0.5	2-3	20-45	4-12
Cisatracurium	4.6	0.15	22-29	0.05	0.15-0.2	2-3	40-60	1-3
Rocuronium	4	0.17-0.29	60-70	0.3	0.6-1.2	1-1.5	31-67	4-16
Vecuronium	4.5	0.16-0.27	51-80	0.05	0.08-0.1	2-3	20-40	0.8-2
Long Duration								
Doxacurium	1-2.5	0.2	100-200	0.025	0.05-0.08	4-6	100-160	n/a
Pancuronium	1-2	0.18-0.26	107-169	0.07	0.08-0.1	3-5	60-100	n/a

[1]ED95: Effective dose causing 95% blockade.

[2]Initial dose (intubation dose) is usually 2 × ED95 with the exception of cisatracurium where the recommended initial dose is 3-4 × ED95.

[3]Prior administration of succinylcholine generally enhances the magnitude and duration of nondepolarizing NMB agents; initial doses should be lower.

[4]Values reflect contribution of cis-trans and trans-trans isomers only.

NONBENZODIAZEPINE ANXIOLYTICS AND HYPNOTICS

Drug	Dosage Forms	Initial Dose	Usual Dosage Range	Onset	Half-Life	Comments
Buspirone (BuSpar®)	Tab	7.5 mg bid	30-60 mg/d	30 min - 1.5 h	2-3 h	Do not use for alcohol or benzodiazepine withdrawal; no sedation or dependence; do not use PRN; use 4 weeks for full therapeutic effect
Chloral hydrate (Aquachloral® Supprettes®, Somnote™)	Cap, rec supp, syr	500 mg - 1 g qhs	500 mg - 2 g/d	30 min	8-11 h	GI irritating; tolerance to hypnotic effect develops rapidly; do not use for alcohol or benzodiazepine withdrawal
Diphenhydramine (Benadryl® Allergy and others)	Sol, cap, tab, cream, lot, syr, elix	25-50 mg qhs	25-200 mg/d	1-3 h	2-8 h	Anticholinergic; max hypnotic dose: 50 mg/d; do not use for alcohol or benzodiazepine withdrawal
Eszopiclone (Lunesta™)	Tab	1-2 mg qhs	1-3 mg qhs	30 min	6-9 h	Use caution in patients with depression especially if suicidal
Hydroxyzine (Atarax®, Vistaril®)	Tab, cap, liq, inj, syr	25-100 mg qid	100-600 mg/d	30 min	3-7 h	Anticholinergic; do not use for alcohol or benzodiazepine withdrawal
Propranolol (Inderal®, Inderal® LA, InnoPran XL™, Propranolol Intensol™)	Tab, cap, sol, inj	10 mg tid	80-160 mg/d	1-2 h	4-6 h	Useful for physical manifestations of anxiety (increased heart rate, tremor); second-line agent; do not use for alcohol or benzodiazepine withdrawal
Zaleplon (Sonata®)	Cap	5-10 mg qhs	5-20 mg qhs	30 min	1 h	Do not use for alcohol or benzodiazepine withdrawal
Zolpidem (Ambien®)	Tab	10 mg qhs	10 mg qhs	30 min	2.5 h	Do not use for alcohol or benzodiazepine withdrawal

NONSTEROIDAL ANTI-INFLAMMATORY DRUGS

Generic Name	Half-Life (hours)	Time to Peak (hours)	Usual Duration (hours)	Maximum Recommended Daily Dose (mg)	Relative Therapeutic Potency	Special Considerations
Celecoxib	11	2-3	24	400	12.5	Less GI distress, COX-2 inhibitor
Diclofenac	1-2	2-3	12	200	7	Less GI distress, less CNS depression
Diflusinal	8-12	2-3	8-12	1500	47	Less hepatic injury
Etodolac	7	1		1200	37.5	Less GI distress
Fenoprofen	3	2	4-6	3200	100	Increased nephrotoxicity, increased antiplatelet activity
Flurbiprofen	3-6	1.5-2		300	10	Increased GI distress
Ibuprofen	2	1-2	4-6	3200	100	Less GI distress, increased nephrotoxicity
Indomethacin	4.5	2	4-6	200	6.25	Increased nephrotoxicity, GI distress, and CNS depression
Ketoprofen	2-4	0.5-2		300	10	
Ketorolac	5-6	2-3	6-8	P.O.: 40; I.M.: 120	1.25	Increased nephrotoxicity and GI distress
Meclofena-mate	1.3	0.5-1.5	2-4	400	12.5	Less hepatic injury, increased GI distress
Mefenamic acid	2	2	4-6	1000	32	Increased GI distress
Meloxicam	15-20	4-5	24	15	0.5	Less GI distress, less hepatic injury
Nabumetone	22.5	6		2000	62.5	Less GI distress
Naproxen (base and sodium salt)	13	2-4	8-12	1500	40	
Oxaprozin	42-50	3-5	24	1800	56	Less GI distress
Piroxicam	50	3-5	24	40	1.25	Less hepatic injury
Rofecoxib	17	2-3	24	50	1.5	Less GI distress, COX-2 inhibitor
Sulindac	7-8	2-4	12	400	12.5	
Tolmetin	2-4	0.5-1	8	2000	56	
Valdecoxib	8-11	2.25-3		40		

NONTOXIC PLANTS

African violet
Air fern
Aluminum plant
Aralia, false
Artillery plant
Baby's tears
Bayberry
Beauty bush
Begonia
Blood leaf
Boston fern
Bridal veil
Burro's tail
Cast iron plant
Chinese evergreen
Chocolate soldier
Christmas begonia
Christmas cactus
Christmas dagger fern
Christmas kalanchoe
Christmas orchid
Christmas palm
Christmas pride
Coleus
Coral bells
Corn plant
Dandelion
Devil's walking stick

Donkey's tail
Dracaena warneckei
Dusty miller
Eggplant
False aralia
Ficus benjamina
Fittonia
Flame violet
Fuchsia
Gardenia
Gloxinia
Goldfish plant
Grape ivy
Hens and chickens
Hibiscus
Honeysuckle
Hoya
Impatiens
Jade plant
Kalonchoe
Lady's slipper
Lilac
Lipstick plant
Marigold
Maternity plant
Monkey grass
Moss
Mountain ash (berries)

Oregon grape
Peperomia
Piggy-back plant
Pilea
Pine cone (seed)
Pink polka dot plant
Plectranthus
Prayer plant
Purple passion
Pussy willow
Pyracantha
Rosary pearls
Rosary plant
Sensitive plant
Snake plant
Spider aralia
Spider plant
Swedish ivy
Tahitian bridal veil
Tin plant
Umbrella plant
Wandering jew
Weeping fig
Wild strawberry
Yucca plant
Zebra plant

OCCUPATIONAL EXPOSURE TO BLOODBORNE PATHOGENS (UNIVERSAL PRECAUTIONS)

Overview and Regulatory Considerations

Every healthcare employee, from nurse to housekeeper, has some (albeit small) risk of exposure to HIV and other viral agents such as hepatitis B and Jakob-Creutzfeldt agent. The incidence of HIV-1 transmission associated with a percutaneous exposure to blood from an HIV-1 infected patient is approximately 0.3% per exposure.[1] In 1989, it was estimated that 12,000 United States healthcare workers acquired hepatitis B annually.[2] An understanding of the appropriate procedures, responsibilities, and risks inherent in the collection and handling of patient specimens is necessary for safe practice and is required by Occupational Safety and Health Administration (OSHA) regulations.

The Occupational Safety and Health Administration published its "Final Rule on Occupational Exposure to Bloodborne Pathogens" in the Federal Register on December 6, 1991. OSHA has chosen to follow the Centers for Disease Control (CDC) definition of universal precautions. The Final Rule provides full legal force to universal precautions and requires employers and employees to treat blood and certain body fluids as if they were infectious. The Final Rule mandates that healthcare workers must avoid parenteral contact and must avoid splattering blood or other potentially infectious material on their skin, hair, eyes, mouth, mucous membranes, or on their personal clothing. Hazard abatement strategies must be used to protect the workers. Such plans typically include, but are not limited to, the following:

safe handling of sharp items ("sharps") and disposal of such into puncture resistant containers

gloves required for employees handling items soiled with blood or equipment contaminated by blood or other body fluids

provisions of protective clothing when more extensive contact with blood or body fluids may be anticipated (eg, surgery, autopsy, or deliveries)

resuscitation equipment to reduce necessity for mouth to mouth resuscitation

restriction of HIV- or hepatitis B-exposed employees to noninvasive procedures

OSHA has specifically defined the following terms: **Occupational exposure** means reasonably anticipated skin, eye mucous membrane, or parenteral contact with blood or other potentially infectious materials that may result from the performance of an employee's duties. **Other potentially infectious materials** are human body fluids including semen, vaginal secretions, cerebrospinal fluid, synovial fluid, pleural fluid, pericardial fluid, peritoneal fluid, amniotic fluid, saliva in dental procedures, and body fluids that are visibly contaminated with blood, and all body fluids in situations where it is difficult or impossible to differentiate between body fluids; any unfixed tissue or organ (other than intact skin) from a human (living or dead); and HIV-containing cell or tissue cultures, organ cultures, and HIV- or HBV-containing culture medium or other solutions, and blood, organs, or other tissues from experimental animals infected with HIV or HBV. An **exposure incident** involves specific eye, mouth, other mucous membrane, nonintact skin, or parenteral contact with blood or other potentially infectious materials that results from the performance of an employee's duties.[3] It is important to understand that some exposures may go unrecognized despite the strictest precautions.

A written Exposure Control Plan is required. Employers must provide copies of the plan to employees and to OSHA upon request. Compliance with OSHA rules may be accomplished by the following methods.

Universal precautions (UPs) means that all human blood and certain body fluids are treated as if known to be infectious for HIV, HBV, and other bloodborne pathogens. UPs do not apply to feces, nasal secretions, saliva, sputum, sweat, tears, urine, or vomitus unless they contain visible blood.

Engineering controls (ECs) are physical devices which reduce or remove hazards from the workplace by eliminating or minimizing hazards or by isolating the worker from exposure. Engineering control devices include sharps disposal containers, self-resheathing syringes, etc.

Work practice controls (WPCs) are practices and procedures that reduce the likelihood of exposure to hazards by altering the way in which a task is performed. Specific examples are the prohibition of two-handed recapping of needles, prohibition of storing food alongside potentially contaminated material, discouragement of pipetting fluids by mouth, encouraging handwashing after removal of gloves, safe handling of contaminated sharps, and appropriate use of sharps containers.

Personal protective equipment (PPE) is specialized clothing or equipment worn to provide protection from occupational exposure. PPE includes gloves, gowns, laboratory coats (the type and characteristics will depend upon the task and degree of exposure anticipated), face shields or masks, and eye protection. Surgical caps or hoods and/or shoe covers or boots are required in instances in which gross contamination can reasonably be anticipated (eg, autopsies, orthopedic surgery). If PPE is penetrated by blood or any contaminated material, the item must be removed immediately or as soon as feasible. **The employer must provide and launder or dispose of all PPE at no cost to the employee**. Gloves must be worn when there is a reasonable anticipation of hand contact with potentially infectious material, including a patient's mucous membranes or nonintact skin. Disposable gloves must be changed as soon as possible after they become torn or punctured. Hands must be washed after gloves are removed. OSHA has revised the PPE standards, effective July 5, 1994, to include the requirement that the employer certify in writing that it has conducted a hazard assessment of the workplace to determine whether hazards are present that will necessitate the use of PPE. Also, verification that the employee has received and understood the PPE training is required.[4]

Housekeeping protocols: OSHA requires that all bins, cans, and similar receptacles intended for reuse, which have a reasonable likelihood for becoming contaminated, be inspected and decontaminated immediately or as soon as feasible upon visible contamination and on a regularly scheduled basis. Broken glass that may be contaminated must not be picked up directly with the hands. Mechanical means (eg, brush, dust pan, tongs, or forceps) must be used. Broken glass must be placed in a proper sharps container.

Employers are responsible for teaching appropriate clean-up procedures for the work area and personal protective equipment. A 1:10 dilution of household bleach is a popular and effective disinfectant. It is prudent for employers to maintain signatures or initials of employees who have been properly educated. If one does not have written proof of education of universal precautions teaching, then by OSHA standards, such education never happened.

Pre-exposure and postexposure protocols: OSHA's Final Rule includes the provision that employees who are exposed to contamination be offered the hepatitis B vaccine at no cost to the employee. Employees may decline; however, a declination form must be signed. The employee must be offered free vaccine if he/she changes his/her mind. Vaccination to prevent the transmission of hepatitis B in the healthcare setting is widely regarded as sound practice.[5] In the event of exposure, a confidential medical evaluation and follow-up must be offered at no cost to the employee. Follow-up must include collection and testing of blood from the source individual for HBV and HIV if permitted by state law if a blood sample is available. If a postexposure specimen must be specially drawn, the individual's consent is usually required. Some states may not require consent for testing of patient blood after accidental exposure. One must refer to state and/or local guidelines for proper guidance.

The employee follow-up must also include appropriate postexposure prophylaxis, counseling, and evaluation of reported illnesses. The employee has the right to decline baseline blood collection and/or testing. If the employee gives consent for the collection but not the testing, the sample must be preserved for 90 days in the event that the employee changes his/her mind within that time. Confidentiality related to blood testing must be ensured. **The employer does not have the right to know the results** of the testing of either the source individual or the exposed employee.

Management of Occupational Exposure to HIV in the Workplace[6]

Likelihood of transmission of HIV-1 from occupational exposure is 0.2% per parenteral exposure (eg, needlestick) to blood from HIV infected patients.

Factors that increase risk for occupational transmission include advanced stages of HIV in source patient, hollow bore needle puncture, a poor state of health, or inexperience of healthcare worker (HCW).

Immediate actions an exposed healthcare worker should take include aggressive first aid at the puncture site (eg, scrubbing site with povidone-iodine solution for 10 minutes) or at mucus membrane site (eg, saline irrigation of eye for 15 minutes). Then immediate reporting to the hospital's occupational medical service. The authors indicate that there is no direct evidence for the efficacy of their recommendations. Other institutions suggest rigorous scrubbing with soap.

After first aid is initiated, the healthcare worker should report exposure to a supervisor and to the institution's occupational medical service for evaluation.

Occupational medicine should perform a thorough investigation including identifying the HIV and hepatitis B status of the source, type of exposure, volume of inoculum, timing of exposure, extent of injury, appropriateness of first aid, as well as psychological status of the healthcare worker. HIV serologies should be performed on the healthcare worker. HIV risk counseling should begin at this point.

All parenteral exposures should be treated equally until they can be evaluated by the occupational medicine service, who will then determine the actual risk of exposure. Follow-up counseling sessions may be necessary.

Although the data are not clear, antiviral prophylaxis may be offered to healthcare workers who are parenterally or mucous membrane exposed. If used, antiretroviral prophylaxis should be initiated within 1-2 hours after exposure.

Counseling regarding risk of exposure, antiviral prophylaxis, plans for follow up, exposure prevention, sexual activity, and providing emotional support and response to concerns are necessary to support the exposed healthcare worker. Follow-up should consist of periodic serologic evaluation and blood chemistries and counts if antiretroviral prophylaxis is initiated. Additional information should be provided to healthcare workers who are pregnant or planning to become pregnant.

Hazardous Communication

Communication regarding the dangers of bloodborne infections through the use of labels, signs, information, and education is required. Storage locations (eg, refrigerators and freezers, waste containers) that are used to store, dispose of, transport, or ship blood or other potentially infectious materials require labels. The label background must be red or bright orange with the biohazard design and the word biohazard in a contrasting color. The label must be part of the container or affixed to the container by permanent means.

Education provided by a qualified and knowledgeable instructor is mandated. The sessions for employees must include:

accessible copies of the regulation

general epidemiology of bloodborne diseases

modes of bloodborne pathogen transmission

an explanation of the exposure control plan and a means to obtain copies of the written plan

an explanation of the tasks and activities that may involve exposure

the use of exposure prevention methods and their limitations (eg, engineering controls, work practices, personal protective equipment)

information on the types, proper use, location, removal, handling, decontamination, and disposal of personal protective equipment

an explanation of the basis for selection of personal protective equipment

information on the HBV vaccine, including information on its efficacy, safety, and method of administration and the benefits of being vaccinated (ie, the employee must understand that the vaccine and vaccination will be offered free of charge)

information on the appropriate actions to take and persons to contact in an emergency involving exposure to blood or other potentially infectious materials

an explanation of the procedure to follow if an exposure incident occurs, including the method of reporting the incident

information on the postexposure evaluation and follow-up that the employer is required to provide for the employee following an exposure incident

an explanation of the signs, labels, and color coding

an interactive question-and-answer period

Record Keeping

The OSHA Final Rule requires that the employer maintain both education and medical records. The medical records must be kept confidential and be maintained for the duration of employment plus 30 years. They must contain a copy of the employee's HBV vaccination status and postexposure incident information. Education records must be maintained for 3 years from the date the program was given.

OSHA has the authority to conduct inspections without notice. Penalties for cited violation may be assessed as follows:

Serious violations. In this situation, there is a substantial probability of death or serious physical harm, and the employer knew, or should have known, of the hazard. A violation of this type carries a mandatory penalty of up to $7000 for each violation.

Other-than-serious violations. The violation is unlikely to result in death or serious physical harm. This type of violation carries a discretionary penalty of up to $7000 for each violation.

Willful violations. These are violations committed knowingly or intentionally by the employer and have penalties of up to $70,000 per violation with a minimum of $5000 per violation. If an employee dies as a result of a willful violation, the responsible party, if convicted, may receive a personal fine of up to $250,000 and/or a 6-month jail term. A corporation may be fined $500,000.

Large fines frequently follow visits to laboratories, physicians' offices, and healthcare facilities by OSHA Compliance Safety and Health Offices (CSHOS). Regulations are vigorously enforced. A working knowledge of the final rule and implementation of appropriate policies and practices is imperative for all those involved in the collection and analysis of medical specimens.

Effectiveness of universal precautions in averting exposure to potentially infectious materials has been documented.[7] Compliance with appropriate rules, procedures, and policies, including reporting exposure incidents, is a matter of personal professionalism and prudent self-preservation.

Footnotes

1. Henderson DK, Fahey BJ, Willy M, et al, "Risk for Occupational Transmission of Human Immunodeficiency Virus Type 1 (HIV-1) Associated with Clinical Exposures. A Prospective Evaluation," *Ann Intern Med*, 1990, 113(10):740-6.

2. Niu MT and Margolis HS, "Moving into a New Era of Government Regulation: Provisions for Hepatitis B Vaccine in the Workplace, *Clin Lab Manage Rev*, 1989, 3:336-40.

3. Bruning LM, "The Bloodborne Pathogens Final Rule — Understanding the Regulation," *AORN Journal*, 1993, 57(2):439-40.

4. "Rules and Regulations," *Federal Register*, 1994, 59(66):16360-3.

5. Schaffner W, Gardner P, and Gross PA, "Hepatitis B Immunization Strategies: Expanding the Target," *Ann Intern Med*, 1993, 118(4):308-9.

6. Fahey BJ, Beekmann SE, Schmitt JM, et al, "Managing Occupational Exposures to HIV-1 in the Healthcare Workplace," *Infect Control Hosp Epidemiol*, 1993, 14(7):405-12.

7. Wong ES, Stotka JL, Chinchilli VM, et al, "Are Universal Precautions Effective in Reducing the Number of Occupational Exposures Among Healthcare Workers?" *JAMA*, 1991, 265(9):1123-8.

References

Brown JW and Blackwell H, "Complying With the New OSHA Regs, Part 1: Teaching Your Staff About Biosafety," *MLO*, 1992, 24(4)24-8. Part 2: "Safety Protocols No Lab Can Ignore," 1992, 24(5):27-9. Part 3: "Compiling Employee Safety Records That Will Satisfy OSHA," 1992, 24(6):45-8.

Buehler JW and Ward JW, "A New Definition for AIDS Surveillance," *Ann Intern Med*, 1993, 118(5):390-2.

Department of Labor, Occupational Safety and Health Administration, "Occupational Exposure to Bloodborne Pathogens; Final Rule (29 CFR Part 1910.1030), " *Federal Register*, December 6, 1991, 64004-182.

Gold JW, "HIV-1 Infection: Diagnosis and Management," *Med Clin North Am*, 1992, 76(1):1-18.

"Hepatitis B Virus: A Comprehensive Strategy for Eliminating Transmission in the United States Through Universal Childhood Vaccination," Recommendations of the Immunization Practices Advisory Committee (ACIP), *MMWR Morb Mortal Wkly Rep*, 1991, 40(RR-13):1-25.

"Mortality Attributable to HIV Infection/AIDS — United States", *MMWR Morb Mortal Wkly Rep*, 1991, 40(3):41-4.

National Committee for Clinical Laboratory Standards, "Protection of Laboratory Workers From Infectious Disease Transmitted by Blood, Body Fluids, and Tissue," NCCLS Document M29-T, Villanova, PA: NCCLS, 1989, 9(1).

"Nosocomial Transmission of Hepatitis B Virus Associated with a Spring-Loaded Fingerstick Device — California," *MMWR Morb Mortal Wkly Rep*, 1990, 39(35):610-3.

Polish LB, Shapiro CN, Bauer F, et al, "Nosocomial Transmission of Hepatitis B Virus Associated with the Use of a Spring-Loaded Fingerstick Device," *N Engl J Med*, 1992, 326(11):721-5.

"Recommendations for Preventing Transmission of Human Immunodeficiency Virus and Hepatitis B Virus to Patients During Exposure-Prone Invasive Procedures," *MMWR Morb Mortal Wkly Rep*, 1991, 40(RR-8):1-9.

"Update: Acquired Immunodeficiency Syndrome — United States," *MMWR Morb Mortal Wkly Rep*, 1992, 41(26):463-8.

"Update: Transmission of HIV Infection During an Invasive Dental Procedure — Florida," *MMWR Morb Mortal Wkly Rep*, 1991, 40(2):21-7, 33.

"Update: Universal Precautions for Prevention of Transmission of Human Immunodeficiency Virus, Hepatitis B Virus, and Other Bloodborne Pathogens in Healthcare Settings," *MMWR Morb Mortal Wkly Rep*, 1988, 37(24):377-82, 387-8.

ORAL MEDICATIONS THAT SHOULD NOT BE CRUSHED OR ALTERED

There are a variety of reasons for crushing tablets or capsule contents prior to administering to the patient. Patients may have nasogastric tubes which do not permit the administration of tablets or capsules; an oral solution for a particular medication may not be available from the manufacturer or readily prepared by pharmacy; patients may have difficulty swallowing capsules or tablets; or mixing of powdered medication with food or drink may make the drug more palatable.

Generally, medications which should not be crushed fall into one of the following categories.

Extended-Release Products. The formulation of some tablets is specialized as to allow the medication within it to be slowly released into the body. This is sometimes accomplished by centering the drug within the core of the tablet, with a subsequent shedding of multiple layers around the core. Wax melts in the GI tract. Slow-K® is an example of this. Capsules may contain beads which have multiple layers which are slowly dissolved with time.

Common Abbreviations for Extended-Release Products

CD	Controlled dose
CR	Controlled release
CRT	Controlled-release tablet
LA	Long-acting
SR	Sustained release
TR	Timed release
TD	Time delay
SA	Sustained action
XL	Extended release
XR	Extended release

Medications Which Are Irritating to the Stomach. Tablets which are irritating to the stomach may be enteric-coated which delays release of the drug until the time when it reaches the small intestine. Enteric-coated aspirin is an example of this.

Foul-Tasting Medication. Some drugs are quite unpleasant to taste so the manufacturer coats the tablet in a sugar coating to increase its palatability. By crushing the tablet, this sugar coating is lost and the patient tastes the unpleasant tasting medication.

Sublingual Medication. Medication intended for use under the tongue should not be crushed. While it appears to be obvious, it is not always easy to determine if a medication is to be used sublingually. Sublingual medications should indicate on the package that they are intended for sublingual use.

Effervescent Tablets. These are tablets which, when dropped into a liquid, quickly dissolve to yield a solution. Many effervescent tablets, when crushed, lose their ability to quickly dissolve.

Recommmendations

It is not advisable to crush certain medications.

Consult individual monographs prior to crushing capsule or tablet.

If crushing a tablet or capsule is contraindicated, consult with your pharmacist to determine whether an oral solution exists or can be compounded.

Drug Product	Dosage Form	Dosage Reasons/Comments
Accuhist®	Tablet	Slow release[8]
Accutane®	Capsule	Mucous membrane irritant
Aciphex™	Tablet	Slow release
Adalat® CC	Tablet	Slow release

(*Continued*)

Drug Product	Dosage Form	Dosage Reasons/Comments
Adderall XR™	Capsule	Slow release[1]
Advicor®	Tablet	Slow release
Afeditab™ CR	Tablet	Slow release
Aggrenox®	Capsule	Slow release **Note:** Capsule may be opened; contents include an aspirin tablet that may be chewed and dipyridamole pellets that may be sprinkled on applesauce
Alavert™ Allergy Sinus 12 Hour	Tablet	Slow release
Allegra-D®	Tablet	Slow release
Altocor™	Tablet	Slow release
Arthritis Bayer® Time Release	Capsule	Slow release
Arthrotec®	Tablet	Enteric-coated
A.S.A.® Enseals®	Tablet	Enteric-coated
Asacol®	Tablet	Slow release
Ascriptin® A/D	Tablet	Enteric-coated
Ascriptin® Extra Strength	Tablet	Enteric-coated
Augmentin XR™	Tablet	Slow release[2,8]
Avinza™	Capsule	Slow release[1] (not pudding)
Avodart™	Capsule	Teratogenic potential[9]
Azulfidine® EN-tabs®	Tablet	Enteric-coated
Bayer® Aspirin EC	Caplet	Enteric-coated
Bayer® Aspirin, Low Adult 81 mg	Tablet	Enteric-coated
Bayer® Aspirin, Regular Strength 325 mg	Caplet	Enteric-coated
Biaxin® XL	Tablet	Slow release
Biltricide®	Tablet	Taste[8]
Bisacodyl	Tablet	Enteric-coated[3]
Bontril® Slow-Release	Capsule	Slow release
Calan® SR	Tablet	Slow release[8]
Carbatrol®	Capsule	Slow release[1]
Cardene® SR	Capsule	Slow release
Cardizem®	Tablet	Slow release
Cardizem® CD	Capsule	Slow release[1]
Cardizem® LA	Tablet	Slow release
Cardizem® SR	Capsule	Slow release[1]
Carter's Little Pills®	Tablet	Enteric-coated
Cartia® XT	Capsule	Slow release
Ceclor® CD	Tablet	Slow release
Ceftin®	Tablet	Taste[2] **Note:** Use suspension for children
CellCept®	Capsule, tablet	Teratogenic potential[9]
Charcoal Plus®	Tablet	Enteric-coated
Chloral Hydrate	Capsule	**Note:** Product is in liquid form within a special capsule[2]
Chlor-Trimeton® 12-Hour	Tablet	Slow release[2]
Cipro™	Tablet	Taste[5]
Cipro® XR	Tablet	Slow release
Claritin-D® 12-Hour	Tablet	Slow release
Claritin-D® 24-Hour	Tablet	Slow release

(*Continued*)

Drug Product	Dosage Form	Dosage Reasons/Comments
Colace®	Capsule	Taste[5]
Colestid®	Tablet	Slow release
Comhist® LA	Capsule	Slow release[1]
Commit™	Lozenge	**Note:** Integrity compromised by chewing or crushing
Compazine® Spansule®	Capsule	Slow release[2]
Concerta®	Tablet	Slow release
Contac® 12-Hour	Tablet	Slow release
Cotazym-S®	Capsule	Enteric-coated[1]
Covera-HS™	Tablet	Slow release
Creon® 5, 10, 20	Capsule	Slow release[1]
Crixivan®	Capsule	Taste **Note:** Capsule may be opened and mixed with fruit puree (eg, banana)
Cymbalta®	Capsule	Enteric-coated
Cytovene®	Capsule	Skin irritant
Cytoxan®	Tablet	**Note:** Drug may be crushed, but maker recommends using injection
Dallergy®	Capsule	Slow release
Dallergy-JR®	Capsule	Slow release
Deconamine® SR	Capsule	Slow release[2]
Defen L.A.®	Tablet	Slow release[8]
Depakene®	Capsule	Slow release mucous membrane irritant[2]
Depakote®	Tablet	Slow release
Depakote® ER	Tablet	Slow release
Desoxyn®	Tablet	Slow release
Desyrel®	Tablet	Taste[5]
Detrol® LA	Capsule	Slow release
Dexedrine® Spansule®	Capsule	Slow release
Diamox® Sequels®	Capsule	Slow release
Dilacor® XR	Capsule	Slow release
Dilatrate-SR®	Capsule	Slow release
Diltia XT®	Capsule	Slow release
Ditropan® XL	Tablet	Slow release
Dolobid®	Tablet	Irritant
Donnatal® Extentab®	Tablet	Slow release[2]
Drisdol®	Capsule	Liquid filled[4]
Drixoral®	Tablet	Slow release[2]
Drixoral® Plus	Tablet	Slow release
Drixoral® Sinus	Tablet	Slow release
Dulcolax®	Capsule	Liquid-filled
Dulcolax®	Tablet	Enteric-coated[3]
Duratuss® G	Tablet	Slow release[9]
Duratuss® GP	Tablet	Slow release[8]
Dynabac®	Tablet	Enteric-coated
DynaCirc® CR	Tablet	Slow release
Easprin®	Tablet	Enteric-coated
EC-Naprosyn®	Tablet	Enteric-coated

(*Continued*)

Drug Product	Dosage Form	Dosage Reasons/Comments
Ecotrin® Adult Low Strength	Tablet	Enteric-coated
Ecotrin® Maximum Strength	Tablet	Enteric-coated
Ecotrin® Regular Strength	Tablet	Enteric-coated
E.E.S.® 400	Tablet	Enteric-coated[2]
Effexor® XR	Capsule	Slow release
Efidac/24® Pseudoephedrine	Tablet	Slow release
Efidac® 24	Tablet	Slow release
E-Mycin®	Tablet	Enteric-coated
Entex® LA	Capsule	Slow release[2]
Entex® PSE	Capsule	Slow release
Entocort™ EC	Capsule	Enteric-coated[1]
Ergomar®	Tablet	Sublingual form[7]
Eryc®	Capsule	Enteric-coated[1]
Ery-Tab®	Tablet	Enteric-coated
Erythrocin Stearate	Tablet	Enteric-coated
Erythromycin Base	Tablet	Enteric-coated
Eskalith CR®	Tablet	Slow release
Evista®	Tablet	Taste; teratogenic potential[9]
Extendryl JR	Capsule	Slow release
Extendryl SR	Capsule	Slow release[2]
Feldene®	Capsule	Mucous membrane irritant
Feosol®	Tablet	Enteric-coated[2]
Feratab®	Tablet	Enteric-coated[2]
Fergon®	Tablet	Enteric-coated
Fero-Grad 500®	Tablet	Slow release
Ferro-Sequels®	Tablet	Slow release
Flagyl ER®	Tablet	Slow release
Flomax®	Capsule	Enteric-coated[1]
Fosamax®	Tablet	Mucous membrane irritant
Fumatinic®	Capsule	Slow release
Geocillin®	Tablet	Taste
Gleevec®	Tablet	Taste[8] **Note:** May be dissolved in mineral oil or apple juice
Glucophage® XR	Tablet	Slow release
Glucotrol® XL	Tablet	Slow release
Gris-PEG®	Tablet	**Note:** Crushing may result in precipitation of larger particles.
Guaifed®	Capsule	Slow release
Guaifed®-PD	Capsule	Slow release
Guaifenex® DM	Tablet	Slow release[8]
Guaifenex® LA	Tablet	Slow release[8]
Guaifenex® PSE	Tablet	Slow release[8]
Guaimax-D®	Tablet	Slow release
Hista-Vent® DA	Tablet	Slow release[8]
Humibid® DM	Tablet	Slow release
Humibid® LA	Tablet	Slow release

(*Continued*)

Drug Product	Dosage Form	Dosage Reasons/Comments
Iberet® Filmtab	Tablet	Slow release[2]
Iberet®-500	Tablet	Slow release[2]
Iberet-Folic-500®	Tablet	Slow release
ICAPS® Time Release	Tablet	Slow release
Imdur™	Tablet	Slow release[8]
Inderal® LA	Capsule	Slow release
Inderide® LA	Capsule	Slow release
Indocin® SR	Capsule	Slow release[1,2]
InnoPran XL™	Capsule	Slow release
Ionamin®	Capsule	Slow release
Isoptin® SR	Tablet	Slow release
Isordil® Sublingual	Tablet	Sublingual form[7]
Isosorbide Dinitrate Sublingual	Tablet	Sublingual form[7]
Isosorbide SR	Tablet	Slow release
K+ 8®	Tablet	Slow release[2]
K+ 10®	Tablet	Slow release[2]
Kadian®	Capsule	Slow release[1] **Note:** Do not give via N/G tubes
Kaon-Cl®	Tablet	Slow release[2]
K-Dur®	Tablet	Slow release
Klor-Con®	Tablet	Slow release[2]
Klor-Con® M	Tablet	Slow release[2]
Klotrix®	Tablet	Slow release[2]
K-Lyte®	Tablet	Effervescent tablet[6]
K-Lyte/Cl®	Tablet	Effervescent tablet[6]
K-Lyte DS®	Tablet	Effervescent tablet[6]
K-Tab®	Tablet	Slow release[2]
Lescol® XL	Tablet	Slow release
Levbid®	Tablet	Slow release[8]
Levsinex® Timecaps®	Capsule	Slow release
Lexxel®	Tablet	Slow release
Lipram 4500	Capsule	Enteric-coated[1]
Lipram-CR	Capsule	Enteric-coated[1]
Lipram-PN	Capsule	Enteric-coated[1]
Lipram-UL	Capsule	Enteric-coated[1]
Lipram (all products)	Capsule	Slow release[1]
Liquibid-PD	Tablet	Slow release[8]
Lithobid®	Tablet	Slow release
Lodine® XL	Tablet	Slow release
Lodrane® LD	Capsule	Slow release[1]
Mag-Tab® SR	Tablet	Slow release
Maxifed®	Tablet	Slow release
Maxifed® DM	Tablet	Slow release
Maxifed-G®	Tablet	Slow release
Mestinon® Timespan®	Tablet	Slow release[2]

(*Continued*)

Drug Product	Dosage Form	Dosage Reasons/Comments
Metadate® CD	Capsule	Slow release[1]
Metadate™ ER	Tablet	Slow release
Methylin™ ER	Tablet	Slow release
Micro-K®	Capsule	Slow release
Motrin®	Tablet	Taste[5]
MS Contin®	Tablet	Slow release[2]
Mucinex®	Tablet	Slow release
Myfortic®	Tablet	Slow release
Naprelan®	Tablet	Slow release
Nasatab® LA	Tablet	Slow release[8]
Nexium®	Capsule	Slow release[1]
Niaspan®	Tablet	Slow release
Nicotinic Acid	Capsule, tablet	Slow release
Nifediac™ CC	Tablet	Slow release
Nitrostat®	Tablet	Sublingual route[7]
Norflex™	Tablet	Slow release
Norpace® CR	Capsule	Slow release form within a special capsule
Oramorph SR®	Tablet	Slow release[2]
Oruvail®	Capsule	Slow release
OxyContin®	Tablet	Slow release
Palgic®-D	Tablet	Slow release[8]
Pancrease®	Capsule	Enteric-coated[1]
Pancrease® MT	Capsule	Enteric-coated[1]
Pancrecarb MS®	Capsule	Enteric-coated[1]
PanMist®-DM	Tablet	Slow release[8]
PanMist®-Jr	Tablet	Slow release[8]
PanMist®-LA	Tablet	Slow release[8]
Pannaz®	Tablet	Slow release[8]
Papaverine Sustained Action	Capsule	Slow release
Paxil CR™	Tablet	Slow release
Pentasa®	Capsule	Slow release
Perdiem® Fiber Therapy	Granules	Wax coated
PhenaVent™ D	Tablet	Slow release
Plendil®	Tablet	Slow release
Prelu-2®	Capsule	Slow release
Prevacid®	Capsule	Slow release
Prevacid®	Suspension	Slow release **Note:** Contains enteric-coated granules
Prilosec®	Capsule	Slow release
Procainamide HCl SR	Tablet	Slow release
Procanbid®	Tablet	Slow release
Procardia®	Capsule	Delays absorption[2,5]
Procardia XL®	Tablet	Slow release **Note:** AUC is unaffected.
Profen II®	Tablet	Slow release[8]
Profen II DM®	Tablet	Slow release[8]

(*Continued*)

Drug Product	Dosage Form	Dosage Reasons/Comments
Profen Forte™ DM	Tablet	Slow release
Pronestyl®-SR	Tablet	Slow release
Propecia®	Tablet	**Note:** Women who are, or may become, pregnant, should not handle crushed or broken tablets
Proscar®	Tablet	**Note:** Women who are, or may become, pregnant, should not handle crushed or broken tablets
Protonix®	Tablet	Slow release
Quibron-T/SR®	Tablet	Slow release[2]
Rescon-Jr	Tablet	Slow release
Respa-DM®	Tablet	Slow release[8]
Respaire®-120 SR	Capsule	Slow release
Ritalin-SR®	Tablet	Slow release
Rondec-TR®	Tablet	Slow release[2]
Rythmol® SR	Capsule	Slow release
Sinemet® CR	Tablet	Slow release
SINUvent® PE	Tablet	Slow release[8]
Slo-Niacin®	Tablet	Slow release[8]
Slow-Mag®	Tablet	Slow release
Somnote™	Capsule	Liquid filled
Sudafed® 12-Hour	Capsule	Slow release[2]
Sular®	Tablet	Slow release
Symax SR	Tablet	Slow release
Taztia XT™	Capsule	Slow release
Tegretol®-XR	Tablet	Slow release
Temodar®	Capsule	**Note:** If capsules are accidentally opened or damaged, rigorous precautions should be taken to avoid inhalation or contact of contents with the skin or mucous membranes[9]
Tessalon®	Capsule	Slow release
Theo-24®	Tablet	Slow release[2]
Theochron®	Tablet	Slow release
Tiazac®	Capsule	Slow release
Topamax®	Capsule	Taste[1]
Topamax®	Tablet	Taste
Touro™ CC	Tablet	Slow release
Touro EX®	Tablet	Slow release
Touro LA®	Tablet	Slow release
Trental®	Tablet	Slow release
TripTone®	Tablet	Slow release
Tylenol® Arthritis Pain	Tablet	Slow release
Tylenol® 8 Hour	Tablet	Slow release
Ultrase®	Capsule	Enteric-coated[1]
Ultrase® MT	Capsule	Enteric-coated[1]
Uniphyl®	Tablet	Slow release
Urocit®-K	Tablet	Wax-coated
Verelan®	Capsule	Slow release[1]
Videx® EC	Capsule	Slow release

(*Continued*)

Drug Product	Dosage Form	Dosage Reasons/Comments
Voltaren®-XR	Tablet	Slow release
VoSpire ER™	Tablet	Slow release
Wellbutrin SR®	Tablet	Slow release
Wellbutrin XL™	Tablet	Slow release
Xanax XR®	Tablet	Slow release
Z-Cof LA	Tablet	Slow release[8]
Zephrex LA®	Tablet	Slow release
ZORprin®	Tablet	Slow release
Zyban®	Tablet	Slow release

[1]Capsule may be opened and the contents taken without crushing or chewing; soft food such as applesauce or pudding may facilitate administration; contents may generally be administered via nasogastric tube using an appropriate fluid, provided entire contents are washed down the tube.

[2]Liquid dosage forms of the product are available; however, dose, frequency of administration, and manufacturers may differ from that of the solid dosage form.

[3]Antacids and/or milk may prematurely dissolve the coating of the tablet.

[4]Capsule may be opened and the liquid contents removed for administration.

[5]The taste of this product in a liquid form would likely be unacceptable to the patient; administration via nasogastric tube should be acceptable.

[6]Effervescent tablets must be dissolved in the amount of diluent recommended by the manufacturer.

[7]Tablets are made to disintegrate under the tongue.

[8]Tablet is scored and may be broken in half without affecting release characteristics.

[9]Skin contact may enhance tumor production; avoid direct contact.

Adapted from Mitchell JF, "Oral Dosage Forms That Should Not Be Crushed—2004," available at: http://www.hospitalpharmacyjournal.com.

PARENTERAL MEDICATION ADMINISTRATION GUIDELINES

There are a number of medications which, by their nature, require significant patient monitoring during their use. The following is a listing of these agents and the suggested special requirements.

1. Intravenous push medications which require a physician's presence during administration:

Adenosine
Antivenoms
Atenolol
Atropine
Bretylium
Calcium salts
Cyanide antidote kit
Digoxin immune Fab
Edrophonium
Ephedrine
Epinephrine
Flumazenil

Ketamine
Labetalol
Metoprolol
Midazolam
Neostigmine
Phentolamine
Physostigmine
Phytonadione (vitamin K)
Propanolol
Quinidine
Thrombolytics
Verapamil

2. Medications which can only be used for anesthesia or in patients with assisted ventilation:

Alfentanil
Cisatracurium
Pancuronium
Propofol
Remifentanil

Rocuronium
Succinylcholine
Sufentanil
Tubocurarine
Vecuronium

3. Patients receiving the following drugs as an infusion on an ongoing basis must be explicitly evaluated for placement in an intensive care unit or its equivalent. In addition to the medical status of the patient, the evaluation should consider the availability of appropriate monitoring equipment for the drug in question, and the availability of adequate nursing staff for the necessary monitoring for the duration of therapy.

Amiodarone
Bretylium
Diltiazem
Dobutamine (>5 mcg/kg/min)
Dopamine (>5 mcg/kg/min)
Enalapril
Epinephrine
Esmolol
Ethyl alcohol
Ibutilide
Inamrinone
Insulin
Intravenous antiarrhythmic agents
Isoproterenol
Labetalol

Lidocaine
Lorazepam
Metaraminol
Midazolam
Milrinone (>0.5 mcg/kg/min)
Naloxone
Nicardipine
Nitroglycerin
Nitroprusside sodium
Norepinephrine
Phenylephrine
Procainamide
Trimethaphan
Verapamil

PEDIATRIC LETHAL INGESTION

Toxins/Medications That Could Kill a Toddler of 10-20 kg With One Tablet, Tablespoon, or Single Dosage Form

(Minimum Potential Fatal Dose in Parenthesis)

Tablets/Capsules

Amantadine
Amoxapine
Amphetamines
Benzonatate
Beta-adrenergic blockers
Buspirone
Calcium channel blockers
Chlorpromazine (25 mg/kg)
Chloroquine (20 mg/kg)
Clonidine
Clozapine
Codeine (7-14 mg/kg)
Colchicine
Cyclobenzaprine
Diflunisal
Diltiazem (15 mg/kg)
Disopyramide (25 mg/kg)
Flecainide (25 mg/kg)
Fluoxetine
Haloperidol
Hydrocodone (1.5 mgkg)
Hydroxychloroquine (20 mg/kg)
Hypoglycemic agents
Imipramine
Isradipine (2.5 mg capsule)

Lithium
Lomotil®
Loxapine (30-70 mg/kg)
LSD
Mefanamic acid
Meprobamate
Methadone (1-2 mg/kg)
Minoxidil
Molindone
Monoamine oxidase inhibitors
Nifedipine (15 mg/kg)
Olanzapine (10 mg)
Phenothiazine
Pramipexole (1 mg tablet)
Prazosin
Procainamide (70 mg/kg)
Quinine (80 mg/kg)
Quinidine (15 mg/kg)
Terazosin
Theophylline (8.4 mg/kg)
Thioridazine (15 mg/kg)
Trazadone
Tricyclic antidepressants (15 mg/kg)
Verapamil (15 mg/kg)

Ointment/Cream

Camphor (100 mg/kg)
Dibucaine (and other local anesthetics)
Doxepin
Lindane

Methylsalicylate (200 mg/kg)
Podophyllin 25% (15-20 mg/kg)
Theophylline

Patches

Clonidine
Fentanyl

Nicotine
Nitroglycerin

Ophthalmic

Atropine

Imidazoline

Nonmedicinal Solutions

Acetonitrile
Ammonia (>10%)
Ammonium fluoride
Benzocaine
Butyrolactone
Diethylene glycol
Ethylene glycol
Formaldehyde
Hydrofluoric acid
Hydrogen peroxide (>10%)

Isopropyl alcohol
Methyl alcohol
Methylene chloride
Nicotine sulfate
Nitroethane
Pennyroyal oil
Selenious acid
Strychnine
Toluene
Zinc chloride

Other

Cigarettes (one entire cigarette or
  three smoked butts)
Boric acid

Bromates (2%)

PHOSPHATE REPLETION GUIDELINES

For Moderate Hypophosphatemia (Serum PO$_4$ <2.0 mg/dL But ≥1.0 mg/dL):

1. Discontinue any phosphate binding antacids.
2. Give 0.08-0.16 mmol/kg I.V. in 250 mL NS or D$_5$W over 4-6 hours via pump.
3. Recheck serum phosphate level.
4. If still <2 mg/dL, repeat.

For Severe Hypophosphatemia (Serum PO$_4$ <1.0 mg/dL):

1. Discontinue any phosphate binding antacids.
2. Give 0.25 mmol/kg I.V. in 250 mL NS or D$_5$W over 4-6 hours via pump.
3. Recheck serum phosphate level.
4. If still <1.0 mg/dL, repeat.
5. If ≥1.0 mg/dL but ≤2.0 mg/dL, use guidelines for moderate hypophosphatemia above.

Dosages as high as 0.5 mmol/kg over 6 hours have been used for patients with serum PO$_4$ levels <0.5 mg/dL. If necessary, dosages may be infused over 2 hours.

Medicinal Chemistry Notes

Inorganic phosphate solutions exist as a mixture of two valence states: HPO_4^{-2} and $H_2PO_4^{-}$. At pH 7.4, the molar ratio of HPO_4^{-2}:$H_2PO_4^{-}$ is 80:20, yielding an average valence of 1.8. Therefore:

1 mmol of phosphate = 1.8 mEq of phosphate = 31 mg elemental P.

For clinical purposes, we round off to a ratio of 1 mmol: 2 mEq.

In K phosphate solutions, the mEq of K$^+$ does not equal the mEq of phosphorus. K phosphate I.V. solution provides:

4 mEq K$^+$/mL

6 mEq phosphorus/mL

3 mmol K$^+$ and phosphorus/mL

Therefore, orders for K phosphate written as mEq are ambiguous and subject to misinterpretation.

Important: Orders for K phosphate written as mEq must be clarified with the prescribing physician.

The compatibility of calcium and phosphates in solution is conditional, dependent on the concentration of both ions. As a rule of thumb, the **sum of the mEq calcium plus the mEq phosphate should not exceed 40.**

References

Kingston M and Al-Siba'l MB, "Treatment of Severe Hypophosphatemia," *Crit Care Med* 1985, 13(1):16-8.

Lent RD, Brown DM, and Kjellstrand CM, "Treatment of Severe Hypophosphatemia," *Ann Intern Med*, 1978, 89:941-4.

PLASMAPHERESIS

Toxicants in Which Plasmapheresis Has Been Shown to Enhance Elimination	
Phenytoin	Diltiazem
Paraquat (decreased level by 80%)	Mercury
Propranolol	Vanadate
Tobramycin	Maprotyline
Verapamil	*Amanita phalloides* (mortality: 18%)

Toxicantsin Which Plasmapheresis is Not Effective in Enhancing Elimination	
Vancomycin	Gentamicin
Thyroxin	Tacrolimus
Digoxin	Organophosphate agents
Carbamazepine (significant rebound effect)	

References

Mokrzycki MH and Kaplan AA, "Therapeutic Plasma Exchange: Complications and Management," *Am J Kidney Dis*, 1994, 23(6):817-27.

Nenov VD, Marinov P, Sabeva J, et al, "Current Applications of Plasmapheresis in Clinical Toxicology," *Nephrol Dial Transplant*, 2003, 18(Suppl 5):56-8.

POSTMORTEM BLOOD-DRUG CONCENTRATIONS

Druid H and Holmgren P, "A Compilation of Fatal and Control Concentrations of Drugs in Postmortem Femoral Blood," *J Forensic Sci*, 1997, 42(1):79-87. Copyright American Society for Testing and Materials (ATSM); reprinted with permission.

Femoral Blood Concentrations of 83 Substances

A compilation of postmortem femoral blood concentrations of drugs is presented. The samples are collected from cases in which the cause of death was:

- **Group A**: Fatal intoxication with the substance exclusively
- **Group B**: Fatal intoxication with the substance in combination with other drugs and/or alcohol
- **Group C**: Other cause of death without incapacitation due to drugs
- **Group D**: Concentrations in whole blood from suspected-drugged drivers

In groups A to C, concentrations refer to femoral blood.

Substance (Synonym)	Molecular Weight§	Case Type	N (mcg/g)	Low (mcg/g)	Median (mcg/g)	High (mcg/g)
Acetaminophen (paracetamol)	151.2	A	0	-	-	-
		B	139	90	170	320
		C	168	1.0	5.0	13
		D	67	0.9	4.0	22
Alimemazine (trimeprazine)	298.4	A	11	1.0	1.6	3.2
		B	9	0.5	0.9	1.2
		C	15	0.1	0.1	0.4
		D	3	0.06	0.1	0.1
Desmethylalimemazine	284.4	A	11	0.2	0.7	1.3
		B	8	0.2	0.3	0.5
		C	9	0.1	0.2	0.2
		D	2	0.07	0.14	0.2
Alprazolam	308.8	A	0	-	-	-
		B	5	0.3	0.3	0.4
		C	6	0.02	0.05	0.05
		D	22	0.02	0.05	0.18
Amitriptyline	277.4	A	49	1.2	3.2	14
		B	39	0.5	1.4	6.0
		C	29	0.1	0.2	0.6
		D	7	0.05	0.09	0.1
Nortriptyline, metabolite	263.4	A	46	0.2	0.8	3.1
		B	33	0.1	0.3	1.2
		C	23	0.1	0.1	0.4
		D	4	0.08	0.09	0.3
Biperiden	311.5	A	0	-	-	-
		B	4	0.25	0.29	0.66
		C	2	0.02	0.04	0.06
		D	0	-	-	-

(*Continued*)

Substance (Synonym)	Molecular Weight§	Case Type	N (mcg/g)	Low (mcg/g)	Median (mcg/g)	High (mcg/g)
Caffeine	194.2	A	0	-	-	-
		B	9	21	30	32
		C	7	12	17	30
		D	0	-	-	-
Carbamazepine	236.3	A	7	35	45	70
		B	9	10	14	19
		C	56	0.5	4.5	10
		D	30	0.9	4.0	8.3
Carisoprodol	260.3	A	14	9.3	25.5	40
		B	16	5.4	11.5	37
		C	7	0.4	0.7	1.8
		D	31	0.4	2.8	8.4
Chlordiazepoxide	299.8	A	1	-	4.4	-
		B	4	2.7	2.9	3.0
		C	12	0.1	0.2	1.3
		D	12	0.3	1.1	6.0
Chlormezanone	273.7	A	1	-	18	-
		B	7	11	14	16
		C	6	0.3	1.3	6.3
		D	17	0.4	1.5	14
Chloroquine	319.9	A	6	1.3	23.5	35.5
		B	3	0.4	1.2	16
		C	9	0.2	0.9	1.7
		D	0	-	-	-
Chlorpromazine	318.9	A	1	-	6.7	-
		B	2	0.8	1.6	2.4
		C	4	0.1	0.1	0.2
		D	0	-	-	-
Desmethylchlorpromazine	304.9	A	1	-	0.1	-
		B	0	-	-	-
		C	0	-	-	-
		D	0	-	-	-
Chlorprothixene	315.9	A	2	1.6	1.6	1.7
		B	2	0.6	3.8	7.0
		C	1	-	0.2	-
		D	0	-	-	-
Chlorzoxazone	169.6	A	0	-	-	-
		B	13	8.0	11	28
		C	8	0.6	1.1	4.6
		D	6	0.3	2.2	3.1
Citalopram	324.4	A	8	3.4	7.0	10.5
		B	13	0.7	1.1	4.7
		C	71	0.1	0.6	1.1
		D	22	0.06	0.15	0.4

(*Continued*)

Substance (Synonym)	Molecular Weight§	Case Type	N (mcg/g)	Low (mcg/g)	Median (mcg/g)	High (mcg/g)
Desmethylcitalopram	310.4	A	8	0.1	0.3	0.7
		B	13	0.1	0.1	0.6
		C	43	0.1	0.2	0.3
		D	9	0.05	0.08	0.1
Clomipramine	314.9	A	9	1.6	1.9	2.4
		B	37	0.6	1.1	5.0
		C	61	0.1	0.2	0.4
		D	17	0.02	0.08	0.4
Desmethylclomipramine	300.9	A	9	0.8	1.4	2.0
		B	37	0.2	0.7	4.9
		C	46	0.1	0.2	0.7
		D	12	0.06	0.3	0.5
7-Amino-clonazepam	285.7	A	0	-	-	-
		+CLO† B	4	0.3	0.6	1.0
		C	6	0.06	0.13	0.18
		D	15	0.02	0.04	0.28
Clozapine	326.8	A	2	1.2	3.2	5.2
		B	0	-	-	-
		C	6	0.1	0.6	1.1
		D	0	-	-	-
Codeine	299.4	A	1	-	0.6	-
		B	25	0.5	1.1	2.6
		C	20	0.02	0.05	0.4
		D	44	0.005	0.04	0.4
Desipramine	266.4	A	0	-	-	-
		B	4	0.9	1.2	1.5
		C	11	0.1	0.2	0.8
		D	2	0.05	0.06	0.06
Diazepam	284.7	A	0	-	-	-
		B	0	-	-	-
		C	90	0.1	0.1	0.3
		D	275	0.1	0.2	0.8
N-Desmethyldiazepam (nordazepam)	270.7	A	0	-	-	-
		B	0	-	-	-
		C	89	0.1	0.1	0.3
		D	251	0.1	0.2	0.7
Diltiazem	414.5	A	0	-	-	-
		B	0	-	-	-
		C	13	0.1	0.2	0.4
		D	0	-	-	-
Dixyrazine	427.6	A	2	5.5	7.5	9.4
		B	12	0.8	2.0	9.0
		C	3	0.2	0.2	0.5
		D	1	-	0.4	-

(*Continued*)

Substance (Synonym)	Molecular Weight§	Case Type	*N* (mcg/g)	Low (mcg/g)	Median (mcg/g)	High (mcg/g)
Ephedrine	174.2	A	0	-	-	-
		B	0	-	-	-
		C	10	0.1	0.2	0.6
		D	16	0.05	0.3	2.0
Ethylmorphine	313.4	A	0	-	-	-
		B	5	0.2	0.4	0.9
		C	0	-	-	-
		D	7	0.01	0.01	0.02
Flunitrazepam	313.3	A	0	-	-	-
		B	0	-	-	-
		C	5	0.02	0.03	0.05
		D	130	0.01	0.01	0.05
7-Amino-flunitrazepam	283.3	+ FLU* A	44	0.16	0.31	0.64
		+ FLU* B	139	0.06	0.14	0.43
		C	73	0.01	0.02	0.12
		D	143	0.01	0.02	0.06
Fluvoxamine	318.4	A	4	3.4	5.0	10.7
		B	10	1.2	3.5	8.1
		C	9	0.2	0.5	0.7
		D	1	-	0.3	-
Hydroxyzine	374.9	A	1	-	2.5	-
		B	8	0.9	1.3	1.5
		C	6	0.1	0.2	0.4
		D	5	0.05	0.2	1.0
Imipramine	280.4	A	0	-	-	-
		B	4	1.2	1.4	2.8
		C	4	0.1	0.2	0.5
		D	1	-	0.1	-
Ketamine	237.7	A	0	-	-	-
		B	0	-	-	-
		C	43	0.3	1.0	3.4
		D	5	0.1	1.0	1.0
Ketobemidone	247.3	A	3	0.2	0.3	0.6
		B	5	0.3	0.4	0.5
		C	5	0.03	0.05	0.12
		D	2	0.05	0.06	0.07
Lidocaine	234.3	A	0	-	-	-
		B	6	1.0	2.1	2.1
		C	113	0.1	0.2	1.2
		D	5	0.06	0.2	0.3
Maprotiline	277.4	A	8	2.7	3.5	5.8
		B	6	1.0	2.7	3.6
		C	11	0.1	0.3	0.9
		D	0	-	-	-

(*Continued*)

Substance (Synonym)	Molecular Weight§	Case Type	N (mcg/g)	Low (mcg/g)	Median (mcg/g)	High (mcg/g)
Melperone	263.4	A	5	1.0	3.7	3.8
		B	7	3.0	5.9	11
		C	6	0.1	0.2	0.2
		D	0	-	-	-
Dihydromelperone	265.3	A	5	0.6	1.1	1.2
		B	7	1.3	2.6	3.0
		C	6	0.1	0.1	0.2
		D	0	-	-	-
Mepivacaine	246.4	A	0	-	-	-
		B	0	-	-	-
		C	21	0.1	0.3	1.3
		D	8	0.2	0.3	0.3
Meprobamate	218.3	A	3	130	245	260
		B	16	22	31	73
		C	5	2.8	3.5	4.6
		D	34	3.7	12.5	3.7
Methadone	309.5	A	6	0.5	0.8	1.1
		B	0	-	-	-
		C	3	0.1	0.1	0.3
		D	24	0.05	0.1	0.2
Methotrimeprazine (levomepromazine)	328.5	A	5	0.8	2.3	3.2
		B	26	0.5	0.9	3.5
		C	15	0.1	0.1	1.7
		D	4	0.04	0.07	0.1
Desmethylmethotrimeprazine	314.5	A	5	0.4	2.3	4.5
		B	21	0.2	0.5	1.7
		C	11	0.1	0.2	1.0
		D	3	0.08	0.1	0.2
Mianserin	264.4	A	3	1.6	2.8	13
		B	8	0.7	0.9	1.3
		C	50	0.03	0.08	0.2
		D	3	0.01	0.02	0.04
Desmethylmianserin	250.4	A	3	1.4	1.5	5.1
		B	5	0.1	0.3	0.4
		C	26	0.03	0.1	0.2
		D	0	-	-	-
Midazolam	325.8	A	0	-	-	-
		B	0	-	-	-
		C	21	0.03	0.05	0.4
		D	0	-	-	-
Moclobemide	268.7	A	0	-	-	-
		B	10	1.9	4.4	21
		C	17	0.2	0.6	2.1
		D	2	0.3	0.4	0.4

(*Continued*)

Substance (Synonym)	Molecular Weight§	Case Type	N (mcg/g)	Low (mcg/g)	Median (mcg/g)	High (mcg/g)
Oxomoclobemide	282.7	A	0	-	-	-
		B	10	0.3	0.9	2.4
		C	18	0.2	0.5	0.8
		D	1	-	0.5	-
Nitrazepam	281.5	A	0	-	-	-
		B	0	-	-	-
		C	12	0.01	0.02	0.03
		D	85	0.02	0.05	0.19
7-Amino-nitrazepam	251.3	+ NIT‡ A	16	0.5	1.2	2.8
		+ NIT‡ B	57	0.2	0.8	1.8
		C	90	0.04	0.08	0.2
		D	83	0.02	0.05	0.2
Nortriptyline	263.4	A	5	1.6	3.8	4.0
		B	8	1.9	2.3	3.3
		C	0	-	-	-
		D	0	-	-	-
Orphenadrine	269.4	A	18	5.3	15	145
		B	10	4.6	8.9	40
		C	17	0.1	0.3	1.6
		D	9	0.1	0.2	0.2
Oxazepam	286.7	A	2	4.4	5.3	6.1
		B	5	2.3	3.6	3.7
		C	20	0.1	0.3	0.7
		D	76	0.2	0.5	1.4
Paroxetine	329.4	A	0	-	-	-
		B	6	0.7	4.5	4.6
		C	15	0.09	0.3	0.5
		D	1	-	0.09	-
Pentobarbital	226.3	A	2	10	34	58
		B	1	-	10	-
		C	11	0.1	0.4	1.4
		D	10	0.1	1.2	4.9
Pethidine	247.3	A	0	-	-	-
		B	0	-	-	-
		C	8	0.2	0.3	0.5
		D	9	0.1	0.2	0.3
Phenazone	188.2	A	0	-	-	-
		B	24	13	31.5	100
		C	10	2.1	6.3	28
		D	22	0.8	2.5	11
Phenobarbital	232.2	A	9	55	75	114
		B	4	25.5	36.5	47
		C	4	2.5	7.0	13
		D	11	1.0	17	90

(*Continued*)

Substance (Synonym)	Molecular Weight§	Case Type	N (mcg/g)	Low (mcg/g)	Median (mcg/g)	High (mcg/g)
Phenylpropanolamine	151.2	A	0	-	-	-
		B	0	-	-	-
		C	5	0.06	0.2	0.3
		D	4	0.09	0.1	0.2
Phenytoin	252.3	A	1	-	43	-
		B	1	-	80	-
		C	14	1.0	5.0	14
		D	5	3.0	11	11.5
Promethazine	284.4	A	3	1.8	2.4	5.4
		B	9	0.6	5.2	11.8
		C	11	0.1	0.1	0.3
		D	6	0.03	0.1	0.1
Desmethylpromethazine	270.4	A	3	0.3	1.4	1.8
		B	9	0.1	0.3	1.6
		C	7	0.1	0.1	0.2
		D	1	-	0.07	-
Propiomazine	340.5	A	24	0.1	0.9	5.4
		B	85	0.08	0.3	1.9
		C	14	0.03	0.05	0.4
		D	4	0.03	0.04	0.08
Dihydropropiomazine	342.5	A	24	0.9	1.9	5.8
		B	85	0.3	0.7	2.0
		C	44	0.03	0.08	0.2
		D	3	0.04	0.09	0.1
Propoxyphene (dextropropoxyphene)	339.5	A	72	1.3	2.8	8.1
		B	223	0.9	2.0	5.9
		C	89	0.1	0.2	0.8
		D	31	0.04	0.1	0.4
Propranolol	259.3	A	7	4.6	11	13
		B	5	3.9	5.8	5.9
		C	2	0.1	1.1	2.0
		D	3	0.1	0.1	1.9
Remoxipride	371.3	A	11	41	65	150
		B	10	3.6	23.5	73
		C	15	0.7	1.6	4.1
		D	4	0.07	0.2	0.1
Salicylate	138.1	A	1	-	94	-
		B	3	150	158	230
		C	5	15	36	39
		D	0	-	-	-

(*Continued*)

Substance (Synonym)	Molecular Weight§	Case Type	N (mcg/g)	Low (mcg/g)	Median (mcg/g)	High (mcg/g)
Theophylline	180.2	A	4	85	110	140
		B	7	20	62	100
		C	27	1.0	4.0	10
		D	3	0.6	2.0	4.0
Thiopental	242.3	A	0	-	-	-
		B	0	-	-	-
		C	36	0.1	0.5	2.1
		D	5	1.2	4.0	4.1
Thioridazine	370.6	A	5	2.4	3.3	3.5
		B	14	1.0	1.8	3.8
		C	19	0.1	0.3	0.7
		D	9	0.1	0.2	0.4
Trichloroethanol	149.4	A	16	60	125	390
		B	6	27	98	109
		C	0	-	-	-
		D	0	-	-	-
Trimethoprim	290.3	A	0	-	-	-
		B	0	-	-	-
		C	6	0.4	2.2	5.9
		D	0	-	-	-
Trimipramine	294.4	A	10	1.7	3.5	8.2
		B	17	0.7	1.9	15
		C	8	0.4	0.5	0.8
		D	2	0.05	0.1	0.2
Desmethyltrimipramine	280.4	A	10	0.3	0.8	2.5
		B	16	0.1	0.5	1.2
		C	7	0.1	0.2	0.5
		D	0	-	-	-
Verapamil	454.6	A	1	-	3.9	-
		B	5	1.6	1.9	3.6
		C	20	0.1	0.2	1.0
		D	0	-	-	-
Norverapamil	440.6	A	1	-	1.3	-
		B	5	0.1	0.8	0.8
		C	17	0.1	0.1	0.3
		D	0	-	-	-
Vinbarbital	224.3	A	2	17	18	19
		B	4	12.1	15.1	18.5
		C	0	-	-	-
		D	0	-	-	-

(*Continued*)

Substance (Synonym)	Molecular Weight§	Case Type	N (mcg/g)	Low (mcg/g)	Median (mcg/g)	High (mcg/g)
Zolpidem	307.4	A	0	-	-	-
		B	9	0.9	1.3	1.3
		C	3	0.08	0.1	0.12
		D	9	0.13	0.16	0.23
Zopiclone	388.5	A	4	0.6	0.7	1.8
		B	16	0.4	1.2	2.3
		C	10	0.06	0.08	0.4
		D	26	0.03	0.11	0.4

*FLU = flunitrazepam.

†CLO = clonazepam.

‡NIT = nitrazepam.

§Molecular weight is given, enabling calculation of molarities.

Low: Lower percentile (N >9), lower quartile (N = 4-9), or minimum value (N <4).

High: Upper percentile (N > 9); upper quartile (N = 4-9), or maximum value (N < 4).

Substance names are given according to Clark's isolation and identification of drugs (3). For some drugs, common synonyms are displayed in brackets.

POSTMORTEM DRUG DATA

Drugs in Which Postmortem Transformation or Redistribution May Occur (Approximate Heart Blood:Peripheral Blood Ratio)

Alfentanil
Alprazolam (1.5)
Amitriptyline (3.1)
Amineptine hydrochloride
Amoxapine (1.8)
Amphetamine
Benztropine (1.3)
Brompheniramine
Bupropion (1.9)
Chloralose
Chloroquine
Chlorpheniramine (3.1)
Chlorpromazine (4.0)
Clomipramine (1.9)
*Clonazepam
Clopenthixol (1.5)
Clothiapine
Clozapine (2.8)
Cocaine (1.5-2.3)
Codeine (1.8)
Cyclobenzaprine (2.2)
D-Methamphetamine (2.1)
Desipramine (2.4)
Dextromethorphan (2)
Diazepam (1.6)
Diltiazem (2.6)
Diphenhydramine (2.3)
Dothiepin (3)
Doxepin (5.5)
Doxylamine
Fentanyl
*Flunitrazepam (3)
Fluoxetine (2.9)
Gamma hydroxybutyrate (1.8)
Haloperidol (3.6)
Imipramine (1.8-2.2)
Ketamine (1.6)
Lidocaine
Maprotiline (3.4)
Mesoridazine (1.3)
Metapramine
Methamphetamine
Methotrimeprazine (1.3)

Methylfentanyl
Methprylon (1.9)
Metoprolol (3.8)
Mexiletine (3.6)
Midazolam (4)
Morphine (heroin) (2.2)
Naproxen (1.5)
N-methylbenzodioxazolybutamine or MBDB (2.5)
Nicotine (3)
*Nitrazepam
Nortriptyline (2.4)
Orphenadrine (1.9)
Oxycodone (3.1)
Paroxetine (1.3)
Pentazocine (2)
Pethidine or Meperidine (2.1)
Phencyclidine (1.8)
Phenylbutazone (2.3)
Phenylpropanolamine (2.4)
Phenytoin (1.4)
Profriptyline
Promethazine (1.6)
Propafenone (2.4)
Propoxyphene (3.5)
Propranolol (2.5)
Pseudoephedrine (1.5)
Quetiapine
Remifentanil
Secobarbital (1.5)
Strychnine (15)
Sufentanil
Temazepam (1.6)
Tetrahydrocannabinol
Timolol (2)
Tranylcypromine (2.2)
Trazadone (1.6)
Triazolam (2.8)
Trichlorethanol (2)
Trimipramine (1.6)
Venlafaxine (1.6)
Verapamil
Zolpidem (2.1)

*Postmortem transformation to 7-amino metabolite may occur.

Toxins/Drugs in Which Postmortem Redistribution Probably Does Not Occur

*Alcohols
Carbamazepine
Carbon monoxide
Chlordiazepoxide
Diflunisal
Ephedrine
Hydrocodone
Hydroxyzine
Lorazepam
Meprobamate

Mirtazapine
Phenelzine
Pheniramine
Phenobarbital
Primidone
Procyclidine
Quinine/Quinidine
Theophylline
Zopiclone

*Ethanol level may increase in decomposed bodies due to postmortem fermentation.

Drugs Which Concentrate in the Bile for Postmortem Analysis (Bile-Blood Ratio in mg/L)

Acebutolol (416-22)
Acetaminophen (560-248)
Amitriptyline (25-2.2)
Amoxapine (61-18)
Anileridine (2.4-0.9)
Antimony (404-4.6)
Barium (6.1-1.9)
Benzoylecyonine (12-2.4)
Bismoth (3.9-0.5)
Buprenorphine (25.3-0.004)
Chlordiazepoxide (4-2.5)
Chlorpromazine (80-1.4)
Chlorprothixene (3.9-0.1)
Clozapine (454-2.8)
Cocaethylene (0.6-0.08)
Cocaine (0.7-0.2)
Cochicine (2.9-0.6)
Codeine (18-2.8)
Colchicine (2.9-0.06)
Cyproheptadine (8.1-0.5)
Desipramine (39-5.6)
Diazepam (2.8-0.9)
Diltiazem (180-11)
Dothiepin (65-3)
Doxepin (108-7.4)
Ecgonine methylester (3.3-1.2)
Ethchlorvynol (382-78)
Fenfluramine (65-6.5)
Fentanyl (0.03-0.01)
Flecainide (290-53)
Fluoxetine (0.013-0.006)
Flurazepam (43-9)
Gamma-Hydroxybutyrate (57-12)
Heroin (morphine) (32-0.43)

Hydromorphone (9.2-0.3)
Hydroxyzine (122-39)
Imipramine (45-3.7)
Isoniazid (900-43)
Levorphanol (24-2.7)
Lidocaine (19-12)
Maprotiline (161-6.2)
Methadone (7.5-1)
Methamphetamine (22-8)
Methapyrilene (25-8)
Methaqualone (83-8)
Methylfentanyl (0.047-0.007)
Methylphenidate (5.7-2.8)
Metoprolol (254-4.7)
Mexiletine (440-38)
Mirtazepine (2.5-0.22)
Norsertraline (57-0.4)
Nortriptyline (11-2)
Oxycodone (28-5)
Para-Methoxyamphetamine (8-1.1)
Perphenazine (40-4)
Phenmetrazine (5-1)
Phenylbutazone (475-400)
Sertraline (11-0.3)
Sodium Azide (651-135)
Sulindac (2810-130)
Thioridazine (9-3)
Tramadol (3.5-1.9)
Trazodone (45-15)
Trichloroethanol (111-79)
Trimipramine (2.4-1.3)
Venlafaxine (195-45)
Zimelidine (1.4-0.7)

Reference

Lemos N and Argarwal A, "Significance of Bile Analysis in Drug Induced Deaths," *J Anal Tox*, 1996, 20:61-3.

Recommended Tissue Sites to Determine Acute Fatal Poisoning

Aconitum alkaloids (liver, kidneys, ileum, feces)
Alimemazine (brain)
Cadmium (liver or renal cortex)
Chloralose (kidney)
Chloroquine (liver >150 mg/kg)
Cocaine (brain – mesolimbic dopamanergic system)
Colchicine (bile)
Copper (liver)
Digoxin (kidney >140 mcg/kg)
Diquat (kidney >2.4 mcg/g)
Edrin (adipose >90 mg/kg)
Ethanol (vitreous)

Gold (renal Cortex)
Heroin (brain/cerebellum)*
Insulin (tissue site injection or femoral blood)
Lidocaine (>15 mg/kg in brain, lung, heart, liver, kidney)†
Platinum (urine or kidney)
Potassium (vitreous: postmortem interval (hours) = $(7.14 \times K^+) - 39.1$)
Silver (brain/liver)
Xylene (liver >1 mg/kg)
Zopiclone (right lobe of liver and blood)

*Cerebellum/blood morphine level ratio is about 1 when death occurs with 1 hour and is 3.5 when death occurs with 2-48 hours of administration; also analyzing 6-Acetylmorphine in CSF can detect 46% more heroin-related cases than blood.

†Absorption of tracheal lidocaine during intubation (CPR) results in a kidney to liver lidocaine ratio less than one whereas absorption during I.V. lidocaine treatment gives a ratio over one.

Autopsy Findings of Toxin-Involved Deaths

Dinitrol-o-cresol (rapid rigor mortis)
Hydrogen sulfide (dark coins)
Carbon monoxide (cherry red? <1% prevalence)
Loperamide (infants <6 months of age - severe abdominal distention)
Diethyltin (interstitial edema of brain white matter)
Methanol (putamen/retinal - photoreceptor cell necrosis; optic nerve degeneration)

Ethylene glycol (oxalate nephrosis)
Benzene/lead acetate (bone marrow fibrosis)
Chronic anthracycline administration (hydropic myocardial degeneration)
Vitamin D (ectopic calcification)
Fentanyl (syringe in vein)

Agents Causing Necrotic Gastroenteritis on Autopsy

Arsenic
Bismuth
Copper
Gold
Iron Salts
Lead
Manganese

Mercury
Nitrites
Nickel
Phosphorous
Thallium
Vanadium
Zinc

General Bibliography

1. Anderson DT and Fritz KL, "Quetiapine (Seroquel®) Concentrations in Seven Post-Mortem Cases," *J Anal Tox*, 2000, 24:300-4.
2. Anderson DT, Fritz KL, and Muto JJ, "Distribution of Mirtazapine (Remeron®) in Thirteen Postmortem Cases," *J Anal Tox*, 1999, 23:544-48.
3. Bailey DN and Shaw RF, "Concentrations of Basic Drugs in Postmortem Human Myocardium," *J Toxicol Clin Tox*, 1982, 19:197-202.
4. Ballantyne B, Marrs T, and Turner P (eds), *General and Applied Toxicology*, New York, NY, Grove, 1993.
5. Barnhart FE, Fogacci JR, and Reed DW, "Methamphetamine - A Study of Postmortem Redistribution," *J Anal Tox*, 1999, 23:69-70.
6. Baselt RC (ed), "Disposition of Toxic Drugs and Chemicals in Man," (5th edition), Chemical Toxicology Institute, Foster City, California, 2000.

7. Braithwaite RA, Elliott SP, and Hale KA, "An Unusual Fatality Due to Abuse of Alfentanil/Midazolam Mixture," *J Toxicol Clin Tox*, 2000, 38:231.

8. Broussard LA, Broussard AK, Pittman TS, et al, "Death Due to Inhalation of Ethyl Chloride," *J Forensic Sci*, 2000, 45(1):223-5.

9. Dalphe-Scott M, Degouffe M, Garbutt D, et al, "A Comparison of Drug Concentrations in Postmortem Cardiac and Peripheral Blood in 320 Cases," *Can Soc For Sei J*, 1995, 28:113-21.

10. Dettling RJ, Briglia EJ, Dal Cortivo LA, et al, "The Production of Amitriptyline from Nortriptyline in Formaldehyde Containing Solutions," *J Anal Tox*, 1990, 14:325-6.

11. Druid H and Holmgren P, "A Compilation of Fatal and Control Concentrations of Drugs in Postmortem Femoral Blood," *J Forensic Sci*, 1997, 42:79-87.

12. Elliott S, "The Presence of Gamma-Hydroxybutyric Acid (GHB) in Postmortem Biological Fluids," *J Anal Toxicol*, 2001, 25:152.

13. Gaulier JM, Marquet P, Lacassie E, et al, "Fatal Intoxication Following Self-Administration of a Massive Dose of Buprenorphine," *J Forensic Sci*, 2000, 45(1):226-8.

14. Gill JR and Stajic M, "Ketamine in Non-Hospital and Hospital Deaths in New York City," *J Forensic Sci*, 2000, 45(3):655-8.

15. Goeringer KE, Raymon L, Christian GD, et al, "Postmortem Forensic Toxicology of Selective Serotonin Reuptake Inhibitors: A Review of Pharmacology and Report of 168 Cases," *J Forensic Sci*, 2000, 45(3):633-48.

16. Hilberg T, Ripel A, Slordal L, et al, "The Extent of Postmortem Drug Redistribution in a Rat Model," *J Forensic Sci*, 1999, 44(5):956-62.

17. Hilberg T, Rogde S, and Marland J, "Postmortem Drug Redistribution - Human Cases Related to Results in Experimental Animals, " *J Forensic Sci*, 1999, 44:3-9.

18. Iten PX and Meier M, "Beta-hydroxybutyric Acid - An Indicator for an Alcoholic Ketoacidosis as Cause of Death in Deceased Alcohol Abusers," *J Forensic Sci*, 2000, 45(3):624-32.

19. Jenkins AJ and Lavins ES, "6-Acetylmorphine Detection in Postmortem Cerebrospinal Fluid," *J Anal Tox*, 1998, 22:173-5.

20. Karch SB, "Alternate Strategies for Postmortem Drug Testing," *J Anal Toxicol*, 2001, 25(5):393-5.

21. Karch SB, Stephens BG, and Ho C, "Methamphetamine-Related Deaths in San Francisco: Demographic, Pathologic, and Toxicologic Profiles," *J Forensic Sci*, 1999, 44(2):359-68.

22. Klintz P, "Interpreting the Results of Medico-Legal Analysis in Cases of Substance Abuse," *J Toxicol Clin Tox*, 2000, 38:197-8.

23. Koves EM, Lawrence K, and Mayer JM, "Stability of Diltiazem in Whole Blood: Forensic Implications," *J Forensic Sci*, 1998, 43(3):587-97.

24. Langford AM, Taylor KK, and Pounder DJ, "Drug Concentration in Selected Skeletal Muscles," *J Forensic Sci*, 1998, 43(1):22-7.

25. Levine B and Smialek JE, "Status of Alcohol Absorption in Drinking Drivers Killed in Traffic Accidents," *J Forensic Sci*, 2000, 45(1):11-15.

26. Levine B, Wu SC, and Smialek JE, "Zolpidem Distribution in Postmortem Cases," *J Forensic Sci*, 1999, 44(2):369-71.

27. Logan BK, Fligner CL, and Haddix T, "Cause and Manner of Death in Fatalities Involving Methamphetamine," *J Forensic Sci*, 1998, 43(1):28-34.

28. Logan BK, Smirnow D, and Gullberg RG, "Lack of Predictable Site-Dependent Differences and Time-Dependent Changes in Postmortem Concentrations of Cocaine Benzolecgonine, and Cocaethylene in Humans," *J Anal Tox*, 1997, 20:23-31.

29. Mackey-Bojack S, Kloss J, and Apple F, "Cocaine, Cocaine Metabolite and Ethanol Concentrations in Postmortem Blood and Vitreous Humor," *J Anal Tox*, 2000, 24:59-65.

30. Moriya F and Hasimoto Y, "Redistribution of Basic Drugs into Cardiac Blood from Surrounding Tissues During Early-Stages Postmortem," *J Forensic Sci*, 1999, 44(1):10-6.

31. Moriya F and Hasimoto Y, "Comparative Studies on Tissue Distributions of Organophosphorus, Carbamate and Organochlorine Pesticides in Decedents Intoxicated with These Chemicals," *J Forensic Sci*, 1999, 44(6):1131-5.

32. Pricone MG, King CV, Drummer OH, et al, "Postmortem Investigation of Lamotrigine Concentrations," *J Forensic Sci*, 2000, 45(1):11-15.

33. Prouty RW and Anderson WH, "The Forensic Science Implications of Site and Temporal Influences on Postmortem Blood-Drug Concentrations," *J Forensic Sci*, 1990, 35:243-70.

34. Robertson MD and Drummer OH, "Postmortem Distribution and Redistribution of Nitrobenzodiazepines in Man," *J Forensic Sci*, 1998, 43(1):9-13.

35. Robertson MD and Drummer OH, "Postmortem Drug Metabolism by Bacteria," *J Forensic Sci*, 1995, 40:382-6.

36. Robertson MD and McMullin MM, "Olanzapine Concentrations in Clinical Serum and Postmortem Blood Specimens - When Does Therapeutic Become Toxic?," *J Forensic Sci*, 2000, 45(2):418-21.

37. Rohrig TP, "Comparison of Fentanyl Concentrations in Unembalmed and Embalmed Liver Samples," *J Anal Tox*, 1998, 22:253.

38. Vesey CJ and Langford RM, "Stabilization of Blood Cyanide," *J Anal Tox*, 1998, 22:176-8.

POUNDS TO KILOGRAMS CONVERSION

1 pound = 0.45359 kilograms

1 kilogram = 2.2 pounds

lb	=	kg	lb	=	kg	lb	=	kg
1		0.45	70		31.75	140		63.50
5		2.27	75		34.02	145		65.77
10		4.54	80		36.29	150		68.04
15		6.80	85		38.56	155		70.31
20		9.07	90		40.82	160		72.58
25		11.34	95		43.09	165		74.84
30		13.61	100		45.36	170		77.11
35		15.88	105		47.63	175		79.38
40		18.14	110		49.90	180		81.65
45		20.41	115		52.16	185		83.92
50		22.68	120		54.43	190		86.18
55		24.95	125		56.70	195		88.45
60		27.22	130		58.91	200		90.72
65		29.48	135		61.24			

PRESCRIPTION PRODUCTS CONTAINING ACETAMINOPHEN

Note: Not a complete list. Other prescription products may contain acetaminophen.

Drug Name	Ingredients	Maximum Recommended 24-Hour No. of Doses	Maximum 24-Hour Acetaminophen Dose
Darvocet-N® 50 Tablets	Propoxyphene napsylate 50 mg Acetaminophen 325 mg	12 tablets	3900 mg
Darvocet-N® 100 Tablets	Propoxyphene napsylate 100 mg Acetaminophen 650 mg	6 tablets	3900 mg
Esgic® Tablets or Capsules	Butalbital 50 mg Acetaminophen 325 mg Caffeine 40 mg	6 tablets 6 capsules	1950 mg
Esgic-Plus® Tablets	Butalbital 50 mg Acetaminophen 500 mg Caffeine 40 mg	6 tablets	3000 mg
Fioricet® Tablets	Butalbital 50 mg Acetaminophen 325 mg Caffeine 40 mg	6 tablets	1950 mg
Fioricet® With Codeine Capsules	Codeine phosphate 30 mg Butalbital 50 mg Caffeine 40 mg Acetaminophen 325 mg	6 capsules	1950 mg
Hycomine® Compound Tablets	Hydrocodone bitartrate 5 mg Chlorpheniramine maleate 2 mg Phenylephrine hydrochloride 10 mg Acetaminophen 250 mg Caffeine 30 mg	Adults: 4 tablets Children (6-12): 2 tablets	Adults: 1000 mg Children: 500 mg
Hydrocet® Capsules	Hydrocodone bitartrate 5 mg Acetaminophen 500 mg	8 capsules	4000 mg
Lorcet®-HD Capsules	Hydrocodone bitartrate 5 mg Acetaminophen 500 mg	8 capsules	4000 mg
Lorcet® 10/650 Tablets	Hydrocodone bitartrate 10 mg Acetaminophen 650 mg	6 tablets	3900 mg
Lortab® 2.5/500 Tablets	Hydrocodone bitartrate 2.5 mg Acetaminophen 500 mg	8 tablets	4000 mg
Lortab® 5/500 Tablets	Hydrocodone bitartrate 5 mg Acetaminophen 500 mg	8 tablets	4000 mg
Lortab® 7.5/500 Tablets	Hydrocodone bitartrate 7.5 mg Acetaminophen 500 mg	6 tablets	3000 mg
Lortab® 10/500 Tablets	Hydrocodone bitartrate 10 mg Acetaminophen 500 mg	6 tablets	3000 mg
Lortab® Elixir	Hydrocodone bitartrate 2.5 mg/5 mL Acetaminophen 167 mg/5 mL	6 tbsp	1002 mg
Midrin® Capsules	Isometheptene mucate 65 mg Dichloralphenazone 100 mg Acetaminophen 325 mg	10 capsules	3250 mg
Norco® Tablets	Hydrocodone bitartrate 10 mg Acetaminophen 325 mg	6 tablets	1950 mg
Percocet® Tablets	Oxycodone hydrochloride 5 mg Acetaminophen 325 mg	4 tablets	1300 mg
Phenaphen® with Codeine No. 3 Capsules	Acetaminophen 325 mg Codeine phosphate 30 mg	12 capsules	3900 mg
Phrenilin® Forte Capsules	Butalbital 50 mg Acetaminophen 650 mg	6 capsules	3900 mg
Phrenilin® Tablets	Butalbital 50 mg Acetaminophen 325 mg	6 tablets	1950 mg
Roxicet® Tablets	Oxycodone hydrochloride 5 mg Acetaminophen 325 mg	4 tablets	1300 mg

(Continued)

Drug Name	Ingredients	Maximum Recommended 24-Hour No. of Doses	Maximum 24-Hour Acetaminophen Dose
Roxicet® 5/500 Caplets	Oxycodone hydrochloride 5 mg Acetaminophen 500 mg	4 caplets	2000 mg
Roxicet® Oral Solution	Oxycodone hydrochloride 5 mg Acetaminophen 325 mg Alcohol 0.4%	20 mL qd	1300 mg
Sedapap® 50/650 Tablets	Butalbital 50 mg Acetaminophen 650 mg	6 tablets	3900 mg
Talacen® Caplets	Pentazocine hydrochloride 25 mg Acetaminophen 650 mg	6 caplets	3900 mg
Tylenol® with Codeine No. 2 Tablets	Codeine phosphate 15 mg Acetaminophen 300 mg Sodium metabisulfite	6 tablets	1800 mg
Tylenol® with Codeine No. 3 Tablets	Codeine phosphate 30 mg Acetaminophen 300 mg Sodium metabisulfite	6 tablets	1800 mg
Tylenol® with Codeine No. 4 Tablets	Codeine phosphate 60 mg Acetaminophen 300 mg Sodium metabisulfite	6 tablets	1800 mg
Tylenol® with Codeine Elixir	Codeine phosphate 12 mg/5 mL Acetaminophen 120 mg/5 mL Alcohol 7%	Adults: 6 tbsp Children (7-12): 8 tsp Children (3-6): 3-4 tsp	2160 mg 960 mg 360-480 mg
Tylox® Capsules	Oxycodone hydrochloride 5 mg Acetaminophen 500 mg	4 capsules	2000 mg
Vicodin® Tablets	Hydrocodone bitartrate 5 mg Acetaminophen 500 mg	8 tablets	4000 mg
Vicodin® ES Tablets	Hydrocodone bitartrate 7.5 mg Acetaminophen 750 mg	5 tablets	3750 mg
Vicodin® HP® Tablets	Hydrocodone bitartrate 10 mg Acetaminophen 660 mg	6 tablets	3960 mg
Wygesic® Tablets	Propoxyphene hydrochloride 65 mg Acetaminophen 650 mg	6 tablets	3900 mg
Zydone® Capsules	Hydrocodone bitartrate 10 mg Acetaminophen 500 mg	8 capsules	4000 mg
Zydone® Tablets	Hydrocodone bitartrate 10 mg Acetaminophen 400 mg	8 tablets	3200 mg

Asian Patent Medicine Herbal Products Containing Phenacetin or Acetaminophen	
Product	**Manufacturer**
Cogent 20	Natural Plants Research Institute
Do Huo Jisheng Wan	Min Kang Drug Manufactory
Saridon	F. Hoffman-LaRoche Ltd
Specific Lumbarglin	Guang Zou Pharmaceutical Industrial Corporation
"Gan Mao Qing" Capsule	Bai Yun Shan Pharmaceutical Factory
Chuifong Toukuwan	Nan-Lien Pharmaceutical Company

RADIATION: BASICS OF EXPOSURE

(Adapted from U.S. Department of Health and Human Services, *Case Studies in Environmental Medicine: Ionizing Radiation*, Agency for Toxic Substances and Diseases Registry, October 1993, 1-48.)

Units of Radiation Measurement		
Characteristic	**Unit**	**Description**
Energy	electron volt (eV) (also ergs, joule)	Kinetic energy of an electron as it moves through a potential difference of 1 volt.
Rate of radioactive decay	curie (Ci)	Radioactivity emitted per unit of time (1 Ci = 3.7×10^{10} disintegrations per second).
Air exposure	roentgen (R)	Amount of X and gamma radiation that causes ionization in air. One roentgen of exposure will produce about 2 billion ion pairs per cubic centimeter of air.
Absorbed dose	rad	Dose resulting from one roentgen of ionizing radiation deposited in any medium, typically water or tissue. One rad results in the absorption of 100 ergs of ionizing radiation per gram of medium.
Biologic effectiveness	rem	Dose of any form of ionizing radiation that produces the same biological effect as 1 roentgen; 1 rem = 1 rad $\times$ radiation weighting factor (RWF), where the value of RWF depends on the type of radiation as follows:
		X radiation = 1
		gamma radiation = 1
		beta = 1
		alpha = 20
		neutrons = 5-20, depending on their energy

Half-Lives of Some Radionuclides in Adult Body Organs				
Radionuclide	**Critical Organ**	**Half-Life**		
		Physical	**Biological**	**Effective**
Uranium-238	Kidney	4,460,000,000 y	4 d	4 d
Hydrogen-3* (tritium)	Whole body	12.3 y	10 d	10 d
Iodine-131	Thyroid	8 d	80 d	7.3 d
Strontium-90	Bone	28 y	50 y	18 y
Plutonium-239	Bone surface	24,400 y	50 y	50 y
	Lung	24,400 y	500 d	500 d
Cobalt-60	Whole body	5.3 y	99.5 d	95 d
Iron-55	Spleen	2.7 Y	600 d	388 d
Iron-59	Spleen	45.1 d	600 d	42 d
Manganese-54	Liver	303 d	25 d	23 d
Cesium-137	Whole body	30 y	70 d	70 d

*Mixed in body water as tritiated water.

Weighting Factors for Calculating Effective Dose Equivalent for Selected Tissues			
Tissue	**Weighting Factor**		
	ICRP60	**NCRP115/ICRP60**	**NRC**
Bladder	0.040	0.05	—
Bone marrow	0.143	0.12	0.12
Bone surface	0.009	0.01	0.03
Breast	0.050	0.05	0.15
Colon	0.141	0.12	—

Weighting Factors for Calculating Effective Dose Equivalent for Selected Tissues (*Continued*)

Tissue	Weighting Factor		
	ICRP60	NCRP115/ICRP60	NRC
Liver	0.022	0.05	—
Lung	0.111	0.12	0.12
Esophagus	0.034	0.05	—
Ovary	0.020	0.05	—
Skin	0.006	0.01	—
Stomach	0.139	0.12	—
Thyroid	0.021	0.05	0.03
Gonads	0.183	0.20	0.25
Subtotal	0.969	1	0.70
Remainder	0.031	0.05	0.30

ICRP60 = International Commission on Radiological Protection, 1990 Recommendations of the ICRP.

NCRP115 = National Council on Radiation Protection and Measurements, 1993, Risk Estimates for Radiation Protection, Report 115, Bethesda, MD.

NRC = Nuclear Regulatory Commission, Title 10, Code of Federal Regulations, Part 20.

Common Diagnostic X-ray Doses*

Examination	Mean KVP	Mean MAS (mrem)	Testes/Ovaries (mrem)	Embryo/Fetus
Chest (PA)	80	12	<0.5	<0.5
Skull (lateral)	72	50	<0.5	<0.5
Abdomen (KUB, AP)	78	601	13.7/146	150
Retrograde pyelogram (AP)	77	91	17.2/161	170
Thoracic spine (AP)	75	82	<0.5/0.7	0.9
Cervical spine (AP)	69	48	<0.5	<0.5
Lumbosacral spine (AP)	77	112	13.2/145	150
Pelvis (AP)	100	30	83/79	133
Barium enema (AP)	120	20	68/132	140

*KVP = kilovolt peak; MAS = milliampere second; PA = posteroanterior view; AP = anteroposterior view; mrem = millirem; KUB = kidney, ureter, bladder.

Background Radiation from Consumer Products

Product	Local Dose (mrem/y)	Portion of Body Considered
Coal combustion (fly ash)	0.03-0.3	Lungs
Oil combustion (soot)	1.6	Lungs
Gas ranges (natural gas)	5	Lungs
Tobacco products*	16,000	Lungs
Dentures and crowns†	700	Superficial layers of tissue in contact with teeth
Ophthalmic glass‡	4000	Cornea
Smoke detectors	0.008	Whole body

*Dose for cigarette smokers only; does not include doses experienced by those subjected to passive smoke.

†Due to the uranium present in glazed dental porcelain.

‡Applies to eyeglasses tinted with uranium or thorium.

Types of Ionizing Radiation

Type	Charge	Atomic Mass (amu)	Source*	Shielding†
Alpha	+2	4	Radium-226 Polonium-210 Uranium-238	Sheet of paper; intact skin
Beta	±1	0.0005	Carbon-14 Strontium-90 Tritium Iodine-131	Lead; aluminium foil; a few centimeters of plastic
Neutron	0	1	Particle accelerator Nuclear reactor	High energy=paraffin Low energy=water
Proton	+1	1	Cosmic radiation Particle accelerator	Air
Gamma	0	0	Cobalt-60 Uranium-238 Iodine-131	A few centimeters of lead; many inches of steel
X	0	0	Diagnostic and therapeutic medicine	A few centimeters of lead; many inches of steel

*Familiar examples of originating source.

†In any given situation, the type and thickness of shielding is dependent on the energy and intensity of the radiation.

The benefit from therapy recommendations in the Immediate Actions to Consider (column 2) and Drugs to Consider (column 3) will be influenced by the route of exposure: ingestion, inhalation, skin absorption, injection, or contaminated wounds. The chemical form and solubility of the radionuclide will also change markedly the efficacy of the recommended treatment. The table below lists therapeutic procedures or drug therapy that may be helpful for the listed elements in favorable circumstances.

Treatment Summary for Internal Contamination by Selected Radioactive Elements

Element	Immediate Actions to Consider	Drugs to Consider	Information and Comment
Americium (Am)	DTPA*	DTPA	Chelation should be started as soon as treatment decision can be made. CaEDTA† may be used if CaDTPA‡ is not immediately available.
Arsenic (As)	Lavage	Dimercaprol	Short-lived isotopes. Use of dimercaprol is not indicated except in massive exposures.
Barium (Ba)	Lavage, purgatives	See column 4	Use of sodium or magnesium sulfate with and after stomach lavage will precipitate insoluble barium sulfate.
Calcium (Ca)	Lavage, purgatives, calcium	Calcium, furosemide	Massive exposure may warrant use of the sodium salt of EDTA§, but with caution over a 3- to 4-hour period to avoid tetany. Furosemide enhances urinary excretion.
Californium (Cf)	DTPA, lavage, purgatives	DTPA	Same as for Americium.
Carbon (C)	(None listed)	No treatment available	Low-energy beta rays of carbon-14 are not detected by survey instruments; collect samples and smears for special low-energy beta counting in laboratory.
Cerium (Ce)	DTPA, lavage, purgatives	DTPA	Same as for Americium.
Cesium (Cs)	Prussian blue, lavage, purgatives	Prussian blue	Ion exchange resins should be as effective as Prussian blue, but have not been used in humans.
Chromium (Cr)	Lavage, purgatives	No treatment available for anionic forms; DTPA or DFOA¶ for cationic forms	Antacids are contraindicated. Adsorbents, such as charcoal, may reduce intestinal tract absorption.
Cobalt (Co)	Lavage, purgatives	See column 4	Penicillamine may be considered for therapeutic trial in large exposures.
Curium (Cm)	DTPA, lavage, purgatives	DTPA	Same as for Americium.
Europium (Eu)	Lavage, purgatives	DTPA	None.

	Treatment Summary for Internal Contamination by Selected Radioactive Elements	*(Continued)*	
Element	**Immediate Actions to Consider**	**Drugs to Consider**	**Information and Comment**
Fission products	Lavage, purgatives	#	Gamma-ray spectroscopy of air or swipe samples may identify prominent radionuclides (mixed). Check also for possible alpha emitters.
Fluorine (F)	Aluminum hydroxide gel	See column 4	Very short half-life. Oral aluminum hydroxide gel will reduce absorption in the gastrointestinal (GI) tract.
Gallium (Ga)	See column 4	See column 4	Short half-life. Penicillamine can be considered for therapeutic trial.
Gold (Au)	None	Dimercaprol and penicillamine are possible therapeutic agents	No known therapy for colloidal gold.
Iodine (I)	Potassium iodide, lavage	Potassium iodide	Success of stable iodine depends on early administration.
Iron (Fe)	Lavage	DFOA	Materials that reduce GI absorption include egg yolk or adsorbents. Oral penicillamine also chelates iron.
Lanthanum (La)	Lavage, purgatives	DTPA	CaEDTA may be used if CaDTPA is not immediately available.
Lead (Pb)	Lavage	EDTA	Dimercaprol and penicillamine are less satisfactory alternative drugs.
Mercury (Hg)	Lavage	Penicillamine	Dimercaprol may be considered for alternative therapy. Gastric lavage with egg white solution or 5% sodium formaldehyde sulfoxide; if unavailable, use a 2% to 5% solution of sodium bicarbonate.
Phosphorus (P)	Lavage, aluminum hydroxide	Phosphates	Severe overdosage may be treated with parathyroid extract (intramuscular) in addition to oral phosphates.
Plutonium (Pu)	DTPA	DTPA	DFOA may be used initially if DTPA is not available. CaEDTA may also be used, but is less effective.
Polonium (Po)	Lavage, purgatives	Dimercaprol	Consider toxicity of dimercaprol before using in cases of low-level exposure. Penicillamine is an alternative treatment.
Potassium (K)	Purgatives, diuretics, aluminum hydroxide	Diuretics	Use aluminum hydroxide antacids first to reduce GI tract absorption. Use oral liquid potassium supplements for dilution.
Promethium (Pm)	DTPA	DTPA	Chelation treatment should be started as soon as possible.
Radium (Ra)	Magnesium sulfate, lavage, purgatives	See column 4	Use 10% magnesium sulfate solution for gastric lavage and as saline cathartic. Oral sulfates reduce intestinal absorption. No effective therapy after absorption.
Rubidium (Rb)	Prussian blue	Prussian blue	Chemical properties are similar to potassium, but efficacy of similar treatments is unknown.
Ruthenium (Ru)	Lavage, purgatives	See column 4	Chlorthalidone causes enhanced urinary excretion. DTPA has variable effectiveness.
Scandium (Sc)	Lavage, purgatives	DTPA	EDTA may be used in place of DTPA.
Sodium (Na)	Lavage	Diuretic	Isotopic dilution (1 L of 0.9% sodium chloride) by intravenous route, followed by furosemide or other diuretic agent.
Strontium (Sr)	Aluminum phosphate, lavage	Strontium or calcium intravenously	Corticosteroid may be considered, but adverse reactions should be balanced against probable limited effectiveness.
Technetium (Tc)	(None listed)	(None listed)	Potassium perchlorate has been used effectively to reduce thyroid dose.
Thorium (Th)	(None listed)	DTPA or DFOA for soluble compounds	Treatment not effective for thorotrast (ThO_2).

	Treatment Summary for Internal Contamination by Selected Radioactive Elements (*Continued*)		
Element	**Immediate Actions to Consider**	**Drugs to Consider**	**Information and Comment**
Tritium (^{3}H)	Forced water	Forced water	Low-energy beta rays of ^{3}H are not detectable by survey instruments; requires samples for special low-energy beta counting in laboratory.
Uranium (U)	DTPA	(None listed)	DTPA must be given within 4 hours to be effective. Sodium bicarbonate protects the kidneys from damage.
Yttrium (Y)	(None listed)	DTPA	CaEDTA may be used if CaDTPA is not immediately available.
Zinc (Zn)	Lavage	DTPA	Zinc sulfate or CaEDTA may be used as a diluting agent if CaDTPA is not immediately available. Penicillamine is another alternative.

*DTPA = diethylenetriaminepentaacetic acid.

†CaEDTA = calcium salt of ethylenediaminetetraacetic acid.

‡CaDTPA = calcium diethylenetriaminepentaacetic acid.

§EDTA = ethylenediaminetetraacetic acid.

¶DFOA = deferoxamine or desferrioxamine.

#Depends on major isotope(s) in mixture, which varies with age of the isotope mixture.

Treatment Scheme for Patients Receiving an Acute High-Dose Radiation Exposure

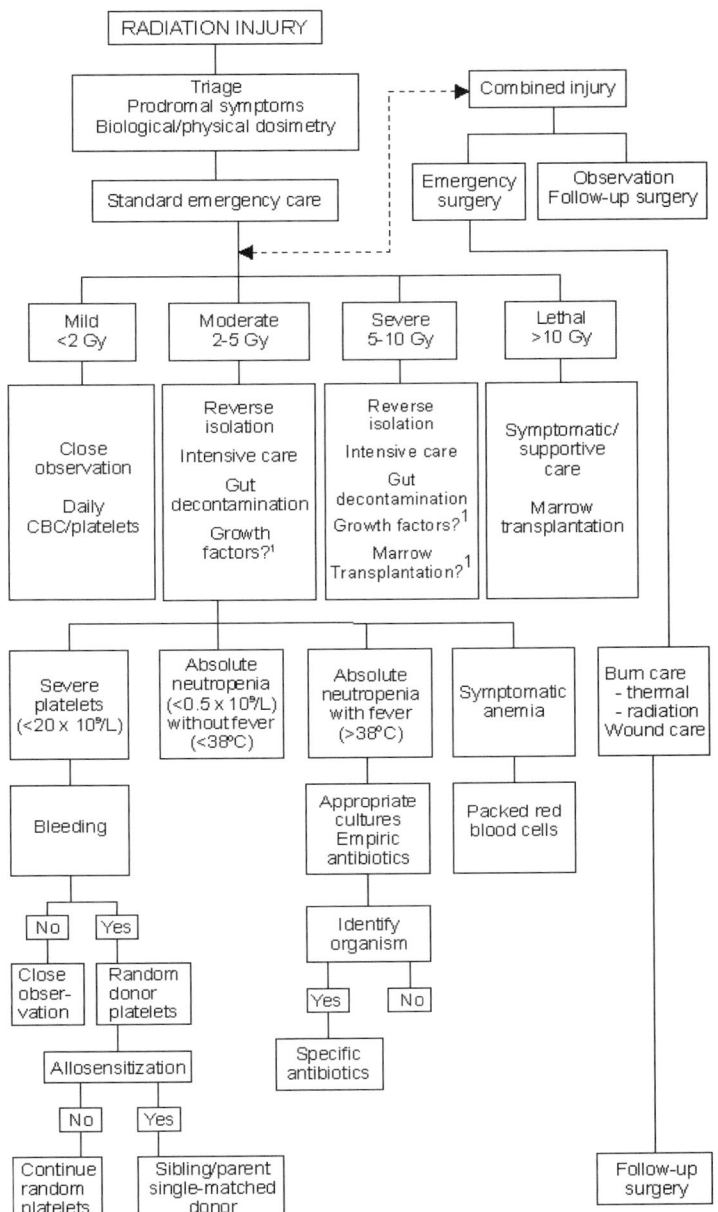

[1]Whole-body exposures >4 Gy may require bone marrow transplantation or administration of colony-stimulating factors or other hematopoietic growth factors that stimulate proliferation of hematopoietic stem cells. However, few data exist to support firm recommendations about the use of these treatments for radiation victims.

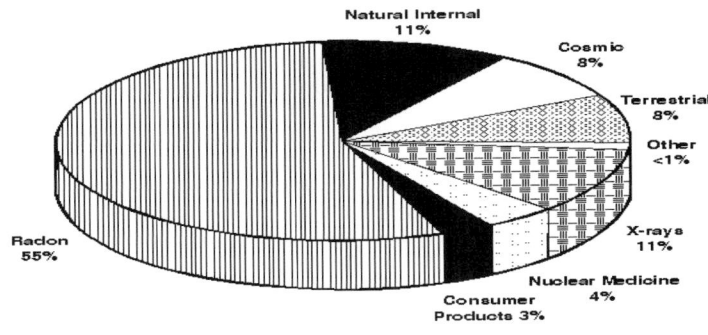

Average Annual Effective Dose Equivalent of Ionizing Radiation of a Member of the U.S. Population*

Source	Effective Dose Equivalent	
	mSv	% of Total Dose
Natural		
Radon†	2.0	55
Cosmic	0.27	8
Terrestrial	0.28	8
Internal	0.39	11
Total natural	3.0	82
Artificial		
Medical		
X-ray	0.39	11
Nuclear	0.14	4
Consumer products	0.10	3
Other		
Occupational	<0.01	<0.3
Nuclear fuel cycle	<0.01	<0.03
Fallout	<0.01	<0.03
Miscellaneous‡	<0.01	<0.03
Total artificial	0.63	18
Total natural and artificial	3.6	100

*Adapted from BEIR V, Washington, DC: National Academy Press, 1990.

†Dose equivalent to bronci from radon daughter products.

‡DOE facilities, smelter, transportation, etc.

Common Analytical Methods for Measuring Radioactive Material Inside and Radiation Outside the Body

Sample Matrix	Preparation Method	Device Used
Whole body, portion of body, or organ (x or γ radiation)	Position individual in front of detector with area of interest shielded from extraneous radiation	Multichannel analyzer with NaI detector for up to a few γ-emitters, a germanium detector for any number of γ-emitters, or a planar germanium detector for α-emitters that also emit x-rays
Urine, blood, or feces	Put any solids into solution; do chemical separation if multiple radioactive elements are present; deposit thin layer on a planchet or mix with liquid scintillation cocktail	Liquid scintillation for α- or β-emitters; alpha spectroscopy for α-emitters; GM counter for high-energy β- or γ-emitters; multichannel analyzer for γ-emitters
Personal monitoring: external radiation dose (β- and γ-radiation)	Heat dosimeter to produce thermoluminescence	TLD
	Develop film	Film badge
	None	Electronic dosimeter
Contamination monitoring: surfaces, skin, clothing, shoes (β- and γ-radiation)	None	GM counter
Contamination monitoring: surfaces, skin, clothing (α-radiation)	None	Proportional counter

GM = Geiger-Mueller; TLD = thermoluminescent dosimeters.

Summary of Some Studies of Humans Exposed to Radiation and Radionuclides

Location	Year(s)	Radionuclide	Purpose of Experiment	Number of People Dosed	Dose and Route of Exposure	Result
ANL	1931-1933	^{226}Ra	Determine the retention time of ^{226}Ra in humans	NA	70-50 mcg; injected	Incomplete
ANL	1943-1946	X-rays; ^{32}P	Determine effects of radiation, process chemicals, and toxic metals in humans	4	X-rays: 30 R ^{32}P; route not specified	White blood cell chemistry was important in assessing the radiation sensitivity of workers exposed to radiation
ANL	1944-1945	^{32}P	Study the metabolism of hemoglobin in cases of polycythemia rubra vera	7	15-40 µCi; route not specified	NA
ANL	1962	^{3}H	Study the uptake of ^{3}H thymidine in tumors and the effects of ^{3}H on tumors	4	10 µCi; injected	Similar growth was noted in both cancerous and non-cancerous cells treated with ^{3}H
ANL	1943-1944	X-ray	Study hematological changes at varying doses of radiation in cancer therapy	14	27-500 R; external exposure	Reduction of white blood cells formed in lymphoid tissue; routine monitoring of blood components not a practical way of assessing the usual occupational radiation exposures
ANL	1948-1953	^{76}As	Determine effects of ^{76}As on hematopoietic tissues in leukemia patients	24	17-90 mCi; intravenous	^{76}As as effective as more commonly used leukemia therapeutic agents
BNL	1950	^{131}I	Determine the usefulness of ^{131}I to treat patients with Grave's disease and metastatic carcinoma of the thyroid	12	4-360 mCi or 6-20 mCi; route not specified	NA
BNL	1951	^{131}I	Study interaction of the thyroid and ^{131}I in children with nephrotic syndrome	8	NA	Maximum uptake of ^{131}I was 30%-60% of administered dose (3-5 µCi); no impairment of I uptake in children with nephrotic syndrome
BNL	1952-1953	^{42}K ^{38}Cl ^{131}I (1 patient)	Examine formation and cycling of cerebrospinal fluid (CSF)	2	NA; injected route not specified	The amount of CSF produced daily is small and fluid production is not solely produced by the choroid plexus
BNL	1963	^{59}Fe	Study iron absorption in women with various menstrual histories	9	1-10 µCi; oral	Menstrual blood loss in women with excessive bleeding was 110-550 mL. Normal women lost 33-59 mL during menstruation. Heavy menstruating women had higher gastrointestinal tract (GIT) absorption of iron than normal women
BNL	1967	^{47}Ca	Study the role of dietary Ca in osteoporosis	7	25 µcCi; intravenous	Diets high in Ca had a small but positive impact on osteoporosis
BNL	Early 1970s	^{82}Br	Study the kinetics of halothane	4	2.5 µCi; inhalation	Concentrations of halothane were initially high in upper parts of the body and low in lower parts of the body; diffusion equilibrium throughout the body was achieved in about 24 minutes

Summary of Some Studies of Humans Exposed to Radiation and Radionuclides (*Continued*)

Location	Year(s)	Radionuclide	Purpose of Experiment	Number of People Dosed	Dose and Route of Exposure	Result
HS	1963	^{131}I	Determine uptake kinetics of ^{131}I in humans	8	NA. Dairy cows consumed 5 mg to 2 g/day of I; volunteers consumed milk produced by the cows exposed to ^{131}I in the diet	Uptake of ^{131}I in humans was characterized
LBL	1942-1946	X-ray	Determine if blood cell changes could be used to indicate exposure in workers on the Manhattan Project.	29	5-50 R, daily dose 100-300 R, total dose; whole body external exposure	Significant deviations in white blood cell counts, anemia formed in relation to dose
LBL	1948-1949	X-ray	Determine the effects of radiation on the pituitary gland during treatment of cancers of other tissues	>1	8000-10,000 rad; external exposure	Pituitary is extremely resistant to x-rays
LBL	1949-1950	X-ray	Effect of radiation on the pituitary gland and its effect on advanced melanoma and breast cancer	3	8500-10,000 rad; external exposure	Pituitary is extremely resistant to x-rays
LBL	Early 1950s	^{60}Co	Determine feasibility of treating bladder cancer using beads labeled with ^{60}Co	35	5000-6000 rad over 7 days. Beads were placed inside the bladder cavity	Noninfiltrating cancers were more successfully treated than were the infiltrating bladder cancers
LBL	1961	^{90}Y	Determine the effectiveness of ^{90}Y in the treatment of acute leukemia in a child	1	200 rad to lymphatic tissue; route not specified	Therapy resulted in temporary remission of leukemia; little effect on peripheral blood cells and red blood cells
LLNL	1980s	^{13}N ^{41}Ar	Determine the uptake and clearance of nitrogen gas in order to better understand "decompression sickness" in deep-sea divers	11	NA; inhalation route of exposure; doses in the mCi range Absorbed dose to the lungs estimated to be 0.3-0.5 rad	NA
LLNL	1955	NA	Obtain information needed to plan for the safe and effective use of military aircraft near "mushroom clouds" during combat operation	4	≤15 R; inhalation and external routes were the likely routes of exposure	No significant internal deposition of fission products or unfissioned Pu were detected in urine or via whole body counting
LLNL	1961-1962	^{85}Sr	Determine the cutaneous absorption kinetics of ^{85}Sr through human skin	2	70 µCi; dermal exposure	Absorption of ^{85}Sr across the skin was low, and ranged from 0.2% to 0.6% total absorption
OR	1956-1973	^{60}Co ^{137}Cs	Study efficacy of total body irradiation on the treatment of leukemia, polycythemia rubra vera, and lymphoma	194	50-300 R, one person received 500 R; external exposure	Higher frequency of remissions after 150 R compared to 250 R. Total body irradiation survived as long, but not longer than, patients treated with nonradiation treatments
OR	1953-1957	^{233}U ^{235}U	Study the distribution and excretion of uranium in humans	NS	4-50 mg; intravenously	99% of injected uranium cleared the blood within 20 hours and the remainder either deposited in the skeleton and kidneys or excreted via the urine

Summary of Some Studies of Humans Exposed to Radiation and Radionuclides *(Continued)*

Location	Year(s)	Radionuclide	Purpose of Experiment	Number of People Dosed	Dose and Route of Exposure	Result
OR	1945	^{32}P	Study effects of beta rays on skin	10	140-1180 rad; external exposure	Threshold dose of beta radiation that resulted in mild tanning was about 200 rad; erythema resulted after a dose of 813 rad
UC	1937-1954	X-rays	Study the effect of x-rays for the treatment of gastric ulcers	116	1100-2930 rad; external exposure	Claimed that moderate irradiation of the stomach reduced acid secretion and was a valuable adjunct to conventional gastric ulcer therapy; therapy was later discontinued due to risks outweighing benefits
UC	1959	^{51}Cr	Determine feasibility of using implanted radiation sources in the treatment of cancer	24	2-5 mCi; implanted within cancerous tissues	16 had good or favorable results; the remainder of patients had questionable or unfavorable results; implants were generally well tolerated
UC	1960s	Various; fallout contains many alpha, beta, and gamma emitting radionuclides; stimulated fallout contained ^{85}Sr, ^{133}Ba, or ^{134}Cs	Gain information in civil defense planning prior to nuclear fallout	10	0.2-0.7 µCi actual fallout;; 0.4-14 µCi simulated fallout; subjects ingested actual fallout from Nevada test site, as well as simulated fallout particles	No gastrointestinal symptoms were reported; studies provided a basis for estimating the systemic uptake and internal radiation dose that could result from the ingestion of fallout after nuclear bomb detonation
UR	1946-1947	^{234}U ^{235}U	Determine dose level at which renal injury is first detectable; measure U elimination and excretion rates	6	6.4-70.9 µCi/kg intravenously	U excretion occurred mainly via the urine and 70%-85% was eliminated with 24 hours; acidosis decreased U excretion; humans tolerated U at doses as high as 70 mcg/kg
UR	1956	^{222}Rn	Determine radiation doses to different parts of the respiratory tract from inhaled ^{222}Rn	2	0.025 µCi; inhalation	Average retention of ^{222}Rn and daughter products in normal atmospheric dust was 25%; retention in filtered air was 75%; radiation exposure to the lungs was due to radon daughter products rather than by ^{222}Rn itself
UR	1966-1967	^{212}Pb	Study absorption of lead from the gastrointestinal tract and determine the radiation hazard and chemical toxicity of ingested lead	4	1 µCi intravenous and/or 5 µCi orally	Lead might be released from binding sites only when red blood cells die
MISC	1950s	^{131}I	Study the transmission of ^{131}I in maternal breast milk to nursing infants	2	100 µCi; oral	^{131}I concentration in maternal milk was high enough to allow significant uptake in the thyroids of nursing infants; ^{131}I tracers should be used with caution when nursing infants
MISC	1953	^{131}I	Study uptake of ^{131}I by the thyroids of human embryos	NA	100-200 µCi (maternal dose); route not specified	Pregnant women were scheduled for abortion prior to receiving ^{131}I; results indicated that it would be unwise to administer ^{131}I for diagnostic or therapeutic purposes while pregnant

Summary of Some Studies of Humans Exposed to Radiation and Radionuclides (*Continued*)

Location	Year(s)	Radionuclide	Purpose of Experiment	Number of People Dosed	Dose and Route of Exposure	Result
MISC	1963-1973	X-rays	Determine the effects of radiation on human testicular function	60	7.5-400 rad; external exposure	Doses of 7.5 rad yielded no adverse effect on testicular function; 27 rad inhibited generation of sperm, and 75 rad destroyed existing sperm cells; doses of 100-400 rad produced temporary sterility; all persons eventually recovered to pre-exposure levels prior to vasectomy

ANL = Argonne National Laboratory; BNL = Brockhaven National Laboratory; HS = Hanford Sites; LBL = Lawrence Berkeley Laboratory; LLNL = Lawrence Livermore National Laboratory; LANL = Los Alamos National Laboratory; ORS = Oak Ridge Sites; UCLA = University of California, Los Angeles; UCACRH = University of Chicago Argonne Cancer Research Hospital; UR = University of Rochester; MISC = other miscellaneous studies performed at other institutions; NA = information not available.

Summary of Some Studies of Humans Exposed to Radiation and Radionuclides (*Continued*)

From Human Radiation Experiments Associated with the U.S. Department of Energy and Its Predecessors; U.S. Department of Energy, Assistant Secretary for Environment, Safety, and Health, Document #DOE/EH-0491, Washington, DC: July, 1995.

Summary of the Dose Response Effects of Ionizing Radiation in Humans

Phase	Feature	Subclinical Range	Sublethal Ranges (100-800 rad)			Lethal Range (over 800 rad)	
		100-200 rad	0-100 rad	200-600 rad	600-800 rad	800-3000 rad	>3000 rad
Initial phase	Incidence of nausea and vomiting	None	5%-50%	50%-100%	75%-100%	90%-100%	100%
	Time of onset		3-6 h	2-4 h	1-2 h	<1 h	<1 h
	Duration		<24 h	<24 h	<48 h	<48 h	48 h
	Mental and physical capabilities	100%	100%	Able to perform routine tasks. Cognitive abilities impaired for 6-20 hours	Able to perform simple and routine tasks. Significant incapacitation in upper part of dose range. Lasts more than 24 hours	Progressive incapacitation	
Latent phase	Duration	>2 wk	7-15 d	0-7 d	0-2 d	None	
Secondary phase	Signs and symptoms	None	Moderate leukopenia	Severe leukopenia; pneumonia; purpura, hemorrhage; infection; hair loss (epilation) at about 300 rads		Diarrhea; fever; disturbance of electrolyte balance	Convulsions; tremor; ataxia; lethargy
	Time of onset after exposure		>2 wk	Several days to 2 weeks		2-3 d	
	Critical period after exposure		None	4-6 wk		5-14 d	1-48 h
	Organ system affected	None		Hematopoietic and respiratory tissues		Gastrointestinal tract; respiratory tissues	Central nervous system
Hospitalization	Percentage	None	<5%	90%	100%	100%	100%

	Duration		45-60 d	60-90 d	90-120 d	2 wk	2 days
Incidence of death		None	None	0% to 80%	90% to 100%	90% to 100%	90% to 100%
Average time to death				3 weeks to 2 months		1-2 wk	2 d
Medical therapy		None	Hematologic surveil-lance	Blood transfusions and antibiotics		Maintenance of electro-lyte bal-ance	Sedatives

Adapted from Academy of Health and Science, 1995.

Summary of Risks of Developing Cancer After Exposure to Ionizing Radiation			
Organ or System	**BEIR Committee Conclusions About Risk**		**Cancer Relative Risk (RR) Factors (low dose/low dose rate) per 10^6 rad (10^4 Gy)***
Mammary/breast	1.	The development of cancer from susceptible mammary cells due to exposure to ionizing radiation depends on the hormonal status of these cells.	92.5
	2.	The age-distribution of radiogenic breast cancers and those breast cancers from unknown causes is similar.	
	3.	Women irradiated at ≤ 20 years of age are at higher risk than those irradiated later in life.	
	4.	There is no evidence to suggest that radiogenic breast cancer will appear during the first 10 years after exposure to ionizing radiation. Peak incidences occur 15-20 years after exposure.	
	5.	The data show little if any decrease in the yield of tumors, when multiple radiation doses are compared to single, brief exposures to ionizing radiation.	
Lung	1.	Absolute risk of lung cancer from exposure to ionizing radiation is similar for both males and females.	75.4
	2.	The data suggest that smoking has a "greater than additive" effect on the development of lung cancer after exposure to ionizing radiation.	
Stomach/digestive system	1.	The incidence of stomach cancers increases with increased exposure to ionizing radiation.	49.3
	2.	Females are at greater risk for developing cancers than are males.	
	3.	The relative risk for developing cancer is higher for those exposed when 30 years of age or younger.	
	4.	The baseline risk for digestive cancers increases with age; most of the excess cancers occur after middle age.	
Thyroid	1.	Susceptibility to radiation-induced thyroid cancer is greater in childhood.	32.1
	2.	Development of thyroid cancer is dependant on the hormonal status of the individual; sustained levels of TSH increase the risk of developing thyroid cancer.	
	3.	For those exposed before puberty, the tumors do not appear until after sexual maturation. The risk is greatest for children exposed within the first 5 years of life.	
	4.	Females are 2-3 times more susceptible than males to radiogenic (and spontaneous) thyroid cancer.	
	5.	Radiogenic cancer of the thyroid is usually preceded by benign thyroid nodules and the frequency of hypothyroidism and goiter is increased in those exposed to large doses when very young.	
Esophagus	1.	Increased incidences of cancer of the esophagus have been observed to occur in humans receiving doses of ionizing radiation.	
	2.	Little human data are available to make strong conclusions about the risk of developing esophageal cancer after exposure to ionizing radiation, although a risk estimate is available.	

Summary of Risks of Developing Cancer After Exposure to Ionizing Radiation *(Continued)*

Organ or System		BEIR Committee Conclusions About Risk	Cancer Relative Risk (RR) Factors (low dose/low dose rate) per 10^6 rad (10^4 Gy)*
Small intestine (duodenum, jejunum, ileum)	1.	Cancers of the small intestine have been produced in laboratory animals exposed to large doses of ionizing radiation.	NR
	2.	None of the human epidemiological studies have conclusively demonstrated an increased risk of developing cancers of the small intestine after exposure to ionizing radiation.	
Large intestine (colon/rectum)	1.	Data imply that there is an increased risk of developing either colon or rectal cancer after exposure to ionizing radiation.	178.5
	2.	Based on human exposure data, the development of colon or rectal cancer is not apparent until 15 years after exposure or longer.	
Skeleton	1.	Large doses of low-LET ionizing radiation can result in the development of bone cancers.	1.3
	2.	The data suggest a threshold of between 4 Gy of low-LET or 13.8 Gy of high-LET radiation before increased bone cancers begin to occur.	
Brain/central nervous system (CNS)	1.	Increased incidences of CNS tumors have been observed in both humans and laboratory animals exposed to ionizing radiation.	NR
	2.	Tumors are both malignant and benign.	
	3.	The brain is considered to be relatively sensitive to developing cancer after exposure to ionizing radiation.	
	4.	Increases have been reported when irradiated during childhood at doses <1-2 Gy.	
Ovary and uterus	1.	There is no clear relationship between exposure to ionizing radiation and the development of uterine or ovarian cancers.	23.8
Testis	1.	There are few human data available for studying the relationship between exposure to ionizing radiation and testicular cancer.	NR
	2.	The existing data suggest that the testis is relatively insensitive to the carcinogenic effects of ionizing radiation.	
Prostate	1.	There is a weak association between cancer of the prostate and exposure to ionizing radiation.	NR
	2.	The relative risk of cancer of the prostate due to exposure to ionizing radiation is small.	
Urinary tract	1.	Exposure to ionizing radiation can cause cancer of the bladder, as well as cancers of the kidney and other urinary structures.	49.7
	2.	Women <55 years old at the time of exposure are at greater risk than older women, with this risk increasing with time after exposure.	
	3.	Gender appears to have little effect on the incidence of bladder cancer mortality.	
Parathyroid glands	1.	Increased incidences of hyperparathyroidism, parathyroid hyperplasia, and parathyroid adenoma occur after exposure to ionizing radiation.	NR
	2.	The data suggest that the incidences of hyperparathyroidism and parathyroid neoplasia increase with increasing doses of ionizing radiation.	
	3.	Time to diagnosis normally is $\geq$30 years.	
Nasal cavity and sinuses	1.	Little human data is available for analysis. Nasal and sinus tumors have been noted after human exposure to internally deposited ^{226}Ra and ^{232}Th.	NR
	2.	The latency of these tumors is at least 10 years.	
	3.	The risk of developing nasal and sinus cavity tumors from routes other than from internalized sources of alpha ion radiation are extremely low.	

Summary of Risks of Developing Cancer After Exposure to Ionizing Radiation *(Continued)*

Organ or System		BEIR Committee Conclusions About Risk	Cancer Relative Risk (RR) Factors (low dose/low dose rate) per 10^6 rad (10^4 Gy)*
Skin	1.	Increased incidences of basal cell and squamous cell carcinomas of the skin have been reported after occupational and therapeutic exposures to ionizing radiation.	1.0
	2.	Incidence from radiation exposure may be 5 times greater if the skin is also exposed to sunlight.	
Bone marrow (leukemia, lymphoma, and multiple myeloma)	1.	Examples include multiple myeloma, non-Hodgkin's lymphoma, and chronic lymphocytic leukemia.	NR
	2.	Multiple myelomas are observed to form after irradiation of the bone marrow.	
	3.	The latent period for multiple myeloma is considerably longer than that of leukemia.	
	4.	In Japanese A-bomb survivors, an excess of multiple myeloma cases did not appear until 20 years after exposure.	
	5.	Excess mortality from multiple myelomas has been observed at doses as low as 0.5-0.99 Gy.	
	6.	No other form for lymphoma has been consistently observed in human populations exposed to excess amounts of ionizing radiation.	
Pharynx, hypopharynx, and larynx	1.	Increased incidences of cancer do arise in these tissues after therapeutic radiation (ie, ankylosing spondylitis) in the 30-60 Gy range. Increases in these cancers were not statistically significant at the $p < 0.05$ level.	NR
	2.	There were no increases in the incidences of these cancers in the Japanese A-bomb survivors exposed to < 1 Gy.	
	3.	The risk of developing cancers of these tissues after exposure to ionizing radiation appears to be very low.	
Salivary gland	1.	The incidence of salivary gland tumors was increased in the Japanese A-bomb survivors, patients treated with x-rays to the head and neck during childhood, and women treated with ^{131}I when middle aged.	NR
	2.	Increases in salivary gland neoplasia are dose-dependent in the Japanese A-bomb survivors, but with no detectable increases in excess immortality.	
	3.	The salivary gland appears to be particularly susceptible to the development of cancer after exposure to ionizing radiation.	
Pancreas	1.	An association between cancer of the pancreas and exposure to ionizing radiation has been suggested in some literature reports.	NR
	2.	Pancreatic cancer has been found in occupationally exposed thorium workers.†	
	3.	The existing data suggest that the pancreas is relatively insensitive to the carcinogenic effects of ionizing radiation.	

LET = linear energy transport; NR = RR factor not reported.

*Values from EPA Report 402-R-96-016, Radiation Exposure and Risk Assessment Manual, June 1996. Sum of all values = 760.6, including a remainder incidence risk of 173.4 for all other organs, including those listed in column 3 as NR.

†Polednak, et al, *Health Physics*, 1980, 44 (Suppl 1):239-51.

Summarized from BEIR V, National Research Council, Washington, DC: National Academy Press, 1990.

Relative Sensitivities of Major Organs and Tissues to the Effects of Ionizing Radiation

Radiosensitivity Category	Organ System	General Cell Type Affected	Frequency of Mitosis
High	Lymphoreticular	Lymphocytes	Very frequent
	Hematological	Immature hematopoietic cells	

Radiosensitivity Category	Organ System	General Cell Type Affected	Frequency of Mitosis
	Reproductive	Spermatogonia	
		Ovarian follicular cells	
	Gastrointestinal	Intestinal epithelium	
		Esophageal epithelium	Frequent
		Gastric mucosa	
	Renal	Urinary bladder epithelium	
	Dermal	Epidermal epithelial cells	
		Mucous membranes	
	Ocular	Epithelium of optic lens	
Medium	Circulatory system	Endothelium	
	Musculoskeletal	Growing bone and cartilaginous tissues	Moderately frequent
	Brain/CNS	Glial cells	
	Dermal	Glandular epithelium of the breast	
	Respiratory	Pulmonary epithelium, tracheobronchial epithelium	
	Renal	Renal epithelium	
	Hepatic	Hepatic epithelium	
	Endocrine	Pancreatic epithelium	
		Thyroid epithelium	
		Adrenal epithelium	
Low	Hematological	Mature hematopoietic cells (erythrocytes, neutrophils, eosinophils, basophils, macrophages)	Infrequently/rarely
	Musculoskeletal	Myocytes, osteocytes	
		Mature connective tissues	
		Mature bone and cartilage	
	Brain and peripheral nervous system	Ganglion cells	

Relative Sensitivities of Major Organs and Tissues to the Effects of Ionizing Radiation (Continued)

Some Internet Sites Related to Ionizing Radiation

Hyper Text Transfer Protocol (HTTP) Address	Web Page Contents
http://www.uic.com/au/ral.htm	A beginner's reference for radiation.
http://www.dne.bnl.gov/CoN/index.html	Radionuclide information on half-life, transformation energies, etc.
http://www.nih.gov/health/chip/od/radiation	Summary information on radiation and its health effects.
http://www.umich.edu/-radinfo/introduction	Introduction to radiation; professional, research, and educational resources.
http://radefx.bcm.tmc.edu/	Baylor College of Medicine Radiation Health Effects Research Resource homepage. Health effects documents, downloadable software, extensive literature searches on Chernobyl health effects, links to other radiation-related sites.
http://www.em.doe.gov/cgi-bin/tc/tindex.html	DOE Environmental Management. Public information access and links to DOE research laboratories.

Some Internet Sites Related to Ionizing Radiation (*Continued*)

Hyper Text Transfer Protocol (HTTP) Address	Web Page Contents
http://www.rerf.or.jp/	Radiation Effects Research Foundation. Atomic bomb survivor studies provided by a joint Japanese-U.S. sponsored research organization. Human health impact of the atomic bomb release on Hiroshima and Nagasaki, Japan.
http://www.ohre.doe.gov/	DOE "cold war" radiation research using human subjects.
http://www.hps.org	Health Physics Society, a scientific organization dealing with radiation safety. Involved in the development, dissemination, and application of radiation protection. Concerned with understanding, evaluating, and controlling the risks from radiation exposure relative to the benefits derived.
http://www.epa.gov/narel/index.html	Reports nationwide radionuclide concentrations in air, drinking water, surface water, precipitation, and milk.
http://www.epa.gov/narel/erd-online.html	
http://www.aapm.org	American Association of Physicists in Medicine. Concerned with the safe use of radiation and radioactive materials in medicine.
http://law.house.gov/4.htm	U.S. House of Representatives internet law library of the Code of Federal Regulations. Provides CFR text.
http://www.nrc.gov/	USNRC. Nuclear waste, nuclear reactors in operation, and rule-making procedures.
http://www.sandia.gov/LabNews/LN01-19-96/palo.html	A newspaper for the employees of Sandia National Laboratories and recounts the Palomares incident.
http://fema.gov/home/fema/radiolo.htm	Federal Emergency Management Agency information on how to prepare for an emergency and what to do if an accident occurs.
http://www.radres.org/intro.htm	Tha Radiation Research Society.
http://www.afrri.usuhs.mil/www/index.html	The Armed Forces Radiobiology Research Institute.
http://cedr.lbl.gov	Comprehensive epidemiologic data resource related to radiological releases from sites.

REFERENCE VALUES FOR ADULTS

Automated Chemistry (CHEMISTRY A)		
Test	Values	Remarks
SERUM/PLASMA		
Acetone	Negative	
Albumin	3.2-5 g/dL	
Alcohol, ethyl	Negative	
Aldolase	1.2-7.6 IU/L	
Ammonia	20-70 mcg/dL	Specimen to be placed on ice as soon as collected.
Amylase	30-110 units/L	
Bilirubin, direct	0-0.3 mg/dL	
Bilirubin, total	0.1-1.2 mg/dL	
Calcium	8.6-10.3 mg/dL	
Calcium, ionized	2.24-2.46 mEq/L	
Chloride	95-108 mEq/L	
Cholesterol, total	$\leq$200 mg/dL	Fasted blood required – normal value affected by dietary habits. This reference range is for a general adult population.
HDL cholesterol	40-60 mg/dL	Fasted blood required – normal value affected by dietary habits.
LDL cholesterol	<160 mg/dL	If triglyceride is >400 mg/dL, LDL cannot be calculated accurately (Friedewald equation). Target LDL-C depends on patient's risk factors.
CO_2	23-30 mEq/L	
Creatine kinase (CK) isoenzymes		
CK-BB	0%	
CK-MB (cardiac)	0%-3.9%	
CK-MM (muscle)	96%-100%	
CK-MB levels must be both $\geq$4% and 10 IU/L to meet diagnostic criteria for CK-MB positive result consistent with myocardial injury.		
Creatine phosphokinase (CPK)	8-150 IU/L	
Creatinine	0.5-1.4 mg/dL	
Ferritin	13-300 ng/mL	
Folate	3.6-20 ng/dL	
GGT (gamma-glutamyltranspeptidase)		
male	11-63 IU/L	
female	8-35 IU/L	
GLDH	To be determined	
Glucose (preprandial)	<115 mg/dL	Goals different for diabetics.
Glucose, fasting	60-110 mg/dL	Goals different for diabetics.
Glucose, nonfasting (2-h postprandial)	<120 mg/dL	Goals different for diabetics.
Hemoglobin A_{1c}	<8	
Hemoglobin, plasma free	<2.5 mg/100 mL	
Hemoglobin, total glycosolated (Hb A_1)	4%-8%	

Automated Chemistry (CHEMISTRY A) *(Continued)*

Test	Values	Remarks
Iron	65-150 mcg/dL	
Iron binding capacity, total (TIBC)	250-420 mcg/dL	
Lactic acid	0.7-2.1 mEq/L	Specimen to be kept on ice and sent to lab as soon as possible.
Lactate dehydrogenase (LDH)	56-194 IU/L	
Lactate dehydrogenase (LDH) isoenzymes		
LD_1	20%-34%	
LD_2	29%-41%	
LD_3	15%-25%	
LD_4	1%-12%	
LD_5	1%-15%	
Flipped LD_1/LD_2 ratios (>1 may be consistent with myocardial injury) particularly when considered in combination with a recent CK-MB positive result.		
Lipase	23-208 units/L	
Magnesium	1.6-2.5 mg/dL	Increased by slight hemolysis.
Osmolality	289-308 mOsm/kg	
Phosphatase, alkaline		
adults 25-60 y	33-131 IU/L	
adults 61 y or older	51-153 IU/L	
infancy-adolescence	Values range up to 3-5 times higher than adults	
Phosphate, inorganic	2.8-4.2 mg/dL	
Potassium	3.5-5.2 mEq/L	Increased by slight hemolysis.
Prealbumin	>15 mg/dL	
Protein, total	6.5-7.9 g/dL	
SGOT (AST)	<35 IU/L (20-48)	
SGPT (ALT) (10-35)	<35 IU/L	
Sodium	134-149 mEq/L	
Transferrin	>200 mg/dL	
Triglycerides	45-155 mg/dL	Fasted blood required.
Troponin I	<1.5 ng/mL	
Urea nitrogen (BUN)	7-20 mg/dL	
Uric acid		
male	2-8 mg/dL	
female	2-7.5 mg/dL	
CEREBROSPINAL FLUID		
Glucose	50-70 mg/dL	
Protein		
adults and children	15-45 mg/dL	CSF obtained by lumbar puncture.

Automated Chemistry (CHEMISTRY A) *(Continued)*

Test	Values	Remarks
newborn infants	60-90 mg/dL.	

On CSF obtained by cisternal puncture: About 25 mg/dL.
On CSF obtained by ventricular puncture: About 10 mg/dL.
Note: Bloody specimen gives erroneously high value due to contamination with blood proteins.

URINE (24-hour specimen is required for all these tests unless specified)		
Amylase	32-641 units/L	The value is in units/L and **not** calculated for total volume.
Amylase, fluid (random samples)		Interpretation of value left for physician, depends on the nature of fluid.
Calcium	Depends upon dietary intake	
Creatine		
male	150 mg/24 h	Higher value on children and during pregnancy.
female	250 mg/24 h	
Creatinine	1000-2000 mg/24 h	
Creatinine clearance (endogenous)		
male female	85-125 mL/min 75-115 mL/min	A blood sample must accompany urine specimen.
Glucose	1 g/24 h	
5-Hydroxyindoleacetic acid	2-8 mg/24 h	
Iron	0.15 mg/24 h	Acid washed container required.
Magnesium	146-209 mg/24 h	
Osmolality	500-800 mOsm/kg	With normal fluid intake.
Oxalate	10-40 mg/24 h	
Phosphate	400-1300 mg/24 h	
Potassium	25-120 mEq/24 h	Varies with diet; the interpretation of urine electrolytes and osmolality should be left for the physician.
Sodium	40-220 mEq/24 h	
Porphobilinogen, qualitative	Negative	
Porphyrins, qualitative	Negative	
Proteins	0.05-0.1 g/24 h	
Salicylate	Negative	
Urea clearance	60-95 mL/min	A blood sample must accompany specimen.
Urea N	10-40 g/24 h	Dependent on protein intake.
Uric acid	250-750 mg/24 h	Dependent on diet and therapy.
Urobilinogen	0.5-3.5 mg/24 h	For qualitative determination on random urine, send sample to urinalysis section in Hematology Lab.
Xylose absorption test		
children	16%-33% of ingested xylose	
FECES		
Fat, 3-day collection	<5 g/d	Value depends on fat intake of 100 g/d for 3 days preceding and during collection.
GASTRIC ACIDITY		
Acidity, total, 12 h	10-60 mEq/L	Titrated at pH 7.

Blood Gases			
	Arterial	**Capillary**	**Venous**
pH	7.35-7.45	7.35-7.45	7.32-7.42
pCO_2 (mm Hg)	35-45	35-45	38-52
pO_2 (mm Hg)	70-100	60-80	24-48
HCO_3 (mEq/L)	19-25	19-25	19-25
TCO_2 (mEq/L)	19-29	19-29	23-33
O_2 saturation (%)	90-95	90-95	40-70
Base excess (mEq/L)	-5 to +5	-5 to +5	-5 to +5

HEMATOLOGY Complete Blood Count				
Age	**Hgb (g/dL)**	**Hct (%)**	**RBC (mill/mm^3)**	**RDW**
0-3 d	15.0-20.0	45-61	4.0-5.9	<18
1-2 wk	12.5-18.5	39-57	3.6-5.5	<17
1-6 mo	10.0-13.0	29-42	3.1-4.3	<16.5
7 mo to 2 y	10.5-13.0	33-38	3.7-4.9	<16
2-5 y	11.5-13.0	34-39	3.9-5.0	<15
5-8 y	11.5-14.5	35-42	4.0-4.9	<15
13-18 y	12.0-15.2	36-47	4.5-5.1	<14.5
Adult male	13.5-16.5	41-50	4.5-5.5	<14.5
Adult female	12.0-15.0	36-44	4.0-4.9	<14.5

Age	**MCV (fL)**	**MCH (pg)**	**MCHC (%)**	**Plts ($\times 10^3$/mm^3)**
0-3 d	95-115	31-37	29-37	250-450
1-2 wk	86-110	28-36	28-38	250-450
1-6 mo	74-96	25-35	30-36	300-700
7 mo to 2 y	70-84	23-30	31-37	250-600
2-5 y	75-87	24-30	31-37	250-550
5-8 y	77-95	25-33	31-37	250-550
13-18 y	78-96	25-35	31-37	150-450
Adult male	80-100	26-34	31-37	150-450
Adult female	80-100	26-34	31-37	150-450

WBC and Differential					
Age	**WBC ($\times 10^3$/mm^3)**	**Segs**	**Bands**	**Lymphs**	**Monos**
0-3 d	9.0-35.0	32-62	10-18	19-29	5-7
1-2 wk	5.0-20.0	14-34	6-14	36-45	6-10
1-6 mo	6.0-17.5	13-33	4-12	41-71	4-7
7 mo to 2 y	6.0-17.0	15-35	5-11	45-76	3-6
2-5 y	5.5-15.5	23-45	5-11	35-65	3-6
5-8 y	5.0-14.5	32-54	5-11	28-48	3-6
13-18 y	4.5-13.0	34-64	5-11	25-45	3-6
Adults	4.5-11.0	35-66	5-11	24-44	3-6

Age	Eosinophils	Basophils	Atypical Lymphs	No. of NRBCs
0-3 d	0-2	0-1	0-8	0-2
1-2 wk	0-2	0-1	0-8	0
1-6 mo	0-3	0-1	0-8	0
7 mo to 2 y	0-3	0-1	0-8	0
2-5 y	0-3	0-1	0-8	0
5-8 y	0-3	0-1	0-8	0
13-18 y	0-3	0-1	0-8	0
Adults	0-3	0-1	0-8	0

Segs = segmented neutrophils.

Bands = band neutrophils.

Lymphs = lymphocytes.

Monos = monocytes.

Erythrocyte Sedimentation Rates and Reticulocyte Counts		
Sedimentation rate, Westergren	Children	0-20 mm/hour
	Adult male	0-15 mm/hour
	Adult female	0-20 mm/hour
Sedimentation rate, Wintrobe	Children	0-13 mm/hour
	Adult male	0-10 mm/hour
	Adult female	0-15 mm/hour
Reticulocyte count	Newborns	2%-6%
	1-6 mo	0%-2.8%
	Adults	0.5%-1.5%

REFERENCE VALUES FOR CHILDREN

	Normal Values	
CHEMISTRY		
Albumin	0-1 y	2-4 g/dL
	1 y to adult	3.5-5.5 g/dL
Ammonia	Newborns	90-150 mcg/dL
	Children	40-120 mcg/dL
	Adults	18-54 mcg/dL
Amylase	Newborns	0-60 units/L
	Adults	30-110 units/L
Bilirubin, conjugated, direct	Newborns	<1.5 mg/dL
	1 mo to adult	0-0.5 mg/dL
Bilirubin, total	0-3 d	2-10 mg/dL
	1 mo to adult	0-1.5 mg/dL
Bilirubin, unconjugated, indirect		0.6-10.5 mg/dL
Calcium	Newborns	7-12 mg/dL
	0-2 y	8.8-11.2 mg/dL
	2 y to adult	9-11 mg/dL
Calcium, ionized, whole blood		4.4-5.4 mg/dL
Carbon dioxide, total		23-33 mEq/L
Chloride		95-105 mEq/L
Cholesterol	Newborns	45-170 mg/dL
	0-1 y	65-175 mg/dL
	1-20 y	120-230 mg/dL
Creatinine	0-1 y	≤0.6 mg/dL
	1 y to adult	0.5-1.5 mg/dL
Glucose	Newborns	30-90 mg/dL
	0-2 y	60-105 mg/dL
	Children to Adults	70-110 mg/dL
Iron		
	Newborns	110-270 mcg/dL
	Infants	30-70 mcg/dL
	Children	55-120 mcg/dL
	Adults	70-180 mcg/dL
Iron binding	Newborns	59-175 mcg/dL
	Infants	100-400 mcg/dL
	Adults	250-400 mcg/dL
Lactic acid, lactate		2-20 mg/dL
Lead, whole blood		<10 mcg/dL
Lipase		

(Continued)

		Normal Values
	Children	20-140 units/L
	Adults	0-190 units/L
Magnesium		1.5-2.5 mEq/L
Osmolality, serum		275-296 mOsm/kg
Osmolality, urine		50-1400 mOsm/kg
Phosphorus	Newborns	4.2-9 mg/dL
	6 wk to 19 mo	3.8-6.7 mg/dL
	19 mo to 3 y	2.9-5.9 mg/dL
	3-15 y	3.6-5.6 mg/dL
	>15 y	2.5-5 mg/dL
Potassium, plasma	Newborns	4.5-7.2 mEq/L
	2 d to 3 mo	4-6.2 mEq/L
	3 mo to 1 y	3.7-5.6 mEq/L
	1-16 y	3.5-5 mEq/L
Protein, total	0-2 y	4.2-7.4 g/dL
	>2 y	6-8 g/dL
Sodium		136-145 mEq/L
Triglycerides	Infants	0-171 mg/dL
	Children	20-130 mg/dL
	Adults	30-200 mg/dL
Urea nitrogen, blood	0-2 y	4-15 mg/dL
	2 y to Adult	5-20 mg/dL
Uric acid	Male	3-7 mg/dL
	Female	2-6 mg/dL
ENZYMES		
Alanine aminotransferase (ALT) (SGPT)	0-2 mo	8-78 units/L
	>2 mo	8-36 units/L
Alkaline phosphatase (ALKP)	Newborns	60-130 units/L
	0-16 y	85-400 units/L
	>16 y	30-115 units/L
Aspartate aminotransferase (AST) (SGOT)	Infants	18-74 units/L
	Children	15-46 units/L
	Adults	5-35 units/L
Creatine kinase (CK)	Infants	20-200 units/L
	Children	10-90 units/L
	Adult male	0-206 units/L
	Adult female	0-175 units/L

(Continued)		
	Normal Values	
Lactate dehydrogenase (LDH)	Newborns	290-501 units/L
	1 mo to 2 y	110-144 units/L
	>16 y	60-170 units/L

Blood Gases			
	Arterial	**Capillary**	**Venous**
pH	7.35-7.45	7.35-7.45	7.32-7.42
pCO_2 (mm Hg)	35-45	35-45	38-52
pO_2 (mm Hg)	70-100	60-80	24-48
HCO_3 (mEq/L)	19-25	19-25	19-25
TCO_2 (mEq/L)	19-29	19-29	23-33
O_2 saturation (%)	90-95	90-95	40-70
Base excess (mEq/L)	−5 to +5	−5 to +5	−5 to +5

Thyroid Function Tests		
T_4 (thyroxine)	1-7 d	10.1-20.9 mcg/dL
	8-14 d	9.8-16.6 mcg/dL
	1 mo to 1 y	5.5-16 mcg/dL
	>1 y	4-12 mcg/dL
FTI	1-3 d	9.3-26.6
	1-4 wk	7.6-20.8
	1-4 mo	7.4-17.9
	4-12 mo	5.1-14.5
	1-6 y	5.7-13.3
	>6 y	4.8-14
T_3 by RIA	Newborns	100-470 ng/dL
	1-5 y	100-260 ng/dL
	5-10 y	90-240 ng/dL
	10 y to Adult	70-210 ng/dL
T_3 uptake		35%-45%
TSH	Cord	3-22 µIU/mL
	1-3 d	<40 µIU/mL
	3-7 d	<25 µIU/mL
	>7 d	0-10 µIU/mL

RENAL FUNCTION TESTS

Endogenous Creatinine Clearance vs Age (timed collection)

Creatinine clearance (mL/min/1.73 m^2) = (Cr$_u$V/Cr$_s$T) (1.73/A)

where:

Cr$_u$	=	urine creatinine concentration (mg/dL)
V	=	total urine collected during sampling period (mL)
Cr$_s$	=	serum creatinine concentration (mg/dL)
T	=	duration of sampling period (min) (24 h = 1440 min)
A	=	body surface area (m^2)

Age-specific normal values

5-7 d	50.6 ± 5.8 mL/min/1.73 m^2
1-2 mo	64.6 ± 5.8 mL/min/1.73 m^2
5-8 mo	87.7 ± 11.9 mL/min/1.73 m^2
9-12 mo	86.9 ± 8.4 mL/min/1.73 m^2
≥18 mo	
male	124 ± 26 mL/min/1.73 m^2
female	109 ± 13.5 mL/min/1.73 m^2
Adults	
male	105 ± 14 mL/min/1.73 m^2
female	95 ± 18 mL/min/1.73 m^2

Note: In patients with renal failure (creatinine clearance <25 mL/min), creatinine clearance may be elevated over GFR because of tubular secretion of creatinine.

Calculation of Creatinine Clearance from a 24-Hour Urine Collection

Equation 1:

$$Cl_{cr} = \frac{U \times V}{P}$$

where:

Cl$_{cr}$	=	creatinine clearance
U	=	urine concentration of creatinine
V	=	total urine volume in the collection
P	=	plasma creatinine concentration

Equation 2:

$$Cl_{cr} = \frac{(\text{total urine volume [mL]}) \times (\text{urine Cr concentration [mg/dL]})}{(\text{serum creatinine [mg/dL]}) \times (\text{time of urine collection [minutes]})}$$

Occasionally, a patient will have a 12- or 24-hour urine collection done for direct calculation of creatinine clearance. Although a urine collection for 24 hours is best, it is difficult to do since many urine collections occur for a much shorter period. A 24-hour urine collection is the desired duration of urine collection because the urine excretion of creatinine is diurnal and thus the measured creatinine clearance will vary throughout the day as the creatinine in the urine varies. When the urine collection is less than 24 hours, the total excreted creatinine will be affected by the time of the day during which the collection is performed. A 24-hour urine collection is sufficient to be able to accurately average the diurnal creatinine excretion variations. If a patient has 24 hours of urine collected for creatinine clearance, equation 1 can be used for calculating the creatinine clearance. To use equation 1 to calculate the creatinine clearance, it will be necessary to know the duration of urine collection, the urine collection volume, the urine creatinine concentration, and the serum creatinine value that reflects the urine collection period. In most cases, a serum creatinine concentration is drawn anytime during the day, but it is best to have the value drawn halfway through the collection period.

Amylase: Creatinine Clearance Ratio

$\dfrac{Amylase_u \times creatinine_p}{Amylase_p \times creatinine_u}$	$\times$	100

u = urine; p = plasma

Serum BUN: Serum Creatinine Ratio

Serum BUN (mg/dL: serum creatinine (mg/dL))

Normal BUN: creatinine ratio is 10-15

BUN: creatinine ratio >20 suggests prerenal azotemia (also seen with high urea-generation states such as GI bleeding)

BUN: creatinine ratio <5 may be seen with disorders affecting urea biosynthesis such as urea cycle enzyme deficiencies and with hepatitis.

Fractional Sodium Excretion

Fractional sodium secretion (FENa) = $Na_u Cr_s / Na_s Cr_u \times 100\%$

where:

Na_u	=	urine sodium (mEq/L)
Na_s	=	serum sodium (mEq/L)
Cr_u	=	urine creatinine (mg/dL)
Cr_s	=	serum creatinine (mg/dL)

FENa <1% suggests prerenal failure

FENa >2% suggest intrinsic renal failure (for newborns, normal FENa is approximately 2.5%)

Note: Disease states associated with a falsely elevated FENa include severe volume depletion (>10%), early acute tubular necrosis, and volume depletion in chronic renal disease. Disorders associated with a lowered FENa include acute glomerulonephritis, hemoglobinuric or myoglobinuric renal failure, nonoliguric acute tubular necrosis, and acute urinary tract obstruction. In addition, FENa may be <1% in patients with acute renal failure **and** a second condition predisposing to sodium retention (eg, burns, congestive heart failure, nephrotic syndrome).

Urine Calcium: Urine Creatinine Ratio (spot sample)

Urine calcium (mg/dL): urine creatinine (mg/dL)

Normal values <0.21 (mean values 0.08 males, 0.06 females)

Premature infants show wide variability of calcium:creatinine ratio, and tend to have lower thresholds for calcium loss than older children. Prematures without nephrolithiasis had mean Ca:Cr ratio of 0.75 ± 0.76. Infants with nephrolithiasis had mean Ca:Cr ratio of 1.32 ± 1.03 (Jacinto JS, Modanlou HD, Crade M, et al, "Renal Calcification Incidence in Very Low Birth Weight Infants," *Pediatrics*, 1988, 81:31.)

Urine Protein: Urine Creatinine Ratio (spot sample)

P_u/Cr_u	Total Protein Excretion ($mg/m^2/d$)
0.1	80
1	800
10	8000

where:

P_u = urine protein concentration (mg/dL)

Cr_u = urine creatinine concentration (mg/dL)

REPRODUCTIVE AND DEVELOPMENTAL HAZARDS

Agents Associated with Adverse Female Reproductive Capacity or Developmental Effects in Human and Animal Studies*

Agent	Human Outcomes	Strength of Association in Humans†	Animal Outcomes	Strength of Association in Animals†
Anesthetic gases‡	Reduced fertility, spontaneous abortion	1,3	Birth defects	1,3
Arsenic	Spontaneous abortion, low birth weight	1	Birth defects, fetal loss	2
Benzo(a)pyrene	None	NA§	Birth defects	1
Cadmium	None	NA	Fetal loss, birth defects	2
Carbon disulfide	Menstrual disorders, spontaneous abortion	1	Birth defects	1
Carbon monoxide	Low birth weight, fetal death (high doses)	1	Birth defects, neonatal mortality	2
Chlordecone	None	NA	Fetal loss	2,3
Chloroform	None	NA	Fetal loss	1
Chloroprene	None	NA	Birth defects	2,3
2,4-Dichlorophenoxy-acetic acid (2,4-D)	Skeletal defects	4	Birth defects	1
Ethylene glycol ethers	Spontaneous abortion	1	Birth defects	2
Ethylene oxide	Spontaneous abortion	1	Fetal loss	1
Formamides	None	NA	Fetal loss, birth defects	2
Inorganic mercury‡	Menstrual disorders, spontaneous abortion	1	Fetal loss, birth defects	1
Lead‡	Spontaneous abortion, prematurity, neurologic dysfunction in child	2	Birth defects, fetal loss	2
Organic mercury	CNS malformation, cerebral palsy	2	Birth defects, fetal loss	2
Physical stress	Prematurity	2	None	NA
Polybrominated biphenyls (PBBs)	None	NA	Fetal loss	2
Polychlorinated biphenyls (PCBs)	Neonatal PCB syndrome (low birth weight, hyperpigmentation, eye abnormalities)	2	Low birth weight, fetal loss	2
Radiation, ionizing	Menstrual disorders, CNS defects, skeletal and eye anomalies, mental retardation, childhood cancer	2	Fetal loss, birth defects	2
Selenium	Spontaneous abortion	3	Low birth weight, birth defects	2
Tellurium	None	NA	Birth defects	2
2,4,5-Trichlorophe-noxy-acetic acid (2,4,5-T)	Skeletal defects	4	Birth defects	1
Video display terminals	Spontaneous abortion	4	Birth defects	1
Vinyl chloride‡	CNS defects	1	Birth defects	1,4
Xylene	Menstrual disorders, fetal loss	1	Fetal loss, birth defects	1

U.S. Department of Health & Human Services, "Reproductive and Developmental Hazards," *Case Studies in Environmental Medicine*, Agency for Toxic Substances and Diseases Registry, September 1993.

*Major studies of the reproductive health effects of exposure to dioxin are currently in progress.

†1 = limited positive data. 2 = strong positive data. 3 = limited negative data. 4 = strong negative data.

‡Symbol used to designate agents that may have male-mediated effects.

§Not applicable because no adverse outcomes were observed.

	Exposure Associated with Male Reproductive Dysfunction				
Agent	Human Outcomes	Strength of Association in Humans*	Animal Outcomes	Strength of Association in Animals*	
Boron	Decreased sperm count	1	Testicular damage	2	
Benzene	None	NA†	Decreased sperm motility, testicular damage	1	
Benzo(a)pyrene	None	NA	Testicular damage	1	
Cadmium	Reduced fertility	1	Testicular damage	2	
Carbon disulfide	Decreased sperm count, decreased sperm motility	2,3	Testicular damage	1	
Carbon monoxide	None	NA	Testicular damage	1	
Carbon tetrachloride	None	NA	Testicular damage	1	
Carbaryl	Abnormal sperm morphology	1	Testicular damage	1	
Chlordecone	Decreased sperm count, decreased sperm motility	2	Testicular damage	2	
Chloroprene	Decreased sperm motility, abnormal morphology, decreased libido	2	Testicular damage	1	
Dibromochloropropane (DBCP)	Decreased sperm count, azoospermia, hormonal changes	2	Testicular damage	2	
Dimethyl dichlorovinyl phosphate (DDVP)	None	NA	Decreased sperm count	2	
Epichlorohydrin	None	NA	Testicular damage	2,3	
Estrogens	Decreased sperm count	2	Decreased sperm count	2	
Ethylene oxide	None	NA	Testicular damage	1	
Ethylene dibromide (EDB)	Abnormal sperm motility	1	Testicular damage	2,3	
Ethylene glycol ethers	Decreased sperm count	1	Testicular damage	2	
Heat	Decreased sperm count	2	Decreased sperm count	2	
Lead	Decreased sperm count	2	Testicular damage, decreased sperm count, decreased sperm motility, abnormal morphology	2	
Manganese	Decreased libido, impotence	1	Testicular damage	1,3	
Polybrominated biphenyls (PBBs)	None	NA	Testicular damage	1	
Polychlorinated biphenyls (PCBs)	None	NA	Testicular damage	1	
Radiation, ionizing	Decreased sperm count	2	Testicular damage	2	

U.S. Department of Health & Human Services, "Reproductive and Developmental Hazards," *Case Studies in Environmental Medicine*, Agency for Toxic Substances and Diseases Registry, September 1993.

*1 = limited positive data. 2 = strong positive data. 3 = limited negative data. 4 = strong negative data.

†Not applicable because no adverse outcomes were observed.

SAFE HANDLING OF HAZARDOUS DRUGS

Due to their inherent toxicity, particularly mutagenicity and carcinogenicity, there has been a concern about the risks of long-term, low-level exposure to antineoplastic agents. The possible risk to healthcare providers who are responsible for preparation and administration of such agents has been a subject of much debate, but few definite answers. Despite more than 20 years, and literally thousands of publications on the topic, there is no definitive evidence of a causal relationship between prolonged exposure to low levels of cytotoxic agents in the workplace and development of malignancies. Neither is there conclusive evidence that such exposure is not hazardous. In the absence of convincing evidence that healthcare personnel are not at risk, prudence requires the presumption that there is some degree of risk, and employees should employ appropriate protective measures.

The potential for many antineoplastic agents to cause secondary malignancies in patients was identified in the 1960s and 1970s. Coupled with evidence of some drugs' carcinogenicity in animals, this information raised the question of possible adverse effects from prolonged low-level exposure. In the late 1970s and 1980s, a large number of anecdotal reports of various side effects and adverse reactions in nurses, pharmacists, and pharmacy technicians involved in preparation and administration of antineoplastic therapy began to appear in the literature. These were followed by reports of increased urine mutagenicity, chromosome abnormalities, changes in immune function, and detectable blood or urine drug levels in personnel who routinely handled antineoplastic agents. As a result of these concerns, a number of groups issued guidelines intended to minimize exposure to antineoplastic agents in the workplace. By the end of the 1980s, the Occupational Safety and Health Administration (OSHA), American Society of Hospital (now Health-System) Pharmacists (ASHP), the National Institutes of Health (NIH), and the National Study Commission on Cytotoxic Exposure had all issued guidelines and policy statements addressing the proper handling of cytotoxic agents by healthcare personnel. Most of the early guidelines acknowledged the paucity and low quality of the available data, and recommended further research to define the actual risks.

During the remainder of the 1980s and 1990s, a number of studies and reports attempting to delineate the nature of the risk, and the appropriate safety measures to be taken were published. The vast majority of these were uncontrolled trials involving very small numbers of individuals, usually at a single institution. The nature and magnitude of the risk has never been properly delineated. Due to the nature of the problem, there has never been a large scale, prospective controlled trial to determine the efficacy of the various protective measures employed. As a result, there is no known threshold of safety for exposure to these agents; nor have any reliable monitoring techniques to assess exposure been developed. Most guidelines are therefore based on an assumption of "zero tolerance" - any exposure is hazardous, and must be avoided. Achieving the appropriate balance between necessary protection for personnel who must work with these agents and over-reaction to the threat remains a challenge.

More recent analysis of the problem has begun to clarify some of the risks, but has also opened previously accepted practices to question. A 1992 report on exposure of healthcare personnel to hazardous agents suggested that the standard biologic safety cabinets recommended for use when compounding hazardous drugs may not provide the desired level of protection. There was evidence suggesting that rather than forming particles or aerosol droplets that could be trapped in a standard HEPA filter, some antineoplastic agents vaporized, yielding vapors that could not be trapped in the filter. This potential for vaporization may be a partial explanation for recent reports indicating detectable contamination of work surfaces in and near hazardous drug preparation areas. This information has led some institutions to begin investigating use of isolator cabinets and sealed preparation systems as replacements for the biologic cabinets.

A 1996 review of 64 studies of workplace exposure to cytotoxic drugs noted numerous methodologic flaws in study design and procedures. The report concluded the methods used to assess exposure in these studies were too nonspecific and insensitive to be reliable measures of exposure. One disturbing aspect of this is the fact that the studies and procedures found to be not sensitive enough to assess routine levels of exposure were the ones used as the basis for development of the existing handling guidelines.

Guidelines and institutional policies for minimizing exposure to hazardous materials have been based on the presumption that environmental exposure to hazardous drugs occurs through three mechanisms:

- **inhalation** of drug dust or aerosolized droplets
- **absorption** through the skin
- **ingestion** of contaminated food or drink

Accordingly, the existing recommendations are heavily weighted toward the use of physical barriers as the primary means of reducing exposure. Among the commonly employed precautions are:

- **Separation:** Hazardous agents are often prepared in a limited number of areas which are separated, to the extent possible, from other drug preparation areas. Almost all institutions have a separate biologic safety cabinet reserved solely for the preparation of antineoplastic agents. Many institutions have a separate "oncology" drug preparation area or satellite pharmacy.

- **Biologic safety cabinets:** Use of a Class IIA or B biologic safety cabinet for the preparation of hazardous agents. Recent reports have questioned the efficacy of these cabinets, and some institutions have adopted the use of Isolator® systems or special closed preparation systems for compounding hazardous agents.

- **Protective clothing:** Another almost universal precaution is the use of protective gloves, gowns, and eye protection while handling antineoplastic agents. If drug preparation is performed in a biologic safety cabinet equipped with a glass front, many institutions dispense with the requirement for wearing safety goggles.

- **Training:** Some of the early reports attributed lower, or undetectable, levels of exposure to hazardous drugs to the experience level, or skill at aseptic technique, of the individual worker. Accordingly, many institutions require some degree of training before personnel are allowed to handle hazardous agents. Although most of the published guidelines recommend personnel who handle hazardous agents have "appropriate" training and experience, none specify what should be included in such a program. Accordingly, the exact nature and length of the required training programs vary widely among institutions.

- **Monitoring:** Appropriate physical parameters for assessing exposure to hazardous drugs are not available. Although some institutions require periodic health monitoring, the definition of what constitutes an appropriate screening program is a matter of some debate. Attempts to monitor the existence of hazardous materials in the work area has been slightly more successful. Assessment of airborne drug levels and surface contamination, in preparation cabinets, "secure" work areas, and areas outside the hazardous drug area has been reported. Additionally, techniques for using ultraviolet light to detect occult drug spills and assess individual's handling technique have been reported. Most of these techniques have not been developed sufficiently to be used in routine practice, and are still limited to the research setting.

Selected Readings

American Society of Hospital Pharmacists, "ASHP Technical Assistance Bulletin on Handling Cytotoxic and Hazardous Drugs," *Am J Hosp Pharm*, 1990, 47:1033-49.

Baker ES and Connor TH, "Monitoring Occupational Exposure to Cancer Chemotherapy Drugs," *Am J Health Syst Pharm*, 1996, 53(22):2713-23.

Bos RP and Sessink PJ, "Biomonitoring of Occupational Exposures to Cytostatic Anticancer Drugs," *Rev Environ Health*, 1997, 12(1):43-58.

Connor TH, "Permeability of Nitrile Rubber, Latex, Polyurethane, and Neoprene Gloves to 18 Antineoplastic Drugs," *Am J Health Syst Pharm*, 1999, 56(23):2450-3.

Connor TH, Anderson RW, Sessink PJ, et al, "Surface Contamination with Antineoplastic Agents in Six Cancer Treatment Centers in Canada and the United States," *Am J Health Syst Pharm*, 1999, 56(14):1427-32.

Sessink PJ, Anzion RB, Van den Broek PH, et al, "Detection of Contamination with Antineoplastic Agents in a Hospital Pharmacy Department, " *Pharm Weekbl Sci*, 1992, 14(1):16-22.

Sessink PJ, Boer KA, Scheefhals AP, et al, "Occupational Exposure to Antineoplastic Agents at Several Departments in a Hospital: Environmental Contamination and Excretion of Cyclophosphamide and Ifosfamide in Urine of Exposed Workers, *Int Arch Occup Environ Health*, 1992, 64(2):105-12.

Sessink PJ and Bos RP, "Drugs Hazardous to Healthcare Workers: Evaluation of Methods for Monitoring Occupational Exposure to Cytostatic Drugs," *Drug Saf*, 1999, 20(4):347-59.

Solimando D and Wilson J, "Demonstration of Skin Fluorescence Following Exposure to Doxorubicin," *Cancer Nursing*, 1983, 6(4):313-5.

Sorsa M and Anderson D, "Monitoring of Occupational Exposure to Cytostatic Anticancer Agents," *Mutat Res*, 1996, 355(1-2):253-61.

Wilson J and Solimando D, "Aseptic Technique as a Safety Precaution in the Preparation of Antineoplastic Agents," *Hospital Pharmacy*, 1981, 16(11):575-81.

SEIZURES, NEONATAL GUIDELINES

Approach to the Treatment of Neonatal Seizures*

Drug	Loading Dose	Maintenance Dose	Half-life	Therapeutic Range
Diazepam	0.25 mg/kg I.V. (in 2 min)	Dose may be repeated several times as clinically needed	25 h preterm 31 h term	35-81 μmol/L
Lorazepam (for refractory seizures)	0.04-1 mg/kg I.V. over 2-5 minutes	May repeat in 15 minutes	10-40 h	50-240 ng/mL
Paraldehyde (rarely used)	0.150-0.200 mL/kg I.V.	0.020 mL/kg/h I.V.	10 h	10-40 mcg/mL
Phenobarbital	20 mg/kg I.V. (in 10 min)	3-4 mg/kg divided (bid), I.V./I.M./P.O.	Age dependant: 100 h by 14 d 20 h by 28 d	16-40 mcg/mL
Phenytoin	20 mg/kg I.V. (1 mg/kg/min)	4-8 mg/kg divided (bid), I.V.	Age dependant: 104 h early neonatal period to 2-7 h late neonatal period	15-20 mcg/mL
Primidone	15-25 mg/kg P.O.	12-20 mg/kg/d	12 h	6-15 mcg/mL

*Incidence: 5 in 1000 live births (occurs in −5% of withdrawal states).

Causes of Neonatal Seizures

1. Trauma
   a. subdural hematoma
   b. intracortical hemorrhage
   c. cortical vein thrombosis
2. Asphyxia — subependymal hemorrhage
3. Congenital abnormalities (cerebral dysgenesis)
   a. lissencephaly
   b. schizencephaly
4. Hypertension
5. Metabolic
   a. hypocalcemia
      - hypomagnesemia
      - high phosphate load
      - IDM (infants of diabetic mothers)
      - hypoparathyroidism
      - maternal hyperparathyroidism
      - idiopathic
      - DiGeorge's syndrome
   b. hypoglycemia
      - galactosemia
      - IUGR (intrauterine growth retardation)
      - IDM (infants of diabetic mothers)
      - glycogen storage disease
      - idiopathic
      - methylmalonic acidemia
      - propionic acidemia
      - maple syrup urine disease
      - asphyxia
   c. electrolyte imbalance
      - hypernatremia

- hypomagnesemia
- hyponatremia

6. Infections
   a. bacterial meningitis
   b. cerebral abscess
   c. herpes encephalitis
   d. Coxsackie meningoencephalitis
   e. cytomegalovirus
   f. toxoplasmosis
   g. syphilis

7. Drug withdrawal
   a. methadone
   b. heroin
   c. barbiturate (short-acting, such as secobarbital and butalbital)
   d. propoxyphene
   e. benzodiazepines (chlordiazepoxide, diazepam)
   f. cocaine
   g. ethanol
   h. codeine
   i. paroxetine

8. Pyridoxine dependency

9. Amino acid disturbances
   a. maple syrup urine disease
   b. urea cycle abnormalities
   c. nonketotic hyperglycinemia
   d. ketotic hyperglycinemia
   e. Leigh disease
   f. isovaleric acidemia

10. Toxins
    a. local anesthetics
    b. isoniazid
    c. lead
    d. indomethacin (from breast feeding)
    e. fentanyl
    f. pyridoxine

11. Familial seizures
    a. neurocutaneous syndromes
       - tuberous sclerosis
       - incontinentia pigmenti
    b. genetic syndromes
       - Zellweger's
       - Smith Lemli Opitz
       - neonatal adrenoleukodystrophy
    c. benign familial epilepsy

12. Cerebral hemorrhage
    a. intraventricular
    b. subarachnoid
    c. subdural

Adapted from Painter MJ, Bergman I, and Crumrie P, "Neonatal Seizures," *Pediatr Clin North Am*, 1986, 33:91-107.

SELECTED PROPERTIES OF BETA-ADRENERGIC BLOCKING DRUGS

Drug	Relative Beta Selectivity	Beta-Blockade Potency Ratio*	ISA	MSA
Acebutolol	*	0.3	*	*
Atenolol	*	1	—	—
Betaxolol	**	1	—	*
Bisoprolol	*		—	—
Carteolol	—		**	0
Esmolol	*	0.02	—	—
Metoprolol	*	1	—	—
Nadolol	—	2-9	—	—
Penbutolol	—		*	0
Pindolol	—	6	**	*
Propranolol	—	1	—	**
Sotalol	—	0.3	—	—
Timolol	—	6	—	—

*Propranolol = 1.

ISA = intrinsic sympathominetic activity; MSA = membrane stabilizing activity.

SELECTIVE SEROTONIN REUPTAKE INHIBITORS (SSRIS) CYP PROFILE

Generic Name (Brand Name)	1A2	2B6	2C8/9	2C19	2D6	3A4
Citalopram (Celexa®)	Weak	Weak	—	Weak	Weak	—
Escitalopram (Lexapro™)	—	—	—	—	Weak	—
Fluoxetine (Prozac®; Prozac® Weekly™; Sarafem™)	Moderate	Weak	Weak	Moderate	**Strong**	Weak
Fluvoxamine	**Strong**	Weak	Weak	**Strong**	Weak	Weak
Paroxetine (Paxil®; Paxil CR™)	Weak	Moderate	Weak	Weak	**Strong**	Weak
Sertraline (Zoloft®)	Weak	Moderate	Weak	Moderate	Moderate	Moderate

Based on a ratio ([I]/Ki) of the serum concentration [I] of drug achieved under typical dosing conditions and a drug's Ki value (inhibitor constant).

Weak = ratio<0.1
Moderate = ratio 0.1-0.99
Strong = ratio≥1

SELECTIVE SEROTONIN REUPTAKE INHIBITORS (SSRIS) FDA-APPROVED INDICATIONS

Generic Name (Brand Name)	Major Depression	Anorexia/Bulimia	Obsessive-Compulsive Disorder (OCD)	Premenstrual Dysphoric Disorder (PMDD)	Panic Disorder	Post-Traumatic Stress Disorder (PTSD)	Social Anxiety Disorder	Generalized Anxiety Disorder (GAD)
Citalopram (Celexa™)	X							X
Escitalopram (Lexapro™)	X							X
Fluoxetine (Prozac®; Prozac® Weekly™; Sarafem™)	X	X	X	X	X			
Fluvoxamine			X					
Paroxetine (Paxil®; Paxil CR™)	X		X	X (Paxil CR™)	X	X	X	X
Sertraline (Zoloft®)	X		X	X	X	X	X	

SELECTIVE SEROTONIN REUPTAKE INHIBITORS (SSRIS) PHARMACOKINETICS

SSRI	Half-life (h)	Metabolite Half-life	Peak Plasma Level (h)	% Protein Bound	Bioavailability (%)	Initial Dose
Citalopram (Celexa™)	35	S-desmethyl-citalopram 59 hours	4	80	80	20 mg qAM
Escitalopram (Lexapro™)	27-32	S-desmethyl-citalopram 59 hours	5	56	80	10 mg qAM
Fluoxetine (Prozac®, Prozac® Weekly™, Sarafem™)	Initial: 24-72 Chronic: 96-144	Norfluoxetine: 4-16 days	6-8	95	72	10-20 mg qAM
Fluvoxamine	16	N/A	3	80	53	50 mg qhs
Paroxetine (Paxil®, Paxil® CR™)	21	N/A	5	95	>90	10-20 mg qAM
Sertraline (Zoloft®)	26	N-desmethyl-sertraline: 62-104 hours	5-8	98	88	25-50 mg qAM

SELECTIVE SEROTONIN REUPTAKE INHIBITORS (SSRIS) RECEPTOR PROFILE[1]

Generic Name (Brand Name)	NE-T	5HT-T	DA-T	M_1	H_1	α_1
Citalopram (Celexa™)	4000	1.16	28,000	2200	476	1890
Escitalopram[2] (Lexapro®)	7841	1.10	27,410	1242	1973	3870
Fluoxetine (Prozac®; Prozac® Weekly™; Sarafem™)	244	0.81	3600	2000	6250	5900
Fluvoxamine	1300	2.22	9100	24,000	>100,000	7700
Paroxetine (Paxil®; Paxil CR™)	40	0.13	500	108	22,000	>100,000
Sertraline (Zoloft®)	417	0.29	25	625	24,000	370

Adapted from Gilman AG, *Goodman and Gilman's The Pharmacological Basis of Therapeutics*, 10th ed, New York, NY: McGraw-Hill, 2001.

[1]Ki (nM; inhibitory constant); NE-T = norepinephrine transporter; 5HT-T = serotonin transporter; DA-T = dopamine transporter; M_1 = muscarinic$_1$ receptor; H_1 = histamine H_1 receptor; α_1 = alpha$_1$ receptor.

[2]Owens MJ, Knight DL, and Nemeroff CB, "Second-Generation SSRIs: Human Monoamine Transporter Binding Profile of Escitalopram and R-Fluoxetine," *Biol Psychiatry*, 2001, 50(5):345-50.

SEROTONIN SYNDROME

Diagnostic Criteria for Serotonin Syndrome

- Recent addition or dosage increase of any agent increasing serotonin activity or availability (usually within 1 day).
- Absence of abused substances, metabolic infectious etiology, or withdrawal.
- No recent addition or dosage increase of a neuroleptic agent prior to onset of signs and symptoms.
- Presence of three or more of the following: (% incidence)

Agitation (34%)	Muscle rigidity (51%)
Abdominal pain (4%)	Mydriasis
Ataxia/incoordination (40%)	Myoclonus (58%)
Diaphoresis (45%)	Nausea (23%)
Diarrhea (8%)	Nystagmus (15%)
Hyperpyrexia (45%)	Restlessness/hyperactivity (48%)
Hypertension/hypotension (35%)	Salivation (2%)
Hyperthermia	Seizures (12%)
Hyperreflexia (52%)	Shivering (26%)
Mental status change-cognitive behavioral changes	Sinus tachycardia (36%)
Anxiety (15%)	Tachypnea (26%)
Euphoria/hypomania (21%)	Tremor (43%)
Confusion (51%)	Unreactive pupils (20%)
Agitation (34%)	
Disorientation	
Coma/unresponsiveness (29%)	

Drugs (as Single Causative Agent) Which Can Induce Serotonin Syndrome

Specific serotonin reuptake inhibitors (SSRI)
Buspirone
Clomipramine
Dextromethorphan
Fentanyl
Granisetron
Linezolide
Lithium
LSD
MAO Inhibitors
MDMA (Ecstasy)
Meperidine
5-Methoxydiisopropyltryptamine ("Foxy Methoxy")
Metoclopramide
Mirtazapine

Nefazodone
Odansetron
Panax Ginseng
Pentazocine
Ritonavir
Sibutramine
St John's Wort
Sumatriptan
Syrian Rue
Tramadol
Trazodone
Tryptophan
Valproate
Venlafaxine

Guidelines for Treatment of Serotonin Syndrome

Approximately 60% of patients present within 6 hours of medication change or overdose. Therapy is primarily supportive with intravenous crystalloid solutions utilized for hypotension and cooling blankets for mild hyperthermia. Norepinephrine is the preferred vasopressor. Chlorpromazine (25 mg I.M.) or dantrolene sodium (1 mg/kg I.V. – maximum dose 10 mg/kg) may have a role in controlling fevers, although there is no proven benefit. Benzodiazepines are the first-line treatment in controlling rigors and thus, limiting fever and rhabdomyolysis, while clonazepam may be specifically useful in treating myoclonus. Endotracheal intubation and paralysis may be required to treat refractory muscular contractions. Tachycardia or tremor can be treated with beta-blocking agents, although due to its blockade of 5-HTIA receptors, the syndrome may worsen. Serotonin blockers such as diphenhydramine (50 mg I.M.), cyproheptadine (adults: 4-8 mg every 2-4 hours up to 0.5 mg/kg/day; children: 0.25 mg/kg/day divided every 6 hours; maximum-12 mg daily), or chlorpromazine (25 mg I.M.) have been used with variable efficacy. Methysergide (2-6 mg/day) and nitroglycerin (I.V. infusion of 2 mg/kg/minute with lorazepam) also have been utilized with variable efficacy in case reports. It appears that cyproheptadine is most consistently beneficial. The syndrome does not resolve spontaneously as long as precipitating agents continue to be administered.

Recovery seen within 1 day in 70% of cases; mortality rate is about 11%.

References

Boyer EW and Shannon M, "The Serotonin Syndrome," *N Engl J Med*, 2005, 352:1112-20.

Christensen RC, "Identifying Serotonin Syndrome in the Emergency Department," *Am J Emerg Med*, 2005, 23(3):406-8.

Gardner DM and Lynd LD, "Sumatriptan Contraindications and the Serotonin Syndrome," *Ann Pharmacother*, 1998, 32(1):33-8

Gitlin MJ, "Venlafaxine, Monoamine Oxidase Inhibitors, and the Serotonin Syndrome," *J Clin Psychopharmacol*, 1997, 17:66-7.

Heisler MA, Guidery JR, and Arnecke B, "Serotonin Syndrome Induced by Administration of Venlafaxine and Phenelzine," *Ann Pharmacother*, 1996, 30:84.

Hodgman MJ, Martin TG, and Krenzelok EP, "Serotonin Syndrome Due to Venlafaxine and Maintenance Tranylcypromine Therapy," *Hum Exp Toxicol*, 1997, 16:14-7.

John L, Perreault MM, Tao T, et al, "Serotonin Syndrome Associated with Nefazodone and Paroxetine," *Ann Emerg Med*, 1997, 29:287-9.

Kious T, Wax P, and Cobaugh D, "Tramadol and Fluoxetine Induced Serotonin Syndrome with Subsequent Severe Hyperpyrexia Despite Cyproheptadine," *J Toxicol Clin Toxicol*, 1999, 37(5):631-2.

LoCurto MJ, "The Serotonin Syndrome," *Emerg Clin North Am*, 1997, 15(3):665-75.

Martin TG, "Serotonin Syndrome," *Ann Emerg Med*, 1996, 28:520-6.

Mills K, "Serotonin Toxicity: A Comprehensive Review for Emergency Medicine," *Top Emerg Med*, 1993, 15:54-73.

Mills KC, "Serotonin Syndrome: A Clinical Update," *Crit Care Clin*, 1997, 13(4):763-83.

Nisijima K, Shimizu M, Abe T, et al, "A Case of Serotonin Syndrome Induced by Concomitant Treatment with Low-Dose Trazodone, and Amitriptyline and Lithium," *Int Clin Psychopharmacol*, 1996, 11:289-90.

Sobanski T, Bagli M, Laux G, et al, "Serotonin Syndrome After Lithium Add-On Medication to Paroxetine," *Pharmacopsychiatry*, 1997, 30:106-7.

Sporer, "The Serotonin Syndrome: Implicated Drugs, Pathophysiology and Management," *Drug Safety*, 1995, 13(2):94-104.

Sternbach H, "The Serotonin Syndrome," *Am J Psychiatry*, 1991, 146:705-7.

Van Berkum MM, Thiel J, Leikin JB, et al, "A Fatality Due to Serotonin Syndrome," *Medical Update for Psychiatrists*, 1997, 2:55-7.

STATUS EPILEPTICUS TREATMENT ALGORITHM

Status Epilepticus Treatment Algorithm

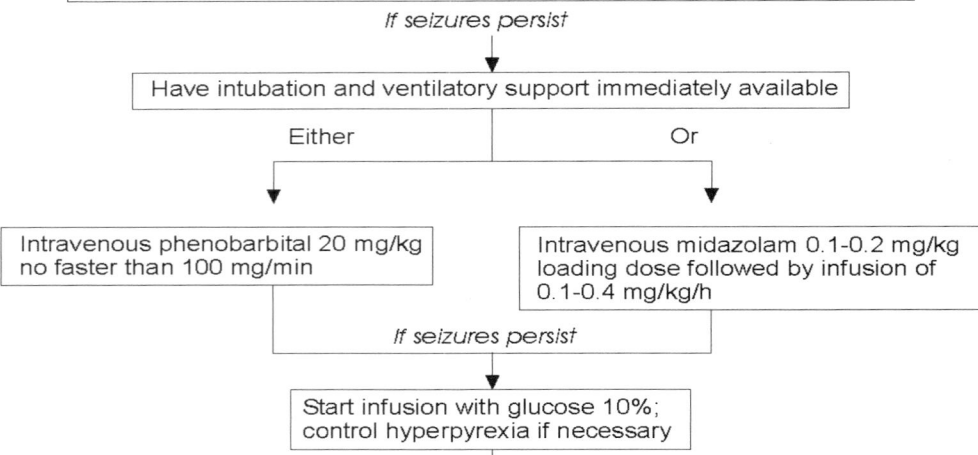

- Assess cardiorespiratory function
- Insert oral airway, administer oxygen 30% to 100%
- Insert indwelling intravenous catheter
- Monitor respiration, blood pressure, body temperature, EKG, and EEG

First-line drugs:
Intravenous diazepam (0.15-0.25 mg/kg) no faster than 2 mg/min or intravenous lorazepam (0.1 mg/kg)
and
Intravenous phenytoin no faster than 50 mg/min to a total of 18 mg/kg; if hypotension develops, slow down infusion rate* or intramuscular fosphenytoin (20 mg/kg). Not usually effective for alcohol withdrawal or some drug-induced seizures.

If seizures persist

Have intubation and ventilatory support immediately available

Either — Or

Intravenous phenobarbital 20 mg/kg no faster than 100 mg/min

Intravenous midazolam 0.1-0.2 mg/kg loading dose followed by infusion of 0.1-0.4 mg/kg/h

If seizures persist

Start infusion with glucose 10%; control hyperpyrexia if necessary

Possible alternatives if anesthesiologist is not immediately available:
- Barbiturate coma: Pentobarbital (4-8 mg/mL in normal saline) loading dose 5-7 mg/kg over 30-60 minutes with a maintenance dose of 2-4 mg/kg/h
- Intravenous paraldehyde 0.05 - 0.1 mL/kg diluted 4% in normal saline
- Intravenous lidocaine (lignocaine) 1-2 mg/kg: If effective, administer additional 50-100 mg in dextrose 5% 250 mL no faster than 2 mg/kg/h
- Intravenous valproic acid: Loading dose of 15-25 mg/kg over 10 minutes to 1 hour followed by an infusion of 1 mg/kg/h
- Valproate rectal suppositories or retention enemas: Dosage of 200-1200 mg every 6 hours in adults or 15-20 mg/kg in pediatric patients
Intravenous valproate sodium dose is 100-200 mg/min; a slower infusion rate of 20 mg/min over 1 hour is associated with fewer side effects
- In children <30 kg, clonazepam (intravenous) at an initial dose of 0.01-0.03 mg/kg/24 h; incremental increase of 0.25-0.5 mg/kg/24 h to a maximum dose of 0.1-0.2 mg/kg/24 h
- Propofol: 1-3 mg/kg as an intravenous bolus followed by an intravenous infusion of 1.5-11.3 mg/kg/h
- Electroconvulsant therapy (investigational)

If seizures persist

General anesthesia (halothane or isoflurane) and neuromuscular blockade.

* May not be effective for xanthine or sympathomimetic overdose

Reprinted with permission from "Induced Seizures in Drug Safety," *Drug Safety*, 1990, 5(2):140.

References

Bebin EM, "Additional Modalities for Treating Acute Seizures in Children: Overview," *J Child Neurol*, 1998, 13(Suppl 1):S23-6.
Brown LA and Levin GM, "Role of Propofol in Refractory Status Epilepticus," *Ann Pharmacother*, 1998, 32(10):1053-9.
Delanty N and French JA, "New Options in Epilepsy Pharmacotherapy," *Formulary*, 1998, 33:1190-206.
Gonzalez C, Palomar M, and Rovira R, "Electroconvulsive Therapy for Status Epilepticus," *Ann Intern Med*, 1997, 127(3): 247-248.
Kendall JL, Reynolds M, and Goldberg R, "Intranasal Midazolam in Patients with Status Epilepticus," *Ann Emerg Med*, 1997, 29:415-7.
Kumar A and Bleck TP, "Intravenous Midazolam for Treatment of Status Epilepticus," *Crit Care Med*, 1992, 20:438.
Rashkin MC, Young C, and Penovich P, "Pentobarbital Treatment of Refractory Status Epilepticus", *Neurology*, 1987, 37:500-3.
Wilder BJ, "The Use of Parenteral Antiepileptic Drugs and the Role for Fosphenytoin," *Neurology*, 1996,(Suppl 1): S1-28.
Yamamoto LG and Yim GK, "The Role of Intravenous Valproic Acid in Status Epilepticus," *Pediatr Emerg Care*, 2000, 16(4):296-8.

Precipitants of Status Epilepticus		
Precipitants	Children ≤16 y, %	Adults >16 y, %
Cerebrovascular	3.3	25.2
Medication change	19.8	18.9
Anoxia	5.3	10.7
Ethanol/drug-related	2.4	12.2
Metabolic	8.2	8.8
Unknown	9.3	8.1
Fever/infection	35.7	4.6
Trauma	3.5	4.6
Tumor	0.7	4.3
Central nervous system infection	4.8	1.8
Congenital	7.0	0.8

Leading Causes of Drug-Induced Seizures

1. Cocaine intoxication
2. Benzodiazepine withdrawal
3. Bupropion

Reference

Pesola GR and Avasarala J, "Bupropion Seizure Proportion Among New-Onset Generalized Seizures and Drug Related Seizures Presenting to an Emergency Department," *J Emerg Med*, 2002, 22(3):235-9.

STRESS REPLACEMENT OF GLUCOCORTICOIDS

Recommendations for stress replacement of glucocorticoids vary. Because of the low risk involved with supplementation, some advocate administration of glucocorticoids for any patient who has received steroids, including topical steroids, within a year. Others reserve glucocorticoid administration for patients who have received more than a 14-day treatment of supraphysiologic steroid therapy within the past year. Yet others consider supplementation in any patient who has received corticosteroid therapy for at least 1 month in the past 6-12 months.

Steroid Status	Prednisone Dose*	Severity of Surgery	Steroid Regimen
Taking steroids	< 10 mg/d	Any surgery	Additional steroid coverage not required; assume normal HPA response
	> 10 mg/d	Minor surgery	25 mg hydrocortisone at induction
		Moderate surgery	Usual preoperative steroids **plus** 25 mg hydrocortisone at induction **plus** 100 mg hydrocortisone per day for 24 hours
		Major surgery	Usual preoperative steroids **plus** 25 mg hydrocortisone at induction **plus** 100 mg hydrocortisone per day for 48-72 hours
	High-dose immuno-suppression	Any surgery	Give usual immunosuppressive doses during perioperative period

*If patient receiving a different corticosteroid, please use the table below to convert to an equivalent prednisone dose.

Steroid Status	Time Off Steroid	Comments
Not currently taking steroids	<3 months	Treat as if on steroids
	>3 months	No perioperative steroids necessary

Please refer to the chart below for potency comparisons and equivalent dosing:

Glucocorticoid	Relative Potency		Equivalent Dose (mg)
	Anti-inflammatory	Mineralocorticoid	
Short Acting			
Cortisone	0.8	2	25
Hydrocortisone	1	2	20
Intermediate Acting			
Prednisone	4	1	5
Prednisolone	4	1	5
Triamcinolone	5	0	4
Methylprednisolone	5	0	4
Long Acting			
Dexamethasone	25-30	0	0.75
Betamethasone	25	0	0.6-0.75

References

Henriques HF III and Lebovic D, "Defining and Focusing Perioperative Steroid Supplementation," *Am Surg*, 1995, 61(9):809-13.

Nicholson G, Burrin JM, and Hall GM, "Peri-Operative Steroid Supplementation," *Anaesthesia*, 1998, 53(11):1091-104.

Salem M, Tainsh RE Jr, Bromberg J, et al, "Perioperative Glucocorticoid Coverage: A Reassessment 42 Years After Emergence of a Problem," *Ann Surg*, 1994, 219(4):416-25.

SUBSTANCE ABUSE AND ANESTHESIA

Substance abuse is a problem that must be considered when evaluating a patient for general surgery under anesthesia. Many agents can potentially interfere with the anesthetics and other agents administered in the perioperative setting. Substances of abuse such as ethanol, central nervous system depressants (opioids, benzodiazepines, barbiturates), and cocaine can all influence the type and the amount of anesthetic administered. Below are brief discussions and tables referring to drugs of abuse and how to perioperatively manage those patients who are abusing the agents.

Ethanol

Chronic Alcohol Abuse

Chronic ethanol abuse results in induction of the cytochrome P-450 system, which can affect many of the anesthetic and other medications used perioperatively. Because of this induction, certain agents may need to be dosed more frequently to achieve the desired effect. Larger doses of many of the anesthetic agents are needed in chronic alcohol abusers because of potential cross tolerance. It has been proven that the doses of certain opioids must be significantly increased in the chronic alcoholic to obtain the desired effect. The following is a list of anesthetic drugs that must be altered in the chronic alcoholic.

Agent	Dose
Volatile agents	Increased
Opioids	Increased
Benzodiazepines	Increased
Barbiturates	Increased

Acute Ethanol Abuse

Acute ethanol intoxication causes significant central nervous system (CNS) depression. For those individuals, including chronic alcoholics undergoing anesthesia while intoxicated, the amount of anesthetic agent used should be decreased.

Agent	Dose
Volatile agents	Decreased
Opioids	Decreased
Benzodiazepines	Decreased
Barbiturates	Decreased

Central Nervous System Depressants

Patients taking CNS depressants on a chronic basis will frequently need increased doses of certain anesthetic agents. Patients who are taking barbiturates chronically will have enzyme induction and may have an increased requirement for some of the anesthetic agents. Patients on chronic opioids will have an increased requirement for opioids perioperatively. In fact, like chronic alcoholics, patients taking opioids and benzodiazepines chronically may have a cross tolerance to other agents, and the dose of many intravenous anesthetic agents may need to be increased. The following is a list of anesthetic drugs that may need to be altered.

Agent	Dose
Barbiturates	Increased barbiturates
Opioids	Increased - opioids, benzodiazepines (?)
Benzodiazepines	Increased - benzodiazepines, opioids, barbiturates

Cocaine

Cocaine addiction is a common problem in our society. The National Institute of Drug Abuse estimated that there was a five-fold increase in cocaine abuse from the mid 1970s to the mid 1980s. This increased prevalence of cocaine use makes it a significant consideration in the perioperative patient. Acute cocaine use places the surgical candidate in jeopardy of systemic adverse effects and drug interactions. Although the incidence of preoperative patients with a positive urine cocaine screen has not been determined, it is not uncommon for patients to arrive for surgery with a positive screen. It is frequently recommended that preoperative patients with a positive urine toxicology screen wait at least 48-72 hours before undergoing a surgical procedure. Although an increase in morbidity and mortality has occurred in the surgical patient following acute cocaine ingestion, many debates and questions remain as to the time delay for surgery and the potential risks of the surgical procedure in patients with a positive screen. Because a positive urine toxicology screen does not yield precise information on the chronicity or the amount of drug used, more emphasis should be focused on the management of the perioperative effects following acute cocaine administration.

The urine toxicology screen for cocaine detects not only the parent compound but also its metabolites. The metabolites of cocaine include ecgonine methyl ether (EME), benzoylecgonine, and norcocaine. A positive urine toxicology screen occurs up to 48-120 hours after cocaine use. This factor must be kept in mind when evaluating patients with a positive cocaine screen.

Perioperative management of the suspected cocaine intoxicated patient should be aimed at cardiovascular stability. It is very important to have an intravenous antihypertensive available or on board in order to blunt acute hyperdynamic responses. Arrhythmia agents must also be readily available.

For the cocaine intoxicated patient, the dose of many anesthetic agents will need to be increased. The following is a list of anesthetic drugs that must be altered in the cocaine intoxicated patient.

Agent	Dose
Volatile agents	Increased
Opioids	Increased
Benzodiazepines	Increased
Barbiturates	Increased

Management of induction of anesthesia for the cocaine intoxicated patient should resemble that of the hypertensive patient and the same techniques should be used. The following measures can be taken to prevent the exaggerated increase in blood pressure during intubation from occurring.

Coadminister opioids during induction
Fentanyl
Alfentanil
Remifentanil
Sufentanil

Administer beta-antagonist during induction
Esmolol
Propranolol
Labetalol
Metoprolol

Administer topical local anesthetic prior to intubation

For maintenance anesthesia, it is important to avoid halothane in this patient population so as not to increase their risks of arrhythmia secondary to the myocardial sensitivity to catecholamines (epinephrine).

Anesthetic management of the cocaine intoxicated patient remains an unresolved issue. The anesthesiologist and the surgeon should consider the risk/benefit analysis of delaying the procedure. If the surgery is elective, it should be delayed for 48-72 hours or until a negative urine toxicology is achieved. If the procedure is emergent, it need not be postponed and the above precautions and techniques should be considered. It is important to remember, however, that if the procedure occurs, events or medications which exacerbate the adrenergic state should be anticipated or avoided.

SULFITE – HYPERSENSITIVITY

Response

Sulfite derivatives are common antioxidant preservatives used in foods and medications. Hypersensitivity reactions to sulfites have been noted with increasing frequency; however, the reaction is still rare. Reactions occur within 2-15 minutes after ingestion or inhalation and include nasal pruritus, rhinorrhea, conjunctivitis, generalized urticaria, dyspnea, wheezing, angioedema, flushing, weakness, and anaphylaxis. Patients frequently have underlying allergic or asthmatic disease and report exacerbations when exposed to air pollution or smog. One study has suggested 5% to 10% of all asthmatics may be at risk for sulfite sensitivity. A more recent study indicates the prevalence rate for nonsteroid-dependent asthmatics is 0.8% and for steroid-dependent asthmatics 8.4%.

The mechanism of hypersensitivity has not been fully elucidated. Available data suggest the reaction is probably IgE mediated; however, IgE antibodies to sulfites have yet to be identified. Accurate diagnosis of sulfite sensitivity is obtained from oral provocative challenge. Skin tests are of no value. There is some evidence that the reaction may be dose related, since more severe reactions have occurred following ingestion of restaurant meals containing 25-100 mg sodium metabisulfite than smaller oral challenge doses. These authors suggested that bisulfites convert to sulfur dioxide in solution, which activates the tracheobronchial irritant receptors and stimulates a cholinergic reflex leading to bronchoconstriction, bradycardia, hypotension, peripheral vasodilation, and diaphoresis.

Sulfite derivatives include sodium bisulfite ($NaHSO_3$), potassium bisulfite ($KHSO_3$), sodium metabisulfite ($Na_2S_2O_5$), sodium sulfite (Na_2SO_3), potassium metabisulfite ($K_2S_2O_5$), and sulfur dioxide (SO_2). The most common food sources are fresh fruits and vegetables (particularly potatoes and green salads), shellfish, soft drinks, beer, wine, dried foods, and fruit drinks. Sympathomimetic medications are very susceptible to oxidation and frequently contain bisulfites in concentrations of 0.3% to 0.75%.

Sulfite Preservatives

Drugs That Contain Sulfite Preservatives	
Drug	**Product**
Amikacin	Amikin® injection
Atropine	Lyopine Vari-Dose®
Bupivacaine	Marcaine® with epinephrine (except dental syringes) Sensorcaine® with epinephrine
Chloroprocaine	Nesacaine® injection
Chlorpromazine	Thorazine® injection
Codeine	Codeine phosphate (Wyeth)
Co-trimoxazole	Bactrim™ injection Septra® injection
Dexamethasone acetate	Decadron®-LA (MSD) Dexone LA® (Kay Phar) Solurex LA® (Hyrex)
Dexamethasone phosphate	AK-Dex® ophthalmic 0.1% solution
Dexamethasone sodium phosphate	Decadron® (MSD) Dexamethasone sodium phosphate (Elkins-Sinns) Solurex® (Hyrex)
Dexamethasone/neomycin	NeoDecadron® solution NeoDecadron® topical cream
Dipivefrin	Propine® solution
Dopamine	Intropin® injection
Epinephrine	Epitrate® 1% solution
Etidocaine	Duranest® with epinephrine injection
Gallamine triethiodide	Flaxedil®

Drugs That Contain Sulfite Preservatives (*Continued*)

Drug	Product
Gentamicin	Apogen® Bristagen® Garamycin® Gentamicin (various)
Hydrocortisone acetate	Hydrocortone® acetate (MSD)
Hydrocortisone acetate/neomycin	Cor-Oticin® suspension
Hydrocortisone sodium phosphate	Hydrocortone® (MSD)
Imipramine	Tofranil® injection
I.V. solutions	Aminosyn® Dialyte® with dextrose Freamine® Hepatamine® Isolyte E with D$_5$W in plastic container Nephramine® 5.4% Normosol® and dextrose 5% in plastic container Procalamine® Renamin® electrolytes Travasol® Veinamine® 8%
Iothalamate sodium	Angio-Conray®
Kanamycin	Klebcil® injection
Lidocaine	Xylocaine® with epinephrine (Astra)
Meperidine	Demerol® injection
Mepivacaine HCl with levonordefrin	Carbocaine® with Neo-Cobefrin®
Metaraminol bitartrate	Aramine® injection
Methotrimeprazine	Levoprome® injection
Methyldopa	Aldomet® injection
Metoclopramide	Reglan® injection
Methoxamine	Vasoxyl® injection
Nalbuphine	Nubain® injection
Netilmicin	Netromycin® injection
Norepinephrine	Levophed® injection
Orphenadrine citrate	Orphenadrine citrate injection (various)
Otic preparations (combination product)	AK-Spore HC® Otic Cortisporin® Otic MY Cort Otic 1-20® Ortega Otic M® Otocort® Otoreid-HC®
Parenteral liver combinations	Reticulogen® Reticulogen Fortified®
Pentazocine	Talwin®
Perphenazine	Trilafon® injection
Phenylephrine/scopolamine	Murocoll-2® ophthalmic drops
Phenylephrine/pyrilaminemaleate/antipyrine	Prefrin™ A ophthalmic
Physostigmine	Eserine sulfate ointment Isopto® eserine 0.25%, 5% solution

Drugs That Contain Sulfite Preservatives (*Continued*)

Drug	Product
Pilocarpine/epinephrine	E-Pilo-1® P$_1$E$_1$® E-Pilo-2® P$_2$E$_1$® E-Pilo-3® P$_3$E$_1$® E-Pilo-4® P$_4$E$_1$® E-Pilo-6® P$_6$E$_1$®
Pilocarpine/physostigmine	Miocel® solution
Prednisolone acetate	Pred Forte® ophthalmic Pred Mild® ophthalmic Prednisolone acetate ophthalmic 1% suspension (Rugby) Predulose® ophthalmic 0.25% suspension
Prednisolone sodium phosphate	AK-Pred® ophthalmic 0.125%, 1% solution Hydeltrasol® (MSD) Key-Pred-SP® (Hyrex) Prednisolone sodium phosphate 0.125%, 1% solution (Rugby) Predulose® ophthalmic 0.25% suspension Solupredalone® (O'Neal)
Prilocaine	Citanest® Forte
Procainamide	Procainamide injection (ASCAT) Pronestyl®
Procaine	Novocain® 1%, 2% injection
Prochlorperazine	Compazine® injection
Promethazine	Anergan® injection Bay Meth® injection Ganphene® injection K-Phene® injection Mallergan® injection Pentazine® injection Phenazine® injection Phencen-50® injection Phenergan® injection Phenoject® injection Prometh® injection Promethazine HCl (various) Prorex® injection Prothazine® injection Provigan® injection V-Gan® injection Zipan® injection
Promethazine/meperidine	Mepergan®
Propiomazine	Largon®
Propoxycaine/procaine	Ravocaine® and Novocain® with Neo-Cobefrin®
Reserpine	Serpasil® injection
Ritodrine	Yutopar® injection
Sodium sulfacetamide	AK-Sulf® Forte Ophthacet®
Streptomycin	Streptomycin sulfate injection (Pfipharmecs)
Sulfisoxazole	Gantrisin® injection
Tetracaine	Pontocaine® 1% injection
Thiethylperazine maleate	Torecan® injection
Tobramycin	Nebcin® injection
Trifluoperazine	Stelazine® concentrate
Tubocurarine chloride	Abbott, Lilly, Squibb

Foods That Contain Preservatives

Artichoke
Asparagus
Canned or dry soup mixes
Cider vinegar
Cornstarch
Dehydrated fruits and vegetables (75 mg)
Flour tortillas
Frozen or dried potatoes
Fruit drinks/soft drinks (25-30 mg)
Horseradish
Instant tea
Jams/jellies

Jelling agents
Molasses
Olives
Pickle/onion relish
Pie crust
Sausages (60 mg)
Seafoods (especially shellfish)
Shredded coconut
Soy protein products
Spinach pasta
Wine/beer (5-10 mg)

TABLE OF WATER-REACTIVE MATERIALS WHICH PRODUCE TOXIC GASES

Materials Which Produce Large Amounts of Toxic-by-Inhalation (TIH) Gas(es) When Spilled in Water

UN/D.O.T. #	Name of Material	TIH Gas(es) Produced
1162	Dimethyldichlorosilane	HCl
1242	Methyldichlorosilane	HCl
1250	Methyltrichlorosilane	HCl
1295	Trichlorosilane	HCl
1298	Trimethylchlorosilane	HCl
1340	Phosphorus pentasulfide, free from yellow and white phosphorus	H_2S
1340	Phosphorus pentasulphide, free from yellow and white phosphorus	H_2S
1360	Calcium phosphide	PH_3
1384	Sodium dithionite	H_2S, SO_2
1384	Sodium hydrosulfite	H_2S, SO_2
1384	Sodium hydrosulphite	H_2S, SO_2
1397	Aluminum phosphide	PH_3
1412	Lithium amide	NH_3
1419	Magnesium aluminum phosphide	PH_3
1432	Sodium phosphide	PH_3
1433	Stannic phosphides	PH_3
1541	Acetone cyanohydrin, stabilized	HCN
1680	Potassium cyanide	HCN
1689	Sodium cyanide	HCN
1714	Zinc phosphide	PH_3
1716	Acetyl bromide	HBr
1717	Acetyl chloride	HCl
1724	Allyl trichlorosilane, stabilized	HCl
1725	Aluminum bromide, anhydrous	HBr
1726	Aluminum chloride, anhydrous	HCl
1728	Amyltrichlorosilane	HCl
1732	Antimony pentafluoride	HF
1736	Benzoyl chloride	HCl
1745	Bromine pentafluoride	HF, HBr, Br_2
1746	Bromine trifluoride	HF, HBr, Br_2
1747	Butyltrichlorosilane	HCl
1752	Chloroacetyl chloride	HCl
1754	Chlorosulfonic acid	HCl
1754	Chlorosulfonic acid and sulfur trioxide mixture	HCl
1754	Chlorosulphonic acid	HCl
1754	Chlorosulphonic acid and sulphur trioxide mixture	HCl
1754	Sulfur trioxide and chlorosulfonic acid	HCl
1754	Sulphur trioxide and chlorosulphonic acid	HCl
1758	Chromium oxychloride	HCl
1777	Fluorosulfonic acid	HF
1777	Fluorosulphonic acid	HF

Materials Which Produce Large Amounts of Toxic-by-Inhalation (TIH) Gas(es) When Spilled in Water (*Continued*)

UN/D.O.T. #	Name of Material	TIH Gas(es) Produced
1801	Octyltrichlorosilane	HCl
1806	Phosphorus pentachloride	HCl
1809	Phosphorus trichloride	HCl
1810	Phosphorus oxychloride	HCl
1818	Silicon tetrachloride	HCl
1828	Sulfur chlorides	HCl, SO_2, H_2S
1828	Sulphur chlorides	HCl, SO_2, H_2S
1834	Sulfuryl chloride	HCl, SO_3
1834	Sulphuryl chloride	HCl, SO_3
1836	Thionyl chloride	HCl, SO_2
1838	Titanium tetrachloride	HCl
1898	Acetyl iodide	HI
1923	Calcium dithionite	H_2S, SO_2
1923	Calcium hydrosulfite	H_2S, SO_2
1923	Calcium hydrosulphite	H_2S, SO_2
1939	Phosphorus oxybromide	HBr
1939	Phosphorus oxybromide, solid	HBr
2004	Magnesium diamide	NH_3
2011	Magnesium phosphide	PH_3
2012	Potassium phosphide	PH_3
2013	Strontium phosphide	PH_3
2442	Trichloroacetyl chloride	HCl
2495	Iodine pentafluoride	HF
2576	Phosphorus oxybromide, molten	HBr
2691	Phosphorus pentabromide	HBr
2692	Boron tribromide	HBr
2806	Lithium nitride	NH_3
2977	Radioactive material, uranium hexafluoride, fissile	HF
2977	Uranium hexafluoride, fissile containing more than 1% uranium-235	HF
2978	Radioactive material, uranium hexafluoride, nonfissile or fissile excepted	HF
2978	Uranium hexafluoride, fissile excepted	HF
2978	Uranium hexafluoride, low specific activity	HF
2978	Uranium hexafluoride, nonfissile	HF
2985	Chlorosilanes, flammable, corrosive, n.o.s.	HCl
2985	Chlorosilanes, n.o.s.	HCl
2986	Chlorosilanes, corrosive, flammable, n.o.s.	HCl
2986	Chlorosilanes, n.o.s.	HCl
2987	Chlorosilanes, corrosive, n.o.s.	HCl
2987	Chlorosilanes, n.o.s.	HCl
2988	Chlorosilanes, n.o.s.	HCl
2988	Chlorosilanes, water-reactive, flammable, corrosive, n.o.s.	HCl
3048	Aluminum phosphide pesticide	PH_3
3049	Metal alkyl halides, n.o.s.	HCl

Materials Which Produce Large Amounts of Toxic-by-Inhalation (TIH) Gas(es) When Spilled in Water (*Continued*)

UN/D.O.T. #	Name of Material	TIH Gas(es) Produced
3049	Metal alkyl halides, water-reactive, n.o.s.	HCl
3049	Metal aryl halides, n.o.s.	HCl
3049	Metal aryl halides, water-reactive, n.o.s.	HCl
3052	Aluminum alkyl halides	HCl
9191	Chlorine dioxide, hydrate, frozen	Cl_2

TERATOGENIC RISKS OF PSYCHOTROPIC MEDICATIONS

Drug	Risk Category	Possible Effects
Antidepressants		
MAOIs	C	Rare fetal malformations; rarely used in pregnancy due to hypertension
SSRIs	C	Increased perinatal complications
TCAs	C/D	Fetal tachycardia, fetal withdrawal, fetal anticholinergic effects, urinary retention, bowel obstruction
Antiparkinsonian		
Amantadine	C	Increase in pregnancy complications
Benztropine	C	Increase in minor malformations
Diphenhydramine	B	Oral clefts
Procyclidine	C	Increase in minor malformations
Trihexyphenidyl	C	Increase in minor malformations
Antipsychotics		
Conventional	C	Rare anomalies, fetal jaundice, fetal anticholinergic effects at birth
Atypical, clozapine	B	Unknown
Atypical, risperidone, quetiapine, olanzapine, ziprasidone	C	Unknown
Anxiolytics		
Benzodiazepines	D	"Floppy baby," withdrawal, cleft lip
Buspirone	B	Unknown
Hypnotic benzodiazepines	X	Decreased intrauterine growth
Mood Stabilizers		
Carbamazepine	D	Neural tube defects, minor anomalies
Lithium	D	Behavioral effects, Epstein's anomaly
Valproate	D	Neural tube defects

Pregnancy categories: A = controlled studies show no risk to humans; B = no evidence of risk in humans, but adequate human studies may not have been performed; C = risk cannot be ruled out; D = positive evidence of risk to humans, risk may be outweighed by potential benefit; X = contraindicated in pregnancy.

TCA = tricyclic antidepressant; MAOI = monoamine oxidase inhibitor; SSRI = selective serotonin reuptake inhibitor.

THERAPEUTIC DRUGS ASSOCIATED WITH HALLUCINATIONS

Drug	Type of Hallucination
Acyclovir	V, T
Alendronate	A
Amantadine	A, V
Aminocaproic Acid	A
Amitriptyline	V
Amoxacillin	V
Amoxapine	V
Amphetamines	T, V
Apomorphine	V
Asparaginase	V
Atropine	A, T, V
Baclofen	A, V
Benztropine	V
Biperiden	V
Bromocriptine	A, V
Bupropion	V
Caffeine (I.V.)	O
Captopril	V
Carbamazepine	V
Chlordiazepoxide	V
Celecoxib	A
Chloroquine	V
Chlorpheniramine	A, V
Chlorpromazine	A, V
Cimetidine	A, V
Clarithromycin	V
Clomipramine	V
Clonazepam	A, V, T
Clonidine	A, V
Corticosteroids	A, V
Cyclizine	V
Cyclobenzaprine	V
Cycloserine	V
Cyclosporine	V
Dantrolene	A, V
Dapsone	V
Dextromethorphan	A, V
Diethylpropion	A
Digoxin	A, V
Dimenhydrinate	A, V
Diphenhydramine	V

(Continued)

Drug	Type of Hallucination
Disopyramide	A, V
Disulfiram	A, V
Doxepin	V
Enalapril	V
Enoxacin	V
Ephedrine (Ma Huang)	A, T, V
Erythropoietin	V
Ethambutol	V
Ethchlorvynol	V
Ethosuximide	V
Fenfluramine	V
Ganciclovir	A, V
Gentamicin	NS
Griseofulvin	A
Hexamethylamine	V
Hydroxytryptophan	V
Hyoscine (scopolamine)	NS
Ifosfamide	A, V
Imipramine	V
Indomethacin	V, O
Isoniazid	A, V
Isosorbide dinitrate	A, V
Isoxsuprine	A
Ketamine	V
Levodopa	A, V
Levothyroxine	V
Lisuride	V
Lithium	V
Lorazepam	V
Maprotiline	V
Methyldopa	V
Methylphenidate	V
Methylprednisolone	V
Minocycline	V
Nalidixic Acid	V
Orciprenaline (Metaproterenol)	V, G
Oxamniquine	V
Oxprenolol	A
Pemoline	A, V, T
Pergolide	A, V
Phenelzine	A, V
Phenobarbital	V
Phenylephrine	A, T, V

(*Continued*)

Drug	Type of Hallucination
Phenytoin	V
Pindolol	A
Piribedil	V
Piroxicam	A, V
Podophyllum	A, V
Primidone	V
Procainamide	V
Promethazine	V
Propoxyphene	A
Propranolol	A, V
Pseudoephedrine/Triprolidine	A, V
Quinacrine	V
Quinapril	V
Quinidine	NS
Ranitidine	A, V
Reserpine	V
Salicylates	V
Selegiline	V
Streptokinase	V
Sulfasalazine	V
Tetracycline	V
Theophylline	V
Timolol	NS
Tocainide	V
Tolterodine	V
Triazolam	A, V, T
Trihexyphenidyl	A, V
Vidarabine	NS
Vigabatrin	A, V
Vincristine	V
Zipeprol	A, V
Zolpidem	A, V
Zonisamide	A

Abbreviations: A = auditory; V = visual; T = tactile; G = gustatory; O = olfactory; NS = not specified.

Reprinted with permission from Leikin JB, et al, "Clinical Feature and Management of Intoxication Due to Hallucinogenic Drugs," *Med Toxicol Adverse Drug Exp*, 1989, 4(5):342; Differential Diagnostic Lists (Dosing and Therapeutic Tools Database, Sullivan CA, Gelman CR, ed); and Micromedex Inc, Englewood, CO.

TOXIC DOSES OF SELECTED DRUGS

Toxic Doses of Selected Drugs Requiring Referral to a Physician or Emergency Department upon Ingestion by Asymptomatic Pediatric Patients* (Home Decontamination and/or Observation Not Sufficient)

Agent	Dose (mg/kg)
Abamectin	20
Acetaminophen#	200
Albuterol	1
Allderal®	4
Amlodipine	0.3
Amoxicillin	300
Ampicillin	300
Aspirin	200
Atenolol	5
Atomexetine	2
Baclofen	5
Barbiturates (short-acting)	5
Benzocaine	100
Borates	200
Caffeine	15
Camphor	30
Captopril	4
Carbachol	0.5
Carbamazepine	20
Carbonyl iron	140
Cetirizine	2
Chloral hydrate	50
Chloramphenicol	1005
Cisapride	0.8
Citalopram	10
Clonazepam	0.05
Clonidine	0.01
Codeine	2
Dextromethorphan#	10
Diazepam	0.5
Diltiazem	1
Digoxin	0.05
Diphenhydramine	7.5
Enalapril	1
Ephedrine	2
Ergot alkaloids	1
Felodipine	0.3
Fenfluramine	10
Fluoride (elemental)	8
Fluoxetine	2.26

(Continued)	
Agent	**Dose (mg/kg)**
Ibuprofen	250
Iron (elemental)	20
Isoniazid	10
Isradipine	0.1
Lidocaine	6
Lisinopril	1
Loperamide	0.4
Metformin	30
Methylene blue	2
Methylphenidate	1
Montelukast	10
Nicardipine	1.25
Ondansetron	1.5
Paroxetine	2
Penicillin products	250
Pentoxifylline	50
Phenobarbital	8
Phentermine	9
Phenylpropanolamine	10
Phenytoin	20
Propranolol (IR)	5
Propranolol (SR)	12
Propoxyphene	10
Pseudoephedrine	11
Ranitidine	50
Senna	15
Sodium chloride	0.5
Sotalol	8
Tacrolimus	1
Theophylline#	10
Thioridazine	3
Tramadol	10
Tricyclic antidepressant	5
Valproic acid	20
Verapamil	2.5
Warfarin	0.5
Zipeprol	8
*Under 6 years of age.	
#Not a long-acting preparation.	

TOXICITY OF COMMON HERBICIDES

Chemical Class	Generic Name	Proprietary Names	Acute Oral LD$_{50}$ (mg/kg)	Known or Suspected Adverse Effects
Acetamides	Metolachlor	Dual, Pennant, others	2780	Irritating to eyes and skin
Aliphatic acids	Trichloroacetic acid Dichloropropionic acid (dalapon)	TCA Dalapon, Revenge	5000 970	Irritating to skin, eyes, and respiratory tract
Anilides	Alachlor Propachlor Propanil	Lasso, Alanox Ramrod, Bexton, Prolex DPA, Chem Rice, Propanex, Riselect, Stam, Stampede	1800 710 >2500	Mild irritant Dermal irritant and sensitizer Irritating to skin, eyes, and respiratory tract
Benzamide	Pronamide	Kerb, Rapier	8350	Moderately irritating to eyes
Benzoic, anisic acid derivatives	Trichlorobenzoic acid Dicamba	TCBA, Tribac, 2,3,6-TBA Banvel	1500 2700	Moderately irritating to skin and respiratory tract
Benzonitriles	Dichlobenil	Casoron, Dyclomec, Barrier	>4460	Minimal toxic, irritant effects
Benzothiadiazinone dioxide	Bentazone	Basagran	>1000	Irritating to eyes and respiratory tract
Carbamates and thiocarbamates (herbicidal)	Asulam Terbucarb Butylate Cycloate Pebulate Vernolate EPTC Diallate Trillate Thiobencarb	Asulox Azac, Azar Sutan Ro-Neet Tillam, PEBC Vernam Eptam, Eradicane Di-allate Fargo Bolero, Saturn	>5000 >34,000 3500 2000 921 1800 1630 395 1675 1300	Some are irritating to eyes, skin, and respiratory tract; particularly in concentrated form. Some may be weak inhibitors of cholinesterase
Carbanilates	Chlorpropham	Sprout-Nip Chloro-IPC	3800	Skin irritants May generate methemoglobin at high dosage
Chloropyridinyl	Triclopyr	Garlon, Turflon	630	Irritating to skin and eyes
Cyclohexenone derivative	Sethoxydim	Poast	3125	Irritating to skin and eyes
Dinitroaminobenzene derivative	Butralin	Amex Tamex	12,600 >5000	May be moderately irritating.
	Pendimethalin	Prowl, Stomp, Accotab, Herbodox, Go-Go-San, Wax Up	2250	These herbicides do not uncouple oxidative phosphorylation or generate methemoglobin
	Oryzalin	Surflan, Dirimal	>10,000	
Fluorodinitrotoluidine compounds	Benfluralin Dinitramin Ethafluralin Fluchoralin Profluralin Trifluralin	Benefin, Balan, Balfin, Quilan Cobex Sonalan Basalin Tolban Treflan	>10,000 3000 >10,000 1550 1808 >10,000	May be mildly irritating. These herbicides do not uncouple phosphorylation or generate methemoglobin
Isoxazolidinone	Clomazone	Command	1369	May be moderately irritating
Nicotinic acid isopropylamine derivative	Imazapyr	Arsenal	>5000	Irritating to eyes and skin; does not contain arsenic
Oxadiazolinone	Oxadiazon	Ronstar	>3500	Minimal toxic and irritant effects
Phosphonates	Glyphosate Fosamine ammonium	Roundup, Glyfonox Krenite	4300 >5000	Irritating to eyes, skin, and upper respiratory tract
Phthalates	Chlorthaldimethyl Endothall	Dachthal, DCPA Aquathol	>10,000 51	Moderately irritating to eyes Free acid is highly toxic; irritating to skin eyes, and respiratory tract
Picolinic acid compound	Picloram	Tordon, Pinene	8200	Irritating to skin, eyes, and respiratory tract. Low systemic toxicity

(*Continued*)

Chemical Class	Generic Name	Proprietary Names	Acute Oral LD$_{50}$ (mg/kg)	Known or Suspected Adverse Effects
Triazines	Ametryn	Ametrex, Evik, Gesapax	1750	Systemic toxicity is unlikely unless large amounts have been ingested. Some triazines are moderately irritating to the eyes, skin, and respiratory tract.
	Atrazine	Aatrex, Atranex, Crisazina	1780	
	Cyanazine	Bladex, Fortrol	288	
	Desmetryn	Semeron	1390	
	Metribuzin	Sencor, Lexone, Sencoral, Sencorex	1100	
	Prometryn	Caparol, Gesagard, Prometrex	5235	
	Propazine	Milo-Pro, Primatol, Prozinex	>7000	
	Simazine	Gesatop, Princep, Caliber 90	>5000	
	Terbuthylazine	Gardoprim, Primatol M	2000	
	Tertutryn	Ternit, Prebane, Terbutrex	2500	
	Prometon	Gesafram 50	2980	
		Pramitol 25E		This particular formulation of prometon is strongly irritating to eyes, skin, and respiratory tract.
Triazole	Amitrole, aminotriazole	Amerol, Azolan, Azole, Weedazol	>10,000	Minimal systemic toxicity; slight irritant effect.
Uracils	Bromacil	Hyvar	5200	Irritant to skin, eyes, and respiratory tract. Moderately irritating.
	Lenacil	Venzar	>11,000	
	Terabacil	Sinbar	>5000	
Urea derivatives	Chlorimuron ethyl	Classic	>4000	Systemic toxicity is unlikely unless large amounts have been ingested. Many substituted ureas are irritating to eyes, skin, and mucous membranes.
	Chlorotoluron	Dicuran, Tolurex	>10,000	
	Diuron	Cekiuron, Crisuron, Dailon, Direx, Diurex, Diuron, Karmex, Unidron, Venduron	>5000	
	Flumeturon	Cotoran, Cottonex	8900	
	Isoproturon	Alon, Arelon, IP50, Tolkan	1826	
	Linuron	Afalon, Linex, Linorox, Linurex, Lorox, Sarclex	1500	
	Methabenzthiazuron	Tribunil	5000	
	Metobromuron	Pattonex	2000	
	Metoxuron	Deftor, Dosaflo, Purivel, Sulerex	3200	
	Monolinuron	Aresin	2100	
	Monuron	Monuron	3600	
	Neburon	Granurex, Neburex	>11,000	
	Siduron	Tupersan	>7500	
	Sulfemeturonmethyl	Oust	5000	
	Tebuthiuron	Spike, Tebusan	644	

From: Reigart JR and Roberts JR, *Recognition and Management of Pesticide Poisonings*, 5th ed, 1999. Available at: http://www.epa.gov/pesticides/safety/healthcare.

TOXICOLOGY FELLOWSHIPS IN THE UNITED STATES AND CANADA

Obtained from American College of Medical Toxicology, 1901 North Roselle Road, Suite 920, Schaumberg, IL 60195

847-885-0674; Fax: 847-885-0393; www.acmt.net

Arizona

Steven C. Curry, MD
Good Samaritan Reg Medical Center
925 E. McDowell Road, 2nd Floor
Phoenix, AZ 85006
Phone: 602-239-6690
Fax: 602-239-4138
Length of fellowship: 2 years
Number of fellowships: 4
Application deadline: N/A
Website:
http://www. rtis.com/pagegen/realtime/toxdept/
Peter Chase, MD, PhD
University of Arizona
Section of Emergency Medicine
1501 N. Campbell
Tucson, AZ 85724
Phone: 520-626-9604
Fax: 520-626-1633
Number of fellowships: 1
Application deadline: November

California

Timothy E. Albertson, MD
University of California, Davis
4150 V Street, Suite 3400
Sacramento, CA 95817
Phone: 916-734-3564
Fax: 916-734-7924
Number of fellowships: 1
Application deadline: March 31
Richard Clark, MD
University of California, SD
Division of Medical Toxicology
Department of Emergency Medicine
200 W. Arbor Drive, #8676
San Diego, CA 92103-8676
Phone: 619-543-6835
Fax: 619-543-3115
Number of fellowships: 2
Application deadline: March 1
Kent R. Olson, MD
University of California, SF

Box 1369
San Francisco, CA 94143-1220
Phone: 415-206-6002
Fax: 415-206-8949
Number of fellowships: Varies
Application deadline: N/A

Colorado

Richard Dart, MD, PhD
Rocky Mountain Poison and Drug Center
777 Bannock Street, Mail Code 0180
Denver, CO 80204
Phone: 303-739-1239
Fax: 303-739-1454
Number of fellowships: 2
Application deadline: September 1
Website: http://www.rmpdc.org

Connecticut

Charles McKay, MD and Marc Boyer, MD
Hartford Hospital
University of Connecticut School of Medicine
Department of Emergency Medicine
80 Seymour Street
Hartford, CT 06102-5037
Phone: 860-545-5411
Fax: 860-545-5132
Number of fellowships: 2
Application deadline: N/A
Website:
http://resprog.uchc.edu/md/emergency/home.html

Georgia

Brent W. Morgan, MD
Emory University &
The Centers for Disease Control (CDC)
Grady Health System
Georgia Poison Center
80 Jesse Hill Jr Drive
PO Box 26066
Atlanta, GA 30335-3050
Phone: 404-616-4620
Fax: 404-616-6657

Length of fellowship: 2 years
Application deadline: N/A
E-mail address: bmorg02@emory.edu

Illinois

Steve Aks, DO
Cook County Hospital
University of Illinois/Rush-Presbyterian
Section of Clinical Toxicology
1900 W. Polk, Room 500
Chicago, IL 60612
Phone: 312-864-5520
Fax: 312-864-9701
Length of fellowship: 2 years
Number of fellowships: 1-2
Application deadline: November 1

Indiana

Daniel Rusyniak, MD
Indiana University School of Medicine
1050 Wishard Blvd.
Room 2200
Indianapolis, IN 46206
Phone: 317-630-7276
Fax: 317-656-4216
Number of fellowships: 2
Application deadline: None

Massachusetts

Edward W. Boyer, MD, PhD
University of Massachusetts
Emergency Medicine Medical Center
55 Lake Avenue
Worcester, MA 01655-0228
Phone: 508-856-4101
Fax: 508-856-6902
Number of fellowships: 1-2 per year
Application deadline: Until filled
Michele Burns, MD
Harvard Medical School
Children's Hospital
Department of Pediatrics, IC Smith Building
300 Longwood Avenue
Boston, MA 02115
Phone: 617-355-6609
Fax: 617-730-0521
Length of fellowship: 2 years
Number of fellowships: 1
Application deadline: Nov 15

Websites:
http://www.childrenshopsital.org/taining/toc.html
http://www.tch.harvard.edu

Michigan

Suzanne White, MD
Childrens Hospital of Michigan
4160 John R., Ste 616
Detroit, MI 48201
Phone: 313-745-5335
Fax: 313-745-5493
Number of fellowships: 2 per year
Application deadline: N/A

New York

Lewis Nelson, MD
New York City Poison Control Center
455 First Avenue, Room 123
New York, NY 10016
Phone: 212-447-8153
Fax: 212-447-8223
Number of fellowships: 1-2
Application deadline: November 30

North Carolina

William "Russ" Kerns II, MD
Carolinas Medical Center
Division of Toxicology
Department of Emergency Medicine
PO Box 32861
Charlotte, NC 28232-2861
Phone: 704-355-5297
Fax: 704-355-8356
Number of fellowships: 1 per year
Application deadline: N/A
E-mail: rkerns@carolinashealthcare.org

Ohio

Curtis P. Snook, MD
University of Cincinnati
Department of Emergency Medicine
231 Bethesda Avenue
Cincinnati, OH 45267-0769
Phone: 513-558-5281
Fax: 513-558-5791
Number of fellowships: 2
Application deadline: N/A

Oregon (Inactive)

B. Zane Horowitz, MD
Oregon Health Sciences University
Oregon Poison Center
Mail Code CB550
3181 SW Sam Jackson Park Road
Portland, OR 97201
Phone: 503-494-7799
Fax: 503-494-4980
Length of fellowship: 2 years
Number of fellowships: 2
Application deadline: Until filled

Pennsylvania

J. Ward Donovan, MD
Pennsylvania State University
Harrisburg Hospital
PO Box 8700
Hershey, PA 17105
Phone: 717-782-5187
Fax: 717-782-5188
Number of fellowships: 1 per year
Application deadline: N/A
E-mail: wdonovan@pinnaclehealth.org
Michael I. Greenberg, MD, MPH
Medical College of Pennsylvania
Division of Toxicology
3300 Henry Avenue
Philadelphia, PA 19143
Phone: 215-842-6545
Fax: 215-843-5121
Number of fellowships: 2
Application deadline: March 1
E-mail address: michael.greenberg@drexel.edu
Daniel Brooks
University of Pittsburgh Medical Center
Toxicology Treatment Program
Suite DL45
200 Lothrop Street
Pittsburgh, PA 15213-2582
Phone: 412-648-6800
Fax: 412-647-5053
Number of fellowships: 1
Application deadline: N/A
E-mail: brooksde@upmc.edu
Fred Harchelroad, MD
Allegheny General Hospital
320 E. North Avenue

Pittsburgh, PA 15212
Phone: 412-359-3368
Fax: 412-359-4963
Length of fellowship: 2 years
Number of fellowships: 1
Application deadline: February 1
Kevin Osterhoudt, MD
Children's Hospital of Pennsylvania
Section of Medical Toxicology
34th Street & Civic Center Boulevard
Philadelphia, PA 19104
Phone: 215-590-1944
Fax: 215-590-2180
Length of fellowship: 2 years
Number of fellowships: 1
Application deadline: September 30
(Linked to Pediatric Emergency Medicine fellowship)

Tennessee

Donna Seger, MD
Vanderbilt University Medical Center
501 Oxford House
Nashville, TN 37205
Phone: 615-936-0760
Fax: 615-936-0756
Number of fellowships: 1
Application deadline: December 1

Texas (Inactive)

Wayne Snodgrass, MD, PhD
University of Texas
Clinical Pharmacology/Toxicology Unit
Poison Control Center
Galveston, TX 77550
Phone: 409-772-9612
Fax: 409-772-9642
Length of fellowship: 2 years
Number of fellowships: 2
Deadline for application: N/A
Kurt Kleinschmidt, MD
University of Texas Southwestern
Emergency Medicine
5323 Harry Hines Boulevard
Dallas, TX 75205
Phone: 214-590-1354
Fax: 214-590-5008
Number of fellowships: 2
Application deadline: Until filled
Website: http://www.swmed.edu/toxicology/

Virginia

Mark A. Kirk, MD
University of Virginia
Division of Medical Toxicology/Department of
 Emergency Medicine
PO Box 800699
Charlottesville, VA 22908-0699
Phone: 434-924-0347
Fax: 434-977-8657
Number of fellowships: 1 per year
Application deadline: N/A
E-mail: mak4z@virginia.edu

Washington (Inactive)

Thomas G. Martin, MD, MPH
University of Washington Medical Center
EMS/UW-TOX Box 356123
1959 NE Pacific Street
Seatlle, WA 98195-6123
Phone: 206-598-4219

Canada

Micheal A. McGuigan, MD, MBA
Hospital for Sick Children
555 University Avenue
Toronto, Ontario M5G IX8 Canada
Phone: 416-813-5821
Fax: 416-813-8001
Length of fellowship: 2 years
Number of fellowships: 1
Deadline for application: N/A

TOXINS WHICH SHOULD BE LAVAGED WITH SOLUTIONS OTHER THAN WATER

GASTRIC	
Aluminum bifluoride	10% calcium gluconate
Aluminum phosphide or zinc phosphide	Avoid water due to release of phosphine
	Lavage with 1:5000 potassium permanganate
Barium carbonate	Magnesium sulfate or sodium sulfate
Bromates	Sodium bicarbonate (isotonic or 5% concentration)
Zinc phosphide	
Shellfish exposure	
Tetrodotoxin	
Cesium	Berlin/Prussian blue
Chlorfenvinphos	2% potassium permangate or 5% sodium bicarbonate
Rubidium	
Chromium	Ascorbic acid 1% solution (10 g in 1 L)
Creosote	Olive oil
DDT	Mannitol
Fluoride	Calcium gluconate (10%)
Iodine	Starch/sodium thiosulfate (1%-5%)
Mercury	Sodium formaldehyde sulfoxylate (20 g in a 5% solution) A 2% to 5% solution of sodium bicarbonate can be used as an alternative therapy
Nicotine	1:5000 to 1:10,000 potassium permanganate (50-100 mg in 1 L water)
Phosphorus	
Physostigmine	
Quinine	
Strychnine	
Paralytic shellfish (saxitoxin)	2% NaHCO$_3$
Paraquat	1-2 g/kg Fullers earth (15%) or bentonite (7%)
Radium	Magnesium sulfate (10%)
Sodium monofluoroacetate	
Strontium	Avoid contact with water due to thermal reaction
Thallium	1% sodium iodine
DERMAL	
Aluminum phosphide, gallium phosphide, zinc phosphide, elemental lithium, sodium, potassium, Rb, Cs, and Fr	Dry wipe (due to explosive hazard), then rinse with water
Calcium oxide	
Chlorosulfonic acid	
Titanium tetrachloride	
Trichlorosilane	
White phosphorus	
Asphalt	Shur-cleanse® or De-solv-it®
Chlorobenzylidene malononitrile (CS)	Alkaline solution
Cyanoacrylate	Acetone with soaking in water or nitromethane
Phenol	Polyethylene glycol (300 or 400) or isopropyl alcohl (water is not contraindicated)
Skunk musk	Irrigate with sodium hypochlorite (5.25%)diluted 1:5 or 1:10 or can use a bath consisting of 1 quart of 3% hydrogen peroxide, ô¥ cup of baking soda, and 1 teaspoon of liquid soap

(Continued)

GASTRIC	
Chloroacetophenone (mace)	Magnesium hydroxide — aluminum hydroxide - simethicone gently blotted over affected area (avoid eyes)

OCULAR	
Aluminum phosphide, gallium phosphide, zinc phosphide, elemental lithium, sodium, potassium, Rb, Cs, and Fr	Dry wipe, then irrigate with water (may react violently with water)
Titanium tetrachloride	
Asphalt	Shur-cleanse® or De-solv-it®
Calcium hydroxide	2% sodium edetate
Calcium oxide	
Mercury fulminate	Water followed by 2% sodium thiosulfate solution
Radioactive materials	Normal saline
White phosphorus (if burns develop during water irrigation)	3% copper sulfate solution (several drops)
Zinc chloride (>1%)	Water followed by (within 2 minutes of exposure) 1.7% (0.5 molar) edetate disodium solution for 15 minutes

TYRAMINE CONTENT OF FOODS

Food	Allowed	Minimize Intake	Not Allowed
Beverages	Milk, decaffeinated coffee, tea, soda	Chocolate beverage, caffeine-containing drinks, clear spirits	Acidophilus milk, beer, ale, wine, malted beverages
Breads/cereals	All except those containing cheese	None	Cheese bread and crackers
Dairy products	Cottage cheese, farmers or pot cheese, cream cheese, ricotta cheese, all milk, eggs, ice cream, pudding (except chocolate)	Yogurt (limit to 4 oz per day)	All other cheeses (aged cheese, American, Camembert, cheddar, Gouda, gruyere, mozzarella, parmesan, provolone, romano, Roquefort, stilton)
Meat, fish, and poultry	All fresh or frozen	Aged meats, hot dogs, canned fish and meat	Chicken and beef liver, dried and pickled fish, summer or dry sausage, pepperoni, dried meats, meat extracts, bologna, liverwurst
Starches — potatoes/rice	All	None	Soybean (including paste)
Vegetables	All fresh, frozen, canned, or dried vegetable juices except those not allowed	Chili peppers, Chinese pea pods	Fava beans, sauerkraut, pickles, olives, Italian broad beans
Fruit	Fresh, frozen, or canned fruits and fruit juices	Avocado, banana, raspberries, figs	Banana peel extract
Soups	All soups not listed to limit or avoid	Commercially canned soups	Soups which contain broad beans, fava beans, cheese, beer, wine, any made with flavor cubes or meat extract, miso soup
Fats	All except fermented	Sour cream	Packaged gravy
Sweets	Sugar, hard candy, honey, molasses, syrups	Chocolate candies	None
Desserts	Cakes, cookies, gelatin, pastries, sherbets, sorbets	Chocolate desserts	Cheese-filled desserts
Miscellaneous	Salt, nuts, spices, herbs, flavorings, Worcestershire sauce	Soy sauce, peanuts	Brewer's yeast, yeast concentrates, all aged and fermented products, monosodium glutamate, vitamins with brewer's yeast

VITAMIN K CONTENT IN SELECTED FOODS

The following lists describe the relative amounts of vitamin K in selected foods. The abbreviations for vitamin K are "H" for high amounts, "M" for medium amounts, and "L" for low amounts.

Foods[1]	Portion Size[2]	Vitamin K Content
Coffee, brewed	10 cups	L
Cola, regular and diet	3½ fl oz	L
Fruit juices, assorted types	3½ fl oz	L
Milk	3½ fl oz	L
Tea, black, brewed	3½ fl oz	L
Bread, assorted types	4 slices	L
Cereal, assorted types	3½ oz	L
Flour, assorted types	1 cup	L
Oatmeal, instant, dry	1 cup	L
Rice, white	½ cup	L
Spaghetti, dry	3½ oz	L
Butter	6 Tbsp	L
Cheddar cheese	3½ oz	L
Eggs	2 large	L
Margarine	7 Tbsp	M
Mayonnaise	7 Tbsp	H
Oils		
Canola, salad, soybean	7 Tbsp	H
Olive	7 Tbsp	M
Corn, peanut, safflower, sesame, sunflower	7 Tbsp	L
Sour cream	8 Tbsp	L
Yogurt	3½ oz	L
Apple	1 medium	L
Banana	1 medium	L
Blueberries	⅔ cup	L
Cantaloupe pieces	⅔ cup	L
Grapes	1 cup	L
Grapefruit	½ medium	L
Lemon	2 medium	L
Orange	1 medium	L
Peach	1 medium	L
Abalone	3½ oz	L
Beef, ground	3½ oz	L
Chicken	3½ oz	L
Mackerel	3½ oz	L
Meatloaf	3½ oz	L
Pork, meat	3½ oz	L
Tuna	3½ oz	L
Turkey, meat	3½ oz	L
Asparagus, raw	7 spears	M
Avocado, peeled	1 small	M

(Continued)

Foods[1]	Portion Size[2]	Vitamin K Content
Beans, pod, raw	1 cup	M
Broccoli, raw and cooked	½ cup	H
Brussel sprout, sprout and top leaf	5 sprouts	H
Cabbage, raw	1½ cups shredded	H
Cabbage, red, raw	1½ cups shredded	M
Carrot	⅔ cup	L
Cauliflower	1 cup	L
Celery	2½ stalks	L
Coleslaw	¾ cup	M
Collard greens	½ cup chopped	H
Cucumber peel, raw	1 cup	H
Cucumber, peel removed	1 cup	L
Eggplant	1¼ cups pieces	L
Endive, raw	2 cups chopped	H
Green scallion, raw	⅔ cup chopped	H
Kale, raw leaf	¾ cup	H
Lettuce, raw, heading, bib, red leaf	1¾ cups shredded	H
Mushroom	1½ cups	L
Mustard greens, raw	1½ cups	H
Onion, white	⅔ cup chopped	L
Parsley, raw and cooked	1½ cups chopped	H
Peas, green, cooked	⅔ cup	M
Pepper, green, raw	1 cup chopped	L
Potato	1 medium	L
Pumpkin	½ cup	L
Spinach, raw leaf	1½ cups	H
Tomato	1 medium	L
Turnip greens, raw	1½ cups chopped	H
Watercress, raw	3 cups chopped	H
Honey	5 Tbsp	L
Jell-O® Gelatin	⅓ cup	L
Peanut butter	6 Tbsp	L
Pickle, dill	1 medium	M
Sauerkraut	1 cup	M
Soybean, dry	½ cup	M

[1]This list is a partial listing of foods. For more complete information, refer to references 1–2.

[2]Portions in chart are calculated from estimated portions provided in reference 4.

References

Booth SL, Sadowski JA, Weihrauch JL, et al, "Vitamin K$_1$ (Phylloquinone) Content of Foods: A Provisional Table," *J Food Comp Anal*, 1993, 6:109-20.

Ferland G, MacDonald DL, and Sadowski JA, "Development of a Diet Low in Vitamin K$_1$ (Phylloquinone)," *J Am Diet Assoc*, 1992, 92, 593-7.

Hogan RP, "Hemorrhagic Diathesis Caused by Drinking an Herbal Tea," *JAMA*, 1983, 249:2679-80.

Pennington JA, *Bowes and Church's Food Values of Portions Commonly Used*, 15th ed, Philadelphia, PA, JP Lippincott Co, 1985.

INDEX

INDEX